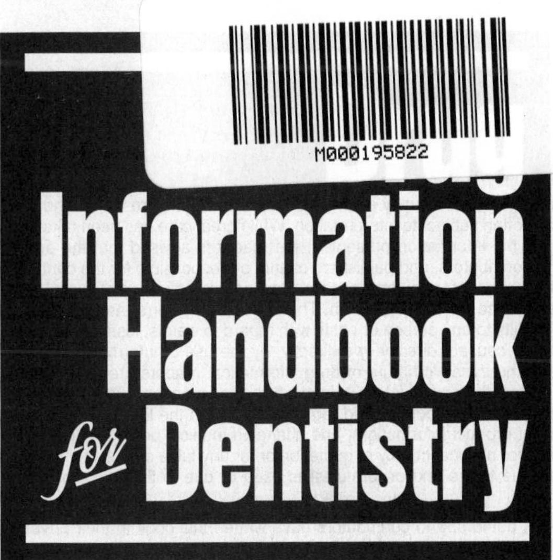

Drug Information Handbook for Dentistry

Oral Medicine for Medically-Compromised Patients & Specific Oral Conditions

9th Edition

Richard L. Wynn, BSPharm, PhD
Professor of Pharmacology
Baltimore College of Dental Surgery
Dental School
University of Maryland Baltimore
Baltimore, Maryland

Timothy F. Meiller, DDS, PhD
Professor
Diagnostic Sciences and Pathology
Baltimore College of Dental Surgery
Professor of Oncology
Greenebaum Cancer Center
University of Maryland Baltimore
Baltimore, Maryland

Harold L. Crossley, DDS, PhD
Associate Professor of Pharmacology
Baltimore College of Dental Surgery
Dental School
University of Maryland Baltimore
Baltimore, Maryland

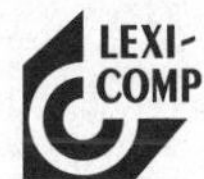

NOTICE

This handbook is intended to serve the user as a handy reference and not as a complete drug information resource. It does not include information on every therapeutic agent available. The publication covers a combination of commonly used drugs in dentistry and medicine and is specifically designed to present important aspects of drug data in a more concise format than is typically found in medical literature, exhaustive drug compendia, or product material supplied by manufacturers.

Drug information is constantly evolving because of ongoing research and clinical experience and is often subject to interpretation. While great care has been taken to ensure the accuracy of the information presented, the reader is advised that the authors, editors, reviewers, contributors, and publishers cannot be responsible for the continued currency of the information or for any errors, omissions, or the application of this information, or for any consequences arising therefrom. Therefore, the author(s) and/or the publisher shall have no liability to any person or entity with regard to claims, loss, or damage caused, or alleged to be caused, directly or indirectly, by the use of information contained herein. Because of the dynamic nature of drug information, readers are advised that decisions regarding drug therapy must be based on the independent judgment of the clinician, changing information about a drug (eg, as reflected in the literature and manufacturer's most current product information), and changing medical practices. The editors are not responsible for any inaccuracy of quotation or for any false or misleading implication that may arise due to the text or formulas as used or due to the quotation of revisions no longer official.

The editors, authors, and contributors have written this book in their private capacities. No official support or endorsement by any federal or state agency or pharmaceutical company is intended or inferred.

The publishers have made every effort to trace the copyright holders for borrowed material. If they have inadvertently overlooked any, they will be pleased to make the necessary arrangements at the first opportunity.

If you have any suggestions or questions regarding any information presented in this handbook, please contact our drug information pharmacist at (330) 650-6506.

This manual was produced using the FormuLex™ Program — a complete publishing service of Lexi-Comp, Inc.

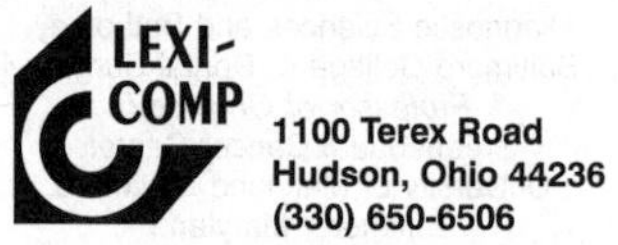

1100 Terex Road
Hudson, Ohio 44236
(330) 650-6506

ISBN 1-59195-055-4

TABLE OF CONTENTS

About the Authors 3
Editorial Advisory Panel 4
Preface to the Ninth Edition 7
Acknowledgments 7
Description of Sections and Fields 8
FDA Pregnancy Categories 10
FDA Tall-Man Project 11
Controlled Substances 12
Prescription Writing 13
Abbreviations, Acronyms, and Symbols Used in Medical Orders 13
Safe Writing Practices 17
Pharmacology of Drug Metabolism and Interactions 18

ALPHABETICAL LISTING OF DRUGS 21

Natural Products: Herbal and Dietary Supplements 1417
ALPHABETICAL LISTING OF NATURAL PRODUCTS 1419
Effects on Various Systems 1452

ORAL MEDICINE TOPICS

Part I: Dental Management and Therapeutic Considerations in Medically-Compromised Patients

Table of Contents 1455
Cardiovascular Diseases 1456
Gastrointestinal Disorders 1474
Respiratory Diseases 1476
Endocrine Disorders and Pregnancy 1479
HIV Infection and AIDS 1482
Rheumatoid Arthritis, Osteoarthritis, and Osteoporosis 1488
Nonviral Infectious Diseases 1493
Antibiotic Prophylaxis, Preprocedural Guidelines for Dental Patients 1507
Systemic Viral Diseases 1517

Part II: Dental Management and Therapeutic Considerations in Patients With Specific Oral Conditions

Table of Contents 1523
Oral Pain 1524
Oral Bacterial Infections 1531
Periodontal Diseases 1540
Oral Fungal Infections 1542
Oral Viral Infections 1545
Oral Nonviral Soft Tissue Ulcerations or Erosions 1549
Dentin Hypersensitivity, High Caries Index, and Xerostomia 1553
Management of Sialorrhea 1555
Temporomandibular Dysfunction (TMD) 1562
Patients Requiring Sedation 1565
Management of Patients Undergoing Cancer Therapy 1567

Part III: Other Oral Medicine Topics

Table of Contents 1571
Dentist's Role in Recognizing Domestic Violence 1572
Chemical Dependency and Smoking Cessation 1574
Animal and Human Bites Guidelines 1580
Dental Office Emergencies 1582
Suggested Readings 1587

APPENDIX

Standard Conversions

Apothecary/Metric Conversions 1596
Pounds/Kilograms Conversion 1597

Calcium Channel Blockers

Calcium Channel Blockers and Gingival Hyperplasia 1598
Calcium Channel Blockers, Comparative Pharmacokinetics 1600

TABLE OF CONTENTS *(Continued)*

Infectious Disease Information
Occupational Exposure to Bloodborne Pathogens (Standard/ Universal Precautions) 1601
Immunizations (Vaccines) 1612

Laboratory Values
Normal Blood Values 1618

Over-the-Counter Dental Products
Dentifrice Products 1619
Denture Adhesive Products 1628
Denture Cleanser Products 1629
Mouth Pain, Cold Sore, and Canker Sore Products 1630
Oral Rinse Products 1634

Miscellaneous
Top 50 Most Prescribed Drugs in 2002 1636
Adult Multivitamin Products 1637
Vitamin B Complex Combination Products 1640

INDEXES
Pharmacologic Category Index 1641
Alphabetical Index 1671

ABOUT THE AUTHORS

Richard L. Wynn, BSPharm, PhD

Richard L. Wynn, PhD, is Professor of Pharmacology at the Baltimore College of Dental Surgery, Dental School, University of Maryland Baltimore. Dr Wynn has served as a dental educator, researcher, and teacher of dental pharmacology and dental hygiene pharmacology for his entire professional career. He holds a BS (pharmacy; registered pharmacist, Maryland), an MS (physiology) and a PhD (pharmacology) from the University of Maryland. Dr Wynn chaired the Department of Pharmacology at the University of Maryland Dental School from 1980 to 1995. Previously, he chaired the Department of Oral Biology at the University of Kentucky College of Dentistry.

Dr Wynn has to his credit over 260 publications including original research articles, textbooks, textbook chapters, monographs, and articles in continuing education journals. He has given over 450 continuing education seminars to dental professionals in the U.S., Canada, and Europe. Dr Wynn has been a consultant to the drug industry for 21 years and his research laboratories have contributed to the development of new analgesics and anesthetics. He is a consultant to the U.S. Pharmacopeia, Dental Drugs and Products section, the Academy of General Dentistry, the American Dental Association, and a former consultant to the Council on Dental Education, Commission on Accreditation. He is a featured columnist and his drug review articles, entitled *Pharmacology Today*, appear in each issue of *General Dentistry*, a journal published by the Academy. One of his primary interests continues to be keeping dental professionals informed on all aspects of drug use in dental practice.

Timothy F. Meiller, DDS, PhD

Dr Meiller is Professor of Diagnostic Sciences and Pathology at the Baltimore College of Dental Surgery and Professor of Oncology in the Program of Oncology at the Greenebaum Cancer Center, University of Maryland Baltimore. He has held his position in Diagnostic Sciences at the Dental School for 26 years and serves as an attending faculty at the Greenebaum Cancer Center.

Dr Meiller is a Diplomate of the American Board of Oral Medicine and a graduate of Johns Hopkins University and the University of Maryland Dental and Graduate Schools, holding a DDS and a PhD in Immunology/Virology. He has over 200 publications to his credit, maintains an active general dental practice, and is a consultant to the National Institutes of Health. He is currently engaged in ongoing investigations into cellular immune dysfunction in oral diseases associated with AIDS, in cancer patients, and in other medically-compromised patients.

Harold L. Crossley, DDS, PhD

Dr Crossley is Associate Professor of Pharmacology at the Baltimore College of Dental Surgery, Dental School, University of Maryland Baltimore. A native of Rhode Island, he received a Bachelor of Science degree in Pharmacy from the University of Rhode Island in 1964. He later was awarded the Master of Science (1970) and Doctorate degrees (1972) in the area of Pharmacology. The University of Maryland Dental School in Baltimore awarded Dr Crossley the DDS degree in 1980. He is the Director of Conjoint Sciences and Preclinical Studies at the School of Dentistry and maintains an intramural part-time private dental practice.

Dr Crossley has coauthored a number of articles dealing with law enforcement on both a local and federal level. This liaison with law enforcement agencies keeps him well-acquainted with the "drug culture." He has been appointed to the Governor's Commission on Prescription Drug Abuse and the Maryland State Dental Association's Well-Being Committee. Drawing on this unique background, Dr Crossley has become nationally and internationally recognized as an expert on street drugs and chemical dependency, as well as the clinical pharmacology of dental drugs.

EDITORIAL ADVISORY PANEL

EDITORIAL ADVISORY PANEL *(Continued)*

PREFACE TO THE NINTH EDITION

The authors of the *Drug Information Handbook for Dentistry* are gratified that the text has received many indicators of success over the years. We wish to thank the practitioners and students that have made each of the previous editions a success. In this new 9th edition, we have endeavored to respond to all of the comments and creative suggestions from our readership.

The philosophy of our book remains the same as in all previous editions. Complete cross-referencing of generic and brand names, medical and oral conditions, along with the therapeutic indication and example prescribing guidelines, have been the basis of the text and our indexing system has been the key to the success of this book. We are confident that dental practitioners and staff members can easily access needed information. Clinicians can cross-reference between an oral medicine problem, a suggested drug regimen, and the important pharmacologic information necessary to move ahead with a treatment selection. The alphabetical index contains over 9,000 entries including generic drug names, natural products, synonyms, and U.S., Canadian, and Mexican brand names.

The first section of monographs contains 1413 drugs including the most recent FDA-approved formulations, many Canadian drugs, and 145 dental-specific drugs. The second section contains monographs for 68 natural products which include the Local Anesthetic/Vasoconstrictor Precautions, like the drug monographs, in addition to the new Effects on Bleeding field.

This 9th edition includes easy-to-use algorithms to help the clinician make treatment decisions in evolving areas of patient care including preprocedural antibiotics related to endocarditis and joint prostheses. Several sections include FAQs, or "Frequently Asked Questions", to help us focus on real-life scenarios.

The following sections in the oral medicine chapter have been updated: Antibiotic prophylaxis; chemical dependency and smoking cessation; odontogenic infections; oral pain; oral bacterial infections; oral fungal infections; oral nonviral soft tissue ulcerations or erosions; nonviral infectious disease; TMD; dentin hypersensitivity, high caries index, and xerostomia. Information on osteoporosis has been added to the rheumatoid arthritis and osteoarthritis section. Updates to the appendix include a completely revised section on infectious disease with a full listing of vaccines, brand names, and their use for convenient, at-a-glance reference; a new list of the top 50 drugs prescribed in 2002 including both generic and names brands; a new table containing various vitamin B complex combination products; a comparison table with pharmacokinetics of calcium channel blockers; and the reinstatement of apothecary/metric and pounds/kilograms conversions (by request).

We know that our text remains an excellent companion to complete oral medicine and medical reference libraries that each clinician should have available. We hope that it compliments the sound foundation that each dental clinician has received during their education and by building on their knowledge of oral and systemic disease we have helped them with this text to focus on therapeutic considerations. Dental office management protocols, along with prescribing guidelines, should aid the busy practitioner. The active general practitioner, the specialist, the dental hygienist, and the advanced student of dentistry or dental hygiene will be better prepared for patient care with this new 9th edition.

Richard L. Wynn

Timothy F. Meiller

Harold L. Crossley

ACKNOWLEDGMENTS

This handbook exists in its present form as a result of the concerted efforts of many individuals, including Jack D. Bolinski, DDS, and Brad F. Bolinski, who recognized the need for a comprehensive dental and medical drug compendium; the publisher and president of Lexi-Comp, Inc, Robert D. Kerscher; Lynn D. Coppinger, managing editor; Barbara F. Kerscher, production manager; Mark F. Bonfiglio, BS, PharmD, RPh, Director of Pharmacotherapy Resources; Brad F. Bolinski, product manager; Sheila L. Digman, project manager; and David C. Marcus, director of information systems.

Much of the material contained in this book was a result of contributions by pharmacists throughout the United States and Canada. Lexi-Comp has assisted many medical institutions in developing hospital-specific formulary manuals that contain clinical drug information, as well as dosing. Working with these clinical pharmacists, hospital pharmacy and therapeutics committees, and hospital drug information centers, Lexi-Comp has developed an evolutionary drug database that reflects the practice of pharmacy in these major institutions.

Special acknowledgment goes out to all Lexi-Comp staff members for their contributions to this handbook. In addition, the authors wish to thank their families, friends, and colleagues who supported them in their efforts to complete this handbook.

DESCRIPTION OF SECTIONS AND FIELDS

The *Drug Information Handbook for Dentistry, 9th Edition* is organized into six sections: Introductory text; drug monographs; natural products; oral medicine topics; appendix; and indexes which include pharmacologic categories and alphabetical listings containing synonyms, as well as U.S., Canadian, and Mexican brand names.

INTRODUCTORY TEXT

Helpful guides to understanding the organization and format of the information in this handbook.

DRUG MONOGRAPHS

This alphabetical listing of drugs contains comprehensive monographs for medications commonly prescribed in dentistry and concise monographs for other popular drugs which dental patients may be taking. *Drug names and cross-references of U.S. brand names and synonyms are printed in red, in addition to the dental-specific fields.* Monographs contain all or most of the following fields:

Generic Name	U.S. adopted name
Pronunciation	Phonetic listing of generic name
Related Information	Cross-reference to other pertinent information found elsewhere in the book
U.S. Brand Names	Common trade names used in the United States
Canadian Brand Names	Trade names found in Canada
Mexican Brand Names	Trade names found in Mexico
Pharmacologic Category	Unique systematic classification of medications
Synonyms	Other names or accepted abbreviations of the generic drug
Use	Information pertaining to appropriate dental and medical indications of the drug; includes Orphan Drug status
Unlabeled/Investigational Use	Information pertaining to non-FDA-approved and investigational indications of the drug
Local Anesthetic/Vasoconstrictor Precautions	Specific information to prevent potential drug interactions related to anesthesia
Effects on Dental Treatment	Includes significant side effects of drug therapy which may directly or indirectly affect dental treatment or diagnosis; may also contain suggested management approaches and patient handling or care
Restrictions	DEA classification for federally scheduled controlled substances and their associated prescribing limits
Dosage	The amount of the drug to be typically given or taken during therapy
Mechanism of Action	How the drug works in the body to elicit a response
Other Adverse Effects	Additional side effects, grouped by percentage of incidence and body systems
Contraindications	Information pertaining to inappropriate use of the drug (dental-specific drugs only)
Warnings/Precautions	Cautions and hazardous conditions related to use of the drug (generally listed for dental-specific drugs only).
Drug Interactions	Identifies agent's role in the hepatic CYP450 system as inhibitor, inducer, or substrate (**bold** isoenzymes are those that appear to be of clinical significance) and lists other agents that, when combined with the drug, may affect therapy. Dental-specific drugs generally have more comprehensive listings.
Dietary/Ethanol/Herb Considerations	Information regarding food, alcohol, herb/nutraceutical interactions with the drug and dietary/nutritional requirements resulting from use of the drug
Pharmacodynamics	May include information on the onset of action and peak effect, duration, absorption, distribution, protein binding, metabolism, bioavailability, half-life elimination, time to peak (serum/plasma), and excretion of drug
Pregnancy Risk Factor	Five categories established by the FDA to indicate the potential of a systemically absorbed drug for causing birth defects
Breast-feeding Considerations	Information pertaining to drug administration while breast-feeding (dental-specific drugs only)
Dosage Forms	Information about the formulation(s), strength(s), and availability (generally listed for dental-specific drugs only)
Generic Available	Indicated by a "yes" or "no"
Comments	Additional pertinent information
Selected Readings	Sources and literature where the user may find additional information

NATURAL PRODUCTS: HERBAL AND DIETARY SUPPLEMENTS

This section is divided into three parts. First, is a brief introduction to popular natural products, followed by an alphabetical listing of monographs. This second section has been expanded and contains concise monographs for products commonly purchased over-the-counter which dental patients may be taking. *Names and synonyms are printed in red, in addition to the dental–specific fields.* Monographs include all or most of the following fields:

Synonyms	Other names or accepted abbreviations of the product
Use	Information pertaining to appropriate medical indications for the product; some include recommendations from Commission E.
Effects on Bleeding	How the product affects bleeding during dental procedures
Local Anesthetic/Vasoconstrictor Precautions	Specific information to prevent potential interactions related to anesthesia
Dosage	The amount of the product to be typically given or taken during therapy
Mechanism of Action/Effect	How the product works in the body to elicit a response
Adverse Reactions	Side effects grouped by percentage of incidence and body systems
Contraindications	Information pertaining to inappropriate use of the product
Warnings	Cautions and hazardous conditions related to use of the product
Potential/Suspected Interactions	A list of drugs and other natural products that may affect therapy

Following the natural product monographs is a description of their known effects on the central nervous system, cardiovascular system, endocrine system, and gastrointestinal system.

ORAL MEDICINE TOPICS

This section is divided into three major parts and contains text on Oral Medicine topics. In each subsection, the systemic condition or the oral disease state is described briefly, followed by the pharmacologic considerations with which the dentist must be familiar.

Part I: **Dental Management and Therapeutic Considerations in Medically-Compromised Patients:** Focuses on common medical conditions and their associated drug therapies with which the dentist must be familiar. Patient profiles with commonly associated drug regimens are described.

Part II: **Dental Management and Therapeutic Considerations in Patients With Specific Oral Conditions:** Focuses on therapies the dentist may choose to prescribe for patients suffering from oral disease or who are in need of special care. Some overlap between these sections has resulted from systemic conditions that have oral manifestations and vice-versa. Cross-references to the descriptions and the monographs for individual drugs described elsewhere in this handbook allow for easy retrieval of information. Example prescriptions of selected drug therapies for each condition are presented so that the clinician can evaluate alternate approaches to treatment. Seldom is there a single drug of choice.

Those drug prescriptions listed represent prototype drugs and popular prescriptions and are examples only. The pharmacologic category index is available for cross-referencing if alternatives or additional drugs are sought.

Part III: **Other Oral Medicine Topics:** Includes protocol for office emergencies, domestic violence, chemical dependency, and animal/human bites, in addition to suggested readings.

APPENDIX

The appendix is broken down into various sections for easy use and offers a compilation of tables and guidelines which can often be helpful when considering patient care. It includes descriptions of most over-the-counter oral care products and dental drug interactions, in addition to, infectious disease information and the top 50 drugs prescribed in 2002.

INDEXES

This section includes a pharmacologic category index with an easy-to-use classification system in alphabetical order and an alphabetical index. The alphabetical index provides a quick reference for major topics within the sections, generic names, synonyms, U.S., Canadian, and Mexican brand names. From this index, the reader can cross-reference to the monographs, oral medicine topics, and appendix information.

FDA PREGNANCY CATEGORIES

Throughout this book there is a field labeled "Pregnancy Risk Factor" and the letter A, B, C, D, or X, immediately following, which signifies a category. The FDA has established these five categories to indicate the potential of a systemically absorbed drug for causing birth defects. The key differentiation among the categories rests upon the reliability of documentation and the risk:benefit ratio. Pregnancy category X is particularly notable in that if any data exists that may implicate a drug as a teratogen and the risk:benefit ratio is clearly negative, the drug is contraindicated during pregnancy.

These categories are summarized as follows:

- A Controlled studies in pregnant women fail to demonstrate a risk to the fetus in the first trimester with no evidence of risk in later trimesters. The possibility of fetal harm appears remote.
- B Either animal-reproductive studies have not demonstrated a fetal risk but there are no controlled studies in pregnant women, or animal-reproduction studies have shown an adverse effect (other than a decrease in fertility) that was not confirmed in controlled studies in women in the first trimester and there is no evidence of a risk in later trimesters.
- C Either studies in animals have revealed adverse effects on the fetus (teratogenic or embryocidal effects or other) and there are no controlled studies in women, or studies in women and animals are not available. Drugs should be given only if the potential benefits justify the potential risk to the fetus.
- D There is positive evidence of human fetal risk, but the benefits from use in pregnant women may be acceptable despite the risk (eg, if the drug is needed in a life-threatening situation or for a serious disease for which safer drugs cannot be used or are ineffective).
- X Studies in animals or human beings have demonstrated fetal abnormalities or there is evidence of fetal risk based on human experience, or both, and the risk of the use of the drug in pregnant women clearly outweighs any possible benefit. The drug is contraindicated in women who are or may become pregnant.

FDA NAME DIFFERENTIATION PROJECT: THE USE OF TALL-MAN LETTERS

Confusion between similar drug names is an important cause of medication errors. For years, The Institute For Safe Medication Practices (ISMP), has urged generic manufacturers use a combination of large and small letters as well as bolding (ie, chlorpro**MAZINE** and chlorpro**PAMIDE**) to help distinguish drugs with look-alike names, especially when they share similar strengths. Recently the FDA's Division of Generic Drugs began to issue recommendation letters to manufacturers suggesting this novel way to label their products to help reduce this drug name confusion. Although this project has had marginal success, the method has successfully eliminated problems with products such as diphenhydr**AMINE** and dimenhy**DRINATE**. Hospitals should also follow suit by making similar changes in their own labels, preprinted order forms, computer screens and printouts, and drug storage location labels.

The following is a list of product names and recommended FDA revisions you will find in this book:

Drug Product	Recommended Revision
acetazolamide	aceta**ZOLAMIDE**
acetohexamide	aceto**HEXAMIDE**
bupropion	bu**PROP**ion
buspirone	bus**PIR**one
chlorpromazine	chlorpro**MAZINE**
chlorpropamide	chlorpro**PAMIDE**
clomiphene	clomi**PHENE**
clomipramine	clomi**PRAMINE**
cycloserine	cyclo**SERINE**
cyclosporine	cyclo**SPORINE**
daunorubicin	**DAUNO**rubicin
dimenhydrinate	dimenhy**DRINATE**
diphenhydramine	diphenhydr**AMINE**
dobutamine	**DOBUT**amine
dopamine	**DOP**amine
doxorubicin	**DOXO**rubicin
glipizide	glipi**ZIDE**
glyburide	gly**BURIDE**
hydralazine	hydr**ALAZINE**
hydroxyzine	hydr**OXY**zine
medroxyprogesterone	medroxy**PROGESTER**one
methylprednisolone	methyl**PREDNIS**olone
methyltestosterone	methyl**TESTOSTER**one
nicardipine	ni**CAR**dipine
nifedipine	**NIFE**dipine
prednisolone	predniso**LONE**
prednisone	predni**SONE**
sulfadiazine	sulfa**DIAZINE**
sulfisoxazole	sulfi**SOXAZOLE**
tolazamide	**TOLAZ**amide
tolbutamide	**TOLBUT**amide
vinblastine	vin**BLAS**tine
vincristine	vin**CRIS**tine

Institute for Safe Medication Practices. "New Tall-Man Lettering Will Reduce Mix-Ups Due to Generic Drug Name Confusion," *ISMP Medication Safety Alert*, September 19, 2001. Available at: http://www.ismp.org.

Institute for Safe Medication Practices. "Prescription Mapping, Can Improve Efficiency While Minimizing Errors With Look-Alike Products," *ISMP Medication Safety Alert*, October 6, 1999. Available at: http://www.ismp.org.

U.S. Pharmacopeia, "USP Quality Review: Use Caution-Avoid Confusion," March 2001, No. 76. Available at: http://www.usp.org.

CONTROLLED SUBSTANCES

Schedule I = C-I

The drugs and other substances in this schedule have no legal medical uses except research. They have a **high** potential for abuse. They include selected opiates such as heroin, opium derivatives, and hallucinogens.

Schedule II = C-II

The drugs and other substances in this schedule have legal medical uses and a **high** abuse potential which may lead to severe dependence. They include former "Class A" narcotics, amphetamines, barbiturates, and other drugs.

Schedule III = C-III

The drugs and other substances in this schedule have legal medical uses and a **lesser** degree of abuse potential which may lead to **moderate** dependence. They include former "Class B" narcotics and other drugs.

Schedule IV = C-IV

The drugs and other substances in this schedule have legal medial uses and **low** abuse potential which may lead to **moderate** dependence. They include barbiturates, benzodiazepines, propoxyphenes, and other drugs.

Schedule V = C-V

The drugs and other substances in this schedule have legal medical uses and **low** abuse potential which may lead to **moderate** dependence. They include narcotic cough preparations, diarrhea preparations, and other drugs.

Note: These are federal classifications. Your individual state may place a substance into a more restricted category. When this occurs, the more restricted category applies. Consult your state law.

PRESCRIPTION WRITING

Doctor's Name
Address
Phone Number

Patient's Name/Date
Patient's Address/Age

Rx

Drug Name/Dosage Size

Disp: Number of tablets, capsules, ounces to be dispensed (roman numerals added as precaution for abused drugs)

Sig: Direction on how drug is to be taken

Doctor's signature
State license number
DEA number (if required)

PRESCRIPTION REQUIREMENTS

1. Date
2. Full name and address of patient
3. Name and address of prescriber
4. Signature of prescriber

If Class II drug, Drug Enforcement Agency (DEA) number necessary.

If Class II and Class III narcotic, a triplicate prescription form (in the state of California) is necessary and it must be handwritten by the prescriber.

Please turn to appropriate oral medicine chapters for examples of prescriptions.

ABBREVIATIONS, ACRONYMS, AND SYMBOLS USED IN MEDICAL ORDERS

Abbreviation	Meaning
$\overline{aa}$, aa	of each
ABG	arterial blood gases
ac	before meals or food
ad	to, up to
a.d.	right ear
ADHD	attention-deficit/hyperactivity disorder
ADLs	activities of daily living
ad lib	at pleasure
AIDS	acquired immune deficiency syndrome
a.l.	left ear
ALS	amyotrophic lateral sclerosis
AM	morning
amp	ampul
amt	amount
aq	water
aq. dest.	distilled water
ARC	AIDS-related complex
ARDS	adult respiratory distress syndrome
ARF	acute renal failure
a.s.	left ear
ASAP	as soon as possible
a.u.	each ear
AUC	area under the curve
bid	twice daily
BLS	basic life support
bm	bowel movement
BMI	body mass index
bp	blood pressure
BPH	benign prostatic hypertrophy/hyperplasia
BSA	body surface area
c	a gallon
$\bar{c}$	with
CA	cancer

PRESCRIPTION WRITING *(Continued)*

Abbreviation	Meaning
CABG	coronary artery bypass graft
CAD	coronary artery disease
cal	calorie
cap	capsule
CBT	cognitive behavioral therapy
cc	cubic centimeter
CCL, Cl_{cr}	creatinine clearance
CF	cystic fibrosis
CIE	chemotherapy-induced emesis
cm	centimeter
CIV	continuous I.V. infusion
CHF	congestive heart failure
CNS	central nervous system
comp	compound
cont	continue
COPD	chronic obstructive pulmonary disease
CRF	chronic renal failure
CT	computed tomography
d	day
DBP	diastolic blood pressure
d/c	discontinue
dil	dilute
disp	dispense
div	divide
DOE	dyspnea on exertion
DTs	delirium tremens
dtd	give of such a dose
DVT	deep vein thrombosis
Dx	diagnosis
ECT	electroconvulsive therapy
EEG	electroencephalogram
EGD	esophagogastroduodenoscopy
EKG	electrocardiogram
elix, el	elixir
emp	as directed
EPS	extrapyramidal symptoms
ESRD	end stage renal disease
et	and
EtOH	alcohol
ex aq	in water
f, ft	make, let be made
FMS	fibromyalgia syndrome
g	gram
GAD	generalized anxiety disorder
GABA	gamma-aminobutyric acid
GE	gastroesophageal
GERD	gastroesophageal reflux disease
GFR	glomerular filtration rate
GI	gastrointestinal
GITS	gastrointestinal therapeutic system
gr	grain
gtt	a drop
GVHD	graft versus host disease
h	hour
HRT	hormone replacement therapy
hs	at bedtime
HSV	herpes simplex virus
HTN	hypertension
IBD	inflammatory bowel disease
IBS	irritable bowel syndrome
ICH	intracranial hemorrhage
IHSS	idiopathic hypertrophic subaortic stenosis
I.M.	intramuscular
IOP	intraocular pressure
IU	international unit
I.V.	intravenous
kcal	kilocalorie
kg	kilogram

Abbreviation	Meaning
KIU	kallikrein inhibitor unit
L	liter
LAMM	L-α-acetyl methadol
liq	liquid, solution
LVH	left ventricular hypertrophy
M	mix; molar
MAOI	monamine oxidase inhibitor
mcg	microgram
MDEA	3,4-methylene-dioxy amphetamine
m. dict	as directed
MDMA	3,4-methylene-dioxy methamphetamine
mEq	milliequivalent
mg	milligram
MI	myocardial infarction
mixt	a mixture
mL	milliliter
mm	millimeter
mM	millimolar
MMSE	mini mental status examination
MPPP	l-methyl-4-proprionoxy-4-phenyl pyridine
MR	mental retardation
MRI	magnetic resonance imaging
MS	multiple sclerosis
NF	National Formulary
NKA	no known allergies
NMS	neuroleptic malignant syndrome
no.	number
noc	in the night
non rep	do not repeat, no refills
NPO	nothing by mouth
NSAID	nonsteroidal anti-inflammatory drug
NV	nausea and vomiting
O, Oct	a pint
OA	osteoarthritis
OC	oral contraceptive
OCD	obsessive-compulsive disorder
o.d.	right eye
o.l.	left eye
o.s.	left eye
OTC	over the counter
o.u.	each eye
PAT	paroxysmal artrial tachycardia
pc, post cib	after meals
PCP	phencyclidine
PD	Parkinson's disease
PE	pulmonary embolus
per	through or by
PID	pelvic inflammatory disease
PM	afternoon or evening
P.O.	by mouth
PONV	postoperative nausea and vomiting
P.R.	rectally
prn	as needed
PSVT	paroxysmal superventricular tachycardia
PTA	prior to admission
PTSD	post-traumatic stress disorder
PUD	peptic ulcer disease
pulv	a powder
PVD	peripheral vascular disease
q	every
qad	every other day
qd	every day
qh	every hour
qid	four times a day
qod	every other day
qs	a sufficient quantity
qs ad	a sufficient quantity to make
qty	quantity
qv	as much as you wish

PRESCRIPTION WRITING *(Continued)*

Abbreviation	Meaning
RA	rheumatoid arthritis
REM	rapid eye movement
Rx	take, a recipe
rep	let it be repeated
$\bar{s}$	without
sa	according to art
SAH	subarachnoid hemorrhage
sat	saturated
SBE	subacute bacterial endocarditis
SBP	systolic blood pressure
S.C.	subcutaneous
SIADH	syndrome of inappropriate antidiuretic hormone secretion
sig	label, or let it be printed
SL	sublingual
SLE	systemic lupus erythematosus
SOB	shortness of breath
sol	solution
solv	dissolve
$\overline{ss}$	one-half
sos	if there is need
SSKI	saturated solution of potassium iodide
SSRI	selective serotonin reuptake inhibitor
stat	at once, immediately
STD	sexually transmitted disease
supp	suppository
SVT	supraventricular tachycardia
Sx	symptom
syr	syrup
tab	tablet
tal	such
TCA	tricyclic antidepressant
TD	tardive dyskinesia
tid	three times a day
TKO	to keep open
TPN	total parenteral nutrition
tr, tinct	tincture
trit	triturate
tsp	teaspoonful
Tx	treatment
ULN	upper limits of normal
ung	ointment
URI	upper respiratory infection
US	ultrasound
UTI	urinary tract infection
u.d., ut dict	as directed
v.o.	verbal order
VTE	venous thromboembolism
VZV	varicella zoster virus
w.a.	while awake
x3	3 times
x4	4 times

SAFE WRITING PRACTICES

Health professionals and their support personnel frequently produce handwritten copies of information they see in print; therefore, such information is subjected to even greater possibilities for error or misinterpretation on the part of others. Thus, particular care must be given to how drug names and strengths are expressed when creating written health-care documents.

The following are a few examples of safe writing rules suggested by the Institute for Safe Medication Practices, Inc.*

1. There should be a space between a number and its units as it is easier to read. There should be no periods after the abbreviations mg or mL.

Correct	Incorrect
10 mg	10mg
100 mg	100mg

2. Never place a decimal and a zero after a whole number (2 mg is correct and 2.0 mg is **incorrect**). If the decimal point is not seen because it falls on a line or because individuals are working from copies where the decimal point is not seen, this causes a tenfold overdose.
3. Just the opposite is true for numbers less than one. Always place a zero before a naked decimal (0.5 mL is correct, .5 mL is **incorrect**).
4. Never abbreviate the word unit. The handwritten U or u, looks like a 0 (zero), and may cause a tenfold overdose error to be made.
5. IU is not a safe abbreviation for international units. The handwritten IU looks like IV. Write out international units or use int. units.
6. Q.D. is not a safe abbreviation for once daily, as when the Q is followed by a sloppy dot, it looks like QID which means four times daily.
7. O.D. is not a safe abbreviation for once daily, as it is properly interpreted as meaning "right eye" and has caused liquid medications such as saturated solution of potassium iodide and Lugol's solution to be administered incorrectly. There is no safe abbreviation for once daily. It must be written out in full.
8. Do not use chemical names such as 6-mercaptopurine or 6-thioguanine, as sixfold overdoses have been given when these were not recognized as chemical names. The proper names of these drugs are mercaptopurine or thioguanine.
9. Do not abbreviate drug names (5FC, 6MP, 5-ASA, MTX, HCTZ, CPZ, PBZ, etc) as they are misinterpreted and cause error.
10. Do not use the apothecary system or symbols.
11. Do not abbreviate microgram as µg; instead use mcg as there is less likelihood of misinterpretation.
12. When writing an outpatient prescription, write a complete prescription. A complete prescription can prevent the prescriber, the pharmacist, and/or the patient from making a mistake and can eliminate the need for further clarification. The legible prescriptions should contain:
    a. patient's full name
    b. for pediatric or geriatric patients: their age (or weight where applicable)
    c. drug name, dosage form and strength; if a drug is new or rarely prescribed, print this information
    d. number or amount to be dispensed
    e. complete instructions for the patient, including the purpose of the medication
    f. when there are recognized contraindications for a prescribed drug, indicate to the pharmacist that you are aware of this fact (ie, when prescribing a potassium salt for a patient receiving an ACE inhibitor, write "K serum leveling being monitored")

*From "Safe Writing" by Davis NM, PharmD and Cohen MR, MS, Lecturers and Consultants for Safe Medication Practices, 1143 Wright Drive, Huntington Valley, PA 19006. Phone: (215) 947-7566.

PHARMACOLOGY OF DRUG METABOLISM AND INTERACTIONS

Most drugs undergo metabolic transformation in the body prior to excretion. Drug metabolism is an enzyme-dependent process that developed as an adaptation to life on earth. Unlike fish, terrestrial vertebrates are unable to excrete lipid soluble compounds because kidney tubular reabsorption favors their retention. Excretion of these substances is accomplished in fish into the surrounding water. Although drug metabolism in humans results in the formation of compounds that are more polar in nature, it does not always result in the initial production of biologlcally inactive compounds. This means that a drug may stay active for some time during this metabolic process. Enzymatic modification of a parent drug can be distinguished by three basic patterns. First, an inactive parent drug may be transformed to an active compound. Second, an active parent drug may be converted to a second active compound which is subsequently converted to an inactive metabolite or byproduct. Third, an inactive compound may be formed directly from an active parent drug.

The most common reaction in drug metabolism is an oxidation reaction in which oxygen in the form of a hydroxyl group is attached to the drug molecule. With oxidation, the original drug molecule is changed just enough so that the drug metabolite will not attach to the receptor that is specific for the original molecule. This chemical change may render the drug inactive and is one mechanism of terminating drug activity. The overall process is called hydroxylation and is the direct incorporation of oxygen into the substrate drug molecule. Although the liver is the primary site for these hydroxylation enzyme reactions, these systems are also present in the kidney and gastrointestinal epithelium. This process is also called oxidative drug metabolism by an oxidative enzyme system.

This oxidative enzyme system relies on a particular cytochrome and numerous isoforms known as the cytochrome P450 system with designations CYP. Cytochrome P450 is a complex of protein and heme that contains an iron atom in its oxidized state. Through an energy transfer cascade, cytochrome P450 is reduced utilizing energy and reducing the iron to a ferrous form. This then binds with molecular oxygen and the cytochrome P450 eventually reverts to its oxidized form. The oxidized drug bound through this process to the cytochrome P450 is then released and the cytochrome is regenerated. The rate of drug biotransformation or metabolism appears to be directly related to the amounts of cytochrome P450 in the microsomal and enzyme cascade. In fact, there is a direct correlation between these systems.

There are five distinct groups of drug metabolizing enzymes which account for the majority of drug metabolism in humans. These enzyme "families", known as isoenzymes, are localized primarily in the liver. The nomenclature of this system has been standardized. Isoenzyme families are identified as a cytochrome (CYP prefix), followed by their numerical designation (eg, 1A2).

Enzymes may be inhibited (slowing metabolism through this pathway) or induced (increased in activity or number). Individual drugs metabolized by a specific enzyme are identified as substrates for the isoenzyme. Considerable effort has been expended in recent years to classify drugs metabolized by this system as either an inhibitor, inducer, or substrate of a specific isoenzyme. It should be noted that a drug may demonstrate complex activity within this scheme, acting as an inhibitor of one isoenzyme while serving as a substrate for another.

By recognizing that a substrate's metabolism may be dramatically altered by concurrent therapy with either an inducer or inhibitor, potential interactions may be identified and addressed. For example, a drug which inhibits CYP1A2 is likely to block metabolism of theophylline (a substrate for this isoenzyme). Because of this interaction, the dose of theophylline required to maintain a consistent level in the patient should be reduced when an inhibitor is added. Failure to make this adjustment may lead to supratherapeutic theophylline concentrations and potential toxicity.

This approach does have limitations. For example, the metabolism of specific drugs may have primary and secondary pathways. The contribution of secondary pathways to the overall metabolism may limit the impact of any given inhibitor. In addition, there may be up to a tenfold variation in the concentration of an isoenzyme across the broad population. In fact, a complete absence of an isoenzyme may occur in some genetic subgroups. Finally, the relative potency of inhibition, relative to the affinity of the enzyme for its substrate, demonstrates a high degree of variability. These issues make it difficult to anticipate whether a theoretical interaction will have a clinically relevant impact in a specific patient.

The details of this enzyme system continue to be investigated and information is expanding daily. However, to be complete, it should be noted that other enzyme systems also influence a drug's pharmacokinetic profile. For example, a key enzyme system regulating absorption of drugs is the p-glycoprotein system. Recent evidence suggests that some interaction originally attributed to the cytochrome system may, in fact, have been the result of inhibition of this enzyme.

The cytochrome P450 information provided in the "Drug Interactions" field of the drug monographs attempts to identify involvement of a particular isoenzyme in the drug's metabolism. Within certain limits, it may be used to identify potential interactions. Many of the drugs used as antivirals, for instance, interfere with specific isoforms of the cytochrome P450 system and may, therefore, interact adversely with the metabolism of other drugs which the patient may be taking.

References

Baker GB, Urichuk CJ, and Coutts RT, "Drug Metabolism and Metabolic Drug-Drug Interactions in Psychiatry," *Child Adolescent Psychopharm News (Suppl).*

DeVane CL, "Pharmacogenetics and Drug Metabolism of Newer Antidepressant Agents," *J Clin Psychiatry*, 1994, 55(Suppl 12):38-45.

Drug Interactions Analysis and Management. Cytochrome (CYP) 450 Isozyme Drug Interactions, Vancouver, WA: Applied Therapeutics, Inc, 523-7.

Ereshefsky L, "Drug-Drug Interactions Involving Antidepressants: Focus on Venlafaxine," *J Clin Psychopharmacol*, 1996, 16(3 Suppl 2):375-535.

Ereshefsky L, *Psychiatr Annal*, 1996, 26:342-50.

Fleishaker JC and Hulst LK, "A Pharmacokinetic and Pharmacodynamic Evaluation of the Combined Administration of Alprazolam and Fluvoxamine," *Eur J Clin Pharmacol*, 1994, 46(1):35-9.

Flockhart DA, et al, *Clin Pharmacol Ther*, 1996, 59:189.

Ketter TA, Flockhart DA, Post RM, et al, "The Emerging Role of Cytochrome P450 3A in Psychopharmacology," *J Clin Psychopharmacol*, 1995, 15(6):387-98.

Michalets EL, "Update: Clinically Significant Cytochrome P450 Drug Interactions," *Pharmacotherapy*, 1998, 18(1):84-112.

Nemeroff CB, DeVane CL, and Pollock BG, "Newer Antidepressants and the Cytochrome P450 System," *Am J Psychiatry*, 1996, 153(3):311-20.

Pollock BG, "Recent Developments in Drug Metabolism of Relevance to Psychiatrists," *Harv Rev Psychiatry*, 1994, 2(4):204-13.

Richelson E, "Pharmacokinetic Drug Interactions of New Antidepressants: A Review of the Effects on the Metabolism of Other Drugs," *Mayo Clin Proc*, 1997, 72(9):835-47.

Riesenman C, "Antidepressant Drug Interactions and the Cytochrome P450 System: A Critical Appraisal," *Pharmacotherapy*, 1995, 15(6 Pt 2):84S-99S.

Schmider J, Greenblatt DJ, von Moltke LL, et al, "Relationship of *In Vitro* Data on Drug Metabolism to *In Vivo* Pharmacokinetics and Drug Interactions: Implications for Diazepam Disposition in Humans," *J Clin Psychopharmacol*, 1996, 16(4):267-72.

Slaughter RL, *Pharm Times*, 1996, 7:6-16.

Watkins PB, "Role of Cytochrome P450 in Drug Metabolism and Hepatotoxicity," *Semin Liver Dis*, 1990, 10(4):235-50.

CONJUGATION REACTIONS IN DRUG METABOLISM

Conjugation reactions involve coupling the drug or polar metabolite with an endogenous chemical compound present in cells such as glucuronic acid, sulfuric acid or acetic acid, or amino acids. The majority of conjugation reactions couple drugs to glucuronic acid. The product formed is called the glucuronide conjugate or glucuronide. The reaction is driven by a family of enzymes known as hepatic glucuronide transferases, found in the endoplasmic reticulum. Conjugation with glucuronic acid also occurs in the kidney and other tissues, but to a much lesser extent.

Conjugation of drugs results in polar, usually more water soluble, compounds that are most often therapeutically inactive. The drug conjugates formed are rapidly excreted in the urine and bile by transport systems favoring these types of water-soluble compounds. Thus, the parent drug is effectively rendered inactive and transported out of the body by this process.

SMOKING AND DRUG METABOLISM

Another area of intense interest involves smoking effects on drug metabolism, as well as, the effects of smoking cessation drugs. A review of the literature suggests that at least a dozen drugs interact with cigarette smoke in a clinically significant manner. Polycyclic aromatic hydrocarbons (PAHs) are largely responsible for enhancing drug metabolism. Cigarette smoke induces an increase in the concentration of CYP1A2, the isoenzyme responsible for metabolism of theophylline. Theophylline is, therefore, eliminated more quickly in smokers than in nonsmokers. As a result of hepatic induction of CYP1A2, serum concentrations of theophylline have been shown to be reduced in smokers. Cigarette smoking may substantially reduce tacrine plasma concentrations. The manufacturer states that mean plasma tacrine concentrations in smokers are about one-third of the concentration in nonsmokers (presumably after multiple doses of tacrine).

Patients with insulin-dependent diabetes who smoke heavily may require a higher dosage of insulin than nonsmokers. Cigarette smoking may also reduce serum concentrations of flecainide. Although the mechanism of this interaction is unknown, enhanced hepatic metabolism is possible. Propoxyphene, a pain reliever, has been found to be less effective in heavy smokers than in nonsmokers. The mechanism for the inefficacy of propoxyphene in smokers compared with nonsmokers may be enhanced biotransformation.

Frankl and Soloff reported in a study of five young, healthy, chronic smokers that propranolol, followed by smoking, significantly decreased cardiac output and significantly increased blood pressure and peripheral resistance compared with smoking alone. Steady-state concentrations of propranolol were found to be lower in smokers than in nonsmokers. Lastly, the incidence of drowsiness associated with the use of diazepam and chlordiazepoxide showed that drowsiness was less likely to occur in smokers than in nonsmokers. Smoking probably acts by producing arousal of the central nervous system rather than by accelerating metabolism and reducing concentrations of these drugs in the brain. Finally, the interaction between smoking and oral contraceptives is complex and may be deadly. Women >35 years of age who smoke >15 cigarettes daily may be at increased risk of myocardial infarction.

The norepinephrine and serotonin reuptake inhibitors, as a new class of smoking cessation drugs, have also received attention relative to metabolic interactions. *In vitro* studies indicate that bupropion is primarily metabolized to hydroxybupropion by the CYP2B6 isoenzyme. Therefore, the potential exists for a drug interaction between Zyban® and drugs that affect the CYP2B6 isoenzyme metabolism (eg, orphenadrine and cyclophosphamide). The hydroxybupropion metabolite of bupropion does not appear to be metabolized by the cytochrome P450 isoenzymes. No systemic data have been collected on the metabolism of Zyban® following concomitant administration with other drugs, or alternatively, the effect of concomitant administration of Zyban® on the metabolism of other drugs.

Animal data, however, indicated that bupropion may be an inducer of drug-metabolizing enzymes in humans. However, following chronic administration of bupropion, 100 mg 3 times/day, to 8 healthy male volunteers for 14 days, there was no evidence of induction of its own metabolism. Because bupropion is extensively metabolized, coadministration of other drugs may affect its clinical activity. Certain drugs may induce the metabolism of bupropion

PHARMACOLOGY OF DRUG METABOLISM AND INTERACTIONS *(Continued)*

(eg, carbamazepine, phenobarbital, phenytoin), while other drugs may inhibit its metabolism (eg, cimetidine). Studies in animals demonstrated that the acute toxicity of bupropion is enhanced by the MAO inhibitor, phenelzine.

Limited clinical data suggest a higher incidence of adverse experiences in patients receiving concurrent administration of bupropion and levodopa. Administration of Zyban® to patients receiving levodopa concurrently should be undertaken with caution, using small initial doses and gradual dosage increases. Concurrent administration of Zyban® and agents that lower the seizure threshold should be undertaken only with extreme caution. Physiological changes resulting from smoking cessation itself, with or without treatment with Zyban®, may alter the pharmacokinetics of some concomitant medications, which may require dosage adjustment.

INTERACTIONS BETWEEN CIGARETTE SMOKE AND DRUGS

Drug	Mechanism	Effect on Cigarette Smokers
Theophylline	Induction of the CYP1A2 isoenzyme	May lead to reduced theophylline serum concentrations and decreased clinical effect; elimination of theophylline is considerably more rapid
Tacrine	Induction of the CYP1A2 isoenzyme	Effectiveness of tacrine may be decreased
Insulin	Decreased insulin absorption; may be related to peripheral vasoconstriction	Insulin-dependent diabetics who smoke heavily may require a 15% to 30% higher dose of insulin than nonsmokers
Flecainide	Unknown	May reduce flecainide serum concentrations
Propoxyphene	Unknown	May require higher dosage of propoxyphene to achieve analgesic effects
Propranolol	Increased release of catacholamines (eg, epinephrine) in smokers	May have increased blood pressure and heart rate relative to nonsmokers; consider effects on prevention of angina pectoris and stroke
Diazepam	Unclear as to whether pharmacokinetics are altered or end-organ responsiveness is decreased	May require larger doses of diazepam and chlordiazepoxide to achieve sedative effects

Adapted from Schein, JR, "Cigarette Smoking and Clinically Significant Drug Interactions," *Ann Pharmacother*, 1995, 29(11):1139-47.

SUMMARY

Once a drug has been metabolized in the liver, it is eliminated through several different mechanisms. One is directly through bile, into the intestine, and eventually excreted in feces. More commonly, the metabolites and the original drug pass back into the liver from the general circulation and are carried to other organs and tissues. Eventually, these metabolites are excreted through the kidney. In the kidney, the drug and its metabolites may be filtered by the glomerulus or secreted by the renal tubules into the urine. From the kidney, some of the drug may be reabsorbed and pass back into the blood. The drug may also be carried to the lung. If the drug or its metabolite is volatile, it can pass from the blood into the alveolar air and be eliminated in the breath. To a minor extent, drugs and metabolites can be excreted by sweat and saliva. In nursing mothers, drugs are also excreted in mother's milk.

The clinical considerations of drug metabolism may affect which other drugs can and should be administered. Drug tolerance may be a consideration, in that larger doses of a drug may be necessary to obtain effect in patients in which the metabolism is extremely rapid. These interactions, via cytochrome P450 or its isoforms, can occasionally be used beneficially to increase/maintain blood levels of one drug by administering a second drug. Dental clinicians should attempt to stay current on this topic of drug interactions as knowledge evolves.

ALPHABETICAL LISTING OF DRUGS

A200® Lice [OTC] *see* Permethrin *on page 1062*

A-200® Maximum Strength [OTC] *see* Pyrethrins and Piperonyl Butoxide *on page 1151*

A and D® Ointment [OTC] *see* Vitamin A and Vitamin D *on page 1392*

Abacavir (a BAK a veer)

Related Information

HIV Infection and AIDS *on page 1482*

U.S. Brand Names Ziagen®

Canadian Brand Names Ziagen®

Pharmacologic Category Antiretroviral Agent, Reverse Transcriptase Inhibitor (Nucleoside)

Use Treatment of HIV infections in combination with other antiretroviral agents

Local Anesthetic/Vasoconstrictor Precautions No information available to require special precautions

Effects on Dental Treatment Hypersensitivity reactions, which may be fatal, occur in ~5% of patients; symptoms may include anaphylaxis, fever, rash (including erythema multiforme), fatigue, diarrhea, abdominal pain, respiratory symptoms (eg, pharyngitis, dyspnea, cough, adult respiratory distress syndrome, or respiratory failure), headache, malaise, lethargy, myalgia, myolysis, arthralgia, edema, paresthesia, nausea and vomiting, oral ulcerations, conjunctivitis, lymphadenopathy, hepatic failure, and renal failure.

>10%:

Adults: Nausea (47%), vomiting (16%), fever (19%), headache (16%), anorexia (11%)

Children: Nausea (38%), vomiting (38%)

1% to 10%: Children: Anorexia (9%)

Frequency not defined: Adults: Weakness, hyperglycemia

Dosage Oral:

Children: 3 months to 16 years: 8 mg/kg body weight twice daily (maximum 300 mg twice daily) in combination with other antiretroviral agents

Adults: 300 mg twice daily in combination with other antiretroviral agents

Mechanism of Action Nucleoside reverse transcriptase inhibitor. Abacavir is a guanosine analogue which is phosphorylated to carbovir triphosphate which interferes with HIV viral RNA dependent DNA polymerase resulting in inhibition of viral replication.

Other Adverse Effects Rates of adverse reactions were defined during combination therapy with lamivudine. Adverse reaction rates attributable to abacavir alone are not available.

Adults:

Central nervous system: Insomnia (7%)

Endocrine & metabolic: Hypertriglyceridemia (25%), **hyperglycemia**

Gastrointestinal: Diarrhea (12%), pancreatitis

Miscellaneous: Transaminases increased, hypersensitivity reaction (5%)

Children:

Dermatologic: Rash (11%)

Gastrointestinal: Diarrhea (16%)

<1%: **Anaphylactoid reaction, pulmonary hypertension**

Postmarketing and/or case reports (adults and children): Erythema multiforme, redistribution/accumulation of body fat, Stevens-Johnson syndrome, toxic epidermal necrolysis

Drug Interactions Increased Effect/Toxicity: Ethanol may increase the risk of toxicity. Abacavir increases the blood levels of amprenavir. Abacavir may decrease the serum concentration of methadone in some patients. Concomitant use of ribavirin and nucleoside analogues may increase the risk of developing lactic acidosis (includes adefovir, didanosine, lamivudine, stavudine, zalcitabine, zidovudine).

Dietary/Ethanol/Herb Considerations

Ethanol may increase risk of toxicity.

Food: May be taken with food.

Pharmacodynamics/Kinetics

Absorption: Rapid and extensive absorption

Distribution: V_d: 0.86 L/kg

Protein binding: 27% to 33%

Metabolism: Hepatic via alcohol dehydrogenase and glucuronyl transferase to inactive carboxylate and glucuronide metabolites

Bioavailability: 83%

Half-life elimination: 1.5 hours

Time to peak: 0.7-1.7 hours

Excretion: Primarily urine (as metabolites, 1.2% as unchanged drug); feces (16% total dose)

Pregnancy Risk Factor C

Generic Available No

Abacavir, Lamivudine, and Zidovudine

(a BAK a veer, la MI vyoo deen, & zye DOE vyoo deen)

Related Information

Abacavir *on page 22*
Lamivudine *on page 773*
Zidovudine *on page 1406*

U.S. Brand Names Trizivir®

Canadian Brand Names Trizivir®

Pharmacologic Category Antiretroviral Agent, Reverse Transcriptase Inhibitor (Nucleoside)

Synonyms Azidothymidine, Abacavir, and Lamivudine; AZT, Abacavir, and Lamivudine; Compound S, Abacavir, and Lamivudine; Lamivudine, Abacavir, and Zidovudine; 3TC, Abacavir, and Zidovudine; ZDV, Abacavir, and Lamivudine; Zidovudine, Abacavir, and Lamivudine

Use Treatment of HIV infection (either alone or in combination with other antiretroviral agents) in patients whose regimen would otherwise contain the components of Trizivir® (based on analyses of surrogate markers in controlled studies with abacavir of up to 24 weeks; there have been no clinical trials conducted with Trizivir®)

Local Anesthetic/Vasoconstrictor Precautions No information available to require special precautions

Effects on Dental Treatment >10%: Nausea (47%), vomiting (16%), hypersensitivity (5%; abacavir)

Dosage Oral:

Adolescents and Adults: 1 tablet twice daily; not recommended for patients <40 kg
Elderly: Use with caution
Dosing comment in renal impairment: Cl_{cr} ≤50 mL/minute: Contraindicated

Mechanism of Action The combination of abacavir, lamivudine, and zidovudine is believed to act synergistically to inhibit reverse transcriptase via DNA chain termination after incorporation of the nucleoside analogue as well as to delay the emergence of mutations conferring resistance

Other Adverse Effects Trizivir®: Fatal hypersensitivity reactions have occurred; if it is to be restarted following an interruption in therapy, first evaluate the patient for previously unsuspected symptoms of hypersensitivity. Do not restart if hypersensitivity is suspected or if hypersensitivity cannot be ruled out.

Based on CNAAB3003 study:
>10%:
- Endocrine & metabolic: Triglycerides increased (25%)
- Gastrointestinal: Diarrhea (12%), loss of appetite/anorexia (11%)

1% to 10%:
- Central nervous system: Insomnia (7%)

Other (frequency unknown): Pancreatitis, GGT increased

Postmarketing and/or case reports (limited to important or life-threatening): Redistribution/accumulation of body fat, **anaphylaxis**, cardiomyopathy, hepatic steatosis, lactic acidosis, Stevens-Johnson syndrome

Dietary/Ethanol/Herb Considerations Food: May be taken with food

Pregnancy Risk Factor C

Generic Available No

ABCD *see* Amphotericin B Cholesteryl Sulfate Complex *on page 97*

Abciximab

(ab SIK si mab)

U.S. Brand Names ReoPro®

Canadian Brand Names Reopro™

Pharmacologic Category Antiplatelet Agent, Glycoprotein IIb/IIIa Inhibitor

Synonyms C7E3; 7E3

Use Prevention of acute cardiac ischemic complications in patients at high risk for abrupt closure of the treated coronary vessel and patients at risk of restenosis; an adjunct with heparin to prevent cardiac ischemic complications in patients with unstable angina not responding to conventional therapy when a percutaneous coronary intervention is scheduled within 24 hours

Local Anesthetic/Vasoconstrictor Precautions No information available to require special precautions

Effects on Dental Treatment As with all anticoagulants, bleeding is a potential adverse effect of abciximab during dental surgery; risk is dependent on multiple variables, including the intensity of anticoagulation and patient susceptibility. **Medical consult is suggested.** It is unlikely that ambulatory patients presenting for dental treatment will be taking I.V. anticoagulant therapy.

>10%: Hypotension (14%), chest pain (11%), nausea (14%), minor bleeding (4% to 17%), bradycardia (5%)

1% to 10%: Headache (7%), vomiting (7%), major bleeding (1% to 14%)

Dosage I.V.: 0.25 mg/kg bolus administered 10-60 minutes before the start of intervention followed by an infusion of 0.125 mcg/kg/minute (to a maximum of 10 mcg/minute) for 12 hours

(Continued)

Abciximab *(Continued)*

Patients with unstable angina not responding to conventional medical therapy and who are planning to undergo percutaneous coronary intervention within 24 hours may be treated with abciximab 0.25 mg/kg intravenous bolus followed by an 18- to 24-hour intravenous infusion of 10 mcg/minute, concluding 1 hour after the percutaneous coronary intervention.

Mechanism of Action Fab antibody fragment of the chimeric human-murine monoclonal antibody 7E3; this agent binds to platelet IIb/IIIa receptors, resulting in steric hindrance, thus inhibiting platelet aggregation

Other Adverse Effects

>10%: Neuromuscular & skeletal: Back pain (18%)

1% to 10%:

Cardiovascular: Peripheral edema (2%)

Gastrointestinal: Abdominal pain (3%)

Hematologic: Thrombocytopenia: <100,000 cells/mm^3 (3% to 6%); <50,000 cells/mm^3 (0.4% to 2%)

Local: Injection site pain (4%)

<1% (Limited to important or life-threatening): **Stroke**, pseudoaneurysm, intracranial hemorrhage, **ventricular tachycardia, palpitation**, arteriovenous fistula, incomplete AV block, nodal arrhythmia, complete AV block, embolism, thrombophlebitis, dyspepsia, diarrhea, ileus, **gastroesophageal reflux**, anemia, leukocytosis, petechiae, **dizziness, agitation, anxiety, abnormal thinking**, hypesthesia, **confusion, muscle contractions, coma**, hypertonia, diplopia, **pneumonia**, pleural effusion, **bronchitis, bronchospasm**, pulmonary embolism, myalgia, urinary retention, dysuria, urinary incontinence, cystalgia, prostatitis, **pain, increased diaphoresis, weakness**, pruritus, **abnormal vision,** cellulitis, peripheral coldness, **xerostomia**, hyperkalemia, **diabetes mellitus**, bullous eruption, **inflammation, allergic reactions/anaphylaxis**

Drug Interactions Increased Effect/Toxicity: The risk of bleeding is increased when abciximab is given with heparin, other anticoagulants, thrombolytics, or antiplatelet drugs. However, aspirin and heparin were used concurrently in the majority of patients in the major clinical studies of abciximab. Allergic reactions may be increased in patients who have received diagnostic or therapeutic monoclonal antibodies due to the presence of HACA antibodies. Concomitant use of other glycoprotein IIb/IIIa antagonists is contraindicated.

Pharmacodynamics/Kinetics Half-life elimination: ~30 minutes

Pregnancy Risk Factor C

Generic Available No

Abelcet® *see* Amphotericin B (Lipid Complex) *on page 100*

Abilify™ *see* Aripiprazole *on page 122*

ABLC *see* Amphotericin B (Lipid Complex) *on page 100*

Abreva® [OTC] *see* Docosanol *on page 463*

Absorbable Cotton *see* Cellulose (Oxidized) *on page 284*

Absorbable Gelatin Sponge *see* Gelatin (Absorbable) *on page 630*

Absorbine Jr.® Antifungal [OTC] *see* Tolnaftate *on page 1322*

Acarbose (AY car bose)

Related Information

Endocrine Disorders and Pregnancy *on page 1479*

U.S. Brand Names Precose®

Canadian Brand Names Prandase®

Mexican Brand Names Glucobay®

Pharmacologic Category Antidiabetic Agent, Alpha-Glucosidase Inhibitor

Use

Monotherapy, as indicated as an adjunct to diet to lower blood glucose in patients with type 2 diabetes mellitus (noninsulin dependent, NIDDM) whose hyperglycemia cannot be managed on diet alone

Combination with a sulfonylurea, metformin, or insulin in patients with type 2 diabetes mellitus (noninsulin dependent, NIDDM) when diet plus acarbose do not result in adequate glycemic control. The effect of acarbose to enhance glycemic control is additive to that of other hypoglycemic agents when used in combination.

Local Anesthetic/Vasoconstrictor Precautions No information available to require special precautions

Effects on Dental Treatment No significant effects or complications reported

Dosage Dosage must be individualized on the basis of effectiveness and tolerance while not exceeding the maximum recommended dose.

Oral:

Adults:

Initial: 25 mg 3 times/day with the first bite of each main meal

Maintenance dose: Should be adjusted at 4- to 8-week intervals based on 1-hour postprandial glucose levels and tolerance. Dosage may be increased from 25 mg 3 times/day to 50 mg 3 times/day. Some patients may benefit from increasing the dose to 100 mg 3 times/day.

Maintenance dose ranges: 50-100 mg 3 times/day.

Maximum dose:

≤60 kg: 50 mg 3 times/day

>60 kg: 100 mg 3 times/day

Patients receiving sulfonylureas: Acarbose given in combination with a sulfonylurea will cause a further lowering of blood glucose and may increase the hypoglycemic potential of the sulfonylurea. If hypoglycemia occurs, appropriate adjustments in the dosage of these agents should be made.

Dosing adjustment in renal impairment: Cl_{cr} <25 mL/minute: Peak plasma concentrations were 5 times higher and AUCs were 6 times larger than in volunteers with normal renal function; however, long-term clinical trials in diabetic patients with significant renal dysfunction have not been conducted and treatment of these patients with acarbose is not recommended.

Mechanism of Action Competitive inhibitor of pancreatic α-amylase and intestinal brush border α-glucosidases, resulting in delayed hydrolysis of ingested complex carbohydrates and disaccharides and absorption of glucose; dose-dependent reduction in postprandial serum insulin and glucose peaks; inhibits the metabolism of sucrose to glucose and fructose

Other Adverse Effects

>10%:

Gastrointestinal: Abdominal pain (21%), flatulence (77%), diarrhea (33%)

Hepatic: Elevated liver transaminases

<1%: **Drowsiness, headache**, vertigo, erythema, urticaria, **severe GI distress, weakness**

Drug Interactions

Increased Effect/Toxicity: Acarbose may increase the risk of hypoglycemia when used with oral hypoglycemics.

Decreased Effect: The effect of acarbose is antagonized/decreased by thiazide and related diuretics, corticosteroids, phenothiazines, thyroid products, estrogens, oral contraceptives, phenytoin, nicotinic acid, sympathomimetics, calcium channel-blocking drugs, isoniazid, intestinal adsorbents (eg, charcoal), and digestive enzyme preparations (eg, amylase, pancreatin). Acarbose decreases the absorption/serum concentration of digoxin.

Dietary/Ethanol/Herb Considerations Ethanol: Avoid use, especially with other diabetic agents; may increase risk of hypoglycemia.

Pharmacodynamics/Kinetics

Absorption: <2% as active drug

Metabolism: Exclusively via GI tract, principally by intestinal bacteria and digestive enzymes; 13 metabolites identified

Bioavailability: Low systemic bioavailability of parent compound; acts locally in GI tract

Excretion: Urine (~34%)

Pregnancy Risk Factor B

Generic Available No

A-Caro-25® *see* Beta-Carotene *on page 176*

Accolate® *see* Zafirlukast *on page 1402*

AccuNeb™ *see* Albuterol *on page 48*

Accupril® *see* Quinapril *on page 1156*

Accuretic™ *see* Quinapril and Hydrochlorothiazide *on page 1158*

Accutane® *see* Isotretinoin *on page 752*

ACE *see* Captopril *on page 238*

Acebutolol (a se BYOO toe lole)

U.S. Brand Names Sectral®

Canadian Brand Names Apo®-Acebutolol; Gen-Acebutolol; Monitan®; Novo-Acebutolol; Nu-Acebutolol; Rhotral; Sectral®

Pharmacologic Category Antiarrhythmic Agent, Class II; Beta Blocker With Intrinsic Sympathomimetic Activity

Synonyms Acebutolol Hydrochloride

Use Treatment of hypertension, ventricular arrhythmias, angina

Local Anesthetic/Vasoconstrictor Precautions No information available to require special precautions

Effects on Dental Treatment Acebutolol is a cardioselective beta-blocker. Local anesthetic with vasoconstrictor can be safely used in patients medicated with acebutolol. Nonselective beta-blockers (ie, propranolol, nadolol) enhance the pressor response to epinephrine, resulting in hypertension and bradycardia; this has not been reported for acebutolol. Many nonsteroidal anti-inflammatory drugs such as ibuprofen and indomethacin can reduce the hypotensive effect of beta-blockers after 3 or more weeks of therapy with the NSAID. Short-term NSAID use (ie, 3 days) requires no special precautions in patients taking beta-blockers.

>10%: Fatigue (11%)

(Continued)

Acebutolol *(Continued)*

1% to 6%: Chest pain (2%), bradycardia, hypotension, CHF, headache (6%), dizziness (6%), anxiety, nausea (4%), vomiting, dyspnea (4%), rhinitis (2%), cough (1%), pharyngitis, wheezing, CNS depression (2%), joint pain

Dosage Oral:

Adults:

Hypertension: 400-800 mg/day (larger doses may be divided); maximum: 1200 mg/day

Ventricular arrhythmias: Initial: 400 mg/day; maintenance: 600-1200 mg/day in divided doses

Elderly: Initial: 200-400 mg/day; dose reduction due to age related decrease in Cl_{cr} will be necessary; do not exceed 800 mg/day

Dosing adjustment in renal impairment:

Cl_{cr} 25-49 mL/minute/1.73 m^2: Reduce dose by 50%.

Cl_{cr} <25 mL/minute/1.73 m^2: Reduce dose by 75%.

Dosing adjustment in hepatic impairment: Use with caution.

Mechanism of Action Competitively blocks $beta_1$-adrenergic receptors with little or no effect on $beta_2$-receptors except at high doses; exhibits membrane stabilizing and intrinsic sympathomimetic activity

Other Adverse Effects

1% to 10%:

Cardiovascular: Edema (2%)

Central nervous system: Insomnia (3%), abnormal dreams (2%), hyperesthesia, hypoesthesia, impotence

Dermatologic: Rash (2%), pruritus

Gastrointestinal: Constipation (4%), diarrhea (4%), dyspepsia (4%), flatulence (3%), abdominal pain

Genitourinary: Micturition frequency (3%), dysuria, nocturia, impotence (2%)

Neuromuscular & skeletal: Arthralgia (2%), myalgia (2%), back pain

Ocular: Abnormal vision (2%), conjunctivitis, dry eyes, eye pain

<1% (Limited to important or life-threatening): Increased transaminases, increased bilirubin, increased alkaline phosphatase, hepatotoxic reaction, **ventricular arrhythmias**, AV block, **facial edema, xerostomia**, anorexia, impotence, urinary retention, cold extremities, systemic lupus erythematosus, **palpitations, exacerbation of pre-existing renal insufficiency**

Postmarketing and/or case reports: Pleurisy, pulmonary granulomas, pneumonitis, lichen planus, lupus erythematosus, drug-induced lupus-like syndrome

Based on experience with other beta-blocking agents: Mental depression (reversible), disorientation, catatonia, short-term memory loss, emotional lability, slightly clouded sensorium, **laryngospasm, respiratory distress, allergic reactions**, erythematous rash, agranulocytosis, purpura, thrombocytopenia, mesenteric artery thrombosis, ischemic colitis, alopecia, Peyronie's disease, claudication

Drug Interactions Inhibits CYP2D6

Increased Effect/Toxicity: Acebutolol may increase the effects of other drugs which slow AV conduction (digoxin, verapamil, diltiazem), alpha-blockers (prazosin, terazosin), and alpha-adrenergic stimulants (epinephrine, phenylephrine). Acebutolol may mask the tachycardia from hypoglycemia caused by insulin and oral hypoglycemics. In patients receiving concurrent therapy, the risk of hypertensive crisis is increased when either clonidine or the beta-blocker is withdrawn. Reserpine has been shown to enhance the effect of acebutolol. Beta-blockers may increase the action or levels of ethanol, disopyramide, nondepolarizing muscle relaxants, and theophylline although the effects are difficult to predict.

Decreased Effect: Decreased effect of acebutolol with aluminum salts, barbiturates, calcium salts, cholestyramine, colestipol, NSAIDs, penicillins (ampicillin), rifampin, and salicylates due to decreased bioavailability and plasma levels. The effect of sulfonylureas may be decreased by beta-blockers; however, the decreased effect has not been shown with tolbutamide.

Dietary/Ethanol/Herb Considerations

Ethanol: Limit use; may increase risk of hypotension or dizziness.

Food: May be taken with meals; food may slightly decrease peak serum concentration.

Herb/Nutraceutical: Avoid black cohosh, dong quai, and evening primrose due to estrogenic activity. Avoid ephedra, ginseng, and yohimbe; may worsen hypertension.

Pharmacodynamics/Kinetics

Onset of action: 1-2 hours

Duration: 12-24 hours

Absorption: Oral: 40%

Protein binding: 5% to 15%

Metabolism: Extensive first-pass effect

Half-life elimination: 6-7 hours

Time to peak: 2-4 hours

Excretion: Feces (~55%); urine (35%)

Pregnancy Risk Factor B (manufacturer); D (2nd and 3rd trimesters - expert analysis)

Generic Available Yes

Selected Readings

Foster CA and Aston SJ, "Propranolol-Epinephrine Interaction: A Potential Disaster," *Plast Reconstr Surg*, 1983, 72(1):74-8.

Wong DG, Spence JD, Lamki L, et al, "Effect of Nonsteroidal Anti-inflammatory Drugs on Control of Hypertension of Beta-Blockers and Diuretics," *Lancet*, 1986, 1(8488):997-1001.

Wynn RL, "Dental Nonsteroidal Anti-inflammatory Drugs and Prostaglandin-Based Drug Interactions, Part Two," *Gen Dent*, 1992, 40(2):104, 106, 108.

Wynn RL, "Epinephrine Interactions With Beta-Blockers," *Gen Dent*, 1994, 42(1):16, 18.

Acebutolol Hydrochloride *see* Acebutolol *on page 25*

Aceon® *see* Perindopril Erbumine *on page 1060*

Acephen® [OTC] *see* Acetaminophen *on page 27*

Acetaminophen (a seet a MIN oh fen)

Related Information

Oral Pain *on page 1524*

Oxycodone and Acetaminophen *on page 1018*

U.S. Brand Names Acephen® [OTC]; Aspirin Free Anacin® Maximum Strength [OTC]; Cetafen® [OTC]; Cetafen Extra® [OTC]; Feverall® [OTC]; Genapap® [OTC]; Genapap® Children [OTC]; Genapap® Extra Strength [OTC]; Genapap® Infant [OTC]; Genebs® [OTC]; Genebs® Extra Strength [OTC]; Infantaire [OTC]; Liquiprin® for Children [OTC]; Mapap® [OTC]; Mapap® Children's [OTC]; Mapap® Extra Strength [OTC]; Mapap® Infants [OTC]; Redutemp® [OTC]; Silapap® Children's [OTC]; Silapap® Infants [OTC]; Tylenol® [OTC]; Tylenol® Arthritis Pain [OTC]; Tylenol® Children's [OTC]; Tylenol® Extra Strength [OTC]; Tylenol® Infants [OTC]; Tylenol® Junior Strength [OTC]; Tylenol® Sore Throat [OTC]; Valorin [OTC]; Valorin Extra [OTC]

Canadian Brand Names Abenol®; Apo®-Acetaminophen; Atasol®; Pediatrix; Tempra®; Tylenol®

Mexican Brand Names Algitrin®; Analphen; Andox®; Cilag®; Datril®; Febrin®; Magnidol®; Minofen®; Neodol®; Neodolito®; Sedalito®; Sinedol®; Sinedol 500; Temperal®; Tempra®; Tylex®; Tylex 750; Winasorb

Pharmacologic Category Analgesic, Miscellaneous

Synonyms APAP; N-Acetyl-P-Aminophenol; Paracetamol

Use

Dental: Treatment of postoperative pain

Medical: Treatment of mild to moderate pain and fever (antipyretic/analgesic); does not have antirheumatic or anti-inflammatory effects

Local Anesthetic/Vasoconstrictor Precautions No information available to require special precautions

Effects on Dental Treatment No significant effects or complications reported

Dosage If fever not controlled with acetaminophen alone, administer with full doses of aspirin on an every 4- to 6-hour schedule, if aspirin is not otherwise contraindicated.

Oral, rectal:

Children <12 years: 10-15 mg/kg/dose every 4-6 hours as needed; do **not** exceed 5 doses (2.6 g) in 24 hours; alternatively, the following age-based doses may be used. See table.

Acetaminophen Dosing

Age	Dosage (mg)	Age	Dosage (mg)
0-3 mo	40	4-5 y	240
4-11 mo	80	6-8 y	320
1-2 y	120	9-10 y	400
2-3 y	160	11 y	480

Adults: 325-650 mg every 4-6 hours or 1000 mg 3-4 times/day; do **not** exceed 4 g/day

Dosing interval in renal impairment:

Cl_{cr} 10-50 mL/minute: Administer every 6 hours

Cl_{cr} <10 mL/minute: Administer every 8 hours (metabolites accumulate)

Hemodialysis: Moderately dialyzable (20% to 50%)

Dosing adjustment/comments in hepatic impairment: Avoid chronic use; limited, low-dose therapy usually well tolerated, however, cases of hepatotoxicity at daily acetaminophen dosages <4 g/day have been reported.

Mechanism of Action Inhibits the synthesis of prostaglandins in the central nervous system and peripherally blocks pain impulse generation; produces antipyresis from inhibition of hypothalamic heat-regulating center

Other Adverse Effects

Frequency not defined:

Endocrine & metabolic: May increase chloride, uric acid, glucose; may decrease sodium, bicarbonate, calcium

Hepatic: May increase bilirubin, alkaline phosphatase

(Continued)

Acetaminophen *(Continued)*

Renal: May increase ammonia

<1%: Rash, **nausea, vomiting**, blood dyscrasias (neutropenia, pancytopenia, leukopenia), anemia, analgesic nephropathy, nephrotoxicity (with chronic overdose), **hypersensitivity reactions (rare)**

Contraindications Hypersensitivity to acetaminophen or any component of the formulation; patients with known G6PD deficiency

Warnings/Precautions May cause severe hepatic toxicity on overdose; use with caution in patients with alcoholic liver disease; chronic daily dosing in adults of 5-8 g of acetaminophen over several weeks or 3-4 g/day of acetaminophen for 1 year have resulted in liver damage

Drug Interactions Substrate of CYP1A2, 2A6, 2C8/9, 2D6, 2E1, 3A4

Decreased Effect: Barbiturates, carbamazepine, hydantoins, rifampin, sulfinpyrazone may decrease the analgesic effect of acetaminophen; cholestyramine may decrease acetaminophen absorption (separate dosing by at least 1 hour)

Increased Toxicity: Barbiturates, carbamazepine, hydantoins, isoniazid, rifampin, sulfinpyrazone may increase the hepatotoxic potential of acetaminophen; chronic ethanol abuse increases risk for acetaminophen toxicity; effect of warfarin may be enhanced

Dietary/Ethanol/Herb Considerations

Ethanol: Avoid use; may cause hepatotoxicity. It has been reported that a combination of two quarts of whiskey a day with 8-10 acetaminophen tablets daily resulted in severe liver toxicity. People who consume ethanol at the same time that they use acetaminophen, even in therapeutic doses, are at risk of developing hepatotoxicity.

Food: Administer oral form with food or milk; may decrease peak serum concentration and slightly delay absorption of extended-release form. Rate of absorption may be decreased with food high in carbohydrates.

Herb/Nutraceutical: Avoid St John's wort; may decrease serum concentration.

Pharmacodynamics/Kinetics

Onset of action: <1 hour

Duration: 4-6 hours

Protein binding: 20% to 50%

Metabolism: At normal therapeutic dosages, hepatic to sulfate and glucuronide metabolites, while a small amount is metabolized by CYP to a highly reactive intermediate (acetylimidoquinone) which is conjugated with glutathione and inactivated; at toxic doses (as little as 4 g daily) glutathione conjugation becomes insufficient to meet the metabolic demand causing an increase in acetylimidoquinone concentration, which may cause hepatic cell necrosis

Half-life elimination:

Neonates: 2-5 hours

Adults: 1-3 hours

Time to peak, serum: Oral: 10-60 minutes; may be delayed in acute overdoses

Excretion: Urine

Pregnancy Risk Factor B

Dosage Forms CAP: 500 mg. **CAPLET:** 500 mg. **CAPLET, extended release:** 650 mg. **ELIX:** 160 mg/5 mL (5 mL, 10 mL, 20 mL, 120 mL, 240 mL, 480 mL, 500 mL, 3780 mL). **GELCAP:** 500 mg. **GELTAB:** 500 mg. **LIQ, oral:** 160 mg/5 mL (120 mL, 240 mL, 480 mL, 3870 mL); 500 mg/15 mL (120 mL, 240 mL). **SOLN, oral drops:** 80 mg/0.8 mL (15 mL, 30 mL); 100 mg/mL (15 mL, 30 mL). **SUPP, rectal:** 80 mg, 120 mg, 325 mg, 650 mg. **SUSP, oral:** 160 mg/5 mL (120 mL, 240 mL). **SUSP, oral drops:** 80 mg/0.8 mL (15 mL, 30 mL); 100 mg/mL (15 mL, 30 mL). **SYR, oral:** 160 mg/5 mL (120 mL). **TAB:** 160 mg, 325 mg, 500 mg. **TAB, chewable:** 80 mg, 160 mg

Generic Available Yes

Comments Doses of acetaminophen >5 g/day for several weeks can produce severe, often fatal liver damage. Hepatotoxicity caused by acetaminophen is potentiated by chronic ethanol consumption.

A study by Hylek, et al, suggested that the combination of acetaminophen with warfarin (Coumadin®) may cause enhanced anticoagulation. The following recommendations have been made by Hylek, et al, and supported by an editorial in *JAMA* by Bell.

Dose and duration of acetaminophen should be as low as possible, individualized and monitored.

For patients who reported taking the equivalent of at least 4 regular strength (325 mg) tablets for longer than a week, the odds of having an INR >6.0 were increased 10-fold above those not taking acetaminophen. Risk decreased with lower intakes of acetaminophen reaching a background level of risk at a dose of 6 or fewer 325 mg tablets per week.

Selected Readings

Ahmad N, Grad HA, Haas DA, et al, "The Efficacy of Nonopioid Analgesics for Postoperative Dental Pain: A Meta-Analysis," *Anesth Prog*, 1997, 44(4):119-26.

Bell WR, "Acetaminophen and Warfarin: Undesirable Synergy," *JAMA*, 1998, 279(9):702-3.

Botting RM, "Mechanism of Action of Acetaminophen: Is There a Cyclooxygenase 3?," *Clin Infect Dis*, 2000, Suppl 5:S202-10.

Dart RC, Kuffner EK, and Rumack BH, "Treatment of Pain or Fever with Paracetamol (Acetaminophen) in the Alcoholic Patient: A Systematic Review," *Am J Ther*, 2000, 7(2):123-34.

Dionne R, "Additive Analgesia Without Opioid Side Effects," *Compend Contin Educ Dent*, 2000, 21(7):572-4, 576-7.

Dionne RA and Berthold CW, "Therapeutic Uses of Nonsteroidal Anti-Inflammatory Drugs in Dentistry," *Crit Rev Oral Biol Med*, 2001, 12(4):315-30.

Dionne RA, Campbell RA, Cooper SA, et al, "Suppression of Postoperative Pain by Preoperative Administration of Ibuprofen in Comparison to Placebo, Acetaminophen, and Acetaminophen Plus Codeine," *J Clin Pharmacol*, 1983, 23(1):37-43.

Grant JA and Weiler JM, "A Report of a Rare Immediate Reaction After Ingestion of Acetaminophen," *Ann Allergy Asthma Immunol*, 2001, 87(3):227-9.

Hylek EM, Heiman H, Skates SJ, et al, "Acetaminophen and Other Risk Factors for Excessive Warfarin Anticoagulation," *JAMA*, 1998, 279(9):657-62.

Kwan D, Bartle WR, and Walker SE, "The Effects of Acetaminophen on Pharmacokinetics and Pharmacodynamics of Warfarin," *J Clin Pharmacol*, 1999, 39(1):68-75.

Lee WM, "Drug-Induced Hepatotoxicity," *N Engl J Med*, 1995, 333(17):1118-27.

Licht H, Seeff LB, and Zimmerman HJ, "Apparent Potentiation of Acetaminophen Hepatotoxicity by Alcohol," *Ann Intern Med*, 1980, 92(4):511.

McClain CJ, Price S, Barve S, et al, "Acetaminophen Hepatotoxicity: An Update," *Curr Gastroenterol Rep*, 1999, 1(1):42-9.

Murphy R, Swartz R, and Watkins PB, "Severe Acetaminophen Toxicity in a Patient Receiving Isoniazid," *Ann Intern Med*, 1990, 113(110):799-800.

Nguyen AM, Graham DY, Gage T, et al, "Nonsteroidal Anti-Inflammatory Drug Use in Dentistry: Gastrointestinal Implications," *Gen Dent*, 1999, 47(6):590-6.

Shek KL, Chan LN, and Nutescu E, "Warfarin-Acetaminophen Drug Interaction Revisited," *Pharmacotherapy*, 1999, 19(10):1153-8.

Tanaka E, Yamazaki K, and Misawa S, "Update: The Clinical Importance of Acetaminophen Hepatotoxicity in Nonalcoholic and Alcoholic Subjects," *J Clin Pharm Ther*, 2000, 25(5):325-32.

Acetaminophen and Chlorpheniramine *see* Chlorpheniramine and Acetaminophen *on page 308*

Acetaminophen and Codeine (a seet a MIN oh fen & KOE deen)

Related Information

Acetaminophen *on page 27*
Codeine *on page 361*

U.S. Brand Names Capital® and Codeine; Phenaphen® With Codeine; Tylenol® With Codeine

Canadian Brand Names Emtec-30; Lenoltec; Triatec-8; Triatec-8 Strong; Triatec-30; Tylenol® with Codeine

Mexican Brand Names Tylex CD

Pharmacologic Category Analgesic, Narcotic

Synonyms Codeine and Acetaminophen

Use

Dental: Treatment of postoperative pain
Medical: Relief of mild to moderate pain

Local Anesthetic/Vasoconstrictor Precautions No information available to require special precautions

Effects on Dental Treatment

>10%: Lightheadedness, dizziness, sedation, vomiting, dyspnea, nausea
1% to 10%: Euphoria, histamine release

Restrictions C-III; C-V

Dosage Doses should be adjusted according to severity of pain and response of the patient. Adult doses ≥60 mg codeine fail to give commensurate relief of pain but merely prolong analgesia and are associated with an appreciably increased incidence of side effects.

Oral:

Children: Analgesic:

Codeine: 0.5-1 mg codeine/kg/dose every 4-6 hours

Acetaminophen: 10-15 mg/kg/dose every 4 hours up to a maximum of 2.6 g/24 hours for children <12 years; **alternatively, the following can be used:**

3-6 years: 5 mL 3-4 times/day as needed of elixir
7-12 years: 10 mL 3-4 times/day as needed of elixir
>12 years: 15 mL every 4 hours as needed of elixir

Adults:

Antitussive: Based on codeine (15-30 mg/dose) every 4-6 hours (maximum: 360 mg/24 hours based on codeine component)

Analgesic: Based on codeine (30-60 mg/dose) every 4-6 hours (maximum: 4000 mg/24 hours based on acetaminophen component)

Mechanism of Action Inhibits the synthesis of prostaglandins in the central nervous system and peripherally blocks pain impulse generation; produces antipyresis from inhibition of hypothalamic heat-regulating center; binds to opiate receptors in the CNS, causing inhibition of ascending pain pathways, altering the perception of and response to pain; causes cough supression by direct central action in the medulla; produces generalized CNS depression

Other Adverse Effects

1% to 10%:

Central nervous system: Dysphoria
Dermatologic: Pruritus
Gastrointestinal: Constipation, abdominal pain

(Continued)

Acetaminophen and Codeine *(Continued)*

<1%: **Palpitations, hypotension, bradycardia, peripheral vasodilation, increased intracranial pressure**, antidiuretic hormone release, **biliary tract spasm**, urinary retention, miosis, **respiratory depression**, physical and psychological dependence, **xerostomia**

Contraindications Hypersensitivity to acetaminophen or any component of the formulation, to codeine phosphate, or similar compounds

Warnings/Precautions Use with caution in patients with hypersensitivity reactions to other phenanthrene derivative opioid agonists (morphine, hydrocodone, hydromorphone, levorphanol, oxycodone, oxymorphone); tablets contain metabisulfite which may cause allergic reactions

Drug Interactions Acetaminophen: Substrate of CYP1A2, 2A6, 2C8/9, 2D6, 2E1, 3A4

Increased Toxicity: CNS depressants, phenothiazines, tricyclic antidepressants, guanabenz, MAO inhibitors (may also decrease blood pressure); effect of warfarin may be enhanced

Dietary/Ethanol/Herb Considerations

Ethanol: Avoid use due to potential hepatotoxicity from acetaminopen component.

Food: May be taken with food

Pregnancy Risk Factor C

Dosage Forms CAP [C-III]: #3: (Phenaphen® With Codeine): Acetaminophen 325 mg and codeine phosphate 30 mg. **ELIX, oral** [C-V]: Acetaminophen 120 mg and codeine phosphate 12 mg per 5 mL (5 mL, 10 mL, 12.5 mL, 15 mL, 120 mL, 480 mL, 3840 mL) (Tylenol® with Codeine): Acetaminophen 120 mg and codeine phosphate 12 mg per 5 mL (480 mL). **SUSP, oral** [C-V] (Capital® and Codeine): Acetaminophen 120 mg and codeine phosphate 12 mg per 5 mL (480 mL). **TAB** [C-III]: #2: Acetaminophen 300 mg and codeine phosphate 15 mg; #3 (Tylenol® with Codeine): Acetaminophen 300 mg and codeine phosphate 30 mg; #4 (Tylenol® with Codeine): Acetaminophen 300 mg and codeine phosphate 60 mg

Generic Available Yes

Comments Codeine products, as with other narcotic analgesics, are recommended only for acute dosing (ie, 3 days or less). The most common adverse effect you will see in your dental patients from codeine is nausea, followed by sedation and constipation. Codeine has narcotic addiction liability, especially when given long-term. Because of the acetaminophen component, this product should be used with caution in patients with alcoholic liver disease.

A study by Hylek, et al, suggested that the combination of acetaminophen with warfarin (Coumadin®) may cause enhanced anticoagulation. The following recommendations have been made by Hylek, et al, and supported by an editorial in *JAMA* by Bell.

Dose and duration of acetaminophen should be as low as possible, individualized and monitored.

For patients who reported taking the equivalent of at least 4 regular strength (325 mg) tablets for longer than a week, the odds of having an INR >6.0 were increased 10-fold above those not taking acetaminophen. Risk decreased with lower intakes of acetaminophen reaching a background level of risk at a dose of 6 or fewer 325 mg tablets per week.

Selected Readings

Change DJ, Fricke JR, Bird SR, et al, "Rofecoxib Versus Codeine/Acetaminophen in Postoperative Dental Pain: A Double-Blind, Randomized, Placebo- and Active Comparator-Controlled Clinical Trial," *Clin Ther*, 2001, 23(9):1446-55.

Dionne RA, "New Approaches to Preventing and Treating Postoperative Pain," *J Am Dent Assoc*, 1992, 123(6):26-34.

Forbes JA, Butterworth GA, Burchfield WH, et al, "Evaluation of Ketorolac, Aspirin, and an Acetaminophen-Codeine Combination in Postoperative Oral Surgery Pain," *Pharmacotherapy*, 1990, 10(6 Pt 2):77S-93S.

Gobetti JP, "Controlling Dental Pain," *J Am Dent Assoc*, 1992, 123(6):47-52.

Mullican WS and Lacy JR, "Tramadol/Acetaminophen Combination Tablets and Codeine/Acetaminophen Combination Capsules for the Management of Chronic Pain: A Comparative Trial," *Clin Ther*, 2001, 23(9):1429-45.

Wynn RL, "Narcotic Analgesics for Dental Pain: Available Products, Strengths, and Formulations," *Gen Dent*, 2001, 49(2):126-8, 130, 132 passim.

Acetaminophen and Diphenhydramine

(a seet a MIN oh fen & dye fen HYE dra meen)

Related Information

Acetaminophen *on page 27*

DiphenhydrAMINE *on page 451*

U.S. Brand Names Anacin PM Aspirin Free [OTC]; Excedrin® P.M. [OTC]; Goody's PM® Powder; Legatrin PM® [OTC]; Tylenol® PM Extra Strength [OTC]; Tylenol® Severe Allergy [OTC]

Pharmacologic Category Analgesic, Miscellaneous

Synonyms Diphenhydramine and Acetaminophen

Use Aid in the relief of insomnia accompanied by minor pain

Local Anesthetic/Vasoconstrictor Precautions No information available to require special precautions

Effects on Dental Treatment 1% to 10%: Xerostomia

Dosage Oral: Adults: 50 mg of diphenhydramine HCl (76 mg diphenhydramine citrate) at bedtime or as directed by physician; do not exceed recommended dosage; not for use in children <12 years of age

Dietary/Ethanol/Herb Considerations Ethanol: Excessive intake may increase risk of acetaminophen-induced hepatotoxicity; avoid use or limit to <3 drinks/day.

Generic Available Yes

Selected Readings

Barker JD Jr, de Carle DJ, and Anuras S, "Chronic Excessive Acetaminophen Use in Liver Damage," *Ann Intern Med*, 1977, 87(3):299-301.

Acetaminophen and Hydrocodone *see* Hydrocodone and Acetaminophen *on page 678*

Acetaminophen and Oxycodone *see* Oxycodone and Acetaminophen *on page 1018*

Acetaminophen and Phenyltoloxamine

(a seet a MIN oh fen & fen il to LOKS a meen)

Related Information

Acetaminophen *on page 27*

U.S. Brand Names Genesec® [OTC]; Percogesic® [OTC]; Phenylgesic® [OTC]

Pharmacologic Category Analgesic, Non-narcotic

Synonyms Phenyltoloxamine and Acetaminophen

Use Relief of mild to moderate pain

Local Anesthetic/Vasoconstrictor Precautions No information available to require special precautions

Effects on Dental Treatment No significant effects or complications reported

Dosage Oral:

Analgesic: Based on acetaminophen component:

Children: 10-15 mg/kg/dose every 4-6 hours as needed; do **not** exceed 5 doses/24 hours

Adults: 325-650 every 4-6 hours as needed; do **not** exceed 4 g/day

Product labeling:

Percogesic®:

Children 6-12 years: 1 tablet every 4 hours; do **not** exceed 4 tablets/24 hours

Adults: 1-2 tablets every 4 hours; do **not** exceed 8 tablets/24 hours

Dietary/Ethanol/Herb Considerations Ethanol: Excessive intake may increase risk of acetaminophen-induced hepatotoxicity; avoid use or limit to <3 drinks/day.

Pregnancy Risk Factor B

Generic Available Yes

Selected Readings

Botting RM, "Mechanism of Action of Acetaminophen: Is There a Cyclooxygenase 3?," *Clin Infect Dis*, 2000, Suppl 5:S202-10.

Dart RC, Kuffner EK, and Rumack BH, "Treatment of Pain or Fever with Paracetamol (Acetaminophen) in the Alcoholic Patient: A Systematic Review," *Am J Ther*, 2000, 7(2):123-34.

Dionne RA, Campbell RA, Cooper SA, et al, "Suppression of Postoperative Pain by Preoperative Administration of Ibuprofen in Comparison to Placebo, Acetaminophen, and Acetaminophen Plus Codeine," *J Clin Pharmacol*, 1983, 23(1):37-43.

Grant JA and Weiler JM, "A Report of a Rare Immediate Reaction After Ingestion of Acetaminophen," *Ann Allergy Asthma Immunol*, 2001, 87(3):227-9.

Kwan D, Bartle WR, and Walker SE, "The Effects of Acetaminophen on Pharmacokinetics and Pharmacodynamics of Warfarin," *J Clin Pharmacol*, 1999, 39(1):68-75.

Licht H, Seeff LB, and Zimmerman HJ, "Apparent Potentiation of Acetaminophen Hepatotoxicity by Alcohol," *Ann Intern Med*, 1980, 92(4):511.

McClain CJ, Price S, Barve S, et al, "Acetaminophen Hepatotoxicity: An Update," *Curr Gastroenterol Rep*, 1999, 1(1):42-9.

Shek KL, Chan LN, and Nutescu E, "Warfarin-Acetaminophen Drug Interaction Revisited," *Pharmacotherapy*, 1999, 19(10):1153-8.

Tanaka E, Yamazaki K, and Misawa S, "Update: The Clinical Importance of Acetaminophen Hepatotoxicity in Nonalcoholic and Alcoholic Subjects," *J Clin Pharm Ther*, 2000, 25(5):325-32.

Acetaminophen and Pseudoephedrine

(a seet a MIN oh fen & soo doe e FED rin)

Related Information

Acetaminophen *on page 27*

Pseudoephedrine *on page 1146*

U.S. Brand Names Alka-Seltzer Plus® Cold and Sinus [OTC]; Children's Tylenol® Sinus [OTC]; Infants Tylenol® Cold [OTC]; Medi-Synal [OTC]; Ornex® [OTC]; Ornex® Maximum Strength [OTC]; Sinus-Relief® [OTC]; Sinutab® Sinus Maximum Strength Without Drowsiness [OTC]; Sudafed® Cold and Sinus [OTC]; Sudafed® Sinus Headache [OTC]; Tylenol® Sinus Non-Drowsy [OTC]

Canadian Brand Names Dristan® N.D.; Dristan® N.D., Extra Strength; Sinutab® Non Drowsy; Sudafed® Head Cold and Sinus Extra Strength; Tylenol® Decongestant; Tylenol® Sinus

Pharmacologic Category Alpha/Beta Agonist; Analgesic, Miscellaneous

Synonyms Pseudoephedrine and Acetaminophen

Use Relief of mild to moderate pain; relief of congestion

(Continued)

Acetaminophen and Pseudoephedrine *(Continued)*

Local Anesthetic/Vasoconstrictor Precautions No information available to require special precautions

Effects on Dental Treatment No significant effects or complications reported

Dosage Oral:

Analgesic: Based on acetaminophen component:

Children: 10-15 mg/kg/dose every 4-6 hours as needed; do **not** exceed 5 doses in 24 hours

Adults: 325-650 mg every 4-6 hours as needed; do **not** exceed 4 g/day

Decongestant: Based on pseudoephedrine component:

Children:

2-6 years: 15 mg every 4 hours; do **not** exceed 90 mg/day

6-12 years: 30 mg every 4 hours; do **not** exceed 180 mg/day

Children >12 years and Adults: 60 mg every 4 hours; do **not** exceed 360 mg/day

Product labeling:

Alka-Seltzer Plus® Cold and Sinus:

Children 6-12 years: 1 dose with water every 4 hours (maximum: 4 doses/24 hours)

Adults: 2 doses with water every 4 hours (maximum: 4 doses/24 hours)

Children's Tylenol® Sinus: Children:

Liquid:

2-5 years (24-47 lbs): 1 teaspoonful every 4-6 hours (maximum: 4 doses/24 hours)

6-11 years (48-95 lbs): 2 teaspoonfuls every 4-6 hours (maximum: 4 doses/24 hours)

Tablet, chewable:

2-5 years (24-47 lbs): 2 tablets every 4-6 hours (maximum: 4 doses/24 hours)

6-11 years (48-95 lbs): 4 tablets every 4-6 hours (maximum: 4 doses/24 hours)

Sine-Aid® Maximum Strength, Tylenol® Sinus Maximum Strength: Children >12 years and Adults: 2 doses every 4-6 hours (maximum: 8 doses/24 hours)

Sinutab® Sinus Maximum Strength Without Drowsiness, Tavist® Sinus: Children >12 years and Adults: 2 doses every 6 hours (maximum: 8 doses/24 hours)

Dietary/Ethanol/Herb Considerations Ethanol: Excessive intake may increase risk of acetaminophen-induced hepatotoxicity; avoid use or limit to <3 drinks/day.

Generic Available Yes

Acetaminophen and Tramadol (a seet a MIN oh fen & TRA ma dole)

Related Information

Acetaminophen *on page 27*

U.S. Brand Names Ultracet™

Pharmacologic Category Analgesic, Non-narcotic; Analgesic, Miscellaneous

Synonyms APAP and Tramadol; Tramadol Hydrochloride and Acetaminophen

Use

Dental: Treatment of postoperative pain (≤5 days)

Medical: Short-term (≤5 days) management of acute pain

Local Anesthetic/Vasoconstrictor Precautions No information available to require special precautions

Effects on Dental Treatment 1% to 10%: Xerostomia, anxiety, confusion, headache, nervousness, weakness, tremors, somnolence (6%), dizziness (3%), hot flashes, nausea (3%), vomiting, increased diaphoresis (4%), euphoria, fatigue

Dosage Oral:

Adults: **Acute pain:** Two tablets every 4-6 hours as needed for pain relief (maximum: 8 tablets/day); treatment should not exceed 5 days

Dosing adjustment in renal impairment: Cl_{cr} <30 mL/minute: Maximum of 2 tablets every 12 hours; treatment should not exceed 5 days

Dosing adjustment in hepatic impairment: Use not recommended

Mechanism of Action

Based on **acetaminophen** component: Inhibits the synthesis of prostaglandins in the central nervous system and peripherally blocks pain impulse generation; produces antipyresis from inhibition of hypothalamic heat-regulating center

Based on **tramadol** component: Binds to μ-opiate receptors in the CNS causing inhibition of ascending pain pathways, altering the perception of and response to pain; also inhibits the reuptake of norepinephrine and serotonin, which also modifies the ascending pain pathway

Other Adverse Effects

1% to 10%:

Central nervous system: Insomnia (2%)

Dermatologic: Pruritus (2%), rash

Gastrointestinal: Constipation (6%), anorexia (3%), diarrhea (3%), abdominal pain, dyspepsia, flatulence

Genitourinary: Prostatic disorder (2%)

<1%: **Abnormal thinking, abnormal vision,** albuminuria, **amnesia,** anemia, **arrhythmia**, ataxia, **chest pain, convulsions**, depersonalization, **dysphagia,**

dyspnea, emotional lability, **hallucination, hypertension, hypotension**, hypertonia, impotence, liver function abnormalities, melena, micturition disorder, **migraine, muscle contractions (involuntary)**, oliguria, **palpitations, paresthesia**, paroniria, **rigors, stupor, [syncope, tachycardia**, tinnitus, **tongue edema**, urinary retention, weight loss, **withdrawal syndrome,** vertigo

Postmarketing and/or case reports: **Agitation, allergic reactions, anaphylactoid reactions, anaphylaxis, cognitive dysfunction, coma**, depression, **diaphoresis**, difficulty concentrating, **fever, GI bleeding**, hepatitis, hyper-reflexia, mental status change, myocardial ischemia, **orthostatic hypotension**, liver failure, pulmonary edema, **seizures, serotonin syndrome,** shivering, Stevens-Johnson syndrome, **suicidal tendency,** toxic epidermal necrolysis, urticaria, **vasodilation**

Contraindications Hypersensitivity to acetaminophen, tramadol, opioids, or any component of the formulation; opioid-dependent patients; acute intoxication with ethanol, hypnotics, narcotics, centrally-acting analgesics, opioids, or psychotropic drugs; hepatic dysfunction

Warnings/Precautions Should be used only with extreme caution in patients receiving MAO inhibitors. Use with caution and reduce dosage when administering to patients receiving other CNS depressants. Seizures may occur when taken within the recommended dosage; risk is increased in patients receiving serotonin reuptake inhibitors (SSRIs or anorectics), tricyclic antidepressants, other cyclic compounds (including cyclobenzaprine, promethazine), neuroleptics, MAO inhibitors, or drugs which may lower seizure threshold. Patients with a history of seizures, or with a risk of seizures (head trauma, metabolic disorders, CNS infection, or malignancy, or during alcohol/drug withdrawal) are also at increased risk. Do not use with ethanol or other acetaminophen- or tramadol-containing products.

Elderly patients and patients with chronic respiratory disorders may be at greater risk of adverse events. Use with caution in patients with increased intracranial pressure or head injury. Use tramadol with caution and reduce dosage in patients with renal dysfunction and in patients with myxedema, hypothyroidism, or hypoadrenalism. Tolerance or drug dependence may result from extended use; abrupt discontinuation should be avoided. Safety and efficacy in pediatric patients have not been established.

Drug Interactions

Acetaminophen: Substrate of CYP1A2, 2A6, 2C8/9, 2D6, 2E1, 3A4

Tramadol: Substrate of **CYP2D6**, 3A4

Amphetamines: May increase the risk of seizures with tramadol.

Anesthetic agents: May increase risk of CNS and respiratory depression; use together with caution and in reduced dosage.

Barbiturates: Barbiturates may increase the hepatotoxic effects of acetaminophen; in addition, acetaminophen levels may be lowered.

Carbamazepine: Carbamazepine decreases half-life of tramadol by 33% to 50%; also have increase risk of seizures; in addition, carbamazepine may increase the hepatotoxic effects and lower serum levels of acetaminophen; concomitant use is not recommended.

CYP2D6 inhibitors: May increase tramadol serum concentrations.

Digoxin: Rare reports of digoxin toxicity with concomitant tramadol use.

Hydantoin anticonvulsants: Phenytoin may increase the hepatotoxic effects of acetaminophen; in addition, acetaminophen levels may be lowered.

SSRIs: May increase the risk of seizures with tramadol by inhibiting CYP metabolism. Includes citalopram, fluoxetine, paroxetine, sertraline.

MAO inhibitors: May increase the risk of seizures. Use extreme caution.

Naloxone: May increase the risk of seizures (if administered in tramadol overdose).

Neuroleptic agents: May increase the risk of tramadol-associated seizures and may have additive CNS depressant effects.

Narcotics: May increase risk of CNS and respiratory depression; use together with caution and in reduced dosage.

Opioids: May increase the risk of seizures, and may have additive CNS depressant effects. Use together with caution and in reduced dosage.

Phenothiazines: May increase risk of CNS and respiratory depression; use together with caution and in reduced dosage.

Rifampin: Rifampin may increase the clearance of acetaminophen.

Quinidine: May increase the tramadol serum concentrations by inhibiting CYP metabolism.

Sulfinpyrazone: Sulfinpyrazone may increase the hepatotoxic effects of acetaminophen; in addition, acetaminophen levels may be lowered.

Tricyclic antidepressants: May increase the risk of seizures.

Warfarin: Acetaminophen and tramadol may lead to an elevation of prothrombin times; monitor.

Dietary/Ethanol/Herb Considerations

Ethanol: Avoid; concomitant use increases liver toxicity.

Food: May be taken with meals; food may delay time to peak plasma concentrations; extent of absorption not affected.

(Continued)

Acetaminophen and Tramadol *(Continued)*

Herb/Nutraceutical:

Based on **acetaminophen** component: Avoid St John's wort; may decrease acetaminophen levels.

Based on **tramadol** component: Avoid gotu kola, kava, SAMe, St John's wort, and valerian; may increase CNS depression.

Pregnancy Risk Factor C

Breast-feeding Considerations Not recommended for post-delivery analgesia in nursing mothers.

Dosage Forms TAB: Acetaminophen 325 mg and tramadol 37.5 mg

Generic Available No

Selected Readings

Wynn RL, "NSAIDS and Cardiovascular Effects, Celecoxib for Dental Pain, and a New Analgesic - Tramadol with Acetaminophen," *Gen Dent*, 2002, 50(3):218-222.

Acetaminophen, Aspirin, and Caffeine

(a seet a MIN oh fen, AS pir in, & KAF een)

Related Information

Acetaminophen *on page 27*

Aspirin *on page 131*

U.S. Brand Names Excedrin® Extra Strength [OTC]; Excedrin® Migraine [OTC]; Genaced [OTC]; Goody's® Extra Strength Headache Powder [OTC]; Vanquish® Extra Strength Pain Reliever [OTC]

Pharmacologic Category Analgesic, Miscellaneous

Synonyms Aspirin, Acetaminophen, and Caffeine; Aspirin, Caffeine and Acetaminophen; Caffeine, Acetaminophen, and Aspirin; Caffeine, Aspirin, and Acetaminophen

Use Relief of mild to moderate pain; mild to moderate pain associated with migraine headache

Local Anesthetic/Vasoconstrictor Precautions No information available to require special precautions

Effects on Dental Treatment No significant effects or complications reported

Dosage Oral: Adults:

Analgesic:

Based on **acetaminophen** component:

Mild to moderate pain: 325-650 mg every 4-6 hours as needed; do **not** exceed 4 g/day

Mild to moderate pain associated with migraine headache: 500 mg/dose (in combination with 500 mg aspirin and 130 mg caffeine) every 6 hours while symptoms persist; do not use for longer than 48 hours

Based on **aspirin** component:

Mild to moderate pain: 325-650 mg every 4-6 hours as needed; do **not** exceed 4 g/day

Mild to moderate pain associated with migraine headache: 500 mg/dose (in combination with 500 mg acetaminophen and 130 mg caffeine) every 6 hours; do not use for longer than 48 hours

Product labeling:

Excedrin® Extra Strength, Excedrin® Migraine: Children >12 years and Adults: 2 doses every 6 hours (maximum: 8 doses/24 hours)

Note: When used for migraine, do not use for longer than 48 hours

Goody's® Extra Strength Headache Powder: Children >12 years and Adults: 1 powder, placed on tongue or dissolved in water, every 4-6 hours (maximum: 4 powders/24 hours)

Goody's® Extra Strength Pain Relief Tablets: Children >12 years and Adults: 2 tablets every 4-6 hours (maximum: 8 tablets/24 hours)

Vanquish® Extra Strength Pain Reliever: Children >12 years and Adults: 2 tablets every 4 hours (maximum: 12 tablets/24 hours)

Dietary/Ethanol/Herb Considerations Ethanol: Excessive intake may increase risk of acetaminophen-induced hepatotoxicity; avoid use or limit to <3 drinks/day.

Pregnancy Risk Factor D

Generic Available Yes

Selected Readings

Desjardins PJ, Cooper SA, Gallegos TL, et al, "The Relative Analgesic Efficacy of Propiram Fumarate, Codeine Aspirin, and Placebo in Postimpaction Dental Pain," *J Clin Pharmacol*, 1984, 24(1):35-42.

Forbes JA, Butterworth GA, Burchfield WH, et al, "Evaluation of Ketorolac, Aspirin, and an Acetaminophen-Codeine Combination in Postoperative Oral Surgery Pain," *Pharmacotherapy*, 1990, 10(6 Pt 2):77S-93S.

Forbes JA, Keller CK, Smith JW, et al, "Analgesic Effect of Naproxen Sodium, Codeine, a Naproxen-Codeine Combination and Aspirin on the Postoperative Pain of Oral Surgery," *Pharmacotherapy*, 1986, 6(5):211-8.

Acetaminophen, Butalbital, and Caffeine *see* Butalbital, Acetaminophen, and Caffeine *on page 214*

Acetaminophen, Caffeine, Codeine, and Butalbital *see* Butalbital, Acetaminophen, Caffeine, and Codeine *on page 215*

Acetaminophen, Caffeine, Hydrocodone, Chlorpheniramine, and Phenylephrine *see* Hydrocodone, Chlorpheniramine, Phenylephrine, Acetaminophen, and Caffeine *on page 686*

Acetaminophen, Chlorpheniramine, and Pseudoephedrine

(a seet a MIN oh fen, klor fen IR a meen, & soo doe e FED rin)

Related Information

Acetaminophen *on page 27*

U.S. Brand Names Alka-Seltzer® Plus Cold Liqui-Gels® [OTC]; Children's Tylenol® Cold [OTC]; Comtrex® Allergy-Sinus [OTC]; Sinutab® Sinus Allergy Maximum Strength [OTC]; Thera-Flu® Flu and Cold; Tylenol® Allergy Sinus [OTC]

Canadian Brand Names Sinutab® Sinus & Allergy; Tylenol® Allergy Sinus; Tylenol® Cold

Pharmacologic Category Analgesic, Miscellaneous; Antihistamine

Synonyms Acetaminophen, Pseudoephedrine, and Chlorpheniramine; Chlorpheniramine, Acetaminophen, and Pseudoephedrine; Chlorpheniramine, Pseudoephedrine, and Acetaminophen; Pseudoephedrine, Acetaminophen, and Chlorpheniramine; Pseudoephedrine, Chlorpheniramine, and Acetaminophen

Use Temporary relief of sinus symptoms

Local Anesthetic/Vasoconstrictor Precautions Use with caution since pseudoephedrine is a sympathomimetic amine which could interact with epinephrine to cause a pressor response

Effects on Dental Treatment

Chlorpheniramine: Significant xerostomia (prolonged use)

Pseudoephedrine: ≤10%: Tachycardia, palpitations, xerostomia (use vasoconstrictor with caution)

Dosage Oral:

Analgesic: Based on **acetaminophen** component:

- Children: 10-15 mg/kg/dose every 4-6 hours as needed; do **not** exceed 5 doses in 24 hours
- Adults: 325-650 mg every 4-6 hours as needed; do **not** exceed 4 g/day

Antihistamine: Based on chlorpheniramine maleate component:

- Children:
  - 2-6 years: 1 mg every 4-6 hours (maximum: 6 mg/24 hours)
  - 6-12 years: 2 mg every 4-6 hours (maximum: 12 mg/24 hours)
- Children >12 years and Adults: 4 mg every 4-6 hours (maximum: 24 mg/24 hours)

Decongestant: Based on **pseudoephedrine** component:

- Children:
  - 2-6 years: 15 mg every 4 hours (maximum: 90 mg/24 hours)
  - 6-12 years: 30 mg every 4 hours (maximum: 180 mg/24 hours)
- Children >12 years and Adults: 60 mg every 4 hours (maximum: 360 mg/24 hours)

Product labeling:

Alka-Seltzer Plus® Cold Medicine Liqui-Gels®:

- Children 6-12 years: 1 softgel every 4 hours with water (maximum: 4 doses/24 hours)
- Children >12 years and Adults: 2 softgels every 4 hours with water (maximum: 4 doses/24 hours)

Sinutab® Sinus Allergy Maximum Strength: Children >12 years and Adults: 2 tablets/caplets every 6 hours (maximum: 8 doses/24 hours)

Thera-Flu® Maximum Strength Flu and Cold Medicine for Sore Throat: Children >12 years and Adults: 1 packet dissolved in hot water every 6 hours (maximum: 4 packets/24 hours)

Dietary/Ethanol/Herb Considerations Ethanol: Excessive intake may increase risk of acetaminophen-induced hepatotoxicity; avoid use or limit to <3 drinks/day.

Pregnancy Risk Factor B

Generic Available Yes

Selected Readings

Barker JD Jr, de Carle DJ, and Anuras S, "Chronic Excessive Acetaminophen Use in Liver Damage," *Ann Intern Med*, 1977, 87(3):299-301.

Acetaminophen, Dextromethorphan, and Pseudoephedrine

(a seet a MIN oh fen, deks troe meth OR fan, & soo doe e FED rin)

Related Information

Acetaminophen *on page 27*

Dextromethorphan *on page 423*

Pseudoephedrine *on page 1146*

U.S. Brand Names Alka-Seltzer® Plus Flu Liqui-Gels® [OTC]; Comtrex® Non-Drowsy Cough and Cold [OTC]; Contac® Severe Cold and Flu/Non-Drowsy [OTC]; Infants' Tylenol® Cold Plus Cough Concentrated Drops [OTC]; Sudafed® Severe Cold [OTC]; Thera-Flu® Non-Drowsy Flu, Cold and Cough [OTC]; Triaminic® Sore Throat Formula [OTC]; Tylenol® Cold Non-Drowsy [OTC]; Tylenol® Flu

(Continued)

Acetaminophen, Dextromethorphan, and Pseudoephedrine *(Continued)*

Non-Drowsy Maximum Strength [OTC]; Vicks® DayQuil® Cold and Flu Non-Drowsy [OTC]

Canadian Brand Names Contac® Cough, Cold and Flu Day & Night™; Sudafed® Cold & Cough Extra Strength; Tylenol® Cold

Pharmacologic Category Antihistamine; Antitussive

Synonyms Dextromethorphan, Acetaminophen, and Pseudoephedrine; Pseudoephedrine, Acetaminophen, and Dextromethorphan; Pseudoephedrine, Dextromethorphan, and Acetaminophen

Use Treatment of mild to moderate pain and fever; symptomatic relief of cough and congestion

Local Anesthetic/Vasoconstrictor Precautions No information available to require special precautions

Effects on Dental Treatment No significant effects or complications reported

Dosage Oral:

Analgesic: Based on acetaminophen component:

Children: 10-15 mg/kg/dose every 4-6 hours as needed; do **not** exceed 5 doses/24 hours

Adults: 325-650 mg every 4-7 hours as needed; do **not** exceed 4 g/day

Cough suppressant: Based on dextromethorphan component:

Children 6-12 years: 15 mg every 6-8 hours; do **not** exceed 60 mg/24 hours

Children >12 years and Adults: 10-20 mg every 4-8 hours **or** 30 mg every 8 hours; do **not** exceed 120 mg/24 hours

Decongestant: Based on pseudoephedrine component:

Children:

2-6 years: 15 mg every 4 hours (maximum: 90 mg/24 hours)

6-12 years: 30 mg every 4 hours (maximum: 180 mg/24 hours)

Children >12 years and Adults: 60 mg every 4 hours (maximum: 360 mg/24 hours)

Product labeling:

Alka-Seltzer Plus® Cold and Flu Liqui-Gels®:

Children 6-12 years: 1 dose every 4 hours (maximum: 4 doses/24 hours)

Children >12 years and Adults: 2 dose every 4 hours (maximum: 4 doses/24 hours)

Infants' Tylenol® Cold Plus Cough Concentrated Drops: Children 2-3 years (24-55 lbs): 2 dropperfuls every 4-6 hours (maximum: 4 doses/24 hours)

Sudafed® Severe Cold, Thera-Flu® Non-Drowsy Maximum Strength (gelcap), Tylenol® Flu Non-Drowsy Maximum Strength: Children >12 years and Adults: 2 doses every 6 hours (maximum: 8 doses/24 hours)

Tylenol® Cold Non-Drowsy:

Children 6-11 years: 1 dose every 6 hours (maximum: 4 doses/24 hours)

Children ≥12 years and Adults: 2 doses every 6 hours (maximum: 8 doses/24 hours)

Thera-Flu® Non-Drowsy Maximum Strength: Children >12 years and Adults: 1 packet dissolved in hot water every 6 hours (maximum: 4 packets/24 hours)

Dietary/Ethanol/Herb Considerations Ethanol: Excessive intake may increase risk of acetaminophen-induced hepatotoxicity; avoid use or limit to <3 drinks/day.

Generic Available Yes

Acetaminophen, Dichloralphenazone, and Isometheptene *see* Acetaminophen, Isometheptene, and Dichloralphenazone *on page 36*

Acetaminophen, Isometheptene, and Dichloralphenazone

(a seet a MIN oh fen, eye soe me THEP teen, & dye KLOR al FEN a zone)

Related Information

Acetaminophen *on page 27*

U.S. Brand Names Midrin®; Migratine®

Pharmacologic Category Analgesic, Miscellaneous

Synonyms Acetaminophen, Dichloralphenazone, and Isometheptene; Dichloralphenazone, Acetaminophen, and Isometheptene; Dichloralphenazone, Isometheptene, and Acetaminophen; Isometheptene, Acetaminophen, and Dichloralphenazone; Isometheptene, Dichloralphenazone, and Acetaminophen

Use Relief of migraine and tension headache

Local Anesthetic/Vasoconstrictor Precautions No information available to require special precautions

Effects on Dental Treatment Frequency not defined: Transient dizziness

Restrictions C-IV

Dosage Oral: Adults:

Migraine headache: 2 capsules to start, followed by 1 capsule every hour until relief is obtained (maximum: 5 capsules/12 hours)

Tension headache: 1-2 capsules every 4 hours (maximum: 8 capsules/24 hours)

Other Adverse Effects Frequency not defined: Dermatological: Rash

Dietary/Ethanol/Herb Considerations Ethanol: Excessive intake may increase risk of acetaminophen-induced hepatotoxicity; avoid use or limit to <3 drinks/day.

Pregnancy Risk Factor B

Generic Available Yes

Comments Should not exceed 5 g in 12 hours; may cause drowsiness; avoid ethanol and other CNS depressants

Acetaminophen, Pseudoephedrine, and Chlorpheniramine *see* Acetaminophen, Chlorpheniramine, and Pseudoephedrine *on page 35*

Acetasol® HC *see* Acetic Acid, Propylene Glycol Diacetate, and Hydrocortisone *on page 38*

AcetaZOLAMIDE (a set a ZOLE a mide)

U.S. Brand Names Diamox®; Diamox Sequels®

Canadian Brand Names Apo®-Acetazolamide; Diamox®

Mexican Brand Names Acetadiazol®

Pharmacologic Category Anticonvulsant, Miscellaneous; Carbonic Anhydrase Inhibitor; Diuretic, Carbonic Anhydrase Inhibitor; Ophthalmic Agent, Antiglaucoma

Use Lowers intraocular pressure to treat glaucoma, also as a diuretic, adjunct treatment of refractory seizures and acute altitude sickness; centrencephalic epilepsies (sustained release not recommended for anticonvulsant)

Local Anesthetic/Vasoconstrictor Precautions No information available to require special precautions

Effects on Dental Treatment

>10%: Metallic taste (resolves upon discontinuation), weakness, malaise

1% to 10%: Drowsiness

Dosage I.M. administration is not recommended because of pain secondary to the alkaline pH.

Neonates and Infants: Hydrocephalus: To slow the progression of hydrocephalus in neonates and infants who may not be good candidates for surgery, acetazolamide I.V. or oral doses of 5 mg/kg/dose every 6 hours increased by 25 mg/kg/day to a maximum of 100 mg/kg/day, if tolerated, have been used. Furosemide was used in combination with acetazolamide.

Children:

- Glaucoma:
  - Oral: 8-30 mg/kg/day or 300-900 mg/m^2/day divided every 8 hours
  - I.M., I.V.: 20-40 mg/kg/24 hours divided every 6 hours, not to exceed 1 g/day
- Edema: Oral, I.M., I.V.: 5 mg/kg or 150 mg/m^2 once every day
- Epilepsy: Oral: 8-30 mg/kg/day in 1-4 divided doses, not to exceed 1 g/day; sustained release capsule is not recommended for treatment of epilepsy

Adults:

- Glaucoma:
  - Chronic simple (open-angle): Oral: 250 mg 1-4 times/day or 500 mg sustained release capsule twice daily
  - Secondary, acute (closed-angle): I.M., I.V.: 250-500 mg, may repeat in 2-4 hours to a maximum of 1 g/day
- Edema: Oral, I.M., I.V.: 250-375 mg once daily
- Epilepsy: Oral: 8-30 mg/kg/day in 1-4 divided doses; **sustained release capsule not recommended**
- Altitude sickness: Oral: 250 mg every 8-12 hours (or 500 mg extended release capsules every 12-24 hours)
  - Therapy should begin 24-48 hours before and continue during ascent and for at least 48 hours after arrival at the high altitude
- Urine alkalinization: Oral: 5 mg/kg/dose repeated 2-3 times over 24 hours

Elderly: Oral: Initial: 250 mg twice daily; use lowest effective dose

Dosing adjustment in renal impairment:

- Cl_{cr} 10-50 mL/minute: Administer every 12 hours
- Cl_{cr} <10 mL/minute: Avoid use → ineffective

Hemodialysis: Moderately dialyzable (20% to 50%)

Peritoneal dialysis: Supplemental dose is unnecessary

Mechanism of Action Reversible inhibition of the enzyme carbonic anhydrase resulting in reduction of hydrogen ion secretion at renal tubule and an increased renal excretion of sodium, potassium, bicarbonate, and water to decrease production of aqueous humor; also inhibits carbonic anhydrase in central nervous system to retard abnormal and excessive discharge from CNS neurons

Other Adverse Effects

>10%:

- Gastrointestinal: Anorexia, diarrhea
- Genitourinary: Polyuria

1% to 10%: Central nervous system: Mental depression

<1%: **Fever**, fatigue, rash, hyperchloremic metabolic acidosis, hypokalemia, **hyperglycemia**, black stools, **GI irritation**, dysuria, bone marrow suppression, blood dyscrasias, **paresthesia, xerostomia,** myopia, renal calculi

Drug Interactions Inhibits CYP3A4

(Continued)

AcetaZOLAMIDE *(Continued)*

Increased Effect/Toxicity: Concurrent use with diflunisal may increase the effect of acetazolamide causing a significant decrease in intraocular pressure. Cyclosporine concentrations may be increased by acetazolamide. Salicylate use may result in carbonic anhydrase inhibitor accumulation and toxicity. Acetazolamide-induced hypokalemia may increase the risk of toxicity with digoxin.

Decreased Effect: Use of acetazolamide may increase lithium excretion and alter excretion of other drugs by alkalinization of urine (eg, amphetamines, quinidine, procainamide, methenamine, phenobarbital, salicylates). Primidone serum concentrations may be decreased.

Dietary/Ethanol/Herb Considerations Food: Administer with food to reduce GI upset; contents of sustained release capsules may be sprinkled on soft food. Short-acting tablets may be crushed and suspended in cherry/chocolate syrup to disguise bitter taste; do not use fruit juices. Drug may alter taste, especially of carbonated beverages. Sodium content of 500 mg injection: 47.2 mg (2.05 mEq).

Pharmacodynamics/Kinetics

Onset of action: Capsule, extended release: 2 hours; I.V.: 2 minutes

Peak effect: Capsule, extended release: 3-6 hours; I.V.: 15 minutes; Tablet: 1-4 hours

Duration: Capsule, extended release: 18-24 hours; I.V.: 4-5 hours; Tablet: 8-12 hours

Distribution: Erythrocytes, kidneys; blood-brain barrier and placenta; distributes into milk (~30% of plasma concentrations)

Protein binding: 95%

Half-life elimination: 2.4-5.8 hours

Excretion: Urine (70% to 100% as unchanged drug)

Pregnancy Risk Factor C

Generic Available Yes

Acetic Acid and Aluminum Acetate Otic *see* Aluminum Acetate and Acetic Acid *on page 67*

Acetic Acid, Hydrocortisone, and Propylene Glycol Diacetate *see* Acetic Acid, Propylene Glycol Diacetate, and Hydrocortisone *on page 38*

Acetic Acid, Propylene Glycol Diacetate, and Hydrocortisone

(a SEE tik AS id, PRO pa leen GLY kole dye AS e tate, & hye droe KOR ti sone)

Related Information

Hydrocortisone *on page 688*

U.S. Brand Names Acetasol® HC; VōSol® HC

Canadian Brand Names VōSol® HC

Pharmacologic Category Otic Agent, Anti-infective

Synonyms Acetic Acid, Hydrocortisone, and Propylene Glycol Diacetate; Hydrocortisone, Acetic Acid, and Propylene Glycol Diacetate; Hydrocortisone, Propylene Glycol Diacetate, and Acetic Acid; Propylene Glycol Diacetate, Acetic Acid, and Hydrocortisone; Propylene Glycol Diacetate, Hydrocortisone, and Acetic Acid

Use Treatment of superficial infections of the external auditory canal caused by organisms susceptible to the action of the antimicrobial, complicated by swelling

Local Anesthetic/Vasoconstrictor Precautions No information available to require special precautions

Effects on Dental Treatment No significant effects or complications reported

Dosage Adults: Otic: Instill 4 drops in ear(s) 3-4 times/day

Other Adverse Effects Frequency not defined: Otic: Transient burning or stinging may be noticed occasionally when the solution is first instilled into the acutely inflamed ear.

Generic Available Yes

AcetoHEXAMIDE (a set oh HEKS a mide)

Related Information

Endocrine Disorders and Pregnancy *on page 1479*

Pharmacologic Category Antidiabetic Agent, Sulfonylurea

Synonyms Dymelor® [DSC]

Use Adjunct to diet for the management of mild to moderately severe, stable, type 2 diabetes mellitus (noninsulin dependent, NIDDM)

Local Anesthetic/Vasoconstrictor Precautions No information available to require special precautions

Effects on Dental Treatment Use salicylates with caution in patients taking acetohexamide due to potential increased hypoglycemia. NSAIDs such as ibuprofen, naproxen and others may be safely used. Acetohexamide-dependent diabetics (noninsulin-dependent, type 1) should be appointed for dental treatment in mornings to minimize chance of stress-induced hypoglycemia.

>10%: Dizziness, headache

Dosage Oral: Adults (elderly patients may be more sensitive and should be started at a lower dosage initially):

Initial: 250 mg/day; increase in increments of 250-500 mg daily at intervals of 5-7 days up to 1.5 g/day. Patients on ≤1 g/day can be controlled with once daily administration. Patients receiving 1.5 g/day usually benefit from twice daily administration before the morning and evening meals. Doses >1.5 g daily are not recommended.

Dosing adjustment in renal impairment: Cl_{cr} <50 mL/minute: Use not recommended due to increased potential for developing hypoglycemia

Dosing adjustment in hepatic impairment: Initiate therapy at lower than recommended doses; further dosage adjustment may be necessary because acetohexamide is extensively metabolized but no specific guidelines are available

Mechanism of Action Believed to cause hypoglycemia by stimulating insulin release from the pancreatic beta cells; reduces glucose output from the liver (decreases gluconeogenesis); insulin sensitivity is increased at peripheral target sites (alters receptor sensitivity/receptor density); potentiates effects of ADH; may produce mild diuresis and significant uricosuric activity

Other Adverse Effects

>10%:

Gastrointestinal: Anorexia, constipation, diarrhea, epigastric fullness, heartburn

1% to 10%: Dermatologic: Photosensitivity, rash, urticaria

<1% (Limited to important or life-threatening): Agranulocytosis, aplastic anemia, bone marrow suppression, cholestatic jaundice, hemolytic anemia, **hypoglycemia,** porphyria, SIADH, thrombocytopenia

Drug Interactions

Increased Effect/Toxicity: Increases hypoglycemia when coadministered with salicylates or beta-adrenergic blockers; MAO inhibitors; oral anticoagulants, NSAIDs, sulfonamides, phenylbutazone, insulin, clofibrate, fluconazole, gemfibrozil, H_2 antagonists, methyldopa, tricyclic antidepressants

Decreased Effect: Decreases hypoglycemic effect when coadministered with cholestyramine, diazoxide, hydantoins, rifampin, thiazides, loop or thiazide diuretics, and phenylbutazone

Dietary/Ethanol/Herb Considerations

Ethanol: Avoid use; may increase risk of hypoglycemia.

Food: May be taken with food.

Pharmacodynamics/Kinetics

Onset of action: 1 hour

Peak effect, hypoglycemic: 8-10 hours

Duration: 12-24 hours; prolonged with renal impairment

Half-life elimination, serum: Parent drug: 0.8-2.4 hours; Metabolite: 5-6 hours

Pregnancy Risk Factor D

Generic Available Yes

Acetohydroxamic Acid (a SEE toe hye droks am ik AS id)

U.S. Brand Names Lithostat®

Canadian Brand Names Lithostat®

Pharmacologic Category Urinary Tract Product

Synonyms AHA

Use Adjunctive therapy in chronic urea-splitting urinary infection

Local Anesthetic/Vasoconstrictor Precautions No information available to require special precautions

Effects on Dental Treatment No significant effects or complications reported

Dosage Oral:

Children: Initial: 10 mg/kg/day

Adults: 250 mg 3-4 times/day for a total daily dose of 10-15 mg/kg/day

Dietary/Ethanol/Herb Considerations

Ethanol: Avoid use; may increase incidence of rash.

Food: Should be taken 1 hour before or 2 hours after meals.

Pregnancy Risk Factor X

Generic Available No

Acetoxymethylprogesterone *see* MedroxyPROGESTERone *on page 849*

Acetylcholine (a se teel KOE leen)

U.S. Brand Names Miochol-E®

Canadian Brand Names Miochol®-E

Pharmacologic Category Cholinergic Agonist; Ophthalmic Agent, Miotic

Synonyms Acetylcholine Chloride

Use Produces complete miosis in cataract surgery, keratoplasty, iridectomy and other anterior segment surgery where rapid miosis is required

Local Anesthetic/Vasoconstrictor Precautions No information available to require special precautions

Effects on Dental Treatment Frequency not defined: Bradycardia, hypotension, flushing, headache, dyspnea, diaphoresis

(Continued)

Acetylcholine *(Continued)*

Dosage Adults: Intraocular: 0.5-2 mL of 1% injection (5-20 mg) instilled into anterior chamber before or after securing one or more sutures

Mechanism of Action Causes contraction of the sphincter muscles of the iris, resulting in miosis and contraction of the ciliary muscle, leading to accommodation spasm

Other Adverse Effects Frequency not defined: Ocular: Altered distance vision, decreased night vision, transient lenticular opacities

Drug Interactions

Increased Effect/Toxicity: Effect may be prolonged or enhanced in patients receiving tacrine.

Decreased Effect: May be decreased with flurbiprofen and suprofen, ophthalmic.

Pharmacodynamics/Kinetics

Onset of action: Rapid

Duration: ~10 minutes

Pregnancy Risk Factor C

Generic Available No

Acetylcholine Chloride *see* Acetylcholine *on page 39*

Acetylcysteine (a se teel SIS teen)

U.S. Brand Names Mucomyst®; Mucosil™

Canadian Brand Names Mucomyst®; Parvolex®

Pharmacologic Category Antidote; Mucolytic Agent

Synonyms Acetylcysteine Sodium; Mercapturic Acid; NAC; *N*-Acetylcysteine; *N*-Acetyl-L-cysteine

Use Adjunctive mucolytic therapy in patients with abnormal or viscid mucous secretions in acute and chronic bronchopulmonary diseases; pulmonary complications of surgery and cystic fibrosis; diagnostic bronchial studies; antidote for acute acetaminophen toxicity

Unlabeled/Investigational Use Prevention of radiocontrast-induced renal dysfunction

Local Anesthetic/Vasoconstrictor Precautions No information available to require special precautions

Effects on Dental Treatment 1% to 10%: Stomatitis, drowsiness, fever, vomiting, nausea, bronchospasm, rhinorrhea, hemoptysis, dizziness

Dosage

Acetaminophen poisoning: Children and Adults: Oral: 140 mg/kg; followed by 17 doses of 70 mg/kg every 4 hours; repeat dose if emesis occurs within 1 hour of administration; therapy should continue until all doses are administered even though the acetaminophen plasma level has dropped below the toxic range

Inhalation: Acetylcysteine 10% and 20% solution (Mucomyst®) (dilute 20% solution with sodium chloride or sterile water for inhalation); 10% solution may be used undiluted

Infants: 1-2 mL of 20% solution or 2-4 mL 10% solution until nebulized given 3-4 times/day

Children: 3-5 mL of 20% solution or 6-10 mL of 10% solution until nebulized given 3-4 times/day

Adolescents: 5-10 mL of 10% to 20% solution until nebulized given 3-4 times/day

Note: Patients should receive an aerosolized bronchodilator 10-15 minutes prior to acetylcysteine

Meconium ileus equivalent: Children and Adults: 100-300 mL of 4% to 10% solution by irrigation or orally

Prevention of radiocontrast-induced renal dysfunction (unlabeled use): Adults: Oral: 600 mg twice daily for 2 days (beginning the day before the procedure); may be given as powder in capsules, some centers use solution (diluted in cola beverage or juice). Hydrate patient with saline concurrently.

Mechanism of Action Exerts mucolytic action through its free sulfhydryl group which opens up the disulfide bonds in the mucoproteins thus lowering mucous viscosity. The exact mechanism of action in acetaminophen toxicity is unknown; thought to act by providing substrate for conjugation with the toxic metabolite.

Other Adverse Effects

Inhalation:

>10%: Unpleasant odor during administration, stickiness on face after nebulization

1% to 10%:

Central nervous system: Chills

Local: Irritation

Miscellaneous: Clamminess

<1% (Limited to important or life-threatening): **Bronchospastic allergic reaction, anaphylactoid reaction, EKG changes (transient)**

Drug Interactions Decreased Effect: Adsorbed by activated charcoal; clinical significance is minimal, though, once a pure acetaminophen ingestion requiring N-acetylcysteine is established; further charcoal dosing is unnecessary once the appropriate initial charcoal dose is achieved (5-10 g:g acetaminophen)

Dietary/Ethanol/Herb Considerations Solution (20%) may be diluted with orange juice or soft drink.

Pharmacodynamics/Kinetics

Onset of action: Inhalation: 5-10 minutes

Duration: Inhalation: >1 hour

Distribution: Oral: 0.33-0.47 L/kg

Protein binding, plasma: Oral: 50%

Half-life elimination: Reduced acetylcysteine: 2 hours; Total acetylcysteine: 5.5 hours

Time to peak, plasma: Oral: 1-2 hours

Excretion: Urine

Pregnancy Risk Factor B

Generic Available Yes

Acetylcysteine Sodium *see* Acetylcysteine *on page 40*

Acetylsalicylic Acid *see* Aspirin *on page 131*

Achromycin® [DSC] *see* Tetracycline *on page 1286*

Aciclovir *see* Acyclovir *on page 42*

Acidulated Phosphate Fluoride *see* Fluoride *on page 586*

Aciphex® *see* Rabeprazole *on page 1162*

Aclovate® *see* Alclometasone *on page 49*

Acrivastine and Pseudoephedrine

(AK ri vas teen & soo doe e FED rin)

Related Information

Pseudoephedrine *on page 1146*

U.S. Brand Names Semprex®-D

Pharmacologic Category Antihistamine

Synonyms Pseudoephedrine and Acrivastine

Use Temporary relief of nasal congestion, decongest sinus openings, running nose, itching of nose or throat, and itchy, watery eyes due to hay fever or other upper respiratory allergies

Local Anesthetic/Vasoconstrictor Precautions Use with caution since pseudoephedrine is a sympathomimetic amine which could interact with epinephrine to cause a pressor response

Effects on Dental Treatment Use vasoconstrictor with caution

>10%: Drowsiness, headache

1% to 10%: Tachycardia, palpitations, xerostomia, nervousness, dizziness, lightheadedness, nausea, vomiting, pharyngitis, cough, diaphoresis, weakness, fatigue

Dosage Oral: Adults: 1 capsule 3-4 times/day

Dosing comments in renal impairment: Do not use

Mechanism of Action Refer to Pseudoephedrine monograph; acrivastine is an analogue of triprolidine and it is considered to be relatively less sedating than traditional antihistamines; believed to involve competitive blockade of H_1-receptor sites resulting in the inability of histamine to combine with its receptor sites and exert its usual effects on target cells

Other Adverse Effects

1% to 10%:

Central nervous system: Insomnia, vertigo

Gastrointestinal: Diarrhea

Genitourinary: Dysuria

<1%: Dysmenorrhea, dyspepsia

Drug Interactions

Increased Effect/Toxicity: Increased risk of hypertensive crisis when acrivastine and pseudoephedrine are given with MAO inhibitors or sympathomimetics. Increased risk of severe CNS depression when given with CNS depressants and ethanol.

Decreased Effect: Decreased effect of guanethidine, reserpine, methyldopa, and beta-blockers when given in conjunction with acrivastine and pseudoephedrine.

Dietary/Ethanol/Herb Considerations

Ethanol: Avoid use; may increase sedation.

Herb/Nutraceutical: Avoid gotu kola, kava, SAMe, St John's wort, and valerian; may increase CNS depression.

Pharmacodynamics/Kinetics

Pseudoephedrine: See Pseudoephedrine monograph.

Acrivastine:

Metabolism: Minimally hepatic

Time to peak: ~1.1 hours

Excretion: Urine (84%); feces (13%)

Pregnancy Risk Factor B

Generic Available No

ACT *see* Dactinomycin *on page 393*

ACT® [OTC] *see* Fluoride *on page 586*

Act-D *see* Dactinomycin *on page 393*

ACTH *see* Corticotropin *on page 372*
Acthar® *see* Corticotropin *on page 372*
ActHIB® *see Haemophilus* b Conjugate Vaccine *on page 656*
Acticin® *see* Permethrin *on page 1062*
Actidose® [OTC] *see* Charcoal *on page 294*
Actidose-Aqua® [OTC] *see* Charcoal *on page 294*
Actifed® Cold and Allergy [OTC] *see* Triprolidine and Pseudoephedrine *on page 1356*
Actigall® *see* Ursodiol *on page 1366*
Actimmune® *see* Interferon Gamma-1b *on page 734*
Actinomycin *see* Dactinomycin *on page 393*
Actinomycin Cl *see* Dactinomycin *on page 393*
Actinomycin D *see* Dactinomycin *on page 393*
Actiq® *see* Fentanyl *on page 565*
Actisite® *see* Tetracycline Periodontal Fibers *on page 1287*
Activase® *see* Alteplase *on page 65*
Activated Carbon *see* Charcoal *on page 294*
Activated Charcoal *see* Charcoal *on page 294*
Activated Dimethicone *see* Simethicone *on page 1222*
Activated Ergosterol *see* Ergocalciferol *on page 508*
Activated Methylpolysiloxane *see* Simethicone *on page 1222*
Activated Protein C, Human, Recombinant *see* Drotrecogin Alfa *on page 483*
Activella™ *see* Estradiol and Norethindrone *on page 525*
Actonel® *see* Risedronate *on page 1186*
Actos® *see* Pioglitazone *on page 1086*
ACU-dyne® [OTC] *see* Povidone-Iodine *on page 1104*
Acular® *see* Ketorolac *on page 765*
Acular® PF *see* Ketorolac *on page 765*
ACV *see* Acyclovir *on page 42*
Acycloguanosine *see* Acyclovir *on page 42*

Acyclovir (ay SYE kloe veer)

Related Information

Oral Viral Infections *on page 1545*
Sexually-Transmitted Diseases *on page 1502*
Systemic Viral Diseases *on page 1517*
Valacyclovir *on page 1367*

U.S. Brand Names Zovirax®

Canadian Brand Names Alti-Acyclovir; Apo®-Acyclovir; Gen-Acyclovir; Nu-Acyclovir; ratio-Acyclovir; Zovirax®

Mexican Brand Names Acifur®; Cicloferon®; Isavir®; Laciken®; Opthavir®; Zovirax®; Zovirax I.V.®

Pharmacologic Category Antiviral Agent

Synonyms Aciclovir; ACV; Acycloguanosine

Use

Dental: Treatment of initial and prophylaxis of recurrent mucosal and cutaneous herpes simplex (HSV-1 and HSV-2) infections

Medical: Treatment of herpes simplex encephalitis, herpes zoster (within 72 hours of appearance; will not prevent postherpetic neuralgia), genital herpes infection, varicella-zoster infections in healthy, nonpregnant persons >13 years of age, children >12 months of age who have a chronic skin or lung disorder or are receiving long-term aspirin therapy, and immunocompromised patients

Local Anesthetic/Vasoconstrictor Precautions No information available to require special precautions

Effects on Dental Treatment 1% to 10%: Lightheadedness (>10% parenteral; 1% to 10% oral), vomiting, nausea (>1% parenteral; 1% to 10% oral)

Dosage Dosing weight should be based on the smaller of lean body weight or total body weight.

Treatment of herpes simplex virus infections: Children >12 years and Adults:

I.V.:

Mucocutaneous HSV or severe initial herpes genitalis infection: 750 mg/m²/day divided every 8 hours or 5 mg/kg/dose every 8 hours for 5-10 days

HSV encephalitis: 1500 mg/m²/day divided every 8 hours or 10 mg/kg/dose for 10 days

Topical: Non-life-threatening mucocutaneous HSV in immunocompromised patients: ½" ribbon of ointment for a 4" square surface area every 3 hours (6 times/day) for 7 days

Treatment of genital herpes simplex virus infections: Adults:

Oral: 200 mg every 4 hours while awake (5 times/day) for 10 days if initial episode; for 5 days if recurrence (begin at earliest signs of disease)

Topical: 1/2" ribbon of ointment for a 4" square surface area every 3 hours (6 times/day) for 7 days

Treatment of varicella-zoster virus (chickenpox) infections:

Oral:

Children: 10-20 mg/kg/dose (up to 800 mg) 4 times/day for 5 days; begin treatment within the first 24 hours of rash onset

Adults: 600-800 mg/dose every 4 hours while awake (5 times/day) for 7-10 days or 1000 mg every 6 hours for 5 days

I.V.: Children and Adults: 1500 mg/m²/day divided every 8 hours or 10 mg/kg/dose every 8 hours for 7 days

Treatment of herpes zoster (shingles) infections:

Oral:

Children (immunocompromised): 250-600 mg/m²/dose 4-5 times/day for 7-10 days

Adults (immunocompromised): 800 mg every 4 hours (5 times/day) for 7-10 days

I.V.:

Children and Adults (immunocompromised): 10 mg/kg/dose or 500 mg/m²/dose every 8 hours

Older Adults (immunocompromised): 7.5 mg/kg/dose every 8 hours

If nephrotoxicity occurs: 5 mg/kg/dose every 8 hours

Prophylaxis in immunocompromised patients:

Varicella zoster or herpes zoster in HIV-positive patients: Adults: Oral: 400 mg every 4 hours (5 times/day) for 7-10 days

Bone marrow transplant recipients: Children and Adults: I.V.:

Allogeneic patients who are HSV seropositive: 150 mg/m²/dose (5 mg/kg) every 12 hours; with clinical symptoms of herpes simplex: 150 mg/m²/dose every 8 hours

Allogeneic patients who are CMV seropositive: 500 mg/m²/dose (10 mg/kg) every 8 hours; for clinically symptomatic CMV infection, consider replacing acyclovir with ganciclovir

Chronic suppressive therapy for recurrent genital herpes simplex virus infections: Adults: 200 mg 3-4 times/day or 400 mg twice daily for up to 12 months, followed by re-evaluation

Dosing adjustment in renal impairment:

Oral: HSV/varicella-zoster:

Cl_{cr} 10-25 mL/minute: Administer dose every 8 hours

Cl_{cr} <10 mL/minute: Administer dose every 12 hours

I.V.:

Cl_{cr} 25-50 mL/minute: 5-10 mg/kg/dose: Administer every 12 hours

Cl_{cr} 10-25 mL/minute: 5-10 mg/kg/dose: Administer every 24 hours

Cl_{cr} <10 mL/minute: 2.5-5 mg/kg/dose: Administer every 24 hours

Hemodialysis: Dialyzable (50% to 100%); administer dose postdialysis

Peritoneal dialysis: Dose as for Cl_{cr} <10 mL/minute

Continuous arteriovenous or venovenous hemofiltration effects: Dose as for Cl_{cr} <10 mL/minute

Mechanism of Action Acyclovir is converted to acyclovir monophosphate by virus-specific thymidine kinase then further converted to acyclovir triphosphate by other cellular enzymes. Acyclovir triphosphate inhibits DNA synthesis and viral replication by competing with deoxyguanosine triphosphate for viral DNA polymerase and being incorporated into viral DNA.

Other Adverse Effects

Systemic (parenteral form):

>10%:

Gastrointestinal: Anorexia, abdominal pain

Local: Inflammation at injection site or phlebitis

1% to 10%: Renal: Acute renal failure

Topical:

>10%: Mild pain, burning, or stinging

1% to 10%: Itching

<1%: **Aggression, agitation**, alopecia, **anaphylaxis**, anemia, angioedema, anorexia, ataxia, **delirium**, diarrhea, elevated LFT, encephalopathy, erythema multiforme, **hallucinations**, hematuria, hepatitis, hyperbilirubinemia, increased BUN, increased serum creatinine, insomnia, jaundice, leukocytoclastic vasculitis, leukopenia, local tissue necrosis (following extravasation), mental depression, myalgia, **paresthesia**, photosensitization, pruritus, **psychosis**, renal failure, **seizures, somnolence, sore throat**, Stevens-Johnson syndrome, thrombocytopenia, thrombocytopenic purpura/hemolytic uremic syndrome (TTP/HUS), toxic epidermal necrolysis, urticaria, **visual disturbances**

Contraindications Hypersensitivity to acyclovir, valacyclovir, or any component of the formulation

Warnings/Precautions Use with caution in patients with pre-existing renal disease or in those receiving other nephrotoxic drugs concurrently; maintain adequate urine output during the first 2 hours after I.V. infusion; use with caution in patients with underlying neurologic abnormalities, serious hepatic or electrolyte abnormalities, or (Continued)

Acyclovir *(Continued)*

substantial hypoxia. Use with caution in immunocompromised patients; thrombocytopenic purpura/hemolytic uremic syndrome (TTP/HUS) has been reported

Drug Interactions Increased CNS side effects with zidovudine and probenecid

Dietary/Ethanol/Herb Considerations Food: Administer oral forms with food to reduce GI upset; does not appear to affect absorption. Injection formulations have a sodium content of 1 g: 96.6 mg (4.2 mEq).

Pharmacodynamics/Kinetics

Absorption: Oral: 15% to 30%

Distribution: Widely (ie, brain, kidney, lungs, liver, spleen, muscle, uterus, vagina, CSF)

Protein binding: <30%

Metabolism: Hepatic (small amounts)

Half-life elimination: Terminal: Neonates: 4 hours; Children 1-12 years: 2-3 hours; Adults: 3 hours

Time to peak, serum: Oral: Within 1.5-2 hours; I.V.: Within 1 hour

Excretion: Urine (30% to 90% as unchanged drug)

Pregnancy Risk Factor B

Dosage Forms CAP: 200 mg. **INJ, powder for reconstitution:** 500 mg, 1000 mg. **INJ, solution** [preservative free]: 50 mg/mL (10 mL, 20 mL). **OINT, topical:** 5% (3 g, 15 g). **SUSP, oral:** 200 mg/5 mL (480 mL). **TAB:** 400 mg, 800 mg

Generic Available Yes

Adagen® *see* Pegademase Bovine *on page 1038*

Adalat® CC *see* NIFEdipine *on page 973*

Adamantanamine Hydrochloride *see* Amantadine *on page 70*

Adapalene (a DAP a leen)

U.S. Brand Names Differin®

Canadian Brand Names Differin®

Mexican Brand Names Adaferin®

Pharmacologic Category Acne Products

Use Treatment of acne vulgaris

Local Anesthetic/Vasoconstrictor Precautions No information available to require special precautions

Effects on Dental Treatment No significant effects or complications reported

Dosage Topical: Children >12 years and Adults: Apply once daily at bedtime; therapeutic results should be noticed after 8-12 weeks of treatment

Mechanism of Action Retinoid-like compound which is a modulator of cellular differentiation, keratinization and inflammatory processes, all of which represent important features in the pathology of acne vulgaris

Other Adverse Effects

>10%: Dermatologic: Erythema, scaling, dryness, pruritus, burning, pruritus or burning immediately after application

≤1%: Skin irritation, stinging sunburn, acne flares; dermatitis, eyelid edema, conjunctivitis, skin discoloration, eczema, rash (topical cream), contact dermatitis

Pharmacodynamics/Kinetics

Absorption: Topical: Minimal

Excretion: Bile

Pregnancy Risk Factor C

Generic Available No

Adderall® *see* Dextroamphetamine and Amphetamine *on page 422*

Adderall XR™ *see* Dextroamphetamine and Amphetamine *on page 422*

Adefovir (a DEF o veer)

U.S. Brand Names Hepsera™

Pharmacologic Category Antiretroviral Agent, Reverse Transcriptase Inhibitor (Nucleoside)

Synonyms Adefovir Dipivoxil

Use Treatment of chronic hepatitis B with evidence of active viral replication (based on persistent elevation of ALT/AST or histologic evidence), including patients with lamivudine-resistant hepatitis B

Local Anesthetic/Vasoconstrictor Precautions No information available to require special precautions

Effects on Dental Treatment 1% to 10%: Fever, headache, nausea, vomiting, cough, sinusitis, pharyngitis, weakness

Dosage Oral:

Adults: 10 mg once daily

Dosing adjustment in renal impairment:

Cl_{cr} 20-49 mL/minute: 10 mg every 48 hours

Cl_{cr} 10-19 mL/minute: 10 mg every 72 hours

Hemodialysis: 10 mg every 7 days (following dialysis)

Mechanism of Action Acyclic nucleotide reverse transcriptase inhibitor which interferes with HBV viral RNA dependent DNA polymerase resulting in inhibition of viral replication

Other Adverse Effects

>10%: Renal: Hematuria (11% vs 10% placebo-treated)

1% to 10%:

Dermatologic: Rash, pruritus

Gastrointestinal: Dyspepsia (3%), flatulence, diarrhea, abdominal pain

Hepatic: AST/ALT increased, abnormal liver function, hepatic failure

Renal: Serum creatinine increased (4%; 26% to 37% in baseline renal dysfunction), renal failure, renal insufficiency

Drug Interactions Increased Effect/Toxicity: Ibuprofen increases the bioavailability of adefovir. Concurrent use of nephrotoxic agents (including aminoglycosides, cyclosporine, NSAIDs, tacrolimus, vancomycin) may increase the risk of nephrotoxicity.

Dietary/Ethanol/Herb Considerations

Ethanol: Should be avoided in hepatitis B infection due to potential hepatic toxicity.

Food: May be taken with food; does not have significant effect on absorption.

Pharmacodynamics/Kinetics

Distribution: 0.35-0.39 L/kg

Protein binding: ≤4%

Metabolism: Prodrug; rapidly converted to adefovir (active metabolite) in intestine

Bioavailability: 59%

Half-life elimination: 7.5 hours; prolonged in renal impairment

Time to peak: 1.75 hours

Excretion: Urine (45% as active metabolite within 24 hours)

Pregnancy Risk Factor C

Generic Available No

Adefovir Dipivoxil *see* Adefovir *on page 44*

Adenine Arabinoside *see* Vidarabine *on page 1384*

Adenocard® *see* Adenosine *on page 45*

Adenoscan® *see* Adenosine *on page 45*

Adenosine (a DEN oh seen)

U.S. Brand Names Adenocard®; Adenoscan®

Canadian Brand Names Adenocard®

Pharmacologic Category Antiarrhythmic Agent, Class IV; Diagnostic Agent

Synonyms 9-Beta-D-ribofuranosyladenine

Use

Adenocard®: Treatment of paroxysmal supraventricular tachycardia (PSVT) including that associated with accessory bypass tracts (Wolff-Parkinson-White syndrome); when clinically advisable, appropriate vagal maneuvers should be attempted prior to adenosine administration; **not effective in atrial flutter, atrial fibrillation, or ventricular tachycardia**

Adenoscan®: Pharmacologic stress agent used in myocardial perfusion thallium-201 scintigraphy

Local Anesthetic/Vasoconstrictor Precautions No information available to require special precautions

Effects on Dental Treatment

>10%: Flushing (18%), palpitations, chest pain, hypotension, headache, dyspnea (12%), diaphoresis

1% to 7%: Dizziness, nausea (3%), paresthesia, chest pressure (7%), numbness

Dosage

Adenocard®: Rapid I.V. push (over 1-2 seconds) via peripheral line:

Neonates: Initial dose: 0.05 mg/kg; if not effective within 2 minutes, increase dose by 0.05 mg/kg increments every 2 minutes to a maximum dose of 0.25 mg/kg or until termination of PSVT

Maximum single dose: 12 mg

Infants and Children: Pediatric advanced life support (PALS): Treatment of SVT: 0.1 mg/kg; if not effective, administer 0.2 mg/kg

Alternatively: Initial dose: 0.05 mg/kg; if not effective within 2 minutes, increase dose by 0.05 mg/kg increments every 2 minutes to a maximum dose of 0.25 mg/kg or until termination of PSVT; medium dose required: 0.15 mg/kg

Maximum single dose: 12 mg

Adults: 6 mg; if not effective within 1-2 minutes, 12 mg may be given; may repeat 12 mg bolus if needed

Maximum single dose: 12 mg

Follow each I.V. bolus of adenosine with normal saline flush

Note: Preliminary results in adults suggest adenosine may be administered via a central line at lower doses (ie, initial adult dose: 3 mg).

Adenoscan®: Continuous I.V. infusion via peripheral line: 140 mcg/kg/minute for 6 minutes using syringe or columetric infusion pump; total dose: 0.84 mg/kg. Thallium-201 is injected at midpoint (3 minutes) of infusion.

(Continued)

Adenosine *(Continued)*

Hemodialysis: Significant drug removal is unlikely based on physiochemical characteristics.

Peritoneal dialysis: Significant drug removal is unlikely based on physiochemical characteristics.

Note: Patients who are receiving concomitant theophylline therapy may be less likely to respond to adenosine therapy.

Note: Higher doses may be needed for administration via peripheral versus central vein.

Mechanism of Action Slows conduction time through the AV node, interrupting the re-entry pathways through the AV node, restoring normal sinus rhythm

Other Adverse Effects <1% (Limited to important or life-threatening): **Intracranial pressure, hyperventilation**

Drug Interactions

Increased Effect/Toxicity: Dipyridamole potentiates effects of adenosine. Use with carbamazepine may increase heart block.

Decreased Effect: Methylxanthines (eg, caffeine, theophylline) antagonize the effect of adenosine.

Dietary/Ethanol/Herb Considerations Food: Avoid food beverages with caffeine; may decrease therapeutic effect of adenosine.

Pharmacodynamics/Kinetics

Onset of action: Rapid

Duration: Very brief

Metabolism: Blood and tissue to inosine then to adenosine monophosphate (AMP) and hypoxanthine

Half-life elimination: <10 seconds

Pregnancy Risk Factor C

Generic Available No

ADH *see* Vasopressin *on page 1379*

Adipex-P® *see* Phentermine *on page 1069*

Adoxa™ *see* Doxycycline *on page 476*

ADR *see* DOXOrubicin *on page 473*

Adrenalin® (Dental) *see* Epinephrine *on page 499*

Adrenocorticotropic Hormone *see* Corticotropin *on page 372*

Adria *see* DOXOrubicin *on page 473*

Adriamycin PFS® *see* DOXOrubicin *on page 473*

Adriamycin RDF® *see* DOXOrubicin *on page 473*

Adrucil® *see* Fluorouracil *on page 588*

Adsorbent Charcoal *see* Charcoal *on page 294*

Advair™ Diskus® *see* Fluticasone and Salmeterol *on page 601*

Advantage-S™ [OTC] *see* Nonoxynol 9 *on page 985*

Advicor™ *see* Niacin and Lovastatin *on page 968*

Advil® [OTC] *see* Ibuprofen *on page 703*

Advil® Children's [OTC] *see* Ibuprofen *on page 703*

Advil® Cold, Children's [OTC] *see* Pseudoephedrine and Ibuprofen *on page 1148*

Advil® Cold & Sinus [OTC] *see* Pseudoephedrine and Ibuprofen *on page 1148*

Advil® Infants' Concentrated Drops [OTC] *see* Ibuprofen *on page 703*

Advil® Junior [OTC] *see* Ibuprofen *on page 703*

Advil® Migraine [OTC] *see* Ibuprofen *on page 703*

AeroBid® *see* Flunisolide *on page 582*

AeroBid®-M *see* Flunisolide *on page 582*

Afrin® [OTC] *see* Oxymetazoline *on page 1022*

Afrin® Extra Moisturizing [OTC] *see* Oxymetazoline *on page 1022*

Afrin® Original [OTC] *see* Oxymetazoline *on page 1022*

Afrin® Severe Congestion [OTC] *see* Oxymetazoline *on page 1022*

Afrin® Sinus [OTC] *see* Oxymetazoline *on page 1022*

Aftate® Antifungal [OTC] *see* Tolnaftate *on page 1322*

Agenerase® *see* Amprenavir *on page 105*

Aggrastat® *see* Tirofiban *on page 1313*

Aggrenox™ *see* Aspirin and Dipyridamole *on page 135*

$AgNO_3$ *see* Silver Nitrate *on page 1221*

Agoral® Maximum Strength Laxative [OTC] *see* Senna *on page 1215*

Agrylin® *see* Anagrelide *on page 108*

AHA *see* Acetohydroxamic Acid *on page 39*

AHF (Human) *see* Antihemophilic Factor (Human) *on page 113*

AHF (Porcine) *see* Antihemophilic Factor (Porcine) *on page 114*

AHF (Recombinant) *see* Antihemophilic Factor (Recombinant) *on page 115*

A-hydroCort® *see* Hydrocortisone *on page 688*

AK-Con™ *see* Naphazoline *on page 952*

AK-Dilate® *see* Phenylephrine *on page 1071*
Akineton® *see* Biperiden *on page 185*
AK-Nefrin® *see* Phenylephrine *on page 1071*
Akne-Mycin® *see* Erythromycin *on page 512*
AK-Pentolate® *see* Cyclopentolate *on page 380*
AK-Poly-Bac® *see* Bacitracin and Polymyxin B *on page 157*
AK-Pred® *see* PrednisoLONE *on page 1110*
AK-Spore® H.C. [DSC] *see* Bacitracin, Neomycin, Polymyxin B, and Hydrocortisone *on page 158*
AK-Sulf® *see* Sulfacetamide *on page 1249*
AK-T-Caine™ *see* Tetracaine *on page 1284*
AKTob® *see* Tobramycin *on page 1315*
AK-Tracin® *see* Bacitracin *on page 156*
AK-Trol® *see* Neomycin, Polymyxin B, and Dexamethasone *on page 962*
Akwa Tears® [OTC] *see* Artificial Tears *on page 128*
Alamast™ *see* Pemirolast *on page 1044*
Alatrofloxacin Mesylate *see* Trovafloxacin/Alatrofloxacin *on page 1361*
Alavert™ [OTC] *see* Loratadine *on page 822*
Albalon® *see* Naphazoline *on page 952*

Albendazole (al BEN da zole)

U.S. Brand Names Albenza®

Mexican Brand Names Bendapar®; Digezanol®; Endoplus®; Eskazole®; Gascop®; Lurdex®; Zentel®

Pharmacologic Category Anthelmintic

Use Treatment of parenchymal neurocysticercosis and cystic hydatid disease of the liver, lung, and peritoneum; albendazole has activity against *Ascaris lumbricoides* (roundworm), *Ancylostoma duodenale* and *Necator americanus* (hookworms), *Enterobius vermicularis* (pinworm), *Hymenolepis nana* and *Taenia* sp (tapeworms), *Opisthorchis sinensis* and *Opisthorchis viverrini* (liver flukes), *Strongyloides stercoralis* and *Trichuris trichiura* (whipworm); activity has also been shown against the liver fluke *Clonorchis sinensis, Giardia lamblia, Cysticercus cellulosae, Echinococcus granulosus, Echinococcus multilocularis,* and *Toxocara* sp.

Local Anesthetic/Vasoconstrictor Precautions No information available to require special precautions

Effects on Dental Treatment Frequency not always defined (N = neurocysticercosis; H = hydatid disease): Headache (11% - N; 1% - H), nausea/vomiting (3% to 6%), dizziness, increased intracranial pressure

Dosage Oral:

Neurocysticercosis:

<60 kg: 15 mg/kg/day in 2 divided doses (maximum: 800 mg/day) with meals for 8-30 days

≥60 kg: 400 mg twice daily for 8-30 days

Note: Give concurrent anticonvulsant and steroid therapy during first week

Hydatid:

<60 kg: 15 mg/kg/day in 2 divided doses with meals (maximum: 800 mg/day) for three 28-day cycles with 14-day drug-free interval in-between

≥60 kg: 400 mg twice daily for 3 cycles as above

Strongyloidiasis/tapeworm: Children >2 years and Adults: 400 mg/day for 3 days; may repeat in 3 weeks

Giardiasis: Adults: 400 mg/day for 3 days

Hookworm, pinworm, roundworm: Children >2 years and Adults: 400 mg as a single dose; may repeat in 3 weeks

Mechanism of Action Active metabolite, albendazole, causes selective degeneration of cytoplasmic microtubules in intestinal and tegmental cells of intestinal helminths and larvae; glycogen is depleted, glucose uptake and cholinesterase secretion are impaired, and desecratory substances accumulate intracellulary. ATP production decreases causing energy depletion, immobilization, and worm death.

Other Adverse Effects Frequency not always defined: N = neurocysticercosis; H = hydatid disease:

Central nervous system: Vertigo

Gastrointestinal: Abdominal pain (6% - H)

Hematologic: Granulocytopenia/agranulocytopenia/pancytopenia (rare)

Hepatic: Increased LFTs (~15% - H, <1% - N)

<1%: **Allergic reactions,** leukopenia (reversible), alopecia/rash/urticaria

Drug Interactions Substrate of CYP1A2, 3A4; inhibits CYP1A2

Increased Effect/Toxicity: Albendazole serum levels are increased when taken with dexamethasone, praziquantel.

Decreased Effect: Cimetidine may increase albendazole metabolism.

Dietary/Ethanol/Herb Considerations Food: Serum levels may be increased if taken with a fatty meal; increases oral bioavailability by 4-5 times.

Pharmacodynamics/Kinetics

Absorption: <5%; may increase up to 4-5 times when administered with a fatty meal

(Continued)

Albendazole *(Continued)*

Distribution: Well inside hydatid cysts and CSF
Protein binding: 70%
Metabolism: Hepatic; extensive first-pass effect; pathways include rapid sulfoxidation (major), hydrolysis, and oxidation
Half-life elimination: 8-12 hours
Time to peak, serum: 2-2.4 hours
Excretion: Urine (<1% as active metabolite); feces

Pregnancy Risk Factor C

Generic Available No

Albenza® *see* Albendazole *on page 47*

Albuterol (al BYOO ter ole)

Related Information

Dental Office Emergencies *on page 1582*
Ipratropium and Albuterol *on page 738*
Respiratory Diseases *on page 1476*

U.S. Brand Names AccuNeb™; Proventil®; Proventil® HFA; Proventil® Repetabs®; Ventolin®; Ventolin® HFA; Volmax®; VoSpire ER™

Canadian Brand Names Airomir; Alti-Salbutamol; Apo®-Salvent; Gen-Salbutamol; PMS-Salbutamol; ratio-Inspra-Sal; ratio-Salbutamol; Rhoxal-salbutamol; Salbu-2; Salbu-4; Ventolin®; Ventolin® Diskus; Ventolin® HFA; Ventrodisk

Mexican Brand Names Inspiryl®; Salbulin; Salbulin Autohaler®; Salbutalan; Ventolin®; Volmax®

Pharmacologic Category Beta$_2$ Agonist

Synonyms Salbutamol

Use Bronchodilator in reversible airway obstruction due to asthma or COPD; prevention of exercise-induced bronchospasm

Local Anesthetic/Vasoconstrictor Precautions No information available to require special precautions

Effects on Dental Treatment

1% to 10%: Xerostomia

Frequency not defined: Angina, atrial fibrillation, chest discomfort, flushing, hypertension, palpitations, tachycardia, CNS stimulation, dizziness, drowsiness, headache, irritability, lightheadedness, migraine, nervousness, tremors, restlessness, gastroenteritis, nausea, unusual taste, tooth discoloration, vomiting, weakness, otitis media, asthma exacerbation, bronchospasm, cough, epistaxis, laryngitis, oropharyngeal dryness/irritation/edema, allergic reaction, lymphadenopathy

Dosage

Oral:
- Children: Bronchospasm (treatment):
  - 2-6 years: 0.1-0.2 mg/kg/dose 3 times/day; maximum dose not to exceed 12 mg/day (divided doses)
  - 6-12 years: 2 mg/dose 3-4 times/day; maximum dose not to exceed 24 mg/day (divided doses)
    - Extended release: 4 mg every 12 hours; maximum dose not to exceed 24 mg/day (divided doses)
- Children >12 years and Adults: Bronchospasm (treatment): 2-4 mg/dose 3-4 times/day; maximum dose not to exceed 32 mg/day (divided doses)
  - Extended release: 8 mg every 12 hours; maximum dose not to exceed 32 mg/day (divided doses). A 4 mg dose every 12 hours may be sufficient in some patients, such as adults of low body weight.
- Elderly: Bronchospasm (treatment): 2 mg 3-4 times/day; maximum: 8 mg 4 times/day

Inhalation: Children ≥4 years and Adults:
- Bronchospasm (treatment):
  - MDI: 90 mcg/spray: 1-2 inhalations every 4-6 hours; maximum: 12 inhalations/day
  - Capsule: 200-400 mcg every 4-6 hours
- Exercise-induced bronchospasm (prophylaxis):
  - MDI-CFC aerosol: 2 inhalations 15 minutes before exercising
  - MDI-HFA aerosol: 2 inhalations 15-30 minutes before exercise
  - Capsule: 200 mcg 15 minutes before exercise

Nebulization:
- Children:
  - Bronchospasm (treatment): 0.01-0.05 mL/kg of 0.5% solution every 4-6 hours
    - 2-12 years: AccuNeb™: 0.63 mg or 1.25 mg 3-4 times/day, as needed, delivered over 5-15 minutes
    - Children >40 kg, patients with more severe asthma, or children 11-12 years: May respond better with a 1.25 mg dose
  - Bronchospasm (acute): 0.01-0.05 mL/kg of 0.5% solution every 4-6 hours; intensive care patients may require more frequent administration; minimum dose: 0.1 mL; maximum dose: 1 mL diluted in 1-2 mL normal saline; continuous nebulized albuterol at 0.3 mg/kg/hour has been used safely in the

treatment of severe status asthmaticus in children; continuous nebulized doses of 3 mg/kg/hour ± 2.2 mg/kg/hour in children whose mean age was 20.7 months resulted in no cardiac toxicity; the optimal dosage for continuous nebulization remains to be determined.

Adults:

Bronchospasm (treatment): 2.5 mg, diluted to a total of 3 mL, 3-4 times/day over 5-15 minutes

Bronchospasm (acute) in intensive care patients: 2.5-5 mg every 20 minutes for 3 doses, then 2.5-10 mg every 1-4 hours as needed, **or** 10-15 mg/hour continuously

Hemodialysis: Not removed

Peritoneal dialysis: Significant drug removal is unlikely based on physiochemical characteristics

Mechanism of Action Relaxes bronchial smooth muscle by action on $beta_2$-receptors with little effect on heart rate

Other Adverse Effects Incidence is dependent upon age of patient, dose, and route of administration; frequency not defined:

Cardiovascular: Extrasystoles

Central nervous system: Nightmares, insomnia

Dermatologic: Angioedema, erythema multiforme, rash, Stevens-Johnson syndrome, urticaria

Endocrine & metabolic: Hypokalemia

Gastrointestinal: Diarrhea

Genitourinary: Micturition difficulty

Warnings/Precautions Use with caution in patients with hyperthyroidism, diabetes mellitus, or sensitivity to sympathomimetic amines; cardiovascular disorders including coronary insufficiency or hypertension; excessive use may result in tolerance. May cause paradoxical bronchospasm. Increased use may indicate a deterioration of condition and requires a re-evaluation of the patient. Excessive use of inhalers has been associated with fatalities.

Because of its minimal effect on $beta_1$-receptors and its relatively long duration of action, albuterol is a rational choice in the elderly when an inhaled beta agonist is indicated. Oral use should be avoided in the elderly due to adverse effects. All patients should utilize a spacer device when using a metered-dose inhaler; spacers and facemasks should be used in children <4 years. Patient response may vary between inhalers that contain chlorofluorocarbons and those which are chlorofluorocarbon-free.

Drug Interactions Substrate of **CYP3A4**

Increased Effect/Toxicity: When used with inhaled ipratropium, an increased duration of bronchodilation may occur. Cardiovascular effects are potentiated in patients also receiving MAO inhibitors, tricyclic antidepressants, and sympathomimetic agents (eg, amphetamine, dopamine, dobutamine). Albuterol may increase the risk of malignant arrhythmias with inhaled anesthetics (eg, enflurane, halothane).

Decreased Effect: When used with nonselective beta-adrenergic blockers (eg, propranolol) the effect of albuterol is decreased.

Dietary/Ethanol/Herb Considerations

Food: Administer oral forms on an empty stomach with water 1 hour before or 2 hours after meals. Avoid food/beverages with caffeine; may cause CNS stimulation.

Herb/Nutraceutical: Avoid ephedra, ginseng, and yohimbe; may cause CNS stimulation.

Pharmacodynamics/Kinetics

Onset of action: Peak effect: Nebulization/oral inhalation: 0.5-2 hours; Oral: 2-3 hours

Duration: Nebulization/oral inhalation: 3-4 hours; Oral: 4-6 hours

Metabolism: Hepatic to an inactive sulfate

Half-life elimination: Inhalation: 3.8 hours; Oral: 3.7-5 hours

Excretion: Urine (30% as unchanged drug)

Pregnancy Risk Factor C

Generic Available Yes: Excludes extended release

Albuterol and Ipratropium *see* Ipratropium and Albuterol *on page 738*

Alcaine® *see* Proparacaine *on page 1132*

Alclometasone (al kloe MET a sone)

U.S. Brand Names Aclovate®

Pharmacologic Category Corticosteroid, Topical

Synonyms Alclometasone Dipropionate

Use Treatment of inflammation of corticosteroid-responsive dermatosis (low potency topical corticosteroid)

Local Anesthetic/Vasoconstrictor Precautions No information available to require special precautions

Effects on Dental Treatment No significant effects or complications reported

(Continued)

Alclometasone *(Continued)*

Dosage Topical: Apply a thin film to the affected area 2-3 times/day. Therapy should be discontinued when control is achieved; if no improvement is seen, reassessment of diagnosis may be necessary.

Mechanism of Action Stimulates the synthesis of enzymes needed to decrease inflammation, suppress mitotic activity, and cause vasoconstriction

Other Adverse Effects

1% to 10%:

Dermatologic: Itching, erythema, dry skin, papular rashes

Local: Burning, irritation

<1%: Hypertrichosis, acneiform eruptions, hypopigmentation, perioral dermatitis, maceration of skin, skin atrophy, striae, miliaria

Pregnancy Risk Factor C

Generic Available No

Alclometasone Dipropionate *see* Alclometasone *on page 49*

Aldactazide® *see* Hydrochlorothiazide and Spironolactone *on page 677*

Aldactone® *see* Spironolactone *on page 1240*

Aldara™ *see* Imiquimod *on page 713*

Aldesleukin (al des LOO kin)

U.S. Brand Names Proleukin®

Canadian Brand Names Proleukin®

Mexican Brand Names Proleukin®

Pharmacologic Category Biological Response Modulator

Synonyms Epidermal Thymocyte Activating Factor; ETAF; IL-2; Interleukin-2; Lymphocyte Mitogenic Factor; NSC-373364; T-Cell Growth Factor; TCGF; Thymocyte Stimulating Factor

Use Treatment of metastatic renal cell cancer, melanoma

Unlabeled/Investigational Use Investigational: Treatment of colorectal cancer, non-Hodgkin's lymphoma, multiple myeloma, HIV infection, and AIDS; may be used in conjunction with lymphokine-activated killer (LAK) cells, tumor-infiltrating lymphocyte (TIL) cells, interleukin-1, and interferons

Local Anesthetic/Vasoconstrictor Precautions No information available to require special precautions

Effects on Dental Treatment

>10%: Stomatitis (32%), hypotension (85%; dose-limiting, possibly fatal), sinus tachycardia (70%), arrhythmias (22%), angina, mental status changes (73%; transient memory loss, confusion, drowsiness), dizziness (17%), somnolence (25%), disorientation (25%), headaches, paranoid delusion, fever, weakness (89%), nausea and vomiting (87%), GI bleeding (13%), congestion (54%), dyspnea (27% to 52%), pain (54%), infection (including sepsis and endocarditis) due to neutrophil impairment (23%), rigors (respond to acetaminophen, diphenhydramine, an NSAID, or meperidine), fatigue (25%), malaise (25%)

1% to 10%: Seizures (1%), coagulation disorders (10%), MI

Dosage Refer to individual protocols; all orders must be written in million International units (million int. units)

I.V.:

Renal cell carcinoma: 600,000 int. units/kg every 8 hours for a maximum of 14 doses; repeat after 9 days of rest for a total of 28 doses per course. Re-evaluate at 4 weeks. Retreat if needed 7 weeks after hospital discharge from previous course.

Melanoma:

Single-agent use: As in renal cell carcinoma

In combination with cytotoxic agents: 24 million int. units/m^2 days 12-16 and 19-23

S.C.:

Single-agent doses: 3-18 million int. units/day for 5 days weekly and repeated weekly up to 6 weeks

In combination with interferon:

5 million int. units/m^2 3 times/week

1.8 million int. units/m^2 twice daily 5 days/week for 6 weeks

Dose modification: In high-dose therapy of RCC, see manufacturer's guidelines for holding and restarting therapy; hold or interrupt a dose - DO NOT REDUCE DOSE; or refer to specific protocol.

Retreatment: Patients should be evaluated for response approximately 4 weeks after completion of a course of therapy and again immediately prior to the scheduled start of the next treatment course; additional courses of treatment may be given to patients only if there is some tumor shrinkage or stable disease following the last course and retreatment is not contraindicated. Each treatment course should be separated by a rest period of at least 7 weeks from the date of hospital discharge; tumors have continued to regress up to 12 months following the initiation of therapy

Investigational regimen: S.C.: 11 million int. units (flat dose) daily x 4 days per week for 4 consecutive weeks; repeat every 6 weeks

Mechanism of Action IL-2 promotes proliferation, differentiation, and recruitment of T and B cells, natural killer (NK) cells, and thymocytes; IL-2 also causes cytolytic activity in a subset of lymphocytes and subsequent interactions between the immune system and malignant cells; IL-2 can stimulate lymphokine-activated killer (LAK) cells and tumor-infiltrating lymphocytes (TIL) cells. LAK cells (which are derived from lymphocytes from a patient and incubated in IL-2) have the ability to lyse cells which are resistant to NK cells; TIL cells (which are derived from cancerous tissue from a patient and incubated in IL-2) have been shown to be 50% more effective than LAK cells in experimental studies.

Other Adverse Effects

>10%:

Cardiovascular: Edema (47%)

Central nervous system: Insomnia, chills (89%)

Dermatologic: Macular erythematous rash (100%; high-dose therapy), pruritus (48%), erythema (41%), rash (26%), exfoliative dermatitis (14%), dry skin (15%)

Endocrine & metabolic: Low electrolyte levels of magnesium, calcium, phosphate, potassium, and sodium (1% to 15%)

Gastrointestinal: Weight gain (23%), anorexia (27%)

Hematologic: Anemia (77%), thrombocytopenia (64%), leukopenia (34%; may be dose-limiting)

Hepatic: Transient elevations of bilirubin (64%) and enzymes (56%), jaundice (11%)

Renal: Oliguria/anuria (63%; 5% to 6% severe), proteinuria (12%), renal failure (dose-limiting toxicity; manifested as oliguria noted within 24-48 hours of initiation of therapy), hypophosphatemia; marked fluid retention, azotemia, and increased serum creatinine (may return to baseline within 7 days of discontinuation of therapy)

1% to 10%:

Cardiovascular: Capillary leak syndrome including peripheral edema, ascites, pulmonary infiltration, and pleural effusion (2% to 4%; may be dose-limiting and potentially fatal)

Endocrine & metabolic: Hypo- and hyperglycemia (2%), increased electrolyte levels of magnesium, calcium, phosphate, potassium, sodium (1%), hypothyroidism

Hepatic: Ascites (4%)

Neuromuscular & skeletal: Arthralgia (6%), myalgia (6%)

Renal: Hematuria (9%), increased creatinine (5%)

Respiratory: Pleural effusions, edema (10%)

<1%: **CHF, coma**, alopecia, pancreatitis, **allergic reactions**, injection site reactions (S.C. doses)

Drug Interactions

Increased Effect/Toxicity:

Aldesleukin may affect central nervous function; therefore, interactions could occur following concomitant administration of psychotropic drugs (eg, narcotics, analgesics, antiemetics, sedatives, tranquilizers).

Concomitant administration of drugs possessing nephrotoxic (eg, aminoglycosides, indomethacin), myelotoxic (eg, cytotoxic chemotherapy), cardiotoxic (eg, doxorubicin), or hepatotoxic (eg, methotrexate, asparaginase) effects with aldesleukin may increase toxicity in these organ systems. The safety and efficacy of aldesleukin in combination with chemotherapies has not been established.

Beta-blockers and other antihypertensives may potentiate the hypotension seen with aldesleukin.

Decreased Effect: Corticosteroids have been shown to decrease toxicity of IL-2, but have not been used since there is concern that they may reduce the efficacy of the lymphokine.

Dietary/Ethanol/Herb Considerations Ethanol: Avoid use due to CNS adverse effects.

Pharmacodynamics/Kinetics

Distribution: V_d: 4-7 L; primarily in plasma and then in the lymphocytes

Bioavailability: I.M.: 37%

Half-life elimination: Initial: 6-13 minutes; Terminal: 80-120 minutes

Pregnancy Risk Factor C

Generic Available No

Comments 22 million units = 1.3 mg

1 Cetus Unit = 6 International Units

1.1 mg = 18 x 10^6 International Units (or 3 x 10^6 Cetus Units)

1 Roche Unit (Teceleukin) = 3 International Units

Aldoclor® *see* Chlorothiazide and Methyldopa *on page 305*

Aldoril® *see* Methyldopa and Hydrochlorothiazide *on page 892*

Aldoril® D *see* Methyldopa and Hydrochlorothiazide *on page 892*

Alefacept (a LE fa sept)

U.S. Brand Names Amevive®

Pharmacologic Category Monoclonal Antibody

Synonyms B 9273; BG 9273; Human LFA-3/IgG(1) Fusion Protein; LFA-3/IgG(1) Fusion Protein, Human

Use Treatment of moderate to severe plaque psoriasis in adults who are candidates for systemic therapy or phototherapy

Local Anesthetic/Vasoconstrictor Precautions No information available to require special precautions

Effects on Dental Treatment 1% to 10%: Dizziness, nausea, pharyngitis, increased cough, infections (1% to 2% requiring hospitalization)

Restrictions Distributed directly to physician offices or to a specialty pharmacy; injections to be administered in physician's office

Dosage Adults:

I.M.: 15 mg once weekly; usual duration of treatment: 12 weeks

I.V.: 7.5 mg once weekly; usual duration of treatment: 12 weeks

A second course of treatment may be initiated at least 12 weeks after completion of the initial course of treatment, provided $CD4^+$ T-lymphocyte counts are within the normal range.

Note: $CD4^+$ T-lymphocyte counts should be monitored before initiation of treatment and weekly during therapy. Dosing should be withheld if $CD4^+$ counts are <250 cells/µL, and dosing should be permanently discontinued if $CD4^+$ lymphocyte counts remain at <250 cell/µL for longer than 1 month.

Dosage adjustment in renal impairment:None

Mechanism of Action Binds to CD2, a receptor on the surface of lymphocytes, inhibiting their interaction with leukocyte functional antigen 3 (LFA-3). Interaction between CD2 and LFA-3 is important for the activation of T-lymphocytes in psoriasis. Activated T-lymphocytes secrete a number of inflammatory mediators, including interferon gamma, which are involved in psoriasis. Since CD2 is primarily expressed on T-lymphocytes, treatment results in a reduction in $CD4^+$ and $CD8^+$ T-lymphocytes, with lesser effects on other cell populations (NK- and B-lymphocytes).

Other Adverse Effects

≥10%:

Hematologic: Lymphopenia (≤10% required temporary discontinuation; ≤17% during a second course of therapy)

Local: Injection site reactions (≤16% of patients; includes pain, inflammation, bleeding, edema, or other reaction)

1% to 10%:

Central nervous system: Chills (6%; primarily during I.V. administration)

Dermatologic: Pruritus

Neuromuscular & skeletal: Myalgia

Miscellaneous: Malignancies (1% vs 0.2% in placebo), antibodies to alefacept (3%; significance unknown)

<1%: Anaphylaxis, allergic reaction, angioedema, headache, MI, transaminase increases (5-10 times ULN), urticaria

Pharmacodynamics/Kinetics

Distribution: V_d: 0.094 L/kg

Bioavailability: 63% (following I.M. administration)

Half-life: 270 hours (following I.V. administration)

Excretion: Clearance: 0.25 mL/hour/kg

Pregnancy Risk Factor B

Generic Available No

Alemtuzumab (ay lem TU zoo mab)

U.S. Brand Names Campath®

Pharmacologic Category Antineoplastic Agent, Monoclonal Antibody

Synonyms Campath-1H; DNA-derived Humanized Monoclonal Antibody; Humanized IgG1 Anti-CD52 Monoclonal Antibody

Use Treatment of B-cell chronic lymphocytic leukemia (B-CLL) in patients treated with alkylating agents and who have failed fludarabine therapy

Unlabeled/Investigational Use Treatment of rheumatoid arthritis, graft versus host disease, multiple myeloma

Local Anesthetic/Vasoconstrictor Precautions No information available to require special precautions

Effects on Dental Treatment

>10%: Hypertension (11%), tachycardia/SVT (11%), headache (13% to 24%), dysthesias (15%), dizziness (12%), neutropenic fever (10%), nausea (47% to 54%), vomiting (33% to 41%), stomatitis/mucositis (14%), cough (25%), bronchitis/pneumonitis (21%), pharyngitis (12%), infection (43% including sepsis, pneumonia, opportunistic infections; received PCP pneumonia and herpes prophylaxis), diaphoresis (19%), pain (24%), weakness (13%)

1% to 10%: Chest pain (10%), somnolence (5%), tremor (7%), bronchospasm (9%), epistaxis (7%), rhinitis (7%)

Dosage Dose escalation is required; usually accomplished in 3-7 days. Do not exceed single doses >30 mg or cumulative doses >90 mg/week. Premedicate with diphenhydramine and acetaminophen 30 minutes before initiation of infusion. Start anti-infective prophylaxis. Discontinue therapy during serious infection, serious hematologic or other serious toxicity until the event resolves. Permanently discontinue if evidence of autoimmune anemia or autoimmune thrombocytopenia occurs.

I.V. infusion: Adults: B-CLL:

Initial: 3 mg/day as a 2-hour infusion; when daily dose is tolerated (eg, infusion-related toxicities at or below Grade 2) increase to 10 mg/day and continue until tolerated; when 10 mg dose tolerated, increase to 30 mg/day

Maintenance: 30 mg/day 3 times/week on alternate days (ie, Monday, Wednesday, Friday) for up to 12 weeks

Dosing adjustment for hematologic toxicity (severe neutropenia or thrombocytopenia, not autoimmune):

First occurrence: ANC <250/µL and/or platelet count ≤25,000/µL: Hold therapy; resume at same dose when ANC ≥500/µL and platelet count ≥50,000/µL. If delay between dosing is ≥7 days, initiate at 3 mg/day and escalate dose as above according to patient tolerance

Second occurrence: ANC <250/µL and/or platelet count ≤25,000/µL: Hold therapy; resume at 10 mg/day when ANC ≥500/µL and platelet count ≥50,000/µL. If delay between dosing is ≥7 days, initiate at 3 mg/day and escalate dose to a maximum of 10 mg/day according to patient tolerance.

Third occurrence: ANC <250/µL and/or platelet count ≤25,000/µL: Permanently discontinue therapy

Patients with a baseline ANC ≤500/µL and/or a baseline platelet count ≤25,000/µL at initiation of therapy: If ANC and/or platelet counts decreased to ≤50% of the baseline value, hold therapy. When ANC and/or platelet count return to baseline, resume therapy. If delay between dosing is ≥7 days, initiate at 3 mg/day and escalate dose as above according to patient tolerance.

Mechanism of Action Recombinant monoclonal antibody binds to CD52, a nonmodulating antigen present on the surface of B and T lymphocytes, a majority of monocytes, macrophages, NK cells and a subpopulation of granulocytes. After binding to leukemic cells, an antibody-dependent lysis occurs.

Other Adverse Effects

>10%:

Cardiovascular: Peripheral edema (13%), hypotension (15% to 32%; infusion related)

Central nervous system (infusion-related): Drug-related fever (83%), fatigue (22% to 34%)

Dermatologic (infusion-related): Rash (30% to 40%), urticaria (22% to 30%), pruritus (14% to 24%)

Gastrointestinal: Anorexia (20%), diarrhea (13% to 22%; infusion-related), abdominal pain (11%)

Hematologic: Lymphopenia, severe neutropenia (64% to 70%), severe anemia (38% to 47%), severe thrombocytopenia (50% to 52%)

Neuromuscular & skeletal: Rigors (89%; infusion-related), myalgia (11%)

Respiratory: Dyspnea (17% to 26%; infusion-related)

1% to 10%:

Central nervous system: Insomnia (10%), malaise (9%), depression (7%), temperature change sensation (5%)

Dermatologic: Purpura (8%)

Gastrointestinal: Dyspepsia (10%), constipation (9%)

Hematologic: Pancytopenia/marrow hypoplasia (6%), positive Coombs' test without hemolysis (2%), autoimmune thrombocytopenia (2%), antibodies to alemtuzumab (2%), autoimmune hemolytic anemia (1%)

Neuromuscular & skeletal: Back pain (10%)

<1%: Abnormal gait, **abnormal thinking**, acidosis, **acute renal failure,** agranulocytosis, alkaline phosphatase elevation, **allergic reactions, anaphylactoid reactions, angina pectoris**, angioedema, anuria, apathy, aphasia, **arthritis, arthritis exacerbation**, arthropathy, ascites, **asthma, biliary pain**, bone fracture, bone marrow aplasia, **bronchitis**, bullous eruption, capillary fragility, **cardiac arrest, cardiac failure**, cellulitis, cerebral hemorrhage, cerebrovascular disorder, cervical dysplasia, **coagulation abnormality**, colitis, **coma, confusion, COPD**, decreased haptoglobin, deep vein thrombosis, **dehydration, diabetes mellitus exacerbation, disseminated intravascular coagulation, duodenal ulcer**, endophthalmitis, **esophagitis, facial edema**, fluid overload, **gingivitis, gastroenteritis, GI hemorrhage, hallucinations**, hearing loss, hematemesis, **hematoma**, hematuria, hemolysis, hemolytic anemia, hemoptysis, hemorrhoids, **hepatic failure,** hepatocellular damage, hyperbilirubinemia, **hyperglycemia**, hyperkalemia, hyperthyroidism, hypoalbuminemia, **hypoglycemia**, hyponatremia, hypovolemia, hypoxia, **influenza-like syndrome**, interstitial pneumonitis, intestinal obstruction, intestinal perforation, intracranial hemorrhage, **lymphadenopathy,** malignant lymphoma, malignant testicular neoplasm, marrow depression, melena, meningitis, **mouth edema, MI**, myositis, **muscle atrophy, nervousness**, osteomyelitis, pancreatitis, **paralysis**, paralytic ileus, paroxysmal

(Continued)

Alemtuzumab *(Continued)*

nocturnal hemoglobinuria-like monocytes, **peptic ulcer**, pericarditis, peritonitis, plasma cell dyscrasia, phlebitis, pleural effusion, pleurisy, pneumothorax, polymyositis, progressive multifocal leukoencephalopathy, prostate cancer, **pseudomembranous colitis,** pulmonary edema, pulmonary embolism, pulmonary fibrosis, pulmonary infiltration, purpuric rash, renal dysfunction, respiratory alkalosis, **respiratory depression, respiratory insufficiency**, secondary leukemia, **seizure (grand mal), sinusitis**, splenic infarction, splenomegaly, squamous cell carcinoma, stridor, subarachnoid hemorrhage, **syncope, loss of taste**, toxic nephropathy, transformation to aggressive lymphoma, transformation to prolymphocytic leukemia, thrombocythemia, thrombophlebitis, **throat tightness**, ureteric obstruction, urinary retention, **ventricular arrhythmia, ventricular tachycardia**

Pharmacodynamics/Kinetics Half-life elimination: 12 days

Pregnancy Risk Factor C

Generic Available No

Alendronate (a LEN droe nate)

Related Information

Rheumatoid Arthritis, Osteoarthritis, and Osteoporosis *on page 1488*

U.S. Brand Names Fosamax®

Canadian Brand Names Fosamax®

Pharmacologic Category Bisphosphonate Derivative

Synonyms Alendronate Sodium

Use Treatment and prevention of osteoporosis in postmenopausal females; treatment of osteoporosis in males; Paget's disease of the bone in patients who are symptomatic, at risk for future complications, or with alkaline phosphatase ≥2 times the upper limit of normal; treatment of glucocorticoid-induced osteoporosis in males and females with low bone mineral density who are receiving a daily dosage ≥7.5 mg of prednisone (or equivalent)

Local Anesthetic/Vasoconstrictor Precautions No information available to require special precautions

Effects on Dental Treatment 1% to 5%: Headache (≤3%), acid reflux (1% to 5%), esophageal ulcer (≤2%), vomiting (≤1%), gastric ulcer (1%), gastritis (≤1%), dysphagia (≤1%), pain (4%), nausea (1% to 4%)

Dosage Must be taken with a full glass (6-8 oz) of plain water first thing in the morning and ≥30 minutes before the first food, beverage, or other medication of the day; instruct patients to stay upright (not to lie down) for at least 30 minutes **and** until after first food of the day (to reduce esophageal irritation). Patients should receive supplemental calcium and vitamin D if dietary intake is inadequate.

Oral:

Adults:

- Osteoporosis:
  - Postmenopausal females:
    - Prophylaxis: 5 mg once daily or 35 mg once weekly
    - Treatment: 10 mg once daily or 70 mg once weekly
  - Males: 10 mg once daily **or** 70 mg once weekly
  - Glucocorticoid-induced osteoporosis: Treatment: 5 mg once daily; a dose of 10 mg once daily should be used in postmenopausal females who are not receiving estrogen. Patients treated with glucocorticoids should receive adequate amounts of calcium and vitamin D.
- Paget's disease of bone: 40 mg once daily for 6 months
  - Retreatment: Relapses during the 12 months following therapy occurred in 9% of patients who responded to treatment. Specific retreatment data are unavailable. Retreatment with alendronate may be considered, following a 6-month post-treatment evaluation period, in patients who have relapsed based on increases in serum alkaline phosphatase, which should be measured periodically. Retreatment may also be considered in those who failed to normalize their serum alkaline phosphatase.

Dosing adjustment in renal impairment:

- Cl_{cr} 35-60 mL/minute: None
- Cl_{cr} <35 mL/minute: Use not recommended due to lack of experience

Mechanism of Action A bisphosphonate which inhibits bone resorption via actions on osteoclasts or on osteoclast precursors; decreases the rate of bone resorption direction, leading to an indirect decrease in bone formation

Other Adverse Effects Incidence increases significantly in Paget's disease at 40 mg/day (mostly GI adverse effects).

>10%: Endocrine & metabolic: Hypocalcemia (18%; transient, mild)

1% to 10%:

- Endocrine & metabolic: Hypophosphatemia (10%; transient, mild)
- Gastrointestinal: Abdominal pain (1% to 7%), dyspepsia (1% to 4%), flatulence (≤4%), diarrhea (≤3%), constipation (≤3%), abdominal distension (≤1%), melena (1%)

Neuromuscular & skeletal: Muscle cramps (≤1%)

<1%, postmarketing, and/or case reports: Angioedema, **duodenal ulcer, esophageal erosions, esophageal perforation, esophageal stricture, esophagitis, hypersensitivity reactions, oropharyngeal ulceration, abnormal taste,** urticaria, uveitis, rash

Warnings/Precautions Use caution in patients with renal impairment; hypocalcemia must be corrected before therapy initiation; ensure adequate calcium and vitamin D intake. May cause irritation to upper GI mucosa. Esophagitis, esophageal ulcers, esophageal erosions, and esophageal stricture (rare) have been reported; risk increases in patients unable to comply with dosing instructions. Use with caution in patients with dysphagia, esophageal disease, gastritis, duodenitis, or ulcers (may worsen underlying condition).

Drug Interactions

Increased Effect/Toxicity: I.V. ranitidine has been shown to double the bioavailability of alendronate. Estrogen replacement therapy, in combination with alendronate, may enhance the therapeutic effects of both agents on the maintenance of bone mineralization. An increased incidence of adverse GI effects has been noted when >10 mg alendronate is used in patients taking aspirin-containing products.

Decreased Effect: Oral medications (especially those containing multivalent cations, including calcium and antacids): May interfere with alendronate absorption; wait at least 30 minutes after taking alendronate before taking any oral medications

Dietary/Ethanol/Herb Considerations

Ethanol: Avoid use

Food: Must be administered first thing in the morning, 30-60 minutes before the first food or drink with 8 oz of **plain water** (not mineral water) to avoid interference with absorption. All food and beverages interfere with alendronate absorption; food decreases absorption by 40%. Caffeine may reduce efficacy. Coffee and orange juice decrease oral bioavailability by 60%. Dairy products decrease absorption through calcium binding. Small, frequent meals may reduce GI upset. Calcium, iron, and multivalent cations may reduce absorption as much as 60%; wait at least 30 minutes before taking any supplement. Take supplemental calcium and vitamin D if dietary intake is inadequate.

Pharmacodynamics/Kinetics

Distribution: 28 L (exclusive of bone)

Protein binding: ~78%

Metabolism: None

Bioavailability: Fasting: Female: 0.7%; Male: 0.6%; reduced 60% with food or drink

Half-life elimination: Exceeds 10 years

Excretion: Urine; feces (as unabsorbed drug)

Pregnancy Risk Factor C

Generic Available No

Alendronate Sodium *see* Alendronate *on page 54*

Aler-Dryl [OTC] *see* DiphenhydrAMINE *on page 451*

Alesse® *see* Combination Hormonal Contraceptives *on page 368*

Aleve® [OTC] *see* Naproxen *on page 953*

Alfenta® *see* Alfentanil *on page 55*

Alfentanil (al FEN ta nil)

U.S. Brand Names Alfenta®

Canadian Brand Names Alfenta®

Mexican Brand Names Rapifen®

Pharmacologic Category Analgesic, Narcotic

Synonyms Alfentanil Hydrochloride

Use Analgesic adjunct given by continuous infusion or in incremental doses in maintenance of anesthesia with barbiturate or N_2O or a primary anesthetic agent for the induction of anesthesia in patients undergoing general surgery in which endotracheal intubation and mechanical ventilation are required

Local Anesthetic/Vasoconstrictor Precautions No information available to require special precautions

Effects on Dental Treatment Erythromycin inhibits the liver metabolism of alfentanil resulting in increased sedation and prolonged respiratory depression.

>10%: Bradycardia, peripheral vasodilation, drowsiness, sedation, increased intracranial pressure, nausea, vomiting

1% to 10%: Arrhythmia, orthostatic hypotension, confusion, CNS depression, blurred vision

Restrictions C-II

Dosage Doses should be titrated to appropriate effects; wide range of doses is dependent upon desired degree of analgesia/anesthesia

Children <12 years: Dose not established

Adults: Dose should be based on ideal body weight; see table on next page:

(Continued)

Alfentanil *(Continued)*

Alfentanil

Indication	Approx Duration of Anesthesia (min)	Induction Period (Initial Dose) (mcg/kg)	Maintenance Period (Increments/ Infusion)	Total Dose (mcg/kg)	Effects
Incremental injection	≤30	8-20	3-5 mcg/kg or 0.5-1 mcg/kg/ min	8-40	Spontaneously breathing or assisted ventilation when required.
	30-60	20-50	5-15 mcg/kg	Up to 75	Assisted or controlled ventilation required. Attenuation of response to laryngoscopy and intubation.
Continuous infusion	>45	50-75	0.5-3 mcg/kg/ min average infusion rate 1-1.5 mcg/kg/ min	Dependent on duration of procedure	Assisted or controlled ventilation required. Some attenuation of response to intubation and incision, with intraoperative stability.
Anesthetic induction	>45	130-245	0.5-1.5 mcg/ kg/min or general anesthetic	Dependent on duration of procedure	Assisted or controlled ventilation required. Administer slowly (over 3 minutes). Concentration of inhalation agents reduced by 30% to 50% for initial hour.

Mechanism of Action Binds with stereospecific receptors at many sites within the CNS, increases pain threshold, alters pain perception, inhibits ascending pain pathways; is an ultra short-acting narcotic

Other Adverse Effects

>10%:

Gastrointestinal: Constipation

Endocrine & metabolic: Antidiuretic hormone release

Ocular: Miosis

<1%: **Convulsions**, mental depression, **paradoxical CNS excitation or delirium, dizziness**, dysesthesia, rash, urticaria, itching, **biliary tract spasm**, urinary tract spasm, **respiratory depression, bronchospasm, laryngospasm, physical and psychological dependence (with prolonged use),** cold/clammy skin

Drug Interactions Substrate of **CYP3A4**

Increased Effect/Toxicity: Dextroamphetamine may enhance the analgesic effect of morphine and other opiate agonists. CNS depressants (eg, benzodiazepines, barbiturates, tricyclic antidepressants), erythromycin, reserpine, beta-blockers may increase the toxic effects of alfentanil.

Pharmacodynamics/Kinetics

Onset of action: Rapid

Duration (dose dependent): 30-60 minutes

Distribution: V_d: Newborns, premature: 1 L/kg; Children: 0.163-0.48 L/kg; Adults: 0.46 L/kg

Half-life elimination: Newborns, premature: 5.33-8.75 hours; Children: 40-60 minutes; Adults: 83-97 minutes

Pregnancy Risk Factor C

Generic Available Yes

Selected Readings

Bartkowski RR, Goldberg ME, Larijani GE, et al, "Inhibition of Alfentanil Metabolism by Erythromycin," *Clin Pharmacol Ther*, 1989, 46(1):99-102.

Bartkowski RR and McDonnell TE, "Prolonged Alfentanil Effect Following Erythromycin Administration," *Anesthesiology*, 1990, 73(3):566-8.

Alfentanil Hydrochloride *see* Alfentanil *on page 55*

Alferon® N *see* Interferon Alfa-n3 *on page 731*

Alglucerase (al GLOO ser ase)

U.S. Brand Names Ceredase®

Pharmacologic Category Enzyme

Synonyms Glucocerebrosidase

Use Orphan drug: Replacement therapy for Gaucher's disease (type 1)

Local Anesthetic/Vasoconstrictor Precautions No information available to require special precautions

Effects on Dental Treatment No significant effects or complications reported

Dosage Usually administered as a 20-60 unit/kg I.V. infusion given with a frequency ranging from 3 times/week to once every 2 weeks

Mechanism of Action Glucocerebrosidase is an enzyme prepared from human placental tissue. Gaucher's disease is an inherited metabolic disorder caused by the defective activity of beta-glucosidase and the resultant accumulation of glucosyl ceramide laden macrophages in the liver, bone, and spleen; acts by replacing the missing enzyme associated with Gaucher's disease.

Other Adverse Effects

>10%: Local: Discomfort, burning, and edema at the site of injection

<1%: **Fever, nausea, vomiting,** chills, abdominal discomfort

Pharmacodynamics/Kinetics Half-life elimination: ~4-20 minutes

Pregnancy Risk Factor C

Generic Available No

Alinia™ *see* Nitazoxanide *on page 978*

Alitretinoin (a li TRET i noyn)

U.S. Brand Names Panretin®

Canadian Brand Names Panretin™

Pharmacologic Category Antineoplastic Agent, Miscellaneous

Use Orphan drug: Topical treatment of cutaneous lesions in AIDS-related Kaposi's sarcoma

Unlabeled/Investigational Use Treatment of cutaneous T-cell lymphomas

Local Anesthetic/Vasoconstrictor Precautions No information available to require special precautions

Effects on Dental Treatment >10%: Paresthesia (3% to 22%), pain (≤34%)

Dosage Topical: Apply gel twice daily to cutaneous Kaposi's sarcoma or T-cell lymphoma (unlabeled use) lesions

Mechanism of Action Binds to retinoid receptors to inhibit growth of Kaposi's sarcoma

Other Adverse Effects

>10%: Dermatologic: Rash (25% to 77%), pruritus (8% to 11%)

3% to 10%:

Cardiovascular: Edema (3% to 8%)

Dermatologic: Exfoliative dermatitis (3% to 9%), skin disorder (≤8%)

Drug Interactions Increased Effect/Toxicity: Increased toxicity of DEET may occur if products containing this compound are used concurrently with alitretinoin. Due to limited absorption after topical application, interaction with systemic medications is unlikely.

Pharmacodynamics/Kinetics Absorption: Not extensive

Pregnancy Risk Factor D

Generic Available No

Alka-Mints® [OTC] *see* Calcium Supplements *on page 229*

Alka-Seltzer® Gas Relief [OTC] *see* Simethicone *on page 1222*

Alka-Seltzer Plus® Cold and Sinus [OTC] *see* Acetaminophen and Pseudoephedrine *on page 31*

Alka-Seltzer® Plus Cold Liqui-Gels® [OTC] *see* Acetaminophen, Chlorpheniramine, and Pseudoephedrine *on page 35*

Alka-Seltzer® Plus Flu Liqui-Gels® [OTC] *see* Acetaminophen, Dextromethorphan, and Pseudoephedrine *on page 35*

Alkeran® *see* Melphalan *on page 855*

Allbee® With C [OTC] *see* Vitamin B Complex and Vitamin C *on page 1392*

Allegra® *see* Fexofenadine *on page 569*

Allegra-D® *see* Fexofenadine and Pseudoephedrine *on page 570*

Aller-Chlor® [OTC] *see* Chlorpheniramine *on page 307*

Allerest® Maximum Strength [OTC] *see* Chlorpheniramine and Pseudoephedrine *on page 308*

Allerfrim® [OTC] *see* Triprolidine and Pseudoephedrine *on page 1356*

Allergen® *see* Antipyrine and Benzocaine *on page 116*

AllerMax® [OTC] *see* DiphenhydrAMINE *on page 451*

Allerphed® [OTC] *see* Triprolidine and Pseudoephedrine *on page 1356*

Allersol® *see* Naphazoline *on page 952*

Allopurinol (al oh PYOOR i nole)

U.S. Brand Names Aloprim™; Zyloprim®

Canadian Brand Names Apo®-Allopurinol; Zyloprim®

Mexican Brand Names Atisuril®; Unizuric 300; Zyloprim®

Pharmacologic Category Xanthine Oxidase Inhibitor

Synonyms Allopurinol Sodium Injection

Use

Oral: Prevention of attack of gouty arthritis and nephropathy; treatment of secondary hyperuricemia which may occur during treatment of tumors or leukemia; prevention of recurrent calcium oxalate calculi

Orphan drug: I.V.: Management of patients with leukemia, lymphoma, and solid tumor malignancies who are receiving cancer chemotherapy which causes elevations of serum and urinary uric acid levels and who cannot tolerate oral therapy

Local Anesthetic/Vasoconstrictor Precautions No information available to require special precautions

(Continued)

Allopurinol *(Continued)*

Effects on Dental Treatment >1%: Nausea (1.3%), vomiting (1.2%), renal failure/impairment (1.2%)

Dosage

Oral:

Children ≤10 years: 10 mg/kg/day in 2-3 divided doses **or** 200-300 mg/m²/day in 2-4 divided doses, maximum: 800 mg/24 hours

Alternative: <6 years: 150 mg/day in 3 divided doses; 6-10 years: 300 mg/day in 2-3 divided doses

Children >10 years and Adults: Daily doses >300 mg should be administered in divided doses

Myeloproliferative neoplastic disorders: 600-800 mg/day in 2-3 divided doses for prevention of acute uric acid nephropathy for 2-3 days starting 1-2 days before chemotherapy

Gout: Mild: 200-300 mg/day; Severe: 400-600 mg/day

Elderly: Initial: 100 mg/day, increase until desired uric acid level is obtained

I.V.: Hyperuricemia secondary to chemotherapy: Intravenous daily dose can be given as a single infusion or in equally divided doses at 6-, 8-, or 12-hour intervals. A fluid intake sufficient to yield a daily urinary output of at least 2 L in adults and the maintenance of a neutral or, preferably, slightly alkaline urine are desirable.

Children: Starting dose: 200 mg/m²/day

Adults: 200-400 mg/m²/day (max: 600 mg/day)

Dosing adjustment in renal impairment: Must be adjusted due to accumulation of allopurinol and metabolites:

Oral: Removed by hemodialysis; adult maintenance doses of allopurinol* (mg) based on creatinine clearance (mL/minute): See table.

Adult Maintenance Doses of Allopurinol*

Creatinine Clearance (mL/min)	Maintenance Dose of Allopurinol (mg)
140	400 qd
120	350 qd
100	300 qd
80	250 qd
60	200 qd
40	150 qd
20	100 qd
10	100 q2d
0	100 q3d

*This table is based on a standard maintenance dose of 300 mg of allopurinol per day for a patient with a creatinine clearance of 100 mL/min.

Hemodialysis: Administer dose posthemodialysis or administer 50% supplemental dose

I.V.:

Cl_{cr} 10-20 mL/minute: 200 mg/day

Cl_{cr} 3-10 mL/minute: 100 mg/day

Cl_{cr} <3 mL/minute: 100 mg/day at extended intervals

Mechanism of Action Allopurinol inhibits xanthine oxidase, the enzyme responsible for the conversion of hypoxanthine to xanthine to uric acid. Allopurinol is metabolized to oxypurinol which is also an inhibitor of xanthine oxidase; allopurinol acts on purine catabolism, reducing the production of uric acid without disrupting the biosynthesis of vital purines.

Other Adverse Effects The most common adverse reaction to allopurinol is a skin rash (usually maculopapular; however, more severe reactions, including Stevens-Johnson syndrome, have also been reported). While some studies cite an incidence of these reactions as high as >10% of cases (often in association with ampicillin or amoxicillin), the product labeling cites a much lower incidence, reflected below.

>1%:

Dermatologic: Rash (1.5%; discontinue at first appearance)

<1%: **Hypersensitivity syndrome**, increased alkaline phosphatase or hepatic transaminases, granulomatous hepatitis, dyspepsia, pancreatitis, gynecomastia, agranulocytosis, aplastic anemia, acute tubular necrosis, interstitial nephritis, nephrolithiasis, vasculitis, toxic epidermal necrolysis, exfoliative dermatitis, Stevens-Johnson syndrome, granuloma annulare, toxic pustuloderma, peripheral neuropathy, neuritis, **paresthesia, bronchospasm**, cataracts, macular retinitis, angioedema, **epistaxis**

Drug Interactions Hepatic enzyme inhibitor; isoenzyme profile not defined

Increased Effect/Toxicity: Allopurinol may increase the effects of azathioprine, chlorpropamide, mercaptopurine, theophylline, and oral anticoagulants. An increased risk of bone marrow suppression may occur when given with myelosuppressive agents (cyclophosphamide, possibly other alkylating agents). Amoxicillin/ampicillin, ACE inhibitors, and thiazide diuretics have been associated with hypersensitivity reactions when combined with allopurinol (rare), and the incidence of rash may be increased with penicillins (ampicillin, amoxicillin). Urinary acidification with large amounts of vitamin C may increase kidney stone formation.

Decreased Effect: Ethanol decreases effectiveness.

Dietary/Ethanol/Herb Considerations

Ethanol: Avoid use; may decrease effectiveness and uricosurics.

Food: Administer tablets after meals with plenty of fluid.

Pharmacodynamics/Kinetics

Onset of action: Peak effect: 1-2 weeks

Absorption: Oral: ~80%; Rectal: Poor and erratic

Distribution: V_d: ~1.6 L/kg; V_{ss}: 0.84-0.87 L/kg; enters breast milk

Protein binding: <1%

Metabolism: ~75% to active metabolites, chiefly oxypurinol

Bioavailability: 49% to 53%

Half-life elimination:

Normal renal function: Parent drug: 1-3 hours; Oxypurinol: 18-30 hours

End-stage renal disease: Prolonged

Time to peak, plasma: Oral: 30-120 minutes

Excretion: Urine (76% as oxypurinol, 12% as unchanged drug)

Allopurinol and oxypurinol are dialyzable

Pregnancy Risk Factor C

Generic Available Yes

Allopurinol Sodium Injection *see* Allopurinol *on page 57*

All-*trans*-Retinoic Acid *see* Tretinoin (Oral) *on page 1338*

Almora® [OTC] *see* Magnesium Supplements *on page 837*

Almora® [OTC], Mag G® [OTC] *see* Magnesium Gluconate *on page 834*

Almotriptan (al moh TRIP tan)

U.S. Brand Names Axert™

Pharmacologic Category Serotonin 5-HT_{1D} Receptor Agonist

Use Acute treatment of migraine with or without aura

Local Anesthetic/Vasoconstrictor Precautions No information available to require special precautions

Effects on Dental Treatment ≥1%: Headache, dizziness, somnolence, nausea (1% to 2%), xerostomia (1%), paresthesia (1%)

Dosage If the first dose is ineffective, diagnosis needs to be re-evaluated. Safety of treating more than 4 migraines/month has not been established.

Oral: Adults:

Migraine: Initial: 6.25-12.5 mg in a single dose; if the headache returns, repeat the dose after 2 hours; no more than 2 doses in 24-hour period

Dosing adjustment in renal impairment: Initial: 6.25 mg in a single dose; maximum daily dose: ≤12.5 mg

Dosing adjustment in hepatic impairment: Initial: 6.25 mg in a single dose; maximum daily dose: ≤12.5 mg

Mechanism of Action Selective agonist for serotonin (5-HT_{1B}, 5-HT_{1D}, 5-HT_{1F} receptors) in cranial arteries; causes vasoconstriction and reduce sterile inflammation associated with antidromic neuronal transmission correlating with relief of migraine

Other Adverse Effects <1%: Abdominal cramps/pain, **incoordination, anxiety**, arthralgia, **arthritis, back pain, bronchitis, chest pain**, chills, colitis, conjunctivitis, **coronary artery vasospasm**, creatine phosphokinase increased, depressive symptoms, dermatitis, **diaphoresis**, diarrhea, diplopia, dream changes, dry eyes, dysmenorrhea, dyspepsia, **dyspnea, ear pain, epistaxis**, erythema, **esophageal reflux, euphoria,** eye irritation, eye pain, **fatigue, fever, gastritis, gastroenteritis**, GGTP increased, hyperacusis, hypercholesterolemia, hypesthesia, **hyperglycemia**, hyper-reflexia, **hypertension**, hypertonia, **hyperventilation**, impaired concentration, insomnia, **laryngismus, laryngitis**, myalgia, myocardial ischemia, **MI**, myopathy, **neck pain, nervousness**, neuropathy, nightmares, nystagmus, **otitis media, palpitations**, smelling disorder, **pharyngitis**, photosensitivity reaction, pruritus, rash, **restlessness, rhinitis, rigid neck, increased salivation**, scotoma, **shakiness, sinusitis, sneezing, syncope, tachycardia, taste alterations, thirst**, tinnitus, **tremor, vasodilation, ventricular fibrillation, ventricular tachycardia**, vertigo, **vomiting, weakness**

Drug Interactions Substrate of CYP2D6, 3A4

Increased Effect/Toxicity: Ergot-containing drugs prolong vasospastic reactions; ketoconazole and CYP3A4 inhibitors increase almotriptan serum concentration; select serotonin reuptake inhibitors may increase symptoms of hyper-reflexia, weakness, and incoordination; MAO inhibitors may increase toxicity

Dietary/Ethanol/Herb Considerations Food: May be taken with food

(Continued)

Almotriptan *(Continued)*

Pharmacodynamics/Kinetics

Absorption: Well absorbed

Distribution: V_d: 180-200 L

Protein binding: ~35%

Metabolism: MAO type A oxidative deamination (~27% of dose); via CYP3A4 and 2D6 (~12% of dose) to inactive metabolites

Bioavailability: 70%

Half-life elimination: 3-4 hours

Time to peak: 1-3 hours

Excretion: Urine (40% as unchanged drug); feces (13% unchanged and metabolized)

Pregnancy Risk Factor C

Generic Available No

Alocril™ *see* Nedocromil *on page 957*

Aloe Vesta® 2-n-1 Antifungal [OTC] *see* Miconazole *on page 906*

Alomide® *see* Lodoxamide *on page 816*

Alophen® [OTC] *see* Bisacodyl *on page 186*

Aloprim™ *see* Allopurinol *on page 57*

Alora® *see* Estradiol *on page 521*

Alosetron (a LOE se tron)

U.S. Brand Names Lotronex®

Pharmacologic Category Selective 5-HT_3 Receptor Antagonist

Use Treatment of irritable bowel syndrome (IBS) in women with severe diarrhea-predominant IBS who have failed to respond to conventional therapy

Unlabeled/Investigational Use Investigational: Alosetron has demonstrated effectiveness as an antiemetic for a wide variety of causes of emesis.

Local Anesthetic/Vasoconstrictor Precautions No information available to require special precautions

Effects on Dental Treatment 1% to 7%: Nausea (7%), hypertension (2%), viral infections (2%), allergic rhinitis (2%), throat and tonsil discomfort and pain (1%), bacterial nose/throat/ear infection (1%), GI discomfort and pain (5%)

Restrictions Only physicians enrolled in GlaxoSmithKline's Prescribing Program for Lotronex® may prescribe this medication. Program stickers must be affixed to all prescriptions; no phone, fax or computerized prescriptions are permitted with this program.

Dosage Discontinue immediately if constipation or signs/symptoms of ischemic colitis occur. Do not reinitiate in patients who develop ischemic colitis.

Oral: Adults: Female: 1 mg once daily for 4 weeks, with or without food; if tolerated, but response is inadequate, may be increased after 4 weeks to 1 mg twice daily. If response is inadequate after 4 weeks of twice daily dosing, discontinue treatment.

Dosing adjustment in hepatic impairment: Specific guidelines unavailable; may increase risk of adverse events

Mechanism of Action Alosetron is a potent and selective antagonist of a subtype of the serotonin receptor, 5-HT_3 receptor. 5-HT_3 receptors are extensively distributed on enteric neurons in the human gastrointestinal tract, as well as other peripheral and central locations. Activation of these channels affect the regulation of visceral pain, colonic transit, and gastrointestinal secretions. In patients with irritable bowel syndrome, improvement in pain, abdominal discomfort, urgency, and diarrhea may occur.

Other Adverse Effects

>10%: Gastrointestinal: Constipation (28%)

1% to 10%:

Central nervous system: Sleep disorders (3%), depression (2%)

Gastrointestinal: Abdominal discomfort and pain (5%), dyspepsia (3%), abdominal distention (2%), hemorrhoids (2%)

<1%: Elevated hepatic transaminases (0.5%), acute ischemic colitis, **arrhythmias**, contusions, **hematomas**, photophobia, proctitis, abnormal bilirubin levels, **breathing disorders, cough, sedation**, abnormal dreams, **allergies, allergic reactions, anxiety**, menstrual disorders, sexual function disorders, acne, folliculitis, urinary infections, polyuria, diuresis, fecal impaction, perforation, toxic megacolon, **abnormal taste**; intestinal obstruction, perforation, or ulceration

Case report: Hepatitis

Drug Interactions Substrate of CYP1A2, **2C8/9**, 3A4; Inhibits CYP1A2, 2E1

Increased Effect/Toxicity: Drugs which decrease GI motility (opiates, anticholinergic agents, tricyclic antidepressants) may increase the risk of constipation and/or severe complications. Inhibitors of CYP2C9, CYP3A4, and CYP1A2 may increase serum levels and toxicity of alosetron (limited data).

Decreased Effect: Inducers of cytochrome P450 isoenzymes may increase the metabolism of alosetron, reducing its efficacy.

Dietary/Ethanol/Herb Considerations Food: May be taken with food

Pharmacodynamics/Kinetics
Distribution: V_d: 65-95 L
Protein binding: 82%
Metabolism: Extensive hepatic metabolism. Alosetron is metabolized by CYP2C9, 3A4, and 1A2. Thirteen metabolites have been detected in the urine. Biological activity of these metabolites in unknown.
Bioavailability: Mean: 50% to 60% (range: 30% to >90%)
Half-life elimination: 1.5 hours for alosetron
Time to peak: 1 hour after oral administration
Excretion: Urine (73%) and feces (24%); 7% as unchanged drug (1% feces, 6% urine)
Pregnancy Risk Factor B
Generic Available No

Alpha$_1$-PI *see* Alpha$_1$-Proteinase Inhibitor *on page 61*

Alpha$_1$-Proteinase Inhibitor (al fa won PRO tee in ase in HI bi tor)

U.S. Brand Names Prolastin®
Canadian Brand Names Prolastin®
Pharmacologic Category Antitrypsin Deficiency Agent
Synonyms Alpha$_1$-PI; Alpha$_1$-Proteinase Inhibitor, Human
Use Treatment of congenital alpha$_1$-antitrypsin deficiency
Local Anesthetic/Vasoconstrictor Precautions No information available to require special precautions
Effects on Dental Treatment No significant effects or complications reported
Dosage I.V.: Adults: 60 mg/kg once weekly (at a rate ≥0.08 mL/kg/minute)
Mechanism of Action Human alpha$_1$-proteinase inhibitor is prepared from the pooled human plasma of normal donors and is intended for use in the therapy of congenital alpha$_1$-antitrypsin deficiency. Alpha$_1$-antitrypsin (AAT) is the principal protease inhibitor in the serum and exists as a single polypeptide glycoprotein. Production of AAT occurs in the liver hepatocyte and secretion occurs at a rate to maintain serum concentrations of 150-200 mg/dL. The major physiologic role of the antiprotease is that of combining with proteolytic enzymes to render them inactive. Several proteases can be inactivated by AAT including trypsin, chymotrypsin, coagulation factor XI, plasmin, thrombin, and neutrophil elastase.
Other Adverse Effects <1%: **Dizziness, lightheadedness**, fever <102°F (delayed ≤12 hours), leukocytosis
Pharmacodynamics/Kinetics Half-life elimination, serum: Parent drug: 4.5-5.2 days
Pregnancy Risk Factor C
Generic Available No

Alpha$_1$-Proteinase Inhibitor, Human *see* Alpha$_1$-Proteinase Inhibitor *on page 61*
Alphagan® [DSC] *see* Brimonidine *on page 197*
Alphagan® P *see* Brimonidine *on page 197*
Alphanate® *see* Antihemophilic Factor (Human) *on page 113*
Alphaquin HP *see* Hydroquinone *on page 693*
Alphatrex® *see* Betamethasone *on page 177*

Alprazolam (al PRAY zoe lam)

Related Information
Patients Requiring Sedation *on page 1565*
Temporomandibular Dysfunction (TMD) *on page 1562*
U.S. Brand Names Alprazolam Intensol®; Xanax®; Xanax XR®
Canadian Brand Names Alti-Alprazolam; Apo®-Alpraz; Gen-Alprazolam; Novo-Alprazol; Nu-Alprax; Xanax®; Xanax TS™
Mexican Brand Names Tafil®
Pharmacologic Category Benzodiazepine
Use Treatment of anxiety disorder (GAD); panic disorder, with or without agoraphobia; anxiety associated with depression
Unlabeled/Investigational Use Treatment of anxiety in children
Local Anesthetic/Vasoconstrictor Precautions No information available to require special precautions
Effects on Dental Treatment
>10%: Significant xerostomia and changes in salivation (normal salivary flow resumes upon discontinuation), drowsiness, lightheadedness, memory impairment, irritability, sedation, fatigue
1% to 10%: Hypotension, confusion, dizziness, akathisia, rigidity, tremors, nasal congestion, derealization, increased salivation, muscle cramps, diaphoresis
Restrictions C-IV
Dosage Oral: Treatment >4 months should be re-evaluated to determine the patient's need for the drug
Children: Anxiety (unlabeled use): Immediate release: Initial: 0.005 mg/kg/dose or 0.125 mg/dose 3 times/day; increase in increments of 0.125-0.25 mg, up to a maximum of 0.02 mg/kg/dose or 0.06 mg/kg/day (0.375-3 mg/day)
(Continued)

Alprazolam *(Continued)*

Adults:

Anxiety: Immediate release: Effective doses are 0.5-4 mg/day in divided doses; the manufacturer recommends starting at 0.25-0.5 mg 3 times/day; titrate dose upward; maximum: 4 mg/day

Anxiety associated with depression: Immediate release: Average dose required: 2.5-3 mg/day in divided doses

Ethanol withdrawal (unlabeled use): Immediate release: Usual dose: 2-2.5 mg/day in divided doses

Panic disorder:

Immediate release: Initial: 0.5 mg 3 times/day; dose may be increased every 3-4 days in increments ≤1 mg/day; many patients obtain relief at 2 mg/day, as much as 10 mg/day may be required

Extended release: 0.5-1 mg once daily; may increase dose every 3-4 days in increments ≤1 mg/day (range: 3-6 mg/day)

Switching from immediate release to extended release: Patients may be switched to extended release tablets by taking the total daily dose of the immediate release tablets and giving it once daily using the extended release preparation.

Dose reduction: Abrupt discontinuation should be avoided. Daily dose may be decreased by 0.5 mg every 3 days, however, some patients may require a slower reduction. If withdrawal symptoms occur, resume previous dose and discontinue on a less rapid schedule.

Elderly: May be more likely to experience ataxia and oversedation; may also have impaired renal function leading to decreased clearance. The smallest effective dose should be used. Titrate gradually, if needed.

Immediate release: Initial 0.25 mg 2-3 times/day

Extended release: Initial: 0.5 mg once daily

Dosing adjustment in hepatic impairment: Reduce dose by 50% to 60% or avoid in cirrhosis

Mechanism of Action Binds to stereospecific benzodiazepine receptors on the postsynaptic GABA neuron at several sites within the central nervous system, including the limbic system, reticular formation. Enhancement of the inhibitory effect of GABA on neuronal excitability results by increased neuronal membrane permeability to chloride ions. This shift in chloride ions results in hyperpolarization (a less excitable state) and stabilization.

Other Adverse Effects

>10%:

Central nervous system: Ataxia dysarthria, depression

Endocrine & metabolic: Libido decreased, menstrual disorders

Gastrointestinal: Appetite increased/decreased, weight gain/loss

Genitourinary: Micturition difficulties

1% to 10%:

Central nervous system: Disinhibition, libido increased, nightmares

Dermatologic: Dermatitis, rash

Gastrointestinal: Dyspepsia

Genitourinary: Sexual dysfunction, incontinence

Neuromuscular & skeletal: Arthralgia

Otic: Tinnitus

Warnings/Precautions Rebound or withdrawal symptoms, including seizures may occur 18 hours to 3 days following abrupt discontinuation or large decreases in dose (more common in patients receiving >4 mg/day or prolonged treatment). Dose reductions or tapering must be approached with extreme caution. Breakthrough anxiety may occur at the end of dosing interval. Use with caution in patients receiving concurrent CYP3A4 inhibitors, particularly when these agents are added to therapy. Has weak uricosuric properties, use with caution in renal impairment or predisposition to urate nephropathy. Use with caution in elderly or debilitated patients, patients with hepatic disease (including alcoholics), renal impairment, or obese patients.

Causes CNS depression (dose-related) resulting in sedation, dizziness, confusion, or ataxia which may impair physical and mental capabilities. Patients must be cautioned about performing tasks which require mental alertness (ie, operating machinery or driving). Use with caution in patients receiving other CNS depressants or psychoactive agents. Effects with other sedative drugs or ethanol may be potentiated. Benzodiazepines have been associated with falls and traumatic injury and should be used with extreme caution in patients who are at risk of these events (especially the elderly). Use with caution in patients with respiratory disease or impaired gag reflex.

Use caution in patients with depression, particularly if suicidal risk may be present. Episodes of mania or hypomania have occurred in depressed patients treated with alprazolam. May cause physical or psychological dependence - use with caution in patients with a history of drug dependence. Acute withdrawal, including seizures, may be precipitated in patients after administration of flumazenil to patients receiving long-term benzodiazepine therapy.

Benzodiazepines have been associated with anterograde amnesia. Paradoxical reactions, including hyperactive or aggressive behavior, have been reported with benzodiazepines, particularly in adolescent/pediatric or psychiatric patients. Does not have analgesic, antidepressant, or antipsychotic properties.

Benzodiazepines have the potential to cause harm to the fetus, particularly when administered during the first trimester. In addition, withdrawal symptoms may occur in the neonate following *in utero* exposure. Use of alprazolam during pregnancy should be avoided. In addition, symptoms of withdrawal, lethargy, and loss of body weight have been reported in infants exposed to alprazolam and/or benzodiazepines while nursing; use during breast-feeding is not recommended.

Drug Interactions Substrate of **CYP3A4**

Increased Effect/Toxicity: Alprazolam potentiates the CNS depressant effects of narcotic analgesics, barbiturates, phenothiazines, ethanol, antihistamines, MAO inhibitors, sedative-hypnotics, and cyclic antidepressants. Serum levels and/or effects of alprazolam may be increased by inhibitors of CYP3A4, including amprenavir, cimetidine, ciprofloxacin, clarithromycin, clozapine, diltiazem, disulfiram, digoxin, erythromycin, ethanol, fluconazole, fluoxetine, fluvoxamine, isoniazid, itraconazole, ketoconazole, labetalol, levodopa, loxapine, metoprolol, metronidazole, miconazole, nefazodone, nelfinavir, omeprazole, rifabutin, troleandomycin, valproic acid, and verapamil.

Decreased Effect: Carbamazepine, rifampin, rifabutin, cigarette smoking, and phenobarbital may enhance the metabolism of alprazolam and decrease its therapeutic effect.

Dietary/Ethanol/Herb Considerations

Ethanol: Avoid use; may increase CNS depression.

Food: Administer with food to reduce GI upset. Grapefruit juice may increase serum concentrations.

Herb/Nutraceutical: Avoid gotu kola, kava, SAMe, and valerian; may increase CNS depression. Avoid St John's wort; may decrease serum concentration and increase CNS depression.

Pharmacodynamics/Kinetics

Distribution: V_d: 0.9-1.2 L/kg; enters breast milk

Protein binding: 80%

Metabolism: Hepatic via CYP3A4; forms 2 active metabolites (4-hydroxyalprazolam and α-hydroxyalprazolam)

Bioavailability: 90%

Half-life elimination:

- Adults: 11.2 hours (range: 6.3-26.9)
- Elderly: 16.3 hours (range: 9-26.9 hours)
- Alcoholic liver disease: 19.7 hours (range: 5.8-65.3 hours)
- Obesity: 21.8 hours (range: 9.9-40.4 hours)

Time to peak, serum: 1-2 hours

Excretion: Urine (as unchanged drug and metabolites)

Pregnancy Risk Factor D

Generic Available Yes: Immediate release tablet

Alprazolam Intensol® *see* Alprazolam *on page 61*

Alprostadil (al PROS ta dill)

U.S. Brand Names Caverject®; Edex®; Muse® Pellet; Prostin VR Pediatric®

Canadian Brand Names Caverject®; Muse® Pellet; Prostin® VR

Mexican Brand Names Caverject®; Muse®

Pharmacologic Category Prostaglandin

Synonyms PGE_1; Prostaglandin E_1

Use

Prostin VR Pediatric®: Temporary maintenance of patency of ductus arteriosus in neonates with ductal-dependent congenital heart disease until surgery can be performed. These defects include cyanotic (eg, pulmonary atresia, pulmonary stenosis, tricuspid atresia, Fallot's tetralogy, transposition of the great vessels) and acyanotic (eg, interruption of aortic arch, coarctation of aorta, hypoplastic left ventricle) heart disease;

Caverject®, Edex®, Muse® Pellet: Treatment of erectile dysfunction of vasculogenic, psychogenic, or neurogenic etiology; adjunct in the diagnosis of erectile dysfunction

Unlabeled/Investigational Use Investigational: Treatment of pulmonary hypertension in infants and children with congenital heart defects with left-to-right shunts

Local Anesthetic/Vasoconstrictor Precautions No information available to require special precautions

Effects on Dental Treatment

>10%: I.V.: Flushing, fever, apnea

1% to 10%: Headache, dizziness, pain, bradycardia, hypotension, hypertension, tachycardia, cardiac arrest, seizures, upper respiratory infection, flu syndrome, sinusitis, nasal congestion, cough leg pain, sepsis

(Continued)

Alprostadil *(Continued)*

Dosage

Patent ductus arteriosus (Prostin VR Pediatric®):

I.V. continuous infusion into a large vein, or alternatively through an umbilical artery catheter placed at the ductal opening: 0.05-0.1 mcg/kg/minute with therapeutic response, rate is reduced to lowest effective dosage; with unsatisfactory response, rate is increased gradually; maintenance: 0.01-0.4 mcg/kg/minute

PGE_1 is usually given at an infusion rate of 0.1 mcg/kg/minute, but it is often possible to reduce the dosage to 1/2 or even 1/10 without losing the therapeutic effect. The mixing schedule is as follows. Infusion rates deliver 0.1 mcg/kg/minute: See table.

Alprostadil

Add 1 Ampul (500 mcg) to:	Concentration (mcg/mL)	Infusion Rate: mL/min/kg Needed to Infuse 0.1 mcg/kg/min	Infusion Rate: mL/kg/24 h
250 mL	2	0.05	72
100 mL	5	0.02	28.8
50 mL	10	0.01	14.4
25 mL	20	0.005	7.2

Therapeutic response is indicated by increased pH in those with acidosis or by an increase in oxygenation (PO_2) usually evident within 30 minutes

Erectile dysfunction:

Caverject®, Edex®: Individualize dose by careful titration; doses >40 mcg (Edex®) or >60 mcg (Caverject®) are not recommended:

Vasculogenic, psychogenic, or mixed etiology: Initiate dosage titration at 2.5 mcg, increasing by 2.5 mcg to a dose of 5 mcg and then in increments of 5-10 mcg depending on the erectile response until the dose produces an erection suitable for intercourse, not lasting >1 hour; if there is absolutely no response to initial 2.5 mcg dose, the second dose may be increased to 7.5 mcg, followed by increments of 5-10 mcg

Neurogenic etiology (eg, spinal cord injury): Initiate dosage titration at 1.25 mcg, increasing to a dose of 2.5 mcg and then 5 mcg; increase further in increments 5 mcg until the dose is reached that produces an erection suitable for intercourse, not lasting >1 hour

Note: Patient must stay in the physician's office until complete detumescence occurs; if there is no response, then the next higher dose may be given within 1 hour; if there is still no response, a 1-day interval before giving the next dose is recommended; increasing the dose or concentration in the treatment of impotence results in increasing pain and discomfort

Muse® Pellet: Intraurethral: Administer as needed to achieve an erection; duration of action is about 30-60 minutes; use only two systems per 24-hour period

Elderly: Greater frequency of renal dysfunction; use lowest effective dose (in clinical studies with Edex®, higher minimally effective doses and a higher rate of lack of effect were noted)

Mechanism of Action Causes vasodilation by means of direct effect on vascular and ductus arteriosus smooth muscle; relaxes trabecular smooth muscle by dilation of cavernosal arteries when injected along the penile shaft, allowing blood flow to and entrapment in the lacunar spaces of the penis (ie, corporeal veno-occlusive mechanism)

Other Adverse Effects

Intraurethral:

>10%: Genitourinary: Penile pain, urethral burning

2% to 10%:

Genitourinary: Vaginal itching (female partner), testicular pain, urethral bleeding (minor)

<2%: Perineal pain

Intracavernosal:

>10%: Genitourinary: Penile pain

1% to 10%:

Genitourinary: Prolonged erection (>4 hours, 4%), penile fibrosis, penis disorder, penile rash, penile edema

Local: Injection site hematoma and/or bruising

<1%: Balanitis, injection site hemorrhage, priapism (0.4%)

Intravenous:

1% to 10%:

Cardiovascular: Edema

Endocrine & metabolic: Hypokalemia

Gastrointestinal: Diarrhea

Hematologic: Disseminated intravascular coagulation

Neuromuscular & skeletal: Back pain

Miscellaneous: Localized pain in structures other than the injection site

<1%: Anemia, anuria, **bleeding, bradypnea, bronchial wheezing**, cerebral bleeding, **CHF, gastric regurgitation**, hematuria, hyperbilirubinemia, hyperemia, **hyperextension of neck, hyperirritability**, hyperkalemia, **hypoglycemia**, hypothermia, **jitteriness, lethargy,** peritonitis, **second degree heart block, shock, stiffness, supraventricular tachycardia**, thrombocytopenia, **ventricular fibrillation**

Drug Interactions Increased Effect/Toxicity: Risk of hypotension and syncope may be increased with antihypertensives.

Dietary/Ethanol/Herb Considerations Ethanol: Avoid use due to vasodilating effect.

Pharmacodynamics/Kinetics

Onset of action: Rapid

Duration: <1 hour

Distribution: Insignificant following penile injection

Protein binding, plasma: 81% to albumin

Metabolism: ~75% by oxidation in one pass via lungs

Half-life elimination: 5-10 minutes

Excretion: Urine (90% as metabolites) within 24 hours

Pregnancy Risk Factor X

Generic Available Yes: Injection 5 mcg/mL

Alrex® *see* Loteprednol *on page 827*

Altace® *see* Ramipril *on page 1166*

Altamist [OTC] *see* Sodium Chloride *on page 1229*

Alteplase (AL te plase)

U.S. Brand Names Activase®; Cathflo™ Activase®

Canadian Brand Names Activase® rt-PA; Cathflo™ Activase®

Mexican Brand Names Actilyse®

Pharmacologic Category Thrombolytic Agent

Synonyms Alteplase, Recombinant; Alteplase, Tissue Plasminogen Activator, Recombinant; tPA

Use Management of acute MI for the lysis of thrombi in coronary arteries; management of acute massive pulmonary embolism (PE) in adults

Acute MI (AMI): Chest pain ≥20 minutes, ≤12-24 hours; S-T elevation ≥0.1 mV in at least two EKG leads

Acute pulmonary embolism (APE): Age ≤75 years: As soon as possible within 5 days of thrombotic event. Documented massive pulmonary embolism by pulmonary angiography or echocardiography or high probability lung scan with clinical shock.

Cathflo™ Activase®: Restoration of central venous catheter function

Unlabeled/Investigational Use Treatment of peripheral arterial thrombotic obstruction

Local Anesthetic/Vasoconstrictor Precautions No information available to require special precautions

Effects on Dental Treatment As with all drugs which may affect hemostasis, bleeding is the major adverse effect associated with alteplase. Hemorrhage may occur at virtually any site; risk is dependent on multiple variables, including the dosage administered, concurrent use of multiple agents which alter hemostasis, and patient predisposition. Rapid lysis of coronary artery thrombi by thrombolytic agents may be associated with reperfusion-related atrial and/or ventricular arrhythmias.

1% to 10%: Hypotension, fever, bruising, GI hemorrhage (5%), nausea, vomiting, bleeding (0.5% major, 7% minor: GUSTO trial)

Dosage

I.V.:

Coronary artery thrombi: Front loading dose (weight-based):

Patients >67 kg: Total dose: 100 mg over 1.5 hours; infuse 15 mg (30 mL) over 1-2 minutes. Infuse 50 mg (100 mL) over 30 minutes. See "Note."

Patients ≤67 kg: Total dose: 1.25 mg/kg; infuse 15 mg I.V. bolus over 1-2 minutes, then infuse 0.75 mg/kg (not to exceed 50 mg) over next 30 minutes, followed by 0.5 mg/kg over next 60 minutes (not to exceed 35 mg). See "Note."

Note: Concurrently, begin heparin 60 units/kg bolus (maximum: 4000 units) followed by continuous infusion of 12 units/kg/hour (maximum: 1000 units/hour) and adjust to aPTT target of 1.5-2 times the upper limit of control. Infuse remaining 35 mg (70 mL) of alteplase over the next hour.

Acute pulmonary embolism: 100 mg over 2 hours.

Acute ischemic stroke: Doses should be given within the first 3 hours of the onset of symptoms; recommended total dose: 0.9 mg/kg (maximum dose should not exceed 90 mg) infused over 60 minutes.

Load with 0.09 mg/kg (10% of the 0.9 mg/kg dose) as an I.V. bolus over 1 minute, followed by 0.81 mg/kg (90% of the 0.9 mg/kg dose) as a continuous

(Continued)

Alteplase *(Continued)*

infusion over 60 minutes. Heparin should not be started for 24 hours or more after starting alteplase for stroke.

Intracatheter: Central venous catheter clearance: Cathflo™ Activase®:

Patients ≥10 to <30 kg: 110% of the internal lumen volume of the catheter (≤2 mg [1 mg/mL]); retain in catheter for ≤2 hours; may instill a second dose if catheter remains occluded

Patients ≥30 kg: 2 mg (1 mg/mL); retain in catheter for ≤2 hours; may instill a second dose if catheter remains occluded

Intra-arterial: Peripheral arterial thrombotic obstruction (unlabeled use): 0.02-0.1 mg/kg/hour for 1-8 hours

Mechanism of Action Initiates local fibrinolysis by binding to fibrin in a thrombus (clot) and converts entrapped plasminogen to plasmin

Other Adverse Effects

1% to 10%:

Genitourinary: GU hemorrhage (4%)

Local: Bleeding at catheter puncture site (15.3%, accelerated administration)

<1% (Limited to important or life-threatening): Intracranial hemorrhage (0.4% to 0.87% when dose is ≤100 mg), retroperitoneal hemorrhage, pericardial hemorrhage, **gingival hemorrhage, epistaxis, allergic reactions: anaphylaxis, anaphylactoid reactions, laryngeal edema**, rash, and urticaria (<0.02%)

Associated with use in MI: AV block, cardiogenic shock, heart failure, cardiac arrest, recurrent ischemia/infarction, myocardial rupture, electromechanical dissociation, pericardial effusion, pericarditis, mitral regurgitation, cardiac tamponade, thromboembolism, pulmonary edema, asystole, ventricular tachycardia, bradycardia, ruptured intracranial AV malformation, seizure, hemorrhagic bursitis, cholesterol crystal embolization

Associated with use in pulmonary embolism: Pulmonary re-embolization, pulmonary edema, pleural effusion, thromboembolism

Associated with use in stroke: Cerebral edema, cerebral herniation, seizure, new ischemic stroke

Drug Interactions

Increased Effect/Toxicity: The potential for hemorrhage with alteplase is increased by oral anticoagulants (warfarin), heparin, low molecular weight heparins, and drugs which affect platelet function (eg, NSAIDs, dipyridamole, ticlopidine, clopidogrel, IIb/IIIa antagonists). Concurrent use with aspirin and heparin may increase the risk of bleeding. However, aspirin and heparin were used concomitantly with alteplase in the majority of patients in clinical studies.

Decreased Effect: Aminocaproic acid (an antifibrinolytic agent) may decrease the effectiveness of thrombolytic therapy. Nitroglycerin may increase the hepatic clearance of alteplase, potentially reducing lytic activity (limited clinical information).

Dietary/Ethanol/Herb Considerations Herb/Nutraceutical: Avoid cat's claw, dong quai, evening primrose, feverfew, red clover, horse chestnut, garlic, green tea, ginseng, and ginkgo due to additional antiplatelet activity.

Pharmacodynamics/Kinetics

Duration: >50% present in plasma cleared ~5 minutes after infusion terminated, ~80% cleared within 10 minutes

Excretion: Clearance: Rapidly from circulating plasma (550-650 mL/minute), primarily hepatic; >50% present in plasma is cleared within 5 minutes after the infusion is terminated, ~80% cleared within 10 minutes

Pregnancy Risk Factor C

Generic Available No

Alteplase, Recombinant *see* Alteplase *on page 65*

Alteplase, Tissue Plasminogen Activator, Recombinant *see* Alteplase *on page 65*

ALternaGel® [OTC] *see* Aluminum Hydroxide *on page 68*

Altinac™ *see* Tretinoin (Topical) *on page 1340*

Altocor™ *see* Lovastatin *on page 828*

Altretamine (al TRET a meen)

U.S. Brand Names Hexalen®

Canadian Brand Names Hexalen®

Pharmacologic Category Antineoplastic Agent, Miscellaneous

Synonyms Hexamethylmelamine; HEXM; HMM; HXM; NSC-13875

Use Palliative treatment of persistent or recurrent ovarian cancer

Local Anesthetic/Vasoconstrictor Precautions No information available to require special precautions

Effects on Dental Treatment

>10%: Nausea/vomiting (50% to 70%)

1% to 10%: Seizures

Dosage Refer to individual protocols. Oral:

Adults: 4-12 mg/kg/day in 3-4 divided doses for 21-90 days

Alternatively: 240-320 mg/m²/day in 3-4 divided doses for 21 days, repeated every 6 weeks

Alternatively: 260 mg/m²/day for 14-21 days of a 28-day cycle in 4 divided doses

Alternatively: 150 mg/m²/day in 3-4 divided doses for 14 days of a 28-day cycle

Mechanism of Action Although altretamine clinical antitumor spectrum resembles that of alkylating agents, the drug has demonstrated activity in alkylator-resistant patients. The drug selectively inhibits the incorporation of radioactive thymidine and uridine into DNA and RNA, inhibiting DNA and RNA synthesis; reactive intermediates covalently bind to microsomal proteins and DNA; can spontaneously degrade to demethylated melamines and formaldehyde which are also cytotoxic.

Other Adverse Effects

>10%:

Central nervous system: Peripheral sensory neuropathy, neurotoxicity (21%; may be dose-limiting and progressive)

Gastrointestinal: Anorexia (48%), diarrhea (48%)

Hematologic: Anemia, thrombocytopenia (31%), leukopenia (62%), neutropenia

1% to 10%:

Gastrointestinal: Stomach cramps

Hepatic: Increased alkaline phosphatase

<1%: **Dizziness**, depression, rash, alopecia, hepatotoxicity, **tremor**

Drug Interactions

Increased Effect/Toxicity: Altretamine may cause severe orthostatic hypotension when administered with MAO inhibitors. Cimetidine may decrease metabolism of altretamine.

Decreased Effect: Phenobarbital may increase metabolism of altretamine which may decrease the effect.

Dietary/Ethanol/Herb Considerations

Ethanol: Avoid use due to GI irritation.

Food: Administer after meals at bedtime.

Pharmacodynamics/Kinetics

Absorption: Well absorbed (75% to 89%)

Distribution: Highly concentrated hepatically and renally; low in other organs

Metabolism: Hepatic; rapid and extensive demethylation; active metabolites

Half-life elimination: 13 hours

Time to peak, plasma: 0.5-3 hours

Excretion: Urine (<1% as unchanged drug)

Pregnancy Risk Factor D

Generic Available No

Alu-Cap® [OTC] *see* Aluminum Hydroxide *on page 68*

Aluminum Acetate and Acetic Acid

(a LOO mi num AS e tate & a SEE tik AS id)

U.S. Brand Names Otic Domeboro®

Pharmacologic Category Antibiotic, Otic

Synonyms Acetic Acid and Aluminum Acetate Otic; Burow's Otic

Use Treatment of superficial infections of the external auditory canal

Local Anesthetic/Vasoconstrictor Precautions No information available to require special precautions

Effects on Dental Treatment No significant effects or complications reported

Dosage Instill 4-6 drops in ear(s) every 2-3 hours; insert saturated wick, keep moist for 24 hours

Other Adverse Effects 1% to 10%: Dermatologic: Irritation

Generic Available Yes

Aluminum Chloride (a LOO mi num KLOR ide)

U.S. Brand Names Gingi-Aid® Gingival Retraction Cord; Gingi-Aid® Solution; Hemodent® Gingival Retraction Cord

Pharmacologic Category Astringent

Use

Dental: Gingival retraction; to control bleeding created during a dental procedure

Medical: Hemostatic agent

Local Anesthetic/Vasoconstrictor Precautions No information available to require special precautions

Effects on Dental Treatment No significant effects or complications reported

Mechanism of Action Precipitates tissue and blood proteins causing a mechanical obstruction to hemorrhage from injured blood vessels

Contraindications No data reported

Warnings/Precautions Since large amounts of astringents may cause tissue irritation and possible damage, only small amounts should be applied

Dosage Forms RETRACTION CORD: [impregnated with aqueous solution]: 1 mg/inch (72 inches); 2 mg/inch (72 inches); [impregnated with aqueous 10% solution and dried]: 0.9 mg/inch (84 inches); 1.8 mg/inch (84 inches). **SOLN, aqueous:** 10 g/100 mL water (15 mL, 30 mL)

Generic Available Yes

Aluminum Hydroxide (a LOO mi num hye DROKS ide)

U.S. Brand Names ALternaGel® [OTC]; Alu-Cap® [OTC]; Alu-Tab® [OTC]; Amphojel® [OTC]; Dialume® [OTC]

Canadian Brand Names Amphojel®; Basaljel®

Pharmacologic Category Antacid; Antidote

Use Treatment of hyperacidity; hyperphosphatemia

Local Anesthetic/Vasoconstrictor Precautions No information available to require special precautions

Effects on Dental Treatment Aluminum and magnesium ions prevent GI absorption of tetracycline by forming a large ionized chelated molecule with the aluminum ion and tetracyclines in the stomach. Aluminum hydroxide prevents GI absorption of ketoconazole and itraconazole by increasing the pH in the GI tract. Any of these drugs should be administered at least 1 hour before $Al(OH)_3$.

>10%: Chalky taste

1% to 10%: Nausea, vomiting

Dosage Oral:

Peptic ulcer disease (dosages empirical):

Children: 5-15 mL/dose every 3-6 hours or 1 and 3 hours after meals and at bedtime

Adults: 15-45 mL every 3-6 hours or 1 and 3 hours after meals and at bedtime

Prophylaxis against GI bleeding:

Infants: 2-5 mL/dose every 1-2 hours

Children: 5-15 mL/dose every 1-2 hours

Adults: 30-60 mL/dose every hour

Titrate to maintain the gastric pH >5

Hyperphosphatemia:

Children: 50-150 mg/kg/24 hours in divided doses every 4-6 hours, titrate dosage to maintain serum phosphorus within normal range

Adults: 500-1800 mg, 3-6 times/day, between meals and at bedtime; best taken with a meal or within 20 minutes of a meal

Antacid: Adults: 30 mL 1 and 3 hours postprandial and at bedtime

Amphojel®: 10 mL suspension or two 300 mg tablets 5-6 times/day between meals and at bedtime

Mechanism of Action Neutralizes hydrochloride in stomach to form $Al (Cl)_3$ salt + H_2O

Other Adverse Effects

>10%: Gastrointestinal: Constipation, stomach cramps, fecal impaction

1% to 10%: Gastrointestinal: Discoloration of feces (white speckles)

<1%: Hypophosphatemia, hypomagnesemia

Drug Interactions Decreased Effect: Aluminum hydroxide decreases the effect of tetracyclines, digoxin, indomethacin, iron salts, isoniazid, allopurinol, benzodiazepines, corticosteroids, penicillamine, phenothiazines, ranitidine, ketoconazole, and itraconazole.

Dietary/Ethanol/Herb Considerations Food: Should be taken 1-3 hours after meals when used as an antacid. When used to decrease phosphorus, should be taken within 20 minutes of a meal.

Pregnancy Risk Factor C

Generic Available Yes

Aluminum Hydroxide and Magnesium Carbonate

(a LOO mi num hye DROKS ide & mag NEE zee um KAR bun nate)

Related Information

Aluminum Hydroxide *on page 68*

U.S. Brand Names Gaviscon® Extra Strength [OTC]; Gaviscon® Liquid [OTC]

Pharmacologic Category Antacid

Synonyms Magnesium Carbonate and Aluminum Hydroxide

Use Temporary relief of symptoms associated with gastric acidity

Local Anesthetic/Vasoconstrictor Precautions No information available to require special precautions

Effects on Dental Treatment Aluminum and magnesium ions prevent GI absorption of tetracycline by forming a large ionized chelated molecule with the tetracyclines in the stomach. Aluminum hydroxide prevents GI absorption of ketoconazole and itraconazole by increasing the pH in the GI tract. Any of these drugs should be administered at least 1 hour before aluminum hydroxide.

Dosage Oral: Adults:

Liquid:

Gaviscon® Regular Strength: 15-30 mL 4 times/day after meals and at bedtime

Gaviscon® Extra Strength Relief: 15-30 mL 4 times/day after meals

Tablet (Gaviscon® Extra Strength Relief): Chew 2-4 tablets 4 times/day

Other Adverse Effects 1% to 10%:

Endocrine & metabolic: Hypermagnesemia, aluminum intoxication (prolonged use and concomitant renal failure), hypophosphatemia

Gastrointestinal: Constipation, diarrhea

Neuromuscular & skeletal: Osteomalacia

Drug Interactions Decreased Effect: Tetracyclines, digoxin, indomethacin, or iron salts, isoniazid, allopurinol, benzodiazepines, corticosteroids, penicillamine, phenothiazines, ranitidine, ketoconazole, itraconazole

Dietary/Ethanol/Herb Considerations Food: Should be taken 1-3 hours after meals with water, milk or juice. Products contain sodium (0.57 mEq/5 mL regular strength liquid, 0.9 mEq/5 mL extra strength liquid, 1.3 mEq extra strength tablet).

Generic Available Yes

Aluminum Hydroxide and Magnesium Hydroxide

(a LOO mi num hye DROKS ide & mag NEE zee um hye DROK side)

Related Information

Aluminum Hydroxide *on page 68*

U.S. Brand Names Maalox® [OTC]; Maalox® TC (Therapeutic Concentrate) [OTC]

Canadian Brand Names Diovol®; Diovol® Ex; Gelusil®; Gelusil® Extra Strength; Mylanta™; Univol®

Pharmacologic Category Antacid

Synonyms Magnesium Hydroxide and Aluminum Hydroxide

Use Antacid, hyperphosphatemia in renal failure

Local Anesthetic/Vasoconstrictor Precautions No information available to require special precautions

Effects on Dental Treatment Aluminum and magnesium ions prevent GI absorption of tetracycline by forming a large ionized chelated molecule with the tetracyclines in the stomach. Aluminum hydroxide prevents GI absorption of ketoconazole and itraconazole by increasing the pH in the GI tract. Any of these drugs should be administered at least 1 hour before aluminum hydroxide.

>10%: Chalky taste
1% to 10%: Nausea, vomiting

Dosage Oral: 5-10 mL 4-6 times/day, between meals and at bedtime; may be used every hour for severe symptoms
Maalox®: 10-20 mL 4 times/day

Other Adverse Effects
>10%: Gastrointestinal: Constipation, stomach cramps, fecal impaction
1% to 10%: Gastrointestinal: Discoloration of feces (white speckles)
<1%: Hypophosphatemia, hypomagnesemia

Drug Interactions Decreased Effect: Tetracyclines, digoxin, indomethacin, or iron salts, isoniazid, allopurinol, benzodiazepines, corticosteroids, penicillamine, phenothiazines, ranitidine, ketoconazole, itraconazole

Dietary/Ethanol/Herb Considerations Food: Should be taken 1-3 hours after meals.

Pregnancy Risk Factor C

Generic Available Yes

Aluminum Hydroxide and Magnesium Trisilicate

(a LOO mi num hye DROKS ide & mag NEE zee um trye SIL i kate)

Related Information

Aluminum Hydroxide *on page 68*

U.S. Brand Names Gaviscon® Tablet [OTC]

Pharmacologic Category Antacid

Synonyms Magnesium Trisilicate and Aluminum Hydroxide

Use Temporary relief of hyperacidity

Local Anesthetic/Vasoconstrictor Precautions No information available to require special precautions

Effects on Dental Treatment Aluminum and magnesium ions prevent GI absorption of tetracycline by forming a large ionized chelated molecule with the tetracyclines in the stomach. Aluminum hydroxide prevents GI absorption of ketoconazole and itraconazole by increasing the pH in the GI tract. Any of these drugs should be administered at least 1 hour before aluminum hydroxide.

Dosage Oral: Adults: Chew 2-4 tablets 4 times/day or as directed by healthcare provider

Drug Interactions Decreased Effect: Tetracyclines, digoxin, indomethacin, or iron salts, isoniazid, allopurinol, benzodiazepines, corticosteroids, penicillamine, phenothiazines, ranitidine, ketoconazole, itraconazole

Dietary/Ethanol/Herb Considerations Food: Should be taken 1-3 hours after meals.

Pregnancy Risk Factor C

Generic Available Yes

Aluminum Hydroxide, Magnesium Hydroxide, and Simethicone

(a LOO mi num hye DROKS ide, mag NEE zee um hye DROKS ide, & sye METH i kone)

Related Information

Aluminum Hydroxide *on page 68*

(Continued)

Aluminum Hydroxide, Magnesium Hydroxide, and Simethicone *(Continued)*

U.S. Brand Names Maalox® Fast Release Liquid [OTC]; Maalox® Max [OTC]; Mylanta® Extra Strength Liquid [OTC]; Mylanta® Liquid [OTC]

Canadian Brand Names Diovol Plus®; Mylanta™ Double Strength; Mylanta™ Extra Strength; Mylanta™ regular Strength

Pharmacologic Category Antacid; Antiflatulent

Synonyms Magnesium Hydroxide, Aluminum Hydroxide, and Simethicone; Simethicone, Aluminum Hydroxide, and Magnesium Hydroxide

Use Temporary relief of hyperacidity associated with gas; may also be used for indications associated with other antacids

Local Anesthetic/Vasoconstrictor Precautions No information available to require special precautions

Effects on Dental Treatment Aluminum and magnesium ions prevent GI absorption of tetracycline by forming a large ionized chelated molecule with the tetracyclines in the stomach. Aluminum hydroxide prevents GI absorption of ketoconazole and itraconazole by increasing the pH in the GI tract. Any of these drugs should be administered at least 1 hour before aluminum hydroxide.

>10%: Chalky taste

1% to 10%: Nausea, vomiting

Dosage Oral: Adults: 10-20 mL or 2-4 tablets 4-6 times/day between meals and at bedtime; may be used every hour for severe symptoms

Other Adverse Effects

>10%: Gastrointestinal: Stomach cramps, constipation, decreased bowel motility, fecal impaction, hemorrhoids

1% to 10%: Gastrointestinal: Discoloration of feces (white speckles)

<1%: Hypophosphatemia, hypomagnesemia, dehydration or fluid restriction

Drug Interactions Decreased Effect: Tetracyclines, digoxin, indomethacin, or iron salts, isoniazid, allopurinol, benzodiazepines, corticosteroids, penicillamine, phenothiazines, ranitidine, ketoconazole, itraconazole

Pregnancy Risk Factor C

Generic Available Yes

Aluminum Sucrose Sulfate, Basic *see* Sucralfate *on page 1247*

Aluminum Sulfate and Calcium Acetate

(a LOO mi num SUL fate & KAL see um AS e tate)

U.S. Brand Names Bluboro® [OTC]; Domeboro® [OTC]; Pedi-Boro® [OTC]

Pharmacologic Category Topical Skin Product

Synonyms Calcium Acetate and Aluminum Sulfate

Use Astringent wet dressing for relief of inflammatory conditions of the skin and to reduce weeping that may occur in dermatitis

Local Anesthetic/Vasoconstrictor Precautions No information available to require special precautions

Effects on Dental Treatment No significant effects or complications reported

Dosage

Topical: Soak affected area in the solution 2-4 times/day for 15-30 minutes or apply wet dressing soaked in the solution 2-4 times/day for 30-minute treatment periods; rewet dressing with solution every few minutes to keep it moist

Domeboro®:

Wet dressing or compress: Saturate dressing and apply to affected area; saturate cloth every 15-30 minutes; repeat as needed

As a soak: Soak for 15-30 minutes 3 times/day

Generic Available Yes

Alupent® *see* Metaproterenol *on page 873*

Alustra™ *see* Hydroquinone *on page 693*

Alu-Tab® [OTC] *see* Aluminum Hydroxide *on page 68*

Amantadine (a MAN ta deen)

Related Information

Respiratory Diseases *on page 1476*

Systemic Viral Diseases *on page 1517*

U.S. Brand Names Symmetrel®

Canadian Brand Names Endantadine®; PMS-Amantadine; Symmetrel®

Pharmacologic Category Anti-Parkinson's Agent, Dopamine Agonist; Antiviral Agent

Synonyms Adamantanamine Hydrochloride; Amantadine Hydrochloride

Use Prophylaxis and treatment of influenza A viral infection; treatment of parkinsonism; treatment of drug-induced extrapyramidal symptoms

Unlabeled/Investigational Use Treatment of Creutzfeldt-Jakob disease

Local Anesthetic/Vasoconstrictor Precautions No information available to require special precautions

Effects on Dental Treatment

>10%: Xerostomia; prolonged use may cause significant xerostomia

1% to 10%: Orthostatic hypotension, anxiety, irritability, headache, somnolence, nervousness, dizziness, hallucinations, confusion, agitation, nausea, nasal dryness, CNS depression

Dosage Oral:

Children: Influenza A treatment:

1-9 years (<45 kg): 5-9 mg/kg/day in 1-2 divided doses to a maximum of 150 mg/day

10-12 years: 100-200 mg/day in 1-2 divided doses

Influenza prophylaxis: Administer for 10-21 days following exposure if the vaccine is concurrently given or for 90 days following exposure if the vaccine is unavailable or contraindicated and re-exposure is possible

Adults:

Drug-induced extrapyramidal symptoms: 100 mg twice daily; may increase to 300-400 mg/day, if needed

Parkinson's disease or Creutzfeldt-Jakob disease (unlabeled use): 100 mg twice daily as sole therapy; may increase to 400 mg/day if needed with close monitoring; initial dose: 100 mg/day if with other serious illness or with high doses of other anti-Parkinson drugs

Influenza A viral infection: 200 mg/day in 1-2 divided doses; initiate within 24-48 hours after onset of symptoms; discontinue as soon as possible based on clinical response (generally within 3-5 days or within 24-48 hours after symptoms disappear)

Influenza prophylaxis: 200 mg/day in 1-2 doses; minimum 10-day course of therapy following exposure if the vaccine is concurrently given or for 90 days following exposure if the vaccine is unavailable or contraindicated and re-exposure is possible

Elderly patients should take the drug in 2 daily doses rather than a single dose to avoid adverse neurologic reactions

Dosing interval in renal impairment:

Cl_{cr} 50-60 mL/minute: Administer 200 mg alternating with 100 mg/day

Cl_{cr} 30-50 mL/minute: Administer 100 mg/day

Cl_{cr} 20-30 mL/minute: Administer 200 mg twice weekly

Cl_{cr} 10-20 mL/minute: Administer 100 mg 3 times/week

Cl_{cr} <10 mL/minute: Administer 200 mg alternating with 100 mg every 7 days

Hemodialysis: Slightly hemodialyzable (5% to 20%); no supplemental dose is needed

Peritoneal dialysis: No supplemental dose is needed

Continuous arterio-venous or venous-venous hemofiltration: No supplemental dose is needed

Mechanism of Action As an antiviral, blocks the uncoating of influenza A virus preventing penetration of virus into host; antiparkinsonian activity may be due to its blocking the reuptake of dopamine into presynaptic neurons or by increasing dopamine release from presynaptic fibers

Other Adverse Effects

1% to 10%:

Cardiovascular: Peripheral edema

Central nervous system: Insomnia, ataxia, dream abnormality, fatigue

Dermatologic: Livedo reticularis

Gastrointestinal: Anorexia, constipation, diarrhea

<1%: Amnesia, **CHF**, decreased libido, **dyspnea**, eczematoid dermatitis, **euphoria**, hyperkinesis, **hypertension, convulsions**, leukopenia, neutropenia, oculogyric episodes, **psychosis**, rash, **slurred speech,** urinary retention, **visual disturbances, vomiting, weakness**

Drug Interactions Increased Effect/Toxicity: Anticholinergics (benztropine and trihexyphenidyl) may potentiate CNS side effects of amantadine. Hydrochlorothiazide, triamterene, and/or trimethoprim may increase toxicity of amantadine; monitor for altered response.

Dietary/Ethanol/Herb Considerations Ethanol: Avoid use; may increase CNS adverse effects.

Pharmacodynamics/Kinetics

Onset of action: Antidyskinetic: Within 48 hours

Absorption: Well absorbed

Distribution: V_d: Normal: 1.5-6.1 L/kg; Renal failure: 5.1 ± 0.2 L/kg; in saliva, tear film, and nasal secretions; in animals, tissue (especially lung) concentrations higher than serum concentrations; crosses blood-brain barrier

Protein binding: Normal renal function: ~67%; Hemodialysis: ~59%

Metabolism: Not appreciable; small amounts of an acetyl metabolite identified

Bioavailability: 86% to 90%

Half-life elimination: Normal renal function: 16 ± 6 hours (9-31 hours); End-stage renal disease: 7-10 days

Excretion: Urine (80% to 90% unchanged) by glomerular filtration and tubular secretion

Total clearance: 2.5-10.5 L/hour

(Continued)

Amantadine *(Continued)*

Pregnancy Risk Factor C

Generic Available Yes

Amantadine Hydrochloride *see* Amantadine *on page 70*

Amaryl® *see* Glimepiride *on page 637*

Ambenonium (am be NOE nee um)

U.S. Brand Names Mytelase®

Canadian Brand Names Mytelase®

Pharmacologic Category Cholinergic Agonist

Synonyms Ambenonium Chloride

Use Treatment of myasthenia gravis

Local Anesthetic/Vasoconstrictor Precautions No information available to require special precautions

Effects on Dental Treatment Frequency not defined: Arrhythmias (especially bradycardia), hypotension, tachycardia, cardiac arrest, syncope, flushing, convulsions, dizziness, loss of consciousness, drowsiness, headache, nausea, vomiting, increased salivation, weakness, muscle cramps, spasms, increased bronchial secretions, laryngospasm, bronchiolar constriction, respiratory muscle paralysis, dyspnea, respiratory depression, respiratory arrest, bronchospasm, diaphoresis (increased), anaphylaxis, allergic reactions, dysphagia

Dosage Oral: Adults: 5-25 mg 3-4 times/day

Other Adverse Effects Frequency not defined:

Cardiovascular: Decreased carbon monoxide, AV block, nodal rhythm, nonspecific EKG changes

Central nervous system: Dysarthria, dysphonia

Dermatologic: Skin rash, thrombophlebitis (I.V.), urticaria

Gastrointestinal: Hyperperistalsis, diarrhea, stomach cramps, flatulence

Genitourinary: Urinary urgency

Neuromuscular & skeletal: Fasciculations, arthralgias

Ocular: Small pupils, lacrimation

Drug Interactions

Increased Effect/Toxicity: Succinylcholine neuromuscular blockade may be prolonged.

Decreased Effect: Corticosteroids antagonize effects of anticholinesterases in myasthenia gravis. Procainamide or quinidine may reverse ambenonium cholinergic effects on muscle.

Pregnancy Risk Factor C

Generic Available No

Ambenonium Chloride *see* Ambenonium *on page 72*

Ambien® *see* Zolpidem *on page 1413*

AmBisome® *see* Amphotericin B (Liposomal) *on page 101*

Amcinonide (am SIN oh nide)

U.S. Brand Names Cyclocort®

Canadian Brand Names Cyclocort®

Pharmacologic Category Corticosteroid, Topical

Use Relief of the inflammatory and pruritic manifestations of corticosteroid-responsive dermatoses (high potency corticosteroid)

Local Anesthetic/Vasoconstrictor Precautions No information available to require special precautions

Effects on Dental Treatment No significant effects or complications reported

Dosage Topical: Adults: Apply in a thin film 2-3 times/day. Therapy should be discontinued when control is achieved; if no improvement is seen, reassessment of diagnosis may be necessary.

Mechanism of Action Stimulates the synthesis of enzymes needed to decrease inflammation, suppress mitotic activity, and cause vasoconstriction

Other Adverse Effects Frequency not defined:

Dermatologic: Acne, hypopigmentation, allergic dermatitis, maceration of the skin, skin atrophy, striae, miliaria, telangiectasia

Endocrine & metabolic: HPA suppression, Cushing's syndrome, growth retardation

Local: Burning, itching, irritation, dryness, folliculitis, hypertrichosis

Systemic: Suppression of HPA axis, Cushing's syndrome, hyperglycemia; these reactions occur more frequently with occlusive dressings

Miscellaneous: **Secondary infection**

Pharmacodynamics/Kinetics

Absorption: Adequate through intact skin; increases with skin inflammation or occlusion

Metabolism: Hepatic

Excretion: Urine and feces

Pregnancy Risk Factor C

Generic Available Yes: Cream

Amerge® *see* Naratriptan *on page 955*
Americaine® [OTC] *see* Benzocaine *on page 169*
Americaine® Anesthetic Lubricant *see* Benzocaine *on page 169*
A-Methapred® *see* MethylPREDNISolone *on page 895*
Amethocaine Hydrochloride *see* Tetracaine *on page 1284*
Amethopterin *see* Methotrexate *on page 884*
Amevive® *see* Alefacept *on page 52*
Amfepramone *see* Diethylpropion *on page 436*
Amibid LA *see* Guaifenesin *on page 650*
Amicar® *see* Aminocaproic Acid *on page 76*
Amidate® *see* Etomidate *on page 549*

Amifostine (am i FOS teen)

U.S. Brand Names Ethyol®

Canadian Brand Names Ethyol®

Mexican Brand Names Ethyol®

Pharmacologic Category Antidote

Synonyms Ethiofos; Gammaphos

Use Reduce the incidence of moderate to severe xerostomia in patients undergoing postoperative radiation treatment for head and neck cancer, where the radiation port includes a substantial portion of the parotid glands. Reduce the cumulative renal toxicity associated with repeated administration of cisplatin in patients with advanced ovarian cancer or nonsmall cell lung cancer. In these settings, the clinical data does not suggest that the effectiveness of cisplatin-based chemotherapy regimens is altered by amifostine.

Local Anesthetic/Vasoconstrictor Precautions No information available to require special precautions

Effects on Dental Treatment >10%: Flushing, hypotension (62%), nausea/vomiting (may be severe), dizziness, somnolence, sneezing, hiccups

Dosage Adults: I.V. (refer to individual protocols): 910 mg/m^2 administered once daily as a 15-minute I.V. infusion, starting 30 minutes prior to chemotherapy

Reduction of xerostomia from head and neck radiation: 200 mg/m^2 I.V. (as a 3-minute infusion) once daily, starting 15-30 minutes before standard fraction radiation therapy

Note: 15-minute infusion is better tolerated than more extended infusions. Further reductions in infusion times have not been systematically investigated. The infusion of amifostine should be interrupted if the systolic blood pressure (mm Hg) decreases significantly from the following baseline values:

Decrease of 20 if baseline systolic blood pressure <100
Decrease of 25 if baseline systolic blood pressure 100-119
Decrease of 30 if baseline systolic blood pressure 120-139
Decrease of 40 if baseline systolic blood pressure 140-179
Decrease of 50 if baseline systolic blood pressure ≥180

Mean onset of hypotension is 14 minutes into the 15-minute infusion and the mean duration was 6 minutes. Hypotension should be treated with fluid infusion and postural management of the patient (supine or Trendelenburg position). If the blood pressure returns to normal within 5 minutes and the patient is asymptomatic, the infusion may be restarted so that the full dose of amifostine may be administered. If the full dose of amifostine cannot be administered, the dose of amifostine for subsequent cycles should be 740 mg/m^2.

Mechanism of Action Prodrug that is dephosphorylated by alkaline phosphatase in tissues to a pharmacologically active free thiol metabolite that can reduce the toxic effects of cisplatin. The free thiol is available to bind to, and detoxify, reactive metabolites of cisplatin; and can also act as a scavenger of free radicals that may be generated in tissues exposed to cisplatin.

Other Adverse Effects

>10%:

Central nervous system: Chills
Miscellaneous: Feeling of warmth/coldness

<1%, postmarketing, and/or case reports: **Apnea, anaphylactoid reactions, anaphylaxis, arrhythmia, atrial fibrillation**, erythema multiforme, **hypersensitivity reactions (fever, rash, hypoxia, dyspnea, laryngeal edema)**, hypocalcemia, mild rashes, myocardial ischemia, **rigors, seizure**, Stevens-Johnson syndrome, toxic epidermal necrolysis

Drug Interactions Increased Effect/Toxicity: Special consideration should be given to patients receiving antihypertensive medications or other drugs that could potentiate hypotension.

Pharmacodynamics/Kinetics

Distribution: V_d: 3.5 L
Metabolism: Hepatic dephosphorylation to two metabolites (active-free thiol and disulfide)
Half-life elimination: 9 minutes
(Continued)

Amifostine *(Continued)*

Excretion: Urine

Clearance, plasma: 2.17 L/minute

Pregnancy Risk Factor C

Generic Available No

Amigesic® *see* Salsalate *on page 1206*

Amikacin (am i KAY sin)

Related Information

Tuberculosis *on page 1493*

U.S. Brand Names Amikin®

Canadian Brand Names Amikin®

Mexican Brand Names Akacin®; Amikafur®; Amikalem®; Amikason's®; Amikayect®; Amikin®; A.M.K.®; Biclin®; Gamikal®; Oprad®; Yectamid®

Pharmacologic Category Antibiotic, Aminoglycoside

Synonyms Amikacin Sulfate

Use Treatment of serious infections due to organisms resistant to gentamicin and tobramycin including *Pseudomonas*, *Proteus*, *Serratia*, and other gram-positive bacilli (bone infections, respiratory tract infections, endocarditis, and septicemia); documented infection of mycobacterial organisms susceptible to amikacin

Local Anesthetic/Vasoconstrictor Precautions No information available to require special precautions

Effects on Dental Treatment No significant effects or complications reported

Dosage Individualization is critical because of the low therapeutic index. Use of ideal body weight (IBW) for determining the mg/kg/dose appears to be more accurate than dosing on the basis of total body weight (TBW). In morbid obesity, dosage requirement may best be estimated using a dosing weight of IBW + 0.4 (TBW - IBW).

Note: Initial and periodic peak and trough plasma drug levels should be determined, particularly in critically ill patients with serious infections or in disease states known to significantly alter aminoglycoside pharmacokinetics (eg, cystic fibrosis, burns, or major surgery)

Infants, Children, and Adults: I.M., I.V.: 5-7.5 mg/kg/dose every 8 hours

Some clinicians suggest a daily dose of 15-20 mg/kg for all patients with normal renal function. This dose is at least as efficacious with similar, if not less, toxicity than conventional dosing.

Dosing interval in renal impairment: Some patients may require larger or more frequent doses if serum levels document the need (ie, cystic fibrosis or febrile granulocytopenic patients)

- Cl_{cr} ≥60 mL/minute: Administer every 8 hours
- Cl_{cr} 40-60 mL/minute: Administer every 12 hours
- Cl_{cr} 20-40 mL/minute: Administer every 24 hours
- Cl_{cr} <20 mL/minute: Loading dose, then monitor levels

Hemodialysis: Dialyzable (50% to 100%); administer dose postdialysis or administer ⅔ normal dose as a supplemental dose postdialysis and follow levels

Peritoneal dialysis: Dose as Cl_{cr} <20 mL/minute: Follow levels

Continuous arteriovenous or venovenous hemodiafiltration effects: Dose as for Cl_{cr} 10-40 mL/minute and follow levels

Mechanism of Action Inhibits protein synthesis in susceptible bacteria by binding to 30S ribosomal subunits

Other Adverse Effects

1% to 10%:

- Central nervous system: Neurotoxicity
- Otic: Ototoxicity (auditory and vestibular)
- Renal: Nephrotoxicity

<1%: **Hypotension, headache, drowsiness, drug fever, nausea, vomiting, paresthesia, tremor, dyspnea, allergic reaction,** rash, arthralgia, **weakness,** eosinophilia

Drug Interactions Increased Effect/Toxicity: Amikacin may increase or prolong the effect of neuromuscular blocking agents. Concurrent use of amphotericin (or other nephrotoxic drugs) may increase the risk of amikacin-induced nephrotoxicity. The risk of ototoxicity from amikacin may be increased with other ototoxic drugs.

Pharmacodynamics/Kinetics

Absorption: I.M.: May be delayed in the bedridden patient

Distribution: Primarily into extracellular fluid (highly hydrophilic); penetrates blood-brain barrier when meninges inflamed; crosses placenta

Relative diffusion of antimicrobial agents from blood into CSF: Good only with inflammation (exceeds usual MICs)

CSF:blood level ratio: Normal meninges: 10% to 20%; Inflamed meninges: 15% to 24%

Half-life elimination (renal function and age dependent):

Infants: Low birth weight (1-3 days): 7-9 hours; Full-term >7 days: 4-5 hours

Children: 1.6-2.5 hours

Adults: Normal renal function: 1.4-2.3 hours; Anuria/end-stage renal disease: 28-86 hours

Time to peak, serum: I.M.: 45-120 minutes

Excretion: Urine (94% to 98%)

Pregnancy Risk Factor C

Generic Available Yes

Amikacin Sulfate *see* Amikacin *on page 74*

Amikin® *see* Amikacin *on page 74*

Amiloride (a MIL oh ride)

U.S. Brand Names Midamor®

Canadian Brand Names Midamor®

Pharmacologic Category Diuretic, Potassium Sparing

Synonyms Amiloride Hydrochloride

Use Counteracts potassium loss induced by other diuretics in the treatment of hypertension or edematous conditions including CHF, hepatic cirrhosis, and hypoaldosteronism; usually used in conjunction with more potent diuretics such as thiazides or loop diuretics

Unlabeled/Investigational Use Investigational: Treatment of cystic fibrosis; reduction of lithium-induced polyuria

Local Anesthetic/Vasoconstrictor Precautions No information available to require special precautions

Effects on Dental Treatment 1% to 10%: Headache, dizziness, dehydration, nausea, vomiting, cough, dyspnea, fatigue, muscle cramps, weakness

Dosage Oral:

Children: Although safety and efficacy in children have not been established by the FDA, a dosage of 0.625 mg/kg/day has been used in children weighing 6-20 kg.

Adults: 5-10 mg/day (up to 20 mg)

Elderly: Initial: 5 mg once daily or every other day

Dosing adjustment in renal impairment:

Cl_{cr} 10-50 mL/minute: Administer at 50% of normal dose.

Cl_{cr} <10 mL/minute: Avoid use.

Mechanism of Action Interferes with potassium/sodium exchange (active transport) in the distal tubule, cortical collecting tubule and collecting duct by inhibiting sodium, potassium-ATPase; decreases calcium excretion; increases magnesium loss

Other Adverse Effects

1% to 10%:

Endocrine & metabolic: Hyperkalemia, hyperchloremic metabolic acidosis, hyponatremia, gynecomastia

Gastrointestinal: Abdominal pain, gas pain, diarrhea, appetite changes, constipation

Genitourinary: Impotence

<1% (Limited to important or life-threatening): **Orthostatic hypotension, arrhythmias, palpitations, chest pain**, alopecia, **GI bleeding**, polyuria, bladder spasms, dysuria, jaundice, **increased intraocular pressure, dyspnea**

Drug Interactions

Increased Effect/Toxicity: Increased risk of amiloride-associated hyperkalemia with triamterene, spironolactone, ACE inhibitors, potassium preparations, cyclosporine, tacrolimus, and indomethacin. Amiloride may increase the toxicity of amantadine and lithium by reduction of renal excretion. Quinidine and amiloride together may increase risk of malignant arrhythmias.

Decreased Effect: Decreased effect of amiloride with use of NSAIDs. Amoxicillin's absorption may be reduced with concurrent use.

Dietary/Ethanol/Herb Considerations Food: Administer with food or milk to avoid GI upset. Hypercalemia may result if taken with potassium; avoid potassium-containing foods (eg, bananas, oranges), salt substitutes, and low-salt milk. Avoid salt substitutes or low salt milk.

Pharmacodynamics/Kinetics

Onset of action: 2 hours

Duration: 24 hours

Absorption: ~15% to 25%

Distribution: V_d: 350-380 L

Protein binding: 23%

Metabolism: No active metabolites

Half-life elimination: Normal renal function: 6-9 hours; End-stage renal disease: 8-144 hours

Time to peak, serum: 6-10 hours

Excretion: Urine and feces (equal amounts as unchanged drug)

Pregnancy Risk Factor B

Generic Available Yes

Amiloride and Hydrochlorothiazide

(a MIL oh ride & hye droe klor oh THYE a zide)

Related Information

Hydrochlorothiazide *on page 675*

U.S. Brand Names Moduretic®

Canadian Brand Names Apo®-Amilzide; Moduret®; Moduretic®; Novamilor; Nu-Amilzide

Pharmacologic Category Diuretic, Combination

Synonyms Hydrochlorothiazide and Amiloride

Use Potassium-sparing diuretic; antihypertensive

Local Anesthetic/Vasoconstrictor Precautions No information available to require special precautions

Effects on Dental Treatment No significant effects or complications reported

Dosage Adults: Oral: Start with 1 tablet/day, then may be increased to 2 tablets/day if needed; usually given in a single dose

Dietary/Ethanol/Herb Considerations Food: May be taken with food

Pregnancy Risk Factor B

Generic Available Yes

Amiloride Hydrochloride *see* Amiloride *on page 75*

2-Amino-6-Mercaptopurine *see* Thioguanine *on page 1296*

2-Amino-6-Trifluoromethoxy-benzothiazole *see* Riluzole *on page 1184*

Aminobenzylpenicillin *see* Ampicillin *on page 103*

Aminocaproic Acid

(a mee noe ka PROE ik AS id)

U.S. Brand Names Amicar®

Canadian Brand Names Amicar®

Pharmacologic Category Hemostatic Agent

Use Treatment of excessive bleeding from fibrinolysis

Local Anesthetic/Vasoconstrictor Precautions No information available to require special precautions

Effects on Dental Treatment 1% to 10%: Hypotension, bradycardia, arrhythmia, dizziness, headache, nasal congestion, nausea, malaise, fatigue, weakness

Dosage In the management of acute bleeding syndromes, oral dosage regimens are the same as the I.V. dosage regimens in adults and children

Chronic bleeding: Oral, I.V.: 5-30 g/day in divided doses at 3- to 6-hour intervals

Acute bleeding syndrome:

- Children: Oral, I.V.: 100 mg/kg or 3 g/m^2 during the first hour, followed by continuous infusion at the rate of 33.3 mg/kg/hour or 1 g/m^2/hour; total dosage should not exceed 18 g/m^2/24 hours
  - Traumatic hyphema: Oral: 100 mg/kg/dose every 6-8 hours
- Adults:
  - Oral: For elevated fibrinolytic activity, administer 5 g during first hour, followed by 1-1.25 g/hour for approximately 8 hours or until bleeding stops
  - I.V.: 4-5 g in 250 mL of diluent during first hour followed by continuous infusion at the rate of 1-1.25 g/hour in 50 mL of diluent, continue for 8 hours or until bleeding stops
  - Maximum daily dose: Oral, I.V.: 30 g

Dosing adjustment in renal impairment: Oliguria or ESRD: Reduce to 15% to 25% of usual dose

Mechanism of Action Competitively inhibits activation of plasminogen to plasmin, also, a lesser antiplasmin effect

Other Adverse Effects

1% to 10%:

- Dermatologic: Rash
- Gastrointestinal: GI irritation, cramps, diarrhea
- Hematologic: Decreased platelet function, elevated serum enzymes
- Neuromuscular & skeletal: Myopathy
- Otic: Tinnitus

<1%: **Convulsions**, ejaculation problems, rhabdomyolysis, renal failure

Drug Interactions Increased Effect/Toxicity: Increased risk of hypercoagulability with oral contraceptives, estrogens. Should not be administered with factor IX complex concentrated or anti-inhibitor complex concentrates due to an increased risk of thrombosis.

Pharmacodynamics/Kinetics

Onset of action: ~1-72 hours

Distribution: Widely through intravascular and extravascular compartments

Metabolism: Minimally hepatic

Half-life elimination: 1-2 hours

Time to peak: Oral: Within 2 hours

Excretion: Urine (68% to 86% as unchanged drug)

Pregnancy Risk Factor C

Generic Available Yes: Injection, syrup

Comments Antifibrinolytic drugs are useful to control bleeding after dental extractions in patients with hemophilia. A clinical trial reported that aminocaproic acid or tranexamic acid reduces both recurrent bleeding and the amount of clotting factor replacement therapy required. In adults, the oral dose was 50-60 mg aminocaproic acid per kg every 4 hours until dental sockets were completely healed.

Extemporaneous solutions incorporating 100 mg aminocaproic acid per 5 mL of oral solution have been used as an oral rinse with some success. Use, however, must be carefully considered since they may not show efficacy in all patients with either drug-induced or hereditary coagulation problems. Studies are ongoing and commercial products may be available in the future.

Amino-Cerv™ *see* Urea *on page 1365*

Aminoglutethimide (a mee noe gloo TETH i mide)

U.S. Brand Names Cytadren®

Pharmacologic Category Antineoplastic Agent, Miscellaneous

Use In postmenopausal patients with breast cancer; third-line salvage agent for metastatic prostate cancer; suppression of adrenal function in selected patients with Cushing's syndrome

Local Anesthetic/Vasoconstrictor Precautions No information available to require special precautions

Effects on Dental Treatment

>10%: Nausea; ~10%: Orthostatic hypotension, headache, dizziness, drowsiness, lethargy, clumsiness

1% to 10%: Hypotension, tachycardia, vomiting

Dosage Adults: Oral:

250 mg every 6 hours may be increased at 1- to 2-week intervals to a total of 2 g/day; administer in divided doses, 2-3 times/day to reduce incidence of nausea and vomiting. Follow adrenal cortical response by careful monitoring of plasma cortisol until the desired level of suppression is achieved.

Mineralocorticoid (fludrocortisone) replacement therapy may be necessary in up to 50% of patients. If glucocorticoid replacement therapy is necessary, 20-30 mg hydrocortisone orally in the morning will replace endogenous secretion.

Dosing adjustment in renal impairment: Dose reduction may be necessary

Mechanism of Action Blocks the enzymatic conversion of cholesterol to delta-5-pregnenolone, thereby reducing the synthesis of adrenal glucocorticoids, mineralocorticoids, estrogens, aldosterone, and androgens

Other Adverse Effects

>10%:

- Dermatologic: Skin rash (36%)
- Gastrointestinal: Anorexia
- Hepatic: Cholestatic jaundice
- Neuromuscular & skeletal: Myalgia
- Renal: Nephrotoxicity
- Respiratory: Pulmonary alveolar damage
- Miscellaneous: Systemic lupus erythematosus

1% to 10%:

- Cardiovascular: Orthostasis
- Dermatologic: Hirsutism, pruritus (5%)
- Endocrine & metabolic: Adrenocortical insufficiency

<1%: Adrenal suppression, hypercholesterolemia, hyperkalemia, hypothyroidism, goiter

Rare: Neutropenia, leukopenia, thrombocytopenia, pancytopenia, agranulocytosis

Drug Interactions Induces **CYP1A2, 2C19, 3A4**

Decreased Effect: Aminoglutethimide may decrease therapeutic effect of dexamethasone, digitoxin (after 3-8 weeks), theophylline, warfarin, and medroxyprogesterone.

Pharmacodynamics/Kinetics

Onset of action: Adrenal suppression: 3-5 days

Absorption: 90%

Distribution: Crosses placenta

Protein binding, plasma: 20% to 25%

Metabolism: Major metabolite is N-acetylaminoglutethimide; induces its own metabolism

Half-life elimination: 7-15 hours; shorter following multiple doses

Excretion: Urine (34% to 50% as unchanged drug, 25% as metabolites)

Pregnancy Risk Factor D

Generic Available No

Aminolevulinic Acid (a MEE noh lev yoo lin ik AS id)

U.S. Brand Names Levulan® Kerastick™

Canadian Brand Names Levulan®

Pharmacologic Category Photosensitizing Agent, Topical; Topical Skin Product

Synonyms Aminolevulinic Acid Hydrochloride

(Continued)

Aminolevulinic Acid *(Continued)*

Use Treatment of nonhyperkeratotic actinic keratoses of the face or scalp; to be used in conjunction with blue light illumination

Local Anesthetic/Vasoconstrictor Precautions No information available to require special precautions

Effects on Dental Treatment Bleeding/hemorrhage (2% to 4%)

Dosage Adults: Topical: Apply to actinic keratoses (**not** perilesional skin) followed 14-18 hours later by blue light illumination. Application/treatment may be repeated at a treatment site after 8 weeks.

Mechanism of Action Aminolevulinic acid is a metabolic precursor of protoporphyrin IX (PpIX), which is a photosensitizer. Photosensitization following application of aminolevulinic acid topical solution occurs through the metabolic conversion to PpIX. When exposed to light of appropriate wavelength and energy, accumulated PpIX produces a photodynamic reaction.

Other Adverse Effects Transient stinging, burning, itching, erythema, and edema result from the photosensitizing properties of this agent. Symptoms subside between 1 minute and 24 hours after turning off the blue light illuminator. Severe stinging or burning was reported in at least 50% of patients from at least 1 lesional site treatment.

>10%: Dermatologic: Severe stinging or burning (50%), scaly or crusted skin (64% to 71%), hyperpigmentation/hypopigmentation (22% to 36%), itching (14% to 25%), erosion (2% to 14%)

1% to 10%:

- Central nervous system: Dysesthesia (≤2%)
- Dermatologic: Skin ulceration (2% to 4%), vesiculation (4% to 5%), pustular drug eruption (≤4%), skin disorder (5% to 12%)
- Local: Wheal/flare (2% to 7%), local pain (1%), tenderness (1%), edema (1%), scabbing (≤2%)

Drug Interactions Increased Effect/Toxicity: Photosensitizing agents such as griseofulvin, thiazide diuretics, sulfonamides, sulfonylureas, phenothiazines, and tetracyclines theoretically may increase the photosensitizing potential of aminolevulinic acid.

Pharmacodynamics/Kinetics

PpIX:

- Peak fluorescence intensity: 11 hours ± 1 hour
- Half-life, mean clearance for lesions: 30 ± 10 hours

Pregnancy Risk Factor C

Generic Available No

Aminolevulinic Acid Hydrochloride *see* Aminolevulinic Acid *on page 77*

Aminophylline (am in OFF i lin)

Related Information

Respiratory Diseases *on page 1476*
Theophylline *on page 1291*

U.S. Brand Names Truphylline®

Canadian Brand Names Phyllocontin®; Phyllocontin®-350

Mexican Brand Names Drafilyn®

Pharmacologic Category Theophylline Derivative

Synonyms Theophylline Ethylenediamine

Use Bronchodilator in reversible airway obstruction due to asthma or COPD; increase diaphragmatic contractility; neonatal idiopathic apnea of prematurity

Local Anesthetic/Vasoconstrictor Precautions No information available to require special precautions

Effects on Dental Treatment Prescribe erythromycin with caution to patients taking theophylline products. Erythromycin will delay the normal metabolic inactivation of theophyllines leading to increased blood levels; this has resulted in nausea, vomiting and CNS restlessness.

1% to 10%: Tachycardia, nervousness, restlessness, nausea, vomiting (uncommon at serum theophylline concentrations ≤15 μg/mL)

Dosage

Neonates: Apnea of prematurity:

- Loading dose: 5 mg/kg for one dose
- Maintenance: I.V.:
  - 0-24 days: Begin at 2 mg/kg/day divided every 12 hours and titrate to desired levels and effects
  - >24 days: 3 mg/kg/day divided every 12 hours; increased dosages may be indicated as liver metabolism matures (usually >30 days of life); monitor serum levels to determine appropriate dosages
- Theophylline levels should be initially drawn after 3 days of therapy; repeat levels are indicated 3 days after each increase in dosage or weekly if on a stabilized dosage

Treatment of acute bronchospasm:

Loading dose (in patients not currently receiving aminophylline or theophylline): 6 mg/kg (based on aminophylline) administered I.V. over 20-30 minutes; administration rate should not exceed 25 mg/minute (aminophylline)

Approximate I.V. maintenance dosages are based upon **continuous infusions**; bolus dosing (often used in children <6 months of age) may be determined by multiplying the hourly infusion rate by 24 hours and dividing by the desired number of doses/day

6 weeks to 6 months: 0.5 mg/kg/hour
6 months to 1 year: 0.6-0.7 mg/kg/hour
1-9 years: 1-1.2 mg/kg/hour
9-12 years and young adult smokers: 0.9 mg/kg/hour
12-16 years: 0.7 mg/kg/hour
Adults (healthy, nonsmoking): 0.7 mg/kg/hour
Older patients and patients with cor pulmonale, patients with CHF or liver failure: 0.25 mg/kg/hour

Dosage should be adjusted according to serum level measurements during the first 12- to 24-hour period; avoid using suppositories due to erratic, unreliable absorption.

Rectal: Adults: 500 mg 3 times/day

Mechanism of Action Causes bronchodilatation, diuresis, CNS and cardiac stimulation, and gastric acid secretion by blocking phosphodiesterase which increases tissue concentrations of cyclic adenine monophosphate (cAMP) which in turn promotes catecholamine stimulation of lipolysis, glycogenolysis, and gluconeogenesis and induces release of epinephrine from adrenal medulla cells

Other Adverse Effects <1%: Insomnia, **irritability, seizures**, skin rash, gastric irritation, **tremor, allergic reactions**

Drug Interactions Substrate of **CYP1A2**, 2E1, 3A4

Dietary/Ethanol/Herb Considerations Food does not appreciably affect absorption; avoid extremes of dietary protein and carbohydrate intake; limit charcoal-broiled foods.

Pharmacodynamics/Kinetics

Theophylline:

Absorption: Oral: Dosage form dependent

Half-life elimination: Highly variable and dependent upon age, liver function, cardiac function, lung disease, and smoking history

Time to peak, serum:

Oral: Liquid: 1 hour; Tablet, enteric-coated: 5 hours; Tablet, uncoated: 2 hours
I.V.: Within 30 minutes

Pregnancy Risk Factor C

Generic Available Yes

Selected Readings

Delaforge M and Sartori E, "*In Vivo* Effects of Erythromycin, Oleandomycin, and Erythralosamine Derivatives on Hepatic Cytochrome P450," *Biochem Pharmacol*, 1990, 40(2):223-8.

Ludden TM, "Pharmacokinetic Interactions of the Macrolide Antibiotics," *Clin Pharmacokinet*, 1985, 10(1):63-79.

Aminosalicylate Sodium *see* Aminosalicylic Acid *on page 79*

Aminosalicylic Acid (a mee noe sal i SIL ik AS id)

Related Information

Nonviral Infectious Diseases *on page 1493*

U.S. Brand Names Paser®

Canadian Brand Names Nemasol® Sodium

Mexican Brand Names Salofalk

Pharmacologic Category Nonsteroidal Anti-inflammatory Agent (NSAID), Oral; Salicylate

Synonyms Aminosalicylate Sodium; 4-Aminosalicylic Acid; Para-Aminosalicylate Sodium; PAS; Sodium PAS

Use Adjunctive treatment of tuberculosis used in combination with other antitubercular agents

Unlabeled/Investigational Use Treatment of Crohn's disease

Local Anesthetic/Vasoconstrictor Precautions No information available to require special precautions

Effects on Dental Treatment NSAIDs are known to reversibly decrease platelet aggregation via mechanisms different than observed with aspirin. The dentist should be aware of the potential of abnormal coagulation. Caution should also be exercised in the use of NSAIDs in patients already on anticoagulant therapy with drugs such as warfarin (Coumadin®).

Frequency not defined: Fever, nausea, vomiting

Dosage Oral:

Children: Tuberculosis: 200-300 mg/kg/day in 3-4 equally divided doses

Adults:

Tuberculosis: 150 mg/kg/day in 2-3 equally divided doses
Crohn's disease (unlabeled use): 1.5 g/day

(Continued)

Aminosalicylic Acid *(Continued)*

Dosing adjustment in renal impairment:

Cl_{cr} 10-50 mL/minute: Administer 50% to 75% of dose

Cl_{cr} <10 mL/minute: Administer 50% of dose

Administer after hemodialysis: Administer 50% of dose

Continuous arteriovenous hemofiltration: Dose for Cl_{cr} <10 mL/minute

Mechanism of Action Aminosalicylic acid (PAS) is a highly specific bacteriostatic agent active against *M. tuberculosis*. Structurally related to para-aminobenzoic acid (PABA) and its mechanism of action is thought to be similar to the sulfonamides, a competitive antagonism with PABA; disrupts plate biosynthesis in sensitive organisms.

Other Adverse Effects Frequency not defined:

Cardiovascular: Pericarditis, vasculitis

Central nervous system: Encephalopathy

Dermatologic: Skin eruptions

Endocrine & metabolic: Goiter (with or without myxedema), hypoglycemia

Gastrointestinal: Abdominal pain, diarrhea

Hematologic: Agranulocytosis, anemia (hemolytic), leukopenia, thrombocytopenia

Hepatic: Hepatitis, jaundice

Ocular: Optic neuritis

Respiratory: Eosinophilic pneumonia

Drug Interactions Decreased Effect: Aminosalicylic acid may decrease serum levels of digoxin and vitamin B_{12}.

Dietary/Ethanol/Herb Considerations Food: May be taken with food; may sprinkle on applesauce or yogurt, or suspend in tomato or orange juice (do not chew granules).

Pharmacodynamics/Kinetics

Absorption: Readily, >90%

Protein binding: 50% to 60%

Metabolism: Hepatic (>50%) via acetylation

Half-life elimination: Reduced with renal impairment

Time to peak, serum: 6 hours

Excretion: Urine (>80% as unchanged drug and metabolites)

Pregnancy Risk Factor C

Generic Available No

Selected Readings

Davidson PT and Le HQ, "Drug Treatment of Tuberculosis - 1992," *Drugs*, 1992, 43(5):651-73.

"Drugs for Tuberculosis," *Med Lett Drugs Ther*, 1993, 35(908):99-101.

Iseman MD, "Treatment of Multidrug-Resistant Tuberculosis," *N Engl J Med*, 1993, 329(11):784-91.

4-Aminosalicylic Acid *see* Aminosalicylic Acid *on page 79*

5-Aminosalicylic Acid *see* Mesalamine *on page 869*

Aminoxin® [OTC] *see* Pyridoxine *on page 1152*

Amiodarone (a MEE oh da rone)

Related Information

Cardiovascular Diseases *on page 1456*

U.S. Brand Names Cordarone®; Pacerone®

Canadian Brand Names Alti-Amiodarone; Cordarone®; Gen-Amiodarone; Novo-Amiodarone; Rhoxal-amiodarone

Mexican Brand Names Braxan®; Cardiorona; Cordarone®

Pharmacologic Category Antiarrhythmic Agent, Class III

Synonyms Amiodarone Hydrochloride

Use

Oral: Management of life-threatening recurrent ventricular fibrillation (VF) or hemodynamically unstable ventricular tachycardia (VT)

I.V.: Initiation of treatment and prophylaxis of frequency recurring VF and unstable VT in patients refractory to other therapy. Also, used for patients when oral amiodarone is indicated, but who are unable to take oral medication.

Unlabeled/Investigational Use Conversion of atrial fibrillation to normal sinus rhythm; maintenance of normal sinus rhythm; prevention of postoperative atrial fibrillation during cardiothoracic surgery; treatment of paroxysmal supraventricular tachycardia (SVT); control of rapid ventricular rate due to accessory pathway conduction in pre-excited atrial arrhythmias [ACLS guidelines]; After defibrillation and epinephrine in cardiac arrest with persistent ventricular tachycardia (VT) or ventricular fibrillation (VF) [ACLS guidelines]; control of hemodynamically stable VT, polymorphic VT or wide-complex tachycardia of uncertain origin [ACLS guidelines]

Local Anesthetic/Vasoconstrictor Precautions No information available to require special precautions

Effects on Dental Treatment

>10%: Nausea, vomiting, hypotension (I.V. 16%)

1% to 10%: Abnormal salivation and taste (oral form), CHF, arrhythmias (including atropine-resistant bradycardia, heart block, sinus arrest, ventricular tachycardia), myocardial depression, flushing, fever, involuntary movements, dizziness, headache, coagulation abnormalities, paresthesia, tremor

Dosage

Oral:

Children (calculate doses for children <1 year on body surface area): Loading dose: 10-15 mg/kg/day or 600-800 mg/1.73 m^2/day for 4-14 days or until adequate control of arrhythmia or prominent adverse effects occur (this loading dose may be given in 1-2 divided doses/day). Dosage should then be reduced to 5 mg/kg/day or 200-400 mg/1.73 m^2/day given once daily for several weeks. If arrhythmia does not recur, reduce to lowest effective dosage possible. Usual daily minimal dose: 2.5 mg/kg/day; maintenance doses may be given for 5 of 7 days/week.

Adults: Ventricular arrhythmias: 800-1600 mg/day in 1-2 doses for 1-3 weeks, then when adequate arrhythmia control is achieved, decrease to 600-800 mg/day in 1-2 doses for 1 month; maintenance: 400 mg/day. Lower doses are recommended for supraventricular arrhythmias.

I.V.:

Children (safety and efficacy of amiodarone use in children has not been fully established): Ventricular arrhythmias: A multicenter study (Perry, 1996; n=40; mean age 5.4 years with 24 of 40 children <2 years of age) used an I.V. loading dose of 5 mg/kg that was divided into five 1 mg/kg aliquots, with each aliquot given over 5-10 minutes. Additional 1-5 mg/kg doses could be administered 30 minutes later in a similar fashion if needed. The mean loading dose was 6.3 mg/kg. A maintenance dose (continuous infusion of 10-15 mg/kg/day) was administered to 21 of the 40 patients. Further studies are needed.

Note: I.V. administration at low flow rates (potentially associated with use in pediatrics) may result in leaching of plasticizers (DEHP) from intravenous tubing. DEHP may adversely affect male reproductive tract development. Alternative means of dosing and administration (1 mg/kg aliquots) may need to be considered.

Adults:

Breakthrough VF or VT: 150 mg supplemental doses in 100 mL D_5W over 10 minutes

Pulseless VF or VT: I.V. push: Initial: 300 mg in 20-30 mL NS or D_5W; if VF or VT recurs, supplemental dose of 150 mg followed by infusion of 1 mg/minute for 6 hours, then 0.5 mg/minute (maximum daily dose: 2.2 g)

Note: When switching from I.V. to oral therapy, use the following as a guide:

<1-week I.V. infusion: 800-1600 mg/day

1- to 3-week I.V. infusion: 600-800 mg/day

>3-week I.V. infusion: 400 mg/day

Recommendations for conversion to intravenous amiodarone after oral administration: During long-term amiodarone therapy (ie, ≥4 months), the mean plasma-elimination halflife of the active metabolite of amiodarone is 61 days. Replacement therapy may not be necessary in such patients if oral therapy is discontinued for a period <2 weeks, since any changes in serum amiodarone concentrations during this period may **not** be clinically significant.

Unlabeled uses:

Prophylaxis of atrial fibrillation following open heart surgery (unlabeled use):

Note: A variety of regimens have been used in clinical trials, including oral and intravenous regimens:

Oral: 400 mg twice daily (starting in postop recovery) for up to 7 days. An alternative regimen of amiodarone 600 mg/day for 7 days prior to surgery, followed by 200 mg/day until hospital discharge, has also been shown to decrease the risk of postoperative atrial fibrillation.

I.V.: 1000 mg infused over 24 hours (starting at postop recovery) for 2 days has been shown to reduce the risk of postoperative atrial fibrillation

Recurrent atrial fibrillation (unlabeled use): No standard regimen defined; examples of regimens include: Oral: Initial: 10 mg/kg/day for 14 days; followed by 300 mg/day for 4 weeks, followed by maintenance dosage of 100-200 mg/day (see Roy D, 2000). Other regimens have been described and are used clinically (ie, 400 mg 3 times/day for 5-7 days, then 400 mg/day for 1 month, then 200 mg/day).

Stable VT or SVT (unlabeled use): First 24 hours: 1000 mg according to following regimen

Step 1: 150 mg (100 mL) over first 10 minutes (mix 3 mL in 100 mL D_5W)

Step 2: 360 mg (200 mL) over next 6 hours (mix 18 mL in 500 mL D_5W): 1 mg/minute

Step 3: 540 mg (300 mL) over next 18 hours: 0.5 mg/minute

Note: After the first 24 hours: 0.5 mg/minute utilizing concentration of 1-6 mg/mL

Elderly: Specific guidelines unavailable; dose selection should be cautious, at low end of dosage range, and titration should be slower to evaluate response.

Dosing adjustment in hepatic impairment: Probably necessary in substantial impairment; specific guidelines unavailable.

Hemodialysis: Not dialyzable (0% to 5%); supplemental dose is unnecessary.

(Continued)

Amiodarone *(Continued)*

Peritoneal dialysis effects: Not dialyzable (0% to 5%); supplemental dose is unnecessary.

Mechanism of Action Class III antiarrhythmic agent which inhibits adrenergic stimulation, prolongs the action potential and refractory period in myocardial tissue; decreases AV conduction and sinus node function

Other Adverse Effects Between 20% and 40% of patients experience some form of neurologic adverse events. With large dosages (>400 mg/day), adverse reactions occur in ~75% of patients and require discontinuance in 5% to 20%.

1% to 10%:

Cardiovascular: Edema

I.V.: Asystole, cardiac arrest, electromechanical dissociation, ventricular tachycardia, cardiogenic shock

Central nervous system: Fatigue, incoordination, malaise, sleep disturbances, ataxia

Dermatologic: Photosensitivity (10%)

Endocrine & metabolic: Hypothyroidism or hyperthyroidism (less common), decreased libido

Gastrointestinal: Constipation, anorexia, abdominal pain,

Hepatic: Abnormal LFTs

Local: Phlebitis (I.V.; concentrations >3 mg/mL)

Neuromuscular & skeletal: Muscular weakness, peripheral neuropathy

Ocular: Visual disturbances, corneal microdeposits (occur in a majority of patients, and lead to visual disturbance in ~10%); other ocular symptoms are listed under the <1% category

Respiratory: Pulmonary toxicity has been estimated to occur at a frequency between 2% and 7% of patients (some reports indicate a frequency as high as 17%). Toxicity may present as hypersensitivity pneumonitis, pulmonary fibrosis (cough, fever, malaise), pulmonary inflammation, interstitial pneumonitis, or alveolar pneumonitis; other rare pulmonary toxicities are listed under the <1% category

Miscellaneous: Abnormal smell (oral form)

<1% (Limited to important or life-threatening): Abnormal renal function, alopecia, ARDS (postoperative), **atrial fibrillation**, brain stem dysfunction, cholestasis, **delirium**, diarrhea, discoloration of skin (slate-blue), dyskinesias, encephalopathy, **hyperglycemia**, hypertriglyceridemia, **hypotension (oral form)**, impotence, increased ALT/AST, increased QT interval, **jaw tremor**, loss of libido, **myoclonic jerks, nodal arrhythmia**, optic neuritis, optic neuropathy, **parkinsonian symptoms**, photophobia, pulmonary edema, rash, **severe hepatotoxicity (potentially fatal hepatitis), sinus bradycardia**, Stevens-Johnson syndrome, **ventricular fibrillation**

Postmarketing and/or case reports: Acute intracranial hypertension (I.V.), **anaphylactic shock**, angioedema, aplastic anemia, bone marrow granuloma, bronchiolitis obliterans organizing pneumonia (BOOP), cholestatic hepatitis, cirrhosis, gynecomastia, hemolytic anemia, hepatitis, leukocytoclastic vasculitis, myopathy, neutropenia, noninfectious epididymitis, pancreatitis, pancytopenia, pleuritis, pseudotumor cerebri, thrombocytopenia, toxic epidermal necrolysis, vasculitis

Drug Interactions Substrate of CYP1A2, **2C8/9**, 2C19, 2D6, 3A4; Inhibits CYP1A2, 2B6, **2C8/9**, 2C19, **2D6, 3A4**

Increased Effect/Toxicity: Due to the long half-life of amiodarone, drug interactions may take 1 or more weeks to develop. Use of amiodarone with diltiazem, verapamil, digoxin, beta-blockers, and other drugs which delay AV conduction may cause excessive AV block (amiodarone may also decrease the metabolism of some of these agents - see below). Amprenavir, cimetidine, nelfinavir, and ritonavir increase amiodarone levels. Amiodarone may increase the levels of digoxin (reduce dose by 50% on initiation), clonazepam, cyclosporine, flecainide (decrease dose up to 33%), metoprolol, phenothiazines, phenytoin, procainamide (reduce dose), propranolol, quinidine, tricyclic antidepressants, and warfarin. Concurrent use of fentanyl may lead to bradycardia, sinus arrest, and hypotension. The effect of drugs which prolong the QT interval, including amitriptyline, astemizole, bepridil, cisapride, disopyramide, erythromycin, gatifloxacin, haloperidol, imipramine, moxifloxacin, quinidine, pimozide, procainamide, sotalol, sparfloxacin, theophylline, and thioridazine may be increased. Cisapride, gatifloxacin, moxifloxacin, and sparfloxacin are contraindicated. Amiodarone may increase lovastatin-induced myopathy; concurrent use not recommended. Amiodarone may alter thyroid function and response to thyroid supplements. Amiodarone enhances the myocardial depressant and conduction defects of inhalation anesthetics (monitor).

Decreased Effect: Amiodarone blood levels may be decreased by phenytoin and rifampin. Amiodarone may alter thyroid function and response to thyroid supplements; monitor closely.

Dietary/Ethanol/Herb Considerations

Ethanol: Avoid use; may increase risk of hypotension or dizziness.

Food increases the rate and extent of absorption; administer consistently with regard to meals. Avoid caffeine (eg, colas, chocolate), garlic, and licorice.

Herb/Nutraceutical: Avoid black cohosh, dong quai, and evening primrose due to estrogenic activity. Avoid ephedra, ginseng, and yohimbe; may cause arrhythmias or hypertension. Avoid garlic; may have increased antihypertensive effect. Avoid ginger due to positive inotropic effects; theoretically, may cause arrhythmia. Avoid hawthorn; may lower peripheral vascular resistance causing additional decrease in BP. Avoid St John's wort; may decrease serum concentration and enhance photosensitization.

Pharmacodynamics/Kinetics

Onset of action: Oral: 3 days to 3 weeks; I.V.: May be more rapid

Peak effect: 1 week to 5 months

Duration after discontinuing therapy: 7-50 days

Note: Mean onset of effect and duration after discontinuation may be shorter in children than adults

Distribution: V_d: 66 L/kg (range: 18-148 L/kg); crosses placenta; enters breast milk in concentrations higher than maternal plasma concentrations

Protein binding: 96%

Metabolism: Hepatic, major metabolite active; possible enterohepatic recirculation

Bioavailability: ~50%

Half-life elimination: 40-55 days (range: 26-107 days); shorter in children than adults

Excretion: Feces; urine (<1% as unchanged drug)

Pregnancy Risk Factor D

Generic Available Yes

Amiodarone Hydrochloride *see* Amiodarone *on page 80*

Amipaque® *see* Radiological/Contrast Media (Nonionic) *on page 1165*

Ami-Tex PSE *see* Guaifenesin and Pseudoephedrine *on page 652*

Amitone® [OTC] *see* Calcium Supplements *on page 229*

Amitriptyline (a mee TRIP ti leen)

Related Information

Temporomandibular Dysfunction (TMD) *on page 1562*

U.S. Brand Names Elavil®; Vanatrip®

Canadian Brand Names Apo®-Amitriptyline; Levate®; PMS-Amitriptyline

Mexican Brand Names Anapsique®; Tryptanol®

Pharmacologic Category Antidepressant, Tricyclic (Tertiary Amine)

Synonyms Amitriptyline Hydrochloride

Use Relief of symptoms of depression

Unlabeled/Investigational Use Analgesic for certain chronic and neuropathic pain; prophylaxis against migraine headaches; treatment of depressive disorders in children

Local Anesthetic/Vasoconstrictor Precautions Use with caution; epinephrine, norepinephrine and levonordefrin have been shown to have an increased pressor response in combination with TCAs

Effects on Dental Treatment Amitriptyline is the most anticholinergic and sedating of the antidepressants; pronounced effects on the cardiovascular system; long-term treatment with TCAs such as amitriptyline increases the risk of caries by reducing salivation and salivary buffer capacity. In a study by Rundergren, et al, pathological alterations were observed in the oral mucosa of 72% of 58 patients; 55% had new carious lesions after taking TCAs for a median of 5½ years. Current research is investigating the use of the salivary stimulant pilocarpine (Salagen®) to overcome the xerostomia from amitriptyline.

>10%: Xerostomia, changes in salivation

Frequency not defined: Orthostatic hypotension, tachycardia, restlessness, dizziness, sedation (moderate to marked), fatigue, anxiety, impaired cognitive function, seizures, extrapyramidal symptoms, blurred vision, diaphoresis

Dosage

Children:

Chronic pain management (unlabeled use): Oral: Initial: 0.1 mg/kg at bedtime, may advance as tolerated over 2-3 weeks to 0.5-2 mg/kg at bedtime

Depressive disorders (unlabeled use): Oral: Initial doses of 1 mg/kg/day given in 3 divided doses with increases to 1.5 mg/kg/day have been reported in a small number of children (n=9) 9-12 years of age; clinically, doses up to 3 mg/kg/day (5 mg/kg/day if monitored closely) have been proposed

Adolescents: Depressive disorders: Oral: Initial: 25-50 mg/day; may administer in divided doses; increase gradually to 100 mg/day in divided doses

Adults:

Depression:

Oral: 50-150 mg/day single dose at bedtime or in divided doses; dose may be gradually increased up to 300 mg/day

I.M.: 20-30 mg 4 times/day

Pain management (unlabeled use): Oral: Initial: 25 mg at bedtime; may increase as tolerated to 100 mg/day

(Continued)

Amitriptyline *(Continued)*

Dosing interval in hepatic impairment: Use with caution and monitor plasma levels and patient response

Hemodialysis: Nondialyzable

Mechanism of Action Increases the synaptic concentration of serotonin and/or norepinephrine in the central nervous system by inhibition of their reuptake by the presynaptic neuronal membrane

Other Adverse Effects Anticholinergic effects may be pronounced (tolerance to these effects usually occurs).

Frequency not defined:

Cardiovascular: Nonspecific EKG changes, changes in AV conduction

Central nervous system: Insomnia

Dermatologic: Allergic rash, urticaria, photosensitivity

Gastrointestinal: Weight gain, constipation

Genitourinary: Urinary retention

Ocular: Mydriasis

Warnings/Precautions Often causes drowsiness/sedation, resulting in impaired performance of tasks requiring alertness (ie, operating machinery or driving). Sedative effects may be additive with other CNS depressants and/or ethanol. The degree of sedation is very high relative to other antidepressants. May worsen psychosis in some patients or precipitate a shift to mania or hypomania in patients with bipolar disease. May cause hyponatremia/SIADH. May increase the risks associated with electroconvulsive therapy. This agent should be discontinued, when possible, prior to elective surgery. Therapy should not be abruptly discontinued in patients receiving high doses for prolonged periods.

May cause orthostatic hypotension; the risk of this problem is very high relative to other antidepressants. Use with caution in patients at risk of hypotension or in patients where transient hypotensive episodes would be poorly tolerated (cardiovascular disease or cerebrovascular disease). The degree of anticholinergic blockade produced by this agent is very high relative to other cyclic antidepressants; use with caution in patients with urinary retention, benign prostatic hyperplasia, narrow-angle glaucoma, xerostomia, visual problems, constipation, or a history of bowel obstruction. May alter glucose control - use with caution in patients with diabetes.

Use caution in patients with depression, particularly if suicidal risk may be present. Use with caution in patients with a history of cardiovascular disease (including previous MI, stroke, tachycardia, or conduction abnormalities). The risk of conduction abnormalities with this agent is high relative to other antidepressants. May lower seizure threshold - use caution in patients with a previous seizure disorder or condition predisposing to seizures such as brain damage, alcoholism, or concurrent therapy with other drugs which lower the seizure threshold. Use with caution in hyperthyroid patients or those receiving thyroid supplementation. Use with caution in patients with hepatic or renal dysfunction and in elderly patients. Not recommended for use in patients <12 years of age.

Drug Interactions Substrate of CYP1A2, 2B6, 2C8/9, 2C19, **2D6**, 3A4; Inhibits CYP1A2, 2C8/9, 2C19, 2D6, 2E1

Increased Effect/Toxicity: Amitriptyline increases the effects of amphetamines, anticholinergics, other CNS depressants (sedatives, hypnotics, or ethanol), carbamazepine, tolazamide, chlorpropamide, and warfarin. When used with MAO inhibitors, hyperpyrexia, hypertension, tachycardia, confusion, seizures, and **deaths have been reported** (serotonin syndrome). Serotonin syndrome has also been reported with ritonavir (rare). The SSRIs (to varying degrees), cimetidine, fenfluramine, grapefruit juice, indinavir, methylphenidate, ritonavir, quinidine, diltiazem, valproate, and verapamil inhibit the metabolism of TCAs and clinical toxicity may result. Use of lithium with a TCA may increase the risk for neurotoxicity. Phenothiazines may increase concentration of some TCAs and TCAs may increase the concentration of phenothiazines. Pressor response to I.V. epinephrine, norepinephrine, and phenylephrine may be enhanced in patients receiving TCAs (**Note:** Effect is unlikely with epinephrine or levonordefrin dosages typically administered as infiltration in combination with local anesthetics). Combined use of beta-agonists or drugs which prolong QT_c (including quinidine, procainamide, disopyramide, cisapride, sparfloxacin, gatifloxacin, moxifloxacin) with TCAs may predispose patients to cardiac arrhythmias.

Decreased Effect: Carbamazepine, phenobarbital, and rifampin may increase the metabolism of amitriptyline resulting in a decreased effect of amitriptyline. Amitriptyline inhibits the antihypertensive response to bethanidine, clonidine, debrisoquin, guanadrel, guanethidine, guanabenz, or guanfacine. Cholestyramine and colestipol may bind TCAs and reduce their absorption.

Dietary/Ethanol/Herb Considerations

Ethanol: Avoid use; may increase CNS depression.

Food: Avoid grapefruit products; may inhibit metabolism of TCAs resulting in clinical toxicity

Herb/Nutraceutical: Avoid gotu kola, kava, SAMe, and valerian; may increase CNS depression. Avoid St John's wort; may decrease serum concentration and increase CNS depression.

Pharmacodynamics/Kinetics

Onset of action: Migraine prophylaxis: 6 weeks, higher dosage may be required in heavy smokers because of increased metabolism; Depression: 4-6 weeks, reduce dosage to lowest effective level

Distribution: Crosses placenta; enters breast milk

Metabolism: Hepatic to nortriptyline (active), hydroxy and conjugated derivatives; may be impaired in the elderly

Half-life elimination: Adults: 9-27 hours (average: 15 hours)

Time to peak, serum: ~4 hours

Excretion: Urine (18% as unchanged drug); feces (small amounts)

Pregnancy Risk Factor D

Generic Available Yes

Selected Readings

Boakes AJ, Laurence DR, Teoh PC, et al, "Interactions Between Sympathomimetic Amines and Antidepressant Agents in Man," *Br Med J*, 1973, 1(849):311-5.

Friedlander AH, Mahler ME, "Major Depressive Disorder. Psychopathology, Medical Management, and Dental Implications," *J Am Dent Assoc*, 201, 132(5):629-38.

Ganzberg S, "Psychoactive Drugs," *ADA Guide to Dental Therapeutics*, 2nd ed, Chicago, IL: ADA Publishing, a Division of ADA Business Enterprises, Inc, 2000, 376-405.

Jastak JT and Yagiela JA, "Vasoconstrictors and Local Anesthesia: A Review and Rationale for Use," *J Am Dent Assoc*, 1983, 107(4):623-30.

Rundegren J, van Dijken J, Mörnstad H, et al, "Oral Conditions in Patients Receiving Long-Term Treatment With Cyclic Antidepressant Drugs," *Swed Dent J*, 1985, 9(2):55-64.

Yagiela JA, "Adverse Drug Interactions in Dental Practice: Interactions Associated With Vasoconstrictors. Part V of a Series," *J Am Dent Assoc*, 1999, 130(5):701-9.

Amitriptyline and Chlordiazepoxide

(a mee TRIP ti leen & klor dye az e POKS ide)

Related Information

Amitriptyline *on page 83*

U.S. Brand Names Limbitrol®; Limbitrol® DS

Canadian Brand Names Limbitrol®

Pharmacologic Category Antidepressant, Tricyclic (Tertiary Amine); Benzodiazepine

Synonyms Chlordiazepoxide and Amitriptyline

Use Treatment of moderate to severe anxiety and/or agitation and depression

Local Anesthetic/Vasoconstrictor Precautions Use with caution; epinephrine, norepinephrine and levonordefrin have been shown to have an increased pressor response in combination with TCAs

Effects on Dental Treatment

Amitriptyline: The most anticholinergic and sedating of the antidepressants; pronounced effects on the cardiovascular system; long-term treatment with TCAs such as amitriptyline increases the risk of caries by reducing salivation and salivary buffer capacity. In a study by Rundergren, et al, pathological alterations were observed in the oral mucosa of 72% of 58 patients; 55% had new carious lesions after taking TCAs for a median of 5½ years. Current research is investigating the use of the salivary stimulant pilocarpine (Salagen®) to overcome the xerostomia from amitriptyline.

Chlordiazepoxide: Over 10% of patients will experience xerostomia which disappears with cessation of drug therapy

Restrictions C-IV

Dosage Initial: 3-4 tablets in divided doses; this may be increased to 6 tablets/day as required; some patients respond to smaller doses and can be maintained on 2 tablets

Dietary/Ethanol/Herb Considerations

Ethanol: Avoid use; may increase CNS depression.

Herb/Nutraceutical: Avoid gotu kola, kava, SAMe, St John's wort, and valerian; may increase CNS depression.

Pregnancy Risk Factor D

Generic Available Yes

Selected Readings

Boakes AJ, Laurence DR, Teoh PC, et al, "Interactions Between Sympathomimetic Amines and Antidepressant Agents in Man," *Br Med J*, 1973, 1(849):311-5.

Jastak JT and Yagiela JA, "Vasoconstrictors and Local Anesthesia: A Review and Rationale for Use," *J Am Dent Assoc*, 1983, 107(4):623-30.

Mitchell JR, "Guanethidine and Related Agents. III Antagonism by Drugs Which Inhibit the Norepinephrine Pump in Man," *J Clin Invest*, 1970, 49(8):1596-604.

Rundegren J, van Dijken J, Mörnstad H, et al, "Oral Conditions in Patients Receiving Long-Term Treatment With Cyclic Antidepressant Drugs," *Swed Dent J*, 1985, 9(2):55-64.

Amitriptyline and Perphenazine

(a mee TRIP ti leen & per FEN a zeen)

Related Information

Amitriptyline *on page 83*

U.S. Brand Names Etrafon®; Triavil®

(Continued)

Amitriptyline and Perphenazine *(Continued)*

Canadian Brand Names Etrafon®; Triavil®

Pharmacologic Category Antidepressant, Tricyclic (Tertiary Amine); Antipsychotic Agent, Phenothiazine, Piperazine

Synonyms Perphenazine and Amitriptyline

Use Treatment of patients with moderate to severe anxiety and depression

Unlabeled/Investigational Use Treatment of depression with psychotic features

Local Anesthetic/Vasoconstrictor Precautions

Amitriptyline: Use with caution; epinephrine, norepinephrine and levonordefrin have been shown to have an increased pressor response in combination with TCAs

Perphenazine: No information available to require special precautions

Effects on Dental Treatment

>10%: Xerostomia

Frequency not defined:

Amitriptyline: Orthostatic hypotension, tachycardia, restlessness, dizziness, sedation (moderate to marked), fatigue, anxiety, impaired cognitive function, seizures, extrapyramidal symptoms, blurred vision, diaphoresis

Perphenazine: Hypotension, orthostatic hypotension, hypertension, tachycardia, bradycardia, dizziness, cardiac arrest, extrapyramidal symptoms (pseudoparkinsonism, akathisia, dystonias, tardive dyskinesia), dizziness, seizures, headache, drowsiness, paradoxical excitement, restlessness, hyperactivity

Amitriptyline: The most anticholinergic and sedating of the antidepressants; pronounced effects on the cardiovascular system; long-term treatment with TCAs such as amitriptyline increases the risk of caries by reducing salivation and salivary buffer capacity. In a study by Rundergren, et al, pathological alterations were observed in the oral mucosa of 72% of 58 patients; 55% had new carious lesions after taking TCAs for a median of 5½ years. Current research is investigating the use of the salivary stimulant pilocarpine (Salagen®) to overcome the xerostomia from amitriptyline.

Perphenazine: Significant hypotension may occur, especially when the drug is administered parenterally; orthostatic hypotension is due to alpha-receptor blockade, the elderly are at greater risk for orthostatic hypotension.

Tardive dyskinesia: Prevalence rate may be 40% in elderly; development of the syndrome and the irreversible nature are proportional to duration and total cumulative dose over time. Extrapyramidal reactions are more common in elderly with up to 50% developing these reactions after 60 years of age; drug-induced **Parkinson's syndrome** occurs often; **Akathisia** is the most common extrapyramidal reaction in elderly.

Increased confusion, memory loss, psychotic behavior, and agitation frequently occur as a consequence of anticholinergic effects. Antipsychotic associated sedation in nonpsychotic patients is extremely unpleasant due to feelings of depersonalization, derealization, and dysphoria.

Dosage Oral: 1 tablet 2-4 times/day

Other Adverse Effects Frequency not defined:

Based on amitriptyline component: Anticholinergic effects may be pronounced (tolerance to these effects usually occurs).

Cardiovascular: Nonspecific EKG changes, changes in AV conduction

Central nervous system: Insomnia

Dermatologic: Allergic rash, urticaria, photosensitivity

Gastrointestinal: Weight gain, constipation

Genitourinary: Urinary retention

Ocular: Mydriasis

Based on perphenazine component:

Central nervous system: Cerebral edema, Neuroleptic malignant syndrome (NMS), impairment of temperature regulation

Dermatologic: Increased sensitivity to sun, rash, discoloration of skin (blue-gray)

Endocrine & metabolic: Lactation, breast enlargement, gynecomastia, menstrual irregularity, amenorrhea, SIADH, changes in libido

Gastrointestinal: Constipation, weight gain, stomach pain, diarrhea, anorexia, ileus

Genitourinary: Difficulty in urination, ejaculatory disturbances, incontinence, polyuria, ejaculating dysfunction, priapism

Hematologic: Agranulocytosis, leukopenia, eosinophilia, hemolytic anemia, thrombocytopenic purpura, pancytopenia

Hepatic: Cholestatic jaundice, hepatotoxicity

Ocular: Pigmentary retinopathy, blurred vision, cornea and lens changes

Dietary/Ethanol/Herb Considerations

Ethanol: Avoid use; may increase CNS depression.

Herb/Nutraceutical: Avoid gotu kola, kava, SAMe, St John's wort, and valerian; may increase CNS depression.

Pregnancy Risk Factor D

Generic Available Yes

Selected Readings

Boakes AJ, Laurence DR, Teoh PC, et al, "Interactions Between Sympathomimetic Amines and Antidepressant Agents in Man," *Br Med J*, 1973, 1(849):311-5.

Jastak JT and Yagiela JA, "Vasoconstrictors and Local Anesthesia: A Review and Rationale for Use," *J Am Dent Assoc*, 1983, 107(4):623-30.

Mitchell JR, "Guanethidine and Related Agents. III Antagonism by Drugs Which Inhibit the Norepinephrine Pump in Man," *J Clin Invest*, 1970, 49(8):1596-604.

Rundegren J, van Dijken J, Mörnstad H, et al, "Oral Conditions in Patients Receiving Long-Term Treatment With Cyclic Antidepressant Drugs," *Swed Dent J*, 1985, 9(2):55-64.

Amitriptyline Hydrochloride *see* Amitriptyline *on page 83*

AmLactin® [OTC] *see* Lactic Acid and Ammonium Hydroxide *on page 771*

Amlexanox (am LEKS an oks)

Related Information

Oral Nonviral Soft Tissue Ulcerations or Erosions *on page 1549*

U.S. Brand Names Aphthasol™

Pharmacologic Category Anti-inflammatory, Locally Applied

Use Dental and Medical: Treatment of aphthous ulcers (ie, canker sores)

Unlabeled/Investigational Use Treatment of allergic disorders

Local Anesthetic/Vasoconstrictor Precautions No information available to require special precautions

Effects on Dental Treatment 1% to 2%: Allergic contact dermatitis, oral irritation; discontinue therapy if rash or contact mucositis (<1%) develops.

Dosage Administer (0.5 cm - ¼") paste directly on ulcers 4 times/day following oral hygiene or meals, and at bedtime

Mechanism of Action As a benzopyrano-bipyridine carboxylic acid derivative, amlexanox has anti-inflammatory and antiallergic properties; it inhibits chemical mediatory release of the slow-reacting substance of anaphylaxis (SRS-A) and may have antagonistic effects on interleukin-3

Contraindications Hypersensitivity to amlexanox or any component of the formulation

Warnings/Precautions Discontinue therapy if rash or contact mucositis develops.

Pharmacodynamics/Kinetics

Absorption: Some from swallowed paste
Metabolism: Hydroxylated and conjugated metabolites
Half-life elimination: 3.5 hours
Time to peak, serum: 2 hours
Excretion: Urine (17% as unchanged drug)

Pregnancy Risk Factor B

Dosage Forms PASTE: 5% (5 g)

Generic Available No

Comments Treatment of canker sores with amlexanox showed a 76% median reduction in ulcer size compared to a 40% reduction with placebo. Greer, et al, reported an overall mean reduction in ulcer size of 1.82 mm² for patients treated with 5% amlexanox versus an average reduction of 0.52 mm² for the control group. Recent studies in over thousands of patients have confirmed that amlexanox accelerates the resolution of pain and healing of aphthous ulcers more significantly than vehicle and no treatment.

Selected Readings

Binnie WH, Curro FA, Khandwala A, et al, "Amlexanox Oral Paste: A Novel Treatment That Accelerates the Healing of Aphthous Ulcers," *Compend Contin Educ Dent*, 1997, 18(11):1116-8, 1120-2, 1124.

Greer RO Jr, Lindenmuth JE, Juarez T, et al, "A Double-Blind Study of Topically Applied 5% Amlexanox in the Treatment of Aphthous Ulcers," *J Oral Maxillofac Surg*, 1993, 51(3):243-8.

Khandwala A, Van Inwegen RG, and Alfano MC, "5% Amlexanox Oral Paste, A New Treatment for Recurrent Minor Aphthous Ulcers: I. Clinical Demonstration of Acceleration of Healing and Resolution of Pain," *Oral Surg Oral Med Oral Pathol Oral Radiol Endod*, 1997, 83(2):222-30.

Khandwala A, Van Inwegen RG, Charney MR, et al, "5% Amlexanox Oral Paste, A New Treatment for Recurrent Minor Aphthous Ulcers: II. Pharmacokinetics and Demonstration of Clinical Safety," *Oral Surg Oral Med Oral Pathol Oral Radiol Endod*, 1997, 83(2):231-8.

Amlodipine (am LOE di peen)

Related Information

Calcium Channel Blockers and Gingival Hyperplasia *on page 1598*
Calcium Channel Blockers, Comparative Pharmacokinetics *on page 1600*
Cardiovascular Diseases *on page 1456*

U.S. Brand Names Norvasc®

Canadian Brand Names Norvasc®

Mexican Brand Names Norvas®

Pharmacologic Category Calcium Channel Blocker

Use Treatment of hypertension and angina

Local Anesthetic/Vasoconstrictor Precautions No information available to require special precautions

Effects on Dental Treatment 1% to 10%: Flushing (0.7% to 2.6%), palpitations (0.7% to 4.5%), headache (7%; similar to placebo), nausea (3%), gingival hyperplasia (~1%; usually resolves upon discontinuation), dyspnea (1% to 2%), muscle cramps (1% to 2%), weakness (1% to 2%)

Dosage Adults: Oral:

Hypertension: Initial dose: 2.5-5 mg once daily; usual dose: 5 mg once daily; (Continued)

Amlodipine *(Continued)*

maximum dose: 10 mg once daily. In general, titrate in 2.5 mg increments over 7-14 days.

Angina: Usual dose: 5-10 mg; use lower doses for elderly or those with hepatic insufficiency (eg, 2.5-5 mg).

Dialysis: Hemodialysis and peritoneal dialysis does not enhance elimination. Supplemental dose is unnecessary.

Elderly: Dosing should start at the lower end of dosing range due to possible increased incidence of hepatic, renal, or cardiac impairment. Elderly patients also show decreased clearance of amlodipine.

Dosing adjustment in hepatic impairment: Administer 2.5 mg once daily.

Mechanism of Action Inhibits calcium ion from entering the "slow channels" or select voltage-sensitive areas of vascular smooth muscle and myocardium during depolarization, producing a relaxation of coronary vascular smooth muscle and coronary vasodilation; increases myocardial oxygen delivery in patients with vasospastic angina

Other Adverse Effects

>10%:

Cardiovascular: Peripheral edema (2% to 15% dose-related)

Respiratory: Pulmonary edema (15% from PRAISE trial, CHF population)

1% to 10%:

Dermatologic: Rash (1% to 2%), pruritus (1% to 2%)

Endocrine & metabolic: Male sexual dysfunction (1% to 2%)

Gastrointestinal: Abdominal pain (1% to 2%), dyspepsia (1% to 2%)

<1%: **Hypotension, bradycardia, arrhythmias, syncope, tachycardia, nervousness, vomiting, xerostomia, tremor, paresthesia, chest pain, hypotension**, insomnia, **malaise,** weight gain, anorexia, diarrhea, pancreatitis, constipation, flatulence, micturition disorder, **joint stiffness,** peripheral neuropathy, tinnitus, peripheral ischemia, **postural hypotension, postural dizziness,** hypoesthesia, vertigo, **dysphagia**, back pain, **hot flashes, pain, rigors**, arthrosis, myalgia, female sexual dysfunction, depression, abnormal dreams, anxiety, depersonalization, **epistaxis**, rash erythematous, angioedema, erythema multiforme, rash maculopapular, **abnormal vision,** conjunctivitis, diplopia, eye pain, micturition frequency, nocturia, **increased diaphoresis, thirst, hyperglycemia**, purpura, **allergic reactions**, leukopenia, thrombocytopenia, vasculitis

Postmarketing and/or case reports: Nonthrombocytopenic purpura, leukocytoclastic vasculitis, **EPS**, gynecomastia, Stevens-Johnson syndrome, erythema multiforme, exfoliative dermatitis, dysosmia, phototoxicity

Drug Interactions Substrate of **CYP3A4**; Inhibits CYP2B6, 2C8/9, 2D6, 3A4

Increased Effect/Toxicity: Azole antifungals (itraconazole, ketoconazole, fluconazole), erythromycin, and other inhibitors of cytochrome P450 isoenzyme 3A4 may inhibit amlodipine's metabolism. Grapefruit juice may modestly increase amlodipine levels. Cyclosporine levels may be increased by amlodipine. Blood pressure-lowering effects of sildenafil are additive with amlodipine.

Decreased Effect: Rifampin (and potentially other enzyme inducers) increase the metabolism of amlodipine. Calcium may reduce the calcium channel blocker's hypotensive effects.

Dietary/Ethanol/Herb Considerations

Ethanol: Avoid use; may increase risk of hypotension or dizziness.

Food: May be taken with meals. Avoid grapefruit products; may modestly increase serum concentration by ~15%. Avoid caffeine (eg, colas, chocolate), garlic, and licorice.

Herb/Nutraceutical: Avoid black cohosh, dong quai, and evening primrose due to estrogenic activity. Avoid ephedra, ginseng, and yohimbe; may worsen hypertension. Avoid garlic; may have increased antihypertensive effects. Avoid ginger due to positive inotropic effects; theoretically, may cause arrhythmia. Avoid hawthorn; may lower peripheral vascular resistance causing additional decrease in BP. Avoid licorice. Avoid St John's wort; may decrease serum concentration.

Pharmacodynamics/Kinetics

Onset of action: 30-50 minutes

Peak effect: 6-12 hours

Duration: 24 hours

Absorption: Oral: Well absorbed

Protein binding: 93%

Metabolism: Hepatic (>90%) to inactive metabolite

Bioavailability: 64% to 90%

Half-life elimination: 30-50 hours

Excretion: Urine

Pregnancy Risk Factor C

Generic Available No

Selected Readings

Jorgensen MG, "Prevalence of Amlodipine-Related Gingival Hyperplasia," *J Periodontol*, 1997, 68(7):676-8.

Wynn RL, "An Update on Calcium Channel Blocker-Induced Gingival Hyp 43(3):218-22.

Wynn RL, "Calcium Channel Blockers and Gingival Hyperplasia," *Ger*

Amlodipine and Benazepril (am LOE di peen & b

Related Information

Amlodipine *on page 87*

U.S. Brand Names Lotrel®

Canadian Brand Names Lotrel®

Pharmacologic Category Antihypertensive Agent Combination

Synonyms Benazepril and Amlodipine

Use Treatment of hypertension

Local Anesthetic/Vasoconstrictor Precautions No information available to require special precautions

Effects on Dental Treatment No significant effects or complications reported

Dosage Adults: Oral: 1 capsule daily

Mechanism of Action The mechanism through which benazepril lowers blood pressure is believed to be primarily suppression of the renin-angiotensin-aldosterone system, benazepril has an antihypertensive effect even in patients with low-renin hypertension; amlodipine is a dihydropyridine calcium antagonist that inhibits the transmembrane influx of calcium ions into vascular smooth muscle and cardiac muscle; amlodipine is a peripheral arterial vasodilator that acts directly on vascular smooth muscle to cause a reduction in peripheral vascular resistance and reduction in blood pressure

Pregnancy Risk Factor C/D (2nd and 3rd trimesters)

Generic Available No

Selected Readings

Wynn RL, "An Update on Calcium Channel Blocker-Induced Gingival Hyperplasia," *Gen Dent,* 1995, 43(3):218-22.

Wynn RL, "Calcium Channel Blockers and Gingival Hyperplasia," *Gen Dent,* 1991, 39(4):240-3.

Ammens® Medicated Deodorant [OTC] *see* Zinc Oxide *on page 1409*

Ammonapse *see* Sodium Phenylbutyrate *on page 1233*

Ammonia Spirit (Aromatic) (a MOE nee ah SPEAR it, air oh MAT ik)

Related Information

Dental Office Emergencies *on page 1582*

Pharmacologic Category Respiratory Stimulant

Synonyms Smelling Salts

Use Respiratory and circulatory stimulant used as "smelling salts" to treat or prevent fainting

Local Anesthetic/Vasoconstrictor Precautions No information available to require special precautions

Effects on Dental Treatment 1% to 10%: Nasal mucosa irritation, coughing, vomiting, nausea

Dosage Vapor should be slowly inhaled about 4" from nostrils and used only until the patient awakens or no longer feels faint; ampul should be held held away from the face and crushed between the fingers

Contraindications Hypersensitivity to ammonia or any component of the formulation

Pregnancy Risk Factor C

Dosage Forms SOLN: 60 mL, 480 mL. **VAPOR, inhalation** [ampul]: 0.33 mL

Generic Available Yes

Ammonium Chloride (a MOE nee um KLOR ide)

Pharmacologic Category Electrolyte Supplement, Parenteral; Urinary Acidifying Agent

Use Diuretic or systemic and urinary acidifying agent; treatment of hypochloremic states

Local Anesthetic/Vasoconstrictor Precautions No information available to require special precautions

Effects on Dental Treatment Frequency not defined: Headache (large doses), coma, confusion, vomiting, gastric irritation, nausea, hyperventilation (large doses)

Dosage Metabolic alkalosis: The following equations represent different methods of correction utilizing either the serum HCO_3^-, the serum chloride, or the base excess

Dosing of mEq NH_4Cl via the chloride-deficit method (hypochloremia):

Dose of mEq NH_4Cl = [0.2 L/kg x body weight (kg)] x [103 - observed serum chloride]; administer 100% of dose over 12 hours, then re-evaluate

Note: 0.2 L/kg is the estimated chloride space and 103 is the average normal serum chloride concentration.

Dosing of mEq NH_4Cl via the bicarbonate-excess method (refractory hypochloremic metabolic alkalosis):

Dose of NH_4Cl = [0.5 L/kg x body weight (kg)] x (observed serum HCO_3^- - 24); administer 50% of dose over 12 hours, then re-evaluate

(Continued)

...nium Chloride *(Continued)*

...ote: 0.5 L/kg is the estimated bicarbonate space and 24 is the average normal serum bicarbonate concentration.

...osing of mEq NH_4Cl via the base-excess method:

Dose of NH_4Cl = [0.3 L/kg x body weight (kg)] x measured base excess (mEq/L); administer 50% of dose over 12 hours, then re-evaluate

Note: 0.3 L/kg is the estimated extracellular bicarbonate and base excess is measured by the chemistry lab and reported with arterial blood gases.

These equations will yield different requirements of ammonium chloride.

Equation #1 is inappropriate to use if the patient has severe metabolic alkalosis without hypochloremia or if the patient has uremia.

Equation #3 is the most useful for the first estimation of ammonium chloride dosage.

Children: Urinary acidifying agents: Oral, I.V.: 75 mg/kg/day in 4 divided doses; maximum daily dose: 6 g

Adults: Urinary acidifying agent/diuretic:

Oral: 1-2 g every 4-6 hours

I.V.: 1.5 g/dose every 6 hours

Mechanism of Action Increases acidity by increasing free hydrogen ion concentration

Other Adverse Effects Frequency not defined:

Dermatologic: Rash

Endocrine & metabolic: Hypokalemia (large doses), metabolic acidosis, hyperchloremia; potassium and sodium may be decreased

Hepatic: Increased ammonia

Local: Pain injection site

Pharmacodynamics/Kinetics

Absorption: Well absorbed; complete within 3-6 hours

Metabolism: Hepatic

Excretion: Urine

Pregnancy Risk Factor C

Generic Available Yes

Ammonium Lactate *see* Lactic Acid and Ammonium Hydroxide *on page 771*

Amnesteen™ *see* Isotretinoin *on page 752*

Amobarbital (am oh BAR bi tal)

U.S. Brand Names Amytal®

Canadian Brand Names Amytal®

Pharmacologic Category Barbiturate

Synonyms Amylobarbitone

Use

Oral: Hypnotic in short-term treatment of insomnia; reduce anxiety and provide sedation preoperatively

I.M., I.V.: Control status epilepticus or acute seizure episodes; control acute episodes of agitated behavior in psychosis and in "Amytal® Interviewing" for narcoanalysis

Local Anesthetic/Vasoconstrictor Precautions No information available to require special precautions

Effects on Dental Treatment

>10%: Dizziness, lightheadedness, "hangover" effect, drowsiness, CNS depression, fever

1% to 10%: Confusion, unusual excitement, nervousness, faint feeling, headache, nausea, vomiting

Restrictions C-II

Dosage

Children: Oral:

Sedation: 6 mg/kg/day divided every 6-8 hours

Insomnia: 2 mg/kg or 70 mg/m^2/day in 4 equally divided doses

Hypnotic: 2-3 mg/kg

Adults:

Insomnia: Oral: 65-200 mg at bedtime

Sedation: Oral: 30-50 mg 2-3 times/day

Preanesthetic: Oral: 200 mg 1-2 hours before surgery

Hypnotic:

Oral: 65-200 mg at bedtime

I.M., I.V.: 65-500 mg, should not exceed 500 mg I.M. or 1000 mg I.V.

Acute episode of agitated behavior:

Oral: 30-50 mg 2-3 times/day

I.M., I.V.: 65-500 mg, should not exceed 500 mg I.M. or 1000 mg I.V.

Status epilepticus/acute seizure episode: I.M., I.V.: 65-500 mg, should not exceed 500 mg I.M. or 1000 mg I.V.

Amobarbital (Amytal®) interview: I.V.: 50 mg/minute for total dose up to 300 mg

Mechanism of Action Interferes with transmission of impulses from the thalamus to the cortex of the brain resulting in an imbalance in central inhibitory and facilitatory mechanisms

Other Adverse Effects

>10%: Local: Pain at injection site

1% to 10%:

Central nervous system: Mental depression, insomnia, nightmares

Gastrointestinal: Constipation

<1%: Agranulocytosis, **apnea**, exfoliative dermatitis, **hallucinations, hypotension, laryngospasm**, megaloblastic anemia, rash, **respiratory depression**, Stevens-Johnson syndrome, thrombocytopenia, thrombophlebitis, urticaria

Drug Interactions Induces **CYP2A6**

Increased Effect/Toxicity: When combined with other CNS depressants, ethanol, narcotic analgesics, antidepressants, or benzodiazepines, additive respiratory and CNS depression may occur. Barbiturates may enhance the hepatotoxic potential of acetaminophen overdoses. Chloramphenicol, MAO inhibitors, valproic acid, and felbamate may inhibit barbiturate metabolism. Barbiturates may impair the absorption of griseofulvin, and may enhance the nephrotoxic effects of methoxyflurane. Concurrent use of meperidine may result in increased CNS depression.

Decreased Effect: Barbiturates are hepatic enzyme inducers, and may increase the metabolism of antipsychotics, some beta-blockers (unlikely with atenolol and nadolol), calcium channel blockers, chloramphenicol, cimetidine, corticosteroids, cyclosporine, disopyramide, doxycycline, ethosuximide, felbamate, furosemide, griseofulvin, lamotrigine, phenytoin, propafenone, quinidine, tacrolimus, TCAs, and theophylline. Barbiturates may increase the metabolism of estrogens and reduce the efficacy of oral contraceptives; an alternative method of contraception should be considered. Barbiturates inhibit the hypoprothrombinemic effects of oral anticoagulants via increased metabolism. Barbiturates may enhance the metabolism of methadone resulting in methadone withdrawal.

Dietary/Ethanol/Herb Considerations

Ethanol: Avoid use; may increase CNS depression.

Herb/Nutraceutical: Avoid gotu kola, kava, SAMe, St John's wort, and valerian; may increase CNS depression.

Pharmacodynamics/Kinetics

Onset of action: Oral: Within 1 hour; I.V.: Within 5 minutes

Distribution: Readily crosses placenta; small amounts enter breast milk

Metabolism: Primarily hepatic via microsomal enzymes

Half-life elimination: Biphasic: Initial: 40 minutes; Terminal: 20 hours

Pregnancy Risk Factor D

Generic Available Yes: Capsule

Amobarbital and Secobarbital

(am oh BAR bi tal & see koe BAR bi tal)

Related Information

Amobarbital *on page 90*

U.S. Brand Names Tuinal®

Pharmacologic Category Barbiturate

Synonyms Secobarbital and Amobarbital

Use Short-term treatment of insomnia

Local Anesthetic/Vasoconstrictor Precautions No information available to require special precautions

Effects on Dental Treatment

>10%: Dizziness, lightheadedness, drowsiness, "hangover" effect

1% to 10%: Confusion, unusual excitement, nervousness, faint feeling, headache, nausea, vomiting

Restrictions C-II

Dosage Adults: Oral: 1-2 capsules at bedtime

Other Adverse Effects

>10%: Local: Pain at injection site

1% to 10%:

Central nervous system: Mental depression, insomnia, nightmares

Gastrointestinal: Constipation

<1%: Agranulocytosis, dermatitis, exfoliative, **hallucinations, hypotension**, megaloblastic anemia, **respiratory depression**, skin rash, Stevens-Johnson syndrome, thrombocytopenia, thrombophlebitis

Pregnancy Risk Factor D

Generic Available No

Amoxapine (a MOKS a peen)

Mexican Brand Names Demolox

Pharmacologic Category Antidepressant, Tricyclic (Secondary Amine)

Synonyms Asendin® [DSC]

(Continued)

Amoxapine *(Continued)*

Use Treatment of depression, psychotic depression, depression accompanied by anxiety or agitation

Local Anesthetic/Vasoconstrictor Precautions Use with caution; epinephrine, norepinephrine and levonordefrin have been shown to have an increased pressor response in combination with TCAs

Effects on Dental Treatment Long-term treatment with TCAs such as amoxapine increases the risk of caries by reducing salivation and salivary buffer capacity.

>10%: Xerostomia, changes in salivation, drowsiness, weakness, blurred vision

1% to 10%: Tremor, nausea, dizziness, headache, confusion, nervousness, restlessness, excitement, anxiety, diaphoresis

Dosage Oral:

Children: Not established in children <16 years of age.

Adolescents: Initial: 25-50 mg/day; increase gradually to 100 mg/day; may administer as divided doses or as a single dose at bedtime

Adults: Initial: 25 mg 2-3 times/day, if tolerated, dosage may be increased to 100 mg 2-3 times/day; may be given in a single bedtime dose when dosage <300 mg/day

Elderly: Initial: 25 mg at bedtime increased by 25 mg weekly for outpatients and every 3 days for inpatients if tolerated; usual dose: 50-150 mg/day, but doses up to 300 mg may be necessary

Maximum daily dose:

Inpatient: 600 mg

Outpatient: 400 mg

Mechanism of Action Reduces the reuptake of serotonin and norepinephrine. The metabolite, 7-OH-amoxapine has significant dopamine receptor blocking activity similar to haloperidol.

Other Adverse Effects

>10%:

Gastrointestinal: Constipation

1% to 10%:

Central nervous system: Insomnia, ataxia

Dermatologic: Edema, skin rash

Endocrine: Elevated prolactin levels

<1%: Abdominal pain, **abnormal taste**, agranulocytosis, **allergic reactions**, breast enlargement, delayed micturition, diarrhea, elevated liver enzymes, **epigastric distress, extrapyramidal symptoms**, flatulence, galactorrhea, **hypertension, hypotension**, impotence, **incoordination, increased intraocular pressure**, increased or decreased libido, lacrimation, leukopenia, menstrual irregularity, mydriasis, **nasal congestion**, neuroleptic malignant syndrome, **numbness**, painful ejaculation, **paresthesia**, photosensitivity, **seizures**, SIADH, **syncope, tachycardia, tardive dyskinesia**, testicular edema, tinnitus, urinary retention, **vomiting**

Drug Interactions Substrate of **CYP2D6**

Increased Effect/Toxicity: Amoxapine increases the effects of amphetamines, anticholinergics, other CNS depressants (sedatives, hypnotics, or ethanol), chlorpropamide, tolazamide, and warfarin. When used with MAO inhibitors, hyperpyrexia, hypertension, tachycardia, confusion, seizures, and **deaths have been reported** (serotonin syndrome). Serotonin syndrome has also been reported with ritonavir (rare). Use of lithium with a TCA may increase the risk for neurotoxicity. Phenothiazines may increase concentration of some TCAs and TCAs may increase the concentration of phenothiazines. Pressor response to I.V. epinephrine, norepinephrine, and phenylephrine may be enhanced in patients receiving TCAs (**Note:** Effect is unlikely with epinephrine or levonordefrin dosages typically administered as infiltration in combination with local anesthetics). Combined use of beta-agonists or drugs which prolong QT_c (including quinidine, procainamide, disopyramide, cisapride, sparfloxacin, gatifloxacin, moxifloxacin) with TCAs may predispose patients to cardiac arrhythmias.

Decreased Effect: Amoxapine inhibits the antihypertensive effects of bethanidine, clonidine, debrisoquin, guanadrel, guanethidine, guanabenz, or guanfacine. Cholestyramine and colestipol may bind TCAs and reduce their absorption.

Dietary/Ethanol/Herb Considerations

Ethanol: Avoid use; may increase CNS depression.

Food: Grapefruit products may inhibit metabolism of TCAs resulting in clinical toxicity. Fruit, fluids, and fiber may reduce constipation.

Herb/Nutraceutical: Avoid gotu kola, kava, SAMe, St John's wort, and valerian; may increase CNS depression.

Pharmacodynamics/Kinetics

Onset of antidepressant effect: Usually occurs after 1-2 weeks, but may require 4-6 weeks

Absorption: Rapid and well absorbed

Distribution: V_d: 0.9-1.2 L/kg; enters breast milk

Protein binding: 80%

Metabolism: Primarily hepatic

Half-life elimination: Parent drug: 11-16 hours; Active metabolite (8-hydroxy): Adults: 30 hours

Time to peak, serum: 1-2 hours

Excretion: Urine (as unchanged drug and metabolites)

Pregnancy Risk Factor C

Generic Available Yes

Selected Readings

Friedlander AH and Mahler ME, "Major Depressive Disorder. Psychopathology, Medical Management, and Dental Implications," *J Am Dent Assoc*, 2001, 132(5):629-38.

Ganzberg S, "Psychoactive Drugs," *ADA Guide to Dental Therapeutics*, 2nd ed, Chicago, IL: ADA Publishing, a Division of ADA Business Enterprises, Inc, 2000, 376-405.

Jastak JT and Yagiela JA, "Vasoconstrictors and Local Anesthesia: A Review and Rationale for Use," *J Am Dent Assoc*, 1983, 107(4):623-30.

Mitchell JR, "Guanethidine and Related Agents. III Antagonism by Drugs Which Inhibit the Norepinephrine Pump in Man," *J Clin Invest*, 1970, 49(8):1596-604.

Rundegren J, van Dijken J, Mörnstad H, et al, "Oral Conditions in Patients Receiving Long-Term Treatment With Cyclic Antidepressant Drugs," *Swed Dent J*, 1985, 9(2):55-64.

Yagiela JA, "Adverse Drug Interactions in Dental Practice: Interactions Associated With Vasoconstrictors. Part V of a Series," *J Am Dent Assoc*, 1999, 130(5):701-9.

Amoxicillin (a moks i SIL in)

Related Information

Animal and Human Bites Guidelines *on page 1580*

Antibiotic Prophylaxis, Preprocedural Guidelines for Dental Patients *on page 1507*

Cardiovascular Diseases *on page 1456*

Gastrointestinal Disorders *on page 1474*

Oral Bacterial Infections *on page 1531*

Periodontal Diseases *on page 1540*

Sexually-Transmitted Diseases *on page 1502*

U.S. Brand Names Amoxil®; Moxilin®; Trimox®

Canadian Brand Names Amoxil®; Apo®-Amoxi; Gen-Amoxicillin; Lin-Amox; Novamoxin®; Nu-Amoxi

Mexican Brand Names Acimox®; Aclimafel®; Acroxil®; Amoxifur®; Amoxil®; Amoxinovag®; Amoxisol®; Ampliron®; Ardine®; Flemoxon®; Gimalxina®; Grunicina®; Hidramox®; Moxlin®; Penamox®; Polymox®; Servamox®; Solciclina®; Xalyn-Or®

Pharmacologic Category Antibiotic, Penicillin

Synonyms Amoxicillin Trihydrate; Amoxycillin; *p*-Hydroxyampicillin

Use

Dental: Treatment of oral-facial infections; prophylaxis of bacterial endocarditis and prophylaxis in total joint replacement patients undergoing dental procedures which produce bacteremia

Medical: Treatment of otitis media, sinusitis, and infections caused by susceptible organisms involving the respiratory tract, skin, and urinary tract; prophylaxis of bacterial endocarditis in patients undergoing surgical procedures; as part of a multidrug regimen for *H. pylori* eradication

Unlabeled/Investigational Use Postexposure prophylaxis for anthrax exposure with documented susceptible organisms

Local Anesthetic/Vasoconstrictor Precautions No information available to require special precautions

Effects on Dental Treatment Prolonged use of penicillins may lead to development of oral candidiasis.

Frequency not defined: Hyperactivity, agitation, anxiety, confusion, convulsions, behavioral changes, dizziness, nausea, vomiting

Dosage Oral:

Children: 20-50 mg/kg/day in divided doses every 8 hours

Prophylaxis of subacute bacterial endocarditis: 50 mg/kg 1 hour before dental procedure with no follow-up dose; total children's dose should not exceed adult dose

Acute otitis media due to highly-resistant strains of *S. pneumoniae*: Doses as high as 80-90 mg/kg/day divided every 12 hours have been used

Anthrax exposure (unlabeled use): **Note:** Postexposure prophylaxis only with documented susceptible organisms:

<40 kg: 15 mg/kg every 8 hours

≥40 kg: 500 mg every 8 hours

Adults: 250-500 mg every 8 hours or 500-875 mg twice daily; maximum dose: 2-3 g/day

Prophylaxis of bacterial endocarditis or joint replacement: 2 g 1 hour before dental procedure with no follow-up dose

Helicobacter pylori eradication: 1000 mg twice daily; requires combination therapy with at least one other antibiotic and an acid-suppressing agent (proton pump inhibitor or H_2 blocker)

Anthrax exposure (unlabeled use): **Note:** Postexposure prophylaxis only with documented susceptible organisms: 500 mg every 8 hours

Dosing interval in renal impairment:

Cl_{cr} 10-50 mL/minute: Administer every 12 hours

Cl_{cr} <10 mL/minute: Administer every 24 hours

(Continued)

Amoxicillin *(Continued)*

Dialysis: Moderately dialyzable (20% to 50%) by hemo- or peritoneal dialysis; approximately 50 mg of amoxicillin per liter of filtrate is removed by continuous arteriovenous or venovenous hemofiltration; dose as per Cl_{cr} <10 mL/minute guidelines

Mechanism of Action Inhibits bacterial cell wall synthesis by binding to one or more of the penicillin binding proteins (PBPs); which in turn inhibits the final transpeptidation step of peptidoglycan synthesis in bacterial cell walls, thus inhibiting cell wall biosynthesis. Bacteria eventually lyse due to ongoing activity of cell wall autolytic enzymes (autolysins and murein hydrolases) while cell wall assembly is arrested.

Other Adverse Effects Frequency not defined:

Central nervous system: Insomnia

Dermatologic: Erythematous maculopapular rashes, erythema multiforme, Stevens-Johnson syndrome, exfoliative dermatitis, toxic epidermal necrolysis, hypersensitivity vasculitis, urticaria

Gastrointestinal: Diarrhea, hemorrhagic colitis, pseudomembranous colitis

Hematologic: Anemia, hemolytic anemia, thrombocytopenia, thrombocytopenia purpura, eosinophilia, leukopenia, agranulocytosis

Hepatic: Elevated AST (SGOT) and ALT (SGPT), cholestatic jaundice, hepatic cholestasis, acute cytolytic hepatitis

Contraindications Hypersensitivity to amoxicillin, penicillin, or any component of the formulation

Warnings/Precautions In patients with renal impairment, doses and/or frequency of administration should be modified in response to the degree of renal impairment; a high percentage of patients with infectious mononucleosis have developed rash during therapy with amoxicillin; a low incidence of cross-allergy with other beta-lactams and cephalosporins exists

Drug Interactions

Allopurinol: Theoretically has an additive potential for amoxicillin rash

Aminoglycosides: May be synergistic against selected organisms

Oral contraceptives: Anecdotal reports suggesting decreased contraceptive efficacy with penicillins have been refuted by more rigorous scientific and clinical data.

Probenecid, disulfiram: May increase levels of penicillins (amoxicillin)

Warfarin: Effects of warfarin may be increased

Dietary/Ethanol/Herb Considerations Food: Administer with food, milk, or juice; does not interfere with absorption. Yogurt, boiled milk, or buttermilk may reduce diarrhea. Fruit, fluids, and fiber may reduce constipation.

Pharmacodynamics/Kinetics

Absorption: Oral: Rapid and nearly complete; food does not interfere

Distribution: Widely to most body fluids and bone; poor penetration into cells, eyes, and across normal meninges

Pleural fluids, lungs, and peritoneal fluid; high urine concentrations are attained; also into synovial fluid, liver, prostate, muscle, and gallbladder; penetrates into middle ear effusions, maxillary sinus secretions, tonsils, sputum, and bronchial secretions; crosses placenta; low concentrations enter breast milk

CSF:blood level ratio: Normal meninges: <1%; Inflamed meninges: 8% to 90%

Protein binding: 17% to 20%

Metabolism: Partially hepatic

Half-life elimination:

Neonates, full-term: 3.7 hours

Infants and Children: 1-2 hours

Adults: Normal renal function: 0.7-1.4 hours

Cl_{cr} <10 mL/minute: 7-21 hours

Time to peak: Capsule: 2 hours; Suspension: 1 hour

Excretion: Urine (80% as unchanged drug); lower in neonates

Pregnancy Risk Factor B

Dosage Forms CAP: 250 mg, 500 mg; (Amoxil®, Moxilin®, Trimox®): 250 mg, 500 mg. **POWDER, oral suspension:** 125 mg/5 mL (80 mL, 100 mL, 150 mL); 250 mg/5 mL (100 mL, 150 mL); (Amoxil®): 125 mg/5 mL (150 mL); 200 mg/5 mL (5 mL, 50 mL, 75 mL, 100 mL); 250 mg/5 mL (100 mL, 150 mL); 400 mg/5 mL (5 mL, 50 mL, 75 mL, 100 mL); (Moxilin®): 250 mg/5 mL (100 mL, 150 mL); (Trimox®): 125 mg/5 mL (80 mL, 100 mL, 150 mL); 250 mg/5 mL (80 mL, 100 mL, 150 mL). **POWDER, oral suspension** (Amoxil®): 50 mg/mL (15 mL, 30 mL). **TAB, chewable:** 125 mg, 200 mg, 250 mg, 400 mg; (Amoxil®): 200 mg, 400 mg. **TAB, film coated** (Amoxil®): 500 mg, 875 mg

Generic Available Yes

Selected Readings

Dajani AS, Taubert KA, Wilson W, et al, "Prevention of Bacterial Endocarditis. Recommendations by the American Heart Association," *JAMA* 1997, 277(22):1794-801.

Dajani AS, Taubert KA, Wilson W, et al, "Prevention of Bacterial Endocarditis: Recommendations by the American Heart Association," *J Am Dent Assoc* 1997, 128(8):1142-51.

Wynn RL, Bergman SA, Meiller TF, et al, "Antibiotics in Treating Oral-Facial Infections of Odontogenic Origin: An Update", *Gen Dent*, 2001, 49(3):238-40, 242, 244 passim.

Amoxicillin and Clavulanate Potassium

(a moks i SIL in & klav yoo LAN ate poe TASS ee um)

Related Information

Amoxicillin *on page 93*

Animal and Human Bites Guidelines *on page 1580*

Oral Bacterial Infections *on page 1531*

U.S. Brand Names Augmentin®; Augmentin ES-600™; Augmentin XR™

Canadian Brand Names Alti-Amoxi-Clav®; Apo®-Amoxi-Clav; Augmentin®; Clavulin®; ratio-AmoxiClav

Mexican Brand Names Clavulin®; Eumetinex

Pharmacologic Category Antibiotic, Penicillin

Synonyms Amoxicillin and Clavulanic Acid

Use

Dental: Treatment of orofacial infections when beta-lactamase-producing staphylococci and beta-lactamase-producing *Bacteroides* are present

Medical: Treatment of otitis media, sinusitis, and infections caused by susceptible organisms involving the lower respiratory tract, skin and skin structure, and urinary tract; spectrum same as amoxicillin with additional coverage of beta-lactamase producing *B. catarrhalis, H. influenzae, N. gonorrhoeae*, and *S. aureus* (not MRSA). The expanded coverage of this combination makes it a useful alternative when penicillinase-producing bacteria are present and patients cannot tolerate alternative treatments.

Local Anesthetic/Vasoconstrictor Precautions No information available to require special precautions

Effects on Dental Treatment Prolonged use of penicillins may lead to development of oral candidiasis.

1% to 10%: Vomiting, nausea

Dosage Dose is based on the amoxicillin component; see "Augmentin® Product-Specific Considerations" table.

Oral:

Infants <3 months: 30 mg/kg/day divided every 12 hours using the 125 mg/5 mL suspension

Children ≥3 months and <40 kg:

Otitis media: 90 mg/kg/day divided every 12 hours for 10 days

Lower respiratory tract infections, severe infections, sinusitis: 45 mg/kg/day divided every 12 hours **or** 40 mg/kg/day divided every 8 hours

Less severe infections: 25 mg/kg/day divided every 12 hours or 20 mg/kg/day divided every 8 hours

Augmentin® Product-Specific Considerations

Strength	Form	Consideration
125 mg	CT, S	q8h dosing
	S	For adults having difficulty swallowing tablets, 125 mg/5 mL suspension may be substituted for 500 mg tablet.
200 mg	CT, S	q12h dosing
	CT	Contains phenylalanine
	S	For adults having difficulty swallowing tablets, 200 mg/5 mL suspension may be substituted for 875 mg tablet.
250 mg	CT, S, T	q8h dosing
	CT	Contains phenylalanine
	T	Not for use in patients <40 kg
	CT, T	Tablet and chewable tablet are not interchangeable due to differences in clavulanic acid.
	S	For adults having difficulty swallowing tablets, 250 mg/5 mL suspension may be substituted for 500 mg tablet.
400 mg	CT, S	q12h dosing
	CT	Contains phenylalanine
	S	For adults having difficulty swallowing tablets, 400 mg/5 mL suspension may be substituted for 875 mg tablet.
500 mg	T	q8h or q12h dosing
600 mg	S	q12 h dosing
		Contains phenylalanine
		Not for use in adults or children ≥40 kg
		600 mg/5 mL suspension is not equivalent to or interchangeable with 200 mg/5 mL or 400 mg/5 mL due to differences in clavulanic acid.
875 mg	T	q12 h dosing; not for use in Cl_{cr} <30 mL/minute
1000 mg	XR	q12h dosing
		Not for use in children <16 years of age
		Not interchangeable with two 500 mg tablets
		Not for use in Cl_{cr} <30 mL/minute or hemodialysis

Legend: CT = chewable tablet, S = suspension, T = tablet, XR = extended release

(Continued)

Amoxicillin and Clavulanate Potassium *(Continued)*

Children >40 kg and Adults: 250-500 mg every 8 hours or 875 mg every 12 hours

Children ≥16 years and Adults:

Acute bacterial sinusitis: Extended release tablet: Two 1000 mg tablets every 12 hours for 10 days

Community-acquired pneumonia: Extended release tablet: Two 1000 mg tablets every 12 hours for 7-10 days

Dosing interval in renal impairment:

Cl_{cr} <30 mL/minute: Do not use 875 mg tablet or extended release tablets

Cl_{cr} 10-30 mL/minute: 250-500 mg every 12 hours

Cl_{cr} <10 mL/minute: 250-500 every 24 hours

Hemodialysis: Moderately dialyzable (20% to 50%)

250-500 mg every 24 hours; administer dose during and after dialysis. Do not use extended release tablets.

Peritoneal dialysis: Moderately dialyzable (20% to 50%)

Amoxicillin: Administer 250 mg every 12 hours

Clavulanic acid: Dose for Cl_{cr} <10 mL/minute

Continuous arteriovenous or venovenous hemofiltration effects:

Amoxicillin: ~50 mg of amoxicillin/L of filtrate is removed

Clavulanic acid: Dose for Cl_{cr} <10 mL/minute

Mechanism of Action Clavulanic acid binds and inhibits beta-lactamases that inactivate amoxicillin resulting in amoxicillin having an expanded spectrum of activity. Amoxicillin inhibits bacterial cell wall synthesis by binding to one or more of the penicillin binding proteins (PBPs); which in turn inhibits the final transpeptidation step of peptidoglycan synthesis in bacterial cell walls, thus inhibiting cell wall biosynthesis. Bacteria eventually lyse due to ongoing activity of cell wall autolytic enzymes (autolysins and murein hydrolases) while cell wall assembly is arrested.

Other Adverse Effects

>10%: Gastrointestinal: Diarrhea (3% to 34%; dose and regimen-dependent)

1% to 10%:

Dermatologic: Diaper rash, skin rash, urticaria

Gastrointestinal: Abdominal discomfort, loose stools

Genitourinary: Vaginitis

Miscellaneous: Moniliasis

<1%: Cholestatic jaundice, flatulence, **headache**, hepatic dysfunction, **PT increased,** thrombocytosis

Reported with ampicillin-class antibiotics: **Agitation**, agranulocytosis, ALT elevated, **anaphylaxis**, anemia, angioedema, **anxiety**, AST elevated, **behavioral changes, black "hairy" tongue, confusion, convulsions, dizziness**, enterocolitis, eosinophilia, erythema multiforme, exanthematous pustulosis, exfoliative dermatitis, **gastritis, glossitis**, hematuria, hemolytic anemia, hemorrhagic colitis, indigestion, insomnia, hyperactivity, interstitial nephritis, leukopenia, **mucocutaneous candidiasis**, pruritus, **pseudomembranous colitis, serum sickness-like reaction**, Stevens-Johnson syndrome, **stomatitis,** thrombocytopenia, thrombocytopenic purpura, **tooth discoloration**, toxic epidermal necrolysis

Contraindications Hypersensitivity to amoxicillin, clavulanic acid, penicillin, or any component of the formulation; history of cholestatic jaundice or hepatic dysfunction with amoxicillin/clavulanate potassium therapy

Warnings/Precautions Prolonged use may result in superinfection; in patients with renal impairment, doses and/or frequency of administration should be modified in response to the degree of renal impairment; high percentage of patients with infectious mononucleosis have developed rash during therapy; a low incidence of cross-allergy with cephalosporins exists; incidence of diarrhea is higher than with amoxicillin alone. Use caution in patients with hepatic dysfunction. Hepatic dysfunction, although rare, is more common in elderly and/or males, and occurs more frequently with prolonged treatment, and may occur after therapy is complete. Due to differing content of clavulanic acid, not all formulations are interchangeable. Some products contain phenylalanine.

Drug Interactions

Allopurinol: Additive potential for amoxicillin rash

Aminoglycosides: May be synergistic against selected organisms

Oral contraceptives: Anecdotal reports suggesting decreased contraceptive efficacy with penicillins have been refuted by more rigorous scientific and clinical data.

Probenecid: May increase levels of penicillins (amoxicillin)

Warfarin: Effects of warfarin may be increased

Dietary/Ethanol/Herb Considerations Food has no affect on amoxicillin absorption but increases clavulanic acid absorption. Administer with meals to increase absorption and reduce GI upset; may mix with milk, formula, or juice. Extended release product should be taken with food. All dosage forms contain potassium.

Pharmacodynamics/Kinetics Amoxicillin pharmacokinetics are not affected by clavulanic acid.

Amoxicillin: See Amoxicillin monograph.

Clavulanic acid:

Metabolism: Hepatic

Excretion: Urine (30% to 40% as unchanged drug)

Pregnancy Risk Factor B

Dosage Forms POWDER, oral suspension: 200: Amoxicillin 200 mg and clavulanate potassium 28.5 mg per 5 mL (100 mL); 400: Amoxicillin 400 mg and clavulanate potassium 57 mg per 5 mL (100 mL); (Augmentin®): 125: Amoxicillin trihydrate 125 mg and clavulanate potassium 31.25 mg per 5 mL (75 mL, 100 mL, 150 mL); 200: Amoxicillin 200 mg and clavulanate potassium 28.5 mg per 5 mL (50 mL, 75 mL, 100 mL); 250: Amoxicillin trihydrate 250 mg and clavulanate potassium 62.5 mg per 5 mL (75 mL, 100 mL, 150 mL); 400: Amoxicillin 400 mg and clavulanate potassium 57 mg per 5 mL (50 mL, 75 mL, 100 mL); (Augmentin ES-600™): Amoxicillin 600 mg and clavulanic potassium 42.9 mg per 5 mL (50 mL, 75 mL, 100 mL, 150 mL). **TAB:** 500: Amoxicillin trihydrate 500 mg and clavulanate potassium 125 mg; 875: Amoxicillin trihydrate 875 mg and clavulanate potassium 125 mg; (Augmentin®): 250: Amoxicillin trihydrate 250 mg and clavulanate potassium 125 mg; 500: Amoxicillin trihydrate 500 mg and clavulanate potassium 125 mg; 875: Amoxicillin trihydrate 875 mg and clavulanate potassium 125 mg. **TAB, chewable:** 200: Amoxicillin trihydrate 200 mg and clavulanate potassium 28.5 mg; 400: Amoxicillin trihydrate 400 mg and clavulanate potassium 57 mg; (Augmentin®): 125: Amoxicillin trihydrate 125 mg and clavulanate potassium 31.25 mg; 200: Amoxicillin trihydrate 200 mg and clavulanate potassium 28.5 mg; 250: Amoxicillin trihydrate 250 mg and clavulanate potassium 62.5 mg; 400: Amoxicillin trihydrate 400 mg and clavulanate potassium 57 mg. **TAB, extended release** (Augmentin XR™): Amoxicillin 1000 mg and clavulanic acid 62.5 mg

Generic Available Yes; Excludes extended release

Comments In maxillary sinus, anterior nasal cavity, and deep neck infections, beta-lactamase-producing staphylococci and beta-lactamase-producing *Bacteroides* usually are present. In these situations, antibiotics that resist the beta-lactamase enzyme are indicated. Amoxicillin and clavulanic acid is administered orally for moderate infections. Ampicillin sodium and sulbactam sodium (Unasyn®) is administered parenterally for more severe infections.

Selected Readings

Wynn RL and Bergman SA, "Antibiotics and Their Use in the Treatment of Orofacial Infections, Part I," *Gen Dent*, 1994, 42(5):398, 400, 402.

Wynn RL and Bergman SA, "Antibiotics and Their Use in the Treatment of Orofacial Infections, Part II," *Gen Dent*, 1994, 42(6):498-502.

Amoxicillin and Clavulanic Acid *see* Amoxicillin and Clavulanate Potassium *on page 95*

Amoxicillin Trihydrate *see* Amoxicillin *on page 93*

Amoxil® *see* Amoxicillin *on page 93*

Amoxycillin *see* Amoxicillin *on page 93*

Amphetamine and Dextroamphetamine *see* Dextroamphetamine and Amphetamine *on page 422*

Amphocin® *see* Amphotericin B (Conventional) *on page 98*

Amphojel® [OTC] *see* Aluminum Hydroxide *on page 68*

Amphotec® *see* Amphotericin B Cholesteryl Sulfate Complex *on page 97*

Amphotericin B Cholesteryl Sulfate Complex

(am foe TER i sin bee ko LES te ril SUL fate KOM pleks)

Related Information

Amphotericin B (Conventional) *on page 98*

U.S. Brand Names Amphotec®

Pharmacologic Category Antifungal Agent, Parenteral

Synonyms ABCD; Amphotericin B Colloidal Dispersion

Use Treatment of invasive aspergillosis in patients who have failed amphotericin B deoxycholate treatment, or who have renal impairment or experience unacceptable toxicity which precludes treatment with amphotericin B deoxycholate in effective doses.

Local Anesthetic/Vasoconstrictor Precautions No information available to require special precautions

Effects on Dental Treatment

>10%: Fever

1% to 10%: Hypotension, tachycardia, nausea, dyspnea, headache

Dosage Children and Adults: I.V.:

Premedication: For patients who experience chills, fever, hypotension, nausea, or other nonanaphylactic infusion-related immediate reactions, premedicate with the following drugs, 30-60 minutes prior to drug administration: a nonsteroidal (eg, ibuprofen, choline magnesium trisalicylate, etc) with or without diphenhydramine; or acetaminophen with diphenhydramine; or hydrocortisone 50-100 mg. If the patient experiences rigors during the infusion, meperidine may be administered.

Range: 3-4 mg/kg/day (infusion of 1 mg/kg/hour); maximum: 7.5 mg/kg/day

(Continued)

Amphotericin B Cholesteryl Sulfate Complex *(Continued)*

Mechanism of Action Binds to ergosterol altering cell membrane permeability in susceptible fungi and causing leakage of cell components with subsequent cell death

Other Adverse Effects

>10%: Central nervous system: Chills

1% to 10%:

Dermatologic: Rash

Endocrine & metabolic: Hypokalemia, hypomagnesemia

Gastrointestinal: Diarrhea, abdominal pain

Hematologic: Thrombocytopenia

Hepatic: LFT changes

Renal: Elevated creatinine

Amphotericin B colloidal dispersion has an improved therapeutic index compared to conventional amphotericin B, and has been used safely in patients with amphotericin B-related nephrotoxicity; however, continued decline of renal function has occurred in some patients.

Drug Interactions

Increased Effect/Toxicity: Toxic effect with other nephrotoxic drugs (eg, cyclosporine and aminoglycosides) may be additive. Corticosteroids may increase potassium depletion caused by amphotericin. Amphotericin B may predispose patients receiving digitalis glycosides or neuromuscular blocking agents to toxicity secondary to hypokalemia.

Decreased Effect: Pharmacologic antagonism may occur with azole antifungals (ketoconazole, miconazole, etc).

Pharmacodynamics/Kinetics

Distribution: V_d: Total volume increases with higher doses, reflects increasing uptake by tissues (with 4 mg/kg/day = 4 L/kg); predominantly distributed in the liver; concentrations in kidneys and other tissues are lower than observed with conventional amphotericin B

Half-life elimination: 28-29 hours; prolonged with higher doses

Pregnancy Risk Factor B

Generic Available No

Amphotericin B Colloidal Dispersion *see* Amphotericin B Cholesteryl Sulfate Complex *on page 97*

Amphotericin B (Conventional)

(am foe TER i sin bee con VEN sha nal)

Related Information

Oral Fungal Infections *on page 1542*

U.S. Brand Names Amphocin®; Fungizone®

Canadian Brand Names Fungizone®

Pharmacologic Category Antifungal Agent, Parenteral; Antifungal Agent, Topical

Synonyms Amphotericin B Desoxycholate

Use Treatment of severe systemic and CNS infections caused by susceptible fungi such as *Candida* species, *Histoplasma capsulatum*, *Cryptococcus neoformans*, *Aspergillus* species, *Blastomyces dermatitidis*, *Torulopsis glabrata*, and *Coccidioides immitis*; fungal peritonitis; irrigant for bladder fungal infections; and topically for cutaneous and mucocutaneous candidal infections; used in fungal infection in patients with bone marrow transplantation, amebic meningoencephalitis, ocular aspergillosis (intraocular injection), candidal cystitis (bladder irrigation), chemoprophylaxis (low-dose I.V.), immunocompromised patients at risk of aspergillosis (intranasal/nebulized), refractory meningitis (intrathecal), coccidioidal arthritis (intra-articular/I.M.).

Low-dose amphotericin B 0.1-0.25 mg/kg/day has been administered after bone marrow transplantation to reduce the risk of invasive fungal disease. Alternative routes of administration and extemporaneous preparations have been used when standard antifungal therapy is not available (eg, inhalation, intraocular injection, subconjunctival application, intracavitary administration into various joints and the pleural space).

Local Anesthetic/Vasoconstrictor Precautions No information available to require special precautions

Effects on Dental Treatment

>10%: Fever, headache, pain, malaise

1% to 10%: Hypotension, hypertension, flushing, nausea, vomiting, delirium, paresthesia (especially with I.T. therapy), renal failure

Dosage

I.V.: Premedication: For patients who experience chills, fever, hypotension, nausea, or other nonanaphylactic infusion-related immediate reactions, premedicate with the following drugs, 30-60 minutes prior to drug administration: a nonsteroidal (eg, ibuprofen, choline magnesium trisalicylate, etc) with or without diphenhydramine; or acetaminophen with diphenhydramine; or hydrocortisone 50-100 mg. If the patient experiences rigors during the infusion, meperidine may be administered.

Infants and Children:

Test dose: I.V.: 0.1 mg/kg/dose to a maximum of 1 mg; infuse over 30-60 minutes. Many clinicians believe a test dose is unnecessary.

Maintenance dose: 0.25-1 mg/kg/day given once daily; infuse over 2-6 hours. Once therapy has been established, amphotericin B can be administered on an every-other-day basis at 1-1.5 mg/kg/dose; cumulative dose: 1.5-2 g over 6-10 week.

Adults:

Test dose: 1 mg infused over 20-30 minutes. Many clinicians believe a test dose is unnecessary.

Maintenance dose: Usual: 0.25-1.5 mg/kg/day; 1-1.5 mg/kg over 4-6 hours every other day may be given once therapy is established; aspergillosis, mucormycosis, rhinocerebral phycomycosis often require 1-1.5 mg/kg/day; do not exceed 1.5 mg/kg/day

Duration of therapy varies with nature of infection: Usual duration is 4-12 weeks or cumulative dose of 1-4 g

I.T.: Meningitis, coccidioidal or cryptococcal:

Children.: 25-100 mcg every 48-72 hours; increase to 500 mcg as tolerated

Adults: Initial: 25-300 mcg every 48-72 hours; increase to 500 mcg to 1 mg as tolerated; maximum total dose: 15 mg has been suggested

Topical: Apply to affected areas 2-4 times/day for 1-4 weeks of therapy depending on nature and severity of infection

Bladder irrigation: Candidal cystitis: Irrigate with 50 mcg/mL solution instilled periodically or continuously for 5-10 days or until cultures are clear

Dosing adjustment in renal impairment: If renal dysfunction is due to the drug, the daily total can be decreased by 50% or the dose can be given every other day; I.V. therapy may take several months

Dialysis: Poorly dialyzed; no supplemental dosage necessary when using hemo- or peritoneal dialysis or continuous arteriovenous or venovenous hemodiafiltration effects

Administration in dialysate: Children and Adults: 1-2 mg/L of peritoneal dialysis fluid either with or without low-dose I.V. amphotericin B (a total dose of 2-10 mg/kg given over 7-14 days). Precipitate may form in ionic dialysate solutions.

Mechanism of Action Binds to ergosterol altering cell membrane permeability in susceptible fungi and causing leakage of cell components with subsequent cell death

Other Adverse Effects

>10%:

Central nervous system: Chills
Endocrine & metabolic: Hypokalemia, hypomagnesemia
Gastrointestinal: Anorexia
Hematologic: Anemia
Renal: Nephrotoxicity

1% to 10%:

Central nervous system: Arachnoiditis, lumbar nerve pain
Genitourinary: Urinary retention
Hematologic: Leukocytosis
Local: Thrombophlebitis
Renal: Renal tubular acidosis

<1%: **Cardiac arrest**, bone marrow suppression, **convulsions**, maculopapular rash, **coagulation defects**, thrombocytopenia, agranulocytosis, leukopenia, acute liver failure, vision changes, hearing loss, anuria, **dyspnea**

Warnings/Precautions Anaphylaxis has been reported with other amphotericin B-containing drugs. During the initial dosing, the drug should be administered under close clinical observation. Avoid additive toxicity with other nephrotoxic drugs; drug-induced renal toxicity usually improves with interrupting therapy, decreasing dosage, or increasing dosing interval. I.V. amphotericin is used primarily for the treatment of patients with progressive and potentially fatal fungal infections; topical preparations may stain clothing. Infusion reactions are most common 1-3 hours after starting the infusion and diminish with continued therapy. Use amphotericin B with caution in patients with decreased renal function. Pulmonary reactions may occur in neutropenic patients receiving leukocyte transfusions; separation of the infusions as much as possible is advised.

Drug Interactions

Increased Effect/Toxicity: Use of amphotericin with other nephrotoxic drugs (eg, cyclosporine and aminoglycosides) may result in additive toxicity. Amphotericin may increase the toxicity of flucytosine. Antineoplastic agents may increase the risk of amphotericin-induced nephrotoxicity, bronchospasms, and hypotension. Corticosteroids may increase potassium depletion caused by amphotericin. Amphotericin B may predispose patients receiving digitalis glycosides or neuromuscular-blocking agents to toxicity secondary to hypokalemia.

Decreased Effect: Pharmacologic antagonism may occur with azole antifungal agents (ketoconazole, miconazole).

(Continued)

Amphotericin B (Conventional) *(Continued)*

Pharmacodynamics/Kinetics

Distribution: Minimal amounts enter the aqueous humor, bile, CSF (inflamed or noninflamed meninges), amniotic fluid, pericardial fluid, pleural fluid, and synovial fluid

Protein binding, plasma: 90%

Half-life elimination: Biphasic: Initial: 15-48 hours; Terminal: 15 days

Time to peak: Within 1 hour following a 4- to 6-hour dose

Excretion: Urine (2% to 5% as biologically active form); ~40% eliminated over a 7-day period and may be detected in urine for at least 7 weeks after discontinued use

Pregnancy Risk Factor B

Generic Available Yes: Powder for reconstitution

Amphotericin B Desoxycholate *see* Amphotericin B (Conventional) *on page 98*

Amphotericin B (Lipid Complex)

(am foe TER i sin bee, LIP id KOM pleks)

Related Information

Amphotericin B (Conventional) *on page 98*

U.S. Brand Names Abelcet®

Canadian Brand Names Abelcet®

Pharmacologic Category Antifungal Agent, Parenteral

Synonyms ABLC

Use Treatment of aspergillosis or any type of progressive fungal infection in patients who are refractory to or intolerant of conventional amphotericin B therapy

Local Anesthetic/Vasoconstrictor Precautions No information available to require special precautions

Effects on Dental Treatment

>10%: Fever, pain

1% to 10%: Hypotension, cardiac arrest, headache, nausea, vomiting, respiratory failure, dyspnea, pneumonia, GI hemorrhage, renal failure

Dosage Children and Adults: I.V.:

Premedication: For patients who experience chills, fever, hypotension, nausea, or other nonanaphylactic infusion-related immediate reactions, premedicate with the following drugs, 30-60 minutes prior to drug administration: a nonsteroidal (eg, ibuprofen, choline magnesium trisalicylate, etc) with or without diphenhydramine; or acetaminophen with diphenhydramine; or hydrocortisone 50-100 mg. If the patient experiences rigors during the infusion, meperidine may be administered.

Range: 2.5-5 mg/kg/day as a single infusion

Dosing adjustment in renal impairment: None; not studied

Hemodialysis: No supplemental dosage necessary

Peritoneal dialysis: No supplemental dosage necessary

Continuous arteriovenous or venovenous hemofiltration: No supplemental dosage necessary

Mechanism of Action Binds to ergosterol altering cell membrane permeability in susceptible fungi and causing leakage of cell components with subsequent cell death

Other Adverse Effects Nephrotoxicity and infusion-related hyperpyrexia, rigors, and chills are reduced relative to amphotericin deoxycholate.

>10%:

Central nervous system: Chills

Renal: Increased serum creatinine

1% to 10%:

Dermatologic: Rash

Endocrine & metabolic: Bilirubinemia, hypokalemia, acidosis

Gastrointestinal: Diarrhea, abdominal pain

Warnings/Precautions Anaphylaxis has been reported with other amphotericin B-containing drugs. Facilities for cardiopulmonary resuscitation should be available during administration due to the possibility of anaphylactic reaction. If severe respiratory distress occurs, the infusion should be immediately discontinued. During the initial dosing, the drug should be administered under close clinical observation. Acute reactions (including fever and chills) may occur 1-2 hours after starting an intravenous infusion. These reactions are usually more common with the first few doses and generally diminish with subsequent doses. Pulmonary reactions may occur in neutropenic patients receiving leukocyte transfusions; separation of the infusions as much as possible is advised.

Drug Interactions

Increased Effect/Toxicity: See Amphotericin B monograph.

Decreased Effect: Pharmacologic antagonism may occur with azole antifungal agents (ketoconazole, miconazole).

Pharmacodynamics/Kinetics

Distribution: V_d: Increases with higher doses; reflects increased uptake by tissues (131 L/kg with 5 mg/kg/day)

Half-life elimination: ~24 hours

Excretion: Clearance: Increases with higher doses (5 mg/kg/day): 400 mL/hour/kg

Pregnancy Risk Factor B

Generic Available No

Amphotericin B (Liposomal) (am foe TER i sin bee lye po SO mal)

Related Information

Amphotericin B (Conventional) *on page 98*

U.S. Brand Names AmBisome®

Canadian Brand Names AmBisome®

Pharmacologic Category Antifungal Agent, Parenteral

Synonyms L-AmB

Use Empirical therapy for presumed fungal infection in febrile, neutropenic patients; treatment of patients with *Aspergillus* species, *Candida* species and/or *Cryptococcus* species infections refractory to amphotericin B desoxycholate, or in patients where renal impairment or unacceptable toxicity precludes the use of amphotericin B desoxycholate; treatment of cryptococcal meningitis in HIV-infected patients; treatment of visceral leishmaniasis

Note: In immunocompromised patients with visceral leishmaniasis treated with amphotericin B (liposomal), relapse rates were high following initial clearance of parasites.

Local Anesthetic/Vasoconstrictor Precautions No information available to require special precautions

Effects on Dental Treatment

>10%: Tachycardia (9% to 18%), hypotension (7% to 14%), hypertension (8% to 20%), chest pain (8% to 12%), headache (9% to 20%), anxiety (7% to 14%), confusion (9% to 13%), nausea (16% to 40%), vomiting (10% to 32%), dyspnea (18% to 23%), lung disorder (14% to 18%), increased cough (2% to 18%), epistaxis (8% to 15%), rhinitis (11%), sepsis (7% to 14%), infection (11% to 12%), pain (14%), weakness (6% to 13%)

1% to 10%: Xerostomia, gum/oral hemorrhage, ulcerative stomatitis, bruising, arrhythmia, atrial fibrillation, bradycardia, cardiac arrest, facial swelling, flushing, postural hypotension, agitation, abnormal thinking, coma, convulsion, dizziness (7% to 8%), hallucinations, nervousness, somnolence, eructation, GI hemorrhage (10%), mucositis, stomatitis, coagulation disorder, hemorrhage, pain, paresthesia, rigors, tremor, asthma, cough, nasal dryness, hemoptysis, hyperventilation, pharyngitis, pneumonia, respiratory insufficiency, respiratory failure, sinusitis, allergic reaction, flu-like syndrome, herpes simplex, hiccup, procedural complication (8% to 10%), diaphoresis (7%)

Dosage Children and Adults: I.V.:

Note: Premedication: For patients who experience chills, fever, hypotension, nausea, or other nonanaphylactic infusion-related immediate reactions, premedicate with the following drugs, 30-60 minutes prior to drug administration: a nonsteroidal (eg, ibuprofen, choline magnesium trisalicylate, etc) with or without diphenhydramine; or acetaminophen with diphenhydramine; or hydrocortisone 50-100 mg. If the patient experiences rigors during the infusion, meperidine may be administered.

Empiric therapy: Recommended initial dose: 3 mg/kg/day

Systemic fungal infections (*Aspergillus, Candida, Cryptococcus*): Recommended initial dose of 3-5 mg/kg/day

Cryptococcal meningitis in HIV-infected patients: 6 mg/kg/day

Treatment of visceral leishmaniasis:

Immunocompetent patients: 3 mg/kg/day on days 1-5, and 3 mg/kg/day on days 14 and 21; a repeat course may be given in patients who do not achieve parasitic clearance

Immunocompromised patients: 4 mg/kg/day on days 1-5, and 4 mg/kg/day on days 10, 17, 24, 31, and 38

Dosing adjustment in renal impairment: None; not studied

Hemodialysis: No supplemental dosage necessary

Peritoneal dialysis effects: No supplemental dosage necessary

Continuous arteriovenous or venovenous hemofiltration: No supplemental dosage necessary

Mechanism of Action Binds to ergosterol altering cell membrane permeability in susceptible fungi and causing leakage of cell components with subsequent cell death

Other Adverse Effects May vary with respect to premedications and underlying illness:

>10%:

Cardiovascular: Peripheral edema (15%), edema (12% to 14%), hypervolemia (8% to 12%)

Central nervous system: Chills (29% to 48%), insomnia (17% to 22%)

Dermatologic: Rash (5% to 25%), pruritus (11%)

(Continued)

Amphotericin B (Liposomal) *(Continued)*

Endocrine & metabolic: Hypokalemia (31% to 51%), hypomagnesemia (15% to 50%), hyperglycemia (8% to 23%), hypocalcemia (5% to 18%), hyponatremia (8% to 12%)

Gastrointestinal: Diarrhea (11% to 30%), abdominal pain (7% to 20%), constipation (15%), anorexia (10% to 14%)

Hematologic: Anemia (27% to 48%), blood transfusion reaction (9% to 18%), leukopenia (15% to 17%), thrombocytopenia (6% to 13%)

Hepatic: Increased alkaline phosphatase (7% to 22%), increased BUN (7% to 21%), bilirubinemia (9% to 18%), increased ALT (15%), increased AST (13%), abnormal LFTs (not specified) (4% to 13%)

Local: Phlebitis (9% to 11%)

Neuromuscular & skeletal: Back pain (12%)

Renal: Increased creatinine (18% to 40%), hematuria (14%)

Respiratory: Lung disorder (14% to 18%), pleural effusion (12%) (11%)

2% to 10%:

Cardiovascular: Valvular heart disease, vascular disorder, cardiomegaly

Central nervous system: Depression, dysesthesia, malaise

Dermatologic: Alopecia, cellulitis, dry skin, maculopapular rash, petechia, purpura, skin discoloration, skin disorder, skin ulcer, urticaria, vesiculobullous rash

Endocrine & metabolic: Acidosis, increased amylase, fluid overload, hypernatremia (4%), hyperchloremia, hyperkalemia, hypermagnesemia, hyperphosphatemia, hypophosphatemia, hypoproteinemia, increased lactate dehydrogenase, increased nonprotein nitrogen

Gastrointestinal: Constipation, enlarged abdomen, fecal incontinence, flatulence, hematemesis, hemorrhoids, ileus, rectal disorder

Genitourinary: Vaginal hemorrhage

Hematologic: Decreased prothrombin, thrombocytopenia

Hepatic: Hepatocellular damage, hepatomegaly, veno-occlusive liver disease

Local: Inflammation at injection site

Neuromuscular & skeletal: Arthralgia, bone pain, dystonia, myalgia

Ocular: Conjunctivitis, dry eyes, eye hemorrhage

Renal: Abnormal renal function, acute kidney failure, dysuria, kidney failure, toxic nephropathy, urinary incontinence

Respiratory: Atelectasis, lung edema, hypoxia (6% to 8%)

Miscellaneous: Cell-mediated immunological reaction, graft versus host disease

Postmarketing and/or case reports: Angioedema, erythema, urticaria, **cyanosis/hypoventilation**, pulmonary edema, agranulocytosis, hemorrhagic cystitis

Warnings/Precautions Anaphylaxis has been reported with amphotericin B desoxycholate and other amphotericin B-containing drugs. Facilities for cardiopulmonary resuscitation should be available during administration due to the possibility of anaphylactic reaction. As with any amphotericin B-containing product the drug should be administered by medically trained personnel. During the initial dosing period, patients should be under close clinical observation. Amphotericin B (liposomal) has been shown to be significantly less toxic than amphotericin B desoxycholate; however, adverse events may still occur. If severe respiratory distress occurs, the infusion should be immediately discontinued and the patient should not receive further infusions. Acute reactions (including fever and chills) may occur 1-2 hours after starting an intravenous infusion. These reactions are usually more common with the first few doses and generally diminish with subsequent doses.

Drug Interactions Increased Effect/Toxicity: Drug interactions have not been studied in a controlled manner; however, drugs that interact with conventional amphotericin B may also interact with amphotericin B liposome for injection. See Drug Interactions - Increased Effect/Toxicity in Amphotericin B (Conventional) monograph.

Pharmacodynamics/Kinetics

Distribution: V_d: 131 L/kg

Half-life elimination: Terminal: 174 hours

Pregnancy Risk Factor B

Generic Available No

Comments Amphotericin B, liposomal is a true single bilayer liposomal drug delivery system. Liposomes are closed, spherical vesicles created by mixing specific proportions of amphophilic substances such as phospholipids and cholesterol so that they arrange themselves into multiple concentric bilayer membranes when hydrated in aqueous solutions. Single bilayer liposomes are then formed by microemulsification of multilamellar vesicles using a homogenizer. Amphotericin B, liposomal consists of these unilamellar bilayer liposomes with amphotericin B intercalated within the membrane. Due to the nature and quantity of amphophilic substances used, and the lipophilic moiety in the amphotericin B molecule, the drug is an integral part of the overall structure of the amphotericin B liposomes. Amphotericin B, liposomal contains true liposomes that are <100 nm in diameter.

Ampicillin (am pi SIL in)

Related Information

Antibiotic Prophylaxis, Preprocedural Guidelines for Dental Patients *on page 1507*

Cardiovascular Diseases *on page 1456*

U.S. Brand Names Marcillin®; Principen®

Canadian Brand Names Apo®-Ampi; Novo-Ampicillin; Nu-Ampi

Mexican Brand Names Anglopen®; Binotal; Dibacilina; Flamicina®; Lampicin®; Marovilina®; Omnipen®; Pentrexyl; Sinaplin®

Pharmacologic Category Antibiotic, Penicillin

Synonyms Aminobenzylpenicillin; Ampicillin Sodium; Ampicillin Trihydrate

Use

Dental: I.V. or I.M. administration for the prevention of bacterial endocarditis in patients not allergic to penicillin and unable to take oral medications

Medical: Treatment of susceptible bacterial infections (nonbeta-lactamase-producing organisms); susceptible bacterial infections caused by streptococci, pneumococci, nonpenicillinase-producing staphylococci, *Listeria*, meningococci; some strains of *H. influenzae, Salmonella, Shigella, E. coli, Enterobacter*, and *Klebsiella*

Local Anesthetic/Vasoconstrictor Precautions No information available to require special precautions

Effects on Dental Treatment 1% to 10%: Vomiting, oral candidiasis, allergic reaction (serum sickness, urticaria, angioedema, bronchospasm, hypotension)

Dosage

Neonates: I.M., I.V.:

Postnatal age ≤7 days:

≤2000 g: Meningitis: 50 mg/kg/dose every 12 hours; other infections: 25 mg/kg/dose every 12 hours

>2000 g: Meningitis: 50 mg/kg/dose every 8 hours; other infections: 25 mg/kg/dose every 8 hours

Postnatal age >7 days:

<1200 g: Meningitis: 50 mg/kg/dose every 12 hours; other infections: 25 mg/kg/dose every 12 hours

1200-2000 g: Meningitis: 50 mg/kg/dose every 8 hours; other infections: 25 mg/kg/dose every 8 hours

>2000 g: Meningitis: 50 mg/kg/dose every 6 hours; other infections: 25 mg/kg/dose every 6 hours

Infants and Children: I.M., I.V.: 100-400 mg/kg/day in doses divided every 4-6 hours

Meningitis: 200 mg/kg/day in doses divided every 4-6 hours; maximum dose: 12 g/day

Children: Oral: 50-100 mg/kg/day in doses divided every 6 hours; maximum dose: 2-3 g/day

Adults:

Oral: 250-500 mg every 6 hours

I.M.: 500 mg to 1.5 g every 4-6 hours

I.V.: 500 mg to 3 g every 4-6 hours; maximum dose: 12 g/day

Sepsis/meningitis: 150-250 mg/kg/24 hours divided every 3-4 hours

Dosing interval in renal impairment:

Cl_{cr} 30-50 mL/minute: Administer every 6-8 hours

Cl_{cr} 10-30 mL/minute: Administer every 8-12 hours

Cl_{cr} <10 mL/minute: Administer every 12 hours

Hemodialysis: Moderately dialyzable (20% to 50%); administer dose after dialysis

Peritoneal dialysis: Moderately dialyzable (20% to 50%)

Administer 250 mg every 12 hours

Continuous arteriovenous or venovenous hemofiltration effects: Dose as for Cl_{cr} 10-50 mL/minute; ~50 mg of ampicillin per liter of filtrate is removed

Mechanism of Action Inhibits bacterial cell wall synthesis by binding to one or more of the penicillin binding proteins (PBPs); which in turn inhibits the final transpeptidation step of peptidoglycan synthesis in bacterial cell walls, thus inhibiting cell wall biosynthesis. Bacteria eventually lyse due to ongoing activity of cell wall autolytic enzymes (autolysins and murein hydrolases) while cell wall assembly is arrested.

Other Adverse Effects

>10%: Local: Pain at injection site

1% to 10%:

Dermatologic: Rash (differentiate, if possible; nonallergic ampicillin rash from hypersensitivity reaction; incidence higher with pre-existing viral infections, *Salmonella* infections, lymphocytic leukemia, or hyperuricemia)

Gastrointestinal: Diarrhea, abdominal cramps

<1%: **Penicillin encephalopathy, seizures** (large I.V. doses or renal dysfunction), anemia, hemolytic anemia, thrombocytopenia, thrombocytopenic purpura, eosinophilia, leukopenia, granulocytopenia, decreased lymphocytes, interstitial nephritis (rare)

Contraindications Hypersensitivity to ampicillin, any component of the formulation, or other penicillins

(Continued)

Ampicillin *(Continued)*

Warnings/Precautions Dosage adjustment may be necessary in patients with renal impairment; a low incidence of cross-allergy with other beta-lactams exists; high percentage of patients with infectious mononucleosis have developed rash during therapy with ampicillin. Appearance of a rash should be carefully evaluated to differentiate a nonallergic ampicillin rash from a hypersensitivity reaction. Ampicillin rash occurs in 5% to 10% of children receiving ampicillin and is a generalized dull red, maculopapular rash, generally appearing 3-14 days after the start of therapy. It normally begins on the trunk and spreads over most of the body. It may be most intense at pressure areas, elbows, and knees.

Drug Interactions

Allopurinol: Theoretically has an additive potential for ampicillin/amoxicillin rash

Aminoglycosides: May be synergistic against selected organisms

Oral contraceptives: Anecdotal reports suggesting decreased contraceptive efficacy with penicillins have been refuted by more rigorous scientific and clinical data.

Probenecid, disulfiram: May increase levels of penicillins (ampicillin)

Warfarin: Effects of warfarin may be increased

Dietary/Ethanol/Herb Considerations Food decreases absorption rate and may decrease serum concentration; administer on an empty stomach 1 hour before or 2 hours after meals.

Pharmacodynamics/Kinetics

Absorption: Oral: 50%

Distribution: Bile, blister, and tissue fluids; penetration into CSF occurs with inflamed meninges only, good only with inflammation (exceeds usual MICs)

Normal meninges: Nil; Inflamed meninges: 5% to 10%

Protein binding: 15% to 25%

Half-life elimination:

Neonates: 2-7 days: 4 hours; 8-14 days: 2.8 hours; 15-30 days: 1.7 hours

Children and Adults: 1-1.8 hours

Anuria/end-stage renal disease: 7-20 hours

Time to peak: Oral: Within 1-2 hours

Excretion: Urine (~90% as unchanged drug) within 24 hours

Pregnancy Risk Factor B

Dosage Forms CAP: 250 mg, 500 mg; (Marcillin®): 500 mg; (Principen®): 250 mg, 500 mg. **INJ, powder for reconstitution:** 125 mg, 250 mg, 500 mg, 1 g, 2 g, 10 g. **POWDER, oral suspension** (Principen®): 125 mg/5 mL (100 mL, 200 mL); 250 mg/5 mL (100 mL, 200 mL)

Generic Available Yes

Selected Readings

Dajani AS, Taubert KA, Wilson W, et al, "Prevention of Bacterial Endocarditis. Recommendations by the American Heart Association," *JAMA* 1997, 277(22):1794-801.

Dajani AS, Taubert KA, Wilson W, et al, "Prevention of Bacterial Endocarditis: Recommendations by the American Heart Association," *J Am Dent Assoc* 1997, 128(8):1142-51.

Wynn RL, Bergman SA, Meiller TF, et al, "Antibiotics in Treating Oral-Facial Infections of Odontogenic Origin: An Update", *Gen Dent*, 2001, 49(3):238-40, 242, 244 passim.

Ampicillin and Sulbactam (am pi SIL in & SUL bak tam)

Related Information

Ampicillin *on page 103*

U.S. Brand Names Unasyn®

Canadian Brand Names Unasyn®

Mexican Brand Names Unasyna; Unasyna Oral

Pharmacologic Category Antibiotic, Penicillin

Synonyms Sulbactam and Ampicillin

Use

Dental: Parenteral beta-lactamase-resistant antibiotic combination in treatment of more severe orofacial infections where beta-lactamase-producing staphylococci and beta-lactamase-producing *Bacteroides* are present

Medical: Treatment of susceptible bacterial infections involved with skin and skin structure, intra-abdominal infections, gynecological infections; spectrum is that of ampicillin plus organisms producing beta-lactamases such as *S. aureus*, *H. influenzae*, *E. coli*, *Klebsiella*, *Acinetobacter*, *Enterobacter*, and anaerobes

Local Anesthetic/Vasoconstrictor Precautions No information available to require special precautions

Effects on Dental Treatment Prolonged use of penicillins may lead to development of oral candidiasis.

>10%: Pain at injection site (I.M.)

1% to 10%: **Allergic reaction (serum sickness, urticaria, bronchospasm, hypotension), pain at injection site (I.V.)**

Dosage Unasyn® (ampicillin/sulbactam) is a combination product. Each 3 g vial contains 2 g of ampicillin and 1 g of sulbactam. Sulbactam has very little antibacterial activity by itself, but effectively extends the spectrum of ampicillin to include beta-lactamase producing strains that are resistant to ampicillin alone. Therefore, dosage recommendations for Unasyn® are based on the ampicillin component.

I.M., I.V.:

Children (3 months to 12 years): 100-200 mg ampicillin/kg/day (150-300 mg Unasyn®) divided every 6 hours; maximum dose: 8 g ampicillin/day (12 g Unasyn®)

Adults: 1-2 g ampicillin (1.5-3 g Unasyn®) every 6-8 hours; maximum dose: 8 g ampicillin/day (12 g Unasyn®)

Dosing interval in renal impairment:

Cl_{cr} 15-29 mL/minute: Administer every 12 hours

Cl_{cr} 5-14 mL/minute: Administer every 24 hours

Mechanism of Action The addition of sulbactam, a beta-lactamase inhibitor, to ampicillin extends the spectrum of ampicillin to include some beta-lactamase producing organisms; inhibits bacterial cell wall synthesis by binding to one or more of the penicillin binding proteins (PBPs); which in turn inhibits the final transpeptidation step of peptidoglycan synthesis in bacterial cell walls, thus inhibiting cell wall biosynthesis. Bacteria eventually lyse due to ongoing activity of cell wall autolytic enzymes (autolysins and murein hydrolases) while cell wall assembly is arrested.

Other Adverse Effects

1% to 10%:

Dermatologic: Rash

Gastrointestinal: Diarrhea

<1%: **Chest pain, fatigue, malaise, headache**, chills, **penicillin encephalopathy, seizures** (large I.V. doses or renal dysfunction), itching, **nausea, vomiting**, enterocolitis, **pseudomembranous colitis, hairy tongue**, dysuria, vaginitis, leukopenia, neutropenia, thrombocytopenia, decreased hemoglobin and hematocrit, increased liver enzymes, thrombophlebitis, increased BUN/creatinine, interstitial nephritis (rare)

Contraindications Hypersensitivity to ampicillin, sulbactam, penicillins, or any component of the formulations

Warnings/Precautions Dosage adjustment may be necessary in patients with renal impairment; a low incidence of cross-allergy with other beta-lactams exists; high percentage of patients with infectious mononucleosis have developed rash during therapy with ampicillin. Appearance of a rash should be carefully evaluated to differentiate a nonallergic ampicillin rash from a hypersensitivity reaction. Ampicillin rash occurs in 5% to 10% of children receiving ampicillin and is a generalized dull red, maculopapular rash, generally appearing 3-14 days after the start of therapy. It normally begins on the trunk and spreads over most of the body. It may be most intense at pressure areas, elbows, and knees.

Drug Interactions

Allopurinol: Theoretically has an additive potential for ampicillin/amoxicillin rash

Aminoglycosides: May be synergistic against selected organisms

Oral contraceptives: Anecdotal reports suggesting decreased contraceptive efficacy with penicillins have been refuted by more rigorous scientific and clinical data.

Probenecid, disulfiram: May increase levels of penicillins (ampicillin)

Warfarin: Effects of warfarin may be increased

Pharmacodynamics/Kinetics

Ampicillin: See Ampicillin monograph.

Sulbactam:

Distribution: Bile, blister, and tissue fluids

Protein binding: 38%

Half-life elimination: Normal renal function: 1-1.3 hours

Excretion: Urine (~75% to 85% as unchanged drug) within 8 hours

Pregnancy Risk Factor B

Dosage Forms INJ, powder for reconstitution: 1.5 g [ampicillin sodium 1 g and sulbactam sodium 0.5 g]; 3 g [ampicillin sodium 2 g and sulbactam sodium 1 g]; 15 g [ampicillin sodium 10 g and sulbactam sodium 5 g] [bulk package]

Generic Available No

Comments In maxillary sinus, anterior nasal cavity, and deep neck infections, beta-lactamase-producing staphylococci and beta-lactamase-producing *Bacteroides* usually are present. In these situations, antibiotics that resist the beta-lactamase enzyme should be administered. Amoxicillin and clavulanic acid is administered orally for moderate infections. Ampicillin sodium and sulbactam sodium (Unasyn®) is administered parenterally for more severe infections.

Selected Readings

Wynn RL and Bergman SA, "Antibiotics and Their Use in the Treatment of Orofacial Infections, Part I," *Gen Dent*, 1994, 42(5):398, 400, 402.

Wynn RL and Bergman SA, "Antibiotics and Their Use in the Treatment of Orofacial Infections, Part II," *Gen Dent*, 1994, 42(6):498-502.

Ampicillin Sodium *see* Ampicillin *on page 103*

Ampicillin Trihydrate *see* Ampicillin *on page 103*

Amprenavir (am PRE na veer)

Related Information

HIV Infection and AIDS *on page 1482*

Tuberculosis *on page 1493*

(Continued)

Amprenavir *(Continued)*

U.S. Brand Names Agenerase®

Canadian Brand Names Agenerase®

Pharmacologic Category Antiretroviral Agent, Protease Inhibitor

Use Treatment of HIV infections in combination with at least two other antiretroviral agents; oral solution should only be used when capsules or other protease inhibitors are not therapeutic options

Local Anesthetic/Vasoconstrictor Precautions No information available to require special precautions

Effects on Dental Treatment

>10%: Perioral tingling/numbness, nausea (38% to 73%), vomiting (20% to 29%)

1% to 10%: Taste disorder, headache, paresthesia, fatigue

Dosage Capsule and oral solution are **not** interchangeable on a mg-per-mg basis.

Oral:

Capsule:

Children 4-12 years and older (<50 kg): 20 mg/kg twice daily or 15 mg/kg 3 times daily; maximum: 2400 mg/day

Children >13 years (>50 kg) and Adults: 1200 mg twice daily

Note: Dosing adjustments for amprenavir when administered in combination therapy:

Efavirenz: Adjustments necessary for both agents:

Amprenavir 1200 mg 3 times/day (single protease inhibitor) **or**

Amprenavir 1200 mg twice daily plus ritonavir 200 mg twice daily

Ritonavir: Adjustments necessary for both agents:

Amprenavir 1200 mg plus ritonavir 200 mg once daily **or**

Amprenavir 600 mg plus ritonavir 100 mg twice daily

Solution:

Children 4-12 years or older (up to 16 years weighing <50 kg): 22.5 mg/kg twice daily or 17 mg/kg 3 times daily; maximum: 2800 mg/day

Children 13-16 years (weighing at least 50 kg) or >16 years and Adults: 1400 mg twice daily

Dosing adjustment in renal impairment: Solution is contraindicated in renal failure.

Dosing adjustment in hepatic impairment:

Child-Pugh score between 5-8:

Capsule: 450 mg twice daily

Solution: 513 mg twice daily; contraindicated in hepatic failure

Child-Pugh score between 9-12:

Capsule: 300 mg twice daily

Solution: 342 mg twice daily; contraindicated in hepatic failure

Mechanism of Action Binds to the protease activity site and inhibits the activity of the enzyme. HIV protease is required for the cleavage of viral polyprotein precursors into individual functional proteins found in infectious HIV. Inhibition prevents cleavage of these polyproteins, resulting in the formation of immature, noninfectious viral particles.

Other Adverse Effects Protease inhibitors cause dyslipidemia which includes elevated cholesterol and triglycerides and a redistribution of body fat centrally to cause "protease paunch," buffalo hump, facial atrophy, and breast enlargement.

>10%:

Central nervous system: Depression (4% to 15%)

Dermatologic: Rash (28%)

Endocrine & metabolic: Hyperglycemia (37% to 41%), hypertriglyceridemia (36% to 47%)

Gastrointestinal: Diarrhea (33% to 56%)

1% to 10%:

Dermatologic: Stevens-Johnson syndrome (1% of total, 4% of patients who develop a rash)

Endocrine & metabolic: Hypercholesterolemia (4% to 9%)

Drug Interactions Substrate of CYP2C8/9, **3A4**; Inhibits CYP2C19, **3A4**

Increased Effect/Toxicity:

Concurrent use of cisapride, pimozide, quinidine, and rifampin is contraindicated. Serum concentrations/effect of many benzodiazepines may be increased; concurrent use of midazolam or triazolam is contraindicated. Concurrent use of ergot alkaloids (dihydroergotamine, ergotamine, ergonovine, methylergonovine) with amprenavir is also contraindicated (may cause vasospasm and peripheral ischemia).

Concurrent use of oral solution with disulfiram or metronidazole is contraindicated (risk of propylene glycol toxicity). Serum concentrations of amiodarone, lidocaine, quinidine and other antiarrhythmics may be increased, potentially leading to toxicity. HMG-CoA reductase inhibitors serum concentrations may be increased by amprenavir, increasing the risk of myopathy/rhabdomyolysis; lovastatin and simvastatin are contraindicated; fluvastatin and pravastatin may be safer alternatives. Serum concentrations/effect of benzodiazepines, calcium channel blockers, cyclosporine, itraconazole, ketoconazole, rifabutin, tacrolimus, tricyclic antidepressants may be increased. May increase warfarin's effects, monitor INR.

Sildenafil serum concentrations may be increased by amprenavir; when used concurrently, do not exceed a maximum sildenafil dose of 25 mg in a 48-hour period. Concurrent therapy with ritonavir may result in increased serum concentrations: dosage adjustment is recommended. Clarithromycin, indinavir, nelfinavir may increase serum concentrations of amprenavir.

Decreased Effect: Enzyme-inducing agents (rifampin, phenobarbital, phenytoin) may decrease serum concentrations/effect of amprenavir; rifampin is contraindicated. The administration of didanosine (buffered formulation) should be separated from amprenavir by 1 hour to limit interaction between formulations. Serum concentrations of estrogen (oral contraceptives) may be decreased, use alternative (nonhormonal) forms of contraception. Dexamethasone may decrease the therapeutic effect of amprenavir. Serum concentrations of delavirdine may be decreased; may lead to loss of virologic response and possible resistance to delavirdine; concomitant use is not recommended. Efavirenz and nevirapine may decrease serum concentrations of amprenavir (dosing for combinations not established). Avoid St John's wort (may lead to subtherapeutic concentrations of amprenavir). Effect of amprenavir may be diminished when administered with methadone (consider alternative antiretroviral); in addition, effect of methadone may be reduced (dosage increase may be required).

Dietary/Ethanol/Herb Considerations

Ethanol: Avoid use with oral solution.

Food: May be taken with food; avoid high-fat meals (levels increased 6-fold). Buttermilk, boiled milk, or yogurt may reduce diarrhea. Formulations contain vitamin E; avoid additional supplements.

Herb/Nutraceutical: Avoid St John's wort; may decrease serum concentration. Capsules contain 109 int. units of vitamin E per capsule; oral solution contains 46 int. units of vitamin E per mL.

Pharmacodynamics/Kinetics

Absorption: 63%

Distribution: 430 L

Protein binding: 90%

Metabolism: Hepatic via CYP (primarily CYP3A4)

Bioavailability: Not established; increased sixfold with high-fat meal

Half-life elimination: 7.1-10.6 hours

Time to peak: 1-2 hours

Excretion: Feces (75%); urine (14% as metabolites)

Pregnancy Risk Factor C

Generic Available No

Selected Readings Kaul DR, Cinti SK, Carver PL, et al, "HIV Protease Inhibitors: Advances in Therapy and Adverse Reactions, Including Metabolic Complications," *Pharmacotherapy*, 1999, 19(3):281-98.

AMPT *see* Metyrosine *on page 905*

Amrinone *see* Inamrinone *on page 716*

Amrinone Lactate *see* Inamrinone *on page 716*

Amyl Nitrite (AM il NYE trite)

Pharmacologic Category Antidote; Vasodilator

Synonyms Isoamyl Nitrite

Use Coronary vasodilator in angina pectoris; adjunct in treatment of cyanide poisoning; produce changes in the intensity of heart murmurs

Local Anesthetic/Vasoconstrictor Precautions No information available to require special precautions

Effects on Dental Treatment 1% to 10%: Postural hypotension, cutaneous flushing of head, neck, and clavicular area, tachycardia, headache, restlessness, nausea, vomiting

Dosage Nasal inhalation:

Cyanide poisoning: Children and Adults: Inhale the vapor from a 0.3 mL crushed ampul every minute for 15-30 seconds until I.V. sodium nitrite infusion is available

Angina: Adults: 1-6 inhalations from 1 crushed ampul; may repeat in 3-5 minutes

Other Adverse Effects <1% (Limited to important or life-threatening): Hemolytic anemia

Drug Interactions Increased Effect/Toxicity: Ethanol taken with amyl nitrite may have additive side effects. Avoid concurrent use of sildenafil - severe reactions may result.

Pharmacodynamics/Kinetics

Onset of action: Angina: Within 30 seconds

Duration: 3-15 minutes

Pregnancy Risk Factor X

Generic Available Yes

Amylobarbitone *see* Amobarbital *on page 90*

Amytal® *see* Amobarbital *on page 90*

Anacin PM Aspirin Free [OTC] *see* Acetaminophen and Diphenhydramine *on page 30*

Anadrol® *see* Oxymetholone *on page 1023*

Anafranil® *see* ClomiPRAMINE *on page 349*

Anagrelide (an A gre lide)

U.S. Brand Names Agrylin®

Canadian Brand Names Agrylin®

Pharmacologic Category Phospholipase A_2 Inhibitor

Synonyms Anagrelide Hydrochloride

Use Treatment of thrombocythemia (ET), secondary to myeloproliferative disorders, to reduce the elevated platelet count and the risk of thrombosis, and to ameliorate associated symptoms (including thrombohemorrhagic events)

Local Anesthetic/Vasoconstrictor Precautions No information available to require special precautions

Effects on Dental Treatment

>10%: Palpitations (27%), headache (44%), dizziness (15%)

1% to 10%: Chest pain (8%), tachycardia (7%), orthostatic hypotension, CHF, angina, atrial fibrillation, hypertension

Dosage Adults: Oral: 0.5 mg 4 times/day or 1 mg twice daily

Maintain for ≥1 week, then adjust to the lowest effective dose to reduce and maintain platelet count <600,000/µL ideally to the normal range; the dose must not be increased by >0.5 mg/day in any 1 week; maximum dose: 10 mg/day or 2.5 mg/dose

Elderly: There are no special requirements for dosing in the elderly

Mechanism of Action Anagrelide appears to inhibit cyclic nucleotide phosphodiesterase and the release of arachidonic acid from phospholipase, possibly by inhibiting phospholipase A_2. It also causes a dose-related reduction in platelet production, which results from decreased megakaryocyte hypermaturation. The drug disrupts the postmitotic phase of maturation.

Other Adverse Effects Frequency not defined:

Cardiovascular: Cardiomyopathy, complete heart block, pericardial perfusion (rare), MI (rare)

Central nervous system: Bad dreams, impaired concentration ability

Dermatologic: Ecchymosis (rare)

Hematologic: Anemia, thrombocytopenia, **lymphadenoma (rare)**

Respiratory: Pleural effusion

Drug Interactions Decreased Effect: There is a single case report that suggests sucralfate may interfere with anagrelide absorption.

Dietary/Ethanol/Herb Considerations Ethanol: Avoid use; may increase CNS adverse effects.

Pharmacodynamics/Kinetics

Duration: 6-24 hours

Metabolism: Hepatic

Half-life elimination, plasma: 1.3 hours

Time to peak, serum: 1 hour

Excretion: Urine (<1% as unchanged drug)

Pregnancy Risk Factor C

Generic Available No

Anagrelide Hydrochloride *see* Anagrelide *on page 108*

Anakinra (an a KIN ra)

U.S. Brand Names Kineret™

Canadian Brand Names Kineret™

Pharmacologic Category Antirheumatic, Disease Modifying; Interleukin-1 Receptor Antagonist

Synonyms IL-1Ra; Interleukin-1 Receptor antagonist

Use Reduction of signs and symptoms of moderately- to severely-active rheumatoid arthritis in adult patients who have failed one or more disease-modifying antirheumatic drugs (DMARDs); may be used alone or in combination with DMARDs (other than tumor necrosis factor-blocking agents)

Local Anesthetic/Vasoconstrictor Precautions No information available to require special precautions

Effects on Dental Treatment

>10%: Headache (12%), infection (40% versus 35% in placebo; serious infections in 2% to 7%); injection site reaction (≤71%; majority are mild, typically lasting 14-28 days) characterized by erythema, ecchymosis, inflammation, and pain

1% to 10%: Nausea (8%), sinusitis (7%), flu-like symptoms (6%)

Dosage Adults: S.C.:

Rheumatoid arthritis: 100 mg once daily (administer at approximately the same time each day)

Dosing adjustment in renal impairment: No specific guidelines for adjustment (clearance decreased by 70% to 75% in patients with Cl_{cr} <30 mL/minute)

Mechanism of Action Binds to the interleukin-1 (IL-1) receptor. IL-1 is induced by inflammatory stimuli and mediates a variety of immunological responses, including degradation of cartilage (loss of proteoglycans) and stimulation of bone resorption.

Other Adverse Effects

1% to 10%

Gastrointestinal: Diarrhea (7%), abdominal pain (5%)

Hematologic: Decreased WBCs (8%)

<1%: Neutropenia (0.3%)

Drug Interactions Increased Effect/Toxicity: Concurrent use of anakinra and etanercept has been associated with an increased risk of serious infection. Use caution with other drugs known to block or decrease the activity of tumor necrosis factor (TNF); includes infliximab and thalidomide.

Pharmacodynamics/Kinetics

Bioavailability: S.C.: 95%

Half-life elimination: Terminal: 4-6 hours

Time to peak: S.C.: 3-7 hours

Pregnancy Risk Factor B

Generic Available No

Ana-Kit® *see* Epinephrine and Chlorpheniramine Insect Sting Kit *on page 500*

Analpram-HC® *see* Pramoxine and Hydrocortisone *on page 1106*

Anamine® [OTC] *see* Chlorpheniramine and Pseudoephedrine *on page 308*

Anaplex® [OTC] *see* Chlorpheniramine and Pseudoephedrine *on page 308*

Anaprox® *see* Naproxen *on page 953*

Anaprox® DS *see* Naproxen *on page 953*

Anaspaz® *see* Hyoscyamine *on page 699*

Anastrozole (an AS troe zole)

U.S. Brand Names Arimidex®

Canadian Brand Names Arimidex®

Mexican Brand Names Arimidex®

Pharmacologic Category Antineoplastic Agent, Miscellaneous

Use Treatment of locally-advanced or metastatic breast cancer (ER-positive or hormone receptor unknown) in postmenopausal women; treatment of advanced breast cancer in postmenopausal women with disease progression following tamoxifen therapy; adjuvant treatment of early ER-positive breast cancer in postmenopausal women

Local Anesthetic/Vasoconstrictor Precautions No information available to require special precautions

Effects on Dental Treatment

>10%: Vasodilatation (25% to 35%), headache (9% to 13%), hot flashes (12% to 35%), cough (7% to 11%), pharyngitis (6% to 12%), pain (11% to 15%), weakness (16% to 17%), arthritis (14%)

1% to 10%: Xerostomia (6%), hypertension (5% to 9%), chest pain (5% to 7%), fever, confusion, nervousness, somnolence, dizziness (6%), anxiety (5%), vomiting (8% to 9%), paresthesia (5% to 6%), dyspnea (6% to 10%), sinusitis, bronchitis, rhinitis, infection (7%), flu-syndrome (5% to 7%), diaphoresis (2% to 4%), lethargy (1%)

Dosage Oral (refer to individual protocols): Adults: Breast cancer: 1 mg once daily (in advanced breast cancer, continue until tumor progression; in early breast cancer, optimal duration of therapy unknown)

Mechanism of Action Potent and selective nonsteroidal aromatase inhibitor. It significantly lowers serum estradiol concentrations and has no detectable effect on formation of adrenal corticosteroids or aldosterone. In postmenopausal women, the principal source of circulating estrogen is conversion of adrenally generated androstenedione to estrone by aromatase in peripheral tissues.

Other Adverse Effects

>10%:

Central nervous system: Depression (5% to 11%)

Neuromuscular & skeletal: Arthralgia (13%), back pain (8% to 12%), bone pain (5% to 11%)

1% to 10%:

Cardiovascular: Peripheral edema (5% to 10%)

Central nervous system: Insomnia (6% to 9%), malaise

Dermatologic: Rash (6% to 10%), alopecia, pruritus

Endocrine & metabolic: Hypercholesteremia (7%)

Gastrointestinal: Constipation (7% to 9%), abdominal pain (7% to 8%), diarrhea (7% to 8%), anorexia (5% to 7%), dyspepsia (5%), weight gain (2% to 8%), weight loss

Genitourinary: Urinary tract infection (6%), vulvovaginitis (6%), vaginal bleeding (5%) leukorrhea (2%), vaginal hemorrhage (2%), vaginal dryness (2%)

Hematologic: Anemia, leukopenia

Hepatic: Liver function tests increased, alkaline phosphatase increased

Local: Deep vein thrombosis, thrombophlebitis

(Continued)

Anastrozole *(Continued)*

Neuromuscular & skeletal: Osteoporosis (7%), fracture (7%), arthrosis (6%), hypertonia (3%), myalgia, arthralgia

Ocular: Cataracts (4%)

Miscellaneous: Lymph edema (9%)

<1%: Angina pectoris, CVA, cerebral ischemia, cerebral infarct, endometrial cancer, erythema multiforme, **MI,** myocardial ischemia, pulmonary embolus, retinal vein thrombosis, Stevens-Johnson syndrome, thrombophlebitis

Postmarketing and/or case reports: **Joint pain or stiffness**

Drug Interactions Inhibits CYP1A2, 2C8/9, 3A4

Decreased Effect: Concurrent use of estrogens may decrease efficacy of anastrozole. Tamoxifen decreases plasma concentration of anastrozole; avoid concurrent use.

Dietary/Ethanol/Herb Considerations Herb/Nutraceutical: Avoid St John's wort; may decrease serum concentration.

Pharmacodynamics/Kinetics

Onset of estradiol reduction: 24 hours

Duration of estradiol reduction: 6 days

Absorption: Well absorbed; not affected by food

Protein binding, plasma: 40%

Metabolism: Extensively hepatic (85%) via N-dealkylation, hydroxylation, and glucuronidation; primary metabolite inactive

Half-life elimination: 50 hours

Excretion: Urine (10% as unchanged drug; 60% as metabolites)

Pregnancy Risk Factor D

Generic Available No

Anatuss LA *see* Guaifenesin and Pseudoephedrine *on page 652*

Anbesol® [OTC] *see* Benzocaine *on page 169*

Anbesol® Baby [OTC] *see* Benzocaine *on page 169*

Anbesol® Maximum Strength [OTC] *see* Benzocaine *on page 169*

Ancef® *see* Cefazolin *on page 263*

Ancobon® *see* Flucytosine *on page 578*

Andehist DM NR Drops *see* Carbinoxamine, Pseudoephedrine, and Dextromethorphan *on page 247*

Andehist NR Drops *see* Carbinoxamine and Pseudoephedrine *on page 247*

Andehist NR Syrup *see* Brompheniramine and Pseudoephedrine *on page 201*

Androderm® *see* Testosterone *on page 1281*

AndroGel® *see* Testosterone *on page 1281*

Android® *see* MethylTESTOSTERone *on page 897*

Anestacon® *see* Lidocaine *on page 801*

Aneurine Hydrochloride *see* Thiamine *on page 1295*

Anexsia® *see* Hydrocodone and Acetaminophen *on page 678*

Anisindione (an is in DY one)

Related Information

Warfarin *on page 1397*

U.S. Brand Names Miradon®

Pharmacologic Category Anticoagulant, Indanedione

Use Prophylaxis and treatment of venous thrombosis, pulmonary embolism, and thromboembolic disorders; atrial fibrillation with risk of embolism; adjunct in the prophylaxis of systemic embolism following MI

Local Anesthetic/Vasoconstrictor Precautions No information available to require special precautions

Effects on Dental Treatment Signs of anisindione overdose may first appear as bleeding from gingival tissue; consultation with prescribing physician is advisable prior to surgery to determine temporary dose reduction or withdrawal of medication.

As with all anticoagulants, bleeding is the major adverse effect of warfarin. Hemorrhage may occur at virtually any site; risk is dependent on multiple variables, including the intensity of anticoagulation and patient susceptibility.

Other adverse effects are often related to idiosyncratic reactions; frequency cannot be accurately estimated:

Fever, headache nausea, GI bleeding, steatorrhea hemorrhage, hemoptysis, epistaxis, pharyngitis, hypersensitivity/allergic reactions

Dosage When discontinuing therapy, manufacturer recommends tapering dose over 3-4 weeks.

Oral: Adults:

Initial: 300 mg on first day, 200 mg on second day, 100 mg on third day

Maintenance dosage: Established by daily PT/INR determinations; range: 25-250 mg/day

Mechanism of Action Interferes with hepatic synthesis of vitamin K-dependent coagulation factors (II, VII, IX, X).

Other Adverse Effects Frequency not defined:

Cardiovascular: Vasculitis, edema, hemorrhagic shock

Dermatologic: Rash, dermatitis, exfoliative dermatitis, urticaria, alopecia

Gastrointestinal: Diarrhea

Genitourinary: Hematuria

Hematologic: Leukopenia, unrecognized bleeding sites (eg, colon cancer) may be uncovered by anticoagulation, retroperitoneal hematoma, agranulocytosis (higher incidence vs warfarin), red cell aplasia, anemia, thrombocytopenia, eosinophilia

Hepatic: Hepatitis, jaundice

Ocular: Paralysis of accommodation

Renal: Renal tubular necrosis, albuminuria, anuria, urine discoloration (red-orange)

Respiratory: Pulmonary hemorrhage

Skin necrosis/gangrene, due to paradoxical local thrombosis, is a known but rare risk of oral anticoagulant therapy. Its onset is usually within the first few days of therapy and is frequently localized to the limbs, breast, or penis. The risk of this effect is increased in patients with protein C or S deficiency. Additional adverse reactions associated with warfarin, but likely to also occur with indanediones, include priapism and skin necrosis ("purple toes" syndrome or cutaneous gangrene).

Drug Interactions

Increased Effect/Toxicity: Refer to Warfarin monograph.

Decreased Effect: Potential drug interactions are generally inferred from documented interactions with warfarin. Since anisindione has not been specifically characterized, it is difficult to extrapolate CYP-mediated interactions to this agent, and interactions based on this mechanism are speculative. Refer to Warfarin monograph.

Dietary/Ethanol/Herb Considerations

Ethanol: Avoid use; acute ingestion (binge drinking) decreases metabolism of oral anticoagulants and increases PT/INR. Chronic daily use (>3 drinks) increases the metabolism of oral anticoagulants and decreases PT/INR.

Food: Anticoagulant effects may be decreased if taken with foods rich in vitamin K; avoid large amounts of alfalfa, asparagus, beef/pork liver, broccoli, Brussels sprouts, cabbage, cauliflower, green tea, kale, lettuce, spinach, turnip greens, and watercress. Many enteral products contain large amounts of vitamin K. Do not change dietary habits once stabilized on oral anticoagulant therapy; a balanced diet with a consistent intake of vitamin K is essential (70-140 mcg/day). Vitamin E may increase anticoagulant effect. Small, frequent meals, frequent oral care, sucking lozenges, or chewing gum may reduce nausea and vomiting.

Herb/Nutraceutical: Avoid cat's claw, dong quai, evening primrose, feverfew, garlic, ginkgo biloba, ginseng, green tea, horse chestnut, and red clover, due to additional antiplatelet activity. Avoid St John's wort; may decrease oral anticoagulant serum concentration. Coenzyme Q_{10}; may decrease response to oral anticoagulants.

Pharmacodynamics/Kinetics

Onset of action: Anticoagulation: 36-72 hours

Peak effect: Full therapeutic effect: 5-7 days; INR may increase in 36-72 hours

Duration: 1-3 days

Metabolism: Hepatic

Pregnancy Risk Factor X

Generic Available No

Ansaid® *see* Flurbiprofen *on page 596*

Ansamycin *see* Rifabutin *on page 1179*

Antabuse® *see* Disulfiram *on page 459*

Antagon® *see* Ganirelix *on page 628*

Antazoline and Naphazoline *see* Naphazoline and Antazoline *on page 952*

Anthra-Derm® *see* Anthralin *on page 111*

Anthralin (AN thra lin)

U.S. Brand Names Anthra-Derm®; Drithocreme®; Drithocreme® HP 1%; Dritho-Scalp®; Micanol®

Canadian Brand Names Anthraforte®; Anthranol®; Anthrascalp®; Micanol®

Mexican Brand Names Anthranol®

Pharmacologic Category Antipsoriatic Agent; Keratolytic Agent

Synonyms Dithranol

Use Treatment of psoriasis (quiescent or chronic psoriasis)

Local Anesthetic/Vasoconstrictor Precautions No information available to require special precautions

Effects on Dental Treatment No significant effects or complications reported

Dosage Adults: Topical: Generally, apply once a day or as directed. The irritant potential of anthralin is directly related to the strength being used and each patient's individual tolerance. Always commence treatment for at least one week using the lowest strength possible.

(Continued)

Anthralin *(Continued)*

Skin application: Apply sparingly only to psoriatic lesions and rub gently and carefully into the skin until absorbed. Avoid applying an excessive quantity which may cause unnecessary soiling and staining of the clothing or bed linen.

Scalp application: Comb hair to remove scalar debris and, after suitably parting, rub cream well into the lesions, taking care to prevent the cream from spreading onto the forehead

Remove by washing or showering; optimal period of contact will vary according to the strength used and the patient's response to treatment. Continue treatment until the skin is entirely clear (ie, when there is nothing to feel with the fingers and the texture is normal)

Mechanism of Action Reduction of the mitotic rate and proliferation of epidermal cells in psoriasis by inhibiting synthesis of nucleic protein from inhibition of DNA synthesis to affected areas

Other Adverse Effects Dermatologic:

1% to 10%: Transient primary irritation of uninvolved skin; temporary discoloration of skin, hair, and fingernails; may also stain fabrics

<1%: Rash, excessive irritation

Drug Interactions Increased Effect/Toxicity: Long-term use of topical corticosteroids may destabilize psoriasis and withdrawal may also give rise to a "rebound" phenomenon. Allow an interval of at least 1 week between the discontinuance of topical corticosteroids and the commencement of therapy.

Pregnancy Risk Factor C

Generic Available No

Anthrax Vaccine (Adsorbed) (AN thraks vak SEEN ad zORBD)

Related Information

Immunizations (Vaccines) *on page 1612*

U.S. Brand Names BioThrax™

Pharmacologic Category Vaccine

Synonyms AVA

Use Immunization against *Bacillus anthracis*. Recommended for individuals who may come in contact with animal products which come from anthrax endemic areas and may be contaminated with *Bacillus anthracis* spores; recommended for high-risk persons such as veterinarians and other handling potentially infected animals. Routine immunization for the general population is not recommended.

The Department of Defense is implementing an anthrax vaccination program against the biological warfare agent anthrax, which will be administered to all active duty and reserve personnel.

Unlabeled/Investigational Use Postexposure prophylaxis in combination with antibiotics

Local Anesthetic/Vasoconstrictor Precautions No information available to require special precautions

Effects on Dental Treatment 1% to 7%: Headache (4% to 7%), fever (≤7%), vomiting (4%), nausea (≤ 4%), respiratory difficulty (4%)

Restrictions Not commercially available in the U.S.; presently, all anthrax vaccine lots are owned by the U.S. Department of Defense. The Centers for Disease Control (CDC) does not currently recommend routine vaccination of the general public. Federal law requires that the date of administration, the vaccine manufacturer, lot number of vaccine, and the administering person's name, title and address be entered into the patient's permanent medical record.

Dosage S.C.:

Children <18 years: Safety and efficacy have not been established

Children ≥18 years and Adults:

Primary immunization: Three injections of 0.5 mL each given 2 weeks apart, followed by three additional injections given at 6-, 12-, and 18 months; it is unnecessary to restart the series if a dose is not given on time; resume as soon as practical

Subsequent booster injections: 0.5 mL at 1-year intervals are recommended for immunity to be maintained

Elderly: Safety and efficacy have not been established for patients >65 years of age

Mechanism of Action Active immunization against *Bacillus anthracis*. The vaccine is prepared from a cell-free filtrate of *B. anthracis*, but no dead or live bacteria.

Other Adverse Effects Local reactions increase in severity by the fifth dose. Moderate local reactions (>5 cm) may be pruritic and may occur if given to a patient with a previous history of anthrax infection.

Includes pre- and postlicensure data; systemic reactions reported more often in women than in men.

>10%:

Central nervous system: Malaise (4% to 11%)

Local: Tenderness (58% to 71%), erythema (12% to 43%), subcutaneous nodule (4% to 39%), induration (8% to 21%), warmth (11% to 19%), local pruritus (7% to 19%)

Neuromuscular & skeletal: Arm motion limitation (7% to 12%)

1% to 10%:

Gastrointestinal: Anorexia (4%)

Local: Mild local reactions (edema/induration <30mm) (9%), edema (8%)

Neuromuscular & skeletal: Myalgia (4% to 7%)

<1%: Chills, body aches, delayed hypersensitivity reaction (started approximately day 17), moderate local reactions (edema/induration >30 mm and <120 mm), severe local reactions (edema/induration >120 mm in diameter or accompanied by marked limitation of arm motion or marked axillary node tenderness)

Postmarketing and/or case reports: **Anaphylaxis**, angioedema, aplastic anemia, arthralgia, aseptic meningitis, **asthma, atrial fibrillation**, cardiomyopathy, cellulitis, cerebrovascular accident, CNS lymphoma, cysts, collagen vascular disease, **dizziness**, encephalitis, **endocarditis, facial palsy**, fatigue, glomerulonephritis, Guillain-Barré syndrome, hearing disorder, idiopathic thrombocytopenia purpura, immune deficiency, inflammatory arthritis, injection site pain/tenderness, leukemia, liver abscess, lymphoma, mental status change, multiple sclerosis, myocarditis, neutropenia, pemphigus vulgaris, peripheral swelling, polyarteritis nodosa, **psychiatric disorders**, renal failure, **seizure, sepsis**, spontaneous abortion, **sudden cardiac arrest**, suicide, **syncope**, transverse myelitis, **tremors**, systemic lupus erythematosus, visual disorder

Drug Interactions Decreased Effect: Effect of vaccine may be decreased with chemotherapy, corticosteroids (high doses, ≥14 days), immunosuppressant agents and radiation therapy; consider waiting at least 3 months between discontinuing therapy and administering vaccine.

Pharmacodynamics/Kinetics Duration: Unknown; may be 1-2 years following two inoculations based on animal data

Pregnancy Risk Factor D

Generic Available No

Selected Readings "Anthrax Vaccine," *Med Lett Drugs Ther*, 1998, May 8;40(1026):52-3.

AntibiOtic® Ear *see* Neomycin, Polymyxin B, and Hydrocortisone *on page 963*

Antidigoxin Fab Fragments, Ovine *see* Digoxin Immune Fab *on page 443*

Antidiuretic Hormone *see* Vasopressin *on page 1379*

Antihemophilic Factor (Human)

(an tee hee moe FIL ik FAK tor HYU man)

U.S. Brand Names Alphanate®; Hemofil® M; Humate-P®; Koāte®-DVI; Monarc® M; Monoclate-P®

Canadian Brand Names Hemofil® M; Humate-P®

Pharmacologic Category Antihemophilic Agent; Blood Product Derivative

Synonyms AHF (Human); Factor VIII (Human)

Use Management of hemophilia A for patients in whom a deficiency in factor VIII has been demonstrated; can be of significant therapeutic value in patients with acquired factor VIII inhibitors not exceeding 10 Bethesda units/mL

Humate-P®: In addition, indicated as treatment of spontaneous bleeding in patients with severe von Willebrand disease and in mild and moderate von Willebrand disease where desmopressin is known or suspected to be inadequate

Orphan drug (Alphanate): Management of von Willebrand disease

Local Anesthetic/Vasoconstrictor Precautions No information available to require special precautions

Effects on Dental Treatment No significant effects or complications reported

Dosage Children and Adults: I.V.: Individualize dosage based on coagulation studies performed prior to treatment and at regular intervals during treatment; 1 AHF unit is the activity present in 1 mL of normal pooled human plasma; dosage should be adjusted to actual vial size currently stocked in the pharmacy. (General guidelines presented; consult individual product labeling for specific dosing recommendations.)

Dosage based on desired factor VIII increase (%):

To calculate dosage needed based on desired factor VIII increase (%):

Body weight (kg) x 0.5 int. units/kg x desired factor VIII increase (%) = int. units factor VIII required

For example:

50 kg x 0.5 int. units/kg x 30 (% increase) = 750 int. units factor VIII

Dosage based on expected factor VIII increase (%):

It is also possible to calculate the **expected** % factor VIII increase:

(# int. units administered x 2%/int. units/kg) divided by body weight (kg) = expected % factor VIII increase

For example:

(1400 int. units x 2%/int. units/kg) divided by 70 kg = 40%

General guidelines:

Minor Hemorrhage: Required peak postinfusion AHF level: 20% to 40% (10-20 int. units/kg), repeat dose every 12-24 hours for 1-3 days until bleeding is

(Continued)

Antihemophilic Factor (Human) *(Continued)*

resolved or healing achieved; mild superficial or early hemorrhages may respond to a single dose

Moderate hemorrhage: Required peak postinfusion AHF level: 30% to 60% (15-30 int. units/kg): Infuse every 12-24 hours for ≥3 days until pain and disability are resolved

Alternatively, a loading dose to achieve 50% (25 int. units/kg) may be given, followed by 10-15 int. units/kg dose given every 8-12 hours; may be needed for >7 days

Severe/life-threatening hemorrhage: Required peak postinfusion AHF level: 60% to 100% (30-50 int. units/kg): Infuse every 8-24 hours until threat is resolved

Alternatively, a loading dose to achieve 80% to 100% (40-50 int. units/kg) may be given, followed by 20-25 int. units/kg dose given every 8-12 hours for ≥14 days

Minor surgery: Required peak postinfusion AHF level: 30% to 80% (15-40 int. units/kg): Highly dependent upon procedure and specific product recommendations; for some procedures, may be administered as a single infusion plus oral antifibrinolytic therapy within 1 hour; in other procedures, may repeat dose every 12-24 hours as needed

Major surgery: Required peak pre- and postsurgery AHF level: 80% to 100% (40-50 int. units/kg): Administer every 6-24 hours until healing is complete (10-14 days)

Prophylaxis: May also be given on a regular schedule to prevent bleeding

If bleeding is not controlled with adequate dose, test for presence of inhibitor. It may not be possible or practical to control bleeding if inhibitor titers >10 Bethesda units/mL; antihemophilic factor (porcine) may be considered as an alternative

von Willebrand disease:

Treatment of hemorrhage in von Willebrand disease (Humate-P®): 1 int. units of factor VIII per kg of body weight would be expected to raise circulating vWF:RC of approximately 3.5-4 int. units/dL

Type 1, mild (if desmopressin is not appropriate): Major hemorrhage:

Loading dose: 40-60 int. units/kg

Maintenance dose: 40-50 int. units/kg every 8-12 hours for 3 days, keeping vWF:RC of nadir >50%; follow with 40-50 int. units/kg daily for up to 7 days

Type 1, moderate or severe:

Minor hemorrhage: 40-50 int. units/kg for 1-2 doses

Major hemorrhage:

Loading dose: 50-75 int. units/kg

Maintenance dose: 40-60 int. units/kg daily for up to 7 days

Types 2 and 3:

Minor hemorrhage: 40-50 int. units/kg for 1-2 doses

Major hemorrhage:

Loading dose: 60-80 int. units/kg

Maintenance dose: 40-60 int. units/kg every 8-12 hours for 3 days, keeping vWF:RC of nadir >50%; follow with 40-60 int. units/kg daily for up to 7 days

Elderly: Response not expected to differ from that of younger patients; dosage should be individualized

Mechanism of Action Protein (factor VIII) in normal plasma which is necessary for clot formation and maintenance of hemostasis; activates factor X in conjunction with activated factor IX; activated factor X converts prothrombin to thrombin, which converts fibrinogen to fibrin, and with factor XIII forms a stable clot

Other Adverse Effects <1%: Acute hemolytic anemia, **allergic reactions (rare), anaphylaxis (rare)**, anemia, blurred vision, **chest tightness**, chills, edema, **fever, headache**, hyperfibrinogenemia, **increased bleeding tendency, itching, jittery feeling**, lethargy, **nausea, paresthesias**, pruritus, **somnolence**, stinging at the infusion site, stomach discomfort, **tachycardia**, tingling, vasomotor reactions (rapid infusion), **vomiting**

Pharmacodynamics/Kinetics Half-life elimination: Mean: 12-17 hours with hemophilia A; consult specific product labeling

Pregnancy Risk Factor C

Generic Available Yes

Antihemophilic Factor (Porcine)

(an tee hee moe FIL ik FAK ter POR seen)

U.S. Brand Names Hyate:C®

Pharmacologic Category Antihemophilic Agent

Synonyms AHF (Porcine); Factor VIII (Porcine)

Use Management of hemophilia A in patients with antibodies to human factor VIII (consider use of human factor VIII in patients with antibody titer of <5 Bethesda units/mL); management of previously nonhemophilic patients with spontaneously-acquired inhibitors to human factor VIII, regardless of initial antihuman inhibitor titer

Local Anesthetic/Vasoconstrictor Precautions No information available to require special precautions

Effects on Dental Treatment 1% to 10%: Fever, headache, nausea, vomiting

Dosage Clinical response should be used to assess efficacy

Initial dose:

Antibody level to human factor VIII <50 Bethesda units/mL: 100-150 porcine units/kg (body weight) is recommended

Antibody level to human factor VIII >50 Bethesda units/mL: Activity of the antibody to antihemophilic (porcine) should be determined; **an antiporcine antibody level** >20 Bethesda units/mL indicates that the patient is unlikely to benefit from treatment; for lower titers, a dose of 100-150 porcine units/kg is recommended

The initial dose may also be calculated using the following method:

1. Determine patient's antibody titer against porcine factor VIII
2. Calculate average plasma volume:
   (body weight kg) (average blood volume) (1 - hematocrit) = plasma volume
   (body weight kg) (80 mL/kg) (1 - hematocrit) = plasma volume
   Note: A hematocrit of 50% = 0.5 for the equation
3. Neutralizing dose:
   (plasma volume mL) (antibody titer Bethesda units/mL) = neutralizing dose units
   This is the predicted dose required to neutralize the circulating antibodies. An incremental dose must be added to the neutralizing dose in order to increase the plasma factor VIII to the desired level.
4. Incremental dose:
   (desired plasma factor VIII level) (body weight) divided by 1.5 = incremental dose units
5. Total dose = neutralizing dose + incremental dose = total dose units

If a patient has previously been treated with Hyate:C®, this may provide a guide to his likely response and, therefore, assist in estimation of the preliminary dose

Subsequent doses: Following administration of the initial dose, if the recovery of factor VIII in the patient's plasma is not sufficient, another larger dose should be administered; if recovery after the second dose is still insufficient, a third and larger dose may prove effective. Once appropriate factor VIII levels are achieved, dosing can be repeated every 6-8 hours.

Mechanism of Action Factor VIII is the coagulation portion of the factor VIII complex in plasma. Factor VIII acts as a cofactor for factor IX to activate factor X in the intrinsic pathway of blood coagulation.

Other Adverse Effects Reactions tend to lessen in frequency and severity as further infusions are given; hydrocortisone and/or antihistamines may help to prevent or alleviate side effects and may be prescribed as precautionary measures.

1% to 10%:

Central nervous system: Chills

Dermatologic: Rashes

<1% and case reports: **Anaphylaxis,** thrombocytopenia

Pharmacodynamics/Kinetics Half-life elimination: 10-11 hours (patients without detectable inhibitors)

Pregnancy Risk Factor C

Generic Available No

Antihemophilic Factor (Recombinant)

(an tee hee moe FIL ik FAK tor ree KOM be nant)

U.S. Brand Names Helixate® FS; Kogenate® FS; Recombinate™; ReFacto®

Canadian Brand Names Kogenate®; Kogenate® FS; Recombinate™; ReFacto®

Pharmacologic Category Antihemophilic Agent

Synonyms AHF (Recombinant); Factor VIII (Recombinant); rAHF

Use Management of hemophilia A for patients in whom a deficiency in factor VIII has been demonstrated; can be of significant therapeutic value in patients with acquired factor VIII inhibitors not exceeding 10 Bethesda units/mL

Orphan drug (ReFacto®): Control and prevention of hemorrhagic episodes; surgical prophylaxis for hemophilia A (congenital factor VIII deficiency or classic hemophilia)

Local Anesthetic/Vasoconstrictor Precautions No information available to require special precautions

Effects on Dental Treatment No significant effects or complications reported

Dosage Children and Adults: I.V.: Individualize dosage based on coagulation studies performed prior to treatment and at regular intervals during treatment; 1 AHF unit is the activity present in 1 mL of normal pooled human plasma; dosage should be adjusted to actual vial size currently stocked in the pharmacy. (General guidelines presented; consult individual product labeling for specific dosing recommendations.)

(Continued)

Antihemophilic Factor (Recombinant) *(Continued)*

Dosage based on desired factor VIII increase (%):

To calculate dosage needed based on desired factor VIII increase (%):

Body weight (kg) x 0.5 int. units/kg x desired factor VIII increase (%) = int. units factor VIII required

For example:

50 kg x 0.5 int. units/kg x 30 (% increase) = 750 int. units factor VIII

Dosage based on expected factor VIII increase (%):

It is also possible to calculate the **expected** % factor VIII increase:

(# int. units administered x 2%/int. units/kg) divided by body weight (kg) = expected % factor VIII increase

For example:

(1400 int. units x 2%/int. units/kg) divided by 70 kg = 40%

General guidelines:

Minor hemorrhage: Required peak postinfusion AHF level: 20% to 40% (10-20 int. units/kg); mild superficial or early hemorrhages may respond to a single dose; may repeat dose every 12-24 hours for 1-3 days until bleeding is resolved or healing achieved

Moderate hemorrhage/minor surgery: Required peak postinfusion AHF level: 30% to 60% (15-30 int. units/kg); repeat dose at 12-24 hours if needed; some products suggest continuing for ≥3 days until pain and disability are resolved

Severe/life-threatening hemorrhage: Required peak postinfusion AHF level: Initial dose: 80% to 100% (40-50 int. units/kg); maintenance dose: 40% to 50% (20-25 int. units/kg) every 8-12 hours until threat is resolved

Major surgery: Required peak pre- and postsurgery AHF level: ~100% (50 int. units/kg) give first dose prior to surgery and repeat every 6-12 hours until healing complete (10-14 days)

Prophylaxis: May also be given on a regular schedule to prevent bleeding

If bleeding is not controlled with adequate dose, test for presence of inhibitor. It may not be possible or practical to control bleeding if inhibitor titers >10 Bethesda units/mL; antihemophilic factor (porcine) may be considered as an alternative

Elderly: Response not expected to differ from that of younger patients; dosage should be individualized

Mechanism of Action Protein (factor VIII) in normal plasma which is necessary for clot formation and maintenance of hemostasis; activates factor X in conjunction with activated factor IX; activated factor X converts prothrombin to thrombin, which converts fibrinogen to fibrin, and with factor XIII forms a stable clot

Other Adverse Effects <1%, postmarketing, and/or case reports: Acne, **allergic reactions**, increased aminotransferase, **anaphylaxis, angina pectoris**, asthenia, increased bilirubin, chest discomfort, chills, cold feet, constipation, **cough**, increased CPK, depersonalization, diarrhea, **dizziness, dyspnea, epistaxis, facial flushing**, fatigue, **fever, headache, hypotension (slight)**, injection site reactions (burning, pruritus, erythema), lethargy, **nausea, increased perspiration,** rash, **rhinitis, somnolence, sore throat, tachycardia, unusual taste,** urticaria, **vasodilation**, abnormal vision, venous catheter access complications, **vomiting**

Pharmacodynamics/Kinetics Half-life elimination: Mean: 14-16 hours

Pregnancy Risk Factor C

Generic Available No

Antihist-1® [OTC] *see* Clemastine *on page 340*

Anti-inhibitor Coagulant Complex

(an tee-in HI bi tor coe AG yoo lant KOM pleks)

U.S. Brand Names Autoplex® T; Feiba VH Immuno®

Canadian Brand Names Feiba® VH Immuno

Pharmacologic Category Antihemophilic Agent; Blood Product Derivative

Synonyms Coagulant Complex Inhibitor

Use Patients with factor VIII inhibitors who are to undergo surgery or those who are bleeding

Local Anesthetic/Vasoconstrictor Precautions No information available to require special precautions

Effects on Dental Treatment No significant effects or complications reported

Dosage Dosage range: 25-100 factor VIII correctional units per kg depending on the severity of hemorrhage

Other Adverse Effects <1%: **Hypotension, flushing, fever, headache**, chills, rash, urticaria, disseminated intravascular coagulation, **anaphylaxis**, indications of protein sensitivity

Pregnancy Risk Factor C

Generic Available No

Antipyrine and Benzocaine (an tee PYE reen & BEN zoe kane)

Related Information

Benzocaine *on page 169*

U.S. Brand Names Allergen®; Auralgan®; Auroto®

Canadian Brand Names Auralgan®

Pharmacologic Category Otic Agent, Analgesic; Otic Agent, Cerumenolytic

Synonyms Benzocaine and Antipyrine

Use Temporary relief of pain and reduction of swelling associated with acute congestive and serous otitis media, swimmer's ear, otitis externa; facilitates ear wax removal

Local Anesthetic/Vasoconstrictor Precautions Information available to require special precautions

Effects on Dental Treatment No significant effects or complications reported

Dosage Otic: Fill ear canal; moisten cotton pledget, place in external ear, repeat every 1-2 hours until pain and congestion are relieved; for ear wax removal instill drops 3-4 times/day for 2-3 days

Other Adverse Effects <1%: **Hypersensitivity reactions**, local burning, edema, stinging, tenderness

Pregnancy Risk Factor C

Generic Available Yes

Antithrombin III (an tee THROM bin three)

U.S. Brand Names Thrombate III™

Canadian Brand Names Thrombate III®

Pharmacologic Category Anticoagulant; Blood Product Derivative

Synonyms AT III; Heparin Cofactor I

Use Agent for hereditary antithrombin III deficiency; has been used effectively for acquired antithrombin III deficiencies related to disseminated intravascular coagulation (DIC); may be useful during acute management of hepatic veno-occlusive disease

Orphan drug:

ATnativ®: Treatment of hereditary antithrombin III deficiency in connection with surgical or obstetrical procedures; treatment of thromboembolism

Thrombate III™: Replacement therapy in congenital deficiency of antithrombin III for prevention and treatment of thrombosis and pulmonary emboli

Local Anesthetic/Vasoconstrictor Precautions No information available to require special precautions

Effects on Dental Treatment Dizziness (2%)

Dosage Adults: After first dose of antithrombin III, level should increase to 120% of normal; thereafter maintain at levels >80%. Generally, achieved by administration of maintenance doses once every 24 hours. Initially and until patient is stabilized, measure antithrombin III level at least twice daily, thereafter once daily and always immediately before next infusion. 1 unit = quantity of antithrombin III in 1 mL of normal pooled human plasma; administration of 1 unit/1 kg raises AT-III level by 1% to 2%; assume plasma volume of 40 mL/kg.

Initial dosage (units) = [desired AT-III level % - baseline AT-III level %] x body weight (kg) divided by 1%/units/kg (eg, if a 70 kg adult patient had a baseline AT-III level of 57%, the initial dose would be (120% - 57%) x 70/1%/units/kg = 4410 units).

Measure antithrombin III preceding and 30 minutes after dose to calculate *in vivo* recovery rate; maintain level within normal range for 2-8 days depending on type of surgery or procedure.

Mechanism of Action Antithrombin III is the primary physiologic inhibitor of *in vivo* coagulation. It is an alpha$_2$-globulin. Its principal actions are the inactivation of thrombin, plasmin, and other active serine proteases of coagulation, including factors IXa, Xa, XIa, XIIa, and VIIa. The inactivation of proteases is a major step in the normal clotting process. The strong activation of clotting enzymes at the site of every bleeding injury facilitates fibrin formation and maintains normal hemostasis. Thrombosis in the circulation would be caused by active serine proteases if they were not inhibited by antithrombin III after the localized clotting process. Patients with congenital deficiency are in a prethrombotic state, even if asymptomatic, as evidenced by elevated plasma levels of prothrombin activation fragment, which are normalized following infusions of antithrombin III concentrate.

Other Adverse Effects <1% (Limited to important or life-threatening): **Lightheadedness, fever, chest tightness, chest pain, vasodilatory effects, edema**, urticaria, fluid overload, nausea, **foul taste in mouth**, cramps, bowel fullness, **hematoma formation**, film over eye, diuretic effects, **dyspnea**, thrombocytopenia, abdominal cramps, hives

Drug Interactions Increased Effect/Toxicity: Heparin's anticoagulant effects are potentiated by antithrombin III. Risk of hemorrhage with antithrombin III may be increased by thrombolytic agents, oral anticoagulants (warfarin), and drugs which affect platelet function (eg, aspirin, NSAIDs, dipyridamole, ticlopidine, clopidogrel, and IIb/IIIa antagonists).

Pregnancy Risk Factor C

Generic Available No

Antithymocyte Globulin (Equine) *see* Lymphocyte Immune Globulin *on page 831*

Antithymocyte Immunoglobulin *see* Lymphocyte Immune Globulin *on page 831*

Antivert® *see* Meclizine *on page 847*
Antizol® *see* Fomepizole *on page 609*
Anucort-HC® *see* Hydrocortisone *on page 688*
Anusol-HC® *see* Hydrocortisone *on page 688*
Anusol® HC-1 [OTC] *see* Hydrocortisone *on page 688*
Anusol® Ointment [OTC] *see* Pramoxine *on page 1105*
Anzemet® *see* Dolasetron *on page 465*
APAP *see* Acetaminophen *on page 27*
APAP and Tramadol *see* Acetaminophen and Tramadol *on page 32*
Apatate® [OTC] *see* Vitamin B Complex *on page 1392*
Aphedrid™ [OTC] *see* Triprolidine and Pseudoephedrine *on page 1356*
Aphrodyne® *see* Yohimbine *on page 1401*
Aphthasol™ *see* Amlexanox *on page 87*
A.P.L.® *see* Chorionic Gonadotropin (Human) *on page 320*
Aplisol® *see* Tuberculin Tests *on page 1362*
Aplonidine *see* Apraclonidine *on page 118*
APPG *see* Penicillin G Procaine *on page 1050*

Apraclonidine (a pra KLOE ni deen)

U.S. Brand Names Iopidine®

Canadian Brand Names Iopidine®

Pharmacologic Category $Alpha_2$ Agonist, Ophthalmic

Synonyms Aplonidine; Apraclonidine Hydrochloride; p-Aminoclonidine

Use Prevention and treatment of postsurgical intraocular pressure elevation

Local Anesthetic/Vasoconstrictor Precautions No information available to require special precautions

Effects on Dental Treatment

1% to 10%: Xerostomia (10%)

<3%: Arrhythmia, chest pain, facial edema, nervousness, somnolence, dizziness, headache, nausea, abnormal taste, paresthesia, asthma, pharyngitis, rhinitis

Dosage Adults: Ophthalmic:

0.5%: Instill 1-2 drops in the affected eye(s) 3 times/day; since apraclonidine 0.5% will be used with other ocular glaucoma therapies, use an approximate 5-minute interval between instillation of each medication to prevent washout of the previous dose

1%: Instill 1 drop in operative eye 1 hour prior to anterior segment laser surgery, second drop in eye immediately upon completion of procedure

Dosing adjustment in renal impairment: Although the topical use of apraclonidine has not been studied in renal failure patients, structurally related clonidine undergoes a significant increase in halflife in patients with severe renal impairment; close monitoring of cardiovascular parameters in patients with impaired renal function is advised if they are candidates for topical apraclonidine therapy

Dosing adjustment in hepatic impairment: Close monitoring of cardiovascular parameters in patients with impaired liver function is advised because the systemic dosage form of clonidine is partially metabolized in the liver

Mechanism of Action Apraclonidine is a potent alpha-adrenergic agent similar to clonidine; relatively selective for $alpha_2$-receptors but does retain some binding to $alpha_1$-receptors; appears to result in reduction of aqueous humor formation; its penetration through the blood-brain barrier is more polar than clonidine which reduces its penetration through the blood-brain barrier and suggests that its pharmacological profile is characterized by peripheral rather than central effects.

Other Adverse Effects

Ocular:

5% to 15%: Discomfort, hyperemia, pruritus 1% to 5%: Blanching, blurred vision, conjunctivitis, discharge, dry eye, foreign body sensation, lid edema, tearing

<1%: Abnormal vision, blepharitis, blepharoconjunctivitis, conjunctival edema, conjunctival follicles, corneal erosion, corneal infiltrate, corneal staining, edema, irritation, keratitis, keratopathy, lid disorder, lid erythema, lid margin crusting, lid retraction, lid scales, pain, photophobia

Systemic:

<3%:

Cardiovascular: Peripheral edema
Central nervous system: Depression, insomnia, malaise
Dermatologic: Contact dermatitis, dermatitis
Gastrointestinal: Constipation
Neuromuscular & skeletal: Abnormal coordination, myalgia, weakness
Respiratory: Parosmia

Postmarketing and/or case reports: **Bradycardia**

Drug Interactions Increased Effect/Toxicity: Topical beta-blockers, pilocarpine may have an additive effect on intraocular pressure.

Pharmacodynamics/Kinetics

Onset of action: 1 hour

Peak effect: Intraocular pressure: 3-5 hours

Pregnancy Risk Factor C
Generic Available No

Apraclonidine Hydrochloride *see* Apraclonidine *on page 118*
Apresazide® [DSC] *see* Hydralazine and Hydrochlorothiazide *on page 675*
Apri® *see* Combination Hormonal Contraceptives *on page 368*
Aprodine® [OTC] *see* Triprolidine and Pseudoephedrine *on page 1356*

Aprotinin (a proe TYE nin)

U.S. Brand Names Trasylol®
Canadian Brand Names Trasylol®
Mexican Brand Names Trasylol®
Pharmacologic Category Blood Product Derivative; Hemostatic Agent
Use Reduction or prevention of blood loss in patients undergoing coronary artery bypass surgery when a high risk of excessive bleeding exists, including open heart reoperation, pre-existing coagulopathies, operations on the great vessels, and when a patient's beliefs prohibit blood transfusions
Local Anesthetic/Vasoconstrictor Precautions No information available to require special precautions
Effects on Dental Treatment 1% to 10%: Atrial fibrillation, myocardial infarction, heart failure, atrial flutter, ventricular tachycardia, hypotension, supraventricular tachycardia, fever, confusion, dyspnea, bronchoconstriction
Dosage Test dose: **All** patients should receive a 1 mL I.V. test dose at least 10 minutes prior to the loading dose to assess the potential for allergic reactions. **Note:** To avoid physical incompatibility with heparin when adding to pump-prime solution, each agent should be added during recirculation to assure adequate dilution.

Regimen A (standard dose):
- 2 million units (280 mg) loading dose I.V. over 20-30 minutes
- 2 million units (280 mg) into pump prime volume
- 500,000 units/hour (70 mg/hour) I.V. during operation

Regimen B (low dose):
- 1 million units (140 mg) loading dose I.V. over 20-30 minutes
- 1 million units (140 mg) into pump prime volume
- 250,000 units/hour (35 mg/hour) I.V. during operation

Mechanism of Action Serine protease inhibitor; inhibits plasmin, kallikrein, and platelet activation producing antifibrinolytic effects; a weak inhibitor of plasma pseudocholinesterase. It also inhibits the contact phase activation of coagulation and preserves adhesive platelet glycoproteins making them resistant to damage from increased circulating plasmin or mechanical injury occurring during bypass

Other Adverse Effects

1% to 10%:
- Local: Phlebitis
- Renal: Increased potential for postoperative renal dysfunction

<1% (Limited to important or life-threatening): Cerebral embolism, cerebrovascular events, **convulsions**, hemolysis, liver damage, pulmonary edema

Drug Interactions

Increased Effect/Toxicity: Heparin and aprotinin prolong ACT; the ACT becomes a poor measure of adequate anticoagulation with the concurrent use of these drugs. Use with succinylcholine or tubocurarine may produce prolonged or recurring apnea.

Decreased Effect: Aprotinin blocks the fibrinolytic activity of thrombolytic agents (alteplase, streptokinase). The antihypertensive effects of captopril (and other ACE inhibitors) may be blocked; avoid concurrent use.

Pharmacodynamics/Kinetics

Half-life elimination: 2.5 hours
Excretion: Urine

Pregnancy Risk Factor B
Generic Available No

Aquacare® [OTC] *see* Urea *on page 1365*
Aquachloral® Supprettes® *see* Chloral Hydrate *on page 295*
Aqua Gem E® [OTC] *see* Vitamin E *on page 1393*
Aqua Lube Plus [OTC] *see* Nonoxynol 9 *on page 985*
AquaMEPHYTON® *see* Phytonadione *on page 1079*
Aquanil™ HC [OTC] *see* Hydrocortisone *on page 688*
Aquaphilic® With Carbamide [OTC] *see* Urea *on page 1365*
AquaSite® [OTC] *see* Artificial Tears *on page 128*
Aquasol A® *see* Vitamin A *on page 1390*
Aquasol E® [OTC] *see* Vitamin E *on page 1393*
Aquatab® *see* Guaifenesin and Pseudoephedrine *on page 652*
Aquatab® C *see* Guaifenesin, Pseudoephedrine, and Dextromethorphan *on page 653*
Aquatab® D Dose Pack *see* Guaifenesin and Pseudoephedrine *on page 652*
Aquatab® DM *see* Guaifenesin and Dextromethorphan *on page 651*

Aquatensen® *see* Methyclothiazide *on page 890*
Aquazide® H *see* Hydrochlorothiazide *on page 675*
Aqueous Procaine Penicillin G *see* Penicillin G Procaine *on page 1050*
Aqueous Testosterone *see* Testosterone *on page 1281*
Ara-A *see* Vidarabine *on page 1384*
Arabinofuranosyladenine *see* Vidarabine *on page 1384*
Arabinosylcytosine *see* Cytarabine *on page 389*
Ara-C *see* Cytarabine *on page 389*
Aralen® Phosphate *see* Chloroquine *on page 303*
Aranesp™ *see* Darbepoetin Alfa *on page 400*
Arava™ *see* Leflunomide *on page 779*
Aredia® *see* Pamidronate *on page 1029*
Arestin™ *see* Minocycline Hydrochloride Periodontal Microspheres *on page 916*

Argatroban (ar GA troh ban)

Pharmacologic Category Anticoagulant, Thrombin Inhibitor

Use Prophylaxis or treatment of thrombosis in adults with heparin-induced thrombocytopenia; adjunct to percutaneous coronary intervention (PCI) in patients who have or are at risk of thrombosis associated with heparin-induced thrombocytopenia

Local Anesthetic/Vasoconstrictor Precautions No information available to require special precautions

Effects on Dental Treatment As with all anticoagulants, bleeding is a potential adverse effect of argatroban during dental surgery; risk is dependent on multiple variables, including the intensity of anticoagulation and patient susceptibility. Medical consult is suggested. It is unlikely that ambulatory patients presenting for dental treatment will be taking intravenous anticoagulant therapy.

>10%: GI bleeding (14%; minor), vasodilation (14% in patients also receiving thrombolytic therapy and/or contrast media)

1% to 10%: Hypotension (7%), cardiac arrest (6%), ventricular tachycardia (5%), atrial fibrillation (3%), fever (7%), nausea (5%), vomiting (4%), dyspnea (8% to 10%), cough (3% to 10%), hemoptysis (minor, 3%), pneumonia (3%), sepsis (6%), infection (4%), GI bleeding (2%; major), pain (5%)

Dosage I.V.: Adults:

Heparin-induced thrombocytopenia:

Initial dose: 2 mcg/kg/minute

Maintenance dose: Measure aPTT after 2 hours, adjust dose until the steady-state aPTT is 1.5-3.0 times the initial baseline value, not exceeding 100 seconds; dosage should not exceed 10 mcg/kg/minute

Conversion to oral anticoagulant: Because there may be a combined effect on the INR when argatroban is combined with warfarin, loading doses of warfarin should not be used. Warfarin therapy should be started at the expected daily dose.

Patients receiving ≤2 mcg/kg/minute of argatroban: Argatroban therapy can be stopped when the combined INR on warfarin and argatroban is >4; repeat INR measurement in 4-6 hours; if INR is below therapeutic level, argatroban therapy may be restarted. Repeat procedure daily until desired INR on warfarin alone is obtained.

Patients receiving >2 mcg/kg/minute of argatroban: Reduce dose of argatroban to 2 mcg/kg/minute; measure INR for argatroban and warfarin 4-6 hours after dose reduction; argatroban therapy can be stopped when the combined INR on warfarin and argatroban is >4. Repeat INR measurement in 4-6 hours; if INR is below therapeutic level, argatroban therapy may be restarted. Repeat procedure daily until desired INR on warfarin alone is obtained.

Percutaneous coronary intervention (PCI):

Initial: Begin infusion of 25 mcg/kg/minute and administer bolus dose of 350 mcg/kg (over 3-5 minutes). ACT should be checked 5-10 minutes after bolus infusion; proceed with procedure if ACT >300 seconds. Following initial bolus:

ACT <300 seconds: Give an additional 150 mcg/kg bolus, and increase infusion rate to 30 mcg/kg/minute (recheck ACT in 5-10 minutes)

ACT >450 seconds: Decrease infusion rate to 15 mcg/kg/minute (recheck ACT in 5-10 minutes)

Once a therapeutic ACT (300-450 seconds) is achieved, infusion should be continued at this dose for the duration of the procedure.

Impending abrupt closure, thrombus formation during PCI, or inability to achieve ACT >300 sec: An additional bolus of 150 mcg/kg, followed by an increase in infusion rate to 40 mcg/kg/minute may be administered.

Dosing adjustment in hepatic impairment: Decreased clearance and increased elimination halflife are seen with hepatic impairment; dose should be reduced. Initial dose for moderate hepatic impairment is 0.5 mcg/kg/minute. **Note:** During PCI, avoid use in patients with elevations of ALT/AST (>3 x ULN); the use of argatroban in these patients has not been evaluated.

Mechanism of Action A direct, highly selective thrombin inhibitor. Reversibly binds to the active thrombin site of free and clot-associated thrombin. Inhibits fibrin formation; activation of coagulation factors V, VIII, and XIII; protein C; and platelet aggregation.

Other Adverse Effects

>10%: Genitourinary: Bleeding and hematuria (12%; minor)

1% to 10%:
- Cardiovascular: Cerebrovascular disorder
- Central nervous system: Intracranial bleeding (1%; only observed in patients also receiving streptokinase or tissue plasminogen activator)
- Gastrointestinal: Diarrhea (6%), abdominal pain (3%)
- Genitourinary: Urinary tract infection (5%)
- Hematologic: Decreased hemoglobin <2 g/dL and hematocrit (minor, 10%)
- Local: Bleeding at injection site (minor, 2% to 5%)
- Renal: Abnormal renal function (3%)

<1% (Limited to important or life-threatening): **Allergic reactions (eg, cough, dyspnea, rash, bullous eruption)**, hemoglobin and hematocrit decreased (major, 0.7%); limb and below-the-knee stump bleed; multisystem hemorrhage and DIC; retroperitoneal bleeding

Drug Interactions Substrate of CYP3A4

Increased Effect/Toxicity:
- Drugs which affect platelet function (eg, aspirin, NSAIDs, dipyridamole, ticlopidine, clopidogrel), anticoagulants, or thrombolytics may potentiate the risk of hemorrhage. Sufficient time must pass after heparin therapy is discontinued; allow heparin's effect on the aPTT to decrease
- Concomitant use of argatroban with warfarin increases PT and INR greater than that of warfarin alone. Argatroban is commonly continued during the initiation of warfarin therapy to assure anticoagulation and to protect against possible transient hypercoagulability.

Pharmacodynamics/Kinetics
- Onset of action: Immediate
- Distribution: 174 mL/kg
- Protein binding: Albumin: 20%; α_1-acid glycoprotein: 35%
- Metabolism: Hepatic via hydroxylation and aromatization. Metabolism via CYP3A4/5 to four known metabolites plays a minor role. Unchanged argatroban is the major plasma component. Plasma concentration of metabolite M1 is 0% to 20% of the parent drug and is three- to fivefold weaker.
- Half-life elimination: 39-51 minutes; Hepatic impairment: ≤181 minutes
- Time to peak: Steady-state: 1-3 hours
- Excretion: Feces (65%); urine (22%); low quantities of metabolites M2-4 in urine

Pregnancy Risk Factor B

Generic Available No

Arginine (AR ji neen)

U.S. Brand Names R-Gene®

Pharmacologic Category Diagnostic Agent

Synonyms Arginine Hydrochloride; L-Arginine

Use Pituitary function test (growth hormone); management of severe, uncompensated, metabolic alkalosis (pH ≥7.55) **after** optimizing therapy with sodium and potassium supplements

Local Anesthetic/Vasoconstrictor Precautions No information available to require special precautions

Effects on Dental Treatment 1% to 10%: Headache, nausea, vomiting, numbness

Dosage I.V.:

Pituitary function test:
- Children: 500 mg kg/dose administered over 30 minutes
- Adults: 30 g (300 mL) administered over 30 minutes

Inborn errors of urea synthesis: Initial: 0.8 g/kg, then 0.2-0.8 g/kg/day as a continuous infusion

Metabolic alkalosis: Children and Adults: ***Arginine hydrochloride is a fourth-line treatment for uncompensated metabolic alkalosis after sodium chloride, potassium chloride, and ammonium chloride supplementation has been optimized.***
- Arginine dose (G) = weight (kg) x 0.1 x (HCO_3^- - 24) where HCO_3^- = the patient's serum bicarbonate concentration in mEq/L
- Give 1/2 to 1/3 dose calculated then re-evaluate
- **Note:** Arginine hydrochloride should never be used as an alternative to chloride supplementation but used in the patient who is unresponsive to sodium chloride or potassium chloride supplementation

Hypochloremia: Children and Adults: Arginine dose (mL) = 0.4 x weight (kg) x (103-Cl^-) where Cl^- = the patient's serum chloride concentration in mEq/L
- Give 1/2 to 1/3 dose calculated then re-evaluate

Mechanism of Action

Stimulates pituitary release of growth hormone and prolactin through origins in the hypothalamus; patients with impaired pituitary function have lower or no increase

(Continued)

Arginine *(Continued)*

in plasma concentrations of growth hormone after administration of arginine. Arginine hydrochloride has been used for severe metabolic alkalosis due to its high chloride content.

Arginine hydrochloride has been used investigationally to treat metabolic alkalosis. Arginine contains 475 mEq of hydrogen ions and 475 mEq of chloride ions/L. Arginine is metabolized by the liver to produce hydrogen ions. It may be used in patients with relative hepatic insufficiency because arginine combines with ammonia in the body to produce urea.

Other Adverse Effects 1% to 10%:

Cardiovascular: Flushing (rapid I.V. infusion)

Local: Venous irritation

Pharmacodynamics/Kinetics

Absorption: Oral: Well absorbed

Time to peak, serum: ~2 hours

Pregnancy Risk Factor C

Generic Available No

Arginine Hydrochloride *see* Arginine *on page 121*

8-Arginine Vasopressin *see* Vasopressin *on page 1379*

Aricept® *see* Donepezil *on page 467*

Arimidex® *see* Anastrozole *on page 109*

Aripiprazole (ay ri PIP ray zole)

U.S. Brand Names Abilify™

Pharmacologic Category Antipsychotic Agent, Quinolone

Synonyms BMS 337039; OPC-14597

Use Treatment of schizophrenia

Unlabeled/Investigational Use Treatment of psychosis, bipolar disorder

Local Anesthetic/Vasoconstrictor Precautions No information available to require special precautions

Effects on Dental Treatment

>10%: Headache (32%), anxiety (25%), lightheadedness (11%), somnolence (11%), nausea (14%), vomiting (12%)

1% to 10%: Chest pain (1%), hypertension (1%), tachycardia (1%), hypotension (1%), bradycardia (1%), akathisia (10%), extrapyramidal symptoms (6%; similar to placebo), fever (2%), nervousness (1%), mania (1%), confusion (1%), tremor (3%), neck pain or rigidity (1%), cogwheel rigidity (1%), weakness (7%), rhinitis (4%), cough (3%), dyspnea (1%), pneumonia (1%), flu-like syndrome (1%), ecchymosis (1%)

Dosage Oral: Adults and Elderly: 10-15 mg once daily; may be increased to a maximum of 30 mg once daily (efficacy at dosages above 10-15 mg has not been shown to be increased). Dosage titration should not be more frequent than every 2 weeks.

Mechanism of Action Aripiprazole exhibits high affinity for D_2, D_3, $5\text{-}HT_{1A}$, and $5\text{-}HT_{2A}$ receptors; moderate affinity for D_4, $5\text{-}HT_{2C}$, $5\text{-}HT_7$, alpha, and H_1 receptors. It also possesses moderate affinity for the serotonin reuptake transporter; has no affinity for muscarinic receptors. Aripiprazole functions as a partial agonist at the D_2 and $5\text{-}HT_{1A}$ receptors, and as an antagonist at the $5\text{-}HT_{2A}$ receptor.

Other Adverse Effects

>10%

Central nervous system: Insomnia (24%)

Endocrine & metabolic: Weight gain (8% to 30%; highest frequency in patients with BMI <23)

1% to 6%

Cardiovascular: Edema (1% peripheral)

Central nervous system: Depression (1%)

Dermatologic: Rash (6%), pruritus (1%)

Endocrine & metabolic: Hypothyroidism (1%), weight loss (1%)

Gastrointestinal: Constipation (10%), anorexia (1%)

Genitourinary: Urinary incontinence (1%)

Hematologic: Anemia (1%)

Neuromuscular & skeletal: CPK increased (1%), muscle cramp (1%)

Ocular: Blurred vision (3%), conjunctivitis (1%)

<1%: Abnormal ejaculation, akinesia, albuminuria, alkaline phosphatase increased, alopecia, ALT increased, amblyopia, amnesia, anorgasmy, apathy, **apnea**, arthralgia, arthritis, aspiration pneumonia, AST increased, **asthma,** ataxia, **atrial fibrillation**, AV block, blunted affect, bradykinesia, buccoglossal syndrome, BUN increased, bursitis, cataract, cerebral ischemia, cholecystitis, cholelithiasis, colitis, cystitis, deafness, **dehydration, delirium, dental caries**, depersonalization, **diabetes mellitus**, dry eyes, **duodenal ulcer, dysphagia,** dystonia, dysuria, edema, eosinophilia, **epistaxis, esophagitis, euphoria,** exfoliative dermatitis, fecal impaction, **gastroenteritis, gastroesophageal reflux, GI hemorrhage, gingival hemorrhage, gingivitis, glossitis**, glycosuria, goiter,

gout, gynecomastia, **heart failure**, hematemesis, hematuria, **hemoptysis**, hepatitis, hepatomegaly, **hiccups**, hypercholesterolemia, hyperglycemia, hyperkalemia, hypernatremia, hyperthyroidism, hyperuricemia, hypoglycemia, hypokinesia, hypotonia, impaired concentration, impotence, incoordination, intestinal obstruction, intestinal perforation, intracranial hemorrhage, lactation (female), laryngitis, LDH increased, leukocytosis, leukopenia, lymphadenopathy, menorrhagia, **MI**, muscle spasm, myasthenia, myoclonus, myopathy, neuroleptic malignant syndrome, neuropathy, nocturia, obsessive thoughts, ocular hemorrhage, oculogyric crisis, pancreatitis, **panic attack, paresthesia, peptic ulcer**, photophobia, photosensitivity, priapism, pulmonary edema, pulmonary embolism, QT prolongation, renal calculus, renal failure, **respiratory failure**, rhabdomyolysis, serum creatinine increased, **stomatitis, stroke, stupor, tardive dyskinesia**, tendonitis, thrombocythemia, thrombocytopenia, tinnitus, **tongue edema**, urinary frequency, urinary retention, urolithiasis, urticaria, vaginal hemorrhage, **vasodilation**, vertigo

Drug Interactions Substrates of **CYP2D6, 3A4**

Increased Effect/Toxicity:

Inhibitors of CYP2D6 may increase serum concentrations of aripiprazole (and metabolite). Manufacturer recommends 50% reduction in aripiprazole dose during concurrent therapy with quinidine. Similar reductions may be required with other potent inhibitors. Inhibitors include amiodarone, cimetidine, delavirdine, fluoxetine, paroxetine, propafenone, quinidine, and ritonavir.

Inhibitors of CYP3A4 may increase serum concentrations of aripiprazole (metabolite concentrations are decreased). Manufacturer recommends a 50% reduction in dose during concurrent ketoconazole therapy. Similar reductions in dose may be required with other potent inhibitors. Inhibitors include amiodarone, cimetidine, clarithromycin, erythromycin, delavirdine, diltiazem, dirithromycin, disulfiram, fluoxetine, fluvoxamine, grapefruit juice, indinavir, itraconazole, ketoconazole, nefazodone, nevirapine, propoxyphene, quinupristin-dalfopristin, ritonavir, saquinavir, verapamil, zafirlukast, zileuton.

Decreased Effect: Enzyme inducers may decrease serum concentrations of aripiprazole (and metabolite). Manufacturer recommends a doubling of the aripiprazole dose when carbamazepine is added. Similar increases may be required with other inducers. Inducers include phenobarbital, phenytoin, rifampin and rifabutin. Withdrawal of an inducing agent may require a decrease in aripiprazole dose.

Dietary/Ethanol/Herb Considerations

Ethanol: Avoid use; may increase CNS depression.

Food: May be taken with food

Herb/Nutraceutical: Avoid kava kava, gotu kola, St John's wort, and valerian; may increase CNS depression. St John's wort may also decrease aripiprazole levels.

Pharmacodynamics/Kinetics

Onset: Initial: 1-3 weeks

Absorption: Well absorbed

Distribution: V_d: 4.9 L/kg

Protein binding: 99%, primarily to albumin

Metabolism: Hepatic, via CYP2D6, CYP3A4 (dehydro-aripiprazole metabolite has affinity for D2 receptors similar to the parent drug and represents 40% of the parent drug exposure in plasma)

Bioavailability: 87%

Half-life: Aripiprazole: 75 hours; dehydro-aripiprazole: 94 hours

Time to peak, plasma: 3-5 hours

Excretion: Feces (55%), urine (25%); primarily as metabolites

Pregnancy Risk Factor C

Generic Available No

Comments Aripiprazole works differently from the classic antipsychotics, such as chlorpromazine, in that it does not appear to block central dopaminergic receptors, but rather seems to be a stabilizer of dopamine-serotonin central systems. The risk of extrapyramidal reactions such as pseudoparkinsonism, acute dystonic reactions, akathisia and tardive dyskinesia are low and the frequencies reported are similar to placebo. Aripiprazole may be associated with neuroleptic malignant syndrome (NMS).

Aristocort® *see* Triamcinolone *on page 1341*

Aristocort® A *see* Triamcinolone *on page 1341*

Aristocort® Forte *see* Triamcinolone *on page 1341*

Aristospan® *see* Triamcinolone *on page 1341*

Arixtra® *see* Fondaparinux *on page 611*

Arlidin® *see* Nylidrin *on page 991*

Armour® Thyroid *see* Thyroid *on page 1303*

Aromasin® *see* Exemestane *on page 552*

Arthropan® [OTC] *see* Choline Salicylate *on page 319*

Arthrotec® *see* Diclofenac and Misoprostol *on page 431*

Articaine Hydrochloride and Epinephrine *see* Articaine Hydrochloride and Epinephrine (Canada) *on page 124*

Articaine Hydrochloride and Epinephrine [Dental] *see* Articaine Hydrochloride and Epinephrine (U.S.) *on page 125*

Articaine Hydrochloride and Epinephrine (Canada)

(AR ti kane hye droe KLOR ide & ep i NEF rin)

Related Information

Articaine Hydrochloride and Epinephrine (U.S.) *on page 125*
Epinephrine *on page 499*
Oral Pain *on page 1524*

Canadian Brand Names Astracaine®; Astracaine® Forte; Ultracaine® DS; Ultracaine® DS Forte

Pharmacologic Category Local Anesthetic, Dental; Local Anesthetic

Synonyms Articaine Hydrochloride and Epinephrine

Use Dental: Anesthesia for infiltration and nerve block anesthesia in clinical dentistry

Local Anesthetic/Vasoconstrictor Precautions No information available to require special precautions

Effects on Dental Treatment Frequency not defined: Arrhythmias, tachycardia, bradycardia, blood pressure changes, excitation, CNS depression, nervousness, dizziness, headache, somnolence, unconsciousness, convulsions, vomiting, nausea, tremors, visual disturbances, blurred vision, allergic reactions (eg, wheezing, acute asthmatic attacks), reactions at site of injection (swelling, burning, ischemia, tissue necrosis)

Dosage

Recommended Ultracaine® DS/Ultracaine® DS Forte Dosages Based on Anesthetic Procedure

Procedure	Injection (4% Solution) Volume (mL)	Total Dose of Articaine HCl (mg)
Infiltration	0.5-2.5	20-100
Nerve Block	0.5-3.4	20-136
Oral Surgery	1.0-5.1	40-204

This table provides dosage guides only. Other dosages may be used; however, do not exceed maximum recommended dose.

Mechanism of Action Blocks nerve conduction by interfering with the permeability of the nerve axonal membrane to sodium ions; this results in the loss of the generation of the nerve axon potential

Other Adverse Effects Frequency not defined:

Cardiovascular: Myocardial depression, edema

Central nervous system: Chills

Dermatologic: Allergic reactions include cutaneous lesions, urticaria, itching, reddening of skin

Gastrointestinal: Diarrhea

Ocular: Blindness, diplopia, pupillary constriction

Otic: Tinnitus

Contraindications Hypersensitivity to any components of the formulation and/or local anesthetics of the amide group; in the presence of inflammation and/or sepsis near the injection site; in patients with severe shock, any degree of heart block, paroxysmal tachycardia, known arrhythmia with rapid heart rate, narrow-angle glaucoma, cholinesterase deficiency, existing neurologic disease, severe hypertension; when articaine with epinephrine is used, the caution required of any vasopressor drug should be followed

Warnings/Precautions Articaine should be used cautiously in persons with known drug allergies or sensitivities, or suspected sensitivity to the amide-type local anesthetics. Avoid excessive premedications with sedatives, tranquilizers, and antiemetic agents. Inject slowly with frequent aspirations and if blood is aspirated, relocate needle. Articaine should be used with extreme caution in patients having a history of thyrotoxicosis or diabetes. Due to the sulfite component of the articaine preparation, hypersensitivity reactions may occur occasionally in patients with bronchial asthma.

Drug Interactions

MAO inhibitors: Administration of local anesthetic solutions containing epinephrine may produce severe, prolonged hypertension

Phenothiazines, butyrophenones: May reduce or reverse the pressor effects of epinephrine; concurrent use of these agents should be avoided; in situations when concurrent therapy is necessary, careful patient monitoring is essential

Tricyclic antidepressants: Pressor response to I.V. epinephrine, norepinephrine, and phenylephrine may be enhanced in patients receiving TCAs (**Note:** Effect is unlikely with epinephrine or levonordefrin dosages typically administered as infiltration in combination with local anesthetics)

Dosage Forms INJ: (Ultracaine DS®): Articaine hydrochloride with epinephrine [1:200,000], sodium metabisulfite [0.5 mg/mL], antioxidant, and water for injection (1.7 mL) [50s]; (Ultracaine® DS Forte): Articaine hydrochloride 4% with epinephrine

[1:100,000], sodium metabisulfite [0.5 mg/mL], antioxidant, and water for injection (1.7 mL) [50s]

Selected Readings

Weaver JM, "Articaine, A New Local Anesthetic for American Dentists: Will It Supersede Lidocaine?" *Anesth Prog*, 1999, 46(4):111-2.

Articaine Hydrochloride and Epinephrine (U.S.)

(AR ti kane hye droe KLOR ide & ep i NEF rin)

Related Information

Articaine Hydrochloride and Epinephrine (Canada) *on page 124*
Epinephrine *on page 499*
Oral Pain *on page 1524*

U.S. Brand Names Septocaine™

Pharmacologic Category Local Anesthetic, Dental; Local Anesthetic

Synonyms Articaine Hydrochloride and Epinephrine [Dental]

Use Dental: Anesthesia agent for infiltration and nerve block anesthesia in clinical dentistry; Septocaine™ is indicated for local, infiltrative, or conductive anesthesia in both simple and complex dental and periodontal procedures

Local Anesthetic/Vasoconstrictor Precautions No information available to require special precautions

Effects on Dental Treatment Adverse reactions are characteristic of those associated with other amide-type local anesthetics; adverse reactions to this group of drugs may also result from excessive plasma levels which may be due to overdosage, unintentional intravascular injection, or slow metabolic degradation.

Controlled trial of 882 patients:

1% to 4%: Headache (4%), paresthesia (1%), gingivitis (1%), facial edema (1%)

≥1%: Pain (13%; whole body)

Dosage These are guidelines for the amount of anesthetic required for most routine procedures. The actual volumes to be used depend upon a number of factors, such as type and extent of surgical procedure, depth of anesthesia, degree of muscular relaxation, and condition of the patient. In all cases, the smallest dose that will produce the desired result should be given. Do not exceed maximum recommended dose; reduce dosage for pediatric patients, elderly, and those with cardiac and/or liver disease.

The following numbers of dental cartridges (1.7 mL) provide the indicated amounts of articaine hydrochloride 4% and epinephrine 1:100,000.

# of Cartridges (1.7 mL)	Articaine HCl (4%) (mg)	Epinephrine 1:100,000 (mg)
1	68	0.017
2	136	0.034
3	204	0.051
4	272	0.068
5	340	0.085
6	408	0.102
7	476	0.119
8	544	0.136

Summary of recommended volumes and concentrations for various types of anesthetic procedures; dosages (administered by submucosal injection and/or nerve block) apply to normal healthy adults:

Recommended Septocaine™ Dosages Based on Anesthetic Procedure

Procedure	Injection (4% Solution) Volume (mL)	Total Dose of Articaine HCl (mg)
Infiltration	0.5-2.5	20-100
Nerve Block	0.5-3.4	20-136
Oral Surgery	1.0-5.1	40-204

This table provides dosage guides only. Other dosages may be used; however, do not exceed maximum recommended dose.

Children <4 years: Safety and efficacy have not been established

Children 4-16 years (dosages in a clinical trial of 61 patients; ~13% required additional injections for complete anesthesia):

Simple procedures: 0.76-5.65 mg/kg (0.9-5.1 mL) was administered safely to 51 patients

Complex procedures: 0.37-7.48 mg/kg (0.7-3.9 mL) was administered safely to 10 patients

(Continued)

Articaine Hydrochloride and Epinephrine (U.S.) *(Continued)*

Elderly (dosages used in a clinical trial; 6% of the patients 65-75 years of age required additional injections for complete anesthesia):

65-75 years

Simple procedures: 0.43-4.76 mg/kg (0.9-11.9 mL) was administered safely to 35 patients

Complex procedures: 1.05-4.27 mg/kg (1.3-6.8 mL) was administered safely to 19 patients

≥75 years:

Simple procedures: 0.78-4.76 mg/kg (1.3-11.9 mL) was administered safely to 7 patients

Complex procedures: 1.12-2.17 mg/kg (1.3-5.1 mL) was administered safely to 4 patients

Maximum recommended dosages:

Children (not recommended in patients <4 years of age): Not to exceed 7 mg/kg (0.175 mL/kg) **or** 3.2 mg/lb (0.0795 mL/lb) of body weight

Adults (normal, healthy): Submucosal infiltration and/or nerve block: Not to exceed 7 mg/kg (0.175 mL/kg) **or** 3.2 mg/lb (0.0795 mL/lb) of body weight

Mechanism of Action Local anesthetics block the generation and conduction of nerve impulses, presumably by increasing the threshold for electrical excitation in the nerve, by slowing the propagation of the nerve impulse, and by reducing the rate of rise of the action potential. In general, the progression of anesthesia is related to the diameter, myelination, and conduction velocity of the affected nerve fibers. Clinically, the order of loss of nerve function is as follows: 1) pain, 2) temperature, 3) touch, 4) proprioception, and 5) skeletal muscle tone.

Other Adverse Effects <1% (≥1 patients in controlled trials; clinically significant): Abdominal pain, **accidental injury,** arthralgia, asthenia, back pain, constipation, diarrhea, **dizziness, xerostomia**, dysmenorrhea, dyspepsia, **ear pain,** ecchymosis, edema, **facial paralysis, glossitis, gum hemorrhage, hemorrhage,** hyperesthesia, **increased salivation, injection site pain, lymphadenopathy, malaise, migraine, oral ulceration**, myalgia, **nausea, neck pain, nervousness**, neuropathy, osteomyelitis, **paresthesia, pharyngitis**, pruritus, **rhinitis**, skin disorder, **somnolence, stomatitis, syncope, tachycardia, abnormal taste, thirst, tongue edema, tooth disorder, vomiting**

Contraindications Hypersensitivity to local anesthetics of the amide type or to sodium metabisulfite

Warnings/Precautions Intravascular injections should be avoided; aspiration should be performed prior to administration of Septocaine™; the needle must be repositioned until no return of blood can be elicited by aspiration; however, absence of blood in the syringe does not guarantee that intravascular injection has been avoided. **Accidental intravascular injection may be associated with convulsions, followed by CNS or cardiorespiratory depression and coma, ultimately progressing to respiratory arrest.** Dental practitioners and/or clinicians using local anesthetic agents should be well trained in diagnosis and management of emergencies that may arise from the use of these agents. Resuscitative equipment, oxygen, and other resuscitative drugs should be available for immediate use.

Because Septocaine™ contains epinephrine, which can cause local tissue necrosis or systemic toxicity, usual precautions for epinephrine administration should be observed. Administration of articaine HCl with epinephrine results in a three- to fivefold increase in plasma epinephrine concentrations compared to baseline; however, in healthy adults, it does not appear to be associated with marked increases in blood pressure or heart rate, except in the case of accidental intravascular injection.

Also contains sodium metabisulfite, which may cause allergic-type reactions (including anaphylactic symptoms, and life-threatening or less severe asthmatic episodes) in certain susceptible patients. The overall prevalence of the sulfite sensitivity in the general population is unknown, and is seen more frequently in asthmatic than in nonasthmatic persons.

To avoid serious adverse effects and high plasma levels, the lowest dosage resulting in effective anesthesia should be administered. Repeated doses may cause significant increases in blood levels with each repeated dose due to the possibility of accumulation of the drug or its metabolites. Tolerance to elevated blood levels varies with patient status. Reduced dosages, commensurate with age and physical condition, should be given to debilitated patients, elderly patients, acutely-ill patients, and pediatric patients. Septocaine™ should also be used with caution in patients with heart block.

Local anesthetic solutions containing a vasoconstrictor (such as Septocaine™) should be used cautiously. Patients with peripheral vascular disease or hypertensive vascular disease may exhibit exaggerated vasoconstrictor response, possibly resulting in ischemic injury or necrosis. It should also be used cautiously in patients during or following the administration of a potent general anesthetic agent, since cardiac arrhythmias may occur under these conditions.

Systemic absorption of local anesthetics may produce CNS and cardiovascular effects. Changes in cardiac conduction, excitability, refractoriness, contractility, and peripheral vascular resistance are minimal at blood concentrations produced by therapeutic doses. However, toxic blood concentrations depress cardiac conduction and excitability, which may lead to AV block, ventricular arrhythmias, and cardiac arrest (sometimes resulting in death). In addition, myocardial contractility is depressed and peripheral vasodilation occurs, leading to decreased cardiac output and arterial blood pressure.

Careful and constant monitoring of cardiovascular and respiratory (adequacy of ventilation) vital signs and the patient's state of consciousness should be done following each local anesthetic injection; at such times, restlessness, anxiety, tinnitus, dizziness, blurred vision, tremors, depression, or drowsiness may be early warning signs of CNS toxicity.

In vitro studies show that ~5% to 10% of articaine is metabolized by the human liver microsomal P450 isoenzyme system; however, no studies have been performed in patient with liver dysfunction, and caution should be used in patients with severe hepatic disease. Use with caution in patients with impaired cardiovascular function, since they may be less able to compensate for function changes associated with prolonged AV conduction produced by these drugs.

Small doses of local anesthetics injected into dental blocks may produce adverse reactions similar to systemic toxicity seen in unintentional intravascular injections at larger doses. Confusion, convulsions, respiratory depression and/or respiratory arrest, and cardiovascular stimulation or depression have been reported. These reactions may be due to intra-arterial injection of the local anesthetic with retrograde flow to the cerebral circulation. Patients receiving such blocks should be observed constantly with resuscitative equipment and personnel trained in treatment of adverse reactions immediately available. Dosage recommendations should not be exceeded; see Dosage

Drug Interactions

MAO inhibitors: Administration of local anesthetic solutions containing epinephrine may produce severe, prolonged hypertension

Phenothiazines, butyrophenones: May reduce or reverse the pressor effects of epinephrine; concurrent use of these agents should be avoided; in situations when concurrent therapy is necessary, careful patient monitoring is essential

Tricyclic antidepressants: Pressor response to I.V. epinephrine, norepinephrine, and phenylephrine may be enhanced in patients receiving TCAs (**Note:** Effect is unlikely with epinephrine or levonordefrin dosages typically administered as infiltration in combination with local anesthetics)

Pharmacodynamics/Kinetics

Onset of action: 1-6 minutes

Duration: Complete anesthesia: ~1 hour

Metabolism: Hepatic via plasma carboxyesterase to articainic acid (inactive)

Half-life elimination: Articaine: 1.8 hours; Articainic acid: 1.5 hours

Excretion: Urine (primarily as metabolites)

Pregnancy Risk Factor C

Breast-feeding Considerations It is not known whether articaine is excreted in human milk. Because many drugs are excreted in human milk, caution should be exercised when Septocaine™ is administered to a nursing woman.

Dosage Forms INJ: (Septocaine™): Articaine hydrochloride 4% with epinephrine (as bitartrate) 1:100,000, sodium chloride 1.6 mg/mL, sodium bisulfite 0.5 mg/mL, and sodium hydroxide (to adjust pH to 5.0) (1.7 mL) [cartridge, 50/box]

Generic Available No

Comments Septocaine™ (articaine hydrochloride 4% and epinephrine 1:100,000) is the first FDA approval in 30 years of a new local dental anesthetic providing complete pulpal anesthesia for approximately 1 hour. Chemically, articaine contains both an amide linkage and an ester linkage, making it chemically unique in the class of local anesthetics. Since it contains the ester linkage, articaine HCl is rapidly metabolized by plasma carboxyesterase to its primary metabolite, articainic acid, which is an inactive product of this metabolism. According to the manufacturer, *in vitro* studies show that the human liver microsomal P450 isoenzyme system metabolizes approximately 5% to 10% of available articaine with nearly quantitative conversion to articainic acid. The elimination half-life of articaine is about 1.8 hours, and that of articainic acid is about 1.5 hours. Articaine is excreted primarily through urine with 53% to 57% of the administered dose eliminated in the first 24 hours following submucosal administration. Articainic acid is the primary metabolite in urine. A minor metabolite, articainic acid glucuronide, is also excreted in the urine. Articaine constitutes only 2% of the total dose excreted in urine.

Selected Readings

Malamed SF, Gagnon S, Leblanc D, "A Comparison Between Articaine HCl and Lidocaine HCl in Pediatric Dental Patients," *Pediatr Dent*, 2000, 22(4):307-11.

Malamed SF, Gagnon S, Leblanc D, "Articaine Hydrochloride: A Study of the Safety of a New Amide Local Anesthetic," *J Am Dent Assoc*, 2001, 132(2):177-85.

Malamed SF, Gagnon S, Leblanc D, "Efficacy of Articaine: A New Amide Local Anesthetic," *J Am Dent Assoc*, 2000, 131(5):635-42.

Schertzer ER Jr, "Articaine vs lidocaine," *J Am Dent Assoc*, 2000, 131(9):1248, 1250.

Weaver JM, "Articaine, A New Local Anesthetic for American Dentists: Will It Supersede Lidocaine?" *Anesth Prog*, 1999, 46(4):111-2.

Artificial Tears (ar ti FISH il teerz)

U.S. Brand Names Akwa Tears® [OTC]; AquaSite® [OTC]; Bion® Tears [OTC]; HypoTears [OTC]; HypoTears PF [OTC]; Isopto® Tears [OTC]; Liquifilm® Tears [OTC]; Moisture® Eyes [OTC]; Moisture® Eyes PM [OTC]; Murine® Tears [OTC]; Murocel® [OTC]; Nature's Tears® [OTC]; Nu-Tears® [OTC]; Nu-Tears® II [OTC]; OcuCoat® [OTC]; OcuCoat® PF [OTC]; Puralube® Tears [OTC]; Refresh® [OTC]; Refresh® Plus [OTC]; Refresh® Tears [OTC]; Teargen® [OTC]; Teargen® II [OTC]; Tearisol® [OTC]; Tears Again® [OTC]; Tears Naturale® [OTC]; Tears Naturale® Free [OTC]; Tears Naturale® II [OTC]; Tears Plus® [OTC]; Tears Renewed® [OTC]; Ultra Tears® [OTC]; Viva-Drops® [OTC]

Canadian Brand Names Teardrops®

Pharmacologic Category Ophthalmic Agent, Miscellaneous

Synonyms Hydroxyethylcellulose; Polyvinyl Alcohol

Use Ophthalmic lubricant; for relief of dry eyes and eye irritation

Local Anesthetic/Vasoconstrictor Precautions No information available to require special precautions

Effects on Dental Treatment No significant effects or complications reported

Dosage Ophthalmic: Use as needed to relieve symptoms, 1-2 drops into eye(s) 3-4 times/day

Other Adverse Effects 1% to 10%: Ocular: Mild stinging or temporary blurred vision

Pregnancy Risk Factor C

Generic Available Yes

ASA *see* Aspirin *on page 131*

5-ASA *see* Mesalamine *on page 869*

Asacol® *see* Mesalamine *on page 869*

Ascorbic Acid (a SKOR bik AS id)

U.S. Brand Names C-500-GR™ [OTC]; Cecon® [OTC]; Cevi-Bid® [OTC]; C-Gram [OTC]; Dull-C® [OTC]; Vita-C® [OTC]

Canadian Brand Names Proflavanol C™; Revitalose C-1000®

Mexican Brand Names Cevalin®; Ce-Vi-Sol®; Redoxon®; Redoxon® Forte

Pharmacologic Category Vitamin, Water Soluble

Synonyms Vitamin C

Use

Dental: Prevention and treatment of scurvy

Medical: Urinary acidification; dietary supplement

Unlabeled/Investigational Use Investigational: Dietary supplement; decrease severity of "colds" (large doses); decrease risk of death by stroke (a 20-year study was recently completed involving 730 individuals receiving ascorbic acid at doses ≥45 mg/day)

Local Anesthetic/Vasoconstrictor Precautions No information available to require special precautions

Effects on Dental Treatment No significant effects or complications reported

Dosage Oral, I.M., I.V., **S.C.:**

Recommended daily allowance (RDA):
- <6 months: 30 mg
- 6 months to 1 year: 35 mg
- 1-3 years: 15 mg; upper limit of intake should not exceed 400 mg/day
- 4-8 years: 25 mg; upper limit of intake should not exceed 650 mg/day
- 9-13 years: 45 mg; upper limit of intake should not exceed 1200 mg/day
- 14-18 years: Upper limit of intake should not exceed 1800 mg/day
  - Male: 75 mg
  - Female: 65 mg
- Adults: Upper limit of intake should not exceed 2000 mg/day
  - Male: 90 mg
  - Female: 75 mg;
- Pregnant female:
  - ≤18 years: 80 mg; upper limit of intake should not exceed 1800 mg/day
  - 19-50 years: 85 mg; upper limit of intake should not exceed 2000 mg/day
- Lactating female:
  - ≤18 years: 15 mg; upper limit of intake should not exceed 1800 mg/day
  - 19-50 years: 20 mg; upper limit of intake should not exceed 2000 mg/day
- Adult smoker: Add an additional 35 mg/day

Children:
- Scurvy: 100-300 mg/day in divided doses for at least 2 weeks
- Urinary acidification: 500 mg every 6-8 hours
- Dietary supplement: 35-100 mg/day

Adults:
- Scurvy: 100-250 mg 1-2 times/day for at least 2 weeks
- Urinary acidification: 4-12 g/day in 3-4 divided doses
- Prevention and treatment of colds: 1-3 g/day
- Dietary supplement: 50-200 mg/day

Mechanism of Action Not fully understood; necessary for collagen formation and tissue repair; involved in some oxidation-reduction reactions as well as other metabolic pathways, such as synthesis of carnitine, steroids, and catecholamines and conversion of folic acid to folinic acid

Other Adverse Effects

1% to 10%: Renal: Hyperoxaluria (large doses)

<1%: **Flushing, faintness, dizziness, headache, fatigue, nausea, vomiting**, heartburn, diarrhea, **flank pain**

Warnings/Precautions Diabetics and patients prone to recurrent renal calculi (eg, dialysis patients) should not take excessive doses for extended periods of time

Drug Interactions

Decreased Effect:
- Aspirin (decreases ascorbate levels, increases aspirin)
- Fluphenazine (decreases fluphenazine levels)
- Warfarin (decreased effect)

Increased Effect:
- Iron (absorption enhanced)
- Oral contraceptives (increased contraceptive effect)

Pharmacodynamics/Kinetics

Absorption: Oral: Readily absorbed; an active process thought to be dose dependent

Distribution: Large

Metabolism: Hepatic via oxidation and sulfation

Excretion: Urine (with high blood levels)

Pregnancy Risk Factor A/C (dose exceeding RDA recommendation)

Dosage Forms CAP: 500 mg, 1000 mg. **CAP, timed release:** 500 mg. **CRYST:** 4 g/teaspoonful (100 g). **INJ, solution:** 250 mg/mL (2 mL, 30 mL); 500 mg/mL (50 mL); (Cenolate®): 500 mg/mL (1 mL, 2 mL). **POWDER, solution:** 4 g/teaspoonful (100 g, 500 g). **SOLN, oral:** 90 mg/mL (50 mL). **TAB:** 100 mg, 250 mg, 500 mg, 1000 mg. **TAB, chewable:** 100 mg, 250 mg, 500 mg. **TAB, timed release:** 500 mg, 1000 mg, 1500 mg

Generic Available Yes

Ascorbic Acid and Ferrous Sulfate *see* Ferrous Sulfate and Ascorbic Acid *on page 569*

Ascriptin® [OTC] *see* Aspirin *on page 131*

Ascriptin® Arthritis Pain [OTC] *see* Aspirin *on page 131*

Ascriptin® Enteric [OTC] *see* Aspirin *on page 131*

Ascriptin® Extra Strength [OTC] *see* Aspirin *on page 131*

Asendin® [DSC] *see* Amoxapine *on page 91*

Asparaginase (a SPIR a ji nase)

U.S. Brand Names Elspar®

Canadian Brand Names Elspar®; Kidrolase®

Mexican Brand Names Leunase®

Pharmacologic Category Antineoplastic Agent, Miscellaneous

Synonyms *E. coli* Asparaginase; *Erwinia* Asparaginase; L-asparaginase; NSC-106977 (*Erwinia*); NSC-109229 (*E. coli*)

Use Treatment of acute lymphocytic leukemia, lymphoma; induction therapy

Local Anesthetic/Vasoconstrictor Precautions No information available to require special precautions

Effects on Dental Treatment

>10%: Somnolence, hallucinations, agitation, disorientation or convulsions (10% to 60%), stupor, confusion, coma (25%), hyperglycemia (10%); acute allergic reactions including fever, rash, urticaria, arthralgia, hypotension, angioedema, bronchospasm, anaphylaxis (15% to 35%; may be dose-limiting or fatal)

1% to 10%: Stomatitis

Dosage Some institutions recommended the following precautions for asparaginase administration: Have parenteral epinephrine, diphenhydramine, and hydrocortisone available at the bedside. Have a freely running I.V. in place. Have a physician readily accessible. Monitor the patient closely for 30-60 minutes. Avoid administering the drug at night.

Some practitioners recommend a desensitization regimen for patients who react to a test dose, or are being retreated following a break in therapy. Doses are doubled and given every 10 minutes until the total daily dose for that day has been administered. For example, if a patient was to receive a total dose of 4000 units, he/she would receive injections 1 through 12 during desensitization. See table on next page.

Refer to individual protocols; dose must be individualized based upon clinical response and tolerance of the patient

(Continued)

Asparaginase *(Continued)*

Asparaginase Desensitization

Injection No.	Elspar Dose (IU)	Accumulated Total Dose
1	1	1
2	2	3
3	4	7
4	8	15
5	16	31
6	32	63
7	64	127
8	128	255
9	256	511
10	512	1023
11	1024	2047
12	2048	4095
13	4096	8191
14	8192	16,383
15	16,384	32,767
16	32,768	65,535
17	65,536	131,071
18	131,072	262,143

Children:

I.V.:

Infusion for induction in combination with vincristine and prednisone: 1000 units/kg/day for 10 days

Consolidation: 6000-10,000 units/m^2/day for 14 days

I.M.: In combination with vincristine and prednisone: 6000 units/m^2 on days 4, 7, 10, 13, 16, 19, 22, 25, 28

Adults:

I.V. infusion single agent for induction:

200 units/kg/day for 28 days **or**

5000-10,000 units/m^2/day for 7 days every 3 weeks **or**

10,000-40,000 units every 2-3 weeks

I.M. as single agent: 6000-12,000 units/m^2; reconstitution to 10,000 units/mL may be necessary. (See pediatric dosage for combination therapy.)

Mechanism of Action Some malignant cells (ie, lymphoblastic leukemia cells and those of lymphocyte derivation) must acquire the amino acid asparagine from surrounding fluid such as blood, whereas normal cells can synthesize their own asparagine. Asparaginase is an enzyme that deaminates asparagine to aspartic acid and ammonia in the plasma and extracellular fluid and therefore deprives tumor cells of the amino acid for protein synthesis.

There are two purified preparations of the enzyme: one from *Escherichia coli* and one from *Erwinia carotovora*. These two preparations vary slightly in the gene sequencing and have slight differences in enzyme characteristics. Both are highly specific for asparagine and have less than 10% activity for the D-isomer. The preparation from *E. coli* has had the most use in clinical and research practice.

Other Adverse Effects

>10%:

Central nervous system: Depression

Endocrine & metabolic: Fever and chills (50% to 60%; infusion-related), hyperglycemia (10%)

Gastrointestinal: Nausea and vomiting (50% to 60%; infusion-related), anorexia, abdominal cramps (70%), acute pancreatitis (15%; may be severe)

Hematologic: Hypofibrinogenemia and depression of clotting factors V and VIII, variable decreased in factors VII and IX, severe protein C deficiency and decrease in antithrombin III (may be dose-limiting or fatal)

Hepatic: Transient elevations of transaminases, bilirubin, and alkaline phosphatase

Renal: Azotemia (66%)

1% to 10%:

Endocrine & metabolic: Hyperuricemia

<1%: **Hypotension, venous thrombosis, Parkinsonian symptoms (tremor, increase muscle tone), disorientation, drowsiness, seizures, coma**, hyperthermia, **hallucinations**, rash, pruritus, urticaria, **insulin-dependent diabetes**, ketoacidosis, weight loss, mild to moderate myelosuppression, leukopenia, anemia, thrombocytopenia

Drug Interactions

Increased Effect/Toxicity: Increased toxicity has been noticed when asparaginase is administered with vincristine (neuropathy) and prednisone (hyperglycemia). Decreased metabolism when used with cyclophosphamide. Increased hepatotoxicity when used with mercaptopurine.

Decreased Effect: Asparaginase terminates methotrexate action.

Pharmacodynamics/Kinetics

Absorption: I.M.: Produces peak blood levels 50% lower than those from I.V. administration

Distribution: V_d: 4-5 L/kg; 70% to 80% of plasma volume; does not penetrate CSF

Metabolism: Systemically degraded

Half-life elimination: 8-30 hours

Excretion: Urine (trace amounts)

Clearance: Unaffected by age, renal or hepatic function

Pregnancy Risk Factor C

Generic Available No

Aspercin [OTC] *see* Aspirin *on page 131*

Aspercin Extra [OTC] *see* Aspirin *on page 131*

Aspergum® [OTC] *see* Aspirin *on page 131*

Aspirin (AS pir in)

Related Information

Butalbital, Aspirin, and Caffeine *on page 216*
Cardiovascular Diseases *on page 1456*
Carisoprodol and Aspirin *on page 252*
Carisoprodol, Aspirin, and Codeine *on page 252*
Oral Pain *on page 1524*
Oxycodone and Aspirin *on page 1020*
Rheumatoid Arthritis, Osteoarthritis, and Osteoporosis *on page 1488*

U.S. Brand Names Ascriptin® [OTC]; Ascriptin® Arthritis Pain [OTC]; Ascriptin® Enteric [OTC]; Ascriptin® Extra Strength [OTC]; Aspercin [OTC]; Aspercin Extra [OTC]; Aspergum® [OTC]; Bayer® Aspirin [OTC]; Bayer® Aspirin Extra Strength [OTC]; Bayer® Aspirin Regimen Adult Low Strength [OTC]; Bayer® Aspirin Regimen Adult Low Strength with Calcium [OTC]; Bayer® Aspirin Regimen Children's [OTC]; Bayer® Aspirin Regimen Regular Strength [OTC]; Bayer® Plus Extra Strength [OTC]; Bufferin® [OTC]; Bufferin® Arthritis Strength [OTC]; Bufferin® Extra Strength [OTC]; Easprin®; Ecotrin® [OTC]; Ecotrin® Low Adult Strength [OTC]; Ecotrin® Maximum Strength [OTC]; Halfprin® [OTC]; St. Joseph® Pain Reliever [OTC]; Sureprin 81™ [OTC]; ZORprin®

Canadian Brand Names Asaphen; Asaphen E.C.; Entrophen®; Novasen

Mexican Brand Names ASA 500®; Aspirina Protect®; Ecotrin®

Pharmacologic Category Salicylate

Synonyms Acetylsalicylic Acid; ASA

Use

Dental: Treatment of postoperative pain

Medical: Treatment of mild to moderate pain, inflammation, and fever; may be used as prophylaxis of MI; prophylaxis of stroke and/or transient ischemic episodes; management of rheumatoid arthritis, rheumatic fever, osteoarthritis, and gout (high dose); adjunctive therapy in revascularization procedures (coronary artery bypass graft [CABG], percutaneous transluminal coronary angioplasty [PTCA], carotid endarterectomy)

Unlabeled/Investigational Use Prevention of pre-eclampsia (low doses), recurrent spontaneous abortions, prematurity, fetal growth retardation (including complications associated with autoimmune disorders such as lupus or antiphospholipid syndrome)

Local Anesthetic/Vasoconstrictor Precautions No information available to require special precautions

Effects on Dental Treatment As with all drugs which may affect hemostasis, bleeding is associated with aspirin. Hemorrhage may occur at virtually any site; risk is dependent on multiple variables including dosage, concurrent use of multiple agents which alter hemostasis, and patient susceptibility. Many adverse effects of aspirin are dose-related, and are rare at low dosages. Other serious reactions are idiosyncratic, related to allergy or individual sensitivity.

Reported for aspirin:

>10%: GI ulceration (6% to 31%)

Frequency unknown: Hypotension, tachycardia, fatigue, nervousness, agitation, confusion, dizziness, headache, lethargy, coma, dehydration, hypoglycemia (children), hyperglycemia, nausea, vomiting, epigastric discomfort, heartburn, gastric erosions, gastric erythema, duodenal ulcers, prolongation of PTs, coagulopathy, bleeding, iron-deficiency anemia, weakness, acetabular bone destruction (OA), asthma, bronchospasm, dyspnea, laryngeal edema, hyperpnea, tachypnea, anaphylaxis

(Continued)

Aspirin *(Continued)*

Case reports: Esophageal stricture, esophagitis with esophageal ulcer, esophageal hematoma, oral mucosal ulcers (aspirin-containing chewing gum), coronary artery spasm, conduction defect and atrial fibrillation (toxicity), delirium periorbital edema, rhinosinusitis

Dosage

Children:

Analgesic and antipyretic: Oral, rectal: 10-15 mg/kg/dose every 4-6 hours, up to a total of 4 g/day

Anti-inflammatory: Oral: Initial: 60-90 mg/kg/day in divided doses; usual maintenance: 80-100 mg/kg/day divided every 6-8 hours; monitor serum concentrations

Antiplatelet effects: Adequate pediatric studies have not been performed; pediatric dosage is derived from adult studies and clinical experience and is not well established; suggested doses have ranged from 3-5 mg/kg/day to 5-10 mg/kg/day given as a single daily dose. Doses are rounded to a convenient amount (eg, 1/2 of 80 mg tablet).

Mechanical prosthetic heart valves: 6-20 mg/kg/day given as a single daily dose (used in combination with an oral anticoagulant in children who have systemic embolism despite adequate oral anticoagulation therapy (INR 2.5-3.5) and used in combination with low-dose anticoagulation (INR 2-3) and dipyridamole when full-dose oral anticoagulation is contraindicated)

Blalock-Taussig shunts: 3-5 mg/kg/day given as a single daily dose

Kawasaki disease: Oral: 80-100 mg/kg/day divided every 6 hours; monitor serum concentrations; after fever resolves: 3-5 mg/kg/day once daily; in patients without coronary artery abnormalities, give lower dose for at least 6-8 weeks or until ESR and platelet count are normal; in patients with coronary artery abnormalities, low-dose aspirin should be continued indefinitely

Antirheumatic: Oral: 60-100 mg/kg/day in divided doses every 4 hours

Adults:

Analgesic and antipyretic: Oral, rectal: 325-650 mg every 4-6 hours up to 4 g/day

Anti-inflammatory: Oral: Initial: 2.4-3.6 g/day in divided doses; usual maintenance: 3.6-5.4 g/day; monitor serum concentrations

Myocardial infarction prophylaxis: 75-325 mg/day; use of a lower aspirin dosage has been recommended in patients receiving ACE inhibitors

Acute MI: 160-325 mg/day

CABG: 325 mg/day starting 6 hours following procedure

PTCA: Initial: 80-325 mg/day starting 2 hours before procedure; longer pretreatment durations (up to 24 hours) should be considered if lower dosages (80-100 mg) are used

Carotid endarterectomy: 81-325 mg/day preoperatively and daily thereafter

Acute stroke : 160-325 mg/day, initiated within 48 hours (in patients who are not candidates for thrombolytics and are not receiving systemic anticoagulation)

Stroke prevention/TIA: 30-325 mg/day (dosages up to 1300 mg/day in 2-4 divided doses have been used in clinical trials)

Pre-eclampsia prevention (unlabeled use): 60-80 mg/day during gestational weeks 13-26 (patient selection criteria not established)

Dosing adjustment in renal impairment: Cl_{cr} <10 mL/minute: Avoid use.

Hemodialysis: Dialyzable (50% to 100%)

Dosing adjustment in hepatic disease: Avoid use in severe liver disease.

Mechanism of Action Inhibits prostaglandin synthesis, acts on the hypothalamus heat-regulating center to reduce fever, blocks prostaglandin synthetase action which prevents formation of the platelet-aggregating substance thromboxane A_2

Other Adverse Effects Reported for aspirin (accurate estimation of frequencies is not possible):

Cardiovascular: Dysrhythmias, edema

Central nervous system: Insomnia, cerebral edema, hyperthermia

Dermatologic: Rash, angioedema, urticaria

Endocrine & metabolic: Acidosis, hyperkalemia, hypernatremia (buffered forms)

Gastrointestinal: Dyspepsia, heartburn, stomach pains

Hematologic: Anemia, disseminated intravascular coagulation, thrombocytopenia, hemolytic anemia

Hepatic: Hepatotoxicity, increased transaminases, hepatitis (reversible)

Neuromuscular & skeletal: Rhabdomyolysis

Otic: Hearing loss, tinnitus

Renal: Interstitial nephritis, papillary necrosis, proteinuria, renal impairment, renal failure (including cases caused by rhabdomyolysis), increased BUN, increased serum creatinine

Respiratory: Respiratory alkalosis, noncardiogenic pulmonary edema

Miscellaneous: Prolonged pregnancy and labor, stillbirths, low birth weight, peripartum bleeding, Reye's syndrome

Postmarketing and/or case reports: Colonic ulceration, coronary artery spasm, ischemic brain infarction, colitis, rectal stenosis (suppository), cholestatic jaundice

Contraindications Hypersensitivity to salicylates, other NSAIDs, or any component of the formulation; asthma; rhinitis; nasal polyps; inherited or acquired bleeding disorders (including factor VII and factor IX deficiency); do not use in children (<16 years of age) for viral infections (chickenpox or flu symptoms), with or without fever, due to a potential association with Reye's syndrome; pregnancy (3rd trimester especially)

Warnings/Precautions Use with caution in patients with platelet and bleeding disorders, renal dysfunction, dehydration, erosive gastritis, or peptic ulcer disease. Heavy ethanol use (>3 drinks/day) can increase bleeding risks. Avoid use in severe renal failure or in severe hepatic failure. Discontinue use if tinnitus or impaired hearing occurs. Caution in mild-moderate renal failure (only at high dosages). Patients with sensitivity to tartrazine dyes, nasal polyps and asthma may have an increased risk of salicylate sensitivity. Avoid aspirin, if possible, for 1- 2 weeks prior to dental or surgical procedures to reduce the risk of excessive bleeding.

Drug Interactions Substrate of CYP2C8/9

ACE inhibitors: The effects of ACE inhibitors may be blunted by aspirin administration, particularly at higher dosages.

Buspirone increases aspirin's free % *in vitro*.

Carbonic anhydrase inhibitors and corticosteroids have been associated with alteration in salicylate serum concentrations.

Heparin and low molecular weight heparins: Concurrent use may increase the risk of bleeding.

Methotrexate serum levels may be increased; consider discontinuing aspirin 2-3 days before high-dose methotrexate treatment or avoid concurrent use.

NSAIDs may increase the risk of gastrointestinal adverse effects and bleeding. Serum concentrations of some NSAIDs may be decreased by aspirin.

Platelet inhibitors (IIb/IIIa antagonists): Risk of bleeding may be increased.

Probenecid effects may be antagonized by aspirin.

Sulfonylureas: The effects of older sulfonylurea agents (tolazamide, tolbutamide) may be potentiated due to displacement from plasma proteins. This effect does not appear to be clinically significant for newer sulfonylurea agents (glyburide, glipizide, glimepiride).

Valproic acid may be displaced from its binding sites which can result in toxicity.

Verapamil may potentiate the prolongation of bleeding time associated with aspirin.

Warfarin and oral anticoagulants may increase the risk of bleeding.

Dietary/Ethanol/Herb Considerations

Ethanol: Avoid use; may enhance gastric mucosal irritation.

Food may decrease the rate but not extent of oral absorption. Administer with food, milk, or large volume of water to reduce GI upset. Fresh fruits containing vitamin C displace drug from binding sites, resulting in increased urinary excretion of aspirin. Limit Benedictine liqueur, curry powder, gherkins, licorice, paprika, prunes, raisins, and tea due to potential salicylate accumulation. Diet may require folic acid and/or iron supplementation; doses of 3-4 g/day may cause iron-deficiency and folic acid deficiency leading to macrocytic anemia. Avoid garlic, ginger, and green tea.

Herb/Nutraceutical: Avoid cat's claw, dong quai, evening primrose, feverfew, garlic, ginger, ginkgo biloba, ginseng, green tea, horse chestnut, and red clover due to additional antiplatelet activity. Limit licorice due to salicylate content.

Pharmacodynamics/Kinetics

Duration: 4-6 hours

Absorption: Rapid

Distribution: V_d: 10 L; readily into most body fluids and tissues

Metabolism: Hydrolyzed to salicylate (active) by esterases in GI mucosa, red blood cells, synovial fluid, and blood; metabolism of salicylate occurs primarily by hepatic conjugation; metabolic pathways are saturable

Bioavailability: 50% to 75% reaches systemic circulation

Half-life elimination: Parent drug: 15-20 minutes; Salicylates (dose dependent): 3 hours at lower doses (300-600 mg), 5-6 hours (after 1 g), 10 hours with higher doses

Time to peak, serum: ~1-2 hours

Excretion: Urine (75% as salicyluric acid, 10% as salicylic acid)

Pregnancy Risk Factor C/D (full-dose aspirin in 3rd trimester - expert analysis)

Dosage Forms CAPLET, buffered: 325 mg, 500 mg. **GELCAP:** 325 mg, 500 mg. **GUM:** 227 mg. **SUPP, rectal:** 60 mg, 120 mg, 125 mg, 200 mg, 300 mg, 325 mg, 600 mg, 650 mg. **TAB:** 325 mg, 500 mg; film coated: 325 mg. **TAB, buffered:** 325 mg, 500 mg. **TAB, chewable:** 81 mg. **TAB, controlled release** (ZORprin®): 800 mg. **TAB, enteric coated:** 81 mg, 162 mg, 325 mg, 500 mg, 650 mg, 975 mg; (Easprin®): 975 mg

Generic Available Yes

Comments Anti-inflammatory actions of aspirin are not seen clinically at doses <3500 mg/day. Patients taking one aspirin tablet daily as an antithrombotic and who require dental surgery should be given special consideration in consultation with the

(Continued)

Aspirin *(Continued)*

physician before removal of the aspirin relative to prevention of postoperative bleeding.

Selected Readings

Desjardins PJ, Cooper SA, Gallegos TL, et al, "The Relative Analgesic Efficacy of Propiram Fumarate, Codeine Aspirin, and Placebo in Post-Impaction Dental Pain," *J Clin Pharmacol*, 1984, 24(1):35-42.

Forbes JA, Butterworth GA, Burchfield WH, et al, "Evaluation of Ketorolac, Aspirin, and an Acetaminophen-Codeine Combination in Postoperative Oral Surgery Pain," *Pharmacotherapy*, 1990, 10(6 Pt 2):77S-93S.

Hurlen M, Erikssen J, Smith P, et al, "Comparison of Bleeding Complications of Warfarin and Warfarin Plus Acetylsalicylic Acid: A Study in 3166 Outpatients," *J Intern Med*, 1994, 236(3):299-304.

Aspirin, Acetaminophen, and Caffeine *see* Acetaminophen, Aspirin, and Caffeine *on page 34*

Aspirin and Carisoprodol *see* Carisoprodol and Aspirin *on page 252*

Aspirin and Codeine (AS pir in & KOE deen)

Related Information

Aspirin *on page 131*
Codeine *on page 361*
Oral Pain *on page 1524*

Canadian Brand Names Coryphen® Codeine

Pharmacologic Category Analgesic, Narcotic

Synonyms Codeine and Aspirin

Use

Dental: Treatment of postoperative pain
Medical: Relief of pain

Local Anesthetic/Vasoconstrictor Precautions No information available to require special precautions

Effects on Dental Treatment Elderly are a high-risk population for adverse effects from NSAIDs due to concomitant disease and drug use; consider renal function decline with age. As much as 60% of elderly patients with GI complications from NSAIDs can develop peptic ulceration and/or hemorrhage asymptomatically; use lowest effective dose for shortest period possible.

Frequency not defined: Palpitations, hypotension, bradycardia, peripheral vasodilation, CNS depression, increased intracranial pressure, nausea, vomiting, respiratory depression, bronchospasm, biliary tract spasm, histamine release, anaphylaxis, physical and psychological dependence

Restrictions C-III

Dosage Oral:

Children:
Aspirin: 10 mg/kg/dose every 4 hours
Codeine: 0.5-1 mg/kg/dose every 4 hours

Adults: 1-2 tablets every 4-6 hours as needed for pain

Dosing adjustment in renal impairment:
Cl_{cr} 10-50 mL/minute: Administer 75% of dose
Cl_{cr} <10 mL/minute: Avoid use

Dosing interval in hepatic disease: Avoid use in severe liver disease

Mechanism of Action Aspirin inhibits prostaglandin synthesis, acts on the hypothalamus heat-regulating center to reduce fever, blocks prostaglandin synthetase action which prevents formation of the platelet-aggregating substance thromboxane A_2; codeine binds to opiate receptors (mu and kappa subtypes) in the CNS causing inhibition of ascending pain pathways, altering the perception of and response to pain

Other Adverse Effects <1%: Xerostomia

Frequency not defined:
Dermatologic: Pruritus, rash, urticaria
Endocrine & metabolic: Antidiuretic hormone release
Gastrointestinal: Constipation
Genitourinary: Urinary tract spasm
Hematologic: Occult bleeding
Hepatic: Hepatotoxicity
Ocular: Miosis

Contraindications Hypersensitivity to aspirin, codeine, or any component of the formulation; premature infants or during labor for delivery of a premature infant; pregnancy

Warnings/Precautions Use with caution in patients with asthma, impaired hepatic function, platelet and bleeding disorders, renal dysfunction, erosive gastritis, or peptic ulcer disease. Previous nonreaction does not guarantee future safe- taking of medication. Do not use aspirin in children <16 years of age for chickenpox or flu symptoms, due to its association with Reye's syndrome. Avoid aspirin-containing products, if possible, for 1-2 weeks prior to dental or surgical procedures to reduce risk of excessive bleeding.

Enhanced analgesia has been seen in elderly patients on therapeutic doses of narcotics; duration of action may be increased; the elderly may be particularly susceptible to the CNS depressant and constipating effects of narcotics.

Dietary/Ethanol/Herb Considerations

Ethanol: Avoid use; may enhance gastric mucosal irritation and increase CNS depression.

Food: Administer with food, milk, or large volume of water to reduce GI upset; food decreases the rate but not extent of oral absorption.

Herb/Nutraceutical: Avoid gotu kola, kava, SAMe, St John's wort, and valerian; may increase CNS depression.

Pregnancy Risk Factor D

Dosage Forms TAB: #3: Aspirin 325 mg and codeine 30 mg; #4: Aspirin 325 mg and codeine 60 mg

Generic Available Yes

Comments Codeine products, as with other narcotic analgesics, are recommended only for limited acute dosing (ie, 3 days or less). The most common adverse effect you will see in your dental patients from codeine is nausea, followed by sedation and constipation. Codeine has narcotic addiction liability, especially when given long-term. The aspirin component has anticoagulant effects and can affect bleeding times.

Selected Readings

Dionne RA, "New Approaches to Preventing and Treating Postoperative Pain," *J Am Dent Assoc*, 1992, 123(6):26-34.

Gobetti JP, "Controlling Dental Pain," *J Am Dent Assoc*, 1992, 123(6):47-52.

Aspirin and Dipyridamole (AS pir in & dye peer ID a mole)

Related Information

Aspirin *on page 131*

Dipyridamole *on page 456*

U.S. Brand Names Aggrenox™

Canadian Brand Names Aggrenox®

Pharmacologic Category Antiplatelet Agent

Synonyms Dipyridamole and Aspirin

Use Reduction in the risk of stroke in patients who have had transient ischemia of the brain or completed ischemic stroke due to thrombosis

Local Anesthetic/Vasoconstrictor Precautions No information available to require special precautions

Effects on Dental Treatment

>10%: Headache (38%), nausea (16%)

1% to 10%: Cardiac failure (2%), pain (6%), seizures (2%), fatigue (6%), malaise (2%), syncope (1%), amnesia (2%), confusion (1%), somnolence (1%) vomiting (8%), GI bleeding (4%), weakness (2%), arthritis (2%), cough (2%), upper respiratory tract infections (1%), epistaxis (2%)

Dosage Oral:

Adults: 1 capsule (dipyridamole 200 mg, aspirin 25 mg) twice daily.

Elderly: Plasma concentrations were 40% higher, but specific dosage adjustments have not been recommended

Dosing adjustment in renal impairment: Not studied; avoid in severe dysfunction (Cl_{cr} <10 mL/minute)

Dosing adjustment in hepatic impairment: Not studied; avoid in severe impairment

Mechanism of Action The antithrombotic action results from additive antiplatelet effects. Dipyridamole inhibits the uptake of adenosine into platelets, endothelial cells, and erythrocytes. Aspirin inhibits platelet aggregation by irreversible inhibition of platelet cyclooxygenase and thus inhibits the generation of thromboxane A2.

Other Adverse Effects

>10%: Gastrointestinal: Dyspepsia, abdominal pain (18%), diarrhea (13%)

1% to 10%:

- Dermatologic: Purpura (1%)
- Gastrointestinal: Rectal bleeding (2%), hemorrhoids (1%), hemorrhage (1%), anorexia (1%)
- Hematologic: Anemia (2%)
- Neuromuscular & skeletal: Back pain (5%), arthralgia (6%), arthrosis (1%), myalgia (1%)

<1% (limited to life-threatening or important symptoms): Intracranial hemorrhage (0.6%), **allergic reaction, fever, hypotension, coma, dizziness, paresthesia,** cerebral hemorrhage, subarachnoid hemorrhage, **gastritis, ulceration, perforation,** tinnitus, deafness, **tachycardia, palpitations, arrhythmia, supraventricular tachycardia,** cholelithiasis, jaundice, hepatic function abnormality, **hyperglycemia, thirst, hematoma, gingival bleeding, agitation,** uterine hemorrhage, **hyperpnea, asthma, bronchospasm,** hemoptysis, pulmonary edema, **loss of taste,** pruritus, urticaria, renal insufficiency and failure, hematuria, **flushing,** hypothermia, **chest pain, angina pectoris,** cerebral edema, pancreatitis, Reye's syndrome, hematemesis, hearing impairment, **anaphylaxis, laryngeal edema**, hepatitis, hepatic failure, rhabdomyolysis, **hypoglycemia,**

(Continued)

Aspirin and Dipyridamole *(Continued)*

dehydration, prolonged PT time, disseminated intravascular coagulation, coagulopathy, thrombocytopenia, prolonged pregnancy and labor, stillbirths, lower weight infants, antepartum and postpartum bleeding, **tachypnea, dyspnea**, rash, alopecia, angioedema, Stevens-Johnson syndrome, interstitial nephritis, papillary necrosis, proteinuria, allergic vasculitis, anemia (aplastic), pancytopenia, thrombocytosis

Dietary/Ethanol/Herb Considerations

Ethanol: Avoid use due to GI irritation.

Food: May be taken with food

Pharmacodynamics/Kinetics

Aggrenox™:

Half-life elimination: Salicylic acid: 1.71 hours

Time to peak: 0.63 hours

Aspirin: See Aspirin monograph.

Dipyridamole:

Distribution: V_d: 92 L

Protein binding: 99%

Metabolism: Hepatic via conjugation with glucuronic acid

Half-life elimination: 13.6 hours

Time to peak: 2 hours

Excretion: Feces (95% as glucuronide metabolite); urine (5%)

Pregnancy Risk Factor B (dipyridamole); D (aspirin)

Generic Available No

Aspirin and Hydrocodone *see* Hydrocodone and Aspirin *on page 680*

Aspirin and Meprobamate (AS pir in & me proe BA mate)

Related Information

Aspirin *on page 131*

Meprobamate *on page 864*

U.S. Brand Names Equagesic®

Canadian Brand Names 292 MEP®

Pharmacologic Category Antianxiety Agent, Miscellaneous

Synonyms Meprobamate and Aspirin

Use Adjunct to treatment of skeletal muscular disease in patients exhibiting tension and/or anxiety

Local Anesthetic/Vasoconstrictor Precautions No information available to require special precautions

Effects on Dental Treatment Use with caution in patients with impaired hepatic function, history of asthma, platelet and bleeding disorders, renal dysfunction, erosive gastritis, or peptic ulcer disease. Previous nonreaction does not guarantee future safe taking of medication. Do not use aspirin in children <16 years of age for chickenpox or flu symptoms due to the association with Reye's syndrome. Avoid aspirin, if possible, for 1 week prior to dental or surgical procedures due to possibility of postoperative bleeding.

Elderly are a high-risk population for adverse effects from nonsteroidal anti-inflammatory agents. As much as 60% of elderly with GI complications from NSAIDs can develop peptic ulceration and/or hemorrhage asymptomatically. Concomitant disease and drug use contribute to the risk of GI adverse effects. Use lowest effective dose for shortest period possible. Consider renal function decline with age.

Restrictions C-IV

Dosage Oral: 1 tablet 3-4 times/day

Dietary/Ethanol/Herb Considerations

Ethanol: Avoid use; may enhance gastric mucosal irritation and increase CNS depression.

Herb/Nutraceutical: Avoid gotu kola, kava, SAMe, St John's wort, and valerian; may increase CNS depression.

Pregnancy Risk Factor D

Generic Available Yes

Comments Abrupt discontinuation after sustained use (generally >10 days) may cause withdrawal symptoms

Selected Readings

Desjardins PJ, Cooper SA, Gallegos TL, et al, "The Relative Analgesic Efficacy of Propiram Fumarate, Codeine Aspirin, and Placebo in Postimpaction Dental Pain," *J Clin Pharmacol*, 1984, 24(1):35-42.

Forbes JA, Butterworth GA, Burchfield WH, et al, "Evaluation of Ketorolac, Aspirin, and an Acetaminophen-Codeine Combination in Postoperative Oral Surgery Pain," *Pharmacotherapy*, 1990, 10(6 Pt 2):77S-93S.

Forbes JA, Keller CK, Smith JW, et al, "Analgesic Effect of Naproxen Sodium, Codeine, a Naproxen-Codeine Combination and Aspirin on the Postoperative Pain of Oral Surgery," *Pharmacotherapy*, 1986, 6(5):211-8.

Aspirin and Oxycodone *see* Oxycodone and Aspirin *on page 1020*

Aspirin, Caffeine and Acetaminophen *see* Acetaminophen, Aspirin, and Caffeine *on page 34*

Aspirin, Caffeine, and Butalbital *see* Butalbital, Aspirin, and Caffeine *on page 216*

Aspirin, Carisoprodol, and Codeine *see* Carisoprodol, Aspirin, and Codeine *on page 252*

Aspirin Free Anacin® Maximum Strength [OTC] *see* Acetaminophen *on page 27*

Aspirin, Orphenadrine, and Caffeine *see* Orphenadrine, Aspirin, and Caffeine *on page 1005*

Astelin® *see* Azelastine *on page 151*

AsthmaNefrin® *see* Epinephrine (Racemic) *on page 500*

Astramorph/PF™ *see* Morphine Sulfate *on page 931*

Atacand® *see* Candesartan *on page 232*

Atacand HCT™ *see* Candesartan and Hydrochlorothiazide *on page 234*

Atarax® *see* HydrOXYzine *on page 697*

Atenolol (a TEN oh lole)

Related Information

Cardiovascular Diseases *on page 1456*

U.S. Brand Names Tenormin®

Canadian Brand Names Apo®-Atenol; Gen-Atenolol; Novo-Atenol; Nu-Atenol; PMS-Atenolol; Rhoxal-atenolol; Tenolin; Tenormin®

Mexican Brand Names Blokium®; Tenormin®

Pharmacologic Category Beta Blocker, Beta$_1$ Selective

Use Treatment of hypertension, alone or in combination with other agents; management of angina pectoris, postmyocardial infarction patients

Unlabeled/Investigational Use Treatment of acute ethanol withdrawal symptoms, supraventricular and ventricular arrhythmias; prophylaxis of migraine headache

Local Anesthetic/Vasoconstrictor Precautions No information available to require special precautions

Effects on Dental Treatment Atenolol is a cardioselective beta-blocker. Local anesthetic with vasoconstrictor can be safely used in patients medicated with atenolol. Nonselective beta-blockers (ie, propranolol, nadolol) enhance the pressor response to epinephrine, resulting in hypertension and bradycardia; this has not been reported for atenolol. Many nonsteroidal anti-inflammatory drugs such as ibuprofen and indomethacin can reduce the hypotensive effect of beta-blockers after 3 or more weeks of therapy with the NSAID. Short-term NSAID use (ie, 3 days) requires no special precautions in patients taking beta-blockers.

1% to 10%: Persistent bradycardia, hypotension, chest pain, heart failure, dizziness, fatigue, confusion, mental impairment, headache, nausea

Dosage

Oral:

- Children: 0.8-1 mg/kg/dose given daily; range of 0.8-1.5 mg/kg/day; maximum dose: 2 mg/kg/day
- Adults:
  - Hypertension: 50 mg once daily, may increase to 100 mg/day. Doses >100 mg are unlikely to produce any further benefit.
  - Angina pectoris: 50 mg once daily, may increase to 100 mg/day. Some patients may require 200 mg/day.
  - Postmyocardial infarction: Follow I.V. dose with 100 mg/day or 50 mg twice daily for 6-9 days

I.V.:

- Hypertension: Dosages of 1.25-5 mg every 6-12 hours have been used in short-term management of patients unable to take oral enteral beta-blockers
- Postmyocardial infarction: Early treatment: 5 mg slow I.V. over 5 minutes; may repeat in 10 minutes. If both doses are tolerated, may start oral atenolol 50 mg every 12 hours or 100 mg/day for 6-9 days

Dosing interval for oral atenolol in renal impairment:

- Cl_{cr} 15-35 mL/minute: Administer 50 mg/day maximum.
- Cl_{cr} <15 mL/minute: Administer 50 mg every other day maximum.

Hemodialysis: Moderately dialyzable (20% to 50%) via hemodialysis; administer dose postdialysis or administer 25-50 mg supplemental dose.

Peritoneal dialysis: Elimination is not enhanced; supplemental dose is unnecessary.

Mechanism of Action Competitively blocks response to beta-adrenergic stimulation, selectively blocks beta$_1$-receptors with little or no effect on beta$_2$-receptors except at high doses

Other Adverse Effects

1% to 10%:

- Cardiovascular: Edema, second- or third-degree AV block, Raynaud's phenomenon
- Central nervous system: Fatigue, insomnia, lethargy, depression, nightmares
- Gastrointestinal: Constipation, diarrhea
- Genitourinary: Impotence
- Miscellaneous: Cold extremities

(Continued)

Atenolol *(Continued)*

<1% (Limited to important or life-threatening): Alopecia, **dyspnea** (especially with large doses), elevated liver enzymes, **hallucinations**, impotence, lupus syndrome, Peyronie's disease, positive ANA, psoriaform rash, **psychosis, thrombocytopenia, wheezing**

Warnings/Precautions Administer cautiously in compensated heart failure and monitor for a worsening of the condition (efficacy of atenolol in heart failure has not been established). Beta-blocker therapy should not be withdrawn abruptly (particularly in patients with CAD), but gradually tapered to avoid acute tachycardia, hypertension, and/or ischemia. Use caution with concurrent use of beta-blockers and either verapamil or diltiazem; bradycardia or heart block can occur. Avoid concurrent I.V. use of both agents. Beta-blockers should be avoided in patients with bronchospastic disease (asthma) and peripheral vascular disease (may aggravate arterial insufficiency). Atenolol, with B1 selectivity, has been used cautiously in bronchospastic disease with close monitoring. Use cautiously in diabetics - may mask hypoglycemic symptoms. May mask signs of thyrotoxicosis. May cause fetal harm when administered in pregnancy. Use cautiously in the renally impaired (dosage adjustment required). Use care with anesthetic agents which decrease myocardial function. Caution in myasthenia gravis.

Drug Interactions

Increased Effect/Toxicity: Atenolol may increase the effects of other drugs which slow AV conduction (digoxin, verapamil, diltiazem), alpha-blockers (prazosin, terazosin), and alpha-adrenergic stimulants (epinephrine, phenylephrine). Atenolol may mask the tachycardia from hypoglycemia caused by insulin and oral hypoglycemics. In patients receiving concurrent therapy, the risk of hypertensive crisis is increased when either clonidine or the beta-blocker is withdrawn. Reserpine has been shown to enhance the effect of atenolol. Beta-blockers may increase the action or levels of ethanol, disopyramide, nondepolarizing muscle relaxants, and theophylline although the effects are difficult to predict.

Decreased Effect: Decreased effect of atenolol with aluminum salts, barbiturates, calcium salts, cholestyramine, colestipol, NSAIDs, penicillins (ampicillin), rifampin, salicylates, and sulfinpyrazone due to decreased bioavailability and plasma levels. Beta-blockers may decrease the effect of sulfonylureas.

Dietary/Ethanol/Herb Considerations

Ethanol: Limit use; may increase risk of hypotension or dizziness.

Food may decrease serum concentration. Avoid caffeine (eg, colas, chocolate), garlic, and licorice.

Herb/Nutraceutical: Avoid black cohosh, dong quai, and evening primrose due to estrogenic activity. Avoid ephedra, ginseng, and yohimbe; may worsen hypertension. Avoid garlic; may have increased antihypertensive effect. Avoid ginger due to positive inotropic effects; theoretically, may cause arrhythmia. Avoid hawthorn; may lower peripheral vascular resistance resulting in additive decrease in BP. Avoid licorice.

Pharmacodynamics/Kinetics

Onset of action: Peak effect: Oral: 2-4 hours

Duration: Normal renal function: 12-24 hours

Absorption: Incomplete

Distribution: Low lipophilicity; does not cross blood-brain barrier

Protein binding: 3% to 15%

Metabolism: Limited hepatic

Half-life elimination: Beta:

- Neonates: ≤35 hours; Mean: 16 hours
- Children: 4.6 hours; children >10 years may have longer half-life (>5 hours) compared to children 5-10 years (<5 hours)
- Adults: Normal renal function: 6-9 hours, prolonged with renal impairment; End-stage renal disease: 15-35 hours

Excretion: Feces (50%); urine (40% as unchanged drug)

Pregnancy Risk Factor D

Generic Available Yes: Tablet

Selected Readings

Foster CA and Aston SJ, "Propranolol-Epinephrine Interaction: A Potential Disaster," *Plast Reconstr Surg*, 1983, 72(1):74-8.

Wong DG, Spence JD, Lamki L, et al, "Effect of Nonsteroidal Anti-inflammatory Drugs on Control of Hypertension of Beta-Blockers and Diuretics," *Lancet*, 1986, 1(8488):997-1001.

Wynn RL, "Dental Nonsteroidal Anti-inflammatory Drugs and Prostaglandin-Based Drug Interactions-Part Two," *Gen Dent*, 1992, 40(2):104, 106, 108.

Wynn RL, "Epinephrine Interactions With Beta-Blockers," *Gen Dent*, 1994, 42(1):16, 18.

Atenolol and Chlorthalidone (a TEN oh lole & klor THAL i done)

Related Information

Atenolol *on page 137*

Chlorthalidone *on page 315*

U.S. Brand Names Tenoretic®

Canadian Brand Names Tenoretic®

Pharmacologic Category Antihypertensive Agent Combination

Synonyms Chlorthalidone and Atenolol

Use Treatment of hypertension with a cardioselective beta-blocker and a diuretic

Local Anesthetic/Vasoconstrictor Precautions No information available to require special precautions

Effects on Dental Treatment Noncardioselective beta-blockers (ie, propranolol, nadolol) enhance the pressor response to epinephrine, resulting in hypertension and bradycardia. This has not been reported for atenolol, a cardioselective beta-blocker. Therefore local anesthetic with vasoconstrictor can be safely used in patients medicated with atenolol. Many nonsteroidal anti-inflammatory drugs such as ibuprofen and indomethacin can reduce the hypotensive effect of beta-blockers after 3 or more weeks of therapy with the NSAID. Short-term NSAID use (ie, 3 days) requires no special precautions in patients taking beta-blockers.

Dosage Adults: Oral: Initial (based on atenolol component): 50 mg once daily, then individualize dose until optimal dose is achieved

Dietary/Ethanol/Herb Considerations Ethanol: Avoid use; may increase risk of hypotension or dizziness.

Pregnancy Risk Factor D

Generic Available Yes

Comments May contain povidone as inactive ingredient

Selected Readings

Foster CA and Aston SJ, "Propranolol-Epinephrine Interaction: A Potential Disaster," *Plast Reconstr Surg*, 1983, 72(1):74-8.

Wong DG, Spence JD, Lamki L, et al, "Effect of Nonsteroidal Anti-inflammatory Drugs on Control of Hypertension of Beta-Blockers and Diuretics," *Lancet*, 1986, 1(8488):997-1001.

Wynn RL, "Dental Nonsteroidal Anti-inflammatory Drugs and Prostaglandin-Based Drug Interactions - Part Two," *Gen Dent*, 1992, 40(2):104, 106, 108.

Wynn RL, "Epinephrine Interactions With Beta-Blockers," *Gen Dent*, 1994, 42(1):16, 18.

ATG *see* Lymphocyte Immune Globulin *on page 831*

Atgam® *see* Lymphocyte Immune Globulin *on page 831*

AT III *see* Antithrombin III *on page 117*

Ativan® *see* Lorazepam *on page 824*

Atomoxetine (AT oh mox e teen)

U.S. Brand Names Strattera™

Pharmacologic Category Norepinephrine Reuptake Inhibitor, Selective

Synonyms Atomoxetine Hydrochloride; LY139603; Tomoxetine

Use Treatment of attention deficit/hyperactivity disorder (ADHD)

Unlabeled/Investigational Use Treatment of depression

Local Anesthetic/Vasoconstrictor Precautions Use vasoconstrictor with caution. Atomoxetine may increase heart rate or blood pressure in the presence of pressor agents. Pressor agents include the vasoconstrictors epinephrine and levonordefrin (Neo-Cobefrin®)

Effects on Dental Treatment

>10%: Headache (17% to 27%), xerostomia (4% to 21%)

1% to 10%: Palpitations (4%), tachycardia (3%), systolic blood pressure increased (2% to 9%), orthostatic hypotension (2%), tachycardia (2%), irritability (8%), somnolence (7%), dizziness (6%), paresthesia (4%), pyrexia (3%), rigors (3%), crying (2%), rhinorrhea (4%), sinus headache (3%), diaphoresis increased (4%), sinusitis (6%), influenza (3%), ear infection (3%), fatigue/lethargy (7% to 9%)

Dosage Oral:

Children and Adolescents ≤70 kg: ADHD: Initial: 0.5 mg/kg/day, increase after minimum of 3 days to ~1.2 mg/kg/day; may administer as either a single daily dose or two evenly divided doses in morning and late afternoon/early evening. Maximum daily dose: 1.4 mg/kg or 100 mg, whichever is less. In patients receiving effective CYP2D6 inhibitors (eg, paroxetine, fluoxetine, quinidine), do not exceed 1.2 mg/kg.

Children and Adolescents >70 kg: Refer to Adults dosing

Adults:

ADHD: Initial: 40 mg/day, increased after minimum of 3 days to ~80 mg/day; may administer as either a single daily dose or two evenly divided doses in morning and late afternoon/early evening. May increase to 100 mg in 2-4 additional weeks to achieve optimal response. In patients receiving effective CYP2D6 inhibitors (eg, paroxetine, fluoxetine, quinidine), do not exceed 80 mg/day.

Depression (unlabeled use): 40-65 mg/day

Dosing adjustment in hepatic impairment:

Moderate hepatic insufficiency (Child-Pugh class B): All doses should be reduced to 50% of normal

Severe hepatic insufficiency (Child-Pugh class C): All doses should be reduced to 25% of normal

Mechanism of Action Selectively inhibits the reuptake of norepinephrine (Ki 4.5nM) with little to no activity at the other neuronal reuptake pumps or receptor sites.

Other Adverse Effects Percentages as reported in children and adults; reactions may be increased in "poor metabolizers" (CYP2D6)

(Continued)

Atomoxetine *(Continued)*

>10%: Gastrointestinal: Abdominal pain (20%), insomnia (16%), appetite decreased (10% to 14%),

1% to 10%:

Central nervous system: Mood swings (5%), abnormal dreams (4%), sleep disturbance (4%)

Dermatologic: Dermatitis (2% to 4%)

Endocrine & metabolic: Dysmenorrhea (7%), libido decreased (6%), menstruation disturbance (3%), orgasm abnormal (2%), weight loss (2%)

Gastrointestinal: Dyspepsia (6% to 8%), diarrhea (4%), flatulence (2%), constipation (3% to 10%)

Genitourinary: Erectile disturbance (7%), ejaculatory disturbance (5%), prostatitis (3%), impotence (3%)

Neuromuscular & skeletal: Myalgia (3%)

Renal: Urinary retention/hesitation (8%)

<1%: Allergy, angioedema, rash, urticaria

Drug Interactions Substrate of CYP2C19, **2D6**

Increased Effect/Toxicity: CYP2D6 inhibitors may increase toxicity of atomoxetine; albuterol may increase risk of cardiovascular toxicity; MAO inhibitors may increase risk of CNS toxicity (combined use is contraindicated)

Dietary/Ethanol/Herb Considerations Food: May be taken with food

Pharmacodynamics/Kinetics

Absorption: Rapid

Distribution: V_d: I.V.: 0.85 L/kg

Protein binding: 98%, primarily albumin

Metabolism: Hepatic, via CYP2D6 and CYP2C19; forms metabolites (4-hydroxyatomoxetine, active, equipotent to atomoxetine; N-desmethylatomoxetine in poor metabolizers, limited activity)

Bioavailability: 63% in extensive metabolizers; 94% in poor metabolizers

Half-life elimination: Atomoxetine: 5 hours (up to 24 hours in poor metabolizers); Active metabolites: 4-hydroxyatomoxetine: 6-8 hours; N-desmethylatomoxetine: 6-8 hours (34-40 hours in poor metabolizers)

Time to peak, plasma: 1-2 hours

Excretion: Urine (80%, as conjugated 4-hydroxy metabolite); feces (17%)

Pregnancy Risk Factor C

Generic Available No

Atomoxetine Hydrochloride *see* Atomoxetine *on page 139*

Atorvastatin (a TORE va sta tin)

U.S. Brand Names Lipitor®

Canadian Brand Names Lipitor®

Mexican Brand Names Lipitor®

Pharmacologic Category Antilipemic Agent, HMG-CoA Reductase Inhibitor

Use Used with dietary therapy for the following:

Hyperlipidemias: To reduce elevations in total cholesterol, LDL-C, apolipoprotein B, and triglycerides in patients with primary hypercholesterolemia (elevations of 1 or more components are present in Fredrickson type IIa, IIb, III, and IV hyperlipidemias); treatment of homozygous familial hypercholesterolemia

Heterozygous familial hypercholesterolemia (HeFH): In adolescent patients (10-17 years of age, females >1 year postmenarche) with HeFH having LDL-C ≥190 mg/dL **or** LDL ≥160 mg/dL with positive family history of premature cardiovascular disease (CVD) or with 2 or more CVD risk factors in the adolescent patient

Local Anesthetic/Vasoconstrictor Precautions No information available to require special precautions

Effects on Dental Treatment

>10%: Headache (3% to 17%)

2% to 10%: Chest pain, dizziness, nausea, sinusitis (≤6%), pharyngitis (≤3%), bronchitis, rhinitis, infection (2% to 10%), flu-like syndrome (≤3%), allergic reaction (≤3%), arthritis, weakness (≤4%)

<2%: Pneumonia, dyspnea, fever, gastroenteritis, vomiting, gastritis, cheilitis, biliary pain, duodenal ulcer, dysphagia, enteritis, gingival hemorrhage, paresthesia, somnolence, torticollis, xerostomia, epistaxis, facial edema, facial paralysis, esophagitis, glossitis, stomatitis, loss of taste, abnormal taste, vasodilation, postural hypotension, hypertension, pharyngitis, rhinitis, migraine, syncope, hypoglycemia, flushing, bruising, incoordination, malaise, lymphadenopathy, leg cramps

Dosage Doses should be individualized according to the baseline LDL-cholesterol levels, the recommended goal of therapy, and patient response; adjustments should be made at intervals of 2-4 weeks.

Oral:

Children 10-17 years (females >1 year postmenarche): HeFH: 10 mg once daily (maximum: 20 mg/day)

Adults: Hyperlipidemias: Initial: 10-20 mg once daily; patients requiring >45% reduction in LDL-C may be started at 40 mg once daily; range: 10-80 mg once daily

Dosing adjustment in renal impairment: No dosage adjustment is necessary.

Dosing adjustment in hepatic impairment: Do not use in active liver disease.

Mechanism of Action Inhibitor of 3-hydroxy-3-methylglutaryl coenzyme A (HMG-CoA) reductase, the rate limiting enzyme in cholesterol synthesis (reduces the production of mevalonic acid from HMG-CoA); this then results in a compensatory increase in the expression of LDL receptors on hepatocyte membranes and a stimulation of LDL catabolism

Other Adverse Effects

2% to 10%:

Cardiovascular: Peripheral edema

Central nervous system: Insomnia

Dermatologic: Rash (≤4%)

Gastrointestinal: Abdominal pain (≤4%), constipation (≤3%), diarrhea (≤4%), dyspepsia (≤3%), flatulence (≤3%)

Genitourinary: Urinary tract infection

Neuromuscular & skeletal: Arthralgia (≤5%), myalgia (≤6%), back pain (≤4%)

<2% (Limited to important or life-threatening): Photosensitivity, edema, elevated transaminases, colitis, rectal hemorrhage, anorexia, increased appetite, tenesmus, hepatitis, pancreatitis, cholestatic jaundice, abnormal dreams, decreased libido, emotional lability, peripheral neuropathy, hyperkinesia, depression, hypesthesia, hypertonia, bursitis, myasthenia, myositis, tendinous contracture, pruritus, alopecia, dry skin, urticaria, acne, eczema, seborrhea, skin ulcer, cystitis, hematuria, impotence, dysuria, nocturia, epididymitis, fibrocystic breast disease, vaginal hemorrhage, nephritis, abnormal urination, amblyopia, tinnitus, deafness, glaucoma, phlebitis, gout, weight gain, anemia, thrombocytopenia, petechiae, myopathy

Postmarketing reports: **Anaphylaxis**, angioneurotic edema, bullous rashes, erythema multiforme, toxic epidermal necrolysis, Stevens-Johnson syndrome, rhabdomyolysis

Class-related events or case reports (not necessarily reported with atorvastatin therapy): Myopathy, increased CPK (>10x normal), rhabdomyolysis, renal failure (secondary to rhabdomyolysis), impaired extraocular muscle movement, **tremor**, memory loss, vertigo, **paresthesia**, peripheral nerve palsy, **anxiety**, depression, psychic disturbance, **hypersensitivity**, angioedema, systemic lupus erythematosus-like syndrome, polymyalgia rheumatica, dermatomyositis, vasculitis, purpura, thrombocytopenia, leukopenia, hemolytic anemia, positive ANA, increased ESR, eosinophilia, arthritis, urticaria, photosensitivity, chills, erythema multiforme, pancreatitis, hepatitis, cholestatic jaundice, fatty liver, cirrhosis, fulminant hepatic necrosis, hepatoma, anorexia, alopecia, nodules, skin discoloration, nail changes, gynecomastia, decreased libido, erectile dysfunction, impotence, cataracts, ophthalmoplegia, elevated transaminases, increased alkaline phosphatase, increased GGT, hyperbilirubinemia, thyroid dysfunction

Warnings/Precautions Secondary causes of hyperlipidemia should be ruled out prior to therapy. Liver function must be monitored by periodic laboratory assessment. Rhabdomyolysis with acute renal failure has occurred. Risk is dose-related and is increased with concurrent use of lipid-lowering agents which may cause rhabdomyolysis (gemfibrozil, fibric acid derivatives, or niacin at doses ≥1 g/day) or during concurrent use with potent CYP3A4 inhibitors (including amiodarone, clarithromycin, cyclosporine, erythromycin, itraconazole, ketoconazole, nefazodone, grapefruit juice in large quantities, verapamil, or protease inhibitors such as indinavir, nelfinavir, or ritonavir). Weigh the risk versus benefit when combining any of these drugs with atorvastatin. Discontinue in any patient experiencing an acute or serious condition predisposing to renal failure secondary to rhabdomyolysis. Use with caution in patients who consume large amounts of ethanol or have a history of liver disease. Safety and efficacy have not been established in patients <10 years or in premenarcheal girls.

Drug Interactions Substrate of **CYP3A4**; Inhibits CYP3A4

Increased Effect/Toxicity: Inhibitors of CYP3A4 (amiodarone, amprenavir, clarithromycin, cyclosporine, diltiazem, fluvoxamine, erythromycin, fluconazole, indinavir, itraconazole, ketoconazole, miconazole, nefazodone, nelfinavir, ritonavir, troleandomycin, and verapamil) may increase atorvastatin blood levels and may increase the risk of atorvastatin-induced myopathy and rhabdomyolysis. The risk of myopathy and rhabdomyolysis due to concurrent use of a CYP3A4 inhibitor with atorvastatin is probably less than lovastatin or simvastatin. Cyclosporine, clofibrate, fenofibrate, gemfibrozil, and niacin also may increase the risk of myopathy and rhabdomyolysis. The effect/toxicity of levothyroxine may be increased by atorvastatin. Levels of digoxin and ethinyl estradiol may be increased by atorvastatin.

Decreased Effect: Colestipol, antacids decreased plasma concentrations but effect on LDL-cholesterol was not altered. Cholestyramine may decrease absorption of atorvastatin when administered concurrently.

(Continued)

Atorvastatin *(Continued)*

Dietary/Ethanol/Herb Considerations

Ethanol: Avoid excessive consumption due to potential hepatic effects.

Food: May be taken with food; Requires a standard cholesterol-lowering diet for 3-6 months prior to and during therapy. Avoid grapefruit products; concurrent intake of large quantities (>1 quart/day) may increase serum concentration.

Herb/Nutraceutical: Avoid St John's wort; may decrease serum concentration.

Pharmacodynamics/Kinetics

Onset of action: Initial changes: 3-5 days; Maximal reduction in plasma cholesterol and triglycerides: 2 weeks

Absorption: Rapid

Protein binding: 98%

Metabolism: Hepatic; forms active ortho- and parahydroxylated derivates and an inactive beta-oxidation product

Half-life elimination: Parent drug: 14 hours

Time to peak, serum: 1-2 hours

Excretion: Bile; urine (2% as unchanged drug)

Pregnancy Risk Factor X

Generic Available No

Selected Readings Siedlik PH, Olson, SC, Yang BB, et al, "Erythromycin Coadministration Increases Plasma Atorvastatin Concentrations," *J Clin Pharmacol*, 1999, 39(5):501-4.

Atovaquone (a TOE va kwone)

Related Information

Systemic Viral Diseases *on page 1517*

U.S. Brand Names Mepron®

Canadian Brand Names Mepron®

Pharmacologic Category Antiprotozoal

Use Acute oral treatment of mild to moderate *Pneumocystis carinii* pneumonia (PCP) in patients who are intolerant to co-trimoxazole; prophylaxis of PCP in patients intolerant to co-trimoxazole; treatment/suppression of *Toxoplasma gondii* encephalitis, primary prophylaxis of HIV-infected persons at high risk for developing *Toxoplasma gondii* encephalitis

Local Anesthetic/Vasoconstrictor Precautions No information available to require special precautions

Effects on Dental Treatment

>10%: Oral moniliasis, headache, fever, anxiety, nausea, vomiting, cough, weakness

1% to 10%: Dizziness, hypoglycemia

Dosage Oral: Adolescents 13-16 years and Adults:

Prevention of PCP: 1500 mg once daily with food

Treatment of mild to moderate PCP: 750 mg twice daily with food for 21 days

Mechanism of Action Has not been fully elucidated; may inhibit electron transport in mitochondria inhibiting metabolic enzymes

Other Adverse Effects Statistics compiled from studies including patients with advanced HIV disease; consequently, it is difficult to distinguish reactions attributed to atovaquone from those caused by the underlying disease or a combination, thereof.

>10%:

- Central nervous system: Insomnia
- Dermatologic: Rash
- Gastrointestinal: Diarrhea

1% to 10%:

- Dermatologic: Pruritus
- Endocrine & metabolic: Hypoglycemia, hyponatremia
- Gastrointestinal: Abdominal pain, constipation, anorexia, dyspepsia, increased amylase
- Hematologic: Anemia, neutropenia, leukopenia
- Hepatic: Elevated liver enzymes
- Renal: Elevated BUN/creatinine

Drug Interactions

Increased Effect/Toxicity: Possible increased toxicity with other highly protein-bound drugs.

Decreased Effect: Rifamycins (rifampin) used concurrently decrease the steady-state plasma concentrations of atovaquone.

Dietary/Ethanol/Herb Considerations Food: High-fat meals may increase absorption up to 3-fold.

Pharmacodynamics/Kinetics

Absorption: Significantly increased with a high-fat meal

Distribution: 3.5 L/kg

Protein binding: >99%

Metabolism: Undergoes enterohepatic recirculation

Bioavailability: Tablet: 23%; Suspension: 47%

Half-life elimination: 2-3 days
Excretion: Feces (94% as unchanged drug)

Pregnancy Risk Factor C

Generic Available No

Atovaquone and Proguanil (a TOE va kwone & pro GWA nil)

Related Information

Atovaquone *on page 142*

U.S. Brand Names Malarone™

Canadian Brand Names Malarone™

Pharmacologic Category Antimalarial Agent

Synonyms Proguanil and Atovaquone

Use Prevention or treatment of acute, uncomplicated *P. falciparum* malaria

Local Anesthetic/Vasoconstrictor Precautions No information available to require special precautions

Effects on Dental Treatment

Reported in ≥5% of adults taking atovaquone/proguanil in treatment doses:
- >10%: Nausea (12%), vomiting (12% adults; 10% to 13% children)
- 1% to 10%: Headache (10%), dizziness (5%), weakness (8%)

Reported in placebo-controlled clinical trials when used for prophylaxis (in general, reactions were similar to or lower than those seen with placebo):
- >10%: Headache (22% adults; 19% children),
- 1% to 10%: Fever (5% adults; 6% children), gastritis (3% adults), vomiting (1% adults; 7% children), upper respiratory tract infection (8% adults), cough (6% adults; 9% children), flu-like syndrome (2% adults; 9% children)

Dosage Oral:

Children (dosage based on body weight):

Prevention of malaria: Start 1-2 days prior to entering a malaria-endemic area, continue throughout the stay and for 7 days after returning. Take as a single dose, once daily.
- 11-20 kg: Atovaquone/proguanil 62.5 mg/25 mg
- 21-30 kg: Atovaquone/proguanil 125 mg/50 mg
- 31-40 kg: Atovaquone/proguanil 187.5 mg/75 mg
- >40 kg: Atovaquone/proguanil 250 mg/100 mg

Treatment of acute malaria: Take as a single dose, once daily for 3 consecutive days.
- 11-20 kg: Atovaquone/proguanil 250 mg/100 mg
- 21-30 kg: Atovaquone/proguanil 500 mg/200 mg
- 31-40 kg: Atovaquone/proguanil 750 mg/300 mg
- >40 kg: Atovaquone/proguanil 1 g/400 mg

Adults:

Prevention of malaria: Atovaquone/proguanil 250 mg/100 mg once daily; start 1-2 days prior to entering a malaria-endemic area, continue throughout the stay and for 7 days after returning

Treatment of acute malaria: Atovaquone/proguanil 1 g/400 mg as a single dose, once daily for 3 consecutive days

Elderly: Use with caution due to possible decrease in renal and hepatic function, as well as possible decreases in cardiac function, concomitant diseases, or other drug therapy.

Dosing adjustment in renal impairment: None in mild to moderate impairment; should not be used as prophylaxis in severe impairment (Cl_{cr} <30 mL/minute). Alternative treatment regimens should be used in patients with Cl_{cr} <30 mL/minute.

Mechanism of Action

Atovaquone: Selectively inhibits parasite mitochondrial electron transport.

Proguanil: The metabolite cycloguanil inhibits dihydrofolate reductase, disrupting deoxythymidylate synthesis. Together, atovaquone/cycloguanil affect the erythrocytic and exoerythrocytic stages of development.

Other Adverse Effects

Reported in ≥5% of adults taking atovaquone/proguanil in treatment doses:
- >10%: Gastrointestinal: Abdominal pain (17%)
- 1% to 10%:
  - Dermatologic: Pruritus (6% children)
  - Gastrointestinal: Diarrhea (8%), anorexia (5%)

Reported in placebo-controlled clinical trials when used for prophylaxis (in general, reactions were similar to or lower than those seen with placebo):
- >10%:
  - Gastrointestinal: Abdominal pain (33% children)
  - Neuromuscular & skeletal: Myalgia (12% adults)
- 1% to 10%:
  - Gastrointestinal: Abdominal pain (9% adults), diarrhea (6% adults, 2% children), dyspepsia (3% adults)
  - Neuromuscular & skeletal: Back pain (8% adults)

(Continued)

Atovaquone and Proguanil *(Continued)*

In addition, 54% of adults in the placebo-controlled trials reported any adverse event (65% for placebo) and 60% of children reported adverse events (62% for placebo).

Case report: Anaphylaxis

Drug Interactions Decreased Effect: Metoclopramide decreases bioavailability of atovaquone. Rifabutin decreases atovaquone levels by 34%. Rifampin decreases atovaquone levels by 50%. Tetracycline decreases plasma concentrations of atovaquone by 40%.

Dietary/Ethanol/Herb Considerations Food: Administer with food or milky beverage; fatty food increases the rate and extent of absorption

Pharmacodynamics/Kinetics

Atovaquone: See Atovaquone monograph.

Proguanil:

Absorption: Extensive

Distribution: 42 L/kg

Protein binding: 75%

Metabolism: Hepatic to active metabolites, cycloguanil (via CYP2C19) and 4-chlorophenylbiguanide

Half-life elimination: 12-21 hours

Excretion: Urine (40% to 60%)

Pregnancy Risk Factor C

Generic Available No

Atridox™ *see* Doxycycline Hyclate Periodontal Extended-Release Liquid *on page 479*

Atromid-S® *see* Clofibrate *on page 347*

Atropine (A troe peen)

Related Information

Cardiovascular Diseases *on page 1456*

U.S. Brand Names Atropine-Care®; Atropisol®; Isopto® Atropine

Canadian Brand Names Dioptic's Atropine Solution; Isopto® Atropine; Minim's Atropine Solution

Mexican Brand Names Lomotil®; Tropyn Z®

Pharmacologic Category Anticholinergic Agent; Anticholinergic Agent, Ophthalmic; Antidote; Antispasmodic Agent, Gastrointestinal; Ophthalmic Agent, Mydriatic

Synonyms Atropine Sulfate

Use Preoperative medication to inhibit salivation and bronchial secretions; treatment of symptomatic sinus bradycardia; antidote for organophosphate pesticide poisoning; to produce mydriasis and cycloplegia for examination of the retina and optic disc and accurate measurement of refractive errors; uveitis; AV block (nodal level); ventricular asystole; treatment of GI disorders (eg, peptic ulcer disease, irritable bowel syndrome, hypermotility of colon)

Local Anesthetic/Vasoconstrictor Precautions No information available to require special precautions

Effects on Dental Treatment

>10%: Xerostomia, changes in salivation, dry throat, nasal dryness

1% to 10%: Dysphagia

Dosage

Neonates, Infants, and Children: Doses <0.1 mg have been associated with paradoxical bradycardia.

Preanesthetic: Oral, I.M., I.V., S.C.:

<5 kg: 0.02 mg/kg/dose 30-60 minutes preop then every 4-6 hours as needed. Use of a minimum dosage of 0.1 mg in neonates <5 kg will result in dosages >0.02 mg/kg. There is no documented minimum dosage in this age group.

>5 kg: 0.01-0.02 mg/kg/dose to a maximum 0.4 mg/dose 30-60 minutes preop; minimum dose: 0.1 mg

Bradycardia: I.V., intratracheal: 0.02 mg/kg, minimum dose 0.1 mg, maximum single dose: 0.5 mg in children and 1 mg in adolescents; may repeat in 5-minute intervals to a maximum total dose of 1 mg in children or 2 mg in adolescents. (**Note:** For intratracheal administration, the dosage must be diluted with normal saline to a total volume of 1-2 mL). When treating bradycardia in neonates, reserve use for those patients unresponsive to improved oxygenation and epinephrine.

Children:

Mydriasis, cycloplegia (preprocedure): Ophthalmic: 0.5% solution: Instill 1-2 drops twice daily for 1-3 days before the procedure

Uveitis: Ophthalmic: 0.5% solution: Instill 1-2 drops up to 3 times/day

Adults (doses <0.5 mg have been associated with paradoxical bradycardia):

Asystole or pulseless electrical activity: I.V.: 1 mg; repeat in 3-5 minutes if asystole persists; total dose of 0.04 mg/kg; may give intratracheally in 10 mL NS (intratracheal dose should be 2-2.5 times the I.V. dose)

Preanesthetic: I.M., I.V., S.C.: 0.4-0.6 mg 30-60 minutes preop and repeat every 4-6 hours as needed

Bradycardia: I.V.: 0.5-1 mg every 5 minutes, not to exceed a total of 3 mg or 0.04 mg/kg; may give intratracheally in 10 mL NS (intratracheal dose should be 2-2.5 times the I.V. dose)

Neuromuscular blockade reversal: I.V.: 25-30 mcg/kg 60 seconds before neostigmine or 7-10 mcg/kg in combination with edrophonium

Organophosphate or carbamate poisoning: I.V.: 1-2 mg/dose every 10-20 minutes until atropine effect (dry flushed skin, tachycardia, mydriasis, fever) is observed, then every 1-4 hours for at least 24 hours; up to 50 mg in first 24 hours and 2 g over several days may be given in cases of severe intoxication

GI disorders: Oral: 0.4-0.6 mg every 4-6 hours

Ophthalmic:

Solution: 1%:

Mydriasis, cycloplegia (preprocedure): Instill 1-2 drops 1 hour before the procedure.

Uveitis: Instill 1-2 drops 4 times/day.

Ointment: Uveitis: Apply a small amount in the conjunctival sac up to 3 times/day. Compress the lacrimal sac by digital pressure for 1-3 minutes after instillation.

Mechanism of Action Blocks the action of acetylcholine at parasympathetic sites in smooth muscle, secretory glands and the CNS; increases cardiac output, dries secretions, antagonizes histamine and serotonin

Other Adverse Effects

>10%:

Dermatologic: Dry/hot skin

Gastrointestinal: Impaired GI motility, constipation

Local: Irritation at injection site

Miscellaneous: Diaphoresis (decreased)

1% to 10%:

Dermatologic: Increased sensitivity to light

Endocrine & metabolic: Decreased flow of breast milk

<1% (Limited to important or life-threatening): Ataxia, blurred vision, **bradycardia (doses <0.5 mg) confusion, delirium, drowsiness, confusion and hallucinations (especially elderly)**, fatigue, **headache**, increased intraocular pain, loss of memory, mydriasis, **orthostatic hypotension, palpitations, restlessness, tachycardia, ventricular fibrillation, ventricular tachycardia**

Drug Interactions

Increased Effect/Toxicity: Amantadine, antihistamines, phenothiazines, and TCAs may increase anticholinergic effects of atropine when used concurrently. Sympathomimetic amines may cause tachyarrhythmias; avoid concurrent use.

Decreased Effect: Effect of some phenothiazines may be antagonized. Levodopa effects may be decreased (limited clinical validation). Drugs with cholinergic mechanisms (metoclopramide, cisapride, bethanechol) decrease anticholinergic effects of atropine.

Pharmacodynamics/Kinetics

Onset of action: I.V.: Rapid

Absorption: Complete

Distribution: Widely throughout the body; crosses placenta; trace amounts enter breast milk; crosses blood-brain barrier

Metabolism: Hepatic

Half-life elimination: 2-3 hours

Excretion: Urine (30% to 50% as unchanged drug and metabolites)

Pregnancy Risk Factor C

Generic Available Yes

Atropine and Difenoxin *see* Difenoxin and Atropine *on page 437*

Atropine and Diphenoxylate *see* Diphenoxylate and Atropine *on page 453*

Atropine-Care® *see* Atropine *on page 144*

Atropine, Hyoscyamine, Scopolamine, and Phenobarbital *see* Hyoscyamine, Atropine, Scopolamine, and Phenobarbital *on page 700*

Atropine Sulfate *see* Atropine *on page 144*

Atropine Sulfate Dental Tablets

(A troe peen SUL fate DEN tal TAB lets)

Related Information

Atropine *on page 144*

Management of Sialorrhea *on page 1555*

U.S. Brand Names Sal-Tropine™

Pharmacologic Category Anticholinergic Agent

Use Dental: Reduction of salivation and bronchial secretions

Local Anesthetic/Vasoconstrictor Precautions No information available to require special precautions

(Continued)

Atropine Sulfate Dental Tablets *(Continued)*

Effects on Dental Treatment Frequency not defined (dose-related):
Children: May produce fever (by inhibiting heat loss by evaporation), scarlitiniform rash
Causes significant xerostomia when used in therapeutic doses:
0.5 mg: **Slight dryness of nose and mouth; bradycardia**
1 mg: **Increased dryness of nose and mouth; thirst; slowing then acceleration of heart rate**; mydriasis
2 mg: **Significant xerostomia; tachycardia with palpitations**; mydriasis; slight blurring of vision; flushing, dry skin
5 mg: **Increase in above symptoms plus disturbance of speech; difficulty swallowing**; headache; hot, dry skin; restlessness with asthenia
10 mg: Above symptoms to **extreme degree plus ataxia, excitement, disorientation, hallucinations, delirium, coma**

Dosage Oral:
Children:
7-16 lbs: 0.1 mg
17-24 lbs: 0.15 mg
24-40 lbs: 0.2 mg
40-65 lbs: 0.3 mg
65-90 lbs: 0.4 mg
>90 lbs: 0.4 mg
Adults: 0.4 mg

Mechanism of Action Blocks the action of acetylcholine at parasympathetic sites in smooth muscle, secretory glands, and the CNS; increases cardiac output, dries secretions, antagonizes histamine and serotonin

Contraindications Hypersensitivity to atropine or any component of the formulation; narrow-angle glaucoma; adhesions between the iris and lens; tachycardia; unstable cardiovascular status in acute hemorrhage; obstructive GI disease; paralytic ileus; intestinal atony of the elderly or debilitated patient; severe ulcerative colitis; toxic megacolon complicating ulcerative colitis; hepatic disease; obstructive uropathy; renal disease; myasthenia gravis (unless used to treat side effects of acetylcholinesterase inhibitor); asthma; thyrotoxicosis; Mobitz type II block

Warnings/Precautions Doses of 0.5-1 mg of atropine are mildly stimulating to the CNS. Larger doses may produce mental disturbances; still larger doses are CNS-depressant. Death from atropine poisoning, though rare, is usually due to paralysis of the medullary centers. Signs and symptoms of atropine overdose include mydriasis, tachycardia, decreased salivation, decreased sweating, diminished bowel sounds, urinary retention, hypertension, and vasodilation. CNS symptoms include anxiety, disorientation, hallucinations, hyperactivity, and convulsions or coma. Hyperthermia may occur. Heat prostration can occur in the presence of a high environmental temperature. Rule out intestinal obstruction before treating diarrhea. Psychosis can occur in sensitive individuals. The elderly may be sensitive to side effects. Use caution in patients with myocardial ischemia. Use caution in hyperthyroidism, autonomic neuropathy, BPH, CHF, tachyarrhythmias, hypertension, and hiatal hernia associated with reflux esophagitis. Use with caution in children with spastic paralysis.

Drug Interactions
Increased Effect: Atropine-induced mouth dryness may be increased if it is given with other drugs that have anticholinergic actions such as tricyclic antidepressants, antipsychotics, some antihistamines, and antiparkinsonism drugs
Decreased Effect: May interfere with absorption of other medications due to its actions on slowing GI motility and gastric emptying

Dosage Forms TAB, as sulfate: 0.4 mg

Generic Available No

Atropisol® *see* Atropine *on page 144*
Atrovent® *see* Ipratropium *on page 737*
A/T/S® *see* Erythromycin *on page 512*

Attapulgite (at a PULL gite)

Related Information
Oral Nonviral Soft Tissue Ulcerations or Erosions *on page 1549*

U.S. Brand Names Children's Kaopectate® [DSC] [OTC]; Diasorb® [OTC]; Kaopectate® Advanced Formula [DSC] [OTC]; Kaopectate® Maximum Strength Caplets [DSC] [OTC]

Canadian Brand Names Kaopectate®

Pharmacologic Category Antidiarrheal

Use Symptomatic treatment of diarrhea

Local Anesthetic/Vasoconstrictor Precautions No information available to require special precautions

Effects on Dental Treatment Frequency not defined: Pneumoconiosis (from chronic inhalation of powder which contains large amounts of silica)
Do not give oral drugs concomitantly with Kaopectate® due to decreased GI absorption.

Restrictions Attapulgite preparations are being discontinued in the U.S., refer to Bismuth monograph for newly-reformulated Kaopectate® products.

Dosage Adequate controlled clinical studies documenting the efficacy of attapulgite are lacking; its usage and dosage has been primarily empiric; the following are manufacturer's recommended dosages

Oral: Give after each bowel movement

Children:

3-6 years: 300-750 mg/dose; maximum dose: 7 doses/day or 2250 mg/day

6-12 years: 600-1500 mg/dose; maximum dose: 7 doses/day or 4500 mg/day

Children >12 years and Adults: 1200-3000 mg/dose; maximum dose: 8 doses/day or 9000 mg/day

Mechanism of Action Controls diarrhea because of its absorbent action

Other Adverse Effects 1% to 10%: Gastrointestinal: Constipation (dose-related)

Drug Interactions Decreased Effect: May decrease GI absorption of orally administered clindamycin, tetracyclines, penicillamine, digoxin.

Pharmacodynamics/Kinetics Absorption: Not absorbed

Pregnancy Risk Factor B

Generic Available Yes

Attenuvax® *see* Measles Virus Vaccine (Live) *on page 845*
Augmentin® *see* Amoxicillin and Clavulanate Potassium *on page 95*
Augmentin ES-600™ *see* Amoxicillin and Clavulanate Potassium *on page 95*
Augmentin XR™ *see* Amoxicillin and Clavulanate Potassium *on page 95*
Auralgan® *see* Antipyrine and Benzocaine *on page 116*

Auranofin (au RANE oh fin)

Related Information

Rheumatoid Arthritis, Osteoarthritis, and Osteoporosis *on page 1488*

U.S. Brand Names Ridaura®

Canadian Brand Names Ridaura®

Pharmacologic Category Gold Compound

Use Management of active stage of classic or definite rheumatoid arthritis in patients that do not respond to or tolerate other agents; psoriatic arthritis; adjunctive or alternative therapy for pemphigus

Local Anesthetic/Vasoconstrictor Precautions No information available to require special precautions

Effects on Dental Treatment 1% to 10%: Glossitis, stomatitis

Dosage Oral:

Children: Initial: 0.1 mg/kg/day divided daily; usual maintenance: 0.15 mg/kg/day in 1-2 divided doses; maximum: 0.2 mg/kg/day in 1-2 divided doses

Adults: 6 mg/day in 1-2 divided doses; after 3 months may be increased to 9 mg/day in 3 divided doses; if still no response after 3 months at 9 mg/day, discontinue drug

Dosing adjustment in renal impairment:

Cl_{cr} 50-80 mL/minute: Reduce dose to 50%

Cl_{cr} <50 mL/minute: Avoid use

Mechanism of Action The exact mechanism of action of gold is unknown; gold is taken up by macrophages which results in inhibition of phagocytosis and lysosomal membrane stabilization; other actions observed are decreased serum rheumatoid factor and alterations in immunoglobulins. Additionally, complement activation is decreased, prostaglandin synthesis is inhibited, and lysosomal enzyme activity is decreased.

Other Adverse Effects

>10%:

Dermatologic: Itching, rash

Ocular: Conjunctivitis

Renal: Proteinuria

1% to 10%:

Dermatologic: Urticaria, alopecia

Hematologic: Eosinophilia, leukopenia, thrombocytopenia

Renal: Hematuria

<1%: Angioedema, ulcerative enterocolitis, **GI hemorrhage, gingivitis, dysphagia, metallic taste**, agranulocytosis, anemia, aplastic anemia, hepatotoxicity, peripheral neuropathy, interstitial pneumonitis

Drug Interactions Increased Effect/Toxicity: Toxicity of penicillamine, antimalarials, hydroxychloroquine, cytotoxic agents, and immunosuppressants may be increased.

Pharmacodynamics/Kinetics

Onset of action: Delayed; therapeutic response may require as long as 3-4 months

Duration: Prolonged

Absorption: Oral: ~20% gold in dose is absorbed

Protein binding: 60%

Half-life elimination (single or multiple dose dependent): 21-31 days

Time to peak, serum: ~2 hours

Excretion: Urine (60% of absorbed gold); remainder in feces

Pregnancy Risk Factor C

Generic Available No

Auro® Ear Drops [OTC] *see* Carbamide Peroxide *on page 244*
Aurolate® *see* Gold Sodium Thiomalate *on page 646*

Aurothioglucose (aur oh thye oh GLOO kose)

Related Information
Rheumatoid Arthritis, Osteoarthritis, and Osteoporosis *on page 1488*

U.S. Brand Names Solganal®

Canadian Brand Names Solganal®

Pharmacologic Category Gold Compound

Use Adjunctive treatment in adult and juvenile active rheumatoid arthritis; alternative or adjunct in treatment of pemphigus; psoriatic patients who do not respond to NSAIDs

Local Anesthetic/Vasoconstrictor Precautions No information available to require special precautions

Effects on Dental Treatment >10%: Gingivitis, glossitis, metallic taste, stomatitis

Dosage I.M.: Doses should initially be given at weekly intervals

Children 6-12 years: Initial: 0.25 mg/kg/dose first week; increment at 0.25 mg/kg/dose increasing with each weekly dose; maintenance: 0.75-1 mg/kg/dose weekly not to exceed 25 mg/dose to a total of 20 doses, then every 2-4 weeks

Adults: 10 mg first week; 25 mg second and third week; then 50 mg/week until 800 mg to 1 g cumulative dose has been given; if improvement occurs without adverse reactions, administer 25-50 mg every 2-3 weeks, then every 3-4 weeks

Mechanism of Action Unknown, may decrease prostaglandin synthesis or may alter cellular mechanisms by inhibiting sulfhydryl systems

Other Adverse Effects

>10%: Dermatologic: Itching, rash, exfoliative dermatitis, reddened skin

1% to 10%: Renal: Proteinuria

<1%: Encephalitis, EEG abnormalities, **fever**, alopecia, ulcerative enterocolitis, vaginitis, agranulocytosis, aplastic anemia, eosinophilia, leukopenia, thrombocytopenia, hepatotoxicity, **pharyngitis, bronchitis**, pulmonary fibrosis, interstitial pneumonitis, peripheral neuropathy, conjunctivitis, corneal ulcers, iritis, glomerulitis, hematuria, nephrotic syndrome, **anaphylactic shock, allergic reaction (severe)**

Drug Interactions Increased Effect/Toxicity: Toxicity of penicillamine, antimalarials, hydroxychloroquine, cytotoxic agents, and immunosuppressants may be increased.

Pharmacodynamics/Kinetics

Absorption: I.M.: Erratic and slow
Distribution: Crosses placenta; enters breast milk
Protein binding: 95% to 99%
Half-life elimination (single or multiple dose dependent): 3-27 days
Time to peak, serum: 4-6 hours
Excretion: Urine (70%); feces (30%)

Pregnancy Risk Factor C

Generic Available No

Auroto® *see* Antipyrine and Benzocaine *on page 116*
Autoplex® T *see* Anti-inhibitor Coagulant Complex *on page 116*
AVA *see* Anthrax Vaccine (Adsorbed) *on page 112*
Avagard™ [OTC] *see* Chlorhexidine Gluconate *on page 300*
Avage™ *see* Tazarotene *on page 1267*
Avalide® *see* Irbesartan and Hydrochlorothiazide *on page 740*
Avandamet™ *see* Rosiglitazone and Metformin *on page 1200*
Avandia® *see* Rosiglitazone *on page 1199*
Avapro® *see* Irbesartan *on page 739*
Avapro® HCT *see* Irbesartan and Hydrochlorothiazide *on page 740*
Avelox® *see* Moxifloxacin *on page 935*
Avelox® I.V. *see* Moxifloxacin *on page 935*
Aventyl® HCl *see* Nortriptyline *on page 989*
Aviane™ *see* Combination Hormonal Contraceptives *on page 368*
Avinza™ *see* Morphine Sulfate *on page 931*
Avita® *see* Tretinoin (Topical) *on page 1340*
Avitene® *see* Microfibrillar Collagen Hemostat *on page 907*
Avodart™ *see* Dutasteride *on page 484*
Avonex® *see* Interferon Beta-1a *on page 732*
Axert™ *see* Almotriptan *on page 59*
Axid® *see* Nizatidine *on page 984*
Axid® AR [OTC] *see* Nizatidine *on page 984*
Aygestin® *see* Norethindrone *on page 986*
Ayr® Baby Saline [OTC] *see* Sodium Chloride *on page 1229*

Ayr® Saline [OTC] *see* Sodium Chloride *on page 1229*
Ayr® Saline Mist [OTC] *see* Sodium Chloride *on page 1229*

Azacitidine (ay za SYE ti deen)

Pharmacologic Category Antineoplastic Agent, Miscellaneous

Synonyms AZA-CR; 5-Azacytidine; 5-AZC; Ladakamycin; NSC-102816

Use Refractory acute lymphocytic and myelogenous leukemia; myelodysplastic syndrome

Unlabeled/Investigational Use Investigational: Treatment of refractory acute lymphocytic and myelogenous leukemia, myelodysplastic syndrome

Local Anesthetic/Vasoconstrictor Precautions No information available to require special precautions

Effects on Dental Treatment

>10%: Coma (300-750 mg/m²), nausea, vomiting, mucositis
1% to 10%: Hypotension, coma

Restrictions Available through NCI (Group C) at 301-496-5725.

Dosage Children and Adults: I.V., S.C.: 50-200 mg/m²/day for 5-10 days, repeated at 2- to 3-week intervals **or** 75 mg/m²/day for 7 days repeated every 4 weeks

Mechanism of Action No precise mechanism of action has been established. The drug appears to interfere with nucleic acid metabolism prior to the steps involving cytidine and uridine, with its major activity in the S phase of the cell cycle. Postulated mechanisms include:

- Phosphorylation to a triphosphate and direct incorporation into DNA
- Phosphorylation to a triphosphate, competition with cytosine triphosphate, and incorporation into RNA, producing defective messenger and transfer RNA
- Competition with uridine and cytidine for uridine kinase
- Inhibition of orotidylic acid decarboxylase, inhibiting pyrimidine synthesis

Other Adverse Effects

>10%:
- Gastrointestinal: Diarrhea
- Hematologic: Leukopenia, thrombocytopenia

1% to 10%:
- Dermatologic: Rash
- Hepatic: Hepatic abnormalities (increased enzyme levels up to coma)
- Renal: Renal toxicity (azotemia, hypophosphatemia, tubular acidosis)

Pharmacodynamics/Kinetics

Absorption: S.C.: Rapid and complete
Distribution: Does not cross blood-brain barrier
Metabolism: Hepatic; hydrolysis to several metabolites
Half-life elimination: ~4 hours
Excretion: Urine (50% to 85%); feces (minor)

Pregnancy Risk Factor C

Generic Available No

AZA-CR *see* Azacitidine *on page 149*
Azactam® *see* Aztreonam *on page 155*
5-Azacytidine *see* Azacitidine *on page 149*

Azatadine (a ZA ta deen)

U.S. Brand Names Optimine®

Canadian Brand Names Optimine®

Mexican Brand Names Idulamine®

Pharmacologic Category Antihistamine

Synonyms Azatadine Maleate

Use Treatment of perennial and seasonal allergic rhinitis and chronic urticaria

Local Anesthetic/Vasoconstrictor Precautions No information available to require special precautions

Effects on Dental Treatment

>10%: Slight to moderate drowsiness, thickening of bronchial secretions
1% to 10%: Xerostomia, dry throat, nasal dryness, headache, nervousness, dizziness, nausea, pharyngitis, fatigue

Dosage Children >12 years and Adults: Oral: 1-2 mg twice daily

Mechanism of Action Azatadine is a piperidine-derivative antihistamine; has both anticholinergic and antiserotonin activity; has been demonstrated to inhibit mediator release from human mast cells *in vitro*; mechanism of this action is suggested to prevent calcium entry into the mast cell through voltage-dependent calcium channels

Other Adverse Effects

1% to 10%:
- Gastrointestinal: Appetite increase, weight gain, diarrhea, abdominal pain
- Neuromuscular & skeletal: Arthralgia

<1%: **Palpitations**, edema, depression, angioedema, photosensitivity, rash, hepatitis, myalgia, **paresthesia, bronchospasm, epistaxis**

Drug Interactions Induces CYP3A4

(Continued)

Azatadine *(Continued)*

Increased Effect/Toxicity: Potential for increased side effects when used with procarbazine, CNS depressants, tricyclic antidepressants, and alcohol.

Dietary/Ethanol/Herb Considerations

Ethanol: Avoid use; may increase CNS depression.

Herb/Nutraceutical: Avoid gotu kola, kava, SAMe, St John's wort, and valerian; may increase CNS depression.

Pharmacodynamics/Kinetics

Onset of action: 1-2 hours

Absorption: Rapid and extensive

Metabolism: Hepatic

Protein binding: Minimally to plasma protein

Half-life elimination: ~8.7 hours

Time to peak: 4 hours

Excretion: Urine (~20% as unchanged drug) within 48 hours

Pregnancy Risk Factor B

Generic Available No

Azatadine and Pseudoephedrine

(a ZA ta deen & soo doe e FED rin)

Related Information

Azatadine *on page 149*

Pseudoephedrine *on page 1146*

U.S. Brand Names Rynatan® Tablet; Trinalin®

Canadian Brand Names Trinalin®

Pharmacologic Category Antihistamine/Decongestant Combination

Synonyms Pseudoephedrine and Azatadine

Use Perennial and seasonal allergic rhinitis and other allergic symptoms including urticaria

Local Anesthetic/Vasoconstrictor Precautions

Azatadine: No information available to require special precautions

Pseudoephedrine: Use with caution since pseudoephedrine is a sympathomimetic amine which could interact with epinephrine to cause a pressor response

Effects on Dental Treatment

Azatadine: Frequency not defined: Drowsiness, xerostomia, dry throat, nasal dryness; due to atropine-like effects

Pseudoephedrine: ≤10%: tachycardia, palpitations, xerostomia; use vasoconstrictor with caution

Dosage Adults: 1 tablet twice daily

Pregnancy Risk Factor C

Generic Available No

Azatadine Maleate *see* Azatadine *on page 149*

Azathioprine (ay za THYE oh preen)

U.S. Brand Names Imuran®

Canadian Brand Names Alti-Azathioprine; Apo®-Azathioprine; Gen-Azathioprine; Imuran®

Mexican Brand Names Azatrilem®; Imuran®

Pharmacologic Category Immunosuppressant Agent

Synonyms Azathioprine Sodium

Use Adjunct with other agents in prevention of rejection of kidney transplants; also used in severe active rheumatoid arthritis unresponsive to other agents; other autoimmune diseases (ITP, SLE, MS, Crohn's disease)

Unlabeled/Investigational Use Adjunct in prevention of rejection of solid organ (nonrenal) transplants

Local Anesthetic/Vasoconstrictor Precautions No information available to require special precautions

Effects on Dental Treatment Frequency not defined: Fever, nausea, vomiting, aphthous stomatitis

Dosage I.V. dose is equivalent to oral dose; dosing should be based on ideal body weight.

Children and Adults: Renal transplantation: Oral, I.V.: 2-5 mg/kg/day to start, then 1-3 mg/kg/day maintenance

Adults: Rheumatoid arthritis: Oral: 1 mg/kg/day for 6-8 weeks; increase by 0.5 mg/kg every 4 weeks until response or up to 2.5 mg/kg/day

Dosing adjustment in renal impairment:

Cl_{cr} 10-50 mL/minute: Administer 75% of normal dose daily

Cl_{cr} <10 mL/minute: Administer 50% of normal dose daily

Hemodialysis: Slightly dialyzable (5% to 20%)

Administer dose posthemodialysis: CAPD effects: Unknown; CAVH effects: Unknown

Mechanism of Action Azathioprine is an imidazolyl derivative of 6-mercaptopurine; antagonizes purine metabolism and may inhibit synthesis of DNA, RNA, and proteins; may also interfere with cellular metabolism and inhibit mitosis

Other Adverse Effects Frequency not defined:

Central nervous system: Chills

Dermatologic: Alopecia, erythematous or maculopapular rash

Gastrointestinal: Anorexia, diarrhea, pancreatitis

Hematologic: Leukopenia, thrombocytopenia, anemia, pancytopenia (bone marrow suppression may be determined, in part, by genetic factors [ie, patients with TPMT deficiency are at higher risk])

Hepatic: Hepatotoxicity, jaundice, hepatic veno-occlusive disease

Neuromuscular & skeletal: Arthralgias

Ocular: Retinopathy

Miscellaneous: **Rare hypersensitivity reactions which include rigors, dyspnea, hypotension**, serum sickness, myalgias, and rash; secondary infections may occur secondary to immunosuppression

Drug Interactions

Increased Effect/Toxicity: Allopurinol may increase serum levels of azathioprine's active metabolite (6-MP). Decrease azathioprine dose to 1/3 to 1/4 of normal dose. Azathioprine and ACE inhibitors may induce severe leukopenia. Aminosalicylates (olsalazine, mesalamine, sulfasalazine) may inhibit TPMT, increasing toxicity/myelosuppression of azathioprine.

Decreased Effect: Azathioprine may result in decreased action of warfarin.

Dietary/Ethanol/Herb Considerations

Food: Administer with food to avoid GI upset.

Herb/Nutraceutical: Avoid cat's claw and echinacea due to immunostimulant properties.

Pharmacodynamics/Kinetics

Distribution: Crosses placenta

Protein binding: ~30%

Metabolism: Extensively hepatic via xanthine oxidase to 6-mercaptopurine (active); 6-MP requires detoxification by thiopurine methyltransferase (TPMT)

Half-life elimination: Parent drug: 12 minutes; 6-mercaptopurine: 0.7-3 hours; End-stage renal disease: Slightly prolonged

Excretion: Urine (primarily as metabolites)

Pregnancy Risk Factor D

Generic Available Yes

Azathioprine Sodium *see* Azathioprine *on page 150*

5-AZC *see* Azacitidine *on page 149*

Azelaic Acid (a zeh LAY ik AS id)

U.S. Brand Names Azelex®; Finacea™; Finevin®

Mexican Brand Names Cutacelan®

Pharmacologic Category Topical Skin Product, Acne

Use Topical treatment of mild to moderate inflammatory acne vulgaris; treatment of mild to moderate rosacea

Local Anesthetic/Vasoconstrictor Precautions No information available to require special precautions

Effects on Dental Treatment 1% to 10%: Paresthesia

Dosage Topical:

Adolescents >12 years and Adults: Acne vulgaris: After skin is thoroughly washed and patted dry, gently but thoroughly massage a thin film of azelaic acid cream into the affected areas twice daily, in the morning and evening. The duration of use can vary and depends on the severity of the acne. In the majority of patients with inflammatory lesions, improvement of the condition occurs within 4 weeks.

Adults: Rosacea: Massage gently into affected areas of the face twice daily

Mechanism of Action Azelaic acid is a dietary constituent normally found in whole grain cereals, can be formed endogenously. Exact mechanism is not known; *in vitro*, azelaic acid possesses antimicrobial activity against *Propionibacterium acnes* and *Staphylococcus epidermidis*; may decrease microcomedo formation

Pharmacodynamics/Kinetics

Absorption: ~3% to 5% penetrates stratum corneum; up to 10% found in epidermis and dermis; 4% systemic

Half-life elimination: Topical: Healthy subjects: 12 hours

Excretion: Urine (as unchanged drug)

Pregnancy Risk Factor B

Generic Available No

Azelastine (a ZEL as teen)

U.S. Brand Names Astelin®; Optivar™

Canadian Brand Names Astelin®

Mexican Brand Names Astelin®; Az®

Pharmacologic Category Antihistamine

Synonyms Azelastine Hydrochloride

(Continued)

Azelastine *(Continued)*

Use

Nasal spray: Treatment of the symptoms of seasonal allergic rhinitis such as rhinorrhea, sneezing, and nasal pruritus in children ≥5 years of age and adults; treatment of the symptoms of vasomotor rhinitis in children ≥12 years of age and adults

Ophthalmic: Treatment of itching of the eye associated with seasonal allergic conjunctivitis in children ≥3 years of age and adults

Local Anesthetic/Vasoconstrictor Precautions No information available to require special precautions

Effects on Dental Treatment Chronic use of antihistamines will inhibit salivary flow, particularly in elderly patients; may contribute to periodontal disease and oral discomfort.

Nasal spray:

>10%: Bitter taste (20%), headache (15%), somnolence (12%)

2% to 10%: Xerostomia, dizziness (2%), nausea (3%), pharyngitis (4%), paroxysmal sneezing (3%), rhinitis (2%), epistaxis (2%), fatigue (2%)

<2%: Aphthous stomatitis, glossitis, flushing, hypertension, tachycardia, drowsiness, nervousness, anxiety, abnormal thinking, vomiting, bronchospasm, cough, burning sensation in throat, laryngitis, allergic reactions, viral infections

Ophthalmic: >10%: Headache (15%), asthma, dyspnea, pharyngitis, flu-like syndrome, bitter taste (10%)

Dosage

Children ≥5-11 years: Seasonal allergic rhinitis: Intranasal: 1 spray each nostril twice daily

Children ≥12 years and Adults: Seasonal allergic rhinitis or vasomotor rhinitis: Intranasal: 2 sprays (137 mcg/spray) each nostril twice daily

Children ≥3 years and Adults: Itching eyes due to seasonal allergic conjunctivitis: Ophthalmic: Instill 1 drop into affected eye(s) twice daily

Mechanism of Action Competes with histamine for H_1-receptor sites on effector cells and inhibits the release of histamine and other mediators involved in the allergic response. When used intranasally, reduces hyper-reactivity of the airways; increases the motility of bronchial epithelial cilia, improving mucociliary transport

Other Adverse Effects

Nasal spray:

2% to 10%:

Gastrointestinal: Weight gain (2%)

Respiratory: Nasal burning (4%)

<2%:

Central nervous system: Fatigue, vertigo, depression, hypoesthesia, depersonalization, sleep disorder, malaise

Dermatologic: Contact dermatitis, eczema, hair and follicle infection, furunculosis

Gastrointestinal: Constipation, increased ALT, gastroenteritis, increased appetite, abdominal pain

Genitourinary: Urinary frequency, hematuria, albuminuria, amenorrhea

Neuromuscular & skeletal: Myalgia, vertigo, temporomandibular dislocation, hypoesthesia, hyperkinesia, back pain, extremity pain

Ocular: Conjunctivitis, watery eyes, eye pain

<1%, postmarketing, and/or reports: **Anaphylactoid reaction, chest pain, nasal congestion, confusion**, diarrhea, **dyspnea, facial edema, involuntary muscle contractions, paresthesia**, parosmia, pruritus, rash, tolerance, urinary retention, visual abnormalities, xerophthalmia

Ophthalmic:

>10%: Ocular: Transient burning/stinging (30%)

1% to 10%:

Central nervous system: Fatigue

Ocular: Conjunctivitis, eye pain, blurred vision (temporary)

Drug Interactions Substrate of CYP1A2, 2C19, 2D6, 3A4; Inhibits CYP2B6, 2C8/9, 2C19, **2D6**, 3A4

Increased Effect/Toxicity: May cause additive sedation when concomitantly administered with other CNS depressant medications. Cimetidine can increase the AUC and C_{max} of azelastine by as much as 65%.

Dietary/Ethanol/Herb Considerations

Ethanol: Avoid use; may cause increased somnolence or fatigue.

Herb/Nutraceutical: Avoid gotu kola, kava, SAMe, St John's wort, and valerian; may increase CNS depression.

Pharmacodynamics/Kinetics

Onset of action: Peak effect: Nasal spray: 3 hours; Ophthalmic solution: 3 minutes

Duration: Nasal spray: 12 hours; Ophthalmic solution: 8 hours

Protein binding: 88%

Metabolism: Hepatic via CYP; active metabolite, desmethylazelastine

Bioavailability: Intranasal: 40%

Half-life elimination: 22 hours

Time to peak, serum: 2-3 hours

Pregnancy Risk Factor C

Generic Available No

Comments Azelastine is absorbed systemically will cause sedation in some patients. Although this agent is clinically effective, the side effects of sedation, bitter taste, and high cost will limits its use in many patients.

Azelastine Hydrochloride *see* Azelastine *on page 151*

Azelex® *see* Azelaic Acid *on page 151*

Azidothymidine *see* Zidovudine *on page 1406*

Azidothymidine, Abacavir, and Lamivudine *see* Abacavir, Lamivudine, and Zidovudine *on page 23*

Azithromycin (az ith roe MYE sin)

Related Information

Antibiotic Prophylaxis, Preprocedural Guidelines for Dental Patients *on page 1507*

Sexually-Transmitted Diseases *on page 1502*

U.S. Brand Names Zithromax®

Canadian Brand Names Zithromax®

Mexican Brand Names Azitrocin®

Pharmacologic Category Antibiotic, Macrolide

Synonyms Azithromycin Dihydrate

Use

Dental: Alternate antibiotic in the treatment of common orofacial infections caused by aerobic gram-positive cocci and susceptible anaerobes; alternate antibiotic for the prevention of bacterial endocarditis in patients undergoing dental procedures

Medical:

Children: Treatment of acute otitis media due to *H. influenzae, M. catarrhalis*, or *S. pneumoniae*; pharyngitis/tonsillitis due to *S. pyogenes*; community-acquired pneumonia due to *C. pneumoniae, H. influenzae, M. pneumoniae*, or *S. pneumoniae*

Adults:

Treatment of mild to moderate upper and lower respiratory tract infections, infections of the skin and skin structure, community-acquired pneumonia, pelvic inflammatory disease (PID), sexually-transmitted diseases (urethritis/cervicitis), pharyngitis/tonsillitis (alternative to first-line therapy), and genital ulcer disease (chancroid) due to susceptible strains of *C. trachomatis, M. catarrhalis, H. influenzae, S. aureus, S. pneumoniae, Mycoplasma pneumoniae*, and *C. psittaci*

Prevention of (or to delay onset of) or treatment of MAC in patients with advanced HIV infection

Prophylaxis of bacterial endocarditis in patients who are allergic to penicillin and undergoing surgical procedures

Acute bacterial exacerbations of chronic obstructive pulmonary disease (COPD) due to *H. influenzae, M. catarrhalis*, or *S. pneumoniae*

Local Anesthetic/Vasoconstrictor Precautions No information available to require special precautions

Effects on Dental Treatment 1% to 10%: Vomiting (especially with high single-dose regimens), nausea

Dosage

Oral:

Children ≥6 months:

Community-acquired pneumonia: 10 mg/kg on day 1 (maximum: 500 mg/day) followed by 5 mg/kg/day once daily on days 2-5 (maximum: 250 mg/day)

Otitis media:

1-day regimen: 30 mg/kg as a single dose (maximum dose: 1500 mg)

3-day regimen: 10 mg/kg once daily for 3 days (maximum: 500 mg/day)

5-day regimen: 10 mg/kg on day 1 (maximum: 500 mg/day) followed by 5 mg/kg/day once daily on days 2-5 (maximum: 250 mg/day)

Children ≥2 years: **Pharyngitis, tonsillitis:** 12 mg/kg/day once daily for 5 days (maximum: 500 mg/day)

Children:

M. avium-infected patients with acquired immunodeficiency syndrome: Not currently FDA approved for use; 10-20 mg/kg/day once daily (maximum: 40 mg/kg/day) has been used in clinical trials; prophylaxis for first episode of MAC: 5-12 mg/kg/day once daily (maximum: 500 mg/day)

Prophylaxis for bacterial endocarditis: 15 mg/kg 1 hour before procedure

Adolescents ≥16 years and Adults:

Respiratory tract, skin and soft tissue infections: 500 mg on day 1 followed by 250 mg/day on days 2-5 (maximum: 500 mg/day)

Alternative regimen for bacterial exacerbation of COPD: 500 mg/day for a total of 3 days

Urethritis/cervicitis:

Due to *C. trachomatis*: 1 g as a single dose

(Continued)

Azithromycin *(Continued)*

Due to *N. gonorrhoeae*: 2 g as a single dose

Chancroid due to *H. ducreyi*: 1 g as a single dose

Prophylaxis of disseminated *M. avium* complex disease in patient with advanced HIV infection: 1200 mg once weekly (may be combined with rifabutin)

Treatment of disseminated *M. avium* complex disease in patient with advanced HIV infection: 600 mg daily (in combination with ethambutol 15 mg/kg)

Prophylaxis for bacterial endocarditis: 500 mg 1 hour prior to the procedure:

I.V.: Adults:

Community-acquired pneumonia: 500 mg as a single dose for at least 2 days, follow I.V. therapy by the oral route with a single daily dose of 500 mg to complete a 7-10 day course of therapy

Pelvic inflammatory disease (PID): 500 mg as a single dose for 1-2 days, follow I.V. therapy by the oral route with a single daily dose of 250 mg to complete a 7-day course of therapy

Dosing adjustment in renal impairment: Use caution in Cl_{cr} <10 mL/minute

Mechanism of Action Inhibits RNA-dependent protein synthesis at the chain elongation step; binds to the 50S ribosomal subunit resulting in blockage of transpeptidation

Other Adverse Effects

1% to 10%: Gastrointestinal: Diarrhea, abdominal pain, cramping

<1%: **Agitation, allergic reaction**, anemia, anorexia, **candidiasis, chest pain**, conjunctivitis, **dermatitis (fungal), dizziness**, dyspepsia, eczema, enteritis, **facial edema, fatigue**, flatulence, **gastritis, headache**, hyperkinesia, **cough**, insomnia, jaundice, leukopenia, **malaise, nervousness, pain, pharyngitis**, pleural effusion, pruritus, rash, **rhinitis**, urticaria

Postmarketing and/or case reports: Acute renal failure, **aggressive behavior, anaphylaxis**, angioedema, **anxiety, arrhythmias (including ventricular tachycardia)**, arthralgia, cholestatic jaundice, deafness, edema, erythema multiforme (rare), hearing loss, hepatic necrosis (rare), hepatitis, hypertrophic pyloric stenosis, **hypotension**, interstitial nephritis, pancreatitis, **paresthesia, pseudomembranous colitis, seizures, somnolence**, Stevens-Johnson syndrome (rare), **syncope, abnormal taste,** thrombocytopenia, tinnitus, **tongue discoloration (rare), torsade de pointes (case report),** vertigo, **weakness**

Contraindications Hypersensitivity to azithromycin, other macrolide antibiotics, or any component of the formulation

Warnings/Precautions Use with caution in patients with hepatic dysfunction; hepatic impairment with or without jaundice has occurred chiefly in older children and adults; it may be accompanied by malaise, nausea, vomiting, abdominal colic, and fever; discontinue use if these occur; may mask or delay symptoms of incubating gonorrhea or syphilis, so appropriate culture and susceptibility tests should be performed prior to initiating azithromycin; pseudomembranous colitis has been reported with use of macrolide antibiotics; use caution with renal dysfunction; safety and efficacy have not been established in children <6 months of age with acute otitis media or community-acquired pneumonia, or in children <2 years of age with pharyngitis/tonsillitis.

Drug Interactions Substrate of CYP3A4; Inhibits CYP3A4

Increased Effect/Toxicity: Azithromycin may increase levels of tacrolimus, phenytoin, ergot alkaloids, alfentanil, astemizole, bromocriptine, carbamazepine, cyclosporine, digoxin, disopyramide, and triazolam; azithromycin did not affect the response to warfarin or theophylline although caution is advised when administered together; nelfinavir may increase azithromycin serum levels (monitor for adverse effects)

Decreased peak serum levels: Aluminum- and magnesium-containing antacids by 24% but not total absorption

Avoid use with pimozide due to significant risk of cardiotoxicity

Dietary/Ethanol/Herb Considerations Food may alter rate and extent of GI absorption depending upon the formulation. Administer suspension and capsules 1 hour before or 2 hours following meals. Oral suspension may be administered with food but absorption is significantly increased (46%). Administer tablet with food to reduce GI upset.

Pharmacodynamics/Kinetics

Absorption: Rapid

Distribution: Extensive tissue; distributes well into skin, lungs, sputum, tonsils, and cervix; penetration into CSF is poor

Protein binding (concentration dependent): 7% to 50%

Metabolism: Hepatic

Bioavailability: 37%; variable effect with food (increased with oral suspension, unchanged with tablet)

Half-life elimination: Terminal: 68 hours

Time to peak, serum: 2.3-4 hours

Excretion: Feces (50% as unchanged drug); urine (~5% to 12%)

Pregnancy Risk Factor B

Breast-feeding Considerations Based on one case report, azithromycin has been shown to accumulate in breast milk.

Dosage Forms INJ, powder for reconstitution: 500 mg. **POWDER, oral suspension:** 100 mg/5 mL (15 mL); 200 mg/5 mL (15 mL, 22.5 mL, 30 mL); 1 g. **TAB:** 250 mg, 500 mg, 600 mg; (Zithromax® TRI-PAK™): 500 mg (3s), (Zithromax® Z-PAK®): 250 mg (6s)

Generic Available No

Comments Although the erythromycins inhibit the hepatic metabolism of theophylline and carbamazepine to enhance their effects, azithromycin has not been shown to inhibit the hepatic metabolism of these drugs. Clauzel, et al, reported that azithromycin did not inhibit the metabolism of theophylline after a standard 5-day regimen (500 mg on day one followed by 250 mg daily). Rapeport, et al, reported that azithromycin did not affect the blood levels of carbamazepine.

Selected Readings

Dajani AS, Taubert KA, Wilson W, et al, "Prevention of Bacterial Endocarditis. Recommendations by the American Heart Association," *JAMA*, 1997, 277(22):1794-801.

Dajani AS, Taubert KA, Wilson W, et al, "Prevention of Bacterial Endocarditis: Recommendations by the American Heart Association," *J Am Dent Assoc*, 1997, 128(8):1142-51.

Wynn RL, "New Erythromycins," *Gen Dent*, 1996, 44(4):304-7.

Wynn RL, Bergman SA, Meiller TF, et al, "Antibiotics in Treating Oral-Facial Infections of Odontogenic Origin: An Update", *Gen Dent*, 2001, 49(3):238-40, 242, 244 passim.

Azithromycin Dihydrate *see* Azithromycin *on page 153*

Azmacort® *see* Triamcinolone *on page 1341*

Azo-Gesic® [OTC] *see* Phenazopyridine *on page 1064*

Azopt® *see* Brinzolamide *on page 198*

Azo-Standard® [OTC] *see* Phenazopyridine *on page 1064*

AZT *see* Zidovudine *on page 1406*

AZT + 3TC *see* Zidovudine and Lamivudine *on page 1407*

AZT, Abacavir, and Lamivudine *see* Abacavir, Lamivudine, and Zidovudine *on page 23*

Azthreonam *see* Aztreonam *on page 155*

Aztreonam (AZ tree oh nam)

U.S. Brand Names Azactam®

Canadian Brand Names Azactam®

Pharmacologic Category Antibiotic, Miscellaneous

Synonyms Azthreonam

Use Treatment of patients with urinary tract infections, lower respiratory tract infections, septicemia, skin/skin structure infections, intra-abdominal infections, and gynecological infections caused by susceptible gram-negative bacilli; often useful in patients with allergies to penicillins or cephalosporins

Local Anesthetic/Vasoconstrictor Precautions No information available to require special precautions

Effects on Dental Treatment 1% to 10%: Adults: Nausea, vomiting

Dosage

Neonates: I.M., I.V.:

- Postnatal age ≤7 days:
  - <2000 g: 30 mg/kg/dose every 12 hours
  - >2000 g: 30 mg/kg/dose every 8 hours
- Postnatal age >7 days:
  - <1200 g: 30 mg/kg/dose every 12 hours
  - 1200-2000 g: 30 mg/kg/dose every 8 hours
  - >2000 g: 30 mg/kg/dose every 6 hours

Children >1 month: I.M., I.V.:

- Mild to moderate infections: 30 mg/kg every 8 hours
- Moderate to severe infections: 30 mg/kg every 6-8 hours
- Cystic fibrosis: 50 mg/kg/dose every 6-8 hours (ie, up to 200 mg/kg/day); maximum: 6-8 g/day

Adults:

- Urinary tract infection: I.M., I.V.: 500 mg to 1 g every 8-12 hours
- Moderately severe systemic infections: 1 g I.V. or I.M. or 2 g I.V. every 8-12 hours
- Severe systemic or life-threatening infections (especially caused by *Pseudomonas aeruginosa*): I.V.: 2 g every 6-8 hours; maximum: 8 g/day

Dosing adjustment in renal impairment: Adults:

- Cl_{cr} >50 mL/minute: 500 mg to 1 g every 6-8 hours
- Cl_{cr} 10-50 mL/minute: 50% to 75% of usual dose given at the usual interval
- Cl_{cr} <10 mL/minute: 25% of usual dosage given at the usual interval

Hemodialysis: Moderately dialyzable (20% to 50%); administer dose postdialysis or supplemental dose of 500 mg after dialysis

Peritoneal dialysis: Administer as for Cl_{cr} <10 mL/minute

Continuous arteriovenous or venovenous hemofiltration: Dose as for Cl_{cr} 10-50 mL/minute

Mechanism of Action Inhibits bacterial cell wall synthesis by binding to one or more of the penicillin binding proteins (PBPs); which in turn inhibits the final transpeptidation step of peptidoglycan synthesis in bacterial cell walls, thus inhibiting cell

(Continued)

Aztreonam *(Continued)*

wall biosynthesis. Bacteria eventually lyse due to ongoing activity of cell wall autolytic enzymes (autolysins and murein hydrolases) while cell wall assembly is arrested. Monobactam structure makes cross-allergenicity with beta-lactams unlikely.

Other Adverse Effects Adults:

1% to 10%:

Dermatologic: Rash

Gastrointestinal: Diarrhea

Local: Thrombophlebitis, pain at injection site

<1%: Abdominal cramps, **abnormal taste, anaphylaxis**, anemia, angioedema, **aphthous ulcer**, breast tenderness, **bronchospasm**, *C. difficile*-associated diarrhea, **chest pain, confusion, diaphoresis**, diplopia, **dizziness, dyspnea**, eosinophilia, erythema multiforme, exfoliative dermatitis, **fever, flushing, halitosis, headache**, hepatitis, **hypotension**, insomnia, jaundice, leukopenia, liver enzymes increased, muscular aches myalgia, neutropenia, **numb tongue**, pancytopenia, **paresthesia**, petechiae, pruritus, pseudomembranous colitis, purpura, **seizures, sneezing, thrombocytopenia**, tinnitus, toxic epidermal necrolysis, urticaria, vaginitis, vertigo, weakness, **wheezing**

Drug Interactions Decreased Effect: Avoid antibiotics that induce beta-lactamase production (cefoxitin, imipenem).

Pharmacodynamics/Kinetics

Absorption: I.M.: Well absorbed; I.M. and I.V. doses produce comparable serum concentrations

Distribution: Widely to most body fluids and tissues; crosses placenta; enters breast milk

V_d: Neonates: 0.26-0.36 L/kg; Children: 0.2-0.29 L/kg; Adults: 0.2 L/kg

Relative diffusion of antimicrobial agents from blood into CSF: Good only with inflammation (exceeds usual MICs)

CSF:blood level ratio: Meninges: Inflamed: 8% to 40%; Normal: ~1%

Protein binding: 56%

Metabolism: Hepatic (minor %)

Half-life elimination:

Neonates: <7 days, ≤2.5 kg: 5.5-9.9 hours; <7 days, >2.5 kg: 2.6 hours; 1 week to 1 month: 2.4 hours

Children 2 months to 12 years: 1.7 hours

Adults: Normal renal function: 1.7-2.9 hours

End-stage renal disease: 6-8 hours

Time to peak: I.M., I.V. push: Within 60 minutes; I.V. infusion: 1.5 hours

Excretion: Urine (60% to 70% as unchanged drug); feces (~13% to 15%)

Pregnancy Risk Factor B

Generic Available No

Azulfidine® *see* Sulfasalazine *on page 1254*

Azulfidine® EN-tabs® *see* Sulfasalazine *on page 1254*

B 9273 *see* Alefacept *on page 52*

Babee® Cof Syrup [OTC] *see* Dextromethorphan *on page 423*

Babee® Teething® [OTC] *see* Benzocaine *on page 169*

Baby Gasz [OTC] *see* Simethicone *on page 1222*

BAC *see* Benzalkonium Chloride *on page 169*

Bacid® [OTC] *see Lactobacillus acidophilus* and *Lactobacillus bulgaricus on page 772*

Baciguent® [OTC] *see* Bacitracin *on page 156*

Baci-IM® *see* Bacitracin *on page 156*

Bacillus Calmette-Guérin (BCG) Live *see* BCG Vaccine *on page 161*

Bacitracin (bas i TRAY sin)

U.S. Brand Names AK-Tracin®; Baciguent® [OTC]; Baci-IM®

Canadian Brand Names Baciguent®

Pharmacologic Category Antibiotic, Ophthalmic; Antibiotic, Topical; Antibiotic, Miscellaneous

Use Treatment of susceptible bacterial infections mainly; has activity against gram-positive bacilli; due to toxicity risks, systemic and irrigant uses of bacitracin should be limited to situations where less toxic alternatives would not be effective; oral administration has been successful in antibiotic-associated colitis and has been used for enteric eradication of vancomycin-resistant enterococci (VRE)

Unlabeled/Investigational Use Oral administration has been successful in antibiotic-associated colitis and has been used for enteric eradication of vancomycin-resistant enterococci (VRE)

Local Anesthetic/Vasoconstrictor Precautions No information available to require special precautions

Effects on Dental Treatment 1% to 10%: Hypotension, facial/lip edema, tightness in chest, nausea, vomiting, diaphoresis

Dosage Do not administer I.V.:
Infants: I.M.:
≤2.5 kg: 900 units/kg/day in 2-3 divided doses
>2.5 kg: 1000 units/kg/day in 2-3 divided doses
Children: I.M.: 800-1200 units/kg/day divided every 8 hours
Adults: Oral:
Antibiotic-associated colitis: 25,000 units 4 times/day for 7-10 days
VRE eradication (unlabeled use): 25,000 units 4 times/day for 7-10 days
Children and Adults:
Topical: Apply 1-5 times/day
Ophthalmic, ointment: Instill 1/4" to 1/2" ribbon every 3-4 hours into conjunctival sac for acute infections, or 2-3 times/day for mild to moderate infections for 7-10 days
Irrigation, solution: 50-100 units/mL in normal saline, lactated Ringer's, or sterile water for irrigation; soak sponges in solution for topical compresses 1-5 times/day or as needed during surgical procedures

Mechanism of Action Inhibits bacterial cell wall synthesis by preventing transfer of mucopeptides into the growing cell wall

Other Adverse Effects 1% to 10%:
Central nervous system: Pain
Dermatologic: Rash, itching
Gastrointestinal: Anorexia, diarrhea, rectal itching
Hematologic: Blood dyscrasias

Drug Interactions Increased Effect/Toxicity: Nephrotoxic drugs, neuromuscular blocking agents, and anesthetics (increased neuromuscular blockade).

Pharmacodynamics/Kinetics
Duration: 6-8 hours
Absorption: Poor from mucous membranes and intact or denuded skin; rapidly following I.M. administration; not absorbed by bladder irrigation, but absorption can occur from peritoneal or mediastinal lavage
Distribution: CSF: Nil even with inflammation
Protein binding, plasma: Minimal
Time to peak, serum: I.M.: 1-2 hours
Excretion: Urine (10% to 40%) within 24 hours

Pregnancy Risk Factor C

Generic Available Yes

Bacitracin and Polymyxin B (bas i TRAY sin & pol i MIKS in bee)

Related Information
Bacitracin *on page 156*
Polymyxin B *on page 1095*

U.S. Brand Names AK-Poly-Bac®; Betadine® First Aid Antibiotics + Moisturizer [OTC]; Polysporin® Ophthalmic; Polysporin® Topical [OTC]

Canadian Brand Names LID-Pack®; Optimyxin®; Optimyxin Plus®; Polycidin® Ophthalmic Ointment

Pharmacologic Category Antibiotic, Ophthalmic; Antibiotic, Topical

Synonyms Polymyxin B and Bacitracin

Use Treatment of superficial infections caused by susceptible organisms

Local Anesthetic/Vasoconstrictor Precautions No information available to require special precautions

Effects on Dental Treatment No significant effects or complications reported

Dosage Children and Adults:
Ophthalmic ointment: Instill 1/2" ribbon in the affected eye(s) every 3-4 hours for acute infections or 2-3 times/day for mild to moderate infections for 7-10 days
Topical ointment/powder: Apply to affected area 1-4 times/day; may cover with sterile bandage if needed

Mechanism of Action See individual monographs for Bacitracin and Polymyxin B

Other Adverse Effects 1% to 10%: Local: Rash, itching, burning, **anaphylactoid reactions**, swelling, conjunctival erythema

Pregnancy Risk Factor C

Generic Available Yes

Bacitracin, Neomycin, and Polymyxin B

(bas i TRAY sin, nee oh MYE sin, & pol i MIKS in bee)

Related Information
Bacitracin *on page 156*
Neomycin *on page 961*
Polymyxin B *on page 1095*

U.S. Brand Names Mycitracin® [OTC]; Neosporin® Ophthalmic Ointment; Neosporin® Topical [OTC]; Triple Antibiotic®

Canadian Brand Names Neosporin® Ophthalmic Ointment; Neotopic®

Pharmacologic Category Antibiotic, Ophthalmic; Antibiotic, Topical

Synonyms Neomycin, Bacitracin, and Polymyxin B; Polymyxin B, Bacitracin, and Neomycin

(Continued)

Bacitracin, Neomycin, and Polymyxin B *(Continued)*

Use Helps prevent infection in minor cuts, scrapes and burns; short-term treatment of superficial external ocular infections caused by susceptible organisms

Local Anesthetic/Vasoconstrictor Precautions No information available to require special precautions

Effects on Dental Treatment No significant effects or complications reported

Dosage Children and Adults:

Ophthalmic: Ointment: Instill 1/2" into the conjunctival sac every 3-4 hours for 7-10 days for acute infections; apply 1/2" 2-3 times/day for mild to moderate infections for 7-10 days

Topical: Apply 1-4 times/day to infected area and cover with sterile bandage as needed

Mechanism of Action Refer to individual monographs for Bacitracin; Neomycin Sulfate; and Polymyxin B Sulfate

Other Adverse Effects 1% to 10%:

Cardiovascular: Edema

Dermatologic: Reddening, allergic contact dermatitis

Local: Itching, failure to heal

Pregnancy Risk Factor C

Generic Available Yes

Bacitracin, Neomycin, Polymyxin B, and Hydrocortisone

(bas i TRAY sin, nee oh MYE sin, pol i MIKS in bee & hye droe KOR ti sone)

Related Information

Bacitracin *on page 156*

Hydrocortisone *on page 688*

Neomycin *on page 961*

Polymyxin B *on page 1095*

U.S. Brand Names AK-Spore® H.C. [DSC]; Cortisporin® Ointment

Canadian Brand Names Cortisporin®

Pharmacologic Category Antibiotic, Ophthalmic; Antibiotic, Otic; Antibiotic, Topical; Corticosteroid, Ophthalmic; Corticosteroid, Otic; Corticosteroid, Topical

Synonyms AK-Spore® H.C. [DSC]; Hydrocortisone, Bacitracin, Neomycin, and Polymyxin B; Neomycin, Bacitracin, Polymyxin B, and Hydrocortisone; Polymyxin B, Bacitracin, Neomycin, and Hydrocortisone

Use Prevention and treatment of susceptible superficial topical infections

Local Anesthetic/Vasoconstrictor Precautions No information available to require special precautions

Effects on Dental Treatment 1% to 10%: Apnea

Dosage Children and Adults:

Ophthalmic: Ointment: Instill 1/2" ribbon to inside of lower lid every 3-4 hours until improvement occurs

Topical: Apply sparingly 2-4 times/day. Therapy should be discontinued when control is achieved; if no improvement is seen, reassessment of diagnosis may be necessary.

Mechanism of Action Refer to individual monographs for Bacitracin, Neomycin, Polymyxin B, and Hydrocortisone

Other Adverse Effects 1% to 10%: Dermatologic: Rash, generalized itching

Pregnancy Risk Factor C

Generic Available Yes

Bacitracin, Neomycin, Polymyxin B, and Lidocaine

(bas i TRAY sin, nee oh MYE sin, pol i MIKS in bee & LYE doe kane)

Related Information

Bacitracin *on page 156*

Lidocaine *on page 801*

Neomycin *on page 961*

Polymyxin B *on page 1095*

U.S. Brand Names Spectrocin Plus® [OTC]

Pharmacologic Category Antibiotic, Topical

Use Prevention and treatment of susceptible superficial topical infections

Local Anesthetic/Vasoconstrictor Precautions No information available to require special precautions

Effects on Dental Treatment No significant effects or complications reported

Dosage Topical: Adults: Apply 1-4 times/day to infected areas; cover with sterile bandage if needed

Generic Available Yes

Baclofen (BAK loe fen)

U.S. Brand Names Lioresal®

Canadian Brand Names Apo®-Baclofen; Gen-Baclofen; Lioresal®; Liotec; Nu-Baclo; PMS-Baclofen

Pharmacologic Category Skeletal Muscle Relaxant

Use Treatment of reversible spasticity associated with multiple sclerosis or spinal cord lesions

Orphan drug: Intrathecal: Treatment of intractable spasticity caused by spinal cord injury, multiple sclerosis, and other spinal disease (spinal ischemia or tumor, transverse myelitis, cervical spondylosis, degenerative myelopathy)

Unlabeled/Investigational Use Treatment of intractable hiccups, intractable pain relief, bladder spasticity, trigeminal neuralgia, cerebral palsy, Huntington's chorea

Local Anesthetic/Vasoconstrictor Precautions No information available to require special precautions

Effects on Dental Treatment

>10%: Drowsiness, psychiatric disturbances, weakness

1% to 10%: Hypotension, confusion, headache, nausea, fatigue

Dosage

Oral (avoid abrupt withdrawal of drug):

Children:

2-7 years: Initial: 10-15 mg/24 hours divided every 8 hours; titrate dose every 3 days in increments of 5-15 mg/day to a maximum of 40 mg/day

≥8 years: Maximum: 60 mg/day in 3 divided doses

Adults: 5 mg 3 times/day, may increase 5 mg/dose every 3 days to a maximum of 80 mg/day

Hiccups: Adults: Usual effective dose: 10-20 mg 2-3 times/day

Intrathecal:

Test dose: 50-100 mcg, doses >50 mcg should be given in 25 mcg increments, separated by 24 hours. A screening dose of 25 mcg may be considered in very small patients. Patients not responding to screening dose of 100 mcg should not be considered for chronic infusion/implanted pump.

Maintenance: After positive response to test dose, a maintenance intrathecal infusion can be administered via an implanted intrathecal pump. Initial dose via pump: Infusion at a 24-hour rate dosed at twice the test dose. Avoid abrupt discontinuation.

Elderly: Oral (the lowest effective dose is recommended): Initial: 5 mg 2-3 times/day, increasing gradually as needed; if benefits are not seen withdraw the drug slowly.

Dosing adjustment in renal impairment: It is necessary to reduce dosage in renal impairment but there are no specific guidelines available

Hemodialysis: Poor water solubility allows for accumulation during chronic hemodialysis. Low-dose therapy is recommended. There have been several case reports of accumulation of baclofen resulting in toxicity symptoms (organic brain syndrome, myoclonia, deceleration and steep potentials in EEG) in patients with renal failure who have received normal doses of baclofen.

Mechanism of Action Inhibits the transmission of both monosynaptic and polysynaptic reflexes at the spinal cord level, possibly by hyperpolarization of primary afferent fiber terminals, with resultant relief of muscle spasticity

Other Adverse Effects

>10%: Central nervous system: Vertigo insomnia, slurred speech, ataxia, hypotonia

1% to 10%:

Dermatologic: Rash

Gastrointestinal: Constipation

Genitourinary: Polyuria

<1%: **Palpitations, chest pain, syncope**, euphoria, excitement, depression, anorexia, **hallucinations, xerostomia, abnormal taste**, abdominal pain, **vomiting**, diarrhea, enuresis, urinary retention, dysuria, impotence, inability to ejaculate, nocturia, **paresthesia**, hematuria, **dyspnea**

Withdrawal reactions have occurred with abrupt discontinuation (particularly severe with intrathecal use).

Drug Interactions Increased Effect/Toxicity: Baclofen may decrease the clearance of ibuprofen or other NSAIDs and increase the potential for renal toxicity. Effects may be additive with CNS depressants.

Dietary/Ethanol/Herb Considerations

Ethanol: Avoid use; may increase CNS depression.

Herb/Nutraceutical: Avoid gotu kola, kava, SAMe, St John's wort, and valerian; may increase CNS depression.

Pharmacodynamics/Kinetics

Onset of action: 3-4 days

Peak effect: 5-10 days

Absorption (dose dependent): Oral: Rapid

Protein binding: 30%

Metabolism: Hepatic (15% of dose)

Half-life elimination: 3.5 hours

Time to peak, serum: Oral: Within 2-3 hours

Excretion: Urine and feces (85% as unchanged drug)

Pregnancy Risk Factor C

Generic Available Yes: Tablets only

BactoShield® CHG [OTC] *see* Chlorhexidine Gluconate *on page 300*

Bactrim™ *see* Sulfamethoxazole and Trimethoprim *on page 1253*
Bactrim™ DS *see* Sulfamethoxazole and Trimethoprim *on page 1253*
Bactroban® *see* Mupirocin *on page 937*
Bactroban® Nasal *see* Mupirocin *on page 937*
Baking Soda *see* Sodium Bicarbonate *on page 1227*
BAL *see* Dimercaprol *on page 449*

Balanced Salt Solution (BAL anced salt soe LOO shun)

U.S. Brand Names BSS®

Canadian Brand Names BSS®; BSS® Plus; Eye-Stream®

Pharmacologic Category Ophthalmic Agent, Miscellaneous

Use Intraocular irrigating solution; also used to soothe and cleanse the eye in conjunction with hard contact lenses

Local Anesthetic/Vasoconstrictor Precautions No information available to require special precautions

Effects on Dental Treatment No significant effects or complications reported

Dosage Use as needed for foreign body removal, gonioscopy and other general ophthalmic office procedures

Generic Available Yes

BAL in Oil® *see* Dimercaprol *on page 449*
Balmex® [OTC] *see* Zinc Oxide *on page 1409*
Balnetar® [OTC] *see* Coal Tar, Lanolin, and Mineral Oil *on page 360*
Bancap HC® *see* Hydrocodone and Acetaminophen *on page 678*
Band-Aid® Hurt-Free™ Antiseptic Wash [OTC] *see* Lidocaine *on page 801*
Banophen® [OTC] *see* DiphenhydrAMINE *on page 451*
Base Ointment *see* Zinc Oxide *on page 1409*

Basiliximab (ba si LIKS i mab)

U.S. Brand Names Simulect®

Canadian Brand Names Simulect®

Mexican Brand Names Simulect®

Pharmacologic Category Monoclonal Antibody

Use Prophylaxis of acute organ rejection in renal transplantation

Local Anesthetic/Vasoconstrictor Precautions No information available to require special precautions

Effects on Dental Treatment Causes gingival hypertrophy (GH) similar to that caused by cyclosporine; early reports indicate that frequency/incidence of basiliximab-induced GH not as high as cyclosporine-induced GH

Reported in 96% of both placebo and basiliximab clinical trial groups:

- >10%: Hypertension, atrial fibrillation, fever, headache, wound complications, nausea, vomiting, tremor, dyspnea, upper respiratory infection, viral infection, pain
- 3% to 10%: Chest pain, cardiac failure, hypotension, arrhythmia, tachycardia, angina pectoris, agitation, anxiety, rigors, dizziness, dehydration, diabetes mellitus, hypoglycemia, gastroenteritis, GI hemorrhage, esophagitis, stomatitis, moniliasis, hematoma, hemorrhage, paresthesia, weakness, bronchitis, bronchospasm, pneumonia, sinusitis, rhinitis, coughing, pharyngitis, facial edema, sepsis, infection, herpes infection, ulcerative stomatitis (3% to 10%)

Dosage Patients previously administered basiliximab should only be re-exposed to a subsequent course of therapy with extreme caution.

I.V.:

- Children <35 kg: Renal transplantation: 10 mg within 2 hours prior to transplant surgery, followed by a second 10 mg dose 4 days after transplantation; the second dose should be withheld if complications occur (including severe hypersensitivity reactions or graft loss)
- Children ≥35 kg and Adults: Renal transplantation: 20 mg within 2 hours prior to transplant surgery, followed by a second 20 mg dose 4 days after transplantation; the second dose should be withheld if complications occur (including severe hypersensitivity reactions or graft loss)

Dosing adjustment in renal/hepatic impairment: No specific recommendations

Mechanism of Action Chimeric (murine/human) monoclonal antibody which blocks the alpha-chain of the interleukin-2 (IL-2) receptor complex; this receptor is expressed on activated T lymphocytes and is a critical pathway for activating cell-mediated allograft rejection

Other Adverse Effects Reported in 96% of both placebo and basiliximab clinical trial groups:

>10%:

- Cardiovascular: Peripheral edema
- Central nervous system: Insomnia
- Dermatologic: Acne
- Endocrine & metabolic: Hypokalemia, hyperkalemia, hyperglycemia, hyperuricemia, hypophosphatemia, hypercholesterolemia

Gastrointestinal: Constipation, diarrhea, abdominal pain, dyspepsia
Genitourinary: Urinary tract infection
Hematologic: Anemia

3% to 10%:

Cardiovascular: Generalized edema, abnormal heart sounds, angina pectoris
Central nervous system: Hypoesthesia, neuropathy, depression, malaise, fatigue,
Dermatologic: Cyst, hypertrichosis, pruritus, rash, skin disorder, skin ulceration
Endocrine & metabolic: Fluid overload, hypercalcemia, hyperlipidemia, hypoglycemia, hypomagnesemia, acidosis, hypertriglyceridemia, hypocalcemia, hyponatremia
Gastrointestinal: Flatulence, melena, enlarged abdomen, weight gain
Genitourinary: Impotence, genital edema, albuminuria, bladder disorder, hematuria, urinary frequency, oliguria, abnormal renal function, renal tubular necrosis, ureteral disorder, urinary retention, dysuria
Hematologic: Purpura, thrombocytopenia, thrombosis, polycythemia, leukopenia
Neuromuscular & skeletal: Arthralgia, arthropathy, cramps, fracture, hernia, myalgia, weakness, back pain, leg pain
Ocular: Cataract, conjunctivitis, abnormal vision
Respiratory: Pulmonary edema
Miscellaneous: Accidental trauma, increased glucocorticoids

Postmarketing and/or case reports: **Severe hypersensitivity reactions (anaphylaxis, hypotension, tachycardia, cardiac failure, dyspnea, bronchospasm, respiratory failure, sneezing**, pruritus, capillary leak syndrome, pulmonary edema, urticaria, rash)

Drug Interactions

Increased Effect/Toxicity: Basiliximab is an immunoglobulin; specific drug interactions have not been evaluated, but are not anticipated.

Decreased Effect: Basiliximab is an immunoglobulin; specific drug interactions have not been evaluated, but are not anticipated. It is not known if the immune response to vaccines will be impaired during or following basiliximab therapy.

Pharmacodynamics/Kinetics

Duration: Mean: 36 days (determined by IL-2R alpha saturation)
Distribution: Mean: V_d: Children: 5.2 ± 2.8 L; Adults: 8.6 ± 4.1 L
Half-life elimination: Children: 9.4 days; Adults: Mean: 7.2 days
Excretion: Clearance: Children: 20 mL/hour; Adults: Mean: 41 mL/hour

Pregnancy Risk Factor B (manufacturer)

Generic Available No

Bausch & Lomb® Computer Eye Drops [OTC] *see* Glycerin *on page 644*
Bayer® Aspirin [OTC] *see* Aspirin *on page 131*
Bayer® Aspirin Extra Strength [OTC] *see* Aspirin *on page 131*
Bayer® Aspirin Regimen Adult Low Strength [OTC] *see* Aspirin *on page 131*
Bayer® Aspirin Regimen Adult Low Strength with Calcium [OTC] *see* Aspirin *on page 131*
Bayer® Aspirin Regimen Children's [OTC] *see* Aspirin *on page 131*
Bayer® Aspirin Regimen Regular Strength [OTC] *see* Aspirin *on page 131*
Bayer® Plus Extra Strength [OTC] *see* Aspirin *on page 131*
BayGam® *see* Immune Globulin (Intramuscular) *on page 713*
BayHep B™ *see* Hepatitis B Immune Globulin *on page 666*
BayRab® *see* Rabies Immune Globulin (Human) *on page 1164*
BayRho-D® Full-Dose *see* Rh_o(D) Immune Globulin *on page 1175*
BayRho-D® Mini-Dose *see* Rh_o(D) Immune Globulin *on page 1175*
BayTet™ *see* Tetanus Immune Globulin (Human) *on page 1283*
Baza® Antifungal [OTC] *see* Miconazole *on page 906*
Baza® Clear [OTC] *see* Vitamin A and Vitamin D *on page 1392*
B-Caro-T™ *see* Beta-Carotene *on page 176*
BCG, Live *see* BCG Vaccine *on page 161*

BCG Vaccine (bee see jee vak SEEN)

Related Information

Immunizations (Vaccines) *on page 1612*

U.S. Brand Names TheraCys®; TICE® BCG

Canadian Brand Names ImmuCyst®; Oncotice™; Pacis™

Pharmacologic Category Biological Response Modulator; Vaccine

Synonyms Bacillus Calmette-Guérin (BCG) Live; BCG, Live

Use Immunization against tuberculosis and immunotherapy for cancer; treatment of bladder cancer

BCG vaccine is not routinely recommended for use in the U.S. for prevention of tuberculosis

BCG vaccine is strongly recommended for infants and children with negative tuberculin skin tests who:

are at high risk of intimate and prolonged exposure to persistently untreated or ineffectively treated patients with infectious pulmonary tuberculosis, and cannot be removed from the source of exposure, and

(Continued)

BCG Vaccine *(Continued)*

cannot be placed on long-term preventive therapy

are continuously exposed with tuberculosis who have bacilli resistant to isoniazid and rifampin

BCG is also recommended for tuberculin-negative infants and children in groups in which the rate of new infections exceeds 1% per year and for whom the usual surveillance and treatment programs have been attempted but are not operationally feasible

BCG should be administered with caution to persons in groups at high risk for HIV infection or persons known to be severely immunocompromised. Although limited data suggest that the vaccine may be safe for use in asymptomatic children infected with HIV, BCG vaccination is not recommended for HIV infected adults or for persons with symptomatic disease. Until further research can clearly define the risks and benefits of BCG vaccination for this population, vaccination should be restricted to persons at exceptionally high risk for tuberculosis infection. HIV infected persons thought to be infected with *Mycobacterium tuberculosis* should be strongly recommended for tuberculosis preventive therapy.

Local Anesthetic/Vasoconstrictor Precautions No information available to require special precautions

Effects on Dental Treatment 1% to 10%: Flu-like syndrome

Restrictions Federal law requires that the date of administration, the vaccine manufacturer, lot number of vaccine, and the administering person's name, title and address be entered into the patient's permanent medical record.

Dosage Children >1 month and Adults:

Immunization against tuberculosis (TICE® BCG): 0.2-0.3 mL percutaneous; initial lesion usually appears after 10-14 days consisting of small red papule at injection site and reaches maximum diameter of 3 mm in 4-6 weeks; conduct postvaccinal tuberculin test (ie, 5 TU of PPD) in 2-3 months; if test is negative, repeat vaccination

Immunotherapy for bladder cancer:

Intravesical treatment: Instill into bladder for 2 hours

TheraCys®: One dose diluted in 50 mL NS (preservative free) instilled into bladder once weekly for 6 weeks followed by one treatment at 3, 6, 12, 18, and 24 months after initial treatment

TICE® BCG: One dose diluted in 50 mL NS (preservative free) instilled into the bladder once weekly for 6 weeks followed by once monthly for 6-12 months

Mechanism of Action BCG live is an attenuated strain of Bacillus Calmette-Guérin used as a biological response modifier; BCG live, when used intravesicular for treatment of bladder carcinoma *in situ*, is thought to cause a local, chronic inflammatory response involving macrophage and leukocyte infiltration of the bladder. By a mechanism not fully understood, this local inflammatory response leads to destruction of superficial tumor cells of the urothelium. Evidence of systemic immune response is also commonly seen, manifested by a positive PPD tuberculin skin test reaction, however, its relationship to clinical efficacy is not well-established. BCG is active immunotherapy which stimulates the host's immune mechanism to reject the tumor.

Other Adverse Effects All serious adverse reactions must be reported to the U.S. Department of Health and Human Services (DHHS) Vaccine Adverse Event Reporting System (VAERS) 1-800-822-7967.

1% to 10%: Genitourinary: Bladder infection, dysuria, polyuria, prostatitis

<1%: Skin ulceration, abscesses, hematuria, anaphylactic shock in infants (rare), lymphadenitis, tuberculosis (in immunosuppressed patients)

Pregnancy Risk Factor C

Generic Available No

Comments Live, attenuated vaccine; live culture preparation of bacillus Calmette-Guérin (BCG) strain of *Mycobacterium bovis* and is a substrain of Pasteur Institute strain designed for use as active immunizing agent against tuberculosis

BCNU *see* Carmustine *on page 253*

B-D™ Glucose [OTC] *see* Glucose (Instant) *on page 641*

Bebulin® VH *see* Factor IX Complex (Human) *on page 553*

Becaplermin (be KAP ler min)

U.S. Brand Names Regranex®

Canadian Brand Names Regranex®

Pharmacologic Category Growth Factor, Platelet-derived; Topical Skin Product

Synonyms Recombinant Human Platelet-Derived Growth Factor B; rPDGF-BB

Use Debridement adjunct for the treatment of diabetic ulcers that occur on the lower limbs and feet

Local Anesthetic/Vasoconstrictor Precautions No information available to require special precautions

Effects on Dental Treatment No significant effects or complications reported

Dosage Topical: Adults: Diabetic ulcers: Apply appropriate amount of gel once daily with a cotton swab or similar tool, as a coating over the ulcer. The amount of becaplermin to be applied will vary depending on the size of the ulcer area. To calculate the length of gel applied to the ulcer, measure the greatest length of the ulcer by the greatest width of the ulcer in inches. Tube size will determine the formula used in the calculation. For a 15 or 7.5 g tube, multiply length x width x 0.6. For a 2 g tube, multiply length x width x 1.3. **Note:** If the ulcer does not decrease in size by ~30% after 10 weeks of treatment or complete healing has not occurred in 20 weeks, continued treatment with becaplermin gel should be reassessed.

Mechanism of Action Recombinant B-isoform homodimer of human platelet-derived growth factor (rPDGF-BB) which enhances formation of new granulation tissue, induces fibroblast proliferation, and differentiation to promote wound healing

Other Adverse Effects <1%: Erythema with purulent discharge, **ulcer infection, tunneling of ulcer**, exuberant granulation tissue, local pain, skin ulceration

Pharmacodynamics/Kinetics

Onset of action: Complete healing: 15% of patients within 8 weeks, 25% at 10 weeks

Absorption: Minimal

Distribution: Binds to PDGF-beta receptors in normal skin and granulation tissue

Pregnancy Risk Factor C

Generic Available No

Beclomethasone (be kloe METH a sone)

Related Information

Respiratory Diseases *on page 1476*

U.S. Brand Names Beconase® [DSC]; Beconase® AQ; QVAR™; Vancenase® AQ 84 mcg [DSC]; Vancenase® Pockethaler® [DSC]; Vanceril® [DSC]

Canadian Brand Names Apo®-Beclomethasone; Gen-Beclo; Nu-Beclomethasone; Propaderm®; QVAR™; Rivanase AQ; Vanceril®

Mexican Brand Names Aerobec; Beconase Aqua; Becotide 100; Becotide 250; Becotide Aerosol

Pharmacologic Category Corticosteroid, Inhalant (Oral); Corticosteroid, Nasal

Synonyms Beclomethasone Dipropionate; Beclovent® [DSC]; Vanceril® [DSC]

Use

Oral inhalation: Maintenance and prophylactic treatment of asthma; includes those who require corticosteroids and those who may benefit from a dose reduction/elimination of systemically administered corticosteroids. Not for relief of acute bronchospasm

Nasal aerosol: Symptomatic treatment of seasonal or perennial rhinitis and to prevent recurrence of nasal polyps following surgery

Local Anesthetic/Vasoconstrictor Precautions No information available to require special precautions

Effects on Dental Treatment Localized infections with *Candida albicans* or *Aspergillus niger* occur frequently in the mouth and pharynx with repetitive use of oral inhaler; may require treatment with appropriate antifungal therapy or discontinuance of inhaler use.

>10%: Oral candidiasis (≤75%)

1% to 10%: Xerostomia, nasal dryness, dry throat

Frequency not defined: Agitation, dizziness, headache, lightheadedness, mental disturbances, hoarseness, loss of taste, nausea, unpleasant taste, vomiting, epistaxis, *Candida* infections, nasal stuffiness, nosebleeds, rhinorrhea, sneezing, cough, paradoxical bronchospasm, pharyngitis, sinusitis, wheezing, anaphylactic/anaphylactoid reactions, death (due to adrenal insufficiency, reported during and after transfer from systemic corticosteroids to aerosol in asthmatic patients), immediate and delayed hypersensitivity reactions

Dosage Nasal inhalation and oral inhalation dosage forms are not to be used interchangeably

Aqueous inhalation, nasal:

Vancenase® AQ, Beconase® AQ: Children ≥6 years and Adults: 1-2 inhalations each nostril twice daily; total dose 168-336 mcg/day

Vancenase® AQ 84 mcg: Children ≥6 years and Adults: 1-2 inhalations in each nostril once daily; total dose 168-336 mcg/day

Intranasal (Vancenase®, Beconase®):

Children 6-12 years: 1 inhalation in each nostril 3 times/day; total dose 252 mcg/day

Children ≥12 years and Adults: 1 inhalation in each nostril 2-4 times/day or 2 inhalations each nostril twice daily (total dose 168-336 mcg/day); usual maximum maintenance: 1 inhalation in each nostril 3 times/day (252 mcg/day)

Oral inhalation (doses should be titrated to the lowest effective dose once asthma is controlled):

Vanceril®:

Children 6-12 years: 1-2 inhalations 3-4 times/day (alternatively: 2-4 inhalations twice daily); maximum dose: 10 inhalations/day (420 mcg)

Children ≥12 years and Adults: 2 inhalations 3-4 times/day (alternatively: 4 inhalations twice daily); maximum dose: 20 inhalations/day (840 mcg/day);

(Continued)

Beclomethasone *(Continued)*

patients with severe asthma: Initial: 12-16 inhalations/day (divided 3-4 times/day); dose should be adjusted downward according to patient's response

Vanceril® 84 mcg double strength:

Children 6-12 years: 2 inhalations twice daily; maximum dose: 5 inhalations/day (420 mcg)

Children ≥12 years and Adults: 2 inhalations twice daily; maximum dose: 10 inhalations/day (840 mcg); patients with severe asthma: Initial: 6-8 inhalations/day (divided twice daily); dose should be adjusted downward according to patient's response

QVAR™:

Children 5-11 years: Initial: 40 mcg twice daily; maximum dose: 80 mcg twice daily

Children ≥12 years and Adults:

Patients previously on bronchodilators only: Initial dose 40-80 mcg twice daily; maximum dose: 320 mcg twice day

Patients previously on inhaled corticosteroids: Initial dose 40-160 mcg twice daily; maximum dose: 320 mcg twice daily

NIH Guidelines (NIH, 1997) (give in divided doses):

Children:

"Low" dose: 84-336 mcg/day (42 mcg/puff: 2-8 puffs/day or 84 mcg/puff: 1-4 puffs/day)

"Medium" dose: 336-672 mcg/day (42 mcg/puff: 8-16 puffs/day or 84 mcg/puff: 4-8 puffs/day)

"High" dose: >672 mcg/day (42 mcg/puff: >16 puffs/day or 84 mcg/puff >8 puffs/day)

Adults:

"Low" dose: 168-504 mcg/day (42 mcg/puff: 4-12 puffs/day or 84 mcg/puff: 2-6 puffs/day)

"Medium" dose: 504-840 mcg/day (42 mcg/puff: 12-20 puffs/day or 84 mcg/puff: 6-10 puffs/day)

"High" dose: >840 mcg/day (42 mcg/puff: >20 puffs/day or 84 mcg/puff: >10 puffs/day)

Mechanism of Action Controls the rate of protein synthesis, depresses the migration of polymorphonuclear leukocytes, fibroblasts, reverses capillary permeability, and lysosomal stabilization at the cellular level to prevent or control inflammation

Other Adverse Effects Frequency not defined:

Central nervous system: Depression, dysphonia

Dermatologic: Acneiform lesions, angioedema, atrophy, **bruising**, pruritus, purpura, striae, rash, urticaria

Endocrine & metabolic: Cushingoid features, growth velocity reduction in children and adolescents, HPA function suppression, weight gain

Gastrointestinal: Loss of smell, unpleasant smell, nasal septum perforation (rare), ulceration of nasal mucosa (rare)

Local: Nasal spray: Burning, transient irritation

Ocular: Cataracts, glaucoma, increased intraocular pressure

Drug Interactions Increased Effect/Toxicity: The addition of salmeterol has been demonstrated to improve response to inhaled corticosteroids (as compared to increasing steroid dosage).

Pharmacodynamics/Kinetics

Onset of action: Therapeutic effect: 1-4 weeks

Absorption: Readily; quickly hydrolyzed by pulmonary esterases prior to absorption

Distribution: Beclomethasone: 20 L; active metabolite: 424 L

Protein binding: 87%

Metabolism: Hepatic via CYP3A4 to active metabolites

Bioavailability: Of active metabolite, 44% following nasal inhalation (43% from swallowed portion)

Half-life elimination: Initial: 3 hours

Excretion: Feces (60%); urine (12%)

Pregnancy Risk Factor C

Generic Available No

Beclomethasone Dipropionate *see* Beclomethasone *on page 163*

Beclovent® [DSC] *see* Beclomethasone *on page 163*

Beconase® [DSC] *see* Beclomethasone *on page 163*

Beconase® AQ *see* Beclomethasone *on page 163*

Behenyl Alcohol *see* Docosanol *on page 463*

Belladonna and Opium (bel a DON a & OH pee um)

Related Information

Opium Tincture *on page 1002*

U.S. Brand Names B&O Supprettes®

Pharmacologic Category Analgesic Combination (Narcotic); Antispasmodic Agent, Urinary

Synonyms Opium and Belladonna

Use Relief of moderate to severe pain associated with rectal or bladder tenesmus that may occur in postoperative states and neoplastic situations; pain associated with ureteral spasms not responsive to non-narcotic analgesics and to space intervals between injections of opiates

Local Anesthetic/Vasoconstrictor Precautions No information available to require special precautions

Effects on Dental Treatment

>10%: Xerostomia, changes in salivation, dry throat and nose

1% to 10%: Dysphagia

Restrictions C-II

Dosage Rectal: Adults: 1 suppository 1-2 times/day, up to 4 doses/day

Mechanism of Action Anticholinergic alkaloids act primarily by competitive inhibition of the muscarinic actions of acetylcholine on structures innervated by postganglionic cholinergic neurons and on smooth muscle; resulting effects include antisecretory activity on exocrine glands and intestinal mucosa and smooth muscle relaxation. Contains many narcotic alkaloids including morphine; its mechanism for gastric motility inhibition is primarily due to this morphine content; it results in a decrease in digestive secretions, an increase in GI muscle tone, and therefore a reduction in GI propulsion.

Other Adverse Effects

>10%:

Dermatologic: Dry skin

Gastrointestinal: Constipation

Miscellaneous: Diaphoresis (decreased)

1% to 10%:

Dermatologic: Increased sensitivity to light

Endocrine & metabolic: Decreased flow of breast milk

<1%: **Orthostatic hypotension, ventricular fibrillation, tachycardia, palpitations, confusion, drowsiness, headache**, loss of memory, fatigue, ataxia, **CNS depression**, rash, antidiuretic hormone release, bloated feeling, **nausea, vomiting, biliary tract spasm**, dysuria, urinary retention, urinary tract spasm, increased intraocular pain, **blurred vision, weakness, respiratory depression, histamine release, physical and psychological dependence**

Drug Interactions

Increased Effect/Toxicity: Additive effects with CNS depressants. May increase effects of digoxin and atenolol. Coadministration with other anticholinergic agents (phenothiazines, tricyclic antidepressants, amantadine, and antihistamines) may increase effects such as dry mouth, constipation, and urinary retention.

Decreased Effect: May decrease effects of drugs with cholinergic mechanisms. Antipsychotic efficacy of phenothiazines may be decreased.

Dietary/Ethanol/Herb Considerations

Ethanol: Avoid use; may increase sedation.

Herb/Nutraceutical: Avoid gotu kola, kava, SAMe, St John's wort, and valerian; may increase CNS depression.

Pharmacodynamics/Kinetics

Opium:

Onset of action: Within 30 minutes

Metabolism: Hepatic, with formation of glucuronide metabolites

Pregnancy Risk Factor C

Generic Available Yes

Belladonna, Phenobarbital, and Ergotamine

(bel a DON a, fee noe BAR bi tal, & er GOT a meen TAR trate)

Related Information

Ergotamine *on page 510*

Phenobarbital *on page 1066*

U.S. Brand Names Bellamine S; Bel-Phen-Ergot S®; Bel-Tabs

Canadian Brand Names Bellergal® Spacetabs®

Pharmacologic Category Ergot Derivative

Synonyms Ergotamine Tartrate, Belladonna, and Phenobarbital; Phenobarbital, Belladonna, and Ergotamine Tartrate

Use Management and treatment of menopausal disorders, GI disorders, and recurrent throbbing headache

Local Anesthetic/Vasoconstrictor Precautions No information available to require special precautions

Effects on Dental Treatment

>10%: Xerostomia, dry throat, nasal dryness, drowsiness, dizziness, nausea, vomiting, weakness in legs

1% to 10%: Difficulty swallowing, precordial distress and pain, transient tachycardia or bradycardia, muscle pains in the extremities

Dosage Oral: 1 tablet each morning and evening

(Continued)

Belladonna, Phenobarbital, and Ergotamine *(Continued)*

Other Adverse Effects

>10%:

Cardiovascular: Peripheral vascular effects (numbness and tingling of fingers and toes)

Dermatologic: Dry skin

Gastrointestinal: Constipation, diarrhea

Miscellaneous: Decreased diaphoresis

1% to 10%:

Dermatologic: Photosensitivity

Endocrine & metabolic: Decreased flow of breast milk

<1% (Limited to important or life-threatening): **Orthostatic hypotension, ventricular fibrillation, palpitations, confusion, headache, loss of memory,** skin rash, increased intraocular pain, **blurred vision**

Drug Interactions

Increased Effect/Toxicity: Combined administration of phenobarbital and CNS depressants such as ethanol, tricyclic depressants, phenothiazines, and narcotic analgesics may result in potentiation of depressant actions. **Phenobarbital taken with warfarin induces liver enzymes that enhance clearance of warfarin. A reduction in phenobarbital dose in patients receiving warfarin has resulted in fatal bleeding episodes.** Griseofulvin, quinidine, doxycycline, and estrogen have been shown to be metabolized at an increased rate. Belladonna and concomitant administration of tricyclic antidepressants may result in additive anticholinergic effects. Valproic acid appears to decrease barbiturate metabolism (increased barbiturate levels). A similar reaction is possible with phenytoin.

Decreased Effect: Phenobarbital may lower plasma levels of dicumarol due to decreased absorption. Possible interaction between ergot alkaloids and beta-blockers.

Pregnancy Risk Factor X

Generic Available Yes

Bellamine S *see* Belladonna, Phenobarbital, and Ergotamine *on page 165*

Bel-Phen-Ergot S® *see* Belladonna, Phenobarbital, and Ergotamine *on page 165*

Bel-Tabs *see* Belladonna, Phenobarbital, and Ergotamine *on page 165*

Benadryl® Allergy [OTC] *see* DiphenhydrAMINE *on page 451*

Benadryl® Allergy and Sinus Fastmelt™ [OTC] *see* Diphenhydramine and Pseudoephedrine *on page 453*

Benadryl® Allergy/Decongestant [OTC] *see* Diphenhydramine and Pseudoephedrine *on page 453*

Benadryl® Children's Allergy and Cold Fastmelt™ [OTC] *see* Diphenhydramine and Pseudoephedrine *on page 453*

Benadryl® Children's Allergy and Sinus [OTC] *see* Diphenhydramine and Pseudoephedrine *on page 453*

Benadryl® Dye-Free Allergy [OTC] *see* DiphenhydrAMINE *on page 451*

Benadryl® Gel [OTC] *see* DiphenhydrAMINE *on page 451*

Benadryl® Gel Extra Strength [OTC] *see* DiphenhydrAMINE *on page 451*

Benadryl® Injection *see* DiphenhydrAMINE *on page 451*

Benazepril (ben AY ze pril)

Related Information

Cardiovascular Diseases *on page 1456*

U.S. Brand Names Lotensin®

Canadian Brand Names Lotensin®

Mexican Brand Names Lotensin®

Pharmacologic Category Angiotensin-Converting Enzyme (ACE) Inhibitor

Synonyms Benazepril Hydrochloride

Use Treatment of hypertension, either alone or in combination with other antihypertensive agents; treatment of left ventricular dysfunction after MI

Local Anesthetic/Vasoconstrictor Precautions No information available to require special precautions

Effects on Dental Treatment 1% to 10%: Headache (6%), dizziness (4%), somnolence (2%), nausea (2%), cough, (1% to 10%), postural dizziness (2%), fatigue

Dosage Oral: Adults: Initial: 10 mg/day in patients not receiving a diuretic; 20-40 mg/day as a single dose or 2 divided doses; base dosage adjustments on peak (2-6 hours after dosing) and trough responses.

Dosing interval in renal impairment: Cl_{cr} <30 mL/minute: Administer 5 mg/day initially; maximum daily dose: 40 mg.

Hemodialysis: Moderately dialyzable (20% to 50%); administer dose postdialysis or administer 25% to 35% supplemental dose.

Peritoneal dialysis: Supplemental dose is unnecessary.

Mechanism of Action Competitive inhibition of angiotensin I being converted to angiotensin II, a potent vasoconstrictor, through the angiotensin I-converting enzyme (ACE) activity, with resultant lower levels of angiotensin II which causes an increase in plasma renin activity and a reduction in aldosterone secretion

Other Adverse Effects

1% to 10%:

Endocrine & metabolic: Hyperkalemia (1%), increased uric acid

Renal: Increased serum creatinine (2%), worsening of renal function may occur in patients with bilateral renal artery stenosis or hypovolemia

<1% (Limited to important or life-threatening): **Hypotension, postural hypotension (0.3%), syncope, angina, palpitation**, peripheral edema, angioedema, **laryngeal edema, shock,** Stevens-Johnson syndrome, pemphigus, **hypersensitivity**, dermatitis, rash, pruritus, photosensitivity, **flushing**, pancreatitis, constipation, **gastritis, vomiting**, melena, thrombocytopenia, hemolytic anemia, **anxiety**, decreased libido, hypertonia, insomnia, **nervousness, paresthesia, asthma, bronchitis, dyspnea, sinusitis**, urinary tract infection, **arthritis,** impotence, alopecia, arthralgia, myalgia, asthenia, **increased diaphoresis**, gynecomastia

Reported with other ACE inhibitors: **Eosinophilic pneumonitis,** neutropenia, **anaphylaxis,** renal insufficiency, renal failure, and a syndrome (including fever, myalgia, arthralgia, interstitial nephritis, vasculitis, rash, eosinophilia, and elevated ESR)

Drug Interactions

Increased Effect/Toxicity: Potassium supplements, co-trimoxazole (high dose), angiotensin II receptor antagonists (candesartan, losartan, irbesartan, etc), or potassium-sparing diuretics (amiloride, spironolactone, triamterene) may result in elevated serum potassium levels when combined with benazepril. ACE inhibitor effects may be increased by phenothiazines or probenecid (increases levels of captopril). ACE inhibitors may increase serum concentrations/effects of digoxin, lithium, and sulfonlyureas. Diuretics have additive hypotensive effects with ACE inhibitors, and hypovolemia increases the potential for adverse renal effects of ACE inhibitors. In patients with compromised renal function, coadministration with NSAIDs may result in further deterioration of renal function. Allopurinol and ACE inhibitors may cause a higher risk of hypersensitivity reaction when taken concurrently.

Decreased Effect: Aspirin (high dose) may reduce the therapeutic effects of ACE inhibitors; at low dosages this does not appear to be significant. Rifampin may decrease the effect of ACE inhibitors. Antacids may decrease the bioavailability of ACE inhibitors (may be more likely to occur with captopril); separate administration times by 1-2 hours. NSAIDs, specifically indomethacin, may reduce the hypotensive effects of ACE inhibitors.

Dietary/Ethanol/Herb Considerations

Ethanol: Avoid use; may increase risk of hypotension or dizziness.

Food: Avoid potassium supplements or salt-substitutes containing potassium. Avoid caffeine (eg, colas, chocolate), garlic, and licorice.

Herb/Nutraceutical: Avoid black cohosh, dong quai, and evening primrose due to estrogenic activity. Avoid ephedra, ginseng, and yohimbe; may worsen hypertension. Avoid garlic; may have increased antihypertensive effect. Avoid ginger due to positive inotropic effects; theoretically, may cause arrhythmia. Avoid hawthorn; may lower peripheral vascular resistance resulting in additive decrease in BP. Avoid licorice.

Pharmacodynamics/Kinetics

Reduction in plasma angiotensin-converting enzyme (ACE) activity:

Onset of action: Peak effect: 1-2 hours after 2-20 mg dose

Duration: >90% inhibition for 24 hours after 5-20 mg dose

Reduction in blood pressure:

Peak effect: Single dose: 2-4 hours; Continuous therapy: 2 weeks

Absorption: Rapid (37%); food does not alter significantly; metabolite (benazeprilat) itself unsuitable for oral administration due to poor absorption

Distribution: V_d: ~8.7 L

Metabolism: Rapidly and extensively hepatic to its active metabolite, benazeprilat, via enzymatic hydrolysis; extensive first-pass effect

Half-life elimination: Effective: 10-11 hours; Benazeprilat: Terminal: 22 hours

Time to peak: Parent drug: 1-1.5 hours

Excretion: Clearance: Nonrenal clearance (ie, biliary, metabolic) appears to contribute to the elimination of benazeprilat (11% to 12%), particularly patients with severe renal impairment; hepatic clearance is the main elimination route of unchanged benazepril

Dialysis: ~6% of metabolite removed in 4 hours of dialysis following 10 mg of benazepril administered 2 hours prior to procedure; parent compound not found in dialysate

Pregnancy Risk Factor C/D (2nd and 3rd trimesters)

Generic Available No

Benazepril and Amlodipine *see* Amlodipine and Benazepril *on page 89*

Benazepril and Hydrochlorothiazide

(ben AY ze pril & hye droe klor oh THYE a zide)

Related Information

Benazepril *on page 166*

Hydrochlorothiazide *on page 675*

(Continued)

Benazepril and Hydrochlorothiazide *(Continued)*

U.S. Brand Names Lotensin® HCT

Canadian Brand Names Lotrel®

Pharmacologic Category Antihypertensive Agent Combination

Synonyms Hydrochlorothiazide and Benazepril

Use Treatment of hypertension

Local Anesthetic/Vasoconstrictor Precautions No information available to require special precautions

Effects on Dental Treatment No significant effects or complications reported

Dosage Dose is individualized

Dietary/Ethanol/Herb Considerations Ethanol: Avoid use; may increase risk of hypotension or dizziness.

Pregnancy Risk Factor C/D (2nd and 3rd trimesters)

Generic Available No

Benazepril Hydrochloride *see* Benazepril *on page 166*

Bendroflumethiazide (ben droe floo meth EYE a zide)

Related Information

Cardiovascular Diseases *on page 1456*

U.S. Brand Names Naturetin®

Pharmacologic Category Diuretic, Thiazide

Use Management of mild to moderate hypertension, edema associated with CHF, pregnancy, or nephrotic syndrome; reportedly does not alter serum electrolyte concentrations appreciably at recommended doses

Local Anesthetic/Vasoconstrictor Precautions No information available to require special precautions

Effects on Dental Treatment 1% to 10%: Orthostatic hypotension

Dosage Oral:

Children: Initial: 0.1-0.4 mg/kg/day in 1-2 doses; maintenance dose: 0.05-0.1 mg/kg/day in 1-2 doses; maximum dose: 20 mg/day

Adults: 2.5-20 mg/day or twice daily in divided doses

Mechanism of Action Like other thiazide diuretics, it inhibits sodium, chloride, and water reabsorption in the renal distal tubules, thereby producing diuresis with a resultant reduction in plasma volume; hypothetically may reduce peripheral resistance through increased prostacyclin synthesis

Other Adverse Effects

1% to 10%:

Endocrine & metabolic: Hyponatremia, hypokalemia

Gastrointestinal: Anorexia, upset stomach, diarrhea

<1% (Limited to important or life-threatening): Agranulocytosis, **allergic reactions**, aplastic anemia, **drowsiness**, hemolytic anemia, hepatic function impairment, hepatitis, hypercalcemia, hyperuricemia, leukopenia, **nausea**, pancreatitis, **paresthesia**, polyuria, thrombocytopenia, uremia, **vomiting**

Drug Interactions

Increased Effect/Toxicity: Increased effect of thiazides with furosemide and other loop diuretics. Increased hypotension and/or renal adverse effects of ACE inhibitors may result in aggressively diuresed patients. Beta-blockers increase hyperglycemic effects of thiazides in type 2 diabetes mellitus. Cyclosporine and thiazides can increase the risk of gout or renal toxicity. Digoxin toxicity can be exacerbated if a thiazide induces hypokalemia or hypomagnesemia. Lithium toxicity can occur with thiazides due to reduced renal excretion of lithium. Thiazides may prolong the duration of action with neuromuscular blocking agents.

Decreased Effect: Effects of oral hypoglycemics may be decreased. Decreased absorption of hydrochlorothiazide with cholestyramine and colestipol. NSAIDs can decrease the efficacy of thiazides, reducing the diuretic and antihypertensive effects.

Pregnancy Risk Factor D

Generic Available No

Benemid [DSC] *see* Probenecid *on page 1119*

Benicar™ *see* Olmesartan *on page 997*

Benoquin® *see* Monobenzone *on page 929*

Bentoquatam (ben to KWA tam)

U.S. Brand Names IvyBlock® [OTC]

Pharmacologic Category Topical Skin Product

Synonyms Quaternium-18 Bentonite

Use Skin protectant for the prevention of allergic contact dermatitis to poison oak, ivy, and sumac

Local Anesthetic/Vasoconstrictor Precautions No information available to require special precautions

Effects on Dental Treatment No significant effects or complications reported

Dosage Children >6 years and Adults: Topical: Apply to skin 15 minutes prior to potential exposure to poison ivy, poison oak, or poison sumac, and reapply every 4 hours

Mechanism of Action An organoclay substance which is capable of absorbing or binding to urushiol, the active principle in poison oak, ivy, and sumac. Bentoquatam serves as a barrier, blocking urushiol skin contact/absorption.

Other Adverse Effects <1%: Erythema

Pharmacodynamics/Kinetics Absorption: Has not been studied

Generic Available No

Bentyl® *see* Dicyclomine *on page 433*

Benylin® Adult [OTC] *see* Dextromethorphan *on page 423*

Benylin® Expectorant [OTC] *see* Guaifenesin and Dextromethorphan *on page 651*

Benylin® Pediatric [OTC] *see* Dextromethorphan *on page 423*

Benza® [OTC] *see* Benzalkonium Chloride *on page 169*

Benzac® *see* Benzoyl Peroxide *on page 171*

Benzac® AC *see* Benzoyl Peroxide *on page 171*

Benzac® AC Wash *see* Benzoyl Peroxide *on page 171*

BenzaClin® *see* Clindamycin and Benzoyl Peroxide *on page 343*

Benzac® W *see* Benzoyl Peroxide *on page 171*

Benzac® W Wash *see* Benzoyl Peroxide *on page 171*

Benzagel® *see* Benzoyl Peroxide *on page 171*

Benzagel® Wash *see* Benzoyl Peroxide *on page 171*

Benzalkonium Chloride (benz al KOE nee um KLOR ide)

Related Information

Periodontal Diseases *on page 1540*

U.S. Brand Names Benza® [OTC]; 3M™ Cavilon™ Skin Cleanser [OTC]; Ony-Clear [OTC]; Zephiran® [OTC]

Pharmacologic Category Antibiotic, Topical

Synonyms BAC

Use Surface antiseptic and germicidal preservative

Local Anesthetic/Vasoconstrictor Precautions No information available to require special precautions

Effects on Dental Treatment 1% to 10%: Hypersensitivity

Dosage Thoroughly rinse anionic detergents and soaps from the skin or other areas prior to use of solutions because they reduce the antibacterial activity of BAC. To protect metal instruments stored in BAC solution, add crushed Anti-Rust Tablets, 4 tablets/quart, to antiseptic solution, change solution at least once weekly. Not to be used for storage of aluminum or zinc instruments, instruments with lenses fastened by cement, lacquered catheters, or some synthetic rubber goods.

Pregnancy Risk Factor C

Generic Available Yes

Benzamycin® *see* Erythromycin and Benzoyl Peroxide *on page 515*

Benzashave® *see* Benzoyl Peroxide *on page 171*

Benzathine Benzylpenicillin *see* Penicillin G Benzathine *on page 1047*

Benzathine Penicillin G *see* Penicillin G Benzathine *on page 1047*

Benzedrex® [OTC] *see* Propylhexedrine *on page 1142*

Benzene Hexachloride *see* Lindane *on page 809*

Benzhexol Hydrochloride *see* Trihexyphenidyl *on page 1351*

Benzmethyzin *see* Procarbazine *on page 1122*

Benzocaine (BEN zoe kane)

Related Information

Mouth Pain, Cold Sore, and Canker Sore Products *on page 1630*

Oral Pain *on page 1524*

U.S. Brand Names Americaine® [OTC]; Americaine® Anesthetic Lubricant; Anbesol® [OTC]; Anbesol® Baby [OTC]; Anbesol® Maximum Strength [OTC]; Babee® Teething® [OTC]; Benzodent® [OTC]; Chiggerex® [OTC]; Chiggertox® [OTC]; Cylex® [OTC]; Detane® [OTC]; Foille® [OTC]; Foille® Medicated First Aid [OTC]; Foille® Plus [OTC]; HDA® Toothache [OTC]; Hurricaine®; Lanacane® [OTC]; Mycinettes® [OTC]; Orabase®-B [OTC]; Orajel® [OTC]; Orajel® Baby [OTC]; Orajel® Baby Nighttime [OTC]; Orajel® Maximum Strength [OTC]; Orasol® [OTC]; Solarcaine® [OTC]; Trocaine® [OTC]; Zilactin®-B [OTC]; Zilactin® Baby [OTC]

Canadian Brand Names Anbesol® Baby; Zilactin-B®; Zilactin Baby®

Mexican Brand Names Graneodin-B

Pharmacologic Category Local Anesthetic, Dental; Local Anesthetic

Synonyms Ethyl Aminobenzoate

Use

Dental: Ester-type topical local anesthetic for temporary relief of pain associated with toothache, minor sore throat pain, and canker sores

(Continued)

Benzocaine *(Continued)*

Medical: Local anesthetic (ester derivative); temporary relief of pain associated with pruritic dermatosis, pruritus, minor burns, acute congestive and serious otitis media, swimmer's ear, otitis externa, hemorrhoids, rectal fissures, anesthetic lubricant for passage of catheters and endoscopic tubes; nonprescription diet aid

Local Anesthetic/Vasoconstrictor Precautions No information available to require special precautions

Effects on Dental Treatment Dose-related (may result from high plasma levels): 1% to 10%: Angioedema, contact dermatitis, burning, stinging

Dosage Dosage for mucous membranes varies depending on area to be anesthetized and vascularity of tissues.

Children and Adults:

Oral mouth/throat preparations: Refer to specific package labeling or as directed by physician; do not administer for >2 days or in children <2 years of age, unless directed by a physician

Topical: Apply to affected area as needed

Mechanism of Action Ester local anesthetic blocks both the initiation and conduction of nerve impulses by decreasing the neuronal membrane's permeability to sodium ions, which results in inhibition of depolarization with resultant blockade of conduction

Other Adverse Effects Dose-related; may result in high plasma levels: <1%: Edema, urticaria, urethritis, methemoglobinemia (risk may be increased in infants), **tenderness**

Contraindications Hypersensitivity to benzocaine, other ester-type local anesthetics, or any component of the formulation; secondary bacterial infection of area; ophthalmic use; see package labeling for specific contraindications

Warnings/Precautions Not intended for use when infections are present

Drug Interactions Decreased Effect: May antagonize actions of sulfonamides

Pharmacodynamics/Kinetics

Absorption: Topical: Poor to intact skin; well absorbed from mucous membranes and traumatized skin

Metabolism: Hepatic (to a lesser extent) and plasma via hydrolysis by cholinesterase

Excretion: Urine (as metabolites)

Pregnancy Risk Factor C

Dosage Forms AERO, oral spray: 20% (60 mL). **AERO, topical spray:** 5% (97.5 mL, 105 mL); 20% (20 mL, 90 mL, 120 mL, 135 mL). **CRM, topical:** 5% (30 g, 454 g); 20% (30 g). **GEL, oral:** 6.3% (7.5 g); 6.5% (15 mL); 7.5% (7.5 g, 10 g, 15 g); 10% (6 g, 7.5 g, 10 g); 20% (6 g, 7 g, 7.5 g, 10 g); (Hurricaine®): 20% (5 g, 30 g). **GEL, topical:** 20% (2.5 g, 28 g). **LIQ, oral:** 6.3% (9 mL, 15 mL, 30 mL); 7.5% (13 mL); 10% (13 mL); 20% (9 mL, 14 mL, 30 mL). **LIQ, topical:** 2% (30 mL). **LOT, oral:** 2.5% (15 mL). **LOZ:** 10 mg, 15 mg. **OINT, oral:** 20% (30 g). **OINT, topical:** 2% (52 g); 5% (3.5 g, 28 g). **PASTE, oral:** 20% (7 g)

Generic Available Yes

Benzocaine and Antipyrine *see* Antipyrine and Benzocaine *on page 116*

Benzocaine and Cetylpyridinium Chloride *see* Cetylpyridinium and Benzocaine *on page 292*

Benzocaine, Butyl Aminobenzoate, Tetracaine, and Benzalkonium Chloride

(BEN zoe kane, BYOO til a meen oh BENZ oh ate, TET ra kane, & benz al KOE nee um KLOR ide)

Related Information

Benzalkonium Chloride *on page 169*
Benzocaine *on page 169*
Tetracaine *on page 1284*

U.S. Brand Names Cetacaine®

Pharmacologic Category Local Anesthetic, Dental; Local Anesthetic

Synonyms Tetracaine Hydrochloride, Benzocaine Butyl Aminobenzoate, and Benzalkonium Chloride

Use Dental: Topical anesthetic to control pain or gagging

Local Anesthetic/Vasoconstrictor Precautions No information available to require special precautions

Effects on Dental Treatment Dose-related (may result from high plasma levels): 1% to 10%: Contact dermatitis, angioedema, burning, stinging

Dosage Apply to affected area for approximately 1 second or less

Other Adverse Effects Dose-related (may result from high plasma levels): <1%: Edema, urticaria, urethritis, methemoglobinemia (risk may be increased in infants), **tenderness**

Contraindications Hypersensitivity to any component of the formulation

Pregnancy Risk Factor C

Dosage Forms AERO, topical: Benzocaine 14%, butyl aminobenzoate 2%, tetracaine 2%, and benzalkonium 0.5% (56 g). **GEL, topical:** Benzocaine 14%, butyl aminobenzoate 2%, tetracaine 2%, and benzalkonium 0.5% (29 g). **LIQ, topical:** Benzocaine 14%, butyl aminobenzoate 2%, tetracaine 2%, and benzalkonium 0.5% (56 mL)

Generic Available No

Benzocaine, Gelatin, Pectin, and Sodium Carboxymethylcellulose

(BEN zoe kane, JEL a tin, PEK tin, & SOW dee um kar box ee meth il SEL yoo lose)

Related Information

Benzocaine *on page 169*

U.S. Brand Names Orabase® With Benzocaine [OTC]

Pharmacologic Category Local Anesthetic, Dental; Local Anesthetic

Use Dental: Topical anesthetic and emollient for oral lesions

Local Anesthetic/Vasoconstrictor Precautions No information available to require special precautions

Effects on Dental Treatment Dose-related (may result from high plasma levels): 1% to 10%: Contact dermatitis, angioedema, burning, stinging

Dosage Apply 2-4 times/day

Other Adverse Effects Dose-related (may result from high plasma levels): <1%: Edema, urticaria, urethritis, methemoglobinemia (risk may be increased in infants), tenderness

Contraindications Hypersensitivity to any component of the formulation

Pregnancy Risk Factor C

Dosage Forms PASTE: Benzocaine 20%, gelatin, pectin, and sodium carboxymethylcellulose (5 g, 15 g)

Generic Available No

Benzodent® [OTC] *see* Benzocaine *on page 169*

Benzoin (BEN zoyn)

U.S. Brand Names TinBen® [OTC]

Pharmacologic Category Antibiotic, Topical; Topical Skin Product

Synonyms Gum Benjamin

Use Protective application for irritations of the skin; sometimes used in boiling water as steam inhalants for their expectorant and soothing action

Local Anesthetic/Vasoconstrictor Precautions No information available to require special precautions

Effects on Dental Treatment No significant effects or complications reported

Dosage Apply 1-2 times/day

Generic Available Yes

Benzonatate (ben ZOE na tate)

Related Information

Management of Patients Undergoing Cancer Therapy *on page 1567*

U.S. Brand Names Tessalon®

Canadian Brand Names Tessalon®

Mexican Brand Names Beknol; Pebegal; Tesalon®; Tusical®; Tusitato®

Pharmacologic Category Antitussive

Use Symptomatic relief of nonproductive cough

Local Anesthetic/Vasoconstrictor Precautions No information available to require special precautions

Effects on Dental Treatment 1% to 10%: Sedation, headache, dizziness, GI upset, numbness in chest, nasal congestion

Dosage Children >10 years and Adults: Oral: 100 mg 3 times/day or every 4 hours up to 600 mg/day

Mechanism of Action Tetracaine congener with antitussive properties; suppresses cough by topical anesthetic action on the respiratory stretch receptors

Other Adverse Effects 1% to 10%:

Dermatologic: Rash

Ocular: Burning sensation in eyes

Pharmacodynamics/Kinetics

Onset of action: Therapeutic: 15-20 minutes

Duration: 3-8 hours

Pregnancy Risk Factor C

Generic Available Yes

Benzoyl Peroxide (BEN zoe il peer OKS ide)

U.S. Brand Names Benzac®; Benzac® AC; Benzac® AC Wash; Benzac® W; Benzac® W Wash; Benzagel®; Benzagel® Wash; Benzashave®; Brevoxyl®; Brevoxyl® Cleansing; Brevoxyl® Wash; Clinac™ BPO; Del Aqua®; Desquam-E™; Desquam-X®; Exact® Acne Medication [OTC]; Fostex® 10% BPO [OTC]; Loroxide®

(Continued)

Benzoyl Peroxide *(Continued)*

[OTC]; Neutrogena® Acne Mask [OTC]; Neutrogena® On The Spot® Acne Treatment [OTC]; Oxy 10® Balanced Medicated Face Wash [OTC]; Palmer's® Skin Success Acne [OTC]; PanOxyl®; PanOxyl®-AQ; PanOxyl® Bar [OTC]; Seba-Gel™; Triaz®; Triaz® Cleanser; Zapzyt® [OTC]

Canadian Brand Names Acetoxyl®; Benoxyl®; Benzac AC®; Benzac W® Gel; Benzac W® Wash; Desquam-X®; Oxyderm™; PanOxyl®; PanOxyl®-AQ; Solugel®

Mexican Brand Names Benoxyl®; Benzac®; Benzaderm®; Solugel®

Pharmacologic Category Topical Skin Product; Topical Skin Product, Acne

Use Adjunctive treatment of mild to moderate acne vulgaris and acne rosacea

Local Anesthetic/Vasoconstrictor Precautions No information available to require special precautions

Effects on Dental Treatment No significant effects or complications reported

Dosage Children and Adults:

Cleansers: Wash once or twice daily; control amount of drying or peeling by modifying dose frequency or concentration

Topical: Apply sparingly once daily; gradually increase to 2-3 times/day if needed. If excessive dryness or peeling occurs, reduce dose frequency or concentration; if excessive stinging or burning occurs, remove with mild soap and water; resume use the next day.

Mechanism of Action Releases free-radical oxygen which oxidizes bacterial proteins in the sebaceous follicles decreasing the number of anaerobic bacteria and decreasing irritating-type free fatty acids

Other Adverse Effects 1% to 10%: Dermatologic: Irritation, contact dermatitis, dry skin, erythema, peeling, stinging

Pharmacodynamics/Kinetics

Absorption: ~5% via skin; gel more penetrating than cream

Metabolism: Converted to benzoic acid in skin

Pregnancy Risk Factor C

Generic Available Yes

Benzoyl Peroxide and Clindamycin *see* Clindamycin and Benzoyl Peroxide *on page 343*

Benzoyl Peroxide and Erythromycin *see* Erythromycin and Benzoyl Peroxide *on page 515*

Benzoyl Peroxide and Hydrocortisone

(BEN zoe il peer OKS ide & hye droe KOR ti sone)

Related Information

Benzoyl Peroxide *on page 171*

Hydrocortisone *on page 688*

U.S. Brand Names Vanoxide-HC®

Canadian Brand Names Vanoxide-HC

Pharmacologic Category Topical Skin Product; Topical Skin Product, Acne

Synonyms Hydrocortisone and Benzoyl Peroxide

Use Treatment of acne vulgaris and oily skin

Local Anesthetic/Vasoconstrictor Precautions No information available to require special precautions

Effects on Dental Treatment No significant effects or complications reported

Dosage Topical: Shake well; apply thin film 1-3 times/day, gently massage into skin

Pregnancy Risk Factor C

Generic Available No

Benzphetamine (benz FET a meen)

U.S. Brand Names Didrex®

Canadian Brand Names Didrex®

Pharmacologic Category Anorexiant

Synonyms Benzphetamine Hydrochloride

Use Short-term adjunct in exogenous obesity

Local Anesthetic/Vasoconstrictor Precautions Use with caution since amphetamines have actions similar to epinephrine and norepinephrine

Effects on Dental Treatment Frequency not defined: Hypertension, palpitations, tachycardia, chest pain, arrhythmias, euphoria, nervousness, restlessness, dizziness, anxiety, headache, agitation, confusion, psychosis, seizure, nausea, vomiting, xerostomia, metallic taste, tremors, blurred vision, bruising

Restrictions C-III

Dosage Adults: Oral: Dose should be individualized based on patient response: Initial: 25-50 mg once daily; titrate to 25-50 mg 1-3 times/day; once-daily dosing should be administered midmorning or midafternoon; maximum dose: 50 mg 3 times/day

Mechanism of Action Noncatechol sympathomimetic amines with pharmacologic actions similar to ephedrine; require breakdown by monoamine oxidase for inactivation; produce central nervous system and respiratory stimulation, a pressor response, mydriasis, bronchodilation, and contraction of the urinary sphincter;

thought to have a direct effect on both alpha- and beta-receptor sites in the peripheral system, as well as release stores of norepinephrine in adrenergic nerve terminals; central nervous system action is thought to occur in the cerebral cortex and reticular activating system; anorexigenic effect is probably secondary to the CNS-stimulating effect; the site of action is probably the hypothalamic feeding center.

Other Adverse Effects Frequency not defined:

Cardiovascular: T-wave changes, pulmonary hypertension, valvulopathy

Central nervous system: Insomnia, mental depression, CVA

Dermatologic: Alopecia, urticaria, skin rash, erythema

Endocrine & metabolic: Changes in libido, gynecomastia, menstrual irregularities, porphyria

Gastrointestinal: Abdominal cramps, constipation

Genitourinary: Impotence

Hematologic: Bone marrow depression, agranulocytosis, leukopenia

Ocular: Mydriasis

Drug Interactions Substrate of CYP2B6, **3A4**

Increased Effect/Toxicity: Amphetamines may precipitate hypertensive crisis or serotonin syndrome in patients receiving MAO inhibitors (selegiline >10 mg/day, isocarboxazid, phenelzine, tranylcypromine, furazolidone). Serotonin syndrome has also been associated with combinations of amphetamines and SSRIs; these combinations should be avoided. TCAs may enhance the effects of amphetamines, potentially leading to hypertensive crisis. Large doses of antacids or urinary alkalinizers increase the half-life and duration of action of amphetamines. May precipitate arrhythmias in patients receiving general anesthetics. Inhibitors of CYP2D6 may increase the effects of amphetamines (includes amiodarone, cimetidine, delavirdine, fluoxetine, paroxetine, propafenone, quinidine, and ritonavir).

Decreased Effect: Amphetamines inhibit the antihypertensive response to guanethidine and guanadrel. Urinary acidifiers decrease the half-life and duration of action of amphetamines. Enzyme inducers (barbiturates, carbamazepine, phenytoin, and rifampin) may decrease serum concentrations of amphetamines.

Pregnancy Risk Factor X

Generic Available No

Benzphetamine Hydrochloride *see* Benzphetamine *on page 172*

Benztropine (BENZ troe peen)

U.S. Brand Names Cogentin®

Canadian Brand Names Apo®-Benztropine; Cogentin®

Pharmacologic Category Anticholinergic Agent; Anti-Parkinson's Agent, Anticholinergic

Synonyms Benztropine Mesylate

Use Adjunctive treatment of Parkinson's disease; treatment of drug-induced extrapyramidal symptoms (except tardive dyskinesia)

Local Anesthetic/Vasoconstrictor Precautions No information available to require special precautions

Effects on Dental Treatment

>10%: Xerostomia, changes in salivation

Frequency not defined: Dry throat and nasal dryness (very prevalent), tachycardia, confusion, disorientation, memory impairment, toxic psychosis, hallucinations, nausea, vomiting, blurred vision, fever

Dosage Use in children ≤3 years of age should be reserved for life-threatening emergencies

Drug-induced extrapyramidal symptom: Oral, I.M., I.V.:

- Children >3 years: 0.02-0.05 mg/kg/dose 1-2 times/day
- Adults: 1-4 mg/dose 1-2 times/day

Acute dystonia: Adults: I.M., I.V.: 1-2 mg

Parkinsonism: Oral:

- Adults: 0.5-6 mg/day in 1-2 divided doses; if one dose is greater, administer at bedtime; titrate dose in 0.5 mg increments at 5- to 6-day intervals
- Elderly: Initial: 0.5 mg once or twice daily; increase by 0.5 mg as needed at 5-6 days; maximum: 4 mg/day

Mechanism of Action Possesses both anticholinergic and antihistaminic effects. *In vitro* anticholinergic activity approximates that of atropine; *in vivo* it is only about half as active as atropine. Animal data suggest its antihistaminic activity and duration of action approach that of pyrilamine maleate. May also inhibit the reuptake and storage of dopamine and thereby, prolong the action of dopamine.

Other Adverse Effects Frequency not defined:

Dermatologic: Rash

Endocrine & metabolic: Heat stroke, hyperthermia

Gastrointestinal: Constipation, ileus

Genitourinary: Urinary retention, dysuria

Ocular: Mydriasis

Drug Interactions Substrate of CYP2D6

(Continued)

Benztropine *(Continued)*

Increased Effect/Toxicity: Central and/or peripheral anticholinergic syndrome can occur when benztropine is administered with amantadine, rimantadine, narcotic analgesics, phenothiazines and other antipsychotics (especially with high anticholinergic activity), tricyclic antidepressants, quinidine and some other antiarrhythmics, and antihistamines. Benztropine may increase the absorption of digoxin.

Decreased Effect: May increase gastric degradation of levodopa and decrease the amount of levodopa absorbed by delaying gastric emptying. Therapeutic effects of cholinergic agents (tacrine, donepezil) and neuroleptics may be antagonized.

Dietary/Ethanol/Herb Considerations

Ethanol: Avoid use; may increase CNS depression.

Herb/Nutraceutical: Avoid gotu kola, kava, SAMe, St John's wort, and valerian; may increase CNS depression.

Pharmacodynamics/Kinetics

Onset of action: Oral: Within 1 hour; Parenteral: Within 15 minutes

Duration: 6-48 hours

Metabolism: Hepatic (N-oxidation, N-dealkylation, and ring hydroxylation)

Bioavailability: 29%

Pregnancy Risk Factor C

Generic Available Yes: Tablet

Benztropine Mesylate *see* Benztropine *on page 173*

Benzylpenicillin Benzathine *see* Penicillin G Benzathine *on page 1047*

Benzylpenicillin Potassium *see* Penicillin G (Parenteral/Aqueous) *on page 1049*

Benzylpenicillin Sodium *see* Penicillin G (Parenteral/Aqueous) *on page 1049*

Benzylpenicilloyl-polylysine (BEN zil pen i SIL oyl-pol i LYE seen)

U.S. Brand Names Pre-Pen®

Pharmacologic Category Diagnostic Agent

Synonyms Penicilloyl-polylysine; PPL

Use Adjunct in assessing the risk of administering penicillin (penicillin or benzylpenicillin) in adults with a history of clinical penicillin hypersensitivity

Local Anesthetic/Vasoconstrictor Precautions No information available to require special precautions

Effects on Dental Treatment Frequency not defined: Hypotension, dyspnea, systemic allergic reactions (rare)

Dosage PPL is administered by a scratch technique or by intradermal injection. For initial testing, PPL should always be applied via the scratch technique. **Do not administer intradermally to patients who have positive reactions to a scratch test.** PPL test alone does not identify those patients who react to a minor antigenic determinant and does not appear to predict reliably the occurrence of late reactions.

Scratch test: Use scratch technique with a 20-gauge needle to make 3-5 mm nonbleeding scratch on epidermis, apply a small drop of solution to scratch, rub in gently with applicator or toothpick. A positive reaction consists of a pale wheal surrounding the scratch site which develops within 10 minutes and ranges from 5-15 mm or more in diameter.

Intradermal test: Use intradermal test with a tuberculin syringe with a 26- to 30-gauge short bevel needle; a dose of 0.01-0.02 mL is injected intradermally. A control of 0.9% sodium chloride should be injected at least 1.5" from the PPL test site. Most skin responses to the intradermal test will develop within 5-15 minutes.

Interpretation:

(-) Negative: No reaction

(±) Ambiguous: Wheal only slightly larger than original bleb with or without erythematous flare and larger than control site

(+) Positive: Itching and marked increase in size of original bleb

Control site should be reactionless

Mechanism of Action Elicits IgE antibodies which produce type I accelerate urticarial reactions to penicillins

Other Adverse Effects Frequency not defined:

Dermatologic: Angioneurotic edema, pruritus, erythema, urticaria

Local: Intense local inflammatory response at skin test site, wheal (locally)

Drug Interactions Decreased Effect: Corticosteroids and other immunosuppressive agents may inhibit the immune response to the skin test.

Pregnancy Risk Factor C

Generic Available No

Bepridil (BE pri dil)

Related Information

Calcium Channel Blockers and Gingival Hyperplasia *on page 1598*

Calcium Channel Blockers, Comparative Pharmacokinetics *on page 1600*

Cardiovascular Diseases *on page 1456*

U.S. Brand Names Vascor®

Canadian Brand Names Vascor®

Pharmacologic Category Calcium Channel Blocker

Synonyms Bepridil Hydrochloride

Use Treatment of chronic stable angina; due to side effect profile, reserve for patients who have been intolerant of other antianginal therapy; bepridil may be used alone or in combination with nitrates or beta-blockers

Local Anesthetic/Vasoconstrictor Precautions No information available to require special precautions

Effects on Dental Treatment

>10%: Nausea, dizziness, headache (7% to 13%)

1% to 10%: Xerostomia, bradycardia, palpitations, CHF (1%), nervousness, drowsiness, psychiatric disturbances (<2%), tremor (<9%), paresthesia (3%), rhinitis, dyspnea (≤9%), cough (≤2%), flu syndrome (≤2%), increased diaphoresis, weakness (7% to 14%), blurred vision

Other drugs of this class can cause gingival hyperplasia (ie, nifedipine) but there have been no reports for bepridil.

Dosage Oral:

Adults: Initial: 200 mg/day, then adjust dose at 10-day intervals until optimal response is achieved; usual dose: 300 mg/day; maximum daily dose: 400 mg

Elderly: Peak concentrations and halflife are markedly increased in the elderly (>74 years); dose selection should be cautious, usually starting at the low end of the dosage range

Dosing adjustment in renal impairment: Risk of toxic reactions is greater in patients with renal impairment; dose selection should be cautious, usually starting at the low end of the dosage range

Mechanism of Action Bepridil, a type 4 calcium antagonist, possesses characteristics of the traditional calcium antagonists, inhibiting calcium ion from entering the "slow channels" or select voltage-sensitive areas of vascular smooth muscle and myocardium during depolarization and producing a relaxation of coronary vascular smooth muscle and coronary vasodilation. However, bepridil may also inhibit fast sodium channels (inward), which may account for some of its side effects (eg, arrhythmias); a direct bradycardia effect of bepridil has been postulated via direct action on the S-A node.

Other Adverse Effects

>10%: Gastrointestinal: Dyspepsia

1% to 10%:

- Cardiovascular: QT prolongation (dose-related; up to 5% with prolongation of ≥25%), edema
- Central nervous system: Insomnia (2% to 3%)
- Dermatologic: Rash (≤2%)
- Endocrine & metabolic: Sexual dysfunction
- Gastrointestinal: Diarrhea, anorexia, constipation, abdominal pain, dyspepsia, flatulence
- Otic: Tinnitus

<1%: Arthritis, **ventricular arrhythmia, torsade de pointes (0.01% to 1%), fever**, leukopenia, neutropenia, altered behavior, **akathisia, abnormal taste, pharyngitis**

Drug Interactions Inhibits CYP2D6

Increased Effect/Toxicity: Use with H_2 blockers may increase bioavailability of bepridil. Use of bepridil with beta-blockers may increase cardiac depressant effects on AV conduction. Bepridil may increase serum levels/effects of carbamazepine, cyclosporine, digitalis, quinidine, and theophylline. Concurrent use of fentanyl with bepridil may increase hypotension. Use with amprenavir, ritonavir, sparfloxacin (possibly also gatifloxacin and moxifloxacin) may increase risk of bepridil toxicity, especially its cardiotoxicity. Use with cisapride may increase the risk of malignant arrhythmias, concurrent use is contraindicated.

Dietary/Ethanol/Herb Considerations

Ethanol: Avoid use; may increase risk of hypotension or dizziness.

Food: Avoid caffeine (eg, colas, chocolate), garlic, and licorice.

Herb/Nutraceutical: Avoid black cohosh, dong quai, and evening primrose due to estrogenic activity. Avoid ephedra, ginseng, and yohimbe; may worsen hypertension. Avoid garlic; may have increased antihypertensive effect. Avoid ginger due to positive inotropic effects; theoretically, may cause arrhythmia. Avoid hawthorn; may lower peripheral vascular resistance causing additional decrease in BP. Avoid licorice. Avoid St John's wort; may decrease serum concentration.

Pharmacodynamics/Kinetics

Onset of action: 1 hour

Absorption: 100%

Protein binding: >99%

Metabolism: Hepatic

Bioavailability: 60%

Half-life elimination: 24 hours

Time to peak: 2-3 hours

Excretion: Urine (as metabolites)

Pregnancy Risk Factor C

Generic Available No

Bepridil Hydrochloride *see* Bepridil *on page 174*

Beractant (ber AKT ant)

U.S. Brand Names Survanta®

Canadian Brand Names Survanta®

Mexican Brand Names Survanta®

Pharmacologic Category Lung Surfactant

Synonyms Bovine Lung Surfactant; Natural Lung Surfactant

Use Prevention and treatment of respiratory distress syndrome (RDS) in premature infants

Prophylactic therapy: Body weight <1250 g in infants at risk for developing or with evidence of surfactant deficiency (administer within 15 minutes of birth)

Rescue therapy: Treatment of infants with RDS confirmed by x-ray and requiring mechanical ventilation (administer as soon as possible - within 8 hours of age)

Local Anesthetic/Vasoconstrictor Precautions No information available to require special precautions

Effects on Dental Treatment No significant effects or complications reported

Dosage

Prophylactic treatment: Administer 100 mg phospholipids (4 mL/kg) intratracheal as soon as possible; as many as 4 doses may be administered during the first 48 hours of life, no more frequently than 6 hours apart. The need for additional doses is determined by evidence of continuing respiratory distress; if the infant is still intubated and requiring at least 30% inspired oxygen to maintain a PaO_2 ≤80 torr.

Rescue treatment: Administer 100 mg phospholipids (4 mL/kg) as soon as the diagnosis of RDS is made; may repeat if needed, no more frequently than every 6 hours to a maximum of 4 doses

Mechanism of Action Replaces deficient or ineffective endogenous lung surfactant in neonates with respiratory distress syndrome (RDS) or in neonates at risk of developing RDS. Surfactant prevents the alveoli from collapsing during expiration by lowering surface tension between air and alveolar surfaces.

Other Adverse Effects During dosing procedure:

>10%: Cardiovascular: Transient bradycardia

1% to 10%: Respiratory: Oxygen desaturation

<1%: Apnea, endotracheal tube blockage, hypercarbia, hypertension, hypocarbia, hypotension, pallor, pulmonary air leaks, pulmonary interstitial emphysema, increased probability of post-treatment nosocomial sepsis, vasoconstriction

Pharmacodynamics/Kinetics Excretion: Clearance: Alveolar clearance is rapid

Generic Available No

Beta-Carotene (BAY tu KAIR oh teen)

U.S. Brand Names A-Caro-25®; B-Caro-T™; Lumitene™

Pharmacologic Category Vitamin, Fat Soluble

Use Prophylaxis and treatment of polymorphous light eruption; prophylaxis against photosensitivity reactions in patients with erythropoietic protoporphyria (EPP)

Unlabeled/Investigational Use Prophylaxis and treatment of polymorphous light eruption; prophylaxis against photosensitivity reactions in erythropoietic protoporphyria

Local Anesthetic/Vasoconstrictor Precautions No information available to require special precautions

Effects on Dental Treatment No significant effects or complications reported

Dosage Oral:

Children <14 years: 30-150 mg/day

Adults: 30-300 mg/day

Mechanism of Action The exact mechanism of action in erythropoietic protoporphyria has not as yet been elucidated; although patient must become carotenemic before effects are observed, there appears to be more than a simple internal light screen responsible for the drug's action. A protective effect was achieved when beta-carotene was added to blood samples. The concentrations of solutions used were similar to those achieved in treated patients. Topically applied beta-carotene is considerably less effective than systemic therapy.

Other Adverse Effects

>10%: Dermatologic: Carotenodermia (yellowing of palms, hands, or soles of feet, and to a lesser extent the face)

<1%: **Dizziness, bruising**, diarrhea, arthralgia

Pharmacodynamics/Kinetics

Metabolism: Prior to absorption, converted to vitamin A in the wall of the small intestine, then oxidized to retinoic acid and retinol in the presence of fat and bile acids; small amounts are then stored in the liver; retinol (active) is conjugated with glucuronic acid

Excretion: Urine and feces

Pregnancy Risk Factor C

Generic Available Yes

Betadine® [OTC] *see* Povidone-Iodine *on page 1104*

Betadine® First Aid Antibiotics + Moisturizer [OTC] *see* Bacitracin and Polymyxin B *on page 157*

Betadine® Ophthalmic *see* Povidone-Iodine *on page 1104*

9-Beta-D-ribofuranosyladenine *see* Adenosine *on page 45*

Betagan® Liquifilm® *see* Levobunolol *on page 789*

Betaine Anhydrous (BAY tayne an HY drus)

U.S. Brand Names Cystadane®

Canadian Brand Names Cystadane™

Pharmacologic Category Homocystinuria, Treatment Agent

Use Orphan drug: Treatment of homocystinuria to decrease elevated homocysteine blood levels; included within the category of homocystinuria are deficiencies or defects in cystathionine beta-synthase (CBS), 5,10-methylenetetrahydrofolate reductase (MTHFR), and cobalamin cofactor metabolism (CBL).

Local Anesthetic/Vasoconstrictor Precautions No information available to require special precautions

Effects on Dental Treatment Frequency not defined: Nausea, GI distress

Dosage

Children <3 years: Dosage may be started at 100 mg/kg/day and then increased weekly by 100 mg/kg increments

Children ≥3 years and Adults: Oral: 6 g/day administered in divided doses of 3 g twice daily. Dosages of up to 20 g/day have been necessary to control homocysteine levels in some patients.

Dosage in all patients can be gradually increased until plasma homocysteine is undetectable or present only in small amounts

Other Adverse Effects Frequency not defined: Gastrointestinal: Diarrhea

Pregnancy Risk Factor C

Generic Available No

Betamethasone (bay ta METH a sone)

Related Information

Respiratory Diseases *on page 1476*

U.S. Brand Names Alphatrex®; Betatrex®; Beta-Val®; Celestone®; Celestone® Phosphate; Celestone® Soluspan®; Diprolene®; Diprolene® AF; Diprosone® [DSC]; Luxiq™; Maxivate®

Canadian Brand Names Betaderm; Betaject™; Betnesol®; Betnovate®; Celestoderm®-EV/2; Celestoderm®-V; Celestone® Soluspan®; Diprolene® Glycol; Diprosone®; Ectosone; Prevex® B; Taro-Sone®; Topilene®; Topisone®; Valisone® Scalp Lotion

Mexican Brand Names Celestone®

Pharmacologic Category Corticosteroid, Systemic; Corticosteroid, Topical

Synonyms Betamethasone Dipropionate; Betamethasone Dipropionate, Augmented; Betamethasone Sodium Phosphate; Betamethasone Valerate; Diprosone® [DSC]; Flubenisolone

Use

Dental: Treatment of a variety of oral diseases of allergic, inflammatory, or autoimmune origin

Medical: Inflammatory dermatoses such as seborrheic or atopic dermatitis, neurodermatitis, anogenital pruritus, psoriasis, inflammatory phase of xerosis

Local Anesthetic/Vasoconstrictor Precautions No information available to require special precautions

Effects on Dental Treatment 1% to 10%:

Systemic: Dizziness or lightheadedness, headache, nervousness (10%), epistaxis, diaphoresis, diabetes

Topical: Itching, allergic contact dermatitis, skin infection (secondary), burning, irritation

Dosage Base dosage on severity of disease and patient response.

Children (use lowest dose listed as initial dose for adrenocortical insufficiency [physiologic replacement]):

I.M.: 0.0175-0.125 mg base/kg/day divided every 6-12 hours **or** 0.5-7.5 mg base/m^2/day divided every 6-12 hours

Oral: 0.0175-0.25 mg/kg/day divided every 6-8 hours **or** 0.5-7.5 mg/m^2/day divided every 6-8 hours

Topical:

≤12 years: Use not recommended.

>12 years: Apply a thin film twice daily; use minimal amount for shortest period of time to avoid HPA axis suppression

Adolescents and Adults:

Oral: 2.4-4.8 mg/day in 2-4 doses; range: 0.6-7.2 mg/day

I.M.: Betamethasone sodium phosphate and betamethasone acetate: 0.6-9 mg/day (generally, 1/3 to 1/2 of oral dose) divided every 12-24 hours

(Continued)

Betamethasone *(Continued)*

Foam: Apply twice daily, once in the morning and once at night to scalp

Adults:

Intrabursal, intra-articular, intradermal: 0.25-2 mL

Intralesional: Rheumatoid arthritis/osteoarthritis:

Very large joints: 1-2 mL

Large joints: 1 mL

Medium joints: 0.5-1 mL

Small joints: 0.25-0.5 mL

Topical: Apply thin film 2-4 times/day. Therapy should be discontinued when control is achieved; if no improvement is seen, reassessment of diagnosis may be necessary.

Dosing adjustment in hepatic impairment: Adjustments may be necessary in patients with liver failure because betamethasone is extensively metabolized in the liver

Mechanism of Action Controls the rate of protein synthesis, depresses the migration of polymorphonuclear leukocytes, fibroblasts, reverses capillary permeability, and lysosomal stabilization at the cellular level to prevent or control inflammation

Other Adverse Effects

Systemic:

>10%:

Central nervous system: Insomnia

Gastrointestinal: Increased appetite, indigestion

1% to 10%:

Dermatologic: Hirsutism, hypopigmentation

Neuromuscular & skeletal: Arthralgia

Ocular: Cataracts, glaucoma

<1% (Limited to important or life-threatening): Vertigo, **seizures, psychoses, pseudotumor cerebri, mood swings, delirium, hallucinations, euphoria,** Cushing's syndrome, pituitary-adrenal axis suppression, growth suppression, glucose intolerance, hypokalemia, alkalosis, amenorrhea, sodium and water retention, **hyperglycemia**

Topical:

1% to 10%: Dermatologic: Erythema, dryness, papular rashes, folliculitis, furunculosis, pustules, pyoderma, vesiculation, hyperesthesia

<1% (Limited to important or life-threatening): Cushing's syndrome, hypokalemic syndrome, glaucoma, cataracts (posterior subcapsular)

Contraindications Hypersensitivity to betamethasone or any component of the formulation; systemic fungal infections

Warnings/Precautions Not to be used in status asthmaticus or for the relief of acute bronchospasm; topical use in patients ≤12 years of age is not recommended. May cause suppression of hypothalamic-pituitary-adrenal (HPA) axis, particularly in younger children or in patients receiving high doses for prolonged periods. Particular care is required when patients are transferred from systemic corticosteroids to inhaled products due to possible adrenal insufficiency or withdrawal from steroids, including an increase in allergic symptoms. Patients receiving 20 mg per day of prednisone (or equivalent) may be most susceptible. Fatalities have occurred due to adrenal insufficiency in asthmatic patients during and after transfer from systemic corticosteroids to aerosol steroids; aerosol steroids do **not** provide the systemic steroid needed to treat patients having trauma, surgery, or infections. Withdrawal and discontinuation of the corticosteroid should be done slowly and carefully

Controlled clinical studies have shown that orally-inhaled and intranasal corticosteroids may cause a reduction in growth velocity in pediatric patients. (In studies of orally-inhaled corticosteroids, the mean reduction in growth velocity was approximately 1 centimeter per year [range 0.3-1.8 cm per year] and appears to be related to dose and duration of exposure.) The growth of pediatric patients receiving inhaled corticosteroids, should be monitored routinely (eg, via stadiometry). To minimize the systemic effects of orally-inhaled and intranasal corticosteroids, each patient should be titrated to the lowest effective dose.

May suppress the immune system, patients may be more susceptible to infection. Use with caution in patients with systemic infections or ocular herpes simplex. Avoid exposure to chickenpox and measles.

Use with caution in patients with hypothyroidism, cirrhosis, ulcerative colitis; do not use occlusive dressings on weeping or exudative lesions and general caution with occlusive dressings should be observed; discontinue if skin irritation or contact dermatitis should occur; do not use in patients with decreased skin circulation

Drug Interactions Inhibits CYP3A4

Phenytoin, phenobarbital, rifampin increase clearance of betamethasone.

Potassium-depleting diuretics increase potassium loss.

Skin test antigens, immunizations: Betamethasone may decrease response and increase potential infections.

Insulin or oral hypoglycemics: Betamethasone may increase blood glucose.

Dietary/Ethanol/Herb Considerations

Ethanol: Avoid use; may enhance gastric mucosal irritation.

Food: Administer with food to reduce GI upset. Betamethasone interferes with calcium absorption. Limit caffeine.

Herb/Nutraceutical: Avoid cat's claw and echinacea due to immunostimulant properties.

Pharmacodynamics/Kinetics

Protein binding: 64%

Metabolism: Hepatic

Half-life elimination: 6.5 hours

Time to peak, serum: I.V.: 10-36 minutes

Excretion: Urine (<5% as unchanged drug)

Pregnancy Risk Factor C

Dosage Forms CRM, topical, as dipropionate: 0.05% (15 g, 45 g, 60 g); (Alphatrex®, Diprosone® [DSC]): 0.05% (15 g, 45 g); (Maxivate®): 0.05% (45 g). **CRM, topical, as dipropionate augmented** (Diprolene® AF): 0.05% (15 g, 50 g). **CRM, topical, as valerate:** 0.1% (15 g, 45 g); (Betatrex®): 0.1% (15 g, 45 g); (Beta-Val®): 0.1% (15 g, 45 g). **FOAM, topical, as valerate** (Luxiq™): 0.12% (50 g, 100 g). **GEL, topical, as dipropionate augmented** (Diprolene®): 0.05% (15 g, 50 g). **INJ, solution, as sodium phosphate** (Celestone® Phosphate): 4 mg/mL (5 mL). **INJ, suspension** (Celestone® Soluspan®): Betamethasone sodium phosphate 3 mg/mL and betamethasone acetate 3 mg/mL [6 mg/mL] (5 mL) **LOT, topical, as dipropionate**: 0.05% (20 mL, 60 mL); (Alphatrex®, Maxivate®): 0.05% (60 mL); (Diprosone® [DSC]): 0.05% (20 mL, 60 mL). **LOT, topical, as dipropionate augmented** (Diprolene®): 0.05% (30 mL, 60 mL). **LOT, topical, as valerate** (Beta-Val®, Betatrex®): 0.1% (60 mL). **OINT, topical, as dipropionate**: 0.05% (15 g, 45 g); (Alphatrex®, Maxivate®): 0.05% (45 g); (Diprosone® [DSC]): 0.05% (15 g, 45 g). **OINT, topical, as dipropionate augmented**: 0.05% (15 g, 45 g, 50 g); (Diprolene®): 0.05% (15 g, 50 g). **OINT, topical, as valerate** (Betatrex®): 0.1% (15 g, 45 g). **SYR, as base** (Celestone®): 0.6 mg/5 mL (118 mL). **TAB, as base** (Celestone®): 0.6 mg

Generic Available Yes

Betamethasone and Clotrimazole

(bay ta METH a sone & kloe TRIM a zole)

Related Information

Betamethasone *on page 177*
Clotrimazole *on page 356*

U.S. Brand Names Lotrisone®

Canadian Brand Names Lotriderm®

Pharmacologic Category Antifungal Agent, Topical; Corticosteroid, Topical

Synonyms Clotrimazole and Betamethasone

Use Topical treatment of various dermal fungal infections (including tinea pedis, cruris, and corpora in patients ≥17 years of age)

Local Anesthetic/Vasoconstrictor Precautions No information available to require special precautions

Effects on Dental Treatment Paresthesia (2%)

Dosage

Children <17 years: Do not use

Children ≥17 years and Adults:

- Tinea corporis, tinea cruris: Topical: Massage into affected area twice daily, morning and evening; do not use for longer than 2 weeks; re-evaluate after 1 week if no clinical improvement; do not exceed 45 g cream/week or 45 mL lotion/week
- Tinea pedis: Topical: Massage into affected area twice daily, morning and evening; do not use for longer than 4 weeks; re-evaluate after 2 weeks if no clinical improvement; do not exceed 45 g cream/week or 45 mL lotion/week

Elderly: Use with caution; skin atrophy and skin ulceration (rare) have been reported in patients with thinning skin; do not use for diaper dermatitis or under occlusive dressings

Mechanism of Action Betamethasone dipropionate is a corticosteroid. Clotrimazole is an antifungal agent.

Other Adverse Effects

1% to 10%:

- Dermatologic: Dry skin (2%)
- Local: Burning (2%)

<1%: Cushing's syndrome, edema, glycosuria, HPA axis suppression (higher in children), **hyperglycemia**, rash, secondary infection, stinging, growth suppression (in children), intracranial hypertension (in children), striae (in children)

Postmarketing/case reports: Skin atrophy, skin ulceration (rare)

Pregnancy Risk Factor C

Generic Available Yes: Cream

Betamethasone Dipropionate *see* Betamethasone *on page 177*
Betamethasone Dipropionate, Augmented *see* Betamethasone *on page 177*
Betamethasone Sodium Phosphate *see* Betamethasone *on page 177*

Betamethasone Valerate *see* Betamethasone *on page 177*

Betapace® *see* Sotalol *on page 1235*

Betapace AF® *see* Sotalol *on page 1235*

Betasept® [OTC] *see* Chlorhexidine Gluconate *on page 300*

Betaseron® *see* Interferon Beta-1b *on page 733*

Betatrex® *see* Betamethasone *on page 177*

Beta-Val® *see* Betamethasone *on page 177*

Betaxolol (be TAKS oh lol)

Related Information

Cardiovascular Diseases *on page 1456*

U.S. Brand Names Betoptic® S; Kerlone®

Canadian Brand Names Betoptic® S

Pharmacologic Category Beta Blocker, $Beta_1$ Selective

Synonyms Betaxolol Hydrochloride

Use Treatment of chronic open-angle glaucoma and ocular hypertension; management of hypertension

Local Anesthetic/Vasoconstrictor Precautions No information available to require special precautions

Effects on Dental Treatment Betaxolol is a cardioselective beta-blocker. Local anesthetic with vasoconstrictor can be safely used in patients medicated with betaxolol. Nonselective beta-blockers (ie, propranolol, nadolol) enhance the pressor response to epinephrine, resulting in hypertension and bradycardia; this has not been reported for betaxolol. Many nonsteroidal anti-inflammatory drugs such as ibuprofen and indomethacin can reduce the hypotensive effect of beta-blockers after 3 or more weeks of therapy with the NSAID. Short-term NSAID use (ie, 3 days) requires no special precautions in patients taking beta-blockers.

Systemic:

>10%: Drowsiness

1% to 10%: Bradycardia, palpitations, CHF, nausea, vomiting, bronchospasm

Dosage

Oral:

Adults: 10 mg/day; may increase dose to 20 mg/day after 7-14 days if desired response is not achieved

Elderly: Initial: 5 mg/day

Dosing adjustment in renal impairment: Administer 5 mg/day; may increase every 2 weeks up to a maximum of 20 mg/day

Cl_{cr} <10 mL/minute: Administer 50% of usual dose.

Ophthalmic: Instill 1 drop twice daily.

Mechanism of Action Competitively blocks $beta_1$-receptors, with little or no effect on $beta_2$-receptors; ophthalmic reduces intraocular pressure by reducing the production of aqueous humor

Other Adverse Effects

Ophthalmic: Ocular:

>10%: Conjunctival hyperemia

1% to 10%: Anisocoria, corneal punctate keratitis, keratitis, corneal staining, decreased corneal sensitivity, eye pain, vision disturbances

Systemic:

>10%:

Central nervous system: Insomnia

Endocrine & metabolic: Decreased sexual ability

1% to 10%:

Cardiovascular: Reduced peripheral, edema circulation

Central nervous system: Mental depression

Gastrointestinal: Diarrhea, constipation, stomach discomfort

Miscellaneous: Cold extremities

<1% (Limited to important or life-threatening): **Chest pain, thrombocytopenia**

Drug Interactions Substrate of **CYP1A2, 2D6**; Inhibits CYP2D6

Increased Effect/Toxicity: The heart rate lowering effects of betaxolol are additive with other drugs which slow AV conduction (digoxin, verapamil, diltiazem). Reserpine increases the effects of betaxolol. Concurrent use of betaxolol may increase the effects of alpha-blockers (prazosin, terazosin), alpha-adrenergic stimulants (epinephrine, phenylephrine), and the vasoconstrictive effects of ergot alkaloids. Betaxolol may mask the tachycardia from hypoglycemia caused by insulin and oral hypoglycemics. In patients receiving concurrent therapy, the risk of hypertensive crisis is increased when either clonidine or the beta-blocker is withdrawn. Beta-blockers may increase the action or levels of ethanol, disopyramide, nondepolarizing muscle relaxants, and theophylline although the effects are difficult to predict.

Decreased Effect: Decreased effect of betaxolol with aluminum salts, barbiturates, calcium salts, cholestyramine, colestipol, NSAIDs, penicillins (ampicillin), rifampin, salicylates, and sulfinpyrazone due to decreased bioavailability and plasma levels. Beta-blockers may decrease the effect of sulfonylureas.

Dietary/Ethanol/Herb Considerations

Ethanol: Avoid use; may increase risk of hypotension or dizziness.

Food: Avoid caffeine (eg, colas, chocolate), garlic, and licorice.

Herb/Nutraceutical: Avoid black cohosh, dong quai, and evening primrose due to estrogenic activity. Avoid ephedra, yohimbe, and ginseng; may worsen hypertension. Avoid garlic; may have increased antihypertensive effect. Avoid ginger due to positive inotropic effects; theoretically, may cause arrhythmia. Avoid hawthorn; may lower peripheral vascular resistance causing additional decrease in BP. Avoid licorice.

Pharmacodynamics/Kinetics

Onset of action: Ophthalmic: 30 minutes; Oral: 1-1.5 hours

Duration: Ophthalmic: ≥12 hours

Absorption: Ophthalmic: Some systemic; Oral: ~100%

Metabolism: Hepatic to multiple metabolites

Protein binding: Oral: 50%

Bioavailability: Oral: 89%

Half-life elimination: Oral: 12-22 hours

Time to peak: Ophthalmic: ~2 hours; Oral: 1.5-6 hours

Excretion: Urine

Pregnancy Risk Factor C (manufacturer); D (2nd and 3rd trimesters - expert analysis)

Generic Available Yes: Solution

Selected Readings

Foster CA and Aston SJ, "Propranolol-Epinephrine Interaction: A Potential Disaster," *Plast Reconstr Surg*, 1983, 72(1):74-8.

Wong DG, Spence JD, Lamki L, et al, "Effect of Nonsteroidal Anti-inflammatory Drugs on Control of Hypertension of Beta-Blockers and Diuretics," *Lancet*, 1986, 1(8488):997-1001.

Wynn RL, "Dental Nonsteroidal Anti-inflammatory Drugs and Prostaglandin-Based Drug Interactions, Part Two," *Gen Dent*, 1992, 40(2):104, 106, 108.

Wynn RL, "Epinephrine Interactions With Beta-Blockers," *Gen Dent*, 1994, 42(1):16, 18.

Betaxolol Hydrochloride *see* Betaxolol *on page 180*

Betaxon® *see* Levobetaxolol *on page 788*

Bethanechol (be THAN e kole)

U.S. Brand Names Urecholine®

Canadian Brand Names Duvoid®; Myotonachol®; PMS-Bethanechol

Pharmacologic Category Cholinergic Agonist

Synonyms Bethanechol Chloride

Use Nonobstructive urinary retention and retention due to neurogenic bladder

Unlabeled/Investigational Use Treatment and prevention of bladder dysfunction caused by phenothiazines; diagnosis of flaccid or atonic neurogenic bladder; gastroesophageal reflux

Local Anesthetic/Vasoconstrictor Precautions No information available to require special precautions

Effects on Dental Treatment This is a cholinergic agent similar to pilocarpine; expect to see salivation and sweating in patients.

Frequency not defined: Hypotension, tachycardia, flushing, headache, nausea, vomiting, eructation, asthmatic attacks, bronchial constriction, headache, malaise

Dosage Oral:

Children:

Urinary retention (unlabeled use): 0.6 mg/kg/day divided 3-4 times/day

Gastroesophageal reflux (unlabeled use): 0.1-0.2 mg/kg/dose given 30 minutes to 1 hour before each meal to a maximum of 4 times/day

Adults:

Urinary retention, neurogenic bladder, and/or bladder atony:

Oral: Initial: 10-50 mg 2-4 times/day (some patients may require dosages of 50-100 mg 4 times/day). To determine effective dose, may initiate at a dose of 5-10 mg, with additional doses of 5-10 mg hourly until an effective cumulative dose is reached. Cholinergic effects at higher oral dosages may be cumulative.

S.C.: Initial: 2.575 mg, may repeat in 15-30 minutes (maximum cumulative initial dose: 10.3 mg); subsequent doses may be given 3-4 times daily as needed (some patients may require more frequent dosing at 2.5- to 3-hour intervals). Chronic neurogenic atony may require doses of 7.5-10 every 4 hours.

Gastroesophageal reflux (unlabeled): Oral: 25 mg 4 times/day

Elderly: Use the lowest effective dose

Mechanism of Action Stimulates cholinergic receptors in the smooth muscle of the urinary bladder and gastrointestinal tract resulting in increased peristalsis, increased GI and pancreatic secretions, bladder muscle contraction, and increased ureteral peristaltic waves

Other Adverse Effects Frequency not defined:

Gastrointestinal: Abdominal cramps, diarrhea

Genitourinary: Urinary urgency

Ocular: Lacrimation, miosis

(Continued)

Bethanechol *(Continued)*

Drug Interactions

Increased Effect/Toxicity: Bethanechol and ganglionic blockers may cause a critical fall in blood pressure. Cholinergic drugs or anticholinesterase agents may have additive effects with bethanechol.

Decreased Effect: Procainamide, quinidine may decrease the effects of bethanechol. Anticholinergic agents (atropine, antihistamines, TCAs, phenothiazines) may decrease effects.

Pharmacodynamics/Kinetics

Onset of action: 30-90 minutes

Duration: Up to 6 hours

Absorption: Variable

Pregnancy Risk Factor C

Generic Available No

Bethanechol Chloride *see* Bethanechol *on page 181*

Betimol® *see* Timolol *on page 1309*

Betoptic® S *see* Betaxolol *on page 180*

Bexarotene (beks AIR oh teen)

U.S. Brand Names Targretin®

Canadian Brand Names Targretin®

Pharmacologic Category Antineoplastic Agent, Miscellaneous

Use

Oral: Treatment of cutaneous manifestations of cutaneous T-cell lymphoma in patients who are refractory to at least one prior systemic therapy

Topical: Treatment of cutaneous lesions in patients with cutaneous T-cell lymphoma (stage 1A and 1B) who have refractory or persistent disease after other therapies or who have not tolerated other therapies

Local Anesthetic/Vasoconstrictor Precautions No information available to require special precautions

Effects on Dental Treatment

>10%: Headache (14% to 42%), weakness (6% to 45%), infection (13% to 23%), fever (5% to 17%), vomiting (4% to 13%), infection (18%), flu-like syndrome (4% to 13%), bacterial infection (1% to 13%), nausea (8% to 16%)

<10%: Xerostomia, gingivitis, hemorrhage, hypertension, angina pectoris, right heart failure, tachycardia, subdural hematoma, syncope, agitation, confusion, dizziness, paresthesia (6%), cough (6%), pharyngitis (6%), diaphoresis (6%), coagulation time increased, pharyngitis, rhinitis, dyspnea, bronchitis, cough, hemoptysis, otitis externa

Dosage

Adults: Oral: 300 mg/m²/day taken as a single daily dose. If there is no tumor response after 8 weeks and the initial dose was well tolerated, then an increase to 400 mg/m²/day can be made with careful monitoring. Maintain as long as the patient is deriving benefit.

If the initial dose is not tolerated, then it may be adjusted to 200 mg/m²/day, then to 100 mg/m²/day or temporarily suspended if necessary to manage toxicity

Dosing adjustment in renal impairment: No studies have been conducted; however, renal insufficiency may result in significant protein binding changes and alter pharmacokinetics of bexarotene

Dosing adjustment in hepatic impairment: No studies have been conducted; however, hepatic impairment would be expected to result in decreased clearance of bexarotene due to the extensive hepatic contribution to elimination

Gel, topical: Apply once every other day for first week, then increase on a weekly basis to once daily, 2 times/day, 3 times/day, and finally 4 times/day, according to tolerance

Mechanism of Action The exact mechanism is unknown. Binds and activates retinoid X receptor subtypes. Once activated, these receptors function as transcription factors that regulate the expression of genes which control cellular differentiation and proliferation. Bexarotene inhibits the growth *in vitro* of some tumor cell lines of hematopoietic and squamous cell origin.

Other Adverse Effects First percentage is at a dose of 300 mg/m²/day; the second percentage is at a dose >300 mg/m²/day. Grade 3 and grade 4 events that occurred more frequently in patients at both doses were hyperlipidemia, hypertriglyceridemia, pruritus, headache, peripheral edema, leukopenia, rash, and hypercholesterolemia. Frequency of events was dose-related.

>10%:

Cardiovascular: Peripheral edema (11% to 13%)

Central nervous system: Chills (10% to 13%), insomnia (5% to 11%)

Dermatologic: Rash (17% to 23%), exfoliative dermatitis (10% to 28%), alopecia (4% to 11%),

Endocrine & metabolic: Hyperlipidemia (~79% in both dosing ranges), hypercholesteremia (32% to 62%), hypothyroidism (29% to 53%)

Gastrointestinal: Abdominal pain (4% to 11%), diarrhea (7% to 42%), anorexia (2% to 23%)
Hematologic: Leukopenia (17% to 47%), hypochromic anemia (4% to 13%), anemia (6% to 25%)
Hepatic: LDH increase (7% to 13%)
Neuromuscular & skeletal: Back pain (2% to 11%)

<10%:

Cardiovascular: Cerebrovascular accident
Central nervous system: Depression, ataxia, hyperesthesia
Dermatologic: Dry skin (~10% for both dosing ranges), skin ulceration, acne, skin nodule, maculopapular rash, serous drainage, vesicular bullous rash, cheilitis
Endocrine & metabolic: Hypoproteinemia, hyperglycemia, weight loss/gain, serum amylase (elevated), breast pain
Gastrointestinal: Constipation, flatulence, colitis, dyspepsia, melena, pancreatitis
Genitourinary: Albuminuria, hematuria, urinary incontinence, urinary tract infection, urinary urgency, dysuria, kidney function abnormality
Hematologic: Eosinophilia, thrombocythemia, lymphocytosis, thrombocytopenia
Hepatic: Hepatic failure
Neuromuscular & skeletal: Arthralgia, myalgia, bone pain, myasthenia, arthrosis, neuropathy
Ocular: Dry eyes, conjunctivitis, blepharitis, corneal lesion, visual field defects, keratitis
Otic: Earache
Renal: Creatinine (elevated)
Respiratory: Pleural effusion, lung edema, hypoxia

Topical:

Cardiovascular: Edema (10%)
Central nervous system: Pain (30%)
Dermatologic: Rash (14% to 72%), pruritus (6% to 40%), contact dermatitis (14%), exfoliative dermatitis (6%)
Hematologic: Leukopenia (6%), lymphadenopathy (6%)

Drug Interactions Substrate of CYP3A4

Increased Effect/Toxicity: Bexarotene plasma concentrations may be increased by azole antifungals, clarithromycin, erythromycin, fluvoxamine, nefazodone, quinine, ritonavir, gemfibrozil, or grapefruit juice.

Decreased Effect: Bexarotene plasma levels may be decreased by rifampin, phenytoin, phenobarbital, or nafcillin.

Dietary/Ethanol/Herb Considerations

Food: Administer with a fat-containing meal. Avoid grapefruit products; may increase serum concentration. Additional vitamin A supplements may lead to vitamin A toxicity (dry skin, irritation, arthralgias, myalgias, abdominal pain, hepatic changes).

Herb/Nutraceutical: Avoid dong quai; may cause photosensitization. Avoid St John's wort; may decrease serum concentration and cause photosensitization.

Pharmacodynamics/Kinetics

Absorption: Significantly improved by a fat-containing meal
Protein binding: >99%
Metabolism: Hepatic via CYP3A4 isoenzyme; four metabolites identified; further metabolized by glucuronidation
Half-life elimination: 7 hours
Time to peak: 2 hours
Excretion: Primarily feces; urine (<1% as unchanged drug and metabolites)

Pregnancy Risk Factor X

Generic Available No

Bextra® *see* Valdecoxib *on page 1368*

BG 9273 *see* Alefacept *on page 52*

Biaxin® *see* Clarithromycin *on page 337*

Biaxin® XL *see* Clarithromycin *on page 337*

Bicalutamide (bye ka LOO ta mide)

U.S. Brand Names Casodex®

Canadian Brand Names Casodex®

Mexican Brand Names Casodex®

Pharmacologic Category Antineoplastic Agent, Antiandrogen

Use In combination therapy with LHRH agonist analogues in treatment of advanced prostatic carcinoma

Local Anesthetic/Vasoconstrictor Precautions No information available to require special precautions

Effects on Dental Treatment

>10%: Hot flashes (49%)

2% to 5%: Xerostomia, angina pectoris, CHF, anxiety, confusion, somnolence, nervousness, fever, diabetes mellitus, dehydration, neck pain, cough, pharyngitis, bronchitis, pneumonia, rhinitis sepsis, pathological fracture, arthritis, leg cramps

(Continued)

Bicalutamide *(Continued)*

Dosage Oral: Adults: 1 tablet once daily (morning or evening), with or without food. It is recommended that bicalutamide be taken at the same time each day; start treatment with bicalutamide at the same time as treatment with an LHRH analog.

Dosing adjustment in liver impairment: Limited data in subjects with severe hepatic impairment suggest that excretion of bicalutamide may be delayed and could lead to further accumulation. Use with caution in patients with moderate to severe hepatic impairment.

Mechanism of Action Pure nonsteroidal antiandrogen that binds to androgen receptors; specifically a competitive inhibitor for the binding of dihydrotestosterone and testosterone; prevents testosterone stimulation of cell growth in prostate cancer

Other Adverse Effects

2% to <5%:

- Cardiovascular: Edema
- Central nervous system: Chills, depression
- Dermatologic: Dry skin, pruritus, alopecia
- Endocrine & metabolic: Breast pain, decreased libido, gout
- Gastrointestinal: Anorexia, dyspepsia, rectal hemorrhage, melena, weight gain
- Genitourinary: Polyuria, urinary impairment, dysuria, urinary retention, urinary urgency
- Hepatic: Alkaline phosphatase increased
- Neuromuscular & skeletal: Myasthenia, myalgia, hypertonia, neuropathy
- Renal: Creatinine increased
- Respiratory: Lung disorder
- Miscellaneous: Neoplasma

<1%: Diarrhea

Drug Interactions Increased Effect/Toxicity: Bicalutamide may displace warfarin from protein binding sites which may result in an increased anticoagulant effect, especially when bicalutamide therapy is started after the patient is already on warfarin.

Pharmacodynamics/Kinetics

- Absorption: Rapid and complete
- Protein binding: 96%
- Metabolism: Extensively hepatic; stereospecific metabolism
- Half-life elimination: Up to 10 days; active enantiomer 5.8 days
- Excretion: Urine and feces (as unchanged drug and metabolites)

Pregnancy Risk Factor X

Generic Available No

Bicillin® C-R *see* Penicillin G Benzathine and Penicillin G Procaine *on page 1048*

Bicillin® C-R 900/300 *see* Penicillin G Benzathine and Penicillin G Procaine *on page 1048*

Bicillin® L-A *see* Penicillin G Benzathine *on page 1047*

Bicitra® *see* Sodium Citrate and Citric Acid *on page 1230*

BiCNU® *see* Carmustine *on page 253*

Biltricide® *see* Praziquantel *on page 1108*

Bimatoprost (bi MAT oh prost)

U.S. Brand Names Lumigan™

Canadian Brand Names Lumigan™

Pharmacologic Category Ophthalmic Agent, Miscellaneous

Use Reduction of intraocular pressure (IOP) in patients with open-angle glaucoma or ocular hypertension; should be used in patients who are intolerant of other IOP-lowering medications or failed treatment with another IOP-lowering medication

Local Anesthetic/Vasoconstrictor Precautions No information available to require special precautions

Effects on Dental Treatment 1% to 10%: Headache (1% to 5%), upper respiratory tract infection (10%), visual disturbance (3% to 10%)

Dosage Ophthalmic: Adult: Open-angle glaucoma or ocular hypertension: Instill 1 drop into affected eye(s) once daily in the evening; do not exceed once-daily dosing (may decrease IOP-lowering effect). If used with other topical ophthalmic agents, separate administration by at least 5 minutes.

Mechanism of Action As a synthetic analog of prostaglandin with ocular hypotensive activity, bimatoprost decreases intraocular pressure by increasing the outflow of aqueous humor.

Other Adverse Effects

>10%: Ocular (15% to 45%): Conjunctival hyperemia, increased eyelash growth, ocular pruritus

1% to 10%:

- Dermatologic: Hirsutism (1% to 5%)
- Hepatic: Abnormal LFTs (1% to 5%)
- Neuromuscular & skeletal: Weakness (1% to 5%)

Ocular:

3% to 10%: Blepharitis, burning, cataract, dryness, eyelid redness, eyelash darkening, foreign body sensation, irritation, pain, pigmentation of periocular skin, superficial punctate keratitis

1% to 3%: Allergic conjunctivitis, asthenopia, conjunctival edema, discharge, increased iris pigmentation, photophobia, tearing

<1%: Iritis

Postmarketing and/or case reports: Bacterial keratitis (caused by inadvertent contamination of multiple-dose ophthalmic solutions), macular edema

Pharmacodynamics/Kinetics

Onset of action: Reduction of IOP: ~4 hours

Peak effect: Maximum reduction of IOP: ~8-12 hours

Distribution: 0.67 L/kg

Protein binding: ~88%

Metabolism: Undergoes oxidation, N-demethylation, and glucuronidation after reaching systemic circulation; forms metabolites

Half-life elimination: I.V.: 45 minutes

Time to peak: 10 minutes

Excretion: Urine (67%); feces (25%)

Pregnancy Risk Factor C

Generic Available No

Biocef *see* Cephalexin *on page 285*

Biofed [OTC] *see* Pseudoephedrine *on page 1146*

Biolon™ *see* Sodium Hyaluronate *on page 1230*

Bion® Tears [OTC] *see* Artificial Tears *on page 128*

Bio-Statin® *see* Nystatin *on page 992*

BioThrax™ *see* Anthrax Vaccine (Adsorbed) *on page 112*

Biperiden (bye PER i den)

U.S. Brand Names Akineton®

Canadian Brand Names Akineton®

Mexican Brand Names Akineton®

Pharmacologic Category Anticholinergic Agent; Anti-Parkinson's Agent, Anticholinergic

Synonyms Biperiden Hydrochloride; Biperiden Lactate

Use Adjunct in the therapy of all forms of Parkinsonism; control of extrapyramidal symptoms secondary to antipsychotics

Local Anesthetic/Vasoconstrictor Precautions No information available to require special precautions

Effects on Dental Treatment Frequency not defined: xerostomia, nasal dryness, and dry throat (very prevalent); orthostatic hypotension, bradycardia, drowsiness, euphoria, disorientation, agitation, blurred vision

Dosage Oral: Adults:

Parkinsonism: 2 mg 3-4 times/day

Extrapyramidal: 2 mg 1-3 times/day

Mechanism of Action Biperiden is a weak peripheral anticholinergic agent with nicotinolytic activity. The beneficial effects in Parkinson's disease and neuroleptic-induced extrapyramidal symptoms are believed to be due to the inhibition of striatal cholinergic receptors.

Other Adverse Effects Frequency not defined:

Central nervous system: Sleep disorder (decreased REM sleep and increased REM latency)

Gastrointestinal: Constipation

Genitourinary: Urinary retention

Neuromuscular & skeletal: Choreic movements

Drug Interactions Inhibits CYP2D6

Increased Effect/Toxicity: Central and/or peripheral anticholinergic syndrome can occur when administered with amantadine (or rimantadine), narcotic analgesics, phenothiazines and other antipsychotics (especially with high anticholinergic activity), tricyclic antidepressants, quinidine and some other antiarrhythmics, and antihistamines. Anticholinergics may increase the bioavailability of atenolol (and possibly other beta-blockers). Anticholinergics may decrease gastric degradation and increase the amount of digoxin or levodopa absorbed by delaying gastric emptying.

Decreased Effect: Anticholinergics may antagonize the therapeutic effect of neuroleptics and cholinergic agents (includes tacrine and donepezil).

Dietary/Ethanol/Herb Considerations

Ethanol: Avoid use; may increase sedation.

Herb/Nutraceutical: Avoid gotu kola, kava, SAMe, St John's wort, and valerian; may increase CNS depression.

Pharmacodynamics/Kinetics

Bioavailability: 29%

Half-life elimination, serum: 18.4-24.3 hours

Time to peak, serum: 1-1.5 hours

(Continued)

Biperiden *(Continued)*

Pregnancy Risk Factor C

Generic Available No

Biperiden Hydrochloride *see* Biperiden *on page 185*

Biperiden Lactate *see* Biperiden *on page 185*

Bisac-Evac™ [OTC] *see* Bisacodyl *on page 186*

Bisacodyl (bis a KOE dil)

U.S. Brand Names Alophen® [OTC]; Bisac-Evac™ [OTC]; Bisacodyl Uniserts® [OTC]; Dulcolax® [OTC]; Feen-A-Mint® [OTC]; Femilax™ [OTC]; Fleet® Bisacodyl Enema [OTC]; Fleet® Stimulant Laxative [OTC]; Modane Tablets® [OTC]

Canadian Brand Names Apo®-Bisacodyl; Dulcolax®

Mexican Brand Names Dulcolan®

Pharmacologic Category Laxative, Stimulant

Use Treatment of constipation; colonic evacuation prior to procedures or examination

Local Anesthetic/Vasoconstrictor Precautions No information available to require special precautions

Effects on Dental Treatment No significant effects or complications reported

Dosage

Children:

- Oral: >6 years: 5-10 mg (0.3 mg/kg) at bedtime or before breakfast
- Rectal suppository:
  - <2 years: 5 mg as a single dose
  - >2 years: 10 mg

Adults:

- Oral: 5-15 mg as single dose (up to 30 mg when complete evacuation of bowel is required)
- Rectal suppository: 10 mg as single dose

Mechanism of Action Stimulates peristalsis by directly irritating the smooth muscle of the intestine, possibly the colonic intramural plexus; alters water and electrolyte secretion producing net intestinal fluid accumulation and laxation

Other Adverse Effects <1%: Vertigo, electrolyte and fluid imbalance (metabolic acidosis or alkalosis, hypocalcemia), mild abdominal cramps, **nausea, vomiting**, rectal burning

Drug Interactions Decreased Effect: Milk or antacids may decrease the effect of bisacodyl. Bisacodyl may decrease the effect of warfarin.

Dietary/Ethanol/Herb Considerations Food: Dairy products may disrupt enteric coating, increasing stomach irritation.

Pharmacodynamics/Kinetics

Onset of action: Oral: 6-10 hours; Rectal: 0.25-1 hour

Absorption: Oral, rectal: Systemic, <5%

Pregnancy Risk Factor C

Generic Available Yes

Bisacodyl Uniserts® [OTC] *see* Bisacodyl *on page 186*

Bishydroxycoumarin *see* Dicumarol *on page 433*

Bismatrol *see* Bismuth *on page 186*

Bismuth (BIZ muth)

Related Information

Gastrointestinal Disorders *on page 1474*

U.S. Brand Names Children's Kaopectate® (reformulation) [OTC]; Colo-Fresh™ [OTC]; Devrom®; Diotame® [OTC]; Kaopectate® [OTC]; Kaopectate® Extra Strength [OTC]; Pepto-Bismol® [OTC]; Pepto-Bismol® Maximum Strength [OTC]

Pharmacologic Category Antidiarrheal

Synonyms Bismatrol; Bismuth Subgallate; Bismuth Subsalicylate; Pink Bismuth

Use Symptomatic treatment of mild, nonspecific diarrhea; indigestion, nausea, control of traveler's diarrhea (enterotoxigenic *Escherichia coli*); as part of a multi-drug regimen for *H. pylori* eradication to reduce the risk of duodenal ulcer recurrence; subgallate formulation to control fecal odors in colostomy, ileostomy, or fecal incontinence

Local Anesthetic/Vasoconstrictor Precautions No information available to require special precautions

Effects on Dental Treatment <10%: Darkening of tongue

Dosage Oral:

Nonspecific diarrhea: Subsalicylate (doses based on 262 mg/5 mL liquid or 262 mg tablets):

Children: Up to 8 doses/24 hours:

- 3-6 years: 1/3 tablet or 5 mL (regular strength) every 30 minutes to 1 hour as needed
- 6-9 years: 2/3 tablet or 10 mL (regular strength) every 30 minutes to 1 hour as needed

9-12 years: 1 tablet or 15 mL (regular strength) every 30 minutes to 1 hour as needed

Adults: 2 tablets or 30 mL every 30 minutes to 1 hour as needed up to 8 doses/24 hours

Prevention of traveler's diarrhea: 2.1 g/day or 2 tablets 4 times/day before meals and at bedtime

Helicobacter pylori eradication: 524 mg 4 times/day with meals and at bedtime; requires combination therapy

Control of fecal odor in ileostomy or colostomy: Subgallate: 1-2 tablets 3 times/day with meals (maximum: 5 tablets/day)

Dosing adjustment in renal impairment: Should probably be avoided in patients with renal failure

Mechanism of Action Bismuth subsalicylate exhibits both antisecretory and antimicrobial action. This agent may provide some anti-inflammatory action as well. The salicylate moiety provides antisecretory effect and the bismuth exhibits antimicrobial directly against bacterial and viral gastrointestinal pathogens. Bismuth has some antacid properties.

Other Adverse Effects

>10%: Gastrointestinal: Grayish black stools

<1%: **Anxiety, confusion, headache**, hearing loss, impaction (in infants and debilitated patients), mental depression, **muscle spasms**, **slurred speech**, tinnitus, **weakness**

Drug Interactions

Increased Effect/Toxicity: Toxicity of aspirin, warfarin, and/or hypoglycemics may be increased.

Decreased Effect: The effects of tetracyclines and uricosurics may be decreased.

Pharmacodynamics/Kinetics

Absorption: Minimal (<1%) across GI tract, salt (eg, salicylate) may be readily absorbed (80%); bismuth subsalicylate is rapidly cleaved to bismuth and salicylic acid in the stomach

Distribution: Salicylate: V_d: 170 mL/kg

Protein binding, plasma: Bismuth and salicylate: >90%

Metabolism: Bismuth: Oral: Salts undergo chemical dissociation; Salicylate: Extensively hepatic

Half-life elimination: Terminal: Bismuth: 21-72 days; Salicylate: 2-5 hours

Excretion: Bismuth: Urine and feces; Salicylate: 10% (as unchanged drug)

Clearance: Bismuth: 50 mL/minute

Pregnancy Risk Factor C/D (3rd trimester)

Generic Available Yes

Bismuth, Metronidazole, and Tetracycline

(BIZ muth, me troe NI da zole, & tet ra SYE kleen)

Related Information

Bismuth *on page 186*

Metronidazole *on page 902*

Tetracycline *on page 1286*

U.S. Brand Names Helidac®

Pharmacologic Category Antibiotic, Tetracycline Derivative; Antidiarrheal

Synonyms Bismuth Subsalicylate, Tetracycline, and Metronidazole; Metronidazole, Bismuth Subsalicylate, and Tetracycline; Metronidazole, Tetracycline, and Bismuth Subsalicylate; Tetracycline, Bismuth Subsalicylate, and Metronidazole; Tetracycline, Metronidazole, and Bismuth Subsalicylate

Use In combination with an H_2 antagonist, as part of a multidrug regimen for *H. pylori* eradication to reduce the risk of duodenal ulcer recurrence

Local Anesthetic/Vasoconstrictor Precautions No information available to require special precautions

Effects on Dental Treatment Tetracyclines are not recommended for use during pregnancy since they can cause enamel hypoplasia and permanent teeth discoloration; long-term use associated with oral candidiasis.

Dosage Adults: Chew 2 bismuth subsalicylate 262.4 mg tablets, swallow 1 metronidazole 250 mg tablet, and swallow 1 tetracycline 500 mg capsule 4 times/day at meals and bedtime, plus an H_2 antagonist (at the appropriate dose) for 14 days; follow with 8 oz of water; the H_2 antagonist should be continued for a total of 28 days

Mechanism of Action Bismuth subsalicylate, metronidazole, and tetracycline individually have demonstrated *in vitro* activity against most susceptible strains of *H. pylori* isolated from patients with duodenal ulcers. Resistance to metronidazole is increasing in the U.S.; an alternative regimen, not containing metronidazole, if *H. pylori* is not eradicated follow therapy.

Other Adverse Effects >1%: **Dizziness, nausea**, diarrhea, abdominal pain, **vomiting**, anal discomfort, anorexia, **paresthesia**

Pregnancy Risk Factor D (tetracycline); B (metronidazole)

Generic Available No

Bismuth Subgallate *see* Bismuth *on page 186*

Bismuth Subsalicylate *see* Bismuth *on page 186*

Bismuth Subsalicylate, Tetracycline, and Metronidazole *see* Bismuth, Metronidazole, and Tetracycline *on page 187*

Bisoprolol (bis OH proe lol)

Related Information

Cardiovascular Diseases *on page 1456*

U.S. Brand Names Zebeta®

Canadian Brand Names Monocor®; Zebeta®

Pharmacologic Category Beta Blocker, $Beta_1$ Selective

Synonyms Bisoprolol Fumarate

Use Treatment of hypertension, alone or in combination with other agents

Unlabeled/Investigational Use Treatment of angina pectoris, supraventricular arrhythmias, PVCs

Local Anesthetic/Vasoconstrictor Precautions No information available to require special precautions

Effects on Dental Treatment Bisoprolol is a cardioselective beta-blocker. Local anesthetic with vasoconstrictor can be safely used in patients medicated with bisoprolol. Nonselective beta-blockers (ie, propranolol, nadolol) enhance the pressor response to epinephrine, resulting in hypertension and bradycardia; this has not been reported for bisoprolol. Many nonsteroidal anti-inflammatory drugs such as ibuprofen and indomethacin can reduce the hypotensive effect of beta-blockers after 3 or more weeks of therapy with the NSAID. Short-term NSAID use (ie, 3 days) requires no special precautions in patients taking beta-blockers.

>10%: Drowsiness

1% to 10%: Bradycardia, palpitations, CHF, nausea, vomiting, bronchospasm

Dosage Oral:

Adults: 5 mg once daily, may be increased to 10 mg, and then up to 20 mg once daily, if necessary

Elderly: Initial dose: 2.5 mg/day; may be increased by 2.5-5 mg/day; maximum recommended dose: 20 mg/day

Dosing adjustment in renal/hepatic impairment: Cl_{cr} <40 mL/minute: Initial: 2.5 mg/day; increase cautiously.

Hemodialysis: Not dialyzable

Mechanism of Action Selective inhibitor of $beta_1$-adrenergic receptors; competitively blocks $beta_1$-receptors, with little or no effect on $beta_2$-receptors at doses <10 mg

Other Adverse Effects

>10%

Central nervous system: Insomnia

Endocrine & metabolic: Decreased sexual ability

1% to 10%:

Cardiovascular: Edema, reduced peripheral circulation

Central nervous system: Mental depression

Gastrointestinal: Diarrhea, constipation, stomach discomfort

Ocular: Mild ocular stinging and discomfort, tearing, photophobia, decreased corneal sensitivity, keratitis

Miscellaneous: Cold extremities

<1% (Limited to important or life-threatening): **Chest pain, arrhythmias, orthostatic hypotension, nervousness, headache**, depression, **hallucinations, confusion (especially in the elderly), dyspnea**, psoriasiform eruption, itching, thrombocytopenia, leukopenia

Drug Interactions Substrate of CYP2D6, **3A4**

Increased Effect/Toxicity: Bisoprolol may increase the effects of other drugs which slow AV conduction (digoxin, verapamil, diltiazem), alpha-blockers (prazosin, terazosin), and alpha-adrenergic stimulants (epinephrine, phenylephrine). Bisoprolol may mask the tachycardia from hypoglycemia caused by insulin and oral hypoglycemics. In patients receiving concurrent therapy, the risk of hypertensive crisis is increased when either clonidine or the beta-blocker is withdrawn. Reserpine has been shown to enhance the effect of beta-blockers. Beta-blockers may increase the action or levels of ethanol, disopyramide, nondepolarizing muscle relaxants, and theophylline although the effects are difficult to predict.

Decreased Effect: Decreased effect of bisoprolol with aluminum salts, barbiturates, calcium salts, cholestyramine, colestipol, NSAIDs, penicillins (ampicillin), rifampin, and salicylates due to decreased bioavailability and plasma levels. The effect of sulfonylureas may be decreased by beta-blockers.

Dietary/Ethanol/Herb Considerations

Food: Avoid caffeine (eg, colas, chocolate), garlic, and licorice.

Herb/Nutraceutical: Avoid black cohosh, dong quai, and evening primrose due to estrogenic activity. Avoid ephedra, ginseng, and yohimbe; may worsen hypertension. Avoid garlic; may have increased antihypertensive effect. Avoid ginger due to positive inotropic effects; theoretically, may cause arrhythmia. Avoid hawthorn; may lower peripheral vascular resistance causing additional decrease in BP. Avoid licorice.

Pharmacodynamics/Kinetics

Onset of action: 1-2 hours
Absorption: Rapid and almost complete
Distribution: Widely; highest concentrations in heart, liver, lungs, and saliva; crosses blood-brain barrier; enters breast milk
Protein binding: 26% to 33%
Metabolism: Extensively hepatic; significant first-pass effect
Half-life elimination: 9-12 hours
Time to peak: 1.7-3 hours
Excretion: Urine (3% to 10% as unchanged drug); feces (<2%)

Pregnancy Risk Factor C (manufacturer); D (2nd and 3rd trimesters - expert analysis)

Generic Available Yes

Selected Readings

Foster CA and Aston SJ, "Propranolol-Epinephrine Interaction: A Potential Disaster," *Plast Reconstr Surg*, 1983, 72(1):74-8.
Wong DG, Spence JD, Lamki L, et al, "Effect of Nonsteroidal Anti-inflammatory Drugs on Control of Hypertension of Beta-Blockers and Diuretics," *Lancet*, 1986, 1(8488):997-1001.
Wynn RL, "Dental Nonsteroidal Anti-inflammatory Drugs and Prostaglandin-Based Drug Interactions, Part Two," *Gen Dent*, 1992, 40(2):104, 106, 108.
Wynn RL, "Epinephrine Interactions With Beta-Blockers," *Gen Dent*, 1994, 42(1):16, 18.

Bisoprolol and Hydrochlorothiazide

(bis OH proe lol & hye droe klor oh THYE a zide)

Related Information

Bisoprolol *on page 188*
Hydrochlorothiazide *on page 675*

U.S. Brand Names Ziac®

Canadian Brand Names Ziac™

Pharmacologic Category Antihypertensive Agent Combination

Synonyms Hydrochlorothiazide and Bisoprolol

Use Treatment of hypertension

Local Anesthetic/Vasoconstrictor Precautions No information available to require special precautions

Effects on Dental Treatment Noncardioselective beta-blockers (ie, propranolol, nadolol) enhance the pressor response to epinephrine, resulting in hypertension and bradycardia. This has not been reported for bisoprolol, a cardioselective beta-blocker. Therefore local anesthetic with vasoconstrictor can be safely used in patients medicated with bisoprolol. Many nonsteroidal anti-inflammatory drugs such as ibuprofen and indomethacin can reduce the hypotensive effect of beta-blockers after 3 or more weeks of therapy with the NSAID. Short-term NSAID use (ie, 3 days) requires no special precautions in patients taking beta-blockers.

>10%: Fatigue
1% to 10%: Chest pain, bradycardia, hypotension, headache, dizziness, hyperglycemia, nausea, rhinitis, cough, dyspnea, abnormal vision

Dosage Oral: Adults: Dose is individualized, given once daily

Other Adverse Effects

1% to 10%:
- Cardiovascular: Edema
- Central nervous system: Depression, abnormal dreams
- Dermatologic: Rash, photosensitivity
- Endocrine & metabolic: Hypokalemia, fluid and electrolyte imbalances (hypocalcemia, hypomagnesemia, hyponatremia), hyperglycemia
- Gastrointestinal: Constipation, diarrhea, dyspepsia, insomnia, flatulence
- Genitourinary: Micturition (frequency)
- Hematologic: Rarely blood dyscrasias
- Neuromuscular & skeletal: Arthralgia, myalgia
- Renal: Prerenal azotemia

<1%: Hypercalcemia, pancreatitis

Pregnancy Risk Factor C/D (2nd and 3rd trimesters)

Generic Available Yes

Bisoprolol Fumarate *see* Bisoprolol *on page 188*
Bistropamide *see* Tropicamide *on page 1360*

Bitolterol

(bye TOLE ter ole)

Related Information

Respiratory Diseases *on page 1476*

Canadian Brand Names Tornalate®

Pharmacologic Category $Beta_2$ Agonist

Synonyms Bitolterol Mesylate; Tornalate® [DSC]

Use Prevention and treatment of bronchial asthma and bronchospasm

Local Anesthetic/Vasoconstrictor Precautions No information available to require special precautions

Effects on Dental Treatment

>10%: Tremors (14%)
(Continued)

Bitolterol *(Continued)*

1% to 10%: Palpitations (3%), chest tightness (1%), nervousness (5%), headache (4%), dizziness (3%), lightheadedness (3%), nausea (3%), bronchial irritation (5%), coughing (4%), xerostomia, unpleasant taste

Dosage Children >12 years and Adults:

Bronchospasm: 2 inhalations at an interval of at least 1-3 minutes, followed by a third inhalation if needed

Prevention of bronchospasm: 2 inhalations every 8 hours; do not exceed 3 inhalations every 6 hours or 2 inhalations every 4 hours

Mechanism of Action Selectively stimulates $beta_2$-adrenergic receptors in the lungs producing bronchial smooth muscle relaxation; minor $beta_1$ activity

Other Adverse Effects <1%: **Arrhythmias, tachycardia**, insomnia, **paradoxical bronchospasm**, hyperkinesia

Drug Interactions

Increased Effect/Toxicity: Increased toxicity with MAO inhibitors, tricyclic antidepressants, sympathomimetic agents (eg, amphetamine, dopamine, dobutamine), inhaled anesthetics (eg, enflurane). Increased toxicity (cardiotoxicity) with aminophylline, theophylline, or oxtriphylline.

Decreased Effect: Decreased effect with beta-adrenergic blockers (eg, propranolol).

Pharmacodynamics/Kinetics

Onset of action: Rapid
Duration: 4-8 hours
Metabolism: Inhalation: Prodrug, hydrolyzed to colterol (active)
Half-life elimination: 3 hours
Time to peak, serum (colterol): Inhalation: ~1 hour
Excretion: Urine and feces

Pregnancy Risk Factor C

Generic Available No

Bitolterol Mesylate *see* Bitolterol *on page 189*
Blenoxane® *see* Bleomycin *on page 190*
Bleo *see* Bleomycin *on page 190*

Bleomycin (blee oh MYE sin)

U.S. Brand Names Blenoxane®

Canadian Brand Names Blenoxane®

Mexican Brand Names Blanoxan®; Bleolem®

Pharmacologic Category Antineoplastic Agent, Antibiotic

Synonyms Bleo; Bleomycin Sulfate; BLM; NSC-125066

Use Treatment of squamous cell carcinomas, melanomas, sarcomas, testicular carcinoma, Hodgkin's lymphoma, and non-Hodgkin's lymphoma

Orphan drug: Sclerosing agent for malignant pleural effusion

Local Anesthetic/Vasoconstrictor Precautions No information available to require special precautions

Effects on Dental Treatment >10%: Fever, stomatitis, nausea, vomiting,

Dosage May be administered I.M., I.V., S.C., or intracavitary; Refer to individual protocols (1 unit = 1 mg)

Adults: Intracavitary injection for malignant pleural effusion: 60 international units (range of 15-120 units; dose generally does not exceed 1 unit/kg) in 50-100 mL SWI

Children and Adults:

Test dose for lymphoma patients: I.M., I.V., S.C.: Because of the possibility of an anaphylactoid reaction, ≤2 units of bleomycin for the first 2 doses; monitor vital signs every 15 minutes; wait a minimum of 1 hour before administering remainder of dose; if no acute reaction occurs, then the regular dosage schedule may be followed

Single-agent therapy:

I.M./I.V./S.C.: Squamous cell carcinoma, lymphoma, testicular carcinoma: 0.25-0.5 units/kg (10-20 units/m^2) 1-2 times/week

CIV: 15 units/m^2 over 24 hours daily for 4 days

Combination-agent therapy:

I.M./I.V.: 3-4 units/m^2

I.V.: ABVD: 10 units/m^2 on days 1 and 15

Maximum cumulative lifetime dose: 400 units

Pleural sclerosing: 60-240 units as a single infusion. Dose may be repeated at intervals of several days if fluid continues to accumulate (mix in 50-100 mL of D_5W, NS, or SWFI); may add lidocaine 100-200 mg to reduce local discomfort.

Dosing adjustment in renal impairment:

Cl_{cr} 10-50 mL/minute: Administer 75% of normal dose

Cl_{cr} <10 mL/minute: Administer 50% of normal dose

Mechanism of Action Inhibits synthesis of DNA; binds to DNA leading to single- and double-strand breaks

Other Adverse Effects

>10%:

Cardiovascular: Raynaud's phenomenon

Central nervous system: Mild febrile reaction, chills, patients may become febrile after intracavitary administration

Dermatologic: Pruritic erythema

Integument: ~50% of patients will develop erythema, induration, and hyperkeratosis and peeling of the skin; hyperpigmentation, alopecia, nailbed changes may occur; this appears to be dose-related and is reversible after cessation of therapy

Irritant chemotherapy

Gastrointestinal: Mucocutaneous toxicity, anorexia

Emetic potential: Moderately low (10% to 30%)

Local: Phlebitis, pain at tumor site

1% to 10%:

Dermatologic: Alopecia

Gastrointestinal: Weight loss

Respiratory: Toxicities (usually pneumonitis) occur in 10% of treated patients; 1% of patients progress to pulmonary fibrosis and death

Miscellaneous: Idiosyncratic: Similar to anaphylaxis and occurs in 1% of lymphoma patients; may include hypotension, confusion, fever, chills, and wheezing. May be immediate or delayed for several hours; symptomatic treatment includes volume expansion, pressor agents, antihistamines, and steroids

<1%: Myocardial infarction, cerebrovascular accident, skin thickening,scleroderma-like skin changes, hepatotoxicity, renal toxicity; respiratory effects are dose-related when total dose is >400 units or with single doses >30 units; pathogenesis is poorly understood, but may be related to damage of pulmonary, vascular, or connective tissue; manifested as an acute or chronic interstitial pneumonitis with interstitial fibrosis, hypoxia, and death; symptoms include cough, dyspnea, and bilateral pulmonary infiltrates noted on CXR; it is controversial whether steroids improve symptoms of bleomycin pulmonary toxicity; tachypnea, rales

Myelosuppressive:

WBC: Rare

Platelets: Rare

Onset: 7 days

Nadir: 14 days

Recovery: 21 days

Drug Interactions

Increased Effect/Toxicity: Lomustine increases severity of leukopenia. Cisplatin may decrease bleomycin elimination.

Decreased Effect: Bleomycin may decrease plasma levels of digoxin. Concomitant therapy with phenytoin results in decreased phenytoin levels.

Pharmacodynamics/Kinetics

Absorption: I.M. and intrapleural administration: 30% to 50% of I.V. serum concentrations; intraperitoneal and S.C. routes produce serum concentrations equal to those of I.V.

Distribution: V_d: 22 L/m^2; highest concentrations in skin, kidney, lung, heart tissues; lowest in testes and GI tract; does not cross blood-brain barrier

Protein binding: 1%

Metabolism: Via several tissues including hepatic, GI tract, skin, pulmonary, renal, and serum

Half-life elimination: Biphasic (renal function dependent):

Normal renal function: Initial: 1.3 hours; Terminal: 9 hours

End-stage renal disease: Initial: 2 hours; Terminal: 30 hours

Time to peak, serum: I.M.: Within 30 minutes

Excretion: Urine (50% to 70% as active drug)

Pregnancy Risk Factor D

Generic Available Yes

Bleomycin Sulfate *see* Bleomycin *on page 190*

Bleph®-10 *see* Sulfacetamide *on page 1249*

Blephamide® *see* Sulfacetamide and Prednisolone *on page 1250*

BLM *see* Bleomycin *on page 190*

Blocadren® *see* Timolol *on page 1309*

Bluboro® [OTC] *see* Aluminum Sulfate and Calcium Acetate *on page 70*

BMS 337039 *see* Aripiprazole *on page 122*

Bonine® [OTC] *see* Meclizine *on page 847*

Bontril PDM® *see* Phendimetrazine *on page 1064*

Bontril® Slow-Release *see* Phendimetrazine *on page 1064*

Boric Acid (BOR ik AS id)

Pharmacologic Category Pharmaceutical Aid; Topical Skin Product

Use

Otic: Prophylaxis of swimmer's ear

(Continued)

Boric Acid *(Continued)*

Topical ointment: Temporary relief of chapped, chafed, or dry skin, diaper rash, abrasions, minor burns, sunburn, insect bites, and other skin irritations

Local Anesthetic/Vasoconstrictor Precautions No information available to require special precautions

Effects on Dental Treatment No significant effects or complications reported

Dosage

Otic: Instill 3-8 drops into each ear

Topical: Apply as needed to affected area 1-2 times/day

Generic Available Yes

Comments Not a corrosive substance

Bosentan (boe SEN tan)

U.S. Brand Names Tracleer™

Canadian Brand Names Tracleer™

Pharmacologic Category Endothelin Antagonist

Use Treatment of pulmonary artery hypertension (PAH) in patients with World Health Organization (WHO) Class III or IV symptoms to improve exercise capacity and decrease the rate of clinical deterioration

Unlabeled/Investigational Use Investigational: Treatment of CHF

Local Anesthetic/Vasoconstrictor Precautions No information available to require special precautions

Effects on Dental Treatment

>10% : Headache (16% to 22%), nasopharyngitis (11%)

1% to 10%: Flushing (7% to 9%), hypotension (7%), palpitations (5%)

Restrictions Bosentan (Tracleer™) is available only through a limited distribution program directly from the manufacturer (Actelion Pharmaceuticals 1-866-228-3546). It will not be available through wholesalers or individual pharmacies.

Dosage When discontinuing treatment, consider a reduction in dosage to 62.5 mg twice daily for 3-7 days (to avoid clinical deterioration).

Oral: Adults:

Initial: 62.5 mg twice daily for 4 weeks; increase to maintenance dose of 125 mg twice daily; adults <40 kg should be maintained at 62.5 mg twice daily

Dosing adjustment in hepatic impairment: Avoid use in patients with **pretreatment** moderate to severe hepatic insufficiency.

Modification based on transaminase elevation:

If any elevation, regardless of degree, is accompanied by clinical symptoms of hepatic injury (unusual fatigue, nausea, vomiting, abdominal pain, fever, or jaundice) or a serum bilirubin ≥2 times the upper limit of normal, treatment should be stopped.

AST/ALT >3 times but ≤5 times upper limit of normal: Confirm with additional test; if confirmed, reduce dose or interrupt treatment. Monitor transaminase levels at least every 2 weeks. May continue or reintroduce treatment, as appropriate, following return to pretreatment values. Begin with initial dose (above) and recheck transaminases within 3 days

AST/ALT >5 times but ≤8 times upper limit of normal: Confirm with additional test; if confirmed, stop treatment. Monitor transaminase levels at least every 2 weeks. May reintroduce treatment, as appropriate, following return to pretreatment values.

AST/ALT >8 times upper limit of normal: Stop treatment

Mechanism of Action Blocks endothelin receptors on vascular endothelium and smooth muscle. Stimulation of these receptors is associated with vasoconstriction. Although bosentan blocks both ET_A and ET_B receptors, the affinity is higher for the A subtype. Improvement in symptoms of pulmonary artery hypertension and a decrease in the rate of clinical deterioration have been demonstrated in clinical trials.

Other Adverse Effects

>10% :

Gastrointestinal: Dyspepsia (4%)

Hematologic: Decreased hemoglobin (≥1 g/dL in up to 57%; typically in first 6 weeks of therapy)

Hepatic: Increased serum transaminases (>3 times upper limit of normal; up to 11%)

1% to 10%:

Cardiovascular: Edema (lower limb, 8%; generalized 4%)

Central nervous system: Fatigue (4%)

Dermatologic: Pruritus (4%)

Hematologic: Anemia (3%)

Hepatic: Abnormal hepatic function (6% to 8%)

Drug Interactions Substrate of **CYP2C8/9, 3A4**; Induces CYP2C8/9, 3A4

Increased Effect/Toxicity:

An increased risk of serum transaminase elevations was observed during concurrent therapy with glyburide; concurrent use is contraindicated. Cyclosporine increases serum concentrations of bosentan (approximately 3-4 times baseline). Concurrent use of cyclosporine is contraindicated. Ketoconazole may increase the serum concentrations of bosentan; concentrations are increased approximately two-fold; monitor for increased effects.

Many interactions have not been specifically evaluated, but may be extrapolated from similar interactions with inducers/inhibitors of CYP3A4 and CYP2C8/9 isoenzymes. Inhibitors of CYP2C9 or CYP3A4 may increase the serum concentrations of bosentan; inhibitors include amiodarone, cimetidine, clarithromycin, erythromycin, delavirdine, diltiazem, dirithromycin, disulfiram, fluoxetine, fluvoxamine, grapefruit juice, indinavir, itraconazole, ketoconazole, nefazodone, nevirapine, propoxyphene, quinupristin-dalfopristin, ritonavir, saquinavir, sulfonamides, verapamil, zafirlukast, zileuton

Decreased Effect: Bosentan may enhance the metabolism of cyclosporine, decreasing its serum concentrations by ~50%; effect on sirolimus and/or tacrolimus has not been specifically evaluated, but may be similar. Concurrent use of cyclosporine is contraindicated. Bosentan may increase the metabolism of selected anticonvulsants (ethosuximide, phenytoin, tiagabine, and zonisamide), antipsychotics, atorvastatin, calcium channel blockers, corticosteroids, doxycycline, estrogens, hormonal contraceptives, lovastatin, protease inhibitors, simvastatin, and warfarin. Bosentan may enhance the metabolism of methadone resulting in methadone withdrawal.

Dietary/Ethanol/Herb Considerations

Food: May be taken with food; bioavailability unaffected.

Herb/Nutraceutical: Avoid St John's wort; may decrease serum concentration.

Pharmacodynamics/Kinetics

Distribution: V_d: 18 L

Protein binding, plasma: >98% to albumin

Metabolism: Hepatic via CYP2C9 and 3A4 to three primary metabolites (one having pharmacologic activity)

Bioavailability: 50%

Half-life elimination: 5 hours; prolonged with heart failure, possibly in PAH

Excretion: Feces (as metabolites); urine (<3% as unchanged drug)

Pregnancy Risk Factor X

Generic Available No

B&O Supprettes® *see* Belladonna and Opium *on page 164*

Botox® *see* Botulinum Toxin Type A *on page 193*

Botox® Cosmetic *see* Botulinum Toxin Type A *on page 193*

Botulinum Toxin Type A (BOT yoo lin num TOKS in type aye)

U.S. Brand Names Botox®; Botox® Cosmetic

Canadian Brand Names Botox®; Botox® Cosmetic

Pharmacologic Category Neuromuscular Blocker Agent, Toxin; Ophthalmic Agent, Toxin

Use Treatment of strabismus and blepharospasm associated with dystonia (including benign essential blepharospasm or VII nerve disorders in patients ≥12 years of age); cervical dystonia (spasmodic torticollis) in patients ≥16 years of age; temporary improvement in the appearance of lines/wrinkles of the face (moderate to severe glabellar lines associated with corrugator and/or procerus muscle activity) in adult patients ≤65 years of age

Orphan drug: Treatment of dynamic muscle contracture in pediatric cerebral palsy patients

Unlabeled/Investigational Use Treatment of oromandibular dystonia, spasmodic dysphonia (laryngeal dystonia) and other dystonias (ie, writer's cramp, focal task-specific dystonias); treatment and prophylaxis of migraine headaches

Local Anesthetic/Vasoconstrictor Precautions No information available to require special precautions

Effects on Dental Treatment Occur in ~1 week; may last up to several months:

>10% : Xerostomia, changes in salivation, headache (11% to 10%), dysphagia (19% in cervical dystonia), neck pain (11% in cervical dystonia), upper respiratory infection (12% in cervical dystonia)

2% to 10%: Dizziness, fever, drowsiness, nausea, facial pain, cough, rhinitis, flu syndrome

<2%: Dyspnea, stiffness, facial weakness, numbness

Dosage I.M.:

Children ≥16 years and Adults: Cervical dystonia: For dosing guidance, the mean dose is 236 units (25th to 75th percentile range 198-300 units) divided among the affected muscles in patients previously treated with botulinum toxin. Initial dose in previously untreated patients should be lower. Sequential dosing should be based on the patient's head and neck position, localization of pain, muscle hypertrophy, patient response, and previous adverse reactions. The total dose injected into the sternocleidomastoid muscles should be ≤100 units to decrease the occurrence of dysphagia.

(Continued)

Botulinum Toxin Type A *(Continued)*

Children ≥12 years and Adults:

Blepharospasm: Initial dose: 1.25-2.5 units injected into the medial and lateral pretarsal orbicularis oculi of the upper and lower lid; dose may be increased up to twice the previous dose if the response from the initial dose lasted ≤2 months; maximum dose per site: 5 units; cumulative dose in a 30-day period: ≤200 units. Tolerance may occur if treatments are given more often than every 3 months, but the effect is not usually permanent.

Strabismus:

Initial dose:

Vertical muscles and for horizontal strabismus <20 prism diopters: 1.25-2.5 units in any one muscle

Horizontal strabismus of 20-50 prism diopters: 2.5-5 units in any one muscle

Persistent VI nerve palsy >1 month: 1.5-2.5 units in the medial rectus muscle

Re-examine patients 7-14 days after each injection to assess the effect of that dose. Subsequent doses for patients experiencing incomplete paralysis of the target may be increased up to twice the previous administered dose. The maximum recommended dose as a single injection for any one muscle is 25 units. Do not administer subsequent injections until the effects of the previous dose are gone.

Adults ≤65 years: Reduction of glabellar lines: An effective dose is determined by gross observation of the patient's ability to activate the superficial muscles injected. The location, size and use of muscles may vary markedly among individuals. Inject 0.1 mL dose into each of five sites, two in each corrugator muscle and one in the procerus muscle (total dose 0.5 mL).

Dosing adjustment for elderly or in renal/hepatic impairment: No specific adjustment recommended

Mechanism of Action Botulinum A toxin is a neurotoxin produced by *Clostridium botulinum*, spore-forming anaerobic bacillus, which appears to affect only the presynaptic membrane of the neuromuscular junction in humans, where it prevents calcium-dependent release of acetylcholine and produces a state of denervation. Muscle inactivation persists until new fibrils grow from the nerve and form junction plates on new areas of the muscle-cell walls.

Other Adverse Effects Occur in ~1 week; may last up to several months:

>10% : Ocular: Ptosis (blepharospasm 10% to 40%, strabismus 1% to 38%, reduction of glabellar lines 1% to 5%); vertical deviation (strabismus 17%)

2% to 10%:

Central nervous system: Speech disorder (cervical dystonia)

Local: Injection site reaction

Neuromuscular & skeletal: Back pain (cervical dystonia); hypertonia (cervical dystonia); weakness (cervical dystonia, reduction of glabellar lines)

Ocular: Dry eyes (blepharospasm 6%), superficial punctate keratitis (blepharospasm 6%)

<2%: Diplopia (cervical dystonia, blepharospasm), ptosis (cervical dystonia), ectropion (blepharospasm), lagophthalmos (blepharospasm), ecchymoses (blepharospasm), eyelid edema (blepharospasm), tearing (blepharospasm), photophobia (blepharospasm), entropion (blepharospasm)

Postmarketing and/or case reports: **Allergic reactions, arrhythmia,** erythema multiforme, **MI,** pruritus, psoriasiform eruption, skin rash, urticaria

Reported following treatment of cervical dystonia: Brachial plexopathy, dysphonia, aspiration

Reported following treatment of blepharospasm: Reduced blinking leading to corneal ulceration, corneal perforation, acute angle-closure glaucoma, focal facial paralysis, exacerbation of myasthenia gravis, syncope, vitreous hemorrhage

Reported following treatment of strabismus: Retrobulbar hemorrhage, ciliary ganglion damage, anterior segment eye ischemia

Reported following reduction of glabellar lines: Exacerbation of myasthenia gravis, retinal vein occlusion, abnormal hearing/hearing loss, glaucoma, vertigo with nystagmus

Warnings/Precautions Higher doses or more frequent administration may result in neutralizing antibody formation and loss of efficacy. Product contains albumin and may carry a remote risk of virus transmission. Use caution if there is inflammation, excessive weakness, or atrophy at the proposed injection site(s). Have appropriate support in case of anaphylactic reaction. Use with caution in patients with neuromuscular diseases (such as myasthenia gravis), neuropathic disorders (such as amyotrophic lateral sclerosis), or patients taking aminoglycosides or other drugs that interfere with neuromuscular transmission. Ensure adequate contraception in women of childbearing years. Long-term effects of chronic therapy unknown.

Cervical dystonia: Dysphagia is common. It may be severe requiring alternative feeding methods. Risk factors include smaller neck muscle mass, bilateral injections into the sternocleidomastoid muscle or injections into the levator scapulae. Dysphasia may be associated with increased risk of upper respiratory infection.

Blepharospasm: Reduced blinking from injection of the orbicularis muscle can lead to corneal exposure and ulceration.

Strabismus: Retrobulbar hemorrhages may occur from needle penetration into orbit. Spatial disorientation, double vision, or past pointing may occur if one or more extraocular muscles are paralyzed. Covering the affected eye may help. Careful testing of corneal sensation, avoidance of lower lid injections, and treatment of epithelial defects necessary.

Temporary reduction in glabellar lines: Do not use more frequently than every 3 months. Patients with marked facial asymmetry, ptosis, excessive dermatochalasis, deep dermal scarring, thick sebaceous skin, or the inability to substantially lessen glabellar lines by physically spreading them apart were excluded from clinical trials. Reduced blinking from injection of the orbicularis muscle can lead to corneal exposure and ulceration. Spatial disorientation, double vision, or past pointing may occur if one or more extraocular muscles are paralyzed.

Drug Interactions Increased Effect/Toxicity: Aminoglycosides, neuromuscular-blocking agents

Pharmacodynamics/Kinetics

Onset of action (improvement):
- Blepharospasm: ~3 days
- Cervical dystonia: ~2 weeks
- Strabismus: ~1-2 days
- Reduction of glabellar lines (Botox® Cosmetic): 1-2 days, increasing in intensity during first week

Duration:
- Blepharospasm: ~3 months
- Cervical dystonia: <3 months
- Strabismus: ~2-6 weeks
- Reduction of glabellar lines (Botox® Cosmetic): Up to 3 months

Absorption: Not expected to be present in peripheral blood at recommended doses

Time to peak:
- Blepharospasm: 1-2 weeks
- Cervical dystonia: ~6 weeks
- Strabismus: Within first week

Pregnancy Risk Factor C (manufacturer)

Generic Available No

Botulinum Toxin Type B (BOT yoo lin num TOKS in type bee)

U.S. Brand Names Myobloc®

Pharmacologic Category Neuromuscular Blocker Agent, Toxin

Use Treatment of cervical dystonia (spasmodic torticollis)

Unlabeled/Investigational Use Treatment of cervical dystonia in patients who have developed resistance to botulinum toxin type A

Local Anesthetic/Vasoconstrictor Precautions No information available to require special precautions

Effects on Dental Treatment

>10%: Xerostomia (3% to 34%), headache (10% to 16%), dysphagia (10% to 25%), neck pain (≤17%; placebo: 16%), infection (13% to 19%; placebo: 15%)

1% to 10%: Chest pain, vasodilation, dizziness (3% to 6%), fever, migraine, anxiety, tremor, somnolence, confusion, bruising, nausea (3% to 10%; placebo: 5%), vomiting, stomatitis, abnormal taste, torticollis (up to 8%; placebo: 7%), cough (3% to 7%; placebo: 3%), rhinitis (1% to 5%; placebo: 6%), dyspnea, pneumonia, flu-syndrome (6% to 9%), allergic reaction, viral infection, abscess, otitis media, weakness, malaise, arthritis, abnormal vision

Dosage

Children: Not established

Adults: Cervical dystonia: I.M.: Initial: 2500-5000 units divided among the affected muscles in patients **previously treated** with botulinum toxin; initial dose in **previously untreated** patients should be lower. Subsequent dosing should be optimized according to patient's response.

Elderly: Limited experience in patients ≥75 years old

Dosing adjustment in renal/hepatic impairment: No specific adjustment recommended

Mechanism of Action Botulinum B toxin is a neurotoxin produced by *Clostridium botulinum,* spore-forming anaerobic bacillus. It cleaves synaptic Vesicle Association Membrane Protein (VAMP; synaptobrevin) which is a component of the protein complex responsible for docking and fusion of the synaptic vesicle to the presynaptic membrane. By blocking neurotransmitter release, botulinum B toxin paralyzes the muscle.

Other Adverse Effects

>10%: Local: Injection site pain (12% to 16%)

1% to 10%:
- Cardiovascular: Peripheral edema
- Central nervous system: Hyperesthesia, vertigo
- Dermatologic: Pruritus

(Continued)

Botulinum Toxin Type B *(Continued)*

Gastrointestinal: Dyspepsia (up to 10%; placebo: 5%)
Genitourinary: Urinary tract infection, cystitis, vaginal moniliasis
Hematologic: Serum neutralizing activity
Neuromuscular & skeletal: Arthralgia (up to 7%; placebo: 5%), back pain (3% to 7%; placebo: 3%), myasthenia (3% to 6%; placebo: 3%)
Ocular: Amblyopia
Otic: Tinnitus
Miscellaneous: Cyst

Drug Interactions Increased Effect/Toxicity: Aminoglycosides, neuromuscular-blocking agents, botulinum toxin type A, other agents which may block neuromuscular transmission

Pharmacodynamics/Kinetics
Duration: 12-16 weeks
Absorption: Not expected to be present in peripheral blood at recommended doses

Pregnancy Risk Factor C (manufacturer)

Generic Available No

Boudreaux's® Butt Paste [OTC] *see* Zinc Oxide *on page 1409*
Bovine Lung Surfactant *see* Beractant *on page 176*
Bravelle™ *see* Follitropins *on page 607*
Breathe Right® Saline [OTC] *see* Sodium Chloride *on page 1229*
Breonesin® [OTC] [DSC] *see* Guaifenesin *on page 650*
Brethaire® [DSC] *see* Terbutaline *on page 1278*
Brethine® *see* Terbutaline *on page 1278*

Bretylium (bre TIL ee um)

Related Information
Cardiovascular Diseases *on page 1456*

Pharmacologic Category Antiarrhythmic Agent, Class III

Synonyms Bretylium Tosylate

Use Treatment of ventricular tachycardia and fibrillation; treatment of other serious ventricular arrhythmias resistant to lidocaine

Local Anesthetic/Vasoconstrictor Precautions No information available to require special precautions

Effects on Dental Treatment
>10%: Hypotension (both postural and supine)
1% to 10%: Nausea, vomiting

Dosage Patients should undergo defibrillation/cardioversion before and after bretylium doses as necessary.

Children (not well established):
I.M.: 2-5 mg/kg as a single dose
I.V.: Acute ventricular fibrillation: Initial: 5 mg/kg, then attempt electrical defibrillation; repeat with 10 mg/kg if ventricular fibrillation persists at 15- to 30-minute intervals to maximum total of 30 mg/kg.
Maintenance dose: I.M., I.V.: 5 mg/kg every 6 hours

Adults:
Immediate life-threatening ventricular arrhythmias (ventricular fibrillation, unstable ventricular tachycardia): Initial dose: I.V.: 5 mg/kg (undiluted) over 1 minute; if arrhythmia persists, administer 10 mg/kg (undiluted) over 1 minute and repeat as necessary (usually at 15- to 30-minute intervals) up to a total dose of 30-35 mg/kg.
Other life-threatening ventricular arrhythmias:
Initial dose: I.M., I.V.: 5-10 mg/kg, may repeat every 1-2 hours if arrhythmia persists; administer I.V. dose (diluted) over 8-10 minutes.
Maintenance dose: I.M.: 5-10 mg/kg every 6-8 hours; I.V. (diluted): 5-10 mg/kg every 6 hours; I.V. infusion (diluted): 1-2 mg/minute (little experience with doses >40 mg/kg/day)
Example dilution: 2 g/250 mL D_5W (infusion pump should be used for I.V. infusion administration)
Rate of I.V. infusion: 1-4 mg/minute
1 mg/minute = 7 mL/hour
2 mg/minute = 15 mL/hour
3 mg/minute = 22 mL/hour
4 mg/minute = 30 mL/hour

Dosing adjustment in renal impairment:
Cl_{cr} 10-50 mL/minute: Administer 25% to 50% of dose.
Cl_{cr} <10 mL/minute: Administer 25% of dose.
Dialysis: Not dialyzable (0% to 5%) via hemo- or peritoneal dialysis; supplemental doses are not needed.

Mechanism of Action Class III antiarrhythmic; after an initial release of norepinephrine at the peripheral adrenergic nerve terminals, inhibits further release by postganglionic nerve endings in response to sympathetic nerve stimulation

Other Adverse Effects <1% (Limited to important or life-threatening): Transient initial hypertension, increase in premature ventricular contractions (PVCs), **bradycardia, chest pain, flushing, syncope, postural hypotension**, renal impairment, **respiratory depression, nasal congestion, dyspnea**

Drug Interactions Increased Effect/Toxicity: Other antiarrhythmic agents may potentiate or antagonize cardiac effects of bretylium. Toxic effects may be additive. The vasopressor effects of catecholamines may be enhanced by bretylium. Toxicity of agents which may prolong QT interval (including cisapride, tricyclic antidepressants, antipsychotics, erythromycin, Class Ia and Class III antiarrhythmics) and specific quinolones (sparfloxacin, gatifloxacin, moxifloxacin) may be increased. Digoxin toxicity may be aggravated by bretylium.

Pharmacodynamics/Kinetics

Onset of action: I.M.: May require 2 hours; I.V.: 6-20 minutes
Peak effect: 6-9 hours
Duration: 6-24 hours
Protein binding: 1% to 6%
Metabolism: None
Half-life elimination: 7-11 hours; Mean: 4-17 hours; End-stage renal disease: 16-32 hours
Excretion: Urine (70% to 80% as unchanged drug) within 24 hours

Pregnancy Risk Factor C

Generic Available Yes

Bretylium Tosylate *see* Bretylium *on page 196*
Brevibloc® *see* Esmolol *on page 518*
Brevicon® *see* Combination Hormonal Contraceptives *on page 368*
Brevital® Sodium *see* Methohexital *on page 882*
Brevoxyl® *see* Benzoyl Peroxide *on page 171*
Brevoxyl® Cleansing *see* Benzoyl Peroxide *on page 171*
Brevoxyl® Wash *see* Benzoyl Peroxide *on page 171*
Bricanyl® [DSC] *see* Terbutaline *on page 1278*

Brimonidine (bri MOE ni deen)

U.S. Brand Names Alphagan® [DSC]; Alphagan® P

Canadian Brand Names Alphagan™; ratio-Brimonidine

Mexican Brand Names Alphagan®

Pharmacologic Category Alpha$_2$ Agonist, Ophthalmic; Ophthalmic Agent, Antiglaucoma

Synonyms Alphagan® [DSC]; Brimonidine Tartrate

Use Lowering of intraocular pressure (IOP) in patients with open-angle glaucoma or ocular hypertension

Local Anesthetic/Vasoconstrictor Precautions No information available to require special precautions

Effects on Dental Treatment

Alphagan®:
>10%: Xerostomia, drowsiness, headache, somnolence and lethargy (≤83% of children 2-6 years of age; 25% of children ≥7 years of age), fatigue
1% to 10%: Arrhythmias (<3%), hypertension (<3%), palpitations (<3%), syncope (<3%), dizziness, anxiety (<3%), upper respiratory symptoms (3% to 9%), nasal dryness (<3%), abnormal taste (3% to 9%), pain, weakness

Alphagan® P: 1% to 10% (unless otherwise noted 1% to 4%): Xerostomia (5% to 9%), hypertension (5& to 9%), dizziness, headache, dyspepsia, bronchitis, cough, dyspnea, pharyngitis, rhinitis, sinus infection, allergic reaction, flu-like syndrome

Dosage Ophthalmic: Children ≥2 years of age and Adults: Glaucoma (Alphagan®, Alphagan® P): Instill 1 drop in affected eye(s) 3 times/day (approximately every 8 hours)

Mechanism of Action Selective for alpha$_2$-receptors; appears to result in reduction of aqueous humor formation and increase uveoscleral outflow

Other Adverse Effects

Alphagan®:
>10%: Ocular: Allergic reactions, blurring, burning, follicular conjunctivitis, foreign body sensation, hyperemia, pruritus, stinging
1% to 10% (unless otherwise noted 3% to 9%):
Central nervous system: Depression (<3%), insomnia (<3%)
Ocular: Corneal staining, corneal erosion, photophobia, eyelid erythema, ocular ache/pain, ocular dryness, tearing, eyelid edema, conjunctival edema, blepharitis, ocular irritation, conjunctival blanching, abnormal vision, lid crusting, conjunctival hemorrhage, conjunctival discharge

Alphagan® P:
>10%: Ocular: Allergic conjunctivitis, conjunctival hyperemia, eye pruritus
1% to 10% (unless otherwise noted 1% to 4%):
Dermatologic: Rash
Gastrointestinal: Dyspepsia

(Continued)

Brimonidine *(Continued)*

Ocular: Burning sensation (5% to 9%), conjunctival folliculosis (5% to 9%), visual disturbance (5% to 9%), blepharitis, conjunctival edema, conjunctival hemorrhage, conjunctivitis, eye discharge, irritation, eyelid edema, eyelid erythema, follicular conjunctivitis, foreign body sensation, pain, photophobia, stinging, superficial punctate keratopathy, visual field defect, vitreous floaters, watery eyes, worsened visual acuity

<1%: Corneal erosion, insomnia, **nasal dryness, somnolence, abnormal taste**

Postmarketing and/or case reports (pediatric patients): **Agitation, apnea, bradycardia, convulsions**, cyanosis, depression, **dyspnea**, emotional instability, **hypotension**, hypothermia, hypotonia, **hypoventilation, irritability**, lethargy, **somnolence, stupor**

Drug Interactions

Increased Effect/Toxicity: CNS depressants (eg, ethanol, barbiturates, opiates, sedatives, anesthetics) may have additive or potentiating effect; topical beta-blockers, pilocarpine may have additive decreased intraocular pressure; antihypertensives, cardiac glycosides may increase effects

Decreased Effect: Tricyclic antidepressants can affect the metabolism and uptake of circulating amines

Dietary/Ethanol/Herb Considerations

Ethanol: Avoid use; may increase CNS depression.

Herb/Nutraceutical: Avoid gotu kola, kava, SAMe, St John's wort, and valerian; may increase CNS depression.

Pharmacodynamics/Kinetics

Onset of action: Peak effect: 2 hours

Metabolism: Hepatic

Half-life elimination: 2-3 hours

Time to peak, plasma: Alphagan®: 1-4 hours; Alphagan® P: 0.5-2.5 hours

Excretion: Urine (74%)

Pregnancy Risk Factor B

Generic Available No

Brimonidine Tartrate *see* Brimonidine *on page 197*

Brinzolamide (brin ZOH la mide)

U.S. Brand Names Azopt®

Canadian Brand Names Azopt™

Pharmacologic Category Carbonic Anhydrase Inhibitor; Ophthalmic Agent, Antiglaucoma

Use Lowers intraocular pressure to treat glaucoma in patients with ocular hypertension or open-angle glaucoma

Local Anesthetic/Vasoconstrictor Precautions No information available to require special precautions

Effects on Dental Treatment 1% to 10%: Taste disturbances, rhinitis, blurred vision (5% to 10%)

Dosage Ophthalmic: Adults: Instill 1 drop in affected eye(s) 3 times/day

Mechanism of Action Inhibition of carbonic anhydrase decreases aqueous humor secretion. This results in a reduction of intraocular pressure.

Other Adverse Effects

1% to 10%:

Dermatologic: Dermatitis (1% to 5%)

Ocular: Blepharitis (1% to 5%), dry eye (1% to 5%), foreign body sensation (1% to 5%), eye discharge (1% to 5%), eye pain (1% to 5%), itching of eye (1% to 5%)

<1%: **Dizziness, headache**, urticaria, alopecia, diarrhea, **nausea, xerostomia**, diplopia, eye fatigue, lid crusting, **dyspnea, pharyngitis, allergic reactions**

Drug Interactions Substrate of CYP3A4

Increased Effect/Toxicity: Concurrent use of oral carbonic anhydrase inhibitors (CAIs) may lead to additive effects and toxicity. High-dose salicylates may result in toxicity from CAIs.

Pharmacodynamics/Kinetics

Onset of action: Peak effect: 2 hours

Duration: 8-12 hours

Absorption: Topical: Into systemic circulation

Distribution: Accumulates in red blood cells, binding to carbonic anhydrase (brinzolamide and metabolite)

Metabolism: To N-desmethyl brinzolamide

Excretion: Urine (as unchanged drug and metabolites)

Pregnancy Risk Factor C

Generic Available No

Brioschi® [OTC] *see* Sodium Bicarbonate *on page 1227*

British Anti-Lewisite *see* Dimercaprol *on page 449*

Brofed® *see* Brompheniramine and Pseudoephedrine *on page 201*

Bromanate® [OTC] *see* Brompheniramine and Pseudoephedrine *on page 201*

Bromazepam (broe MA ze pam)

Canadian Brand Names Apo®-Bromazepam; Gen-Bromazepam; Lectopam®; Novo-Bromazepam; Nu-Bromazepam

Pharmacologic Category Benzodiazepine

Use Short-term, symptomatic treatment of anxiety

Local Anesthetic/Vasoconstrictor Precautions No information available to require special precautions

Effects on Dental Treatment Paradoxical reactions (including excitation, agitation, hallucinations, and psychosis) are known to occur with benzodiazepines.

Frequency not defined: Hypotension, palpitations, tachycardia, drowsiness, dizziness, confusion, euphoria, lethargy, slurred speech, stupor, headache, seizures, anterograde amnesia, hyperglycemia, hypoglycemia, xerostomia, nausea, vomiting, weakness, muscle spasms, blurred vision, depth perception decreased

Restrictions CDSA IV

Dosage Oral:

Adults: Initial: 6-18 mg/day in equally divided doses; initial course of treatment should not last longer than 1 week; optimal dosage range: 6-30 mg/day

Elderly/debilitated: Initial dose: 3 mg/day in divided doses

Mechanism of Action Binds to stereospecific benzodiazepine receptors on the postsynaptic GABA neuron at several sites within the central nervous system, including the limbic system, reticular formation. Enhancement of the inhibitory effect of GABA on neuronal excitability results by increased neuronal membrane permeability to chloride ions. This shift in chloride ions results in hyperpolarization (a less excitable state) and stabilization.

Other Adverse Effects Frequency not defined:

Central nervous system: Ataxia, depression

Dermatologic: Rash, pruritus

Genitourinary: Incontinence, libido decreased

Hematologic: Hemoglobin decreased, hematocrit decreased, WBCs increased/decreased

Hepatic: Transaminases increased, alkaline phosphatase increased, bilirubin increased

Drug Interactions Substrate of **CYP3A4**; Inhibits CYP2E1

Increased Effect/Toxicity: Benzodiazepines potentiate the CNS depressant effects of narcotic analgesics, barbiturates, phenothiazines, ethanol, antihistamines, MAO inhibitors, sedative-hypnotics, and cyclic antidepressants. Serum levels and/or effects of benzodiazepines may be increased by inhibitors of CYP3A4 including amiodarone, amprenavir, cimetidine, clarithromycin, erythromycin, delavirdine, diltiazem, dirithromycin, disulfiram, fluoxetine, fluvoxamine, grapefruit juice, indinavir, itraconazole, ketoconazole, nefazodone, nevirapine, propoxyphene, quinupristin-dalfopristin, ritonavir, saquinavir, verapamil, zafirlukast, zileuton.

Decreased Effect: Carbamazepine, rifampin, rifabutin may enhance the metabolism of benzodiazepines and decrease its therapeutic effect.

Dietary/Ethanol/Herb Considerations

Ethanol: Avoid ethanol; may increase CNS depression.

Food: May be taken with food; small, frequent meals, chewing gum, or sucking lozenges may reduce nausea and vomiting. Fluids, fruit, and fiber may reduce constipation. Avoid grapefruit products; may increase serum concentration.

Herb/Nutraceutical: Avoid gotu kola, kava, SAMe, and valerian; may increase CNS depression. Avoid St John's wort; may decrease serum concentration and increase CNS depression.

Pharmacodynamics/Kinetics

Protein binding: 70%

Metabolism: Hepatic

Bioavailability: 60%

Half-life elimination: 20 hours

Excretion: Urine (69%), as metabolites

Pregnancy Risk Factor D (based on other benzodiazepines)

Generic Available Yes

Bromfed® [OTC] *see* Brompheniramine and Pseudoephedrine *on page 201*

Bromfed-PD® [OTC] *see* Brompheniramine and Pseudoephedrine *on page 201*

Bromfenex® *see* Brompheniramine and Pseudoephedrine *on page 201*

Bromfenex® PD *see* Brompheniramine and Pseudoephedrine *on page 201*

Bromocriptine (broe moe KRIP teen)

U.S. Brand Names Parlodel®

Canadian Brand Names Apo® Bromocriptine; Parlodel®; PMS-Bromocriptine

Mexican Brand Names Cryocriptina; Parlodel®; Serocryptin®

Pharmacologic Category Anti-Parkinson's Agent, Dopamine Agonist; Ergot Derivative

Synonyms Bromocriptine Mesylate

(Continued)

Bromocriptine *(Continued)*

Use

Amenorrhea with or without galactorrhea; infertility or hypogonadism; prolactin-secreting adenomas; acromegaly; Parkinson's disease

A previous indication for prevention of postpartum lactation was withdrawn voluntarily by Sandoz Pharmaceuticals Corporation

Unlabeled/Investigational Use Treatment of neuroleptic malignant syndrome (NMS)

Local Anesthetic/Vasoconstrictor Precautions No information available to require special precautions

Effects on Dental Treatment

>10%: Headache, dizziness, nausea, fatigue

1% to 10%: Orthostatic hypotension, lightheadedness, drowsiness, vomiting, nasal congestion

Dosage Oral: Adults:

Parkinsonism: 1.25 mg 2 times/day, increased by 2.5 mg/day in 2- to 4-week intervals (usual dose range is 30-90 mg/day in 3 divided doses), though elderly patients can usually be managed on lower doses

Neuroleptic malignant syndrome: 2.5-5 mg 3 times/day

Hyperprolactinemia: 2.5 mg 2-3 times/day

Acromegaly: Initial: 1.25-2.5 mg increasing as necessary every 3-7 days; usual dose: 20-30 mg/day

Prolactin-secreting adenomas: Initial: 1.25-2.5 mg/day; daily range 2.5-10 mg.

Dosing adjustment in hepatic impairment: No guidelines are available, however, may be necessary

Mechanism of Action Semisynthetic ergot alkaloid derivative and a dopamine receptor agonist which activates postsynaptic dopamine receptors in the tuberoinfundibular and nigrostriatal pathways

Other Adverse Effects

1% to 10%: Gastrointestinal: Anorexia, abdominal cramps, constipation

<1%: **Arrhythmias**, hair loss, insomnia, **paranoia, visual hallucinations**

Drug Interactions Substrate of **CYP3A4**; Inhibits **CYP3A4**

Increased effect with antifungals (azole derivatives); CYP3A4 inhibitors (eg, amiodarone, cimetidine, erythromycin, ritonavir); macrolide antibiotics; protease inhibitors; MAO inhibitors. Bromocriptine may increase the effects of CYP3A4 substrates (eg, benzodiazepines, buspirone, calcium channel blockers); sibutramine; and other serotonin agonists (serotonin syndrome).

Decreased effect with antipsychotics, metoclopramide.

Dietary/Ethanol/Herb Considerations

Ethanol: Avoid use; may increase GI side effects or ethanol intolerance.

Food: Administer with food to reduce GI upset, before meals if dry mouth occurs, and after meals if drooling occurs. Avoid grapefruit products may increase serum levels/toxicity.

Herb/Nutraceutical: Avoid St John's wort; may decrease serum concentration.

Pharmacodynamics/Kinetics

Protein binding: 90% to 96%

Metabolism: Primarily hepatic

Half-life elimination: Biphasic: Initial: 6-8 hours; Terminal: 50 hours

Time to peak, serum: 1-2 hours

Excretion: Feces; urine (2% to 6% as unchanged drug)

Pregnancy Risk Factor B

Generic Available No

Bromocriptine Mesylate *see* Bromocriptine *on page 199*

Bromodiphenhydramine and Codeine

(brome oh dye fen HYE dra meen & KOE deen)

Related Information

Codeine *on page 361*

Pharmacologic Category Antihistamine/Antitussive

Synonyms Codeine and Bromodiphenhydramine

Use Relief of upper respiratory symptoms and cough associated with allergies or common cold

Local Anesthetic/Vasoconstrictor Precautions No information available to require special precautions

Effects on Dental Treatment Bromodiphenhydramine: 1% to 10%: Xerostomia

Restrictions C-V

Dosage Oral: Adults: 5-10 mL every 4-6 hours

Other Adverse Effects Codeine: **<1%: Xerostomia**

Pregnancy Risk Factor C

Generic Available Yes

Brompheniramine and Pseudoephedrine

(brome fen IR a meen & soo doe e FED rin)

Related Information

Pseudoephedrine *on page 1146*

U.S. Brand Names Andehist NR Syrup; Brofed®; Bromanate® [OTC]; Bromfed® [OTC]; Bromfed-PD® [OTC]; Bromfenex®; Bromfenex® PD; Children's Dimetapp® Elixir Cold & Allergy [OTC]; Rondec® Syrup; Touro™ Allergy

Pharmacologic Category Antihistamine/Decongestant Combination

Synonyms Pseudoephedrine and Brompheniramine

Use Temporary relief of symptoms of seasonal and perennial allergic rhinitis, and vasomotor rhinitis, including nasal obstruction

Local Anesthetic/Vasoconstrictor Precautions Use with caution since pseudoephedrine is a sympathomimetic amine which could interact with epinephrine to cause a pressor response

Effects on Dental Treatment

Brompheniramine: Prolonged use may decrease salivary flow

Pseudoephedrine: ≤10%: Tachycardia, palpitations, and xerostomia; use vasoconstrictor with caution

Frequency not defined: Arrhythmias, flushing, hypertension, convulsions, CNS stimulation, dizziness, excitability (children; rare), giddiness, hallucinations, headache, irritability, nervousness, sedation, nausea, vomiting, tremors, weakness, respiratory difficulty

Dosage Oral:

Capsule, sustained release:

Based on 60 mg pseudoephedrine:

Children 6-12 years: 1 capsule every 12 hours

Children ≥12 years and Adults: 1-2 capsules every 12 hours

Based on 120 mg pseudoephedrine: Children ≥12 years and Adults: 1 capsule every 12 hours

Elixir: Maximum: 4 doses in 24 hours:

Children:

6-11 months (6-8 kg): Brompheniramine 1 mg/pseudoephedrine 15 mg per 5 mL: 2.5 mL every 6-8 hours

12-23 months (8-10 kg): Brompheniramine 1 mg/pseudoephedrine 15 mg per 5 mL: 3.75 mL every 6-8 hours

2-6 years: Brompheniramine 1 mg/pseudoephedrine 15 mg per 5 mL: 5 mL every 4 hours

6-12 years: Brompheniramine 1 mg/pseudoephedrine 15 mg per 5 mL: 10 mL every 4 hours

Children >12 years and Adults: Brompheniramine 1 mg/pseudoephedrine 15 mg per 5 mL: 20 mL every 4 hours

Syrup:

Children 2-6 years:

Brompheniramine 4 mg/pseudoephedrine 30 mg: 2.5 mL 3 times/day

Brompheniramine 4 mg/pseudoephedrine 45 mg per 5 mL: 2.5 mL 4 times/day

Children >6 years and adults:

Brompheniramine 4 mg/pseudoephedrine 30 mg: 5 mL 3 times/day

Brompheniramine 4 mg/pseudoephedrine 45 mg per 5 mL: 5 mL 4 times/day

Mechanism of Action Brompheniramine maleate is an antihistamine with H_1-receptor activity; pseudoephedrine, a sympathomimetic amine and isomer of ephedrine, acts as a decongestant in respiratory tract mucous membranes with less vasoconstrictor action than ephedrine in normotensive individuals.

Other Adverse Effects Frequency not defined:

Cardiovascular: Pallor

Central nervous system: Insomnia, lassitude

Gastrointestinal: Anorexia, diarrhea, dyspepsia

Ocular: Diplopia

Renal: Dysuria, polyuria, urinary retention (with BPH)

Dietary/Ethanol/Herb Considerations Ethanol: Avoid ethanol (may increase CNS depression).

Pharmacodynamics/Kinetics

See Pseudoephedrine monograph.

Brompheniramine:

Metabolism: Hepatic

Time to peak: Syrup: 5 hours

Excretion: Urine

Pregnancy Risk Factor C

Generic Available No

Broncho Saline® [OTC] *see* Sodium Chloride *on page 1229*

Brontex® *see* Guaifenesin and Codeine *on page 650*

BSS® *see* Balanced Salt Solution *on page 160*

B-type Natriuretic Peptide (Human) *see* Nesiritide *on page 964*

Budesonide (byoo DES oh nide)

U.S. Brand Names Entocort™ EC; Pulmicort Respules™; Pulmicort Turbuhaler®; Rhinocort® [DSC]; Rhinocort® Aqua™

Canadian Brand Names Entocort®; Gen-Budesonide AQ; Pulmicort®; Rhinocort® Turbuhaler®

Mexican Brand Names Pulmicort®; Rhinocort®

Pharmacologic Category Corticosteroid, Inhalant (Oral); Corticosteroid, Nasal; Corticosteroid, Systemic

Synonyms Rhinocort® [DSC]

Use

Intranasal: Children ≥6 years of age and Adults: Management of symptoms of seasonal or perennial rhinitis

Nebulization: Children 12 months to 8 years: Maintenance and prophylactic treatment of asthma

Oral capsule: Treatment of active Crohn's disease (mild to moderate) involving the ileum and/or ascending colon

Oral inhalation: Maintenance and prophylactic treatment of asthma; includes patients who require corticosteroids and those who may benefit from systemic dose reduction/elimination

Local Anesthetic/Vasoconstrictor Precautions No information available to require special precautions

Effects on Dental Treatment Localized infections with *Candida albicans* or *Aspergillus niger* have occurred frequently in the mouth and pharynx with repetitive use of oral inhaler of corticosteroids. These infections may require treatment with appropriate antifungal therapy or discontinuance of treatment with corticosteroid inhaler.

Severity varies by dose and duration:

>10%: Headache (≤21%; capsule) nausea (≤11%; capsule), respiratory infection, rhinitis

1% to 10%: Syncope, hypertension, chest pain, fever, migraine, neck pain, nervousness, dizziness, bruising, gastroenteritis, vomiting, xerostomia, nasal dryness, dry throat, abnormal taste, dysphonia, paresthesia, oral candidiasis, bronchitis, bronchospasm, cough, epistaxis, nasal pharyngitis, sinusitis, allergic reaction, flu-like syndrome, herpes simplex, infection, viral infection, ear infection, external ear infection, fatigue

Dosage

Nasal inhalation: Children ≥6 years and Adults:

Rhinocort®: Initial: 8 sprays (4 sprays/nostril) per day (256 mcg/day), given as either 2 sprays in each nostril in the morning and evening or as 4 sprays in each nostril in the morning; after symptoms decrease (usually by 3-7 days), reduce dose slowly every 2-4 weeks to the smallest amount needed to control symptoms

Rhinocort® Aqua™: 64 mcg/day as a single 32 mcg spray in each nostril. Some patients who do not achieve adequate control may benefit from increased dosage. A reduced dosage may be effective after initial control is achieved.

Maximum dose: Children <12 years: 128 mcg/day; Adults: 256 mcg/day

Nebulization: Children 12 months to 8 years: Pulmicort Respules™: Titrate to lowest effective dose once patient is stable; start at 0.25 mg/day or use as follows:

Previous therapy of bronchodilators alone: 0.5 mg/day administered as a single dose or divided twice daily (maximum daily dose: 0.5 mg)

Previous therapy of inhaled corticosteroids: 0.5 mg/day administered as a single dose or divided twice daily (maximum daily dose: 1 mg)

Previous therapy of oral corticosteroids: 1 mg/day administered as a single dose or divided twice daily (maximum daily dose: 1 mg)

Oral inhalation:

Children ≥6 years:

Previous therapy of bronchodilators alone: 200 mcg twice initially which may be increased up to 400 mcg twice daily

Previous therapy of inhaled corticosteroids: 200 mcg twice initially which may be increased up to 400 mcg twice daily

Previous therapy of oral corticosteroids: The highest recommended dose in children is 400 mcg twice daily

Adults:

Previous therapy of bronchodilators alone: 200-400 mcg twice initially which may be increased up to 400 mcg twice daily

Previous therapy of inhaled corticosteroids: 200-400 mcg twice initially which may be increased up to 800 mcg twice daily

Previous therapy of oral corticosteroids: 400-800 mcg twice daily which may be increased up to 800 mcg twice daily

NIH Guidelines (NIH, 1997) (give in divided doses twice daily):

Children:

"Low" dose: 100-200 mcg/day

"Medium" dose: 200-400 mcg/day (1-2 inhalations/day)

"High" dose: >400 mcg/day (>2 inhalation/day)

Adults:
"Low" dose: 200-400 mcg/day (1-2 inhalations/day)
"Medium" dose: 400-600 mcg/day (2-3 inhalations/day)
"High" dose: >600 mcg/day (>3 inhalation/day)

Oral: Adults: Treatment may be tapered to 6 mg once daily for 2 weeks prior to complete cessation. Patients receiving CYP3A4 inhibitors should be monitored closely for signs and symptoms of hypercorticism; dosage reduction may be required.

Crohn's disease: 9 mg once daily in the morning; safety and efficacy have not been established for therapy duration >8 weeks; recurring episodes may be treated with a repeat 8-week course of treatment

Dosing adjustment in hepatic impairment: Reduction may be required; monitor closely for signs and symptoms of hypercorticism

Mechanism of Action Controls the rate of protein synthesis, depresses the migration of polymorphonuclear leukocytes, fibroblasts, reverses capillary permeability, and lysosomal stabilization at the cellular level to prevent or control inflammation

Other Adverse Effects Severity varies with dose and duration:

>10%: Symptoms of HPA axis suppression and/or hypercorticism (acne, easy bruising, fat redistribution, striae, edema) may occur in >10% of patients following administration of dosage forms which result in higher systemic exposure (ie, oral capsule), but may be less frequent than rates observed with comparator drugs (prednisolone). These symptoms may be rare (<1%) following administration via methods which result in lower exposures (topical).

1% to 10%:
Cardiovascular: Edema
Central nervous system: Emotional lability, insomnia, pain, vertigo
Dermatologic: Contact dermatitis, eczema, pruritus, pustular rash, rash
Endocrine & metabolic: Hypokalemia, adrenal insufficiency
Gastrointestinal: Abdominal pain, anorexia, diarrhea, dyspepsia, weight gain, flatulence
Hematologic: Cervical lymphadenopathy, purpura, leukocytosis
Neuromuscular & skeletal: Arthralgia, fracture, hyperkinesis, hypertonia, myalgia, weakness, back pain
Ocular: Conjunctivitis, eye infection
Otic: Earache
Respiratory: Nasal irritation, stridor
Miscellaneous: Moniliasis, voice alteration

<1%: **Aggressive reactions**, alopecia, angioedema, avascular necrosis of the femoral head, depression, **dyspnea**, hoarseness, hypersensitivity reactions (immediate and delayed: rash, contact dermatitis, angioedema, **bronchospasm**), intermenstrual bleeding, **irritability, nasal septum perforation, psychosis, somnolence, osteoporosis**

Postmarketing and/or case reports: Growth suppression, benign intracranial hypertension

Drug Interactions Substrate of CYP3A4

Increased Effect/Toxicity: Cimetidine may decrease the clearance and increase the bioavailability of budesonide, increasing its serum concentrations. In addition, CYP3A4 inhibitors may increase the serum level and/or toxicity of budesonide this effect was shown with ketoconazole, but not erythromycin. Other potential inhibitors include amiodarone, cimetidine, clarithromycin, delavirdine, diltiazem, dirithromycin, disulfiram, fluoxetine, fluvoxamine, grapefruit juice, indinavir, itraconazole, ketoconazole, nefazodone, nevirapine, propoxyphene, quinupristin-dalfopristin, ritonavir, saquinavir, verapamil, zafirlukast, zileuton. The addition of salmeterol has been demonstrated to improve response to inhaled corticosteroids (as compared to increasing steroid dosage).

Decreased Effect: CYP3A4 inducers (including carbamazepine, phenytoin, phenobarbital, rifampin) may decrease budesonide levels and/or effects. Theoretically, proton pump inhibitors (omeprazole, pantoprazole) alter gastric pH may affect the rate of dissolution of enteric-coated capsules. Administration with omeprazole did not alter kinetics of budesonide capsules.

Dietary/Ethanol/Herb Considerations

Food: Capsule administration with a high-fat meal delays peak concentration, but does not alter the extent of absorption. Avoid grapefruit products with oral form; may double systemic exposure.

Herb/Nutraceutical: Avoid St John's wort; may decrease serum concentration.

Pharmacodynamics/Kinetics

Onset of action: Respules®: 2-8 days; Rhinocort® Aqua™: ~10 hours; Turbuhaler®: 24 hours
Peak effect: Respules®: 4-6 weeks; Rhinocort® Aqua™: ~2 weeks; Turbuhaler®: 1-2 weeks
Absorption: Capsule: Rapid and complete
Distribution: 2.2-3.9 L/kg
Protein binding: 85% to 90%
Metabolism: Hepatic via CYP3A4 to two metabolites: 16 alpha-hydroxyprednisolone and 6 beta-hydroxybudesonide; minor activity

(Continued)

Budesonide *(Continued)*

Bioavailability: Limited by high first-pass effect; Capsule: 9% to 21%; Respules®: 6%; Turbuhaler®: 6% to 13%; Nasal: 34%

Half-life elimination: 2-3.6 hours

Time to peak: Capsule: 30-600 minutes (variable in Crohn's disease); Respules®: 10-30 minutes; Turbuhaler®: 1-2 hours; Nasal: 1 hour

Excretion: Urine (60%) and feces as metabolites

Pregnancy Risk Factor C/B (Pulmicort Turbuhaler®)

Generic Available No

Bufferin® [OTC] *see* Aspirin *on page 131*

Bufferin® Arthritis Strength [OTC] *see* Aspirin *on page 131*

Bufferin® Extra Strength [OTC] *see* Aspirin *on page 131*

Bumetanide (byoo MET a nide)

Related Information

Cardiovascular Diseases *on page 1456*

U.S. Brand Names Bumex®

Canadian Brand Names Bumex®; Burinex®

Mexican Brand Names Bumedyl®; Drenural®; Miccil®

Pharmacologic Category Diuretic, Loop

Use Management of edema secondary to CHF or hepatic or renal disease including nephrotic syndrome; may be used alone or in combination with antihypertensives in the treatment of hypertension; can be used in furosemide-allergic patients

Local Anesthetic/Vasoconstrictor Precautions No information available to require special precautions

Effects on Dental Treatment 1%: Dizziness, muscle cramps

Dosage

Oral, I.M., I.V.:

- Neonates: 0.01-0.05 mg/kg/dose every 24-48 hours
- Infants and Children: 0.015-0.1 mg/kg/dose every 6-24 hours (maximum dose: 10 mg/day)

Adults:

- Edema:
  - Oral: 0.5-2 mg/dose (maximum dose: 10 mg/day) 1-2 times/day
  - I.M., I.V.: 0.5-1 mg/dose; may repeat in 2-3 hours for up to 2 doses if needed (maximum dose: 10 mg/day)
  - Continuous I.V. infusion: 0.9-1 mg/hour
- Hypertension: Oral: 0.5 mg daily (range: 1-4 mg/day, maximum dose: 5 mg/day); for larger doses, divide into 2-3 doses daily

Mechanism of Action Inhibits reabsorption of sodium and chloride in the ascending loop of Henle and proximal renal tubule, interfering with the chloride-binding cotransport system, thus causing increased excretion of water, sodium, chloride, magnesium, phosphate and calcium; it does not appear to act on the distal tubule

Other Adverse Effects

>10%:

- Endocrine & metabolic: Hyperuricemia (18%), hypochloremia (15%), hypokalemia (15%)
- Renal: Azotemia (11%)

1% to 10%:

- Endocrine & metabolic: Hyponatremia (9%), hyperglycemia (7%), variations in phosphorus (5%), CO_2 content (4%), bicarbonate (3%), and calcium (2%)
- Otic: Ototoxicity (1%)
- Renal: Increased serum creatinine (7%)

<1% (Limited to important or life-threatening): **Hypotension, orthostatic hypotension, headache, nausea**, encephalopathy (in patients with pre-existing liver disease), impaired hearing, pruritus, **weakness, hives, abdominal pain, arthritic pain, musculoskeletal pain,** rash, **vomiting**, vertigo, **chest pain**, ear discomfort, fatigue, **dehydration, diaphoresis, hyperventilation**, upset stomach, renal failure, asterixis, itching, nipple tenderness, diarrhea, premature ejaculation, hypernatremia, **xerostomia**

Drug Interactions

Increased Effect/Toxicity:

Bumetanide-induced hypokalemia may predispose to digoxin toxicity and may increase the risk of arrhythmia with drugs which may prolong QT interval, including type Ia and type III antiarrhythmic agents, cisapride, and some quinolones (sparfloxacin, gatifloxacin, and moxifloxacin). The risk of toxicity from lithium and salicylates (high dose) may be increased by loop diuretics. Hypotensive effects and/or adverse renal effects of ACE inhibitors and NSAIDs are potentiated by bumetanide-induced hypovolemia. The effects of peripheral adrenergic-blocking drugs or ganglionic blockers may be increased by bumetanide.

Bumetanide may increase the risk of ototoxicity with other ototoxic agents (aminoglycosides, cis-platinum), especially in patients with renal dysfunction.

Synergistic diuretic effects occur with thiazide-type diuretics. Diuretics tend to be synergistic with other antihypertensive agents, and hypotension may occur.

Decreased Effect: Glucose tolerance may be decreased by loop diuretics, requiring adjustment of hypoglycemic agents. Cholestyramine or colestipol may reduce bioavailability of bumetanide. Indomethacin (and other NSAIDs) may reduce natriuretic and hypotensive effects of diuretics. Hypokalemia may reduce the efficacy of some antiarrhythmics.

Dietary/Ethanol/Herb Considerations

Ethanol: Avoid use; has diuretic properties and may increase risk of dizziness or lightheadedness.

Food: Administer tablets with food to reduce GI upset. Increase intake of potassium-rich foods (citrus fruits, bananas); may cause a potassium loss requiring a potassium supplement or medication to help prevent potassium loss. Avoid caffeine (eg, colas, chocolate), garlic, and licorice.

Herb/Nutraceutical: Avoid black cohosh, dong quai, and evening primrose due to estrogenic activity. Avoid ephedra, ginseng, and yohimbe; may worsen hypertension. Avoid escin (from the horse chestnut seed); may have additive diuretic effects. Avoid garlic; may have increased antihypertensive effect. Avoid ginger due to positive inotropic effects; theoretically, may cause arrhythmia. Ginseng may decrease the effectiveness of loop diuretics (1 case report). Avoid hawthorn; may lower peripheral vascular resistance causing additional decrease in BP. Avoid licorice.

Pharmacodynamics/Kinetics

Onset of action: Oral, I.M.: 0.5-1 hour; I.V.: 2-3 minutes

Duration: 6 hours

Distribution: V_d: 13-25 L/kg

Protein binding: 95%

Metabolism: Partially hepatic

Half-life elimination: Infants <6 months: Possibly 2.5 hours; Children and Adults: 1-1.5 hours

Excretion: Primarily urine (as unchanged drug and metabolites)

Pregnancy Risk Factor C (manufacturer); D (expert analysis)

Generic Available Yes

Bumex® *see* Bumetanide *on page 204*

Buphenyl® *see* Sodium Phenylbutyrate *on page 1233*

Bupivacaine (byoo PIV a kane)

Related Information

Oral Pain *on page 1524*

U.S. Brand Names Marcaine®; Marcaine® Spinal; Sensorcaine®; Sensorcaine®-MPF

Canadian Brand Names Marcaine®; Sensorcaine®

Mexican Brand Names Buvacaina®

Pharmacologic Category Local Anesthetic

Synonyms Bupivacaine Hydrochloride

Use

Dental: Local anesthetic (injectable) for infiltration

Medical: Local anesthetic (injectable) for peripheral nerve block, infiltration, sympathetic block, caudal or epidural block, retrobulbar block

Local Anesthetic/Vasoconstrictor Precautions No information available to require special precautions

Effects on Dental Treatment Most effects are dose-related; CNS symptoms may be an early indication of more significant toxicity (seizures). Frequency not defined: Hypotension, heart block, bradycardia, palpitations, ventricular arrhythmias, cardiac arrest, restlessness, anxiety, dizziness, seizures, nausea, vomiting, weakness, blurred vision, apnea, allergic and anaphylactoid reactions, hypoventilation

Dosage Dose varies with procedure, depth of anesthesia, vascularity of tissues, duration of anesthesia and condition of patient. Some formulations contain metabisulfites (in epinephrine-containing injection); do not use solutions containing preservatives for caudal or epidural block.

Local anesthesia: Infiltration: 0.25% infiltrated locally; maximum: 175 mg

Caudal block (with or without epinephrine, preservative free):

Children: 1-3.7 mg/kg

Adults: 15-30 mL of 0.25% or 0.5%

Epidural block (other than caudal block - with or without epinephrine, preservative free):

Administer in 3-5 mL increments, allowing sufficient time to detect toxic manifestations of inadvertent I.V. or I.T. administration:

Children: 1.25 mg/kg/dose

Adults: 10-20 mL of 0.25% or 0.5%

Surgical procedures requiring a high degree of muscle relaxation and prolonged effects **only**: 10-20 mL of 0.75% (**Note:** Not to be used in obstetrical cases)

(Continued)

Bupivacaine *(Continued)*

Maxillary and mandibular infiltration and nerve block: 9 mg (1.8 mL) of 0.5% (with epinephrine) per injection site; a second dose may be administered if necessary to produce adequate anesthesia after allowing up to 10 minutes for onset, up to a maximum of 90 mg per dental appointment

Obstetrical anesthesia: Incremental dose: 3-5 mL of 0.5% (not exceeding 50-100 mg in any dosing interval); allow sufficient time to detect toxic manifestations or inadvertent I.V. or I.T. injection

Peripheral nerve block: 5 mL of 0.25 or 0.5%; maximum: 400 mg/day

Sympathetic nerve block: 20-50 mL of 0.25%

Retrobulbar anesthesia: 2-4 mL of 0.75%

Spinal anesthesia: Solution of 0.75% bupivacaine in 8.25% dextrose is used:
- Lower extremity and perineal procedures: 1 mL
- Lower abdominal procedures: 1.6 mL
- Obstetrical:
  - Normal vaginal delivery: 0.8 mL (higher doses may be required in some patients)
  - Cesarean section: 1-1.4 mL

Mechanism of Action Blocks both the initiation and conduction of nerve impulses by decreasing the neuronal membrane's permeability to sodium ions, which results in inhibition of depolarization with resultant blockade of conduction

Other Adverse Effects Most effects are dose-related and often due to accelerated absorption from the injection site, unintentional intravascular injection, or slow metabolic degradation. Frequency not defined:

Ocular: Pupillary constriction

Otic: Tinnitus

Rare symptoms (usually associated with unintentional subarachnoid injection during high spinal anesthesia):
- Cardiovascular: Persistent anesthesia, paresthesia, paralysis, headache, septic meningitis, and cranial nerve palsies
- Gastrointestinal: Fecal incontinence and loss of sphincter control
- Genitourinary: Urinary incontinence, loss of perineal sensation, and loss of sexual function

Contraindications Hypersensitivity to bupivacaine hydrochloride, amide-type local anesthetics (etidocaine, lidocaine, mepivacaine, prilocaine, ropivacaine) or any component of the formulation (para-aminobenzoic acid or parabens in specific formulations); not to be used for obstetrical paracervical block anesthesia

Warnings/Precautions Use with caution in patients with hepatic impairment. Some commercially available formulations contain sodium metabisulfite, which may cause allergic-type reactions; not recommended for use in children <12 years of age. The solution for spinal anesthesia should not be used in children <18 years of age. **Do not use solutions containing preservatives for caudal or epidural block**. Local anesthetics have been associated with rare occurrences of sudden respiratory arrest; convulsions due to systemic toxicity leading to cardiac arrest have also been reported, presumably following unintentional intravascular injection. The 0.75% is **not** recommended for obstetrical anesthesia. A test dose is recommended prior to epidural administration (prior to initial dose) and all reinforcing doses with continuous catheter technique.

Drug Interactions Substrate of CYP1A2, 2C19, 2D6, 3A4

Increased Effect: Hyaluronidase

Increased Toxicity: Beta-blockers, ergot-type oxytocics, MAO inhibitors, TCAs, phenothiazines, vasopressors

Pharmacodynamics/Kinetics

Onset of action: Anesthesia (route dependent): 4-10 minutes

Duration: 1.5-8.5 hours

Metabolism: Hepatic

Half-life elimination (age dependent): Neonates: 8.1 hours; Adults: 1.5-5.5 hours

Excretion: Urine (~6%)

Pregnancy Risk Factor C

Dosage Forms INJ, solution [preservative free]: 0.25% [2.5 mg/mL] (20 mL, 30 mL, 50 mL), 0.5% [5 mg/mL] (20 mL, 30 mL), 0.75% [7.5 mg/mL] (20 mL, 30 mL); (Marcaine®): 0.25% [2.5 mg/mL] (10 mL, 30 mL, 50 mL), 0.5% [5 mg/mL] (10 mL, 30 mL), 0.75% [7.5 mg/mL] (10 mL, 30 mL); (Marcaine® Spinal): 0.75% [7.5 mg/mL] (2 mL); (Sensorcaine®-MPF): 0.25% [2.5 mg/mL] (10 mL, 30 mL), 0.5% [5 mg/mL] (10 mL, 30 mL), 0.75% [7.5 mg/mL] (10 mL, 30 mL). **INJ, solution:** 0.25% [2.5 mg/mL] (10 mL, 30 mL, 50 mL), 0.5% [5 mg/mL] (10 mL, 30 mL, 50 mL), 0.75% [7.5 mg/mL] (10 mL, 30 mL); (Marcaine®, Sensorcaine®): 0.25% [2.5 mg/mL] (50 mL), 0.5% [5 mg/mL] (50 mL). **INJ, solution, with epinephrine 1:200,000** [preservative free]: (Marcaine®): 0.25% [2.5 mg/mL] (10 mL, 30 mL, 50 mL), 0.5% [5 mg/mL] (3 mL, 10 mL, 30 mL), 0.75% [7.5 mg/mL] (30 mL); (Sensorcaine®-MPF): 0.25% [2.5 mg/mL] (10 mL, 30 mL), 0.5% [5 mg/mL] (5 mL, 10 mL, 30 mL). **INJ, solution, with epinephrine 1:200,000** (Marcaine®, Sensorcaine®): 0.25% [2.5 mg/mL] (50 mL); 0.5% [5 mg/mL] (50 mL)

Generic Available Yes

Bupivacaine and Epinephrine (byoo PIV a kane & ep i NEF rin)

Related Information

Bupivacaine *on page 205*
Epinephrine *on page 499*
Oral Pain *on page 1524*

U.S. Brand Names Marcaine® with Epinephrine

Canadian Brand Names Sensorcaine® With Epinephrine

Pharmacologic Category Local Anesthetic, Dental; Local Anesthetic

Use Dental and Medical: Local anesthesia

Local Anesthetic/Vasoconstrictor Precautions No information available to require special precautions

Effects on Dental Treatment It is common to misinterpret psychogenic responses to local anesthetic injection as an allergic reaction. Intraoral injections are perceived by many patients as a stressful procedure in dentistry. Common symptoms to this stress are diaphoresis, palpitations, hyperventilation. Patients may exhibit hypersensitivity to bisulfites contained in local anesthetic solution to prevent oxidation of epinephrine. In general, patients reacting to bisulfites have a history of asthma and their airways are hyper-reactive to asthmatic syndrome.

Degree of adverse effects in the CNS and cardiovascular system is directly related to the blood levels of bupivacaine. (frequency not defined): Bradycardia, hypersensitivity reactions (rare; may be manifest as dermatologic reactions and edema at injection site), asthmatic syndromes

High blood levels: Anxiety, restlessness, disorientation, confusion, dizziness, tremors, seizures, CNS depression (resulting in somnolence, unconsciousness and possible respiratory arrest), nausea, vomiting

Dosage The effective anesthetic dose varies with procedure, intensity of anesthesia needed, duration of anesthesia required, and physical condition of the patient; always use the lowest effective dose along with careful aspiration.

The following numbers of dental carpules (1.8 mL) provide the indicated amounts of bupivacaine hydrochloride 0.5% and vasoconstrictor (epinephrine 1:200,000): See table.

# of Cartridges (1.8 mL)	Bupivacaine HCl (0.5%) (mg)	Epinephrine 1:200,000 (mg)
1	9	0.009
2	18	0.018
3	27	0.027
4	36	0.036
5	45	0.045
6	54	0.054
7	63	0.063
8	72	0.072
9	81	0.081
10	90	0.090

Children <10 years: Not established

Children >10 years and Adults: **Infiltration and nerve block in maxillary and mandibular area:** 9 mg (1.8 mL) of bupivacaine as a 0.5% solution with epinephrine 1:200,000 per injection site. A second dose may be administered if necessary to produce adequate anesthesia after allowing up to 10 minutes for onset; up to a maximum of 90 mg of bupivacaine hydrochloride per dental appointment.

Mechanism of Action Local anesthetics bind selectively to the intracellular surface of sodium channels to block influx of sodium into the axon. As a result, depolarization necessary for action potential propagation and subsequent nerve function is prevented. The block at the sodium channel is reversible. When drug diffuses away from the axon, sodium channel function is restored and nerve propagation returns.

Epinephrine prolongs the duration of the anesthetic actions of bupivacaine by causing vasoconstriction (alpha adrenergic receptor agonist) of the vasculature surrounding the nerve axons. This prevents the diffusion of bupivacaine away from the nerves resulting in a longer retention in the axon

Contraindications Hypersensitivity to bupivacaine or any component of the formulation

Warnings/Precautions Should be avoided in patients with uncontrolled hyperthyroidism

Pharmacodynamics/Kinetics

Onset of action: Infiltration and nerve block: 2-20 minutes
Duration: Infiltration: 1 hour; Nerve block: 5-7 hours
Half-life elimination, serum: Adults: 1.5-5.5 hours

Pregnancy Risk Factor C

Dosage Forms INJ: Bupivacaine hydrochloride 0.5% with epinephrine 1:200,000 (1.8 mL) [cartridge, 50/box]

(Continued)

Bupivacaine and Epinephrine *(Continued)*

Generic Available Yes

Selected Readings

Ayoub ST and Coleman AE, "A Review of Local Anesthetics," *Gen Dent*, 1992, 40(4):285-7, 289-90.
Jastak JT and Yagiela JA, "Vasoconstrictors and Local Anesthesia: A Review and Rationale for Use," *J Am Dent Assoc*, 1983, 107(4):623-30.
MacKenzie TA and Young ER, "Local Anesthetic Update," *Anesth Prog*, 1993, 40(2):29-34.
Wynn RL, "Epinephrine Interactions With Beta-Blockers," *Gen Dent*, 1994, 42(1):16, 18.
Yagiela JA, "Local Anesthetics," *Anesth Prog*, 1991, 38(4-5):128-41.

Bupivacaine Hydrochloride *see* Bupivacaine *on page 205*

Buprenex® *see* Buprenorphine *on page 208*

Buprenorphine (byoo pre NOR feen)

U.S. Brand Names Buprenex®; Subutex®

Canadian Brand Names Buprenex®

Mexican Brand Names Temgesic®

Pharmacologic Category Analgesic, Narcotic

Synonyms Buprenorphine Hydrochloride

Use

Injection: Management of moderate to severe pain

Tablet: Treatment of opioid dependence

Unlabeled/Investigational Use Injection: Treatment of heroin and opioid withdrawal symptoms

Local Anesthetic/Vasoconstrictor Precautions No information available to require special precautions

Effects on Dental Treatment

Injection:

>10%: Sedation

1% to 10%: Hypotension, respiratory depression, dizziness, headache, vomiting, nausea, diaphoresis

Tablet:

>10%: Headache (30%), anxiety (12%), nausea (10% to 14%), rhinitis (11%), infection (12% to 20%), diaphoresis (12% to 13%), pain (24%), weakness (14%)

1% to 10%: Nervousness (6%), somnolence (5%), dizziness (4%), fever (3%), vomiting (5% to 8%), cough (4%), pharyngitis (4%), flu-like syndrome (6%)

Restrictions Injection: C-V; Tablet: C-III

Prescribing of tablets for opioid dependence is limited to physicians who have met the qualification criteria and have received a DEA number specific to prescribing this product. Tablets will be available through pharmacies and wholesalers which normally provide controlled substances.

Dosage These are guidelines and do not represent the maximum doses that may be required in all patients. Doses should be titrated to pain relief/prevention. In high-risk patients (eg, elderly, debilitated, presence of respiratory disease) and/or concurrent CNS depressant use, reduce dose by one-half. Long-term use is not recommended; has an analgesic "ceiling".

Acute pain (moderate to severe):

Children 2-12 years: I.M., slow I.V.: 2-6 mcg/kg every 4-6 hours

Children ≥13 years and Adults:

I.M.: Initial: Opiate-naive: 0.3 mg every 6-8 hours as needed; initial dose (up to 0.3 mg) may be repeated once in 30-60 minutes after the initial dose if needed; usual dosage range: 0.15-0.6 mg every 4-8 hours as needed

Slow I.V.: Initial: Opiate-naive: 0.3 mg every 6-8 hours as needed; initial dose (up to 0.3 mg) may be repeated once in 30-60 minutes after the initial dose if needed

Elderly: 0.15 mg every 6 hours; elderly patients are more likely to suffer from confusion and drowsiness compared to younger patients

Heroin or opiate withdrawal (unlabeled use): Children ≥13 years and Adults: I.M., slow I.V.: Variable; 0.1-0.4 mg every 6 hours

Sublingual: Children ≥16 years and Adults: Opioid dependence:

Induction: Range: 12-16 mg/day (doses during an induction study used 8 mg on day 1, followed by 16 mg on day 2; induction continued over 3-4 days). Treatment should begin at least 4 hours after last use of heroin or short-acting opioid, preferably when first signs of withdrawal appear. Titrating dose to clinical effectiveness should be done as rapidly as possible to prevent undue withdrawal symptoms and patient drop-out during the induction period.

Maintenance: Target dose: 16 mg/day; range: 4-24 mg/day; patients should be switched to the buprenorphine/naloxone combination product for maintenance and unsupervised therapy

Mechanism of Action Buprenorphine exerts its analgesic effect via high affinity binding to μ opiate receptors in the CNS; displays both agonist and antagonist activity

Other Adverse Effects

Injection:

1% to 10%:

Ocular: Miosis

Otic: Vertigo

<1%: **Agitation, apnea**, appetite decreased, blurred vision, **bradycardia, confusion**, constipation, **convulsion, coma**, cyanosis, depersonalization, depression, diplopia, **dyspnea**, dysphoria, **euphoria, fatigue,** flatulence, **flushing, hallucinations, hypertension**, injection site reaction, malaise, **nervousness**, pallor, **paresthesia**, pruritus, **psychosis**, rash, slurred speech, **tachycardia**, tinnitus, **tremor**, urinary retention, urticaria, **weakness,** Wenckebach block, **xerostomia**

Tablet:

>10:

Central nervous system: Insomnia (21% to 25%), depression (11%),

Gastrointestinal: Abdominal pain (12%), constipation (8% to 11%)

Neuromuscular & skeletal: Back pain (14%)

Miscellaneous: Withdrawal syndrome (19%; placebo 37%)

1% to 10%:

Central nervous system: Chills (6%)

Gastrointestinal: Dyspepsia (3%)

Ocular: Lacrimation (5%)

Drug Interactions Substrate of **CYP3A4**

Increased Effect/Toxicity: Barbiturate anesthetics and other CNS depressants may produce additive respiratory and CNS depression. Respiratory and CV collapse was reported in a patient who received diazepam and buprenorphine. Effects may be additive with other CNS depressants. CYP3A4 inhibitors may increase serum levels/toxicity of buprenorphine (inhibitors include amiodarone, cimetidine, clarithromycin, erythromycin, delavirdine, diltiazem, dirithromycin, disulfiram, fluoxetine, fluvoxamine, grapefruit juice, indinavir, itraconazole, ketoconazole, nefazodone, nevirapine, propoxyphene, quinupristin-dalfopristin, ritonavir, saquinavir, verapamil, zafirlukast, and zileuton); monitor for altered effects; a decrease in buprenorphine dosage may be required.

Decreased Effect: Enzyme inducers may reduce serum concentrations of buprenorphine, resulting in loss of efficacy (includes barbiturates, carbamazepine, phenytoin rifabutin, and rifampin). Naltrexone may antagonize the effect of narcotic analgesics; concurrent use or use within 7-10 days of injection for pain relief is contraindicated.

Dietary/Ethanol/Herb Considerations

Ethanol: Avoid use; may increase CNS depression.

Herb/Nutraceutical: Avoid gotu kola, kava, SAMe, St John's wort, and valerian; may increase CNS depression.

Pharmacodynamics/Kinetics

Onset of action: Analgesic: 10-30 minutes

Duration: 6-8 hours

Absorption: I.M., S.C.: 30% to 40%

Distribution: V_d: 97-187 L/kg

Protein binding: High

Metabolism: Primarily hepatic; extensive first-pass effect

Half-life elimination: 2.2-3 hours

Excretion: Feces (70%); urine (20% as unchanged drug)

Pregnancy Risk Factor C

Generic Available Yes: Injection

Buprenorphine Hydrochloride *see* Buprenorphine *on page 208*

BuPROPion (byoo PROE pee on)

Related Information

Chemical Dependency and Smoking Cessation *on page 1574*

U.S. Brand Names Wellbutrin®; Wellbutrin SR®; Zyban®

Canadian Brand Names Wellbutrin®; Zyban®

Mexican Brand Names Wellbutrin®

Pharmacologic Category Antidepressant, Dopamine-Reuptake Inhibitor; Smoking Cessation Aid

Use Treatment of depression; adjunct in smoking cessation

Unlabeled/Investigational Use Treatment of attention-deficit/hyperactivity disorder (ADHD)

Local Anesthetic/Vasoconstrictor Precautions Although this is not a tricyclic antidepressant, it can cause hypertensive episodes and should be used with caution in the presence of a vasoconstrictor.

Effects on Dental Treatment

>10%: Significant xerostomia; normal salivary flow resumes with discontinuation

Frequency not defined: Arrhythmias, chest pain, flushing, hypertension (may be severe), hypotension, palpitations, syncope, tachycardia, agitation, anxiety, confusion, dizziness, euphoria, headache, hostility, irritability, decreased

(Continued)

BuPROPion *(Continued)*

memory, migraine, nervousness, somnolence, sweating, hot flashes, dysphagia, nausea, vomiting, abnormal taste, arthritis, neck pain, paresthesia, tremor, twitching, blurred vision, increased cough, pharyngitis, sinusitis, allergic reaction (anaphylaxis, pruritus, urticaria), infection

Dosage Oral:

Children and Adolescents: ADHD (unlabeled use): 1.4-6 mg/kg/day

Adults:

Depression:

Immediate release: 100 mg 3 times/day; begin at 100 mg twice daily; may increase to a maximum dose of 450 mg/day

Sustained release: Initial: 150 mg/day in the morning; may increase to 150 mg twice daily by day 4 if tolerated; target dose: 300 mg/day given as 150 mg twice daily; maximum dose: 400 mg/day given as 200 mg twice daily

Smoking cessation (Zyban®): Initiate with 150 mg once daily for 3 days; increase to 150 mg twice daily; treatment should continue for 7-12 weeks

Elderly: Depression: 50-100 mg/day, increase by 50-100 mg every 3-4 days as tolerated; there is evidence that the elderly respond at 150 mg/day in divided doses, but some may require a higher dose

Dosing comment in renal impairment: Reduction in initial dose required in renal failure; monitor patient closely (elimination of the major metabolites may be affected by reduced renal function; not studied)

Dosing adjustment in hepatic impairment:

Note: The mean AUC increased by ~1.5-fold for hydroxybupropion and ~2.5-fold for erythro/threohydrobupropion; median T_{max} was observed 19 hours later for hydroxybupropion, 31 hours later for erythro/threohydrobupropion; mean halflife for hydroxybupropion increased fivefold, and increased twofold for erythro/threohydrobupropion in patients with severe hepatic cirrhosis compared to healthy volunteers.

Mild to moderate hepatic impairment: Use with caution and/or reduced dose/frequency

Severe hepatic cirrhosis: Use with extreme caution; maximum dose:

Wellbutrin®: 75 mg/day

Wellbutrin SR®: 100 mg/day or 150 mg every other day

Zyban®: 150 mg every other day

Mechanism of Action Aminoketone antidepressant structurally different from all other previously marketed antidepressants; like other antidepressants the mechanism of bupropion's activity is not fully understood; weak inhibitor of the neuronal uptake of serotonin, norepinephrine, and dopamine, and does not inhibit monoamine oxidase.

Other Adverse Effects Frequency not defined:

Central nervous system: Insomnia, sleep disturbance

Dermatologic: Pruritus, rash, urticaria

Endocrine & metabolic: Libido decreased, menstrual complaints

Gastrointestinal: Abdominal pain, anorexia, appetite increased, constipation, diarrhea, dyspepsia

Genitourinary: Urinary frequency

Neuromuscular & skeletal: Arthralgia, arthritis, myalgia

Ocular: Amblyopia

Otic: Auditory disturbance, tinnitus

Postmarketing and/or case reports: Accommodation abnormality, akinesia, alopecia, amnesia, anemia, angioedema, aphasia, ataxia, atrioventricular block, **bronchospasm, bruxism**, chills, colitis, **coma, coordination abnormal,** cystitis, deafness, delirium, depersonalization, derealization, diplopia, dry eyes, dry skin, dysarthria, dyskinesia, dyspareunia, dysphoria, **dyspnea**, dystonia, dysuria, **ecchymosis,** edema, EEG abnormality, ejaculation abnormality, emotional lability, enuresis, **epistaxis, esophagitis**, exfoliative dermatitis, **extrapyramidal syndrome, extrasystoles, facial edema, fever with rash (and other symptoms suggestive of delayed hypersensitivity resembling serum sickness), flushing, frigidity, gastric reflux, GI hemorrhage, gingivitis, glossitis**, glycosuria, **gum hemorrhage**, gynecomastia, hepatic damage, hepatitis, hirsutism, **hyperglycemia**, hyperkinesia, hypertonia, hypesthesia, **hypoglycemia**, hypokinesia, hypomania, impotence, intestinal perforation, jaundice, **leg cramps,** leukocytosis, leukopenia, libido increased, **lymphadenopathy,** maculopapular rash, **malaise, manic reaction, oral ulceration, muscle rigidity, muscle weakness, musculoskeletal chest pain**, mydriasis, **MI, myoclonus,** neuralgia, neuropathy, nocturia, painful erection, pallor, pancreatitis, pancytopenia, paranoia, **paranoid reaction**, peripheral edema, phlebitis, photosensitivity, polyuria, **postural hypotension**, prostate disorder, pulmonary embolism, rhabdomyolysis, **increase in salivation**, salpingitis, **sciatica, seizure**, SIADH, **stomach ulcer, stomatitis, stroke, suicidal ideation, tardive dyskinesia**, testicular swelling, **thirst, tongue edema**, thrombocytopenia, urinary incontinence, urinary retention, vaginal irritation, vaginitis, **vasodilation**, vertigo

Drug Interactions Substrate of CYP1A2, 2A6, **2B6**, 2C8/9, 2D6, 2E1, 3A4; Inhibits **CYP2D6**

Increased Effect/Toxicity: Treatment-emergent hypertension may occur in patients treated with bupropion and nicotine patch. Cimetidine may inhibit the metabolism (increase clinical/adverse effects) of bupropion. Toxicity of bupropion is enhanced by levodopa and phenelzine (MAO inhibitors). Risk of seizures may be increased with agents that may lower seizure threshold (antipsychotics, antidepressants, theophylline, abrupt discontinuation of benzodiazepines, systemic steroids). Effect of warfarin may be altered by bupropion. Concurrent use with amantadine appears to result in a higher incidence of adverse effects; use caution.

Decreased Effect: Carbamazepine, phenobarbital, and phenytoin may increase the metabolism (decrease clinical effect) of bupropion. Effect of warfarin may be altered by bupropion.

Dietary/Ethanol/Herb Considerations

Ethanol: Avoid use; may lower seizure threshold and increase CNS depression.

Herb/Nutraceutical: Avoid gotu kola, kava, SAMe, St John's wort, and valerian; may increase CNS depression.

Pharmacodynamics/Kinetics

Absorption: Rapid

Distribution: V_d: 19-21 L/kg

Protein binding: 82% to 88%

Metabolism: Extensively hepatic to 3 active metabolites: Hydroxybupropion, erythrohydrobupropion, threohydrobupropion

Bioavailability: 5% to 20% in animals

Half-life:

Distribution: 3-4 hours

Elimination: 21 ± 9 hours; Metabolites: Hydroxybupropion: 20 ± 5 hours; Erythrohydrobupropion: 33 ± 10 hours; Threohydrobupropion: 37 ± 13 hours

Time to peak, serum: Bupropion: ~3 hours

Metabolites: Hydroxybupropion, erythrohydrobupropion, threohydrobupropion: 6 hours

Excretion: Urine (87%); feces (10%)

Pregnancy Risk Factor B

Generic Available Yes: Wellbutrin® strength only

Burnamycin [OTC] *see* Lidocaine *on page 801*

Burn Jel [OTC] *see* Lidocaine *on page 801*

Burn-O-Jel [OTC] *see* Lidocaine *on page 801*

Burow's Otic *see* Aluminum Acetate and Acetic Acid *on page 67*

BuSpar® *see* BusPIRone *on page 211*

BusPIRone (byoo SPYE rone)

Related Information

Patients Requiring Sedation *on page 1565*

U.S. Brand Names BuSpar®

Canadian Brand Names Apo®-Buspirone; BuSpar®; Buspirex; Gen-Buspirone; Lin-Buspirone; Novo-Buspirone; Nu-Buspirone; PMS-Buspirone

Mexican Brand Names Neurosine®

Pharmacologic Category Antianxiety Agent, Miscellaneous

Synonyms Buspirone Hydrochloride

Use Management of generalized anxiety disorder (GAD)

Unlabeled/Investigational Use Management of aggression in mental retardation and secondary mental disorders; treatment of major depression, premenstrual syndrome; potential augmenting agent for antidepressants

Local Anesthetic/Vasoconstrictor Precautions No information available to require special precautions

Effects on Dental Treatment

>10%: Dizziness

1% to 10%: Drowsiness, EPS, serotonin syndrome, confusion, nervousness, lightheadedness, excitement, anger, hostility, headache, nausea, paresthesia, tremor, diaphoresis, allergic reactions, xerostomia, weakness, numbness, incoordination, blurred vision, tunnel vision

Dosage Oral:

Generalized anxiety disorder:

Children and Adolescents: Initial: 5 mg daily; increase in increments of 5 mg/day at weekly intervals as needed, to a maximum dose of 60 mg/day divided into 2-3 doses

Adults: 15 mg/day (7.5 mg twice daily); may increase in increments of 5 mg/day every 2-4 days to a maximum of 60 mg/day; target dose for most people is 30 mg/day (15 mg twice daily)

Dosing adjustment in renal or hepatic impairment: Buspirone is metabolized by the liver and excreted by the kidneys. Patients with impaired hepatic or renal function demonstrated increased plasma levels and a prolonged halflife of buspirone. Therefore, use in patients with severe hepatic or renal impairment cannot be recommended.

(Continued)

BusPIRone *(Continued)*

Mechanism of Action The mechanism of action of buspirone is unknown. Buspirone has a high affinity for serotonin 5-HT_{1A} and 5-HT_2 receptors, without affecting benzodiazepine-GABA receptors; buspirone has moderate affinity for dopamine D_2 receptors

Other Adverse Effects 1% to 10%:

Dermatologic: Rash

Gastrointestinal: Diarrhea

Drug Interactions Substrate of CYP2D6, **3A4**

Increased Effect/Toxicity: Concurrent use of buspirone with SSRIs or trazodone may cause serotonin syndrome. Erythromycin, clarithromycin, diltiazem, itraconazole, ketoconazole, verapamil, and grapefruit juice may result in increases in buspirone concentrations. Buspirone should not be used concurrently with an MAO inhibitor due to reports of increased blood pressure; theoretically, a selective MAO type B inhibitors (selegiline) has a lower risk of this reaction. Concurrent use of buspirone with nefazodone may increase risk of CNS adverse events; limit buspirone initial dose (eg, 2.5 mg/day).

Decreased Effect: Enzyme inducers (phenobarbital, carbamazepine, phenytoin, rifampin) may reduce serum concentrations of buspirone resulting in loss of efficacy.

Dietary/Ethanol/Herb Considerations

Ethanol: Avoid use; may increase CNS depression.

Food may decrease absorption but may also decrease first-pass metabolism, thereby increasing bioavailability. Avoid grapefruit products; may cause increased serum concentration.

Herb/Nutraceutical: Avoid gotu kola, kava, SAMe, and valerian; may increase CNS depression. Avoid St John's wort; may decrease serum concentration and increase CNS depression.

Pharmacodynamics/Kinetics

Protein binding: 95%

Metabolism: Hepatic via oxidation; extensive first-pass effect

Half-life elimination: 2-3 hours

Time to peak, serum: Within 0.7-1.5 hours

Pregnancy Risk Factor B

Generic Available Yes

Buspirone Hydrochloride *see* BusPIRone *on page 211*

Busulfan (byoo SUL fan)

U.S. Brand Names Busulfex®; Myleran®

Canadian Brand Names Busulfex®; Myleran®

Mexican Brand Names Myleran®

Pharmacologic Category Antineoplastic Agent, Alkylating Agent

Use

Oral: Chronic myelogenous leukemia and bone marrow disorders, such as polycythemia vera and myeloid metaplasia, conditioning regimens for bone marrow transplantation

I.V.: Combination therapy with cyclophosphamide as a conditioning regimen prior to allogeneic hematopoietic progenitor cell transplantation for chronic myelogenous leukemia

Local Anesthetic/Vasoconstrictor Precautions No information available to require special precautions

Effects on Dental Treatment >10%: Nausea, vomiting 1% to 10%: Weakness

Dosage Busulfan should be based on adjusted ideal body weight because actual body weight, ideal body weight, or other factors can produce significant differences in busulfan clearance among lean, normal, and obese patients; refer to individual protocols

Children:

For remission induction of CML: Oral: 0.06-0.12 mg/kg/day **OR** 1.8-4.6 mg/m^2/day; titrate dosage to maintain leukocyte count above 40,000/mm^3; reduce dosage by 50% if the leukocyte count reaches 30,000-40,000/mm^3; discontinue drug if counts fall to ≤20,000/mm^3

BMT marrow-ablative conditioning regimen:

Oral: 1 mg/kg/dose (ideal body weight) every 6 hours for 16 doses

I.V.:

≤12 kg: 1.1 mg/kg/dose (ideal body weight) every 6 hours for 16 doses

>12 kg: 0.8 mg/kg/dose (ideal body weight) every 6 hours for 16 doses

Adjust dose to desired AUC [1125 μmol(min)] using the following formula:

Adjusted dose (mg) = Actual dose (mg) x [target AUC μmol(min) / actual AUC μmol(min)]

Adults:

For remission induction of CML: Oral: 4-8 mg/day (may be as high as 12 mg/day); Maintenance doses: Controversial, range from 1-4 mg/day to 2 mg/week; treatment is continued until WBC reaches 10,000-20,000 cells/mm^3 at which time drug is discontinued; when WBC reaches 50,000/mm^3, maintenance dose is resumed

BMT marrow-ablative conditioning regimen:

Oral: 1 mg/kg/dose (ideal body weight) every 6 hours for 16 doses

I.V.: 0.8 mg/kg (ideal body weight or actual body weight, whichever is lower) every 6 hours for 4 days (a total of 16 doses)

I.V. dosing in morbidly obese patients: Dosing should be based on adjusted ideal body weight (AIBW) which should be calculated as ideal body weight (IBW) + 0.25 times (actual weight minus ideal body weight)

AIBW = IBW + 0.25 x (AW - IBW)

Cyclophosphamide, in combination with busulfan, is given on each of two days as a 1-hour infusion at a dose of 160 mg/m^2 beginning on BMT day -3, 6 hours following the 16th dose of busulfan

Unapproved use:

Polycythemia vera: 2-6 mg/day

Thrombocytosis: 4-6 mg/day

Mechanism of Action Reacts with N-7 position of guanosine and interferes with DNA replication and transcription of RNA. Busulfan has a more marked effect on myeloid cells (and is, therefore, useful in the treatment of CML) than on lymphoid cells. The drug is also very toxic to hematopoietic stem cells (thus its usefulness in high doses in BMT preparative regimens). Busulfan exhibits little immunosuppressive activity. Interferes with the normal function of DNA by alkylation and cross-linking the strands of DNA.

Other Adverse Effects

>10%: Hematologic: Severe pancytopenia, leukopenia, thrombocytopenia, anemia, and bone marrow suppression are common and patients should be monitored closely while on therapy. Since this is a delayed effect (busulfan affects the stem cells), the drug should be discontinued temporarily at the first sign of a large or rapid fall in any blood element. Some patients may develop bone marrow fibrosis or chronic aplasia which is probably due to the busulfan toxicity. In large doses, busulfan is myeloablative and is used for this reason in BMT. Myelosuppressive:

WBC: Moderate

Platelets: Moderate

Onset: 7-10 days

Nadir: 14-21 days

Recovery: 28 days

1% to 10%:

Dermatologic: Hyperpigmentation skin (busulfan tan), urticaria, erythema, alopecia

Endocrine & metabolic: Amenorrhea

Gastrointestinal: Diarrhea

<1%: Endocardial fibrosis, adrenal suppression, gynecomastia, hyperuricemia, hemorrhagic cystitis (rare), hepatic dysfunction, blurred vision, cataracts, **"busulfan lung syndrome" (after long-term or high-dose therapy; manifested by a diffuse interstitial pulmonary fibrosis and persistent cough, fever, rales, dyspnea and may be relieved by corticosteroids)**

Frequency not defined: Fertility/carcinogenesis: Sterility, ovarian suppression, amenorrhea, azoospermia, testicular atrophy, malignant tumors

Drug Interactions Substrate of **CYP3A4**

Increased Effect/Toxicity: Itraconazole or other cytotoxic agents may increase risk of pulmonary toxicity. CYP3A4 inhibitors, itraconazole, or other cytotoxic agents may increase risk of pulmonary toxicity.

Dietary/Ethanol/Herb Considerations

Ethanol: Avoid use due to GI irritation.

Herb/Nutraceutical: Avoid St John's wort; may decrease serum concentration.

Pharmacodynamics/Kinetics

Duration: 28 days

Absorption: Rapid and complete

Distribution: V_d: ~1 L/kg; into CSF and saliva with levels similar to plasma

Protein binding: ~14%

Metabolism: Extensively hepatic (may increase with multiple doses)

Half-life elimination: After first dose: 3.4 hours; After last dose: 2.3 hours

Time to peak, serum: Oral: Within 4 hours; I.V.: Within 5 minutes

Excretion: Urine (10% to 50% as metabolites) within 24 hours (<2% as unchanged drug)

Pregnancy Risk Factor D

Generic Available No

Busulfex® *see* Busulfan *on page 212*

Butabarbital Sodium (byoo ta BAR bi tal)

U.S. Brand Names Butisol Sodium®

Pharmacologic Category Barbiturate

Use Sedative; hypnotic

Local Anesthetic/Vasoconstrictor Precautions No information available to require special precautions

(Continued)

Butabarbital Sodium *(Continued)*

Effects on Dental Treatment

>10%: Dizziness, lightheadedness, drowsiness, "hangover" effect,

1% to 10%: Confusion, unusual excitement, nervousness, faint feeling, headache, nausea, vomiting

Restrictions C-III

Dosage Oral:

Children: Preoperative sedation: 2-6 mg/kg/dose (maximum: 100 mg)

Adults:

Sedative: 15-30 mg 3-4 times/day

Hypnotic: 50-100 mg

Preop: 50-100 mg 1-1½ hours before surgery

Mechanism of Action Interferes with transmission of impulses from the thalamus to the cortex of the brain resulting in an imbalance in central inhibitory and facilitatory mechanisms

Other Adverse Effects

1% to 10%:

Central nervous system: Mental depression, insomnia, nightmares

Gastrointestinal: Constipation

<1%: Agranulocytosis, angioedema, dependence, exfoliative dermatitis, **hallucinations, hypotension**, megaloblastic anemia, rash, **respiratory depression**, Stevens-Johnson syndrome, thrombocytopenia, thrombophlebitis

Drug Interactions Barbiturates are cytochrome P450 enzyme inducers. Patients should be monitored when these drugs are started or stopped for a decreased or increased therapeutic effect respectively.

Increased Effect/Toxicity: When butabarbital is combined with other CNS depressants, ethanol, narcotic analgesics, antidepressants, or benzodiazepines, additive respiratory and CNS depression may occur. Barbiturates may enhance the hepatotoxic potential of acetaminophen overdoses. Chloramphenicol, MAO inhibitors, valproic acid, and felbamate may inhibit barbiturate metabolism. Barbiturates may impair the absorption of griseofulvin, and may enhance the nephrotoxic effects of methoxyflurane.

Decreased Effect: Barbiturates such as butabarbital are hepatic enzyme inducers, and may increase the metabolism of antipsychotics, some beta-blockers (unlikely with atenolol and nadolol), calcium channel blockers, chloramphenicol, cimetidine, corticosteroids, cyclosporine, disopyramide, doxycycline, ethosuximide, felbamate, furosemide, griseofulvin, lamotrigine, phenytoin, propafenone, quinidine, tacrolimus, TCAs, and theophylline. Barbiturates may increase the metabolism of estrogens and reduce the efficacy of oral contraceptives; an alternative method of contraception should be considered. Barbiturates inhibit the hypoprothrombinemic effects of oral anticoagulants via increased metabolism. Barbiturates may enhance the metabolism of methadone resulting in methadone withdrawal.

Dietary/Ethanol/Herb Considerations

Ethanol: Avoid use; may increase CNS depression.

Herb/Nutraceutical: Avoid gotu kola, kava, SAMe, St John's wort, and valerian; may increase CNS depression.

Pharmacodynamics/Kinetics

Distribution: V_d: 0.8 L/kg

Protein binding: 26%

Metabolism: Hepatic

Half-life elimination: 1.6 days to 5.8 days

Time to peak, serum: 40-60 minutes

Excretion: Urine (as metabolites)

Pregnancy Risk Factor D

Generic Available Yes

Butalbital, Acetaminophen, and Caffeine

(byoo TAL bi tal, a seet a MIN oh fen, & KAF een)

Related Information

Acetaminophen *on page 27*

U.S. Brand Names Esgic®; Esgic-Plus™; Fioricet®; Repan®

Pharmacologic Category Barbiturate

Synonyms Acetaminophen, Butalbital, and Caffeine

Use Relief of the symptomatic complex of tension or muscle contraction headache

Local Anesthetic/Vasoconstrictor Precautions No information available to require special precautions

Effects on Dental Treatment

>10%: Dizziness, lightheadedness, drowsiness, "hangover" effect, nausea, epigastric discomfort

1% to 10%: Confusion, unusual excitement, nervousness, faint feeling, headache, vomiting, GI ulceration, troubled breathing, anaphylactic shock, weakness, fatigue

Dosage Oral:

Adults: 1-2 tablets or capsules every 4 hours; not to exceed 6/day

Dosing interval in renal or hepatic impairment: Should be reduced

Other Adverse Effects

>10%: Gastrointestinal: Heartburn, stomach pains, dyspepsia

1% to 10%:

Central nervous system: Mental depression, insomnia, nightmares

Dermatologic: Skin rash

Gastrointestinal: Constipation

Hematologic: Hemolytic anemia

Drug Interactions

Increased Effect/Toxicity: MAO inhibitors may enhance CNS effects of butalbital. Increased effect (CNS depression) with narcotic analgesics, ethanol, general anesthetics, tranquilizers such as chlordiazepoxide, sedative hypnotics, or other CNS depressants.

Decreased Effect: Butalbital may diminish effects of uricosuric agents such as probenecid and sulfinpyrazone.

Dietary/Ethanol/Herb Considerations

Ethanol: Avoid use; may increase CNS depression.

Herb/Nutraceutical: Avoid gotu kola, kava, SAMe, St John's wort, and valerian; may increase CNS depression.

Pregnancy Risk Factor D

Generic Available Yes

Selected Readings

Botting RM, "Mechanism of Action of Acetaminophen: Is There a Cyclooxygenase 3?," *Clin Infect Dis*, 2000, Suppl 5:S202-10.

Dart RC, Kuffner EK, and Rumack BH, "Treatment of Pain or Fever with Paracetamol (Acetaminophen) in the Alcoholic Patient: A Systematic Review," *Am J Ther*, 2000, 7(2):123-34.

Grant JA and Weiler JM, "A Report of a Rare Immediate Reaction After Ingestion of Acetaminophen," *Ann Allergy Asthma Immunol*, 2001, 87(3):227-9.

Kwan D, Bartle WR, and Walker SE, "The Effects of Acetaminophen on Pharmacokinetics and Pharmacodynamics of Warfarin," *J Clin Pharmacol*, 1999, 39(1):68-75.

McClain CJ, Price S, Barve S, et al, "Acetaminophen Hepatotoxicity: An Update," *Curr Gastroenterol Rep*, 1999, 1(1):42-9.

Shek KL, Chan LN, and Nutescu E, "Warfarin-Acetaminophen Drug Interaction Revisited," *Pharmacotherapy*, 1999, 19(10):1153-8.

Tanaka E, Yamazaki K, and Misawa S, "Update: The Clinical Importance of Acetaminophen Hepatotoxicity in Nonalcoholic and Alcoholic Subjects," *J Clin Pharm Ther*, 2000, 25(5):325-32.

Butalbital, Acetaminophen, Caffeine, and Codeine

(byoo TAL bi tal, a seet a MIN oh fen, KAF een, & KOE deen)

Related Information

Acetaminophen *on page 27*

Codeine *on page 361*

U.S. Brand Names Fioricet® with Codeine

Pharmacologic Category Analgesic Combination (Narcotic); Barbiturate

Synonyms Acetaminophen, Caffeine, Codeine, and Butalbital; Caffeine, Acetaminophen, Butalbital, and Codeine; Codeine, Acetaminophen, Butalbital, and Caffeine

Use Dental and Medical: Relief of symptoms of complex tension (muscle contraction) headache

Local Anesthetic/Vasoconstrictor Precautions No information available to require special precautions

Effects on Dental Treatment Frequency not defined: Tachycardia, palpitations, hypotension, syncope, drowsiness, fatigue, mental confusion, disorientation, nervousness, hallucination, euphoria, seizure, headache, agitation, fainting, excitement, fever, nausea, xerostomia, GI spasm, leg pain, weakness, numbness, allergic reaction, anaphylaxis, agranulocytosis, irritability, nausea, thrombocytopenia, tremors, vomiting

Restrictions C-III

Dosage Oral: Adults: 1-2 capsules every 4 hours; total daily dosage should not exceed 6 capsules.

Dosing comment in hepatic impairment: Avoid chronic use; limited, low-dose therapy usually well tolerated, however, cases of hepatotoxicity at daily acetaminophen dosages <4 g/day have been reported.

Mechanism of Action Combination product for the treatment of tension headache. Contains codeine (narcotic analgesic), butalbital (barbiturate), caffeine (CNS stimulant), and acetaminophen (nonopiate, nonsalicylate analgesic).

Other Adverse Effects Frequency not defined:

Cardiovascular: Edema

Central nervous system: Depression

Dermatologic: Rash, erythema, pruritus, urticaria, erythema multiforme, exfoliative dermatitis, toxic epidermal necrolysis

Gastrointestinal: Constipation heartburn, flatulence

Genitourinary: Urinary retention, diuresis

Otic: Tinnitus

(Continued)

Butalbital, Acetaminophen, Caffeine, and Codeine *(Continued)*

Contraindications Hypersensitivity to butalbital, codeine, caffeine, acetaminophen, or any component of the formulation; porphyria; known G6PD deficiency; pregnancy (prolonged use or high doses at term)

Warnings/Precautions May cause severe hepatic toxicity on overdose; use with caution in patients with alcoholic liver disease; chronic daily dosing in adults of 5-8 g of acetaminophen over several weeks or 3-4 g/day of acetaminophen for 1 year have resulted in liver damage. Use with caution in patients with hypersensitivity reactions to other phenanthrene derivative opioid agonists (eg, morphine, hydrocodone, oxycodone). Use caution with Addison's disease, severe renal or hepatic impairment. Use caution in patients with head injury or other intracranial lesions, acute abdominal conditions, urethral stricture of BPH, or in patients with respiratory diseases. Elderly and/or debilitated patients may be more susceptible to CNS depressants, as well as constipating effects of narcotics. Tolerance or drug dependence may result from extended use. Safety and efficacy in pediatric patients have not been established.

Dietary/Ethanol/Herb Considerations

Ethanol: Avoid use; may increase CNS depression.

Herb/Nutraceutical: Avoid gotu kola, kava, SAMe, St John's wort, and valerian; may increase CNS depression.

Pregnancy Risk Factor C (per manufacturer)/D (prolonged use or high doses at term)

Breast-feeding Considerations Codeine, caffeine, barbiturates, and acetaminophen are excreted in breast milk in small amounts. Discontinuation of breast-feeding or discontinuation of the drug should be considered.

Dosage Forms CAP: Butalbital 50 mg, caffeine 40 mg, acetaminophen 325 mg, and codeine phosphate 30 mg

Generic Available Yes

Selected Readings

Botting RM, "Mechanism of Action of Acetaminophen: Is There a Cyclooxygenase 3?," *Clin Infect Dis*, 2000, Suppl 5:S202-10.

Dart RC, Kuffner EK, and Rumack BH, "Treatment of Pain or Fever with Paracetamol (Acetaminophen) in the Alcoholic Patient: A Systematic Review," *Am J Ther*, 2000, 7(2):123-34.

Grant JA and Weiler JM, "A Report of a Rare Immediate Reaction After Ingestion of Acetaminophen," *Ann Allergy Asthma Immunol*, 2001, 87(3):227-9.

Kwan D, Bartle WR, and Walker SE, "The Effects of Acetaminophen on Pharmacokinetics and Pharmacodynamics of Warfarin," *J Clin Pharmacol*, 1999, 39(1):68-75.

McClain CJ, Price S, Barve S, et al, "Acetaminophen Hepatotoxicity: An Update," *Curr Gastroenterol Rep*, 1999, 1(1):42-9.

Shek KL, Chan LN, and Nutescu E, "Warfarin-Acetaminophen Drug Interaction Revisited," *Pharmacotherapy*, 1999, 19(10):1153-8.

Tanaka E, Yamazaki K, and Misawa S, "Update: The Clinical Importance of Acetaminophen Hepatotoxicity in Nonalcoholic and Alcoholic Subjects," *J Clin Pharm Ther*, 2000, 25(5):325-32.

Butalbital, Aspirin, and Caffeine

(byoo TAL bi tal, AS pir in, & KAF een)

Related Information

Aspirin *on page 131*

U.S. Brand Names Fiorinal®

Canadian Brand Names Fiorinal®

Pharmacologic Category Barbiturate

Synonyms Aspirin, Caffeine, and Butalbital; Butalbital Compound

Use Relief of the symptomatic complex of tension or muscle contraction headache

Local Anesthetic/Vasoconstrictor Precautions No information available to require special precautions

Effects on Dental Treatment

>10%: Dizziness, lightheadedness, drowsiness, "hangover" effect, nausea, epigastric discomfort

1% to 10%: Confusion, unusual excitement, nervousness, faint feeling, headache, vomiting, GI ulceration, troubled breathing, anaphylactic shock, weakness, fatigue

Avoid aspirin products, if possible, for 1 week prior to surgery due to possibility of postoperative bleeding.

Restrictions C-III

Dosage Oral:

Adults: 1-2 tablets or capsules every 4 hours; not to exceed 6/day

Dosing interval in renal or hepatic impairment: Should be reduced

Other Adverse Effects

>10%: Gastrointestinal: Heartburn, stomach pains, dyspepsia

1% to 10%:

- Central nervous system: Mental depression, insomnia, nightmares
- Dermatologic: Skin rash
- Gastrointestinal: Constipation
- Hematologic: Hemolytic anemia

Drug Interactions

Increased Effect/Toxicity: Enhanced effect/toxicity with oral anticoagulants (warfarin), oral antidiabetic agents, insulin, 6-mercaptopurine, methotrexate, NSAIDs, narcotic analgesics (propoxyphene, meperidine, etc), benzodiazepines, sedative-hypnotics, other CNS depressants. The CNS effects of butalbital may be enhanced by MAO inhibitors.

Decreased Effect: May decrease the effect of uricosuric agents (probenecid and sulfinpyrazone) reducing their effect on gout.

Dietary/Ethanol/Herb Considerations

Ethanol: Avoid use; may increase CNS depression.

Herb/Nutraceutical: Avoid gotu kola, kava, SAMe, St John's wort, and valerian; may increase CNS depression.

Pregnancy Risk Factor C/D (prolonged use or high doses at term)

Generic Available Yes

Butalbital, Aspirin, Caffeine, and Codeine

(byoo TAL bi tal, AS pir in, KAF een, & KOE deen)

Related Information

Aspirin *on page 131*

Codeine *on page 361*

U.S. Brand Names Fiorinal® With Codeine

Canadian Brand Names Fiorinal®-C 1/2; Fiorinal®-C 1/4; Tecnal C 1/2; Tecnal C 1/4

Pharmacologic Category Analgesic Combination (Narcotic); Barbiturate

Synonyms Codeine and Butalbital Compound; Codeine, Butalbital, Aspirin, and Caffeine

Use Mild to moderate pain when sedation is needed

Local Anesthetic/Vasoconstrictor Precautions No information available to require special precautions

Effects on Dental Treatment

>10%: Dizziness, lightheadedness, drowsiness, nausea, epigastric discomfort

1% to 10%: Confusion, unusual excitement, nervousness, faint feeling GI ulceration

Restrictions C-III

Dosage Adults: Oral: 1-2 capsules every 4 hours as needed for pain; up to 6/day

Other Adverse Effects

>10%:

Gastrointestinal: Heartburn, stomach pains, dyspepsia

1% to 10%:

Central nervous system: Mental depression, insomnia, nightmares, intoxicated feeling

Dermatologic: Rash

Gastrointestinal: Constipation

<1% (Limited to important or life-threatening): **Tachycardia, chest pain, palpitations, syncope, hallucinations, nervousness, jitters**, exfoliative dermatitis, Stevens-Johnson syndrome, agranulocytosis, megaloblastic anemia, thrombocytopenia, occult bleeding, **prolongation of bleeding time**, leukopenia, iron-deficiency anemia, hepatotoxicity, thrombophlebitis, impaired renal function, **respiratory depression, bronchospasm, epistaxis, allergic reaction**

Drug Interactions

Increased Effect/Toxicity: MAO inhibitors may enhance the CNS effects of butalbital. In patients receiving concomitant corticosteroids during the chronic use of ASA, withdrawal of corticosteroids may result in salicylism. Butalbital compound and codeine may enhance effects of oral anticoagulants. Increased effect with oral antidiabetic agents and insulin, 6-mercaptopurine and methotrexate, NSAIDs, other narcotic analgesics, ethanol, general anesthetics, tranquilizers such as chlordiazepoxide, sedative hypnotics, or other CNS depressants.

Decreased Effect: Aspirin, butalbital, caffeine, and codeine may diminish effects of uricosuric agents such as probenecid and sulfinpyrazone.

Dietary/Ethanol/Herb Considerations

Ethanol: Avoid use; may increase CNS depression.

Herb/Nutraceutical: Avoid gotu kola, kava, SAMe, St John's wort, and valerian; may increase CNS depression.

Pregnancy Risk Factor C/D (prolonged use or high doses at term)

Generic Available Yes

Comments Abrupt discontinuation after sustained use (generally >10 days) may cause withdrawal symptoms

Butalbital Compound *see* Butalbital, Aspirin, and Caffeine *on page 216*

Butenafine (byoo TEN a fine)

U.S. Brand Names Lotrimin® Ultra™ [OTC]; Mentax®

Pharmacologic Category Antifungal Agent, Topical

Synonyms Butenafine Hydrochloride

Use Topical treatment of tinea pedis (athlete's foot), tinea cruris (jock itch), tinea corporis (ringworm), and tinea versicolor

(Continued)

Butenafine *(Continued)*

Local Anesthetic/Vasoconstrictor Precautions No information available to require special precautions

Effects on Dental Treatment No significant effects or complications reported

Dosage Children >12 years and Adults: Topical:

Tinea corporis, tinea cruris, or tinea versicolor: Apply once daily for 2 weeks to affected area and surrounding skin

Tinea pedis: Apply once daily for 4 weeks or twice daily for 7 days to affected area and surrounding skin (7-day regimen may have lower efficacy)

Mechanism of Action Butenafine exerts antifungal activity by blocking squalene epoxidation, resulting in inhibition of ergosterol synthesis (antidermatophyte and *Sporothrix schenckii* activity). In higher concentrations, the drug disrupts fungal cell membranes (anticandidal activity).

Other Adverse Effects

>1%: Dermatologic: Burning, stinging, irritation, erythema, pruritus (2%)

<1%: Contact dermatitis

Pharmacodynamics/Kinetics

Absorption: Minimal systemic

Metabolism: Hepatic via hydroxylation

Half-life elimination: 35 hours

Time to peak, serum: 6 hours

Pregnancy Risk Factor B

Generic Available No

Butenafine Hydrochloride *see* Butenafine *on page 217*

Butisol Sodium® *see* Butabarbital Sodium *on page 213*

Butoconazole (byoo toe KOE na zole)

U.S. Brand Names Gynazole-1™; Mycelex®-3 [OTC]

Canadian Brand Names Femstat® One

Mexican Brand Names Femstal®

Pharmacologic Category Antifungal Agent, Vaginal

Synonyms Butoconazole Nitrate

Use Local treatment of vulvovaginal candidiasis

Local Anesthetic/Vasoconstrictor Precautions No information available to require special precautions

Effects on Dental Treatment No significant effects or complications reported

Dosage Adults: Female:

Femstat®-3 [OTC]: Insert 1 applicatorful (~5 g) intravaginally at bedtime for 3 consecutive days

Gynazole-1™: Insert 1 applicatorful (~5 g) intravaginally as a single dose; treatment may need to be extended for up to 6 days in pregnant women (use in pregnancy during 2nd or 3rd trimester only)

Mechanism of Action Increases cell membrane permeability in susceptible fungi (*Candida*)

Other Adverse Effects Frequency not defined:

Gastrointestinal: Abdominal pain or cramping

Genitourinary: Pelvic pain; vulvar/vaginal burning, itching, soreness, and swelling

Pharmacodynamics/Kinetics

Absorption: 2%

Metabolism: Not reported

Time to peak: 12-24 hours

Pregnancy Risk Factor C (use only in 2nd or 3rd trimester)

Generic Available No

Butoconazole Nitrate *see* Butoconazole *on page 218*

Butorphanol (byoo TOR fa nole)

U.S. Brand Names Stadol®; Stadol® NS

Canadian Brand Names Apo®-Butorphanol; Stadol NS™

Pharmacologic Category Analgesic, Narcotic

Synonyms Butorphanol Tartrate

Use

Parenteral: Management of moderate to severe pain; preoperative medication; supplement to balanced anesthesia; management of pain during labor

Nasal spray: Management of moderate to severe pain, including migraine headache pain

Local Anesthetic/Vasoconstrictor Precautions No information available to require special precautions

Effects on Dental Treatment

>10%: Drowsiness (≤43%), dizziness (19%), nausea (13%), vomiting (13%), nasal congestion (Stadol® NS)

1% to 10%: Vasodilation, palpitations, lightheadedness, headache, anxiety, confusion, tremor, paresthesia, bronchitis, cough, dyspnea, epistaxis, pharyngitis, rhinitis, sinus congestion, sinusitis, upper respiratory infection, increased diaphoresis, xerostomia, unpleasant aftertaste, weakness, lethargy, euphoria

Restrictions C-IV

Dosage These are guidelines and do not represent the maximum doses that may be required in all patients. Doses should be titrated to pain relief/prevention. Long-term use is not recommended; has an analgesic "ceiling".

Adults:

Parenteral:

Acute pain (moderate to severe):

I.M.: Initial: 2 mg, may repeat every 3-4 hours as needed; usual range: 1-4 mg every 3-4 hours as needed

I.V.: Initial: 1 mg, may repeat every 3-4 hours as needed; usual range: 0.5-2 mg every 3-4 hours as needed

Preoperative medication: I.M.: 2 mg 60-90 minutes before surgery

Supplement to balanced anesthesia: I.V.: 2 mg shortly before induction and/or an incremental dose of 0.5-1 mg (up to 0.06 mg/kg), depending on previously administered sedative, analgesic, and hypnotic medications

Pain during labor (fetus >37 weeks gestation and no signs of fetal distress):

I.M., I.V.: 1-2 mg; may repeat in 4 hours

Note: Alternative analgesia should be used for pain associated with delivery or if delivery is anticipated within 4 hours

Nasal spray:

Moderate to severe pain (including migraine headache pain): Initial: 1 spray (~1 mg per spray) in 1 nostril; if adequate pain relief is not achieved within 60-90 minutes, an additional 1 spray in 1 nostril may be given; may repeat initial dose sequence in 3-4 hours after the last dose as needed

Alternatively, an initial dose of 2 mg (1 spray in each nostril) may be used in patients who will be able to remain recumbent (in the event drowsiness or dizziness occurs); additional 2 mg doses should not be given for 3-4 hours

Note: In some clinical trials, an initial dose of 2 mg (as 2 doses 1 hour apart or 2 mg initially - 1 spray in each nostril) has been used, followed by 1 mg in 1 hour; side effects were greater at these dosages

Dosage adjustment in renal impairment:

I.M., I.V.: Initial dosage should generally be 1/2 of the recommended dose; repeated dosing must be based on initial response rather than fixed intervals, but generally should be at least 6 hours apart

Nasal spray: Initial dose should not exceed 1 mg; a second dose may be given after 90-120 minutes

Dosage adjustment in hepatic impairment:

I.M., I.V.: Initial dosage should generally be 1/2 of the recommended dose; repeated dosing must be based on initial response rather than fixed intervals, but generally should be at least 6 hours apart

Nasal spray: Initial dose should not exceed 1 mg; a second dose may be given after 90-120 minutes

Elderly:

I.M., I.V.: Initial dosage should generally be 1/2 of the recommended dose; repeated dosing must be based on initial response rather than fixed intervals, but generally should be at least 6 hours apart

Nasal Spray: Initial dose should not exceed 1 mg; a second dose may be given after 90-120 minutes

Mechanism of Action Mixed narcotic agonist-antagonist with central analgesic actions; binds to opiate receptors in the CNS, causing inhibition of ascending pain pathways, altering the perception of and response to pain; produces generalized CNS depression

Other Adverse Effects

>10%: Central nervous system: Insomnia (Stadol® NS)

1% to 10%:

Dermatologic: Pruritus

Gastrointestinal: Anorexia, constipation, stomach pain

Ocular: Blurred vision

Otic: Ear pain, tinnitus

Respiratory: Nasal irritation

<1%: **Bradycardia, tachycardia, hypertension, paradoxical CNS stimulation, hallucinations**, mental depression, malaise, **restlessness**, nightmares, **CNS depression**, decreased urination, rash, stomach cramps, painful urination, blurred vision, tinnitus, **dyspnea, respiratory depression**, dependence (with prolonged use), difficulty speaking (transient), **hypotension, syncope, agitation**, dysphoria, **hostility**, vertigo, **withdrawal symptoms, hives**

Stadol® NS: **Edema, chest pain, hypertension, tachycardia, convulsions, delusions,** depression, **apnea, shallow breathing**

Drug Interactions Increased Effect/Toxicity: Increased toxicity with CNS depressants, phenothiazines, barbiturates, skeletal muscle relaxants, alfentanil, guanabenz, and MAO inhibitors.

(Continued)

Butorphanol *(Continued)*

Dietary/Ethanol/Herb Considerations

Ethanol: Avoid use; may increase CNS depression.

Herb/Nutraceutical: Avoid gotu kola, kava, SAMe, St John's wort, and valerian; may increase CNS depression.

Pharmacodynamics/Kinetics

Onset of action: I.M.: 5-10 minutes; I.V.: <10 minutes; Nasal: Within 15 minutes

Peak effect: I.M.: 0.5-1 hour; I.V.: 4-5 minutes

Duration: I.M., I.V.: 3-4 hours; Nasal: 4-5 hours

Absorption: Rapid and well absorbed

Protein binding: 80%

Metabolism: Hepatic

Bioavailability: Nasal: 60% to 70%

Half-life elimination: 2.5-4 hours

Excretion: Primarily urine

Pregnancy Risk Factor C/D (prolonged use or high doses at term)

Generic Available Yes: Injection

Butorphanol Tartrate *see* Butorphanol *on page 218*

BW-430C *see* Lamotrigine *on page 774*

C2B8 *see* Rituximab *on page 1190*

C7E3 *see* Abciximab *on page 23*

C8-CCK *see* Sincalide *on page 1225*

311C90 *see* Zolmitriptan *on page 1411*

C-500-GR™ [OTC] *see* Ascorbic Acid *on page 128*

Cabergoline (ca BER go leen)

U.S. Brand Names Dostinex®

Canadian Brand Names Dostinex®

Pharmacologic Category Ergot Derivative

Use Treatment of hyperprolactinemic disorders, either idiopathic or due to pituitary adenomas

Unlabeled/Investigational Use Adjunct for the treatment of Parkinson's disease

Local Anesthetic/Vasoconstrictor Precautions No information available to require special precautions

Effects on Dental Treatment

>10%: Headache (26%), dizziness (17%), nausea (29%)

1% to 10%: Syncope (1%), flu-like symptoms (1%), weakness (6%), hot flashes (3%), hypotension (1%), palpitations (1%), somnolence (2%), anxiety (1%), nervousness (1%), vomiting (4%), paresthesias (2%), rhinitis (1%), xerostomia (2%), throat irritation (1%), toothache (1%) fatigue (5%), malaise (1%), periorbital edema (1%), pain (2%), abnormal vision (1%)

Dosage Initial dose: Oral: 0.25 mg twice weekly; the dose may be increased by 0.25 mg twice weekly up to a maximum of 1 mg twice weekly according to the patient's serum prolactin level. Dosage increases should not occur more rapidly than every 4 weeks. Once a normal serum prolactin level is maintained for 6 months, the dose may be discontinued and prolactin levels monitored to determine if cabergoline is still required. The durability of efficacy beyond 24 months of therapy has not been established.

Elderly: No dosage recommendations suggested, but start at the low end of the dosage range

Mechanism of Action Cabergoline is a long-acting dopamine receptor agonist with a high affinity for D_2 receptors; prolactin secretion by the anterior pituitary is predominantly under hypothalamic inhibitory control exerted through the release of dopamine

Other Adverse Effects 1% to 10%:

Cardiovascular: Dependent edema (1%), peripheral edema (1%)

Central nervous system: Vertigo (4%), depression (3%), insomnia (1%), impaired concentration (1%)

Dermatologic: Acne (1%), pruritus (1%)

Endocrine: Breast pain (2%), dysmenorrhea (1%)

Gastrointestinal: Constipation (7%), abdominal pain (5%), dyspepsia (5%), anorexia, (1%) diarrhea (2%), flatulence (2%)

Neuromuscular & skeletal: Arthralgia (1%)

Drug Interactions

Increased effect with antifungals (azole derivatives); CYP3A4 inhibitors (eg, amiodarone, cimetidine, erythromycin, ritonavir); macrolide antibiotics; protease inhibitors; MAO inhibitors. Cabergoline may increase the effects of sibutramine and other serotonin agonists (serotonin syndrome).

Decreased effect with antipsychotics, metoclopramide.

Pharmacodynamics/Kinetics

Distribution: Extensive, particularly to the pituitary

Protein binding: 40% to 42%

Metabolism: Extensively hepatic; minimal CYP

Half-life elimination: 63-69 hours
Time to peak: 2-3 hours

Pregnancy Risk Factor B

Generic Available No

Cafergot® *see* Ergotamine *on page 510*

Caffeine, Acetaminophen, and Aspirin *see* Acetaminophen, Aspirin, and Caffeine *on page 34*

Caffeine, Acetaminophen, Butalbital, and Codeine *see* Butalbital, Acetaminophen, Caffeine, and Codeine *on page 215*

Caffeine and Sodium Benzoate

(KAF een & SOW dee um BEN zoe ate)

Pharmacologic Category Diuretic, Miscellaneous

Synonyms Sodium Benzoate and Caffeine

Use Emergency stimulant in acute circulatory failure, diuretic, relief of spinal puncture headache

Local Anesthetic/Vasoconstrictor Precautions No information available to require special precautions

Effects on Dental Treatment Frequency not defined: Tachycardia, palpitations, restlessness, nervousness, mild delirium, headache, anxiety, nausea, vomiting, gastric irritation

Dosage

Children: Stimulant: I.M., I.V., S.C.: 8 mg/kg every 4 hours as needed
Adults:
- Stimulant/diuretic: I.M., I.V.: 500 mg, maximum single dose: 1 g
- Spinal puncture headaches:
  - I.V.: 500 mg in 1000 mL NS infused over 1 hour, followed by 1000 mL NS infused over 1 hour; a second course of caffeine can be given for unrelieved headache pain in 4 hours.
  - Oral: 300 mg

Other Adverse Effects Frequency not defined:

Cardiovascular: Extrasystoles
Central nervous system: Insomnia
Neuromuscular & skeletal: Muscle tension (following abrupt cessation of drug after regular consumption of 500-600 mg/day)
Renal: Diuresis

Pregnancy Risk Factor C

Generic Available Yes

Caffeine, Aspirin, and Acetaminophen *see* Acetaminophen, Aspirin, and Caffeine *on page 34*

Caffeine, Hydrocodone, Chlorpheniramine, Phenylephrine, and Acetaminophen *see* Hydrocodone, Chlorpheniramine, Phenylephrine, Acetaminophen, and Caffeine *on page 686*

Caffeine, Orphenadrine, and Aspirin *see* Orphenadrine, Aspirin, and Caffeine *on page 1005*

Calan® *see* Verapamil *on page 1382*

Calan® SR *see* Verapamil *on page 1382*

Cal Carb-HD® [OTC] *see* Calcium Supplements *on page 229*

Calcibind® *see* Cellulose Sodium Phosphate *on page 284*

Calci-Chew™ [OTC] *see* Calcium Supplements *on page 229*

Calciday-667® [OTC] *see* Calcium Supplements *on page 229*

Calcifediol (kal si fe DYE ole)

U.S. Brand Names Calderol®

Canadian Brand Names Calderol®

Pharmacologic Category Vitamin D Analog

Synonyms 25-HCC; 25-Hydroxycholecalciferol; 25-Hydroxyvitamin D_3

Use Treatment and management of metabolic bone disease associated with chronic renal failure or hypocalcemia in patients on chronic renal dialysis

Local Anesthetic/Vasoconstrictor Precautions No information available to require special precautions

Effects on Dental Treatment Frequency not defined: Hypotension, arrhythmias, hypertension, irritability, headache, somnolence, seizures, (rare), nausea, vomiting, metallic taste, xerostomia

Dosage Oral: Hepatic osteodystrophy:

Infants: 5-7 mcg/kg/day
Children and Adults: Usual dose: 20-100 mcg/day or 20-200 mcg every other day; titrate to obtain normal serum calcium/phosphate levels; increase dose at 4-week intervals; initial dose: 300-350 mcg/week, administered daily or on alternate days

Mechanism of Action Vitamin D analog that (along with calcitonin and parathyroid hormone) regulates serum calcium homeostasis by promoting absorption of calcium and phosphorus in the small intestine; promotes renal tubule resorption of phosphate; increases rate of accretion and resorption in bone minerals

(Continued)

Calcifediol *(Continued)*

Other Adverse Effects Frequency not defined:
Dermatologic: Pruritus
Endocrine & metabolic: Hypercalcemia, polydipsia, hypermagnesemia
Gastrointestinal: Constipation, anorexia, pancreatitis,
Hepatic: Elevated LFTs
Neuromuscular & skeletal: Myalgia, bone pain
Ocular: Conjunctivitis, photophobia
Renal: Polyuria

Drug Interactions
Increased Effect/Toxicity: The effect of calcifediol is increased with thiazide diuretics. Additive effect with antacids (magnesium).
Decreased Effect: The effect of calcifediol is decreased when taken with cholestyramine or colestipol.

Pharmacodynamics/Kinetics
Absorption: Rapid from small intestines
Distribution: Activated in kidneys; stored in liver and fat depots
Half-life elimination: 12-22 days
Time to peak: Within 4 hours
Excretion: Feces

Pregnancy Risk Factor C (manufacturer); A/D (dose exceeding RDA recommendation) (expert analysis)

Generic Available No

Calciferol™ *see* Ergocalciferol *on page 508*
Calcijex™ *see* Calcitriol *on page 223*
Calcimar® *see* Calcitonin *on page 222*
Calci-Mix™ [OTC] *see* Calcium Supplements *on page 229*

Calcipotriene (kal si POE try een)

U.S. Brand Names Dovonex®
Pharmacologic Category Topical Skin Product; Vitamin D Analog
Use Treatment of moderate plaque psoriasis
Local Anesthetic/Vasoconstrictor Precautions No information available to require special precautions
Effects on Dental Treatment No significant effects or complications reported
Dosage Topical: Adults: Apply in a thin film to the affected skin twice daily and rub in gently and completely
Mechanism of Action Synthetic vitamin D_3 analog which regulates skin cell production and proliferation
Other Adverse Effects
Dermatologic:
>10%: Burning, itching, skin irritation, erythema, dry skin, peeling, rash, worsening of psoriasis
1% to 10%: Dermatitis
<1%: Skin atrophy, hyperpigmentation, folliculitis, hypercalcemia
Pregnancy Risk Factor C
Generic Available No

Calcitonin (kal si TOE nin)

Related Information
Rheumatoid Arthritis, Osteoarthritis, and Osteoporosis *on page 1488*
U.S. Brand Names Calcimar®; Miacalcin®
Canadian Brand Names Calcimar®; Caltine®; Miacalcin® NS
Mexican Brand Names Miacalcic®; Oseum®; Tonocalcin®
Pharmacologic Category Antidote
Synonyms Calcitonin (Salmon)
Use Calcitonin (salmon): Treatment of Paget's disease of bone (osteitis deformans); adjunctive therapy for hypercalcemia; used in postmenopausal osteoporosis and osteogenesis imperfecta
Local Anesthetic/Vasoconstrictor Precautions No information available to require special precautions
Effects on Dental Treatment
>10%: Flushing, nausea
1% to 10%: Back/joint pain
Dosage Salmon calcitonin:
Children: Dosage not established
Adults:
Paget's disease: I.M., S.C.: Initial: 100 units/day; maintenance: 50 units/day or 50-100 units every 1-3 days
Hypercalcemia: Initial: I.M., S.C.: 4 units/kg every 12 hours; may increase up to 8 units/kg every 12 hours to a maximum of every 6 hours
Osteogenesis imperfecta: I.M., S.C.: 2 units/kg 3 times/week

Postmenopausal osteoporosis:
I.M., S.C.: 100 units/day
Intranasal: 200 units (1 spray)/day

Mechanism of Action Structurally similar to human calcitonin; it directly inhibits osteoclastic bone resorption; promotes the renal excretion of calcium, phosphate, sodium, magnesium and potassium by decreasing tubular reabsorption; increases the jejunal secretion of water, sodium, potassium, and chloride

Other Adverse Effects
>10%:
Gastrointestinal: Diarrhea, anorexia
Local: Edema at injection site
1% to 10%:
Genitourinary: Polyuria
Respiratory: Nasal bleeding/crusting (following intranasal administration)
<1% (Limited to important or life-threatening): **Dyspnea**

Drug Interactions Decreased Effect: Calcitonin may be antagonized by calcium and vitamin D in treating hypercalcemia.

Dietary/Ethanol/Herb Considerations
Ethanol: Avoid use; may increase risk of osteoporosis.
Food: Adequate vitamin D and calcium intake is essential due to risk of osteoporosis. Patients with Paget's disease and hypercalcemia should follow a low calcium diet as prescribed.

Pharmacodynamics/Kinetics
Hypercalcemia:
Onset of action: ~2 hours
Duration: 6-8 hours
Distribution: Does not cross placenta
Half-life elimination: S.C.: 1.2 hours
Excretion: Urine (as inactive metabolites)

Pregnancy Risk Factor C

Generic Available No

Calcitonin (Salmon) *see* Calcitonin *on page 222*
Cal-Citrate® 250 [OTC] *see* Calcium Citrate *on page 224*
Cal-citrate® 250 [OTC] *see* Calcium Supplements *on page 229*

Calcitriol (kal si TRYE ole)

U.S. Brand Names Calcijex™; Rocaltrol®

Canadian Brand Names Rocaltrol®

Mexican Brand Names Rocaltrol®; Tirocal®

Pharmacologic Category Vitamin D Analog

Synonyms 1,25 Dihydroxycholecalciferol

Use Management of hypocalcemia in patients on chronic renal dialysis; management of secondary hyperparathyroidism in moderate to severe chronic renal failure; management of hypocalcemia in hypoparathyroidism and pseudohypoparathyroidism

Unlabeled/Investigational Use Decrease severity of psoriatic lesions in psoriatic vulgaris; treatment of vitamin D-resistant rickets

Local Anesthetic/Vasoconstrictor Precautions No information available to require special precautions

Effects on Dental Treatment Frequency not defined: Cardiac arrhythmias, hypertension, hypotension, headache, irritability, seizures (rare), somnolence, psychosis, metallic taste, nausea, vomiting, xerostomia, soft tissue calcification

Dosage Individualize dosage to maintain calcium levels of 9-10 mg/dL
Renal failure:
Children:
Oral: 0.25-2 mcg/day have been used (with hemodialysis); 0.014-0.041 mcg/kg/day (not receiving hemodialysis); increases should be made at 4- to 8-week intervals
I.V.: 0.01-0.05 mcg/kg 3 times/week if undergoing hemodialysis
Adults:
Oral: 0.25 mcg/day or every other day (may require 0.5-1 mcg/day); increases should be made at 4- to 8-week intervals
I.V.: 0.5 mcg/day 3 times/week (may require from 0.5-3 mcg/day given 3 times/week) if undergoing hemodialysis
Hypoparathyroidism/pseudohypoparathyroidism: Oral (evaluate dosage at 2- to 4-week intervals):
Children:
<1 year: 0.04-0.08 mcg/kg once daily
1-5 years: 0.25-0.75 mcg once daily
Children >6 years and Adults: 0.5-2 mcg once daily
Vitamin D-dependent rickets: Children and Adults: Oral: 1 mcg once daily
Vitamin D-resistant rickets (familial hypophosphatemia): Children and Adults: Oral: Initial: 0.015-0.02 mcg/kg once daily; maintenance: 0.03-0.06 mcg/kg once daily; maximum dose: 2 mcg once daily
(Continued)

Calcitriol *(Continued)*

Hypocalcemia in premature infants: Oral: 1 mcg once daily for 5 days

Hypocalcemic tetany in premature infants: I.V.: 0.05 mcg/kg once daily for 5-12 days

Elderly: No dosage recommendations, but start at the lower end of the dosage range

Mechanism of Action Promotes absorption of calcium in the intestines and retention at the kidneys thereby increasing calcium levels in the serum; decreases excessive serum phosphatase levels, parathyroid hormone levels, and decreases bone resorption; increases renal tubule phosphate resorption

Other Adverse Effects

>10%: Endocrine & metabolic: Hypercalcemia (33%)

Frequency not defined:

Dermatologic: Pruritus, erythema multiforme

Endocrine & metabolic: Hypermagnesemia, polydipsia

Gastrointestinal: Anorexia, constipation, pancreatitis

Hepatic: Elevated LFTs

Neuromuscular & skeletal: Bone pain, myalgia, dystrophy

Ocular: Conjunctivitis, photophobia

Renal: Polyuria

Drug Interactions Induces CYP3A4

Increased Effect/Toxicity: Risk of hypercalcemia with thiazide diuretics. Risk of hypermagnesemia with magnesium-containing antacids. Risk of digoxin toxicity may be increased (if hypercalcemia occurs).

Decreased Effect: Cholestyramine and colestipol decrease absorption/effect of calcitriol. Thiazide diuretics, enzyme inducers (phenytoin, phenobarbital), and corticosteroids may reduce the effect of calcitriol.

Pharmacodynamics/Kinetics

Onset of action: ~2-6 hours

Duration: 3-5 days

Absorption: Oral: Rapid

Protein binding: 99.9%

Metabolism: Primarily to 1,24,25-trihydroxycholecalciferol and 1,24,25-trihydroxy ergocalciferol

Half-life elimination: 3-8 hours

Excretion: Primarily feces; urine (4% to 6%)

Pregnancy Risk Factor C (manufacturer); A/D (dose exceeding RDA recommendation) (expert analysis)

Generic Available Yes

Calcium Acetate *see* Calcium Supplements *on page 229*

Calcium Acetate and Aluminum Sulfate *see* Aluminum Sulfate and Calcium Acetate *on page 70*

Calcium Carbonate *see* Calcium Supplements *on page 229*

Calcium Carbonate and Simethicone

(KAL see um KAR bun ate & sye METH i kone)

U.S. Brand Names Titralac® Plus Liquid [OTC]

Pharmacologic Category Antacid; Antiflatulent

Synonyms Simethicone and Calcium Carbonate

Use Relief of acid indigestion, heartburn, peptic esophagitis, hiatal hernia, and gas

Local Anesthetic/Vasoconstrictor Precautions No information available to require special precautions

Effects on Dental Treatment Do not give tetracyclines concomitantly.

Dosage Oral: 0.5-2 g 4-6 times/day

Dietary/Ethanol/Herb Considerations Ethanol: Avoid use; may enhance gastric mucosal irritation and significant consumption can increase risk of osteoporosis.

Pregnancy Risk Factor C

Generic Available Yes

Calcium Carbonate, Magnesium Hydroxide, and Famotidine *see* Famotidine, Calcium Carbonate, and Magnesium Hydroxide *on page 557*

Calcium Chloride *see* Calcium Supplements *on page 229*

Calcium Citrate (KAL see um SIT rate)

U.S. Brand Names Cal-Citrate® 250 [OTC]; Citracal® [OTC]

Pharmacologic Category Calcium Salt

Use Antacid; treatment and prevention of calcium deficiency or hyperphosphatemia (eg, osteoporosis, osteomalacia, mild/moderate renal insufficiency, hypoparathyroidism, postmenopausal osteoporosis, rickets)

Local Anesthetic/Vasoconstrictor Precautions No information available to require special precautions

Effects on Dental Treatment No significant effects or complications reported

Dosage Oral: Dosage is in terms of **elemental calcium:**
- Dietary Reference Intake:
  - 0-6 months: 210 mg/day
  - 7-12 months: 270 mg/day
  - 1-3 years: 500 mg/day
  - 4-8 years: 800 mg/day
  - Adults, Male/Female:
    - 9-18 years: 1300 mg/day
    - 19-50 years: 1000 mg/day
    - ≥51 years: 1200 mg/day
  - Female: Pregnancy: Same as for Adults, Male/Female
  - Female: Lactating: Same as for Adults, Male/Female
- Dietary supplement: Usual dose: 500 mg to 2 g 2-4 times/day

Mechanism of Action Moderates nerve and muscle performance via action potential excitation threshold regulation

Other Adverse Effects
- <1%: **Headache**, hypophosphatemia, hypercalcemia, **nausea**, anorexia, **vomiting**, abdominal pain, constipation, **thirst**
- Frequency not defined:
  - Mild hypercalcemia (calcium: >10.5 mg/dL); may be asymptomatic or manifest itself as constipation, anorexia, **nausea, vomiting**
  - More severe hypercalcemia (calcium: >12 mg/dL); associated with **confusion, delirium, stupor, coma**

Drug Interactions
- Increased Effect/Toxicity: High doses of calcium with thiazide diuretics may result in milk-alkali syndrome and hypercalcemia; monitor response. Calcium salts may decrease T_4 absorption; separate dose from levothyroxine by at least 4 hours. Calcium acetate may potentiate digoxin toxicity.
- Decreased Effect: Absorption of tetracycline, atenolol (and potentially other beta-blockers), iron, quinolone antibiotics, alendronate, sodium fluoride, and zinc absorption may be significantly decreased; space administration times. Effects of calcium channel blockers (eg, verapamil) effects may be diminished. Polystyrene sulfonate's potassium-binding ability may be reduced; avoid concurrent administration.

Dietary/Ethanol/Herb Considerations Ethanol: Avoid use may increase risk of osteoporosis.

Pharmacodynamics/Kinetics Absorption: Requires vitamin D

Pregnancy Risk Factor C

Generic Available No

Calcium Citrate *see* Calcium Supplements *on page 229*
Calcium Disodium Edetate *see* Edetate Calcium Disodium *on page 486*
Calcium Disodium Versenate® *see* Edetate Calcium Disodium *on page 486*
Calcium EDTA *see* Edetate Calcium Disodium *on page 486*

Calcium Glubionate (KAL see um gloo BYE oh nate)

U.S. Brand Names Neo-Calglucon® [OTC]

Mexican Brand Names Calcium-Sandoz®

Pharmacologic Category Calcium Salt

Use Adjunct in treatment and prevention of postmenopausal osteoporosis; treatment and prevention of calcium depletion or hyperphosphatemia (eg, osteoporosis, osteomalacia, mild/moderate renal insufficiency, hypoparathyroidism, rickets)

Local Anesthetic/Vasoconstrictor Precautions No information available to require special precautions

Effects on Dental Treatment No significant effects or complications reported

Dosage Dosage is in terms of **elemental** calcium
- Dietary Reference Intake:
  - 0-6 months: 210 mg/day
  - 7-12 months: 270 mg/day
  - 1-3 years: 500 mg/day
  - 4-8 years: 800 mg/day
  - Adults, Male/Female:
    - 9-18 years: 1300 mg/day
    - 19-50 years: 1000 mg/day
    - ≥51 years: 1200 mg/day
  - Female: Pregnancy: Same as for Adults, Male/Female
  - Female: Lactating: Same as for Adults, Male/Female
- Syrup is a hyperosmolar solution; dosage is in terms of calcium glubionate, elemental calcium is in parentheses
- Neonatal hypocalcemia: 1200 mg (77 mg Ca^{++})/kg/day in 4-6 divided doses
  - Maintenance: Infants and Children: 600-2000 mg (38-128 mg Ca^{++})/kg/day in 4 divided doses up to a maximum of 9 g (575 mg Ca^{++})/day
- Adults: 6-18 g (~0.5-1 g Ca^{++})/day in divided doses
- Dosing adjustment in renal impairment: Cl_{cr} <25 mL/minute: Adjustments may be necessary depending on the serum calcium levels

(Continued)

Calcium Glubionate *(Continued)*

Mechanism of Action As dietary supplement, used to prevent or treat negative calcium balance; in osteoporosis, it helps to prevent or decrease the rate of bone loss. The calcium in calcium salts moderates nerve and muscle performance and allows normal cardiac function.

Other Adverse Effects

<1%: **Headache**, hypophosphatemia, hypercalcemia, **nausea, anorexia, vomiting, thirst**, abdominal pain, constipation

Frequency not defined:

Mild hypercalcemia (calcium: >10.5 mg/dL); may be asymptomatic or manifest itself as constipation, anorexia, **nausea, vomiting**

More severe hypercalcemia (calcium: >12 mg/dL); associated with **confusion, delirium, stupor, coma**

Drug Interactions

Increased Effect/Toxicity: High doses of calcium with thiazide diuretics may result in milk-alkali syndrome and hypercalcemia; monitor response. Calcium salts may decrease T_4 absorption; separate dose from levothyroxine by at least 4 hours. Calcium acetate may potentiate digoxin toxicity.

Decreased Effect: Absorption of tetracycline, atenolol (and potentially other beta-blockers), iron, quinolone antibiotics, alendronate, sodium fluoride, and zinc absorption may be significantly decreased; space administration times. Effects of calcium channel blockers (eg, verapamil) effects may be diminished. Polystyrene sulfonate's potassium-binding ability may be reduced; avoid concurrent administration.

Dietary/Ethanol/Herb Considerations

Ethanol: Avoid use; may increase risk of osteoporosis.

Food: Food may increase absorption. Calcium may decrease iron absorption. Bran, foods high in oxalates, or whole grain cereals may decrease calcium absorption.

Pharmacodynamics/Kinetics

Absorption: Requires vitamin D; minimal unless chronic, high doses are given; calcium is absorbed in soluble, ionized form; solubility of calcium is increased in an acid environment

Distribution: Crosses placenta; enters breast milk

Excretion: Primarily feces (as unabsorbed calcium); urine (20%)

Pregnancy Risk Factor C

Generic Available No

Calcium Glubionate *see* Calcium Supplements *on page 229*

Calcium Gluceptate (KAL see um gloo SEP tate)

Pharmacologic Category Calcium Salt

Use Treatment of cardiac disturbances of hyperkalemia, hypocalcemia, or calcium channel blocker toxicity; cardiac resuscitation when epinephrine fails to improve myocardial contractions; treatment of hypermagnesemia and hypocalcemia

Local Anesthetic/Vasoconstrictor Precautions No information available to require special precautions

Effects on Dental Treatment No significant effects or complications reported

Dosage Dose expressed in mg of calcium gluceptate (elemental calcium is in parentheses)

Cardiac resuscitation in the presence of hypocalcemia, hyperkalemia, magnesium toxicity, or calcium channel blocker toxicity: I.V.:

Children: 110 mg (9 mg Ca^{++})/kg/dose

Adults: 1.1-1.5 g (90-123 mg Ca^{++})

Hypocalcemia:

I.M.:

Children: 200-500 mg (16.4-41 mg Ca^{++})/kg/day divided every 6 hours

Adults: 500 mg to 1.1 g/dose as needed

I.V.: Adults: 1.1-4.4 g (90-360 mg Ca^{++}) administered slowly as needed (≤2 mL/minute)

After citrated blood administration: Children and Adults: I.V.: 0.45 mEq Ca^{++}/100 mL blood infused

Dosing adjustment in renal impairment: Cl_{cr} <25 mL/minute: Adjustments may be necessary depending on the serum calcium levels

Mechanism of Action Moderates nerve and muscle performance via action potential excitation threshold regulation

Other Adverse Effects <1%: **Vasodilation, hypotension, bradycardia, cardiac arrhythmias, ventricular fibrillation, syncope**, lethargy, **mania, coma**, erythema, hypomagnesemia, hypercalcemia, elevated serum amylase, tissue necrosis, muscle weakness, hypercalciuria

Drug Interactions

Increased Effect/Toxicity: High doses of calcium with thiazide diuretics may result in milk-alkali syndrome and hypercalcemia; monitor response. Calcium may potentiate digoxin toxicity.

Decreased Effect: Effects of calcium channel blockers (eg, verapamil) effects may be diminished.

Pharmacodynamics/Kinetics

Distribution: Crosses placenta; enters breast milk

Excretion: Primarily feces (as unabsorbed calcium); urine (20%)

Pregnancy Risk Factor C

Generic Available Yes

Calcium Gluceptate *see* Calcium Supplements *on page 229*

Calcium Gluconate *see* Calcium Supplements *on page 229*

Calcium Lactate (KAL see um LAK tate)

Pharmacologic Category Calcium Salt

Use Adjunct in prevention of postmenopausal osteoporosis; treatment and prevention of calcium depletion

Local Anesthetic/Vasoconstrictor Precautions No information available to require special precautions

Effects on Dental Treatment No significant effects or complications reported

Dosage Oral: Dosage in terms of **calcium lactate:**

Dietary Reference Intake (in terms of elemental calcium):

- 0-6 months: 210 mg/day
- 7-12 months: 270 mg/day
- 1-3 years: 500 mg/day
- 4-8 years: 800 mg/day
- Adults, Male/Female:
  - 9-18 years: 1300 mg/day
  - 19-50 years: 1000 mg/day
  - ≥51 years: 1200 mg/day
- Female: Pregnancy: Same as Adults, Male/Female
- Female: Lactating: Same as Adults, Male/Female

Children: 500 mg/kg/day divided every 6-8 hours; maximum daily dose: 9 g

Adults: 1.5-3 g divided every 8 hours

Mechanism of Action As dietary supplement, used to prevent or treat negative calcium balance; in osteoporosis, it helps to prevent or decrease the rate of bone loss. The calcium in calcium salts moderates nerve and muscle performance and allows normal cardiac function.

Other Adverse Effects <1%: Constipation, **dizziness, headache**, hypercalcemia, hypercalciuria, hypomagnesemia, hypophosphatemia, **confusion**, milk-alkali syndrome, **nausea, vomiting, xerostomia**

Drug Interactions

Increased Effect/Toxicity: High doses of calcium with thiazide diuretics may result in milk-alkali syndrome and hypercalcemia; monitor response. Calcium salts may decrease T_4 absorption; separate dose from levothyroxine by at least 4 hours. Calcium acetate may potentiate digoxin toxicity.

Decreased Effect: Absorption of tetracycline, atenolol (and potentially other beta-blockers), iron, quinolone antibiotics, alendronate, sodium fluoride, and zinc absorption may be significantly decreased; space administration times. Effects of calcium channel blockers (eg, verapamil) effects may be diminished. Polystyrene sulfonate's potassium-binding ability may be reduced; avoid concurrent administration.

Dietary/Ethanol/Herb Considerations Ethanol: Avoid use; may increase risk of osteoporosis.

Pharmacodynamics/Kinetics Absorption: Requires vitamin D

Pregnancy Risk Factor C

Generic Available Yes

Calcium Lactate *see* Calcium Supplements *on page 229*

Calcium Leucovorin *see* Leucovorin *on page 783*

Calcium Pantothenate *see* Pantothenic Acid *on page 1033*

Calcium Phosphate (Tribasic) (KAL see um FOS fate, tri BAY sik)

U.S. Brand Names Posture® [OTC]

Pharmacologic Category Calcium Salt

Synonyms Tricalcium Phosphate

Use Adjunct in prevention of postmenopausal osteoporosis; treatment and prevention of calcium depletion

Local Anesthetic/Vasoconstrictor Precautions No information available to require special precautions

Effects on Dental Treatment No significant effects or complications reported

Dosage Oral (dosage is in terms of **elemental calcium**):

Dietary Reference Intake:

- 0-6 months: 210 mg/day
- 7-12 months: 270 mg/day
- 1-3 years: 500 mg/day
- 4-8 years: 800 mg/day
- Adults, Male/Female:
  - 9-18 years: 1300 mg/day

(Continued)

Calcium Phosphate (Tribasic) *(Continued)*

19-50 years: 1000 mg/day
≥51 years: 1200 mg/day
Female: Pregnancy: Same as for Adults, Male/Female
Female: Lactating: Same as for Adults, Male/Female
Prevention of osteoporosis:
Children: 45-65 mg/kg/day
Adults: 1-2 g/day

Mechanism of Action As dietary supplement, used to prevent or treat negative calcium balance; in osteoporosis, it helps to prevent or decrease the rate of bone loss. The calcium in calcium salts moderates nerve and muscle performance and allows normal cardiac function.

Other Adverse Effects <1%: Constipation, hypercalcemia, hypophosphatemia, milk-alkali syndrome, **nausea, xerostomia**

Drug Interactions

Increased Effect/Toxicity: High doses of calcium with thiazide diuretics may result in milk-alkali syndrome and hypercalcemia; monitor response. Calcium salts may decrease T_4 absorption; separate dose from levothyroxine by at least 4 hours. Calcium acetate may potentiate digoxin toxicity.

Decreased Effect: Absorption of tetracycline, atenolol (and potentially other beta-blockers), iron, quinolone antibiotics, alendronate, sodium fluoride, and zinc absorption may be significantly decreased; space administration times. Effects of calcium channel blockers (eg, verapamil) effects may be diminished. Polystyrene sulfonate's potassium-binding ability may be reduced; avoid concurrent administration.

Dietary/Ethanol/Herb Considerations Ethanol: Avoid use; may increase risk of osteoporosis.

Pregnancy Risk Factor C

Generic Available No

Calcium Phosphate, Tribasic *see* Calcium Supplements *on page 229*

Calcium Polycarbophil (KAL see um pol i KAR boe fil)

U.S. Brand Names Equalactin® Chewable Tablet [OTC]; Fiberall® Chewable Tablet [OTC]; FiberCon® Tablet [OTC]; Fiber-Lax® Tablet [OTC]; Mitrolan® Chewable Tablet [OTC]

Pharmacologic Category Antidiarrheal; Laxative, Bulk-Producing

Use Treatment of constipation or diarrhea by restoring a more normal moisture level and providing bulk in the patient's intestinal tract

Local Anesthetic/Vasoconstrictor Precautions No information available to require special precautions

Effects on Dental Treatment Oral medication should be given at least 1 hour prior to taking the bulk-producing laxative in order to prevent decreased absorption of medication.

Dosage Oral:

General dosing guidelines:
Children:
2-6 years: 500 mg (1 tablet) 1-2 times/day, up to 1.5 g/day
6-12 years: 500 mg (1 tablet) 1-3 times/day, up to 3 g/day
Adults: 1 g 4 times/day, up to 6 g/day

Mitrolan® product labeling:
Children:
3-6 years: 1 tablet twice daily; maximum: 3 tablets/24 hours
6-12 years: 1 tablet 3 times/day; maximum: 6 tablets/24 hours
Adults: 2 tablets 4 times/day; maximum: 12 tablets/24 hours

FiberCon® product labeling: Adults: 2 tablets once daily; maximum: 2 tablets 4 times/day

Mechanism of Action Restoring a more normal moisture level and providing bulk in the patient's intestinal tract

Other Adverse Effects 1% to 10%: Gastrointestinal: Abdominal fullness

Drug Interactions

Increased Effect/Toxicity: High doses of calcium with thiazide diuretics may result in milk-alkali syndrome and hypercalcemia; monitor response. Calcium salts may decrease T_4 absorption; separate dose from levothyroxine by at least 4 hours. Calcium acetate may potentiate digoxin toxicity.

Decreased Effect: Absorption of tetracycline, atenolol (and potentially other beta-blockers), iron, quinolone antibiotics, alendronate, sodium fluoride, and zinc absorption may be significantly decreased; space administration times. Effects of calcium channel blockers (eg, verapamil) effects may be diminished. Polystyrene sulfonate's potassium-binding ability may be reduced; avoid concurrent administration.

Pregnancy Risk Factor C

Generic Available Yes

Calcium Supplements (KAL see um SUP le ments)

Related Information

Rheumatoid Arthritis, Osteoarthritis, and Osteoporosis *on page 1488*

U.S. Brand Names Alka-Mints® [OTC]; Amitone® [OTC]; Cal Carb-HD® [OTC]; Calci-Chew™ [OTC]; Calciday-667® [OTC]; Calci-Mix™ [OTC]; Cal-citrate® 250 [OTC]; Calphron®; Cal-Plus® [OTC]; Caltrate® 600 [OTC]; Caltrate, Jr.® [OTC]; Chooz® [OTC]; Citracal® [OTC]; Dicarbosil® [OTC]; Equilet® [OTC]; Florical® [OTC]; Gencalc® 600 [OTC]; Mallamint® [OTC]; Neo-Calglucon® [OTC]; Nephro-Calci® [OTC]; Os-Cal® 500 [OTC]; Oyst-Cal 500 [OTC]; Oystercal® 500; PhosLo®; Posture® [OTC]; Rolaids® Calcium Rich [OTC]; Tums® [OTC]; Tums® E-X Extra Strength Tablet [OTC]; Tums® Ultra® [OTC]

Pharmacologic Category Electrolyte Supplement; Electrolyte Supplement, Parenteral

Synonyms Calcium Acetate; Calcium Carbonate; Calcium Chloride; Calcium Citrate; Calcium Glubionate; Calcium Gluceptate; Calcium Gluconate; Calcium Lactate; Calcium Phosphate, Tribasic

Use Treatment and prevention of calcium deficiency, hyperphosphatemia, osteoporosis; relief of acid indigestion, heartburn; emergency treatment of hypocalcemic tetany; treatment of hypermagnesemia, cardiac disturbances of hyperkalemia, hypocalcemia, or calcium channel blocking agent toxicity; topical treatment of hydrofluoric acid burns; control of hyperphosphatemia in endstage renal failure

Local Anesthetic/Vasoconstrictor Precautions No information available to require special precautions

Effects on Dental Treatment Frequency not defined: Vasodilation, hypotension, bradycardia, cardiac arrhythmias, ventricular fibrillation, syncope, headache, confusion, dizziness, lethargy, coma, hypercalcemia, nausea, vomiting, xerostomia, muscle weakness

Dosage Multiple salt forms of calcium exist; close attention must be paid to the salt form when ordering and administering calcium; incorrect selection or substitution of one salt for another without proper dosage adjustment may result in serious over- or underdosing. See table.

Elemental Calcium Content of Calcium Salts

Calcium Salt	Elemental Calcium (mg/ 1 g of salt form)	mEq Calcium Per Gram	Approximate Equivalent Doses (mg of calcium salt)
Calcium acetate	250	12.7	354
Calcium carbonate	400	20	225
Calcium chloride	270	13.5	330
Calcium citrate	211	10.6	425
Calcium glubionate	64	3.2	1400
Calcium gluceptate	82	4.1	1100
Calcium gluconate	90	4.5	1000
Calcium lactate	130	6.5	700
Calcium phosphate, tribasic	390	19.3	233

Children:

Oral: Dosage is in terms of **elemental calcium:**

Recommended daily allowance (RDA):

- <6 months: 400 mg/day
- 6-12 months: 600 mg/day
- 1-10 years: 800 mg/day
- 11-24 years: 1200 mg/day

Adequate intake (per 1997 National Academy of Science recommendations):

- <6 months: 210 mg/day
- 7-12 months: 270 mg/day
- 1-3 years: 500 mg/day
- 4-8 years: 800 mg/day
- 9-18 years: 1300 mg/day
- 19-50 years: 1000 mg/day
- ≥51 years: 1200 mg/day

Hypocalcemia (dose depends on clinical condition and serum calcium level):

Oral:

Dose expressed in mg of **elemental calcium:**

- Neonates: 50-150 mg/kg/day in 4-6 divided doses; not to exceed 1 g/day
- Children: 45-65 mg/kg/day in 4 divided doses

Dose expressed in mg of **calcium gluconate:**

- Neonates: 500-1500 mg/kg/day in 4-6 divided doses
- Infants and Children: 500-725 mg/kg/day in 3-4 divided doses

(Continued)

Calcium Supplements *(Continued)*

- Dose expressed in mg of **calcium glubionate:**
  - Neonates: 1200 mg/kg/day in 4-6 divided doses
  - Infants and Children: 600-2000 mg/kg/day in 4 divided up to a maximum of 9 g/day
- Dose expressed in mg of **calcium lactate:**
  - Neonates and Infants: 400-500 mg/kg/day divided every 4-6 hours
  - Children: 500 mg/kg/day divided every 6-8 hours; maximum daily dose 9 g

I.V.:

- Dosage expressed in mg of **calcium chloride:**
  - Children (Manufacturer's recommendation): 2.7-5 mg/kg/dose every 4-6 hours
  - Neonates, Infants, and Children (alternative dosing): 10-20 mg/kg/dose (infants <1 mEq; children 1-7mEq), repeat every 4-6 hours if needed
- Dose expressed in mg of **calcium gluceptate:**
  - Infants and Children: 200-500 mg/kg/day divided every 6 hours
- Dose expressed in mg of **calcium gluconate:**
  - Neonates: 200-800 mg/kg/day as a continuous infusion or in 4 divided doses
  - Infants and Children: 200-500 mg/kg/day as a continuous infusion or in 4 divided doses

Cardiac arrest in the presence of hyperkalemia or hypocalcemia, magnesium toxicity, or calcium antagonist toxicity: I.V.:

- Dosage expressed in mg of **calcium chloride:**
  - Neonates, Infants, and Children: 20 mg/kg; may repeat in 10 minutes if necessary
- Dose expressed in mg of **calcium gluceptate:** Infants and Children: 110 mg/kg/dose
- Dosage expressed in mg of **calcium gluconate:** (Note: Calcium chloride is the recommended salt):
  - Infants and Children: 60-100 mg/kg/dose (maximum 3 g/dose)

Tetany: I.V.:

- Dose expressed in mg of **calcium chloride:** Neonates, Infants, and Children: 10 mg/kg over 5-10 minutes; may repeat after 6 hours or follow with an infusion with a maximum dose of 200 mg/kg/day
- Dose expressed in mg of **calcium gluconate:**
  - Neonates: 100-200 mg/kg/dose; may follow with 500 mg/kg/day in 3-4 divided doses or as a continuous infusion
  - Infants and Children: 100-200 mg/kg/dose over 5-10 minutes; may repeat after 6 hours or follow with an infusion of 500 mg/kg/day

Adults:

Oral:

- Antacid (calcium carbonate): Dosage is in terms of **elemental calcium:** 0.5 - 1.5 g as needed
  - Recommended daily allowance (RDA): >24 years: 800 mg/day
  - Adequate intake (per 1997 National Academy of Science recommendations):
    - 19-50 years: 1000 mg/day
    - >50 years: 1200 mg/day
- Prevention of osteoporosis: 1000-1500 mg/day (divided in 500 mg increments)
  - Women >65 years of age receiving estrogen supplements: 1000 mg/day in divided doses
  - Women >65 years of age who are **not** receiving estrogen supplements or men >55 years of age: 1500 mg/day in divided doses
- Hypocalcemia (dose depends on clinical condition and serum calcium level):
  - Dose expressed in mg of **elemental calcium:** 1-2 g or more per day in 3-4 divided doses
  - Dose expressed in mg of **calcium gluconate:** 10-20 g daily in 3-4 divided doses
  - Dose expressed in mg of **calcium glubionate:** 6-18 g/day in divided doses
  - Dose expressed in mg of **calcium lactate:** 1.5-3 g divided every 8 hours

I.V.:

- Dosage expressed in mg of **calcium chloride:** 500 mg to 1 g/dose every 6 hours
- Dose expressed in mg of **calcium gluceptate:** 500 mg to 1.1 g/dose as needed
- Dose expressed in mg of **calcium gluconate:** 2-15 g/day as a continuous infusion or in divided doses

Cardiac arrest in the presence of hyperkalemia or hypocalcemia, magnesium toxicity, or calcium antagonist toxicity: I.V.:

- Dosage expressed in mg of **calcium chloride:** 2-4 mg/kg; may repeat in 10 minutes if necessary
- Dose expressed in mg of **calcium gluceptate:** 1.1-1.54 g/dose
- Dosage expressed in mg of **calcium gluconate:** 500-800 mg (maximum 3 g/dose) **Note:** Calcium chloride is the recommended salt.

Hypocalcemia secondary to citrated blood infusion: I.V.: Give 0.45 mEq **elemental** calcium for each 100 mL citrated blood infused

Tetany: I.V.:

- Dose expressed in mg of **calcium chloride:** 1 g over 10-30 minutes; may repeat after 6 hours

Dose expressed in mg of **calcium gluconate:** 1-3 g may be administered until therapeutic response occurs

Topical: Hydrofluoric acid (HF) burns (HF concentration <20%): Both calcium gluconate and carbonate have been used at concentrations ranging from 2.5% to 33%: Massage calcium gluconate gel or slurry into exposed area for 15 minutes.

Calcium gluconate gel: Crush 3.5 g calcium gluconate tablets into a fine powder; add to 5 oz tube of water-soluble surgical lubricant (eg, K-Y® Jelly) or add 3.5 g calcium gluconate injection to 5 oz of water-soluble surgical lubricant (calcium carbonate may be substituted; do not use calcium chloride due to potential for irritation)

Calcium carbonate slurry: 32.5% slurry can be prepared by triturating ten 650 mg tablets into a fine powder and adding 20 mL of water-soluble lubricant gel (eg, K-Y® Jelly).

Mechanism of Action Moderates nerve and muscle performance via action potential excitation threshold regulation; neutralizes acidity of stomach (carbonate salt); combines with dietary phosphate to form insoluble calcium phosphate which is excreted in feces and reduces phosphate absorption (acetate and carbonate salts)

Other Adverse Effects Frequency not defined:

Dermatologic: Erythema

Endocrine & metabolic: Milk-alkali syndrome, hypophosphatemia, hypercalciuria, hypomagnesemia

Gastrointestinal: Constipation, elevated serum amylase

Local: Tissue necrosis (I.V. administration)

Drug Interactions

Increased Effect/Toxicity: May potentiate digoxin toxicity; high doses of calcium with thiazide diuretics may result in milk-alkali syndrome and hypercalcemia

Decreased Effect: May antagonize the effects of calcium channel blockers (eg, verapamil); when administered orally, calcium decreases the absorption of tetracycline, atenolol, iron salts, quinolone antibiotics, alendronate, salicylates, sodium fluoride, and zinc; decreases potassium-binding ability of polystyrene sulfonate.

Dietary/Ethanol/Herb Considerations Food: Oral forms must be taken with food or large volume of juice to be affective. Large intakes of dietary fiber may decrease calcium absorption due to a decreased GI transit time and the formation of fiber-calcium complexes. Do not give orally with bran, foods high in oxalates (eg, spinach, rhubarb), or whole grain cereals; may decrease calcium absorption. Some products may contain tartrazine which may cause allergic reactions in susceptible individuals.

Pregnancy Risk Factor C

Dosage Forms Elemental calcium listed in brackets:

Calcium acetate:

Capsule (PhosLo®): 333.5 mg [84.5 mg]; 667 mg [169 mg]

Gelcap (PhosLo®): 667 mg [169 mg]

Injection: 0.5 mEq calcium/mL [calcium acetate/mL 39.55 mg] (10 mL, 50 mL, 100 mL)

Calcium carbonate:

Capsule: 1500 mg [600 mg]

Calci-Mix™: 1250 mg [500 mg]

Florical®: 364 mg [145.6 mg] with sodium fluoride 8.3 mg

Powder (Cal Carb-HD®): 6.5 g/packet [2.6 g]

Suspension, oral: 1250 mg/5 mL [500 mg]

Tablet: 650 mg [260 mg], 1500 mg [600 mg]

Calciday-667®: 667 mg [267 mg]

Cal-Plus®, Caltrate® 600, Gencalc® 600, Nephro-Calci®: 1500 mg [600 mg]

Florical®: 364 mg [145.6 mg] with sodium fluoride 8.3 mg

Os-Cal® 500, Oyst-Cal 500, Oystercal® 500: 1250 mg [500 mg]

Tablet, chewable:

Alka-Mints®: 850 mg [340 mg]

Amitone®: 350 mg [140 mg] ®

Caltrate, Jr.®: 750 mg [300 mg]

Chooz®, Dicarbosil®, Equilet®, Tums®: 500 mg [200 mg]

Mallamint®: 420 mg [168 mg]

Rolaids® Calcium Rich: 550 mg [220 mg]

Tums® E-X Extra Strength: 750 mg [300 mg]

Tums® Ultra®: 1000 mg [400 mg]

Calcium chloride:

Injection: 10% = 100 mg/mL [27.2 mg/mL, 1.36 mEq/mL] (10 mL)

Calcium citrate:

Tablet: 950 mg [200 mg]

Cal-Citrate®: 250 mg [100% calcium citrate]

Tablet, effervescent: 2376 mg [500 mg]

Calcium glubionate: Syrup: 1.8 g/5 mL [115 mg/5mL] (480 mL)

Calcium gluceptate: Injection: 220 mg/mL [18 mg/mL, 0.9 mEq/mL] (5 mL)

Calcium gluconate:

Injection: 10% = 100 mg/mL [9 mg/mL] (10 mL, 50 mL, 100 mL, 200 mL)

(Continued)

Calcium Supplements *(Continued)*

Tablet: 500 mg [45 mg], 650 mg [58.5 mg], 975 mg [87.75 mg], 1 g [90 mg]

Calcium lactate:

Capsule: 500 mg [90 mg]

Tablet: 325 mg [42.25 mg], 650 mg [84.5 mg]

Calcium phosphate, tribasic: Tablet [sugar free]: 1565.2 mg [600 mg]

Generic Available Yes

CaldeCORT® [OTC] *see* Hydrocortisone *on page 688*

Calderol® *see* Calcifediol *on page 221*

Calfactant (cal FAC tant)

U.S. Brand Names Infasurf®

Pharmacologic Category Lung Surfactant

Use Prevention of respiratory distress syndrome (RDS) in premature infants at high risk for RDS and for the treatment ("rescue") of premature infants who develop RDS

Prophylaxis: Therapy at birth with calfactant is indicated for premature infants <29 weeks of gestational age at significant risk for RDS. Should be administered as soon as possible, preferably within 30 minutes after birth.

Treatment: For infants ≤72 hours of age with RDS (confirmed by clinical and radiologic findings) and requiring endotracheal intubation.

Local Anesthetic/Vasoconstrictor Precautions No information available to require special precautions

Effects on Dental Treatment >10%: Bradycardia (34%), reflux (21%)

Dosage Intratracheal administration **only**: Each dose is 3 mL/kg body weight at birth; should be administered every 12 hours for a total of up to 3 doses

Mechanism of Action Endogenous lung surfactant is essential for effective ventilation because it modifies alveolar surface tension, thereby stabilizing the alveoli. Lung surfactant deficiency is the cause of respiratory distress syndrome (RDS) in premature infants and lung surfactant restores surface activity to the lungs of these infants.

Other Adverse Effects

Cardiovascular: Cyanosis (65%)

Respiratory: Airway obstruction (39%), requirement for manual ventilation (16%), reintubation (1% to 10%)

Pharmacodynamics/Kinetics No human studies of absorption, biotransformation, or excretion have been performed

Generic Available No

Calphron® *see* Calcium Supplements *on page 229*

Cal-Plus® [OTC] *see* Calcium Supplements *on page 229*

Caltrate® 600 [OTC] *see* Calcium Supplements *on page 229*

Caltrate, Jr.® [OTC] *see* Calcium Supplements *on page 229*

Camila™ *see* Norethindrone *on page 986*

Campath® *see* Alemtuzumab *on page 52*

Campath-1H *see* Alemtuzumab *on page 52*

Campho-Phenique® [OTC] *see* Camphor and Phenol *on page 232*

Camphor and Phenol (KAM for & FEE nole)

U.S. Brand Names Campho-Phenique® [OTC]

Pharmacologic Category Topical Skin Product

Synonyms Phenol and Camphor

Use Relief of pain and for minor infections

Local Anesthetic/Vasoconstrictor Precautions No information available to require special precautions

Effects on Dental Treatment No significant effects or complications reported

Dosage Apply as needed

Pregnancy Risk Factor C

Generic Available Yes

Camphorated Tincture of Opium *see* Paregoric *on page 1034*

Camptosar® *see* Irinotecan *on page 740*

Camptothecin-11 *see* Irinotecan *on page 740*

Canasa™ *see* Mesalamine *on page 869*

Cancidas® *see* Caspofungin *on page 258*

Candesartan (kan de SAR tan)

U.S. Brand Names Atacand®

Canadian Brand Names Atacand®

Mexican Brand Names Atacand®

Pharmacologic Category Angiotensin II Receptor Blocker

Synonyms Candesartan Cilexetil

Use Alone or in combination with other antihypertensive agents in treating essential hypertension; may have an advantage over losartan due to minimal metabolism requirements and consequent use in mild to moderate hepatic impairment

Local Anesthetic/Vasoconstrictor Precautions No information available to require special precautions

Effects on Dental Treatment Frequency not defined: Flushing, tachycardia, palpitations, angina, MI, dizziness, lightheadedness, drowsiness, headache, anxiety, depression, somnolence, fever, hyperglycemia, weakness, upper respiratory tract infection, bronchitis, epistaxis, increased diaphoresis

Dosage Adults: Oral: Usual dose is 4-32 mg once daily; dosage must be individualized. Blood pressure response is dose-related over the range of 2-32 mg. The usual recommended starting dose of 16 mg once daily when it is used as monotherapy in patients who are not volume depleted. It can be administered once or twice daily with total daily doses ranging from 8-32 mg. Larger doses do not appear to have a greater effect and there is relatively little experience with such doses.

Elderly: No initial dosage adjustment is necessary for elderly patients (although higher concentrations (C_{max}) and AUC were observed in these populations), for patients with mildly impaired renal function, or for patients with mildly impaired hepatic function.

Dosing adjustment in hepatic impairment: No initial adjustment required in mild hepatic impairment; consider initiation at lower dosages in moderate hepatic impairment (AUC increased by 145%). No data available concerning dosing in severe hepatic impairment.

Mechanism of Action Candesartan is an angiotensin receptor antagonist. Angiotensin II acts as a vasoconstrictor. In addition to causing direct vasoconstriction, angiotensin II also stimulates the release of aldosterone. Once aldosterone is released, sodium as well as water are reabsorbed. The end result is an elevation in blood pressure. Candesartan binds to the AT1 angiotensin II receptor. This binding prevents angiotensin II from binding to the receptor thereby blocking the vasoconstriction and the aldosterone secreting effects of angiotensin II.

Other Adverse Effects May be associated with worsening of renal function in patients dependent on renin-angiotensin-aldosterone system.

Frequency not defined:
Central nervous system: Depression, vertigo
Dermatologic: Angioedema, rash
Endocrine & metabolic: Hypertriglyceridemia
Genitourinary: Hyperuricemia, hematuria
Neuromuscular & skeletal: Back pain, increased CPK

<1%, postmarketing, and/or case reports: Abnormal hepatic function, agranulocytosis, arthralgia, **cough, chest pain**, diarrhea, dyspepsia, **dyspnea, epistaxis**, fatigue, **gastroenteritis**, hepatitis, leukopenia, myalgia, **nausea**, neutropenia, **paresthesias**, peripheral edema, **pharyngitis**, pruritus, **rhinitis, sinusitis**, urticaria, **vomiting**

Drug Interactions Substrate of CYP2C8/9; Inhibits CYP2C8/9

Increased Effect/Toxicity: The risk of lithium toxicity may be increased by candesartan; monitor lithium levels. Concurrent use with potassium-sparing diuretics (amiloride, spironolactone, triamterene), potassium supplements, or trimethoprim (high-dose) may increase the risk of hyperkalemia.

Dietary/Ethanol/Herb Considerations

Ethanol: Avoid use; may increase risk of hypotension or dizziness.

Food reduces the time to maximal concentration and increases the C_{max}. Avoid caffeine (eg, colas, chocolate), garlic, and licorice.

Herb/Nutraceutical: Avoid black cohosh, dong quai, and evening primrose due to estrogenic activity. Avoid ephedra, ginseng, and yohimbe; may worsen hypertension. Avoid garlic; may have increased antihypertensive effect. Avoid ginger due to positive inotropic effects; theoretically, may cause arrhythmia. Avoid hawthorn; may lower peripheral vascular resistance causing additional decrease in BP. Avoid licorice.

Pharmacodynamics/Kinetics

Onset of action: 2-3 hours
Peak effect: 6-8 hours
Duration: >24 hours
Distribution: V_d: 0.13 L/kg
Protein binding: 99%
Metabolism: To candesartan by the intestinal wall cells
Bioavailability: 15%
Half-life elimination (dose dependent): 5-9 hours
Time to peak: 3-4 hours
Excretion: Urine (26%)
Clearance: Total body: 0.37 mL/kg/minute; Renal: 0.19 mL/kg/minute

Pregnancy Risk Factor C/D (2nd and 3rd trimesters)

Generic Available No

Candesartan and Hydrochlorothiazide

(kan de SAR tan & hye droe klor oh THYE a zide)

Related Information

Candesartan *on page 232*

Hydrochlorothiazide *on page 675*

U.S. Brand Names Atacand HCT™

Canadian Brand Names Atacand® Plus

Pharmacologic Category Angiotensin II Receptor Blocker Combination

Synonyms Candesartan Cilexetil and Hydrochlorothiazide

Use Treatment of hypertension; combination product should not be used for initial therapy

Local Anesthetic/Vasoconstrictor Precautions No information available to require special precautions

Effects on Dental Treatment 1% to 10%: Dizziness (3%), headache (3%, placebo 5%), upper respiratory tract infection (4%), flu-like symptoms (2%)

Dosage Oral:

Adults: Replacement therapy: Combination product can be substituted for individual agents; maximum therapeutic effect would be expected within 4 weeks

Usual dosage range:

Candesartan: 8-32 mg/day, given once daily or twice daily in divided doses

Hydrochlorothiazide: 12.5-50 mg once daily

Elderly: No initial adjustment in normal renal and hepatic function; some patients may have increased sensitivity

Dosing adjustment in renal impairment: Serum levels of candesartan are increased and the halflife of hydrochlorothiazide is prolonged in patients with renal impairment. Do not use if Cl_{cr} <30 mL/minute

Dosing adjustment in hepatic impairment: Use with caution

Mechanism of Action

Candesartan: Candesartan is an angiotensin receptor antagonist. Angiotensin II acts as a vasoconstrictor. In addition to causing direct vasoconstriction, angiotensin II also stimulates the release of aldosterone. Once aldosterone is released, sodium as well as water are reabsorbed. The end result is an elevation in blood pressure. Candesartan binds to the AT1 angiotensin II receptor. This binding prevents angiotensin II from binding to the receptor, thereby blocking the vasoconstriction and the aldosterone-secreting effects of angiotensin II.

Hydrochlorothiazide: Inhibits sodium reabsorption in the distal tubules causing increased excretion of sodium and water as well as potassium and hydrogen ions

Other Adverse Effects

1% to 10%: Neuromuscular & skeletal: Back pain (3%)

<1%: Abdominal pain, abnormal EKG, abnormal hepatic function, agranulocytosis, **angina pectoris**, angioedema (<0.5%), **anxiety**, arthralgia, **arthritis**, arthrosis, **asthenia, bradycardia, bronchitis, chest pain**, conjunctivitis, **cough**, cystitis, depression, dermatitis, diarrhea, dyspepsia, **dyspnea**, eczema, elevated BUN, elevated CPK, elevated transaminases, **epistaxis**, extrasystoles, **fatigue, gastritis, gastroenteritis**, hematuria, hepatitis, hypesthesia, **hyperglycemia**, hyperuricemia, hypokalemia, **increased diaphoresis, infection**, insomnia, **leg cramps**, leukopenia, myalgia, **MI (<0.5%), nausea**, neutropenia, **pain, palpitations, paresthesia**, peripheral edema, **pharyngitis**, pruritus, rash, **rhinitis, sciatica, sinusitis, tachycardia,** tinnitus, urinary tract infection, urticaria, vertigo, **viral infection, vomiting**

Dietary/Ethanol/Herb Considerations Ethanol: Avoid use; may potentiate orthostatic hypotension.

Pregnancy Risk Factor C/D (2nd and 3rd trimesters)

Generic Available No

Candesartan Cilexetil *see* Candesartan *on page 232*

Candesartan Cilexetil and Hydrochlorothiazide *see* Candesartan and Hydrochlorothiazide *on page 234*

C. angustifolia *see* Senna *on page 1215*

Cantharidin (kan THAR e din)

U.S. Brand Names Verr-Canth™

Canadian Brand Names Canthacur®; Cantharone®

Pharmacologic Category Keratolytic Agent

Use Removal of ordinary and periungual warts

Local Anesthetic/Vasoconstrictor Precautions No information available to require special precautions

Effects on Dental Treatment 1% to 10%: Syncope, GI hemorrhage, rectal bleeding, dysphagia, burning of oropharynx, delirium

Dosage Apply directly to lesion, cover with nonporous tape, remove tape in 24 hours, reapply if necessary

Other Adverse Effects 1% to 10%:

Central nervous system: Ataxia

Dermatologic: Dermal irritation, dermal burns, acantholysis

Genitourinary: Priapism
Hepatic: Fatty degeneration
Neuromuscular & skeletal: Hyper-reflexia
Ocular: Conjunctivitis, iritis, keratitis
Renal: Proteinuria, hematuria

Pregnancy Risk Factor C
Generic Available No

Cantil® *see* Mepenzolate *on page 858*
Capastat® Sulfate *see* Capreomycin *on page 237*

Capecitabine (ka pe SITE a been)

U.S. Brand Names Xeloda®
Canadian Brand Names Xeloda®
Mexican Brand Names Xeloda®
Pharmacologic Category Antineoplastic Agent, Antimetabolite
Use

Treatment of metastatic colorectal cancer.

Treatment of metastatic breast cancer in combination with docetaxel after failure of prior anthracycline therapy.

Monotherapy treatment of metastatic breast cancer resistant to both paclitaxel and an anthracycline-containing chemotherapy regimen or resistant to paclitaxel and for whom further anthracycline therapy is not indicated (eg, patients who have received cumulative doses of 400 mg/m^2 of doxorubicin or doxorubicin equivalents). Resistance is defined as progressive disease while on treatment, with or without an initial response, or relapse within 6 months of completing treatment with an anthracycline-containing adjuvant regimen.

Local Anesthetic/Vasoconstrictor Precautions No information available to require special precautions

Effects on Dental Treatment As reported in monotherapy trials:

>10%: Fever (12% to 18%), mild to moderate nausea (43% to 53%), vomiting (27% to 37%), paresthesia (21%), dyspnea (14% in colorectal cancer), stomatitis (~25%), fatigue (~40%), pain (12% in colorectal cancer), paresthesia (21%)

5% to 10%: Chest pain (6% in colorectal cancer), abnormal taste (6% in colorectal cancer), headache (-10%), dizziness (-8%), dehydration (7%), oral discomfort (10% in colorectal cancer), upper GI inflammatory disorders (8% in colorectal cancer), hemorrhage (6% in colorectal cancer), taste disturbance (6% in colorectal cancer), cough (7%), viral infection (5% in colorectal cancer)

<5%: Angina, asthma, atrial fibrillation, bronchitis, bradycardia, oral candidiasis, bronchopneumonia, bronchospasm, cardiac arrest, cardiac failure, confusion, diaphoresis increased, duodenitis, dysphagia, esophagitis, fungal infection, gastric ulcer, gastritis, gastroenteritis, GI hemorrhage, hemoptysis, hot flashes, hypotension, hypersensitivity, hypertension, impaired balance, infection, flu-like illness, irritability, laryngitis, loss of consciousness, myocardial infarction, pneumonia, respiratory distress, sedation, sepsis, tachycardia, thirst, tremor, sore throat (2%), epistaxis (3%)

Dosage Oral:

Adults: 2500 mg/m^2/day in 2 divided doses (~12 hours apart) at the end of a meal for 2 weeks followed by a 1-week rest period given as 3-week cycles

Capecitabine dose calculation according to BSA table: The following can be used to determine the total daily dose (mg) based on a dosing level of 2500 mg/m^2/day. (The number of tablets per dose, given morning and evening, are also listed): See table.

Capecitabine Dose Calculation According to BSA Table

Dose Level 2500 mg/m^2/day		# of tablets per dose (morning and evening)	
Surface Area (m^2)	**Total Daily Dose (mg)**	**150 mg**	**500 mg**
≤1.25	3000	0	3
1.26-1.37	3300	1	3
1.38-1.51	3600	2	3
1.52-1.65	4000	0	4
1.66-1.77	4300	1	4
1.78-1.91	4600	2	4
1.92-2.05	5000	0	5
2.06-2.17	5300	1	5
≥2.18	5600	2	5

Elderly: Specific recommendations unavailable; use with caution and monitor; elderly patients are pharmacodynamically more sensitive to the toxic effects of 5-fluorouracil

(Continued)

Capecitabine *(Continued)*

Dosing adjustment in renal impairment: Baseline calculation of creatinine clearance is required (Cockroft-Gault per manufacturer); carefully monitor and interrupt therapy if grade 2-, 3-, or 4 toxicity develops.

Cl_{cr} 50-80 mL/minute: No adjustment of initial dose

Cl_{cr} 30-50 mL/minute: Reduce initial dose to 1900 mg/m^2/day (25% reduction in dose)

Cl_{cr} <30 mL/minute: Do not use

Dosing adjustment in hepatic impairment: Carefully monitor patients; no starting dose adjustment is necessary for mild to moderate impairment; severe impairment not studied

Dosage modification guidelines: Carefully monitor patients for toxicity. Toxicity caused by capecitabine administration may be managed by symptomatic treatment, dose interruptions, and adjustment of dose. Once the dose has been reduced, it should not be increased at a later time.

Dosage reduction for toxicity: The starting dose may be reduced by 25% in patients experiencing significant adverse effects at the full starting dose if symptoms persist, a further reduction (to 50% of the starting dose) may be considered. These recommendations were based on clinical studies reported at the 36th Annual Meeting of the American Society of Clinical Oncology (ASCO). See table.

Recommended Dose Modifications

Toxicity NCI Grades	During a Course of Therapy	Dose Adjustment for Next Cycle (% of starting dose)
Grade 1	Maintain dose level	Maintain dose level
Grade 2		
1st appearance	Interrupt until resolved to grade 0-1	100%
2nd appearance	Interrupt until resolved to grade 0-1	75%
3rd appearance	Interrupt until resolved to grade 0-1	50%
4th appearance	Discontinue treatment permanently	
Grade 3		
1st appearance	Interrupt until resolved to grade 0-1	75%
2nd appearance	Interrupt until resolved to grade 0-1	50%
3rd appearance	Discontinue treatment permanently	
Grade 4		
1st appearance	Discontinue permanently OR If physician deems it to be in the patient's best interest to continue, interrupt until resolved to grade 0-1	50%

Mechanism of Action Capecitabine is a prodrug of fluorouracil. It undergoes hydrolysis in the liver and tissues to form fluorouracil which is the active moiety. Fluorouracil is a fluorinated pyrimidine antimetabolite that inhibits thymidylate synthetase, blocking the methylation of deoxyuridylic acid to thymidylic acid, interfering with DNA, and to a lesser degree, RNA synthesis. Fluorouracil appears to be phase specific for the G_1 and S phases of the cell cycle.

Other Adverse Effects As reported in monotherapy trials:

>10%:

Cardiovascular: Edema (9% to 15%)

Dermatologic: Palmar-plantar erythrodysesthesia (hand-and-foot syndrome) (~55%, may be dose limiting), dermatitis (27% to 37%)

Gastrointestinal: Diarrhea (~55%; may be dose limiting), decreased appetite (26% in colorectal cancer), anorexia (23%), abdominal pain (20% to 35%), constipation (~15%)

Hematologic: Lymphopenia (94%), anemia (72% to 80%; Grade 3/4: <1% to 3%), neutropenia (13% to 26%; Grade 3/4: 1% to 2%), thrombocytopenia (24%; Grade 3/4: 1% to 3%)

Hepatic: Increased bilirubin (22% to 48%)

Ocular: Eye irritation (~15%)

5% to 10%:

Cardiovascular: Venous thrombosis (85 in colorectal cancer)

Central nervous system: Insomnia (8%), mood alteration (colorectal cancer: 5%), depression (colorectal cancer: 5%)

Dermatologic: Nail disorders (7%), skin discoloration (colorectal cancer: 7%), alopecia (colorectal cancer: 6%)

Gastrointestinal: Motility disorder (colorectal cancer: 10%), dyspepsia (8%), ileus (colorectal cancer: 6%)

Neuromuscular & skeletal: Back pain (colorectal cancer: 10%), myalgia (9%), neuropathy (colorectal cancer: 10%), arthralgia (colorectal cancer: 8%), limb pain (colorectal cancer: 6%)

Ocular: Abnormal vision (colorectal cancer: 5%)

<5%: Abdominal distension, appetite increased, arthritis, ascites, ataxia, bone pain, cachexia, cardiomyopathy, cerebral vascular accident, cholestasis, colitis, conjunctivitis, deep vein thrombosis, dysarthria, dysrhythmia, ecchymoses, EKG changes, encephalopathy, fibrosis, hematemesis, hepatitis, hepatic failure, hepatic fibrosis, hoarseness, hypokalemia, hypomagnesemia, hypertriglyceridemia, idiopathic thrombocytopenia purpura, ileus, keratoconjunctivitis, leukopenia, lymphedema, myocardial ischemia, myocarditis, necrotizing enterocolitis, nocturia, pericardial effusion, thrombocytopenic purpura, pancytopenia, photosensitivity reaction, pneumonia, proctalgia, pruritus, pulmonary embolism, radiation recall syndrome, renal impairment, skin ulceration, toxic dilation of intestine, thrombophlebitis, weight gain, ventricular extrasystoles, vertigo

Drug Interactions Increased Effect/Toxicity: Taking capecitabine immediately before an aluminum hydroxide/magnesium hydroxide antacid or a meal increases the absorption of capecitabine. The concentration of capecitabine's active metabolite (5-fluorouracil) is increased and its toxicity may be enhanced by leucovorin. Deaths from severe enterocolitis, diarrhea, and dehydration have been reported in elderly patients receiving weekly leucovorin and fluorouracil. Response to warfarin may be increased by capecitabine; changes may occur days to months after starting or stopping capecitabine therapy.

Dietary/Ethanol/Herb Considerations Food: Administer with with food; reduces the rate and absorption of capecitabine but current safety and efficacy data are based on administration with food (taken within 30 minutes after meal in all clinical trials).

Pharmacodynamics/Kinetics

Absorption: Rapid and extensive

Protein binding: <60%; 35% to albumin

Metabolism: Hepatic: Inactive metabolites: 5′-deoxy-5-fluorocytidine, 5′-deoxy-5-fluorouridine; Tissue: Active metabolite: 5-fluorouracil

Half-life elimination: 0.5-1 hour

Time to peak: 1.5 hours; Fluorouracil: 2 hours

Excretion: Urine (96%, 50% as α-fluoro-β-alanine)

Pregnancy Risk Factor D

Generic Available No

Capex™ *see* Fluocinolone *on page 584*

Capital® and Codeine *see* Acetaminophen and Codeine *on page 29*

Capitrol® *see* Chloroxine *on page 306*

Capoten® *see* Captopril *on page 238*

Capozide® *see* Captopril and Hydrochlorothiazide *on page 240*

Capreomycin (kap ree oh MYE sin)

Related Information

Nonviral Infectious Diseases *on page 1493*

U.S. Brand Names Capastat® Sulfate

Pharmacologic Category Antibiotic, Miscellaneous; Antitubercular Agent

Synonyms Capreomycin Sulfate

Use Treatment of tuberculosis in conjunction with at least one other antituberculosis agent

Local Anesthetic/Vasoconstrictor Precautions No information available to require special precautions

Effects on Dental Treatment No significant effects or complications reported

Dosage I.M.:

Infants and Children: 15 mg/kg/day, up to 1 g/day maximum

Adults: 15-20 mg/kg/day up to 1 g/day for 60-120 days, followed by 1 g 2-3 times/week

Dosing interval in renal impairment: Adults:

Cl_{cr} >100 mL/minute: Administer 13-15 mg/kg every 24 hours

Cl_{cr} 80-100 mL/minute: Administer 10-13 mg/kg every 24 hours

Cl_{cr} 60-80 mL/minute: Administer 7-10 mg/kg every 24 hours

Cl_{cr} 40-60 mL/minute: Administer 11-14 mg/kg every 48 hours

Cl_{cr} 20-40 mL/minute: Administer 10-14 mg/kg every 72 hours

Cl_{cr} <20 mL/minute: Administer 4-7 mg/kg every 72 hours

Mechanism of Action Capreomycin is a cyclic polypeptide antimicrobial. It is administered as a mixture of capreomycin IA and capreomycin IB. The mechanism of action of capreomycin is not well understood. Mycobacterial species that have become resistant to other agents are usually still sensitive to the action of capreomycin. However, significant cross-resistance with viomycin, kanamycin, and neomycin occurs.

Other Adverse Effects

>10%:

Otic: Ototoxicity [subclinical hearing loss (11%), clinical loss (3%)], tinnitus

(Continued)

Capreomycin *(Continued)*

Renal: Nephrotoxicity (36%, increased BUN)

1% to 10%: Hematologic: Eosinophilia (dose-related, mild)

<1%: Vertigo, hypokalemia, leukocytosis, thrombocytopenia (rare); pain, induration, and bleeding at injection site; hypersensitivity (urticaria, rash, fever)

Drug Interactions

Increased effect/duration of nondepolarizing neuromuscular blocking agents.

Increased toxicity (nephrotoxicity and ototoxicity, respiratory paralysis) may occur with aminoglycosides (eg, streptomycin)

Pharmacodynamics/Kinetics

Half-life elimination: Normal renal function: 4-6 hours

Time to peak, serum: I.M.: ~1 hour

Excretion: Urine (as unchanged drug)

Pregnancy Risk Factor C

Generic Available No

Capreomycin Sulfate *see* Capreomycin *on page 237*

Capsaicin (kap SAY sin)

Related Information

Cayenne *on page 1424*

U.S. Brand Names Capsin® [OTC]; Capzasin-P® [OTC]; Dolorac™ [OTC]; No Pain-HP® [OTC]; R-Gel® [OTC]; Zostrix® [OTC]; Zostrix®-HP [OTC]

Canadian Brand Names Antiphogistine Rub A-535 Capsaicin; Zostrix®; Zostrix® H.P.

Pharmacologic Category Analgesic, Topical; Topical Skin Product

Use Topical treatment of pain associated with postherpetic neuralgia, rheumatoid arthritis, osteoarthritis, diabetic neuropathy; postsurgical pain

Unlabeled/Investigational Use Treatment of pain associated with psoriasis, chronic neuralgias unresponsive to other forms of therapy, and intractable pruritus

Local Anesthetic/Vasoconstrictor Precautions No information available to require special precautions

Effects on Dental Treatment 1% to 10%: Cough

Dosage Children ≥2 years and Adults: Topical: Apply to affected area at least 3-4 times/day; application frequency less than 3-4 times/day prevents the total depletion, inhibition of synthesis, and transport of substance P resulting in decreased clinical efficacy and increased local discomfort

Mechanism of Action Induces release of substance P, the principal chemomediator of pain impulses from the periphery to the CNS, from peripheral sensory neurons; after repeated application, capsaicin depletes the neuron of substance P and prevents reaccumulation

Other Adverse Effects

>10%: Local: Transient burning on application which usually diminishes with repeated use (≥30%)

1% to 10%: Dermatologic: Itching, stinging sensation, erythema

Drug Interactions Substrate of CYP2E1

Pharmacodynamics/Kinetics

Onset of action: 14-28 days

Peak effect: 4-6 weeks of continuous therapy

Duration: Several hours

Pregnancy Risk Factor C

Generic Available Yes

Capsin® [OTC] *see* Capsaicin *on page 238*

Captopril (KAP toe pril)

Related Information

Cardiovascular Diseases *on page 1456*

U.S. Brand Names Capoten®

Canadian Brand Names Alti-Captopril; Apo®-Capto; Capoten™; Gen-Captopril; Novo-Captopril; Nu-Capto®; PMS-Captopril®

Mexican Brand Names Capitral®; Capoten®; Capotena; Captral®; Cardipril®; Cryopril®; Ecapresan; Ecaten®; Kenolan®; Lenpryl®; Precaptil; Romir®

Pharmacologic Category Angiotensin-Converting Enzyme (ACE) Inhibitor

Synonyms ACE

Use Management of hypertension; treatment of CHF, left ventricular dysfunction after MI, diabetic nephropathy

Unlabeled/Investigational Use Treatment of hypertensive crisis, hypertension secondary to scleroderma renal crisis or Takayasu's disease, rheumatoid arthritis, idiopathic edema, Bartter's syndrome; diagnosis of anatomic renal artery stenosis or aldosteronism; postmyocardial infarction for prevention of ventricular failure; increase circulation in Raynaud's phenomenon

Local Anesthetic/Vasoconstrictor Precautions No information available to require special precautions

Effects on Dental Treatment

1% to 10%: Hypotension (1% to 3%), tachycardia (1%), chest pain (1%), palpitations (1%), (≤2%), hypersensitivity reactions (rash, pruritus, fever, arthralgia, and eosinophilia --4% to 7%; dependent on dose and renal function), loss or diminished perception of taste (2% to 4%)

Frequency not defined: Cardiac arrest, orthostatic hypotension, syncope, flushing, angina, MI, CHF, confusion, nervousness, somnolence, glossitis, blurred vision, bronchospasm, eosinophilic pneumonitis, rhinitis, anaphylactoid reactions

Dosage Dosage must be titrated according to patient's response; use lowest effective dose.

Oral:

Infants: Initial: 0.15-0.3 mg/kg/dose; titrate dose upward to maximum of 6 mg/kg/day in 1-4 divided doses; usual required dose: 2.5-6 mg/kg/day

Children: Initial: 0.5 mg/kg/dose; titrate upward to maximum of 6 mg/kg/day in 2-4 divided doses

Older Children: Initial: 6.25-12.5 mg/dose every 12-24 hours; titrate upward to maximum of 6 mg/kg/day

Adolescents: Initial: 12.5-25 mg/dose given every 8-12 hours; increase by 25 mg/dose to maximum of 450 mg/day

Adults:

Acute hypertension (urgency/emergency): 12.5-25 mg, may repeat as needed (may be given sublingually, but no therapeutic advantage demonstrated)

Hypertension:

Initial dose: 12.5-25 mg 2-3 times/day; may increase by 12.5-25 mg/dose at 1- to 2-week intervals up to 50 mg 3 times/day; add diuretic before further dosage increases

Maximum dose: 150 mg 3 times/day

Congestive heart failure:

Initial dose: 6.25-12.5 mg 3 times/day in conjunction with cardiac glycoside and diuretic therapy; initial dose depends upon patient's fluid/electrolyte status

Target dose: 50 mg 3 times/day

Maximum dose: 150 mg 3 times/day

LVD after MI: Initial dose: 6.25 mg followed by 12.5 mg 3 times/day; then increase to 25 mg 3 times/day during next several days and then over next several weeks to target dose of 50 mg 3 times/day

Diabetic nephropathy: 25 mg 3 times/day; other antihypertensives often given concurrently

Dosing adjustment in renal impairment:

Cl_{cr} 10-50 mL/minute: Administer at 75% of normal dose.

Cl_{cr} <10 mL/minute: Administer at 50% of normal dose.

Dysfunction: Smaller doses every 8-12 hours; renal function and leukocyte count should be carefully monitored during therapy.

Hemodialysis: Moderately dialyzable (20% to 50%); administer dose postdialysis or administer 25% to 35% supplemental dose.

Peritoneal dialysis: Supplemental dose is unnecessary.

Mechanism of Action Competitive inhibitor of angiotensin-converting enzyme (ACE); prevents conversion of angiotensin I to angiotensin II, a potent vasoconstrictor; results in lower levels of angiotensin II which causes an increase in plasma renin activity and a reduction in aldosterone secretion

Other Adverse Effects

1% to 10%:

Dermatologic: Rash (maculopapular or urticarial) (4% to 7%), pruritus (2%); in patients with rash, a positive ANA and/or eosinophilia has been noted in 7% to 10%.

Endocrine & metabolic: Hyperkalemia (1% to 11%)

Hematologic: Neutropenia may occur in up to 4% of patients with renal insufficiency or collagen-vascular disease.

Renal: Proteinuria (1%), increased serum creatinine, worsening of renal function (may occur in patients with bilateral renal artery stenosis or hypovolemia)

Frequency not defined:

Cardiovascular: Angioedema, cerebrovascular insufficiency, rhythm disturbances, pallor, Raynaud's syndrome

Central nervous system: Ataxia, depression

Dermatologic: Bullous pemphigus, erythema multiforme, Stevens-Johnson syndrome, exfoliative dermatitis

Endocrine & metabolic: Serum transaminases, serum bilirubin, alkaline phosphatase increased; gynecomastia

Gastrointestinal: Pancreatitis, dyspepsia

Genitourinary: Urinary frequency, impotence

Hematologic: Anemia, thrombocytopenia, pancytopenia, agranulocytosis, anemia

Hepatic: Jaundice, hepatitis, hepatic necrosis (rare), cholestasis, hyponatremia (symptomatic)

Neuromuscular & skeletal: Asthenia, myalgia, myasthenia

Renal: Renal insufficiency, renal failure, nephrotic syndrome, polyuria, oliguria

(Continued)

Captopril *(Continued)*

<1% (Limited to important or life-threatening symptoms; frequency ≤ to placebo): Gastric irritation, abdominal pain, **nausea, vomiting**, diarrhea, anorexia, constipation, **aphthous ulcers, peptic ulcer, dizziness, headache**, malaise, fatigue, insomnia, **xerostomia, dyspnea**, alopecia, **paresthesia, angina**, glomerulonephritis, cholestatic jaundice, psoriasis, hyperthermia, myalgia, arthralgia

Postmarketing and/or case reports: Aplastic anemia, hemolytic anemia, **bronchospasm**, alopecia, systemic lupus erythematosus, Kaposi's sarcoma, pericarditis, exacerbations of Huntington's disease, Guillain-Barré syndrome, **seizures** (in premature infants), syndrome (may include fever, myalgia, arthralgia, interstitial nephritis, vasculitis, rash, eosinophilia, and elevated ESR)

Drug Interactions Substrate of **CYP2D6**

Increased Effect/Toxicity:

The following drugs may result in elevated serum potassium levels when combined with captopril: Potassium supplements, sulfamethoxazole and trimethoprim (high dose), angiotensin II receptor antagonists (candesartan, losartan, irbesartan, etc), or potassium-sparing diuretics (amiloride, spironolactone, triamterene). ACE inhibitor effects may be increased by phenothiazines or probenecid (increases levels of captopril). ACE inhibitors may increase serum concentrations/effects of digoxin, lithium, and sulfonlyureas.

Diuretics have additive hypotensive effects with ACE inhibitors, and hypovolemia increases the potential for adverse renal effects of ACE inhibitors. In patients with compromised renal function, coadministration with NSAIDs may result in further deterioration of renal function. Allopurinol and ACE inhibitors may cause a higher risk of hypersensitivity reaction when taken concurrently.

Decreased Effect: Aspirin (high dose) may reduce the therapeutic effects of ACE inhibitors; at low dosages this does not appear to be significant. Rifampin may decrease the effect of ACE inhibitors. Antacids may decrease the bioavailability of ACE inhibitors (may be more likely to occur with captopril); separate administration times by 1-2 hours. NSAIDs, specifically indomethacin, may reduce the hypotensive effects of ACE inhibitors. More likely to occur in low renin or volume dependent hypertensive patients.

Dietary/Ethanol/Herb Considerations

Ethanol: Avoid use; may increase risk of hypotension or dizziness.

Food: Administer on an empty stomach 1 hour before or 2 hours after meals; food may decrease serum concentration. Long-term use may result in zinc deficiency resulting in decreased taste perception. Increased dietary intake of potassium or potassium supplements may increase the risk of hyperkalemia. Avoid caffeine (eg, colas, chocolate), garlic, and licorice.

Herb/Nutraceutical: Avoid black cohosh, dong quai, and evening primrose due to estrogenic activity. Avoid ephedra, yohimbe, and ginseng; may worsen hypertension. Avoid garlic; may have increased antihypertensive effect. Avoid ginger due to positive inotropic effects; theoretically, may cause arrhythmia. Avoid hawthorn; may lower peripheral vascular resistance resulting in additive decrease in BP. Avoid licorice.

Pharmacodynamics/Kinetics

Onset of action: Peak effect: Blood pressure reduction: 1-1.5 hours after dose

Duration: Dose related, may require several weeks of therapy before full hypotensive effect

Absorption: 60% to 75%; reduced 30% to 40% by food

Protein binding: 25% to 30%

Metabolism: 50%

Half-life elimination (renal and cardiac function dependent):

Adults, healthy volunteers: 1.9 hours; Congestive heart failure: 2.06 hours; Anuria: 20-40 hours

Excretion: Urine (95%) within 24 hours

Pregnancy Risk Factor C/D (2nd and 3rd trimesters)

Generic Available Yes

Captopril and Hydrochlorothiazide

(KAP toe pril & hye droe klor oh THYE a zide)

Related Information

Captopril *on page 238*

Cardiovascular Diseases *on page 1456*

Hydrochlorothiazide *on page 675*

U.S. Brand Names Capozide®

Canadian Brand Names Capozide®

Pharmacologic Category Antihypertensive Agent Combination

Synonyms Hydrochlorothiazide and Captopril

Use Management of hypertension and treatment of CHF

Local Anesthetic/Vasoconstrictor Precautions No information available to require special precautions

Effects on Dental Treatment No significant effects or complications reported

Dosage Oral: Adults: Hypertension, CHF: May be substituted for previously titrated dosages of the individual components; alternatively, may initiate as follows:

Initial: Single tablet (captopril 25 mg/hydrochlorothiazide 15 mg) taken once daily; daily dose of captopril should not exceed 150 mg; daily dose of hydrochlorothiazide should not exceed 50 mg

Mechanism of Action Captopril is a competitive inhibitor of angiotensin-converting enzyme (ACE); prevents conversion of angiotensin I to angiotensin II, a potent vasoconstrictor. This results in lower levels of angiotensin II which causes an increase in plasma renin activity and a reduction in aldosterone secretion. Hydrochlorothiazide inhibits sodium reabsorption in the distal tubules causing increased excretion of sodium and water as well as potassium and hydrogen ions.

Dietary/Ethanol/Herb Considerations Ethanol: Avoid use; may increase risk of hypotension or dizziness.

Pregnancy Risk Factor C/D (2nd and 3rd trimesters)

Generic Available Yes

Capzasin-P® [OTC] *see* Capsaicin *on page 238*

Carac™ *see* Fluorouracil *on page 588*

Carafate® *see* Sucralfate *on page 1247*

Carbachol (KAR ba kole)

U.S. Brand Names Carbastat®; Carboptic®; Isopto® Carbachol; Miostat®

Canadian Brand Names Carbastat®; Isopto® Carbachol; Miostat®

Pharmacologic Category Cholinergic Agonist; Ophthalmic Agent, Antiglaucoma; Ophthalmic Agent, Miotic

Synonyms Carbacholine; Carbamylcholine Chloride

Use Lowers intraocular pressure in the treatment of glaucoma; cause miosis during surgery

Local Anesthetic/Vasoconstrictor Precautions No information available to require special precautions

Effects on Dental Treatment Frequency not defined: Arrhythmia, flushing, hypotension, syncope, headache epigastric distress, vomiting, increased salivation, asthma, diaphoresis

Dosage Adults:

Ophthalmic: Instill 1-2 drops up to 3 times/day

Intraocular: 0.5 mL instilled into anterior chamber before or after securing sutures

Mechanism of Action Synthetic direct-acting cholinergic agent that causes miosis by stimulating muscarinic receptors in the eye

Other Adverse Effects Frequency not defined:

Gastrointestinal: Abdominal cramps, diarrhea

Genitourinary: Urinary bladder tightness

Ocular: Bullous keratopathy, burning (transient), ciliary spasm, conjunctival injection, corneal clouding, irritation, postoperative iritis (following cataract extraction), retinal detachment, stinging (transient)

Drug Interactions Decreased Effect: NSAIDs may reduce carbachol's effect.

Pharmacodynamics/Kinetics

Ophthalmic instillation:

Onset of action: Miosis: 10-20 minutes

Duration: Reduction in intraocular pressure: 4-8 hours

Intraocular administration:

Onset of action: Miosis: 2-5 minutes

Duration: 24 hours

Pregnancy Risk Factor C

Generic Available No

Carbacholine *see* Carbachol *on page 241*

Carbamazepine (kar ba MAZ e peen)

U.S. Brand Names Carbatrol®; Epitol®; Tegretol®; Tegretol®-XR

Canadian Brand Names Apo®-Carbamazepine; Apo®-Carbamazepine CR; Gen-Carbamazepine CR; Novo-Carbamaz; Nu-Carbamazepine®; PMS-Carbamazepine; Taro-Carbamazepine Chewable; Tegretol®

Mexican Brand Names Carbazep®; Carbazina®; Clostedal®; Neugeron®; Tegretol®

Pharmacologic Category Anticonvulsant, Miscellaneous

Synonyms CBZ

Use

Dental: Relief of pain in trigeminal or glossopharyngeal neuralgia

Medical: Prophylaxis of partial seizures with complex symptomatology (psychomotor, temporal lobe), generalized tonic-clonic seizures (grand mal), mixed seizure patterns

Unlabeled/Investigational Use Treatment of bipolar disorders and other affective disorders, resistant schizophrenia, ethanol withdrawal symptoms, restless leg syndrome, psychotic behavior associated with dementia, post-traumatic stress disorders

(Continued)

Carbamazepine *(Continued)*

Local Anesthetic/Vasoconstrictor Precautions No information available to require special precautions

Effects on Dental Treatment Frequency not defined: CHF, syncope, bradycardia, hyper- or hypotension, arrhythmias, lymphadenopathy, sedation, dizziness, fatigue, confusion, headache, slurred speech, fever, nausea, vomiting, gastric distress, sore throat, oral ulceration, blurred vision, hypersensitivity (including multiorgan reactions), diaphoresis

Dosage Dosage must be adjusted according to patient's response and serum concentrations.

Oral:

Children:

<6 years: Initial: 5 mg/kg/day; dosage may be increased every 5-7 days to 10 mg/kg/day; then up to 20 mg/kg/day if necessary; administer in 2-4 divided doses

6-12 years: Initial: 100 mg twice daily or 10 mg/kg/day in 2 divided doses; increase by 100 mg/day at weekly intervals depending upon response; usual maintenance: 20-30 mg/kg/day in 2-4 divided doses (maximum dose: 1000 mg/day)

Children >12 years and Adults: 200 mg twice daily to start, increase by 200 mg/day at weekly intervals until therapeutic levels achieved; usual dose: 400-1200 mg/day in 2-4 divided doses; maximum dose: 12-15 years: 1000 mg/day, >15 years: 1200 mg/day; some patients have required up to 1.6-2.4 g/day

Trigeminal or glossopharyngeal neuralgia: Initial: 100 mg twice daily with food, gradually increasing in increments of 100 mg twice daily as needed; usual maintenance: 400-800 mg daily in 2 divided doses; maximum dose: 1200 mg/day

Elderly: 100 mg 1-2 times daily, increase in increments of 100 mg/day at weekly intervals until therapeutic level is achieved; usual dose: 400-1000 mg/day

Dosing adjustment in renal impairment: Cl_{cr} <10 mL/minute: Administer 75% of dose

Mechanism of Action In addition to anticonvulsant effects, carbamazepine has anticholinergic, antineuralgic, antidiuretic, muscle relaxant and antiarrhythmic properties; may depress activity in the nucleus ventralis of the thalamus or decrease synaptic transmission or decrease summation of temporal stimulation leading to neural discharge by limiting influx of sodium ions across cell membrane or other unknown mechanisms; stimulates the release of ADH and potentiates its action in promoting reabsorption of water; chemically related to tricyclic antidepressants

Other Adverse Effects Frequency not defined:

Cardiovascular: Edema, thrombophlebitis, thromboembolism

Central nervous system: Ataxia, aseptic meningitis (case report)

Dermatologic: Rash, urticaria, toxic epidermal necrolysis, Stevens-Johnson syndrome, photosensitivity reaction, alterations in skin pigmentation, exfoliative dermatitis, erythema multiforme, purpura, alopecia

Endocrine & metabolic: Hyponatremia, SIADH, chills

Gastrointestinal: Abdominal pain, diarrhea, constipation, anorexia, pancreatitis

Genitourinary: Urinary retention, urinary frequency, azotemia, renal failure, impotence

Hematologic: Aplastic anemia, agranulocytosis, eosinophilia, leukopenia, pancytopenia, thrombocytopenia, bone marrow suppression, acute intermittent porphyria, leukocytosis

Hepatic: Hepatitis, abnormal LFTs, jaundice, hepatic failure

Neuromuscular & skeletal: Peripheral neuritis

Ocular: Nystagmus, lens opacities, conjunctivitis

Otic: Tinnitus, hyperacusis

Miscellaneous: Disorders mimicking lymphoma, eosinophilia, hepatosplenomegaly

Contraindications Hypersensitivity to carbamazepine or any component of the formulation; may have cross-sensitivity with tricyclic antidepressants; marrow depression; MAO inhibitor use; pregnancy (may harm fetus)

Warnings/Precautions MAO inhibitors should be discontinued for a minimum of 14 days before carbamazepine is begun; administer with caution to patients with history of cardiac damage, hepatic or renal disease; potentially fatal blood cell abnormalities have been reported following treatment; patients with a previous history of adverse hematologic reaction to any drug may be at increased risk; early detection of hematologic change is important; advise patients of early signs and symptoms including fever, sore throat, mouth ulcers, infections, easy bruising, petechial or purpuric hemorrhage; carbamazepine is not effective in absence, myoclonic or akinetic seizures; exacerbation of certain seizure types have been seen after initiation of carbamazepine therapy in children with mixed seizure disorders. Elderly may have increased risk of SIADH-like syndrome. Carbamazepine has mild anticholinergic activity; use with caution in patients with increased intraocular pressure (monitor closely), or sensitivity to anticholinergic effects (urinary retention, constipation). Drug should be discontinued if there are any signs of hypersensitivity.

Drug Interactions Substrate of CYP2C8/9, **3A4**; Induces **CYP1A2, 2B6, 2C8/9, 2C19, 3A4**

Acetaminophen: Carbamazepine may enhance hepatotoxic potential of acetaminophen; risk is greater in acetaminophen overdose

Antipsychotics: Carbamazepine may enhance the metabolism (decrease the efficacy) of antipsychotics; monitor for altered response; dose adjustment may be needed

Barbiturates: May reduce serum concentrations of carbamazepine; monitor

Benzodiazepines: Serum concentrations and effect of benzodiazepines may be reduced by carbamazepine; monitor for decreased effect

Calcium channel blockers: Diltiazem and verapamil may increase carbamazepine levels, due to enzyme inhibition (see below); other calcium channel blockers (felodipine) may be decreased by carbamazepine due to enzyme induction

Chlorpromazine: **Note:** Carbamazepine suspension is incompatible with chlorpromazine solution. Schedule carbamazepine suspension at least 1-2 hours apart from other liquid medicinals.

Corticosteroids: Metabolism may be increased by carbamazepine

Cyclosporine (and other immunosuppressants): Carbamazepine may enhance the metabolism of immunosuppressants, decreasing its clinical effect; includes both cyclosporine and tacrolimus

CYP3A4 inhibitors: Serum level and/or toxicity of carbamazepine may be increased; inhibitors include amiodarone, cimetidine, clarithromycin, erythromycin, delavirdine, diltiazem, dirithromycin, disulfiram, fluoxetine, fluvoxamine, grapefruit juice, indinavir, itraconazole, ketoconazole, metronidazole, nefazodone, nevirapine, propoxyphene, quinine, quinupristin-dalfopristin, ritonavir, saquinavir, ticlopidine, verapamil, zafirlukast, zileuton; monitor for altered effects; a decrease in carbamazepine dosage may be required

Danazol: May increase serum concentrations of carbamazepine; monitor

Doxycycline: Carbamazepine may enhance the metabolism of doxycycline, decreasing its clinical effect

Ethosuximide: Serum levels may be reduced by carbamazepine

Felbamate: May increase carbamazepine levels and toxicity (increased epoxide metabolite concentrations); carbamazepine may decrease felbamate levels due to enzyme induction

Immunosuppressants: Carbamazepine may enhance the metabolism of immunosuppressants, decreasing its clinical effect; includes both cyclosporine and tacrolimus

Isoniazid: May increase the serum concentrations and toxicity of carbamazepine; in addition, carbamazepine may increase the hepatic toxicity of isoniazid (INH)

Isotretinoin: May decrease the effect of carbamazepine

Lamotrigine: Increases the epoxide metabolite of carbamazepine resulting in toxicity; carbamazepine increases the metabolism of lamotrigine

Lithium: Neurotoxicity may result in patients receiving concurrent carbamazepine

Loxapine: May increase concentrations of epoxide metabolite and toxicity of carbamazepine

Mefloquine: Concomitant use with carbamazepine may reduce seizure control by lowering plasma levels. Monitor.

Methadone: Carbamazepine may enhance the metabolism of methadone resulting in methadone withdrawal

Methylphenidate: concurrent use of carbamazepine may reduce the therapeutic effect of methylphenidate; limited documentation; monitor for decreased effect

Neuromuscular blocking agents, nondepolarizing: Effects may be of shorter duration when administered to patients receiving carbamazepine

Oral contraceptives: Metabolism may be increased by carbamazepine, resulting in a loss of efficacy

Phenytoin: Carbamazepine levels may be decreased by phenytoin; metabolism may be altered by carbamazepine

SSRIs: Metabolism may be increased by carbamazepine (due to enzyme induction)

Theophylline: Serum levels may be reduced by carbamazepine

Thioridazine: **Note:** Carbamazepine suspension is incompatible with thioridazine liquid. Schedule carbamazepine suspension at least 1-2 hours apart from other liquid medicinals.

Thyroid: Serum levels may be reduced by carbamazepine

Tramadol: Tramadol's risk of seizures may be increased with TCAs (carbamazepine may be associated with similar risk due to chemical similarity to TCAs)

Tricyclic antidepressants: May increase serum concentrations of carbamazepine; carbamazepine may decrease concentrations of tricyclics due to enzyme induction

Valproic acid: Serum levels may be reduced by carbamazepine; carbamazepine levels may also be altered by valproic acid

Warfarin: Carbamazepine may inhibit the hypoprothrombinemic effects of oral anticoagulants via increased metabolism; this combination should generally be avoided

Dietary/Ethanol/Herb Considerations

Ethanol: Avoid use; may increase CNS depression.

(Continued)

Carbamazepine *(Continued)*

Food: Administer with food to reduce GI upset; food may increase serum concentration. Avoid grapefruit products; may increase serum concentration.

Herb/Nutraceutical: Avoid evening primrose; decreases seizure threshold. Avoid gotu kola, kava, SAMe, St John's wort, and valerian; may increase CNS depression.

Pharmacodynamics/Kinetics

Absorption: Slow

Distribution: V_d: Neonates: 1.5 L/kg; Children: 1.9 L/kg; Adults: 0.59-2 L/kg

Protein binding: 75% to 90%; may be decreased in newborns

Metabolism: Hepatic to active epoxide metabolite; induces hepatic enzymes to increase metabolism

Bioavailability: 85%

Half-life elimination: Initial: 18-55 hours; Multiple doses: Children: 8-14 hours; Adults: 12-17 hours

Time to peak, serum: Unpredictable, 4-8 hours

Excretion: Urine (1% to 3% as unchanged drug)

Pregnancy Risk Factor D

Breast-feeding Considerations Crosses into breast milk. AAP considers **compatible** with breast-feeding.

Dosage Forms CAP, extended release: 200 mg, 300 mg. **SUSP, oral:** 100 mg/5 mL (450 mL). **TAB:** 200 mg. **TAB, chewable:** 100 mg. **TAB, extended release:** 100 mg, 200 mg, 400 mg

Generic Available Yes

Carbamide *see* Urea *on page 1365*

Carbamide Peroxide (KAR ba mide per OKS ide)

Related Information

Oral Rinse Products *on page 1634*

U.S. Brand Names Auro® Ear Drops [OTC]; Debrox® Otic [OTC]; E•R•O Ear [OTC]; Gly-Oxide® Oral [OTC]; Mollifene® Ear Wax Removing Formula [OTC]; Murine® Ear Drops [OTC]; Orajel® Perioseptic® [OTC]; Proxigel® Oral [OTC]

Pharmacologic Category Otic Agent, Cerumenolytic

Synonyms Urea Peroxide

Use

Dental: Relief of minor swelling of gums, oral mucosal surfaces, and lips, including canker sores and dental irritation

Medical: Emulsify and disperse ear wax

Local Anesthetic/Vasoconstrictor Precautions No information available to require special precautions

Effects on Dental Treatment 1% to 10%: Superinfections, rash, irritation, redness

Dosage Children and Adults:

Oral:

Gel: Gently massage on affected area 4 times/day; do not drink or rinse mouth for 5 minutes after use

Solution (should not be used for >7 days): Oral preparation should not be used in children <3 years of age; apply several drops undiluted on affected area 4 times/day after meals and at bedtime; expectorate after 2-3 minutes **or** place 10 drops onto tongue, mix with saliva, swish for several minutes, expectorate

Otic:

Children <12 years: Tilt head sideways and individualize the dose according to patient size; 3 drops (range: 1-5 drops) twice daily for up to 4 days, tip of applicator should not enter ear canal; keep drops in ear for several minutes by keeping head tilted and placing cotton in ear

Children ≥12 years and Adults: Tilt head sideways and instill 5-10 drops twice daily up to 4 days, tip of applicator should not enter ear canal; keep drops in ear for several minutes by keeping head tilted and placing cotton in ear

Mechanism of Action Carbamide peroxide releases hydrogen peroxide which serves as a source of nascent oxygen upon contact with catalase; deodorant action is probably due to inhibition of odor-causing bacteria; softens impacted cerumen due to its foaming action

Contraindications Otic preparation should not be used in patients with a perforated tympanic membrane; ear drainage, ear pain or rash in the ear; do not use in the eye; do not use otic preparation longer than 4 days; oral preparation should not be used in children <3 years

Warnings/Precautions

Oral: With prolonged use of oral carbamide peroxide, there is a potential for overgrowth of opportunistic organisms; damage to periodontal tissues; delayed wound healing; should not be used for longer than 7 days

Otic: Do not use if ear drainage or discharge, ear pain, irritation, or rash in ear; should not be used for longer than 4 days

Pharmacodynamics/Kinetics Onset of action: ~24 hours

Pregnancy Risk Factor C

Dosage Forms GEl, oral: 10% (34 g). **SOLN, oral:** 10% (15 mL, 60 mL); 15% (13.3 mL). **SOLN, otic:** 6.5% (15 mL, 30 mL)

Generic Available Yes

Carbamylcholine Chloride *see* Carbachol *on page 241*

Carbastat® *see* Carbachol *on page 241*

Carbatrol® *see* Carbamazepine *on page 241*

Carbaxefed DM RF *see* Carbinoxamine, Pseudoephedrine, and Dextromethorphan *on page 247*

Carbaxefed RF *see* Carbinoxamine and Pseudoephedrine *on page 247*

Carbenicillin (kar ben i SIL in)

U.S. Brand Names Geocillin®

Mexican Brand Names Carbecin Inyectable

Pharmacologic Category Antibiotic, Penicillin

Synonyms Carbenicillin Indanyl Sodium; Carindacillin

Use Treatment of serious urinary tract infections and prostatitis caused by susceptible gram-negative aerobic bacilli

Local Anesthetic/Vasoconstrictor Precautions No information available to require special precautions

Effects on Dental Treatment 1% to 10%: Unpleasant taste, glossitis, nausea, vomiting

Prolonged use of penicillins may lead to development of oral candidiasis.

Dosage Oral:

Children: 30-50 mg/kg/day divided every 6 hours; maximum dose: 2-3 g/day

Adults: 1-2 tablets every 6 hours for urinary tract infections or 2 tablets every 6 hours for prostatitis

Dosing interval in renal impairment: Adults:

Cl_{cr} 10-50 mL/minute: Administer 382-764 mg every 12-24 hours

Cl_{cr} <10 mL/minute: Administer 382-764 mg every 24-48 hours

Moderately dialyzable (20% to 50%)

Mechanism of Action Inhibits bacterial cell wall synthesis by binding to one or more of the penicillin binding proteins (PBPs); which in turn inhibits the final transpeptidation step of peptidoglycan synthesis in bacterial cell walls, thus inhibiting cell wall biosynthesis. Bacteria eventually lyse due to ongoing activity of cell wall autolytic enzymes (autolysins and murein hydrolases) while cell wall assembly is arrested.

Other Adverse Effects

>10%: Gastrointestinal: Diarrhea

<1%: **Headache**, skin rash, urticaria, anemia, thrombocytopenia, leukopenia, neutropenia, eosinophilia, hyperthermia, itchy eyes, vaginitis, hypokalemia, hematuria, thrombophlebitis

Drug Interactions

Increased Effect/Toxicity: Increased bleeding effects if taken with high doses of heparin or oral anticoagulants. Aminoglycosides may be synergistic against selected organisms. Probenecid and disulfiram may increase levels of penicillins (carbenicillin).

Decreased Effect: Decreased effectiveness with tetracyclines. Although anecdotal reports suggest oral contraceptive efficacy could be reduced by penicillins, this has been refuted by more rigorous scientific and clinical data.

Pharmacodynamics/Kinetics

Absorption: 30% to 40%

Distribution: Crosses placenta; small amounts enter breast milk; distributes into bile; low concentrations attained in CSF

Protein binding: ~50%

Half-life elimination: Children: 0.8-1.8 hours; Adults: 1-1.5 hours, prolonged to 10-20 hours with renal insufficiency

Time to peak, serum: Normal renal function: 0.5-2 hours; concentrations are inadequate for treatment of systemic infections

Excretion: Urine (~80% to 99% as unchanged drug)

Pregnancy Risk Factor B

Generic Available No

Carbenicillin Indanyl Sodium *see* Carbenicillin *on page 245*

Carbetapentane and Chlorpheniramine

(kar bay ta PEN tane & klor fen IR a meen)

Related Information

Chlorpheniramine *on page 307*

U.S. Brand Names Tannic-12; Tannic-12 S; Tussi-12®; Tussi-12 S™

Pharmacologic Category Antihistamine/Antitussive

Synonyms Carbetapentane Tannate and Chlorpheniramine Tannate; Chlorpheniramine and Carbetapentane

Use Symptomatic relief of cough associated with upper respiratory tract conditions, such as the common cold, bronchitis, bronchial asthma

(Continued)

Carbetapentane and Chlorpheniramine *(Continued)*

Local Anesthetic/Vasoconstrictor Precautions No information available to require special precautions

Effects on Dental Treatment Chronic use of antihistamines will inhibit salivary flow, particularly in elderly patients; this may contribute to periodontal disease and oral discomfort.

Frequency not defined: Drowsiness, excitation (children), sedation, dry mucous membranes

Dosage Oral:

Children: Based on carbetapentane 30 mg and chlorpheniramine 4 mg per 5 mL suspension:

2-6 years: 2.5-5 mL every 12 hours

>6 years: 5-10 mL every 12 hours

Adults: Based on carbetapentane 60 mg and chlorpheniramine 5 mg per tablet: 1-2 tablets every 12 hours

Mechanism of Action Carbetapentane is a nonopiod cough suppressant; chlorpheniramine, is an H_1-receptor antagonist

Other Adverse Effects Frequency not defined: Gastrointestinal: GI motility decreased

Drug Interactions Increased Effect/Toxicity: Sedative effects of CNS depressants may be potentiated; MAO inhibitors may increase and prolong anticholinergic effects; avoid use with and within 14 days of treatment with MAO inhibitors

Dietary/Ethanol/Herb Considerations

Ethanol: Avoid use; may increase CNS depression.

Food: Tussi-12 S™ contains tartrazine.

Pregnancy Risk Factor C

Generic Available No

Carbetapentane Tannate and Chlorpheniramine Tannate *see* Carbetapentane and Chlorpheniramine *on page 245*

Carbidopa (kar bi DOE pa)

U.S. Brand Names Lodosyn®

Pharmacologic Category Anti-Parkinson's Agent, Dopamine Agonist

Use Given with levodopa in the treatment of parkinsonism to enable a lower dosage of levodopa to be used and a more rapid response to be obtained and to decrease side-effects; for details of administration and dosage, see Levodopa; has no effect without levodopa

Local Anesthetic/Vasoconstrictor Precautions No information available to require special precautions

Effects on Dental Treatment Dopaminergic therapy in Parkinson's disease includes the use of carbidopa in combination with levodopa. Carbidopa/levodopa combination is associated with orthostatic hypotension. Patients medicated with this drug combination should be carefully assisted from the chair and observed for signs of orthostatic hypotension.

Dosage Oral: Adults: 70-100 mg/day; maximum daily dose: 200 mg

Mechanism of Action Carbidopa is a peripheral decarboxylase inhibitor with little or no pharmacological activity when given alone in usual doses. It inhibits the peripheral decarboxylation of levodopa to dopamine; and as it does not cross the blood-brain barrier, unlike levodopa, effective brain concentrations of dopamine are produced with lower doses of levodopa. At the same time, reduced peripheral formation of dopamine reduces peripheral side-effects, notably nausea and vomiting, and cardiac arrhythmias, although the dyskinesias and adverse mental effects associated with levodopa therapy tend to develop earlier.

Other Adverse Effects Administration with levodopa:

>10%: Central nervous system: Anxiety, confusion, nervousness, mental depression

1% to 10%:

Cardiovascular: Orthostatic hypotension, palpitations, cardiac arrhythmias

Central nervous system: Memory loss, nervousness, insomnia, fatigue, hallucinations, ataxia, dystonic movements

Gastrointestinal: Nausea, vomiting, GI bleeding

Ocular: Blurred vision

<1%: Hypertension, duodenal ulcer, hemolytic anemia

Pharmacodynamics/Kinetics

Absorption: 40% to 70%

Distribution: Does not cross the blood-brain barrier; in rats, reported to cross placenta and be excreted in milk

Protein binding: 36%

Half-life elimination: 1-2 hours

Excretion: Urine (as unchanged drug and metabolites)

Pregnancy Risk Factor C

Generic Available No

Carbidopa and Levodopa *see* Levodopa and Carbidopa *on page 793*

Carbinoxamine and Pseudoephedrine

(kar bi NOKS a meen & soo doe e FED rin)

Related Information

Pseudoephedrine *on page 1146*

U.S. Brand Names Andehist NR Drops; Carbaxefed RF; Hydro-Tussin™-CBX; Palgic®-D; Palgic®-DS; Rondec® Drops; Rondec® Tablets; Rondec-TR®

Pharmacologic Category Adrenergic Agonist Agent; Antihistamine, H_1 Blocker; Decongestant

Synonyms Pseudoephedrine and Carbinoxamine

Use Seasonal and perennial allergic rhinitis; vasomotor rhinitis

Local Anesthetic/Vasoconstrictor Precautions Pseudoephedrine is a sympathomimetic which has potential to enhance vasoconstrictor effects of epinephrine; use local anesthetic with vasoconstrictor with caution

Effects on Dental Treatment

1% to 10%: Xerostomia (normal salivary flow resumes upon discontinuation)

Frequency not defined: Arrhythmias, cardiovascular collapse, hypertension, tachycardia, anxiety, convulsions, CNS stimulation, dizziness, excitability (children; rare), fear, hallucinations, headache, nervousness, restlessness, sedation, nausea, vomiting, tremor, weakness, respiratory difficulty

Dosage Oral:

Children:

Drops (Andehist NR, Carbaxefed RF, Rondec®):
- 1-3 months: 0.25 mL 4 times/day
- 3-6 months: 0.5 mL 4 times/day
- 6-12 months: 0.75 mL 4 times/day
- 12-24 months: 1 mL 4 times/day

Syrup (Hydro-Tussin™-CBX, Palgic®-DS):
- 1-3 months: 1.25 mL up to 4 times/day
- 3-6 months: 2.5 mL up to 4 times/day
- 6-9 months: 3.75 mL up to 4 times/day
- 9-18 months: 3.75-5 mL up to 4 times/day
- 18 months to 6 years: 5 mL 3-4 times/day
- >6 years: Refer to adult dosing.

Tablet (Rondec®): ≥6 years: Refer to adult dosing.

Tablet, sustained release:
- 6-12 years (Palgic®-D): One-half tablet every 12 hours
- ≥12 years (Palgic®-D, Rondec-TR®): Refer to adult dosing.

Adults:
- Syrup (Hydro-Tussin™-CBX, Palgic®-DS): 10 mL 4 times/day
- Tablet (Rondec®): 1 tablet 4 times a day
- Tablets, sustained release (Palgic®-D, Rondec-TR®): 1 tablet every 12 hours

Mechanism of Action Carbinoxamine competes with histamine for H_1-receptor sites on effector cells in the gastrointestinal tract, blood vessels, and respiratory tract; pseudoephedrine, a sympathomimetic amine and isomer of ephedrine, acts as a decongestant in respiratory tract mucous membranes with less vasoconstrictor action than ephedrine in normotensive individuals

Other Adverse Effects Frequency not defined:

Cardiovascular: Pallor

Central nervous system: Insomnia

Gastrointestinal: Anorexia, diarrhea, dyspepsia

Ocular: Diplopia

Renal: Dysuria, polyuria, urinary retention (with BPH)

Drug Interactions

Increased Effect/Toxicity: Increased sedation/CNS depression with barbiturates and other CNS depressants; anticholinergic effects may be increased by MAO inhibitors, tricyclic antidepressants

Decreased Effect: May decrease effects of antihypertensive agents.

Dietary/Ethanol/Herb Considerations

Ethanol: Avoid use; may increase CNS depression.

Herb/Nutraceutical: Avoid gotu kola, kava, SAMe, St John's wort, and valerian; may increase CNS depression.

Pregnancy Risk Factor C

Generic Available No

Carbinoxamine, Dextromethorphan, and Pseudoephedrine *see* Carbinoxamine, Pseudoephedrine, and Dextromethorphan *on page 247*

Carbinoxamine, Pseudoephedrine, and Dextromethorphan

(kar bi NOKS a meen, soo doe e FED rin, & deks troe meth OR fan)

Related Information

Dextromethorphan *on page 423*

Pseudoephedrine *on page 1146*

U.S. Brand Names Andehist DM NR Drops; Carbaxefed DM RF; Rondec®-DM Drops

(Continued)

Carbinoxamine, Pseudoephedrine, and Dextromethorphan *(Continued)*

Pharmacologic Category Antihistamine/Decongestant/Antitussive

Synonyms Carbinoxamine, Dextromethorphan, and Pseudoephedrine; Dextromethorphan, Carbinoxamine, and Pseudoephedrine; Dextromethorphan, Pseudoephedrine, and Carbinoxamine; Pseudoephedrine, Carbinoxamine, and Dextromethorphan; Pseudoephedrine, Dextromethorphan, and Carbinoxamine

Use Relief of coughs and upper respiratory symptoms, including nasal congestion, associated with allergy or the common cold

Local Anesthetic/Vasoconstrictor Precautions Use with caution since pseudoephedrine is a sympathomimetic amine which could interact with epinephrine to cause a pressor response

Effects on Dental Treatment

≤10%: Tachycardia, palpitations, xerostomia; use vasoconstrictor with caution

Frequency not defined: Arrhythmias, cardiovascular collapse, hypertension, anxiety, convulsions, CNS stimulation, dizziness, drowsiness, excitability (children; rare), fear, hallucinations, headache, nervousness, restlessness, sedation, GI upset, nausea, vomiting, tremors, weakness, respiratory difficulty

Dosage Infants: Drops:

1-3 months: 1/4 mL 4 times/day
3-6 months: 1/2 mL 4 times/day
6-12 months: 3/4 mL 4 times/day
12-24 months: 1 mL 4 times/day

Mechanism of Action Carbinoxamine competes with histamine for H_1-receptor sites on effector cells in the gastrointestinal tract, blood vessels, and respiratory tract; pseudoephedrine, a sympathomimetic amine and isomer of ephedrine, acts as a decongestant in respiratory tract mucous membranes with less vasoconstrictor action than ephedrine in normotensive individuals; dextromethorphan, a non-narcotic antitussive, increases cough threshold by its activity on the medulla oblongata.

Other Adverse Effects Frequency not defined:

Cardiovascular: Pallor
Central nervous system: Insomnia
Gastrointestinal: Anorexia, diarrhea, dyspepsia
Ocular: Diplopia
Renal: Dysuria, polyuria, urinary retention (with BPH)

Dietary/Ethanol/Herb Considerations

Ethanol: Avoid use; may increase CNS depression.

Herb/Nutraceutical: Avoid gotu kola, kava, SAMe, St John's wort, and valerian; may increase CNS depression.

Pregnancy Risk Factor C

Generic Available No

Carbocaine® [DSC] *see* Mepivacaine *on page 861*

Carbocaine® 2% with Neo-Cobefrin® *see* Mepivacaine and Levonordefrin *on page 862*

Carbocaine® 3% *see* Mepivacaine Dental Anesthetic *on page 863*

Carbol-Fuchsin Solution (kar bol-FOOK sin soe LOO shun)

U.S. Brand Names Castellani Paint Modified

Pharmacologic Category Antifungal Agent, Topical

Synonyms Castellani Paint

Use Treatment of superficial mycotic infections

Local Anesthetic/Vasoconstrictor Precautions No information available to require special precautions

Effects on Dental Treatment No significant effects or complications reported

Dosage Topical: Apply to affected area 2-4 times/day

Generic Available No

Carbolic Acid *see* Phenol *on page 1068*

Carboplatin (KAR boe pla tin)

U.S. Brand Names Paraplatin®

Canadian Brand Names Paraplatin-AQ

Mexican Brand Names Blastocarb®; Carboplat; Carbotec®; Paraplatin®

Pharmacologic Category Antineoplastic Agent, Alkylating Agent

Synonyms CBDCA

Use Initial treatment of ovarian cancer; secondary treatment of advanced ovarian cancer

Unlabeled/Investigational Use Treatment of lung, head and neck, endometrial, esophageal, bladder, breast, and cervical cancers, CNS and germ cell tumors, osteogenic sarcoma, and high-dose therapy with stem cell/bone marrow support

Local Anesthetic/Vasoconstrictor Precautions No information available to require special precautions

Effects on Dental Treatment >10%: Stomatitis, nausea, vomiting

Dosage IVPB, I.V. infusion, intraperitoneal (refer to individual protocols):

Children:

Solid tumor: 300-600 mg/m^2 once every 4 weeks

Brain tumor: 175 mg/m^2 once weekly for 4 weeks with a 2-week recovery period between courses; dose is then adjusted on platelet count and neutrophil count values

Adults:

Ovarian cancer: Usual doses range from 360 mg/m^2 I.V. every 3 weeks single agent therapy to 300 mg/m^2 every 4 weeks as combination therapy

In general, however, single intermittent courses of carboplatin should not be repeated until the neutrophil count is at least 2000 and the platelet count is at least 100,000

The following dose adjustments are modified from a controlled trial in previously treated patients with ovarian carcinoma. Blood counts were done weekly, and the recommendations are based on the lowest post-treatment platelet or neutrophil value.

Carboplatin dosage adjustment based on pretreatment platelet counts:

- Platelets >100,000 cells/mm^3 and neutrophils >2000 cells/mm^3: Adjust dose 125% from prior course
- Platelets 50-100,000 cells/mm^3 and neutrophils 500-2000 cells/mm^3: No dose adjustment
- Platelets <50,000 cells/mm^3 and neutrophils <500 cells/mm^3: Adjust dose 75% from prior course

Carboplatin dosage adjustment based on the Egorin formula (based on platelet counts):

Previously untreated patients:

$$\text{dosage (mg/m}^2) = (0.091) \frac{(Cl_{cr})}{(BSA)} \frac{(\text{Pretreat Plt count - Plt nadir count desired} \times 100)}{(\text{Pretreatment Plt count})} + 86$$

Previously treated patients with heavily myelosuppressive agents:

$$\text{dosage (mg/m}^2) = (0.091) \frac{(Cl_{cr})}{(BSA)} \frac{[(\text{Pretreat Plt count - Plt nadir count desired} \times 100) - 17]}{(\text{Pretreatment Plt count})} + 86$$

Autologous BMT: I.V.: 1600 mg/m^2 (total dose) divided over 4 days **requires BMT (ie, FATAL without BMT)**

Dosing adjustment in hepatic impairment: There are no published studies available on the dosing of carboplatin in patients with impaired liver function. Human data regarding the biliary elimination of carboplatin are unavailable; however, pharmacokinetic studies in rabbits and rats reflect a biliary excretion of 0.4% to 0.7% of the dose (ie, 0.05 mL/minute/kg biliary clearance).

Dosing adjustment in renal impairment: These dosing recommendations apply to the initial course of treatment. Subsequent dosages should be adjusted according to the patient's tolerance based on the degree of bone marrow suppression.

Cl_{cr} <60 mL/minute: Increased risk of severe bone marrow suppression. In renally impaired patients who received single agent carboplatin therapy, the incidence of severe leukopenia, neutropenia, or thrombocytopenia has been about 25% when the following dosage modifications have been used:

Cl_{cr} 41-59 mL/minute: Recommended dose on day 1 is 250 mg/m^2

Cl_{cr} 16-40 mL/minute: Recommended dose on day 1 is 200 mg/m^2

Cl_{cr} <15 mL/minute: The data available for patients with severely impaired kidney function are too limited to permit a recommendation for treatment

or

Dosing adjustment in renal impairment: CALVERT FORMULA

Total dose (mg) = Target AUC (mg/mL/minute) x (GFR [mL/minute] + 25)

Note: The dose of carboplatin calculated is TOTAL mg DOSE **not** mg/m^2. AUC is the area under the concentration versus time curve.

Target AUC value will vary depending upon:

Number of agents in the regimen

Treatment status (ie, previously untreated or treated)

For single agent carboplatin/no prior chemotherapy: Total dose (mg): 6-8 (GFR + 25)

For single agent carboplatin/prior chemotherapy: Total dose (mg): 4-6 (GFR + 25)

For combination chemotherapy/no prior chemotherapy: Total dose (mg): 4.5-6 (GFR + 25)

For combination chemotherapy/prior chemotherapy: A reasonable approach for these patients would be to use a target AUC value <5 for the initial cycle

Note: The Jelliffe formula (below) substantially underestimates the creatinine clearance in patients with a serum creatinine <1.5 mg/dL. However, the Jelliffe formula is more accurate in estimating creatinine clearance in patients with significant renal impairment than the Cockroft and Gault formula.

Cl_{cr} (mL/minute/1.73 m^2) for males = 98 - [(0.8) (Age - 20)]/S_{cr}

(Continued)

Carboplatin *(Continued)*

Cl_{cr} (mL/minute/1.73 m^2) for females = 98 - [(0.8) (Age - 20)]/S_{cr} multiplied by 90%

Intraperitoneal: 200-650 mg/m^2 in 2 L of dialysis fluid have been administered into the peritoneum of ovarian cancer patients

Mechanism of Action Analogue of cisplatin which covalently binds to DNA; possible cross-linking and interference with the function of DNA

Other Adverse Effects

>10%:

Dermatologic: Alopecia (includes other agents in combination with carboplatin)

Endocrine & metabolic: Hypomagnesemia, hypokalemia, hyponatremia, hypocalcemia; less severe than those seen after cisplatin (usually asymptomatic)

Hematologic: Myelosuppression is dose-related and is the dose-limiting toxicity; thrombocytopenia is the predominant manifestation, with a reported incidence of 37% in patients receiving 400 mg/m^2 as a single agent and 80% in patients receiving 520 mg/m^2; leukopenia has been reported in 27% to 38% of patients receiving carboplatin as a single agent

Nadir: ~21 days following a single dose

Hepatic: Increased alkaline phosphatase, AST (usually mild and reversible)

Otic: Hearing loss at high tones (above speech ranges) has been reported in up to 19% in one series; clinically important ototoxicity is not usually seen; routine audiometric testing is not recommended

Renal: Elevations in creatinine and BUN have been reported; most of them are mild and they are commonly reversible; considerably less nephrotoxic than cisplatin

1% to 10%: Neuromuscular & skeletal: Peripheral neuropathy (4% to 6%; up to 10% in older and/or previously-treated patients)

<1% (Limited to important or life-threatening): Neurotoxicity has only been noted in patients previously treated with cisplatin; urticaria, rash, nephrotoxicity (uncommon), secondary malignancies, anaphylaxis, malaise, hypertension

Drug Interactions Increased Effect/Toxicity: Nephrotoxic drugs; aminoglycosides increase risk of ototoxicity. When administered as sequential infusions, observational studies indicate a potential for increased toxicity when platinum derivatives (carboplatin, cisplatin) are administered before taxane derivatives (docetaxel, paclitaxel).

Dietary/Ethanol/Herb Considerations Herb/Nutraceutical: Avoid black cohosh and dong quai in estrogen-dependent tumors.

Pharmacodynamics/Kinetics

Distribution: V_d: 16 L/kg; Into liver, kidney, skin, and tumor tissue

Protein binding: 0%; platinum is 30% irreversibly bound

Metabolism: Minimally hepatic to aquated and hydroxylated compounds

Half-life elimination: Terminal: 22-40 hours; Cl_{cr} >60 mL/minute: 2.5-5.9 hours

Excretion: Urine (~60% to 90%) within 24 hours

Pregnancy Risk Factor D

Generic Available No

Carboprost *see* Carboprost Tromethamine *on page 250*

Carboprost Tromethamine (KAR boe prost tro METH a meen)

U.S. Brand Names Hemabate™

Canadian Brand Names Hemabate™

Pharmacologic Category Abortifacient; Prostaglandin

Synonyms Carboprost

Use Termination of pregnancy and refractory postpartum uterine bleeding

Unlabeled/Investigational Use Investigational: Treatment of hemorrhagic cystitis

Local Anesthetic/Vasoconstrictor Precautions No information available to require special precautions

Effects on Dental Treatment

>10%: Nausea (33%)

1% to 10%: Flushing (7%)

Dosage I.M.: Adults:

Abortion: Initial: 250 mcg, then 250 mcg at 1½-hour to 3½-hour intervals depending on uterine response; a 500 mcg dose may be given if uterine response is not adequate after several 250 mcg doses; do not exceed 12 mg total dose or continuous administration for >2 days

Refractory postpartum uterine bleeding: Initial: 250 mcg; may repeat at 15- to 90-minute intervals to a total dose of 2 mg

Bladder irrigation for hemorrhagic cystitis (refer to individual protocols): [0.4-1.0 mg/dL as solution] 50 mL instilled into bladder 4 times/day for 1 hour

Mechanism of Action Carboprost tromethamine is a prostaglandin similar to prostaglandin F_2 alpha (dinoprost) except for the addition of a methyl group at the C-15 position. This substitution produces longer duration of activity than dinoprost; carboprost stimulates uterine contractility which usually results in expulsion of the products of conception and is used to induce abortion between 13-20 weeks of pregnancy. Hemostasis at the placentation site is achieved through the myometrial contractions produced by carboprost.

Other Adverse Effects <1%: **Hypertension, hypotension, drowsiness**, vertigo, **nervousness, fever, headache**, dystonia, vasovagal syndrome, breast tenderness, **xerostomia, vomiting**, diarrhea, hematemesis, **abnormal taste**, bladder spasms, myalgia, **blurred vision, cough, asthma, respiratory distress, septic shock, hiccups**

Drug Interactions Increased Effect/Toxicity: Toxicity may be increased by oxytocic agents.

Pregnancy Risk Factor X

Generic Available No

Carboptic® *see* Carbachol *on page 241*

Carbose D *see* Carboxymethylcellulose *on page 251*

Carboxymethylcellulose (kar boks ee meth il SEL yoo lose)

U.S. Brand Names Cellufresh® [OTC]; Celluvisc® [OTC]

Canadian Brand Names Celluvisc™; Refresh Plus™; Refresh Tears™

Pharmacologic Category Ophthalmic Agent, Miscellaneous

Synonyms Carbose D; Carboxymethylcellulose Sodium

Use Preservative-free artificial tear substitute

Local Anesthetic/Vasoconstrictor Precautions No information available to require special precautions

Effects on Dental Treatment No significant effects or complications reported

Dosage Ophthalmic: Adults: Instill 1-2 drops into eye(s) 3-4 times/day

Generic Available Yes

Carboxymethylcellulose Sodium *see* Carboxymethylcellulose *on page 251*

Cardene® *see* NiCARdipine *on page 969*

Cardene® I.V. *see* NiCARdipine *on page 969*

Cardene® SR *see* NiCARdipine *on page 969*

Cardizem® *see* Diltiazem *on page 447*

Cardizem® CD *see* Diltiazem *on page 447*

Cardizem® LA *see* Diltiazem *on page 447*

Cardizem® SR *see* Diltiazem *on page 447*

Cardura® *see* Doxazosin *on page 470*

Carimune™ *see* Immune Globulin (Intravenous) *on page 714*

Carindacillin *see* Carbenicillin *on page 245*

Carisoprodate *see* Carisoprodol *on page 251*

Carisoprodol (kar i soe PROE dole)

Related Information

Carisoprodol and Aspirin *on page 252*

Carisoprodol, Aspirin, and Codeine *on page 252*

U.S. Brand Names Soma®

Canadian Brand Names Soma®

Pharmacologic Category Skeletal Muscle Relaxant

Synonyms Carisoprodate; Isobamate

Use

Dental: Treatment of muscle spasms and pain associated with acute temporomandibular joint pain

Medical: Skeletal muscle relaxant

Local Anesthetic/Vasoconstrictor Precautions No information available to require special precautions

Effects on Dental Treatment

>10%: Drowsiness

1% to 10%: Tachycardia, tightness in chest, facial flushing, syncope, allergic fever, dizziness, lightheadedness, headache, paradoxical CNS stimulation, nausea, vomiting, trembling, dyspnea, hiccups

Dosage Oral: Adults: 350 mg 3-4 times/day; take last dose at bedtime; compound: 1-2 tablets 4 times/day

Mechanism of Action Precise mechanism is not yet clear, but many effects have been ascribed to its central depressant actions

Other Adverse Effects

1% to 10%:

Central nervous system: Mental depression

Dermatologic: Angioedema

Gastrointestinal: Stomach cramps

Ocular: Burning eyes

<1%: Ataxia, rash, urticaria, erythema multiforme, aplastic anemia, leukopenia, eosinophilia, **blurred vision**

Contraindications Hypersensitivity to carisoprodol, meprobamate or any component of the formulation; acute intermittent porphyria

Warnings/Precautions May cause CNS depression, which may impair physical or mental abilities. Effects with other sedative drugs or ethanol may be potentiated.

(Continued)

Carisoprodol *(Continued)*

Use with caution in patients with hepatic/renal dysfunction. Tolerance or drug dependence may result from extended use.

Drug Interactions Substrate of **CYP2C19**

Increased Toxicity: Ethanol, CNS depressants, phenothiazines

Dietary/Ethanol/Herb Considerations

Ethanol: Avoid use; may increase CNS depression.

Herb/Nutraceutical: Avoid gotu kola, kava, SAMe, St John's wort, and valerian; may increase CNS depression.

Pharmacodynamics/Kinetics

Onset of action: ~30 minutes

Duration: 4-6 hours

Distribution: Crosses placenta; high concentrations enter breast milk

Metabolism: Hepatic

Half-life elimination: 8 hours

Excretion: Urine

Pregnancy Risk Factor C

Dosage Forms TAB: 350 mg

Generic Available Yes

Carisoprodol and Aspirin (kar i soe PROE dole & AS pir in)

Related Information

Aspirin *on page 131*

Carisoprodol *on page 251*

U.S. Brand Names Soma® Compound

Pharmacologic Category Skeletal Muscle Relaxant

Synonyms Aspirin and Carisoprodol

Use

Dental: Treatment of muscle spasms and pain associated with acute temporomandibular joint pain

Medical: Skeletal muscle relaxant

Local Anesthetic/Vasoconstrictor Precautions No information available to require special precautions

Effects on Dental Treatment Elderly are a high-risk population for adverse effects from nonsteroidal anti-inflammatory agents. As much as 60% of elderly patients with GI complications from NSAIDs can develop peptic ulceration and/or hemorrhage asymptomatically. Concomitant disease and drug use contribute to the risk of GI adverse effects. Use lowest effective dose for shortest period possible. Consider renal function decline with age.

Dosage Oral: Adults: 1-2 tablets 4 times/day

Contraindications Hypersensitivity to any component of the formulation

Warnings/Precautions Avoid aspirin, if possible, for 1 week prior to dental or surgical procedures due to possibility of postoperative bleeding. Use with caution in impaired hepatic function; use with caution in patients with platelet and bleeding disorders, renal dysfunction, erosive gastritis, or peptic ulcer disease, previous nonreaction does not guarantee future safe taking of medication; do not use aspirin in children <16 years of age for chickenpox or flu symptoms due to the association with Reye's syndrome. Use with caution in patients with history of asthma.

Dietary/Ethanol/Herb Considerations

Ethanol: Avoid use; may enhance gastric mucosal irritation and increase CNS depression.

Herb/Nutraceutical: Avoid gotu kola, kava, SAMe, St John's wort, and valerian; may increase CNS depression.

Pregnancy Risk Factor C/D (full-dose aspirin in 3rd trimester)

Dosage Forms TAB: Carisoprodol 200 mg and aspirin 325 mg

Generic Available Yes

Carisoprodol, Aspirin, and Codeine

(kar i soe PROE dole, AS pir in, & KOE deen)

Related Information

Aspirin *on page 131*

Carisoprodol *on page 251*

Codeine *on page 361*

U.S. Brand Names Soma® Compound w/Codeine

Pharmacologic Category Skeletal Muscle Relaxant

Synonyms Aspirin, Carisoprodol, and Codeine; Codeine, Aspirin, and Carisoprodol

Use

Dental: Treatment of muscle spasms and pain associated with acute temporomandibular joint pain

Medical: Skeletal muscle relaxant

Local Anesthetic/Vasoconstrictor Precautions No information available to require special precautions

Effects on Dental Treatment Elderly are a high-risk population for adverse effects from nonsteroidal anti-inflammatory agents. As much as 60% of elderly patients with GI complications from NSAIDs can develop peptic ulceration and/or hemorrhage asymptomatically. Concomitant disease and drug use contribute to the risk of GI adverse effects. Use lowest effective dose for shortest period possible. Consider renal function decline with age.

Restrictions C-III

Dosage Oral: Adults: 1 or 2 tablets 4 times/day

Contraindications Hypersensitivity to any component of the formulation

Warnings/Precautions Avoid aspirin, if possible, for 1 week prior to dental or surgical procedures due to possibility of postoperative bleeding. Use with caution in impaired hepatic function; use with caution in patients with platelet and bleeding disorders, renal dysfunction, erosive gastritis, or peptic ulcer disease, previous nonreaction does not guarantee future safe taking of medication; do not use aspirin in children <16 years of age for chickenpox or flu symptoms due to the association with Reye's syndrome. Use with caution in patients with history of asthma.

Dietary/Ethanol/Herb Considerations

Ethanol: Avoid use; may enhance gastric mucosal irritation and increase CNS depression.

Herb/Nutraceutical: Avoid gotu kola, kava, SAMe, St John's wort, and valerian; may increase CNS depression.

Pregnancy Risk Factor C/D (full-dose aspirin in 3rd trimester)

Dosage Forms TAB: Carisoprodol 200 mg, aspirin 325 mg, and codeine 16 mg

Generic Available Yes

Carmol® 10 [OTC] *see* Urea *on page 1365*

Carmol® 20 [OTC] *see* Urea *on page 1365*

Carmol® 40 *see* Urea *on page 1365*

Carmol® Deep Cleaning *see* Urea *on page 1365*

Carmol-HC® *see* Urea and Hydrocortisone *on page 1365*

Carmol® Scalp *see* Sulfacetamide *on page 1249*

Carmustine (kar MUS teen)

U.S. Brand Names BiCNU®; Gliadel®

Canadian Brand Names BiCNU®

Mexican Brand Names Bicnu®

Pharmacologic Category Antineoplastic Agent, Alkylating Agent

Synonyms BCNU

Use Treatment of brain tumors (glioblastoma, brainstem glioma, medulloblastoma, astrocytoma, ependymoma, and metastatic brain tumors), multiple myeloma, Hodgkin's disease, non-Hodgkin's lymphomas, melanoma, lung cancer, colon cancer

Gliadel®: Adjunct to surgery in patients with recurrent glioblastoma multiforme

Local Anesthetic/Vasoconstrictor Precautions No information available to require special precautions

Effects on Dental Treatment

>10%: Hypotension (from high dose therapy due to alcohol content of diluent), dizziness

1% to 10% (wafer form): Amnesia, confusion, convulsion, headache, somnolence, stupor, stomatitis

Dosage I.V. (refer to individual protocols):

Children: 200-250 mg/m² every 4-6 weeks as a single dose

Adults: Usual dosage (per manufacturer labeling): 150-200 mg/m² every 6-8 weeks as a single dose or divided into daily injections on 2 successive days

Next dose is to be determined based on hematologic response to the previous dose. Repeat dose should not be administered until circulating blood elements have returned to acceptable levels (leukocytes >4000, platelets >100,000), usually 6 weeks

Listed are the suggested carmustine doses, based upon the nadir after the prior dose.

- Leukocytes >4000 mm³ and platelets >100,000 mm³: Give 100% of prior dose
- Leukocytes 3000-3999 mm³ and platelets 75,000-99,999 mm³: Give 100% of prior dose
- Leukocytes 2000-2999 mm³ and platelets 25,000-74,999 mm³: Give 70% of prior dose
- Leukocytes <2000 mm³ and platelets <25,000 mm³: Give 50% of prior dose

Primary brain cancer:

150-200 mg/m² every 6-8 weeks as a single dose or divided into daily injections on 2 successive days

20-65 mg/m² every 4-6 weeks

0.5-1 mg/kg every 4-6 weeks

40-80 mg/m²/day for 3 days every 6-8 weeks

Autologous BMT: ALL OF THE FOLLOWING DOSES ARE FATAL WITHOUT BMT

Combination therapy: Up to 300-900 mg/m²

(Continued)

Carmustine *(Continued)*

Single-agent therapy: Up to 1200 mg/m^2 (fatal necrosis is associated with doses >2 g/m^2)

Adjunct to surgery in patients with recurrent glioblastoma multiforme (Gliadel®): Implantation: Up to 8 wafers may be placed in the resection cavity (total dose 62.6 mg); should the size and shape not accommodate 8 wafers, the maximum number of wafers allowed should be placed

Hemodialysis: Supplemental dosing is not required

Dosing adjustment in hepatic impairment: Dosing adjustment may be necessary; however, no specific guidelines are available

Mechanism of Action Interferes with the normal function of DNA by alkylation and cross-linking the strands of DNA, and by possible protein modification

Other Adverse Effects

>10%:

Central nervous system: Ataxia, seizures (54%; postoperatively from wafer form)

Dermatologic: Pain and burning at the injection site (may be relieved by diluting the drug and infusing it through a fast-running dextrose or saline infusion); phlebitis

Gastrointestinal: Severe nausea and vomiting (usually begins within 2-4 hours and lasts 4-6 hours; patients should receive a prophylactic antiemetic regimen including a serotonin (5-HT$_3$) antagonist and dexamethasone)

Hematologic: Myelosuppression - cumulative, dose-related, delayed, thrombocytopenia is usually more common and more severe than leukopenia

Onset (days): 7-14

Nadir (days): 21-35

Recovery (days): 42-56

Hepatic: Reversible increases in bilirubin, alkaline phosphatase, and SGOT occur in 20% to 25% of patients

Ocular: Ocular toxicities (transient conjunctival flushing and blurred vision), retinal hemorrhages

Respiratory: Interstitial fibrosis occurs in up to 50% of patients receiving a cumulative dose >1400 mg/m^2, or bone marrow transplantation doses; may be delayed up to 3 years; rare in patients receiving lower doses. A history of lung disease or concomitant bleomycin therapy may increase the risk of this reaction. Patients should have baseline and periodic pulmonary function tests, patients with forced vital capacity (FVC) or carbon monoxide diffusing capacity of the lungs (DLCO) <70% of predicted are at higher risk.

1% to 10%:

Central nervous system: Wafers: Aphasia, ataxia, cerebral edema, depression, diplopia, hemiplegia, hydrocephalus, insomnia, meningitis

Dermatologic: Flushing (probably due to alcohol in diluent), alopecia

Gastrointestinal: Anorexia, constipation, diarrhea

Hematologic: Anemia

<1%: Azotemia, cerebral hemorrhage infarction (wafer formulation), dermatitis, hepatic coma, hyperpigmentation, painless jaundice, subacute hepatitis

Drug Interactions Increased Effect/Toxicity: Carmustine given in combination with cimetidine is reported to cause bone marrow depression. Carmustine given in combination with etoposide is reported to cause severe hepatic dysfunction with hyperbilirubinemia, ascites, and thrombocytopenia.

Dietary/Ethanol/Herb Considerations Ethanol: Avoid use due to GI irritation.

Pharmacodynamics/Kinetics

Distribution: Readily crosses blood-brain barrier producing CSF levels equal to 15% to 70% of blood plasma levels; enters breast milk; highly lipid soluble

Metabolism: Rapidly hepatic

Half-life elimination: Biphasic: Initial: 1.4 minutes; Secondary: 20 minutes (active metabolites: plasma half-life of 67 hours)

Excretion: Urine (~60% to 70%) within 96 hours; lungs (6% to 10% as CO_2)

Pregnancy Risk Factor D

Generic Available No

Carnitor® *see* Levocarnitine *on page 791*

Carrington Antifungal [OTC] *see* Miconazole *on page 906*

Carteolol (KAR tee oh lole)

Related Information

Cardiovascular Diseases *on page 1456*

U.S. Brand Names Cartrol® Oral; Ocupress® Ophthalmic

Canadian Brand Names Cartrol® Oral; Ocupress® Ophthalmic

Pharmacologic Category Beta Blocker With Intrinsic Sympathomimetic Activity; Ophthalmic Agent, Antiglaucoma

Synonyms Carteolol Hydrochloride

Use Management of hypertension; treatment of chronic open-angle glaucoma and intraocular hypertension

Local Anesthetic/Vasoconstrictor Precautions No information available to require special precautions

Effects on Dental Treatment Carteolol is a nonselective beta-blocker and may enhance the pressor response to epinephrine, resulting in hypertension and bradycardia. Many nonsteroidal anti-inflammatory drugs such as ibuprofen and indomethacin can reduce the hypotensive effect of beta-blockers after 3 or more weeks of therapy with the NSAID. Short-term NSAID use (ie, 3 days) requires no special precautions in patients taking beta-blockers.

1% to 10%: Bradycardia, palpitations, CHF, nausea, vomiting, bronchospasm, drowsiness (≥10%)

Dosage Adults:

Oral: 2.5 mg as a single daily dose, with a maintenance dose normally 2.5-5 mg once daily; doses >10 mg do not increase response and may in fact decrease effect.

Ophthalmic: Instill 1 drop in affected eye(s) twice daily.

Dosing interval in renal impairment: Oral:

Cl_{cr} >60 mL/minute/1.73 m^2: Administer every 24 hours.

Cl_{cr} 20-60 mL/minute/1.73 m^2: Administer every 48 hours.

Cl_{cr} <20 mL/minute/1.73 m^2: Administer every 72 hours.

Mechanism of Action Blocks both $beta_1$- and $beta_2$-receptors and has mild intrinsic sympathomimetic activity; has negative inotropic and chronotropic effects and can significantly slow AV nodal conduction

Other Adverse Effects

Ophthalmic:

>10%: Ocular: Conjunctival hyperemia

1% to 10%: Ocular: Anisocoria, corneal punctate keratitis, corneal staining, decreased corneal sensitivity, eye pain, vision disturbances

Systemic:

>10%:

Central nervous system: Insomnia

Endocrine & metabolic: Decreased sexual ability

1% to 10%:

Cardiovascular: Edema, reduced peripheral circulation

Central nervous system: Mental depression

Gastrointestinal: Diarrhea or constipation, stomach discomfort

Miscellaneous: Cold extremities

<1% (Limited to important or life-threatening): **Chest pain, arrhythmias, dyspnea, orthostatic hypotension, nervousness, headache, hallucinations, confusion (especially in elderly)**, psoriasiform eruption, itching, polyuria, thrombocytopenia, leukopenia, depression

Drug Interactions Substrate of CYP2D6

Increased Effect/Toxicity: Carteolol may increase the effects of other drugs which slow AV conduction (digoxin, verapamil, diltiazem), alpha-blockers (prazosin, terazosin), and alpha-adrenergic stimulants (epinephrine, phenylephrine). Carteolol may mask the tachycardia from hypoglycemia caused by insulin and oral hypoglycemics. In patients receiving concurrent therapy, the risk of hypertensive crisis is increased when either clonidine or the beta-blocker is withdrawn. Reserpine has been shown to enhance the effect of beta-blockers. Beta-blockers may increase the action or levels of ethanol, disopyramide, nondepolarizing muscle relaxants, and theophylline although the effects are difficult to predict.

Decreased Effect: Decreased effect of beta-blockers with aluminum salts, barbiturates, calcium salts, cholestyramine, colestipol, NSAIDs, penicillins (ampicillin), rifampin, salicylates, and sulfinpyrazone due to decreased bioavailability and plasma levels. Beta-blockers may decrease the effect of sulfonylureas (possibly hyperglycemia). Nonselective beta-blockers blunt the effect of beta-2 adrenergic agonists (albuterol).

Dietary/Ethanol/Herb Considerations

Ethanol: Avoid use; may increase risk of hypotension or dizziness.

Food: Avoid caffeine (eg, colas, chocolate), garlic, and licorice.

Herb/Nutraceutical: Avoid black cohosh, dong quai, and evening primrose due to estrogenic activity. Avoid ephedra, ginseng, and yohimbe; may worsen hypertension. Avoid garlic; may have increased antihypertensive effect. Avoid hawthorn; may lower peripheral vascular resistance causing additional decrease in BP. Avoid licorice.

Pharmacodynamics/Kinetics

Onset of action: Oral: 1-1.5 hours

Peak effect: 2 hours

Duration: 12 hours

Absorption: Oral: 80%

Protein binding: 23% to 30%

Metabolism: 30% to 50%

Half-life elimination: 6 hours

Excretion: Urine (as metabolites)

Pregnancy Risk Factor C (manufacturer); D (2nd and 3rd trimesters - expert analysis)

Generic Available Yes: Drops

(Continued)

Carteolol *(Continued)*

Selected Readings

Foster CA and Aston SJ, "Propranolol-Epinephrine Interaction: A Potential Disaster," *Plast Reconstr Surg*, 1983, 72(1):74-8.

Wong DG, Spence JD, Lamki L, et al, "Effect of Nonsteroidal Anti-inflammatory Drugs on Control of Hypertension of Beta-Blockers and Diuretics," *Lancet*, 1986, 1(8488):997-1001.

Wynn RL, "Dental Nonsteroidal Anti-inflammatory Drugs and Prostaglandin-Based Drug Interactions, Part Two," *Gen Dent*, 1992, 40(2):104, 106, 108.

Wynn RL, "Epinephrine Interactions With Beta-Blockers," *Gen Dent*, 1994, 42(1):16, 18.

Carteolol Hydrochloride *see* Carteolol *on page 254*

Cartia XT™ *see* Diltiazem *on page 447*

Cartrol® Oral *see* Carteolol *on page 254*

Carvedilol (KAR ve dil ole)

Related Information

Cardiovascular Diseases *on page 1456*

U.S. Brand Names Coreg®

Canadian Brand Names Coreg®

Mexican Brand Names Dilatrend®

Pharmacologic Category Beta Blocker With Alpha-Blocking Activity

Use Management of hypertension; can be used alone or in combination with other agents, especially thiazide-type diuretics; mild to severe heart failure of ischemic or cardiomyopathic origin usually in addition to standardized therapy.

Unlabeled/Investigational Use Treatment of angina pectoris

Local Anesthetic/Vasoconstrictor Precautions Use with caution, epinephrine has interacted with noncardioselective beta-blockers to result in initial hypertensive episode followed by bradycardia

Effects on Dental Treatment Noncardioselective beta-blockers enhance the pressor response to epinephrine, resulting in hypertension and bradycardia. Many nonsteroidal anti-inflammatory drugs, such as ibuprofen and indomethacin, can reduce the hypotensive effect of beta-blockers after 3 or more weeks of therapy with the NSAID. Short-term NSAID use (ie, 3 days) requires no special precautions in patients taking beta-blockers.

>10%: Dizziness (6% to 32%), weakness (11%), upper respiratory tract infection (14% to 18%), hypotension (9% to 14%), pain fatigue (4% to 24%)

1% to 10%: Bradycardia (2% to 10%), hypertension (3%), angina (2% to 6%), postural hypotension (2%), syncope (3% to 8%), palpitations, headache (5% to 8%), fever (3%), paresthesia (2%), somnolence (2%), dehydration (2%), hypoglycemia, nausea (4% to 9%), vomiting (6%), melena, periodontitis, sinusitis (5%), bronchitis (5%), pharyngitis (2% to 3%), rhinitis (2%), increased cough (5%), infection (2%), increased diaphoresis (3%), viral infection (2%), allergy, sudden death, pain (9%), muscle cramps, blurred vision (3% to 5%)

Dosage Oral: Adults: Reduce dosage if heart rate drops to <55 beats/minute.

Hypertension: 6.25 mg twice daily; if tolerated, dose should be maintained for 1-2 weeks, then increased to 12.5 mg twice daily. Dosage may be increased to a maximum of 25 mg twice daily after 1-2 weeks. Maximum dose: 50 mg/day

CHF: 3.125 mg twice daily for 2 weeks; if this dose is tolerated, may increase to 6.25 mg twice daily. Double the dose every 2 weeks to the highest dose tolerated by patient. (Prior to initiating therapy, other heart failure medications should be stabilized and fluid retention minimized.)

Maximum recommended dose:

- Mild to moderate heart failure:
  - <85 kg: 25 mg twice daily
  - >85 kg: 50 mg twice daily
- Severe heart failure: 25 mg twice daily

Angina pectoris (unlabeled use): 25-50 mg twice daily

Dosing comment in hepatic impairment: Contraindicated in dysfunction

Mechanism of Action As a racemic mixture, carvedilol has nonselective beta-adrenoreceptor and alpha-adrenergic blocking activity. No intrinsic sympathomimetic activity has been documented. Associated effects in hypertensive patients include reduction of cardiac output, exercise- or beta agonist-induced tachycardia, reduction of reflex orthostatic tachycardia, vasodilation, decreased peripheral vascular resistance (especially in standing position), decreased renal vascular resistance, reduced plasma renin activity, and increased levels of atrial natriuretic peptide. In CHF, associated effects include decreased pulmonary capillary wedge pressure, decreased pulmonary artery pressure, decreased heart rate, decreased systemic vascular resistance, increased stroke volume index, and decreased right arterial pressure (RAP).

Other Adverse Effects Includes data from hypertension and heart failure trials. Higher rates of adverse reactions have generally been noted in patients with CHF. However, the frequency of adverse effects associated with placebo is also increased in this population. Events occurring at a frequency > placebo in clinical trials:

>10%:
- Endocrine & metabolic: Weight gain (10% to 12%)
- Gastrointestinal: Diarrhea (2% to 12%)

1% to 10%:
- Cardiovascular: AV block (3%), dependent edema (4%), peripheral edema (1% to 7%), generalized edema (5% to 6%)
- Central nervous system: Insomnia (2%), malaise, hypesthesia, vertigo
- Endocrine & metabolic: Gout (6%), hypercholesterolemia (4%), hyperkalemia (3%), hypervolemia (2%), hypertriglyceridemia (1%), hyperuricemia, hyponatremia
- Genitourinary: Urinary tract infection (2% to 3%), hematuria (3%), impotence
- Hematologic: Thrombocytopenia (1% to 2%), decreased prothrombin, purpura
- Hepatic: Increased transaminases, increased alkaline phosphatase
- Neuromuscular & skeletal: Back pain (2% to 7%), arthralgia (6%), myalgia (3%)
- Renal: Increased BUN (6%), abnormal renal function, albuminuria, glycosuria, increased creatinine (3%), kidney failure

<1%: Peripheral ischemia, **tachycardia**, hypokinesis, bilirubinemia, **nervousness**, sleep disorder, aggravated depression, impaired concentration, **abnormal thinking, paranoia**, emotional lability, **asthma**, decreased libido (male), pruritus, erythematous rash, maculopapular rash, psoriaform rash, photosensitivity, tinnitus, micturition (increased), **xerostomia, diabetes mellitus**, anemia, leukopenia, AV block (complete), bundle branch block, hypokalemia, myocardial ischemia, cerebrovascular disorder, **convulsions, migraine, neuralgia, paresis, anaphylactoid reaction**, alopecia, exfoliative dermatitis, **amnesia, GI hemorrhage, bronchospasm**, pulmonary edema, hearing loss, respiratory alkalosis, decreased HDL-cholesterol, pancytopenia, atypical lymphocytes

Additional events from clinical trials in heart failure patients occurring at a frequency >2% but equal to or less than the frequency reported in patients receiving placebo: **Asthenia, cardiac failure**, flatulence, dyspepsia, **arthritis,** depression, anemia, rash, **leg cramps, chest pain, headache**

Drug Interactions Substrate of CYP1A2, **2C8/9, 2D6**, 2E1, 3A4

Increased Effect/Toxicity: Clonidine and cimetidine increase the serum levels and effects of carvedilol. Carvedilol may increase the levels of cyclosporine. Carvedilol may increase the effects of other drugs which slow AV conduction (digoxin, verapamil, diltiazem), alpha-blockers (prazosin, terazosin), and alpha-adrenergic stimulants (epinephrine, phenylephrine). Carvedilol may mask the tachycardia from hypoglycemia caused by insulin and oral hypoglycemics. In patients receiving concurrent therapy, the risk of hypertensive crisis is increased when either clonidine or the beta-blocker is withdrawn. Reserpine has been shown to enhance the effect of beta-blockers. Beta-blockers may increase the action or levels of disopyramide, and theophylline although the effects are difficult to predict.

Decreased Effect: Rifampin may reduce the plasma concentration of carvedilol by up to 70%. Decreased effect of beta-blockers has also occurred with antacids, barbiturates, calcium channel blockers, cholestyramine, colestipol, NSAIDs, penicillins (ampicillin), and salicylates due to decreased bioavailability and plasma levels. Beta-blockers may decrease the effect of sulfonylureas. Nonselective beta-blockers blunt the effect of beta-2 adrenergic agonists (albuterol).

Dietary/Ethanol/Herb Considerations

Ethanol: Avoid use; may increase risk of hypotension or dizziness.

Food: Administer with food to minimize risk of hypotension; food decreases rate but not extent of absorption. Fluids, fruit, and fiber may reduce constipation. Avoid caffeine (eg, colas, chocolate), garlic, and licorice.

Herb/Nutraceutical: Avoid black cohosh, dong quai, and evening primrose due to estrogenic activity. Avoid ephedra, ginseng, and yohimbe; may worsen hypertension. Avoid garlic; may have increased antihypertensive effect. Avoid hawthorn; may lower peripheral vascular resistance causing additional decrease in BP. Avoid licorice.

Pharmacodynamics/Kinetics

Onset of action: 1-2 hours
- Peak antihypertensive effect: ~1-2 hours

Absorption: Rapid; food decreases rate but not extent of absorption; administration with food minimizes risks of orthostatic hypotension

Distribution: V_d: 115 L

Protein binding: <98%, primarily to albumin

Metabolism: Extensively hepatic, primarily by aromatic ring oxidation and glucuronidation (2% excreted unchanged); three active metabolites (4-hydroxyphenyl metabolite is 13 times more potent than parent drug for beta-blockade); first-pass effect; plasma concentrations in the elderly and those with cirrhotic liver disease are 50% and 4-7 times higher, respectively

Bioavailability: 25% to 35%

Half-life elimination: 7-10 hours

Excretion: Primarily feces

Pregnancy Risk Factor C (manufacturer); D (2nd and 3rd trimesters - expert analysis)

(Continued)

Carvedilol *(Continued)*

Generic Available No

Selected Readings

Foster CA and Aston SJ, "Propranolol-Epinephrine Interaction: A Potential Disaster," *Plast Reconstr Surg*, 1983, 72(1):74-8.

Wong DG, Spence JD, Lamki L, et al, "Effect of Nonsteroidal Anti-inflammatory Drugs on Control of Hypertension of Beta-Blockers and Diuretics," *Lancet*, 1986, 1(8488):997-1001.

Wynn RL, "Dental Nonsteroidal Anti-inflammatory Drugs and Prostaglandin-Based Drug Interactions, Part Two," *Gen Dent*, 1992, 40(2):104, 106, 108.

Wynn RL, "Epinephrine Interactions With Beta-Blockers," *Gen Dent*, 1994, 42(1):16, 18.

Casanthranol and Docusate *see* Docusate and Casanthranol *on page 464*

Cascara (kas KAR a)

Pharmacologic Category Laxative, Stimulant

Synonyms Cascara Sagrada

Use Temporary relief of constipation; sometimes used with milk of magnesia ("black and white" mixture)

Local Anesthetic/Vasoconstrictor Precautions No information available to require special precautions

Effects on Dental Treatment 1% to 10%: Faintness, nausea

Dosage Fluid extract is 5 times more potent than aromatic fluid extract.

Oral (aromatic fluid extract):
- Infants: 1.25 mL/day (range: 0.5-1.5 mL) as needed
- Children 2-11 years: 2.5 mL/day (range: 1-3 mL) as needed
- Children ≥12 years and Adults: 5 mL/day (range: 2-6 mL) as needed at bedtime (1 tablet as needed at bedtime)

Mechanism of Action Direct chemical irritation of the intestinal mucosa resulting in an increased rate of colonic motility and change in fluid and electrolyte secretion

Other Adverse Effects 1% to 10%:
- Endocrine & metabolic: Electrolyte and fluid imbalance
- Gastrointestinal: Abdominal cramps, diarrhea
- Genitourinary: Discoloration of urine (reddish pink or brown)

Drug Interactions Decreased Effect: Decreased effect of oral anticoagulants.

Pharmacodynamics/Kinetics
- Onset of action: 6-10 hours
- Absorption: Oral: Poor, from small intestine
- Metabolism: Hepatic

Pregnancy Risk Factor C

Generic Available Yes

Cascara Sagrada *see* Cascara *on page 258*

Casodex® *see* Bicalutamide *on page 183*

Caspofungin (kas poe FUN jin)

U.S. Brand Names Cancidas®

Canadian Brand Names Cancidas®

Mexican Brand Names Cancidas®

Pharmacologic Category Antifungal Agent, Parenteral

Synonyms Caspofungin Acetate

Use Treatment of invasive *Aspergillus* infection, candidemia, and other *Candida* infections (abscesses, esophageal, intra-abdominal, peritonitis, pleural space)

Local Anesthetic/Vasoconstrictor Precautions No information available to require special precautions

Effects on Dental Treatment
- >10%: Headache (≤11%), fever (3% to 26%)
- 1% to 6%: Flushing (3%), facial edema (≤3%), dizziness (2%), paresthesia (1% to 3%), nausea (2% to 6%), vomiting (1% to 4%), flu-like syndrome (3%), pain (1% to 5%) paresthesia (1% to 3%), tremors (2%) diaphoresis (≤1%)

Dosage I.V.:
- Children: Safety and efficacy not established
- Adults: Duration of caspofungin treatment should be determined by patient status and clinical response.
  - **Invasive *Aspergillus*: Initial dose: 70 mg infused slowly; subsequent dosing: 50 mg/day**
  - **Invasive candidiasis:** Initial dose: 70 mg infused slowly; subsequent dosing: 50 mg/day
  - **Esophageal candidiasis:** 50 mg/day; **Note:** The majority of patients studied for this indication also had oropharyngeal involvement.
  - Concomitant use of an enzyme inducer:
    - Patients receiving rifampin: 70 mg caspofungin daily
    - Patients receiving carbamazepine, dexamethasone, efavirenz, nevirapine, **or** phenytoin (and possibly other enzyme inducers) may require an increased daily dose of caspofungin (70 mg/day).
- Dosage adjustment in hepatic impairment:
  - Mild hepatic insufficiency (Child-Pugh score 5-6): No adjustment necessary

Moderate hepatic insufficiency (Child-Pugh score 7-9): 35 mg/day; initial 70 mg loading dose should still be administered in treatment of invasive infections

Mechanism of Action Inhibits synthesis of β(1,3)-D-glucan, an essential component of the cell wall of susceptible fungi. Highest activity in regions of active cell growth. Mammalian cells do not require β(1,3)-D-glucan, limiting potential toxicity.

Other Adverse Effects

>10%:

Hematologic: Hemoglobin decreased (3% to 12%)

Hepatic: Serum alkaline phosphatase (3% to 11%) increased, transaminases increased (up to 13%)

Local: Infusion site reactions (2% to 12%), phlebitis (up to 16%)

1% to 10%:

Central nervous system: Chills (up to 5%), insomnia (1%)

Dermatologic: Rash (<1% to 5%), pruritus (1% to 3%), erythema (1% to 2%)

Endocrine & metabolic: Hypokalemia (10%)

Gastrointestinal: Abdominal pain (2% to 4%), diarrhea (1% to 4%), anorexia (1%)

Hematologic: Eosinophils increased (3%), neutrophils decreased (2% to 3%), WBC decreased (5% to 6%), anemia (up to 4%), platelet count decreased (2% to 3%)

Hepatic: Bilirubin increased (3%)

Local: Phlebitis/thrombophlebitis (4% to 6%), induration (up to 3%)

Neuromuscular & skeletal: Myalgia (up to 3%), paresthesia (1% to 3%), tremor (2%)

Renal: Nephrotoxicity (8%)*, proteinuria (5%), hematuria (2%), serum creatinine increased (<1% to 4%), urinary WBCs increased (up to 8%), urinary RBCs increased (1% to 4%), blood urea nitrogen increased (1%)

*Nephrotoxicity defined as serum creatinine ≥2X baseline value or ≥1 mg/dL in patients with serum creatinine above ULN range (patients with Cl_{cr} <30 mL/minute were excluded)

<1%: **Adult respiratory distress syndrome (ARDS),** jaundice, pulmonary edema, renal insufficiency, serum bicarbonate decreased, **tachypnea**

Postmarketing and/or case reports: **Anaphylaxis, dyspnea,** dystonia, **facial swelling,** hepatic dysfunction, hypercalcemia, peripheral edema, swelling, stridor

Drug Interactions

Increased Effect/Toxicity: Concurrent administration of cyclosporine may increase caspofungin concentrations. In limited experience, a high frequency of elevated hepatic serum transaminases was observed.

Decreased Effect: Caspofungin may decrease blood concentrations of tacrolimus. In limited experience, some enzyme inducers decreased the serum concentrations of caspofungin. Dosage adjustment of caspofungin to 70 mg is required for patients on rifampin and should be considered when used with other inducers; includes carbamazepine, dexamethasone, efavirenz, nevirapine, and phenytoin.

Pharmacodynamics/Kinetics

Protein binding: 97% to albumin

Metabolism: Slowly, via hydrolysis and *N*-acetylation as well as by spontaneous degradation, with subsequent metabolism to component amino acids

Half-life elimination: Beta (distribution): 9-11 hours; Terminal: 40-50 hours

Excretion: Urine (41%) and feces (35%) as unchanged drug and metabolites

Pregnancy Risk Factor C

Generic Available No

Caspofungin Acetate *see* Caspofungin *on page 258*

Cassia acutifolia *see* Senna *on page 1215*

Castellani Paint *see* Carbol-Fuchsin Solution *on page 248*

Castellani Paint Modified *see* Carbol-Fuchsin Solution *on page 248*

Castor Oil (KAS tor oyl)

U.S. Brand Names Emulsoil® [OTC]; Neoloid® [OTC]; Purge® [OTC]

Pharmacologic Category Laxative, Miscellaneous

Synonyms Oleum Ricini

Use Preparation for rectal or bowel examination or surgery; rarely used to relieve constipation; also applied to skin as emollient and protectant

Local Anesthetic/Vasoconstrictor Precautions No information available to require special precautions

Effects on Dental Treatment 1% to 10%: Dizziness, nausea

Dosage Oral:

Liquid:

Children 2-11 years: 5-15 mL as a single dose

Children ≥12 years and Adults: 15-60 mL as a single dose

Emulsified:

36.4%:

Children <2 years: 5-15 mL/dose

Children 2-11 years: 7.5-30 mL/dose

Children ≥12 years and Adults: 30-60 mL/dose

(Continued)

Castor Oil *(Continued)*

95%, mix with ½ to 1 full glass liquid:
Children: 5-10 mL/day
Adults: 15-60 mL/day

Mechanism of Action Acts primarily in the small intestine; hydrolyzed to ricinoleic acid which reduces net absorption of fluid and electrolytes and stimulates peristalsis

Other Adverse Effects

1% to 10%:
Endocrine & metabolic: Electrolyte disturbance
Gastrointestinal: Abdominal cramps, diarrhea

<1%: Pelvic congestion

Pharmacodynamics/Kinetics Onset of action: 2-6 hours

Pregnancy Risk Factor X

Generic Available Yes

Cataflam® *see* Diclofenac *on page 429*
Catapres® *see* Clonidine *on page 351*
Catapres-TTS®-1 *see* Clonidine *on page 351*
Catapres-TTS®-2 *see* Clonidine *on page 351*
Catapres-TTS®-3 *see* Clonidine *on page 351*
Cathflo™ Activase® *see* Alteplase *on page 65*
Caverject® *see* Alprostadil *on page 63*
CB-1348 *see* Chlorambucil *on page 296*
CBDCA *see* Carboplatin *on page 248*
CBZ *see* Carbamazepine *on page 241*
CCNU *see* Lomustine *on page 818*
2-CdA *see* Cladribine *on page 336*
CDDP *see* Cisplatin *on page 332*
Ceclor® *see* Cefaclor *on page 260*
Ceclor® CD *see* Cefaclor *on page 260*
Cecon® [OTC] *see* Ascorbic Acid *on page 128*
Cedax® *see* Ceftibuten *on page 276*
CeeNU® *see* Lomustine *on page 818*

Cefaclor (SEF a klor)

U.S. Brand Names Ceclor®; Ceclor® CD

Canadian Brand Names Apo®-Cefaclor; Ceclor®; Novo-Cefaclor; Nu-Cefaclor; PMS-Cefaclor

Mexican Brand Names Ceclor®

Pharmacologic Category Antibiotic, Cephalosporin (Second Generation)

Use

Dental: An alternate antibiotic in treatment of orofacial infections in patients allergic to penicillins; susceptible bacteria including aerobic gram-positive bacteria and anaerobes

Medical: Infections caused by susceptible organisms including *Staphylococcus aureus* and *H. influenzae*; treatment of otitis media, sinusitis, and infections involving the respiratory tract, skin and skin structure, bone and joint, and urinary tract

Local Anesthetic/Vasoconstrictor Precautions No information available to require special precautions

Effects on Dental Treatment No significant effects or complications reported

Dosage Oral:

Children >1 month: 20-40 mg/kg/day divided every 8-12 hours; maximum dose: 2 g/day (total daily dose may be divided into two doses for treatment of otitis media or pharyngitis)

Adults: 250-500 mg every 8 hours

Extended release tablets:

500 mg every 12 hours for 7 days for acute bacterial exacerbations of or secondary infections with chronic bronchitis

375 mg every 12 hours for 10 days for pharyngitis or tonsillitis, or for uncomplicated skin and skin structure infections

Dosing adjustment in renal impairment: Cl_{cr} <50 mL/minute: Administer 50% of dose

Hemodialysis: Moderately dialyzable (20% to 50%)

Mechanism of Action Inhibits bacterial cell wall synthesis by binding to one or more of the penicillin-binding proteins (PBPs) which in turn inhibits the final transpeptidation step of peptidoglycan synthesis in bacterial cell walls, thus inhibiting cell wall biosynthesis. Bacteria eventually lyse due to ongoing activity of cell wall autolytic enzymes (autolysins and murein hydrolases) while cell wall assembly is arrested.

Other Adverse Effects

1% to 10%:

Dermatologic: Rash (maculopapular, erythematous, or morbilliform) (1% to 2%)
Gastrointestinal: Diarrhea (2%)
Hematologic: Eosinophilia (2%)
Hepatic: Elevated transaminases (3%)

<1%: **Anaphylaxis,** urticaria, pruritus, angioedema, **serum-sickness,** arthralgia, hepatitis, cholestatic jaundice, Stevens-Johnson syndrome, **nausea, vomiting, pseudomembranous colitis,** vaginitis, hemolytic anemia, neutropenia, interstitial nephritis, **CNS irritability, hyperactivity, agitation, nervousness**, insomnia, **confusion, dizziness, hallucinations, somnolence, seizures, prolonged PT**

Reported with other cephalosporins: **Fever,** abdominal pain, **superinfection, renal dysfunction, toxic nephropathy, hemorrhage,** cholestasis

Contraindications Hypersensitivity to cefaclor, any component of the formulation, or other cephalosporins

Warnings/Precautions Modify dosage in patients with severe renal impairment; prolonged use may result in superinfection; a low incidence of cross-hypersensitivity to penicillins exists

Drug Interactions

Increased Effect: Probenecid may decrease cephalosporin elimination

Increased Toxicity: Furosemide, aminoglycosides may be a possible additive to nephrotoxicity

Dietary/Ethanol/Herb Considerations Administer with food to reduce GI upset; serum concentration may slightly decrease.

Pharmacodynamics/Kinetics

Absorption: Well absorbed, acid stable

Distribution: Widely throughout the body and reaches therapeutic concentration in most tissues and body fluids, including synovial, pericardial, pleural, peritoneal fluids; bile, sputum, and urine; bone, myocardium, gallbladder, skin and soft tissue; crosses placenta; enters breast milk

Protein binding: 25%

Metabolism: Partially hepatic

Half-life elimination: 0.5-1 hour; prolonged with renal impairment

Time to peak: Capsule: 60 minutes; Suspension: 45 minutes

Excretion: Urine (80% as unchanged drug)

Pregnancy Risk Factor B

Breast-feeding Considerations Theoretically, drug absorbed by nursing infant may change bowel flora or affect fever work-up result. **Note:** As a class, cephalosporins are used to treat infections in infants.

Dosage Forms CAP (Ceclor®) 250 mg, 500 mg. **POWDER, oral suspension:** 125 mg/5 mL (75 mL, 150 mL); 187 mg/5 mL (50 mL, 100 mL); 250 mg/5 mL (75 mL, 150 mL); 375 mg/5 mL (50 mL, 100 mL); (Ceclor®): 125 mg/5 mL (150 mL); 187 mg/5 mL (100 mL); 250 mg/5 mL (75 mL, 150 mL); 375 mg/5 mL (100 mL). **TAB, extended release** (Ceclor® CD): 375 mg, 500 mg

Generic Available Yes

Comments Patients allergic to penicillins can use a cephalosporin; the incidence of cross-reactivity between penicillins and cephalosporins is 1% when the allergic reaction to penicillin is delayed. Cefaclor is effective against anaerobic bacteria, but the sensitivity of alpha-hemolytic *Streptococcus* vary; approximately 10% of strains are resistant. Nearly 70% are intermediately sensitive. If the patient has a history of immediate reaction to penicillin, the incidence of cross-reactivity is 20%; cephalosporins are contraindicated in these patients.

Selected Readings Saxon A, Beall GN, Rohr AS, et al, "Immediate Hypersensitivity Reactions to Beta-Lactam Antibiotics," *Ann Intern Med*, 1987, 107(2):204-15.

Cefadroxil (sef a DROKS il)

Related Information

Antibiotic Prophylaxis, Preprocedural Guidelines for Dental Patients *on page 1507*

U.S. Brand Names Duricef®

Canadian Brand Names Apo®-Cefadroxil; Duricef™; Novo-Cefadroxil

Mexican Brand Names Cefamox®; Duracef®

Pharmacologic Category Antibiotic, Cephalosporin (First Generation)

Synonyms Cefadroxil Monohydrate

Use

Dental: Alternative antibiotic for prevention of bacterial endocarditis

Note: Individuals allergic to amoxicillin (penicillins) may receive cefadroxil provided they have not had an immediate, local, or systemic IgE-mediated anaphylactic allergic reaction to penicillin.

Medical: Treatment of susceptible bacterial infections, including those caused by group A beta-hemolytic *Streptococcus*

Local Anesthetic/Vasoconstrictor Precautions No information available to require special precautions

Effects on Dental Treatment No significant effects or complications reported

(Continued)

Cefadroxil *(Continued)*

Dosage Oral:

Children: 30 mg/kg/day divided twice daily up to a maximum of 2 g/day

Adults: 1-2 g/day in 2 divided doses

Prophylaxis against bacterial endocarditis:

Children: 50 mg/kg 1 hour prior to the procedure

Adults: 2 g 1 hour prior to the procedure

Dosing interval in renal impairment:

Cl_{cr} 10-25 mL/minute: Administer every 24 hours

Cl_{cr} <10 mL/minute: Administer every 36 hours

Mechanism of Action Inhibits bacterial cell wall synthesis by binding to one or more of the penicillin-binding proteins (PBPs) which in turn inhibits the final transpeptidation step of peptidoglycan synthesis in bacterial cell walls, thus inhibiting cell wall biosynthesis. Bacteria eventually lyse due to ongoing activity of cell wall autolytic enzymes (autolysins and murein hydrolases) while cell wall assembly is arrested.

Other Adverse Effects

1% to 10%: Gastrointestinal: Diarrhea

<1%: **Anaphylaxis,** rash (maculopapular and erythematous), erythema multiforme, Stevens-Johnson syndrome, **serum sickness,** arthralgia, urticaria, pruritus, angioedema, **pseudomembranous colitis,** abdominal pain, dyspepsia, **nausea, vomiting,** elevated transaminases, cholestasis, vaginitis, neutropenia, agranulocytosis, thrombocytopenia, **fever**

Reported with other cephalosporins: Toxic epidermal necrolysis, **superinfection,** renal dysfunction, toxic nephropathy, aplastic anemia, hemolytic anemia, **hemorrhage, prolonged PT,** increased BUN, increased creatinine, eosinophilia, pancytopenia, **seizures**

Contraindications Hypersensitivity to cefadroxil, other cephalosporins, or any component of the formulation

Warnings/Precautions Modify dosage in patients with severe renal impairment; prolonged use may result in superinfection; use with caution in patients with a history of penicillin allergy especially IgE-mediated reactions (eg, anaphylaxis, angioedema, urticaria); may cause antibiotic-associated colitis or colitis secondary to *C. difficile*

Drug Interactions

Increased Effect: Probenecid may decrease cephalosporin elimination

Increased Toxicity: Furosemide, aminoglycosides may be a possible additive to nephrotoxicity

Dietary/Ethanol/Herb Considerations Food: Administration with food, infant formula, or cow's milk does **not** significantly affect absorption.

Pharmacodynamics/Kinetics

Absorption: Rapid and well absorbed

Distribution: Widely throughout the body and reaches therapeutic concentrations in most tissues and body fluids, including synovial, pericardial, pleural, and peritoneal fluids; bile, sputum, and urine; bone, myocardium, gallbladder, skin and soft tissue; crosses placenta; enters breast milk

Protein binding: 20%

Half-life elimination: 1-2 hours; Renal failure: 20-24 hours

Time to peak, serum: 70-90 minutes

Excretion: Urine (>90% as unchanged drug)

Pregnancy Risk Factor B

Breast-feeding Considerations Theoretically, drug absorbed by nursing infant may change bowel flora or affect fever work-up result. **Note:** As a class, cephalosporins are used to treat infections in infants.

Dosage Forms CAP: 500 mg. **SUSP, oral:** 125 mg/5 mL, 250 mg/5 mL, 500 mg/5 mL (50 mL, 100 mL). **TAB:** 1 g

Generic Available Yes

Selected Readings

"Advisory Statement. Antibiotic Prophylaxis for Dental Patients With Total Joint Replacements. American Dental Association; American Academy of Orthopedic Surgeons," *J Am Dent Assoc*, 1997, 128(7):1004-8.

Dajani AS, Taubert KA, Wilson W, et al, "Prevention of Bacterial Endocarditis. Recommendations by the American Heart Association," *JAMA*, 1997, 277(22):1794-801.

Dajani AS, Taubert KA, Wilson W, et al, "Prevention of Bacterial Endocarditis: Recommendations by the American Heart Association," *J Am Dent Assoc*, 1997, 128(8):1142-51.

Donowitz GR and Mandell GL, "Drug Therapy. Beta-Lactam Antibiotics (1)," *N Engl J Med*, 1988, 318(7):419-26.

Donowitz GR and Mandell GL, "Drug Therapy. Beta-Lactam Antibiotics (2)," *N Engl J Med*, 1988, 318(8):490-500.

Gustaferro CA and Steckelberg JM, "Cephalosporin Antimicrobial Agents and Related Compounds," *Mayo Clin Proc*, 1991, 66(10):1064-73.

Cefadroxil Monohydrate *see* Cefadroxil *on page 261*

Cefadyl® *see* Cephapirin *on page 287*

Cefamandole (sef a MAN dole)

U.S. Brand Names Mandol® [DSC]

Pharmacologic Category Antibiotic, Cephalosporin (Second Generation)

Synonyms Cefamandole Nafate

Use Treatment of susceptible bacterial infection; mainly respiratory tract, skin and skin structure, bone and joint, urinary tract and gynecologic, septicemia; surgical prophylaxis. Active against methicillin-sensitive staphylococci, many streptococci, and various gram-negative bacilli including *E. coli*, some *Klebsiella*, *P. mirabilis*, *H. influenzae*, and *Moraxella*.

Local Anesthetic/Vasoconstrictor Precautions No information available to require special precautions

Effects on Dental Treatment No significant effects or complications reported

Dosage I.M., I.V.:

Children: 50-150 mg/kg/day in divided doses every 4-8 hours

Adults: Usual dose: 500-1000 mg every 4-8 hours; in life-threatening infections: 2 g every 4 hours may be needed

Dosing interval in renal impairment:

Cl_{cr} 25-50 mL/minute: 1-2 g every 8 hours

Cl_{cr} 10-25 mL/minute: 1 g every 8 hours

Cl_{cr} <10 mL/minute: 1 g every 12 hours

Hemodialysis: Moderately dialyzable (20% to 50%)

Mechanism of Action Inhibits bacterial cell wall synthesis by binding to one or more of the penicillin-binding proteins (PBPs) which in turn inhibits the final transpeptidation step of peptidoglycan synthesis in bacterial cell walls, thus inhibiting cell wall biosynthesis. Bacteria eventually lyse due to ongoing activity of cell wall autolytic enzymes (autolysins and murein hydrolases) while cell wall assembly is arrested.

Other Adverse Effects Contains MTT side chain which may lead to increased risk of hypoprothrombinemia and **bleeding**.

1% to 10%:

Gastrointestinal: Diarrhea

Local: Thrombophlebitis

<1%: **Anaphylaxis**, rash (maculopapular and erythematous), urticaria, pseudomembranous colitis, **nausea**, **vomiting**, elevated transaminases, cholestasis, eosinophilia, neutropenia, thrombocytopenia, increased BUN, increased creatinine, **fever**, prolonged PT

Reported with other cephalosporins: Toxic epidermal necrolysis, Stevens-Johnson syndrome, abdominal pain, **superinfection,** renal dysfunction, toxic nephropathy, aplastic anemia, hemolytic anemia, **hemorrhage**, pancytopenia, vaginitis, **seizures**

Drug Interactions Increased Effect/Toxicity: Disulfiram-like reaction has been reported when taken within 72 hours of ethanol consumption. Increased cefamandole plasma levels when taken with probenecid. Aminoglycosides, furosemide when taken with cefamandole may increase nephrotoxicity. Increase in hypoprothrombinemic effect with warfarin or heparin and cefamandole.

Dietary/Ethanol/Herb Considerations Ethanol: Avoid use; may cause a disulfiram-like reaction.

Pharmacodynamics/Kinetics

Distribution: Well throughout the body, except CSF; poor penetration even with inflamed meninges

Protein binding: 56% to 78%

Metabolism: Extensive enterohepatic recirculation

Half-life elimination: 30-60 minutes

Time to peak, serum: I.M.: 1-2 hours

Excretion: Primarily urine (as unchanged drug); feces (high concentrations)

Pregnancy Risk Factor B

Generic Available No

Cefamandole Nafate *see* Cefamandole *on page 263*

Cefazolin (sef A zoe lin)

Related Information

Animal and Human Bites Guidelines *on page 1580*

Antibiotic Prophylaxis, Preprocedural Guidelines for Dental Patients *on page 1507*

U.S. Brand Names Ancef®; Kefzol® [DSC]

Canadian Brand Names Kefzol®

Mexican Brand Names Cefamezin

Pharmacologic Category Antibiotic, Cephalosporin (First Generation)

Synonyms Cefazolin Sodium

Use

Dental: Alternative antibiotic for prevention of bacterial endocarditis when parenteral administration is needed. Individuals allergic to amoxicillin (penicillins) may receive cefazolin provided they have not had an immediate, local, or systemic

(Continued)

Cefazolin *(Continued)*

IgE-mediated anaphylactic allergic reaction to penicillin. Alternate antibiotic for premedication in patients not allergic to penicillin who may be at potential increased risk of hematogenous total joint infection when parenteral administration is needed.

Medical: Treatment of gram-positive bacilli and cocci (except enterococcus); some gram-negative bacilli including *E. coli*, *Proteus*, and *Klebsiella* may be susceptible

Local Anesthetic/Vasoconstrictor Precautions No information available to require special precautions

Effects on Dental Treatment No significant effects or complications reported

Dosage I.M., I.V.:

Children >1 month: 25-100 mg/kg/day divided every 6-8 hours; maximum: 6 g/day

Adults: 250 mg to 2 g every 6-12 (usually 8) hours, depending on severity of infection; maximum dose: 12 g/day

Prophylaxis against bacterial endocarditis:

Infants and Children: 25 mg/kg 30 minutes before procedure; maximum dose: 1 g

Adults: 1 g 1 hour before procedure

Dosing adjustment in renal impairment:

Cl_{cr} 10-30 mL/minute: Administer every 12 hours

Cl_{cr} <10 mL/minute: Administer every 24 hours

Hemodialysis: Moderately dialyzable (20% to 50%); administer dose postdialysis or administer supplemental dose of 0.5-1 g after dialysis

Peritoneal dialysis: Administer 0.5 g every 12 hours

Continuous arteriovenous or venovenous hemofiltration: Dose as for Cl_{cr} 10-30 mL/minute; removes 30 mg of cefazolin per liter of filtrate per day

Mechanism of Action Inhibits bacterial cell wall synthesis by binding to one or more of the penicillin-binding proteins (PBPs) which in turn inhibits the final transpeptidation step of peptidoglycan synthesis in bacterial cell walls, thus inhibiting cell wall biosynthesis. Bacteria eventually lyse due to ongoing activity of cell wall autolytic enzymes (autolysins and murein hydrolases) while cell wall assembly is arrested.

Other Adverse Effects

1% to 10%:

Gastrointestinal: Diarrhea

Local: Pain at injection site

<1%: **Anaphylaxis**, rash, pruritus, Stevens-Johnson syndrome, **oral candidiasis, nausea, vomiting**, abdominal cramps, anorexia, **pseudomembranous colitis,** eosinophilia, neutropenia, leukopenia, thrombocytopenia, thrombocytosis, elevated transaminases, phlebitis, vaginitis, **fever, seizures**

Reported with other cephalosporins: Toxic epidermal necrolysis, abdominal pain, cholestasis, **superinfection**, renal dysfunction, toxic nephropathy, aplastic anemia, hemolytic anemia, **hemorrhage, prolonged PT,** pancytopenia

Contraindications Hypersensitivity to cefazolin sodium, any component of the formulation, or other cephalosporins

Warnings/Precautions Modify dosage in patients with severe renal impairment; prolonged use may result in superinfection; use with caution in patients with a history of penicillin allergy especially IgE-mediated reactions (eg, anaphylaxis, angioedema, urticaria); may cause antibiotic-associated colitis or colitis secondary to *C. difficile*

Drug Interactions

Increased Effect: High-dose probenecid decreases clearance

Increased Toxicity: Aminoglycosides increase nephrotoxic potential

Pharmacodynamics/Kinetics

Distribution: Widely into most body tissues and fluids including gallbladder, liver, kidneys, bone, sputum, bile, pleural, and synovial; CSF penetration is poor; crosses placenta; enters breast milk

Protein binding: 74% to 86%

Metabolism: Minimally hepatic

Half-life elimination: 90-150 minutes; prolonged with renal impairment

Time to peak, serum: I.M.: 0.5-2 hours

Excretion: Urine (80% to 100% as unchanged drug)

Pregnancy Risk Factor B

Breast-feeding Considerations Theoretically, drug absorbed by nursing infant may change bowel flora or affect fever work-up result. **Note:** As a class, cephalosporins are used to treat infections in infants.

Dosage Forms INF [premixed in D_5W, frozen] (Ancef®): 500 mg (50 mL); 1 g (50 mL). **Injection, powder for reconstitution** (Ancef®, Kefzol®): 500 mg, 1 g, 10 g, 20 g. **Injection, powder for reconstitution:** 500 mg, 1 g [with 50 mL D_5W in DUPLEX™ container]

Generic Available Yes

Selected Readings

"Advisory Statement. Antibiotic Prophylaxis for Dental Patients With Total Joint Replacements. American Dental Association; American Academy of Orthopedic Surgeons," *J Am Dent Assoc*, 1997, 128(7):1004-8.

Dajani AS, Taubert KA, Wilson W, et al, "Prevention of Bacterial Endocarditis. Recommendations by the American Heart Association," *JAMA*, 1997, 277(22):1794-801.

Dajani AS, Taubert KA, Wilson W, et al, "Prevention of Bacterial Endocarditis: Recommendations by the American Heart Association," *J Am Dent Assoc*, 1997, 128(8):1142-51.

Donowitz GR and Mandell GL, "Drug Therapy. Beta-Lactam Antibiotics (1)," *N Engl J Med*, 1988, 318(7):419-26.

Donowitz GR and Mandell GL, "Drug Therapy. Beta-Lactam Antibiotics (2)," *N Engl J Med*, 1988, 318(8):490-500.

Gustaferro CA and Steckelberg JM, "Cephalosporin Antimicrobial Agents and Related Compounds," *Mayo Clin Proc*, 1991, 66(10):1064-73.

Cefazolin Sodium *see* Cefazolin *on page 263*

Cefdinir (SEF di ner)

U.S. Brand Names Omnicef®

Canadian Brand Names Omnicef®

Pharmacologic Category Antibiotic, Cephalosporin (Third Generation)

Synonyms CFDN

Use Treatment of community-acquired pneumonia, acute exacerbations of chronic bronchitis, acute bacterial otitis media, acute maxillary sinusitis, pharyngitis/tonsillitis, and uncomplicated skin and skin structure infections.

Local Anesthetic/Vasoconstrictor Precautions No information available to require special precautions

Effects on Dental Treatment No significant effects or complications reported

Dosage Oral:

Children: 7 mg/kg/dose twice daily for 5-10 days or 14 mg/kg/dose once daily for 10 days (maximum: 600 mg/day)

Adolescents and Adults: 300 mg twice daily or 600 mg once daily for 10 days

Dosing adjustment in renal impairment: Cl_{cr} <30 mL/minute: 300 mg once daily

Hemodialysis removes cefdinir; recommended initial dose: 300 mg (or 7 mg/kg/dose) every other day. At the conclusion of each hemodialysis session, 300 mg (or 7 mg/kg/dose) should be given. Subsequent doses (300 mg or 7 mg/kg/dose) should be administered every other day.

Mechanism of Action Inhibits bacterial cell wall synthesis by binding to one or more of the penicillin-binding proteins (PBPs) which in turn inhibits the final transpeptidation step of peptidoglycan synthesis in bacterial cell walls, thus inhibiting cell wall biosynthesis. Bacteria eventually lyse due to ongoing activity of cell wall autolytic enzymes (autolysins and murein hydrolases) while cell wall assembly is arrested.

Other Adverse Effects

1% to 10%

Dermatologic: Cutaneous moniliasis (1%)

Gastrointestinal: Diarrhea (8%), rash (3%), increased GGT (1%)

<1% (Limited to important or life-threatening): Leukopenia, **nausea**, vaginal moniliasis, rash, Stevens-Johnson syndrome, exfoliative dermatitis, erythema multiforme, toxic epidermal necrolysis, erythema nodosum, hepatitis, cholestasis, hepatic failure, jaundice, **anaphylaxis, shock**, edema, **laryngeal edema**, hemorrhagic colitis, enterocolitis, pseudomembranous colitis, pancytopenia, granulocytopenia, leukopenia, thrombocytopenia, ITP, hemolytic anemia, **respiratory failure, asthma exacerbation, eosinophilic pneumonia, idiopathic interstitial pneumonia, fever**, acute renal failure, nephropathy, **coagulopathy**, DIC, **upper GI bleeding, peptic ulcer**, ileus, **loss of consciousness**, vasculitis, **cardiac failure, chest pain, MI, hypertension, involuntary movements**, rhabdomyolysis

Reported with other cephalosporins: **Dizziness, headache**, encephalopathy, asterixis, **neuromuscular excitability, seizures**, aplastic anemia, interstitial nephritis, toxic nephropathy, angioedema, **hemorrhage, prolonged PT, serum-sickness reactions, superinfection**

Drug Interactions

Increased Effect/Toxicity: Probenecid increases the effects of cephalosporins by decreasing the renal elimination in those which are secreted by tubular secretion. Anticoagulant effects may be increased when administered with cephalosporins.

Decreased Effect: Coadministration with iron or antacids reduces the rate and extent of cefdinir absorption.

Dietary/Ethanol/Herb Considerations Food: May be taken with food.

Pharmacodynamics/Kinetics

Protein binding: 60% to 70%

Metabolism: Minimally hepatic

Bioavailability: Capsule: 16% to 21%; suspension 25%

Half-life elimination: 100 minutes

Excretion: Primarily urine

Pregnancy Risk Factor B

Generic Available No

Cefditoren (sef de TOR en)

U.S. Brand Names Spectracef™

Pharmacologic Category Antibiotic, Cephalosporin

(Continued)

Cefditoren *(Continued)*

Synonyms Cefditoren Pivoxil

Use Dental and Medical: Treatment of acute bacterial exacerbation of chronic bronchitis (due to susceptible organisms including *Haemophilus influenzae, Haemophilus parainfluenzae, Streptococcus pneumoniae*-penicillin susceptible only, *Moraxella catarrhalis*); pharyngitis or tonsillitis (*Streptococcus pyogenes*); and uncomplicated skin and skin structure infections (*Staphylococcus aureus*-not MRSA, *Streptococcus pyogenes*)

Local Anesthetic/Vasoconstrictor Precautions No information available to require special precautions

Effects on Dental Treatment 1% to 6%: Headache (2% to 3%), nausea (4% to 6%), vomiting (1%)

Dosage Oral: Children ≥12 years, Adults:

Acute bacterial exacerbation of chronic bronchitis: 400 mg twice daily for 10 days

Community-acquired pneumonia: 400 mg twice daily for 14 days

Pharyngitis, tonsillitis, uncomplicated skin and skin structure infections: 200 mg twice daily for 10 days

Dosing adjustment in renal impairment:

Cl_{cr} 30-49 mL/minute: Maximum dose: 200 mg twice daily

Cl_{cr} <30 mL/minute: Maximum dose: 200 mg once daily

Endstage renal disease: Not established

Mechanism of Action Inhibits bacterial cell wall synthesis by binding to one or more of the penicillin binding proteins (PBPs); which in turn inhibits the final transpeptidation step of peptidoglycan synthesis in bacterial cell walls, thus inhibiting cell wall biosynthesis. Bacteria eventually lyse due to ongoing activity of cell wall autolytic enzymes (autolysins and murein hydrolases) while cell wall assembly is arrested.

Other Adverse Effects

>10%: Gastrointestinal: Diarrhea (11% to 15%)

1% to 10%:

Endocrine & metabolic: Glucose increased (1%)

Gastrointestinal: Abdominal pain (2%), dyspepsia (1% to 2%)

Genitourinary: Vaginal moniliasis (3% to 6%)

Hematologic: Hematocrit decreased (2%)

Renal: Hematuria (3%), urinary white blood cells increased (2%)

<1%: Abnormal dreams, decreased serum albumin, **allergic reaction**, anorexia, increased appetite, BUN increased, **decreased serum calcium,** decreased serum chloride, increased serum cholesterol, **coagulation time increased**, constipation, **diaphoresis, dizziness, xerostomia, eructation,** eosinophils increased, **fever**, flatulence, **fungal infection, gastritis, GI disorder, hemoglobin decreased, hyperglycemia**, inorganic phosphorus decreased, insomnia, leukopenia, lymphocytes increased, **oral ulceration**, myalgia, **nervousness,** neutrophils decreased, **oral moniliasis, pain**, peripheral edema, **pharyngitis, platelet count increased**, positive direct Coombs' test, potassium increased, **pseudomembranous colitis,** proteinuria, pruritus, rash, **rhinitis**, SGOT increased, SGPT increased, **sinusitis, somnolence, stomatitis, abnormal taste**, thrombocytopenia, urinary frequency, urticaria, vaginitis, **weakness**, weight loss, white blood cell increase/decrease

Reported with cephalosporin antibiotics: **Anaphylaxis**, aplastic anemia, cholestasis, erythema multiforme, **hemorrhage,** hemolytic anemia, renal dysfunction, **hyperactivity (reversible), serum sickness-like reaction**, Stevens-Johnson syndrome, toxic epidermal necrolysis, toxic nephropathy

Contraindications Hypersensitivity to cefditoren, other cephalosporins, milk protein, or any component of the formulation; carnitine deficiency

Warnings/Precautions Use with caution in patients with a history of penicillin allergy, especially IgE-mediated reactions (eg, anaphylaxis, urticaria); may cause antibiotic-associated colitis or colitis secondary to *C. difficile*. Use caution in patients with renal or hepatic impairment. Cefditoren causes renal excretion of carnitine, do not use in patients with carnitine deficiency; not for long-term therapy due to the possible development of carnitine deficiency over time. Cefditoren tablets contain sodium caseinate, which may cause hypersensitivity reactions in patients with milk protein hypersensitivity; this does not affect patients with lactose intolerance. Safety and efficacy have not been established in children <12 years of age.

Drug Interactions

Antacids: Aluminum- and magnesium-containing antacids decrease oral absorption; concomitant use should be avoided.

Histamine H_2 antagonists: Famotidine decreases oral absorption; concomitant use should be avoided.

Probenecid: Serum concentration of cefditoren may be increased.

Dietary/Ethanol/Herb Considerations Food: Administer with food; moderate- to high-fat meals increase bioavailability and maximum plasma concentration. Plasma carnitine levels are decreased during therapy (39% with 200 mg dosing, 63% with 400 mg dosing); Boiled milk, buttermilk, or yogurt may reduce diarrhea.

Pharmacodynamics/Kinetics

Distribution: 9.3 ± 1.6 L

Protein binding: 88% (*in vitro*), primarily to albumin

Metabolism: Cefditoren pivoxil is hydrolyzed to cefditoren (active) and pivalate

Bioavailability: ~14% to 16%, increased by moderate to high-fat meal

Half-life elimination: 1.6 ± 0.4 hours

Time to peak: 1.5-3 hours

Excretion: Urine (as cefditoren and pivaloylcarnitine)

Pregnancy Risk Factor B

Dosage Forms TAB: 200 mg

Generic Available No

Cefditoren Pivoxil *see* Cefditoren *on page 265*

Cefepime (SEF e pim)

U.S. Brand Names Maxipime®

Canadian Brand Names Maxipime™

Mexican Brand Names Maxipime®

Pharmacologic Category Antibiotic, Cephalosporin (Fourth Generation)

Synonyms Cefepime Hydrochloride

Use Treatment of uncomplicated and complicated urinary tract infections, including pyelonephritis caused by typical urinary tract pathogens; monotherapy for febrile neutropenia; uncomplicated skin and skin structure infections caused by *Streptococcus pyogenes*; moderate to severe pneumonia caused by pneumococcus, *Pseudomonas aeruginosa*, and other gram-negative organisms; complicated intra-abdominal infections (in combination with metronidazole). Also active against methicillin-susceptible staphylococci, *Enterobacter* sp, and many other gram-negative bacilli.

Children 2 months to 16 years: Empiric therapy of febrile neutropenia patients, uncomplicated skin/soft tissue infections, pneumonia, and uncomplicated/complicated urinary tract infections.

Local Anesthetic/Vasoconstrictor Precautions No information available to require special precautions

Effects on Dental Treatment 1% to 10%: Fever (1%), headache (1%), nausea, vomiting

Dosage I.V.:

Children:

Febrile neutropenia: 50 mg/kg every 8 hours for 7-10 days

Uncomplicated skin/soft tissue infections, pneumonia, and complicated/uncomplicated UTI: 50 mg/kg twice daily

Adults:

Most infections: 1-2 g every 12 hours for 5-10 days; higher doses or more frequent administration may be required in pseudomonal infections

Urinary tract infections, uncomplicated: 500 mg every 12 hours

Monotherapy for febrile neutropenic patients: 2 g every 8 hours for 7 days or until the neutropenia resolves

Dosing adjustment in renal impairment: Adults: Recommended maintenance schedule based on creatinine clearance (mL/minute), compared to normal dosing schedule: See table.

Cefepime Hydrochloride

Creatinine Clearance (mL/minute)	Recommended Maintenance Schedule			
>60 Normal recommended dosing schedule	500 mg every 12 hours	1 g every 12 hours	2 g every 12 hours	2 g every 8 hours
30-60	500 mg every 24 hours	1 g every 24 hours	2 g every 24 hours	2 g every 12 hours
11-29	500 mg every 24 hours	500 mg every 24 hours	1 g every 24 hours	2 g every 24 hours
<11	250 mg every 24 hours	250 mg every 24 hours	500 mg every 24 hours	1 g every 24 hours

Hemodialysis: Removed by dialysis; administer supplemental dose of 250 mg after each dialysis session

Peritoneal dialysis: Removed to a lesser extent than hemodialysis; administer 250 mg every 48 hours

Continuous arteriovenous or venovenous hemofiltration: Dose as normal Cl_{cr} (eg, >30 mL/minute)

Mechanism of Action Inhibits bacterial cell wall synthesis by binding to one or more of the penicillin-binding proteins (PBPs) which in turn inhibits the final transpeptidation step of peptidoglycan synthesis in bacterial cell walls, thus inhibiting cell

(Continued)

Cefepime *(Continued)*

wall biosynthesis. Bacteria eventually lyse due to ongoing activity of cell wall autolytic enzymes (autolysis and murein hydrolases) while cell wall assembly is arrested.

Other Adverse Effects

>10%: Hematologic: Positive Coombs' test without hemolysis

1% to 10%:

Dermatologic: Rash, pruritus

Gastrointestinal: Diarrhea

Local: Pain, erythema at injection site

<1%: **Anaphylactic shock, anaphylaxis**, agranulocytosis, **coma**, encephalopathy, **hallucinations**, leukopenia, myoclonus, **neuromuscular excitability**, neutropenia, **seizures**, thrombocytopenia

Reported with other cephalosporins: Aplastic anemia, erythema multiforme, hemolytic anemia, **hemorrhage,** pancytopenia, **prolonged PT,** renal dysfunction, Stevens-Johnson syndrome, **superinfection,** toxic epidermal necrolysis, toxic nephropathy, vaginitis

Drug Interactions Increased Effect/Toxicity: High-dose probenecid decreases clearance and increases effect of cefepime. Aminoglycosides increase nephrotoxic potential when taken with cefepime.

Pharmacodynamics/Kinetics

Absorption: I.M.: Rapid and complete

Distribution: V_d: Adults: 14-20 L; penetrates into inflammatory fluid at concentrations ~80% of serum levels and into bronchial mucosa at levels ~60% of those reached in the plasma; crosses blood-brain barrier

Protein binding, plasma: 16% to 19%

Metabolism: Minimally hepatic

Half-life elimination: 2 hours

Time to peak: 0.5-1.5 hours

Excretion: Urine (85% as unchanged drug)

Pregnancy Risk Factor B

Generic Available No

Cefepime Hydrochloride *see* Cefepime *on page 267*

Cefixime (sef IKS eem)

Related Information

Nonviral Infectious Diseases *on page 1493*

Sexually-Transmitted Diseases *on page 1502*

U.S. Brand Names Suprax® [DSC]

Canadian Brand Names Suprax®

Mexican Brand Names Denvar®; Novacef

Pharmacologic Category Antibiotic, Cephalosporin (Third Generation)

Synonyms Suprax® [DSC]

Use Treatment of urinary tract infections, otitis media, respiratory infections due to susceptible organisms including *S. pneumoniae* and *S. pyogenes, H. influenzae* and many Enterobacteriaceae; documented poor compliance with other oral antimicrobials; outpatient therapy of serious soft tissue or skeletal infections due to susceptible organisms; single-dose oral treatment of uncomplicated cervical/urethral gonorrhea due to *N. gonorrhoeae*

Local Anesthetic/Vasoconstrictor Precautions No information available to require special precautions

Effects on Dental Treatment 1% to 10%: Nausea

Dosage Oral:

Children: 8 mg/kg/day divided every 12-24 hours

Adolescents and Adults: 400 mg/day divided every 12-24 hours

Uncomplicated cervical/urethral gonorrhea due to *N. gonorrhoeae*: 400 mg as a single dose

For *S. pyogenes* infections, treat for 10 days; use suspension for otitis media due to increased peak serum levels as compared to tablet form

Dosing adjustment in renal impairment:

Cl_{cr} 21-60 mL/minute or with renal hemodialysis: Administer 75% of the standard dose

Cl_{cr} <20 mL/minute or with CAPD: Administer 50% of the standard dose

Moderately dialyzable (10%)

Mechanism of Action Inhibits bacterial cell wall synthesis by binding to one or more of the penicillin binding proteins (PBPs); which in turn inhibits the final transpeptidation step of peptidoglycan synthesis in bacterial cell walls, thus inhibiting cell wall biosynthesis. Bacteria eventually lyse due to ongoing activity of cell wall autolytic enzymes (autolysins and murein hydrolases) while cell wall assembly is arrested.

Other Adverse Effects

>10%: Gastrointestinal: Diarrhea (16%)

1% to 10%: Gastrointestinal: Abdominal pain, dyspepsia, flatulence

<1%: Rash, urticaria, pruritus, erythema multiforme, Stevens-Johnson syndrome, serum sickness-like reaction, **fever, vomiting**, pseudomembranous colitis, transaminase elevations, increased BUN, increased creatinine, **headache, dizziness**, thrombocytopenia, leukopenia, eosinophilia, **prolonged PT**, vaginitis, **candidiasis**

Reported with other cephalosporins: **Anaphylaxis, seizures**, toxic epidermal necrolysis, renal dysfunction, toxic nephropathy, interstitial nephritis, cholestasis, aplastic anemia, hemolytic anemia, **hemorrhage,** pancytopenia, neutropenia, agranulocytosis, colitis, **superinfection**

Drug Interactions Increased Effect/Toxicity: Probenecid increases cefixime concentration. Cefixime may increase carbamazepine.

Dietary/Ethanol/Herb Considerations Food: Administer with food to reduce GI upset; food delays absorption.

Pharmacodynamics/Kinetics

Absorption: 40% to 50%

Distribution: Widely throughout the body and reaches therapeutic concentration in most tissues and body fluids, including synovial, pericardial, pleural, peritoneal; bile, sputum, and urine; bone, myocardium, gallbladder, and skin and soft tissue

Protein binding: 65%

Half-life elimination: Normal renal function: 3-4 hours; Renal failure: Up to 11.5 hours

Time to peak, serum: 2-6 hours (15% to 50% higher for oral suspension vs tablets); delayed with food

Excretion: Urine (50% of absorbed dose as active drug); feces (10%)

Pregnancy Risk Factor B

Generic Available No

Cefizox® *see* Ceftizoxime *on page 277*

Cefobid® *see* Cefoperazone *on page 270*

Cefonicid (se FON i sid)

U.S. Brand Names Monocid® [DSC]

Mexican Brand Names Monocidur

Pharmacologic Category Antibiotic, Cephalosporin (Second Generation)

Synonyms Cefonicid Sodium; Monocid® [DSC]

Use Treatment of susceptible bacterial infection; mainly respiratory tract, skin and skin structure, bone and joint, urinary tract and gynecologic, septicemia; active against methicillin-sensitive staphylococci, many streptococci, and various gram-negative bacilli including *E. coli*, some *Klebsiella*, *P. mirabilis*, *H. influenzae*, and *Moraxella*.

Local Anesthetic/Vasoconstrictor Precautions No information available to require special precautions

Effects on Dental Treatment No significant effects or complications reported

Dosage Adults: I.M., I.V.: 0.5-2 g every 24 hours

Prophylaxis: Preop: 1 g/hour

Dosing interval in renal impairment: Dosing based on Cl_{cr} (mL/minute/1.73 m^2)

Cl_{cr} 60-79: 10-24 mg/kg every 24 hours

Cl_{cr} 40-59: 8-20 mg/kg every 24 hours

Cl_{cr} 20-39: 4-15 mg/kg every 24 hours

Cl_{cr} 10-19: 4-15 mg/kg every 48 hours

Cl_{cr} 5-9: 4-15 mg/kg every 3-5 days

Cl_{cr} <5: 3-4 mg/kg every 3-5 days

Mechanism of Action Inhibits bacterial cell wall synthesis by binding to one or more of the penicillin-binding proteins (PBPs) which in turn inhibits the final transpeptidation step of peptidoglycan synthesis in bacterial cell walls, thus inhibiting cell wall biosynthesis. Bacteria eventually lyse due to ongoing activity of cell wall autolytic enzymes (autolysins and murein hydrolases) while cell wall assembly is arrested.

Other Adverse Effects

1% to 10%:

Hematologic: Increased eosinophils (3%), increased platelets (2%)

Hepatic: Altered LFTs (increased transaminases, LDH, alkaline phosphatase) (2%)

Local: Pain, burning at injection site (6%)

<1%: **Fever**, rash, pruritus, erythema, **anaphylactoid reactions,** diarrhea, pseudomembranous colitis, abdominal pain, increased transaminases, increased BUN, increased creatinine, interstitial nephritis, neutropenia, decreased WBC, thrombocytopenia

Reported with other cephalosporins: **Anaphylaxis, seizures**, Stevens-Johnson syndrome, toxic epidermal necrolysis, renal dysfunction, toxic nephropathy, cholestasis, aplastic anemia, hemolytic anemia, **hemorrhage,** pancytopenia, agranulocytosis, colitis, **superinfection**

Drug Interactions Increased Effect/Toxicity: Probenecid may decrease cephalosporin elimination. Furosemide, aminoglycosides in combination with cefonicid may result in additive nephrotoxicity.

(Continued)

Cefonicid *(Continued)*

Pharmacodynamics/Kinetics

Absorption: I.M.: Well absorbed

Distribution: Widely into most body tissues; low concentrations in CSF and eye

Protein binding: 98%

Metabolism: None

Half-life elimination: 3.5-5.8 hours

Excretion: Urine (as unchanged drug)

Pregnancy Risk Factor B

Generic Available No

Cefonicid Sodium *see* Cefonicid *on page 269*

Cefoperazone (sef oh PER a zone)

U.S. Brand Names Cefobid®

Canadian Brand Names Cefobid®

Pharmacologic Category Antibiotic, Cephalosporin (Third Generation)

Synonyms Cefoperazone Sodium

Use Treatment of susceptible bacterial infection; mainly respiratory tract, skin and skin structure, bone and joint, urinary tract and gynecologic as well as septicemia. Active against a variety of gram-negative bacilli, some gram-positive cocci, and has some activity against *Pseudomonas aeruginosa*.

Local Anesthetic/Vasoconstrictor Precautions No information available to require special precautions

Effects on Dental Treatment No significant effects or complications reported

Dosage I.M., I.V.:

Children (not approved): 100-150 mg/kg/day divided every 8-12 hours; up to 12 g/day

Adults: 2-4 g/day in divided doses every 12 hours; up to 12 g/day

Dosing adjustment in hepatic impairment: Reduce dose 50% in patients with advanced liver cirrhosis; maximum daily dose: 4 g

Mechanism of Action Inhibits bacterial cell wall synthesis by binding to one or more of the penicillin-binding proteins (PBPs) which in turn inhibits the final transpeptidation step of peptidoglycan synthesis in bacterial cell walls, thus inhibiting cell wall biosynthesis. Bacteria eventually lyse due to ongoing activity of cell wall autolytic enzymes (autolysins and murein hydrolases) while cell wall assembly is arrested.

Other Adverse Effects Contains MTT side chain which may lead to increased risk of hypoprothrombinemia and bleeding.

1% to 10%:

Dermatologic: Rash (maculopapular or erythematous) (2%)

Gastrointestinal: Diarrhea (3%)

Hematologic: Decreased neutrophils (2%), decreased hemoglobin or hematocrit (5%), eosinophilia (10%)

Hepatic: Increased transaminases (5% to 10%)

<1%: Hypoprothrombinemia, **bleeding**, pseudomembranous colitis, **nausea, vomiting**, elevated BUN, elevated creatinine, pain at injection site, induration at injection site, phlebitis, drug fever

Reported with other cephalosporins: **Anaphylaxis, seizures**, Stevens-Johnson syndrome, toxic epidermal necrolysis, renal dysfunction, toxic nephropathy, cholestasis, aplastic anemia, hemolytic anemia, pancytopenia, agranulocytosis, colitis, **superinfection**

Drug Interactions Increased Effect/Toxicity: Probenecid may decrease cephalosporin elimination resulting in increased levels. Furosemide, aminoglycosides in combination with cefoperazone may result in additive nephrotoxicity.

Dietary/Ethanol/Herb Considerations

Ethanol: Avoid use; disulfiram-like reaction reported within 72 hours.

Food may decrease vitamin K synthesis by suppressing GI flora; resulting in increased risk of hemorrhage. Monitor prothrombin time and administer vitamin K as needed. Patients at risk are those with malabsorption states (eg, cystic fibrosis) or poor nutritional status.

Pharmacodynamics/Kinetics

Distribution: Widely in most body tissues and fluids; highest concentrations in bile; low penetration in CSF; variable when meninges are inflamed; crosses placenta; small amounts enter breast milk

Half-life elimination: 2 hours; prolonged with hepatic disease or biliary obstruction

Time to peak, serum: I.M.: 1-2 hours

Excretion: Feces via the biliary tract (70% to 75%); urine (20% to 30% as unchanged drug)

Pregnancy Risk Factor B

Generic Available No

Cefoperazone Sodium *see* Cefoperazone *on page 270*

Cefotan® *see* Cefotetan *on page 272*

Cefotaxime (sef oh TAKS eem)

Related Information

Sexually-Transmitted Diseases *on page 1502*

U.S. Brand Names Claforan®

Canadian Brand Names Claforan®

Mexican Brand Names Alfotax; Benaxima®; Biosint®; Cefaxim; Cefoclin; Cefradil® Claforan®; Fotexina®; Taporin®; Viken®

Pharmacologic Category Antibiotic, Cephalosporin (Third Generation)

Synonyms Cefotaxime Sodium

Use Treatment of susceptible infection in respiratory tract, skin and skin structure, bone and joint, urinary tract, gynecologic as well as septicemia, and documented or suspected meningitis. Active against most gram-negative bacilli (not *Pseudomonas*) and gram-positive cocci (not enterococcus). Active against many penicillin-resistant pneumococci.

Local Anesthetic/Vasoconstrictor Precautions No information available to require special precautions

Effects on Dental Treatment 1% to 10%: Nausea, vomiting

Dosage

Infants and Children 1 month to 12 years: I.M., I.V.: <50 kg: 50-180 mg/kg/day in divided doses every 4-6 hours

Meningitis: 200 mg/kg/day in divided doses every 6 hours

Children >12 years and Adults:

Uncomplicated infections: I.M., I.V.: 1 g every 12 hours

Moderate/severe infections: I.M., I.V.: 1-2 g every 8 hours

Infections commonly needing higher doses (eg, septicemia): I.V.: 2 g every 6-8 hours

Life-threatening infections: I.V.: 2 g every 4 hours

Preop: I.M., I.V.: 1 g 30-90 minutes before surgery

C-section: 1 g as soon as the umbilical cord is clamped, then 1 g I.M., I.V. at 6- and 12-hour intervals

Dosing interval in renal impairment:

Cl_{cr} 10-50 mL/minute: Administer every 8-12 hours

Cl_{cr} <10 mL/minute: Administer every 24 hours

Hemodialysis: Moderately dialyzable

Dosing adjustment in hepatic impairment: Moderate dosage reduction is recommended in severe liver disease

Continuous arteriovenous or venovenous hemodiafiltration effects: Administer 1 g every 12 hour

Mechanism of Action Inhibits bacterial cell wall synthesis by binding to one or more of the penicillin-binding proteins (PBPs) which in turn inhibits the final transpeptidation step of peptidoglycan synthesis in bacterial cell walls, thus inhibiting cell wall biosynthesis. Bacteria eventually lyse due to ongoing activity of cell wall autolytic enzymes (autolysins and murein hydrolases) while cell wall assembly is arrested.

Other Adverse Effects

1% to 10%:

Dermatologic: Rash, pruritus

Gastrointestinal: Diarrhea, colitis

Local: Pain at injection site

<1%: Anaphylaxis, arrhythmias (after rapid IV injection via candidiasis, central catheter), eosinophilia, erythema multiforme, fever, headache, increased BUN, increased creatinine, increased transaminases, interstitial nephritis, neutropenia, phlebitis, pseudomembranous colitis, Stevens-Johnson syndrome, thrombocytopenia, toxic epidermal necrolysis, transaminase elevations, urticaria, vaginitis

Reported with other cephalosporins: Agranulocytosis, aplastic anemia, cholestasis, hemolytic anemia, **hemorrhage**, pancytopenia, renal dysfunction, **seizures, superinfection,** toxic nephropathy

Drug Interactions Increased Effect/Toxicity: Probenecid may decrease cephalosporin elimination resulting in increased levels. Furosemide, aminoglycosides in combination with cefotaxime may result in additive nephrotoxicity.

Pharmacodynamics/Kinetics

Distribution: Widely to body tissues and fluids including aqueous humor, ascitic and prostatic fluids, bone; penetrates CSF best when meninges are inflamed; crosses placenta; enters breast milk

Metabolism: Partially hepatic to active metabolite, desacetylcefotaxime

Half-life elimination:

Cefotaxime: Premature neonates <1 week: 5-6 hours; Full-term neonates <1 week: 2-3.4 hours; Adults: 1-1.5 hours; prolonged with renal and/or hepatic impairment

Desacetylcefotaxime: 1.5-1.9 hours; prolonged with renal impairment

Time to peak, serum: I.M.: Within 30 minutes

Excretion: Urine (as unchanged drug and metabolites)

Pregnancy Risk Factor B

Generic Available Yes

Cefotaxime Sodium *see* Cefotaxime *on page 271*

Cefotetan (SEF oh tee tan)

Related Information

Animal and Human Bites Guidelines *on page 1580*

U.S. Brand Names Cefotan®

Canadian Brand Names Cefotan®

Pharmacologic Category Antibiotic, Cephalosporin (Second Generation)

Synonyms Cefotetan Disodium

Use Less active against staphylococci and streptococci than first generation cephalosporins, but active against anaerobes including *Bacteroides fragilis*; active against gram-negative enteric bacilli including *E. coli*, *Klebsiella*, and *Proteus*; used predominantly for respiratory tract, skin and skin structure, bone and joint, urinary tract and gynecologic as well as septicemia; surgical prophylaxis; intra-abdominal infections and other mixed infections

Local Anesthetic/Vasoconstrictor Precautions No information available to require special precautions

Effects on Dental Treatment No significant effects or complications reported

Dosage I.M., I.V.:

Children: 20-40 mg/kg/dose every 12 hours

Adults: 1-6 g/day in divided doses every 12 hours; usual dose: 1-2 g every 12 hours for 5-10 days; 1-2 g may be given every 24 hours for urinary tract infection

Dosing interval in renal impairment:

Cl_{cr} 10-30 mL/minute: Administer every 24 hours

Cl_{cr} <10 mL/minute: Administer every 48 hours

Hemodialysis: Slightly dialyzable (5% to 20%); administer 1/4 the usual dose every 24 hours on days between dialysis; administer 1/2 the usual dose on the day of dialysis.

Continuous arteriovenous or venovenous hemodiafiltration effects: Administer 750 mg every 12 hours

Mechanism of Action Inhibits bacterial cell wall synthesis by binding to one or more of the penicillin-binding proteins (PBPs) which in turn inhibits the final transpeptidation step of peptidoglycan synthesis in bacterial cell walls, thus inhibiting cell wall biosynthesis. Bacteria eventually lyse due to ongoing activity of cell wall autolytic enzymes (autolysins and murein hydrolases) while cell wall assembly is arrested.

Other Adverse Effects Contains MTT side chain which may lead to increased risk of hypoprothrombinemia and **bleeding**.

1% to 10%:

Gastrointestinal: Diarrhea (1.3%)

Hepatic: Increased transaminases (1.2%)

Miscellaneous: Hypersensitivity reactions (1.2%)

<1%: **Anaphylaxis**, urticaria, rash, pruritus, pseudomembranous colitis, **nausea, vomiting**, eosinophilia, thrombocytosis, agranulocytosis, hemolytic anemia, leukopenia, thrombocytopenia, prolonged PT, **bleeding**, elevated BUN, elevated creatinine, nephrotoxicity, phlebitis, **fever**

Reported with other cephalosporins: **Seizures**, Stevens-Johnson syndrome, toxic epidermal necrolysis, renal dysfunction, toxic nephropathy, cholestasis, aplastic anemia, hemolytic anemia, **hemorrhage,** pancytopenia, agranulocytosis, colitis, **superinfection**

Drug Interactions Increased Effect/Toxicity: Probenecid may decrease cephalosporin elimination. Furosemide, aminoglycosides in combination with cefotetan may result in additive nephrotoxicity. May cause disulfiram-like reaction with concomitant ethanol use. Effects of warfarin may be enhanced by cefotetan (due to effects on gastrointestinal flora).

Dietary/Ethanol/Herb Considerations Ethanol: Avoid use; disulfiram-like reaction reported within 72 hours.

Pharmacodynamics/Kinetics

Distribution: Widely to body tissues and fluids including bile, sputum, prostatic, peritoneal; low concentrations enter CSF; crosses placenta; enters breast milk

Protein binding: 76% to 90%

Half-life elimination: 3-5 hours

Time to peak, serum: I.M.: 1.5-3 hours

Excretion: Primarily urine (as unchanged drug); feces (20%)

Pregnancy Risk Factor B

Generic Available Yes

Cefotetan Disodium *see* Cefotetan *on page 272*

Cefoxitin (se FOKS i tin)

U.S. Brand Names Mefoxin®

Canadian Brand Names Mefoxin®

Pharmacologic Category Antibiotic, Cephalosporin (Second Generation)

Synonyms Cefoxitin Sodium

Use Less active against staphylococci and streptococci than first generation cephalosporins, but active against anaerobes including *Bacteroides fragilis*; active against gram-negative enteric bacilli including *E. coli*, *Klebsiella*, and *Proteus*; used predominantly for respiratory tract, skin and skin structure, bone and joint, urinary tract and gynecologic as well as septicemia; surgical prophylaxis; intra-abdominal infections and other mixed infections; indicated for bacterial *Eikenella corrodens* infections

Local Anesthetic/Vasoconstrictor Precautions No information available to require special precautions

Effects on Dental Treatment No significant effects or complications reported

Dosage

Infants >3 months and Children: I.M., I.V.:

- Mild to moderate infection: 80-100 mg/kg/day in divided doses every 4-6 hours
- Severe infection: 100-160 mg/kg/day in divided doses every 4-6 hours; maximum dose: 12 g/day
- Perioperative prophylaxis: 30-40 mg/kg 30-60 minutes prior to surgery followed by 30-40 mg/kg/dose every 6 hours for no more than 24 hours after surgery depending on the procedure

Adolescents and Adults: I.M., I.V.: Perioperative prophylaxis: 1-2 g 30-60 minutes prior to surgery followed by 1-2 g every 6-8 hours for no more than 24 hours after surgery depending on the procedure

Adults: I.M., I.V.: 1-2 g every 6-8 hours (I.M. injection is painful); up to 12 g/day

- Pelvic inflammatory disease:
  - Inpatients: I.V.: 2 g every 6 hours **plus** doxycycline 100 mg I.V. or 100 mg orally every 12 hours until improved, followed by doxycycline 100 mg orally twice daily to complete 14 days
  - Outpatients: I.M.: 2 g **plus** probenecid 1 g orally as a single dose, followed by doxycycline 100 mg orally twice daily for 14 days

Dosing interval in renal impairment:

- Cl_{cr} 30-50 mL/minute: Administer 1-2 g every 8-12 hours
- Cl_{cr} 10-29 mL/minute: Administer 1-2 g every 12-24 hours
- Cl_{cr} 5-9 mL/minute: Administer 0.5-1 g every 12-24 hours
- Cl_{cr} <5 mL/minute: Administer 0.5-1 g every 24-48 hours

Hemodialysis: Moderately dialyzable (20% to 50%); administer a loading dose of 1-2 g after each hemodialysis; maintenance dose as noted above based on Cl_{cr}

Continuous arteriovenous or venovenous hemodiafiltration effects: Dose as for Cl_{cr} 10-50 mL/minute

Mechanism of Action Inhibits bacterial cell wall synthesis by binding to one or more of the penicillin-binding proteins (PBPs) which in turn inhibits the final transpeptidation step of peptidoglycan synthesis in bacterial cell walls, thus inhibiting cell wall biosynthesis. Bacteria eventually lyse due to ongoing activity of cell wall autolytic enzymes (autolysins and murein hydrolases) while cell wall assembly is arrested.

Other Adverse Effects

1% to 10%: Gastrointestinal: Diarrhea

<1%: **Anaphylaxis, dyspnea, fever**, rash, exfoliative dermatitis, toxic epidermal necrolysis, pruritus, angioedema, **nausea, hypotension, vomiting, dyspnea**, pseudomembranous colitis, phlebitis, interstitial nephritis, increased BUN, increased creatinine, leukopenia, thrombocytopenia, hemolytic anemia, bone marrow suppression, eosinophilia, increased transaminases, jaundice, thrombophlebitis, increased nephrotoxicity (with aminoglycosides), exacerbation of myasthenia gravis, **prolonged PT**

Reported with other cephalosporins: **Seizures**, Stevens-Johnson syndrome, toxic epidermal necrolysis, erythema multiforme, urticaria, **serum-sickness reactions,** renal dysfunction, toxic nephropathy, cholestasis, aplastic anemia, hemolytic anemia, **hemorrhage,** pancytopenia, agranulocytosis, colitis, vaginitis, **superinfection**

Drug Interactions Increased Effect/Toxicity: Probenecid may decrease cephalosporin elimination. Furosemide, aminoglycosides in combination with cefoxitin may result in additive nephrotoxicity.

Pharmacodynamics/Kinetics

Distribution: Widely to body tissues and fluids including pleural, synovial, ascitic, bile; poorly penetrates into CSF even with inflammation of the meninges; crosses placenta; small amounts enter breast milk

Protein binding: 65% to 79%

Half-life elimination: 45-60 minutes; significantly prolonged with renal impairment

Time to peak, serum: I.M.: 20-30 minutes

Excretion: Urine (85% as unchanged drug)

Pregnancy Risk Factor B

Generic Available No

Cefoxitin Sodium *see* Cefoxitin *on page 272*

Cefpodoxime (sef pode OKS eem)

U.S. Brand Names Vantin®

Canadian Brand Names Vantin®

(Continued)

Cefpodoxime *(Continued)*

Mexican Brand Names Orelox®

Pharmacologic Category Antibiotic, Cephalosporin (Third Generation)

Synonyms Cefpodoxime Proxetil

Use Treatment of susceptible acute, community-acquired pneumonia caused by *S. pneumoniae* or nonbeta-lactamase producing *H. influenzae*; acute uncomplicated gonorrhea caused by *N. gonorrhoeae*; uncomplicated skin and skin structure infections caused by *S. aureus* or *S. pyogenes*; acute otitis media caused by *S. pneumoniae, H. influenzae*, or *M. catarrhalis*; pharyngitis or tonsillitis; and uncomplicated urinary tract infections caused by *E. coli, Klebsiella*, and *Proteus*

Local Anesthetic/Vasoconstrictor Precautions No information available to require special precautions

Effects on Dental Treatment Headache (1%), nausea (4%)

Dosage Oral:

Children 2 months to 12 years:

Acute otitis media: 10 mg/kg/day divided every 12 hours (400 mg/day) for 5 days (maximum: 200 mg/dose)

Acute maxillary sinusitis: 10 mg/kg/day divided every 12 hours for 10 days (maximum: 200 mg/dose)

Pharyngitis/tonsillitis: 10 mg/kg/day in 2 divided doses for 5-10 days (maximum: 100 mg/dose)

Children ≥12 years and Adults:

Acute community-acquired pneumonia and bacterial exacerbations of chronic bronchitis: 200 mg every 12 hours for 14 days and 10 days, respectively

Acute maxillary sinusitis: 200 mg every 12 hours for 10 days

Skin and skin structure: 400 mg every 12 hours for 7-14 days

Uncomplicated gonorrhea (male and female) and rectal gonococcal infections (female): 200 mg as a single dose

Pharyngitis/tonsillitis: 100 mg every 12 hours for 5-10 days

Uncomplicated urinary tract infection: 100 mg every 12 hours for 7 days

Dosing adjustment in renal impairment: Cl_{cr} <30 mL/minute: Administer every 24 hours

Hemodialysis: Administer dose 3 times/week following hemodialysis

Mechanism of Action Inhibits bacterial cell wall synthesis by binding to one or more of the penicillin-binding proteins (PBPs) which in turn inhibits the final transpeptidation step of peptidoglycan synthesis in bacterial cell walls, thus inhibiting cell wall biosynthesis. Bacteria eventually lyse due to ongoing activity of cell wall autolytic enzymes (autolysins and murein hydrolases) while cell wall assembly is arrested.

Other Adverse Effects

>10%:

Dermatologic: Diaper rash (12%)

Gastrointestinal: Diarrhea (infants/toddlers) (15%)

1% to 10%:

Dermatologic: Rash (1%)

Gastrointestinal: Diarrhea (7%), abdominal pain (2%), vomiting (1% to 2%)

Genitourinary: Vaginal infections (3%)

<1%: **Anaphylaxis, chest pain, hypotension, fungal skin infection**, pseudomembranous colitis, vaginal candidiasis, pruritus, flatulence, **xerostomia, fever, cough, epistaxis, dizziness, anxiety, weakness, flushing, taste alteration,** malaise, decreased appetite, **fatigue,** insomnia, nightmares, eye itching, tinnitus, purpuric nephritis

Reactions reported with other cephalosporins: **Seizures**, Stevens-Johnson syndrome, toxic epidermal necrolysis, erythema multiforme, urticaria, **serum-sickness reactions,** renal dysfunction, interstitial nephritis toxic nephropathy, cholestasis, aplastic anemia, hemolytic anemia, **hemorrhage**, pancytopenia, agranulocytosis, colitis, vaginitis, **superinfection**

Drug Interactions

Increased Effect/Toxicity: Probenecid may decrease cephalosporin elimination. Furosemide, aminoglycosides in combination with cefpodoxime may result in additive nephrotoxicity.

Decreased Effect: Antacids and H_2-receptor antagonists reduce absorption and serum concentration of cefpodoxime.

Dietary/Ethanol/Herb Considerations Food: May be taken with food but delays absorption and may increase serum concentration.

Pharmacodynamics/Kinetics

Absorption: Rapid and well absorbed (50%), acid stable; enhanced in the presence of food or low gastric pH

Distribution: Good tissue penetration, including lung and tonsils; penetrates into pleural fluid

Protein binding: 18% to 23%

Metabolism: De-esterified in GI tract to active metabolite, cefpodoxime

Half-life elimination: 2.2 hours; prolonged with renal impairment

Time to peak: Within 1 hour

Excretion: Urine (80% as unchanged drug) in 24 hours

Pregnancy Risk Factor B

Generic Available No

Cefpodoxime Proxetil *see* Cefpodoxime *on page 273*

Cefprozil (sef PROE zil)

U.S. Brand Names Cefzil®

Canadian Brand Names Cefzil®

Mexican Brand Names Procef®

Pharmacologic Category Antibiotic, Cephalosporin (Second Generation)

Use Treatment of otitis media and infections involving the respiratory tract and skin and skin structure; active against methicillin-sensitive staphylococci, many streptococci, and various gram-negative bacilli including *E. coli*, some *Klebsiella*, *P. mirabilis*, *H. influenzae*, and *Moraxella*.

Local Anesthetic/Vasoconstrictor Precautions No information available to require special precautions

Effects on Dental Treatment 1% to 4%: Dizziness nausea (4%), vomiting, superinfection

Dosage Oral:

Infants and Children >6 months to 12 years: Otitis media: 15 mg/kg every 12 hours for 10 days

Pharyngitis/tonsillitis:

Children 2-12 years: 7.5 -15 mg/kg/day divided every 12 hours for 10 days (administer for >10 days if due to *S. pyogenes*); maximum: 1 g/day

Children >13 years and Adults: 500 mg every 24 hours for 10 days

Uncomplicated skin and skin structure infections:

Children 2-12 years: 20 mg/kg every 24 hours for 10 days; maximum: 1 g/day

Children >13 years and Adults: 250 mg every 12 hours, or 500 mg every 12-24 hours for 10 days

Secondary bacterial infection of acute bronchitis or acute bacterial exacerbation of chronic bronchitis: 500 mg every 12 hours for 10 days

Dosing adjustment in renal impairment: Cl_{cr} <30 mL/minute: Reduce dose by 50%

Hemodialysis: Reduced by hemodialysis; administer dose after the completion of hemodialysis

Mechanism of Action Inhibits bacterial cell wall synthesis by binding to one or more of the penicillin-binding proteins (PBPs) which in turn inhibits the final transpeptidation step of peptidoglycan synthesis in bacterial cell walls, thus inhibiting cell wall biosynthesis. Bacteria eventually lyse due to ongoing activity of cell wall autolytic enzymes (autolysins and murein hydrolases) while cell wall assembly is arrested.

Other Adverse Effects

1% to 10%:

Dermatologic: Diaper rash (2%)

Gastrointestinal: Diarrhea (3%), abdominal pain (1%)

Genitourinary: Vaginitis, genital pruritus (2%)

Hepatic: Increased transaminases (2%)

<1%: **Anaphylaxis**, angioedema, pseudomembranous colitis, rash, urticaria, erythema multiforme, serum sickness, Stevens-Johnson syndrome, **hyperactivity, headache**, insomnia, **confusion, somnolence**, leukopenia, eosinophilia, thrombocytopenia, elevated BUN, elevated creatinine, arthralgia, cholestatic jaundice, **fever**

Reported with other cephalosporins: **Seizures**, toxic epidermal necrolysis, renal dysfunction, interstitial nephritis, toxic nephropathy, aplastic anemia, hemolytic anemia, **hemorrhage,** pancytopenia, agranulocytosis, colitis, vaginitis

Drug Interactions Increased Effect/Toxicity: Probenecid may decrease cephalosporin elimination. Furosemide, aminoglycosides in combination with cefprozil may result in additive nephrotoxicity.

Dietary/Ethanol/Herb Considerations Food: May be taken with food but delays absorption and may decrease serum concentration.

Pharmacodynamics/Kinetics

Absorption: Well absorbed (94%)

Distribution: Low amounts enter breast milk

Protein binding: 35% to 45%

Half-life elimination: Normal renal function: 1.3 hours

Time to peak, serum: Fasting: 1.5 hours

Excretion: Urine (61% as unchanged drug)

Pregnancy Risk Factor B

Generic Available No

Ceftazidime (SEF tay zi deem)

U.S. Brand Names Ceptaz®; Fortaz®; Tazicef®; Tazidime®

Canadian Brand Names Fortaz®; Tazidime®

Mexican Brand Names Ceftazim; Fortum®; Izadima®; Tagal®; Taloken; Taxifur®; Waytrax

(Continued)

Ceftazidime *(Continued)*

Pharmacologic Category Antibiotic, Cephalosporin (Third Generation)

Use Treatment of documented susceptible *Pseudomonas aeruginosa* infection and infections due to other susceptible aerobic gram-negative organisms; empiric therapy of a febrile, granulocytopenic patient

Local Anesthetic/Vasoconstrictor Precautions No information available to require special precautions

Effects on Dental Treatment No significant effects or complications reported

Dosage

Infants and Children 1 month to 12 years: I.V.: 30-50 mg/kg/dose every 8 hours; maximum dose: 6 g/day

Adults: I.M., I.V.: 500 mg to 2 g every 8-12 hours

Urinary tract infections: 250-500 mg every 12 hours

Dosing interval in renal impairment:

Cl_{cr} 30-50 mL/minute: Administer every 12 hours

Cl_{cr} 10-30 mL/minute: Administer every 24 hours

Cl_{cr} <10 mL/minute: Administer every 48-72 hours

Hemodialysis: Dialyzable (50% to 100%)

Continuous arteriovenous or venovenous hemodiafiltration effects: Dose as for Cl_{cr} 30-50 mL/minute

Mechanism of Action Inhibits bacterial cell wall synthesis by binding to one or more of the penicillin-binding proteins (PBPs) which in turn inhibits the final transpeptidation step of peptidoglycan synthesis in bacterial cell walls, thus inhibiting cell wall biosynthesis. Bacteria eventually lyse due to ongoing activity of cell wall autolytic enzymes (autolysins and murein hydrolases) while cell wall assembly is arrested.

Other Adverse Effects

1% to 10%:

Gastrointestinal: Diarrhea (1%)

Local: Pain at injection site (1%)

Miscellaneous: Hypersensitivity reactions (2%)

<1%: **Anaphylaxis**, angioedema, asterixis, increased BUN and creatinine, **candidiasis, dizziness**, encephalopathy, eosinophilia, erythema multiforme, **fever, headache**, hemolytic anemia, hyperbilirubinemia, jaundice, leukopenia, myoclonus, **nausea, neuromuscular excitability, paresthesia**, phlebitis, pruritus, pseudomembranous colitis, rash, Stevens-Johnson syndrome, thrombocytosis, toxic epidermal necrolysis, transaminases increased, vaginitis, **vomiting**

Reported with other cephalosporins: **Seizures**, urticaria, serum-sickness reactions, renal dysfunction, interstitial nephritis, toxic nephropathy, elevated BUN, elevated creatinine, cholestasis, aplastic anemia, hemolytic anemia, pancytopenia, agranulocytosis, colitis, **prolonged PT, hemorrhage, superinfection**

Drug Interactions Increased Effect/Toxicity: Probenecid may decrease cephalosporin elimination. Aminoglycosides: *in vitro* studies indicate additive or synergistic effect against some strains of Enterobacteriaceae and *Pseudomonas aeruginosa*. Furosemide, aminoglycosides in combination with ceftazidime may result in additive nephrotoxicity.

Pharmacodynamics/Kinetics

Distribution: Widely throughout the body including bone, bile, skin, CSF (higher concentrations achieved when meninges are inflamed), endometrium, heart, pleural and lymphatic fluids

Protein binding: 17%

Half-life elimination: 1-2 hours, prolonged with renal impairment; Neonates <23 days: 2.2-4.7 hours

Time to peak, serum: I.M.: ~1 hour

Excretion: Urine (80% to 90% as unchanged drug)

Pregnancy Risk Factor B

Generic Available No

Ceftibuten (sef TYE byoo ten)

Related Information

Oral Bacterial Infections *on page 1531*

U.S. Brand Names Cedax®

Mexican Brand Names Cedax®

Pharmacologic Category Antibiotic, Cephalosporin (Third Generation)

Use Oral cephalosporin for treatment of bronchitis, otitis media, and pharyngitis/tonsillitis due to *H. influenzae* and *M. catarrhalis*, both beta-lactamase-producing and nonproducing strains, as well as *S. pneumoniae* (weak) and *S. pyogenes*

Local Anesthetic/Vasoconstrictor Precautions No information available to require special precautions

Effects on Dental Treatment 1% to 3%: Headache (3%), dizziness, nausea, vomiting

Dosage Oral:

Children <12 years: 9 mg/kg/day for 10 days; maximum daily dose: 400 mg

Children ≥12 years and Adults: 400 mg once daily for 10 days; maximum: 400 mg

Dosing adjustment in renal impairment:

Cl_{cr} 30-49 mL//minute: Administer 4.5 mg/kg or 200 mg every 24 hours

Cl_{cr} <29 mL/minute: Administer 2.25 mg/kg or 100 mg every 24 hours

Mechanism of Action Inhibits bacterial cell wall synthesis by binding to one or more of the penicillin-binding proteins (PBPs) which in turn inhibits the final transpeptidation step of peptidoglycan synthesis in bacterial cell walls, thus inhibiting cell wall biosynthesis. Bacteria eventually lyse due to ongoing activity of cell wall autolytic enzymes (autolysins and murein hydrolases) while cell wall assembly is arrested.

Other Adverse Effects

1% to 10%:

Gastrointestinal: Diarrhea (3%), dyspepsia (2%), abdominal pain (1%)

Hematologic: Increased eosinophils (3%), decreased hemoglobin (2%), thrombocytosis

Hepatic: Increased ALT (1%), increased bilirubin (1%)

Renal: Increased BUN (4%)

<1%: Anorexia, **agitation**, constipation, diaper rash, **dyspnea**, dysuria, **fatigue, candidiasis**, rash, urticaria, **irritability, paresthesia, nasal congestion**, insomnia, **rigors**, increased transaminases, increased creatinine, leukopenia, **xerostomia**

Reported with other cephalosporins: **Anaphylaxis, fever, paresthesia**, pruritus, Stevens-Johnson syndrome, toxic epidermal necrolysis, erythema multiforme, angioedema, pseudomembranous colitis, hemolytic anemia, vaginitis, encephalopathy, asterixis, **neuromuscular excitability, seizures, serum-sickness reactions**, renal dysfunction, interstitial nephritis, toxic nephropathy, cholestasis, aplastic anemia, hemolytic anemia, pancytopenia, agranulocytosis, colitis, **prolonged PT, hemorrhage, superinfection**

Drug Interactions Increased Effect/Toxicity: High-dose probenecid decreases clearance. Aminoglycosides in combination with ceftibuten may increase nephrotoxic potential.

Dietary/Ethanol/Herb Considerations Food: May be taken with food; food decreases peak concentrations, delays T_{max}, and lowers AUC. Administer suspension 1 hour before or 2 hours after meals. Capsules may be taken with food.

Pharmacodynamics/Kinetics

Absorption: Rapid; food decreases peak concentrations, delays T_{max}, and lowers AUC

Distribution: V_d: Children: 0.5 L/kg; Adults: 0.21 L/kg

Half-life elimination: 2 hours

Time to peak: 2-3 hours

Excretion: Urine

Pregnancy Risk Factor B

Generic Available No

Comments In clinical trials, ceftibuten once or twice daily was at least as effective as cefaclor or ciprofloxacin for treatment of acute bacterial exacerbations of bronchitis, as effective as amoxicillin/clavulanic acid or cefaclor for otitis media, as effective as penicillin for pharyngitis, and as effective as trimethoprim-sulfamethoxazole for urinary tract infections

Ceftin® *see* Cefuroxime *on page 279*

Ceftizoxime (sef ti ZOKS eem)

Related Information

Sexually-Transmitted Diseases *on page 1502*

U.S. Brand Names Cefizox®

Canadian Brand Names Cefizox®

Mexican Brand Names Ultracef®

Pharmacologic Category Antibiotic, Cephalosporin (Third Generation)

Synonyms Ceftizoxime Sodium

Use Treatment of susceptible bacterial infection, mainly respiratory tract, skin and skin structure, bone and joint, urinary tract and gynecologic, as well as septicemia; active against many gram-negative bacilli (not *Pseudomonas*), some gram-positive cocci (not *Enterococcus*), and some anaerobes

Local Anesthetic/Vasoconstrictor Precautions No information available to require special precautions

Effects on Dental Treatment 1% to 10%: Fever

Dosage I.M., I.V.:

Children ≥6 months: 150-200 mg/kg/day divided every 6-8 hours (maximum of 12 g/24 hours)

Adults: 1-2 g every 8-12 hours, up to 2 g every 4 hours or 4 g every 8 hours for life-threatening infections

Dosing adjustment in renal impairment: Adults:

Cl_{cr} 10-30 mL/minute: Administer 1 g every 12 hours

Cl_{cr} <10 mL/minute: Administer 1 g every 24 hours

Moderately dialyzable (20% to 50%)

(Continued)

Ceftizoxime *(Continued)*

Continuous arteriovenous or venovenous hemodiafiltration effects: Dose as for Cl_{cr} 10-50 mL/minute

Mechanism of Action Inhibits bacterial cell wall synthesis by binding to one or more of the penicillin-binding proteins (PBPs) which in turn inhibits the final transpeptidation step of peptidoglycan synthesis in bacterial cell walls, thus inhibiting cell wall biosynthesis. Bacteria eventually lyse due to ongoing activity of cell wall autolytic enzymes (autolysins and murein hydrolases) while cell wall assembly is arrested.

Other Adverse Effects

1% to 10%:

- Dermatologic: Rash, pruritus
- Hematologic: Eosinophilia, thrombocytosis
- Hepatic: Elevated transaminases, alkaline phosphatase
- Local: Pain, burning at injection site

<1%: **Anaphylaxis**, diarrhea, **nausea, vomiting**, injection site reactions, phlebitis, **paresthesia, numbness**, increased bilirubin, increased BUN, increased creatinine, anemia, leukopenia, neutropenia, thrombocytopenia, vaginitis

Reported with cephalosporins: Stevens-Johnson syndrome, toxic epidermal necrolysis, erythema multiforme, pseudomembranous colitis, angioedema, hemolytic anemia, **candidiasis,** encephalopathy, asterixis, **neuromuscular excitability, seizures, serum-sickness reactions,** renal dysfunction, interstitial nephritis, toxic nephropathy, cholestasis, aplastic anemia, hemolytic anemia, pancytopenia, agranulocytosis, colitis, **prolonged PT, hemorrhage, superinfection**

Drug Interactions Increased Effect/Toxicity: Probenecid may decrease cephalosporin elimination. Furosemide, aminoglycosides in combination with ceftizoxime may result in additive nephrotoxicity.

Pharmacodynamics/Kinetics

Distribution: V_d: 0.35-0.5 L/kg; widely into most body tissues and fluids including gallbladder, liver, kidneys, bone, sputum, bile, pleural and synovial fluids; has good CSF penetration; crosses placenta; small amounts enter breast milk

Protein binding: 30%

Half-life elimination: 1.6 hours; Cl_{cr} <10 mL/minute: 25 hours

Time to peak, serum: I.M.: 0.5-1 hour

Excretion: Urine (as unchanged drug)

Pregnancy Risk Factor B

Generic Available No

Ceftizoxime Sodium *see* Ceftizoxime *on page 277*

Ceftriaxone (sef trye AKS one)

Related Information

Animal and Human Bites Guidelines *on page 1580*

Nonviral Infectious Diseases *on page 1493*

Sexually-Transmitted Diseases *on page 1502*

U.S. Brand Names Rocephin®

Canadian Brand Names Rocephin®

Mexican Brand Names Benaxona®; Cefaxona®; Ceftrex®; Rocephin®; Tacex®; Terbac®; Triaken®

Pharmacologic Category Antibiotic, Cephalosporin (Third Generation)

Synonyms Ceftriaxone Sodium

Use Treatment of lower respiratory tract infections, skin and skin structure infections, bone and joint infections, intra-abdominal and urinary tract infections, sepsis and meningitis due to susceptible organisms; documented or suspected infection due to susceptible organisms in home care patients and patients without I.V. line access; treatment of documented or suspected gonococcal infection or chancroid; emergency room management of patients at high risk for bacteremia, periorbital or buccal cellulitis, salmonellosis or shigellosis, and pneumonia of unestablished etiology (<5 years of age); treatment of Lyme disease, depends on the stage of the disease (used in Stage II and Stage III, but not stage I; doxycycline is the drug of choice for Stage I)

Local Anesthetic/Vasoconstrictor Precautions No information available to require special precautions

Effects on Dental Treatment No significant effects or complications reported

Dosage I.M., I.V.:

Neonates:

- Postnatal age ≤7 days: 50 mg/kg/day given every 24 hours
- Postnatal age >7 days:
  - ≤2000 g: 50 mg/kg/day given every 24 hours
  - >2000 g: 50-75 mg/kg/day given every 24 hours
- Gonococcal prophylaxis: 25-50 mg/kg as a single dose (dose not to exceed 125 mg)
- Gonococcal infection: 25-50 mg/kg/day (maximum dose: 125 mg) given every 24 hours for 10-14 days

Infants and Children: 50-75 mg/kg/day in 1-2 divided doses every 12-24 hours; maximum: 2 g/24 hours

Meningitis: 100 mg/kg/day divided every 12-24 hours, up to a maximum of 4 g/24 hours; loading dose of 75 mg/kg/dose may be given at start of therapy

Otitis media: I.M.: 50 mg/kg as a single dose (maximum: 1 g)

Uncomplicated gonococcal infections, sexual assault, and STD prophylaxis: I.M.: 125 mg as a single dose plus doxycycline

Complicated gonococcal infections:

Infants: I.M., I.V.: 25-50 mg/kg/day in a single dose (maximum: 125 mg/dose); treat for 7 days for disseminated infection and 7-14 days for documented meningitis

<45 kg: 50 mg/kg/day once daily; maximum: 1 g/day; for ophthalmia, peritonitis, arthritis, or bacteremia: 50-100 mg/kg/day divided every 12-24 hours; maximum: 2 g/day for meningitis or endocarditis

>45 kg: 1 g/day once daily for disseminated gonococcal infections; 1-2 g dose every 12 hours for meningitis or endocarditis

Acute epididymitis: I.M.: 250 mg in a single dose

Adults: 1-2 g every 12-24 hours (depending on the type and severity of infection); maximum dose: 2 g every 12 hours for treatment of meningitis

Uncomplicated gonorrhea: I.M.: 250 mg as a single dose

Surgical prophylaxis: 1 g 30 minutes to 2 hours before surgery

Dosing adjustment in renal or hepatic impairment: No change necessary

Hemodialysis: Not dialyzable (0% to 5%); administer dose postdialysis

Peritoneal dialysis: Administer 750 mg every 12 hours

Continuous arteriovenous or venovenous hemofiltration: Removes 10 mg of ceftriaxone per liter of filtrate per day

Mechanism of Action Inhibits bacterial cell wall synthesis by binding to one or more of the penicillin-binding proteins (PBPs) which in turn inhibits the final transpeptidation step of peptidoglycan synthesis in bacterial cell walls, thus inhibiting cell wall biosynthesis. Bacteria eventually lyse due to ongoing activity of cell wall autolytic enzymes (autolysins and murein hydrolases) while cell wall assembly is arrested.

Other Adverse Effects

1% to 10%:

Dermatologic: Rash (2%)

Gastrointestinal: Diarrhea (3%)

Hematologic: Eosinophilia (6%), thrombocytosis (5%), leukopenia (2%)

Hepatic: Elevated transaminases (3.1% to 3.3%)

Local: Pain, induration at injection site (I.V. 1%); warmth, tightness, induration (5% to 17%) following I.M. injection

Renal: Increased BUN (1%)

<1%: Agranulocytosis, **anaphylaxis**, anemia, basophilia, **bronchospasm, candidiasis,** chills, **diaphoresis, dizziness, dysgeusia, flushing,** gallstones, glycosuria, **headache,** hematuria, hemolytic anemia, jaundice, leukocytosis, lymphocytosis, lymphopenia, monocytosis, **nausea**, neutropenia, phlebitis, **prolonged or decreased PT,** pruritus, renal stones, **serum sickness,** thrombocytopenia, urinary casts, vaginitis, **vomiting**; increased alkaline phosphatase, bilirubin, and creatinine

Postmarketing and/or case reports: Nephrolithiasis, renal precipitations

Reported with other cephalosporins: Angioedema, aplastic anemia, asterixis, cholestasis, colitis, encephalopathy, erythema multiforme, **hemorrhage**, interstitial nephritis, neuromuscular excitability, pancytopenia, **paresthesia**, pseudomembranous colitis, renal dysfunction, **seizures**, Stevens-Johnson syndrome, **superinfection,** toxic epidermal necrolysis, toxic nephropathy

Drug Interactions Increased Effect/Toxicity: Aminoglycosides may result in synergistic antibacterial activity. High-dose probenecid decreases clearance. Aminoglycosides increase nephrotoxic potential.

Pharmacodynamics/Kinetics

Absorption: I.M.: Well absorbed

Distribution: Widely throughout the body including gallbladder, lungs, bone, bile, CSF (higher concentrations achieved when meninges are inflamed); crosses placenta; enters amniotic fluid and breast milk

Protein binding: 85% to 95%

Half-life elimination: Normal renal and hepatic function: 5-9 hours

Neonates: Postnatal: 1-4 days old: 16 hours; 9-30 days old: 9 hours

Time to peak, serum: I.M.: 1-2 hours

Excretion: Urine (33% to 65% as unchanged drug); feces

Pregnancy Risk Factor B

Generic Available No

Ceftriaxone Sodium *see* Ceftriaxone *on page 278*

Cefuroxime (se fyoor OKS eem)

U.S. Brand Names Ceftin®; Kefurox® [DSC]; Zinacef®

Canadian Brand Names Apo®-Cefuroxime; Ceftin®; Kefurox®; Zinacef®

Mexican Brand Names Cefuracet®; Cetoxil®; Froxal®; Zinnat®

(Continued)

Cefuroxime *(Continued)*

Pharmacologic Category Antibiotic, Cephalosporin (Second Generation)

Synonyms Cefuroxime Axetil; Cefuroxime Sodium

Use Treatment of infections caused by staphylococci, group B streptococci, *H. influenzae* (type A and B), *E. coli*, *Enterobacter*, *Salmonella*, and *Klebsiella*; treatment of susceptible infections of the lower respiratory tract, otitis media, urinary tract, skin and soft tissue, bone and joint, sepsis and gonorrhea

Local Anesthetic/Vasoconstrictor Precautions No information available to require special precautions

Effects on Dental Treatment No significant effects or complications reported

Dosage Cefuroxime axetil film-coated tablets and oral suspension are not bioequivalent and are not substitutable on a mg/mg basis.

Children ≥3 months to 12 years:

Pharyngitis, tonsillitis: Oral:

Suspension: 20 mg/kg/day (maximum: 500 mg/day) in 2 divided doses for 10 days

Tablet: 125 mg every 12 hours for 10 days

Acute otitis media, impetigo: Oral:

Suspension: 30 mg/kg/day (maximum: 1 g/day) in 2 divided doses for 10 days

Tablet: 250 mg twice daily for 10 days

I.M., I.V.: 75-150 mg/kg/day divided every 8 hours; maximum dose: 6 g/day

Meningitis: Not recommended (doses of 200-240 mg/kg/day divided every 6-8 hours have been used); maximum dose: 9 g/day

Acute bacterial maxillary sinusitis:

Suspension: 30 mg/kg/day in 2 divided doses for 10 days; maximum dose: 1 g/day

Tablet: 250 mg twice daily for 10 days

Children ≥13 years and Adults:

Oral: 250-500 mg twice daily for 10 days (5 days in selected patients with acute bronchitis)

Uncomplicated urinary tract infection: 125-250 mg every 12 hours for 7-10 days

Uncomplicated gonorrhea: 1 g as a single dose

Early Lyme disease: 500 mg twice daily for 20 days

I.M., I.V.: 750 mg to 1.5 g/dose every 8 hours or 100-150 mg/kg/day in divided doses every 6-8 hours; maximum: 6 g/24 hours

Dosing adjustment in renal impairment:

Cl_{cr} 10-20 mL/minute: Administer every 12 hours

Cl_{cr} <10 mL/minute: Administer every 24 hours

Hemodialysis: Dialyzable (25%)

Continuous arteriovenous or venovenous hemodiafiltration effects: Dose as for Cl_{cr} 10-20 mL/minute

Mechanism of Action Inhibits bacterial cell wall synthesis by binding to one or more of the penicillin-binding proteins (PBPs) which in turn inhibits the final transpeptidation step of peptidoglycan synthesis in bacterial cell walls, thus inhibiting cell wall biosynthesis. Bacteria eventually lyse due to ongoing activity of cell wall autolytic enzymes (autolysins and murein hydrolases) while cell wall assembly is arrested.

Other Adverse Effects

1% to 10%:

Hematologic: Eosinophilia (7%), decreased hemoglobin and hematocrit (10%)

Hepatic: Increased transaminases (4%), increased alkaline phosphatase (2%)

Local: Thrombophlebitis (2%)

<1%: **Anaphylaxis**, angioedema, cholestasis, colitis, diarrhea, **dizziness**, erythema multiforme, **fever, GI bleeding, headache**, hemolytic anemia, increased BUN, increased creatinine, interstitial nephritis, leukopenia, **nausea**, neutropenia, pain at injection site, pancytopenia, **prolonged PT/INR,** pseudomembranous colitis, rash, **seizures,** stomach cramps, thrombocytopenia, toxic epidermal necrolysis, vaginitis, **vomiting**

Reported with other cephalosporins: Agranulocytosis, aplastic anemia, asterixis, encephalopathy, **hemorrhage, neuromuscular excitability, serum-sickness reactions, superinfection**, toxic nephropathy

Drug Interactions Increased Effect/Toxicity: High-dose probenecid decreases clearance. Aminoglycosides in combination with cefuroxime may result in additive nephrotoxicity.

Dietary/Ethanol/Herb Considerations Food: May be taken with food but food increases bioavailability. Dairy products may increase serum concentration. Boiled milk, buttermilk, or yogurt may reduce diarrhea.

Pharmacodynamics/Kinetics

Absorption: Oral (cefuroxime axetil): Increases with food

Distribution: Widely to body tissues and fluids; crosses blood-brain barrier; therapeutic concentrations achieved in CSF even when meninges are not inflamed; crosses placenta; enters breast milk

Protein binding: 33% to 50%

Bioavailability: Tablet: Fasting: 37%; Following food: 52%

Half-life elimination:
- Neonates: ≤3 days old : 5.1-5.8 hours; 6-14 days old: 2-4.2 hours; 3-4 weeks old: 1-1.5 hours
- Adults: 1-2 hours; prolonged with renal impairment

Time to peak, serum: I.M.: ~15-60 minutes; I.V.: 2-3 minutes

Excretion: Urine (66% to 100% as unchanged drug)

Pregnancy Risk Factor B

Generic Available Yes: Tablet, powder for injection

Cefuroxime Axetil *see* Cefuroxime *on page 279*
Cefuroxime Sodium *see* Cefuroxime *on page 279*
Cefzil® *see* Cefprozil *on page 275*
Celebrex® *see* Celecoxib *on page 281*

Celecoxib (ce le COX ib)

Related Information

Rheumatoid Arthritis, Osteoarthritis, and Osteoporosis *on page 1488*

U.S. Brand Names Celebrex®

Canadian Brand Names Celebrex®

Mexican Brand Names Celebrex®

Pharmacologic Category Nonsteroidal Anti-inflammatory Drug (NSAID), COX-2 Selective

Use

Dental: Management of acute pain

Relief of the signs and symptoms of osteoarthritis; relief of the signs and symptoms of rheumatoid arthritis in adults; decreasing intestinal polyps in familial adenomatous polyposis (FAP); management of acute pain; treatment of primary dysmenorrhea

Local Anesthetic/Vasoconstrictor Precautions No information available to require special precautions

Effects on Dental Treatment Nonselective NSAIDs are known to reversibly decrease platelet aggregation via mechanisms different than observed with aspirin. According to the manufacturer, celecoxib, at single doses up to 800 mg and multiple doses of 600 mg twice daily, had no effect on platelet aggregation or bleeding time. Comparative NSAIDs (naproxen 500 mg twice daily, ibuprofen 800 mg three times daily or diclofenac 75 mg twice daily) significantly reduced platelet aggregation and prolonged the bleeding times.

>10%: Headache (16%)

2% to 5%: Dizziness (2%), nausea (4%), upper respiratory tract infection (8%), sinusitis (5%), pharyngitis (2%), rhinitis (2%), accidental injury (3%)

≤2%: Hypertension (aggravated), chest pain, MI, palpitations, tachycardia, facial edema, migraine, fever, anxiety, nervousness, somnolence, hot flashes, diabetes mellitus, hyperglycemia, eructation, esophagitis, gastroenteritis, vomiting, gastroesophageal reflux, hiatal hernia, stomatitis, abnormal taste, xerostomia, tooth disorder, neck stiffness, paresthesia, weakness, bronchitis, bronchospasm, cough, dyspnea, laryngitis, pneumonia, epistaxis, allergic reactions, flu-like syndrome, herpes infection, bacterial infection, moniliasis, viral infection, increased diaphoresis, otitis media, fatigue, pain, leg cramps, blurred vision, bruising, earache

Dosage Adults: Oral:

Acute pain or primary dysmenorrhea: Initial dose: 400 mg, followed by an additional 200 mg if needed on day 1; maintenance dose: 200 mg twice daily as needed

Familial adenomatous polyposis (FAP): 400 mg twice daily

Osteoarthritis: 200 mg/day as a single dose or in divided dose twice daily

Rheumatoid arthritis: 100-200 mg twice daily

Elderly: No specific adjustment is recommended, however, AUC may be increased by 50%, compared to younger subjects. Use the lowest recommended dose in patients weighing <50 kg.

Dosing adjustment in renal impairment: No specific recommendations; not recommended in patients with advanced renal disease

Dosing adjustment in hepatic impairment: AUC may be increased by 40% to 180%; decrease dose by 50% in patients with moderate impairment (Child-Pugh Class II)

Mechanism of Action Inhibits prostaglandin synthesis by decreasing the activity of the enzyme, cyclooxygenase-2 (COX-2), which results in decreased formation of prostaglandin precursors. Celecoxib does not inhibit cyclooxygenase-1 (COX-1) at therapeutic concentrations.

Other Adverse Effects

2% to 10%:
- Cardiovascular: Peripheral edema (2%)
- Central nervous system: Insomnia (2%)
- Dermatologic: Skin rash (2%)
- Gastrointestinal: Dyspepsia (9%), diarrhea (6%), abdominal pain (4%), flatulence (2%)

(Continued)

Celecoxib *(Continued)*

Neuromuscular & skeletal: Back pain (3%)

≤2%:

Central nervous system: Vertigo, hypoesthesia, hypotonia, depression,

Dermatologic: Alopecia, dermatitis, photosensitivity, pruritus, rash (maculopapular), rash (erythematous), dry skin, urticaria

Endocrine & metabolic: Hypercholesterolemia, breast pain, dysmenorrhea, menstrual disturbances, hypokalemia

Gastrointestinal: Constipation, tenesmus, diverticulitis, hemorrhoids, anorexia, increased appetite, weight gain, melena

Genitourinary: Prostate disorder, vaginal bleeding, vaginitis, monilial vaginitis, dysuria, cystitis, urinary frequency, incontinence, urinary tract infection

Hematologic: Anemia, thrombocytopenia

Hepatic: Elevated transaminases, increased alkaline phosphatase

Neuromuscular & skeletal: Increased CPK, arthralgia, myalgia, bone disorder, fracture, synovitis, tendonitis, neuralgia, neuropathy

Ocular: Glaucoma, cataract, conjunctivitis, eye pain

Otic: Deafness, tinnitus

Renal: Increased BUN, increased creatinine, albuminuria, hematuria, renal calculi

Miscellaneous: Breast cancer

<0.1% (Limited to important or life-threatening): **CHF, ventricular fibrillation**, pulmonary embolism, **syncope**, cerebrovascular accident, **gangrene,** thrombophlebitis, thrombocytopenia, ataxia, acute renal failure, intestinal obstruction, pancreatitis, intestinal perforation, **GI bleeding**, colitis, **esophageal perforation, sepsis, sudden death**

Postmarketing and/or case reports: Agranulocytosis, **anaphylactoid reactions**, angioedema, aplastic anemia, aseptic meningitis, erythema multiforme, exfoliative dermatitis, hepatic failure, hepatitis, hypoglycemia, hyponatremia, interstitial nephritis, jaundice, leukopenia, pancytopenia, Stevens-Johnson syndrome, toxic epidermal necrolysis, vasculitis

Contraindications Hypersensitivity to celecoxib, any component of the formulation, sulfonamides, aspirin, or other NSAIDs; pregnancy (3rd trimester)

Warnings/Precautions GI irritation, ulceration, bleeding, and perforation may occur with NSAIDs (it is unclear whether celecoxib is associated with rates of these events which are similar to nonselective NSAIDs). Use with caution in patients with a history of GI disease (bleeding or ulcers), use lowest dose for shortest time possible. Use with caution in patients with decreased renal function, hepatic disease, CHF, hypertension, or asthma. Anaphylactoid reactions may occur, even with no prior exposure to celecoxib. Use caution in patients with known or suspected deficiency of cytochrome P450 isoenzyme 2C9. Safety and efficacy have not been established in patients <18 years of age.

Drug Interactions Substrate of CYP2C8/9, 3A4; Inhibits CYP2D6

ACE inhibitors: Antihypertensive effect may be diminished by celecoxib.

Aspirin: Low-dose aspirin may be used with celecoxib, however, monitor for GI complications.

CYP2C9 inhibitors (ie, amiodarone, fluoxetine, sulfonamides, ritonavir, zafirlukast): Theoretically, may result in significant increases in celecoxib concentrations.

Fluconazole: Fluconazole increases celecoxib concentrations twofold. Lowest dose of celecoxib should be used.

Lithium: Plasma levels of lithium are increased by ~17% when used with celecoxib. Monitor lithium levels closely when treatment with celecoxib is started or withdrawn.

Loop diuretics (bumetanide, furosemide, torsemide): Natriuretic effect of furosemide and other loop diuretics may be decreased by celecoxib.

Methotrexate: Severe bone marrow suppression, aplastic anemia, and GI toxicity have been reported with concomitant NSAID therapy. Selective COX-2 inhibitors appear to have a lower risk of this toxicity, however, caution is warranted.

Thiazide diuretics: Natriuretic effects of thiazide diuretics may be decreased by celecoxib.

Warfarin: Bleeding events and increased prothrombin time have been reported with concomitant use. Monitor closely, especially in the elderly.

Dietary/Ethanol/Herb Considerations

Ethanol: Avoid use due to increased GI irritation.

Food: Administer with food to reduce GI upset; peak concentrations are delayed and AUC is increased by 10% to 20% when taken with a high-fat meal. Larger doses (>200 mg twice daily) should be taken with food to improve absorption.

Pharmacodynamics/Kinetics

Distribution: V_d (apparent): 400 L

Protein binding: 97% to albumin

Metabolism: Hepatic via CYP2C9; forms inactive metabolites

Bioavailability: Absolute: Unknown

Half-life elimination: 11 hours

Time to peak: 3 hours

Excretion: Urine (as metabolites, <3% as unchanged drug)

Pregnancy Risk Factor C/D (3rd trimester)

Breast-feeding Considerations In animal studies, celecoxib has been found to be excreted in milk; it is not known whether celecoxib is excreted in human milk. Because many drugs are excreted in milk, and the potential for serious adverse reactions exists, a decision should be made whether to discontinue nursing or discontinue the drug, taking into account the importance of the drug to the mother.

Dosage Forms CAP: 100 mg, 200 mg, 400 mg

Generic Available No

Comments According to the manufacturer, two out of 5,285 patients (0.04%) experienced significant upper GI bleeding, at 14 and 32 days after initiation of dosing. Approximately 40% of the 5,285 patients were in studies that required them to be free of ulcers by endoscopy at entry into the study. As a result, the manufacturer stressed that it is unclear if the study population is representative of the general population. As of this printing, long-term studies comparing the incidence of serious upper GI adverse effects in patients taking celecoxib compared to other nonselective NSAIDs had not been reported. Celecoxib does not appear to inhibit platelet aggregation at recommended doses. Reports have shown that celecoxib does not generally affect platelet counts, prothrombin time or partial thromboplastin time (PTT).

Cross-reactivity, including bronchospasm, between aspirin and other NSAIDs has been reported in aspirin-sensitive patients. The manufacturer suggests that celecoxib should not be administered to patients with this type of aspirin sensitivity and should be used with caution in patients with pre-existing asthma.

The manufacturer studied the effect of celecoxib on the anticoagulant effect of warfarin and found no alteration of anticoagulant effect, as determined by prothrombin time, in patients taking 2 mg to 5 mg daily. However, the manufacturer has issued a caution when using celecoxib with warfarin since those patients are at increased risk of bleeding complications.

A literature report suggested that the enzyme COX-2 (cyclo-oxygenase type 2) is a major source of systemic prostacyclin biosynthesis in humans. Prostacyclin is involved in blood vessel dilation and inhibition of blood clotting. In view of the fact that celecoxib inhibits the COX-2 enzyme, prostacyclin production could be suppressed. The resultant effects on hemostasis are unknown at this time.

Recent news reports have noted an association between selective COX-2 inhibitors and increased cardiovascular risk. This was prompted by publication of a meta-analysis entitled "Risk of Cardiovascular Events Associated With Selective COX-2 Inhibitors" in the August 22, 2001, edition of the *Journal of the American Medical Association* (JAMA), viewable at http://jama.ama-assn.org/issues/v286n8/rfull/jsc10193.html. The researchers reanalyzed four previously published trials, assessing cardiovascular events in patients receiving either celecoxib or rofecoxib. They found an association between the use of COX-2 inhibitors and cardiovascular events (including MI and ischemic stroke). The annualized MI rate was found to be significantly higher in patients receiving celecoxib or rofecoxib than in the control (placebo) group from a recent meta-analysis of primary prevention trials. Although cause and effect cannot be established (these trials were originally designed to assess GI effects, not cardiovascular ones), the authors believe the available data raise a cautionary flag concerning the risk of cardiovascular events with the use of COX-2 inhibitors. The manufacturers of these agents, as well as other healthcare professionals, dispute the methods and validity of the study's conclusions. To date, the FDA has not required any change in the labeling of these agents. Further study is required before any potential risk may be defined.

Selected Readings

Everts B, Wahrborg P, Hedner T, "COX-2 Specific Inhibitors - The Emergence of a New Class of Analgesic and Anti-inflammatory Drugs," *Clin Rheumatol*, 2000, 19(5):331-43.

Jouzeau JY, Terlain B, Abid A, et al, "Cyclo-oxygenase Isoenzymes. How Recent Findings Affect Thinking About Nonsteroidal Anti-inflammatory Drugs," *Drugs*, 1997, 53(4):563-82.

Kaplan-Machlis B and Klostermeyer BS, "The Cyclo-oxygenase-2 Inhibitors: Safety and Effectiveness," *Ann Pharmacother*, 1999, 33(9):979-88.

Kurumbail RG, Stevens AM, Gierse JK, et al, "Structural Basis for Selective Inhibition of Cyclo-oxygenase-2 By Anti-inflammatory Agents," *Nature*, 1996, 384(6610):644-8.

Malmstrom K, Daniels S, Kotey P, et al, "Comparison of Rofecoxib and Celecoxib, two Cyclooxygenase-2 Inhibitors, in Postoperative Dental Pain: A Randomized Placebo- and Active-Comparator-Controlled Clinical Trial," *Clin Ther*, 1999, 21(10):1653-63.

McAdam BF, Catella-Lawson F, Mardini IA, et al, "Systemic Biosynthesis of Prostacyclin by Cyclo-oxygenase (COX)-2: The Human Pharmacology of a Selective Inhibitor of COX-2," *Proc Natl Acad Sci U S A*, 1999, 96(1):272-7.

Moore PA and Hersh EV, "Celecoxib and Rofecoxib. The Role of COX-2 Inhibitors in Dental Practice," *J Am Dent Assoc*, 2001, 132(4):451-6.

Needleman P and Isakson PC, "The Discovery and Function of COX-2," *J Rheumatol*, 1997, 24(S49):6-8.

Whelton A, Maurath CJ, Verburg KM, et al, "Renal Safety and Tolerability of Celecoxib, a Novel Cyclo-oxygenase-2 Inhibitor," *Am J Ther*, 2000, 7(3):159-75.

Wynn RL, "The New COX-2 Inhibitors: Celecoxib and Rofecoxib," *Home Health Care Consultant*, 2001, 8(10):24-31.

Wynn RL, "The New COX-2 Inhibitors: Rofecoxib (Vioxx®) and Celecoxib (Celebrex™)," *Gen Dent*, 2000, 48(1):16-20.

Wynn RL, "NSAIDS and Cardiovascular Effects, Celecoxib for Dental Pain, and a New Analgesic - Tramadol with Acetaminophen," *Gen Dent*, 2002, 50(3):218-222.

Celestone® *see* Betamethasone *on page 177*

Celestone® Phosphate *see* Betamethasone *on page 177*
Celestone® Soluspan® *see* Betamethasone *on page 177*
Celexa™ *see* Citalopram *on page 334*
CellCept® *see* Mycophenolate *on page 939*
Cellufresh® [OTC] *see* Carboxymethylcellulose *on page 251*

Cellulose (Oxidized) (SEL yoo lose, OKS i dyzed)

Related Information
Cellulose (Oxidized/Regenerated) *on page 284*

U.S. Brand Names Oxycel®; Surgicel®

Pharmacologic Category Hemostatic Agent

Synonyms Absorbable Cotton

Use Dental and Medical: Temporary packing for the control of capillary, venous, or small arterial hemorrhage

Local Anesthetic/Vasoconstrictor Precautions No information available to require special precautions

Effects on Dental Treatment 1% to 10%: Headache, encapsulation of fluid, foreign body reactions (with or without) infection

Dosage Minimal amounts of an appropriate size are laid on the bleeding site.

Other Adverse Effects 1% to 10%: Respiratory: Nasal burning or stinging, sneezing (rhinological procedures)

Contraindications Do not apply as packing or wadding as a hemostatic agents; do not use for packing or implantation in fractures or laminectomies; do not use to control hemorrhage from large arteries or on nonhemorrhagic serous oozing surfaces

Warnings/Precautions By swelling, oxidized cellulose may cause nerve damage by pressure in bony confine (ie, optic nerve and chiasm); always remove from these sites of application or do not use at all (see Contraindications); do not autoclave, do not moisten with water or saline (lessens hemostatic effect). Avoid wadding or packing tightly; do not use after application of $AgNO_3$ or other escharotic agents.

Pregnancy Risk Factor No data reported

Dosage Forms PAD (Oxycel®): 3" x 3" (8 ply). **PLEDGET** (Oxycel®): 2" x 1" x 1". **STRIP:** (Oxycel®): 5" x 1/2" (4 ply), 18" x 2" (4 ply), 36" x 1/2" (4 ply); (Surgicel®): 1/2" x 2", 2" x 3", 2" x 14", 4" x 8"

Generic Available No

Cellulose (Oxidized/Regenerated)

(SEL yoo lose, OKS i dyzed re JEN er aye ted)

Related Information
Cellulose (Oxidized) *on page 284*

U.S. Brand Names Surgicel® Absorbable Hemostat

Pharmacologic Category Hemostatic Agent

Use
Dental: To control bleeding created during a dental procedure
Medical: Hemostatic agent

Local Anesthetic/Vasoconstrictor Precautions No information available to require special precautions

Effects on Dental Treatment No significant effects or complications reported

Dosage Minimal amounts of the fabric strip are laid on the bleeding site or held firmly against the tissues until hemostasis occurs.

Mechanism of Action Cellulose, oxidized regenerated is saturated with blood at the bleeding site and swells into a brownish or black gelatinous mass which aids in the formation of a clot. When used in small amounts, it is absorbed from the sites of implantation with little or no tissue reaction.

Contraindications Not to be used as packing or wadding unless it is removed after hemostasis occurs; not to be used for implantation in bone defects

Warnings/Precautions Autoclaving causes physical breakdown of the product. Closing the material in a contaminated wound without drainage may lead to complications. The material should not be moistened before insertion since the hemostatic effect is greater when applied dry. The material should not be impregnated with anti-infective agents. Its hemostatic effect is not enhanced by the addition of thrombin. The material may be left *in situ* when necessary but it is advisable to remove it once hemostasis is achieved.

Dosage Forms STRIP, knitted fabric: 1/2" x 2" envelopes

Generic Available No

Comments Oxidized regenerated cellulose is prepared by the controlled oxidation of regenerated cellulose. The fabric is white with a pale yellow cast and has a faint, caramel-like aroma. A slight discoloration may occur with age but this does not effect its hemostatic actions.

Cellulose Sodium Phosphate (sel yoo lose SOW dee um FOS fate)

U.S. Brand Names Calcibind®

Canadian Brand Names Calcibind®

Pharmacologic Category Urinary Tract Product

Synonyms CSP; Sodium Cellulose Phosphate

Use Adjunct to dietary restriction to reduce renal calculi formation in absorptive hypercalciuria type I

Local Anesthetic/Vasoconstrictor Precautions No information available to require special precautions

Effects on Dental Treatment No significant effects or complications reported

Dosage Adults: Oral: 5 g 3 times/day with meals; decrease dose to 5 g with main meal and 2.5 g with each of two other meals when urinary calcium declines to <150 mg/day

Pregnancy Risk Factor C

Generic Available No

Celluvisc® [OTC] *see* Carboxymethylcellulose *on page 251*

Celontin® *see* Methsuximide *on page 889*

Cenestin® *see* Estrogens (Conjugated A/Synthetic) *on page 528*

Centrum® [OTC] *see* Vitamins (Multiple/Oral) *on page 1394*

Centrum® Performance™ [OTC] *see* Vitamins (Multiple/Oral) *on page 1394*

Centrum® Silver® [OTC] *see* Vitamins (Multiple/Oral) *on page 1394*

Cēpacol® Anesthetic Troches [OTC] *see* Cetylpyridinium and Benzocaine *on page 292*

Cēpacol® Mouthwash/Gargle [OTC] *see* Cetylpyridinium *on page 292*

Cēpacol Viractin® [OTC] *see* Tetracaine *on page 1284*

Cēpastat® [OTC] *see* Phenol *on page 1068*

Cēpastat® Extra Strength [OTC] *see* Phenol *on page 1068*

Cephalexin (sef a LEKS in)

Related Information

Antibiotic Prophylaxis, Preprocedural Guidelines for Dental Patients *on page 1507*

Oral Bacterial Infections *on page 1531*

U.S. Brand Names Biocef; Keflex®; Keftab®

Canadian Brand Names Apo®-Cephalex; Keftab®; Novo-Lexin®; Nu-Cephalex®

Mexican Brand Names Ceporex; Naxifelar

Pharmacologic Category Antibiotic, Cephalosporin (First Generation)

Synonyms Cephalexin Hydrochloride; Cephalexin Monohydrate

Use

Dental: Prophylaxis in total joint replacement patients undergoing dental procedures which produce bacteremia; alternative antibiotic for prevention of bacterial endocarditis

Note: Individuals allergic to amoxicillin (penicillins) may receive cefadroxil provided they have not had an immediate, local, or systemic IgE-mediated anaphylactic allergic reaction to penicillin.

Medical: Treatment of susceptible bacterial infections, including those caused by group A beta-hemolytic *Streptococcus*, *Staphylococcus*, *Klebsiella pneumoniae*, *E. coli*, *Proteus mirabilis*, and *Shigella*; predominantly used for lower respiratory tract, urinary tract, skin and soft tissue, and bone and joint; prophylaxis against bacterial endocarditis in high-risk patients undergoing surgical procedures who are allergic to penicillin

Local Anesthetic/Vasoconstrictor Precautions No information available to require special precautions

Effects on Dental Treatment No significant effects or complications reported

Dosage Oral:

Children: 25-50 mg/kg/day every 6 hours; severe infections: 50-100 mg/kg/day in divided doses every 6 hours; maximum: 3 g/24 hours

Adults: 250-1000 mg every 6 hours; maximum: 4 g/day

Prophylaxis of bacterial endocarditis (dental, oral, respiratory tract, or esophageal procedures):

Children: 50 mg/kg 1 hour prior to procedure

Adults: 2 g 1 hour prior to procedure

Dosing adjustment in renal impairment: Adults:

Cl_{cr} 10-40 mL/minute: 250-500 mg every 8-12 hours

Cl_{cr} <10 mL/minute: 250 mg every 12-24 hours

Hemodialysis: Moderately dialyzable (20% to 50%)

Mechanism of Action Inhibits bacterial cell wall synthesis by binding to one or more of the penicillin-binding proteins (PBPs) which in turn inhibits the final transpeptidation step of peptidoglycan synthesis in bacterial cell walls, thus inhibiting cell wall biosynthesis. Bacteria eventually lyse due to ongoing activity of cell wall autolytic enzymes (autolysins and murein hydrolases) while cell wall assembly is arrested.

Other Adverse Effects

1% to 10%: Gastrointestinal: Diarrhea

<1%: **Dizziness, fatigue, headache**, rash, urticaria, angioedema, **anaphylaxis**, erythema multiforme, toxic epidermal necrolysis, Stevens-Johnson syndrome,

(Continued)

Cephalexin *(Continued)*

serum-sickness reaction, nausea, vomiting, dyspepsia, **gastritis**, abdominal pain, **pseudomembranous colitis,** interstitial nephritis, **agitation, hallucinations, confusion**, arthralgia, eosinophilia, neutropenia, thrombocytopenia, anemia, increased transaminases, hepatitis, cholestasis

Reported with other cephalosporins: **Vomiting,** agranulocytosis, colitis, pancytopenia, aplastic anemia, hemolytic anemia, **hemorrhage, prolonged PT,** encephalopathy, asterixis, **neuromuscular excitability, seizures, superinfection**

Contraindications Hypersensitivity to cephalexin, any component of the formulation, or other cephalosporins

Warnings/Precautions Modify dosage in patients with severe renal impairment, prolonged use may result in superinfection; use with caution in patients with a history of penicillin allergy, especially IgE-mediated reactions (eg, anaphylaxis, urticaria); may cause antibiotic-associated colitis or colitis secondary to *C. difficile*

Drug Interactions

Increased Effect: High-dose probenecid decreases clearance

Increased Toxicity: Aminoglycosides increase nephrotoxic potential

Dietary/Ethanol/Herb Considerations Food: Administer with food to reduce GI upset; food may decrease serum concentration. Administer 1 hour before or 2 hours after meals to increase total absorption.

Pharmacodynamics/Kinetics

Absorption: Delayed in young children; may be decreased up to 50% in neonates

Distribution: Widely into most body tissues and fluids, including gallbladder, liver, kidneys, bone, sputum, bile, and pleural and synovial fluids; CSF penetration is poor; crosses placenta; enters breast milk

Protein binding: 6% to 15%

Half-life elimination: Neonates: 5 hours old; Children 3-12 months: 2.5 hours; Adults: 0.5-1.2 hours; prolonged with renal impairment

Time to peak, serum: ~1 hour

Excretion: Urine (80% to 100% as unchanged drug) within 8 hours

Pregnancy Risk Factor B

Breast-feeding Considerations Theoretically, drug absorbed by nursing infant may change bowel flora or affect fever work-up result. **Note:** As a class, cephalosporins are used to treat infections in infants.

Dosage Forms CAP, as monohydrate: 250 mg, 500 mg. **POWDER, oral suspension, as monohydrate:** 125 mg/5 mL (5 mL unit dose, 60 mL, 100 mL, 200 mL); 250 mg/5 mL (5 mL unit dose, 100 mL, 200 mL). **TAB, as hydrochloride:** 500 mg. **TAB, as monohydrate:** 250 mg, 500 mg, 1 g.

Generic Available Yes

Comments Cephalexin is effective against anaerobic bacteria, but the sensitivity of alpha-hemolytic *Streptococcus* vary; approximately 10% of strains are resistant. Nearly 70% are intermediately sensitive. Patients allergic to penicillins can use a cephalosporin; the incidence of cross-reactivity between penicillins and cephalosporins is 1% when the allergic reaction to penicillin is delayed. If the patient has a history of immediate reaction to penicillin, the incidence of cross-reactivity is 20%; cephalosporins are contraindicated in these patients.

Selected Readings

"Advisory Statement. Antibiotic Prophylaxis for Dental Patients With Total Joint Replacements. American Dental Association; American Academy of Orthopedic Surgeons," *J Am Dent Assoc*, 1997, 128(7):1004-8.

Dajani AS, Taubert KA, Wilson W, et al, "Prevention of Bacterial Endocarditis. Recommendations by the American Heart Association," *JAMA* 1997, 277(22):1794-801.

Dajani AS, Taubert KA, Wilson W, et al, "Prevention of Bacterial Endocarditis: Recommendations by the American Heart Association," *J Am Dent Assoc* 1997, 128(8):1142-51.

Saxon A, Beall GN, Rohr AS, et al, "Immediate Hypersensitivity Reactions to Beta-Lactam Antibiotics," *Ann Intern Med*, 1987, 107(2):204-15.

Wynn RL, Bergman SA, Meiller TF, et al, "Antibiotics in Treating Oral-Facial Infections of Odontogenic Origin: An Update", *Gen Dent*, 2001, 49(3):238-40, 242, 244 passim.

Cephalexin Hydrochloride *see* Cephalexin *on page 285*

Cephalexin Monohydrate *see* Cephalexin *on page 285*

Cephalothin (sef A loe thin)

Pharmacologic Category Antibiotic, Cephalosporin (First Generation)

Synonyms Cephalothin Sodium

Use Treatment of infections when caused by susceptible strains in respiratory, genitourinary, GI, skin and soft tissue, bone and joint infections; septicemia; treatment of susceptible gram-positive bacilli and cocci (never enterococcus); some gram-negative bacilli including *E. coli, Proteus,* and *Klebsiella* may be susceptible

Local Anesthetic/Vasoconstrictor Precautions No information available to require special precautions

Effects on Dental Treatment 1% to 10%: Nausea, vomiting

Dosage I.M., I.V.:

Neonates:

Postnatal age <7 days:

<2000 g: 20 mg every 12 hours

>2000 g: 20 mg every 8 hours
Postnatal age >7 days:
<2000 g: 20 mg every 8 hours
>2000 g: 20 mg every 6 hours
Children: 75-125 mg/kg/day divided every 4-6 hours; maximum dose: 10 g in a 24-hour period
Adults: 500 mg to 2 g every 4-6 hours
Dosing interval in renal impairment:
Cl_{cr} 10-50 mL/minute: Administer every 6-8 hours
Cl_{cr} <10 mL/minute: Administer every 12 hours
Continuous arteriovenous or venovenous hemodiafiltration effects: Administer 1 g every 8 hours

Mechanism of Action Inhibits bacterial cell wall synthesis by binding to one or more of the penicillin-binding proteins (PBPs) which in turn inhibits the final transpeptidation step of peptidoglycan synthesis in bacterial cell walls, thus inhibiting cell wall biosynthesis. Bacteria eventually lyse due to ongoing activity of cell wall autolytic enzymes (autolysins and murein hydrolases) while cell wall assembly is arrested.

Other Adverse Effects
1% to 10%: Gastrointestinal: Diarrhea
<1%: Maculopapular and erythematous rash, dyspepsia, pseudomembranous colitis; bleeding, pain, and induration at injection site
Reported with other cephalosporins: **Anaphylaxis**, erythema multiforme, toxic epidermal necrolysis, Stevens-Johnson syndrome, **dizziness, fever, headache, CNS irritability, seizures**, decreased hemoglobin, neutropenia, leukopenia, agranulocytosis, pancytopenia, aplastic anemia, hemolytic anemia, interstitial nephritis, toxic nephropathy, vaginitis, angioedema, cholestasis, **hemorrhage, prolonged PT, serum-sickness reactions, superinfection**

Pharmacodynamics/Kinetics
Distribution: Does not penetrate CSF unless meninges are inflamed; crosses placenta; small amounts enter breast milk
Protein binding: 65% to 80%
Metabolism: Partially hepatic and renal via deacetylation
Half-life elimination: 30-60 minutes
Time to peak, serum: I.M.: ~30 minutes
Excretion: Urine (50% to 75% as unchanged drug)

Pregnancy Risk Factor B

Generic Available Yes

Cephalothin Sodium *see* Cephalothin *on page 286*

Cephapirin (sef a PYE rin)

U.S. Brand Names Cefadyl®

Canadian Brand Names Cefadyl®

Pharmacologic Category Antibiotic, Cephalosporin (First Generation)

Synonyms Cephapirin Sodium

Use Treatment of infections when caused by susceptible strains in respiratory, genitourinary, GI, skin and soft tissue, bone and joint infections, septicemia; treatment of susceptible gram-positive bacilli and cocci (never enterococcus); some gram-negative bacilli including *E. coli*, *Proteus*, and *Klebsiella* may be susceptible

Local Anesthetic/Vasoconstrictor Precautions No information available to require special precautions

Effects on Dental Treatment No significant effects or complications reported

Dosage I.M., I.V.:
Children: 10-20 mg/kg/dose every 6 hours up to 4 g/24 hours
Adults: 500 mg to 1 g every 6 hours up to 12 g/day
Perioperative prophylaxis: 1-2 g 30 minutes to 1 hour prior to surgery and every 6 hours as needed for 24 hours following
Dosing interval in renal impairment:
Cl_{cr} 10-50 mL/minute: Administer every 6-8 hours
Cl_{cr} <10 mL/minute: Administer every 12 hours
Continuous arteriovenous or venovenous hemodiafiltration effects: Administer 1 g every 8 hours

Mechanism of Action Inhibits bacterial cell wall synthesis by binding to one or more of the penicillin-binding proteins (PBPs) which in turn inhibits the final transpeptidation step of peptidoglycan synthesis in bacterial cell walls, thus inhibiting cell wall biosynthesis. Bacteria eventually lyse due to ongoing activity of cell wall autolytic enzymes (autolysins and murein hydrolases) while cell wall assembly is arrested.

Other Adverse Effects
1% to 10%: Gastrointestinal: Diarrhea
<1%: **CNS irritation, seizures, fever,** rash, urticaria, leukopenia, thrombocytopenia, increased transaminases
Reported with other cephalosporins: **Anaphylaxis**, erythema multiforme, toxic epidermal necrolysis, Stevens-Johnson syndrome, **dizziness, fever, headache**,

(Continued)

Cephapirin *(Continued)*

encephalopathy, asterixis, **neuromuscular excitability, seizures, nausea, vomiting**, pseudomembranous colitis, decreased hemoglobin, agranulocytosis, pancytopenia, aplastic anemia, hemolytic anemia, interstitial nephritis, toxic nephropathy, pain at injection site, vaginitis, angioedema, cholestasis, **hemorrhage, prolonged PT, serum-sickness reactions, superinfection**

Drug Interactions Increased Effect/Toxicity: High-dose probenecid decreases clearance of cephapirin. Aminoglycosides in combination with cephapirin may result in additive nephrotoxicity.

Pharmacodynamics/Kinetics

Distribution: Widely into most body tissues and fluids including gallbladder, liver, kidneys, bone, sputum, bile, and pleural and synovial fluids; CSF penetration is poor; crosses placenta; small amounts enter breast milk

Protein binding: 22% to 25%

Metabolism: Partially hepatic, renal, and in plasma to metabolites (50% active)

Half-life elimination: 36-60 minutes

Time to peak, serum: I.M.: ~30 minutes; I.V.: ~5 minutes

Excretion: Urine (60% to 85% as unchanged drug)

Pregnancy Risk Factor B

Generic Available No

Cephapirin Sodium *see* Cephapirin *on page 287*

Cephradine (SEF ra deen)

Related Information

Antibiotic Prophylaxis, Preprocedural Guidelines for Dental Patients *on page 1507*

U.S. Brand Names Velosef®

Mexican Brand Names Veracef

Pharmacologic Category Antibiotic, Cephalosporin (First Generation)

Use

Dental: Prophylaxis in total joint replacement patients undergoing dental procedures which produce bacteremia

Medical: Treatment of infections when caused by susceptible strains in respiratory, genitourinary, GI, skin and soft tissue, bone and joint infections; treatment of susceptible gram-positive bacilli and cocci (never enterococcus); some gram-negative bacilli including *E. coli*, *Proteus*, and *Klebsiella* may be susceptible

Local Anesthetic/Vasoconstrictor Precautions No information available to require special precautions

Effects on Dental Treatment No significant effects or complications reported

Dosage Oral:

Children ≥9 months: 25-50 mg/kg/day in divided doses every 6 hours

Adults: 250-500 mg every 6-12 hours

Prophylaxis: 2 g taken 1 hour prior to dental procedure

Dosing adjustment in renal impairment: Adults:

Cl_{cr} 10-50 mL/minute: 250 mg every 6 hours

Cl_{cr} <10 mL/minute: 125 mg every 6 hours

Mechanism of Action Inhibits bacterial cell wall synthesis by binding to one or more of the penicillin-binding proteins (PBPs) which in turn inhibits the final transpeptidation step of peptidoglycan synthesis in bacterial cell walls, thus inhibiting cell wall biosynthesis. Bacteria eventually lyse due to ongoing activity of cell wall autolytic enzymes (autolysins and murein hydrolases) while cell wall assembly is arrested.

Other Adverse Effects

1% to 10%: Gastrointestinal: Diarrhea

<1%: Rash, **nausea, vomiting, pseudomembranous colitis,** increased BUN, increased creatinine

Reported with other cephalosporins: **Anaphylaxis**, erythema multiforme, toxic epidermal necrolysis, Stevens-Johnson syndrome, **dizziness, fever, headache**, encephalopathy, asterixis, **neuromuscular excitability, seizures**, neutropenia, leukopenia, agranulocytosis, pancytopenia, aplastic anemia, hemolytic anemia, interstitial nephritis, toxic nephropathy, vaginitis, angioedema, cholestasis, **hemorrhage, prolonged PT, serum-sickness reactions, superinfection**

Contraindications Hypersensitivity to cephradine, any component of the formulation, or cephalosporins

Warnings/Precautions Modify dosage in patients with severe renal impairment, prolonged use may result in superinfection; use with caution in patients with a history of penicillin allergy, especially IgE-mediated reactions (eg, anaphylaxis, urticaria); may cause antibiotic-associated colitis or colitis secondary to *C. difficile*

Drug Interactions

Increased Effect: High-dose probenecid decreases clearance

Increased Toxicity: Aminoglycosides may increase nephrotoxic potential

Dietary/Ethanol/Herb Considerations Food: Administer with food to reduce GI upset; absorption is delayed but absorption unaffected; Boiled milk, buttermilk, or yogurt may reduce diarrhea.

Pharmacodynamics/Kinetics

Absorption: Well absorbed

Distribution: Widely into most body tissues and fluids including gallbladder, liver, kidneys, bone, sputum, bile, and pleural and synovial fluids; CSF penetration is poor; crosses placenta; enters breast milk

Protein binding: 18% to 20%

Half-life elimination: 1-2 hours; prolonged with renal impairment

Time to peak, serum: 1-2 hours

Excretion: Urine (~80% to 90% as unchanged drug) within 6 hours

Pregnancy Risk Factor B

Breast-feeding Considerations Theoretically, drug absorbed by nursing infant may change bowel flora or affect fever work-up result. **Note:** As a class, cephalosporins are used to treat infections in infants.

Dosage Forms CAP: 250 mg, 500 mg. **POWDER, oral suspension:** 125 mg/5 mL (5 mL, 100 mL, 200 mL); 250 mg/5 mL (5 mL, 100 mL, 200 mL)

Generic Available Yes

Selected Readings

"Advisory Statement. Antibiotic Prophylaxis for Dental Patients With Total Joint Replacements. American Dental Association; American Academy of Orthopedic Surgeons," *J Am Dent Assoc*, 1997, 128(7):1004-8.

Donowitz GR and Mandell GL, "Drug Therapy. Beta-Lactam Antibiotics (1)," *N Engl J Med*, 1988, 318(7):419-26.

Donowitz GR and Mandell GL, "Drug Therapy. Beta-Lactam Antibiotics (2)," *N Engl J Med*, 1988, 318(8):490-500.

Gustaferro CA and Steckelberg JM, "Cephalosporin Antimicrobial Agents and Related Compounds," *Mayo Clin Proc*, 1991, 66(10):1064-73.

Ceptaz® *see* Ceftazidime *on page 275*

Cerebyx® *see* Fosphenytoin *on page 618*

Ceredase® *see* Alglucerase *on page 56*

Cerezyme® *see* Imiglucerase *on page 709*

Cerose-DM® [OTC] *see* Chlorpheniramine, Phenylephrine, and Dextromethorphan *on page 309*

Cerubidine® *see* DAUNOrubicin Hydrochloride *on page 402*

Cerumenex® *see* Triethanolamine Polypeptide Oleate-Condensate *on page 1348*

Cervidil® *see* Dinoprostone *on page 450*

C.E.S. *see* Estrogens (Conjugated/Equine) *on page 529*

Cetacaine® *see* Benzocaine, Butyl Aminobenzoate, Tetracaine, and Benzalkonium Chloride *on page 170*

Cetacort® *see* Hydrocortisone *on page 688*

Cetafen® [OTC] *see* Acetaminophen *on page 27*

Cetafen Extra® [OTC] *see* Acetaminophen *on page 27*

Ceta-Plus® *see* Hydrocodone and Acetaminophen *on page 678*

Cetirizine (se TI ra zeen)

U.S. Brand Names Zyrtec®

Canadian Brand Names Apo®-Cetirizine; Reactine™

Mexican Brand Names Virlix®; Zyrtec®

Pharmacologic Category Antihistamine

Synonyms Cetirizine Hydrochloride; P-071; UCB-P071

Use Perennial and seasonal allergic rhinitis and other allergic symptoms including urticaria; chronic idiopathic urticaria

Local Anesthetic/Vasoconstrictor Precautions No information available to require special precautions

Effects on Dental Treatment

>10%: Headache (11% to 14% children; 12% placebo), somnolence (14% adults; 2% to 4% children)

2% to 10%: Dizziness (2%; adults), nausea (2% to 3% children; 2% placebo), vomiting (2% to 3%; children), epistaxis (2% to 4% children; 3% placebo), pharyngitis (3% to 6% children; 3% placebo), bronchospasm (2% to 3% children; 2% placebo), xerostomia (5%), fatigue (6%; adults), malaise (4%)

<2% (as reported in adults and/or children): Facial edema, flushing, orofacial dyskinesia, hyperventillation, respiratory disorder, rhinitis, increased salivation, sinusitis, sputum increased, stomatitis, sweating, syncope, tachycardia, loss of taste, abnormal taste, tongue discoloration and edema, twitching, ulcerative stomatitis, upper respiratory tract infection, amnesia, anaphylaxis, anxiety, bronchitis, cardiac failure, chest pain, confusion, dehydration, diabetes mellitus, dyspnea, eructation, fever, fussiness, gastritis, hot flashes, hypertension, hypotension, irritability, melena, migraine, nervousness, paralysis, paresthesia, pneumonia, rigors, abnormal thinking, tremor, weakness, visual field defect, pain

Dosage Oral:

Children:

6-12 months: Chronic urticaria, perennial allergic rhinitis: 2.5 mg once daily

12 months to <2 years: Chronic urticaria, perennial allergic rhinitis: 2.5 mg once daily; may increase to 2.5 mg every 12 hours if needed

(Continued)

Cetirizine *(Continued)*

2-5 years: Chronic urticaria, perennial or seasonal allergic rhinitis: Initial: 2.5 mg once daily; may be increased to 2.5 mg every 12 hours **or** 5 mg once daily

Children ≥6 years and Adults: Chronic urticaria, perennial or seasonal allergic rhinitis: 5-10 mg once daily, depending upon symptom severity

Elderly: Initial: 5 mg once daily; may increase to 10 mg/day; adjust for renal impairment

Dosing adjustment in renal/hepatic impairment:

Children <6 years: Use not recommended

Children 6-11 years: <2.5 mg once daily

Children ≥12 and Adults:

Cl_{cr} 11-31 mL/minute, hemodialysis, or hepatic impairment: Administer 5 mg once daily

Cl_{cr} <11 mL/minute, not on dialysis: Use not recommended

Mechanism of Action Competes with histamine for H_1-receptor sites on effector cells in the gastrointestinal tract, blood vessels, and respiratory tract

Other Adverse Effects

2% to 10%:

Central nervous system: Insomnia (children 9%, adults <2%)

Gastrointestinal: Abdominal pain (children 4% to 6%), diarrhea (children 2% to 3%)

<2% (as reported in adults and/or children): Abdomen enlarged, accommodation loss, acne, alopecia, angioedema, anorexia, appetite increased, arthralgia, arthritis, arthrosis, ataxia, back pain, bilirubin increased, blindness, breast pain (female), bullous eruption, cholestasis, concentration impaired, conjunctivitis, constipation, abnormal coordination, cystitis, deafness, depersonalization, depression, dermatitis, dry skin, dysmenorrhea, dyspepsia, dysphonia, dysuria, earache, eczema, edema, emotional lability, erythematosus rash, euphoria, eye pain, flatulence, furunculosis, glaucoma, glomerulonephritis, hematuria, hemolytic anemia, hemorrhoids, hepatitis, hyperesthesia, hyperkeratosis, hyperkinesia, hypertonia, hypertrichosis, hypoesthesia, intermenstrual bleeding, leg cramps, leg edema, leukorrhea, libido decreased, liver enzymes elevated (transient), abnormal liver function, lymphadenopathy, maculopapular rash, menorrhagia, micturition frequency, myalgia, myelitis, nasal polyp, ocular hemorrhage, ototoxicity, pallor, paroniria, parosmia, periorbital edema, photosensitivity, pneumonia, polyuria, pruritus, ptosis, purpura, rash, rectal hemorrhage, seborrhea, skin disorder, skin nodule, sleep disorder, thrombocytopenia, tinnitus, urinary incontinence, urinary retention, urinary tract infection, urticaria, vaginitis, vertigo, weight gain

Drug Interactions Substrate of CYP3A4

Increased Effect/Toxicity: Increased toxicity with CNS depressants and anticholinergics.

Dietary/Ethanol/Herb Considerations

Ethanol: Avoid use; may increase CNS depression.

Herb/Nutraceutical: Avoid gotu kola, kava, SAMe, St John's wort, and valerian; may increase CNS depression.

Pharmacodynamics/Kinetics

Onset of action: 15-30 minutes

Absorption: Rapid

Protein binding, plasma: Mean: 93%

Metabolism: Limited hepatic

Half-life elimination: 8 hours

Time to peak, serum: 1 hour

Excretion: Urine (70%); feces (10%)

Pregnancy Risk Factor B

Generic Available No

Cetirizine and Pseudoephedrine

(se TI ra zeen & soo doe e FED rin)

Related Information

Cetirizine *on page 289*

Pseudoephedrine *on page 1146*

U.S. Brand Names Zyrtec-D 12 Hour™

Pharmacologic Category Antihistamine/Decongestant Combination

Synonyms Cetirizine Hydrochloride and Pseudoephedrine Hydrochloride; Pseudoephedrine Hydrochloride and Cetirizine Hydrochloride

Use Treatment of symptoms of seasonal or perennial allergic rhinitis

Local Anesthetic/Vasoconstrictor Precautions No information available to require special precautions

Effects on Dental Treatment

Based on cetirizine component:

>10%: Headache (10% to 12%), drowsiness (26%; high doses)

1% to 10%: Dizziness, drowsiness, xerostomia, fatigue

Based on pseudoephedrine component (frequency not defined): Tachycardia, palpitations, arrhythmias, nervousness, excitability, dizziness, drowsiness, convulsions, hallucinations, headache, transient stimulation, nausea, vomiting, dysuria, weakness, tremors, dyspnea, diaphoresis

Dosage Oral:

Children ≥12 years and Adults: Seasonal/perennial allergic rhinitis: 1 tablet twice daily

Elderly: Adjust dose according to renal dysfunction

Dosing adjustment in renal impairment: Cl_{cr} 11-31 mL/minute or if patient is on hemodialysis: 1 tablet once daily

Dosing adjustment in hepatic impairment: 1 tablet once daily

Mechanism of Action Cetirizine is an antihistamine; exhibits selective inhibition of H_1 receptors. Pseudoephedrine is a sympathomimetic and exerts a decongestant action on nasal mucosa.

Other Adverse Effects

Based on cetirizine component: <1%: Depression

Based on pseudoephedrine component (frequency not defined): Central nervous system: Insomnia

Dietary/Ethanol/Herb Considerations

Ethanol: Avoid use; may increase CNS depression.

Food: May be taken with food but absorption and maximal concentration are reduced

Herb/Nutraceutical: Avoid ephedra, ginseng, and yohimbe; may cause hypertension. Avoid gotu kola, kava, SAMe, St John's wort, and valerian; may increase CNS depression.

Pharmacodynamics/Kinetics

Zyrtec-D 12 Hour™:

Half-life elimination: Cetirizine: 7.9 hours; Pseudoephedrine: 6 hours

Time to peak: Cetirizine: 2.2 hours; Pseudoephedrine: 4.4 hours

Excretion: Urine (70%); feces (10%)

Pregnancy Risk Factor C

Generic Available No

Cetirizine Hydrochloride *see* Cetirizine *on page 289*

Cetirizine Hydrochloride and Pseudoephedrine Hydrochloride *see* Cetirizine and Pseudoephedrine *on page 290*

Cetrorelix (se troh REE liks)

U.S. Brand Names Cetrotide™

Pharmacologic Category Antigonadotropic Agent

Synonyms Cetrorelix Acetate

Use Inhibits premature luteinizing hormone (LH) surges in women undergoing controlled ovarian stimulation

Local Anesthetic/Vasoconstrictor Precautions No information available to require special precautions

Effects on Dental Treatment 1%: Headache, nausea

Dosage S.C.: Adults: Female: Used in conjunction with controlled ovarian stimulation therapy using gonadotropins (FSH, HMG):

Single-dose regimen: 3 mg given when serum estradiol levels show appropriate stimulation response, usually stimulation day 7 (range days 5-9). If hCG is not administered within 4 days, continue cetrorelix at 0.25 mg/day until hCG is administered

Multiple-dose regimen: 0.25 mg morning or evening of stimulation day 5, or morning of stimulation day 6; continue until hCG is administered.

Elderly: Not intended for use in women ≥65 years of age (Phase 2 and Phase 3 studies included women 19-40 years of age)

Dosing adjustment in renal impairment: No specific guidelines are available.

Dosing adjustment in hepatic impairment: No specific guidelines are available.

Mechanism of Action Competes with naturally occurring GnRH for binding on receptors of the pituitary. This delays luteinizing hormone surge, preventing ovulation until the follicles are of adequate size.

Other Adverse Effects

1% to 10%:

Endocrine & metabolic: Ovarian hyperstimulation syndrome, WHO grade II or III (3%)

Hepatic: Increased ALT, AST, GGT, and alkaline phosphatase (1% to 2%)

Postmarketing and/or case reports: Severe anaphylactic reaction (cough, rash, hypotension) occurred in one patient (following several months of treatment in a study not related to fertility). Congenital abnormalities and stillbirths have been reported, however, the relationship to cetrorelix treatment has not been established. Local injection site reactions (bruising, erythema, itching, pruritus, redness, swelling) have also been reported.

Drug Interactions No formal studies have been performed.

Pharmacodynamics/Kinetics

Onset of action: 0.25 mg dose: 2 hours; 3 mg dose: 1 hour

(Continued)

Cetrorelix *(Continued)*

Duration: 3 mg dose (single dose): 4 days
Absorption: Rapid
Protein binding: 86%
Metabolism: Transformed by peptidases; cetrorelix and peptides (1-9), (1-7), (1-6), and (1-4) are found in the bile; peptide (1-4) is the predominant metabolite
Bioavailability: 85%
Half-life elimination: 0.25 mg dose: 5 hours; 0.25 mg multiple doses: 20.6 hours; 3 mg dose: 62.8 hours
Time to peak: 0.25 mg dose: 1 hour; 3 mg dose: 1.5 hours
Excretion: Feces (5% to 10% as unchanged drug and metabolites); urine (2% to 4% as unchanged drug); within 24 hours

Pregnancy Risk Factor X

Generic Available No

Cetrorelix Acetate *see* Cetrorelix *on page 291*

Cetrotide™ *see* Cetrorelix *on page 291*

Cetylpyridinium (SEE til peer i DI nee um)

U.S. Brand Names Cēpacol® Mouthwash/Gargle [OTC]

Pharmacologic Category Local Anesthetic

Synonyms Cetylpyridinium Chloride

Use Dental and Medical: Antiseptic

Local Anesthetic/Vasoconstrictor Precautions No information available to require special precautions

Effects on Dental Treatment No significant effects or complications reported

Dosage Children >6 years and Adults: **Oral:** Rinse or gargle to freshen mouth; may be used before or after brushing; may be used every 2-3 hours

Pregnancy Risk Factor C

Dosage Forms MOUTHWASH, as chloride: 0.05% and alcohol 14% (120 mL, 180 mL, 720 mL, 960 mL)

Generic Available No

Cetylpyridinium and Benzocaine

(SEE til peer i DI nee um & BEN zoe kane)

Related Information

Benzocaine *on page 169*
Cetylpyridinium *on page 292*

U.S. Brand Names Cēpacol® Anesthetic Troches [OTC]

Pharmacologic Category Local Anesthetic

Synonyms Benzocaine and Cetylpyridinium Chloride; Cetylpyridinium Chloride and Benzocaine

Use Dental and Medical: Symptomatic relief of sore throat

Local Anesthetic/Vasoconstrictor Precautions No information available to require special precautions

Effects on Dental Treatment No significant effects or complications reported

Dosage Antiseptic/anesthetic: Oral: Dissolve in mouth as needed for sore throat

Contraindications Hypersensitivity to any component of the formulation

Pregnancy Risk Factor C

Dosage Forms TROCHE: Cetylpyridinium 1:1500 and benzocaine 10 mg (18s)

Generic Available Yes

Cetylpyridinium Chloride *see* Cetylpyridinium *on page 292*

Cetylpyridinium Chloride and Benzocaine *see* Cetylpyridinium and Benzocaine *on page 292*

Cevi-Bid® [OTC] *see* Ascorbic Acid *on page 128*

Cevimeline (se vi ME leen)

Related Information

Management of Patients Undergoing Cancer Therapy *on page 1567*

U.S. Brand Names Evoxac™

Canadian Brand Names Evoxac™

Pharmacologic Category Cholinergic Agonist

Synonyms Cevimeline Hydrochloride

Use Dental and Medical: Treatment of symptoms of xerostomia in patients with Sjögren's syndrome

Local Anesthetic/Vasoconstrictor Precautions No information available to require special precautions

Effects on Dental Treatment May cause decreased visual acuity (particularly at night and in patients with central lens changes) and impaired depth perception; patients should be cautioned about driving at night or performing hazardous activities in reduced lighting.

>10%: Headache (14%; placebo 20%), nausea (14%), rhinitis (11%), sinusitis (12%), upper respiratory infection (11%), increased diaphoresis (19%)

1% to 10%: Abnormal vision, chest pain, palpitations, dizziness (4%), anxiety (1%), fever, migraine, hot flashes (2%), vomiting (5%), belching, rigors (1%), tremor, earache, otitis media, cough (6%), bronchitis (4%), pneumonia, epistaxis, flu-like syndrome, infection, fungal infection, allergy, hiccups, excessive salivation (2%), salivary gland pain, xerostomia, sialoadenitis, gastroesophageal reflux, ulcerative stomatitis, tooth disorder, fatigue (3%), pain (3%), CNS depression, leg cramps, skeletal pain (3%)

Dosage Oral: Adults: 30 mg 3 times/day

Mechanism of Action Binds to muscarinic (cholinergic) receptors, causing an increase in secretion of exocrine glands (including salivary glands)

Other Adverse Effects

>10%: Gastrointestinal: Diarrhea (10%)

1% to 10%:

Cardiovascular: Peripheral edema, edema

Central nervous system: Insomnia (2%), hypoesthesia, vertigo

Dermatologic: Rash (4%; placebo 6%), pruritus, skin disorder, erythematous rash

Gastrointestinal: Dyspepsia (8%; placebo 9%), abdominal pain (8%), constipation, flatulence, increased amylase, anorexia

Genitourinary: Urinary tract infection (6%), vaginitis, cystitis

Hematologic: Anemia

Local: Abscess

Neuromuscular & skeletal: Back pain (5%), arthralgia (4%), hypertonia, myalgia, hyporeflexia

Ocular: Conjunctivitis (4%), eye pain, eye abnormality, xerophthalmia

<1%: **Syncope, malaise, substernal chest pain, abnormal ECG, hypertension, hypotension, arrhythmia**, T-wave inversion, **angina, MI**, pericarditis, pulmonary embolism, peripheral ischemia, thrombophlebitis, vasculitis, **dysphagia**, enterocolitis, **gastric ulcer, GI hemorrhage**, ileus, **melena, mucositis, esophageal stricture, esophagitis, peptic ulcer, stomatitis, tongue discoloration, tongue ulceration**, hypothyroidism, thrombocytopenic purpura, thrombocytopenia, anemia, eosinophilia, granulocytopenia, leukopenia, leukocytosis, **lymphadenopathy,** cholelithiasis, increased transaminases, arthropathy, avascular necrosis (femoral head), bursitis, costochondritis, synovitis, tendonitis, tenosynovitis, **coma, dyskinesia,** dysphonia, aggravated **MS,** neuralgia, neuropathy, **paresthesia, agitation, confusion**, depersonalization, emotional lability, **manic reaction, paranoia, somnolence**, hyperkinesia, **hallucination, falling, sepsis, bronchospasm, nasal ulcer**, pleural effusion, pulmonary fibrosis, systemic lupus erythematosus, alopecia, dermatitis, eczema, photosensitivity reaction, dry skin, skin ulceration, bullous eruption, deafness, motion sickness, parosmia, **taste perversion**, blepharitis, cataract, corneal ulceration, diplopia, glaucoma, anterior chamber hemorrhage, retinal disorder, scleritis, tinnitus, epididymitis, menstrual disorder, genital pruritus, dysuria, hematuria, renal calculus, abnormal renal function, decreased urine flow, **postural hypotension, aphasia, convulsions, paralysis, gingival hyperplasia**, intestinal obstruction, bundle branch block, increased CPK, electrolyte abnormality, **aggressive behavior, delirium**, impotence, **apnea**, oliguria, urinary retention, lymphocytosis

Contraindications Hypersensitivity to cevimeline or any component of the formulation; uncontrolled asthma; narrow-angle glaucoma; acute iritis; other conditions where miosis is undesirable

Warnings/Precautions May alter cardiac conduction and/or heart rate; use caution in patients with significant cardiovascular disease, including angina, MI, or conduction disturbances. Cevimeline has the potential to increase bronchial smooth muscle tone, airway resistance, and bronchial secretions; use with caution in patients with controlled asthma, COPD, or chronic bronchitis. May cause decreased visual acuity (particularly at night and in patients with central lens changes) and impaired depth perception. Patients should be cautioned about driving at night or performing hazardous activities in reduced lighting. May cause a variety of parasympathomimetic effects, which may be particularly dangerous in elderly patients; excessive sweating may lead to dehydration in some patients.

Use with caution in patients with a history of biliary stones or nephrolithiasis; cevimeline may induce smooth muscle spasms, precipitating cholangitis, cholecystitis, biliary obstruction, renal colic, or ureteral reflux in susceptible patients. Patients with a known or suspected deficiency of CYP2D6 may be at higher risk of adverse effects. Safety and efficacy has not been established in pediatric patients.

Drug Interactions Substrate of CYP2D6, CYP3A4

Increased Effect: Drugs which inhibit CYP2D6 (including amiodarone, fluoxetine, paroxetine, quinidine, ritonavir) or CYP3A4 (including diltiazem, erythromycin, itraconazole, ketoconazole, verapamil) may increase levels of cevimeline. The effects of other cholinergic agents may be increased during concurrent administration with cevimeline. Concurrent use of cevimeline and beta-blockers may increase the potential for conduction disturbances.

Decreased Effect: Anticholinergic agents (atropine, TCAs, phenothiazines) may antagonize the effects of cevimeline

Dietary/Ethanol/Herb Considerations Food: May be taken with food to reduce GI upset: boiled milk, buttermilk, or yogurt may reduce diarrhea.

(Continued)

Cevimeline *(Continued)*

Pharmacodynamics/Kinetics

Distribution: V_d: 6 L/kg

Protein binding: <20%

Metabolism: Hepatic via CYP2D6 and CYP3A4

Half-life elimination: 5 hours

Time to peak: 1.5-2 hours

Excretion: Urine (as metabolites and unchanged drug)

Pregnancy Risk Factor C

Dosage Forms CAP: 30 mg

Generic Available No

Cevimeline Hydrochloride *see* Cevimeline *on page 292*

CFDN *see* Cefdinir *on page 265*

CG *see* Chorionic Gonadotropin (Human) *on page 320*

CGP-42446 *see* Zoledronic Acid *on page 1410*

C-Gram [OTC] *see* Ascorbic Acid *on page 128*

CharcoAid® [OTC] *see* Charcoal *on page 294*

Charcoal (CHAR kole)

U.S. Brand Names Actidose® [OTC]; Actidose-Aqua® [OTC]; CharcoAid® [OTC]; Charcocaps® [OTC]; Liqui-Char® [OTC]

Canadian Brand Names Charcadole®; Charcadole®, Aqueous; Charcadole® TFS

Pharmacologic Category Antidiarrheal; Antidote; Antiflatulent

Synonyms Activated Carbon; Activated Charcoal; Adsorbent Charcoal; Liquid Antidote; Medicinal Carbon; Medicinal Charcoal

Use Emergency treatment in poisoning by drugs and chemicals; repetitive doses for gastric dialysis in uremia to adsorb various waste products, and repetitive doses have proven useful to enhance the elimination of certain drugs (eg, theophylline, phenobarbital, and aspirin)

Local Anesthetic/Vasoconstrictor Precautions No information available to require special precautions

Effects on Dental Treatment >10%: Vomiting

Dosage Oral:

Acute poisoning:

Charcoal with sorbitol: Single-dose:

Children 1-12 years: 1-2 g/kg/dose or 15-30 g or approximately 5-10 times the weight of the ingested poison; 1 g adsorbs 100-1000 mg of poison; the use of repeat oral charcoal with sorbitol doses is not recommended. In young children, sorbitol should be repeated no more than 1-2 times/day.

Adults: 30-100 g

Charcoal in water:

Single-dose:

Infants <1 year: 1 g/kg

Children 1-12 years: 15-30 g or 1-2 g/kg

Adults: 30-100 g or 1-2 g/kg

Multiple-dose:

Infants <1 year: 0.5 g/kg every 4-6 hours

Children 1-12 years: 20-60 g or 0.5-1 g/kg every 2-6 hours until clinical observations, serum drug concentration have returned to a subtherapeutic range, or charcoal stool apparent

Adults: 20-60 g or 0.5-1 g/kg every 2-6 hours

Gastric dialysis: Adults: 20-50 g every 6 hours for 1-2 days

Intestinal gas, diarrhea, GI distress: Adults: 520-975 mg after meals or at first sign of discomfort; repeat as needed to a maximum dose of 4.16 g/day

Mechanism of Action Adsorbs toxic substances or irritants, thus inhibiting GI absorption; adsorbs intestinal gas; the addition of sorbitol results in hyperosmotic laxative action causing catharsis

Other Adverse Effects

>10%: Gastrointestinal: Diarrhea (sorbitol), constipation, black stools

<1%: Swelling of abdomen

Drug Interactions Decreased Effect: Charcoal decreases the effect of ipecac syrup. Charcoal effect is reduced when taken with milk, ice cream, or sherbet.

Dietary/Ethanol/Herb Considerations Food: Avoid milk, ice cream, sherbet, or marmalade; may reduce charcoal's effectiveness; Flavoring agents (eg, chocolate) and sorbitol can enhance palatability.

Pharmacodynamics/Kinetics Excretion: Feces (as charcoal)

Pregnancy Risk Factor C

Generic Available Yes

Charcocaps® [OTC] *see* Charcoal *on page 294*

Chenix® *see* Chenodiol *on page 295*

Chenodeoxycholic Acid *see* Chenodiol *on page 295*

Chenodiol (kee noe DYE ole)

U.S. Brand Names Chenix®

Pharmacologic Category Bile Acid

Synonyms Chenodeoxycholic Acid

Use Orphan drug: Oral dissolution of cholesterol gallstones in selected patients

Local Anesthetic/Vasoconstrictor Precautions No information available to require special precautions

Effects on Dental Treatment No significant effects or complications reported

Dosage Adults:

Oral: 13-16 mg/kg/day in 2 divided doses, starting with 250 mg twice daily the first 2 weeks and increasing by 250 mg/day each week thereafter until the recommended or maximum tolerated dose is achieved

Dosing comments in hepatic impairment: Contraindicated in the presence of known hepatocyte dysfunction or bile ductal abnormalities

Mechanism of Action Chenodiol is a primary acid excreted into bile, normally constituting one-third of the total biliary bile acids. Synthesis of chenodiol is regulated by the relative composition and flux of cholesterol and bile acids through the hepatocyte by a negative feedback effect on the rate-limiting enzymes for synthesis of cholesterol (HMG-CoA reductase) and bile acids (cholesterol 7 alpha-hydroxyl).

Other Adverse Effects

>10%:

Gastrointestinal: Diarrhea (mild), biliary pain

Miscellaneous: Aminotransferase increases

1% to 10%:

Endocrine & metabolic: Increases in cholesterol and LDL-cholesterol

Gastrointestinal: Dyspepsia

<1%: Diarrhea (severe), cramps, **nausea, vomiting**, flatulence, constipation, leukopenia, intrahepatic cholestasis, higher cholecystectomy rates

Drug Interactions Decreased Effect: Antacids, cholestyramine, colestipol, and oral contraceptives exhibit decreased effectiveness when taken with chenodiol.

Pregnancy Risk Factor X

Generic Available No

Cheracol® *see* Guaifenesin and Codeine *on page 650*

Cheracol® D [OTC] *see* Guaifenesin and Dextromethorphan *on page 651*

Cheracol® Plus [OTC] *see* Guaifenesin and Dextromethorphan *on page 651*

Cheratussin DAC *see* Guaifenesin, Pseudoephedrine, and Codeine *on page 653*

Chiggerex® [OTC] *see* Benzocaine *on page 169*

Chiggertox® [OTC] *see* Benzocaine *on page 169*

Children's Dimetapp® Elixir Cold & Allergy [OTC] *see* Brompheniramine and Pseudoephedrine *on page 201*

Children's Kaopectate® [DSC] [OTC] *see* Attapulgite *on page 146*

Children's Kaopectate® (reformulation) [OTC] *see* Bismuth *on page 186*

Children's Sudafed® Cough & Cold [OTC] *see* Pseudoephedrine and Dextromethorphan *on page 1147*

Children's Tylenol® Cold [OTC] *see* Acetaminophen, Chlorpheniramine, and Pseudoephedrine *on page 35*

Children's Tylenol® Sinus [OTC] *see* Acetaminophen and Pseudoephedrine *on page 31*

Chirocaine® *see* Levobupivacaine *on page 789*

Chlo-Amine® [OTC] *see* Chlorpheniramine *on page 307*

Chlorafed® [OTC] *see* Chlorpheniramine and Pseudoephedrine *on page 308*

Chloral *see* Chloral Hydrate *on page 295*

Chloral Hydrate (KLOR al HYE drate)

U.S. Brand Names Aquachloral® Supprettes®

Canadian Brand Names PMS-Chloral Hydrate

Pharmacologic Category Hypnotic, Miscellaneous

Synonyms Chloral; Hydrated Chloral; Trichloroacetaldehyde Monohydrate

Use

Dental: Short-term sedative and hypnotic for dental procedures

Medical: Short-term sedative and hypnotic (<2 weeks); sedative/hypnotic for diagnostic procedures; sedative prior to EEG evaluations

Local Anesthetic/Vasoconstrictor Precautions No information available to require special precautions

Effects on Dental Treatment Frequency not defined: Disorientation, sedation, excitement (paradoxical), dizziness, fever, headache, confusion, lightheadedness, hallucinations, drowsiness, "hangover" effect, gastric irritation, nausea, vomiting, physical and psychological dependence (prolonged use of large doses)

Restrictions C-IV

(Continued)

Chloral Hydrate *(Continued)*

Dosage

Children:

Sedation or anxiety: Oral, rectal: 5-15 mg/kg/dose every 8 hours (maximum: 500 mg/dose)

Hypnotic: Oral, rectal: 20-40 mg/kg/dose up to a maximum of 50 mg/kg/24 hours or 1 g/dose or 2 g/24 hours

Conscious sedation: Oral: 50-75 mg/kg/dose 30-60 minutes prior to procedure; may repeat 30 minutes after initial dose if needed, to a total maximum dose of 120 mg/kg or 1 g total

Prior to EEG: Oral, rectal: 20-25 mg/kg/dose, 30-60 minutes prior to EEG; may repeat in 30 minutes to maximum of 100 mg/kg or 2 g total

Adults: Oral, rectal:

Sedation, anxiety: 250 mg 3 times/day

Hypnotic: 500-1000 mg at bedtime or 30 minutes prior to procedure, not to exceed 2 g/24 hours

Dosing comment in renal impairment: Cl_{cr} <50 mL/minute: Avoid use

Hemodialysis: Dialyzable (50% to 100%); supplemental dose is unnecessary

Dosing comment in hepatic impairment: Avoid use in severe impairment

Mechanism of Action Central nervous system depressant effects are due to its active metabolite trichloroethanol, mechanism unknown

Other Adverse Effects Frequency not defined:

Central nervous system: Ataxia nightmares

Dermatologic: Rash, urticaria

Gastrointestinal: Diarrhea, flatulence

Hematologic: Leukopenia, eosinophilia, acute intermittent porphyria

Contraindications Hypersensitivity to chloral hydrate or any component of the formulation; hepatic or renal impairment; gastritis or ulcers; severe cardiac disease

Warnings/Precautions Use with caution in patients with porphyria; use with caution in neonates, drug may accumulate with repeated use, prolonged use in neonates associated with hyperbilirubinemia; tolerance to hypnotic effect develops, therefore, not recommended for use >2 weeks; taper dosage to avoid withdrawal with prolonged use; trichloroethanol (TCE), a metabolite of chloral hydrate, is a carcinogen in mice; there is no data in humans. Chloral hydrate is considered a second line hypnotic agent in the elderly. Recent interpretive guidelines from the Centers for Medicare and Medicaid Services (CMS) discourage the use of chloral hydrate in residents of long-term care facilities.

Drug Interactions

CNS depressants: Sedative effects and/or respiratory depression with chloral hydrate may be additive with other CNS depressants; monitor for increased effect; includes ethanol, sedatives, antidepressants, narcotic analgesics, and benzodiazepines

Furosemide: Diaphoresis, flushing, and hypertension have occurred in patients who received I.V. furosemide within 24 hours after administration of chloral hydrate; consider using a benzodiazepine

Phenytoin: Half-life may be decreased by chloral hydrate; limited documentation (small, single-dose study); monitor

Warfarin: Effect of oral anticoagulants may be increased by chloral hydrate; monitor INR; warfarin dosage may require adjustment. Chloral hydrate's metabolite may displace warfarin from its protein binding sites resulting in an increase in the hypoprothrombinemic response to warfarin.

Dietary/Ethanol/Herb Considerations

Ethanol: Avoid use; may increase CNS depression.

Food: Administer with chilled liquid to mask taste.

Herb/Nutraceutical: Avoid gotu kola, kava, melatonin, SAMe, St John's wort, and valerian; may increase CNS depression.

Pharmacodynamics/Kinetics

Onset of action: Peak effect: 0.5-1 hour

Duration: 4-8 hours

Absorption: Oral, rectal: Well absorbed

Distribution: Crosses placenta; negligible amounts enter breast milk

Metabolism: Rapidly hepatic to trichloroethanol (active metabolite); variable amounts hepatically and renally to trichloroacetic acid (inactive)

Half-life elimination: Active metabolite: 8-11 hours

Excretion: Urine (as metabolites); feces (small amounts)

Pregnancy Risk Factor C

Dosage Forms CAP: 500 mg. **SUPP, rectal:** 324 mg, 500 mg, 648 mg. **SYR:** 500 mg/5 mL (5 mL, 10 mL, 480 mL)

Generic Available Yes

Chlorambucil (klor AM byoo sil)

U.S. Brand Names Leukeran®

Canadian Brand Names Leukeran®

Mexican Brand Names Leukeran®

Pharmacologic Category Antineoplastic Agent, Alkylating Agent

Synonyms CB-1348; Chlorambucilum; Chloraminophene; Chlorbutinum; NSC-3088; WR-139013

Use Management of chronic lymphocytic leukemia, Hodgkin's and non-Hodgkin's lymphoma; breast and ovarian carcinoma; Waldenström's macroglobulinemia, testicular carcinoma, thrombocythemia, choriocarcinoma

Local Anesthetic/Vasoconstrictor Precautions No information available to require special precautions

Effects on Dental Treatment 1% to 10%: Nausea (mild), vomiting, stomatitis

Dosage Oral (refer to individual protocols):

Children:

General short courses: 0.1-0.2 mg/kg/day **OR** 4.5 mg/m²/day for 3-6 weeks for remission induction (usual: 4-10 mg/day); maintenance therapy: 0.03-0.1 mg/kg/day (usual: 2-4 mg/day)

Nephrotic syndrome: 0.1-0.2 mg/kg/day every day for 5-15 weeks with low-dose prednisone

Chronic lymphocytic leukemia (CLL):

Biweekly regimen: Initial: 0.4 mg/kg/dose every 2 weeks; increase dose by 0.1 mg/kg every 2 weeks until a response occurs and/or myelosuppression occurs

Monthly regimen: Initial: 0.4 mg/kg, increase dose by 0.2 mg/kg every 4 weeks until a response occurs and/or myelosuppression occurs

Malignant lymphomas:

Non-Hodgkin's lymphoma: 0.1 mg/kg/day

Hodgkin's lymphoma: 0.2 mg/kg/day

Adults: 0.1-0.2 mg/kg/day **or**

3-6 mg/m²/day for 3-6 weeks, then adjust dose on basis of blood counts **or**

0.4 mg/kg and increased by 0.1 mg/kg biweekly or monthly **or**

14 mg/m²/day for 5 days, repeated every 21-28 days

Hemodialysis: Supplemental dosing unnecessary

Peritoneal dialysis: Supplemental dosing unnecessary

Mechanism of Action Interferes with DNA replication and RNA transcription by alkylation and cross-linking the strands of DNA

Other Adverse Effects

>10%:

Dermatologic: Skin rashes

Hematologic: Myelosuppression (common, dose-limiting)

Onset: 7 days

Nadir: 14 days

Recovery: 28 days; may be prolonged to 6-8 weeks in some patients

Hepatic: Transient elevations in liver enzymes

1% to 10%:

Endocrine & metabolic: Hyperuricemia, menstrual cramps

Gastrointestinal: Diarrhea

<1%: **Agitation**, amenorrhea, angioneurotic edema, ataxia, chromosomal damage, **confusion, fever, hallucination**, hepatic necrosis, hepatotoxicity, infertility (may be irreversible in some patients), **muscular twitching**, myoclonia, neuropathy, primary AML, secondary malignancies, **seizures** (rare), skin hypersensitivity, **tremors, weakness**; interstitial pneumonitis or fibrosis including **cough, dyspnea, fever**, hypoxia, pulmonary dysplasia (related to long-term [>6 months] or high-dose [>2000 mg] therapy), rales, **respiratory distress**, urticaria

Drug Interactions Decreased Effect: Patients may experience impaired immune response to vaccines; possible infection after administration of live vaccines in patients receiving immunosuppressants.

Dietary/Ethanol/Herb Considerations

Ethanol: Avoid use; may increase GI irritation.

Food: Avoid spices and acidic or hot foods. Do not mix with milk, ice cream, or sherbet.

Pharmacodynamics/Kinetics

Absorption: 70% to 80% with meals

Distribution: V_d: 0.14-0.24 L/kg

Protein binding: ~99%

Metabolism: Hepatic; active metabolite, phenylacetic acid mustard

Bioavailability: Reduced 10% to 20% with food

Half-life elimination: 1.5 hours; Phenylacetic acid mustard: 2.5 hours

Excretion: Urine (60% primarily as metabolites, <1% as unchanged drug)

Pregnancy Risk Factor D

Generic Available No

Chlorambucilum *see* Chlorambucil *on page 296*

Chloraminophene *see* Chlorambucil *on page 296*

Chloramphenicol (klor am FEN i kole)

U.S. Brand Names Chloromycetin®; Chloroptic®; Ocu-Chlor®

Canadian Brand Names Chloromycetin®; Diochloram®; Pentamycetin®

(Continued)

Chloramphenicol *(Continued)*

Mexican Brand Names Cetina; Chloromycetin®; Clorafen®; Cloramfeni®; Cloran®; Clordil®; Paraxin; Quemicetina®

Pharmacologic Category Antibiotic, Ophthalmic; Antibiotic, Otic; Antibiotic, Miscellaneous

Use Treatment of serious infections due to organisms resistant to other less toxic antibiotics or when its penetrability into the site of infection is clinically superior to other antibiotics to which the organism is sensitive; useful in infections caused by *Bacteroides*, *H. influenzae*, *Neisseria meningitidis*, *Salmonella*, and *Rickettsia*; active against many vancomycin-resistant enterococci

Local Anesthetic/Vasoconstrictor Precautions No information available to require special precautions

Effects on Dental Treatment No significant effects or complications reported

Dosage

Meningitis: I.V.: Infants >30 days and Children: 50-100 mg/kg/day divided every 6 hours

Other infections: I.V.:

Infants >30 days and Children: 50-75 mg/kg/day divided every 6 hours; maximum daily dose: 4 g/day

Adults: 50-100 mg/kg/day in divided doses every 6 hours; maximum daily dose: 4 g/day

Ophthalmic: Children and Adults: Instill 1-2 drops 4-6 times/day or 1.25 cm (½" of ointment every 3-4 hours); increase interval between applications after 72 hours to 2-3 times/day; treatment should continue for ~7 days

Otic solution: Instill 2-3 drops into ear 3 times/day

Topical: Gently rub into the affected area 1-4 times/day

Dosing comment in hepatic impairment: Avoid use in severe impairment as increased toxicity may occur.

Hemodialysis: Slightly dialyzable (5% to 20%) via hemo- and peritoneal dialysis; no supplemental doses needed in dialysis or continuous arteriovenous or veno-venous hemofiltration

Mechanism of Action Reversibly binds to 50S ribosomal subunits of susceptible organisms preventing amino acids from being transferred to growing peptide chains thus inhibiting protein synthesis

Other Adverse Effects Frequency not defined:

Aplastic anemia, an idiosyncratic reaction which can occur with any route of administration; usually occurs 3 weeks to 12 months after initial exposure to chloramphenicol

Bone marrow suppression is thought to be dose-related with serum concentrations >25 µg/mL and reversible once chloramphenicol is discontinued; anemia and neutropenia may occur during the first week of therapy

Gray syndrome is characterized by circulatory collapse, cyanosis, acidosis, abdominal distention, myocardial depression, coma, and death; reaction appears to be associated with serum levels ≥50 µg/mL; may result from drug accumulation in patients with impaired hepatic or renal function

Additional reactions include allergic sensitization (topical), angioneurotic edema, urticaria, vesicular dermatitis, maculopapular dermatitis, conjunctival hyperemia and ocular burning/stinging (ophthalmic)

<1%: Nightmares, **headache**, rash, diarrhea, **stomatitis**, enterocolitis, **nausea, vomiting**, peripheral neuropathy, optic neuritis

Drug Interactions Inhibits CYP2C8/9, 3A4

Increased Effect/Toxicity: Chloramphenicol increases serum concentrations of chlorpropamide, phenytoin, and oral anticoagulants.

Decreased Effect: Phenobarbital and rifampin may decrease serum concentrations of chloramphenicol.

Dietary/Ethanol/Herb Considerations

Ethanol: Use with caution; may cause a mild disulfiram-like reaction.

Food may decrease intestinal absorption of vitamin B_{12} and increase dietary need for riboflavin, pyridoxine, and vitamin B_{12}.

Pharmacodynamics/Kinetics

Distribution: To most tissues and body fluids; readily crosses placenta; enters breast milk

CSF:blood level ratio: Normal meninges: 66%; Inflamed meninges: >66%

Protein binding: 60%

Metabolism: Extensively hepatic (90%) to inactive metabolites, principally by glucuronidation; chloramphenicol palmitate is hydrolyzed by lipases in GI tract to the active base; chloramphenicol sodium succinate is hydrolyzed by esterases to active base

Half-life elimination

Normal renal function: 1.6-3.3 hours

End-stage renal disease: 3-7 hours

Cirrhosis: 10-12 hours

Neonates: Postnatal: 1-2 days old: 24 hours; 10-16 days old: 10 hours

Time to peak: Oral: Within 0.5-3 hours

Excretion: Urine (5% to 15%); Neonates: Urine (6% to 80% as unchanged drug), feces (4%)

Pregnancy Risk Factor C

Generic Available Yes

Chloramphenicol and Prednisolone

(klor am FEN i kole & pred NIS oh lone)

Related Information

Chloramphenicol *on page 297*

U.S. Brand Names Chloroptic-P®

Pharmacologic Category Antibiotic, Ophthalmic; Corticosteroid, Ophthalmic

Synonyms Prednisolone and Chloramphenicol

Use Topical anti-infective and corticosteroid for treatment of ocular infections

Local Anesthetic/Vasoconstrictor Precautions No information available to require special precautions

Effects on Dental Treatment No significant effects or complications reported

Dosage Ophthalmic: Instill 1-2 drops in eye(s) 2-4 times/day

Pregnancy Risk Factor C

Generic Available No

Chloramphenicol, Hydrocortisone, and Polymyxin B *see* Chloramphenicol, Polymyxin B, and Hydrocortisone *on page 299*

Chloramphenicol, Polymyxin B, and Hydrocortisone

(klor am FEN i kole, pol i MIKS in bee, & hye droe KOR ti sone)

Related Information

Chloramphenicol *on page 297*

Hydrocortisone *on page 688*

Pharmacologic Category Antibiotic, Ophthalmic; Corticosteroid, Ophthalmic

Synonyms Chloramphenicol, Hydrocortisone, and Polymyxin B; Hydrocortisone, Chloramphenicol, and Polymyxin B; Hydrocortisone, Polymyxin B, and Chloramphenicol; Polymyxin B, Chloramphenicol, and Hydrocortisone; Polymyxin B, Hydrocortisone, and Chloramphenicol

Use Topical anti-infective and corticosteroid for treatment of ocular infections

Local Anesthetic/Vasoconstrictor Precautions No information available to require special precautions

Effects on Dental Treatment No significant effects or complications reported

Dosage Apply 1/2" ribbon every 3-4 hours until improvement occurs

Pregnancy Risk Factor C

Generic Available No

ChloraPrep® [OTC] *see* Chlorhexidine Gluconate *on page 300*

Chloraseptic® Gargle [OTC] *see* Phenol *on page 1068*

Chloraseptic® Mouth Pain Spray [OTC] *see* Phenol *on page 1068*

Chloraseptic® Rinse [OTC] *see* Phenol *on page 1068*

Chloraseptic® Spray [OTC] *see* Phenol *on page 1068*

Chloraseptic® Spray for Kids [OTC] *see* Phenol *on page 1068*

Chlorbutinum *see* Chlorambucil *on page 296*

Chlordiazepoxide (klor dye az e POKS ide)

U.S. Brand Names Librium®

Canadian Brand Names Apo®-Chlordiazepoxide

Pharmacologic Category Benzodiazepine

Synonyms Methaminodiazepoxide Hydrochloride

Use Management of anxiety disorder or for the short-term relief of symptoms of anxiety; withdrawal symptoms of acute alcoholism; preoperative apprehension and anxiety

Local Anesthetic/Vasoconstrictor Precautions No information available to require special precautions

Effects on Dental Treatment

>10%: Xerostomia (normal salivary flow resumes upon discontinuation), drowsiness, lightheadedness, irritability, fatigue, memory impairment

1% to 10%: Hypotension, confusion, dizziness, akathisia, rigidity, tremor, muscle cramps, nasal congestion

Restrictions C-IV

Dosage

Children:

- <6 years: Use not recommended
- >6 years: Anxiety: Oral, I.M.: 0.5 mg/kg/24 hours divided every 6-8 hours

Adults:

- Anxiety:
  - Oral: 15-100 mg divided 3-4 times/day
  - I.M., I.V.: Initial: 50-100 mg followed by 25-50 mg 3-4 times/day as needed
- Preoperative anxiety: I.M.: 50-100 mg prior to surgery

(Continued)

Chlordiazepoxide *(Continued)*

Ethanol withdrawal symptoms: Oral, I.V.: 50-100 mg to start, dose may be repeated in 2-4 hours as necessary to a maximum of 300 mg/24 hours

Note: Up to 300 mg may be given I.M. or I.V. during a 6-hour period, but not more than this in any 24-hour period.

Dosing adjustment in renal impairment: Cl_{cr} <10 mL/minute: Administer 50% of dose

Hemodialysis: Not dialyzable (0% to 5%)

Dosing comment in hepatic impairment: Avoid use

Mechanism of Action Binds to stereospecific benzodiazepine receptors on the postsynaptic GABA neuron at several sites within the central nervous system, including the limbic system, reticular formation. Enhancement of the inhibitory effect of GABA on neuronal excitability results by increased neuronal membrane permeability to chloride ions. This shift in chloride ions results in hyperpolarization (a less excitable state) and stabilization.

Other Adverse Effects

>10%:

Central nervous system: Ataxia, dysarthria
Dermatologic: Rash
Endocrine & metabolic: Decreased libido, menstrual disorders
Gastrointestinal: Increased or decreased appetite, weight gain/loss
Genitourinary: Micturition difficulties

1% to 10%:

Central nervous system: Disinhibition, increased libido
Dermatologic: Dermatitis
Genitourinary: Sexual dysfunction, incontinence
Otic: Tinnitus

Drug Interactions Substrate of **CYP3A4**

Increased Effect/Toxicity: Chlordiazepoxide potentiates the CNS depressant effects of narcotic analgesics, barbiturates, phenothiazines, ethanol, antihistamines, MAO inhibitors, sedative-hypnotics, and cyclic antidepressants. Serum concentrations/effects of chlordiazepoxide may be increased by inhibitors of CYP3A4, including cimetidine, ciprofloxacin, clarithromycin, clozapine, diltiazem, disulfiram, digoxin, erythromycin, ethanol, fluconazole, fluoxetine, fluvoxamine, grapefruit juice, isoniazid, itraconazole, ketoconazole, labetalol, levodopa, loxapine, metoprolol, metronidazole, miconazole, nefazodone, omeprazole, phenytoin, rifabutin, rifampin, troleandomycin, valproic acid, and verapamil.

Decreased Effect: Carbamazepine, rifampin, rifabutin may enhance the metabolism of chlordiazepoxide and decrease its therapeutic effect.

Dietary/Ethanol/Herb Considerations

Ethanol: Avoid use; may increase CNS depression.

Food: Grapefruit products may increase serum concentration (unlikely because of high oral bioavailability of chlordiazepoxide).

Herb/Nutraceutical: Avoid gotu kola, kava, SAMe, St John's wort, and valerian; may increase CNS depression.

Pharmacodynamics/Kinetics

Distribution: V_d: 3.3 L/kg; crosses placenta; enters breast milk

Protein binding: 90% to 98%

Metabolism: Extensively hepatic to desmethyldiazepam (active and long-acting)

Half-life elimination: 6.6-25 hours; End-stage renal disease: 5-30 hours; Cirrhosis: 30-63 hours

Time to peak, serum: Oral: Within 2 hours; I.M.: Results in lower peak plasma levels than oral

Excretion: Urine (minimal as unchanged drug)

Pregnancy Risk Factor D

Generic Available Yes

Chlordiazepoxide and Amitriptyline *see* Amitriptyline and Chlordiazepoxide *on page 85*

Chlordiazepoxide and Clidinium *see* Clidinium and Chlordiazepoxide *on page 341*

Chloresium® [OTC] *see* Chlorophyll *on page 302*

Chlorhexidine Gluconate (klor HEKS i deen GLOO koe nate)

Related Information

Antiplaque Agents *on page 1554*
Dentin Hypersensitivity, High Caries Index, and Xerostomia *on page 1553*
Management of Patients Undergoing Cancer Therapy *on page 1567*
Oral Bacterial Infections *on page 1531*
Oral Nonviral Soft Tissue Ulcerations or Erosions *on page 1549*
Periodontal Diseases *on page 1540*

U.S. Brand Names Avagard™ [OTC]; BactoShield® CHG [OTC]; Betasept® [OTC]; ChloraPrep® [OTC]; Chlorostat® [OTC]; Dyna-Hex® [OTC]; Hibiclens® [OTC]; Peridex®; PerioChip®; PerioGard®; Stat Touch 2 [OTC] [DSC]

Canadian Brand Names Apo®-Chlorhexadine; Hibidil® 1:2000; ORO-Clense; SpectroGram 2™

Pharmacologic Category Antibiotic, Oral Rinse; Antibiotic, Topical

Synonyms Stat Touch 2 [OTC] [DSC]

Use

Dental:

Antimicrobial dental rinse: Active against gram-positive and gram-negative organisms, facultative anaerobes, aerobes, and yeast

Chip, for periodontal pocket insertion: Adjunct to scaling and root planing procedures for reduction of pocket depth in patients with adult periodontitis; may be used as part of a periodontal maintenance program

Medical: Cleanser for surgical scrub and skin wounds, germicidal hand rinse; active against gram-positive and gram-negative organisms, facultative anaerobes, aerobes, and yeast

Local Anesthetic/Vasoconstrictor Precautions No information available to require special precautions

Effects on Dental Treatment Staining may be visible as soon as 1 week after therapy begins and is more pronounced when there is a heavy accumulation of unremoved plaque and when teeth fillings have rough surfaces. Stain does not have a clinically adverse effect but because removal may not be possible, patient with frontal restoration should be advised of the potential permanency of the stain.

>10%: Increased tartar on teeth, altered taste perception, staining of oral surfaces (mucosa, teeth, dorsum of tongue)

1% to 10%: Oral/tongue irritation

Dosage Adults:

Oral rinse (Peridex®, PerioGard®):

First floss and brush teeth, completely rinse toothpaste from mouth and swish 15 mL (one capful) undiluted oral rinse around in mouth for 30 seconds, then expectorate. Caution patient not to swallow the medicine and instruct not to eat for 2-3 hours after treatment.

Treatment of gingivitis: Oral prophylaxis: Swish for 30 seconds with 15 mL chlorhexidine, then expectorate; repeat twice daily (morning and evening). Patient should have a re-evaluation followed by a dental prophylaxis every 6 months.

Periodontal chip: Periodontal chip: Adults: One chip is inserted into a periodontal pocket with a probing pocket depth ≥5 mm. Up to 8 chips may be inserted in a single visit. Treatment is recommended every 3 months in pockets with a remaining depth ≥5 mm. If dislodgment occurs 7 days or more after placement, the subject is considered to have had the full course of treatment. If dislodgment occurs within 48 hours, a new chip should be inserted. The chip biodegrades completely and does not need to be removed. Patients should avoid dental floss at the site of PerioChip® insertion for 10 days after placement because flossing might dislodge the chip.

Insertion of periodontal chip: Pocket should be isolated and surrounding area dried prior to chip insertion. The chip should be grasped using forceps with the rounded edges away from the forceps. The chip should be inserted into the periodontal pocket to its maximum depth. It may be maneuvered into position using the tips of the forceps or a flat instrument.

Antimicrobial dressing (Biopatch®): Replace device dressing at intervals ≤7 days

Cleanser:

Surgical scrub: Scrub 3 minutes and rinse thoroughly, wash for an additional 3 minutes

Hand sanitizer (Avagard™): Dispense 1 pumpful in palm of one hand; dip fingertips of opposite hand into solution and work it under nails. Spread remainder evenly over hand and just above elbow, covering all surfaces. Repeat on other hand. Dispense another pumpful in each hand and reapply to each hand up to the wrist. Allow to dry before gloving.

Hand wash: Wash for 15 seconds and rinse

Hand rinse: Rub 15 seconds and rinse

Mechanism of Action The bactericidal effect of chlorhexidine is a result of the binding of this cationic molecule to negatively charged bacterial cell walls and extramicrobial complexes. At low concentrations, this causes an alteration of bacterial cell osmotic equilibrium and leakage of potassium and phosphorous resulting in a bacteriostatic effect. At high concentrations of chlorhexidine, the cytoplasmic contents of the bacterial cell precipitate and result in cell death.

Other Adverse Effects

Oral: <1%: **Facial edema, nasal congestion, dyspnea**

Topical: Skin erythema and roughness, dryness, **sensitization, allergic reactions**

Contraindications Hypersensitivity to chlorhexidine gluconate or any component of the formulation

Warnings/Precautions

Oral: Staining of oral surfaces (mucosa, teeth, tooth restorations, dorsum of tongue) may occur; may be visible as soon as 1 week after therapy begins and is more pronounced when there is a heavy accumulation of unremoved plaque and when teeth fillings have rough surfaces. Stain does not have a clinically adverse effect,

(Continued)

Chlorhexidine Gluconate *(Continued)*

but because removal may not be possible, patient with frontal restoration should be advised of the potential permanency of the stain.

Topical: For topical use only. Keep out of eyes and ears. May stain fabric. There have been case reports of anaphylaxis following chlorhexidine disinfection. Not for preoperative preparation of face or head; avoid contact with meninges.

Pharmacodynamics/Kinetics

Topical hand sanitizer (Avagard™): Duration of antimicrobial protection: 6 hours

Oral rinse (Peridex®, PerioGard®):

Absorption: ~30% retained in the oral cavity following rinsing and slowly released into oral fluids; poorly absorbed

Time to peak, plasma: Oral rinse: Detectable levels not present after 12 hours

Excretion: Feces (~90%); urine (<1%)

Pregnancy Risk Factor B

Dosage Forms CHIP, periodontal pocket insertion (PerioChip®): 2.5 mg. **LIQ, topical** [surgical scrub] (3M™ Avagard™): 1% (500 mL); (BactoShield® CHG): 2% (120 mL, 480 mL, 750 mL, 1000 mL, 3800 mL); 4% (120 mL, 480 mL, 750 mL, 1000 mL, 3800 mL); (Betasept®): 4% (120 mL, 240 mL, 480 mL, 960 mL, 3840 mL); (ChloraPrep®): 2% (0.67 mL, 1.5 mL, 3 mL, 10.5 mL); (Chlorostat®): 2% (360 mL, 3840 mL); (Dyna-Hex): 2% (120 mL, 960 mL, 3840 mL); 4% (120 mL, 960 mL, 3840 mL); (Hibiclens®): 4% (15 mL, 120 mL, 240 mL, 480 mL, 960 mL, 3840 mL); (Stat Touch 2 [DSC]): 2% (946 mL, 3800 mL). **LIQ, oral rinse**: 0.12% (480 mL); (Peridex®): 0.12% (480 mL); (PerioGard®): 0.12% (480 mL). **SPONGE/BRUSH** (BactoShield® CHG, Hibiclens®): 4% per sponge/brush

Generic Available Yes: Oral liquid

Selected Readings

al-Tannir MA and Goodman HS, "A Review of Chlorhexidine and Its Use in Special Populations," *Spec Care Dentist*, 1994, 14(3):116-22.

Emerson D and Pierce C, "A Case of a Single Ingestion of 4% Hibiclens®," *Vet Hum Toxicol*, 1988, 30(6):583.

Ferretti GA, Brown AT, Raybould TP, et al, "Oral Antimicrobial Agents - Chlorhexidine," *NCI Monogr*, 1990, 9:51-5.

Greenstein G, Berman C, and Jaffin R, "Chlorhexidine. An Adjunct to Periodontal Therapy," *J Periodontol*, 1986, 57(6):370-7.

Johnson BT, "Uses of Chlorhexidine in Dentistry," *Gen Dent*, 1995, 43(2):126-32, 134-40.

Massano G, Ciocatto E, Rosabianca C, et al, "Striking Aminotransferase Rise After Chlorhexidine Self-Poisoning," *Lancet*, 1982, 1(8266):289.

Quinn MW and Bini RM, "Bradycardia Associated With Chlorhexidine Spray," *Arch Dis Child*, 1989, 64(6):892-3.

Yong D, Parker FC, and Foran SM, "Severe Allergic Reactions and Intra-Urethral Chlorhexidine Gluconate," *Med J Aust*, 1995, 162(5):257-8.

Yusof ZA, "Chlorhexidine Mouthwash: A Review of Its Pharmacological Activity, Clinical Effects, Uses and Abuses," *Dent J Malays*, 1988, 10(1):9-16.

2-Chlorodeoxyadenosine *see* Cladribine *on page 336*

Chloroethane *see* Ethyl Chloride *on page 544*

Chloromag® *see* Magnesium Chloride *on page 833*

Chloromag® *see* Magnesium Supplements *on page 837*

Chloromycetin® *see* Chloramphenicol *on page 297*

Chlorophyll (KLOR oh fil)

U.S. Brand Names Chloresium® [OTC]; Derifil® [OTC]; Nullo® [OTC]; PALS® [OTC]

Pharmacologic Category Gastrointestinal Agent, Miscellaneous

Synonyms Chlorophyllin

Use

Oral: Control fecal and urinary odors in colostomy, ileostomy, or incontinence

Topical: Promotes normal healing, relieves pain and swelling, and reduces malodors in wounds, burns, surface ulcers, abrasions and skin irritations

Local Anesthetic/Vasoconstrictor Precautions No information available to require special precautions

Effects on Dental Treatment No significant effects or complications reported

Dosage

Topical: Apply generously and cover with gauze, linen, or other appropriate dressing; do not change dressings more often than every 48-72 hours

Oral: Children >12 years and Adults: 1-2 tablets/day; may increase to 3 tablets/day

Ostomy: Take tablets orally or place in the appliance

Other Adverse Effects 1% to 10%: Gastrointestinal: Mild diarrhea, green stools

Generic Available Yes

Chlorophyllin *see* Chlorophyll *on page 302*

Chloroprocaine (klor oh PROE kane)

Related Information

Oral Pain *on page 1524*

U.S. Brand Names Nesacaine®; Nesacaine®-MPF

Canadian Brand Names Nesacaine®-CE

Pharmacologic Category Local Anesthetic

Synonyms Chloroprocaine Hydrochloride

Use Infiltration anesthesia and peripheral and epidural anesthesia

Local Anesthetic/Vasoconstrictor Precautions No information available to require special precautions

Effects on Dental Treatment No significant effects or complications reported

Dosage Dosage varies with anesthetic procedure, the area to be anesthetized, the vascularity of the tissues, depth of anesthesia required, degree of muscle relaxation required, and duration of anesthesia; range: 1.5-25 mL of 2% to 3% solution; single adult dose should not exceed 800 mg

Infiltration and peripheral nerve block: 1% to 2%

Infiltration, peripheral and central nerve block, including caudal and epidural block: 2% to 3%, without preservatives

Mechanism of Action Chloroprocaine HCl is benzoic acid, 4-amino-2-chloro-2-(diethylamino) ethyl ester monohydrochloride. Chloroprocaine is an ester-type local anesthetic, which stabilizes the neuronal membranes and prevents initiation and transmission of nerve impulses thereby affecting local anesthetic actions. Local anesthetics including chloroprocaine, reversibly prevent generation and conduction of electrical impulses in neurons by decreasing the transient increase in permeability to sodium. The differential sensitivity generally depends on the size of the fiber; small fibers are more sensitive than larger fibers and require a longer period for recovery. Sensory pain fibers are usually blocked first, followed by fibers that transmit sensations of temperature, touch, and deep pressure. High concentrations block sympathetic somatic sensory and somatic motor fibers. The spread of anesthesia depends upon the distribution of the solution. This is primarily dependent on the volume of drug injected.

Other Adverse Effects <1%: Myocardial depression, **hypotension, bradycardia, cardiovascular collapse**, edema, **anxiety, restlessness, disorientation, confusion, seizures, drowsiness, unconsciousness**, chills, urticaria, **nausea, vomiting**, transient stinging or burning at injection site, **tremor, blurred vision**, tinnitus, **respiratory arrest, anaphylactoid reactions**

Drug Interactions

Increased Effect/Toxicity: Avoid concurrent use of bupivacaine due to safety and efficacy concerns.

Decreased Effect: The para-aminobenzoic acid metabolite of chloroprocaine may decrease the efficacy of sulfonamide antibiotics.

Pharmacodynamics/Kinetics

Onset of action: 6-12 minutes

Duration: 30-60 minutes

Metabolism: Plasma cholinesterases

Excretion: Urine

Pregnancy Risk Factor C

Generic Available Yes

Selected Readings

Freeman DW and Arnold NI, "Paracervical Block With Low Doses of Chloroprocaine: Fetal and Maternal Effects," *JAMA*, 1975, 231(1):56-7.

Jankowsky EC, "Pharmacologic Aspects of Local Anesthetic Use," *Anesth Clin North Am*, 1990, 8:1-25.

Chloroprocaine Hydrochloride *see* Chloroprocaine *on page 302*

Chloroptic® *see* Chloramphenicol *on page 297*

Chloroptic-P® *see* Chloramphenicol and Prednisolone *on page 299*

Chloroquine (KLOR oh kwin)

U.S. Brand Names Aralen® Phosphate

Canadian Brand Names Aralen®

Pharmacologic Category Aminoquinoline (Antimalarial)

Synonyms Chloroquine Phosphate

Use Suppression or chemoprophylaxis of malaria; treatment of uncomplicated or mild to moderate malaria; extraintestinal amebiasis

Unlabeled/Investigational Use Treatment of rheumatoid arthritis, discoid lupus erythematosus, scleroderma, pemphigus

Local Anesthetic/Vasoconstrictor Precautions No information available to require special precautions

Effects on Dental Treatment Frequency not defined: Fatigue, personality changes, headache, nausea, vomiting, stomatitis, blurred vision

Dosage

Suppression or prophylaxis of malaria: Oral (dosage expressed in terms of mg of base):

Children: Administer 5 mg base/kg/week on the same day each week (not to exceed 300 mg base/dose); begin 1-2 weeks prior to exposure; continue for 4-6 weeks after leaving endemic area; if suppressive therapy is not begun prior to exposure, double the initial loading dose to 10 mg base/kg and administer in 2 divided doses 6 hours apart, followed by the usual dosage regimen

(Continued)

Chloroquine *(Continued)*

Adults: 300 mg/week (base) on the same day each week; begin 1-2 weeks prior to exposure; continue for 4-6 weeks after leaving endemic area; if suppressive therapy is not begun prior to exposure, double the initial loading dose to 600 mg base and administer in 2 divided doses 6 hours apart, followed by the usual dosage regimen

Acute attack:

Oral:

Children: 10 mg/kg on day 1, followed by 5 mg/kg 6 hours later and 5 mg/kg on days 2 and 3

Adults: 600 mg on day 1, followed by 300 mg 6 hours later, followed by 300 mg on days 2 and 3

I.M. (as hydrochloride):

Children: 5 mg/kg, repeat in 6 hours

Adults: Initial: 160-200 mg, repeat in 6 hours if needed; maximum: 800 mg first 24 hours; begin oral dosage as soon as possible and continue for 3 days until 1.5 g has been given

Extraintestinal amebiasis:

Children: Oral: 10 mg/kg once daily for 2-3 weeks (up to 300 mg base/day)

Adults:

Oral: 600 mg base/day for 2 days followed by 300 mg base/day for at least 2-3 weeks

I.M., as hydrochloride: 160-200 mg/day for 10 days; resume oral therapy as soon as possible

Dosing adjustment in renal impairment: Cl_{cr} <10 mL/minute: Administer 50% of dose

Hemodialysis: Minimally removed

Mechanism of Action Binds to and inhibits DNA and RNA polymerase; interferes with metabolism and hemoglobin utilization by parasites; inhibits prostaglandin effects; chloroquine concentrates within parasite acid vesicles and raises internal pH resulting in inhibition of parasite growth; may involve aggregates of ferriprotoporphyrin IX acting as chloroquine receptors causing membrane damage; may also interfere with nucleoprotein synthesis

Other Adverse Effects Frequency not defined:

Cardiovascular: **Hypotension** (rare), EKG changes (rare)

Dermatologic: Pruritus, hair bleaching, pleomorphic skin eruptions, alopecia, lichen planus eruptions, alopecia, mucosal pigmentary changes (blue-black)

Gastrointestinal: Diarrhea, anorexia

Hematologic: Blood dyscrasias

Ocular: Retinopathy (including irreversible changes in some patients long-term or high dose)

Otic: Nerve deafness, tinnitus

Drug Interactions Substrate of **CYP2D6, 3A4**; Inhibits CYP2D6

Increased Effect/Toxicity: Chloroquine serum concentrations may be elevated with concomitant cimetidine use.

Decreased Effect: Decreased absorption if administered concomitantly with kaolin and magnesium trisilicate.

Dietary/Ethanol/Herb Considerations Ethanol: Avoid use; may increase GI irritation.

Pharmacodynamics/Kinetics

Duration: Small amounts may be present in urine months following discontinuation of therapy

Absorption: Oral: Rapid (~89%)

Distribution: Widely in body tissues (eg, eyes, heart, kidneys, liver, lungs) where retention prolonged; crosses placenta; enters breast milk

Metabolism: Partially hepatic

Half-life elimination: 3-5 days

Time to peak, serum: 1-2 hours

Excretion: Urine (~70% as unchanged drug); acidification of urine increases elimination

Pregnancy Risk Factor C

Generic Available Yes

Chloroquine Phosphate *see* Chloroquine *on page 303*

Chlorostat® [OTC] *see* Chlorhexidine Gluconate *on page 300*

Chlorothiazide (klor oh THYE a zide)

Related Information

Cardiovascular Diseases *on page 1456*

U.S. Brand Names Diuril®

Canadian Brand Names Diuril®

Pharmacologic Category Diuretic, Thiazide

Use Management of mild to moderate hypertension, or edema associated with CHF or nephrotic syndrome in patients unable to take oral hydrochlorothiazide; when a thiazide is the diuretic of choice

Local Anesthetic/Vasoconstrictor Precautions No information available to require special precautions

Effects on Dental Treatment 1% to 10%: Orthostatic hypotension, epigastric distress

Dosage The manufacturer states that I.V. and oral dosing are equivalent. Some clinicians may use lower I.V. doses, however, because of chlorothiazide's poor oral absorption.

Infants <6 months:
 Oral: 20-40 mg/kg/day in 2 divided doses
 I.V.: 2-8 mg/kg/day in 2 divided doses
Infants >6 months and Children:
 Oral: 20 mg/kg/day in 2 divided doses
 I.V.: 4 mg/kg/day
Adults:
 Oral: 500 mg to 2 g/day divided in 1-2 doses
 I.V.: 100-500 mg/day (for edema only)
Elderly: Oral: 500 mg once daily **or** 1 g 3 times/week

Mechanism of Action Inhibits sodium reabsorption in the distal tubules causing increased excretion of sodium and water as well as potassium and hydrogen ions, magnesium, phosphate, calcium

Other Adverse Effects

1% to 10%:
 Dermatologic: Photosensitivity
 Endocrine & metabolic: Hypokalemia
 Gastrointestinal: Anorexia

<1% (Limited to important or life-threatening): Agranulocytosis, alopecia, aplastic anemia, cholecystitis, cutaneous vasculitis, diarrhea or constipation, **dizziness**, electrolyte imbalance, exfoliative dermatitis (I.V.), glycosuria, **headache**, hematuria (I.V.), hemolytic anemia, hypercalcemia, hyperglycemia, hyperuricemia or gout, hyponatremia, leukopenia, **muscle cramps or spasm, nausea**, necrotizing angiitis, pancreatitis, **paresthesia**, polyuria, pulmonary edema, purpura, rash, renal failure, **restlessness**, sexual ability (decreased), Stevens-Johnson syndrome, thrombocytopenia, toxic epidermal necrolysis (I.V.), uremia, urticaria, vasculitis, **vomiting, weakness**

Drug Interactions

Increased Effect/Toxicity: Increased effect of chlorothiazide with furosemide and other loop diuretics. Increased hypotension and/or renal adverse effects of ACE inhibitors may result in aggressively diuresed patients. Beta-blockers increase hyperglycemic effects of thiazides in Type 2 diabetes mellitus. Cyclosporine and thiazides can increase the risk of gout or renal toxicity. Digoxin toxicity can be exacerbated if a thiazide induces hypokalemia or hypomagnesemia. Lithium toxicity can occur with thiazides due to reduced renal excretion of lithium. Thiazides may prolong the duration of action with neuromuscular blocking agents.

Decreased Effect: Effects of oral hypoglycemics may be decreased. Decreased absorption of chlorothiazide with cholestyramine and colestipol. NSAIDs can decrease the efficacy of thiazides, reducing the diuretic and antihypertensive effects.

Dietary/Ethanol/Herb Considerations

Ethanol: Avoid use; may increase risk of hypotension or dizziness.

Food may increase serum concentration; May require decrease in dietary sodium and calcium and increase in potassium, zinc, magnesium, and riboflavin. Avoid caffeine, garlic and licorice.

Herb/Nutraceutical: Avoid black cohosh, dong quai, and evening primrose due to estrogenic activity. Dong quai and St John's wort may cause additional photosensitization. Avoid ephedra, ginseng, and yohimbe; may worsen hypertension. Avoid escin (from the horse chestnut seed); may have additive diuretic effects. Avoid garlic; may have increased antihypertensive effect. Avoid ginger due to positive inotropic effects; theoretically, may cause arrhythmia. Avoid hawthorn; may lower peripheral vascular resistance and cause more BP reductions. Avoid licorice due to mineralocorticoid activity.

Pharmacodynamics/Kinetics

Onset of action: Diuresis: Oral: 2 hours
Duration of diuretic action: Oral: 6-12 hours; I.V.: ~2 hours
Absorption: Oral: Poor
Half-life elimination: 1-2 hours
Time to peak, serum: Oral: ~4 hours

Pregnancy Risk Factor C (manufacturer); D (expert analysis)

Generic Available Yes: Tablet

Chlorothiazide and Methyldopa

(klor oh THYE a zide & meth il DOE pu)

Related Information

Chlorothiazide *on page 304*
Methyldopa *on page 891*

U.S. Brand Names Aldoclor®

(Continued)

Chlorothiazide and Methyldopa *(Continued)*

Canadian Brand Names Aldoclor®

Pharmacologic Category Antihypertensive Agent Combination

Synonyms Methyldopa and Chlorothiazide

Use Treatment of hypertension

Local Anesthetic/Vasoconstrictor Precautions No information available to require special precautions

Effects on Dental Treatment No significant effects or complications reported

Dosage Oral: 1 tablet 2-3 times/day for first 48 hours, then adjust

Dietary/Ethanol/Herb Considerations

Ethanol: Avoid use; may increase CNS depression.

Herb/Nutraceutical: Avoid gotu kola, kava, SAMe, St John's wort, and valerian; may increase CNS depression.

Pregnancy Risk Factor D

Generic Available No

Chlorothiazide and Reserpine (klor oh THYE a zide & re SER peen)

Related Information

Chlorothiazide *on page 304*

Reserpine *on page 1173*

U.S. Brand Names Diupres®

Pharmacologic Category Antihypertensive Agent Combination

Synonyms Reserpine and Chlorothiazide

Use Management of hypertension

Local Anesthetic/Vasoconstrictor Precautions No information available to require special precautions

Effects on Dental Treatment No significant effects or complications reported

Dosage Oral: 1-2 tablets 1-2 times/day

Dietary/Ethanol/Herb Considerations

Ethanol: Avoid use; may increase CNS depression.

Herb/Nutraceutical: Avoid gotu kola, kava, SAMe, St John's wort, and valerian; may increase CNS depression.

Pregnancy Risk Factor D

Generic Available Yes

Chloroxine (klor OKS een)

U.S. Brand Names Capitrol®

Canadian Brand Names Capitrol®

Pharmacologic Category Topical Skin Product

Use Treatment of dandruff or seborrheic dermatitis of the scalp

Local Anesthetic/Vasoconstrictor Precautions No information available to require special precautions

Effects on Dental Treatment No significant effects or complications reported

Dosage Use twice weekly, massage into wet scalp, avoid contact with eyes, lather should remain on the scalp for approximately 3 minutes, then rinsed; application should be repeated and the scalp rinsed thoroughly

Pregnancy Risk Factor C

Generic Available No

Chlorphenesin (klor FEN e sin)

U.S. Brand Names Maolate®

Canadian Brand Names Mycil®

Pharmacologic Category Skeletal Muscle Relaxant

Synonyms Chlorphenesin Carbamate

Use Adjunctive treatment of discomfort in short-term, acute, painful musculoskeletal conditions

Local Anesthetic/Vasoconstrictor Precautions No information available to require special precautions

Effects on Dental Treatment Frequency not defined: Drowsiness, confusion, increased nervousness, dizziness, paradoxical stimulation, headache, nausea, anaphylactoid reactions, drug fever

Dosage Adults: Oral: 800 mg 3 times/day, then adjusted to lowest effective dosage, usually 400 mg 4 times/day for up to a maximum of 2 months

Other Adverse Effects Frequency not defined:

Central nervous system: Insomnia

Gastrointestinal: Stomach cramps

Hematologic: Leukopenia, thrombocytopenia, agranulocytosis, pancytopenia (rare)

Dietary/Ethanol/Herb Considerations

Ethanol: Avoid use; may increase CNS depression.

Herb/Nutraceutical: Avoid gotu kola, kava, SAMe, St John's wort, and valerian; may increase CNS depression.

Pregnancy Risk Factor C

Generic Available No

Chlorphenesin Carbamate *see* Chlorphenesin *on page 306*

Chlorpheniramine (klor fen IR a meen)

Related Information

Oral Bacterial Infections *on page 1531*

U.S. Brand Names Aller-Chlor® [OTC]; Chlo-Amine® [OTC]; Chlor-Trimeton® [OTC]

Canadian Brand Names Chlor-Tripolon®

Pharmacologic Category Antihistamine

Synonyms Chlorpheniramine Maleate; CTM

Use Perennial and seasonal allergic rhinitis and other allergic symptoms including urticaria

Local Anesthetic/Vasoconstrictor Precautions No information available to require special precautions

Effects on Dental Treatment Chronic use of antihistamines will inhibit salivary flow, particularly in elderly patients; this may contribute to periodontal disease and oral discomfort.

>10%: Slight to moderate drowsiness, thickening of bronchial secretions

1% to 10%: Headache, excitability, nervousness, dizziness, nausea, weakness, pharyngitis, xerostomia, fatigue

Dosage

Children: Oral: 0.35 mg/kg/day in divided doses every 4-6 hours

2-6 years: 1 mg every 4-6 hours, not to exceed 6 mg in 24 hours

6-12 years: 2 mg every 4-6 hours, not to exceed 12 mg/day or sustained release 8 mg at bedtime

Children >12 years and Adults: Oral: 4 mg every 4-6 hours, not to exceed 24 mg/day or sustained release 8-12 mg every 8-12 hours, not to exceed 24 mg/day

Adults: Allergic reactions: I.M., I.V., S.C.: 10-20 mg as a single dose; maximum recommended dose: 40 mg/24 hours

Elderly: Oral: 4 mg once or twice daily. **Note:** Duration of action may be 36 hours or more when serum concentrations are low.

Hemodialysis: Supplemental dose is unnecessary

Mechanism of Action Competes with histamine for H_1-receptor sites on effector cells in the gastrointestinal tract, blood vessels, and respiratory tract

Other Adverse Effects 1% to 10%:

Gastrointestinal: Diarrhea, abdominal pain, appetite increase, weight gain

Genitourinary: Urinary retention

Neuromuscular & skeletal: Arthralgia

Ocular: Diplopia

Renal: Polyuria

Warnings/Precautions Causes sedation, caution must be used in performing tasks which require alertness (ie, operating machinery or driving). Sedative effects of CNS depressants or ethanol are potentiated. Use with caution in patients with angle-closure glaucoma, pyloroduodenal obstruction (including stenotic peptic ulcer), urinary tract obstruction (including bladder neck obstruction and symptomatic prostatic hyperplasia), hyperthyroidism, increased intraocular pressure, and cardiovascular disease (including hypertension and tachycardia). High sedative and anticholinergic properties, therefore may not be considered the antihistamine of choice for prolonged use in the elderly. May cause paradoxical excitation in pediatric patients, and can result in hallucinations, coma, and death in overdose.

Drug Interactions Substrate of CYP2D6, **3A4**; Inhibits **CYP2D6**

Increased Effect/Toxicity: CNS depressants may increase the degree of sedation and respiratory depression with antihistamines. May increase the absorption of digoxin. Central and/or peripheral anticholinergic syndrome can occur when administered with amantadine, rimantadine, narcotic analgesics, phenothiazines and other antipsychotics (especially with high anticholinergic activity), tricyclic antidepressants, quinidine, disopyramide, procainamide, and antihistamines.

Decreased Effect: May increase gastric degradation of levodopa and decrease the amount of levodopa absorbed by delaying gastric emptying. Therapeutic effects of cholinergic agents (tacrine, donepezil) and neuroleptics may be antagonized.

Dietary/Ethanol/Herb Considerations

Ethanol: Avoid use; may increase CNS depression.

Food: May be taken with food

Herb/Nutraceutical: Avoid gotu kola, kava, SAMe, St John's wort, and valerian; may increase CNS depression.

Pharmacodynamics/Kinetics Half-life elimination, serum: 20-24 hours

Pregnancy Risk Factor B

Generic Available Yes

Chlorpheniramine, Acetaminophen, and Pseudoephedrine *see* Acetaminophen, Chlorpheniramine, and Pseudoephedrine *on page 35*

Chlorpheniramine and Acetaminophen

(klor fen IR a meen & a seet a MIN oh fen)

Related Information

Acetaminophen *on page 27*
Chlorpheniramine *on page 307*

U.S. Brand Names Coricidin® [OTC]

Pharmacologic Category Antihistamine/Analgesic

Synonyms Acetaminophen and Chlorpheniramine

Use Symptomatic relief of congestion, headache, aches and pains of colds and flu

Local Anesthetic/Vasoconstrictor Precautions No information available to require special precautions

Effects on Dental Treatment Chronic use of antihistamines will inhibit salivary flow, particularly in elderly patients; this may contribute to periodontal disease and oral discomfort.

Dosage Adults: Oral: 2 tablets every 4 hours

Dietary/Ethanol/Herb Considerations

Ethanol: Avoid use; may increase CNS depression.
Herb/Nutraceutical: Avoid gotu kola, kava, SAMe, St John's wort, and valerian; may increase CNS depression.

Generic Available Yes

Selected Readings

Botting RM, "Mechanism of Action of Acetaminophen: Is There a Cyclooxygenase 3?," *Clin Infect Dis*, 2000, Suppl 5:S202-10.
Dart RC, Kuffner EK, and Rumack BH, "Treatment of Pain or Fever with Paracetamol (Acetaminophen) in the Alcoholic Patient: A Systematic Review," *Am J Ther*, 2000, 7(2):123-34.
Grant JA and Weiler JM, "A Report of a Rare Immediate Reaction After Ingestion of Acetaminophen," *Ann Allergy Asthma Immunol*, 2001, 87(3):227-9.
Kwan D, Bartle WR, and Walker SE, "The Effects of Acetaminophen on Pharmacokinetics and Pharmacodynamics of Warfarin," *J Clin Pharmacol*, 1999, 39(1):68-75.
McClain CJ, Price S, Barve S, et al, "Acetaminophen Hepatotoxicity: An Update," *Curr Gastroenterol Rep*, 1999, 1(1):42-9.
Shek KL, Chan LN, and Nutescu E, "Warfarin-Acetaminophen Drug Interaction Revisited," *Pharmacotherapy*, 1999, 19(10):1153-8.
Tanaka E, Yamazaki K, and Misawa S, "Update: The Clinical Importance of Acetaminophen Hepatotoxicity in Nonalcoholic and Alcoholic Subjects," *J Clin Pharm Ther*, 2000, 25(5):325-32.

Chlorpheniramine and Carbetapentane *see* Carbetapentane and Chlorpheniramine *on page 245*

Chlorpheniramine and Hydrocodone *see* Hydrocodone and Chlorpheniramine *on page 682*

Chlorpheniramine and Phenylephrine

(klor fen IR a meen & fen il EF rin)

Related Information

Chlorpheniramine *on page 307*

U.S. Brand Names Dallergy-D®; Ed A-Hist®; Histatab® Plus [OTC]; Histor-D®; Rolatuss® Plain; Ru-Tuss®

Pharmacologic Category Antihistamine/Decongestant Combination

Synonyms Phenylephrine and Chlorpheniramine

Use Temporary relief of nasal congestion and eustachian tube congestion as well as runny nose, sneezing, itching of nose or throat, itchy and watery eyes

Local Anesthetic/Vasoconstrictor Precautions Use with caution since phenylephrine is a sympathomimetic amine which could interact with epinephrine to cause a pressor response

Effects on Dental Treatment

Chlorpheniramine: Prolonged use will cause significant xerostomia
Phenylephrine: Up to 10% of patients could experience tachycardia, palpitations, and xerostomia (prolonged use worsens); use vasoconstrictor with caution

Dosage Oral:

Children:
2-5 years: 2.5 mL every 4 hours
6-12 years: 5 mL every 4 hours
Adults: 10 mL every 4 hours

Dietary/Ethanol/Herb Considerations

Ethanol: Avoid use; may increase CNS depression.
Herb/Nutraceutical: Avoid gotu kola, kava, SAMe, St John's wort, and valerian; may increase CNS depression.

Pregnancy Risk Factor C

Generic Available Yes

Chlorpheniramine and Pseudoephedrine

(klor fen IR a meen & soo doe e FED rin)

Related Information

Chlorpheniramine *on page 307*
Pseudoephedrine *on page 1146*

U.S. Brand Names Allerest® Maximum Strength [OTC]; Anamine® [OTC]; Anaplex® [OTC]; Chlorafed® [OTC]; Chlor-Trimeton® Allergy/Decongestant [OTC];

Codimal-LA® [OTC]; Codimal-LA® Half [OTC]; Co-Pyronil® 2 Pulvules® [OTC]; Deconamine® [OTC]; Deconamine® SR [OTC]; Fedahist® [OTC]; Hayfebrol® [OTC]; Histalet® [OTC]; Klerist-D® [OTC]; Pseudo-Gest Plus® [OTC]; Rhinosyn® [OTC]; Rhinosyn-PD® [OTC]; Ryna® [OTC]; Sudafed® Cold & Allergy [OTC]

Canadian Brand Names Triaminic® Cold & Allergy

Pharmacologic Category Antihistamine/Decongestant Combination

Synonyms Pseudoephedrine and Chlorpheniramine

Use Relief of nasal congestion associated with the common cold, hay fever, and other allergies, sinusitis, eustachian tube blockage, and vasomotor and allergic rhinitis

Local Anesthetic/Vasoconstrictor Precautions Use with caution since pseudoephedrine is a sympathomimetic amine which could interact with epinephrine to cause a pressor response

Effects on Dental Treatment

Chlorpheniramine: Prolonged use will cause significant xerostomia

Pseudoephedrine: Up to 10% of patients could experience tachycardia, palpitations, and xerostomia (prolonged use worsens); use vasoconstrictor with caution

Dosage Oral:

Capsule: One every 12 hours

Tablet: One 3-4 times/day

Dietary/Ethanol/Herb Considerations

Ethanol: Avoid use; may increase CNS depression.

Herb/Nutraceutical: Avoid gotu kola, kava, SAMe, St John's wort, and valerian; may increase CNS depression.

Pregnancy Risk Factor C

Generic Available Yes

Chlorpheniramine, Ephedrine, Phenylephrine, and Carbetapentane

(klor fen IR a meen, e FED rin, fen il EF rin, & kar bay tu PEN tane)

Related Information

Chlorpheniramine *on page 307*

U.S. Brand Names Rentamine® [OTC]; Rynatuss® [OTC]; Rynatuss® Pediatric Suspension [OTC]; Tri-Tannate Plus® [OTC]

Pharmacologic Category Antihistamine/Decongestant/Antitussive

Use Symptomatic relief of cough with a decongestant and an antihistamine

Local Anesthetic/Vasoconstrictor Precautions

Ephedrine: Use vasoconstrictors with caution since ephedrine may enhance cardiostimulation and vasopressor effects of sympathomimetics

Phenylephrine: Use with caution since phenylephrine is a sympathomimetic amine which could interact with epinephrine to cause a pressor response

Effects on Dental Treatment

Chlorpheniramine: Prolonged use will cause significant xerostomia

Ephedrine: No significant effects or complications reported

Phenylephrine: Up to 10% of patients could experience tachycardia, palpitations, and xerostomia; use vasoconstrictor with caution

Dosage Oral:

Children:

<2 years: Titrate dose individually

2-6 years: 2.5-5 mL every 12 hours

>6 years: 5-10 mL every 12 hours

Adults: 1-2 tablets every 12 hours

Dietary/Ethanol/Herb Considerations

Ethanol: Avoid use; may increase CNS depression.

Herb/Nutraceutical: Avoid gotu kola, kava, SAMe, St John's wort, and valerian; may increase CNS depression.

Pregnancy Risk Factor C

Generic Available Yes: Liquid

Chlorpheniramine, Hydrocodone, Phenylephrine, Acetaminophen, and Caffeine *see* Hydrocodone, Chlorpheniramine, Phenylephrine, Acetaminophen, and Caffeine *on page 686*

Chlorpheniramine Maleate *see* Chlorpheniramine *on page 307*

Chlorpheniramine, Phenylephrine, and Dextromethorphan

(klor fen IR a meen, fen il EF rin, & deks troe meth OR fan)

Related Information

Chlorpheniramine *on page 307*

Dextromethorphan *on page 423*

U.S. Brand Names Cerose-DM® [OTC]

Pharmacologic Category Antihistamine/Decongestant/Antitussive

Use Temporary relief of cough due to minor throat and bronchial irritation; relieves nasal congestion, runny nose and sneezing

(Continued)

Chlorpheniramine, Phenylephrine, and Dextromethorphan *(Continued)*

Local Anesthetic/Vasoconstrictor Precautions

Chlorpheniramine, Dextromethorphan: No information available to require special precautions

Phenylephrine: Use with caution since phenylephrine is a sympathomimetic amine which could interact with epinephrine to cause a pressor response

Effects on Dental Treatment

Chlorpheniramine: Prolonged use will cause significant xerostomia

Dextromethorphan: No significant effects or complications reported

Phenylephrine: Up to 10% of patients could experience tachycardia, palpitations, and xerostomia (prolonged use worsens); use vasoconstrictor with caution

Dosage Oral:

Children 6-12 years: 1/2 teaspoonful every 4 hour as needed; maximum: 6 doses/24 hours

Children >12 years and Adults: 1 teaspoonful every 4 hours as needed; maximum: 6 doses/24 hours

Dietary/Ethanol/Herb Considerations

Ethanol: Avoid use; may increase CNS depression.

Herb/Nutraceutical: Avoid gotu kola, kava, SAMe, St John's wort, and valerian; may increase CNS depression.

Generic Available No

Chlorpheniramine, Phenylephrine, and Methscopolamine

(klor fen IR a meen, fen il EF rin, & meth skoe POL a meen)

Related Information

Chlorpheniramine *on page 307*

U.S. Brand Names D.A.II™; Dallergy®; Dura-Vent®/DA; Extendryl; Extendryl JR; Extendryl SR

Pharmacologic Category Antihistamine/Decongestant/Anticholinergic

Use Treatment of upper respiratory symptoms such as respiratory congestion, allergic rhinitis, vasomotor rhinitis, sinusitis, and allergic skin reactions of urticaria and angioedema

Local Anesthetic/Vasoconstrictor Precautions Use with caution since phenylephrine is a sympathomimetic amine which could interact with epinephrine to cause a pressor response

Effects on Dental Treatment

Chlorpheniramine: Significant xerostomia (prolonged use)

Methscopolamine: Anticholinergic side effects can cause a reduction of saliva production or secretion contributes to discomfort and dental disease (ie, caries, oral candidiasis and periodontal disease)

Phenylephrine: ≤10%: Tachycardia, palpitations, and xerostomia; use vasoconstrictor with caution

Frequency not defined: Arrhythmias, bradycardia, cardiovascular collapse, flushing, hypotension, anxiety, convulsions, CNS depression, dizziness, drowsiness, excitability, fear, giddiness, hallucinations, headache, irritability, restlessness, tenseness, tremor, dysphagia, gastric irritation, nausea, weakness, blurred vision, nasal dryness, dry throat, respiratory difficulty

Dosage Oral: Relief of respiratory symptoms:

Children 6-11 years:

- D.A.II™: One tablet every 12 hours
- D.A. Chewable®, Extendryl chewable tablet: One tablet every 4 hours; do not exceed 4 doses in 24 hours
- Dallergy®: One-half caplet every 12 hours
- Dura-Vent®/DA: One-half tablet every 12 hours
- Extendryl JR: One capsule every 12 hours
- Extendryl syrup: 2.5-5 mL, may repeat up to every 4 hours depending on age and body weight

Children ≥12 years and Adults (if disturbances in urination occur in patients without renal impairment, medication should be discontinued for 1-2 days and should then be restarted at a lower dose):

- D.A.II™: Two tablets every 12 hours
- Dallergy®, Extendryl SR: 1 capsule every 12 hours
- Dura-Vent®/DA: One tablet every 12 hours
- D.A. Chewable®, Extendryl: 1-2 chewable tablets every 4 hours
- Extendryl syrup: 5-10 mL every 3-4 hours (4 times/day)

Elderly: Use with caution; population may have increased adverse reactions

Dosing adjustment in renal impairment: Use not recommended

Mechanism of Action

Chlorpheniramine maleate: Antihistamine

Phenylephrine hydrochloride: Sympathomimetic agent (primarily alpha), decongestant

Methscopolamine nitrate: Derivative of scopolamine, antisecretory effects

Other Adverse Effects Frequency not defined:

Cardiovascular: Pallor

Central nervous system: Insomnia, lassitude

Gastrointestinal: Constipation

Genitourinary: Dysuria, urinary retention

Ocular: Mydriasis

Drug Interactions

Increased Effect/Toxicity: Increased effects/toxicity seen with concomitant use of antihistamines, beta-adrenergic blockers, CNS depressants, and MAO inhibitors

Decreased Effect: Decreased effects of antihypertensive agents seen with concomitant use

Dietary/Ethanol/Herb Considerations

Ethanol: Avoid use; may increase CNS depression.

Herb/Nutraceutical: Avoid gotu kola, kava, SAMe, St John's wort, and valerian; may increase CNS depression.

Pregnancy Risk Factor C

Generic Available Yes

Chlorpheniramine, Phenylephrine, and Phenyltoloxamine

(klor fen IR a meen, fen il EF rin, & fen il tole LOKS a meen)

Related Information

Chlorpheniramine *on page 307*

U.S. Brand Names Comhist®; Comhist® LA

Pharmacologic Category Antihistamine/Decongestant Combination

Use Symptomatic relief of rhinitis and nasal congestion due to colds or allergy

Local Anesthetic/Vasoconstrictor Precautions Use with caution since phenylephrine is a sympathomimetic amine which could interact with epinephrine to cause a pressor response

Effects on Dental Treatment

Chlorpheniramine: Prolonged use will cause significant xerostomia

Phenylephrine: Up to 10% of patients could experience tachycardia, palpitations, and xerostomia; use vasoconstrictor with caution

Dosage Oral: 1 capsule every 8-12 hours or 1-2 tablets 3 times/day

Dietary/Ethanol/Herb Considerations

Ethanol: Avoid use; may increase CNS depression.

Herb/Nutraceutical: Avoid gotu kola, kava, SAMe, St John's wort, and valerian; may increase CNS depression.

Pregnancy Risk Factor C

Generic Available No

Chlorpheniramine, Phenylephrine, Codeine, and Potassium Iodide

(klor fen IR a meen, fen il EF rin, KOE deen & poe TASS ee um EYE oh dide)

Related Information

Chlorpheniramine *on page 307*

Codeine *on page 361*

U.S. Brand Names Pediacof®; Pedituss®

Pharmacologic Category Antihistamine/Decongestant/Antitussive/Expectorant

Use Symptomatic relief of rhinitis, nasal congestion and cough due to colds or allergy

Local Anesthetic/Vasoconstrictor Precautions Use with caution since phenylephrine is a sympathomimetic amine which could interact with epinephrine to cause a pressor response

Effects on Dental Treatment

Chlorpheniramine: Prolonged use will cause significant xerostomia

Phenylephrine: Up to 10% of patients could experience tachycardia, palpitations, and xerostomia (prolonged use worsens); use vasoconstrictor with caution

Restrictions C-V

Dosage Children 6 months to 12 years: 1.25-10 mL every 4-6 hours

Other Adverse Effects Codeine: <1%: **Xerostomia**

Dietary/Ethanol/Herb Considerations

Ethanol: Avoid use; may increase CNS depression.

Herb/Nutraceutical: Avoid gotu kola, kava, SAMe, St John's wort, and valerian; may increase CNS depression.

Generic Available No

Chlorpheniramine, Pseudoephedrine, and Acetaminophen *see* Acetaminophen, Chlorpheniramine, and Pseudoephedrine *on page 35*

Chlorpheniramine, Pseudoephedrine, and Codeine

(klor fen IR a meen, soo doe e FED rin, & KOE deen)

Related Information

Chlorpheniramine *on page 307*

Pseudoephedrine *on page 1146*

U.S. Brand Names Codehist® DH; Decohistine® DH; Dihistine® DH; Ryna-C®

(Continued)

Chlorpheniramine, Pseudoephedrine, and Codeine *(Continued)*

Pharmacologic Category Antihistamine/Decongestant/Antitussive

Use Temporary relief of cough associated with minor throat or bronchial irritation or nasal congestion due to common cold, allergic rhinitis, or sinusitis

Local Anesthetic/Vasoconstrictor Precautions Use with caution since pseudoephedrine is a sympathomimetic amine which could interact with epinephrine to cause a pressor response

Effects on Dental Treatment

≤10%: Pseudoephedrine: Tachycardia, palpitations, and xerostomia; use vasoconstrictor with caution

1% to 10%: Hypotension, sedation, dizziness, drowsiness, increased intracranial pressure, biliary tract spasm, physical or psychological dependence (prolonged use)

Frequency not defined: Chlorpheniramine: Significant xerostomia (prolonged use)

Restrictions C-V

Dosage Oral:

Children:

25-50 lb: 1.25-2.50 mL every 4-6 hours, up to 4 doses in 24-hour period

50-90 lb: 2.5-5 mL every 4-6 hours, up to 4 doses in 24-hour period

Adults: 10 mL every 4-6 hours, up to 4 doses in 24-hour period

Other Adverse Effects 1% to 10%:

Gastrointestinal: Constipation

Genitourinary: Urinary tract spasm

Dietary/Ethanol/Herb Considerations

Ethanol: Avoid use; may increase CNS depression.

Herb/Nutraceutical: Avoid gotu kola, kava, SAMe, St John's wort, and valerian; may increase CNS depression.

Pregnancy Risk Factor C

Generic Available Yes

Chlorpheniramine, Pyrilamine, and Phenylephrine

(klor fen IR a meen, pye RIL a meen, & fen il EF rin)

Related Information

Chlorpheniramine *on page 307*

U.S. Brand Names Rhinatate®; R-Tannamine®; R-Tannate®; Rynatan® Pediatric Suspension; Tanoral®; Triotann®; Tri-Tannate®

Pharmacologic Category Antihistamine/Decongestant Combination

Use Symptomatic relief of nasal congestion associated with upper respiratory tract condition

Local Anesthetic/Vasoconstrictor Precautions Use with caution since phenylephrine is a sympathomimetic amine which could interact with epinephrine to cause a pressor response

Effects on Dental Treatment

Chlorpheniramine: Prolonged use will cause significant xerostomia

Phenylephrine: Up to 10% of patients could experience tachycardia, palpitations, and xerostomia; use vasoconstrictor with caution

Dosage

Children:

2-6 years: 2.5-5 mL (pediatric suspension) every 12 hours

>6 years: 5-10 mL (pediatric suspension) every 12 hours

Adults: 1-2 tablets every 12 hours

Dietary/Ethanol/Herb Considerations

Ethanol: Avoid use; may increase CNS depression.

Herb/Nutraceutical: Avoid gotu kola, kava, SAMe, St John's wort, and valerian; may increase CNS depression.

Pregnancy Risk Factor C

Generic Available Yes

ChlorproMAZINE (klor PROE ma zeen)

U.S. Brand Names Thorazine®

Canadian Brand Names Apo®-Chlorpromazine; Largactil®; Novo-Chlorpromazine

Mexican Brand Names Largactil®

Pharmacologic Category Antipsychotic Agent, Phenothiazine, Aliphatic

Synonyms Chlorpromazine Hydrochloride; CPZ

Use Control of mania; treatment of schizophrenia; control of nausea and vomiting; relief of restlessness and apprehension before surgery; acute intermittent porphyria; adjunct in the treatment of tetanus; intractable hiccups; combativeness and/or explosive hyperexcitable behavior in children 1-12 years of age and in short-term treatment of hyperactive children

Unlabeled/Investigational Use Management of psychotic disorders

Local Anesthetic/Vasoconstrictor Precautions Most pharmacology textbooks state that in presence of phenothiazines, systemic doses of epinephrine paradoxically decrease the blood pressure. This is the so called "epinephrine reversal" phenomenon. This has never been observed when epinephrine is given by infiltration as part of the anesthesia procedure.

Effects on Dental Treatment

Significant hypotension may occur, especially when the drug is administered parenterally. Orthostatic hypotension is due to alpha-receptor blockade; elderly are at greater risk.

Tardive dyskinesia: Prevalence rate may be 40% in elderly; development of the syndrome and the irreversible nature are proportional to duration and total cumulative dose over time. Extrapyramidal reactions are more common in elderly with up to 50% developing these reactions after 60 years of age; drug-induced **Parkinson's syndrome** occurs often; **Akathisia** is the most common extrapyramidal reaction in elderly.

Increased confusion, memory loss, psychotic behavior, and agitation frequently occur as a consequence of anticholinergic effects. Antipsychotic associated sedation in nonpsychotic patients is extremely unpleasant due to feelings of depersonalization, derealization, and dysphoria

Frequency not defined: Postural hypotension, tachycardia, dizziness, drowsiness, dystonias, akathisia, pseudoparkinsonism, tardive dyskinesia, neuroleptic malignant syndrome, seizures, hyper- or hypoglycemia, nausea, xerostomia, blurred vision

Dosage

Children ≥6 months:

Schizophrenia/psychoses:

Oral: 0.5-1 mg/kg/dose every 4-6 hours; older children may require 200 mg/day or higher

I.M., I.V.: 0.5-1 mg/kg/dose every 6-8 hours

<5 years (22.7 kg): Maximum: 40 mg/day

5-12 years (22.7-45.5 kg): Maximum: 75 mg/day

Nausea and vomiting:

Oral: 0.5-1 mg/kg/dose every 4-6 hours as needed

I.M., I.V.: 0.5-1 mg/kg/dose every 6-8 hours

<5 years (22.7 kg): Maximum: 40 mg/day

5-12 years (22.7-45.5 kg): Maximum: 75 mg/day

Rectal: 1 mg/kg/dose every 6-8 hours as needed

Adults:

Schizophrenia/psychoses:

Oral: Range: 30-2000 mg/day in 1-4 divided doses, initiate at lower doses and titrate as needed; usual dose: 400-600 mg/day; some patients may require 1-2 g/day

I.M., I.V.: Initial: 25 mg, may repeat (25-50 mg) in 1-4 hours, gradually increase to a maximum of 400 mg/dose every 4-6 hours until patient is controlled; usual dose: 300-800 mg/day

Intractable hiccups: Oral, I.M.: 25-50 mg 3-4 times/day

Nausea and vomiting:

Oral: 10-25 mg every 4-6 hours

I.M., I.V.: 25-50 mg every 4-6 hours

Rectal: 50-100 mg every 6-8 hours

Elderly: Behavioral symptoms associated with dementia: Initial: 10-25 mg 1-2 times/day; increase at 4- to 7-day intervals by 10-25 mg/day. Increase dose intervals (bid, tid, etc) as necessary to control behavior response or side effects; maximum daily dose: 800 mg; gradual increases (titration) may prevent some side effects or decrease their severity.

Hemodialysis: Not dialyzable (0% to 5%)

Dosing comment in hepatic impairment: Avoid use in severe dysfunction

Mechanism of Action Blocks postsynaptic mesolimbic dopaminergic receptors in the brain; exhibits a strong alpha-adrenergic blocking effect and depresses the release of hypothalamic and hypophyseal hormones; believed to depress the reticular activating system, thus affecting basal metabolism, body temperature, wakefulness, vasomotor tone, and emesis

Other Adverse Effects Frequency not defined:

Cardiovascular: Nonspecific QT changes

Central nervous system: Neuroleptic malignant syndrome

Dermatologic: Photosensitivity, dermatitis, skin pigmentation (slate gray)

Endocrine & metabolic: Lactation, breast engorgement, false-positive pregnancy test, amenorrhea, gynecomastia, hyper- or hypoglycemia

Gastrointestinal: Constipation

Genitourinary: Urinary retention, ejaculatory disorder, impotence

Hematologic: Agranulocytosis, eosinophilia, leukopenia, hemolytic anemia, aplastic anemia, thrombocytopenic purpura

Hepatic: Jaundice

Ocular: Corneal and lenticular changes, epithelial keratopathy, pigmentary retinopathy

(Continued)

ChlorproMAZINE *(Continued)*

Drug Interactions Substrate of CYP1A2, **2D6**, 3A4; Inhibits CYP2D6, 2E1

Increased Effect/Toxicity: Effects on CNS depression may be additive when chlorpromazine is combined with CNS depressants (narcotic analgesics, ethanol, barbiturates, cyclic antidepressants, antihistamines, or sedative-hypnotics). Chlorpromazine may increase the effects/toxicity of anticholinergics, antihypertensives, lithium (rare neurotoxicity), trazodone, or valproic acid. Concurrent use with TCA may produce increased toxicity or altered therapeutic response. Chloroquine and propranolol may increase chlorpromazine concentrations. Hypotension may occur when chlorpromazine is combined with epinephrine. May increase the risk of arrhythmia when combined with antiarrhythmics, cisapride, pimozide, sparfloxacin, or other drugs which prolong QT interval. Metoclopramide may increase risk of extrapyramidal symptoms (EPS).

Decreased Effect: Phenothiazines inhibit the ability of bromocriptine to lower serum prolactin concentrations. Benztropine (and other anticholinergics) may inhibit the therapeutic response to chlorpromazine and excess anticholinergic effects may occur. Cigarette smoking and barbiturates may enhance the hepatic metabolism of chlorpromazine. Antihypertensive effects of guanethidine and guanadrel may be inhibited by chlorpromazine. Chlorpromazine may inhibit the antiparkinsonian effect of levodopa. Chlorpromazine and possibly other low potency antipsychotics may reverse the pressor effects of epinephrine.

Dietary/Ethanol/Herb Considerations

Ethanol: Avoid use; may increase CNS depression.

Food: Administer capsules and tablets with food to reduce GI upset; oral solution may be mixed with 2-4 oz of water, milk, or juice; avoid grapefruit juice (may increase serum levels) and caffeine-containing beverages.

Herb/Nutraceutical: Avoid dong quai; may enhance photosensitization. Avoid kava, gotu kola, SAMe, and valerian; may increase CNS depression. Avoid St John's wort; may decrease chlorpromazine levels, increase photosensitization, or enhance sedative effect.

Pharmacodynamics/Kinetics

Onset of action: I.M.: 15 minutes; Oral: 30-60 minutes

Absorption: Rapid

Distribution: V_d: 20 L/kg; crosses the placenta; enters breast milk

Protein binding: 92% to 97%

Metabolism: Extensively hepatic to active and inactive metabolites

Bioavailability: 20%

Half-life, biphasic: Initial: 2 hours; Terminal: 30 hours

Excretion: Urine (<1% as unchanged drug) within 24 hours

Pregnancy Risk Factor C

Generic Available Yes

Chlorpromazine Hydrochloride *see* ChlorproMAZINE *on page 312*

ChlorproPAMIDE (klor PROE pa mide)

Related Information

Endocrine Disorders and Pregnancy *on page 1479*

U.S. Brand Names Diabinese®

Canadian Brand Names Apo®-Chlorpropamide; Novo-Propamide

Mexican Brand Names Deavynfar; Diabinese®; Insogen®

Pharmacologic Category Antidiabetic Agent, Sulfonylurea

Use Management of blood sugar in type 2 diabetes mellitus (noninsulin dependent, NIDDM)

Unlabeled/Investigational Use Treatment of neurogenic diabetes insipidus

Local Anesthetic/Vasoconstrictor Precautions No information available to require special precautions

Effects on Dental Treatment Chlorpropamide-dependent diabetics (noninsulin dependent, Type 2) should be appointed for dental treatment in morning in order to minimize chance of stress-induced hypoglycemia.

>10%: Headache, dizziness, nausea, vomiting

Dosage Oral: The dosage of chlorpropamide is variable and should be individualized based upon the patient's response

Initial dose:

Adults: 250 mg/day in mild to moderate diabetes in middle-aged, stable diabetic

Elderly: 100-125 mg/day in older patients

Subsequent dosages may be increased or decreased by 50-125 mg/day at 3- to 5-day intervals

Maintenance dose: 100-250 mg/day; severe diabetics may require 500 mg/day; avoid doses >750 mg/day

Dosing comment in renal impairment: Cl_{cr} <50 mL/minute: Avoid use

Hemodialysis: Removed with hemoperfusion

Peritoneal dialysis: Supplemental dose is unnecessary

Dosing adjustment in hepatic impairment: Reduction recommended; conservative initial and maintenance doses are recommended because chlorpropamide undergoes extensive hepatic metabolism.

Mechanism of Action Stimulates insulin release from the pancreatic beta cells; reduces glucose output from the liver; insulin sensitivity is increased at peripheral target sites

Other Adverse Effects

>10%: Gastrointestinal: Anorexia, constipation, heartburn, epigastric fullness, diarrhea

1% to 10%: Dermatologic: Skin rash, urticaria, photosensitivity

<1%: Edema, hypoglycemia, hyponatremia, SIADH, blood dyscrasias, aplastic anemia, hemolytic anemia, bone marrow suppression, thrombocytopenia, agranulocytosis, cholestatic jaundice

Drug Interactions Substrate of CYP2C8/9

Increased Effect/Toxicity: A possible interaction between chlorpropamide and fluoroquinolone antibiotics has been reported resulting in a potentiation of hypoglycemic action of chlorpropamide. Toxic potential is increased when given concomitantly with other highly protein bound drugs (ie, phenylbutazone, oral anticoagulants, hydantoins, salicylates, NSAIDs, beta-blockers, sulfonamides) - increase hypoglycemic effect. Ethanol may be associated with disulfiram reactions. Phenylbutazone may increase hypoglycemic effects. Possible interactions between chlorpropamide and coumarin derivatives have been reported that may either potentiate or weaken the effects of coumarin derivatives.

Decreased Effect: Certain drugs tend to produce hyperglycemia and may lead to loss of control (ie, thiazides and other diuretics, corticosteroids, phenothiazines, thyroid products, estrogens, oral contraceptives, phenytoin, nicotinic acid, sympathomimetics, calcium channel blocking drugs, and isoniazid). Possible interactions between chlorpropamide and coumarin derivatives have been reported that may either potentiate or weaken the effects of coumarin derivatives.

Dietary/Ethanol/Herb Considerations

Ethanol: Avoid use; possible disulfiram-like reaction may occur.

Food: Administer consistently in regard to meals; dietary modification, based on ADA recommendations, is part of therapy. Hypoglycemia may occur; decrease blood glucose concentration.

Herb/Nutraceutical: Black cohosh can potentiate hypoglycemic effects of certain medications. Garlic can increase blood insulin levels increasing the risk of hypoglycemia.

Pharmacodynamics/Kinetics

Onset of action: Peak effect: ~6-8 hours

Distribution: V_d: 0.13-0.23 L/kg; enters breast milk

Protein binding: 60% to 90%

Metabolism: Extensively hepatic (~80%)

Half-life elimination: 30-42 hours; prolonged in elderly or with renal impairment

End-stage renal disease: 50-200 hours

Time to peak, serum: 3-4 hours

Excretion: Urine (10% to 30% as unchanged drug)

Pregnancy Risk Factor C

Generic Available Yes

Chlorthalidone (klor THAL i done)

Related Information

Cardiovascular Diseases *on page 1456*

U.S. Brand Names Thalitone®

Canadian Brand Names Apo®-Chlorthalidone

Mexican Brand Names Higroton 50

Pharmacologic Category Diuretic, Thiazide

Synonyms Hygroton® [DSC]

Use Management of mild to moderate hypertension when used alone or in combination with other agents; treatment of edema associated with CHF or nephrotic syndrome. Recent studies have found chlorthalidone effective in the treatment of isolated systolic hypertension in the elderly.

Local Anesthetic/Vasoconstrictor Precautions No information available to require special precautions

Effects on Dental Treatment 1% to 10%: Epigastric distress

Dosage Oral:

Children (nonapproved): 2 mg/kg/dose 3 times/week or 1-2 mg/kg/day

Adults: 25-100 mg/day or 100 mg 3 times/week

Elderly: Initial: 12.5-25 mg/day or every other day; there is little advantage to using doses >25 mg/day

Dosing adjustment in renal impairment: Cl_{cr} <10 mL/minute: Administer every 48 hours

Mechanism of Action Sulfonamide-derived diuretic that inhibits sodium and chloride reabsorption in the cortical-diluting segment of the ascending loop of Henle

(Continued)

Chlorthalidone *(Continued)*

Other Adverse Effects

1% to 10%:

Dermatologic: Photosensitivity

Endocrine & metabolic: Hypokalemia

Gastrointestinal: Anorexia

<1% (Limited to important or life-threatening): Agranulocytosis, aplastic anemia, cholecystitis, constipation, cutaneous vasculitis, diarrhea, **dizziness**, glycosuria, **headache**, hepatic function impairment, hypercalcemia, **hyperglycemia**, hyperuricemia or gout, hyponatremia, insomnia, leukopenia, **muscle cramps or spasm, nausea**, necrotizing angiitis, pancreatitis, paresthesia, polyuria, purpura, rash, **restlessness**, sexual ability (decreased), thrombocytopenia, urticaria, **vomiting**, vasculitis, **weakness**

Drug Interactions

Increased Effect/Toxicity: Increased effect of chlorthalidone with furosemide and other loop diuretics. Increased hypotension and/or renal adverse effects of ACE inhibitors may result in aggressively diuresed patients. Beta-blockers increase hyperglycemic effects of thiazides in Type 2 diabetes mellitus. Cyclosporine and thiazides can increase the risk of gout or renal toxicity. Digoxin toxicity can be exacerbated if a thiazide induces hypokalemia or hypomagnesemia. Lithium toxicity can occur with thiazides due to reduced renal excretion of lithium. Thiazides may prolong the duration of action with neuromuscular blocking agents.

Decreased Effect: Effects of oral hypoglycemics may be decreased. Decreased absorption of chlorthalidone with cholestyramine and colestipol. NSAIDs can decrease the efficacy of chlorthalidone, reducing the diuretic and antihypertensive effects.

Dietary/Ethanol/Herb Considerations

Food: Administer with food early in the day. Include potassium-rich foods in diet (citrus fruits, bananas); may cause a potassium loss requiring potassium supplement or medication to help prevent potassium loss.

Herb/Nutraceutical: Avoid black cohosh, dong quai, and evening primrose due to estrogenic activity. Dong quai and St John's Wort may cause photosensitization. Avoid ephedra, yohimbe, and ginseng; may worsen hypertension. Avoid escin (from the horse chestnut seed); may have additive diuretic effects. Avoid hawthorn; may lower peripheral vascular resistance and cause increased BP reductions.

Pharmacodynamics/Kinetics

Onset of action: Peak effect: 2-6 hours

Absorption: 65%

Distribution: Crosses placenta; enters breast milk

Metabolism: Hepatic

Half-life elimination: 35-55 hours; may be prolonged with renal impairment; Anuria: 81 hours

Excretion: Urine (~50% to 65% as unchanged drug)

Pregnancy Risk Factor B (manufacturer); D (expert analysis)

Generic Available Yes

Chlorthalidone and Atenolol *see* Atenolol and Chlorthalidone *on page 138*

Chlorthalidone and Clonidine *see* Clonidine and Chlorthalidone *on page 353*

Chlor-Trimeton® [OTC] *see* Chlorpheniramine *on page 307*

Chlor-Trimeton® Allergy/Decongestant [OTC] *see* Chlorpheniramine and Pseudoephedrine *on page 308*

Chlorzoxazone (klor ZOKS a zone)

Related Information

Temporomandibular Dysfunction (TMD) *on page 1562*

U.S. Brand Names Parafon Forte® DSC

Canadian Brand Names Parafon Forte®; Strifon Forte®

Pharmacologic Category Skeletal Muscle Relaxant

Use

Dental: Treatment of muscle spasm associated with acute temporomandibular joint pain

Medical: Treatment of muscle spasm associated with acute painful musculoskeletal conditions

Local Anesthetic/Vasoconstrictor Precautions No information available to require special precautions

Effects on Dental Treatment Frequency not defined: Dizziness, drowsiness, lightheadedness, paradoxical stimulation, malaise, nausea, vomiting

Dosage Oral:

Children: 20 mg/kg/day or 600 mg/m^2/day in 3-4 divided doses

Adults: 250-500 mg 3-4 times/day up to 750 mg 3-4 times/day

Mechanism of Action Acts on the spinal cord and subcortical levels by depressing polysynaptic reflexes

Other Adverse Effects Frequency not defined:

Dermatologic: Rash, petechiae, ecchymoses (rare), angioneurotic edema
Gastrointestinal: Stomach cramps
Genitourinary: Urine discoloration
Hepatic: Liver dysfunction
Miscellaneous: **Anaphylaxis (very rare)**

Contraindications Hypersensitivity to chlorzoxazone or any component of the formulation; impaired liver function

Drug Interactions Substrate of CYP1A2, 2A6, 2D6, **2E1**, 3A4; Inhibits CYP2E1, 3A4

Increased Effect/Toxicity: Alcohol, CNS depressants

Dietary/Ethanol/Herb Considerations

Ethanol: Avoid use; may increase CNS depression.
Herb/Nutraceutical: Avoid gotu kola, kava, SAMe, St John's wort, and valerian; may increase CNS depression.

Pharmacodynamics/Kinetics

Onset of action: ~1 hour
Duration: 6-12 hours
Absorption: Readily absorbed
Metabolism: Extensively hepatic via glucuronidation
Excretion: Urine (as conjugates)

Pregnancy Risk Factor C

Dosage Forms CAPLET (Parafon Forte® DSC): 500 mg. **TAB:** 250 mg

Generic Available Yes

Cholac® *see* Lactulose *on page 772*

Cholecalciferol (kole e kal SI fer ole)

U.S. Brand Names Delta-D®

Canadian Brand Names D-Vi-Sol®

Pharmacologic Category Vitamin D Analog

Synonyms D_3

Use Dietary supplement, treatment of vitamin D deficiency, or prophylaxis of deficiency

Local Anesthetic/Vasoconstrictor Precautions No information available to require special precautions

Effects on Dental Treatment Frequency not defined: Hypotension, arrhythmias, hypertension, irritability, headache, somnolence, nausea, vomiting, metallic taste, xerostomia, weakness, pain

Dosage Adults: Oral: 400-1000 units/day

Other Adverse Effects Frequency not defined:

Central nervous system: Overt psychosis (rare)
Dermatologic: Pruritus
Endocrine & metabolic: Polydipsia
Gastrointestinal: Anorexia, pancreatitis, constipation, weight loss
Genitourinary: Albuminuria, polyuria
Hepatic: Increased LFTs
Neuromuscular & skeletal: Bone pain, myalgia
Ocular: Conjunctivitis, photophobia
Renal: Azotemia, nephrocalcinosis

Drug Interactions Inhibits CYP2C8/9, 2C19, 2D6

Pregnancy Risk Factor C

Generic Available No

Comments Cholecalciferol 1 mg = 40,000 units of vitamin D activity

Cholera Vaccine (KOL er a vak SEEN)

Related Information

Immunizations (Vaccines) *on page 1612*

Canadian Brand Names Mutacol Berna®

Pharmacologic Category Vaccine

Use The World Health Organization no longer recommends cholera vaccination for travel to or from cholera-endemic areas. Some countries may still require evidence of a complete primary series or a booster dose given within 6 months of arrival. Vaccination should not be considered as an alternative to continued careful selection of foods and water. Ideally, cholera and yellow fever vaccines should be administered at least 3 weeks apart.

Local Anesthetic/Vasoconstrictor Precautions No information available to require special precautions

Effects on Dental Treatment >10%: Fever, headache

Restrictions Federal law requires that the date of administration, the vaccine manufacturer, lot number of vaccine, and the administering person's name, title and address be entered into the patient's permanent medical record.
(Continued)

Cholera Vaccine *(Continued)*

Dosage

Children:

6 months to 4 years: Two 0.2 mL doses I.M./S.C. 1 week to 1 month apart; booster doses (0.2 mL I.M./S.C.) every 6 months

5-10 years: Two 0.3 mL doses I.M./S.C. or two 0.2 mL intradermal doses 1 week to 1 month apart; booster doses (0.3 mL I.M./S.C. or 0.2 mL I.D.) every 6 months

Children ≥10 years and Adults: Two 0.5 mL doses given I.M./S.C. or two 0.2 mL doses I.D. 1 week to 1 month apart; booster doses (0.5 mL I.M. or S.C. or 0.2 mL I.D.) every 6 months

Mechanism of Action Inactivated vaccine producing active immunization

Other Adverse Effects All serious adverse reactions must be reported to the U.S. Department of Health and Human Services (DHHS) Vaccine Adverse Event Reporting System (VAERS) 1-800-822-7967.

>10%:

Central nervous system: Malaise

Local: Pain, edema, tenderness, erythema, and induration at injection site

Pregnancy Risk Factor C

Generic Available No

Comments Inactivated bacteria vaccine

Cholestyramine Resin (koe LES tir a meen REZ in)

Related Information

Cardiovascular Diseases *on page 1456*

U.S. Brand Names LoCHOLEST®; LoCHOLEST® Light; Prevalite®; Questran®; Questran® Light

Canadian Brand Names Novo-Cholamine; Novo-Cholamine Light; PMS-Cholestyramine; Questran®; Questran® Light Sugar Free

Pharmacologic Category Antilipemic Agent, Bile Acid Sequestrant

Use Adjunct in the management of primary hypercholesterolemia; pruritus associated with elevated levels of bile acids; diarrhea associated with excess fecal bile acids; binding toxicologic agents; pseudomembraneous colitis

Local Anesthetic/Vasoconstrictor Precautions No information available to require special precautions

Effects on Dental Treatment

>10%: Nausea, vomiting,

1% to 10%: Headache, belching

Dosage Oral (dosages are expressed in terms of anhydrous resin):

Powder:

Children: 240 mg/kg/day in 3 divided doses; need to titrate dose depending on indication

Adults: 4 g 1-2 times/day to a maximum of 24 g/day and 6 doses/day

Dialysis: Not removed by hemo- or peritoneal dialysis; supplemental doses unnecessary with dialysis or continuous arteriovenous or venovenous hemofiltration

Mechanism of Action Forms a nonabsorbable complex with bile acids in the intestine, releasing chloride ions in the process; inhibits enterohepatic reuptake of intestinal bile salts and thereby increases the fecal loss of bile salt-bound low density lipoprotein cholesterol

Other Adverse Effects

>10%: Gastrointestinal: Constipation, heartburn, stomach pain

1% to 10%: Gastrointestinal: Bloating, diarrhea

<1% (Limited to important or life-threatening): Hyperchloremic acidosis, gallstones or pancreatitis, **GI bleeding, peptic ulcer**, steatorrhea or malabsorption syndrome, hypoprothrombinemia (secondary to vitamin K deficiency)

Drug Interactions Decreased Effect: Cholestyramine resin may cause decreased absorption of digitalis glycosides (oral), warfarin, thyroid hormones, thiazide diuretics, propranolol, phenobarbital, amiodarone, methotrexate, NSAIDs, and other drugs.

Dietary/Ethanol/Herb Considerations

Food: Mix powder with applesauce, fluid, jello, or pudding. High doses or long-term therapy may decrease the absorption of folic acid, calcium, iron, and fat-soluble vitamins A, D, E, and K. Supplementation may be required.

Pharmacodynamics/Kinetics

Onset of action: Peak effect: 21 days

Absorption: None

Excretion: Feces (as insoluble complex with bile acids)

Pregnancy Risk Factor C

Generic Available Yes

Choline Magnesium Trisalicylate

(KOE leen mag NEE zee um trye sa LIS i late)

Related Information

Rheumatoid Arthritis, Osteoarthritis, and Osteoporosis *on page 1488*
Temporomandibular Dysfunction (TMD) *on page 1562*

U.S. Brand Names Tricosal®; Trilisate®

Pharmacologic Category Salicylate

Use Management of osteoarthritis, rheumatoid arthritis, and other arthritis; salicylate salts may not inhibit platelet aggregation and, therefore, should not be substituted for aspirin in the prophylaxis of thrombosis; acute painful shoulder

Local Anesthetic/Vasoconstrictor Precautions No information available to require special precautions

Effects on Dental Treatment NSAID formulations are known to reversibly decrease platelet aggregation via mechanisms different than observed with aspirin. The dentist should be aware of the potential of abnormal coagulation. Caution should also be exercised in the use of NSAIDs in patients already on anticoagulant therapy with drugs such as warfarin (Coumadin®).

<20%: Nausea, vomiting, epigastric pain
<2%: Headache, lightheadedness, dizziness, drowsiness, lethargy

Dosage Oral (based on total salicylate content):

Children <37 kg: 50 mg/kg/day given in 2 divided doses
Adults: 500 mg to 1.5 g 2-3 times/day; usual maintenance dose: 1-4.5 g/day
Dosing comment in renal impairment: Avoid use in severe impairment.

Mechanism of Action Inhibits prostaglandin synthesis; acts on the hypothalamus heat-regulating center to reduce fever; blocks the generation of pain impulses

Other Adverse Effects

<20%:
Gastrointestinal: Diarrhea, heartburn, dyspepsia, constipation
Otic: Tinnitus

<2%: Otic: Hearing impairment

<1%: **Gastric ulceration**, occult bleeding, increased BUN and creatinine, rash, pruritus, anorexia, weight gain, edema, **epistaxis, dysgeusia**

Drug Interactions

Increased Effect/Toxicity: Choline magnesium trisalicylate may increase the hypoprothrombinemic effect of warfarin.

Decreased Effect: Antacids may decrease choline magnesium trisalicylate absorption/ salicylate concentrations.

Dietary/Ethanol/Herb Considerations

Ethanol: Avoid use; may enhance gastric mucosal irritation and cause bleeding.

Administer with food or milk; may decrease rate but not extent of oral absorption. Limit Benedictine liqueur, curry powder, licorice, paprika, prunes, raisins, tea, and gherkins; may cause salicylate accumulation. Also limit intake of foods containing vitamin C. Avoid magnesium or use with caution in renal insufficiency; may cause hypermagnesemia. Avoid garlic, ginger, and green tea.

Herb/Nutraceutical: Avoid cat's claw, dong quai, evening primrose, feverfew, garlic, ginger, ginkgo biloba, ginseng, green tea, horse chestnut, and red clover due to additional antiplatelet activity. Limit licorice due to salicylate content.

Pharmacodynamics/Kinetics

Onset of action: Peak effect: ~2 hours
Absorption: Stomach and small intestines
Distribution: Readily into most body fluids and tissues; crosses placenta; enters breast milk
Half-life elimination (dose dependent): Low dose: 2-3 hours; High dose: 30 hours
Time to peak, serum: ~2 hours

Pregnancy Risk Factor C/D (3rd trimester)

Generic Available Yes

Choline Salicylate (KOE leen sa LIS i late)

Related Information

Rheumatoid Arthritis, Osteoarthritis, and Osteoporosis *on page 1488*
Temporomandibular Dysfunction (TMD) *on page 1562*

U.S. Brand Names Arthropan® [OTC]

Canadian Brand Names Teejel®

Pharmacologic Category Salicylate

Use Temporary relief of pain of rheumatoid arthritis, rheumatic fever, osteoarthritis, and other conditions for which oral salicylates are recommended; useful in patients in which there is difficulty in administering doses in a tablet or capsule dosage form, because of the liquid dosage form

Local Anesthetic/Vasoconstrictor Precautions No information available to require special precautions

Effects on Dental Treatment NSAID formulations are known to reversibly decrease platelet aggregation via mechanisms different than observed with aspirin. The dentist should be aware of the potential of abnormal coagulation. Caution

(Continued)

Choline Salicylate *(Continued)*

should also be exercised in the use of NSAIDs in patients already on anticoagulant therapy with drugs such as warfarin (Coumadin®).

>10%: Nausea, epigastric discomfort

1% to 10%: Gastrointestinal ulceration, weakness, dyspnea, anaphylactic shock, fatigue

Dosage

Children >12 years and Adults: Oral: 5 mL (870 mg) every 3-4 hours, if necessary, but not more than 6 doses in 24 hours

Rheumatoid arthritis: 870-1740 mg (5-10 mL) up to 4 times/day

Dosing comment in renal impairment: Avoid use in severe impairment.

Mechanism of Action Inhibits prostaglandin synthesis; acts on the hypothalamus heat-regulating center to reduce fever; blocks the generation of pain impulses

Other Adverse Effects

>10%: Gastrointestinal: Heartburn, stomach pains, dyspepsia

1% to 10%:

Dermatologic: Rash

Hematologic: Hemolytic anemia

<1%: Insomnia, **nervousness, jitters**, occult bleeding, **prolongation of bleeding time**, leukopenia, thrombocytopenia, iron-deficiency anemia, hepatotoxicity, impaired renal function, **bronchospasm**

Drug Interactions

Increased Effect/Toxicity: Effect of warfarin may be increased.

Decreased Effect: Decreased effect of salicylates with antacids. Effect of ACE-inhibitors and diuretics may be decreased by concurrent therapy with NSAIDs.

Pharmacodynamics/Kinetics

Absorption: Stomach and small intestines in ~2 hours

Distribution: Readily into most body fluids and tissues; crosses placenta; enters breast milk

Protein binding: 75% to 90%

Metabolism: Hepatically hydrolyzed to salicylate

Half-life elimination (dose dependent): Low dose: 2-3 hours; High dose: 30 hours

Time to peak, serum: 1-2 hours

Excretion: Urine

Pregnancy Risk Factor C/D (3rd trimester)

Generic Available No

Chondroitin Sulfate and Sodium Hyaluronate

(kon DROY tin SUL fate and SOW de um hye al yoor ON ate)

U.S. Brand Names Viscoat®

Pharmacologic Category Ophthalmic Agent, Viscoelastic

Synonyms Sodium Hyaluronate-Chrondroitin Sulfate

Use Surgical aid in anterior segment procedures, protects corneal endothelium and coats intraocular lens thus protecting it

Local Anesthetic/Vasoconstrictor Precautions No information available to require special precautions

Effects on Dental Treatment No significant effects or complications reported

Dosage Carefully introduce (using a 27-gauge needle or cannula) into anterior chamber after thoroughly cleaning the chamber with a balanced salt solution

Mechanism of Action Functions as a tissue lubricant and is thought to play an important role in modulating the interactions between adjacent tissues

Other Adverse Effects 1% to 10%: Ocular: Increased intraocular pressure

Pharmacodynamics/Kinetics

Absorption: Intravitreous injection: Diffusion occurs slowly

Excretion: By Canal of Schlemm

Pregnancy Risk Factor C

Generic Available No

Chooz® [OTC] *see* Calcium Supplements *on page 229*

Chorex® *see* Chorionic Gonadotropin (Human) *on page 320*

Choriogonadotropin Alfa *see* Chorionic Gonadotropin (Recombinant) *on page 321*

Chorionic Gonadotropin (Human)

(kor ee ON ik goe NAD oh troe pin)

Related Information

Chorionic Gonadotropin (Recombinant) *on page 321*

U.S. Brand Names A.P.L.®; Chorex®; Choron®; Gonic®; Novarel™; Pregnyl®; Profasi®

Canadian Brand Names Humegon®; Pregnyl®; Profasi® HP

Pharmacologic Category Ovulation Stimulator

Synonyms CG; hCG

Use Induces ovulation and pregnancy in anovulatory, infertile females; treatment of hypogonadotropic hypogonadism, prepubertal cryptorchidism; spermatogenesis induction with follitropin alfa or follitropin beta

Local Anesthetic/Vasoconstrictor Precautions No information available to require special precautions

Effects on Dental Treatment No significant effects or complications reported

Dosage I.M.:

Children:

Prepubertal cryptorchidism: 1000-2000 units/m^2/dose 3 times/week for 3 weeks **OR** 4000 units 3 times/week for 3 weeks **OR** 5000 units every second day for 4 injections **OR** 500 units 3 times/week for 4-6 weeks

Hypogonadotropic hypogonadism: 500-1000 units 3 times/week for 3 weeks, followed by the same dose twice weekly for 3 weeks **OR** 1000-2000 units 3 times/week **OR** 4000 units 3 times/week for 6-9 months; reduce dosage to 2000 units 3 times/week for additional 3 months

Adults:

Induction of ovulation: Female: 5000-10,000 units one day following last dose of menotropins

Spermatogenesis induction: Male: Initial: 1500 int. units twice weekly to normalize serum testosterone levels. If no response in 8 weeks, increase dose to 3000 int. units twice weekly. After normalization of testosterone levels, combine with follitropin beta (Follistim®). Continue hCG at same dose used to normalize testosterone levels. Treatment response was noted at up to 12 months.

Mechanism of Action Stimulates production of gonadal steroid hormones by causing production of androgen by the testis; as a substitute for luteinizing hormone (LH) to stimulate ovulation

Other Adverse Effects

1% to 10%:

Central nervous system: Mental depression

Endocrine & metabolic: Pelvic pain, ovarian cysts, enlargement of breasts, precocious puberty

Local: Pain at the injection site

Neuromuscular & skeletal: Premature closure of epiphyses

<1%: Peripheral edema, **irritability, restlessness, headache**, ovarian hyperstimulation syndrome, gynecomastia

Pharmacodynamics/Kinetics

Half-life elimination: Biphasic: Initial: 11 hours; Terminal: 23 hours

Excretion: Urine (as unchanged drug) within 3-4 days

Pregnancy Risk Factor C

Generic Available Yes

Chorionic Gonadotropin (Recombinant)

(kor ee ON ik goe NAD oh troe pin ree KOM be nant)

Related Information

Chorionic Gonadotropin (Human) *on page 320*

U.S. Brand Names Ovidrel®

Pharmacologic Category Gonadotropin; Ovulation Stimulator

Synonyms Choriogonadotropin Alfa; r-hCG

Use As part of an assisted reproductive technology (ART) program, induces ovulation in infertile females who have been pretreated with follicle stimulating hormones (FSH); induces ovulation and pregnancy in infertile females when the cause of infertility is functional

Local Anesthetic/Vasoconstrictor Precautions No information available to require special precautions

Effects on Dental Treatment

3%: Nausea, vomiting

<2%: Arrhythmia, dizziness, fever, headache, hot flashes, hyperglycemia, paresthesias, cough, pharyngitis, upper respiratory tract infection, hiccups, malaise

Dosage S.C.:

Adults: Female: Assisted reproductive technologies (ART) and ovulation induction: 250 mcg given 1 day following the last dose of follicle stimulating agent. Use only after adequate follicular development has been determined. Hold treatment when there is an excessive ovarian response.

Dosing adjustment for elderly or in renal/hepatic impairment: Safety and efficacy not established

Mechanism of Action Luteinizing hormone analogue produced by recombinant DNA techniques; stimulates rupture of the ovarian follicle once follicular development has occurred.

Other Adverse Effects

2% to 10%:

Endocrine & metabolic: Ovarian cyst (3%), ovarian hyperstimulation (<2% to 3%)

Gastrointestinal: Abdominal pain (3% to 4%)

Local: Injection site: Pain (8%), bruising (3% to 5%), reaction (<2% to 3%), inflammation (<2% to 2%)

Miscellaneous: Postoperative pain (5%)

(Continued)

Chorionic Gonadotropin (Recombinant) *(Continued)*

<2%:

Cardiovascular: Heart murmur

Central nervous system: Emotional lability, insomnia

Dermatologic: Pruritus, rash

Endocrine & metabolic: Breast pain, intermenstrual bleeding, vaginal hemorrhage

Gastrointestinal: Abdominal enlargement, diarrhea, flatulence

Genitourinary: Cervical carcinoma, cervical lesion, dysuria, genital herpes, genital moniliasis, leukorrhea, urinary incontinence, urinary tract infection, vaginitis

Hematologic: Leukocytosis

Neuromuscular & skeletal: Back pain

Renal: Albuminuria

Miscellaneous: Ectopic pregnancy

In addition, the following have been reported with menotropin therapy: Adnexal torsion, hemoperitoneum, mild to moderate ovarian enlargement, pulmonary and vascular complications. Ovarian neoplasms have also been reported (rare) with multiple drug regimens used for ovarian induction (relationship not established).

Pharmacodynamics/Kinetics

Distribution: V_d: 5.9 ± 1 L

Bioavailability: 40%

Half-life elimination: Initial: 4 hours; Terminal: 29 hours

Time to peak: 12-24 hours

Excretion: Urine ($^1/_{10}{}^{th}$ of dose)

Pregnancy Risk Factor X

Generic Available No

Choron® *see* Chorionic Gonadotropin (Human) *on page 320*

Chromium *see* Trace Metals *on page 1328*

Chymodiactin® *see* Chymopapain *on page 322*

Chymopapain (KYE moe pa pane)

U.S. Brand Names Chymodiactin®

Pharmacologic Category Enzyme

Use Alternative to surgery in patients with herniated lumbar intervertebral discs

Local Anesthetic/Vasoconstrictor Precautions No information available to require special precautions

Effects on Dental Treatment 1% to 10%: Dizziness, headache, nausea, weakness in legs

Dosage Adults: 2000-4000 units/disc with a maximum cumulative dose not to exceed 8000 units for patients with multiple disc herniations

Mechanism of Action Chymopapain, when injected into the disc center, causes hydrolysis of the mucal mucopolysaccharide protein complex into acid polysaccharide, polypeptides, and amino acids. Subsequently, the water trapping properties of the nucleus pulposus are destroyed which permanently diminishes the pressure within the disc. The adjacent structures including the annulus fibrosus are not affected by chymopapain.

Other Adverse Effects >10%: Neuromuscular & skeletal: Back pain

Pregnancy Risk Factor C

Generic Available No

Ciclopirox (sye kloe PEER oks)

Related Information

Oral Fungal Infections *on page 1542*

U.S. Brand Names Loprox®; Penlac™

Canadian Brand Names Loprox®; Penlac™

Mexican Brand Names Loprox®

Pharmacologic Category Antifungal Agent, Topical

Synonyms Ciclopirox Olamine

Use

Cream/lotion: Treatment of tinea pedis (athlete's foot), tinea cruris (jock itch), tinea corporis (ringworm), cutaneous candidiasis, and tinea versicolor (pityriasis)

Lacquer: Topical treatment of mild to moderate onychomycosis of the fingernails and toenails due to *Trichophyton rubrum*

Local Anesthetic/Vasoconstrictor Precautions No information available to require special precautions

Effects on Dental Treatment No significant effects or complications reported

Dosage Children >10 years and Adults:

Cream/lotion: Apply twice daily, gently massage into affected areas; if no improvement after 4 weeks of treatment, re-evaluate the diagnosis

Lacquer: Apply to affected nails daily (as a part of a comprehensive management program for onychomycosis)

Mechanism of Action Inhibiting transport of essential elements in the fungal cell causing problems in synthesis of DNA, RNA, and protein

Other Adverse Effects 1% to 10%:
Dermatologic: Pruritus
Local: Irritation, redness, burning, or pain

Pharmacodynamics/Kinetics
Absorption: <2% through intact skin
Distribution: To epidermis, corium (dermis), including hair, hair follicles, and sebaceous glands
Protein binding: 94% to 98%
Half-life elimination: 1.7 hours
Excretion: Urine and feces (small amounts)

Pregnancy Risk Factor B

Generic Available No

Ciclopirox Olamine *see* Ciclopirox *on page 322*

Cidofovir (si DOF o veer)

Related Information
Systemic Viral Diseases *on page 1517*

U.S. Brand Names Vistide®

Pharmacologic Category Antiviral Agent

Use Treatment of cytomegalovirus (CMV) retinitis in patients with acquired immunodeficiency syndrome (AIDS). **Note:** Should be administered with probenecid.

Local Anesthetic/Vasoconstrictor Precautions No information available to require special precautions

Effects on Dental Treatment
>10%: Infection, fever, headache, amnesia, anxiety, confusion, seizures, nausea, vomiting, gastritis, weakness, paresthesia, asthma, bronchitis, cough, dyspnea, pharyngitis
1% to 10%: Hypotension, syncope, tachycardia, dizziness, hallucinations, somnolence, hyperglycemia, dehydration, stomatitis, abnormal taste, pneumonia, rhinitis, sinusitis, diaphoresis, allergic reactions

Dosage
Induction: 5 mg/kg I.V. over 1 hour once weekly for 2 consecutive weeks
Maintenance: 5 mg/kg over 1 hour once every other week
Administer with probenecid - 2 g orally 3 hours prior to each cidofovir dose and 1 g at 2 and 8 hours after completion of the infusion (total: 4 g)
Hydrate with 1 L of 0.9% NS I.V. prior to cidofovir infusion; a second liter may be administered over a 1- to 3-hour period immediately following infusion, if tolerated
Dosing adjustment in renal impairment:
Cl_{cr} 41-55 mL/minute: 2 mg/kg
Cl_{cr} 30-40 mL/minute: 1.5 mg/kg
Cl_{cr} 20-29 mL/minute: 1 mg/kg
Cl_{cr} <19 mL/minute: 0.5 mg/kg
If the creatinine increases by 0.3-0.4 mg/dL, reduce the cidofovir dose to 3 mg/kg; discontinue therapy for increases ≥0.5 mg/dL or development of ≥3+ proteinuria

Mechanism of Action Cidofovir is converted to cidofovir diphosphate which is the active intracellular metabolite; cidofovir diphosphate suppresses CMV replication by selective inhibition of viral DNA synthesis. Incorporation of cidofovir into growing viral DNA chain results in reductions in the rate of viral DNA synthesis.

Other Adverse Effects
>10%:
Central nervous system: Chills, amnesia, insomnia
Dermatologic: Alopecia, rash, acne, skin discoloration
Gastrointestinal: Diarrhea, anorexia, abdominal pain, constipation, dyspepsia
Hematologic: Thrombocytopenia, neutropenia, anemia
Ocular: Amblyopia, conjunctivitis, ocular hypotony
Renal: Tubular damage, proteinuria, elevated creatinine
1% to 10%:
Cardiovascular: Pallor
Central nervous system: Depression, malaise
Dermatologic: Pruritus, urticaria
Endocrine & metabolic: Hyperlipidemia, hypocalcemia, hypokalemia
Genitourinary: Glycosuria, urinary incontinence, urinary tract infections
Neuromuscular & skeletal: Skeletal pain
Ocular: Retinal detachment, iritis, uveitis, abnormal vision
Renal: Hematuria
<1% (Limited to life-threatening or significant reactions): Fanconi syndrome, increased bicarbonate excretion, metabolic acidosis, hepatic failure, pancreatitis, uveitis, iritis

Drug Interactions Increased Effect/Toxicity: Drugs with nephrotoxic potential (eg, amphotericin B, aminoglycosides, foscarnet, and I.V. pentamidine) should be avoided during cidofovir therapy.

Dietary/Ethanol/Herb Considerations Administer with food to reduce GI upset.

Pharmacodynamics/Kinetics The following pharmacokinetic data is based on a combination of cidofovir administered with probenecid
(Continued)

Cidofovir *(Continued)*

Distribution: V_d: 0.54 L/kg; does not cross significantly into CSF
Protein binding: <6%
Metabolism: Minimal; phosphorylation occurs intracellularly
Half-life elimination, plasma: ~2.6 hours
Excretion: Urine

Pregnancy Risk Factor C

Generic Available No

Comments Cidofovir preparation should be performed in a class two laminar flow biologic safety cabinet and personnel should be wearing surgical gloves and a closed front surgical gown with knit cuffs; appropriate safety equipment is recommended for preparation, administration, and disposal of cidofovir. If cidofovir contacts skin, wash and flush thoroughly with water.

Selected Readings Hitchcock MJ, Jaffe HS, Martin JC, et al, "Cidofovir, A New Agent With Potent Antiherpesvirus Activity," *Antiviral Chemistry & Chemotherapy*, 1996, 7:115-27.

Cilazapril (sye LAY za pril)

Canadian Brand Names Inhibace®

Pharmacologic Category Angiotensin-Converting Enzyme (ACE) Inhibitor

Synonyms Cilazapril Monohydrate

Use Management of hypertension; treatment of CHF

Local Anesthetic/Vasoconstrictor Precautions No information available to require special precautions

Effects on Dental Treatment 1% to 8%: Palpitations (1%), hypotension (1%; CHF), orthostatic hypotension (2%), headache (3% to 5%), dizziness (3% to 8%), nausea (1% to 3%), weakness (≤2%), cough (2% in hypertension; ≤7.5% in CHF), fatigue (2% to 3%)

Dosage Oral:

Hypertension: 2.5-5 mg once daily (maximum dose: 10 mg/day)
CHF: Initial: 0.5 mg once daily; if tolerated, after 5 days increase to 1 mg/day (lowest maintenance dose); may increase to maximum of 2.5 mg once daily
Elderly: Initial: 1.25 mg once daily; titrate slowly as tolerated
Dosing adjustment in renal impairment:
Hypertension:
Cl_{cr} 10-40 mL/minute: Initial: 0.5 mg once daily (maximum dose: 2.5 mg once daily)
Cl_{cr} <10 mL/minute: 0.25-0.5 mg once or twice weekly
CHF:
Cl_{cr} 10-40 mL/minute: Initial: 0.25-0.5 mg once daily (maximum dose: 2.5 mg once daily)
Cl_{cr} <10 mL/minute: 0.25-0.5 mg once or twice weekly
Dosing adjustment in hepatic impairment: Initial: ≤0.5 mg once daily (with caution)

Mechanism of Action Competitive inhibitor of angiotensin-converting enzyme (ACE); prevents conversion of angiotensin I to angiotensin II, a potent vasoconstrictor; results in lower levels of angiotensin II which causes an increase in plasma renin activity and a reduction in aldosterone secretion.

Other Adverse Effects

1% to 10% Renal: Increased serum creatinine

<1%: **Angina**, angioedema, anorexia, **anxiety, arrhythmia**, ataxia, **atrial fibrillation, AV block, bradycardia, bronchospasm, cardiogenic shock, confusion**, constipation, depression, diarrhea, dyspepsia, **dyspnea**, dysuria, gout, hemolytic anemia, hyperbilirubinemia, **hyperglycemia**, hyperkalemia, insomnia, leukopenia, **MI**, neutropenia, **nervousness**, pancreatitis, **paresthesia**, pemphigus, polyuria, proteinuria, pruritus, purpura, rash, renal failure, **rhinitis, somnolence**, Stevens-Johnson syndrome, **stroke, syncope, abnormal taste**, thrombocytopenic purpura, tinnitus, transaminases increased, **tremor**, urticaria, **vomiting**

Drug Interactions

Increased Effect/Toxicity:

Potassium supplements, sulfamethoxazole/trimethoprim (high dose), angiotensin II receptor antagonists (candesartan, losartan, irbesartan, etc), or potassium-sparing diuretics (amiloride, spironolactone, triamterene) may result in elevated serum potassium levels when combined with cilazapril. ACE inhibitor effects may be increased by phenothiazines or probenecid (increases levels of other ACE-inhibitors). ACE inhibitors may increase serum concentrations/effects of digoxin, lithium, and sulfonlyureas.

Diuretics have additive hypotensive effects with ACE inhibitors, and hypovolemia increases the potential for adverse renal effects of ACE inhibitors. In patients with compromised renal function, coadministration with nonsteroidal anti-inflammatory drugs may result in further deterioration of renal function. Allopurinol and ACE inhibitors may cause a higher risk of hypersensitivity reaction when taken concurrently

Decreased Effect: Aspirin (high dose) may reduce the therapeutic effects of ACE inhibitors; at low dosages this does not appear to be significant. Rifampin may decrease the effect of ACE inhibitors. Antacids may decrease the bioavailability of ACE inhibitors (may be more likely to occur with captopril); separate administration times by 1-2 hours. NSAIDs, specifically indomethacin, may reduce the hypotensive effects of ACE inhibitors. More likely to occur in low renin or volume-dependent hypertensive patients.

Dietary/Ethanol/Herb Considerations

Ethanol: Avoid use; may increase risk of hypotension or dizziness.

Food: May be taken with food; serum concentration may decrease (no apparent effect on activity). Long-term use may result in zinc deficiency resulting in decreased taste perception. Avoid caffeine (eg, colas, chocolate), garlic, and licorice.

Herb/Nutraceutical: Avoid black cohosh, dong quai, and evening primrose due to estrogenic activity. Avoid ephedra, ginseng, and yohimbe; may worsen hypertension. Avoid garlic; may have increased antihypertensive effect. Avoid ginger due to positive inotropic effects; theoretically, may cause arrhythmia. Avoid hawthorn; may lower peripheral vascular resistance causing additional decrease in BP. Avoid licorice.

Pharmacodynamics/Kinetics

Onset: Antihypertensive: ~1 hour

Duration: Therapeutic effect: 24 hours

Absorption: Rapid

Metabolism: To active form (cilazaprilat)

Bioavailability: 57%

Half-life elimination: Cilazaprilat: Terminal: 36-49 hours

Time to peak: 3-7 hours

Excretion: In urine (91%)

Pregnancy Risk Factor Not assigned; C/D (2nd and 3rd trimesters) based on other ACE-inhibitors

Cilazapril Monohydrate *see* Cilazapril *on page 324*

Cilostazol (sil OH sta zol)

U.S. Brand Names Pletal®

Canadian Brand Names Pletal®

Pharmacologic Category Antiplatelet Agent; Phosphodiesterase Enzyme Inhibitor

Synonyms OPC13013

Use Symptomatic management of peripheral vascular disease, primarily intermittent claudication; currently being investigated for the treatment of acute coronary syndromes and for graft patency improvement in percutaneous coronary interventions with or without stenting

Unlabeled/Investigational Use Investigational: Treatment of acute coronary syndromes and for graft patency improvement in percutaneous coronary interventions with or without stenting

Local Anesthetic/Vasoconstrictor Precautions No information available to require special precautions

Effects on Dental Treatment If a patient is to undergo elective surgery and an antiplatelet effect is not desired, a medical consult is suggested to consider reduction or discontinuation of cilostazol dose prior to surgery.

>10%: Headache (27% to 34%), infection (10% to 14%), rhinitis (7% tp 12%)

3% to 10%: Palpitations (5% to 10%), tachycardia (4%), dizziness (9% to 10%), nausea (6% to 7%), pharyngitis (7% to 10%), cough (3% to 4%)

<2%: Facial edema, fever, CHF, cardiac arrest, hemorrhage, hypotension, myocardial infarction/ischemia, postural hypotension, ventricular arrhythmia, supraventricular arrhythmia, syncope, duodenitis, peptic ulcer, duodenal ulcer, esophagitis, esophageal hemorrhage, gastritis, diabetes mellitus, anxiety, malaise, tongue edema (per manufacturer), bruising

Dosage Adults: Oral: 100 mg twice daily taken at least one-half hour before or 2 hours after breakfast and dinner; dosage should be reduced to 50 mg twice daily during concurrent therapy with inhibitors of CYP3A4 or CYP2C19 (see Drug Interactions)

Mechanism of Action Cilostazol and its metabolites are inhibitors of phosphodiesterase III. As a result cyclic AMP is increased leading to inhibition of platelet aggregation and vasodilation. Other effects of phosphodiesterase III inhibition include increased cardiac contractility, accelerated AV nodal conduction, increased ventricular automaticity, heart rate, and coronary blood flow.

Other Adverse Effects

>10%: Gastrointestinal: Abnormal stools (12% to 15%), diarrhea (12% to 19%)

2% to 10%:

Cardiovascular: Peripheral edema (7% to 9%)

Gastrointestinal: Dyspepsia (6%), abdominal pain (4% to 5%), flatulence (2% to 3%)

Neuromuscular & skeletal: Back pain (6% to 7%), myalgia (2% to 3%)

<2%: Chills, edema, nuchal rigidity, pelvic pain, retroperitoneal hemorrhage, cerebral infarction/ischemia, anorexia, cholelithiasis, colitis, hematemesis, anemia,

(Continued)

Cilostazol *(Continued)*

polycythemia, purpura, increased creatinine, gout, hyperlipidemia, hyperuricemia, arthralgia, bone pain, bursitis, insomnia, neuralgia, dry skin, urticaria, amblyopia, blindness, conjunctivitis, diplopia, retinal hemorrhage, cystitis, albuminuria, vaginitis, vaginal hemorrhage, urinary frequency

Drug Interactions Substrate of CYP1A2, 2C19, 2D6, 3A4

Increased Effect/Toxicity: Cilostazol serum concentrations may be increased by erythromycin, diltiazem, and omeprazole. Increased concentrations of cilostazol may be anticipated during concurrent therapy with other inhibitors of CYP3A4 (ie, clarithromycin, ketoconazole, itraconazole, fluconazole, miconazole, fluvoxamine, fluoxetine, nefazodone, and sertraline) or inhibitors of CYP2C19. Aspirin-induced inhibition of platelet aggregation is potentiated by concurrent cilostazol. The effect on platelet aggregation with other antiplatelet drugs is unknown.

Dietary/Ethanol/Herb Considerations Food: Administer with a high-fat meal may increase peak concentration by 90%. Avoid grapefruit products.

Pharmacodynamics/Kinetics

Onset of action: 2-4 weeks; may require up to 12 weeks

Protein binding: 97% to 98%

Metabolism: Hepatic via CYP3A4 (primarily), 1A2, 2C19, and 2D6; at least one metabolite has significant activity

Half-life elimination: 11-13 hours

Excretion: Urine (74%) and feces (20%) as metabolites

Pregnancy Risk Factor C

Generic Available No

Ciloxan® *see* Ciprofloxacin *on page 328*

Cimetidine (sye MET i deen)

Related Information

Gastrointestinal Disorders *on page 1474*

U.S. Brand Names Tagamet®; Tagamet® HB 200 [OTC]

Canadian Brand Names Apo®-Cimetidine; Gen-Cimetidine; Novo-Cimetidine; Nu-Cimet®; PMS-Cimetidine; Tagamet® HB

Mexican Brand Names Blocan; Cimetase®; Cimetigal; Columina; Tagamet®; Ulcedine; Zymerol

Pharmacologic Category Histamine H_2 Antagonist

Use Short-term treatment of active duodenal ulcers and benign gastric ulcers; long-term prophylaxis of duodenal ulcer; gastric hypersecretory states; gastroesophageal reflux; prevention of upper GI bleeding in critically ill patients

Unlabeled/Investigational Use Part of a multidrug regimen for *H. pylori* eradication to reduce the risk of duodenal ulcer recurrence

Local Anesthetic/Vasoconstrictor Precautions No information available to require special precautions

Effects on Dental Treatment 1% to 10%: Dizziness, agitation, headache, drowsiness, nausea, vomiting

Dosage

Children: Oral, I.M., I.V.: 20-40 mg/kg/day in divided doses every 6 hours

Adults:

Short-term treatment of active ulcers:

Oral: 300 mg 4 times/day or 800 mg at bedtime or 400 mg twice daily for up to 8 weeks

I.M., I.V.: 300 mg every 6 hours or 37.5 mg/hour by continuous infusion; I.V. dosage should be adjusted to maintain an intragastric pH ≥5

Patients with an active bleed: Administer cimetidine as a continuous infusion (see above)

Duodenal ulcer prophylaxis: Oral: 400-800 mg at bedtime

Gastric hypersecretory conditions: Oral, I.M., I.V.: 300-600 mg every 6 hours; dosage not to exceed 2.4 g/day

Helicobacter pylori eradication (unlabeled use): 400 mg twice daily; requires combination therapy with antibiotics

Dosing adjustment/interval in renal impairment: Children and Adults:

Cl_{cr} 20-40 mL/minute: Administer every 8 hours or 75% of normal dose

Cl_{cr} 0-20 mL/minute: Administer every 12 hours or 50% of normal dose

Hemodialysis: Slightly dialyzable (5% to 20%)

Dosing adjustment/comments in hepatic impairment: Usual dose is safe in mild disease; use with caution reduce dosage in severe disease; increased risk of CNS toxicity in cirrhosis suggested by enhanced penetration of CNS

Mechanism of Action Competitive inhibition of histamine at H_2-receptors of the gastric parietal cells resulting in reduced gastric acid secretion, gastric volume and hydrogen ion concentration reduced

Other Adverse Effects

1% to 10%: Gastrointestinal: Diarrhea

<1%: **Bradycardia, hypotension, tachycardia, confusion, fever**, rash, gynecomastia, edema of the breasts, decreased sexual ability, neutropenia, agranulocytosis, thrombocytopenia, increased AST/ALT, myalgia, elevated creatinine

Drug Interactions Inhibits **CYP1A2**, 2C8/9, 2C19, **2D6**, 2E1, **3A4**

Increased Effect/Toxicity: Cimetidine increases warfarin's effect in a dose-related manner. Cimetidine may increase serum concentrations of alfentanil, amiodarone, benzodiazepines (except lorazepam, oxazepam, temazepam), beta-blockers (except atenolol, betaxolol, bisoprolol, nadolol, penbutolol), calcium channel blockers, carbamazepine, cisapride (avoid concurrent use), citalopram, flecainide, lidocaine, melphalan, meperidine, metronidazole, moricizine, paroxetine, phenytoin, procainamide, propafenone, quinidine, quinolone antibiotics, tacrine, TCAs, theophylline, and triamterene. Cimetidine increases carmustine's myelotoxicity; avoid concurrent use.

Decreased Effect: Ketoconazole, fluconazole, itraconazole (especially capsule) decrease serum concentration; avoid concurrent use with H_2 antagonists. Delavirdine's absorption is decreased; avoid concurrent use with H_2 antagonists.

Dietary/Ethanol/Herb Considerations

Ethanol: Avoid use; may enhance gastric mucosal irritation.

Food: Administer with food; may decrease peak serum concentration. Limit xanthine-containing foods/beverages; may decrease iron absorption. Avoid caffeine; may increase serum caffeine concentration.

Herb/Nutraceutical: Avoid St John's wort; may decrease serum concentration.

Pharmacodynamics/Kinetics

Onset of action: 1 hour

Duration: 6 hours

Distribution: Crosses placenta; enters breast milk

Protein binding: 20%

Metabolism: Partially hepatic

Bioavailability: 60% to 70%

Half-life elimination: Neonates: 3.6 hours; Children: 1.4 hours; Adults: Normal renal function: 2 hours

Time to peak, serum: Oral: 1-2 hours

Excretion: Primarily urine (as unchanged drug); feces (some)

Pregnancy Risk Factor B

Generic Available Yes

Cinobac® *see* Cinoxacin *on page 327*

Cinoxacin (sin OKS a sin)

U.S. Brand Names Cinobac®

Canadian Brand Names Cinobac®

Mexican Brand Names Gugecin

Pharmacologic Category Antibiotic, Quinolone

Use Treatment and prevention of urinary tract infections (UTIs)

Local Anesthetic/Vasoconstrictor Precautions No information available to require special precautions

Effects on Dental Treatment 1% to 10%: Headache, dizziness, GI bleeding, belching, nausea, vomiting

Dosage Adults: Oral:

Treatment of UTI: 1 g/day in 2-4 doses for 7-14 days

Prophylaxis against recurrent UTI: 250 mg once daily at bedtime (has been used up to 5 months)

Dosing adjustment in renal impairment:

- Cl_{cr} >50-80 mL/minute: 250 mg 3 times/day
- Cl_{cr} 20-50 mL/minute: 250 mg twice daily
- Cl_{cr} <20 mL/minute: 250 mg/day

Mechanism of Action Inhibits microbial synthesis of DNA with resultant inhibition of protein synthesis

Other Adverse Effects

1% to 10%:

- Cardiovascular: Edema, angioedema
- Dermatologic: Rash, urticaria
- Gastrointestinal: Heartburn, abdominal pain, flatulence, anorexia, diarrhea

<1%: Alkaline phosphatase increased, ALT/AST increased, **anaphylactic reactions**, BUN increased, **confusion, drowsiness**, erythema multiforme, insomnia, hemoglobin/hematocrit decreased, photophobia, perianal burning, **seizures** (rare), serum creatinine increased, Stevens-Johnson syndrome, thrombocytopenia, tingling sensation, tinnitus, toxic epidermal necrolysis; quinolones have been associated with tendonitis and tendon rupture

Drug Interactions

Increased Effect/Toxicity: Quinolones may cause increased levels of azlocillin, cyclosporine, and caffeine/theophylline. Azlocillin, cimetidine, loop diuretics (furosemide, torsemide), and probenecid increase quinolone levels (decreased renal secretion). An increased incidence of seizures may occur with foscarnet or NSAIDs. The hypoprothrombinemic effect of warfarin is enhanced by some quinolone antibiotics. Concurrent use of corticosteroids may increase risk of tendon rupture.

(Continued)

Cinoxacin *(Continued)*

Decreased Effect: Metal cations (magnesium, aluminum, iron, and zinc) bind quinolones in the gastrointestinal tract and inhibit absorption (by up to 98%). Due to electrolyte content, antacids, electrolyte supplements, sucralfate, quinapril, and some didanosine formulations should be avoided. Levofloxacin should be administered 4 hours before or 8 hours (a minimum of 2 hours before and 2 hours after) after these agents. Antineoplastic agents may decrease the absorption of quinolones.

Dietary/Ethanol/Herb Considerations Food: Administer with food; decreases peak serum concentration by 30% but not extent of absorption.

Pharmacodynamics/Kinetics

Absorption: Oral: Rapid and complete; food decreases peak levels by 30% but not total amount absorbed

Distribution: Crosses placenta; concentrates in prostate tissue

Protein binding: 60% to 80%

Half-life elimination: 1.5 hours; prolonged with renal impairment

Time to peak, serum: 2-3 hours

Excretion: Urine (~60% as unchanged drug)

Pregnancy Risk Factor C

Generic Available No

Cipro® *see* Ciprofloxacin *on page 328*

Ciprofloxacin (sip roe FLOKS a sin)

Related Information

Antibiotic Prophylaxis, Preprocedural Guidelines for Dental Patients *on page 1507*

Nonviral Infectious Diseases *on page 1493*

Sexually-Transmitted Diseases *on page 1502*

Tuberculosis *on page 1493*

U.S. Brand Names Ciloxan®; Cipro®; Cipro® XR

Canadian Brand Names Ciloxan®; Cipro®

Mexican Brand Names Cimogal®; Ciprobiotic®; Ciproflox®; Ciprofur®; Ciproxina®; Eni®; Italnik®; Kenzoflex®; Microrgan®; Mitroken®; Nivoflox®; Novoquin®; Opthaflox®; Quinoflox®; Sophixin®; Sophixin Ofteno; Suiflox®; Zipra®

Pharmacologic Category Antibiotic, Ophthalmic; Antibiotic, Quinolone

Synonyms Ciprofloxacin Hydrochloride

Use

Dental: Useful as a single agent or in combination with metronidazole in the treatment of periodontitis associated with the presence of *Actinobacillus actinomycetemcomitans*, (AA) as well as enteric rods/pseudomonads

Medical: Treatment of documented or suspected infections of the lower respiratory tract, sinuses, skin and skin structure, bone/joints, and urinary tract (including prostatitis) due to susceptible bacterial strains; especially indicated for pseudomonal infections and those due to multidrug-resistant gram-negative organisms, chronic bacterial prostatitis, infectious diarrhea, complicated gram-negative and anaerobic intra-abdominal infections (with metronidazole) due to *E. coli* (enteropathic strains), *B. fragilis, P. mirabilis, K. pneumoniae, P. aeruginosa, Campylobacter jejuni* or *Shigella*; approved for acute sinusitis caused by *H. influenzae* or *M. catarrhalis*; also used in treatment of typhoid fever due to *Salmonella typhi* (although eradication of the chronic typhoid carrier state has not been proven), osteomyelitis when parenteral therapy is not feasible, acute uncomplicated cystitis in females, to reduce incidence or progression of disease following exposure to aerolized *Bacillus anthracis*, febrile neutropenia (with piperacillin), and sexually-transmitted diseases such as uncomplicated cervical and urethral gonorrhea due to *Neisseria gonorrhoeae*; used ophthalmologically for superficial ocular infections (corneal ulcers, conjunctivitis) due to susceptible strains

Local Anesthetic/Vasoconstrictor Precautions No information available to require special precautions

Effects on Dental Treatment 1% to 5%: Headache (1%), restlessness (1%) nausea (5%), vomiting (2%)

Dosage

Children (see Warnings/Precautions):

Oral: 20-30 mg/kg/day in 2 divided doses; maximum: 1.5 g/day

Cystic fibrosis: 20-40 mg/kg/day divided every 12 hours

Anthrax:

Inhalational (postexposure prophylaxis): 15 mg/kg/dose every 12 hours for 60 days; maximum: 500 mg/dose

Cutaneous (treatment): 10-15 mg/kg every 12 hours for 60 days; amoxicillin 80 mg/kg/day divided every 8 hours is an option for completion of treatment after clinical improvement. **Note:** In the presence of systemic involvement, extensive edema, lesions on head/neck, refer to I.V. dosing for treatment of inhalational/GI/oropharyngeal anthrax

I.V.: 15-20 mg/kg/day divided every 12 hours

Cystic fibrosis: 15-30 mg/kg/day divided every 8-12 hours
Anthrax:
Inhalational (postexposure prophylaxis): 10 mg/kg/dose every 12 hours for 60 days; do **not** exceed 400 mg/dose (800 mg/day)
Inhalational/GI/oropharyngeal (treatment): Initial: 10-15 mg/kg every 12 hours for 60 days (maximum: 500 mg/dose); switch to oral therapy when clinically appropriate; refer to Adults dosing for notes on combined therapy and duration

Adults: Oral:
Lower respiratory tract, skin/skin structure infections: 500-750 mg twice daily for 7-14 days depending on severity and susceptibility
Chancroid: 500 mg twice daily for 3 days
Sinusitis (acute): 500 mg every 12 hours for 10 days
Bone/joint infections: 500-750 mg twice daily for 4-6 weeks, depending on severity and susceptibility
Infectious diarrhea: 500 mg every 12 hours for 5-7 days
Intra-abdominal (in combination with metronidazole): 500 mg every 12 hours for 7-14 days
Typhoid fever: 500 mg every 12 hours for 10 days
Urethral/cervical gonococcal infections: 250-500 mg as a single dose (CDC recommends concomitant doxycycline or azithromycin due to developing resistance; avoid use in Asian or Western Pacific travelers)
Disseminated gonococcal infection: 500 mg twice daily to complete 7 days of therapy (initial treatment with ceftriaxone 1 g I.M./I.V. daily for 24-48 hours after improvement begins)
Urinary tract infection:
Acute uncomplicated: Immediate release formulation: 100 mg or 250 mg every 12 hours for 3 days
Uncomplicated/acute cystitis: Extended release formulation: 500 mg every 24 hours for 3 days
Mild/moderate: Immediate release formulation: 250 mg every 12 hours for 7-14 days
Severe/complicated: Immediate release formulation: 500 mg every 12 hours for 7-14 days
Chronic bacterial prostatitis: 500 mg every 12 hours for 28 days
Anthrax:
Inhalational (postexposure prophylaxis): 500 mg every 12 hours for 60 days
Cutaneous (treatment): 500 mg every 12 hours for 60 days. **Note:** In the presence of systemic involvement, extensive edema, lesions on head/neck, refer to I.V. dosing for treatment of inhalational/GI/oropharyngeal anthrax

Adults: I.V.:
Bone/joint infections:
Mild to moderate: 400 mg every 12 hours for 4-6 weeks
Severe or complicated: 400 mg every 8 hours for 4-6 weeks
Lower respiratory tract, skin/skin structure infections:
Mild to moderate: 400 mg every 12 hours for 7-14 days
Severe or complicated: 400 mg every 8 hours for 7-14 days
Nosocomial pneumonia (mild to moderate to severe): 400 mg every 8 hours for 10-14 days
Prostatitis (chronic, bacterial): 400 mg every 12 hours for 28 days
Sinusitis (acute): 400 mg every 12 hours for 10 days
Urinary tract infection:
Mild to moderate: 200 mg every 12 hours for 7-14 days
Severe or complicated: 400 mg every 12 hours for 7-14 days
Febrile neutropenia (with piperacillin): 400 mg every 8 hours for 7-14 days
Intra-abdominal infection (with metronidazole): 400 mg every 12 hours for 7-14 days
Anthrax:
Inhalational (postexposure prophylaxis): 400 mg every 12 hours for 60 days
Inhalational/GI/oropharyngeal (treatment): 400 mg every 12 hours. **Note:** Initial treatment should include two or more agents predicted to be effective (per CDC recommendations). Agents suggested for use in conjunction with ciprofloxacin or doxycycline include rifampin, vancomycin, imipenem, penicillin, ampicillin, chloramphenicol, clindamycin, and clarithromycin. May switch to oral antimicrobial therapy when clinically appropriate. Continue combined therapy for 60 days.

Elderly: No dosage adjustment in normal renal function

Ophthalmic:
Solution: Children >1 year and Adults: Instill 1-2 drops in eye(s) every 2 hours while awake for 2 days and 1-2 drops every 4 hours while awake for the next 5 days
Ointment: Children >2 years and Adults: Apply a 1/2" ribbon into the conjunctival sac 3 times/day for the first 2 days, followed by a 1/2" ribbon applied twice daily for the next 5 days

(Continued)

Ciprofloxacin *(Continued)*

Dosing adjustment in renal impairment:

Cl_{cr} 30-50 mL/minute: Oral: 250-500 mg every 12 hours

Cl_{cr} 5-29 mL/minute:

Oral: 250-500 mg every 18 hours

I.V.: 200-400 mg every 18-24 hours

Dialysis: Only small amounts of ciprofloxacin are removed by hemo- or peritoneal dialysis (<10%); usual dose: Oral: 250-500 mg every 24 hours following dialysis

Continuous arteriovenous or venovenous hemodiafiltration effects: Administer 200-400 mg I.V. every 12 hours

Mechanism of Action Inhibits DNA-gyrase in susceptible organisms; inhibits relaxation of supercoiled DNA and promotes breakage of double-stranded DNA

Other Adverse Effects

1% to 10%:

Dermatologic: Rash (1%)

Gastrointestinal: Diarrhea (2%), abdominal pain (2%)

Hepatic: ALT/AST increased (2%)

Renal: Serum creatinine increased (1%)

<1% and postmarketing reports (limited to important or life-threatening): Acute renal failure, agranulocytosis, **allergic reactions, anaphylaxis,** anemia, angina pectoris, arthralgia, **cardiopulmonary arrest,** cholestatic jaundice, **confusion, delirium, dizziness, drowsiness, dyspnea**, edema, erythema multiforme, **GI bleeding, hallucinations**, hepatic necrosis, **hypertension, joint pain**, liver enzymes increased, methemoglobinemia, **myasthenia gravis (exacerbation), MI,** nightmares, **palpitations**, pancreatitis, photosensitivity, **prolongation of PT, pseudomembranous colitis, seizures**, Stevens-Johnson syndrome, **syncope**, tendon rupture, toxic epidermal necrolysis, **tremor**, vasculitis, **visual disturbance, painful oral mucosa, oral candidiasis, oral ulceration, xerostomia**

Contraindications Hypersensitivity to ciprofloxacin, any component of the formulation, or other quinolones

Warnings/Precautions Not recommended in children <18 years of age (exception - postexposure treatment of inhalational anthrax); has caused transient arthropathy in children. CNS stimulation may occur (tremor, restlessness, confusion, and very rarely hallucinations or seizures). Use with caution in patients with known or suspected CNS disorder. Green discoloration of teeth in newborns has been reported; prolonged use may result in superinfection. Tendon inflammation and/or rupture have been reported with ciprofloxacin and other quinolone antibiotics. Risk may be increased with concurrent corticosteroids, particularly in the elderly. Discontinue at first sign of tendon inflammation or pain.

Severe hypersensitivity reactions, including anaphylaxis, have occurred with quinolone therapy. If an allergic reaction occurs (itching, urticaria, dyspnea, facial edema, loss of consciousness, tingling, cardiovascular collapse), discontinue drug immediately. Quinolones may exacerbate myasthenia gravis, use with caution (rare, potentially life-threatening weakness of respiratory muscles may occur).

Drug Interactions Inhibits **CYP1A2, 3A4**

Enteral feedings may decrease plasma concentrations of ciprofloxacin probably by >30% inhibition of absorption. Ciprofloxacin should not be administered with enteral feedings. The feeding would need to be discontinued for 1-2 hours prior to and after ciprofloxacin administration. Nasogastric administration produces a greater loss of ciprofloxacin bioavailability than does nasoduodenal administration.

Aluminum/magnesium products, didanosine, quinapril, and sucralfate may decrease absorption of ciprofloxacin by ≥90% if administered concurrently. Administer ciprofloxacin at least 4 hours and preferably 6 hours after the dose of these agents or change to an H_2 antagonist or omeprazole.

Calcium, iron, zinc, and multivitamins with minerals products may decrease absorption of ciprofloxacin significantly if administered concurrently. Administer ciprofloxacin 2 hours before dose or at least 6 hours after the dose of these agents.

Antineoplastic agents may decrease the absorption of quinolones.

Cimetidine, and other H_2 antagonists may inhibit renal elimination of quinolones. No effect on bioavailability demonstrated with ciprofloxacin.

Corticosteroids: Concurrent use may increase the risk of tendon rupture, particularly in elderly patients (overall incidence rare).

Cyclosporine: Ciprofloxacin may increase serum levels.

Foscarnet has been associated with an increased risk of seizures with some quinolones.

Loop diuretics: Serum levels of some quinolones are increased by loop diuretic administration. May diminish renal excretion.

NSAIDs: The CNS stimulating effect of some quinolones may be enhanced, resulting in neuroexcitation and/or seizures.

Probenecid: Blocks renal secretion of quinolones, increasing concentrations.

Theophylline (and caffeine): Serum levels may be increased by ciprofloxacin; in addition, CNS stimulation/seizures may occur at lower theophylline serum levels due to additive CNS effects.

Warfarin: The hypoprothrombinemic effect of warfarin is enhanced by ciprofloxacin; monitor INR closely during therapy.

Dietary/Ethanol/Herb Considerations

Food: Administer with food to reduce GI upset (manufacturer recommends administration 2 hours after meals). Food decreases rate, but not extent of absorption. Administration with caffeine may increase caffeine levels; restrict caffeine intake if excessive cardiac or CNS stimulation occurs.

Extended release tablet may be taken with meals containing dairy products (with <800 mg calcium content) but not with dairy products alone; dairy products may be taken 6 hours before or 2 hours following a dose of ciprofloxacin. The manufacturer states that the usual dietary intake of calcium (including meals which include dairy products) has not been shown to interfere with ciprofloxacin absorption.

Enteral feedings may decrease plasma concentrations of ciprofloxacin probably by >30% inhibition of absorption. Ciprofloxacin should not be administered with enteral feedings. The feeding would need to be discontinued for 1-2 hours prior to and after ciprofloxacin administration. Nasogastric administration produces a greater loss of ciprofloxacin bioavailability than does nasoduodenal administration.

Oral multivitamins, and mineral supplements: Absorption of ciprofloxacin is decreased by divalent and trivalent cations. The manufacturer states that the usual dietary intake of calcium has not been shown to interfere with ciprofloxacin absorption. These products may be taken 6 hours before or 2 hours following a dose of ciprofloxacin.

Herb/Nutraceutical: Avoid dong quai and St John's wort; may increase photosensitization.

Pharmacodynamics/Kinetics

Absorption: Oral: Immediate release tablet: Rapid (~50% to 85%)

Distribution: V_d: 2.1-2.7 L/kg; tissue concentrations often exceed serum concentrations especially in kidneys, gallbladder, liver, lungs, gynecological tissue, and prostatic tissue; CSF concentrations: 10% of serum concentrations (noninflamed meninges), 14% to 37% (inflamed meninges); crosses placenta; enters breast milk

Protein binding: 20% to 40%

Metabolism: Partially hepatic; forms 4 metabolites (limited activity)

Half-life elimination: Children: 2.5 hours; Adults: Normal renal function: 3-5 hours

Time to peak: Oral: Immediate release tablet: 0.5-2 hours; Extended release tablet: 1-2.5 hours

Excretion: Urine (30% to 50% as unchanged drug); feces (20% to 40%)

Pregnancy Risk Factor C

Breast-feeding Considerations Not compatible; can resume breast-feeding 48 hours after the last dose. Theoretically, may affect cartilage in weight-bearing joints.

Dosage Forms INF [premixed in D_5W] (Cipro®): 200 mg (100mL); 400 mg (200 mL). **INJ, solution** (Cipro®): 200 mg (20 mL); 400 mg (40 mL). **OINT, ophthalmic, as hydrochloride** (Ciloxan®): 3.33 mg/g [0.3% base] (3.5 g). **SOLN, ophthalmic as hydrochloride** (Ciloxan®): 3.33 mg/g [0.3% base] (2.5 mL, 5 mL, 10 mL). **SUSP, oral** (Cipro®): 250 mg/5 mL (100 mL); 500 mg/5 mL (100 mL). **TAB** [film coated] (Cipro®): 100 mg, 250 mg, 500 mg, 750 mg. **TAB, extended release** [film coated] (Cipro® XR): 500 mg

Generic Available No

Selected Readings

Rams TE and Slots J, "Antibiotics in Periodontal Therapy: An Update," *Compendium*, 1992, 13(12):1130, 1132, 1134.

Wynn RL, Bergman SA, Meiller TF, et al, "Antibiotics in Treating Oral-Facial Infections of Odontogenic Origin: An Update", *Gen Dent*, 2001, 49(3):238-40, 242, 244 passim.

Ciprofloxacin and Hydrocortisone

(sip roe FLOKS a sin & hye droe KOR ti sone)

Related Information

Ciprofloxacin *on page 328*

Hydrocortisone *on page 688*

U.S. Brand Names Cipro® HC Otic

Canadian Brand Names Cipro® HC

Pharmacologic Category Antibiotic/Corticosteroid, Otic

Synonyms Hydrocortisone and Ciprofloxacin

Use Treatment of acute otitis externa, sometimes known as "swimmer's ear"

Local Anesthetic/Vasoconstrictor Precautions No information available to require special precautions

Effects on Dental Treatment No significant effects or complications reported

Dosage Children >1 year of age and Adults: Otic: The recommended dosage for all patients is three drops of the suspension in the affected ear twice daily for seven day; twice-daily dosing schedule is more convenient for patients than that of existing treatments with hydrocortisone, which are typically administered three or four times a day; a twice-daily dosage schedule may be especially helpful for parents and caregivers of young children

Generic Available No

Ciprofloxacin Hydrochloride *see* Ciprofloxacin *on page 328*

Cipro® HC Otic *see* Ciprofloxacin and Hydrocortisone *on page 331*

Cipro® XR *see* Ciprofloxacin *on page 328*

Cisapride (SIS a pride)

Related Information

Endocrine Disorders and Pregnancy *on page 1479*

U.S. Brand Names Propulsid®

Mexican Brand Names Enteropride; Kinestase®; Unamol

Pharmacologic Category Gastrointestinal Agent, Prokinetic

Use Treatment of nocturnal symptoms of gastroesophageal reflux disease (GERD); has demonstrated effectiveness for gastroparesis, refractory constipation, and nonulcer dyspepsia

Local Anesthetic/Vasoconstrictor Precautions No information available to require special precautions

Effects on Dental Treatment

>5%: Xerostomia, headache, nausea, rhinitis

<5%: Tachycardia, extrapyramidal effects, somnolence, seizures, anxiety, sinusitis, cough, upper respiratory tract infection, increased incidence of viral infection

Restrictions In U.S., available via limited-access protocol only.

Dosage Oral:

Children: 0.15-0.3 mg/kg/dose 3-4 times/day; maximum: 10 mg/dose

Adults: Initial: 10 mg 4 times/day at least 15 minutes before meals and at bedtime; in some patients the dosage will need to be increased to 20 mg to obtain a satisfactory result

Mechanism of Action Enhances the release of acetylcholine at the myenteric plexus. *In vitro* studies have shown cisapride to have serotonin-4 receptor agonistic properties which may increase gastrointestinal motility and cardiac rate; increases lower esophageal sphincter pressure and lower esophageal peristalsis; accelerates gastric emptying of both liquids and solids.

Other Adverse Effects

>5%:

Dermatologic: Rash

Gastrointestinal: Diarrhea, GI cramping, dyspepsia, flatulence,

<5%:

Central nervous system: Fatigue, insomnia

Hematologic: Thrombocytopenia, increased LFTs, pancytopenia, leukopenia, granulocytopenia, aplastic anemia

Drug Interactions Substrate of 1A2, 2A6, 2B6, 2C8/9, 2C19, **3A4**; Inhibits CYP2D6

Increased Effect/Toxicity: Cisapride may increase blood levels of warfarin, diazepam, cimetidine, ranitidine, and CNS depressants. The risk of cisapride-induced malignant arrhythmias may be increased by azole antifungals (fluconazole, itraconazole, ketoconazole, miconazole), antiarrhythmics (Class Ia; quinidine, procainamide, and Class III; amiodarone, sotalol), bepridil, cimetidine, maprotiline, macrolide antibiotics (erythromycin, clarithromycin, troleandomycin), molindone, nefazodone, protease inhibitors (amprenavir, indinavir, nelfinavir, ritonavir), phenothiazines (eg, prochlorperazine, promethazine), sertindole, tricyclic antidepressants (eg amitriptyline), and some quinolone antibiotics (sparfloxacin, gatifloxacin, moxifloxacin). Cardiovascular disease or electrolyte imbalances (potentially due to diuretic therapy) increase the risk of malignant arrhythmias.

Decreased Effect: Cisapride may decrease the effect of atropine and digoxin.

Dietary/Ethanol/Herb Considerations

Ethanol: Avoid use; cisapride increases ethanol absorption.

Food: Avoid grapefruit products due to increased bioavailability of cisapride.

Herb/Nutraceutical: Avoid St John's wort; may decrease serum concentration.

Pharmacodynamics/Kinetics

Onset of action: 0.5-1 hour

Protein binding: 97.5% to 98%

Metabolism: Extensively hepatic to norcisapride

Bioavailability: 35% to 40%

Half-life elimination: 6-12 hours

Excretion: Urine and feces (<10%)

Pregnancy Risk Factor C

Generic Available No

Cisplatin (SIS pla tin)

U.S. Brand Names Platinol®; Platinol®-AQ

Mexican Brand Names Blastolem®; Medsaplatin; Niyaplat; Platinol®; Tecnoplatin®

Pharmacologic Category Antineoplastic Agent, Alkylating Agent

Synonyms CDDP

Use Treatment of head and neck, breast, testicular, and ovarian cancer; Hodgkin's and non-Hodgkin's lymphoma; neuroblastoma; sarcomas, bladder, gastric, lung, esophageal, cervical, and prostate cancer; myeloma, melanoma, mesothelioma, small cell lung cancer, and osteosarcoma

Local Anesthetic/Vasoconstrictor Precautions No information available to require special precautions

Effects on Dental Treatment Frequency not defined: Bradycardia, arrhythmias, seizures, anaphylactoid reactions (bronchoconstriction, tachycardia, hypotension, facial edema)

Dosage It is recommended that a 24-hour urine creatinine clearance be checked prior to a patient's first dose of cisplatin and periodically thereafter (ie, after every 2-3 cycles of cisplatin) An estimated Cl_{cr} should be on all cisplatin chemotherapy orders along with other patient parameters (ie, patient's height, weight, and body surface area). Pharmacy and nursing staff should check the Cl_{cr} on the order and determine the appropriateness of cisplatin dosing. The manufacturer recommends that subsequent cycles should only be given when serum creatinine <1.5 mg/dL, WBC ≥4,000/mm³, platelets ≥ 100,000/mm³, and BUN <25.

Pretreatment hydration with 1-2 L of chloride-containing fluid is recommended prior to cisplatin administration; adequate hydration and urinary output (>100 mL/hour) should be maintained for 24 hours after administration. **Note:** If the dose prescribed is a reduced dose, then this should be indicated on the chemotherapy order.

I.V. (refer to individual protocols):

Children: Various dosage schedules range from 30-100 mg/m² once every 2-3 weeks; may also dose similar to adult dosing

Recurrent brain tumors: 60 mg/m² once daily for 2 consecutive days every 3-4 weeks

Adults:

Advanced bladder cancer: 50-70 mg/m² every 3-4 weeks

Head and neck cancer: 100-120 mg/m² every 3-4 weeks

Testicular cancer: 10-20 mg/m²/day for 5 days repeated every 3-4 weeks

Metastatic ovarian cancer: 75-100 mg/m² every 3 weeks

Intraperitoneal: cisplatin has been administered intraperitoneal with systemic sodium thiosulfate for ovarian cancer; doses up to 90-270 mg/m² have been administered and retained for 4 hours before draining

Dosing adjustment in renal impairment:

Cl_{cr} 10-50 mL/minute: Administer 50% of normal dose

Cl_{cr} <10 mL/minute: Do not administer

Hemodialysis: Partially cleared by hemodialysis; administer dose posthemodialysis

CAPD effects: Unknown

CAVH effects: Unknown

Mechanism of Action Inhibits DNA synthesis by the formation of DNA cross-links; denatures the double helix; covalently binds to DNA bases and disrupts DNA function; may also bind to proteins; the *cis*-isomer is 14 times more cytotoxic than the *trans*-isomer; both forms cross-link DNA but cis-platinum is less easily recognized by cell enzymes and, therefore, not repaired. Cisplatin can also bind two adjacent guanines on the same strand of DNA producing intrastrand cross-linking and breakage.

Other Adverse Effects Frequency not defined:

Cardiovascular: Raynaud's phenomenon

Central nervous system: Encephalopathy

Dermatologic: Mild alopecia

Endocrine & metabolic: Hypomagnesemia, hypocalcemia, hypokalemia, hypophosphatemia, hyperuricemia

Gastrointestinal: **Nausea and vomiting (76% to 100%; dose-related)**

Hematologic: Myelosuppression

Hepatic: Elevated liver enzymes

Local: Phlebitis, tissue sloughing and necrosis if infiltrated

Neuromuscular & skeletal: Peripheral neuropathy (related to cumulative doses >200 mg/m2)

Ocular: Papilledema, optic neuritis

Otic: Ototoxicity (especially pronounced in children; hearing loss in the high-frequency range is related to a cumulative dose of cisplatin >400 mg/m2)

Renal: Nephrotoxicity (damage to the proximal tubules), azotemia, elevated BUN and serum creatinine

Drug Interactions

Increased Effect/Toxicity: Cisplatin and ethacrynic acid have resulted in severe ototoxicity in animals. Delayed bleomycin elimination with decreased glomerular filtration rate. When administered as sequential infusions, observational studies indicate a potential for increased toxicity when platinum derivatives (carboplatin, cisplatin) are administered before taxane derivatives (docetaxel, paclitaxel).

Decreased Effect: Sodium thiosulfate theoretically inactivates drug systemically; has been used clinically to reduce systemic toxicity with intraperitoneal administration of cisplatin.

(Continued)

Cisplatin *(Continued)*

Dietary/Ethanol/Herb Considerations Herb/Nutraceutical: Avoid black cohosh and dong quai in estrogen-dependent tumors.

Pharmacodynamics/Kinetics

Distribution: I.V.: Rapidly into tissue; high concentrations in kidneys, liver, ovaries, uterus, and lungs

Protein binding: >90%

Metabolism: Nonenzymatic; inactivated (in both cell and bloodstream) by sulfhydryl groups; covalently binds to glutathione and thiosulfate

Half-life elimination: Initial: 20-30 minutes; Beta: 60 minutes; Terminal: ~24 hours; Secondary half-life: 44-73 hours

Excretion: Urine (>90%); feces (10%)

Pregnancy Risk Factor D

Generic Available Yes

13-*cis*-Retinoic Acid *see* Isotretinoin *on page 752*

Citalopram (sye TAL oh pram)

Related Information

Escitalopram *on page 516*

U.S. Brand Names Celexa™

Canadian Brand Names Celexa®

Mexican Brand Names Seropram®

Pharmacologic Category Antidepressant, Selective Serotonin Reuptake Inhibitor

Synonyms Citalopram Hydrobromide; Nitalapram

Use Treatment of depression

Unlabeled/Investigational Use Investigational: Treatment of dementia, smoking cessation, ethanol abuse symptoms, obsessive-compulsive disorder (OCD) in children, diabetic neuropathy

Local Anesthetic/Vasoconstrictor Precautions Although caution should be used in patients taking tricyclic antidepressants, no interactions have been reported with vasoconstrictors and citalopram, a nontricyclic antidepressant which acts to increase serotonin

Effects on Dental Treatment

>10%: Xerostomia; Somnolence, nausea, diaphoresis

<10%: Agitation, yawning, vomiting, tremor, cough, rhinitis, sinusitis

Premarketing trials reported abnormal taste.

Dosage Oral:

Children and Adolescents: OCD (unlabeled use): 10-40 mg/day

Adults: Depression: Initial: 20 mg/day, generally with an increase to 40 mg/day; doses of more than 40 mg are not usually necessary. Should a dose increase be necessary, it should occur in 20 mg increments at intervals of no less than 1 week. Maximum dose: 60 mg/day; reduce dosage in elderly or those with hepatic impairment.

Mechanism of Action A bicyclic phthalane derivative, citalopram selectively inhibits serotonin reuptake in the presynaptic neurons

Other Adverse Effects

>10%: Central nervous system: Insomnia

<10%:

Central nervous system: Anorexia

Dermatologic: Rash, pruritus

Endocrine & metabolic: Sexual dysfunction

Gastrointestinal: Diarrhea, dyspepsia, abdominal pain, weight gain

Neuromuscular & skeletal: Arthralgia, myalgia

<1%, postmarketing, and/or case reports: SIADH

Drug Interactions Substrate of **CYP2C19**, 2D6, **3A4**; Inhibits CYP1A2, 2B6, 2C19, 2D6

Increased Effect/Toxicity:

MAO inhibitors: Citalopram should not be used with nonselective MAO inhibitors (phenelzine, isocarboxazid) or other drugs with MAO inhibition (linezolid); fatal reactions have been reported. Wait 5 weeks after stopping citalopram before starting a nonselective MAO inhibitor and 2 weeks after stopping an MAO inhibitor before starting citalopram. Concurrent selegiline has been associated with mania, hypertension, or serotonin syndrome (risk may be reduced relative to nonselective MAO inhibitors).

Combined used of SSRIs and amphetamines, buspirone, meperidine, nefazodone, serotonin agonists (such as sumatriptan), sibutramine, other SSRIs, sympathomimetics, ritonavir, tramadol, and venlafaxine may increase the risk of serotonin syndrome. Risk of hyponatremia may increase with concurrent use of loop diuretics (bumetanide, furosemide, torsemide). Citalopram may increase the hypoprothrombinemic response to warfarin. Inhibitors of CYP3A4 or CYP2C19 may increase serum levels/effects of citalopram.

Combined use of sumatriptan (and other serotonin agonists) may result in toxicity; weakness, hyper-reflexia, and incoordination have been observed with sumatriptan and SSRIs. In addition, concurrent use may theoretically increase the risk of serotonin syndrome; includes sumatriptan, naratriptan, rizatriptan, and zolmitriptan.

Decreased Effect: Cyproheptadine may inhibit the effects of serotonin reuptake inhibitors.

Dietary/Ethanol/Herb Considerations

Ethanol: Avoid use; may cause CNS depression.

Food: Administer with food to reduce GI upset; avoid grapefruit products (may increase serum) and caffeine.

Herb/Nutraceutical: Avoid gotu kola, kava, SAMe, and St John's wort; may increase risk for serotonin syndrome, avoid valerian; may increase CNS depression. Avoid melatonin; may cause acute psychosis. Avoid tryptophan; may cause serotonin syndrome.

Pharmacodynamics/Kinetics

Distribution: V_d: 12 L/kg

Protein binding, plasma: ~80%

Metabolism: Extensively hepatic, including CYP, to N-demethylated, N-oxide, and deaminated metabolites

Bioavailability: 80%

Half-life elimination: 24-48 hours; average 35 hours (doubled with hepatic impairment)

Time to peak, serum: 1-6 hours, average within 4 hours

Excretion: Urine (10% as unchanged drug)

Note: Clearance was decreased, while AUC and half-life were significantly increased in elderly patients and in patients with hepatic impairment. Mild to moderate renal impairment may reduce clearance of citalopram (17% reduction noted in trials). No pharmacokinetic information is available concerning patients with severe renal impairment.

Pregnancy Risk Factor C

Generic Available No

Comments Problems with SSRI-induced bruxism have been reported and may preclude their use; clinicians attempting to evaluate any patient with bruxism or involuntary muscle movement, who is simultaneously being treated with an SSRI drug, should be aware of the potential association.

Selected Readings Gerber PE and Lynd LD, "Selective Serotonin Reuptake Inhibitor-induced Movement Disorders," *Ann Pharmacother*, 1998, 32(6):692-8.

Citalopram Hydrobromide *see* Citalopram *on page 334*

Citanest® Forte *see* Prilocaine and Epinephrine *on page 1116*

Citanest® Plain *see* Prilocaine *on page 1114*

Citracal® [OTC] *see* Calcium Citrate *on page 224*

Citracal® [OTC] *see* Calcium Supplements *on page 229*

Citrate of Magnesia *see* Magnesium Citrate *on page 834*

Citrate of Magnesia (Magnesium Citrate) *see* Magnesium Supplements *on page 837*

Citric Acid and d-gluconic Acid Irrigant *see* Citric Acid Bladder Mixture *on page 335*

Citric Acid and Potassium Citrate *see* Potassium Citrate and Citric Acid *on page 1101*

Citric Acid Bladder Mixture (SI trik AS id BLAD dur MIKS chur)

U.S. Brand Names Renacidin®

Pharmacologic Category Urinary Tract Product

Synonyms Citric Acid and d-gluconic Acid Irrigant; Citric Acid, Magnesium Hydroxycarbonate, D-Gluconic Acid, Magnesium Acid Citrate, and Calcium Carbonate; Hemiacidrin

Use Preparing solutions for irrigating indwelling urethral catheters; to dissolve or prevent formation of calcifications

Orphan drug: Treatment of renal and bladder calculi of the apatite or struvite type

Local Anesthetic/Vasoconstrictor Precautions No information available to require special precautions

Effects on Dental Treatment No significant effects or complications reported

Dosage 30-60 mL of 10% (sterile) solution 2-3 times/day by means of a rubber syringe

Pregnancy Risk Factor C

Generic Available Yes

Citric Acid, Magnesium Hydroxycarbonate, D-Gluconic Acid, Magnesium Acid Citrate, and Calcium Carbonate *see* Citric Acid Bladder Mixture *on page 335*

Citric Acid, Sodium Citrate, and Potassium Citrate

(SI trik AS id, SOW dee um SIT rate, & poe TASS ee um SIT rate)

Related Information

Potassium Citrate *on page 1100*

U.S. Brand Names Cytra-3; Polycitra®

(Continued)

Citric Acid, Sodium Citrate, and Potassium Citrate *(Continued)*

Pharmacologic Category Alkalinizing Agent

Synonyms Potassium Citrate, Citric Acid, and Sodium Citrate; Potassium Citrate Mixture and Sodium Citrate; Sodium Citrate and Potassium Citrate Mixture; Sodium Citrate, Citric Acid, and Potassium Citrate

Use Conditions where long-term maintenance of an alkaline urine is desirable as in control and dissolution of uric acid and cystine calculi of the urinary tract

Local Anesthetic/Vasoconstrictor Precautions No information available to require special precautions

Effects on Dental Treatment No significant effects or complications reported

Dosage Oral:

Children: 5-15 mL diluted in water after meals and at bedtime

Adults: 15-30 mL diluted in water after meals and at bedtime

Drug Interactions

Increased Effect/Toxicity: Increased toxicity/levels of amphetamines, ephedrine, pseudoephedrine, flecainide, quinidine, and quinine due to urinary alkalinization.

Decreased Effect: Decreased effect/levels of lithium, chlorpropamide, and salicylates due to urinary alkalinization.

Dietary/Ethanol/Herb Considerations Food: Administer after meals.

Pregnancy Risk Factor Not established

Generic Available No

Citrovorum Factor *see* Leucovorin *on page 783*

Citrucel® [OTC] *see* Methylcellulose *on page 891*

CI-719 *see* Gemfibrozil *on page 631*

CL184116 *see* Porfimer *on page 1098*

Cla *see* Clarithromycin *on page 337*

Cladribine (KLA dri been)

U.S. Brand Names Leustatin®

Canadian Brand Names Leustatin®

Pharmacologic Category Antineoplastic Agent, Antimetabolite

Synonyms 2-CdA; 2-Chlorodeoxyadenosine

Use Treatment of hairy cell leukemia, chronic lymphocytic leukemia, non-Hodgkin's lymphomas, progressive multiple sclerosis

Local Anesthetic/Vasoconstrictor Precautions No information available to require special precautions

Effects on Dental Treatment

>10%: Fever (70%), headache (13%), fatigue (17%)

1% to 10%: Tachycardia, dizziness, pain, severe infections (possibly related to thrombocytopenia), nausea (mild to moderate; usually not seen at doses <0.3 mg/kg/day), weakness, diaphoresis, malaise

Dosage I.V.: Refer to individual protocols.

Pediatrics: Acute leukemias: Optimum dose not determined; 6.2-7.5 mg/m^2/day continuous infusion for days 1-5; maximum tolerated dose was 8.9 mg/m^2/day.

Adults:

Hairy cell leukemia: Continuous infusion:

0.09-0.1 mg/kg/day days 1-7; may be repeated every 28-35 days **or**

3.4 mg/m^2/day S.C. days 1-7

Chronic lymphocytic leukemia: Continuous infusion:

0.1 mg/kg/day days 1-7 **or**

0.028-0.14 mg/kg/day as a 2-hour infusion days 1-5

Chronic myelogenous leukemia: 15 mg/m^2/day as a 1-hour infusion days 1-5; if no response increase second course to 20 mg/m^2/day.

Mechanism of Action A purine nucleoside analogue; prodrug which is activated via phosphorylation by deoxycytidine kinase to a 5'-triphosphate derivative. This active form incorporates into susceptible cells and into DNA to result in the breakage of DNA strand and shutdown of DNA synthesis. This also results in a depletion of nicotinamide adenine dinucleotide and adenosine triphosphate (ATP). The induction of strand breaks results in a drop in the cofactor nicotinamide adenine dinucleotide and disruption of cell metabolism. ATP is depleted to deprive cells of an important source of energy. Cladribine effectively kills resting as well as dividing cells.

Other Adverse Effects

>10%:

Allergic: Chills (18%); skin reactions (erythema, itching) at catheter site (18%)

Dermatologic: Rash

Hematologic: Myelosuppression (common, dose-limiting), leukopenia (70%), anemia (37%), thrombocytopenia (12%)

Nadir: 5-10 days

Recovery: 4-8 weeks

1% to 10%:
Cardiovascular: Edema
Central nervous system: Chills
Dermatologic: Pruritus, erythema
Gastrointestinal: Constipation, abdominal pain
Neuromuscular & skeletal: Myalgia, arthralgia
Renal: Renal failure at high (>0.3 mg/kg/day) doses
Miscellaneous: Delayed herpes zoster infections, tumor lysis syndrome

<1%: Neuromuscular & skeletal: **Paraparesis, quadriplegia (high doses)**

Miscellaneous: One report of opportunistic infection, possibly due to decreased CD4 counts.

Dietary/Ethanol/Herb Considerations Ethanol: Avoid use due to GI irritation.

Pharmacodynamics/Kinetics

Distribution: V_d: 4.52 ± 2.82 L/kg
Protein binding, plasma: 20%
Half-life elimination: Biphasic: Alpha: 25 minutes; Beta: 6.7 hours; Terminal, mean: Normal renal function: 5.4 hours
Excretion: Urine
Clearance: Estimated systemic: 640 mL/hour/kg

Pregnancy Risk Factor D

Generic Available Yes

Claforan® *see* Cefotaxime *on page 271*
Clarinex® *see* Desloratadine *on page 410*
Claripel™ *see* Hydroquinone *on page 693*

Clarithromycin (kla RITH roe mye sin)

Related Information

Antibiotic Prophylaxis, Preprocedural Guidelines for Dental Patients *on page 1507*
Gastrointestinal Disorders *on page 1474*
Oral Bacterial Infections *on page 1531*
Respiratory Diseases *on page 1476*

U.S. Brand Names Biaxin®; Biaxin® XL

Canadian Brand Names Biaxin®; Biaxin® XL

Mexican Brand Names Adel®; Klaricid®; Mabicrol®

Pharmacologic Category Antibiotic, Macrolide

Synonyms Cla

Use

Dental: Alternate antibiotic in the treatment of common orofacial infections caused by aerobic gram-positive cocci and susceptible anaerobes; alternate antibiotic for the prevention of bacterial endocarditis in patients undergoing dental procedures

Medical:

Adults:

Pharyngitis/tonsillitis due to susceptible *S. pyogenes*

Acute maxillary sinusitis and acute exacerbation of chronic bronchitis due to susceptible *H. influenzae, M. catarrhalis,* or *S. pneumoniae*;

Pneumonia due to susceptible *H. influenzae, Mycoplasma pneumoniae, S. pneumoniae,* or *Chlamydia pneumoniae* (TWAR);

Uncomplicated skin/skin structure infections due to susceptible *S. aureus, S. pyogenes*;

Disseminated mycobacterial infections due to *M. avium* or *M. intracellulare*

Prevention of disseminated mycobacterial infections due to *M. avium* complex (MAC) disease (eg, patients with advanced HIV infection)

Duodenal ulcer disease due to *H. pylori* in regimens with other drugs including amoxicillin and lansoprazole or omeprazole, ranitidine bismuth citrate, bismuth subsalicylate, tetracycline and/or an H_2 antagonist

Alternate antibiotic for prophylaxis of bacterial endocarditis in patients who are allergic to penicillin and undergoing surgical or dental procedures

Children:

Pharyngitis/tonsillitis, acute maxillary sinusitis, uncomplicated skin/skin structure infections, and mycobacterial infections due to the above organisms

Acute otitis media (*H. influenzae, M. catarrhalis,* or *S. pneumoniae*)

Prevention of disseminated mycobacterial infections due to MAC disease in patients with advanced HIV infection

Local Anesthetic/Vasoconstrictor Precautions No information available to require special precautions

Effects on Dental Treatment 1% to 7%: Headache (2%), vomiting (6%; children), nausea (3%; adults), abnormal taste (7%; adults), increased PT (1%)

Dosage Oral:

Children ≥6 months: 15 mg/kg/day divided every 12 hours for 10 days

Mycobacterial infection (prevention and treatment): 7.5 mg/kg twice daily, up to 500 mg twice daily

Prophylaxis of bacterial endocarditis: 15 mg/kg 1 hour before procedure (maximum dose: 500 mg)

(Continued)

Clarithromycin *(Continued)*

Adults:

Usual dose: 250-500 mg every 12 hours **or** 1000 mg (two 500 mg extended release tablets) once daily for for 7-14 days

Upper respiratory tract: 250-500 mg every 12 hours for 10-14 days

Pharyngitis/tonsillitis: 250 mg every 12 hours for 10 days

Acute maxillary sinusitis: 500 mg every 12 hours **or** 1000 mg (two 500 mg extended release tablets) once daily for 14 days

Lower respiratory tract: 250-500 mg every 12 hours for 7-14 days

Acute exacerbation of chronic bronchitis due to:

M. catarrhalis and *S. pneumoniae*: 250 mg every 12 hours **or** 1000 mg (two 500 mg extended release tablets) once daily for 7-14 days

H. influenzae: 500 mg every 12 hours for 7-14 days

Pneumonia due to:

C. pneumoniae, *M. pneumoniae*, and *S. pneumoniae*: 250 mg every 12 hours for 7-14 days **or** 1000 mg (two 500 mg extended release tablets) once daily for 7 days

H. influenzae: 250 mg every 12 hours for 7 days **or** 1000 mg (two 500 mg extended release tablets) once daily for 7 days

Mycobacterial infection (prevention and treatment): 500 mg twice daily (use with other antimycobacterial drugs, eg, ethambutol, clofazimine, or rifampin)

Prophylaxis of bacterial endocarditis: 500 mg 1 hour prior to procedure

Uncomplicated skin and skin structure: 250 mg every 12 hours for 7-14 days

Helicobacter pylori: Combination regimen with bismuth subsalicylate, tetracycline, clarithromycin, and an H_2-receptor antagonist; or combination of omeprazole and clarithromycin; 250 mg twice daily to 500 mg 3 times/day

Dosing adjustment in renal impairment:

Cl_{cr} <30 mL/minute: Half the normal dose or double the dosing interval

In combination with ritonavir:

Cl_{cr} 30-60 mL/minute: Decrease clarithromycin dose by 50%

Cl_{cr} <30 mL/minute: Decrease clarithromycin dose by 75%

Dosing adjustment in hepatic impairment: No dosing adjustment is needed as long as renal function is normal

Elderly: Pharmacokinetics are similar to those in younger adults; may have age-related reductions in renal function; monitor and adjust dose if necessary

Mechanism of Action Exerts its antibacterial action by binding to 50S ribosomal subunit resulting in inhibition of protein synthesis. The 14-OH metabolite of clarithromycin is twice as active as the parent compound against certain organisms.

Other Adverse Effects

1% to 10%:

Dermatologic: Rash (3%; children)

Gastrointestinal: Diarrhea (%), heartburn (2%; adults); abdominal pain (2% adults; 3% children)

Renal: Elevated BUN (4%)

<1% (Limited to important or life-threatening): *Clostridium difficile* colitis, alkaline phosphatase increased, **anaphylaxis,** anorexia, **anxiety,** AST increased, bilirubin increased, **dizziness, dyspnea, glossitis, hallucinations,** hepatic dysfunction, hepatitis, **hypoglycemia,** jaundice, leukopenia, **manic behavior, neuromuscular blockade (case reports),** neutropenia, pancreatitis, **psychosis,** QT prolongation, **seizures,** serum creatinine increased, Stevens-Johnson syndrome, thrombocytopenia; **tongue discoloration, torsade de pointes**, toxic epidermal necrolysis, **tremor, ventricular tachycardia**, vertigo, **vomiting**

Contraindications Hypersensitivity to clarithromycin, erythromycin, or any macrolide antibiotic; use with ergot derivatives, pimozide, astemizole, cisapride; combination with ranitidine bismuth citrate should not be used in patients with history of acute porphyria or Cl_{cr} <25 mL/minute

Warnings/Precautions Dosage adjustment required with severe renal impairment, decreased dosage or prolonged dosing interval may be appropriate; antibiotic-associated colitis has been reported with use of clarithromycin. Macrolides (including clarithromycin) have been associated with rare QT prolongation and ventricular arrhythmias, including torsade de pointes. Safety and efficacy in children <6 months of age have not been established.

Drug Interactions Substrate of **CYP3A4**; Inhibits CYP1A2, **3A4**

Alfentanil (and possibly other narcotic analgesics): Serum levels may be increased by clarithromycin; monitor for increased effect.

Antipsychotic agents (particularly mesoridazine and thioridazine): Risk of QT_c prolongation and malignant arrhythmias may be increased.

Astemizole: Concomitant use is contraindicated; may lead to QT_c prolongation or torsade de pointes.

Benzodiazepines (those metabolized by CYP3A4, including alprazolam, midazolam, triazolam): Serum levels may be increased by clarithromycin; somnolence and confusion have been reported.

Bromocriptine: Serum levels may be increased by clarithromycin; monitor for increased effect.

Buspirone: Serum levels may be increased by clarithromycin; monitor.

Calcium channel blockers (felodipine, verapamil, and potentially others metabolized by CYP3A4): Serum levels may be increased by clarithromycin; monitor.

Carbamazepine: Serum levels may be increased by clarithromycin; monitor.

Cilostazol: Serum levels may be increased by clarithromycin; monitor.

Cisapride: Serum levels may be increased by clarithromycin; serious arrhythmias have occurred; concurrent use contraindicated.

Clindamycin (and lincomycin): Use with clarithromycin may result in pharmacologic antagonism; manufacturer recommends avoiding this combination.

Clozapine: Serum levels may be increased by clarithromycin; monitor.

Colchicine: serum levels/toxicity may be increased by clarithromycin; monitor.

Cyclosporine: Serum levels may be increased by clarithromycin; monitor serum levels.

Delavirdine: Serum levels may be increased by clarithromycin; monitor.

Digoxin: Serum levels may be increased by clarithromycin; digoxin toxicity and potentially fatal arrhythmias have been reported; monitor digoxin levels.

Disopyramide: Serum levels may be increased by clarithromycin; in addition, QT_c prolongation and risk of malignant arrhythmia may be increased; avoid combination.

Ergot alkaloids: Concurrent use may lead to acute ergot toxicity (severe peripheral vasospasm and dysesthesia).

Fluconazole: Increases clarithromycin levels and AUC by ~25%

HMG-CoA reductase inhibitors (atorvastatin, lovastatin, and simvastatin); Clarithromycin may increase serum levels of "statins" metabolized by CYP3A4, increasing the risk of myopathy/rhabdomyolysis (does not include fluvastatin and pravastatin). Switch to pravastatin/fluvastatin or suspend treatment during course of clarithromycin therapy.

Loratadine: Serum levels may be increased by clarithromycin; monitor.

Methylprednisolone: Serum levels may be increased by clarithromycin; monitor.

Neuromuscular-blocking agents: May be potentiated by clarithromycin (case reports).

Phenytoin: Serum levels may be increased by clarithromycin; other evidence suggested phenytoin levels may be decreased in some patients; monitor.

Pimozide: Serum levels may be increased, leading to malignant arrhythmias; concomitant use is contraindicated.

Protease inhibitors (amprenavir, nelfinavir, and ritonavir): May increase serum levels of clarithromycin.

QT_c-prolonging agents: Concomitant use may increase the risk of malignant arrhythmias.

Quinidine: Serum levels may be increased by clarithromycin; in addition, the risk of QT_c prolongation and malignant arrhythmias may be increased during concurrent use.

Quinolone antibiotics (sparfloxacin, gatifloxacin, or moxifloxacin): Concurrent use may increase the risk of malignant arrhythmias.

Rifabutin: Serum levels may be increased by clarithromycin; monitor.

Sildenafil: Serum levels may be increased by clarithromycin; monitor.

Tacrolimus: Serum levels may be increased by clarithromycin; monitor serum concentration.

Theophylline: Serum levels may be increased by clarithromycin; monitor.

Valproic acid (and derivatives): Serum levels may be increased by clarithromycin; monitor.

Vinblastine (and vincristine): Serum levels may be increased by clarithromycin.

Warfarin: Effects may be potentiated; monitor INR closely and adjust warfarin dose as needed or choose another antibiotic

Zafirlukast: Serum levels may be decreased by clarithromycin; monitor.

Zidovudine: Peak levels (but not AUC) of zidovudine may be increased; other studies suggest levels may be decreased.

Zopiclone: Serum levels may be increased by clarithromycin; monitor.

Dietary/Ethanol/Herb Considerations

Ethanol: Use with caution; may increase CNS depression.

Administer with food or milk to reduce GI upset; extended release tablets should be taken with food; food or milk delays absorption but total absorption unaffected. Buttermilk, boiled milk, or yogurt may reduce diarrhea.

Herb/Nutraceutical: Avoid St John's wort; may decrease serum concentration.

Pharmacodynamics/Kinetics

Absorption: Highly stable in presence of gastric acid (unlike erythromycin); food delays but does not affect extent of absorption

Distribution: Widely into most body tissues except CNS

Metabolism: Partially hepatic; converted to 14-OH clarithromycin (active metabolite)

Bioavailability: 50%

Half-life elimination: 5-7 hours

Time to peak: 2-4 hours

Excretion: Primarily urine

Clearance: Approximates normal GFR

Pregnancy Risk Factor C

(Continued)

Clarithromycin *(Continued)*

Breast-feeding Considerations Erythromycins may be taken while breast-feeding. Use caution.

Dosage Forms GRAN, oral suspension: 125 mg/5 mL (50 mL, 100 mL); 187.5 mg/5 mL (100 mL); 250 mg/5 mL (50 mL, 100 mL). **TAB, film coated:** 250 mg, 500 mg. **TAB, film coated, extended release:** 500 mg

Generic Available No

Comments *Helicobacter pylori* induced gastric ulcers: Combination regimen with bismuth subsalicylate, tetracycline, clarithromycin, and an H_2-receptor antagonist; or combination of omeprazole and clarithromycin. Adult dosage: Oral: 250 mg twice daily to 500 mg 3 times/day.

Selected Readings

Amsden GW, "Erythromycin, Clarithromycin, and Azithromycin: Are the Differences Real?" *Clin Ther,* 1996, 18(1):56-72.

Dajani AS, Taubert KA, Wilson W, et al, "Prevention of Bacterial Endocarditis. Recommendations by the American Heart Association," *JAMA* 1997, 277(22):1794-801.

Dajani AS, Taubert KA, Wilson W, et al, "Prevention of Bacterial Endocarditis: Recommendations by the American Heart Association," *J Am Dent Assoc* 1997, 128(8):1142-51.

"Pimozide (Orap) Contraindicated With Clarithromycin (Biaxin®) and Other Macrolide Antibiotics," *FDA Medical Bulletin,* October 1996, 26 (3).

Wynn RL, "New Erythromycins," *Gen Dent,* 1996, 44(4):304-7.

Wynn RL, Bergman SA, Meiller TF, et al, "Antibiotics in Treating Oral-Facial Infections of Odontogenic Origin: An Update", *Gen Dent,* 2001, 49(3):238-40, 242, 244 passim.

Claritin® [OTC] *see* Loratadine *on page 822*

Claritin-D® 12-Hour [OTC] *see* Loratadine and Pseudoephedrine *on page 823*

Claritin-D® 24-Hour [OTC] *see* Loratadine and Pseudoephedrine *on page 823*

Clear Eyes® [OTC] *see* Naphazoline *on page 952*

Clear Eyes® ACR [OTC] *see* Naphazoline *on page 952*

Clemastine (KLEM as teen)

U.S. Brand Names Antihist-1® [OTC]; Tavist®; Tavist®-1 [OTC]

Mexican Brand Names Tavist®

Pharmacologic Category Antihistamine

Synonyms Clemastine Fumarate

Use Perennial and seasonal allergic rhinitis and other allergic symptoms including urticaria

Local Anesthetic/Vasoconstrictor Precautions No information available to require special precautions

Effects on Dental Treatment

>10%: Slight to moderate drowsiness, thickening of bronchial secretions

1% to 10%: Headache, nervousness, increased dizziness, xerostomia, nausea, pharyngitis, fatigue

Dosage Oral:

Infants and Children <6 years: 0.05 mg/kg/day as **clemastine base** or 0.335-0.67 mg/day clemastine fumarate (0.25-0.5 mg base/day) divided into 2 or 3 doses; maximum daily dosage: 1.34 mg (1 mg base)

Children 6-12 years: 0.67-1.34 mg clemastine fumarate (0.5-1 mg base) twice daily; do not exceed 4.02 mg/day (3 mg/day base)

Children ≥12 years and Adults: 1.34 mg clemastine fumarate (1 mg base) twice daily to 2.68 mg (2 mg base) 3 times/day; do not exceed 8.04 mg/day (6 mg base)

Elderly: Consider lower doses in patients >60 years

Mechanism of Action Competes with histamine for H_1-receptor sites on effector cells in the gastrointestinal tract, blood vessels, and respiratory tract

Other Adverse Effects

1% to 10%:

Gastrointestinal: Appetite increase, weight gain, diarrhea, abdominal pain

Neuromuscular & skeletal: Arthralgia

<1%: Edema, **palpitations**, depression, angioedema, photosensitivity, rash, hepatitis, myalgia, **paresthesia, bronchospasm, epistaxis**

Drug Interactions Inhibits **CYP2D6**, 3A4

Increased Effect/Toxicity: CNS depressants may increase the degree of sedation and respiratory depression with antihistamines. May increase the absorption of digoxin. Central and/or peripheral anticholinergic syndrome can occur when administered with amantadine, rimantadine, narcotic analgesics, phenothiazines and other antipsychotics (especially with high anticholinergic activity), tricyclic antidepressants, quinidine, disopyramide, procainamide, and antihistamines.

Decreased Effect: May increase gastric degradation of levodopa and decrease the amount of levodopa absorbed by delaying gastric emptying. Therapeutic effects of cholinergic agents (tacrine, donepezil) and neuroleptics may be antagonized.

Dietary/Ethanol/Herb Considerations

Ethanol: Avoid use; may increase CNS depression.

Herb/Nutraceutical: Avoid gotu kola, kava, SAMe, St John's wort, and valerian; may increase CNS depression.

Pharmacodynamics/Kinetics

Onset of action: Peak effect: Therapeutic: 5-7 hours

Duration: 8-16 hours

Absorption: Almost complete

Metabolism: Hepatic

Excretion: Urine

Pregnancy Risk Factor B

Generic Available Yes

Clemastine Fumarate *see* Clemastine *on page 340*

Cleocin® *see* Clindamycin *on page 341*

Cleocin HCl® *see* Clindamycin *on page 341*

Cleocin Pediatric® *see* Clindamycin *on page 341*

Cleocin Phosphate® *see* Clindamycin *on page 341*

Cleocin T® *see* Clindamycin *on page 341*

Clidinium and Chlordiazepoxide

(kli DI nee um & klor dye az e POKS ide)

U.S. Brand Names Librax®

Canadian Brand Names Apo®-Chlorax; Librax®

Pharmacologic Category Antispasmodic Agent, Gastrointestinal; Benzodiazepine

Synonyms Chlordiazepoxide and Clidinium

Use Adjunct treatment of peptic ulcer; treatment of irritable bowel syndrome

Local Anesthetic/Vasoconstrictor Precautions No information available to require special precautions

Effects on Dental Treatment

>10%: Xerostomia, changes in salivation

1% to 10%: Drowsiness, confusion, anticholinergic side effects, nausea

Dosage Oral: 1-2 capsules 3-4 times/day, before meals or food and at bedtime

Other Adverse Effects 1% to 10%:

Central nervous system: Ataxia

Gastrointestinal: Constipation

Drug Interactions Increased Effect/Toxicity: Additive effects may result from concomitant benzodiazepine and/or anticholinergic therapy.

Dietary/Ethanol/Herb Considerations

Ethanol: Avoid use; may increase CNS depression.

Herb/Nutraceutical: Avoid gotu kola, kava, SAMe, St John's wort, and valerian; may increase CNS depression.

Pregnancy Risk Factor D

Generic Available Yes

Comments After extended therapy, abrupt discontinuation should be avoided and a gradual dose tapering schedule followed

Climara® *see* Estradiol *on page 521*

Clinac™ BPO *see* Benzoyl Peroxide *on page 171*

Clindagel™ *see* Clindamycin *on page 341*

Clindamycin (klin da MYE sin)

Related Information

Animal and Human Bites Guidelines *on page 1580*

Antibiotic Prophylaxis, Preprocedural Guidelines for Dental Patients *on page 1507*

Cardiovascular Diseases *on page 1456*

Oral Bacterial Infections *on page 1531*

Periodontal Diseases *on page 1540*

Sexually-Transmitted Diseases *on page 1502*

U.S. Brand Names Cleocin®; Cleocin HCl®; Cleocin Pediatric®; Cleocin Phosphate®; Cleocin T®; Clindagel™; Clindets®

Canadian Brand Names Alti-Clindamycin; Dalacin® C; Dalacin® T; Dalacin® Vaginal

Mexican Brand Names Clindazyn®; Cutaclin®; Dalacin C®; Dalacin T®; Dalacin V®; Galecin®; Klyndaken®

Pharmacologic Category Antibiotic, Miscellaneous

Synonyms Clindamycin Hydrochloride; Clindamycin Phosphate

Use

Dental: Alternate antibiotic, when amoxicillin cannot be used, for the standard regimen for prevention of bacterial endocarditis in patients undergoing dental procedures; alternate antibiotic in the treatment of common oral-facial infections caused by aerobic gram-positive cocci and susceptible anaerobes; alternate antibiotic for prophylaxis for dental patients with total joint replacement

Medical: Treatment against aerobic and anaerobic streptococci (except enterococci), most staphylococci, *Bacteroides* sp and *Actinomyces*; treatment of *Gardnerella, PCP, vaginalis*, severe acne; alternate treatment for toxoplasmosis

(Continued)

Clindamycin *(Continued)*

Local Anesthetic/Vasoconstrictor Precautions No information available to require special precautions

Effects on Dental Treatment Systemic: 1% to 10%: Hypotension, nausea, vomiting, fungal overgrowth, dizziness, headache, hypersensitivity, pseudomembranous colitis **(has never occurred with the 1-dose regimen of clindamycin used to prevent bacterial endocarditis)**

Dosage

Infants and Children (avoid in neonates; contains benzyl alcohol):

Oral: 8-20 mg/kg/day as hydrochloride; 8-25 mg/kg/day as palmitate in 3-4 divided doses; minimum dose of palmitate: 37.5 mg 3 times/day

I.M., I.V.:

<1 month: 15-20 mg/kg/day

>1 month: 20-40 mg/kg/day in 3-4 divided doses

Children: **Prevention of bacterial endocarditis:** Oral: 20 mg/kg 1 hour before procedure with no follow-up dose needed; for patients allergic to penicillin and unable to take oral medications: 20 mg/kg I.V. within 30 minutes before procedure

Children ≥12 years and Adults: Topical: Apply a thin film twice daily

Adults:

Oral: 150-450 mg/dose every 6-8 hours; maximum dose: 1.8 g/day

Prevention of bacterial endocarditis in patients unable to take amoxicillin: Oral: 600 mg 1 hour before procedure with no follow-up dose needed; for patients allergic to penicillin and unable to take oral medications: 600 mg I.V. within 30 minutes before procedure

I.M., I.V.: 1.2-1.8 g/day in 2-4 divided doses; maximum dose: 4.8 g/day

Pelvic inflammatory disease: I.V.: 900 mg every 8 hours with gentamicin 2 mg/kg, then 1.5 mg/kg every 8 hours; continue after discharge with doxycycline 100 mg twice daily to complete 14 days of total therapy

Pneumocystis carinii pneumonia:

Oral: 300-450 mg 4 times/day with primaquine

I.M., I.V.: 1200-2400 mg/day with pyrimethamine

I.V.: 600 mg 4 times/day with primaquine

Bacterial vaginosis:

Oral: 300 mg twice daily for 7 days

Intravaginal:

Suppositories: Insert one ovule (100 mg clindamycin) daily into vagina at bedtime for 3 days

Cream: One full applicator inserted intravaginally once daily before bedtime for 3 or 7 consecutive days

Dosing adjustment in hepatic impairment: Adjustment recommended in patients with severe hepatic disease

Mechanism of Action Reversibly binds to 50S ribosomal subunits preventing peptide bond formation thus inhibiting bacterial protein synthesis; bacteriostatic or bactericidal depending on drug concentration, infection site, and organism

Other Adverse Effects

Systemic:

>10%: Gastrointestinal: Diarrhea, abdominal pain

1% to 10%:

Dermatologic: Urticaria, rashes, Stevens-Johnson syndrome

Local: Thrombophlebitis, sterile abscess at I.M. injection site

<1% (Limited to important or life-threatening): Renal dysfunction (rare), neutropenia, granulocytopenia, thrombocytopenia, polyarthritis

Topical:

>10%: Dermatologic: Dryness, burning, itching, scaliness, erythema, or peeling of skin (lotion, solution); oiliness (gel, lotion)

<1% (Limited to important or life-threatening): Pseudomembranous colitis, **nausea, vomiting**, diarrhea (severe), abdominal pain, folliculitis, **hypersensitivity reactions**

Vaginal:

>10%: Genitourinary: Vaginitis or vulvovaginal pruritus (from *Candida albicans*), painful intercourse

1% to 10%: Gastrointestinal: Diarrhea, stomach cramps

Contraindications Hypersensitivity to clindamycin or any component of the formulation; previous pseudomembranous colitis; hepatic impairment

Warnings/Precautions Dosage adjustment may be necessary in patients with severe hepatic dysfunction; can cause severe and possibly fatal colitis; use with caution in patients with a history of pseudomembranous colitis; discontinue drug if significant diarrhea, abdominal cramps, or passage of blood and mucus occurs. Avoid in neonates (contains benzyl alcohol).

Drug Interactions Increased duration of neuromuscular blockade from tubocurarine, pancuronium

Dietary/Ethanol/Herb Considerations

Food: Oral form may be taken with food but may delay peak concentration.

Herb/Nutraceutical: Avoid St John's wort; may decrease serum concentration.

Pharmacodynamics/Kinetics

Absorption: Topical: ~10%; Oral: Rapid (90%)

Distribution: High concentrations in bone and urine; no significant levels in CSF, even with inflamed meninges; crosses placenta; enters breast milk

Metabolism: Hepatic

Bioavailability: Topical: <1%

Half-life elimination: Neonates: Premature: 8.7 hours; Full-term: 3.6 hours; Adults: 1.6-5.3 hours (average: 2-3 hours)

Time to peak, serum: Oral: Within 60 minutes; I.M.: 1-3 hours

Excretion: Urine (10%) and feces (~4%) as active drug and metabolites

Pregnancy Risk Factor B

Dosage Forms CAP, as hydrochloride (Cleocin HCl®): 75 mg, 150 mg, 300 mg. **CRM, vaginal, as phosphate** (Cleocin®): 2% (40 g) **GEL, topical, as phosphate** (Cleocin T®): 1% [10 mg/g] (30 g, 60 g); (Clindagel™): 1% [10 mg/g] (42 g, 77 g). **GRAN, oral solution, as palmitate** (Cleocin Pediatric®): 75 mg/5 mL (100 mL). **INF, as phosphate** [premixed in D_5W] (Cleocin Phosphate®): 300 mg (50 mL); 600 mg (50 mL); 900 mg (50 mL). **INJ, solution, as phosphate** (Cleocin Phosphate®): 150 mg/mL (2 mL, 4 mL, 6 mL, 60 mL). **LOTION, as phosphate** (Cleocin T®): 1% (60 mL). **PLEDGET, topical**: (Clindets®): 1% (69s); (Cleocin T®): 1% (60s). **SOLN, topical, as phosphate** (Cleocin T®): 1% (30 mL, 60 mL). **SUPP, vaginal, as phosphate** (Cleocin®): 100 mg

Generic Available Yes

Comments Has not been shown to interfere with oral contraceptive activity; however, it however, it reduces GI microflora, thus, oral contraceptive users should be advised to use additional methods of birth control.

Selected Readings

"Advisory Statement. Antibiotic Prophylaxis for Dental Patients With Total Joint Replacements. American Dental Association; American Academy of Orthopedic Surgeons," *J Am Dent Assoc*, 1997, 128(7):1004-8.

Dajani AS, Taubert KA, Wilson W, et al, "Prevention of Bacterial Endocarditis. Recommendations by the American Heart Association," *JAMA* 1997, 277(22):1794-801.

Dajani AS, Taubert KA, Wilson W, et al, "Prevention of Bacterial Endocarditis: Recommendations by the American Heart Association," *J Am Dent Assoc* 1997, 128(8):1142-51.

Wynn RL, "Clindamycin: An Often Forgotten but Important Antibiotic," *AGD Impact*, 1994, 22:10.

Wynn RL and Bergman SA, "Antibiotics and Their Use in the Treatment of Orofacial Infections, Part I," *Gen Dent*, 1994, 42(5):398, 400, 402.

Wynn RL and Bergman SA, "Antibiotics and Their Use in the Treatment of Orofacial Infections, Part II," *Gen Dent*, 1994, 42(6):498-502.

Wynn RL, Bergman SA, Meiller TF, et al, "Antibiotics in Treating Oral-Facial Infections of Odontogenic Origin: An Update", *Gen Dent*, 2001, 49(3):238-40, 242, 244 passim.

Clindamycin and Benzoyl Peroxide

(klin da MYE sin & BEN zoe il peer OKS ide)

Related Information

Benzoyl Peroxide *on page 171*

Clindamycin *on page 341*

U.S. Brand Names BenzaClin®; Duac™

Pharmacologic Category Topical Skin Product; Topical Skin Product, Acne

Synonyms Benzoyl Peroxide and Clindamycin

Use Topical treatment of acne vulgaris

Local Anesthetic/Vasoconstrictor Precautions No information available to require special precautions

Effects on Dental Treatment No significant effects or complications reported

Dosage Topical: Children ≥12 years and Adults: Apply to affected areas after skin has been cleansed and dried; avoid applying to inside nose, mouth, eyes, and mucous membranes

BenzaClin®: Acne: Apply twice daily (morning and evening)

Duac™: Inflammatory acne: Apply once daily in the evening

Mechanism of Action Clindamycin and benzoyl peroxide have activity against *Propionibacterium acnes in vitro.* This organism has been associated with acne vulgaris. Benzoyl peroxide releases free-radical oxygen which oxidizes bacterial proteins in the sebaceous follicles decreasing the number of anaerobic bacteria and decreasing irritating-type free fatty acids. Clindamycin reversibly binds to 50S ribosomal subunits preventing peptide bond formation thus inhibiting bacterial protein synthesis; bacteriostatic or bactericidal depending on drug concentration, infection site, and organism.

Other Adverse Effects Frequency not defined: Dermatologic: Dry skin, pruritus, peeling, erythema, sunburn, redness, burning

Postmarketing and/or case reports: Colitis, diarrhea, pseudomembranous colitis

Drug Interactions

Increased Effect/Toxicity: Tretinoin may cause increased adverse events with concurrent use.

Decreased Effect: Erythromycin may antagonize clindamycin's effects.

Pharmacodynamics/Kinetics

Absorption: Benzoyl peroxide: <2% systemically absorbed

Metabolism: Benzoyl peroxide: Converted to benzoic acid in the skin

Pregnancy Risk Factor C

Generic Available No

Clindamycin Hydrochloride *see* Clindamycin *on page 341*

Clindamycin Phosphate *see* Clindamycin *on page 341*

Clindets® *see* Clindamycin *on page 341*

Clinoril® *see* Sulindac *on page 1257*

Clobazam (KLOE ba zam)

Canadian Brand Names Alti-Clobazam; Frisium®; Novo-Clobazam; PMS-Clobazam

Pharmacologic Category Benzodiazepine

Use Adjunctive treatment of epilepsy

Unlabeled/Investigational Use Monotherapy for epilepsy or intermittent seizures

Local Anesthetic/Vasoconstrictor Precautions No information available to require special precautions

Effects on Dental Treatment Paradoxical reactions (including excitation, agitation, hallucinations, and psychosis) are known to occur with benzodiazepines.

>10%: Drowsiness (17%)

1% to 10%: Dizziness (2%), behavior disorder (1%), blurred vision (1%)

Frequency not defined: Confusion, lethargy, slurred speech, tremor, anterograde amnesia, nausea, xerostomia, muscle spasm

Dosage Oral:

Children:

<2 years: Initial 0.5-1 mg/kg/day

2-16 years: Initial: 5 mg/day; may be increased (no more frequently than every 5 days) to a maximum of 40 mg/day

Adults: Initial: 5-15 mg/day; may be gradually adjusted (based on tolerance and seizure control) to a maximum of 80 mg/day; daily doses of up to 30 mg may be taken as a single dose at bedtime (higher doses should be divided)

Dosing adjustment in hepatic impairment: Avoid use in severe impairment. Use lower doses in mild-moderate impairment and monitor closely.

Mechanism of Action Clobazam is a 1,5 benzodiazepine which binds to stereospecific benzodiazepine receptors on the postsynaptic GABA neuron at several sites within the central nervous system, including the limbic system, reticular formation. Enhancement of the inhibitory effect of GABA on neuronal excitability results by increased neuronal membrane permeability to chloride ions. This shift in chloride ions results in hyperpolarization (a less excitable state) and stabilization.

Other Adverse Effects Decreased WBCs and other hematologic abnormalities have been rarely associated with benzodiazepines.

Frequency not always defined:

Central nervous system: Ataxia (4%), depression

Dermatologic: Rash, pruritus, urticaria

Gastrointestinal: Weight gain (2%)

Dose-related: Constipation

Drug Interactions Substrate of **CYP3A4**

Increased Effect/Toxicity: Benzodiazepines potentiate the CNS depressant effects of narcotic analgesics, barbiturates, phenothiazines, ethanol, antihistamines, MAO inhibitors, sedative-hypnotics, and cyclic antidepressants. Serum levels and/or effects of benzodiazepines may be increased by inhibitors of CYP3A4, including amiodarone, amprenavir, cimetidine, clarithromycin, erythromycin, delavirdine, diltiazem, dirithromycin, disulfiram, fluoxetine, fluvoxamine, grapefruit juice, indinavir, itraconazole, ketoconazole, nefazodone, nevirapine, propoxyphene, quinupristin-dalfopristin, ritonavir, saquinavir, verapamil, zafirlukast, zileuton.

Decreased Effect: Carbamazepine, rifampin, rifabutin may enhance the metabolism of benzodiazepines and decrease its therapeutic effect.

Dietary/Ethanol/Herb Considerations

Ethanol: Avoid use; may increase bioavailability of clobazam by 50% and increase CNS depression.

Food: Administer with food to reduce GI upset. Small, frequent meals, chewing gum, or sucking lozenges may reduce nausea and vomiting. Fluids, fruit, and fiber may reduce constipation. Avoid grapefruit products; may increase serum concentration.

Herb/Nutraceutical: Avoid gotu kola, kava, SAMe, and valerian; may increase CNS depression. Avoid St John's wort; may decrease serum concentration and increase CNS depression.

Pharmacodynamics/Kinetics

Absorption: Rapid

Protein binding: 85% to 91%

Metabolism: Hepatic via N-dealkylation (likely via CYP) to active metabolite (N-desmethyl), and glucuronidation

Bioavailability: 87%

Half-life elimination: 18 hours; N-desmethyl (active): 42 hours

Time to peak: 15 minutes to 4 hours
Excretion: Urine (90%), as metabolites

Pregnancy Risk Factor Not assigned; similar agents rated D. Contraindicated in 1st trimester (per manufacturer).

Generic Available Yes

Comments Clobazam is a 1,5 benzodiazepine; other benzodiazepines are typically 1,4 substituted.

Clobetasol (kloe BAY tu sol)

Related Information

Oral Nonviral Soft Tissue Ulcerations or Erosions *on page 1549*

U.S. Brand Names Cormax®; Embeline™ E; Olux®; Temovate®; Temovate E®

Canadian Brand Names Dermovate®; Gen-Clobetasol; Novo-Clobetasol®

Mexican Brand Names Dermatovate®

Pharmacologic Category Corticosteroid, Topical

Synonyms Clobetasol Propionate

Use Short-term relief of inflammation of moderate to severe corticosteroid-responsive dermatoses (very high potency topical corticosteroid)

Local Anesthetic/Vasoconstrictor Precautions No information available to require special precautions

Effects on Dental Treatment No significant effects or complications reported

Dosage Topical: Discontinue when control achieved; if improvement not seen within 2 weeks, reassessment of diagnosis may be necessary.

Children <12 years: Use not recommended

Children ≥12 years and Adults:

Steroid-responsive dermatoses:

Cream, emollient cream, gel, ointment: Apply twice daily for up to 2 weeks (maximum dose: 50 g/week)

Foam, solution: Apply to affected scalp twice daily for up to 2 weeks (maximum dose: 50 g/week or 50 mL/week)

Mild to moderate plaque-type psoriasis of nonscalp areas: Foam: Apply to affected area twice daily for up to 2 weeks (maximum dose: 50 g/week); do not apply to face or intertriginous areas

Children ≥16 years and Adults: Moderate to severe plaque-type psoriasis: Emollient cream: Apply twice daily for up to 2 weeks, has been used for up to 4 weeks when application is <10% of body surface area; use with caution (maximum dose: 50 g/week)

Mechanism of Action Stimulates the synthesis of enzymes needed to decrease inflammation, suppress mitotic activity, and cause vasoconstriction

Other Adverse Effects May depend upon formulation used, length of application, surface area covered, and the use of occlusive dressings. Frequency not defined;

Endocrine & metabolic: Adrenal suppression, Cushing's syndrome, hyperglycemia

Local: Application site: Burning, cracking/fissuring of the skin, dryness, erythema, folliculitis, irritation, numbness, pruritus, skin atrophy, stinging, telangiectasia

Renal: Glucosuria

Reported with other high-potency topical steroids: Acneiform eruptions, allergic contact dermatitis, hypertrichosis, hypopigmentation, maceration of the skin, miliaria, perioral dermatitis, secondary infection

Pharmacodynamics/Kinetics

Absorption: Percutaneous absorption is variable and dependent upon many factors including vehicle used, integrity of epidermis, dose, and use of occlusive dressings

Metabolism: Hepatic

Excretion: Urine and feces

Pregnancy Risk Factor C

Generic Available Yes: Excludes foam

Clobetasol Propionate *see* Clobetasol *on page 345*

Clocort™ *see* Hydrocortisone *on page 688*

Clocortolone (kloe KOR toe lone)

U.S. Brand Names Cloderm®

Canadian Brand Names Cloderm®

Pharmacologic Category Corticosteroid, Topical

Synonyms Clocortolone Pivalate

Use Inflammation of corticosteroid-responsive dermatoses (intermediate-potency topical corticosteroid)

Local Anesthetic/Vasoconstrictor Precautions No information available to require special precautions

Effects on Dental Treatment No significant effects or complications reported

Dosage Adults: Apply sparingly and gently; rub into affected area from 1-4 times/day. Therapy should be discontinued when control is achieved; if no improvement is seen, reassessment of diagnosis may be necessary.

(Continued)

Clocortolone *(Continued)*

Mechanism of Action Stimulates the synthesis of enzymes needed to decrease inflammation, suppress mitotic activity, and cause vasoconstriction

Other Adverse Effects

1% to 10%:

Dermatologic: Itching, erythema

Local: Burning, dryness, irritation, papular rashes

<1%: Hypertrichosis, acneiform eruptions, maceration of skin, skin atrophy, striae, hypopigmentation, perioral dermatitis, miliaria

Pharmacodynamics/Kinetics

Absorption: Percutaneous absorption is variable and dependent upon many factors including vehicle used, integrity of epidermis, dose, and use of occlusive dressings; small amounts enter circulatory system via skin

Metabolism: Hepatic

Excretion: Urine and feces

Pregnancy Risk Factor C

Generic Available No

Clocortolone Pivalate *see* Clocortolone *on page 345*

Clocream [OTC] *see* Vitamin A and Vitamin D *on page 1392*

Cloderm® *see* Clocortolone *on page 345*

Clofazimine (kloe FA zi meen)

Related Information

Tuberculosis *on page 1493*

U.S. Brand Names Lamprene®

Canadian Brand Names Lamprene®

Pharmacologic Category Leprostatic Agent

Synonyms Clofazimine Palmitate

Use Orphan drug: Treatment of dapsone-resistant leprosy; multibacillary dapsone-sensitive leprosy; erythema nodosum leprosum; *Mycobacterium avium-intracellulare* (MAI) infections

Local Anesthetic/Vasoconstrictor Precautions No information available to require special precautions

Effects on Dental Treatment

>10%: Nausea, vomiting

1% to 10%: Elevated blood sugar

Dosage Oral:

Children: Leprosy: 1 mg/kg/day every 24 hours in combination with dapsone and rifampin

Adults:

Dapsone-resistant leprosy: 100 mg/day in combination with one or more antileprosy drugs for 3 years; then alone 100 mg/day

Dapsone-sensitive multibacillary leprosy: 100 mg/day in combination with two or more antileprosy drugs for at least 2 years and continue until negative skin smears are obtained, then institute single drug therapy with appropriate agent

Erythema nodosum leprosum: 100-200 mg/day for up to 3 months or longer then taper dose to 100 mg/day when possible

Pyoderma gangrenosum: 300-400 mg/day for up to 12 months

Dosing adjustment in hepatic impairment: Should be considered in severe hepatic dysfunction

Mechanism of Action Binds preferentially to mycobacterial DNA to inhibit mycobacterial growth; also has some anti-inflammatory activity through an unknown mechanism

Other Adverse Effects

>10%:

Dermatologic: Dry skin

Gastrointestinal: Abdominal pain, diarrhea

Miscellaneous: Pink to brownish-black discoloration of the skin and conjunctiva

1% to 10%:

Dermatologic: Rash, pruritus

Gastrointestinal: Fecal discoloration

Genitourinary: Discoloration of urine

Ocular: Irritation of the eyes

Miscellaneous: Discoloration of sputum, sweat

<1%: Edema, vascular pain, **dizziness, drowsiness**, fatigue, **headache**, giddiness, **taste disorder, fever**, erythroderma, acneiform eruptions, monilial cheilosis, phototoxicity, hypokalemia, bowel obstruction, **GI bleeding**, anorexia, constipation, weight loss, eosinophilic enteritis, cystitis, eosinophilia, anemia, hepatitis, jaundice, enlarged liver, increased albumin/ serum bilirubin/AST, bone pain, neuralgia, **diminished vision, lymphadenopathy**

Drug Interactions Inhibits CYP3A4

Decreased Effect: Combined use may decrease effect with dapsone (unconfirmed).

Dietary/Ethanol/Herb Considerations Food increases the extent of absorption.

Pharmacodynamics/Kinetics

Absorption: Slow (45% to 70%)

Distribution: Highly lipophilic; deposited primarily in fatty tissue and cells of the reticuloendothelial system; taken up by macrophages throughout the body; distributed to breast milk, mesenteric lymph nodes, adrenal glands, subcutaneous fat, liver, bile, gallbladder, spleen, small intestine, muscles, bones, and skin; does not appear to cross blood-brain barrier; remains in tissues for prolonged periods

Metabolism: Partially hepatic to two metabolites

Half-life elimination: Terminal: 8 days; Tissue: 70 days

Time to peak, serum: Chronic therapy: 1-6 hours

Excretion: Primarily feces; urine (negligible amounts as unchanged drug); sputum, saliva, and sweat (small amounts)

Pregnancy Risk Factor C

Generic Available No

Clofazimine Palmitate *see* Clofazimine *on page 346*

Clofibrate (kloe FYE brate)

U.S. Brand Names Atromid-S®

Pharmacologic Category Antilipemic Agent, Fibric Acid

Use Adjunct to dietary therapy in the management of hyperlipidemias associated with high triglyceride levels (types III, IV, V); primarily lowers triglycerides and very low density lipoprotein

Local Anesthetic/Vasoconstrictor Precautions No information available to require special precautions

Effects on Dental Treatment Frequency not defined: Nausea, diarrhea, fever, chest pain, cardiac arrhythmias, stomatitis, gastritis, peptic ulcer arthritis, tremors, flu-like syndrome, increased diaphoresis

Dosage Adults: Oral: 500 mg 4 times/day; some patients may respond to lower doses

Dosing interval in renal impairment:

Cl_{cr} >50 mL/minute: Administer every 6-12 hours

Cl_{cr} 10-50 mL/minute: Administer every 12-18 hours

Cl_{cr} <10 mL/minute: Avoid use

Hemodialysis: Elimination is not enhanced via hemodialysis; supplemental dose is unnecessary

Mechanism of Action Mechanism is unclear but thought to reduce cholesterol synthesis and triglyceride hepatic-vascular transference

Other Adverse Effects

Frequency not defined: Less common:

Central nervous system: **Headache, dizziness**, fatigue

Gastrointestinal: **Vomiting**, loose stools, heartburn, flatulence, abdominal distress, **epigastric pain**

Neuromuscular & skeletal: **Muscle cramping, aching, weakness**, myalgia

Frequency unknown:

Dermatologic: Rash, urticaria, pruritus, alopecia, toxic epidermal necrolysis, erythema multiforme, Stevens-Johnson syndrome; dry, brittle hair

Endocrine & metabolic: Polyphagia, gynecomastia, hyperkalemia

Gastrointestinal: Gallstones, pancreatitis, weight gain

Genitourinary: Impotence, decreased libido

Hematologic: Leukopenia, anemia, eosinophilia, agranulocytosis, thrombocytopenic purpura

Hepatic: Increased LFTs, hepatomegaly, jaundice

Local: Thrombophlebitis

Neuromuscular & skeletal: Myalgia, myopathy, myositis, arthralgia, rhabdomyolysis, increased creatinine phosphokinase (CPK)

Ocular: Photophobic

Renal: Dysuria, hematuria, proteinuria, renal toxicity (allergic), rhabdomyolysis-induced renal failure

Miscellaneous: Systemic lupus erythematosus

Drug Interactions Substrate of CYP3A4; Inhibits CYP2A6; Induces CYP2B6, 2E1, 3A4

Increased Effect/Toxicity: Clofibrate may increase effects of warfarin, insulin, and sulfonylureas. Clofibrate's levels may be increased with probenecid. HMG-CoA reductase inhibitors (atorvastatin, cerivastatin, fluvastatin, lovastatin, pravastatin, simvastatin) may increase the risk of myopathy and rhabdomyolysis. The manufacturer warns against the concomitant use. However, combination therapy with statins has been used in some patients with resistant hyperlipidemias (with great caution).

Decreased Effect: Rifampin (and potentially other inducers of CYP3A4) may reduce blood levels of clofibrate.

Dietary/Ethanol/Herb Considerations Food: Administer with food or milk to reduce GI upset. Adherence to prescribed diet is a very important part of the cardiac risk reduction program.

(Continued)

Clofibrate *(Continued)*

Pharmacodynamics/Kinetics

Absorption: Complete

Distribution: V_d: 5.5 L/kg; crosses placenta

Protein binding: 95%

Metabolism: Hepatic to an inactive glucuronide ester; intestinal transformation required to activate drug

Half-life elimination: 6-24 hours, significantly prolonged with renal impairment; Anuria: 110 hours

Time to peak, serum: 3-6 hours

Excretion: Urine (40% to 70%)

Pregnancy Risk Factor C

Generic Available Yes

Clomid® *see* ClomiPHENE *on page 348*

ClomiPHENE (KLOE mi feen)

U.S. Brand Names Clomid®; Milophene®; Serophene®

Canadian Brand Names Clomid®; Milophene®; Serophene®

Mexican Brand Names Omifin

Pharmacologic Category Ovulation Stimulator

Synonyms Clomiphene Citrate

Use Treatment of ovulatory failure in patients desiring pregnancy

Unlabeled/Investigational Use Treatment of male infertility

Local Anesthetic/Vasoconstrictor Precautions No information available to require special precautions

Effects on Dental Treatment

>10%: Hot flashes

1% to 10%: Headache, nausea, vomiting, blurred vision

Dosage Adults: Oral:

Male (infertility): 25 mg/day for 25 days with 5 days rest, or 100 mg every Monday, Wednesday, Friday

Female (ovulatory failure): 50 mg/day for 5 days (first course); start the regimen on or about the fifth day of cycle. The dose should be increased only in those patients who do not ovulate in response to cyclic 50 mg Clomid®. A low dosage or duration of treatment course is particularly recommended if unusual sensitivity to pituitary gonadotropin is suspected, such as in patients with polycystic ovary syndrome.

If ovulation does not appear to occur after the first course of therapy, a second course of 100 mg/day (two 50 mg tablets given as a single daily dose) for 5 days should be given. This course may be started as early as 30 days after the previous one after precautions are taken to exclude the presence of pregnancy. Increasing the dosage or duration of therapy beyond 100 mg/day for 5 days is not recommended. The majority of patients who are going to ovulate will do so after the first course of therapy. If ovulation does not occur after 3 courses of therapy, further treatment is not recommended and the patient should be re-evaluated. If 3 ovulatory responses occur, but pregnancy has not been achieved, further treatment is not recommended. If menses does not occur after an ovulatory response, the patient should be re-evaluated. Long-term cyclic therapy is not recommended beyond a total of about 6 cycles.

Mechanism of Action Induces ovulation by stimulating the release of pituitary gonadotropins

Other Adverse Effects

>10%: Endocrine & metabolic: Ovarian enlargement

1% to 10%:

Cardiovascular: Thromboembolism

Central nervous system: Mental depression

Endocrine & metabolic: Breast enlargement (males), breast discomfort (females), abnormal menstrual flow

Gastrointestinal: Distention, bloating

Hepatic: Hepatotoxicity

Ocular: Diplopia, floaters, after-images, phosphenes, photophobia

<1%: Insomnia, fatigue, alopecia (reversible), weight gain, polyuria

Drug Interactions Decreased Effect: Decreased response when used with danazol. Decreased estradiol response when used with clomiphene.

Pharmacodynamics/Kinetics

Metabolism: Undergoes enterohepatic recirculation

Half-life elimination: 5-7 days

Excretion: Primarily feces; urine (small amounts)

Pregnancy Risk Factor X

Generic Available Yes

Clomiphene Citrate *see* ClomiPHENE *on page 348*

ClomiPRAMINE (kloe MI pra meen)

U.S. Brand Names Anafranil®

Canadian Brand Names Anafranil®; Apo®-Clomipramine; Gen-Clomipramine; Novo-Clopramine

Mexican Brand Names Anafranil®

Pharmacologic Category Antidepressant, Tricyclic (Tertiary Amine)

Synonyms Clomipramine Hydrochloride

Use Treatment of obsessive-compulsive disorder (OCD)

Unlabeled/Investigational Use Treatment of depression, panic attacks, chronic pain

Local Anesthetic/Vasoconstrictor Precautions Use with caution; epinephrine, norepinephrine and levonordefrin have been shown to have an increased pressor response in combination with TCAs

Effects on Dental Treatment Long-term treatment with TCAs such as clomipramine increases the risk of caries by reducing salivation and salivary buffer capacity.

>10%: Xerostomia, changes in salivation, dizziness, drowsiness, headache, nervousness, nausea, tremor, increased diaphoresis, fatigue

1% to 10%: Hypotension, palpitations, tachycardia, confusion, yawning, paresthesia, memory impairment, anxiety, twitching, agitation, migraine, flushing, fever, vomiting, blurred vision

Dosage Oral: Initial:

Children:

<10 years: Safety and efficacy have not been established.

≥10 years: OCD: 25 mg/day; gradually increase, as tolerated, to a maximum of 3 mg/kg/day or 200 mg/day (whichever is smaller)

Adults: OCD: 25 mg/day and gradually increase, as tolerated, to 100 mg/day the first 2 weeks, may then be increased to a total of 250 mg/day maximum

Mechanism of Action Clomipramine appears to affect serotonin uptake while its active metabolite, desmethylclomipramine, affects norepinephrine uptake

Other Adverse Effects

>10%:

Central nervous system: Insomnia

Endocrine & metabolic: Libido changes

Gastrointestinal: Constipation, increased appetite, weight gain, dyspepsia, anorexia, abdominal pain

Neuromuscular & skeletal: Myoclonus

1% to 10%:

Central nervous system: Hypertonia, sleep disorder, speech disorder, abnormal dreaming, memory impairment, impaired coordination, depersonalization, emotional lability

Dermatologic: Rash, pruritus, dermatitis

Gastrointestinal: Diarrhea

Genitourinary: Difficult urination

Ocular: Eye pain

<1%: Abnormal accommodation, alopecia, breast enlargement, **decreased lower esophageal sphincter tone (may cause GE reflux)**, galactorrhea, hyperacusis, increased liver enzymes, marrow depression, photosensitivity, prostatic disorder, **seizures**, SIADH, **gum disorder**

Drug Interactions Substrate of **CYP1A2, 2C19, 2D6**, 3A4; Inhibits **CYP2D6**

Increased Effect/Toxicity: Clomipramine increases the effects of amphetamines, anticholinergics, lithium, other CNS depressants (sedatives, hypnotics, ethanol), chlorpropamide, tolazamide, phenothiazines, and warfarin. When used with MAO inhibitors or other serotonergic drugs, serotonin syndrome may occur. Serotonin syndrome has also been reported with ritonavir (rare). Clomipramine serum concentrations/toxicity may be increased by SSRIs (to varying degrees), cimetidine, grapefruit juice, indinavir, methylphenidate, ritonavir, quinidine, diltiazem, phenothiazines, and verapamil. Pressor response to I.V. epinephrine, norepinephrine, and phenylephrine may be enhanced in patients receiving TCAs (**Note:** Effect is unlikely with epinephrine or levonordefrin dosages typically administered as infiltration in combination with local anesthetics). Combined use of beta-agonists or drugs which prolong QT_c (including quinidine, procainamide, disopyramide, cisapride, sparfloxacin, gatifloxacin, moxifloxacin) with TCAs may predispose patients to cardiac arrhythmias.

Decreased Effect: Clomipramine serum concentrations/effect may be decreased by carbamazepine, cholestyramine, colestipol, phenobarbital, and rifampin. Clomipramine inhibits the antihypertensive response to bethanidine, clonidine, debrisoquin, guanadrel, guanethidine, guanabenz, and guanfacine.

Dietary/Ethanol/Herb Considerations

Ethanol: Avoid use; may increase sedation.

Food: Avoid grapefruit products; may increase serum concentration/toxicity.

Herb/Nutraceutical: Avoid gotu kola, kava, SAMe, St John's wort, and valerian; may increase CNS depression.

Pharmacodynamics/Kinetics

Absorption: Rapid

(Continued)

ClomiPRAMINE *(Continued)*

Metabolism: Hepatic to desmethylclomipramine (active); extensive first-pass effect
Half-life elimination: 20-30 hours

Pregnancy Risk Factor C

Generic Available Yes

Selected Readings

Boakes AJ, Laurence DR, Teoh PC, et al, "Interactions Between Sympathomimetic Amines and Antidepressant Agents in Man," *Br Med J*, 1973, 1(849):311-5.
Friedlander AH, Mahler ME, "Major Depressive Disorder. Psychopathology, Medical Management, and Dental Implications," *J Am Dent Assoc*, 201, 132(5):629-38.
Ganzberg S, "Psychoactive Drugs," *ADA Guide to Dental Therapeutics*, 2nd ed, Chicago, IL: ADA Publishing, a Division of ADA Business Enterprises, Inc, 2000, 376-405.
Jastak JT and Yagiela JA, "Vasoconstrictors and Local Anesthesia: A Review and Rationale for Use," *J Am Dent Assoc*, 1983, 107(4):623-30.
Mitchell JR, "Guanethidine and Related Agents. III Antagonism by Drugs Which Inhibit the Norepinephrine Pump in Man," *J Clin Invest*, 1970, 49(8):1596-604.
Rundegren J, van Dijken J, Mörnstad H, et al, "Oral Conditions in Patients Receiving Long-Term Treatment With Cyclic Antidepressant Drugs," *Swed Dent J*, 1985, 9(2):55-64.
Yagiela JA, "Adverse Drug Interactions in Dental Practice: Interactions Associated With Vasoconstrictors. Part V of a Series," *J Am Dent Assoc*, 1999, 130(5):701-9.

Clomipramine Hydrochloride *see* ClomiPRAMINE *on page 349*

Clonazepam (kloe NA ze pam)

U.S. Brand Names Klonopin™

Canadian Brand Names Alti-Clonazepam; Apo®-Clonazepam; Clonapam; Gen-Clonazepam; Klonopin™; Novo-Clonazepam; Nu-Clonazepam; PMS-Clonazepam; Rho-Clonazepam; Rivotril®

Mexican Brand Names Kenoket®; Rivotril®

Pharmacologic Category Benzodiazepine

Use Alone or as an adjunct in the treatment of petit mal variant (Lennox-Gastaut), akinetic, and myoclonic seizures; petit mal (absence) seizures unresponsive to succimides; panic disorder with or without agoraphobia

Unlabeled/Investigational Use Treatment of restless legs syndrome, neuralgia, multifocal tic disorder, parkinsonian dysarthria, bipolar disorder; adjunct therapy for schizophrenia

Local Anesthetic/Vasoconstrictor Precautions No information available to require special precautions

Effects on Dental Treatment

>10%: Xerostomia, changes in salivation, drowsiness
1% to 10%: Dizziness, allergic reactions, upper respiratory tract infection, sinusitis, rhinitis, cough, fatigue, incoordination

Restrictions C-IV

Dosage Oral:

Children <10 years or 30 kg: Seizure disorders:
- Initial daily dose: 0.01-0.03 mg/kg/day (maximum: 0.05 mg/kg/day) given in 2-3 divided doses; increase by no more than 0.5 mg every third day until seizures are controlled or adverse effects seen
- Usual maintenance dose: 0.1-0.2 mg/kg/day divided 3 times/day, not to exceed 0.2 mg/kg/day

Adults:
- Seizure disorders:
  - Initial daily dose not to exceed 1.5 mg given in 3 divided doses; may increase by 0.5-1 mg every third day until seizures are controlled or adverse effects seen (maximum: 20 mg/day)
  - Usual maintenance dose: 0.05-0.2 mg/kg; do not exceed 20 mg/day
- Panic disorder: 0.25 mg twice daily; increase in increments of 0.125-0.25 mg twice daily every 3 days; target dose: 1 mg/day (maximum: 4 mg/day)

Elderly: Initiate with low doses and observe closely
Hemodialysis: Supplemental dose is unnecessary

Mechanism of Action The exact mechanism is unknown, but believed to be related to its ability to enhance the activity of GABA; suppresses the spike-and-wave discharge in absence seizures by depressing nerve transmission in the motor cortex

Other Adverse Effects

1% to 10%:
- Central nervous system: Ataxia, dysarthria, depression
- Dermatologic: Dermatitis
- Endocrine & metabolic: Decreased libido
- Gastrointestinal: Anorexia, constipation, diarrhea

<1%: Blood dyscrasias, menstrual irregularities

Drug Interactions Substrate of **CYP3A4**

Increased Effect/Toxicity: Combined use of clonazepam and valproic acid has been associated with absence seizures. Clonazepam potentiates the CNS depressant effects of narcotic analgesics, barbiturates, phenothiazines, ethanol, antihistamines, MAO inhibitors, sedative-hypnotics, and cyclic antidepressants. Serum levels and/or toxicity of clonazepam may be increased by inhibitors of CYP3A4, including cimetidine, ciprofloxacin, clarithromycin, clozapine, delavirdine, diltiazem, disulfiram, digoxin, erythromycin, ethanol, fluconazole, fluoxetine, fluvoxamine, grapefruit juice, indinavir, isoniazid, itraconazole, ketoconazole, loxapine, metoprolol, metronidazole, miconazole, nefazodone, nevirapine, quinupristin/dalfopristin, omeprazole, phenytoin, rifabutin, rifampin, ritonavir, saquinavir, troleandomycin, verapamil, zafirlukast, and zileuton.

Decreased Effect: The combined use of clonazepam and valproic acid has been associated with absence seizures. Carbamazepine, rifampin, rifabutin may enhance the metabolism of clonazepam and decrease its therapeutic effect.

Dietary/Ethanol/Herb Considerations

Ethanol: Avoid use; may increase CNS depression.

Food: Avoid grapefruit products; may increase serum concentration.

Herb/Nutraceutical: Avoid gotu kola, kava, SAMe, and valerian; may increase CNS depression. Avoid St John's wort; may decrease serum concentration and increase CNS depression. Melatonin may enhance activity of clonazepam; use cautiously.

Pharmacodynamics/Kinetics

Onset of action: 20-60 minutes

Duration: Infants and young children: 6-8 hours; Adults: ≤12 hours

Absorption: Well absorbed

Distribution: Adults: V_d: 1.5-4.4 L/kg

Protein binding: 85%

Metabolism: Extensively hepatic via glucuronide and sulfate conjugation

Half-life elimination: Children: 22-33 hours; Adults: 19-50 hours

Time to peak, serum: 1-3 hours; Steady-state: 5-7 days

Excretion: Urine (<2% as unchanged drug); metabolites excreted as glucuronide or sulfate conjugates

Pregnancy Risk Factor D

Generic Available Yes

Clonidine (KLOE ni deen)

Related Information

Cardiovascular Diseases *on page 1456*

U.S. Brand Names Catapres®; Catapres-TTS®-1; Catapres-TTS®-2; Catapres-TTS®-3; Duraclon™

Canadian Brand Names Apo®-Clonidine; Carapres®; Dixarit®; Novo-Clonidine®; Nu-Clonidine®

Mexican Brand Names Catapresan-100®

Pharmacologic Category $Alpha_2$-Adrenergic Agonist

Synonyms Clonidine Hydrochloride

Use Management of mild to moderate hypertension; either used alone or in combination with other antihypertensives

Orphan drug (Duraclon™): For continuous epidural administration as adjunctive therapy with intraspinal opiates for treatment of cancer pain in patients tolerant to or unresponsive to intraspinal opiates

Unlabeled/Investigational Use Treatment of heroin or nicotine withdrawal symptoms, severe pain, dysmenorrhea, vasomotor symptoms associated with menopause, ethanol dependence, glaucoma, diabetes-associated diarrhea, impulse control disorder, attention-deficit/hyperactivity disorder (ADHD), clozapine-induced sialorrhea; prophylaxis of migraines

Local Anesthetic/Vasoconstrictor Precautions No information available to require special precautions

Effects on Dental Treatment

>10%: Significant xerostomia (40% oral; 25% transdermal), drowsiness (35% oral; 12% transdermal), dizziness (16% oral)

1% to 10%: Orthostatic hypotension (3% oral), headache (1% oral, 5% transdermal), sedation (3% transdermal), nervousness (3% oral, 1% transdermal), weakness (10% transdermal), nausea (5% oral, 1% transdermal), vomiting (5% oral), dry throat (2% transdermal), abnormal taste (1% transdermal), dizziness (2% transdermal), fatigue (6% transdermal), lethargy (3% transdermal), allergic contact sensitivity (5% transdermal), malaise (1% oral), withdrawal syndrome (1% oral)

Dosage

Children:

Oral:

Hypertension: Initial: 5-10 mcg/kg/day in divided doses every 8-12 hours; increase gradually at 5- to 7-day intervals to 25 mcg/kg/day in divided doses every 6 hours; maximum: 0.9 mg/day

Clonidine tolerance test (test of growth hormone release from pituitary): 0.15 mg/m² or 4 mcg/kg as single dose

ADHD (unlabeled use): Initial: 0.05 mg/day; increase every 3-7 days by 0.05 mg/day to 3-5 mcg/kg/day given in divided doses 3-4 times/day (maximum dose: 0.3-0.4 mg/day)

(Continued)

Clonidine *(Continued)*

Epidural infusion: Pain management: Reserved for patients with severe intractable pain, unresponsive to other analgesics or epidural or spinal opiates: Initial: 0.5 mcg/kg/hour; adjust with caution, based on clinical effect

Adults:

Oral:

Acute hypertension (urgency): Initial 0.1-0.2 mg; may be followed by additional doses of 0.1 mg every hour, if necessary, to a maximum total dose of 0.6 mg

Hypertension: Initial dose: 0.1 mg twice daily, usual maintenance dose: 0.2-1.2 mg/day in 2-4 divided doses; maximum recommended dose: 2.4 mg/day

Nicotine withdrawal symptoms: 0.1 mg twice daily to maximum of 0.4 mg/day for 3-4 weeks

Transdermal: Hypertension: Apply once every 7 days; for initial therapy start with 0.1 mg and increase by 0.1 mg at 1- to 2-week intervals; dosages >0.6 mg do not improve efficacy

Epidural infusion: Pain management: Starting dose: 30 mcg/hour; titrate as required for relief of pain or presence of side effects; minimal experience with doses >40 mcg/hour; should be considered an adjunct to intraspinal opiate therapy

Elderly: Initial: 0.1 mg once daily at bedtime, increase gradually as needed

Dosing adjustment in renal impairment: Cl_{cr} <10 mL/minute: Administer 50% to 75% of normal dose initially

Dialysis: Not dialyzable (0% to 5%) via hemo- or peritoneal dialysis; supplemental dose unnecessary

Mechanism of Action Stimulates alpha$_2$-adrenoceptors in the brain stem, thus activating an inhibitory neuron, resulting in reduced sympathetic outflow from the CNS, producing a decrease in peripheral resistance, renal vascular resistance, heart rate, and blood pressure; epidural clonidine may produce pain relief at spinal presynaptic and postjunctional alpha$_2$-adrenoceptors by preventing pain signal transmission; pain relief occurs only for the body regions innervated by the spinal segments where analgesic concentrations of clonidine exist

Other Adverse Effects Incidence is not always reported:

>10%: Dermatologic: Transient localized skin reactions characterized by pruritus, and erythema (15% to 50% transdermal)

1% to 10%:

Central nervous system: Insomnia (2% transdermal), mental depression (1% oral)

Dermatologic: Rash (1% oral), allergic contact sensitivity (5% transdermal), localized vesiculation (7%), hyperpigmentation (5% at application site), edema (3%), excoriation (3%), burning (3%), throbbing, blanching (1%), papules (1%), and generalized macular rash (1%) has occurred in patients receiving transdermal clonidine.

Endocrine & metabolic: Sodium and water retention, sexual dysfunction (3% oral, 2% transdermal), impotence (3% oral, 2% transdermal)

Gastrointestinal: Anorexia and malaise (1% oral), constipation (10% oral, 1% transdermal), weight gain (1% oral)

Genitourinary: Nocturia (1% oral)

Hepatic: Liver function test (mild abnormalities, 1% oral)

<1% (Limited to important or life-threatening): Hepatitis (oral), difficulty in micturition (oral, transdermal), urinary retention (oral), hives (oral, transdermal), angioedema (oral, transdermal), urticaria (oral, transdermal), alopecia (oral, transdermal), parotid pain (oral), gynecomastia (oral, transdermal), transient elevation of blood glucose (oral), elevation of creatinine phosphokinase (oral), **palpitations (oral, transdermal), tachycardia (oral, transdermal), bradycardia (oral), sinus bradycardia (oral, transdermal), atrioventricular block (oral, transdermal), CHF (oral, transdermal)**, EKG abnormalities (oral, transdermal), **flushing**, pallor, Raynaud's phenomenon (oral, transdermal), **chest pain (transdermal), increase in blood pressure (transdermal), weakness, muscle or joint pain (0.6% oral), leg cramps (0.3% oral), fever (oral, transdermal)**, malaise (transdermal), vivid dreams (oral, transdermal), nightmares (oral, transdermal), insomnia (oral), **behavioral changes (transdermal), restlessness (oral, transdermal), anxiety (oral, transdermal)**, mental depression (transdermal), **visual and auditory hallucinations (oral, transdermal), delirium (transdermal), CVA (transdermal), irritability (transdermal),** weight gain (transdermal), rash (transdermal), **orthostatic symptoms (transdermal), syncope (oral, transdermal), agitation (transdermal) , contact dermatitis (transdermal),** localized hypo- or hyperpigmentation (transdermal), anorexia (transdermal), vomiting (transdermal), loss of libido (transdermal), decreased sexual activity (transdermal), **blurred vision (transdermal),** burning of the eyes (transdermal), dryness of the eyes (transdermal), weakly positive Coombs' test (oral), increased sensitivity to ethanol (oral), thrombocytopenia (oral), abdominal pain (oral), pseudo-obstruction (oral)

Drug Interactions

Increased Effect/Toxicity: Concurrent use with antipsychotics (especially low potency), narcotic analgesics, or nitroprusside may produce additive hypotensive effects. Clonidine may decrease the symptoms of hypoglycemia with oral hypoglycemic agents or insulin. Alcohol, barbiturates, and other CNS depressants may have additive CNS effects when combined with clonidine. Epidural clonidine may prolong the sensory and motor blockade of local anesthetics. Clonidine may increase cyclosporine (and perhaps tacrolimus) serum concentrations. Beta-blockers may potentiate bradycardia in patients receiving clonidine and may increase the rebound hypertension of withdrawal. Tricyclic antidepressants may also enhance the hypertensive response associated with abrupt clonidine withdrawal.

Decreased Effect: Tricyclic antidepressants (TCAs) antagonize the hypotensive effects of clonidine.

Dietary/Ethanol/Herb Considerations

Ethanol: Avoid use; may increase CNS depression.

Food: Hypertensive patients may need to decrease sodium and calorie intake. Avoid caffeine, garlic and licorice.

Herb/Nutraceutical: Avoid black cohosh, dong quai, and evening primrose due to estrogenic activity. Avoid ephedra, ginseng, and yohimbe; may worsen hypertension. Avoid garlic; may increase antihypertensive effect. Avoid gotu kola, kava, SAMe, St John's wort, and valerian; may increase CNS depression. Avoid ginger due to positive inotropic effects; theoretically, may cause arrhythmia. Avoid hawthorn; may decrease peripheral vascular resistance and cause additive decrease in BP. Avoid licorice.

Pharmacodynamics/Kinetics

Onset of action: Oral: 0.5-1 hour

Duration: 6-10 hours

Distribution: V_d: Adults: 2.1 L/kg; highly lipid soluble; distributes readily into extravascular sites

Protein binding: 20% to 40%

Metabolism: Extensively hepatic to inactive metabolites; undergoes enterohepatic recirculation

Bioavailability: 75% to 95%

Half-life elimination: Adults: Normal renal function: 6-20 hours; Renal impairment: 18-41 hours

Time to peak: 2-4 hours

Excretion: Urine (65%, 32% as unchanged drug); feces (22%)

Pregnancy Risk Factor C

Generic Available Yes: Tablet

Clonidine and Chlorthalidone (KLOE ni deen & klor THAL i done)

Related Information

Chlorthalidone *on page 315*

Clonidine *on page 351*

U.S. Brand Names Combipres®

Pharmacologic Category Antihypertensive Agent Combination

Synonyms Chlorthalidone and Clonidine

Use Management of mild to moderate hypertension

Local Anesthetic/Vasoconstrictor Precautions No information available to require special precautions

Effects on Dental Treatment No significant effects or complications reported

Dosage Oral: 1 tablet 1-2 times/day; maximum: 0.6 mg clonidine and 30 mg chlorthalidone

Pregnancy Risk Factor C

Generic Available Yes

Clonidine Hydrochloride *see* Clonidine *on page 351*

Clopidogrel (kloe PID oh grel)

Related Information

Cardiovascular Diseases *on page 1456*

U.S. Brand Names Plavix®

Canadian Brand Names Plavix®

Pharmacologic Category Antiplatelet Agent

Synonyms Clopidogrel Bisulfate

Use Reduce atherosclerotic events (MI, stroke, vascular deaths) in patients with atherosclerosis documented by recent MI (MI), recent stroke, or established peripheral arterial disease; prevention of thrombotic complications after coronary stenting; acute coronary syndrome (unstable angina or non-Q-wave MI)

Unlabeled/Investigational Use In aspirin-allergic patients, prevention of coronary artery bypass graft closure (saphenous vein)

Local Anesthetic/Vasoconstrictor Precautions No information available to require special precautions

Effects on Dental Treatment If a patient is to undergo elective surgery and an antiplatelet effect is not desired, clopidogrel should be discontinued 7 days prior to surgery. As with all drugs which may affect hemostasis, bleeding is associated with clopidogrel. Hemorrhage may occur at virtually any site; risk is dependent on

(Continued)

Clopidogrel *(Continued)*

multiple variables, including the concurrent use of multiple agents which alter hemostasis and patient susceptibility.

>10%: Vomiting

2% to 10%: Chest pain (8%), hypertension (4%), headache (3% to 8%), dizziness (2% to 6%), pain (6%), nausea (3%), epistaxis (3%) dyspnea (5%), rhinitis (4%), bronchitis (4%), cough(3%), upper respiratory infections (9%), flu-like syndrome (8%), fatigue (3% to 10%)

1% to 3%: Anxiety, atrial fibrillation, cardiac failure, fever, GI hemorrhage, leg cramps, palpitations, paresthesia, syncope, vomiting, weakness

Dosage Oral: Adults:

Recent MI, recent stroke, or established arterial disease: 75 mg once daily

Acute coronary syndrome: Initial: 300 mg loading dose, followed by 75 mg once daily (in combination with aspirin 75-325 mg once daily)

Prevention of coronary artery bypass graft closure (saphenous vein): Aspirin-allergic patients (unlabeled use): Loading dose: 300 mg 6 hours following procedure; maintenance: 50-100 mg/day

Mechanism of Action Blocks the ADP receptors, which prevent fibrinogen binding at that site and thereby reduce the possibility of platelet adhesion and aggregation

Other Adverse Effects

>10%: Gastrointestinal: Abdominal pain, dyspepsia, constipation (27% compared to 30% in patients receiving aspirin)

3% to 10%:

Cardiovascular: Edema (4%)
Central nervous system: Depression (4%)
Dermatologic: Rash (4%), pruritus (3%)
Endocrine & metabolic: Hypercholesterolemia (4%)
Gastrointestinal: Abdominal pain (2% to 6%), dyspepsia (2% to 5%), diarrhea (2% to 5%)
Genitourinary: Urinary tract infection (3%)
Hematologic: Purpura (5%)
Hepatic: Liver function test abnormalities (<3%; discontinued in 0.11%)
Neuromuscular & skeletal: Arthralgia (6%), back pain (6%)

1% to 3%:

Central nervous system: Insomnia, vertigo
Dermatologic: Eczema
Endocrine & metabolic: Hyperuricemia, gout
Gastrointestinal: Constipation
Genitourinary: Cystitis
Hematologic: Anemia, hematoma
Neuromuscular & skeletal: Arthritis, neuralgia
Ocular: Cataract, conjunctivitis

<1% (Limited to important or life-threatening): Agranulocytosis, **allergic reaction, anaphylactoid reaction**, angioedema, aplastic anemia, bilirubinemia, **bronchospasm**, bullous eruption, fatty liver, granulocytopenia, hematuria, hemoptysis, hemothorax, hepatitis, hypochromic anemia, intracranial hemorrhage (0.4%), ischemic necrosis, leukopenia, maculopapular rash, menorrhagia, neutropenia (0.05%), ocular hemorrhage, pulmonary hemorrhage, purpura, retroperitoneal bleeding, thrombocytopenia, thrombotic thrombocytopenic purpura, urticaria

Warnings/Precautions Use with caution in patients who may be at risk of increased bleeding, including patients with peptic ulcer disease, trauma, or surgery. Consider discontinuing 5 days before elective surgery. Use caution in mixing with other antiplatelet drugs. Use with caution in patients with severe liver disease (experience is limited). Cases of thrombotic thrombocytopenic purpura (usually occurring within the first 2 weeks of therapy) have been reported.

Drug Interactions Substrate of CYP1A2, 3A4; Inhibits CYP2C8/9

Increased Effect/Toxicity: At high concentrations, clopidogrel may interfere with the metabolism of amiodarone, cisapride, cyclosporine, diltiazem, fluvastatin, irbesartan, losartan, oral hypoglycemics, paclitaxel, phenytoin, quinidine, sildenafil, tamoxifen, torsemide, verapamil, and some NSAIDs which may result in toxicity. Clopidogrel and naproxen resulted in an increase of GI occult blood loss. Anticoagulants (warfarin, thrombolytics, drotrecogin alfa) or other antiplatelet agents may increase the risk of bleeding.

Dietary/Ethanol/Herb Considerations

Food: May be taken with food; avoid garlic, ginger, and green tea

Herb/Nutraceutical: Avoid cat's claw, dong quai, evening primrose, feverfew, garlic, ginger, ginkgo biloba, ginseng, green tea, horse chestnut, and red clover due to additional antiplatelet activity.

Pharmacodynamics/Kinetics

Onset of action: Inhibition of platelet aggregation detected: 2 hours after 300 mg administered; after second day of treatment with 50-100 mg/day

Peak effect: 50-100 mg/day: Bleeding time: 5-6 days; Platelet function: 3-7 days

Absorption: Well absorbed

Metabolism: Extensively hepatic via hydrolysis; biotransformation to carboxyl acid derivative (active metabolite that inhibits platelet aggregation)
Half-life elimination: ~8 hours
Time to peak, serum: ~1 hour
Excretion: Urine

Pregnancy Risk Factor B

Generic Available No

Selected Readings Wynn RL, "Clopidogrel (Plavix): Dental Considerations of an Antiplatelet Drug," *Gen Dent*, 2001, 49(6):564-8.

Clopidogrel Bisulfate *see* Clopidogrel *on page 353*

Clorazepate (klor AZ e pate)

U.S. Brand Names Tranxene®

Canadian Brand Names Apo®-Clorazepate; Novo-Clopate®

Mexican Brand Names Tranxene®

Pharmacologic Category Benzodiazepine

Synonyms Clorazepate Dipotassium

Use Treatment of generalized anxiety disorder; management of ethanol withdrawal; adjunct anticonvulsant in management of partial seizures

Local Anesthetic/Vasoconstrictor Precautions No information available to require special precautions

Effects on Dental Treatment Many patients will experience drowsiness; orthostatic hypotension is possible. It is suggested that narcotic analgesics not be given for pain control to patients taking clorazepate due to enhanced sedation.

>10%: Xerostomia (normal salivary flow resumes upon discontinuation)
Frequency not defined: Hypotension, drowsiness, fatigue, lightheadedness, memory impairment, anxiety, headache, slurred speech, confusion, nervousness, dizziness, irritability, nausea, vomiting, tremors, blurred vision

Restrictions C-IV

Dosage Oral:

Children 9-12 years: Anticonvulsant: Initial: 3.75-7.5 mg/dose twice daily; increase dose by 3.75 mg at weekly intervals, not to exceed 60 mg/day in 2-3 divided doses
Children >12 years and Adults: Anticonvulsant: Initial: Up to 7.5 mg/dose 2-3 times/day; increase dose by 7.5 mg at weekly intervals, not to exceed 90 mg/day
Adults:
- Anxiety:
  - Regular release tablets (Tranxene® T-Tab®): 7.5-15 mg 2-4 times/day
  - Sustained release (Tranxene®-SD): 11.25 or 22.5 mg once daily at bedtime
- Ethanol withdrawal: Initial: 30 mg, then 15 mg 2-4 times/day on first day; maximum daily dose: 90 mg; gradually decrease dose over subsequent days

Mechanism of Action Binds to stereospecific benzodiazepine receptors on the postsynaptic GABA neuron at several sites within the central nervous system, including the limbic system, reticular formation. Enhancement of the inhibitory effect of GABA on neuronal excitability results by increased neuronal membrane permeability to chloride ions. This shift in chloride ions results in hyperpolarization (a less excitable state) and stabilization.

Other Adverse Effects Frequency not defined:

Central nervous system: Ataxia, insomnia, depression
Dermatologic: Rash
Endocrine & metabolic: Decreased libido
Gastrointestinal: Constipation, diarrhea, increased or decreased appetite
Ocular: Diplopia

Drug Interactions Substrate of **CYP3A4**

Increased Effect/Toxicity: Clorazepate potentiates the CNS depressant effects of narcotic analgesics, barbiturates, phenothiazines, ethanol, antihistamines, MAO inhibitors, sedative-hypnotics, and cyclic antidepressants. Serum concentrations/toxicity of clorazepate may be increased by inhibitors of CYP3A4, including amprenavir, cimetidine, ciprofloxacin, clarithromycin, clozapine, diltiazem, disulfiram, digoxin, erythromycin, ethanol, fluconazole, fluoxetine, fluvoxamine, grapefruit juice, isoniazid, itraconazole, ketoconazole, labetalol, levodopa, loxapine, metoprolol, metronidazole, miconazole, nefazodone, nelfinavir, omeprazole, phenytoin, rifabutin, rifampin, ritonavir, troleandomycin, valproic acid, and verapamil.

Decreased Effect: Carbamazepine, rifampin, rifabutin may enhance the metabolism of clorazepate and decrease its therapeutic effect.

Dietary/Ethanol/Herb Considerations

Ethanol: Avoid use; may increase CNS depression.
Food: Avoid grapefruit products; may increase serum concentration/toxicity.
Herb/Nutraceutical: Avoid gotu kola, kava, SAMe, St John's wort, and valerian; may increase CNS depression. Melatonin may enhance activity of clorazepate; use cautiously.

Pharmacodynamics/Kinetics

Onset of action: 1-2 hours
(Continued)

Clorazepate *(Continued)*

Duration: Variable, 8-24 hours
Distribution: Crosses placenta; appears in urine
Metabolism: Rapidly decarboxylated to desmethyldiazepam (active) in acidic stomach prior to absorption; hepatically to oxazepam (active)
Half-life elimination: Adults: Desmethyldiazepam: 48-96 hours; Oxazepam: 6-8 hours
Time to peak, serum: ~1 hour
Excretion: Primarily urine

Pregnancy Risk Factor D

Generic Available Yes

Clorazepate Dipotassium *see* Clorazepate *on page 355*
Clorpactin® WCS-90 [OTC] *see* Oxychlorosene *on page 1017*

Clotrimazole (kloe TRIM a zole)

Related Information

Oral Fungal Infections *on page 1542*

U.S. Brand Names Cruex® [OTC]; Gyne-Lotrimin® [OTC]; Gyne-Lotrimin® 3 [OTC]; Gynix® [OTC]; Lotrimin®; Lotrimin® AF [OTC]; Mycelex®; Mycelex®-3; Mycelex®-7 [OTC]; Mycelex® Twin Pack [OTC]; Trivagizole 3™

Canadian Brand Names Canesten® Topical, Canesten® Vaginal; Clotrimaderm; Trivagizole-3®

Mexican Brand Names Candimon®; Lotrimin®

Pharmacologic Category Antifungal Agent, Oral Nonabsorbed; Antifungal Agent, Topical; Antifungal Agent, Vaginal

Use

Dental: Treatment of susceptible fungal infections, including oropharyngeal candidiasis; limited data suggests that the use of clotrimazole troches may be effective for prophylaxis against oropharyngeal candidiasis in neutropenic patients

Medical: Treatment of susceptible fungal infections including dermatophytoses, superficial mycoses, cutaneous candidiasis, and vulvovaginal candidiasis

Local Anesthetic/Vasoconstrictor Precautions No information available to require special precautions

Effects on Dental Treatment 1% to 10%: Oral troche: Nausea, vomiting

Dosage

Children >3 years and Adults:

Oral:

Prophylaxis: 10 mg troche dissolved 3 times/day for the duration of chemotherapy or until steroids are reduced to maintenance levels

Treatment: 10 mg troche dissolved slowly 5 times/day for 14 consecutive days

Topical (cream, lotion, solution): Apply twice daily; if no improvement occurs after 4 weeks of therapy, re-evaluate diagnosis

Children >12 years and Adults:

Vaginal:

Cream:

1%: Insert 1 applicatorful vaginal cream daily (preferably at bedtime) for 7 consecutive days

2%: Insert 1 applicatorful vaginal cream daily (preferably at bedtime) for 3 consecutive days

Tablet: Insert 100 mg/day for 7 days or 500 mg single dose

Topical (cream, lotion, solution): Apply to affected area twice daily (morning and evening) for 7 consecutive days

Mechanism of Action Binds to phospholipids in the fungal cell membrane altering cell wall permeability resulting in loss of essential intracellular elements

Other Adverse Effects

Oral: >10%: Hepatic: Abnormal LFTs

Vaginal: 1% to 10%: Local: Mild burning, irritation, stinging

<1% (Limited to important or life-threatening): Vulvar itching, soreness, edema, or discharge; polyuria; burning or itching of penis of sexual partner

Contraindications Hypersensitivity to clotrimazole or any component of the formulation

Warnings/Precautions Clotrimazole should not be used for treatment of systemic fungal infection; safety and effectiveness of clotrimazole lozenges (troches) in children <3 years of age have not been established; when using topical formulation, avoid contact with eyes

Drug Interactions Inhibits CYP2A6, 2C8/9, 2E1, 3A4

Pharmacodynamics/Kinetics

Absorption: Topical: Negligible through intact skin

Time to peak, serum:

Oral topical: Salivary levels occur within 3 hours following 30 minutes of dissolution time

Vaginal cream: High vaginal levels: 8-24 hours

Vaginal tablet: High vaginal levels: 1-2 days

Excretion: Feces (as metabolites)

Pregnancy Risk Factor B (topical); C (troches)

Dosage Forms COMBO PACK: Vaginal tablet 100 mg (7s) and vaginal cream 1% (7 g); vaginal tablet 200 mg (3s) and vaginal cream 1%; vaginal tablet 500 mg (1s) and vaginal cream 1% (7 g). **CRM** (Lotrimin®, Mycelex®): 1% (15 g, 30 g, 45 g, 90 g). **CRM, vaginal:** 1% (45 g, 90 g); (Mycelex®-3, Trivagizole 3™): 2% (25 g). **LOTION** (Lotrimin®): 1% (30 mL). **SOLN, topical** (Lotrimin®, Mycelex®): 1% (10 mL, 30 mL). **TAB, vaginal:** 100 mg (7s); 500 mg (1s). **TROCHE** (Mycelex®): 10 mg

Generic Available Yes

Clotrimazole and Betamethasone *see* Betamethasone and Clotrimazole *on page 179*

Cloxacillin (kloks a SIL in)

U.S. Brand Names Cloxapen®

Canadian Brand Names Apo®-Cloxi; Novo-Cloxin®; Nu-Cloxi®

Pharmacologic Category Antibiotic, Penicillin

Synonyms Cloxacillin Sodium

Use

Dental: Treatment of susceptible orofacial infections causing respiratory tract, skin, and skin structure infections

Medical: Treatment of susceptible bacterial infections, notably penicillinase-producing staphylococci causing respiratory tract, skin and skin structure, bone and joint, and urinary tract infections

Local Anesthetic/Vasoconstrictor Precautions No information available to require special precautions

Effects on Dental Treatment Prolonged use of penicillins may lead to development of oral candidiasis.

Dosage Oral:

Children >1 month (<20 kg): 50-100 mg/kg/day in divided doses every 6 hours; up to a maximum of 4 g/day

Children (>20 kg) and Adults: 250-500 mg every 6 hours

Hemodialysis: Not dialyzable (0% to 5%)

Mechanism of Action Inhibits bacterial cell wall synthesis by binding to one or more of the penicillin-binding proteins (PBPs) which in turn inhibits the final transpeptidation step of peptidoglycan synthesis in bacterial cell walls, thus inhibiting cell wall biosynthesis. Bacteria eventually lyse due to ongoing activity of cell wall autolytic enzymes (autolysins and murein hydrolases) while cell wall assembly is arrested.

Other Adverse Effects

1% to 10%: Gastrointestinal: Diarrhea, abdominal pain

<1%: **Fever, seizures** (extremely high doses and/or renal failure), rash (maculopapular to exfoliative), **vomiting, pseudomembranous colitis,** vaginitis, eosinophilia, leukopenia, neutropenia, thrombocytopenia, agranulocytosis, anemia, hemolytic anemia, **prolonged PT,** hepatotoxicity, transient elevated LFTs, hematuria, interstitial nephritis, increased BUN/creatinine, **serum sickness-like reactions, hypersensitivity**

Contraindications Hypersensitivity to cloxacillin, any component of the formulation, or penicillins

Warnings/Precautions Monitor PT if patient concurrently on warfarin, elimination of drug is slow in renally impaired; use with caution in patients allergic to cephalosporins due to a low incidence of cross-hypersensitivity

Drug Interactions

Oral contraceptives: Anecdotal reports suggesting decreased contraceptive efficacy with penicillins have been refuted by more rigorous scientific and clinical data.

Probenecid, disulfiram: May increase levels of penicillins (cloxacillin)

Warfarin: Effects of warfarin may be increased

Dietary/Ethanol/Herb Considerations Food: Administer on an empty stomach.

Pharmacodynamics/Kinetics

Absorption: Oral: ~50%

Distribution: Widely to most body fluids and bone; penetration into cells, into eye, and across normal meninges is poor; crosses placenta; enters breast milk; inflammation increases amount that crosses blood-brain barrier

Protein binding: 90% to 98%

Metabolism: Extensively hepatic to active and inactive metabolites

Half-life elimination: 0.5-1.5 hours; prolonged with renal impairment and in neonates

Time to peak, serum: 0.5-2 hours

Excretion: Urine and feces

Pregnancy Risk Factor B

Breast-feeding Considerations No data reported; however, other penicillins may be taken while breast-feeding.

Dosage Forms CAP: 250 mg, 500 mg. **POWDER, oral suspension:** 125 mg/5 mL (100 mL, 200 mL)

(Continued)

Cloxacillin *(Continued)*

Generic Available Yes

Comments Although cloxacillin is a penicillin antibiotic indicated for infections caused by penicillinase-secreting staph, amoxicillin with clavulanic acid is considered the drug of choice for these types of orofacial infections

Cloxacillin Sodium *see* Cloxacillin *on page 357*

Cloxapen® *see* Cloxacillin *on page 357*

Clozapine (KLOE za peen)

U.S. Brand Names Clozaril®

Canadian Brand Names Clozaril®; Rhoxal-clozapine

Mexican Brand Names Clopsine®; Leponex®

Pharmacologic Category Antipsychotic Agent, Dibenzodiazepine

Use Treatment-refractory schizophrenia; reduce risk of recurrent suicidal behavior in schizophrenia or schizoaffective disorder

Unlabeled/Investigational Use Treatment of schizoaffective or bipolar disorders, childhood psychosis

Local Anesthetic/Vasoconstrictor Precautions Most pharmacology textbooks state that in presence of phenothiazines, systemic doses of epinephrine paradoxically decrease the blood pressure. This is the so called "epinephrine reversal" phenomenon. This has never been observed when epinephrine is given by infiltration as part of the anesthesia procedure.

Effects on Dental Treatment Many patients may experience orthostatic hypotension with clozapine; precautions should be taken; do not use atropine-like drugs for xerostomia in patients taking clozapine due to significant potentiation.

>10%: Sialorrhea, tachycardia, drowsiness, dizziness

1% to 10%: Xerostomia, hypertension, hypotension, syncope, akathisia, seizures, headache, akinesia, confusion, myoclonic jerks, nausea, vomiting, tremor, fever, increased diaphoresis, angina, restlessness, agitation, anxiety, weakness, rhinorrhea, tremors, rigidity, fatigue, lethargy, visual disturbances

Dosage In the event of planned termination of clozapine, gradual reduction in dose over a 1- to 2-week period is recommended. If conditions warrant abrupt discontinuation (leukopenia), monitor patient for psychosis and cholinergic rebound (headache, nausea, vomiting, diarrhea). If dosing is interrupted for >48 hours, therapy must be reinitiated at 12.5-25 mg/day; may be increased more rapidly than with initial titration.

Children and Adolescents: Childhood psychosis (unlabeled use): Initial: 25 mg/day; increase to a target dose of 25-400 mg/day

Adults: Schizophrenia: Initial: 25 mg once or twice daily; increased, as tolerated to a target dose of 300-450 mg/day after 2-4 weeks, but may require doses as high as 600-900 mg/day

Elderly: Schizophrenia: Dose selection and titration should be cautious

Mechanism of Action Clozapine is a weak $dopamine_1$ and $dopamine_2$ receptor blocker, but blocks D_1-D_5 receptors; in addition, it blocks the $serotonin_2$, alpha-adrenergic, histamine H_1, and cholinergic receptors

Other Adverse Effects

>10%:
- Gastrointestinal: Constipation, weight gain, diarrhea
- Genitourinary: Urinary incontinence

1% to 10%:
- Cardiovascular: EKG changes
- Central nervous system: Nightmares, akinesia, insomnia, ataxia, depression
- Dermatologic: Rash
- Gastrointestinal: Abdominal discomfort, heartburn, anorexia, diarrhea
- Hematologic: Eosinophilia, leukopenia, leukocytosis
- Hepatic: Abnormal LFTs
- Neuromuscular & skeletal: Hyperkinesia

<1% (limited to important or life-threatening): Agranulocytosis, **arrhythmias**, blurred vision, cardiomyopathy (usually dilated), **CHF, diabetes mellitus**, difficult urination, granulocytopenia, **hyperglycemia**, impotence, **MI**, myocarditis, neuroleptic malignant syndrome, pericardial effusion, pericarditis, **tardive dyskinesia,** thrombocytopenia, thromboembolism, pulmonary embolism, **stroke**

Postmarketing and/or case reports: Aspiration, cholestasis, ESR increased, fecal impaction, hepatitis, intestinal obstruction, jaundice, narrow-angle glaucoma, paralytic ileus, photosensitivity, **salivary gland swelling, status epilepticus**

Drug Interactions Substrate of **CYP1A2**, 2A6, 2C8/9, 2C19, 2D6, 3A4; Inhibits CYP2C8/9, 2D6, 3A4

Increased Effect/Toxicity: May potentiate anticholinergic and hypotensive effects of other drugs. Benzodiazepines in combination with clozapine may produce respiratory depression and hypotension, especially during the first few weeks of therapy. May potentiate effect/toxicity of risperidone. Clozapine serum concentrations may be increased by inhibitors of CYP1A2, CYP2D6, and CYP3A4. The list of inhibitors is extensive, but includes amiodarone, cimetidine, ciprofloxacin, clarithromycin, delavirdine, diltiazem, erythromycin, fluoxetine, fluvoxamine, indinavir, isoniazid, itraconazole, ketoconazole, nefazodone, paroxetine, quinidine, ritonavir, saquinavir, sertraline, verapamil, zafirlukast, and zileuton. Metoclopramide may increase risk of extrapyramidal symptoms (EPS).

Decreased Effect: Carbamazepine, phenytoin, primidone, and valproic acid may increase the hepatic metabolism (decrease serum levels) of clozapine. Cigarette smoking (nicotine) may enhance the metabolism of clozapine. Clozapine may reverse the pressor effect of epinephrine (avoid in treatment of drug-induced hypotension).

Dietary/Ethanol/Herb Considerations

Ethanol: Avoid use; may increase CNS depression.

Food: May be taken with food; avoid caffeine. Avoid grapefruit products; may increase serum concentration.

Herb/Nutraceutical: Avoid gotu kola, kava, SAMe, and valerian; may increase CNS depression. Avoid St John's wort; may decrease serum concentration and increase CNS depression.

Pharmacodynamics/Kinetics

Protein binding: 97% to serum proteins

Metabolism: Extensively hepatic; forms metabolites

Half-life elimination: 12 hours (range: 4-66 hours)

Time to peak: 2.5 hours

Excretion: Urine (~50%) and feces (30%) with trace amounts of unchanged drug

Pregnancy Risk Factor B

Generic Available Yes

Clozaril® *see* Clozapine *on page 358*

Coagulant Complex Inhibitor *see* Anti-inhibitor Coagulant Complex *on page 116*

Coagulation Factor VIIa *see* Factor VIIa (Recombinant) *on page 554*

Coal Tar (KOLE tar)

U.S. Brand Names Denorex® [OTC]; DHS® Tar [OTC]; Duplex® T [OTC]; Estar® [OTC]; Fototar® [OTC]; Neutrogena® T/Derm; Oxipor® VHC [OTC]; Pentrax® [OTC]; Polytar® [OTC]; psoriGel® [OTC]; Tegrin® Dandruff Shampoo [OTC]; T/Gel® [OTC]; Zetar® [OTC]

Canadian Brand Names Balnetar®; Estar®; SpectroTar Skin Wash™; Targel®; Zetar®

Pharmacologic Category Topical Skin Product

Synonyms Crude Coal Tar; LCD; Pix Carbonis

Use Topically for controlling dandruff, seborrheic dermatitis, or psoriasis

Local Anesthetic/Vasoconstrictor Precautions No information available to require special precautions

Effects on Dental Treatment No significant effects or complications reported

Dosage

Bath: Add appropriate amount to bath water, for adults usually 60-90 mL of a 5% to 20% solution or 15-25 mL of 30% lotion; soak 5-20 minutes, then pat dry; use once daily to 3 days

Shampoo: Rub shampoo onto wet hair and scalp, rinse thoroughly; repeat; leave on 5 minutes; rinse thoroughly; apply twice weekly for the first 2 weeks then once weekly or more often if needed

Skin: Apply to the affected area 1-4 times/day; decrease frequency to 2-3 times/week once condition has been controlled

Scalp psoriasis: Tar oil bath or coal tar solution may be painted sparingly to the lesions 3-12 hours before each shampoo

Psoriasis of the body, arms, legs: Apply at bedtime; if thick scales are present, use product with salicylic acid and apply several times during the day

Other Adverse Effects 1% to 10%: Dermatologic: Dermatitis, folliculitis

Pregnancy Risk Factor C

Generic Available Yes

Comments Avoid exposure to sunlight for 24 hours after use; may stain clothing and skin

Coal Tar and Salicylic Acid (KOLE tar & sal i SIL ik AS id)

Related Information

Coal Tar *on page 359*

Salicylic Acid *on page 1204*

U.S. Brand Names Neutrogena® T/Sal [OTC]; P & S Plus® [OTC]; X-Seb™ T [OTC]

Canadian Brand Names Sebcur/T®

Pharmacologic Category Topical Skin Product

Synonyms Salicylic Acid and Coal Tar

Use Seborrheal dermatitis, dandruff, psoriasis

Local Anesthetic/Vasoconstrictor Precautions No information available to require special precautions

Effects on Dental Treatment No significant effects or complications reported

Dosage

Seborrheal dermatitis or dandruff: Shampoo twice weekly

(Continued)

Coal Tar and Salicylic Acid *(Continued)*

Psoriasis of the body, arms, legs: Gel: Apply at bedtime; if thick scales are present, apply several times during the day

Pregnancy Risk Factor C

Generic Available Yes

Coal Tar, Lanolin, and Mineral Oil

(KOLE tar, LAN oh lin, & MIN er al oyl)

Related Information

Coal Tar *on page 359*

U.S. Brand Names Balnetar® [OTC]

Pharmacologic Category Topical Skin Product

Synonyms Coal Tar, Mineral Oil, and Lanolin; Lanolin, Coal Tar, and Mineral Oil; Lanolin, Mineral Oil, and Coal Tar; Mineral Oil, Coal Tar, and Lanolin; Mineral Oil, Lanolin, and Coal Tar

Use Psoriasis; seborrheal dermatitis; atopic dermatitis; eczematoid dermatitis

Local Anesthetic/Vasoconstrictor Precautions No information available to require special precautions

Effects on Dental Treatment No significant effects or complications reported

Dosage Add to bath water, soak for 5-20 minutes then pat dry

Generic Available No

Coal Tar, Mineral Oil, and Lanolin *see* Coal Tar, Lanolin, and Mineral Oil *on page 360*

Cocaine (koe KANE)

Pharmacologic Category Local Anesthetic

Synonyms Cocaine Hydrochloride

Use Topical anesthesia for mucous membranes

Local Anesthetic/Vasoconstrictor Precautions Although plain local anesthetic is not contraindicated, vasoconstrictor is absolutely contraindicated in any patient under the influence of or within 2 hours of cocaine use

Effects on Dental Treatment See "Comments"

>10%: Loss of taste perception, CNS stimulation, rhinitis, nasal congestion

1% to 10%: Decreased heart rate (low doses), tachycardia (moderate doses), hypertension, ventricular and cardiac arrhythmias, atrial flutter and fibrillation, CHF, pulmonary hypertension, sinus tachycardia, tachycardia (supraventricular), vasoconstriction, fever, nervousness, restlessness, excitation, headache, psychosis, hallucinations, agitation, seizures, dystonic reactions, vasculitis, clonic-tonic reactions, paranoia, nausea, paresthesia, tremors, tachypnea, nasal mucosa damage (when snorting), bronchiolitis obliterans organizing pneumonia, euphoria, slurred speech

Restrictions C-II

Dosage Dosage depends on the area to be anesthetized, tissue vascularity, technique of anesthesia, and individual patient tolerance; use the lowest dose necessary to produce adequate anesthesia should be used, not to exceed 1 mg/kg. Use reduced dosages for children, elderly, or debilitated patients.

Topical application (ear, nose, throat, bronchoscopy): Concentrations of 1% to 4% are used. Concentrations >4% are not recommended because of potential for increased incidence and severity of systemic toxic reactions.

Mechanism of Action Ester local anesthetic blocks both the initiation and conduction of nerve impulses by decreasing the neuronal membrane's permeability to sodium ions, which results in inhibition of depolarization with resultant blockade of conduction; interferes with the uptake of norepinephrine by adrenergic nerve terminals producing vasoconstriction

Other Adverse Effects

>10%: Loss of smell

1% to 10%:

Cardiovascular: Cardiomyopathy, myocarditis, QRS prolongation, Raynaud's phenomenon, cerebral vasculitis, thrombosis,

Central nervous system: Hyperthermia, cerebral vascular accident, vasculitis, sympathetic storm

Dermatologic: Skin infarction, pruritus, madarosis

Gastrointestinal: Anorexia, colonic ischemia, spontaneous bowel perforation

Genitourinary: Priapism, uterine rupture

Hematologic: Thrombocytopenia

Neuromuscular & skeletal: Chorea (extrapyramidal), fasciculations

Ocular: Mydriasis (peak effect at 45 minutes; may last up to 12 hours), sloughing of the corneal epithelium, ulceration of the cornea, iritis, mydriasis, chemosis

Renal: Myoglobinuria, necrotizing vasculitis

Respiratory: Hyposmia

Miscellaneous: "Washed-out" syndrome

Drug Interactions Substrate of **CYP3A4**; Inhibits **CYP2D6**, 3A4

Increased Effect/Toxicity: Increased toxicity with MAO inhibitors. Use with epinephrine may cause extreme hypertension and/or cardiac arrhythmias.

Pharmacodynamics/Kinetics Following topical administration to mucosa:

Onset of action: ~1 minute

Peak effect: ~5 minutes

Duration (dose dependent): ≥30 minutes; cocaine metabolites may appear in urine of neonates up to 5 days after birth due to maternal cocaine use shortly before birth

Absorption: Well absorbed through mucous membranes; limited by drug-induced vasoconstriction; enhanced by inflammation

Distribution: Enters breast milk

Metabolism: Hepatic; major metabolites are ecgonine methyl ester and benzoyl ecgonine

Half-life elimination: 75 minutes

Excretion: Primarily urine (<10% as unchanged drug and metabolites)

Pregnancy Risk Factor C/X (nonmedicinal use)

Generic Available Yes

Comments The cocaine user, regardless of how the cocaine was administered, presents a potential life-threatening situation in the dental operatory. A patient under the influence of cocaine could be compared to a car going 100 mph. Blood pressure is elevated, heart rate is likely increased, and the use of a local anesthetic with epinephrine may result in a medical emergency. Such patients can be identified by their jitteriness, irritability, talkativeness, tremors, and short, abrupt speech patterns. These same signs and symptoms may also be seen in a normal dental patient with preoperative dental anxiety; therefore, the dentist must be particularly alert in order to identify the potential cocaine abuser. If cocaine use is suspected, the patient should never be given a local anesthetic with vasoconstrictor, for fear of exacerbating the cocaine-induced sympathetic response. Life-threatening episodes of cardiac arrhythmias and hypertensive crises have been reported when local anesthetic with vasoconstrictor was administered to a patient under the influence of cocaine. No local anesthetic, used by any dentist, can interfere with, nor test positive by cocaine in any urine testing screen. Therefore, the dentist does not need to be concerned with any false drug-use accusations associated with dental anesthesia.

Cocaine Hydrochloride *see* Cocaine *on page 360*

Codafed® Expectorant *see* Guaifenesin, Pseudoephedrine, and Codeine *on page 653*

Codafed® Pediatric Expectorant *see* Guaifenesin, Pseudoephedrine, and Codeine *on page 653*

Codehist® DH *see* Chlorpheniramine, Pseudoephedrine, and Codeine *on page 311*

Codeine (KOE deen)

Related Information

Carisoprodol, Aspirin, and Codeine *on page 252*

Oral Pain *on page 1524*

Pharmacologic Category Analgesic, Narcotic; Antitussive

Synonyms Codeine Phosphate; Codeine Sulfate; Methylmorphine

Use

Dental: Treatment of postoperative pain

Medical: Treatment of mild to moderate pain; antitussive in lower doses

Note: Dextromethorphan has equivalent antitussive activity but has much lower toxicity in accidental overdose.

Local Anesthetic/Vasoconstrictor Precautions No information available to require special precautions

Effects on Dental Treatment

>10%: Drowsiness

1% to 10%: Tachycardia, bradycardia, hypotension, dizziness, lightheadedness, malaise, headache, restlessness, paradoxical CNS stimulation, confusion nausea, vomiting, weakness, blurred vision, dyspnea, histamine release, xerostomia

Restrictions C-II

Dosage These are guidelines and do not represent the maximum doses that may be required in all patients. Doses should be titrated to pain relief/prevention. Doses >1.5 mg/kg body weight are not recommended.

Analgesic:

Children: Oral, I.M., S.C.: 0.5-1 mg/kg/dose every 4-6 hours as needed; maximum: 60 mg/dose

Adults:

Oral: 30 mg every 4-6 hours as needed; patients with prior opiate exposure may require higher initial doses. Usual range: 15-120 mg every 4-6 hours as needed

I.M., S.C.: 30 mg every 4-6 hours as needed; patients with prior opiate exposure may require higher initial doses. Usual range: 15-120 mg every 4-6 hours as needed; more frequent dosing may be needed

(Continued)

Codeine *(Continued)*

Antitussive: Oral (for nonproductive cough):

Children: 1-1.5 mg/kg/day in divided doses every 4-6 hours as needed: Alternative dose according to age:

2-6 years: 2.5-5 mg every 4-6 hours as needed; maximum: 30 mg/day

6-12 years: 5-10 mg every 4-6 hours as needed; maximum: 60 mg/day

Adults: 10-20 mg/dose every 4-6 hours as needed; maximum: 120 mg/day

Dosing adjustment in renal impairment:

Cl_{cr} 10-50 mL/minute: Administer 75% of dose

Cl_{cr} <10 mL/minute: Administer 50% of dose

Dosing adjustment in hepatic impairment: Probably necessary

Mechanism of Action Binds to opiate receptors in the CNS, causing inhibition of ascending pain pathways, altering the perception of and response to pain; causes cough supression by direct central action in the medulla; produces generalized CNS depression

Other Adverse Effects

>10%: Gastrointestinal: Constipation

1% to 10%:

Central nervous system: False feeling of well-being

Dermatologic: Rash, urticaria

Gastrointestinal: Anorexia

Genitourinary: Decreased urination, ureteral spasm

Hepatic: Increased LFTs

Local: Burning at injection site

<1%: **Convulsions, hallucinations**, mental depression, nightmares, insomnia, paralytic ileus, **biliary spasm, stomach cramps, muscle rigidity, trembling**

Frequency not defined: Increased AST, ALT

Contraindications Hypersensitivity to codeine or any component of the formulation; pregnancy (prolonged use or high doses at term)

Warnings/Precautions An opioid-containing analgesic regimen should be tailored to each patient's needs and based upon the type of pain being treated (acute versus chronic), the route of administration, degree of tolerance for opioids (naive versus chronic user), age, weight, and medical condition. The optimal analgesic dose varies widely among patients. Doses should be titrated to pain relief/prevention.

Use with caution in patients with hypersensitivity reactions to other phenanthrene derivative opioid agonists (morphine, hydrocodone, hydromorphone, levorphanol, oxycodone, oxymorphone); respiratory diseases including asthma, emphysema, COPD, or severe liver or renal insufficiency; some preparations contain sulfites which may cause allergic reactions; tolerance or drug dependence may result from extended use

Not recommended for use for cough control in patients with a productive cough; not recommended as an antitussive for children <2 years of age; the elderly may be particularly susceptible to the CNS depressant and confusion as well as constipating effects of narcotics

Not approved for I.V. administration (although this route has been used clinically). If given intravenously, must be given slowly and the patient should be lying down. Rapid intravenous administration of narcotics may increase the incidence of serious adverse effects, in part due to limited opportunity to assess response prior to administration of the full dose. Access to respiratory support should be immediately available

Drug Interactions Substrate of **CYP2D6**, 3A4; Inhibits CYP2D6

Increased Toxicity: CNS depressants, phenothiazines, TCAs, other narcotic analgesics, guanabenz, MAO inhibitors, neuromuscular blockers

Decreased effect with cigarette smoking

Dietary/Ethanol/Herb Considerations

Ethanol: Avoid or limit use; may increase CNS depression.

Food: Administer with food to reduce GI upset.

Herb/Nutraceutical: Avoid gotu kola, kava, SAMe, and valerian; may increase CNS depression. Avoid St John's wort; may decrease serum concentration and increase CNS depression.

Pharmacodynamics/Kinetics

Onset of action: Oral: 0.5-1 hour; I.M.: 10-30 minutes

Peak effect: Oral: 1-1.5 hours; I.M.: 0.5-1 hour

Duration: 4-6 hours

Absorption: Oral: Adequate

Distribution: Crosses placenta; enters breast milk

Protein binding: 7%

Metabolism: Hepatic to morphine (active)

Half-life elimination: 2.5-3.5 hours

Excretion: Urine (3% to 16% as unchanged drug, norcodeine, and free and conjugated morphine)

Pregnancy Risk Factor C/D (prolonged use or high doses at term)

Dosage Forms INJ, as phosphate: 30 mg (1 mL, 2 mL); 60 mg (1 mL, 2 mL). **SOLN, oral, as phosphate:** 15 mg/5 mL. **TAB, as phosphate, soluble:** 30 mg, 60 mg. **TAB, as sulfate:** 15 mg, 30 mg, 60 mg. **TAB, soluble, as sulfate:** 15 mg, 30 mg, 60 mg

Generic Available Yes

Comments It is recommended that codeine not be used as the sole entity for analgesia because of moderate efficacy along with relatively high incidence of nausea, sedation, and constipation. In addition, codeine has some narcotic addiction liability. Codeine in combination with acetaminophen or aspirin is recommended. Maximum effective analgesic dose of codeine is 60 mg (1 grain). Beyond 60 mg increases respiratory depression only. Sodium thiosulfate is an effective chemical antidote for codeine poisoning.

Selected Readings

Desjardins PJ, Cooper SA, Gallegos TL, et al, "The Relative Analgesic Efficacy of Propiram Fumarate, Codeine, Aspirin, and Placebo in Postimpaction Dental Pain," *J Clin Pharmacol*, 1984, 24(1):35-42.

Forbes JA, Keller CK, Smith JW, et al, "Analgesic Effect of Naproxen Sodium, Codeine, a Naproxen-Codeine Combination and Aspirin on the Postoperative Pain of Oral Surgery," *Pharmacotherapy*, 1986, 6(5):211-8.

Codeine, Acetaminophen, Butalbital, and Caffeine *see* Butalbital, Acetaminophen, Caffeine, and Codeine *on page 215*

Codeine and Acetaminophen *see* Acetaminophen and Codeine *on page 29*

Codeine and Aspirin *see* Aspirin and Codeine *on page 134*

Codeine and Bromodiphenhydramine *see* Bromodiphenhydramine and Codeine *on page 200*

Codeine and Butalbital Compound *see* Butalbital, Aspirin, Caffeine, and Codeine *on page 217*

Codeine and Guaifenesin *see* Guaifenesin and Codeine *on page 650*

Codeine and Promethazine *see* Promethazine and Codeine *on page 1129*

Codeine, Aspirin, and Carisoprodol *see* Carisoprodol, Aspirin, and Codeine *on page 252*

Codeine, Butalbital, Aspirin, and Caffeine *see* Butalbital, Aspirin, Caffeine, and Codeine *on page 217*

Codeine, Guaifenesin, and Pseudoephedrine *see* Guaifenesin, Pseudoephedrine, and Codeine *on page 653*

Codeine Phosphate *see* Codeine *on page 361*

Codeine, Promethazine, and Phenylephrine *see* Promethazine, Phenylephrine, and Codeine *on page 1130*

Codeine, Pseudoephedrine, and Triprolidine *see* Triprolidine, Pseudoephedrine, and Codeine *on page 1357*

Codeine Sulfate *see* Codeine *on page 361*

Codiclear® DH *see* Hydrocodone and Guaifenesin *on page 683*

Codimal-LA® [OTC] *see* Chlorpheniramine and Pseudoephedrine *on page 308*

Codimal-LA® Half [OTC] *see* Chlorpheniramine and Pseudoephedrine *on page 308*

Cod Liver Oil *see* Vitamin A and Vitamin D *on page 1392*

Cogentin® *see* Benztropine *on page 173*

Co-Gesic® *see* Hydrocodone and Acetaminophen *on page 678*

Cognex® *see* Tacrine *on page 1260*

Colace® [OTC] *see* Docusate *on page 463*

ColBenemid® [DSC] *see* Colchicine and Probenecid *on page 364*

Colchicine (KOL chi seen)

Canadian Brand Names ratio-Colchicine

Mexican Brand Names Colchiquim®; Colchiquim-30

Pharmacologic Category Colchicine

Use Treatment of acute gouty arthritis attacks and prevention of recurrences of such attacks; management of familial Mediterranean fever

Unlabeled/Investigational Use Treatment of primary biliary cirrhosis

Local Anesthetic/Vasoconstrictor Precautions No information available to require special precautions

Effects on Dental Treatment >10%: Nausea, vomiting

Dosage

Familial Mediterranean fever: Prophylaxis: Oral:

Children:

≤5 years: 0.5 mg/day

>5 years: 1-1.5 mg/day in 2-3 divided doses

Adults: 1-2 mg daily in divided doses (occasionally reduced to 0.6 mg/day in patients with GI intolerance)

Gouty arthritis, acute attacks: Adults:

Oral: Initial: 0.5-1.2 mg, then 0.5-0.6 mg every 1-2 hours or 1-1.2 mg every 2 hours until relief or GI side effects (nausea, vomiting, or diarrhea) occur to a maximum total dose of 8 mg; wait 3 days before initiating another course of therapy

(Continued)

Colchicine *(Continued)*

I.V.: Initial: 1-3 mg, then 0.5 mg every 6 hours until response, not to exceed total dose of 4 mg. If pain recurs, it may be necessary to administer additional daily doses; the amount of colchicine administered intravenously in an acute treatment period (generally ~1 week) should not exceed a total dose of 4 mg. Do not administer more colchicine by any route for at least 7 days after a full course of I.V. therapy (4 mg); transfer to oral colchicine in a dose similar to that being given I.V.

Gouty arthritis, prophylaxis of recurrent attacks: Adults: Oral: 0.5-0.6 mg/day or every other day; patients who are to undergo surgical procedures may receive 0.5-0.6 mg 3 times/day for 3 days before and 3 days after surgery

Dosing adjustment in renal impairment:

Cl_{cr} <50 mL/minute: Avoid chronic use or administration

Cl_{cr} <10 mL/minute: Decrease dose by 75% for treatment of acute attacks

Hemodialysis: Not dialyzable (0% to 5%); supplemental dose is unnecessary

Peritoneal dialysis: Supplemental dose is unnecessary

Mechanism of Action Decreases leukocyte motility, decreases phagocytosis in joints and lactic acid production, thereby reducing the deposition of urate crystals that perpetuates the inflammatory response

Other Adverse Effects

>10%: Gastrointestinal: Diarrhea, abdominal pain

1% to 10%:

Dermatologic: Alopecia

Gastrointestinal: Anorexia

<1%: Rash, azoospermia, agranulocytosis, aplastic anemia, bone marrow suppression, hepatotoxicity, myopathy, peripheral neuritis

Drug Interactions Substrate of **CYP3A4**; Induces CYP2C8/9, 2E1, 3A4

Increased Effect/Toxicity: Increased toxicity may be seen when taken with sympathomimetic agents or CNS depressant (effects are enhanced). Alkalizing agents potentiate effects of colchicine.

Decreased Effect: Vitamin B_{12} absorption may be decreased with colchicine. Acidifying agents inhibit action of colchicine.

Dietary/Ethanol/Herb Considerations

Ethanol: Avoid use; may enhance gastric mucosal irritation.

Food: Vitamin B_{12}: Malabsorption of the substrate; may result in macrocytic anemia or neurologic dysfunction.

Pharmacodynamics/Kinetics

Onset of action: Oral: Pain relief: ~12 hours if adequately dosed

Distribution: Concentrates in leukocytes, kidney, spleen, and liver; does not distribute in heart, skeletal muscle, and brain

Protein binding: 10% to 31%

Metabolism: Partially hepatic via deacetylation

Half-life elimination: 12-30 minutes; End-stage renal disease: 45 minutes

Time to peak, serum: Oral: 0.5-2 hours, declining for the next 2 hours before increasing again due to enterohepatic recycling

Excretion: Primarily feces; urine (10% to 20%)

Pregnancy Risk Factor C (oral); D (parenteral)

Generic Available Yes

Colchicine and Probenecid (KOL chi seen & proe BEN e sid)

Related Information

Colchicine *on page 363*

Pharmacologic Category Antigout Agent; Anti-inflammatory Agent; Uricosuric Agent

Synonyms ColBenemid® [DSC]; Probenecid and Colchicine

Use Treatment of chronic gouty arthritis when complicated by frequent, recurrent acute attacks of gout

Local Anesthetic/Vasoconstrictor Precautions No information available to require special precautions

Effects on Dental Treatment 1% to 10%: Flushing, headache, dizziness, nausea, vomiting, hypersensitivity reactions

Dosage Adults: Oral: 1 tablet daily for 1 week, then 1 tablet twice daily thereafter

Other Adverse Effects 1% to 10%:

Dermatologic: Rash, alopecia

Gastrointestinal: Anorexia, diarrhea, abdominal pain

Hematologic: Anemia, leukopenia, aplastic anemia, agranulocytosis

Hepatic: Hepatic necrosis, hepatotoxicity

Neuromuscular & skeletal: Peripheral neuritis, myopathy

Renal: Nephrotic syndrome, uric acid stones, polyuria

Dietary/Ethanol/Herb Considerations Ethanol: Avoid use; may enhance gastric mucosal irritation.

Pregnancy Risk Factor C

Generic Available Yes

Comments Do not initiate therapy until an acute gouty attack has subsided.

Colesevelam (koe le SEV a lam)

U.S. Brand Names WelChol™

Canadian Brand Names WelChol™

Pharmacologic Category Antilipemic Agent, Bile Acid Sequestrant

Use Adjunctive therapy to diet and exercise in the management of elevated LDL in primary hypercholesterolemia (Fredrickson type IIa) when used alone or in combination with an HMG-CoA reductase inhibitor

Local Anesthetic/Vasoconstrictor Precautions No information available to require special precautions

Effects on Dental Treatment 1% to 5%: Weakness (4%), myalgia (2%), pharyngitis (3%)

Dosage Adult: Oral:

Monotherapy: 3 tablets twice daily with meals or 6 tablets once daily with a meal; maximum dose: 7 tablets/day

Combination therapy with an HMG-CoA reductase inhibitor: 4-6 tablets daily; maximum dose: 6 tablets/day

Mechanism of Action Colesevelam binds bile acids including glycocholic acid in the intestine, impeding their reabsorption. Increases the fecal loss of bile salt-bound LDL-C

Other Adverse Effects

>10%: Gastrointestinal: Constipation (11%)

2% to 10%:

Gastrointestinal: Dyspepsia (8%)

Neuromuscular & skeletal: Myalgia (2%)

Incidence ≤placebo: **Infection, headache, pain**, back pain, abdominal pain, **flu syndrome**, flatulence, diarrhea, **nausea, sinusitis, rhinitis, cough**

Drug Interactions Decreased Effect: Sustained-release verapamil AUC and C_{max} were reduced (clinical significance unknown). Digoxin, lovastatin, metoprolol, quinidine, valproic acid, or warfarin absorption was not significantly affected with concurrent administration.

Dietary/Ethanol/Herb Considerations Food: Administer with food; follow dietary guidelines.

Pharmacodynamics/Kinetics

Onset of action: Peak effect: Therapeutic: ~2 weeks

Absorption: Insignificant

Excretion: Urine (0.05%) after 1 month of chronic dosing

Pregnancy Risk Factor B

Generic Available No

Colestid® *see* Colestipol *on page 365*

Colestipol (koe LES ti pole)

Related Information

Cardiovascular Diseases *on page 1456*

U.S. Brand Names Colestid®

Canadian Brand Names Colestid®

Pharmacologic Category Antilipemic Agent, Bile Acid Sequestrant

Synonyms Colestipol Hydrochloride

Use Adjunct in management of primary hypercholesterolemia; regression of arteriolosclerosis; relief of pruritus associated with elevated levels of bile acids; possibly used to decrease plasma half-life of digoxin in toxicity

Local Anesthetic/Vasoconstrictor Precautions No information available to require special precautions

Effects on Dental Treatment 1% to 10%: Headache, dizziness, anxiety, drowsiness, belching, nausea, vomiting, fatigue

Dosage Adults: Oral:

Granules: 5-30 g/day given once or in divided doses 2-4 times/day; initial dose: 5 g 1-2 times/day; increase by 5 g at 1- to 2-month intervals

Tablets: 2-16 g/day; initial dose: 2 g 1-2 times/day; increase by 2 g at 1- to 2-month intervals

Mechanism of Action Binds with bile acids to form an insoluble complex that is eliminated in feces; it thereby increases the fecal loss of bile acid-bound low density lipoprotein cholesterol

Other Adverse Effects

>10%: Gastrointestinal: Constipation

1% to 10%:

Central nervous system: Vertigo

Gastrointestinal: Abdominal pain and distention, flatulence, diarrhea

<1% (Limited to important or life-threatening): **Peptic ulceration**, gallstones, **GI irritation and bleeding**, anorexia, steatorrhea or malabsorption syndrome, cholelithiasis, cholecystitis, **dyspnea**

Drug Interactions Decreased Effect: Colestipol can reduce the absorption of numerous medications when used concurrently. Give other medications 1 hour before or 4 hours after giving colestipol. Medications which may be affected include

(Continued)

Colestipol *(Continued)*

HMG-CoA reductase inhibitors, thiazide diuretics, propranolol (and potentially other beta-blockers), corticosteroids, thyroid hormones, digoxin, valproic acid, NSAIDs, loop diuretics, sulfonylureas, troglitazone (and potentially other agents in this class - pioglitazone and rosiglitazone). Absorption of warfarin and other oral anticoagulants is reduced by cholestyramine and may also be reduced by colestipol; separate administration times (as detailed above).

Dietary/Ethanol/Herb Considerations Administer with 3-4 oz water or juice.

Pharmacodynamics/Kinetics

Absorption: None

Excretion: Feces

Pregnancy Risk Factor C

Generic Available No

Colestipol Hydrochloride *see* Colestipol *on page 365*

Colfosceril Palmitate (kole FOS er il PALM i tate)

U.S. Brand Names Exosurf Neonatal®

Mexican Brand Names Exosurf®

Pharmacologic Category Lung Surfactant

Synonyms Dipalmitoylphosphatidylcholine; DPPC; Synthetic Lung Surfactant

Use Neonatal respiratory distress syndrome:

Prophylactic therapy: Body weight <1350 g in infants at risk for developing RDS; body weight >1350 g in infants with evidence of pulmonary immaturity

Rescue therapy: Treatment of infants with RDS based on respiratory distress not attributable to any other causes and chest radiographic findings consistent with RDS

Local Anesthetic/Vasoconstrictor Precautions No information available to require special precautions

Effects on Dental Treatment 1% to 10%: Apnea, mucous plugging

Dosage For intratracheal use only. Neonates:

Prophylactic treatment: Administer 5 mL/kg (as two 2.5 mL/kg half-doses) as soon as possible; the second and third doses should be administered at 12 and 24 hours later to those infants remaining on ventilators

Rescue treatment: Administer 5 mL/kg (as two 2.5 mL/kg half-doses) as soon as the diagnosis of RDS is made; the second 5 mL/kg (as two 2.5 mL/kg half-doses) dose should be administered 12 hours later

Mechanism of Action Replaces deficient or ineffective endogenous lung surfactant in neonates with respiratory distress syndrome (RDS) or in neonates at risk of developing RDS; reduces surface tension and stabilizes the alveoli from collapsing

Other Adverse Effects 1% to 10%: Respiratory: Pulmonary hemorrhage, decrease in transcutaneous O_2 of >20%

Pharmacodynamics/Kinetics

Absorption: Intratracheal: From alveolus

Metabolism: Catabolized and reutilized for further synthesis and secretion in pulmonary tissue

Generic Available No

Colgate Total® Toothpaste *see* Triclosan and Fluoride *on page 1348*

Colistimethate (koe lis ti METH ate)

U.S. Brand Names Coly-Mycin® M

Canadian Brand Names Coly-Mycin® M

Pharmacologic Category Antibiotic, Miscellaneous

Synonyms Colistimethate Sodium

Use Treatment of infections due to sensitive strains of certain gram-negative bacilli which are resistant to other antibacterials or in patients allergic to other antibacterials

Unlabeled/Investigational Use Inhalation: Prevention of *Pseudomonas aeruginosa* respiratory tract infections in immunocompromised patients, adjunct agent for treatment of *P. aeruginosa* infections in patients with cystic fibrosis and other seriously ill or chronically ill patients

Local Anesthetic/Vasoconstrictor Precautions No information available to require special precautions

Effects on Dental Treatment 1% to 10%: Respiratory arrest, slurred speech, GI upset

Dosage Children and Adults:

I.M., I.V.: 2.5-5 mg/kg/day in 2-4 divided doses

Inhalation: 75 mg in 3 mL NS (4 mL total) via nebulizer twice daily

Dosing interval in renal impairment: Adults:

S_{cr} 0.7-1.2 mg/dL: 100-125 mg 2-4 times/day

S_{cr} 1.3-1.5 mg/dL: 75-115 mg twice daily

S_{cr} 1.6-2.5 mg/dL: 66-150 mg once or twice daily

S_{cr} 2.6-4 mg/dL: 100-150 mg every 36 hours

Mechanism of Action Hydrolyzed to colistin, which acts as a cationic detergent which damages the bacterial cytoplasmic membrane causing leaking of intracellular substances and cell death

Other Adverse Effects 1% to 10%:
Central nervous system: Vertigo
Dermatologic: Urticaria
Renal: Nephrotoxicity

Drug Interactions Increased Effect/Toxicity: Other nephrotoxic drugs, neuromuscular blocking agents.

Pharmacodynamics/Kinetics
Distribution: Widely, except for CNS, synovial, pleural, and pericardial fluids
Half-life elimination: 1.5-8 hours; Anuria: ≤2-3 days
Time to peak: ~2 hours
Excretion: Primarily urine (as unchanged drug)

Pregnancy Risk Factor B

Generic Available No

Colistimethate Sodium *see* Colistimethate *on page 366*

Colistin, Neomycin, and Hydrocortisone

(koe LIS tin, nee oh MYE sin & hye droe KOR ti sone)

Related Information
Hydrocortisone *on page 688*

U.S. Brand Names Coly-Mycin® S Otic; Cortisporin®-TC Otic

Pharmacologic Category Antibiotic/Corticosteroid, Otic

Synonyms Hydrocortisone, Colistin, and Neomycin; Neomycin, Colistin, and Hydrocortisone

Use Treatment of superficial and susceptible bacterial infections of the external auditory canal; for treatment of susceptible bacterial infections of mastoidectomy and fenestration cavities

Local Anesthetic/Vasoconstrictor Precautions No information available to require special precautions

Effects on Dental Treatment No significant effects or complications reported

Dosage
Children: 3 drops in affected ear 3-4 times/day
Adults: 4 drops in affected ear 3-4 times/day

Pregnancy Risk Factor C

Generic Available No

CollaCote® *see* Collagen (Absorbable) *on page 367*

Collagen *see* Microfibrillar Collagen Hemostat *on page 907*

Collagen (Absorbable) (KOL la jen, ab ZORB abul)

U.S. Brand Names CollaCote®; CollaPlug®; CollaTape®

Pharmacologic Category Hemostatic Agent

Use
Dental: To control bleeding created during dental surgery
Medical: Hemostatic agent

Local Anesthetic/Vasoconstrictor Precautions No information available to require special precautions

Effects on Dental Treatment No significant effects or complications reported

Dosage Children and Adults: A sufficiently large dressing should be selected so as to completely cover the oral wound. The dressing should be applied over the wound and held in place with moderate pressure. The period of time necessary to apply pressure will vary with the degree of bleeding. In general, 2-5 minutes should be sufficient to achieve hemostasis. At the end of the procedure, the dressing can be removed, replaced or left *in situ*, any excess dressing should be removed prior to wound closure.

Mechanism of Action The highly porous sponge structure absorbs blood and wound exudate. The collagen component causes aggregation of platelets which bind to collagen fibrils. The aggregated platelets degranulate, releasing coagulation factors that promote the formation of fibrin.

Contraindications No data reported

Warnings/Precautions Should not be used on infected or contaminated wounds

Dosage Forms **DRESSING, wound:** 3/8" x 3/4"; 3/4" x 1 1/2"; 1" x 3"

Generic Available Yes

Collagenase (KOL la je nase)

U.S. Brand Names Santyl®

Canadian Brand Names Santyl®

Pharmacologic Category Enzyme, Topical Debridement

Use Promotes debridement of necrotic tissue in dermal ulcers and severe burns
Orphan drug: Injection: Treatment of Peyronie's or Dupytren's disease

Local Anesthetic/Vasoconstrictor Precautions No information available to require special precautions

(Continued)

Collagenase *(Continued)*

Effects on Dental Treatment No significant effects or complications reported

Dosage Topical: Apply once daily (or more frequently if the dressing becomes soiled)

Mechanism of Action Collagenase is an enzyme derived from the fermentation of *Clostridium histolyticum* and differs from other proteolytic enzymes in that its enzymatic action has a high specificity for native and denatured collagen. Collagenase will not attack collagen in healthy tissue or newly formed granulation tissue. In addition, it does not act on fat, fibrin, keratin, or muscle.

Other Adverse Effects Frequency not defined:
Local: Irritation, pain, and burning at site of application
Postmarketing and/or case reports: Hypersensitivity reaction

Drug Interactions Decreased Effect: Enzymatic activity is inhibited by detergents, benzalkonium chloride, hexachlorophene, nitrofurazone, tincture of iodine, and heavy metal ions (silver and mercury).

Pregnancy Risk Factor C

Generic Available No

CollaPlug® *see* Collagen (Absorbable) *on page 367*
CollaTape® *see* Collagen (Absorbable) *on page 367*
Colo-Fresh™ [OTC] *see* Bismuth *on page 186*
Coly-Mycin® M *see* Colistimethate *on page 366*
Coly-Mycin® S Otic *see* Colistin, Neomycin, and Hydrocortisone *on page 367*
Colyte® *see* Polyethylene Glycol-Electrolyte Solution *on page 1094*

Combination Hormonal Contraceptives

(KOM bi na shun HOR mo nal kon tru SEP tivz)

Related Information
Estradiol *on page 521*
Rheumatoid Arthritis, Osteoarthritis, and Osteoporosis *on page 1488*

U.S. Brand Names Alesse®; Apri®; Aviane™; Brevicon®; Cryselle™; Cyclessa®; Demulen®; Desogen®; Enpresse™; Estrostep® 21 [DSC]; Estrostep® Fe; femhrt®; Kariva™; Lessina™; Levlen®; Levlite™; Levora®; Loestrin®; Loestrin® Fe; Lo/Ovral®; Low-Ogestrel®; Microgestin™ Fe; Mircette®; Modicon®; Necon® 0.5/35; Necon® 1/35; Necon® 7/7/7; Necon® 10/11; Nordette®; Norinyl® 1+35; Nortrel™; Nortrel™ 7/7/7; NuvaRing®; Ogestrel®; Ortho-Cept®; Ortho-Cyclen® Lo; Ortho Evra™; Ortho-Novum®; Ortho Sprintec™; Ovcon®; Ovral®; Portia™; PREVEN®; Tri-Cyclen®; Tri-Levlen®; Tri-Norinyl®; Triphasil®; Trivora®; Yasmin®; Zovia™

Pharmacologic Category Contraceptive; Estrogen and Progestin Combination

Synonyms Ethinyl Estradiol and Desogestrel; Ethinyl Estradiol and Drospirenone; Ethinyl Estradiol and Ethynodiol Diacetate; Ethinyl Estradiol and Etonogestrel; Ethinyl Estradiol and Levonorgestrel; Ethinyl Estradiol and Norelgestromin; Ethinyl Estradiol and Norethindrone; Ethinyl Estradiol and Norgestimate; Ethinyl Estradiol and Norgestrel

Use Labeled indications are product specific and may include the following: Prevention of pregnancy; postcoital contraception; treatment of acne; moderate to severe vasomotor symptoms associated with menopause; prevention of osteoporosis

Unlabeled/Investigational Use Treatment of hypermenorrhea, endometriosis, female hypogonadism

Local Anesthetic/Vasoconstrictor Precautions No information available to require special precautions

Effects on Dental Treatment No significant effects or complications reported

Dosage
Children ≥15 years and Adults: Female: Oral: Acne (Estrostep®, Ortho Tri-Cyclen®): Refer to dosing for contraception
Adults: Female: Contraception: Oral: (Abbreviated/refer to package insert):
Schedule 1 (Sunday starter): Dose begins on first Sunday after onset of menstruation; if the menstrual period starts on Sunday, take first tablet that very same day. With a Sunday start, an additional method of contraception should be used until after the first 7 days of consecutive administration:
For 21-tablet package: 1 tablet/day for 21 consecutive days, followed by 7 days off of the medication; a new course begins on the 8th day after the last tablet is taken
For 28-tablet package: 1 tablet/day without interruption
Schedule 2 (Day-1 starter): Dose starts on first day of menstrual cycle taking 1 tablet/day:
For 21-tablet package: 1 tablet/day for 21 consecutive days, followed by 7 days off of the medication; a new course begins on the 8th day after the last tablet is taken
For 28-tablet package: 1 tablet/day without interruption
Missed doses **monophasic formulations** (refer to package insert for complete information):
One dose missed: Take as soon as remembered or take 2 tablets next day

Two consecutive doses missed in the first 2 weeks: Take 2 tablets as soon as remembered or 2 tablets next 2 days. An additional method of contraception should be used for 7 days after missed dose.

Two consecutive doses missed in week 3 or three consecutive doses missed at any time: An additional method of contraception must be used for 7 days after a missed dose.

Missed doses **biphasic/triphasic formulations** (refer to package insert for complete information):

One dose missed: Take as soon as remembered or take 2 tablets next day.

Two consecutive doses missed in week 1 or week 2 of the pack: Take 2 tablets as soon as remembered and 2 tablets the next day. Resume taking 1 tablet/day until the pack is empty. An additional method of contraception should be used for 7 days after a missed dose.

Two consecutive doses missed in week 3 of the pack: An additional method of contraception must be used for 7 days after a missed dose.

Three or more consecutive doses missed: An additional method of contraception must be used for 7 days after a missed dose.

Topical patch: (Abbreviated labeling/refer to package insert): Apply one patch each week for 3 weeks (21 total days); followed by one week that is patch-free. Each patch should be applied on the same day each week ("patch change day") and only one patch should be worn at a time. No more than 7 days should pass during the patch-free interval.

If a patch becomes partially or completely detached for <24 hours: Try to reapply to same place, or replace with a new patch immediately. Do not reapply if patch is no longer sticky, if it is sticking to itself or another surface, or if it has material sticking to it.

If a patch becomes partially or completely detached for >24 hours (or time period is unknown): Apply a new patch and use this day of the week as the new "patch change day" from this point on. **An additional method of contraception (nonhormonal) should be used until after the first 7 days of consecutive administration.**

Vaginal ring: (Abbreviated labeling/refer to package insert): One ring, inserted vaginally and left in place for 3 consecutive weeks, then removed for 1 week. A new ring is inserted 7 days after the last was removed (even if bleeding is not complete) and should be inserted at ~ the same time of day the ring was removed the previous week.

If the ring is accidentally removed from the vagina at anytime during the 3-week period of use, it may be rinsed with cool or lukewarm water (not hot) and reinserted as soon as possible. If the ring is not reinserted within 3 hours, contraceptive effectiveness will be decreased. **An additional form of contraception should be used until the ring has been inserted for 7 continuous days.*** If the ring has been removed for longer than 1 week, pregnancy must be ruled out prior to restarting therapy. **An additional form of contraception should be used for the following 7 days.***

If the ring has been left in place for >3 weeks, a new ring should be inserted following a 1-week (ring-free) interval. Pregnancy must be ruled out prior to insertion and **an additional form of contraception should be used for the following 7 days.***

*Note: Diaphragms may interfere with proper ring placement, and therefore, are not recommended for use as an additional form of contraception.

Adults: Female: Postcoital contraception: Oral:

Ethinyl estradiol 0.03 mg and norgestrel 0.3 mg formulation: 4 tablets within 72 hours of unprotected intercourse and 4 tablets 12 hours after first dose

Ethinyl estradiol 0.05 mg and norgestrel 0.5 mg formulation: 2 tablets within 72 hours of unprotected intercourse and 2 tablets 12 hours after first dose

PREVEN™: Initial: 2 tablets as soon as possible (but within 72 hours of unprotected intercourse), followed by a second dose of 2 tablets 12 hours later.

Adults: Female: Moderate to severe vasomotor symptoms associated with menopause: Oral: femhrt® 1/5: 1 tablet/day; patients should be re-evaluated at 3- to 6-month intervals to determine if treatment is still necessary

Adults: Female: Prevention of osteoporosis: Oral: femhrt® 1/5: 1 tablet/day

Mechanism of Action Combination hormonal contraceptives inhibit ovulation via a negative feedback mechanism on the hypothalamus, which alters the normal pattern of gonadotropin secretion of a follicle-stimulating hormone (FSH) and luteinizing hormone by the anterior pituitary. The follicular phase FSH and midcycle surge of gonadotropins are inhibited. In addition, combination hormonal contraceptives produce alterations in the genital tract, including changes in the cervical mucus, rendering it unfavorable for sperm penetration even if ovulation occurs. Changes in the endometrium may also occur, producing an unfavorable environment for nidation. Combination hormonal contraceptive drugs may alter the tubal transport of the ova through the fallopian tubes. Progestational agents may also alter sperm fertility. Drospirenone is a spironolactone analogue with antimineralocorticoid and antiandrogenic activity.

Other Adverse Effects Adverse reactions associated with oral combination hormonal contraceptive agents are also likely to appear with vaginally-administered rings and topically-administered patches (frequency difficult to anticipate).

(Continued)

Combination Hormonal Contraceptives *(Continued)*

Cardiovascular: Arterial thromboembolism, cerebral hemorrhage, cerebral thrombosis, edema, hypertension, mesenteric thrombosis, MI
Central nervous system: Depression, dizziness, headache, migraine, nervousness, premenstrual syndrome, stroke
Dermatologic: Acne, erythema multiforme, erythema nodosum, hirsutism, loss of scalp hair, melasma (may persist), rash (allergic)
Endocrine & metabolic: Amenorrhea, breakthrough bleeding, breast enlargement, breast secretion, breast tenderness, carbohydrate intolerance, lactation decreased (postpartum), glucose tolerance decreased, libido changes, menstrual flow changes, sex hormone-binding globulins (SHBG) increased, spotting, temporary infertility (following discontinuation), thyroid-binding globulin increased, triglycerides increased
Gastrointestinal: Abdominal cramps, appetite changes, bloating, colitis, gallbladder disease, nausea, vomiting, weight gain/loss
Genitourinary: Cervical erosion changes, cervical secretion changes, cystitis-like syndrome, vaginal candidiasis, vaginitis
Hematologic: Antithrombin III decreased, folate levels decreased, hemolytic uremic syndrome, norepinephrine-induced platelet aggregability increased, porphyria, prothrombin increased; factors VII, VIII, IX, and X increased
Hepatic: Benign liver tumors, Budd-Chiari syndrome, cholestasis, cholestatic jaundice, hepatic adenomas, jaundice
Local: Thrombophlebitis
Ocular: Cataracts, change in corneal curvature (steepening), contact lens intolerance, optic neuritis, retinal thrombosis
Renal: Impaired renal function
Respiratory: Pulmonary thromboembolism
Miscellaneous: Hemorrhagic eruption
Vaginal ring: Coital problems, device expulsion, emotional lability, foreign body sensation, vaginal discomfort

9% to 22%: Topical patch:
Central nervous system: Headache
Dermatologic: Application site reaction
Endocrine & metabolic: Breast symptoms
Gastrointestinal: Abdominal pain, nausea
Genitourinary: Menstrual cramps
Respiratory: Upper respiratory infection

Drug Interactions Desogestrel: CYP2C9 and CYP2C19 enzyme substrate; Drospirenone: CYP3A4 enzyme substrate; CYP1A1, CYP2C9, CYP2C19, and CYP3A4 enzyme inhibitor (weak); Ethinyl estradiol, etonogestrel, levonorgestrel, and norgestrel are CYP3A4 enzyme substrates

Dietary/Ethanol/Herb Considerations
Ethanol: Avoid use; increases estrogen concentration and risk of breast cancer; may also increase risk of osteoporosis.
Food: CNS effects of caffeine may be enhanced if taken with combination hormonal contraceptives. Grapefruit juice increases ethinyl estradiol concentrations and would be expected to increase progesterone; clinical implications unclear. Small, frequent meals may help concentration with loss of appetite. Fruit, fluids, and fiber may reduce constipation.
Herb/nutraceutical: Avoid black cohosh and dong quai due to estrogenic activity. Avoid ginseng, red clover, and saw palmetto. Avoid St John's wort; may decrease effectiveness by inducing hepatic enzymes.

Pharmacodynamics/Kinetics
Absorption:
Topical patch: Absorption is therapeutically equivalent when applied to the abdomen, buttock, upper outer arm, and upper torso
Ethinyl estradiol: Rapid; reaches plateau by ~48 hours
Norelgestromin: Rapid; reaches plateau by ~48 hours
Duration: Intravaginal ring: Serum levels (contraceptive effectiveness) decrease after 3 weeks of continuous use

Dosage Forms
Intravaginal ring: NuvaRing®: Ethinyl estradiol and etonogestrel [3-week duration]
Patch, topical: Ortho Evra™: Ethinyl estradiol and norelgestromin [7 day duration]
Tablets: femhrt® 1/5: Ethinyl estradiol and norethindrone acetate PREVEN™: Ethinyl estradiol and levonorgestrel
Low-dose formulations:
Alesse® 21: Ethinyl estradiol and levonorgestrel
Alesse® 28: Ethinyl estradiol and levonorgestrel
Aviane™ 28: Ethinyl estradiol and levonorgestrel
Kariva™: Ethinyl estradiol and desogestrel
Lessina™: Ethinyl estradiol and levonorgestrel
Levlite™ 21: Ethinyl estradiol and levonorgestrel
Levlite™ 28: Ethinyl estradiol and levonorgestrel
Mircette®: Ethinyl estradiol and desogestrel

Monophasic formulations:
- Apri® 28: Ethinyl estradiol and desogestrel
- Brevicon®: Ethinyl estradiol and norethindrone
- Cryselle™: Ethinyl estradiol and norgestrel
- Demulin® 1/35-21: Ethinyl estradiol and ethynodiol diacetate
- Demulin® 1/35-28: Ethinyl estradiol and ethynodiol diacetate
- Demulin® 1/50-21: Ethinyl estradiol and ethynodiol diacetate
- Demulin® 1/50-28: Ethinyl estradiol and ethynodiol diacetate
- Desogen®: Ethinyl estradiol and desogestrel
- Levlen® 21: Ethinyl estradiol and levonorgestrel
- Levlen® 28: Ethinyl estradiol and levonorgestrel
- Levora® 21: Ethinyl estradiol and levonorgestrel
- Levora® 28: Ethinyl estradiol and levonorgestrel
- Loestrin® 21 1/20: Ethinyl estradiol and norethindrone acetate
- Loestrin® 21 1.5/30: Ethinyl estradiol and norethindrone acetate
- Loestrin® Fe 1/20: Ethinyl estradiol and norethindrone acetate
- Loestrin® Fe 1.5/30: Ethinyl estradiol and norethindrone acetate
- Lo/Ovral®: Ethinyl estradiol and norgestrel
- Low-Ogestrel® 21: Ethinyl estradiol and norgestrel
- Low-Ogestrel® 28: Ethinyl estradiol and norgestrel
- Lo/Ovral® 28: Ethinyl estradiol and norgestrel
- Microgestin™ Fe 1/20: Ethinyl estradiol and norethindrone acetate
- Microgestin™ Fe 1.5/30: Ethinyl estradiol and norethindrone acetate
- Nordette® 21: Ethinyl estradiol and levonorgestrel
- Nordette® 28: Ethinyl estradiol and levonorgestrel
- Modicon® 21: Ethinyl estradiol norethindrone
- Modicon® 28: Ethinyl estradiol and norethindrone
- Necon® 0.5/35-21: Ethinyl estradiol and norethindrone
- Necon® 0.5/35-28: Ethinyl estradiol and norethindrone
- Necon® 1/35-21: Ethinyl estradiol and norethindrone
- Necon® 1/35-28: Ethinyl estradiol and norethindrone
- Norinyl® 1+35: Ethinyl estradiol and norethindrone
- Nortrel™ 0.5/35 mg: Ethinyl estradiol and norethindrone
- Nortrel™ 1/35 mg: Ethinyl estradiol and norethindrone
- Ogestrel® 21: Ethinyl estradiol and norgestrel
- Ogestrel® 28: Ethinyl estradiol and norgestrel
- Ortho-Cept® 28: Ethinyl estradiol desogestrel
- Ortho-Cyclen®: Ethinyl estradiol and norgestimate
- Ortho-Novum® 1/35 21: Ethinyl estradiol and norethindrone
- Ortho-Novum® 1/35 28: Ethinyl estradiol and norethindrone
- Ovcon® 35 21-day: Ethinyl estradiol and norethindrone
- Ovcon® 35 28-day: Ethinyl estradiol and norethindrone
- Ovcon® 50: Ethinyl estradiol and norethindrone
- Ovral® 21: Ethinyl estradiol and norgestrel
- Ovral® 28: Ethinyl estradiol and norgestrel
- Zovia™ 1/35-21: Ethinyl estradiol and ethynodiol diacetate
- Zovia™ 1/35-28: Ethinyl estradiol and ethynodiol diacetate
- Zovia™ 1/50-21: Ethinyl estradiol and ethynodiol diacetate
- Zovia™ 1/50-28: Ethinyl estradiol and ethynodiol diacetate
- Yasmin®: Ethinyl estradiol and drospirenone

Biphasic formulations:
- Jenest™-28: Ethinyl estradiol and norethindrone
- Necon® 10/11-21: Ethinyl estradiol and norethindrone
- Necon® 10/11-28: Ethinyl estradiol and norethindrone
- Ortho-Novum® 10/11-21: Ethinyl estradiol and norethindrone
- Ortho-Novum® 10/11-28: Ethinyl estradiol and norethindrone

Triphasic formulations:
- Cyclessa®: Ethinyl estradiol desogestrel
- Enpresse™: Ethinyl estradiol and levonorgestrel
- Estrostep® 21: Ethinyl estradiol and norethindrone
- Estrostep® Fe: Ethinyl estradiol and norethindrone
- Ortho-Novum® 7/7/7 21: Ethinyl estradiol and norethindrone
- Ortho-Novum® 7/7/7 28: Ethinyl estradiol and norethindrone
- Ortho Tri-Cyclen®: Ethinyl estradiol and norgestimate
- Tri-Levlen® 21: Ethinyl estradiol and levonorgestrel
- Tri-Norinyl® 28: Ethinyl estradiol and norethindrone
- Triphasil® 21: Ethinyl estradiol and levonorgestrel
- Trivora® 21: Ethinyl estradiol levonorgestrel
- Tri-Levlen® 28: Ethinyl estradiol and levonorgestrel
- Triphasil® 28: Ethinyl estradiol and levonorgestrel
- Trivora® 28: Ethinyl estradiol and levonorgestrel

CombiPatch® *see* Estradiol and Norethindrone *on page 525*

Combipres® *see* Clonidine and Chlorthalidone *on page 353*

Combivent® *see* Ipratropium and Albuterol *on page 738*

Combivir® *see* Zidovudine and Lamivudine *on page 1407*

Comhist® *see* Chlorpheniramine, Phenylephrine, and Phenyltoloxamine *on page 311*
Comhist® LA *see* Chlorpheniramine, Phenylephrine, and Phenyltoloxamine *on page 311*
Commit™ [OTC] *see* Nicotine *on page 971*
Compazine® *see* Prochlorperazine *on page 1123*
Compound E *see* Cortisone Acetate *on page 373*
Compound F *see* Hydrocortisone *on page 688*
Compound S *see* Zidovudine *on page 1406*
Compound S, Abacavir, and Lamivudine *see* Abacavir, Lamivudine, and Zidovudine *on page 23*
Compound W® [OTC] *see* Salicylic Acid *on page 1204*
Compound W® One Step Wart Remover [OTC] *see* Salicylic Acid *on page 1204*
Compoz® Nighttime Sleep Aid [OTC] *see* DiphenhydrAMINE *on page 451*
Compro™ *see* Prochlorperazine *on page 1123*
Comtan® *see* Entacapone *on page 497*
Comtrex® Allergy-Sinus [OTC] *see* Acetaminophen, Chlorpheniramine, and Pseudoephedrine *on page 35*
Comtrex® Non-Drowsy Cough and Cold [OTC] *see* Acetaminophen, Dextromethorphan, and Pseudoephedrine *on page 35*
Conceptrol® [OTC] *see* Nonoxynol 9 *on page 985*
Concerta® *see* Methylphenidate *on page 893*
Condylox® *see* Podofilox *on page 1093*
Congestac® *see* Guaifenesin and Pseudoephedrine *on page 652*
Conjugated Estrogen and Methyltestosterone *see* Estrogens (Esterified) and Methyltestosterone *on page 534*
Constilac® *see* Lactulose *on page 772*
Constulose® *see* Lactulose *on page 772*
Contac® Severe Cold and Flu/Non-Drowsy [OTC] *see* Acetaminophen, Dextromethorphan, and Pseudoephedrine *on page 35*
Copaxone® *see* Glatiramer Acetate *on page 636*
Copegus™ *see* Ribavirin *on page 1176*
Copolymer-1 *see* Glatiramer Acetate *on page 636*
Copper *see* Trace Metals *on page 1328*
Co-Pyronil® 2 Pulvules® [OTC] *see* Chlorpheniramine and Pseudoephedrine *on page 308*
Cordarone® *see* Amiodarone *on page 80*
Cordran® *see* Flurandrenolide *on page 594*
Cordran® SP *see* Flurandrenolide *on page 594*
Coreg® *see* Carvedilol *on page 256*
Corgard® *see* Nadolol *on page 943*
Coricidin® [OTC] *see* Chlorpheniramine and Acetaminophen *on page 308*
Corlopam® *see* Fenoldopam *on page 562*
Cormax® *see* Clobetasol *on page 345*
CortaGel® Maximum Strength [OTC] *see* Hydrocortisone *on page 688*
Cortaid® Intensive Therapy [OTC] *see* Hydrocortisone *on page 688*
Cortaid® Maximum Strength [OTC] *see* Hydrocortisone *on page 688*
Cortaid® Sensitive Skin With Aloe [OTC] *see* Hydrocortisone *on page 688*
Cortef® *see* Hydrocortisone *on page 688*
Corticool® [OTC] *see* Hydrocortisone *on page 688*

Corticotropin (kor ti koe TROE pin)

U.S. Brand Names Acthar®; H.P. Acthar® Gel

Pharmacologic Category Corticosteroid, Systemic

Synonyms ACTH; Adrenocorticotropic Hormone; Corticotropin, Repository

Use Acute exacerbations of multiple sclerosis; diagnostic aid in adrenocortical insufficiency, severe muscle weakness in myasthenia gravis

Cosyntropin is preferred over corticotropin for diagnostic test of adrenocortical insufficiency (cosyntropin is less allergenic and test is shorter in duration)

Local Anesthetic/Vasoconstrictor Precautions No information available to require special precautions

Effects on Dental Treatment

>10%: Nervousness

1% to 10%: Diabetes mellitus, epistaxis

Dosage Injection has a rapid onset and duration of activity of approximately 2 hours; the repository injection has a slower onset, but may sustain effects for ≤3 days

Children:

Anti-inflammatory/immunosuppressant:

I.M., I.V., S.C. (aqueous): 1.6 units/kg/day or 50 units/m²/day divided every 6-8 hours

I.M. (gel): 0.8 units/kg/day or 25 units/m²/day divided every 12-24 hours

Infantile spasms: Various regimens have been used. Some neurologists recommend low-dose ACTH (5-40 units/day) for short periods (1-6 weeks), while others recommend larger doses of ACTH (40-160 units/day) for long periods of treatment (3-12 months). Well designed comparative dosing studies are needed. Example of low dose regimen:

Initial: I.M. (gel): 20 units/day for 2 weeks, if patient responds, taper and discontinue; if patient does not respond, increase dose to 30 units/day for 4 weeks then taper and discontinue

I.M. usual dose (gel): 20-40 units/day or 5-8 units/kg/day in 1-2 divided doses; range: 5-160 units/day

Oral prednisone (2 mg/kg/day) was as effective as I.M. ACTH gel (20 units/day) in controlling infantile spasms

Adults: Acute exacerbation of MS: I.M.: 80-120 units/day for 2-3 weeks

Diagnostic purposes: I.V.: 10-25 units in 500 mL 5% dextrose in water infused over 8 hours

Repository injection: I.M., S.C.: 40-80 units every 24-72 hours

Mechanism of Action Stimulates the adrenal cortex to secrete adrenal steroids (including hydrocortisone, cortisone), androgenic substances, and a small amount of aldosterone

Other Adverse Effects

>10%:

Central nervous system: Insomnia

Gastrointestinal: Increased appetite, indigestion

1% to 10%:

Dermatologic: Hirsutism

Neuromuscular & skeletal: Arthralgia

Ocular: Cataracts

Pregnancy Risk Factor C

Generic Available Yes

Corticotropin, Repository *see* Corticotropin *on page 372*

Cortifoam® *see* Hydrocortisone *on page 688*

Cortisol *see* Hydrocortisone *on page 688*

Cortisone Acetate (KOR ti sone AS e tate)

Related Information

Respiratory Diseases *on page 1476*

Triamcinolone *on page 1341*

Canadian Brand Names Cortone®

Pharmacologic Category Corticosteroid, Systemic

Synonyms Compound E

Use Management of adrenocortical insufficiency

Local Anesthetic/Vasoconstrictor Precautions No information available to require special precautions

Effects on Dental Treatment A compromised immune response may occur if patient has been taking systemic cortisone. The need for corticosteroid coverage in these patients should be considered before any dental treatment; consult with physician.

>10%: Nervousness

1% to 10%: Diabetes mellitus, epistaxis

Dosage If possible, administer glucocorticoids before 9 AM to minimize adrenocortical suppression. Dosing depends upon the condition being treated and the response of the patient. Supplemental doses may be warranted during times of stress in the course of withdrawing therapy.

Children:

Anti-inflammatory or immunosuppressive: Oral: 2.5-10 mg/kg/day **or** 20-300 mg/m^2/day in divided doses every 6-8 hours

Physiologic replacement: Oral: 0.5-0.75 mg/kg/day **or** 20-25 mg/m^2/day in divided doses every 8 hours

Adults:

Anti-inflammatory or immunosuppressive: Oral: 25-300 mg/day in divided doses every 12-24 hours

Physiologic replacement: Oral: 25-35 mg/day

Hemodialysis: Supplemental dose is unnecessary

Peritoneal dialysis: Supplemental dose is unnecessary

Mechanism of Action Decreases inflammation by suppression of migration of polymorphonuclear leukocytes and reversal of increased capillary permeability

Other Adverse Effects

>10%:

Central nervous system: Insomnia

Gastrointestinal: Increased appetite, indigestion

1% to 10%:

Dermatologic: Hirsutism

Neuromuscular & skeletal: Arthralgia

(Continued)

Cortisone Acetate *(Continued)*

Ocular: Cataracts, glaucoma

<1%: Edema, **hypertension,** vertigo, **seizures, headache, psychoses, pseudotumor cerebri, mood swings, delirium, hallucinations, euphoria,** acne, **skin atrophy, bruising,** hyperpigmentation, Cushing's syndrome, pituitary-adrenal axis suppression, growth suppression, glucose intolerance, hypokalemia, alkalosis, amenorrhea, sodium and water retention, **hyperglycemia, peptic ulcer, nausea, vomiting,** abdominal distention, ulcerative esophagitis, pancreatitis, myalgia, **osteoporosis, fractures, muscle wasting, hypersensitivity reactions**

Drug Interactions CYP3A3/4 enzyme substrate

Increased Effect/Toxicity: Estrogens may increase cortisone effects. Cortisone may increase ulcerogenic potential of NSAIDs, and may increase potassium deletion due to diuretics.

Decreased Effect: Enzyme inducers (barbiturates, phenytoin, rifampin) may decrease cortisone effects. Effect of live virus vaccines may be decreased. Anticholinesterase agents may decrease effect of cortisone.

Cortisone may decrease effects of warfarin and salicylates.

Dietary/Ethanol/Herb Considerations Food: Administer with food to reduce GI upset. Limit caffeine. Interferes with calcium absorption; May require increased intake of potassium, pyridoxine, vitamin C, vitamin D, folate, calcium, and phosphorus may require a decrease in sodium.

Pharmacodynamics/Kinetics

Onset of action: Peak effect: Oral: ~2 hours; I.M.: 20-48 hours

Duration: 30-36 hours

Absorption: Slow

Distribution: Muscles, liver, skin, intestines, and kidneys; crosses placenta; enters breast milk

Metabolism: Hepatic to inactive metabolites

Half-life elimination: 0.5-2 hours; End-stage renal disease: 3.5 hours

Excretion: Urine and feces

Pregnancy Risk Factor D

Generic Available Yes

Cortisporin® Cream *see* Neomycin, Polymyxin B, and Hydrocortisone *on page 963*

Cortisporin® Ointment *see* Bacitracin, Neomycin, Polymyxin B, and Hydrocortisone *on page 158*

Cortisporin® Ophthalmic *see* Neomycin, Polymyxin B, and Hydrocortisone *on page 963*

Cortisporin® Otic *see* Neomycin, Polymyxin B, and Hydrocortisone *on page 963*

Cortisporin®-TC Otic *see* Colistin, Neomycin, and Hydrocortisone *on page 367*

Cortizone®-5 [OTC] *see* Hydrocortisone *on page 688*

Cortizone®-10 Maximum Strength [OTC] *see* Hydrocortisone *on page 688*

Cortizone®-10 Plus Maximum Strength [OTC] *see* Hydrocortisone *on page 688*

Cortizone® 10 Quick Shot [OTC] *see* Hydrocortisone *on page 688*

Cortizone® for Kids [OTC] *see* Hydrocortisone *on page 688*

Cortrosyn® *see* Cosyntropin *on page 374*

Corvert® *see* Ibutilide *on page 706*

Cosmegen® *see* Dactinomycin *on page 393*

Cosyntropin (koe sin TROE pin)

U.S. Brand Names Cortrosyn®

Canadian Brand Names Cortrosyn®

Pharmacologic Category Diagnostic Agent

Synonyms Synacthen; Tetracosactide

Use Diagnostic test to differentiate primary adrenal from secondary (pituitary) adrenocortical insufficiency

Local Anesthetic/Vasoconstrictor Precautions No information available to require special precautions

Effects on Dental Treatment 1% to 10%: Flushing, fever

Dosage

Adrenocortical insufficiency: I.M., I.V. (over 2 minutes): Peak plasma cortisol concentrations usually occur 45-60 minutes after cosyntropin administration

Neonates: 0.015 mg/kg/dose

Children <2 years: 0.125 mg

Children >2 years and Adults: 0.25-0.75 mg

When greater cortisol stimulation is needed, an I.V. infusion may be used:

Children >2 years and Adults: 0.25 mg administered at 0.04 mg/hour over 6 hours

Congenital adrenal hyperplasia evaluation: 1 mg/m^2/dose up to a maximum of 1 mg

Mechanism of Action Stimulates the adrenal cortex to secrete adrenal steroids (including hydrocortisone, cortisone), androgenic substances, and a small amount of aldosterone

Other Adverse Effects

1% to 10%:

Dermatologic: Pruritus

Gastrointestinal: Chronic pancreatitis

<1%: **Hypersensitivity reactions**

Pharmacodynamics/Kinetics

Distribution: Crosses placenta

Time to peak, serum: I.M., IVP: ~1 hour; plasma cortisol levels rise in healthy individuals within 5 minutes

Pregnancy Risk Factor C

Generic Available No

Co-Trimoxazole *see* Sulfamethoxazole and Trimethoprim *on page 1253*

Coumadin® *see* Warfarin *on page 1397*

Covera-HS® *see* Verapamil *on page 1382*

Cozaar® *see* Losartan *on page 825*

CP-99,219-27 *see* Trovafloxacin/Alatrofloxacin *on page 1361*

CPM *see* Cyclophosphamide *on page 381*

CPT-11 *see* Irinotecan *on page 740*

CPZ *see* ChlorproMAZINE *on page 312*

Creomulsion® Cough [OTC] *see* Dextromethorphan *on page 423*

Creomulsion® for Children [OTC] *see* Dextromethorphan *on page 423*

Creon® *see* Pancrelipase *on page 1030*

Creo-Terpin® [OTC] *see* Dextromethorphan *on page 423*

Cresylate® *see* m-Cresyl Acetate *on page 844*

Crinone® *see* Progesterone *on page 1125*

Critic-Aid Skin Care® [OTC] *see* Zinc Oxide *on page 1409*

Crixivan® *see* Indinavir *on page 718*

Crolom® *see* Cromolyn Sodium *on page 375*

Cromoglycic Acid *see* Cromolyn Sodium *on page 375*

Cromolyn Sodium (KROE moe lin SOW dee um)

Related Information

Respiratory Diseases *on page 1476*

U.S. Brand Names Crolom®; Gastrocrom®; Intal®; Nasalcrom® [OTC]; Opticrom®

Canadian Brand Names Apo®-Cromolyn; Intal®; Nalcrom®; Nu-Cromolyn; Opticrom®

Pharmacologic Category Mast Cell Stabilizer

Synonyms Cromoglycic Acid; Disodium Cromoglycate; DSCG

Use

Inhalation: May be used as an adjunct in the prophylaxis of allergic disorders, including rhinitis, asthma; prevention of exercise-induced bronchospasm

Oral: Systemic mastocytosis

Ophthalmic: Treatment of vernal keratoconjunctivitis, vernal conjunctivitis, and vernal keratitis

Unlabeled/Investigational Use Oral: Treatment of food allergy symptoms, inflammatory bowel disease (IBS)

Local Anesthetic/Vasoconstrictor Precautions No information available to require special precautions

Effects on Dental Treatment

>10%:

Inhalation: Unpleasant taste

Intranasal: Increase in sneezing, burning, stinging, nasal irritation

1% to 10%: Intranasal: Headache, cough, postnasal drip, xerostomia, unpleasant taste, hoarseness

Frequency not defined:

Ophthalmic: Dyspnea

Systemic: Chest pain, flushing, palpitations, tachycardia, anxiety, behavior changes, convulsions, dizziness, fatigue, hallucinations, headache, irritability, lethargy, migraine, nervousness, postprandial lightheadedness, psychosis, dysphagia, esophagospasm, glossitis, nausea, stomatitis, unpleasant taste, vomiting, leg stiffness or weakness, paresthesia, dyspnea, pharyngitis

Dosage

Oral (once desired effect is achieved, dose may be tapered to lowest effective dose):

Systemic mastocytosis:

Children 2-12 years: 100 mg 4 times/day; not to exceed 40 mg/kg/day; given 1/2 hour prior to meals and at bedtime

Children >12 years and Adults: 200 mg 4 times/day; given 1/2 hour prior to meals and at bedtime; if control of symptoms is not seen within 2-3 weeks, dose may be increased to a maximum 40 mg/kg/day

Food allergy and inflammatory bowel disease (unlabeled use):

Children <2 years: Use not recommended

(Continued)

Cromolyn Sodium *(Continued)*

Children 2-12 years: Initial dose: 100 mg 4 times/day; may double the dose if effect is not satisfactory within 2-3 weeks; not to exceed 40 mg/kg/day

Children >12 years and Adults: Initial: 200 mg 4 times/day; may double the dose if effect is not satisfactory within 2-3 weeks; up to 400 mg 4 times/day

Dosing adjustment in renal/hepatic impairment: Specific guidelines unavailable; consider lower dose

Inhalation:

Chronic asthma: Taper frequency to the lowest effective dose (ie, 4 times/day to 3 times/day to twice daily]):

Nebulization solution: Children >2 years and Adults: Initial: 20 mg 4 times/day; usual dose: 20 mg 3-4 times/day

Metered spray:

Children 5-12 years: Initial: 2 inhalations 4 times/day; usual dose: 1-2 inhalations 3-4 times/day

Children ≥12 years and Adults: Initial: 2 inhalations 4 times/day; usual dose: 2-4 inhalations 3-4 times/day

Prevention of allergen- or exercise-induced bronchospasm (administer 10-15 minutes prior to exercise or allergen exposure but no longer than 1 hour before):

Nebulization solution: Children >2 years and Adults: Single dose of 20 mg

Metered spray: Children >5 years and Adults: Single dose of 2 inhalations

Ophthalmic: Children >4 years and Adults: 1-2 drops in each eye 4-6 times/day

Nasal: Allergic rhinitis (treatment and prophylaxis): Children ≥2 years and Adults: 1 spray into each nostril 3-4 times/day; may be increased to 6 times/day (symptomatic relief may require 2-4 weeks)

Mechanism of Action Prevents the mast cell release of histamine, leukotrienes and slow-reacting substance of anaphylaxis by inhibiting degranulation after contact with antigens

Other Adverse Effects

Intranasal: <1% (Limited to important or life-threatening): **Anaphylactic reactions, epistaxis**

Frequency not defined:

Ophthalmic: Ocular: Conjunctival injection, dryness around the eye, edema, eye irritation, immediate hypersensitivity reactions, itchy eyes, puffy eyes, styes, rash, watery eyes

Systemic:

Cardiovascular: Angioedema, edema, premature ventricular contractions

Central nervous system: Depression, insomnia, hypoesthesia

Dermatologic: Erythema, photosensitivity, pruritus, purpura, rash, urticaria

Gastrointestinal: Abdominal pain, constipation, diarrhea, dyspepsia, flatulence

Genitourinary: Dysuria, urinary frequency

Hematologic: Neutropenia, pancytopenia, polycythemia

Hepatic: Liver function test abnormal

Local: Burning

Neuromuscular & skeletal: Arthralgia, myalgia,

Otic: Tinnitus

Miscellaneous: Lupus erythematosus

Pharmacodynamics/Kinetics

Onset: Response to treatment:

Nasal spray: May occur at 1-2 weeks

Ophthalmic: May be seen within a few days; treatment for up to 6 weeks is often required

Oral: May occur within 2-6 weeks

Absorption:

Inhalation: ~8% reaches lungs upon inhalation; well absorbed

Oral: <1% of dose absorbed

Half-life elimination: 80-90 minutes

Time to peak, serum: Inhalation: ~15 minutes

Excretion: Urine and feces (equal amounts as unchanged drug); exhaled gases (small amounts)

Pregnancy Risk Factor B

Generic Available Yes: Solution for inhalation, ophthalmic drops

Crotamiton (kroe TAM i ton)

U.S. Brand Names Eurax® Topical

Mexican Brand Names Eurax®

Pharmacologic Category Scabicidal Agent

Use Treatment of scabies (*Sarcoptes scabiei*) and symptomatic treatment of pruritus

Local Anesthetic/Vasoconstrictor Precautions No information available to require special precautions

Effects on Dental Treatment No significant effects or complications reported

Dosage Topical:

Scabicide: Children and Adults: Wash thoroughly and scrub away loose scales, then towel dry; apply a thin layer and massage drug onto skin of the entire body from the neck to the toes (with special attention to skin folds, creases, and interdigital spaces). Repeat application in 24 hours. Take a cleansing bath 48 hours after the final application. Treatment may be repeated after 7-10 days if live mites are still present.

Pruritus: Massage into affected areas until medication is completely absorbed; repeat as necessary

Mechanism of Action Crotamiton has scabicidal activity against *Sarcoptes scabiei*; mechanism of action unknown

Other Adverse Effects <1%: Local irritation, pruritus, contact dermatitis, warm sensation

Pregnancy Risk Factor C

Generic Available No

Crude Coal Tar *see* Coal Tar *on page 359*
Cruex® [OTC] *see* Clotrimazole *on page 356*
Cryselle™ *see* Combination Hormonal Contraceptives *on page 368*
Crystalline Penicillin *see* Penicillin G (Parenteral/Aqueous) *on page 1049*
Crystal Violet *see* Gentian Violet *on page 636*
Crystamine® *see* Cyanocobalamin *on page 377*
Crysti 1000® *see* Cyanocobalamin *on page 377*
Crystodigin® [DSC] *see* Digitoxin *on page 440*
CSA *see* CycloSPORINE *on page 383*
CSP *see* Cellulose Sodium Phosphate *on page 284*
CTM *see* Chlorpheniramine *on page 307*
CTX *see* Cyclophosphamide *on page 381*
Cuprimine® *see* Penicillamine *on page 1046*
Curosurf® *see* Poractant Alfa *on page 1097*
Cutivate® *see* Fluticasone *on page 599*
CyA *see* CycloSPORINE *on page 383*

Cyanocobalamin (sye an oh koe BAL u min)

U.S. Brand Names Crystamine®; Crysti 1000®; Cyanoject®; Cyomin®; Ener-B®; Nascobal®

Canadian Brand Names Scheinpharm B12

Pharmacologic Category Vitamin, Water Soluble

Synonyms Vitamin B_{12}

Use

Dental: Treatment of vitamin B_{12} deficiency

Medical: Treatment of pernicious anemia; dietary supplement for increased B_{12} requirements due to pregnancy, thyrotoxicosis, hemorrhage, malignancy, liver or kidney disease

Local Anesthetic/Vasoconstrictor Precautions No information available to require special precautions

Effects on Dental Treatment

>10%: Headache (2% to 11%)

1% to 10%: Anxiety, dizziness, pain, nervousness, hypoesthesia, sore throat, nausea, vomiting, weakness (1% to 4%), arthritis, paresthesia, abnormal gait, dyspnea, rhinitis

Dosage

Recommended daily allowance (RDA):

Children: 0.3-2 mcg

Adults: 2 mcg

Nutritional deficiency:

Intranasal gel: 500 mcg once weekly

Oral: 25-250 mcg/day

Anemias: I.M. or deep S.C. (oral is not generally recommended due to poor absorption and I.V. is not recommended due to more rapid elimination):

Pernicious anemia, congenital (if evidence of neurologic involvement): 1000 mcg/day for at least 2 weeks; maintenance: 50-100 mcg/month or 100 mcg for 6-7 days; if there is clinical improvement, give 100 mcg every other day for 7 doses, then every 3-4 days for 2-3 weeks; follow with 100 mcg/month for life. Administer with folic acid if needed.

Children: 30-50 mcg/day for 2 or more weeks (to a total dose of 1000-5000 mcg), then follow with 100 mcg/month as maintenance dosage

Adults: 100 mcg/day for 6-7 days; if improvement, administer same dose on alternate days for 7 doses; then every 3-4 days for 2-3 weeks; once hematologic values have returned to normal, maintenance dosage: 100 mcg/month. **Note:** Use only parenteral therapy as oral therapy is not dependable.

Hematologic remission (without evidence of nervous system involvement): Intranasal gel: 500 mcg once weekly

(Continued)

Cyanocobalamin *(Continued)*

Vitamin B_{12} deficiency:
- Children:
  - Neurologic signs: 100 mcg/day for 10-15 days (total dose of 1-1.5 mg), then once or twice weekly for several months; may taper to 60 mcg every month
  - Hematologic signs: 10-50 mcg/day for 5-10 days, followed by 100-250 mcg/dose every 2-4 weeks
- Adults: Initial: 30 mcg/day for 5-10 days; maintenance: 100-200 mcg/month

Schilling test: I.M.: 1000 mcg

Mechanism of Action Coenzyme for various metabolic functions, including fat and carbohydrate metabolism and protein synthesis, used in cell replication and hematopoiesis

Other Adverse Effects

1% to 10%:
- Central nervous system: Hypoesthesia
- Dermatologic: Itching
- Gastrointestinal: Dyspepsia, diarrhea
- Neuromuscular & skeletal: Back pain, myalgia

<1%: Peripheral vascular thrombosis, urticaria, **anaphylaxis, CHF**, pulmonary edema

Contraindications Hypersensitivity to cyanocobalamin or any component of the formulation, cobalt; patients with hereditary optic nerve atrophy, Leber's disease

Warnings/Precautions I.M. route used to treat pernicious anemia; vitamin B_{12} deficiency for >3 months results in irreversible degenerative CNS lesions; treatment of vitamin B_{12} megaloblastic anemia may result in severe hypokalemia, sometimes, fatal, when anemia corrects due to cellular potassium requirements. B_{12} deficiency masks signs of polycythemia vera; vegetarian diets may result in B_{12} deficiency; pernicious anemia occurs more often in gastric carcinoma than in general population. Patients with Leber's disease may suffer rapid optic atrophy when treated with vitamin B_{12}.

Drug Interactions Decreased Effect: Neomycin, colchicine, and anticonvulsants may decrease absorption. Chloramphenicol may decrease B_{12} effects.

Dietary/Ethanol/Herb Considerations Ethanol decreases B_{12} absorption.

Pharmacodynamics/Kinetics

Absorption: From the terminal ileum in presence of calcium; gastric "intrinsic factor" must be present to transfer the compound across the intestinal mucosa

Distribution: Principally stored in the liver, also stored in the kidneys and adrenals

Protein binding: To transcobalamin II

Metabolism: Converted in tissues to active coenzymes, methylcobalamin and deoxyadenosylcobalamin

Pregnancy Risk Factor A/C (dose exceeding RDA recommendation); C (nasal gel)

Dosage Forms GEL, intranasal (Nascobal®): 500 mcg/0.1 mL (5 mL). **INJ:** 100 mcg/mL (1 mL, 10 mL, 30 mL); 1000 mcg/mL (1 mL, 10 mL, 30 mL). **TAB [OTC]:** 25 mcg, 50 mcg, 100 mcg, 250 mcg, 500 mcg, 1000 mcg

Generic Available Yes

Cyanocobalamin, Folic Acid, and Pyridoxine *see* Folic Acid, Cyanocobalamin, and Pyridoxine *on page 607*

Cyanoject® *see* Cyanocobalamin *on page 377*

Cyclandelate (sye KLAN de late)

Pharmacologic Category Vasodilator

Use Considered as "possibly effective" for adjunctive therapy in peripheral vascular disease and possibly senility due to cerebrovascular disease or multi-infarct dementia; migraine prophylaxis, vertigo, tinnitus, and visual disturbances secondary to cerebrovascular insufficiency and diabetic peripheral polyneuropathy

Local Anesthetic/Vasoconstrictor Precautions No information available to require special precautions

Effects on Dental Treatment May enhance action of drugs causing vasodilation.

Dosage Adults: Oral: Initial: 1.2-1.6 g/day in divided doses before meals and at bedtime until response; maintenance therapy: 400-800 mg/day in 2-4 divided doses; start with lowest dose in elderly due to hypotensive potential; decrease dose by 200 mg decrements to achieve minimal maintenance dose; improvement can usually be seen over weeks of therapy and prolonged use; short courses of therapy are usually ineffective and not recommended

Mechanism of Action Cyclandelate, 3,3,5-trimethylcyclohexyl mandelate is a vasodilator that exerts a direct, papaverine-like action on smooth muscles, particularly that found within the blood vessels. Animal data indicate that cyclandelate also has antispasmodic properties; exhibits no adrenergic stimulation or blocking action; action exceeds that of papaverine; mild calcium channel blocking agent, may benefit in mild hypercalcemia; calcium channel blocking activity may explain some of its pharmacologic effects (enhanced blood flow) and inhibition of platelet aggregation.

Other Adverse Effects <1%: **Facial flushing, tachycardia, headache, pain, dizziness; tingling sensation in face, fingers, or toes; belching, heartburn; weakness**

Drug Interactions Increased Effect/Toxicity: May enhance action of drugs causing vasodilation/hypotension.

Pregnancy Risk Factor C

Generic Available Yes

Cyclessa® *see* Combination Hormonal Contraceptives *on page 368*

Cyclizine (SYE kli zeen)

U.S. Brand Names Marezine® [OTC]

Pharmacologic Category Antihistamine

Synonyms Cyclizine Hydrochloride; Cyclizine Lactate

Use Prevention and treatment of nausea, vomiting, and vertigo associated with motion sickness; control of postoperative nausea and vomiting

Local Anesthetic/Vasoconstrictor Precautions No information available to require special precautions

Effects on Dental Treatment

>10%: Xerostomia, drowsiness

1% to 10%: Headache, nausea

Dosage Oral:

Children 6-12 years: 25 mg up to 3 times/day

Adults: 50 mg taken 30 minutes before departure, may repeat in 4-6 hours if needed, up to 200 mg/day

Mechanism of Action Cyclizine is a piperazine derivative with properties of histamines. The precise mechanism of action in inhibiting the symptoms of motion sickness is not known. It may have effects directly on the labyrinthine apparatus and central actions on the labyrinthine apparatus and on the chemoreceptor trigger zone. Cyclizine exerts a central anticholinergic action.

Other Adverse Effects 1% to 10%:

Dermatologic: Dermatitis

Genitourinary: Urinary retention

Ocular: Diplopia

Renal: Polyuria

Drug Interactions Increased Effect/Toxicity: Increased effect/toxicity with CNS depressants, alcohol.

Dietary/Ethanol/Herb Considerations

Ethanol: Avoid use; may increase CNS depression.

Herb/Nutraceutical: Avoid gotu kola, kava, SAMe, St John's wort, and valerian; may increase CNS depression.

Pregnancy Risk Factor B

Generic Available No

Cyclizine Hydrochloride *see* Cyclizine *on page 379*

Cyclizine Lactate *see* Cyclizine *on page 379*

Cyclobenzaprine (sye kloe BEN za preen)

Related Information

Temporomandibular Dysfunction (TMD) *on page 1562*

U.S. Brand Names Flexeril®

Canadian Brand Names Apo®-Cyclobenzaprine; Flexeril®; Flexitec; Gen-Cyclobenzaprine; Novo-Cycloprine®; Nu-Cyclobenzaprine

Pharmacologic Category Skeletal Muscle Relaxant

Synonyms Cyclobenzaprine Hydrochloride

Use

Dental: Treatment of muscle spasm associated with acute temporomandibular joint pain

Medical: Treatment of muscle spasm associated with acute painful musculoskeletal conditions; supportive therapy in tetanus

Local Anesthetic/Vasoconstrictor Precautions No information available to require special precautions

Effects on Dental Treatment

>10%: Xerostomia (21% to 32%), changes in salivation, drowsiness (29% to 39%), dizziness (1% to 11%), fatigue

1% to 3%: Confusion, headache, irritability, mental acuity decreased, nervousness, nausea, weakness, pharyngitis, blurred vision

Dosage Oral (do not use longer than 2-3 weeks):

Adults: Initial: 5 mg 3 times/day; may increase to 10 mg 3 times/day if needed

Elderly: 5 mg 3 times/day; plasma concentration and incidence of adverse effects are increased; dose should be titrated slowly

Dosage adjustment in hepatic impairment:

Mild: 5 mg 3 times/day; use with caution and titrate slowly

Moderate to severe: Use not recommended

(Continued)

Cyclobenzaprine *(Continued)*

Mechanism of Action Centrally-acting skeletal muscle relaxant pharmacologically related to tricyclic antidepressants; reduces tonic somatic motor activity influencing both alpha and gamma motor neurons

Other Adverse Effects

1% to 10%: Gastrointestinal: Abdominal pain (1% to 3%), constipation (1% to 3%), diarrhea (1% to 3%), dyspepsia (1% to 3%)

<1% (Limited to important or life-threatening): Ageusia, **agitation, anaphylaxis**, angioedema, anorexia, **arrhythmia**, cholestasis, diplopia, facial edema, **gastritis, hallucinations**, hepatitis (rare), hypertonia, **hypotension**, insomnia, jaundice, abnormal LFTS, malaise, **palpitations, paresthesia**, pruritus, **psychosis**, rash, **seizures, tachycardia, thinking abnormal**, tinnitus, **tongue edema, tremors**, urinary frequency, urinary retention, urticaria, vertigo, **vomiting**

Contraindications Hypersensitivity to cyclobenzaprine or any component of the formulation; do not use concomitantly or within 14 days of MAO inhibitors; hyperthyroidism; CHF; arrhythmias

Warnings/Precautions Cyclobenzaprine shares the toxic potentials of the tricyclic antidepressants and the usual precautions of tricyclic antidepressant therapy should be observed; use with caution in patients with urinary hesitancy, angle-closure glaucoma, hepatic impairment, or in the elderly. Do not use concomitantly or within 14 days after MAO inhibitors; combination may cause hypertensive crisis, severe convulsions. Safety and efficacy have not been established in patients <15 years of age.

Drug Interactions Substrate of **CYP1A2**, 2D6, 3A4

Anticholinergics: Because of cyclobenzaprine's anticholinergic action, use with caution in patients receiving these agents.

CNS depressants: Effects may be enhanced by cyclobenzaprine.

Guanethidine: Antihypertensive effect of guanethidine may be decreased; effect seen with tricyclic antidepressants.

MAO inhibitors: Do not use concomitantly or within 14 days after MAO inhibitors.

Tramadol: May increase risk of seizure; effect seen with tricyclic antidepressants and tramadol.

Dietary/Ethanol/Herb Considerations

Ethanol: Avoid use; may increase CNS depression.

Herb/Nutraceutical: Avoid gotu kola, kava, SAMe, St John's wort, and valerian; may increase CNS depression.

Pharmacodynamics/Kinetics

Onset of action: ~1 hour

Duration: 12-24 hours

Absorption: Complete

Metabolism: Hepatic via CYP3A4, 1A2, and 2D6; may undergo enterohepatic recirculation

Bioavailability: 33% to 55%

Half-life elimination: 18 hours (range: 8-37 hours)

Time to peak, serum: 3-8 hours

Excretion: Urine (as inactive metabolites); feces (as unchanged drug)

Pregnancy Risk Factor B

Dosage Forms TAB: 10 mg; (Flexeril®) 5 mg, 10 mg

Generic Available Yes

Cyclobenzaprine Hydrochloride *see* Cyclobenzaprine *on page 379*
Cyclocort® *see* Amcinonide *on page 72*
Cyclogyl® *see* Cyclopentolate *on page 380*
Cyclomydril® *see* Cyclopentolate and Phenylephrine *on page 381*

Cyclopentolate (sye kloe PEN toe late)

U.S. Brand Names AK-Pentolate®; Cyclogyl®; I-Pentolate®

Canadian Brand Names Cyclogyl®; Diopentolate®

Pharmacologic Category Anticholinergic Agent, Ophthalmic

Synonyms Cyclopentolate Hydrochloride

Use Diagnostic procedures requiring mydriasis and cycloplegia

Local Anesthetic/Vasoconstrictor Precautions No information available to require special precautions

Effects on Dental Treatment 1% to 10%: Tachycardia, restlessness, hallucinations, psychosis, hyperactivity, seizures, allergic reaction

Dosage Ophthalmic:

Neonates and Infants: **Note:** Cyclopentolate and phenylephrine combination formulation is the preferred agent for use in neonates and infants due to lower cyclopentolate concentration and reduced risk for systemic reactions.

Children: Instill 1 drop of 0.5%, 1%, or 2% in eye followed by 1 drop of 0.5% or 1% in 5 minutes, if necessary

Adults: Instill 1 drop of 1% followed by another drop in 5 minutes; 2% solution in heavily pigmented iris

Mechanism of Action Prevents the muscle of the ciliary body and the sphincter muscle of the iris from responding to cholinergic stimulation, causing mydriasis and cycloplegia

Other Adverse Effects 1% to 10%:

Central nervous system: Incoherent speech, ataxia

Dermatologic: Burning sensation

Ocular: Increase in intraocular pressure, loss of visual accommodation

Drug Interactions Decreased Effect: Carbachol and/or cholinesterase inhibitor effects may be decreased with concurrent use.

Pharmacodynamics/Kinetics

Onset of action: Peak effect: Cycloplegia: 25-75 minutes; Mydriasis: 30-60 minutes

Duration: ≤24 hours

Pregnancy Risk Factor C

Generic Available Yes

Cyclopentolate and Phenylephrine

(sye kloe PEN toe late & fen il EF rin)

Related Information

Cyclopentolate *on page 380*

U.S. Brand Names Cyclomydril®

Pharmacologic Category Ophthalmic Agent, Antiglaucoma

Synonyms Phenylephrine and Cyclopentolate

Use Induce mydriasis greater than that produced with cyclopentolate HCl alone

Local Anesthetic/Vasoconstrictor Precautions No information available to require special precautions

Effects on Dental Treatment No significant effects or complications reported

Dosage Ophthalmic: Neonates, Infants, Children, and Adults: Instill 1 drop into the eye every 5-10 minutes, for up to 3 doses, approximately 40-50 minutes before the examination

Pregnancy Risk Factor C

Generic Available No

Cyclopentolate Hydrochloride *see* Cyclopentolate *on page 380*

Cyclophosphamide (sye kloe FOS fa mide)

U.S. Brand Names Cytoxan®; Neosar®

Canadian Brand Names Cytoxan®; Procytox®

Mexican Brand Names Genoxal®; Ledoxina®

Pharmacologic Category Antineoplastic Agent, Alkylating Agent

Synonyms CPM; CTX; CYT; NSC-26271

Use

Oncologic: Treatment of Hodgkin's and non-Hodgkin's lymphoma, Burkitt's lymphoma, chronic lymphocytic leukemia (CLL), chronic myelocytic leukemia (CML), acute myelocytic leukemia (AML), acute lymphocytic leukemia (ALL), mycosis fungoides, multiple myeloma, neuroblastoma, retinoblastoma, rhabdomyosarcoma, Ewing's sarcoma; breast, testicular, endometrial, ovarian, and lung cancers, and in conditioning regimens for bone marrow transplantation

Nononcologic: Prophylaxis of rejection for kidney, heart, liver, and bone marrow transplants, severe rheumatoid disorders, nephrotic syndrome, Wegener's granulomatosis, idiopathic pulmonary hemosideroses, myasthenia gravis, multiple sclerosis, systemic lupus erythematosus, lupus nephritis, autoimmune hemolytic anemia, idiopathic thrombocytic purpura (ITP), macroglobulinemia, and antibody-induced pure red cell aplasia

Local Anesthetic/Vasoconstrictor Precautions No information available to require special precautions

Effects on Dental Treatment

>10%: Mucositis, stomatitis

1% to 10%: Headache, facial flushing

Dosage Patients with compromised bone marrow function may require a 33% to 50% reduction in initial loading dose. Refer to individual protocols.

Children: I.V.

SLE: 500-750 mg/m^2 every month; maximum dose: 1 g/m^2

JRA/vasculitis: 10 mg/kg every 2 weeks

Children and Adults:

Oral: 50-100 mg/m^2/day as continuous therapy or 400-1000 mg/m^2 in divided doses over 4-5 days as intermittent therapy

I.V.:

Single Doses: 400-1800 mg/m^2 (30-50 mg/kg) per treatment course (1-5 days) which can be repeated at 2-4 week intervals

MAXIMUM SINGLE DOSE WITHOUT BMT is 7 g/m^2 (190 mg/kg) SINGLE AGENT THERAPY

Continuous daily doses: 60-120 mg/m^2 (1-2.5 mg/kg) per day

Autologous BMT: IVPB: 50 mg/kg/dose x 4 days or 60 mg/kg/dose for 2 days; total dose is usually divided over 2-4 days

(Continued)

Cyclophosphamide *(Continued)*

Nephrotic syndrome: Oral: 2-3 mg/kg/day every day for up to 12 weeks when corticosteroids are unsuccessful

Dosing adjustment in renal impairment: A large fraction of cyclophosphamide is eliminated by hepatic metabolism; some authors recommend no adjustment unless severe insufficiency (Cl_{cr} <20 mL/minute)

Cl_{cr} >10 mL/minute: Administer 100% of normal dose

Cl_{cr} <10 mL/minute: Administer 75% of normal dose

Hemodialysis: Moderately dialyzable (20% to 50%); administer dose posthemodialysis or administer supplemental 50% dose

CAPD/CAVH effects: Unknown

Dosing adjustment in hepatic impairment: Some authors recommend dosage reductions (of up to 30%); however, the pharmacokinetics of cyclophosphamide are not significantly altered in the presence of hepatic insufficiency. Cyclophosphamide undergoes hepatic transformation in the liver to its 4-hydroxycyclophosphamide, which breaks down to its active form, phosphoramide mustard.

Mechanism of Action Cyclophosphamide is an alkylating agent that prevents cell division by cross-linking DNA strands and decreasing DNA synthesis. It is a cell cycle phase nonspecific agent. Cyclophosphamide also possesses potent immunosuppressive activity. Cyclophosphamide is a prodrug that must be metabolized to active metabolites in the liver.

Other Adverse Effects

>10%:

Dermatologic: Alopecia (40% to 60%; usually regrows but may be different color/texture, loss usually begins 3-6 weeks after start of therapy)

Endocrine & metabolic: Sterility (interferes with oogenesis and spermatogenesis; may be irreversible), gonadal suppression (amenorrhea)

Gastrointestinal: Nausea and vomiting (higher doses; 6-10 hours postadministration), anorexia, diarrhea

Genitourinary: Severe, potentially fatal acute hemorrhagic cystitis or urinary fibrosis, believed to be a result of chemical irritation of the bladder by acrolein, a cyclophosphamide metabolite, occurs in 7% to 12% of patients and has been reported in up to 40% of patients in some series. Patients should be encouraged to drink plenty of fluids during therapy (most adults will require at least 2 L/day), void frequently, and avoid taking the drug at night. With large I.V. doses, I.V. hydration is usually recommended. The use of mesna and/or continuous bladder irrigation is rarely needed for doses <2 g/m^2.

Hematologic: Thrombocytopenia and anemia are less common than leukopenia

Onset: 7 days

Nadir: 10-14 days

Recovery: 21 days

1% to 10%:

Dermatologic: Skin rash

Renal: SIADH (>50 mg/kg or 1 g/m^2), renal tubular necrosis (usually resolves upon discontinuation)

Respiratory: Nasal congestion (when large I.V. doses are administered too rapidly); during or postinfusion: runny eyes, rhinorrhea, sinus congestion, sneezing (decongestant or decongestant/antihistamine can be used to prevent or relieve these symptoms)

<1%: **CHF (high doses),** cardiac necrosis or hemorrhagic myocarditis (rare but fatal), potentiation of cardiac toxicity of anthracyclines, **anaphylactic reactions, dizziness,** darkening of skin/fingernails, hyperglycemia, hypokalemia, hyperuricemia, hepatotoxicity, jaundice, secondary malignancy, Stevens-Johnson syndrome, toxic epidermal necrolysis, hemorrhagic colitis, hemorrhagic ureteritis, renal tubular necrosis, interstitial pneumonitis, pulmonary fibrosis (high doses)

Drug Interactions Substrate of CYP2A6, **2B6**, 2C8/9, **2C19**, 3A4; Inhibits CYP3A4; Induces CYP2B6, 2C8/9

Increased Effect/Toxicity: Allopurinol may cause an increase in bone marrow depression and may result in significant elevations of cyclophosphamide cytotoxic metabolites. Cyclophosphamide reduces serum pseudocholinesterase concentrations and may prolong the neuromuscular blocking activity of succinylcholine. **Use with caution with halothane, nitrous oxide, and succinylcholine.** Chloramphenicol causes prolonged cyclophosphamide half-life and increased toxicity. Cimetidine inhibits hepatic metabolism of drugs and may decrease the activation of cyclophosphamide. Cyclophosphamide may enhance cardiac toxicity of anthracyclines (doxorubicin). Phenobarbital and phenytoin induce hepatic enzymes and cause a more rapid production of cyclophosphamide metabolites with a concurrent decrease in the serum half-life of the parent compound. Tetrahydrocannabinol results in enhanced immunosuppression in animal studies. Leukopenia may be prolonged with thiazide diuretics.

Decreased Effect: Cyclophosphamide may decrease digoxin serum levels.

Dietary/Ethanol/Herb Considerations Herb/Nutraceutical: Avoid black cohosh and dong quai in estrogen-dependent tumors. Avoid St John's wort; may decrease serum concentration.

Pharmacodynamics/Kinetics

Absorption: Oral: Well absorbed

Distribution: V_d: 0.48-0.71 L/kg; crosses placenta; crosses into CSF (not in high enough concentrations to treat meningeal leukemia)

Protein binding: 10% to 56%

Metabolism: Hepatic to active metabolites acrolein, 4-aldophosphamide, 4-hydroperoxycyclophosphamide, and nor-nitrogen mustard

Bioavailability: >75%

Half-life elimination: 4-8 hours

Time to peak, serum: Oral: ~1 hour

Excretion: Urine (<30% as unchanged drug, 85% to 90% as metabolites)

Pregnancy Risk Factor D

Generic Available Yes

CycloSERINE (sye kloe SER een)

Related Information

Nonviral Infectious Diseases *on page 1493*

Tuberculosis *on page 1493*

U.S. Brand Names Seromycin® Pulvules®

Pharmacologic Category Antibiotic, Miscellaneous; Antitubercular Agent

Use Adjunctive treatment in pulmonary or extrapulmonary tuberculosis; has been studied for use in Gaucher's disease

Unlabeled/Investigational Use Treatment of Gaucher's disease

Local Anesthetic/Vasoconstrictor Precautions No information available to require special precautions

Effects on Dental Treatment Frequency not defined: Cardiac arrhythmias, drowsiness, headache, dizziness, seizures, confusion, psychosis, paresis, coma, tremors

Dosage Some of the neurotoxic effects may be relieved or prevented by the concomitant administration of pyridoxine

Tuberculosis: Oral:

- Children: 10-20 mg/kg/day in 2 divided doses up to 1000 mg/day for 18-24 months
- Adults: Initial: 250 mg every 12 hours for 14 days, then administer 500 mg to 1 g/day in 2 divided doses for 18-24 months (maximum daily dose: 1 g)

Dosing interval in renal impairment:

- Cl_{cr} 10-50 mL/minute: Administer every 24 hours
- Cl_{cr} <10 mL/minute: Administer every 36-48 hours

Mechanism of Action Inhibits bacterial cell wall synthesis by competing with amino acid (D-alanine) for incorporation into the bacterial cell wall; bacteriostatic or bactericidal

Other Adverse Effects Frequency not defined:

Central nervous system: Vertigo

Dermatologic: Rash

Endocrine & metabolic: Vitamin B_{12} deficiency

Hematologic: Folate deficiency

Hepatic: Liver enzymes increased

Drug Interactions Increased Effect/Toxicity: Alcohol, isoniazid, and ethionamide increase toxicity of cycloserine. Cycloserine inhibits the hepatic metabolism of phenytoin and may increase risk of epileptic seizures.

Dietary/Ethanol/Herb Considerations

Ethanol: Avoid use; may increase CNS depression.

Food: May require increased intake of folic acid and vitamin B_{12}.

Herb/Nutraceutical: Avoid gotu kola, kava, SAMe, St John's wort, and valerian; may increase CNS depression.

Pharmacodynamics/Kinetics

Absorption: ~70% to 90%

Distribution: Widely to most body fluids and tissues including CSF, breast milk, bile, sputum, lymph tissue, lungs, and ascitic, pleural, and synovial fluids; crosses placenta

Half-life elimination: Normal renal function: 10 hours

Metabolism: Hepatic

Time to peak, serum: 3-4 hours

Excretion: Urine (60% to 70% as unchanged drug) within 72 hours; feces (small amounts); remainder metabolized

Pregnancy Risk Factor C

Generic Available No

Cyclosporin A *see* CycloSPORINE *on page 383*

CycloSPORINE (SYE kloe spor een)

U.S. Brand Names Gengraf™; Neoral®; Restasis™; Sandimmune®

Canadian Brand Names Neoral®; Rhoxal-cyclosporine; Sandimmune® I.V.

Mexican Brand Names Consupren; Sandimmun Neoral®

Pharmacologic Category Immunosuppressant Agent

Synonyms CSA; CyA; Cyclosporin A

(Continued)

CycloSPORINE *(Continued)*

Use Prophylaxis of organ rejection in kidney, liver, and heart transplants, has been used with azathioprine and/or corticosteroids; severe, active rheumatoid arthritis (RA) not responsive to methotrexate alone; severe, recalcitrant plaque psoriasis in nonimmunocompromised adults unresponsive to or unable to tolerate other systemic therapy

Ophthalmic emulsion (Restasis™): Increase tear production when suppressed tear production is presumed to be due to keratoconjunctivitis sicca-associated ocular inflammation (in patients not already using topical anti-inflammatory drugs or punctal plugs)

Unlabeled/Investigational Use Short-term, high-dose cyclosporine as a modulator of multidrug resistance in cancer treatment; allogenic bone marrow transplants for prevention and treatment of graft-versus-host disease; treatment of severe autoimmune disease (ie, SLE, myasthenia gravis) resistant to corticosteroids and other therapy, focal segmental glomerulosclerosis

Local Anesthetic/Vasoconstrictor Precautions No information available to require special precautions

Effects on Dental Treatment

>10%: Gingival hypertrophy (4% to 16%), hypertension (13% to 53%; psoriasis 25% to 27%), headache (2% to 15%; RA 17%, psoriasis 14% to 16%), nausea (RA 23%), tremor (12% to 55%), upper respiratory infection (psoriasis 8% to 11%), infection (psoriasis 24% to 25%)

2% to 10% (kidney/liver/heart transplant patients): Flushing (<1% to 4%), myocardial infarction, convulsions (1% to 5%), anxiety, confusion, fever, hyperglycemia, nausea (2% to 10%), vomiting (2% to 10%), gastritis, mouth sores, swallowing difficulty, upper GI bleeding, paresthesia (1% to 3%), tingling, weakness, sinusitis (≤7%), allergic reactions, hiccups,

1% to 10%

RA patients (<3% unless otherwise noted): Hypertension (8%), chest pain (4%), arrhythmia (2%), cardiac failure, myocardial infarction, dizziness (8%), pain (6%), migraine (2%), anxiety, nervousness, paranoia, somnolence, diabetes mellitus, hot flashes, hypoglycemia, vomiting (9%), gingivitis (4%), gum hyperplasia (2%), xerostomia, dysphagia, enanthema, eructation, esophagitis, gastric ulcer, gastritis, gastroenteritis, gingival bleeding, glossitis, salivary gland enlargement, abnormal taste, tongue disorder, tooth disorder, peptic ulcer paresthesia (8%), tremor (8%), leg cramps/muscle contractions (2%), weakness, cough (5%), dyspnea (5%), sinusitis (4%), bronchospasm, epistaxis, infection (9%), abscess, allergy, bacterial infection, carcinoma, fungal infection, herpes simplex, moniliasis, diaphoresis increased, tonsillitis, viral infection

Psoriasis patients (<3% unless otherwise noted): Chest pain, flushing, psychiatric events (4% to 5%), pain (3% to 4%), dizziness, fever, nervousness, hot flashes, nausea (5% to 6%), gum hyperplasia (4% to 6%), gingival bleeding, bleeding disorder, clotting disorder, platelet disorder, red blood cell disorder, paresthesia (5% to 7%), bronchospasm (5%), cough (5%), dyspnea (5%), rhinitis (5%), respiratory infection, flu-like symptoms (8% to 10%)

Dosage Neoral® and Sandimmune® are not bioequivalent and cannot be used interchangeably.

Conversion to cyclosporine (modified) from cyclosporine (nonmodified): Start with daily dose previously used and adjust to obtain preconversion cyclosporine trough concentration. Plasma concentrations should be monitored every 4-7 days and dose adjusted as necessary, until desired trough level is obtained. When transferring patients with previously poor absorption of cyclosporine (nonmodified), monitor trough levels at least twice weekly (especially if initial dose exceeds 10 mg/kg/day); high plasma levels are likely to occur.

Adults: Oral: Cyclosporine (modified):

Note: Increase the frequency of blood pressure monitoring after each alteration in dosage of cyclosporine. Cyclosporine dosage should be decreased by 25% to 50% in patients with no history of hypertension who develop sustained hypertension during therapy and, if hypertension persists, treatment with cyclosporine should be discontinued.

Rheumatoid arthritis: Initial: 2.5 mg/kg/day, divided twice daily; salicylates, NSAIDs, and oral glucocorticoids may be continued (refer to Drug Interactions)

Dose may be increased by 0.5-0.75 mg/kg/day if insufficient response is seen after 8 weeks of treatment. Additional dosage increases may be made again at 12 weeks (maximum dose: 4 mg/kg/day). Discontinue if no benefit is seen by 16 weeks of therapy.

Psoriasis: Initial: 2.5 mg/kg/day, divided twice daily

Dose may be increased by 0.5 mg/kg/day if insufficient response is seen after 4 weeks of treatment. Additional dosage increases may be made every 2 weeks if needed (maximum dose: 4 mg/kg/day). Discontinue if no benefit is seen by 6 weeks of therapy. Once patients are adequately controlled, the dose should be decreased to the lowest effective dose. Doses lower than 2.5 mg/kg/day may be effective. Treatment longer than 1 year is not recommended.

Dosing adjustment in renal impairment: For severe psoriasis:

Serum creatinine levels ≥25% above pretreatment levels: Take another sample within 2 weeks; if the level remains ≥25% above pretreatment levels, decrease dosage of cyclosporine (modified) by 25% to 50%. If two dosage adjustments do not reverse the increase in serum creatinine levels, treatment should be discontinued.

Serum creatinine levels ≥50% above pretreatment levels: Decrease cyclosporine dosage by 25% to 50%. If two dosage adjustments do not reverse the increase in serum creatinine levels, treatment should be discontinued.

Autoimmune diseases: 1-3 mg/kg/day

Focal segmental glomerulosclerosis: Initial: 3 mg/kg/day divided every 12 hours

Keratoconjunctivitis sicca: Ophthalmic: Children ≥16 years and Adults: Instill 1 drop in each eye every 12 hours

Newly-transplanted patients (adjunct therapy with corticosteroids is recommended):

Children: Refer to adult dosing; children may require, and are able to tolerate, larger doses than adults.

Adults:

Oral (dose is dependent upon type of transplant and formulation): Initial: Should be given 4-12 hours prior to transplant or may be given postoperatively; adjust initial dose to achieve desired plasma concentration

Cyclosporine (modified):

Renal: 9 ± 3 mg/kg/day, divided twice daily

Liver: 8 ± 4 mg/kg/day, divided twice daily

Heart: 7 ± 3 mg/kg/day, divided twice daily

Cyclosporine (nonmodified): Initial dose: 15 mg/kg/day as a single dose (range 14-18 mg/kg); lower doses of 10-14 mg/kg/day have been used for renal transplants. Continue initial dose daily for 1-2 weeks; taper by 5% per week to a maintenance dose of 5-10 mg/kg/day; some renal transplant patients may be dosed as low as 3 mg/kg/day

When using the nonmodified formulation, cyclosporine levels may increase in liver transplant patients when the T-tube is closed; dose may need decreased

I.V.: Cyclosporine (nonmodified): Initial dose: 5-6 mg/kg/day as a single dose (1/3 the oral dose), infused over 2-6 hours; use should be limited to patients unable to take capsules or oral solution; patients should be switched to an oral dosage form as soon as possible

Hemodialysis: Supplemental dose is unnecessary.

Peritoneal dialysis: Supplemental dose is unnecessary.

Dosing adjustment in hepatic impairment: Probably necessary; monitor levels closely

Mechanism of Action Inhibition of production and release of interleukin II and inhibits interleukin II-induced activation of resting T-lymphocytes.

Other Adverse Effects Adverse reactions reported with kidney, liver, and heart transplantation, unless otherwise noted. Although percentage is reported for specific condition, reaction may occur in anyone taking cyclosporine. [Reactions reported for rheumatoid arthritis (RA) are based on cyclosporine (modified) 2.5 mg/kg/day versus placebo.]

>10%:

Dermatologic: Hirsutism (21% to 45%), hypertrichosis (RA 19%)

Endocrine & metabolic: Increased triglycerides (psoriasis 15%), female reproductive disorder (psoriasis 8% to 11%)

Gastrointestinal: Abdominal discomfort (RA 15%), dyspepsia (RA 12%)

Renal: Renal dysfunction/nephropathy (25% to 38%; RA 10%, psoriasis 21%), creatinine elevation ≥50% (RA 24%), increased creatinine (psoriasis 16% to 20%)

Kidney, liver, and heart transplants (≤2% unless otherwise noted):

Central nervous system: Lethargy

Dermatologic: Acne (1% to 6%), brittle fingernails, hair breaking, pruritus

Endocrine & metabolic: Gynecomastia (<4%)

Gastrointestinal: Diarrhea (3% to 8%), abdominal discomfort (<7%), cramps (≤4%), anorexia, constipation, pancreatitis, weight loss

Hematologic: Leukopenia (<6%), anemia, thrombocytopenia

Hepatic: Hepatotoxicity (<7%)

Neuromuscular & skeletal: Joint pain, muscle pain

Ocular: Conjunctivitis, visual disturbance

Otic: Hearing loss, tinnitus

Renal: Hematuria

Miscellaneous: Lymphoma (<6%), night sweats

RA **only** (<3% unless otherwise noted):

Cardiovascular: Edema (5%), abnormal heart sounds, peripheral ischemia

Central nervous system: Insomnia (4%), depression (3%), hypoesthesia, emotional lability, impaired concentration, malaise, vertigo

(Continued)

CycloSPORINE *(Continued)*

Dermatologic: Purpura (3%), abnormal pigmentation, angioedema, cellulitis, dermatitis, dry skin, eczema, folliculitis, nail disorder, pruritus, skin disorder, urticaria

Endocrine & metabolic: Menstrual disorder (3%), breast fibroadenosis, breast pain, goiter, hyperkalemia, hyperuricemia, libido increased/decreased

Gastrointestinal: Flatulence (5%), constipation, weight loss/gain

Genitourinary: Leukorrhea (1%), abnormal urine, micturition urgency, nocturia, polyuria, pyelonephritis, urinary incontinence, uterine hemorrhage

Hematologic: Anemia, leukopenia

Hepatic: Bilirubinemia

Neuromuscular & skeletal: Arthralgia, bone fracture, joint dislocation, myalgia, neuropathy, stiffness, synovial cyst, tendon disorder

Ocular: Abnormal vision, cataract, conjunctivitis, eye pain

Otic: Tinnitus, deafness, vestibular disorder

Renal: Increased BUN, hematuria, renal abscess

Miscellaneous: Herpes zoster, lymphadenopathy

Psoriasis (1% to <3% unless otherwise noted):

Central nervous system: Insomnia, vertigo

Dermatologic: Hypertrichosis (5% to 7%), acne, dry skin, folliculitis, keratosis, pruritus, rash, skin malignancies

Gastrointestinal: Diarrhea (5% to 6%), abdominal discomfort (3% to 6%), dyspepsia (2% to 3%), abdominal distention, appetite increased, constipation

Genitourinary: Micturition increased

Hepatic: Hyperbilirubinemia

Neuromuscular & skeletal: Arthralgia (1% to 6%)

Ocular: Abnormal vision

Postmarketing and/or case reports (any indication): Death (due to renal deterioration), mild hypomagnesemia, hyperkalemia, increased uric acid, gout, hyperbilirubinemia, increased cholesterol, encephalopathy, impaired consciousness, neurotoxicity

Ophthalmic emulsion (Restasis™): Ocular:

>10%: Burning (17%)

1% to 10%: Hyperemia (conjunctival 5%), eye pain, pruritus, stinging

Drug Interactions Substrate of **CYP3A4**; Inhibits CYP2C8/9, 3A4

Increased Toxicity: Voriconazole may increase cyclosporine serum concentrations; decrease cyclosporine dosage by 50% when initiating voriconazole. Cyclosporine increases toxicity of digoxin, diuretics, methotrexate, and nifedipine.

Drugs that increase cyclosporine concentrations: Allopurinol, metoclopramide, nicardipine, octreotide, CYP3A4 inhibitors (amiodarone, bromocriptine, cimetidine, clarithromycin, danazol, erythromycin, delavirdine, diltiazem, disulfiram, fluconazole, fluoxetine, fluvoxamine, indinavir, itraconazole, ketoconazole, nefazodone, nevirapine, propoxyphene, quinupristin-dalfopristin, ritonavir, saquinavir, verapamil, zafirlukast, zileuton)

Drugs that enhance nephrotoxicity of cyclosporine: Aminoglycosides, amphotericin B, acyclovir, cimetidine, ketoconazole, lovastatin, melphalan, NSAIDs, ranitidine, trimethoprim and sulfamethoxazole, tacrolimus

Decreased Effect: Decreases effect of live vaccines. Orlistat may decrease absorption of cyclosporine; avoid concomitant use.

Drugs that decrease cyclosporine concentrations: Carbamazepine, nafcillin, phenobarbital, phenytoin, rifampin, isoniazid, ticlopidine

Dietary/Ethanol/Herb Considerations

Food may elevate peak serum concentration. Avoid grapefruit products; absorption increased which may result in renal toxicity. Diluting oral solution improves flavor. May dilute Neoral® oral solution with orange juice or apple juice; may dilute Sandimmune® oral solution with milk, chocolate milk, or orange juice. Mix thoroughly.

Herb/Nutraceutical: Avoid cat's claw and echinacea due to immunostimulant properties. Avoid St John's wort; may increase metabolism and decrease plasma concentration. Ginkgo biloba and milk thistle have been reported to protect the liver.

Pharmacodynamics/Kinetics

Absorption:

Ophthalmic emulsion: Serum concentrations not detectable.

Oral:

Cyclosporine (non-modified): Erratic and incomplete; dependent on presence of food, bile acids, and GI motility; larger oral doses are needed in pediatrics due to shorter bowel length and limited intestinal absorption

Cyclosporine (modified): Erratic and incomplete; increased absorption, up to 30% when compared to cyclosporine (non-modified); less dependent on food, bile acids, or GI motility when compared to cyclosporine (non-modified)

Distribution: Widely in tissues and body fluids including the liver, pancreas, and lungs; crosses placenta; enters breast milk

V_{dss}: 4-6 L/kg in renal, liver, and marrow transplant recipients (slightly lower values in cardiac transplant patients; children <10 years have higher values)
Protein binding: 90% to 98% to lipoproteins
Metabolism: Extensively hepatic via CYP; forms at least 25 metabolites; extensive first-pass effect following oral administration
Bioavailability: Oral:
Cyclosporine (non-modified): Dependent on patient population and transplant type (<10% in adult liver transplant patients and as high as 89% in renal transplant patients); bioavailability of Sandimmune® capsules and oral solution are equivalent; bioavailability of oral solution is ~30% of the I.V. solution
Children: 28% (range: 17% to 42%); gut dysfunction common in BMT patients and oral bioavailability is further reduced
Cyclosporine (modified): Bioavailability of Neoral® capsules and oral solution are equivalent:
Children: 43% (range: 30% to 68%)
Adults: 23% greater than with cyclosporine (non-modified) in renal transplant patients; 50% greater in liver transplant patients
Half-life elimination: Oral: May be prolonged in patients with hepatic impairment and shorter in pediatric patients due to the higher metabolism rate
Cyclosporine (non-modified): Biphasic: Alpha: 1.4 hours; Terminal: 19 hours (range: 10-27 hours)
Cyclosporine (modified): Biphasic: Terminal: 8.4 hours (range: 5-18 hours)
Time to peak, serum: Oral:
Cyclosporine (non-modified): 2-6 hours; some patients have a second peak at 5-6 hours
Cyclosporine (modified): Renal transplant: 1.5-2 hours
Excretion: Primarily feces; urine (6%, 0.1% as unchanged drug and metabolites)

Pregnancy Risk Factor C

Generic Available Yes

Comments Cyclosporine serum levels are likely to be increased with clarithromycin or erythromycin administration. Toxic cyclosporine concentrations and renal toxicity may result. Clarithromycin inhibits the CYP3A4 enzyme which metabolizes cyclosporine. Azithromycin (Zithromax®) and dirithromycin (Dynabac®) are unlikely to interact with cyclosporine.

Selected Readings

Ferrari SL, Goffin E, Mourad M, et al, "The Interaction Between Clarithromycin and Cyclosporine in Kidney Transplant Recipients," *Transplantation*, 1994, 58(6):725-7.
Harnett JD, Parfrey PS, Paul MD, et al, "Erythromycin-Cyclosporine Interaction in Renal Transplant Recipients," *Transplantation*, 1987, 43(2):316-8.

Cyklokapron® *see* Tranexamic Acid *on page 1333*
Cylert® *see* Pemoline *on page 1044*
Cylex® [OTC] *see* Benzocaine *on page 169*
Cyomin® *see* Cyanocobalamin *on page 377*

Cyproheptadine (si proe HEP ta deen)

U.S. Brand Names Periactin®

Canadian Brand Names Periactin®

Mexican Brand Names Viternum®

Pharmacologic Category Antihistamine

Synonyms Cyproheptadine Hydrochloride

Use Perennial and seasonal allergic rhinitis and other allergic symptoms including urticaria

Unlabeled/Investigational Use Appetite stimulation; treatment of blepharospasm, cluster or migraine headaches, Nelson's syndrome, pruritus, schizophrenia, spinal cord damage associated spasticity, tardive dyskinesia

Local Anesthetic/Vasoconstrictor Precautions No information available to require special precautions

Effects on Dental Treatment
>10%: Slight to moderate drowsiness, thickening of bronchial secretions
1% to 10%: Xerostomia, headache, nervousness, dizziness, nausea, pharyngitis, fatigue

Dosage Oral:
Children:
Allergic conditions: 0.25 mg/kg/day or 8 mg/m²/day in 2-3 divided doses **or**
2-6 years: 2 mg every 8-12 hours (not to exceed 12 mg/day)
7-14 years: 4 mg every 8-12 hours (not to exceed 16 mg/day)
Migraine headaches: 4 mg 2-3 times/day
Children ≥12 years and Adults: Spasticity associated with spinal cord damage: 4 mg at bedtime; increase by a 4 mg dose every 3-4 days; average daily dose: 16 mg in divided doses; not to exceed 36 mg/day
Children >13 years and Adults: Appetite stimulation (anorexia nervosa): 2 mg 4 times/day; may be increased gradually over a 3-week period to 8 mg 4 times/day
Adults:
Allergic conditions: 4-20 mg/day divided every 8 hours (not to exceed 0.5)
Cluster headaches: 4 mg 4 times/day
(Continued)

Cyproheptadine *(Continued)*

Migraine headaches: 4-8 mg 3 times/day

Dosing adjustment in hepatic impairment: Reduction required in significant dysfunction

Mechanism of Action A potent antihistamine and serotonin antagonist, competes with histamine for H_1-receptor sites on effector cells in the gastrointestinal tract, blood vessels, and respiratory tract

Other Adverse Effects

1% to 10%:

Gastrointestinal: Appetite stimulation, diarrhea, abdominal pain,

Neuromuscular & skeletal: Arthralgia

<1%: **Tachycardia, palpitations,** edema, **sedation, CNS stimulation, seizures,** depression, photosensitivity, rash, angioedema, hemolytic anemia, leukopenia, thrombocytopenia, hepatitis, myalgia, **paresthesia, bronchospasm, epistaxis, allergic reactions**

Drug Interactions Increased Effect/Toxicity: Cyproheptadine may potentiate the effect of CNS depressants. MAO inhibitors may cause hallucinations when taken with cyproheptadine.

Dietary/Ethanol/Herb Considerations

Ethanol: Avoid use; may increase CNS depression.

Herb/Nutraceutical: Avoid gotu kola, kava, SAMe, St John's wort, and valerian; may increase CNS depression.

Pharmacodynamics/Kinetics

Absorption: Completely

Metabolism: Almost completely hepatic

Excretion: Urine (>50% primarily as metabolites); feces (~25%)

Pregnancy Risk Factor B

Generic Available Yes

Cyproheptadine Hydrochloride *see* Cyproheptadine *on page 387*

Cystadane® *see* Betaine Anhydrous *on page 177*

Cystagon® *see* Cysteamine *on page 388*

Cysteamine (sis TEE a meen)

U.S. Brand Names Cystagon®

Pharmacologic Category Anticystine Agent; Urinary Tract Product

Synonyms Cysteamine Bitartrate

Use Orphan drug: Treatment of nephropathic cystinosis

Local Anesthetic/Vasoconstrictor Precautions No information available to require special precautions

Effects on Dental Treatment

>5%: Fever, vomiting (35%), lethargy (11%)

<5%: Hypertension, somnolence, headache, seizures, confusion, dizziness, jitteriness, nervousness, hallucinations, dehydration, bad breath, gastroenteritis, duodenitis, duodenal ulceration, tremor

Dosage Oral: Initiate therapy with $^1/_4$ to $^1/_8$ of maintenance dose; titrate slowly upward over 4-6 weeks

Children <12 years: Maintenance: 1.3 g/m²/day divided into 4 doses

Children >12 years and Adults (>110 lbs): 2 g/day in 4 divided doses; dosage may be increased to 1.95 g/m²/day if cystine levels are <1 nmol/$^1/_2$ cystine/mg protein, although intolerance and incidence of adverse events may be increased

Mechanism of Action Reacts with cystine in the lysosome to convert it to cysteine and to a cysteine-cysteamine mixed disulfide, both of which can then exit the lysosome in patients with cystinosis, an inherited defect of lysosomal transport

Other Adverse Effects

>7%:

Dermatologic: Rash (7%)

Gastrointestinal: Anorexia (31%), diarrhea (16%)

<5%:

Central nervous system: Encephalopathy, ataxia, impaired cognition, emotional changes, nightmares

Dermatologic: Urticaria

Gastrointestinal: Abdominal pain, dyspepsia, constipation

Hematologic: Anemia, leukopenia

Hepatic: Abnormal LFTs

Neuromuscular & skeletal: Hyperkinesia

Otic: Decreased hearing

Pregnancy Risk Factor C

Generic Available No

Cysteamine Bitartrate *see* Cysteamine *on page 388*

Cysteine (SIS teen)

Pharmacologic Category Dietary Supplement

Synonyms Cysteine Hydrochloride

Use Supplement to crystalline amino acid solutions, in particular the specialized pediatric formulas (eg, Aminosyn® PF, TrophAmine®) to meet the intravenous amino acid nutritional requirements of infants receiving parenteral nutrition (PN)

Local Anesthetic/Vasoconstrictor Precautions No information available to require special precautions

Effects on Dental Treatment Frequency not defined: Fever, nausea

Dosage Neonates and Infants: I.V.: Added as a fixed ratio to crystalline amino acid solution: 40 mg cysteine per g of amino acids; dosage will vary with the daily amino acid dosage (eg, 0.5-2.5 g/kg/day amino acids would result in 20-100 mg/kg/day cysteine); individual doses of cysteine of 0.8-1 mmol/kg/day have also been added directly to the daily PN solution; the duration of treatment relates to the need for PN; patients on chronic PN therapy have received cysteine until 6 months of age and in some cases until 2 years of age

Mechanism of Action Cysteine is a sulfur-containing amino acid synthesized from methionine via the transulfuration pathway. It is a precursor of the tripeptide glutathione and also of taurine. Newborn infants have a relative deficiency of the enzyme necessary to affect this conversion. Cysteine may be considered an essential amino acid in infants.

Other Adverse Effects Frequency not defined:

Endocrine & metabolic: Metabolic acidosis

Renal: Elevated BUN, azotemia

Generic Available Yes

Cysteine Hydrochloride *see* Cysteine *on page 388*

Cystospaz® *see* Hyoscyamine *on page 699*

Cystospaz-M® *see* Hyoscyamine *on page 699*

CYT *see* Cyclophosphamide *on page 381*

Cytadren® *see* Aminoglutethimide *on page 77*

Cytarabine (sye TAIR a been)

U.S. Brand Names Cytosar-U®

Canadian Brand Names Cytosar®

Mexican Brand Names Laracit®

Pharmacologic Category Antineoplastic Agent, Antimetabolite

Synonyms Arabinosylcytosine; Ara-C; Cytarabine Hydrochloride; Cytosine Arabinosine Hydrochloride

Use Ara-C is one of the most active agents in leukemia; also active against lymphoma, meningeal leukemia, and meningeal lymphoma; has little use in the treatment of solid tumors

Local Anesthetic/Vasoconstrictor Precautions No information available to require special precautions

Effects on Dental Treatment

>10%: Fever (>80%), nausea, vomiting, mucositis

1% to 10%: Dizziness, headache, somnolence, confusion, syndrome of sudden respiratory distress

Dosage I.V. bolus, IVPB, and CIV doses of cytarabine are very different. Bolus doses are relatively well tolerated since the drug is rapidly metabolized; but are associated with greater neurotoxicity. Continuous infusion uniformly results in myelosuppression. Refer to individual protocols. Children and Adults:

Remission induction:

I.V.: 100-200 mg/m²/day for 5-10 days; a second course, beginning 2-4 weeks after the initial therapy, may be required in some patients.

I.T.: 5-75 mg/m² every 2-7 days until CNS findings normalize; or age-based dosing:

<1 year: 20 mg

1-2 years: 30 mg

2-3 years: 50 mg

>3 years: 75 mg

Remission maintenance:

I.V.: 70-200 mg/m²/day for 2-5 days at monthly intervals

I.M., S.C.: 1-1.5 mg/kg single dose for maintenance at 1- to 4-week intervals

High-dose therapies:

Doses as high as 1-3 g/m² have been used for refractory or secondary leukemias or refractory non-Hodgkin's lymphoma.

Doses of 3 g/m² every 12 hours for up to 12 doses have been used

Bone marrow transplant: 1.5 g/m² continuous infusion over 48 hours

Hemodialysis: Supplemental dose is unnecessary.

Peritoneal dialysis: Supplemental dose is unnecessary.

Dosing adjustment in hepatic impairment: Dose may need to be adjusted since cytarabine is partially detoxified in the liver.

Mechanism of Action Inhibition of DNA synthesis. Cytosine gains entry into cells by a carrier process, and then must be converted to its active compound, aracytidine triphosphate. Cytosine is a purine analog and is incorporated into DNA; however, the primary action is inhibition of DNA polymerase resulting in decreased

(Continued)

Cytarabine *(Continued)*

DNA synthesis and repair. The degree of cytotoxicity correlates linearly with incorporation into DNA; therefore, incorporation into the DNA is responsible for drug activity and toxicity. Cytarabine is specific for the S phase of the cell cycle.

Other Adverse Effects

>10%:

Dermatologic: Alopecia

Gastrointestinal: Diarrhea (subsides quickly after discontinuing the drug; GI effects may be more pronounced with divided I.V. bolus doses than with continuous infusion)

Hematologic: Myelosuppression; neutropenia and thrombocytopenia are severe, anemia may also occur

Onset: 4-7 days

Nadir: 14-18 days

Recovery: 21-28 days

Hepatic: Hepatic dysfunction, mild jaundice, and acute increases in transaminases can be produced

Ocular: Tearing, ocular pain, foreign body sensation, photophobia, and blurred vision may occur with high-dose therapy; ophthalmic corticosteroids usually prevent or relieve the condition

1% to 10%:

Cardiovascular: Thrombophlebitis, cardiomegaly

Central nervous system: Malaise; a severe cerebellar toxicity occurs in about 8% of patients receiving a high dose >36-48 g/m^2/cycle (irreversible or fatal in about 1%)

Dermatologic: Skin freckling, itching, cellulitis at injection site; rash, pain, erythema, and skin sloughing of the palmar and plantar surfaces may occur with high-dose therapy. Prophylactic topical steroids and/or skin moisturizers may be useful.

Genitourinary: Urinary retention

Neuromuscular & skeletal: Myalgia, bone pain

Respiratory: Syndrome of sudden respiratory distress, including tachypnea, hypoxemia, interstitial and alveolar infiltrates progressing to pulmonary edema, pneumonia

<1%: Increases in amylase and lipase levels; isolated cases of pancreatitis have been reported; **dysphagia (intrathecal use);** peripheral neuropathy, neuritis; accessory nerve paralysis (intrathecal use); diplopia (reported with intrathecal use); **cough, hoarseness (intrathecal use);** aphonia (reported with intrathecal use)

Drug Interactions

Increased Effect/Toxicity: Alkylating agents and radiation, purine analogs, and methotrexate when coadministered with cytarabine result in increased toxic effects.

Decreased Effect: Decreased effect of gentamicin, flucytosine. Decreased digoxin oral tablet absorption.

Pharmacodynamics/Kinetics

Distribution: V_d: Total body water; widely and rapidly since it enters the cells readily; crosses blood-brain barrier with CSF levels of 40% to 50% of plasma level

Metabolism: Primarily hepatic; aracytidine triphosphate is the active moiety; about 86% to 96% of dose is metabolized to inactive uracil arabinoside

Half-life elimination: Initial: 7-20 minutes; Terminal: 0.5-2.6 hours

Excretion: Urine (~80% as metabolites) within 24-36 hours

Pregnancy Risk Factor D

Generic Available Yes

Cytarabine Hydrochloride *see* Cytarabine *on page 389*

Cytarabine (Liposomal) (sye TARE a been li pu SOE mol)

U.S. Brand Names DepoCyt™

Canadian Brand Names DepoCyt™

Pharmacologic Category Antineoplastic Agent, Antimetabolite

Use Treatment of neoplastic (lymphomatous) meningitis

Local Anesthetic/Vasoconstrictor Precautions No information available to require special precautions

Effects on Dental Treatment Chemical arachnoiditis is commonly observed, and may include neck pain, neck rigidity, headache, fever, nausea, vomiting, and back pain (may occur in up to 100% of cycles without dexamethasone prophylaxis; incidence reduced to 33% when dexamethasone is used concurrently).

>10%: Headache (28%), confusion (14%), somnolence (12%), fever (11%), pain (11%), vomiting (12%), nausea (11%)

1% to 10%: Weakness (19%), abnormal gait (4%)

Dosage Adults:

Induction: 50 mg intrathecally every 14 days for a total of 2 doses (weeks 1 and 3)

Consolidation: 50 mg intrathecally every 14 days for 3 doses (weeks 5, 7, and 9), followed by an additional dose at week 13

Maintenance: 50 mg intrathecally every 28 days for 4 doses (weeks 17, 21, 25, and 29)

If drug-related neurotoxicity develops, the dose should be reduced to 25 mg. If toxicity persists, treatment with liposomal cytarabine should be discontinued.

Note: Patients should be started on dexamethasone 4 mg twice daily (oral or I.V.) for 5 days, beginning on the day of liposomal cytarabine injection

Mechanism of Action This is a sustained-release formulation of the active ingredient cytarabine, which acts through inhibition of DNA synthesis; cell cycle-specific for the S phase of cell division; cytosine gains entry into cells by a carrier process, and then must be converted to its active compound; cytosine acts as an analog and is incorporated into DNA; however, the primary action is inhibition of DNA polymerase resulting in decreased DNA synthesis and repair; degree of its cytotoxicity correlates linearly with its incorporation into DNA; therefore, incorporation into the DNA is responsible for drug activity and toxicity

Other Adverse Effects

1% to 10%:

- Cardiovascular: Peripheral edema (7%)
- Gastrointestinal: Constipation (7%)
- Genitourinary: Incontinence (3%)
- Hematologic: Neutropenia (9%), thrombocytopenia (8%), anemia (1%)
- Neuromuscular & skeletal: Back pain (7%)

<1%: **Anaphylaxis, neck pain**

Drug Interactions No formal studies of interactions with other medications have been conducted. The limited systemic exposure minimizes the potential for interaction between liposomal cytarabine and other medications.

Pharmacodynamics/Kinetics

Absorption: Systemic exposure following intrathecal administration is negligible since transfer rate from CSF to plasma is slow

Metabolism: In plasma to ara-U (inactive)

Half-life elimination, CSF: 100-263 hours

Time to peak, CSF: Intrathecal: ~5 hours

Excretion: Primarily urine (as metabolites - ara-U)

Pregnancy Risk Factor D

Generic Available No

Cytomel® *see* Liothyronine *on page 810*

Cytosar-U® *see* Cytarabine *on page 389*

Cytosine Arabinosine Hydrochloride *see* Cytarabine *on page 389*

Cytotec® *see* Misoprostol *on page 920*

Cytovene® *see* Ganciclovir *on page 626*

Cytoxan® *see* Cyclophosphamide *on page 381*

Cytra-2 *see* Sodium Citrate and Citric Acid *on page 1230*

Cytra-3 *see* Citric Acid, Sodium Citrate, and Potassium Citrate *on page 335*

Cytra-K *see* Potassium Citrate and Citric Acid *on page 1101*

D_3 *see* Cholecalciferol *on page 317*

D-3-Mercaptovaline *see* Penicillamine *on page 1046*

d4T *see* Stavudine *on page 1242*

Dacarbazine (da KAR ba zeen)

U.S. Brand Names DTIC-Dome®

Canadian Brand Names DTIC®

Pharmacologic Category Antineoplastic Agent, Alkylating Agent

Synonyms DIC; Dimethyl Triazeno Imidazol Carboxamide; DTIC; Imidazole Carboxamide

Use Treatment of malignant melanoma, Hodgkin's disease, soft-tissue sarcomas, fibrosarcomas, rhabdomyosarcoma, islet cell carcinoma, medullary carcinoma of the thyroid, and neuroblastoma

Local Anesthetic/Vasoconstrictor Precautions No information available to require special precautions

Effects on Dental Treatment

>10%: Nausea and vomiting (>90%; can be severe)

1% to 10%: Flu-like syndrome, metallic taste

Dosage Refer to individual protocols. Some dosage regimens include:

Intra-arterial: 50-400 mg/m² for 5-10 days

I.V.:

- ABVD for Hodgkin's disease: 375 mg/m² days 1 and 15 every 4 weeks
- Metastatic melanoma (alone or in combination with other agents): 150-250 mg/m² days 1-5 every 3-4 weeks
- Metastatic melanoma: 850 mg/m² every 3 weeks

High dose: Bone marrow/blood cell transplantation: I.V.: 1-3 g/m²; maximum dose as a single agent: 3.38 g/m²; generally combined with other high-dose chemotherapeutic drugs

Dosing adjustment in renal/hepatic impairment: No guidelines exist

(Continued)

Dacarbazine *(Continued)*

Mechanism of Action Alkylating agent which forms methylcarbonium ions that attack nucleophilic groups in DNA; cross-links strands of DNA resulting in the inhibition of DNA, RNA, and protein synthesis, but the exact mechanism of action is still unclear; originally developed as a purine antimetabolite, but it does not interfere with purine synthesis; metabolism by the host is necessary for activation of dacarbazine, then the methylated species acts by alkylation of nucleic acids; dacarbazine is active in all phases of the cell cycle

Other Adverse Effects

>10%:

Hematologic: Myelosuppression, leukopenia, thrombocytopenia; dose-limiting

Onset: 5-7 days

Nadir: 7-10 days

Recovery: 21-28 days

Local: Pain on infusion, may be minimized by administration through a central line, or by administration as a short infusion (eg, 1-2 hours as opposed to bolus injection)

1% to 10%:

Dermatologic: Alopecia, rash, photosensitivity

Gastrointestinal: Anorexia

<1%: **Headache**, diarrhea (following high-dose bolus injection), transient elevation in liver enzymes, hepatic vein occlusion, hepatic necrosis, **paresthesias, anaphylactic reactions**, eosinophilia

Drug Interactions Substrate of **CYP1A2, 2E1**

Decreased Effect: Metabolism may be increased by drugs that induce hepatic enzymes (carbamazepine, phenytoin, phenobarbital, and rifampin), potentially leading to decreased efficacy. Patients may experience impaired immune response to vaccines; possible infection after administration of live vaccines in patients receiving immunosuppressants.

Dietary/Ethanol/Herb Considerations

Ethanol: Avoid use due to GI irritation.

Herb/Nutraceutical: Avoid dong quai and St John's wort; may cause photosensitization.

Pharmacodynamics/Kinetics

Onset of action: I.V.: 18-24 days

Distribution: V_d: 0.6 L/kg, exceeding total body water; suggesting binding to some tissue (probably liver)

Protein binding: 5%

Metabolism: Extensively hepatic; hepatobiliary excretion is probably of some importance; metabolites may also have an antineoplastic effect

Half-life elimination: Biphasic: Initial: 20-40 minutes; Terminal: 5 hours

Excretion: Urine (~30% to 50% as unchanged drug)

Pregnancy Risk Factor C

Generic Available Yes

Daclizumab (dac KLYE zue mab)

U.S. Brand Names Zenapax®

Canadian Brand Names Zenapax®

Pharmacologic Category Immunosuppressant Agent

Use Part of an immunosuppressive regimen (including cyclosporine and corticosteroids) for the prophylaxis of acute organ rejection in patients receiving renal transplant

Unlabeled/Investigational Use Treatment of graft-versus-host disease

Local Anesthetic/Vasoconstrictor Precautions No information available to require special precautions

Effects on Dental Treatment

≥5%: Chest pain, hypertension, hypotension, tachycardia, dizziness, fever, headache, pain, post-traumatic pain, tremor, epigastric pain, nausea, pyrosis, vomiting, bleeding, cough, dyspnea, wound infection, impaired wound healing, fatigue

≥2% to <5%: Anxiety, dehydration, diabetes mellitus, gastritis, leg cramps, weakness, congestion, hypoxia, pharyngitis, rhinitis

Dosage Daclizumab is used adjunctively with other immunosuppressants (eg, cyclosporine, corticosteroids, mycophenolate mofetil, and azathioprine): I.V.:

Children: Use same weight-based dose as adults

Adults:

Immunoprophylaxis against acute renal allograft rejection: 1 mg/kg infused over 15 minutes within 24 hours before transplantation (day 0), then every 14 days for 4 additional doses

Treatment of graft-versus-host disease (unlabeled use, limited data): 0.5-1.5 mg/kg, repeat same dosage for transient response. Repeat doses have been administered 11-48 days following the initial dose.

Mechanism of Action Daclizumab is a chimeric (90% human, 10% murine) monoclonal IgG antibody produced by recombinant DNA technology. Daclizumab inhibits immune reactions by binding and blocking the alpha-chain of the interleukin-2 receptor (CD25) located on the surface of activated lymphocytes.

Other Adverse Effects Although reported adverse events are frequent, when daclizumab is compared with placebo the incidence of adverse effects is similar between the two groups. Many of the adverse effects reported during clinical trial use of daclizumab may be related to the patient population, transplant procedure, and concurrent transplant medications. Diarrhea, fever, postoperative pain, pruritus, respiratory tract infections, urinary tract infections, and vomiting occurred more often in children than adults.

≥5%:
- Cardiovascular: Edema, thrombosis
- Central nervous system: Insomnia
- Dermatologic: Acne, cellulitis
- Gastrointestinal: Abdominal distention, abdominal pain, constipation, diarrhea, dyspepsia
- Genitourinary: Dysuria
- Neuromuscular & skeletal: Back pain, musculoskeletal pain
- Renal: Oliguria, renal tubular necrosis
- Respiratory: Pulmonary edema
- Miscellaneous: Lymphocele

≥2% to <5%:
- Central nervous system: Depression, shivering
- Dermatologic: Hirsutism, pruritus, rash
- Endocrine & metabolic: Fluid overload
- Gastrointestinal: Flatulence, hemorrhoids
- Genitourinary: Urinary retention, urinary tract bleeding
- Local: Application site reaction
- Neuromuscular & skeletal: Arthralgia, myalgia
- Ocular: Vision blurred
- Renal: Hydronephrosis, renal damage, renal insufficiency
- Respiratory: Atelectasis, hypoxia, pleural effusion, rales
- Miscellaneous: Night sweats, prickly sensation

<1%: **Severe hypersensitivity reactions (rare)**

Pharmacodynamics/Kinetics

Distribution: V_d:
- Adults: Central compartment: 0.031 L/kg; Peripheral compartment: 0.043 L/kg
- Children: Central compartment: 0.067 L/kg; Peripheral compartment: 0.047 L/kg

Half-life elimination (estimated): Adults: Terminal: 20 days; Children: 13 days

Pregnancy Risk Factor C

Generic Available No

DACT *see* Dactinomycin *on page 393*

Dactinomycin (dak ti noe MYE sin)

U.S. Brand Names Cosmegen®

Canadian Brand Names Cosmegen®

Mexican Brand Names Ac-De®

Pharmacologic Category Antineoplastic Agent, Antibiotic

Synonyms ACT; Act-D; Actinomycin; Actinomycin Cl; Actinomycin D; DACT; NSC-3053

Use Treatment of testicular tumors, melanoma, choriocarcinoma, Wilms' tumor, neuroblastoma, retinoblastoma, rhabdomyosarcoma, uterine sarcomas, Ewing's sarcoma, Kaposi's sarcoma, sarcoma botryoides, and soft tissue sarcoma

Local Anesthetic/Vasoconstrictor Precautions No information available to require special precautions

Effects on Dental Treatment

>10%: Fever, stomatitis, esophagitis, dysphagia, GI ulceration, pharyngitis, unusual fatigue, malaise, lethargy

1% to 10%: Mucositis

Dosage Almost ALWAYS expressed in MICROGRAMS rather than milligrams; some practitioners recommend calculation of the dosage for obese or edematous patients on the basis of body surface area in an effort to relate dosage to lean body mass.

Refer to individual protocols: I.V.:

Children >6 months: 15 mcg/kg/day **or** 400-600 mcg/m²/day for 5 days every 3-6 weeks

Adults: 2.5 mg/m² in divided doses over 1 week, repeated every 2 weeks **or**
0.75-2 mg/m² every 1-4 weeks **or**
400-600 mcg/m²/day for 5 days, repeated every 3-6 weeks

Mechanism of Action Binds to the guanine portion of DNA intercalating between guanine and cytosine base pairs inhibiting DNA and RNA synthesis and protein synthesis

Other Adverse Effects

>10%:
- Dermatologic: Alopecia (reversible), skin eruptions, acne, increased pigmentation of previously irradiated skin, cheilitis, maculopapular rash

(Continued)

Dactinomycin *(Continued)*

Endocrine & metabolic: Hypocalcemia
Gastrointestinal: Severe nausea and vomiting (within 2-5 hours, persists up to 24 hours), anorexia, abdominal pain, diarrhea
Hematologic: Myelosuppression, anemia
Hepatic: Liver toxicity, ascites, hepatomegaly, hepatitis
Local: Extravasation: An irritant and should be administered through a rapidly running I.V. line; extravasation can lead to tissue necrosis, pain, and ulceration
Vesicant chemotherapy

<1%: **Anaphylactoid reaction**, hepatitis, hyperuricemia, LFT abnormalities

Drug Interactions Increased Effect/Toxicity: Dactinomycin potentiates the effects of radiation therapy.

Dietary/Ethanol/Herb Considerations Ethanol: Avoid use due to GI irritation.

Pharmacodynamics/Kinetics

Distribution: High concentrations found in bone marrow and tumor cells, submaxillary gland, liver, and kidney; crosses placenta; poor CSF penetration
Metabolism: Hepatic, minimal
Half-life elimination: 36 hours
Time to peak, serum: I.V.: 2-5 minutes
Excretion: Bile (50%); feces (14%); urine (~10% as unchanged drug)

Pregnancy Risk Factor C

Generic Available No

D.A.II™ *see* Chlorpheniramine, Phenylephrine, and Methscopolamine *on page 310*

Dakin's Solution *see* Sodium Hypochlorite Solution *on page 1231*

Dallergy® *see* Chlorpheniramine, Phenylephrine, and Methscopolamine *on page 310*

Dallergy-D® *see* Chlorpheniramine and Phenylephrine *on page 308*

Dalmane® *see* Flurazepam *on page 595*

***d*-Alpha Tocopherol** *see* Vitamin E *on page 1393*

Dalteparin (dal TE pa rin)

U.S. Brand Names Fragmin®

Canadian Brand Names Fragmin®

Pharmacologic Category Low Molecular Weight Heparin

Use Prevention of deep vein thrombosis which may lead to pulmonary embolism, in patients requiring abdominal surgery who are at risk for thromboembolism complications (ie, patients >40 years of age, obesity, patients with malignancy, history of deep vein thrombosis or pulmonary embolism, and surgical procedures requiring general anesthesia and lasting longer than 30 minutes); prevention of DVT in patients undergoing hip surgery; acute treatment of unstable angina or non-Q-wave MI; prevention of ischemic complications in patients on concurrent aspirin therapy

Unlabeled/Investigational Use Active treatment of deep vein thrombosis

Local Anesthetic/Vasoconstrictor Precautions No information available to require special precautions

Effects on Dental Treatment No significant effects or complications reported

Dosage Adults: S.C.:

Low-moderate risk patients undergoing abdominal surgery: 2500 int. units 1-2 hours prior to surgery, then once daily for 5-10 days postoperatively
High-risk patients undergoing abdominal surgery: 5000 int. units 1-2 hours prior to surgery and then once daily for 5-10 days postoperatively
Patients undergoing total hip surgery: **Note:** Three treatment options are currently available. Dose is given for 5-10 days, although up to 14 days of treatment have been tolerated in clinical trials:
Postoperative start:
Initial: 2500 int. units 4-8 hours* after surgery
Maintenance: 5000 int. units once daily; start at least 6 hours after postsurgical dose
Preoperative (starting day of surgery):
Initial: 2500 int. units within 2 hours before surgery
Adjustment: 2500 int. units 4-8 hours* after surgery
Maintenance: 5000 int. units once daily; start at least 6 hours after postsurgical dose
Preoperative (starting evening prior to surgery):
Initial: 5000 int. units 10-14 hours before surgery
Adjustment: 5000 int. units 4-8 hours* after surgery
Maintenance: 5000 int. units once daily, allowing 24 hours between doses.
Dose may be delayed if hemostasis is not yet achieved.
Patients with unstable angina or non-Q-wave MI: 120 int. units/kg body weight (maximum dose: 10,000 int. units) every 12 hours for 5-8 days with concurrent aspirin therapy. Discontinue dalteparin once patient is clinically stable.
Dosing adjustment in renal impairment: Use with caution, accumulation can be expected; halflife is increased with chronic failure (no specific recommendations)

Dosing adjustment in hepatic impairment: Use with caution; no specific recommendations

Mechanism of Action Low molecular weight heparin analog with a molecular weight of 4000-6000 daltons; the commercial product contains 3% to 15% heparin with a molecular weight <3000 daltons, 65% to 78% with a molecular weight of 3000-8000 daltons and 14% to 26% with a molecular weight >8000 daltons; while dalteparin has been shown to inhibit both factor Xa and factor IIa (thrombin), the antithrombotic effect of dalteparin is characterized by a higher ratio of antifactor Xa to antifactor IIa activity (ratio = 4)

Other Adverse Effects

1% to 10%

Hematologic: Wound hematoma (0.1% to 3%), bleeding (3% to 5%)

Local: Pain at injection site (up to 12%), injection site hematoma (0.2% to 7%)

<1% (Limited to important or life-threatening): Thrombocytopenia (including heparin-induced thrombocytopenia), **allergic reaction (fever,** pruritus, rash, injections site reaction, bullous eruption), **anaphylactoid reaction,** operative site bleeding, **GI bleeding,** skin necrosis

Spinal or epidural hematomas can occur following neuraxial anesthesia or spinal puncture, resulting in paralysis. Risk is increased in patients with indwelling epidural catheters or concomitant use of other drugs affecting hemostasis.

Drug Interactions Increased Effect/Toxicity: The risk of bleeding with dalteparin may be increased by drugs which affect platelet function (eg, aspirin, NSAIDs, dipyridamole, ticlopidine, clopidogrel), oral anticoagulants, and thrombolytic agents. Although the risk of bleeding may be increased during concurrent warfarin therapy, dalteparin is commonly continued during the initiation of warfarin therapy to assure anticoagulation and to protect against possible transient hypercoagulability.

Dietary/Ethanol/Herb Considerations

Food: Avoid garlic, ginger, and green tea.

Herb/Nutraceutical: Avoid cat's claw, dong quai, evening primrose, feverfew, garlic, ginger, ginkgo biloba, ginseng, horse chestnut, and red clover due to additional antiplatelet activity.

Pharmacodynamics/Kinetics

Onset of action: 1-2 hours

Duration: >12 hours

Half-life elimination (route dependent): 2-5 hours

Time to peak, serum: 4 hours

Pregnancy Risk Factor B

Generic Available No

Damason-P® *see* Hydrocodone and Aspirin *on page 680*

Danaparoid (da NAP a roid)

U.S. Brand Names Orgaran® [DSC]

Canadian Brand Names Orgaran®

Pharmacologic Category Anticoagulant

Synonyms Danaparoid Sodium; Orgaran® [DSC]

Use Prevention of postoperative deep vein thrombosis following elective hip replacement surgery

Unlabeled/Investigational Use Systemic anticoagulation for patients with heparin-induced thrombocytopenia: factor Xa inhibition is used to monitor degree of anticoagulation if necessary

Local Anesthetic/Vasoconstrictor Precautions No information available to require special precautions

Effects on Dental Treatment As with all anticoagulants, bleeding is the major adverse effect of danaparoid. Hemorrhage may occur at virtually any site; risk is dependent on multiple variables.

>10%: Fever (22%), nausea (4% to 14%)

1% to 10%: Headache (3%), asthenia (2%), dizziness (2%), pain (9%), vomiting (3%), infection (2%)

Dosage S.C.:

Children: Safety and effectiveness have not been established.

Adults:

Prevention of DVT following hip replacement: S.C.: 750 anti-Xa units twice daily; beginning 1-4 hours before surgery and then not sooner than 2 hours after surgery and every 12 hours until the risk of DVT has diminished. The average duration of therapy is 7-10 days.

Adults: Treatment (unlabeled uses): Based on diagnosis/indication: See table on next page.

Dosing adjustment in elderly and severe renal impairment: Adjustment may be necessary. Patients with serum creatinine levels ≥2.0 mg/dL should be carefully monitored.

Hemodialysis: See table on next page.

(Continued)

Adult Danaparoid Treatment Dosing Regimens (Not FDA Approved)

	Body Weight (kg)	I.V. Bolus aFXaU	Long-Term Infusion aFXaU	Level of aFXaU/mL	Monitoring
Deep Vein Thrombosis OR Acute Pulmonary Embolism	<55 55-90 >90	1250 2500 3750	400 units/h over 4 h then 300 units/h over 4 h, then 150-200 units/h maintenance dose	0.5-0.8	Days 1-3 daily, then every alternate day
Deep Vein Thrombosis OR Pulmonary Embolism >5 d old	<90 >90	1250 1250	S.C.: 3 x 750/d S.C.: 3 x 1250/d	<0.5	Not necessary
Embolectomy	<90 >90 and high risk	2500 preoperatively 2500 preoperatively	S.C.: 2 x 1250/d postoperatively 150-200 units/hour I.V.; perioperative arterial irrigation, if necessary: 750 units/20 mL NaCl	<0.4 0.5-0.8	Not necessary Days 1-3 daily, then every alternate day
Peripheral Arterial Bypass		2500 preoperatively	150-200 units/h	0.5-0.8	Days 1-3 daily, then every alternate day
Cardiac Catheter	<90 >90	2500 preoperatively 3750 preoperatively			
Surgery (excluding vascular)			S.C.: 750, 1-4 h preoperatively S.C.: 750, 2-5 h postoperatively, then 2 x 750/d	<0.35	Not necessary

Hemodialysis With Danaparoid Sodium

Dialysis on alternate days	Dosage prior to dialysis in aFXaU (dosage for body wt <55 kg)	
First dialysis	3750 (<55 kg 2500)	
Second dialysis	3750 (<55 kg 2000)	
Further dialysis:		
aFXa level before dialysis (eg, day 5)	**Bolus before next dialysis, aFXaU (eg, day 7)**	**aFXa level during dialysis**
<0.3	3000 (<55 kg 2000)	0.5-0.8
0.3-0.35	2500 (<55 kg 2000)	
0.35-0.4	2000 (<55 kg 1500)	
>0.4	No bolus; if fibrin strands occur, 1500 aFXaU I.V.	
Monitoring: 30 minutes before dialysis and after 4 hours of dialysis		
Daily Dialysis		
First dialysis	3750 (<55 kg 2500)	
Second dialysis	2500 (<55 kg 2000)	
Further dialyses	See above	
As with "dialysis on alternate days", always take the aFXa activity preceding the previous dialysis as a basis for the current dosage.		

Mechanism of Action Prevents fibrin formation in coagulation pathway via thrombin generation inhibition by anti-Xa and anti-IIa effects.

Other Adverse Effects

>10%: Gastrointestinal: Constipation (4% to 11%)

1% to 10%:

Cardiovascular: Peripheral edema (3%), edema (3%)
Central nervous system: Insomnia (3%)
Dermatologic: Rash (2% to 5%), pruritus (4%)
Genitourinary: Urinary tract infection (3% to 4%), urinary retention (2%)
Hematologic: Anemia (2%)
Local: Injection site pain (8% to 14%), injection site hematoma (5%)

Neuromuscular & skeletal: Joint disorder (3%)

<1% (Limited to important or life-threatening): Spinal or epidural hematomas can occur following neuraxial anesthesia or spinal puncture, resulting in paralysis. Risk is increased in patients with indwelling epidural catheters or concomitant use of other drugs affecting hemostasis, thrombocytopenia, hyperkalemia, wound infection, skin rash, allergic reaction.

Drug Interactions Increased Effect/Toxicity: The risk of hemorrhage associated with danaparoid may be increased with thrombolytic agents, oral anticoagulants (warfarin) and drugs which affect platelet function (eg, aspirin, NSAIDs, dipyridamole, ticlopidine, clopidogrel).

Dietary/Ethanol/Herb Considerations

Food: Avoid garlic, ginger, and green tea.

Herb/Nutraceutical: Avoid cat's claw, dong quai, evening primrose, feverfew, garlic, ginger, ginkgo biloba, ginseng, green tea, horse chestnut, and red clover due to additional antiplatelet activity.

Pharmacodynamics/Kinetics

Onset of action: Peak effect: S.C.: Maximum antifactor Xa and antithrombin (antifactor IIa) activities occur in 2-5 hours

Half-life elimination, plasma: Mean: Terminal: ~24 hours

Excretion: Primarily urine

Pregnancy Risk Factor B

Generic Available No

Danaparoid Sodium *see* Danaparoid *on page 395*

Danazol (DA na zole)

U.S. Brand Names Danocrine®

Canadian Brand Names Cyclomen®; Danocrine®

Mexican Brand Names Ladogal®; Norciden®; Zoldan-A

Pharmacologic Category Androgen

Use Treatment of endometriosis, fibrocystic breast disease, and hereditary angioedema

Local Anesthetic/Vasoconstrictor Precautions No information available to require special precautions

Effects on Dental Treatment Frequency not defined: Flushing, hypertension, dizziness, fainting, headache, nervousness, tremor, gastroenteritis, nausea, vomiting, muscle cramps, neck pain, paresthesias, spasms, weakness, visual disturbances, hoarseness, sore throat, diaphoresis; joint lockup, swelling, or pain

Dosage Adults: Oral:

Female: Endometriosis: Initial: 200-400 mg/day in 2 divided doses for mild disease; individualize dosage. Usual maintenance dose: 800 mg/day in 2 divided doses to achieve amenorrhea and rapid response to painful symptoms. Continue therapy uninterrupted for 3-6 months (up to 9 months).

Female: Fibrocystic breast disease: Range: 100-400 mg/day in 2 divided doses

Male/Female: Hereditary angioedema: Initial: 200 mg 2-3 times/day; after favorable response, decrease the dosage by 50% or less at intervals of 1-3 months or longer if the frequency of attacks dictates. If an attack occurs, increase the dosage by up to 200 mg/day.

Mechanism of Action Suppresses pituitary output of follicle-stimulating hormone and luteinizing hormone that causes regression and atrophy of normal and ectopic endometrial tissue; decreases rate of growth of abnormal breast tissue; reduces attacks associated with hereditary angioedema by increasing levels of C4 component of complement

Other Adverse Effects Frequency not defined:

Cardiovascular: Benign intracranial hypertension (rare), edema

Central nervous system: **Anxiety (rare)**, chills (rare), **convulsions (rare)**, depression, emotional lability, **fever (rare)**, Guillain-Barré syndrome, sleep disorders

Dermatologic: Acne, hair loss, mild hirsutism, maculopapular rash, papular rash, petechial rash, pruritus, purpuric rash, seborrhea, Stevens-Johnson syndrome (rare), photosensitivity (rare), urticaria, vesicular rash

Endocrine & metabolic: Amenorrhea (which may continue post therapy), breast size reduction, clitoris hypertrophy, glucose intolerance, HDL decreased, LDL increased, libido changes, nipple discharge, menstrual disturbances (spotting, altered timing of cycle), semen abnormalities (changes in volume, viscosity, sperm count/motility), spermatogenesis reduction

Gastrointestinal: Appetite changes (rare), **bleeding gums (rare)**, constipation, pancreatitis (rare), weight gain

Genitourinary: Vaginal dryness, vaginal irritation, pelvic pain

Hematologic: Eosinophilia, erythrocytosis (reversible), leukocytosis, leukopenia, platelet count increased, polycythemia, RBC increased, thrombocytopenia

Hepatic: Cholestatic jaundice, hepatic adenoma, jaundice, liver enzymes (elevated), malignant tumors (after prolonged use), peliosis hepatis

Neuromuscular & skeletal: Back pain, carpal tunnel syndrome (rare), extremity pain

Ocular: Cataracts (rare)

Renal: Hematuria

(Continued)

Danazol *(Continued)*

Respiratory: **Nasal congestion (rare)**
Miscellaneous: Voice change or instability (deepening of pitch)

Drug Interactions Inhibits CYP3A4

Increased Effect/Toxicity: Danazol may increase serum levels of carbamazepine, cyclosporine, tacrolimus, and warfarin leading to toxicity; dosage adjustment may be needed; monitor. Concomitant use of danazol and HMG-CoA reductase inhibitors may lead to severe myopathy or rhabdomyolysis. Danazol may enhance the glucose-lowering effect of hypoglycemic agents.

Decreased Effect: Danazol may decrease effectiveness of hormonal contraceptives. Nonhormonal birth control methods are recommended.

Dietary/Ethanol/Herb Considerations Food delays time to peak serum concentration; high-fat meals increase plasma concentration.

Pharmacodynamics/Kinetics

Onset of action: Therapeutic: ~4 weeks
Metabolism: Extensively hepatic, primarily to 2-hydroxymethylethisterone
Half-life elimination: 4.5 hours (variable)
Time to peak, serum: Within 2 hours
Excretion: Urine

Pregnancy Risk Factor X

Generic Available Yes

Danocrine® *see* Danazol *on page 397*
Dantrium® *see* Dantrolene *on page 398*

Dantrolene (DAN troe leen)

U.S. Brand Names Dantrium®

Canadian Brand Names Dantrium®

Pharmacologic Category Skeletal Muscle Relaxant

Synonyms Dantrolene Sodium

Use Treatment of spasticity associated with spinal cord injury, stroke, cerebral palsy, or multiple sclerosis; treatment of malignant hyperthermia

Unlabeled/Investigational Use Treatment of neuroleptic malignant syndrome (NMS)

Local Anesthetic/Vasoconstrictor Precautions No information available to require special precautions

Effects on Dental Treatment

>10%: Drowsiness, dizziness, lightheadedness, nausea, vomiting, weakness, fatigue

1% to 10%: Fever, headache, nervousness, respiratory depression, blurred vision

Dosage

Spasticity: Oral:

Children: Initial: 0.5 mg/kg/dose twice daily, increase frequency to 3-4 times/day at 4- to 7-day intervals, then increase dose by 0.5 mg/kg to a maximum of 3 mg/kg/dose 2-4 times/day up to 400 mg/day

Adults: 25 mg/day to start, increase frequency to 2-4 times/day, then increase dose by 25 mg every 4-7 days to a maximum of 100 mg 2-4 times/day or 400 mg/day

Malignant hyperthermia: Children and Adults:

Preoperative prophylaxis:

Oral: 4-8 mg/kg/day in 4 divided doses, begin 1-2 days prior to surgery with last dose 3-4 hours prior to surgery

I.V.: 2.5 mg/kg ~1¼ hours prior to anesthesia and infused over 1 hour with additional doses as needed and individualized

Crisis: I.V.: 2.5 mg/kg; may repeat dose up to cumulative dose of 10 mg/kg; if physiologic and metabolic abnormalities reappear, repeat regimen

Postcrisis follow-up: Oral: 4-8 mg/kg/day in 4 divided doses for 1-3 days; I.V. dantrolene may be used when oral therapy is not practical; individualize dosage beginning with 1 mg/kg or more as the clinical situation dictates

Neuroleptic malignant syndrome (unlabeled use): I.V.: 1 mg/kg; may repeat dose up to maximum cumulative dose of 10 mg/kg, then switch to oral dosage

Mechanism of Action Acts directly on skeletal muscle by interfering with release of calcium ion from the sarcoplasmic reticulum; prevents or reduces the increase in myoplasmic calcium ion concentration that activates the acute catabolic processes associated with malignant hyperthermia

Other Adverse Effects

>10%:

Dermatologic: Rash
Gastrointestinal: Diarrhea (mild)

1% to 10%:

Cardiovascular: Pleural effusion with pericarditis
Central nervous system: Chills, insomnia, mental depression
Gastrointestinal: Diarrhea (severe), constipation, anorexia, stomach cramps

<1%: **Seizures, confusion**, hepatitis, hepatic necrosis

Drug Interactions Substrate of **CYP3A4**

Increased Effect/Toxicity: Increased toxicity with estrogens (hepatotoxicity), CNS depressants (sedation), MAO inhibitors, phenothiazines, clindamycin (increased neuromuscular blockade), verapamil (hyperkalemia and cardiac depression), warfarin, clofibrate, and tolbutamide.

Dietary/Ethanol/Herb Considerations

Ethanol: Avoid use; may increase CNS depression.

Herb/Nutraceutical: Avoid gotu kola, kava, SAMe, St John's wort, and valerian; may increase CNS depression.

Pharmacodynamics/Kinetics

Absorption: Oral: Slow and incomplete

Metabolism: Hepatic

Half-life elimination: 8.7 hours

Excretion: Feces (45% to 50%); urine (25% as unchanged drug and metabolites)

Pregnancy Risk Factor C

Generic Available No

Dantrolene Sodium *see* Dantrolene *on page 398*

Dapiprazole (DA pi pray zole)

U.S. Brand Names Rēv-Eyes™

Pharmacologic Category Alpha$_1$ Blocker, Ophthalmic

Synonyms Dapiprazole Hydrochloride

Use Reverse dilation due to drugs (adrenergic or parasympathomimetic) after eye exams

Local Anesthetic/Vasoconstrictor Precautions No information available to require special precautions

Effects on Dental Treatment

>10%: Headache

1% to 10%: Blurred vision

Dosage Adults: Ophthalmic: Instill 2 drops followed 5 minutes later by an additional 2 drops into the conjunctiva of each eye; should not be used more frequently than once a week in the same patient

Mechanism of Action Dapiprazole is a selective alpha-adrenergic blocking agent, exerting effects primarily on alpha$_1$-adrenoreceptors. It induces miosis via relaxation of the smooth dilator (radial) muscle of the iris, which causes pupillary constriction. It is devoid of cholinergic effects. Dapiprazole also partially reverses the cycloplegia induced with parasympatholytic agents such as tropicamide. Although the drug has no significant effect on the ciliary muscle *per se*, it may increase accommodative amplitude, therefore relieving the symptoms of paralysis of accommodation.

Other Adverse Effects Ocular:

>10%: Conjunctival injection, burning and itching eyes, lid edema, ptosis, lid erythema, chemosis, punctate keratitis, corneal edema, photophobia

1% to 10%: Dry eyes, tearing of eye

Pregnancy Risk Factor B

Generic Available No

Dapiprazole Hydrochloride *see* Dapiprazole *on page 399*

Dapsone (DAP sone)

Related Information

HIV Infection and AIDS *on page 1482*

Mexican Brand Names Dapsoderm-X®

Pharmacologic Category Antibiotic, Miscellaneous

Synonyms Diaminodiphenylsulfone

Use Treatment of leprosy and dermatitis herpetiformis (infections caused by *Mycobacterium leprae*); prophylaxis of toxoplasmosis in severely immunocompromised patients; alternative agent for *Pneumocystis carinii* pneumonia prophylaxis (given alone) and treatment (given with trimethoprim); may be useful in relapsing polychondritis, prophylaxis of malaria, inflammatory bowel disorders, leishmaniasis, rheumatic/connective tissue disorders, brown recluse spider bites

Unlabeled/Investigational Use May be useful in relapsing polychondritis, prophylaxis of malaria, inflammatory bowel disorders, leishmaniasis, rheumatic/connective tissue disorders, brown recluse spider bites

Local Anesthetic/Vasoconstrictor Precautions No information available to require special precautions

Effects on Dental Treatment No significant effects or complications reported

Dosage Oral:

Leprosy:

Children: 1-2 mg/kg/24 hours, up to a maximum of 100 mg/day

Adults: 50-100 mg/day for 3-10 years

Dermatitis herpetiformis: Adults: Start at 50 mg/day, increase to 300 mg/day, or higher to achieve full control, reduce dosage to minimum level as soon as possible

(Continued)

Dapsone *(Continued)*

Pneumocystis carinii pneumonia:

Prophylaxis:

Children >1 month: 2 mg/kg/day once daily (maximum dose: 100 mg/day) or 4 mg/kg/dose once weekly (maximum dose: 200 mg)

Adults: 100 mg/day

Treatment: Adults: 100 mg/day in combination with trimethoprim (15-20 mg/kg/day) for 21 days

Dosing in renal impairment: No specific guidelines are available

Mechanism of Action Competitive antagonist of para-aminobenzoic acid (PABA) and prevents normal bacterial utilization of PABA for the synthesis of folic acid

Other Adverse Effects

1% to 10%: Hematologic: Hemolysis, methemoglobinemia

<1%: Reactional states (ie, abrupt changes in clinical activity occurring during any leprosy treatment; classified as reversal of erythema nodosum leprosum reactions); insomnia, headache, exfoliative dermatitis, photosensitivity, nausea, vomiting, anemia, leukopenia, agranulocytosis, hepatitis, cholestatic jaundice, peripheral neuropathy (usually in nonleprosy patients), **blurred vision,** tinnitus, SLE

Drug Interactions Substrate of CYP2C8/9, 2C19, 2E1, **3A4**

Increased Effect/Toxicity: Folic acid antagonists (methotrexate) may increase the risk of hematologic reactions of dapsone; probenecid decreases dapsone excretion; trimethoprim with dapsone may increase toxic effects of both drugs Dapsone levels may be increased by protease inhibitors (amprenavir, nelfinavir, ritonavir).

Decreased Effect: Para-aminobenzoic acid and rifampin levels are decreased when given with dapsone.

Dietary/Ethanol/Herb Considerations

Food: Do not administer with alkaline foods; may decrease absorption.

Herb/Nutraceutical: Avoid St John's wort; may decrease serum concentration.

Pharmacodynamics/Kinetics

Absorption: Well absorbed

Distribution: V_d: 1.5 L/kg; throughout total body water and present in all tissues, especially liver and kidney

Metabolism: Hepatic

Half-life elimination: 30 hours (range: 10-50 hours)

Excretion: Urine

Pregnancy Risk Factor C

Generic Available Yes

Daranide® *see* Dichlorphenamide *on page 428*

Daraprim® *see* Pyrimethamine *on page 1152*

Darbepoetin Alfa (dar be POE e tin AL fu)

U.S. Brand Names Aranesp™

Canadian Brand Names Aranesp™

Pharmacologic Category Colony Stimulating Factor; Growth Factor; Recombinant Human Erythropoietin

Synonyms Erythropoiesis Stimulating Protein

Use Treatment of anemia associated with chronic renal failure (CRF), including patients on dialysis (ESRD) and patients not on dialysis; anemia associated with chemotherapy for nonmyeloid malignancies

Local Anesthetic/Vasoconstrictor Precautions No information available to require special precautions

Effects on Dental Treatment

>10%: Hypertension (4% to 23%), hypotension (22%), edema (21%), arrhythmia (10%), fever (9% to 19%), headache (12% to 16%), dizziness (8% to 14%), vomiting (15%), nausea (14%), upper respiratory infection (14%), dyspnea (12%), cough (10%), infection (27%)

1% to 10%: Limb pain (10%), angina/chest pain (6% to 8%), CHF (6%), MI (2%), seizure (1%), stroke (1%), dehydration (5%), weakness (5%), bronchitis (6%), influenza-like symptoms

Dosage

I.V., S.C.: Correction of anemia associated with CRF:

Initial: 0.45 mcg/kg once weekly; dosage should be titrated to limit increases in hemoglobin to <1 g/dL over any 2-week interval, with a target concentration of <12 g/dL.

Maintenance: Titrated to hematologic response. Some patients may require doses <0.45 mcg/kg once weekly. Selected patients may be managed by administering S.C. doses every 2 weeks.

Conversion from epoetin alfa to darbepoetin alfa: Initial: Estimate dosage based on weekly epoetin alfa dosage; see table on next page.

Dosing adjustment: Goal: Dose should be adjusted to achieve and maintain a target hemoglobin not to exceed 12 g/dL.

Conversion From Epoetin Alfa to Darbepoetin Alfa

Previous Dosage of Epoetin Alfa (units/week)	Darbepoetin Alfa Dosage (mcg/week)
<2500	6.25
2500-4999	12.5
5000-10,999	25
11,000-17,999	40
18,000-33,999	60
34,000-89,999	100
≥90,000	200

Note: In patients receiving epoetin alfa 2-3 times per week, darbepoetin alfa is administered once weekly. In patients receiving epoetin alfa once weekly, darbepoetin alfa is administered once every 2 weeks.

Inadequate response: Hemoglobin increases <1 g/dL over 4 weeks and iron stores are adequate: Increase by ~25% of the previous dose; increases should not be made more frequently than once monthly.

Excessive response:

Hemoglobin increases >1 g/dL in any 2-week period: Decrease dose

Hemoglobin increases and approaches the target value of 12 g/dL: Decrease weekly dosage by ~25%. If hemoglobin continues to increase, hold dose temporarily until hemoglobin begins to decrease, then restart at a dose 25% below the previous dose.

S.C.: Correction of anemia associated with cancer patients receiving chemotherapy: Initial: 2.25 mcg/kg once weekly; adjust dose as follows to achieve and maintain a target hemoglobin:

Inadequate response: Hemoglobin increases <1 g/dL after 6 weeks of therapy: Increase dose to 4.5 mcg/kg

Excessive responses:

Hemoglobin increases >1 g/dL in a 2-week period **OR** if hemoglobin exceeds 12 g/dL: Reduce dose by 25%

Hemoglobin >13 g/dL: Withhold dose until hemoglobin falls to 12 g/dL, then reinitiate at 25% less than previous dose.

Dosing adjustment in renal impairment: Dosage requirements for patients with chronic renal failure who do not require dialysis may be lower than in dialysis patients. Monitor patients closely during the time period in which a dialysis regimen is initiated, dosage requirement may increase.

Mechanism of Action Induces erythropoiesis by stimulating the division and differentiation of committed erythroid progenitor cells; induces the release of reticulocytes from the bone marrow into the bloodstream, where they mature to erythrocytes. There is a dose response relationship with this effect. This results in an increase in reticulocyte counts followed by a rise in hematocrit and hemoglobin levels. When administered S.C. or I.V., darbepoetin's half-life is ~3 times that of epoetin alfa concentrations.

Other Adverse Effects Frequency in patients with CRF or cancer may be, in part, a reflection of population in which the drug is used and/or associated with dialysis procedures.

>10%:

Cardiovascular: Edema (21%), peripheral edema (11%)

Central nervous system: Fatigue (9% to 33%)

Gastrointestinal: Diarrhea (16% to 22%), constipation (5% to 18%), abdominal pain (12%)

Neuromuscular & skeletal: Myalgia (21%), arthralgia (11% to 13%)

1% to 10%:

Cardiovascular: Fluid overload (6%), thrombosis (6%)

Central nervous system: TIA (1%)

Dermatologic: Pruritus (8%), rash (7%)

Local: Injection site pain (7%)

Neuromuscular & skeletal: Back pain (8%)

Respiratory: Bronchitis (6%), pulmonary embolism (1%)

Miscellaneous: Vascular access thrombosis (8%, annualized rate 0.22 events per patient year), vascular access infection (6%), (6%), vascular access hemorrhage (6%)

Dietary/Ethanol/Herb Considerations Ethanol: Avoid use due to adverse effects on erythropoiesis.

Pharmacodynamics/Kinetics

Onset of action: Increased hemoglobin levels not generally observed until 2-6 weeks after initiating treatment

Absorption: S.C.: Slow

Distribution: V_d: 0.06 L/kg

Bioavailability: CRF: S.C.: ~37% (range: 30% to 50%)

(Continued)

Darbepoetin Alfa *(Continued)*

Half-life elimination: CRF: Terminal: I.V.: 21 hours, S.C.: 49 hours; **Note:** Half-life is ~3 times as long as epoetin alfa

Time to peak: S.C.: CRF: 34 hours (range: 24-72 hours); Cancer: 90 hours (range: 71-123 hours)

Pregnancy Risk Factor C

Generic Available No

Darvocet-N® 50 *see* Propoxyphene and Acetaminophen *on page 1136*

Darvocet-N® 100 *see* Propoxyphene and Acetaminophen *on page 1136*

Darvon® *see* Propoxyphene *on page 1135*

Darvon® Compound-65 Pulvules® *see* Propoxyphene and Aspirin *on page 1137*

Darvon-N® *see* Propoxyphene *on page 1135*

Daunomycin *see* DAUNOrubicin Hydrochloride *on page 402*

DAUNOrubicin Citrate (Liposomal)

(daw noe ROO bi sin SI trate li pu SOE mol)

U.S. Brand Names DaunoXome®

Pharmacologic Category Antineoplastic Agent, Anthracycline

Use First-line cytotoxic therapy for advanced HIV-associated Kaposi's sarcoma

Local Anesthetic/Vasoconstrictor Precautions No information available to require special precautions

Effects on Dental Treatment

>10%: Headache (28%), vomiting, nausea (55%), cough (28%), dyspnea (26%), rhinitis, allergic reactions (24%), fatigue (51%)

1% to 10%: Hypertension, palpitations, syncope, tachycardia, chest pain, hot flashes, stomatitis (10%), sinusitis

Dosage Refer to individual protocols. Adults: I.V.:

20-40 mg/m² every 2 weeks

100 mg/m² every 3 weeks

Dosing adjustment in renal impairment: Serum creatinine >3 mg/dL: Administer 50% of normal dose

Dosing adjustment in hepatic impairment:

Bilirubin 1.2-3 mg/dL: Administer 75% of normal dose

Bilirubin >3 mg/dL: Administer 50% of normal dose

Mechanism of Action Liposomes have been shown to penetrate solid tumors more effectively, possibly because of their small size and longer circulation time. Once in tissues, daunorubicin is released. Daunorubicin inhibits DNA and RNA synthesis by intercalation between DNA base pairs and by steric obstruction; and intercalates at points of local uncoiling of the double helix. Although the exact mechanism is unclear, it appears that direct binding to DNA (intercalation) and inhibition of DNA repair (topoisomerase II inhibition) result in blockade of DNA and RNA synthesis and fragmentation of DNA.

Other Adverse Effects

>10%:

Central nervous system: Neuropathy (13%)

Hematologic: Myelosuppression, neutropenia (51%), thrombocytopenia, anemia

Onset: 7 days

Nadir: 14 days

Recovery: 21 days

Gastrointestinal: Abdominal pain, anorexia (23%), diarrhea (38%)

1% to 10%:

Cardiovascular: Edema

Dermatologic: Alopecia (8%), pruritus (7%)

Gastrointestinal: Constipation (7%)

Neuromuscular & skeletal: Arthralgia (7%), myalgia (7%)

Ocular: Conjunctivitis, eye pain (5%)

Drug Interactions Decreased Effect: Patients may experience impaired immune response to vaccines; possible infection after administration of live vaccines in patients receiving immunosuppressants.

Dietary/Ethanol/Herb Considerations Ethanol: Avoid use due to GI irritation.

Pharmacodynamics/Kinetics

Distribution: V_d: 3-6.4 L

Metabolism: Similar to daunorubicin, but metabolite plasma levels are low

Half-life elimination: Distribution: 4.4 hours; Terminal: 3-5 hours

Excretion: Primarily feces; some urine

Clearance, plasma: 17.3 mL/minute

Pregnancy Risk Factor D

Generic Available No

DAUNOrubicin Hydrochloride

(do noe ROO bi sin hye droe KLOR ide)

U.S. Brand Names Cerubidine®

Canadian Brand Names Cerubidine®

Mexican Brand Names Rubilem®; Trixilem

Pharmacologic Category Antineoplastic Agent, Anthracycline

Synonyms Daunomycin; DNR; Rubidomycin Hydrochloride

Use Treatment of acute lymphocytic (ALL) and nonlymphocytic (ANLL) leukemias

Local Anesthetic/Vasoconstrictor Precautions No information available to require special precautions

Effects on Dental Treatment

>10%: Mild nausea or vomiting, stomatitis

1% to 10%: Discoloration of saliva, sweat, or tears; GI ulceration

Dosage I.V. (refer to individual protocols):

Children:

ALL combination therapy: Remission induction: 25-45 mg/m^2 on day 1 every week for 4 cycles **or** 30-45 mg/m^2/day for 3 days

AML combination therapy: Induction: I.V. continuous infusion: 30-60 mg/m^2/day on days 1-3 of cycle

In children <2 years or <0.5 m^2, daunorubicin should be based on weight - mg/kg: 1 mg/kg per protocol with frequency dependent on regimen employed. Cumulative dose should not exceed 300 mg/m^2 in children >2 years or 10 mg/kg in children <2 years.

Adults:

Range: 30-60 mg/m^2/day for 3-5 days, repeat dose in 3-4 weeks

AML: Single agent induction: 60 mg/m^2/day for 3 days; repeat every 3-4 weeks

AML: Combination therapy induction: 45 mg/m^2/day for 3 days of the first course of induction therapy; subsequent courses: Every day for 2 days

ALL combination therapy: 45 mg/m^2/day for 3 days

Cumulative dose should not exceed 400-600 mg/m^2.

Dosing adjustment in renal impairment:

Cl_{cr} <10 mL/minute: Administer 75% of normal dose

Cl_{cr} >3 mg/dL: Administer 50% of normal dose

Dosing adjustment in hepatic impairment:

Serum bilirubin 1.2-3 mg/dL or AST 60-180 int. units: Reduce dose to 75%

Serum bilirubin 3.1-5 mg/dL or AST >180 int. units: Reduce dose to 50%

Serum bilirubin >5 mg/dL: Omit use

Mechanism of Action Inhibition of DNA and RNA synthesis, by intercalating between DNA base pairs and by steric obstruction; is not cell cycle-specific for the S phase of cell division; daunomycin is preferred over doxorubicin for the treatment of ANLL because of its dose-limiting toxicity (myelosuppression) is not of concern in the therapy of this disease; has less mucositis associated with its use

Other Adverse Effects

>10%:

Cardiovascular: Transient EKG abnormalities (supraventricular tachycardia, S-T wave changes, atrial or ventricular extrasystoles; generally asymptomatic and self-limiting), CHF (dose-related, may be delayed for 7-8 years after treatment; cumulative dose, radiation therapy, age, and use of cyclophosphamide increase risk)

Dermatologic: Alopecia, radiation recall

Genitourinary: Discoloration of urine (red)

Hematologic: Myelosuppression (primarily leukopenia), thrombocytopenia, anemia

Onset: 7 days

Nadir: 10-14 days

Recovery: 21-28 days

1% to 10%:

Dermatologic: Skin "flare" at injection site

Endocrine & metabolic: Hyperuricemia

Gastrointestinal: Diarrhea

<1%: Systemic hypersensitivity (including urticaria, pruritus, angioedema, dysphagia, dyspnea), pericarditis, myocarditis, MI, skin rash, pigmentation of nail beds, nail banding, onycholysis, infertility, sterility, elevated bilirubin and transaminases, hepatitis

Drug Interactions Decreased Effect: Patients may experience impaired immune response to vaccines; possible infection after administration of live vaccines in patients receiving immunosuppressants.

Dietary/Ethanol/Herb Considerations Ethanol: Avoid use due to GI irritation.

Pharmacodynamics/Kinetics

Distribution: Many body tissues, particularly the liver, kidneys, lung, spleen, and heart; not into CNS; crosses placenta; V_d: 40 L/kg

Metabolism: Primarily hepatic to daunorubicinol (active), then to inactive aglycones, conjugated sulfates, and glucuronides

Half-life elimination: Distribution: 2 minutes; Elimination: 14-20 hours; Terminal: 18.5 hours; Daunorubicinol plasma half-life: 24-48 hours

Excretion: Feces (40%); urine (~25% as unchanged drug and metabolites)

Pregnancy Risk Factor D

Generic Available Yes

DaunoXome® *see* DAUNOrubicin Citrate (Liposomal) *on page 402*
1-Day™ [OTC] *see* Tioconazole *on page 1312*
Daypro® *see* Oxaprozin *on page 1010*
DCF *see* Pentostatin *on page 1057*
DDAVP® *see* Desmopressin *on page 410*
ddC *see* Zalcitabine *on page 1403*
ddI *see* Didanosine *on page 434*
1-Deamino-8-D-Arginine Vasopressin *see* Desmopressin *on page 410*
Debacterol® *see* Sulfonated Phenolics in Aqueous Solution *on page 1257*
Debrox® Otic [OTC] *see* Carbamide Peroxide *on page 244*
Decadron® *see* Dexamethasone *on page 413*
Decadron® Phosphate *see* Dexamethasone *on page 413*
Deca-Durabolin® [DSC] *see* Nandrolone *on page 951*
Declomycin® *see* Demeclocycline *on page 406*
Decofed® [OTC] *see* Pseudoephedrine *on page 1146*
Decohistine® DH *see* Chlorpheniramine, Pseudoephedrine, and Codeine *on page 311*
Deconamine® [OTC] *see* Chlorpheniramine and Pseudoephedrine *on page 308*
Deconamine® SR [OTC] *see* Chlorpheniramine and Pseudoephedrine *on page 308*
Deconsal® II *see* Guaifenesin and Pseudoephedrine *on page 652*
Defen-LA® *see* Guaifenesin and Pseudoephedrine *on page 652*

Deferoxamine (de fer OKS a meen)

U.S. Brand Names Desferal®

Canadian Brand Names Desferal®; PMS-Deferoxamine

Pharmacologic Category Antidote

Synonyms Deferoxamine Mesylate

Use Acute iron intoxication when serum iron is >450-500 µg/dL or when clinical signs of significant iron toxicity exist; chronic iron overload secondary to multiple transfusions; diagnostic test for iron overload; iron overload secondary to congenital anemias; hemochromatosis; removal of corneal rust rings following surgical removal of foreign bodies

Unlabeled/Investigational Use Investigational: Treatment of aluminum accumulation in renal failure, aluminum-induced bone disease

Local Anesthetic/Vasoconstrictor Precautions No information available to require special precautions

Effects on Dental Treatment Frequency not defined: Flushing, hypotension, tachycardia, shock, convulsions, fever, dizziness, paresthesia, seizures, headache, CNS depression, coma, agitation, leg cramps, blurred vision, impaired vision, acute respiratory distress syndrome (with dyspnea, cyanosis), anaphylaxis

Dosage

Children and Adults:

Acute iron toxicity: I.V. route is used when severe toxicity is evidenced by systemic symptoms (coma, shock, metabolic acidosis, or severe GI bleeding) or potentially severe intoxications (serum iron level >500 µg/dL). When severe symptoms are not present, the I.M. route may be preferred; however, the use of deferoxamine in situations where the serum iron concentration is <500 µg/dL or when severe toxicity is not evident is a subject of some clinical debate.

Dose: For the first 1000 mg, infuse at 15 mg/kg/hour (although rates up to 40-50 mg/kg/hour have been given in patients with massive iron intoxication); may be followed by 500 mg every 4 hours for up to 2 doses; subsequent doses of 500 mg have been administered every 4-12 hours

Maximum recommended dose: 6 g/day (however, doses as high as 16-37 g have been administered)

Children:

Chronic iron overload: S.C.: 20-40 mg/kg/day over 8-12 hours (via a portable, controlled infusion device)

Aluminum-induced bone disease: 20-40 mg/kg every hemodialysis treatment, frequency dependent on clinical status of the patient

Adults: Chronic iron overload:

I.M.: 500-1000 mg/day; in addition, 2000 mg should be given with each unit of blood transfused (administer separately from blood)

I.V.: 2 g after each unit of blood infusion at 15 mg/kg/hour

S.C.: 1-2 g every day over 8-24 hours

Dosing adjustment in renal impairment: Cl_{cr} <10 mL/minute: Administer 50% of dose

Has been used investigationally as a single 40 mg/kg I.V. dose over 2 hours, to promote mobilization of aluminum from tissue stores as an aid in the diagnosis of aluminum-associated osteodystrophy

Mechanism of Action Complexes with trivalent ions (ferric ions) to form ferrioxamine, which are removed by the kidneys

Other Adverse Effects Frequency not defined:

Cardiovascular: Edema

Central nervous system: Neuropathy, exacerbation of aluminum-related encephalopathy (dialysis), aphasia

Dermatologic: Erythema, urticaria, pruritus, rash, cutaneous wheal formation

Endocrine & metabolic: Hypocalcemia

Gastrointestinal: Abdominal discomfort, diarrhea

Genitourinary: Dysuria

Hematologic: Thrombocytopenia, leukopenia

Local: Pain and induration at injection site

Ocular: Visual loss, scotoma, visual field defects, optic neuritis, cataracts, retinal pigmentary abnormalities

Otic: Hearing loss, tinnitus

Renal: Renal impairment, acute renal failure

Drug Interactions Increased Effect/Toxicity: May cause loss of consciousness when administered with prochlorperazine. Concomitant treatment with vitamin C (>500 mg/day) has been associated with cardiac impairment.

Pharmacodynamics/Kinetics

Absorption: Oral: <15%

Metabolism: Hepatic to ferrioxamine

Half-life elimination: Parent drug: 6.1 hours; Ferrioxamine: 5.8 hours

Excretion: Urine (as unchanged drug and metabolites)

Pregnancy Risk Factor C

Generic Available No

Deferoxamine Mesylate *see* Deferoxamine *on page 404*

Del Aqua® *see* Benzoyl Peroxide *on page 171*

Delatestryl® *see* Testosterone *on page 1281*

Delavirdine (de la VIR deen)

Related Information

HIV Infection and AIDS *on page 1482*

Tuberculosis *on page 1493*

U.S. Brand Names Rescriptor®

Canadian Brand Names Rescriptor®

Mexican Brand Names Rescriptor®

Pharmacologic Category Antiretroviral Agent, Reverse Transcriptase Inhibitor (Non-nucleoside)

Synonyms U-90152S

Use Treatment of HIV-1 infection in combination with at least two additional antiretroviral agents

Local Anesthetic/Vasoconstrictor Precautions No information available to require special precautions

Effects on Dental Treatment 1% to 10%: Headache, nausea, vomiting, fatigue

Dosage Adults: Oral: 400 mg 3 times/day

Mechanism of Action Delavirdine binds directly to reverse transcriptase, blocking RNA-dependent and DNA-dependent DNA polymerase activities

Other Adverse Effects

>10%: Dermatologic: Rash (3.2% required discontinuation)

1% to 10%:

- Dermatologic: Pruritus
- Gastrointestinal: Diarrhea
- Metabolic: Increased ALT (SGPT), increased AST (SGOT)

<1%: **Incoordination, ethanol intolerance, allergic reaction,** alopecia, anemia, angioedema, **bradycardia,** calculi of kidney, **chest pain, confusion,** dermal leukocytoblastic vasculitis, desquamation, **dyspnea, ecchymosis,** edema, eosinophilia, **epistaxis,** erythema multiforme, granulocytosis, **hallucinations,** hematuria, hemospermia, hyperkalemia, hyperuricemia, hypocalcemia, hyponatremia, hypophosphatemia, increased lipase, increased serum alkaline phosphatase, increased serum creatine phosphokinase, increased serum creatinine, kidney pain, **malaise, myalgia, neck rigidity,** neuropathy, neutropenia, nonspecific hepatitis, nystagmus, **palpitations,** pancytopenia, **paralysis, paranoid symptoms, postural hypotension,** proteinuria, Stevens-Johnson syndrome, **syncope, tachycardia,** thrombocytopenia, **vasodilation,** vertigo, vesiculobullous rash

Postmarketing and/or case reports: **Hepatic failure,** hemolytic anemia, rhabdomyolysis, **acute renal failure**

Drug Interactions Substrate of CYP2D6, **3A4**; Inhibits CYP1A2, 2C8/9, 2C19, 2D6, 3A4

Increased Effect/Toxicity: Delavirdine concentrations may be increased by clarithromycin, ketoconazole, and fluoxetine. Delavirdine increases plasma concentrations of alprazolam, amiodarone, amphetamines, amprenavir, astemizole,

(Continued)

Delavirdine *(Continued)*

bepridil, calcium channel blockers (dihydropyridine-type), cisapride, clarithromycin, dapsone, dexamethasone, ergot alkaloids, flecainide, HMG-CoA reductase inhibitors, indinavir, methadone, midazolam, pimozide, propafenone, quinidine, rifabutin, saquinavir, sildenafil, triazolam, and warfarin.

Decreased Effect: Decreased plasma concentrations of delavirdine with amprenavir, carbamazepine, dexamethasone, phenobarbital, phenytoin, rifabutin, rifampin, didanosine, and saquinavir. Decreased absorption of delavirdine with antacids, histamine-2 receptor antagonists, proton pump inhibitors (omeprazole, lansoprazole), and didanosine. Delavirdine decreases plasma concentrations of didanosine.

Dietary/Ethanol/Herb Considerations

Food: May be taken with food

Herb/Nutraceutical: Avoid St John's wort; may decrease serum concentration.

Pharmacodynamics/Kinetics

Absorption: Rapid

Distribution: Low concentration in saliva and semen; CSF 0.4% concurrent plasma concentration

Protein binding: ~98%, primarily albumin

Metabolism: Hepatic via CYP3A4 and 2D6 (**Note:** May reduce CYP3A activity and inhibit its own metabolism.)

Bioavailability: 85%

Half-life elimination: 2-11 hours

Time to peak, plasma: 1 hour

Excretion: Urine (51%, <5% as unchanged drug); feces (44%); nonlinear kinetics exhibited

Pregnancy Risk Factor C

Generic Available No

Delestrogen® *see* Estradiol *on page 521*

Delfen® [OTC] *see* Nonoxynol 9 *on page 985*

Delsym® [OTC] *see* Dextromethorphan *on page 423*

Delta-9-tetrahydro-cannabinol *see* Dronabinol *on page 480*

Delta-9 THC *see* Dronabinol *on page 480*

Deltacortisone *see* PredniSONE *on page 1112*

Delta-D® *see* Cholecalciferol *on page 317*

Deltadehydrocortisone *see* PredniSONE *on page 1112*

Deltahydrocortisone *see* PrednisoLONE *on page 1110*

Deltasone® *see* PredniSONE *on page 1112*

Demadex® *see* Torsemide *on page 1327*

Demeclocycline (dem e kloe SYE kleen)

U.S. Brand Names Declomycin®

Canadian Brand Names Declomycin®

Mexican Brand Names Ledermicina

Pharmacologic Category Antibiotic, Tetracycline Derivative

Synonyms Demeclocycline Hydrochloride; Demethylchlortetracycline

Use Treatment of susceptible bacterial infections (acne, gonorrhea, pertussis and urinary tract infections) caused by both gram-negative and gram-positive organisms; used when penicillin is contraindicated (other agents are preferred)

Unlabeled/Investigational Use Treatment of chronic syndrome of inappropriate secretion of antidiuretic hormone (SIADH)

Local Anesthetic/Vasoconstrictor Precautions No information available to require special precautions

Effects on Dental Treatment Tetracyclines are not recommended for use during pregnancy or in children ≤8 years of age since they have been reported to cause enamel hypoplasia and permanent teeth discoloration. The use of tetracyclines should only be used in these patients if other agents are contraindicated or alternative antimicrobials will not eradicate the organism. Long-term use associated with oral candidiasis.

1% to 10%: Nausea, diarrhea

Dosage Oral:

Children ≥8 years: 8-12 mg/kg/day divided every 6-12 hours

Adults: 150 mg 4 times/day or 300 mg twice daily

Uncomplicated gonorrhea (penicillin sensitive): 600 mg stat, 300 mg every 12 hours for 4 days (3 g total)

SIADH: 900-1200 mg/day or 13-15 mg/kg/day divided every 6-8 hours initially, then decrease to 600-900 mg/day

Dosing comments in renal/hepatic impairment: Should be avoided

Mechanism of Action Inhibits protein synthesis by binding with the 30S and possibly the 50S ribosomal subunit(s) of susceptible bacteria; may also cause alterations in the cytoplasmic membrane; inhibits the action of ADH in patients with chronic SIADH

Other Adverse Effects

1% to 10%: Dermatologic: Photosensitivity

<1%: Pericarditis, **increased intracranial pressure,** bulging fontanels in infants, dermatologic effects, pruritus, exfoliative dermatitis, **diabetes insipidus syndrome, vomiting, esophagitis,** anorexia, abdominal cramps, **paresthesia,** acute renal failure, azotemia, **superinfections, anaphylaxis,** pigmentation of nails

Drug Interactions

Increased Effect/Toxicity: Increased effect of warfarin, digoxin when taken with demeclocycline.

Decreased Effect: Decreased effect with antacids (aluminum, calcium, zinc, or magnesium), bismuth salts, sodium bicarbonate, barbiturates, carbamazepine, and hydantoins. Decreased effect of penicillins. Although anecdotal reports suggest oral contraceptive efficacy could be reduced by tetracyclines, this has been refuted by more rigorous scientific and clinical data.

Dietary/Ethanol/Herb Considerations

Food (especially dairy products) may decrease serum concentration; administer on an empty stomach.

Herb/Nutraceutical: Avoid dong quai and St John's wort; may cause photosensitization.

Pharmacodynamics/Kinetics

Onset of action: SIADH: Several days

Absorption: ~50% to 80%; reduced by food and dairy products

Protein binding: 41% to 50%

Metabolism: Hepatic (small amounts) to inactive metabolites; undergoes enterohepatic recirculation

Half-life elimination: Reduced renal function: 10-17 hours

Time to peak, serum: 3-6 hours

Excretion: Urine (42% to 50% as unchanged drug)

Pregnancy Risk Factor D

Generic Available No

Demeclocycline Hydrochloride *see* Demeclocycline *on page 406*

Demerol® *see* Meperidine *on page 858*

4-demethoxydaunorubicin *see* Idarubicin *on page 706*

Demethylchlortetracycline *see* Demeclocycline *on page 406*

Demser® *see* Metyrosine *on page 905*

Demulen® *see* Combination Hormonal Contraceptives *on page 368*

Denavir® *see* Penciclovir *on page 1046*

Denileukin Diftitox (de ne LU kin DEFT e tox)

U.S. Brand Names ONTAK®

Pharmacologic Category Antineoplastic Agent, Miscellaneous

Use Treatment of patients with persistent or recurrent cutaneous T-cell lymphoma whose malignant cells express the CD25 component of the IL-2 receptor

Local Anesthetic/Vasoconstrictor Precautions No information available to require special precautions

Effects on Dental Treatment

>10%: Hypotension (36%), chest pain (24%), vasodilation (22%), tachycardia (12%), fever (81%), headache (26%), pain (48%), dizziness (22%), nervousness (11%), nausea/vomiting (64%), dyspnea (29%), increased cough (26%), pharyngitis (17%), rhinitis (13%), hypersensitivity (69%), infection (48%), increased diaphoresis (10%), paresthesia (13%), infusion-related hypersensitivity reactions (69%; may include hypotension, back pain, dyspnea, vasodilation, rash, chest pain, tachycardia, dysphagia, syncope, anaphylaxis), flu-like syndrome (91%; beginning several hours to days postinfusion)

1% to 10%: Hypertension (6%), arrhythmias (6%), myocardial infarction (1%), confusion (8%), dehydration (9%), confusion (8%), dysphagia (6%)

Dosage Adults: I.V.: A treatment cycle consists of 9 or 18 mcg/kg/day for 5 consecutive days administered every 21 days. The optimal duration of therapy has not been determined. Only 2% of patients who failed to demonstrate a response (at least a 25% decrease in tumor burden) prior to the fourth cycle responded to subsequent treatment.

Mechanism of Action Denileukin diftitox is a fusion protein (a combination of amino acid sequences from diphtheria toxin and interleukin-2) which selectively delivers the cytotoxic activity of diphtheria toxin to targeted cells. It interacts with the high-affinity IL-2 receptor on the surface of malignant cells to inhibit intracellular protein synthesis, rapidly leading to cell death.

Other Adverse Effects Occurrence diminishes after the first two treatment courses. Reported during treatment (includes all levels of severity):

>10%:

Cardiovascular: Edema (47%)

Central nervous system: Chills (81%)

Dermatologic: Rash (34%), pruritus (20%)

(Continued)

Denileukin Diftitox *(Continued)*

Endocrine & metabolic: Hypoalbuminemia (83%), hypocalcemia (17%), weight loss (14%)
Gastrointestinal: Anorexia (36%), diarrhea (29%)
Hematologic: Decreased lymphocyte count (34%), anemia (18%)
Hepatic: Increased transaminases (61%)
Neuromuscular & skeletal: Asthenia (66%), myalgia (17%)
Miscellaneous: Vascular leak syndrome (27%; hypotension, edema, or hypoalbuminemia usually developed within the first 2 weeks of infusion, 6% required hospitalization as symptoms may persist or even worsen despite cessation of denileukin diftitox)

1% to 10%:
Cardiovascular: Hypertension (6%), arrhythmias (6%), MI (1%)
Central nervous system: Insomnia (9%), confusion (8%)
Endocrine & metabolic: Dehydration (9%), hypokalemia (6%), hyperthyroidism (<5%), hypothyroidism (<5%)
Gastrointestinal: Constipation (9%), dyspepsia (7%), dysphagia (6%), pancreatitis (<5%)
Genitourinary: Hematuria (10%), albuminuria (10%), pyuria (10%)
Hematologic: Thrombotic events (7%), thrombocytopenia (8%), leukopenia (6%)
Local: Injection site reaction (8%), anaphylaxis (1%)
Neuromuscular & skeletal: Arthralgia (8%)
Renal: Increased creatinine (7%), acute renal insufficiency (<5%), microscopic hematuria (<5%)
Respiratory: Lung disorder (8%)

Pharmacodynamics/Kinetics
Distribution: V_d = 0.06-0.08 L/kg
Metabolism: Hepatic via proteolytic degradation (animal studies)
Half-life elimination: Distribution: 2-5 minutes; Terminal: 70-80 minutes

Pregnancy Risk Factor C

Generic Available No

Denorex® [OTC] *see* Coal Tar *on page 359*
DentiPatch® *see* Lidocaine (Transoral) *on page 807*
Deoxycoformycin *see* Pentostatin *on page 1057*
2′-deoxycoformycin *see* Pentostatin *on page 1057*
Depacon® *see* Valproic Acid and Derivatives *on page 1371*
Depakene® *see* Valproic Acid and Derivatives *on page 1371*
Depakote® Delayed Release *see* Valproic Acid and Derivatives *on page 1371*
Depakote® ER *see* Valproic Acid and Derivatives *on page 1371*
Depakote® Sprinkle® *see* Valproic Acid and Derivatives *on page 1371*
Depen® *see* Penicillamine *on page 1046*
DepoCyt™ *see* Cytarabine (Liposomal) *on page 390*
Depo®-Estradiol *see* Estradiol *on page 521*
Depo-Medrol® *see* MethylPREDNISolone *on page 895*
Deponit® [DSC] *see* Nitroglycerin *on page 981*
Depo-Provera® *see* MedroxyPROGESTERone *on page 849*
Depo-Provera® Contraceptive *see* MedroxyPROGESTERone *on page 849*
Depo-Testadiol® *see* Estradiol and Testosterone *on page 527*
Depo®-Testosterone *see* Testosterone *on page 1281*
Deprenyl *see* Selegiline *on page 1213*
Derifil® [OTC] *see* Chlorophyll *on page 302*
Dermarest Dricort® [OTC] *see* Hydrocortisone *on page 688*
Derma-Smoothe/FS® *see* Fluocinolone *on page 584*
Dermatop® *see* Prednicarbate *on page 1110*
Dermazene® *see* Iodoquinol and Hydrocortisone *on page 736*
Dermtex® HC [OTC] *see* Hydrocortisone *on page 688*
DES *see* Diethylstilbestrol *on page 437*
Deserpidine and Methyclothiazide *see* Methyclothiazide and Deserpidine *on page 890*
Desferal® *see* Deferoxamine *on page 404*
Desiccated Thyroid *see* Thyroid *on page 1303*

Desipramine (des IP ra meen)

U.S. Brand Names Norpramin®

Canadian Brand Names Alti-Desipramine; Apo®-Desipramine; Norpramin®; Novo-Desipramine; Nu-Desipramine; PMS-Desipramine

Pharmacologic Category Antidepressant, Tricyclic (Secondary Amine)

Synonyms Desipramine Hydrochloride; Desmethylimipramine Hydrochloride

Use Treatment of depression

Unlabeled/Investigational Use Analgesic adjunct in chronic pain, peripheral neuropathies; treatment of substance-related disorders, attention-deficit/hyperactivity disorder (ADHD)

Local Anesthetic/Vasoconstrictor Precautions Use with caution; epinephrine, norepinephrine and levonordefrin have been shown to have an increased pressor response in combination TCAs

Effects on Dental Treatment Long-term treatment with TCAs increases the risk of caries by reducing salivation and salivary buffer capacity.

>10%: Xerostomia, changes in salivation

Frequency not defined: Arrhythmias, hypotension, hypertension, palpitations, tachycardia, dizziness, drowsiness, headache, confusion, delirium, hallucinations, nervousness, restlessness, parkinsonian syndrome, disorientation, anxiety, agitation, hypomania, exacerbation of psychosis, incoordination, seizures, extrapyramidal symptoms, decreased lower esophageal sphincter tone (may cause GE reflux), nausea, unpleasant taste, weakness, numbness, tingling, paresthesia of extremities, blurred vision, excessive diaphoresis, allergic reactions

Dosage Oral (dose is generally administered at bedtime):

Children 6-12 years: Depression: 10-30 mg/day or 1-3 mg/kg/day in divided doses; do not exceed 5 mg/kg/day

Adolescents: Depression: Initial: 25-50 mg/day; gradually increase to 100 mg/day in single or divided doses (maximum: 150 mg/day)

Adults: Depression: Initial: 75 mg/day in divided doses; increase gradually to 150-200 mg/day in divided or single dose (maximum: 300 mg/day)

Elderly: Depression: Initial dose: 10-25 mg/day; increase by 10-25 mg every 3 days for inpatients and every week for outpatients if tolerated; usual maintenance dose: 75-100 mg/day, but doses up to 150 mg/day may be necessary

Hemodialysis/peritoneal dialysis: Supplemental dose is unnecessary

Mechanism of Action Traditionally believed to increase the synaptic concentration of norepinephrine (and to a lesser extent, serotonin) in the central nervous system by inhibition of its reuptake by the presynaptic neuronal membrane. However, additional receptor effects have been found including desensitization of adenyl cyclase, down regulation of beta-adrenergic receptors, and down regulation of serotonin receptors.

Other Adverse Effects Frequency not defined:

Cardiovascular: Heart block

Central nervous system: Insomnia

Dermatologic: Alopecia, photosensitivity, skin rash, urticaria

Endocrine & metabolic: Breast enlargement, galactorrhea, SIADH

Gastrointestinal: Constipation, weight gain/loss, anorexia, abdominal cramps, diarrhea, heartburn

Genitourinary: Difficult urination, sexual dysfunction, testicular edema

Hematologic: Agranulocytosis, eosinophilia, purpura, thrombocytopenia

Hepatic: Cholestatic jaundice, increased liver enzyme

Neuromuscular & skeletal: Fine muscle tremors, ataxia

Ocular: Disturbances of accommodation, mydriasis, increased intraocular pressure

Drug Interactions Substrate of CYP1A2, **2D6**; Inhibits CYP2D6, 2E1

Increased Effect/Toxicity: Desipramine increases the effects of amphetamines, anticholinergics, other CNS depressants (sedatives, hypnotics, or ethanol), chlorpropamide, tolazamide, and warfarin. When used with MAO inhibitors, serotonin syndrome may occur. Serotonin syndrome has also been reported with ritonavir (rare). The SSRIs (to varying degrees), cimetidine, grapefruit juice, indinavir, methylphenidate, ritonavir (and other protease inhibitors), quinidine, diltiazem, and verapamil inhibit the metabolism of TCAs and clinical toxicity may result. Use of lithium with a TCA may increase the risk for neurotoxicity. Phenothiazines may increase concentration of some TCAs and TCAs may increase concentration of phenothiazines. Pressor response to I.V. epinephrine, norepinephrine, and phenylephrine may be enhanced in patients receiving TCAs (**Note:** Effect is unlikely with epinephrine or levonordefrin dosages typically administered as infiltration in combination with local anesthetics). Combined use of beta-agonists or drugs which prolong QT_c (including quinidine, procainamide, disopyramide, cisapride, sparfloxacin, gatifloxacin, moxifloxacin) with TCAs may predispose patients to cardiac arrhythmias.

Decreased Effect: Desipramine's serum levels/effect may be decreased by carbamazepine, cholestyramine, colestipol, phenobarbital, and rifampin. Desipramine inhibits the antihypertensive effect of to bethanidine, clonidine, debrisoquin, guanadrel, guanethidine, guanabenz, or guanfacine.

Dietary/Ethanol/Herb Considerations

Ethanol: Avoid use; may increase CNS depression.

Food: Avoid grapefruit products; may inhibit the metabolism resulting in toxicity.

Herb/Nutraceutical: Avoid gotu kola, kava, SAMe, St John's wort, tryptophan, and valerian; may increase risk of serotonin syndrome and/or excessive sedation.

Pharmacodynamics/Kinetics

Onset of action: 1-3 weeks; Maximum antidepressant effect: >2 weeks

Absorption: Well absorbed

Metabolism: Hepatic

(Continued)

Desipramine *(Continued)*

Half-life elimination: Adults: 7-60 hours
Time to peak, plasma: 4-6 hours
Excretion: Urine (70%)

Pregnancy Risk Factor C

Generic Available Yes

Selected Readings

Boakes AJ, Laurence DR, Teoh PC, et al, "Interactions Between Sympathomimetic Amines and Antidepressant Agents in Man," *Br Med J*, 1973, 1(849):311-5.

Friedlander AH, Mahler ME, "Major Depressive Disorder. Psychopathology, Medical Management, and Dental Implications," *J Am Dent Assoc*, 201, 132(5):629-38.

Ganzberg S, "Psychoactive Drugs," *ADA Guide to Dental Therapeutics*, 2nd ed, Chicago, IL: ADA Publishing, a Division of ADA Business Enterprises, Inc, 2000, 376-405.

Jastak JT and Yagiela JA, "Vasoconstrictors and Local Anesthesia: A Review and Rationale for Use," *J Am Dent Assoc*, 1983, 107(4):623-30.

Mitchell JR, "Guanethidine and Related Agents. III Antagonism by Drugs Which Inhibit the Norepinephrine Pump in Man," *J Clin Invest*, 1970, 49(8):1596-604.

Rundegren J, van Dijken J, Mörnstad H, et al, "Oral Conditions in Patients Receiving Long-Term Treatment With Cyclic Antidepressant Drugs," *Swed Dent J*, 1985, 9(2):55-64.

Yagiela JA, "Adverse Drug Interactions in Dental Practice: Interactions Associated With Vasoconstrictors. Part V of a Series," *J Am Dent Assoc*, 1999, 130(5):701-9.

Desipramine Hydrochloride *see* Desipramine *on page 408*

Desitin® [OTC] *see* Zinc Oxide *on page 1409*

Desitin® Creamy [OTC] *see* Zinc Oxide *on page 1409*

Desloratadine (des lor AT a deen)

U.S. Brand Names Clarinex®

Canadian Brand Names Aerius®

Pharmacologic Category Antihistamine, Nonsedating

Use Relief of nasal and non-nasal symptoms of seasonal allergic rhinitis (SAR) and perennial allergic rhinitis (PAR); treatment of chronic idiopathic urticaria (CIU)

Local Anesthetic/Vasoconstrictor Precautions No information available to require special precautions

Effects on Dental Treatment

>10%: Headache (14%)

1% to 10%: Xerostomia (3%), somnolence (2%), dizziness (4%), nausea (5%), pharyngitis (3% to 4%), fatigue (2% to 5%)

Dosage Oral:

Adults and Children ≥12 years: 5 mg once daily

Dosing adjustment in renal/hepatic impairment: 5 mg every other day

Mechanism of Action Desloratadine, a major metabolite of loratadine, is a long-acting tricyclic antihistamine with selective peripheral histamine H_1 receptor antagonistic activity and additional anti-inflammatory properties.

Other Adverse Effects

1% to 10%:

Endocrine & metabolic: Dysmenorrhea (2%)
Gastrointestinal: Dyspepsia (3%)
Neuromuscular & skeletal: Myalgia (3%)

Postmarketing and/or case reports: **Anaphylaxis,** bilirubin increased, **dyspnea,** edema, **hypersensitivity reactions,** liver enzymes increased, pruritus, rash, **tachycardia,** urticaria

Drug Interactions Increased Effect/Toxicity: With concurrent use of desloratadine and erythromycin or ketoconazole, the C_{max} and AUC of desloratadine and its metabolite are increased; however, no clinically-significant changes in the safety profile of desloratadine were observed in clinical studies.

Dietary/Ethanol/Herb Considerations Food: May be taken with food; bioavailability unaffected.

Pharmacodynamics/Kinetics

Protein binding: Desloratadine: 82% to 87%; 3-hydroxydesloratadine: 85% to 89%

Metabolism: Hepatic to active metabolite, 3-hydroxydesloratadine (specific enzymes not identified); undergoes glucuronidation. Decreased in slow metabolizers of desloratadine. Not expected to affect or be affected by medications metabolized by CYP with normal doses.

Half-life elimination: 27 hours

Time to peak: 3 hours

Excretion: Urine and feces (as metabolites)

Pregnancy Risk Factor C

Generic Available No

Desmethylimipramine Hydrochloride *see* Desipramine *on page 408*

Desmopressin (des moe PRES in)

U.S. Brand Names DDAVP®; Stimate™

Canadian Brand Names Apo®-Desmopressin; DDAVP®; Minirin®; Octostim®

Mexican Brand Names Minirin®

Pharmacologic Category Antihemophilic Agent; Hemostatic Agent; Vasopressin Analog, Synthetic

Synonyms 1-Deamino-8-D-Arginine Vasopressin; Desmopressin Acetate

Use Treatment of diabetes insipidus; control of bleeding in hemophilia A, and mild-to-moderate classic von Willebrand disease (type I); primary nocturnal enuresis

Local Anesthetic/Vasoconstrictor Precautions No information available to require special precautions

Effects on Dental Treatment Frequency not defined (may be dose- or route-related): Acute MI, blood pressure increased/decreased, chest pain, facial flushing, palpitations, agitation, coma, dizziness, headache, somnolence, nausea, sore throat, vomiting, cough, nasal congestion, epistaxis

Dosage

Children:

Diabetes insipidus:

Intranasal (using 100 mcg/mL nasal solution): 3 months to 12 years: Initial: 5 mcg/day (0.05 mL/day) divided 1-2 times/day; range: 5-30 mcg/day (0.05-0.3 mL/day) divided 1-2 times/day; adjust morning and evening doses separately for an adequate diurnal rhythm of water turnover; doses <10 mcg should be administered using the rhinal tube system

Oral: ≥4 years: Initial: 0.05 mg twice daily; total daily dose should be increased or decreased as needed to obtain adequate antidiuresis (range: 0.1-1.2 mg divided 2-3 times/day)

Hemophilia A and von Willebrand disease (type I):

I.V.: >3 months: 0.3 mcg/kg by slow infusion; may repeat dose if needed; begin 30 minutes before procedure

Intranasal: ≥11 months: Refer to adult dosing.

Nocturnal enuresis:

Intranasal (using 100 mcg/mL nasal solution): ≥6 years: Initial: 20 mcg (0.2 mL) at bedtime; range: 10-40 mcg; it is recommended that 1/2 of the dose be given in each nostril

Oral: 0.2 mg at bedtime; dose may be titrated up to 0.6 mg to achieve desired response. Patients previously on intranasal therapy can begin oral tablets 24 hours after the last intranasal dose.

Children ≥12 years and Adults:

Diabetes insipidus:

I.V., S.C.: 2-4 mcg/day (0.5-1 mL) in 2 divided doses or 1/10 of the maintenance intranasal dose

Intranasal (using 100 mcg/mL nasal solution): 10-40 mcg/day (0.1-0.4 mL) divided 1-3 times/day; adjust morning and evening doses separately for an adequate diurnal rhythm of water turnover. **Note:** The nasal spray pump can only deliver doses of 10 mcg (0.1 mL) or multiples of 10 mcg (0.1 mL); if doses other than this are needed, the rhinal tube delivery system is preferred.

Oral: Initial: 0.05 mg twice daily; total daily dose should be increased or decreased as needed to obtain adequate antidiuresis (range: 0.1-1.2 mg divided 2-3 times/day)

Hemophilia A and mild to moderate von Willebrand disease (type I):

I.V.: 0.3 mcg/kg by slow infusion, begin 30 minutes before procedure

Intranasal: Using high concentration spray (1.5 mg/mL): <50 kg: 150 mcg (1 spray); >50 kg: 300 mcg (1 spray each nostril); repeat use is determined by the patient's clinical condition and laboratory work; if using preoperatively, administer 2 hours before surgery

Mechanism of Action Enhances reabsorption of water in the kidneys by increasing cellular permeability of the collecting ducts; possibly causes smooth muscle constriction with resultant vasoconstriction; raises plasma levels of von Willebrand factor and factor VIII

Other Adverse Effects Frequency not defined (may be dose- or route-related):

Cardiovascular: Acute cerebrovascular thrombosis, edema

Central nervous system: Chills, insomnia

Endocrine & metabolic: Hyponatremia, water intoxication

Gastrointestinal: Abdominal cramps, dyspepsia

Genitourinary: Balanitis, vulval pain

Local: Injection: Burning pain, erythema, and swelling at the injection site

Miscellaneous: **Allergic reactions (rare), anaphylaxis (rare)**

Drug Interactions

Increased Effect/Toxicity: Chlorpropamide, fludrocortisone may increase ADH response.

Decreased Effect: Demeclocycline and lithium may decrease ADH response.

Dietary/Ethanol/Herb Considerations Ethanol: Avoid use; may decrease antidiuretic effect.

Pharmacodynamics/Kinetics

Intranasal administration: Onset of increased factor VIII activity: 30 minutes (dose related)

Peak effect 1.5 hours

(Continued)

Desmopressin *(Continued)*

I.V. infusion:
Onset of increased factor VIII activity: 30 minutes (dose related)
Peak effect: 1.5-2 hours
Half-life elimination: Terminal: 75 minutes
Oral tablets:
Onset of action: ADH: ~1 hour
Peak effect: 4-7 hours
Half-life elimination: 1.5-2.5 hours
Bioavailability: 5% compared to intranasal; 0.16% compared to I.V.

Pregnancy Risk Factor B

Generic Available Yes: Injection only

Desmopressin Acetate *see* Desmopressin *on page 410*

Desogen® *see* Combination Hormonal Contraceptives *on page 368*

Desonide (DES oh nide)

U.S. Brand Names DesOwen®; Tridesilon®

Canadian Brand Names Desocort®

Mexican Brand Names Desowen®

Pharmacologic Category Corticosteroid, Topical

Use Adjunctive therapy for inflammation in acute and chronic corticosteroid responsive dermatosis (low potency corticosteroid)

Local Anesthetic/Vasoconstrictor Precautions No information available to require special precautions

Effects on Dental Treatment No significant effects or complications reported

Dosage Corticosteroid responsive dermatoses: Topical: Apply 2-4 times/day sparingly. Therapy should be discontinued when control is achieved; if no improvement is seen, reassessment of diagnosis may be necessary.

Mechanism of Action Stimulates the synthesis of enzymes needed to decrease inflammation, suppress mitotic activity, and cause vasoconstriction

Other Adverse Effects <1%: Itching; dry skin; folliculitis; hypertrichosis; acneiform eruptions; hypopigmentation; perioral dermatitis; allergic contact dermatitis; skin maceration; skin atrophy; striae; local burning, irritation, miliaria; secondary infection

Pharmacodynamics/Kinetics
Onset of action: ~7 days
Absorption: Extensive from scalp, face, axilla, and scrotum; adequate through epidermis on appendages; may be increased with occlusion or addition of penetrants (eg, urea, DMSO)
Metabolism: Hepatic
Excretion: Primarily urine

Pregnancy Risk Factor C

Generic Available Yes

DesOwen® *see* Desonide *on page 412*

Desoximetasone (des oks i MET a sone)

U.S. Brand Names Topicort®; Topicort®-LP

Canadian Brand Names Desoxi®; Taro-Desoximetasone; Topicort®

Pharmacologic Category Corticosteroid, Topical

Use Relieves inflammation and pruritic symptoms of corticosteroid-responsive dermatosis (intermediate- to high-potency topical corticosteroid)

Local Anesthetic/Vasoconstrictor Precautions No information available to require special precautions

Effects on Dental Treatment No significant effects or complications reported

Dosage Desoximetasone is a potent fluorinated topical corticosteroid. Therapy should be discontinued when control is achieved; if no improvement is seen, reassessment of diagnosis may be necessary.

Children: Apply sparingly in a very thin film to affected area 1-2 times/day
Adults: Apply sparingly to affected area in a thin film twice daily

Mechanism of Action Stimulates the synthesis of enzymes needed to decrease inflammation, suppress mitotic activity, and cause vasoconstriction

Other Adverse Effects <1%: Itching; dry skin; folliculitis; hypertrichosis; acneiform eruptions; hypopigmentation; perioral dermatitis; allergic contact dermatitis; skin maceration; skin atrophy; striae; local burning, irritation, miliaria; secondary infection

Pharmacodynamics/Kinetics
Absorption: Extensive from the scalp, face, axilla, and scrotum; adequate through epidermis on appendages; may be increased with occlusion or addition of penetrants
Distribution: Small amounts reach systemic circulation and dermal layers

Pregnancy Risk Factor C

Generic Available Yes

Desoxyephedrine Hydrochloride *see* Methamphetamine *on page 877*
Desoxyn® *see* Methamphetamine *on page 877*
Desoxyphenobarbital *see* Primidone *on page 1118*
Desquam-E™ *see* Benzoyl Peroxide *on page 171*
Desquam-X® *see* Benzoyl Peroxide *on page 171*
Desyrel® *see* Trazodone *on page 1336*
Detane® [OTC] *see* Benzocaine *on page 169*
Detrol® *see* Tolterodine *on page 1322*
Detrol® LA *see* Tolterodine *on page 1322*
Devrom® *see* Bismuth *on page 186*
Dex4 Glucose [OTC] *see* Glucose (Instant) *on page 641*
Dexacidin® *see* Neomycin, Polymyxin B, and Dexamethasone *on page 962*
Dexacine™ *see* Neomycin, Polymyxin B, and Dexamethasone *on page 962*
Dexalone® [OTC] *see* Dextromethorphan *on page 423*

Dexamethasone (deks a METH a sone)

Related Information

Dental Office Emergencies *on page 1582*
Neomycin, Polymyxin B, and Dexamethasone *on page 962*
Oral Nonviral Soft Tissue Ulcerations or Erosions *on page 1549*
Respiratory Diseases *on page 1476*

U.S. Brand Names Decadron®; Decadron® Phosphate; Dexamethasone Intensol®; Dexasone®; Dexasone® L.A.; DexPak® TaperPak®; Maxidex®; Solurex®; Solurex L.A.®

Canadian Brand Names Decadron®; Dexasone®; Diodex®; Maxidex®; PMS-Dexamethasone

Mexican Brand Names Alin®; Alin Depot®; Decadron®; Decadronal®; Decorex; Dexagrin®; Dibasona®; Indarzona®

Pharmacologic Category Antiemetic; Anti-inflammatory Agent; Anti-inflammatory Agent, Ophthalmic; Corticosteroid, Nasal; Corticosteroid, Ophthalmic; Corticosteroid, Systemic; Corticosteroid, Topical

Synonyms Dexamethasone Acetate; Dexamethasone Sodium Phosphate

Use

Dental: Treatment of a variety of oral diseases of allergic, inflammatory, or autoimmune origin

Medical: Systemically and locally for chronic inflammatory, allergic, hematologic, neoplastic, and autoimmune diseases; management of cerebral edema, septic shock; diagnostic agent; antiemetic

Unlabeled/Investigational Use General indicator consistent with depression; diagnosis of Cushing's syndrome

Local Anesthetic/Vasoconstrictor Precautions No information available to require special precautions

Effects on Dental Treatment Systemic:

>10%: Nervousness

1% to 10%: Diabetes mellitus, epistaxis

Dosage

Children:

Antiemetic (prior to chemotherapy): I.V. (should be given as sodium phosphate): 5-20 mg given 15-30 minutes before treatment

Anti-inflammatory immunosuppressant: Oral, I.M., I.V. (injections should be given as sodium phosphate): 0.08-0.3 mg/kg/day **or** 2.5-10 mg/m²/day in divided doses every 6-12 hours

Extubation or airway edema: Oral, I.M., I.V. (injections should be given as sodium phosphate): 0.5-2 mg/kg/day in divided doses every 6 hours beginning 24 hours prior to extubation and continuing for 4-6 doses afterwards

Cerebral edema: I.V. (should be given as sodium phosphate): Loading dose: 1-2 mg/kg/dose as a single dose; maintenance: 1-1.5 mg/kg/day (maximum: 16 mg/day) in divided doses every 4-6 hours for 5 days then taper for 5 days, then discontinue

Bacterial meningitis in infants and children >2 months: I.V. (should be given as sodium phosphate): 0.6 mg/kg/day in 4 divided doses every 6 hours for the first 4 days of antibiotic treatment; start dexamethasone at the time of the first dose of antibiotic

Physiologic replacement: Oral, I.M., I.V.: 0.03-0.15 mg/kg/day **or** 0.6-0.75 mg/m²/day in divided doses every 6-12 hours

Adults:

Antiemetic:

Prophylaxis: Oral, I.V.: 10-20 mg 15-30 minutes before treatment on each treatment day

Continuous infusion regimen: Oral or I.V.: 10 mg every 12 hours on each treatment day

Mildly emetogenic therapy: Oral, I.M., I.V.: 4 mg every 4-6 hours

Delayed nausea/vomiting: Oral: 4-10 mg 1-2 times/day for 2-4 days **or**

(Continued)

Dexamethasone *(Continued)*

8 mg every 12 hours for 2 days; then
4 mg every 12 hours for 2 days **or**
20 mg 1 hour before chemotherapy; then
10 mg 12 hours after chemotherapy; then
8 mg every 12 hours for 4 doses; then
4 mg every 12 hours for 4 doses

Anti-inflammatory:

Oral, I.M., I.V. (injections should be given as sodium phosphate): 0.75-9 mg/day in divided doses every 6-12 hours

I.M. (as acetate): 8-16 mg; may repeat in 1-3 weeks

Intralesional (as acetate): 0.8-1.6 mg

Intra-articular/soft tissue (as acetate): 4-16 mg; may repeat in 1-3 weeks

Intra-articular, intralesional, or soft tissue (as sodium phosphate): 0.4-6 mg/day

Ophthalmic:

Ointment: Apply thin coating into conjunctival sac 3-4 times/day; gradually taper dose to discontinue

Suspension: Instill 2 drops into conjunctival sac every hour during the day and every other hour during the night; gradually reduce dose to every 3-4 hours, then to 3-4 times/day

Topical: Apply 1-4 times/day. Therapy should be discontinued when control is achieved; if no improvement is seen, reassessment of diagnosis may be necessary.

Chemotherapy: Oral, I.V.: 40 mg every day for 4 days, repeated every 4 weeks (VAD regimen)

Cerebral edema: I.V. 10 mg stat, 4 mg I.M./I.V. (should be given as sodium phosphate) every 6 hours until response is maximized, then switch to oral regimen, then taper off if appropriate; dosage may be reduced after 24 days and gradually discontinued over 5-7 days

Dexamethasone suppression test (depression indicator) or diagnosis for Cushing's syndrome (unlabeled uses): Oral: 1 mg at 11 PM, draw blood at 8 AM the following day for plasma cortisol determination

Physiological replacement: Oral, I.M., I.V. (should be given as sodium phosphate): 0.03-0.15 mg/kg/day **or** 0.6-0.75 mg/m^2/day in divided doses every 6-12 hours

Treatment of shock:

Addisonian crisis/shock (ie, adrenal insufficiency/responsive to steroid therapy): I.V. (given as sodium phosphate): 4-10 mg as a single dose, which may be repeated if necessary

Unresponsive shock (ie, unresponsive to steroid therapy): I.V. (given as sodium phosphate): 1-6 mg/kg as a single I.V. dose or up to 40 mg initially followed by repeat doses every 2-6 hours while shock persists

Hemodialysis: Supplemental dose is unnecessary

Peritoneal dialysis: Supplemental dose is unnecessary

Mechanism of Action Decreases inflammation by suppression of migration of polymorphonuclear leukocytes and reversal of increased capillary permeability; suppresses normal immune response. Dexamethasone's mechanism of antiemetic activity is unknown.

Other Adverse Effects

Systemic:

>10%:

Central nervous system: Insomnia
Gastrointestinal: Increased appetite, indigestion

1% to 10%:

Dermatologic: Hirsutism
Neuromuscular & skeletal: Arthralgia
Ocular: Cataracts

<1% and/or case reports: **Seizures, mood swings, headache, delirium, hallucinations, euphoria, skin atrophy, bruising**, hyperpigmentation, acne, amenorrhea, sodium and water retention, Cushing's syndrome, hyperglycemia, bone growth suppression, abdominal distention, **ulcerative esophagitis**, pancreatitis, **muscle wasting, hypersensitivity reactions**

Topical: <1%: Itching, dryness, folliculitis, hypertrichosis, acneiform eruptions, hypopigmentation, **perioral dermatitis, allergic contact dermatitis, skin maceration, skin atrophy,** striae, miliaria, **local burning, irritation, secondary infection**

Contraindications Hypersensitivity to dexamethasone or any component of the formulation; active untreated infections; ophthalmic use in viral, fungal, or tuberculosis diseases of the eye

Warnings/Precautions Use with caution in patients with hypothyroidism, cirrhosis, hypertension, CHF, ulcerative colitis, thromboembolic disorders. Corticosteroids should be used with caution in patients with diabetes, osteoporosis, peptic ulcer, glaucoma, cataracts, or tuberculosis. Use caution in hepatic impairment. Because of the risk of adverse effects, systemic corticosteroids should be used cautiously in the elderly in the smallest possible dose and for the shortest possible time.

May cause suppression of hypothalamic-pituitary-adrenal (HPA) axis, particularly in younger children or in patients receiving high doses for prolonged periods. Particular care is required when patients are transferred from systemic corticosteroids to inhaled products due to possible adrenal insufficiency or withdrawal from steroids, including an increase in allergic symptoms. Patients receiving 20 mg per day of prednisone (or equivalent) may be most susceptible. Fatalities have occurred due to adrenal insufficiency in asthmatic patients during and after transfer from systemic corticosteroids to aerosol steroids; aerosol steroids do **not** provide the systemic steroid needed to treat patients having trauma, surgery, or infections

Controlled clinical studies have shown that orally-inhaled and intranasal corticosteroids may cause a reduction in growth velocity in pediatric patients. (In studies of orally-inhaled corticosteroids, the mean reduction in growth velocity was approximately 1 centimeter per year [range 0.3-1.8 cm per year] and appears to be related to dose and duration of exposure.) The growth of pediatric patients receiving inhaled corticosteroids, should be monitored routinely (eg, via stadiometry). To minimize the systemic effects of orally-inhaled and intranasal corticosteroids, each patient should be titrated to the lowest effective dose.

May suppress the immune system, patients may be more susceptible to infection. Use with caution in patients with systemic infections or ocular herpes simplex. Avoid exposure to chickenpox and measles.

Drug Interactions Substrate of CYP3A4; Induces CYP2A6, 2B6, 2C8/9, 3A4

Increased Effect: Salmeterol: The addition of salmeterol has been demonstrated to improve response to inhaled corticosteroids (as compared to increasing steroid dosage).

Decreased Effect: Barbiturates, phenytoin, rifampin may decrease dexamethasone effects; dexamethasone decreases effect of salicylates, vaccines, toxoids

Dietary/Ethanol/Herb Considerations

Ethanol: Avoid use; may enhance gastric mucosal irritation.

Food: Administer with food to reduce GI upset. Limit caffeine. Interferes with calcium absorption; may require increased intake of calcium, folate, phosphorus. potassium, pyridoxine, vitamin C, and vitamin D.

Herb/Nutraceutical: Avoid cat's claw and echinacea due to immunostimulant properties.

Pharmacodynamics/Kinetics

Onset of action: Acetate: Prompt

Duration of metabolic effect: 72 hours; acetate is a long-acting repository preparation

Metabolism: Hepatic

Half-life elimination: Normal renal function: 1.8-3.5 hours; Biological half-life: 36-54 hours

Time to peak, serum: Oral: 1-2 hours; I.M.: ~8 hours

Excretion: Urine and feces

Pregnancy Risk Factor C

Dosage Forms ELIXIR, as base: 0.5 mg/5 mL (100 mL, 240 mL). **INJ, suspension, as acetate** (Dexasone® LA, Solurex LA®): 8 mg/mL (5 mL). **INJ, solution, as sodium phosphate:** 4 mg/mL (1 mL, 5 mL, 10 mL, 25 mL, 30 mL); 10 mg/mL (1 mL, 10 mL); (Decadron® Phosphate): 4 mg/mL (5 mL, 25 mL); 24 mg/mL (5 mL); (Dexasone®): 4 mg/mL (5 mL); (Solurex®): 4 mg/mL (5 mL, 10 mL, 30 mL). **OINT, ophthalmic, as sodium phosphate:** 0.05% (3.5 g). **SOLN, oral:** 0.5 mg/5 mL (5 mL, 500 mL). **SOLN, oral concentrate** (Dexamethasone Intensol®): 1 mg/mL (30 mL). **SUSP, ophthalmic** (Maxidex®): 0.1% (5 mL, 15 mL). **TAB:** 0.25 mg, 0.5 mg, 0.75 mg, 1 mg, 1.5 mg, 2 mg, 4 mg, 6 mg; (Decadron®): 0.5 mg, 0.75 mg, 4 mg; (DexPak® TaperPak®): 1.5 mg

Generic Available Yes

Dexamethasone Acetate *see* Dexamethasone *on page 413*

Dexamethasone and Neomycin *see* Neomycin and Dexamethasone *on page 961*

Dexamethasone and Tobramycin *see* Tobramycin and Dexamethasone *on page 1317*

Dexamethasone Intensol® *see* Dexamethasone *on page 413*

Dexamethasone, Neomycin, and Polymyxin B *see* Neomycin, Polymyxin B, and Dexamethasone *on page 962*

Dexamethasone Sodium Phosphate *see* Dexamethasone *on page 413*

Dexasone® *see* Dexamethasone *on page 413*

Dexasone® L.A. *see* Dexamethasone *on page 413*

Dexbrompheniramine and Pseudoephedrine

(deks brom fen EER a meen & soo doe e FED rin)

Related Information

Pseudoephedrine *on page 1146*

U.S. Brand Names Drixomed®; Drixoral® Cold & Allergy [OTC]

Canadian Brand Names Drixoral®

Pharmacologic Category Antihistamine/Decongestant Combination

Synonyms Pseudoephedrine and Dexbrompheniramine

(Continued)

Dexbrompheniramine and Pseudoephedrine *(Continued)*

Use Relief of symptoms of upper respiratory mucosal congestion in seasonal and perennial nasal allergies, acute rhinitis, rhinosinusitis and eustachian tube blockage

Local Anesthetic/Vasoconstrictor Precautions Use with caution since pseudoephedrine is a sympathomimetic amine which could interact with epinephrine to cause a pressor response

Effects on Dental Treatment ≤10%: Tachycardia, palpitations, xerostomia; use vasoconstrictor with caution

Dosage Children >12 years and Adults: Oral: 1 timed release tablet every 12 hours, may require 1 tablet every 8 hours

Pregnancy Risk Factor B

Generic Available Yes

Dexchlorpheniramine (deks klor fen EER a meen)

U.S. Brand Names Polaramine® [DSC]

Pharmacologic Category Antihistamine

Synonyms Dexchlorpheniramine Maleate; Polaramine® [DSC]

Use Perennial and seasonal allergic rhinitis and other allergic symptoms including urticaria

Local Anesthetic/Vasoconstrictor Precautions No information available to require special precautions

Effects on Dental Treatment

>10%: Slight to moderate drowsiness, thickening of bronchial secretions

1% to 10%: Significant xerostomia (≤10%; resolves upon discontinuation), drowsiness (≤10%), headache, nervousness, dizziness, nausea, pharyngitis, fatigue

Dosage Oral:

Children:

2-5 years: 0.5 mg every 4-6 hours (do not use timed release)

6-11 years: 1 mg every 4-6 hours or 4 mg timed release at bedtime

Adults: 2 mg every 4-6 hours or 4-6 mg timed release at bedtime or every 8-10 hours

Mechanism of Action Competes with histamine for H_1-receptor sites on effector cells in the gastrointestinal tract, blood vessels, and respiratory tract

Other Adverse Effects 1% to 10%:

Gastrointestinal: Appetite increase, weight gain, diarrhea, abdominal pain

Neuromuscular & skeletal: Arthralgia

Drug Interactions

Increased Effect/Toxicity: CNS depressants may increase the degree of sedation and respiratory depression with antihistamines. May increase the absorption of digoxin. Central and/or peripheral anticholinergic syndrome can occur when administered with amantadine, rimantadine, narcotic analgesics, phenothiazines and other antipsychotics (especially with high anticholinergic activity), tricyclic antidepressants, quinidine, disopyramide, procainamide, and antihistamines.

Decreased Effect: May increase gastric degradation of levodopa and decrease the amount of levodopa absorbed by delaying gastric emptying. Therapeutic effects of cholinergic agents (tacrine, donepezil) and neuroleptics may be antagonized.

Dietary/Ethanol/Herb Considerations

Ethanol: Avoid use; may increase CNS depression.

Herb/Nutraceutical: Avoid gotu kola, kava, SAMe, St John's wort, and valerian; may increase CNS depression.

Pharmacodynamics/Kinetics

Onset of action: ~1 hour

Duration: 3-6 hours

Absorption: Well absorbed

Metabolism: Hepatic

Pregnancy Risk Factor B

Generic Available Yes: Sustained action tablet, syrup

Dexchlorpheniramine Maleate *see* Dexchlorpheniramine *on page 416*

Dexedrine® *see* Dextroamphetamine *on page 420*

Dexferrum® *see* Iron Dextran Complex *on page 743*

Dexmedetomidine (deks MED e toe mi deen)

U.S. Brand Names Precedex™

Canadian Brand Names Precedex™

Pharmacologic Category $Alpha_2$-Adrenergic Agonist; Sedative

Synonyms Dexmedetomidine Hydrochloride

Use Sedation of initially intubated and mechanically ventilated patients during treatment in an intensive care setting; duration of infusion should not exceed 24 hours

Unlabeled/Investigational Use Unlabeled: Premedication prior to anesthesia induction with thiopental; premedication to attenuate the cardiostimulatory and postanesthetic delirium of ketamine; relief of pain and reduction of opioid dose following laparoscopic tubal ligation; adjunct anesthetic in ophthalmic surgery; treatment of shivering

Local Anesthetic/Vasoconstrictor Precautions No information available to require special precautions

Effects on Dental Treatment

>10%: Xerostomia, changes in salivation, hypotension (30%), nausea (11%)

1% to 10%: Bradycardia (8%), atrial fibrillation (7%), pain (3%), infection (2%), thirst (2%)

Dosage Individualize and titrate to desired clinical effect.

Adults: I.V.: Solution must be diluted prior to administration. Initial: Loading infusion of 1 mcg/kg over 10 minutes, followed by a maintenance infusion of 0.2-0.7 mcg/kg/hour; not indicated for infusions lasting >24 hours

Elderly (>65 years of age): Consider dose reduction; no specific guidelines available. Dose selections should be cautious, at the low end of dosage range; titration should be slower, allowing adequate time to evaluate response.

Dosing adjustment in hepatic impairment: Consider reduction; no specific guidelines available

Mechanism of Action Selective $alpha_2$-adrenoceptor agonist with sedative properties; $alpha_1$ activity was observed at high doses or after rapid infusions

Other Adverse Effects 1% to 10%:

Hematologic: Anemia (3%), leukocytosis (2%)

Renal: Oliguria (2%)

Respiratory: Hypoxia (6%), pulmonary edema (2%), pleural effusion (3%)

Drug Interactions Substrate of **CYP2A6**; Inhibits CYP1A2, 2C8/9, **2D6**, 3A4

Increased Effect/Toxicity: Possible enhanced effects and pharmacodynamic interaction with sedatives, hypnotics, opioids, and anesthetics; monitor and decrease the dose as necessary of each agent and/or dexmedetomidine. Enhanced effects may occur with sevoflurane, isoflurane, propofol, alfentanil, and midazolam. Hypotension and/or bradycardia may be increased by vasodilators and heart rate-lowering agents.

Pharmacodynamics/Kinetics

Onset of action: Rapid

Distribution: V_{ss}: Approximately 118 L; rapid

Protein binding: 94%

Metabolism: Hepatic via glucuronidation and CYP2A6

Half-life elimination: 6 minutes; Terminal: 2 hours

Excretion: Urine (95%); feces (4%)

Pregnancy Risk Factor C

Generic Available No

Dexmedetomidine Hydrochloride *see* Dexmedetomidine *on page 416*

Dexmethylphenidate (dex meth il FEN i date)

U.S. Brand Names Focalin™

Pharmacologic Category Central Nervous System Stimulant

Synonyms Dexmethylphenidate Hydrochloride

Use Treatment of attention-deficit/hyperactivity disorder (ADHD)

Local Anesthetic/Vasoconstrictor Precautions No information available to require special precautions

Effects on Dental Treatment

1% to 10%: Fever (5%), nausea (9%)

>10%: Gastrointestinal: Abdominal pain (15%)

1% to 10%:

Gastrointestinal: Anorexia (6%)

Adverse effects seen with methylphenidate (frequency not defined):

Cardiovascular: **Angina, cardiac arrhythmias**, cerebral arteritis, cerebral occlusion, **hypertension, hypotension, palpitations, pulse increase/decrease, tachycardia**

Central nervous system: Depression, **dizziness, drowsiness, fever, headache**, insomnia, **nervousness**, neuroleptic malignant syndrome (NMS), Tourette's syndrome, toxic psychosis

Dermatologic: Erythema multiforme, exfoliative dermatitis, hair loss, rash, urticaria

Endocrine & metabolic: Growth retardation

Gastrointestinal: Abdominal pain, anorexia, **nausea, vomiting**, weight loss

Hematologic: Anemia, leukopenia, thrombocytopenic purpura

Hepatic: Abnormal LFTs, hepatic coma, transaminase elevation

Neuromuscular & skeletal: Arthralgia, dyskinesia

Ocular: Blurred vision

Renal: Necrotizing vasculitis

Restrictions C-II

Dosage Oral: Children ≥6 years and Adults: Treatment of ADHD: Initial: 2.5 mg twice daily in patients not currently taking methylphenidate; dosage may be adjusted in 2.5-5 mg increments at weekly intervals (maximum dose: 20 mg/day); doses should be taken at least 4 hours apart

(Continued)

Dexmethylphenidate *(Continued)*

When switching from methylphenidate to dexmethylphenidate, the starting dose of dexmethylphenidate should be half that of methylphenidate (maximum dose: 20 mg/day)

Safety and efficacy for long-term use of dexmethylphenidate have not yet been established. Patients should be re-evaluated at appropriate intervals to assess continued need of the medication.

Dose reductions and discontinuation: Reduce dose or discontinue in patients with paradoxical aggravation. Discontinue if no improvement is seen after one month of treatment.

Mechanism of Action Dexmethylphenidate is the more active, *d-threo*-enantiomer, of racemic methylphenidate. It is a CNS stimulant; blocks the reuptake of norepinephrine and dopamine, and increases their release into the extraneuronal space.

Other Adverse Effects

>10%: Gastrointestinal: Abdominal pain (15%)

1% to 10%:

Gastrointestinal: Anorexia (6%)

Adverse effects seen with methylphenidate (frequency not defined):

Cardiovascular: **Angina, cardiac arrhythmias**, cerebral arteritis, cerebral occlusion, **hypertension, hypotension, palpitations, pulse increase/decrease, tachycardia**

Central nervous system: Depression, **dizziness, drowsiness, fever, headache**, insomnia, **nervousness**, neuroleptic malignant syndrome (NMS), Tourette's syndrome, toxic psychosis

Dermatologic: Erythema multiforme, exfoliative dermatitis, hair loss, rash, urticaria

Endocrine & metabolic: Growth retardation

Gastrointestinal: Abdominal pain, anorexia, **nausea, vomiting**, weight loss

Hematologic: Anemia, leukopenia, thrombocytopenic purpura

Hepatic: Abnormal LFTs, hepatic coma, transaminase elevation

Neuromuscular & skeletal: Arthralgia, dyskinesia

Ocular: Blurred vision

Renal: Necrotizing vasculitis

Respiratory: **Cough increased, pharyngitis, sinusitis, upper respiratory tract infection**

Miscellaneous: **Hypersensitivity reactions**

Drug Interactions

Increased Effect/Toxicity: Methylphenidate may cause hypertensive effects when used in combination with MAO inhibitors or drugs with MAO-inhibiting activity (linezolid). Risk may be less with selegiline (MAO type B selective at low doses); it is best to avoid this combination. NMS has been reported in a patient receiving methylphenidate and venlafaxine. Methylphenidate may increase levels of phenytoin, phenobarbital, TCAs, and warfarin. Increased toxicity with clonidine and sibutramine.

Decreased Effect: Effectiveness of antihypertensive agents may be decreased. Carbamazepine may decrease the effect of methylphenidate.

Dietary/Ethanol/Herb Considerations

Ethanol: Avoid use; may cause CNS depression.

Food: May be taken with food; high-fat meal may increase time to peak concentration. Avoid caffeine

Herb/Nutraceutical: Avoid ephedra, ginseng, and yohimbe; may cause hypertension. Avoid gotu kola, kava, SAMe, St John's wort, and valerian; may increase CNS depression.

Pharmacodynamics/Kinetics

Absorption: Rapid

Metabolism: Via de-esterification to inactive metabolite, *d*-α-phenyl-piperidine acetate (*d*-ritalinic acid)

Half-life elimination: 2.2 hours

Time to peak: Fasting: 1-1.5 hours

Excretion: Urine (90%)

Pregnancy Risk Factor C

Generic Available No

Dexmethylphenidate Hydrochloride *see* Dexmethylphenidate *on page 417*

DexPak® TaperPak® *see* Dexamethasone *on page 413*

Dexpanthenol (deks PAN the nole)

U.S. Brand Names Panthoderm® [OTC]

Pharmacologic Category Gastrointestinal Agent, Stimulant; Topical Skin Product

Synonyms Pantothenyl Alcohol

Use Prophylactic use to minimize paralytic ileus; treatment of postoperative distention; topical to relieve itching and to aid healing of minor dermatoses

Local Anesthetic/Vasoconstrictor Precautions No information available to require special precautions

Effects on Dental Treatment Frequency not defined: Agitation, vomiting, paresthesia, dyspnea, allergic reactions

Dosage

Children and Adults: Relief of itching and aid in skin healing: Topical: Apply to affected area 1-2 times/day

Adults:

Prevention of postoperative ileus: I.M.: 250-500 mg stat, repeat in 2 hours, followed by doses every 6 hours until danger passes

Paralytic ileus: I.M.: 500 mg stat, repeat in 2 hours, followed by doses every 6 hours, if needed

Mechanism of Action A pantothenic acid B vitamin analog that is converted to coenzyme A internally; coenzyme A is essential to normal fatty acid synthesis, amino acid synthesis and acetylation of choline in the production of the neurotransmitter, acetylcholine

Other Adverse Effects Frequency not defined.

Cardiovascular: Slight drop in blood pressure

Dermatologic: Dermatitis, irritation, itching, urticaria

Gastrointestinal: Diarrhea, hyperperistalsis, vomiting

Drug Interactions Increased Effect/Toxicity: Increased/prolonged effect when dexpanthenol injection is given with succinylcholine; do not give dexpanthenol within 1 hour of succinylcholine.

Pharmacodynamics/Kinetics Absorption: Well absorbed

Pregnancy Risk Factor C

Generic Available Yes: Injection

Dexrazoxane (deks ray ZOKS ane)

U.S. Brand Names Zinecard®

Canadian Brand Names Zinecard®

Pharmacologic Category Cardioprotectant

Synonyms ICRF-187

Use Reduction of the incidence and severity of cardiomyopathy associated with doxorubicin administration in women with metastatic breast cancer who have received a cumulative doxorubicin dose of 300 mg/m^2 and who would benefit from continuing therapy with doxorubicin. It is not recommended for use with the initiation of doxorubicin therapy.

Local Anesthetic/Vasoconstrictor Precautions No information available to require special precautions

Effects on Dental Treatment No significant effects or complications reported

Dosage Adults: I.V.: The recommended dosage ratio of dexrazoxane:doxorubicin is 10:1 (eg, 500 mg/m^2 dexrazoxane:50 mg/m^2 doxorubicin). Administer the reconstituted solution by slow I.V. push or rapid I.V. infusion from a bag. After completing the infusion, and prior to a total elapsed time of 30 minutes (from the beginning of the dexrazoxane infusion), administer the I.V. injection of doxorubicin.

Mechanism of Action Derivative of EDTA and potent intracellular chelating agent. The mechanism of cardioprotectant activity is not fully understood. Appears to be converted intracellularly to a ring-opened chelating agent that interferes with iron-mediated free radical generation thought to be responsible, in part, for anthracycline-induced cardiomyopathy.

Other Adverse Effects Effects are likely attributable to the FAC regimen, except pain on injection observed mainly with dexrazoxane. Patients receiving FAC with dexrazoxane experienced more severe leukopenia, granulocytopenia, and thrombocytopenia at nadir than patients receiving FAC without dexrazoxane; but recovery counts were similar for the two groups.

1% to 2%: Dermatologic: Urticaria, recall skin reaction, extravasation

Drug Interactions Decreased Effect: The use of dexrazoxane concurrently with the initiation of FAC therapy may interfere with the antitumor efficacy of the regimen, and this use is not recommended.

Pharmacodynamics/Kinetics

Distribution: V_d: 22-22.4 L/m^2

Protein binding: None

Half-life elimination: 2.1-2.5 hours

Excretion: Urine (42%)

Clearance, renal: 3.35 L/hour/m^2; Plasma: 6.25-7.88 L/hour/m^2

Pregnancy Risk Factor C

Generic Available No

Dextran (DEKS tran)

Related Information

Dextran 1 *on page 420*

U.S. Brand Names Gentran®; LMD®

Canadian Brand Names Gentran®

Mexican Brand Names Alpha-Dextrano"40"; Rheomacrodex®

Pharmacologic Category Plasma Volume Expander

(Continued)

Dextran *(Continued)*

Synonyms Dextran 40; Dextran 70; Dextran, High Molecular Weight; Dextran, Low Molecular Weight

Use Blood volume expander used in treatment of shock or impending shock when blood or blood products are not available; dextran 40 is also used as a priming fluid in cardiopulmonary bypass and for prophylaxis of venous thrombosis and pulmonary embolism in surgical procedures associated with a high risk of thromboembolic complications

Local Anesthetic/Vasoconstrictor Precautions No information available to require special precautions

Effects on Dental Treatment No significant effects or complications reported

Dosage Dose and infusion rate are dependent upon the patient's fluid status and must be individualized.

I.V. (requires an infusion pump):

Volume expansion/shock:

Children: Total dose should not exceed 20 mL/kg during first 24 hours

Adults: 500-1000 mL at a rate of 20-40 mL/minute; maximum daily dose: 20 mL/kg for first 24 hours; 10 mL/kg/day thereafter; therapy should not be continued beyond 5 days

Pump prime (Dextran 40): Varies with the volume of the pump oxygenator; generally, the 10% solution is added in a dose of 1-2 g/kg

Prophylaxis of venous thrombosis/pulmonary embolism (Dextran 40): Begin during surgical procedure and give 50-100 g on the day of surgery; an additional 50 g (500 mL) should be administered every 2-3 days during the period of risk (up to 2 weeks postoperatively); usual maximum infusion rate for nonemergency use: 4 mL/minute

Dosing in renal and/or hepatic impairment: Use with extreme caution

Mechanism of Action Produces plasma volume expansion by virtue of its highly colloidal starch structure, similar to albumin; average molecular weight: dextran 40 = 40,000; dextran 70 = 70,000

Other Adverse Effects <1% (Limited to important or life-threatening): **Mild hypotension, tightness of chest, wheezing**

Pharmacodynamics/Kinetics

Onset of action: Minutes to 1 hour (depending upon the molecular weight polysaccharide administered)

Excretion: Urine (~75%) within 24 hours

Pregnancy Risk Factor C

Generic Available Yes

Dextran 1 (DEKS tran won)

Related Information

Dextran *on page 419*

U.S. Brand Names Promit®

Pharmacologic Category Plasma Volume Expander

Use Prophylaxis of serious anaphylactic reactions to I.V. infusion of dextran

Local Anesthetic/Vasoconstrictor Precautions No information available to require special precautions

Effects on Dental Treatment No significant effects or complications reported

Dosage I.V. (time between dextran 1 and dextran solution should not exceed 15 minutes):

Children: 0.3 mL/kg 1-2 minutes before I.V. infusion of dextran

Adults: 20 mL 1-2 minutes before I.V. infusion of dextran

Mechanism of Action Binds to dextran-reactive immunoglobulin without bridge formation and no formation of large immune complexes

Other Adverse Effects <1% (Limited to important or life-threatening): **Mild hypotension, tightness of chest, wheezing**

Pregnancy Risk Factor C

Generic Available No

Dextran 40 *see* Dextran *on page 419*

Dextran 70 *see* Dextran *on page 419*

Dextran, High Molecular Weight *see* Dextran *on page 419*

Dextran, Low Molecular Weight *see* Dextran *on page 419*

Dextroamphetamine (deks troe am FET a meen)

Related Information

Dextroamphetamine and Amphetamine *on page 422*

U.S. Brand Names Dexedrine®; Dextrostat®

Canadian Brand Names Dexedrine®

Pharmacologic Category Stimulant

Synonyms Dextroamphetamine Sulfate

Use Narcolepsy; attention-deficit/hyperactivity disorder (ADHD)

Unlabeled/Investigational Use Treatment of exogenous obesity, depression, abnormal behavioral syndrome in children (minimal brain dysfunction)

Local Anesthetic/Vasoconstrictor Precautions Use vasoconstriction with caution in patients taking dextroamphetamine. Amphetamines enhance the sympathomimetic response of epinephrine and norepinephrine leading to potential hypertension and cardiotoxicity.

Effects on Dental Treatment Up to 10% of patients taking dextroamphetamines may present with hypertension. The use of local anesthetic without vasoconstrictor is recommended in these patients.

1% to 10%: Xerostomia

Frequency not defined: Palpitations, tachycardia, hypertension, exacerbation of motor and phonic tics, restlessness, dizziness, headache, psychosis, Tourette's syndrome, unpleasant taste, tremors, euphoria, overstimulation

Restrictions C-II

Dosage Oral:

Children:

Narcolepsy: 6-12 years: Initial: 5 mg/day; may increase at 5 mg increments in weekly intervals until side effects appear (maximum dose: 60 mg/day)

ADHD:

3-5 years: Initial: 2.5 mg/day given every morning; increase by 2.5 mg/day in weekly intervals until optimal response is obtained; usual range: 0.1-0.5 mg/kg/dose every morning with maximum of 40 mg/day

≥6 years: 5 mg once or twice daily; increase in increments of 5 mg/day at weekly intervals until optimal response is obtained; usual range: 0.1-0.5 mg/kg/dose every morning (5-20 mg/day) with maximum of 40 mg/day

Children >12 years and Adults:

Narcolepsy: Initial: 10 mg/day, may increase at 10 mg increments in weekly intervals until side effects appear; maximum: 60 mg/day

Exogenous obesity (unlabeled use): 5-30 mg/day in divided doses of 5-10 mg 30-60 minutes before meals

Mechanism of Action Blocks reuptake of dopamine and norepinephrine from the synapse, thus increases the amount of circulating dopamine and norepinephrine in cerebral cortex to reticular activating system; inhibits the action of monoamine oxidase and causes catecholamines to be released. Peripheral actions include elevated blood pressure, weak bronchodilator, and respiratory stimulant action.

Other Adverse Effects Frequency not defined:

Cardiovascular: Cardiomyopathy

Central nervous system: Dyskinesia, dysphoria,

Dermatologic: Rash, urticaria

Endocrine & metabolic: Changes in libido

Gastrointestinal: Diarrhea, constipation, anorexia, weight loss,

Genitourinary: Impotence

Drug Interactions Substrate of **CYP2D6**

Increased Effect/Toxicity: Dextroamphetamine may precipitate hypertensive crisis or serotonin syndrome in patients receiving MAO inhibitors (selegiline >10 mg/day, isocarboxazid, phenelzine, tranylcypromine, furazolidone). Serotonin syndrome has also been associated with combinations of amphetamines and SSRIs; these combinations should be avoided. TCAs may enhance the effects of amphetamines. Large doses of antacids or urinary alkalinizers increase the half-life and duration of action of amphetamines. May precipitate arrhythmias in patients receiving general anesthetics.

Decreased Effect: Amphetamines inhibit the antihypertensive response to guanethidine and guanadrel. Urinary acidifiers decrease the half-life and duration of action of amphetamines.

Dietary/Ethanol/Herb Considerations

Ethanol: Avoid use; may increase CNS depression.

Food: Avoid acidic food, juices, or vitamin C; may alter serum concentration. Do not mix with fruit juice or other acid-containing liquid. Avoid caffeine (eg, colas, chocolate).

Herb/Nutraceutical: Avoid ephedra, ginseng, and yohimbe; may cause arrhythmias or hypertension.

Herb/Nutraceutical: Avoid gotu kola, kava, SAMe, St John's wort, and valerian; may increase CNS depression.

Pharmacodynamics/Kinetics

Onset of action: 1-1.5 hours

Distribution: V_d: Adults: 3.5-4.6 L/kg; distributes into CNS; mean CSF concentrations are 80% of plasma; enters breast milk

Metabolism: Hepatic via CYP monooxygenase and glucuronidation

Half-life elimination: Adults: 10-13 hours

Time to peak, serum: T_{max}: Immediate release: 3 hours; sustained release: 8 hours

Excretion: Urine (as unchanged drug and inactive metabolites)

Pregnancy Risk Factor C

Generic Available Yes

Dextroamphetamine and Amphetamine

(deks troe am FET a meen & am FET a meen)

Related Information

Dextroamphetamine *on page 420*

U.S. Brand Names Adderall®; Adderall XR™

Pharmacologic Category Stimulant

Synonyms Amphetamine and Dextroamphetamine

Use Attention-deficit/hyperactivity disorder (ADHD); narcolepsy

Local Anesthetic/Vasoconstrictor Precautions Use vasoconstriction with caution in patients taking dextroamphetamine. Amphetamines enhance the sympathomimetic response of epinephrine and norepinephrine leading to potential hypertension and cardiotoxicity.

Effects on Dental Treatment Up to 10% of patients taking dextroamphetamines may present with hypertension. The use of local anesthetic without vasoconstrictor is recommended in these patients.

Adderall XR™: 1% to 10%: Nervousness (6%), fever (4%), dizziness (2%), weakness (2%), vomiting (7%), nausea (5%), infection (2% to 4%)

Restrictions C-II

Dosage Use lowest effective individualized dose; administer first dose as soon as patient is awake.

Oral:

ADHD:

Children: <3 years: Use not recommended

Children: 3-5 years (Adderall®): Initial 2.5 mg/day given every morning; increase daily dose in 2.5 mg increments at weekly intervals until optimal response is obtained (maximum dose: 40 mg/day given in 1-3 divided doses); use intervals of 4-6 hours between additional doses

Children: ≥6 years:

Adderall®: Initial: 5 mg 1-2 times/day; increase daily dose in 5 mg increments at weekly intervals until optimal response is obtained (usual maximum dose: 40 mg/day given in 1-3 divided doses); use intervals of 4-6 hours between additional doses

Adderall XR™: 5-10 mg once daily in the morning; if needed, may increase daily dose in 5-10 mg increments at weekly intervals (maximum dose: 30 mg/day)

Narcolepsy: Adderall®

Children: 6-12 years: Initial: 5 mg/day; increase daily dose in 5 mg at weekly intervals until optimal response is obtained (maximum dose: 60 mg/day given in 1-3 divided doses)

Children >12 years and Adults: Initial: 10 mg/day; increase daily dose in 10 mg increments at weekly intervals until optimal response is obtained (maximum dose: 60 mg/day given in 1-3 divided doses)

Mechanism of Action Blocks reuptake of dopamine and norepinephrine from the synapse, thus increases the amount of circulating dopamine and norepinephrine in cerebral cortex to reticular activating system; inhibits the action of monoamine oxidase and causes catecholamines to be released. Peripheral actions include elevated blood pressure, weak bronchodilator, and respiratory stimulant action.

Other Adverse Effects

Adderall XR™:

>10%:

Central nervous system: Insomnia (1% to 17%)

Gastrointestinal: Appetite decreased (22%), abdominal pain (14%)

1% to 10%:

Central nervous system: Emotional lability (1% to 9%)

Gastrointestinal: Anorexia (3%), diarrhea (2%), dyspepsia (2%), weight loss (1%)

<1%: Depression

Reported with amphetamine use (frequency not defined):

Cardiovascular: **Palpitations, tachycardia, hypertension**, cardiomyopathy

Central nervous system: Overstimulation, euphoria, dyskinesia, dysphoria, exacerbation of motor and phonic tics, restlessness, insomnia, **headache, psychosis**, exacerbation of Tourette's syndrome

Dermatologic: Rash, urticaria

Endocrine & metabolic: Changes in libido

Gastrointestinal: Constipation, **xerostomia, unpleasant taste**

Genitourinary: Impotence

Neuromuscular & skeletal: **Tremor**

Drug Interactions

Increased Effect/Toxicity: Dextroamphetamine and amphetamine may precipitate hypertensive crisis or serotonin syndrome in patients receiving MAO inhibitors (selegiline >10 mg/day, isocarboxazid, phenelzine, tranylcypromine, furazolidone). Serotonin syndrome has also been associated with combinations of amphetamines and SSRIs; these combinations should be avoided. TCAs may enhance the effects of amphetamines, potentially leading to hypertensive crisis.

Large doses of antacids or urinary alkalinizers increase the half-life and duration of action of amphetamines. May precipitate arrhythmias in patients receiving general anesthetics. Inhibitors of CYP2D6 may increase the effects of amphetamines (includes amiodarone, cimetidine, delavirdine, fluoxetine, paroxetine, propafenone, quinidine, and ritonavir).

Decreased Effect: Amphetamines inhibit the antihypertensive response to guanethidine and guanadrel. Urinary acidifiers decrease the half-life and duration of action of amphetamines. Enzyme inducers (barbiturates, carbamazepine, phenytoin, and rifampin) may decrease serum concentrations of amphetamines.

Dietary/Ethanol/Herb Considerations

Ethanol: Avoid use; may increase CNS depression.

Food: Avoid acidic food or juices and vitamin C; may alter serum concentration. Avoid caffeine (eg, colas, chocolate).

Herb/Nutraceutical: Avoid ephedra, ginseng, and yohimbe; may cause arrhythmias or hypertension. Avoid gotu kola, kava, SAMe, St John's wort, and valerian; may increase CNS depression.

Pharmacodynamics/Kinetics

Onset: 30-60 minutes

Duration: 4-6 hours

Absorption: Well-absorbed

Distribution: V_d: Adults: 3.5-4.6 L/kg; concentrates in breast milk (avoid breast-feeding); distributes into CNS, mean CSF concentrations are 80% of plasma

Half-life elimination:

- Children: D-amphetamine: 9 hours; L-amphetamine: 11 hours
- Adults: D-amphetamine: 10 hours; L-amphetamine: 13 hours

Metabolism: Hepatic via cytochrome P450 monooxygenase and glucuronidation

Time to peak: T_{max}: Adderall®: 3 hours; Adderall XR™: 7 hours

Excretion: 70% of a single dose is eliminated within 24 hours; excreted as unchanged amphetamine (30%), benzoic acid, hydroxyamphetamine, hippuric acid, norephedrine, and *p*-hydroxynorephedrine

Pregnancy Risk Factor C

Generic Available Yes: Tablet

Dextroamphetamine Sulfate *see* Dextroamphetamine *on page 420*

Dextromethorphan (deks troe meth OR fan)

Related Information

Codeine *on page 361*

Guaifenesin, Pseudoephedrine, and Dextromethorphan *on page 653*

U.S. Brand Names Babee® Cof Syrup [OTC]; Benylin® Adult [OTC]; Benylin® Pediatric [OTC]; Creomulsion® Cough [OTC]; Creomulsion® for Children [OTC]; Creo-Terpin® [OTC]; Delsym® [OTC]; Dexalone® [OTC]; Diabe-Tuss DM [OTC]; Hold® DM [OTC]; Pertussin® DM [OTC]; Robitussin® Maximum Strength Cough [OTC]; Robitussin® Pediatric Cough [OTC]; Scot-Tussin DM® Cough Chasers [OTC]; Silphen DM® [OTC]; Simply Cough™ [OTC]; Vicks® 44® Cough Relief [OTC]

Mexican Brand Names Athos®; Bekidiba Dex®; Neopulmonier®; Romilar®

Pharmacologic Category Antitussive

Use Symptomatic relief of coughs caused by minor viral upper respiratory tract infections or inhaled irritants; most effective for a chronic nonproductive cough

Unlabeled/Investigational Use *N*-methyl-D-aspartate (NMDA) antagonist in cerebral injury

Local Anesthetic/Vasoconstrictor Precautions No information available to require special precautions

Effects on Dental Treatment No significant effects or complications reported

Dosage Oral:

Children:

- <2 years: Use only as directed by a physician
- 2-6 years (syrup): 2.5-7.5 mg every 4-8 hours; extended release is 15 mg twice daily (maximum: 30 mg/24 hours)
- 6-12 years: 5-10 mg every 4 hours or 15 mg every 6-8 hours; extended release is 30 mg twice daily (maximum: 60 mg/24 hours)

Children >12 years and Adults: 10-20 mg every 4 hours or 30 mg every 6-8 hours; extended release: 60 mg twice daily; maximum: 120 mg/day

Mechanism of Action Chemical relative of morphine lacking narcotic properties except in overdose; controls cough by depressing the medullary cough center

Other Adverse Effects <1%: **Drowsiness, dizziness, coma, respiratory depression, nausea, GI upset,** constipation, abdominal discomfort

Drug Interactions Substrate of CYP2B6, 2C8/9, 2C19, **2D6**, 2E1, 3A4; Inhibits CYP2D6

Increased Effect/Toxicity: May increase effect/toxicity of MAO inhibitors.

Pharmacodynamics/Kinetics

Onset of action: Antitussive: 15-30 minutes

Duration: ≤6 hours

Pregnancy Risk Factor C

Generic Available Yes

Dextromethorphan, Acetaminophen, and Pseudoephedrine *see* Acetaminophen, Dextromethorphan, and Pseudoephedrine *on page 35*

Dextromethorphan and Guaifenesin *see* Guaifenesin and Dextromethorphan *on page 651*

Dextromethorphan and Promethazine *see* Promethazine and Dextromethorphan *on page 1129*

Dextromethorphan and Pseudoephedrine *see* Pseudoephedrine and Dextromethorphan *on page 1147*

Dextromethorphan, Carbinoxamine, and Pseudoephedrine *see* Carbinoxamine, Pseudoephedrine, and Dextromethorphan *on page 247*

Dextromethorphan, Guaifenesin, and Pseudoephedrine *see* Guaifenesin, Pseudoephedrine, and Dextromethorphan *on page 653*

Dextromethorphan, Pseudoephedrine, and Carbinoxamine *see* Carbinoxamine, Pseudoephedrine, and Dextromethorphan *on page 247*

Dextropropoxyphene *see* Propoxyphene *on page 1135*

Dextrose and Tetracaine *see* Tetracaine and Dextrose *on page 1285*

Dextrose, Levulose and Phosphoric Acid *see* Phosphorated Carbohydrate Solution *on page 1078*

Dextrostat® *see* Dextroamphetamine *on page 420*

DFMO *see* Eflornithine *on page 489*

DHAD *see* Mitoxantrone *on page 923*

DHE *see* Dihydroergotamine *on page 445*

D.H.E. 45® *see* Dihydroergotamine *on page 445*

DHPG Sodium *see* Ganciclovir *on page 626*

DHS™ Sal [OTC] *see* Salicylic Acid *on page 1204*

DHS® Tar [OTC] *see* Coal Tar *on page 359*

DHS™ Zinc [OTC] *see* Pyrithione Zinc *on page 1154*

DHT™ *see* Dihydrotachysterol *on page 446*

DHT™ Intensol™ *see* Dihydrotachysterol *on page 446*

Diaβeta® *see* GlyBURIDE *on page 642*

Diabetic Tussin® DM [OTC] *see* Guaifenesin and Dextromethorphan *on page 651*

Diabetic Tussin® DM Maximum Strength [OTC] *see* Guaifenesin and Dextromethorphan *on page 651*

Diabetic Tussin® EX [OTC] *see* Guaifenesin *on page 650*

Diabe-Tuss DM [OTC] *see* Dextromethorphan *on page 423*

Diabinese® *see* ChlorproPAMIDE *on page 314*

Dialume® [OTC] *see* Aluminum Hydroxide *on page 68*

Diaminocyclohexane Oxalatoplatinum *see* Oxaliplatin *on page 1008*

Diaminodiphenylsulfone *see* Dapsone *on page 399*

Diamox® *see* AcetaZOLAMIDE *on page 37*

Diamox Sequels® *see* AcetaZOLAMIDE *on page 37*

Diasorb® [OTC] *see* Attapulgite *on page 146*

Diastat® Rectal Delivery System *see* Diazepam *on page 424*

Diazepam (dye AZ e pam)

Related Information

Dental Office Emergencies *on page 1582*

Patients Requiring Sedation *on page 1565*

Temporomandibular Dysfunction (TMD) *on page 1562*

U.S. Brand Names Diastat® Rectal Delivery System; Diazepam Intensol®; Valium®

Canadian Brand Names Apo®-Diazepam; Diastat®; Diazemuls®; Valium®

Mexican Brand Names Alboral®; Diatex; Ortopsique®; Pacitran®; Valium®

Pharmacologic Category Benzodiazepine

Use

Dental: Oral medication for preoperative dental anxiety; sedative component in I.V. conscious sedation in oral surgery patients; skeletal muscle relaxant

Medical: Management of anxiety disorders, ethanol withdrawal symptoms; skeletal muscle relaxant; treatment of convulsive disorders

Orphan drug: Viscous solution for rectal administration: Management of selected, refractory epilepsy patients on stable regimens of antiepileptic drugs (AEDs) requiring intermittent use of diazepam to control episodes of increased seizure activity

Unlabeled/Investigational Use Treatment of amnesia, panic disorders; preoperative sedation, light anesthesia

Local Anesthetic/Vasoconstrictor Precautions No information available to require special precautions

Effects on Dental Treatment

>10%: Xerostomia, changes in salivation

Frequency not defined: Hypotension, drowsiness, amnesia, slurred speech, paradoxical excitement or rage, fatigue, memory impairment, headache, anxiety, confusion, nausea, tremors, blurred vision, decreased respiratory rate, apnea

Restrictions C-IV

Dosage Oral absorption is more reliable than I.M.

Children:

Conscious sedation for procedures: Oral: 0.2-0.3 mg/kg (maximum: 10 mg) 45-60 minutes prior to procedure

Sedation/muscle relaxant/anxiety:

Oral: 0.12-0.8 mg/kg/day in divided doses every 6-8 hours

I.M., I.V.: 0.04-0.3 mg/kg/dose every 2-4 hours to a maximum of 0.6 mg/kg within an 8-hour period if needed

Status epilepticus:

Infants 30 days to 5 years: I.V.: 0.05-0.3 mg/kg/dose given over 2-3 minutes, every 15-30 minutes to a maximum total dose of 5 mg; repeat in 2-4 hours as needed **or** 0.2-0.5 mg/dose every 2-5 minutes to a maximum total dose of 5 mg

>5 years: I.V.: 0.05-0.3 mg/kg/dose given over 2-3 minutes every 15-30 minutes to a maximum total dose of 10 mg; repeat in 2-4 hours as needed **or** 1 mg/dose given over 2-3 minutes, every 2-5 minutes to a maximum total dose of 10 mg

Rectal: 0.5 mg/kg, then 0.25 mg/kg in 10 minutes if needed

Anticonvulsant (acute treatment): Rectal gel formulation:

Infants <6 months: Use not recommended

Children <2 years: Safety and efficacy not studied

Children 2-5 years: 0.5 mg/kg

Children 6-11 years: 0.3 mg/kg

Children ≥12 years and Adults: 0.2 mg/kg

Note: Dosage should be rounded upward to the next available dose, 2.5, 5, 10, 15, and 20 mg/dose; dose may be repeated in 4-12 hours if needed; do not use more than 5 times per month or more than once every 5 days

Adolescents: **Conscious sedation for procedures:**

Oral: 10 mg

I.V.: 5 mg, may repeat with 1/2 dose if needed

Adults:

Anxiety/sedation/skeletal muscle relaxant:

Oral: 2-10 mg 2-4 times/day

I.M., I.V.: 2-10 mg, may repeat in 3-4 hours if needed

Status epilepticus: I.V.: 5-10 mg every 10-20 minutes, up to 30 mg in an 8-hour period; may repeat in 2-4 hours if necessary

Rapid tranquilization of agitated patient (administer every 30-60 minutes): Oral: 5-10 mg; average total dose for tranquilization: 20-60 mg

Elderly: Oral: Initial:

Anxiety: 1-2 mg 1-2 times/day; increase gradually as needed, rarely need to use >10 mg/day (watch for hypotension and excessive sedation)

Skeletal muscle relaxant: 2-5 mg 2-4 times/day

Hemodialysis: Not dialyzable (0% to 5%); supplemental dose is unnecessary

Dosing adjustment in hepatic impairment: Reduce dose by 50% in cirrhosis and avoid in severe/acute liver disease

Mechanism of Action Binds to stereospecific benzodiazepine receptors on the postsynaptic GABA neuron at several sites within the central nervous system, including the limbic system, reticular formation. Enhancement of the inhibitory effect of GABA on neuronal excitability results by increased neuronal membrane permeability to chloride ions. This shift in chloride ions results in hyperpolarization (a less excitable state) and stabilization.

Other Adverse Effects Frequency not defined:

Central nervous system: Ataxia, insomnia, depression, vertigo

Dermatologic: Rash

Endocrine & metabolic: Changes in libido

Gastrointestinal: Constipation

Genitourinary: Incontinence, urinary retention

Hepatic: Jaundice

Local: Phlebitis, pain with injection

Neuromuscular & skeletal: Dysarthria

Ocular: Diplopia

Contraindications Hypersensitivity to diazepam or any component of the formulation (cross-sensitivity with other benzodiazepines may exist); narrow-angle glaucoma; not for use in children <6 months of age (oral) or <30 days of age (parenteral); pregnancy

Warnings/Precautions Diazepam has been associated with increasing the frequency of grand mal seizures. Withdrawal has also been associated with an increase in the seizure frequency. Use with caution with drugs which may decrease diazepam metabolism. Use with caution in elderly or debilitated patients, patients with hepatic disease (including alcoholics), or renal impairment. Active metabolites

(Continued)

Diazepam *(Continued)*

with extended half-lives may lead to delayed accumulation and adverse effects. Use with caution in patients with respiratory disease or impaired gag reflex.

Acute hypotension, muscle weakness, apnea, and cardiac arrest have occurred with parenteral administration. Acute effects may be more prevalent in patients receiving concurrent barbiturates, narcotics, or ethanol. Appropriate resuscitative equipment and qualified personnel should be available during administration and monitoring. Avoid use of the injection in patients with shock, coma, or acute ethanol intoxication. Intra-arterial injection or extravasation of the parenteral formulation should be avoided. Parenteral formulation contains propylene glycol, which has been associated with toxicity when administered in high dosages.

Causes CNS depression (dose-related) resulting in sedation, dizziness, confusion, or ataxia which may impair physical and mental capabilities. Patients must be cautioned about performing tasks which require mental alertness (ie, operating machinery or driving). Use with caution in patients receiving other CNS depressants or psychoactive agents. Effects with other sedative drugs or ethanol may be potentiated. The dosage of narcotics should be reduced by approximately 1/3 when diazepam is added. Benzodiazepines have been associated with falls and traumatic injury and should be used with extreme caution in patients who are at risk of these events (especially the elderly).

Use caution in patients with depression, particularly if suicidal risk may be present. Use with caution in patients with a history of drug dependence. Benzodiazepines have been associated with dependence and acute withdrawal symptoms on discontinuation or reduction in dose. Acute withdrawal, including seizures, may be precipitated in patients after administration of flumazenil to patients receiving long-term benzodiazepine therapy.

Diazepam has been associated with anterograde amnesia. Paradoxical reactions, including hyperactive or aggressive behavior, have been reported with benzodiazepines, particularly in adolescent/pediatric or psychiatric patients. Does not have analgesic, antidepressant, or antipsychotic properties.

Drug Interactions Substrate of CYP1A2, 2B6, 2C8/9, **2C19, 3A4**; Inhibits CYP2C19, 3A4

CNS depressants: Sedative effects and/or respiratory depression may be additive with CNS depressants; includes ethanol, barbiturates, narcotic analgesics, and other sedative agents; monitor for increased effect

Enzyme inducers: Metabolism of some benzodiazepines may be increased, decreasing their therapeutic effect; consider using an alternative sedative/hypnotic agent; potential inducers include phenobarbital, phenytoin, carbamazepine, rifampin, and rifabutin

Levodopa: Therapeutic effects may be diminished in some patients following the addition of a benzodiazepine; limited/inconsistent data

Oral contraceptives: May decrease the clearance of some benzodiazepines (those which undergo oxidative metabolism); monitor for increased benzodiazepine effect

Theophylline: May partially antagonize some of the effects of benzodiazepines; monitor for decreased response; may require higher doses for sedation

Dietary/Ethanol/Herb Considerations

Ethanol: Avoid use; may increase CNS depression.

Food: May be taken with food but may increase serum concentration. Avoid grapefruit products; may increase serum concentration/toxicity.

Herb/Nutraceutical: Avoid gotu kola, kava, SAMe, and valerian; may increase CNS depression. Avoid St John's wort; may decrease serum concentration and increase CNS depression. Melatonin may enhance diazepam activity; use cautiously.

Pharmacodynamics/Kinetics

I.V.: Status epilepticus:

Onset of action: Almost immediate

Duration: 20-30 minutes

Absorption: Oral: 85% to 100%, more reliable than I.M.

Protein binding: 98%

Metabolism: Hepatic

Half-life elimination: Parent drug: Adults: 20-50 hours; increased half-life in neonates, elderly, and those with severe hepatic disorders; Active major metabolite (desmethyldiazepam): 50-100 hours; may be prolonged in neonates

Pregnancy Risk Factor D

Breast-feeding Considerations Clinical effects on the infant include sedation; AAP reports that USE MAY BE OF CONCERN.

Dosage Forms GEL, rectal delivery system (Diastat®): Adult rectal tip [6 cm]: 5 mg/mL (15 mg, 20 mg); pediatric rectal tip [4.4 cm]: 5 mg/mL (2.5 mg, 5 mg); universal rectal tip [pediatric/adult 4.4 cm]: 5 mg/mL (10 mg). **INJ, solution:** 5 mg/mL (2 mL, 10 mL). **SOLN, oral:** 5 mg/5 mL (5 mL, 10 mL, 500 mL). **SOLN, oral concentrate** (Diazepam Intensol®): 5 mg/mL (30 mL). **TAB** (Valium®): 2 mg, 5 mg, 10 mg

Generic Available Yes: Injection, tablet, solution only

Diazepam Intensol® *see* Diazepam *on page 424*

Diazoxide (dye az OKS ide)

U.S. Brand Names Hyperstat®; Proglycem®

Canadian Brand Names Hyperstat® I.V.; Proglycem®

Mexican Brand Names Hyperstat I.V.®; Sefulken®

Pharmacologic Category Antihypertensive; Antihypoglycemic Agent

Use

Oral: Hypoglycemia related to islet cell adenoma, carcinoma, hyperplasia, or adenomatosis, nesidioblastosis, leucine sensitivity, or extrapancreatic malignancy

I.V.: Severe hypertension

Local Anesthetic/Vasoconstrictor Precautions No information available to require special precautions

Effects on Dental Treatment 1% to 10%: Hypotension, dizziness, nausea, vomiting, weakness

Dosage

Hypertension: Children and Adults: I.V.: 1-3 mg/kg up to a maximum of 150 mg in a single injection; repeat dose in 5-15 minutes until blood pressure adequately reduced; repeat administration at intervals of 4-24 hours; monitor the blood pressure closely; do not use longer than 10 days

Hyperinsulinemic hypoglycemia: Oral: **Note:** Use lower dose listed as initial dose
Newborns and Infants: 8-15 mg/kg/day in divided doses every 8-12 hours
Children and Adults: 3-8 mg/kg/day in divided doses every 8-12 hours

Dialysis: Elimination is not enhanced via hemo- or peritoneal dialysis; supplemental dose is unnecessary

Mechanism of Action Inhibits insulin release from the pancreas; produces direct smooth muscle relaxation of the peripheral arterioles which results in decrease in blood pressure and reflex increase in heart rate and cardiac output

Other Adverse Effects <1%: **Tachycardia, flushing, angina, MI, seizures, headache, extrapyramidal symptoms** and development of abnormal facies with chronic oral use; cerebral infarction, rash, hirsutism, cellulitis, hyperglycemia, ketoacidosis, sodium and water retention, hyperuricemia, inhibition of labor, anorexia, constipation, leukopenia, thrombocytopenia, pain, burning, phlebitis upon extravasation

Drug Interactions

Increased Effect/Toxicity: Diuretics and hypotensive agents may potentiate diazoxide adverse effects. Diazoxide may decrease warfarin protein binding.

Decreased Effect: Diazoxide may increase phenytoin metabolism or free fraction.

Pharmacodynamics/Kinetics

Onset of action: Hyperglycemic: Oral: ~1 hour
Peak effect: Hypotensive: I.V.: ~5 minutes

Duration: Hyperglycemic: Oral: Normal renal function: 8 hours; Hypotensive: I.V.: Usually 3-12 hours

Protein binding: 90%

Half-life elimination: Children: 9-24 hours; Adults: 20-36 hours; End-stage renal disease: >30 hours

Excretion: Urine (50% as unchanged drug)

Pregnancy Risk Factor C

Generic Available No

Dibenzyline® *see* Phenoxybenzamine *on page 1068*

Dibucaine (DYE byoo kane)

U.S. Brand Names Nupercainal® [OTC]

Pharmacologic Category Local Anesthetic, Dental; Local Anesthetic

Use

Dental: Amide derivative topical local anesthetic for minor skin conditions

Medical: Fast, temporary relief of pain and itching due to hemorrhoids, minor burns

Local Anesthetic/Vasoconstrictor Precautions No information available to require special precautions

Effects on Dental Treatment 1% to 10%: Angioedema, contact dermatitis, burning

Dosage Children and Adults: Topical: Apply gently to the affected areas; no more than 30 g for adults or 7.5 g for children should be used in any 24-hour period

Mechanism of Action Local anesthetics bind selectively to the intracellular surface of sodium channels to block influx of sodium into the axon. As a result, depolarization necessary for action potential propagation and subsequent nerve function is prevented. The block at the sodium channel is reversible. When drug diffuses away from the axon, sodium channel function is restored and nerve propagation returns.

Contraindications Hypersensitivity to amide-type anesthetics, ophthalmic use

Warnings/Precautions Avoid use in sensitive individuals

Pharmacodynamics/Kinetics

Onset of action: ~15 minutes

(Continued)

Dibucaine *(Continued)*

Duration: 2-4 hours

Absorption: Poor through intact skin; well absorbed through mucous membranes and excoriated skin

Pregnancy Risk Factor C

Breast-feeding Considerations No data reported; probably compatible

Dosage Forms OINT 1% (30 g, 60 g, 454 g); (Nupercainal®): 1% (30 g, 60g)

Generic Available Yes

DIC *see* Dacarbazine *on page 391*

Dicarbosil® [OTC] *see* Calcium Supplements *on page 229*

Dichloralphenazone, Acetaminophen, and Isometheptene *see* Acetaminophen, Isometheptene, and Dichloralphenazone *on page 36*

Dichloralphenazone, Isometheptene, and Acetaminophen *see* Acetaminophen, Isometheptene, and Dichloralphenazone *on page 36*

Dichlorodifluoromethane and Trichloromonofluoromethane

(dye klor oh dye flor oh METH ane & tri klor oh mon oh flor oh METH ane)

Related Information

Temporomandibular Dysfunction (TMD) *on page 1562*

U.S. Brand Names Fluori-Methane®

Pharmacologic Category Analgesic, Topical

Synonyms Trichloromonofluoromethane and Dichlorodifluoromethane

Use

Dental: Topical application in the management of myofascial pain, restricted motion, and muscle spasm

Medical: For the control of pain associated with injections

Local Anesthetic/Vasoconstrictor Precautions No information available to require special precautions

Effects on Dental Treatment No significant effects or complications reported

Dosage Invert bottle over treatment area approximately 12" away from site of application; open dispenseal spring valve completely, allowing liquid to flow in a stream from the bottle. The rate of spraying is approximately 10 cm/second and should be continued until entire muscle has been covered.

Contraindications Hypersensitivity to dichlorofluoromethane and/or trichloromonofluoromethane, or any component of the formulation; patients having vascular impairment of the extremities

Warnings/Precautions For external use only; care should be taken to minimize inhalation of vapors, especially with application to head and neck; avoid contact with eyes; should not be applied to the point of frost formation

Pharmacodynamics/Kinetics No data reported

Dosage Forms AERO, topical: Dichlorodifluoromethane 15% and trichloromonofluoromethane 85% (103 mL)

Generic Available No

Comments Dichlorodifluoromethane and trichloromonofluoromethane are not classified as carcinogens; based on animal studies and human experience, these fluorocarbons pose no hazard to man relative to systemic toxicity, carcinogenicity, mutagenicity, or teratogenicity when occupational exposures are <1000 ppm over an 8-hour time weighted average.

Dichlorotetrafluoroethane and Ethyl Chloride *see* Ethyl Chloride and Dichlorotetrafluoroethane *on page 545*

Dichlorphenamide (dye klor FEN a mide)

U.S. Brand Names Daranide®

Canadian Brand Names Daranide®

Pharmacologic Category Carbonic Anhydrase Inhibitor; Diuretic, Carbonic Anhydrase Inhibitor; Ophthalmic Agent, Antiglaucoma

Synonyms Diclofenamide

Use Adjunct in treatment of open-angle glaucoma and perioperative treatment for angle-closure glaucoma

Local Anesthetic/Vasoconstrictor Precautions No information available to require special precautions

Effects on Dental Treatment

>10%: Metallic taste, fatigue, malaise

1% to 10%: Drowsiness

Dosage Adults: Oral: 100-200 mg to start followed by 100 mg every 12 hours until desired response is obtained; maintenance dose: 25-50 mg 1-3 times/day

Other Adverse Effects

>10%:

Gastrointestinal: Diarrhea, anorexia

Genitourinary: Polyuria

1% to 10%:

Central nervous system: Mental depression

Renal: Renal calculi

Drug Interactions Decreased Effect: Increased lithium excretion and altered excretion of other drugs by alkalinization of the urine.

Pregnancy Risk Factor C

Generic Available No

Dichysterol *see* Dihydrotachysterol *on page 446*

Diclofenac (dye KLOE fen ak)

Related Information

Rheumatoid Arthritis, Osteoarthritis, and Osteoporosis *on page 1488*

Temporomandibular Dysfunction (TMD) *on page 1562*

U.S. Brand Names Cataflam®; Solaraze™; Voltaren®; Voltaren Ophthalmic®; Voltaren®-XR

Canadian Brand Names Apo®-Diclo; Apo®-Diclo Rapide; Apo®-Diclo SR; Cataflam®; Diclotec; Novo-Difenac®; Novo-Difenac K; Novo-Difenac-SR®; Nu-Diclo; Nu-Diclo-SR; PMS-Diclofenac; PMS-Diclofenac SR; Riva-Diclofenac; Riva-Diclofenac-K; Voltaren®; Voltaren Ophtha®; Voltaren Rapide®

Mexican Brand Names 3-A Ofteno®; Artrenac®; Cataflam®; Cataflam Dispersible®; Clonodifen®; Deflox®; Dicloran®; Dolaren®; Dolflam®; Dolo Pangavit-D; Fustaren®; Fustaren Retard; Galedol®; Lifenac®; Lifenal; Liroken®; Logesic®; Merxil®; Selectofen®; Volfenac Gel®; Volfenac Retard®; Voltaren®; Voltaren Emulgel®

Pharmacologic Category Nonsteroidal Anti-inflammatory Drug (NSAID)

Synonyms Diclofenac Potassium; Diclofenac Sodium

Use

Dental:

Immediate-release tablets: Acute treatment of mild to moderate pain; ankylosing spondylitis; primary dysmenorrhea; acute and chronic treatment of rheumatoid arthritis, osteoarthritis

Medical:

Delayed-release tablets: Acute and chronic treatment of rheumatoid arthritis, osteoarthritis, ankylosing spondylitis

Extended-release tablets: Chronic treatment of osteoarthritis, rheumatoid arthritis

Ophthalmic solution: Postoperative inflammation following cataract extraction; temporary relief of pain and photophobia in patients undergoing corneal refractive surgery

Topical gel: Actinic keratosis (AK) in conjunction with sun avoidance

Unlabeled/Investigational Use Treatment of juvenile rheumatoid arthritis

Local Anesthetic/Vasoconstrictor Precautions No information available to require special precautions

Effects on Dental Treatment NSAID formulations are known to reversibly decrease platelet aggregation via mechanisms different than observed with aspirin. The dentist should be aware of the potential of abnormal coagulation. Caution should also be exercised in the use of NSAIDs in patients already on anticoagulant therapy with drugs such as warfarin (Coumadin®).

>10%: Application site reactions (gel): Contact dermatitis (19% to 33%), pain (15% to 26%), paresthesia (8% to 20%)

1% to 10%: Headache (7%), dizziness (3%) nausea (3% to 9%), peptic ulcer/GI bleed (≤2%), abnormal vision, blurred vision

Dosage Adults:

Oral:

Analgesia/primary dysmenorrhea: Starting dose: 50 mg 3 times/day; maximum dose: 150 mg/day

Rheumatoid arthritis: 150-200 mg/day in 2-4 divided doses (100 mg/day of sustained release product)

Osteoarthritis: 100-150 mg/day in 2-3 divided doses (100-200 mg/day of sustained release product)

Ankylosing spondylitis: 100-125 mg/day in 4-5 divided doses

Elderly: No specific recommendations; may demonstrate adverse effects at lower doses than younger adults, and >60% may develop asymptomatic peptic ulceration with or without hemorrhage; monitor renal function

Dosing adjustment in renal impairment: Monitor closely in significant impairment

Dosing adjustment in hepatic impairment: No specific recommendations

Ophthalmic:

Cataract surgery: Instill 1 drop into affected eye 4 times/day beginning 24 hours after cataract surgery and continuing for 2 weeks

Corneal refractive surgery: Instill 1-2 drops into affected eye within the hour prior to surgery, within 15 minutes following surgery, and then continue for 4 times/day, up to 3 days

Topical: Apply gel to lesion area twice daily for 60-90 days

(Continued)

Diclofenac *(Continued)*

Mechanism of Action Inhibits prostaglandin synthesis by decreasing the activity of the enzyme, cyclooxygenase, which results in decreased formation of prostaglandin precursors. Mechanism of action for the treatment of AK has not been established.

Other Adverse Effects

>10%:

Local: Application site reactions (gel): Pruritus (31% to 52%), rash (35% to 46%), dry skin (25% to 27%), exfoliation (6% to 24%)

Ocular: Ophthalmic drops (incidence may be dependent upon indication): Lacrimation (30%), keratitis (28%), elevated IOP (15%), transient burning/stinging (15%)

1% to 10%:

Dermatologic: Pruritus (1% to 3%), rash (1% to 3%)

Endocrine & metabolic: Fluid retention (1% to 3%)

Gastrointestinal: Abdominal cramps (3% to 9%), abdominal pain (3% to 9%), constipation (3% to 9%), diarrhea (3% to 9%), flatulence (3% to 9%), indigestion (3% to 9%), abdominal distention (1% to 3%)

Hepatic: Increased ALT/AST (2%)

Local: Application site reactions (gel): Edema (4%)

Ocular: Ophthalmic drops: Acute elevated IOP, conjunctivitis, corneal deposits, corneal edema, corneal opacity, corneal lesions, discharge, eyelid swelling, injection, iritis, irritation, itching, lacrimation disorder, ocular allergy

Otic: Tinnitus (1% to 3%)

<1%, postmarketing, and case reports (limited): Oral forms: **Acute renal failure,** agranulocytosis, allergic purpura, alopecia, **anaphylactoid reactions, anaphylaxis,** angioedema, **aphthous stomatitis,** aplastic anemia, appetite changes, aseptic meningitis, **asthma,** azotemia, bloody diarrhea, bullous eruption, cirrhosis, colitis, **CHF, dermatitis, xerostomia, dry mucous membranes, eczema, eosinophilia, epistaxis, erythema multiforme major, esophageal lesions, GI hemorrhage,** hearing loss, decreased hemoglobin, hemolytic anemia, hepatic necrosis, hepatitis, hepatorenal syndrome, **hypertension,** interstitial nephritis, jaundice, **laryngeal edema,** leukopenia, **malaise,** melena, nephrotic syndrome, oliguria, pancreatitis, papillary necrosis, photosensitivity, proteinuria, purpura, Stevens-Johnson syndrome, **swelling of lips and tongue, taste disorder,** thrombocytopenia, urticaria, **visual changes, vomiting**

Contraindications Hypersensitivity to diclofenac, any component of the formulation, aspirin or other NSAIDs, including patients who experience bronchospasm, asthma, rhinitis, or urticaria following NSAID or aspirin; porphyria; pregnancy (3rd trimester)

Warnings/Precautions Use with caution in patients with CHF, dehydration, hypertension, decreased renal or hepatic function, history of GI disease, active GI ulceration or bleeding, or those receiving anticoagulants. Anaphylactoid reactions have been reported with NSAID use, even without prior exposure; may be more common in patients with the aspirin triad. Use with caution in patients with pre-existing asthma. Rare cases of severe hepatic reactions (including necrosis, jaundice, fulminant hepatitis) have been reported. Vision changes (including changes in color) have been rarely reported with oral diclofenac.

Topical gel should not be applied to the eyes, open wounds, infected areas, or to exfoliative dermatitis. Monitor patients for 1 year following application of ophthalmic drops for corneal refractive procedures. Patients using ophthalmic drops should not wear soft contact lenses. Ophthalmic drops may slow/delay healing or prolong bleeding time following surgery. Elderly are at a high risk for adverse effects from NSAIDs. As many as 60% of elderly can develop peptic ulceration and/or hemorrhage asymptomatically.

Use lowest effective dose for shortest period possible. Use of NSAIDs can compromise existing renal function especially when Cl_{cr} is <30 mL/minute. CNS adverse effects such as confusion, agitation, and hallucination are generally seen in overdose or high-dose situations; however, elderly may demonstrate these adverse effects at lower doses than younger adults. Withhold for at least 4-6 half-lives prior to surgical or dental procedures.

Drug Interactions Substrate of CYP1A2, 2B6, 2C8/9, 2C19, 2D6, 3A4; Inhibits CYP2C8/9, 2E1

ACE inhibitors: Antihypertensive effects may be decreased by concurrent therapy with NSAIDs; monitor blood pressure

Angiotensin II antagonists: Antihypertensive effects may be decreased by concurrent therapy with NSAIDs; monitor blood pressure

Anticoagulants (warfarin, heparin, LMWHs) in combination with NSAIDs can cause increased risk of bleeding.

Other antiplatelet drugs (ticlopidine, clopidogrel, aspirin, abciximab, dipyridamole, eptifibatide, tirofiban) can cause an increased risk of bleeding.

Cholestyramine and colestipol reduce the bioavailability of diclofenac; separate administration times.

Corticosteroids may increase the risk of GI ulceration; avoid concurrent use.

Cyclosporine: NSAIDs may increase serum creatinine, potassium, blood pressure, and cyclosporine levels; monitor cyclosporine levels and renal function carefully.

Gentamicin and amikacin serum concentrations are increased by indomethacin in premature infants. Results may apply to other aminoglycosides and NSAIDs.

Hydralazine's antihypertensive effect is decreased; avoid concurrent use.

Lithium levels can be increased; avoid concurrent use if possible or monitor lithium levels and adjust dose. Sulindac may have the least effect. When NSAID is stopped, lithium will need adjustment again.

Loop diuretics efficacy (diuretic and antihypertensive effect) is reduced. Indomethacin reduces this efficacy, however, it may be anticipated with any NSAID.

Methotrexate: Severe bone marrow suppression, aplastic anemia, and GI toxicity have been reported with concomitant NSAID therapy. Avoid use during moderate or high-dose methotrexate (increased and prolonged methotrexate levels). NSAID use during low-dose treatment of rheumatoid arthritis has not been fully evaluated; extreme caution is warranted.

Thiazides antihypertensive effects are decreased; avoid concurrent use.

Verapamil plasma concentration is decreased by diclofenac; avoid concurrent use.

Warfarin's INRs may be increased by piroxicam. Other NSAIDs may have the same effect depending on dose and duration. Monitor INR closely. Use the lowest dose of NSAIDs possible and for the briefest duration.

Dietary/Ethanol/Herb Considerations

Ethanol: Avoid use; may enhance gastric mucosal irritation.

Food: Administer with 8 oz water and food or milk to reduce GI upset. Avoid garlic, ginger, and green tea.

Herb/Nutraceutical: Avoid cat's claw, dong quai, evening primrose, feverfew, garlic, ginger, ginkgo biloba, ginseng, green tea, horse chestnut, and red clover due to additional antiplatelet activity. Avoid kava and valerian; may enhance benzodiazepine activity.

Pharmacodynamics/Kinetics

Onset of action: Cataflam® is more rapid than sodium salt (Voltaren®) because it dissolves in the stomach instead of the duodenum

Absorption: Topical gel: 10%

Protein binding: 99% to albumin

Metabolism: Hepatic to several metabolites

Half-life elimination: 2 hours

Time to peak, serum: Cataflam®: ~1 hour; Voltaren®: ~2 hours

Excretion: Urine (65%); feces (35%)

Pregnancy Risk Factor B/D (3rd trimester)

Dosage Forms GEL, as sodium (Solaraze™): 30 mg/g (50 g). **SOLN, ophthalmic, as sodium** (Voltaren Ophthalmic®): 0.1% (2.5 mL, 5 mL). **TAB, as potassium** (Cataflam®): 50 mg. **TAB, delayed release, enteric coated, as sodium** (Voltaren®): 25 mg, 50 mg, 75 mg. **TAB, extended release, as sodium** (Voltaren®-XR): 100 mg

Generic Available Yes

Diclofenac and Misoprostol (dye KLOE fen ak & mye soe PROST ole)

Related Information

Diclofenac *on page 429*

Rheumatoid Arthritis, Osteoarthritis, and Osteoporosis *on page 1488*

U.S. Brand Names Arthrotec®

Canadian Brand Names Arthrotec®

Pharmacologic Category Nonsteroidal Anti-inflammatory Drug (NSAID); Prostaglandin

Synonyms Misoprostol and Diclofenac

Use The diclofenac component is indicated for the treatment of osteoarthritis and rheumatoid arthritis; the misoprostol component is indicated for the prophylaxis of NSAID-induced gastric and duodenal ulceration

Local Anesthetic/Vasoconstrictor Precautions No information available to require special precautions

Effects on Dental Treatment Nausea (11%), anaphylactic reactions (1% to 10%)

Dosage Oral: If not tolerated, dose may be reduced to 1 tablet twice daily.

Adults:

Arthrotec® 50:

Osteoarthritis: 1 tablet 2-3 times/day

Rheumatoid arthritis: 1 tablet 3-4 times/day

Arthrotec® 75: Patients who cannot tolerate full daily Arthrotec® 50 regimens: 1 tablet twice daily (may not be as effective at preventing GI ulceration)

Elderly: No specific adjustment is recommended; may require reduced dosage due to lower body weight; monitor renal function

Mechanism of Action See individual agents.

Other Adverse Effects

>10%: Gastrointestinal: Abdominal pain (21%), diarrhea (19%), dyspepsia (14%)

1% to 10%:

Endocrine & metabolic: Elevated transaminase levels

Gastrointestinal: Flatulence (9%)

(Continued)

Diclofenac and Misoprostol *(Continued)*

Hematologic: Anemia

Postmarketing and/or case reports (associated with misoprostol): Uterine rupture, fetal or infant death (when used during pregnancy)

Drug Interactions

Increased Effect/Toxicity: Aspirin (shared toxicity), digoxin (elevated digoxin levels), warfarin (synergistic bleeding potential), methotrexate (increased methotrexate levels), cyclosporine (increased nephrotoxicity), lithium (increased lithium levels)

Decreased Effect: Aspirin (displaces diclofenac from binding sites), antihypertensive agents (decreased blood pressure control), antacids (may decrease absorption). Antihypertensive effects of ACE-inhibitors and angiotensin antagonists may be decreased by concurrent therapy with NSAIDs.

Dietary/Ethanol/Herb Considerations Ethanol: Avoid use; may enhance gastric mucosal irritation.

Pregnancy Risk Factor X

Generic Available No

Diclofenac Potassium *see* Diclofenac *on page 429*

Diclofenac Sodium *see* Diclofenac *on page 429*

Diclofenamide *see* Dichlorphenamide *on page 428*

Dicloxacillin (dye kloks a SIL in)

Related Information

Oral Bacterial Infections *on page 1531*

Canadian Brand Names Dycill®; Pathocil®

Mexican Brand Names Brispen; Cilpen®; Ditterolina®; Posipen®

Pharmacologic Category Antibiotic, Penicillin

Synonyms Dicloxacillin Sodium

Use

Dental: Treatment of susceptible orofacial infections, notably penicillinase-producing staphylococci

Medical: Treatment of systemic infections such as pneumonia, skin and soft tissue infections, and osteomyelitis caused by penicillinase-producing staphylococci

Local Anesthetic/Vasoconstrictor Precautions No information available to require special precautions

Effects on Dental Treatment Prolonged use of penicillins may lead to development of oral candidiasis.

1% to 10%: Nausea

Dosage Oral:

Newborns: Use not recommended

Children <40 kg: 12.5-25 mg/kg/day divided every 6 hours; doses of 50-100 mg/kg/day in divided doses every 6 hours have been used for therapy of osteomyelitis

Children >40 kg and Adults: 125-250 mg every 6 hours

Hemodialysis: Not dialyzable (0% to 5%); supplemental dosage unnecessary

Peritoneal dialysis: Supplemental dosage unnecessary

Continuous arteriovenous or venovenous hemofiltration: Supplemental dosage unnecessary

Mechanism of Action Inhibits bacterial cell wall synthesis by binding to one or more of the penicillin binding proteins (PBPs); which in turn inhibits the final transpeptidation step of peptidoglycan synthesis in bacterial cell walls, thus inhibiting cell wall biosynthesis. Bacteria eventually lyse due to ongoing activity of cell wall autolytic enzymes (autolysins and murein hydrolases) while cell wall assembly is arrested.

Other Adverse Effects

1% to 10%: Gastrointestinal: Diarrhea, abdominal pain

<1%: **Fever, seizures** (extremely high doses and/or renal failure), rash (maculopapular to exfoliative), **vomiting, pseudomembranous colitis,** vaginitis, eosinophilia, leukopenia, neutropenia, thrombocytopenia, agranulocytosis, anemia, hemolytic anemia, **prolonged PT,** hepatotoxicity, transient elevated LFTs, hematuria, interstitial nephritis, increased BUN/creatinine, **serum sickness-like reactions, hypersensitivity**

Contraindications Hypersensitivity to dicloxacillin, penicillin, or any component of the formulation

Warnings/Precautions Monitor PT if patient concurrently on warfarin; elimination of drug is slow in neonates; use with caution in patients allergic to cephalosporins

Drug Interactions Induces CYP3A4

Oral contraceptives: Anecdotal reports suggesting decreased contraceptive efficacy with penicillins have been refuted by more rigorous scientific and clinical data.

Probenecid, disulfiram: May increase levels of penicillins (dicloxacillin)

Warfarin: Concurrent use may decrease effect of warfarin

Dietary/Ethanol/Herb Considerations Food: Administer on an empty stomach; food decreases absorption rate and serum concentration.

Pharmacodynamics/Kinetics

Absorption: 35% to 76%; rate and extent reduced by food

Distribution: Throughout body with highest concentrations in kidney and liver; CSF penetration is low; crosses placenta; enters breast milk

Protein binding: 96%

Half-life elimination: 0.6-0.8 hour; slightly prolonged with renal impairment

Time to peak, serum: 0.5-2 hours

Excretion: Feces; urine (56% to 70% as unchanged drug); prolonged in neonates

Pregnancy Risk Factor B

Breast-feeding Considerations No data reported; however, other penicillins may be taken while breast-feeding.

Dosage Forms CAP: 250 mg, 500 mg

Generic Available Yes

Comments Although dicloxacillin is a penicillin antibiotic indicated for infections caused by penicillinase secreting staph, amoxicillin with clavulanic acid is considered the drug of choice for these types of orofacial infections

Dicloxacillin Sodium *see* Dicloxacillin *on page 432*

Dicumarol (dye KOO ma role)

Related Information

Cardiovascular Diseases *on page 1456*

Warfarin *on page 1397*

Pharmacologic Category Anticoagulant, Coumarin Derivative

Synonyms Bishydroxycoumarin

Use Prophylaxis and treatment of thromboembolic disorders

Local Anesthetic/Vasoconstrictor Precautions No information available to require special precautions

Effects on Dental Treatment Signs of dicumarol overdose may first appear as bleeding from gingival tissue; consultation with prescribing physician is advisable prior to surgery to determine temporary dose reduction or withdrawal of medication.

1% to 10%: Nausea, vomiting

Dosage Adults: Oral: 25-200 mg/day based on PT (PT) determinations

Mechanism of Action Interferes with hepatic synthesis of vitamin K-dependent coagulation factors (II, VII, IX, X)

Other Adverse Effects 1% to 10%:

Dermatologic: Alopecia

Gastrointestinal: Stomach cramps, diarrhea

Hematologic: Leukopenia

Drug Interactions Substrate of **2C8/9**

Increased Effect/Toxicity: May accentuate toxicities of oral hypoglycemics and anticonvulsants. The following will decrease prothrombin time: Antacids, antihistamines, phenobarbital, carbamazepine, cholestyramine, meprobamate, glutethimide, ethchlorvynol, oral contraceptives, ranitidine, chloral hydrate, diuretics. Increased prothrombin time due to allopurinol, amiodarone, cimetidine, clofibrate, dextran, diazoxide, diflunisal, diuretics, disulfiram, fenoprofen, ibuprofen, indomethacin, influenza virus vaccine, methyldopa, methylphenidate, MAO inhibitors, naproxen, nortriptyline, phenytoin, propylthiouracil, salicylates, quinidine, quinine, ranitidine, tolbutamide, thyroid drugs, sulindac, co-trimoxazole.

Dietary/Ethanol/Herb Considerations Food: Avoid proteolytic enzymes (eg, papain), fried/boiled onions, and soybean oil.

Pregnancy Risk Factor D

Generic Available Yes

Dicyclomine (dye SYE kloe meen)

U.S. Brand Names Bentyl®

Canadian Brand Names Bentylol®; Formulex®; Lomine

Pharmacologic Category Anticholinergic Agent

Synonyms Dicyclomine Hydrochloride; Dicycloverine Hydrochloride

Use Treatment of functional disturbances of GI motility such as irritable bowel syndrome

Unlabeled/Investigational Use Treatment of urinary incontinence

Local Anesthetic/Vasoconstrictor Precautions No information available to require special precautions

Effects on Dental Treatment

>10%: Xerostomia, changes in salivation

Reported for pharmacologically similar drugs with anticholinergic/antispasmodic action; frequency not defined: Syncope, tachycardia, palpitations, dizziness, lightheadedness, tingling, headache, drowsiness, nervousness, numbness, mental confusion and/or excitement, lethargy, speech disturbance, severe allergic reaction or drug idiosyncrasies including anaphylaxis, nausea, vomiting, loss of taste, weakness, blurred vision, dyspnea, apnea, asphyxia, nasal stuffiness or congestion, sneezing, throat congestion

(Continued)

Dicyclomine *(Continued)*

Dosage

Oral:

Infants >6 months: 5 mg/dose 3-4 times/day

Children: 10 mg/dose 3-4 times/day

Adults: Begin with 80 mg/day in 4 equally divided doses, then increase up to 160 mg/day

I.M. **(should not be used I.V.)**: Adults: 80 mg/day in 4 divided doses (20 mg/dose)

Mechanism of Action Blocks the action of acetylcholine at parasympathetic sites in smooth muscle, secretory glands and the CNS

Other Adverse Effects Reported for pharmacologically similar drugs with anticholinergic/antispasmodic action; frequency not defined:

Central nervous system: Insomnia

Dermatologic: Rash, urticaria, itching, and other dermal manifestations; severe allergic reaction or drug idiosyncrasies including anaphylaxis

Endocrine & metabolic: Suppression of lactation

Gastrointestinal: Constipation, bloated feeling, abdominal pain, anorexia

Genitourinary: Urinary hesitancy, urinary retention, impotence

Ocular: Diplopia, mydriasis, cycloplegia, increased ocular tension

Miscellaneous: Decreased diaphoresis

Drug Interactions

Increased Effect/Toxicity: Dicyclomine taken with anticholinergics, amantadine, narcotic analgesics, Type I antiarrhythmics, antihistamines, phenothiazines, tricyclic antidepressants may result in increased toxicity.

Decreased Effect: Decreased effect with phenothiazines, anti-Parkinson's drugs, haloperidol, sustained release dosage forms, and with antacids.

Dietary/Ethanol/Herb Considerations

Ethanol: Avoid use; may increase CNS depression.

Herb/Nutraceutical: Avoid gotu kola, kava, SAMe, St John's wort, and valerian; may increase CNS depression.

Pharmacodynamics/Kinetics

Onset of action: 1-2 hours

Duration: ≤4 hours

Absorption: Oral: Well absorbed

Metabolism: Extensive

Half-life elimination: Initial: 1.8 hours; Terminal: 9-10 hours

Excretion: Urine (small amounts as unchanged drug)

Pregnancy Risk Factor B

Generic Available Yes

Dicyclomine Hydrochloride *see* Dicyclomine *on page 433*

Dicycloverine Hydrochloride *see* Dicyclomine *on page 433*

Didanosine (dye DAN oh seen)

Related Information

HIV Infection and AIDS *on page 1482*

U.S. Brand Names Videx®; Videx® EC

Canadian Brand Names Videx®; Videx® EC

Mexican Brand Names Videx®

Pharmacologic Category Antiretroviral Agent, Reverse Transcriptase Inhibitor (Nucleoside)

Synonyms ddI; Dideoxyinosine

Use Treatment of HIV infection; always to be used in combination with at least two other antiretroviral agents

Local Anesthetic/Vasoconstrictor Precautions No information available to require special precautions

Effects on Dental Treatment 1% to 10%: Xerostomia

Dosage Treatment of HIV infection: Oral (administer on an empty stomach):

Children:

2 weeks to 8 months: 100 mg/m² twice daily

>8 months: 120 mg/m² twice daily

Children <1 year should receive 1 tablet per dose and children >1 year should receive 2-4 tablets per dose for adequate buffering and absorption; tablets should be chewed or dispersed

Adults: Dosing based on patient weight:

Note: Preferred dosing frequency is twice daily for didanosine tablets

Tablets:

<60 kg: 125 mg twice daily or 250 mg once daily

≥60 kg: 200 mg twice daily or 400 mg once daily

Note: Adults should receive 2-4 tablets per dose for adequate buffering and absorption; tablets should be chewed or dispersed; didanosine has also been used as 300 mg once daily

Buffered Powder:

<60 kg: 167 mg twice daily

≥60 kg; 250 mg twice daily

Sustained release capsule:

<60 kg: 250 mg once daily

≥60 kg; 400 mg once daily

Elderly patients have a higher frequency of pancreatitis (10% versus 5% in younger patients); monitor renal function and dose accordingly

Dosing adjustment in renal impairment: Dosing based on patient weight, creatinine clearance, and dosage form: See table.

Recommended Dose (mg) of Didanosine by Body Weight

Creatinine Clearance (mL/min)	≥60 kg			<60 kg		
	Tablet* (mg)	Buffered Powder† (mg)	Sustained Release Capsule (mg)	Tablet* (mg)	Buffered Powder† (mg)	Sustained Release Capsule (mg)
≥60	400 qd or 200 bid	250 bid	400 qd	250 qd or 125 bid	167 bid	250 qd
30-59	200 qd or 100 bid	100 bid	200 qd	150 qd or 75 bid	100 bid	125 qd
10-29	150 qd	167 qd	125 qd	100 qd	100 qd	125 qd
<10	100 qd	100 qd	125 qd	75 qd	100 qd	‡

*Chewable/dispersible buffered tablet; 2 tablets must be taken with each dose; different strengths of tablets may be combined to yield the recommended dose.

†Buffered powder for oral solution

‡Not suitable for use in patients <60 kg with Cl_{cr} <10 mL/minute; use alternate formulation

Hemodialysis: Removed by hemodialysis (40% to 60%)

Dosing adjustment in hepatic impairment: Should be considered; monitor for toxicity

Mechanism of Action Didanosine, a purine nucleoside analogue and the deamination product of dideoxyadenosine (ddA), inhibits HIV replication *in vitro* in both T cells and monocytes. Didanosine is converted within the cell to the mono-, di-, and triphosphates of ddA. These ddA triphosphates act as substrate and inhibitor of HIV reverse transcriptase substrate and inhibitor of HIV reverse transcriptase thereby blocking viral DNA synthesis and suppressing HIV replication.

Other Adverse Effects As reported in monotherapy studies; risk of toxicity may increase when combined with other agents.

>10%:

Gastrointestinal: Increased amylase (15% to 17%), abdominal pain (7% to 13%), diarrhea (19% to 28%)

Neuromuscular & skeletal: Peripheral neuropathy (17% to 20%)

1% to 10%:

Dermatologic: Rash, pruritus

Endocrine & metabolic: Increased uric acid

Gastrointestinal: Pancreatitis; patients >65 years of age had a higher frequency of pancreatitis than younger patients

Hepatic: Increased SGOT, increased SGPT, increased alkaline phosphatase

Postmarketing reports: Alopecia, **anaphylactoid reaction,** anemia, anorexia, arthralgia, chills/**fever, diabetes mellitus,** dyspepsia, flatulence, granulocytopenia, hepatitis, hyperlactatemia (symptomatic), **hypersensitivity,** lactic acidosis/hepatomegaly, leukopenia, liver failure, myalgia, myopathy, neuritis, optic renal impairment, pain, retinal depigmentation, rhabdomyolysis, **seizures,** thrombocytopenia, **weakness**

Drug Interactions

Increased Effect/Toxicity: Concomitant administration of other drugs which have the potential to cause peripheral neuropathy or pancreatitis may increase the risk of these toxicities Allopurinol may increase didanosine concentration; avoid concurrent use. Concomitant use of antacids with buffered tablet or pediatric didanosine solution may potentiate adverse effects of aluminum- or magnesium-containing antacids. Ganciclovir may increase didanosine concentration; monitor. Hydroxyurea may precipitate didanosine-induced pancreatitis if added to therapy; concomitant use is not recommended. Coadministration with ribavirin or tenofovir may increase exposure to didanosine and/or its active metabolite increasing the risk or severity of didanosine toxicities, including pancreatitis, lactic acidosis, and peripheral neuropathy; monitor closely and suspend therapy if signs or symptoms of toxicity are noted.

Decreased Effect: Didanosine buffered tablets and buffered pediatric solution may decrease absorption of quinolones or tetracyclines (administer 2 hours prior to didanosine buffered formulations). Didanosine should be held during PCP treatment with pentamidine. Didanosine may decrease levels of indinavir. Drugs whose absorption depends on the level of acidity in the stomach such as ketoconazole, itraconazole, and dapsone should be administered at least 2 hours prior to the buffered formulations of didanosine (not affected by sustained release capsules). Methadone may decrease didanosine concentrations.

Dietary/Ethanol/Herb Considerations

Ethanol: Avoid use; increases risk of pancreatitis.

(Continued)

Didanosine *(Continued)*

Food decreases AUC and C_{max}; may decrease serum concentration by 55%. Administer at least 1 hour before or 2 hours after meal. Do not mix with fruit juice or other acid-containing liquid. Each chewable tablet contains 8.6 mEq magnesium. Each single-dose powder packet (for oral solution) contains 1380 mg sodium.

Pharmacodynamics/Kinetics

Absorption: Subject to degradation by acidic pH of stomach; some formulations are buffered to resist acidic pH; ≤50% reduction in peak plasma concentration is observed in presence of food. Sustained release capsules contain enteric-coated beadlets which dissolve in the small intestine.

Distribution: V_d: Children: 35.6 L/m²; Adults: 1.08 L/kg

Protein binding: <5%

Metabolism: Has not been evaluated in humans; studies conducted in dogs show extensive metabolism with allantoin, hypoxanthine, xanthine, and uric acid being the major metabolites found in urine

Bioavailability: 42%

Half-life elimination:

Children and Adolescents: 0.8 hour

Adults: Normal renal function: 1.5 hours; active metabolite, ddATP, has an intracellular half-life >12 hours *in vitro*; Renal impairment: 2.5-5 hours

Time to peak: Buffered tablets: 0.67 hours; Sustained release capsules: 2 hours

Excretion: Urine (~55% as unchanged drug)

Clearance: Total body: Averages 800 mL/minute

Pregnancy Risk Factor B

Generic Available No

Dideoxycytidine *see* Zalcitabine *on page 1403*

Dideoxyinosine *see* Didanosine *on page 434*

Didrex® *see* Benzphetamine *on page 172*

Didronel® *see* Etidronate Disodium *on page 546*

Diethylpropion (dye eth il PROE pee on)

U.S. Brand Names Tenuate®; Tenuate® Dospan®

Canadian Brand Names Tenuate®; Tenuate® Dospan®

Mexican Brand Names Ifa Norex®; Neobes®

Pharmacologic Category Anorexiant

Synonyms Amfepramone; Diethylpropion Hydrochloride

Use Short-term adjunct in a regimen of weight reduction based on exercise, behavioral modification, and caloric reduction in the management of exogenous obesity for patients with an initial body mass index ≥30 kg/m² or ≥27 kg/m² in the presence of other risk factors (diabetes, hypertension)

Unlabeled/Investigational Use Treatment of migraine headaches

Local Anesthetic/Vasoconstrictor Precautions Use vasoconstrictor with caution in patients taking diethylpropion. Amphetamine-like drugs such as diethylpropion enhance the sympathomimetic response of epinephrine and norepinephrine leading to potential hypertension and cardiotoxicity.

Effects on Dental Treatment

>10%: Xerostomia, changes in salivation, hypertension (the use of local anesthetic without vasoconstrictor is recommended in these patients)

Frequency not defined: Palpitations, tachycardia, chest pain, euphoria, arrhythmias, nervousness, restlessness, dizziness, anxiety, headache, agitation, confusion, psychosis, seizure, nausea, vomiting, metallic taste, tremor, blurred vision, bruising

Restrictions C-IV

Dosage Adults: Oral:

Tablet: 25 mg 3 times/day before meals or food

Tablet, controlled release: 75 mg at midmorning

Mechanism of Action Diethylpropion is used as an anorexiant agent possessing pharmacological and chemical properties similar to those of amphetamines. The mechanism of action of diethylpropion in reducing appetite appears to be secondary to CNS effects, specifically stimulation of the hypothalamus to release catecholamines into the central nervous system; anorexiant effects are mediated via norepinephrine and dopamine metabolism. An increase in physical activity and metabolic effects (inhibition of lipogenesis and enhancement of lipolysis) may also contribute to weight loss.

Other Adverse Effects Frequency not defined:

Cardiovascular: T-wave changes, pulmonary hypertension, valvulopathy

Central nervous system: Insomnia, mental depression, CVA

Dermatologic: Alopecia, urticaria, skin rash, erythema

Endocrine & metabolic: Changes in libido, gynecomastia, menstrual irregularities, porphyria

Gastrointestinal: Abdominal cramps, constipation

Genitourinary: Impotence

Hematologic: Bone marrow depression, agranulocytosis, leukopenia
Ocular: Mydriasis

Drug Interactions
Increased Effect/Toxicity: Concurrent use or use within 14 days following the administration of a MAO inhibitor is contraindicated (hypertensive crisis). Concurrent use of sibutramine and diethylpropion is contraindicated (severe hypertension, tachycardia). Concurrent use with TCAs may result in enhanced toxicity. Concurrent use with other anorectic agents may cause serious cardiac problems and is contraindicated.
Decreased Effect: Diethylpropion may displace guanethidine from the neuron and antagonize its antihypertensive effects; discontinue diethylpropion or use alternative antihypertensive.

Dietary/Ethanol/Herb Considerations
Ethanol: Avoid use; may increase CNS depression.
Herb/Nutraceutical: Avoid gotu kola, kava, SAMe, St John's wort, and valerian; may increase CNS depression.

Pharmacodynamics/Kinetics
Onset of action: 1 hour
Duration: 12-24 hours

Pregnancy Risk Factor B
Generic Available Yes

Diethylpropion Hydrochloride *see* Diethylpropion *on page 436*

Diethylstilbestrol (dye eth il stil BES trole)

Pharmacologic Category Estrogen Derivative
Synonyms DES; Diethylstilbestrol Diphosphate Sodium; Stilbestrol
Use Palliative treatment of inoperable metastatic prostatic carcinoma and postmenopausal, inoperable, progressing breast cancer
Local Anesthetic/Vasoconstrictor Precautions No information available to require special precautions
Effects on Dental Treatment
>10% Nausea
1% to 10%: Headache, migraine, vomiting
Dosage Adults:
Male:
Prostate carcinoma (inoperable, progressing): Oral: 1-3 mg/day
Diphosphate: Inoperable progressing prostate cancer:
Oral: 50 mg 3 times/day; increase up to 200 mg or more 3 times/day; maximum daily dose: 1 g
I.V.: Give 0.5 g, dissolved in 250 mL of saline or D_5W, administer slowly the first 10-15 minutes then adjust rate so that the entire amount is given in 1 hour; repeat for ≥5 days depending on patient response, then repeat 0.25-0.5 g 1-2 times for 1 week or change to oral therapy
Female: Postmenopausal inoperable, progressing breast carcinoma: Oral: 15 mg/day
Mechanism of Action Competes with estrogenic and androgenic compounds for binding onto tumor cells and thereby inhibits their effects on tumor growth
Other Adverse Effects
>10%:
Cardiovascular: Peripheral edema
Endocrine & metabolic: Enlargement of breasts (female and male), breast tenderness
Gastrointestinal: Anorexia, bloating
1% to 10%:
Endocrine & metabolic: Increased libido (female), decreased libido (male)
Gastrointestinal: Diarrhea

Diethylstilbestrol Diphosphate Sodium *see* Diethylstilbestrol *on page 437*

Difenoxin and Atropine (dye fen OKS in & A troe peen)

Related Information
Atropine *on page 144*
U.S. Brand Names Motofen®
Pharmacologic Category Antidiarrheal
Synonyms Atropine and Difenoxin
Use Treatment of diarrhea
Local Anesthetic/Vasoconstrictor Precautions No information available to require special precautions
Effects on Dental Treatment 1% to 10%: Xerostomia, dizziness, drowsiness, lightheadedness, headache, nausea, vomiting, epigastric distress
Restrictions C-IV
Dosage Adults: Oral: Initial: 2 tablets, then 1 tablet after each loose stool; 1 tablet every 3-4 hours, up to 8 tablets in a 24-hour period; if no improvement after 48 hours, continued administration is not indicated
(Continued)

Difenoxin and Atropine *(Continued)*

Drug Interactions Increased Effect/Toxicity: Concurrent use with MAO inhibitors may precipitate hypertensive crisis. May potentiate action of barbiturates, tranquilizers, narcotics, and alcohol. Difenoxin has the potential to prolong biological half-life of drugs for which the rate of elimination is dependent on the microsomal drug metabolizing enzyme system.

Dietary/Ethanol/Herb Considerations Ethanol: Avoid use; ethanol effects may be potentiated.

Pharmacodynamics/Kinetics
Absorption: Rapid and well absorbed
Metabolism: To inactive hydroxylated metabolite
Time to peak, plasma: Within 40-60 minutes
Excretion: Urine and feces (primarily as conjugates)

Pregnancy Risk Factor C

Generic Available No

Differin® *see* Adapalene *on page 44*

Diflorasone (dye FLOR a sone)

U.S. Brand Names Maxiflor®; Psorcon®; Psorcon® e™

Canadian Brand Names Florone®; Psorcon®

Pharmacologic Category Corticosteroid, Topical

Synonyms Diflorasone Diacetate

Use Relieves inflammation and pruritic symptoms of corticosteroid-responsive dermatosis (high to very high potency topical corticosteroid)

Maxiflor®: High potency topical corticosteroid
Psorcon™: Very high potency topical corticosteroid

Local Anesthetic/Vasoconstrictor Precautions No information available to require special precautions

Effects on Dental Treatment No significant effects or complications reported

Dosage Topical: Apply ointment sparingly 1-3 times/day; apply cream sparingly 2-4 times/day. Therapy should be discontinued when control is achieved; if no improvement is seen, reassessment of diagnosis may be necessary.

Mechanism of Action Decreases inflammation by suppression of migration of polymorphonuclear leukocytes and reversal of increased capillary permeability

Other Adverse Effects <1%: Itching, folliculitis, maceration, burning, dryness, muscle atrophy, arthralgia, secondary infection

Pharmacodynamics/Kinetics
Absorption: Negligible, around 1% reaches dermal layers or systemic circulation; occlusive dressings increase absorption percutaneously
Metabolism: Primarily hepatic

Pregnancy Risk Factor C

Generic Available Yes

Diflorasone Diacetate *see* Diflorasone *on page 438*
Diflucan® *see* Fluconazole *on page 576*

Diflunisal (dye FLOO ni sal)

Related Information
Oral Pain *on page 1524*
Rheumatoid Arthritis, Osteoarthritis, and Osteoporosis *on page 1488*
Temporomandibular Dysfunction (TMD) *on page 1562*

U.S. Brand Names Dolobid®

Canadian Brand Names Apo®-Diflunisal; Novo-Diflunisal; Nu-Diflunisal

Mexican Brand Names Dolobid®

Pharmacologic Category Nonsteroidal Anti-inflammatory Drug (NSAID)

Use
Dental: Treatment of postoperative pain
Medical: Management of pain and inflammatory disorders usually including rheumatoid arthritis and osteoarthritis

Local Anesthetic/Vasoconstrictor Precautions No information available to require special precautions

Effects on Dental Treatment NSAID formulations are known to reversibly decrease platelet aggregation via mechanisms different than observed with aspirin. The dentist should be aware of the potential of abnormal coagulation. Caution should also be exercised in the use of NSAIDs in patients already on anticoagulant therapy with drugs such as warfarin (Coumadin®).

>10%: Headache
1% to 10%: Arrhythmias, angina pectoris, dizziness, GI ulceration

Dosage Adults: **Oral:**
Pain: Initial: 500-1000 mg followed by 250-500 mg every 8-12 hours; maximum daily dose: 1.5 g
Inflammatory condition: 500-1000 mg/day in 2 divided doses; maximum daily dose: 1.5 g

Dosing adjustment in renal impairment: Cl_{cr} <50 mL/minute: Administer 50% of normal dose

Mechanism of Action Inhibits prostaglandin synthesis by decreasing the activity of the enzyme, cyclooxygenase, which results in decreased formation of prostaglandin precursors

Other Adverse Effects

>10%: Endocrine & metabolic: Fluid retention

1% to 10%:

Dermatologic: Rash

Genitourinary: Vaginal bleeding

Otic: Tinnitus

<1%: **Chest pain**, vasculitis, **tachycardia, convulsions, hallucinations,** mental depression, **drowsiness, nervousness**, insomnia, toxic epidermal necrolysis, urticaria, exfoliative dermatitis, itching, erythema multiforme, Stevens-Johnson syndrome, angioedema, **stomatitis, esophagitis or gastritis,** cystitis, hemolytic anemia, agranulocytosis, thrombocytopenia, hepatitis, peripheral neuropathy, **trembling, weakness, blurred vision, change in vision**, decreased hearing, interstitial nephritis, nephrotic syndrome, renal impairment, **wheezing, dyspnea, anaphylaxis, diaphoresis (increased)**

Contraindications Hypersensitivity to diflunisal or any component of the formulation; may be a cross-sensitivity with other NSAIDs including aspirin; should not be used in patients with active GI bleeding; pregnancy (3rd trimester)

Warnings/Precautions Peptic ulceration and GI bleeding have been reported; platelet function and bleeding time are inhibited; ophthalmologic effects; impaired renal function, use lower dosage; dehydration; peripheral edema; possibility of Reye's syndrome; elevation in liver tests. Withhold for at least 4-6 half-lives prior to surgical or dental procedures.

Drug Interactions

ACE inhibitors: Antihypertensive effects may be decreased by concurrent therapy with NSAIDs; monitor blood pressure

Angiotensin II antagonists: Antihypertensive effects may be decreased by concurrent therapy with NSAIDs; monitor blood pressure

Antacids: Decreased effect (may decrease absorption)

Increased effect/toxicity: Digoxin, anticoagulants, phenytoin, sulfonylureas, sulfonamides, lithium, hydrochlorothiazide, acetaminophen (levels)

Methotrexate: Severe bone marrow suppression, aplastic anemia, and GI toxicity have been reported with concomitant NSAID therapy. Avoid use during moderate or high-dose methotrexate (increased and prolonged methotrexate levels). NSAID use during low-dose treatment of rheumatoid arthritis has not been fully evaluated; extreme caution is warranted.

Dietary/Ethanol/Herb Considerations

Ethanol: Avoid use; may enhance gastric mucosal irritation.

Food: Administer with food or milk to reduce GI upset. Avoid excessive amounts of fruit juices, vitamin C or salicylate-containing foods (curry powder, prunes, raisins, tea, or licorice).

Herb/Nutraceutical: Avoid cat's claw, dong quai, evening primrose, feverfew, garlic, ginger, ginkgo biloba, ginseng, green tea, horse chestnut, and red clover due to additional antiplatelet activity. Avoid kava and valerian; may enhance benzodiazepine activity. Limit licorice due to salicylate content.

Pharmacodynamics/Kinetics

Onset of action: Analgesic: ~1 hour

Duration: 8-12 hours

Absorption: Well absorbed

Distribution: Enters breast milk

Metabolism: Extensively hepatic

Half-life elimination: 8-12 hours; prolonged with renal impairment

Time to peak, serum: 2-3 hours

Excretion: Urine (~3% as unchanged drug, 90% as glucuronide conjugates) within 72-96 hours

Pregnancy Risk Factor C (1st and 2nd trimesters); D (3rd trimester)

Dosage Forms TAB: 250 mg, 500 mg

Generic Available Yes

Comments The advantage of diflunisal as a pain reliever is its 12-hour duration of effect. In many cases, this long effect will ensure a full night sleep during the postoperative pain period.

Selected Readings

Ahmad N, Grad HA, Haas DA, et al, "The Efficacy of Nonopioid Analgesics for Postoperative Dental Pain: A Meta-Analysis," *Anesth Prog*, 1997, 44(4):119-26.

Brooks PM and Day RO, "Nonsteroidal Anti-inflammatory Drugs - Differences and Similarities," *N Engl J Med*, 1991, 324(24):1716-25.

Dionne R, "Additive Analgesia Without Opioid Side Effects," *Compend Contin Educ Dent*, 2000, 21(7):572-4, 576-7.

Dionne RA, "New Approaches to Preventing and Treating Postoperative Pain," *J Am Dent Assoc*, 1992, 123(6):26-34.

Dionne RA and Berthold CW, "Therapeutic Uses of Nonsteroidal Anti-Inflammatory Drugs in Dentistry," *Crit Rev Oral Biol Med*, 2001, 12(4):315-30.

(Continued)

Diflunisal *(Continued)*

Forbes JA, Calderazzo JP, Bowser MW, et al, "A 12-Hour Evaluation of the Analgesic Efficacy of Diflunisal, Aspirin, and Placebo in Postoperative Dental Pain," *J Clin Pharmacol*, 1982, 22(2-3):89-96.
Gobetti JP, "Controlling Dental Pain," *J Am Dent Assoc*, 1992, 123(6):47-52.
Nguyen AM, Graham DY, Gage T, et al, "Nonsteroidal Anti-Inflammatory Drug Use in Dentistry: Gastrointestinal Implications," *Gen Dent*, 1999, 47(6):590-6.

Digibind® *see* Digoxin Immune Fab *on page 443*
DigiFab™ *see* Digoxin Immune Fab *on page 443*
Digitek® *see* Digoxin *on page 441*

Digitoxin (di ji TOKS in)

Related Information

Cardiovascular Diseases *on page 1456*
Digoxin *on page 441*
Digoxin Immune Fab *on page 443*

Pharmacologic Category Antiarrhythmic Agent, Class IV

Synonyms Crystodigin® [DSC]

Use Treatment of CHF, atrial fibrillation, atrial flutter, paroxysmal atrial tachycardia, and cardiogenic shock

Local Anesthetic/Vasoconstrictor Precautions Use vasoconstrictors with caution due to risk of cardiac arrhythmias with digitoxin.

Effects on Dental Treatment Sensitive gag reflex may cause difficulty in taking a dental impression.

1% to10%: Nausea, vomiting

Dosage Oral:

Children: Doses are very individualized; **when recommended**, digitalizing dose is as follows:
- <1 year: 0.045 mg/kg
- 1-2 years: 0.04 mg/kg
- >2 years: 0.03 mg/kg which is equivalent to 0.75 mg/m^2
- Maintenance: Approximately $^1/_{10}$ of the digitalizing dose

Adults: Oral:
- Rapid loading dose: Initial: 0.6 mg followed by 0.4 mg and then 0.2 mg at intervals of 4-6 hours
- Slow loading dose: 0.2 mg twice daily for a period of 4 days followed by a maintenance dose
- Maintenance: 0.05-0.3 mg/day
- Most common dose: 0.15 mg/day

Dosing adjustment in renal impairment: Cl_{cr} <10 mL/minute: Administer 50% to 75% of normal dose.

Hemodialysis: Not dialyzable (0% to 5%)

Dosing adjustment in hepatic impairment: Necessary in severe liver disease.

Mechanism of Action Digitalis binds to and inhibits magnesium and adenosine triphosphate dependent sodium and potassium ATPase thereby increasing the influx of calcium ions, from extracellular to intracellular cytoplasm due to the inhibition of sodium and potassium ion movement across the myocardial membranes; this increase in calcium ions results in a potentiation of the activity of the contractile heart muscle fibers and an increase in the force of myocardial contraction (positive inotropic effect); digitalis may also increase intracellular entry of calcium via slow calcium channel influx; stimulates release and blocks re-uptake of norepinephrine; decreases conduction through the SA and AV nodes

Other Adverse Effects

1% to 10%: Gastrointestinal: Anorexia

<1% (Limited to important or life-threatening): Sinus bradycardia, AV block, SA block, atrial or nodal ectopic beats, ventricular arrhythmias, bigeminy, trigeminy, atrial tachycardia with AV block, drowsiness, headache, fatigue, lethargy, vertigo, disorientation, hyperkalemia with acute toxicity, feeding intolerance, abdominal pain, diarrhea, neuralgia, blurred vision, halos, yellow or green vision, diplopia, photophobia, flashing lights

Drug Interactions Substrate of **CYP3A4**

Dietary/Ethanol/Herb Considerations

Food may delay, but does not affect extent of absorption. Increased fiber (bran) or foods high in pectin may decrease oral absorption. May require increased intake of potassium to avoid digitoxin toxicity. Avoid licorice.

Herb/Nutraceutical: Avoid aloe, horsetail, and licorice; may increase risk of digitoxin toxicity due to potassium loss. Avoid ephedra, ginseng, and yohimbe due to risk of cardiac stimulation. Avoid hawthorn; may increase effects. Avoid St John's wort.

Pharmacodynamics/Kinetics

Absorption: 90% to 100%
Distribution: V_d: 7 L/kg
Protein binding: 90% to 97%
Metabolism: Hepatic (50% to 70%)
Half-life elimination: 7-8 days

Time to peak: 8-12 hours
Excretion: Urine and feces (30% to 50% as unchanged drug)

Pregnancy Risk Factor C

Generic Available No

Digoxin (di JOKS in)

Related Information

Cardiovascular Diseases *on page 1456*
Digitoxin *on page 440*
Digoxin Immune Fab *on page 443*

U.S. Brand Names Digitek®; Lanoxicaps®; Lanoxin®

Canadian Brand Names Digoxin CSD; Lanoxicaps®; Lanoxin®; Novo-Digoxin

Mexican Brand Names Lanoxin®; Mapluxin®

Pharmacologic Category Antiarrhythmic Agent, Class IV; Cardiac Glycoside

Use Treatment of CHF and to slow the ventricular rate in tachyarrhythmias such as atrial fibrillation, atrial flutter, and supraventricular tachycardia (paroxysmal atrial tachycardia); cardiogenic shock

Local Anesthetic/Vasoconstrictor Precautions Use vasoconstrictor with caution due to risk of cardiac arrhythmias with digoxin

Effects on Dental Treatment Sensitive gag reflex may cause difficulty in taking a dental impression.

2% to 5%: Headache (3%), dizziness (5%), nausea (3%), vomiting (2%) mental disturbances (4%)

Frequency not defined: Visual disturbances (blurred or yellow vision), weakness, apathy, confusion, anxiety, delirium, hallucinations, fever, laryngeal edema, facial edema

Dosage When changing from oral (tablets or liquid) or I.M. to I.V. therapy, dosage should be reduced by 20% to 25% (refer to the following table).

Dosage Recommendations for Digoxin

Age	Total Digitalizing Dose† (mcg/kg*)		Daily Maintenance Dose‡ (mcg/kg*)	
	P.O.	I.V. or I.M.	P.O.	I.V. or I.M.
Preterm infant*	20-30	15-25	5-7.5	4-6
Full-term infant*	25-35	20-30	6-10	5-8
1 mo - 2 y*	35-60	30-50	10-15	7.5-12
2-5 y*	30-40	25-35	7.5-10	6-9
5-10 y*	20-35	15-30	5-10	4-8
>10 y*	10-15	8-12	2.5-5	2-3
Adults	0.75-1.5 mg	0.5-1 mg	0.125-0.5 mg	0.1-0.4 mg

*Based on lean body weight and normal renal function for age. Decrease dose in patients with ↓ renal function; digitalizing dose often not recommended in infants and children.

†Give one-half of the total digitalizing dose (TDD) in the initial dose, then give one-quarter of the TDD in each of two subsequent doses at 8- to 12-hour intervals. Obtain EKG 6 hours after each dose to assess potential toxicity.

‡Divided every 12 hours in infants and children <10 years of age. Given once daily to children >10 years of age and adults.

Dosing adjustment in renal impairment:
- Cl_{cr} 10-50 mL/minute: Administer 25% to 75% of dose or every 36 hours
- Cl_{cr} <10 mL/minute: Administer 10% to 25% of dose or every 48 hours
- Reduce loading dose by 50% in ESRD

Hemodialysis: Not dialyzable (0% to 5%)

Mechanism of Action

Congestive heart failure: Inhibition of the sodium/potassium ATPase pump which acts to increase the intracellular sodium-calcium exchange to increase intracellular calcium leading to increased contractility

Supraventricular arrhythmias: Direct suppression of the AV node conduction to increase effective refractory period and decrease conduction velocity - positive inotropic effect, enhanced vagal tone, and decreased ventricular rate to fast atrial arrhythmias. Atrial fibrillation may decrease sensitivity and increase tolerance to higher serum digoxin concentrations.

Other Adverse Effects Incidence not always reported; frequency not always defined:

Cardiovascular: Heart block; first-, second- (Wenckebach), or third-degree heart block; asystole; atrial tachycardia with block; AV dissociation; accelerated junctional rhythm; ventricular tachycardia or ventricular fibrillation; PR prolongation; ST segment depression

Central nervous system: Depression

Dermatologic: Maculopapular rash (2%), erythematous, scarlatiniform, papular, vesicular or bullous rashes, urticaria, pruritus, angioneurotic edema, shedding of fingernails or toenails, alopecia

Gastrointestinal: Diarrhea (3%), abdominal pain

(Continued)

Digoxin *(Continued)*

<1% (Limited to important or life-threatening): Gynecomastia, thrombocytopenia, **palpitations,** unifocal or multiform ventricular premature contractions (especially bigeminy or trigeminy), anorexia, abdominal pain, intestinal ischemia, hemorrhagic necrosis of the intestines, increase plasma estrogen and decreased serum luteinizing hormone in men and postmenopausal women and decreased plasma testosterone in men, vaginal cornification, eosinophilia, sexual dysfunction, **diaphoresis**

Children are more likely to experience cardiac arrhythmias as a sign of excessive dosing. The most common are conduction disturbances or tachyarrhythmias (atrial tachycardia with or without block) and junctional tachycardia. Ventricular tachyarrhythmias are less common. In infants, sinus bradycardia may be a sign of digoxin toxicity. Any arrhythmia seen in a child on digoxin should be considered as digoxin toxicity. The gastrointestinal and central nervous system symptoms are not frequently seen in children.

Drug Interactions Substrate of CYP3A4

Increased Effect/Toxicity: Beta-blocking agents (propranolol), verapamil, and diltiazem may have additive effects on heart rate. Carvedilol has additive effects on heart rate and inhibits the metabolism of digoxin. Digoxin levels may be increased by amiodarone (reduce digoxin dose 50%), bepridil, cyclosporine, diltiazem, indomethacin, itraconazole, some macrolides (erythromycin, clarithromycin), methimazole, nitrendipine, propafenone, propylthiouracil, quinidine (reduce digoxin dose 33% to 50% on initiation), tetracyclines, and verapamil. Moricizine may increase the toxicity of digoxin (mechanism undefined). Spironolactone may interfere with some digoxin assays, but may also increase blood levels directly. Succinylcholine administration to patients on digoxin has been associated with an increased risk of arrhythmias. Rare cases of acute digoxin toxicity have been associated with parenteral calcium (bolus) administration. The following medications have been associated with increased digoxin blood levels which appear to be of limited clinical significance: Famciclovir, flecainide, ibuprofen, fluoxetine, nefazodone, cimetidine, famotidine, ranitidine, omeprazole, trimethoprim.

Decreased Effect: Amiloride and spironolactone may reduce the inotropic response to digoxin. Cholestyramine, colestipol, kaolin-pectin, and metoclopramide may reduce digoxin absorption. Levothyroxine (and other thyroid supplements) may decrease digoxin blood levels. Penicillamine has been associated with reductions in digoxin blood levels The following reported interactions appear to be of limited clinical significance: Aminoglutethimide, aminosalicylic acid, aluminum-containing antacids, sucralfate, sulfasalazine, neomycin, ticlopidine.

Dietary/Ethanol/Herb Considerations

Food may delay, but does not affect extent of absorption. Increased fiber (bran) or foods high in pectin may decrease oral absorption. May require increased intake of potassium digitoxin toxicity. Avoid licorice.

Herb/Nutraceutical: Avoid aloe, horsetail, and licorice; may increase risk of digitoxin toxicity due to potassium loss. Avoid ephedra, ginseng, and yohimbe due to risk of cardiac stimulation. Avoid hawthorn; may increase effects. Avoid St John's wort.

Pharmacodynamics/Kinetics

Onset of action: Oral: 1-2 hours; I.V.: 5-30 minutes

Peak effect: Oral: 2-8 hours; I.V.: 1-4 hours

Duration: Adults: 3-4 days both forms

Absorption: By passive nonsaturable diffusion in the upper small intestine; food may delay, but does not affect extent of absorption

Distribution:

Normal renal function: 6-7 L/kg

V_d: Extensive to peripheral tissues, with a distinct distribution phase which lasts 6-8 hours; concentrates in heart, liver, kidney, skeletal muscle, and intestines. Heart/serum concentration is 70:1. Pharmacologic effects are delayed and do not correlate well with serum concentrations during distribution phase.

Hyperthyroidism: Increased V_d

Hyperkalemia, hyponatremia: Decreased digoxin distribution to heart and muscle

Hypokalemia: Increased digoxin distribution to heart and muscles

Concomitant quinidine therapy: Decreased V_d

Chronic renal failure: 4-6 L/kg

Decreased sodium/potassium ATPase activity - decreased tissue binding

Neonates, full-term: 7.5-10 L/kg

Children: 16 L/kg

Adults: 7 L/kg, decreased with renal disease

Protein binding: 30%; in uremic patients, digoxin is displaced from plasma protein binding sites

Metabolism: Via sequential sugar hydrolysis in the stomach or by reduction of lactone ring by intestinal bacteria (in ~10% of population, gut bacteria may metabolize up to 40% of digoxin dose); metabolites may contribute to therapeutic and toxic effects of digoxin; metabolism is reduced with CHF

Bioavailability: Oral (formulation dependent): Elixir: 75% to 85%; Tablet: 70% to 80%

Half-life elimination (age, renal and cardiac function dependent):
Neonates: Premature: 61-170 hours; Full-term: 35-45 hours
Infants: 18-25 hours
Children: 35 hours
Adults: 38-48 hours
Adults, anephric: 4-6 days
Half-life elimination: Parent drug: 38 hours; Metabolites: Digoxigenin: 4 hours; Monodigitoxoside: 3-12 hours
Time to peak, serum: Oral: ~1 hour
Excretion: Urine (50% to 70% as unchanged drug)

Pregnancy Risk Factor C

Generic Available Yes; Excludes capsule

Digoxin Immune Fab (di JOKS in i MYUN fab)

Related Information

Digitoxin *on page 440*
Digoxin *on page 441*

U.S. Brand Names Digibind®; DigiFab™

Canadian Brand Names Digibind®

Pharmacologic Category Antidote

Synonyms Antidigoxin Fab Fragments, Ovine

Use Treatment of life-threatening or potentially life-threatening digoxin intoxication, including:

- acute digoxin ingestion (ie, >10 mg in adults or >4 mg in children)
- chronic ingestions leading to steady-state digoxin concentrations > 6 ng/mL in adults or >4 ng/mL in children
- manifestations of digoxin toxicity due to overdose (life-threatening ventricular arrhythmias, progressive bradycardia, second- or third-degree heart block not responsive to atropine, serum potassium >5 mEq/L in adults or >6 mEq in children)

Local Anesthetic/Vasoconstrictor Precautions No information available to require special precautions

Effects on Dental Treatment Frequency not defined: Exacerbation of low cardiac output states and CHF, rapid ventricular response in patients with atrial fibrillation, postural hypotension, allergic reactions, serum sickness

Dosage Each vial of Digibind® 38 mg or DigiFab™ 40 mg will bind ~0.5 mg of digoxin or digitoxin.

Estimation of the dose is based on the body burden of digitalis. This may be calculated if the amount ingested is known or the postdistribution serum drug level is known (round dose to the nearest whole vial). See table.

Digoxin Immune Fab

Tablets Ingested (0.25 mg)	Fab Dose (vials)
5	2
10	4
25	10
50	20
75	30
100	40
150	60
200	80

Fab dose based on serum drug level postdistribution:
Digoxin: No. of vials = level (ng/mL) x body weight (kg) divided by 100
Digitoxin: No. of vials = digitoxin (ng/mL) x body weight (kg) divided by 1000

If neither amount ingested nor drug level are known, dose empirically as follows:
For acute toxicity: 20 vials, administered in 2 divided doses to decrease the possibility of a febrile reaction, and to avoid fluid overload in small children.
For chronic toxicity: 6 vials; for infants and small children (≤20kg), a single vial may be sufficient

Mechanism of Action Digoxin immune antigen-binding fragments (Fab) are specific antibodies for the treatment of digitalis intoxication in carefully selected patients; binds with molecules of digoxin or digitoxin and then is excreted by the kidneys and removed from the body

Other Adverse Effects Frequency not defined:
Endocrine & metabolic: Hypokalemia
Local: Phlebitis

Drug Interactions Increased Effect/Toxicity: Digoxin: Following administration of digoxin immune Fab, serum digoxin levels are markedly increased due to bound complexes (may be clinically misleading, since bound complex cannot interact with receptors).

(Continued)

Digoxin Immune Fab *(Continued)*

Pharmacodynamics/Kinetics

Onset of action: I.V.: Improvement in 2-30 minutes for toxicity

Half-life elimination: 15-20 hours; prolonged with renal impairment

Excretion: Urine; undetectable amounts within 5-7 days

Pregnancy Risk Factor C

Generic Available No

Dihematoporphyrin Ether *see* Porfimer *on page 1098*

Dihistine® DH *see* Chlorpheniramine, Pseudoephedrine, and Codeine *on page 311*

Dihistine® Expectorant *see* Guaifenesin, Pseudoephedrine, and Codeine *on page 653*

Dihydrocodeine, Aspirin, and Caffeine

(dye hye droe KOE deen, AS pir in, & KAF een)

Related Information

Aspirin *on page 131*

Oral Pain *on page 1524*

U.S. Brand Names Synalgos®-DC

Pharmacologic Category Analgesic, Narcotic

Synonyms Dihydrocodeine Compound

Use

Dental: Treatment of postoperative pain

Medical: Management of mild to moderate pain that requires relaxation

Local Anesthetic/Vasoconstrictor Precautions No information available to require special precautions

Effects on Dental Treatment Elderly are a high-risk population for adverse effects from nonsteroidal anti-inflammatory agents. As much as 60% of elderly patients with GI complications from NSAIDs can develop peptic ulceration and/or hemorrhage asymptomatically. Concomitant disease and drug use contribute to the risk of GI adverse effects. Use lowest effective dose for shortest period possible. Consider renal function decline with age.

The most common adverse effect you will see in your dental patients from dihydrocodeine is nausea, followed by sedation and constipation.

>10%: Lightheadedness, dizziness, drowsiness, sedation nausea, vomiting

1% to 10%: Hypotension, palpitations, bradycardia, peripheral vasodilation, increased intracranial pressure, biliary tract spasm, respiratory depression, histamine release, physical and psychological dependence (prolonged use)

Restrictions C-III

Dosage Oral: Adults: 1-2 capsules every 4-6 hours as needed for pain

Elderly: Initial dosing should be cautious (low end of adult dosing range)

Mechanism of Action Binds to opiate receptors in the CNS, causing inhibition of ascending pain pathways, altering the perception of and response to pain; causes cough suppression by direct central action in the medulla; produces generalized CNS depression

Other Adverse Effects

>10%:

Dermatologic: Pruritus, skin reactions

Gastrointestinal: Constipation

1% to 10%:

Endocrine & metabolic: Antidiuretic hormone release

Genitourinary: Urinary tract spasm

Ocular: Miosis

Contraindications Hypersensitivity to dihydrocodeine or any component of the formulation; pregnancy (prolonged use or high doses at term)

Warnings/Precautions Use with caution in patients with hypersensitivity reactions to other phenanthrene derivative opioid agonists (morphine, hydrocodone, hydromorphone, levorphanol, oxycodone, oxymorphone); respiratory diseases including asthma, emphysema, COPD, or severe liver or renal insufficiency. Some preparations contain sulfites which may cause allergic reactions. Tolerance or drug dependence may result from extended use. Use with caution in patients with platelet and bleeding disorders, erosive gastritis, or peptic ulcer disease, previous nonreaction does not guarantee future safe taking of medication. Do not use aspirin in children <16 years of age for chickenpox or flu symptoms due to the association with Reye's syndrome. Avoid aspirin, if possible, for 1 week prior to dental or surgical procedures due to possibility of postoperative bleeding.

Drug Interactions Substrate of **CYP2D6**

Increased Toxicity: MAO inhibitors may increase adverse symptoms

Dietary/Ethanol/Herb Considerations

Ethanol: Avoid use; may increase CNS depression.

Food: Administer with food. Fruit, fluids, and fiber may reduce constipation.

Herb/Nutraceutical: Avoid gotu kola, kava, SAMe, St John's wort, and valerian; may increase CNS depression.

Pharmacodynamics/Kinetics

Onset of action: 10-30 minutes

Duration: 4-6 hours

Metabolism: Hepatic

Half-life elimination, serum: 3.8 hours

Time to peak, serum: 30-60 minutes

Pregnancy Risk Factor B/D (prolonged use or high doses at term)

Breast-feeding Considerations

Acetaminophen: May be taken while breast-feeding.

Aspirin: Use cautiously due to potential adverse effects in nursing infants.

Dihydrocodeine: No data reported.

Dosage Forms CAP (Synalgos®-DC): Dihydrocodeine 16 mg, aspirin 356.4 mg, and caffeine 30 mg

Generic Available Yes

Comments Dihydrocodeine products, as with other narcotic analgesics, are recommended only for acute dosing (ie, 3 days or less); use with caution in patients with alcoholic liver disease. Dextromethorphan has equivalent antitussive activity but has much lower toxicity in accidental overdose.

Selected Readings "Drugs for Pain," *Med Lett Drugs Ther*, 1998, 40(1033):79-84.

Dihydrocodeine Compound *see* Dihydrocodeine, Aspirin, and Caffeine *on page 444*

Dihydroergotamine (dye hye droe er GOT a meen)

U.S. Brand Names D.H.E. 45®; Migranal®

Canadian Brand Names Migranal®

Pharmacologic Category Ergot Derivative

Synonyms DHE; Dihydroergotamine Mesylate

Use Treatment of migraine headache with or without aura; injection also indicated for treatment of cluster headaches

Unlabeled/Investigational Use Adjunct for DVT prophylaxis for hip surgery, for orthostatic hypotension, xerostomia secondary to antidepressant use, and pelvic congestion with pain

Local Anesthetic/Vasoconstrictor Precautions No information available to require special precautions

Effects on Dental Treatment Nasal spray:

>10%: Rhinitis (26%)

1% to 10%: Dizziness (4%), somnolence (3%), hot flashes (1%), nausea (10%), abnormal taste (8%), vomiting (4%), weakness (1%), stiffness (1%), pharyngitis (3%)

Dosage Adults:

I.M., S.C.: 1 mg at first sign of headache; repeat hourly to a maximum dose of 3 mg total; maximum dose: 6 mg/week

I.V.: 1 mg at first sign of headache; repeat hourly up to a maximum dose of 2 mg total; maximum dose: 6 mg/week

Intranasal: 1 spray (0.5 mg) of nasal spray should be administered into each nostril; if needed, repeat after 15 minutes, up to a total of 4 sprays. **Note:** Do not exceed 3 mg (6 sprays) in a 24-hour period and no more than 8 sprays in a week.

Elderly: Patients >65 years of age were not included in controlled clinical studies

Dosing adjustment in renal impairment: Contraindicated in severe renal impairment

Dosing adjustment in hepatic impairment: Reductions are probably necessary but specific guidelines are unavailable; contraindicated in severe hepatic dysfunction

Mechanism of Action Ergot alkaloid alpha-adrenergic blocker directly stimulates vascular smooth muscle to vasoconstrict peripheral and cerebral vessels; also has effects on serotonin receptors

Other Adverse Effects

1% to 10%: Nasal spray:

Gastrointestinal: Diarrhea (2%)

Local: Application site reaction (6%)

<1% (Limited to important or life-threatening): Injection and nasal spray: Abdominal pain, **anxiety,** cerebral hemorrhage, **coronary artery vasospasm,** cramps, diarrhea, **dizziness,** edema, **flushing, headache,** hyperkinesis, **hypertension, increased diaphoresis, muscular weakness, myalgia, MI, myocardial ischemia, palpitation, paresthesia,** peripheral ischemia, peripheral cyanosis, rash, **stroke,** subarachnoid hemorrhage, **transient ventricular tachycardia, tremor, ventricular fibrillation, xerostomia**

Postmarketing and/or case reports: Injection: Pleural and retroperitoneal fibrosis have been reported following prolonged use; cardiac valvular fibrosis has been associated with ergot alkaloids

Drug Interactions Substrate of **CYP3A4**; Inhibits CYP3A4

Increased effect with antifungals (azole derivatives); CYP3A4 inhibitors (eg, amiodarone, cimetidine, erythromycin, ritonavir); macrolide antibiotics; nitroglycerin; protease inhibitors; MAO inhibitors; beta blockers (vasoconstriction); sumatriptan (vasospasm); vasoconstrictors. Dihydroergotamine may increase the effects of

(Continued)

Dihydroergotamine *(Continued)*

heparin (injection site hematoma), sibutramine, and other serotonin agonists (serotonin syndrome)

Decreased effect with antipsychotics, metoclopramide.

Dietary/Ethanol/Herb Considerations Ethanol: Avoid use; may cause or worsen headaches.

Pharmacodynamics/Kinetics

Onset of action: 15-30 minutes
Duration: 3-4 hours
Distribution: V_d: 14.5 L/kg
Protein binding: 93%
Metabolism: Extensively hepatic
Half-life elimination: 1.3-3.9 hours
Time to peak, serum: I.M.: 15-30 minutes
Excretion: Primarily feces; urine (10% mostly as metabolites)

Pregnancy Risk Factor X

Generic Available No

Dihydroergotamine Mesylate *see* Dihydroergotamine *on page 445*
Dihydroergotoxine *see* Ergoloid Mesylates *on page 509*
Dihydrogenated Ergot Alkaloids *see* Ergoloid Mesylates *on page 509*
Dihydrohydroxycodeinone *see* Oxycodone *on page 1017*
Dihydromorphinone *see* Hydromorphone *on page 691*

Dihydrotachysterol (dye hye droe tak IS ter ole)

U.S. Brand Names DHT™; DHT™ Intensol™; Hytakerol®

Canadian Brand Names Hytakerol®

Pharmacologic Category Vitamin D Analog

Synonyms Dichysterol

Use Treatment of hypocalcemia associated with hypoparathyroidism; prophylaxis of hypocalcemic tetany following thyroid surgery

Local Anesthetic/Vasoconstrictor Precautions No information available to require special precautions

Effects on Dental Treatment No significant effects or complications reported

Dosage Oral:

Hypoparathyroidism:
- Infants and young Children: Initial: 1-5 mg/day for 4 days, then 0.1-0.5 mg/day
- Older Children and Adults: Initial: 0.8-2.4 mg/day for several days followed by maintenance doses of 0.2-1 mg/day

Nutritional rickets: 0.5 mg as a single dose or 13-50 mcg/day until healing occurs

Renal osteodystrophy: Maintenance: 0.25-0.6 mg/24 hours adjusted as necessary to achieve normal serum calcium levels and promote bone healing

Mechanism of Action Synthetic analogue of vitamin D with a faster onset of action; stimulates calcium and phosphate absorption from the small intestine, promotes secretion of calcium from bone to blood; promotes renal tubule resorption of phosphate

Other Adverse Effects

>10%:
- Endocrine & metabolic: Hypercalcemia
- Renal: Elevated serum creatinine, hypercalciuria

<1%: **Convulsions,** polydipsia, **nausea, vomiting,** anorexia, weight loss, polyuria, anemia, **weakness,** metastatic calcification, renal damage

Drug Interactions

Increased Effect/Toxicity: Thiazide diuretics may increase calcium levels.

Decreased Effect: Decreased effect/levels of vitamin D if taken with cholestyramine, colestipol, or mineral oil. Phenytoin and phenobarbital may inhibit activation leading to decreased effectiveness.

Pharmacodynamics/Kinetics

Onset of action: Peak effect: Calcium: 2-4 weeks
Duration: ≤9 weeks
Absorption: Well absorbed
Distribution: Stored in liver, fat, skin, muscle, and bone
Excretion: Feces

Pregnancy Risk Factor A/D (dose exceeding RDA recommendation)

Generic Available Yes

1,25 Dihydroxycholecalciferol *see* Calcitriol *on page 223*
Dihydroxypropyl Theophylline *see* Dyphylline *on page 485*
Diiodohydroxyquin *see* Iodoquinol *on page 735*
Dilacor® XR *see* Diltiazem *on page 447*
Dilantin® *see* Phenytoin *on page 1073*
Dilatrate®-SR *see* Isosorbide Dinitrate *on page 750*
Dilaudid® *see* Hydromorphone *on page 691*
Dilaudid-HP® *see* Hydromorphone *on page 691*

Dilor® *see* Dyphylline *on page 485*
Diltia XT® *see* Diltiazem *on page 447*

Diltiazem (dil TYE a zem)

Related Information

Calcium Channel Blockers and Gingival Hyperplasia *on page 1598*
Calcium Channel Blockers, Comparative Pharmacokinetics *on page 1600*
Cardiovascular Diseases *on page 1456*

U.S. Brand Names Cardizem®; Cardizem® CD; Cardizem® LA; Cardizem® SR; Cartia XT™; Dilacor® XR; Diltia XT®; Tiazac®

Canadian Brand Names Alti-Diltiazem CD; Apo®-Diltiaz; Apo®-Diltiaz CD; Apo®-Diltiaz SR; Cardizem®; Cardizem® CD; Cardizem® SR; Gen-Diltiazem; Gen-Diltiazem SR; Med-Diltiazem; Novo-Diltazem; Novo-Diltazem-CD; Novo-Diltazem SR; Nu-Diltiaz; Nu-Diltiaz-CD; ratio-Diltiazem CD; Rhoxal-diltiazem CD; Rhoxal-diltiazem SR; Syn-Diltiazem®; Tiazac®

Mexican Brand Names Angiotrofin®; Angiotrofin A.P.; Angiotrofin Retard; Presoken; Presoquim; Tilazem®

Pharmacologic Category Calcium Channel Blocker

Synonyms Diltiazem Hydrochloride

Use

Oral: Treatment of essential hypertension, chronic stable angina, or angina from coronary artery spasm

Injection: Treatment of atrial fibrillation or atrial flutter, paroxysmal supraventricular tachycardia (PSVT)

Unlabeled/Investigational Use Investigational: Treatment of Duchenne muscular dystrophy

Local Anesthetic/Vasoconstrictor Precautions No information available to require special precautions

Effects on Dental Treatment Diltiazem has been reported to cause >10% incidence of gingival hyperplasia; usually disappears with discontinuation (consultation with physician is suggested).

>10%: Headache (5% to 12%)

2% to 10%: Pain (6%), bradycardia (2% to 6%), hypotension (<2% to 4%), vasodilation (2% to 3%), flushing (1% to 2%), palpitations (1% to 2%), dizziness (3% to 10%), nervousness (2%), vomiting (2%), weakness (1% to 4%), rhinitis (<2% to 10%), pharyngitis (2% to 6%), dyspnea (1% to 6%), bronchitis (1% to 4%), sinus congestion (1% to 2%)

<2%: Allergic reaction, amnesia, angina, anorexia, arrhythmia, bruising, CHF, dysgeusia, xerostomia, epistaxis, gait abnormality, hallucinations, hyperglycemia, muscle cramps, nausea, neck rigidity, pain, paresthesia, personality change, somnolence, syncope, tachycardia, thirst, tremor

Dosage Adults:

Oral:

Angina:

Capsule, extended release (Cardizem® CD, Cartia XT™, Dilacor XR®, Diltia XT™, Tiazac®): Initial: 120-180 mg once daily (maximum dose: 480 mg/day)

Tablet, immediate release (Cardizem®): Usual starting dose: 30 mg 4 times/day; usual range: 180-360 mg/day

Hypertension:

Capsule, extended release (Cardizem® CD, Cartia XT™, Dilacor XR®, Diltia XT™, Tiazac®): Initial: 180-240 mg once daily; dose adjustment may be made after 14 days; usual range: 180-480 mg/day (maximum dose: 540 mg/day)

Capsule, sustained release (Cardizem® SR): Initial: 60-120 mg twice daily; dose adjustment may be made after 14 days; usual range: 240-360 mg/day

Tablet, extended release (Cardizem® LA): Initial: 180-240 mg once daily; dose adjustment may be made after 14 days; usual range: 180-480 mg/day (maximum dose: 540 mg/day)

Elderly: Patients ≥60 years may respond to a lower initial dose (ie, 120 mg once daily using extended release capsule)

I.V.: Atrial fibrillation, atrial flutter, PSVT:

- Initial bolus dose: 0.25 mg/kg actual body weight over 2 minutes (average adult dose: 20 mg)
- Repeat bolus dose (may be administered after 15 minutes if the response is inadequate.): 0.35 mg/kg actual body weight over 2 minutes (average adult dose: 25 mg)
- Continuous infusion (requires an infusion pump; infusions >24 hours or infusion rates >15 mg/hour are not recommended.): Initial infusion rate of 10 mg/hour; rate may be increased in 5 mg/hour increments up to 15 mg/hour as needed; some patients may respond to an initial rate of 5 mg/hour.

If diltiazem injection is administered by continuous infusion for >24 hours, the possibility of decreased diltiazem clearance, prolonged elimination half-life, and increased diltiazem and/or diltiazem metabolite plasma concentrations should be considered.

Conversion from I.V. diltiazem to oral diltiazem: Start oral approximately 3 hours after bolus dose.

(Continued)

Diltiazem *(Continued)*

Oral dose (mg/day) is approximately equal to [rate (mg/hour) x 3 + 3] x 10.
3 mg/hour = 120 mg/day
5 mg/hour = 180 mg/day
7 mg/hour = 240 mg/day
11 mg/hour = 360 mg/day

Dosing comments in renal/hepatic impairment: Use with caution as extensively metabolized by the liver and excreted in the kidneys and bile.

Dialysis: Not removed by hemo- or peritoneal dialysis; supplemental dose is not necessary.

Mechanism of Action Inhibits calcium ion from entering the "slow channels" or select voltage-sensitive areas of vascular smooth muscle and myocardium during depolarization, producing a relaxation of coronary vascular smooth muscle and coronary vasodilation; increases myocardial oxygen delivery in patients with vasospastic angina

Other Adverse Effects Various dosage forms:

>10%: Cardiovascular: Edema (2% to 15%)

2% to 10%:

Cardiovascular: AV block (first degree 2% to 8%), edema, lower limb (2% to 8%), extrasystoles (2%)

Dermatologic: Rash (1% to 4%)

Endocrine & metabolic: Gout (1% to 2%)

Gastrointestinal: Dyspepsia (1% to 6%), constipation (<2% to 4%), diarrhea (1% to 2%)

Local: Injection site reactions: Burning, itching (4%)

Neuromuscular & skeletal: Myalgia (2%)

<2%: Albuminuria, alkaline phosphatase increased, amblyopia, anorexia, AV block (second or third degree), bundle branch block, CPK elevated, crystalluria, depression, dreams abnormal, EKG abnormalities, gynecomastia, hyperuricemia, impotence, insomnia, LDH increased, nocturia, petechiae, photosensitivity, polyuria, pruritus, SGOT increased, SGPT increased, tinnitus, ventricular extrasystoles, weight gain

Postmarketing and/or case reports: Alopecia, angioedema, asystole, **bleeding time increased,** erythema multiforme, exfoliative dermatitis, **extrapyramidal symptoms, gingival hyperplasia,** hemolytic anemia, leukopenia, purpura, retinopathy, Stevens-Johnson syndrome, thrombocytopenia, toxic epidermal necrolysis

Drug Interactions Substrate of CYP2C8/9, 2D6, **3A4**; Inhibits CYP2C8/9, 2D6, **3A4**

Increased Effect/Toxicity: Diltiazem effects may be additive with amiodarone, beta-blockers, or digoxin, which may lead to bradycardia, other conduction delays, and decreased cardiac output. Serum concentrations/toxicity of diltiazem may be increased by inhibitors of CYP3A4, including amprenavir, cimetidine, ciprofloxacin, clarithromycin, clozapine, diltiazem, disulfiram, digoxin, erythromycin, ethanol, fluconazole, fluoxetine, fluvoxamine, isoniazid, itraconazole, ketoconazole, labetalol, levodopa, loxapine, metoprolol, metronidazole, miconazole, nefazodone, nelfinavir, omeprazole, phenytoin, rifabutin, rifampin, ritonavir, troleandomycin, valproic acid, and verapamil. Diltiazem may increase serum levels/toxicity of alfentanil (possibly fentanyl and sufentanil), some benzodiazepines (specifically midazolam and triazolam), carbamazepine, cisapride (QT prolongation, arrhythmia), cyclosporine, digoxin, HMG-CoA reductase inhibitors, lithium (neurotoxicity), midazolam, moricizine, and tacrolimus.

Decreased Effect: Rifampin markedly reduces diltiazem serum levels resulting in decreased diltiazem effect. Coadministration with other cytochrome P450 enzyme inducers should be avoided (includes phenytoin, barbiturates, and carbamazepine).

Dietary/Ethanol/Herb Considerations

Ethanol: Avoid use; may increase risk of hypotension or vasodilation.

Food may increase serum concentration; avoid caffeine, garlic, and grapefruit products.

Herb/Nutraceutical: Avoid black cohosh, dong quai, and evening primrose due to estrogenic activity. Avoid ephedra, ginseng, and yohimbe; may worsen arrhythmia or hypertension. Avoid garlic; may have increased antihypertensive effect. Avoid ginger due to positive inotropic effects; theoretically, may cause arrhythmia. Avoid hawthorn; may lower peripheral vascular resistance and enhance reductions in BP. Avoid St John's wort; may decrease serum concentration.

Pharmacodynamics/Kinetics

Onset of action: Oral: Immediate release tablet: 30-60 minutes

Absorption: 70% to 80%

Distribution: V_d: 3-13 L/kg; enters breast milk

Protein binding: 77% to 85%

Metabolism: Hepatic; extensive first-pass effect; following single I.V. injection, plasma concentrations of N-monodesmethyldiltiazem and desacetyldiltiazem are typically undetectable; however, these metabolites accumulate to detectable concentrations following 24-hour constant rate infusion.

N-monodesmethyldiltiazem appears to have 20% of the potency of diltiazem; desacetyldiltiazem is about 50% as potent as the parent compound.

Bioavailability: Oral: ~40% to 60%

Half-life elimination: Immediate release tablet: 3-4.5 hours, may be prolonged with renal impairment

Time to peak, serum: Immediate release tablet: 2-3 hours

Excretion: Urine and feces (primarily as metabolites)

Pregnancy Risk Factor C

Generic Available Yes

Diltiazem Hydrochloride *see* Diltiazem *on page 447*

DimenhyDRINATE (dye men HYE dri nate)

U.S. Brand Names Dramamine® [OTC]; Hydrate® [DSC]; TripTone® [OTC]

Canadian Brand Names Apo®-Dimenhydrinate; Gravol®

Mexican Brand Names Dramamine®; Vomisin®

Pharmacologic Category Antihistamine

Use Treatment and prevention of nausea, vertigo, and vomiting associated with motion sickness

Local Anesthetic/Vasoconstrictor Precautions No information available to require special precautions

Effects on Dental Treatment

>10%: Thickening of bronchial secretions

≤10%: Significant xerostomia and drowsiness; resolves upon discontinuation

1% to 10%: Headache, fatigue, nervousness, dizziness, nausea, pharyngitis

Dosage

Children:

Oral:

2-5 years: 12.5-25 mg every 6-8 hours, maximum: 75 mg/day

6-12 years: 25-50 mg every 6-8 hours, maximum: 150 mg/day

I.M.: 1.25 mg/kg or 37.5 mg/m^2 4 times/day, not to exceed 300 mg/day

Adults: Oral, I.M., I.V.: 50-100 mg every 4-6 hours, not to exceed 400 mg/day

Mechanism of Action Competes with histamine for H_1-receptor sites on effector cells in the gastrointestinal tract, blood vessels, and respiratory tract; blocks chemoreceptor trigger zone, diminishes vestibular stimulation, and depresses labyrinthine function through its central anticholinergic activity

Other Adverse Effects

1% to 10%:

Gastrointestinal: Appetite increase, weight gain, diarrhea, abdominal pain

Neuromuscular & skeletal: Arthralgia

Drug Interactions

Increased Effect/Toxicity: CNS depressants may increase the degree of sedation and respiratory depression with antihistamines. May increase the absorption of digoxin. Central and/or peripheral anticholinergic syndrome can occur when administered with amantadine, rimantadine, narcotic analgesics, phenothiazines and other antipsychotics (especially with high anticholinergic activity), tricyclic antidepressants, quinidine, disopyramide, procainamide, and antihistamines.

Decreased Effect: May increase gastric degradation of levodopa and decrease the amount of levodopa absorbed by delaying gastric emptying. Therapeutic effects of cholinergic agents (tacrine, donepezil) and neuroleptics may be antagonized.

Dietary/Ethanol/Herb Considerations

Ethanol: Avoid use; may increase CNS depression.

Herb/Nutraceutical: Avoid gotu kola, kava, SAMe, St John's wort, and valerian; may increase CNS depression.

Pharmacodynamics/Kinetics

Onset of action: Oral: ~15-30 minutes

Absorption: Oral: Well absorbed

Pregnancy Risk Factor B

Generic Available Yes

Dimercaprol (dye mer KAP role)

U.S. Brand Names BAL in Oil®

Pharmacologic Category Antidote

Synonyms BAL; British Anti-Lewisite; Dithioglycerol

Use Antidote to gold, arsenic (except arsine), and mercury poisoning (except nonalkyl mercury); adjunct to edetate calcium disodium in lead poisoning; possibly effective for antimony, bismuth, chromium, copper, nickel, tungsten, or zinc

Local Anesthetic/Vasoconstrictor Precautions No information available to require special precautions

Effects on Dental Treatment

>10%: Hypertension, tachycardia (dose-related), headache

1% to 10%: Nausea, vomiting

(Continued)

Dimercaprol *(Continued)*

Dosage Children and Adults: Deep I.M.:

Arsenic, mercury, and gold poisoning: 3 mg/kg every 4-6 hours for 2 days, then every 12 hours for 7-10 days or until recovery (initial dose may be up to 5 mg if severe poisoning)

Lead poisoning (in conjunction with calcium EDTA): For symptomatic acute encephalopathy or blood level >100 mcg/dL: 4-5 mg/kg every 4 hours for 3-5 days

Mechanism of Action Sulfhydryl group combines with ions of various heavy metals to form relatively stable, nontoxic, soluble chelates which are excreted in urine

Other Adverse Effects <1%: **Nervousness, fever, convulsions, salivation,** transient neutropenia, thrombocytopenia, **increased PT,** pain at the injection site, abscess formation, myalgia, **paresthesia,** blepharospasm, burning eyes, nephrotoxicity, dysuria, **burning sensation of the lips, mouth, throat,** and penis

Drug Interactions Increased Effect/Toxicity: Toxic complexes with iron, cadmium, selenium, or uranium

Pharmacodynamics/Kinetics

Distribution: To all tissues including the brain

Metabolism: Rapidly hepatic to inactive metabolites

Time to peak, serum: 0.5-1 hour

Excretion: Urine

Pregnancy Risk Factor C

Generic Available No

Dimetapp® 12-Hour Non-Drowsy Extentabs® [OTC] *see* Pseudoephedrine *on page 1146*

Dimetapp® Decongestant [OTC] *see* Pseudoephedrine *on page 1146*

β,β-Dimethylcysteine *see* Penicillamine *on page 1046*

Dimethyl Triazeno Imidazol Carboxamide *see* Dacarbazine *on page 391*

Dinoprostone (dye noe PROST one)

U.S. Brand Names Cervidil®; Prepidil®; Prostin E_2®

Canadian Brand Names Cervidil®; Prepidil®; Prostin E2®

Mexican Brand Names Prepidil®; Propess®

Pharmacologic Category Abortifacient; Prostaglandin

Synonyms PGE_2; Prostaglandin E_2

Use

Gel: Promote cervical ripening prior to labor induction; usage for gel include any patient undergoing induction of labor with an unripe cervix, most commonly for pre-eclampsia, eclampsia, postdates, diabetes, intrauterine growth retardation, and chronic hypertension

Suppositories: Terminate pregnancy from 12th through 28th week of gestation; evacuate uterus in cases of missed abortion or intrauterine fetal death; manage benign hydatidiform mole

Vaginal insert: Initiation and/or cervical ripening in patients at or near term in whom there is a medical or obstetrical indication for the induction of labor

Local Anesthetic/Vasoconstrictor Precautions No information available to require special precautions

Effects on Dental Treatment

>10%: Headache, vomiting, nausea

1% to 10%: Bradycardia, fever

Dosage

Abortifacient: Insert 1 suppository high in vagina, repeat at 3- to 5-hour intervals until abortion occurs up to 240 mg (maximum dose); continued administration for longer than 2 days is not advisable

Cervical ripening:

Gel:

Intracervical: 0.25-1 mg

Intravaginal: 2.5 mg

Suppositories: Intracervical: 2-3 mg

Vaginal Insert (Cervidil®): 10 mg (to be removed at the onset of active labor or after 12 hours)

Mechanism of Action A synthetic prostaglandin E_2 abortifacient that stimulates uterine contractions similar to those seen during natural labor

Other Adverse Effects

>10%: Gastrointestinal: Diarrhea,

1% to 10%: Neuromuscular & skeletal: Back pain

<1%: **Hypotension, cardiac arrhythmias, syncope, flushing, tightness of the chest, vasomotor and vasovagal reactions, dizziness,** chills, **pain, hot flashes, wheezing, dyspnea, coughing, bronchospasm,** shivering

Drug Interactions Increased effect of oxytocics

Pharmacodynamics/Kinetics

Onset of action (uterine contractions): Within 10 minutes

Duration: Up to 2-3 hours

Absorption: Vaginal: Slow

Metabolism: In many tissues including renal, pulmonary, and splenic systems
Excretion: Primarily urine; feces (small amounts)

Pregnancy Risk Factor C

Generic Available No

Diocto® [OTC] *see* Docusate *on page 463*

Diocto C® [OTC] *see* Docusate and Casanthranol *on page 464*

Dioctyl Calcium Sulfosuccinate *see* Docusate *on page 463*

Dioctyl Sodium Sulfosuccinate *see* Docusate *on page 463*

Diotame® [OTC] *see* Bismuth *on page 186*

Diovan® *see* Valsartan *on page 1374*

Diovan HCT® *see* Valsartan and Hydrochlorothiazide *on page 1375*

Dipalmitoylphosphatidylcholine *see* Colfosceril Palmitate *on page 366*

Dipentum® *see* Olsalazine *on page 999*

Diphen® [OTC] *see* DiphenhydrAMINE *on page 451*

Diphen® AF [OTC] *see* DiphenhydrAMINE *on page 451*

Diphen® Cough [OTC] *see* DiphenhydrAMINE *on page 451*

Diphenhist [OTC] *see* DiphenhydrAMINE *on page 451*

DiphenhydrAMINE (dye fen HYE dra meen)

Related Information

Dental Office Emergencies *on page 1582*
Diphenhydramine and Pseudoephedrine *on page 453*
Management of Patients Undergoing Cancer Therapy *on page 1567*
Oral Nonviral Soft Tissue Ulcerations or Erosions *on page 1549*
Oral Viral Infections *on page 1545*

U.S. Brand Names Aler-Dryl [OTC]; AllerMax® [OTC]; Banophen® [OTC]; Benadryl® Allergy [OTC]; Benadryl® Dye-Free Allergy [OTC]; Benadryl® Gel [OTC]; Benadryl® Gel Extra Strength [OTC]; Benadryl® Injection; Compoz® Nighttime Sleep Aid [OTC]; Diphen® [OTC]; Diphen® AF [OTC]; Diphen® Cough [OTC]; Diphenhist [OTC]; Genahist® [OTC]; Hydramine® [OTC]; Hydramine® Cough [OTC]; Hyrexin-50®; Nytol® [OTC]; Nytol® Maximum Strength [OTC]; Siladryl® Allergy [OTC]; Silphen® [OTC]; Sleepinal® [OTC]; Sominex® [OTC]; Sominex® Maximum Strength [OTC]; Tusstat®; Twilite® [OTC]; Unisom® Maximum Strength SleepGels® [OTC]

Canadian Brand Names Allerdryl®; Allernix; Benadryl®; Nytol®; Nytol® Extra Strength; PMS-Diphenhydramine; Simply Sleep®

Pharmacologic Category Antihistamine

Synonyms Diphenhydramine Hydrochloride

Use

Dental: Symptomatic relief of nasal mucosal congestion

Medical: Symptomatic relief of allergic symptoms caused by histamine release which include nasal allergies and allergic dermatosis; mild nighttime sedation; prevention of motion sickness and as an antitussive; has antinauseant and topical anesthetic properties; treatment of antipsychotic-induced extrapyramidal symptoms

Local Anesthetic/Vasoconstrictor Precautions No information available to require special precautions

Effects on Dental Treatment Chronic use of antihistamines will inhibit salivary flow, particularly in elderly patients; may contribute to periodontal disease and oral discomfort.

1% to 10%: Xerostomia

Frequency not defined: Hypotension, palpitations, tachycardia, sedation, sleepiness, dizziness, disturbed coordination, headache, fatigue, nervousness, paradoxical excitement, insomnia, euphoria, confusion, nausea, vomiting, diarrhea, dry mucous membranes, tremors, paresthesia, blurred vision, thickening of bronchial secretions

Dosage

Children:

Oral, I.M., I.V.:

Treatment of moderate to severe allergic reactions: 5 mg/kg/day or 150 mg/m²/day in divided doses every 6-8 hours, not to exceed 300 mg/day

Minor allergic rhinitis or motion sickness:
- 2 to <6 years: 6.25 mg every 4-6 hours; maximum: 37.5 mg/day
- 6 to <12 years: 12.5-25 mg every 4-6 hours; maximum: 150 mg/day
- ≥12 years: 25-50 mg every 4-6 hours; maximum: 300 mg/day

Night-time sleep aid: 30 minutes before bedtime:
- 2 to <12 years: 1 mg/kg/dose; maximum: 50 mg/dose
- ≥12 years: 50 mg

Oral: **Antitussive:**
- 2 to <6 years: 6.25 mg every 4 hours; maximum 37.5 mg/day
- 6 to <12 years: 12.5 mg every 4 hours; maximum 75 mg/day
- ≥12 years: 25 mg every 4 hours; maximum 150 mg/day

I.M., I.V.: Treatment of dystonic reactions: 0.5-1 mg/kg/dose

(Continued)

DiphenhydrAMINE *(Continued)*

Adults:

Oral: 25-50 mg every 6-8 hours

Minor allergic rhinitis or motion sickness: 25-50 mg every 4-6 hours; maximum: 300 mg/day

Moderate to severe allergic reactions: 25-50 mg every 4 hours, not to exceed 400 mg/day

Nighttime sleep aid: 50 mg at bedtime

I.M., I.V.: 10-50 mg in a single dose every 2-4 hours, not to exceed 400 mg/day

Dystonic reaction: 50 mg in a single dose; may repeat in 20-30 minutes if necessary

Topical: For external application, not longer than 7 days

Mechanism of Action Competes with histamine for H_1-receptor sites on effector cells in the gastrointestinal tract, blood vessels, and respiratory tract; anticholinergic and sedative effects are also seen

Other Adverse Effects Frequency not defined:

Dermatologic: Photosensitivity, rash, angioedema, urticaria

Gastrointestinal: Diarrhea, abdominal pain, appetite increase, weight gain, anorexia

Genitourinary: Urinary retention, urinary frequency, difficult urination

Hematologic: Hemolytic anemia, thrombocytopenia, agranulocytosis

Contraindications Hypersensitivity to diphenhydramine or any component of the formulation; acute asthma; not for use in neonates

Warnings/Precautions Causes sedation, caution must be used in performing tasks which require alertness (ie, operating machinery or driving). Sedative effects of CNS depressants or ethanol are potentiated. Use with caution in patients with angle-closure glaucoma, pyloroduodenal obstruction (including stenotic peptic ulcer), urinary tract obstruction (including bladder neck obstruction and symptomatic prostatic hyperplasia), hyperthyroidism, increased intraocular pressure, and cardiovascular disease (including hypertension and tachycardia). Diphenhydramine has high sedative and anticholinergic properties, so it may not be considered the antihistamine of choice for prolonged use in the elderly. May cause paradoxical excitation in pediatric patients, and can result in hallucinations, coma, and death in overdose. Some preparations contain sodium bisulfite; syrup formulations may contain alcohol.

Drug Interactions Inhibits CYP2D6

Amantadine, rimantadine: Central and/or peripheral anticholinergic syndrome can occur when administered with amantadine or rimantadine

Anticholinergic agents: Central and/or peripheral anticholinergic syndrome can occur when administered with narcotic analgesics, phenothiazines and other antipsychotics (especially with high anticholinergic activity), tricyclic antidepressants, quinidine and some other antiarrhythmics, and antihistamines

Atenolol: Drugs with high anticholinergic activity may increase the bioavailability of atenolol (and possibly other beta-blockers); monitor for increased effect

Cholinergic agents: Drugs with high anticholinergic activity may antagonize the therapeutic effect of cholinergic agents; includes donepezil, rivastigmine, and tacrine

CNS depressants: Sedative effects may be additive with CNS depressants; includes ethanol, benzodiazepines, barbiturates, narcotic analgesics, and other sedative agents; monitor for increased effect

Digoxin: Drugs with high anticholinergic activity may decrease gastric degradation and increase the amount of digoxin absorbed by delaying gastric emptying

Ethanol: Syrup should not be given to patients taking drugs that can cause disulfiram reactions (ie, metronidazole, chlorpropamide) due to high alcohol content

Levodopa: Drugs with high anticholinergic activity may increase gastric degradation and decrease the amount of levodopa absorbed by delaying gastric emptying

Neuroleptics: Drugs with high anticholinergic activity may antagonize the therapeutic effects of neuroleptics

Dietary/Ethanol/Herb Considerations

Ethanol: Avoid use; may increase CNS depression.

Food: May be taken with food

Herb/Nutraceutical: Avoid gotu kola, kava, SAMe, St John's wort, and valerian; may increase CNS depression.

Pharmacodynamics/Kinetics

Onset of action: Maximum sedative effect: 1-3 hours

Duration: 4-7 hours

Protein binding: 78%

Metabolism: Extensively hepatic; smaller degrees in pulmonary and renal systems; significant first-pass effect

Bioavailability: Oral: 40% to 60%

Half-life elimination: 2-8 hours; Elderly: 13.5 hours

Time to peak, serum: 2-4 hours

Excretion: Urine (as unchanged drug)

Pregnancy Risk Factor B

Breast-feeding Considerations Infants may be more sensitive to the effects of antihistamines.

Dosage Forms CAP: 25 mg, 50 mg; (Banophen®, Diphen®, Diphenhist®, Genahist®): 25 mg; (Nytol® Maximum Strength, Sleepinal®): 50 mg. **ELIX:** 12.5 mg/5 mL (5 mL, 10 mL, 20 mL, 120 mL, 480 mL, 3780 mL); (Banophen®): 12.5 mg/5 mL (120 mL, 480 mL, 3840 mL); (Diphen AF): 12.5 mg/5 mL (120 mL, 240 mL, 480 mL, 3840 mL); (Genahist®, Hydramine®): 12.5 mg/5 mL (120 mL). **GEL, topical** (Benadryl®): 1% (120 mL); (Benadryl® Extra Strength): 2% (120 mL). **INJ, solution:** 10 mg/mL (30 mL); 50 mg/mL (1 mL, 10 mL); (Benadryl®): 50 mg/mL (1 mL, 10 mL); (Hyrexin®): 50 mg/mL (10 mL). **LIQ:** (Benadryl® Allergy): 12.5 mg/5 mL (120 mL, 240 mL); (Benadryl® Dye-Free Allergy): 12.5 mg/5 mL (120 mL). **SOFTGEL:** (Benadryl® Dye-Free Allergy): 25 mg; (Unisom® Maximum Strength SleepGels®): 50 mg. **SOLN, oral** (AllerMax®): 12.5 mg/5 mL (120 mL); (Diphenhist®): 12.5 mg/5 mL (120 mL, 480 mL). **SOLN, topical:** 1% (60 mL); 2%. **SYR:** 12.5 mg/5 mL (120 mL, 240 mL, 480 mL); (Diphen® Cough, Siladryl® Allergy, Silphen® Cough): 12.5 mg/5 mL (120 mL, 240 mL, 480 mL); (Diphenhist®): 12.5 mg/5 mL (120 mL); (Hydramine® Cough): 12.5 mg/5 mL (120 mL, 480 mL); (Tusstat®): 12.5 mg/5 mL (120 mL, 240 mL, 3840 mL). **TAB:** 25 mg, 50 mg; (Aler-Dryl, AllerMax®, Compoz® Nighttime Sleep Aid, Sominex® Maximum Strength, Twilite®): 50 mg; (Banophen®, Benadryl® Allergy, Diphenhist®, Genahist®, Nytol®, Sominex®): 25 mg. **TAB, chewable** (Benadryl® Allergy): 12.5 mg

Generic Available Yes

Comments 25-50 mg of diphenhydramine orally every 4-6 hours can be used to treat mild dermatologic manifestations of allergic reactions to penicillin and other antibiotics. Diphenhydramine is not recommended as local anesthetic for either infiltration route or nerve block since the vehicle has caused local necrosis upon injection. A 50:50 mixture of diphenhydramine liquid (12.5 mg/5 mL) in Kaopectate® or Maalox® is used as a local application for recurrent aphthous ulcers; swish 1 tablespoonful for 2 minutes 4 times/day.

Diphenhydramine and Acetaminophen *see* Acetaminophen and Diphenhydramine *on page 30*

Diphenhydramine and Pseudoephedrine

(dye fen HYE dra meen & soo doe e FED rin)

Related Information

DiphenhydrAMINE *on page 451*

Pseudoephedrine *on page 1146*

U.S. Brand Names Benadryl® Allergy and Sinus Fastmelt™ [OTC]; Benadryl® Allergy/Decongestant [OTC]; Benadryl® Children's Allergy and Cold Fastmelt™ [OTC]; Benadryl® Children's Allergy and Sinus [OTC]

Pharmacologic Category Antihistamine/Decongestant Combination

Synonyms Pseudoephedrine and Diphenhydramine

Use Relief of symptoms of upper respiratory mucosal congestion in seasonal and perennial nasal allergies, acute rhinitis, rhinosinusitis, and eustachian tube blockage

Local Anesthetic/Vasoconstrictor Precautions Use with caution since pseudoephedrine is a sympathomimetic amine which could interact with epinephrine to cause a pressor response

Effects on Dental Treatment Chronic use of antihistamines will inhibit salivary flow, particularly in elderly patients; may contribute to periodontal disease and oral discomfort.

Dosage Based on **pseudoephedrine** component:

Adults: Oral: 60 mg every 4-6 hours, maximum: 240 mg/day

Generic Available Yes

Diphenhydramine Hydrochloride *see* DiphenhydrAMINE *on page 451*

Diphenoxylate and Atropine (dye fen OKS i late & A troe peen)

Related Information

Atropine *on page 144*

U.S. Brand Names Lomocot®; Lomotil®; Lonox®

Canadian Brand Names Lomotil®

Pharmacologic Category Antidiarrheal

Synonyms Atropine and Diphenoxylate

Use Treatment of diarrhea

Local Anesthetic/Vasoconstrictor Precautions No information available to require special precautions

Effects on Dental Treatment

1% to 10%: Significant xerostomia (normal salivary flow resumes upon discontinuation), drowsiness, nervousness, restlessness, dizziness, headache, blurred vision, respiratory depression

Restrictions C-V

Dosage Oral:

Children (use with caution in young children due to variable responses): Liquid: 0.3-0.4 mg of diphenoxylate/kg/day in 2-4 divided doses **or**

(Continued)

Diphenoxylate and Atropine *(Continued)*

<2 years: Use not recommended
2-5 years: 2 mg of diphenoxylate 3 times/day
5-8 years: 2 mg of diphenoxylate 4 times/day
8-12 years: 2 mg of diphenoxylate 5 times/day

Adults: 15-20 mg/day of diphenoxylate in 3-4 divided doses; maintenance: 5-15 mg/day in 2-3 divided doses

Mechanism of Action Diphenoxylate inhibits excessive GI motility and GI propulsion; commercial preparations contain a subtherapeutic amount of atropine to discourage abuse

Other Adverse Effects

1% to 10%:
Central nervous system: Mental depression
Gastrointestinal: Paralytic ileus
Genitourinary: Urinary retention and dysuria

<1%: **Tachycardia, sedation, euphoria,** hyperthermia, pruritus, urticaria, **nausea, vomiting,** abdominal discomfort, pancreatitis, stomach cramps, **muscle cramps, weakness, diaphoresis (increased)**

Drug Interactions Increased Effect/Toxicity: MAO inhibitors (hypertensive crisis), CNS depressants when taken with diphenoxylate may result in increased adverse effects, antimuscarinics (paralytic ileus). May prolong half-life of drugs metabolized in liver.

Dietary/Ethanol/Herb Considerations

Ethanol: Avoid use; may increase CNS depression.

Herb/Nutraceutical: Avoid gotu kola, kava, SAMe, St John's wort, and valerian; may increase CNS depression.

Pharmacodynamics/Kinetics

Atropine: See Atropine monograph.

Diphenoxylate:

Onset of action: Antidiarrheal: 45-60 minutes
Peak effect: Antidiarrheal: ~2 hours
Duration: Antidiarrheal: 3-4 hours
Absorption: Well absorbed
Metabolism: Extensively hepatic to diphenoxylic acid (active)
Half-life elimination: 2.5 hours
Time to peak, serum: 2 hours
Excretion: Primarily feces (as metabolites); urine (~14%, <1% as unchanged drug)

Pregnancy Risk Factor C

Generic Available Yes

Diphenylhydantoin *see* Phenytoin *on page 1073*

Diphtheria and Tetanus Toxoids and Acellular Pertussis Adsorbed, Hepatitis B (Recombinant) and Inactivated Poliovirus Vaccine Combined *see* Diphtheria, Tetanus Toxoids, Acellular Pertussis, Hepatitis B (Recombinant), and Poliovirus (Inactivated) Vaccine *on page 454*

Diphtheria CRM$_{197}$ Protein *see* Pneumococcal Conjugate Vaccine (7-Valent) *on page 1091*

Diphtheria CRM$_{197}$ Protein Conjugate *see Haemophilus* b Conjugate Vaccine *on page 656*

Diphtheria, Tetanus Toxoids, Acellular Pertussis, Hepatitis B (Recombinant), and Poliovirus (Inactivated) Vaccine

(dip THEER ee a, TET a nus TOKS oyds, ay CEL yoo lar per TUS sis, hep a TYE tis bee ree KOM be nant, & POE lee oh VYE rus vak SEEN, in ak ti VAY ted)

Related Information

Immunizations (Vaccines) *on page 1612*
Poliovirus Vaccine (Inactivated) *on page 1093*
Tetanus Toxoid (Adsorbed) *on page 1283*
Tetanus Toxoid (Fluid) *on page 1284*

U.S. Brand Names Pediarix™

Pharmacologic Category Vaccine

Synonyms Diphtheria and Tetanus Toxoids and Acellular Pertussis Adsorbed, Hepatitis B (Recombinant) and Inactivated Poliovirus Vaccine Combined

Use Combination vaccine for the active immunization against diphtheria, tetanus, pertussis, hepatitis B virus (all known subtypes), and poliomyelitis (caused by poliovirus types 1, 2, and 3)

Local Anesthetic/Vasoconstrictor Precautions No information available to require special precautions

Effects on Dental Treatment No significant effects or complications reported

Restrictions Federal law requires that the date of administration, the vaccine manufacturer, lot number of vaccine, and the administering person's name, title and address be entered into the patient's permanent medical record.

Dosage I.M.: Children:

Immunization: 0.5 mL; repeat in 6-8 week intervals (preferably 8-week intervals) for a total of 3 doses. Vaccination usually begins at 2 months, but may be started as early as 6 weeks of age.

Use in children previously vaccinated with one or more component, and who are also scheduled to receive all vaccine components:

Hepatitis B vaccine: Infants born of HBsAg-negative mothers who received 1 dose of hepatitis B vaccine at birth may be given Pediarix™ (safety data limited); use in infants who received more than 1 dose of hepatitis B vaccine has not been studied. Infants who received 1 or more doses of hepatitis B vaccine (recombinant) may be given Pediarix™ to complete the hepatitis B series (safety and efficacy not established).

Diphtheria and tetanus toxoids, and acellular pertussis vaccine (DTaP): Infants previously vaccinated with 1 or 2 doses of Infanrix® may use Pediarix™ to complete the first 3 doses of the series (safety and efficacy not established); use of Pediarix™ to complete DTaP vaccination started with products other than Infanrix® is not recommended.

Inactivated polio vaccine (IPV): Infants previously vaccinated with 1 or 2 doses of IPV may use Pediarix™ to complete the first 3 doses of the series (safety and efficacy not established).

Mechanism of Action Promotes active immunity to diphtheria, tetanus, pertussis, hepatitis B and poliovirus (types 1, 2 and 3) by inducing production of specific antibodies and antitoxins.

Other Adverse Effects All serious adverse reactions must be reported to the U.S. Department of Health and Human Services (DHHS) Vaccine Adverse Event Reporting System (VAERS) 1-800-822-7967.

As reported in a U.S. lot Consistency Study: >10%:

Central nervous system:
- Sleeping increased (28% to 47%, grade 3: <1% to 2%)
- Restlessness (28% to 30%, grade 3: ≤1%)
- Fever ≥100.4°F (26% to 31%); >103.1°F (<1%); incidence of fever is higher than reported with separately administered vaccines

Gastrointestinal: Appetite decreased (19% to 22%, grade 3: <1%)

Local: Injection site:
- Redness (25% to 36%, >20 mm: ≤1%)
- Pain (23% to 30%, grade 3: ≤1%)
- Swelling (15% to 22%; >20 mm: 1%)

Miscellaneous: Fussiness (57% to 64%; grade 3: 2% to 3%)

Drug Interactions Decreased Effect: Immunosuppressant medications or therapies (eg, antimetabolites, alkylating agents, cytotoxic drugs, corticosteroids, irradiation) may decrease vaccine effectiveness; consider deferring vaccination for 3 months after immunosuppressant therapy is discontinued.

Pharmacodynamics/Kinetics Onset of action: Immune response observed to all components 1 month following the 3-dose series

Pregnancy Risk Factor C

Generic Available No

Diphtheria Toxoid Conjugate *see Haemophilus* b Conjugate Vaccine *on page 656*

Dipivalyl Epinephrine *see* Dipivefrin *on page 455*

Dipivefrin (dye PI ve frin)

U.S. Brand Names Propine®

Canadian Brand Names Apo®-Dipivefrin; Ophtho-Dipivefrin™; PMS-Dipivefrin; Propine®

Pharmacologic Category Alpha/Beta Agonist; Ophthalmic Agent, Antiglaucoma; Ophthalmic Agent, Vasoconstrictor

Synonyms Dipivalyl Epinephrine; Dipivefrin Hydrochloride; DPE

Use Reduces elevated intraocular pressure in chronic open-angle glaucoma; also used to treat ocular hypertension, low tension, and secondary glaucomas

Local Anesthetic/Vasoconstrictor Precautions No information available to require special precautions

Effects on Dental Treatment 1% to 10%: Headache

Dosage Adults: Ophthalmic: Instill 1 drop every 12 hours into the eyes

Mechanism of Action Dipivefrin is a prodrug of epinephrine which is the active agent that stimulates alpha- and/or beta-adrenergic receptors increasing aqueous humor outflow

Other Adverse Effects

1% to 10%:

Local: Burning, stinging

Ocular: Ocular congestion, photophobia, mydriasis, blurred vision, ocular pain, bulbar conjunctival follicles, blepharoconjunctivitis, cystoid macular edema

(Continued)

Dipivefrin *(Continued)*

<1%: **Arrhythmias, hypertension**

Drug Interactions Increased Effect/Toxicity: Increased or synergistic effect when used with other agents to lower intraocular pressure.

Pharmacodynamics/Kinetics

Ocular pressure effect:

Onset of action: ~30 minutes

Duration: ≥12 hours

Mydriasis:

Onset of action: ~30 minutes

Duration: Several hours

Absorption: Rapid into aqueous humor

Metabolism: Converted to epinephrine

Pregnancy Risk Factor B

Generic Available Yes

Dipivefrin Hydrochloride *see* Dipivefrin *on page 455*
Diprivan® *see* Propofol *on page 1133*
Diprolene® *see* Betamethasone *on page 177*
Diprolene® AF *see* Betamethasone *on page 177*
Dipropylacetic Acid *see* Valproic Acid and Derivatives *on page 1371*
Diprosone® [DSC] *see* Betamethasone *on page 177*

Dipyridamole (dye peer ID a mole)

U.S. Brand Names Persantine®

Canadian Brand Names Apo®-Dipyridamole FC; Novo-Dipiradol; Persantine®

Mexican Brand Names Dirinol; Lodimol; Trompersantin

Pharmacologic Category Antiplatelet Agent; Vasodilator

Use Maintains patency after surgical grafting procedures including coronary artery bypass; used with warfarin to decrease thrombosis in patients after artificial heart valve replacement; used with aspirin to prevent coronary artery thrombosis; in combination with aspirin or warfarin to prevent other thromboembolic disorders. Dipyridamole may also be given 2 days prior to open heart surgery to prevent platelet activation by extracorporeal bypass pump and as a diagnostic agent in CAD.

Unlabeled/Investigational Use Treatment of proteinuria in pediatric renal disease

Local Anesthetic/Vasoconstrictor Precautions No information available to require special precautions

Effects on Dental Treatment

>10%: Dizziness (14% oral)

1% to 10%: Hypotension (5%), hypertension (2%), blood pressure lability (2%), chest pain

Dosage

Children: Oral: 3-6 mg/kg/day in 3 divided doses

Doses of 4-10 mg/kg/day have been used investigationally to treat proteinuria in pediatric renal disease

Mechanical prosthetic heart valves: Oral: 2-5 mg/kg/day (used in combination with an oral anticoagulant in children who have systemic embolism despite adequate oral anticoagulant therapy, and used in combination with low-dose oral anticoagulation (INR 2-3) plus aspirin in children in whom full-dose oral anticoagulation is contraindicated)

Adults:

Oral: 75-400 mg/day in 3-4 divided doses

Evaluation of coronary artery disease: I.V.: 0.14 mg/kg/minute for 4 minutes; maximum dose: 60 mg

Hemodialysis: Significant drug removal is unlikely based on physiochemical characteristics

Mechanism of Action Inhibits the activity of adenosine deaminase and phosphodiesterase, which causes an accumulation of adenosine, adenine nucleotides, and cyclic AMP; these mediators then inhibit platelet aggregation and may cause vasodilation; may also stimulate release of prostacyclin or PGD_2; causes coronary vasodilation

Other Adverse Effects

>10%:

Cardiovascular: Exacerbation of angina pectoris (20% I.V.)

Central nervous system: Headache (12% I.V.)

1% to 10%:

Cardiovascular: EKG abnormalities (ST-T changes, extrasystoles), tachycardia (3% I.V.)

Central nervous system: Headache (2% I.V.), flushing (3% I.V.), fatigue (1% I.V.)

Dermatologic: Rash (2% oral)

Gastrointestinal: Abdominal distress (6% oral), nausea (5% I.V.)

Neuromuscular & skeletal: Paresthesia (1% I.V.)

Respiratory: Dyspnea (3% I.V.)

<1% (Limited to important or life-threatening):

I.V.: EKG abnormalities, arrhythmias (ventricular tachycardia, bradycardia, AV block, SVT, atrial fibrillation, asystole), palpitations, MI, syncope, orthostatic hypotension, cardiomyopathy, edema, hypertonia, tremors, abnormal coordination, vertigo, dyspepsia, xerostomia, abdominal pain, flatulence, vomiting, eructation, dysphagia, tenesmus, increased appetite, pharyngitis, bronchospasm, hyperventilation, rhinitis, coughing, pleural pain, myalgia, back pain, injection site reaction, diaphoresis, asthenia, malaise, arthralgia, rigor, dysgeusia, leg cramping, earache, tinnitus, vision abnormalities, thirst, depersonalization, renal pain, perineal pain, breast pain, intermittent claudication

Oral: Diarrhea, **vomiting, flushing,** pruritus, **angina pectoris, liver dysfunction**

Postmarketing and/or case reports: Rapidly progressive glomerulonephritis, thrombotic thrombocytopenic purpura, **esophageal hematoma,** gallstones, **epistaxis, pharyngeal bleeding,** respiratory arrest (I.V.)

Drug Interactions

Increased Effect/Toxicity: Dipyridamole enhances the risk of bleeding with aspirin (and other antiplatelet agents), heparin, low-molecular weight heparins, and warfarin. Adenosine blood levels and pharmacologic effects are increased with dipyridamole; consider reduced doses of adenosine.

Decreased Effect: Decreased vasodilation from I.V. dipyridamole when given to patients taking theophylline. Theophylline may reduce the pharmacologic effects of dipyridamole (hold theophylline preparations for 36-48 hours before dipyridamole facilitated stress test).

Dietary/Ethanol/Herb Considerations

Food: Avoid garlic, ginger, and green tea.

Herb/Nutraceutical: Avoid cat's claw, dong quai, evening primrose, feverfew, garlic, ginger, ginkgo biloba, ginseng, green tea, horse chestnut, and red clover due to additional antiplatelet activity.

Pharmacodynamics/Kinetics

Absorption: Readily, but variable

Distribution: Adults: V_d: 2-3 L/kg

Protein binding: 91% to 99%

Metabolism: Hepatic

Half-life elimination: Terminal: 10-12 hours

Time to peak, serum: 2-2.5 hours

Excretion: Feces (as glucuronide conjugates and unchanged drug)

Pregnancy Risk Factor B

Generic Available Yes

Dipyridamole and Aspirin *see* Aspirin and Dipyridamole *on page 135*

Dirithromycin (dye RITH roe mye sin)

U.S. Brand Names Dynabac®

Pharmacologic Category Antibiotic, Macrolide

Use Treatment of mild to moderate upper and lower respiratory tract infections due to *Moraxella catarrhalis*, *Streptococcus pneumoniae*, *Legionella pneumophila*, *H. influenzae*, or *S. pyogenes*, ie, acute exacerbation of chronic bronchitis, secondary bacterial infection of acute bronchitis, community-acquired pneumonia, pharyngitis/tonsillitis, and uncomplicated infections of the skin and skin structure due to *Staphylococcus aureus*

Local Anesthetic/Vasoconstrictor Precautions No information available to require special precautions

Effects on Dental Treatment 1% to 10%: Headache, dizziness, nausea, vomiting, weakness, pain, increased cough, dyspnea

Dosage Adults: Oral: 500 mg once daily for 5-14 days (14 days required for treatment of community-acquired pneumonia due to *Legionella*, *Mycoplasma*, or *S. pneumoniae*; 10 days is recommended for treatment of *S. pyogenes* pharyngitis/tonsillitis)

Mechanism of Action After being converted during intestinal absorption to its active form, erythromycylamine, dirithromycin inhibits protein synthesis by binding to the 50S ribosomal subunits of susceptible microorganisms

Other Adverse Effects

1% to 10%:

Central nervous system: Vertigo, insomnia

Dermatologic: Rash, pruritus, urticaria

Endocrine & metabolic: Hyperkalemia

Gastrointestinal: Abdominal pain, nausea, diarrhea, vomiting, dyspepsia, flatulence

Hematologic: Thrombocytosis, eosinophilia, segmented neutrophils

Neuromuscular & skeletal: Increased CPK

<1%: **Palpitations, vasodilation, syncope**, edema, **anxiety,** depression, **somnolence, fever, malaise,** dysmenorrhea, hypochloremia, hypophosphatemia, increased uric acid, **dehydration,** abnormal stools, anorexia, **gastritis,** abdominal pain, constipation, **abnormal taste, xerostomia, oral ulceration,** polyuria, vaginitis, neutropenia, thrombocytopenia, decreased hemoglobin/hematocrit; increased alkaline phosphatase, bands, basophils; leukocytosis, monocytosis,

(Continued)

Dirithromycin *(Continued)*

Increased ALT/AST, GGT, hyperbilirubinemia, **paresthesia, tremor,** myalgia, amblyopia, tinnitus, increased creatinine, phosphorus, **epistaxis, hemoptysis, hyperventilation,** hypoalbuminemia, **flu-like syndrome, diaphoresis, thirst**

Drug Interactions Substrate of CYP3A4

Increased Effect/Toxicity: Absorption of dirithromycin is slightly enhanced with concomitant antacids and H_2 antagonists. Dirithromycin may, like erythromycin, increase the effect of alfentanil, anticoagulants, bromocriptine, carbamazepine, cyclosporine, digoxin, disopyramide, ergots, methylprednisolone, cisapride, astemizole, and triazolam. Interactions with nonsedating antihistamines (eg, astemizole) or theophylline are not known to occur; however, caution is advised with coadministration.

Dietary/Ethanol/Herb Considerations Administer with food or within 1 hour of meal.

Pharmacodynamics/Kinetics

Absorption: Rapid

Distribution: V_d: 800 L; rapidly and widely (higher levels in tissues than plasma)

Protein binding: 14% to 30%

Metabolism: Hydrolyzed to erythromycylamine

Bioavailability: 10%

Half-life elimination: 8 hours (range: 2-36 hours)

Time to peak: 4 hours

Excretion: Feces (81% to 97%)

Pregnancy Risk Factor C

Generic Available No

Selected Readings "Pimozide (Orap) Contraindicated With Clarithromycin (Biaxin®) and Other Macrolide Antibiotics," *FDA Medical Bulletin*, October 1996, 26(3).

Disalcid® [DSC] *see* Salsalate *on page 1206*

Disalicylic Acid *see* Salsalate *on page 1206*

Disodium Cromoglycate *see* Cromolyn Sodium *on page 375*

***d*-Isoephedrine Hydrochloride** *see* Pseudoephedrine *on page 1146*

Disopyramide (dye soe PEER a mide)

Related Information

Cardiovascular Diseases *on page 1456*

U.S. Brand Names Norpace®; Norpace® CR

Canadian Brand Names Norpace®; Rythmodan®; Rythmodan®-LA

Mexican Brand Names Dimodan

Pharmacologic Category Antiarrhythmic Agent, Class Ia

Synonyms Disopyramide Phosphate

Use Suppression and prevention of unifocal and multifocal atrial and premature, ventricular premature complexes, coupled ventricular tachycardia; effective in the conversion of atrial fibrillation, atrial flutter, and paroxysmal atrial tachycardia to normal sinus rhythm and prevention of the recurrence of these arrhythmias after conversion by other methods

Local Anesthetic/Vasoconstrictor Precautions No information available to require special precautions

Effects on Dental Treatment

>10%: Xerostomia (32%)

1% to 10%: CHF, hypotension, syncope, chest pain, fatigue, headache, malaise, dizziness, nervousness, dry throat, nausea, vomiting, weakness, muscular pain, blurred vision, dyspnea

Dosage Oral:

Children:

- <1 year: 10-30 mg/kg/24 hours in 4 divided doses
- 1-4 years: 10-20 mg/kg/24 hours in 4 divided doses
- 4-12 years: 10-15 mg/kg/24 hours in 4 divided doses
- 12-18 years: 6-15 mg/kg/24 hours in 4 divided doses

Adults:

- <50 kg: 100 mg every 6 hours or 200 mg every 12 hours (controlled release)
- >50 kg: 150 mg every 6 hours or 300 mg every 12 hours (controlled release); if no response, increase to 200 mg every 6 hours. Maximum dose required for patients with severe refractory ventricular tachycardia is 400 mg every 6 hours.

Elderly: Dose with caution, starting at the lower end of dosing range

Dosing adjustment in renal impairment: 100 mg (nonsustained release) given at the following intervals, based on creatinine clearance (mL/minute):

- Cl_{cr} 30-40 mL/minute: Administer every 8 hours
- Cl_{cr} 15-30 mL/minute: Administer every 12 hours
- Cl_{cr} <15 mL/minute: Administer every 24 hours

or alter the dose as follows:

- Cl_{cr} 30-<40 mL/minute: Reduce dose 50%
- Cl_{cr} 15-30 mL/minute: Reduce dose 75%

Dialysis: Not dialyzable (0% to 5%) by hemo- or peritoneal methods; supplemental dose is unnecessary.

Dosing interval in hepatic impairment: 100 mg every 6 hours or 200 mg every 12 hours (controlled release)

Mechanism of Action Class Ia antiarrhythmic: Decreases myocardial excitability and conduction velocity; reduces disparity in refractory between normal and infarcted myocardium; possesses anticholinergic, peripheral vasoconstrictive, and negative inotropic effects

Other Adverse Effects

>10%:

Gastrointestinal: Constipation (11%)

Genitourinary: Urinary hesitancy (14% to 23%)

1% to 10%:

Cardiovascular: Cardiac conduction disturbance, edema

Dermatologic: Rash, generalized dermatoses, pruritus

Endocrine & metabolic: Hypokalemia, elevated cholesterol, elevated triglycerides

Gastrointestinal: Abdominal distension, flatulence, abdominal bloating, anorexia, diarrhea, weight gain

Genitourinary: Urinary retention, urinary frequency, urinary urgency, impotence (1% to 3%)

Ocular: Dry eyes

<1% (Limited to important or life-threatening): **New or worsened arrhythmias (proarrhythmic effect), hypoglycemia,** cholestatic jaundice, **fever, respiratory distress,** thrombocytopenia, agranulocytosis, gynecomastia, **psychotic reaction,** depression, insomnia, dysuria, **numbness, tingling, paresthesia,** elevated transaminases, AV block, increased serum creatinine, increased BUN, elevated creatinine, decreased hemoglobin, decreased hematocrit, hepatotoxicity. Rare cases of lupus have been reported (generally in patients previously receiving procainamide).

Postmarketing and/or case reports: Peripheral neuropathy, **psychosis,** pupillary dilation, toxic cutaneous blisters

Drug Interactions Substrate of **CYP3A4**

Increased Effect/Toxicity:

Disopyramide may increase the effects/toxicity of anticholinergics, beta-blockers, flecainide, procainamide, quinidine, or propafenone. Digoxin and quinidine serum concentrations may be increased by disopyramide. Erythromycin and clarithromycin may increase disopyramide serum concentrations, increasing toxicity (widening QT interval).

Disopyramide effect/toxicity may be additive with drugs which may prolong the QT interval - amiodarone, amitriptyline, astemizole, bepridil, cisapride (use is contraindicated), disopyramide, erythromycin, haloperidol, imipramine, pimozide, quinidine, sotalol, and thioridazine. In addition concurrent use with sparfloxacin, gatifloxacin, and moxifloxacin may result in additional prolongation of the QT interval; concurrent use is contraindicated.

Decreased Effect: Hepatic microsomal enzyme inducing agents (eg, phenytoin, phenobarbital, rifampin) may increase metabolism of disopyramide leading to a decreased effect. Anticoagulants may have decreased prothrombin times after discontinuation of disopyramide.

Dietary/Ethanol/Herb Considerations

Ethanol: Avoid use; may increase CNS depression.

Food: Administer on an empty stomach. Avoid caffeine.

Herb/Nutraceutical: Avoid ephedra, ginseng, and yohimbe; may worsen arrhythmia. Avoid St John's wort; may decrease serum concentration. Ginger has positive inotropic effects and theoretically could affect antiarrhythmic activity. Avoid gotu kola, kava, SAMe, St John's wort, and valerian; may increase CNS depression.

Pharmacodynamics/Kinetics

Onset of action: 0.5-3.5 hours

Duration: 1.5-8.5 hours

Absorption: 60% to 83%

Protein binding (concentration dependent): 20% to 60%

Metabolism: Hepatic to inactive metabolites

Half-life elimination: Adults: 4-10 hours; prolonged with hepatic or renal impairment

Excretion: Urine (40% to 60% as unchanged drug); feces (10% to 15%)

Pregnancy Risk Factor C

Generic Available Yes

Disopyramide Phosphate *see* Disopyramide *on page 458*

Disulfiram (dye SUL fi ram)

U.S. Brand Names Antabuse®

Pharmacologic Category Aldehyde Dehydrogenase Inhibitor

Use Management of chronic alcoholism

Local Anesthetic/Vasoconstrictor Precautions No information available to require special precautions

Effects on Dental Treatment Frequency not defined: Drowsiness, headache, fatigue, psychosis, allergic dermatitis, metallic or garlic-like aftertaste

(Continued)

Disulfiram *(Continued)*

Dosage Adults: Oral: Do not administer until the patient has abstained from ethanol for at least 12 hours

Initial: 500 mg/day as a single dose for 1-2 weeks; maximum daily dose is 500 mg

Average maintenance dose: 250 mg/day; range: 125-500 mg; duration of therapy is to continue until the patient is fully recovered socially and a basis for permanent self control has been established; maintenance therapy may be required for months or even years

Mechanism of Action Disulfiram is a thiuram derivative which interferes with aldehyde dehydrogenase. When taken concomitantly with alcohol, there is an increase in serum acetaldehyde levels. High acetaldehyde causes uncomfortable symptoms including flushing, nausea, thirst, palpitations, chest pain, vertigo, and hypotension. This reaction is the basis for disulfiram use in postwithdrawal long-term care of alcoholism.

Other Adverse Effects Frequency not defined:

Dermatologic: Rash, acneiform eruptions

Genitourinary: Impotence

Hepatic: Hepatitis (cholestatic and fulminant), hepatic failure (multiple case reports)

Neuromuscular & skeletal: Peripheral neuritis, polyneuritis, peripheral neuropathy

Ocular: Optic neuritis

Drug Interactions Substrate of CYP1A2, 2A6, 2B6, 2D6, 2E1, 3A4; Inhibits CYP1A2, 2A6, 2B6, 2C8/9, 2D6, **2E1**, 3A4

Increased Effect/Toxicity: Disulfiram may increase serum concentrations of benzodiazepines that undergo oxidative metabolism (all but oxazepam, lorazepam, temazepam). Disulfiram increases phenytoin and theophylline serum concentrations; toxicity may occur. Disulfiram inhibits the metabolism of warfarin resulting in an increased hypoprothrombinemic response. Disulfiram results in severe ethanol intolerance (disulfiram reaction) secondary to disulfiram's ability to inhibit aldehyde dehydrogenase; this combination should be avoided. Combined use with isoniazid, metronidazole, or MAO inhibitors may result in adverse CNS effects; this combination should be avoided. Some pharmaceutic dosage forms include ethanol, including elixirs and intravenous trimethoprim-sulfamethoxazole (contains 10% ethanol as a solubilizing agent); these may inadvertently provoke a disulfiram reaction.

Dietary/Ethanol/Herb Considerations Ethanol: Avoid use; usual metabolism is inhibited and may cause a disulfiram reaction (abdominal or chest pain, headache, nausea, or vomiting)

Pharmacodynamics/Kinetics

Onset of action: Full effect: 12 hours

Duration: ~1-2 weeks after last dose

Absorption: Rapid

Metabolism: To diethylthiocarbamate

Excretion: Feces and exhaled gases (as metabolites)

Pregnancy Risk Factor C

Generic Available No

Dithioglycerol *see* Dimercaprol *on page 449*

Dithranol *see* Anthralin *on page 111*

Ditropan® *see* Oxybutynin *on page 1016*

Ditropan® XL *see* Oxybutynin *on page 1016*

Diupres® *see* Chlorothiazide and Reserpine *on page 306*

Diuril® *see* Chlorothiazide *on page 304*

Divalproex Sodium *see* Valproic Acid and Derivatives *on page 1371*

***dl*-Alpha Tocopherol** *see* Vitamin E *on page 1393*

4-dmdr *see* Idarubicin *on page 706*

DNA-derived Humanized Monoclonal Antibody *see* Alemtuzumab *on page 52*

DNase *see* Dornase Alfa *on page 467*

DNR *see* DAUNOrubicin Hydrochloride *on page 402*

Doan's® [OTC] *see* Magnesium Salicylate *on page 837*

Doan's® Extra Strength [OTC] *see* Magnesium Salicylate *on page 837*

DOBUTamine (doe BYOO ta meen)

U.S. Brand Names Dobutrex®

Canadian Brand Names Dobutrex®

Mexican Brand Names Dobuject®; Dobutrex®; Oxiken®

Pharmacologic Category Adrenergic Agonist Agent

Synonyms Dobutamine Hydrochloride

Use Short-term management of patients with cardiac decompensation

Unlabeled/Investigational Use Postive inotropic agent for use in myocardial dysfunction of sepsis

Local Anesthetic/Vasoconstrictor Precautions No information available to require special precautions

Effects on Dental Treatment Frequency not defined: Increased heart rate and blood pressure, hypotension, anginal pain (1% to 3%), nonspecific chest pain (1% to 3%), palpitations (1% to 3%), fever (1% to 3%), headache (1% to 3%), paresthesia, nausea (1% to 3%), dyspnea (1% to 3%)

Dosage Administration requires the use of an infusion pump; I.V. infusion:

Neonates: 2-15 mcg/kg/minute, titrate to desired response

Children and Adults: 2.5-20 mcg/kg/minute; maximum: 40 mcg/kg/minute, titrate to desired response. See table.

Infusion Rates of Various Dilutions of Dobutamine

Desired Delivery Rate (mcg/kg/min)	Infusion Rate (mL/kg/min)	
	500 mcg/mL*	1000 mcg/mL†
2.5	0.005	0.0025
5.0	0.01	0.005
7.5	0.015	0.0075
10.0	0.02	0.01
12.5	0.025	0.0125
15.0	0.03	0.015

* 500 mg per liter or 250 mg per 500 mL of diluent.

†1000 mg per liter or 250 mg per 250 mL of diluent.

Mechanism of Action Stimulates beta$_1$-adrenergic receptors, causing increased contractility and heart rate, with little effect on beta$_2$- or alpha-receptors

Other Adverse Effects Frequency not defined:

Cardiovascular: Increased ventricular ectopic activity, premature ventricular beats (5%, dose-related)

Endocrine & metabolic: Slight decrease in serum potassium

Hematologic: Thrombocytopenia (isolated cases)

Local: Phlebitis, local inflammatory changes and pain from infiltration, cutaneous necrosis (isolated cases)

Neuromuscular & skeletal: Mild leg cramps

Drug Interactions

Increased Effect/Toxicity: General anesthetics (eg, halothane or cyclopropane) and usual doses of dobutamine have resulted in ventricular arrhythmias in animals. Bretylium and may potentiate dobutamine's effects. Beta-blockers (nonselective ones) may increase hypertensive effect; avoid concurrent use. Cocaine may cause malignant arrhythmias. Guanethidine, MAO inhibitors, methyldopa, reserpine, and tricyclic antidepressants can increase the pressor response to sympathomimetics.

Decreased Effect: Beta-adrenergic blockers may decrease effect of dobutamine and increase risk of severe hypotension.

Pharmacodynamics/Kinetics

Onset of action: I.V.: 1-10 minutes

Peak effect: 10-20 minutes

Metabolism: In tissues and hepatically to inactive metabolites

Half-life elimination: 2 minutes

Excretion: Urine (as metabolites)

Pregnancy Risk Factor B

Generic Available Yes

Dobutamine Hydrochloride *see* DOBUTamine *on page 460*

Dobutrex® *see* DOBUTamine *on page 460*

Docetaxel (doe se TAKS el)

U.S. Brand Names Taxotere®

Canadian Brand Names Taxotere®

Mexican Brand Names Taxotere®

Pharmacologic Category Antineoplastic Agent, Natural Source (Plant) Derivative

Use Treatment of patients with locally-advanced or metastatic breast cancer, after failure of prior chemotherapy; treatment of patients with locally advanced or metastatic nonsmall cell lung cancer (NSCLC) after failure of prior platinum-based chemotherapy; in combination with cisplatin in treatment of patients who have not previously received chemotherapy for unresected NSCLC

Unlabeled/Investigational Use Investigational: Treatment of gastric, pancreatic, head and neck, and ovarian cancers, soft tissue sarcoma, and melanoma

Local Anesthetic/Vasoconstrictor Precautions No information available to require special precautions

Effects on Dental Treatment

>10%: Mucositis/stomatitis (26% to 42%, severe in 6% to 7%; premedication may reduce frequency and severity), nausea and vomiting (40% to 80%, severe in 1% to 5%), paresthesia and pain (23% to 49%; severe in up to 6%),

1% to 10%: Taste perversion (6%), hypotension (3%)

(Continued)

Docetaxel *(Continued)*

Dosage Corticosteroids (oral dexamethasone 8 mg twice daily for 3 days or 5 days starting 1 day prior to docetaxel administration) are necessary to reduce the potential for hypersensitivity and severe fluid retention

Adults: I.V. infusion: Refer to individual protocols:

Breast cancer (locally advanced or metastatic): 60-100 mg/m^2 over 1 hour every 3 weeks; patients initially started at 60 mg/m^2 who do not develop toxicity may tolerate higher doses

Nonsmall-cell lung cancer: I.V.: 75 mg/m^2 over 1 hour every 3 weeks

Dosing adjustment for toxicity:

Note: Toxicity includes febrile neutropenia, neutrophils ≤500/mm^3 for >1 week, severe or cumulative cutaneous reactions; in nonsmall cell lung cancer, this may also include other grade 3/4 nonhematologic toxicities.

Breast cancer: Patients dosed initially at 100 mg/m^2; reduce dose to 75 mg/m^2; **Note:** If the patient continues to experience these adverse reactions, the dosage should be reduced to 55 mg/m^2 or therapy should be discontinued

Nonsmall cell lung cancer:

Monotherapy: Patients dosed initially at 75 mg/m^2 should have dose held until toxicity is resolved, then resume at 55 mg/m^2; discontinue patients who develop ≥ grade 3 peripheral neuropathy.

Combination therapy: Patients dosed initially at 75 mg/m^2, in combination with cisplatin, should have the docetaxel dosage reduced to 65 mg/m^2 in subsequent cycles; if further adjustment is required, dosage may be reduced to 50 mg/m^2

Dosing adjustment in hepatic impairment:

Total bilirubin ≥ the upper limit of normal (ULN), or AST/ALT >1.5 times the ULN concomitant with alkaline phosphatase >2.5 times the ULN: Docetaxel **should not be administered** secondary to increased incidence of treatment-related mortality

Mechanism of Action Docetaxel promotes the assembly of microtubules from tubulin dimers, and inhibits the depolymerization of tubulin which stabilizes microtubules in the cell. This results in inhibition of DNA, RNA, and protein synthesis. Most activity occurs during the M phase of the cell cycle.

Other Adverse Effects Frequencies cited for nonsmall cell lung cancer and breast cancer treatment. Exact frequency may vary based on tumor type, prior treatment, premedication, and dosage of docetaxel.

>10%:

Cardiovascular: Fluid retention, including peripheral edema, pleural effusions, and ascites (33% to 47%); may be more common at cumulative doses ≥400 mg/m^2. Up to 64% in breast cancer patients with dexamethasone premedication.

Dermatologic: Alopecia (56% to 76%); nail disorder (11% to 31%, banding, onycholysis, hypo- or hyperpigmentation)

Gastrointestinal: Diarrhea (33% to 43%)

Hematologic: Myelosuppression, neutropenia (75% to 85%), thrombocytopenia, anemia

Onset: 4-7 days

Nadir: 5-9 days

Recovery: 21 days

Hepatic: Transaminase levels increased (18%)

Miscellaneous: Hypersensitivity reactions (6% to 13%; angioedema, rash, flushing, fever, hypotension); frequency substantially reduced by premedication with dexamethasone starting one day prior to docetaxel administration.

1% to 10%:

Dermatologic: Rash and skin eruptions (6%)

Hepatic: Bilirubin increased (9%)

Neuromuscular & skeletal: Myalgia (6% to 91%), arthralgia (3% to 9%)

Miscellaneous: Infusion site reactions (up to 4%)

<1%, postmarketing and/or case reports (Limited to important or life-threatening): **Atrial fibrillation, acute respiratory distress syndrome (ARDS), dehydration,** erythema multiforme, **GI hemorrhage, GI obstruction, GI perforation,** hepatitis, ileus, interstitial pneumonia, ischemic colitis, lacrimal duct obstruction, **MI,** neutropenic enterocolitis, pulmonary edema, pulmonary embolism, radiation recall, **seizures,** Stevens-Johnson syndrome

Drug Interactions Substrate of **CYP3A4**; Inhibits CYP3A4

Increased Effect/Toxicity: Increased toxicity with cytochrome P450 substrate agents. Possibility of an inhibition of metabolism of docetaxel in patients treated with ketoconazole, erythromycin, astemizole, or cyclosporine. When administered as sequential infusions, observational studies indicate a potential for increased toxicity when platinum derivatives (carboplatin, cisplatin) are administered before taxane derivatives (docetaxel, paclitaxel).

Dietary/Ethanol/Herb Considerations

Ethanol: Avoid use due to GI irritation.

Herb/Nutraceutical: Avoid St John's wort; may decrease serum concentration.

Pharmacodynamics/Kinetics Exhibits linear pharmacokinetics at the recommended dosage range

Distribution: Extensive extravascular distribution and/or tissue binding; V_d: 80-90 L/m^2, V_{dss}: 113 L (mean steady state)

Protein binding: 94%, primarily to alpha$_1$-acid glycoprotein, albumin, and lipoproteins

Metabolism: Hepatic; oxidation via CYP3A4 to metabolites

Half-life elimination: Alpha, beta, gamma: 4 minutes, 36 minutes, and 10-18 hours, respectively

Excretion: Feces (75%); urine (6%); ~80% within 48 hours

Clearance: Total body: Mean: 21 L/hour/m^2

Pregnancy Risk Factor D

Generic Available No

Docosanol (doe KOE san ole)

U.S. Brand Names Abreva® [OTC]

Pharmacologic Category Antiviral Agent, Topical

Synonyms Behenyl Alcohol; *n*-Docosanol

Use Treatment of herpes simplex of the face or lips

Local Anesthetic/Vasoconstrictor Precautions No information available to require special precautions

Effects on Dental Treatment No significant effects or complications reported

Dosage Children ≥12 years and Adults: Topical: Wash hands before and after applying cream. Apply 5 times/day to affected area of face or lips. Begin treatment at first "tingle" of cold sore or fever blister and continue until healed. Rub into area gently, but completely. Do not apply directly to inside of mouth or around eyes.

Mechanism of Action Prevents viral entry and replication at the cellular level

Contraindications Hypersensitivity to docosanol or any component of the formulation

Warnings/Precautions For external use only. Do not apply to inside of mouth or around eyes. Not for use in children <12 years of age.

Dosage Forms CRM: 10% (2 g)

Generic Available No

Comments Inform patient to contact healthcare provider if sore gets worse or does not heal within 10 days. Advise patient not to share product with others; may spread infection. Before prescribing, ask female patients of childbearing age if pregnant or breast-feeding.

Docusate (DOK yoo sate)

U.S. Brand Names Colace® [OTC]; Diocto® [OTC]; Docusoft-S™ [OTC]; DOS® [OTC]; D-S-S® [OTC]; Ex-Lax® Stool Softener [OTC]; Fleet® Sof-Lax® [OTC]; Genasoft® [OTC]; Phillips'® Stool Softener Laxative [OTC]; Surfak® [OTC]

Canadian Brand Names Albert® Docusate; Colace®; Colax-C®; PMS-Docusate Calcium; PMS-Docusate Sodium; Regulex®; Selax®; Soflax™

Pharmacologic Category Stool Softener

Synonyms Dioctyl Calcium Sulfosuccinate; Dioctyl Sodium Sulfosuccinate; Docusate Calcium; Docusate Potassium; Docusate Sodium; DOSS; DSS

Use Stool softener in patients who should avoid straining during defecation and constipation associated with hard, dry stools; prophylaxis for straining (Valsalva) following MI. A safe agent to be used in elderly; some evidence that doses <200 mg are ineffective; stool softeners are unnecessary if stool is well hydrated or "mushy" and soft; shown to be ineffective used long-term.

Unlabeled/Investigational Use Ceruminolytic

Local Anesthetic/Vasoconstrictor Precautions No information available to require special precautions

Effects on Dental Treatment 1% to 10%: Throat irritation

Dosage Docusate salts are interchangeable; the amount of sodium or calcium per dosage unit is clinically insignificant

Infants and Children <3 years: Oral: 10-40 mg/day in 1-4 divided doses

Children: Oral:

- 3-6 years: 20-60 mg/day in 1-4 divided doses
- 6-12 years: 40-150 mg/day in 1-4 divided doses

Adolescents and Adults: Oral: 50-500 mg/day in 1-4 divided doses

Older Children and Adults: Rectal: Add 50-100 mg of docusate liquid to enema fluid (saline or water); administer as retention or flushing enema

Ceruminolytic (unlabeled use): Intra-aural: Administer 1 mL of docusate sodium in 2 mL syringes; if no clearance in 15 minutes, irrigate with 50-100 mL normal saline (this method is 80% effective)

Mechanism of Action Reduces surface tension of the oil-water interface of the stool resulting in enhanced incorporation of water and fat allowing for stool softening

Other Adverse Effects 1% to 10%: Gastrointestinal: Intestinal obstruction, diarrhea, abdominal cramping

(Continued)

Docusate *(Continued)*

Drug Interactions

Increased Effect/Toxicity: Increased toxicity with mineral oil, phenolphthalein.

Decreased Effect: Decreased effect of warfarin with high doses of docusate.

Pharmacodynamics/Kinetics

Onset of action: 12-72 hours

Excretion: Feces

Pregnancy Risk Factor C

Generic Available Yes

Docusate and Casanthranol (DOK yoo sate & ka SAN thra nole)

Related Information

Docusate *on page 463*

U.S. Brand Names Diocto C® [OTC]; Docusoft Plus™ [OTC]; Doxidan® [OTC]; Fleet® Sof-Lax® Overnight [OTC]; Genasoft® Plus [OTC]; Peri-Colace® [OTC]

Canadian Brand Names Peri-Colace®

Pharmacologic Category Laxative/Stool Softener

Synonyms Casanthranol and Docusate; DSS With Casanthranol

Use Treatment of constipation generally associated with dry, hard stools and decreased intestinal motility

Local Anesthetic/Vasoconstrictor Precautions No information available to require special precautions

Effects on Dental Treatment 1% to 10%: Throat irritation

Dosage Oral:

Children: 5-15 mL of syrup at bedtime or 1 capsule at bedtime

Adults: 1-2 capsules or 15-30 mL syrup at bedtime, may be increased to 2 capsules or 30 mL twice daily or 3 capsules at bedtime

Other Adverse Effects 1% to 10%:

Dermatologic: Rash

Gastrointestinal: Intestinal obstruction, diarrhea, abdominal cramping

Pregnancy Risk Factor C

Generic Available Yes

Docusate Calcium *see* Docusate *on page 463*

Docusate Potassium *see* Docusate *on page 463*

Docusate Sodium *see* Docusate *on page 463*

Docusoft Plus™ [OTC] *see* Docusate and Casanthranol *on page 464*

Docusoft-S™ [OTC] *see* Docusate *on page 463*

Dofetilide (doe FET il ide)

U.S. Brand Names Tikosyn™

Canadian Brand Names Tikosyn™

Pharmacologic Category Antiarrhythmic Agent, Class III

Use Maintenance of normal sinus rhythm in patients with chronic atrial fibrillation/atrial flutter of longer than 1-week duration who have been converted to normal sinus rhythm; conversion of atrial fibrillation and atrial flutter to normal sinus rhythm

Local Anesthetic/Vasoconstrictor Precautions No information available to require special precautions

Effects on Dental Treatment

>10%: Headache (11%)

2% to 10%: Dizziness (8%), ventricular tachycardia (2.6% to 3.7%), chest pain (10%), nausea (5%), dyspnea (6%), respiratory tract infection (7%), flu syndrome (4%)

<2%: Facial paralysis, flaccid paralysis, migraine, paralysis, ventricular fibrillation, heart arrest, myocardial infarction, sudden death, syncope, paresthesia, cough

Dosage Adults: Oral:

Note: QT or QT_c must be determined prior to first dose. If QT_c >440 msec (>500 msec in patients with ventricular conduction abnormalities), dofetilide is contraindicated.

Initial: 500 mcg orally twice daily. Initial dosage must be adjusted in patients with estimated Cl_{cr} <60 mL/minute (see Dosage Adjustment in Renal Impairment). Dofetilide may be initiated at lower doses than recommended based on physician discretion.

Modification of dosage in response to initial dose:

QT_c interval should be measured 2-3 hours after the initial dose. If the QT_c >15% of baseline, or if the QT_c is >500 msec (550 msec in patients with ventricular conduction abnormalities) dofetilide should be adjusted. If the starting dose is 500 mcg twice daily, then adjust to 250 mcg twice daily. If the starting dose was 250 mcg twice daily, then adjust to 125 mcg twice daily. If the starting dose was 125 mcg twice daily then adjust to 125 mcg every day.

Continued monitoring for doses 2-5:

QT_c interval must be determined 2-3 hours after each subsequent dose of dofetilide for in-hospital doses 2-5. If the measured QT_c is >500 msec (550 msec in patients with ventricular conduction abnormalities) at any time, dofetilide should be discontinued.

Chronic therapy (following the 5th dose):

QT or QT_c and creatinine clearance should be evaluated every 3 months. If QT_c >500 msec (>550 msec in patients with ventricular conduction abnormalities), dofetilide should be discontinued.

Elderly: No specific dosage adjustments recommended but careful assessment of renal function is critical

Dosing adjustment in renal impairment:

Cl_{cr} >60 mL/minute: Administer 500 mcg twice daily.
Cl_{cr} 40-60 mL/minute: Administer 250 mcg twice daily.
Cl_{cr} 20-39 mL/minute: Administer 125 mcg twice daily.
Cl_{cr} <20 mL/minute: Contraindicated in this group.

Mechanism of Action Vaughan Williams Class III antiarrhythmic activity. Blockade of the cardiac ion channel carrying the rapid component of the delayed rectifier potassium current. Dofetilide has no effect on sodium channels, adrenergic alpha-receptors, or adrenergic beta-receptors. It increases the monophasic action potential duration due to delayed repolarization. The increase in the QT interval is a function of prolongation of both effective and functional refractory periods in the His-Purkinje system and the ventricles. Changes in cardiac conduction velocity and sinus node function have not been observed in patients with or without structural heart disease. PR and QRS width remain the same in patients with pre-existing heart block and or sick sinus syndrome.

Other Adverse Effects Supraventricular arrhythmia patients (incidence > placebo):

2% to 10%:

Central nervous system: Insomnia (4%)
Dermatologic: Rash (3%)
Gastrointestinal: Diarrhea (3%), abdominal pain (3%)
Neuromuscular & skeletal: Back pain (3%)

<2%:

Cardiovascular: AV block (≤1.5%), bundle branch block, heart block, edema,
Dermatologic: Angioedema
Gastrointestinal: Liver damage

Drug Interactions Substrate of CYP3A4

Increased Effect/Toxicity: Dofetilide concentrations are increased by cimetidine, verapamil, ketoconazole, and trimethoprim (concurrent use of these agents is contraindicated). Dofetilide levels may also be increased by renal cationic transport inhibitors (including triamterene, metformin, amiloride, and megestrol) or inhibitors of cytochrome P450 isoenzyme 3A4 (including amiodarone, azole antifungal agents, clarithromycin, cannabinoids, diltiazem, erythromycin, nefazodone, norfloxacin, protease inhibitors, quinidine, serotonin reuptake inhibitors. verapamil, and zafirlukast). Diuretics and other drugs which may deplete potassium and/or magnesium (aminoglycoside antibiotics, amphotericin, cyclosporine) may increase dofetilide's toxicity (torsade de pointes).

Dietary/Ethanol/Herb Considerations

Food: May be taken with food

Herb/Nutraceutical: Avoid ephedra, ginseng, and yohimbe; may worsen arrhythmia. Avoid St John's wort; may decrease serum concentration.

Pharmacodynamics/Kinetics

Absorption: >90%
Distribution: V_d: 3 L/kg
Protein binding: 60% to 70%
Metabolism: Hepatic via CYP3A4, but low affinity for it; metabolites formed by N-dealkylation and N-oxidation
Bioavailability: >90%
Half-life elimination: 10 hours
Time to peak: Fasting: 2-3 hours
Excretion: Urine (80%, 80% as unchanged drug, 20% as inactive or minimally active metabolites); renal elimination consists of glomerular filtration and active tubular secretion via cationic transport system

Pregnancy Risk Factor C

Generic Available No

Selected Readings

Buxton AE, Lee KL, Fisher JD, et al, "A Randomized Study of the Prevention of Sudden Death in Patients With Coronary Artery Disease," *N Engl J Med*, 1999, 341(25):1882-90.

Prystowsky EN, Benson DW Jr, Fuster V, et al, "Management of Patients With Atrial Fibrillation: A Statement for Healthcare Professionals. From the Subcommittee on Electrocardiography and Electrophysiology, American Heart Association," *Circulation*, 1996, 93(6):1262-77.

Wynn RL, "Atrial Fibrillation: Medications and Dental Considerations," *Gen Dent*, 1999, 47(6):548-51.

Dolasetron (dol A se tron)

U.S. Brand Names Anzemet®

Canadian Brand Names Anzemet®

Mexican Brand Names Anzemet®

Pharmacologic Category Antiemetic; Selective 5-HT_3 Receptor Antagonist

Synonyms Dolasetron Mesylate; MDL 73,147EF

(Continued)

Dolasetron *(Continued)*

Use Prevention of nausea and vomiting associated with emetogenic cancer chemotherapy, including initial and repeat courses; prevention of postoperative nausea and vomiting and treatment of postoperative nausea and vomiting (injectable form only)

Generally **not** recommended for treatment of existing chemotherapy-induced emesis (CIE) or for prophylaxis of nausea from agents with a low emetogenic potential.

Local Anesthetic/Vasoconstrictor Precautions No information available to require special precautions

Effects on Dental Treatment

>10%: Headache (31%), dizziness, lightheadedness (23%), taste alterations (12%)

1% to 10%: Hypertension, hypotension (6%), sedation (8%), nervousness (3%), fatigue (2%), listlessness, grogginess, nausea (6%), paresthesia, visual disturbances (mostly blurred vision) (9%)

Dosage Oral administration of I.V. solution is equivalent to tablets.

Children <2 years: Use not recommended

Nausea and vomiting associated with chemotherapy (including initial and repeat courses):

- Children 2-16 years:
  - Oral: 1.8 mg/kg within 1 hour before chemotherapy; maximum: 100 mg/dose
  - I.V.: 1.8 mg/kg ~30 minutes before chemotherapy; maximum: 100 mg/dose
- Adults:
  - Oral: 200 mg single dose
  - I.V.:
    - 0.6-5 mg/kg as a single dose
    - 50 mg 1-2 minute bolus
    - 2.4-3 mg/kg 20-minute infusion

Prevention of postoperative nausea and vomiting:

- Children 2-16 years:
  - Oral: 1.2 mg/kg within 2 hours before surgery; maximum: 100 mg/dose
  - I.V.: 0.35 mg/kg (maximum: 12.5 mg) ~15 minutes before stopping anesthesia
- Adults:
  - Oral: 100 mg within 2 hours before surgery
  - I.V.: 12.5 mg ~15 minutes before stopping anesthesia

Treatment of postoperative nausea and vomiting: I.V. (only):

- Children: 0.35 mg/kg (maximum: 12.5 mg) as soon as needed
- Adults: 12.5 mg as soon as needed

Mechanism of Action Selective serotonin receptor (5-HT_3) antagonist, blocking serotonin both peripherally (primary site of action) and centrally at the chemoreceptor trigger zone

Other Adverse Effects

>10%:

- Gastrointestinal: Loose stools/diarrhea (50%); increased appetite (27%);

1% to 10%:

- Cardiovascular: EKG abnormalities, prolonged P-R, QRS, and QT_c intervals
- Central nervous system: Slow movement (3%)
- Gastrointestinal: Constipation (3%), diarrhea, abdominal pain, flatulence
- Hepatic: Mild elevations of serum aminotransferases (7%)
- Local: Pain at injection site (1%)
- Ocular: Photosensitivity (2%)

Drug Interactions Substrate of CYP2C8/9, 3A4; Inhibits CYP2D6

Increased Effect/Toxicity: Increased blood levels of active metabolite may occur during concurrent administration of cimetidine and atenolol. Inhibitors of this isoenzyme may increase blood levels of active metabolite. Due to the potential to potentiate QT_c prolongation, drugs which may prolong QT interval directly (eg, antiarrhythmics) or by causing alterations in electrolytes (eg, diuretics) should be used with caution.

Decreased Effect: Blood levels of active metabolite are decreased during coadministration of rifampin.

Dietary/Ethanol/Herb Considerations

Food: I.V. injection may be diluted in apple or apple-grape juice and taken orally.

Herb/Nutraceutical: Avoid St John's wort; may decrease serum concentration.

Pharmacodynamics/Kinetics

Metabolism: Hepatic to a reduced alcohol (active metabolite MDL 74,156)

Half-life elimination: Dolasetron: 10 minutes; MDL 74,156: 8 hours

Excretion: Urine (as unchanged drug)

Pregnancy Risk Factor B

Generic Available No

Dolasetron Mesylate *see* Dolasetron *on page 465*

Dolobid® *see* Diflunisal *on page 438*

Dolophine® *see* Methadone *on page 876*

Dolorac™ [OTC] *see* Capsaicin *on page 238*

Domeboro® [OTC] *see* Aluminum Sulfate and Calcium Acetate *on page 70*

Dome Paste Bandage *see* Zinc Gelatin *on page 1409*

Donepezil (doe NEP e zil)

U.S. Brand Names Aricept®

Canadian Brand Names Aricept®

Mexican Brand Names Eranz®

Pharmacologic Category Acetylcholinesterase Inhibitor (Central)

Synonyms E2020

Use Treatment of mild to moderate dementia of the Alzheimer's type

Unlabeled/Investigational Use Treatment of attention-deficit/hyperactivity disorder (ADHD)

Local Anesthetic/Vasoconstrictor Precautions No information available to require special precautions

Effects on Dental Treatment

>10%: Headache, nausea

1% to 10%: Syncope, chest pain, hypertension, atrial fibrillation, hypotension, hot flashes, dizziness, fatigue, somnolence, bruising, vomiting, GI bleeding, epigastric pain, muscle cramps, arthritis, body pain

Dosage Oral:

Children: ADHD (unlabeled use): 5 mg/day

Adults: Dementia of Alzheimer's type: Initial: 5 mg/day at bedtime; may increase to 10 mg/day at bedtime after 4-6 weeks

Mechanism of Action Alzheimer's disease is characterized by cholinergic deficiency in the cortex and basal forebrain, which contributes to cognitive deficits. Donepezil reversibly and noncompetitively inhibits centrally-active acetylcholinesterase, the enzyme responsible for hydrolysis of acetylcholine. This appears to result in increased concentrations of acetylcholine available for synaptic transmission in the central nervous system.

Other Adverse Effects

>10%: Gastrointestinal: Diarrhea

1% to 10%:

Central nervous system: Abnormal dreams, depression, insomnia

Gastrointestinal: Anorexia, weight loss, fecal incontinence, bloating

Genitourinary: Frequent urination

<1%: **CHF, delusions,** dysarthria, **dysphasia, dyspnea,** eosinophilia, intracranial hemorrhage, **paresthesia,** pruritus, thrombocytopenia, **tremors**

Postmarketing and/or case reports: Abdominal pain, **agitation,** cholecystitis, **confusion, convulsions, hallucinations,** heart block, hemolytic anemia, hyponatremia, neuroleptic malignant syndrome, pancreatitis, rash

Drug Interactions Substrate of CYP2D6, 3A4

Increased Effect/Toxicity: Ketoconazole and quinidine inhibit donepezil's metabolism *in vitro* and may increase toxicity. A synergistic effect may be seen with concurrent administration of succinylcholine or cholinergic agonists (bethanechol).

Decreased Effect: Donepezil levels may be decreased by enzyme inducers (phenytoin, carbamazepine, dexamethasone, rifampin, and phenobarbital). Anticholinergic agents (benztropine) may inhibit the effects of donepezil.

Dietary/Ethanol/Herb Considerations Herb/Nutraceutical: Avoid St John's wort; may decrease serum concentration.

Pharmacodynamics/Kinetics

Absorption: Well absorbed

Protein binding: 96%, primarily to albumin (75%) and α_1-acid glycoprotein (21%)

Metabolism: Extensively to four major metabolites (two are active) via CYP2D6 and 3A4; undergoes glucuronidation

Bioavailability: 100%

Half-life elimination: 70 hours; time to steady-state: 15 days

Time to peak, plasma: 3-4 hours

Excretion: Urine (as unchanged drug)

Pregnancy Risk Factor C

Generic Available No

Donnapectolin-PG® *see* Hyoscyamine, Atropine, Scopolamine, Kaolin, Pectin, and Opium *on page 701*

Donnatal® [DSC] *see* Hyoscyamine, Atropine, Scopolamine, and Phenobarbital *on page 700*

Dopar® *see* Levodopa *on page 792*

Dopram® *see* Doxapram *on page 469*

Doral® *see* Quazepam *on page 1154*

Dornase Alfa (DORE nase AL fu)

U.S. Brand Names Pulmozyme®

Canadian Brand Names Pulmozyme™

Mexican Brand Names Pulmozyme®

Pharmacologic Category Enzyme

(Continued)

Dornase Alfa *(Continued)*

Synonyms DNase; Recombinant Human Deoxyribonuclease

Use Management of cystic fibrosis patients to reduce the frequency of respiratory infections that require parenteral antibiotics, and to improve pulmonary function

Unlabeled/Investigational Use Treatment of chronic bronchitis

Local Anesthetic/Vasoconstrictor Precautions No information available to require special precautions

Effects on Dental Treatment

>10%: Pharyngitis

1% to 10%: Chest pain laryngitis, cough, dyspnea, hemoptysis, rhinitis, hoarseness, wheezing

Dosage Inhalation:

Children >3 months to Adults: 2.5 mg once daily through selected nebulizers; experience in children <5 years is limited

Patients unable to inhale or exhale orally throughout the entire treatment period may use Pari-Baby™ nebulizer. Some patients may benefit from twice daily administration.

Mechanism of Action The hallmark of cystic fibrosis lung disease is the presence of abundant, purulent airway secretions composed primarily of highly polymerized DNA. The principal source of this DNA is the nuclei of degenerating neutrophils, which is present in large concentrations in infected lung secretions. The presence of this DNA produces a viscous mucous that may contribute to the decreased mucociliary transport and persistent infections that are commonly seen in this population. Dornase alfa is a deoxyribonuclease (DNA) enzyme produced by recombinant gene technology. Dornase selectively cleaves DNA, thus reducing mucous viscosity and as a result, airflow in the lung is improved and the risk of bacterial infection may be decreased.

Other Adverse Effects

>10%: Miscellaneous: Voice alteration

1% to 10%:

Dermatologic: Rash

Ocular: Conjunctivitis

Pharmacodynamics/Kinetics

Onset of action: Nebulization: Enzyme levels are measured in sputum in ~15 minutes

Duration: Rapidly declines

Pregnancy Risk Factor B

Generic Available No

Doryx® *see* Doxycycline *on page 476*

Dorzolamide (dor ZOLE a mide)

U.S. Brand Names Trusopt®

Canadian Brand Names Trusopt®

Mexican Brand Names Trusopt®

Pharmacologic Category Carbonic Anhydrase Inhibitor; Ophthalmic Agent, Antiglaucoma

Synonyms Dorzolamide Hydrochloride

Use Lowers intraocular pressure to treat glaucoma in patients with ocular hypertension or open-angle glaucoma

Local Anesthetic/Vasoconstrictor Precautions No information available to require special precautions

Effects on Dental Treatment No significant effects or complications reported

Dosage Adults: Glaucoma: Instill 1 drop in the affected eye(s) 3 times/day

Mechanism of Action Reversible inhibition of the enzyme carbonic anhydrase resulting in reduction of hydrogen ion secretion at renal tubule and an increased renal excretion of sodium, potassium, bicarbonate, and water to decrease production of aqueous humor; also inhibits carbonic anhydrase in central nervous system to retard abnormal and excessive discharge from CNS neurons

Other Adverse Effects

>10%:

Gastrointestinal: Bitter taste following administration (25%)

Ocular: Burning, stinging or discomfort immediately following administration (33%); superficial punctate keratitis (10% to 15%); signs and symptoms of ocular allergic reaction (10%)

1% to 5%: Ocular: Blurred vision, conjunctivitis, dryness, lid reactions, photophobia, tearing

<1%: Choriodal detachment (following filtration procedures), fatigue, headache, iridocyclitis (rare), nausea, rashes (rare), urolithiasis, weakness, xerostomia

Postmarketing and/or case reports: Allergic reaction (systemic), angioedema, **bronchospasm, dyspnea, epistaxis,** eyelid crusting, myopia, **paresthesia, pharyngitis,** pruritus, urticaria

Drug Interactions Substrate of CYP2C8/9, 3A4

Increased Effect/Toxicity: Salicylate use may result in carbonic anhydrase inhibitor accumulation and toxicity including CNS depression and metabolic acidosis

Pharmacodynamics/Kinetics

Onset of action: Peak effect: 2 hours

Duration: 8-12 hours

Absorption: Topical: Reaches systemic circulation where it accumulates in RBCs during chronic dosing as a result of binding to CA-11

Distribution: In RBCs during chronic administration

Protein binding: 33%

Metabolism: To N-desethyl metabolite (less potent than parent drug)

Half-life elimination: Terminal RBC: 147 days; washes out of RBCs nonlinearly, resulting in a rapid decline of drug concentration initially, followed by a slower elimination phase with a half-life of about 4 months

Excretion: Urine (as unchanged drug and metabolite, N-desethyl)

Pregnancy Risk Factor C

Generic Available No

Dorzolamide Hydrochloride *see* Dorzolamide *on page 468*

DOS® [OTC] *see* Docusate *on page 463*

DOSS *see* Docusate *on page 463*

Dostinex® *see* Cabergoline *on page 220*

Dovonex® *see* Calcipotriene *on page 222*

Doxapram (DOKS a pram)

U.S. Brand Names Dopram®

Pharmacologic Category Respiratory Stimulant; Stimulant

Synonyms Doxapram Hydrochloride

Use Respiratory and CNS stimulant for respiratory depression secondary to anesthesia, drug-induced CNS depression; acute hypercapnia secondary to COPD

Local Anesthetic/Vasoconstrictor Precautions No information available to require special precautions

Effects on Dental Treatment 1% to 10%: Angina, hypotension, palpitations, tachycardia, vasoconstriction, headache, nausea, vomiting, dyspnea

Dosage Contains a significant amount of benzyl alcohol (0.9%); I.V.: Adults:

Respiratory depression following anesthesia:

Intermittent injection: Initial: 0.5-1 mg/kg; may repeat at 5-minute intervals (only in patients who demonstrate initial response); maximum total dose: 2 mg/kg

I.V. infusion: Initial: 5 mg/minute until adequate response or adverse effects seen; decrease to 1-3 mg/minute; maximum total dose: 4 mg/kg

Drug-induced CNS depression:

Intermittent injection: Initial: 1-2 mg/kg, repeat after 5 minutes; may repeat at 1-2 hour intervals (until sustained consciousness); maximum 3 g/day

I.V. infusion: Initial: Bolus dose of 2 mg/kg, repeat after 5 minutes. If no response, wait 1-2 hours and repeat. If some stimulation is noted, initiate infusion at 1-3 mg/minute (depending on size of patient/depth of CNS depression); suspend infusion if patient begins to awaken. Infusion should not be continued for >2 hours. May reinstitute infusion as described above, including bolus, after rest interval of 30 minutes to 2 hours; maximum: 3 g/day

Acute hypercapnia secondary to COPD: I.V. infusion: Initial: Initiate infusion at 1-2 mg/minute (depending on size of patient/depth of CNS depression); may increase to maximum rate of 3 mg/minute; infusion should not be continued for >2 hours. Monitor arterial blood gases prior to initiation of infusion and at 30-minute intervals during the infusion (to identify possible development of acidosis/CO_2 retention). Additional infusions are not recommended (per manufacturer).

Hemodialysis: Not dialyzable

Mechanism of Action Stimulates respiration through action on respiratory center in medulla or indirectly on peripheral carotid chemoreceptors

Other Adverse Effects

1% to 10%: Cardiovascular: Ectopic beats

<1%: Abdominal distension, **arrhythmias, CNS stimulation, coughing, diaphoresis, feeling of warmth, fever, flushing, hallucinations,** hemolysis, hyper-reflexia, **hypertension (dose-related), irritability, jitters,** lacrimation, **laryngospasm, lightheadedness,** mydriasis, phlebitis, **restlessness, retching, seizures, tremor**; premature neonates exposed to doxapram have developed severe adverse reactions including CNS and cardiovascular events

Drug Interactions Increased Effect/Toxicity: Increased blood pressure with sympathomimetics, MAO inhibitors. Halothane, cyclopropane, and enflurane may sensitize the myocardium to catecholamine and epinephrine which is released at the initiation of doxapram, hence, separate discontinuation of anesthetics and start of doxapram until the volatile agent has been excreted.

Pharmacodynamics/Kinetics

Onset of action: Respiratory stimulation: I.V.: 20-40 seconds

Peak effect: 1-2 minutes

Duration: 5-12 minutes

Half-life elimination, serum: Adults: Mean: 3.4 hours

(Continued)

Doxapram *(Continued)*

Pregnancy Risk Factor B

Generic Available No

Comments Initial studies suggest a therapeutic range of at least 1.5 mg/L; toxicity becomes frequent at serum levels >5 mg/L

Doxapram Hydrochloride *see* Doxapram *on page 469*

Doxazosin (doks AYE zoe sin)

Related Information

Cardiovascular Diseases *on page 1456*

U.S. Brand Names Cardura®

Canadian Brand Names Alti-Doxazosin; Apo®-Doxazosin; Cardura-1™; Cardura-2™; Cardura-4™; Gen-Doxazosin; Novo-Doxazosin

Mexican Brand Names Cardura®

Pharmacologic Category Alpha$_1$ Blocker

Use Treatment of hypertension alone or in conjunction with diuretics, cardiac glycosides, ACE inhibitors, or calcium antagonists (particularly appropriate for those with hypertension and other cardiovascular risk factors such as hypercholesterolemia and diabetes mellitus); treatment of urinary outflow obstruction and/or obstructive and irritative symptoms associated with benign prostatic hyperplasia (BPH), particularly useful in patients with troublesome symptoms who are unable or unwilling to undergo invasive procedures, but who require rapid symptomatic relief

Local Anesthetic/Vasoconstrictor Precautions No information available to require special precautions

Effects on Dental Treatment

>10%: Dizziness (16% to 19%), headache (10% to 14%)

1% to 10%: Xerostomia, orthostatic hypotension (dose-related; 0.3% up to 10%), hypotension (2%), palpitations (1% to 2%), chest pain (1% to 2%), arrhythmia (1%), syncope (2%), flushing (1%), fatigue (8% to 12%), somnolence (3% to 5%), nervousness (2%), pain (2%), vertigo (2%), anxiety (1%), paresthesia (1%), weakness (1%), nausea (2% to 3%), arthritis (1%), weakness, muscle cramps (1%), abnormal vision (1% to 2%), rhinitis (3%), dyspnea (1% to 3%), respiratory disorder (1%), epistaxis (1%), flu-like syndrome (1%), increased diaphoresis (1%)

Dosage Oral:

Adults: 1 mg once daily in morning or evening; may be increased to 2 mg once daily. Thereafter titrate upwards, if needed, over several weeks, balancing therapeutic benefit with doxazosin-induced postural hypotension

Hypertension: Maximum dose: 16 mg/day

BPH: Maximum dose: 8 mg/day

Elderly: Initial: 0.5 mg once daily

Mechanism of Action Competitively inhibits postsynaptic alpha-adrenergic receptors which results in vasodilation of veins and arterioles and a decrease in total peripheral resistance and blood pressure; approximately 50% as potent on a weight by weight basis as prazosin

Other Adverse Effects

1% to 10%:

Cardiovascular: Edema (3% to 4%)

Central nervous system: Vertigo (2%), insomnia (1%), movement disorder (1%), ataxia (1%), hypertonia (1%), depression (1%)

Dermatologic: Rash (1%), pruritus (1%)

Endocrine & metabolic: Sexual dysfunction (2%)

Gastrointestinal: Abdominal pain (2%), diarrhea (2%), dyspepsia (1% to 2%), constipation (1%), flatulence (1%)

Genitourinary: Urinary tract infection (1%), impotence (1%), polyuria (2%), incontinence (1%)

Neuromuscular & skeletal: Back pain (2%) myalgia (1%)

Ocular: Conjunctivitis (1%)

Otic: Tinnitus (1%)

<1% (Limited to important or life-threatening): Abnormal lacrimation, **abnormal thinking, agitation,** alopecia, **amnesia, angina,** anorexia, **bradycardia,** breast pain, **bronchospasm, confusion, coughing,** depersonalization, dry skin, earache, eczema, emotional lability, fecal incontinence, **fever, gastroenteritis,** gout, **hot flashes,** hypoesthesia, hypokalemia, impaired concentration, **infection, lymphadenopathy, migraine, MI,** pallor, **paranoia, paresis,** parosmia, peripheral ischemia, **pharyngitis,** photophobia, purpura, renal calculus, **rigors, sinusitis, stroke, syncope, tachycardia, abnormal taste, thirst, twitching,** weight gain/loss

Postmarketing and/or case reports: **Allergic reaction, bradycardia, bronchospasm,** cataplexy, cholestasis, enuresis, gynecomastia, hematuria, hepatitis, leukopenia, micturition abnormality, nocturia, priapism, systemic lupus erythematosus, thrombocytopenia, urticaria, **vomiting**

Drug Interactions

Increased Effect/Toxicity: Increased hypotensive effect with beta-blockers, diuretics, ACE inhibitors, calcium channel blockers, and other antihypertensive medications.

Decreased Effect: Decreased hypotensive effect with NSAIDs.

Dietary/Ethanol/Herb Considerations

Ethanol: Use with caution; may increase risk of hypotension or dizziness.

Food: Avoid caffeine (eg, colas, chocolate), garlic, and licorice.

Herb/Nutraceutical: Avoid black cohosh, dong quai, and evening primrose due to estrogenic activity. Avoid ephedra, ginseng, and yohimbe; may worsen hypertension. Avoid garlic; may have increased antihypertensive effect. Avoid ginger due to positive inotropic effects; theoretically, may cause arrhythmia. Avoid hawthorn; may lower peripheral vascular resistance causing additional decrease in BP. Avoid licorice. Avoid saw palmetto when used for BPH due to limited experience with this combination.

Pharmacodynamics/Kinetics Not significantly affected by increased age

Duration: >24 hours

Metabolism: Extensively hepatic

Half-life elimination: 22 hours

Time to peak, serum: 2-3 hours

Excretion: Feces (63%); urine (9%)

Pregnancy Risk Factor C

Generic Available Yes

Doxepin (DOKS e pin)

U.S. Brand Names Prudoxin™; Sinequan®; Zonalon®

Canadian Brand Names Apo®-Doxepin; Novo-Doxepin; Sinequan™; Zonalon

Pharmacologic Category Antidepressant, Tricyclic (Tertiary Amine); Topical Skin Product

Synonyms Doxepin Hydrochloride

Use

Oral: Depression, pruritis

Topical: Short-term (<8 days) management of moderate pruritus in adults with atopic dermatitis or lichen simplex chronicus

Unlabeled/Investigational Use Analgesic for certain chronic and neuropathic pain; treatment of anxiety

Local Anesthetic/Vasoconstrictor Precautions Use with caution; epinephrine, norepinephrine and levonordefrin have been shown to have an increased pressor response in combination with TCAs

Effects on Dental Treatment Long-term treatment with TCAs increases the risk of caries by reducing salivation and salivary buffer capacity.

>10%: Xerostomia, changes in salivation

Frequency not defined: Hypotension, hypertension, tachycardia, drowsiness, dizziness, headache, disorientation, confusion, seizure, vomiting, aphthous stomatitis, unpleasant taste, trouble with gums, decreased lower esophageal sphincter tone (may cause GE reflux), nausea, weakness, tremors, numbness, paresthesia, extrapyramidal symptoms, tardive dyskinesia, blurred vision, diaphoresis (excessive), allergic reactions

Dosage

Oral (entire daily dose may be given at bedtime):

- Depression or anxiety (unlabeled use):
  - Children: 1-3 mg/kg/day in single or divided doses
  - Adolescents: Initial: 25-50 mg/day in single or divided doses; gradually increase to 100 mg/day
  - Adults: Initial: 30-150 mg/day at bedtime or in 2-3 divided doses; may gradually increase up to 300 mg/day; single dose should not exceed 150 mg; select patients may respond to 25-50 mg/day
  - Elderly: Use a lower dose and adjust gradually; preferred agent for sedation
  - Dosing adjustment in hepatic impairment: Lower dose and adjust gradually
- Pruritis (systemic effects increased as compared to topical route): 25-50 mg

Topical: Adults: Pruritis: Apply a thin film 4 times/day with at least 3- to 4-hour interval between applications; should not be used for >8 days

Mechanism of Action Increases the synaptic concentration of serotonin and norepinephrine in the central nervous system by inhibition of their reuptake by the presynaptic neuronal membrane

Other Adverse Effects Frequency not defined:

Central nervous system: Ataxia

Dermatologic: Alopecia, photosensitivity, rash, pruritus

Endocrine & metabolic: Breast enlargement, galactorrhea, SIADH, increase or decrease in blood sugar, increased or decreased libido

Gastrointestinal: Constipation, indigestion, anorexia, weight gain, diarrhea

Genitourinary: Urinary retention, testicular edema

Hematologic: Agranulocytosis, leukopenia, eosinophilia, thrombocytopenia, purpura

(Continued)

Doxepin *(Continued)*

Otic: Tinnitus

Drug Interactions Substrate of **CYP1A2, 2D6, 3A4**

Increased Effect/Toxicity: Doxepin increases the effects of amphetamines, anticholinergics, other CNS depressants (sedatives, hypnotics, or ethanol), chlorpropamide, tolazamide, and warfarin. When used with MAO inhibitors, hyperpyrexia, hypertension, tachycardia, confusion, seizures, and **deaths have been reported** (serotonin syndrome). Serotonin syndrome has also been reported with ritonavir (rare). The SSRIs (to varying degrees), cimetidine, grapefruit juice, indinavir, methylphenidate, ritonavir, quinidine, diltiazem, and verapamil inhibit the metabolism of TCAs and clinical toxicity may result. Use of lithium with a TCA may increase the risk for neurotoxicity. Phenothiazines may increase concentration of some TCAs and TCAs may increase concentration of phenothiazines. Pressor response to I.V. epinephrine, norepinephrine, and phenylephrine may be enhanced in patients receiving TCAs (**Note:** Effect is unlikely with epinephrine or levonordefrin dosages typically administered as infiltration in combination with local anesthetics). Combined use of beta-agonists or drugs which prolong QT_c (including quinidine, procainamide, disopyramide, cisapride, sparfloxacin, gatifloxacin, moxifloxacin) with TCAs may predispose patients to cardiac arrhythmias.

Decreased Effect: Carbamazepine, phenobarbital, and rifampin may increase the metabolism of doxepin resulting in decreased effect of doxepin. Doxepin inhibits the antihypertensive response to bethanidine, clonidine, debrisoquin, guanadrel, guanethidine, guanabenz, and guanfacine. Cholestyramine and colestipol may bind TCAs and reduce their absorption.

Dietary/Ethanol/Herb Considerations

Ethanol: Avoid use; may increase CNS depression.

Food: Avoid grapefruit products; may inhibit metabolism of some TCAs resulting in toxicity.

Herb/Nutraceutical: Avoid kava, SAMe, St John's wort, triptophan, and valerian; may increase risk of serotonin syndrome and/or excessive sedation.

Pharmacodynamics/Kinetics

Onset of action: Peak effect: Antidepressant: Usually >2 weeks; Anxiolytic: may occur sooner

Distribution: Crosses placenta; enters breast milk

Protein binding: 80% to 85%

Metabolism: Hepatic; metabolites include desmethyldoxepin (active)

Half-life elimination: Adults: 6-8 hours

Excretion: Urine

Pregnancy Risk Factor C

Generic Available Yes: Capsule, solution

Selected Readings

Friedlander AH, Mahler ME, "Major Depressive Disorder. Psychopathology, Medical Management, and Dental Implications," *J Am Dent Assoc*, 201, 132(5):629-38.

Ganzberg S, "Psychoactive Drugs," *ADA Guide to Dental Therapeutics*, 2nd ed, Chicago, IL: ADA Publishing, a Division of ADA Business Enterprises, Inc, 2000, 376-405.

Jastak JT and Yagiela JA, "Vasoconstrictors and Local Anesthesia: A Review and Rationale for Use," *J Am Dent Assoc*, 1983, 107(4):623-30.

Mitchell JR, "Guanethidine and Related Agents. III Antagonism by Drugs Which Inhibit the Norepinephrine Pump in Man," *J Clin Invest*, 1970, 49(8):1596-604.

Rundegren J, van Dijken J, Mörnstad H, et al, "Oral Conditions in Patients Receiving Long-Term Treatment With Cyclic Antidepressant Drugs," *Swed Dent J*, 1985, 9(2):55-64.

Yagiela JA, "Adverse Drug Interactions in Dental Practice: Interactions Associated With Vasoconstrictors. Part V of a Series," *J Am Dent Assoc*, 1999, 130(5):701-9.

Doxepin Hydrochloride *see* Doxepin *on page 471*

Doxercalciferol (doks er kal si FEER ole)

U.S. Brand Names Hectorol®

Canadian Brand Names Hectorol®

Pharmacologic Category Vitamin D Analog

Use Reduction of elevated intact parathyroid hormone (iPTH) in the management of secondary hyperparathyroidism in patients on chronic hemodialysis

Local Anesthetic/Vasoconstrictor Precautions No information available to require special precautions

Effects on Dental Treatment Some of the signs and symptoms of hypercalcemia include anorexia, nausea, vomiting, constipation, polyuria, weakness, fatigue, confusion, stupor, and coma.

>10%: Headache (28%), malaise (28%), dizziness (11.5%), nausea/vomiting (34%), dyspnea (11.5%)

1% to 10%: Bradycardia (6.6%)

Dosage

Oral:

If the iPTH >400 pg/mL, then the initial dose is 10 mcg 3 times/week at dialysis. The dose is adjusted at 8-week intervals based upon the iPTH levels.

If the iPTH level is decreased by 50% and >300 pg/mL, then the dose can be increased to 12.5 mcg 3 times/week for 8 more weeks. This titration process can continue at 8-week intervals up to a maximum dose of 20 mcg 3 times/week. Each increase should be by 2.5 mcg/dose.

If the iPTH is between 150-300 pg/mL, maintain the current dose.

If the iPTH is <100 pg/mL, then suspend the drug for 1 week; resume doxercalciferol at a reduced dose. Decrease each dose (not weekly dose) by at least 2.5 mcg.

I.V.:

If the iPTH >400 pg/mL, then the initial dose is 4 mcg 3 times/week after dialysis, administered as a bolus dose

If the iPTH level is decreased by 50% and >300 pg/mL, then the dose can be increased by 1-2 mcg at 8-week intervals as necessary

If the iPTH is between 150-300 pg/mL, maintain the current dose.

If the iPTH is <100 pg/mL, then suspend the drug for 1 week; resume doxercalciferol at a reduced dose (at least 1 mcg lower)

Mechanism of Action Doxercalciferol is metabolized to the active form of vitamin D. The active form of vitamin D controls the intestinal absorption of dietary calcium, the tubular reabsorption of calcium by the kidneys, and in conjunction with PTH, the mobilization of calcium from the skeleton.

Other Adverse Effects

>10%: Cardiovascular: Edema (34.4%)

1% to 10%:

Central nervous system: Sleep disorder (3.3%)
Dermatologic: Pruritus (8.2%)
Gastrointestinal: Anorexia (4.9%), constipation (3.3%), dyspepsia (4.9%)
Neuromuscular & skeletal: Arthralgia (4.9%)
Miscellaneous: Abscess (3.3%)

Drug Interactions

Increased Effect/Toxicity: Doxercalciferol toxicity may be increased by concurrent use of other vitamin D supplements or magnesium-containing antacids and supplements.

Decreased Effect: Absorption of doxercalciferol is reduced with mineral oil and cholestyramine.

Pharmacodynamics/Kinetics

Metabolism: Hepatic via CYP27

Half-life elimination: Active metabolite: 32-37 hours; up to 96 hours

Pregnancy Risk Factor B

Generic Available No

Doxidan® [OTC] *see* Docusate and Casanthranol *on page 464*

Doxil® *see* DOXOrubicin (Liposomal) *on page 475*

DOXOrubicin (doks oh ROO bi sin)

Related Information

DOXOrubicin (Liposomal) *on page 475*

U.S. Brand Names Adriamycin PFS®; Adriamycin RDF®; Rubex®

Canadian Brand Names Adriamycin®

Mexican Brand Names Adriblastina®; Doxolem®; Doxotec®

Pharmacologic Category Antineoplastic Agent, Anthracycline

Synonyms ADR; Adria; Doxorubicin Hydrochloride; Hydroxydaunomycin Hydrochloride; Hydroxyldaunorubicin Hydrochloride; NSC-123127

Use Treatment of leukemias, lymphomas, multiple myeloma, osseous and nonosseous sarcomas, mesotheliomas, germ cell tumors of the ovary or testis, and carcinomas of the head and neck, thyroid, lung, breast, stomach, pancreas, liver, ovary, bladder, prostate, uterus, and neuroblastoma

Local Anesthetic/Vasoconstrictor Precautions No information available to require special precautions

Effects on Dental Treatment

>10%: Nausea, vomiting, stomatitis, GI ulceration, CHF (dose-related; may be delayed for 7-8 years after treatment),

Dosage Refer to individual protocols. I.V.:

Children:

35-75 mg/m² as a single dose, repeat every 21 days **or**
20-30 mg/m² once weekly **or**
60-90 mg/m² given as a continuous infusion over 96 hours every 3-4 weeks

Adults:

Usual or typical dose: 60-75 mg/m² as a single dose, repeat every 21 days **or** other dosage regimens like 20-30 mg/m²/day for 2-3 days, repeat in 4 weeks **or** 20 mg/m² once weekly

The lower dose regimen should be given to patients with decreased bone marrow reserve, prior therapy or marrow infiltration with malignant cells

Dosing adjustment in renal impairment:

Cl_{cr} <10 mL/minute: Administer 75% of normal dose

Hemodialysis: Supplemental dose unnecessary

(Continued)

DOXOrubicin *(Continued)*

Dosing adjustment in hepatic impairment:

Bilirubin 1.2-3 mg/dL: Administer 50% of dose

Bilirubin 3.1-5 mg/dL: Administer 25% of dose

Bilirubin >5 mg/dL: Do not administer drug

Mechanism of Action Inhibition of DNA and RNA synthesis by intercalation between DNA base pairs by inhibition of topoisomerase II and by steric obstruction. Doxorubicin intercalates at points of local uncoiling of the double helix. Although the exact mechanism is unclear, it appears that direct binding to DNA (intercalation) and inhibition of DNA repair (topoisomerase II inhibition) result in blockade of DNA and RNA synthesis and fragmentation of DNA. Doxorubicin is also a powerful iron chelator; the iron-doxorubicin complex can bind DNA and cell membranes and produce free radicals that immediately cleave the DNA and cell membranes.

Other Adverse Effects

>10%:

Dermatologic: Alopecia, radiation recall

Gastrointestinal: Anorexia, diarrhea

Genitourinary: Discoloration of urine, mild dysuria, urinary frequency, hematuria, bladder spasms, cystitis following bladder instillation

Hematologic: Myelosuppression, primarily leukopenia (75%); thrombocytopenia and anemia

Onset: 7 days

Nadir: 10-14 days

Recovery: 21-28 days

1% to 10%:

Cardiovascular: Transient EKG abnormalities (supraventricular tachycardia, S-T wave changes, atrial or ventricular extrasystoles); generally asymptomatic and self-limiting.

Recommended maximum cumulative doses:

No risk factors: 550 mg/m^2

Concurrent radiation: 450 mg/m^2

Note: Regardless of cumulative dose, if the left ventricular ejection fraction is <30% to 40%, the drug is usually not given.

Dermatologic: Skin "flare" at injection site; discoloration of saliva, sweat, or tears

Endocrine & metabolic: Hyperuricemia

<1%: Pericarditis, myocarditis, myocardial infection, skin rash, pigmentation of nail beds, nail banding, onycholysis, urticaria, infertility, sterility, elevations of bilirubin and transaminases, hepatitis, **systemic hypersensitivity (including urticaria, pruritus, angioedema, dysphagia, and dyspnea)**

Drug Interactions Substrate of **CYP2D6, 3A4**; Inhibits CYP2D6, 3A4

Increased Effect/Toxicity: Allopurinol may enhance the antitumor activity of doxorubicin (animal data only). Cyclosporine may increase doxorubicin levels, enhancing hematologic toxicity or may induce coma or seizures. Cyclophosphamide enhances the cardiac toxicity of doxorubicin by producing additional myocardial cell damage. Mercaptopurine increases doxorubicin toxicities. Streptozocin greatly enhances leukopenia and thrombocytopenia. Verapamil alters the cellular distribution of doxorubicin and may result in increased cell toxicity by inhibition of the P-glycoprotein pump. Paclitaxel reduces doxorubicin clearance and increases toxicity if administered prior to doxorubicin. High doses of progesterone enhance toxicity (neutropenia and thrombocytopenia). Based on mouse studies, cardiotoxicity may be enhanced by verapamil. Concurrent therapy with actinomycin-D may result in recall pneumonitis following radiation.

Decreased Effect: Doxorubicin may decrease plasma levels and effectiveness of digoxin and phenytoin. Phenobarbital increases elimination (decreases effect) of doxorubicin. Doxorubicin may decrease the antiviral activity of zidovudine.

Dietary/Ethanol/Herb Considerations Herb/Nutraceutical: Avoid black cohosh and dong quai in estrogen-dependent tumors. Avoid St John's wort; may decrease serum concentration.

Pharmacodynamics/Kinetics

Absorption: Oral: Poor (<50%)

Distribution: V_d: 25 L/kg; to many body tissues, particularly liver, spleen, kidney, lung, heart; does not distribute into the CNS; crosses placenta

Protein binding, plasma: 70%

Metabolism: Primarily hepatic to doxorubicinol (active), then to inactive aglycones, conjugated sulfates, and glucuronides

Half-life elimination:

Distribution: 10 minutes

Elimination: Doxorubicin: 1-3 hours; Metabolites: 3-3.5 hours

Terminal: 17-30 hours

Male: 54 hours; Female: 35 hours

Excretion: Feces (~40% to 50% as unchanged drug); urine (~3% to 10% as metabolites, 1% doxorubicinol, <1% adrimycine aglycones, and unchanged drug)

Clearance: Male: 113 L/hour; Female: 44 L/hour

Pregnancy Risk Factor D

Generic Available Yes

Doxorubicin Hydrochloride *see* DOXOrubicin *on page 473*

Doxorubicin Hydrochloride (Liposomal) *see* DOXOrubicin (Liposomal) *on page 475*

DOXOrubicin (Liposomal) (doks oh ROO bi sin lip pah SOW mal)

Related Information

DOXOrubicin *on page 473*

U.S. Brand Names Doxil®

Canadian Brand Names Caelyx®

Pharmacologic Category Antineoplastic Agent, Anthracycline

Synonyms Doxorubicin Hydrochloride (Liposomal)

Use Treatment of AIDS-related Kaposi's sarcoma, breast cancer, ovarian cancer, solid tumors

Local Anesthetic/Vasoconstrictor Precautions No information available to require special precautions

Effects on Dental Treatment

>10%: Nausea (18%)

1% to 10%: Mucositis (7%), arrhythmias, tachycardia, CHF (1%), vomiting (8%)

Dosage Refer to individual protocols.

I.V. (patient's ideal weight should be used to calculate body surface area): 20 mg/m^2 over 30 minutes, once every 3 weeks, for as long as patients respond satisfactorily and tolerate treatment.

AIDS-KS patients: I.V.: 20 mg/m^2/dose over 30 minutes once every 3 weeks for as long as patients respond satisfactorily and tolerate treatment

Breast cancer: I.V.: 20-80 mg/m^2/dose has been studied in a limited number of phase I/II trials

Ovarian cancer: I.V.: 50 mg/m^2/dose repeated every 4 weeks (minimum of 4 courses is recommended)

Solid tumors: I.V.: 50-60 mg/m^2/dose repeated every 3-4 weeks has been studied in a limited number of phase I/II trials

See table.

Recommended Dose Modification Guidelines

Toxicity Grade	Dose Adjustment
PALMAR-PLANTAR ERYTHRODYSESTHESIA	
1 (Mild erythema, swelling, or desquamation not interfering with daily activities)	Redose unless patient has experienced previous Grade 3 or 4 toxicity. If so, delay up to 2 weeks and decrease dose by 25%; return to original dosing interval.
2 (Erythema, desquamation, or swelling interfering with, but not precluding, normal physical activities; small blisters or ulcerations <2 cm in diameter)	Delay dosing up to 2 weeks or until resolved to Grade 0-1. If after 2 weeks there is no resolution, liposomal doxorubicin should be discontinued.
3 (Blistering, ulceration, or swelling interfering with walking or normal daily activities; cannot wear regular clothing)	Delay dosing up to 2 weeks or until resolved to Grade 0-1. Decrease dose by 25% and return to original dosing interval; if after 2 weeks there is no resolution, liposomal doxorubicin should be discontinued.
4 (Diffuse or local process causing infectious complications, or a bed-ridden state or hospitalization)	Delay dosing up to 2 weeks or until resolved to Grade 0-1. Decrease dose by 25% and return to original dosing interval. If after 2 weeks there is no resolution, liposomal doxorubicin should be discontinued.
STOMATITIS	
1 (Painless ulcers, erythema, or mild soreness)	Redose unless patient has experienced previous Grade 3 or 4 toxicity. If so, delay up to 2 weeks and decrease by 25%. Return to original dosing interval.
2 (Painful erythema, edema, or ulcers, but can eat)	Delay dosing up to 2 weeks or until resolved to Grade 0-1. If after 2 weeks there is no resolution, liposomal doxorubicin should be discontinued.
3 (Painful erythema, edema, or ulcers, but cannot eat)	Delay dosing up to 2 weeks or until resolved to Grade 0-1. Decrease dose by 25% and return to original dosing interval. If after 2 weeks there is no resolution, liposomal doxorubicin should be discontinued.
4 (Requires parenteral or enteral support)	Delay dosing up to 2 weeks or until resolved to Grade 0-1. Decrease dose by 25% and return to original dosing interval. If after 2 weeks there is no resolution, liposomal doxorubicin should be discontinued.

(Continued)

DOXOrubicin (Liposomal) *(Continued)*

Dosing adjustment in hepatic impairment:

Bilirubin 1.2-3 mg/dL or AST 60-180 units/L: Administer 50% of dose

Bilirubin >3 mg/dL: Administer 25% of dose

See table.

Hematological Toxicity

Grade	ANC	Platelets	Modification
1	1500 - 1900	75,000 - 150,000	Resume treatment with no dose reduction
2	1000 - <1500	50,000 - <75,000	Wait until ANC ≥1500 and platelets ≥75,000; redose with no dose reduction
3	500 - 999	25,000 - <50,000	Wait until ANC ≥1500 and platelets ≥75,000; redose with no dose reduction
4	<500	<25,000	Wait until ANC ≥1500 and platelets ≥75,000; redose at 25% dose reduction or continue full dose with cytokine support

Mechanism of Action Doxil® is doxorubicin hydrochloride encapsulated in long-circulating STEALTH® liposomes. Liposomes are microscopic vesicles composed of a phospholipid bilayer that are capable of encapsulating active drugs. Doxorubicin works through inhibition of topoisomerase-II at the point of DNA cleavage. A second mechanism of action is the production of free radicals (the hydroxy radical OH) by doxorubicin, which in turn can destroy DNA and cancerous cells. Doxorubicin is also a very powerful iron chelator, equal to deferoxamine. The iron-doxorubicin complex can bind DNA and cell membranes rapidly and produce free radicals that immediately cleave the DNA and cell membranes. Inhibits DNA and RNA synthesis by intercalating between DNA base pairs and by steric obstruction; active throughout entire cell cycle.

Other Adverse Effects

>10%: Hematologic: Myelosuppression, leukopenia (60% to 80%), thrombocytopenia (6% to 24%), anemia (6% to 53%)

1% to 10%:

Cardiovascular: Pericardial effusion, cardiomyopathy

Dermatologic: Hyperpigmentation of nail beds; erythematous streaking of vein; alopecia (9%)

Miscellaneous: Infusion-related reactions (bronchospasm, chest tightness, chills, dyspnea, facial edema, flushing, headache, hypotension, pruritus) have occurred (up to 10%)

<1%: Conjunctivitis, fever, serious infusion reactions (anaphylactic or anaphylactoid reactions), urticaria

Drug Interactions Substrate of **CYP2D6, 3A4**; Inhibits CYP2D6, 3A4

Increased Effect/Toxicity: Allopurinol may enhance the antitumor activity of doxorubicin (animal data only). Cyclosporine may induce coma or seizures. Cyclophosphamide enhances the cardiac toxicity of doxorubicin by producing additional myocardial cell damage. Mercaptopurine increases toxicities. Streptozocin greatly enhances leukopenia and thrombocytopenia. Verapamil alters the cellular distribution of doxorubicin and may result in increased cell toxicity by inhibition of the P-glycoprotein pump.

Decreased Effect: Doxorubicin may decrease plasma levels and effectiveness of digoxin and phenytoin. Phenobarbital increases elimination (decreases effect) of doxorubicin. Doxorubicin may decrease the antiviral activity of zidovudine.

Dietary/Ethanol/Herb Considerations

Ethanol: Avoid use due to GI irritation.

Herb/Nutraceutical: Avoid black cohosh and dong quai in estrogen-dependent tumors. Avoid St John's wort; may decrease serum concentration.

Pharmacodynamics/Kinetics

Distribution: V_{dss}: Confined mostly to the vascular fluid volume

Protein binding, plasma: Doxorubicin: 70%

Metabolism: Hepatic and in plasma to both active and inactive metabolites

Excretion: Urine (5% as doxorubicin or doxorubicinol)

Clearance: Mean: 0.041 L/hour/m^2

Pregnancy Risk Factor D

Generic Available No

Doxy-100® *see* Doxycycline *on page 476*

Doxycycline (doks i SYE kleen)

Related Information

Animal and Human Bites Guidelines *on page 1580*

Nonviral Infectious Diseases *on page 1493*

Periodontal Diseases *on page 1540*

Sexually-Transmitted Diseases *on page 1502*

U.S. Brand Names Adoxa™; Doryx®; Doxy-100®; Monodox®; Vibramycin®; Vibra-Tabs®

Canadian Brand Names Apo®-Doxy; Apo®-Doxy Tabs; Doxycin; Doxytec; Novo-Doxylin; Nu-Doxycycline; Vibra-Tabs®

Mexican Brand Names Vibramicina®

Pharmacologic Category Antibiotic, Tetracycline Derivative

Synonyms Doxycycline Calcium; Doxycycline Hyclate; Doxycycline Monohydrate

Use

Dental: Treatment of periodontitis associated with presence of *Actinobacillus actinomycetemcomitans* AA

Medical: Principally in the treatment of infections caused by susceptible *Rickettsia*, *Chlamydia*, and *Mycoplasma*; alternative to mefloquine for malaria prophylaxis; treatment for syphilis, uncomplicated *Neisseria gonorrhoeae*, *Listeria*, *Actinomyces israelii*, and *Clostridium* infections in penicillin-allergic patients; for community-acquired pneumonia and other common infections due to susceptible organisms; anthrax due to *Bacillus anthracis*, including inhalational anthrax (postexposure); treatment of infections caused by uncommon susceptible gram-negative and gram-positive organisms including *Borrelia recurrentis*, *Ureaplasma urealyticum*, *Haemophilus ducreyi*, *Yersinia pestis*, *Francisella tularensis*, *Vibrio cholerae*, *Campylobacter fetus*, *Brucella* spp, *Bartonella bacilliformis*, and *Calymmatobacterium granulomatis*

Unlabeled/Investigational Use Sclerosing agent for pleural effusion injection; treatment of vancomycin-resistant enterococci (VRE)

Local Anesthetic/Vasoconstrictor Precautions No information available to require special precautions

Effects on Dental Treatment Opportunistic "superinfection" with *Candida albicans*; tetracyclines are not recommended for use during pregnancy or in children ≤8 years of age since they have been reported to cause enamel hypoplasia and permanent teeth discoloration. The use of tetracyclines should only be used in these patients if other agents are contraindicated or alternative antimicrobials will not eradicate the organism.

Frequency not defined: Dysphagia, esophagitis (rare), esophageal ulcerations (rare), glossitis, tooth discoloration (children) anaphylaxis, oral candidiasis (long-term use)

Dosage

Children:

Anthrax: Doxycycline should be used in children if antibiotic susceptibility testing, exhaustion of drug supplies, or allergic reaction preclude use of penicillin or ciprofloxacin. For treatment, the consensus recommendation does not include a loading dose for doxycycline.

Inhalational (postexposure prophylaxis) (*MMWR*, 2001, 50:889-893): Oral, I.V. (use oral route when possible):

≤8 years: 2.2 mg/kg every 12 hours for 60 days

>8 years and ≤45 kg: 2.2 mg/kg every 12 hours for 60 days

>8 years and >45 kg: 100 mg every 12 hours for 60 days

Cutaneous (treatment): Oral: See dosing for "Inhalational (postexposure prophylaxis)"

Note: In the presence of systemic involvement, extensive edema, and/or lesions on head/neck, doxycycline should initially be administered I.V.

Inhalational/GI/oropharyngeal (treatment): I.V.: Refer to dosing for inhalational anthrax (postexposure prophylaxis); switch to oral therapy when clinically appropriate; refer to Adults dosing for "Note" on combined therapy and duration

Children ≥8 years (<45 kg): **Susceptible infections:** Oral, I.V.: 2-5 mg/kg/day in 1-2 divided doses, not to exceed 200 mg/day

Children >8 years (>45 kg) and Adults: **Susceptible infections:** Oral, I.V.: 100-200 mg/day in 1-2 divided doses

Acute gonococcal infection (PID) in combination with another antibiotic: 100 mg every 12 hours until improved, followed by 100 mg orally twice daily to complete 14 days

Community-acquired pneumonia: 100 mg twice daily

Lyme disease: Oral: 100 mg twice daily for 14-21 days

Early syphilis: 200 mg/day in divided doses for 14 days

Late syphilis: 200 mg/day in divided doses for 28 days

Uncomplicated chlamydial infections: 100 mg twice daily for ≥7 days

Endometritis, salpingitis, parametritis, or peritonitis: 100 mg I.V. twice daily with cefoxitin 2 g every 6 hours for 4 days and for ≥48 hours after patient improves; then continue with oral therapy 100 mg twice daily to complete a 10- to 14-day course of therapy

Sclerosing agent for pleural effusion injection (unlabeled use): 500 mg as a single dose in 30-50 mL of NS or SWI

(Continued)

Doxycycline *(Continued)*

Adults:

Anthrax:

Inhalational (postexposure prophylaxis): Oral, I.V. (use oral route when possible): 100 mg every 12 hours for 60 days (*MMWR*, 2001, 50:889-93); **Note:** Preliminary recommendation, FDA review and update is anticipated.

Cutaneous (treatment): Oral: 100 mg every 12 hours for 60 days. **Note:** In the presence of systemic involvement, extensive edema, lesions on head/neck, refer to I.V. dosing for treatment of inhalational/GI/oropharyngeal anthrax

Inhalational/GI/oropharyngeal (treatment): I.V.: Initial: 100 mg every 12 hours; switch to oral therapy when clinically appropriate; some recommend initial loading dose of 200 mg, followed by 100 mg every 8-12 hours (*JAMA*, 1997, 278:399-411). **Note:** Initial treatment should include two or more agents predicted to be effective (per CDC recommendations). Agents suggested for use in conjunction with doxycycline or ciprofloxacin include rifampin, vancomycin, imipenem, penicillin, ampicillin, chloramphenicol, clindamycin, and clarithromycin. May switch to oral antimicrobial therapy when clinically appropriate. Continue combined therapy for 60 days

Dialysis: Not dialyzable; 0% to 5% by hemo- and peritoneal methods or by continuous arteriovenous or venovenous hemofiltration: No supplemental dosage necessary

Mechanism of Action Inhibits protein synthesis by binding with the 30S and possibly the 50S ribosomal subunit(s) of susceptible bacteria; may also cause alterations in the cytoplasmic membrane

Doxycycline inhibits collagenase *in vitro* and has been shown to inhibit collagenase in the gingival crevicular fluid in adults with periodontitis

Other Adverse Effects Frequency not defined:

Cardiovascular: Intracranial hypertension, pericarditis

Dermatologic: Angioneurotic edema, exfoliative dermatitis (rare), photosensitivity, rash, urticaria

Endocrine & metabolic: Brown/black discoloration of thyroid gland (no dysfunction reported)

Gastrointestinal: Anorexia, diarrhea, enterocolitis, inflammatory lesions in anogenital region

Hematologic: Eosinophilia, hemolytic anemia, neutropenia, thrombocytopenia

Renal: Increased BUN

Miscellaneous: Anaphylactoid purpura, bulging fontanels (infants), SLE exacerbation

Contraindications Hypersensitivity to doxycycline, tetracycline or any component of the formulation; children <8 years of age, except in treatment of anthrax (including inhalational anthrax postexposure prophylaxis); severe hepatic dysfunction; pregnancy

Warnings/Precautions Do not use during pregnancy; use of tetracyclines during tooth development may cause permanent discoloration of the teeth and enamel hypoplasia. Prolonged use may result in superinfection, including oral or vaginal candidiasis. Photosensitivity reaction may occur with this drug; avoid prolonged exposure to sunlight or tanning equipment. Avoid in children ≤8 years of age.

Drug Interactions Substrate of **CYP3A4**; Inhibits CYP3A4

Antacids (containing aluminum, calcium, or magnesium): Decreased absorption of tetracyclines

Anticoagulants: Tetracyclines may decrease plasma thrombin activity; monitor

Barbiturates: Decreased half-life of doxycycline

Bismuth subsalicylate: Decreased absorption of tetracyclines

Carbamazepine: Decreased half-life of doxycycline

Iron-containing products: Decreased absorption of tetracyclines

Methoxyflurane: Concomitant use may cause fatal renal toxicity.

Oral contraceptives: Anecdotal reports suggesting decreased contraceptive efficacy with tetracyclines have been refuted by more rigorous scientific and clinical data.

Phenytoin: Decreased half-life of doxycycline

Dietary/Ethanol/Herb Considerations

Ethanol: Avoid or limit use (<3 drinks/day); chronic ingestion may decrease serum concentration.

Food: Administer with food or milk due to GI intolerance; may decrease absorption up to 20%. Of currently available tetracyclines, doxycycline has the least affinity for calcium; may decrease absorption of amino acids, calcium, iron, magnesium, and zinc. Administration with calcium or iron may decrease doxycycline absorption. Boiled milk, buttermilk, or yogurt may reduce diarrhea.

Herb/Nutraceutical: Avoid dong quai; may cause additional photosensitization. Avoid St John's wort; may decrease serum concentration and cause additional photosensitization.

Pharmacodynamics/Kinetics

Absorption: Oral: Almost complete; reduced by food or milk by 20%

Distribution: Widely into body tissues and fluids including synovial, pleural, prostatic, seminal fluids, and bronchial secretions; saliva, aqueous humor, and CSF penetration is poor; readily crosses placenta; enters breast milk

Protein binding: 90%

Metabolism: Not hepatic; partially inactivated in GI tract by chelate formation

Half-life elimination: 12-15 hours (usually increases to 22-24 hours with multiple doses); End-stage renal disease: 18-25 hours

Time to peak, serum: 1.5-4 hours

Excretion: Feces (30%); urine (23%)

Pregnancy Risk Factor D

Dosage Forms CAP, as hyclate (Vibramycin®): 50 mg, 100 mg. **CAP, as monohydrate** (Monodox®): 50 mg, 100 mg. **CAP, coated pellets, as hyclate** (Doryx®): 100 mg. **INJ, powder for reconstitution, as hyclate** (Doxy-100®): 100 mg. **POWDER, oral suspension, as monohydrate** (Vibramycin®): 25 mg/5 mL (60 mL). **SYR, as calcium** (Vibramycin®): 50 mg/5 mL (480 mL). **TAB, as hyclate** (Vibra-Tabs®): 100 mg. **TAB, as monohydrate** (Adoxa™): 50 mg, 100 mg

Generic Available Yes

Doxycycline Calcium *see* Doxycycline *on page 476*

Doxycycline Hyclate *see* Doxycycline *on page 476*

Doxycycline Hyclate Periodontal Extended-Release Liquid

(doks i SYE kleen HI klayt pair ee oh DON tol eks TEN did ri LEES LI kwid)

Related Information

Doxycycline *on page 476*

U.S. Brand Names Atridox™

Pharmacologic Category Antibiotic, Tetracycline Derivative

Use Dental: Treatment of chronic adult periodontitis for gain in clinical attachment, reduction in probing depth, and reduction in bleeding on probing

Local Anesthetic/Vasoconstrictor Precautions No information available to require special precautions

Effects on Dental Treatment Mechanical oral hygiene procedures (ie, toothbrushing, flossing) should be avoided in any treated area for 7 days.

Effects reported in clinical trials were similar in incidence between doxycycline-containing product and vehicle alone; comparable to standard therapies including scaling and root planing or oral hygiene. Although there is no known relationship between doxycycline and hypertension, unspecified essential hypertension was noted in 1.6% of the doxycycline gel group, as compared to 0.2% in the vehicle group (allergic reactions to the vehicle were also reported in two patients).

Local/Oral:

- >10%: Discoloration of teeth (in children), gum discomfort (18%), toothache (14%)
- 1% to 10%: Periodontal abscess (10%), tooth sensitivity (8%), broken tooth (5%), tooth mobility (2%), endodontic abscess (2%), jaw pain (1%)

Systemic:

- >10%: Headache (27%)
- 1% to 10%: Muscle aches (7%), nausea (2%), GI upset (4%)

Dosage Subgingival: Dose depends on size, shape and number of pockets treated. Application may be repeated four months after initial treatment. The delivery system consists of 2 separate syringes in a single pouch. Syringe A contains 450 mg of a bioabsorbable polymer gel; syringe B contains doxycycline hyclate 50 mg. To prepare for instillation, couple syringe A to syringe B. Inject contents of syringe A (purple stripe) into syringe B, then push contents back into syringe A. Repeat this mixing cycle at a rate of one cycle per second for 100 cycles. If syringes are stored prior to use (a maximum of 3 days), repeat mixing cycle 10 times before use. After appropriate mixing, contents should be in syringe A. Holding syringes vertically, with syringe A at the bottom, pull back on the syringe A plunger, allowing contents to flow down barrel for several seconds. Uncouple syringes and attach enclosed blunt cannula to syringe A. Local anesthesia is not required for placement. Cannula tip may be bent to resemble periodontal probe and used to explore pocket. Express product from syringe until pocket is filled. To separate tip from formulation, turn tip towards the tooth and press against tooth surface to achieve separation. An appropriate dental instrument may be used to pack gel into the pocket. Pockets may be covered with either Coe-pak™ or Octyldent™ dental adhesive.

Mechanism of Action Inhibits protein synthesis by binding with the 30S and possibly the 50S ribosomal subunit(s) of susceptible bacteria; may also cause alterations in the cytoplasmic membrane

Doxycycline inhibits collagenase *in vitro* and has been shown to inhibit collagenase in the gingival crevicular fluid in adults with periodontitis

Other Adverse Effects Systemic: Gastrointestinal: Diarrhea (3%)

Contraindications Hypersensitivity to doxycycline, tetracycline or any component of the formulation; children <8 years of age; severe hepatic dysfunction; pregnancy

(Continued)

Doxycycline Hyclate Periodontal Extended-Release Liquid *(Continued)*

Warnings/Precautions Do not use during pregnancy; use of tetracyclines during tooth development may cause permanent discoloration of the teeth and enamel hypoplasia. Prolonged use may result in superinfection, including oral or vaginal candidiasis. Photosensitivity may occur; avoid prolonged exposure to sunlight or tanning equipment. Atridox™ has not been evaluated or tested in immunocompromised patients, those with oral candidiasis, or conditions characterized by severe periodontal defects with little remaining periodontium. May result in overgrowth of nonsusceptible organisms, including fungi. Effects of treatment >6 months have not been evaluated; has not been evaluated for use in regeneration of alveolar bone.

Pharmacodynamics/Kinetics Systemic absorption from dental subgingival gel may occur, but is limited by the slow rate of dissolution from this formulation over 7 days.

Pregnancy Risk Factor D

Dosage Forms GEL, subgingival (Atridox™): 50 mg in each 500 mg of blended formulation [doxycycline syringe (50 mg)]

Generic Available No

Doxycycline Monohydrate *see* Doxycycline *on page 476*

Doxycycline Subantimicrobial

(doks i SYE kleen sub an tee mye CROE bee ul)

Related Information

Doxycycline *on page 476*

U.S. Brand Names Periostat®

Pharmacologic Category Antibiotic, Tetracycline Derivative

Use Dental: Adjunct to scaling and root planing to promote attachment level gain and to reduce pocket depth in adult periodontitis (systemic levels are subinhibitory against bacteria)

Local Anesthetic/Vasoconstrictor Precautions No information available to require special precautions

Effects on Dental Treatment No significant effects or complications reported

Dosage Adults: **Adjunctive treatment for periodontitis:** Oral: 20 mg twice daily at least 1 hour before or 2 hours after morning and evening meals for up to 9 months

Mechanism of Action Has been shown to inhibit collagenase activity *in vitro*; has been noted to reduce elevated collagenase activity in the gingival crevicular fluid of patients with periodontal disease; systemic levels do not reach inhibitory concentrations against bacteria.

Contraindications Hypersensitivity to doxycycline, tetracycline or any component of the formulation; children <8 years of age; pregnancy

Warnings/Precautions Do not use during pregnancy; use of tetracyclines during tooth development may cause permanent discoloration of the teeth and enamel hypoplasia. Prolonged use may result in superinfection, including oral or vaginal candidiasis. Photosensitivity may occur; avoid prolonged exposure to sunlight or tanning equipment. Effectiveness has not been established in patients with coexisting oral candidiasis; use with caution in patients with a history or predisposition to oral candidiasis.

Dosage Forms TAB (Periostat®): 20 mg

Generic Available No

DPA *see* Valproic Acid and Derivatives *on page 1371*

DPE *see* Dipivefrin *on page 455*

D-Penicillamine *see* Penicillamine *on page 1046*

DPH *see* Phenytoin *on page 1073*

DPPC *see* Colfosceril Palmitate *on page 366*

Dramamine® [OTC] *see* DimenhyDRINATE *on page 449*

Dramamine® Less Drowsy Formula [OTC] *see* Meclizine *on page 847*

Drisdol® *see* Ergocalciferol *on page 508*

Dristan® Sinus [OTC] *see* Pseudoephedrine and Ibuprofen *on page 1148*

Drithocreme® *see* Anthralin *on page 111*

Drithocreme® HP 1% *see* Anthralin *on page 111*

Dritho-Scalp® *see* Anthralin *on page 111*

Drixomed® *see* Dexbrompheniramine and Pseudoephedrine *on page 415*

Drixoral® Cold & Allergy [OTC] *see* Dexbrompheniramine and Pseudoephedrine *on page 415*

Dronabinol (droe NAB i nol)

Related Information

Chemical Dependency and Smoking Cessation *on page 1574*

U.S. Brand Names Marinol®

Canadian Brand Names Marinol®

Pharmacologic Category Antiemetic; Appetite Stimulant

Synonyms Delta-9-tetrahydro-cannabinol; Delta-9 THC; Tetrahydrocannabinol; THC

Use Treatment of chemotherapy-associated nausea and vomiting refractory to other antiemetic; AIDS- and cancer-related anorexia

Local Anesthetic/Vasoconstrictor Precautions No information available to require special precautions

Effects on Dental Treatment

>10%: Xerostomia (38% to 50%), drowsiness (48%), sedation (53%), confusion (30%), dizziness (21%), anxiety,

1% to 10%: Orthostatic hypotension, tachycardia, headache, hallucinations (5%), memory lapse (4%), paresthesia, weakness

Restrictions C-III

Dosage Refer to individual protocols. Oral:

Antiemetic:

Children: 5 mg/m^2 starting 6-8 hours before chemotherapy and every 4-6 hours after to be continued for 12 hours after chemotherapy is discontinued

Adults: 5 mg/m^2 1-3 hours before chemotherapy, then 5 mg/m^2/dose every 2-4 hours after chemotherapy for a total of 4-6 doses/day; increase doses in increments of 2.5 mg/m^2 to a maximum of 15 mg/m^2/dose.

Appetite stimulant: Initial: 2.5 mg twice daily (before lunch and dinner); titrate up to a maximum of 20 mg/day.

Mechanism of Action Unknown, may inhibit endorphins in the emetic center, suppress prostaglandin synthesis, and/or inhibit medullary activity through an unspecified cortical action

Other Adverse Effects

>10%:

Central nervous system: Detachment, difficulty concentrating, mood change

Gastrointestinal: Increased appetite (when used as antiemetic)

1% to 10%:

Central nervous system: Ataxia (4%), depression (7%), vertigo

<1%: **Syncope,** nightmares, diarrhea, myalgia, tinnitus, **diaphoresis**

Drug Interactions CYP2C18 and 3A3/4 enzyme substrate

Increased Effect/Toxicity: Increased toxicity (drowsiness) with alcohol, barbiturates, and benzodiazepines.

Dietary/Ethanol/Herb Considerations

Ethanol: Avoid use; may increase CNS depression.

Food: Administration with high-lipid meals may increase absorption.

Herb/Nutraceutical: Avoid gotu kola, kava, SAMe, and valerian; may increase CNS depression. Avoid St John's wort; may decrease serum concentration.

Pharmacodynamics/Kinetics

Onset of action: Within 1 hour

Absorption: Oral: 90% to 95%; ~5% to 10% of dose gets into systemic circulation

Distribution: V_d: 2.5-6.4 L; tetrahydrocannabinol is highly lipophilic and distributes to adipose tissue

Protein binding: 97% to 99%

Metabolism: Hepatic to at least 50 metabolites, some of which are active; 11-hydroxytetrahydrocannabinol (11-OH-THC) is the major metabolite; extensive first-pass effect

Half-life elimination: THC: 19-24 hours; THC metabolites: 49-53 hours

Time to peak, serum: 2-3 hours

Excretion: Feces (35% as unconjugated metabolites); urine (10% to 15% as acid metabolites and conjugates)

Pregnancy Risk Factor C

Generic Available No

Droperidol (droe PER i dole)

U.S. Brand Names Inapsine®

Mexican Brand Names Dehydrobenzperidol®

Pharmacologic Category Antiemetic; Antipsychotic Agent, Butyrophenone

Use Antiemetic in surgical and diagnostic procedures; preoperative medication in patients when other treatments are ineffective or inappropriate

Local Anesthetic/Vasoconstrictor Precautions Manufacturer's information states that droperidol may block vasopressor activity of epinephrine. This has not been observed during use of epinephrine as a vasoconstrictor in local anesthesia.

Effects on Dental Treatment See Warnings/Precautions

>10%: Restlessness, anxiety, extrapyramidal symptoms, dystonic reactions, pseudoparkinsonian signs and symptoms, tardive dyskinesia, seizures, altered central temperature regulation, akathisia

1% to 10%: Hypotension (especially orthostatic), tachycardia, hallucinations, sedation, drowsiness, persistent tardive dyskinesia, nausea, vomiting

Dosage Titrate carefully to desired effect

Children 2-12 years: Nausea and vomiting: I.M., I.V.: 0.05-0.06 mg/kg (maximum initial dose: 0.1 mg/kg); additional doses may be repeated to achieve effect; administer additional doses with caution

(Continued)

Droperidol *(Continued)*

Adults: Nausea and vomiting: I.M., I.V.: Initial: 2.5 mg; additional doses of 1.25 mg may be administered to achieve desired effect; administer additional doses with caution

Mechanism of Action Antiemetic effect is a result of blockade of dopamine stimulation of the chemoreceptor trigger zone. Other effects include alpha-adrenergic blockade, peripheral vascular dilation, and reduction of the pressor effect of epinephrine resulting in hypotension and decreased peripheral vascular resistance; may also reduce pulmonary artery pressure

Other Adverse Effects EKG changes, retinal pigmentation are more common than with chlorpromazine. Relative to other neuroleptics, droperidol has a low potency of cholinergic blockade.

>10%:

Cardiovascular: QT_c prolongation (dose dependent)
Endocrine & metabolic: Swelling of breasts
Gastrointestinal: Weight gain, constipation

1% to 10%:

Cardiovascular: Abnormal T waves with prolonged ventricular repolarization
Genitourinary: Dysuria

<1%: Adynamic ileus, agranulocytosis, alopecia, amenorrhea, arrhythmia, **blurred vision,** cholestatic jaundice, **contact dermatitis,** galactorrhea, gynecomastia, heat stroke, hyperpigmentation, laryngospasm, leukopenia (usually with large doses for prolonged periods), neuroleptic malignant syndrome (NMS), obstructive jaundice, overflow incontinence, photosensitivity (rare), priapism, pruritus, rash, **respiratory depression,** retinal pigmentation, sexual dysfunction, tardive dystonia, torsade de pointes, urinary retention, ventricular tachycardia, visual acuity decreased (may be irreversible), **xerostomia**

Warnings/Precautions May alter cardiac conduction. Cases of QT prolongation and torsade de pointes, including some fatal cases, have been reported. Use extreme caution in patients with bradycardia (<50 bpm), cardiac disease, concurrent MAOI therapy, Class I and Class III antiarrhythmics or other drugs known to prolong QT interval, and electrolyte disturbances (hypokalemia or hypomagnesemia), including concomitant drugs which may alter electrolytes (diuretics).

Use with caution in patients with seizures, bone marrow suppression, or severe liver disease. May be sedating, use with caution in disorders where CNS depression is a feature. Caution in patients with hemodynamic instability, predisposition to seizures, subcortical brain damage, renal or respiratory disease. Esophageal dysmotility and aspiration have been associated with antipsychotic use - use with caution in patients at risk of pneumonia (ie, Alzheimer's disease). Caution in breast cancer or other prolactin-dependent tumors (may elevate prolactin levels). May alter temperature regulation or mask toxicity of other drugs due to antiemetic effects. May cause orthostatic hypotension - use with caution in patients at risk of this effect or those who would tolerate transient hypotensive episodes (cerebrovascular disease, cardiovascular disease, or other medications which may predispose). Significant hypotension may occur; injection contains benzyl alcohol; injection also contains sulfites which may cause allergic reaction.

May cause anticholinergic effects (confusion, agitation, constipation, xerostomia, blurred vision, urinary retention). Therefore, they should be used with caution in patients with decreased GI motility, urinary retention, BPH, xerostomia, or visual problems. Conditions which also may be exacerbated by cholinergic blockade include narrow-angle glaucoma (screening is recommended) and worsening of myasthenia gravis. Relative to other neuroleptics, droperidol has a low potency of cholinergic blockade.

May cause extrapyramidal symptoms, including pseudoparkinsonism, acute dystonic reactions, akathisia, and tardive dyskinesia (risk of these reactions is high relative to other neuroleptics). May be associated with neuroleptic malignant syndrome (NMS) or pigmentary retinopathy. Safety in children <6 months of age has not been established.

Drug Interactions Increased Effect/Toxicity: Droperidol in combination with certain forms of conduction anesthesia may produce peripheral vasodilitation and hypotension. Droperidol and CNS depressants will likely have additive CNS effects. Droperidol and cyclobenzaprine may have an additive effect on prolonging the QT interval. Use caution with other agents known to prolong QT interval (Class I or Class III antiarrhythmics, some quinolone antibiotics, cisapride, some phenothiazines, pimozide, tricyclic antidepressants). Potassium- or magnesium-depleting agents (diuretics, aminoglycosides, amphotericin B, cyclosporine) may increase risk of arrhythmias. Metoclopramide may increase risk of extrapyramidal symptoms (EPS).

Dietary/Ethanol/Herb Considerations Avoid ethanol; increases sedative effect.

Pharmacodynamics/Kinetics

Onset of action: Peak effect: Parenteral: ~30 minutes
Duration: Parenteral: 2-4 hours, may extend to 12 hours
Absorption: I.M.: Rapid

Distribution: Crosses blood-brain barrier and placenta
V_d: Children: ~0.25-0.9 L/kg; Adults: ~2 L/kg
Protein binding: Extensive
Metabolism: Hepatic, to *p*-fluorophenylacetic acid, benzimidazolone, *p*-hydroxypiperidine
Half-life elimination: Adults: 2.3 hours
Excretion: Urine (75%, <1% as unchanged drug); feces (22%, 11% to 50% as unchanged drug)

Pregnancy Risk Factor C

Generic Available Yes

Drotrecogin Alfa (dro TRE coe jin AL fu)

U.S. Brand Names Xigris®

Pharmacologic Category Protein C (Activated)

Synonyms Activated Protein C, Human, Recombinant; Drotrecogin Alfa, Activated; Protein C (Activated), Human, Recombinant

Use Reduction of mortality from severe sepsis (associated with organ dysfunction) in adults at high risk of death (eg, APACHE II score ≥25)

Local Anesthetic/Vasoconstrictor Precautions No information available to require special precautions

Effects on Dental Treatment As with all drugs which may affect hemostasis, bleeding is the major adverse effect associated with drotrecogin alfa. Hemorrhage may occur at virtually any site; risk is dependent on multiple variables, including the dosage administered, concurrent use of multiple agents which alter hemostasis, and patient predisposition.

>10%: Bruising, GI bleeding

Dosage I.V.:

Adults: 24 mcg/kg/hour for a total of 96 hours; stop infusion **immediately** if clinically-important bleeding is identified

Dosing adjustment in renal impairment: No specific recommendations

Mechanism of Action Inhibits factors Va and VIIIa, limiting thrombotic effects. Additional *in vitro* data suggest inhibition of plasminogen activator inhibitor-1 (PAF-1) resulting in profibrinolytic activity, inhibition of macrophage production of tumor necrosis factor, blocking of leukocyte adhesion, and limitation of thrombin-induced inflammatory responses. Relative contribution of effects on the reduction of mortality from sepsis is not completely understood.

Other Adverse Effects

1% to 10%: Hematologic: Bleeding (serious 2.4% during infusion vs 3.5% during 28-day study period; individual events listed as <1%)

<1%: **Gastrointestinal hemorrhage,** intrathoracic hemorrhage, retroperitoneal bleeding, genitourinary bleeding, intracranial hemorrhage (0.2%; frequencies up to 2% noted in a previous trial without placebo control), **skin/soft tissue bleeding**, immune reaction (antibody production)

Drug Interactions Increased Effect/Toxicity: Concurrent use of antiplatelet agents, including aspirin (>650 mg/day, recent use within 7 days), cilostazol, clopidogrel, dipyridamole, ticlopidine, NSAIDs, or glycoprotein IIb/IIIa antagonists (recent use within 7 days) may increase risk of bleeding. Concurrent use of low molecular weight heparins or heparin at therapeutic rates of infusion may increase the risk of bleeding. However, the use of low-dose prophylactic heparin does not appear to affect safety. Recent use of thrombolytic agents (within 3 days) may increase the risk of bleeding. Recent use of warfarin (within 7 days or elevation of INR ≥3) may increase the risk of bleeding. Other drugs which interfere with coagulation may increase risk of bleeding (including antithrombin III, danaparoid, direct thrombin inhibitors)

Dietary/Ethanol/Herb Considerations

Food: Avoid garlic, ginger, and green tea.

Herb/Nutraceutical: Recent use/intake of herbs with anticoagulant activity may increase the risk of bleeding. Avoid cat's claw, dong quai, evening primrose, feverfew, garlic, ginger, ginkgo biloba, ginseng, green tea, horse chestnut, and red clover due to additional antiplatelet activity.

Pharmacodynamics/Kinetics

Duration: Plasma nondetectable within 2 hours of discontinuation
Metabolism: Inactivated by endogenous plasma protease inhibitors; mean clearance: 40 L/hour; increased with severe sepsis (~50%)
Half-life elimination: 1.6 hours

Pregnancy Risk Factor C

Generic Available No

Drotrecogin Alfa, Activated *see* Drotrecogin Alfa *on page 483*

Droxia™ *see* Hydroxyurea *on page 696*

Dr. Scholl's® Callus Remover [OTC] *see* Salicylic Acid *on page 1204*

Dr. Scholl's® Clear Away [OTC] *see* Salicylic Acid *on page 1204*

DSCG *see* Cromolyn Sodium *on page 375*

D-S-S® [OTC] *see* Docusate *on page 463*

DSS With Casanthranol *see* Docusate and Casanthranol *on page 464*
DTIC *see* Dacarbazine *on page 391*
DTIC-Dome® *see* Dacarbazine *on page 391*
DTO *see* Opium Tincture *on page 1002*
Duac™ *see* Clindamycin and Benzoyl Peroxide *on page 343*
Dulcolax® [OTC] *see* Bisacodyl *on page 186*
Dull-C® [OTC] *see* Ascorbic Acid *on page 128*
DuoFilm® [OTC] *see* Salicylic Acid *on page 1204*
DuoNeb™ *see* Ipratropium and Albuterol *on page 738*
DuoPlant® [DSC] [OTC] *see* Salicylic Acid *on page 1204*
DuP 753 *see* Losartan *on page 825*
Duplex® T [OTC] *see* Coal Tar *on page 359*
Duraclon™ *see* Clonidine *on page 351*
Duragesic® *see* Fentanyl *on page 565*
Duramist® Plus [OTC] *see* Oxymetazoline *on page 1022*
Duramorph® *see* Morphine Sulfate *on page 931*
Duranest® [DSC] *see* Etidocaine and Epinephrine *on page 545*
Duration® [OTC] *see* Oxymetazoline *on page 1022*
Duratuss™ *see* Guaifenesin and Pseudoephedrine *on page 652*
Duratuss® DM *see* Guaifenesin and Dextromethorphan *on page 651*
Duratuss-G® *see* Guaifenesin *on page 650*
Duratuss™ GP *see* Guaifenesin and Pseudoephedrine *on page 652*
Duratuss® HD *see* Hydrocodone, Pseudoephedrine, and Guaifenesin *on page 687*
Dura-Vent®/DA *see* Chlorpheniramine, Phenylephrine, and Methscopolamine *on page 310*
Duricef® *see* Cefadroxil *on page 261*

Dutasteride (doo TAS teer ide)

U.S. Brand Names Avodart™

Pharmacologic Category 5 Alpha-Reductase Inhibitor

Use Treatment of symptomatic benign prostatic hyperplasia (BPH)

Unlabeled/Investigational Use Treatment of male patterned baldness

Local Anesthetic/Vasoconstrictor Precautions No information available to require special precautions

Effects on Dental Treatment No significant effects or complications reported

Dosage Oral: Adults: Male: 0.5 mg once daily

Mechanism of Action Dutasteride is a 4-azo analog of testosterone and is a competitive, selective inhibitor of both reproductive tissues (type 2) and skin and hepatic (type 1) 5α-reductase. This results in inhibition of the conversion of testosterone to dihydrotestosterone and markedly suppresses serum dihydrotestosterone levels.

Other Adverse Effects Frequency of adverse events (except gynecomastia) tends to decrease with continued use (>6 months).

>10%: Endocrine & metabolic: Serum testosterone increased, thyroid-stimulating hormone increased

1% to 10%: Endocrine & metabolic: Impotence (5%), libido decreased (3%), ejaculation disorders (2%), gynecomastia (including breast tenderness, breast enlargement) (1% to 2%)

Drug Interactions Substrate of CYP3A4

Increased Effect/Toxicity: Diltiazem and verapamil and other CYP3A4 inhibitors increase dutasteride levels because of CYP3A4 inhibition.

Dietary/Ethanol/Herb Considerations

Food: May be taken with food; maximum serum concentration reduced by 10% to 15% (not clinically significant).

Herb/Nutraceutical: Avoid St John's wort; may decrease serum concentration. Avoid saw palmetto; concurrent use has not been adequately studied.

Pharmacodynamics/Kinetics

Absorption: Via skin when handling capsules

Distribution: ~12% of serum concentrations partitioned into semen

Protein binding: 99% to albumin; ~97% to α_1-acid glycoprotein; >96% to semen protein

Metabolism: Hepatic via CYP3A4 isoenzyme; forms metabolites: 6-hydroxydutasteride has activity similar to parent compound, 4′-hydroxydutasteride and 1,2-dihydrodutasteride are much less potent than parent *in vitro*

Bioavailability: 60% (range: 40% to 94%)

Half-life elimination: Terminal: ~5 weeks

Time to peak: 2-3 hours

Excretion: Feces (40% as metabolites, 5% as unchanged drug); urine (<1% as unchanged drug); 55% of dose unaccounted for

Pregnancy Risk Factor X

Generic Available No

Dyazide® *see* Hydrochlorothiazide and Triamterene *on page 677*
Dymelor® [DSC] *see* AcetoHEXAMIDE *on page 38*
Dynabac® *see* Dirithromycin *on page 457*
Dynacin® *see* Minocycline *on page 915*
DynaCirc® *see* Isradipine *on page 754*
DynaCirc® CR *see* Isradipine *on page 754*
Dyna-Hex® [OTC] *see* Chlorhexidine Gluconate *on page 300*

Dyphylline (DYE fi lin)

U.S. Brand Names Dilor®; Lufyllin®

Canadian Brand Names Dilor®; Lufyllin®

Pharmacologic Category Theophylline Derivative

Synonyms Dihydroxypropyl Theophylline

Use Bronchodilator in reversible airway obstruction due to asthma or COPD

Local Anesthetic/Vasoconstrictor Precautions No information available to require special precautions

Effects on Dental Treatment Do not prescribe any erythromycin product to patients taking theophylline products. Erythromycin will delay the normal metabolic inactivation of theophyllines leading to increased blood levels; this has resulted in nausea, vomiting and CNS restlessness.

1% to 10%: Tachycardia, nervousness, restlessness, nausea, vomiting

Dosage

Children: I.M.: 4.4-6.6 mg/kg/day in divided doses

Adults:

Oral: Up to 15 mg/kg 4 times/day, individualize dosage

I.M.: 250-500 mg, do not exceed total dosage of 15 mg/kg every 6 hours

Dosing adjustment in renal impairment:

Cl_{cr} 50-80 mL/minute: Administer 75% of normal dose

Cl_{cr} 10-50 mL/minute: Administer 50% of normal dose

Cl_{cr} <10 mL/minute: Administer 25% of normal dose

Drug Interactions

Increased Effect/Toxicity: Dyphylline may have synergistic toxicity with sympathomimetics. Cimetidine, ranitidine, allopurinol, beta-blockers (nonspecific), erythromycin, influenza virus vaccine, corticosteroids, ephedrine, quinolones, thyroid hormones, oral contraceptives, amiodarone, troleandomycin, clindamycin, carbamazepine, isoniazid, loop diuretics, and lincomycin may increase dyphylline concentrations. Tetracyclines may enhance dyphylline toxicity.

Decreased Effect: Cigarette and marijuana smoking, rifampin, barbiturates, hydantoins, ketoconazole, sulfinpyrazone, sympathomimetics, isoniazid, loop diuretics, carbamazepine, and aminoglutethimide may decrease dyphylline concentrations. Dyphylline may antagonize benzodiazepine's sedative action and may decrease the effects of phenytoin, lithium, and neuromuscular blocking agents. Cigarette smoking may require an increase of dosage by 50% to 100%.

Dietary/Ethanol/Herb Considerations Food: Charcoal-broiled foods may increase elimination, reducing half-life by 50%.

Pregnancy Risk Factor C

Generic Available No

Comments This drug is rarely used today. Requires a special laboratory measuring procedure rather than the standard theophylline assay. Saliva levels are approximately equal to 60% of plasma levels.

Dyrenium® *see* Triamterene *on page 1344*
E_2C and MPA *see* Estradiol and Medroxyprogesterone *on page 523*
7E3 *see* Abciximab *on page 23*
E2020 *see* Donepezil *on page 467*
EarSol® HC *see* Hydrocortisone *on page 688*
Easprin® *see* Aspirin *on page 131*

Echothiophate Iodide (ek oh THYE oh fate EYE oh dide)

U.S. Brand Names Phospholine Iodide®

Pharmacologic Category Ophthalmic Agent, Antiglaucoma; Ophthalmic Agent, Miotic

Synonyms Ecostigmine Iodide

Use Used as miotic in treatment of open-angle glaucoma; may be useful in specific case of narrow-angle glaucoma; accommodative esotropia

Local Anesthetic/Vasoconstrictor Precautions No information available to require special precautions

Effects on Dental Treatment No significant effects or complications reported

Dosage Adults:

Ophthalmic: Glaucoma: Instill 1 drop twice daily into eyes with 1 dose just prior to bedtime; some patients have been treated with 1 dose daily or every other day

(Continued)

Echothiophate Iodide *(Continued)*

Accommodative esotropia:

Diagnosis: Instill 1 drop of 0.125% once daily into both eyes at bedtime for 2-3 weeks

Treatment: Use lowest concentration and frequency which gives satisfactory response, with a maximum dose of 0.125% once daily, although more intensive therapy may be used for short periods of time

Mechanism of Action Produces miosis and changes in accommodation by inhibiting cholinesterase, thereby preventing the breakdown of acetylcholine; acetylcholine is, therefore, allowed to continuously stimulate the iris and ciliary muscles of the eye

Other Adverse Effects

1% to 10%: Ocular: Stinging, burning eyes, myopia, visual blurring

<1%: **Bradycardia, hypotension, flushing, nausea, vomiting,** diarrhea, **muscle weakness,** retinal detachment, **diaphoresis,** browache, miosis, twitching eyelids, watering eyes, **dyspnea**

Pharmacodynamics/Kinetics

Onset of action: Miosis: 10-30 minutes; Intraocular pressure decrease: 4-8 hours

Peak effect: Intraocular pressure decrease: 24 hours

Duration: 1-4 weeks

Pregnancy Risk Factor C

Generic Available No

EC-Naprosyn® *see* Naproxen *on page 953*

E. coli **Asparaginase** *see* Asparaginase *on page 129*

Econazole (e KONE a zole)

U.S. Brand Names Spectazole®

Canadian Brand Names Ecostatin®; Spectazole™

Mexican Brand Names Micostyl®; Pevaryl Lipogel®

Pharmacologic Category Antifungal Agent, Topical

Synonyms Econazole Nitrate

Use Topical treatment of tinea pedis (athlete's foot), tinea cruris (jock itch), tinea corporis (ringworm), tinea versicolor, and cutaneous candidiasis

Local Anesthetic/Vasoconstrictor Precautions No information available to require special precautions

Effects on Dental Treatment No significant effects or complications reported

Dosage Children and Adults: Topical:

Tinea pedis, tinea cruris, tinea corporis, tinea versicolor: Apply sufficient amount to cover affected areas once daily

Cutaneous candidiasis: Apply sufficient quantity twice daily (morning and evening)

Duration of treatment: Candidal infections and tinea cruris, versicolor, and corporis should be treated for 2 weeks and tinea pedis for 1 month; occasionally, longer treatment periods may be required

Mechanism of Action Alters fungal cell wall membrane permeability; may interfere with RNA and protein synthesis, and lipid metabolism

Other Adverse Effects

1% to 10%: Genitourinary: Vulvar/vaginal burning

<1% (Limited to important or life-threatening): Vulvar itching, soreness, edema, or discharge; polyuria; burning or itching of penis of sexual partner

Drug Interactions Inhibits CYP2E1

Pharmacodynamics/Kinetics

Absorption: <10%

Metabolism: Hepatic to more than 20 metabolites

Excretion: Urine; feces (<1%)

Pregnancy Risk Factor C

Generic Available Yes

Econazole Nitrate *see* Econazole *on page 486*

Econopred® *see* PrednisoLONE *on page 1110*

Econopred® Plus *see* PrednisoLONE *on page 1110*

Ecostigmine Iodide *see* Echothiophate Iodide *on page 485*

Ecotrin® [OTC] *see* Aspirin *on page 131*

Ecotrin® Low Adult Strength [OTC] *see* Aspirin *on page 131*

Ecotrin® Maximum Strength [OTC] *see* Aspirin *on page 131*

Ed A-Hist® *see* Chlorpheniramine and Phenylephrine *on page 308*

Edathamil Disodium *see* Edetate Disodium *on page 488*

Edecrin® [DSC] *see* Ethacrynic Acid *on page 538*

Edetate Calcium Disodium (ED e tate KAL see um dye SOW dee um)

U.S. Brand Names Calcium Disodium Versenate®

Pharmacologic Category Chelating Agent

Synonyms Calcium Disodium Edetate; Calcium EDTA

Use Treatment of symptomatic acute and chronic lead poisoning or for symptomatic patients with high blood lead levels; used as an aid in the diagnosis of lead poisoning; possibly useful in poisoning by zinc, manganese, and certain heavy radioisotopes

Local Anesthetic/Vasoconstrictor Precautions No information available to require special precautions

Effects on Dental Treatment Frequency not defined: Arrhythmias, hypotension, fever, headache, GI upset, nausea, vomiting, numbness, tremor, paresthesia, nasal congestion, sneezing

Dosage Several regimens have been recommended:

Diagnosis of lead poisoning: Mobilization test (not recommended by AAP guidelines): I.M., I.V.:

Children: 500 mg/m^2/dose (maximum dose: 1 g) as a single dose or divided into 2 doses

Adults: 500 mg/m^2/dose

Note: Urine is collected for 24 hours after first EDTA dose and analyzed for lead content; if the ratio of mcg of lead in urine to mg calcium EDTA given is >1, then test is considered positive; for convenience, an 8-hour urine collection may be done after a single 50 mg/kg I.M. (maximum dose: 1 g) or 500 mg/m^2 I.V. dose; a positive test occurs if the ratio of lead excretion to mg calcium EDTA >0.5-0.6.

Treatment of lead poisoning: Children and Adults (each regimen is specific for route):

Symptoms of lead encephalopathy and/or blood lead level >70 mcg/dL: Treat 5 days; give in conjunction with dimercaprol; wait a minimum of 2 days with no treatment before considering a repeat course:

I.M.: 250 mg/m^2/dose every 4 hours

I.V.: 50 mg/kg/day as 24-hour continuous I.V. infusion **or** 1-1.5 g/m^2 I.V. as either an 8- to 24-hour infusion or divided into 2 doses every 12 hours

Symptomatic lead poisoning **without** encephalopathy **or** asymptomatic with blood lead level >70 mcg/dL: Treat 3-5 days; treatment with dimercaprol is recommended until the blood lead level concentration <50 mcg/dL:

I.M.: 167 mg/m^2 every 4 hours

I.V.: 1 g/m^2 as an 8- to 24-hour infusion or divided every 12 hours

Asymptomatic **children** with blood lead level 45-69 mcg/dL: I.V.: 25 mg/kg/day for 5 days as an 8- to 24-hour infusion or divided into 2 doses every 12 hours

Depending upon the blood lead level, additional courses may be necessary; repeat at least 2-4 days and preferably 2-4 weeks apart

Adults with lead nephropathy: An alternative dosing regimen reflecting the reduction in renal clearance is based upon the serum creatinine. Refer to the following:

Dose of Ca EDTA based on serum creatinine:

S_{cr} ≤2 mg/dL: 1 g/m^2/day for 5 days*

S_{cr} 2-3 mg/dL: 500 mg/m^2/day for 5 days*

S_{cr} 3-4 mg/dL: 500 mg/m^2/dose every 48 hours for 3 doses*

S_{cr} >4 mg/dL: 500 mg/m^2/week*

*Repeat these regimens monthly until lead excretion is reduced toward normal.

Mechanism of Action Calcium is displaced by divalent and trivalent heavy metals, forming a nonionizing soluble complex that is excreted in urine

Other Adverse Effects Frequency not defined:

Cardiovascular: EKG changes

Central nervous system: Chills

Dermatologic: Cheilosis, skin lesions

Endocrine & metabolic: Hypercalcemia

Gastrointestinal: Anorexia

Hematologic: Anemia, bone marrow suppression (transient)

Hepatic: Liver function test increased (mild)

Local: Thrombophlebitis following I.V. infusion (when concentration >5 mg/mL), pain at injection site following I.M. injection

Neuromuscular & skeletal: Arthralgia

Ocular: Lacrimation

Renal: Renal tubular necrosis, microscopic hematuria, proteinuria

Miscellaneous: Zinc deficiency

Drug Interactions Decreased Effect: Do not use simultaneously with zinc insulin preparations; do not mix in the same syringe with dimercaprol.

Pharmacodynamics/Kinetics

Onset of action: Chelation of lead: I.V.: 1 hour

Absorption: I.M., S.C.: Well absorbed

Distribution: Into extracellular fluid; minimal CSF penetration

Half-life elimination, plasma: I.M.: 1.5 hours; I.V.: 20 minutes

Excretion: Urine (as metal chelates or unchanged drug); decreased GFR decreases elimination

Pregnancy Risk Factor B

Generic Available No

Edetate Disodium (ED e tate dye SOW dee um)

U.S. Brand Names Endrate®

Pharmacologic Category Chelating Agent

Synonyms Edathamil Disodium; EDTA; Sodium Edetate

Use Emergency treatment of hypercalcemia; control digitalis-induced cardiac dysrhythmias (ventricular arrhythmias)

Local Anesthetic/Vasoconstrictor Precautions No information available to require special precautions

Effects on Dental Treatment 1% to 10%: Nausea, vomiting

Dosage Hypercalcemia: I.V.:

Children: 40-70 mg/kg/day slow infusion over 3-4 hours or more to a maximum of 3 g/24 hours; administer for 5 days and allow 5 days between courses of therapy

Adults: 50 mg/kg/day over 3 or more hours to a maximum of 3 g/24 hours; a suggested regimen of 5 days followed by 2 days without drug and repeated courses up to 15 total doses

Digitalis-induced arrhythmias: Children and Adults: 15 mg/kg/hour (maximum dose: 60 mg/kg/day) as continuous infusion

Mechanism of Action Chelates with divalent or trivalent metals to form a soluble complex that is then eliminated in urine

Other Adverse Effects Rapid I.V. administration or excessive doses may cause a sudden drop in serum calcium concentration which may lead to hypocalcemic tetany, seizures, arrhythmias, and death from respiratory arrest. Do **not** exceed recommended dosage and rate of administration.

1% to 10%: Gastrointestinal: Abdominal cramps, diarrhea

<1%: **Arrhythmias, transient hypotension,** acute tubular necrosis, **seizures, fever, headache,** tetany, chills, eruptions, dermatologic lesions, hypomagnesemia, hypokalemia, anemia, thrombophlebitis, pain at the site of injection, **paresthesia, back pain, muscle cramps,** nephrotoxicity, **death from respiratory arrest**

Drug Interactions Increased Effect/Toxicity: Increased effect of insulin (edetate disodium may decrease blood glucose concentrations and reduce insulin requirements in diabetic patients treated with insulin).

Pharmacodynamics/Kinetics

Metabolism: None

Half-life elimination: 20-60 minutes

Time to peak: I.V.: 24-48 hours

Excretion: Following chelation: Urine (95%); chelates within 24-48 hours

Pregnancy Risk Factor C

Generic Available Yes

Edex® *see* Alprostadil *on page 63*

EDTA *see* Edetate Disodium *on page 488*

E.E.S.® *see* Erythromycin *on page 512*

Efavirenz (e FAV e renz)

Related Information

HIV Infection and AIDS *on page 1482*

Tuberculosis *on page 1493*

U.S. Brand Names Sustiva®

Canadian Brand Names Sustiva®

Pharmacologic Category Antiretroviral Agent, Reverse Transcriptase Inhibitor (Non-nucleoside)

Use Treatment of HIV-1 infections in combination with at least two other antiretroviral agents. Also has some activity against hepatitis B virus and herpes viruses.

Local Anesthetic/Vasoconstrictor Precautions No information available to require special precautions

Effects on Dental Treatment *Reported in ≥10% of patients 3-16 years of age:

>10%: Dizziness* (2% to 28%), anxiety (1% to 11%), pain* (1% to 13%) nausea* (2% to 12%)

1% to 10% Headache* (2% to 7%), somnolence (2% to 7%), fatigue (2% to 7%), nervousness (2% to 6%), hallucinations (1%), diaphoresis increased (1% to 2%), vomiting* (6% to 7%)

<2%: Xerostomia and abnormal taste

Dosage Oral: Dosing at bedtime is recommended to limit central nervous system effects; should not be used as single-agent therapy

Children: Dosage is based on body weight
- 10 kg to <15 kg: 200 mg once daily
- 15 kg to <20 kg: 250 mg once daily
- 20 kg to <25 kg: 300 mg once daily
- 25 kg to <32.5 kg: 350 mg once daily
- 32.5 kg to <40 kg: 400 mg once daily
- ≥40 kg: 600 mg once daily

Adults: 600 mg once daily

Mechanism of Action As a non-nucleoside reverse transcriptase inhibitor, efavirenz has activity against HIV-1 by binding to reverse transcriptase. It consequently blocks the RNA-dependent and DNA-dependent DNA polymerase activities including HIV-1 replication. It does not require intracellular phosphorylation for antiviral activity.

Other Adverse Effects *Reported in ≥10% of patients 3-16 years of age:

>10%:

Central nervous system: Depression (1% to 16%), insomnia (6% to 16%)
Dermatologic: Rash* (NCI grade 1: 9% to 11%; NCI grade 2: 15% to 32%)
Endocrine & metabolic: HDL increased (25% to 35%), total cholesterol increased (20% to 40%)
Gastrointestinal: Diarrhea* (3% to 14%)

1% to 10%

Central nervous system: Impaired concentration (2% to 8%), abnormal dreams (1% to 6%), severe depression (2%)
Dermatologic: Pruritus (1% to 9%), diaphoresis increased (1% to 2%)
Gastrointestinal: Dyspepsia (3%), abdominal pain (1% to 3%), anorexia (1% to 2%)

<1%: **Aggressive behavior, manic reaction,** rash (NCI grades 3 or 4), **paranoid reaction, suicide attempts, suicidal ideation**

Postmarketing and/or case reports: **Allergic reaction, aggressive reaction, agitation,** arthralgia, ataxia, body fat accumulation/redistribution, constipation, **convulsions, coordination abnormal, delusions, dyspnea,** emotional lability, erythema multiforme, **flushing,** gynecomastia, hepatitis, hypertriglyceridemia, hypoesthesia, liver failure, liver enzyme elevations, malabsorption, mania, myalgia, myopathy, nail disorder, neuropathy, neurosis, **palpitations, paranoia, paresthesia, psychosis,** skin discoloration, Stevens-Johnson syndrome, suicide, tinnitus, **tremor, visual abnormality, weakness**

Drug Interactions Substrate of **CYP2B6, 3A4**; Inhibits CYP2C8/9, 2C19, 3A4; Induces CYP2B6, 3A4

Increased Effect/Toxicity: Coadministration with medications metabolized by these enzymes may lead to increased concentration-related effects. Cisapride, midazolam, triazolam, and ergot alkaloids may result in life-threatening toxicities; concurrent use is contraindicated. The AUC of nelfinavir is increased (20%); AUC of both ritonavir and efavirenz are increased by 20% during concurrent therapy. The AUC of ethinyl estradiol is increased 37% by efavirenz (clinical significance unknown). May increase (or decrease) effect of warfarin.

Decreased Effect: Other inducers of this enzyme (including phenobarbital, rifampin, rifabutin, and St John's wort) may decrease serum concentrations of efavirenz. Concentrations of indinavir may be reduced; dosage increase to 1000 mg 3 times/day is recommended. Concentrations of saquinavir may be decreased (use as sole protease inhibitor is not recommended). The AUC of amprenavir may be decreased (36%). Plasma concentrations of clarithromycin are decreased (clinical significance unknown). Serum concentrations of methadone are decreased; monitor for withdrawal. May decrease (or increase) effect of warfarin.

Dietary/Ethanol/Herb Considerations

Ethanol: Avoid use due to hepatic and CNS adverse effects.
Food: Administer on an empty stomach; high-fat meals increases absorption. Boiled milk, buttermilk, or yogurt may reduce diarrhea.
Herb/Nutraceutical: Avoid St John's wort; may decrease serum concentration.

Pharmacodynamics/Kinetics

Absorption: Increased 50% by fatty meals
Distribution: CSF concentrations exceed free fraction in serum
Protein binding: >99%, primarily to albumin
Metabolism: Hepatic
Half-life elimination: Single dose: 52-76 hours; Multiple doses: 40-55 hours
Time to peak: 3-8 hours
Excretion: Feces (16% to 41% primarily as unchanged drug); urine (14% to 34% as metabolites)

Pregnancy Risk Factor C

Generic Available No

Effer-K™ *see* Potassium Supplements *on page 1102*
Effexor® *see* Venlafaxine *on page 1380*
Effexor® XR *see* Venlafaxine *on page 1380*
Eflone® *see* Fluorometholone *on page 587*

Eflornithine (ee FLOR ni theen)

U.S. Brand Names Vaniqa™

Pharmacologic Category Antiprotozoal; Topical Skin Product

Synonyms DFMO; Eflornithine Hydrochloride

Use Cream: Females ≥12 years: Reduce unwanted hair from face and adjacent areas under the chin

Orphan drug: Injection: Treatment of meningoencephalitic stage of *Trypanosoma brucei gambiense* infection (sleeping sickness)

(Continued)

Eflornithine *(Continued)*

Local Anesthetic/Vasoconstrictor Precautions No information available to require special precautions

Effects on Dental Treatment 1% to 10%:

Injection: Seizures (may be due to the disease) (8%), dizziness, vomiting

Topical: Headache (4% to 5%), dizziness (1%), facial edema (≤3%)

Dosage

Children ≥12 years and Adults: Females: Topical: Apply thin layer of cream to affected areas of face and adjacent chin twice daily, at least 8 hours apart

Adults: I.V. infusion: 100 mg/kg/dose given every 6 hours (over at least 45 minutes) for 14 days

Dosing adjustment in renal impairment: Injection: Should be adjusted; no specific guidelines available

Mechanism of Action Eflornithine exerts antitumor and antiprotozoal effects through specific, irreversible ("suicide") inhibition of the enzyme ornithine decarboxylase (ODC). ODC is the rate-limiting enzyme in the biosynthesis of putrescine, spermine, and spermidine, the major polyamines in nucleated cells. Polyamines are necessary for the synthesis of DNA, RNA, and proteins and are, therefore, necessary for cell growth and differentiation. Although many microorganisms and higher plants are able to produce polyamines from alternate biochemical pathways, all mammalian cells depend on ornithine decarboxylase to produce polyamines. Eflornithine inhibits ODC and rapidly depletes animal cells of putrescine and spermidine; the concentration of spermine remains the same or may even increase. Rapidly dividing cells appear to be most susceptible to the effects of eflornithine. Topically, the inhibition of ODC in the skin leads to a decreased rate of hair growth.

Other Adverse Effects

Injection: >10%: Hematologic (reversible): Anemia (55%), leukopenia (37%), thrombocytopenia (14%)

1% to 10%:

Dermatologic: Alopecia

Gastrointestinal: Diarrhea

Hematologic: Eosinophilia

Otic: Hearing impairment

<1%: Abdominal pain, anorexia, facial edema, headache, weakness

Topical:

>10%: Dermatologic: Acne (11% to 21%), pseudofolliculitis barbae (5% to 15%)

1% to 10%:

Central nervous system: Vertigo (≤1%)

Dermatologic: Pruritus (3% to 4%), burning skin (2% to 4%), tingling skin (1% to 4%), dry skin (2% to 3%), rash (1% to 3%), alopecia (1% to 2%), skin irritation (1% to 2%), erythema (≤2%), ingrown hair (≤2%), folliculitis (≤1%)

Gastrointestinal: Dyspepsia (2%), anorexia (≤2%)

<1%: **Bleeding, herpes simplex, lip swelling, nausea, numbness,** rosacea, **weakness,** cheilitis, **contact dermatitis**

Drug Interactions Cream: Possible interactions with other topical products have not been studied.

Pharmacodynamics/Kinetics

Absorption: Topical: <1%

Half-life elimination: I.V.: 3-3.5 hours; Topical: 8 hours

Excretion: Primarily urine (as unchanged drug)

Pregnancy Risk Factor C

Generic Available No

Eflornithine Hydrochloride *see* Eflornithine *on page 489*

Efudex® *see* Fluorouracil *on page 588*

E-Gems® [OTC] *see* Vitamin E *on page 1393*

EHDP *see* Etidronate Disodium *on page 546*

ELA-Max® [OTC] *see* Lidocaine *on page 801*

ELA-Max® 5 [OTC] *see* Lidocaine *on page 801*

Elavil® *see* Amitriptyline *on page 83*

Eldepryl® *see* Selegiline *on page 1213*

Eldopaque® [OTC] *see* Hydroquinone *on page 693*

Eldopaque Forte® *see* Hydroquinone *on page 693*

Eldoquin® [OTC] *see* Hydroquinone *on page 693*

Eldoquin Forte® *see* Hydroquinone *on page 693*

Electrolyte Lavage Solution *see* Polyethylene Glycol-Electrolyte Solution *on page 1094*

Eletriptan (el e TRIP tan)

U.S. Brand Names Relpax®

Pharmacologic Category Serotonin $5\text{-}HT_{1B, 1D}$ Receptor Agonist

Synonyms Eletriptan Hydrobromide

Use Acute treatment of migraine, with or without aura

Local Anesthetic/Vasoconstrictor Precautions No information available to require special precautions

Effects on Dental Treatment 1% to 10%: Chest pain/tightness (1% to 4%; placebo 1%), palpitations, dizziness (3% to 7%; placebo 3%), somnolence (3% to 7%; placebo 4%), headache (3% to 4%; placebo 3%), pain, nausea (4% to 8%; placebo 5%), xerostomia (2% to 4%, placebo 2%), dysphagia (1% to 2%), abdominal pain/discomfort (1% to 2%; placebo 1%), weakness (4% to 10%), paresthesia (3% to 4%), pharyngitis, diaphoresis

Dosage Oral: Adults: Acute migraine: 20-40 mg; if the headache improves but returns, dose may be repeated after 2 hours have elapsed since first dose; maximum 80 mg/day.

Note: If the first dose is ineffective, diagnosis needs to be re-evaluated. Safety of treating >3 headaches/month has not been established.

Dosage adjustment in renal impairment: No dosing adjustment needed; monitor for increased blood pressure

Dosage adjustment in hepatic impairment:

Mild to moderate impairment: No adjustment necessary

Severe impairment: Use is contraindicated

Mechanism of Action Selective agonist for serotonin (5-HT_{1B}, 5-HT_{1D}, 5-HT_{1F} receptors) in cranial arteries; causes vasoconstriction and reduce sterile inflammation associated with antidromic neuronal transmission correlating with relief of migraine

Other Adverse Effects

1% to 10%:

Central nervous system: Chills, vertigo

Gastrointestinal: Dyspepsia (1% to 2%; placebo 1%)

Neuromuscular & skeletal: Back pain, hypertonia, hypesthesia

<1% (Limited to important and/or life-threatening): **Agitation, allergic reaction, angina, arrhythmia,** ataxia, **confusion,** constipation, CPK increased, depersonalization, depression, diarrhea, dreams (abnormal), dyspnea, edema, emotional lability, **esophagitis, euphoria,** hyperesthesia, hyperkinesia, **hypertension,** impotence, **incoordination,** insomnia, lacrimation disorder, LFTs abnormal, myalgia, myasthenia, **nervousness,** peripheral vascular disorder, photophobia, polyuria, pruritus, rash, **salivation increased, shock, speech disorder, stupor, tachycardia, taste perversion,** thrombophlebitis, tinnitus, **tongue edema, tremor,** urinary frequency, **vasospasm, abnormal vision**

Drug Interactions Substrate of **CYP3A4**

Increased Effect/Toxicity: CYP3A4 inhibitors increase serum concentration and half-life of eletriptan; do not use eletriptan within 72 hours of potent CYP3A4 inhibitors (ie, erythromycin, fluconazole, ketoconazole, and verapamil). Ergot-containing drugs prolong vasospastic reactions; do not use within 24 hours of eletriptan.

Dietary/Ethanol/Herb Considerations Food: High-fat meal increases bioavailability.

Pharmacodynamics/Kinetics

Absorption: Well absorbed

Distribution: V_d: 138 L

Protein binding: ~85%

Metabolism: Hepatic via CYP3A4; forms one metabolite (active)

Bioavailability: ~50%, increased with high-fat meal

Half-life elimination: 4 hours (Elderly: 4.4-5.7 hours); Metabolite: ~13 hours

Time to peak, plasma: 1.5-2 hours

Pregnancy Risk Factor C

Generic Available No

Eletriptan Hydrobromide *see* Eletriptan *on page 490*

Elidel® *see* Pimecrolimus *on page 1083*

Eligard™ *see* Leuprolide *on page 784*

Elimite® *see* Permethrin *on page 1062*

Elitek™ *see* Rasburicase *on page 1169*

Elixophyllin® *see* Theophylline *on page 1291*

Elixophyllin-GG® *see* Theophylline and Guaifenesin *on page 1293*

Ellence® *see* Epirubicin *on page 501*

Elmiron® *see* Pentosan Polysulfate Sodium *on page 1056*

Elocon® *see* Mometasone Furoate *on page 928*

Eloxatin™ *see* Oxaliplatin *on page 1008*

Elspar® *see* Asparaginase *on page 129*

Embeline™ E *see* Clobetasol *on page 345*

Emcyt® *see* Estramustine *on page 527*

Emetrol® [OTC] *see* Phosphorated Carbohydrate Solution *on page 1078*

Emgel® *see* Erythromycin *on page 512*

Emko® [OTC] *see* Nonoxynol 9 *on page 985*

EMLA® *see* Lidocaine and Prilocaine *on page 806*

Emulsoil® [OTC] *see* Castor Oil *on page 259*

ENA 713 *see* Rivastigmine *on page 1192*

Enalapril (e NAL a pril)

Related Information

Cardiovascular Diseases *on page 1456*

Enalapril and Felodipine *on page 494*

U.S. Brand Names Vasotec®; Vasotec® I.V.

Canadian Brand Names Vasotec®; Vasotec® I.V.

Mexican Brand Names Enaladil®; Feliberal®; Glioten®; Kenopril®; Norpril®; Palane®; Pulsol®; Renitec®

Pharmacologic Category Angiotensin-Converting Enzyme (ACE) Inhibitor

Synonyms Enalaprilat; Enalapril Maleate

Use Management of mild to severe hypertension; treatment of CHF, left ventricular dysfunction after MI

Unlabeled/Investigational Use

Unlabeled: Treatment of hypertensive crisis, hypertension secondary to scleroderma renal crisis, idiopathic edema, Bartter's syndrome, diabetic nephropathy, rheumatoid arthritis; diagnosis of anatomic renal artery stenosis, or aldosteronism; postmyocardial infarction for prevention of ventricular failure

Investigational: Treatment of severe CHF in infants, neonatal hypertension, acute pulmonary edema

Local Anesthetic/Vasoconstrictor Precautions No information available to require special precautions

Effects on Dental Treatment 1% to 10%: Abnormal taste, hypotension (0.9% to 7%), chest pain (2%), syncope (0.5% to 2%), orthostasis (2%), orthostatic hypotension (2%), headache (2% to 5%), dizziness (4% to 8%), fatigue, (2% to 3%), weakness (2%), vomiting, nausea, weakness, bronchitis (1% to 2%), cough (1% to 2%), dyspnea (1% to 2%)

Dosage Use lower listed initial dose in patients with hyponatremia, hypovolemia, severe CHF, decreased renal function, or in those receiving diuretics.

Oral: **Enalapril**: Children 1 month to 16 years: Hypertension: Initial: 0.08 mg/kg (up to 5 mg) once daily; adjust dosage based on patient response; doses >0.58 mg/kg (40 mg) have not been evaluated in pediatric patients

Investigational: Congestive heart failure: Initial oral doses of **enalapril**: 0.1 mg/kg/day increasing as needed over 2 weeks to 0.5 mg/kg/day have been used in infants

Investigational: Neonatal hypertension: I.V. doses of **enalaprilat**: 5-10 mcg/kg/dose administered every 8-24 hours have been used; monitor patients carefully; select patients may require higher doses

Adults:

Oral: **Enalapril**

Hypertension: 2.5-5 mg/day then increase as required, usual therapeutic dose for hypertension: 10-40 mg/day in 1-2 divided doses. **Note:** Initiate with 2.5 mg if patient is taking a diuretic which cannot be discontinued. May add a diuretic if blood pressure cannot be controlled with enalapril alone.

Heart failure: As standard therapy alone or with diuretics, beta-blockers, and digoxin, initiate with 2.5 mg once or twice daily (usual range: 5-20 mg/day in 2 divided doses; target: 40 mg)

Asymptomatic left ventricular dysfunction: 2.5 mg twice daily, titrated as tolerated to 20 mg/day

I.V.: **Enalaprilat**

Hypertension: 1.25 mg/dose, given over 5 minutes every 6 hours; doses as high as 5 mg/dose every 6 hours have been tolerated for up to 36 hours. **Note:** If patients are concomitantly receiving diuretic therapy, begin with 0.625 mg I.V. over 5 minutes; if the effect is not adequate after 1 hour, repeat the dose and administer 1.25 mg at 6-hour intervals thereafter; if adequate, administer 0.625 mg I.V. every 6 hours.

Heart failure: Avoid I.V. administration in patients with unstable heart failure or those suffering acute MI.

Conversion from I.V. to oral therapy if not concurrently on diuretics: 5 mg once daily; subsequent titration as needed; if concurrently receiving diuretics and responding to 0.625 mg I.V. every 6 hours, initiate with 2.5 mg/day.

Dosing adjustment in renal impairment:

Oral: Enalapril:

Cl_{cr} 30-80 mL/minute: Administer 5 mg/day titrated upwards to maximum of 40 mg.

Cl_{cr} <30 mL/minute: Administer 2.5 mg day; titrated upward until blood pressure is controlled.

For heart failure patients with sodium <130 mEq/L or serum creatinine >1.6 mg/dL, initiate dosage with 2.5 mg/day, increasing to twice daily as needed. Increase further in increments of 2.5 mg/dose at >4-day intervals to a maximum daily dose of 40 mg.

I.V.: Enalaprilat:

Cl_{cr} >30 mL/minute: Initiate with 1.25 mg every 6 hours and increase dose based on response.

Cl_{cr} <30 mL/minute: Initiate with 0.625 mg every 6 hours and increase dose based on response.

Hemodialysis: Moderately dialyzable (20% to 50%); administer dose postdialysis (eg, 0.625 mg I.V. every 6 hours) or administer 20% to 25% supplemental dose following dialysis; Clearance: 62 mL/minute.

Peritoneal dialysis: Supplemental dose is unnecessary, although some removal of drug occurs.

Dosing adjustment in hepatic impairment: Hydrolysis of enalapril to enalaprilat may be delayed and/or impaired in patients with severe hepatic impairment, but the pharmacodynamic effects of the drug do not appear to be significantly altered; no dosage adjustment.

Mechanism of Action Competitive inhibitor of angiotensin-converting enzyme (ACE); prevents conversion of angiotensin I to angiotensin II, a potent vasoconstrictor; results in lower levels of angiotensin II which causes an increase in plasma renin activity and a reduction in aldosterone secretion

Other Adverse Effects Includes data from hypertension and heart failure trials; higher rates noted in CHF (frequency of adverse effects associated with placebo is also increased in this population):

1% to 10%:

Dermatologic: Rash (2%)

Gastrointestinal: Abdominal pain, diarrhea, anorexia, constipation

Renal: Increased serum creatinine (0.2% to 20%), worsening of renal function (in patients with bilateral renal artery stenosis or hypovolemia)

<1% (Limited to important or life-threatening): Agranulocytosis, alopecia, anemia, angina pectoris, angioedema, **cardiac arrest, asthma,** ataxia, **blurred vision, bronchospasm, confusion,** conjunctivitis, CVA, depression, **diaphoresis, drowsiness,** dysrhythmias, dyspepsia, erythema multiforme, **glossitis,** gynecomastia, hemolysis with G6PD, hepatitis, hyperkalemia, **hypoglycemia,** ileus, impotence, insomnia, jaundice, **MI, nervousness,** neutropenia, oliguria, **palpitations,** pancreatitis, **paresthesia,** pemphigus, pruritus, pulmonary edema, renal dysfunction, Stevens-Johnson syndrome, **stomatitis,** tinnitus, **upper respiratory infection,** urinary tract infection, urticaria, vertigo, **xerostomia**; worsening of renal function may occur in patients with bilateral renal artery stenosis or in hypovolemic patients

Postmarketing and/or case reports: Depression, exfoliative dermatitis, giant cell arteritis, **hallucinations,** Henoch-Schönlein purpura, lichen-form reaction, ototoxicity, pemphigus foliaceus, photosensitivity, **psychosis,** sicca syndrome, systemic lupus erythematosus, toxic epidermal necrolysis, toxic pustuloderma; a syndrome which may include arthralgia, elevated ESR, eosinophilia and positive ANA, fever, interstitial nephritis, myalgia, rash, and vasculitis has been reported for enalapril and other ACE inhibitors

Drug Interactions Substrate of **CYP3A4**

Increased Effect/Toxicity:

Potassium supplements, co-trimoxazole (high dose), angiotensin II receptor antagonists (candesartan, losartan, irbesartan, etc), or potassium-sparing diuretics (amiloride, spironolactone, triamterene) may result in elevated serum potassium levels when combined with enalapril. ACE inhibitor effects may be increased by phenothiazines or probenecid (increases levels of captopril). ACE inhibitors may increase serum concentrations/effects of digoxin, lithium, and sulfonlyureas.

Diuretics have additive hypotensive effects with ACE inhibitors, and hypovolemia increases the potential for adverse renal effects of ACE inhibitors. In patients with compromised renal function, coadministration with NSAIDs may result in further deterioration of renal function. Allopurinol and ACE inhibitors may cause a higher risk of hypersensitivity reaction when taken concurrently.

Decreased Effect: Aspirin (high dose) may reduce the therapeutic effects of ACE inhibitors; at low dosages this does not appear to be significant. Rifampin may decrease the effect of ACE inhibitors. Antacids may decrease the bioavailability of ACE inhibitors (may be more likely to occur with captopril); separate administration times by 1-2 hours. NSAIDs may reduce the hypotensive effects of ACE inhibitors. More likely to occur in low renin or volume dependent hypertensive patients.

Dietary/Ethanol/Herb Considerations

Ethanol: Avoid or limit use; may increase risk of hypotension or dizziness.

Food: Administer with food to reduce GI upset; limit salt substitutes and potassium-rich foods. Avoid caffeine, garlic, and licorice.

Herb/Nutraceutical: Avoid black cohosh, dong quai, and evening primrose due to estrogenic activity. Avoid ephedra, ginseng, and yohimbe; may worsen hypertension. Avoid garlic; may have increased antihypertensive effect. Avoid ginger due to positive inotropic effects; theoretically, may cause arrhythmia. Avoid hawthorn; may lower peripheral vascular resistance resulting in additive decrease in BP.

(Continued)

Enalapril *(Continued)*

Avoid licorice; causes sodium and water retention and increases potassium loss. Avoid St John's wort; may decrease serum concentration.

Pharmacodynamics/Kinetics

Onset of action: Oral: ~1 hour
Duration: Oral: 12-24 hours
Absorption: Oral: 55% to 75%
Protein binding: 50% to 60%
Metabolism: Prodrug, undergoes hepatic biotransformation to enalaprilat
Half-life elimination:
Enalapril: Adults: Healthy: 2 hours; Congestive heart failure: 3.4-5.8 hours
Enalaprilat: Infants 6 weeks to 8 months old: 6-10 hours; Adults: 35-38 hours
Time to peak, serum: Oral: Enalapril: 0.5-1.5 hours; Enalaprilat (active): 3-4.5 hours
Excretion: Urine (60% to 80%); some feces

Pregnancy Risk Factor C/D (2nd and 3rd trimesters)

Generic Available Yes

Enalapril and Felodipine (e NAL a pril & fe LOE di peen)

Related Information

Enalapril *on page 492*
Felodipine *on page 560*

U.S. Brand Names Lexxel®

Canadian Brand Names Lexxel™

Pharmacologic Category Antihypertensive Agent Combination

Synonyms Felodipine and Enalapril

Use Treatment of hypertension, however, not indicated for initial treatment of hypertension; replacement therapy in patients receiving separate dosage forms (for patient convenience); when monotherapy with one component fails to achieve desired antihypertensive effect, or when dose-limiting adverse effects limit upward titration of monotherapy

Local Anesthetic/Vasoconstrictor Precautions No information available to require special precautions

Effects on Dental Treatment ~1%: Gingival hyperplasia (fewer reports with felodipine than with other CCBs); resolves upon discontinuation (consultation with physician is suggested)

Dosage Adults: Oral: 1 tablet daily

Mechanism of Action See individual agents.

Dietary/Ethanol/Herb Considerations Ethanol: Avoid or limit use; may increase risk of hypotension or dizziness.

Pregnancy Risk Factor C/D (2nd and 3rd trimesters)

Generic Available No

Enalapril and Hydrochlorothiazide

(e NAL a pril & hye droe klor oh THYE a zide)

Related Information

Cardiovascular Diseases *on page 1456*
Enalapril *on page 492*
Hydrochlorothiazide *on page 675*

U.S. Brand Names Vaseretic®

Canadian Brand Names Vaseretic®

Pharmacologic Category Antihypertensive Agent Combination

Synonyms Hydrochlorothiazide and Enalapril

Use Treatment of hypertension

Local Anesthetic/Vasoconstrictor Precautions No information available to require special precautions

Effects on Dental Treatment No significant effects or complications reported

Dosage Oral: Dose is individualized

Dietary/Ethanol/Herb Considerations Ethanol: Avoid or limit use; may increase risk of hypotension or dizziness.

Pregnancy Risk Factor C/D (2nd and 3rd trimesters)

Generic Available No

Enalaprilat *see* Enalapril *on page 492*
Enalapril Maleate *see* Enalapril *on page 492*
Enbrel® *see* Etanercept *on page 537*
Encare® [OTC] *see* Nonoxynol 9 *on page 985*
Endal® *see* Guaifenesin and Phenylephrine *on page 652*
Endocet® *see* Oxycodone and Acetaminophen *on page 1018*
Endodan® *see* Oxycodone and Aspirin *on page 1020*
Endrate® *see* Edetate Disodium *on page 488*
Enduron® *see* Methyclothiazide *on page 890*
Enduronyl® *see* Methyclothiazide and Deserpidine *on page 890*
Enduronyl® Forte *see* Methyclothiazide and Deserpidine *on page 890*

Ener-B® *see* Cyanocobalamin *on page 377*

Enfuvirtide (en FYOO vir tide)

U.S. Brand Names Fuzeon™

Pharmacologic Category Antiretroviral Agent, Fusion Protein Inhibitor

Synonyms T-20

Use Treatment of HIV-1 infection in combination with other antiretroviral agents

Local Anesthetic/Vasoconstrictor Precautions No information available to require special precautions

Effects on Dental Treatment 1% to 10%: Anxiety (6%) taste disturbance (2%) weakness (6%), cough (7%), pneumonia, sinusitis (6%), infections (4% to 6%), flu-like symptoms (2%), lymphadenopathy (2%)

Restrictions Roche and Trimeris have committed to make Fuzeon™ available for distribution before the end of March. When the drug becomes commercially available, it is expected that the demand for this product may exceed supply. The companies are finalizing a U. S. Progressive Distribution Plan to provide Fuzeon™ to patients, emphasizing the need to ensure uninterrupted supply to patients once they begin therapy. The details of this plan are expected to be announced soon.

Dosage S.C.:

Children ≥6 years: 2 mg/kg twice daily (maximum dose: 90 mg twice daily)

Adults: 90 mg twice daily

Mechanism of Action Binds to the first heptad-repeat (HR1) in the gp41 subunit of the viral envelope glycoprotein. Inhibits the fusion of HIV-1 virus with CD4 cells by blocking the conformational change in gp41 required for membrane fusion and entry into CD4 cells; lowers viral load in patients with evidence of HIV-1 replication despite ongoing antiretroviral therapy

Other Adverse Effects

>10%:

- Central nervous system: Insomnia (11%)
- Local: Injection site reactions (98%; pain, erythema, induration, pruritus, ecchymosis, nodule or cyst formation)

1% to 10%:

- Central nervous system: Depression (9%)
- Dermatologic: Pruritus (5%)
- Endocrine & metabolic: Weight loss (7%), anorexia (3%)
- Gastrointestinal: Triglycerides increased (9%), appetite decreased (6%), constipation (4%), abdominal pain (3%), pancreatitis (2%), taste disturbance (2%), serum amylase increased (6%)
- Hematologic: Eosinophilia (8%), anemia (2%)
- Hepatic: Serum transaminases increased (4%)
- Local: Injection site infection (1%)
- Neuromuscular & skeletal: Neuropathy (9%), myalgia (5%)
- Ocular: Conjunctivitis (2%)

<1%: **Hypersensitivity reactions (eg, rash, fever, nausea, vomiting, hypotension, and/or hepatic transaminases increased); worsening of abacavir hypersensitivity, renal insufficiency, renal failure,** thrombocytopenia, neutropenia, **hyperglycemia,** Guillain-Barré syndrome, sixth nerve palsy

Pharmacodynamics/Kinetics

Distribution: V_d: 5.5 L

Protein binding: 92%

Metabolism : Proteolytic hydrolysis (CYP isoenzymes do not appear to contribute to metabolism); clearance: 24.8 mL/hour/kg

Half-life elimination: 3.8 hours

Time to peak: 8 hours

Pregnancy Risk Factor B

Generic Available No

Engerix-B® *see* Hepatitis B Vaccine *on page 666*

Engerix-B® and Havrix® *see* Hepatitis A (Inactivated) and Hepatitis B (Recombinant) Vaccine *on page 664*

Enhanced-potency Inactivated Poliovirus Vaccine *see* Poliovirus Vaccine (Inactivated) *on page 1093*

Enoxaparin (ee noks a PA rin)

U.S. Brand Names Lovenox®

Canadian Brand Names Lovenox®; Lovenox® HP

Mexican Brand Names Clexane®

Pharmacologic Category Low Molecular Weight Heparin

Synonyms Enoxaparin Sodium

Use

Prevention of deep vein thrombosis following hip or knee replacement surgery or abdominal surgery in patients at risk for thromboembolic complications (high-risk patients include those with one or more of the following risk factors: >40 years of age, obese, general anesthesia lasting >30 minutes, malignancy, history of deep vein thrombosis or pulmonary embolism)

(Continued)

Enoxaparin *(Continued)*

Prevention of deep vein thrombosis in medical patients at risk for thromboembolic complications due to severely restricted mobility during acute illness

Inpatient treatment of acute deep vein thrombosis with and without pulmonary embolism when administered in conjunction with warfarin sodium

Outpatient treatment of acute deep vein thrombosis without pulmonary embolism when administered in conjunction with warfarin sodium

Prevention of ischemic complications of unstable angina and non-Q wave MI (when administered with aspirin)

Local Anesthetic/Vasoconstrictor Precautions No information available to require special precautions

Effects on Dental Treatment As with all anticoagulants, bleeding is the major adverse effect of enoxaparin. Hemorrhage may occur at virtually any site; risk is dependent on multiple variables. At the recommended doses, single injections of enoxaparin do not significantly influence platelet aggregation or affect global clotting time (ie, PT or aPTT).

1% to 10%: Fever (5% to 8%), confusion, pain, bruising, nausea (3%), hemorrhage (5% to 13%)

Dosage S.C.:

Children: Prophylaxis of DVT following abdominal, hip replacement or knee replacement surgery: Safety and effectiveness have not been established. Few studies have been conducted; the Fifth American College of Chest Physicians Consensus Conference on Antithrombotic Therapy (Michelson, 1998) recommends low molecular weight heparin as an alternative to heparin therapy in children ≥2 months with DVT or pulmonary embolism; the following initial doses and titration schedule, based on therapeutic antifactor Xa levels of 0.5-1 unit/mL, are recommended. **Note:** For treatment of DVT or pulmonary embolism in children ≥2 months of age, enoxaparin should be continued for 5-10 days and oral anticoagulation should be overlapped for 4-5 days (Michelson, 1998)

Infants >2 months and Children ≤18 years: Prophylaxis: Initial: 0.5 mg/kg every 12 hours; treatment: Initial: 1 mg/kg every 12 hours

Dosage titration:

Antifactor Xa <0.35 units/mL: Increase dose by 25%; repeat antifactor Xa level 4 hour after next dose

Antifactor Xa 0.35-0.49 units/mL: Increase dose by 10%; repeat antifactor Xa level 4 hour after next dose

Antifactor Xa 0.5-1 unit/mL: Keep same dosage; repeat antifactor Xa level next day, then 1 week later (4 hour after dose)

Antifactor Xa 1.1-1.5 units/mL: Decrease dose by 20%; repeat antifactor Xa level before next dose

Antifactor Xa 1.6-2 units/mL: Hold dose for 3 hour and decrease dose by 30%; repeat antifactor Xa level before next dose, then 4 hour after next dose

Antifactor Xa >2 units/mL: Hold all doses until antifactor Xa is 0.5 units/mL, then decrease dose by 40%; repeat antifactor Xa level before next dose and every 12 hour until antifactor Xa <0.5 units/mL

Adults:

DVT prophylaxis in hip replacement:

30 mg twice daily: First dose within 12-24 hours after surgery and every 12 hours until risk of deep vein thrombosis has diminished or the patient is adequately anticoagulated on warfarin. Average duration of therapy: 7-10 days.

40 mg once daily: First dose within 9-15 hours before surgery and daily until risk of deep vein thrombosis has diminished or the patient is adequately anticoagulated on warfarin. Average duration of therapy: 7-10 days unless warfarin is not given concurrently, then 40 mg S.C. once daily should be continued for 3 more weeks (4 weeks total).

DVT prophylaxis in knee replacement: 30 mg twice daily: First dose within 12-24 hours after surgery and every 12 hours until risk of deep vein thrombosis has diminished. Average duration of therapy: 7-10 days; maximum course: 14 days.

DVT prophylaxis in high-risk patients undergoing abdominal surgery: 40 mg once daily, with initial dose given 2 hours prior to surgery; usual duration: 7-10 days and up to 12 days has been tolerated in clinical trials.

DVT prophylaxis in medical patients with severely restricted mobility during acute illness: 40 mg once daily; usual duration: 6-11 days; up to 14 days was used in clinical trial

Treatment of acute proximal DVT: Start warfarin within 72 hours and continue enoxaparin until INR is between 2.0 and 3.0 (usually 7 days).

Inpatient treatment of DVT with or without pulmonary embolism: 1 mg/kg/dose every 12 hours or 1.5 mg/kg once daily.

Outpatient treatment of DVT without pulmonary embolism: 1 mg/kg/dose every 12 hours.

Prevention of ischemic complications with unstable angina or non-Q-wave MI: 1 mg/kg twice daily in conjunction with oral aspirin therapy (100-325 mg once daily); treatment should be continued for a minimum of 2 days and continued until clinical stabilization (usually 2-8 days).

Elderly: Increased incidence of bleeding with doses of 1.5 mg/kg/day or 1 mg/kg every 12 hours; injection-associated bleeding and serious adverse reactions are also increased in the elderly. Careful attention should be paid to elderly patients <45 kg.

Dosing adjustment in renal impairment: Total clearance is lower and elimination is delayed in patients with renal failure; adjustment may be necessary in elderly and patients with severe renal impairment.

Hemodialysis: Supplemental dose is unnecessary.

Peritoneal dialysis: Significant drug removal is unlikely based on physiochemical characteristics.

Mechanism of Action Standard heparin consists of components with molecular weights ranging from 4000-30,000 daltons with a mean of 16,000 daltons. Heparin acts as an anticoagulant by enhancing the inhibition rate of clotting proteases by antithrombin III impairing normal hemostasis and inhibition of factor Xa. Low molecular weight heparins have a small effect on the activated partial thromboplastin time and strongly inhibit factor Xa. Enoxaparin is derived from porcine heparin that undergoes benzylation followed by alkaline depolymerization. The average molecular weight of enoxaparin is 4500 daltons which is distributed as (≤20%) 2000 daltons (≥68%) 2000-8000 daltons, and (≤15%) >8000 daltons. Enoxaparin has a higher ratio of antifactor Xa to antifactor IIa activity than unfractionated heparin.

Other Adverse Effects

1% to 10%:

Dermatologic: Erythema

Gastrointestinal: Diarrhea

Hematologic: Thrombocytopenia (2%), hypochromic anemia (2%)

Hepatic: Increased ALT/AST

Local: Injection site hematoma (9%), local reactions (irritation, pain, ecchymosis, erythema)

<1% and/or postmarketing case reports (limited to important or life-threatening): Hyperlipidemia, hypertriglyceridemia, pruritus, **allergic reaction,** urticaria, **anaphylactoid reaction,** vesicobullous rash, purpura, thrombocytosis, skin necrosis, eczematous plaques, itchy erythematous patches. Retroperitoneal or intracranial bleed (some fatal). Spinal or epidural hematomas can occur following neuraxial anesthesia or spinal puncture, resulting in paralysis. Risk is increased in patients with indwelling epidural catheters or concomitant use of other drugs affecting hemostasis. Prosthetic valve thrombosis, including fatal cases, has been reported in pregnant women receiving enoxaparin as thromboprophylaxis.

Thrombocytopenia with thrombosis: Cases of heparin-induced thrombocytopenia (some complicated by organ infarction, limb ischemia, or death) have been reported.

Drug Interactions Increased Effect/Toxicity: Risk of bleeding with enoxaparin may be increased with thrombolytic agents, oral anticoagulants (warfarin), drugs which affect platelet function (eg, aspirin, NSAIDs, dipyridamole, ticlopidine, clopidogrel, and IIb/IIIa antagonists). Although the risk of bleeding may be increased during concurrent therapy with warfarin, enoxaparin is commonly continued during the initiation of warfarin therapy to assure anticoagulation and to protect against possible transient hypercoagulability. Some cephalosporins and penicillins may block platelet aggregation, theoretically increasing the risk of bleeding.

Dietary/Ethanol/Herb Considerations

Food: Avoid garlic, ginger, and green tea.

Herb/Nutraceutical: Avoid cat's claw, dong quai, evening primrose, feverfew, garlic, ginger, ginkgo biloba, ginseng, green tea, horse chestnut, and red clover due to additional antiplatelet activity.

Pharmacodynamics/Kinetics

Onset of action: Peak effect: S.C.: Antifactor Xa and antithrombin (antifactor IIa): 3-5 hours

Duration: 40 mg dose: Antifactor Xa activity: ~12 hours

Protein binding: Does not bind to heparin binding proteins

Half-life elimination, plasma: 2-4 times longer than standard heparin, independent of dose

Excretion: Urine

Pregnancy Risk Factor B

Generic Available No

Enoxaparin Sodium *see* Enoxaparin *on page 495*

Enpresse™ *see* Combination Hormonal Contraceptives *on page 368*

Entacapone (en TA ka pone)

U.S. Brand Names Comtan®

Canadian Brand Names Comtan®

Pharmacologic Category Anti-Parkinson's Agent, COMT Inhibitor

Use Adjunct to levodopa/carbidopa therapy in patients with idiopathic Parkinson's disease who experience "wearing-off" symptoms at the end of a dosing interval

(Continued)

Entacapone *(Continued)*

Local Anesthetic/Vasoconstrictor Precautions No information available to require special precautions

Effects on Dental Treatment Dopaminergic therapy in Parkinson's disease (ie, treatment with levodopa) is associated with orthostatic hypotension. Entacapone enhances levodopa bioavailability and may increase the occurrence of hypotension/syncope in the dental patient. The patient should be carefully assisted from the chair and observed for signs of orthostatic hypotension.

>10%: Nausea (14%)

1% to 10%: Orthostatic hypotension (4%), syncope (1%), dizziness (8%), fatigue (6%), hallucinations (4%), anxiety (2%), somnolence (2%), agitation (1%), vomiting (4%), gastritis (1%), weakness (2%), dyspnea (3%), increased diaphoresis (2%), bacterial infection (1%), xerostomia (3%), abnormal taste (1%)

Dosage Oral:

Adults: 200 mg dose, up to a maximum of 8 times/day; maximum daily dose: 1600 mg/day. Always administer with levodopa/carbidopa. To optimize therapy, the levodopa/carbidopa dosage must be reduced, usually by 25%. This reduction is usually necessary when the patient is taking more than 800 mg of levodopa daily.

Dosing adjustment in hepatic impairment: Treat with caution and monitor carefully; AUC and C_{max} can be possibly doubled

Mechanism of Action Entacapone is a reversible and selective inhibitor of catechol-O-methyltransferase (COMT). When entacapone is taken with levodopa, the pharmacokinetics are altered, resulting in more sustained levodopa serum levels compared to levodopa taken alone. The resulting levels of levodopa provide for increased concentrations available for absorption across the blood-brain barrier, thereby providing for increased CNS levels of dopamine, the active metabolite of levodopa.

Other Adverse Effects

>10%: Neuromuscular & skeletal: Dyskinesia (25%), placebo (15%)

1% to 10%:

- Dermatologic: Purpura (2%)
- Gastrointestinal: Diarrhea (10%), abdominal pain (8%), constipation (6%), dyspepsia (2%), flatulence (2%),
- Genitourinary: Brown-orange urine discoloration (10%)
- Neuromuscular & skeletal: Hyperkinesia (10%), hypokinesia (9%), back pain (4%)

<1%: Hyperpyrexia and confusion (resembling neuroleptic malignant syndrome), pulmonary fibrosis, rhabdomyolysis, retroperitoneal fibrosis

Note: Approximately 14% of the 603 patients given entacapone in the double-blind, placebo-controlled trials discontinued treatment due to adverse events compared to 9% of the 400 patients who received placebo.

Drug Interactions Inhibits CYP1A2, 2A6, 2C8/9, 2C19, 2D6, 2E1, 3A4

Increased Effect/Toxicity: Cardiac effects with drugs metabolized by COMT (eg, epinephrine, isoproterenol, dopamine, apomorphine, bitolterol, dobutamine, methyldopa) increased other CNS depressants; nonselective MAO inhibitors are not recommended; chelates iron. Caution with drugs that interfere with glucuronidation, intestinal, biliary excretion, intestinal beta-glucuronidase (eg, probenecid, cholestyramine, erythromycin, chloramphenicol, rifampicin, ampicillin).

Decreased Effect: Entacapone is an iron chelator and an iron supplement should not be administered concurrently with this medicine.

Dietary/Ethanol/Herb Considerations

Ethanol: Avoid use; may increase CNS adverse effects.

Food: May be taken with food

Pharmacodynamics/Kinetics

Onset of action: Rapid

Peak effect: 1 hour

Absorption: Rapid

Distribution: I.V.: V_{dss}: 20 L

Protein binding: 98%, primarily to albumin

Metabolism: Isomerization to the *cis*-isomer, followed by direct glucuronidation of the parent and *cis*-isomer

Bioavailability: 35%

Half-life elimination: B phase: 0.4-0.7 hours; Y phase: 2.4 hours

Time to peak, serum: 1 hour

Excretion: Feces (90%); urine (10%)

Pregnancy Risk Factor C

Generic Available No

Entertainer's Secret® [OTC] *see* Saliva Substitute *on page 1205*

Entex® LA *see* Guaifenesin and Phenylephrine *on page 652*

Entex® PSE *see* Guaifenesin and Pseudoephedrine *on page 652*

Entocort™ EC *see* Budesonide *on page 202*

Entsol® [OTC] *see* Sodium Chloride *on page 1229*

Enulose® *see* Lactulose *on page 772*

Enzone® *see* Pramoxine and Hydrocortisone *on page 1106*

Ephedrine (e FED rin)

Related Information

Ephedra *on page 1430*

U.S. Brand Names Pretz-D® [OTC]

Pharmacologic Category Alpha/Beta Agonist

Synonyms Ephedrine Sulfate

Use Treatment of bronchial asthma, nasal congestion, acute bronchospasm, idiopathic orthostatic hypotension

Local Anesthetic/Vasoconstrictor Precautions Use vasoconstrictors with caution since ephedrine may enhance cardiostimulation and vasopressor effects of sympathomimetics such as epinephrine

Effects on Dental Treatment

1% to 10%: Xerostomia

Frequency not defined: Hypertension, tachycardia, palpitations, elevation or depression of blood pressure, chest pain, arrhythmias, CNS stimulating effects, nervousness, anxiety, apprehension, fear, tension, agitation, excitation, restlessness, irritability, insomnia, hyperactivity, dizziness, headache, nausea, GI upset, vomiting, tremor (more common in elderly), weakness, dyspnea, increased diaphoresis

Dosage

Children:

Oral, S.C.: 3 mg/kg/day or 25-100 mg/m^2/day in 4-6 divided doses every 4-6 hours

I.M., slow I.V. push: 0.2-0.3 mg/kg/dose every 4-6 hours

Adults:

Oral: 25-50 mg every 3-4 hours as needed

I.M., S.C.: 25-50 mg, parenteral adult dose should not exceed 150 mg in 24 hours

I.V.: 5-25 mg/dose slow I.V. push repeated after 5-10 minutes as needed, then every 3-4 hours not to exceed 150 mg/24 hours

Nasal spray:

Children 6-12 years: 1-2 sprays into each nostril, not more frequently than every 4 hours

Children ≥12 years and Adults: 2-3 sprays into each nostril, not more frequently than every 4 hours

Mechanism of Action Releases tissue stores of epinephrine and thereby produces an alpha- and beta-adrenergic stimulation; longer-acting and less potent than epinephrine

Other Adverse Effects Frequency not defined:

Cardiovascular: Unusual pallor

Gastrointestinal: Anorexia

Genitourinary: Painful urination

Neuromuscular & skeletal: Trembling

Drug Interactions

Increased Effect/Toxicity: Increased (toxic) cardiac stimulation with other sympathomimetic agents, theophylline, cardiac glycosides, or general anesthetics. Increased blood pressure with atropine or MAO inhibitors.

Decreased Effect: Alpha- and beta-adrenergic blocking agents decrease ephedrine vasopressor effects.

Dietary/Ethanol/Herb Considerations

Food: Avoid caffeine.

Herb/Nutraceutical: Avoid ephedra, ginseng, and yohimbe; may cause CNS stimulation.

Pharmacodynamics/Kinetics

Onset of action: Oral: Bronchodilation: 0.25-1 hour

Duration: Oral: 3-6 hours

Distribution: Crosses placenta; enters breast milk

Metabolism: Minimally hepatic

Half-life elimination: 2.5-3.6 hours

Excretion: Urine (60% to 77% as unchanged drug) within 24 hours

Pregnancy Risk Factor C

Generic Available Yes

Ephedrine Sulfate *see* Ephedrine *on page 499*

Epidermal Thymocyte Activating Factor *see* Aldesleukin *on page 50*

Epifoam® *see* Pramoxine and Hydrocortisone *on page 1106*

Epinephrine (ep i NEF rin)

Related Information

Dental Office Emergencies *on page 1582*

Respiratory Diseases *on page 1476*

U.S. Brand Names Adrenalin® (Dental); Sus-Phrine® (Dental)

(Continued)

Epinephrine *(Continued)*

Pharmacologic Category Adrenergic Agonist Agent; Alpha/Beta Agonist; Antidote; Bronchodilator; Vasoconstrictor

Use Dental: Emergency drug for treatment of anaphylactic reactions; used as vasoconstrictor to prolong local anesthesia

Local Anesthetic/Vasoconstrictor Precautions No information available to require special precautions

Effects on Dental Treatment No significant effects or complications reported

Dosage Hypersensitivity reaction:

Children: S.C.: 0.01 mg/kg every 15 minutes for 2 doses then every 4 hours as needed (single doses not to exceed 0.5 mg)

Adults: I.M., S.C.: 0.2-0.5 mg every 20 minutes to 4 hours (single dose maximum: 1 mg)

Mechanism of Action Stimulates alpha-, $beta_1$-, and $beta_2$-adrenergic receptors resulting in relaxation of smooth muscle of the bronchial tree, cardiac stimulation, and dilation of skeletal muscle vasculature; small doses can cause vasodilation via $beta_2$-vascular receptors; large doses may produce constriction of skeletal and vascular smooth muscle; decreases production of aqueous humor and increases aqueous outflow; dilates the pupil by contracting the dilator muscle

Contraindications Hypersensitivity to epinephrine or any component of the formulation; cardiac arrhythmias, angle-closure glaucoma

Warnings/Precautions Use with caution in elderly patients, patients with diabetes mellitus, cardiovascular diseases (angina, tachycardia, MI), thyroid disease, or cerebral arteriosclerosis, Parkinson's; some products contain sulfites as antioxidants. Rapid I.V. infusion may cause death from cerebrovascular hemorrhage or cardiac arrhythmias. Oral inhalation of epinephrine is **not** the preferred route of administration.

Drug Interactions Increased cardiac irritability if administered concurrently with halogenated inhalational anesthetics, beta-blocking agents, alpha-blocking agents

Dietary/Ethanol/Herb Considerations

Food: Avoid caffeine.

Herb/Nutraceutical: Avoid ephedra, ginseng, and yohimbe; may cause CNS stimulation. Ginger is a positive inotrope and could affect inotropic agents.

Pharmacodynamics/Kinetics Absorption: None

Pregnancy Risk Factor C

Breast-feeding Considerations Usual infiltration doses of epinephrine given to nursing mothers has not been shown to affect the health of the nursing infant.

Dosage Forms INJ: (Adrenalin®): 1 mg/mL [1:1000] (1 mL, 30 mL). **INJ, suspension for:** (Sus-Phrine®): 5 mg/mL [1:200] (0.3 mL, 5 mL)

Generic Available Yes

Epinephrine and Chlorpheniramine Insect Sting Kit

(ep i NEF rin & klor fen IR a meen IN sekt sting kit)

U.S. Brand Names Ana-Kit®

Pharmacologic Category Antidote

Use Anaphylaxis emergency treatment of insect bites or stings by the sensitive patient that may occur within minutes of insect sting or exposure to an allergic substance

Local Anesthetic/Vasoconstrictor Precautions No information available to require special precautions

Effects on Dental Treatment No significant effects or complications reported

Dosage Children and Adults: I.M. or S.C.:

Epinephrine:
- <2 years: 0.05-0.1 mL
- 2-6 years: 0.15 mL
- 6-12 years: 0.2 mL
- >12 years : 0.3 mL

Chlorpheniramine:
- <6 years: 1 tablet
- 6-12 years: 2 tablets
- >12 years: 4 tablets

Generic Available No

Epinephrine and Lidocaine *see* Lidocaine and Epinephrine *on page 804*

Epinephrine (Racemic) (ep i NEF rin, ra SEE mik)

U.S. Brand Names AsthmaNefrin®; microNefrin®; S-2®; Vaponefrin®

Pharmacologic Category Alpha/Beta Agonist; Vasoconstrictor

Local Anesthetic/Vasoconstrictor Precautions No information available to require special precautions

Effects on Dental Treatment No significant effects or complications reported

Pharmacodynamics/Kinetics

Onset of action: Bronchodilation: S.C.: 5-10 minutes; Inhalation: ~1 minute

Absorption: Oral: None

Dosage Forms INH, solution for, oral: (AsthmaNefrin®, microNefrin®, S-2®): Racepinephrine 2.25% [epinephrine base 1.125%] (7.5 mL, 15 mL, 30 mL)

Generic Available Yes

Epinephrine (Racemic) and Aluminum Potassium Sulfate

(ep i NEF rin ra SEE mik & a LOO mi num poe TASS ee um SUL fate)

Related Information

Epinephrine (Racemic) *on page 500*

U.S. Brand Names Van R Gingibraid®

Pharmacologic Category Adrenergic Agonist Agent; Alpha/Beta Agonist; Astringent; Vasoconstrictor

Use Dental: Gingival retraction

Local Anesthetic/Vasoconstrictor Precautions No information available to require special precautions

Effects on Dental Treatment Tissue retraction around base of the tooth (therapeutic effect)

Dosage Pass the impregnated yarn around the neck of the tooth and place into gingival sulcus; normal tissue moisture, water, or gingival retraction solutions activate impregnated yarn. Limit use to one quadrant of the mouth at a time; recommended use is for 3-8 minutes in the mouth.

Mechanism of Action Epinephrine stimulates $alpha_1$ adrenergic receptors to cause vasoconstriction in blood vessels in gingiva; aluminum potassium sulfate, precipitates tissue and blood proteins

Contraindications Hypersensitivity to epinephrine or any component of the formulation; cardiovascular disease, hyperthyroidism, or diabetes; do not apply to areas of heavy or deep bleeding or over exposed bone

Warnings/Precautions Caution should be exercised whenever using gingival retraction cords with epinephrine since it delivers vasoconstrictor doses of racemic epinephrine to patients; the general medical history should be thoroughly evaluated before using in any patient

Pharmacodynamics/Kinetics No data reported

Dosage Forms YARN [saturated in solution of 8% racemic epinephrine and 7% aluminum potassium sulfate]: Type "0e": 0.20 ±0.10 mg epinephrine/inch; Type "1e": 0.40 ±0.20 mg epinephrine/inch; Type "2e": 0.60 ±0.20 mg epinephrine/inch

Generic Available No

Epipodophyllotoxin *see* Etoposide *on page 549*

Epirubicin

(ep i ROO bi sin)

U.S. Brand Names Ellence®

Canadian Brand Names Ellence®; Pharmorubicin®

Mexican Brand Names Epilem®; Farmorubicin®

Pharmacologic Category Antineoplastic Agent, Anthracycline

Use As a component of adjuvant therapy following primary resection of primary breast cancer in patients with evidence of axillary node tumor involvement

Local Anesthetic/Vasoconstrictor Precautions No information available to require special precautions

Effects on Dental Treatment

>10%: Mucositis (9% to 59%), lethargy (1% to 46%), hot flashes (5% to 39%), nausea, vomiting (83% to 92%), infection (15% to 21%)

1% to 10%: CHF (0.4% to 1.5%), fever (1% to 5%), hypersensitivity, anaphylaxis

Dosage

Adults: I.V.:

Recommended starting dose: 100-120 mg/m^2. Epirubicin is given in repeated 3- to 4-week cycles with the total dose given on day 1 of each cycle or divided equally and given on days 1 and 8 of each cycle. Patients receiving the 120 mg/m^2 regimen should also receive prophylactic antibiotics with TMP-SMX or a fluoroquinolone.

As a component of adjuvant therapy in patients with axillary-node positive breast cancer:

CEF-120: 60 mg/m^2 on days 1 and 8 of cycle (in combination with cyclophosphamide and 5-fluorouracil); cycle is repeated every 28 days for 6 cycles

FEC-100: 100 mg/m^2 on day 1 of cycle (in combination with 5-fluorouracil and cyclophosphamide); cycle is repeated every 21 days for 6 cycles

Dosing adjustment in bone marrow dysfunction:

Patients with heavy pretreatment, pre-existing bone marrow depression, or the presence of neoplastic bone marrow infiltration: Consider lower starting doses of 75-90 mg/m^2

Dosage modifications after the first treatment cycle: Nadir platelet counts <50,000/mm^3, ANC <250/mm^3, neutropenic fever, or grades 3/4 nonhematologic toxicity: Reduce day 1 dose in subsequent cycles to 75% of the current cycle. Day 1 chemotherapy in subsequent courses of treatment should be delayed until platelet counts are ≥100,000/mm^3, ANC ≥1500/mm^3, and nonhematologic toxicities have recovered to ≤ grade 1.

(Continued)

Epirubicin *(Continued)*

In addition, for patients receiving divided dose (day 1 and day 8) regimen:

Day 8 platelet counts 75,000-100,000/mm^3 and ANC 1000-1499/mm^3: Day 8 dose should be 75% of the day 1 dose

Day 8 platelet counts <75,000/mm^3, ANC <1000/mm^3, or grade 3 or 4 nonhematologic toxicity: Omit day 8 dose

Dosing adjustment in renal impairment: Severe renal impairment (serum creatinine >5 mg/dL): Lower doses should be considered

Dosing adjustment in hepatic impairment:

Bilirubin 1.2-3 mg/dL or AST 2-4 times the upper limit of normal: 50% of recommended starting dose

Bilirubin >3 mg/dL or AST >4 times the upper limit of normal: 25% of recommended starting dose

Elderly: Plasma clearance of epirubicin in elderly female patients was noted to be reduced by 35%. Although no initial dosage reduction is specifically recommended, particular care should be exercised in monitoring toxicity and adjusting subsequent dosage in elderly patients (particularly females >70 years).

Mechanism of Action Epirubicin is an anthracycline cytotoxic agent. The precise mechanism of its cytotoxic and antiproliferative effect has not been elucidated. Epirubicin is known to inhibit DNA and RNA synthesis by steric obstruction after intercalating between DNA base pairs; active throughout entire cell cycle. Intercalation triggers DNA cleavage by topoisomerase II, resulting in cytocidal activity. Epirubicin also inhibits DNA helicase, and generates cytotoxic free radicals.

Other Adverse Effects Vesicant chemotherapy. Epirubicin infiltration can cause severe inflammation, tissue necrosis, and ulceration. If the drug is infiltrated, consult institutional policy, apply ice to the area, and elevate the limb. Can have ongoing tissue destruction secondary to propagation of free radicals; may require debridement.

Grade 3 and 4 leukopenia may occur in 1.5% to 58.6% of patients, depending on the protocol and dosage of epirubicin. Grade 3 or 4 gastrointestinal toxicity was noted to occur in 22% to 25% of patients.

>10%:

Dermatologic: Alopecia (69% to 95%)

Endocrine & metabolic: Amenorrhea (69% to 72%)

Gastrointestinal: Diarrhea (7% to 25%)

Hematologic: Leukopenia (49% to 80%), neutropenia (54% to 80%), anemia (13% to 72%), thrombocytopenia (5% to 49%)

Local: Injection site reactions (3% to 20%)

Ocular: Conjunctivitis (1% to 15%)

1% to 10%:

Cardiovascular: Decreased LVEF (asymptomatic) (1.4% to 1.8%)

Dermatologic: Rash (1% to 9%), skin changes (0.7% to 5%)

Gastrointestinal: Anorexia (2% to 3%)

Other reactions (percentage not specified): Acute myelogenous leukemia (0.2% at 3 years), acute lymphoid leukemia, increased transaminases, radiation recall, skin and nail hyperpigmentation, photosensitivity reaction, urticaria, premature menopause in women

Drug Interactions Increased Effect/Toxicity: Cimetidine increased the blood levels of epirubicin (AUC increased by 50%).

Dietary/Ethanol/Herb Considerations

Ethanol: Avoid use due to GI irritation.

Herb/Nutraceutical: Avoid black cohosh and dong quai in estrogen-dependent tumors. Avoid St John's wort; may decrease serum concentration.

Pharmacodynamics/Kinetics

Distribution: V_{ss} 21-27 L/kg

Protein binding: 77% to albumin

Metabolism: Extensively via hepatic and extrahepatic (including RBCs) routes

Half-life elimination: Triphasic; Mean terminal: 33 hours

Excretion: Feces; urine (lesser extent)

Pregnancy Risk Factor D

Generic Available No

Epitol® *see* Carbamazepine *on page 241*

Epivir® *see* Lamivudine *on page 773*

Epivir-HBV® *see* Lamivudine *on page 773*

Eplerenone (e PLER en one)

U.S. Brand Names Inspra™

Pharmacologic Category Antihypertensive; Selective Aldosterone Blocker

Use Treatment of hypertension; may be used alone or in combination with other antihypertensive agents

Local Anesthetic/Vasoconstrictor Precautions No information available to require special precautions

Effects on Dental Treatment

1% to 10%: Dizziness (3%), fatigue (2%), cough (2%), flu-like syndrome (2%)

Dosage Oral:

Adults: Hypertension: Initial: 50 mg once daily; may increase to 50 mg twice daily if response is not adequate; may take up to 4 weeks for full therapeutic response. Doses >100 mg/day are associated with increased risk of hyperkalemia and no greater therapeutic effect.

Concurrent use with weak CYP3A4 inhibitors: Initial: 25 mg once daily

Elderly: Use with caution due to possible increased risk of hyperkalemia.

Dosing adjustment in renal impairment: Contraindicated with Cl_{cr} <50 mL/minute or serum creatinine >2.0 mg/dL in males or >1.8 mg/dL in females; risk of hyperkalemia increases with decreased renal function

Mechanism of Action Aldosterone increases blood pressure primarily by inducing sodium reabsorption. Eplerenone reduces blood pressure by blocking aldosterone binding at mineralocorticoid receptors found in the kidney, heart, blood vessels and brain.

Other Adverse Effects

>10%: Endocrine & metabolic: Hypertriglyceridemia (1% to 15%, dose-related)

1% to 10%:

Endocrine & metabolic: Hyponatremia (2%, dose-related), hypercholesterolemia (<1% to 1%), hyperkalemia (dose-related, up to 1% at maximum recommended dose), breast pain (males <1% to 1%), gynecomastia (males <1% to 1%)

Gastrointestinal: Diarrhea (2%), abdominal pain (1%)

Genitourinary: Abnormal vaginal bleeding (<1% to 2%)

Renal: Albuminuria (1%)

<1%: BUN increased, LFTs increased, serum creatinine increased, uric acid increased

Drug Interactions Substrate of **CYP3A4**

Increased Effect/Toxicity: ACE inhibitors, angiotensin II receptor antagonists, NSAIDs, potassium supplements, and potassium-sparing diuretics increase the risk of hyperkalemia; concomitant use with potassium supplements and potassium sparing diuretics is contraindicated; monitor potassium levels with ACE inhibitors and angiotensin II receptor antagonists. Potent CYP3A3/4 inhibitors (ie, itraconazole, ketoconazole) lead to five-fold increase in eplerenone; concurrent use is contraindicated. Less potent CYP3A3/4 inhibitors (ie, erythromycin, fluconazole, saquinavir, verapamil) lead to approximately two-fold increase in eplerenone; starting dose should be decreased to 25 mg/day. Although interaction studies have not been conducted, monitoring of lithium levels is recommended.

Decreased Effect: NSAIDs may decrease the antihypertensive effects of eplerenone.

Dietary/Ethanol/Herb Considerations

Food: May be taken with food. Grapefruit juice increases eplerenone AUC ~25%. Do not use salt substitutes containing potassium.

Herb/Nutraceutical: St John's wort decreases eplerenone AUC ~30%.

Pharmacodynamics/Kinetics

Distribution: V_d: 43-90 L

Protein binding: ~50%; primarily to $alpha_1$-acid glycoproteins

Metabolism: Primarily hepatic via CYP3A4; metabolites inactive

Half-life elimination: 4-6 hours

Time to peak, plasma: 1.5 hours; may take up to 4 weeks for full therapeutic effect

Excretion: Urine (67%; <5% as unchanged drug), feces (32%)

Pregnancy Risk Factor B

Generic Available No

EPO *see* Epoetin Alfa *on page 503*

Epoetin Alfa (e POE e tin AL fu)

U.S. Brand Names Epogen®; Procrit®

Canadian Brand Names Eprex®

Mexican Brand Names Epomax®; Eprex®

Pharmacologic Category Colony Stimulating Factor

Synonyms EPO; Erythropoietin; *r*HuEPO-α

Use

Treatment of anemia related to zidovudine therapy in HIV-infected patients; in patients when the endogenous erythropoietin level is ≤500 mU/mL and the dose of zidovudine is ≤4200 mg/week

Treatment of anemia in cancer patients on chemotherapy; in patients with nonmyeloid malignancies where anemia is caused by the effect of the concomitantly administered chemotherapy; to decrease the need for transfusions in patients who will be receiving chemotherapy for a minimum of 2 months

Reduction of allogeneic block transfusion in surgery patients scheduled to undergo elective, noncardiac, nonvascular surgery

Orphan drug (Epogen®): Treatment of anemia associated with end-stage renal disease; treatment of anemia associated with HIV infection or HIV treatment

(Continued)

Epoetin Alfa *(Continued)*

Unlabeled/Investigational Use Treatment of anemia associated with rheumatic disease, hypogenerative anemia of Rh hemolytic disease, sickle cell anemia, acute renal failure, Gaucher's disease, Castleman's disease, paroxysmal nocturnal hemoglobinuria

Local Anesthetic/Vasoconstrictor Precautions No information available to require special precautions

Effects on Dental Treatment

>10%: Hypertension, fatigue, headache, fever

1% to 10%: Chest pain, seizures, nausea, vomiting

Dosage

Chronic renal failure patients: I.V., S.C.:

Initial dose: 50-100 units/kg 3 times/week

Reduce dose by 25 units/kg when

1) hematocrit approaches 36% **or**

2) when hematocrit increases >4 points in any 2-week period

Increase dose if hematocrit does not increase by 5-6 points after 8 weeks of therapy and hematocrit is below suggested target range

Suggested target hematocrit range: 30% to 36%

Maintenance dose: Individualize to target range

Dialysis patients: Median dose: 75 units/kg 3 times/week

Nondialysis patients: Doses of 75-150 units/kg

Zidovudine-treated, HIV-infected patients: Patients with erythropoietin levels >500 mU/mL are **unlikely** to respond

Initial dose: I.V., S.C.: 100 units/kg 3 times/week for 8 weeks

Increase dose by 50-100 units/kg 3 times/week if response is not satisfactory in terms of reducing transfusion requirements or increasing hematocrit after 8 weeks of therapy

Evaluate response every 4-8 weeks thereafter and adjust the dose accordingly by 50-100 units/kg increments 3 times/week

If patients have not responded satisfactorily to a 300 unit/kg dose 3 times/week, it is unlikely that they will respond to higher doses

Stop dose if hematocrit exceeds 40% and resume treatment at a 25% dose reduction when hematocrit drops to 36%

Cancer patients on chemotherapy: Treatment of patients with erythropoietin levels >200 mU/mL is **not recommended**

Initial dose: S.C.: 150 units/kg 3 times/week

Dose adjustment: If response is not satisfactory in terms of reducing transfusion requirement or increasing hematocrit after 8 weeks of therapy, the dose may be increased up to 300 units/kg 3 times/week. If patients do not respond, it is unlikely that they will respond to higher doses.

If hematocrit exceeds 40%, hold the dose until it falls to 36% and reduce the dose by 25% when treatment is resumed

Surgery patients: Prior to initiating treatment, obtain a hemoglobin to establish that is >10 mg/dL or ≤13 mg/dL

Initial dose: S.C.: 300 units/kg/day for 10 days before surgery, on the day of surgery, and for 4 days after surgery

Alternative dose: S.C.: 600 units/kg in once weekly doses (21, 14, and 7 days before surgery) plus a fourth dose on the day of surgery

Mechanism of Action Induces erythropoiesis by stimulating the division and differentiation of committed erythroid progenitor cells; induces the release of reticulocytes from the bone marrow into the bloodstream, where they mature to erythrocytes. There is a dose response relationship with this effect. This results in an increase in reticulocyte counts followed by a rise in hematocrit and hemoglobin levels.

Other Adverse Effects

1% to 10%:

Cardiovascular: Edema

Gastrointestinal: Diarrhea

Hematologic: Clotted access

Neuromuscular & skeletal: Arthralgias, asthenia

<1%: **MI,** CVA/TIA, rash, **hypersensitivity reactions,** thrombosis, **flu-like syndrome,** hyperkalemia

Pharmacodynamics/Kinetics

Onset of action: Several days

Peak effect: 2-3 weeks

Distribution: V_d: 9 L; rapid in the plasma compartment; concentrated in liver, kidneys, and bone marrow

Metabolism: Some degradation does occur

Bioavailability: S.C.: ~21% to 31%; intraperitoneal epoetin: 3% (a few patients)

Half-life elimination: Circulating: Chronic renal failure: 4-13 hours; Healthy volunteers: 20% shorter

Time to peak, serum: S.C.: 2-8 hours

Excretion: Feces (majority); urine (small amounts, 10% unchanged in normal volunteers)

Pregnancy Risk Factor C
Generic Available No
Comments

Professional Services:
Amgen (Epogen®): 1-800-772-6436
Ortho Biotech (Procrit®): 1-800-325-7504

Reimbursement Assistance:
Amgen: 1-800-272-9376
Ortho Biotech: 1-800-553-3851

Epogen® *see* Epoetin Alfa *on page 503*

Epoprostenol (e poe PROST en ole)

U.S. Brand Names Flolan®
Canadian Brand Names Flolan®
Pharmacologic Category Prostaglandin
Synonyms Epoprostenol Sodium; PGI_2; PGX; Prostacyclin
Use Orphan drug: Treatment of primary pulmonary hypertension; treatment of secondary pulmonary hypertension due to intrinsic precapillary pulmonary vascular disease
Unlabeled/Investigational Use Treatment of atherosclerosis, peripheral vascular disorders, neonatal pulmonary hypertension, neonatal purpura fulminans, and pulmonary hypertension associated with ARDS, SLE, or CHF; cardiopulmonary bypass surgery; hemodialysis
Local Anesthetic/Vasoconstrictor Precautions No information available to require special precautions
Effects on Dental Treatment No significant effects or complications reported
Restrictions Orders for epoprostenol are distributed by two sources in the United States. Information on orders or reimbursement assistance may be obtained from either Accredo Health, Inc (1-800-935-6526) or TheraCom, Inc (1-877-356-5264).
Dosage The drug is administered by continuous intravenous infusion via a central venous catheter using an ambulatory infusion pump. During dose ranging it may be administered peripherally.

I.V.:

Acute dose ranging: The initial infusion rate should be 2 ng/kg/minute by continuous I.V. and increased in increments of 2 ng/kg/minute every 15 minutes or longer until dose-limiting effects are elicited (such as chest pain, anxiety, dizziness, changes in heart rate, dyspnea, nausea, vomiting, headache, hypotension and/or flushing)

Continuous chronic infusion: Initial: 4 ng/kg/minute **less** than the maximum-tolerated infusion rate determined during acute dose ranging

If maximum-tolerated infusion rate is <5 ng/kg/minute, the chronic infusion rate should be $1/2$ the maximum-tolerated acute infusion rate

Dosing adjustments: Adjustments in the chronic infusion rate should be based on persistence, recurrence, or worsening of patient symptoms of pulmonary hypertension. If symptoms persist or recur after improving, the infusion rate should be increased by 1-2 ng/kg/minute increments, every 15 minutes or greater; following establishment of a new chronic infusion rate, the patient should be observed and vital signs monitored.

Mechanism of Action Epoprostenol is also known as prostacyclin and PGI_2. It is a strong vasodilator of all vascular beds. In addition, it is a potent endogenous inhibitor of platelet aggregation. The reduction in platelet aggregation results from epoprostenol's activation of intracellular adenylate cyclase and the resultant increase in cyclic adenosine monophosphate concentrations within the platelets. Additionally, it is capable of decreasing thrombogenesis and platelet clumping in the lungs by inhibiting platelet aggregation.
Other Adverse Effects <1%, postmarketing, and/or case reports: Anemia, hypersplenism, hyperthyroidism, pancytopenia, splenomegaly
Drug Interactions Increased Effect/Toxicity: The hypotensive effects of epoprostenol may be exacerbated by other vasodilators, diuretics, or by using acetate in dialysis fluids. Patients treated with anticoagulants (heparins, warfarin, thrombin inhibitors) or antiplatelet agents (ticlopidine, clopidogrel, IIb/IIIa antagonists, aspirin) and epoprostenol should be monitored for increased bleeding risk.
Pharmacodynamics/Kinetics

Metabolism: Rapidly hydrolyzed at neutral pH in blood and subject to some enzymatic degradation to one active metabolite and 13 inactive metabolites

Half-life elimination: 2.7-6 minutes; Continuous infusion: ~15 minutes

Excretion: Urine (12% as unchanged drug)

Pregnancy Risk Factor B
Generic Available No

Epoprostenol Sodium *see* Epoprostenol *on page 505*

Eprosartan (ep roe SAR tan)

U.S. Brand Names Teveten®

Canadian Brand Names Teveten®

Pharmacologic Category Angiotensin II Receptor Blocker

Use Treatment of hypertension; may be used alone or in combination with other antihypertensives

Local Anesthetic/Vasoconstrictor Precautions No information available to require special precautions

Effects on Dental Treatment 1% to 10%: Fatigue (2%), upper respiratory tract infection (8%), rhinitis (4%), pharyngitis (4%), cough (4%), viral infection (2%), injury (2%)

Dosage Oral:

Adults: Dosage must be individualized; can administer once or twice daily with total daily doses of 400-800 mg. Usual starting dose is 600 mg once daily as monotherapy in patients who are euvolemic. Limited clinical experience with doses >800 mg.

Dosing adjustment for elderly or in renal/hepatic impairment: No starting dosage adjustment required; monitor carefully

Mechanism of Action Angiotensin II is formed from angiotensin I in a reaction catalyzed by angiotensin-converting enzyme (ACE, kininase II). Angiotensin II is the principal pressor agent of the renin-angiotensin system, with effects that include vasoconstriction, stimulation of synthesis and release of aldosterone, cardiac stimulation, and renal reabsorption of sodium. Eprosartan blocks the vasoconstrictor and aldosterone-secreting effects of angiotensin II by selectively blocking the binding of angiotensin II to the AT1 receptor in many tissues, such as vascular smooth muscle and the adrenal gland. Its action is therefore independent of the pathways for angiotensin II synthesis. Blockade of the renin-angiotensin system with ACE inhibitors, which inhibit the biosynthesis of angiotensin II from angiotensin I, is widely used in the treatment of hypertension. ACE inhibitors also inhibit the degradation of bradykinin, a reaction also catalyzed by ACE. Because eprosartan does not inhibit ACE (kininase II), it does not affect the response to bradykinin. Whether this difference has clinical relevance is not yet known. Eprosartan does not bind to or block other hormone receptors or ion channels known to be important in cardiovascular regulation.

Other Adverse Effects

1% to 10%:

Central nervous system: Depression (1%)

Endocrine & metabolic: Hypertriglyceridemia (1%)

Gastrointestinal: Abdominal pain (2%)

Genitourinary: Urinary tract infection (1%)

<1% (Limited to important or life-threatening): Ethanol intolerance, **weakness, substernal chest pain, facial edema**, peripheral edema, **fatigue, fever, hot flashes, influenza-like symptoms, malaise, rigors, pain, angina pectoris, bradycardia,** abnormal EKG, extrasystoles, **atrial fibrillation, hypotension, tachycardia, palpitations,** anorexia, constipation, **esophagitis,** flatulence, **gastritis, gastroenteritis, gingivitis nausea, periodontitis, toothache, vomiting,** anemia, purpura, increased transaminases, increased creatine phosphokinase, **diabetes mellitus,** glycosuria, gout, hypercholesterolemia, **hyperglycemia,** hyperkalemia, hypokalemia, hyponatremia, **arthritis, aggravated arthritis,** arthrosis, skeletal pain, tendonitis, back pain, **anxiety,** ataxia, insomnia, **migraine,** neuritis, **nervousness, paresthesia, somnolence, tremor,** vertigo, **herpes simplex, otitis externa, otitis media, asthma, epistaxis**, eczema, furunculosis, pruritus, rash, maculopapular rash, **increased diaphoresis,** conjunctivitis, **abnormal vision,** xerophthalmia, tinnitus, albuminuria, cystitis, hematuria, micturition frequency, polyuria, renal calculus, urinary incontinence, **leg cramps,** peripheral ischemia, increases in BUN or creatinine, leukopenia, neutropenia, thrombocytopenia, **xerostomia**

Drug Interactions Inhibits CYP2C8/9

Increased Effect/Toxicity: Eprosartan may increase risk of lithium toxicity. May increase risk of hyperkalemia with potassium-sparing diuretics (eg, amiloride, potassium, spironolactone, triamterene), potassium supplements, or high doses of trimethoprim.

Dietary/Ethanol/Herb Considerations

Ethanol: Avoid use; may increase risk of hypotension or dizziness.

Food: Avoid caffeine and garlic.

Herb/Nutraceutical: Avoid black cohosh, dong quai, and evening primrose due to estrogenic activity. Avoid ephedra, ginseng, and yohimbe; may worsen hypertension. Avoid garlic; may have increased antihypertensive effect. Avoid ginger due to positive inotropic effects; theoretically, may cause arrhythmia. Avoid hawthorn; may lower peripheral vascular resistance resulting in additive decrease in BP.

Pharmacodynamics/Kinetics

Protein binding: 98%

Metabolism: Minimally hepatic

Bioavailability: 300 mg dose: 13%

Half-life elimination: Terminal: 5-9 hours

Time to peak, serum: Fasting: 1-2 hours
Excretion: Feces (90%); urine (7%, mostly as unchanged drug)
Clearance: 7.9 L/hour

Pregnancy Risk Factor C (1st trimester); D (2nd and 3rd trimesters)

Generic Available No

Epsom Salts (Magnesium Sulfate) *see* Magnesium Supplements *on page 837*

EPT *see* Teniposide *on page 1274*

Eptifibatide (ep TIF i ba tide)

Related Information

Cardiovascular Diseases *on page 1456*

U.S. Brand Names Integrilin®

Canadian Brand Names Integrilin®

Pharmacologic Category Antiplatelet Agent, Glycoprotein IIb/IIIa Inhibitor

Synonyms Intrifiban

Use Treatment of patients with acute coronary syndrome (UA/NQMI), including patients who are to be managed medically and those undergoing percutaneous coronary intervention (PCI including PTCA; intracoronary stenting)

Local Anesthetic/Vasoconstrictor Precautions No information available to require special precautions

Effects on Dental Treatment

>10%: Bleeding (4.4% to 10.8% major; 10.5% to 14.2% minor); patients weighing <70 kg may have an increased risk of major bleeding

Frequency not defined: Hypotension

Dosage I.V.: Adults:

Acute coronary syndrome: Bolus of 180 mcg/kg (maximum: 22.6 mg) over 1-2 minutes, begun as soon as possible following diagnosis, followed by a continuous infusion of 2 mcg/kg/minute (maximum: 15 mg/hour) until hospital discharge or initiation of CABG surgery, up to 72 hours. Concurrent aspirin (160-325 mg initially and daily thereafter) and heparin therapy (target aPTT 50-70 seconds) are recommended.

Percutaneous coronary intervention (PCI) with or without stenting: Bolus of 180 mcg/kg (maximum: 22.6 mg) administered immediately before the initiation of PCI, followed by a continuous infusion of 2 mcg/kg/minute (maximum: 15 mg/hour). A second 180 mcg/kg bolus (maximum: 22.6 mg) should be administered 10 minutes after the first bolus. Infusion should be continued until hospital discharge or for up to 18-24 hours, whichever comes first; minimum of 12 hours of infusion is recommended. Concurrent aspirin (160-325 mg 1-24 hours before PCI and daily thereafter) and heparin therapy (ACT 200-300 seconds during PCI) are recommended. Heparin infusion after PCI is discouraged. In patients who undergo coronary artery bypass graft surgery, discontinue infusion prior to surgery.

Dosing adjustment in renal impairment:

Acute coronary syndrome: S_{cr} >2 mg/dL and <4 mg/dL: Use 180 mcg/kg bolus (maximum: 22.6 mg) and 1 mcg/kg/minute infusion (maximum: 7.5 mg/hour)

Percutaneous coronary intervention (PCI) with or without stenting: Adults: S_{cr} >2 mg/dL and <4 mg/dL: Use 180 mcg/kg bolus (maximum: 22.6 mg) administered immediately before the initiation of PCI and followed by a continuous infusion of 1 mcg/kg/minute (maximum: 7.5 mg/hour). A second 180 mcg/kg (maximum: 22.6 mg) bolus should be administered 10 minutes after the first bolus.

Mechanism of Action Eptifibatide is a cyclic heptapeptide which blocks the platelet glycoprotein IIb/IIIa receptor, the binding site for fibrinogen, von Willebrand factor, and other ligands. Inhibition of binding at this final common receptor reversibly blocks platelet aggregation and prevents thrombosis.

Other Adverse Effects

Local: Injection site reaction

Neuromuscular & skeletal: Back pain

1% to 10%: Hematologic: Thrombocytopenia (1.2% to 3.2%)

<1% (Limited to important or life-threatening): Intracranial hemorrhage (0.5% to 0.7%), **anaphylaxis**

Postmarketing and/or case reports: **GI hemorrhage,** pulmonary hemorrhage

Drug Interactions Increased Effect/Toxicity: Eptifibatide effect may be increased by other drugs which affect hemostasis include thrombolytics, oral anticoagulants, NSAIDs, dipyridamole, heparin, low molecular weight heparins, ticlopidine, and clopidogrel. Avoid concomitant use of other IIb/IIIa inhibitors. Cephalosporins which contain the MTT side chain may theoretically increase the risk of hemorrhage. Use with aspirin and heparin may increase bleeding over aspirin and heparin alone. However, aspirin and heparin were used concurrently in the majority of patients in the major clinical studies of eptifibatide.

Pharmacodynamics/Kinetics

Onset of action: Within 1 hour

Duration: Platelet function restored ~4 hours following discontinuation

Protein binding: ~25%

Half-life elimination: 2.5 hours

(Continued)

Eptifibatide *(Continued)*

Excretion: Primarily urine (as eptifibatide and metabolites); significant renal impairment may alter disposition of this compound

Clearance: Total body: 55-58 mL/kg/hour; Renal: ~50% of total in healthy subjects

Pregnancy Risk Factor B

Generic Available No

Equagesic® *see* Aspirin and Meprobamate *on page 136*
Equalactin® Chewable Tablet [OTC] *see* Calcium Polycarbophil *on page 228*
Equilet® [OTC] *see* Calcium Supplements *on page 229*
Ergamisol® *see* Levamisole *on page 786*

Ergocalciferol (er goe kal SIF e role)

U.S. Brand Names Calciferol™; Drisdol®

Canadian Brand Names Drisdol®; Ostoforte®

Pharmacologic Category Vitamin D Analog

Synonyms Activated Ergosterol; Viosterol; Vitamin D_2

Use Treatment of refractory rickets, hypophosphatemia, hypoparathyroidism

Local Anesthetic/Vasoconstrictor Precautions No information available to require special precautions

Effects on Dental Treatment Frequency not defined: Hypotension, cardiac arrhythmias, hypertension (late), irritability, headache, somnolence, nausea, vomiting, metallic taste, xerostomia, weakness

Dosage Oral dosing is preferred; I.M. therapy required with GI, liver, or biliary disease associated with malabsorption

Dietary supplementation (each mcg = 40 USP units):
- Premature infants: 10-20 mcg/day (400-800 units), up to 750 mcg/day (30,000 units)
- Infants and healthy Children: 10 mcg/day (400 units)
- Adults: 10 mcg/day (400 units)

Renal failure:
- Children: 100-1000 mcg/day (4000-40,000 units)
- Adults: 500 mcg/day (20,000 units)

Hypoparathyroidism:
- Children: 1.25-5 mg/day (50,000-200,000 units) and calcium supplements
- Adults: 625 mcg to 5 mg/day (25,000-200,000 units) and calcium supplements

Vitamin D-dependent rickets:
- Children: 75-125 mcg/day (3000-5000 units); maximum: 1500 mcg/day
- Adults: 250 mcg to 1.5 mg/day (10,000-60,000 units)

Nutritional rickets and osteomalacia:
- Children and Adults (with normal absorption): 25-125 mcg/day (1000-5000 units)
- Children with malabsorption: 250-625 mcg/day (10,000-25,000 units)
- Adults with malabsorption: 250-7500 mcg (10,000-300,000 units)

Vitamin D-resistant rickets:
- Children: Initial: 1000-2000 mcg/day (40,000-80,000 units) with phosphate supplements; daily dosage is increased at 3- to 4-month intervals in 250-500 mcg (10,000-20,000 units) increments
- Adults: 250-1500 mcg/day (10,000-60,000 units) with phosphate supplements

Familial hypophosphatemia: 10,000-80,000 units daily plus 1-2 g/day elemental phosphorus

Osteoporosis prophylaxis: Adults:
- 51-70 years: 400 units/day
- >70 years: 600 units/day
- Maximum daily dose: 2000 units/day

Mechanism of Action Stimulates calcium and phosphate absorption from the small intestine, promotes secretion of calcium from bone to blood; promotes renal tubule phosphate resorption

Other Adverse Effects Frequency not defined:
- Central nervous system: **Psychoses (rare)**, hyperthermia (late)
- Dermatologic: Pruritus
- Endocrine & metabolic: Polydipsia, hypermagnesemia, decreased libido (late), hypercholesterolemia, mild acidosis (late), polydipsia (late)
- Gastrointestinal: Constipation, anorexia, pancreatitis, weight loss (rare), constipation
- Genitourinary: Polyuria (late)
- Hepatic: Increased LFTs
- Neuromuscular & skeletal: Myalgia, bone pain
- Ocular: Conjunctivitis, photophobia (late)
- Renal: Increased BUN (late), vascular/nephrocalcinosis (rare)

Drug Interactions

Increased Effect/Toxicity: Thiazide diuretics may increase vitamin D effects. Cardiac glycosides may increase toxicity.

Decreased Effect: Cholestyramine, colestipol, mineral oil may decrease oral absorption.

Pharmacodynamics/Kinetics

Onset of action: Peak effect: ~1 month following daily doses

Absorption: Readily; requires bile

Metabolism: Inactive until hydroxylated hepatically and renally to calcifediol and then to calcitriol (most active form)

Pregnancy Risk Factor A/C (dose exceeding RDA recommendation)

Generic Available Yes

Ergoloid Mesylates (ER goe loid MES i lates)

Canadian Brand Names Hydergine®

Pharmacologic Category Ergot Derivative

Synonyms Dihydroergotoxine; Dihydrogenated Ergot Alkaloids

Use Treatment of cerebrovascular insufficiency in primary progressive dementia, Alzheimer's dementia, and senile onset

Local Anesthetic/Vasoconstrictor Precautions No information available to require special precautions

Effects on Dental Treatment Frequency not defined: Orthostatic hypotension, bradycardia, flushing, GI disturbances, transient nausea, blurred vision, nasal congestion, sublingual irritation (SL tablets)

Dosage Adults: Oral: 1 mg 3 times/day up to 4.5-12 mg/day; up to 6 months of therapy may be necessary

Mechanism of Action Ergoloid mesylates do not have the vasoconstrictor effects of the natural ergot alkaloids; exact mechanism in dementia is unknown; originally classed as peripheral and cerebral vasodilator, now considered a "metabolic enhancer"; there is no specific evidence which clearly establishes the mechanism by which ergoloid mesylate preparations produce mental effects, nor is there conclusive evidence that the drug particularly affects cerebral arteriosclerosis or cerebrovascular insufficiency

Other Adverse Effects Frequency not defined: Dermatologic: Skin rash

Drug Interactions Substrate of **CYP3A4**

Increased effect with antifungals (azole derivatives); CYP3A4 inhibitors (eg, amiodarone, cimetidine, erythromycin, ritonavir); macrolide antibiotics; protease inhibitors; MAO inhibitors; beta blockers (vasoconstriction); sumatriptan (vasospasm); vasoconstrictors. Ergoloid mesylates may increase the effects of sibutramine and other serotonin agonists (serotonin syndrome).

Decreased effect with antipsychotics, metoclopramide.

Pharmacodynamics/Kinetics

Absorption: Rapid yet incomplete

Half-life elimination, serum: 3.5 hours

Time to peak, serum: ~1 hour

Pregnancy Risk Factor C

Generic Available Yes

Ergomar® *see* Ergotamine *on page 510*

Ergometrine Maleate *see* Ergonovine *on page 509*

Ergonovine (er goe NOE veen)

Pharmacologic Category Ergot Derivative

Synonyms Ergometrine Maleate; Ergonovine Maleate

Use Prevention and treatment of postpartum and postabortion hemorrhage caused by uterine atony or subinvolution

Unlabeled/Investigational Use Treatment of migraine headaches; diagnosis of Prinzmetal's angina

Local Anesthetic/Vasoconstrictor Precautions No information available to require special precautions

Effects on Dental Treatment 1% to 10%: Nausea, vomiting

Dosage Adults: I.M., I.V. (I.V. should be reserved for emergency use only): 0.2 mg, repeat dose in 2-4 hours as needed

Mechanism of Action Ergot alkaloid alpha-adrenergic agonist directly stimulates vascular smooth muscle to vasoconstrict peripheral and cerebral vessels; may also have antagonist effects on serotonin

Other Adverse Effects <1%: **Palpitations, bradycardia, transient chest pain, hypertension (sometimes extreme - treat with I.V. chlorpromazine),** cerebrovascular accidents, **shock, MI,** ergotism, **seizures, dizziness, headache,** thrombophlebitis, tinnitus, **dyspnea, diaphoresis**

Drug Interactions Substrate of **CYP3A4**

Increased effect with antifungals (azole derivatives); CYP3A4 inhibitors (eg, amiodarone, cimetidine, erythromycin, ritonavir); macrolide antibiotics; protease inhibitors; MAO inhibitors; beta blockers (vasoconstriction); sumatriptan (vasospasm); vasoconstrictors. Ergonovine may increase the effects of sibutramine and other serotonin agonists (serotonin syndrome).

Decreased effect with antipsychotics, metoclopramide.

(Continued)

Ergonovine *(Continued)*

Pharmacodynamics/Kinetics

Onset of action: I.M.: ~2-5 minutes

Duration: I.M.: Uterine effect: 3 hours; I.V.: ~45 minutes

Metabolism: Hepatic

Excretion: Primarily feces; urine

Pregnancy Risk Factor X

Generic Available No

Ergonovine Maleate *see* Ergonovine *on page 509*

Ergotamine (er GOT a meen)

U.S. Brand Names Cafergot®; Ergomar®; Wigraine®

Canadian Brand Names Cafergor®

Mexican Brand Names Ergocaf; Sydolil

Pharmacologic Category Ergot Derivative

Synonyms Ergotamine Tartrate; Ergotamine Tartrate and Caffeine

Use Abort or prevent vascular headaches, such as migraine, migraine variants, or so-called "histaminic cephalalgia"

Local Anesthetic/Vasoconstrictor Precautions No information available to require special precautions

Effects on Dental Treatment

>10%: Xerostomia, changes in salivation

Frequency not defined: Bradycardia, hypertension, tachycardia, vasospasm, nausea, vomiting, muscle pain, numbness, paresthesias, weakness

Dosage

Oral (Cafergot®, Wigraine®): 2 tablets at onset of attack; then 1 tablet every 30 minutes as needed; maximum: 6 tablets per attack; do not exceed 10 tablets/week.

Sublingual (Ergomar®): 1 tablet under tongue at first sign, then 1 tablet every 30 minutes if needed; maximum dose: 3 tablets/24 hours, 5 tablets/week

Rectal (Cafergot®): 1 suppository rectally at first sign of an attack; follow with second dose after 1 hour, if needed; maximum: 2 per attack; do not exceed 5/week.

Mechanism of Action Has partial agonist and/or antagonist activity against tryptaminergic, dopaminergic and alpha-adrenergic receptors depending upon their site; is a highly active uterine stimulant; it causes constriction of peripheral and cranial blood vessels and produces depression of central vasomotor centers

Other Adverse Effects Frequency not defined:

Cardiovascular: Absence of pulse, cardiac valvular fibrosis, cyanosis, edema, EKG changes, gangrene, ischemia, precordial distress and pain

Central nervous system: Vertigo

Dermatologic: Itching

Gastrointestinal: Anal or rectal ulcer (with overuse of suppository), nausea, vomiting

Genitourinary: Retroperitoneal fibrosis

Respiratory: Pleuropulmonary fibrosis

Miscellaneous: Cold extremities

Drug Interactions

Ergotamine: Substrate of **CYP3A4**; Inhibits 3A4

Caffeine: Substrate of **1A2**, 2C8/9, 2D6, 2E1, 3A4; Inhibits **1A2**

Increased effect with antifungals (azole derivatives); CYP3A4 inhibitors (eg, amiodarone, cimetidine, erythromycin, ritonavir); macrolide antibiotics; protease inhibitors; MAO inhibitors; beta blockers (vasoconstriction); sumatriptan (vasospasm); vasoconstrictors. Ergotamine may increase the effects of sibutramine and other serotonin agonists (serotonin syndrome). Effects of caffeine may be increased by quinolone antibiotics, CYP1A2 inhibitors (eg, cimetidine, fluvoxamine, ticlopidine); the effects of CYP1A2 substrates (eg, clozapine, doxepin, theophylline) may be increased by caffeine.

Decreased effect with antipsychotics, metoclopramide.

Dietary/Ethanol/Herb Considerations

Ethanol: Avoid use; may cause or worsen headaches.

Food: Caffeine increases GI absorption.

Pharmacodynamics/Kinetics

Absorption: Ergotamine: Oral, rectal: Erratic; enhanced by caffeine coadministration

Metabolism: Extensively hepatic

Time to peak, serum: Ergotamine: 0.5-3 hours

Half-life elimination: 2 hours

Excretion: Feces (90% as metabolites)

Pregnancy Risk Factor X

Generic Available Yes

Ergotamine Tartrate *see* Ergotamine *on page 510*

Ergotamine Tartrate and Caffeine *see* Ergotamine *on page 510*

Ergotamine Tartrate, Belladonna, and Phenobarbital *see* Belladonna, Phenobarbital, and Ergotamine *on page 165*

E•R•O Ear [OTC] *see* Carbamide Peroxide *on page 244*

Errin™ *see* Norethindrone *on page 986*

Ertapenem (er ta PEN em)

U.S. Brand Names Invanz®

Pharmacologic Category Antibiotic, Carbapenem

Synonyms Ertapenem Sodium; L-749,345; MK-0826

Use Treatment of moderate-severe, complicated intra-abdominal infections, skin and skin structure infections, pyelonephritis, acute pelvic infections, and community-acquired pneumonia. Antibacterial coverage includes aerobic gram-positive organisms, aerobic gram-negative organisms, anaerobic organisms.

Methicillin-resistant *Staphylococcus*, *Enterococcus* spp, penicillin-resistant strains of *Streptococcus pneumoniae,* beta-lactamase-positive strains of *Haemophilus influenzae* are **resistant** to ertapenem, as are most *Pseudomonas aeruginosa.*

Local Anesthetic/Vasoconstrictor Precautions No information available to require special precautions

Effects on Dental Treatment

1% to 10%: Chest pain (1%), hypertension (0.7% to 2%), hypotension (1% to 2%), tachycardia (1% to 2%), Headache (6% to 7%), altered mental status (ie, agitation, confusion, disorientation, decreased mental acuity, changed mental status, somnolence, stupor) (3% to 5%), fever (2% to 5%), dizziness (2%), fatigue (1%), anxiety (0.8% to 1%), nausea (6% to 9%), (4%), vomiting (4%), acid regurgitation (1% to 2%), oral candidiasis (0.1% to 1%), leg pain (0.4% to 1%), dyspnea (1% to 3%), cough (1% to 2%), pharyngitis (0.7% to 1%), rales/rhonchi (0.5% to 1%), respiratory distress (0.2% to 1%)

Dosage I.V. therapy may be administered for up to 14 days; I.M. for up to 7 days

Adults: I.V., I.M.:

- Intra-abdominal infection: 1 g/day for 5-14 days
- Skin and skin structure infections: 1 g/day for 7-14 days
- Community-acquired pneumonia: 1 g/day; duration of total antibiotic treatment: 10-14 days
- Urinary tract infections/pyelonephritis: 1 g/day; duration of total antibiotic treatment: 10-14 days
- Acute pelvic infections: 1 g/day for 3-10 days

Dosing adjustment in renal impairment: Cl_{cr} <30 mL/minute: 500 mg/day

Hemodialysis: When the daily dose is given within 6 hours prior to hemodialysis, a supplementary dose of 150 mg is required following hemodialysis.

Dosing adjustment in hepatic impairment: Not studied

Mechanism of Action Inhibits bacterial cell wall synthesis by binding to one or more of the penicillin binding proteins; which in turn inhibits the final transpeptidation step of peptidoglycan synthesis in bacterial cell walls, thus inhibiting cell wall biosynthesis. Bacteria eventually lyse due to ongoing activity of cell wall autolytic enzymes (autolysins and murein hydrolases) while cell wall assembly is arrested.

Other Adverse Effects

1% to 10%:

- Cardiovascular: Swelling/edema (3%)
- Central nervous system: Insomnia (3%)
- Dermatologic: Rash (2% to 3%), pruritus (1% to 2%), erythema (1% to 2%)
- Gastrointestinal: Diarrhea (9% to 10%), abdominal pain constipation (3% to 4%), dyspepsia (1%)
- Genitourinary: Vaginitis (1% to 3%)
- Hematologic: Platelet count increased (4% to 7%), eosinophils increased (1% to 2%)
- Hepatic: Hepatic enzyme elevations (7% to 9%), alkaline phosphatase increase (4% to 7%)
- Local: Infused vein complications (5% to 7%), phlebitis/thrombophlebitis (1.5% to 2%), extravasation (0.7% to 2%)

<1%: Abdominal distention, aggressive behavior, anorexia, **arrhythmia, asthma,** asystole, **atrial fibrillation,** bicarbonate (serum) decreased, bilirubin (direct and indirect) increased, bladder dysfunction, BUN increased, **bradycardia, bronchoconstriction, candidiasis, cardiac arrest,** chills, cholelithiasis, *C. difficile*-associated diarrhea, **dehydration,** depression, dermatitis, desquamation, **duodenitis, dysphagia, epistaxis,** epithelial (urine) cells increased, **esophagitis, facial edema, flank pain,** flatulence, **flushing, gastritis, GI hemorrhage,** gout, jaundice, **heart failure,** heart murmur, hematoma, hematuria, hemoptysis, hemorrhoids, **hiccups,** hypesthesia, hypoxemia, ileus, injection site induration, injection site pain, **malaise,** monocytes increased, **mouth ulcer,** necrosis, **nervousness,** oliguria/anuria, **pain,** pancreatitis, **paresthesia, PTT increased, pharyngeal discomfort,** pleural effusion, pleuritic pain, pseudomembranous colitis, pyloric stenosis, renal insufficiency, **seizures (0.5%),** sodium (serum) **increased, spasm, stomatitis,** subdural hemorrhage, **sweating, syncope, abnormal taste, tremor,** urinary retention, urticaria, vaginal candidiasis, vaginal

(Continued)

Ertapenem *(Continued)*

pruritus, vulvovaginitis, weight loss, ventricular tachycardia, vertigo, voice disturbance

Drug Interactions Increased Effect/Toxicity: Probenecid decreases the renal clearance of ertapenem.

Pharmacodynamics/Kinetics

Absorption: I.M.: Almost complete
Distribution: V_{dss}: 8.2 L
Protein binding (concentration dependent): 85% at 300 mcg/mL, 95% at <100 mcg/mL
Metabolism: Hydrolysis to inactive metabolite
Bioavailability: I.M.: 90%
Half-life elimination: 4 hours
Time to peak: I.M.: 2.3 hours
Excretion: Urine (80% as unchanged drug and metabolite); feces (10%)

Pregnancy Risk Factor B

Generic Available No

Ertapenem Sodium *see* Ertapenem *on page 511*
Erwinia **Asparaginase** *see* Asparaginase *on page 129*
Eryc® *see* Erythromycin *on page 512*
Erycette® *see* Erythromycin *on page 512*
Eryderm® *see* Erythromycin *on page 512*
Erygel® *see* Erythromycin *on page 512*
EryPed® *see* Erythromycin *on page 512*
Ery-Tab® *see* Erythromycin *on page 512*
Erythra-Derm™ *see* Erythromycin *on page 512*
Erythrocin® *see* Erythromycin *on page 512*

Erythromycin (er ith roe MYE sin)

Related Information

Cardiovascular Diseases *on page 1456*
Oral Bacterial Infections *on page 1531*
Oral Viral Infections *on page 1545*
Respiratory Diseases *on page 1476*
Sexually-Transmitted Diseases *on page 1502*

U.S. Brand Names Akne-Mycin®; A/T/S®; E.E.S.®; Emgel®; Eryc®; Erycette®; Eryderm®; Erygel®; EryPed®; Ery-Tab®; Erythra-Derm™; Erythrocin®; PCE®; Romycin®; Staticin®; Theramycin Z®; T-Stat®

Canadian Brand Names Apo®-Erythro Base; Apo®-Erythro E-C; Apo®-Erythro-ES; Apo®-Erythro-S; Diomycin®; EES®; Erybid™; Eryc®; Erythromid®; Nu-Erythromycin-S; PCE®; PMS-Erythromycin

Mexican Brand Names Eritroquim; Ilosone®; Latotryd®; Lauricin®; Lauritran®; Lederpax; Luritran®; Optomicin®; Pantomicina®; Procephal®; Tromigal

Pharmacologic Category Antibiotic, Macrolide; Antibiotic, Ophthalmic; Antibiotic, Topical; Topical Skin Product; Topical Skin Product, Acne

Synonyms Erythromycin Base; Erythromycin Estolate; Erythromycin Ethylsuccinate; Erythromycin Gluceptate; Erythromycin Lactobionate; Erythromycin Stearate

Use

Dental: An alternative to penicillin VK for treating orofacial infections

Medical:

Systemic: Treatment of susceptible bacterial infections including *S. pyogenes*, some *S. pneumoniae*, some *S. aureus*, *M. pneumoniae*, *Legionella pneumophila*, diphtheria, pertussis, chancroid, *Chlamydia*, erythrasma, *N. gonorrhoeae*, *E. histolytica*, syphilis and nongonococcal urethritis, and *Campylobacter* gastroenteritis; used in conjunction with neomycin for decontaminating the bowel

Ophthalmic: Treatment of superficial eye infections involving the conjunctiva or cornea; neonatal ophthalmia

Topical: Treatment of acne vulgaris

Unlabeled/Investigational Use Systemic: Treatment of gastroparesis

Local Anesthetic/Vasoconstrictor Precautions No information available to require special precautions

Effects on Dental Treatment

1% to 8%: Oral candidiasis, headache (8%), vomiting (3%), dyspnea (1%), cough (3%), pain (2%), nausea (8%), weakness (2%)

Frequency not defined: Fever, seizures, hypersensitivity reactions, allergic reactions, ventricular arrhythmias, torsade de pointes (rare), ventricular tachycardia (rare), pseudomembranous colitis

Dosage

Neonates: Ophthalmic: Prophylaxis of neonatal gonococcal or chlamydial conjunctivitis: 0.5-1 cm ribbon of ointment should be instilled into each conjunctival sac

Infants and Children (**Note:** 400 mg ethylsuccinate = 250 mg base, stearate, or estolate salts):

Oral: 30-50 mg/kg/day divided every 6-8 hours; may double doses in severe infections

Orofacial infections: Base and ethylsuccinate: 30-50 mg/kg/day divided every 6-8 hours; do not exceed 2 g/day

Preop bowel preparation: 20 mg/kg erythromycin base at 1, 2, and 11 PM on the day before surgery combined with mechanical cleansing of the large intestine and oral neomycin

I.V.: Lactobionate: 20-40 mg/kg/day divided every 6 hours

Adults:

Oral:

Base: 250-500 mg every 6-12 hours

Ethylsuccinate: 400-800 mg every 6-12 hours

Orofacial infections:

Stearate or base: 250-500 mg every 6 hours for at least 7 days

Ethylsuccinate: 400-800 mg every 6 hours for at least 7 days

Preop bowel preparation: Oral: 1 g erythromycin base at 1, 2, and 11 PM on the day before surgery combined with mechanical cleansing of the large intestine and oral neomycin

I.V.: Lactobionate: 15-20 mg/kg/day divided every 6 hours or 500 mg to 1 g every 6 hours, or given as a continuous infusion over 24 hours (maximum: 4 g/24 hours)

Children and Adults:

Ophthalmic: Instill 1/2" (1.25 cm) 2-6 times/day depending on the severity of the infection

Topical: Apply over the affected area twice daily after the skin has been thoroughly washed and patted dry

Dialysis: Slightly dialyzable (5% to 20%); no supplemental dosage necessary in hemo or peritoneal dialysis or in continuous arteriovenous or venovenous hemofiltration

Prokinetic agent to improve gastric emptying time and intestinal motility: I.V.:

Adults: 200 mg was infused initially followed by 250 mg orally 3 times/day 30 minutes before meals.

Children: 3 mg/kg infused over 60 minutes initially followed by 20 mg/kg/day orally in 3-4 divided doses before meals or before meals and at bedtime

Mechanism of Action Inhibits RNA-dependent protein synthesis at the chain elongation step; binds to the 50S ribosomal subunit resulting in blockage of transpeptidation

Other Adverse Effects Frequency not always defined:

Systemic:

Cardiovascular: QT_c prolongation

Dermatitis: Rash (3%), pruritus (1%)

Gastrointestinal: Abdominal pain (8%), cramping, diarrhea (7%), dyspepsia (2%), flatulence (2%), anorexia, hypertrophic pyloric stenosis (including cases in infants or IHPS), pancreatitis

Hematologic: Eosinophilia (1%)

Hepatic: Cholestatic jaundice (most common with estolate), increased LFTs (2%)

Local: Phlebitis at the injection site, thrombophlebitis

Topical: 1% to 10%: Dermatologic: Erythema, desquamation, dryness, pruritus

Contraindications Hypersensitivity to erythromycin or any component of the formulation

Systemic: Pre-existing liver disease (erythromycin estolate); concomitant use with ergot derivatives, pimozide, astemizole, or cisapride; hepatic impairment

Warnings/Precautions Systemic: Hepatic impairment with or without jaundice has occurred, it may be accompanied by malaise, nausea, vomiting, abdominal colic, and fever; discontinue use if these occur; avoid using erythromycin lactobionate in neonates since formulations may contain benzyl alcohol which is associated with toxicity in neonates; observe for superinfections. Use in infants has been associated with infantile hypertrophic pyloric stenosis (IHPS). Macrolides have been associated with rare QT prolongation and ventricular arrhythmias, including torsade de pointes. Elderly may be at increased risk of adverse events, including hearing loss and/or torsade de pointes when dosage ≥4 g/day, particularly if concurrent renal/hepatic impairment.

Drug Interactions Substrate of CYP2B6, **3A4**; Inhibits CYP1A2, **3A4**

Alfentanil (and possibly other narcotic analgesics): Serum levels may be increased by erythromycin; monitor for increased effect.

Antipsychotic agents (particularly mesoridazine and thioridazine): Risk of QT_c prolongation and malignant arrhythmias may be increased.

Astemizole: Concomitant use is contraindicated; may lead to QT_c prolongation or torsade de pointes.

Benzodiazepines (those metabolized by CYP3A4, including alprazolam and triazolam): Serum levels may be increased by erythromycin; somnolence and confusion have been reported.

(Continued)

Erythromycin *(Continued)*

Bromocriptine: Serum levels may be increased by erythromycin; monitor for increased effect.
Buspirone: Serum levels may be increased by erythromycin; monitor.
Calcium channel blockers (felodipine, verapamil, and potentially others metabolized by CYP3A4): Serum levels may be increased by erythromycin; monitor.
Carbamazepine: Serum levels may be increased by erythromycin; monitor.
Cilostazol: Serum levels may be increased by erythromycin.
Cisapride: Serum levels may be increased by erythromycin; serious arrhythmias have occurred; concurrent use contraindicated.
Clindamycin (and lincomycin): Use with erythromycin may result in pharmacologic antagonism; manufacturer recommends avoiding this combination.
Clozapine: Serum levels may be increased by erythromycin; monitor.
Colchicine: serum levels/toxicity may be increased by erythromycin; monitor.
Cyclosporine: Serum levels may be increased by erythromycin; monitor serum levels.
Delavirdine: Serum levels of erythromycin may be increased; also, serum levels of delavirdine may increased by erythromycin (low risk); monitor.
Digoxin: Serum levels may be increased by erythromycin; monitor digoxin levels.
Disopyramide: Serum levels may be increased by erythromycin; in addition, QT_c prolongation and risk of malignant arrhythmia may be increased; avoid combination.
Ergot alkaloids: Concurrent use may lead to acute ergot toxicity (severe peripheral vasospasm and dysesthesia).
HMG-CoA reductase inhibitors (atorvastatin, lovastatin, and simvastatin); Erythromycin may increase serum levels of "statins" metabolized by CYP3A4, increasing the risk of myopathy/rhabdomyolysis (does not include fluvastatin and pravastatin). Switch to pravastatin/fluvastatin or suspend treatment during course of erythromycin therapy.
Loratadine: Serum levels may be increased by erythromycin; monitor.
Methylprednisolone: Serum levels may be increased by erythromycin; monitor.
Neuromuscular-blocking agents: May be potentiated by erythromycin (case reports).
Phenytoin: Serum levels may be increased by erythromycin; other evidence suggested phenytoin levels may be decreased in some patients; monitor.
Pimozide: Serum levels may be increased, leading to malignant arrhythmias; concomitant use is contraindicated.
Protease inhibitors (amprenavir, nelfinavir, and ritonavir): May increase serum levels of erythromycin.
QT_c-prolonging agents: Concomitant use may increase the risk of malignant arrhythmias.
Quinidine: Serum levels may be increased by erythromycin; in addition, the risk of QT_c prolongation and malignant arrhythmias may be increased during concurrent use.
Quinolone antibiotics (sparfloxacin, gatifloxacin, and moxifloxacin): Concurrent use may increase the risk of malignant arrhythmias.
Rifabutin: Serum levels may be increased by erythromycin; monitor.
Sildenafil: Serum levels may be increased by erythromycin; consider reduction in sildenafil dosage.
Tacrolimus: Serum levels may be increased by erythromycin; monitor serum concentration.
Theophylline: Serum levels may be increased by erythromycin; monitor.
Valproic acid (and derivatives): Serum levels may be increased by erythromycin; monitor.
Vinblastine (and vincristine): Serum levels may be increased by erythromycin.
Warfarin: Effects may be potentiated; monitor INR closely and adjust warfarin dose as needed or choose another antibiotic.
Zafirlukast: Serum levels may be decreased by erythromycin; monitor.
Zopiclone: Serum levels may be increased by erythromycin; monitor.

Dietary/Ethanol/Herb Considerations

Ethanol: Avoid use; ethanol effects may be enhanced and absorption of erythromycin may be decreased.
Food increases absorption and may alter serum concentration. Avoid milk and acidic beverages 1 hour before or after a dose. Ethylsuccinate, estolate, and enteric-coated products are **not** affected by food; ethylsuccinate may be better absorbed with food.
Herb/Nutraceutical: Avoid St John's wort; may decrease serum concentration.

Pharmacodynamics/Kinetics

Absorption: Oral: Variable but better with salt forms than with base form; 18% to 45%; ethylsuccinate may be better absorbed with food
Distribution: Crosses placenta; enters breast milk
  Relative diffusion from blood into CSF: Minimal even with inflammation
  CSF:blood level ratio: Normal meninges: 1% to 12%; Inflamed meninges: 7% to 25%
Protein binding: 75% to 90%

Metabolism: Hepatic via demethylation

Half-life elimination: Peak: 1.5-2 hours; End-stage renal disease: 5-6 hours

Time to peak, serum: Base: 4 hours; Ethylsuccinate: 0.5-2.5 hours; delayed with food due to differences in absorption

Excretion: Primarily feces; urine (2% to 15% as unchanged drug)

Pregnancy Risk Factor B

Dosage Forms CAP, delayed release, enteric-coated pellets, as base (Eryc®): 250 mg. **GEL, topical:** 2% (30 g, 60 g); (A/T/S®): 2% (30 g); (Emgel®): 2% (27 g, 50 g); (Erygel®): 2% (30 g, 60 g). **GRAN, for oral suspension, as ethylsuccinate** (E.E.S.®): 200 mg/5 mL (100 mL, 200 mL). **INJ, powder for reconstitution, as lactobionate** (Erythrocin®): 500 mg, 1 g. **OINT, ophthalmic:** 0.5% [5 mg/g] (1 g, 3.5 g); (Romycin®): 0.5% [5 mg/g] (3.5 g). **OINT, topical** (Akne-Mycin®): 2% (25 g). **POWDER, for oral suspension, as ethylsuccinate** (Ery-Ped®): 200 mg/5 mL (5 mL, 100 mL, 200 mL); 400 mg/5 mL (5 mL, 60 mL, 100 mL, 200 mL). **POWDER, for oral suspension, as ethylsuccinate** [drops] (Ery-Ped®): 100 mg/2.5 mL (50 mL). **SOLN, topical:** 1.5% (60 mL); 2% (60 mL); (A/T/S/®, Eryderm®, Erythra-Derm™, T-Stat®, Theramycin™ Z): 2% (60 mL); (Staticin®): 1.5% (60 mL). **SUSP, oral, as estolate**: 125 mg/5 mL (480 mL); 250 mg/5 mL (480 mL). **SUSP, oral, as ethylsuccinate**: 200 mg/5 mL (480 mL); 400 mg/5 mL (480 mL); (E.E.S.®): 200 mg/5 mL (100 mL, 480 mL); 400 mg/5 mL (100 mL, 480 mL). **Swab** (Erycette®, T-Stat®): 2% (60s). **TAB, chewable, as ethylsuccinate** (EryPed®): 200 mg. **TAB, delayed release, enteric coated, as base** (Ery-Tab®): 250 mg, 333 mg, 500 mg. **TAB, film coated, as base:** 250 mg, 500 mg. **TAB**, film coated, as ethylsuccinate (E.E.S.®): 400 mg. **TAB, film coated, as stearate** (Erythrocin®): 250 mg, 500 mg. **TAB, polymer-coated particles, as base** (PCE®): 333 mg, 500 mg

Generic Available Yes

Comments Many patients cannot tolerate erythromycin because of abdominal pain and nausea; the mechanism of this adverse effect appears to be the motilin agonistic properties of erythromycin in the GI tract. For these patients, clindamycin is indicated as the alternative antibiotic for treatment of orofacial infections.

Erythromycin has been used as a prokinetic agent to improve gastric emptying time and intestinal motility. In adults, 200 mg was infused I.V. initially followed by 250 mg orally 3 times/day 30 minutes before meals. In children, erythromycin 3 mg/kg I.V. has been infused over 60 minutes initially followed by 20 mg/kg/day orally in 3-4 divided doses before meals or before meals and at bedtime.

HMG-CoA reductase inhibitors, also known as the statins, effectively decrease the hepatic cholesterol biosynthesis resulting in the reduction of blood LDL-cholesterol concentrations. The AUC of atorvastatin (Lipitor®) was increased 33% by erythromycin administration. Combination of erythromycin and lovastatin (Mevacor®) has been associated with rhabdomyolysis (Ayanian, et al). The administration of erythromycin with cerivastatin (Baycol®) produced a 50% increase in area under the concentration curve for cerivastatin. The mechanism of erythromycin is inhibiting the CYP3A4 metabolism of atorvastatin, lovastatin, and cerivastatin. Simvastatin (Zocor®) would likely be affected in a similar manner by the coadministration of erythromycin. Clarithromycin (Biaxin®) may exert a similar effect as erythromycin on atorvastatin, lovastatin, cerivastatin, and simvastatin. Erythromycin 3 times/day had no effect on pravastatin (Pravachol®) plasma concentrations (Bottorff, et al).

Selected Readings

Ayanian JZ, Fuchs CS, and Stone RM, "Lovastatin and Rhabdomyolysis," *Ann Intern Med*, 1988, 109(8):682-3.

"Pimozide (Orap) Contraindicated With Clarithromycin (Biaxin®) and Other Macrolide Antibiotics," *FDA Medical Bulletin*, October 1996, 26(3).

Wynn RL and Bergman SA, "Antibiotics and Their Use in the Treatment of Orofacial Infections, Part I," *Gen Dent*, 1994, 42(5):398, 400, 402.

Wynn RL and Bergman SA, "Antibiotics and Their Use in the Treatment of Orofacial Infections, Part II," *Gen Dent*, 1994, 42(6):498-502.

Wynn RL, "Current Concepts of the Erythromycins," *Gen Dent*, 1991, 39(6):408,10-1.

Erythromycin and Benzoyl Peroxide

(er ith roe MYE sin & BEN zoe il per OKS ide)

Related Information

Benzoyl Peroxide *on page 171*

Erythromycin *on page 512*

U.S. Brand Names Benzamycin®

Pharmacologic Category Topical Skin Product; Topical Skin Product, Acne

Synonyms Benzoyl Peroxide and Erythromycin

Use Topical control of acne vulgaris

Local Anesthetic/Vasoconstrictor Precautions No information available to require special precautions

Effects on Dental Treatment No significant effects or complications reported

Dosage Apply twice daily, morning and evening

Pregnancy Risk Factor C

Generic Available No

Erythromycin and Sulfisoxazole

(er ith roe MYE sin & sul fi SOKS a zole)

Related Information

Erythromycin *on page 512*

U.S. Brand Names Eryzole®; Pediazole®

Canadian Brand Names Pediazole®

Pharmacologic Category Antibiotic, Macrolide; Antibiotic, Macrolide Combination; Antibiotic, Sulfonamide Derivative

Synonyms Sulfisoxazole and Erythromycin

Use Treatment of susceptible bacterial infections of the upper and lower respiratory tract, otitis media in children caused by susceptible strains of *Haemophilus influenzae*, and many other infections in patients allergic to penicillin

Local Anesthetic/Vasoconstrictor Precautions No information available to require special precautions

Effects on Dental Treatment Frequency not defined: Ventricular arrhythmias, headache, fever, nausea, vomiting, oral candidiasis, hypersensitivity reactions

Dosage Dosage recommendation is based on erythromycin content.

Oral:

Children ≥2 months: 50 mg/kg/day erythromycin and 150 mg/kg/day sulfisoxazole in divided doses every 6 hours; not to exceed 2 g erythromycin/day or 6 g sulfisoxazole/day for 10 days

Adults >45 kg: 400 mg erythromycin and 1200 mg sulfisoxazole every 6 hours

Dosing adjustment in renal impairment (sulfisoxazole must be adjusted):

Cl_{cr} 10-50 mL/minute: Administer every 8-12 hours

Cl_{cr} <10 mL/minute: Administer every 12-24 hours

Mechanism of Action Erythromycin inhibits bacterial protein synthesis; sulfisoxazole competitively inhibits bacterial synthesis of folic acid from para-aminobenzoic acid

Other Adverse Effects Frequency not defined:

Dermatologic: Rash, Stevens-Johnson syndrome, toxic epidermal necrolysis

Gastrointestinal: Abdominal pain, cramping, hypertrophic pyloric stenosis, diarrhea, pseudomembranous colitis

Hematologic: Agranulocytosis, aplastic anemia, eosinophilia

Hepatic: Hepatic necrosis, cholestatic jaundice

Local: Phlebitis at the injection site, thrombophlebitis

Renal: Toxic nephrosis, crystalluria

Pregnancy Risk Factor C

Generic Available Yes

Erythromycin Base *see* Erythromycin *on page 512*

Erythromycin Estolate *see* Erythromycin *on page 512*

Erythromycin Ethylsuccinate *see* Erythromycin *on page 512*

Erythromycin Gluceptate *see* Erythromycin *on page 512*

Erythromycin Lactobionate *see* Erythromycin *on page 512*

Erythromycin Stearate *see* Erythromycin *on page 512*

Erythropoiesis Stimulating Protein *see* Darbepoetin Alfa *on page 400*

Erythropoietin *see* Epoetin Alfa *on page 503*

Eryzole® *see* Erythromycin and Sulfisoxazole *on page 516*

Escitalopram (es sye TAL oh pram)

Related Information

Citalopram *on page 334*

U.S. Brand Names Lexapro™

Pharmacologic Category Antidepressant, Selective Serotonin Reuptake Inhibitor

Synonyms Escitalopram Oxalate; Lu-26-054; S-Citalopram

Use Treatment of major depressive disorder

Unlabeled/Investigational Use Treatment of anxiety disorders

Local Anesthetic/Vasoconstrictor Precautions Although caution should be used in patients taking tricyclic antidepressants, no interactions have been reported with vasoconstrictors and escitalopram, a nontricyclic antidepressant which acts to increase serotonin.

Effects on Dental Treatment

>10%: Nausea (15%)

1% to 10%: Xerostomia (6%), toothache (~1%), chest pain, hypertension, palpitations, somnolence (6%), dizziness (5%), fatigue (5%), fever, irritability, lethargy, lightheadedness, migraine, yawning, gastroenteritis, gastroesophageal reflux, heartburn, vomiting, limb pain, muscle cramp, neck/shoulder pain, paresthesia, tremors, blurred vision, earache, rhinitis (5%), sinusitis (3%), bronchitis, coughing, nasal or sinus congestion, sinus headache, diaphoresis (5%), flu-like syndrome (5%), allergy

Dosage Escitalopram is the S-enantiomer of the racemic derivative citalopram; 20 mg escitalopram is equipotent to 40 mg citalopram.

Oral:

Adults: Depression: Initial: 10 mg/day; dose may be increased to 20 mg/day after at least 1 week

Elderly: 10 mg/day

Dosing adjustment in renal impairment:

Severe impairment: Cl_{cr} <20 mL/minute: Use caution

Dosing adjustment in hepatic impairment: 10 mg/day

Mechanism of Action Escitalopram is the S-enantiomer of citalopram, which selectively inhibits the reuptake of serotonin with little to no effect on norepinephrine or dopamine reuptake.

Other Adverse Effects

1% to 10%:

Central nervous system: Insomnia (9%), dreaming abnormal, concentration impaired, vertigo

Dermatologic: Rash

Endocrine & metabolic: Libido decreased (3%), anorgasmia (2%), hot flashes, menstrual cramps

Gastrointestinal: Diarrhea (8%), appetite decreased (3%), constipation (3%), indigestion (3%), abdominal pain (2%), abdominal cramps, appetite increased, flatulence, heartburn, weight gain/loss

Genitourinary: Ejaculation disorder (9%), impotence (3%), urinary tract infection, urinary frequency

Neuromuscular & skeletal: Arthralgia, myalgia,

Otic: Tinnitus

<1%: Abdominal discomfort, acne, **agitation,** alopecia, **amnesia, anaphylaxis,** anemia, **anxiety attack,** apathy, **arthritis,** arthropathy, **asthma, auditory hallucination,** back discomfort, **belching,** bilirubin increased, bloating, **bradycardia, bruising, bruxism**, carbohydrate craving, carpal tunnel syndrome, **chest tightness,** chills, **confusion,** conjunctivitis, abnormal crying, depersonalization, depression aggravated, depression, dermatitis, dry eyes, dry skin, dysequilibrium, dyspepsia, dysuria, EKG abnormal, eczema, edema, emotional lability, **excitability,** eye infection, eye irritation, **faintness,** feeling unreal, **flushing,** folliculitis, **forgetfulness,** furunculosis, **gagging, gastritis,** gout, **hematoma,** hemorrhoids, hypercholesterolemia, **hyperglycemia,** hyper-reflexia, **jaw pain, jaw stiffness, jitteriness, joint stiffness,** kidney stone, **laryngitis, leg pain,** lipoma, **malaise,** menorrhagia, **muscle contractions (involuntary), muscle stiffness, muscle weakness,** muscular tone increased, **nervousness, nosebleed, panic reaction,** pelvic inflammation, pneumonia, pruritus, pupils dilated, **restless legs, restlessness aggravated, shaking, shortness of breath,** spotting between menses, stool frequency increased, **suicidal tendency, suicide attempt, syncope, tachycardia, taste alteration, tics, tracheitis, tremulousness nervous, twitching,** urinary frequency, varicose vein, **vision abnormal, visual disturbance, weakness**

Postmarketing and/or case reports: Acute renal failure, akathisia, angioedema, choreoathetosis, delirium, dyskinesia, epidermal necrolysis, erythema multiforme, grand mal seizures, hemolytic anemia, nystagmus, pancreatitis, priapism, prolactinemia, prothrombin decreased, QT prolonged, rhabdomyolysis, serotonin syndrome, thrombocytopenia, thrombosis, **torsade de pointes, ventricular arrhythmia, withdrawal syndrome**

Drug Interactions Substrate of **CYP2C19, 3A4**; Inhibits CYP2D6

Increased Effect/Toxicity:

MAO inhibitors: Escitalopram should not be used with nonselective MAO inhibitors (phenelzine, isocarboxazid) or other drugs with MAO inhibition (linezolid); fatal reactions have been reported. Wait 5 weeks after stopping escitalopram before starting a nonselective MAO inhibitor and 2 weeks after stopping an MAO inhibitor before starting escitalopram. Concurrent selegiline has been associated with mania, hypertension, or serotonin syndrome (risk may be reduced relative to nonselective MAO inhibitors).

Combined used of SSRIs and buspirone, meperidine, moclobemide, nefazodone, other SSRIs, tramadol, trazodone, and venlafaxine may increase the risk of serotonin syndrome. Escitalopram increases serum levels/effects of CYP2D6 substrates (tricyclic antidepressants)

Combined use of sumatriptan (and other serotonin agonists) may result in toxicity; weakness, hyper-reflexia, and incoordination have been observed with sumatriptan and SSRIs. In addition, concurrent use may theoretically increase the risk of serotonin syndrome; includes sumatriptan, naratriptan, rizatriptan, and zolmitriptan.

Dietary/Ethanol/Herb Considerations

Ethanol: Avoid use; may increase CNS depression.

Food: May be taken with food

Herb/Nutraceutical: Avoid gotu kola, kava kava, SAMe, St John's wort, and valerian; may increase CNS depression.

Pharmacodynamics/Kinetics

Onset: 1-2 weeks

Protein binding: 56% to plasma proteins

(Continued)

Escitalopram *(Continued)*

Metabolism: Hepatic via CYP2D6, 2C19, and 3A4 to an active metabolite, S-desmethylcitalopram (S-DCT); S-DCT is metabolized to S-didesmethylcitalopram (active) via CYP2D6

Half-life elimination: Escitalopram: 27-32 hours; S-desmethylcitalopram: 59 hours

Time to peak: Escitalopram: 5 ± 1.5 hours; S-desmethylcitalopram: 14 hours

Excretion: Urine (Escitalopram: 8%; S-DCT: 10%)

Clearance: Total body: 37-40 L/hour; Renal: Escitalopram: 2.7 L/hour; S-desmethylcitalopram: 6.9 L/hour

Pregnancy Risk Factor C

Generic Available No

Escitalopram Oxalate *see* Escitalopram *on page 516*

Esclim® *see* Estradiol *on page 521*

Eserine Salicylate *see* Physostigmine *on page 1078*

Esgic® *see* Butalbital, Acetaminophen, and Caffeine *on page 214*

Esgic-Plus™ *see* Butalbital, Acetaminophen, and Caffeine *on page 214*

Eskalith® *see* Lithium *on page 815*

Eskalith CR® *see* Lithium *on page 815*

Esmolol (ES moe lol)

U.S. Brand Names Brevibloc®

Canadian Brand Names Brevibloc®

Mexican Brand Names Brevibloc®

Pharmacologic Category Antiarrhythmic Agent, Class II; Beta Blocker, $Beta_1$ Selective

Synonyms Esmolol Hydrochloride

Use Treatment of supraventricular tachycardia and atrial fibrillation/flutter (primarily to control ventricular rate); treatment of tachycardia and/or hypertension (especially intraoperative or postoperative)

Local Anesthetic/Vasoconstrictor Precautions No information available to require special precautions

Effects on Dental Treatment Esmolol is a cardioselective beta-blocker. Local anesthetic with vasoconstrictor can be safely used in patients medicated with esmolol. Nonselective beta-blockers (ie, propranolol, nadolol) enhance the pressor response to epinephrine, resulting in hypertension and bradycardia; this has not been reported for esmolol. Many nonsteroidal anti-inflammatory drugs such as ibuprofen and indomethacin can reduce the hypotensive effect of beta-blockers after 3 or more weeks of therapy with the NSAID. Short-term NSAID use (ie, 3 days) requires no special precautions in patients taking beta-blockers.

>10%: Symptomatic hypotension (12%), diaphoresis (10%)

1% to 10%: Dizziness (3%), somnolence (3%), confusion (2%), headache (2%), agitation (2%), fatigue (1%), nausea (7%), vomiting (1%)

Dosage I.V. infusion requires an infusion pump (must be adjusted to individual response and tolerance):

Children: A limited amount of information regarding esmolol use in pediatric patients is currently available. Some centers have utilized doses of 100-500 mcg/kg given over 1 minute for control of supraventricular tachycardias.

Loading doses of 500 mcg/kg/minute over 1 minute with maximal doses of 50-250 mcg/kg/minute (mean = 173) have been used in addition to nitroprusside to treat postoperative hypertension after coarctation of aorta repair.

Adults:

Intraoperative tachycardia and/or hypertension (immediate control): Initial bolus: 80 mg (~1 mg/kg) over 30 seconds, followed by a 150 mcg/kg/minute infusion, if necessary. Adjust infusion rate as needed to maintain desired heart rate and/or blood pressure, up to 300 mcg/kg/minute.

Supraventricular tachycardia or gradual control of postoperative tachycardia/hypertension: Loading dose: 500 mcg/kg over 1 minute; follow with a 50 mcg/kg/minute infusion for 4 minutes; response to this initial infusion rate may be a rough indication of the responsiveness of the ventricular rate.

Infusion may be continued at 50 mcg/kg/minute or, if the response is inadequate, titrated upward in 50 mcg/kg/minute increments (increased no more frequently than every 4 minutes) to a maximum of 200 mcg/kg/minute.

To achieve more rapid response, following the initial loading dose and 50 mcg/kg/minute infusion, rebolus with a second 500 mcg/kg loading dose over 1 minute, and increase the maintenance infusion to 100 mcg/kg/minute for 4 minutes. If necessary, a third (and final) 500 mcg/kg loading dose may be administered, prior to increasing to an infusion rate of 150 mcg/minute. After 4 minutes of the 150 mcg/kg/minute infusion, the infusion rate may be increased to a maximum rate of 200 mcg/kg/minute (without a bolus dose).

Usual dosage range (SVT): 50-200 mcg/kg/minute with average dose of 100 mcg/kg/minute. For control of postoperative hypertension, as many as one-third of patients may require higher doses (250-300 mcg/kg/minute) to control blood pressure; the safety of doses >300 mcg/kg/minute has not been studied.

Esmolol: Hemodynamic effects of beta-blockade return to baseline within 20-30 minutes after discontinuing esmolol infusions.

Guidelines for withdrawal of therapy:

Transfer to alternative antiarrhythmic drug (propranolol, digoxin, verapamil).

Infusion should be reduced by 50% 30 minutes following the first dose of the alternative agent.

Following the second dose of the alternative drug, patient's response should be monitored and if control is adequate for the first hours, esmolol may be discontinued.

Dialysis: Not removed by hemo- or peritoneal dialysis; supplemental dose is unnecessary.

Mechanism of Action Class II antiarrhythmic: Competitively blocks response to $beta_1$-adrenergic stimulation with little or no effect of $beta_2$-receptors except at high doses, no intrinsic sympathomimetic activity, no membrane stabilizing activity

Other Adverse Effects

>10%: Cardiovascular: Asymptomatic hypotension (25%)

1% to 10%:

Cardiovascular: Peripheral ischemia (1%)

Local: Pain on injection (8%)

<1% (Limited to important or life-threatening): Pallor, **flushing, bradycardia, severe bradycardia/asystole (rare), chest pain, syncope,** heart block, edema, depression, **abnormal thinking, anxiety, fever, lightheadedness, seizures,** erythema, skin discoloration, anorexia, dyspepsia, constipation, **xerostomia,** abdominal discomfort, urinary retention, thrombophlebitis, infusion site reactions, **paresthesia, rigors,** midcapsular pain, **weakness, abnormal vision, bronchospasm, wheezing, dyspnea, nasal congestion,** pulmonary edema, **CHF, abnormal taste,** depression, acne, eczema, psoriasis, skin irritation, pruritus, **flushing,** alopecia, exfoliative dermatitis, skin necrosis (from extravasation)

Drug Interactions

Increased Effect/Toxicity: Esmolol may increase the effect/toxicity of verapamil, and may increase potential for hypertensive crisis after or during withdrawal of either agent when combined with clonidine. Esmolol may extend the effect of neuromuscular blocking agents (succinylcholine). Esmolol may increase digoxin serum levels by 10% to 20% and may increase theophylline concentrations. Morphine may increase esmolol blood concentrations.

Decreased Effect: Decreased effect of beta-blockers with aluminum salts, barbiturates, calcium salts, cholestyramine, colestipol, NSAIDs, penicillins (ampicillin), rifampin, salicylates, and sulfinpyrazone due to decreased bioavailability and plasma levels. Beta-blockers may decrease the effect of sulfonylureas. Xanthines (eg, theophylline, caffeine) may decrease effects of esmolol.

Dietary/Ethanol/Herb Considerations

Ethanol: Avoid use; may increase risk of hypotension or dizziness.

Food: Avoid caffeine, garlic, ginger, and xanthine-containing foods or beverages.

Herb/Nutraceutical: Avoid black cohosh, dong quai, and evening primrose due to estrogenic activity. Avoid ephedra, ginseng, and yohimbe; may cause arrhythmias or hypertension. Avoid garlic; may increase antihypertensive effect. Avoid ginger due to positive inotropic effects; theoretically, may cause arrhythmia. Avoid hawthorn; may lower peripheral vascular resistance resulting in additive decrease in BP.

Pharmacodynamics/Kinetics

Onset of action: Beta-blockade: I.V.: 2-10 minutes (quickest when loading doses are administered)

Duration: 10-30 minutes; prolonged following higher cumulative doses, extended duration of use

Protein binding: 55%

Metabolism: In blood by esterases

Half-life elimination: Adults: 9 minutes

Excretion: Urine (~69% as metabolites, 2% unchanged drug)

Pregnancy Risk Factor C (manufacturer); D (2nd and 3rd trimesters - expert analysis)

Generic Available No

Selected Readings

Foster CA and Aston SJ, "Propranolol-Epinephrine Interaction: A Potential Disaster," *Plast Reconstr Surg*, 1983, 72(1):74-8.

Wong DG, Spence JD, Lamki L, et al, "Effect of Nonsteroidal Anti-inflammatory Drugs on Control of Hypertension of Beta-Blockers and Diuretics," *Lancet*, 1986, 1(8488):997-1001.

Wynn RL, "Dental Nonsteroidal Anti-inflammatory Drugs and Prostaglandin-Based Drug Interactions, Part Two," *Gen Dent*, 1992, 40(2):104, 106, 108.

Wynn RL, "Epinephrine Interactions With Beta-Blockers," *Gen Dent*, 1994, 42(1):16, 18.

Esmolol Hydrochloride *see* Esmolol *on page 518*

Esomeprazole (es oh ME pray zol)

U.S. Brand Names Nexium®

Canadian Brand Names Nexium®

(Continued)

Esomeprazole *(Continued)*

Pharmacologic Category Proton Pump Inhibitor

Synonyms Esomeprazole Magnesium

Use Short-term (4-8 weeks) treatment of erosive esophagitis; maintaining symptom resolution and healing of erosive esophagitis; treatment of symptomatic gastroesophageal reflux disease; as part of a multidrug regimen for *Helicobacter pylori* eradication in patients with duodenal ulcer disease (active or history of within the past 5 years)

Local Anesthetic/Vasoconstrictor Precautions No information available to require special precautions

Effects on Dental Treatment 1% to 10%: Xerostomia, headache (4% to 6%), nausea

Dosage Oral (delayed-release capsules should be swallowed whole and taken at least 1 hour before eating):

Children: Safety and efficacy not established

Adults: Oral:

Erosive esophagitis (healing): 20-40 mg once daily for 4-8 weeks; maintenance: 20 mg once daily

Symptomatic GERD: 20 mg once daily for 4 weeks

Helicobacter pylori eradication: 40 mg once daily; requires combination therapy

Dosing adjustment in hepatic impairment:

Mild to moderate liver impairment (Child-Pugh Class A or B): None

Severe liver impairment (Child-Pugh Class C): Dose should not exceed 20 mg/day

Mechanism of Action Proton pump inhibitor suppresses gastric acid secretion by inhibition of the H^+/K^+-ATPase in the gastric parietal cell

Other Adverse Effects

1% to 10%: Gastrointestinal: Diarrhea (4%), flatulence, abdominal pain (4%), constipation

<1%: Acne, albuminuria, alkaline phosphatase elevations, **allergic reactions,** anemia, angioedema, anorexia, apathy, arthralgia, **arthritis exacerbation,** arthropathy, asthenia, **asthma exacerbation,** back pain, bilirubinemia, cervical lymphadenopathy, **chest pain, confusion,** conjunctivitis, **cough,** cramps, cystitis, depression exacerbation, dermatitis, **dizziness,** dysmenorrhea, dyspepsia, **dysphagia, dyspnea,** dysuria, **earache,** edema, **epigastric pain, epistaxis, eructation, facial edema,** fibromyalgia syndrome, **fungal infection,** hematuria, hepatic enzyme elevations, hernia, **hot flashes, hypertonia, fatigue, fever, flu-like syndrome, flushing, gastroenteritis, GI dysplasia, GI hemorrhage,** genital moniliasis, glycosuria, goiter, **hiccup, hypertension,** hyperuricemia, hypochromic anemia, hypoesthesia, hyponatremia, impotence, increased appetite, increased creatinine, increased total bilirubin, insomnia, **larynx edema,** leukocytosis, leukopenia, maculopapular rash, **malaise,** melena, **migraine, migraine exacerbation, moniliasis, nervousness, otitis media, pain, paresthesia,** peripheral edema, parosmia, **pharyngitis,** polymyalgia rheumatica, polyuria, pruritus, pruritus ani, rash, **rhinitis, rigors,** serum gastrin elevation, **sinusitis,** skin inflammation, **somnolence, substernal chest pain, diaphoresis, tachycardia, loss of taste, abnormal taste, thirst,** thrombocytopenia, thyroid stimulating hormone elevation, tinnitus, **tongue edema, tremor, ulcerative stomatitis,** urticaria, vaginitis, vertigo, **visual field defect,** vision change, **vitamin B_{12}** deficiency, vomiting, weight changes (loss/gain)

Postmarketing and/or case reports: **Anaphylaxis**

Drug Interactions Substrate of **CYP2C19,** 3A4

Increased Effect/Toxicity: Increased serum concentration of diazepam, digoxin, penicillins

Decreased Effect: Decreased absorption of dapsone, iron, itraconazole, ketoconazole and other drugs where an acidic stomach is required for absorption.

Dietary/Ethanol/Herb Considerations Food decreases absorption by 33% to 53%; administer ≥1 hour before meals. The contents of the capsule remain intact when exposed to tap water, orange and apple juice, or yogurt; may be mixed with 1 tablespoon of applesauce.

Pharmacodynamics/Kinetics

Distribution: V_{dss}: 16 L

Protein binding: 97%

Metabolism: Hepatic via CYP2C19 and 3A4 enzymes to hydroxy, desmethyl, and sulfone metabolites (all inactive)

Bioavailability: 90% with repeat dosing

Half-life elimination: 1-1.5 hours

Time to peak: 1.5 hours

Excretion: Urine (80%); feces (20%)

Pregnancy Risk Factor B

Generic Available No

Esomeprazole Magnesium *see* Esomeprazole *on page 519*

Esoterica® Regular [OTC] *see* Hydroquinone *on page 693*

Especol® [OTC] *see* Phosphorated Carbohydrate Solution *on page 1078*

Estar® [OTC] *see* Coal Tar *on page 359*

Estazolam (es TA zoe lam)

U.S. Brand Names ProSom®

Mexican Brand Names Tasedan®

Pharmacologic Category Benzodiazepine

Use Short-term management of insomnia

Local Anesthetic/Vasoconstrictor Precautions No information available to require special precautions

Effects on Dental Treatment

>10%: Significant xerostomia (normal salivary flow resumes upon discontinuation) somnolence, weakness

1% to 10%: Flushing, palpitations, anxiety, confusion, dizziness, incoordination, hangover effect, agitation, amnesia, euphoria, hostility, seizure, stupor, gastritis, taste perversion, paresthesia, cough, dyspnea, asthma, rhinitis, sinusitis, diaphoresis

Restrictions C-IV

Dosage Oral:

Adults: 1 mg at bedtime, some patients may require 2 mg; start at doses of 0.5 mg in debilitated or small elderly patients

Dosing adjustment in hepatic impairment: May be necessary

Mechanism of Action Binds to stereospecific benzodiazepine receptors on the postsynaptic GABA neuron at several sites within the central nervous system, including the limbic system, reticular formation. Enhancement of the inhibitory effect of GABA on neuronal excitability results by increased neuronal membrane permeability to chloride ions. This shift in chloride ions results in hyperpolarization (a less excitable state) and stabilization.

Other Adverse Effects

1% to 10%:

Central nervous system: Hypokinesia, apathy, emotional lability, sleep disorder, twitch

Dermatologic: Dermatitis, pruritus, rash, urticaria

Gastrointestinal: Constipation, decreased/increased appetite, flatulence

Genitourinary: Frequent urination, menstrual cramps, urinary hesitancy, urinary frequency, vaginal discharge/itching

Ocular: Photophobia, eye pain, eye swelling

<1%: **Allergic reactions,** chills, **drug dependence, fever, muscle spasm, myalgia, neck pain**

Drug Interactions Substrate of CYP3A4

Increased Effect/Toxicity: Serum levels and/or toxicity of estazolam may be increased by cimetidine, ciprofloxacin, clarithromycin, clozapine, CNS depressants, diltiazem, disulfiram, digoxin, erythromycin, ethanol, fluconazole, fluoxetine, fluvoxamine, grapefruit juice, isoniazid, itraconazole, ketoconazole, labetalol, levodopa, loxapine, metoprolol, metronidazole, miconazole, nefazodone, omeprazole, phenytoin, rifabutin, rifampin, troleandomycin, valproic acid, and verapamil.

Decreased Effect: Carbamazepine, rifampin, rifabutin may enhance the metabolism of estazolam and decrease its therapeutic effect.

Dietary/Ethanol/Herb Considerations

Ethanol: Avoid use; may increase CNS depression.

Food: Administer with milk to reduce GI upset; absorption is decreased 33% to 53% when taken with food. Avoid grapefruit products; may increase serum concentration/toxicity.

Herb/Nutraceutical: Avoid gotu kola, kava, melatonin, SAMe, St John's wort, and valerian; may increase CNS depression.

Pharmacodynamics/Kinetics

Onset of action: ~1 hour

Duration: Variable

Metabolism: Extensively hepatic

Half-life elimination: 10-24 hours (no significant changes in elderly)

Time to peak, serum: 0.5-1.6 hours

Excretion: Urine (<5% as unchanged drug)

Pregnancy Risk Factor X

Generic Available Yes

Esterified Estrogen and Methyltestosterone *see* Estrogens (Esterified) and Methyltestosterone *on page 534*

Esterified Estrogens *see* Estrogens (Esterified) *on page 533*

Estinyl® *see* Ethinyl Estradiol *on page 541*

Estrace® *see* Estradiol *on page 521*

Estraderm® *see* Estradiol *on page 521*

Estradiol (es tra DYE ole)

Related Information

Endocrine Disorders and Pregnancy *on page 1479*

(Continued)

Estradiol *(Continued)*

Rheumatoid Arthritis, Osteoarthritis, and Osteoporosis *on page 1488*

U.S. Brand Names Alora®; Climara®; Delestrogen®; Depo®-Estradiol; Esclim®; Estrace®; Estraderm®; Estring®; Gynodiol®; Vagifem®; Vivelle®; Vivelle-Dot®

Canadian Brand Names Climara®; Delestrogen®; Depo®-Estradiol; Estrace®; Estraderm®; Estradot®; Estring®; Estrogel®; Oesclim®; Vagifem®; Vivelle®

Mexican Brand Names Climaderm®; Estraderm TTS®; Ginedisc®; Oestrogel; Systen®

Pharmacologic Category Estrogen Derivative

Synonyms Estradiol Cypionate; Estradiol Hemihydrate; Estradiol Transdermal; Estradiol Valerate

Use Treatment of moderate to severe vasomotor symptoms associated with menopause; treatment of vulvar and vaginal atrophy; hypoestrogenism (due to hypogonadism, castration, or primary ovarian failure); prostatic cancer (palliation), breast cancer (palliation), osteoporosis (prophylaxis); abnormal uterine bleeding due to hormonal imbalance; postmenopausal urogenital symptoms of the lower urinary tract (urinary urgency, dysuria)

Local Anesthetic/Vasoconstrictor Precautions No information available to require special precautions

Effects on Dental Treatment Frequency not defined: Hypertension, dizziness, headache, migraine, nausea, vomiting

Dosage All dosage needs to be adjusted based upon the patient's response

Oral:

- Prostate cancer (androgen-dependent, inoperable, progressing): 10 mg 3 times/day for at least 3 months
- Breast cancer (inoperable, progressing in appropriately selected patients): 10 mg 3 times/day for at least 3 months
- Osteoporosis prophylaxis in postmenopausal females: 0.5 mg/day in a cyclic regimen (3 weeks on and 1 week off)
- Female hypoestrogenism (due to hypogonadism, castration, or primary ovarian failure): 1-2 mg/day; titrate as necessary to control symptoms using minimal effective dose for maintenance therapy
- Treatment of moderate to severe vasomotor symptoms associated with menopause: 1-2 mg/day, adjusted as necessary to limit symptoms; administration should be cyclic (3 weeks on, 1 week off). Patients should be re-evaluated at 3- to 6-month intervals to determine if treatment is still necessary.

I.M.

- Prostate cancer: Valerate: ≥30 mg or more every 1-2 weeks
- Moderate to severe vasomotor symptoms associated with menopause:
  - Cypionate: 1-5 mg every 3-4 weeks
  - Valerate: 10-20 mg every 4 weeks
- Female hypoestrogenism (due to hypogonadism):
  - Cypionate: 1.5-2 mg monthly
  - Valerate: 10-20 mg every 4 weeks

Transdermal: Indicated dose may be used continuously in patients without an intact uterus. May be given continuously or cyclically (3 weeks on, 1 week off) in patients with an intact uterus. When changing patients from oral to transdermal therapy, start transdermal patch 1 week after discontinuing oral hormone (may begin sooner if symptoms reappear within 1 week):

- Once-weekly patch:
  - Moderate to severe vasomotor symptoms associated with menopause (Climara®): Apply 0.025 mg/day patch once weekly. Adjust dose as necessary to control symptoms. Patients should be re-evaluated at 3- to 6-month intervals to determine if treatment is still necessary.
  - Osteoporosis prophylaxis in postmenopausal women (Climara®): Apply patch once weekly; minimum effective dose 0.025 mg/day; adjust response to therapy by biochemical markers and bone mineral density
- Twice-weekly patch:
  - Moderate to severe vasomotor symptoms associated with menopause, vulvar/vaginal atrophy, female hypogonadism: Titrate to lowest dose possible to control symptoms, adjusting initial dose after the first month of therapy; re-evaluate therapy at 3- to 6-month intervals to taper or discontinue medication:
    - Alora®, Esclim®, Estraderm®, Vivelle-Dot®: Apply 0.05 mg patch twice weekly
    - Vivelle®: Apply 0.0375 mg patch twice weekly
  - Prevention of osteoporosis in postmenopausal women:
    - Alora®, Vivelle®, Vivelle-Dot®: Apply 0.025 mg patch twice weekly, increase dose as necessary
    - Estraderm®: Apply 0.05 mg patch twice weekly

Vaginal cream: Vulvar and vaginal atrophy: Insert 2-4 g/day intravaginally for 2 weeks, then gradually reduce to ½ the initial dose for 2 weeks, followed by a maintenance dose of 1 g 1-3 times/week

Vaginal ring: Postmenopausal vaginal atrophy, urogenital symptoms: Estring®: Following insertion, Estring® should remain in place for 90 days

Vaginal tablets: Atrophic vaginitis: Vagifem®: Initial: Insert 1 tablet once daily for 2 weeks; maintenance: Insert 1 tablet twice weekly; attempts to discontinue or taper medication should be made at 3- to 6-month intervals

Dosing adjustment in hepatic impairment: Reduction recommended in mild-moderate impairment; use not recommended in severe impairment

Mechanism of Action Estrogens are responsible for the development and maintenance of the female reproductive system and secondary sexual characteristics. Estradiol is the principle intracellular human estrogen and is more potent than estrone and estriol at the receptor level; it is the primary estrogen secreted prior to menopause. Following menopause, estrone and estrone sulfate are more highly produced. Estrogens modulate the pituitary secretion of gonadotropins, luteinizing hormone, and follicle-stimulating hormone through a negative feedback system; estrogen replacement reduces elevated levels of these hormones in postmenopausal women.

Other Adverse Effects Frequency not defined:

Cardiovascular: Edema, venous thromboembolism

Central nervous system: Mental depression

Dermatologic: Chloasma, erythema multiforme, erythema nodosum, hemorrhagic eruption, hirsutism, loss of scalp hair, melasma

Endocrine & metabolic: Breast enlargement, breast tenderness, changes in libido, increased thyroid-binding globulin, increased total thyroid hormone (T_4), increased serum triglycerides/phospholipids, increased HDL-cholesterol, decreased LDL-cholesterol, impaired glucose tolerance, hypercalcemia

Gastrointestinal: Abdominal cramps, bloating, cholecystitis, cholelithiasis, gallbladder disease, pancreatitis, weight gain/loss

Genitourinary: Alterations in frequency and flow of menses, changes in cervical secretions, endometrial cancer, increased size of uterine leiomyomata, vaginal candidiasis

Vaginal: Trauma from applicator insertion may occur in women with severely atrophic vaginal mucosa

Hematologic: Aggravation of porphyria, decreased antithrombin III and antifactor Xa, increased levels of fibrinogen, increased platelet aggregability and platelet count; increased prothrombin and factors VII, VIII, IX, X

Hepatic: Cholestatic jaundice

Local: Transdermal patches: Burning, erythema, irritation, pruritus, rash

Neuromuscular & skeletal: Chorea

Ocular: Intolerance to contact lenses, steeping of corneal curvature

Respiratory: Pulmonary thromboembolism

Miscellaneous: Carbohydrate intolerance

Postmarketing and/or case reports: Vivelle®; **Anaphylaxis** (isolated reports), elevated LFTs (rare), **leg pain**

Drug Interactions Substrate of **CYP1A2**, 2A6, 2B6, 2C8/9, 2C19, 2D6, 2E1, **3A4**; Inhibits CYP1A2; Induces CYP3A4

Increased Effect/Toxicity: Estradiol with hydrocortisone increases corticosteroid toxic potential. Anticoagulants and estradiol increase the potential for thromboembolic events.

Decreased Effect: Rifampin, nelfinavir, and ritonavir decrease estradiol serum concentrations. Anticonvulsants which are enzyme inducers (barbiturates, carbamazepine, phenobarbital, phenytoin, primidone) may potentially decrease estrogen levels.

Dietary/Ethanol/Herb Considerations

Ethanol: Avoid use; increases estrogen level and risk of breast cancer; may also increase risk of osteoporosis.

Food: Estradiol may decrease folic acid absorption. Avoid grapefruit products; may increase serum concentration. Ascorbic acid (>1 g/day) may increase serum concentration of estradiol.

Herb/Nutraceutical: Avoid black cohosh, dong quai, and evening primrose due to estrogenic activity. Avoid ginseng, red clover, and saw palmetto due to potential hormonal effects. Avoid St John's wort; may decrease estradiol concentration.

Pharmacodynamics/Kinetics

Absorption: Oral, topical: Well absorbed

Distribution: Crosses placenta; enters breast milk

Protein binding: 37% to sex-hormone-binding globulin; 61% to albumin

Metabolism: Oral: Hepatic via oxidation and conjugation in GI tract; hydroxylated via CYP3A4 to metabolites; first-pass effect; enterohepatic recirculation

Excretion: Primarily urine (as metabolites); feces (small amounts)

Pregnancy Risk Factor X

Generic Available Yes

Estradiol and Medroxyprogesterone

(es tra DYE ole & me DROKS ee proe JES te rone)

Related Information

Estradiol *on page 521*

U.S. Brand Names Lunelle™

Pharmacologic Category Contraceptive

(Continued)

Estradiol and Medroxyprogesterone *(Continued)*

Synonyms E_2C and MPA; Estradiol Cypionate and Medroxyprogesterone Acetate; Medroxyprogesterone Acetate and Estradiol Cypionate

Use Prevention of pregnancy

Local Anesthetic/Vasoconstrictor Precautions No information available to require special precautions

Effects on Dental Treatment Since this is a combination estrogen-progesterone product, when prescribing antibiotics, patient must be warned to use additional methods of birth control if on hormonal contraceptives.

Dosage Adults: Female: I.M.: 0.5 mL

First dose: Within first 5 days of menstrual period or within 5 days of a complete 1st trimester abortion; do not administer <4 weeks postpartum **if not breast-feeding** or <6 weeks postpartum **if breast-feeding**

Maintenance dose: Monthly, every 28-30 days following previous injection; do not exceed 33 days; pregnancy must be ruled out if >33 days have past between injections; bleeding episodes cannot be used to guide injection schedule; shortening schedule may lead to menstrual pattern changes

Switching from other forms of contraception: First injection should be given within 7 days of last active oral contraceptive pill; when switching from other methods, timing of injection should ensure continuous contraceptive coverage

Elderly: Not for postmenopausal use

Dosing adjustment in renal impairment: Not studied; adjustment not anticipated due to hepatic metabolism

Dosing adjustment in hepatic impairment: Contraindicated in dysfunction

Mechanism of Action Inhibits secretion of gonadotropins, leading to prevention of follicular maturation and ovulation. Also leads to thickening and reduction in volume of cervical mucus (decreases sperm penetration) and thinning of endometrium (reduces possibility of implantation).

Other Adverse Effects Frequency not defined:

Cardiovascular: Arterial thromboembolism, cerebral hemorrhage, cerebral thrombosis, edema, **hypertension**, mesenteric thrombosis, **MI**

Central nervous system: **Dizziness**, emotional lability, **headache**, mental depression, **migraine, nervousness**, premenstrual syndrome

Dermatologic: Acne, alopecia, erythema multiforme, erythema nodosum, hirsutism, melasma, rash (allergic)

Endocrine & metabolic: Amenorrhea, breast enlargement, breast secretion, breast tenderness/pain, decreased lactation (immediately postpartum), decreased libido/libido changes, dysmenorrhea, menorrhagia, metrorrhagia, temporary infertility following discontinuation

Gastrointestinal: Abdominal pain, appetite changes, enlarged abdomen, colitis, gallbladder disease, nausea, weight gain/loss (weight gain was the most common reason for discontinuing medication)

Genitourinary: Cervical changes, cystitis-like syndrome, vaginal moniliasis, vaginitis, vulvovaginal disorder

Hematologic: Hemolytic uremic syndrome, hemorrhagic eruption, porphyria

Hepatic: Budd-Chiari syndrome, hepatic adenoma, benign hepatic tumor

Local: Thrombophlebitis

Neuromuscular & skeletal: Weakness

Ocular: Cataracts, intolerance to contact lenses, retinal thrombosis

Renal: Impaired renal function

Respiratory: Pulmonary thromboembolism

Miscellaneous: **Anaphylaxis**, carbohydrate intolerance

Drug Interactions

Increased Effect/Toxicity: Estradiol may inhibit metabolism of cyclosporine, prednisolone, and theophylline, leading to increased plasma levels.

Decreased Effect: Estradiol may decrease plasma levels of acetaminophen, clofibrate, morphine, salicylic acid, and temazepam. Enzyme inducers (carbamazepine, phenobarbital, phenytoin, and rifampin) may increase the metabolism of estradiol, resulting in decreased effect, leading to pregnancy. Griseofulvin, penicillins, and tetracyclines have been shown to alter pharmacokinetics of oral contraceptives leading to pregnancy; effects are not consistent with synthetic steroids. Aminoglutethimide and phenylbutazone may decrease contraceptive effectiveness and increase menstrual irregularities. St John's wort may induce hepatic enzymes resulting in decreased effect of contraceptive and breakthrough bleeding.

Dietary/Ethanol/Herb Considerations

Food: Ascorbic acid (>1 g/day) may increase serum concentration of estradiol. Estradiol may decrease folic acid absorption. Avoid grapefruit products; may increase serum concentration.

Herb/Nutraceutical: Avoid black cohosh, dong quai, and evening primrose due to estrogenic activity. Avoid ginseng, red clover, and saw palmetto due to potential hormonal effects. Avoid St John's wort; may decrease estradiol concentration.

Pharmacodynamics/Kinetics

Absorption: Prolonged

Protein binding: 17-β-estradiol: 97% to sex-hormone-binding globulin and albumin; MPA: 86% to albumin

Metabolism: Hepatic; estradiol via CYP1A2, 3A4, and 3A5-7 to estrone and estriol

Half-life elimination: Mean: 17 β-estradiol: 8.4 days; MPA: 14.7 days

Time to peak: 17 β-estradiol: 1-7 days; MPA: 1-10 days

Excretion: Urine

Pregnancy Risk Factor X

Estradiol and NGM *see* Estradiol and Norgestimate *on page 526*

Estradiol and Norethindrone (es tra DYE ole & nor eth IN drone)

Related Information

Estradiol *on page 521*
Norethindrone *on page 986*

U.S. Brand Names Activella™; CombiPatch®

Pharmacologic Category Estrogen Derivative

Synonyms Norethindrone and Estradiol

Use Women with an intact uterus:

Tablet: Treatment of moderate to severe vasomotor symptoms associated with menopause; treatment of vulvar and vaginal atrophy; prophylaxis for postmenopausal osteoporosis

Transdermal patch: Treatment of moderate to severe vasomotor symptoms associated with menopause; treatment of vulvar and vaginal atrophy; treatment of hypoestrogenism due to hypogonadism, castration, or primary ovarian failure

Local Anesthetic/Vasoconstrictor Precautions No information available to require special precautions

Effects on Dental Treatment Frequency not defined: Dizziness, fatigue, headache, migraine, nervousness, nausea, vomiting, weakness, pharyngitis, rhinitis, allergic reaction, flu-like syndrome

Dosage Adults:

Oral: 1 tablet daily

Transdermal patch:

Continuous combined regimen: Apply one patch twice weekly

Continuous sequential regimen: Apply estradiol-only patch for first 14 days of cycle, followed by one CombiPatch™ applied twice weekly for the remaining 14 days of a 28-day cycle

Other Adverse Effects Frequency not defined:

Cardiovascular: Altered blood pressure, cardiovascular accident, edema, venous thromboembolism

Central nervous system: Insomnia, mental depression

Dermatologic: Chloasma, erythema multiforme, erythema nodosum, hemorrhagic eruption, hirsutism, itching, loss of scalp hair, melasma, pruritus, skin rash

Endocrine & metabolic: Breast enlargement, breast tenderness, breast pain, changes in libido

Gastrointestinal: Abdominal pain, bloating, changes in appetite, flatulence, gallbladder disease, pancreatitis, weight gain/loss

Genitourinary: Alterations in frequency and flow of menses, changes in cervical secretions, cystitis-like syndrome, increased size of uterine leiomyomata, premenstrual-like syndrome, vaginal candidiasis, vaginitis

Hematologic: Aggravation of porphyria

Hepatic: Cholestatic jaundice

Local: Application site reaction (transdermal patch)

Neuromuscular & skeletal: Arthralgia, back pain, chorea, myalgia,

Ocular: Intolerance to contact lenses, steeping of corneal curvature

Respiratory: Pulmonary thromboembolism

Miscellaneous: Carbohydrate intolerance

Dietary/Ethanol/Herb Considerations

Ethanol: Avoid use; increases estrogen concentration and risk of breast cancer; may also increase risk of osteoporosis.

Food: Ascorbic acid (>1 g/day) may increase serum concentration of estradiol. Avoid grapefruit products; may increase estradiol concentration. Estradiol may decrease folic acid absorption.

Herb/Nutraceutical: Avoid black cohosh, dong quai, and evening primrose due to estrogenic activity. Avoid ginseng, red clover, and saw palmetto due to potential hormonal effects. Avoid St John's wort; may decrease estradiol concentration.

Pharmacodynamics/Kinetics

Activella™:

Bioavailability: Estradiol: 50%; Norethindrone: 100%

Half-life elimination: Estradiol: 12-14 hours; Norethindrone: 8-11 hours

Time to peak: Estradiol: 5-8 hours

Pregnancy Risk Factor X

Generic Available No

Estradiol and Norgestimate (es tra DYE ole & nor JES ti mate)

Related Information

Estradiol *on page 521*

U.S. Brand Names Ortho-Prefest®

Pharmacologic Category Estrogen and Progestin Combination

Synonyms Estradiol and NGM; Norgestimate and Estradiol

Use Women with an intact uterus: Treatment of moderate to severe vasomotor symptoms associated with menopause; treatment of atrophic vaginitis; prevention of osteoporosis

Local Anesthetic/Vasoconstrictor Precautions No information available to require special precautions

Effects on Dental Treatment

>10: Headache (23%), upper respiratory tract infection (21%), flu-like symptoms (11%)

1% to 10%: Fatigue (6%), pain (6%), dizziness (5%), nausea (6%), sinusitis (8%), pharyngitis (7%), coughing (5%), viral infection (6%)

Dosage Oral: Adults: Females with an intact uterus:

Treatment of menopausal symptoms, atrophic vaginitis: Treatment is cyclical and consists of the following: One tablet of estradiol 1 mg (pink tablet) once daily for 3 days, followed by 1 tablet of estradiol 1 mg and norgestimate 0.09 mg (white tablet) once daily for 3 days; repeat sequence continuously. **Note:** This dose may not be the lowest effective combination for these indications. In case of a missed tablet, restart therapy with next available tablet in sequence (taking only 1 tablet each day).

Prevention of osteoporosis: See "Treatment of menopausal symptoms"

Mechanism of Action Estrogens are responsible for the development and maintenance of the female reproductive system and secondary sexual characteristics. Estradiol is the principle intracellular human estrogen and is more potent than estrone and estriol at the receptor level; it is the primary estrogen secreted prior to menopause. Following menopause, estrone and estrone sulfate are more highly produced. Estrogens modulate the pituitary secretion of gonadotropins, luteinizing hormone, and follicle-stimulating hormone through a negative feedback system; estrogen replacement reduces elevated levels of these hormones in postmenopausal women.

Progestins inhibit gonadotropin production which then prevents follicular maturation and ovulation. In women with adequate estrogen, progestins transform a proliferative endometrium into a secretory endometrium; when administered with estradiol, reduces the incidence of endometrial hyperplasia and risk of adenocarcinoma.

Other Adverse Effects

>10:

Endocrine & metabolic: Breast pain (16%)

Gastrointestinal: Abdominal pain (12%)

Neuromuscular & skeletal: Back pain (12%)

1% to 10%:

Central nervous system: Depression (5%)

Endocrine & metabolic: Vaginal bleeding (9%), dysmenorrhea (8%), vaginitis (7%)

Gastrointestinal: Flatulence (5%)

Neuromuscular & skeletal: Arthralgia (9%), myalgia (5%)

Associated with estrogens (frequency not defined): Edema, **migraine, vomiting,** chloasma, melasma, erythema multiforme, hemorrhagic eruptions, loss of scalp hair, hirsutism, breast tenderness, breast enlargement, galactorrhea, decreased carbohydrate tolerance, changes in libido, abdominal cramps, bloating, gallbladder disease, weight gain/loss, changes in vaginal bleeding, abnormal withdrawal bleeding/flow, breakthrough bleeding, spotting, increase in size of uterine leiomyomata, vaginal candidiasis, changes in cervical secretion, porphyria, cholestatic jaundice, chorea, steepening of corneal curvature, intolerance to contact lenses

Drug Interactions

Increased Effect/Toxicity: Acetaminophen and ascorbic acid may increase plasma levels of estrogen component. Atorvastatin and indinavir increase plasma levels of estrogen/progestin combinations. Estrogen/progestin combinations increase the plasma levels of alprazolam, chlordiazepoxide, cyclosporine, diazepam, prednisolone, selegiline, theophylline, tricyclic antidepressants. Estrogen/progestin combinations may increase (or decrease) the effects of coumarin derivatives.

Decreased Effect: Estrogen/progestin combinations may decrease plasma levels of acetaminophen, clofibric acid, lorazepam, morphine, oxazepam, salicylic acid, temazepam. Estrogen/progestin levels decreased by aminoglutethimide, amprenavir, anticonvulsants, griseofulvin, lopinavir, nelfinavir, nevirapine, rifampin, and ritonavir. Estrogen/progestin combinations may decrease (or increase) the effects of coumarin derivatives.

Dietary/Ethanol/Herb Considerations

Ethanol: Avoid use; increases estrogen concentration and risk of breast cancer; may also increase risk of osteoporosis.

Food: CNS effects of caffeine may be enhanced. Ascorbic acid (>1 g/day) may increase serum concentration of estradiol. Estradiol may decrease folic acid. Avoid grapefruit products; may increase estradiol concentration. Ensure adequate calcium and vitamin D intake when used for the prevention of osteoporosis.

Herb/Nutraceutical: Avoid black cohosh, dong quai, and evening primrose due to estrogenic activity. Avoid ginseng, red clover, and saw palmetto due to potential hormonal effects. Avoid St John's wort; may decrease the plasma concentration.

Pharmacodynamics/Kinetics

Estradiol: See Estradiol monograph.

Norgestimate:

Protein binding: 17-deacetylnorgestimate: 99%

Metabolism: Forms 17-deacetylnorgestimate (major active metabolite) and other metabolites; first-pass effect

Half-life elimination: 17-deacetylnorgestimate: 37 hours

Excretion: Norgestimate metabolites: Urine and feces

Pregnancy Risk Factor X

Generic Available No

Estradiol and Testosterone (es tra DYE ole & tes TOS ter one)

Related Information

Estradiol *on page 521*

U.S. Brand Names Depo-Testadiol®

Canadian Brand Names Climacteron®

Pharmacologic Category Estrogen Derivative

Synonyms Estradiol Cypionate and Testosterone Cypionate; Estradiol Valerate and Testosterone Enanthate; Testosterone and Estradiol

Use Vasomotor symptoms associated with menopause

Local Anesthetic/Vasoconstrictor Precautions No information available to require special precautions

Effects on Dental Treatment Frequency not defined: Hypertension, MI, stroke, dizziness, anxiety, headache, migraine, nausea, GI distress, increased susceptibility to *Candida* infection

Dosage Adults: All dosage needs to be adjusted based upon the patient's response

Other Adverse Effects Frequency not defined:

Cardiovascular: Edema, thromboembolism

Central nervous system: Depression

Dermatologic: Chloasma, melasma, rash

Endocrine & metabolic: Alterations in frequency and flow of menses, breast tenderness or enlargement, decreased glucose tolerance, increased triglycerides and LDL

Hepatic: Cholestatic jaundice

Dietary/Ethanol/Herb Considerations

Ethanol: Avoid use; increases estrogen concentration and risk of breast cancer.

Food: Ascorbic acid (>1 g/day) may increase serum concentration of estradiol. Estradiol may decrease folic acid absorption. Avoid grapefruit products; may increase serum concentration.

Herb/Nutraceutical: Avoid black cohosh, dong quai, and evening primrose due to estrogenic activity. Avoid ginseng, red clover, and saw palmetto due to potential hormonal effects. Avoid St John's wort; may decrease estradiol concentration.

Pregnancy Risk Factor X

Generic Available No

Estradiol Cypionate *see* Estradiol *on page 521*

Estradiol Cypionate and Medroxyprogesterone Acetate *see* Estradiol and Medroxyprogesterone *on page 523*

Estradiol Cypionate and Testosterone Cypionate *see* Estradiol and Testosterone *on page 527*

Estradiol Hemihydrate *see* Estradiol *on page 521*

Estradiol Transdermal *see* Estradiol *on page 521*

Estradiol Valerate *see* Estradiol *on page 521*

Estradiol Valerate and Testosterone Enanthate *see* Estradiol and Testosterone *on page 527*

Estramustine (es tra MUS teen)

U.S. Brand Names Emcyt®

Canadian Brand Names Emcyt®

Pharmacologic Category Antineoplastic Agent, Alkylating Agent

Synonyms Estramustine Phosphate Sodium

Use Palliative treatment of prostatic carcinoma (progressive or metastatic)

Local Anesthetic/Vasoconstrictor Precautions No information available to require special precautions

Effects on Dental Treatment

>10%: Nausea, vomiting, dyspnea

(Continued)

Estramustine *(Continued)*

1% to 10%: MI, lethargy, leg cramps

Dosage Refer to individual protocols.

Oral: 10-16 mg/kg/day (14 mg/kg/day is most common) or 140 mg 4 times/day (some patients have been maintained for >3 years on therapy)

I.V.: 300 mg/day for 3-4 weeks, then 300-450 mg/week for 3-8 weeks (investigational)

Mechanism of Action Mechanism is not completely clear, thought to act as an alkylating agent and as estrogen

Other Adverse Effects

>10%:

Cardiovascular: Impaired arterial circulation; ischemic heart disease; venous thromboembolism; cardiac decompensation (58%), about 50% of complications occur within the first 2 months of therapy, 85% occur within the first year; edema

Endocrine & metabolic: Sodium and water retention, gynecomastia, breast tenderness, decreased libido

Hematologic: Thrombocytopenia

Local: Thrombophlebitis (nearly 100% with I.V. administration)

1% to 10%:

Central nervous system: Insomnia

Gastrointestinal: Diarrhea, anorexia, flatulence

Hematologic: Leukopenia

Hepatic: Increases in serum transaminases, jaundice

Respiratory: Pulmonary embolism

<1%: **Allergic reactions,** angioedema, **cardiac arrest,** depression, gynecomastia, hypercalcemia, hyperpigmentation, **hot flashes,** impotence, rash, urticaria

Drug Interactions Decreased Effect: Milk products and calcium-rich foods/drugs may impair the oral absorption of estramustine phosphate sodium.

Dietary/Ethanol/Herb Considerations Food: Dairy products and calcium-rich foods may impair oral absorption.

Pharmacodynamics/Kinetics

Absorption: Oral: 75%

Metabolism:

GI tract: Initial dephosphorylation

Hepatic: Oxidation and hydrolysis; metabolites include estramustine, estrone, estradiol, nitrogen mustard

Half-life elimination: Terminal: 20-24 hours

Time to peak, serum: 2-3 hours

Excretion: Feces (2.9% to 4.8% as unchanged drug)

Pregnancy Risk Factor C

Generic Available No

Estramustine Phosphate Sodium *see* Estramustine *on page 527*

Estratab® [DSC] *see* Estrogens (Esterified) *on page 533*

Estratest® *see* Estrogens (Esterified) and Methyltestosterone *on page 534*

Estratest® H.S. *see* Estrogens (Esterified) and Methyltestosterone *on page 534*

Estring® *see* Estradiol *on page 521*

Estrogenic Substance Aqueous *see* Estrone *on page 535*

Estrogenic Substances, Conjugated *see* Estrogens (Conjugated/Equine) *on page 529*

Estrogens (Conjugated A/Synthetic)

(ES troe jenz, KON joo gate ed, aye, sin THET ik)

Related Information

Endocrine Disorders and Pregnancy *on page 1479*

U.S. Brand Names Cenestin®

Pharmacologic Category Estrogen Derivative

Synonyms Estrogens, Conjugated, A (Synthetic)

Use Treatment of moderate to severe vasomotor symptoms of menopause; treatment of vulvar and vaginal atrophy

Local Anesthetic/Vasoconstrictor Precautions No information available to require special precautions

Effects on Dental Treatment Associated with estrogen therapy; frequency not defined: Hypertension, dizziness, headache, migraine, nausea, vomiting

Dosage The lowest dose that will control symptoms should be used; medication should be discontinued as soon as possible. Oral:

Adults:

Moderate to severe vasomotor symptoms: 0.625 mg/day; may be titrated up to 1.25 mg/day. Attempts to discontinue medication should be made at 3- to 6-month intervals.

Vulvar and vaginal atrophy: 0.3 mg/day

Elderly: Refer to Adults dosing. A higher incidence of stroke and invasive breast cancer were observed in women >75 years in a WHI substudy using conjugated equine estrogen.

Mechanism of Action Conjugated A/synthetic estrogens contain a mixture of 9 synthetic estrogen substances, including sodium estrone sulfate, sodium equilin sulfate, sodium 17 alpha-dihydroequilin, sodium 17 alpha-estradiol and sodium 17 beta-dihydroequilin. Estrogens are responsible for the development and maintenance of the female reproductive system and secondary sexual characteristics. Estradiol is the principle intracellular human estrogen and is more potent than estrone and estriol at the receptor level; it is the primary estrogen secreted prior to menopause. Following menopause, estrone and estrone sulfate are more highly produced. Estrogens modulate the pituitary secretion of gonadotropins, luteinizing hormone, and follicle-stimulating hormone through a negative feedback system; estrogen replacement reduces elevated levels of these hormones in postmenopausal women.

Other Adverse Effects Associated with estrogen therapy; frequency not defined:

Cardiovascular: Edema, venous thromboembolism

Central nervous system: Mental depression

Dermatologic: Chloasma, erythema multiforme, erythema nodosum, hemorrhagic eruption, hirsutism, loss of scalp hair, melasma

Endocrine & metabolic: Breast enlargement, breast tenderness, changes in libido, thyroid-binding globulin increased, total thyroid hormone (T_4) increased, serum triglycerides/phospholipids increased, HDL-cholesterol increased, LDL-cholesterol decreased, impaired glucose tolerance, hypercalcemia

Gastrointestinal: Abdominal cramps, bloating, cholecystitis, cholelithiasis, gallbladder disease, pancreatitis, weight gain/loss

Genitourinary: Alterations in frequency and flow of menses, changes in cervical secretions, endometrial cancer, increased size of uterine leiomyomata, vaginal candidiasis

Hematologic: Aggravation of porphyria, antithrombin III and antifactor Xa decreased, levels of fibrinogen decreased, platelet aggregability and platelet count increased; prothrombin and factors VII, VIII, IX, X increased

Hepatic: Cholestatic jaundice

Neuromuscular & skeletal: Chorea

Ocular: Intolerance to contact lenses, steeping of corneal curvature

Respiratory: Pulmonary thromboembolism

Miscellaneous: Carbohydrate intolerance

Drug Interactions Based on estradiol and estrone: Substrate of **1A2**, 2A6, 2B6, 2C8/9, 2C19, 2D6, 2E1, **3A4**; Inhibits 1A2; Induces 3A4

Increased Effect/Toxicity: CYP3A4 enzyme inhibitors may increase estrogen plasma concentrations leading to increased incidence of adverse effects; examples of CYP3A4 enzyme inhibitors include clarithromycin, erythromycin, itraconazole, ketoconazole, and ritonavir. Anticoagulants increase the potential for thromboembolic events Estrogens may enhance the effects of hydrocortisone and prednisone

Decreased Effect: CYP3A4 enzyme inducers may decrease estrogen plasma concentrations leading to decreased therapeutic effect or changes in uterine bleeding profile; examples of CYP3A4 enzyme inducers include carbamazepine, phenobarbital, and rifampin

Dietary/Ethanol/Herb Considerations

Ethanol: Avoid use; increases estrogen concentration and risk of breast cancer.

Food: Ascorbic acid (>1 g/day) may increase serum concentration. Estrogen decreases folic acid absorption. Avoid grapefruit products; may increase serum concentration.

Herb/Nutraceutical: Avoid black cohosh, dong quai, and evening primrose due to estrogenic activity. Avoid ginseng, red clover, and saw palmetto due to potential hormonal effects. Avoid St John's wort; may decrease serum concentration.

Pharmacodynamics/Kinetics

Absorption: Readily absorbed

Protein-binding: Sex hormone-binding globulin (SHBG) and albumin

Metabolism: Hepatic to metabolites

Time to peak: 4-16 hours

Excretion: Urine

Pregnancy Risk Factor X

Generic Available No

Comments Not biologically equivalent to conjugated estrogens from equine source. Contains 9 unique estrogenic compounds (equine source contains at least 10 active estrogenic compounds).

Estrogens (Conjugated/Equine)

(ES troe jenz, KON joo gay ted, E kwine)

Related Information

Endocrine Disorders and Pregnancy *on page 1479*

U.S. Brand Names Premarin®

Canadian Brand Names Cenestin; C.E.S.®; Congest; Premarin®

(Continued)

Estrogens (Conjugated/Equine) *(Continued)*

Pharmacologic Category Estrogen Derivative

Synonyms C.E.S.; Estrogenic Substances, Conjugated

Use Treatment of moderate to severe vasomotor symptoms associated with menopause; treatment of vulvar and vaginal atrophy; hypoestrogenism (due to hypogonadism, castration, or primary ovarian failure); prostatic cancer (palliation); breast cancer (palliation); osteoporosis (prophylaxis, women at significant risk only)

Unlabeled/Investigational Use Treatment of uremic or abnormal uterine bleeding

Local Anesthetic/Vasoconstrictor Precautions No information available to require special precautions

Effects on Dental Treatment Frequency not defined: Dizziness, headache, migraine, nausea, vomiting, hypertension

Dosage Adults:

Male: Androgen-dependent prostate cancer: Oral: 1.25-2.5 mg 3 times/day

Female:

Prevention of osteoporosis in postmenopausal women: Oral: 0.625 mg/day, cyclically* or daily, depending on medical assessment of patient

Moderate to severe vasomotor symptoms associated with menopause: Oral: The lowest dose that will control symptoms should be used. Medication should be discontinued as soon as possible. 0.625 mg/day was previously recommended. May be given cyclically* or daily, depending on medical assessment of patient

Vulvar and vaginal atrophy:

Oral: The lowest dose that will control symptoms should be used. Medication should be discontinued as soon as possible. 0.3-1.25 mg (or more) daily, depending on tissue response of the patient, was previously recommended. May be given cyclically* or daily, depending on medical assessment of patient.

Vaginal cream: Intravaginal: $^1/_2$ to 2 g/day given cyclically*

Abnormal uterine bleeding:

Acute/heavy bleeding:

Oral: 1.25 mg, may repeat every 4 hours for 24 hours, followed by 1.25 mg once daily for 7-10 days

I.V.: 25 mg, may repeat every 4 hours up to 3 doses

Note: Oral/I.V.: Treatment should be followed by a low-dose oral contraceptive; medroxyprogesterone acetate along with or following estrogen therapy can also be given

Nonacute/lesser bleeding: Oral: 1.25 mg once daily for 7-10 days

Female hypogonadism: Oral: 0.3-0.625 mg/day given cyclically*; adjust dose in response to symptoms and endometrium response; progestin treatment should be added to maintain bone mineral density

Female castration, primary ovarian failure: Oral: 1.25 mg/day given cyclically*; adjust according to severity of symptoms and patient response. For maintenance, adjust to the lowest effective dose.

***Cyclic administration:** Either 3 weeks on, 1 week off **or** 25 days on, 5 days off

Male and Female:

Breast cancer palliation, metastatic disease in selected patients: Oral: 10 mg 3 times/day for at least 3 months

Uremic bleeding: I.V.: 0.6 mg/kg/day for 5 days

Elderly: Refer to Adults dosing; a higher incidence of stroke and invasive breast cancer was observed in women >75 years in a WHI substudy.

Mechanism of Action Conjugated estrogens contain a mixture of estrone sulfate, equilin sulfate, 17 alpha-dihydroequilin, 17 alpha-estradiol and 17 beta-dihydroequilin. Estrogens are responsible for the development and maintenance of the female reproductive system and secondary sexual characteristics. Estradiol is the principle intracellular human estrogen and is more potent than estrone and estriol at the receptor level; it is the primary estrogen secreted prior to menopause. Following menopause, estrone and estrone sulfate are more highly produced. Estrogens modulate the pituitary secretion of gonadotropins, luteinizing hormone, and follicle-stimulating hormone through a negative feedback system; estrogen replacement reduces elevated levels of these hormones in postmenopausal women.

Other Adverse Effects Frequency not defined:

Cardiovascular: Edema, venous thromboembolism

Central nervous system: Mental depression

Dermatologic: Chloasma, erythema multiforme, erythema nodosum, hemorrhagic eruption, hirsutism, loss of scalp hair, melasma

Endocrine & metabolic: Breast enlargement, breast tenderness, changes in libido, increased thyroid-binding globulin, increased total thyroid hormone (T_4), increased serum triglycerides/phospholipids, increased HDL-cholesterol, decreased LDL-cholesterol, impaired glucose tolerance, hypercalcemia

Gastrointestinal: Abdominal cramps, bloating, cholecystitis, cholelithiasis, gallbladder disease, pancreatitis, weight gain/loss

Genitourinary: Alterations in frequency and flow of menses, changes in cervical secretions, endometrial cancer, increased size of uterine leiomyomata, vaginal candidiasis

Hematologic: Aggravation of porphyria, decreased antithrombin III and antifactor Xa, increased levels of fibrinogen, increased platelet aggregability and platelet count; increased prothrombin and factors VII, VIII, IX, X

Hepatic: Cholestatic jaundice

Neuromuscular & skeletal: Chorea

Ocular: Intolerance to contact lenses, steeping of corneal curvature

Respiratory: Pulmonary thromboembolism

Miscellaneous: Carbohydrate intolerance

Warnings/Precautions Should not be used to prevent coronary heart disease. May increase the risks of MI, stroke, pulmonary emboli, and deep vein thrombosis; incidence of these effects was shown to be significantly increased in postmenopausal women using conjugated equine estrogens (CEE) in combination with medroxyprogesterone acetate (MPA). Unopposed estrogens may increase the risk of endometrial carcinoma in postmenopausal women. Estrogens may increase the risk of breast cancer (controversial/currently under study; increased risk of invasive breast cancer observed in postmenopausal women using CEE in combination with MPA). Use with caution in patients with diseases which may be exacerbated by fluid retention, including asthma, epilepsy, migraine, diabetes, cardiac or renal dysfunction. Use with caution in patients with a history of hypercalcemia, cardiovascular disease, and gallbladder disease. May increase blood pressure. Use with caution in patients with hepatic disease. Estrogen compounds are generally associated with lipid effects such as increased HDL-cholesterol and decreased LDL-cholesterol. Triglycerides may also be increased; use with caution in patients with familial defects of lipoprotein metabolism. Estrogens may cause premature closure of the epiphyses in young individuals. May increase size of pre-existing uterine leiomyomata. Before prescribing estrogen therapy to postmenopausal women, the risks and benefits must be weighed for each patient. Women should be informed of these risks and benefits, as well as possible effects of progestin when added to estrogen therapy. Use for shortest duration possible consistent with treatment goals. Conduct periodic risk:benefit assessments. When used solely for the treatment of vulvar and vaginal atrophy, topical vaginal products should be considered. When used solely for prevention of osteoporosis in women at significant risk, nonestrogen treatment options should be considered. Safety and efficacy in pediatric patients have not been established.

Drug Interactions Based on estradiol and estrone: Substrate of **1A2**, 2A6, 2B6, 2C8/9, 2C19, 2D6, 2E1, **3A4**; Inhibits 1A2; Induces 3A4

Increased Effect/Toxicity: Hydrocortisone taken with estrogen may cause corticosteroid-induced toxicity. Increased potential for thromboembolic events with anticoagulants.

Decreased Effect: Rifampin, nelfinavir, and ritonavir decrease estradiol serum concentrations. Anticonvulsants which are enzyme inducers (barbiturates, carbamazepine, phenobarbital, phenytoin, primidone) may potentially decrease estrogen levels.

Dietary/Ethanol/Herb Considerations

Ethanol: Avoid use; increases estrogen concentration and risk of breast cancer; may also increase risk of osteoporosis.

Food: Ascorbic acid (>1 g/day) may increase serum concentration. Estrogen decreases folic acid absorption. Avoid grapefruit products; may increase serum concentration.

Herb/Nutraceutical: Avoid black cohosh, dong quai, and evening primrose due to estrogenic activity. Avoid ginseng, red clover, and saw palmetto due to potential hormonal effects. Avoid St John's wort; may decrease serum concentration.

Pharmacodynamics/Kinetics

Absorption: Well absorbed

Metabolism: Hepatic to inactive compounds

Excretion: Urine and feces

Pregnancy Risk Factor X

Generic Available No

Estrogens (Conjugated/Equine) and Medroxyprogesterone

(ES troe jenz, KON joo gay ted, E kwine, & me DROKS ee proe JES te rone)

Related Information

Endocrine Disorders and Pregnancy *on page 1479*

U.S. Brand Names Premphase®; Prempro™

Canadian Brand Names Premphase®; Premplus®; Prempro™

Pharmacologic Category Estrogen Derivative

Synonyms Medroxyprogesterone and Estrogens (Conjugated); MPA and Estrogens (Conjugated)

Use Women with an intact uterus: Treatment of moderate to severe vasomotor symptoms associated with menopause; treatment of atrophic vaginitis; osteoporosis (prophylaxis)

(Continued)

Estrogens (Conjugated/Equine) and Medroxyprogesterone *(Continued)*

Local Anesthetic/Vasoconstrictor Precautions No information available to require special precautions

Effects on Dental Treatment

>10%: Headache (28% to 37%), pain (11% to 13%), nausea (9% to 11%), pharyngitis (11% to 13%), Infection (16% to 18%), flu-like syndrome (10% to 13%)

1% to 10%: Dizziness (3% to 5%), weakness (6% to 10%), cramps (3% to 5%), sinusitis (7% to 8%), rhinitis (6% to 8%)

Dosage Oral: Adults:

Treatment of moderate to severe vasomotor symptoms associated with menopause or treatment of atrophic vaginitis in females with an intact uterus. (The lowest dose that will control symptoms should be used; medication should be discontinued as soon as possible):

Premphase®: One maroon conjugated estrogen 0.625 mg tablet daily on days 1 through 14 and one light blue conjugated estrogen 0.625 mg/MPA 5 mg tablet daily on days 15 through 28; re-evaluate patients at 3- and 6-month intervals to determine if treatment is still necessary; monitor patients for signs of endometrial cancer; rule out malignancy if unexplained vaginal bleeding occurs

Prempro™: One conjugated estrogen 0.625 mg/MPA 2.5 mg tablet daily; re-evaluate at 3-and 6-month intervals to determine if therapy is still needed; dose may be increased to one conjugated estrogen 0.625 mg/MPA 5 mg tablet daily in patients with bleeding or spotting, once malignancy has been ruled out

Osteoporosis prophylaxis in females with an intact uterus:

Premphase®: One maroon conjugated estrogen 0.625 tablet daily on days 1 through 14 and one light blue conjugated estrogen 0.625 mg/MPA 5 mg tablet daily on days 15 through 28; monitor patients for signs of endometrial cancer; rule out malignancy if unexplained vaginal bleeding occurs

Prempro™: One conjugated estrogen 0.625 mg/MPA 2.5 mg tablet daily; dose may be increased to one conjugated estrogen 0.625 mg/MPA 5 mg tablet daily; in patients with bleeding or spotting, once malignancy has been ruled out

Elderly: Refer to Adults dosing; a higher incidence of stroke and invasive breast cancer was observed in women >75 years in a WHI substudy.

Mechanism of Action

Conjugated estrogens contain a mixture of estrone sulfate, equilin sulfate, 17 alpha-dihydroequilin, 17 alpha-estradiol, and 17 beta-dihydroequilin. Estrogens are responsible for the development and maintenance of the female reproductive system and secondary sexual characteristics. Estradiol is the principle intracellular human estrogen and is more potent than estrone and estriol at the receptor level; it is the primary estrogen secreted prior to menopause. Following menopause, estrone and estrone sulfate are more highly produced. Estrogens modulate the pituitary secretion of gonadotropins, luteinizing hormone, and follicle-stimulating hormone through a negative feedback system; estrogen replacement reduces elevated levels of these hormones in postmenopausal women.

MPA inhibits gonadotropin production which then prevents follicular maturation and ovulation. In women with adequate estrogen, MPA transforms a proliferative endometrium into a secretory endometrium; when administered with conjugated estrogens, reduces the incidence of endometrial hyperplasia and risk of adenocarcinoma.

Other Adverse Effects

>10%:

Central nervous system: Depression (6% to 11%)
Endocrine & metabolic: Breast pain (32% to 38%), dysmenorrhea (8% to 13%)
Gastrointestinal: Abdominal pain (16% to 23%)
Neuromuscular & skeletal: Back pain (13% to 16%)

1% to 10%:

Cardiovascular: Peripheral edema (3% to 4%)
Dermatologic: Pruritus (5% to 10%), rash (4% to 6%)
Endocrine & metabolic: Leukorrhea (5% to 9%)
Gastrointestinal: Flatulence (8% to 9%), diarrhea (5% to 6%), dyspepsia (5% to 6%)
Genitourinary: Vaginitis (5% to 7%), cervical changes (4% to 5%), vaginal hemorrhage (1% to 3%)
Neuromuscular & skeletal: Arthralgia (7% to 9%), hypertonia (3% to 4%)

Reported with conjugated estrogens and/or progestins: Abdominal cramps, acne, abnormal uterine bleeding, aggravation of porphyria, amenorrhea, **anaphylactoid reactions, anaphylaxis,** antifactor Xa decreased, antithrombin III decreased, appetite changes, bloating, breast enlargement, breast tenderness, cerebral embolism, cerebral thrombosis, chloasma, cholestatic jaundice, cholecystitis, cholelithiasis, chorea, contact lens intolerance, cystitis-like syndrome, decreased carbohydrate tolerance, dizziness; factors VII, VIII, IX, X, XII, VII-X complex, and II-VII-X complex increased; endometrial hyperplasia, erythema multiforme, erythema nodosum, galactorrhea, hemorrhagic eruption, **fatigue,** fibrinogen increased, impaired glucose tolerance, HDL-cholesterol increased, hirsutism, hypertension, increase in size of uterine leiomyomata, gallbladder disease, insomnia, LDL-cholesterol decreased, libido changes, loss of scalp hair, melasma, **migraine, nervousness,** optic neuritis, pancreatitis, platelet aggregability and platelet count increased, premenstrual like syndrome, PT and PTT accelerated, pulmonary embolism, pyrexia, retinal thrombosis, **somnolence,** steepening of corneal curvature, thrombophlebitis, thyroid-binding globulin increased, total thyroid hormone (T_4) increased, triglycerides increased, urticaria, vaginal candidiasis, **vomiting,** weight gain/loss

Drug Interactions

Increased Effect/Toxicity: Hydrocortisone taken with estrogen may cause corticosteroid-induced toxicity. Increased potential for thromboembolic events with anticoagulants.

Decreased Effect: Conjugated estrogens: Anticonvulsants which are enzyme inducers (barbiturates, carbamazepine, phenobarbital, phenytoin, primidone) may potentially decrease estrogen levels. Rifampin, nelfinavir, and ritonavir decrease estradiol serum concentrations. Aminoglutethimide may decrease effects by increasing hepatic metabolism.

Dietary/Ethanol/Herb Considerations

Ethanol: Avoid use; increases estrogen concentration and risk of breast cancer; may also increase risk of osteoporosis.

Food: Ascorbic acid (>1 g/day) may increase serum concentration. Estrogen decreases folic acid absorption. Avoid grapefruit products; may increase serum concentration.

Herb/Nutraceutical: Avoid black cohosh, dong quai, and evening primrose due to estrogenic activity. Avoid ginseng, red clover, and saw palmetto due to potential hormonal effects. Avoid St John's wort; may decrease serum concentration.

Pharmacodynamics/Kinetics

Premphase®, Prempro™:

Half-life elimination: 10-24 hours

Time to peak: 4-10 hours

Pregnancy Risk Factor X

Generic Available No

Estrogens (Esterified) (ES troe jenz, es TER i fied)

Related Information

Endocrine Disorders and Pregnancy *on page 1479*

U.S. Brand Names Estratab® [DSC]; Menest®

Canadian Brand Names Estratab®; Menest®

Pharmacologic Category Estrogen Derivative

Synonyms Esterified Estrogens; Estratab® [DSC]

Use Treatment of moderate to severe vasomotor symptoms associated with menopause; treatment of vulvar and vaginal atrophy; hypoestrogenism (due to hypogonadism, castration, or primary ovarian failure); prostatic cancer (palliation); breast cancer (palliation); osteoporosis (prophylaxis, in women at significant risk only)

Local Anesthetic/Vasoconstrictor Precautions No information available to require special precautions

Effects on Dental Treatment Frequency not defined: Hypertension, dizziness, headache, migraine, nausea, vomiting

Dosage Oral: Adults:

Prostate cancer (palliation): 1.25-2.5 mg 3 times/day

Female hypogonadism: 2.5-7.5 mg of estrogen daily for 20 days followed by a 10-day rest period. Administer cyclically (3 weeks on and 1 week off). If bleeding does not occur by the end of the 10-day period, repeat the same dosing schedule; the number of courses is dependent upon the responsiveness of the endometrium. If bleeding occurs before the end of the 10-day period, begin an estrogen-progestin cyclic regimen of 2.5-7.5 mg esterified estrogens daily for 20 days. During the last 5 days of estrogen therapy, give an oral progestin. If bleeding occurs before regimen is concluded, discontinue therapy and resume on the fifth day of bleeding.

Moderate to severe vasomotor symptoms associated with menopause: 1.25 mg/day administered cyclically (3 weeks on and 1 week off). If patient has not menstruated within the last 2 months or more, cyclic administration is started arbitrary. If the patient is menstruating, cyclical administration is started on day 5 of the bleeding. For short-term use only and should be discontinued as soon as possible. Re-evaluate at 3- to 6-month intervals for tapering or discontinuation of therapy.

Atopic vaginitis and kraurosis vulvae: 0.3 to ≥1.25 mg/day, depending on the tissue response of the individual patient. Administer cyclically. For short-term use only and should be discontinued as soon as possible. Re-evaluate at 3- to 6-month intervals for tapering or discontinuation of therapy.

Breast cancer (palliation): 10 mg 3 times/day for at least 3 months

Osteoporosis in postmenopausal women: Initial: 0.3 mg/day and increase to a maximum daily dose of 1.25 mg/day; initiate therapy as soon as possible after menopause; cyclically or daily, depending on medical assessment of patient.

(Continued)

Estrogens (Esterified) *(Continued)*

Monitor patients with an intact uterus for signs of endometrial cancer; rule out malignancy if unexplained vaginal bleeding occurs

Female castration and primary ovarian failure: 1.25 mg/day, cyclically. Adjust dosage upward or downward, according to the severity of symptoms and patient response. For maintenance, adjust dosage to lowest level that will provide effective control.

Elderly: Refer to Adults dosing. A higher incidence of stroke and invasive breast cancer were observed in women >75 years in a WHI substudy using conjugated equine estrogen.

Dosing adjustment in hepatic impairment: Reduction recommended in mild to moderate impairment; use not recommended in severe impairment

Mechanism of Action Esterified estrogens contain a mixture of estrogenic substances; the principle component is estrone. Preparations contain 75% to 85% sodium estrone sulfate and 6% to 15% sodium equilin sulfate such that the total is not <90%. Estrogens are responsible for the development and maintenance of the female reproductive system and secondary sexual characteristics. Estradiol is the principle intracellular human estrogen and is more potent than estrone and estriol at the receptor level; it is the primary estrogen secreted prior to menopause. In males and following menopause in females, estrone and estrone sulfate are more highly produced. Estrogens modulate the pituitary secretion of gonadotropins, luteinizing hormone, and follicle-stimulating hormone through a negative feedback system; estrogen replacement reduces elevated levels of these hormones.

Other Adverse Effects Frequency not defined:

Cardiovascular: Edema, venous thromboembolism

Central nervous system: Mental depression

Dermatologic: Chloasma, erythema multiforme, erythema nodosum, hemorrhagic eruption, hirsutism, loss of scalp hair, melasma

Endocrine & metabolic: Breast enlargement, breast tenderness, changes in libido, increased thyroid-binding globulin, increased total thyroid hormone (T_4), increased serum triglycerides/phospholipids, increased HDL-cholesterol, decreased LDL-cholesterol, impaired glucose tolerance, hypercalcemia

Gastrointestinal: Abdominal cramps, bloating, cholecystitis, cholelithiasis, gallbladder disease, pancreatitis, weight gain/loss

Genitourinary: Alterations in frequency and flow of menses, changes in cervical secretions, endometrial cancer, increased size of uterine leiomyomata, vaginal candidiasis

Hematologic: Aggravation of porphyria, decreased antithrombin III and antifactor Xa, increased levels of fibrinogen, increased platelet aggregability and platelet count; increased prothrombin and factors VII, VIII, IX, X

Hepatic: Cholestatic jaundice

Neuromuscular & skeletal: Chorea

Ocular: Intolerance to contact lenses, steeping of corneal curvature

Respiratory: Pulmonary thromboembolism

Miscellaneous: Carbohydrate intolerance

Drug Interactions Based on estrone: Substrate of **1A2**, 2B6, 2C8/9, 2E1, **3A4**

Increased Effect/Toxicity: Hydrocortisone taken with estrogen may cause corticosteroid-induced toxicity. Increased potential for thromboembolic events with anticoagulants.

Decreased Effect: Rifampin, nelfinavir, and ritonavir decrease estradiol serum concentrations. Anticonvulsants which are enzyme inducers (barbiturates, carbamazepine, phenobarbital, phenytoin, primidone) may potentially decrease estrogen levels.

Dietary/Ethanol/Herb Considerations

Ethanol: Avoid use; increases estrogen concentration and risk of breast cancer; may also increase risk of osteoporosis.

Food: Ascorbic acid (>1 g/day) may increase serum concentration. Estrogen decreases folic acid absorption. Avoid grapefruit products; may increase serum concentration.

Herb/Nutraceutical: Avoid black cohosh, dong quai, and evening primrose due to estrogenic activity. Avoid ginseng, red clover, and saw palmetto due to potential hormonal effects. Avoid St John's wort; may decrease serum concentration.

Pharmacodynamics/Kinetics

Absorption: Readily

Metabolism: Rapidly hepatic to estrone sulfate, conjugated and unconjugated metabolites; first-pass effect

Excretion: Urine (as unchanged drug and as glucuronide and sulfate conjugates)

Pregnancy Risk Factor X

Generic Available No

Estrogens (Esterified) and Methyltestosterone

(ES troe jenz, es TER i fied, & meth il tes TOS te rone)

Related Information

Endocrine Disorders and Pregnancy *on page 1479*

U.S. Brand Names Estratest®; Estratest® H.S.

Canadian Brand Names Estratest®

Pharmacologic Category Estrogen Derivative

Synonyms Conjugated Estrogen and Methyltestosterone; Esterified Estrogen and Methyltestosterone

Use Vasomotor symptoms of menopause

Local Anesthetic/Vasoconstrictor Precautions No information available to require special precautions

Effects on Dental Treatment 1% to 10%: Nausea, vomiting, headache

Dosage Adults: Female: Oral: Lowest dose that will control symptoms should be chosen, normally given 3 weeks on and 1 week off

Mechanism of Action

Conjugated estrogens: Activate estrogen receptors (DNA protein complex) located in estrogen-responsive tissues. Once activated, regulate transcription of certain genes leading to observed effects.

Testosterone: Increases synthesis of DNA, RNA, and various proteins in target tissues

Other Adverse Effects 1% to 10%:

Cardiovascular: Increase in blood pressure, edema, thromboembolic disorder

Central nervous system: Depression

Dermatologic: Chloasma, melasma

Endocrine & metabolic: Breast tenderness, change in menstrual flow, hypercalcemia

Hepatic: Cholestatic jaundice

Drug Interactions Estrone: Substrate of **1A2**, 2B6, 2C8/9, 2E1, **3A4**

Dietary/Ethanol/Herb Considerations

Ethanol: Avoid use; increases estrogen concentration and risk of breast cancer.

Food: Ascorbic acid (>1 g/day) may increase serum concentration. Estrogen decreases folic acid absorption. Avoid grapefruit products; may increase serum concentration

Herb/Nutraceutical: Avoid black cohosh, dong quai, and evening primrose due to estrogenic activity. Avoid ginseng, red clover, and saw palmetto due to potential hormonal effects. Avoid St John's wort; may decrease concentration.

Pregnancy Risk Factor X

Generic Available No

Estrone (ES trone)

Related Information

Endocrine Disorders and Pregnancy *on page 1479*

Pharmacologic Category Estrogen Derivative

Synonyms Estrogenic Substance Aqueous

Use Hypogonadism; primary ovarian failure; vasomotor symptoms of menopause; prostatic carcinoma; inoperable breast cancer, kraurosis vulvae, abnormal uterine bleeding due to hormone imbalance

Local Anesthetic/Vasoconstrictor Precautions No information available to require special precautions

Effects on Dental Treatment

>10%: Nausea

1% to 10%: Headache, vomiting

Dosage Adults: I.M.:

Male: Prostatic carcinoma: 2-4 mg 2-3 times/week

Female:

Senile vaginitis and kraurosis vulvae: 0.1-0.5 mg 2-3 times/week

Breast cancer (inoperable, progressing): 5 mg 3 or more times/week

Primary ovarian failure, hypogonadism: 0.1-1 mg/week, up to 2 mg/week in single or divided doses

Abnormal uterine bleeding: 2.5 mg/day for several days

Mechanism of Action A natural ovarian estrogenic hormone available as an aqueous mixture of water insoluble estrone and water soluble estrone potassium sulfate; all estrogens, including estrone, act in a similar manner; there is no evidence that there are biological differences among various estrogen preparations other than their ability to bind to cellular receptors inside the target cells.

Other Adverse Effects

>10%:

Cardiovascular: Peripheral edema

Endocrine & metabolic: Enlargement of breasts, breast tenderness

Gastrointestinal: Anorexia, bloating

1% to 10%:

Endocrine & metabolic: Increased libido

Gastrointestinal: Diarrhea

Dietary/Ethanol/Herb Considerations

Ethanol: Avoid use; increases estrogen level and risk of breast cancer.

(Continued)

Estrone *(Continued)*

Food: Ascorbic acid (>1 g/day) may increase serum concentration. Estrogen decreases folic acid absorption. Avoid grapefruit products; may increase serum concentration.

Herb/Nutraceutical: Avoid black cohosh, dong quai, and evening primrose due to estrogenic activity. Avoid ginseng, red clover, and saw palmetto due to potential hormonal effects. Avoid St John's wort; may decrease estradiol concentration.

Pharmacodynamics/Kinetics Absorption: Readily absorbed from the GI tract

Estropipate (ES troe pih pate)

Related Information

Endocrine Disorders and Pregnancy *on page 1479*

U.S. Brand Names Ogen®; Ortho-Est®

Canadian Brand Names Ogen®

Mexican Brand Names Ogen®

Pharmacologic Category Estrogen Derivative

Synonyms Piperazine Estrone Sulfate

Use Treatment of moderate to severe vasomotor symptoms associated with menopause; treatment of vulvar and vaginal atrophy; hypoestrogenism (due to hypogonadism, castration, or primary ovarian failure); osteoporosis (prophylaxis, in women at significant risk only)

Local Anesthetic/Vasoconstrictor Precautions No information available to require special precautions

Effects on Dental Treatment Frequency not defined: Hypertension, dizziness, headache, migraine, nausea, vomiting

Dosage Adults:

Oral:

Moderate to severe vasomotor symptoms associated with menopause: Usual dosage range: 0.75-6 mg estropipate daily; use the lowest dose and regimen that will control symptoms, and discontinue as soon as possible. Attempt to discontinue or taper medication at 3- to 6-month intervals. If a patient with vasomotor symptoms has not menstruated within the last ≥2 months, start the cyclic administration arbitrarily. If the patient has menstruated, start cyclic administration on day 5 of bleeding.

Female hypogonadism: 1.5-9 mg estropipate daily for the first 3 weeks, followed by a rest period of 8-10 days; use the lowest dose and regimen that will control symptoms. Repeat if bleeding does not occur by the end of the rest period. The duration of therapy necessary to product the withdrawal bleeding will vary according to the responsiveness of the endometrium. If satisfactory withdrawal bleeding does not occur, give an oral progestin in addition to estrogen during the third week of the cycle.

Female castration or primary ovarian failure: 1.5-9 mg estropipate daily for the first 3 weeks of a theoretical cycle, followed by a rest period of 8-10 days; use the lowest dose and regimen that will control symptoms

Osteoporosis prophylaxis: 0.75 mg estropipate daily for 25 days of a 31-day cycle

Atrophic vaginitis or kraurosis vulvae: 0.75-6 mg estropipate daily; administer cyclically. Use the lowest dose and regimen that will control symptoms; discontinue as soon as possible.

Intravaginal: Atrophic vaginitis or kraurosis vulvae: Instill 2-4 g/day intravaginally; use the lowest dose and regimen that will control symptoms; attempt to discontinue or taper medication at 3- to 6-month intervals

Elderly: Refer to Adult dosing. A higher incidence of stroke and invasive breast cancer were observed in women >75 years in a WHI substudy using conjugated equine estrogen.

Dosing adjustment in hepatic impairment: Reduction recommended in mild to moderate impairment; use not recommended in severe impairment

Mechanism of Action Estrogens are responsible for the development and maintenance of the female reproductive system and secondary sexual characteristics. Estradiol is the principle intracellular human estrogen and is more potent than estrone and estriol at the receptor level; it is the primary estrogen secreted prior to menopause. In males and following menopause in females, estrone and estrone sulfate are more highly produced. Estrogens modulate the pituitary secretion of gonadotropins, luteinizing hormone, and follicle-stimulating hormone through a negative feedback system; estrogen replacement reduces elevated levels of these hormones. Estropipate is prepared from purified crystalline estrone that has been solubilized as the sulfate and stabilized with piperazine.

Other Adverse Effects Frequency not defined:

Cardiovascular: Edema, venous thromboembolism

Central nervous system: Mental depression

Dermatologic: Chloasma, erythema multiforme, erythema nodosum, hemorrhagic eruption, hirsutism, loss of scalp hair, melasma

Endocrine & metabolic: Breast enlargement, breast tenderness, changes in libido, increased thyroid-binding globulin, increased total thyroid hormone (T_4), increased serum triglycerides/phospholipids, increased HDL-cholesterol, decreased LDL-cholesterol, impaired glucose tolerance, hypercalcemia

Gastrointestinal: Abdominal cramps, bloating, cholecystitis, cholelithiasis, gallbladder disease, pancreatitis, weight gain/loss

Genitourinary: Alterations in frequency and flow of menses, changes in cervical secretions, endometrial cancer, increased size of uterine leiomyomata, vaginal candidiasis

Hematologic: Aggravation of porphyria, decreased antithrombin III and antifactor Xa, increased levels of fibrinogen, increased platelet aggregability and platelet count; increased prothrombin and factors VII, VIII, IX, X

Hepatic: Cholestatic jaundice

Neuromuscular & skeletal: Chorea

Ocular: Intolerance to contact lenses, steeping of corneal curvature

Respiratory: Pulmonary thromboembolism

Miscellaneous: Carbohydrate intolerance

Drug Interactions Based on estrone: Substrate of **CYP1A2**, 2B6, 2C8/9, 2E1, **3A4**

Increased Effect/Toxicity: Hydrocortisone taken with estrogen may cause corticosteroid-induced toxicity. Increased potential for thromboembolic events with anticoagulants.

Decreased Effect: Rifampin, nelfinavir, and ritonavir decrease estradiol serum concentrations. Anticonvulsants which are enzyme inducers (barbiturates, carbamazepine, phenobarbital, phenytoin, primidone) may potentially decrease estrogen levels.

Dietary/Ethanol/Herb Considerations

Ethanol: Avoid use; increases estrogen concentration and risk of breast cancer; may also increase risk of osteoporosis.

Food: Folic acid absorption may be decreased.

Herb/Nutraceutical: Avoid black cohosh and dong quai due to estrogenic activity. Avoid ginseng, red clover, and saw palmetto due to potential hormonal effects. Avoid St John's wort; may decrease serum concentration.

Pharmacodynamics/Kinetics

Absorption: Well absorbed

Metabolism: Hepatic and in target tissues; first-pass effect

Pregnancy Risk Factor X

Generic Available Yes: Tablet

Estrostep® 21 [DSC] *see* Combination Hormonal Contraceptives *on page 368*

Estrostep® Fe *see* Combination Hormonal Contraceptives *on page 368*

ETAF *see* Aldesleukin *on page 50*

Etanercept (et a NER cept)

Related Information

Rheumatoid Arthritis, Osteoarthritis, and Osteoporosis *on page 1488*

U.S. Brand Names Enbrel®

Canadian Brand Names Enbrel®

Pharmacologic Category Antirheumatic, Disease Modifying

Use Reduction in signs and symptoms of moderately to severely active rheumatoid arthritis, moderately to severely active polyarticular juvenile arthritis, or psoriatic arthritis in patients who have had an inadequate response to one or more disease-modifying antirheumatic drugs (DMARDs)

Unlabeled/Investigational Use Treatment of Crohn's disease

Local Anesthetic/Vasoconstrictor Precautions No information available to require special precautions

Effects on Dental Treatment Includes those >3% with incidence higher than placebo:

>10%: Headache (17%) respiratory tract infection (38%), upper respiratory tract infection (29%), rhinitis (12%), infection (35%)

≥3% to 10%: Dizziness (7%), nausea (9%), vomiting (3%), weakness (5%), pharyngitis (7%), respiratory disorder (5%), sinusitis (3%), cough (6%)

<3%: Dyspnea, GI hemorrhage, heart failure, infection (serious), MI,

Dosage S.C.:

Children 4-17 years: Juvenile rheumatoid arthritis: 0.4 mg/kg (maximum: 25 mg dose) twice weekly; doses should be separated by 72-96 hours

Adult: Rheumatoid arthritis, psoriatic arthritis: 25 mg given twice weekly; doses should be separated by 72-96 hours; if the physician determines that it is appropriate, patients may self-inject after proper training in injection technique

Alternative dosing (unlabeled): 50 mg once weekly

Elderly: Although greater sensitivity of some elderly patients cannot be ruled out, no overall differences in safety or effectiveness were observed

Mechanism of Action Etanercept is a recombinant DNA-derived protein composed of tumor necrosis factor receptor (TNFR) linked to the Fc portion of human IgG1. Etanercept binds tumor necrosis factor (TNF) and blocks its interaction with cell surface receptors. TNF plays an important role in the inflammatory processes of rheumatoid arthritis (RA) and the resulting joint pathology.

(Continued)

Etanercept *(Continued)*

Other Adverse Effects Includes those >3% with incidence higher than placebo:

>10%:

Local: Injection site reaction (37%)

Miscellaneous: Positive ANA (11%), positive antidouble-stranded DNA antibodies (15% by RIA, 3% by *Crithidia luciliae* assay)

≥3% to 10%:

Dermatologic: Rash (5%)

Gastrointestinal: Abdominal pain (5%), dyspepsia (4%)

<3%: Alopecia, cerebral ischemia, cholecystitis, deep vein thrombosis, depression, malignancies, membranous glomerulopathy, myocardial ischemia, pancreatitis, polymyositis, pulmonary embolism, thrombophlebitis, vasculitis (cutaneous)

Pediatric patients (JRA): The percentages of patients reporting abdominal pain (17%) and vomiting (14.5%) was higher than in adult RA. Two patients developed varicella infection associated with aseptic meningitis which resolved without complications.

Postmarketing and/or case reports: Angioedema, anorexia, aplastic anemia, chest pain, cutaneous vasculitis, demyelinating CNS disorders, diarrhea, **fatigue, flu syndrome, joint pain,** optic neuritis, pancytopenia, **paresthesia,** pruritus, pulmonary disease, seizures, stroke, subcutaneous nodules, thrombocytopenia, tuberculosis, urticaria, xerophthalmia, **xerostomia**

Pharmacodynamics/Kinetics

Onset of action: ~2-3 weeks

Half-life elimination: 115 hours (range: 98-300 hours)

Time to peak: 72 hours (range: 48-96 hours)

Excretion: Clearance: Children: 45.9 mL/hour/m^2; Adults: 89 mL/hour (52 mL/hour/m^2)

Pregnancy Risk Factor B

Generic Available No

Ethacrynate Sodium *see* Ethacrynic Acid *on page 538*

Ethacrynic Acid (eth a KRIN ik AS id)

Related Information

Cardiovascular Diseases *on page 1456*

U.S. Brand Names Edecrin® [DSC]

Canadian Brand Names Edecrin®

Pharmacologic Category Diuretic, Loop

Synonyms Edecrin® [DSC]; Ethacrynate Sodium

Use Management of edema associated with CHF; hepatic cirrhosis or renal disease; short-term management of ascites due to malignancy, idiopathic edema, and lymphedema

Local Anesthetic/Vasoconstrictor Precautions No information available to require special precautions

Effects on Dental Treatment Frequency not defined: Headache, fatigue, apprehension, confusion, fever, hyperglycemia, malaise, dysphagia, nausea, vomiting, GI bleeding, blurred vision

Dosage

Children: Oral: 1 mg/kg/dose once daily; increase at intervals of 2-3 days as needed, to a maximum of 3 mg/kg/day.

Adults:

Oral: 50-200 mg/day in 1-2 divided doses; may increase in increments of 25-50 mg at intervals of several days; doses up to 200 mg twice daily may be required with severe, refractory edema.

I.V. (dilute in D_5W or NS (1 mg/mL) and infuse over several minutes): 0.5-1 mg/kg/dose (maximum: 100 mg/dose); repeat doses not routinely recommended; however, if indicated, repeat doses every 8-12 hours.

Dosing comment in renal impairment: Cl_{cr} <10 mL/minute: Avoid use

Dialysis: Not removed by hemo- or peritoneal dialysis; supplemental dose is unnecessary.

Mechanism of Action Inhibits reabsorption of sodium and chloride in the ascending loop of Henle and distal renal tubule, interfering with the chloride-binding cotransport system, thus causing increased excretion of water, sodium, chloride, magnesium, and calcium

Other Adverse Effects Frequency not defined:

Central nervous system: Chills, encephalopathy (patients with pre-existing liver disease), vertigo

Dermatologic: Skin rash, Henoch-Schönlein purpura (in patient with rheumatic heart disease)

Endocrine & metabolic: Hyponatremia, variations in phosphorus, CO_2 content, bicarbonate, and calcium; reversible hyperuricemia, gout, hyperglycemia, hypoglycemia (occurred in two uremic patients who received doses above those recommended)

Gastrointestinal: Anorexia, abdominal discomfort or pain, dysphagia, diarrhea, acute pancreatitis (rare)

Genitourinary: Hematuria
Hepatic: Jaundice, abnormal LFTs
Hematologic: Agranulocytosis, severe neutropenia, thrombocytopenia
Local: Thrombophlebitis (with intravenous use), local irritation and pain,
Otic: Tinnitus, temporary or permanent deafness
Renal: Increased serum creatinine

Drug Interactions

Increased Effect/Toxicity:

Ethacrynic acid-induced hypokalemia may predispose to digoxin toxicity and may increase the risk of arrhythmia with drugs which may prolong QT interval, including type Ia and type III antiarrhythmic agents, cisapride, and some quinolones (sparfloxacin, gatifloxacin, and moxifloxacin). The risk of toxicity from lithium and salicylates (high dose) may be increased by loop diuretics. Hypotensive effects and/or adverse renal effects of ACE inhibitors and NSAIDs are potentiated by ethacrynic acid-induced hypovolemia. The effects of peripheral adrenergic-blocking drugs or ganglionic blockers may be increased by ethacrynic acid.

Ethacrynic acid may increase the risk of ototoxicity with other ototoxic agents (aminoglycosides, cis-platinum), especially in patients with renal dysfunction. Synergistic diuretic effects occur with thiazide-type diuretics. Diuretics tend to be synergistic with other antihypertensive agents, and hypotension may occur. Nephrotoxicity has been associated with concomitant use of cephaloridine or cephalexin.

Decreased Effect: Probenecid decreases diuretic effects of ethacrynic acid. Glucose tolerance may be decreased by loop diuretics, requiring adjustment of hypoglycemic agents. Cholestyramine or colestipol may reduce bioavailability of ethacrynic acid. Indomethacin (and other NSAIDs) may reduce natriuretic and hypotensive effects of diuretics.

Dietary/Ethanol/Herb Considerations

Food: Administer tablets with food early in the day. Increase intake of potassium-rich foods (citrus fruits, bananas); may cause a potassium loss requiring a potassium supplement or medication to help prevent potassium loss. Instruct patients not to alter diet without consultation especially if potassium supplements or medications to reduce potassium loss have been prescribed; too much potassium can be as harmful as too little.

Herb/Nutraceutical: Ginseng may decrease the effectiveness of loop diuretics (1 case report). Avoid escin (from the horse chestnut seed); may have additive diuretic effects. Avoid hawthorn; may lower peripheral vascular resistance resulting in additive decrease in BP.

Pharmacodynamics/Kinetics

Onset of action: Diuresis: Oral: ~30 minutes; I.V.: 5 minutes
Peak effect: Oral: 2 hours; I.V.: 30 minutes
Duration: Oral: 12 hours; I.V.: 2 hours
Absorption: Oral: Rapid
Protein binding: >90%
Metabolism: Hepatic (35% to 40%) to active cysteine conjugate
Half-life elimination: Normal renal function: 2-4 hours
Excretion: Feces and urine (30% to 60% as unchanged drug)

Pregnancy Risk Factor B

Generic Available No

Ethambutol (e THAM byoo tole)

Related Information

Nonviral Infectious Diseases *on page 1493*
Tuberculosis *on page 1493*

U.S. Brand Names Myambutol®

Canadian Brand Names Etibi®

Pharmacologic Category Antitubercular Agent

Synonyms Ethambutol Hydrochloride

Use Treatment of tuberculosis and other mycobacterial diseases in conjunction with other antituberculosis agents

Local Anesthetic/Vasoconstrictor Precautions No information available to require special precautions

Effects on Dental Treatment Frequency not defined: Headache, confusion, disorientation, malaise, fever, dizziness, hallucinations, nausea, vomiting, anaphylaxis

Dosage Oral:

Ethambutol is generally not recommended in children whose visual acuity cannot be monitored. However, ethambutol should be considered for all children with organisms resistant to other drugs, when susceptibility to ethambutol has been demonstrated, or susceptibility is likely.

Note: A four-drug regimen (isoniazid, rifampin, pyrazinamide, and either streptomycin or ethambutol) is preferred for the initial, empiric treatment of TB. When the drug susceptibility results are available, the regimen should be altered as appropriate.

(Continued)

Ethambutol *(Continued)*

Children and Adults:

Daily therapy: 15-25 mg/kg/day (maximum: 2.5 g/day)

Directly observed therapy (DOT): Twice weekly: 50 mg/kg (maximum: 2.5 g)

DOT: 3 times/week: 25-30 mg/kg (maximum: 2.5 g)

Adults: Treatment of disseminated *Mycobacterium avium* complex (MAC) in patients with advanced HIV infection: 15 mg/kg ethambutol in combination with azithromycin 600 mg daily

Dosing interval in renal impairment:

Cl_{cr} 10-50 mL/minute: Administer every 24-36 hours

Cl_{cr} <10 mL/minute: Administer every 48 hours

Hemodialysis: Slightly dialyzable (5% to 20%); Administer dose postdialysis

Peritoneal dialysis: Dose for Cl_{cr} <10 mL/minute

Continuous arteriovenous or venovenous hemofiltration: Administer every 24-36 hours

Mechanism of Action Suppresses mycobacteria multiplication by interfering with RNA synthesis

Other Adverse Effects Frequency not defined:

Dermatologic: Rash, pruritus

Endocrine & metabolic: Acute gout or hyperuricemia

Gastrointestinal: Abdominal pain, anorexia

Hematologic: Leukopenia, thrombocytopenia, eosinophilia

Hepatic: Abnormal LFTs

Neuromuscular & skeletal: Peripheral neuritis

Ocular: Optic neuritis; symptoms may include decreased acuity, scotoma, color blindness, or visual defects (usually reversible with discontinuation, irreversible blindness has been described)

Drug Interactions Decreased Effect: Ethambutol absorption is decreased when taken with aluminum salts.

Dietary/Ethanol/Herb Considerations Food: Administer with food to reduce GI upset; absorption unaffected

Pharmacodynamics/Kinetics

Absorption: ~80%

Distribution: Widely throughout body; concentrated in kidneys, lungs, saliva, and red blood cells

Relative diffusion from blood into CSF: Adequate with or without inflammation (exceeds usual MICs)

CSF:blood level ratio: Normal meninges: 0%; Inflamed meninges: 25%

Protein binding: 20% to 30%

Metabolism: Hepatic (20%) to inactive metabolite

Half-life elimination: 2.5-3.6 hours; End-stage renal disease: 7-15 hours

Time to peak, serum: 2-4 hours

Excretion: Urine (~50%) and feces (20%) as unchanged drug

Pregnancy Risk Factor C

Generic Available Yes

Ethambutol Hydrochloride *see* Ethambutol *on page 539*

Ethamolin® *see* Ethanolamine Oleate *on page 540*

ETH and C *see* Terpin Hydrate and Codeine *on page 1281*

Ethanolamine Oleate (ETH a nol a meen OH lee ate)

U.S. Brand Names Ethamolin®

Pharmacologic Category Sclerosing Agent

Synonyms Monoethanolamine

Use Orphan drug: Sclerosing agent used for bleeding esophageal varices

Local Anesthetic/Vasoconstrictor Precautions No information available to require special precautions

Effects on Dental Treatment Esophageal ulcer (2%), esophageal stricture (1.3%)

Dosage Adults: 1.5-5 mL per varix, up to 20 mL total or 0.4 mL/kg for a 50 kg patient; doses should be decreased in patients with severe hepatic dysfunction and should receive less than recommended maximum dose

Mechanism of Action Derived from oleic acid and similar in physical properties to sodium morrhuate; however, the exact mechanism of the hemostatic effect used in endoscopic injection sclerotherapy is not known. Intravenously injected ethanolamine oleate produces a sterile inflammatory response resulting in fibrosis and occlusion of the vein; a dose-related extravascular inflammatory reaction occurs when the drug diffuses through the venous wall. Autopsy results indicate that variceal obliteration occurs secondary to mural necrosis and fibrosis. Thrombosis appears to be a transient reaction.

Other Adverse Effects

1% to 10%:

Central nervous system: Pyrexia (1.8%)

Respiratory: Pleural effusion (2%), pneumonia (1.2%)

Miscellaneous: Retrosternal pain (1.6%)

<1%: **Esophagitis,** perforation, injection necrosis, acute renal failure, **anaphylaxis**

Pregnancy Risk Factor C

Generic Available No

Ethaverine (eth AV er een)

Pharmacologic Category Vasodilator

Synonyms Ethaverine Hydrochloride

Use Peripheral and cerebral vascular insufficiency associated with arterial spasm

Local Anesthetic/Vasoconstrictor Precautions No information available to require special precautions

Effects on Dental Treatment Frequency not defined: Tachycardia, hypotension, dizziness, drowsiness, sedation, lethargy, headache, xerostomia, facial flushing, nausea, diaphoresis

Dosage Adults: Oral: 100 mg 3 times/day

Other Adverse Effects Frequency not defined:

Central nervous system: Vertigo

Dermatologic: Pruritus

Gastrointestinal: Constipation

Hepatic: Hepatic hypersensitivity

Ethaverine Hydrochloride *see* Ethaverine *on page 541*

Ethinyl Estradiol (ETH in il es tra DYE ole)

Related Information

Endocrine Disorders and Pregnancy *on page 1479*

Estradiol *on page 521*

U.S. Brand Names Estinyl®

Pharmacologic Category Estrogen Derivative

Use Treatment of moderate to severe vasomotor symptoms associated with menopause; hypogonadism; prostatic cancer (palliation); breast cancer (palliation)

Local Anesthetic/Vasoconstrictor Precautions No information available to require special precautions

Effects on Dental Treatment Frequency not defined: Hypertension, dizziness, headache, migraine, nausea, vomiting

Dosage Oral: Adults:

Prostatic cancer (palliation): 0.15-2 mg/day

Female hypogonadism: 0.05 mg 1-3 times/day during the first 2 weeks of a theoretical menstrual cycle; follow with a progesterone during the last half of the arbitrary cycle; continue for 3-6 months. The patient should not be treated for the following 2 months to determine if additional therapy is needed.

Vasomotor symptoms associated with menopause: Usual dosage range: 0.02-0.05 mg/day; give cyclically for short-term use only and use the lowest dose that will control symptoms. Discontinue as soon as possible and administer cyclically (3 weeks on and 1 week off). Attempt to discontinue or taper medication at 3- to 6-month intervals. In severe cases (due to surgery or roentgenologic castration), doses of 0.05 mg 3 times/day may be needed initially; clinical improvement may be seen within a few weeks, decrease to lowest dose which will control symptoms

Breast cancer (palliation in appropriately selected postmenopausal women): 1 mg 3 times/day

Dosing adjustment in hepatic impairment: Reduction recommended in mild to moderate impairment; use not recommended in severe impairment

Mechanism of Action Estrogens are responsible for the development and maintenance of the female reproductive system and secondary sexual characteristics. Estradiol is the principle intracellular human estrogen and is more potent than estrone and estriol at the receptor level; it is the primary estrogen secreted prior to menopause. In males and following menopause in females, estrone and estrone sulfate are more highly produced. Estrogens modulate the pituitary secretion of gonadotropins, luteinizing hormone, and follicle-stimulating hormone through a negative feedback system; estrogen replacement reduces elevated levels of these hormones. Ethinyl estradiol is a synthetic derivative of estradiol. The addition of the ethinyl group prevents rapid degradation by the liver.

Other Adverse Effects Frequency not defined:

Cardiovascular: Edema, venous thromboembolism

Central nervous system: Mental depression

Dermatologic: Chloasma, erythema multiforme, erythema nodosum, hemorrhagic eruption, hirsutism, loss of scalp hair, melasma

Endocrine & metabolic: Breast enlargement, breast tenderness, changes in libido, increased thyroid-binding globulin, increased total thyroid hormone (T_4), increased serum triglycerides/phospholipids, increased HDL-cholesterol, decreased LDL-cholesterol, impaired glucose tolerance, hypercalcemia

Gastrointestinal: Abdominal cramps, bloating, cholecystitis, cholelithiasis, gallbladder disease, pancreatitis, weight gain/loss

(Continued)

Ethinyl Estradiol *(Continued)*

Genitourinary: Alterations in frequency and flow of menses, changes in cervical secretions, endometrial cancer, increased size of uterine leiomyomata, vaginal candidiasis

Hematologic: Aggravation of porphyria, decreased antithrombin III and antifactor Xa, increased levels of fibrinogen, increased platelet aggregability and platelet count; increased prothrombin and factors VII, VIII, IX, X

Hepatic: Cholestatic jaundice

Neuromuscular & skeletal: Chorea

Ocular: Intolerance to contact lenses, steeping of corneal curvature

Respiratory: Pulmonary thromboembolism

Miscellaneous: Carbohydrate intolerance

Drug Interactions Substrate of **CYP3A4**, 3A5-7; Inhibits CYP1A2, 2B6, 2C19, 3A4

Increased Effect/Toxicity: Hydrocortisone taken with estrogen may cause corticosteroid-induced toxicity. Increased potential for thromboembolic events with anticoagulants.

Decreased Effect: Rifampin, nelfinavir, and ritonavir decrease estradiol serum concentrations. Anticonvulsants which are enzyme inducers (barbiturates, carbamazepine, phenobarbital, phenytoin, primidone) may potentially decrease estrogen levels.

Dietary/Ethanol/Herb Considerations

Ethanol: Avoid use; increases estrogen concentration and risk of breast cancer.

Food: Ascorbic acid (>1 g/day) may increase serum concentration of estradiol. Estradiol may decrease folic acid absorption. Avoid grapefruit products; may increase serum concentration.

Herb/Nutraceutical: Avoid black cohosh, dong quai, and evening primrose due to estrogenic activity. Avoid ginseng, red clover, and saw palmetto due to potential hormonal effects. Avoid St John's wort; may decrease serum concentration.

Pharmacodynamics/Kinetics

Absorption: Oral: Rapid and complete

Distribution: V_d: 2-4 L/kg

Protein binding: 50% to 97%, primarily to albumin

Metabolism: Primarily hepatic via CYP3A4; less first-pass effect than with estradiol; extensive enterohepatic recirculation; converted to estrone and estriol

Bioavailability: 38% to 55%

Half-life elimination: ~8-25 hours

Time to peak: Initial: 2-3 hours; Secondary: 12 hours

Excretion: Urine and feces (as metabolites)

Pregnancy Risk Factor X

Generic Available No

Ethinyl Estradiol and Desogestrel *see* Combination Hormonal Contraceptives *on page 368*

Ethinyl Estradiol and Drospirenone *see* Combination Hormonal Contraceptives *on page 368*

Ethinyl Estradiol and Ethynodiol Diacetate *see* Combination Hormonal Contraceptives *on page 368*

Ethinyl Estradiol and Etonogestrel *see* Combination Hormonal Contraceptives *on page 368*

Ethinyl Estradiol and Levonorgestrel *see* Combination Hormonal Contraceptives *on page 368*

Ethinyl Estradiol and Norelgestromin *see* Combination Hormonal Contraceptives *on page 368*

Ethinyl Estradiol and Norethindrone *see* Combination Hormonal Contraceptives *on page 368*

Ethinyl Estradiol and Norgestimate *see* Combination Hormonal Contraceptives *on page 368*

Ethinyl Estradiol and Norgestrel *see* Combination Hormonal Contraceptives *on page 368*

Ethiofos *see* Amifostine *on page 73*

Ethionamide (e thye on AM ide)

Related Information

Nonviral Infectious Diseases *on page 1493*

Tuberculosis *on page 1493*

U.S. Brand Names Trecator®-SC

Canadian Brand Names Trecator®-SC

Pharmacologic Category Antitubercular Agent

Use Treatment of tuberculosis and other mycobacterial diseases, in conjunction with other antituberculosis agents, when first-line agents have failed or resistance has been demonstrated

Local Anesthetic/Vasoconstrictor Precautions No information available to require special precautions

Effects on Dental Treatment Frequency not defined: Postural hypotension, psychiatric disturbances, drowsiness, dizziness, seizures, headache, hypoglycemia, metallic taste, nausea, vomiting, stomatitis, weakness (common), blurred vision

Dosage Oral:

Children: 15-20 mg/kg/day in 2 divided doses, not to exceed 1 g/day

Adults: 500-1000 mg/day in 1-3 divided doses

Dosing adjustment in renal impairment: Cl_{cr} <50 mL/minute: Administer 50% of dose

Mechanism of Action Inhibits peptide synthesis

Other Adverse Effects Frequency not defined:

Dermatologic: Rash, alopecia

Endocrine & metabolic: Hypothyroidism or goiter, gynecomastia

Gastrointestinal: Diarrhea, anorexia, abdominal pain

Hematologic: Thrombocytopenia

Hepatic: Hepatitis (5%), jaundice

Neuromuscular & skeletal: Peripheral neuritis, weakness (common)

Ocular: Optic neuritis

Respiratory: Olfactory disturbances

Drug Interactions Increased Effect/Toxicity: Cycloserine and isoniazid; increased hepatotoxicity with rifampin

Pharmacodynamics/Kinetics

Absorption: Rapid

Distribution: Crosses placenta

Protein binding: 10%

Metabolism: Extensively hepatic

Bioavailability: 80%

Half-life elimination: 2-3 hours

Time to peak, serum: ~3 hours

Excretion: Urine (as unchanged drug and active and inactive metabolites)

Pregnancy Risk Factor C

Generic Available No

Ethmozine® *see* Moricizine *on page 931*

Ethosuximide (eth oh SUKS i mide)

U.S. Brand Names Zarontin®

Canadian Brand Names Zarontin®

Pharmacologic Category Anticonvulsant, Succinimide

Use Management of absence (petit mal) seizures

Local Anesthetic/Vasoconstrictor Precautions No information available to require special precautions

Effects on Dental Treatment Frequency not defined: Drowsiness, sedation, dizziness, lethargy, euphoria, headache, irritability, hyperactivity, fatigue, aggressiveness, mental depression (with cases of overt suicidal intentions), paranoid psychosis, GI upset, epigastric pain, diarrhea, nausea, vomiting, gum hypertrophy, tongue swelling, hiccups

Dosage Oral:

Children 3-6 years: Initial: 250 mg/day (or 15 mg/kg/day) in 2 divided doses; increase every 4-7 days; usual maintenance dose: 15-40 mg/kg/day in 2 divided doses

Children >6 years and Adults: Initial: 250 mg twice daily; increase by 250 mg as needed every 4-7 days, up to 1.5 g/day in 2 divided doses; usual maintenance dose: 20-40 mg/kg/day in 2 divided doses

Dosing comment in renal/hepatic dysfunction: Use with caution

Mechanism of Action Increases the seizure threshold and suppresses paroxysmal spike-and-wave pattern in absence seizures; depresses nerve transmission in the motor cortex

Other Adverse Effects Frequency not defined:

Central nervous system: Ataxia night terrors, disturbance in sleep, inability to concentrate

Dermatologic: Stevens-Johnson syndrome, SLE, rash, hirsutism

Endocrine & metabolic: Increased libido

Gastrointestinal: Weight loss, diarrhea, anorexia, abdominal pain

Genitourinary: Vaginal bleeding, microscopic hematuria

Hematologic: Leukopenia, agranulocytosis, pancytopenia, eosinophilia

Ocular: Myopia

Drug Interactions Substrate of **CYP3A4**

Increased Effect/Toxicity: Isoniazid may inhibit hepatic metabolism of ethosuximide with a resultant increase in ethosuximide serum concentrations. Ethosuximide may elevate phenytoin levels. Valproate acid has been reported to both increase and decrease ethosuximide levels.

Decreased Effect: Enzyme inducers (phenobarbital, rifampin, phenytoin, valproic acid) may decrease levels of ethosuximide.

(Continued)

Ethosuximide *(Continued)*

Dietary/Ethanol/Herb Considerations

Ethanol: Avoid use; may increase CNS depression.

Food: Administer with food or milk to reduce GI upset. Increase dietary intake of folate. Avoid grapefruit products; may increase serum concentration.

Herb/Nutraceutical: Avoid gotu kola, kava, SAMe, and valerian; may increase CNS depression. Avoid St John's wort; may decrease serum concentration and increase CNS depression.

Pharmacodynamics/Kinetics

Distribution: Adults: V_d: 0.62-0.72 L/kg

Metabolism: Hepatic (~80% to 3 inactive metabolites)

Half-life elimination, serum: Children: 30 hours; Adults: 50-60 hours

Time to peak, serum: Capsule: ~2-4 hours; Syrup: <2-4 hours

Excretion: Urine, slowly (50% as metabolites, 10% to 20% as unchanged drug); feces (small amounts)

Pregnancy Risk Factor C

Generic Available Yes

Ethotoin (ETH oh toyn)

U.S. Brand Names Peganone®

Canadian Brand Names Peganone®

Pharmacologic Category Anticonvulsant, Hydantoin

Synonyms Ethylphenylhydantoin

Use Generalized tonic-clonic or complex-partial seizures

Local Anesthetic/Vasoconstrictor Precautions No information available to require special precautions

Effects on Dental Treatment

>10%: Psychiatric changes, slurred speech, dizziness, drowsiness, nausea, vomiting

1% to 10%: Headache

Dosage Oral:

Children: 30-60 mg/kg/day or 250 mg twice daily, may be increased up to 2-3 g/day

Adults: 250 mg 4 times/day after meals, may be increased up to 3 g/day in divided doses 4 times/day

Other Adverse Effects

>10%: Gastrointestinal: Constipation

1% to 10%:

- Central nervous system: Insomnia
- Dermatologic: Skin rash
- Gastrointestinal: Anorexia, weight loss
- Hematologic: Leukopenia
- Hepatic: Hepatitis
- Renal: Increase in serum creatinine

<1% (Limited to important or life-threatening): **Arrhythmias,** ataxia, blood dyscrasias, cardiovascular collapse, **gingival hyperplasia, lymphadenopathy,** nystagmus, **paresthesia,** peripheral neuropathy, SLE-like syndrome, Stevens-Johnson syndrome, thrombophlebitis, venous irritation and pain

Drug Interactions Inhibits CYP2C19

Dietary/Ethanol/Herb Considerations

Ethanol: Avoid use; may increase CNS depression.

Herb/Nutraceutical: Avoid gotu kola, kava, SAMe, St John's wort, and valerian; may increase CNS depression.

Pregnancy Risk Factor D

Generic Available No

Ethoxynaphthamido Penicillin Sodium *see* Nafcillin *on page 945*

Ethyl Aminobenzoate *see* Benzocaine *on page 169*

Ethyl Chloride (ETH il KLOR ide)

Pharmacologic Category Local Anesthetic

Synonyms Chloroethane

Use Local anesthetic in minor operative procedures and to relieve pain caused by insect stings and burns, and irritation caused by myofascial and visceral pain syndromes

Local Anesthetic/Vasoconstrictor Precautions No information available to require special precautions

Effects on Dental Treatment 1% to 10%: Mucous membrane irritation; freezing may alter skin pigment

Dosage Dosage varies with use

Pregnancy Risk Factor C

Generic Available Yes

Comments Spray for a few seconds to the point of frost formation when the tissue becomes white; avoid prolonged spraying of skin beyond this point

Ethyl Chloride and Dichlorotetrafluoroethane

(ETH il KLOR ide & dye klor oh te tra flore oh ETH ane)

Related Information

Ethyl Chloride *on page 544*

U.S. Brand Names Fluro-Ethyl®

Pharmacologic Category Local Anesthetic

Synonyms Dichlorotetrafluoroethane and Ethyl Chloride

Use Topical refrigerant anesthetic to control pain associated with minor surgical procedures, dermabrasion, injections, contusions, and minor strains

Local Anesthetic/Vasoconstrictor Precautions No information available to require special precautions

Effects on Dental Treatment No significant effects or complications reported

Dosage Press gently on side of spray valve allowing the liquid to emerge as a fine mist approximately 2" to 4" from site of application

Pregnancy Risk Factor C

Generic Available No

Ethylphenylhydantoin *see* Ethotoin *on page 544*

Ethyol® *see* Amifostine *on page 73*

Etidocaine and Epinephrine (e TI doe kane & ep i NEF rin)

Related Information

Epinephrine *on page 499*

Oral Pain *on page 1524*

U.S. Brand Names Duranest® [DSC]

Canadian Brand Names Duranest®

Pharmacologic Category Local Anesthetic, Dental; Local Anesthetic

Synonyms Duranest® [DSC]; Etidocaine Hydrochloride

Use

Dental: An amide-type local anesthetic for local infiltration anesthesia; injection near nerve trunks to produce nerve block

Medical: Infiltration anesthesia, peripheral nerve blocks, central neural blocks

Local Anesthetic/Vasoconstrictor Precautions No information available to require special precautions

Effects on Dental Treatment Frequency not defined: Hypotension, bradycardia, cardiovascular collapse, anxiety, restlessness, disorientation, confusion, seizures, drowsiness, unconsciousness, nausea, vomiting, tremors, blurred vision, respiratory arrest, anaphylactoid reactions, transient stinging or burning at injection site

Dosage The effective anesthetic dose varies with procedure, intensity of anesthesia needed, duration of anesthesia required, and physical condition of the patient. Always use the lowest effective dose along with careful aspiration.

Children <10 years: Dosage has not been established

Children >10 years and Adults: **Dental infiltration and nerve block:** 15-75 mg (1-5 mL) as a 1.5% solution; up to a maximum of 5.5 mg/kg of body weight but not to exceed 400 mg/injection of etidocaine hydrochloride with epinephrine 1:200,000.

The numbers of dental carpules (1.8 mL) in the table provide the indicated amounts of etidocaine hydrochloride 1.5% and epinephrine 1:200,000.

# of Cartridges (1.8 mL)	Etidocaine (1.5%) (mg)	Epinephrine 1:200,000 (mg)
1	27	0.009
2	54	0.018
3	81	0.027
4	108	0.036
5	135	0.045
6	162	0.054
7	189	0.063
8	216	0.072
9	243	0.081
10	270	0.090

Mechanism of Action Blocks nervous conduction through the stabilization of neuronal membranes. By preventing the transient increase in membrane permeability to sodium, the ionic fluxes necessary for initiation and transmission of electrical impulses are inhibited and local anesthesia is induced.

Other Adverse Effects Frequency not defined:

Cardiovascular: Myocardial depression

Central nervous system: Chills

Dermatologic: Urticaria

Otic: Tinnitus

(Continued)

Etidocaine and Epinephrine *(Continued)*

Contraindications Hypersensitivity to etidocaine, other amide local anesthetics, or any component of the formulation; heart block, severe hemorrhage, severe hypotension

Warnings/Precautions Use with caution in patients with cardiac disease and hyperthyroidism; fetal bradycardia may occur up to 20% of the time; use with caution in areas of inflammation or sepsis, in debilitated or elderly patients, and those with severe cardiovascular disease or hepatic dysfunction; some products may contain sulfites

Drug Interactions Due to epinephrine component, use with tricyclic antidepressants or MAO inhibitors could result in increased pressor response; use with nonselective beta-blockers (ie, propranolol) could result in serious hypertension and reflex bradycardia

Pharmacodynamics/Kinetics

Onset of action: Anesthetic: 2-5 minutes
Duration: ~4-10 hours
Absorption: Rapid
Distribution: Wide V_d into neuronal tissues
Protein binding: High
Metabolism: Extensively hepatic
Excretion: Urine (small amounts)

Pregnancy Risk Factor B

Breast-feeding Considerations Usual infiltration doses of etidocaine hydrochloride with epinephrine given to nursing mothers has not been shown to affect the health of the nursing infant.

Dosage Forms INJ, solution: 1% [10 mg/mL] (30 mL). **INJ, solution**, with epinephrine 1:200,000: 1% [10 mg/mL] (30 mL); 1.5% [15 mg/mL] (1.8 mL, 20 mL)

Generic Available No

Selected Readings

Ayoub ST and Coleman AE, "A Review of Local Anesthetics," *Gen Dent*, 1992, 40(4):285-7, 289-90.
Jastak JT and Yagiela JA, "Vasoconstrictors and Local Anesthesia: A Review and Rationale for Use," *J Am Dent Assoc*, 1983, 107(4):623-30.
MacKenzie TA and Young ER, "Local Anesthetic Update," *Anesth Prog*, 1993, 40(2):29-34.
Wynn RL, "Epinephrine Interactions With Beta-Blockers," *Gen Dent*, 1994, 42(1):16, 18.
Wynn RL, "Recent Research on Mechanisms of Local Anesthetics," *Gen Dent*, 1995, 43(4):316-8.
Yagiela JA, "Local Anesthetics," *Anesth Prog*, 1991, 38(4-5):128-41.

Etidocaine Hydrochloride *see* Etidocaine and Epinephrine *on page 545*

Etidronate Disodium (e ti DROE nate dye SOW dee um)

Related Information

Rheumatoid Arthritis, Osteoarthritis, and Osteoporosis *on page 1488*

U.S. Brand Names Didronel®

Canadian Brand Names Didronel®

Pharmacologic Category Bisphosphonate Derivative

Synonyms EHDP; Sodium Etidronate

Use Symptomatic treatment of Paget's disease and heterotopic ossification due to spinal cord injury or after total hip replacement, hypercalcemia associated with malignancy

Local Anesthetic/Vasoconstrictor Precautions No information available to require special precautions

Effects on Dental Treatment 1% to 9%: Fever (9%), convulsions (3%), abnormal taste (3%), dyspnea (3%), nausea (7% to 30%; dose-related)

Dosage Adults: Oral formulation should be taken on an empty stomach 2 hours before any meal.

Paget's disease: Oral
- Initial: 5-10 mg/kg/day (not to exceed 6 months) or 11-20 mg/kg/day (not to exceed 3 months). Doses >10 mg/kg/day are **not** recommended.
- Retreatment: Initiate only after etidronate-free period ≥90 days. Monitor patients every 3-6 months. Retreatment regimens are the same as for initial treatment.

Heterotopic ossification: Oral:
- Caused by spinal cord injury: 20 mg/kg/day for 2 weeks, then 10 mg/kg/day for 10 weeks; total treatment period: 12 weeks
- Complicating total hip replacement: 20 mg/kg/day for 1 month preoperatively then 20 mg/kg/day for 3 months postoperatively; total treatment period is 4 months

Hypercalcemia associated with malignancy:
- I.V. (dilute dose in at least 250 mL NS): 7.5 mg/kg/day for 3 days; there should be at least 7 days between courses of treatment
- Oral: Start 20 mg/kg/day on the last day of infusion and continue for 30-90 days

Dosing adjustment in renal impairment:
- S_{cr} 2.5-5 mg/dL: Use with caution
- S_{cr} >5 mg/dL: Use not recommended

Mechanism of Action Decreases bone resorption by inhibiting osteocystic osteolysis; decreases mineral release and matrix or collagen breakdown in bone

Other Adverse Effects

>10%: Neuromuscular & skeletal: Bone pain (10% to 20%, Paget's)

1% to 10%:

Endocrine & metabolic: Hypophosphatemia (3%), hypomagnesemia (3%), fluid overload (6%), hypercalcemia of malignancy

Gastrointestinal: Diarrhea (7% to 30%; dose-related), constipation (3%)

Hepatic: LFT changes (3%)

Renal: Increased serum creatinine (10%)

<1%: **Pain**, angioedema, rash, occult blood in stools, **increased risk of fractures**, nephrotoxicity, **hypersensitivity reactions**, urticaria

Drug Interactions Increased Effect/Toxicity: Foscarnet and plicamycin may have additive hypocalcemic effect.

Dietary/Ethanol/Herb Considerations Administer with black coffee, tea, or fruit juice on an empty stomach; food decreases absorption and bioavailability. Avoid food or supplements with calcium, iron, or magnesium within 2 hours of administration; maintain adequate intake of calcium and vitamin D.

Pharmacodynamics/Kinetics

Onset of action: 1-3 months

Duration: Can persist for 12 months without continuous therapy

Absorption: Dose dependent

Metabolism: None

Excretion: Primarily urine (as unchanged drug); feces (as unabsorbed drug)

Pregnancy Risk Factor B (oral); C (parenteral)

Generic Available No

Etodolac (ee toe DOE lak)

Related Information

Rheumatoid Arthritis, Osteoarthritis, and Osteoporosis *on page 1488*

Temporomandibular Dysfunction (TMD) *on page 1562*

U.S. Brand Names Lodine®; Lodine® XL

Canadian Brand Names Apo®-Etodolac; Lodine®; Utradol™

Mexican Brand Names Lodine® Retard

Pharmacologic Category Nonsteroidal Anti-inflammatory Drug (NSAID)

Synonyms Etodolic Acid

Use

Dental: Treatment of postoperative pain

Medical: Acute and long-term use in management of osteoarthritis; management of pain

Unlabeled/Investigational Use Treatment of rheumatoid arthritis

Local Anesthetic/Vasoconstrictor Precautions No information available to require special precautions

Effects on Dental Treatment NSAID formulations are known to reversibly decrease platelet aggregation via mechanisms different than observed with aspirin. The dentist should be aware of the potential of abnormal coagulation. Caution should also be exercised in the use of NSAIDs in patients already on anticoagulant therapy with drugs such as warfarin (Coumadin®).

1% to 9%: Nausea (3% to 9%), vomiting (1% to 3%), gastritis (1% to 3%), weakness (3% to 9%), blurred vision (1% to 3%), CNS depression (1% to 3%)

Dosage Single dose of 76-100 mg is comparable to the analgesic effect of aspirin 650 mg.

Adults: Oral:

Acute pain: 200-400 mg every 6-8 hours, as needed, not to exceed total daily doses of 1200 mg; for patients weighing <60 kg, total daily dose should not exceed 20 mg/kg/day

Osteoarthritis: Initial: 800-1200 mg/day given in divided doses: 400 mg 2 or 3 times/day; 300 mg 2, 3, or 4 times/day; 200 mg 3 or 4 times/day; total daily dose should not exceed 1200 mg; for patients weighing <60 kg, total daily dose should not exceed 20 mg/kg/day

Lodine® XL: 400-1000 mg once daily

Elderly: No substantial differences in the pharmacokinetics or side-effects profile were seen in patients ≥65 years, compared with the general population.

Mechanism of Action Inhibits prostaglandin synthesis by decreasing the activity of the enzyme, cyclooxygenase, which results in decreased formation of prostaglandin precursors

Other Adverse Effects

1% to 10%:

Dermatologic: Rash (1% to 3%), pruritus (1% to 3%)

Gastrointestinal: Abdominal cramps (3% to 9%), (1% to 3%), dyspepsia (10%), diarrhea (3% to 9%), constipation (1% to 3%), flatulence (3% to 9%), melena (1% to 3%)

Genitourinary: Polyuria (1% to 3%)

Otic: Tinnitus (1% to 3%)

<1%: **CHF, hypertension, arrhythmia, tachycardia, confusion, hallucinations**, aseptic meningitis, mental depression, **drowsiness,** insomnia, urticaria, erythema multiforme, toxic epidermal necrolysis, Stevens-Johnson syndrome, angioedema, polydipsia, **hot flashes, GI ulceration,** cystitis, agranulocytosis,

(Continued)

Etodolac *(Continued)*

anemia, hemolytic anemia, bone marrow suppression, leukopenia, thrombocytopenia, hepatitis, peripheral neuropathy, toxic amblyopia, conjunctivitis, dry eyes, decreased hearing, acute renal failure, **allergic rhinitis, dyspnea, epistaxis**, anorexia, **stomatitis**

Contraindications Hypersensitivity to etodolac, aspirin, other NSAIDs, or any component of the formulation; active gastric/duodenal ulcer disease; pregnancy (3rd trimester)

Warnings/Precautions Use with caution in patients with CHF, hypertension, dehydration, decreased renal or hepatic function, history of GI disease (bleeding or ulcers), or those receiving anticoagulants. Elderly are at a high risk for adverse effects from NSAIDs. As many as 60% of elderly can develop peptic ulceration and/or hemorrhage asymptomatically.

Use lowest effective dose for shortest period possible. Use of NSAIDs can compromise existing renal function especially when Cl_{cr} is <30 mL/minute. CNS adverse effects such as confusion, agitation, and hallucination are generally seen in overdose or high-dose situations; however, elderly may demonstrate these adverse effects at lower doses than younger adults. Withhold for at least 4-6 half-lives prior to surgical or dental procedures.

Drug Interactions

ACE inhibitors: Antihypertensive effects may be decreased by concurrent therapy with NSAIDs; monitor blood pressure.

Angiotensin II antagonists: Antihypertensive effects may be decreased by concurrent therapy with NSAIDs; monitor blood pressure.

Anticoagulants (warfarin, heparin, LMWHs) in combination with NSAIDs can cause increased risk of bleeding.

Other antiplatelet drugs (ticlopidine, clopidogrel, aspirin, abciximab, dipyridamole, eptifibatide, tirofiban) can cause an increased risk of bleeding.

Cholestyramine and colestipol reduce the bioavailability of some NSAIDs; separate administration times.

Corticosteroids may increase the risk of GI ulceration; avoid concurrent use.

Cyclosporine: NSAIDs may increase serum creatinine, potassium, blood pressure, and cyclosporine levels; monitor cyclosporine levels and renal function carefully.

Hydralazine's antihypertensive effect is decreased; avoid concurrent use.

Lithium levels can be increased; avoid concurrent use if possible or monitor lithium levels and adjust dose. Sulindac may have the least effect. When NSAID is stopped, lithium will need adjustment again.

Loop diuretics efficacy (diuretic and antihypertensive effect) is reduced. Indomethacin reduces this efficacy, however, it may be anticipated with any NSAID.

Methotrexate: Severe bone marrow suppression, aplastic anemia, and GI toxicity have been reported with concomitant NSAID therapy. Avoid use during moderate or high-dose methotrexate (increased and prolonged methotrexate levels). NSAID use during low-dose treatment of rheumatoid arthritis has not been fully evaluated; extreme caution is warranted.

Thiazides antihypertensive effects are decreased; avoid concurrent use.

Verapamil plasma concentration is decreased by some NSAIDs; avoid concurrent use.

Warfarin's INRs may be increased by piroxicam. Other NSAIDs may have the same effect depending on dose and duration. Monitor INR closely. Use the lowest dose of NSAIDs possible and for the briefest duration.

Dietary/Ethanol/Herb Considerations

Ethanol: Avoid use; may enhance gastric mucosal irritation.

Food: Administer with food or milk to reduce GI upset; may decrease peak serum concentration. Avoid garlic, ginger, and green tea.

Herb/Nutraceutical: Avoid cat's claw, dong quai, evening primrose, feverfew, garlic, ginger, ginkgo biloba, ginseng, green tea, horse chestnut, and red clover due to additional antiplatelet activity. Avoid kava and valerian; may enhance benzodiazepine activity.

Pharmacodynamics/Kinetics

Onset of action: Analgesic: 2-4 hours; Maximum anti-inflammatory effect: A few days

Absorption: Well absorbed

Distribution: V_d: 0.4 L/kg

Protein binding: High

Metabolism: Hepatic

Half-life elimination: 7 hours

Time to peak, serum: 1 hour

Excretion: Urine

Pregnancy Risk Factor C/D (3rd trimester)

Dosage Forms CAP (Lodine®): 200 mg, 300 mg. **TAB** (Lodine®): 400 mg, 500 mg. **TAB, extended release** (Lodine® XL): 400 mg, 500 mg, 600 mg

Generic Available Yes

Selected Readings

Brooks PM and Day RO, "Nonsteroidal Anti-inflammatory Drugs - Differences and Similarities," *N Engl J Med*, 1991, 324(24):1716-25.

Tucker PW, Smith JR, and Adams DF, "A Comparison of 2 Analgesic Regimens for the Control of Postoperative Periodontal Discomfort," *J Periodontol*, 1996, 67(2):125-9.

Etodolic Acid *see* Etodolac *on page 547*

Etomidate (e TOM i date)

U.S. Brand Names Amidate®

Canadian Brand Names Amidate®

Pharmacologic Category General Anesthetic

Use Induction and maintenance of general anesthesia

Unlabeled/Investigational Use Sedation for diagnosis of seizure foci

Local Anesthetic/Vasoconstrictor Precautions No information available to require special precautions

Effects on Dental Treatment 1% to 10%: Hiccups

Dosage Children >10 years and Adults: I.V.: Initial: 0.2-0.6 mg/kg over 30-60 seconds for induction of anesthesia; maintenance: 5-20 mcg/kg/minute

Mechanism of Action Ultrashort-acting nonbarbiturate hypnotic (benzylimidazole) used for the induction of anesthesia; chemically, it is a carboxylated imidazole which produces a rapid induction of anesthesia with minimal cardiovascular effects; produces EEG burst suppression at high doses

Other Adverse Effects

>10%:

- Endocrine & metabolic: Adrenal suppression
- Gastrointestinal: Nausea and vomiting (on emergence from anesthesia)
- Local: Pain at injection site (30% to 80%)
- Neuromuscular & skeletal: Myoclonus (33%), transient skeletal movements, uncontrolled eye movements

<1%: Decreased cortisol synthesis, apnea, **arrhythmias, bradycardia, hypertension, hyperventilation, hypotension, hypoventilation, laryngospasm, tachycardia**

Drug Interactions Increased Effect/Toxicity: Fentanyl decreases etomidate elimination. Verapamil may increase the anesthetic and respiratory depressant effects of etomidate.

Pharmacodynamics/Kinetics

Onset of action: 30-60 seconds

Peak effect: 1 minute

Duration: 3-5 minutes; terminated by redistribution

Distribution: V_d: 2-4.5 L/kg

Protein binding: 76%;

Metabolism: Hepatic and plasma esterases

Half-life elimination: Terminal: 2.6 hours

Pregnancy Risk Factor C

Generic Available Yes

Etopophos® *see* Etoposide Phosphate *on page 551*

Etoposide (e toe POE side)

U.S. Brand Names Toposar®; VePesid®

Canadian Brand Names VePesid®

Mexican Brand Names Etopos®; Lastet®; Medsaposide; Serozide®; VePesid®; Vp-Tec®

Pharmacologic Category Antineoplastic Agent, Podophyllotoxin Derivative

Synonyms Epipodophyllotoxin; VP-16; VP-16-213

Use Treatment of lung, testicular, bladder, prostate, and uterine carcinomas; lymphomas, ANLL, hepatoma, rhabdomyosarcoma, neuroblastoma, histiocytosis, gestational trophoblastic disease, mycosis fungoides, Kaposi's or Ewing's sarcoma, Wilms' tumor, and brain tumors

Local Anesthetic/Vasoconstrictor Precautions No information available to require special precautions

Effects on Dental Treatment >10%: Mucositis (especially at high doses)

Dosage Refer to individual protocols:

Children: I.V.: 60-120 mg/m²/day for 3-5 days every 3-6 weeks

- AML:
  - Remission induction: 150 mg/m²/day for 2-3 days for 2-3 cycles
  - Intensification or consolidation: 250 mg/m²/day for 3 days, courses 2-5
- Brain tumor: 150 mg/m²/day on days 2 and 3 of treatment course
- Neuroblastoma: 100 mg/m²/day over 1 hour on days 1-5 of cycle; repeat cycle every 4 weeks
- BMT conditioning regimen used in patients with rhabdomyosarcoma or neuroblastoma: I.V. continuous infusion: 160 mg/m²/day for 4 days
- Conditioning regimen for allogenic BMT: 60 mg/kg/dose as a single dose

(Continued)

Etoposide *(Continued)*

Adults:

Small cell lung cancer:

Oral: Twice the I.V. dose rounded to the nearest 50 mg given once daily if total dose ≤400 mg or in divided doses if >400 mg

I.V.: 35 mg/m²/day for 4 days or 50 mg/m²/day for 5 days every 3-4 weeks total dose ≤400 mg/day or in divided doses if >400 mg/day

IVPB: 60-100 mg/m²/day for 3 days (with cisplatin)

CIV: 500 mg/m² over 24 hours every 3 weeks

Testicular cancer:

IVPB: 50-100 mg/m²/day for 5 days repeated every 3-4 weeks

I.V.: 100 mg/m² every other day for 3 doses repeated every 3-4 weeks

BMT/relapsed leukemia: I.V.: 2.4-3.5 g/m² or 25-70 mg/kg administered over 4-36 hours

Dosing adjustment in renal impairment:

Cl_{cr} 10-50 mL/minute: Administer 75% of normal dose

Cl_{cr} <10 mL minute: Administer 50% of normal dose

Hemodialysis: Supplemental dose is unnecessary

Peritoneal dialysis: Supplemental dose is unnecessary

CAPD effects: Unknown

CAVH effects: Unknown

Dosing adjustment in hepatic impairment:

Bilirubin 1.5-3 mg/dL or AST 60-180 units: Reduce dose by 50%

Bilirubin 3-5 mg/dL or AST >180 units: Reduce by 75%

Bilirubin >5 mg/dL: Do not administer

Mechanism of Action Etoposide does not inhibit microtubular assembly. It has been shown to delay transit of cells through the S phase and arrest cells in late S or early G_2 phase. The drug may inhibit mitochondrial transport at the NADH dehydrogenase level or inhibit uptake of nucleosides into HeLa cells. Etoposide is a topoisomerase II inhibitor and appears to cause DNA strand breaks.

Other Adverse Effects

>10%:

Cardiovascular: Hypotension (rapid infusion)

Dermatologic: Alopecia (22% to 93%)

Endocrine & metabolic: Ovarian failure (38%), amenorrhea

Gastrointestinal: Mild to moderate nausea and vomiting, anorexia (10% to 13%)

Hematologic: Myelosuppression, leukopenia (91%), thrombocytopenia (41%), anemia

Onset: 5-7 days

Nadir: 7-14 days

Recovery: 21-28 days

1% to 10%:

Gastrointestinal: Stomatitis (1% to 6%), diarrhea (1% to 13%), abdominal pain

Neuromuscular & skeletal: Peripheral neuropathies (0.7% to 2%)

<1%: **Tachycardia, CHF, MI, somnolence, fatigue, headache,** anovulatory cycles, hypomenorrhea, hepatitis, thrombophlebitis, **anaphylactoid reactions** (chills, fever, bronchospasm, dyspnea, hypotension); possibly related to rapid infusion (0.7% to 2%)

Drug Interactions Substrate of CYP1A2, 2E1, **3A4**; Inhibits CYP2C8/9, 3A4

Increased Effect/Toxicity: The effects of etoposide may be increased by calcium antagonists (increased effects noted *in vitro*). Cyclosporine may increase the levels of etoposide. Etoposide may increase the effects/toxicity of methotrexate and warfarin. There have been reports of frequent hepatic dysfunction with hyperbilirubinemia, ascites, and thrombocytopenia when etoposide is combined with carmustine.

Dietary/Ethanol/Herb Considerations

Ethanol: Avoid use; may increase GI irritation.

Food does not affect GI absorption with doses ≤200 mg of injection.

Herb/Nutraceutical: Avoid St John's wort; may decrease serum concentration.

Pharmacodynamics/Kinetics

Absorption: Oral: 25% to 75%; significant inter- and intrapatient variation

Distribution: Average V_d: 3-36 L/m²; poor penetration across the blood-brain barrier; CSF concentrations <10% of plasma concentrations

Protein binding: 94% to 97%

Metabolism: Hepatic to hydroxy acid and cislactone metabolites

Half-life elimination: Terminal: 4-15 hours; Children: Normal renal/hepatic function: 6-8 hours

Time to peak, serum: Oral: 1-1.5 hours

Excretion:

Children: Urine (≤55% as unchanged drug)

Adults: Urine (42% to 67%; 8% to 35% as unchanged drug) within 24 hours; feces (up to 16%)

Pregnancy Risk Factor D

Generic Available Yes

Etoposide Phosphate (e toe POE side FOS fate)

Related Information

Etoposide *on page 549*

U.S. Brand Names Etopophos®

Mexican Brand Names Etopos; Medsaposide; Serozide®

Pharmacologic Category Antineoplastic Agent, Podophyllotoxin Derivative

Use Treatment of refractory testicular tumors and small cell lung cancer

Local Anesthetic/Vasoconstrictor Precautions No information available to require special precautions

Effects on Dental Treatment

>10%: Mucositis (especially at high doses)

1% to 6%: Stomatitis

Dosage Refer to individual protocols. Adults:

Small cell lung cancer: I.V. (in combination with other approved chemotherapeutic drugs): **Equivalent doses of etoposide phosphate to an etoposide dosage** range of 35 mg/m²/day for 4 days to 50 mg/m²/day for 5 days. Courses are repeated at 3- to 4-week intervals after adequate recovery from any toxicity.

Testicular cancer: I.V. (in combination with other approved chemotherapeutic agents): **Equivalent dose of etoposide phosphate to etoposide dosage** range of 50-100 mg/m²/day on days 1-5 to 100 mg/m²/day on days 1, 3, and 5. Courses are repeated at 3- to 4-week intervals after adequate recovery from any toxicity.

Dosing adjustment in renal impairment:

- Cl_{cr} 15-50 mL/minute: Administer 75% of normal dose
- Cl_{cr} <15 mL minute: Data unavailable; consider further dose reduction

Hemodialysis: Supplemental dose unnecessary

Peritoneal dialysis: Supplemental dose unnecessary

CAPD/CAVH effects: Unknown

Dosing adjustment in hepatic impairment:

- Bilirubin 1.5-3 mg/dL or AST 60-180 units: Reduce dose by 50%
- Bilirubin 3-5 mg/dL or AST >180 units: Reduce by 75%
- Bilirubin >5 mg/dL: Do not administer

Mechanism of Action Etoposide phosphate is converted *in vivo* to the active moiety, etoposide, by dephosphorylation. Etoposide inhibits mitotic activity; inhibits cells from entering prophase; inhibits DNA synthesis. Initially thought to be mitotic inhibitors similar to podophyllotoxin, but actually have no effect on microtubule assembly. However, later shown to induce DNA strand breakage and inhibition of topoisomerase II (an enzyme which breaks and repairs DNA); etoposide acts in late S or early G2 phases.

Other Adverse Effects Based on **etoposide**:

>10%:

- Cardiovascular: Hypotension (rapid infusion)
- Dermatologic: Alopecia (22% to 93%)
- Endocrine & metabolic: Ovarian failure (38%), amenorrhea
- Gastrointestinal: Mild to moderate nausea and vomiting, anorexia (10% to 13%)
- Hematologic: Myelosuppression, leukopenia (91%), thrombocytopenia (41%), anemia
  - Onset: 5-7 days
  - Nadir: 7-14 days
  - Recovery: 21-28 days

1% to 10%:

- Gastrointestinal: Diarrhea (1% to 13%), abdominal pain
- Neuromuscular & skeletal: Peripheral neuropathies (0.7% to 2%)

<1%: **Tachycardia, CHF, MI, somnolence, fatigue, headache,** anovulatory cycles, hypomenorrhea, hepatitis, thrombophlebitis, **anaphylactoid reactions** (chills, fever, bronchospasm, dyspnea, hypotension); possibly related to rapid infusion (0.7% to 2%)

Drug Interactions Substrate of CYP1A2, 2E1, **3A4**; Inhibits CYP2C8/9, 3A4

Increased Effect/Toxicity: Etoposide taken with warfarin may result in prolongation of bleeding times. Alteration of MTX transport has been found as a slow efflux of MTX and its polyglutamated form out of the cell, leading to intercellular accumulation of MTX. Calcium antagonists increase the rate of VP-16-induced DNA damage and cytotoxicity *in vitro*. Use with carmustine has shown reports of frequent hepatic dysfunction with hyperbilirubinemia, ascites, and thrombocytopenia. Cyclosporine may cause additive cytotoxic effects on tumor cells.

Dietary/Ethanol/Herb Considerations

Ethanol: Avoid use; may increase GI irritation.

Food does not affect GI absorption with doses ≤200 mg of injection.

Herb/Nutraceutical: Avoid St John's wort; may decrease serum concentration.

Pharmacodynamics/Kinetics

Distribution: Average V_d: 3-36 L/m²; poor penetration across blood-brain barrier; concentrations in CSF being <10% that of plasma

Protein binding: 94% to 97%

Metabolism: Hepatic (with a biphasic decay)

(Continued)

Etoposide Phosphate *(Continued)*

Half-life elimination: Terminal: 4-15 hours; Children: Normal renal/hepatic function: 6-8 hours

Excretion: Urine (as unchanged drug and metabolites), feces (2% to 16%); Children: I.V.: Urine (≤55% as unchanged drug)

Pregnancy Risk Factor D

Generic Available No

Etrafon® *see* Amitriptyline and Perphenazine *on page 85*

Eudal®-SR *see* Guaifenesin and Pseudoephedrine *on page 652*

Eulexin® *see* Flutamide *on page 598*

Eurax® Topical *see* Crotamiton *on page 376*

Evac-U-Gen [OTC] *see* Senna *on page 1215*

Evista® *see* Raloxifene *on page 1165*

Evoxac™ *see* Cevimeline *on page 292*

Exact® Acne Medication [OTC] *see* Benzoyl Peroxide *on page 171*

Excedrin® Extra Strength [OTC] *see* Acetaminophen, Aspirin, and Caffeine *on page 34*

Excedrin® Migraine [OTC] *see* Acetaminophen, Aspirin, and Caffeine *on page 34*

Excedrin® P.M. [OTC] *see* Acetaminophen and Diphenhydramine *on page 30*

Exelderm® *see* Sulconazole *on page 1249*

Exelon® *see* Rivastigmine *on page 1192*

Exemestane (eks e MES tane)

U.S. Brand Names Aromasin®

Canadian Brand Names Aromasin®

Pharmacologic Category Antineoplastic Agent, Miscellaneous

Use Treatment of advanced breast cancer in postmenopausal women whose disease has progressed following tamoxifen therapy

Local Anesthetic/Vasoconstrictor Precautions No information available to require special precautions

Effects on Dental Treatment

>10%: Fatigue (22%), pain (13%), anxiety (10%), hot flashes (13%), nausea (18%)

1% to 10%: Hypertension (5%), chest pain dizziness (8%), headache (8%), fever (5%), confusion, vomiting (7%), weakness, paresthesia, pathological fracture, dyspnea (10%), cough (6%), bronchitis, sinusitis, pharyngitis, rhinitis, flu-like symptoms (6%), diaphoresis (6%), lymphedema, infection

Dosage Oral:

Adults: 25 mg once daily after a meal; treatment should continue until tumor progression is evident

Dosing adjustment in renal/hepatic impairment: Safety of chronic doses has not been studied

Mechanism of Action Exemestane is an irreversible, steroidal aromatase inactivator. It prevents conversion of androgens to estrogens by tying up the enzyme aromatase. In breast cancers where growth is estrogen-dependent, this medicine will lower circulating estrogens.

Other Adverse Effects

>10%: Central nervous system: Depression (13%)

1% to 10%:

Cardiovascular: Edema (7%)

Central nervous system: Hypoesthesia

Dermatologic: Rash, itching, alopecia

Gastrointestinal: Abdominal pain (6%), anorexia (6%), constipation (5%), diarrhea (4%), increased appetite (3%), dyspepsia

Genitourinary: Urinary tract infection

Neuromuscular & skeletal: Arthralgia

<1%: GGT increased, transaminases increased

A dose-dependent decrease in sex hormone-binding globulin has been observed with daily doses of 25 mg or more. Serum luteinizing hormone and follicle-stimulating hormone levels have increased with this medicine.

Drug Interactions Substrate of CYP3A4

Increased Effect/Toxicity: Although exemestane is a CYP3A4 substrate, ketoconazole, a CYP3A4 inhibitor, did not change the pharmacokinetics of exemestane. No other potential drug interactions have been evaluated.

Dietary/Ethanol/Herb Considerations

Food: High-fat meal increases plasma concentration by 40%.

Herb/Nutraceutical: Avoid black cohosh and dong quai in estrogen-dependent tumors. Avoid St John's wort; may decrease serum concentration.

Pharmacodynamics/Kinetics

Absorption: Rapid and moderate (~42%) following oral administration; absorption increases ~40% following high-fat meal

Distribution: Extensive

Protein binding: 90%, primarily to albumin and α_1-acid glycoprotein

Metabolism: Extensively hepatic; oxidation (CYP3A4) of methylene group, reduction of 17-keto group with formation of many secondary metabolites; metabolites are inactive

Half-life elimination: 24 hours

Time to peak: Women with breast cancer: 1.2 hours

Excretion: Urine (<1% as unchanged drug, 39% to 45% as metabolites); feces (36% to 48%)

Pregnancy Risk Factor D

Generic Available No

ex-lax® [OTC] *see* Senna *on page 1215*

ex-lax® Maximum Strength [OTC] *see* Senna *on page 1215*

Ex-Lax® Stool Softener [OTC] *see* Docusate *on page 463*

Exosurf Neonatal® *see* Colfosceril Palmitate *on page 366*

Extendryl *see* Chlorpheniramine, Phenylephrine, and Methscopolamine *on page 310*

Extendryl JR *see* Chlorpheniramine, Phenylephrine, and Methscopolamine *on page 310*

Extendryl SR *see* Chlorpheniramine, Phenylephrine, and Methscopolamine *on page 310*

Eye-Sine™ [OTC] *see* Tetrahydrozoline *on page 1288*

Ezetimibe (ez ET i mibe)

U.S. Brand Names Zetia™

Pharmacologic Category Antilipemic Agent, 2-Azetidinone

Use Use in combination with dietary therapy for the treatment of primary hypercholesterolemia (as monotherapy or in combination with HMG-CoA reductase inhibitors); homozygous sitosterolemia; homozygous familial hypercholesterolemia (in combination with atorvastatin or simvastatin)

Local Anesthetic/Vasoconstrictor Precautions No information available to require special precautions

Effects on Dental Treatment 1% to 10%: Sinusitis (4% to 5%), pharyngitis (2% to 3%; placebo 2%), chest pain (3%), dizziness (3%), fatigue (2%), headache (8%)

Dosage Oral: Hyperlipidemias:

Children ≥10 years and Adults: 10 mg/day

Elderly: No dosage adjustment required

Dosing adjustment in renal impairment: None; bioavailability increased with severe impairment

Dosing adjustment in hepatic impairment: Bioavailability increased

Moderate to severe impairment (Child-Pugh score 7-15): Use not recommended

Mechanism of Action Inhibits absorption of cholesterol at the brush border of the small intestine, leading to a decreased delivery of cholesterol to the liver, reduction of hepatic cholesterol stores and an increased clearance of cholesterol from the blood; decreases total C, LDL-C, ApoB, and triglycerides while increasing HDL-C

Other Adverse Effects 1% to 10%:

Gastrointestinal: Diarrhea (3% to 4%), abdominal pain (3%)

Neuromuscular & skeletal: Arthralgia (4%)

Drug Interactions

Increased Effect/Toxicity: Cyclosporine may increase plasma levels of ezetimibe. Fibric acid derivatives may increase bioavailability of ezetimibe (safety and efficacy of concomitant use not established).

Decreased Effect: Bile acid sequestrants may decrease ezetimibe bioavailability; administer ezetimibe ≥2 hours before or ≥4 hours after bile acid sequestrants.

Dietary/Ethanol/Herb Considerations Food: May be taken with food. Patients should be placed on a standard cholesterol-lowering diet for 6 weeks prior to and during therapy.

Pharmacodynamics/Kinetics

Protein binding: >90% to plasma proteins

Metabolism: Undergoes conjugation in the small intestine and liver; forms metabolite (active); may undergo enterohepatic recycling

Bioavailability: Variable

Half-life: 22 hours (ezetimibe and metabolite)

Time to peak, plasma: 4-12 hours

Excretion: Feces (78%, 69% as ezetimibe); urine (11%, 9% as metabolite)

Pregnancy Risk Factor C

Generic Available No

F_3T *see* Trifluridine *on page 1350*

Factor IX Complex (Human) (FAK ter nyne KOM pleks HYU man)

U.S. Brand Names Bebulin® VH; Profilnine® SD; Proplex® T

Pharmacologic Category Antihemophilic Agent; Blood Product Derivative

Synonyms Prothrombin Complex Concentrate

(Continued)

Factor IX Complex (Human) *(Continued)*

Use

Control bleeding in patients with factor IX deficiency (hemophilia B or Christmas disease) **Note:** Factor IX concentrate containing **only** factor IX is also available and preferable for this indication.

Prevention/control of bleeding in hemophilia A patients with inhibitors to factor VIII

Prevention/control of bleeding in patients with factor VII deficiency

Emergency correction of the coagulopathy of warfarin excess in critical situations.

Local Anesthetic/Vasoconstrictor Precautions No information available to require special precautions

Effects on Dental Treatment 1% to 10%: Fever, headache

Dosage Children and Adults: Dosage is expressed in units of factor IX activity and must be individualized. I.V. only:

Formula for units required to raise blood level %:

Total blood volume (mL blood/kg) = 70 mL/kg (adults), 80 mL/kg (children)

Plasma volume = total blood volume (mL) x [1 - Hct (in decimals)]

For example, for a 70 kg adult with a Hct = 40%: Plasma volume = [70 kg x 70 mL/kg] x [1 - 0.4] = 2940 mL

To calculate number of units needed to increase level to desired range (highly individualized and dependent on patient's condition): Number of units = desired level increase [desired level - actual level] x plasma volume (in mL)

For example, for a 100% level in the above patient who has an actual level of 20%: Number of units needed = [1 (for a 100% level) - 0.2] x 2940 mL = 2352 units

As a general rule, the level of factor IX required for treatment of different conditions is listed below:

Minor Spontaneous Hemorrhage, Prophylaxis:

Desired levels of factor IX for hemostasis: 15% to 25%

Initial loading dose to achieve desired level: <20-30 units/kg

Frequency of dosing: Once; repeated in 24 hours if necessary

Duration of treatment: Once; repeated if necessary

Major Trauma or Surgery:

Desired levels of factor IX for hemostasis: 25% to 50%

Initial loading dose to achieve desired level: <75 units/kg

Frequency of dosing: Every 18-30 hours, depending on halflife and measured factor IX levels

Duration of treatment: Up to 10 days, depending upon nature of insult

Factor VIII inhibitor patients: 75 units/kg/dose; may be given every 6-12 hours

Anticoagulant overdosage: I.V.: 15 units/kg

Mechanism of Action Replaces deficient clotting factor including factor X; hemophilia B, or Christmas disease, is an X-linked recessively inherited disorder of blood coagulation characterized by insufficient or abnormal synthesis of the clotting protein factor IX. Factor IX is a vitamin K-dependent coagulation factor which is synthesized in the liver. Factor IX is activated by factor XIa in the intrinsic coagulation pathway. Activated factor IX (IXa), in combination with factor VII:C activates factor X to Xa, resulting ultimately in the conversion of prothrombin to thrombin and the formation of a fibrin clot. The infusion of exogenous factor IX to replace the deficiency present in hemophilia B temporarily restores hemostasis.

Other Adverse Effects

1% to 10%:

Central nervous system: Chills

Neuromuscular & skeletal: Tingling

Miscellaneous: Transient fever (following rapid administration)

<1%: Disseminated intravascular coagulation (DIC), **flushing, nausea, somnolence,** thrombosis following high dosages because of presence of activated clotting factors, **tightness in chest or neck,** urticaria, **vomiting**

Drug Interactions Increased Effect/Toxicity: Do not coadminister with aminocaproic acid; may increase risk for thrombosis.

Pharmacodynamics/Kinetics

Half-life elimination:

VII component: Initial: 4-6 hours; Terminal: 22.5 hours

IX component: 24 hours

Pregnancy Risk Factor C

Generic Available No

Factor VIIa (Recombinant) (FAK ter SEV en ree KOM be nant)

U.S. Brand Names Novo-Seven®

Pharmacologic Category Antihemophilic Agent; Blood Product Derivative

Synonyms Coagulation Factor VIIa; rFVIIa

Use Treatment of bleeding episodes in patients with hemophilia A or B when inhibitors to factor VIII or factor IX are present

Local Anesthetic/Vasoconstrictor Precautions No information available to require special precautions

Effects on Dental Treatment 1% to 10%: Hypertension

Dosage Children and Adults: I.V. administration only: 90 mcg/kg every 2 hours until hemostasis is achieved or until the treatment is judged ineffective. The dose and interval may be adjusted based upon the severity of bleeding and the degree of hemostasis achieved. The duration of therapy following hemostasis has not been fully established; for patients experiencing severe bleeds, dosing should be continued at 3-6 hour intervals after hemostasis has been achieved and the duration of dosing should be minimized.

In clinical trials, dosages have ranged from 35-120 mcg/kg and a decision on the final therapeutic dosages was reached within 8 hours in the majority of patients

Mechanism of Action Recombinant factor VIIa, a vitamin K-dependent glycoprotein, promotes hemostasis by activating the extrinsic pathway of the coagulation cascade. It replaces deficient activated coagulation factor VII, which complexes with tissue factor and may activate coagulation factor X to Xa and factor IX to IXa. When complexed with other factors, coagulation factor Xa converts prothrombin to thrombin, a key step in the formation of a fibrin-platelet hemostatic plug.

Other Adverse Effects

1% to 10%:

Hematologic: Hemorrhage, decreased plasma fibrinogen

Musculoskeletal: Hemarthrosis

<1%: Abnormal renal function, **allergic reactions,** arthrosis, **bradycardia, coagulation disorder,** disseminated intravascular coagulation (DIC), edema, fibrinolysis increased, **headache, hypotension,** injection-site reactions, prothrombin decreased, pneumonia, pruritus, purpura, rash, **vomiting**

Pharmacodynamics/Kinetics

Distribution: V_d: 103 mL/kg (78-139)

Half-life elimination: 2.3 hours (1.7-2.7)

Excretion: Clearance: 33 mL/kg/hour (27-49)

Pregnancy Risk Factor C

Generic Available No

Factor VIII (Human) *see* Antihemophilic Factor (Human) *on page 113*

Factor VIII (Porcine) *see* Antihemophilic Factor (Porcine) *on page 114*

Factor VIII (Recombinant) *see* Antihemophilic Factor (Recombinant) *on page 115*

Famciclovir (fam SYE kloe veer)

Related Information

Sexually-Transmitted Diseases *on page 1502*

Systemic Viral Diseases *on page 1517*

U.S. Brand Names Famvir®

Canadian Brand Names Famvir®

Pharmacologic Category Antiviral Agent

Use Management of acute herpes zoster (shingles) and recurrent episodes of genital herpes; treatment of recurrent herpes simplex in immunocompetent patients

Local Anesthetic/Vasoconstrictor Precautions No information available to require special precautions

Effects on Dental Treatment 1% to 10%: Fatigue (4% to 6%), fever (1% to 3%), dizziness (3% to 5%), somnolence (1% to 2%), headache, vomiting (1% to 5%), (1% to 5%), nausea, paresthesia (1% to 3%), sinusitis/pharyngitis (2%)

Dosage Initiate therapy as soon as herpes zoster is diagnosed.

Adults: Oral:

Acute herpes zoster: 500 mg every 8 hours for 7 days

Recurrent herpes simplex in immunocompetent patients: 125 mg twice daily for 5 days

Genital herpes:

First episode: 250 mg 3 times/day for 7-10 days

Recurrent episodes: 125 mg twice daily for 5 days

Prophylaxis: 250 mg twice daily

Severe (hospitalized patients): 250 mg twice daily

Dosing interval in renal impairment:

Herpes zoster:

Cl_{cr} ≥60 mL/minute: Administer 500 mg every 8 hours

Cl_{cr} 40-59 mL/minute: Administer 500 mg every 12 hours

Cl_{cr} 20-39 mL/minute: Administer 500 mg every 24 hours

Cl_{cr} <20 mL/minute: Administer 250 mg every 24 hours

Recurrent genital herpes:

Cl_{cr} ≥40 mL/minute: Administer 125 mg every 12 hours

Cl_{cr} 20-39 mL/minute: Administer 125 mg every 24 hours

Cl_{cr} <20 mL/minute: Administer 125 mg every 48 hours

Suppression of recurrent genital herpes:

Cl_{cr} ≥40 mL/minute: Administer 250 mg every 12 hours

Cl_{cr} 20-39 mL/minute: Administer 125 mg every 12 hours

Cl_{cr} <20 mL/minute: Administer 125 mg every 24 hours

(Continued)

Famciclovir *(Continued)*

Recurrent orolabial or genital herpes in HIV-infected patients:

Cl_{cr} ≥40 mL/minute: Administer 500 mg every 12 hours

Cl_{cr} 20-39 mL/minute: Administer 500 mg every 24 hours

Cl_{cr} <20 mL/minute: Administer 250 mg every 24 hours

Mechanism of Action After undergoing rapid biotransformation to the active compound, penciclovir, famciclovir is phosphorylated by viral thymidine kinase in HSV-1, HSV-2, and VZV-infected cells to a monophosphate form; this is then converted to penciclovir triphosphate and competes with deoxyguanosine triphosphate to inhibit HSV-2 polymerase (ie, herpes viral DNA synthesis/replication is selectively inhibited)

Other Adverse Effects

1% to 10%:

Dermatologic: Pruritus (1% to 4%)

Gastrointestinal: Diarrhea (4% to 8%), constipation (1% to 5%), anorexia (1% to 3%), abdominal pain (1% to 4%)

<1%: **Rigors,** arthralgia, **upper respiratory infection**

Drug Interactions Increased Effect/Toxicity:

Cimetidine: Penciclovir AUC may increase due to impaired metabolism.

Digoxin: C_{max} of digoxin increases by ~19%.

Probenecid: Penciclovir serum levels significantly increase.

Theophylline: Penciclovir AUC/C_{max} may increase and renal clearance decrease, although not clinically significant.

Dietary/Ethanol/Herb Considerations Food: May be taken with food; reduces peak concentration and rate of absorption (conversion to penciclovir); bioavailability unaffected

Pharmacodynamics/Kinetics

Absorption: Food decreases maximum peak concentration and delays time to peak; AUC remains the same

Distribution: V_{dss}: 0.98-1.08 L/kg

Protein binding: 20%

Metabolism: Rapidly deacetylated and oxidized to penciclovir; not via CYP

Bioavailability: 77%

Half-life elimination: Penciclovir: 2-3 hours (10, 20, and 7 hours in HSV-1, HSV-2, and VZV-infected cells, respectively); prolonged with renal impairment

Time to peak: 0.9 hours; C_{max} and T_{max} are decreased and prolonged with noncompensated hepatic impairment

Excretion: Urine (>90% as unchanged drug)

Pregnancy Risk Factor B

Generic Available No

Famotidine (fa MOE ti deen)

Related Information

Gastrointestinal Disorders *on page 1474*

U.S. Brand Names Pepcid®; Pepcid® AC [OTC]

Canadian Brand Names Apo®-Famotidine; Gen-Famotidine; Novo-Famotidine; Nu-Famotidine; Pepcid®; Pepcid AC®; Pepcid® I.V.; ratio-Famotidine; Rhoxal-famotidine; Riva-Famotidine

Mexican Brand Names Durater®; Famoxal®; Farmotex®; Pepcidine®; Sigafam®

Pharmacologic Category Histamine H_2 Antagonist

Use

Pepcid®: Therapy and treatment of duodenal ulcer, gastric ulcer, control gastric pH in critically ill patients, symptomatic relief in gastritis, gastroesophageal reflux, active benign ulcer, and pathological hypersecretory conditions

Pepcid® AC: Relief of heartburn, acid indigestion, and sour stomach

Unlabeled/Investigational Use Part of a multidrug regimen for *H. pylori* eradication to reduce the risk of duodenal ulcer recurrence

Local Anesthetic/Vasoconstrictor Precautions No information available to require special precautions

Effects on Dental Treatment

>10% (pediatric patients <1 year of age): Agitation (≤14%), vomiting (≤14%)

1% to 10%: Dizziness (1%), headache (5%)

Dosage

Children (dose and duration of treatment should be individualized):

Peptic ulcer: 1-16 years:

Oral: 0.5 mg/kg/day at bedtime or divided twice daily (maximum dose: 40 mg/day); doses of up to 1 mg/kg/day have been used in clinical studies

I.V.: 0.25 mg/kg every 12 hours (maximum dose: 40 mg/day); doses of up to 0.5 mg/kg have been used in clinical studies

GERD: Oral:

<3 months: 0.5 mg/kg once daily

3-12 months: 0.5 mg/kg twice daily

1-16 years: 1 mg/kg/day divided twice daily (maximum dose: 40 mg twice daily); doses of up to 2 mg/kg/day have been used in clinical studies

Adults:

Duodenal ulcer: Oral: Acute therapy: 40 mg/day at bedtime for 4-8 weeks; maintenance therapy: 20 mg/day at bedtime

Helicobacter pylori eradication (unlabeled use): 40 mg once daily; requires combination therapy with antibiotics

Gastric ulcer: Oral: Acute therapy: 40 mg/day at bedtime

Hypersecretory conditions: Oral: Initial: 20 mg every 6 hours, may increase in increments up to 160 mg every 6 hours

GERD: Oral: 20 mg twice daily for 6 weeks

Esophagitis and accompanying symptoms due to GERD: Oral: 20 mg or 40 mg twice daily for up to 12 weeks

Patients unable to take oral medication: I.V.: 20 mg every 12 hours

Heartburn, indigestion, sour stomach: Pepcid® AC [OTC]: Oral: 10 mg every 12 hours; dose may be taken 15-60 minutes before eating foods known to cause heartburn

Dosing adjustment in renal impairment:

Cl_{cr} <50 mL/minute: Manufacturer recommendation: Administer 50% of dose **or** increase the dosing interval to every 36-48 hours (to limit potential CNS adverse effects).

Cl_{cr} <10 mL/minute: Administer 50% of dose **or** increase dosing interval to every 36-48 hours.

Mechanism of Action Competitive inhibition of histamine at H_2 receptors of the gastric parietal cells, which inhibits gastric acid secretion

Other Adverse Effects

1% to 10%: Gastrointestinal: Constipation (1%), diarrhea (2%)

<1%: Abdominal discomfort, acne, agranulocytosis, **allergic reaction,** anorexia, **belching, bradycardia, bronchospasm, drowsiness,** dry skin, **fatigue, fever,** flatulence, **hypertension,** increased AST/ALT, increased BUN/creatinine, insomnia, neutropenia, **palpitations, paresthesia,** proteinuria, pruritus, **seizures, tachycardia,** thrombocytopenia, urticaria, **weakness**

Drug Interactions Decreased serum levels of ketoconazole and itraconazole due to reduced absorption.

Dietary/Ethanol/Herb Considerations

Ethanol: Avoid use; may cause gastric mucosal irritation.

Food may increase bioavailability.

Pharmacodynamics/Kinetics

Onset of action: GI: Oral: Within 1 hour

Duration: 10-12 hours

Protein binding: 15% to 20%

Bioavailability: Oral: 40% to 50%

Half-life elimination: 2.5-3.5 hours; prolonged with renal impairment; Oliguria: 20 hours

Time to peak, serum: Oral: ~1-3 hours

Excretion: Urine (as unchanged drug)

Pregnancy Risk Factor B

Generic Available Yes: Injection, tablet

Famotidine, Calcium Carbonate, and Magnesium Hydroxide

(fa MOE ti deen, KAL see um KAR bun ate, & mag NEE zee um hye DROKS ide)

U.S. Brand Names Pepcid® Complete [OTC]

Canadian Brand Names Pepcid® Complete [OTC]

Pharmacologic Category Antacid; Histamine H_2 Antagonist

Synonyms Calcium Carbonate, Magnesium Hydroxide, and Famotidine; Magnesium Hydroxide, Famotidine, and Calcium Carbonate

Use Relief of heartburn due to acid indigestion

Local Anesthetic/Vasoconstrictor Precautions No information available to require special precautions

Effects on Dental Treatment No significant effects or complications reported

Dosage Children ≥12 years and Adults: Relief of heartburn due to acid indigestion: Oral: Pepcid® Complete: 1 tablet as needed; no more than 2 tablets in 24 hours; do **not** swallow whole, chew tablet completely before swallowing; do not use for longer than 14 days (see Additional Information for dosing ranges for individual ingredients)

Mechanism of Action

Famotidine: H_2 antagonist

Calcium carbonate: Antacid

Magnesium hydroxide: Antacid

Generic Available No

Famvir® *see* Famciclovir *on page 555*

Fansidar® *see* Sulfadoxine and Pyrimethamine *on page 1252*

Fareston® *see* Toremifene *on page 1326*

Faslodex® *see* Fulvestrant *on page 621*

Fat Emulsion (fat e MUL shun)

U.S. Brand Names Intralipid®; Liposyn® III

Canadian Brand Names Intralipid®

Mexican Brand Names Emulsan 20%; Lyposyn; Lipocin

Pharmacologic Category Caloric Agent

Synonyms Intravenous Fat Emulsion

Use Source of calories and essential fatty acids for patients requiring parenteral nutrition of extended duration

Local Anesthetic/Vasoconstrictor Precautions No information available to require special precautions

Effects on Dental Treatment Frequency not defined: Flushing, chest pain, headache, dizziness, nausea, vomiting, dyspnea, sepsis, diaphoresis

Dosage Fat emulsion should not exceed 60% of the total daily calories

Premature Infants: Initial dose: 0.25-0.5 g/kg/day, increase by 0.25-0.5 g/kg/day to a maximum of 3 g/kg/day depending on needs/nutritional goals; limit to 1 g/kg/day if on phototherapy; maximum rate of infusion: 0.15 g/kg/hour (0.75 mL/kg/hour of 20% solution)

Infants and Children: Initial dose: 0.5-1 g/kg/day, increase by 0.5 g/kg/day to a maximum of 3 g/kg/day depending on needs/nutritional goals; maximum rate of infusion: 0.25 g/kg/hour (1.25 mL/kg/hour of 20% solution)

Adolescents and Adults: Initial dose: 1 g/kg/day, increase by 0.5-1 g/kg/day to a maximum of 2.5 g/kg/day of 10% and 3 g/kg/day of 20% depending on needs/nutritional goals; maximum rate of infusion: 0.25 g/kg/hour (1.25 mL/kg/hour of 20% solution); do not exceed 50 mL/hour (20%) or 100 mL/hour (10%)

Prevention of essential fatty acid deficiency (8% to 10% of total caloric intake): 0.5-1 g/kg/24 hours

Children: 5-10 mL/kg/day at 0.1 mL/minute then up to 100 mL/hour

Adults: 500 mL (10%) twice weekly at rate of 1 mL/minute for 30 minutes, then increase to 42 mL/hour (500 mL over 12 hours)

Note: At the onset of therapy, the patient should be observed for any immediate allergic reactions such as dyspnea, cyanosis, and fever; slower initial rates of infusion may be used for the first 10-15 minutes of the infusion (eg, 0.1 mL/minute of 10% or 0.05 mL/minute of 20% solution)

Mechanism of Action Essential for normal structure and function of cell membranes

Other Adverse Effects Frequency not defined:

Cardiovascular: Cyanosis

Endocrine & metabolic: Hyperlipemia

Gastrointestinal: Diarrhea

Hematologic: Hypercoagulability, thrombocytopenia in neonates (rare)

Hepatic: Hepatomegaly

Local: Thrombophlebitis

Pharmacodynamics/Kinetics

Metabolism: Undergoes lipolysis to free fatty acids which are utilized by reticuloendothelial cells

Half-life elimination: 0.5-1 hour

Pregnancy Risk Factor B/C

Generic Available No

5-FC *see* Flucytosine *on page 578*

FC1157a *see* Toremifene *on page 1326*

Fedahist® [OTC] *see* Chlorpheniramine and Pseudoephedrine *on page 308*

Feen-A-Mint® [OTC] *see* Bisacodyl *on page 186*

Feiba VH Immuno® *see* Anti-inhibitor Coagulant Complex *on page 116*

Felbamate (FEL ba mate)

U.S. Brand Names Felbatol®

Pharmacologic Category Anticonvulsant, Miscellaneous

Use Not as a first-line antiepileptic treatment; only in those patients who respond inadequately to alternative treatments and whose epilepsy is so severe that a substantial risk of aplastic anemia and/or liver failure is deemed acceptable in light of the benefits conferred by its use. Patient must be fully advised of risk and provide signed written informed consent. Felbamate can be used as either monotherapy or adjunctive therapy in the treatment of partial seizures (with and without generalization) and in adults with epilepsy.

Orphan drug: Adjunctive therapy in the treatment of partial and generalized seizures associated with Lennox-Gastaut syndrome in children

Local Anesthetic/Vasoconstrictor Precautions No information available to require special precautions

Effects on Dental Treatment

>10%: Somnolence, headache, fatigue, dizziness, nausea, vomiting

1% to 10%: Xerostomia, abnormal taste, chest pain, palpitations, tachycardia, sinusitis, pharyngitis, nervousness, anxiety, stupor, malaise, agitation, psychological disturbances, aggressive reaction, tremors, abnormal gait, paresthesia, abnormal vision

Restrictions A patient "informed consent" form should be completed and signed by the patient and physician. Copies are available from Wallace Pharmaceuticals by calling 609-655-6147.

Dosage Anticonvulsant:

Monotherapy: Children >14 years and Adults:

Initial: 1200 mg/day in divided doses 3 or 4 times/day; titrate previously untreated patients under close clinical supervision, increasing the dosage in 600 mg increments every 2 weeks to 2400 mg/day based on clinical response and thereafter to 3600 mg/day as clinically indicated

Conversion to monotherapy: Initiate at 1200 mg/day in divided doses 3 or 4 times/day, reduce the dosage of the concomitant anticonvulsant(s) by 20% to 33% at the initiation of felbamate therapy; at week 2, increase the felbamate dosage to 2400 mg/day while reducing the dosage of the other anticonvulsant(s) up to an additional 33% of their original dosage; at week 3, increase the felbamate dosage up to 3600 mg/day and continue to reduce the dosage of the other anticonvulsant(s) as clinically indicated

Adjunctive therapy: Children with Lennox-Gastaut and ages 2-14 years:

Week 1:

Felbamate: 15 mg/kg/day divided 3-4 times/day

Concomitant anticonvulsant(s): Reduce original dosage by 20% to 30%

Week 2:

Felbamate: 30 mg/kg/day divided 3-4 times/day

Concomitant anticonvulsant(s): Reduce original dosage up to an additional 33%

Week 3:

Felbamate: 45 mg/kg/day divided 3-4 times/day

Concomitant anticonvulsant(s): Reduce dosage as clinically indicated

Adjunctive therapy: Children >14 years and Adults:

Week 1:

Felbamate: 1200 mg/day initial dose

Concomitant anticonvulsant(s): Reduce original dosage by 20% to 33%

Week 2:

Felbamate: 2400 mg/day (therapeutic range)

Concomitant anticonvulsant(s): Reduce original dosage by up to an additional 33%

Week 3:

Felbamate: 3600 mg/day (therapeutic range)

Concomitant anticonvulsant(s): Reduce original dosage as clinically indicated

Dosing adjustment in renal impairment: Use caution; reduce initial and maintenance doses by 50% (halflife prolonged by 9-15 hours)

Mechanism of Action Mechanism of action is unknown but has properties in common with other marketed anticonvulsants; has weak inhibitory effects on GABA-receptor binding, benzodiazepine receptor binding, and is devoid of activity at the MK-801 receptor binding site of the NMDA receptor-ionophore complex.

Other Adverse Effects

>10%: Gastrointestinal: Anorexia, constipation

1% to 10%:

Central nervous system: Depression or behavior changes, ataxia

Dermatologic: Skin rash, acne, pruritus

Gastrointestinal: Diarrhea, abdominal pain, weight gain,

Neuromuscular & skeletal: Myalgia

Ocular: Diplopia

Miscellaneous: ALT increase

<1%: **Euphoria, hallucinations,** leukocytosis, leukopenia, **lymphadenopathy, migraine, suicide attempts,** thrombocytopenia, urticaria, aplastic anemia

Drug Interactions Substrate of CYP2E1, **3A4**; Inhibits CYP2C19; Induces CYP3A4

Increased Effect/Toxicity: Felbamate increases serum phenytoin, phenobarbital, and valproic acid concentrations which may result in toxicity; consider decreasing phenytoin or phenobarbital dosage by 25%. A decrease in valproic acid dosage may also be necessary.

Decreased Effect: Carbamazepine, phenytoin may decrease serum felbamate concentrations. Felbamate may decrease carbamazepine levels and increase levels of the active metabolite of carbamazepine (10,11-epoxide) resulting in carbamazepine toxicity; monitor for signs of carbamazepine toxicity (dizziness, ataxia, nystagmus, drowsiness).

Dietary/Ethanol/Herb Considerations

Ethanol: Avoid use; may increase CNS depression.

Food does not affect absorption of tablet.

Herb/Nutraceutical: Avoid evening primrose; decreases seizure threshold. Avoid gotu kola, kava, SAMe, St John's wort, and valerian; may increase CNS depression.

(Continued)

Felbamate *(Continued)*

Pharmacodynamics/Kinetics

Absorption: Rapid and almost complete; food has no effect upon the tablet's absorption

Distribution: V_d: 0.7-1 L/kg

Protein binding: 22% to 25%, primarily to albumin

Half-life elimination: 20-23 hours (average)

Time to peak, serum: ~3 hours

Excretion: Urine (40% to 50% as unchanged drug, 40% as inactive metabolites)

Pregnancy Risk Factor C

Generic Available No

Felbatol® *see* Felbamate *on page 558*

Feldene® *see* Piroxicam *on page 1090*

Felodipine (fe LOE di peen)

Related Information

Calcium Channel Blockers and Gingival Hyperplasia *on page 1598*

Calcium Channel Blockers, Comparative Pharmacokinetics *on page 1600*

Cardiovascular Diseases *on page 1456*

Enalapril and Felodipine *on page 494*

U.S. Brand Names Plendil®

Canadian Brand Names Plendil®; Renedil®

Mexican Brand Names Logimax; Munobal; Plendil®

Pharmacologic Category Calcium Channel Blocker

Use Treatment of hypertension, CHF

Local Anesthetic/Vasoconstrictor Precautions No information available to require special precautions

Effects on Dental Treatment

>10%: Headache (11% to 15%)

1% to 10%: Gingival hyperplasia (~1%; fewer reports than other CCBs, resolves upon discontinuation, consultation with physician is suggested), tachycardia (0.4% to 2.5%), flushing (4% to 7%), pharyngitis, pneumonia, sinusitis

Dosage Oral:

Adults: 2.5-10 mg once daily; usual initial dose: 5 mg; increase by 5 mg at 2-week intervals, as needed; maximum: 10 mg

Elderly: Begin with 2.5 mg/day

Dosing adjustment/comments in hepatic impairment: May require reduction (initial: 2.5 mg/day); monitor blood pressure

Mechanism of Action Inhibits calcium ions from entering the "slow channels" or select voltage-sensitive areas of vascular smooth muscle and myocardium during depolarization, producing a relaxation of coronary vascular smooth muscle and coronary vasodilation; increases myocardial oxygen delivery in patients with vasospastic angina

Other Adverse Effects

2% to 10%: Cardiovascular: Peripheral edema (2% to 17%)

<1% (Limited to important or life-threatening): Abdominal pain, **acid regurgitation,** anemia, angioedema, angina pectoris, **anxiety disorders, arrhythmia,** arthralgia, back pain, **bronchitis, chest pain, joint pain CHF,** constipation, **contusion,** CVA, decreased libido, depression, diarrhea, **dizziness, dyspnea,** dysuria, **epistaxis,** erythema, **facial edema**, flatulence, **flu-like illness, flushing,** gynecomastia, **hypotension,** impotence, **influenza,** insomnia, **irritability, leg/foot pain,** leukocytoclastic vasculitis, **MI, muscle cramps,** myalgia, **MI, nausea, nervousness, palpitations, paresthesias, pharyngitis,** polyuria, premature beats, **respiratory infection, sinusitis, somnolence, syncope,** urinary frequency, urinary urgency, urticaria, **visual disturbances, vomiting, xerostomia**

Drug Interactions Substrate of **CYP3A4**; Inhibits CYP2C8/9, 2D6, 3A4

Increased Effect/Toxicity: Inhibitors of CYP3A4, including azole antifungals (ketoconazole, itraconazole) and erythromycin, may inhibit calcium channel blocker metabolism, increasing the effects of felodipine. Beta-blockers may have increased pharmacokinetic or pharmacodynamic interactions with felodipine. Cyclosporine increases felodipine's serum concentration. Ethanol increases felodipine's absorption; watch for a greater hypotensive effect.

Decreased Effect: Felodipine may decrease pharmacologic actions of theophylline. Calcium may reduce the calcium channel blocker's effects, particularly hypotension. Carbamazepine significantly reduces felodipine's bioavailability; avoid this combination. Nafcillin decreases plasma concentration of felodipine; avoid this combination. Rifampin increases the metabolism of felodipine. Felodipine may decrease pharmacologic actions of theophylline.

Dietary/Ethanol/Herb Considerations

Ethanol increases absorption; watch for a greater hypotensive effect.

Food: Administer on an empty stomach; high-fat/carbohydrate meals increase C_{max} by 60%. Avoid grapefruit products; may increase therapeutic and vasodilator effects resulting in severe hypotension and myocardial ischemia; grapefruit juice increases C_{mac} by 2-fold. Fluids, fruit, and fiber may reduce constipation. Avoid caffeine (eg, colas, chocolate), garlic, and licorice.

Herb/Nutraceutical: Avoid black cohosh, dong quai, and evening primrose due to estrogenic activity. Avoid ephedra, ginseng, and yohimbe; may worsen hypertension. Avoid garlic; may have increased antihypertensive effect. Avoid ginger due to positive inotropic effects; theoretically, may cause arrhythmia. Avoid hawthorn; may lower peripheral and vascular resistance causing additional decrease in BP. Avoid licorice. Avoid St John's wort; may decrease serum concentration.

Pharmacodynamics/Kinetics

Onset of action: 2-5 hours

Duration: 16-24 hours

Absorption: 100%; Absolute: 20% due to first-pass effect

Protein binding: >99%

Metabolism: Hepatic; extensive first-pass effect

Half-life elimination: 11-16 hours

Excretion: Urine (as metabolites)

Pregnancy Risk Factor C

Generic Available No

Selected Readings

Lombardi T, Fiore-Donno G, Belser U, et al, "Felodipine-Induced Gingival Hyperplasia: A Clinical and Histologic Study," *J Oral Pathol Med*, 1991, 20(2):89-92.

Young PC, Turiansky GW, Sau P, et al, "Felodipine-Induced Gingival Hyperplasia," *Cutis*, 1998, 62(1):41-3.

Felodipine and Enalapril *see* Enalapril and Felodipine *on page 494*

Femara® *see* Letrozole *on page 782*

femhrt® *see* Combination Hormonal Contraceptives *on page 368*

Femilax™ [OTC] *see* Bisacodyl *on page 186*

Femiron® [OTC] *see* Iron Supplements *on page 745*

Femizol-M™ [OTC] *see* Miconazole *on page 906*

Fenesin™ [DSC] *see* Guaifenesin *on page 650*

Fenesin™ DM *see* Guaifenesin and Dextromethorphan *on page 651*

Fenofibrate (fen oh FYE brate)

U.S. Brand Names TriCor®

Canadian Brand Names Apo®-Fenofibrate; Apo®-Feno-Micro; Gen-Fenofibrate Micro; Lipidil Micro®; Lipidil Supra®; Novo-Fenofibrate; Nu-Fenofibrate; PMS-Fenofibrate Micro; TriCor®

Mexican Brand Names Controlip®; Lipidil®

Pharmacologic Category Antilipemic Agent, Fibric Acid

Synonyms Procetofene; Proctofene

Use Adjunct to dietary therapy for the treatment of adults with very high elevations of serum triglyceride levels (types IV and V hyperlipidemia) who are at risk of pancreatitis and who do not respond adequately to a determined dietary effort; safety and efficacy may be greater than that of clofibrate; adjunct to dietary therapy for the reduction of low density lipoprotein cholesterol (LDL-C), total cholesterol (total-C), triglycerides, and apolipoprotein B (apo B) in adult patients with primary hypercholesterolemia or mixed dyslipidemia (Fredrickson types IIa and IIb); its efficacy can be enhanced by combination with other hypolipidemic agents that have a different mechanism of action

Local Anesthetic/Vasoconstrictor Precautions No information available to require special precautions

Effects on Dental Treatment

1% to 10%: Otitis media, respiratory disorder (6%), rhinitis (2%)

Frequency not defined: Angina pectoris, arrhythmias, atrial fibrillation, cardiovascular disorder, chest pain, hypertension, hypotension, migraine, MI, palpitations, tachycardia, vasodilatation, anxiety, depression, dizziness, fever, malaise, nervousness, pain, somnolence, bruising, contact dermatitis, fungal dermatitis, diabetes mellitus, hypoglycemia, duodenal ulcer, eructation, esophagitis, gastroenteritis, gastritis, GI disorder, nausea, peptic ulcer, tooth disorder, vomiting, xerostomia, lymphadenopathy, arthritis, leg cramps, paresthesia, abnormal vision, ear pain, asthma, bronchitis, cough increased, dyspnea, laryngitis, asthma, bronchitis, cough increased, dyspnea, laryngitis, pharyngitis, pneumonia, sinusitis, accidental injury, allergic reaction, diaphoresis, herpes simplex, infection

Dosage Oral:

Adults:

Hypertriglyceridemia: Initial:

Capsule: 67 mg/day with meals, up to 200 mg/day

Tablet: 54 mg/day with meals, up to 160 mg/day

Hypercholesterolemia or mixed hyperlipidemia: Initial:

Capsule: 200 mg/day with meals

Tablet: 160 mg/day with meals

Elderly: Initial: 67 mg/day (capsule) or 54 mg/day (tablet)

(Continued)

Fenofibrate *(Continued)*

Dosing adjustment in renal impairment: Decrease dose or increase dosing interval in renal failure: Initial: 67 mg/day (capsule) or 54 mg/day (tablet)

Hemodialysis has no effect on removal of fenofibric acid from the plasma.

Mechanism of Action Fenofibric acid is believed to increase VLDL catabolism by enhancing the synthesis of lipoprotein lipase; as a result of a decrease in VLDL levels, total plasma triglycerides are reduced by 30% to 60%; modest increase in HDL occurs in some hypertriglyceridemic patients

Other Adverse Effects

1% to 10%:

Gastrointestinal: Abdominal pain (5%), constipation (2%)

Hepatic: Abnormal LFTs (7%), creatine phosphokinase increased (3%), ALT increased (3%), AST increased (3%)

Neuromuscular & skeletal: Back pain (3%)

Frequency not defined:

Cardiovascular: Coronary artery disorder, edema, electrocardiogram abnormality, extrasystoles, peripheral edema, peripheral vascular disorder, phlebitis, varicose veins

Central nervous system: Depression, insomnia, neuralgia, vertigo

Dermatologic: Acne, alopecia, eczema, maculopapular rash, nail disorder, photosensitivity reaction, pruritus, skin disorder, skin ulcer, urticaria

Endocrine & metabolic: Gout, gynecomastia, hyperuricemia

Gastrointestinal: Anorexia, appetite increased, colitis, diarrhea, dyspepsia, flatulence, rectal disorder, rectal hemorrhage, weight gain/loss

Genitourinary: Cystitis, dysuria, prostatic disorder, libido decreased, pregnancy (unintended), urinary frequency, urolithiasis, vaginal moniliasis

Hematologic: Anemia, eosinophilia, leukopenia, lymphadenopathy, thrombocytopenia

Hepatic: Cholelithiasis, cholecystitis, fatty liver deposits

Neuromuscular & skeletal: Arthralgia, arthritis, arthrosis, bursitis, hypertonia, joint disorder, myalgia, myasthenia, myositis, tenosynovitis

Ocular: Amblyopia, cataract, conjunctivitis, eye disorder, refraction disorder

Renal: Creatinine increased, kidney function abnormality

Miscellaneous: Cyst, herpes zoster

Drug Interactions Substrate of CYP3A4

Increased Effect/Toxicity: The hypolipidemic effect of fenofibrate is increased when used with cholestyramine or colestipol. Fenofibrate may increase the effect of chlorpropamide and warfarin. Concurrent use of fenofibrate with HMG-CoA reductase inhibitors (atorvastatin, cerivastatin, fluvastatin, lovastatin, pravastatin, simvastatin) may increase the risk of myopathy and rhabdomyolysis. The manufacturer warns against concomitant use. However, combination therapy with statins has been used in some patients with resistant hyperlipidemias (with great caution).

Decreased Effect: Rifampin (and potentially other enzyme inducers) may decrease levels of fenofibrate.

Dietary/Ethanol/Herb Considerations Food: Administer with food.

Pharmacodynamics/Kinetics

Absorption: 60% to 90% with meals

Distribution: Widely to most tissues except brain or eye; concentrates in liver, kidneys, and gut

Protein binding: >99%

Metabolism: Tissue and plasma via esterases to active form, fenofibric acid; undergoes inactivation by glucuronidation hepatically or renally

Half-life elimination: 21 hours; Elderly: 30 hours; Hepatic impairment: 44-54 hours

Time to peak: 4-6 hours

Excretion: Urine (60% to 93% as metabolites); feces (5% to 25%); hemodialysis has no effect on removal of fenofibric acid from plasma

Pregnancy Risk Factor C

Generic Available No

Fenoldopam (fe NOL doe pam)

U.S. Brand Names Corlopam®

Canadian Brand Names Corlopam®

Pharmacologic Category Dopamine Agonist

Synonyms Fenoldopam Mesylate

Use Treatment of severe hypertension particularly I.V. and in patients with renal compromise; potential use for CHF

Local Anesthetic/Vasoconstrictor Precautions No information available to require special precautions

Effects on Dental Treatment

>10%: Xerostomia, changes in salivation

Frequency not defined: Fibrillation (atrial), hypotension, tachycardia, facial flushing, pain, angina, headache, dizziness, nausea, vomiting, blurred vision

Dosage I.V.:

Severe hypertension: Initial: 0.1 mcg/kg/minute; may be increased in increments of 0.05-0.2 mcg/kg/minute until target blood pressure is achieved; average rate: 0.25-0.5 mcg/kg/minute; usual length of treatment is 1-6 hours with tapering of 12% every 15-30 minutes

Mechanism of Action A selective postsynaptic dopamine agonist (D_1-receptors) which exerts hypotensive effects by decreasing peripheral vasculature resistance with increased renal blood flow, diuresis, and natriuresis; 6 times as potent as dopamine in producing renal vasodilitation; has minimal adrenergic effects

Other Adverse Effects Frequency not defined:

Cardiovascular: Edema, asymptomatic T wave flattening on EKG

Gastrointestinal: Diarrhea

Ocular: Intraocular pressure (increased)

Drug Interactions Increased Effect/Toxicity: Concurrent acetaminophen may increase fenoldopam levels (30% to 70%). Beta-blockers increase the risk of hypotension.

Pharmacodynamics/Kinetics

Onset of action: I.V.: 10 minutes

Duration: Oral: 2-4 hours; I.V.: 1 hour

Absorption: Oral: Good; peak serum levels at 1 hour

Distribution: V_d: 0.6 L/kg

Half-life elimination: I.V.: 9.8 minutes

Metabolism: Hepatic to multiple metabolites; the 8-sulfate metabolite may have some activity; extensive first-pass effect

Excretion: Urine (80%); feces (20%)

Generic Available No

Fenoldopam Mesylate *see* Fenoldopam *on page 562*

Fenoprofen (fen oh PROE fen)

Related Information

Rheumatoid Arthritis, Osteoarthritis, and Osteoporosis *on page 1488*

Temporomandibular Dysfunction (TMD) *on page 1562*

U.S. Brand Names Nalfon®

Canadian Brand Names Nalfon®

Pharmacologic Category Nonsteroidal Anti-inflammatory Drug (NSAID)

Synonyms Fenoprofen Calcium

Use Symptomatic treatment of acute and chronic rheumatoid arthritis and osteoarthritis; relief of mild to moderate pain

Local Anesthetic/Vasoconstrictor Precautions No information available to require special precautions

Effects on Dental Treatment NSAID formulations are known to reversibly decrease platelet aggregation via mechanisms different than observed with aspirin. The dentist should be aware of the potential of abnormal coagulation. Caution should also be exercised in the use of NSAIDs in patients already on anticoagulant therapy with drugs such as warfarin (Coumadin®).

>10%: Dizziness (7% to 15%), somnolence (9% to 15%), nausea (8% to 14%), vomiting (3% to 14%)

1% to 10%: Headache (9%)

Dosage Adults: Oral:

Rheumatoid arthritis: 300-600 mg 3-4 times/day up to 3.2 g/day

Mild to moderate pain: 200 mg every 4-6 hours as needed

Mechanism of Action Inhibits prostaglandin synthesis by decreasing the activity of the enzyme, cyclooxygenase, which results in decreased formation of prostaglandin precursors

Other Adverse Effects

>10%:

Gastrointestinal: Abdominal cramps (2% to 4%), heartburn, indigestion, dyspepsia (10% to 14%), flatulence (14%), anorexia (14%), constipation (7% to 14%), occult blood in stool (14%), diarrhea (2% to 14%)

1% to 10%:

Dermatologic: Itching

Endocrine & metabolic: Fluid retention

<1%: **CHF, hypertension, arrhythmias, tachycardia, confusion, hallucinations,** aseptic meningitis, mental depression, **drowsiness,** insomnia, urticaria, erythema multiforme, toxic epidermal necrolysis, Stevens-Johnson syndrome, angioedema, polydipsia, **hot flashes, gastritis, GI ulceration**, cystitis, polyuria, agranulocytosis, anemia, hemolytic anemia, bone marrow suppression, leukopenia, thrombocytopenia, hepatitis, peripheral neuropathy, toxic amblyopia, **blurred vision,** conjunctivitis, dry eyes, decreased hearing, acute renal failure, **allergic rhinitis, dyspnea, epistaxis,** rash, pruritus

Drug Interactions

Increased effect/toxicity of phenytoin, sulfonamides, sulfonylureas, salicylates, and oral anticoagulants. Serum concentration/toxicity of methotrexate may be increased.

(Continued)

Fenoprofen *(Continued)*

Decreased effect with phenobarbital.

Dietary/Ethanol/Herb Considerations

Ethanol: Avoid use; may enhance gastric mucosal irritation.

Food: Administer with food or milk to reduce GI upset; may decrease peak serum concentration. Avoid garlic, ginger, and green tea.

Herb/Nutraceutical: Avoid cat's claw, dong quai, evening primrose, feverfew, garlic, ginger, ginkgo biloba, ginseng, green tea, horse chestnut, and red clover due to additional antiplatelet activity. Avoid kava and valerian; may enhance benzodiazepine activity.

Pharmacodynamics/Kinetics

Onset of action: A few days

Absorption: Rapid, 80%

Distribution: Does not cross the placenta

Protein binding: 99%

Metabolism: Extensively hepatic

Half-life elimination: 2.5-3 hours

Time to peak, serum: ~2 hours

Excretion: Urine (2% to 5% as unchanged drug); feces (small amounts)

Pregnancy Risk Factor B/D (3rd trimester)

Generic Available Yes: Tablet

Fenoprofen Calcium *see* Fenoprofen *on page 563*

Fenoterol (fen oh TER ole)

Canadian Brand Names Berotec®

Pharmacologic Category Beta$_2$ Agonist

Synonyms Fenoterol Hydrobromide

Use Treatment and prevention of symptoms of reversible obstructive pulmonary disease (including asthma and acute bronchospasm), chronic bronchitis, emphysema

Local Anesthetic/Vasoconstrictor Precautions No information available to require special precautions

Effects on Dental Treatment May be dose-related:

>10% (in treatment of acute bronchospasm with high-dose nebulization): Tachycardia (≤21%), headache (≤12%), tremors (32%)

1% to 10%: Palpitations, tachycardia, headache, dizziness, nervousness, muscle cramps pharyngeal irritation, cough

Dosage Inhalation: Children ≥12 years of age and Adults:

MDI:

Acute treatment: 1 puff initially; may repeat in 5 minutes; if relief is not evident, additional doses and/or other therapy may be necessary

Intermittent/long-term treatment: 1-2 puffs 3-4 times/day (maximum of 8 puffs/24 hours)

Solution: 0.5-1 mg (up to maximum of 2.5 mg)

Mechanism of Action Relaxes bronchial smooth muscle by action on beta$_2$ receptors with little effect on heart rate.

Other Adverse Effects <1%: **Agitation, allergic reaction, arrhythmia, bronchospasm (paradoxical),** hypokalemia, **hyperglycemia, hypertension, nausea,** pruritus, rash, **restlessness,** sleep disorder, **tachycardia,** urticaria, **vomiting**

Drug Interactions

Increased Effect/Toxicity: When used with inhaled ipratropium, an increased duration of bronchodilation may occur. Cardiovascular effects are potentiated in patients also receiving MAO inhibitors, tricyclic antidepressants, and sympathomimetic agents (eg, amphetamine, dopamine, dobutamine). Fenoterol may increase the risk of malignant arrhythmias with inhaled anesthetics (eg, enflurane, halothane). Concurrent use with diuretics may increase the risk of hypokalemia.

Decreased Effect: When used with nonselective beta-adrenergic blockers (eg, propranolol), the effect of fenoterol is decreased.

Dietary/Ethanol/Herb Considerations

Food: Avoid or limit caffeine; may cause CNS stimulation. Small, frequent meals, chewing gum, or sucking lozenges may reduce nausea.

Herb/Nutraceutical: Avoid ephedra, ginseng, and yohimbe; may cause CNS stimulation.

Pharmacodynamics/Kinetics

Onset of action: 5 minutes

Peak effect: 30-60 minutes

Duration: 3-4 hours (up to 6-8 hours)

Pregnancy Risk Factor Not available; similar agents rated C

Fenoterol Hydrobromide *see* Fenoterol *on page 564*

Fentanyl (FEN ta nil)

U.S. Brand Names Actiq®; Duragesic®; Sublimaze®

Canadian Brand Names Actiq®; Duragesic®

Mexican Brand Names Durogesic®; Fentanest®

Pharmacologic Category Analgesic, Narcotic; General Anesthetic

Synonyms Fentanyl Citrate

Use

Dental: Adjunct in preoperative I.V. conscious sedation in patients undergoing dental surgery

Medical: Sedation, relief of pain, preoperative medication, adjunct to general or regional anesthesia, management of chronic pain (transdermal product)

Actiq® is indicated only for management of breakthrough cancer pain in patients who are tolerant to and currently receiving opioid therapy for persistent cancer pain.

Local Anesthetic/Vasoconstrictor Precautions No information available to require special precautions

Effects on Dental Treatment Actiq® may contribute to dental carries due to sugar content of oral lozenge; advise patients to maintain good oral hygiene.

>10%: Xerostomia, changes in salivation, hypotension, bradycardia, CNS depression, drowsiness, sedation, nausea, vomiting, respiratory depression

1% to 10%: Cardiac arrhythmias, orthostatic hypotension, confusion, biliary tract spasm

Restrictions C-II

Dosage These are guidelines and do not represent the maximum doses that may be required in all patients. Doses should be titrated to pain relief/prevention. Monitor vital signs routinely. Single I.M. doses have a duration of 1-2 hours, single I.V. doses last 0.5-1 hour.

Children 1-12 years:

Sedation for minor procedures/analgesia: I.M., I.V.: 1-2 mcg/kg/dose; may repeat at 30- to 60-minute intervals. **Note:** Children 18-36 months of age may require 2-3 mcg/kg/dose

Continuous sedation/analgesia: Initial I.V. bolus: 1-2 mcg/kg then 1 mcg/kg/hour; titrate upward; usual: 1-3 mcg/kg/hour

Pain control: Transdermal: Use not recommended

Children >12 years and Adults: **Sedation for minor procedures/analgesia:** I.M., I.V.: 0.5-1 mcg/kg/dose; higher doses are used for major procedures

Adults:

Premedication: I.M., slow I.V.: 50-100 mcg/dose 30-60 minutes prior to surgery

Adjunct to regional anesthesia: I.M., slow I.V.: 50-100 mcg/dose; if I.V. used, give over 1-2 minutes

Severe pain: I.M.: 50-100 mcg/dose every 1-2 hours as needed; patients with prior opiate exposure may tolerate higher initial doses

Adjunct to general anesthesia: Slow I.V.:

Low dose: Initial: 2 mcg/kg/dose; Maintenance: Additional doses infrequently needed

Moderate dose: Initial: 2-20 mcg/kg/dose; Maintenance: 25-100 mcg/dose may be given slow I.V. or I.M. as needed

High dose: Initial: 20-50 mcg/kg/dose; Maintenance: 25 mcg to one-half the initial loading dose may be given as needed

General anesthesia without additional anesthetic agents: Slow I.V.: 50-100 mcg/kg with O_2 and skeletal muscle relaxant

Mechanically-ventilated patients (based on 70 kg patient): Slow I.V.: 0.35-1.5 mcg/kg every 30-60 minutes as needed; infusion: 0.7-10 mcg/kg/hour

Patient-controlled analgesia (PCA): I.V.: Usual concentration: 50 mcg/mL

Demand dose: Usual: 10 mcg; range: 10-50 mcg

Lockout interval: 5-8 minutes

Equianalgesic Doses of Opioid Agonists

Drug	Equianalgesic Dose (mg)	
	I.M.	P.O.
Codeine	75	130
Hydromorphone	1.5	7.5
Levorphanol	2 (acute)	4 (acute)
Meperidine	75	300
Methadone	10 (acute)	20 (acute)
Morphine	10	30
Oxycodone	—	20
Oxymorphone	1	10 (PR)

From "Principles of Analgesic Use," *Am Pain Soc*, 1999.

(Continued)

Fentanyl *(Continued)*

Pain control: Transdermal: Initial: 25 mcg/hour system; if currently receiving opiates, convert to fentanyl equivalent and administer equianalgesic dosage titrated to minimize the adverse effects and provide analgesia. The dosage should not be titrated more frequently than every 3 days after the initial dose or every 6 days thereafter. The majority of patients are controlled on every 72-hour administration, however, a small number of patients require every 48-hour administration.

To convert patients from oral or parenteral opioids to Duragesic®, the previous 24-hour analgesic requirement should be calculated. This analgesic requirement should be converted to the equianalgesic oral morphine dose (see tables on previous page and below).

Corresponding Doses of Oral/Intramuscular Morphine and Duragesic™

P.O. 24-Hour Morphine (mg/d)	I.M. 24-Hour Morphine (mg/d)	Duragesic™ Dose (mcg/h)
45-134	8-22	25
135-224	28-37	50
225-314	38-52	75
315-404	53-67	100
405-494	68-82	125
495-584	83-97	150
585-674	98-112	175
675-764	113-127	200
765-854	128-142	225
855-944	143-157	250
945-1034	158-172	275
1035-1124	173-187	300

Product information, Duragesic™ — Janssen Pharmaceutica, January, 1991.

Breakthrough cancer pain: Transmucosal (Actiq®): Dosing should be individually titrated to provide adequate analgesia with minimal side effects. It is indicated only for management of breakthrough cancer pain in patients who are tolerant to and currently receiving opioid therapy for persistent cancer pain. An initial starting dose of 200 mcg should be used for the treatment of breakthrough cancer pain. Patients should be monitored closely in order to determine the proper dose. If redosing for the same episode is necessary, the second dose may be started 15 minutes after completion of the first dose. Dosing should be titrated so that the patient's pain can be treated with one single dose. Generally, 1-2 days is required to determine the proper dose of analgesia with limited side effects. Once the dose has been determined, consumption should be limited to 4 units/day or less. Patients needing more than 4 units/day should have the dose of their long-term opioid re-evaluated. If signs of excessive opioid effects occur before a dose is complete, the unit should be removed from the patient's mouth immediately, and subsequent doses decreased.

Elderly >65 years: Dose should be reduced to 2.5-5 mcg/kg; elderly have been found to be twice as sensitive as younger patients to the effects of fentanyl. Patients in this age group generally require smaller doses of Actiq® than younger patients

Dosing adjustment in renal impairment:

Cl_{cr} 10-50 mL/minute: Administer at 75% of normal dose

Cl_{cr} <10 mL/minute: Administer at 50% of normal dose

Dosing adjustment in renal/hepatic impairment: Actiq®: Although fentanyl kinetics may be altered in renal/hepatic disease, Actiq® can be used successfully in the management of breakthrough cancer pain. Doses should be titrated to reach clinical effect with careful monitoring of patients with severe renal/hepatic disease.

Mechanism of Action Binds with stereospecific receptors at many sites within the CNS, increases pain threshold, alters pain reception, inhibits ascending pain pathways

Other Adverse Effects

>10%:

Gastrointestinal: Constipation

Neuromuscular & skeletal: Chest wall rigidity (high dose I.V.)

Ocular: Miosis

<1%: ADH release, **bronchospasm, circulatory depression, CNS excitation or delirium, cold/clammy skin, convulsions**, dysesthesia, erythema, itching, **laryngospasm, paradoxical dizziness, physical and psychological dependence (prolonged use)**, pruritus, rash, urinary tract spasm, urticaria

Postmarketing and/or case reports: **Blurred vision**, edema, **tachycardia**, weight loss

Contraindications Hypersensitivity to fentanyl or any component of the formulation; increased intracranial pressure; severe respiratory depression; severe liver or renal insufficiency; pregnancy (prolonged use or high doses near term)

Actiq® must not be used in patients who are intolerant to opioids. Patients are considered opioid-tolerant if they are taking at least 60 mg morphine/day, 50 mcg transdermal fentanyl/hour, or an equivalent dose of another opioid for ≥1 week.

Warnings/Precautions An opioid-containing analgesic regimen should be tailored to each patient's needs and based upon the type of pain being treated (acute versus chronic), the route of administration, degree of tolerance for opioids (naive versus chronic user), age, weight, and medical condition. The optimal analgesic dose varies widely among patients. Doses should be titrated to pain relief/prevention.

Fentanyl shares the toxic potentials of opiate agonists, and precautions of opiate agonist therapy should be observed; use with caution in patients with bradycardia; rapid I.V. infusion may result in skeletal muscle and chest wall rigidity leading to respiratory distress and/or apnea, bronchoconstriction, laryngospasm; inject slowly over 3-5 minutes; nondepolarizing skeletal muscle relaxant may be required. Tolerance of drug dependence may result from extended use. The elderly may be particularly susceptible to the CNS depressant and constipating effects of narcotics.

Actiq® should be used only for the care of cancer patients and is intended for use by specialists who are knowledgeable in treating cancer pain. For patients who have received transmucosal product within 6-12 hours, it is recommended that if other narcotics are required, they should be used at starting doses 1/4 to 1/3 those usually recommended. Actiq® preparations contain an amount of medication that can be fatal to children. Keep all units out of the reach of children and discard any open units properly. Patients and caregivers should be counseled on the dangers to children including the risk of exposure to partially-consumed units. Safety and efficacy have not been established in children <16 years of age.

Topical patches: Serum fentanyl concentrations may increase approximately one-third for patients with a body temperature of 40°C secondary to a temperature-dependent increase in fentanyl release from the system and increased skin permeability. Patients who experience adverse reactions should be monitored for at least 12 hours after removal of the patch.

Drug Interactions Substrate of **CYP3A4**; Inhibits CYP3A4

CNS depressants: Increased sedation with CNS depressants, phenothiazines

CYP3A4 inducers (including carbamazepine, phenytoin, phenobarbital, rifampin): May decrease serum levels of fentanyl by increasing metabolism.

CYP3A4 inhibitors (including erythromycin, clarithromycin, ketoconazole, itraconazole, protease inhibitors): May increase serum concentration of fentanyl.

MAO inhibitors: Not recommended to use Actiq® within 14 days. Severe and unpredictable potentiation by MAO Inhibitors has been reported with opioid analgesics.

Dietary/Ethanol/Herb Considerations

Ethanol: Avoid use; may increase CNS depression.

Food: Glucose may cause hyperglycemia.

Herb/Nutraceutical: Avoid gotu kola, kava, SAMe, and valerian; may increase CNS depression. Avoid St John's wort; may decrease serum concentration.

Pharmacodynamics/Kinetics

Onset of action: Analgesic: I.M.: 7-15 minutes; I.V.: Almost immediate; Transmucosal: 5-15 minutes

Peak effect: Transmucosal: Analgesic: 20-30 minutes

Duration: I.M.: 1-2 hours; I.V.: 0.5-1 hour; Transmucosal: Related to blood level; respiratory depressant effect may last longer than analgesic effect

Absorption: Transmucosal: Rapid, ~25% from the buccal mucosa; 75% swallowed with saliva and slowly absorbed from GI tract

Distribution: Highly lipophilic, redistributes into muscle and fat

Metabolism: Hepatic

Bioavailability: Transmucosal: ~50% (range: 36% to 71%)

Half-life elimination: 2-4 hours; Transmucosal: 6.6 hours (range: 5-15 hours)

Excretion: Urine (primarily as metabolites, 10% as unchanged drug)

Pregnancy Risk Factor C/D (prolonged use or high doses at term)

Dosage Forms INJ, solution, as citrate [preservative free]: 0.05 mg/mL (2 mL, 5 mL, 10 mL, 20 mL, 30 mL, 50 mL); (Sublimaze®): 0.05 mg/mL (2 mL, 5 mL, 10 mL, 20 mL). **LOZ, oral transmucosal, as citrate** (Actiq®): 200 mcg, 400 mcg, 600 mcg, 800 mcg, 1200 mcg, 1600 mcg. **Transdermal system** (Duragesic®): 25 mcg/hour [10 cm^2] (5s); 50 mcg/hour [20 cm^2] (5s); 75 mcg/hour [30 cm^2]; 100 mcg/hour [40 cm^2] (5s)

Generic Available Yes: Injection only

Comments Transdermal fentanyl should not be used as a pain reliever in dentistry due to danger of hypoventilation

(Continued)

Fentanyl *(Continued)*

Selected Readings Dionne RA, Yagiela JA, Moore PA, et al, "Comparing Efficacy and Safety of Four Intravenous Sedation Regimens in Dental Outpatients," *Am Dent Assoc*, 2001, 132(6):740-51.

Fentanyl Citrate *see* Fentanyl *on page 565*
Feostat® [OTC] *see* Iron Supplements *on page 745*
Feratab® [OTC] *see* Iron Supplements *on page 745*
Fer-Gen-Sol [OTC] *see* Iron Supplements *on page 745*
Fergon® [OTC] *see* Iron Supplements *on page 745*
Fer-In-Sol® [OTC] *see* Iron Supplements *on page 745*
Fer-Iron® [OTC] *see* Iron Supplements *on page 745*
Fero-Grad 500® [OTC] *see* Ferrous Sulfate and Ascorbic Acid *on page 569*
Ferretts [OTC] *see* Iron Supplements *on page 745*

Ferric Gluconate (FER ik GLOO koe nate)

U.S. Brand Names Ferrlecit®

Pharmacologic Category Iron Salt

Synonyms Sodium Ferric Gluconate

Use Repletion of total body iron content in patients with iron-deficiency anemia who are undergoing hemodialysis in conjunction with erythropoietin therapy

Local Anesthetic/Vasoconstrictor Precautions No information available to require special precautions

Effects on Dental Treatment Do not prescribe tetracyclines simultaneously with iron since GI tract absorption of both tetracycline and iron may be inhibited. Major reactions include serious hypotension (1%) and hypersensitivity (ie, pruritus, chest pain, hypotension, nausea, abdominal pain, flank pain, fatigue, and rash).

Frequency not defined: Hypotension, chest pain, hypertension, syncope, tachycardia, angina, MI, headache, fatigue, fever, malaise, dizziness, paresthesia, insomnia, agitation, somnolence, pain, hypoglycemia, nausea, vomiting, epigastric pain, lymphadenopathy, weakness, leg cramps, paresthesia, blurred vision, dyspnea, cough, rhinitis, upper respiratory infection, pneumonia, hypersensitivity reactions, infection, rigors, xerostomia, flu-like syndrome, sepsis, carcinoma, increased diaphoresis, hemorrhage, nervousness

Dosage Adults: A test dose of 2 mL diluted in 50 mL 0.9% sodium chloride over 60 minutes was previously recommended (not in current manufacturer labeling).

Repletion of iron in hemodialysis patients: I.V.: 125 mg elemental iron per 10 mL (either by I.V. infusion or slow I.V. injection). Most patients will require a cumulative dose of 1 g elemental iron over approximately 8 sequential dialysis treatments to achieve a favorable response.

Mechanism of Action Supplies a source to elemental iron necessary to the function of hemoglobin, myoglobin and specific enzyme systems; allows transport of oxygen via hemoglobin

Other Adverse Effects

Frequency not defined:

Cardiovascular: Pulmonary edema, hypovolemia, peripheral edema
Central nervous system: Insomnia
Dermatologic: Pruritus, rash
Endocrine & metabolic: Hyperkalemia, hypokalemia
Gastrointestinal: Abdominal pain, diarrhea, rectal disorder, dyspepsia, flatulence, melena,
Genitourinary: Urinary tract infection
Hematologic: Anemia, abnormal erythrocytes
Local: Injection site reactions, injection site pain
Neuromuscular & skeletal: Myalgia, arthralgia, groin pain
Ocular: Conjunctivitis

Drug Interactions Decreased Effect: Chloramphenicol may decrease effect of ferric gluconate injection; ferric gluconate injection may decrease the absorption of oral iron

Dietary/Ethanol/Herb Considerations Food: Milk may decrease absorption of iron.

Pharmacodynamics/Kinetics Half-life elimination: Bound: 1 hour

Pregnancy Risk Factor B

Generic Available No

Comments Contains benzyl alcohol 9 mg/mL

Ferrlecit® *see* Ferric Gluconate *on page 568*
Ferro-Sequels® [OTC] *see* Iron Supplements *on page 745*
Ferrous Fumarate *see* Iron Supplements *on page 745*
Ferrous Gluconate *see* Iron Supplements *on page 745*
Ferrous Salts *see* Iron Supplements *on page 745*
Ferrous Sulfate *see* Iron Supplements *on page 745*

Ferrous Sulfate and Ascorbic Acid

(FER us SUL fate & a SKOR bik AS id)

Related Information

Ascorbic Acid *on page 128*

U.S. Brand Names Fero-Grad 500® [OTC]; Vitelle™ Irospan® [OTC]

Pharmacologic Category Iron Salt; Vitamin

Synonyms Ascorbic Acid and Ferrous Sulfate

Use Treatment of iron deficiency in nonpregnant adults; treatment and prevention of iron deficiency in pregnant adults

Local Anesthetic/Vasoconstrictor Precautions No information available to require special precautions

Effects on Dental Treatment Do not prescribe tetracyclines simultaneously with iron since GI tract absorption of both tetracycline and iron may be inhibited. Liquid preparations may temporarily stain the teeth.

Based on **ferrous sulfate** component: >10%: GI irritation, epigastric pain, nausea, vomiting

Dosage Adults: Oral: 1 tablet daily

Other Adverse Effects Based on **ferrous sulfate** component:

>10%: Gastrointestinal: Dark stool, stomach cramping, constipation

1% to 10%:

Gastrointestinal: Heartburn, diarrhea

Genitourinary: Discoloration of urine

<1%: Contact irritation

Drug Interactions

Increased Effect/Toxicity: Concurrent administration of ≥200 mg vitamin C per 30 mg elemental iron increases absorption of oral iron.

Decreased Effect: Absorption of oral preparation of iron and tetracyclines are decreased when both of these drugs are given together. Absorption of quinolones may be decreased due to formation of a ferric ion-quinolone complex when given concurrently. Concurrent administration of antacids and H_2 blockers (cimetidine) may decrease iron absorption. Iron may decrease absorption of levodopa, methyldopa, penicillamine when given at the same time. Response to iron therapy may be delayed by chloramphenicol.

Dietary/Ethanol/Herb Considerations Food decreases absorption (especially cereals, coffee, dietary fiber, eggs, milk, and tea).

Generic Available No

Fertinex® *see* Follitropins *on page 607*

$FeSO_4$ (Ferrous Sulfate) *see* Iron Supplements *on page 745*

Fe-Tinic™ 150 [OTC] *see* Polysaccharide-Iron Complex *on page 1096*

Feverall® [OTC] *see* Acetaminophen *on page 27*

Fexofenadine (feks oh FEN a deen)

U.S. Brand Names Allegra®

Canadian Brand Names Allegra®

Mexican Brand Names Allegra®

Pharmacologic Category Antihistamine, Nonsedating

Synonyms Fexofenadine Hydrochloride

Use Relief of symptoms associated with seasonal allergic rhinitis; treatment of chronic idiopathic urticaria

Local Anesthetic/Vasoconstrictor Precautions No information available to require special precautions

Effects on Dental Treatment

Otitis media (3%)

>10%: Headache (7% to 11%)

1% to 10%: Fever (2%), dizziness (2%), pain (2%), drowsiness (1% to 2%), fatigue (1%), nausea (2%), otitis media (2%), cough (4%), upper respiratory tract infection (3% to 4%), sinusitis (2%), viral infection (3%)

Dosage Oral:

Children 6-11 years: 30 mg twice daily

Children ≥12 years and Adults:

Seasonal allergic rhinitis: 60 mg twice daily **or** 180 mg once daily

Chronic idiopathic urticaria: 60 mg twice daily

Dosing adjustment in renal impairment: Cl_{cr} <40 mL/minute:

Children 6-11 years: Initial: 30 mg once daily

Children ≥12 years and Adults: Initial: 60 mg once daily

Mechanism of Action Fexofenadine is an active metabolite of terfenadine and like terfenadine it competes with histamine for H_1-receptor sites on effector cells in the gastrointestinal tract, blood vessels and respiratory tract; it appears that fexofenadine does not cross the blood brain barrier to any appreciable degree, resulting in a reduced potential for sedation

Other Adverse Effects

1% to 10%:

Endocrine & metabolic: Dysmenorrhea (2%)

(Continued)

Fexofenadine *(Continued)*

Gastrointestinal: Nausea (2%), dyspepsia (1%)
Neuromuscular & skeletal: Back pain (2% to 3%)

<1%, postmarketing, and/or case reports: **Hypersensitivity reactions (anaphylaxis, angioedema, dyspnea, flushing, pruritus, rash, urticaria)**, insomnia, **nervousness,** sleep disorders, paroniria (terrifying dreams)

Drug Interactions Substrate of CYP3A4; Inhibits CYP2D6

Increased Effect/Toxicity: Erythromycin and ketoconazole increased the levels of fexofenadine; however, no increase in adverse events or QT_c intervals was noted. The effect of other macrolide agents or azoles has not been investigated.

Decreased Effect: Aluminum- and magnesium-containing antacids decrease plasma levels of fexofenadine; separate administration is recommended.

Dietary/Ethanol/Herb Considerations

Ethanol: Avoid use; although limited with fexofenadine, may increase risk of sedation.

Herb/Nutraceutical: Avoid St John's wort; may decrease serum concentration.

Pharmacodynamics/Kinetics

Onset of action: 60 minutes
Duration: Antihistaminic effect: ≥12 hours
Protein binding: 60% to 70%, primarily albumin and $alpha_1$-acid glycoprotein
Metabolism: ~5% mostly by gut flora; 0.5% to 1.5% by CYP
Half-life elimination: 14.4 hours
Time to peak, serum: ~2.6 hours
Excretion: Feces (~80%) and urine (~11%) as unchanged drug

Pregnancy Risk Factor C

Generic Available No

Selected Readings

"Fexofenadine," *Med Lett Drugs Ther*, 1996, 38(986):95-6.
Markham A and Wagstaff AJ, "Fexofenadine," *Drugs*, 1998, 55(2):269-74 (discussion 275-6).
Simons FE, Bergman JN, Watson WT, et al, "The Clinical Pharmacology of Fexofenadine in Children," *J Allergy Clin Immunol*, 1996, 98(6 Pt 1):1062-4.

Fexofenadine and Pseudoephedrine

(feks oh FEN a deen & soo doe e FED rin)

Related Information

Fexofenadine *on page 569*
Pseudoephedrine *on page 1146*

U.S. Brand Names Allegra-D®

Canadian Brand Names Allegra-D®

Pharmacologic Category Antihistamine/Decongestant Combination

Synonyms Pseudoephedrine and Fexofenadine

Use Relief of symptoms associated with seasonal allergic rhinitis in adults and children ≥12 years of age

Local Anesthetic/Vasoconstrictor Precautions Pseudoephedrine component: Use with caution since pseudoephedrine is a sympathomimetic amine which could interact with epinephrine to cause a pressor response

Effects on Dental Treatment Pseudoephedrine: Up to 10% of patients could experience tachycardia, palpitations, and xerostomia; use vasoconstrictor with caution.

Dosage Oral:

Children ≥12 years and Adults: One tablet twice daily; it is recommended that the administration with food should be avoided.

Dosage adjustment in renal impairment: One tablet once daily

Pregnancy Risk Factor C

Generic Available No

Fexofenadine Hydrochloride *see* Fexofenadine *on page 569*
Fiberall® *see* Psyllium *on page 1149*
Fiberall® Chewable Tablet [OTC] *see* Calcium Polycarbophil *on page 228*
FiberCon® Tablet [OTC] *see* Calcium Polycarbophil *on page 228*
FiberEase™ [OTC] *see* Methylcellulose *on page 891*
Fiber-Lax® Tablet [OTC] *see* Calcium Polycarbophil *on page 228*

Fibrin Sealant Kit (FI brin SEEL ent kit)

U.S. Brand Names Tisseel® VH

Canadian Brand Names Tisseel® VH

Pharmacologic Category Hemostatic Agent

Synonyms FS

Use Adjunct to hemostasis in cardiopulmonary bypass surgery and splenic injury (due to blunt or penetrating trauma to the abdomen) when the control of bleeding by conventional surgical techniques is ineffective or impractical; adjunctive sealant for closure of colostomies; hemostatic agent in heparinized patients undergoing cardiopulmonary bypass

Local Anesthetic/Vasoconstrictor Precautions No information available to require special precautions

Effects on Dental Treatment No significant effects or complications reported

Dosage Adjunct to hemostasis: Adults: Apply topically; actual dose is based on size of surface to be covered:

Maximum area to be sealed: 4 cm^2
Required size of Tisseel® VH kit: 0.5 mL
Maximum area to be sealed: 8 cm^2
Required size of Tisseel® VH kit: 1 mL
Maximum area to be sealed: 16 cm^2
Required size of Tisseel® VH kit: 2 mL
Maximum area to be sealed: 40 cm^2
Required size of Tisseel® VH kit: 5 mL

Apply in thin layers to avoid excess formation of granulation tissue and slow absorption of the sealant. Following application, hold the sealed parts in the desired position for 3-5 minutes. To prevent sealant from adhering to gloves or surgical instruments, wet them with saline prior to contact.

Mechanism of Action Formation of a biodegradable adhesive is done by duplicating the last step of the coagulation cascade, the formation of fibrin from fibrinogen. Fibrinogen is the main component of the sealant solution. The solution also contains thrombin, which transforms fibrinogen from the sealer protein solution into fibrin, and fibrinolysis inhibitor (aprotinin), which prevents the premature degradation of fibrin. When mixed as directed, a viscous solution forms that sets into an elastic coagulum.

Other Adverse Effects No adverse events were reported in clinical trials. Anaphylactoid or anaphylactic reactions have occurred with other plasma-derived products.

Drug Interactions Decreased Effect: Decreased effect: Local concentrations/applications of alcohol, heavy-metal ions, iodine; oxycellulose preparations

Pharmacodynamics/Kinetics Onset of action: Final prepared sealant: 70% strength: ~10 minutes; Full strength: ~2 hours

Pregnancy Risk Factor C

Filgrastim (fil GRA stim)

U.S. Brand Names Neupogen®

Canadian Brand Names Neupogen®

Mexican Brand Names Neupogen®

Pharmacologic Category Colony Stimulating Factor

Synonyms G-CSF; Granulocyte Colony Stimulating Factor

Use Stimulation of granulocyte production in patients with malignancies, including myeloid malignancies; receiving myelosuppressive therapy associated with a significant risk of neutropenia; severe chronic neutropenia (SCN); receiving bone marrow transplantation (BMT); undergoing peripheral blood progenitor cell (PBPC) collection

Local Anesthetic/Vasoconstrictor Precautions No information available to require special precautions

Effects on Dental Treatment

>10%: Chest pain, fever, nausea, vomiting, mucositis, pain
1% to 10%: Headache dyspnea, cough, weakness, sore throat

Dosage Dosing, even in morbidly obese patients, should be based on actual body weight. Rounding doses to the nearest vial size often enhances patient convenience and reduces costs without compromising clinical response. Refer to individual protocols.

Myelosuppressive therapy: 5 mcg/kg/day - doses may be increased by 5 mcg/kg according to the duration and severity of the neutropenia.

Bone marrow transplantation: 5-10 mcg/kg/day - doses may be increased by 5 mcg/kg according to the duration and severity of neutropenia; recommended steps based on neutrophil response:

When ANC >1000/mm^3 for 3 consecutive days: Reduce filgrastim dose to 5 mcg/kg/day
If ANC remains >1000/mm^3 for 3 more consecutive days: Discontinue filgrastim
If ANC decreases to <1000/mm^3: Resume at 5 mcg/kg/day
If ANC decreases <1000/mm^3 during the 5 mcg/kg/day dose, increase filgrastim to 10 mcg/kg/day and follow the above steps

Peripheral blood progenitor cell (PBPC) collection: 10 mcg/kg/day **or** 5-8 mcg/kg twice daily in donors. The optimal timing and duration of growth factor stimulation has not been determined.

Severe chronic neutropenia:
Congenital: 6 mcg/kg twice daily
Idiopathic/cyclic: 5 mcg/kg/day

Hemodialysis: Not removed

Mechanism of Action Stimulates the production, maturation, and activation of neutrophils, G-CSF activates neutrophils to increase both their migration and cytotoxicity. See table on next page.

(Continued)

Filgrastim *(Continued)*

Comparative Effects — G-CSF vs. GM-CSF

Proliferation/Differentiation	G-CSF (Filgrastim)	GM-CSF (Sargramostim)
Neutrophils	Yes	Yes
Eosinophils	No	Yes
Macrophages	No	Yes
Neutrophil migration	Enhanced	Inhibited

Other Adverse Effects

>10%:

Dermatologic: Alopecia
Endocrine & metabolic: Fluid retention
Gastrointestinal: Diarrhea, splenomegaly (up to 33% of patients with cyclic neutropenia/congenital agranulocytosis receiving filgrastim for ≥14 days; rare in other patients)
Neuromuscular & skeletal: Bone pain (24%); commonly in the lower back, posterior iliac crest, and sternum

1% to 10%:

Cardiovascular: S-T segment depression (3%)
Dermatologic: Rash
Gastrointestinal: Anorexia, constipation
Hematologic: Leukocytosis
Local: Pain at injection site

<1%: **Transient supraventricular arrhythmias,** pericarditis, **hypotension,** thrombophlebitis, **hypersensitivity reactions**

Drug Interactions Increased Effect/Toxicity: Drugs which may potentiate the release of neutrophils (eg, lithium) should be used with caution.

Pharmacodynamics/Kinetics

Onset of action: ~24 hours; plateaus in 3-5 days
Duration: ANC decreases by 50% within 2 days after discontinuing G-CSF; white counts return to the normal range in 4-7 days; peak plasma levels can be maintained for up to 12 hours
Absorption: S.C.: 100%
Distribution: V_d: 150 mL/kg; no evidence of drug accumulation over a 11- to 20-day period
Metabolism: Systemically degraded
Half-life elimination: 1.8-3.5 hours
Time to peak, serum: S.C.: 2-6 hours

Pregnancy Risk Factor C

Generic Available No

Comments

Reimbursement Hotline: 1-800-272-9376
Professional Services [Amgen]: 1-800-77-AMGEN

Finacea™ *see* Azelaic Acid *on page 151*

Finasteride (fi NAS teer ide)

U.S. Brand Names Propecia®; Proscar®

Canadian Brand Names Propecia®; Proscar®

Mexican Brand Names Propeshia®; Proscar®

Pharmacologic Category 5 Alpha-Reductase Inhibitor

Use

Propecia®: Treatment of male pattern hair loss in **men only**. Safety and efficacy were demonstrated in men between 18-41 years of age.
Proscar®: Treatment of symptomatic benign prostatic hyperplasia (BPH)

Unlabeled/Investigational Use Adjuvant monotherapy after radical prostatectomy in the treatment of prostatic cancer; treatment of female hirsutism

Local Anesthetic/Vasoconstrictor Precautions No information available to require special precautions

Effects on Dental Treatment No significant effects or complications reported

Dosage Oral: Adults:

Male:

Benign prostatic hyperplasia (Proscar®): 5 mg/day as a single dose; clinical responses occur within 12 weeks to 6 months of initiation of therapy; long-term administration is recommended for maximal response
Male pattern baldness (Propecia®): 1 mg daily

Female: Hirsutism: 5 mg/day

Dosing adjustment in hepatic impairment: Use with caution in patients with liver function abnormalities because finasteride is metabolized extensively in the liver

Mechanism of Action Finasteride is a 4-azo analog of testosterone and is a competitive inhibitor of both tissue and hepatic 5-alpha reductase. This results in inhibition of the conversion of testosterone to dihydrotestosterone and markedly suppresses serum dihydrotestosterone levels; depending on dose and duration, serum testosterone concentrations may or may not increase. Testosterone-dependent processes such as fertility, muscle strength, potency, and libido are not affected by finasteride.

Other Adverse Effects

1% to 10%:

Endocrine & metabolic: Libido decreased

Genitourinary: <4% incidence of erectile dysfunction, decreased volume of ejaculate

<1%, postmarketing and/or case reports: **Hypersensitivity** (pruritus, rash, urticaria, swelling of face/lips), testicular pain, breast tenderness, breast enlargement

Drug Interactions Substrate of CYP3A4

Dietary/Ethanol/Herb Considerations

Food: Administer on an empty stomach; food may reduce extent of oral absorption.

Herb/Nutraceutical: Avoid saw palmetto; concurrent use has not been adequately studied. Avoid St John's wort; may decrease serum concentration.

Pharmacodynamics/Kinetics

Onset of action: 3-6 months of ongoing therapy

Duration:

After a single oral dose as small as 0.5 mg: 65% depression of plasma dihydrotestosterone levels persists 5-7 days

After 6 months of treatment with 5 mg/day: Circulating dihydrotestosterone levels are reduced to castrate levels without significant effects on circulating testosterone; levels return to normal within 14 days of discontinuation of treatment

Absorption: May be reduced with food

Protein binding: 90%

Metabolism: Hepatic; two active metabolites identified

Bioavailability: Mean: 63%

Half-life elimination, serum: Parent drug: ~5-17 hours (mean: 1.9 fasting, 4.2 with breakfast); Elderly: 8 hours; Adults: 6 hours (3-16); rate decreased in elderly, but no dosage adjustment needed

Time to peak, serum: 2-6 hours

Excretion: Feces (57%) and urine (39%) as metabolites

Pregnancy Risk Factor X

Generic Available No

Finevin® *see* Azelaic Acid *on page 151*

Fioricet® *see* Butalbital, Acetaminophen, and Caffeine *on page 214*

Fioricet® with Codeine *see* Butalbital, Acetaminophen, Caffeine, and Codeine *on page 215*

Fiorinal® *see* Butalbital, Aspirin, and Caffeine *on page 216*

Fiorinal® With Codeine *see* Butalbital, Aspirin, Caffeine, and Codeine *on page 217*

Fisalamine *see* Mesalamine *on page 869*

FK506 *see* Tacrolimus *on page 1261*

Flagyl® *see* Metronidazole *on page 902*

Flagyl ER® *see* Metronidazole *on page 902*

Flarex® *see* Fluorometholone *on page 587*

Flatulex® [OTC] *see* Simethicone *on page 1222*

Flavoxate (fla VOKS ate)

U.S. Brand Names Urispas®

Canadian Brand Names Urispas®

Mexican Brand Names Bladuril®

Pharmacologic Category Antispasmodic Agent, Urinary

Synonyms Flavoxate Hydrochloride

Use Antispasmodic to provide symptomatic relief of dysuria, nocturia, suprapubic pain, urgency, and incontinence due to detrusor instability and hyper-reflexia in elderly with cystitis, urethritis, urethrocystitis, urethrotrigonitis, and prostatitis

Local Anesthetic/Vasoconstrictor Precautions No information available to require special precautions

Effects on Dental Treatment

>10%: Xerostomia, changes in salivation, dry throat

Frequency not defined: Tachycardia, palpitations, drowsiness, confusion (especially in elderly), nervousness, fatigue, headache, nausea, vomiting, blurred vision

Dosage Children >12 years and Adults: Oral: 100-200 mg 3-4 times/day; reduce the dose when symptoms improve

Mechanism of Action Synthetic antispasmotic with similar actions to that of propantheline; it exerts a direct relaxant effect on smooth muscles via phosphodiesterase inhibition, providing relief to a variety of smooth muscle spasms; it is especially useful for the treatment of bladder spasticity, whereby it produces an increase in urinary capacity

(Continued)

Flavoxate *(Continued)*

Other Adverse Effects Frequency not defined:

Central nervous system: Vertigo, hyperpyrexia
Dermatologic: Rash, urticaria
Gastrointestinal: Constipation
Genitourinary: Dysuria
Hematologic: Leukopenia
Ocular: Increased intraocular pressure

Dietary/Ethanol/Herb Considerations

Ethanol: Avoid use; may increase CNS depression.
Herb/Nutraceutical: Avoid gotu kola, kava, SAMe, St John's wort, and valerian; may increase CNS depression.

Pharmacodynamics/Kinetics

Onset of action: 55-60 minutes
Metabolism: To methyl; flavone carboxylic acid active
Excretion: Urine (10% to 30%) within 6 hours

Pregnancy Risk Factor B

Generic Available No

Flavoxate Hydrochloride *see* Flavoxate *on page 573*

Flecainide (fle KAY nide)

Related Information

Cardiovascular Diseases *on page 1456*

U.S. Brand Names Tambocor™

Canadian Brand Names Tambocor™

Mexican Brand Names Tambocor®

Pharmacologic Category Antiarrhythmic Agent, Class Ic

Synonyms Flecainide Acetate

Use Prevention and suppression of documented life-threatening ventricular arrhythmias (eg, sustained ventricular tachycardia); controlling symptomatic, disabling supraventricular tachycardias in patients without structural heart disease in whom other agents fail

Local Anesthetic/Vasoconstrictor Precautions No information available to require special precautions

Effects on Dental Treatment

>10%: Dizziness (19% to 30%), visual disturbances (16%), dyspnea (~10%)
4% to 10%: Palpitations (6%), chest pain (5%), headache (4% to 10%), fatigue (8%), nervousness (5%), nausea (9%), tremors (5%), weakness (5%)
1% to 3%: Tachycardia (1% to 3%), malaise, paresis, vertigo, syncope, somnolence, anxiety, paresthesias (1%), blurred vision

Dosage Oral:

Children:
Initial: 3 mg/kg/day or 50-100 mg/m^2/day in 3 divided doses
Usual: 3-6 mg/kg/day or 100-150 mg/m^2/day in 3 divided doses; up to 11 mg/kg/day or 200 mg/m^2/day for uncontrolled patients with subtherapeutic levels

Adults:
Life-threatening ventricular arrhythmias:
Initial: 100 mg every 12 hours
Increase by 50-100 mg/day (given in 2 doses/day) every 4 days; maximum: 400 mg/day.
Use of higher initial doses and more rapid dosage adjustments have resulted in an increased incidence of proarrhythmic events and CHF, particularly during the first few days. Do not use a loading dose. Use very cautiously in patients with history of CHF or MI.
Prevention of paroxysmal supraventricular arrhythmias in patients with disabling symptoms but no structural heart disease:
Initial: 50 mg every 12 hours
Increase by 50 mg twice daily at 4-day intervals; maximum: 300 mg/day.

Dosing adjustment in severe renal impairment: Cl_{cr} <35 mL/minute: Decrease initial dose to 50 mg every 12 hours; increase doses at intervals >4 days monitoring EKG levels closely.

Dialysis: Not dialyzable (0% to 5%) via hemo- or peritoneal dialysis; no supplemental dose necessary.

Dosing comment in hepatic impairment: Monitoring of plasma levels is recommended because of significantly increased halflife.

When transferring from another antiarrhythmic agent, allow for 2-4 half-lives of the agent to pass before initiating flecainide therapy.

Mechanism of Action Class Ic antiarrhythmic; slows conduction in cardiac tissue by altering transport of ions across cell membranes; causes slight prolongation of refractory periods; decreases the rate of rise of the action potential without affecting its duration; increases electrical stimulation threshold of ventricle, His-Purkinje system; possesses local anesthetic and moderate negative inotropic effects

Other Adverse Effects

>1% to 10%:

Cardiovascular: Edema (3.5%), proarrhythmic (4% to 12%), sinus node dysfunction (1.2%)

1% and 3%: Hypoesthesia, paresis, ataxia, vertigo, tinnitus, insomnia, depression, rash constipation (1%), abdominal pain (3%), anorexia (1% to 3%), diarrhea (0.7% to 3%), diplopia (1% to 3%)

<1% (Limited to important or life-threatening): **Bradycardia, paradoxical increase in ventricular rate in atrial fibrillation/flutter,** heart block, increased P-R, QRS duration, **ventricular arrhythmias, CHF, flushing,** AV block, **angina, hypertension, hypotension, amnesia, confusion,** decreased libido, depersonalization, **euphoria,** apathy, **nervousness,** twitching, neuropathy, **weakness, abnormal taste,** urticaria, exfoliative dermatitis, pruritus, alopecia, flatulence, **xerostomia,** blood dyscrasias, possible hepatic dysfunction, **paresthesia,** eye pain, photophobia, **bronchospasm, pneumonitis, swollen lips/tongue/mouth,** arthralgia, myalgia, polyuria, urinary retention, leukopenia, granulocytopenia, thrombocytopenia, **metallic taste,** alters pacing threshold

Postmarketing and/or case reports: **Tardive dyskinesia,** corneal deposits

Drug Interactions Substrate of CYP1A2, **2D6**; Inhibits CYP2D6

Increased Effect/Toxicity: Flecainide concentrations may be increased by amiodarone (reduce flecainide 25% to 33%), amprenavir, cimetidine, digoxin, propranolol, quinidine, and ritonavir. Beta-adrenergic blockers, disopyramide, verapamil may enhance flecainide's negative inotropic effects. Alkalinizing agents (ie, high-dose antacids, cimetidine, carbonic anhydrase inhibitors, sodium bicarbonate) may decrease flecainide clearance, potentially increasing toxicity. Propranolol blood levels are increased by flecainide.

Decreased Effect: Smoking and acid urine increase flecainide clearance.

Dietary/Ethanol/Herb Considerations

Food: Clearance may be decreased in those with strict vegetarian diets due to urinary pH ≥8. Dairy products (milk, infant formula, yogurt) may interfere with absorption in infants; one case report of a neonate (GA 34 weeks PNA >6 days) who required extremely large doses of oral flecainide when administered every 8 hours with "milk feeds"; changing the feedings from "milk feeds" to 5% glucose feeds alone resulted in a doubling of flecainide serum concentration and toxicity.

Herb/Nutraceutical: Ginger has positive inotropic effects and theoretically could affect antiarrhythmic activity. Avoid hawthorn; may increase QT interval.

Pharmacodynamics/Kinetics

Absorption: Oral: Rapid

Distribution: Adults: V_d: 5-13.4 L/kg

Protein binding: Alpha$_1$ glycoprotein: 40% to 50%

Metabolism: Hepatic

Bioavailability: 85% to 90%

Half-life elimination: Infants: 11-12 hours; Children: 8 hours; Adults: 7-22 hours, increased with congestive heart failure or renal dysfunction; End-stage renal disease: 19-26 hours

Time to peak, serum: ~1.5-3 hours

Excretion: Urine (80% to 90%, 10% to 50% as unchanged drug and metabolites)

Pregnancy Risk Factor C

Generic Available No

Flecainide Acetate *see* Flecainide *on page 574*

Fleet® Babylax® [OTC] *see* Glycerin *on page 644*

Fleet® Bisacodyl Enema [OTC] *see* Bisacodyl *on page 186*

Fleet® Enema [OTC] *see* Phosphate Supplements *on page 1076*

Fleet® Glycerin Suppositories [OTC] *see* Glycerin *on page 644*

Fleet® Glycerin Suppositories Maximum Strength [OTC] *see* Glycerin *on page 644*

Fleet® Liquid Glycerin Suppositories [OTC] *see* Glycerin *on page 644*

Fleet® Phospho®-Soda [OTC] *see* Phosphate Supplements *on page 1076*

Fleet® Sof-Lax® [OTC] *see* Docusate *on page 463*

Fleet® Sof-Lax® Overnight [OTC] *see* Docusate and Casanthranol *on page 464*

Fleet® Stimulant Laxative [OTC] *see* Bisacodyl *on page 186*

Fletcher's® Castoria® [OTC] *see* Senna *on page 1215*

Flexeril® *see* Cyclobenzaprine *on page 379*

Flolan® *see* Epoprostenol *on page 505*

Flomax® *see* Tamsulosin *on page 1266*

Flonase® *see* Fluticasone *on page 599*

Florical® [OTC] *see* Calcium Supplements *on page 229*

Florinef® *see* Fludrocortisone *on page 580*

Flovent® *see* Fluticasone *on page 599*

Flovent® Rotadisk® *see* Fluticasone *on page 599*

Floxin® *see* Ofloxacin *on page 995*

Floxuridine (floks YOOR i deen)

U.S. Brand Names FUDR®

Canadian Brand Names FUDR®

Pharmacologic Category Antineoplastic Agent, Antimetabolite

Synonyms Fluorodeoxyuridine; FUDR

Use Management of hepatic metastases of colorectal and gastric cancers

Local Anesthetic/Vasoconstrictor Precautions No information available to require special

Effects on Dental Treatment >10%: Stomatitis

Dosage Refer to individual protocols.

Intra-arterial:
- 0.1-0.6 mg/kg/day
- 4-20 mg/day

I.V.:
- 0.15 mg/kg/day for 7-14 days
- 0.5-1 mg/kg/day for 6-15 days
- 30 mg/kg/day for 5 days, then 15 mg/kg/day every other day, up to 11 days

Mechanism of Action Mechanism of action and pharmacokinetics are very similar to 5-FU; FUDR® is the deoxyribonucleotide of 5-FU. Inhibits DNA and RNA synthesis via formation of carbonium ions; cross-links strands of DNA, causing an imbalance of growth and cell death

Other Adverse Effects

>10%:
- Gastrointestinal: Diarrhea (may be dose-limiting)
- Hematologic: Myelosuppression, may be dose-limiting; leukopenia, thrombocytopenia, anemia

1% to 10%:
- Dermatologic: Alopecia, photosensitivity, hyperpigmentation of the skin, localized erythema, dermatitis
- Gastrointestinal: Anorexia
- Hepatic: Biliary sclerosis, cholecystitis, jaundice

<1%: **Nausea, vomiting,** intrahepatic abscess

Drug Interactions

Increased Effect/Toxicity: Any form of therapy which adds to the stress of the patient, interferes with nutrition, or depresses bone marrow function will increase the toxicity of floxuridine. Pentostatin and floxuridine administered together has resulted in fatal pulmonary toxicity.

Decreased Effect: Patients may experience impaired immune response to vaccines; possible infection after administration of live vaccines in patients receiving immunosuppressants.

Dietary/Ethanol/Herb Considerations Ethanol: Avoid use due to GI irritation.

Pharmacodynamics/Kinetics

Metabolism: Hepatic; Active metabolites: Floxuridine monophosphate (FUDR-MP) and fluorouracil; Inactive metabolites: Urea, CO_2, α-fluoro-β-alanine, α-fluoro-β-guanidopropionic acid, α-fluoro-β-ureidopropionic acid, and dihydrofluorouracil

Excretion: Urine: Fluorouracil, urea, α-fluoro-β-alanine, α-fluoro-β-guanidopropionic acid, α-fluoro-β-ureidopropionic acid, and dihydrofluorouracil; exhaled gases (CO_2)

Pregnancy Risk Factor D

Generic Available Yes

Flubenisolone *see* Betamethasone *on page 177*

Flucaine® *see* Proparacaine and Fluorescein *on page 1133*

Fluconazole (floo KOE na zole)

Related Information

Oral Fungal Infections *on page 1542*

Sexually-Transmitted Diseases *on page 1502*

U.S. Brand Names Diflucan®

Canadian Brand Names Apo®-Fluconazole; Diflucan®

Mexican Brand Names Afungil®; Diflucan®; Neofomiral®; Oxifungol®; Zonal®

Pharmacologic Category Antifungal Agent, Oral; Antifungal Agent, Parenteral

Use

Dental: Treatment of susceptible fungal infections in the oral cavity including candidiasis, oral thrush, and chronic mucocutaneous candidiasis; treatment of esophageal and oropharyngeal candidiasis caused by *Candida* species

Medical: Treatment of oral or vaginal candidiasis unresponsive to nystatin or clotrimazole, non-life-threatening *Candida* infections (eg, cystitis, esophagitis), hepatosplenic candidiasis, and other *Candida* infections in persons unable to tolerate amphotericin B; treatment of cryptococcal infections; secondary prophylaxis for cryptococcal meningitis in persons with AIDS; antifungal prophylaxis in allogeneic bone marrow transplant recipients

Local Anesthetic/Vasoconstrictor Precautions No information available to require special precautions

Effects on Dental Treatment

>10%: Headache (2% to 13%)

1% to 7%: Nausea (4% to 7%), vomiting (2%)

Frequency not defined: Seizures, dizziness, abnormal taste, dyspnea

Dosage The daily dose of fluconazole is the same for oral and I.V. administration. Oral formulations should be used in persons able to tolerate oral medications. Parenteral formulation should be reserved for patients who are both unable to take oral medications and unable to tolerate amphotericin B (eg, due to hypersensitivity or renal insufficiency).

Neonates: First 2 weeks of life, especially premature neonates: Same dose as older children every 72 hours

Children: Once-daily dosing by indication: See table.

Fluconazole — Once-Daily Dosing — Children

Indication	Day 1	Daily Therapy	Minimum Duration of Therapy
Oropharyngeal candidiasis	6 mg/kg	3 mg/kg	14 d
Esophageal candidiasis	6 mg/kg	3-12 mg/kg	21 d and for at least 2 wks following resolution of symptoms
Systemic candidiasis	—	6-12 mg/kg	28 d
Cryptococcal meningitis acute	12 mg/kg	6-12 mg/kg	10-12 wk after CSF culture becomes negative
relapse suppression	6 mg/kg	6 mg/kg	N/A

N/A = Not applicable

Adults: **Oral,** I.V.: Once-daily dosing by indication: See table.

Fluconazole — Once-Daily Dosing — Adults

Indication	Day 1	Daily Therapy	Minimum Duration of Therapy
Oropharyngeal candidiasis	200 mg	100 mg	14 d
Esophageal candidiasis	200 mg	100 mg	21 d and for at least 14 d following resolution of symptoms
Prevention of candidiasis in bone marrow transplant	400 mg	400 mg	3 d before neutropenia, 7 d after neutrophils >1000 cells/mm^3
Candidiasis UTIs, peritonitis	50-200 mg	50-200 mg	N/A
Systemic candidiasis	400 mg	200 mg	28 d
Cryptococcal meningitis acute	400 mg	200 mg	10-12 wk after CSF culture becomes negative
relapse suppression	200 mg	200 mg	N/A
Vaginal candidiasis	150 mg	Single dose	N/A

N/A = Not applicable

Dosing adjustment/interval in renal impairment:

Vaginal candidiasis single-dose therapy: No adjustment

Multiple dosing: Administer usual load then adjust daily doses

Cl_{cr} 11-50 mL/minute: Administer 50% of recommended dose or administer every 48 hours

Hemodialysis: One dose after each dialysis

Continuous arteriovenous or venovenous hemodiafiltration effects: Dose as for Cl_{cr} 10-50 mL/minute

Mechanism of Action Interferes with cytochrome P450 activity, decreasing ergosterol synthesis (principal sterol in fungal cell membrane) and inhibiting cell membrane formation

Other Adverse Effects Frequency not always defined:

Cardiovascular: Pallor, angioedema

Dermatologic: Rash (2%), alopecia, toxic epidermal necrolysis, Stevens-Johnson syndrome

Endocrine & metabolic: Hypertriglyceridemia, hypokalemia

Gastrointestinal: Abdominal pain (2% to 6%), diarrhea (2% to 3%)

Hematologic: Leukopenia, thrombocytopenia

Hepatic: Hepatic failure (rare), hepatitis, cholestasis, jaundice, increased ALT/AST, increased alkaline phosphatase

Miscellaneous: **Anaphylactic reactions (rare)**

(Continued)

Fluconazole *(Continued)*

Contraindications Hypersensitivity to fluconazole, other azoles, or any component of the formulation; concomitant administration with cisapride or astemizole

Warnings/Precautions Should be used with caution in patients with renal and hepatic dysfunction or previous hepatotoxicity from other azole derivatives. Patients who develop abnormal LFTs during fluconazole therapy should be monitored closely and discontinued if symptoms consistent with liver disease develop.

Drug Interactions Inhibits CYP1A2, **2C8/9, 2C19, 3A4**

Alprazolam, triazolam, midazolam, and diazepam serum concentrations are increased; consider a benzodiazepine not metabolized by CYP3A4 or another antifungal that is metabolized by CYP3A4.

Calcium channel blockers may have increased serum concentrations; consider another agent instead of a calcium channel blocker, another antifungal, or reduce the dose of the calcium channel blocker. Monitor blood pressure.

Losartan's active metabolite is reduced in concentration; consider another antihypertensive agent unaffected by the azole antifungals, another antifungal, or monitor blood pressure closely.

HMG-CoA reductase inhibitors (except pravastatin and fluvastatin) have increased serum concentrations; switch to pravastatin/fluvastatin or monitor for development of myopathy.

Caffeine's metabolism is decreased; monitor for tachycardia, nervousness, and anxiety.

Cisapride's serum concentration is increased which may lead to malignant arrhythmias; concurrent use is contraindicated.

Tacrolimus's serum concentration is increased; monitor tacrolimus's serum concentration and renal function.

Cyclosporine's serum concentration is increased; monitor cyclosporine's serum concentration and renal function.

Rifampin decreases fluconazole's serum concentration; monitor infection status.

Warfarin's effects are increased; monitor INR and adjust warfarin's dose as needed.

Phenytoin's serum concentration is increased; monitor phenytoin levels and adjust dose as needed.

Dietary/Ethanol/Herb Considerations Food: Administer with food to reduce GI upset.

Pharmacodynamics/Kinetics

Distribution: Widely throughout body with good penetration into CSF, eye, peritoneal fluid, sputum, skin, and urine

Relative diffusion blood into CSF: Adequate with or without inflammation (exceeds usual MICs)

CSF:blood level ratio: Normal meninges: 70% to 80%; Inflamed meninges: >70% to 80%

Protein binding, plasma: 11% to 12%

Bioavailability: Oral: >90%

Half-life elimination: Normal renal function: 25-30 hours

Time to peak, serum: Oral: ~2-4 hours

Excretion: Urine (80% as unchanged drug)

Pregnancy Risk Factor C

Dosage Forms INF [premixed in sodium chloride or dextrose]: 2 mg/mL (100 mL, 200 mL). **POWDER, oral suspension:** 10 mg/mL (35 mL); 40 mg/mL (35 mL). **TAB:** 50 mg, 100 mg, 150 mg, 200 mg

Generic Available No

Flucytosine (floo SYE toe seen)

U.S. Brand Names Ancobon®

Canadian Brand Names Ancobon®

Pharmacologic Category Antifungal Agent, Oral

Synonyms 5-FC; 5-Flurocytosine

Use Adjunctive treatment of susceptible fungal infections (usually *Candida* or *Cryptococcus*); synergy with amphotericin B for certain fungal infections (*Cryptococcus* spp., *Candida* spp.)

Local Anesthetic/Vasoconstrictor Precautions No information available to require special precautions

Effects on Dental Treatment Frequency not defined: Confusion, headache, hallucinations, dizziness, drowsiness, psychosis, parkinsonism, sedation, hypoglycemia, nausea, vomiting, paresthesia, weakness, respiratory arrest, anaphylaxis

Dosage Oral:

Children and Adults: 50-150 mg/kg/day in divided doses every 6 hours

Dosing interval in renal impairment: Use lower initial dose:

Cl_{cr} 20-40 mL/minute: Administer every 12 hours

Cl_{cr} 10-20 mL/minute: Administer every 24 hours

Cl_{cr} <10 mL/minute: Administer every 24-48 hours

Hemodialysis: Dialyzable (50% to 100%); administer dose posthemodialysis

Continuous arteriovenous or venovenous hemodiafiltration effects: Dose as for Cl_{cr} 10-50 mL/minute

Peritoneal dialysis: Adults: Administer 0.5-1 g every 24 hours

Mechanism of Action Penetrates fungal cells and is converted to fluorouracil which competes with uracil interfering with fungal RNA and protein synthesis

Other Adverse Effects Frequency not defined:

Central nervous system: Ataxia
Dermatologic: Rash, photosensitivity, pruritus, urticaria
Endocrine & metabolic: Temporary growth failure, hypokalemia
Gastrointestinal: Diarrhea, abdominal pain, loss of appetite
Hematologic: Bone marrow suppression, anemia, leukopenia, thrombocytopenia
Hepatic: Elevated liver enzymes, hepatitis, jaundice, azotemia
Neuromuscular & skeletal: Peripheral neuropathy
Otic: Hearing loss
Renal: Elevated BUN and serum creatinine, renal failure

Drug Interactions Increased effect with amphotericin B. Amphotericin B-induced renal dysfunction may predispose patient to flucytosine accumulation and myelosuppression.

Dietary/Ethanol/Herb Considerations Food: Administer with food to reduce GI upset; decreases rate but not extent of absorption.

Pharmacodynamics/Kinetics

Absorption: 75% to 90%
Distribution: Into CSF, aqueous humor, joints, peritoneal fluid, and bronchial secretions
Protein binding: 2% to 4%
Metabolism: Minimally hepatic
Half-life elimination: 3-8 hours; Anuria: Up to 200 hours; End-stage renal disease: 75-200 hours
Time to peak, serum: ~2-6 hours
Excretion: Urine (75% to 90% as unchanged drug)

Pregnancy Risk Factor C

Generic Available No

Fludara® *see* Fludarabine *on page 579*

Fludarabine (floo DAIR a been)

U.S. Brand Names Fludara®

Canadian Brand Names Fludara®

Mexican Brand Names Fludara®

Pharmacologic Category Antineoplastic Agent, Antimetabolite

Synonyms Fludarabine Phosphate

Use Salvage therapy of non-Hodgkin's lymphoma and acute leukemias

Orphan drug: Treatment of chronic lymphocytic leukemia (CLL), including refractory CLL

Local Anesthetic/Vasoconstrictor Precautions No information available to require special precautions

Effects on Dental Treatment

>10%: Fatigue, somnolence (30%), paresthesia, weakness

1% to 10%: CHF, malaise, headache, hyperglycemia, stomatitis (1.5%), nausea/vomiting (3% to 10%)

Dosage I.V.:

Children:

Acute leukemia: 10 mg/m² bolus over 15 minutes followed by continuous infusion of 30.5 mg/m²/day over 5 days **or**

10.5 mg/m² bolus over 15 minutes followed by 30.5 mg/m²/day over 48 hours followed by cytarabine has been used in clinical trials

Solid tumors: 9 mg/m² bolus followed by 27 mg/m²/day continuous infusion over 5 days

Adults:

Chronic lymphocytic leukemia: 25 mg/m²/day over a 30-minute period for 5 days; 5-day courses are repeated every 28 days days

Non-Hodgkin's lymphoma: Loading dose: 20 mg/m² followed by 30 mg/m²/day for 48 hours

Dosing in renal impairment:

Cl_{cr} 30-70 mL/minute: Reduce dose by 20%

Cl_{cr} <30 mL/minute: Use not recommended

Mechanism of Action Fludarabine is analogous to that of Ara-C and Ara-A. Following systemic administration, FAMP is rapidly dephosphorylated to 2-fluoro-Ara-A. 2-Fluoro-Ara-A enters the cell by a carrier-mediated transport process, then is phosphorylated intracellularly by deoxycytidine kinase to form the active metabolite 2-fluoro-Ara-ATP. 2-Fluoro-Ara-ATP inhibits DNA synthesis by inhibition of DNA polymerase and ribonucleotide reductase.

Other Adverse Effects

>10%:

Cardiovascular: Edema

(Continued)

Fludarabine *(Continued)*

Central nervous system: Chills
Dermatologic: Rash
Hematologic: Myelosuppression, common, dose-limiting toxicity, primarily leukopenia and thrombocytopenia
Nadir: 10-14 days
Recovery: 5-7 weeks
Neuromuscular & skeletal: Myalgia

1% to 10%:
Dermatologic: Alopecia
Gastrointestinal: Anorexia, diarrhea (1.8%)
Hematologic: Eosinophilia, hemolytic anemia, may be dose-limiting, possibly fatal in some patients

<1%: **Muscle weakness**; a syndrome characterized by cortical blindness, coma, and paralysis - 36% at doses >96 mg/m^2 for 5-7 days; <0.2% at doses <125 mg/m^2/cycle (onset of neurologic symptoms may be delayed for 3-4 weeks); metabolic acidosis, metallic taste, blurred vision, diplopia, photophobia (primarily in patients receiving high doses), increased risk for opportunistic infections due to decreased CD4 counts

Postmarketing and/or case reports: Pulmonary toxicity (including interstitial pneumonitis, pulmonary fibrosis, pulmonary hemorrhage, respiratory failure, or ARDS) has been reported; may improve with steroid administration.

Drug Interactions Increased Effect/Toxicity: Cytarabine when administered with or prior to a fludarabine dose competes for deoxycytidine kinase decreasing the metabolism of F-ara-A to the active F-ara-ATP (inhibits the antineoplastic effect of fludarabine); however, administering fludarabine prior to cytarabine may stimulate activation of cytarabine.

Dietary/Ethanol/Herb Considerations Ethanol: Avoid use due to GI irritation.

Pharmacodynamics/Kinetics
Distribution: V_d: 38-96 L/m^2; widely with extensive tissue binding
Metabolism: I.V.: Fludarabine phosphate is rapidly dephosphorylated to 2-fluoro-vidarabine, which subsequently enters tumor cells and is phosphorylated to the active triphosphate derivative; rapidly dephosphorylated in the serum
Bioavailability: 75%
Half-life elimination: 2-fluoro-vidarabine: 9 hours
Excretion: Urine (60%, 23% as 2-fluoro-vidarabine) within 24 hours

Pregnancy Risk Factor D
Generic Available No

Fludarabine Phosphate *see* Fludarabine *on page 579*

Fludrocortisone (floo droe KOR ti sone)

U.S. Brand Names Florinef®
Canadian Brand Names Florinef®
Pharmacologic Category Corticosteroid, Systemic
Synonyms Fluohydrisone Acetate; Fluohydrocortisone Acetate; 9α-Fluorohydrocortisone Acetate
Use Partial replacement therapy for primary and secondary adrenocortical insufficiency in Addison's disease; treatment of salt-losing adrenogenital syndrome
Local Anesthetic/Vasoconstrictor Precautions No information available to require special precautions
Effects on Dental Treatment Frequency not defined: Hypertension, CHF, convulsions, headache, dizziness, bruising hyperglycemia, peptic ulcer, muscle weakness, diaphoresis, anaphylaxis (generalized)

Dosage Oral:
Infants and Children: 0.05-0.1 mg/day
Adults: 0.1-0.2 mg/day with ranges of 0.1 mg 3 times/week to 0.2 mg/day
Addison's disease: Initial: 0.1 mg/day; if transient hypertension develops, reduce the dose to 0.05 mg/day. Preferred administration with cortisone (10-37.5 mg/day) or hydrocortisone (10-30 mg/day).
Salt-losing adrenogenital syndrome: 0.1-0.2 mg/day

Mechanism of Action Promotes increased reabsorption of sodium and loss of potassium from renal distal tubules

Other Adverse Effects Frequency not defined:
Cardiovascular: Edema
Dermatologic: Acne, rash
Endocrine & metabolic: Hypokalemic alkalosis, suppression of growth, HPA suppression
Ocular: Cataracts

Drug Interactions Decreased Effect: Anticholinesterases effects are antagonized. Decreased corticosteroid effects by rifampin, barbiturates, and hydantoins. May decrease salicylate levels.

Dietary/Ethanol/Herb Considerations Food: Administer with or after meals; once daily dose should be taken with food in the morning. Systemic use of mineralocorticoids/corticosteroids may require intake of increased calcium, folate, phosphorus, potassium, vitamins A, B_6, C, D, and zinc, and decreased sodium (often not required, as the increased retention of sodium is usually the desired therapeutic effect); may need to give salt tablets to effectively increase BP in patients with postural hypotension

Pharmacodynamics/Kinetics

Absorption: Rapid and complete

Protein binding: 42%

Metabolism: Hepatic

Half-life elimination, plasma: 30-35 minutes; Biological: 18-36 hours

Time to peak, serum: ~1.7 hours

Pregnancy Risk Factor C

Generic Available Yes

Flumadine® *see* Rimantadine *on page 1185*

Flumazenil (FLOO may ze nil)

Related Information

Dental Office Emergencies *on page 1582*

U.S. Brand Names Romazicon®

Canadian Brand Names Anexate®; Romazicon™

Mexican Brand Names Lanexat®

Pharmacologic Category Antidote

Use Benzodiazepine antagonist - reverses sedative effects of benzodiazepines used in general anesthesia; for management of benzodiazepine overdose; flumazenil does **not** antagonize the CNS effects of other GABA agonists (eg, ethanol, barbiturates, or general anesthetics), **does not** reverse narcotics

Flumazenil

Pediatric Dosage Further studies are needed	
Pediatric dosage for **reversal of conscious sedation:** Intravenously through a freely running intravenous infusion into a large vein to minimize pain at the injection site	
Initial dose	0.01 mg/kg over 15 seconds (maximum dose of 0.2 mg)
Repeat doses	0.005-0.01 mg/kg (maximum dose of 0.2 mg) repeated at 1-minute intervals
Maximum total cumulative dose	1 mg
Pediatric dosage for **management of benzodiazepine overdose:** Intravenously through a freely running intravenous infusion into a large vein to minimize pain at the injection site	
Initial dose	0.01 mg/kg (maximum dose: 0.2 mg)
Repeat doses	0.01 mg/kg (maximum dose of 0.2 mg) repeated at 1-minute intervals
Maximum total cumulative dose	1 mg
In place of repeat bolus doses, follow-up continuous infusions of 0.005-0.01 mg/kg/hour have been used; further studies are needed.	
Adult Dosage	
Adult dosage for **reversal of conscious sedation:** Intravenously through a freely running intravenous infusion into a large vein to minimize pain at the injection site	
Initial dose	0.2 mg intravenously over 15 seconds
Repeat doses	If desired level of consciousness is not obtained, 0.2 mg may be repeated at 1-minute intervals.
Maximum total cumulative dose	1 mg (usual dose 0.6-1 mg) **In the event of resedation:** Repeat doses may be given at 20-minute intervals with maximum of 1 mg/dose and 3 mg/hour
Adult dosage for **suspected benzodiazepine overdose:** Intravenously through a freely running intravenous infusion into a large vein to minimize pain at the injection site	
Initial dose	0.2 mg intravenously over 30 seconds
Repeat doses	0.5 mg over 30 seconds repeated at 1-minute intervals
Maximum total cumulative dose	3 mg (usual dose 1-3 mg) Patients with a partial response at 3 mg may require additional titration up to a total dose of 5 mg. If a patient has not responded 5 minutes after cumulative dose of 5 mg, the major cause of sedation is not likely due to benzodiazepines. **In the event of resedation:** May repeat doses at 20-minute intervals with maximum of 1 mg/dose and 3 mg/hour

(Continued)

Flumazenil *(Continued)*

Local Anesthetic/Vasoconstrictor Precautions No information available to require special precautions

Effects on Dental Treatment

>10%: Vomiting, nausea

1% to 10%: Xerostomia, palpitations, headache, anxiety, nervousness, crying, euphoria, agitation, dizziness, paranoia, hot flashes, tremors, weakness, paresthesia, blurred vision, abnormal vision, dyspnea, hyperventilation, diaphoresis

Dosage

Children and Adults: I.V.: See table on previous page.

Resedation: Repeated doses may be given at 20-minute intervals as needed; repeat treatment doses of 1 mg (at a rate of 0.5 mg/minute) should be given at any time and no more than 3 mg should be given in any hour. After intoxication with high doses of benzodiazepines, the duration of a single dose of flumazenil is not expected to exceed 1 hour; if desired, the period of wakefulness may be prolonged with repeated low intravenous doses of flumazenil, or by an infusion of 0.1-0.4 mg/hour. Most patients with benzodiazepine overdose will respond to a cumulative dose of 1-3 mg and doses >3 mg do not reliably produce additional effects. Rarely, patients with a partial response at 3 mg may require additional titration up to a total dose of 5 mg. **If a patient has not responded 5 minutes after receiving a cumulative dose of 5 mg, the major cause of sedation is not likely to be due to benzodiazepines.**

Elderly: No differences in safety or efficacy have been reported. However, increased sensitivity may occur in some elderly patients.

Dosing in renal impairment: Not significantly affected by renal failure (Cl_{cr} <10 mL/minute) or hemodialysis beginning 1 hour after drug administration

Dosing in hepatic impairment: Initial dose of flumazenil used for initial reversal of benzodiazepine effects is not changed; however, subsequent doses in liver disease patients should be reduced in size or frequency

Mechanism of Action Competitively inhibits the activity at the benzodiazepine recognition site on the GABA/benzodiazepine receptor complex. Flumazenil does not antagonize the CNS effect of drugs affecting GABA-ergic neurons by means other than the benzodiazepine receptor (ethanol, barbiturates, general anesthetics) and does not reverse the effects of opioids

Other Adverse Effects

1% to 10%:

Central nervous system: Insomnia, abnormal crying, depression, emotional lability, ataxia, depersonalization, increased tears, dysphoria

Local: Pain at injection site

<1%: Abnormal hearing, altered blood pressure (increases and decreases), sensation of coldness, **bradycardia, chest pain, generalized convulsions, hiccups, hypertension, shivering, somnolence, tachycardia, thick tongue, ventricular extrasystoles, withdrawal syndrome**

Drug Interactions Increased Effect/Toxicity: Use with caution in overdosage involving mixed drug overdose. Toxic effects may emerge (especially with cyclic antidepressants) with the reversal of the benzodiazepine effect by flumazenil.

Pharmacodynamics/Kinetics

Onset of action: 1-3 minutes; 80% response within 3 minutes

Peak effect: 6-10 minutes

Duration: Resedation: ~1 hour; duration related to dose given and benzodiazepine plasma concentrations; reversal effects of flumazenil may wear off before effects of benzodiazepine

Distribution: Initial V_d: 0.5 L/kg; V_{dss} 0.77-1.6 L/kg

Protein binding: 40% to 50%

Metabolism: Hepatic; dependent upon hepatic blood flow

Half-life elimination: Adults: Alpha: 7-15 minutes; Terminal: 41-79 minutes

Excretion: Feces; urine (0.2% as unchanged drug)

Pregnancy Risk Factor C

Generic Available No

Flunisolide (floo NIS oh lide)

Related Information

Respiratory Diseases *on page 1476*

U.S. Brand Names AeroBid®; AeroBid®-M; Nasalide®; Nasarel®

Canadian Brand Names Alti-Flunisolide; Apo®-Flunisolide; Nasalide®; Rhinalar®

Pharmacologic Category Corticosteroid, Inhalant (Oral); Corticosteroid, Nasal

Use Steroid-dependent asthma; nasal solution is used for seasonal or perennial rhinitis

Local Anesthetic/Vasoconstrictor Precautions No information available to require special precautions

Effects on Dental Treatment

>10%: *Candida* infections of the nose or pharynx, atrophic rhinitis, sore throat, bitter taste, palpitations, dizziness, headache, nervousness, GI irritation, sneezing,

coughing, upper respiratory tract infection, bronchitis, nasal congestion, nasal dryness and burning, increased susceptibility to infections

1% to 10%: Xerostomia, dry throat, loss of taste, epistaxis, diaphoresis

Dosage

Children >6 years:

Oral inhalation: 2 inhalations twice daily (morning and evening) up to 4 inhalations/day

Nasal: 1 spray each nostril twice daily (morning and evening), not to exceed 4 sprays/day each nostril

Adults:

Oral inhalation: 2 inhalations twice daily (morning and evening) up to 8 inhalations/day maximum

Nasal: 2 sprays each nostril twice daily (morning and evening); maximum dose: 8 sprays/day in each nostril

Mechanism of Action Decreases inflammation by suppression of migration of polymorphonuclear leukocytes and reversal of increased capillary permeability; does not depress hypothalamus

Other Adverse Effects

>10%:

Dermatologic: Itching, rash

Endocrine & metabolic: Adrenal suppression, menstrual problems

Gastrointestinal: Anorexia

1% to 10%:

Central nervous system: Insomnia, psychic changes

Dermatologic: Acne, urticaria

Gastrointestinal: Increased appetite

Ocular: Cataracts

Miscellaneous: Loss of smell

<1%, postmarketing and/or case reports: Abdominal fullness, **bronchospasm, dyspnea,** growth suppression

Drug Interactions Expect interactions similar to other corticosteroids.

Increased Effect: The addition of salmeterol has been demonstrated to **improve** response to inhaled corticosteroids (as compared to increasing steroid dosage).

Pharmacodynamics/Kinetics

Absorption: Nasal inhalation: ~50%

Metabolism: Rapidly hepatic to active metabolites

Bioavailability: 40% to 50%

Half-life elimination: 1.8 hours

Excretion: Urine and feces (equal amounts)

Pregnancy Risk Factor C

Generic Available No

Flunitrazepam (floo nye TRAZ e pam)

Pharmacologic Category Benzodiazepine

Synonyms RO5-420; Rohypnol

Use Europe: Treatment of insomnia and sedation (short-term therapy) and anesthesia induction or supplementation

Local Anesthetic/Vasoconstrictor Precautions No information available to require special precautions

Effects on Dental Treatment Illegal drug of abuse, not currently marketed in the U.S.; look for signs and symptoms of drug abuse (eg, euphoric effects, cognitive dysfunction, lethargy, dizziness, headache).

Dosage

Anesthesia induction: I.V.: 0.015-0.03 mg/kg slowly over 30-60 seconds

Premedication for anesthesia: I.M.: 0.015-0.03 mg/kg slowly over 30-60 seconds

Anesthesia maintenance: I.V.: 0.2-0.5 mg (0.005-0.01 mg/kg) 2-3 hours after anesthesia induction

Insomnia: Oral: 0.5-2 mg nightly; in elderly, 0.5 mg dose should be initiated

Elderly: Reduce dosage

Mechanism of Action Intermediate to long-acting benzodiazepine; facilitates the gamma-aminobutyric acid-mediated neuroreceptors, producing sedative and muscle-relaxing effects which slow the response time of the central nervous system

Other Adverse Effects Frequency not defined:

Cardiovascular: **Tachycardia**, myocardial depression, **shock, CHF**, sinus tachycardia, night terrors, **amnesia (anterograde), drowsiness, confusion, decreased blood pressure**

Central nervous system: **Slurred speech, disorientation, anxiety, panic attacks, incoordination**

Gastrointestinal: **Nausea**, diarrhea

Hematologic: Porphyria

Neuromuscular & skeletal: **Tremor**

Ophthalmic: Visual disturbances

Renal: Urinary retention

Respiratory: **Cough, apnea**

Miscellaneous: **Hiccups**

(Continued)

Flunitrazepam *(Continued)*

Contraindications Hypersensitivity to flunitrazepam, nitrazepam, or clonazepam

Drug Interactions

Increased Effect/Toxicity: Enhances sedative effects of ethanol and general anesthesia; increased intraovular pressure can occur with succinylcholine.

Decreased Effect: Theophylline antagonizes sedative effects.

Dietary/Ethanol/Herb Considerations Insoluble in water

Ethanol: Avoid use; aggravates sedative and toxic effects of flunitrazepam

Food can reduce absorption by 50%

Pharmacodynamics/Kinetics

Onset of action: Sedation: 20 minutes

Peak effect: 1-2 hours

Duration: 8-12 hours

Distribution: V_d: 3.4-5.5 L/kg

Protein binding: 80% to 90%

Metabolism: Hepatic to 7-aminoflunitrazepam and other metabolites

Bioavailability: 80% to 90%

Half-life elimination: 9-25 hours

Excretion: Renal

Comments Several tablets are required to produce euphoric effect; tolerance to sedatives develops quickly. Signs and symptoms of acute overdose include hypotension, apnea, coma, and ataxia; oral dose of 28 mg associated with fatality. Psychomotor effects from 1 mg last 8-12 hours. Serum flunitrazepam levels >0.01 mg/L are associated with driving impairment. Withdrawal symptoms include seizures, sweating, palpitations, hallucinations, and abdominal cramps.

Fluocinolone (floo oh SIN oh lone)

U.S. Brand Names Capex™; Derma-Smoothe/FS®; Synalar®

Canadian Brand Names Capex™; Derma-Smoothe/FS®; Fluoderm; Synalar®

Mexican Brand Names Synalar®

Pharmacologic Category Corticosteroid, Topical

Synonyms Fluocinolone Acetonide

Use Relief of susceptible inflammatory dermatosis [low, medium, high potency topical corticosteroid]; psoriasis of the scalp; atopic dermatitis in children ≥2 years of age

Local Anesthetic/Vasoconstrictor Precautions No information available to require special precautions

Effects on Dental Treatment No significant effects or complications reported

Dosage Topical:

Children ≥2 years: Atopic dermatitis (Derma-Smoothe/FS®): Moisten skin; apply to affected area twice daily; do not use for longer than 4 weeks

Children and Adults: Corticosteroid-responsive dermatoses: Cream, ointment, solution: Apply a thin layer to affected area 2-4 times/day; may use occlusive dressings to manage psoriasis or recalcitrant conditions

Adults:

Atopic dermatitis (Derma-Smoothe/FS®): Apply thin film to affected area 3 times/day

Scalp psoriasis (Derma-Smoothe/FS®): Massage thoroughly into wet or dampened hair/scalp; cover with shower cap. Leave on overnight (or for at least 4 hours). Remove by washing hair with shampoo and rinsing thoroughly.

Seborrheic dermatitis of the scalp (Capex™): Apply no more than 1 ounce to scalp once daily; work into lather and allow to remain on scalp for ~5 minutes. Remove from hair and scalp by rinsing thoroughly with water.

Mechanism of Action A synthetic corticosteroid which differs structurally from triamcinolone acetonide in the presence of an additional fluorine atom in the 6-alpha position on the steroid nucleus. The mechanism of action for all topical corticosteroids is not well defined, however, is believed to be a combination of anti-inflammatory, antipruritic, and vasoconstrictive properties.

Other Adverse Effects Frequency not defined:

Dermatologic: Acneiform eruptions, allergic contact dermatitis, burning, dryness, folliculitis, irritation, itching, hypertrichosis, hypopigmentation, miliaria, perioral dermatitis, skin atrophy, striae

Endocrine & metabolic: Cushing's syndrome, HPA axis suppression

Miscellaneous: **Secondary infection**

Pharmacodynamics/Kinetics

Absorption: Dependent on strength of preparation, amount applied, nature of skin at application site, vehicle, and use of occlusive dressing; increased in areas of skin damage, inflammation, or occlusion

Distribution: Throughout local skin; absorbed drug is distributed rapidly into muscle, liver, skin, intestines, and kidneys

Metabolism: Primarily in skin; small amount absorbed into systemic circulation is primarily hepatic to inactive compounds

Excretion: Urine (primarily as glucuronide and sulfate, also as unconjugated products); feces (small amounts)

Pregnancy Risk Factor C
Generic Available Yes; Excludes oil, shampoo

Fluocinolone Acetonide *see* Fluocinolone *on page 584*

Fluocinolone, Hydroquinone, and Tretinoin

(floo oh SIN oh lone, HYE droe kwin one, & TRET i noyn)

Related Information
Fluocinolone *on page 584*

U.S. Brand Names Tri-Luma™

Pharmacologic Category Corticosteroid, Topical; Depigmenting Agent; Retinoic Acid Derivative

Synonyms Hydroquinone, Fluocinolone Acetonide, and Tretinoin; Tretinoin, Fluocinolone Acetonide, and Hydroquinone

Use Short-term treatment of moderate to severe melasma of the face

Local Anesthetic/Vasoconstrictor Precautions No information available to require special precautions

Effects on Dental Treatment Xerostomia (1%)

Dosage Topical: Adults: Melasma: Apply a thin film once daily to hyperpigmented areas of melasma (including ½ inch of normal-appearing surrounding skin). Apply 30 minutes prior to bedtime; not indicated for use beyond 8 weeks. Do not use occlusive dressings.

Mechanism of Action Not clearly defined. Hydroquinone may interrupt melanin synthesis (tyrosine-tyrosinase pathway); reduces hyperpigmentation.

Other Adverse Effects

>10%

Dermatologic: Erythema (41%), desquamation (38%), burning (18%), dry skin (14%), pruritus (11%)

1% to 10%

Cardiovascular: Telangiectasia (3%)

Central nervous system: **Paresthesia (3%),** hyperesthesia (2%)

Dermatologic: Acne (5%), pigmentation change (2%), irritation (2%), papules (1%), rash (1%), rosacea (1%), vesicles (1%)

<1%: Other reactions reported with one or more components: Acneiform eruptions, allergic contact dermatitis, burning, Cushing's syndrome, folliculitis, HPA axis suppression, hypertrichosis, hypopigmentation, irritation, itching, miliaria, ochronosis (exogenous), perioral dermatitis, secondary infection, skin atrophy, striae

Drug Interactions Tretinoin: Substrate of CYP2A6, 2B6, 2C8/9; Inhibits CYP2C8/9; Induces CYP2E1

Increased Effect/Toxicity: Avoid soaps/cosmetic preparations which are medicated, abrasive, irritating, or any product with strong drying effects (including alcohol, astringent, benzoyl peroxide, resorcinol, salicylic acid, sulfur). Drugs with photosensitizing effects should also be avoided (includes tetracyclines, thiazides, fluoroquinolones, phenothiazines, sulfonamides).

Dietary/Ethanol/Herb Considerations

Food: Avoid excessive intake of vitamin A (cod liver oil, halibut fish oil).

Herb/Nutraceutical: Avoid dong quai and St John's wort; may cause additional photosensitization.

Pharmacodynamics/Kinetics

Absorption: Minimal

Metabolism: Hepatic for the small amount absorbed

Excretion: Urine and feces

Pregnancy Risk Factor C
Generic Available No

Fluocinonide (floo oh SIN oh nide)

Related Information
Oral Nonviral Soft Tissue Ulcerations or Erosions *on page 1549*

U.S. Brand Names Lidex®; Lidex-E®

Canadian Brand Names Lidemol®; Lidex®; Lyderm®; Lydonide; Tiamol®; Topsyn®

Mexican Brand Names Topsyn®

Pharmacologic Category Corticosteroid, Topical

Use Anti-inflammatory, antipruritic, relief of inflammatory and pruritic manifestations [high potency topical corticosteroid]

Local Anesthetic/Vasoconstrictor Precautions No information available to require special precautions

Effects on Dental Treatment No significant effects or complications reported

Dosage Children and Adults: Topical: Apply thin layer to affected area 2-4 times/day depending on the severity of the condition. Therapy should be discontinued when control is achieved; if no improvement is seen, reassessment of diagnosis may be necessary.

Mechanism of Action Fluorinated topical corticosteroid considered to be of high potency. The mechanism of action for all topical corticosteroids is not well defined, however, is felt to be a combination of three important properties: anti-inflammatory activity, immunosuppressive properties, and antiproliferative actions.

(Continued)

Fluocinonide *(Continued)*

Other Adverse Effects Frequency not defined:

Cardiovascular: Intracranial hypertension

Dermatologic: Acne, hypopigmentation, allergic dermatitis, maceration of the skin, skin atrophy, striae, miliaria, telangiectasia, folliculitis, hypertrichosis

Endocrine & metabolic: HPA suppression, Cushing's syndrome, growth retardation

Local: Burning, itching, irritation, dryness,

Miscellaneous: **Secondary infection**

Pharmacodynamics/Kinetics

Absorption: Dependent on strength of product, amount applied, and nature of skin at application site; ranges from ~1% in areas of thick stratum corneum (palms, soles, elbows, etc) to 36% in areas of thin stratum corneum (face, eyelids, etc); increased in areas of skin damage, inflammation, or occlusion

Distribution: Throughout local skin; absorbed drug into muscle, liver, skin, intestines, and kidneys

Metabolism: Primarily in skin; small amount absorbed into systemic circulation is primarily hepatic to inactive compounds

Excretion: Urine (primarily as glucuronide and sulfate, also as unconjugated products); feces (small amounts as metabolites)

Pregnancy Risk Factor C

Generic Available Yes

Fluohydrisone Acetate *see* Fludrocortisone *on page 580*

Fluohydrocortisone Acetate *see* Fludrocortisone *on page 580*

Fluoracaine® *see* Proparacaine and Fluorescein *on page 1133*

Fluor-A-Day [OTC] *see* Fluoride *on page 586*

Fluoride (FLOR ide)

Related Information

Dentin Hypersensitivity, High Caries Index, and Xerostomia *on page 1553*
Management of Patients Undergoing Cancer Therapy *on page 1567*

U.S. Brand Names ACT® [OTC]; Fluor-A-Day [OTC]; Fluorigard® [OTC]; Fluorinse®; Flura-Drops®; Flura-Loz®; Gel-Kam® [OTC]; Gel-Kam® Rinse; Lozi-Flur™; Luride®; Luride® Lozi-Tab®; NeutraCare®; NeutraGard® [OTC]; Pediaflor®; Pharmaflur®; Pharmaflur® 1.1; Phos-Flur®; Phos-Flur® Rinse [OTC]; PreviDent®; PreviDent® 5000 Plus™; Stan-gard®; Stop®; Thera-Flur-N®

Canadian Brand Names Fluor-A-Day®; Fluotic®

Mexican Brand Names Audifluor®

Pharmacologic Category Fluoride; Mineral (Oral/Topical)

Synonyms Acidulated Phosphate Fluoride; Sodium Fluoride; Stannous Fluoride

Use Dental: Prevention of dental caries

Local Anesthetic/Vasoconstrictor Precautions No information available to require special precautions

Effects on Dental Treatment Products containing stannous fluoride may stain teeth.

Dosage

Dental rinse or gel:

Children 6-12 years: 5-10 mL rinse or apply to teeth and spit daily after brushing
Adults: 10 mL rinse or apply to teeth and spit daily after brushing

PreviDent® rinse: Children >6 years and Adults: Once weekly, rinse 10 mL vigorously around and between teeth for 1 minute, then spit; this should be done preferably at bedtime, after thoroughly brushing teeth; for maximum benefit, do

Fluoride Ion

Fluoride Content of Drinking Water	Daily Dose, Oral (mg)
<0.3 ppm	
Birth - 6 months	None
6 months - 3 years	0.25
3-6 years	0.5
6-16 years	1.0
0.3-0.6 ppm	
Birth - 6 months	0
6 months - 3 years	0
3-6 years	0.25
6-16 years	0.5

Table from: Recommended dosage schedule of The American Dental Association, The American Academy of Pediatric Dentistry, and The American Academy of Pediatrics

not eat, drink, or rinse mouth for at least 30 minutes after treatment; do not swallow

Fluorinse®: Children >6 years and Adults: Once weekly, vigorously swish 5-10 mL in mouth for 1 minute, then spit

The previous table shows the recommended daily dose of oral fluoride supplement (mg), based on fluoride ion content (ppm) in drinking water (2.2 mg of sodium fluoride is equivalent to 1 mg of fluoride ion).

Mechanism of Action Promotes remineralization of decalcified enamel; inhibits the cariogenic microbial process in dental plaque; increases tooth resistance to acid dissolution

Other Adverse Effects <1%: Rash, **nausea, vomiting**

Contraindications Hypersensitivity to fluoride, tartrazine, or any component of the formulation; when fluoride content of drinking water exceeds 0.7 ppm; low sodium or sodium-free diets; do not use 1 mg tablets in children <3 years of age or when drinking water fluoride content is ≥0.3 ppm; do not use 1 mg/5 mL rinse (as supplement) in children <6 years of age

Warnings/Precautions Prolonged ingestion with excessive doses may result in dental fluorosis and osseous changes; do **not** exceed recommended dosage; some products contain tartrazine

Drug Interactions Decreased effect/absorption with magnesium-, aluminum-, and calcium-containing products

Dietary/Ethanol/Herb Considerations Food: Do not administer with milk; do **not** allow eating or drinking for 30 minutes after use.

Pharmacodynamics/Kinetics

Absorption: Oral: Rapid and complete; sodium fluoride; other soluble fluoride salts; calcium, iron, or magnesium may delay absorption

Distribution: 50% of fluoride is deposited in teeth and bone after ingestion; topical application works superficially on enamel and plaque; crosses placenta; enters breast milk

Excretion: Urine and feces

Pregnancy Risk Factor C

Dosage Forms **CRM, topical**, as sodium (PreviDent® 5000 Plus™): 1.1% (51 g). **GEL-DROPS**, as sodium fluoride (Thera-Flur-N®): 1.1% (24 mL). **GEL, topical**, as acidulated phosphate fluoride (Phos-Flur®): 1.1% (60 g). **GEL, topical**, as sodium fluoride (NeutraCare®): 1.1% (60 g); (PreviDent®): 1.1% (60 g). **GEL, topical**, as stannous fluoride (Gel-Kam®): 0.4% (129 g); (Stan-Gard®): 0.4% (122 g); (Stop®): 0.4% (120 g). **LOZ, as sodium** (Flura-Loz®, Fluor-A-Day): 2.2 mg; (Lozi-Flur™): 2.21 mg. **SOLN, oral drops**, as sodium (Flura-Drops®): 0.55 mg/drop (24 mL); (Luride®, Pediaflor®): 1.1 mg/mL (50 mL). **SOLN, oral rinse**, as sodium (ACT®): 0.05% (530 mL); (Fluorigard®, NeutraGard®): 0.05% (480 mL); (Fluorinse®): 0.2% (480 mL); (Phos-Flur®): 0.44% (500 mL); (PreviDent®): 0.2% (250 mL). **SOLN, oral rinse concentrate**, as stannous fluoride (Gel-Kam®): 0.63% (300 mL). **TAB, chewable**, as sodium (Fluor-A-Day): 0.56 mg, 1.1 mg, 2.21 mg; (Luride® Lozi-Tabs®): 0.55 mg, 1.1 mg, 2.2 mg; (Pharmaflur®): 2.2 mg; (Pharmaflur® 1.1): 1.1 mg

Generic Available Yes

Comments Neutral pH fluoride preparations are preferred in patients with oral mucositis to reduce tissue irritation; long-term use of acidulated fluorides has been associated with enamel demineralization and damage to porcelain crowns

Selected Readings Wynn RC, "Fluoride: After 50 Years, a Clearer Picture of Its Mechanism," *Gen Dent*, 2002, 50(2):118-22, 124, 126.

Fluoride and Triclosan (Dental) *see* Triclosan and Fluoride *on page 1348*

Fluorigard® [OTC] *see* Fluoride *on page 586*

Fluori-Methane® *see* Dichlorodifluoromethane and Trichloromonofluoromethane *on page 428*

Fluorinse® *see* Fluoride *on page 586*

Fluorodeoxyuridine *see* Floxuridine *on page 576*

9α-Fluorohydrocortisone Acetate *see* Fludrocortisone *on page 580*

Fluorometholone (flore oh METH oh lone)

U.S. Brand Names Eflone®; Flarex®; Fluor-Op®; FML®; FML® Forte

Canadian Brand Names Flarex®; FML®; FML Forte®; PMS-Fluorometholone

Pharmacologic Category Corticosteroid, Ophthalmic

Use Treatment of steroid-responsive inflammatory conditions of the eye

Local Anesthetic/Vasoconstrictor Precautions No information available to require special precautions

Effects on Dental Treatment No significant effects or complications reported

Dosage Children >2 years and Adults: Ophthalmic: Re-evaluate therapy if improvement is not seen within 2 days; use care not to discontinue prematurely; in chronic conditions, gradually decrease dosing frequency prior to discontinuing treatment

Ointment: Apply small amount (~½ inch ribbon) to conjunctival sac every 4 hours in severe cases; 1-3 times/day in mild to moderate cases

Solution: Instill 1-2 drops into conjunctival sac every hour during day, every 2 hours at night until favorable response is obtained, then use 1 drop every 4 hours; for

(Continued)

Fluorometholone *(Continued)*

mild to moderate inflammation, instill 1-2 drops into conjunctival sac 2-4 times/day

Mechanism of Action Decreases inflammation by suppression of migration of polymorphonuclear leukocytes and reversal of increased capillary permeability

Other Adverse Effects Frequency not defined:

Ocular: Anterior uveitis, burning upon application, cataract formation, conjunctival hyperemia, conjunctivitis, corneal ulcers, glaucoma with optic nerve damage, perforation of the globe, secondary ocular infection (bacterial, fungal, viral), intraocular pressure elevation, visual acuity and field defects, keratitis, mydriasis, stinging upon application, delayed wound healing

Miscellaneous: Systemic hypercorticoidism (rare), **abnormal taste**

Pharmacodynamics/Kinetics Absorption: Into aqueous humor with slight systemic absorption

Pregnancy Risk Factor C

Generic Available Yes: Suspension (as base)

Fluorometholone and Sulfacetamide *see* Sulfacetamide and Fluorometholone *on page 1250*

Fluor-Op® *see* Fluorometholone *on page 587*

Fluoroplex® *see* Fluorouracil *on page 588*

Fluorouracil (flure oh YOOR a sil)

U.S. Brand Names Adrucil®; Carac™; Efudex®; Fluoroplex®

Canadian Brand Names Adrucil®; Efudex®

Mexican Brand Names Efudix; Fluoro-uracil

Pharmacologic Category Antineoplastic Agent, Antimetabolite

Synonyms 5-Fluorouracil; 5-FU

Use Treatment of carcinomas of the breast, colon, head and neck, pancreas, rectum, or stomach; topically for the management of actinic or solar keratoses and superficial basal cell carcinomas

Local Anesthetic/Vasoconstrictor Precautions No information available to require special precautions

Effects on Dental Treatment Toxicity depends on route and duration of treatment (frequency not defined):

I.V.: Angina, confusion, disorientation, euphoria, headache, bleeding, esophagopharyngitis, nausea, stomatitis, ulceration, vomiting epistaxis, anaphylaxis, generalized allergic reactions

Topical: Headache, allergic contact dermatitis

Dosage Adults:

Carcinoma of the breast, colon, pancreas, rectum, and stomach: Refer to individual protocols: All dosages are based on the patient's actual weight. However, the estimated lean body mass (dry weight) is used if the patient is obese or if there has been a spurious weight gain due to edema, ascites, or other forms of abnormal fluid retention.

I.V.: Manufacturers suggested dosing:

Initial sequence: 12 mg/kg once daily on days 1-4 (maximum daily dose: 800 mg); no treatment is given on day 5; if no toxicity is observed, administer 6 mg/kg on days 6, 8, 10, and 12; no treatment is given on days 7, 9, or 11

Poor risk patients/patients with poor nutritional status: 6 mg/kg once daily on days 1-3 (maximum dose: 400 mg); no therapy is given on day 4; if no toxicity is observed, administer 3 mg/kg on days 5, 7, and 9; no treatment is given on days 6 or 8

Maintenance: Repeat initial sequence every 30 days after last day of previous treatment **or** 10-15 mg/kg/week as a single dose (maximum 1 g/week, begin when toxic signs from initial course of treatment have subsided); further duration of treatment and dosage are dependent upon patient response; treatment has ranged from 9-45 courses over 12-60 months

Examples of other dosing regimens include:

Intermittent bolus dose in combination with other agents: 600 mg/m^2 every 3-4 weeks

Continuous infusion in combination with other agents: 1000 mg/m^2/day for 4-5 days every 3-4 weeks

Bolus dose in combination with leucovorin: 425 mg/m^2/day for 5 days every 4 weeks

Continuous protracted infusion: 200-300 mg/m^2/day

Actinic keratoses: Topical:

Carac™: Apply thin film to lesions once daily for up to 4 weeks, as tolerated

Efudex®: Apply cream or solution to lesions twice daily for 2-4 weeks; complete healing may not be evident for 1-2 months following treatment

Fluoroplex®: Apply to lesions twice daily for 2-6 weeks

Basal cell carcinoma: Topical: Efudex®: Apply 5% cream or solution to affected lesions twice daily for 3-6 weeks; treatment may be continued for up to 10-12 weeks

Mechanism of Action A pyrimidine antimetabolite that interferes with DNA synthesis by blocking the methylation of deoxyuridylic acid; 5-FU rapidly enters the cell and is activated to the nucleotide level; there it inhibits thymidylate synthetase (TS), or is incorporated into RNA (most evident during the GI phase of the cell cycle). The reduced folate cofactor is required for tight binding to occur between the 5-FdUMP and TS.

Other Adverse Effects Toxicity depends on route and duration of treatment (frequency not defined):

I.V.:

Cardiovascular: Myocardial ischemia, nail changes

Central nervous system: Acute cerebellar syndrome, nystagmus

Dermatologic: Alopecia, dermatitis, dry skin, fissuring, palmar-plantar erythrodysesthesia syndrome, pruritic maculopapular rash, photosensitivity, vein pigmentations

Gastrointestinal: Anorexia, diarrhea, sloughing

Hematologic: Agranulocytosis, anemia, leukopenia, pancytopenia, thrombocytopenia

Myelosuppression:

Onset: 7-10 days

Nadir: 9-14 days

Recovery: 21-28 days

Local: Thrombophlebitis

Ocular: Lacrimation, lacrimal duct stenosis, photophobia, visual changes

Miscellaneous: Loss of nails

Topical:

Central nervous system: Telangiectasia

Dermatologic: Photosensitivity, pruritus, rash, scarring

Hematologic: Leukocytosis

Local: Burning, crusting, dryness, edema, erosion, erythema, hyperpigmentation, irritation, pain, soreness, ulceration

Ocular: Eye irritation (burning, watering, sensitivity, stinging, itching)

Miscellaneous: Birth defects, miscarriage

Drug Interactions

Increased Effect/Toxicity: Leucovorin increases the folate pool and, in certain tumors, may promote TS inhibition and increase 5-FU activity. Leucovorin must be given before or with the 5-FU to prime the cells; it is not used as a rescue agent in this case. Allopurinol inhibits thymidine phosphorylase (an enzyme that activates 5-FU). The antitumor effect of 5-FU appears to be unaltered, but the toxicity is increased. Cimetidine results in increased plasma levels of 5-FU due to drug metabolism inhibition and reduction of liver blood flow induced by cimetidine.

Decreased Effect: Methotrexate: This interaction is schedule dependent; **5-FU should be given following MTX, not prior to.** If 5-FU is given first: 5-FU inhibits the TS binding and thus the reduced folate pool is not depleted, thereby negating the effect of MTX.

Dietary/Ethanol/Herb Considerations

Ethanol: Avoid use due to GI irritation.

Herb/Nutraceutical: Avoid black cohosh and dong quai in estrogen-dependent tumors.

Pharmacodynamics/Kinetics

Duration: ~3 weeks

Distribution: V_d: ~22% of total body water; penetrates extracellular fluid, CSF, and third space fluids (eg, pleural effusions and ascitic fluid)

Metabolism: Hepatic (90%); via a dehydrogenase enzyme; 5-FU must be metabolized to be active; dose may need to be omitted in patients with hepatic failure (bilirubin >5 mg/dL)

Bioavailability: <75%, erratic and undependable

Half-life elimination: Biphasic: Initial: 6-20 minutes; doses of 400-600 mg/m^2 produce drug concentrations above the threshold for cytotoxicity for normal tissue and remain there for 6 hours; two metabolites, FdUMP and FUTP, have prolonged half-lives depending on the type of tissue; the clinical effect of these metabolites has not been determined

Excretion: Lung (large amounts as CO_2); urine (5% as unchanged drug) in 6 hours

Pregnancy Risk Factor D (injection); X (topical)

Generic Available Yes: Injection

5-Fluorouracil *see* Fluorouracil *on page 588*

Fluoxetine (floo OKS e teen)

U.S. Brand Names Prozac®; Prozac® Weekly™; Sarafem™

Canadian Brand Names Alti-Fluoxetine; Apo®-Fluoxetine; CO Fluoxetine; Gen-Fluoxetine; Novo-Fluoxetine; Nu-Fluoxetine; PMS-Fluoxetine; Prozac®; Rhoxal-fluoxetine

Mexican Brand Names Fluoxac®; Prozac®; Siquial®

Pharmacologic Category Antidepressant, Selective Serotonin Reuptake Inhibitor

Synonyms Fluoxetine Hydrochloride

(Continued)

Fluoxetine *(Continued)*

Use Treatment of major depressive disorder; treatment of binge-eating and vomiting in patients with moderate-to-severe bulimia nervosa; obsessive-compulsive disorder (OCD); premenstrual dysphoric disorder (PMDD); panic disorder with or without agoraphobia

Unlabeled/Investigational Use Treatment of selective mutism

Local Anesthetic/Vasoconstrictor Precautions Although caution should be used in patients taking tricyclic antidepressants, no interactions have been reported with vasoconstrictors and fluoxetine, a nontricyclic antidepressant which acts to increase serotonin

Effects on Dental Treatment Problems with SSRI-induced bruxism have been reported and may preclude their use; clinicians attempting to evaluate any patient with bruxism or involuntary muscle movement, who is simultaneously being treated with an SSRI drug, should be aware of this potential association.

>10%: Xerostomia (4% to 12%), changes in salivation, headache (21%), anxiety (6% to 15%), nervousness (8% to 14%), somnolence (5% to 17%), nausea (12% to 29%), weakness (7% to 21%), tremors (3% to 13%), pharyngitis (3% to 11%), yawning (≤11%)

1% to 10%: Vasodilation (1% to 5%), fever (2%), chest pain, hemorrhage, hypertension, palpitations, dizziness (9%), abnormal thinking (2%), agitation, amnesia, confusion, vomiting (3%), taste perversion, abnormal vision (2%), ear pain, sinusitis (1% to 6%), flu-like syndrome (3% to 10%), diaphoresis (2% to 8%)

Dosage Oral:

Children:

Depression: 8-18 years: 10-20 mg/day; lower-weight children can be started at 10 mg/day, may increase to 20 mg/day after 1 week if needed

OCD: 7-18 years: Initial: 10 mg/day; in adolescents and higher-weight children, dose may be increased to 20 mg/day after 2 weeks. Range: 10-60 mg/day

Selective mutism (unlabeled use):

<5 years: No dosing information available

5-18 years: Initial: 5-10 mg/day; titrate upwards as needed (usual maximum dose: 60 mg/day)

Adults: 20 mg/day in the morning; may increase after several weeks by 20 mg/day increments; maximum: 80 mg/day; doses >20 mg should be divided into morning and noon doses. **Note:** Lower doses of 5-10 mg/day have been used for initial treatment.

Usual dosage range:

Bulimia nervosa: 60-80 mg/day

Depression: 20-40 mg/day; patients maintained on Prozac® 20 mg/day may be changed to Prozac® Weekly™ 90 mg/week, starting dose 7 days after the last 20 mg/day dose

Obesity: 20-60 mg/day

OCD: 40-80 mg/day

Panic disorder: Initial: 10 mg/day; after 1 week, increase to 20 mg/day; may increase after several weeks; doses >60 mg/day have not been evaluated

PMDD (Sarafem™): 20 mg/day continuously, **or** 20 mg/day starting 14 days prior to menstruation and through first full day of menses (repeat with each cycle)

Elderly: Depression: Some patients may require an initial dose of 10 mg/day with dosage increases of 10 and 20 mg every several weeks as tolerated; should not be taken at night unless patient experiences sedation

Dosing adjustment in renal impairment:

Single dose studies: Pharmacokinetics of fluoxetine and norfluoxetine were similar among subjects with all levels of impaired renal function, including anephric patients on chronic hemodialysis

Chronic administration: Additional accumulation of fluoxetine or norfluoxetine may occur in patients with severely impaired renal function

Hemodialysis: Not removed by hemodialysis; use of lower dose or less frequent dosing is not usually necessary.

Dosing adjustment in hepatic impairment: Elimination halflife of fluoxetine is prolonged in patients with hepatic impairment; a lower or less frequent dose of fluoxetine should be used in these patients

Cirrhosis patients: Administer a lower dose or less frequent dosing interval

Compensated cirrhosis without ascites: Administer 50% of normal dose

Mechanism of Action Inhibits CNS neuron serotonin reuptake; minimal or no effect on reuptake of norepinephrine or dopamine; does not significantly bind to alpha-adrenergic, histamine, or cholinergic receptors

Other Adverse Effects Percentages as reported in placebo-controlled trials (generally similar in adults and children); actual frequency may be dependent upon diagnosis and in some cases the range presented may be lower than or equal to placebo for a particular disorder

>10%:

Central nervous system: Insomnia (10% to 33%)

Endocrine & metabolic: Libido decreased (1% to 11%)

Gastrointestinal: Diarrhea (8% to 18%), anorexia (4% to 11%)

1% to 10%:

Central nervous system: Dream abnormality (1% to 5%), chills, emotional lability, sleep disorder

Dermatologic: Rash (2% to 6%), pruritus (4%)

Endocrine & metabolic: Ejaculation abnormal (<1% to 7%), impotence (<1% to 7%)

Gastrointestinal: Dyspepsia (6% to 10%), constipation (5%), flatulence (3%), weight loss (2%), appetite increased, weight gain

Genitourinary: Urinary frequency

Otic: Tinnitus

<1%, postmarketing and/or case reports: Acne, albuminuria, **allergies,** alopecia, amenorrhea, **anaphylactoid reactions,** anemia, **angina, aphthous stomatitis, arrhythmia, arthritis, asthma, bone pain, bruising,** bursitis, cataract, **CHF,** cholelithiasis, cholestatic jaundice, colitis, **dehydration, dyskinesia, dysphagia, ecchymosis,** edema, **eosinophilic pneumonia, epistaxis,** erythema nodosum, **esophagitis, euphoria,** exfoliative dermatitis, **extrapyramidal symptoms (rare), gastritis, glossitis,** gout, gynecomastia, **hallucinations,** hepatic failure/necrosis, **hemorrhage, hiccup, hostility,** hypercholesteremia, hyperprolactinemia, **hyperventilation, hypoglycemia,** hypokalemia, **hypotension,** hypothyroidism, immune-related hemolytic anemia, kidney failure, **laryngospasm, leg cramps,** abnormal LFTs, **lupus-like syndrome, malaise, migraine, misuse/abuse, MI,** neuroleptic malignant syndrome (NMS), optic neuritis, pancreatitis, pancytopenia, photosensitivity reaction, **postural hypotension,** priapism, pulmonary embolism, pulmonary hypertension, QT prolongation, **serotonin syndrome,** Stevens-Johnson syndrome, **suicidal ideation, syncope, tachycardia,** tinnitus, thrombocytopenia, thrombocytopenic purpura, vasculitis, **ventricular tachycardia (including torsade de pointes)**

Warnings/Precautions Potential for severe reaction when used with MAO inhibitors - serotonin syndrome (hyperthermia, muscular rigidity, mental status changes/agitation, autonomic instability) may occur. Fluoxetine may elevate plasma levels of thioridazine and increase the risk of QT_c interval prolongation. This may lead to serious ventricular arrhythmias such as torsade de pointes-type arrhythmias and sudden death. Fluoxetine use has been associated with occurrences of significant rash and allergic events, including vasculitis, lupus-like syndrome, laryngospasm, anaphylactoid reactions, and pulmonary inflammatory disease. May precipitate a shift to mania or hypomania in patients with bipolar disease. May cause insomnia, anxiety, nervousness or anorexia. Use with caution in patients where weight loss is undesirable. May impair cognitive or motor performance - caution operating hazardous machinery or driving. Use caution in patients with depression, particularly if suicidal risk may be present. Use caution in patients with a previous seizure disorder or condition predisposing to seizures such as brain damage, alcoholism, or concurrent therapy with other drugs which lower the seizure threshold. Use with caution in patients with hepatic or renal dysfunction and in elderly patients. May cause hyponatremia/SIADH. May increase the risks associated with electroconvulsive treatment. Use with caution in patients at risk of bleeding or receiving concurrent anticoagulant therapy - may cause impairment in platelet function. May alter glycemic control in patients with diabetes. Due to the long half-life of fluoxetine and its metabolites, the effects and interactions noted may persist for prolonged periods following discontinuation. May cause or exacerbate sexual dysfunction.

Drug Interactions Substrate of 1A2, 2B6, **2C8/9**, 2C19, **2D6**, 2E1, 3A4; Inhibits 1A2, **2B6**, 2C8/9, 2C19, **2D6**, 3A4

Increased Effect/Toxicity:

MAO inhibitors: Fluoxetine should not be used with nonselective MAO inhibitors (phenelzine, isocarboxazid) or other drugs with MAO inhibition (linezolid); fatal reactions have been reported. Wait 5 weeks after stopping fluoxetine before starting a nonselective MAO inhibitor and 2 weeks after stopping an MAO inhibitor before starting fluoxetine. Concurrent selegiline has been associated with mania, hypertension, or serotonin syndrome (risk may be reduced relative to nonselective MAO inhibitors).

Phenothiazines: Fluoxetine may inhibit the metabolism of thioridazine or mesoridazine, resulting in increased plasma levels and increasing the risk of QT_c interval prolongation. This may lead to serious ventricular arrhythmias, such as torsade de pointes-type arrhythmias and sudden death. Do not use together. Wait at least 5 weeks after discontinuing fluoxetine prior to starting thioridazine.

Combined used of SSRIs and amphetamines, buspirone, meperidine, nefazodone, serotonin agonists (such as sumatriptan), sibutramine, other SSRIs, sympathomimetics, ritonavir, tramadol, and venlafaxine may increase the risk of serotonin syndrome. Fluoxetine may increase serum levels/effects of benzodiazepines (alprazolam and diazepam), beta-blockers (except atenolol or nadolol), carbamazepine, carvedilol, clozapine, cyclosporine (and possibly tacrolimus), dextromethorphan, digoxin, haloperidol, HMG-CoA reductase inhibitors (lovastatin and simvastatin - increasing the risk of rhabdomyolysis), phenytoin, propafenone, trazodone, tricyclic antidepressants, and valproic acid. Concurrent lithium may increase risk of neurotoxicity, and lithium levels may be increased. Risk of hyponatremia may increase with concurrent use of loop

(Continued)

Fluoxetine *(Continued)*

diuretics (bumetanide, furosemide, torsemide). Fluoxetine may increase the hypoprothrombinemic response to warfarin.

Combined use of sumatriptan (and other serotonin agonists) may result in toxicity; weakness, hyper-reflexia, and incoordination have been observed with sumatriptan and SSRIs. In addition, concurrent use may theoretically increase the risk of serotonin syndrome; includes sumatriptan, naratriptan, rizatriptan, and zolmitriptan.

Decreased Effect: Cyproheptadine may inhibit the effects of serotonin reuptake inhibitors. Lithium levels may be decreased by fluoxetine (in addition to reports of increased lithium levels).

Dietary/Ethanol/Herb Considerations

Ethanol: Avoid ethanol; may increase CNS depression

Food: May be taken with food; avoid caffeine

Herb/Nutraceutical: Avoid gotu kola, kava, SAMe, St John's wort, and valerian; may increase CNS depression. Avoid melatonin; may cause acute psychosis. Avoid tryptophan; may cause serotonin syndrome.

Pharmacodynamics/Kinetics

Absorption: Well absorbed; delayed 1-2 hours with weekly formulation

Protein binding: 95%

Metabolism: Hepatic to norfluoxetine (active; equal to fluoxetine)

Half-life elimination: Adults:

Parent drug: 1-3 days (acute), 4-6 days (chronic), 7.6 days (cirrhosis)

Metabolite (norfluoxetine): 9.3 days (range: 4-16 days), 12 days (cirrhosis)

Due to long half-life, resolution of adverse reactions after discontinuation may be slow

Time to peak: 6-8 hours

Excretion: Urine (10% as norfluoxetine, 2.5% to 5% as fluoxetine)

Note: Weekly formulation results in greater fluctuations between peak and trough concentrations of fluoxetine and norfluoxetine compared to once-daily dosing (24% daily/164% weekly; 17% daily/43% weekly, respectively). Trough concentrations are 76% lower for fluoxetine and 47% lower for norfluoxetine than the concentrations maintained by 20 mg once-daily dosing. Steady-state fluoxetine concentrations are ~50% lower following the once-weekly regimen compared to 20 mg once daily. Average steady-state concentrations of once-daily dosing were highest in children ages 6 to <13 (fluoxetine 171 ng/mL; norfluoxetine 195 ng/mL), followed by adolescents ages 13 to <18 (fluoxetine 86 ng/mL; norfluoxetine 113 ng/mL); concentrations were considered to be within the ranges reported in adults (fluoxetine 91-302 ng/mL; norfluoxetine 72-258 ng/mL).

Pregnancy Risk Factor C

Generic Available Yes; Excludes delayed release capsule

Selected Readings

Friedlander AH and Mahler ME, "Major Depressive Disorder. Psychopathology, Medical Management, and Dental Implications," *J Am Dent Assoc*, 2001, 132(5):629-38.

Gerber PE and Lynd LD, "Selective Serotonin Reuptake Inhibitor-induced Movement Disorders," *Ann Pharmacother*, 1998, 32(6):692-8.

Wynn RL, "New Antidepressant Medications," *Gen Dent*, 1997, 45(1):24-8.

Fluoxetine Hydrochloride *see* Fluoxetine *on page 589*

Fluoxymesterone (floo oks i MES te rone)

U.S. Brand Names Halotestin®

Canadian Brand Names Halotestin®

Mexican Brand Names Stenox®

Pharmacologic Category Androgen

Use Replacement of endogenous testicular hormone; in females, used as palliative treatment of breast cancer

Unlabeled/Investigational Use Stimulation of erythropoiesis; treatment of angioneurotic edema

Local Anesthetic/Vasoconstrictor Precautions No information available to require special precautions

Effects on Dental Treatment 1% to 10%: GI irritation, nausea, vomiting

Restrictions C-III

Dosage Adults: Oral:

Male:

Hypogonadism: 5-20 mg/day

Delayed puberty: 2.5-20 mg/day for 4-6 months

Female: Inoperable breast carcinoma: 10-40 mg/day in divided doses for 1-3 months

Mechanism of Action Synthetic androgenic anabolic hormone responsible for the normal growth and development of male sex hormones and development of male sex organs and maintenance of secondary sex characteristics; synthetic testosterone derivative with significant androgen activity; stimulates RNA polymerase activity resulting in an increase in protein production; increases bone development;

halogenated derivative of testosterone with up to 5 times the activity of methyltestosterone

Other Adverse Effects

>10%:

Male: Priapism

Female: Menstrual problems (amenorrhea), virilism, breast soreness

Cardiovascular: Edema

Dermatologic: Acne

1% to 10%:

Male: Prostatic carcinoma, hirsutism (increase in pubic hair growth), impotence, testicular atrophy

Cardiovascular: Edema

Genitourinary: Prostatic hyperplasia

Hepatic: Hepatic dysfunction

<1%:

Male: Gynecomastia

Female: Amenorrhea

Hypercalcemia, leukopenia, polycythemia, hepatic necrosis, cholestatic hepatitis, **hypersensitivity reactions**

Drug Interactions

Increased Effect/Toxicity: Fluoxymesterone may suppress clotting factors II, V, VII, and X; therefore, bleeding may occur in patients on anticoagulant therapy May elevate cyclosporine serum levels. May enhance hypoglycemic effect of insulin therapy; may decrease blood glucose concentrations and insulin requirements in patients with diabetes. Lithium may potentiate EPS and other CNS effect. May potentiate the effects of narcotics including respiratory depression

Decreased Effect: May decrease barbiturate levels and fluphenazine effectiveness.

Pharmacodynamics/Kinetics

Absorption: Rapid

Protein binding: 98%

Metabolism: Hepatic; enterohepatic recirculation

Half-life elimination: 10-100 minutes

Excretion: Urine (90%)

Pregnancy Risk Factor X

Generic Available Yes

Fluphenazine (floo FEN a zeen)

U.S. Brand Names Prolixin®; Prolixin Decanoate®; Prolixin Enanthate® [DSC]

Canadian Brand Names Apo®-Fluphenazine; Apo®-Fluphenazine Decanoate; Modecate®; Moditen® Enanthate; Moditen® HCl; PMS-Fluphenazine Decanoate

Pharmacologic Category Antipsychotic Agent, Phenothiazine, Piperazine

Synonyms Fluphenazine Decanoate; Fluphenazine Enanthate; Fluphenazine Hydrochloride; Prolixin Enanthate® [DSC]

Use Management of manifestations of psychotic disorders and schizophrenia; depot formulation may offer improved outcome in individuals with psychosis who are nonadherent with oral antipsychotics

Unlabeled/Investigational Use Treatment of pervasive developmental disorder

Local Anesthetic/Vasoconstrictor Precautions Most pharmacology textbooks state that in presence of phenothiazines, systemic doses of epinephrine paradoxically decrease the blood pressure. This is the so called "epinephrine reversal" phenomenon. This has never been observed when epinephrine is given by infiltration as part of the anesthesia procedure.

Effects on Dental Treatment Orthostatic hypotension and nasal congestion are possible and since the drug is a dopamine antagonist, extrapyramidal symptoms of the TMJ are a possibility.

Frequency not defined: Hypotension, tachycardia, fluctuations in blood pressure, hypertension, arrhythmias, Parkinsonian symptoms, akathisia, dystonias, tardive dyskinesia, dizziness, headache, drowsiness, lethargy, restlessness, excitement, seizures, increased salivation, xerostomia, laryngeal edema, blurred vision, asthma

Dosage

Children: Oral: Childhood-onset pervasive developmental disorder (unlabeled use): 0.04 mg/kg/day

Adults: Psychoses:

Oral: 0.5-10 mg/day in divided doses at 6- to 8-hour intervals; some patients may require up to 40 mg/day

I.M.: 2.5-10 mg/day in divided doses at 6- to 8-hour intervals (parenteral dose is $1/3$ to $1/2$ the oral dose for the hydrochloride salts)

I.M. (decanoate): 12.5 mg every 2 weeks

Conversion from hydrochloride to decanoate I.M. 0.5 mL (12.5 mg) decanoate every 3 weeks is approximately equivalent to 10 mg hydrochloride/day

I.M. (enanthate): 12.5-25 mg every 2 weeks

Hemodialysis: Not dialyzable (0% to 5%)

(Continued)

Fluphenazine *(Continued)*

Mechanism of Action Blocks postsynaptic mesolimbic dopaminergic D_1 and D_2 receptors in the brain; depresses the release of hypothalamic and hypophyseal hormones; believed to depress the reticular activating system thus affecting basal metabolism, body temperature, wakefulness, vasomotor tone, and emesis

Other Adverse Effects Frequency not defined:

Cardiovascular: Edema

Central nervous system: Hyper-reflexia, cerebral edema, bizarre dreams, EEG changes, depression, NMS, altered central temperature regulation

Dermatologic: Increased sensitivity to sun, rash, skin pigmentation, itching, erythema, urticaria, seborrhea, eczema, dermatitis

Endocrine & metabolic: Changes in menstrual cycle, breast pain, amenorrhea, galactorrhea, gynecomastia, changes in libido, elevated prolactin, SIADH

Gastrointestinal: Weight gain, loss of appetite, constipation, paralytic ileus

Genitourinary: Ejaculatory disturbances, impotence, polyuria, bladder paralysis, enuresis

Hematologic: Agranulocytosis, leukopenia, thrombocytopenia, nonthrombocytopenic purpura, eosinophilia, pancytopenia

Hepatic: Cholestatic jaundice, hepatotoxicity

Neuromuscular & skeletal: Trembling of fingers, SLE, facial hemispasm

Ocular: Pigmentary retinopathy, cornea and lens changes glaucoma

Drug Interactions Substrate of **CYP2D6**; Inhibits CYP1A2, 2D6, 2E1

Increased Effect/Toxicity: Effects on CNS depression may be additive when fluphenazine is combined with CNS depressants (narcotic analgesics, ethanol, barbiturates, cyclic antidepressants, antihistamines, sedative-hypnotics). Fluphenazine may increase the effects/toxicity of anticholinergics, antihypertensives, lithium (rare neurotoxicity), trazodone, or valproic acid. Concurrent use with TCA may produce increased toxicity or altered therapeutic response. Chloroquine and propranolol may increase chlorpromazine concentrations. Hypotension may occur when fluphenazine is combined with epinephrine. May increase the risk of arrhythmia when combined with antiarrhythmics, cisapride, pimozide, sparfloxacin, or other drugs which prolong QT interval. Metoclopramide may increase risk of extrapyramidal symptoms (EPS).

Decreased Effect: Phenothiazines inhibit the activity of guanethidine, guanadrel, levodopa, and bromocriptine. Barbiturates and cigarette smoking may enhance the hepatic metabolism of fluphenazine. Fluphenazine and possibly other low potency antipsychotics may reverse the pressor effects of epinephrine.

Dietary/Ethanol/Herb Considerations

Ethanol: Avoid use; may increase CNS depression.

Herb/Nutraceutical: Avoid dong quai; may cause additional photosensitization. Avoid gotu kola, kava, SAMe, and valerian; may increase CNS depression. Avoid St John's wort; may cause additional photosensitization and increase CNS depression.

Pharmacodynamics/Kinetics

Onset of action: I.M., S.C. (derivative dependent): Hydrochloride salt: ~1 hour

Peak effect: Neuroleptic: Decanoate: 48-96 hours

Duration: Hydrochloride salt: 6-8 hours; Decanoate (lasts the longest): 24-72 hours

Absorption: Oral: Erratic and variable

Distribution: Crosses placenta; enters breast milk

Protein binding: 91% and 99%

Metabolism: Hepatic

Half-life elimination (derivative dependent): Enanthate: 84-96 hours; Hydrochloride: 33 hours; Decanoate: 163-232 hours

Excretion: Urine (as metabolites)

Pregnancy Risk Factor C

Generic Available Yes: Injection, tablet

Fluphenazine Decanoate *see* Fluphenazine *on page 593*

Fluphenazine Enanthate *see* Fluphenazine *on page 593*

Fluphenazine Hydrochloride *see* Fluphenazine *on page 593*

Flura-Drops® *see* Fluoride *on page 586*

Flura-Loz® *see* Fluoride *on page 586*

Flurandrenolide (flure an DREN oh lide)

U.S. Brand Names Cordran®; Cordran® SP

Canadian Brand Names Cordran®

Pharmacologic Category Corticosteroid, Topical

Synonyms Flurandrenolone

Use Inflammation of corticosteroid-responsive dermatoses [medium potency topical corticosteroid]

Local Anesthetic/Vasoconstrictor Precautions No information available to require special precautions

Effects on Dental Treatment No significant effects or complications reported

Dosage Topical: Therapy should be discontinued when control is achieved; if no improvement is seen, reassessment of diagnosis may be necessary.

Children:

Ointment, cream: Apply sparingly 1-2 times/day

Tape: Apply once daily

Adults: Cream, lotion, ointment: Apply sparingly 2-3 times/day

Mechanism of Action Decreases inflammation by suppression of migration of polymorphonuclear leukocytes and reversal of increased capillary permeability

Other Adverse Effects Frequency not defined:

Cardiovascular: Intracranial hypertension

Dermatologic: Itching, dry skin, folliculitis, hypertrichosis, acneiform eruptions, hyperpigmentation, perioral dermatitis, allergic contact dermatitis, skin atrophy, striae, miliaria, acne, maceration of the skin

Endocrine & metabolic: Cushing's syndrome, growth retardation, HPA suppression

Local: Burning, irritation

Miscellaneous: **Secondary infection**

Pharmacodynamics/Kinetics

Absorption: Adequate with intact skin; repeated applications lead to depot effects on skin, potentially resulting in enhanced percutaneous absorption

Metabolism: Hepatic

Excretion: Urine; feces (small amounts)

Pregnancy Risk Factor C

Generic Available No

Flurandrenolone *see* Flurandrenolide *on page 594*

Flurazepam (flure AZ e pam)

U.S. Brand Names Dalmane®

Canadian Brand Names Apo®-Flurazepam; Dalmane®

Pharmacologic Category Benzodiazepine

Synonyms Flurazepam Hydrochloride

Use Short-term treatment of insomnia

Local Anesthetic/Vasoconstrictor Precautions No information available to require special precautions

Effects on Dental Treatment

>10%: Xerostomia, changes in salivation

Frequency not defined: Palpitations, chest pain, drowsiness, lightheadedness, memory impairment, headache, hangover effect, confusion, nervousness, dizziness, falling, apprehension, irritability, euphoria, slurred speech, restlessness, hallucinations, nausea, vomiting, bitter taste, blurred vision, apnea, dyspnea, diaphoresis, drug dependence

Restrictions C-IV

Dosage Guidelines from CMS (Centers for Medicare and Medicaid Services), formerly known as HCFA, discourage use in residents of long-term care facilities.

Oral:

Children: Insomnia:

≤15 years: Dose not established

>15 years: 15 mg at bedtime

Adults: Insomnia: 15-30 mg at bedtime

Elderly: Insomnia: 15 mg at bedtime **Note:** Avoid use if possible

Mechanism of Action Binds to stereospecific benzodiazepine receptors on the postsynaptic GABA neuron at several sites within the central nervous system, including the limbic system, reticular formation. Enhancement of the inhibitory effect of GABA on neuronal excitability results by increased neuronal membrane permeability to chloride ions. This shift in chloride ions results in hyperpolarization (a less excitable state) and stabilization.

Other Adverse Effects Frequency not defined:

Central nervous system: Ataxia, depression, talkativeness

Dermatologic: Rash, pruritus

Gastrointestinal: Constipation, increased/excessive salivation, heartburn, upset stomach, diarrhea, increased or decreased appetite, weight gain/loss

Hematologic: Granulocytopenia

Hepatic: Elevated AST/ALT, total bilirubin, alkaline phosphatase, cholestatic jaundice

Neuromuscular & skeletal: Dysarthria, body/joint pain, reflex slowing, weakness

Ocular: Burning eyes, difficulty focusing

Otic: Tinnitus

Drug Interactions Substrate of **CYP3A4**; Inhibits CYP2E1

Increased Effect/Toxicity: Serum levels and response to flurazepam may be increased by amprenavir, cimetidine, ciprofloxacin, clarithromycin, clozapine, CNS depressants, diltiazem, disulfiram, digoxin, erythromycin, ethanol, fluconazole, fluoxetine, fluvoxamine, grapefruit juice, isoniazid, itraconazole, ketoconazole, labetalol, levodopa, loxapine, metoprolol, metronidazole, miconazole, nefazodone, nelfinavir, omeprazole, phenytoin, rifabutin, rifampin, ritonavir, troleandomycin, valproic acid, and verapamil.

(Continued)

Flurazepam *(Continued)*

Decreased Effect: Carbamazepine, rifampin, and rifabutin may enhance the metabolism of flurazepam and decrease its therapeutic effect; consider using an alternative sedative/hypnotic agent.

Dietary/Ethanol/Herb Considerations

Ethanol: Avoid use; may increase CNS depression.

Food: Administer with food to reduce GI upset. Serum concentration and response to flurazepam may be increased by grapefruit products, but unlikely because of flurazepam's high oral bioavailability.

Herb/Nutraceutical: Avoid gotu kola, kava, SAMe, St John's wort, and valerian; may increase CNS depression. Melatonin may enhance activity of clonazepam; use cautiously.

Pharmacodynamics/Kinetics

Onset of action: Hypnotic: 15-20 minutes

Peak effect: 3-6 hours

Duration: 7-8 hours

Metabolism: Hepatic to N-desalkylflurazepam (active)

Half-life elimination: Desalkylflurazepam:

Adults: Single dose: 74-90 hours; Multiple doses: 111-113 hours

Elderly (61-85 years): Single dose: 120-160 hours; Multiple doses: 126-158 hours

Pregnancy Risk Factor X

Generic Available Yes

Flurazepam Hydrochloride *see* Flurazepam *on page 595*

Flurbiprofen (flure BI proe fen)

Related Information

Rheumatoid Arthritis, Osteoarthritis, and Osteoporosis *on page 1488*

Temporomandibular Dysfunction (TMD) *on page 1562*

U.S. Brand Names Ansaid®; Ocufen®

Canadian Brand Names Alti-Flurbiprofen; Ansaid®; Apo®-Flurbiprofen; Froben®; Froben-SR®; Novo-Flurprofen; Nu-Flurprofen; Ocufen™

Mexican Brand Names Ansaid®

Pharmacologic Category Nonsteroidal Anti-inflammatory Drug (NSAID)

Synonyms Flurbiprofen Sodium

Use

Dental: Treatment of postoperative pain

Medical:

Oral: Acute or long-term treatment of signs and symptoms of rheumatoid arthritis and osteoarthritis

Ophthalmic: Inhibition of intraoperative miosis; prevention and management of postoperative ocular inflammation and postoperative cystoid macular edema remains to be determined

Local Anesthetic/Vasoconstrictor Precautions No information available to require special precautions

Effects on Dental Treatment NSAID formulations are known to reversibly decrease platelet aggregation via mechanisms different than observed with aspirin. The dentist should be aware of the potential of abnormal coagulation. Caution should also be exercised in the use of NSAIDs in patients already on anticoagulant therapy with drugs such as warfarin (Coumadin®).

Oral:

1% to 10%: Headache (3% to 9%), dizziness (1% to 10%), vomiting (1% to 3%), nausea (3% to 9%)

<1%: Stomatitis, xerostomia

Frequency not defined: CHF, hypertension, arrhythmias, tachycardia, nervousness, confusion, hallucinations, drowsiness, hot flashes, gastritis, GI ulceration, blurred vision, dyspnea, allergic rhinitis, epistaxis

Dosage

Oral:

Dental: 100 mg every 12 hours

Rheumatoid arthritis and osteoarthritis: 200-300 mg/day in 2-, 3-, or 4 divided doses

Ophthalmic: Instill 1 drop every 30 minutes, 2 hours prior to surgery (total of 4 drops to each affected eye)

Mechanism of Action Inhibits prostaglandin synthesis by decreasing the activity of the enzyme, cyclooxygenase, which results in decreased formation of prostaglandin precursors

Other Adverse Effects Frequency not always defined:

Oral:

Cardiovascular: Angioedema

Central nervous system: Aseptic meningitis, mental depression, insomnia

Dermatologic: Itching, rash, urticaria, erythema multiforme, toxic epidermal necrolysis, Stevens-Johnson syndrome

Endocrine & metabolic: Fluid retention (3% to 9%), polydipsia

Gastrointestinal: Diarrhea (3% to 9%), constipation (1% to 3%), flatulence (1% to 3%), abdominal cramps (3% to 9%), heartburn, indigestion, dyspepsia (3% to 9%)
Genitourinary: Urinary tract infection (3% to 9%), cystitis, polyuria
Hematologic: Agranulocytosis, anemia, hemolytic anemia, bone marrow suppression, leukopenia, thrombocytopenia
Hepatic: Increased LFTs (1% to 3%), hepatitis
Neuromuscular & skeletal: Peripheral neuropathy
Ocular: Toxic amblyopia, conjunctivitis, dry eyes
Otic: Decreased hearing, tinnitus
Renal: Acute renal failure
Ophthalmic: Ocular:
>10%: Slowing of corneal wound healing, mild ocular stinging, itching and burning eyes, irritation
1% to 10%: Eye redness

Contraindications Hypersensitivity to flurbiprofen or any component of the formulation; dendritic keratitis; pregnancy (3rd trimester)

Warnings/Precautions Use with caution in patients with CHF, dehydration, hypertension, decreased renal or hepatic function, history of GI disease (bleeding or ulcers), or those receiving anticoagulants. Elderly are at a high risk for adverse effects from NSAIDs. As many as 60% of elderly can develop peptic ulceration and/or hemorrhage asymptomatically.

Use lowest effective dose for shortest period possible. Use of NSAIDs can compromise existing renal function especially when Cl_{cr} is <30 mL/minute. CNS adverse effects such as confusion, agitation, and hallucination are generally seen in overdose or high-dose situations; however, elderly may demonstrate these adverse effects at lower doses than younger adults. Withhold for at least 4-6 half-lives prior to surgical or dental procedures. Ophthalmic solution contains thimerosal.

Drug Interactions Substrate of CYP2C8/9; Inhibits CYP2C8/9
ACE inhibitors: Antihypertensive effects may be decreased by concurrent therapy with NSAIDs; monitor blood pressure.
Angiotensin II antagonists: Antihypertensive effects may be decreased by concurrent therapy with NSAIDs; monitor blood pressure.
Anticoagulants (warfarin, heparin, LMWHs) in combination with NSAIDs can cause increased risk of bleeding.
Other antiplatelet drugs (ticlopidine, clopidogrel, aspirin, abciximab, dipyridamole, eptifibatide, tirofiban) can cause an increased risk of bleeding.
Loop diuretics efficacy (diuretic and antihypertensive effect) is reduced. Indomethacin reduces this efficacy, however, it may be anticipated with any NSAID.
Cholestyramine and colestipol reduce the bioavailability of some NSAIDs; separate administration times.
Corticosteroids may increase the risk of GI ulceration; avoid concurrent use.
Cyclosporine: NSAIDs may increase serum creatinine, potassium, blood pressure, and cyclosporine levels; monitor cyclosporine levels and renal function carefully.
Gentamicin and amikacin serum concentrations are increased by indomethacin in premature infants. Results may apply to other aminoglycosides and NSAIDs.
Hydralazine's antihypertensive effect is decreased; avoid concurrent use.
Lithium levels can be increased; avoid concurrent use if possible or monitor lithium levels and adjust dose. Sulindac may have the least effect. When NSAID is stopped, lithium will need adjustment again.
Methotrexate: Severe bone marrow suppression, aplastic anemia, and GI toxicity have been reported with concomitant NSAID therapy. Avoid use during moderate or high-dose methotrexate (increased and prolonged methotrexate levels). NSAID use during low-dose treatment of rheumatoid arthritis has not been fully evaluated; extreme caution is warranted.
Thiazides antihypertensive effects are decreased; avoid concurrent use.
Warfarin's INRs may be increased by piroxicam. Other NSAIDs may have the same effect depending on dose and duration. Monitor INR closely. Use the lowest dose of NSAIDs possible and for the briefest duration.
Verapamil plasma concentration is decreased by some NSAIDs; avoid concurrent use.

Dietary/Ethanol/Herb Considerations
Ethanol: Avoid use; may enhance gastric mucosal irritation.
Food: Administer with food or milk to reduce GI upset; may decrease rate but not extent of absorption. Avoid garlic, ginger, and green tea.
Herb/Nutraceutical: Avoid cat's claw, dong quai, evening primrose, feverfew, garlic, ginger, ginkgo biloba, ginseng, green tea, horse chestnut, and red clover due to additional antiplatelet activity.

Pharmacodynamics/Kinetics
Onset of action: ~1-2 hours
Metabolism: Hepatic via CYP2C9
Half-life elimination: 5.7 hours
Time to peak: 1.5 hours
Excretion: Urine

Pregnancy Risk Factor C/D (3rd trimester)
(Continued)

Flurbiprofen *(Continued)*

Dosage Forms SOLN, ophthalmic (Ocufen®): 0.03% (2.5 mL). **TAB** (Ansaid®): 50 mg, 100 mg

Generic Available Yes

Comments Flurbiprofen is a chiral NSAID with the S-(+) enantiomer possessing most of the beneficial anti-inflammatory activity; both the S-(+) and R-(-) enantiomers possess analgesic activity. All flurbiprofen preparations are marketed as the racemic mixture (equal parts of each enantiomer). Flurbiprofen may be effective in the treatment of periodontal disease. Animal studies have shown flurbiprofen in topical form to be effective in reducing loss of attachment and bone loss. Flurbiprofen as with other NSAIDs can be administered preoperatively in the patient undergoing dental surgery in order to delay the onset and severity of postoperative pain. Doses which have been used are 100 mg twice daily the day before procedure, and 50-100 mg 30 minutes before the procedure.

Selected Readings

Ahmad N, Grad HA, Haas DA, et al, "The Efficacy of Nonopioid Analgesics for Postoperative Dental Pain: A Meta-Analysis," *Anesth Prog*, 1997, 44(4):119-26.

Bragger U, Muhle T, Fourmousis I, et al, "Effect of the NSAID Flurbiprofen on Remodeling After Periodontal Surgery," *J Periodontal Res*, 1997, 32(7):575-82.

Cooper SA and Kupperman A, "The Analgesic Efficacy of Flurbiprofen Compared to Acetaminophen With Codeine," *J Clin Dent*, 1991, 2(3):70-4.

Dionne R, "Additive Analgesia Without Opioid Side Effects," *Compend Contin Educ Dent*, 2000, 21(7):572-4, 576-7.

Dionne RA, "Suppression of Dental Pain by the Preoperative Administration of Flurbiprofen," *Am J Med*, 1986, 80(3A):41-9.

Dionne RA and Berthold CW, "Therapeutic Uses of Nonsteroidal Anti-Inflammatory Drugs in Dentistry," *Crit Rev Oral Biol Med*, 2001, 12(4):315-30.

Dionne RA, Snyder J, and Hargreaves KM, "Analgesic Efficacy of Flurbiprofen in Comparison With Acetaminophen, Acetaminophen Plus Codeine, and Placebo After Impacted Third Molar Removal," *J Oral Maxillofac Surg*, 1994, 52(9):919-24.

Forbes JA, Yorio CC, Selinger LR, et al, "An Evaluation of Flurbiprofen, Aspirin, and Placebo in Postoperative Oral Surgery Pain," *Pharmacotherapy*, 1989, 9(2):66-73.

Gallardo F and Rossi E, "Analgesic Efficacy of Flurbiprofen as Compared to Acetaminophen and Placebo After Periodontal Surgery," *J Periodontol*, 1990, 61(4):224-7.

Jeffcoat MK, Reddy MS, Haigh S, et al, "A Comparison of Topical Ketorolac, Systemic Flurbiprofen, and Placebo for the Inhibition of Bone Loss in Adult Periodontitis," *J Periodontol*, 1995, 66(5):329-38.

Jeffcoat MK, Reddy MS, Wang IC, et al, "The Effect of Systemic Flurbiprofen on Bone Supporting Dental Implants," *J Am Dent Assoc*, 1995, 126(3):305-11.

Malmberg AB and Yaksh TL, "Antinociception Produced by Spinal Delivery of the S and R Enantiomers of Flurbiprofen in the Formalin Test," *Eur J Pharmacol*, 1994, 256(2):205-9.

Nguyen AM, Graham DY, Gage T, et al, "Nonsteroidal Anti-Inflammatory Drug Use in Dentistry: Gastrointestinal Implications," *Gen Dent*, 1999, 47(6):590-6.

Flurbiprofen Sodium *see* Flurbiprofen *on page 596*

5-Flurocytosine *see* Flucytosine *on page 578*

Fluro-Ethyl® *see* Ethyl Chloride and Dichlorotetrafluoroethane *on page 545*

FluShield® *see* Influenza Virus Vaccine *on page 722*

Flutamide (FLOO ta mide)

U.S. Brand Names Eulexin®

Canadian Brand Names Apo®-Flutamide; Euflex®; Eulexin®; Novo-Flutamide; PMS-Flutamide

Mexican Brand Names Eulexin®; Fluken®; Flulem®

Pharmacologic Category Antineoplastic Agent, Antiandrogen

Use In combination therapy with LHRH agonist analogues in treatment of metastatic prostatic carcinoma. A study has shown that the addition of flutamide to leuprolide therapy in patients with advanced prostatic cancer increased median actuarial survival time to 34.9 months versus 27.9 months with leuprolide alone. To achieve benefit to combination therapy, both drugs need to be started simultaneously.

Unlabeled/Investigational Use Treatment of female hirsutism

Local Anesthetic/Vasoconstrictor Precautions No information available to require special precautions

Effects on Dental Treatment

>10%: Hot flashes, nausea, vomiting (11% to 12%)

1% to 10%: Hypertension (1%), drowsiness, confusion, anxiety, nervousness, headache, dizziness, weakness (1%), bruising

Dosage Oral: Adults:

Prostatic carcinoma: 2 capsules every 8 hours for a total daily dose of 750 mg

Female hirsutism: 250 mg daily

Mechanism of Action Nonsteroidal antiandrogen that inhibits androgen uptake or inhibits binding of androgen in target tissues

Other Adverse Effects

>10%:

Endocrine & metabolic: Gynecomastia, breast tenderness, galactorrhea (9% to 42%); impotence; decreased libido; tumor flare

Hepatic: Increased AST (SGOT) and LDH levels, transient, mild

1% to 10%:

Cardiovascular: Edema

Central nervous system: Insomnia

Dermatologic: Pruritus, photosensitivity, herpes zoster
Gastrointestinal: Anorexia, increased appetite, constipation, indigestion, upset stomach (4% to 6%); diarrhea
Hematologic: Anemia (6%), leukopenia (3%), thrombocytopenia (1%)
<1%: Discoloration of urine (yellow), hepatitis, hepatic failure, jaundice, sulfhemoglobinemia, thrombophlebitis, malignant breast neoplasm (male), **MI,** pulmonary embolism

Drug Interactions Substrate of **CYP1A2, 3A4**; Inhibits CYP1A2
Increased Effect/Toxicity: Warfarin effects may be increased.

Dietary/Ethanol/Herb Considerations
Food: May be taken with food; bioavailability unaffected
Herb/Nutraceutical: Avoid St John's wort; may decrease serum concentration.

Pharmacodynamics/Kinetics
Absorption: Oral: Rapid and complete
Protein binding: Parent drug: 94% to 96%; 2-hydroxyflutamide: 92% to 94%
Metabolism: Extensively hepatic to more than 10 metabolites, primarily 2-hydroxyflutamide (active)
Half-life elimination: 5-6 hours (2-hydroxyflutamide)
Excretion: Primarily urine (as metabolites)

Pregnancy Risk Factor D

Generic Available Yes

Comments To achieve benefit to combination therapy, both drugs need to be started simultaneously

Fluticasone (floo TIK a sone)

Related Information
Fluticasone and Salmeterol *on page 601*
Respiratory Diseases *on page 1476*

U.S. Brand Names Cutivate®; Flonase®; Flovent®; Flovent® Rotadisk®

Canadian Brand Names Cutivate™; Flonase®; Flovent®; Flovent® HFA

Mexican Brand Names Cutivate®; Flixonase®; Flixotide®

Pharmacologic Category Corticosteroid, Inhalant (Oral); Corticosteroid, Nasal; Corticosteroid, Topical; Corticosteroid, Topical (Medium Potency)

Synonyms Fluticasone Propionate

Use
Inhalation: Maintenance treatment of asthma as prophylactic therapy. It is also indicated for patients requiring oral corticosteroid therapy for asthma to assist in total discontinuation or reduction of total oral dose. NOT indicated for the relief of acute bronchospasm.
Intranasal: Management of seasonal and perennial allergic rhinitis and nonallergic rhinitis in patients ≥4 years of age
Topical: Relief of inflammation and pruritus associated with corticosteroid-responsive dermatoses in patients ≥3 months of age

Local Anesthetic/Vasoconstrictor Precautions No information available to require special precautions

Effects on Dental Treatment Localized infections with *Candida albicans* or *Aspergillus niger* have occurred frequently in the mouth and pharynx with repetitive use of oral inhaler of corticosteroids. These infections may require treatment with appropriate antifungal therapy or discontinuance of treatment with corticosteroid inhaler.
Oral inhalation (dose-dependent):
>10%: Headache (2% to 22%), upper respiratory tract infection (14% to 22%), throat irritation (3% to 22%), nasal congestion (4% to 16%), pharyngitis (6% to 14%), oral candidiasis (≤11%)
1% to 10%: Nausea/vomiting (1% to 8%), viral GI infection (3% to 5%), GI discomfort/pain (1% to 4%), fever (1% to 7%), sinusitis/sinus infection (3% to 10%), rhinitis (1% to 9%), influenza (3% to 8%), bronchitis (1% to 8%), upper respiratory inflammation (5%), allergic rhinitis (3% to 5%), cough (1% to 5%), nasal discharge (1% to 5%), viral respiratory infection (1% to 5%), viral infection (2% to 5%), pain (1% to 5%)
1% to 3%: Otitis, chest symptoms, palpitations, dizziness, fatigue, malaise, migraine, mood disorders, nervousness, paralysis of cranial nerves, giddiness, fungal skin infection, gastroenteritis, GI infections, mouth/tongue disorder, oral erythema, oral rash, oral ulcerations, stomach disorder, viral gastroenteritis, hematoma, local irritation from inhalant, limb pain, muscle cramps/spasms, musculoskeletal inflammation, earache, chest congestion, dyspnea, epistaxis, laryngitis, lower respiratory infections, mouth irritation, nasal pain, nasopharyngitis, nose/throat polyps, oropharyngeal plaques, sneezing, throat constriction bacterial infections, dental discomfort/pain, dental problems, pressure-induced disorders, postoperative complications, soft tissue injury, tonsillitis, tooth decay, wounds/lacerations
Postmarketing and/or case reports: Agitation, aggression, asthma exacerbation, bronchospasm, chest tightness, hoarseness, hyperglycemia, paradoxical bronchospasm, pneumonia, restlessness, vasculitis, wheezing
Nasal inhalation:
>10%: Headache (7% to 16%), pharyngitis (6% to 8%)
(Continued)

Fluticasone *(Continued)*

1% to 7%: Dizziness (1% to 3%), fever (1% to 3%), nausea/vomiting (3% to 5%), epistaxis (6% to 7%), asthma symptoms (3% to 7%), cough (4%), blood in nasal mucous (1% to 3%), runny nose (1% to 3%), bronchitis (1% to 3%), aches and pains (1% to 3%), flu-like symptoms (1% to 3%)

Dosage

Children:

Asthma: Inhalation, oral:

Flovent®: Children ≥12 years: Refer to adult dosing.

Flovent® Diskus® and Rotadisk®: **Note:** Titrate to the lowest effective dose once asthma stability is achieved; children previously maintained on Flovent® Rotadisk® may require dosage adjustments when transferred to Flovent® Diskus®

Children ≥4-11 years: Dosing based on previous therapy

Bronchodilator alone: Recommended starting dose: 50 mcg twice daily; highest recommended dose: 100 mcg twice daily

Inhaled corticosteroids: Recommended starting dose: 50 mcg twice daily; highest recommended dose: 100 mcg twice daily; a higher starting dose may be considered in patients previously requiring higher doses of inhaled corticosteroids

Children ≥11 years: Refer to adult dosing.

Inflammation/pruritus associated with corticosteroid-responsive dermatoses: Topical: Children ≥3 months: Apply sparingly in a thin film twice daily; therapy should be discontinued when control is achieved. If no improvement is seen within 2 weeks, reassessment of diagnosis may be necessary. Safety and efficacy for use in pediatric patients <3 months have not been established.

Rhinitis: Intranasal: Children ≥4 years and Adolescents: Initial: 1 spray (50 mcg/spray) per nostril once daily; patients not adequately responding or patients with more severe symptoms may use 2 sprays (100 mcg) per nostril. Depending on response, dosage may be reduced to 100 mcg daily. Total daily dosage should not exceed 2 sprays in each nostril (200 mcg)/day. Dosing should be at regular intervals.

Adults:

Asthma: Inhalation, oral (titrate to the lowest effective dose once asthma stability is achieved):

Flovent®: Dosing based on previous therapy

Bronchodilator alone: Recommended starting dose: 88 mcg twice daily; highest recommended dose: 440 mcg twice daily

Inhaled corticosteroids: Recommended starting dose: 88-220 mcg twice daily; highest recommended dose: 440 mcg twice daily; a higher starting dose may be considered in patients previously requiring higher doses of inhaled corticosteroids

Oral corticosteroids: Recommended starting dose: 880 mcg twice daily; highest recommended dose: 880 mcg twice daily; starting dose is patient dependent. In patients on chronic oral corticosteroids therapy, reduce prednisone dose no faster than 2.5 mg/day on a weekly basis; begin taper after ≥1 week of fluticasone therapy

Flovent® Diskus® and Rotadisk®: Dosing based on previous therapy

Bronchodilator alone: Recommended starting dose 100 mcg twice daily; highest recommended dose: 500 mcg twice daily

Inhaled corticosteroids: 100-250 mcg twice daily; highest recommended dose: 500 mcg twice daily; a higher starting dose may be considered in patients previously requiring higher doses of inhaled corticosteroids

Oral corticosteroids: 500-1000 mcg twice daily; highest recommended dose: 1000 mcg twice daily; starting dose is patient dependent. In patients on chronic oral corticosteroids therapy, reduce prednisone dose no faster than 2.5 mg/day on a weekly basis; begin taper after ≥1 week of fluticasone therapy

Inflammation/pruritus associated with corticosteroid-responsive dermatoses: Topical: Apply sparingly in a thin film twice daily; therapy should be discontinued when control is achieved. If no improvement is seen within 2 weeks, reassessment of diagnosis may be necessary.

Rhinitis: Intranasal: Initial: 2 sprays (50 mcg/spray) per nostril once daily; may also be divided into 100 mcg twice a day. After the first few days, dosage may be reduced to 1 spray per nostril once daily for maintenance therapy. Dosing should be at regular intervals.

Dosing adjustment in hepatic impairment: Fluticasone is primarily cleared in the liver; plasma levels may be increased in patients with impairment; use with caution and monitor.

Mechanism of Action Fluticasone belongs to a new group of corticosteroids which utilizes a fluorocarbothioate ester linkage at the 17 carbon position; extremely potent vasoconstrictive and anti-inflammatory activity; has a weak HPA inhibitory potency when applied topically, which gives the drug a high therapeutic index. The effectiveness of inhaled fluticasone is due to its direct local effect. The mechanism of action for all topical corticosteroids is believed to be a combination of three important properties: anti-inflammatory activity, immunosuppressive properties, and antiproliferative actions.

Other Adverse Effects

Oral inhalation (dose-dependent):

>3%:

Gastrointestinal: Diarrhea (1% to 4%)

Neuromuscular & skeletal: Muscle injury (1% to 5%), musculoskeletal pain (1% to 5%), back problems (<1% to 4%)

1% to 3%:

Cardiovascular: Edema

Central nervous system: Sleep disorders

Dermatologic: Acne, dermatitis/dermatosis, eczema, folliculitis, photodermatitis, pruritus, skin rash, urticaria

Endocrine & metabolic: Dysmenorrhea, fluid disturbances, goiter, uric acid metabolism disorder

Gastrointestinal: Abdominal discomfort/pain, appetite disturbances, colitis, dyspepsia, weight gain

Genitourinary: Urinary tract infection

Hematologic: Hematoma

Hepatic: Cholecystitis

Neuromuscular & skeletal: Arthralgia/articular rheumatism

Ocular: Blepharoconjunctivitis, conjunctivitis, irritation, keratitis

Otic: Ear polyps

Miscellaneous: Burns, contusion, cysts lumps, masses

Postmarketing and/or case reports: Aphonia, cataracts, Churg-Strauss syndrome, Cushingoid features, depression, ecchymoses, eosinophilic conditions, glaucoma, growth velocity reduction in children/adolescents, increased intraocular pressure

Nasal inhalation:

1% to 10%: Gastrointestinal: Abdominal pain (1% to 3%), diarrhea (1% to 3%)

<1% and postmarketing reports: **Alteration or loss of sense of taste** and/or smell, **anaphylaxis/anaphylactoid reactions**, angioedema, **blurred vision, bronchospasm,** cataracts, conjunctivitis, dry/irritated eyes, **dry throat, dyspnea, facial and tongue edema,** glaucoma, **hypersensitivity reactions**, increased intraocular pressure, **nasal septal perforation (rare), nasal ulcer,** pruritus, skin rash, **sore throat, throat irritation,** urticaria, voice changes, **wheezing**

Topical:

Dermatologic: Pruritus (3%), skin irritation (3%), exacerbation of eczema (2%), dry skin (1%)

Neuromuscular & skeletal: Numbness of fingers (1%)

Reported with other topical corticosteroids (in decreasing order of occurrence): **Irritation,** folliculitis, acneiform eruptions, hypopigmentation, perioral dermatitis, **allergic contact dermatitis, secondary infection, skin atrophy,** striae, miliaria, pustular psoriasis from chronic plaque psoriasis

Drug Interactions Substrate of CYP3A4

Increased Effect/Toxicity:

CYP3A4 inhibitors: Serum level and/or toxicity of fluticasone may be increased; this effect was shown with ketoconazole, but not erythromycin. Other potential inhibitors include amiodarone, cimetidine, clarithromycin, delavirdine, diltiazem, dirithromycin, disulfiram, fluoxetine, fluvoxamine, grapefruit juice, indinavir, itraconazole, ketoconazole, nefazodone, nevirapine, propoxyphene, quinupristin-dalfopristin, ritonavir, saquinavir, verapamil, zafirlukast, zileuton.

Salmeterol: The addition of salmeterol has been demonstrated to improve response to inhaled corticosteroids (as compared to increasing steroid dosage).

Dietary/Ethanol/Herb Considerations Herb/Nutraceutical: In theory, St John's wort may decrease serum concentration by inducing CYP3A3/4 isoenzymes.

Pharmacodynamics/Kinetics

Absorption:

Cream: 5% (increased with inflammation)

Oral inhalation: Primarily via lungs, minimal GI absorption due to presystemic metabolism

Distribution: 4.2 L/kg

Protein binding: 91%

Metabolism: Hepatic via CYP3A4 to 17β-carboxylic acid (negligible activity)

Bioavailability: Oral inhalation: 14% to 30%

Excretion: Feces (as parent drug and metabolites); urine (<5% as metabolites)

Pregnancy Risk Factor C

Generic Available No

Fluticasone and Salmeterol (floo TIK a sone & sal ME te role)

Related Information

Fluticasone *on page 599*

Salmeterol *on page 1205*

(Continued)

Fluticasone and Salmeterol *(Continued)*

U.S. Brand Names Advair™ Diskus®

Canadian Brand Names Advair™ Diskus®

Pharmacologic Category $Beta_2$ Agonist; Corticosteroid, Inhalant (Oral)

Synonyms Salmeterol and Fluticasone

Use Maintenance treatment of asthma in adults and children ≥12 years; **not** for use for relief of acute bronchospasm

Local Anesthetic/Vasoconstrictor Precautions No information to require special precautions

Effects on Dental Treatment Localized infections with *Candida albicans* or *Aspergillus niger* have occurred frequently in the mouth and pharynx with repetitive use of oral inhaler of corticosteroids. These infections may require treatment with appropriate antifungal therapy or discontinuance of treatment with corticosteroid inhaler.

>10%: Upper respiratory tract infection (21% to 27%), pharyngitis (10% to 13%),headache (12% to 13%)

1% to 10%: Oral candidiasis (1% to 4%), palpitations, bronchitis (2% to 8%), upper respiratory tract inflammation (6% to 7%), cough (3% to 6%), sinusitis (4% to 5%), hoarseness/dysphonia (2% to 5%), viral respiratory tract infections (4%) GI infections, oral discomfort/pain, oral erythema/rash, oral ulcerations, unusual taste, viral GI infections (≤3%), nasal congestion, ear/nose/throat infections, lower respiratory tract infections, nasal sinus disorders, pneumonia, rhinitis, rhinorrhea/post nasal drip, sneezing, wheezing, ear signs and symptoms (nonspecified) fractures, muscle injuries, muscle stiffness, muscle tightness/rigidity, musculoskeletal pain (2% to 4%) blood in nasal mucosa, congestion, lower respiratory signs and symptoms (nonspecified), nasal irritation, nasal signs and symptoms (nonspecified), allergies/allergic reactions, bacterial infections, candidiasis (≤3%), diaphoresis, viral infections

Dosage Oral inhalation (do not use to transfer patients from systemic corticosteroid therapy):

Children ≥12 and Adults: One inhalation twice daily, morning and evening, 12 hours apart

Advair™ Diskus® is available in 3 strengths, initial dose prescribed should be based upon previous asthma therapy. Dose should be increased after 2 weeks if adequate response is not achieved. Patients should be titrated to lowest effective dose once stable. (Because each strength contains salmeterol 50 mcg/inhalation, dose adjustments should be made by changing inhaler strength. No more than 1 inhalation of any strength should be taken more than twice a day). Maximum dose: Fluticasone 500 mcg/salmeterol 50 mcg, one inhalation twice daily.

Patients not currently on inhaled corticosteroids: Fluticasone 100 mcg/salmeterol 50 mcg

Patients currently using inhaled beclomethasone dipropionate:
- ≤420 mcg/day: Fluticasone 100 mcg/salmeterol 50 mcg
- 462-840 mcg/day: Fluticasone 250 mcg/salmeterol 50 mcg

Patients currently using inhaled budesonide:
- ≤400 mcg/day: Fluticasone 100 mcg/salmeterol 50 mcg
- 800-1200 mcg/day: Fluticasone 250 mcg/salmeterol 50 mcg
- 1600 mcg/day: Fluticasone 500 mcg/salmeterol 50 mcg

Patients currently using inhaled flunisolide:
- ≤1000 mcg/day: Fluticasone 100 mcg/salmeterol 50 mcg
- 1250-2000 mcg/day: Fluticasone 250 mcg/salmeterol 50 mcg

Patients currently using inhaled fluticasone propionate aerosol:
- ≤176 mcg/day: Fluticasone 100 mcg/salmeterol 50 mcg
- 440 mcg/day: Fluticasone 250 mcg/salmeterol 50 mcg
- 660-880 mcg/day: Fluticasone 500 mcg/salmeterol 50 mcg

Patients currently using inhaled fluticasone propionate powder:
- ≤200 mcg/day: Fluticasone 100 mcg/salmeterol 50 mcg
- 500 mcg/day: Fluticasone 250 mcg/salmeterol 50 mcg
- 1000 mcg/day: Fluticasone 500 mcg/salmeterol 50 mcg

Patients currently using inhaled triamcinolone acetonide:
- ≤1000 mcg/day: Fluticasone 100 mcg/salmeterol 50 mcg
- 1100-1600 mcg/day: Fluticasone 250 mcg/salmeterol 50 mcg

Mechanism of Action Combination of fluticasone (corticosteroid) and salmeterol (long-acting $beta_2$ agonist) designed to improve pulmonary function and control over what is produced by either agent when used alone. Because fluticasone and salmeterol act locally in the lung, plasma levels do not predict therapeutic effect.

Fluticasone: The mechanism of action for all topical corticosteroids is believed to be a combination of three important properties: Anti-inflammatory activity, immunosuppressive properties, and antiproliferative actions. Fluticasone has extremely potent vasoconstrictive and anti-inflammatory activity.

Salmeterol: Relaxes bronchial smooth muscle by selective action on $beta_2$-receptors with little effect on heart rate

Other Adverse Effects

1% to 10%:

Cardiovascular: Chest symptoms, fluid retention

Central nervous system: Compressed nerve syndromes, hypnagogic effects, pain, sleep disorders, tremors

Dermatologic: Hives, skin flakiness/ichthyosis, urticaria, viral skin infections

Gastrointestinal: Appendicitis, constipation, GI disorder, infection, signs and symptoms (nonspecified), nausea/vomiting (4% to 6%), diarrhea (2% to 4%), pain/discomfort (1% to 4%)

Hematologic: Contusions/hematomas, lymphatic signs and symptoms (nonspecified)

Hepatic: Abnormal LFTs

Neuromuscular & skeletal: Arthralgia, articular rheumatism, bone/cartilage disorders, fractures, muscle injuries, muscle stiffness, muscle tightness/rigidity, musculoskeletal pain (2% to 4%)

Ocular: Conjunctivitis, eye redness, keratitis

Miscellaneous: Burns, sweat/sebum disorders, wounds and lacerations

Postmarketing and/or case reports: Serious exacerbations of asthma (some fatal), abdominal pain, **agitation, aggression,** aphonia, **arrhythmias,** back pain, **bronchospasm and immediate bronchospasm, chest congestion, chest tightness, choking, contact dermatitis, contusions,** cramps, Cushing syndrome, Cushingoid features, depression, dysmenorrhea, **dyspnea,** dyspepsia, **earache,** ecchymoses, growth velocity reduction in children/adolescents, hypercorticism, **hyperglycemia, hypersensitivity reaction (immediate and delayed), influenza, laryngeal spasm/irritation,** irregular menstruation, **muscle spasm,** myositis, pallor, **paresthesia,** paradoxical tracheitis, paranasal sinus pain, photodermatitis, PID, restlessness, stridor, vaginal candidiasis, vaginitis, vulvovaginitis, rare cases of vasculitis (Churg-Strauss syndrome), **ventricular tachycardia,** weight gain, **xerostomia**

Drug Interactions

Increased Effect/Toxicity: Diuretics (loop, thiazide): Hypokalemia from diuretics may be worsened by beta-agonists (dose related); use with caution. Ketoconazole and other CYP3A4 inhibitors may increase levels and/or effects of fluticasone. May cause increased cardiovascular toxicity with MAO inhibitors or tricyclic antidepressants; wait at least 2 weeks after discontinuing these agents to start fluticasone/salmeterol.

Decreased Effect: Beta-adrenergic blockers (eg, propranolol) may decreased the effect of salmeterol component and may cause bronchospasm in asthmatics; use with caution.

Pharmacodynamics/Kinetics

Advair™ Diskus®:

Onset of action: 30-60 minutes

Peak effect: ≥1 week for full effect

Duration: 12 hours

Pregnancy Risk Factor C

Generic Available No

Fluticasone Propionate *see* Fluticasone *on page 599*

Fluvastatin (FLOO va sta tin)

Related Information

Cardiovascular Diseases *on page 1456*

U.S. Brand Names Lescol®; Lescol® XL

Canadian Brand Names Lescol®

Mexican Brand Names Canef®; Lescol®

Pharmacologic Category Antilipemic Agent, HMG-CoA Reductase Inhibitor

Use To be used as a component of multiple risk factor intervention in patients at risk for atherosclerosis vascular disease due to hypercholesterolemia

Adjunct to dietary therapy to reduce elevated total cholesterol (total-C), LDL-C, triglyceride, and apolipoprotein B (apo-B) levels and to increase HDL-C in primary hypercholesterolemia and mixed dyslipidemia (Fredrickson types IIa and IIb); to slow the progression of coronary atherosclerosis in patients with coronary heart disease

Local Anesthetic/Vasoconstrictor Precautions No information available to require special precautions

Effects on Dental Treatment 1% to 10%: Headache (9%), fatigue (3%), nausea (3%), sinusitis (3%), bronchitis (2%)

Dosage Adults: Oral:

Patients requiring ≥25% decrease in LDL-C: 40 mg capsule or 80 mg extended release tablet once daily in the evening; may also use 40 mg capsule twice daily

Patients requiring <25% decrease in LDL-C: 20 mg capsule once daily in the evening

Note: Dosing range: 20-80 mg/day; adjust dose based on response to therapy; maximum response occurs within 4-6 weeks

(Continued)

Fluvastatin *(Continued)*

Dosing adjustment in renal impairment: Less than 6% excreted renally; no adjustment required in mild to moderate impairment; use with caution in severe impairment

Dosing adjustment in hepatic impairment: Levels may accumulate in patients with liver disease (increased AUC and C_{max}); use caution with severe hepatic impairment or heavy ethanol ingestion; contraindicated in active liver disease or unexplained transaminase elevations; decrease dose and monitor effects carefully in patients with hepatic insufficiency

Mechanism of Action Acts by competitively inhibiting 3-hydroxyl-3-methylglutaryl-coenzyme A (HMG-CoA) reductase, the enzyme that catalyzes the reduction of HMG-CoA to mevalonate; this is an early rate-limiting step in cholesterol biosynthesis. HDL is increased while total, LDL and VLDL cholesterols, apolipoprotein B, and plasma triglycerides are decreased.

Other Adverse Effects As reported with capsules (in general, reactions with extended release tablet were similar, but less frequent):

1% to 10%:

Central nervous system: Insomnia (3%)

Gastrointestinal: Dyspepsia (8%), diarrhea (5%), abdominal pain (5%)

Genitourinary: Urinary tract infection (2%)

Neuromuscular & skeletal: Myalgia (5%)

<1% including additional class-related events (not necessarily reported with fluvastatin therapy) and postmarketing case reports: Myopathy, arthralgia, muscle cramps, increased CPK (>10x normal), rhabdomyolysis, renal failure (secondary to rhabdomyolysis), blurred vision, alteration in taste, impaired extraocular muscle movement, facial paresis, tremor, dizziness, memory loss, vertigo, paresthesia, peripheral neuropathy, peripheral nerve palsy, anxiety, depression, psychic disturbance, hypersensitivity reaction, angioedema, anaphylaxis, systemic lupus erythematosus-like syndrome, polymyalgia rheumatica, dermatomyositis, vasculitis, purpura, thrombocytopenia, leukopenia, hemolytic anemia, positive ANA, increased ESR, eosinophilia, arthritis, urticaria, photosensitivity, fever, chills, flushing, malaise, dyspnea, rash, toxic epidermal necrolysis, erythema multiforme, Stevens-Johnson syndrome, pancreatitis, hepatitis, cholestatic jaundice, fatty liver, cirrhosis, fulminant hepatic necrosis, hepatoma, anorexia, vomiting, alopecia, pruritus, nodules, skin discoloration, dryness of skin/mucous membranes, nail changes, gynecomastia, decreased libido, erectile dysfunction, impotence, cataracts, ophthalmoplegia, elevated transaminases, increased alkaline phosphatase, increased GGT, hyperbilirubinemia, thyroid dysfunction

Drug Interactions Substrate of CYP2C8/9, 2D6, 3A4; Inhibits CYP1A2, **2C8/9**, 2D6, 3A4

Increased Effect/Toxicity: Cimetidine, omeprazole, ranitidine, and ritonavir may increase fluvastatin blood levels. Clofibrate, erythromycin, gemfibrozil, fenofibrate, and niacin may increase the risk of myopathy and rhabdomyolysis. Anticoagulant effect of warfarin may be increased by fluvastatin. Cholestyramine effect will be additive with fluvastatin if administration times are separated. Fluvastatin may increase C_{max} and decrease clearance of digoxin.

Decreased Effect: Administration of cholestyramine at the same time with fluvastatin reduces absorption and clinical effect of fluvastatin. Separate administration times by at least 4 hours. Rifampin and rifabutin may decrease fluvastatin blood levels.

Dietary/Ethanol/Herb Considerations

Ethanol: Avoid excessive consumption due to potential hepatic effects.

Food: May be taken with food; reduces rate but not the extent of absorption. Requires standard cholesterol-lowering diet for 3-6 months prior to and during therapy.

Herb/Nutraceutical: St John's wort is a CYP3A/34 isoenzyme inducer and may decrease serum concentration.

Pharmacodynamics/Kinetics

Distribution: V_d: 0.35 L/kg

Protein binding: >98%

Metabolism: To inactive and active metabolites [oxidative metabolism via CYP2C9 (75%), 2C8 (~5%), and 3A4 (~20%) isoenzymes]; active forms do not circulate systemically; extensive first-pass hepatic extraction

Bioavailability: Absolute: Capsule: 24%; Extended release tablet: 29%

Half-life elimination: Capsule: <3 hours; Extended release tablet: 9 hours

Excretion: Feces (90%): urine (5%)

Pregnancy Risk Factor X

Generic Available No

Fluvirin® *see* Influenza Virus Vaccine *on page 722*

Fluvoxamine (floo VOKS ah meen)

U.S. Brand Names Luvox® [DSC]

Canadian Brand Names Alti-Fluvoxamine; Apo®-Fluvoxamine; Luvox®; Novo-Fluvoxamine; Nu-Fluvoxamine; PMS-Fluvoxamine

Mexican Brand Names Luvox®

Pharmacologic Category Antidepressant, Selective Serotonin Reuptake Inhibitor

Synonyms Luvox® [DSC]

Use Treatment of obsessive-compulsive disorder (OCD) in children ≥8 years of age and adults

Unlabeled/Investigational Use Treatment of major depression, panic disorder, anxiety disorders in children

Local Anesthetic/Vasoconstrictor Precautions Although caution should be used in patients taking tricyclic antidepressants, no interactions have been reported with vasoconstrictors and fluvoxamine, a nontricyclic antidepressant which acts to increase serotonin

Effects on Dental Treatment Problems with SSRI-induced bruxism have been reported and may preclude their use; clinicians attempting to evaluate any patient with bruxism or involuntary muscle movement, who is simultaneously being treated with an SSRI drug, should be aware of the potential association.

>10%: Xerostomia (14%), headache (22%), somnolence (22%), nervousness (12%), dizziness (11%), nausea (40%), weakness (14%)

1% to 10%: Abnormal taste, vomiting, palpitations, somnolence, mania, hypomania, abnormal thinking, agitation, anxiety, malaise, amnesia, yawning, CNS stimulation, tremors, blurred vision, dyspnea, diaphoresis

Dosage Oral (divide into 2 doses when total daily dose exceeds 50 mg):

Children 8-17 years: Initial: 25 mg at bedtime; adjust in 25 mg increments at 4- to 7-day intervals, as tolerated, to maximum therapeutic benefit: Range: 50-200 mg/day

Maximum: Children: 8-11 years: 200 mg/day, adolescents: 300 mg/day; lower doses may be effective in female versus male patients

Adults: Initial: 50 mg at bedtime; adjust in 50 mg increments at 4- to 7-day intervals; usual dose range: 100-300 mg/day; divide total daily dose into 2 doses; administer larger portion at bedtime

Dosing adjustment for elderly or in hepatic impairment: Reduce dose; titrate slowly

Mechanism of Action Inhibits CNS neuron serotonin uptake; minimal or no effect on reuptake of norepinephrine or dopamine; does not significantly bind to alpha-adrenergic, histamine or cholinergic receptors

Other Adverse Effects

>10%:

Central nervous system: Insomnia (21%)

Gastrointestinal: Diarrhea (11%)

1% to 10%:

Central nervous system: Vertigo, hypertonia

Endocrine & metabolic: Decreased libido

Gastrointestinal: Abdominal pain, dyspepsia, constipation, anorexia, flatulence, weight gain

Genitourinary: Delayed ejaculation, impotence, anorgasmia, urinary frequency, urinary retention

<1%: Acne, alopecia, anemia, angina, ataxia, bradycardia, delayed menstruation, dermatitis, dry skin, dysuria, elevated liver transaminases, extrapyramidal symptoms, hyponatremia, lactation, leukocytosis, nocturia, priapism, seizures, serotonin syndrome, SIADH, thrombocytopenia, urticaria

Postmarketing and/or case reports (causal relationship not established): Agranulocytosis, akinesia with fever, anaphylaxis, angioedema, aplastic anemia, Henoch-Schönlein purpura, hepatitis, neuropathy, pancreatitis, Stevens-Johnson syndrome, torsade de pointes, toxic epidermal necrolysis, vasculitis, ventricular tachycardia

Drug Interactions Substrate of **CYP1A2, 2D6**; Inhibits **CYP1A2, 2B6**, 2C8/9, **2C19**, 2D6, **3A4**

Increased Effect/Toxicity:

MAO inhibitors: Fluvoxamine should not be used with nonselective MAO inhibitors (phenelzine, isocarboxazid) and drugs with MAO inhibitor properties (linezolid); fatal reactions have been reported. Wait 5 weeks after stopping fluvoxamine before starting a nonselective MAO inhibitor and 2 weeks after stopping an MAO inhibitor before starting fluvoxamine. Concurrent selegiline has been associated with mania, hypertension, or serotonin syndrome (risk may be reduced relative to nonselective MAO inhibitors).

Phenothiazines: Fluvoxamine may inhibit the metabolism of thioridazine or mesoridazine, resulting in increased plasma levels and increasing the risk of QT_c interval prolongation. This may lead to serious ventricular arrhythmias, such as torsade de pointes-type arrhythmias and sudden death. Do not use together. Wait at least 5 weeks after discontinuing fluvoxamine prior to starting thioridazine.

(Continued)

Fluvoxamine *(Continued)*

Combined used of SSRIs and amphetamines, buspirone, meperidine, nefazodone, serotonin agonists (such as sumatriptan), sibutramine, other SSRIs, sympathomimetics, ritonavir, tramadol, and venlafaxine may increase the risk of serotonin syndrome. Fluvoxamine may increase serum levels/effects of benzodiazepines (alprazolam and diazepam), beta-blockers (except atenolol or nadolol), carbamazepine, carvedilol, clozapine, cyclosporin (and possibly tacrolimus), dextromethorphan, digoxin, haloperidol, HMG-CoA reductase inhibitors (lovastatin and simvastatin - increasing the risk of rhabdomyolysis), mexiletine, phenytoin, propafenone, quinidine, tacrine, theophylline, trazodone, tricyclic antidepressants, and valproic acid. Concurrent lithium may increase risk of nephrotoxicity. Risk of hyponatremia may increase with concurrent use of loop diuretics (bumetanide, furosemide, torsemide). Fluvoxamine may increase the hypoprothrombinemic response to warfarin.

Combined use of sumatriptan (and other serotonin agonists) may result in toxicity; weakness, hyper-reflexia, and incoordination have been observed with sumatriptan and SSRIs. In addition, concurrent use may theoretically increase the risk of serotonin syndrome; includes sumatriptan, naratriptan, rizatriptan, and zolmitriptan.

Decreased Effect: Cyproheptadine, a serotonin antagonist, may inhibit the effects of serotonin reuptake inhibitors (fluvoxamine); monitor for altered antidepressant response.

Dietary/Ethanol/Herb Considerations

Ethanol: Although ethanol may not cause much CNS depression here, depressed patients should avoid/limit intake.

Food: Fluids, fruit, and fiber may reduce constipation. Buttermilk, boiled milk, or yogurt may reduce diarrhea. Avoid caffeine.

Herb/Nutraceutical: Avoid kava, SAMe, St John's wort, and valerian; may increase risk of serotonin syndrome and/or excessive sedation. The bioavailability of melatonin has been reported to be increased by fluvoxamine; acute psychosis may result. Avoid tryptophan; may cause serotonin syndrome.

Pharmacodynamics/Kinetics

Absorption: Steady-state plasma concentrations have been noted to be 2-3 times higher in children than those in adolescents; female children demonstrated a significantly higher AUC than males

Distribution: V_d: ~25 L/kg

Protein binding: ~80%, primarily to albumin

Metabolism: Hepatic

Bioavailability: 53%; not significantly affected by food

Half-life elimination: ~15 hours

Time to peak, plasma: 3-8 hours

Excretion: Urine

Pregnancy Risk Factor C

Generic Available Yes

Selected Readings

Friedlander AH, Mahler ME, "Major Depressive Disorder. Psychopathology, Medical Management, and Dental Implications," *J Am Dent Assoc*, 2001, 132(5):629-38.

Gerber PE and Lynd LD, "Selective Serotonin Reuptake Inhibitor-induced Movement Disorders," *Ann Pharmacother*, 1998, 32(6):692-8.

Wynn RL, "New Antidepressant Medications," *Gen Dent*, 1997, 45(1):24-8.

Fluzone® *see* Influenza Virus Vaccine *on page 722*

FML® *see* Fluorometholone *on page 587*

FML® Forte *see* Fluorometholone *on page 587*

FML-S® *see* Sulfacetamide and Fluorometholone *on page 1250*

Focalin™ *see* Dexmethylphenidate *on page 417*

Foille® [OTC] *see* Benzocaine *on page 169*

Foille® Medicated First Aid [OTC] *see* Benzocaine *on page 169*

Foille® Plus [OTC] *see* Benzocaine *on page 169*

Folacin *see* Folic Acid *on page 606*

Folacin, Vitamin B_{12}, and Vitamin B_6 *see* Folic Acid, Cyanocobalamin, and Pyridoxine *on page 607*

Folate *see* Folic Acid *on page 606*

Folgard® [OTC] *see* Folic Acid, Cyanocobalamin, and Pyridoxine *on page 607*

Folic Acid (FOE lik AS id)

Canadian Brand Names Apo®-Folic

Mexican Brand Names A.f. Valdecasas®; Flynoken®; Folitab

Pharmacologic Category Vitamin, Water Soluble

Synonyms Folacin; Folate; Pteroylglutamic Acid

Use

Dental: Treatment of megaloblastic and macrocytic anemias due to folate deficiency

Medical: Dietary supplement in prevention of neural tube defects

Local Anesthetic/Vasoconstrictor Precautions No information available to require special precautions

Effects on Dental Treatment Frequency not defined: Flushing, irritability, confusion, malaise, GI upset, bronchospasm, hypersensitivity reactions

Dosage Oral, I.M., I.V., **S.C.:**

Infants: 0.1 mg/day

Children: Initial: 1 mg/day

Deficiency: 0.5-1 mg/day

Maintenance dose:

<4 years: Up to 0.3 mg/day

>4 years: 0.4 mg/day

Adults: Initial: 1 mg/day

Deficiency: 1-3 mg/day

Maintenance dose: 0.5 mg/day

Women of childbearing age, pregnant, and lactating women: 0.8 mg/day

RDA:

Adult male: 0.15-0.2 mg/day

Adult female: 400 mcg/day

Mechanism of Action Folic acid is necessary for formation of a number of coenzymes in many metabolic systems, particularly for purine and pyrimidine synthesis; required for nucleoprotein synthesis and maintenance in erythropoiesis; stimulates WBC and platelet production in folate deficiency anemia

Other Adverse Effects Frequency not defined:

Central nervous system: Difficulty sleeping

Dermatologic: Pruritus, rash

Contraindications Pernicious, aplastic, or normocytic anemias

Warnings/Precautions Doses >0.1 mg/day may obscure pernicious anemia with continuing irreversible nerve damage progression; the dose that masks anemia is controversial, but doses of 400 mcg daily (or even less) have been reported. Resistance to treatment may occur with depressed hematopoiesis, alcoholism, deficiencies of other vitamins. Injection contains benzyl alcohol (1.5%) as preservative (use care in administration to neonates).

Drug Interactions Decreased Effect: In folate-deficient patients, folic acid therapy (>15 mg/day) may increase phenytoin metabolism. Phenytoin, primidone, para-aminosalicylic acid, and sulfasalazine may decrease serum folate concentrations and cause deficiency. Oral contraceptives may also impair folate metabolism producing depletion, but the effect is unlikely to cause anemia or megaloblastic changes. Concurrent administration of chloramphenicol and folic acid may result in antagonism of the hematopoietic response to folic acid; dihydrofolate reductase inhibitors (eg, methotrexate, trimethoprim) may interfere with folic acid utilization.

Pharmacodynamics/Kinetics

Onset of effect: Peak effect: Oral: 0.5-1 hour

Absorption: Proximal part of small intestine

Pregnancy Risk Factor A/C (dose exceeding RDA recommendation)

Dosage Forms INJ, solution: 5 mg/mL (10 mL). **TAB:** 0.4 mg, 0.8 mg, 1 mg

Generic Available Yes

Folic Acid, Cyanocobalamin, and Pyridoxine

(FOE lik AS id, sye an oh koe BAL a min, & peer i DOKS een)

Related Information

Folic Acid *on page 606*

U.S. Brand Names Folgard® [OTC]; Foltx®

Pharmacologic Category Vitamin

Synonyms Cyanocobalamin, Folic Acid, and Pyridoxine; Folacin, Vitamin B_{12}, and Vitamin B_6; Pyridoxine, Folic Acid, and Cyanocobalamin

Use Nutritional supplement in end-stage renal failure, dialysis, hyperhomocysteinemia, homocystinuria, malabsorption syndromes, dietary deficiencies

Local Anesthetic/Vasoconstrictor Precautions No information available to require special precautions

Effects on Dental Treatment No significant effects or complications reported

Dosage Oral: Adults: 1 tablet daily

Generic Available No

Folinic Acid *see* Leucovorin *on page 783*

Follistim® *see* Follitropins *on page 607*

Follitropin Alfa *see* Follitropins *on page 607*

Follitropin Alpha *see* Follitropins *on page 607*

Follitropin Beta *see* Follitropins *on page 607*

Follitropins (foe li TRO pins)

U.S. Brand Names Bravelle™; Fertinex®; Follistim®; Gonal-F®

Canadian Brand Names Gonal-F®; Puregon™

Mexican Brand Names Gonal-F®; Puregon®

Pharmacologic Category Gonadotropin; Ovulation Stimulator

(Continued)

Follitropins *(Continued)*

Synonyms Follitropin Alfa; Follitropin Alpha; Follitropin Beta; Recombinant Human Follicle Stimulating Hormone; rFSH-alpha; rFSH-beta; rhFSH-alpha; rhFSH-beta; Urofollitropin

Use

Urofollitropin:

Bravelle™: Ovulation induction in patients who previously received pituitary suppression; Assisted Reproductive Technologies (ART)

Fertinex®: Ovulation induction in patients with polycystic ovary syndrome and infertility who have not responded to clomiphene citrate therapy; ART

Follitropin alfa (Gonal-F®), Follitropin beta (Follistim®): Ovulation induction in patients in whom the cause of infertility is functional and not caused by primary ovarian failure; ART; spermatogenesis induction

Local Anesthetic/Vasoconstrictor Precautions No information available to require special precautions

Effects on Dental Treatment Frequency varies by specific product and route of administration.

2% to 10%: Headache, dizziness, fever hives, nausea, vomiting, exacerbation of asthma, sinusitis, pharyngitis, joint pains, malaise, headache, fatigue, flu-like symptoms

<2% and/or postmarketing reports (limited to important or life-threatening): Asthma, atelectasis, hypotension, migraine, paresthesia, respiratory distress

Dosage Use the lowest dose consistent with the expectation of good results. Over the course of treatment, doses may vary depending on individual patient response. When used for ovulation induction, if response to follitropin is appropriate, hCG is given 1 day following the last dose. Withhold hCG if serum estradiol is >2000 pg/mL, if the ovaries are abnormally enlarged, or if abdominal pain occurs.

Adults:

Urofollitropin: Female:

Bravelle™: Ovulation induction: I.M., S.C.: Initial: 150 int. units daily for the first 5 days of treatment. Dose adjustments of ≤75-150 int. units can be made every ≥2 days; maximum daily dose: 450 int. units; treatment >12 days is not recommended

ART: S.C.: 225 int. units for the first 5 days; dose may be adjusted based on patient response, but adjustments should not be made more frequently than once every 2 days; maximum adjustment: 75-150 int. units; maximum daily dose: 450 int. units; maximum duration of treatment: 12 days

Fertinex®: S.C.:

Ovulation induction: Initial: 75 int. units/day; consider dose adjustment after 5-7 days. Do not increase more than twice in any cycle or by more than 75 int. units per adjustment; dosage range: 75-300 int. units/day

ART: Initiate therapy in the early follicular phase (cycle day 2 or day 3) at a dose of 150 int. units/day, until sufficient follicular development is attained; in most cases, therapy should not exceed 10 days

Follitropin alfa (Gonal-F®): S.C.:

Ovulation induction: Female: Initial: 75 int. units/day; consider dose adjustment after 5-7 days; additional dose adjustments of up to 37.5 int. units may be considered after 14 days; further dose increases of the same magnitude can be made, if necessary, every 7 days (maximum dose: 300 int. units)

ART: Female: Initiate therapy with follitropin alfa in the early follicular phase (cycle day 2 or day 3) at a dose of 150 int. units/day, until sufficient follicular development is attained. In most cases, therapy should not exceed 10 days. In patients whose endogenous gonadotropin levels are suppressed, initiate follitropin alfa at a dose of 225 int. units/day. Continue treatment until adequate follicular development is indicated as determined by ultrasound in combination with measurement of serum estradiol levels. Consider adjustments to dose after 5 days based on the patient's response; adjust subsequent dosage every 3-5 days by ≤75-150 int. units additionally at each adjustment. Doses >450 int. units/day are not recommended. Once adequate follicular development is evident, administer hCG (5000-10,000 units) to induce final follicular maturation in preparation for oocyte.

Spermatogenesis induction: Male: Therapy should begin with hCG pretreatment until serum testosterone is in normal range, then 150 int. units 3 times/week with hCG 3 times/week; continue with lowest dose needed to induce spermatogenesis (maximum dose: 300 int. units 3 times/week); may be given for up to 18 months

Follitropin beta (Follistim®):

Female: I.M., S.C.:

Ovulation induction: Stepwise approach: Initiate therapy with 75 int. units/day for up to 14 days. Increase by 37.5 int. units at weekly intervals until follicular growth or serum estradiol levels indicate an adequate response. The maximum, individualized, daily dose that has been safely used for ovulation induction in patients during clinical trials is 300 int. units.

ART: A starting dose of 150-225 int. units of follitropin beta is recommended for at least the first 4 days of treatment. The dose may be adjusted for the individual patient based upon their ovarian response. Daily maintenance doses ranging from 75-300 int. units for 6-12 days are usually sufficient, although longer treatment may be necessary. Maintenance doses of up to 375-600 int. units may be necessary according to individual response. The maximum daily dose used in clinical studies is 600 int. units. When a sufficient number of follicles of adequate size are present, the final maturation of the follicles is induced by administering hCG at a dose of 5000-10,000 int. units. Oocyte retrieval is performed 34-36 hours later. Withhold hCG in cases where the ovaries are abnormally enlarged on the last day of follitropin beta therapy.

Male: S.C.: Spermatogenesis induction: **Note:** Begin therapy with hCG pretreatment to normalize serum testosterone levels. Once normal levels are reached, follitropin beta therapy is initiated, and must be administered concurrently with hCG treatment.

450 int. units/week given as 225 int. units twice weekly or 150 int. units 3 times/week with hCG; treatment response was noted at up to 12 months

Mechanism of Action Urofollitropin is a preparation of highly purified follicle-stimulating hormone (FSH) extracted from the urine of postmenopausal women. Follitropin alfa and follitropin beta are human FSH preparations of recombinant DNA origin. Follitropins stimulate ovarian follicular growth in women who do not have primary ovarian failure, and stimulate spermatogenesis in men with hypogonadotrophic hypogonadism. FSH is required for normal follicular growth, maturation, gonadal steroid production, and spermatogenesis.

Other Adverse Effects Frequency varies by specific product and route of administration.

2% to 10%:

Dermatologic: Acne (male), dermoid cyst (male), dry skin, body rash, hair loss,

Endocrine & metabolic: Ovarian hyperstimulation syndrome, adnexal torsion, mild to moderate ovarian enlargement, abdominal pain, ovarian cysts, breast tenderness, gynecomastia (male)

Gastrointestinal: Diarrhea, abdominal cramps, bloating, flatulence, dyspepsia

Genitourinary: Urinary tract infection, menstrual disorder, intermenstrual bleeding, dysmenorrhea, cervical lesion

Local: Pain, rash, swelling, or irritation at the site of injection

Neuromuscular & skeletal: Back pain, varicose veins (male)

Miscellaneous: Febrile reactions

<2% and/or postmarketing reports (limited to important or life-threatening): Adnexal torsion, atelectasis, congenital abnormalities (incidence not greater than in general population), hemoperitoneum, vaginal hemorrhage

Pharmacodynamics/Kinetics

Onset of action: Peak effect: Spermatogenesis, median: 165 days (range: 25-327 days); Follicle development: Within cycle

Absorption: Rate limited: I.M., S.C.: Slower than elimination rate

Distribution: Mean V_d: Follitropin alfa: 10 L; Follitropin beta: 8 L

Metabolism: Total clearance of follitropin alfa was 0.6 L/hour following I.V. administration

Bioavailability: Ranges from ~66% to 82% depending on agent

Half-life elimination:

Mean: S.C.: Follitropin alfa: 24-32 hours; Follitropin beta: ~30 hours; Urofollitropin: 32-37 hours

Mean terminal: Multiple doses: I.M. follitropin alfa, S.C. follitropin beta: ~30 hours; I.M. urofollitropin: 15 hours, S.C. urofollitropin: 21 hours

Time to peak:

Follitropin alfa: S.C.: 16 hours; I.M.: 25 hours

Follitropin beta: I.M.: 27 hours

Urofollitropin: Single dose: S.C.: 15-20 hours, I.M.: 10-17 hours; Multiple doses: I.M., S.C.: 10 hours

Excretion: Clearance: Follitropin alfa: I.V.: 0.6 L/hour

Pregnancy Risk Factor X

Generic Available No

Foltx® *see* Folic Acid, Cyanocobalamin, and Pyridoxine *on page 607*

Fomepizole (foe ME pi zole)

U.S. Brand Names Antizol®

Pharmacologic Category Antidote

Synonyms 4-Methylpyrazole; 4-MP

Use Orphan drug: Treatment of methanol or ethylene glycol poisoning alone or in combination with hemodialysis

Unlabeled/Investigational Use Treatment of known or suspected propylene glycol toxicity

Local Anesthetic/Vasoconstrictor Precautions No information available to require special precautions

(Continued)

Fomepizole *(Continued)*

Effects on Dental Treatment

>10%: Headache (14%), nausea (11%)

6%: Bad/metallic taste, dizziness, drowsiness

≤3%: Increased agitation, anxiety, lightheadedness, seizure, vomiting, lymphangitis, transient blurred vision, visual disturbances, hiccups, pharyngitis, bradycardia, facial flush, hypotension, tachycardia

Dosage Adults:

Ethylene glycol and methanol toxicity: I.V.: A loading dose of 15 mg/kg should be administered, followed by doses of 10 mg/kg every 12 hours for 4 doses, then 15 mg/kg every 12 hours thereafter until ethylene glycol levels have been reduced <20 mg/dL and patient is asymptomatic with normal pH

Dosing adjustment in renal impairment: Fomepizole and its metabolites are excreted in the urine; dialysis should be considered in addition to fomepizole in the case of renal failure, significant or worsening metabolic acidosis, or a measured ethylene glycol level of ≥50 mg/dL. Patients should be dialyzed to correct metabolic abnormalities and to lower the ethylene glycol level <50 mg/dL; fomepizole is dialyzable and the frequency of dosing should be increased to every 4 hours during hemodialysis

Hemodialysis: Fomepizole is dialyzable and frequency of dosing should be increased to every 4 hours during hemodialysis.

Dose at the beginning of hemodialysis:

If <6 hours since last fomepizole dose: Do not administer dose

If ≥6 hours since last fomepizole dose: Administer next scheduled dose

Dosing during hemodialysis: Dose every 4 hours

Dosing at the time hemodialysis is complete, based on time between last dose and the end of hemodialysis:

<1 hour: Do not administer dose at the end of hemodialysis

1-3 hours: Administer 1/2 of next scheduled dose

>3 hours: Administer next scheduled dose

Maintenance dose when off hemodialysis: Give next scheduled dose 12 hours from last dose administered.

Dosing adjustment in hepatic impairment: Fomepizole is metabolized in the liver; specific dosage adjustments have not been determined in patients with hepatic impairment

Mechanism of Action Fomepizole competitively inhibits alcohol dehydrogenase, an enzyme which catalyzes the metabolism of ethanol, ethylene glycol, and methanol to their toxic metabolites. Ethylene glycol is metabolized to glycoaldehyde, then oxidized to glycolate, glyoxylate, and oxalate. Glycolate and oxalate are responsible for metabolic acidosis and renal damage. Methanol is metabolized to formaldehyde, then oxidized to formic acid. Formic acid is responsible for metabolic acidosis and visual disturbances.

Other Adverse Effects

1% to 3%:

Cardiovascular: Phlebosclerosis,

Central nervous system: Vertigo

Dermatologic: Rash

Gastrointestinal: Abdominal pain, decreased appetite, diarrhea, heartburn,

Hematologic: Anemia, disseminated intravascular coagulation, eosinophilia, lymphangitis

Hepatic: Increased LFTs

Local: Application site reaction, inflammation at the injection site, pain during injection, phlebitis

Neuromuscular & skeletal: Backache

Ocular: Nystagmus

Renal: Anuria

Respiratory: Abnormal smell

Miscellaneous: Multiorgan failure, speech disturbances

Postmarketing and/or case reports: Mild allergic reactions (mild rash, eosinophilia)

Drug Interactions Inhibits **CYP2A6**

Dietary/Ethanol/Herb Considerations Ethanol decreases the rate of fomepizole elimination by ~50%; conversely, fomepizole decreases the rate of elimination of ethanol by ~40%.

Pharmacodynamics/Kinetics

Onset of effect: Peak effect: Maximum: 1.5-2 hours

Absorption: Oral: Readily absorbed

Distribution: V_d: 0.6-1.02 L/kg; rapidly into total body water

Protein binding: Negligible

Metabolism: Hepatic to 4-carboxypyrazole (80% to 85% of dose), 4-hydroxymethylpyrazole, and their N-glucuronide conjugates; following multiple doses, induces its own metabolism via CYP oxidases after 30-40 hours

Half-life elimination: Has not been calculated; varies with dose

Excretion: Urine (1% to 3.5% as unchanged drug and metabolites)

Pregnancy Risk Factor C

Generic Available No

Selected Readings

Borron SW and Baud FJ, "Intravenous 4-Methylpyrazole as an Antidote for Diethylene Glycol and Triethylene Glycol Poisoning: A Case Report," *Vet Hum Toxicol*, 1997, 37(1): 26-8.

Brent J, McMartin K, Phillips S, et al, "4-Methylpyrazole (Fomepizole) Therapy of Ethylene Glycol Poisoning: Preliminary Results of the Meta Trial," *J Toxicol Clin Toxicol*, 1997, 35(5):507.

Brent J, McMartin K, Phillips SP, et al, "4-Methylpyrazole (Fomepizole) Therapy of Methanol Poisoning: Preliminary Results of the Meta Trial," *J Toxicol Clin Toxicol*, 1997, 35(5):507.

Hung O, Kaplan J, Hoffman R, et al, "Improved Understanding of the Ethanol-Chloral Hydrate Interaction Using 4-MP," *J Toxicol Clin Toxicol*, 1997, 35(5):507-8.

Jacobsen D and McMartin KE, "Antidotes for Methanol and Ethylene Glycol Poisoning," *J Toxicol Clin Toxicol*, 1997, 35(2):127-43.

Jacobsen D and McMartin K, "4-Methylpyrazole - Present Status," *J Toxicol Clin Toxicol*, 1996, 34(4):379-81.

Jacobsen D, Ostensen J, Bredesen L, et al, "4-Methylpyrazole (4-MP) Is Effectively Removed by Haemodialysis in the Pig Model," *Hum Exp Toxicol*, 1996, 15(6):494-6.

Jacobsen D, Sebastian CS, Barron SK, et al, "Effects of 4-Methylpyrazole, Methanol/Ethylene Glycol Antidote in Healthy Humans," *J Emerg Med*, 1990, 8(4):455-61.

Jobard E, Harry P, Turcant A, et al, "4-Methylpyrazole and Hemodialysis in Ethylene Glycol Poisoning," *J Toxicol Clin Toxicol*, 1996, 34(4):373-7.

McMartin KE and Heath A, "Treatment of Ethylene Glycol Poisoning With Intravenous 4-Methylpyrazole," *N Engl J Med*, 1989, 320(2):125.

Fomivirsen (foe MI vir sen)

Related Information

Systemic Viral Diseases *on page 1517*

U.S. Brand Names Vitravene™

Canadian Brand Names Vitravene™

Pharmacologic Category Antiviral Agent, Ophthalmic

Synonyms Fomivirsen Sodium

Use Local treatment of cytomegalovirus (CMV) retinitis in patients with acquired immunodeficiency syndrome who are intolerant or insufficiently responsive to other treatments for CMV retinitis or when other treatments for CMV retinitis are contraindicated

Local Anesthetic/Vasoconstrictor Precautions No information available to require special precautions

Effects on Dental Treatment

5% to 10%: Fever, headache, nausea, vomiting, pneumonia, sinusitis, sepsis, infection

2% to 5%: Chest pain, confusion, dizziness, pain, dehydration, allergic reaction, diaphoresis

Dosage Adults: Intravitreal injection: Induction: 330 mcg (0.05 mL) every other week for 2 doses, followed by maintenance dose of 330 mcg (0.05 mL) every 4 weeks

If progression occurs during maintenance, a repeat of the induction regimen may be attempted to establish resumed control. Unacceptable inflammation during therapy may be managed by temporary interruption, provided response has been established. Topical corticosteroids have been used to reduce inflammation.

Mechanism of Action Inhibits synthesis of viral protein by binding to mRNA which blocks replication of cytomegalovirus through an antisense mechanism

Other Adverse Effects

5% to 10%:
- Gastrointestinal: Abdominal pain, diarrhea
- Hematologic: Anemia
- Neuromuscular & skeletal: Asthenia
- Ocular: Uveitis, abnormal vision, anterior chamber inflammation, blurred vision, cataract, conjunctival hemorrhage, decreased visual acuity, loss of color vision, eye pain, increased intraocular pressure, photophobia, retinal detachment, retinal edema, retinal hemorrhage, retinal pigment changes, vitreitis
- Miscellaneous: Systemic CMV

2% to 5%:
- Central nervous system: Depression, neuropathy
- Gastrointestinal: Abnormal LFTs, pancreatitis, anorexia, weight loss
- Hematologic: Thrombocytopenia, lymphoma
- Neuromuscular & skeletal: Back pain, cachexia
- Ocular: Application site reaction, conjunctival hyperemia, conjunctivitis, corneal edema, decreased peripheral vision, eye irritation, keratic precipitates, optic neuritis, photopsia, retinal vascular disease, visual field defect, vitreous hemorrhage, vitreous opacity
- Renal: Kidney failure

Pharmacodynamics/Kinetics Pharmacokinetic studies have not been conducted in humans. In animal models, the drug is cleared from the eye after 7-10 days. It is metabolized by sequential nucleotide removal, with a small amount of the radioactivity from a dose appearing in the urine.

Generic Available No

Fomivirsen Sodium *see* Fomivirsen *on page 611*

Fondaparinux (fon de PAIR i nuks)

U.S. Brand Names Arixtra®

Canadian Brand Names Arixtra®

(Continued)

Fondaparinux *(Continued)*

Pharmacologic Category Factor Xa Inhibitor

Synonyms Fondaparinux Sodium

Use Prophylaxis of deep vein thrombosis (DVT) in patients undergoing surgery for hip fracture or hip or knee replacement

Unlabeled/Investigational Use Treatment of DVT

Local Anesthetic/Vasoconstrictor Precautions No information available to require special precautions

Effects on Dental Treatment No significant effects or complications reported

Dosage S.C.:

Adults: ≥50 kg: Usual dose: 2.5 mg once daily. **Note:** Initiate dose after hemostasis has been established, 6-8 hours postoperatively.

Elderly: Use caution, elimination may be prolonged; assess renal function before initiating therapy

Dosing adjustment in renal impairment:

Cl_{cr} 30-50 mL/minute: Use caution

Cl_{cr} <30 mL/minute: Contraindicated

Mechanism of Action Fondaparinux is a synthetic pentasaccharide that causes an antithrombin III-mediated selective inhibition of factor Xa. Neutralization of factor Xa interrupts the blood coagulation cascade and inhibits thrombin formation and thrombus development.

Other Adverse Effects Hemorrhage may occur at any site; risk appears increased by a number of factors including renal dysfunction, age (>75 years), and weight (<50 kg).

>10%:

Central nervous system: Fever (14%)

Gastrointestinal: Nausea (11%)

Hematologic: Anemia (20%)

1% to 10%:

Cardiovascular: Edema (9%), hypotension (4%), confusion (3%)

Central nervous system: Insomnia (5%), dizziness (4%), headache (2%), pain (2%)

Dermatologic: Rash (8%), purpura (4%), bullous eruption (3%)

Endocrine & metabolic: Hypokalemia (4%)

Gastrointestinal: Constipation (9%), vomiting (6%), diarrhea (3%), dyspepsia (2%)

Genitourinary: Urinary tract infection (4%), urinary retention (3%)

Hematologic: Moderate thrombocytopenia (50,000-100,000/mm^3: 3%), major bleeding (2% to 3%), minor bleeding (3% to 4%), hematoma (3%); risk of major bleeding increased as high as 5% in patients receiving initial dose <6 hours postsurgery

Hepatic: SGOT increased (2%), SGPT increased (3%)

Local: Injection site reaction (bleeding, rash, pruritus)

Miscellaneous: Wound drainage increased (5%)

<1%: Severe thrombocytopenia (<50,000/mm^3)

Drug Interactions Increased Effect/Toxicity: Anticoagulants, antiplatelet agents, drotrecogin alfa, NSAIDs, salicylates, and thrombolytic agents may enhance the anticoagulant effect and/or increase the risk of bleeding.

Dietary/Ethanol/Herb Considerations

Food: Avoid alfalfa, garlic, ginger, green tea, and licorice.

Herb/Nutraceutical: Avoid alfalfa, anise, bilberry, bladderwrack, bromelain, cat's claw, celery, coleus, cordyceps, dong quai, evening primrose oil, fenugreek, feverfew, garlic, ginger, ginkgo biloba, ginseng (American/Panax/Siberian), grape seed, green tea, guggul, horse chestnut seed, horseradish, licorice, prickly ash, red clover, reishi, sweet clover, turmeric, and white willow due to anticoagulant/antiplatelet activity.

Pharmacodynamics/Kinetics

Absorption: Rapid and complete

Distribution: V_d: 7-11 L; mainly in blood

Protein binding: ≥94% to antithrombin III

Bioavailability: 100%

Half-life elimination: 17-21 hours; prolonged with worsening renal impairment

Time to peak: 2-3 hours

Excretion: Urine (as unchanged drug)

Pregnancy Risk Factor B

Generic Available No

Fondaparinux Sodium *see* Fondaparinux *on page 611*

Foradil® Aerolizer™ *see* Formoterol *on page 612*

Formoterol (for MOE te rol)

U.S. Brand Names Foradil® Aerolizer™

Canadian Brand Names Foradil®; Oxeze® Turbuhaler®

Mexican Brand Names Foradil®; Oxis®

Pharmacologic Category Beta$_2$ Agonist

Synonyms Formoterol Fumarate

Use Maintenance treatment of asthma and prevention of bronchospasm in patients ≥5 years of age with reversible obstructive airway disease, including patients with symptoms of nocturnal asthma, who require regular treatment with inhaled, short-acting beta$_2$ agonists; maintenance treatment of bronchoconstriction in patients with COPD; prevention of exercise-induced bronchospasm in patients ≥12 years of age

Local Anesthetic/Vasoconstrictor Precautions No information available to require special precautions

Effects on Dental Treatment 1% to 10%: Xerostomia

Dosage Inhalation:

Children ≥5 years and Adults: Asthma maintenance: 12 mcg capsule every 12 hours

Children ≥12 years and Adults: Exercise-induced bronchospasm: 12 mcg capsule at least 15 minutes before exercise on an "as needed" basis; additional doses should not be used for another 12 hours. **Note:** If already using for asthma maintenance then should not use additional doses for exercise-induced bronchospasm.

Adults: Maintenance treatment for COPD: 12 mcg capsule every 12 hours

Elderly: No specific recommendations

Dosing adjustment in renal/hepatic impairment: Not studied

Mechanism of Action Relaxes bronchial smooth muscle by selective action on beta$_2$ receptors with little effect on heart rate. Formoterol has a long-acting effect.

Other Adverse Effects Children are more likely to have infection, inflammation, abdominal pain, nausea, and dyspepsia.

>10%: Miscellaneous: Viral infection (17%)

1% to 10%:

Cardiovascular: Chest pain (2%)

Central nervous system: Tremor (2%), dizziness (2%), insomnia (2%), dysphonia (1%)

Dermatologic: Rash (1%)

Respiratory: Bronchitis (5%), infection (3%), dyspnea (2%), tonsillitis (1%)

<1%: Anaphylactic reactions (severe hypotension, angioedema), asthma exacerbation, cramps, hypokalemia, increase in plasma glucose, tachycardia

Drug Interactions Substrate of CYP2A6, 2C8/9, 2C19, 2D6

Increased Effect/Toxicity: Adrenergic agonists, antidepressants (tricyclic), beta-blockers, corticosteroids, diuretics, drugs that prolong QT_c interval, MAO inhibitors, theophylline derivatives

Pharmacodynamics/Kinetics

Duration: Improvement in FEV_1 observed for 12 hours in most patients

Absorption: Rapidly into plasma

Protein binding: 61% to 64% *in vitro* at higher concentrations than achieved with usual dosing

Metabolism: Hepatic via direct glucuronidation and O-demethylation; CYP2D6, CYP2C8/9, CYP2C19, CYP2A6 involved in O-demethylation

Half-life elimination: ~10-14 hours

Time to peak: Maximum improvement in FEV_1 in 1-3 hours

Excretion:

Children 5-12 years: Urine (7% to 9% as direct glucuronide metabolites, 6% as unchanged drug)

Adults: Urine (15% to 18% as direct glucuronide metabolites, 10% as unchanged drug)

Pregnancy Risk Factor C

Generic Available No

Formoterol Fumarate *see* Formoterol *on page 612*

Formulation R™ [OTC] *see* Phenylephrine *on page 1071*

5-Formyl Tetrahydrofolate *see* Leucovorin *on page 783*

Fortaz® *see* Ceftazidime *on page 275*

Forteo™ *see* Teriparatide *on page 1280*

Fortovase® *see* Saquinavir *on page 1207*

Fosamax® *see* Alendronate *on page 54*

Foscarnet (fos KAR net)

Related Information

Systemic Viral Diseases *on page 1517*

U.S. Brand Names Foscavir®

Canadian Brand Names Foscavir®

Pharmacologic Category Antiviral Agent

Synonyms PFA; Phosphonoformate; Phosphonoformic Acid

(Continued)

Foscarnet *(Continued)*

Use

Herpes virus infections suspected to be caused by acyclovir - (HSV, VZV) or ganciclovir - (CMV) resistant strains (this occurs almost exclusively in immunocompromised persons, eg, with advanced AIDS), who have received prolonged treatment for a herpes virus infection

CMV retinitis in persons with AIDS; other CMV infections in persons unable to tolerate ganciclovir; may be given in combination with ganciclovir in patients who relapse after monotherapy with either drug

Local Anesthetic/Vasoconstrictor Precautions No information available to require special precautions

Effects on Dental Treatment No significant effects or complications reported

Dosage

CMV retinitis: I.V.:

Induction treatment: 60 mg/kg/dose every 8 hours **or** 100 mg/kg every 12 hours for 14-21 days

Maintenance therapy: 90-120 mg/kg/day as a single infusion

Acyclovir-resistant HSV induction treatment: I.V.: 40 mg/kg/dose every 8-12 hours for 14-21 days

Dosing adjustment in renal impairment:

Induction and maintenance dosing schedules based on creatinine clearance (mL/minute/kg): See tables.

Induction Dosing of Foscarnet in Patients with Abnormal Renal Function

Cl_{cr} (mL/min/kg)	HSV Equivalent to 40 mg/kg q12h	HSV Equivalent to 40 mg/kg q8h	CMV Equivalent to 60 mg/kg q8h	CMV Equivalent to 90 mg/kg q12h
<0.4	not recommended	not recommended	not recommended	not recommended
≥0.4-0.5	20 mg/kg every 24 hours	35 mg/kg every 24 hours	50 mg/kg every 24 hours	50 mg/kg every 24 hours
>0.5-0.6	25 mg/kg every 24 hours	40 mg/kg every 24 hours	60 mg/kg every 24 hours	60 mg/kg every 24 hours
>0.6-0.8	35 mg/kg every 24 hours	25 mg/kg every 12 hours	40 mg/kg every 12 hours	80 mg/kg every 24 hours
>0.8-1.0	20 mg/kg every 12 hours	35 mg/kg every 12 hours	50 mg/kg every 12 hours	50 mg/kg every 12 hours
>1.0-1.4	30 mg/kg every 12 hours	30 mg/kg every 8 hours	45 mg/kg every 8 hours	70 mg/kg every 12 hours
>1.4	40 mg/kg every 12 hours	40 mg/kg every 8 hours	60 mg/kg every 8 hours	90 mg/kg every 12 hours

Maintenance Dosing of Foscarnet in Patients with Abnormal Renal Function

Cl_{cr} (mL/min/kg)	CMV Equivalent to 90 mg/kg q24h	CMV Equivalent to 120 mg/kg q24h
<0.4	not recommended	not recommended
≥0.4-0.5	50 mg/kg every 48 hours	65 mg/kg every 48 hours
>0.5-0.6	60 mg/kg every 48 hours	80 mg/kg every 48 hours
>0.6-0.8	80 mg/kg every 48 hours	105 mg/kg every 48 hours
>0.8-1.0	50 mg/kg every 24 hours	65 mg/kg every 24 hours
>1.0-1.4	70 mg/kg every 24 hours	90 mg/kg every 24 hours
>1.4	90 mg/kg every 24 hours	120 mg/kg every 24 hours

Hemodialysis:

Foscarnet is highly removed by hemodialysis (30% in 4 hours HD)

Doses of 50 mg/kg/dose posthemodialysis have been found to produce similar serum concentrations as doses of 90 mg/kg twice daily in patients with normal renal function

Doses of 60-90 mg/kg/dose loading dose (posthemodialysis) followed by 45 mg/kg/dose posthemodialysis (3 times/week) with the monitoring of weekly plasma concentrations to maintain peak plasma concentrations in the range of 400-800 μMolar has been recommended by some clinicians

Continuous arteriovenous or venovenous hemodiafiltration effects: Dose as for Cl_{cr} 10-50 mL/minute

Mechanism of Action Pyrophosphate analogue which acts as a noncompetitive inhibitor of many viral RNA and DNA polymerases as well as HIV reverse transcriptase. Similar to ganciclovir, foscarnet is a virostatic agent. Foscarnet does not require activation by thymidine kinase.

Other Adverse Effects

>10%:

Central nervous system: Fever (65%), headache (26%), seizures (10%)
Gastrointestinal: Nausea (47%), diarrhea (30%), vomiting
Hematologic: Anemia (33%)
Renal: Abnormal renal function/decreased creatinine clearance (27%)

1% to 10%:

Central nervous system: Fatigue, malaise, dizziness, hypoesthesia, depression/confusion/anxiety (≥5%)
Dermatologic: Rash
Endocrine & metabolic: Electrolyte imbalance (especially potassium, calcium, magnesium, and phosphorus)
Gastrointestinal: Anorexia
Hematologic: Granulocytopenia, leukopenia (≥5%), thrombocytopenia, thrombosis
Local: Injection site pain
Neuromuscular & skeletal: Paresthesia, involuntary muscle contractions, rigors, neuropathy (peripheral), weakness
Ocular: Vision abnormalities
Respiratory: Coughing, dyspnea (≥5%)
Miscellaneous: Sepsis, diaphoresis (increased)

<1%: Cardiac failure, bradycardia, arrhythmias, cerebral edema, leg edema, peripheral edema, syncope, substernal chest pain, hypothermia, abnormal crying, malignant hyperpyrexia, vertigo, coma, speech disorders, gynecomastia, decreased gonadotropins, cholecystitis, cholelithiasis, hepatitis, hepatosplenomegaly, ascites, abnormal gait, dyskinesia, hypertonia, nystagmus, vocal cord paralysis

Drug Interactions Increased Effect/Toxicity: Concurrent use with ciprofloxacin (or other fluoroquinolone) increases seizure potential. Acute renal failure (reversible) has been reported with cyclosporine due most likely to a synergistic toxic effect. Nephrotoxic drugs (amphotericin B, I.V. pentamidine, aminoglycosides, etc) should be avoided, if possible, to minimize additive renal risk with foscarnet. Concurrent use of pentamidine also increases the potential for hypocalcemia. Protease inhibitors (ritonavir, saquinavir) have been associated with an increased risk of renal impairment during concurrent use of foscarnet

Pharmacodynamics/Kinetics

Distribution: Up to 28% of cumulative I.V. dose may be deposited in bone
Metabolism: Biotransformation does not occur
Half-life elimination: ~3 hours
Excretion: Urine (≤28% as unchanged drug)

Pregnancy Risk Factor C

Generic Available No

Foscavir® *see* Foscarnet *on page 613*

Fosfomycin (fos foe MYE sin)

U.S. Brand Names Monurol™

Canadian Brand Names Monurol™

Mexican Brand Names Fosfocil®; Monurol®

Pharmacologic Category Antibiotic, Miscellaneous

Synonyms Fosfomycin Tromethamine

Use A single oral dose in the treatment of uncomplicated urinary tract infections in women due to susceptible strains of *E. coli* and *Enterococcus*; multiple doses have been investigated for complicated urinary tract infections in men; may have an advantage over other agents since it maintains high concentration in the urine for up to 48 hours

Local Anesthetic/Vasoconstrictor Precautions No information available to require special precautions

Effects on Dental Treatment No significant effects or complications reported

Dosage Adults: Urinary tract infections: Oral:

Female: Single dose of 3 g in 4 oz of water
Male: 3 g once daily for 2-3 days for complicated urinary tract infections
Dosing adjustment in renal impairment: Decrease dose; 80% removed by dialysis, repeat dose after dialysis

Mechanism of Action As a phosphonic acid derivative, fosfomycin inhibits bacterial wall synthesis (bactericidal) by inactivating the enzyme, pyruvyl transferase, which is critical in the synthesis of cell walls by bacteria; the tromethamine salt is preferable to the calcium salt due to its superior absorption

Other Adverse Effects

>1%:

Central nervous system: Headache
Dermatologic: Rash
Gastrointestinal: Diarrhea (2% to 8%), nausea, vomiting, epigastric discomfort, anorexia

<1%: Dizziness, drowsiness, fatigue, pruritus

(Continued)

Fosfomycin *(Continued)*

Drug Interactions Decreased Effect: Antacids or calcium salts may cause precipitate formation and decrease fosfomycin absorption. Increased gastrointestinal motility due to metoclopramide may lower fosfomycin tromethamine serum concentrations and urinary excretion. This drug interaction possibly could be extrapolated to other medications which increase gastrointestinal motility.

Pharmacodynamics/Kinetics

Absorption: Well absorbed

Distribution: V_d: 2 L/kg; high concentrations in urine; well into other tissues; crosses maximally into CSF with inflamed meninges

Protein binding: <3%

Bioavailability: 34% to 58%

Half-life elimination: 4-8 hours; Cl_{cr} <10 mL/minute: 50 hours

Time to peak, serum: 2 hours

Excretion: Urine (as unchanged drug); high urinary levels (100 mcg/mL) persist for >48 hours

Pregnancy Risk Factor B

Generic Available No

Fosfomycin Tromethamine *see* Fosfomycin *on page 615*

Fosinopril (foe SIN oh pril)

Related Information

Cardiovascular Diseases *on page 1456*

U.S. Brand Names Monopril®

Canadian Brand Names Monopril™

Pharmacologic Category Angiotensin-Converting Enzyme (ACE) Inhibitor

Use Treatment of hypertension, either alone or in combination with other antihypertensive agents; treatment of CHF, left ventricular dysfunction after MI

Local Anesthetic/Vasoconstrictor Precautions No information available to require special precautions

Effects on Dental Treatment No significant effects or complications reported

Dosage Adults: Oral:

Hypertension: Initial: 10 mg/day; most patients are maintained on 20-40 mg/day. May need to divide the dose into two if trough effect is inadequate; discontinue the diuretic, if possible 2-3 days before initiation of therapy; resume diuretic therapy carefully, if needed.

Heart failure: Initial: 10 mg/day (5 mg if renal dysfunction present) and increase, as needed, to a maximum of 40 mg once daily over several weeks; usual dose: 20-40 mg/day. If hypotension, orthostasis, or azotemia occur during titration, consider decreasing concomitant diuretic dose, if any.

Hemodialysis: Moderately dialyzable (20% to 50%)

Mechanism of Action Competitive inhibitor of angiotensin-converting enzyme (ACE); prevents conversion of angiotensin I to angiotensin II, a potent vasoconstrictor; results in lower levels of angiotensin II which causes an increase in plasma renin activity and a reduction in aldosterone secretion; a CNS mechanism may also be involved in hypotensive effect as angiotensin II increases adrenergic outflow from CNS; vasoactive kallikreins may be decreased in conversion to active hormones by ACE inhibitors, thus reducing blood pressure

Other Adverse Effects Includes data from hypertension and heart failure trials; patients with CHF generally reported increased frequency but also with placebo.

>10%: Central nervous system: Dizziness (2% to 12%)

1% to 10%:

- Cardiovascular: Orthostatic hypotension (1% to 2%), palpitation (1%)
- Central nervous system: Dizziness (1% to 2%; up to 12% in CHF patients), headache (3%), weakness (1%), fatigue (1% to 2%)
- Endocrine & metabolic: Hyperkalemia (2.6%)
- Gastrointestinal: Diarrhea (2%), nausea/vomiting (1.2% to 2.2%)
- Hepatic: Increased transaminases
- Neuromuscular & skeletal: Musculoskeletal pain (<1% to 3%), noncardiac chest pain (<1% to 2%)
- Renal: Increased serum creatinine, worsening of renal function (in patients with bilateral renal artery stenosis or hypovolemia)
- Respiratory: Cough (2% to 10%)
- Miscellaneous: Upper respiratory infection (2%)

>1% but ≤ frequency in patients receiving placebo: Sexual dysfunction, fever, flu-like syndrome, dyspnea, rash, headache, insomnia

<1% (Limited to important or life-threatening): Angina, MI, cerebrovascular accident, syncope, hypotension, hypertensive crisis, claudication, flushing, edema, vertigo, insomnia, memory disturbance, drowsiness, angioedema, urticaria, rash, photosensitivity, pruritus, gout, decreased libido, pancreatitis, hepatitis, dysphagia, abdominal distension, flatulence, constipation, heartburn, xerostomia, lymphadenopathy, arthralgia, myalgia, memory disturbance, tremor, mood

change, confusion, paresthesia, sleep disturbance, vertigo, drowsiness, bronchospasm, pharyngitis, laryngitis, epistaxis. tinnitus, vision, abnormal taste, eye irritation, renal insufficiency, urinary frequency, weight gain, hyperhydrosis, lower extremity edema, shock, sudden death, hypertension, bradycardia, tachycardia, hepatomegaly, TIA, cerebral infarction, numbness, behavioral change, sinus abnormality, tracheobronchitis, pleuritic chest pain, anaphylactoid reaction. In a small number of patients, a symptom complex of cough, bronchospasm, and eosinophilia has been observed with fosinopril.

Postmarketing and/or case reports: Gynecomastia, scleroderma, eosinophilic vasculitis

Other events reported with ACE inhibitors: Neutropenia, agranulocytosis, eosinophilic pneumonitis, cardiac arrest, pancytopenia, hemolytic anemia, anemia, aplastic anemia, thrombocytopenia, acute renal failure, hepatic failure, jaundice, symptomatic hyponatremia, bullous pemphigus, exfoliative dermatitis, Stevens-Johnson syndrome. In addition, a syndrome which may include fever, myalgia, arthralgia, interstitial nephritis, vasculitis, rash, eosinophilia and positive ANA, and elevated ESR has been reported for other ACE inhibitors.

Drug Interactions

Increased Effect/Toxicity:

Potassium supplements, co-trimoxazole (high dose), angiotensin II receptor antagonists (candesartan, losartan, irbesartan, etc), or potassium-sparing diuretics (amiloride, spironolactone, triamterene) may result in elevated serum potassium levels when combined with fosinopril. ACE inhibitor effects may be increased by phenothiazines or probenecid (increases levels of captopril). ACE inhibitors may increase serum concentrations/effects of digoxin, lithium, and sulfonlyureas.

Diuretics have additive hypotensive effects with ACE inhibitors, and hypovolemia increases the potential for adverse renal effects of ACE inhibitors. In patients with compromised renal function, coadministration with NSAIDs may result in further deterioration of renal function. Allopurinol and ACE inhibitors may cause a higher risk of hypersensitivity reaction when taken concurrently.

Decreased Effect: Aspirin (high dose) may reduce the therapeutic effects of ACE inhibitors; at low dosages this does not appear to be significant. Rifampin may decrease the effect of ACE inhibitors. Antacids may decrease the bioavailability of ACE inhibitors (may be more likely to occur with captopril); separate administration times by 1-2 hours. NSAIDs, specifically indomethacin, may reduce the hypotensive effects of ACE inhibitors. More likely to occur in low renin or volume dependent hypertensive patients.

Dietary/Ethanol/Herb Considerations

Ethanol: Avoid use; may increase risk of hypotension or dizziness.

Food: Avoid salt substitutes and potassium supplements.

Herb/Nutraceutical: Avoid black cohosh, dong quai, and evening primrose due to estrogenic activity. Avoid ephedra, garlic, ginseng, and yohimbe; may worsen hypertension. Avoid hawthorn; may lower peripheral vascular resistance resulting in additive decrease in BP.

Pharmacodynamics/Kinetics

Onset of action: 1 hour

Duration: 24 hours

Absorption: 36%

Protein binding: 95%

Metabolism: Prodrug, hydrolyzed to its active metabolite fosinoprilat by intestinal wall and hepatic esterases

Bioavailability: 36%

Half-life elimination, serum (fosinoprilat): 12 hours

Time to peak, serum: ~3 hours

Excretion: Urine and feces (as fosinoprilat and other metabolites in roughly equal proportions, 45% to 50%)

Pregnancy Risk Factor C/D (2nd and 3rd trimesters)

Generic Available No

Fosinopril and Hydrochlorothiazide

(foe SIN oh pril & hye droe klor oh THYE a zide)

Related Information

Fosinopril *on page 616*

Hydrochlorothiazide *on page 675*

U.S. Brand Names Monopril-HCT®

Canadian Brand Names Monopril-HCT®

Pharmacologic Category Antihypertensive Agent Combination

Synonyms Hydrochlorothiazide and Fosinopril

Use Treatment of hypertension; not indicated for first-line treatment

Local Anesthetic/Vasoconstrictor Precautions No information available to require special precautions

Effects on Dental Treatment No significant effects or complications reported

(Continued)

Fosinopril and Hydrochlorothiazide *(Continued)*

Dosage A patient whose blood pressure is not adequately controlled with fosinopril or hydrochlorothiazide monotherapy may be switched to combination therapy; **not** for initial treatment.

Oral:

Adults: Hypertension: Fosinopril 10-80 mg per day, hydrochlorothiazide 12.5-50 mg per day

Dosing adjustment in renal impairment:

Cl_{cr} <30 mL/minute or serum creatinine ≥3 mg/dL: Use not recommended

Dosing adjustment in hepatic impairment: Use caution in patients with progressive liver disease. Metabolism of fosinopril to its active metabolite, fosinoprilat, will be reduced as will clearance of fosinoprilat.

Mechanism of Action Fosinopril is a competitive inhibitor of angiotensin-converting enzyme (ACE); prevents conversion of angiotensin I to angiotensin II, a potent vasoconstrictor; results in lower levels of angiotensin II which causes an increase in plasma renin activity and a reduction in aldosterone secretion; a CNS mechanism may also be involved in hypotensive effect as angiotensin II increases adrenergic outflow from CNS; vasoactive kallikreins may be decreased in conversion to active hormones by ACE inhibitors, thus reducing blood pressure. Hydrochlorothiazide inhibits sodium reabsorption in the distal tubules causing increased excretion of sodium and water as well as potassium and hydrogen ions.

Other Adverse Effects

2% to 10%:

Central nervous system: Headache (7%, less than placebo), fatigue (4%), dizziness (3%), orthostatic hypotension (2%)

Neuromuscular & skeletal: Musculoskeletal pain (2%)

Respiratory: Cough (6%), upper respiratory infection (2%, less than placebo)

<2%: Abdominal pain, angioedema, breast mass, BUN elevation (similar to placebo), chest pain, creatinine elevation (similar to placebo), depression, diarrhea, dyspepsia, dysuria, edema, eosinophilia, esophagitis, fever, flushing, gastritis, gout, heartburn, hepatic necrosis, leukopenia, libido change, LFTs elevations (transaminases, LDH, alkaline phosphatase, serum bilirubin), muscle cramps, myalgia, nausea, neutropenia, numbness, paresthesia, pharyngitis, pruritus, rash, rhinitis, sexual dysfunction, sinus congestion, somnolence, syncope, tinnitus, urinary frequency, urinary tract infection, viral infection, vomiting, weakness

Other adverse events reported with ACE inhibitors: Aplastic anemia, bullous pemphigus, cardiac arrest, cholestatic jaundice, exfoliative dermatitis, hemolytic anemia, hyperkalemia, pancreatitis, pancytopenia, photosensitivity; syndrome that may include one or more of arthralgia/arthritis, vasculitis, serositis, myalgia, fever, rash or other dermopathy, positive ANA titer, leukocytosis, eosinophilia, and elevated ESR; thrombocytopenia

Other adverse events reported with hydrochlorothiazide: Agranulocytosis, anaphylactic reactions, anorexia, blurred vision (transient), constipation, cramping, glucosuria, hemolytic anemia, hypercalcemia, hyperglycemia, hyperuricemia, hypokalemia, jaundice (intrahepatic cholestatic), lightheadedness, muscle spasm, necrotizing angiitis, pancreatitis, photosensitivity, pneumonitis, pulmonary edema, purpura, respiratory distress, restlessness, sialadenitis, SLE, Stevens-Johnson syndrome, urticaria, vertigo, xanthopsia

Drug Interactions

Increased Effect/Toxicity: $Alpha_1$ blockers, diuretics increase hypotension. Beta blockers may increase hyperglycemic effect. Cyclosporine may increase risk of gout or renal toxicity. Risk of lithium toxicity may be increased. Mercaptopurine may increase risk of neutropenia. Digoxin and neuromuscular-blocking agents: Effects may be increased with hypokalemia. Potassium-sparing diuretics, potassium supplements, trimethoprim may increase risk of hyperkalemia.

Decreased Effect: Aspirin, NSAIDs may decrease antihypertensive effect. Antacids, cholestyramine, colestipol may decrease absorption.

Dietary/Ethanol/Herb Considerations

Ethanol: Avoid use; may increase risk of hypotension or dizziness.

Food may decrease peak serum concentration. Avoid caffeine (eg, colas, chocolate), garlic, and licorice.

Herb/Nutraceutical: Avoid black cohosh, dong quai, and evening primrose due to estrogenic activity; dong quai may also cause photosensitization. Avoid ephedra, ginseng, and yohimbe; may worsen hypertension. Avoid garlic; may have increased antihypertensive effect. Avoid ginger due to positive inotropic effects; theoretically, may cause arrhythmia. Avoid hawthorn; may lower peripheral vascular resistance causing additional decrease in BP. Avoid licorice.

Pregnancy Risk Factor C (1st trimester)/D (2nd and 3rd trimester)

Generic Available No

Fosphenytoin (FOS fen i toyn)

Related Information

Phenytoin *on page 1073*

U.S. Brand Names Cerebyx®

Canadian Brand Names Cerebyx®

Pharmacologic Category Anticonvulsant, Hydantoin

Synonyms Fosphenytoin Sodium

Use Indicated for short-term parenteral administration when other means of phenytoin administration are unavailable, inappropriate or deemed less advantageous; the safety and effectiveness of fosphenytoin in this use has not been systematically evaluated for more than 5 days; may be used for the control of generalized convulsive status epilepticus and prevention and treatment of seizures occurring during neurosurgery

Local Anesthetic/Vasoconstrictor Precautions No information available to require special precautions

Effects on Dental Treatment No significant effects or complications reported

Dosage The dose, concentration in solutions, and infusion rates for fosphenytoin are expressed as phenytoin sodium equivalents. Fosphenytoin should always be prescribed and dispensed in phenytoin sodium equivalents.

Children 5-18 years: I.V.: A limited number of children have been studied. Seven children received a single I.V. loading dose of fosphenytoin 10-20 mg **PE**/kg for the treatment of acute generalized convulsive status epilepticus (Pellock, 1996). Some centers are using the phenytoin dosing guidelines in children and dosing fosphenytoin using **PE** doses equal to the phenytoin doses (ie, phenytoin 1 mg = fosphenytoin 1 mg **PE**). Further pediatric studies are needed.

Adults:

Status epilepticus: I.V.: Loading dose: Phenytoin equivalent: 15-20 mg/kg I.V. administered at 100-150 mg/minute

Nonemergent loading and maintenance dosing: I.V. or I.M.:

Loading dose: Phenytoin equivalent: 10-20 mg/kg I.V. or I.M. (maximum I.V. rate: 150 mg/minute)

Initial daily maintenance dose: Phenytoin equivalent: 4-6 mg/kg/day I.V. or I.M.

I.M. or I.V. substitution for oral phenytoin therapy: May be substituted for oral phenytoin sodium at the same total daily dose, however, Dilantin® capsules are ~90% bioavailable by the oral route; phenytoin, supplied as fosphenytoin, is 100% bioavailable by both the I.M. and I.V. routes; for this reason, plasma phenytoin concentrations may increase when I.M. or I.V. fosphenytoin is substituted for oral phenytoin sodium therapy; in clinical trials I.M. fosphenytoin was administered as a single daily dose utilizing either 1 or 2 injection sites; some patients may require more frequent dosing

Dosing adjustments in renal/hepatic impairment: Phenytoin clearance may be substantially reduced in cirrhosis and plasma level monitoring with dose adjustment advisable; free phenytoin levels should be monitored closely in patients with renal or hepatic disease or in those with hypoalbuminemia; furthermore, fosphenytoin clearance to phenytoin may be increased without a similar increase in phenytoin in these patients leading to increase frequency and severity of adverse events

Mechanism of Action Diphosphate ester salt of phenytoin which acts as a water soluble prodrug of phenytoin; after administration, plasma esterases convert fosphenytoin to phosphate, formaldehyde and phenytoin as the active moiety; phenytoin works by stabilizing neuronal membranes and decreasing seizure activity by increasing efflux or decreasing influx of sodium ions across cell membranes in the motor cortex during generation of nerve impulses

Other Adverse Effects

>10%:

Central nervous system: Dizziness (31%), somnolence (21%), ataxia (11%)

Dermatologic: Pruritus (49%)

Ocular: Nystagmus (44%)

1% to 10%:

Cardiovascular: Hypotension (8%), vasodilation (>1%), tachycardia (2%)

Central nervous system: Stupor (8%), incoordination (4%), paresthesia (4%), choreoathetosis (4%), tremor (3%), agitation (3%)

Gastrointestinal: Nausea (>5%), vomiting (2%)

Ocular: Blurred vision (2%), diplopia (3%)

<1%: Rash, exfoliative dermatitis, erythema multiforme, acne, diabetes insipidus, lymphadenopathy, neutropenia, thrombocytopenia, anemia (megaloblastic)

Frequency not defined:

Central nervous system: Sensory paresthesia (long-term treatment)

Local: Pain on injection

Renal: Nephrotic syndrome

Drug Interactions As phenytoin: Substrate of **CYP2C8/9, 2C19**, 3A4; Induces **CYP2B6, 2C8/9, 2C19, 3A4**

Increased Effect/Toxicity: Phenytoin may increase phenobarbital and primidone levels. Protein binding of phenytoin can be affected by valproic acid or salicylates. Serum phenytoin concentrations may be increased by cimetidine, felbamate, ethosuximide, methsuximide, chloramphenicol, disulfiram, fluconazole, omeprazole, isoniazid, trimethoprim, or sulfonamides.

(Continued)

Fosphenytoin *(Continued)*

Decreased Effect: No drugs are known to interfere with the conversion of fosphenytoin to phenytoin. Phenytoin may decrease the serum concentration or effectiveness of valproic acid, ethosuximide, felbamate, benzodiazepines, carbamazepine, lamotrigine, primidone, warfarin, oral contraceptives, corticosteroids, cyclosporine, theophylline, chloramphenicol, rifampin, doxycycline, quinidine, mexiletine, disopyramide, dopamine, or nondepolarizing skeletal muscle relaxants. Serum phenytoin concentrations may be decreased by rifampin, cisplatin, vinblastine, bleomycin, and folic acid.

Pharmacodynamics/Kinetics

Onset of action: May be more rapid due to more rapid infusion

Protein binding: 95% to 99% to albumin; can displace phenytoin and increase free fraction (up to 30% unbound) during the period required for conversion of fosphenytoin to phenytoin

Metabolism: Converted via hydrolysis to phenytoin

Bioavailability: I.M.: 100%

Half-life elimination: Variable (mean: 12-29 hours); kinetics of phenytoin are saturable

Time to peak: Conversion to phenytoin: Following I.V. administration conversion half-life elimination is 15 minutes; following I.M. administration, peak phenytoin levels are reached in 3 hours

Excretion: Urine (as inactive metabolites)

See Phenytoin monograph for additional information.

Pregnancy Risk Factor D

Generic Available No

Fosphenytoin Sodium *see* Fosphenytoin *on page 618*

Fostex® 10% BPO [OTC] *see* Benzoyl Peroxide *on page 171*

Fototar® [OTC] *see* Coal Tar *on page 359*

Fragmin® *see* Dalteparin *on page 394*

Freezone® [OTC] *see* Salicylic Acid *on page 1204*

Frova® *see* Frovatriptan *on page 620*

Frovatriptan (froe va TRIP tan)

U.S. Brand Names Frova®

Pharmacologic Category Antimigraine Agent; Serotonin 5-$HT_{1B,\ 1D}$ Receptor Agonist

Synonyms Frovatriptan Succinate

Use Acute treatment of migraine with or without aura in adults

Local Anesthetic/Vasoconstrictor Precautions No information available to require special precautions

Effects on Dental Treatment 1% to 10%: Xerostomia (3%), rhinitis (1%), sinusitis (1%), flushing (4%), palpitation (1%), diaphoresis (1%)

Dosage Oral: Adults: Migraine: 2.5 mg; if headache recurs, a second dose may be given if first dose provided some relief and at least 2 hours have elapsed since the first dose (maximum daily dose: 7.5 mg)

Dosing adjustment in hepatic impairment: None required in mild to moderate impairment; use with caution in severe impairment

Mechanism of Action Selective agonist for serotonin (5-HT_{1B} and 5-HT_{1D} receptor) in cranial arteries to cause vasoconstriction and reduces sterile inflammation associated with antidromic neuronal transmission correlating with relief of migraine.

Other Adverse Effects

1% to 10%:

Cardiovascular: Chest pain (2%)

Central nervous system: Dizziness (8%), fatigue (5%), headache (4%), hot or cold sensation (3%), anxiety (1%), dysesthesia (1%), hypoesthesia (1%), insomnia (1%), pain (1%)

Gastrointestinal: Dyspepsia (2%), abdominal pain (1%), diarrhea (1%), vomiting (1%)

Neuromuscular & skeletal: Paresthesia (4%), skeletal pain (3%)

Ocular: Visual abnormalities (1%)

Otic: Tinnitus (1%)

<1%: Abnormal dreaming, abnormal gait, abnormal lacrimation, abnormal reflexes, abnormal urine, agitation, amnesia, arthralgia, arthrosis, ataxia, back pain, bradycardia, bullous eruption, cheilitis, confusion, conjunctivitis, constipation, dehydration, depersonalization, depression, dysphagia, dyspnea, ear ache, EKG changes, emotional lability, epistaxis, eructation, esophagospasm, euphoria, eye pain, fever, gastroesophageal reflux, hiccup, hot flashes, hyperacusis, hyperesthesia, hypertonia, hyperventilation, hypocalcemia, hypoglycemia, hypotonia, impaired concentration, involuntary muscle contractions, laryngitis, leg cramps, malaise, micturition, muscle weakness, myalgia, nervousness, nocturia, peptic ulcer, personality disorder, pharyngitis, polyuria, pruritus, purpura, renal pain, rigors, **increased saliva, salivary gland pain, speech disorder, stomatitis,**

syncope, tachycardia, abnormal taste, thirst, tongue paralysis, toothache, tremor, unspecified pain, urinary frequency, vertigo, weakness

Drug Interactions Substrate of CYP1A2

Increased Effect/Toxicity: The effects of frovatriptan may be increased by CYP1A2 inhibitors (eg, cimetidine, ciprofloxacin, erythromycin), estrogen derivatives, propranolol. Ergot derivatives may increase the effects of frovatriptan (do not use within 24 hours of each other). SSRIs may exhibit additive toxicity with frovatriptan or other serotonin agonists (eg, antidepressants, dextromethorphan, tramadol) leading to serotonin syndrome.

Decreased Effect: The effects of frovatriptan may be decreased by CYP1A2 inducers (eg, carbamazepine, phenobarbital, phenytoin, ritonavir), ergotamine.

Dietary/Ethanol/Herb Considerations Food does not affect bioavailability.

Pharmacodynamics/Kinetics

Distribution: Male: 4.2 L/kg; Female: 3.0 L/kg

Protein binding: 15%

Metabolism: Primarily hepatic via CYP1A2

Bioavailability: 20% to 30%

Half-life elimination: 26 hours

Time to peak: 2-4 hours

Excretion: Feces (62%); urine (32%)

Pregnancy Risk Factor C

Generic Available No

Frovatriptan Succinate *see* Frovatriptan *on page 620*

Frusemide *see* Furosemide *on page 622*

FS *see* Fibrin Sealant Kit *on page 570*

5-FU *see* Fluorouracil *on page 588*

FUDR® *see* Floxuridine *on page 576*

Fulvestrant (fool VES trant)

U.S. Brand Names Faslodex®

Pharmacologic Category Antineoplastic Agent, Estrogen Receptor Antagonist

Synonyms ICI 182,780

Use Treatment of hormone receptor positive metastatic breast cancer in postmenopausal women with disease progression following antiestrogen therapy.

Local Anesthetic/Vasoconstrictor Precautions No information available to require special precautions

Effects on Dental Treatment Vasodilation (18%)

Dosage I.M.: Adults (postmenopausal women): 250 mg at 1-month intervals

Mechanism of Action Steroidal compound which competitively binds to estrogen receptors on tumors and other tissue targets, producing a nuclear complex that decreases DNA synthesis and inhibits estrogen effects. Fulvestrant has no estrogen-receptor agonist activity. Causes down-regulation of estrogen receptors and inhibits tumor growth.

Other Adverse Effects

>10%:

Central nervous system: Pain (19%), headache (15%)

Gastrointestinal: Nausea (26%), vomiting (13%), constipation (13%), diarrhea (12%), abdominal pain (12%)

Local: Injection site reaction (11%)

Neuromuscular & skeletal: Weakness (23%), bone pain (16%), back pain (14%)

Respiratory: Pharyngitis (16%), dyspnea (15%)

1% to 10%:

Cardiovascular: Edema (9%), chest pain (7%)

Central nervous system: Dizziness (7%), insomnia (7%), paresthesia (6%), fever (6%), depression (6%), anxiety (5%)

Dermatologic: Rash (7%)

Gastrointestinal: Anorexia (9%)

Genitourinary: Pelvic pain (10%), urinary tract infection (6%)

Hematologic: Anemia (5%)

Neuromuscular & skeletal: Arthritis (3%)

Respiratory: Cough (10%)

Miscellaneous: Increased diaphoresis (5%)

<1%: Leukopenia, myalgia, thrombosis, vaginal bleeding, vertigo

Drug Interactions Substrate of **CYP3A4**

Increased Effect/Toxicity: Serum level and/or toxicity of fulvestrant may be increased by CYP3A4 inhibitors; inhibitors include amiodarone, cimetidine, clarithromycin, erythromycin, delavirdine, diltiazem, dirithromycin, disulfiram, fluoxetine, fluvoxamine, grapefruit juice, indinavir, itraconazole, ketoconazole, nefazodone, nevirapine, propoxyphene, quinupristin-dalfopristin, ritonavir, saquinavir, verapamil, zafirlukast, zileuton

Decreased Effect: Serum level of fulvestrant may be increased by enzyme-inducing agents, decreasing its therapeutic effect; potential inducers include phenobarbital, phenytoin, carbamazepine, rifampin, and rifabutin. However, a clinical study with rifampin did not demonstrate an effect on fulvestrant pharmacokinetics.

(Continued)

Fulvestrant *(Continued)*

Dietary/Ethanol/Herb Considerations Food: Serum concentration and/or toxicity may be increased by CYP3A3/4 inhibitor, grapefruit juice; avoid grapefruit products.

Pharmacodynamics/Kinetics

Duration: I.M.: Plasma levels maintained for at least 1 month

Distribution: V_d: 3-5 L/kg

Protein binding: 99%

Metabolism: Hepatic via multiple pathways (CYP3A4 substrate, relative contribution to metabolism unknown)

Bioavailability: Oral: Poor

Half-life elimination: ~40 days

Time to peak, plasma: I.M.: 7-9 days

Excretion: Feces (>90%); urine (<1%)

Pregnancy Risk Factor D

Generic Available No

Fulvicin® P/G *see* Griseofulvin *on page 649*

Fulvicin-U/F® *see* Griseofulvin *on page 649*

Fungi-Guard [OTC] *see* Tolnaftate *on page 1322*

Fungi-Nail® [OTC] *see* Undecylenic Acid and Derivatives *on page 1365*

Fungizone® *see* Amphotericin B (Conventional) *on page 98*

Fung-O® [OTC] *see* Salicylic Acid *on page 1204*

Fungoid® Tincture [OTC] *see* Miconazole *on page 906*

Furadantin® *see* Nitrofurantoin *on page 980*

Furazolidone (fyoor a ZOE li done)

Canadian Brand Names Furoxone®

Mexican Brand Names Furoxona®; Furoxona Gotas; Furoxona Tabletas; Fuxol®; Salmocide®

Pharmacologic Category Antiprotozoal

Synonyms Tri-Luma

Use Treatment of bacterial or protozoal diarrhea and enteritis caused by susceptible organisms *Giardia lamblia* and *Vibrio cholerae*

Local Anesthetic/Vasoconstrictor Precautions No information available to require special precautions

Effects on Dental Treatment No significant effects or complications reported

Dosage Oral:

Children >1 month: 5-8 mg/kg/day in 4 divided doses for 7 days, not to exceed 400 mg/day or 8.8 mg/kg/day

Adults: 100 mg 4 times/day for 7 days

Mechanism of Action Inhibits several vital enzymatic reactions causing antibacterial and antiprotozoal action

Other Adverse Effects

>10%: Genitourinary: Discoloration of urine (dark yellow to brown)

1% to 10%:

Central nervous system: Headache

Gastrointestinal: Abdominal pain, diarrhea, nausea, vomiting

<1%: Agranulocytosis, arthralgia, disulfiram-like reaction after ethanol ingestion, dizziness, drowsiness, fever, hemolysis in patients with G6PD deficiency, hypoglycemia, leukopenia, malaise, orthostatic hypotension, rash

Drug Interactions Increased Effect/Toxicity: Increased effect with sympathomimetic amines, tricyclic antidepressants, tyramine-containing foods, MAO inhibitors, meperidine, anorexiants, dextromethorphan, fluoxetine, paroxetine, sertraline, and trazodone. Increased effect/toxicity of levodopa. Disulfiram-like reaction with alcohol.

Dietary/Ethanol/Herb Considerations

Food: Ethanol: Avoid use; may contain tyramine (eg, Chianti, hearty red wine, and beer).

Food: Avoid food/beverages high in tyramine (eg, avocadoes, bananas, broad bean pods, canned figs, cheese, chicken liver, pickled herring, raisins, sour cream, soy sauce, yeast extracts, yogurt, pods, meats prepared with tenderizers, and foods aged to improve flavor); may cause sudden and severe high BP or hemorrhagic stroke.

Pharmacodynamics/Kinetics

Absorption: Poor

Excretion: Urine (33% as active drug and metabolites)

Pregnancy Risk Factor C

Generic Available No

Furazosin *see* Prazosin *on page 1108*

Furosemide (fyoor OH se mide)

Related Information

Cardiovascular Diseases *on page 1456*

U.S. Brand Names Lasix®

Canadian Brand Names Apo®-Furosemide; Lasix®; Lasix® Special

Mexican Brand Names Edenol®; Henexal; Lasix®; Selectofur®; Zafimida®

Pharmacologic Category Diuretic, Loop

Synonyms Frusemide

Use Management of edema associated with CHF and hepatic or renal disease; alone or in combination with antihypertensives in treatment of hypertension

Local Anesthetic/Vasoconstrictor Precautions No information available to require special precautions

Effects on Dental Treatment No significant effects or complications reported

Dosage

Infants and Children:

Oral: 1-2 mg/kg/dose increased in increments of 1 mg/kg/dose with each succeeding dose until a satisfactory effect is achieved to a maximum of 6 mg/kg/dose no more frequently than 6 hours.

I.M., I.V.: 1 mg/kg/dose, increasing by each succeeding dose at 1 mg/kg/dose at intervals of 6-12 hours until a satisfactory response up to 6 mg/kg/dose.

Adults:

Oral: 20-80 mg/dose initially increased in increments of 20-40 mg/dose at intervals of 6-8 hours; usual maintenance dose interval is twice daily or every day; may be titrated up to 600 mg/day with severe edematous states.

I.M., I.V.: 20-40 mg/dose, may be repeated in 1-2 hours as needed and increased by 20 mg/dose until the desired effect has been obtained. Usual dosing interval: 6-12 hours; for acute pulmonary edema, the usual dose is 40 mg I.V. over 1-2 minutes. If not adequate, may increase dose to 80 mg.

Continuous I.V. infusion: Initial I.V. bolus dose of 0.1 mg/kg followed by continuous I.V. infusion doses of 0.1 mg/kg/hour doubled every 2 hours to a maximum of 0.4 mg/kg/hour if urine output is <1 mL/kg/hour have been found to be effective and result in a lower daily requirement of furosemide than with intermittent dosing. Other studies have used a rate of ≤4 mg/minute as a continuous I.V. infusion.

Elderly: Oral, I.M., I.V.: Initial: 20 mg/day; increase slowly to desired response.

Refractory heart failure: Oral, I.V.: Doses up to 8 g/day have been used.

Dosing adjustment/comments in renal impairment: Acute renal failure: High doses (up to 1-3 g/day - oral/I.V.) have been used to initiate desired response; avoid use in oliguric states.

Dialysis: Not removed by hemo- or peritoneal dialysis; supplemental dose is unnecessary.

Dosing adjustment/comments in hepatic disease: Diminished natriuretic effect with increased sensitivity to hypokalemia and volume depletion in cirrhosis; monitor effects, particularly with high doses.

Mechanism of Action Inhibits reabsorption of sodium and chloride in the ascending loop of Henle and distal renal tubule, interfering with the chloride-binding cotransport system, thus causing increased excretion of water, sodium, chloride, magnesium, and calcium

Other Adverse Effects Frequency not defined:

Cardiovascular: Orthostatic hypotension, necrotizing angiitis, thrombophlebitis, chronic aortitis, acute hypotension, sudden death from cardiac arrest (with I.V. or I.M. administration)

Central nervous system: Paresthesias, vertigo, dizziness, lightheadedness, headache, blurred vision, xanthopsia , fever, restlessness

Dermatologic: Exfoliative dermatitis, erythema multiforme, purpura, photosensitivity, urticaria, rash, pruritus, cutaneous vasculitis

Endocrine & metabolic: Hyperglycemia, hyperuricemia, hypokalemia, hypochloremia, metabolic alkalosis, hypocalcemia, hypomagnesemia, gout, hypernatremia

Gastrointestinal: Nausea, vomiting, anorexia, **oral and gastric irritation**, cramping, diarrhea, constipation, pancreatitis, intrahepatic cholestatic jaundice, ischemia hepatitis

Genitourinary: Urinary bladder spasm, urinary frequency

Hematological: Aplastic anemia (rare), thrombocytopenia, agranulocytosis (rare), hemolytic anemia, leukopenia, anemia, purpura

Neuromuscular & skeletal: Muscle spasm, weakness

Otic: Hearing impairment (reversible or permanent with rapid I.V. or I.M. administration), tinnitus, reversible deafness (with rapid I.V. or I.M. administration)

Renal: Vasculitis, allergic interstitial nephritis, glycosuria, fall in glomerular filtration rate and renal blood flow (due to overdiuresis), transient rise in BUN

Miscellaneous: Anaphylaxis (rare), exacerbate or activate systemic lupus erythematosus

Drug Interactions

Increased Effect/Toxicity:

Furosemide-induced hypokalemia may predispose to digoxin toxicity and may increase the risk of arrhythmia with drugs which may prolong QT interval, including type Ia and type III antiarrhythmic agents, cisapride, and some quinolones (sparfloxacin, gatifloxacin, and moxifloxacin). The risk of toxicity from

(Continued)

Furosemide *(Continued)*

lithium and salicylates (high dose) may be increased by loop diuretics. Hypotensive effects and/or adverse renal effects of ACE inhibitors and NSAIDs are potentiated by furosemide-induced hypovolemia. The effects of peripheral adrenergic-blocking drugs or ganglionic blockers may be increased by furosemide.

Furosemide may increase the risk of ototoxicity with other ototoxic agents (aminoglycosides, cis-platinum), especially in patients with renal dysfunction. Synergistic diuretic effects occur with thiazide-type diuretics. Diuretics tend to be synergistic with other antihypertensive agents, and hypotension may occur.

Decreased Effect: Indomethacin, aspirin, phenobarbital, phenytoin, and NSAIDs may reduce natriuretic and hypotensive effects of furosemide. Colestipol, cholestyramine, and sucralfate may reduce the effect of furosemide; separate administration by 2 hours. Furosemide may antagonize the effect of skeletal muscle relaxants (tubocurarine). Glucose tolerance may be decreased by furosemide, requiring an adjustment in the dose of hypoglycemic agents. Metformin may decrease furosemide concentrations.

Dietary/Ethanol/Herb Considerations

Ethanol: Avoid use; has diuretic properties and may increase risk of dizziness and hypotension.

Food: Administer on an empty stomach if possible; may be taken with food or milk to reduce GI upset but may decrease serum concentration. Do not mix with acidic solutions. Avoid caffeine (eg, colas, chocolate) and garlic; limit licorice. May cause a potassium loss requiring a potassium supplement, medication to help prevent potassium loss, or a dietary increase in foods high in potassium (citrus fruits). Limit licorice.

Herb/Nutraceutical: Avoid black cohosh, dong quai, and evening primrose due to estrogenic activity. Avoid ephedra, ginseng, and yohimbe; may worsen hypertension. Avoid escin (from the horse chestnut seed); may have additive diuretic effects. Avoid garlic; may have increased antihypertensive effect. Avoid ginger due to positive inotropic effects; theoretically, may cause arrhythmia. Avoid ginseng; may decrease effectiveness of loop diuretics (1 case report). Avoid hawthorn; may lower peripheral vascular resistance resulting in additive decrease in BP. Limit licorice.

Pharmacodynamics/Kinetics

Onset of action: Diuresis: Oral: 30-60 minutes; I.M.: 30 minutes; I.V.: ~5 minutes

Peak effect: Oral: 1-2 hours

Duration: Oral: 6-8 hours; I.V.: 2 hours

Absorption: Oral: 60% to 67%

Protein binding: >98%

Metabolism: Minimally hepatic

Half-life elimination: Normal renal function: 0.5-1.1 hours; End-stage renal disease: 9 hours

Excretion: Urine (Oral: 50%, I.V.: 80%) within 24 hours; feces (as unchanged drug); nonrenal clearance prolonged in renal impairment

Pregnancy Risk Factor C

Generic Available Yes

Fuzeon™ *see* Enfuvirtide *on page 495*

Gabapentin (GA ba pen tin)

U.S. Brand Names Neurontin®

Canadian Brand Names Apo®-Gabapentin; Neurontin®; Novo-Gabapentin; PMS-Gabapentin

Mexican Brand Names Neurontin®

Pharmacologic Category Anticonvulsant, Miscellaneous

Use Adjunct for treatment of partial seizures with and without secondary generalized seizures in patients >12 years of age with epilepsy; adjunct for treatment of partial seizures in pediatric patients 3-12 years of age; management of postherpetic neuralgia (PHN) in adults

Unlabeled/Investigational Use Treatment of bipolar disorder, social phobia, chronic pain

Local Anesthetic/Vasoconstrictor Precautions No information available to require special precautions

Effects on Dental Treatment

Children 3-12 years:

>10%: Viral infection (11%)

1% to 10%: Bronchitis (3%), respiratory infection (2%), fever (10%), hostility (8%), somnolence (8%), fatigue (3%), abnormal thinking (2%), dizziness (2%), nausea/vomiting (8%)

Children >12 years and Adults:

>10%: Somnolence (20%), fatigue (11%), dizziness (17%)

1% to 7%: Pharyngitis (3%), coughing (2%), abnormal thinking (2%), amnesia (2%), blurred vision (4%), CNS depression (2%), xerostomia (2%), dry throat

(2%), dental abnormalities (1%), twitching (1%), rhinitis (4%), nervousness (2%), incoordination (1%), tremors (7%)

Dosage Oral:

Children: Anticonvulsant:

3-12 years: Initial: 10-15 mg/kg/day in 3 divided doses; titrate to effective dose over ~3 days; dosages of up to 50 mg/kg/day have been tolerated in clinical studies

3-4 years: Effective dose: 40 mg/kg/day in 3 divided doses

≥5-12 years: Effective dose: 25-35 mg/kg/day in 3 divided doses

Note: If gabapentin is discontinued or if another anticonvulsant is added to therapy, it should be done slowly over a minimum of 1 week

Children >12 years and Adults:

Anticonvulsant: Initial: 300 mg 3 times/day; if necessary the dose may be increased using 300 mg or 400 mg capsules 3 times/day up to 1800 mg/day

Dosage range: 900-1800 mg administered in 3 divided doses at 8-hour intervals

Pain (unlabeled use): 300-1800 mg/day given in 3 divided doses has been the most common dosage range

Bipolar disorder (unlabeled use): 300-3000 mg/day given in 3 divided doses; **Note:** Does not appear to be effective as an adjunctive treatment for bipolar disorder (Pande AC, 2000)

Adults: **Postherpetic neuralgia:** Day 1: 300 mg, Day 2: 300 mg twice daily, Day 3: 300 mg 3 times/day; dose may be titrated as needed for pain relief (range: 1800-3600 mg/day, daily doses >1800 mg do not generally show greater benefit)

Elderly: Studies have shown a decrease in clearance as age increases. This is most likely due to age-related decreases in renal function; dose reductions may be needed.

Dosing adjustment in renal impairment: Children ≥12 years and Adults: See table.

Neurontin® Dosing Adjustments in Renal Impairment

Creatinine Clearance (mL/min)	Total Daily Dose Range (mg/day)	Dosage Regimens Based on Renal Function (mg)				
≥60	900-3600	300 tid	400 tid	600 tid	800 tid	1200 tid
>30-59	400-1400	200 bid	300 bid	400 bid	500 bid	700 bid
>15-29	200-700	200 qd	300 qd	400 qd	500 qd	700 qd
15[1]	100-300	100 qd	125 qd	150 qd	200 qd	300 qd
Hemodialysis[2]		Post-Hemodialysis Supplemental Dose				
		125 mg	150 mg	200 mg	250 mg	350 mg

[1]Cl_{cr}<15 mL/minute: Reduce daily dose in proportion to creatinine clearance.

[2]Supplemental dose administered after each 4 hours of hemodialysis (maintenance doses based on renal function).

Mechanism of Action Exact mechanism of action is not known, but does have properties in common with other anticonvulsants; although structurally related to GABA, it does not interact with GABA receptors

Other Adverse Effects >12 years of age (unless otherwise noted):

>10%: Central nervous system: Ataxia (12%)

1% to 10%:

Cardiovascular: Peripheral edema (2%)

Central nervous system: Emotional lability (4% to 6% in children 3-12 years), dysarthria (2%)

Dermatologic: Pruritus (1%)

Gastrointestinal: Weight gain (3% in adults and children), dyspepsia (2%), appetite stimulation (1%), constipation (1%)

Genitourinary: Impotence (1%)

Hematologic: Leukopenia (1%), decreased WBC (1%)

Neuromuscular & skeletal: Hyperkinesia (3% to 5% in children 3-12 years), back pain (2%), myalgia (2%)

Ocular: Nystagmus (8%), diplopia (6%)

Postmarketing and additional clinical reports (limited): **Allergy,** alopecia, **angina pectoris,** angioedema, anorexia, **coagulation defect**, erythema multiforme, ethanol intolerance, **facial edema**, flatulence, **gingivitis**, blood glucose fluctuation, subdural hematoma, hepatitis, hypercholesterolemia, hyperlipidemia, **hypertension,** hyponatremia, intracranial hemorrhage, jaundice, elevated LFTs, **malaise, palpitation**, pancreatitis, peripheral vascular disorder, pneumonia, purpura, Stevens-Johnson syndrome, new (or exacerbation of) tumors, vertigo, **weakness**

Warnings/Precautions Avoid abrupt withdrawal, may precipitate seizures; may be associated with a slight incidence (0.6%) of status epilepticus and sudden deaths (0.0038 deaths/patient year); use cautiously in patients with severe renal dysfunction; rat studies demonstrated an association with pancreatic adenocarcinoma in male rats; clinical implication unknown. May cause CNS depression, which may impair physical or mental abilities. Patients must be cautioned about performing tasks which require mental alertness (ie, operating machinery or driving). Effects

(Continued)

Gabapentin *(Continued)*

with other sedative drugs or ethanol may be potentiated. Pediatric patients (3-12 years of age) have shown increased incidence of CNS-related adverse effects, including emotional lability, hostility, thought disorder, and hyperkinesia. Safety and efficacy in children <3 years of age have not been established.

Drug Interactions

Increased Effect/Toxicity: Cimetidine may increased gabapentin levels. Gabapentin may increase peak concentrations of norethindrone. Morphine may increase gabapentin serum concentrations.

Decreased Effect: Gabapentin does not modify plasma concentrations of standard anticonvulsant medications (eg, valproic acid, carbamazepine, phenytoin, or phenobarbital). Antacids reduce the bioavailability of gabapentin by 20%.

Dietary/Ethanol/Herb Considerations

Ethanol: Avoid use; may increase CNS depression.

Food: Administer with food; rate/extent of absorption unaffected. Avoid caffeine.

Herb/Nutraceutical: Avoid evening primrose; decreases seizure threshold. Avoid gotu kola, kava, SAMe, St John's wort, and valerian; may increase CNS depression.

Pharmacodynamics/Kinetics

Absorption: 50% to 60%

Distribution: V_d: 0.6-0.8 L/kg

Protein binding: 0%

Half-life elimination: 5-6 hours

Excretion: Urine (56% to 80%)

Pregnancy Risk Factor C

Generic Available No

Comments With its recent successful use in chronic pain (unlabeled), gabapentin has become popular in TMD treatment.

Selected Readings

Laird MA and Gidal BE, "Use of Gabapentin in the Treatment of Neuropathic Pain," *Ann Pharmacother*, 2000, 34(6):802-7.

Rose MA and Kam PCA, "Gabapentin: Pharmacology and Its Use in Pain Management," *Anaesthesia*, 2002, 57:451-62.

Rosenberg JM, Harrell C, Ristic H, et al, "The Effect of Gabapentin on Neuropathic Pain," *Clin J Pain*, 1997, 13(3):251-5.

Rowbotham M, Harden N, Stacey B, et al, "Gabapentin for the Treatment of Postherpetic Neuralgia: A Randomized Controlled Trial," *JAMA*, 1998, 280(21):1837-42.

Gabitril® *see* Tiagabine *on page 1304*

Gadoteridol *see* Radiological/Contrast Media (Nonionic) *on page 1165*

Gamimune® N *see* Immune Globulin (Intravenous) *on page 714*

Gamma Benzene Hexachloride *see* Lindane *on page 809*

Gammagard® S/D *see* Immune Globulin (Intravenous) *on page 714*

Gamma Globulin *see* Immune Globulin (Intramuscular) *on page 713*

Gamma Hydroxybutyric Acid *see* Sodium Oxybate *on page 1231*

Gammaphos *see* Amifostine *on page 73*

Gammar®-P I.V. *see* Immune Globulin (Intravenous) *on page 714*

Ganciclovir (gan SYE kloe veer)

Related Information

Systemic Viral Diseases *on page 1517*

Valganciclovir *on page 1370*

U.S. Brand Names Cytovene®; Vitrasert®

Canadian Brand Names Cytovene®; Vitrasert®

Mexican Brand Names Cymevene®

Pharmacologic Category Antiviral Agent

Synonyms DHPG Sodium; GCV Sodium; Nordeoxyguanosine

Use

Parenteral: Treatment of CMV retinitis in immunocompromised individuals, including patients with acquired immunodeficiency syndrome; prophylaxis of CMV infection in transplant patients; may be given in combination with foscarnet in patients who relapse after monotherapy with either drug

Oral: Alternative to the I.V. formulation for maintenance treatment of CMV retinitis in immunocompromised patients, including patients with AIDS, in whom retinitis is stable following appropriate induction therapy and for whom the risk of more rapid progression is balanced by the benefit associated with avoiding daily I.V. infusions.

Implant: Treatment of CMV retinitis

Local Anesthetic/Vasoconstrictor Precautions No information available to require special precautions

Effects on Dental Treatment 1% to 10%: Xerostomia

Dosage

CMV retinitis: Slow I.V. infusion (dosing is based on total body weight):

Children >3 months and Adults:

Induction therapy: 5 mg/kg/dose every 12 hours for 14-21 days followed by maintenance therapy

Maintenance therapy: 5 mg/kg/day as a single daily dose for 7 days/week or 6 mg/kg/day for 5 days/week

CMV retinitis: Oral: 1000 mg 3 times/day with food **or** 500 mg 6 times/day with food

Prevention of CMV disease in patients with advanced HIV infection and normal renal function: Oral: 1000 mg 3 times/day with food

Prevention of CMV disease in transplant patients: Same initial and maintenance dose as CMV retinitis except duration of initial course is 7-14 days, duration of maintenance therapy is dependent on clinical condition and degree of immunosuppression

Intravitreal implant: One implant for 5- to 8-month period; following depletion of ganciclovir, as evidenced by progression of retinitis, implant may be removed and replaced

Elderly: Dose selection should be cautious, reflecting greater frequency of organ impairment

Dosing adjustment in renal impairment:

I.V. (Induction):

Cl_{cr} 50-69 mL/minute: Administer 2.5 mg/kg/dose every 12 hours

Cl_{cr} 25-49 mL/minute: Administer 2.5 mg/kg/dose every 24 hours

Cl_{cr} 10-24 mL/minute: Administer 1.25 mg/kg/dose every 24 hours

Cl_{cr} <10 mL/minute: Administer 1.25 mg/kg/dose 3 times/week following hemodialysis

I.V. (Maintenance):

Cl_{cr} 50-69 mL/minute: Administer 2.5 mg/kg/dose every 24 hours

Cl_{cr} 25-49 mL/minute: Administer 1.25 mg/kg/dose every 24 hours

Cl_{cr} 10-24 mL/minute: Administer 0.625 mg/kg/dose every 24 hours

Cl_{cr} <10 mL/minute: Administer 0.625 mg/kg/dose 3 times/week following hemodialysis

Oral:

Cl_{cr} 50-69 mL/minute: Administer 1500 mg/day or 500 mg 3 times/day

Cl_{cr} 25-49 mL/minute: Administer 1000 mg/day or 500 mg twice daily

Cl_{cr} 10-24 mL/minute: Administer 500 mg/day

Cl_{cr} <10 mL/minute: Administer 500 mg 3 times/week following hemodialysis

Hemodialysis effects: Dialyzable (50%) following hemodialysis; administer dose postdialysis. During peritoneal dialysis, dose as for Cl_{cr} <10 mL/minute. During continuous arteriovenous or venovenous hemofiltration, administer 2.5 mg/kg/dose every 24 hours.

Mechanism of Action Ganciclovir is phosphorylated to a substrate which competitively inhibits the binding of deoxyguanosine triphosphate to DNA polymerase resulting in inhibition of viral DNA synthesis

Other Adverse Effects

>10%:

Central nervous system: Fever (38% to 48%)

Dermatologic: Rash (15% oral, 10% I.V.)

Gastrointestinal: Abdominal pain (17% to 19%), diarrhea (40%), nausea (25%), anorexia (15%), vomiting (13%)

Hematologic: Anemia (20% to 25%), leukopenia (30% to 40%)

1% to 10%:

Central nervous system: Confusion, neuropathy (8% to 9%), headache (4%)

Dermatologic: Pruritus (5%)

Hematologic: Thrombocytopenia (6%), neutropenia with ANC <500/mm^3 (5% oral, 14% I.V.)

Neuromuscular & skeletal: Paresthesia (6% to 10%), weakness (6%)

Ocular: Retinal detachment (8% oral, 11% I.V.; relationship to ganciclovir not established)

Miscellaneous: Sepsis (4% oral, 15% I.V.)

<1% (Limited to important or life-threatening): Alopecia, arrhythmia, ataxia, bronchospasm, coma, dyspnea, encephalopathy, exfoliative dermatitis, extrapyramidal symptoms, nervousness, pancytopenia, psychosis, seizures, urticaria, eosinophilia, hemorrhage, Stevens-Johnson syndrome, torsade de pointes, renal failure, SIADH, visual loss

Drug Interactions

Increased Effect/Toxicity: Immunosuppressive agents may increase hematologic toxicity of ganciclovir. Imipenem/cilastatin may increase seizure potential. Oral ganciclovir increases blood levels of zidovudine, although zidovudine decreases steady-state levels of ganciclovir. Since both drugs have the potential to cause neutropenia and anemia, some patients may not tolerate concomitant therapy with these drugs at full dosage. Didanosine levels are increased with concurrent ganciclovir. Other nephrotoxic drugs (eg, amphotericin and cyclosporine) may have additive nephrotoxicity with ganciclovir.

Decreased Effect: A decrease in blood levels of ganciclovir AUC may occur when used with didanosine.

(Continued)

Ganciclovir *(Continued)*

Dietary/Ethanol/Herb Considerations Food: Absorption of oral form under fasting conditions is absolute.

Pharmacodynamics/Kinetics

Distribution: V_d: 15.26 L/1.73 m^2; widely to all tissues including CSF and ocular tissue

Protein binding: 1% to 2%

Bioavailability: Oral: Fasting: 5%; Following food: 6% to 9%; Following fatty meal: 28% to 31%

Half-life elimination: 1.7-5.8 hours; prolonged with renal impairment; End-stage renal disease: 5-28 hours

Excretion: Urine (80% to 99% as unchanged drug)

Pregnancy Risk Factor C

Generic Available No

Ganirelix (ga ni REL ix)

U.S. Brand Names Antagon®

Canadian Brand Names Antagon®; Orgalutran®

Pharmacologic Category Antigonadotropic Agent

Synonyms Ganirelix Acetate

Use Inhibits premature luteinizing hormone (LH) surges in women undergoing controlled ovarian hyperstimulation in fertility clinics.

Local Anesthetic/Vasoconstrictor Precautions No information available to require special precautions

Effects on Dental Treatment No significant effects or complications reported

Dosage Adult: S.C.: 250 mcg/day during the mid-to-late phase after initiating follicle-stimulating hormone on day 2 or 3 of cycle. Treatment should be continued daily until the day of chorionic gonadotropin administration.

Mechanism of Action Competitively blocks the gonadotropin-release hormone receptors on the pituitary gonadotroph and transduction pathway. This suppresses gonadotropin secretion and luteinizing hormone secretion preventing ovulation until the follicles are of adequate size.

Other Adverse Effects

1% to 10%:

- Central nervous system: Headache (3%)
- Endocrine & metabolic: Ovarian hyperstimulation syndrome (2%)
- Gastrointestinal: Abdominal pain (5%), nausea (1%), abdominal pain (1%)
- Genitourinary: Vaginal bleeding (2%)
- Local: Injection site reaction (1%)

<1%: Congenital abnormalities

Pharmacodynamics/Kinetics

Absorption: S.C.: Rapid

Distribution: Mean V_d: 43.7 L

Protein binding: 81.9%

Metabolism: Hepatic to two primary metabolites (1-4 and 1-6 peptide)

Bioavailability: 91.1%

Half-life elimination: 16.2 hours

Time to peak: 1.1 hours

Excretion: Feces (75%) within 288 hours; urine (22%) within 24 hours

Pregnancy Risk Factor X

Generic Available No

Ganirelix Acetate *see* Ganirelix *on page 628*

Gani-Tuss® NR *see* Guaifenesin and Codeine *on page 650*

Gantrisin® *see* SulfiSOXAZOLE *on page 1256*

Garamycin® *see* Gentamicin *on page 634*

Gastrocrom® *see* Cromolyn Sodium *on page 375*

Gas-X® [OTC] *see* Simethicone *on page 1222*

Gas-X® Extra Strength [OTC] *see* Simethicone *on page 1222*

Gatifloxacin (ga ti FLOKS a sin)

Related Information

Oral Bacterial Infections *on page 1531*

Respiratory Diseases *on page 1476*

Sexually-Transmitted Diseases *on page 1502*

U.S. Brand Names Tequin®

Canadian Brand Names Tequin®

Pharmacologic Category Antibiotic, Quinolone

Use Treatment of the following infections when caused by susceptible bacteria: Acute bacterial exacerbation of chronic bronchitis due to *S. pneumoniae, H. influenzae, H. parainfluenzae, M. catarrhalis*, or *S. aureus*; acute sinusitis due to *S. pneumoniae, H. influenzae*; community-acquired pneumonia due to *S. pneumoniae, H. influenzae, H. parainfluenzae, M. catarrhalis, S. aureus, M. pneumoniae, C. pneumoniae*, or *L. pneumophilia*; uncomplicated skin and skin structure infection due to *S. aureus* or *S. pyogenes;* uncomplicated urinary tract infections (cystitis) due to *E. coli, K. pneumoniae*, or *P. mirabilis*; complicated urinary tract infections due to *E. coli, K. pneumoniae*, or *P. mirabilis*; pyelonephritis due to *E. coli*; uncomplicated urethral and cervical gonorrhea; acute, uncomplicated rectal infections in women due to *N. gonorrhoeae*

Local Anesthetic/Vasoconstrictor Precautions No information available to require special precautions

Effects on Dental Treatment No significant effects or complications reported

Dosage Adults: Oral, I.V.:

Acute bacterial exacerbation of chronic bronchitis: 400 mg every 24 hours for 5 days

Acute sinusitis: 400 mg every 24 hours for 10 days

Community-acquired pneumonia: 400 mg every 24 hours for 7-14 days

Uncomplicated skin/skin structure infections: 400 mg every 24 hours for 7-10 days

Uncomplicated urinary tract infections (cystitis): 400 mg single dose or 200 mg every 24 hours for 3 days

Complicated urinary tract infections: 400 mg every 24 hours for 7-10 days

Acute pyelonephritis: 400 mg every 24 hours for 7-10 days

Uncomplicated urethral gonorrhea in men, cervical or rectal gonorrhea in women: 400 mg single dose

Dosing adjustment in renal impairment: Creatinine clearance <40 mL/minute (or patients on hemodialysis/CAPD) should receive an initial dose of 400 mg, followed by a subsequent dose of 200 mg every 24 hours. Patients receiving single-dose or 3-day therapy for appropriate indications do not require dosage adjustment. Administer after hemodialysis.

Mechanism of Action Gatifloxacin is a DNA gyrase inhibitor, and also inhibits topoisomerase IV. DNA gyrase (topoisomerase II) is an essential bacterial enzyme that maintains the superhelical structure of DNA. DNA gyrase is required for DNA replication and transcription, DNA repair, recombination, and transposition; inhibition is bactericidal.

Other Adverse Effects

3% to 10%:

Central nervous system: Headache (3%), dizziness (3%)

Gastrointestinal: Nausea (8%), diarrhea (4%)

Genitourinary: Vaginitis (6%)

Local: Injection site reactions (5%)

0.1% to 3%: Abdominal pain, abnormal dreams, abnormal vision, agitation, alkaline phosphatase increased, allergic reaction, anorexia, anxiety, arthralgia, back pain, chest pain, chills, confusion, constipation, diaphoresis, dry skin, dyspepsia, dyspnea, dysuria, facial edema, fever, flatulence, gastritis, glossitis, hematuria, hyperglycemia, hypertension, insomnia, leg cramps, oral ulceration, nervousness, oral candidiasis, palpitation, paresthesia, peripheral edema, pharyngitis, pruritus, rash, serum amylase increased, serum bilirubin increased, serum transaminases increased, somnolence, **stomatitis, abnormal taste, thirst**, tinnitus, tremor, weakness, vasodilation, vertigo, vomiting

<0.1%: Abnormal thinking, arthritis, asthenia, ataxia, bone pain, bradycardia, breast pain, bronchospasm, cheilitis, colitis, cyanosis, depersonalization, depression, diabetes mellitus, dysphagia, ear pain, ecchymosis, edema, epistaxis, ethanol intolerance, euphoria, eye pain, gastrointestinal hemorrhage, gingivitis, halitosis, hallucination, hematemesis, hematuria, hostility, hyperesthesia, hypertonia, hyperventilation, hypoglycemia, lymphadenopathy, maculopapular rash, metrorrhagia, migraine, myalgia, myasthenia, neck pain, panic attacks, paranoia, parosmia, photophobia, pseudomembranous colitis, psychosis, ptosis, rectal hemorrhage, **seizures, stress, tachycardia, abnormal taste, tongue edema**, vesiculobullous rash

Postmarketing and/or case reports: Anaphylactic reaction, angioneurotic edema, hepatitis, increased INR, increased PT, severe hyper-/hypoglycemia, nonketotic hyperglycemia, tendon rupture, thrombocytopenia, torsade de pointes

Drug Interactions

Increased Effect/Toxicity: Drugs which prolong QT interval (including Class Ia and Class III antiarrhythmics, erythromycin, cisapride, antipsychotics, and cyclic antidepressants) are contraindicated with gatifloxacin. Drugs which may induce bradycardia (eg, beta-blockers, amiodarone) should be avoided. Gatifloxacin may alter glucose control in patients receiving hypoglycemic agents with or without insulin. Cases of severe disturbances (including symptomatic hypoglycemia) have been reported, typically within 1-3 days of gatifloxacin initiation. Probenecid, loop diuretics, and cimetidine (possibly other H_2 antagonists) may increase the serum concentrations of gatifloxacin (based on experience with other quinolones). Digoxin levels may be increased in some patients by gatifloxacin. NSAIDs and foscarnet have been associated with an increased risk of seizures with some quinolones (not reported with gatifloxacin). The hypoprothrombinemic effect of warfarin is enhanced by some quinolone antibiotics. Monitoring of the INR during concurrent therapy is recommended by the manufacturer. Concurrent use of corticosteroids may increase risk of tendon rupture.

(Continued)

Gatifloxacin *(Continued)*

Decreased Effect: Metal cations (magnesium, aluminum, iron, and zinc) inhibit intestinal absorption of gatifloxacin (by up to 98%). Antacids, electrolyte supplements, sucralfate, quinapril, and some didanosine formulations should be avoided. Gatifloxacin should be administered 4 hours before or 8 hours after these agents. Calcium carbonate was not found to alter the absorption of gatifloxacin. Antineoplastic agents, H_2 antagonists, and proton pump inhibitors may also decrease absorption of some quinolones. Gatifloxacin may alter glucose control in patients receiving hypoglycemic agents with or without insulin.

Dietary/Ethanol/Herb Considerations

Food: May be taken with food or milk; administer 4 hours before supplements containing iron, zinc, or magnesium (including multivitamins).

Herb/Nutraceutical: Avoid dong quai and St John's wort; may cause photosensitization.

Pharmacodynamics/Kinetics

Absorption: Oral: Well absorbed

Distribution: V_d: 1.5-2.0 L/kg; concentrates in alveolar macrophages and lung parenchyma

Protein binding: 20%

Metabolism: Only 1%; no interaction with CYP

Bioavailability: 96%

Half-life elimination: 7.1-13.9 hours; ESRD/CAPD: 30-40 hours

Time to peak: Oral: 1 hour

Excretion: Urine (as unchanged drug); feces (5%)

Pregnancy Risk Factor C

Generic Available No

Gaviscon® Extra Strength [OTC] *see* Aluminum Hydroxide and Magnesium Carbonate *on page 68*

Gaviscon® Liquid [OTC] *see* Aluminum Hydroxide and Magnesium Carbonate *on page 68*

Gaviscon® Tablet [OTC] *see* Aluminum Hydroxide and Magnesium Trisilicate *on page 69*

G-CSF *see* Filgrastim *on page 571*

G-CSF (PEG Conjugate) *see* Pegfilgrastim *on page 1040*

GCV Sodium *see* Ganciclovir *on page 626*

Gelatin (Absorbable) (JEL a tin, ab ZORB a bul)

U.S. Brand Names Gelfilm®; Gelfoam®

Pharmacologic Category Hemostatic Agent

Synonyms Absorbable Gelatin Sponge

Use

Dental and Medical: Adjunct to provide hemostasis in surgery

Medical: Open prostatic surgery

Local Anesthetic/Vasoconstrictor Precautions No information available to require special precautions

Effects on Dental Treatment 1% to 10%: Local infection and abscess formation

Dosage Hemostasis: Apply packs or sponges dry or saturated with sodium chloride. When applied dry, hold in place with moderate pressure. When applied wet, squeeze to remove air bubbles. The powder is applied as a paste prepared by adding approximately 4 mL of sterile saline solution to the powder.

Contraindications Should not be used in closure of skin incisions since they may interfere with the healing of skin edges

Warnings/Precautions Do not sterilize by heat; do not use in the presence of infection

Pregnancy Risk Factor No data reported

Dosage Forms **FILM, ophthalmic** (Gelfilm®): 25 mm x 50 mm (6s). **FILM, topical** (Gelfilm®): 100 mm x 125 mm (1s). **POWDER, topical** (Gelfoam®): 1 g. **SPONGE, dental** (Gelfoam®): Size 4 (12s). **SPONGE, topical** (Gelfoam®): Size 50 (4s), size 100 (6s), size 200 (6s), size 2 cm (1s), size 6 cm (6s), size 12-7 mm (12s)

Generic Available No

Gelclair™ *see* Maltodextrin *on page 840*

Gelfilm® *see* Gelatin (Absorbable) *on page 630*

Gelfoam® *see* Gelatin (Absorbable) *on page 630*

Gel-Kam® [OTC] *see* Fluoride *on page 586*

Gel-Kam® Rinse *see* Fluoride *on page 586*

Gelucast® *see* Zinc Gelatin *on page 1409*

Gemcitabine (jem SIT a been)

U.S. Brand Names Gemzar®

Canadian Brand Names Gemzar®

Mexican Brand Names Gemzar®

Pharmacologic Category Antineoplastic Agent, Antimetabolite

Synonyms Gemcitabine Hydrochloride

Use Adenocarcinoma of the pancreas; first-line therapy for patients with locally advanced (nonresectable stage II or stage III) or metastatic (stage IV) adenocarcinoma of the pancreas (indicated for patients previously treated with 5-FU); combination with cisplatin for the first-line treatment of patients with inoperable, locally advanced (stage IIIA or IIIB) or metastatic (stage IV) nonsmall-cell lung cancer

Local Anesthetic/Vasoconstrictor Precautions No information available to require special precautions

Effects on Dental Treatment No significant effects or complications reported

Dosage Refer to individual protocols. I.V.:

Pancreatic cancer: 1000 mg/m^2 over 30 minutes weekly for 7 weeks followed by 1 week rest; repeat cycles 3 out of every 4 weeks.

Nonsmall cell lung cancer (in combination with cisplatin): 1000 mg/m^2 over 30 minutes on days 1, 8, 15; repeat every 28 days **or** 1250 mg/m^2 over 30 minutes on days 1, 8; repeat every 21 days.

Dosing reductions based on hematologic function: Patients who complete an entire 7-week initial cycle of gemcitabine therapy or a subsequent 3-week cycle at a dose of 1000 mg/m^2 may have the dose for subsequent cycles increased by 25% (1250 mg/m^2), provided that the absolute granulocyte count (AGC) and platelet nadirs exceed 1500 x 10^6/L and 100,000 x 10^6/L, respectively, and if nonhematologic toxicity has not been more than World Health Organization Grade 1

For patients who tolerate the subsequent course, at a dose of 1250 mg/m^2, the dose for the next cycle can be increased to 1500 mg/m^2, provided again that the AGC and platelet nadirs exceed 1500 x 10^6/L and 100,000 x 10^6/L, respectively, and again, if nonhematologic toxicity has not been greater than WHO Grade 1

Dosing adjustment in renal/hepatic impairment: Use with caution; not studied in patients with significant dysfunction

Mechanism of Action Nucleoside analogue that primarily kills cells undergoing DNA synthesis (S-phase) and blocks the progression of cells through the G1/S-phase boundary

Other Adverse Effects

>10%:

- Central nervous system: Fatigue, fever (40%), lethargy, pain (10% to 48%), somnolence (5% to 11%)
- Dermatologic: Alopecia (15%); mild to moderate rashes (5% to 32%)
- Endocrine & metabolic: Increased serum transaminase levels (~66%), mild, transient
- Gastrointestinal: Mild nausea, vomiting, anorexia (20% to 70%); stomatitis (10% to 14%)
- Hematologic: Myelosuppression (20% to 30%), primarily leukopenia, may be dose-limiting
- Neuromuscular & skeletal: Weakness (15% to 25%)
- Renal: Proteinuria, hematuria (45%), elevation of BUN
- Respiratory: Mild to moderate dyspnea (10% to 23%)
- Miscellaneous: Flu-like syndrome (myalgia, fever, chills, fatigue) (20% to 100%), may be dose-limiting

1% to 10%:

- Dermatologic: Pruritus (8%)
- Gastrointestinal: Mild diarrhea (7%), constipation (6%)
- Hematologic: Thrombocytopenia (~10%), anemia (6%)
- Hepatic: Elevated bilirubin (10%)
- Neuromuscular & skeletal: Paresthesia (2% to 10%), peripheral neuropathies (paresthesias, decreased tendon reflexes) (3.5%)
- Respiratory: Severe dyspnea (3%)
- Miscellaneous: Allergic reactions (4%), mild, usually edema, bronchospasm

<1% (Limited to important of life-threatening): Hemolytic-uremic syndrome, adult respiratory distress syndrome (ARDS), pulmonary edema, interstitial pneumonia

Dietary/Ethanol/Herb Considerations Ethanol: Avoid use due to GI irritation.

Pharmacodynamics/Kinetics

Distribution: V_d: Male: 15.6 mL mL/m^2; Female: 11.3 L/m^2

Protein binding: Low

Metabolism: Hepatic, metabolites: di- and triphosphates (active); uridine derivative (inactive)

Half-life elimination: Infusion time: ≤1 hour: 32-94 minutes; Infusion time: 3-4 hours: 4-10.5 hours

Time to peak: 30 minutes

Excretion: Urine (99%, 92% to 98% as intact drug or inactive uridine metabolite); feces (<1%)

Pregnancy Risk Factor D

Generic Available No

Gemcitabine Hydrochloride *see* Gemcitabine *on page 630*

Gemfibrozil (jem FI broe zil)

Related Information

Cardiovascular Diseases *on page 1456*

(Continued)

Gemfibrozil *(Continued)*

U.S. Brand Names Lopid®

Canadian Brand Names Apo®-Gemfibrozil; Gen-Gemfibrozil; Lopid®; Novo-Gemfibrozil; Nu-Gemfibrozil; PMS-Gemfibrozil

Mexican Brand Names Lopid®

Pharmacologic Category Antilipemic Agent, Fibric Acid

Synonyms CI-719

Use Treatment of hypertriglyceridemia in types IV and V hyperlipidemia for patients who are at greater risk for pancreatitis and who have not responded to dietary intervention

Local Anesthetic/Vasoconstrictor Precautions No information available to require special precautions

Effects on Dental Treatment No significant effects or complications reported

Dosage Adults: Oral: 1200 mg/day in 2 divided doses, 30 minutes before breakfast and dinner

Hemodialysis: Not removed by hemodialysis; supplemental dose is unnecessary

Mechanism of Action The exact mechanism of action of gemfibrozil is unknown, however, several theories exist regarding the VLDL effect; it can inhibit lipolysis and decrease subsequent hepatic fatty acid uptake as well as inhibit hepatic secretion of VLDL; together these actions decrease serum VLDL levels; increases HDL-cholesterol; the mechanism behind HDL elevation is currently unknown

Other Adverse Effects

>10% Gastrointestinal: Dyspepsia (20%)

1% to 10%:

Central nervous system: Fatigue (4%), vertigo (2%), headache (1%)

Dermatologic: Eczema (2%), rash (2%)

Gastrointestinal: Abdominal pain (10%), diarrhea (7%), nausea/vomiting (3%), constipation (1%)

<1% or case reports with probable causation (limited to important or life-threatening): Hypoesthesia, paresthesia, abnormal taste, cataracts, intracranial hemorrhage, peripheral vascular disease, cholestatic jaundice, dizziness, somnolence, peripheral neuritis, decreased libido, depression, headache, blurred vision, impotence, myopathy, myasthenia, myalgia, arthralgia, synovitis, rhabdomyolysis, increased creatinine phosphokinase, increased bilirubin, increased transaminases, increased alkaline phosphatase, anemia, leukopenia, bone marrow hypoplasia, eosinophilia, angioedema, laryngeal edema, urticaria, exfoliative dermatitis, rash, dermatitis, pruritus, vasculitis, Raynaud's phenomenon, hypokalemia, nephrotoxicity, dermatomyositis/polymyositis

Reports where causal relationship has not been established: Weight loss, extrasystoles, pancreatitis, hepatoma, colitis, confusion, seizures, syncope, retinal edema, decreased fertility (male), renal dysfunction, positive ANA, drug-induced lupus-like syndrome, thrombocytopenia, anaphylaxis, vasculitis, alopecia, photosensitivity

Drug Interactions Substrate of CYP3A4

Increased Effect/Toxicity: Gemfibrozil may potentiate the effects of bexarotene (avoid concurrent use), sulfonylureas (including glyburide, chlorpropamide), and warfarin. HMG-CoA reductase inhibitors (atorvastatin, fluvastatin, lovastatin, pravastatin, simvastatin) may increase the risk of myopathy and rhabdomyolysis. The manufacturer warns against the concurrent use of lovastatin (if unavoidable, limit lovastatin to <20 mg/day). Combination therapy with statins has been used in some patients with resistant hyperlipidemias (with great caution).

Decreased Effect: Cyclosporine's blood levels may be reduced during concurrent therapy. Rifampin may decreased gemfibrozil blood levels.

Dietary/Ethanol/Herb Considerations

Ethanol: Avoid use; may increase triglyceride levels.

Food: Administer with food or milk to reduce GI upset; should be taken 30 minutes before meals if possible.

Pharmacodynamics/Kinetics

Onset of action: May require several days

Absorption: Well absorbed

Protein binding: 99%

Metabolism: Hepatic via oxidation to two inactive metabolites; undergoes enterohepatic recycling

Half-life elimination: 1.4 hours

Time to peak, serum: 1-2 hours

Excretion: Urine (70% primarily as unchanged drug)

Pregnancy Risk Factor C

Generic Available Yes

Gemtuzumab Ozogamicin (gem TUZ yoo mab oh zog a MYE sin)

U.S. Brand Names Mylotarg®

Canadian Brand Names Mylotarg™

Pharmacologic Category Antineoplastic Agent, Monoclonal Antibody

Use Treatment of acute myeloid leukemia (CD33 positive) in first relapse in patients who are ≥60 years of age and who are not considered candidates for cytotoxic chemotherapy.

Local Anesthetic/Vasoconstrictor Precautions No information available to require special precautions

Effects on Dental Treatment Adults >60 years of age:

>10%: Hypertension (20%), hypotension (16%), fever (80%), headache (26%), pain (25%), dizziness (11%), nausea (64%), vomiting (55%), anorexia (31%), bleeding (15%), lymphopenia, weakness (45%), dyspnea (36%), epistaxis (29%; severe 3%), cough (19%), pharyngitis (14%), infection (28%), sepsis (24%), neutropenic fever (20%), stomatitis/mucositis (25%), ecchymosis (15%)

1% to 10%: Tachycardia (10%), CNS depression (10%), hyperglycemia (2%), hemorrhage (8%), elevated PT, rhinitis (10%), pneumonia (10%)

Dosage I.V.:

Adults ≥60 years: 9 mg/m², infused over 2 hours. The patient should receive diphenhydramine 50 mg orally and acetaminophen 650-1000 mg orally 1 hour prior to administration of each dose. Acetaminophen dosage should be repeated as needed every 4 hours for two additional doses. A full treatment course is a total of two doses administered with 14 days between doses. Full hematologic recovery is unnecessary for administration of the second dose. There has been only limited experience with repeat courses of gemtuzumab ozogamicin.

Dosing adjustment in renal/hepatic impairment: Not studied

Mechanism of Action Antibody to CD33 antigen, which is expressed on leukemic blasts in >80% of patients with acute myeloid leukemia (AML), as well as normal myeloid cells. Binding results in internalization of the antibody-antigen complex. Following internalization, the calicheamicin derivative is released inside the myeloid cell. The calicheamicin derivative binds to DNA resulting in double strand breaks and cell death. Pluripotent stem cells and nonhematopoietic cells are not affected.

Other Adverse Effects Adults >60 years of age:

>10%:

- Cardiovascular: Peripheral edema (21%)
- Central nervous system: Chills (66%), insomnia (18%)
- Dermatologic: Rash (23%), petechiae (21%)
- Endocrine & metabolic: Hypokalemia (30%)
- Gastrointestinal: Diarrhea (38%), abdominal pain (29%), constipation (28%), abdominal distention (11%), dyspepsia (11%)
- Hematologic: Neutropenia (98%; median recovery 40.5 days), thrombocytopenia (99%; median recovery 39 days); anemia (47%)
- Hepatic: Hyperbilirubinemia (23%) increased LDH (18%), increased transaminases (9% to 17%)
- Local: Local reaction (25%)
- Neuromuscular & skeletal: Back pain (18%)

1% to 10%:

- Central nervous system: Cerebral hemorrhage (2%), intracranial hemorrhage (2%)
- Endocrine & metabolic: Hypomagnesemia (4%)
- Genitourinary: Hematuria (10%; severe 1%), vaginal hemorrhage (7%)
- Hematologic: Disseminated intravascular coagulation (DIC) (2%)
- Neuromuscular & skeletal: Arthralgia (10%)
- Respiratory: Hypoxia (6%)

<1% (Limited to important or life threatening symptoms): **Hepatic failure,** jaundice, hepatosplenomegaly, veno-occlusive disease

Postmarketing and/or case reports: **Acute respiratory distress syndrome, anaphylaxis, hypersensitivity reactions, noncardiogenic pulmonary edema, renal failure**

Dietary/Ethanol/Herb Considerations Ethanol: Avoid use due to GI irritation.

Pharmacodynamics/Kinetics Half-life elimination: Calicheamicin: Total: Initial: 45 hours, Repeat dose: 60 hours; Unconjugated: 100 hours (no change noted in repeat dosing)

Pregnancy Risk Factor D

Generic Available No

Gemzar® *see* Gemcitabine *on page 630*
Genac® [OTC] *see* Triprolidine and Pseudoephedrine *on page 1356*
Genaced [OTC] *see* Acetaminophen, Aspirin, and Caffeine *on page 34*
Genahist® [OTC] *see* DiphenhydrAMINE *on page 451*
Genapap® [OTC] *see* Acetaminophen *on page 27*
Genapap® Children [OTC] *see* Acetaminophen *on page 27*
Genapap® Extra Strength [OTC] *see* Acetaminophen *on page 27*
Genapap® Infant [OTC] *see* Acetaminophen *on page 27*
Genaphed® [OTC] *see* Pseudoephedrine *on page 1146*
Genasal [OTC] *see* Oxymetazoline *on page 1022*
Genasoft® [OTC] *see* Docusate *on page 463*
Genasoft® Plus [OTC] *see* Docusate and Casanthranol *on page 464*

Genasyme® [OTC] *see* Simethicone *on page 1222*
Genatuss DM® [OTC] *see* Guaifenesin and Dextromethorphan *on page 651*
Gencalc® 600 [OTC] *see* Calcium Supplements *on page 229*
Genebs® [OTC] *see* Acetaminophen *on page 27*
Genebs® Extra Strength [OTC] *see* Acetaminophen *on page 27*
Generlac *see* Lactulose *on page 772*
Genesec® [OTC] *see* Acetaminophen and Phenyltoloxamine *on page 31*
Geneye® [OTC] *see* Tetrahydrozoline *on page 1288*
Genfiber® [OTC] *see* Psyllium *on page 1149*
Gengraf™ *see* CycloSPORINE *on page 383*
Genoptic® *see* Gentamicin *on page 634*
Genotropin® *see* Human Growth Hormone *on page 671*
Genotropin Miniquick® *see* Human Growth Hormone *on page 671*
Genpril® [OTC] *see* Ibuprofen *on page 703*
Gentacidin® *see* Gentamicin *on page 634*
Gentak® *see* Gentamicin *on page 634*

Gentamicin (jen ta MYE sin)

Related Information

Cardiovascular Diseases *on page 1456*

U.S. Brand Names Garamycin®; Genoptic®; Gentacidin®; Gentak®

Canadian Brand Names Alcomicin®; Diogent®; Garamycin®; Minim's Gentamicin 0.3%; SAB-Gentamicin

Mexican Brand Names Garalen; Garamicina®; Genemicin®; Genenicina®; Genkova®; Genrex®; Gentabac®; Gentacin®; Genta Grin®; Gentarim®; Gentazaf®; G.I.®; Ikatin®; Nozolon; Quilagen; Servigenta®; Tondex®; Yectamicina®

Pharmacologic Category Antibiotic, Aminoglycoside; Antibiotic, Ophthalmic; Antibiotic, Topical

Synonyms Gentamicin Sulfate

Use

Dental: Prevention of bacterial endocarditis; treatment of respiratory tract, skin, and soft tissue infections prior to dental procedures

Medical: Treatment of susceptible bacterial infections, normally gram-negative organisms including *Pseudomonas*, *Proteus*, *Serratia*, and gram-positive *Staphylococcus*; treatment of bone, respiratory tract, skin, soft tissue, abdominal, ophthalmic, and urinary tract infections; treatment of endocarditis and septicemia

Local Anesthetic/Vasoconstrictor Precautions No information available to require special precautions

Effects on Dental Treatment No significant effects or complication reported

Dosage Individualization is critical because of the low therapeutic index. Use of ideal body weight (IBW) for determining the mg/kg/dose appears to be more accurate than dosing on the basis of total body weight (TBW). Dosage requirement in patients with morbid obesity may best be estimated using a dosing weight of IBW + 0.4 (TBW - IBW). Some patients may require larger or more frequent doses (eg, every 6 hours) if serum levels document the need; initial and periodic peak and trough plasma drug levels should be determined, particularly in critically ill patients with serious infections or in disease states known to significantly alter aminoglycoside pharmacokinetics (eg, cystic fibrosis, burns, or major surgery). Some clinicians suggest a daily dose of 4-7 mg/kg for all patients with normal renal function, which is at least as efficacious, with similar if not less, toxicity than conventional dosing.

Newborns: Intrathecal: 1 mg every day

Infants >3 months: Intrathecal: 1-2 mg/day

Infants and Children <5 years: I.M., I.V.: 2.5 mg/kg/dose every 8 hours

- Treatment of cystic fibrosis: 2.5 mg/kg/dose every 6 hours

Children >5 years: I.M., I.V.: 1.5-2.5 mg/kg/dose every 8 hours

- **Prevention of bacterial endocarditis:** Dental, oral, upper respiratory procedures, GI/GU procedures: 2 mg/kg with ampicillin (50 mg/kg) 30 minutes prior to procedure

Adults: I.M., I.V.:

- Severe life-threatening infections: 2-2.5 mg/kg/dose
- Urinary tract infections: 1.5 mg/kg/dose
- Synergy (for gram-positive infections): 1 mg/kg/dose
- **Prevention of bacterial endocarditis:**
  - Dental, oral, or upper respiratory procedures: 1.5 mg/kg not to exceed 80 mg with ampicillin (1-2 g) 30 minutes prior to procedure
  - GI/GU surgery: 1.5 mg/kg not to exceed 80 mg with ampicillin (2 g) 30 minutes prior to procedure

Children and Adults:

- Intrathecal: 4-8 mg/day
- Ophthalmic:
  - Ointment: Instill 1/2" (1.25 cm) 2-3 times/day to every 3-4 hours
  - Solution: Instill 1-2 drops every 2-4 hours, up to 2 drops every hour for severe infections

Topical: Apply 3-4 times/day to affected area

Dosing interval in renal impairment:

Cl_{cr} ≥60 mL/minute: Administer every 8 hours

Cl_{cr} 40-60 mL/minute: Administer every 12 hours

Cl_{cr} 20-40 mL/minute: Administer every 24 hours

Cl_{cr} <20 mL/minute: Loading dose, then monitor levels

Hemodialysis: Dialyzable; removal by hemodialysis: 30% removal of aminoglycosides occurs during 4 hours of HD; administer dose after dialysis and follow levels

Removal by continuous ambulatory peritoneal dialysis (CAPD):

Administration via CAPD fluid:

Gram-negative infection: 4-8 mg/L (4-8 mcg/mL) of CAPD fluid

Gram-positive infection (ie, synergy): 3-4 mg/L (3-4 mcg/mL) of CAPD fluid

Administration via I.V., I.M. route during CAPD: Dose as for Cl_{cr} <10 mL/minute and follow levels

Removal via continuous arteriovenous or venovenous hemofiltration: Dose as for Cl_{cr} 10-40 mL/minute and follow levels

Dosing comment in hepatic disease: Monitor plasma concentrations

Mechanism of Action Interferes with bacterial protein synthesis by binding to 30S and 50S ribosomal subunits resulting in a defective bacterial cell membrane

Other Adverse Effects

>10%:

Central nervous system: Neurotoxicity (vertigo, ataxia)

Neuromuscular & skeletal: **Gait instability**

Otic: Ototoxicity (auditory and vestibular)

Renal: Nephrotoxicity, decreased creatinine clearance

1% to 10%:

Cardiovascular: Edema

Dermatologic: Skin itching, reddening of skin, rash

<1%: **Drowsiness, headache, pseudomotor cerebri,** photosensitivity, **allergic reaction,** erythema, anorexia, **nausea, vomiting,** weight loss, **increased salivation,** enterocolitis, granulocytopenia, agranulocytosis, thrombocytopenia, elevated LFTs, **burning, stinging, tremors, muscle cramps, weakness, dyspnea**

Contraindications Hypersensitivity to gentamicin or other aminoglycosides

Warnings/Precautions Not intended for long-term therapy due to toxic hazards associated with extended administration; pre-existing renal insufficiency, vestibular or cochlear impairment, myasthenia gravis, hypocalcemia, conditions which depress neuromuscular transmission

Parenteral aminoglycosides have been associated with significant nephrotoxicity or ototoxicity; the ototoxicity may be directly proportional to the amount of drug given and the duration of treatment; tinnitus or vertigo are indications of vestibular injury and impending hearing loss; renal damage is usually reversible

Drug Interactions

Increased Toxicity:

Aminoglycosides may potentiate the effects of neuromuscular-blocking agents.

Penicillins, cephalosporins, amphotericin B, loop diuretics may increase nephrotoxic potential

Decreased Effect: Gentamicin's efficacy reduced when given concurrently with carbenicillin, ticarcillin, or piperacillin to patients with severe renal impairment (inactivation). Separate administration.

Pharmacodynamics/Kinetics

Absorption: Oral: None

Distribution: Crosses placenta

V_d: Increased by edema, ascites, fluid overload; decreased with dehydration

Neonates: 0.4-0.6 L/kg

Children: 0.3-0.35 L/kg

Adults: 0.2-0.3 L/kg

Relative diffusion from blood into CSF: Minimal even with inflammation

CSF:blood level ratio: Normal meninges: Nil; Inflamed meninges: 10% to 30%

Protein binding: <30%

Half-life elimination

Infants: <1 week old: 3-11.5 hours; 1 week to 6 months old: 3-3.5 hours

Adults: 1.5-3 hours; End-stage renal disease: 36-70 hours

Time to peak, serum: I.M.: 30-90 minutes; I.V.: 30 minutes after 30-minute infusion

Excretion: Urine (as unchanged drug)

Clearance: Directly related to renal function

Pregnancy Risk Factor C

Breast-feeding Considerations No data reported; however, gentamicin is not absorbed orally and other aminoglycosides may be taken while breast-feeding.

Dosage Forms CRM, topical (Garamycin®): 0.1% (15 g). **INF** [premixed in NS]: 40 mg (50 mL); 60 mg (50 mL, 100 mL); 70 mg (50 mL); 80 mg (50 mL, 100 mL); 90 mg (100 mL); 100 mg (50 mL, 100 mL); 120 mg (100 mL). **INJ, solution** [ADD-Vantage® vial]: 10 mg/mL (6 mL, 8 mL, 10 mL). **INJ, solution:** 40 mg/mL (2 mL, 20 mL); (Garamycin®): 40 mg/mL (2 mL). **INJ, solution, pediatric:** 10 mg/mL (2 mL). **INJ, solution, pediatric** [preservative free]: 10 mg/mL (2 mL). **OINT,**

(Continued)

Gentamicin *(Continued)*

ophthalmic: 0.3% [3 mg/g] (3.5 g). **OINT, topical** (Garamycin®): 0.1% (15 g). **SOLN, ophthalmic:** 0.3% (5 mL, 15 mL); (Garamycin®, Gentacidin®): 0.3% (5 mL); (Genoptic®): 0.3% (1 mL, 5 mL); (Gentak®): 0.3% (5 mL, 15 mL)

Generic Available Yes

Gentamicin and Prednisolone *see* Prednisolone and Gentamicin *on page 1112*
Gentamicin Sulfate *see* Gentamicin *on page 634*
GenTeal® [OTC] *see* Hydroxypropyl Methylcellulose *on page 696*
GenTeal® Mild [OTC] *see* Hydroxypropyl Methylcellulose *on page 696*

Gentian Violet (JEN shun VYE oh let)

Pharmacologic Category Antibiotic, Topical; Antifungal Agent, Topical

Synonyms Crystal Violet; Methylrosaniline Chloride

Use Treatment of cutaneous or mucocutaneous infections caused by *Candida albicans* and other superficial skin infections

Local Anesthetic/Vasoconstrictor Precautions No information available to require special precautions

Effects on Dental Treatment No significant effects or complications reported

Dosage Children and Adults: Topical: Apply 0.5% to 2% locally with cotton to lesion 2-3 times/day for 3 days, do not swallow and avoid contact with eyes

Mechanism of Action Topical antiseptic/germicide effective against some vegetative gram-positive bacteria, particularly *Staphylococcus* sp, and some yeast; it is much less effective against gram-negative bacteria and is ineffective against acid-fast bacteria

Other Adverse Effects Frequency not defined:
Dermatologic: Vesicle formation
Gastrointestinal: **Esophagitis, ulceration of mucous membranes**
Local: Burning, irritation
Respiratory: **Laryngitis, laryngeal obstruction, tracheitis**
Miscellaneous: Sensitivity reactions

Pregnancy Risk Factor C

Generic Available Yes

Gentran® *see* Dextran *on page 419*
Geocillin® *see* Carbenicillin *on page 245*
Geref® [DSC] *see* Sermorelin Acetate *on page 1215*
Geref® Diagnostic *see* Sermorelin Acetate *on page 1215*
Geritol® Tonic [OTC] *see* Vitamins (Multiple/Oral) *on page 1394*
German Measles Vaccine *see* Rubella Virus Vaccine (Live) *on page 1202*
Gevrabon® [OTC] *see* Vitamin B Complex *on page 1392*
GG *see* Guaifenesin *on page 650*
GHB *see* Sodium Oxybate *on page 1231*
GI87084B *see* Remifentanil *on page 1171*
Gingi-Aid® Gingival Retraction Cord *see* Aluminum Chloride *on page 67*
Gingi-Aid® Solution *see* Aluminum Chloride *on page 67*

Glatiramer Acetate (gla TIR a mer AS e tate)

U.S. Brand Names Copaxone®

Canadian Brand Names Copaxone®

Pharmacologic Category Biological, Miscellaneous

Synonyms Copolymer-1

Use Treatment of relapsing-remitting type multiple sclerosis; studies indicate that it reduces the frequency of attacks and the severity of disability; appears to be most effective for patients with minimal disability

Local Anesthetic/Vasoconstrictor Precautions No information available to require special precautions

Effects on Dental Treatment Reported in >2% of patients in placebo-controlled trials:

>10%: Dyspnea (19%), rhinitis (14%), palpitations (17%), vasodilation (27%), flu-like syndrome (19%), chest pain (21%), pain (28%), anxiety (23%), diaphoresis (15%) nausea (22%), weakness (41%), infection (50%), lymphadenopathy (12%)

1% to 10%: Facial edema (6%), tachycardia (5%), hypertension (1%), syncope (5%), herpes simplex (4%), neck pain (8%) fever (8%), migraine (5%), agitation (4%), confusion (2%), nervousness (2%), speech disorder (2%), stupor (1%), bruising (8%), vomiting (6%), vomiting (6%), GI disorder (5%), gastroenteritis (3%), oral moniliasis (1%), ulcerative stomatitis (1%), salivary gland enlargement, tremor (7%), ear pain (7%), bronchitis (9%), laryngismus (5%), bacterial infection (5%)

Dosage Adults: S.C.: 20 mg daily

Mechanism of Action Glatiramer is a mixture of random polymers of four amino acids; L-alanine, L-glutamic acid, L-lysine and L-tyrosine, the resulting mixture is antigenically similar to myelin basic protein, which is an important component of the myelin sheath of nerves; glatiramer is thought to suppress T-lymphocytes specific for a myelin antigen, it is also proposed that glatiramer interferes with the antigen-presenting function of certain immune cells opposing pathogenic T-cell function

Other Adverse Effects Reported in >2% of patients in placebo-controlled trials:

>10%:

- Dermatologic: Pruritus (18%), rash (18%)
- Gastrointestinal: Diarrhea (12%)
- Local: Injection site reactions: Pain (73%), erythema (66%), inflammation (49%), pruritus (40%), mass (27%), induration (13%), welt (11%)
- Neuromuscular & skeletal: Arthralgia (24%), hypertonia (22%), back pain (16%)

1% to 10%:

- Cardiovascular: Peripheral edema (7%), edema (3%)
- Central nervous system: Vertigo (6%), chills (4%), abnormal dreams (1%), emotional lability (1%)
- Dermatologic: Erythema (4%), urticaria (4%), skin nodule (2%), eczema, pustular rash, skin atrophy
- Endocrine & metabolic: Dysmenorrhea (6%), amenorrhea (1%), menorrhagia (1%), vaginal hemorrhage (1%)
- Gastrointestinal: Anorexia (8%), weight gain (3%)
- Genitourinary: Urinary urgency (10%), vaginal moniliasis (8%), hematuria (1%), impotence (1%)
- Local: Injection site reactions: Hemorrhage (5%), urticaria (5%), edema (1%), atrophy (1%), abscess (1%), hypersensitivity (1%)
- Neuromuscular & skeletal: Foot drop (3%)
- Ocular: Eye disorder (4%), nystagmus (2%), visual field defect (1%)
- Otic: Ear pain (7%)
- Miscellaneous: Cyst (2%)

<1% (Limited to important or life-threatening): Angioedema, aphasia, **atrial fibrillation**, cholecystitis, **coma**, corneal ulcer, **esophageal ulcer, esophagitis, ethanol intolerance, GI hemorrhage, GI carcinoma**, gout, **hallucinations**, hematemesis, hepatomegaly, **hypotension**, injection site abscess or fibrosis, leukopenia, **manic reaction**, optic neuritis, pancreatitis, pancytopenia, paraplegia, photosensitivity reaction, **postural hypotension,** priapism, rash, **seizures, serum sickness**, splenomegaly, suicide attempt

Postmarketing and/or case reports (limited to important or life-threatening): **Sepsis, lupus erythematosus, allergic reaction, anaphylactoid reaction**, thrombosis, pericardial effusion, **MI, CHF,** cardiomyopathy, **arrhythmia, angina**, hepatitis, cirrhosis, cholelithiasis, thrombocytopenia, **rheumatoid arthritis**, meningitis, CNS neoplasm, **stroke, seizure**, neuralgia, pulmonary embolism, glaucoma, blindness, renal failure, carcinoma (breast, bladder, lung)

Pharmacodynamics/Kinetics

Distribution: Small amounts of intact and partial hydrolyzed drug enter lymphatic circulation

Metabolism: S.C.: Large percentage hydrolyzed locally

Pregnancy Risk Factor B

Generic Available No

Gliadel® *see* Carmustine *on page 253*

Glibenclamide *see* GlyBURIDE *on page 642*

Glimepiride (GLYE me pye ride)

Related Information

Endocrine Disorders and Pregnancy *on page 1479*

U.S. Brand Names Amaryl®

Canadian Brand Names Amaryl®

Mexican Brand Names Amaryl®

Pharmacologic Category Antidiabetic Agent, Sulfonylurea

Use Management of type 2 diabetes mellitus (noninsulin dependent, NIDDM) as an adjunct to diet and exercise to lower blood glucose or in combination with metformin; use in combination with insulin to lower blood glucose in patients whose hyperglycemia cannot be controlled by diet and exercise in conjunction with an oral hypoglycemic agent

Local Anesthetic/Vasoconstrictor Precautions No information available to require special precautions

Effects on Dental Treatment Glimepiride-dependent diabetics (noninsulin dependent, type 2) should be appointed for dental treatment in morning in order to minimize chance of stress-induced hypoglycemia

Dosage Oral (allow several days between dose titrations):

Adults: Initial: 1-2 mg once daily, administered with breakfast or the first main meal; usual maintenance dose: 1-4 mg once daily; after a dose of 2 mg once daily, increase in increments of 2 mg at 1- to 2-week intervals based upon the patient's blood glucose response to a maximum of 8 mg once daily

(Continued)

Glimepiride *(Continued)*

Combination with insulin therapy (fasting glucose level for instituting combination therapy is in the range of >150 mg/dL in plasma or serum depending on the patient): initial recommended dose: 8 mg once daily with the first main meal

After starting with low-dose insulin, upward adjustments of insulin can be done approximately weekly as guided by frequent measurements of fasting blood glucose. Once stable, combination-therapy patients should monitor their capillary blood glucose on an ongoing basis, preferably daily.

Elderly: Initial: 1 mg/day; dose titration and maintenance dosing should be conservative to avoid hypoglycemia

Dosing adjustment/comments in renal impairment: Cl_{cr} <22 mL/minute: Initial starting dose should be 1 mg and dosage increments should be based on fasting blood glucose levels

Dosing adjustment in hepatic impairment: Data unavailable

Mechanism of Action Stimulates insulin release from the pancreatic beta cells; reduces glucose output from the liver; insulin sensitivity is increased at peripheral target sites

Other Adverse Effects

1% to 10%: Central nervous system: Headache

<1%: Agranulocytosis, anorexia, aplastic anemia, blood dyscrasias, bone marrow suppression, cholestatic jaundice, constipation, diarrhea, diuretic effect, edema, epigastric fullness, erythema, heartburn, hemolytic anemia, hepatitis, hypoglycemia, hyponatremia, nausea, photosensitivity, pruritus, rash, thrombocytopenia, urticaria, vomiting

Other reactions reported with sulfonylureas: Porphyria, vasculitis

Drug Interactions Substrate of **CYP2C8/9**

Increased Effect/Toxicity: Anticoagulants, androgens, fluconazole, miconazole, salicylates, gemfibrozil, sulfonamides, tricyclic antidepressants, probenecid, MAO inhibitors, beta-blockers, methyldopa, digitalis glycosides, urinary acidifiers may increase the hypoglycemic effects of glimepiride.

Decreased Effect: There may be a decreased effect of glimepiride with corticosteroids, cholestyramine, estrogens, oral contraceptives, phenytoin, rifampin, thiazide and other diuretics, phenothiazines, NSAIDs, thyroid products, nicotinic acid, isoniazid, sympathomimetics, urinary alkalinizers, and charcoal. **Note:** However, data from pooled data did **not** demonstrate drug interactions with calcium channel blockers, estrogens, NSAIDs, HMG-CoA reductase inhibitors, sulfonamides, or thyroid hormone.

Dietary/Ethanol/Herb Considerations

Ethanol: Use with caution; may increase risk of hypoglycemia.

Food: Administer with breakfast or first main meal of the day. Dietary modification, based on ADA recommendations, is part of therapy. Hypoglycemia may occur (decreases blood glucose concentration); patients must be able to recognize symptoms (palpitations, sweaty palms, lightheadedness). Food delays absorption.

Herb/Nutraceutical: Use caution with chromium, garlic, gymnema, and horse chestnut; may cause hypoglycemia. Black cohosh may enhance effects of antidiabetic agents.

Pharmacodynamics/Kinetics

Onset of action: Peak effect: Blood glucose reductions: 2-3 hours
Duration: 24 hours
Absorption: 100%; delayed when given with food
Protein binding: >99.5%
Metabolism: Completely hepatic
Half-life elimination: 5-9 hours
Excretion: Urine and feces (as metabolites)

Pregnancy Risk Factor C

Generic Available No

GlipiZIDE (GLIP i zide)

Related Information

Endocrine Disorders and Pregnancy *on page 1479*
Glipizide and Metformin *on page 639*

U.S. Brand Names Glucotrol®; Glucotrol® XL

Mexican Brand Names Glupitel®; Minodiab®

Pharmacologic Category Antidiabetic Agent, Sulfonylurea

Synonyms Glydiazinamide

Use Management of type 2 diabetes mellitus (noninsulin dependent, NIDDM)

Local Anesthetic/Vasoconstrictor Precautions No information available to require special precautions

Effects on Dental Treatment Glipizide-dependent diabetics (noninsulin dependent, type 2) should be appointed for dental treatment in morning in order to minimize chance of stress-induced hypoglycemia.

Dosage Give ~30 minutes before a meal to obtain the greatest reduction in postprandial hyperglycemia.

Oral (allow several days between dose titrations):

Adults: Initial: 5 mg/day; adjust dosage at 2.5-5 mg daily increments as determined by blood glucose response at intervals of several days. Maximum recommended once-daily dose: 15 mg; maximum recommended total daily dose: 40 mg; extended release (Glucotrol® XL) maximum recommended dose: 20 mg.

Elderly: Initial: 2.5 mg/day; increase by 2.5-5 mg/day at 1- to 2-week intervals

Dosing adjustment/comments in renal impairment: Cl_{cr} <10 mL/minute: Some investigators recommend not using

Dosing adjustment in hepatic impairment: Initial dosage should be 2.5 mg/day

Mechanism of Action Stimulates insulin release from the pancreatic beta cells; reduces glucose output from the liver; insulin sensitivity is increased at peripheral target sites

Other Adverse Effects Frequency not defined:

Cardiovascular: Edema

Central nervous system: Headache

Dermatologic: Rash, urticaria, photosensitivity

Endocrine & metabolic: Hypoglycemia, hyponatremia, SIADH (rare)

Gastrointestinal: Anorexia, nausea, vomiting, diarrhea, epigastric fullness, constipation, heartburn

Hematologic: Blood dyscrasias, aplastic anemia, hemolytic anemia, bone marrow suppression, thrombocytopenia, agranulocytosis

Hepatic: Cholestatic jaundice, hepatic porphyria

Renal: Diuretic effect (minor)

Miscellaneous: Disulfiram-like reaction

Drug Interactions Substrate of **2C8/9**

Increased Effect/Toxicity: Increased effects/hypoglycemic effects of glipizide with H_2 antagonists, anticoagulants, androgens, cimetidine, fluconazole, salicylates, gemfibrozil, sulfonamides, tricyclic antidepressants, probenecid, MAO inhibitors, methyldopa, digitalis glycosides, and urinary acidifiers.

Decreased Effect: Decreased effect of glipizide with beta-blockers, cholestyramine, hydantoins, rifampin, thiazide diuretics, urinary alkalinizers, and charcoal.

Dietary/Ethanol/Herb Considerations

Ethanol: Use with caution; may cause hypoglycemia or rare disulfiram reaction.

Food may delay release of insulin; administer at the same time each day 30 minutes before meals to avoid erratic absorption. Dietary modification, based on ADA recommendations, is part of therapy. Hypoglycemia may occur; decreases blood glucose concentration.

Herb/Nutraceutical: Use caution with chromium, garlic, gymnema, and horse chestnut; may cause hypoglycemia. Black cohosh may enhance effects of antidiabetic agents.

Pharmacodynamics/Kinetics

Onset of action: Peak effect: Blood glucose reductions: 1.5-2 hours

Duration: 12-24 hours

Absorption: Delayed with food

Protein binding: 92% to 99%

Metabolism: Hepatic with metabolites

Half-life elimination: 2-4 hours

Excretion: Urine (60% to 80%, 91% to 97% as metabolites); feces (11%)

Pregnancy Risk Factor C

Generic Available Yes: Not extended release formulation

Glipizide and Metformin (GLIP i zide & met FOR min)

Related Information

GlipiZIDE *on page 638*

Metformin *on page 874*

U.S. Brand Names Metaglip™

Pharmacologic Category Antidiabetic Agent, Biguanide; Antidiabetic Agent, Sulfonylurea

Synonyms Glipizide and Metformin Hydrochloride; Metformin and Glipizide

Use Initial therapy for management of type 2 diabetes mellitus (noninsulin dependent, NIDDM) when hyperglycemia cannot be managed with diet and exercise alone. Second-line therapy for management of type 2 diabetes (NIDDM) when hyperglycemia cannot be managed with a sulfonylurea or metformin along with diet and exercise.

Local Anesthetic/Vasoconstrictor Precautions No information available to require special precautions

Effects on Dental Treatment Upper respiratory tract infection (8% to 10%)

Dependent diabetics (noninsulin dependent, type 2) should be appointed in the morning in order to minimize chance of stress-induced hypoglycemia.

Dosage Oral:

Adults:

Type 2 diabetes, first-line therapy: Initial: Glipizide 2.5 mg/metformin 250 mg once daily with a meal. Dose adjustment: Increase dose by 1 tablet/day every 2 weeks, up to a maximum of glipizide 10 mg/metformin 1000 mg daily

(Continued)

Glipizide and Metformin *(Continued)*

Patients with fasting plasma glucose (FPG) 280-320 mg/dL: Consider glipizide 2.5 mg/metformin 500 mg twice daily. Dose adjustment: Increase dose by 1 tablet/day every 2 weeks, up to a maximum of glipizide 10 mg/metformin 2000 mg daily in divided doses

Type 2 diabetes, second-line therapy: Glipizide 2.5 mg/metformin 500 mg **or** glipizide 5 mg/metformin 500 mg twice daily with morning and evening meals; starting dose should not exceed current daily dose of glipizide (or sulfonylurea equivalent) or metformin. Dose adjustment: Titrate dose in increments of no more than glipizide 5 mg/metformin 500 mg, up to a maximum dose of glipizide 20 mg/metformin 2000 mg daily.

Elderly: Conservative doses recommended due to potentially decreased renal function; **do not titrate to maximum dose**; should not be used in patients ≥80 years unless renal function is verified as normal

Dosing adjustment in renal impairment: Risk of lactic acidosis increases with degree of renal impairment; contraindicated in renal disease or dysfunction.

Dosing adjustment in hepatic impairment: Use should be avoided; liver disease is a risk factor for the development of lactic acidosis during metformin therapy.

Mechanism of Action The combination of glipizide and metformin is used to improve glycemic control in patients with type 2 diabetes mellitus (noninsulin dependent, NIDDM) by using two different, but complementary, mechanisms of action:

Glipizide: Stimulates insulin release from the pancreatic beta cells; reduces glucose output from the liver; insulin sensitivity is increased at peripheral target sites

Metformin: Decreases hepatic glucose production, decreasing intestinal absorption of glucose and improves insulin sensitivity (increases peripheral glucose uptake and utilization)

Other Adverse Effects

>10%:

- Central nervous system: Headache (12%)
- Endocrine & metabolic: Hypoglycemia (8% to 13%)
- Gastrointestinal: Diarrhea (2% to 18%)

1% to 10%:

- Cardiovascular: Hypertension (3%)
- Central nervous system: Dizziness (2% to 5%)
- Gastrointestinal: Nausea/vomiting (<1% to 8%), abdominal pain (6%)
- Neuromuscular & skeletal: Musculoskeletal pain (8%)
- Renal: Urinary tract infection (1%)

Dietary/Ethanol/Herb Considerations

Ethanol: Avoid use; may increase risk of lactic acidosis and hypoglycemia.

Food: Administer at the same time each day with food to reduce GI upset; food decreases the extent and slightly delays the absorption. Dietary modification, based on ADA recommendations, is a part of therapy. Metformin may decrease absorption of vitamin B_{12} and/or folic acid; may require supplementation. Hypoglycemia may occur; decreases blood glucose concentration; must be able to recognize symptoms of hypoglycemia (palpitations, sweaty palms, lightheadedness).

Herb/Nutraceutical: Use caution with chromium, garlic, gymnema, and horse chestnut; may cause hypoglycemia. Black cohosh may enhance effects of antidiabetic agents.

Pregnancy Risk Factor C

Generic Available No

Glipizide and Metformin Hydrochloride *see* Glipizide and Metformin *on page 639*

GlucaGen® *see* Glucagon *on page 640*

GlucaGen® Diagnostic Kit *see* Glucagon *on page 640*

Glucagon (GLOO ka gon)

U.S. Brand Names GlucaGen®; GlucaGen® Diagnostic Kit; Glucagon Diagnostic Kit; Glucagon Emergency Kit

Pharmacologic Category Antidote; Diagnostic Agent

Use Management of hypoglycemia; diagnostic aid in the radiologic examination of GI tract when a hypnotic state is needed

Unlabeled/Investigational Use Cardiac stimulant in management of severe cases of beta-adrenergic blocking agent overdosage

Local Anesthetic/Vasoconstrictor Precautions No information available to require special precautions

Effects on Dental Treatment No significant effects or complications reported

Dosage

Hypoglycemia or insulin shock therapy: I.M., I.V., S.C.:

Children: 0.025-0.1 mg/kg/dose, not to exceed 1 mg/dose, repeated in 20 minutes as needed

Adults: 0.5-1 mg, may repeat in 20 minutes as needed

If patient fails to respond to glucagon, I.V. dextrose must be given

Beta-blocker overdose (unlabeled use): I.V.: 3-10 mg **or** initially 0.5-5 mg bolus followed by continuous infusion 1-5 mg/hour

Diagnostic aid: Adults: I.M., I.V.: 0.25-2 mg 10 minutes prior to procedure

Mechanism of Action Stimulates adenylate cyclase to produce increased cyclic AMP, which promotes hepatic glycogenolysis and gluconeogenesis, causing a raise in blood glucose levels

Other Adverse Effects Frequency not defined:

Gastrointestinal: Nausea, vomiting (high incidence with rapid administration of high doses)

Miscellaneous: Hypersensitivity reactions (hypotension, respiratory distress, urticaria)

Drug Interactions Increased Effect/Toxicity: Hypoprothrombinemic effects of glucagon and warfarin may be increased, possibly with bleeding.

Pharmacodynamics/Kinetics

Onset of action: Peak effect: Blood glucose levels: Parenteral: 5-20 minutes

Duration: 60-90 minutes

Metabolism: Primarily hepatic; some inactivation occurring renally and in plasma

Half-life elimination, plasma: 3-10 minutes

Pregnancy Risk Factor B

Generic Available No

Comments 1 unit = 1 mg

Glucagon Diagnostic Kit *see* Glucagon *on page 640*

Glucagon Emergency Kit *see* Glucagon *on page 640*

Glucocerebrosidase *see* Alglucerase *on page 56*

Glucophage® *see* Metformin *on page 874*

Glucophage® XR *see* Metformin *on page 874*

Glucose *see* Glucose (Instant) *on page 641*

Glucose (Instant) (GLOO kose, IN stant)

Related Information

Dental Office Emergencies *on page 1582*

U.S. Brand Names B-D™ Glucose [OTC]; Dex4 Glucose [OTC]; Glutol™ [OTC]; Glutose™ [OTC]; Insta-Glucose® [OTC]

Pharmacologic Category Antihypoglycemic Agent

Synonyms Glucose

Use Management of hypoglycemia

Local Anesthetic/Vasoconstrictor Precautions No information available to require special precautions

Effects on Dental Treatment No significant effects or complications reported

Dosage Adults: Oral: 10-20 g

Other Adverse Effects Frequency not defined: Gastrointestinal: Nausea, diarrhea

Pregnancy Risk Factor A

Generic Available Yes

Comments 4 calories/g

Glucose Polymers (GLOO kose POL i merz)

U.S. Brand Names Moducal® [OTC]; Polycose® [OTC]

Pharmacologic Category Dietary Supplement

Use Calorie supplement for those not able to meet the caloric requirement with usual food intake

Local Anesthetic/Vasoconstrictor Precautions No information available to require special precautions

Effects on Dental Treatment No significant effects or complications reported

Dosage Adults: Oral: Add to foods or beverages or mix in water

Dietary/Ethanol/Herb Considerations Food: May be added to foods or beverages

Generic Available No

Glucotrol® *see* GlipiZIDE *on page 638*

Glucotrol® XL *see* GlipiZIDE *on page 638*

Glucovance® *see* Glyburide and Metformin *on page 643*

Glu-K® [OTC] *see* Potassium Supplements *on page 1102*

Glutamic Acid (gloo TAM ik AS id)

Pharmacologic Category Gastrointestinal Agent, Miscellaneous

Synonyms Glutamic Acid Hydrochloride

Use Treatment of hypochlorhydria and achlorhydria

Local Anesthetic/Vasoconstrictor Precautions No information available to require special precautions

Effects on Dental Treatment No significant effects or complications reported

Dosage Adults: Oral:

Tablet/powder: 500-1000 mg/day before meals or food

Capsule: 1-3 capsules 3 times/day before meals

(Continued)

Glutamic Acid *(Continued)*

Other Adverse Effects Frequency not defined: Endocrine & metabolic: Systemic acidosis (massive overdosage)

Pregnancy Risk Factor C

Generic Available Yes

Glutamic Acid Hydrochloride *see* Glutamic Acid *on page 641*

Glutol™ [OTC] *see* Glucose (Instant) *on page 641*

Glutose™ [OTC] *see* Glucose (Instant) *on page 641*

Glybenclamide *see* GlyBURIDE *on page 642*

Glybenzcyclamide *see* GlyBURIDE *on page 642*

GlyBURIDE (GLYE byoor ide)

Related Information

Endocrine Disorders and Pregnancy *on page 1479*

U.S. Brand Names Diaβeta®; Glynase® PresTab®; Micronase®

Canadian Brand Names Albert® Glyburide; Apo®-Glyburide; Diaβeta®; Euglucon®; Gen-Glybe; Novo-Glyburide; Nu-Glyburide; PMS-Glyburide; ratio-Glyburide

Mexican Brand Names Daonil®; Euglucon®; Glibenil®; Glucal®; Glucoven®; Nadib®; Norboral®

Pharmacologic Category Antidiabetic Agent, Sulfonylurea

Synonyms Diabeta; Glibenclamide; Glybenclamide; Glybenzcyclamide

Use Management of type 2 diabetes mellitus (noninsulin dependent, NIDDM)

Unlabeled/Investigational Use Alternative to insulin in women for the treatment of gestational diabetes (11-33 weeks gestation)

Local Anesthetic/Vasoconstrictor Precautions No information available to require special precautions

Effects on Dental Treatment Glyburide-dependent diabetics (noninsulin dependent, type 2) should be appointed for dental treatment in morning in order to minimize chance of stress-induced hypoglycemia.

Dosage Oral:

Adults:

Initial: 2.5-5 mg/day, administered with breakfast or the first main meal of the day. In patients who are more sensitive to hypoglycemic drugs, start at 1.25 mg/day.

Increase in increments of no more than 2.5 mg/day at weekly intervals based on the patient's blood glucose response

Maintenance: 1.25-20 mg/day given as single or divided doses; maximum: 20 mg/day

Elderly: Initial: 1.25-2.5 mg/day, increase by 1.25-2.5 mg/day every 1-3 weeks

Micronized tablets (Glynase™ PresTab™): Adults:

Initial: 1.5-3 mg/day, administered with breakfast or the first main meal of the day in patients who are more sensitive to hypoglycemic drugs, start at 0.75 mg/day. Increase in increments of no more than 1.5 mg/day in weekly intervals based on the patient's blood glucose response.

Maintenance: 0.75-12 mg/day given as a single dose or in divided doses. Some patients (especially those receiving >6 mg/day) may have a more satisfactory response with twice-daily dosing.

Dosing comment in renal impairment: Cl_{cr} <50 mL/minute: Use not recommended

Dosing adjustment in hepatic impairment: Use conservative initial and maintenance doses and avoid use in severe disease

Mechanism of Action Stimulates insulin release from the pancreatic beta cells; reduces glucose output from the liver; insulin sensitivity is increased at peripheral target sites

Other Adverse Effects Frequency not defined:

Central nervous system: Headache, dizziness

Dermatologic: Pruritus, rash, urticaria, photosensitivity reaction

Endocrine & metabolic: Hypoglycemia, hyponatremia (SIADH reported with other sulfonylureas)

Gastrointestinal: Nausea, epigastric fullness, heartburn, constipation, diarrhea, anorexia

Genitourinary: Nocturia

Hematologic: Leukopenia, thrombocytopenia, hemolytic anemia, aplastic anemia, bone marrow suppression, agranulocytosis

Hepatic: Cholestatic jaundice, hepatitis

Neuromuscular & skeletal: Arthralgia, paresthesia

Ocular: Blurred vision

Renal: Diuretic effect (minor)

Drug Interactions CYP3A3/4 enzyme substrate

Increased Effect/Toxicity: Increased hypoglycemic effects of glyburide may occur with oral anticoagulants (warfarin), phenytoin, other hydantoins, salicylates, NSAIDs, sulfonamides, and beta-blockers. Ethanol ingestion may cause disulfiram reactions.

Decreased Effect: Thiazides and other diuretics, corticosteroids may decrease effectiveness of glyburide.

Dietary/Ethanol/Herb Considerations

Ethanol: Use with caution; may increase risk of hypoglycemia and cause disulfiram reactions.

Food: Administer at the same time each day, 30 minutes before meals, to avoid erratic absorption; a delayed release of insulin may occur if taken with food. Dietary modification, based on ADA recommendations, is part of therapy. Hypoglycemia may occur; decreases blood glucose concentration.

Herb/Nutraceutical: Use caution with chromium, garlic, gymnema, and horse chestnut; may cause hypoglycemia. Black cohosh may enhance effects of antidiabetic agents.

Pharmacodynamics/Kinetics

Onset of action: Serum insulin levels begin to increase 15-60 minutes after a single dose

Duration: ≤24 hours

Protein binding, plasma: >99%

Metabolism: To one moderately active and several inactive metabolites

Half-life elimination: 5-16 hours; may be prolonged with renal or hepatic impairment

Time to peak, serum: Adults: 2-4 hours

Excretion: Feces (50%) and urine (50%) as metabolites

Pregnancy Risk Factor C

Generic Available Yes

Glyburide and Metformin (GLYE byoor ide & met FOR min)

Related Information

GlyBURIDE *on page 642*

Metformin *on page 874*

U.S. Brand Names Glucovance®

Pharmacologic Category Antidiabetic Agent, Biguanide; Antidiabetic Agent, Sulfonylurea

Synonyms Glyburide and Metformin Hydrochloride

Use Initial therapy for management of type 2 diabetes mellitus (noninsulin dependent, NIDDM). Second-line therapy for management of type 2 diabetes (NIDDM) when hyperglycemia cannot be managed with a sulfonylurea or metformin; combination therapy with a thiazolidinedione may be required to achieve additional control.

Local Anesthetic/Vasoconstrictor Precautions No information available to require special precautions

Effects on Dental Treatment Glyburide-dependent diabetics (noninsulin dependent, type 2) should be appointed for dental treatment in morning in order to minimize chance of stress-induced hypoglycemia. Metformin-dependent diabetics (noninsulin dependent, type 2) should be appointed for dental treatment in morning in order to minimize chance of stress-induced hypoglycemia.

Dosage Dose must be individualized. Dosages expressed as glyburide/metformin components.

Oral:

Adults:

Initial therapy (no prior treatment with sulfonylurea or metformin): 1.25 mg/250 mg once daily with a meal; patients with Hb A_{1c} >9% or fasting plasma glucose (FPG) >200 mg/dL may start with 1.25 mg/250 mg twice daily

Dosage may be increased in increments of 1.25 mg/250 mg, at intervals of not less than 2 weeks; maximum daily dose: 10 mg/2000 mg (limited experience with higher doses)

Previously treated with a sulfonylurea or metformin alone: Initial: 2.5 mg/500 mg or 5 mg/500 mg twice daily; increase in increments no greater than 5 mg/500 mg; maximum daily dose: 20 mg/2000 mg

When switching patients previously on a sulfonylurea and metformin together, do not exceed the daily dose of glyburide (or glyburide equivalent) or metformin.

Note: May combine with a thiazolidinedione in patients with an inadequate response to glyburide/metformin therapy (risk of hypoglycemia may be increased).

Elderly: Conservative doses are recommended due to potentially decreased renal function; **do not titrate to maximum dose**; should not be used in patients ≥80 years of age unless renal function is verified as normal

Dosing adjustment in renal impairment: Risk of lactic acidosis increases with degree of impairment; contraindicated in renal disease or dysfunction

Dosing adjustment in hepatic impairment: Use conservative initial and maintenance doses and avoid use in severe disease

Mechanism of Action The combination of glyburide and metformin is used to improve glycemic control in patients with type 2 diabetes mellitus by using two different, but complementary, mechanisms of action:

Glyburide: Stimulates insulin release from the pancreatic beta cells; reduces glucose output from the liver; insulin sensitivity is increased at peripheral target sites

(Continued)

Glyburide and Metformin *(Continued)*

Metformin: Decreases hepatic glucose production, decreasing intestinal absorption of glucose and improves insulin sensitivity (increases peripheral glucose uptake and utilization)

Other Adverse Effects

>10%:

Endocrine & metabolic: Hypoglycemia (11% to 38%, effects higher when increased doses were used as initial therapy)

Gastrointestinal: Diarrhea (17%)

Respiratory: Upper respiratory infection (17%)

1% to 10%:

Central nervous system: Headache (9%), dizziness (6%)

Gastrointestinal: Nausea (8%), vomiting (8%), abdominal pain (7%) (combined GI effects increased to 38% in patients taking high doses as initial therapy)

<1%: Disulfuram-like reactions (rare) reported in patients taking glyburide

Dietary/Ethanol/Herb Considerations

Ethanol: Avoid or limit use; may cause hypoglycemia and increase incidence of lactic acidosis. Disulfiram-like reaction (flushing, headache, nausea, vomiting, sweating, or tachycardia) reported with sulfonylureas.

Food: Administer with food to reduce GI upset. Drug decreases absorption of folic acid and vitamin B_{12}; monitor for signs and symptoms of deficiency. Drug decreases blood glucose concentration; monitor. Hypoglycemia does not usually occur unless a patient is predisposed (eg, cases of reduced caloric intake, strenuous exercise without repletion of calories, alcohol ingestion) or when metformin is combined with another oral antidiabetic agent.

Pharmacodynamics/Kinetics

Glucovance®:

Bioavailability: 18% with 2.5 mg glyburide/500 mg metformin dose; 7% with 5 mg glyburide/500 mg metformin dose; bioavailability is greater than that of Micronase® brand of glyburide and therefore not bioequivalent

Time to peak: 2.75 hours when taken with food

Glyburide: See Glyburide monograph.

Metformin: This component of Glucovance® is bioequivalent to metformin coadministration with glyburide.

Pregnancy Risk Factor B (manufacturer); C (expert analysis)

Generic Available No

Comments

Glyburide: Symptoms of overdose include severe hypoglycemia, seizures, cerebral damage, tingling of lips and tongue, nausea, yawning, confusion, agitation, tachycardia, sweating, convulsions, stupor, and coma. Intoxications with sulfonylureas can cause hypoglycemia and are best managed with glucose administration (orally for milder hypoglycemia or by injection in more severe forms).

Metformin: Lactic acidosis may occur. Hemodialysis may be used in suspected cases of overdose.

Glyburide and Metformin Hydrochloride *see* Glyburide and Metformin *on page 643*

Glycerin (GLIS er in)

U.S. Brand Names Bausch & Lomb® Computer Eye Drops [OTC]; Fleet® Babylax® [OTC]; Fleet® Glycerin Suppositories [OTC]; Fleet® Glycerin Suppositories Maximum Strength [OTC]; Fleet® Liquid Glycerin Suppositories [OTC]; Osmoglyn®; Sani-Supp® [OTC]

Mexican Brand Names Supositorios Senosiain®

Pharmacologic Category Laxative; Ophthalmic Agent, Miscellaneous

Synonyms Glycerol

Use Constipation; reduction of intraocular pressure; reduction of corneal edema; glycerin has been administered orally to reduce intracranial pressure

Local Anesthetic/Vasoconstrictor Precautions No information available to require special precautions

Effects on Dental Treatment No significant effects or complications reported

Dosage

Constipation: Rectal:

Children <6 years: 1 infant suppository 1-2 times/day as needed or 2-5 mL as an enema

Children >6 years and Adults: 1 adult suppository 1-2 times/day as needed or 5-15 mL as an enema

Children and Adults:

Reduction of intraocular pressure: Oral: 1-1.8 g/kg 1-1½ hours preoperatively; additional doses may be administered at 5-hour intervals

Reduction of intracranial pressure: Oral: 1.5 g/kg/day divided every 4 hours; 1 g/kg/dose every 6 hours has also been used

Reduction of corneal edema: Ophthalmic solution: Instill 1-2 drops in eye(s) prior to examination OR for lubricant effect, instill 1-2 drops in eye(s) every 3-4 hours

Mechanism of Action Osmotic dehydrating agent which increases osmotic pressure; draws fluid into colon and thus stimulates evacuation

Other Adverse Effects Frequency not defined:

Cardiovascular: Arrhythmias

Central nervous system: Headache, confusion, dizziness, hyperosmolar nonketotic coma

Endocrine: Polydipsia, hyperglycemia, dehydration

Gastrointestinal: Nausea, vomiting, tenesmus, rectal irritation, cramping pain, diarrhea, **xerostomia**

Pharmacodynamics/Kinetics

Onset of action:

- Decrease in intraocular pressure: Oral: 10-30 minutes
- Reduction of intracranial pressure: Oral: 10-60 minutes
- Constipation: Suppository: 15-30 minutes
- Peak effect:
  - Decrease in intraocular pressure: Oral: 60-90 minutes
  - Reduction of intracranial pressure: Oral: 60-90 minutes

Duration:

- Decrease in intraocular pressure: Oral: 4-8 hours
- Reduction of intracranial pressure: Oral: ~2-3 hours

Absorption: Oral: Well absorbed; Rectal: Poorly absorbed

Half-life elimination, serum: 30-45 minutes

Pregnancy Risk Factor C

Generic Available Yes

Glycerol *see* Glycerin *on page 644*

Glycerol Guaiacolate *see* Guaifenesin *on page 650*

Glycerol Triacetate *see* Triacetin *on page 1340*

Glyceryl Trinitrate *see* Nitroglycerin *on page 981*

Glycopyrrolate (glye koe PYE roe late)

U.S. Brand Names Robinul®; Robinul® Forte

Pharmacologic Category Anticholinergic Agent

Synonyms Glycopyrronium Bromide

Use Inhibit salivation and excessive secretions of the respiratory tract preoperatively; reversal of neuromuscular blockade; control of upper airway secretions; adjunct in treatment of peptic ulcer

Local Anesthetic/Vasoconstrictor Precautions No information available to require special precautions

Effects on Dental Treatment

>10%: Significant xerostomia, dry throat; normal salivary flow resumes upon discontinuation

1% to 10%: Dysphagia

Dosage

Children:

- Control of secretions:
  - Oral: 40-100 mcg/kg/dose 3-4 times/day
  - I.M., I.V.: 4-10 mcg/kg/dose every 3-4 hours; maximum: 0.2 mg/dose or 0.8 mg/24 hours
- Intraoperative: I.V.: 4 mcg/kg not to exceed 0.1 mg; repeat at 2- to 3-minute intervals as needed
- Preoperative: I.M.:
  - <2 years: 4.4-8.8 mcg/kg 30-60 minutes before procedure
  - >2 years: 4.4 mcg/kg 30-60 minutes before procedure

Children and Adults: Reverse neuromuscular blockade: I.V.: 0.2 mg for each 1 mg of neostigmine or 5 mg of pyridostigmine administered or 5-15 mcg/kg glycopyrrolate with 25-70 mcg/kg of neostigmine or 0.1-0.3 mg/kg of pyridostigmine (agents usually administered simultaneously, but glycopyrrolate may be administered first if bradycardia is present)

Adults:

- Intraoperative: I.V.: 0.1 mg repeated as needed at 2- to 3-minute intervals
- Preoperative: I.M.: 4.4 mcg/kg 30-60 minutes before procedure
- Peptic ulcer:
  - Oral: 1-2 mg 2-3 times/day
  - I.M., I.V.: 0.1-0.2 mg 3-4 times/day

Mechanism of Action Blocks the action of acetylcholine at parasympathetic sites in smooth muscle, secretory glands, and the CNS

Other Adverse Effects

>10%:

- Dermatologic: Dry skin
- Gastrointestinal: Constipation
- Local: Irritation at injection site
- Respiratory: Dry nose
- Miscellaneous: Diaphoresis (decreased)

(Continued)

Glycopyrrolate *(Continued)*

1% to 10%:
Dermatologic: Increased sensitivity to light
Endocrine & metabolic: Decreased flow of breast milk

<1%: **Orthostatic hypotension, ventricular fibrillation, tachycardia, palpitations**, confusion, drowsiness, headache, loss of memory, fatigue, ataxia, rash, bloated feeling, nausea, vomiting, dysuria, weakness, increased intraocular pain, blurred vision

Drug Interactions
Increased effects of other anticholinergic agents.
Increased toxicity with amantadine and cyclopropane.
Decreased effect of levodopa.

Pharmacodynamics/Kinetics
Onset of action: Oral: 50 minutes; I.M.: 20-40 minutes; I.V.: ~1 minute
Peak effect: Oral: ~1 hour
Duration: Vagal effect: 2-3 hours; Inhibition of salivation: Up to 7 hours; Anticholinergic: Oral: 8-12 hours
Absorption: Oral: Poor and erratic
Metabolism: Hepatic (minimal)
Bioavailability: ~10%
Half-life elimination: 20-40 minutes

Pregnancy Risk Factor B
Generic Available Yes: Injection

Glycopyrronium Bromide *see* Glycopyrrolate *on page 645*
Glydiazinamide *see* GlipiZIDE *on page 638*
Glynase® PresTab® *see* GlyBURIDE *on page 642*
Gly-Oxide® Oral [OTC] *see* Carbamide Peroxide *on page 244*
Glyquin® *see* Hydroquinone *on page 693*
Glyset® *see* Miglitol *on page 913*
Glytuss® [OTC] *see* Guaifenesin *on page 650*
GM-CSF *see* Sargramostim *on page 1209*

Gold Sodium Thiomalate (gold SOW dee um thye oh MAL ate)

U.S. Brand Names Aurolate®
Canadian Brand Names Myochrysine®
Pharmacologic Category Gold Compound
Use Treatment of progressive rheumatoid arthritis
Local Anesthetic/Vasoconstrictor Precautions No information available to require special precautions
Effects on Dental Treatment >10%: Stomatitis, gingivitis, glossitis
Dosage I.M.:
Children: Initial: Test dose of 10 mg is recommended, followed by 1 mg/kg/week for 20 weeks; maintenance: 1 mg/kg/dose at 2- to 4-week intervals thereafter for as long as therapy is clinically beneficial and toxicity does not develop. Administration for 2-4 months is usually required before clinical improvement is observed.
Adults: 10 mg first week; 25 mg second week; then 25-50 mg/week until 1 g cumulative dose has been given; if improvement occurs without adverse reactions, administer 25-50 mg every 2-3 weeks for 2-20 weeks, then every 3-4 weeks indefinitely
Dosing adjustment in renal impairment:
Cl_{cr} 50-80 mL/minute: Administer 50% of normal dose
Cl_{cr} <50 mL/minute: Avoid use

Mechanism of Action Unknown, may decrease prostaglandin synthesis or may alter cellular mechanisms by inhibiting sulfhydryl systems

Other Adverse Effects
>10%:
Dermatologic: Itching, rash
Ocular: Conjunctivitis

1% to 10%:
Dermatologic: Urticaria, alopecia
Hematologic: Eosinophilia, leukopenia, thrombocytopenia
Renal: Proteinuria, hematuria

<1%: Angioedema, ulcerative enterocolitis, GI hemorrhage, dysphagia, **metallic taste**, agranulocytosis, anemia, aplastic anemia, hepatotoxicity, peripheral neuropathy, interstitial pneumonitis

Drug Interactions Decreased Effect: Penicillamine and acetylcysteine may decrease effect of gold sodium thiomalate.

Pharmacodynamics/Kinetics
Onset of action: Delayed; may require up to 3 months
Half-life elimination: 5 days; may be prolonged with multiple doses
Time to peak, serum: 4-6 hours
Excretion: Urine (60% to 90%); feces (10% to 40%)

Pregnancy Risk Factor C

Generic Available No

Comments Approximately 50% gold

GoLYTELY® *see* Polyethylene Glycol-Electrolyte Solution *on page 1094*

Gonak™ [OTC] *see* Hydroxypropyl Methylcellulose *on page 696*

Gonal-F® *see* Follitropins *on page 607*

Gonic® *see* Chorionic Gonadotropin (Human) *on page 320*

Gonioscopic Ophthalmic Solution *see* Hydroxypropyl Methylcellulose *on page 696*

Goniosol® [OTC] *see* Hydroxypropyl Methylcellulose *on page 696*

Goody's® Extra Strength Headache Powder [OTC] *see* Acetaminophen, Aspirin, and Caffeine *on page 34*

Goody's PM® Powder *see* Acetaminophen and Diphenhydramine *on page 30*

Gordofilm® [OTC] *see* Salicylic Acid *on page 1204*

Gormel® [OTC] *see* Urea *on page 1365*

Goserelin (GOE se rel in)

U.S. Brand Names Zoladex®

Canadian Brand Names Zoladex®; Zoladex® LA

Mexican Brand Names Prozoladex; Zoladex®

Pharmacologic Category Antineoplastic Agent, Miscellaneous; Gonadotropin Releasing Hormone Analog; Luteinizing Hormone-Releasing Hormone Analog

Synonyms Goserelin Acetate

Use

Prostate carcinoma: Palliative treatment of advanced carcinoma of the prostate. An alternative treatment of prostatic cancer when orchiectomy or estrogen administration are either not indicated or unacceptable to the patient. Combination with flutamide for the management of locally confined stage T2b-T4 (stage B2-C) carcinoma of the prostate.

3.6 mg implant **only**:

Endometriosis: Management of endometriosis, including pain relief and reduction of endometriotic lesions for the duration of therapy

Advanced breast cancer: Palliative treatment of advanced breast cancer in pre- and perimenopausal women. Estrogen and progesterone receptor values may help to predict whether goserelin therapy is likely to be beneficial.

Note: The 10.8 mg implant is not indicated in women as the data are insufficient to support reliable suppression of serum estradiol

Local Anesthetic/Vasoconstrictor Precautions No information available to require special precautions

Effects on Dental Treatment 1% to 10%: Abnormal taste

Dosage Adults: S.C.:

Monthly implant: 3.6 mg injected into upper abdomen every 28 days; while a delay of a few days is permissible, attempt to adhere to the 28-day schedule

3-month implant: 10.8 mg injected into the upper abdominal wall every 12 weeks; while a delay of a few days is permissible, attempt to adhere to the 12-week schedule

Prostate carcinoma: Intended for long-term administration

Endometriosis: Recommended duration: 6 months; retreatment is not recommended since safety data is unavailable. If symptoms recur after a course of therapy, and further treatment is contemplated, consider monitoring bone mineral density. Currently, there are no clinical data on the effect of treatment of benign gynecological conditions with goserelin for periods >6 months.

Mechanism of Action LHRH synthetic analog of luteinizing hormone-releasing hormone also known as gonadotropin-releasing hormone (GnRH) incorporated into a biodegradable depot material which allows for continuous slow release over 28 days; mechanism of action is similar to leuprolide

Other Adverse Effects Hormone replacement therapy may decrease vasomotor symptoms and loss of bone mineral density. Adverse reaction profile varies with gender and therapeutic use.

>10%:

Central nervous system: Headache (11%)

Endocrine & metabolic: Hot flashes (53% to 62% of men, 100% of women), sexual dysfunction (15% to 21%), decreased libido, impotence, impaired erection (16% to 18%), tumor flare, bone pain (23% of women, 1% to 10% of men), vaginal dryness (10% to 14%)

1% to 10%:

Cardiovascular: Anginal pain, arrhythmias, hypertension, thromboembolic events, CHF, MI (1% to 5%), edema

Central nervous system: Lethargy (5% to 8%), anxiety, depression, dizziness, insomnia

Dermatologic: Urticaria, maculopapular rashes (10%)

Endocrine & metabolic: Gynecomastia, breast swelling (3% to 5%), bone loss, diaphoresis

Gastrointestinal: Abdominal pain, diarrhea, nausea, vomiting (5%), anorexia

(Continued)

Goserelin *(Continued)*

<1%: Spinal cord compression, ovarian cyst formation, pituitary apoplexy (following initiation in patients with functional pituitary adenoma)

Changes in blood pressure (usually transient) have been associated with goserelin use. Osteoporosis, decreased bone mineral density, and fracture have been reported rarely in men treated with goserelin.

Pharmacodynamics/Kinetics

Absorption: S.C.: Rapid and can be detected in serum in 10 minutes

Distribution: V_d: Males: 44.1 L; Females: 20.3 L

Time to peak, serum: S.C.: 12-15 days

Half-life elimination: S.C. dose: 5 hours; Renal impairment: 12 hours

Excretion: Urine (90%)

Pregnancy Risk Factor X

Generic Available No

Goserelin Acetate *see* Goserelin *on page 647*

GP 47680 *see* Oxcarbazepine *on page 1012*

G-Phed *see* Guaifenesin and Pseudoephedrine *on page 652*

G-Phed-PD *see* Guaifenesin and Pseudoephedrine *on page 652*

Gramicidin, Neomycin, and Polymyxin B *see* Neomycin, Polymyxin B, and Gramicidin *on page 963*

Granisetron (gra NI se tron)

U.S. Brand Names Kytril®

Canadian Brand Names Kytril®

Mexican Brand Names Kytril®

Pharmacologic Category Selective 5-HT_3 Receptor Antagonist

Use

Oral: Prophylaxis of chemotherapy-related emesis; prophylaxis of nausea and vomiting associated with radiation therapy, including total body irradiation and fractionated abdominal radiation

I.V.: Prophylaxis of chemotherapy-related emesis; prophylaxis and treatment of postoperative nausea and vomiting (PONV)

Local Anesthetic/Vasoconstrictor Precautions No information available to require special precautions

Effects on Dental Treatment No significant effects or complications reported

Dosage

Oral: Adults:

Prophylaxis of chemotherapy-related emesis: 2 mg once daily up to 1 hour before chemotherapy or 1 mg twice daily; the first 1 mg dose should be given up to 1 hour before chemotherapy. **Note:** Administer granisetron on day(s) of chemotherapy.

Prophylaxis of radiation therapy-associated emesis: 2 mg once daily given 1 hour before radiation therapy.

I.V.:

Children ≥2 years and Adults: Prophylaxis of chemotherapy-related emesis:

Within U.S.: 10 mcg/kg/dose (or 1 mg/dose) administered IVPB over 5 minutes given within 30 minutes of chemotherapy: for some drugs (eg, carboplatin, cyclophosphamide) with a later onset of emetic action, 10 mcg/kg every 12 hours may be necessary.

Outside U.S.: 40 mcg/kg/dose (or 3 mg/dose); maximum: 9 mg/24 hours

Breakthrough: Repeat the dose 2-3 times within the first 24 hours as necessary (suggested by anecdotal information; not based on controlled trials, or generally recommended).

Note: Administer granisetron on the day(s) of chemotherapy

Adults: PONV:

Prevention: 1 mg given undiluted over 30 seconds; administer before induction of anesthesia or before reversal of anesthesia

Treatment: 1 mg given undiluted over 30 seconds

Dosing interval in hepatic impairment: Kinetic studies in patients with hepatic impairment showed that total clearance was approximately halved, however, standard doses were very well tolerated

Mechanism of Action Selective 5-HT_3-receptor antagonist, blocking serotonin, both peripherally on vagal nerve terminals and centrally in the chemoreceptor trigger zone

Other Adverse Effects

>10%:

Central nervous system: Headache (8% to 21%)

Gastrointestinal: Constipation (3% to 18%)

1% to 10%:

Cardiovascular: Hypertension (1% to 2%)

Central nervous system: Dizziness, insomnia, anxiety, somnolence, fever (3% to 8%), pain (10%)

Gastrointestinal: Abdominal pain, diarrhea (1% to 9%), dyspepsia

Hepatic: Elevated liver enzymes (5% to 6%)
Neuromuscular & skeletal: Weakness (5% to 18%)

<1%: Arrhythmias, agitation, angina, atrial fibrillation, anaphylaxis, allergic reactions, **syncope, hypotension, hot flashes**

Drug Interactions Substrate of CYP3A4

Dietary/Ethanol/Herb Considerations Herb/Nutraceutical: Avoid St John's wort; may decrease serum concentration.

Pharmacodynamics/Kinetics

Duration: Generally up to 24 hours

Distribution: V_d: 2-4 L/kg; widely throughout body

Protein binding: 65%

Metabolism: Hepatic via N-demethylation, oxidation, and conjugation; some metabolites may have 5-HT_3 antagonist activity

Half-life elimination: Cancer patients: 10-12 hours; Healthy volunteers: 4-5 hours; PONV: 9 hours

Excretion: Urine (12% as unchanged drug, 49% as metabolites); feces (34% as metabolites)

Pregnancy Risk Factor B

Generic Available No

Granulex® *see* Trypsin, Balsam Peru, and Castor Oil *on page 1362*

Granulocyte Colony Stimulating Factor *see* Filgrastim *on page 571*

Granulocyte Colony Stimulating Factor (PEG Conjugate) *see* Pegfilgrastim *on page 1040*

Granulocyte-Macrophage Colony Stimulating Factor *see* Sargramostim *on page 1209*

Grifulvin® V *see* Griseofulvin *on page 649*

Griseofulvin (gri see oh FUL vin)

U.S. Brand Names Fulvicin® P/G; Fulvicin-U/F®; Grifulvin® V; Gris-PEG®

Canadian Brand Names Fulvicin® U/F

Mexican Brand Names Fulvina® P/G; Grisovin®; Grisovin-FP

Pharmacologic Category Antifungal Agent, Oral

Synonyms Griseofulvin Microsize; Griseofulvin Ultramicrosize

Use Treatment of susceptible tinea infections of the skin, hair, and nails

Local Anesthetic/Vasoconstrictor Precautions No information available to require special precautions

Effects on Dental Treatment May cause soreness or irritation of mouth or tongue

Dosage Oral:

Children >2 years:
- Microsize: 10-20 mg/kg/day in single or 2 divided doses
- Ultramicrosize: >2 years: 5-10 mg/kg/day in single or 2 divided doses

Adults:
- Microsize: 500-1000 mg/day in single or divided doses
- Ultramicrosize: 330-375 mg/day in single or divided doses; doses up to 750 mg/day have been used for infections more difficult to eradicate such as tinea unguium

Duration of therapy depends on the site of infection:
- Tinea corporis: 2-4 weeks
- Tinea capitis: 4-6 weeks or longer
- Tinea pedis: 4-8 weeks
- Tinea unguium: 3-6 months or longer

Mechanism of Action Inhibits fungal cell mitosis at metaphase; binds to human keratin making it resistant to fungal invasion

Other Adverse Effects Frequency not defined:

Central nervous system: Headache, fatigue, dizziness, insomnia, mental confusion

Dermatologic: Rash (most common), urticaria (most common), photosensitivity, angioneurotic edema (rare)

Gastrointestinal: Nausea, vomiting, epigastric distress, diarrhea, GI bleeding

Genitourinary: Menstrual irregularities (rare)

Hematologic: Leukopenia

Neuromuscular & skeletal: Paresthesia (rare)

Renal: Hepatotoxicity, proteinuria, nephrosis

Miscellaneous: **Oral thrush**, drug-induced lupus-like syndrome (rare)

Drug Interactions Induces CYP1A2, 2C8/9, 3A4

Increased Effect/Toxicity: Increased toxicity with ethanol, may cause tachycardia and flushing.

Decreased Effect: Barbiturates may decrease levels. Decreased warfarin activity. Decreased oral contraceptive effectiveness.

Dietary/Ethanol/Herb Considerations

Ethanol: Avoid use; may increase CNS depression; causes disulfiram-like reaction (flushing, headache, nausea, and in some patients, vomiting and chest and/or abdominal pain).

Food may increase serum concentration, especially high-fat meals.

(Continued)

Griseofulvin *(Continued)*

Herb/Nutraceutical: Avoid gotu kola, kava, SAMe, St John's wort, and valerian; may increase CNS depression.

Pharmacodynamics/Kinetics

Absorption: Ultramicrosize griseofulvin absorption is almost complete; absorption of microsize griseofulvin is variable (25% to 70% of an oral dose); enhanced by ingestion of a fatty meal (GI absorption of ultramicrosize is ~1.5 times that of microsize)

Distribution: Crosses placenta

Metabolism: Extensively hepatic

Half-life elimination: 9-22 hours

Excretion: Urine (<1% as unchanged drug); feces; perspiration

Pregnancy Risk Factor C

Generic Available Yes: Ultramicrosized product

Griseofulvin Microsize *see* Griseofulvin *on page 649*

Griseofulvin Ultramicrosize *see* Griseofulvin *on page 649*

Gris-PEG® *see* Griseofulvin *on page 649*

Growth Hormone *see* Human Growth Hormone *on page 671*

Guaifed® [OTC] *see* Guaifenesin and Pseudoephedrine *on page 652*

Guaifed-PD® *see* Guaifenesin and Pseudoephedrine *on page 652*

Guaifenesin (gwye FEN e sin)

Related Information

Guaifenesin and Phenylephrine *on page 652*

Guaifenesin, Pseudoephedrine, and Dextromethorphan *on page 653*

U.S. Brand Names Amibid LA; Breonesin® [OTC] [DSC]; Diabetic Tussin® EX [OTC]; Duratuss-G®; Fenesin™ [DSC]; Glytuss® [OTC]; Guaifenex® G; Guaifenex® LA; Guiatuss® [OTC]; Humibid® L.A.; Humibid® Pediatric; Hytuss® [OTC]; Hytuss-2X® [OTC]; Liquibid®; Liquibid® 1200; Mucinex™ [OTC]; Organidin® NR; Phanasin [OTC]; Respa-GF®; Robitussin® [OTC]; Scot-Tussin® Sugar Free Expectorant [OTC]; Touro Ex®

Canadian Brand Names Balminil Expectorant; Benylin® E Extra Strength; Koffex Expectorant; Robitussin®

Mexican Brand Names Formula E; Tukol®

Pharmacologic Category Expectorant

Synonyms GG; Glycerol Guaiacolate

Use Temporary control of cough due to minor throat and bronchial irritation

Local Anesthetic/Vasoconstrictor Precautions No information available to require special precautions

Effects on Dental Treatment No significant effects or complications reported

Dosage Oral:

Children:

- <2 years: 12 mg/kg/day in 6 divided doses
- 2-5 years: 50-100 mg every 4 hours, not to exceed 600 mg/day
- 6-11 years: 100-200 mg every 4 hours, not to exceed 1.2 g/day

Children >12 years and Adults: 200-400 mg every 4 hours to a maximum of 2.4 g/day

Mechanism of Action Thought to act as an expectorant by irritating the gastric mucosa and stimulating respiratory tract secretions, thereby increasing respiratory fluid volumes and decreasing phlegm viscosity

Other Adverse Effects Frequency not defined:

Central nervous system: Drowsiness, headache

Dermatologic: Rash

Gastrointestinal: Nausea, vomiting, stomach pain

Drug Interactions Increased Effect/Toxicity: May increase toxicity/effect of disulfiram, MAO inhibitors, metronidazole, and procarbazine.

Dietary/Ethanol/Herb Considerations Some products contain ethanol.

Pharmacodynamics/Kinetics

Absorption: Well absorbed

Metabolism: Hepatic (60%)

Half-life elimination: ~1 hour

Excretion: Urine (as unchanged drug and metabolites)

Pregnancy Risk Factor C

Generic Available Yes

Guaifenesin and Codeine (gwye FEN e sin & KOE deen)

Related Information

Codeine *on page 361*

Guaifenesin *on page 650*

U.S. Brand Names Brontex®; Cheracol®; Gani-Tuss® NR; Guaituss AC®; Mytussin® AC; Robafen® AC; Robitussin® A-C [DSC]; Romilar® AC; Tussi-Organidin® NR; Tussi-Organidin® S-NR

Pharmacologic Category Antitussive; Cough Preparation; Expectorant

Synonyms Codeine and Guaifenesin; Robitussin® A-C [DSC]

Use Temporary control of cough due to minor throat and bronchial irritation

Local Anesthetic/Vasoconstrictor Precautions No information available to require special precautions

Effects on Dental Treatment 1% to 10%: Xerostomia, dyspnea, tachycardia, bradycardia, hypotension

Restrictions C-V

Dosage Oral:

Children:

2-6 years: 1-1.5 mg/kg codeine/day divided into 4 doses administered every 4-6 hours (maximum: 30 mg/24 hours)

6-12 years: 5 mL every 4 hours, not to exceed 30 mL/24 hours

Children >12 years and Adults: 5-10 mL every 6 hours not to exceed 60 mL/24 hours

Mechanism of Action

Guaifenesin is thought to act as an expectorant by irritating the gastric mucosa and stimulating respiratory tract secretions, thereby increasing respiratory fluid volumes and decreasing phlegm viscosity

Codeine is an antitussive that controls cough by depressing the medullary cough center

Other Adverse Effects

Based on guaifenesin component:

Central nervous system: Drowsiness, headache

Dermatologic: Rash

Gastrointestinal: Nausea, vomiting, stomach pain

Based on codeine component:

>10%:

Central nervous system: Drowsiness

Gastrointestinal: Constipation

1% to 10%:

Central nervous system: Dizziness, lightheadedness, false feeling of well being, malaise, headache, restlessness, paradoxical CNS stimulation, confusion

Dermatologic: Rash, urticaria

Gastrointestinal: Anorexia, nausea, vomiting,

Genitourinary: Decreased urination, ureteral spasm

Hepatic: Increased LFTs

Local: Burning at injection site

Neuromuscular & skeletal: Weakness

Ocular: Blurred vision

Miscellaneous: Histamine release

<1%: Convulsions, hallucinations, mental depression, nightmares, insomnia, paralytic ileus, biliary spasm, stomach cramps, muscle rigidity, trembling

Frequency not defined: Hepatic: Increased AST, ALT

Dietary/Ethanol/Herb Considerations

Ethanol: Avoid or limit use; may increase CNS depression.

Herb/Nutraceutical: Avoid gotu kola, kava, SAMe, St John's wort, and valerian; may increase CNS depression.

Pregnancy Risk Factor C

Generic Available Yes

Guaifenesin and Dextromethorphan

(gwye FEN e sin & deks troe meth OR fan)

Related Information

Dextromethorphan *on page 423*

Guaifenesin *on page 650*

U.S. Brand Names Aquatab® DM; Benylin® Expectorant [OTC]; Cheracol® D [OTC]; Cheracol® Plus [OTC]; Diabetic Tussin® DM [OTC]; Diabetic Tussin® DM Maximum Strength [OTC]; Duratuss® DM; Fenesin™ DM; Genatuss DM® [OTC]; Guaifenex® DM; Guiatuss-DM® [OTC]; Humibid® DM; Hydro-Tussin™ DM; Kolephrin® GG/DM [OTC]; Mytussin® DM [OTC]; Respa® DM; Robitussin® DM [OTC]; Robitussin® Sugar Free Cough [OTC]; Safe Tussin® 30 [OTC]; Silexin® [OTC]; Tolu-Sed® DM [OTC]; Touro® DM; Tussi-Organidin® DM NR; Vicks® 44E [OTC]; Vicks® Pediatric Formula 44E [OTC]

Canadian Brand Names Balminil DM E; Benylin® DM-E; Koffex DM-Expectorant; Robitussin® DM

Pharmacologic Category Antitussive; Cough Preparation; Expectorant

Synonyms Dextromethorphan and Guaifenesin

Use Temporary control of cough due to minor throat and bronchial irritation

Local Anesthetic/Vasoconstrictor Precautions No information available to require special precautions

Effects on Dental Treatment No significant effects or complications reported

Dosage Oral:

Children: Dextromethorphan: 1-2 mg/kg/24 hours divided 3-4 times/day

Children >12 years and Adults: 5 mL every 4 hours or 10 mL every 6-8 hours not to exceed 40 mL/24 hours

(Continued)

Guaifenesin and Dextromethorphan *(Continued)*

Mechanism of Action

Guaifenesin is thought to act as an expectorant by irritating the gastric mucosa and stimulating respiratory tract secretions, thereby increasing respiratory fluid volumes and decreasing phlegm viscosity

Dextromethorphan is a chemical relative of morphine lacking narcotic properties except in overdose; controls cough by depressing the medullary cough center

Other Adverse Effects Frequency not defined:

Central nervous system: Drowsiness, headache
Dermatologic: Rash
Gastrointestinal: Nausea, vomiting

Pharmacodynamics/Kinetics Onset of action: Oral: Antitussive: 15-30 minutes

Pregnancy Risk Factor C

Generic Available Yes

Guaifenesin and Hydrocodone *see* Hydrocodone and Guaifenesin *on page 683*

Guaifenesin and Phenylephrine (gwye FEN e sin & fen il EF rin)

Related Information

Guaifenesin *on page 650*
Phenylephrine *on page 1071*

U.S. Brand Names Endal®; Entex® LA; Liquibid-D; Prolex-D

Pharmacologic Category Decongestant; Expectorant

Synonyms Phenylephrine and Guaifenesin

Use Symptomatic relief of those respiratory conditions where tenacious mucous plugs and congestion complicate the problem such as sinusitis, pharyngitis, bronchitis, asthma, and as an adjunctive therapy in serous otitis media

Local Anesthetic/Vasoconstrictor Precautions Use with caution since phenylephrine is a sympathomimetic amine which could interact with epinephrine to cause a pressor response

Effects on Dental Treatment

Guaifenesin: No significant effects or complications reported

Phenylephrine: Up to 10% of patients could experience tachycardia, palpitations, and xerostomia; use vasoconstrictor with caution

Dosage Oral: Adults: 1 or 2 every 12 hours

Product labeling: Adults: Endal®: 1-2 timed release tablets every 12 hours

Mechanism of Action See individual agents.

Generic Available Yes

Guaifenesin and Pseudoephedrine

(gwye FEN e sin & soo doe e FED rin)

Related Information

Guaifenesin *on page 650*
Pseudoephedrine *on page 1146*

U.S. Brand Names Ami-Tex PSE; Anatuss LA; Aquatab®; Aquatab® D Dose Pack; Congestac®; Deconsal® II; Defen-LA®; Duratuss™; Duratuss™ GP; Entex® PSE; Eudal®-SR; G-Phed; G-Phed-PD; Guaifed® [OTC]; Guaifed-PD®; Guaifenex® GP; Guaifenex® PSE; Guaifen PSE; Guai-Vent™/PSE; Maxifed®; Maxifed-G®; Miraphen PSE; PanMist® Jr.; PanMist® LA; PanMist® S; Pseudo GG TR; Pseudovent™, Pseudovent™-Ped; Respa-1st®; Respaire®-60 SR; Respaire®-120 SR; Robitussin-PE® [OTC]; Robitussin® Severe Congestion [OTC]; Touro LA®; V-Dec-M®; Versacaps®; Zephrex®; Zephrex LA®

Canadian Brand Names Novahistex® Expectorant with Decongestant

Pharmacologic Category Decongestant; Expectorant

Synonyms Pseudoephedrine and Guaifenesin

Use Enhance the output of respiratory tract fluid and reduce mucosal congestion and edema in the nasal passage

Local Anesthetic/Vasoconstrictor Precautions Use with caution since pseudoephedrine is a sympathomimetic amine which could interact with epinephrine to cause a pressor response

Effects on Dental Treatment

Guaifenesin: No significant effects or complications reported

Pseudoephedrine: Up to 10% of patients could experience tachycardia, palpitations, and xerostomia; use vasoconstrictor with caution

Dosage Oral:

Children:

2-6 years: 2.5 mL every 4 hours not to exceed 15 mL/24 hours
6-12 years: 5 mL every 4 hours not to exceed 30 mL/24 hours

Children >12 years and Adults: 10 mL every 4 hours not to exceed 60 mL/24 hours

Pregnancy Risk Factor C

Generic Available Yes

Guaifenesin and Theophylline *see* Theophylline and Guaifenesin *on page 1293*

Guaifenesin, Hydrocodone, and Pseudoephedrine *see* Hydrocodone, Pseudoephedrine, and Guaifenesin *on page 687*

Guaifenesin, Pseudoephedrine, and Codeine

(gwye FEN e sin, soo doe e FED rin, & KOE deen)

Related Information

Codeine *on page 361*
Guaifenesin *on page 650*
Pseudoephedrine *on page 1146*

U.S. Brand Names Cheratussin DAC; Codafed® Expectorant; Codafed® Pediatric Expectorant; Dihistine® Expectorant; Guiatuss™ DAC®; Halotussin® DAC; Mytussin® DAC; Nucofed® Expectorant; Nucofed® Pediatric Expectorant; Nucotuss®; Robitussin®-DAC [DSC]

Canadian Brand Names Benylin® 3.3 mg-D-E; Calmylin with Codeine

Pharmacologic Category Antitussive/Decongestant/Expectorant

Synonyms Codeine, Guaifenesin, and Pseudoephedrine; Pseudoephedrine, Guaifenesin, and Codeine; Robitussin®-DAC [DSC]

Use Temporarily relieves nasal congestion and controls cough due to minor throat and bronchial irritation; helps loosen phlegm and thin bronchial secretions to make coughs more productive

Local Anesthetic/Vasoconstrictor Precautions Use with caution since pseudoephedrine is a sympathomimetic amine which could interact with epinephrine to cause a pressor response

Effects on Dental Treatment

Codeine: <1%: Xerostomia
Guaifenesin: No significant effects or complications reported
Pseudoephedrine: Up to 10% of patients could experience tachycardia, palpitations, and xerostomia; use vasoconstrictor with caution

Restrictions C-III; C-V

Dosage Oral:

Children 6-12 years: 5 mL every 4 hours, not to exceed 40 mL/24 hours
Children >12 years and Adults: 10 mL every 4 hours, not to exceed 40 mL/24 hours

Pregnancy Risk Factor C

Generic Available Yes

Guaifenesin, Pseudoephedrine, and Dextromethorphan

(gwye FEN e sin, soo doe e FED rin, & deks troe meth OR fan)

Related Information

Dextromethorphan *on page 423*
Guaifenesin *on page 650*
Pseudoephedrine *on page 1146*

U.S. Brand Names Aquatab® C; Guiatuss™ CF; Maxifed® DM; PanMist®-DM; Robitussin® CF [OTC]; Robitussin® Cold and Congestion [OTC]; Robitussin® Cough and Cold Infant [OTC]; Touro™ CC

Canadian Brand Names Balminil DM + Decongestant + Expectorant; Benylin® DM-D-E; Koffex DM + Decongestant + Expectorant; Novahistex® DM Decongestant Expectorant; Novahistine® DM Decongestant Expectorant; Robitussin® Cough & Cold®

Pharmacologic Category Antitussive/Decongestant/Expectorant

Synonyms Dextromethorphan, Guaifenesin, and Pseudoephedrine; Pseudoephedrine, Dextromethorphan, and Guaifenesin

Use Temporarily relieves nasal congestion and controls cough due to minor throat and bronchial irritation; helps loosen phlegm and thin bronchial secretions to make coughs more productive

Local Anesthetic/Vasoconstrictor Precautions Use with caution since pseudoephedrine is a sympathomimetic amine which could interact with epinephrine to cause a pressor response

Effects on Dental Treatment

Guaifenesin: No significant effects or complications reported
Pseudoephedrine: Up to 10% of patients could experience tachycardia, palpitations, and xerostomia; use vasoconstrictor with caution
Dextromethorphan: No significant effects or complications reported

Dosage Adults: Oral: 2 capsules or 10 mL every 4 hours

Mechanism of Action See individual agents.

Generic Available Yes: Syrup; Tablet, extended release

Guaifenex® DM *see* Guaifenesin and Dextromethorphan *on page 651*
Guaifenex® G *see* Guaifenesin *on page 650*
Guaifenex® GP *see* Guaifenesin and Pseudoephedrine *on page 652*
Guaifenex® LA *see* Guaifenesin *on page 650*
Guaifenex® PSE *see* Guaifenesin and Pseudoephedrine *on page 652*
Guaifen PSE *see* Guaifenesin and Pseudoephedrine *on page 652*
Guaituss AC® *see* Guaifenesin and Codeine *on page 650*
Guai-Vent™/PSE *see* Guaifenesin and Pseudoephedrine *on page 652*

Guanabenz (GWAHN a benz)

Related Information

Cardiovascular Diseases *on page 1456*

U.S. Brand Names Wytensin® [DSC]

Canadian Brand Names Wytensin®

Pharmacologic Category Alpha$_2$-Adrenergic Agonist

Synonyms Guanabenz Acetate; Wytensin® [DSC]

Use Management of hypertension

Local Anesthetic/Vasoconstrictor Precautions No information available to require special precautions

Effects on Dental Treatment

28% to 38%: Significant xerostomia; normal salivary flow resumes upon discontinuation

≤3%: Taste disorder nasal congestion, dyspnea

Dosage Oral:

Adults: Initial: 4 mg twice daily; increase in increments of 4-8 mg/day every 1-2 weeks to a maximum of 32 mg twice daily.

Dosing adjustment in hepatic impairment: Probably necessary

Mechanism of Action Stimulates alpha$_2$-adrenoreceptors in the brain stem, thus activating an inhibitory neuron, resulting in reduced sympathetic outflow, producing a decrease in vasomotor tone and heart rate

Other Adverse Effects Higher rates with larger doses:

>5% (at doses of 16 mg/day):
- Cardiovascular: Orthostasis
- Central nervous system: Drowsiness or sedation (39%), dizziness (12% to 17%), headache (5%)
- Neuromuscular & skeletal: Weakness (~10%)

≤3% (may be similar to placebo):
- Cardiovascular: Arrhythmias, palpitations, chest pain, edema
- Central nervous system: Anxiety, ataxia, depression, sleep disturbances
- Dermatologic: Rash, pruritus
- Endocrine & metabolic: Disturbances of sexual function, gynecomastia, decreased sexual function
- Gastrointestinal: Diarrhea, vomiting, constipation, nausea
- Genitourinary: Polyuria
- Neuromuscular & skeletal: Myalgia
- Ocular: Blurring of vision

Drug Interactions Substrate of **CYP1A2**

Increased Effect/Toxicity:

Nitroprusside and guanabenz have additive hypotensive effects. Noncardioselective beta-blockers (nadolol, propranolol, timolol) may exacerbate rebound hypertension when guanabenz is withdrawn. The beta-blocker should be withdrawn first. The gradual withdrawal of guanabenz or a cardioselective beta-blocker could be substituted.

Hypoglycemic agents: Hypoglycemic symptoms may be reduced. Educate patient about decreased signs and symptoms of hypoglycemia or avoid use in patients with frequent episodes of hypoglycemia.

Decreased Effect: TCAs decrease the hypotensive effect of guanabenz.

Pharmacodynamics/Kinetics

Onset of action: Antihypertensive: ~1 hour

Absorption: ~75%

Half-life elimination, serum: 7-10 hours

Pregnancy Risk Factor C

Generic Available Yes

Guanabenz Acetate *see* Guanabenz *on page 654*

Guanadrel (GWAHN a drel)

Related Information

Cardiovascular Diseases *on page 1456*

U.S. Brand Names Hylorel®

Canadian Brand Names Hylorel®

Pharmacologic Category False Neurotransmitter

Synonyms Guanadrel Sulfate

Use Considered a second line agent in the treatment of hypertension, usually with a diuretic

Local Anesthetic/Vasoconstrictor Precautions

Manufacturer's information states that guanadrel may block vasopressor activity of epinephrine. This has not been observed during use of epinephrine as a vasoconstrictor in local anesthesia.

Effects on Dental Treatment

>10%: Palpitations (30%), dyspnea at rest (18%), coughing (27%)

1% to 10%: Xerostomia, glossitis (8%), orthostatic hypotension

Dosage Oral:

Adults: Initial: 10 mg/day (5 mg twice daily); adjust dosage weekly or monthly until blood pressure is controlled, usual dosage: 20-75 mg/day, given twice daily. For larger dosage, 3-4 times/day dosing may be needed.

Elderly: Initial: 5 mg once daily

Dosing interval in renal impairment:

Cl_{cr} 10-50 mL/minute: Administer every 12-24 hours.

Cl_{cr} <10 mL/minute: Administer every 24-48 hours.

Mechanism of Action Acts as a false neurotransmitter that blocks the adrenergic actions of norepinephrine; it displaces norepinephrine from its presynaptic storage granules and thus exposes it to degradation; it thereby produces a reduction in total peripheral resistance and, therefore, blood pressure

Other Adverse Effects

>10%:

Cardiovascular: Chest pain (28%), peripheral edema (29%)

Central nervous system: Fatigue (64%), headache (58%), faintness (47% to 49%), drowsiness (45%), confusion (15%)

Gastrointestinal: Increased bowel movements (31%), gas pain (24% to 32%), constipation (21%), anorexia (19%), weight gain/loss (42% to 44%)

Genitourinary: Nocturia (48%), polyuria (34%), ejaculation disturbances (18%)

Neuromuscular & skeletal: Paresthesia (25%), aching limbs (43%), leg cramps (20% to 26%)

Ocular: Visual disturbances (29%)

1% to 10%:

Central nervous system: Psychological problems (4%), depression (2%), sleep disorders (2%)

Gastrointestinal: Nausea/vomiting (4%)

Genitourinary: Impotence (5%)

Renal: Hematuria (2%)

<1% (Limited to important or life-threatening): **Syncope, angina**

Drug Interactions

Increased Effect/Toxicity: Increased toxicity of direct-acting amines (epinephrine, norepinephrine) by guanadrel; the hypotensive effect of guanadrel may be potentiated. Increased effect of beta-blockers, vasodilators. Norepinephrine/phenylephrine have exaggerated pressor response; monitor blood pressure closely. MAO inhibitors may cause severe hypertension; give at least 1 week apart.

Decreased Effect: TCAs decrease hypotensive effect of guanadrel. Phenothiazines may inhibit the antihypertensive response to guanadrel; consider an alternative antihypertensive with different mechanism of action. Amphetamines, related sympathomimetics, and methylphenidate decrease the antihypertensive response to guanadrel; consider an alternative antihypertensive with different mechanism of action. Reassess the need for amphetamine, related sympathomimetic, or methylphenidate; consider alternatives. Ephedrine may inhibit the antihypertensive response to guanadrel; consider an alternative antihypertensive with different mechanism of action. Reassess the need for ephedrine.

Dietary/Ethanol/Herb Considerations

Ethanol: Avoid use; may increase CNS depression or orthostasis.

Herb/Nutraceutical: Avoid gotu kola, kava, SAMe, St John's wort, and valerian; may increase CNS depression.

Pharmacodynamics/Kinetics

Onset of action: Peak effect: 4-6 hours

Duration: 4-14 hours

Absorption: Rapid

Half-life elimination, serum: Biphasic: Initial: 1-4 hours; Terminal: 5-45 hours

Time to peak, serum: 1.5-2 hours

Pregnancy Risk Factor B

Generic Available No

Guanadrel Sulfate *see* Guanadrel *on page 654*

Guanfacine (GWAHN fa seen)

Related Information

Cardiovascular Diseases *on page 1456*

U.S. Brand Names Tenex®

Canadian Brand Names Tenex®

Pharmacologic Category $Alpha_2$-Adrenergic Agonist

Synonyms Guanfacine Hydrochloride

Use Management of hypertension

Local Anesthetic/Vasoconstrictor Precautions No information available to require special precautions

Effects on Dental Treatment >10%: Xerostomia (up to 54%), changes in salivation

Dosage Adults: Oral: Hypertension: 1 mg usually at bedtime, may increase if needed at 3- to 4-week intervals; 1 mg/day is most common dose

(Continued)

Guanfacine *(Continued)*

Mechanism of Action Stimulates $alpha_2$-adrenoreceptors in the brain stem, thus activating an inhibitory neuron, resulting in reduced sympathetic outflow, producing a decrease in vasomotor tone and heart rate

Other Adverse Effects

>10%:

Central nervous system: Somnolence (5% to 40%), headache (3% to 13%), dizziness (2% to 15%)

Gastrointestinal: Constipation (2% to 15%)

1% to 10%:

Central nervous system: Fatigue (2% to 10%)

Endocrine & metabolic: Impotence (up to 7%)

<1% (Limited to important or life-threatening): Agitation, alopecia, amnesia, blurred vision, **bradycardia**, chest pain, confusion, depression, dermatitis, diaphoresis, dysphagia, **dyspnea**, edema, exfoliative dermatitis, hypokinesia, **hypotension**, insomnia, leg cramps, malaise, nervousness, orthostasis, palpitations, paresthesia, pruritus, rash, **rebound hypertension, syncope**, tinnitus, urinary incontinence, vertigo

Note: Mania and aggressive behavior have been reported in pediatric patients with ADHD who received guanfacine.

Drug Interactions

Increased Effect/Toxicity:

Nitroprusside and guanfacine have additive hypotensive effects. Noncardioselective beta-blockers (nadolol, propranolol, timolol) may exacerbate rebound hypertension when guanfacine is withdrawn. The beta-blocker should be withdrawn first. The gradual withdrawal of guanfacine or a cardioselective beta-blocker could be substituted.

Hypoglycemic agents: Hypoglycemic symptoms may be decreased. Educate patient about decreased signs and symptoms of hypoglycemia or avoid use in patients with frequent episodes of hypoglycemia.

Decreased Effect: TCAs decrease the hypotensive effect of guanfacine.

Dietary/Ethanol/Herb Considerations

Ethanol: Avoid use; may increase CNS depression.

Herb/Nutraceutical: Avoid gotu kola, kava, SAMe, St John's wort, and valerian; may increase CNS depression.

Pharmacodynamics/Kinetics

Onset of action: Peak effect: 8-11 hours

Duration: 24 hours following single dose

Half-life elimination, serum: 17 hours

Time to peak, serum: 1-4 hours

Pregnancy Risk Factor B

Generic Available No

Guanfacine Hydrochloride *see* Guanfacine *on page 655*

Guiatuss® [OTC] *see* Guaifenesin *on page 650*

Guiatuss™ CF *see* Guaifenesin, Pseudoephedrine, and Dextromethorphan *on page 653*

Guiatuss™ DAC® *see* Guaifenesin, Pseudoephedrine, and Codeine *on page 653*

Guiatuss-DM® [OTC] *see* Guaifenesin and Dextromethorphan *on page 651*

Gum Benjamin *see* Benzoin *on page 171*

Gynazole-1™ *see* Butoconazole *on page 218*

Gyne-Lotrimin® [OTC] *see* Clotrimazole *on page 356*

Gyne-Lotrimin® 3 [OTC] *see* Clotrimazole *on page 356*

Gynix® [OTC] *see* Clotrimazole *on page 356*

Gynodiol® *see* Estradiol *on page 521*

Gynol II® [OTC] *see* Nonoxynol 9 *on page 985*

Haemophilus b Conjugate Vaccine

(he MOE fi lus bee KON joo gate vak SEEN)

Related Information

Immunizations (Vaccines) *on page 1612*

U.S. Brand Names ActHIB®; HibTITER®; PedvaxHIB®

Canadian Brand Names ActHIB®; PedvaxHIB®

Pharmacologic Category Vaccine

Synonyms Diphtheria CRM_{197} Protein Conjugate; Diphtheria Toxoid Conjugate; *Haemophilus* b Oligosaccharide Conjugate Vaccine; *Haemophilus* b Polysaccharide Vaccine; HbCV; Hib Polysaccharide Conjugate; PRP-D

Use Routine immunization of children 2 months to 5 years of age against invasive disease caused by *H. influenzae*

Unimmunized children ≥5 years of age with a chronic illness known to be associated with increased risk of *Haemophilus influenzae* type b disease, specifically, persons with anatomic or functional asplenia or sickle cell anemia or those who have undergone splenectomy, should receive Hib vaccine.

Haemophilus b conjugate vaccines are not indicated for prevention of bronchitis or other infections due to *H. influenzae* in adults; adults with specific dysfunction or certain complement deficiencies who are at especially high risk of *H. influenzae* type b infection (HIV-infected adults); patients with Hodgkin's disease (vaccinated at least 2 weeks before the initiation of chemotherapy or 3 months after the end of chemotherapy)

Local Anesthetic/Vasoconstrictor Precautions No information available to require special precautions

Effects on Dental Treatment No significant effects or complications reported

Restrictions Federal law requires that the date of administration, the vaccine manufacturer, lot number of vaccine, and the administering person's name, title and address be entered into the patient's permanent medical record.

Dosage Children: I.M.: 0.5 mL as a single dose should be administered according to one of the following "brand-specific" schedules; do not inject I.V. (see table)

Vaccination Schedule for *Haemophilus* b Conjugate Vaccines

Age at 1st Dose (mo)	HibTITER®		PedvaxHIB®		ProHIBiT®	
	Primary Series	Booster	Primary Series	Booster	Primary Series	Booster
2-6*	3 doses, 2 months apart	15 mo†	2 doses, 2 months apart	12 mo†		
7-11	2 doses, 2 months apart	15 mo†	2 doses, 2 months apart	15 mo†		
12-14	1 dose	15 mo†	1 dose	15 mo†		
15-60	1 dose	—	1 dose	—	1 dose	—

*It is not currently recommended that the various *Haemophilus* b conjugate vaccines be interchanged (ie, the same brand should be used throughout the entire vaccination series). If the health care provider does not know which vaccine was previously used, it is prudent that an infant, 2-6 months of age, be given a primary series of three doses.

†At least 2 months after previous dose.

Mechanism of Action Stimulates production of anticapsular antibodies and provides active immunity to *Haemophilus influenzae*

Other Adverse Effects When administered during the same visit that DTP vaccine is given, the rates of systemic reactions do not differ from those observed only when DTP vaccine is administered. All serious adverse reactions must be reported to the U.S. Department of Health and Human Services (DHHS) Vaccine Adverse Event Reporting System (VAERS) 1-800-822-7967.

25%:
- Cardiovascular: Edema
- Dermatologic: Local erythema
- Local: Increased risk of *Haemophilus* b infections in the week after vaccination
- Miscellaneous: Warmth

>10%: Acute febrile reactions

1% to 10%:
- Central nervous system: Fever (up to 102.2°F), irritability, lethargy
- Gastrointestinal: Anorexia, diarrhea
- Local: Irritation at injection site

<1%: **Edema of the eyes/face, convulsions, fever (>102.2°F)**, unusual fatigue, urticaria, itching, **vomiting**, weakness, **dyspnea**

Drug Interactions Decreased Effect: Immunosuppressive agents and/or immunoglobulins within 1 month may decrease antibody production.

Pharmacodynamics/Kinetics Seroconversion following one dose of Hib vaccine for children 18 months or 24 months of age or older is 75% to 90% respectively.

Onset of action: Serum antibody response: 1-2 weeks
Duration: Immunity: 1.5 years

Pregnancy Risk Factor C

Generic Available No

Comments Federal law requires that the date of administration, the vaccine manufacturer, lot number of vaccine, and the administering person's name, title and address be entered into the patient's permanent medical record

***Haemophilus* b Oligosaccharide Conjugate Vaccine** *see Haemophilus* b Conjugate Vaccine *on page 656*

***Haemophilus* b Polysaccharide Vaccine** *see Haemophilus* b Conjugate Vaccine *on page 656*

Halcinonide (hal SIN oh nide)

U.S. Brand Names Halog®; Halog®-E

Canadian Brand Names Halog®

Mexican Brand Names Dermalog®

Pharmacologic Category Corticosteroid, Topical

(Continued)

Halcinonide *(Continued)*

Use Inflammation of corticosteroid-responsive dermatoses [high potency topical corticosteroid]

Local Anesthetic/Vasoconstrictor Precautions No information available to require special precautions

Effects on Dental Treatment No significant effects or complications reported

Dosage Children and Adults: Topical: Steroid-responsive dermatoses: Apply sparingly 1-3 times/day, occlusive dressing may be used for severe or resistant dermatoses; a thin film is effective; do not overuse. Therapy should be discontinued when control is achieved; if no improvement is seen, reassessment of diagnosis may be necessary.

Mechanism of Action Decreases inflammation by suppression of migration of polymorphonuclear leukocytes and reversal of increased capillary permeability

Other Adverse Effects Frequency not defined:

Dermatologic: Itching, dry skin, folliculitis, hypertrichosis, acneiform eruptions, hypopigmentation, perioral dermatitis, allergic contact dermatitis, skin maceration, skin atrophy, striae

Local: Burning, irritation, miliaria

Miscellaneous: Secondary infection

Pharmacodynamics/Kinetics

Absorption: Percutaneous absorption varies by location of topical application and use of occlusive dressings

Metabolism: Primarily hepatic

Excretion: Urine

Pregnancy Risk Factor C

Generic Available No

Halcion® *see* Triazolam *on page 1345*

Haldol® *see* Haloperidol *on page 659*

Haldol® Decanoate *see* Haloperidol *on page 659*

Halfprin® [OTC] *see* Aspirin *on page 131*

Halobetasol (hal oh BAY ta sol)

U.S. Brand Names Ultravate®

Canadian Brand Names Ultravate™

Pharmacologic Category Corticosteroid, Topical

Synonyms Halobetasol Propionate

Use Relief of inflammatory and pruritic manifestations of corticosteroid-response dermatoses [very high potency topical corticosteroid]

Local Anesthetic/Vasoconstrictor Precautions No information available to require special precautions

Effects on Dental Treatment No significant effects or complications reported

Dosage Children and Adults: Topical: Steroid-responsive dermatoses: Apply sparingly to skin twice daily, rub in gently and completely; treatment should not exceed 2 consecutive weeks and total dosage should not exceed 50 g/week. Therapy should be discontinued when control is achieved; if no improvement is seen, reassessment of diagnosis may be necessary.

Mechanism of Action Corticosteroids inhibit the initial manifestations of the inflammatory process (ie, capillary dilation and edema, fibrin deposition, and migration and diapedesis of leukocytes into the inflamed site) as well as later sequelae (angiogenesis, fibroblast proliferation)

Other Adverse Effects Frequency not defined:

Dermatologic: Itching, dry skin, folliculitis, hypertrichosis, acneiform eruptions, hypopigmentation, perioral dermatitis, allergic contact dermatitis, skin maceration, skin atrophy, striae

Local: Burning, irritation, miliaria

Miscellaneous: Secondary infection

Pharmacodynamics/Kinetics

Absorption: Percutaneous absorption varies by location of topical application and use of occlusive dressings; ~3% of a topically applied dose of ointment enters circulation within 96 hours

Metabolism: Primarily hepatic

Excretion: Urine

Pregnancy Risk Factor C

Generic Available No

Halobetasol Propionate *see* Halobetasol *on page 658*

Halofantrine (ha loe FAN trin)

Pharmacologic Category Antimalarial Agent

Synonyms Halofantrine Hydrochloride

Use Treatment of mild to moderate acute malaria caused by susceptible strains of *Plasmodium falciparum* and *Plasmodium vivax*

Local Anesthetic/Vasoconstrictor Precautions No information available to require special precautions

Effects on Dental Treatment No significant effects or complications reported

Dosage Oral:

Children (unlabeled):

<40 kg: 8 mg/kg every 6 hours for 3 doses; repeat in 1 week

≥40 kg: 500 mg every 6 hours for 3 doses; repeat in 1 week

Adults: 500 mg every 6 hours for 3 doses; repeat in 1 week

Mechanism of Action Exact mechanism unknown; destruction of asexual blood forms, possible inhibition of proton pump

Other Adverse Effects

1% to 10%:

Cardiovascular: Edema

Central nervous system: Malaise, headache (3%), dizziness (5%)

Dermatologic: Pruritus (3%)

Gastrointestinal: Nausea (3%), vomiting (4%), abdominal pain (9%), diarrhea (6%), anorexia (5%)

Hematologic: Leukocytosis

Hepatic: Elevated LFTs

Local: Tenderness

Neuromuscular & skeletal: Myalgia (1%), rigors (2%)

Respiratory: Cough

Miscellaneous: Lymphadenopathy

<1%: **Tachycardia, hypotension**, hypoglycemia, sterile abscesses, asthma, anaphylactic shock, chest pain, **palpitations**, orthostasis, weakness, confusion, depression, paresthesias, constipation, abnormal vision, tinnitus, **facial edema**, urticaria

Postmarketing and/or case reports: Anaphylaxis, CVA, hemolytic anemia, hypertensive crisis, pulmonary edema, QT_c prolongation, seizures, tetany, ventricular arrhythmia

Drug Interactions Substrate of CYP2C8/9, 2D6, **3A4**; Inhibits CYP2D6

Increased Effect/Toxicity: CYP3A4 inhibitors (potent) may increase serum levels/toxicity of halofantrine. Increased toxicity (QT_c interval prolongation) with other agents that cause QT_c interval prolongation, especially mefloquine.

Dietary/Ethanol/Herb Considerations Food: Absorption may be increased 60% with high-fat meals.

Pharmacodynamics/Kinetics

Absorption: Erratic and variable; serum levels are proportional to dose up to 1000 mg; smaller doses should be divided; may be increased 60% with high fat meals

Distribution: V_d: 570 L/kg; widely to most tissues

Metabolism: Hepatic to active metabolite

Half-life elimination: 6-10 days; Metabolite: 3-4 days; may be prolonged in active disease

Excretion: Primarily in feces (hepatobiliary)

Clearance: Parasite: Mean: 40-84 hours

Pregnancy Risk Factor C

Generic Available No

Halofantrine Hydrochloride *see* Halofantrine *on page 658*

Halog® *see* Halcinonide *on page 657*

Halog®-E *see* Halcinonide *on page 657*

Haloperidol (ha loe PER i dole)

U.S. Brand Names Haldol®; Haldol® Decanoate

Canadian Brand Names Apo®-Haloperidol; Apo®-Haloperidol LA; Haloperidol-LA Omega; Haloperidol Long Acting; Novo-Peridol; Peridol; PMS-Haloperidol LA

Mexican Brand Names Haldol®; Haldol decanoas®; Haloperil®

Pharmacologic Category Antipsychotic Agent, Butyrophenone

Synonyms Haloperidol Decanoate; Haloperidol Lactate

Use Management of schizophrenia; control of tics and vocal utterances of Tourette's disorder in children and adults; severe behavioral problems in children

Unlabeled/Investigational Use Treatment of psychosis; emergency sedation of severely agitated or delirious patients; adjunctive treatment of ethanol dependence; antiemetic

Local Anesthetic/Vasoconstrictor Precautions Manufacturer's information states that haloperidol may block vasopressor activity of epinephrine. This has not been observed during use of epinephrine as a vasoconstrictor in local anesthesia.

Effects on Dental Treatment Orthostatic hypotension and nasal congestion are possible; since the drug is a dopamine antagonist, extrapyramidal symptoms of the TMJ are a possibility.

Dosage

Children: 3-12 years (15-40 kg): Oral:

Initial: 0.05 mg/kg/day or 0.25-0.5 mg/day given in 2-3 divided doses; increase by 0.25-0.5 mg every 5-7 days; maximum: 0.15 mg/kg/day

(Continued)

Haloperidol *(Continued)*

Usual maintenance:
Agitation or hyperkinesia: 0.01-0.03 mg/kg/day once daily
Nonpsychotic disorders: 0.05-0.075 mg/kg/day in 2-3 divided doses
Psychotic disorders: 0.05-0.15 mg/kg/day in 2-3 divided doses

Children 6-12 years: Sedation/psychotic disorders: I.M. (as lactate): 1-3 mg/dose every 4-8 hours to a maximum of 0.15 mg/kg/day; change over to oral therapy as soon as able

Adults:
Psychosis:
Oral: 0.5-5 mg 2-3 times/day; usual maximum: 30 mg/day
I.M. (as lactate): 2-5 mg every 4-8 hours as needed
I.M. (as decanoate): Initial: 10-20 times the daily oral dose administered at 4-week intervals
Maintenance dose: 10-15 times initial oral dose; used to stabilize psychiatric symptoms

Sedation in the intensive care unit:
I.M., IVP, IVPB: May repeat bolus doses after 30 minutes until calm achieved then administer 50% of the maximum dose every 6 hours
Mild agitation: 0.5-2 mg
Moderate agitation: 2.5-5 mg
Severe agitation: 10-20 mg
Oral: Agitation: 5-10 mg
Continuous intravenous infusion (100 mg/100 mL D_5W): Rates of 1-40 mg/hour have been used

Rapid tranquilization of severely-agitated patient (unlabeled use): Administer every 30-60 minutes:
Oral: 5-10 mg
I.M.: 5 mg
Average total dose (oral or I.M.) for tranquilization: 10-20 mg

Elderly: Initial: Oral: 0.25-0.5 mg 1-2 times/day; increase dose at 4- to 7-day intervals by 0.25-0.5 mg/day; increase dosing intervals (twice daily, 3 times/day, etc) as necessary to control response or side effects

Hemodialysis/peritoneal dialysis: Supplemental dose is unnecessary

Mechanism of Action Blocks postsynaptic mesolimbic dopaminergic D_1 and D_2 receptors in the brain; depresses the release of hypothalamic and hypophyseal hormones; believed to depress the reticular activating system thus affecting basal metabolism, body temperature, wakefulness, vasomotor tone, and emesis

Other Adverse Effects Frequency not defined:

Cardiovascular: **Hypotension, hypertension, tachycardia, arrhythmias**, abnormal T waves with prolonged ventricular repolarization

Central nervous system: Restlessness, anxiety, **extrapyramidal symptoms, dystonic reactions, pseudoparkinsonian signs and symptoms, tardive dyskinesia**, neuroleptic malignant syndrome (NMS), altered central temperature regulation, akathisia, tardive dystonia, insomnia, euphoria, agitation, drowsiness, depression, lethargy, headache, confusion, vertigo, **seizures**

Dermatologic: Hyperpigmentation, pruritus, rash, contact dermatitis, alopecia, photosensitivity (rare)

Endocrine & metabolic: Amenorrhea, galactorrhea, gynecomastia, sexual dysfunction, lactation, breast engorgement, mastalgia, menstrual irregularities, hyperglycemia, hypoglycemia, hyponatremia

Gastrointestinal: Nausea, vomiting, anorexia, constipation, diarrhea, **increased salivation, dyspepsia, xerostomia**

Genitourinary: Urinary retention, priapism

Hematologic: Cholestatic jaundice, obstructive jaundice

Ocular: Blurred vision

Respiratory: **Laryngospasm, bronchospasm**

Miscellaneous: Heat stroke, diaphoresis

Drug Interactions Substrate of CYP1A2, **2D6, 3A4**; Inhibits **CYP2D6**

Increased Effect/Toxicity: Haloperidol concentrations/effects may be increased by chloroquine, fluoxetine, paroxetine, propranolol, quinidine, and sulfadoxine-pyridoxine. Haloperidol may increase the effects of antihypertensives, CNS depressants (ethanol, narcotics, sedative-hypnotics), lithium, trazodone, and TCAs. Haloperidol in combination with indomethacin may result in drowsiness, tiredness, and confusion. Metoclopramide may increase risk of extrapyramidal symptoms (EPS).

Decreased Effect: Haloperidol may inhibit the ability of bromocriptine to lower serum prolactin concentrations. Benztropine (and other anticholinergics) may inhibit the therapeutic response to haloperidol and excess anticholinergic effects may occur. Barbiturates, carbamazepine, and cigarette smoking may enhance the hepatic metabolism of haloperidol. Haloperidol may inhibit the antiparkinsonian effect of levodopa; avoid this combination.

Dietary/Ethanol/Herb Considerations

Ethanol: Avoid use; may increase CNS depression.

Food: Dilute oral concentration with water or juice. Avoid grapefruit products; may increase serum concentration/toxicity. Avoid caffeine.

Herb/Nutraceutical: Avoid gotu kola, kava, SAMe, St John's wort, and valerian; may increase CNS depression.

Pharmacodynamics/Kinetics

Onset of action: Sedation: I.V.: ~1 hour

Duration: Decanoate: ~3 weeks

Distribution: Crosses placenta; enters breast milk

Protein binding: 90%

Metabolism: Hepatic to inactive compounds

Bioavailability: Oral: 60%

Half-life elimination: 20 hours

Time to peak, serum: 20 minutes

Excretion: Urine (33% to 40% as metabolites) within 5 days; feces (15%)

Pregnancy Risk Factor C

Generic Available Yes

Haloperidol Decanoate *see* Haloperidol *on page 659*

Haloperidol Lactate *see* Haloperidol *on page 659*

Halotestin® *see* Fluoxymesterone *on page 592*

Halotussin® DAC *see* Guaifenesin, Pseudoephedrine, and Codeine *on page 653*

Haltran® [OTC] *see* Ibuprofen *on page 703*

Havrix® *see* Hepatitis A Vaccine *on page 665*

Havrix® and Engerix-B® *see* Hepatitis A (Inactivated) and Hepatitis B (Recombinant) Vaccine *on page 664*

Hayfebrol® [OTC] *see* Chlorpheniramine and Pseudoephedrine *on page 308*

HbCV *see Haemophilus* b Conjugate Vaccine *on page 656*

HBIG *see* Hepatitis B Immune Globulin *on page 666*

hBNP *see* Nesiritide *on page 964*

25-HCC *see* Calcifediol *on page 221*

hCG *see* Chorionic Gonadotropin (Human) *on page 320*

HCTZ *see* Hydrochlorothiazide *on page 675*

HCTZ and Telmisartan *see* Telmisartan and Hydrochlorothiazide *on page 1270*

HDA® Toothache [OTC] *see* Benzocaine *on page 169*

HDCV *see* Rabies Virus Vaccine *on page 1164*

Head & Shoulders® Classic Clean [OTC] *see* Pyrithione Zinc *on page 1154*

Head & Shoulders® Classic Clean 2-In-1 [OTC] *see* Pyrithione Zinc *on page 1154*

Head & Shoulders® Dry Scalp Care [OTC] *see* Pyrithione Zinc *on page 1154*

Head & Shoulders® Extra Fullness [OTC] *see* Pyrithione Zinc *on page 1154*

Head & Shoulders® Refresh [OTC] *see* Pyrithione Zinc *on page 1154*

Head & Shoulders® Smooth & Silky 2-In-1 [OTC] *see* Pyrithione Zinc *on page 1154*

Healon® *see* Sodium Hyaluronate *on page 1230*

Healon®5 *see* Sodium Hyaluronate *on page 1230*

Healon GV® *see* Sodium Hyaluronate *on page 1230*

Hectorol® *see* Doxercalciferol *on page 472*

Helidac® *see* Bismuth, Metronidazole, and Tetracycline *on page 187*

Helistat® *see* Microfibrillar Collagen Hemostat *on page 907*

Helixate® FS *see* Antihemophilic Factor (Recombinant) *on page 115*

Hemabate™ *see* Carboprost Tromethamine *on page 250*

Hemiacidrin *see* Citric Acid Bladder Mixture *on page 335*

Hemin (HEE min)

U.S. Brand Names Panhematin®

Pharmacologic Category Blood Modifiers

Use Orphan drug: Treatment of recurrent attacks of acute intermittent porphyria (AIP) only after an appropriate period of alternate therapy has been tried

Local Anesthetic/Vasoconstrictor Precautions No information available to require special precautions

Effects on Dental Treatment No significant effects or complications reported

Dosage I.V.: 1-4 mg/kg/day administered over 10-15 minutes for 3-14 days; may be repeated no earlier than every 12 hours; not to exceed 6 mg/kg in any 24-hour period

Other Adverse Effects Frequency not defined:

Central nervous system: Mild pyrexia

Hematologic: Leukocytosis

Local: Phlebitis

Case report: Coagulopathy

Generic Available No

Hemocyte® [OTC] *see* Iron Supplements *on page 745*

Hemodent® Gingival Retraction Cord *see* Aluminum Chloride *on page 67*
Hemofil® M *see* Antihemophilic Factor (Human) *on page 113*
Hemril-HC® *see* Hydrocortisone *on page 688*

Heparin (HEP a rin)

U.S. Brand Names Hep-Lock®

Canadian Brand Names Hepalean®; Hepalean® Leo; Hepalean®-LOK

Mexican Brand Names Dixaparine; Helberina; Inhepar; Proparin®

Pharmacologic Category Anticoagulant

Synonyms Heparin Calcium; Heparin Lock Flush; Heparin Sodium

Use Prophylaxis and treatment of thromboembolic disorders

Local Anesthetic/Vasoconstrictor Precautions No information available to require special precautions

Effects on Dental Treatment Heparin, being a potent antithrombin agent, has caused bleeding from the gums.

Dosage

Children:

Intermittent I.V.: Initial: 50-100 units/kg, then 50-100 units/kg every 4 hours

I.V. infusion: Initial: 50 units/kg, then 15-25 units/kg/hour; increase dose by 2-4 units/kg/hour every 6-8 hours as required

Adults:

Prophylaxis (low-dose heparin): S.C.: 5000 units every 8-12 hours

Intermittent I.V.: Initial: 10,000 units, then 50-70 units/kg (5000-10,000 units) every 4-6 hours

I.V. infusion (weight-based dosing per institutional nomogram recommended):

Acute coronary syndromes: MI: Fibrinolytic therapy:

Alteplase or reteplase with first or second bolus: Concurrent bolus of 60 units/kg (maximum: 4000 units), then 12 units/kg/hour (maximum: 1000 units/hour) as continuous infusion. Check aPTT every 4-6 hours; adjust to target of 1.5-2 times the upper limit of control (50-70 seconds in clinical trials); usual range 10-30 units/kg/hour. Duration of heparin therapy depends on concurrent therapy and the specific patient risks for systemic or venous thromboembolism.

Streptokinase: Heparin use optional depending on concurrent therapy and specific patient risks for systemic or venous thromboembolism (anterior MI, CHF, previous embolus, atrial fibrillation, LV thrombus): If heparin is administered, start when aPTT <2 times the upper limit of control; do not use a bolus, but initiate infusion adjusted to a target aPTT of 1.5-2 times the upper limit of control (50-70 seconds in clinical trials). If heparin is not administered by infusion, 7500-12,500 units S.C. every 12 hours (when aPTT <2 times the upper limit of control) is recommended.

Percutaneous coronary intervention: Heparin bolus and infusion may be administered to an activated clotting time (ACT) of 300-350 seconds if no concurrent GPIIb/IIIa receptor antagonist is administered or 200-250 seconds if a GPIIb/IIIa receptor antagonist is administered.

Treatment of unstable angina (high-risk and some intermediate-risk patients): Initial bolus of 60-70 units/kg (maximum: 5000 units), followed by an initial infusion of 12-15 units/kg/hour (maximum: 1000 units/hour). The American College of Chest Physicians consensus conference has recommended dosage adjustments to correspond to a therapeutic range equivalent to heparin levels of 0.3-0.7 units/mL by antifactor Xa determinations, which correlates with aPTT values between 60 and 80 seconds

Treatment of venous thromboembolism (DVT/PE): 80 units/kg I.V. push followed by continuous infusion of 18 units/kg/hour

Line flushing: When using daily flushes of heparin to maintain patency of single and double lumen central catheters, 10 units/mL is commonly used for younger infants (eg, <10 kg) while 100 units/mL is used for older infants, children, and adults. Capped PVC catheters and peripheral heparin locks require flushing more frequently (eg, every 6-8 hours). Volume of heparin flush is usually similar to volume of catheter (or slightly greater). Additional flushes should be given when stagnant blood is observed in catheter, after catheter is used for drug or blood administration, and after blood withdrawal from catheter.

Addition of heparin (0.5-1 unit/mL) to peripheral and central TPN has been shown to increase duration of line patency. The final concentration of heparin used for TPN solutions may need to be decreased to 0.5 units/mL in small infants receiving larger amounts of volume in order to avoid approaching therapeutic amounts. Arterial lines are heparinized with a final concentration of 1 unit/mL.

Using a standard heparin solution (25,000 units/500 mL D_5W), the following infusion rates can be used to achieve the listed doses.

For a dose of:

400 units/hour: Infuse at 8 mL/hour

500 units/hour: Infuse at 10 mL/hour

600 units/hour: Infuse at 12 mL/hour
700 units/hour: Infuse at 14 mL/hour
800 units/hour: Infuse at 16 mL/hour
900 units/hour: Infuse at 18 mL/hour
1000 units/hour: Infuse at 20 mL/hour
1100 units/hour: Infuse at 22 mL/hour
1200 units/hour: Infuse at 24 mL/hour
1300 units/hour: Infuse at 26 mL/hour
1400 units/hour: Infuse at 28 mL/hour
1500 units/hour: Infuse at 30 mL/hour
1600 units/hour: Infuse at 32 mL/hour
1700 units/hour: Infuse at 34 mL/hour
1800 units/hour: Infuse at 36 mL/hour
1900 units/hour: Infuse at 38 mL/hour
2000 units/hour: Infuse at 40 mL/hour

Dosing adjustments in the elderly: Patients >60 years of age may have higher serum levels and clinical response (longer aPTTs) as compared to younger patients receiving similar dosages; lower dosages may be required

Mechanism of Action Potentiates the action of antithrombin III and thereby inactivates thrombin (as well as activated coagulation factors IX, X, XI, XII, and plasmin) and prevents the conversion of fibrinogen to fibrin; heparin also stimulates release of lipoprotein lipase (lipoprotein lipase hydrolyzes triglycerides to glycerol and free fatty acids)

Other Adverse Effects Frequency not defined:

Cardiovascular: Chest pain, vasospasm (possibly related to thrombosis), hemorrhagic shock

Central nervous system: Fever, headache, chills

Dermatologic: Unexplained bruising, urticaria, alopecia, dysesthesia pedis, purpura, eczema, cutaneous necrosis (following deep S.C. injection), erythematous plaques (case reports)

Endocrine & metabolic: Hyperkalemia (supression of aldosterone), rebound hyperlipidemia on discontinuation

Gastrointestinal: Nausea, vomiting, constipation, hematemesis

Genitourinary: Frequent or persistent erection

Hematologic: Hemorrhage, blood in urine, bleeding from gums, epistaxis, adrenal hemorrhage, ovarian hemorrhage, retroperitoneal hemorrhage, thrombocytopenia (see note)

Hepatic: Elevated liver enzymes (AST/ALT) Local: Irritation, ulceration, cutaneous necrosis have been rarely reported with deep S.C. injections, I.M. injection (not recommended) is associated with a high incidence of these effects

Neuromuscular & skeletal: Peripheral neuropathy, osteoporosis (chronic therapy effect)

Ocular: Conjunctivitis (allergic reaction)

Respiratory: Hemoptysis, pulmonary hemorrhage, asthma, rhinitis, bronchospasm (case reports)

Miscellaneous: Allergic reactions, anaphylactoid reactions

Note: Thrombocytopenia has been reported to occur at an incidence between 0% and 30%. It is often of no clinical significance. However, immunologically mediated heparin-induced thrombocytopenia has been estimated to occur in 1% to 2% of patients, and is marked by a progressive fall in platelet counts and, in some cases, thromboembolic complications (skin necrosis, pulmonary embolism, gangrene of the extremities, stroke or MI); daily platelet counts for 5-7 days at initiation of therapy may help detect the onset of this complication.

Drug Interactions

Increased Effect/Toxicity: The risk of hemorrhage associated with heparin may be increased by oral anticoagulants (warfarin), thrombolytics, dextran, and drugs which affect platelet function (eg, aspirin, NSAIDs, dipyridamole, ticlopidine, clopidogrel, IIb/IIIa antagonists). However, heparin is often used in conjunction with thrombolytic therapy or during the initiation of warfarin therapy to assure anticoagulation and to protect against possible transient hypercoagulability. Cephalosporins which contain the MTT side chain and parenteral penicillins (may inhibit platelet aggregation) may increase the risk of hemorrhage. Other drugs reported to increase heparin's anticoagulant effect include antihistamines, tetracycline, quinine, nicotine, and cardiac glycosides (digoxin).

Decreased Effect: Nitroglycerin (I.V.) may decrease heparin's anticoagulant effect. This interaction has not been validated in some studies, and may only occur at high nitroglycerin dosages.

Dietary/Ethanol/Herb Considerations

Food: Heparin may interfere with calcium absorption when taken for >6 months. Avoid garlic, ginger, and green tea.

Herb/Nutraceutical: Avoid cat's claw, dong quai, evening primrose, feverfew, garlic, ginger, ginkgo biloba, ginseng, green tea, horse chestnut, and red clover due to additional antiplatelet activity.

Pharmacodynamics/Kinetics

Onset of action: Anticoagulation: I.V.: Immediate; S.C.: ~20-30 minutes

(Continued)

Heparin *(Continued)*

Absorption: Oral, rectal, I.M.: Erratic at best from all these routes of administration; S.C. absorption is also erratic, but considered acceptable for prophylactic use

Distribution: Does not cross placenta; does not enter breast milk

Metabolism: Hepatic; may be partially metabolized in the reticuloendothelial system

Half-life elimination: Mean: 1.5 hours; Range: 1-2 hours; affected by obesity, renal function, hepatic function, malignancy, presence of pulmonary embolism, and infections

Excretion: Urine (small amounts as unchanged drug)

Pregnancy Risk Factor C

Generic Available Yes

Heparin Calcium *see* Heparin *on page 662*

Heparin Cofactor I *see* Antithrombin III *on page 117*

Heparin Lock Flush *see* Heparin *on page 662*

Heparin Sodium *see* Heparin *on page 662*

Hepatitis A (Inactivated) and Hepatitis B (Recombinant) Vaccine

(hep u TYE tis ay, in ak ti VAY ted, & hep u TYE tis bee, ree KOM bi nent, vak SEEN)

Related Information

Immunizations (Vaccines) *on page 1612*

Systemic Viral Diseases *on page 1517*

U.S. Brand Names Twinrix®

Canadian Brand Names Twinrix™

Pharmacologic Category Vaccine

Synonyms Engerix-B® and Havrix®; Havrix® and Engerix-B®; Hepatitis B (Recombinant) and Hepatitis A Inactivated Vaccine

Use Active immunization against disease caused by hepatitis A virus and hepatitis B virus (all known subtypes) in populations desiring protection against or at high risk of exposure to these viruses.

Populations include travelers to areas of intermediate/high endemicity for **both** HAV and HBV; those at increased risk of HBV infection due to behavioral or occupational factors; patients with chronic liver disease; laboratory workers who handle live HAV and HBV; healthcare workers, police, and other personnel who render firstaid or medical assistance; workers who come in contact with sewage; employees of day care centers and correctional facilities; patients/staff of hemodialysis units; male homosexuals; patients frequently receiving blood products; military personnel; users of injectable illicit drugs; close household contacts of patients with hepatitis A and hepatitis B infection.

Local Anesthetic/Vasoconstrictor Precautions No information available to require special precautions

Effects on Dental Treatment >10%: Flu-like syndrome, upper respiratory tract infection

Restrictions Federal law requires that the date of administration, the vaccine manufacturer, lot number of vaccine, and the administering person's name, title, and address be entered into the patient's permanent medical record.

Dosage I.M.: Adults: Primary immunization: Three doses (1 mL each) given on a 0-, 1-, and 6-month schedule

Mechanism of Action

Hepatitis A vaccine (Havrix®), an inactivated virus vaccine, offers active immunization against hepatitis A virus infection at an effective immune response rate in up to 99% of subjects.

Recombinant hepatitis B vaccine (Engerix-B®) is a noninfectious subunit viral vaccine. The vaccine is derived from hepatitis B surface antigen (HB_sAg) produced through recombinant DNA techniques from yeast cells. The portion of the hepatitis B gene which codes for HB_sAg is cloned into yeast which is then cultured to produce hepatitis B vaccine.

In immunocompetent people, Twinrix® provides active immunization against hepatitis A virus infection (at an effective immune response rate >99% of subjects) and against hepatitis B virus infection (at an effective immune response rate of 93% to 97%) 30 days after completion of the 3-dose series. This is comparable to using hepatitis A vaccine (Havrix®) and hepatitis B vaccine (Engerix-B®) concomitantly.

Other Adverse Effects All serious adverse reactions must be reported to the U.S. Department of Health and Human Services (DHHS) Vaccine Adverse Event Reporting System (VAERS) 1-800-822-7967. Incidence of adverse effects of the combination product were similar to those occurring after administration of hepatitis A vaccine and hepatitis B vaccine alone. (Incidence reported is not versus placebo.)

>10%:

Central nervous system: Headache (13% to 22%), fatigue (11% to 14%)

Local: Injection site reaction: Soreness (37% to 41%), redness (9% to 11%)

1% to 10%:

Central nervous system: Fever (2% to 3%)

Gastrointestinal: Diarrhea (4% to 6%), nausea (2% to 4%), vomiting (≤1%)

Local: Injection site reaction: Swelling (4% to 6%), induration

<1%: Abdominal pain, agitation, anorexia, arthralgia, back pain, bruising at the injection site, diaphoresis, dizziness, erythema, **flushing**, insomnia, irritability, migraine, myalgia, paresthesia, petechia, pruritus at the injection site, rash, somnolence, **syncope**, urticaria, vertigo, vomiting, weakness

Postmarketing and/or case reports (as reported with hepatitis A vaccine and hepatitis B vaccine; also see individual agents): Allergic reactions, alopecia, anaphylaxis, anaphylactoid reactions, angioedema, arthritis, Bell's palsy, bronchospasm, congenital abnormality, conjunctivitis, convulsions, dyspepsia, dyspnea, earache, eczema, encephalopathy, erythema multiforme, erythema nodosum, Guillain-Barré syndrome, hepatitis, herpes zoster, hyperhydrosis, jaundice, keratitis, LFT abnormalities, myelitis, neuropathy, optic neuritis, paresis, serum sickness like syndrome, Stevens-Johnson syndrome, thrombocytopenia, tinnitus, visual disturbances

Drug Interactions Decreased Effect: Immunosuppressant agents may decrease immune response to vaccine.

Pharmacodynamics/Kinetics

Onset of action: Seroconversion for antibodies against HAV and HBV were detected 1 month after completion of the 3-dose series.

Duration: Patients remained seropositive for at least 4 years during clinical studies.

Pregnancy Risk Factor C

Generic Available No

Hepatitis A Vaccine (hep u TYE tis ay vak SEEN)

Related Information

Immunizations (Vaccines) *on page 1612*

Systemic Viral Diseases *on page 1517*

U.S. Brand Names Havrix®; VAQTA®

Canadian Brand Names Avaxim®; Avaxim®-Pediatric; Epaxal Berna®; Havrix™; VAQTA®

Pharmacologic Category Vaccine

Use For populations desiring protection against hepatitis A or for populations at high risk of exposure to hepatitis A virus (travelers to developing countries, household and sexual contacts of persons infected with hepatitis A), child day care employees, patients with chronic liver disease, illicit drug users, male homosexuals, institutional workers (eg, institutions for the mentally and physically handicapped persons, prisons, etc), and healthcare workers who may be exposed to hepatitis A virus (eg, laboratory employees); protection lasts for approximately 15 years

Local Anesthetic/Vasoconstrictor Precautions No information available to require special precautions

Effects on Dental Treatment No significant effects or complications reported

Restrictions Federal law requires that the date of administration, the vaccine manufacturer, lot number of vaccine, and the administering person's name, title, and address be entered into the patient's permanent medical record.

Dosage I.M.:

Havrix®:

Children 2-18 years: 720 ELISA units (administered as 2 injections of 360 ELISA units [0.5 mL]) 15-30 days prior to travel with a booster 6-12 months following primary immunization; the deltoid muscle should be used for I.M. injection

Adults: 1440 ELISA units(1 mL) 15-30 days prior to travel with a booster 6-12 months following primary immunization; injection should be in the deltoid

VAQTA®:

Children 2-17 years: 25 units (0.5 mL) with 25 units (0.5 mL) booster to be given 6-18 months after primary immunization

Adults: 50 units (1 mL) with 50 units (1 mL) booster to be given 6 months after primary immunization

Mechanism of Action As an inactivated virus vaccine, hepatitis A vaccine offers active immunization against hepatitis A virus infection at an effective immune response rate in up to 99% of subjects

Other Adverse Effects All serious adverse reactions must be reported to the U.S. Department of Health and Human Services (DHHS) Vaccine Adverse Event Reporting System (VAERS) 1-800-822-7967.

>10%:

Central nervous system: Headache

Local: Pain, tenderness, and warmth

1% to 10%:

Endocrine & metabolic: Pharyngitis (1%)

Gastrointestinal: Abdominal pain (1%)

Local: Cutaneous reactions at the injection site (soreness, edema, and redness)

Frequency not defined:

Central nervous system: Fever (rare), fatigue

(Continued)

Hepatitis A Vaccine *(Continued)*

Hepatic: Transient LFT abnormalities

Pharmacodynamics/Kinetics

Onset of action (protection): 3 weeks after a single dose

Duration: Neutralizing antibodies have persisted for >3 years; unconfirmed evidence indicates that antibody levels may persist for 5-10 years

Pregnancy Risk Factor C

Generic Available No

Selected Readings Centers for Disease Control, "Recommendations of the Advisory Committee on Immunization Practices (ACIP): General Recommendations on Immunization," *MMWR*, 1994, 43(RR-1):23.

Hepatitis B Immune Globulin

(hep a TYE tis bee i MYUN GLOB yoo lin)

Related Information

Immunizations (Vaccines) *on page 1612*

Occupational Exposure to Bloodborne Pathogens (Standard/Universal Precautions) *on page 1601*

Systemic Viral Diseases *on page 1517*

U.S. Brand Names BayHep B™; Nabi-HB®

Canadian Brand Names BayHep B™

Pharmacologic Category Immune Globulin

Synonyms HBIG

Use Provide prophylactic passive immunity to hepatitis B infection to those individuals exposed; newborns of mothers known to be hepatitis B surface antigen positive; hepatitis B immune globulin is not indicated for treatment of active hepatitis B infections and is ineffective in the treatment of chronic active hepatitis B infection

Local Anesthetic/Vasoconstrictor Precautions No information available to require special precautions

Effects on Dental Treatment No significant effects or complications reported

Dosage I.M.:

Newborns: Hepatitis B: 0.5 mL as soon after birth as possible (within 12 hours); may repeat at 3 months in order for a higher rate of prevention of the carrier state to be achieved; at this time an active vaccination program with the vaccine may begin

Adults: Postexposure prophylaxis: 0.06 mL/kg as soon as possible after exposure (ie, within 24 hours of needlestick, ocular, or mucosal exposure or within 14 days of sexual exposure); usual dose: 3-5 mL; repeat at 28-30 days after exposure

Note: HBIG may be administered at the same time (but at a different site) or up to 1 month preceding hepatitis B vaccination without impairing the active immune response

Note: Has been administered intravenously in hepatitis-B-positive liver transplant patients.

Mechanism of Action Hepatitis B immune globulin (HBIG) is a nonpyrogenic sterile solution containing 10% to 18% protein of which at least 80% is monomeric immunoglobulin G (IgG). HBIG differs from immune globulin in the amount of anti-HB_s. Immune globulin is prepared from plasma that is not preselected for anti-HB_s content. HBIG is prepared from plasma preselected for high titer anti-HB_s. In the U.S., HBIG has an anti-HB_s high titer >1:100,000 by IRA. There is no evidence that the causative agent of AIDS (HTLV-III/LAV) is transmitted by HBIG.

Other Adverse Effects Frequency not defined:

Central nervous system: Dizziness, malaise, fever, lethargy, chills

Dermatologic: Urticaria, angioedema, rash, erythema

Gastrointestinal: Vomiting, nausea

Genitourinary: Nephrotic syndrome

Local: Pain, tenderness, and muscular stiffness at injection site

Neuromuscular & skeletal: Arthralgia, myalgia

Miscellaneous: Anaphylaxis

Pharmacodynamics/Kinetics

Absorption: Slow

Time to peak, serum: 1-6 days

Pregnancy Risk Factor C

Generic Available No

Hepatitis B Inactivated Virus Vaccine (plasma derived) *see* Hepatitis B Vaccine *on page 666*

Hepatitis B Inactivated Virus Vaccine (recombinant DNA) *see* Hepatitis B Vaccine *on page 666*

Hepatitis B (Recombinant) and Hepatitis A Inactivated Vaccine *see* Hepatitis A (Inactivated) and Hepatitis B (Recombinant) Vaccine *on page 664*

Hepatitis B Vaccine

(hep a TYE tis bee vak SEEN)

Related Information

Diphtheria, Tetanus Toxoids, Acellular Pertussis, Hepatitis B (Recombinant), and Poliovirus (Inactivated) Vaccine *on page 454*

Immunizations (Vaccines) *on page 1612*
Systemic Viral Diseases *on page 1517*

U.S. Brand Names Engerix-B®; Recombivax HB®

Canadian Brand Names Engerix-B®; Recombivax HB®

Pharmacologic Category Vaccine

Synonyms Hepatitis B Inactivated Virus Vaccine (plasma derived); Hepatitis B Inactivated Virus Vaccine (recombinant DNA)

Use Immunization against infection caused by all known subtypes of hepatitis B virus, in individuals considered at high risk of potential exposure to hepatitis B virus or HB_sAg-positive materials: See table.

Pre-exposure Prophylaxis for Hepatitis B
Health care workers[1]
Special patient groups (eg, adolescents, infants born to HB_sAg–positive mothers, children born after 11/21/91, military personnel, etc)
Hemodialysis patients[2](see dosing recommendations)
Recipients of certain blood products[3]
Lifestyle factors
Homosexual and bisexual men
Intravenous drug abusers
Heterosexually active persons with multiple sexual partners or recently acquired sexually transmitted diseases
Environmental factors
Household and sexual contacts of HBV carriers
Prison inmates
Clients and staff of institutions for the mentally handicapped
Residents, immigrants and refugees from areas with endemic HBV infection
International travelers at increased risk of acquiring HBV infection

[1]The risk of hepatitis B virus (HBV) infection for health care workers varies both between hospitals and within hospitals. Hepatitis B vaccination is recommended for all health care workers with blood exposure.

[2]Hemodialysis patients often respond poorly to hepatitis B vaccination; higher vaccine doses or increased number of doses are required. A special formulation of one vaccine is now available for such persons (Recombivax HB®, 40 mcg/mL). The anti-Hb_s(antibody to hepatitis B surface antigen) response of such persons should be tested after they are vaccinated, and those who have not responded should be revaccinated with 1-3 additional doses.

Patients with chronic renal disease should be vaccinated as early as possible, ideally before they require hemodialysis. In addition, their anti-HB_s levels should be monitored at 6-12 month intervals to assess the need for revaccination.

[3]Patients with hemophilia should be immunized subcutaneously, not intramuscularly.

Local Anesthetic/Vasoconstrictor Precautions No information available to require special precautions

Effects on Dental Treatment No significant effects or complications reported

Restrictions Federal law requires that the date of administration, the vaccine manufacturer, lot number of vaccine, and the administering person's name, title, and address be entered into the patient's permanent medical record.

Dosage I.M.:

Immunization regimen: Regimen consists of 3 doses (0, 1, and 6 months): First dose given on the elected date, second dose given 1 month later, third dose given 6 months after the first dose; see table.

Routine Immunization Regimen of Three I.M. Hepatitis B Vaccine Doses

Age	Initial		1 mo		6 mo	
	Recombivax HB® (mL)	Engerix-B® (mL)	Recombivax HB® (mL)	Engerix-B® (mL)	Recombivax HB® (mL)	Engerix-B® (mL)
Birth[1]- 19 y	0.5[2]	0.5[3]	0.5[2]	0.5[3]	0.5[2]	0.5[3]
≥20 y	1[4]	1[5]	1[4]	1[5]	1[4]	1[5]
Dialysis or immunocompromised patients[6]	1[7]	2[8]	1[7]	2[8]	1[7]	2[8]

[1]Infants born of HB_s Ag **negative**mothers.

[2]5 mcg/0.5 mL pediatric/adolescent formulation

[3]10 mcg/0.5 mL formulation

[4]10 mcg/mL adult formulation

[5]20 mcg/mL formulation

[6]Revaccinate if anti-HB_s <10 mIU/mL ≥1-2 months after third dose.

[7]40 mcg/mL dialysis formulation

[8]Two 1 mL doses given at different sites using the 40 mcg/2 mL dialysis formulation

Alternative dosing schedule for **Recombivax HB®:** Children 11-15 years (10 mcg/mL adult formulation): First dose of 1 mL given on the elected date, second dose given 4-6 months later

(Continued)

Hepatitis B Vaccine *(Continued)*

Alternative dosing schedules for **Engerix-B®**:

Children ≤10 years (10 mcg/0.5 mL formulation): High-risk children: 0.5 mL at 0, 1, 2, and 12 months; lower-risk children ages 5-10 who are candidates for an extended administration schedule may receive an alternative regimen of 0.5 mL at 0, 12, and 24 months. If booster dose is needed, revaccinate with 0.5 mL.

Adolescents 11-19 years (20 mcg/mL formulation): 1 mL at 0, 1, and 6 months. High-risk adolescents: 1 mL at 0, 1, 2, and 12 months; lower-risk adolescents 11-16 years who are candidates for an extended administration schedule may receive an alternative regimen of 0.5 mL (using the 10 mcg/0.5 mL) formulation at 0, 12, and 24 months. If booster dose is needed, revaccinate with 20 mcg.

Adults ≥20 years: High-risk adults (20 mcg/mL formulation): 1 mL at 0, 1, 2, and 12 months. If booster dose is needed, revaccinate with 1 mL.

Postexposure prophylaxis: See table.

Postexposure Prophylaxis Recommended Dosage for Infants Born to HB_sAg-Positive Mothers

Treatment	Birth	Within 7 d	1 mo	6 mo
Engerix-B® (pediatric formulation 10 mcg/0.5 mL)[1]	Note[2]	0.5 mL[2]	0.5 mL	0.5 mL
Recombivax HB® (pediatric/adolescent formulation 5 mcg/0.5 mL)	Note[2]	0.5 mL[2]	0.5 mL	0.5 mL
Hepatitis B immune globulin	0.5 mL	—	—	—

[1]Note: An alternate regimen is administration of the vaccine at birth, within 7 days of birth, and 1, 2, and 12 months later.

[2]Note: The first dose may be given at birth at the same time as HBIG, but give in the opposite anterolateral thigh. This may better ensure vaccine absorption.

Mechanism of Action Recombinant hepatitis B vaccine is a noninfectious subunit viral vaccine. The vaccine is derived from hepatitis B surface antigen (HB_sAg) produced through recombinant DNA techniques from yeast cells. The portion of the hepatitis B gene which codes for HB_sAg is cloned into yeast which is then cultured to produce hepatitis B vaccine.

Other Adverse Effects All serious adverse reactions must be reported to the U.S. Department of Health and Human Services (DHHS) Vaccine Adverse Event Reporting System (VAERS) 1-800-822-7967.

>10%: Injection site reactions

Frequency not defined:

Cardiovascular: **Hypotension**

Central nervous system: Agitation, chills, dizziness, fatigue, fever (≥37.5°C/ 100°F), flushing, headache, insomnia, irritability, lightheadedness, malaise, vertigo

Dermatologic: Angioedema, petechiae, pruritus, rash, urticaria

Gastrointestinal: Abdominal pain, appetite decreased, cramps, diarrhea, dyspepsia, nausea, vomiting

Genitourinary: Dysuria

Local: Injection site reactions: Ecchymosis, erythema, induration, pain, nodule formation, soreness, swelling, tenderness, warmth

Neuromuscular & skeletal: Achiness, arthralgia, back pain, myalgia, neck pain, neck stiffness, paresthesia, shoulder pain, weakness

Otic: Earache

Respiratory: **Cough, pharyngitis, rhinitis, upper respiratory tract infection**

Miscellaneous: Lymphadenopathy, diaphoresis

Postmarketing and/or case reports: Alopecia, anaphylaxis, arthritis, Bell's palsy, **bronchospasm**, conjunctivitis, constipation, eczema, encephalitis, erythema nodosum, erythema multiforme, erythrocyte sedimentation rate increased, Guillain-Barré syndrome, herpes zoster, hypoesthesia, keratitis, liver enzyme elevation, migraine, multiple sclerosis, optic neuritis, palpitations, paresis, paresthesia, purpura, seizures, serum-sickness like syndrome (may be delayed days to weeks), Stevens-Johnson syndrome, syncope, tachycardia, thrombocytopenia, transverse myelitis, visual disturbances, vertigo

Drug Interactions Decreased Effect: Immunosuppressive agents

Pharmacodynamics/Kinetics Duration of action: Following a 3-dose series, immunity lasts ~5-7 years

Pregnancy Risk Factor C

Generic Available No

Selected Readings

Centers for Disease Control, "Recommendations of the Advisory Committee on Immunization Practices (ACIP): General Recommendations on Immunization," *MMWR*, 1994, 43(RR-1):23.

Gardner P and Schaffner W, "Immunization of Adults," *N Engl J Med*, 1993, 328(17):1252-8.

Hep-Lock® *see* Heparin *on page 662*
Hepsera™ *see* Adefovir *on page 44*
Herceptin® *see* Trastuzumab *on page 1335*
HES *see* Hetastarch *on page 669*
Hespan® *see* Hetastarch *on page 669*

Hetastarch (HET a starch)

U.S. Brand Names Hespan®; Hextend®

Mexican Brand Names HAES-steril®

Pharmacologic Category Plasma Volume Expander, Colloid

Synonyms HES; Hydroxyethyl Starch

Use Blood volume expander used in treatment of hypovolemia

Hespan®: Adjunct in leukapheresis to improve harvesting and increasing the yield of granulocytes by centrifugal means

Unlabeled/Investigational Use Hextand®: Priming fluid in pump oxygenators during cardiopulmonary bypass, and as a plasma volume expander during cardiopulmonary bypass

Local Anesthetic/Vasoconstrictor Precautions No information available to require special precautions

Effects on Dental Treatment No significant effects or complications reported

Dosage

Children: Safety and efficacy not established

Adults: I.V. infusion (requires infusion pump):

Plasma volume expansion: 500-1000 mL (up to 1500 mL/day) or 20 mL/kg/day (up to 1500 mL/day); larger volumes (15,000 mL/24 hours) have been used safely in small numbers of patients

Leukapheresis: 250-700 mL; **Note:** Citrate anticoagulant is added before use.

Dosing adjustment in renal impairment: Cl_{cr} <10 mL/minute: Initial dose is the same but subsequent doses should be reduced by 20% to 50% of normal

Mechanism of Action A synthetic polymer derived from a waxy starch composed of amylopectin; average molecular weight = 450,000; produces plasma volume expansion by virtue of its highly colloidal starch structure, similar to albumin; does not have oxygen-carrying capacity and is not a substitute for blood or plasma; large volumes may interfere with platelet function and prolong PT and PTT times

Other Adverse Effects Frequency not defined:

Cardiovascular: Circulatory overload, heart failure, peripheral edema

Central nervous system: Chills, fever, headache, intracranial bleeding

Dermatologic: Itching, pruritus, rash

Endocrine & metabolic: Amylase levels increased, parotid gland enlargement, indirect bilirubin increased, metabolic acidosis

Gastrointestinal: Vomiting

Hematologic: Bleeding, factor VIII:C plasma levels decreased, decreased plasma aggregation decreased, von Willebrand factor decreased, dilutional coagulopathy; prolongation of PT, PTT, clotting time, and bleeding time; thrombocytopenia, anemia, disseminated intravascular coagulopathy (rare), hemolysis (rare)

Neuromuscular & skeletal: Myalgia

Miscellaneous: Anaphylactoid reactions, hypersensitivity, **flu-like symptoms (mild)**

Pharmacodynamics/Kinetics

Onset of action: Volume expansion: I.V.: ~30 minutes

Duration: 24-36 hours

Metabolism: Molecules >50,000 daltons require enzymatic degradation by the reticuloendothelial system or amylases in the blood

Excretion: Urine (~40%) within 24 hours; smaller molecular weight molecules readily excreted

Pregnancy Risk Factor C

Generic Available Yes: Sodium chloride infusion

Hexachlorocyclohexane *see* Lindane *on page 809*

Hexachlorophene (heks a KLOR oh feen)

U.S. Brand Names pHisoHex®

Canadian Brand Names pHisoHex®

Pharmacologic Category Antibiotic, Topical

Use Surgical scrub and as a bacteriostatic skin cleanser; control an outbreak of gram-positive infection when other procedures have been unsuccessful

Local Anesthetic/Vasoconstrictor Precautions No information available to require special precautions

Effects on Dental Treatment No significant effects or complications reported

Dosage Children and Adults: Topical: Apply 5 mL cleanser and water to area to be cleansed; lather and rinse thoroughly under running water

Mechanism of Action Bacteriostatic polychlorinated biphenyl which inhibits membrane-bound enzymes and disrupts the cell membrane

(Continued)

Hexachlorophene *(Continued)*

Other Adverse Effects <1%: CNS injury, **seizures**, irritability, photosensitivity, dermatitis, redness, dry skin

Pharmacodynamics/Kinetics

Absorption: Percutaneously through inflamed, excoriated, and intact skin
Distribution: Crosses placenta
Half-life elimination: Infants: 6.1-44.2 hours

Pregnancy Risk Factor C

Generic Available No

Hexalen® *see* Altretamine *on page 66*

Hexamethylenetetramine *see* Methenamine *on page 879*

Hexamethylmelamine *see* Altretamine *on page 66*

HEXM *see* Altretamine *on page 66*

Hextend® *see* Hetastarch *on page 669*

Hexylresorcinol (heks il re ZOR si nole)

U.S. Brand Names Sucrets® Original [OTC]

Pharmacologic Category Local Anesthetic

Use Minor antiseptic and local anesthetic for sore throat

Local Anesthetic/Vasoconstrictor Precautions No information available to require special precautions

Effects on Dental Treatment No significant effects or complications reported

Dosage May be used as needed, allow to dissolve slowly in mouth

Generic Available Yes

Hibiclens® [OTC] *see* Chlorhexidine Gluconate *on page 300*

Hib Polysaccharide Conjugate *see Haemophilus* b Conjugate Vaccine *on page 656*

HibTITER® *see Haemophilus* b Conjugate Vaccine *on page 656*

Hiprex® *see* Methenamine *on page 879*

Histalet® [OTC] *see* Chlorpheniramine and Pseudoephedrine *on page 308*

Histatab® Plus [OTC] *see* Chlorpheniramine and Phenylephrine *on page 308*

Histor-D® *see* Chlorpheniramine and Phenylephrine *on page 308*

Hi-Vegi-Lip® [OTC] *see* Pancreatin *on page 1030*

Hivid® *see* Zalcitabine *on page 1403*

HMM *see* Altretamine *on page 66*

HMS Liquifilm® *see* Medrysone *on page 850*

Hold® DM [OTC] *see* Dextromethorphan *on page 423*

Homatropine (hoe MA troe peen)

U.S. Brand Names Isopto® Homatropine

Pharmacologic Category Anticholinergic Agent, Ophthalmic; Ophthalmic Agent, Mydriatic

Synonyms Homatropine Hydrobromide

Use Producing cycloplegia and mydriasis for refraction; treatment of acute inflammatory conditions of the uveal tract

Local Anesthetic/Vasoconstrictor Precautions No information available to require special precautions

Effects on Dental Treatment 1% to 10%: Nasal congestion

Dosage Ophthalmic:

Children:
- Mydriasis and cycloplegia for refraction: Instill 1 drop of 2% solution immediately before the procedure; repeat at 10-minute intervals as needed
- Uveitis: Instill 1 drop of 2% solution 2-3 times/day

Adults:
- Mydriasis and cycloplegia for refraction: Instill 1-2 drops of 2% solution or 1 drop of 5% solution before the procedure; repeat at 5- to 10-minute intervals as needed; maximum of 3 doses for refraction
- Uveitis: Instill 1-2 drops of 2% or 5% 2-3 times/day up to every 3-4 hours as needed

Mechanism of Action Blocks response of iris sphincter muscle and the accommodative muscle of the ciliary body to cholinergic stimulation resulting in dilation and loss of accommodation

Other Adverse Effects

>10%: Ocular: Blurred vision, photophobia

1% to 10%:
- Local: Stinging, local irritation
- Ocular: Increased intraocular pressure

<1%: Vascular congestion, edema, drowsiness, exudate, eczematoid dermatitis, follicular conjunctivitis

Pharmacodynamics/Kinetics
Onset of action: Accommodation and pupil effect: Ophthalmic:
Maximum mydriatic effect: Within 10-30 minutes
Maximum cycloplegic effect: Within 30-90 minutes
Duration:
Mydriasis: 6 hours to 4 days
Cycloplegia: 10-48 hours

Pregnancy Risk Factor C

Generic Available No

Homatropine and Hydrocodone *see* Hydrocodone and Homatropine *on page 684*
Homatropine Hydrobromide *see* Homatropine *on page 670*
Horse Antihuman Thymocyte Gamma Globulin *see* Lymphocyte Immune Globulin *on page 831*
H.P. Acthar® Gel *see* Corticotropin *on page 372*
HTF919 *see* Tegaserod *on page 1268*
Humalog® *see* Insulin Preparations *on page 723*
Humalog® Mix 75/25™ *see* Insulin Preparations *on page 723*
Human Diploid Cell Cultures Rabies Vaccine *see* Rabies Virus Vaccine *on page 1164*

Human Growth Hormone (HYU man grothe HOR mone)

U.S. Brand Names Genotropin®; Genotropin Miniquick®; Humatrope®; Norditropin®; Norditropin® Cartridges; Nutropin®; Nutropin AQ®; Nutropin Depot®; Protropin®; Saizen®; Serostim®

Canadian Brand Names Humatrope®; Nutropin® AQ; Nutropine®; Protropine®; Saizen®; Serostim®

Pharmacologic Category Growth Hormone

Synonyms Growth Hormone; Somatrem; Somatropin

Use
Children:
Long-term treatment of growth failure due to lack of adequate endogenous growth hormone secretion (Genotropin®, Humatrope®, Norditropin®, Nutropin®, Nutropin AQ®, Nutropin Depot®, Protropin®, Saizen®)
Long-term treatment of short stature associated with Turner syndrome (Humatrope®, Nutropin®, Nutropin AQ®)
Treatment of Prader-Willi syndrome (Genotropin®)
Treatment of growth failure associated with chronic renal insufficiency (CRI) up until the time of renal transplantation (Nutropin®, Nutropin AQ®)
Long-term treatment of growth failure in children born small for gestational age who fail to manifest catch-up growth by 2 years of age (Genotropin®)
Adults:
AIDS wasting or cachexia with concomitant antiviral therapy (Serostim®)
Replacement of endogenous growth hormone in patients with adult growth hormone deficiency who meet both of the following criteria (Genotropin®, Humatrope®, Nutropin®, Nutropin AQ®):
Biochemical diagnosis of adult growth hormone deficiency by means of a subnormal response to a standard growth hormone stimulation test (peak growth hormone ≤5 μg/L)
and
Adult-onset: Patients who have adult growth hormone deficiency whether alone or with multiple hormone deficiencies (hypopituitarism) as a result of pituitary disease, hypothalamic disease, surgery, radiation therapy, or trauma
or
Childhood-onset: Patients who were growth hormone deficient during childhood, confirmed as an adult before replacement therapy is initiated

Unlabeled/Investigational Use Investigational: Treatment of CHF

Local Anesthetic/Vasoconstrictor Precautions No information available to require special precautions

Effects on Dental Treatment No significant effects or complications reported

Dosage
Children (individualize dose):
Growth hormone deficiency:
Somatrem: Protropin®: I.M., S.C.: Weekly dosage: 0.3 mg/kg divided into daily doses
Somatropin:
Genotropin®: S.C.: Weekly dosage: 0.16-0.24 mg/kg divided into 6-7 doses
Humatrope®: I.M., S.C.: Weekly dosage: 0.18 mg/kg; maximum replacement dose: 0.3 mg/kg/week; dosing should be divided into equal doses given 3 times/week on alternating days, 6 times/week, or daily
Norditropin®: S.C.: Weekly dosage: 0.024-0.034 mg/kg administered in the evening, divided into doses 6-7 times/week; cartridge and vial formulations are bioequivalent; cartridge formulation does not need to be reconstituted prior to use; cartridges must be administered using the corresponding color-coded NordiPen® injection pen

(Continued)

Human Growth Hormone *(Continued)*

Nutropin Depot®: S.C.:

Once-monthly injection: 1.5 mg/kg administered on the same day of each month; patients >15 kg will require more than 1 injection per dose

Twice-monthly injection: 0.75 mg/kg administered twice each month on the same days of each month (eg, days 1 and 15 of each month); patients >30 kg will require more than 1 injection per dose

Nutropin®, Nutropin® AQ: S.C.: Weekly dosage: 0.3 mg/kg divided into daily doses; pubertal patients: ≤0.7 mg/kg/week divided daily

Saizen®: I.M., S.C.: Weekly dosage: 0.06 mg/kg administered 3 times/week

Note: Therapy should be discontinued when patient has reached satisfactory adult height, when epiphyses have fused, or when the patient ceases to respond. Growth of 5 cm/year or more is expected, if growth rate does not exceed 2.5 cm in a 6-month period, double the dose for the next 6 months; if there is still no satisfactory response, discontinue therapy

Chronic renal insufficiency (CRI): Nutropin®, Nutropin® AQ: S.C.: Weekly dosage: 0.35 mg/kg divided into daily injections; continue until the time of renal transplantation

Dosage recommendations in patients treated for CRI who require dialysis:

Hemodialysis: Administer dose at night prior to bedtime or at least 3-4 hours after hemodialysis to prevent hematoma formation from heparin

CCPD: Administer dose in the morning following dialysis

CAPD: Administer dose in the evening at the time of overnight exchange

Turner syndrome: Humatrope®, Nutropin®, Nutropin® AQ: S.C.: Weekly dosage: ≤0.375 mg/kg divided into equal doses 3-7 times per week

Prader-Willi syndrome: Genotropin®: S.C.: Weekly dosage: 0.24 mg/kg divided into 6-7 doses

Small for gestational age: Genotropin®: S.C.: Weekly dosage: 0.48 mg/kg divided into 6-7 doses

Adults:

Growth hormone deficiency: To minimize adverse events in older or overweight patients, reduced dosages may be necessary. During therapy, dosage should be decreased if required by the occurrence of side effects or excessive IGF-I levels.

Somatropin:

Nutropin®, Nutropin® AQ: S.C.: ≤0.006 mg/kg/day; dose may be increased according to individual requirements, up to a maximum of 0.025 mg/kg/day in patients <35 years of age, or up to a maximum of 0.0125 mg/kg/day in patients ≥35 years of age

Humatrope®: S.C.: ≤0.006 mg/kg/day; dose may be increased according to individual requirements, up to a maximum of 0.0125 mg/kg/day

Genotropin®: S.C.: Weekly dosage: ≤0.04 mg/kg divided into 6-7 doses; dose may be increased at 4- to 8-week intervals according to individual requirements, to a maximum of 0.08 mg/kg/week

AIDS wasting or cachexia:

Serostim®: S.C.: Dose should be given once daily at bedtime; patients who continue to lose weight after 2 weeks should be re-evaluated for opportunistic infections or other clinical events; rotate injection sites to avoid lipodystrophy

Daily dose based on body weight:

<35 kg: 0.1 mg/kg
35-45 kg: 4 mg
45-55 kg: 5 mg
>55 kg: 6 mg

Elderly: Patients ≥65 years of age may be more sensitive to the action of growth hormone and more prone to adverse effects; in general, dosing should be cautious, beginning at low end of dosing range.

Dosing adjustment in renal impairment: Specific recommendations unavailable; reports indicate patients with chronic renal failure tend to have decreased clearance.

Dosing adjustment in hepatic impairment: Specific recommendations unavailable; clearance may be reduced in severe dysfunction

Mechanism of Action Somatropin and somatrem are purified polypeptide hormones of recombinant DNA origin; somatropin contains the identical sequence of amino acids found in human growth hormone while somatrem's amino acid sequence is identical plus an additional amino acid, methionine; human growth hormone stimulates growth of linear bone, skeletal muscle, and organs; stimulates erythropoietin which increases red blood cell mass; exerts both insulin-like and diabetogenic effects

Other Adverse Effects

Growth hormone deficiency: Antigrowth hormone antibodies, carpal tunnel syndrome (rare), fluid balance disturbances, glucosuria, gynocomastia (rare), headache, hematuria, hyperglycemia (mild), hypoglycemia, hypothyroidism, leukemia, lipoatrophy, muscle pain, increased growth of pre-existing nevi (rare), pain/ local reactions at the injection site, pancreatitis (rare), peripheral edema, exacerbation of psoriasis, seizures

Prader-Willi syndrome: Aggressiveness, arthralgia, edema, hair loss, headache, benign intracranial hypertension, myalgia

Turner syndrome: Humatrope®: Surgical procedures (45%), otitis media (43%), ear disorders (18%), hypothyroidism (13%), increased nevi (11%), peripheral edema (7%)

Adult growth hormone replacement: Increased ALT, increased AST, arthralgia, back pain, carpal tunnel syndrome, diabetes mellitus, fatigue, flu-like syndrome, generalized edema, gastritis, gynocomastia (rare), headache, hypoesthesia, joint disorder, myalgia, increased growth of pre-existing nevi, pain, pancreatitis (rare), paresthesia, peripheral edema, pharyngitis, rhinitis, stiffness in extremities, weakness

AIDS wasting or cachexia (limited): Serostim®: Musculoskeletal discomfort (54%), increased tissue turgor (27%), diarrhea (26%), neuropathy (26%), nausea (26%), fatigue (17%), albuminuria (15%), increased diaphoresis (14%), anorexia (12%), anemia (12%), increased AST (12%), insomnia (11%), tachycardia (11%), hyperglycemia (10%), increased ALT (10%)

Postmarketing and/or case reports: Diabetes, diabetic ketoacidosis, glucose intolerance

Small for gestational age: Mild, transient hyperglycemia; benign intracranial hypertension (rare); central precocious puberty; jaw prominence (rare); aggravation of pre-existing scoliosis (rare); injection site reactions; progression of pigmented nevi

Drug Interactions

Increased Effect/Toxicity: Limited data suggest somatropin may increase clearance of medications metabolized via CYP2B6, 2C, and 3A3/4.

Decreased Effect: Glucocorticoid therapy may inhibit growth-promoting effects. Growth hormone may induce insulin resistance in patients with diabetes mellitus; monitor glucose and adjust insulin dose as necessary.

Pharmacodynamics/Kinetics Somatrem and somatropin have equivalent pharmacokinetic properties

Duration: Maintains supraphysiologic levels for 18-20 hours
Absorption: I.M., S.C.: Well absorbed
Metabolism: Hepatic and renal (~90%)
Half-life elimination: Preparation and route of administration dependent
Excretion: Urine

Pregnancy Risk Factor B/C (depending upon manufacturer)

Generic Available No

Humanized IgG1 Anti-CD52 Monoclonal Antibody *see* Alemtuzumab *on page 52*

Human LFA-3/IgG(1) Fusion Protein *see* Alefacept *on page 52*

Human Thyroid Stimulating Hormone *see* Thyrotropin Alpha *on page 1304*

Humate-P® *see* Antihemophilic Factor (Human) *on page 113*

Humatin® *see* Paromomycin *on page 1035*

Humatrope® *see* Human Growth Hormone *on page 671*

Humibid® DM *see* Guaifenesin and Dextromethorphan *on page 651*

Humibid® L.A. *see* Guaifenesin *on page 650*

Humibid® Pediatric *see* Guaifenesin *on page 650*

Humulin® 50/50 *see* Insulin Preparations *on page 723*

Humulin® 70/30 *see* Insulin Preparations *on page 723*

Humulin® L *see* Insulin Preparations *on page 723*

Humulin® N *see* Insulin Preparations *on page 723*

Humulin® R *see* Insulin Preparations *on page 723*

Humulin® R (Concentrated) U-500 *see* Insulin Preparations *on page 723*

Humulin® U *see* Insulin Preparations *on page 723*

Hurricaine® *see* Benzocaine *on page 169*

HXM *see* Altretamine *on page 66*

Hyalgan® *see* Sodium Hyaluronate *on page 1230*

Hyaluronic Acid *see* Sodium Hyaluronate *on page 1230*

Hyate:C® *see* Antihemophilic Factor (Porcine) *on page 114*

Hycamptamine *see* Topotecan *on page 1325*

Hycamtin® *see* Topotecan *on page 1325*

Hycodan® *see* Hydrocodone and Homatropine *on page 684*

Hycomine® Compound *see* Hydrocodone, Chlorpheniramine, Phenylephrine, Acetaminophen, and Caffeine *on page 686*

Hycosin *see* Hydrocodone and Guaifenesin *on page 683*

Hycotuss® *see* Hydrocodone and Guaifenesin *on page 683*

HydrALAZINE (hye DRAL a zeen)

Related Information

Cardiovascular Diseases *on page 1456*

Canadian Brand Names Apo®-Hydralazine; Apresoline®; Novo-Hylazin; Nu-Hydral

Mexican Brand Names Apresolina

(Continued)

HydrALAZINE *(Continued)*

Pharmacologic Category Vasodilator

Synonyms Hydralazine Hydrochloride

Use Management of moderate to severe hypertension, CHF, hypertension secondary to pre-eclampsia/eclampsia; treatment of primary pulmonary hypertension

Local Anesthetic/Vasoconstrictor Precautions No information available to require special precautions

Effects on Dental Treatment No significant effects or complications reported

Dosage

Children:

Oral: Initial: 0.75-1 mg/kg/day in 2-4 divided doses; increase over 3-4 weeks to maximum of 7.5 mg/kg/day in 2-4 divided doses; maximum daily dose: 200 mg/day

I.M., I.V.: 0.1-0.2 mg/kg/dose (not to exceed 20 mg) every 4-6 hours as needed, up to 1.7-3.5 mg/kg/day in 4-6 divided doses

Adults:

Oral:

Hypertension:

Initial dose: 10 mg 4 times/day for first 2-4 days; increase to 25 mg 4 times/day for the balance of the first week

Increase by 10-25 mg/dose gradually to 50 mg 4 times/day; 300 mg/day may be required for some patients

Congestive heart failure:

Initial dose: 10-25 mg 3-4 times/day

Adjustment: Dosage must be adjusted based on individual response

Target dose: 75 mg 4 times/day in combination with isosorbide dinitrate (40 mg 4 times/day)

Range: Typically 200-600 mg daily in 2-4 divided doses; dosages as high as 3 g/day have been used in some patients for symptomatic and hemodynamic improvement. Hydralazine 75 mg 4 times/day combined with isosorbide dinitrate 40 mg 4 times/day were shown in clinical trials to provide a mortality benefit in the treatment of CHF. Higher doses may be used for symptomatic and hemodynamic improvement following optimization of standard therapy.

I.M., I.V.:

Hypertension: Initial: 10-20 mg/dose every 4-6 hours as needed, may increase to 40 mg/dose; change to oral therapy as soon as possible.

Pre-eclampsia/eclampsia: 5 mg/dose then 5-10 mg every 20-30 minutes as needed.

Elderly: Oral: Initial: 10 mg 2-3 times/day; increase by 10-25 mg/day every 2-5 days.

Dosing interval in renal impairment:

Cl_{cr} 10-50 mL/minute: Administer every 8 hours.

Cl_{cr} <10 mL/minute: Administer every 8-16 hours in fast acetylators and every 12-24 hours in slow acetylators.

Hemodialysis: Supplemental dose is unnecessary.

Peritoneal dialysis: Supplemental dose is unnecessary.

Mechanism of Action Direct vasodilation of arterioles (with little effect on veins) with decreased systemic resistance

Other Adverse Effects Frequency not defined:

Cardiovascular: Tachycardia, angina pectoris, orthostatic hypotension (rare), dizziness (rare), paradoxical hypertension, peripheral edema, vascular collapse (rare), flushing

Central nervous system: Increased intracranial pressure (I.V., in patient with pre-existing increased intracranial pressure), fever (rare), chills (rare), anxiety*, disorientation*, depression*, coma*

Dermatologic: Rash (rare), urticaria (rash), pruritus (rash)

Gastrointestinal: Anorexia, nausea, vomiting, diarrhea, constipation, adynamic ileus

Genitourinary: Difficulty in micturition, impotence

Hematologic: Hemolytic anemia (rare), eosinophilia (rare), decreased hemoglobin concentration (rare), reduced erythrocyte count (rare), leukopenia (rare), agranulocytosis (rare), thrombocytopenia (rare)

Neuromuscular & skeletal: Rheumatoid arthritis, muscle cramps, weakness, tremors, peripheral neuritis (rare)

Ocular: Lacrimation, conjunctivitis

Respiratory: Nasal congestion, dyspnea

Miscellaneous: Drug-induced lupus-like syndrome (dose-related; fever, arthralgia, splenomegaly, lymphadenopathy, asthenia, myalgia, malaise, pleuritic chest pain, edema, positive ANA, positive LE cells, maculopapular facial rash, positive direct Coombs' test, pericarditis, pericardial tamponade), diaphoresis

*Seen in uremic patients and severe hypertension where rapidly escalating doses may have caused hypotension leading to these effects.

Drug Interactions Inhibits CYP3A4

Increased Effect/Toxicity: Hydralazine may increase levels of beta-blockers (metoprolol, propranolol). Some beta-blockers (acebutolol, atenolol, and nadolol) are unlikely to be affected due to limited hepatic metabolism. Concurrent use of hydralazine with MAO inhibitors may cause a significant decrease in blood pressure. Propranolol may increase hydralazine serum concentrations.

Decreased Effect: NSAIDs (eg, indomethacin) may decrease the hemodynamic effects of hydralazine.

Dietary/Ethanol/Herb Considerations

Ethanol: Avoid use; may increase CNS depression.

Food enhances bioavailability. Avoid caffeine (eg, colas, chocolate), garlic, and licorice.

Herb/Nutraceutical: Avoid black cohosh, dong quai, and evening primrose due to estrogenic activity. Avoid ephedra, ginseng, and yohimbe; may worsen hypertension. Avoid garlic; may have increased antihypertensive effect. Avoid ginger due to positive inotropic effects; theoretically, may cause arrhythmia. Avoid gotu kola, kava, SAMe, St John's wort, and valerian; may increase CNS depression. Avoid hawthorn; may lower peripheral vascular resistance resulting in additive decrease in BP. Avoid licorice.

Pharmacodynamics/Kinetics

Onset of action: Oral: 20-30 minutes; I.V.: 5-20 minutes

Duration: Oral: 2-4 hours; I.V.: 2-6 hours

Distribution: Crosses placenta; enters breast milk

Protein binding: 85% to 90%

Metabolism: Hepatically acetylated; extensive first-pass effect (oral)

Bioavailability: 30% to 50%; increased with food

Half-life elimination: Normal renal function: 2-8 hours; End-stage renal disease: 7-16 hours

Excretion: Urine (14% as unchanged drug)

Pregnancy Risk Factor C

Generic Available Yes

Hydralazine and Hydrochlorothiazide

(hye DRAL a zeen & hye droe klore oh THYE a zide)

Related Information

HydrALAZINE *on page 673*

Hydrochlorothiazide *on page 675*

Pharmacologic Category Antihypertensive Agent Combination

Synonyms Apresazide® [DSC]; Hydrochlorothiazide and Hydralazine

Use Management of moderate to severe hypertension and treatment of CHF

Local Anesthetic/Vasoconstrictor Precautions No information available to require special precautions

Effects on Dental Treatment No significant effects or complications reported

Dosage Adults: Oral: Take as directed; not to exceed 50 mg hydrochlorothiazide per day

Pregnancy Risk Factor C

Generic Available Yes

Hydralazine Hydrochloride *see* HydrALAZINE *on page 673*

Hydralazine, Hydrochlorothiazide, and Reserpine

(hye DRAL a zeen, hye droe klore oh THYE a zide, & re ZER peen)

Related Information

HydrALAZINE *on page 673*

Hydrochlorothiazide *on page 675*

Pharmacologic Category Antihypertensive Agent Combination

Synonyms Hydrochlorothiazide, Hydralazine, and Reserpine; Reserpine, Hydralazine, and Hydrochlorothiazide

Use Treatment of hypertensive disorders

Local Anesthetic/Vasoconstrictor Precautions No information available to require special precautions

Effects on Dental Treatment No significant effects or complications reported

Dosage Adults: Oral: 1-2 tablets 3 times/day

Pregnancy Risk Factor C

Generic Available Yes

Hydramine® [OTC] *see* DiphenhydrAMINE *on page 451*

Hydramine® Cough [OTC] *see* DiphenhydrAMINE *on page 451*

Hydrate® [DSC] *see* DimenhyDRINATE *on page 449*

Hydrated Chloral *see* Chloral Hydrate *on page 295*

Hydrea® *see* Hydroxyurea *on page 696*

Hydrisalic™ [OTC] *see* Salicylic Acid *on page 1204*

Hydrocet® *see* Hydrocodone and Acetaminophen *on page 678*

Hydrochlorothiazide (hye droe klore oh THYE a zide)

Related Information

Cardiovascular Diseases *on page 1456*

Moexipril and Hydrochlorothiazide *on page 927*

(Continued)

Hydrochlorothiazide *(Continued)*

U.S. Brand Names Aquazide® H; Microzide™; Oretic®

Canadian Brand Names Apo®-Hydro; Novo-Hydrazide

Mexican Brand Names Diclotride®

Pharmacologic Category Diuretic, Thiazide

Synonyms HCTZ

Use Management of mild to moderate hypertension; treatment of edema in CHF and nephrotic syndrome

Unlabeled/Investigational Use Treatment of lithium-induced diabetes insipidus

Local Anesthetic/Vasoconstrictor Precautions No information available to require special precautions

Effects on Dental Treatment 1% to 10%: Orthostatic hypotension, hypotension

Dosage Effect of drug may be decreased when used every day.

Oral:

Children (in pediatric patients, chlorothiazide may be preferred over hydrochlorothiazide as there are more dosage formulations [eg, suspension] available):

<6 months: 2-3 mg/kg/day in 2 divided doses

>6 months: 2 mg/kg/day in 2 divided doses

Adults:

Edema: 25-100 mg/day in 1-2 doses; maximum: 200 mg/day

Hypertension: 25-50 mg/day; minimal increase in response and more electrolyte disturbances are seen with doses >50 mg/day

Elderly: 12.5-25 mg once daily

Dosing comment in renal impairment: Cl_{cr} 25-50 mL/minute: Not effective

Mechanism of Action Inhibits sodium reabsorption in the distal tubules causing increased excretion of sodium and water as well as potassium and hydrogen ions

Other Adverse Effects

1% to 10%:

Dermatologic: Photosensitivity

Endocrine & metabolic: Hypokalemia

Gastrointestinal: Anorexia, epigastric distress

<1% (Limited to important or life-threatening): Agranulocytosis, allergic myocarditis, allergic reactions (possibly with life-threatening anaphylactic shock), alopecia, aplastic anemia, eosinophilic pneumonitis, erythema multiforme, exfoliative dermatitis, hemolytic anemia, hepatic function impairment, hypercalcemia, interstitial nephritis, leukopenia, pancreatitis, renal failure, **respiratory distress**, Stevens-Johnson syndrome, thrombocytopenia, toxic epidermal necrolysis

Drug Interactions

Increased Effect/Toxicity: Increased effect of hydrochlorothiazide with furosemide and other loop diuretics. Increased hypotension and/or renal adverse effects of ACE inhibitors may result in aggressively diuresed patients. Beta-blockers increase hyperglycemic effects of thiazides in type 2 diabetes mellitus. Cyclosporine and thiazides can increase the risk of gout or renal toxicity. Digoxin toxicity can be exacerbated if a thiazide induces hypokalemia or hypomagnesemia. Lithium toxicity can occur with thiazides due to reduced renal excretion of lithium. Thiazides may prolong the duration of action with neuromuscular blocking agents.

Decreased Effect: Effects of oral hypoglycemics may be decreased. Decreased absorption of hydrochlorothiazide with cholestyramine and colestipol. NSAIDs can decrease the efficacy of thiazides, reducing the diuretic and antihypertensive effects.

Dietary/Ethanol/Herb Considerations

Food: Administer with first meal early in the day; food may decrease peak serum concentration. Increase intake of potassium-rich foods (eg, bananas and citrus fruit); may require a potassium supplement or medication to prevent potassium loss; may also deplete sodium and magnesium. Avoid caffeine (eg, colas, chocolate), garlic, and licorice.

Herb/Nutraceutical: Avoid black cohosh, dong quai, and evening primrose due to estrogenic activity; dong quai may also cause photosensitization. Avoid ephedra, ginseng, and yohimbe; may worsen hypertension. Avoid garlic; may have increased antihypertensive effect. Avoid ginger due to positive inotropic effects; theoretically, may cause arrhythmia. Avoid hawthorn; may lower peripheral vascular resistance causing additional decrease in BP. Avoid licorice.

Pharmacodynamics/Kinetics

Onset of action: Diuresis: ~2 hours

Peak effect: 4-6 hours

Duration: 6-12 hours

Absorption: ~50% to 80%

Distribution: 3.6-7.8 L/kg

Protein binding: 68%

Metabolism: Not metabolized

Bioavailability: 50% to 80%

Half-life elimination: 5.6-14.8 hours

Time to peak: 1-2.5 hours

Excretion: Urine (as unchanged drug)

Pregnancy Risk Factor B (manufacturer); D (expert analysis)

Generic Available Yes

Hydrochlorothiazide and Amiloride *see* Amiloride and Hydrochlorothiazide *on page 76*

Hydrochlorothiazide and Benazepril *see* Benazepril and Hydrochlorothiazide *on page 167*

Hydrochlorothiazide and Bisoprolol *see* Bisoprolol and Hydrochlorothiazide *on page 189*

Hydrochlorothiazide and Captopril *see* Captopril and Hydrochlorothiazide *on page 240*

Hydrochlorothiazide and Enalapril *see* Enalapril and Hydrochlorothiazide *on page 494*

Hydrochlorothiazide and Fosinopril *see* Fosinopril and Hydrochlorothiazide *on page 617*

Hydrochlorothiazide and Hydralazine *see* Hydralazine and Hydrochlorothiazide *on page 675*

Hydrochlorothiazide and Irbesartan *see* Irbesartan and Hydrochlorothiazide *on page 740*

Hydrochlorothiazide and Lisinopril *see* Lisinopril and Hydrochlorothiazide *on page 814*

Hydrochlorothiazide and Losartan *see* Losartan and Hydrochlorothiazide *on page 827*

Hydrochlorothiazide and Methyldopa *see* Methyldopa and Hydrochlorothiazide *on page 892*

Hydrochlorothiazide and Moexipril *see* Moexipril and Hydrochlorothiazide *on page 927*

Hydrochlorothiazide and Propranolol *see* Propranolol and Hydrochlorothiazide *on page 1142*

Hydrochlorothiazide and Quinapril *see* Quinapril and Hydrochlorothiazide *on page 1158*

Hydrochlorothiazide and Spironolactone

(hye droe klore oh THYE a zide & speer on oh LAK tone)

Related Information

Cardiovascular Diseases *on page 1456*

Hydrochlorothiazide *on page 675*

U.S. Brand Names Aldactazide®

Canadian Brand Names Aldactazide 25®; Aldactazide 50®; Novo-Spirozine

Pharmacologic Category Antihypertensive Agent Combination

Synonyms Spironolactone and Hydrochlorothiazide

Use Management of mild to moderate hypertension; treatment of edema in CHF and nephrotic syndrome, and cirrhosis of the liver accompanied by edema and/or ascites

Local Anesthetic/Vasoconstrictor Precautions No information available to require special precautions

Effects on Dental Treatment No significant effects or complications reported

Dosage Oral:

Children: 1.66-3.3 mg/kg/day (of spironolactone) in 2-4 divided doses

Adults:

Hydrochlorothiazide 25 mg and spironolactone 25 mg: ½-8 tablets daily

Hydrochlorothiazide 50 mg and spironolactone 50 mg: ½-4 tablets daily in 1-2 doses

Dietary/Ethanol/Herb Considerations

Food: Avoid food with high potassium content and potassium-containing salt substitutes.

Herb/Nutraceutical: Avoid licorice; causes sodium and water retention and increases potassium loss.

Pregnancy Risk Factor C

Generic Available Yes

Hydrochlorothiazide and Telmisartan *see* Telmisartan and Hydrochlorothiazide *on page 1270*

Hydrochlorothiazide and Triamterene

(hye droe klore oh THYE a zide & trye AM ter een)

Related Information

Cardiovascular Diseases *on page 1456*

Hydrochlorothiazide *on page 675*

U.S. Brand Names Dyazide®; Maxzide®; Maxzide®-25

Canadian Brand Names Apo®-Triazide; Novo-Triamzide; Nu-Triazide; Penta-Triamterene HCTZ; Riva-Zide

Pharmacologic Category Antihypertensive Agent Combination; Diuretic, Potassium Sparing; Diuretic, Thiazide

Synonyms Triamterene and Hydrochlorothiazide

(Continued)

Hydrochlorothiazide and Triamterene *(Continued)*

Use Management of mild to moderate hypertension; treatment of edema in CHF and nephrotic syndrome

Local Anesthetic/Vasoconstrictor Precautions No information available to require special precautions

Effects on Dental Treatment No significant effects or complications reported

Dosage Adults: Oral:

Hydrochlorothiazide 25 mg and triamterene 37.5 mg: 1-2 tablets/capsules once daily

Hydrochlorothiazide 50 mg and triamterene 75 mg: 1/2-1 tablet daily

Mechanism of Action

Based on **triamterene** component: Competes with aldosterone for receptor sites in the distal renal tubules, increasing sodium, chloride, and water excretion while conserving potassium and hydrogen ions; may block the effect of aldosterone on arteriolar smooth muscle as well

Based on **hydrochlorothiazide** component: Inhibits sodium reabsorption in the distal tubules causing increased excretion of sodium and water as well as potassium and hydrogen ions

Other Adverse Effects Frequency not defined:

Central nervous system: Dizziness, fatigue

Dermatologic: Purpura, **cracked corners of mouth**

Endocrine & metabolic: Electrolyte disturbances

Gastrointestinal: **Bright orange tongue, burning of tongue**, loss of appetite, nausea, vomiting, stomach cramps, diarrhea, upset stomach

Hematologic: Aplastic anemia, agranulocytosis, hemolytic anemia, leukopenia, thrombocytopenia, megaloblastic anemia

Neuromuscular & skeletal: Muscle cramps

Ocular: Xanthopsia, transient blurred vision

Respiratory: Allergic pneumonitis, pulmonary edema, **respiratory distress**

Dietary/Ethanol/Herb Considerations Food may decrease peak serum concentration. Avoid food with high potassium content and potassium-containing salt substitutes.

Pregnancy Risk Factor C (per manufacturer)

Generic Available Yes

Hydrochlorothiazide and Valsartan *see* Valsartan and Hydrochlorothiazide *on page 1375*

Hydrochlorothiazide, Hydralazine, and Reserpine *see* Hydralazine, Hydrochlorothiazide, and Reserpine *on page 675*

Hydrocil® [OTC] *see* Psyllium *on page 1149*

Hydrocodone and Acetaminophen

(hye droe KOE done & a seet a MIN oh fen)

Related Information

Acetaminophen *on page 27*

Oral Pain *on page 1524*

U.S. Brand Names Anexsia®; Bancap HC®; Ceta-Plus®; Co-Gesic®; Hydrocet®; Hydrogesic® [DSC]; Lorcet® 10/650; Lorcet®-HD; Lorcet® Plus; Lortab®; Margesic® H; Maxidone™; Norco®; Stagesic®; Vicodin®; Vicodin® ES; Vicodin® HP; Zydone®

Pharmacologic Category Analgesic Combination (Narcotic)

Synonyms Acetaminophen and Hydrocodone; Hydrogesic® [DSC]

Use

Dental: Treatment of postoperative pain; relief of moderate to moderately severe pain

Medical: Relief of moderate to severe pain; antitussive (hydrocodone)

Local Anesthetic/Vasoconstrictor Precautions No information available to require special precautions

Effects on Dental Treatment Frequency not defined: Hypotension, bradycardia, lightheadedness, dizziness, sedation, drowsiness, fatigue, confusion, nausea, vomiting, weakness, dyspnea

Restrictions C-III

Dosage Doses should be titrated to appropriate analgesic effect. For children ≥12 years of age and adults, the dosage of acetaminophen should be limited to ≤4 g/day (and possibly less in patients with hepatic impairment or ethanol use).

Oral:

Children:

Analgesic (acetaminophen): Refer to Acetaminophen monograph

Antitussive (hydrocodone): 0.6 mg/kg/day in 3-4 divided doses; even though dosing by hydrocodone, make sure to keep within age-specific acetaminophen doses as well

A single dose should not exceed 10 mg in children >12 years, 5 mg in children 2-12 years, and 1.25 mg in children <2 years of age

Adults: **Analgesic:** 1-2 tablets or capsules every 4-6 hours or 5-10 mL solution every 4-6 hours as needed for pain; do not exceed 4 g/day of acetaminophen

Hydrocodone 2.5-5 mg and acetaminophen 400-500 mg; maximum: 8 tablets/capsules per day

Hydrocodone 7.5 mg and acetaminophen: 400-650 mg; maximum: 6 tablets/capsules per day

Hydrocodone 2.5 mg and acetaminophen: 167 mg/5 mL (elixir/solution); maximum: 6 tablespoonfuls/day

Hydrocodone 7.5 mg and acetaminophen 750 mg; maximum: 5 tablets/capsules per day

Hydrocodone 10 mg and acetaminophen: 350-660 mg; maximum: 6 tablets/day per product labeling

Mechanism of Action Hydrocodone, as with other narcotic (opiate) analgesics, blocks pain perception in the cerebral cortex by binding to specific receptor molecules (opiate receptors) within the neuronal membranes of synapses. This binding results in a decreased synaptic chemical transmission throughout the CNS thus inhibiting the flow of pain sensations into the higher centers. Mu and kappa are the two subtypes of the opiate receptor which hydrocodone binds to cause analgesia.

Acetaminophen inhibits the synthesis of prostaglandins in the CNS and peripherally blocks pain impulse generation; produces antipyresis from inhibition of hypothalamic heat-regulating center.

Other Adverse Effects

Frequency not defined: Genitourinary: Decreased urination

<1%: **Hypertension, hallucinations**, anorexia, **biliary tract spasm**, urinary tract spasm, diplopia, miosis, **histamine release, physical and psychological dependence (prolonged use), xerostomia**

Contraindications Hypersensitivity to hydrocodone, acetaminophen, or any component of the formulation; CNS depression; severe respiratory depression

Warnings/Precautions Use with caution in patients with hypersensitivity reactions to other phenanthrene derivative opioid agonists (morphine, hydrocodone, hydromorphone, levorphanol, oxycodone, oxymorphone); tablets contain metabisulfite which may cause allergic reactions; tolerance or drug dependence may result from extended use

Drug Interactions

Hydrocodone: Substrate of **CYP2D6**

Acetaminophen: Substrate of CYP1A2, 2A6, 2C8/9, 2D6, 2E1, 3A4

Decreased effect with phenothiazines

Increased effect with dextroamphetamine

Increased toxicity with CNS depressants, TCAs; effect of warfarin may be enhanced by acetaminophen

Dietary/Ethanol/Herb Considerations

Ethanol: Avoid use or limit to <3 drinks/day; may increase acetaminophen toxicity and cause CNS depression.

Food: Rate of absorption of acetaminophen may be decreased when administered with food high in carbohydrates.

Herb/Nutraceutical: Avoid kava, SAMe, St John's wort, and valerian; may increase risk of excessive sedation.

Pharmacodynamics/Kinetics

Acetaminophen: See Acetaminophen monograph.

Hydrocodone:

Onset of action: Narcotic analgesic: 10-20 minutes

Duration: 4-8 hours

Distribution: Crosses placenta

Metabolism: Hepatic; O-demethylation; N-demethylation and 6-ketosteroid reduction

Half-life elimination: 3.3-4.4 hours

Excretion: Urine

Pregnancy Risk Factor C

Breast-feeding Considerations

Hydrocodone: No data reported.

Acetaminophen: May be taken while breast-feeding.

Dosage Forms CAP (Bancap HC®, Ceta-Plus®, Hydrocet®, Hydrogesic®, Lorcet®-HD, Margesic® H, Stagesic®): Hydrocodone 5 mg and acetaminophen 500 mg. **ELIX** (Lortab®): Hydrocodone 2.5 mg and acetaminophen 167 mg per 5 mL (480 mL). **TAB:** Hydrocodone 2.5 mg and acetaminophen 500 mg; hydrocodone 5 mg and acetaminophen 500 mg; hydrocodone 7.5 mg and acetaminophen 500 mg; hydrocodone 7.5 mg and acetaminophen 650 mg; hydrocodone 7.5 mg and acetaminophen 750 mg; hydrocodone 10 mg and acetaminophen 325 mg; hydrocodone 10 mg and acetaminophen 500 mg; hydrocodone 10 mg and acetaminophen 650 mg; (Anexsia®): 5/325: Hydrocodone 5 mg and acetaminophen 325 mg; 5/500: Hydrocodone 5 mg and acetaminophen 500 mg; 7.5/325: Hydrocodone 7.5 mg and acetaminophen 325 mg; 7.5/650: Hydrocodone 7.5 mg and acetaminophen 650 mg; 10/660: Hydrocodone 10 mg and acetaminophen 660 mg; (Co-Gesic® 5/500): Hydrocodone 5 mg and acetaminophen 500 mg; (Lorcet® 10/650): Hydrocodone 10 mg and acetaminophen 650 mg; (Lorcet® Plus): Hydrocodone 7.5 mg and acetaminophen 650 mg; (Lortab®): 2.5/500: Hydrocodone 2.5 mg and acetaminophen

(Continued)

Hydrocodone and Acetaminophen *(Continued)*

500 mg; 5/500: Hydrocodone 5 mg and acetaminophen 500 mg; 7.5/500: Hydrocodone 7.5 mg and acetaminophen 500 mg; 10/500: Hydrocodone 10 mg and acetaminophen 500 mg; (Maxidone™): Hydrocodone 10 mg and acetaminophen 750 mg; (Norco®): Hydrocodone 5 mg and acetaminophen 325 mg; Hydrocodone 7.5 mg and acetaminophen 325 mg; Hydrocodone 10 mg and acetaminophen 325 mg; (Vicodin®): Hydrocodone 5 mg and acetaminophen 500 mg; (Vicodin® ES): Hydrocodone 7.5 mg and acetaminophen 750 mg; (Vicodin® HP): Hydrocodone 10 mg and acetaminophen 660 mg; (Zydone®): Hydrocodone 5 mg and acetaminophen 400 mg; Hydrocodone 7.5 mg and acetaminophen 400 mg; Hydrocodone 10 mg and acetaminophen 400 mg

Generic Available Yes

Comments Neither hydrocodone nor acetaminophen elicit anti-inflammatory effects. Because of addiction liability of opiate analgesics, the use of hydrocodone should be limited to 2-3 days postoperatively for treatment of dental pain. Nausea is the most common adverse effect seen after use in dental patients; sedation and constipation are second. Nausea elicited by narcotic analgesics is centrally mediated and the presence or absence of food will not affect the degree nor incidence of nausea.

Acetaminophen:

A study by Hylek, et al, suggested that the combination of acetaminophen with warfarin (Coumadin®) may cause enhanced anticoagulation. The following recommendations have been made by Hylek, et al, and supported by an editorial in *JAMA* by Bell.

Dose and duration of acetaminophen should be as low as possible, individualized and monitored

The study by Hylek reported the following:

For patients who reported taking the equivalent of at least 4 regular strength (325 mg) tablets for longer than a week, the odds of having an INR >6.0 were increased 10-fold above those not taking acetaminophen. Risk decreased with lower intakes of acetaminophen reaching a background level of risk at a dose of 6 or fewer 325 mg tablets per week.

Selected Readings

Bell WR, "Acetaminophen and Warfarin: Undesirable Synergy," *JAMA*, 1998, 279(9):702-3.

Botting RM, "Mechanism of Action of Acetaminophen: Is There a Cyclooxygenase 3?," *Clin Infect Dis*, 2000, Suppl 5:S202-10.

Dart RC, Kuffner EK, and Rumack BH, "Treatment of Pain or Fever with Paracetamol (Acetaminophen) in the Alcoholic Patient: A Systematic Review," *Am J Ther*, 2000, 7(2):123-34.

Dionne RA, "New Approaches to Preventing and Treating Postoperative Pain," *J Am Dent Assoc*, 1992, 123(6):26-34.

Gobetti JP, "Controlling Dental Pain," *J Am Dent Assoc*, 1992, 123(6):47-52.

Grant JA and Weiler JM, "A Report of a Rare Immediate Reaction After Ingestion of Acetaminophen," *Ann Allergy Asthma Immunol*, 2001, 87(3):227-9.

Hylek EM, Heiman H, Skates SJ, et al, "Acetaminophen and Other Risk factors for excessive warfarin anticoagulation, " *JAMA*, 1998, 279(9):657-62.

Kwan D, Bartle WR, and Walker SE, "The Effects of Acetaminophen on Pharmacokinetics and Pharmacodynamics of Warfarin," *J Clin Pharmacol*, 1999, 39(1):68-75.

McClain CJ, Price S, Barve S, et al, "Acetaminophen Hepatotoxicity: An Update," *Curr Gastroenterol Rep*, 1999, 1(1):42-9.

Shek KL, Chan LN, and Nutescu E, "Warfarin-Acetaminophen Drug Interaction Revisited," *Pharmacotherapy*, 1999, 19(10):1153-8.

Tanaka E, Yamazaki K, and Misawa S, "Update: The Clinical Importance of Acetaminophen Hepatotoxicity in Nonalcoholic and Alcoholic Subjects," *J Clin Pharm Ther*, 2000, 25(5):325-32.

Wynn RL, "Narcotic Analgesics for Dental Pain: Available Products, Strengths, and Formulations," *Gen Dent*, 2001, 49(2):126-8, 130, 132 passim.

Hydrocodone and Aspirin (hye droe KOE done & AS pir in)

Related Information

Aspirin *on page 131*

U.S. Brand Names Damason-P®

Pharmacologic Category Analgesic Combination (Narcotic)

Synonyms Aspirin and Hydrocodone

Use Dental and Medical: Relief of moderate to moderately severe pain

Local Anesthetic/Vasoconstrictor Precautions No information available to require special precautions

Effects on Dental Treatment Nausea is the most common adverse effect seen after use in dental patients. Sedation and constipation are second. Aspirin component affects bleeding times and could influence wound-healing time. Elderly are a high-risk population for adverse effects from NDSAIDs. As much as 60% of elderly patients with GI complications from NSAIDs can develop peptic ulceration and/or hemorrhage asymptomatically. Concomitant disease and drug use contribute to the risk of GI adverse effects.

>10%: Hypotension, lightheadedness, dizziness, sedation, drowsiness, fatigue, nausea, epigastric discomfort, weakness

1% to 10%: Bradycardia, confusion, vomiting, GI ulceration, dyspnea, anaphylactic shock

Restrictions C-III

Dosage Adults: **Oral:** 1-2 tablets every 4-6 hours as needed for pain

Mechanism of Action

Based on **hydrocodone** component: Binds to opiate receptors in the CNS, altering the perception of and response to pain; suppresses cough in medullary center; produces generalized CNS depression

Based on **aspirin** component: Inhibits prostaglandin synthesis, acts on the hypothalamus heat-regulating center to reduce fever, blocks prostaglandin synthetase action which prevents formation of the platelet-aggregating substance thromboxane A_2

Other Adverse Effects

>10%: Gastrointestinal: Heartburn, stomach pains, dyspepsia

1% to 10%:

Dermatologic: Rash

Genitourinary: Decreased urination

Hematologic: Hemolytic anemia

<1%: **Hypertension, hallucinations**, insomnia, **nervousness, jitters, anorexia, biliary tract spasm**, urinary tract spasm, occult bleeding, **prolongated bleeding time**, leukopenia, thrombocytopenia, iron-deficiency anemia, hepatotoxicity, diplopia, miosis, impaired renal function, **bronchospasm, histamine release, physical and psychological dependence (prolonged use), xerostomia**

Contraindications

Based on **hydrocodone** component: Hypersensitivity to hydrocodone or any component of the formulation

Based on **aspirin** component: Hypersensitivity to salicylates, other NSAIDs, or any component of the formulation; asthma; rhinitis; nasal polyps; inherited or acquired bleeding disorders (including factor VII and factor IX deficiency); pregnancy (in 3rd trimester especially); do not use in children (<16 years) for viral infections (chickenpox or flu symptoms), with or without fever, due to a potential association with Reye's syndrome

Warnings/Precautions Use with caution in patients with impaired renal function, erosive gastritis, or peptic ulcer disease. Children and teenagers should not use for chickenpox or flu symptoms before a physician is consulted about Reye's syndrome. Tolerance or drug dependence may result from extended use.

Based on **hydrocodone** component: Use with caution in patients with hypersensitivity reactions to other phenanthrene-derivative opioid agonists (morphine, codeine, hydromorphone, levorphanol, oxycodone, oxymorphone); should be used with caution in elderly or debilitated patients, and those with severe impairment of hepatic or renal function, prostatic hyperplasia, or urethral stricture. Also use caution in patients with head injury, increased intracranial pressure, acute abdomen, or impaired thyroid function. Hydrocodone suppresses the cough reflex; caution should be exercised when this agent is used postoperatively and in patients with pulmonary diseases (including asthma, emphysema, COPD)

Based on **aspirin** component: Use with caution in patients with platelet and bleeding disorders, renal dysfunction, dehydration, erosive gastritis, or peptic ulcer disease. Heavy ethanol use (>3 drinks/day) can increase bleeding risks. Avoid use in severe renal failure or in severe hepatic failure. Discontinue use if tinnitus or impaired hearing occurs. Caution in mild-moderate renal failure (only at high dosages). Patients with sensitivity to tartrazine dyes, nasal polyps and asthma may have an increased risk of salicylate sensitivity. Patients should avoid ASA if possible, for 1-2 weeks prior to dental or surgical procedures to reduce the risk of excessive bleeding.

Drug Interactions

Based on **hydrocodone** component: Substrate of **CYP2D6**

Increased Toxicity: CNS depressants, MAO inhibitors, general anesthetics, and tricyclic antidepressants may potentiate the effects of opiate agonists; dextroamphetamine may enhance the analgesic effect of opiate agonists

Based on **aspirin** component: Substrate of CYP2C8/9

ACE inhibitors: The effects of ACE inhibitors may be blunted by aspirin administration, particularly at higher dosages.

Buspirone increases aspirin's free % *in vitro.*

Carbonic anhydrase inhibitors and corticosteroids have been associated with alteration in salicylate serum concentrations.

Heparin and low molecular weight heparins: Concurrent use may increase the risk of bleeding

Methotrexate serum levels may be increased; consider discontinuing aspirin 2-3 days before high-dose methotrexate treatment or avoid concurrent use.

NSAIDs may increase the risk of gastrointestinal adverse effects and bleeding. Serum concentrations of some NSAIDs may be decreased by aspirin.

Platelet inhibitors (IIb/IIIa antagonists): Risk of bleeding may be increased.

Probenecid effects may be antagonized by aspirin.

Sulfonylureas: The effects of older sulfonylurea agents (tolazamide, tolbutamide) may be potentiated due to displacement from plasma proteins. This effect does not appear to be clinically significant for newer sulfonylurea agents (glyburide, glipizide, glimepiride).

Valproic acid may be displaced from its binding sites which can result in toxicity.

(Continued)

Hydrocodone and Aspirin *(Continued)*

Verapamil may potentiate the prolongation of bleeding time associated with aspirin.

Warfarin and oral anticoagulants may increase the risk of bleeding.

Dietary/Ethanol/Herb Considerations

Ethanol: Avoid use; may increase risk of bleeding, gastric mucosal irritation, and CNS depression; watch for sedation (based on hydrocodone component)

Food may decrease the rate but not the extent of oral absorption. Based on **aspirin** component, administer with food or milk to reduce GI upset. Avoid garlic, ginger, and green tea.

Herb/Nutraceutical: Avoid cat's claw, dong quai, evening primrose, feverfew, garlic, ginger, ginkgo biloba, ginseng, green tea, horse chestnut, and red clover due to additional antiplatelet activity. Avoid gotu kola, kava, SAMe, St John's wort, and valerian; may increase CNS depression.

Pharmacodynamics/Kinetics

Aspirin: See Aspirin monograph.

Hydrocodone:

Onset of action: Narcotic analgesic: 10-20 minutes

Duration: 4-8 hours

Distribution: Crosses placenta

Metabolism: Hepatic; O-demethylation; N-demethylation and 6-ketosteroid reduction

Half-life elimination: 3.3-4.4 hours

Excretion: Urine

Pregnancy Risk Factor D

Breast-feeding Considerations

Hydrocodone: No data reported.

Aspirin: Cautious use due to potential adverse effects in nursing infants.

Dosage Forms TAB: Hydrocodone 5 mg and aspirin 500 mg

Generic Available No

Comments Because of addiction liability of opiate analgesics, the use of hydrocodone should be limited to 2-3 days postoperatively for treatment of dental pain.

Selected Readings

Dionne RA, "New Approaches to Preventing and Treating Postoperative Pain," *J Am Dent Assoc*, 1992, 123(6):26-34.

Gobetti JP, "Controlling Dental Pain," *J Am Dent Assoc*, 1992, 123(6):47-52.

Wynn RL, "Narcotic Analgesics for Dental Pain: Available Products, Strengths, and Formulations," *Gen Dent*, 2001, 49(2):126-8, 130, 132 passim.

Hydrocodone and Chlorpheniramine

(hye droe KOE done & klor fen IR a meen)

Related Information

Chlorpheniramine *on page 307*

U.S. Brand Names Tussionex®

Pharmacologic Category Antihistamine/Antitussive

Synonyms Chlorpheniramine and Hydrocodone

Use Symptomatic relief of cough and allergy

Local Anesthetic/Vasoconstrictor Precautions No information available to require special precautions

Effects on Dental Treatment Prolonged use will cause significant xerostomia.

Restrictions C-III

Dosage Oral:

Children 6-12 years: 2.5 mL every 12 hours; do not exceed 5 mL/24 hours

Adults: 5 mL every 12 hours; do not exceed 10 mL/24 hours

Mechanism of Action

Based on **hydrocodone** component: Binds to opiate receptors in the CNS, altering the perception of and response to pain; suppresses cough in medullary center; produces generalized CNS depression

Based on **chlorpheniramine** component: Competes with histamine for H_1-receptor sites on effector cells in the gastrointestinal tract, blood vessels, and respiratory tract

Other Adverse Effects Frequency not defined (limited to important or life-threatening):

Central nervous system: Anxiety, drowsiness, sedation, lethargy

Dermatologic: Facial pruritus

Gastrointestinal: Constipation, nausea

Genitourinary: Ureteral spasms

Respiratory: **Respiratory depression, pharynx dryness**

Drug Interactions

Hydrocodone: Substrate of **CYP2D6**

Chlorpheniramine: Substrate of CYP2D6, **3A4**; Inhibits **CYP2D6**

Increased Toxicity:

Based on **hydrocodone** component: CNS depressants, MAO inhibitors, general anesthetics, and tricyclic antidepressants may potentiate the effects of opiate agonists; dextroamphetamine may enhance the analgesic effect of opiate agonists

Based on **chlorpheniramine** component: CYP2D6 enzyme substrate; CNS depressants, MAO inhibitors, tricyclic antidepressants, phenothiazines increase CNS depression.

Dietary/Ethanol/Herb Considerations Ethanol: Based on **hydrocodone** component, avoid or limit use; may increase CNS depression (watch for sedation).

Pharmacodynamics/Kinetics

Chlorpheniramine: See Chlorpheniramine monograph.

Hydrocodone:

Onset of action: Narcotic analgesic: 10-20 minutes

Duration: 4-8 hours

Distribution: Crosses placenta

Metabolism: Hepatic; O-demethylation; N-demethylation and 6-ketosteroid reduction

Half-life elimination: 3.3-4.4 hours

Excretion: Urine

Pregnancy Risk Factor C

Generic Available No

Hydrocodone and Guaifenesin

(hye droe KOE done & gwe FEN e sin)

Related Information

Guaifenesin *on page 650*

U.S. Brand Names Codiclear® DH; Hycosin; Hycotuss®; Kwelcof®; Pneumotussin®; Vicodin Tuss®; Vitussin

Pharmacologic Category Antitussive/Expectorant

Synonyms Guaifenesin and Hydrocodone

Use Symptomatic relief of nonproductive coughs associated with upper and lower respiratory tract congestion

Local Anesthetic/Vasoconstrictor Precautions No information available to require special precautions

Effects on Dental Treatment No significant effects or complications reported

Restrictions C-III

Dosage Oral:

Children:

<2 years: 0.3 mg/kg/day (hydrocodone) in 4 divided doses

2-12 years: 2.5 mL every 4 hours, after meals and at bedtime

>12 years: 5 mL every 4 hours, after meals and at bedtime

Adults: 5 mL every 4 hours, after meals and at bedtime, not >30 mL in a 24-hour period

Mechanism of Action

Based on **hydrocodone** component: Binds to opiate receptors in the CNS, altering the perception of and response to pain; suppresses cough in medullary center; produces generalized CNS depression

Based on **guaifenesin** component: Thought to act as an expectorant by irritating the gastric mucosa and stimulating respiratory tract secretions, thereby increasing respiratory fluid volumes and decreasing phlegm viscosity

Other Adverse Effects Frequency not defined:

Cardiovascular: **Hypertension, postural hypotension, palpitations**

Central nervous system: Drowsiness, sedation, mental clouding, mental and physical impairment, anxiety, fear, dysphoria, dizziness, psychotic dependence, mood changes

Gastrointestinal: Nausea, vomiting, constipation (with prolonged use)

Genitourinary: Ureteral spasm, urinary retention

Ocular: Blurred vision

Respiratory: **Respiratory depression (dose-related)**

Drug Interactions Hydrocodone: Substrate of **CYP2D6**

Increased Effect/Toxicity:

Based on **hydrocodone** component: CNS depressants, MAO inhibitors, general anesthetics, and tricyclic antidepressants may potentiate the effects of opiate agonists. Dextroamphetamine may enhance the analgesic effect of opiate agonists.

Based on **guaifenesin** component: Disulfiram, MAO inhibitors, metronidazole, procarbazine

Dietary/Ethanol/Herb Considerations

Ethanol: Avoid or limit use; may increase CNS depression.

Herb/Nutraceutical: Avoid gotu kola, kava, SAMe, St John's wort, and valerian; may increase CNS depression.

Pharmacodynamics/Kinetics

Guaifenesin: See Guaifenesin monograph.

Hydrocodone:

Onset of action: Narcotic analgesic: 10-20 minutes

Duration: 4-8 hours

Distribution: Crosses placenta

(Continued)

Hydrocodone and Guaifenesin *(Continued)*

Metabolism: Hepatic; O-demethylation; N-demethylation and 6-ketosteroid reduction
Half-life elimination: 3.3-4.4 hours
Excretion: Urine

Pregnancy Risk Factor C
Generic Available Yes: Liquid

Hydrocodone and Homatropine

(hye droe KOE done & hoe MA troe peen)

Related Information
Homatropine *on page 670*

U.S. Brand Names Hycodan®; Hydromet®; Hydropane®; Tussigon®
Pharmacologic Category Antitussive
Synonyms Homatropine and Hydrocodone
Use Symptomatic relief of cough
Local Anesthetic/Vasoconstrictor Precautions No information available to require special precautions
Effects on Dental Treatment Xerostomia
Restrictions C-III
Dosage Oral (based on hydrocodone component):
Children: 0.6 mg/kg/day in 3-4 divided doses; do not administer more frequently than every 4 hours
A single dose should not exceed 1.25 mg in children <2 years of age, 5 mg in children 2-12 years, and 10 mg in children >12 years
Adults: 10 mg every 4-6 hours, a single dose should not exceed 15 mg; do not administer more frequently than every 4 hours

Mechanism of Action
Based on **hydrocodone** component: Binds to opiate receptors in the CNS, altering the perception of and response to pain; suppresses cough in medullary center; produces generalized CNS depression
Based on **homatropine** component: Blocks response of iris sphincter muscle and the accommodative muscle of the ciliary body to cholinergic stimulation resulting in dilation and loss of accommodation

Other Adverse Effects Frequency not defined:
Cardiovascular: **Bradycardia, tachycardia, hypotension, hypertension**
Central nervous system: Lightheadedness, dizziness, sedation, drowsiness, fatigue, confusion, hallucinations
Gastrointestinal: Nausea, vomiting, anorexia, impaired GI motility
Genitourinary: Decreased urination, urinary tract spasm
Hepatic: Biliary tract spasm
Neuromuscular & skeletal: Weakness
Ocular: Diplopia, miosis, mydriasis, blurred vision
Respiratory: Dyspnea
Miscellaneous: Histamine release, physical and psychological dependence (with prolonged use)

Drug Interactions Hydrocodone: Substrate of **CYP2D6**
Increased Toxicity:
Based on **hydrocodone** component: CNS depressants, MAO inhibitors, general anesthetics, and tricyclic antidepressants may potentiate the effects of opiate agonists. Dextroamphetamine may enhance the analgesic effect of opiate agonists.
Based on **homatropine** component: Phenothiazine and TCAs may increase anticholinergic effects when used concurrently. Sympathomimetic amines may cause tachyarrhythmias; avoid concurrent use.

Dietary/Ethanol/Herb Considerations
Ethanol: Avoid or limit use; may increase CNS depression.
Herb/Nutraceutical: Avoid gotu kola, kava, SAMe, St John's wort, and valerian; may increase CNS depression.

Pharmacodynamics/Kinetics Duration: Hydrocodone: 4-6 hours
Pregnancy Risk Factor C
Generic Available Yes: Syrup

Hydrocodone and Ibuprofen

(hye droe KOE done & eye byoo PROE fen)

Related Information
Ibuprofen *on page 703*
Oral Pain *on page 1524*

U.S. Brand Names Vicoprofen®
Canadian Brand Names Vicoprofen®
Pharmacologic Category Analgesic, Narcotic
Synonyms Ibuprofen and Hydrocodone
Use
Dental: Relief of moderate to moderately severe pain

Medical: Short-term (generally <10 days) management of moderate to severe acute pain, excluding osteoarthritis or rheumatoid arthritis

Local Anesthetic/Vasoconstrictor Precautions No information available to require special precautions

Effects on Dental Treatment

>10%: Xerostomia (3% to 9%), oral ulceration (<3%), headache (27%), dizziness (14%), sedation (22%), nausea (21%)

1% to 9%: Bradycardia, palpitations (<3%), vasodilation (<3%), nervousness, confusion, fever (<3%), pain (3% to 9%), anxiety (3% to 9%), abnormal thoughts, vomiting (3% to 9%), gastritis (<3%), weakness (3% to 9%), dyspnea, hiccups, pharyngitis, rhinitis, flu syndrome (<3%), infection (3% to 9%)

Restrictions C-III

Dosage Adults: **Oral:** 1-2 tablets every 4-6 hours as needed for pain; maximum: 5 tablets/day

Mechanism of Action

Based on **hydrocodone** component: Binds to opiate receptors in the CNS, altering the perception of and response to pain; suppresses cough in medullary center; produces generalized CNS depression

Based on **ibuprofen** component: Inhibits prostaglandin synthesis by decreasing the activity of the enzyme, cyclooxygenase, which results in decreased formation of prostaglandin precursors

Other Adverse Effects

>10%:

Dermatologic: Rash, urticaria

Gastrointestinal: Constipation (22%), dyspepsia (12%)

1% to 9%:

Cardiovascular: Edema (3% to 9%)

Dermatologic: Itching (3% to 9%)

Endocrine & metabolic: Fluid retention

Gastrointestinal: Anorexia, diarrhea (3% to 9%), flatulence (3% to 9%), melena (<3%)

Genitourinary: Polyuria (<3%)

Otic: Tinnitus

<1%: **CHF, arrhythmias, tachycardia, hypertension, hallucinations,** mental depression, insomnia, aseptic meningitis, urticaria, erythema multiforme, toxic epidermal necrolysis, Stevens-Johnson syndrome, polydipsia, **hot flashes, biliary tract spasm**, cystitis, urinary tract spasm, neutropenia, anemia, agranulocytosis, **inhibition of platelet aggregation,** hemolytic anemia, bone marrow suppression, leukopenia, thrombocytopenia, hepatitis, peripheral neuropathy, **vision changes, blurred vision**, conjunctivitis, dry eyes, toxic amblyopia, diplopia, miosis, decreased hearing, **acute renal failure,** polyuria, **allergic rhinitis, epistaxis, histamine release, physical and psychological dependence (prolonged use)**

Contraindications Hypersensitivity to hydrocodone, ibuprofen, aspirin, other NSAIDs, or any component of the formulation; pregnancy (3rd trimester)

Warnings/Precautions As with any opioid analgesic agent, this agent should be used with caution in elderly or debilitated patients, and those with severe impairment of hepatic or renal function, hypothyroidism, Addison's disease, prostatic hyperplasia, or urethral stricture. The usual precautions should be observed and the possibility of respiratory depression should be kept in mind. Patients with head injury, increased intracranial pressure, acute abdomen, active peptic ulcer disease, history of upper GI disease, impaired thyroid function, asthma, hypertension, edema, heart failure, and any bleeding disorder should use this agent cautiously. Hydrocodone suppresses the cough reflex; as with opioids, caution should be exercised when this agent is used postoperatively and in patients with pulmonary disease.

Drug Interactions

Based on **hydrocodone** component: Substrate of **CYP2D6**

Increased Toxicity Potential: Aspirin, other CNS depressants, alcohol, MAO inhibitors, ACE inhibitors, tricyclic antidepressants, lithium, anticoagulants, anticholinergics, methotrexate

Decreased Effect: May decrease efficacy of ACE inhibitors and diuretics

Based on **ibuprofen** component: Substrate of CYP2C8/9, 2C19; Inhibits CYP2C8/9

ACE-inhibitors: Antihypertensive effects may be decreased by concurrent therapy with NSAIDs; monitor blood pressure.

Angiotensin II antagonists: Antihypertensive effects may be decreased by concurrent therapy with NSAIDs; monitor blood pressure.

Anticoagulants (warfarin, heparin, LMWHs) in combination with NSAIDs can cause increased risk of bleeding.

Antiplatelet drugs (ticlopidine, clopidogrel, aspirin, abciximab, dipyridamole, eptifibatide, tirofiban) can cause an increased risk of bleeding.

Loop diuretics efficacy (diuretic and antihypertensive effect) is reduced. Indomethacin reduces this efficacy, however, it may be anticipated with any NSAID.

Cholestyramine and colestipol reduce the bioavailability of diclofenac; separate administration times.

(Continued)

Hydrocodone and Ibuprofen *(Continued)*

Cyclosporine: NSAIDs may increase serum creatinine, potassium, blood pressure, and cyclosporine levels; monitor cyclosporine levels and renal function carefully.

Lithium levels can be increased; avoid concurrent use if possible or monitor lithium levels and adjust dose. Sulindac may have the least effect. When NSAID is stopped, lithium will need adjustment again.

Verapamil plasma concentration is decreased by diclofenac; avoid concurrent use.

Gentamicin and amikacin serum concentrations are increased by indomethacin in premature infants. Results may apply to other aminoglycosides and NSAIDs.

Hydralazine's antihypertensive effect is decreased; avoid concurrent use.

Warfarin's INRs may be increased by piroxicam. Other NSAIDs may have the same effect depending on dose and duration. Monitor INR closely. Use the lowest dose of NSAIDs possible and for the briefest duration.

Corticosteroids may increase the risk of GI ulceration; avoid concurrent use.

Thiazides antihypertensive effects are decreased; avoid concurrent use.

Vancomycin's serum concentration is increased by indomethacin in neonates.

Dietary/Ethanol/Herb Considerations

Ethanol: Based on **hydrocodone** component, avoid use; may increase CNS depression (watch for sedation)

Food may decrease ibuprofen peak serum concentration. Avoid garlic, ginger, and green tea.

Herb/Nutraceutical: Avoid cat's claw, dong quai, evening primrose, feverfew, garlic, ginger, ginkgo biloba, ginseng, green tea, horse chestnut, and red clover due to additional antiplatelet activity.

Pharmacodynamics/Kinetics

Ibuprofen: See Ibuprofen monograph.

Hydrocodone:

Onset of action: Narcotic analgesic: 10-20 minutes

Duration: 4-8 hours

Distribution: Crosses placenta

Protein binding: 19% to 45%

Metabolism: Hepatic; O-demethylation; N-demethylation and 6-ketosteroid reduction

Half-life elimination: 3.3-4.4 hours

Time to peak: 1.7 hours

Excretion: Urine

Pregnancy Risk Factor C/D (3rd trimester)

Dosage Forms TAB: Hydrocodone 7.5 mg and ibuprofen 200 mg

Generic Available No

Comments The combination of 15 mg hydrocodone bitartrate with 400 mg ibuprofen was compared to 400 mg ibuprofen alone and placebo for the ability to diminish postoperative pain (pain after cesarean section or gynecologic surgery, 120 patients). Analgesia was measured during a 6-hour period after dosing based on onset of relief, hourly and summary variables, and duration of effect. A significantly greater proportion of patients treated with the hydrocodone/ibuprofen combination reported onset of relief compared with ibuprofen or placebo. Time to onset of relief did not differ among treatments. Hydrocodone with ibuprofen and ibuprofen alone were significantly more effective than placebo for all measures. The combination of hydrocodone with ibuprofen was significantly superior to ibuprofen for all hourly analgesic evaluations, weighted sum of pain intensity differences, total pain relief, and global rating of study medications. This report demonstrated an analgesic superiority of 15 mg hydrocodone bitartrate combined with 400 mg ibuprofen compared to 400 mg ibuprofen alone.

Selected Readings

Dionne R, "To Tame the Pain?" *Compend Contin Educ Dent*, 1998, 19(4):426-8, 430-1.

Hargreaves KM, "Management of Pain in Endodontic Patients," *Tex Dent J*, 1997, 114(10):27-31.

Sunshine A, Olson NZ, O'Neill E, et al, "Analgesic Efficacy of a Hydrocodone With Ibuprofen Combination Compared With Ibuprofen Alone for the Treatment of Acute Postoperative Pain," *J Clin Pharmacol*, 1997, 37(10):908-15.

Wynn RL, "Narcotic Analgesics for Dental Pain: Available Products, Strengths, and Formulations," *Gen Dent*, 2001, 49(2):126-8, 130, 132 passim.

Hydrocodone, Chlorpheniramine, Phenylephrine, Acetaminophen, and Caffeine

(hye droe KOE done, klor fen IR a meen, fen il EF rin, a seet a MIN oh fen, & KAF een)

Related Information

Acetaminophen *on page 27*

Chlorpheniramine *on page 307*

Phenylephrine *on page 1071*

U.S. Brand Names Hycomine® Compound

Pharmacologic Category Antitussive/Decongestant

Synonyms Acetaminophen, Caffeine, Hydrocodone, Chlorpheniramine, and Phenylephrine; Caffeine, Hydrocodone, Chlorpheniramine, Phenylephrine, and Acetaminophen; Chlorpheniramine, Hydrocodone, Phenylephrine, Acetaminophen, and Caffeine; Phenylephrine, Hydrocodone, Chlorpheniramine, Acetaminophen, and Caffeine

Use Symptomatic relief of cough and symptoms of upper respiratory infection

Local Anesthetic/Vasoconstrictor Precautions Use with caution since phenylephrine is a sympathomimetic amine which could interact with epinephrine to cause a pressor response

Effects on Dental Treatment

Acetaminophen: No significant effects or complications reported

Chlorpheniramine: Prolonged use will cause significant xerostomia

Phenylephrine: Up to 10% of patients could experience tachycardia, palpitations, and xerostomia; use vasoconstrictor with caution

Restrictions C-III

Dosage Adults: Oral: 1 tablet every 4 hours, up to 4 times/day

Other Adverse Effects Frequency not defined:

Cardiovascular: **Hypertension, postural hypotension**

Central nervous system: Sedation, drowsiness, mental clouding, lethargy, impairment of mental and physical performance, anxiety, fear, dysphoria, dizziness, psychic dependence, mood changes

Dermatologic: Rash, pruritus

Gastrointestinal: Nausea, vomiting, constipation (with prolonged use)

Genitourinary: Ureteral spasms, spasm of vesical sphincters and urinary retention

Ocular: Blurred vision

Respiratory: **Respiratory depression**

Dietary/Ethanol/Herb Considerations

Ethanol: Avoid use; may increase CNS depression. Excessive intake may increase the risk of acetaminophen-induced hepatotoxicity.

Herb/Nutraceutical: Avoid gotu kola, kava, SAMe, St John's wort, and valerian; may increase CNS depression.

Pharmacodynamics/Kinetics

See Chlorpheniramine, Phenylephrine, and Acetaminophen monographs.

Hydrocodone:

Onset of action: Narcotic analgesic: 10-20 minutes

Duration: 4-8 hours

Distribution: Crosses placenta

Metabolism: Hepatic; O-demethylation; N-demethylation and 6-ketosteroid reduction

Half-life elimination: 3.3-4.4 hours

Excretion: Urine

Pregnancy Risk Factor C

Generic Available No

Selected Readings

Barker JD Jr, de Carle DJ, and Anuras S, "Chronic Excessive Acetaminophen Use in Liver Damage," *Ann Intern Med*, 1977, 87(3):299-301.

Botting RM, "Mechanism of Action of Acetaminophen: Is There a Cyclooxygenase 3?," *Clin Infect Dis*, 2000, Suppl 5:S202-10.

Dart RC, Kuffner EK, and Rumack BH, "Treatment of Pain or Fever with Paracetamol (Acetaminophen) in the Alcoholic Patient: A Systematic Review," *Am J Ther*, 2000, 7(2):123-34.

Dionne RA, Campbell RA, Cooper SA, et al, "Suppression of Postoperative Pain by Preoperative Administration of Ibuprofen in Comparison to Placebo, Acetaminophen, and Acetaminophen Plus Codeine," *J Clin Pharmacol*, 1983, 23(1):37-43.

Grant JA and Weiler JM, "A Report of a Rare Immediate Reaction After Ingestion of Acetaminophen," *Ann Allergy Asthma Immunol*, 2001, 87(3):227-9.

Kwan D, Bartle WR, and Walker SE, "The Effects of Acetaminophen on Pharmacokinetics and Pharmacodynamics of Warfarin," *J Clin Pharmacol*, 1999, 39(1):68-75.

Licht H, Seeff LB, and Zimmerman HJ, "Apparent Potentiation of Acetaminophen Hepatotoxicity by Alcohol," *Ann Intern Med*, 1980, 92(4):511.

McClain CJ, Price S, Barve S, et al, "Acetaminophen Hepatotoxicity: An Update," *Curr Gastroenterol Rep*, 1999, 1(1):42-9.

Shek KL, Chan LN, and Nutescu E, "Warfarin-Acetaminophen Drug Interaction Revisited," *Pharmacotherapy*, 1999, 19(10):1153-8.

Tanaka E, Yamazaki K, and Misawa S, "Update: The Clinical Importance of Acetaminophen Hepatotoxicity in Nonalcoholic and Alcoholic Subjects," *J Clin Pharm Ther*, 2000, 25(5):325-32.

Hydrocodone, Pseudoephedrine, and Guaifenesin

(hye droe KOE done, soo doe e FED rin, & gwe FEN e sin)

Related Information

Guaifenesin *on page 650*

Pseudoephedrine *on page 1146*

U.S. Brand Names Duratuss® HD; Hydro-Tussin™ HD; Hydro-Tussin™ XP; Pancof®-XP; Su-Tuss®-HD; Tussend® Expectorant

Pharmacologic Category Antitussive/Decongestant/Expectorant

Synonyms Guaifenesin, Hydrocodone, and Pseudoephedrine; Pseudoephedrine, Hydrocodone, and Guaifenesin

(Continued)

Hydrocodone, Pseudoephedrine, and Guaifenesin *(Continued)*

Use Symptomatic relief of irritating, nonproductive cough associated with respiratory conditions such as bronchitis, bronchial asthma, tracheobronchitis, and the common cold

Local Anesthetic/Vasoconstrictor Precautions Use with caution since pseudoephedrine is a sympathomimetic amine which could interact with epinephrine to cause a pressor response

Effects on Dental Treatment

Guaifenesin: No significant effects or complications reported

Pseudoephedrine: Up to 10% of patients could experience tachycardia, palpitations, and xerostomia; use vasoconstrictor with caution

Restrictions C-III

Dosage Adults: Oral: 5 mL every 4-6 hours

Other Adverse Effects Frequency not defined:

Cardiovascular: **Arrhythmias, hypertension**

Central nervous system: Drowsiness, fear, anxiety, tenseness, restlessness, pallor, insomnia, hallucinations, CNS depression

Gastrointestinal: GI upset, nausea, constipation (with prolonged use)

Genitourinary: Dysuria

Hepatic: Slight elevation in serum transaminase levels

Neuromuscular & skeletal: Weakness, tremor

Respiratory: Respiratory difficulty

Patients hyper-reactive to pseudoephedrine may display ephedrine-like reactions such as **tachycardia, palpitations**, headache, dizziness, or nausea; patient idiosyncrasy to adrenergic agents may be manifested by insomnia, dizziness, weakness, tremor, or arrhythmias.

Dietary/Ethanol/Herb Considerations

Ethanol: Avoid use; may increase CNS depression.

Herb/Nutraceutical: Avoid gotu kola, kava, SAMe, St John's wort, and valerian; may increase CNS depression.

Pharmacodynamics/Kinetics

See Guaifenesin and Pseudoephedrine monographs.

Hydrocodone:

Onset of action: Narcotic analgesic: 10-20 minutes

Duration: 4-8 hours

Distribution: Crosses placenta

Metabolism: Hepatic; O-demethylation; N-demethylation and 6-ketosteroid reduction

Half-life elimination: 3.3-4.4 hours

Excretion: Urine

Pregnancy Risk Factor C

Generic Available Yes

Hydrocortisone (hye droe KOR ti sone)

Related Information

Dental Office Emergencies *on page 1582*

U.S. Brand Names A-hydroCort®; Anucort-HC®; Anusol-HC®; Anusol® HC-1 [OTC]; Aquanil™ HC [OTC]; CaldeCORT® [OTC]; Cetacort®; Clocort™; CortaGel® Maximum Strength [OTC]; Cortaid® Intensive Therapy [OTC]; Cortaid® Maximum Strength [OTC]; Cortaid® Sensitive Skin With Aloe [OTC]; Cortef®; Corticool® [OTC]; Cortifoam®; Cortizone®-5 [OTC]; Cortizone®-10 Maximum Strength [OTC]; Cortizone®-10 Plus Maximum Strength [OTC]; Cortizone® 10 Quick Shot [OTC]; Cortizone® for Kids [OTC]; Dermarest Dricort® [OTC]; Dermtex® HC [OTC]; EarSol® HC; Hemril-HC®; Hydrocortone®; Hydrocortone® Phosphate; Hytone®; Lacti-Care-HC®; Locoid®; Locoid Lipocream®; Nupercainal® Hydrocortisone Cream [OTC]; Nutracort®; Pandel®; Post Peel Healing Balm [OTC]; Preparation H® Hydrocortisone [OTC]; Proctocort®; ProctoCream® HC; Proctosol-HC®; Sarnol®-HC [OTC]; Solu-Cortef®; Summer's Eve® SpecialCare™ Medicated Anti-Itch Cream [OTC]; Texacort®; Theracort® [OTC]; Westcort®

Canadian Brand Names Aquacort®; Cortamed®; Cortate®; Cortef®; Cortenema®; Cortifoam™; Cortoderm; Emo-Cort®; Hycort™; Hyderm; HydroVal®; Locoid®; Prevex® HC; Sarna® HC; Solu-Cortef®; Westcort®

Mexican Brand Names Aquanil HC®; Flebocortid; LactiCare-HC®; Nositrol; Nutracort®

Pharmacologic Category Corticosteroid, Rectal; Corticosteroid, Systemic; Corticosteroid, Topical

Synonyms Compound F; Cortisol; Hydrocortisone Acetate; Hydrocortisone Buteprate; Hydrocortisone Butyrate; Hydrocortisone Cypionate; Hydrocortisone Sodium Phosphate; Hydrocortisone Sodium Succinate; Hydrocortisone Valerate

Use

Dental: Treatment of a variety of oral diseases of allergic, inflammatory or autoimmune origin

Medical: Management of adrenocortical insufficiency; relief of inflammation of corticosteroid-responsive dermatoses (low and medium potency topical corticosteroid); adjunctive treatment of ulcerative colitis

Local Anesthetic/Vasoconstrictor Precautions No information available to require special precautions

Effects on Dental Treatment

>10%: Nervousness

1% to 10%: Diabetes mellitus, epistaxis

Dosage Dose should be based on severity of disease and patient response.

Acute adrenal insufficiency: I.M., I.V.:

Infants and young Children: Succinate: 1-2 mg/kg/dose bolus, then 25-150 mg/day in divided doses every 6-8 hours

Older Children: Succinate: 1-2 mg/kg bolus then 150-250 mg/day in divided doses every 6-8 hours

Adults: Succinate: 100 mg I.V. bolus, then 300 mg/day in divided doses every 8 hours or as a continuous infusion for 48 hours; once patient is stable change to oral, 50 mg every 8 hours for 6 doses, then taper to 30-50 mg/day in divided doses

Chronic adrenal corticoid insufficiency: Adults: Oral: 20-30 mg/day

Anti-inflammatory or immunosuppressive:

Infants and Children:

Oral: 2.5-10 mg/kg/day **or** 75-300 mg/m²/day every 6-8 hours

I.M., I.V.: Succinate: 1-5 mg/kg/day **or** 30-150 mg/m²/day divided every 12-24 hours

Adolescents and Adults: Oral, I.M., I.V.: Succinate: 15-240 mg every 12 hours

Congenital adrenal hyperplasia: Oral: Initial: 10-20 mg/m²/day in 3 divided doses; a variety of dosing schedules have been used. **Note:** Inconsistencies have occurred with liquid formulations; tablets may provide more reliable levels. Doses must be individualized by monitoring growth, bone age, and hormonal levels. Mineralocorticoid and sodium supplementation may be required based upon electrolyte regulation and plasma renin activity.

Physiologic replacement: Children:

Oral: 0.5-0.75 mg/kg/day **or** 20-25 mg/m²/day every 8 hours

I.M.: Succinate: 0.25-0.35 mg/kg/day **or** 12-15 mg/m²/day once daily

Shock: I.M., I.V.: Succinate:

Children: Initial: 50 mg/kg, then repeated in 4 hours and/or every 24 hours as needed

Adolescents and Adults: 500 mg to 2 g every 2-6 hours

Status asthmaticus: Children and Adults: I.V.: Succinate: 1-2 mg/kg/dose every 6 hours for 24 hours, then maintenance of 0.5-1 mg/kg every 6 hours

Adults:

Rheumatic diseases:

Intralesional, intra-articular, soft tissue injection: Acetate:

Large joints: 25 mg (up to 37.5 mg)

Small joints: 10-25 mg

Tendon sheaths: 5-12.5 mg

Soft tissue infiltration: 25-50 mg (up to 75 mg)

Bursae: 25-37.5 mg

Ganglia: 12.5-25 mg

Stress dosing (surgery) in patients known to be adrenally-suppressed or on chronic systemic steroids: I.V.:

Minor stress (ie, inguinal herniorrhaphy): 25 mg/day for 1 day

Moderate stress (ie, joint replacement, cholecystectomy): 50-75 mg/day (25 mg every 8-12 hours) for 1-2 days

Major stress (pancreatoduodenectomy, esophagogastrectomy, cardiac surgery): 100-150 mg/day (50 mg every 8-12 hours) for 2-3 days

Dermatosis: Children >2 years and Adults: Topical: Apply to affected area 3-4 times/day (Buteprate: Apply once or twice daily). Therapy should be discontinued when control is achieved; if no improvement is seen, reassessment of diagnosis may be necessary.

Ulcerative colitis: Adults: Rectal: 10-100 mg 1-2 times/day for 2-3 weeks

Mechanism of Action Decreases inflammation by suppression of migration of polymorphonuclear leukocytes and reversal of increased capillary permeability

Other Adverse Effects

>10%:

Central nervous system: Insomnia

Gastrointestinal: Increased appetite, indigestion

1% to 10%:

Dermatologic: Hirsutism

Neuromuscular & skeletal: Arthralgia

Ocular: Cataracts

<1%: **Hypertension**, edema, **euphoria, headache, delirium, hallucinations, seizures, mood swings**, acne, dermatitis, **skin atrophy, bruising,** hyperpigmentation, hypokalemia, **hyperglycemia**, Cushing's syndrome, sodium and water retention, bone growth suppression, amenorrhea, **peptic ulcer,** abdominal

(Continued)

Hydrocortisone *(Continued)*

distention, **ulcerative esophagitis,** pancreatitis, **muscle wasting, hypersensitivity reactions, immunosuppression**

Contraindications Hypersensitivity to hydrocortisone or any component of the formulation; serious infections, except septic shock or tuberculous meningitis; viral, fungal, or tubercular skin lesions

Warnings/Precautions

Use with caution in patients with hyperthyroidism, cirrhosis, nonspecific ulcerative colitis, hypertension, osteoporosis, thromboembolic tendencies, CHF, convulsive disorders, myasthenia gravis, thrombophlebitis, peptic ulcer, diabetes, glaucoma, cataracts, or tuberculosis. Use caution in hepatic impairment.

May cause HPA axis suppression. Acute adrenal insufficiency may occur with abrupt withdrawal after long-term therapy or with stress; young pediatric patients may be more susceptible to adrenal axis suppression from topical therapy. Avoid use of topical preparations with occlusive dressings or on weeping or exudative lesions.

Because of the risk of adverse effects, systemic corticosteroids should be used cautiously in the elderly, in the smallest possible dose, and for the shortest possible time

Drug Interactions Substrate of CYP3A4; Induces CYP3A4

Increased Toxicity:

Oral anticoagulants change prothrombin time

Potassium-depleting diuretics increase risk of hypokalemia

Cardiac glucosides increase risk of arrhythmias or digitalis toxicity secondary to hypokalemia

Decreased Effect:

Insulin decreases hypoglycemic effect

Phenytoin, phenobarbital, ephedrine, and rifampin increase metabolism of hydrocortisone and decrease steroid blood level

Dietary/Ethanol/Herb Considerations

Ethanol: Avoid use; may enhance gastric mucosal irritation.

Food: Administer with food to reduce GI upset. Systemic use interferes with calcium absorption; requires diet rich in pyridoxine, vitamins A, B_6, C, D, folate, calcium, phosphorus, potassium, and zinc. Limit caffeine and sodium.

Herb/Nutraceutical: Avoid cat's claw and echinacea due to immunostimulant properties. Avoid St John's wort; may decrease serum concentration.

Pharmacodynamics/Kinetics

Onset of action:

Hydrocortisone acetate: Slow

Hydrocortisone sodium phosphate (water soluble): Rapid

Hydrocortisone sodium succinate (water soluble): Rapid

Duration:

Hydrocortisone acetate: Long

Hydrocortisone sodium phosphate (water soluble): Short

Absorption: Rapid by all routes, except rectally

Metabolism: Hepatic

Half-life elimination: Biologic: 8-12 hours

Excretion: Urine (primarily as 17-hydroxysteroids and 17-ketosteroids)

Pregnancy Risk Factor C

Breast-feeding Considerations It is not known if hydrocortisone is excreted in breast milk, however, other corticosteroids are excreted. Prednisone and prednisolone are excreted in breast milk; the AAP considers them to be "usually compatible" with breast-feeding. Hypertension was reported in a nursing infant when a topical corticosteroid was applied to the nipples of the mother.

Dosage Forms AERO, rectal, as acetate (Cortifoam®): 10% (15 g). **AERO, topical spray, as base** (Cortizone® 10 Quick Shot): 1% (44 mL); (Dermtex® HC): 1% (52 mL). **CRM, rectal, as acetate** (Nupercainal® Hydrocortisone Cream): 1% (30 g). **CRM, rectal, as base**: (Cortizone®-10): 1% (30 g); (Preparation H® Hydrocortisone): 1% (27 g). **CRM, topical, as acetate**: 0.5% (30 g); 1% (30 g); (Cortaid® Maximum Strength): 1% (15 g, 30 g, 40 g); (Cortaid® Sensitive Skin With Aloe): 0.5% (15 g). **CRM, topical, as base**: 0.5% (30 g); 1% (1.5 g, 30 g, 454 g); 2.5% (20 g, 30 g, 454 g); (Anusol-HC®): 2.5% (30 g); (CaldeCORT®): 1% (15 g, 30 g); (Cortaid® Intensive Therapy): 1% (60 g); (Cortaid® Maximum Strength): 1% (15 g, 30 g, 40 g, 60 g); (Cortizone®-5): 0.5% (30 g, 60 g); (Cortizone®-10 Maximum Strength): 1% (30 g, 60 g); (Cortizone®-10 Plus Maximum Strength): 1% (30 g, 60 g); (Cortizone® for Kids): 0.5% (30 g); (Dermarest® Dri-Cort): 1% (15 g, 30 g); (Hytone®): 2.5% (30 g, 60 g); (Post Peel Healing Balm): 1% (23 g); (ProctoCream® HC): 2.5% (30 g); (Proctocort®): 1% (30 g); (Proctosol-HC®): 2.5% (30 g); (Summer's Eve® SpecialCare™ Medicated Anti-Itch Cream): 1% (30 g). **CRM, topical, as butyrate** (Locoid®, Locoid Lipocream®): 0.1% (15 g, 45 g). **CRM, topical, as probutate** (Pandel®): 0.1% (15 g, 45 g, 80 g). **CRM, topical, as valerate** (Westcort®): 0.2% (15 g, 45 g, 60 g). **GEL, topical, as base**: (Corticool®): 1% (45 g); (Cortagel® Maximum Strength): 1% (15 g, 30 g). **INJ, powder for reconstitution, as sodium succinate**: (A-Hydrocort®): 100 mg, 250 mg;

(Solu-Cortef®): 100 mg, 250 mg, 500 mg, 1 g. **INJ, solution, as sodium phosphate** (Hydrocortone® Phosphate): 50 mg/mL (2 mL). **LOTION, topical, as base**: 1% (120 mL); 2.5% (60 mL); (Aquanil™ HC): 1% (120 mL); (Cetacort®, Sarnol®-HC): 1% (60 mL); (Hytone®): 1% (30 mL, 120 mL); 2.5% (60 mL); (Lacti-Care-HC®): 1% (120 mL); 2.5% (60 mL, 120 mL); (Nutracort®): 1% (60 mL, 120 mL); 2.5% (60 mL, 120 mL); (Theracort®): 1% (120 mL). **OINT, topical, as acetate**: 1% (30 g); (Anusol® HC-1): 1% (21 g); (Cortaid® Maximum Strength): 1% (15 g, 30 g). **OINT, topical, as base**: 0.5% (30 g); 1% (30 g, 454 g); 2.5% (20 g, 30 g, 454 g); (Cortizone®-5): 0.5% (30 g); (Cortizone®-10 Maximum Strength): 1% (30 g, 60 g); (Hytone®): 2.5% (30 g). **OINT, topical, as base** [in Orabase®]: 1% (25 g, 110 g, 454 g). **OINT, topical, as butyrate** (Locoid®): 0.1% (15 g, 45 g). **OINT, topical, as valerate** (Westcort®): 0.2% (15 g, 45 g, 60 g). **SOLN, otic, as base** (EarSol® HC): 1% (30 mL). **SOLN, rectal, as base** (Colocort™): 100 mg/60 mL (7s). **SOLN, topical, as base** (Texacort®): 1% (30 mL) [DSC]; 2.5% (30 mL). **SOLN, topical, as butyrate** (Locoid®): 0.1% (20 mL, 60 mL). **SUPP, rectal**: 25 mg (12s, 24s); (Anucort™ HC): 25 mg (12s, 24s, 100s); (Anusol-HC®, Proctosol-HC®): 25 mg (12s, 24s); (Hemril® HC): 25 mg (12s); (Proctocort®): 30 mg (12s, 24s); **SUSP, oral, as cypionate** (Cortef®): 10 mg/5 mL (120 mL) [DSC]. **TAB, as base**: 20 mg; (Cortef®): 5 mg, 10 mg, 20 mg; (Hydrocortone®): 10 mg

Generic Available Yes

Hydrocortisone Acetate *see* Hydrocortisone *on page 688*

Hydrocortisone, Acetic Acid, and Propylene Glycol Diacetate *see* Acetic Acid, Propylene Glycol Diacetate, and Hydrocortisone *on page 38*

Hydrocortisone and Benzoyl Peroxide *see* Benzoyl Peroxide and Hydrocortisone *on page 172*

Hydrocortisone and Ciprofloxacin *see* Ciprofloxacin and Hydrocortisone *on page 331*

Hydrocortisone and Iodoquinol *see* Iodoquinol and Hydrocortisone *on page 736*

Hydrocortisone and Lidocaine *see* Lidocaine and Hydrocortisone *on page 805*

Hydrocortisone and Oxytetracycline *see* Oxytetracycline and Hydrocortisone *on page 1025*

Hydrocortisone and Pramoxine *see* Pramoxine and Hydrocortisone *on page 1106*

Hydrocortisone and Urea *see* Urea and Hydrocortisone *on page 1365*

Hydrocortisone, Bacitracin, Neomycin, and Polymyxin B *see* Bacitracin, Neomycin, Polymyxin B, and Hydrocortisone *on page 158*

Hydrocortisone Buteprate *see* Hydrocortisone *on page 688*

Hydrocortisone Butyrate *see* Hydrocortisone *on page 688*

Hydrocortisone, Chloramphenicol, and Polymyxin B *see* Chloramphenicol, Polymyxin B, and Hydrocortisone *on page 299*

Hydrocortisone, Colistin, and Neomycin *see* Colistin, Neomycin, and Hydrocortisone *on page 367*

Hydrocortisone Cypionate *see* Hydrocortisone *on page 688*

Hydrocortisone, Neomycin, and Polymyxin B *see* Neomycin, Polymyxin B, and Hydrocortisone *on page 963*

Hydrocortisone, Polymyxin B, and Chloramphenicol *see* Chloramphenicol, Polymyxin B, and Hydrocortisone *on page 299*

Hydrocortisone, Propylene Glycol Diacetate, and Acetic Acid *see* Acetic Acid, Propylene Glycol Diacetate, and Hydrocortisone *on page 38*

Hydrocortisone Sodium Phosphate *see* Hydrocortisone *on page 688*

Hydrocortisone Sodium Succinate *see* Hydrocortisone *on page 688*

Hydrocortisone Valerate *see* Hydrocortisone *on page 688*

Hydrocortone® *see* Hydrocortisone *on page 688*

Hydrocortone® Phosphate *see* Hydrocortisone *on page 688*

Hydrogesic® [DSC] *see* Hydrocodone and Acetaminophen *on page 678*

Hydromet® *see* Hydrocodone and Homatropine *on page 684*

Hydromorphone (hye droe MOR fone)

Related Information

Oxymorphone *on page 1024*

U.S. Brand Names Dilaudid®; Dilaudid-HP®

Canadian Brand Names Dilaudid®; Dilaudid-HP®; Dilaudid-HP-Plus®; Dilaudid® Sterile Powder; Dilaudid-XP®; Hydromorph Contin®; Hydromorphone HP; PMS-Hydromorphone

Pharmacologic Category Analgesic, Narcotic

Synonyms Dihydromorphinone; Hydromorphone Hydrochloride

Use Management of moderate to severe pain; antitussive at lower doses

Local Anesthetic/Vasoconstrictor Precautions No information available to require special precautions

Effects on Dental Treatment 10%: Xerostomia and nausea

Frequency not defined: Palpitations, hypotension, peripheral vasodilation, tachycardia, bradycardia, facial flushing, CNS depression, increased intracranial pressure, fatigue, headache, nervousness, restlessness, dizziness, lightheadedness,

(Continued)

Hydromorphone *(Continued)*

drowsiness, hallucinations, seizures, vomiting, biliary tract spasm, trembling, weakness, myoclonus, respiratory depression, dyspnea, histamine release, physical and psychological dependence

Restrictions C-II

Dosage

Acute pain (moderate to severe): **Note:** These are guidelines and do not represent the maximum doses that may be required in all patients. Doses should be titrated to pain relief/prevention.

Young Children ≥6 months and <50 kg:

Oral: 0.03-0.08 mg/kg/dose every 3-4 hours as needed

I.V.: 0.015 mg/kg/dose every 3-6 hours as needed

Older Children >50 kg and Adults:

Oral: Initial: Opiate-naive: 2-4 mg every 3-4 hours as needed; patients with prior opiate exposure may require higher initial doses; usual dosage range: 2-8 mg every 3-4 hours as needed

I.V.: Initial: Opiate-naive: 0.2-0.6 mg every 2-3 hours as needed; patients with prior opiate exposure may tolerate higher initial doses

Note: More frequent dosing may be needed.

Mechanically-ventilated patients (based on 70 kg patient): 0.7-2 mg every 1-2 hours as needed; infusion (based on 70 kg patient): 0.5-1 mg/hour

Patient-controlled analgesia (PCA): (Opiate-naive: Consider lower end of dosing range)

Usual concentration: 0.2 mg/mL

Demand dose: Usual: 0.1-0.2 mg; range: 0.05-0.5 mg

Lockout interval: 5-15 minutes

4-hour limit: 4-6 mg

Epidural:

Bolus dose: 1-1.5 mg

Infusion concentration: 0.05-0.075 mg/mL

Infusion rate: 0.04-0.4 mg/hour

Demand dose: 0.15 mg

Lockout interval: 30 minutes

I.M., S.C.: **Note:** I.M. use may result in variable absorption and a lag time to peak effect.

Initial: Opiate-naive: 0.8-1 mg every 4-6 hours as needed; patients with prior opiate exposure may require higher initial doses; usual dosage range: 1-2 mg every 3-6 hours as needed

Rectal: 3 mg every 4-8 hours as needed

Chronic pain: Patients taking opioids chronically may become tolerant and require doses higher than the usual dosage range to maintain the desired effect. Tolerance can be managed by appropriate dose titration. There is no optimal or maximal dose for hydromorphone in chronic pain. The appropriate dose is one that relieves pain throughout its dosing interval without causing unmanageable side effects.

Antitussive: Oral:

Children 6-12 years: 0.5 mg every 3-4 hours as needed

Children >12 years and Adults: 1 mg every 3-4 hours as needed

Dosing adjustment in hepatic impairment: Should be considered

Mechanism of Action Binds to opiate receptors in the CNS, causing inhibition of ascending pain pathways, altering the perception of and response to pain; causes cough supression by direct central action in the medulla; produces generalized CNS depression

Other Adverse Effects Frequency not defined:

Central nervous system: Mental depression

Dermatologic: Pruritus, rash, urticaria

Endocrine & metabolic: Antidiuretic hormone release

Gastrointestinal: Constipation, stomach cramps, anorexia, paralytic ileus

Genitourinary: Decreased urination, ureteral spasm, urinary tract spasm

Hepatic: LFTs increased, AST increased, ALT increased

Local: Pain at injection site (I.M.)

Ocular: Miosis

Drug Interactions Increased Effect/Toxicity: CNS depressants, phenothiazines, and tricyclic antidepressants may potentiate the adverse effects of hydromorphone.

Dietary/Ethanol/Herb Considerations

Ethanol: Avoid use; may increase CNS depression.

Food: Administer with food or milk to reduce GI upset.

Herb/Nutraceutical: Avoid gotu kola, kava, SAMe, St John's wort, and valerian; may increase CNS depression.

Pharmacodynamics/Kinetics

Onset of action: Analgesic: Oral: 15-30 minutes

Peak effect: Oral: 30-60 minutes

Duration: 4-5 hours

Absorption: I.M.: Variable and delayed

Metabolism: Hepatic; no active metabolites

Bioavailability: 62%
Half-life elimination: 1-3 hours
Excretion: Urine (primarily as glucuronide conjugates)

Pregnancy Risk Factor B/D (prolonged use or high doses at term)
Generic Available Yes

Hydromorphone Hydrochloride *see* Hydromorphone *on page 691*
Hydropane® *see* Hydrocodone and Homatropine *on page 684*
Hydroquinol *see* Hydroquinone *on page 693*

Hydroquinone (HYE droe kwin one)

U.S. Brand Names Alphaquin HP; Alustra™; Claripel™; Eldopaque® [OTC]; Eldopaque Forte®; Eldoquin® [OTC]; Eldoquin Forte®; Esoterica® Regular [OTC]; Glyquin®; Lustra®; Lustra-AF™; Melanex®; Melpaque HP®; Melquin-3® [OTC]; Melquin HP®; NeoStrata AHA [OTC]; Nuquin HP®; Palmer's® Skin Success Fade Cream™ [OTC]; Solaquin® [OTC]; Solaquin Forte®

Canadian Brand Names Eldopaque™; Eldoquin™; Lustra®; NeoStrata® HQ; Solaquin™; Solaquin Forte™; Ultraquin™

Mexican Brand Names Crema Blanca®; Crema Blanca Bustillos; Eldopaque®; Eldoquin®; Hidroquin®

Pharmacologic Category Depigmenting Agent

Synonyms Hydroquinol; Quinol

Use Gradual bleaching of hyperpigmented skin conditions

Local Anesthetic/Vasoconstrictor Precautions No information available to require special precautions

Effects on Dental Treatment No significant effects or complications reported

Dosage Children >12 years and Adults: Topical: Apply thin layer and rub in twice daily

Mechanism of Action Produces reversible depigmentation of the skin by suppression of melanocyte metabolic processes, in particular the inhibition of the enzymatic oxidation of tyrosine to DOPA (3,4-dihydroxyphenylalanine); sun exposure reverses this effect and will cause repigmentation.

Other Adverse Effects Frequency not defined:
Dermatologic: Dermatitis, dryness, erythema, stinging, inflammatory reaction, sensitization
Local: Irritation

Pharmacodynamics/Kinetics Onset and duration of depigmentation produced by hydroquinone varies among individuals

Pregnancy Risk Factor C

Generic Available Yes: 4% cream

Hydroquinone, Fluocinolone Acetonide, and Tretinoin *see* Fluocinolone, Hydroquinone, and Tretinoin *on page 585*
Hydro-Tussin™-CBX *see* Carbinoxamine and Pseudoephedrine *on page 247*
Hydro-Tussin™ DM *see* Guaifenesin and Dextromethorphan *on page 651*
Hydro-Tussin™ HD *see* Hydrocodone, Pseudoephedrine, and Guaifenesin *on page 687*
Hydro-Tussin™ XP *see* Hydrocodone, Pseudoephedrine, and Guaifenesin *on page 687*

Hydroxocobalamin (hye droks oh koe BAL a min)

Mexican Brand Names Axofor®; Duradoce®

Pharmacologic Category Vitamin, Water Soluble

Synonyms Vitamin B_{12}

Use Treatment of pernicious anemia, vitamin B_{12} deficiency, increased B_{12} requirements due to pregnancy, thyrotoxicosis, hemorrhage, malignancy, liver or kidney disease

Unlabeled/Investigational Use Treatment of neuropathies, multiple sclerosis (MS)

Local Anesthetic/Vasoconstrictor Precautions No information available to require special precautions

Effects on Dental Treatment No significant effects or complications reported

Dosage Vitamin B_{12} deficiency: I.M.:
Children: 1-5 mg given in single doses of 100 mcg over 2 or more weeks, followed by 30-50 mcg/month
Adults: 30 mcg/day for 5-10 days, followed by 100-200 mcg/month

Mechanism of Action Coenzyme for various metabolic functions, including fat and carbohydrate metabolism and protein synthesis, used in cell replication and hematopoiesis

Other Adverse Effects Frequency not defined:
Cardiovascular: Peripheral vascular thrombosis
Dermatologic: Itching, urticaria
Gastrointestinal: Diarrhea
Miscellaneous: Hypersensitivity reactions

Pregnancy Risk Factor A/C (dose exceeding RDA recommendation)

Generic Available Yes

Hydroxyamphetamine and Tropicamide

(hye droks ee am FET a meen & troe PIK a mide)

U.S. Brand Names Paremyd®

Pharmacologic Category Adrenergic Agonist Agent, Ophthalmic

Synonyms Tropicamide and Hydroxyamphetamine

Use Short-term pupil dilation for diagnostic procedures and exams

Local Anesthetic/Vasoconstrictor Precautions No information available to require special precautions

Effects on Dental Treatment No significant effects or complications reported

Dosage Ophthalmic: Adults: Instill 1-2 drops into conjunctival sac(s)

Mechanism of Action Hydroxyamphetamine hydrobromide is an indirect acting sympathomimetic agent which causes the release of norepinephrine from adrenergic nerve terminals, resulting in mydriasis. Tropicamide is a parasympatholytic agent which produces mydriasis and paralysis by blocking the sphincter muscle in the iris and the ciliary muscle.

Other Adverse Effects Frequency not defined (as reported with Paremyd® or similar medications):

Cardiovascular: **Hypotension, MI, tachycardia, ventricular fibrillation**, pallor

Central nervous system: Behavioral disturbances, headache, psychotic reactions

Gastrointestinal: Dry mouth, nausea, vomiting

Neuromuscular & skeletal: Muscle rigidity

Ocular: Blurred vision, intraocular pressure increased, photophobia, transient stinging

Miscellaneous: Allergic reaction, **cardiorespiratory collapse, vasomotor collapse**

Pharmacodynamics/Kinetics

Onset: 15 minutes

Duration: 3 hours; complete recovery usually occurs in 6-8 hours, but may take up to 24 hours

Time to peak: 60 minutes

Pregnancy Risk Factor C

Generic Available No

4-Hydroxybutyrate *see* Sodium Oxybate *on page 1231*

Hydroxycarbamide *see* Hydroxyurea *on page 696*

Hydroxychloroquine

(hye droks ee KLOR oh kwin)

Related Information

Rheumatoid Arthritis, Osteoarthritis, and Osteoporosis *on page 1488*

U.S. Brand Names Plaquenil®

Canadian Brand Names Plaquenil®

Pharmacologic Category Aminoquinoline (Antimalarial)

Synonyms Hydroxychloroquine Sulfate

Use Suppression and treatment of acute attacks of malaria; treatment of systemic lupus erythematosus and rheumatoid arthritis

Unlabeled/Investigational Use Treatment of porphyria cutanea tarda, polymorphous light eruptions

Local Anesthetic/Vasoconstrictor Precautions No information available to require special precautions

Effects on Dental Treatment No significant effects or complications reported

Dosage Note: Hydroxychloroquine sulfate 200 mg is equivalent to 155 mg hydroxychloroquine base and 250 mg chloroquine phosphate. Oral:

Children:

Chemoprophylaxis of malaria: 5 mg/kg (base) once weekly; should not exceed the recommended adult dose; begin 2 weeks before exposure; continue for 4-6 weeks after leaving endemic area; if suppressive therapy is not begun prior to the exposure, double the initial dose and give in 2 doses, 6 hours apart

Acute attack: 10 mg/kg (base) initial dose; followed by 5 mg/kg at 6, 24, and 48 hours

JRA or SLE: 3-5 mg/kg/day divided 1-2 times/day; avoid exceeding 7 mg/kg/day

Adults:

Chemoprophylaxis of malaria: 310 mg base weekly on same day each week; begin 2 weeks before exposure; continue for 4-6 weeks after leaving endemic area; if suppressive therapy is not begun prior to the exposure, double the initial dose and give in 2 doses, 6 hours apart

Acute attack: 620 mg first dose day 1; 310 mg in 6 hours day 1; 310 mg in 1 dose day 2; and 310 mg in 1 dose on day 3

Rheumatoid arthritis: 310-465 mg/day to start taken with food or milk; increase dose until optimum response level is reached; usually after 4-12 weeks dose should be reduced by $1/2$ and a maintenance dose of 155-310 mg/day given

Lupus erythematosus: 310 mg every day or twice daily for several weeks depending on response; 155-310 mg/day for prolonged maintenance therapy

Mechanism of Action Interferes with digestive vacuole function within sensitive malarial parasites by increasing the pH and interfering with lysosomal degradation of hemoglobin; inhibits locomotion of neutrophils and chemotaxis of eosinophils; impairs complement-dependent antigen-antibody reactions

Other Adverse Effects Frequency not defined:

Cardiovascular: Cardiomyopathy (rare, relationship to hydroxychloroquine unclear)

Central nervous system: Irritability, nervousness, emotional changes, nightmares, psychosis, headache, dizziness, vertigo, **seizures**, ataxia, lassitude

Dermatologic: Bleaching of hair, alopecia, pigmentation changes (skin and mucosal; black-blue color), rash (urticarial, morbilliform, lichenoid, maculopapular, purpuric, erythema annulare centrifugum, Stevens-Johnson syndrome, acute generalized exanthematous pustulosis, and exfoliative dermatitis)

Endocrine & metabolic: Weight loss

Gastrointestinal: Anorexia, nausea, vomiting, diarrhea, abdominal cramping

Hematologic: Aplastic anemia, agranulocytosis, leukopenia, thrombocytopenia, hemolysis (in patients with glucose-6-phosphate deficiency)

Hepatic: Abnormal liver function/hepatic failure (isolated cases)

Neuromuscular & skeletal: Myopathy, palsy, or neuromyopathy leading to progressive weakness and atrophy of proximal muscle groups (may be associated with mild sensory changes, loss of deep tendon reflexes, abnormal nerve conduction)

Ocular: Disturbance in accommodation, keratopathy, corneal changes/deposits (visual disturbances, blurred vision, photophobia - reversible on discontinuation), macular edema, atrophy, abnormal pigmentation, retinopathy (early changes reversible - may progress despite discontinuation if advanced), optic disc pallor/atrophy, attenuation of retinal arterioles, pigmentary retinopathy, scotoma, decreased visual acuity, nystagmus

Otic: Tinnitus, deafness

Miscellaneous: Exacerbation of porphyria and nonlight sensitive psoriasis

Drug Interactions

Increased Effect/Toxicity: Cimetidine increases levels of chloroquine and probably other 4-aminoquinolones.

Decreased Effect: Chloroquine and other 4-aminoquinolones absorption may be decreased due to GI binding with kaolin or magnesium trisilicate.

Dietary/Ethanol/Herb Considerations Ethanol: Avoid use due to GI irritation.

Pharmacodynamics/Kinetics

Onset of action: Rheumatic disease: May require 4-6 weeks to respond

Absorption: Complete

Protein binding: 55%

Metabolism: Hepatic

Half-life elimination: 32-50 days

Time to peak: Rheumatic disease: Several months

Excretion: Urine (as metabolites and unchanged drug); may be enhanced by urinary acidification

Pregnancy Risk Factor C

Generic Available Yes

Hydroxychloroquine Sulfate *see* Hydroxychloroquine *on page 694*

25-Hydroxycholecalciferol *see* Calcifediol *on page 221*

Hydroxydaunomycin Hydrochloride *see* DOXOrubicin *on page 473*

Hydroxyethylcellulose *see* Artificial Tears *on page 128*

Hydroxyethyl Starch *see* Hetastarch *on page 669*

Hydroxyldaunorubicin Hydrochloride *see* DOXOrubicin *on page 473*

Hydroxypropyl Cellulose (hye droks ee PROE pil SEL yoo lose)

Related Information

Hydroxypropyl Methylcellulose *on page 696*

U.S. Brand Names Lacrisert®

Canadian Brand Names Lacrisert®

Pharmacologic Category Ophthalmic Agent, Miscellaneous

Use Dry eyes (moderate to severe)

Local Anesthetic/Vasoconstrictor Precautions No information available to require special precautions

Effects on Dental Treatment No significant effects or complications reported

Dosage Adults: Ophthalmic: Apply once daily into the inferior cul-de-sac beneath the base of tarsus, not in apposition to the cornea nor beneath the eyelid at the level of the tarsal plate

Other Adverse Effects Frequency not defined:

Local: Irritation

Ocular: Blurred vision, edema of the eyelids

Generic Available No

Hydroxypropyl Methylcellulose

(hye droks ee PROE pil meth il SEL yoo lose)

Related Information

Hydroxypropyl Cellulose *on page 695*

U.S. Brand Names GenTeal® [OTC]; GenTeal® Mild [OTC]; Gonak™ [OTC]; Goniosol® [OTC]; Isopto® Tears [OTC]; Tearisol® [OTC]

Canadian Brand Names Genteal®; Isopto® Tears; Ocucoat®

Pharmacologic Category Ophthalmic Agent, Miscellaneous

Synonyms Gonioscopic Ophthalmic Solution

Use Ophthalmic surgical aid in cataract extraction and intraocular implantation; gonioscopic examinations

Local Anesthetic/Vasoconstrictor Precautions No information available to require special precautions

Effects on Dental Treatment No significant effects or complications reported

Dosage Introduced into anterior chamber of eye with 20-gauge or larger cannula

Other Adverse Effects Frequency not defined: Local: Irritation

Pregnancy Risk Factor C

Generic Available No

Hydroxyurea

(hye droks ee yoor EE a)

U.S. Brand Names Droxia™; Hydrea®; Mylocel™

Canadian Brand Names Gen-Hydroxyurea; Hydrea®

Mexican Brand Names Hydrea®

Pharmacologic Category Antineoplastic Agent, Antimetabolite

Synonyms Hydroxycarbamide

Use Treatment of CML in chronic phase; radiosensitizing agent in the treatment of primary brain tumors, head and neck tumors, uterine cervix and nonsmall cell lung cancer, and psoriasis; treatment of hematologic conditions such as essential thrombocythemia, polycythemia vera, hypereosinophilia, and hyperleukocytosis due to acute leukemia. Has shown activity against renal cell cancer, melanoma, ovarian cancer, head and neck cancer (excluding lip cancer), and prostate cancer.

Orphan drug (Droxia™): Sickle cell anemia: Specifically for patients >18 years of age who have had at least three "painful crises" in the previous year - to reduce frequency of these crises and the need for blood transfusions

Local Anesthetic/Vasoconstrictor Precautions No information available to require special precautions

Effects on Dental Treatment No significant effects or complications reported

Dosage All dosage should be based on ideal or actual body weight, whichever is less.

Oral (refer to individual protocols):

Children:

- No FDA-approved dosage regimens have been established; dosages of 1500-3000 mg/m² as a single dose in combination with other agents every 4-6 weeks have been used in the treatment of pediatric astrocytoma, medulloblastoma, and primitive neuroectodermal tumors
- CML: Initial: 10-20 mg/kg/day once daily; adjust dose according to hematologic response

Adults: Dose should always be titrated to patient response and WBC counts; usual oral doses range from 10-30 mg/kg/day or 500-3000 mg/day; if WBC count falls to <2500 cells/mm³, or the platelet count to <100,000/mm³, therapy should be stopped for at least 3 days and resumed when values rise toward normal

- Solid tumors:
  - Intermittent therapy: 80 mg/kg as a single dose every third day
  - Continuous therapy: 20-30 mg/kg/day given as a single dose/day
- Concomitant therapy with irradiation: 80 mg/kg as a single dose every third day starting at least 7 days before initiation of irradiation
- Resistant chronic myelocytic leukemia: Continuous therapy: 20-30 mg/kg as a single daily dose
- HIV: 1000-1500 mg daily in a single dose or divided doses
- Sickle cell anemia (moderate/severe disease): Initial: 15 mg/kg/day, increased by 5 mg/kg every 12 weeks if blood counts are in an acceptable range until the maximum tolerated dose of 35 mg/kg/day is achieved or the dose that does not produce toxic effects
  - *Acceptable range:*
    - Neutrophils ≥2500 cells/mm³
    - Platelets ≥95,000/mm³
    - Hemoglobin >5.3 g/dL, and
    - Reticulocytes ≥95,000/mm³ if the hemoglobin concentration is <9 g/dL
  - *Toxic range:*
    - Neutrophils <2000 cells/mm³
    - Platelets <80,000/mm³
    - Hemoglobin <4.5 g/dL
    - Reticulocytes <80,000/mm³ if the hemoglobin concentration is <9 g/dL

Monitor for toxicity every 2 weeks; if toxicity occurs, stop treatment until the bone marrow recovers; restart at 2.5 mg/kg/day less than the dose at which toxicity occurs; if no toxicity occurs over the next 12 weeks, then the subsequent dose should be increased by 2.5 mg/kg/day; reduced dosage of hydroxyurea alternating with erythropoietin may decrease myelotoxicity and increase levels of fetal hemoglobin in patients who have not been helped by hydroxyurea alone

Dosing adjustment in renal impairment:

Cl_{cr} 10-50 mL/minute: Administer 50% of normal dose

Cl_{cr} <10 mL/minute: Administer 20% of normal dose

Hemodialysis: Supplemental dose is unnecessary. Hydroxyurea is a low molecular weight compound with high aqueous solubility that may be freely dialyzable, however, clinical studies confirming this hypothesis have not been performed; peak serum concentrations are reached within 2 hours after oral administration and by 24 hours, the concentration in the serum is zero

CAPD effects: Unknown

CAVH effects: Dose for GFR 10-50 mL/minute

Mechanism of Action Thought to interfere (unsubstantiated hypothesis) with synthesis of DNA, during the S phase of cell division, without interfering with RNA synthesis; inhibits ribonucleoside diphosphate reductase, preventing conversion of ribonucleotides to deoxyribonucleotides; cell-cycle specific for the S phase and may hold other cells in the G_1 phase of the cell cycle.

Other Adverse Effects Frequency not defined:

Cardiovascular: Edema

Central nervous system: Drowsiness (with high doses), hallucinations, headache, dizziness, disorientation, **seizures**, fever, chills

Dermatologic: Erythema of the hands and face, maculopapular rash, pruritus, dry skin, dermatomyositis-like skin changes, hyperpigmentation, atrophy of skin and nails, scaling and violet papules (long-term use), nail banding, skin cancer

Endocrine & metabolic: Hyperuricemia

Gastrointestinal: Nausea, vomiting, stomatitis, anorexia, diarrhea, constipation, mucositis (potentiated in patients receiving radiation), pancreatitis, ulceration of buccal mucosa and GI epithelium (severe intoxication)

Emetic potential: Low (10% to 30%)

Genitourinary: Dysuria

Hematologic: Myelosuppression (primarily leukopenia); Dose-limiting toxicity, causes a rapid drop in leukocyte count (seen in 4-5 days in nonhematologic malignancy and more rapidly in leukemia); thrombocytopenia and anemia occur less often

Onset: 24-48 hours

Nadir: 10 days

Recovery: 7 days after stopping drug (reversal of WBC count occurs rapidly but the platelet count may take 7-10 days to recover)

Other hematologic effects include megaloblastic erythropoiesis, macrocytosis, hemolysis, decreased serum iron, persistent cytopenias, secondary leukemias (long-term use)

Hepatic: Elevation of hepatic enzymes, hepatotoxicity, hyperbilirubinemia (polycythemia vera)

Neuromuscular & skeletal: Weakness, peripheral neuropathy

Renal: Increased creatinine and BUN due to impairment of renal tubular function

Respiratory: Acute diffuse pulmonary infiltrates (rare), **dyspnea**, pulmonary fibrosis

Drug Interactions Increased Effect/Toxicity: Zidovudine, zalcitabine, didanosine may increase synergy. The potential for neurotoxicity may increase with concomitant administration with fluorouracil. Hydroxyurea modulates the metabolism and cytotoxicity of cytarabine; dose reduction is recommended. Hydroxyurea may precipitate didanosine- or stavudine-induced pancreatitis, hepatotoxicity, or neuropathy; concomitant use is not recommended.

Pharmacodynamics/Kinetics

Absorption: Readily (≥80%)

Distribution: Readily crosses blood-brain barrier; well into intestine, brain, lung, kidney tissues, effusions and ascites; enters breast milk

Metabolism: Hepatic and via GI tract; 50% degradation by enzymes of intestinal bacteria

Half-life elimination: 3-4 hours

Time to peak: ~2 hours

Excretion: Urine (80%, 50% as unchanged drug, 30% as urea); exhaled gases (as CO_2)

Pregnancy Risk Factor D

Generic Available Yes: Capsule

25-Hydroxyvitamin D_3 *see* Calcifediol *on page 221*

HydrOXYzine (hye DROKS i zeen)

Related Information

Patients Requiring Sedation *on page 1565*

U.S. Brand Names Atarax®; Vistaril®

(Continued)

HydrOXYzine *(Continued)*

Canadian Brand Names Apo®-Hydroxyzine; Atarax™; Novo-Hydroxyzin; PMS-Hydroxyzine; Vistaril®

Pharmacologic Category Antiemetic; Antihistamine

Synonyms Hydroxyzine Hydrochloride; Hydroxyzine Pamoate

Use Dental and Medical: Treatment of anxiety; preoperative sedative; antipruritic

Unlabeled/Investigational Use Antiemetic; treatment of ethanol withdrawal symptoms

Local Anesthetic/Vasoconstrictor Precautions No information available to require special precautions

Effects on Dental Treatment

1% to 10%: Xerostomia

Frequency not defined: Drowsiness, headache, fatigue, nervousness, dizziness, tremors, paresthesia, seizure, blurred vision, thickening of bronchial secretions

Dosage

Children:

Oral: 0.6 mg/kg/dose every 6 hours

I.M.: 0.5-1.1 mg/kg/dose every 4-6 hours as needed

Adults:

Antiemetic: I.M.: 25-100 mg/dose every 4-6 hours as needed

Anxiety: Oral: 25-100 mg 4 times/day; maximum dose: 600 mg/day

Preoperative sedation:

Oral: 50-100 mg

I.M.: 25-100 mg

Management of pruritus: Oral: 25 mg 3-4 times/day

Dosing interval in hepatic impairment: Change dosing interval to every 24 hours in patients with primary biliary cirrhosis

Mechanism of Action Competes with histamine for H_1-receptor sites on effector cells in the gastrointestinal tract, blood vessels, and respiratory tract. Possesses skeletal muscle relaxing, bronchodilator, antihistamine, antiemetic, and analgesic properties.

Contraindications Hypersensitivity to hydroxyzine or any component of the formulation

Warnings/Precautions Causes sedation, caution must be used in performing tasks which require alertness (ie, operating machinery or driving). Sedative effects of CNS depressants or ethanol are potentiated. S.C., intra-arterial, and I.V. administration are not recommended since thrombosis and digital gangrene can occur; extravasation can result in sterile abscess and marked tissue induration; should be used with caution in patients with narrow-angle glaucoma, prostatic hyperplasia, and bladder neck obstruction; should also be used with caution in patients with asthma or COPD.

Anticholinergic effects are not well tolerated in the elderly. Hydroxyzine may be useful as a short-term antipruritic, but it is not recommended for use as a sedative or anxiolytic in the elderly.

Drug Interactions Inhibits CYP2D6

Amantadine, rimantadine: Central and/or peripheral anticholinergic syndrome can occur when administered with amantadine or rimantadine

Anticholinergic agents: Central and/or peripheral anticholinergic syndrome can occur when administered with narcotic analgesics, phenothiazines and other antipsychotics (especially with high anticholinergic activity), tricyclic antidepressants, quinidine and some other antiarrhythmics, and antihistamines

Antipsychotics: Hydroxyzine may antagonize the therapeutic effects of antipsychotics

CNS depressants: Sedative effects of hydroxyzine may be additive with CNS depressants; includes ethanol, benzodiazepines, barbiturates, narcotic analgesics, and other sedative agents; monitor for increased effect

Dietary/Ethanol/Herb Considerations

Ethanol: Avoid use; may increase CNS depression.

Herb/Nutraceutical: Avoid gotu kola, kava, SAMe, St John's wort, and valerian; may increase CNS depression.

Pharmacodynamics/Kinetics

Onset of action: 15-30 minutes

Duration: 4-6 hours

Absorption: Oral: Rapid

Metabolism: Exact fate unknown

Half-life elimination: 3-7 hours

Time to peak: ~2 hours

Pregnancy Risk Factor C

Dosage Forms CAP, as pamoate (Vistaril®): 25 mg, 50 mg, 100 mg. **INJ, solution**, as hydrochloride: 25 mg/mL (1 mL); 50 mg/mL (1 mL, 2 mL, 10 mL); (Vistaril®): 50 mg/mL (10 mL). **SUSP, oral**, as pamoate (Vistaril®): 25 mg/5 mL (120 mL, 480 mL). **SYR**, as hydrochloride: 10 mg/5 mL (120 mL, 480 mL, 4000 mL); (Atarax®): 10 mg/5 mL (480 mL). **TAB**, as hydrochloride: 10 mg, 25 mg, 50 mg; (Atarax®): 10 mg, 25 mg, 50 mg, 100 mg

Generic Available Yes

Hydroxyzine Hydrochloride *see* HydrOXYzine *on page 697*

Hydroxyzine Pamoate *see* HydrOXYzine *on page 697*

Hygroton® [DSC] *see* Chlorthalidone *on page 315*

Hylorel® *see* Guanadrel *on page 654*

Hyoscine *see* Scopolamine *on page 1210*

Hyoscyamine (hye oh SYE a meen)

U.S. Brand Names Anaspaz®; Cystospaz®; Cystospaz-M®; Hyosine; Levbid®; Levsin®; Levsinex®; Levsin/SL®; NuLev™; Spacol; Spacol T/S; Symax SL; Symax SR

Canadian Brand Names Cystospaz®; Levsin®

Pharmacologic Category Anticholinergic Agent

Synonyms Hyoscyamine Sulfate; *l*-Hyoscyamine Sulfate

Use

Oral: Adjunctive therapy for peptic ulcers, irritable bowel, neurogenic bladder/bowel; treatment of infant colic, GI tract disorders caused by spasm; to reduce rigidity, tremors, sialorrhea, and hyperhidrosis associated with parkinsonism; as a drying agent in acute rhinitis

Injection: Preoperative antimuscarinic to reduce secretions and block cardiac vagal inhibitory reflexes; to improve radiologic visibility of the kidneys; symptomatic relief of biliary and renal colic; reduce GI motility to facilitate diagnostic procedures (ie, endoscopy, hypotonic duodenography); reduce pain and hypersecretion in pancreatitis, certain cases of partial heart block associated with vagal activity; reversal of neuromuscular blockade

Local Anesthetic/Vasoconstrictor Precautions No information available to require special precautions

Effects on Dental Treatment >10%: Xerostomia; normal salivary flow resumes upon discontinuation

Dosage

Oral: Children: Gastrointestinal disorders: Dose as listed, based on age and weight (kg) using 0.125 mg/mL drops; repeat dose every 4 hours as needed:

Children <2 years:

3.4 kg: 4 drops; maximum: 24 drops/24 hours

5 kg: 5 drops; maximum: 30 drops/24 hours

7 kg: 6 drops; maximum: 36 drops/24 hours

10 kg: 8 drops; maximum: 48 drops/24 hours

Oral, S.L.:

Children 2-12 years: Gastrointestinal disorders: Dose as listed, based on age and weight (kg); repeat dose every 4 hours as needed:

10 kg: 0.031-0.033 mg; maximum: 0.75 mg/24 hours

20 kg: 0.0625 mg; maximum: 0.75 mg/24 hours

40 kg: 0.0938 mg; maximum: 0.75 mg/24 hours

50 kg: 0.125 mg; maximum: 0.75 mg/24 hours

Children >12 years and Adults: Gastrointestinal disorders: 0.125-0.25 mg every 4 hours or as needed (before meals or food); maximum: 1.5 mg/24 hours

Cystospaz®: 0.15-0.3 mg up to 4 times/day

Oral (timed release): Children >12 years and Adults: Gastrointestinal disorders: 0.375-0.75 mg every 12 hours; maximum: 1.5 mg/24 hours

I.M., I.V., S.C.: Children >12 years and Adults: Gastrointestinal disorders: 0.25-0.5 mg; may repeat as needed up to 4 times/day, at 4-hour intervals

I.V.: Children >2 year and Adults: I.V.: Preanesthesia: 5 mcg/kg given 30-60 minutes prior to induction of anesthesia or at the time preoperative narcotics or sedatives are administered

I.V.: Adults: Diagnostic procedures: 0.25-0.5 mg given 5-10 minutes prior to procedure

To reduce drug-induced bradycardia during surgery: 0.125 mg; repeat as needed

To reverse neuromuscular blockade: 0.2 mg for every 1 mg neostigmine (or the physostigmine/pyridostigmine equivalent)

Mechanism of Action Blocks the action of acetylcholine at parasympathetic sites in smooth muscle, secretory glands and the CNS; increases cardiac output, dries secretions, antagonizes histamine and serotonin

Other Adverse Effects Frequency not defined:

Cardiovascular: **Palpitations, tachycardia**

Central nervous system: Ataxia, dizziness, drowsiness, headache, insomnia, mental confusion/excitement, nervousness, speech disorder, weakness

Dermatologic: Urticaria

Endocrine & metabolic: Lactation suppression

Gastrointestinal: Bloating, constipation, **loss of taste**, nausea, vomiting

Genitourinary: Impotence, urinary hesitancy, urinary retention

Ocular: Blurred vision, cycloplegia, increased ocular tension, mydriasis

Miscellaneous: Allergic reactions, sweating decreased

(Continued)

Hyoscyamine *(Continued)*

Drug Interactions

Increased toxicity with amantadine, antihistamines, antimuscarinics, haloperidol, phenothiazines, tricyclic antidepressants, and MAO inhibitors.

Decreased effect with antacids.

Pharmacodynamics/Kinetics

Onset of action: 2-3 minutes
Duration: 4-6 hours
Absorption: Well absorbed
Distribution: Crosses placenta; small amounts enter breast milk
Protein binding: 50%
Metabolism: Hepatic
Half-life elimination: 3-5 hours
Excretion: Urine

Pregnancy Risk Factor C

Generic Available Yes

Hyoscyamine, Atropine, Scopolamine, and Phenobarbital

(hye oh SYE a meen, A troe peen, skoe POL a meen & fee noe BAR bi tal)

Related Information

Atropine *on page 144*
Hyoscyamine *on page 699*
Phenobarbital *on page 1066*
Scopolamine *on page 1210*

U.S. Brand Names Donnatal® [DSC]

Canadian Brand Names Donnatal®

Pharmacologic Category Anticholinergic Agent; Antispasmodic Agent, Gastrointestinal

Synonyms Atropine, Hyoscyamine, Scopolamine, and Phenobarbital; Donnatal® [DSC]; Phenobarbital, Hyoscyamine, Atropine, and Scopolamine; Scopolamine, Hyoscyamine, Atropine, and Phenobarbital

Use Adjunct in treatment of peptic ulcer disease, irritable bowel, spastic colitis, spastic bladder, and renal colic

Local Anesthetic/Vasoconstrictor Precautions No information available to require special precautions

Effects on Dental Treatment >10%: Xerostomia, dry throat; normal salivary flow resumes upon discontinuation

Dosage Oral:

Children 2-12 years: Kinesed® dose: ½ to 1 tablet 3-4 times/day

Children: Donnatal® elixir: 0.1 mL/kg/dose every 4 hours; maximum dose: 5 mL **OR** alternatively, dose (mL) based on weight (kg):
- 4.5 kg: 0.5 mL every 4 hours OR 0.75 mL every 6 hours
- 10 kg: 1 mL every 4 hours OR 1.5 mL every 6 hours
- 14 kg: 1.5 mL every 4 hours OR 2 mL every 6 hours
- 23 kg: 2.5 mL every 4 hours OR 3.8 mL every 6 hours
- 34 kg: 3.8 mL every 4 hours OR 5 mL every 6 hours
- ≥45 kg: 5 mL every 4 hours OR 7.5 mL every 6 hours

Adults: 1-2 capsules or tablets 3-4 times/day; or 1 Donnatal® Extentab® in sustained release form every 12 hours; or 5-10 mL elixir 3-4 times/day or every 8 hours

Mechanism of Action See individual agents.

Other Adverse Effects

>10%:
- Dermatologic: Dry skin
- Gastrointestinal: Constipation
- Local: Irritation at injection site
- Respiratory: Dry nose
- Miscellaneous: Diaphoresis (decreased)

1% to 10%:
- Dermatologic: Increased sensitivity to light
- Endocrine & metabolic: Decreased flow of breast milk
- Gastrointestinal: Dysphagia

<1%: **Orthostatic hypotension, ventricular fibrillation, tachycardia, palpitations**, confusion, drowsiness, headache, loss of memory, fatigue, ataxia, rash, bloated feeling, nausea, vomiting, dysuria, increased intraocular pain, blurred vision

Drug Interactions Phenobarbital: Substrate of CYP2C8/9, **2C19**, 2E1; Induces **CYP1A2, 2A6, 2B6, 2C8/9, 3A4**

Increased Effect/Toxicity: Toxicity of CNS depressants, coumarin anticoagulants, amantadine, antihistamine, phenothiazides, antidiarrheal suspensions, corticosteroids, digitalis, griseofulvin, tetracyclines, anticonvulsants, MAO inhibitors, and tricyclic antidepressants may be increased.

Pharmacodynamics/Kinetics Absorption: Well absorbed

Pregnancy Risk Factor C
Generic Available No

Hyoscyamine, Atropine, Scopolamine, Kaolin, and Pectin

(hye oh SYE a meen, A troe peen, skoe POL a meen, KAY oh lin & PEK tin)

Related Information
Atropine *on page 144*
Hyoscyamine *on page 699*
Kaolin and Pectin *on page 760*
Scopolamine *on page 1210*

Pharmacologic Category Anticholinergic Agent; Antidiarrheal

Use Antidiarrheal; also used in gastritis, enteritis, colitis, and acute GI upsets, and nausea which may accompany any of these conditions

Local Anesthetic/Vasoconstrictor Precautions No information available to require special precautions

Effects on Dental Treatment >10%: Xerostomia; normal salivary flow resumes upon discontinuation

Dosage Oral:
Children:
- 10-20 lb: 2.5 mL
- 20-30 lb: 5 mL
- >30 lb: 5-10 mL

Adults:
- Diarrhea: 30 mL at once and 15-30 mL with each loose stool
- Other conditions: 15 mL every 3 hours as needed

Pregnancy Risk Factor C
Generic Available Yes

Hyoscyamine, Atropine, Scopolamine, Kaolin, Pectin, and Opium

(hye oh SYE a meen, A troe peen, skoe POL a meen, KAY oh lin, PEK tin, & OH pee um)

Related Information
Atropine *on page 144*
Hyoscyamine *on page 699*
Kaolin and Pectin *on page 760*
Opium Tincture *on page 1002*
Scopolamine *on page 1210*

U.S. Brand Names Donnapectolin-PG®; Kapectolin PG®

Pharmacologic Category Anticholinergic Agent; Antidiarrheal

Use Treatment of diarrhea

Local Anesthetic/Vasoconstrictor Precautions No information available to require special precautions

Effects on Dental Treatment >10%: Xerostomia; normal salivary flow resumes upon discontinuation

Restrictions C-V

Dosage Oral:
Children 6-12 years: Initial: 10 mL, then, 5-10 mL every 3 hours thereafter
- Alternate children's dosing recommendations based on body weight:
  - 10 lb: 2.5 mL
  - 20 lb: 5 mL
  - ≥30 lb: 5-10 mL
- Do not administer more than 4 doses in any 24-hour period

Children >12 years and Adults: Initial: 30 mL (1 fluid oz) followed by 15 mL every 3 hours

Pregnancy Risk Factor C
Generic Available Yes
Comments Hyoscyamine is dialyzable

Hyoscyamine, Methenamine, Sodium Biphosphate, Phenyl Salicylate, and Methylene Blue *see* Methenamine, Sodium Biphosphate, Phenyl Salicylate, Methylene Blue, and Hyoscyamine *on page 880*
Hyoscyamine Sulfate *see* Hyoscyamine *on page 699*
Hyosine *see* Hyoscyamine *on page 699*
Hyperstat® *see* Diazoxide *on page 427*
HypoTears [OTC] *see* Artificial Tears *on page 128*
HypoTears PF [OTC] *see* Artificial Tears *on page 128*
Hyrexin-50® *see* DiphenhydrAMINE *on page 451*
Hytakerol® *see* Dihydrotachysterol *on page 446*
Hytinic® [OTC] *see* Polysaccharide-Iron Complex *on page 1096*
Hytone® *see* Hydrocortisone *on page 688*
Hytrin® *see* Terazosin *on page 1276*

Hytuss® [OTC] *see* Guaifenesin *on page 650*
Hytuss-2X® [OTC] *see* Guaifenesin *on page 650*
Hyzaar® *see* Losartan and Hydrochlorothiazide *on page 827*
Iberet® [OTC] *see* Vitamins (Multiple/Oral) *on page 1394*
Iberet®-500 [OTC] *see* Vitamins (Multiple/Oral) *on page 1394*
Iberet-Folic-500® *see* Vitamins (Multiple/Oral) *on page 1394*
Ibidomide Hydrochloride *see* Labetalol *on page 769*

Ibritumomab (ib ri TYOO mo mab)

U.S. Brand Names Zevalin™

Pharmacologic Category Antineoplastic Agent, Monoclonal Antibody; Radiopharmaceutical

Synonyms Ibritumomab Tiuxetan; In-111 Zevalin; Y-90 Zevalin

Use Treatment of relapsed or refractory low-grade, follicular, or transformed B-cell non-Hodgkin's lymphoma (including rituximab-refractory follicular non-Hodgkin's lymphoma) as part of a therapeutic regimen with rituximab (Zevalin™ therapeutic regimen); **not to be used as single-agent therapy**; must be radiolabeled prior to use

Local Anesthetic/Vasoconstrictor Precautions No information available to require special precautions

Effects on Dental Treatment 1% to 10%: Hypotension (6%), flushing (6%), cough (10%), throat irritation (10%), rhinitis (6%), bronchospasm (5%), epistaxis (3%), apnea (1%)

Dosage I.V.: Adults: Ibritumomab is administered **only** as part of the Zevalin™ therapeutic regimen (a combined treatment regimen with rituximab). The regimen consists of two steps:

Step 1:

Rituximab infusion: 250 mg/m² at an initial rate of 50 mg/hour. If hypersensitivity or infusion-related events do not occur, increase infusion in increments of 50 mg/hour every 30 minutes, to a maximum of 400 mg/hour. Infusions should be temporarily slowed or interrupted if hypersensitivity or infusion-related events occur. The infusion may be resumed at one-half the previous rate upon improvement of symptoms.

In-111 ibritumomab infusion: Within 4 hours of the completion of rituximab infusion, inject 5 mCi (1.6 mg total antibody dose) over 10 minutes.

Biodistribution of In-111 ibritumomab should be assessed by imaging at 2-24 hours and at 48-72 hours postinjection. An optional third imaging may be performed 90-120 hours following injection. If biodistribution is not acceptable, the patient should not proceed to Step 2.

Step 2 (initiated 7-9 days following Step 1):

Rituximab infusion: 250 mg/m² at an initial rate of 100 mg/hour (50 mg/hour if infusion-related events occurred with the first infusion). If hypersensitivity or infusion-related events do not occur, increase infusion in increments of 100 mg/hour every 30 minutes, to a maximum of 400 mg/hour, as tolerated.

Y-90 ibritumomab infusion: Within 4 hours of the completion of rituximab infusion:

Platelet count >150,000 cells/mm³: Inject 4 mCi (14.8 MBq/kg actual body weight) over 10 minutes

Platelet count between 100,000-149,000 cells/mm³: Inject 3 mCi (11.1 MBq/kg actual body weight) over 10 minutes

Platelet count <100,000 cells/mm³: Do **not** administer

Maximum dose: The prescribed, measured, and administered dose of Y-90 ibritumomab must not exceed 32 mCi (1184 MBq), regardless of the patient's body weight

Mechanism of Action Ibritumomab is a monoclonal antibody directed against the CD20 antigen found on B lymphocytes (normal and malignant). Ibritumomab binding induces apoptosis in B lymphocytes *in vitro*. It is combined with the chelator tiuxetan, which acts as a specific chelation site for either Indium-111 (In-111) or Yttrium-90 (Y-90). The monoclonal antibody acts as a delivery system to direct the radioactive isotope to the targeted cells, however, binding has been observed in lymphoid cells throughout the body and in lymphoid nodules in organs such as the large and small intestines. Indium-111 is a gamma-emitter used to assess biodistribution of ibritumomab, while Y-90 emits beta particles. Beta-emission induces cellular damage through the formation of free radicals (in both target cells and surrounding cells).

Other Adverse Effects Severe, potentially life-threatening allergic reactions have occurred in association with infusions.

>10%:

Central nervous system: Chills (24%), fever (17%), pain (13%), headache (12%)
Gastrointestinal: Nausea (31%), abdominal pain (16%), vomiting (12%)
Hematologic: Thrombocytopenia (95%), neutropenia (77%), anemia (61%)
Myelosuppressive:
WBC: Severe
Platelets: Severe

Nadir: 7-9 weeks
Recovery: 22-35 days
Neuromuscular & skeletal: Weakness (43%)
Respiratory: Dyspnea (14%)
Miscellaneous: Infection (29%)

1% to 10%:
Cardiovascular: Peripheral edema (8%), angioedema (5%)
Central nervous system: Dizziness (10%), insomnia (5%), anxiety (4%)
Dermatologic: Pruritus (9%), rash (8%), urticaria (4%), petechia (3%)
Gastrointestinal: Diarrhea (9%), anorexia (8%), abdominal distension (5%), constipation (5%), dyspepsia (4%), melena (2%; life threatening in 1%), gastrointestinal hemorrhage (1%)
Hematologic: Bruising (7%), pancytopenia (2%), secondary malignancies (2%)
Neuromuscular & skeletal: Back pain (8%), arthralgia (7%), myalgia (7%)
Miscellaneous: Diaphoresis (4%), allergic reaction (2%; life-threatening in 1%)

<1%: Arthritis, encephalopathy, hematemesis, pulmonary edema, pulmonary embolism, stroke (hemorrhagic), subdural hematoma, tachycardia, urticaria, vaginal hemorrhage. Myeloid malignancies and dysplasia have also been reported in patients who had received treatment with ibritumomab.

Drug Interactions

Increased Effect/Toxicity: Due to the high incidence of thrombocytopenia associated with ibritumomab, the use of agents which decrease platelet function may be associated with a higher risk of bleeding (includes aspirin, NSAIDs, glycoprotein IIb/IIIa antagonists, clopidogrel and ticlopidine). In addition, the risk of bleeding may be increased with anticoagulant agents, including heparin, low molecular weight heparins, thrombolytics, and warfarin. The safety of live viral vaccines has not been established.

Decreased Effect: Response to vaccination may be impaired.

Dietary/Ethanol/Herb Considerations

Food: Avoid garlic, ginger, and green tea.

Herb/Nutraceutical: Avoid cat's claw, dong quai, evening primrose, feverfew, garlic, ginger, ginkgo biloba, ginseng, green tea, horse chestnut, and red clover due to antiplatelet activity.

Pharmacodynamics/Kinetics

Duration: Beta cell recovery begins in ~12 weeks; generally in normal range within 9 months

Distribution: To lymphoid cells throughout the body and in lymphoid nodules in organs such as the large and small intestines, spleen, testes, and liver

Metabolism: Has not been characterized; the product of yttrium-90 radioactive decay is zirconium-90 (nonradioactive); Indium-111 decays to cadmium-111 (nonradioactive)

Half-life elimination: Y-90 ibritumomab: 30 hours; Indium-111 decays with a physical half-life of 67 hours; Yttrium-90 decays with a physical half-life of 64 hours

Excretion: A median of 7.2% of the radiolabeled activity was excreted in urine over 7 days

Pregnancy Risk Factor D

Generic Available No

Ibritumomab Tiuxetan *see* Ibritumomab *on page 702*

Ibuprofen (eye byoo PROE fen)

Related Information

Oral Pain *on page 1524*
Rheumatoid Arthritis, Osteoarthritis, and Osteoporosis *on page 1488*
Temporomandibular Dysfunction (TMD) *on page 1562*

U.S. Brand Names Advil® [OTC]; Advil® Children's [OTC]; Advil® Infants' Concentrated Drops [OTC]; Advil® Junior [OTC]; Advil® Migraine [OTC]; Genpril® [OTC]; Haltran® [OTC]; Ibu-Tab®; I-Prin [OTC]; Menadol® [OTC]; Midol® Maximum Strength Cramp Formula [OTC]; Motrin®; Motrin® Children's [OTC]; Motrin® IB [OTC]; Motrin® Infants' [OTC]; Motrin® Junior Strength [OTC]; Motrin® Migraine Pain [OTC]

Canadian Brand Names Advil®; Apo®-Ibuprofen; Motrin®; Motrin® (Children's); Motrin® IB; Novo-Profen®; Nu-Ibuprofen

Mexican Brand Names Advil®; Algidol®; Butacortelone; Citalgan®; Days®; Dibufen®; Diprodol®; Flexafen®; Kedvil; Motrin®; Proartinal®; Quadrax®; Tabalon®

Pharmacologic Category Nonsteroidal Anti-inflammatory Drug (NSAID)

Synonyms *p*-Isobutylhydratropic Acid

Use

Dental: Management of pain and swelling

Medical: Inflammatory diseases and rheumatoid disorders including juvenile rheumatoid arthritis, mild to moderate pain, fever, dysmenorrhea, gout, ankylosing spondylitis, acute migraine headache

Unlabeled/Investigational Use Treatment of cystic fibrosis

Local Anesthetic/Vasoconstrictor Precautions No information available to require special precautions

(Continued)

Ibuprofen *(Continued)*

Effects on Dental Treatment NSAID formulations are known to reversibly decrease platelet aggregation via mechanisms different than observed with aspirin. The dentist should be aware of the potential of abnormal coagulation. Caution should also be exercised in the use of NSAIDs in patients already on anticoagulant therapy with drugs such as warfarin (Coumadin®).

1% to 10%: Headache (1% to 3%), nervousness (<3%), fatigue (<3%), vomiting (1% to 3%), abdominal pain/cramps/distress (1% to 3%), peptic ulcer, GI bleeding or perforation, nausea (3% to 9%)

Dosage Oral:

Children:

Analgesic: 4-10 mg/kg/dose every 6-8 hours

Antipyretic: 6 months to 12 years: Temperature <102.5°F (39°C): 5 mg/kg/dose; temperature >102.5°F: 10 mg/kg/dose given every 6-8 hours; maximum daily dose: 40 mg/kg/day

Juvenile rheumatoid arthritis: 30-70 mg/kg/24 hours divided every 6-8 hours

<20 kg: Maximum: 400 mg/day

20-30 kg: Maximum: 600 mg/day

30-40 kg: Maximum: 800 mg/day

>40 kg: Use adult dosage

Start at lower end of dosing range and titrate upward; maximum: 2.4 g/day

Adults:

Inflammatory disease: 400-800 mg/dose 3-4 times/day; maximum dose: 3.2 g/day

Analgesia, treatment of fever or dysmenorrhea: 200-400 mg/dose every 4-6 hours; maximum daily dose: 1.2 g (unless directed by physician)

Dosing comment in severe hepatic impairment: Avoid use

Mechanism of Action Inhibits prostaglandin synthesis by decreasing the activity of the enzyme, cyclooxygenase, which results in decreased formation of prostaglandin precursors

Other Adverse Effects

1% to 9%:

Dermatologic: Itching (1% to 3%), rash (3% to 9%), urticaria

Endocrine & metabolic: Fluid retention

Gastrointestinal: Dyspepsia (1% to 3%), heartburn, diarrhea (1% to 3%), constipation (1% to 3%), flatulence (1% to 3%), indigestion (1% to 3%)

Otic: Tinnitus

<1%: Edema, **CHF, arrhythmias, tachycardia, hypertension, confusion, hallucinations,** mental depression, **drowsiness,** insomnia, aseptic meningitis, erythema multiforme, toxic epidermal necrolysis, Stevens-Johnson syndrome, polydipsia, **hot flashes, gastritis, GI ulceration,** cystitis, polyuria, neutropenia, anemia, agranulocytosis, **inhibition of platelet aggregation,** hemolytic anemia, bone marrow suppression, leukopenia, thrombocytopenia, hepatitis, peripheral neuropathy, **vision changes, blurred vision,** conjunctivitis, dry eyes, toxic amblyopia, decreased hearing, acute renal failure, **allergic rhinitis, dyspnea, epistaxis, xerostomia**

Contraindications Hypersensitivity to ibuprofen, any component of the formulation, aspirin, or other NSAIDs; patients with "aspirin triad" (bronchial asthma, aspirin intolerance, rhinitis); pregnancy (3rd trimester)

Warnings/Precautions Use with caution in patients with CHF, hypertension, dehydration, decreased renal or hepatic function, history of GI disease (bleeding or ulcers), or those receiving anticoagulants. Elderly are at a high risk for adverse effects from NSAIDs. As many as 60% of elderly can develop peptic ulceration and/or hemorrhage asymptomatically. Fatal asthmatic and anaphylactoid reactions have occurred in patients with "aspirin triad" (see Contraindications).

Use lowest effective dose for shortest period possible. Use of NSAIDs can compromise existing renal function especially when Cl_{cr} is <30 mL/minute. CNS adverse effects such as confusion, agitation, and hallucination are generally seen in overdose or high-dose situations; however, elderly may demonstrate these adverse effects at lower doses than younger adults. Do not exceed 3200 mg/day. Withhold for at least 4-6 half-lives prior to surgical or dental procedures.

Drug Interactions Substrate of CYP2C8/9, 2C19; Inhibits CYP2C8/9

ACE inhibitors: Antihypertensive effects may be decreased by concurrent therapy with NSAIDs; monitor blood pressure.

Angiotensin II antagonists: Antihypertensive effects may be decreased by concurrent therapy with NSAIDs; monitor blood pressure.

Anticoagulants (warfarin, heparin, LMWHs) in combination with NSAIDs can cause increased risk of bleeding.

Antiplatelet drugs (ticlopidine, clopidogrel, aspirin, abciximab, dipyridamole, eptifibatide, tirofiban) can cause an increased risk of bleeding.

Corticosteroids: May increase the risk of GI ulceration; avoid concurrent use

Cyclosporine: NSAIDs may increase serum creatinine, potassium, blood pressure, and cyclosporine levels; monitor cyclosporine levels and renal function carefully.

Hydralazine's antihypertensive effect is decreased; avoid concurrent use

Lithium levels can be increased; avoid concurrent use if possible or monitor lithium levels and adjust dose. Sulindac may have the least effect. When NSAID is stopped, lithium will need adjustment again.

Loop diuretics efficacy (diuretic and antihypertensive effect) is reduced. Indomethacin reduces this efficacy, however, it may be anticipated with any NSAID.

Methotrexate: Severe bone marrow suppression, aplastic anemia, and GI toxicity have been reported with concomitant NSAID therapy. Avoid use during moderate or high-dose methotrexate (increased and prolonged methotrexate levels). NSAID use during low-dose treatment of rheumatoid arthritis has not been fully evaluated; extreme caution is warranted.

Warfarin's INRs may be increased by piroxicam. Other NSAIDs may have the same effect depending on dose and duration. Monitor INR closely. Use the lowest dose of NSAIDs possible and for the briefest duration. May alter the anticoagulant effects of warfarin; concurrent use with other antiplatelet agents or anticoagulants may increase risk of bleeding.

Dietary/Ethanol/Herb Considerations

Ethanol: Avoid use; may enhance gastric mucosal irritation.

Food: Administer with with food or milk to reduce GI upset. Food decreases rate of absorption but not extent; may decrease ibuprofen peak serum concentration. Limit salicylate-containing foods (curry powder, prunes, raisins, tea, or licorice); avoid excessive amounts of vitamin C. Avoid garlic, ginger, and green tea.

Herb/Nutraceutical: Avoid cat's claw, dong quai, evening primrose, feverfew, garlic, ginger, ginkgo biloba, ginseng, green tea, horse chestnut, and red clover due to additional antiplatelet activity. Avoid kava and valerian; may enhance benzodiazepine activity.

Pharmacodynamics/Kinetics

Onset of action: Analgesic: 30-60 minutes; Anti-inflammatory: ≤7 days

Peak effect: 1-2 weeks

Duration: 4-6 hours

Absorption: Oral: Rapid (85%)

Protein binding: 90% to 99%

Metabolism: Hepatic via oxidation

Half-life elimination: 2-4 hours; End-stage renal disease: Unchanged

Time to peak: ~1-2 hours

Excretion: Urine (1% as free drug); some feces

Pregnancy Risk Factor B/D (3rd trimester)

Breast-feeding Considerations Limited data suggests minimal excretion in breast milk.

Dosage Forms CAPLET 200 mg [OTC]; (Motrin® Junior Strength): 100 mg; (Advil®, Menadol®, Motrin® IB, Motrin® Migraine Pain): 200 mg. **CAP, liqui-gel** (Advil®, Advil® Migraine): 200 mg. **GELCAP** (Advil®, Motrin® IB): 200 mg. **SUSP, oral:** 100 mg/5 mL (5 mL, 120 mL, 480 mL); (Advil® Children's, Motrin® Children's): 100 mg/5 mL (60 mL, 120 mL). **SUSP, oral drops** (Advil® Infants' Concentrated Drops, Motrin® Infants'): 40 mg/mL (15 mL). **TAB:** 200 mg [OTC], 400 mg, 600 mg, 800 mg; (Advil® Junior): 100 mg; (Advil®, Genpril®, Haltran®, I-Prin, Midol®, Maximum Strength Cramp Formula, Motrin® IB): 200 mg; (Ibu-Tab®, Motrin®): 400 mg, 600 mg, 800 mg. **TAB, chewable** (Advil® Children's, Motrin® Children's): 50 mg; (Advil® Junior, Motrin® Junior Strength): 100 mg.

Generic Available Yes: Caplet, suspension, tablet

Comments Preoperative use of ibuprofen at a dose of 400-600 mg every 6 hours 24 hours before the appointment decreases postoperative edema and hastens healing time.

Selected Readings

Ahmad N, Grad HA, Haas DA, et al, "The Efficacy of Nonopioid Analgesics for Postoperative Dental Pain: A Meta-Analysis," *Anesth Prog*, 1997, 44(4):119-26.

Brooks PM and Day RO, "Nonsteroidal Anti-inflammatory Drugs - Differences and Similarities," *N Engl J Med*, 1991, 324(24):1716-25.

Dionne R, "Additive Analgesia Without Opioid Side Effects," *Compend Contin Educ Dent*, 2000, 21(7):572-4, 576-7.

Dionne RA, "New Approaches to Preventing and Treating Postoperative Pain," *J Am Dent Assoc*, 1992, 123(6):26-34.

Dionne RA and Berthold CW, "Therapeutic Uses of Nonsteroidal Anti-Inflammatory Drugs in Dentistry," *Crit Rev Oral Biol Med*, 2001, 12(4):315-30.

Gobetti JP, "Controlling Dental Pain," *J Am Dent Assoc*, 1992, 123(6):47-52.

Hersh EV, Levin LM, Cooper SA, et al, "Ibuprofen Liquigel for Oral Surgery Pain," *Clin Ther*, 2000, 22(11):1306-18.

Pearlman B, Boyatzis S, Daly C, et al, "The Analgesic Efficacy of Ibuprofen in Periodontal Surgery: A Multicentre Study," *Aust Dent J*, 1997, 42(5):328-34.

Winter L Jr, Bass E, Recant B, et al, "Analgesic Activity of Ibuprofen (Motrin®) in Postoperative Oral Surgical Pain," *Oral Surg Oral Med Oral Pathol*, 1978, 45(2):159-66.

Wynn RL, "NSAIDS and Cardiovascular Effects, Celecoxib for Dental Pain, and a New Analgesic - Tramadol with Acetaminophen," *Gen Dent*, 2002, 50(3):218-222.

Nguyen AM, Graham DY, Gage T, et al, "Nonsteroidal Anti-Inflammatory Drug Use in Dentistry: Gastrointestinal Implications," *Gen Dent*, 1999, 47(6):590-6.

Ibuprofen and Hydrocodone *see* Hydrocodone and Ibuprofen *on page 684*

Ibuprofen and Pseudoephedrine *see* Pseudoephedrine and Ibuprofen *on page 1148*

Ibu-Tab® *see* Ibuprofen *on page 703*

Ibutilide (i BYOO ti lide)

U.S. Brand Names Corvert®

Pharmacologic Category Antiarrhythmic Agent, Class III

Synonyms Ibutilide Fumarate

Use Acute termination of atrial fibrillation or flutter of recent onset; the effectiveness of ibutilide has not been determined in patients with arrhythmias >90 days in duration

Local Anesthetic/Vasoconstrictor Precautions No information available to require special precautions

Effects on Dental Treatment No significant effects or complications reported

Dosage I.V.: Initial:

Adults:

<60 kg: 0.01 mg/kg over 10 minutes

≥60 kg: 1 mg over 10 minutes

If the arrhythmia does not terminate within 10 minutes after the end of the initial infusion, a second infusion of equal strength may be infused over a 10-minute period

Elderly: Dose selection should be cautious, usually starting at the lower end of the dosing range.

Mechanism of Action Exact mechanism of action is unknown; prolongs the action potential in cardiac tissue

Other Adverse Effects

1% to 10%:

Cardiovascular: Sustained polymorphic ventricular tachycardia (ie, torsade de pointes) (1.7%, often requiring cardioversion), nonsustained polymorphic ventricular tachycardia (2.7%), nonsustained monomorphic ventricular tachycardia (4.9%), ventricular extrasystoles (5.1%), nonsustained monomorphic VT (4.9%), tachycardia/supraventricular tachycardia (2.7%), hypotension (2%), bundle branch block (1.9%), AV block (1.5%), bradycardia (1.2%), QT segment prolongation, hypertension (1.2%), palpitations (1%)

Central nervous system: Headache (3.6%)

Gastrointestinal: Nausea (>1%)

<1% (Limited to important or life-threatening): Supraventricular extrasystoles (0.9%), nodal arrhythmia (0.7%), CHF (0.5%), syncope (0.3%, not > placebo), idioventricular rhythm (0.2%), sustained monomorphic ventricular tachycardia (0.2%), renal failure (0.3%)

Postmarketing and/or case reports: Erythematous bullous lesions

Drug Interactions Increased Effect/Toxicity: Class Ia antiarrhythmic drugs (disopyramide, quinidine, and procainamide) and other class III drugs such as amiodarone and sotalol should not be given concomitantly with ibutilide due to their potential to prolong refractoriness. Signs of digoxin toxicity may be masked when coadministered with ibutilide. Toxicity of ibutilide is potentiated by concurrent administration of other drugs which may prolong QT interval: phenothiazines, tricyclic and tetracyclic antidepressants, cisapride, sparfloxacin, gatifloxacin, moxifloxacin, erythromycin, and astemizole.

Dietary/Ethanol/Herb Considerations Herb/Nutraceutical: Ginger has positive inotropic effects and theoretically could affect antiarrhythmic activity. Avoid hawthorn due to similar effects on cardiac electrophysiology.

Pharmacodynamics/Kinetics

Onset of action: ~90 minutes after start of infusion (1/2 of conversions to sinus rhythm occur during infusion)

Distribution: V_d: 11 L/kg

Protein binding: 40%

Metabolism: Extensively hepatic; oxidation

Half-life elimination: 2-12 hours (average: 6 hours)

Excretion: Urine (82%, 7% as unchanged drug and metabolites); feces (19%)

Pregnancy Risk Factor C

Generic Available No

Ibutilide Fumarate *see* Ibutilide *on page 706*

IC-Green® *see* Indocyanine Green *on page 719*

ICI 182,780 *see* Fulvestrant *on page 621*

ICI 204, 219 *see* Zafirlukast *on page 1402*

ICRF-187 *see* Dexrazoxane *on page 419*

Idamycin® [DSC] *see* Idarubicin *on page 706*

Idamycin PFS® *see* Idarubicin *on page 706*

Idarubicin (eye da ROO bi sin)

U.S. Brand Names Idamycin® [DSC]; Idamycin PFS®

Canadian Brand Names Idamycin®

Mexican Brand Names Idamycin®

Pharmacologic Category Antineoplastic Agent, Anthracycline

Synonyms 4-demethoxydaunorubicin; 4-dmdr; Idamycin® [DSC]; Idarubicin Hydrochloride

Use Treatment of acute leukemias (AML, ANLL, ALL), accelerated phase or blast crisis of chronic myelogenous leukemia (CML), breast cancer

Local Anesthetic/Vasoconstrictor Precautions No information available to require special precautions

Effects on Dental Treatment

>10%: Stomatitis (11%), GI hemorrhage (30%)

1% to 10%: Seizures

Dosage Refer to individual protocols. I.V.:

Children:

Leukemia: 10-12 mg/m^2/day for 3 days every 3 weeks

Solid tumors: 5 mg/m^2/day for 3 days every 3 weeks

Adults:

Leukemia induction: 12 mg/m^2/day for 3 days

Leukemia consolidation: 10-12 mg/m^2/day for 2 days

Dosing adjustment in renal/hepatic impairment: No specific dosage adjustment is recommended

Hemodialysis: Significant drug removal is unlikely based on physiochemical characteristics

Peritoneal dialysis: Significant drug removal is unlikely based on physiochemical characteristics

Mechanism of Action Derivative of daunorubicin; the only structural difference between idarubicin and the parent compound, daunorubicin, is lack of the methoxyl group at the C4 position of the aglycone. Similar to daunorubicin, idarubicin exhibits inhibitory effects on DNA and RNA polymerase *in vitro*. Idarubicin has an affinity for DNA similar to the parent compound and somewhat higher efficacy than daunorubicin in stabilizing the DNA double helix against heat denaturation.

Other Adverse Effects

>10%:

Cardiovascular: CHF (dose-related), transient EKG abnormalities (supraventricular tachycardia, S-T wave changes, atrial or ventricular extrasystoles); generally asymptomatic and self-limiting.

The relative cardiotoxicity of idarubicin compared to doxorubicin is unclear. Some investigators report no increase in cardiac toxicity at cumulative oral idarubicin doses up to 540 mg/m^2. Other reports suggest a maximum cumulative intravenous dose of 150 mg/m^2.

Central nervous system: Headache

Dermatologic: Alopecia (25% to 30%), radiation recall, skin rash (11%), urticaria

Gastrointestinal: Nausea/vomiting (30% to 60%), diarrhea (9% to 22%)

Genitourinary: Discoloration of urine (reddish)

Hematologic (effects generally less severe with oral form): Myelosuppression (primarily leukopenia), thrombocytopenia, anemia

Nadir: 10-15 days

Recovery: 21-28 days

Hepatic: Elevations of bilirubin and transaminases (44%)

1% to 10%: Neuromuscular & skeletal: Peripheral neuropathy

<1%: Hyperuricemia

Drug Interactions Decreased Effect: Patients may experience impaired immune response to vaccines; possible infection after administration of live vaccines in patients receiving immunosuppressants.

Pharmacodynamics/Kinetics

Absorption: Oral: Variable (4% to 77%; mean: ~30%)

Distribution: V_d: 64 L/kg (some reports indicate 2250 L); extensive tissue binding; CSF

Protein binding: 94% to 97%

Metabolism: Hepatic to idarubicinol (pharmacologically active)

Half-life elimination: Oral: 14-35 hours; I.V.: 12-27 hours

Time to peak, serum: 1-5 hours

Excretion:

Oral: Urine (~5% of dose; 0.5% to 0.7% as unchanged drug, 4% as idarubicinol); hepatic (8%)

I.V.: Urine (13% as idarubicinol, 3% as unchanged drug); hepatic (17%)

Pregnancy Risk Factor D

Generic Available No

Idarubicin Hydrochloride *see* Idarubicin *on page 706*

Ifex® *see* Ifosfamide *on page 707*

IFLrA *see* Interferon Alfa-2a *on page 726*

Ifosfamide (eye FOSS fa mide)

U.S. Brand Names Ifex®

Canadian Brand Names Ifex®

Mexican Brand Names Ifolem®; Ifoxan®

Pharmacologic Category Antineoplastic Agent, Alkylating Agent

(Continued)

Ifosfamide *(Continued)*

Use Treatment of lung cancer, Hodgkin's and non-Hodgkin's lymphoma, breast cancer, acute and chronic lymphocytic leukemias, ovarian cancer, sarcomas, pancreatic and gastric carcinomas

Orphan drug: Treatment of testicular cancer

Local Anesthetic/Vasoconstrictor Precautions No information available to require special precautions

Effects on Dental Treatment No significant effects or complications reported

Dosage Refer to individual protocols. To prevent bladder toxicity, ifosfamide should be given with the urinary protector mesna and hydration of at least 2 L of oral or I.V. fluid per day.

I.V.:

Children:

1200-1800 mg/m²/day for 3-5 days every 21-28 days **or**
5 g/m² once every 21-28 days **or**
3 g/m²/day for 2 days every 21-28 days

Adults:

50 mg/kg/day or 700-2000 mg/m² for 5 days every 3-4 weeks
Alternatives: 2400 mg/m²/day for 3 days or 5000 mg/m² as a single dose every 3-4 weeks

Dosing adjustment in renal impairment:

S_{cr} >3.0 mg/dL: Withhold drug
S_{cr} 2.1-3.0 mg/dL: Reduce dose by 25% to 50%

Dosing adjustment in hepatic impairment: Although no specific guidelines are available, it is possible that adjusted doses are indicated in hepatic disease. One author (Falkson G, et al, "An Extended Phase II Trial of Ifosfamide Plus Mesna in Malignant Mesothelioma," *Invest New Drugs*, 1992, 10:337-43.) recommended the following dosage adjustments:

AST >300 or bilirubin >3.0 mg/dL: Decrease ifosfamide dose by 75%

Mechanism of Action Causes cross-linking of strands of DNA by binding with nucleic acids and other intracellular structures; inhibits protein synthesis and DNA synthesis; an analogue of cyclophosphamide, and like cyclophosphamide, it undergoes activation by microsomal enzymes in the liver. Ifosfamide is metabolized to active compounds, ifosfamide mustard, and acrolein

Other Adverse Effects

>10%:

Central nervous system: Somnolence, confusion, hallucinations (12%)
Dermatologic: Alopecia (75% to 100%)
Endocrine & metabolic: Metabolic acidosis (31%)
Gastrointestinal: Constipation, nausea/vomiting (58%; may be more common with higher doses or bolus infusions)
Genitourinary: Hemorrhagic cystitis (40% to 50%); patients should be vigorously hydrated (at least 2 L/day) and receive mesna
Hematologic: Myelosuppression, leukopenia (65% to 100%), thrombocytopenia (10%) - dose-related
Onset: 7-14 days
Nadir: 21-28 days
Recovery: 21-28 days
Renal: Hematuria (6% to 92%)

1% to 10%:

Central nervous system: Hallucinations, depressive psychoses, polyneuropathy
Dermatologic: Dermatitis, nail banding/ridging, hyperpigmentation
Endocrine & metabolic: SIADH, sterility, elevated transaminases (3%)
Hematologic: Anemia
Local: Phlebitis
Renal: Increased creatinine/BUN (6%)
Respiratory: Nasal stuffiness

<1%: Anorexia, **cardiotoxicity**, diarrhea, **stomatitis**, acute tubular necrosis, pulmonary fibrosis

Drug Interactions Substrate of CYP2A6, **2B6, 2C8/9, 2C19, 3A4**; Inhibits CYP3A4; Induces CYP2C8/9

Increased Effect/Toxicity: Activation by microsomal enzymes may be enhanced during therapy with enzyme inducers such as phenobarbital, carbamazepine, and phenytoin.

Dietary/Ethanol/Herb Considerations Herb/Nutraceutical: Avoid St John's wort; may decrease serum concentration.

Pharmacodynamics/Kinetics Pharmacokinetics are dose dependent

Distribution: V_d: 5.7-49 L; does penetrate CNS, but not in therapeutic levels
Protein binding: Negligible
Metabolism: Hepatic to active metabolites phosphoramide mustard, acrolein, and inactive dichloroethylated and carboxy metabolites; acrolein is the agent implicated in development of hemorrhagic cystitis
Bioavailability: Estimated at 100%

Half-life elimination: Beta: High dose: 11-15 hours (3800-5000 mg/m^2); Lower dose: 4-7 hours (1800 mg/m^2)
Time to peak, plasma: Oral: Within 1 hour
Excretion: Urine (15% to 50% as unchanged drug, 41% as metabolites)

Pregnancy Risk Factor D

Generic Available No

Comments Usually used in combination with mesna, a prophylactic agent for hemorrhagic cystitis

IG *see* Immune Globulin (Intramuscular) *on page 713*

IGIM *see* Immune Globulin (Intramuscular) *on page 713*

IL-1Ra *see* Anakinra *on page 108*

IL-2 *see* Aldesleukin *on page 50*

IL-11 *see* Oprelvekin *on page 1003*

Imdur® *see* Isosorbide Mononitrate *on page 751*

Imidazole Carboxamide *see* Dacarbazine *on page 391*

Imiglucerase (imi GLOO ser ase)

U.S. Brand Names Cerezyme®

Pharmacologic Category Enzyme

Use Orphan drug: Long-term enzyme replacement therapy for patients with Type 1 Gaucher's disease

Local Anesthetic/Vasoconstrictor Precautions No information available to require special precautions

Effects on Dental Treatment 1% to 10%: Hypotension (<1.5%), hypersensitivity reaction (7%; pruritus, flushing, urticaria, angioedema, bronchospasm), anaphylactoid reaction (2%), headache, dizziness, nausea

Dosage I.V.: Children ≥2 years and Adults: 2.5 units/kg 3 times/week up to as much as 60 units/kg administered as frequently as once a week or as infrequently as every 4 weeks; 60 units/kg administered every 2 weeks is the most common dose

Other Adverse Effects

<1.5%:
- Cardiovascular: Cyanosis
- Dermatologic: Rash, pruritus
- Gastrointestinal: Abdominal discomfort
- Genitourinary: Urinary frequency decreased

Postmarketing and/or case reports: Peripheral edema, pulmonary hypertension

Pregnancy Risk Factor C

Generic Available No

Imipemide *see* Imipenem and Cilastatin *on page 709*

Imipenem and Cilastatin (i mi PEN em & sye la STAT in)

Related Information

Animal and Human Bites Guidelines *on page 1580*

U.S. Brand Names Primaxin®

Canadian Brand Names Primaxin®

Mexican Brand Names Tienam®

Pharmacologic Category Antibiotic, Carbapenem

Synonyms Imipemide

Use Treatment of respiratory tract, urinary tract, intra-abdominal, gynecologic, bone and joint, skin structure, and polymicrobic infections as well as bacterial septicemia and endocarditis. Antibacterial activity includes resistant gram-negative bacilli (*Pseudomonas aeruginosa* and *Enterobacter* sp), gram-positive bacteria (methicillin-sensitive *Staphylococcus aureus* and *Streptococcus* sp) and anaerobes.

Note: I.M. administration is not intended for severe or life-threatening infections (eg, septicemia, endocarditis, shock)

Local Anesthetic/Vasoconstrictor Precautions No information available to require special precautions

Effects on Dental Treatment No significant effects or complications reported

Dosage Dosage based on **imipenem** content:

Neonates: Non-CNS infections: I.V.:
- <1 week: 25 mg/kg every 12 hours
- 1-4 weeks: 25 mg/kg every 8 hours
- 4 weeks to 3 months: 25 mg/kg every 6 hours

Children: >3 months: Non-CNS infections: I.V.: 15-25 mg/kg every 6 hours
- Maximum dosage: Susceptible infections: 2 g/day; moderately susceptible organisms: 4 g/day

Children: Cystic fibrosis: I.V.: Doses up to 90 mg/kg/day have been used

Adults:
- Mild infections:
  - I.M.: 500 mg every 12 hours; intra-abdominal infections: 750 mg every 12 hours
  - I.V.:
    - Fully-susceptible organisms: 250 mg every 6 hours (1g/day)
    - Moderately-susceptible organisms: 500 mg every 6 hours (2 g/day)

(Continued)

Imipenem and Cilastatin *(Continued)*

Moderate infections:
- I.M.: 750 mg every 12 hours
- I.V.:
  - Fully-susceptible organisms: 500 mg every 6-8 hours (1.5-2 g/day)
  - Moderately-susceptible organisms: 500 mg every 6 hours or 1 g every 8 hours (2-3 g/day)

Severe infections: I.V.: **Note:** I.M. administration is not intended for severe or life-threatening infections (eg, septicemia, endocarditis, shock):
- Fully-susceptible organisms: 500 mg every 6 hours (2 g/day)
- Moderately-susceptible organisms: 1 g every 6-8 hours (3-4 g/day)
- Maximum daily dose should not exceed 50 mg/kg or 4 g/day, whichever is lower

Urinary tract infection, uncomplicated: I.V.: 250 mg every 6 hours (1 g/day)

Urinary tract infection, complicated: I.V.: 500 mg every 6 hours (2 g/day)

Dosing adjustment in renal impairment: I.V.: **Note:** Adjustments have not been established for I.M. dosing:
- Patients with a Cl_{cr} <5 mL/minute/1.73 m^2 should not receive imipenem/cilastatin unless hemodialysis is instituted within 48 hours.
- Patients weighing <30 kg with impaired renal function should not receive imipenem/cilastatin.
- Hemodialysis: Use the dosing recommendation for patients with a Cl_{cr} 6-20 mL/minute
- Peritoneal dialysis: Dose as for Cl_{cr} <10 mL/minute

Imipenem and Cilastatin Dosage in Renal Impairment

Reduced I.V. Dosage Regimen Based on Creatinine Clearance (mL/minute/1.73 m^2) and Body Weight (kg)					
	Body Weight (kg)				
	≥70	60	50	40	30
Total daily dose for normal renal function: 1 g/day					
Cl_{cr} ≥71	250 mg q6h	250 mg q8h	125 mg q6h	125 mg q6h	125 mg q8h
Cl_{cr} 41-70	250 mg q8h	125 mg q6h	125 mg q6h	125 mg q8h	125 mg q8h
Cl_{cr} 21-40	250 mg q12h	250 mg q12h	125 mg q8h	125 mg q12h	125 mg q12h
Cl_{cr} 6-20	250 mg q12h	125 mg q12h	125 mg q12h	125 mg q12h	125 mg q12h
Total daily dose for normal renal function: 1.5 g/day					
Cl_{cr} ≥71	500 mg q8h	250 mg q6h	250 mg q6h	250 mg q8h	125 mg q6h
Cl_{cr} 41-70	250 mg q6h	250 mg q8h	250 mg q8h	125 mg q6h	125 mg q8h
Cl_{cr} 21-40	250 mg q8h	250 mg q8h	250 mg q12h	125 mg q8h	125 mg q8h
Cl_{cr} 6-20	250 mg q12h	250 mg q12h	250 mg q12h	125 mg q12h	125 mg q12h
Total daily dose for normal renal function: 2 g/day					
Cl_{cr} ≥71	500 mg q6h	500 mg q8h	250 mg q6h	250 mg q6h	250 mg q8h
Cl_{cr} 41-70	500 mg q8h	250 mg q6h	250 mg q6h	250 mg q8h	125 mg q6h
Cl_{cr} 21-40	250 mg q6h	250 mg q8h	250 mg q8h	250 mg q12h	125 mg q8h
Cl_{cr} 6-20	250 mg q12h	250 mg q12h	250 mg q12h	250 mg q12h	125 mg q12h
Total daily dose for normal renal function: 3 g/day					
Cl_{cr} ≥71	1000 mg q8h	750 mg q8h	500 mg q6h	500 mg q8h	250 mg q6h
Cl_{cr} 41-70	500 mg q6h	500 mg q8h	500 mg q8h	250 mg q6h	250 mg q8h
Cl_{cr} 21-40	500 mg q8h	500 mg q8h	250 mg q6h	250 mg q8h	250 mg q8h
Cl_{cr} 6-20	500 mg q12h	500 mg q12h	250 mg q12h	250 mg q12h	250 mg q12h
Total daily dose for normal renal function: 4 g/day					
Cl_{cr} ≥71	1000 mg q6h	1000 mg q8h	750 mg q8h	500 mg q6h	500 mg q8h
Cl_{cr} 41-70	750 mg q8h	750 mg q8h	500 mg q6h	500 mg q8h	250 mg q6h
Cl_{cr} 21-40	500 mg q6h	500 mg q8h	500 mg q8h	250 mg q6h	250 mg q8h
Cl_{cr} 6-20	500 mg q12h	500 mg q12h	500 mg q12h	250 mg q12h	250 mg q12h

Continuous arteriovenous or venovenous hemofiltration: Dose as for Cl_{cr} 20-30 mL/minute; monitor for seizure activity; imipenem is well removed by CAVH but cilastatin is not; removes 20 mg of imipenem per liter of filtrate per day

See table on previous page.

Mechanism of Action Inhibits bacterial cell wall synthesis by binding to one or more of the penicillin binding proteins (PBPs); which in turn inhibits the final transpeptidation step of peptidoglycan synthesis in bacterial cell walls, thus inhibiting cell wall biosynthesis. Bacteria eventually lyse due to ongoing activity of cell wall autolytic enzymes (autolysins and murein hydrolases) while cell wall assembly is arrested. Cilastatin prevents renal metabolism of imipenem by competitive inhibition of dehydropeptidase along the brush border of the renal tubules.

Other Adverse Effects

1% to 10%:

Gastrointestinal: Nausea/diarrhea/vomiting (1% to 2%)

Local: Phlebitis (3%), pain at I.M. injection site (1.2%)

<1%: Abnormal urinalysis, anaphylaxis, anemia, confusion (acute), dizziness, emergence of resistant strains of *P. aeruginosa* eosinophilia, fever, hypersensitivity, hypotension, increased BUN/creatine, increased LFTs, increased PT, neutropenia (including agranulocytosis), pain at injection site, palpitations, positive Coombs' test, pruritus, pseudomembranous colitis, rash, seizures, somnolence, thrombocytopenia, urticaria

Postmarketing reports and/or case reports: Hemorrhagic colitis, hepatitis, jaundice, abdominal pain, **staining of teeth, glossitis**, pancytopenia, leukopenia, hemolytic anemia, encephalopathy, tremor, confusion, myoclonus, paresthesia, vertigo, headache, psychic disturbances, hallucinations, tinnitus, **abnormal taste, dyspnea**, thoracic spine pain, **tachycardia**, Stevens-Johnson syndrome, toxic epidermal necrolysis, erythema multiforme, angioneurotic edema, **flushing**, cyanosis, hyperhidrosis, candidiasis, pruritus vulvae, polyarthralgia, drug fever, asthenia, acute renal failure, polyuria, urine discoloration

Drug Interactions Increased toxicity with Beta-lactam antibiotics and probenecid.

Pharmacodynamics/Kinetics

Absorption: I.M.: Imipenem: 60% to 75%; cilastatin: 95% to 100%

Distribution: Rapidly and widely to most tissues and fluids including sputum, pleural fluid, peritoneal fluid, interstitial fluid, bile, aqueous humor, reproductive organs, and bone; highest concentrations in pleural fluid, interstitial fluid, peritoneal fluid, and reproductive organs; low concentrations in CSF; crosses placenta; enters breast milk

Metabolism: Renally by dehydropeptidase; activity is blocked by cilastatin; cilastatin is partially metabolized renally

Half-life elimination: Both drugs: 60 minutes; prolonged with renal impairment

Excretion: Both drugs: Urine (~70% as unchanged drug)

Pregnancy Risk Factor C

Generic Available No

Imipramine (im IP ra meen)

U.S. Brand Names Tofranil®; Tofranil-PM®

Canadian Brand Names Apo®-Imipramine; Tofranil®

Mexican Brand Names Talpramin®; Tofranil®; Tofranil-PM®

Pharmacologic Category Antidepressant, Tricyclic (Tertiary Amine)

Synonyms Imipramine Hydrochloride; Imipramine Pamoate

Use Treatment of various forms of depression

Unlabeled/Investigational Use Treatment of enuresis in children, panic disorder, attention-deficit/hyperactivity disorder (ADHD); analgesic for certain chronic and neuropathic pain

Local Anesthetic/Vasoconstrictor Precautions Use with caution; epinephrine, norepinephrine and levonordefrin have been shown to have an increased pressor response in combination with TCAs

Effects on Dental Treatment >10%: Xerostomia, changes in salivation

Long-term treatment with TCAs such as imipramine increases the risk of caries by reducing salivation and salivary buffer capacity. In a study by Rundergren, et al, pathological alterations were observed in the oral mucosa of 72% of 58 patients; 55% had new carious lesions after taking TCAs for a median of 5½ years. Current research is investigating the use of the salivary stimulant pilocarpine to overcome the xerostomia from imipramine.

Dosage Oral:

Children:

Depression: 1.5 mg/kg/day with dosage increments of 1 mg/kg every 3-4 days to a maximum dose of 5 mg/kg/day in 1-4 divided doses; monitor carefully especially with doses ≥3.5 mg/kg/day

Enuresis: ≥6 years: Initial: 10-25 mg at bedtime, if inadequate response still seen after 1 week of therapy, increase by 25 mg/day; dose should not exceed 2.5 mg/kg/day or 50 mg at bedtime if 6-12 years of age or 75 mg at bedtime if ≥12 years of age

(Continued)

Imipramine *(Continued)*

Adjunct in the treatment of cancer pain: Initial: 0.2-0.4 mg/kg at bedtime; dose may be increased by 50% every 2-3 days up to 1-3 mg/kg/dose at bedtime

Adolescents: Initial: 25-50 mg/day; increase gradually; maximum: 100 mg/day in single or divided doses

Adults: Initial: 25 mg 3-4 times/day, increase dose gradually, total dose may be given at bedtime; maximum: 300 mg/day

Elderly: Initial: 10-25 mg at bedtime; increase by 10-25 mg every 3 days for inpatients and weekly for outpatients if tolerated; average daily dose to achieve a therapeutic concentration: 100 mg/day; range: 50-150 mg/day

Mechanism of Action Traditionally believed to increase the synaptic concentration of serotonin and/or norepinephrine in the central nervous system by inhibition of their reuptake by the presynaptic neuronal membrane. However, additional receptor effects have been found including desensitization of adenyl cyclase, down regulation of beta-adrenergic receptors, and down regulation of serotonin receptors.

Other Adverse Effects

<1%: Agranulocytosis, alopecia, cholestatic jaundice, eosinophilia, increased liver enzymes, itching, petechiae, photosensitivity, purpura, rash, thrombocytopenia, urticaria

Frequency not defined:

Cardiovascular: **Orthostatic hypotension, arrhythmias, tachycardia, hypertension, palpitations, MI, heart block, EKG changes, CHF, stroke**

Central nervous system: Dizziness, drowsiness, headache, agitation, insomnia, nightmares, hypomania, psychosis, fatigue, confusion, hallucinations, disorientation, delusions, **anxiety, restlessness, seizures**

Endocrine & metabolic: Gynecomastia, breast enlargement, galactorrhea, increase or decrease in libido, increase/decrease in blood sugar, SIADH

Gastrointestinal: Nausea, **unpleasant taste**, weight gain/loss, constipation, ileus, stomatitis, abdominal cramps, vomiting, anorexia, **epigastric disorders**, diarrhea, **black tongue**

Genitourinary: Urinary retention, impotence

Neuromuscular & skeletal: Weakness, numbness, tingling, paresthesias, incoordination, ataxia, tremor, peripheral neuropathy, **extrapyramidal symptoms**

Ocular: Blurred vision, disturbances of accommodation, mydriasis

Otic: Tinnitus

Miscellaneous: Diaphoresis

Drug Interactions Substrate of CYP1A2, 2B6, **2C19, 2D6**, 3A4; Inhibits CYP1A2, 2C19, 2D6, 2E1

Increased Effect/Toxicity: Imipramine increases the effects of amphetamines, anticholinergics, other CNS depressants (sedatives, hypnotics, or ethanol), chlorpropamide, tolazamide, and warfarin. When used with MAO inhibitors, hyperpyrexia, hypertension, tachycardia, confusion, seizures, and **deaths have been reported** (serotonin syndrome). Serotonin syndrome has also been reported with ritonavir (rare). The SSRIs (to varying degrees), cimetidine, grapefruit juice, indinavir, methylphenidate, ritonavir, quinidine, diltiazem, and verapamil inhibit the metabolism of TCAs and clinical toxicity may result. Use of lithium with a TCA may increase the risk for neurotoxicity. Phenothiazines may increase concentration of some TCAs and TCAs may increase concentration of phenothiazines. Pressor response to I.V. epinephrine, norepinephrine, and phenylephrine may be enhanced in patients receiving TCAs (**Note:** Effect is unlikely with epinephrine or levonordefrin dosages typically administered as infiltration in combination with local anesthetics). Combined use of beta-agonists or drugs which prolong QT_c (including quinidine, procainamide, disopyramide, cisapride, sparfloxacin, gatifloxacin, moxifloxacin) with TCAs may predispose patients to cardiac arrhythmias.

Decreased Effect: Carbamazepine, phenobarbital, and rifampin may increase the metabolism of imipramine resulting in decreased effect of imipramine. Imipramine inhibits the antihypertensive response to bethanidine, clonidine, debrisoquin, guanadrel, guanethidine, guanabenz, and guanfacine. Cholestyramine and colestipol may bind TCAs and reduce their absorption; monitor for altered response.

Dietary/Ethanol/Herb Considerations

Ethanol: Avoid use; increases CNS depression.

Food: Avoid grapefruit products; may inhibit metabolism resulting in clinical toxicity. Avoid caffeine.

Herb/Nutraceutical: Avoid kava, SAMe, St John's wort, tryptophan, and valerian; may increase risk of serotonin syndrome and/or excessive sedation.

Pharmacodynamics/Kinetics

Onset of action: Peak antidepressant effect: Usually after ≥2 weeks

Absorption: Well absorbed

Distribution: Crosses placenta

Metabolism: Hepatic via CYP to desipramine (active) and other metabolites; significant first-pass effect

Half-life elimination: 6-18 hours

Excretion: Urine (as metabolites)

Pregnancy Risk Factor D

Generic Available Yes: Tablet

Selected Readings

Friedlander AH, Mahler ME, "Major Depressive Disorder. Psychopathology, Medical Management, and Dental Implications," *J Am Dent Assoc*, 201, 132(5):629-38.

Ganzberg S, "Psychoactive Drugs," *ADA Guide to Dental Therapeutics*, 2nd ed, Chicago, IL: ADA Publishing, a Division of ADA Business Enterprises, Inc, 2000, 376-405.

Jastak JT and Yagiela JA, "Vasoconstrictors and Local Anesthesia: A Review and Rationale for Use," *J Am Dent Assoc*, 1983, 107(4):623-30.

Mitchell JR, "Guanethidine and Related Agents. III Antagonism by Drugs Which Inhibit the Norepinephrine Pump in Man," *J Clin Invest*, 1970, 49(8):1596-604.

Rundegren J, van Dijken J, Mörnstad H, et al, "Oral Conditions in Patients Receiving Long-Term Treatment With Cyclic Antidepressant Drugs," *Swed Dent J*, 1985, 9(2):55-64.

Wynn RL, "New Antidepressant Medications," *Gen Dent*, 1997, 45(1):24-8.

Yagiela JA, "Adverse Drug Interactions in Dental Practice: Interactions Associated With Vasoconstrictors. Part V of a Series," *J Am Dent Assoc*, 1999, 130(5):701-9.

Imipramine Hydrochloride *see* Imipramine *on page 711*

Imipramine Pamoate *see* Imipramine *on page 711*

Imiquimod (i mi KWI mod)

Related Information

Oral Viral Infections *on page 1545*

Systemic Viral Diseases *on page 1517*

U.S. Brand Names Aldara™

Canadian Brand Names Aldara™

Pharmacologic Category Skin and Mucous Membrane Agent; Topical Skin Product

Use Treatment of external genital and perianal warts/condyloma acuminata in children ≥12 years of age and adults

Local Anesthetic/Vasoconstrictor Precautions No information available to require special precautions

Effects on Dental Treatment No significant effects or complications reported

Dosage Children ≥12 years and Adults: Topical: Apply 3 times/week prior to normal sleeping hours and leave on the skin for 6-10 hours. Following treatment period, remove cream by washing the treated area with mild soap and water. Examples of 3 times/week application schedules are: Monday, Wednesday, Friday; or Tuesday, Thursday, Saturday. Continue imiquimod treatment until there is total clearance of the genital/perianal warts for ≤16 weeks. A rest period of several days may be taken if required by the patient's discomfort or severity of the local skin reaction. Treatment may resume once the reaction subsides.

Mechanism of Action Mechanism of action is unknown; however, induces cytokines, including interferon-alpha and others

Other Adverse Effects

>10%: Local (mild/moderate): Erythema (54% to 61%), itching (22% to 32%), erosion (21% to 32%), burning (9% to 26%), excoriation/flaking (18% to 25%), edema (12% to 17%), scabbing (9% to 13%)

1% to 10%:

- Central nervous system: Pain (2% to 8%), headache (4% to 5%)
- Local (severe): Erythema (4%), erosion (1%), edema (1%)
- Local (mild/moderate): Pain, induration, ulceration (5% to 7%), vesicles (2% to 3%), soreness (<1% to 3%)
- Neuromuscular & skeletal: Myalgia (1%)
- Miscellaneous: **Influenza-like symptoms (1% to 3%), fungal infections (2% to 11%)**

Drug Interactions Substrate of CYP1A2, 3A4

Pharmacodynamics/Kinetics

Absorption: Minimal

Excretion: Urine and feces (<0.9%)

Pregnancy Risk Factor B

Generic Available No

Imitrex® *see* Sumatriptan *on page 1258*

Immune Globulin (Intramuscular)

(i MYUN GLOB yoo lin, IN tra MUS kyoo ler)

Related Information

Immunizations (Vaccines) *on page 1612*

Systemic Viral Diseases *on page 1517*

U.S. Brand Names BayGam®

Canadian Brand Names Baygam™

Pharmacologic Category Immune Globulin

Synonyms Gamma Globulin; IG; IGIM; Immune Serum Globulin; ISG

Use Household and sexual contacts of persons with hepatitis A, measles, varicella, and possibly rubella; travelers to high-risk areas outside tourist routes; staff, attendees, and parents of diapered attendees in day-care center outbreaks

(Continued)

Immune Globulin (Intramuscular) *(Continued)*

For travelers, IG is not an alternative to careful selection of foods and water; immune globulin can interfere with the antibody response to parenterally administered live virus vaccines. Frequent travelers should be tested for hepatitis A antibody, immune hemolytic anemia, and neutropenia (with ITP, I.V. route is usually used).

Local Anesthetic/Vasoconstrictor Precautions No information available to require special precautions

Effects on Dental Treatment No significant effects or complications reported

Dosage I.M.:

Hepatitis A:

Pre-exposure prophylaxis upon travel into endemic areas (hepatitis A vaccine preferred):

0.02 mL/kg for anticipated risk 1-3 months

0.06 mL/kg for anticipated risk >3 months

Repeat approximate dose every 4-6 months if exposure continues

Postexposure prophylaxis: 0.02 mL/kg given within 7 days of exposure

Measles:

Prophylaxis: 0.25 mL/kg/dose (maximum dose: 15 mL) given within 6 days of exposure followed by live attenuated measles vaccine in 3 months or at 15 months of age (whichever is later)

For patients with leukemia, lymphoma, immunodeficiency disorders, generalized malignancy, or receiving immunosuppressive therapy: 0.5 mL/kg (maximum dose: 15 mL)

Poliomyelitis: Prophylaxis: 0.3 mL/kg/dose as a single dose

Rubella: Prophylaxis: 0.55 mL/kg/dose within 72 hours of exposure

Varicella:: Prophylaxis: 0.6-1.2 mL/kg (varicella zoster immune globulin preferred) within 72 hours of exposure

IgG deficiency: 1.3 mL/kg, then 0.66 mL/kg in 3-4 weeks

Hepatitis B: Prophylaxis: 0.06 mL/kg/dose (HBIG preferred)

Mechanism of Action Provides passive immunity by increasing the antibody titer and antigen-antibody reaction potential

Other Adverse Effects Frequency not defined:

Cardiovascular: **Flushing**, angioedema

Central nervous system: Chills, lethargy, fever

Dermatologic: Urticaria, erythema

Gastrointestinal: Nausea, vomiting

Local: Pain, tenderness, muscle stiffness at I.M. site

Neuromuscular & skeletal: Myalgia

Miscellaneous: Hypersensitivity reactions

Pharmacodynamics/Kinetics

Duration: Immune effect: Usually 3-4 weeks

Half-life elimination: 23 days

Time to peak, serum: I.M.: ~24-48 hours

Pregnancy Risk Factor C

Generic Available No

Immune Globulin (Intravenous)

(i MYUN GLOB yoo lin, IN tra VEE nus)

Related Information

Systemic Viral Diseases *on page 1517*

U.S. Brand Names Carimune™; Gamimune® N; Gammagard® S/D; Gammar®-P I.V.; Iveegam EN; Panglobulin®; Polygam® S/D; Venoglobulin®-S

Canadian Brand Names Gamimune® N; Gammagard® S/D; Iveegam Immuno®

Mexican Brand Names Citax; Intacglobin; Sandoglobulina®

Pharmacologic Category Immune Globulin

Synonyms IVIG

Use

Treatment of primary immunodeficiency syndromes (congenital agammaglobulinemia, severe combined immunodeficiency syndromes [SCIDS], common variable immunodeficiency, X-linked immunodeficiency, Wiskott-Aldrich syndrome); idiopathic thrombocytopenic purpura (ITP); Kawasaki disease (in combination with aspirin)

Prevention of bacterial infection in B-cell chronic lymphocytic leukemia (CLL); pediatric HIV infection; bone marrow transplant (BMT)

Unlabeled/Investigational Use Treatment of autoimmune diseases (eg, myasthenia gravis, SLE, bullous pemphigoid, severe rheumatoid arthritis), Guillain-Barré syndrome, autoimmune hemolytic anemia or neutropenia, refractory dermatomyositis/polymyositis; adjunct in appropriate anti-infective therapy to prevent or modify acute bacterial or viral infections in patients with iatrogenically-induced or disease-associated immunodepression

Local Anesthetic/Vasoconstrictor Precautions No information available to require special precautions

Effects on Dental Treatment No significant effects or complications reported

Dosage Approved doses and regimens may vary between brands; check manufacturer guidelines. **Note:** Some clinicians dose IVIG on ideal body weight or an adjusted ideal body weight in morbidly obese patients. The volume of distribution of IVIG preparations in healthy subjects is similar to that observed with endogenous IgG. IVIG remains primarily in the intravascular space. Patients with congenital humoral immunodeficiencies appear to have about 70% of the IVIG available in the intravascular space.

Infants and Children: Prevention of gastroenteritis (unlabeled use): Oral: 50 mg/kg/day divided every 6 hours

Children: I.V.:

Pediatric HIV: 400 mg/kg every 28 days

Severe systemic viral and bacterial infections (unlabeled use): 500-1000 mg/kg/week

Children and Adults: I.V.:

Primary immunodeficiency disorders: 200-400 mg/kg every 4 weeks or as per monitored serum IgG concentrations

B-cell chronic lymphocytic leukemia (CLL): 400 mg/kg/dose every 3 weeks

Idiopathic thrombocytopenic purpura (ITP):

Acute: 400 mg/kg/day for 5 days or 1000 mg/kg/day for 1-2 days

Chronic: 400 mg/kg as needed to maintain platelet count >30,000/mm^3; may increase dose to 800 mg/kg (1000 mg/kg if needed)

Kawasaki disease: Initiate therapy within 10 days of disease onset: 2 g/kg as a single dose administered over 10 hours, or 400 mg/kg/day for 4 days. **Note:** Must be used in combination with aspirin: 80-100 mg/kg/day in 4 divided doses for 14 days; when fever subsides, dose aspirin at 3-5 mg/kg once daily for ≥6-8 weeks

Acquired immunodeficiency syndrome (patients must be symptomatic) (unlabeled use): Various regimens have been used, including:

200-250 mg/kg/dose every 2 weeks

or

400-500 mg/kg/dose every month or every 4 weeks

Autoimmune hemolytic anemia and neutropenia (unlabeled use): 1000 mg/kg/dose for 2-3 days

Autoimmune diseases (unlabeled use): 400 mg/kg/day for 4 days

Bone marrow transplant: 500 mg/kg beginning on days 7 and 2 pretransplant, then 500 mg/kg/week for 90 days post-transplant

Adjuvant to severe cytomegalovirus infections (unlabeled use): 500 mg/kg/dose every other day for 7 doses

Guillain-Barré syndrome (unlabeled use): Various regimens have been used, including:

400 mg/kg/day for 4 days

or

1000 mg/kg/day for 2 days

or

2000 mg/kg/day for one day

Refractory dermatomyositis (unlabeled use): 2 g/kg/dose every month x 3-4 doses

Refractory polymyositis (unlabeled use): 1 g/kg/day x 2 days every month x 4 doses

Chronic inflammatory demyelinating polyneuropathy (unlabeled use): Various regimens have been used, including:

400 mg/kg/day for 5 doses once each month

or

800 mg/kg/day for 3 doses once each month

or

1000 mg/kg/day for 2 days once each month

Dosing adjustment in renal impairment: Cl_{cr} <10 mL/minute: Avoid use

Mechanism of Action Replacement therapy for primary and secondary immunodeficiencies; interference with F_c receptors on the cells of the reticuloendothelial system for autoimmune cytopenias and ITP; possible role of contained antiviral-type antibodies

Other Adverse Effects Frequency not defined:

Cardiovascular: Flushing of the face, tachycardia, hypertension, hypotension, chest tightness, angioedema, lightheadedness, chest pain, MI, CHF, pulmonary embolism

Central nervous system: Anxiety, chills, dizziness, drowsiness, fatigue, fever, headache, irritability, lethargy, malaise, aseptic meningitis syndrome

Dermatologic: Pruritus, rash, urticaria

Gastrointestinal: Abdominal cramps, nausea, vomiting

Hematologic: Autoimmune hemolytic anemia, mild hemolysis

Local: Pain or irritation at infusion site

Neuromuscular & skeletal: Arthralgia, back or hip pain, myalgia, nuchal rigidity

Ocular: Photophobia, painful eye movements

(Continued)

Immune Globulin (Intravenous) *(Continued)*

Renal: Acute renal failure, acute tubular necrosis, anuria, BUN elevated, creatinine elevated, nephrotic syndrome, oliguria, proximal tubular nephropathy, osmotic nephrosis

Respiratory: **Dyspnea, wheezing, infusion-related lung injury**

Miscellaneous: Diaphoresis, hypersensitivity reactions, anaphylaxis

Drug Interactions Decreased Effect: Decreases effect of live virus vaccines (eg, measles, mumps, rubella); separate administration by at least 3 months

Pharmacodynamics/Kinetics

Onset of action: I.V.: Provides immediate antibody levels

Duration: Immune effect: 3-4 weeks (variable)

Distribution: V_d: 0.09-0.13 L/kg

Intravascular portion: Healthy subjects: 41% to 57%; Patients with congenital humoral immunodeficiencies: ~70%

Half-life elimination: IgG (variable among patients): Healthy subjects: 14-24 days; Patients with congenital humoral immunodeficiencies: 26-35 days; hypermetabolism associated with fever and infection have coincided with a shortened half-life

Pregnancy Risk Factor C

Generic Available No

Immune Serum Globulin *see* Immune Globulin (Intramuscular) *on page 713*

Imodium® A-D [OTC] *see* Loperamide *on page 819*

Imogam® *see* Rabies Immune Globulin (Human) *on page 1164*

Imovax® Rabies *see* Rabies Virus Vaccine *on page 1164*

Imuran® *see* Azathioprine *on page 150*

In-111 Zevalin *see* Ibritumomab *on page 702*

Inamrinone (eye NAM ri none)

Pharmacologic Category Phosphodiesterase Enzyme Inhibitor

Synonyms Amrinone; Amrinone Lactate

Use Infrequently used as a last resort, short-term therapy in patients with intractable heart failure

Local Anesthetic/Vasoconstrictor Precautions No information available to require special precautions

Effects on Dental Treatment 1% to 10%: Arrhythmias (3%; especially in high-risk patients), hypotension (1% to 2%; may be infusion rate-related), nausea (1% to 2%)

Dosage Dosage is based on clinical response and should not exceed 10 mg/kg/24 hours.

Infants, Children, and Adults: 0.75 mg/kg I.V. bolus over 2-3 minutes followed by maintenance infusion of 5-10 mcg/kg/minute; I.V. bolus may need to be repeated in 30 minutes.

Dosing adjustment in renal failure: Cl_{cr} <10 mL/minute: Administer 50% to 75% of dose.

Mechanism of Action Inhibits myocardial cyclic adenosine monophosphate (cAMP) phosphodiesterase activity and increases cellular levels of cAMP resulting in a positive inotropic effect and increased cardiac output; also possesses systemic and pulmonary vasodilator effects resulting in pre- and afterload reduction; slightly increases atrioventricular conduction

Other Adverse Effects

1% to 10%: Hematologic: Thrombocytopenia (may be dose-related)

<1% (Limited to important or life-threatening): **Chest pain, fever, vomiting**, abdominal pain, anorexia, hepatotoxicity, pain or burning at injection site, **hypersensitivity** (especially with prolonged therapy); contains sulfites resulting in allergic reactions in susceptible people

Drug Interactions Increased Effect/Toxicity: Diuretics may cause significant hypovolemia and decrease filling pressure. Inotropic effects with digitalis are additive.

Pharmacodynamics/Kinetics

Onset of action: I.V.: 2-5 minutes

Peak effect: ~10 minutes

Duration (dose dependent): Low dose: ~30 minutes; Higher doses: ~2 hours

Half-life elimination, serum: Adults: Healthy volunteers: 3.6 hours, Congestive heart failure: 5.8 hours

Pregnancy Risk Factor C

Generic Available Yes

Inapsine® *see* Droperidol *on page 481*

Indapamide (in DAP a mide)

Related Information

Cardiovascular Diseases *on page 1456*

U.S. Brand Names Lozol®

Canadian Brand Names Apo®-Indapamide; Gen-Indapamide; Lozide®; Lozol®; Novo-Indapamide; Nu-Indapamide; PMS-Indapamide

Pharmacologic Category Diuretic, Thiazide-Related

Use Management of mild to moderate hypertension; treatment of edema in CHF and nephrotic syndrome

Local Anesthetic/Vasoconstrictor Precautions No information available to require special precautions

Effects on Dental Treatment 1% to 10%: Orthostatic hypotension, palpitations (<5%), flushing, xerostomia, rhinorrhea

Dosage Adults: Oral:

Edema: 2.5-5 mg/day. **Note:** There is little therapeutic benefit to increasing the dose >5 mg/day; there is, however, an increased risk of electrolyte disturbances

Hypertension: 1.25 mg in the morning, may increase to 5 mg/day by increments of 1.25-2.5 mg; consider adding another antihypertensive and decreasing the dose if response is not adequate

Mechanism of Action Diuretic effect is localized at the proximal segment of the distal tubule of the nephron; it does not appear to have significant effect on glomerular filtration rate nor renal blood flow; like other diuretics, it enhances sodium, chloride, and water excretion by interfering with the transport of sodium ions across the renal tubular epithelium

Other Adverse Effects

1% to 10%:

Central nervous system: Dizziness (<5%), lightheadedness (<5%), vertigo (<5%), headache (≥5%), depression, drowsiness (<5%), fatigue, lethargy, malaise, lassitude, **anxiety, agitation, nervousness, restlessness (<5%)** (≥5%)

Dermatologic: Rash (<5%), pruritus (<5%), hives (<5%)

Endocrine & metabolic: Hyperglycemia (<5%), hyperuricemia (<5%)

Gastrointestinal: Anorexia, gastric irritation, nausea, vomiting, abdominal pain, cramping, bloating, diarrhea, constipation, weight loss

Genitourinary: Nocturia, frequent urination, polyuria, impotence (<5%), reduced libido (<5%), glycosuria (<5%)

Neuromuscular & skeletal: Muscle cramps, spasm, weakness (≥5%)

Ocular: Blurred vision (<5%)

Renal: Necrotizing angiitis, vasculitis, cutaneous vasculitis (<5%)

<1% (Limited to important or life-threatening symptoms, and/or postmarketing reports): Hepatitis, hypercalcemia, jaundice, LFTs abnormality, pancreatitis, purpura

Drug Interactions

Increased Effect/Toxicity: The diuretic effect of indapamide is synergistic with furosemide and other loop diuretics. Increased hypotension and/or renal adverse effects of ACE inhibitors may result in aggressively diuresed patients. Cyclosporine and thiazide-type diuretics can increase the risk of gout or renal toxicity. Digoxin toxicity can be exacerbated if a diuretic induces hypokalemia or hypomagnesemia. Lithium toxicity can occur with thiazide-type diuretics due to reduced renal excretion of lithium. Thiazide-type diuretics may prolong the duration of action of neuromuscular blocking agents.

Decreased Effect: Effects of oral hypoglycemics may be decreased. Decreased absorption of indapamide with cholestyramine and colestipol. NSAIDs can decrease the efficacy of thiazide-type diuretics, reducing the diuretic and antihypertensive effects.

Dietary/Ethanol/Herb Considerations

Ethanol: Avoid use; may increase risk of hypotension or dizziness.

Food: Administer with food or milk to reduce GI upset. Avoid caffeine (eg, colas, chocolate), garlic, and licorice.

Herb/Nutraceutical: Avoid black cohosh, dong quai, and evening primrose due to estrogenic activity. Avoid ephedra, ginseng, and yohimbe; may worsen hypertension. Avoid escin (from the horse chestnut seed); may have additive diuretic effects. Avoid garlic; may have increased antihypertensive effect. Avoid ginger due to positive inotropic effects; theoretically, may cause arrhythmia. Avoid hawthorn; may lower peripheral vascular resistance and cause more BP reductions. Avoid licorice.

Pharmacodynamics/Kinetics

Onset of action: 1-2 hours

Duration: ≤36 hours

Absorption: Complete

Protein binding, plasma: 71% to 79%

Metabolism: Extensively hepatic

Half-life elimination: 14-18 hours

Time to peak: 2-2.5 hours

Excretion: Urine (~60%) within 48 hours; feces (~16% to 23%)

Pregnancy Risk Factor B (manufacturer); D (expert analysis)

Generic Available Yes

Inderal® *see* Propranolol *on page 1139*

Inderal® LA *see* Propranolol *on page 1139*

Inderide® *see* Propranolol and Hydrochlorothiazide *on page 1142*

Indinavir (in DIN a veer)

Related Information

HIV Infection and AIDS *on page 1482*
Tuberculosis *on page 1493*

U.S. Brand Names Crixivan®

Canadian Brand Names Crixivan®

Mexican Brand Names Crixivan®

Pharmacologic Category Antiretroviral Agent, Protease Inhibitor

Use Treatment of HIV infection; should always be used as part of a multidrug regimen (at least three antiretroviral agents)

Local Anesthetic/Vasoconstrictor Precautions No information available to require special precautions

Effects on Dental Treatment Abnormal taste (3%)

Dosage

Children (investigational): 500 mg/m^2 every 8 hours (patients with smaller BSA may require lower doses of 300-400 mg/m^2 every 8 hours)

Adults: Oral: 800 mg every 8 hours

Dosing adjustments for indinavir when administered in combination therapy:

Delavirdine, itraconazole, or ketoconazole: Reduce indinavir dose to 600 mg every 8 hours

Efavirenz: Increase indinavir dose to 1000 mg every 8 hours

Lopinavir and ritonavir (Kaletra™): Indinavir 600 mg twice daily

Nevirapine: Increase indinavir dose to 1000 mg every 8 hours

Rifabutin: Reduce rifabutin to ½ the standard dose plus increase indinavir to 1000 mg every 8 hours

Ritonavir: Adjustments necessary for both agents:

Ritonavir 100-200 mg twice daily plus indinavir 800 mg twice daily **or**

Ritonavir 400 mg twice daily plus indinavir 400 mg twice daily

Dosing adjustment in hepatic impairment: Mild-moderate impairment due to cirrhosis: 600 mg every 8 hours or with ketoconazole coadministration

Mechanism of Action Indinavir is a human immunodeficiency virus protease inhibitor, binding to the protease activity site and inhibiting the activity of this enzyme. HIV protease is an enzyme required for the cleavage of viral polyprotein precursors into individual functional proteins found in infectious HIV. Inhibition prevents cleavage of these polyproteins resulting in the formation of immature noninfectious viral particles.

Other Adverse Effects Protease inhibitors cause dyslipidemia which includes elevated cholesterol and triglycerides and a redistribution of body fat centrally to cause "protease paunch", buffalo hump, facial atrophy, and breast enlargement. These agents also cause hyperglycemia (exacerbation or new-onset diabetes).

10%:

Hepatic: Hyperbilirubinemia (14%)

Renal: Nephrolithiasis/urolithiasis (29%, pediatric patients)

1% to 10%:

Central nervous system: Headache (6%), insomnia (3%)

Gastrointestinal: Abdominal pain (9%), nausea (12%), diarrhea/vomiting (4% to 5%)

Neuromuscular & skeletal: Weakness (4%), flank pain (3%)

Renal: Nephrolithiasis/urolithiasis (12%, adult patients), hematuria

<1%: Malaise, dizziness, somnolence, anorexia, decreased hemoglobin, pancreatitis, urticaria, depression, increased serum cholesterol, **fever, MI, angina, xerostomia**

Postmarketing and/or case reports: Acute renal failure, alopecia, anaphylactoid reactions, crystalluria, depression, dysuria, erythema multiforme, hemolytic anemia, hepatic failure, hepatitis, interstitial nephritis, new-onset diabetes, paresthesia (oral), pruritus, pyelonephritis, Stevens-Johnson syndrome, vasculitis

Drug Interactions Substrate of CYP2D6, **3A4**; Inhibits CYP2C8/9, 2C19, 2D6, **3A4**

Increased Effect/Toxicity: Levels of indinavir are increased by delavirdine, itraconazole, ketoconazole, nelfinavir, sildenafil, and ritonavir. Cisapride, pimozide, and astemizole should be avoided with indinavir due to life-threatening cardiotoxicity. Concurrent use of indinavir with lovastatin and simvastatin may increase the risk of myopathy or rhabdomyolysis. Cautious use of atorvastatin and cerivastatin may be possible. Benzodiazepines with indinavir may result in prolonged sedation and respiratory depression (midazolam and triazolam are contraindicated). Concurrent use of ergot alkaloids is contraindicated. Amprenavir and rifabutin concentrations are increased during concurrent therapy with indinavir. Other medications metabolized by cytochrome P450 isoenzyme 3A4 (including calcium channel blockers) may be affected. Concurrent sildenafil is associated with increased risk of hypotension, visual changes, and priapism. Clarithromycin and quinidine may increase serum concentrations of indinavir. Serum concentrations of these drugs may also be increased. Other CYP3A4 inhibitors may have similar effects.

Decreased Effect: Concurrent use of efavirenz, rifampin, and rifabutin may decrease the effectiveness of indinavir (dosage increase of indinavir is recommended); concurrent use of rifampin is not recommended; dosage decrease of rifabutin is recommended. The efficacy of protease inhibitors may be decreased when given with nevirapine. Gastric pH is lowered and absorption may be decreased when didanosine and indinavir are taken <1 hour apart. Fluconazole may decrease serum concentration of indinavir.

Dietary/Ethanol/Herb Considerations

Food: Administer on an empty stomach; food may decrease bioavailability (may be taken with food if taken with ritonavir). Administration with a high fat, high calorie diet resulted in a reduction in AUC and in maximum serum concentration (77% and 84% respectively). Administration with lighter meals (eg, dry toast, skim milk, corn flakes) resulted in little/no change in indinavir concentration. Avoid coadministration with grapefruit products; may decrease indinavir serum concentration.

Herb/Nutraceutical: Avoid St John's wort; appears to induce CYP3A enzymes and has lead to 57% reductions in indinavir AUCs and 81% reductions in trough serum concentration, which may lead to treatment failures.

Pharmacodynamics/Kinetics

Absorption: Administration with a high fat, high calorie diet resulted in a reduction in AUC and in maximum serum concentration (77% and 84% respectively); lighter meal resulted in little or no change in these parameters.

Protein binding, plasma: 60%

Metabolism: Hepatic via CYP3A4; seven metabolites of indinavir identified

Bioavailability: Good

Half-life elimination: 1.8 ± 0.4 hour

Time to peak: 0.8 ± 0.3 hour

Excretion: Urine and feces

Pregnancy Risk Factor C

Generic Available No

Indocin® *see* Indomethacin *on page 719*

Indocin® I.V. *see* Indomethacin *on page 719*

Indocin® SR *see* Indomethacin *on page 719*

Indocyanine Green (in doe SYE a neen green)

U.S. Brand Names IC-Green®

Pharmacologic Category Diagnostic Agent

Use Determining hepatic function, cardiac output and liver blood flow and for ophthalmic angiography

Local Anesthetic/Vasoconstrictor Precautions No information available to require special precautions

Effects on Dental Treatment 1% to 10%: Diaphoresis, anaphylactoid reactions

Dosage

Angiography: Use 40 mg of dye in 2 mL of aqueous solvent, in some patients, half the volume (1 mL) has been found to produce angiograms of comparable resolution; immediately following the bolus dose of dye, a bolus of sodium chloride 0.9% is given; this regimen will deliver a spatially limited dye bolus of optimal concentration to the choroidal vasculature following I.V. injection

Determination of cardiac output: Dye is injected as rapidly as possible into the right atrium, right ventricle, or pulmonary artery through a cardiac catheter; the usual dose is 1.25 mg for infants, 2.5 mg for children, and 5 mg for adults; total dose should not exceed 2 mg/kg; the dye is diluted with sterile water for injection or sodium chloride 0.9% to make a final volume of 1 mL; doses are repeated periodically to obtain several dilution curves; the dye should be flushed from the catheter with sodium chloride 0.9% to prevent hemolysis

Other Adverse Effects 1% to 10%:

Central nervous system: Headache

Dermatologic: Pruritus, skin discoloration

Pregnancy Risk Factor C

Generic Available No

Indometacin *see* Indomethacin *on page 719*

Indomethacin (in doe METH a sin)

Related Information

Rheumatoid Arthritis, Osteoarthritis, and Osteoporosis *on page 1488*

Temporomandibular Dysfunction (TMD) *on page 1562*

U.S. Brand Names Indocin®; Indocin® I.V.; Indocin® SR

Canadian Brand Names Apo®-Indomethacin; Indocid®; Indocid® P.D.A.; Indocin®; Indo-Lemmon; Indotec; Novo-Methacin; Nu-Indo; Rhodacine®

Mexican Brand Names Antalgin®; Antalgin® Dialicels; Indocid®; Malival®; Malival AP

Pharmacologic Category Nonsteroidal Anti-inflammatory Drug (NSAID)

Synonyms Indometacin; Indomethacin Sodium Trihydrate

(Continued)

Indomethacin *(Continued)*

Use Management of inflammatory diseases and rheumatoid disorders; moderate pain; acute gouty arthritis, acute bursitis/tendonitis, moderate to severe osteoarthritis, rheumatoid arthritis, ankylosing spondylitis; I.V. form used as alternative to surgery for closure of patent ductus arteriosus in neonates

Local Anesthetic/Vasoconstrictor Precautions No information available to require special precautions

Effects on Dental Treatment NSAID formulations are known to reversibly decrease platelet aggregation via mechanisms different than observed with aspirin. The dentist should be aware of the potential of abnormal coagulation. Caution should also be exercised in the use of NSAIDs in patients already on anticoagulant therapy with drugs such as warfarin (Coumadin®).

Dosage

Patent ductus arteriosus:

Neonates: I.V.: Initial: 0.2 mg/kg, followed by 2 doses depending on postnatal age (PNA):

PNA **at time of first dose** <48 hours: 0.1 mg/kg at 12- to 24-hour intervals
PNA **at time of first dose** 2-7 days: 0.2 mg/kg at 12- to 24-hour intervals
PNA **at time of first dose** >7 days: 0.25 mg/kg at 12- to 24-hour intervals

In general, may use 12-hour dosing interval if urine output >1 mL/kg/hour after prior dose; use 24-hour dosing interval if urine output is <1 mL/kg/hour but >0.6 mL/kg/hour; doses should be withheld if patient has oliguria (urine output <0.6 mL/kg/hour) or anuria

Inflammatory/rheumatoid disorders: Oral:

Children: 1-2 mg/kg/day in 2-4 divided doses; maximum dose: 4 mg/kg/day; not to exceed 150-200 mg/day

Adults: 25-50 mg/dose 2-3 times/day; maximum dose: 200 mg/day; extended release capsule should be given on a 1-2 times/day schedule

Mechanism of Action Inhibits prostaglandin synthesis by decreasing the activity of the enzyme, cyclooxygenase, which results in decreased formation of prostaglandin precursors

Other Adverse Effects

>10%: Central nervous system: Headache (12%)

1% to 10%:

Central nervous system: Dizziness (3% to 9%), fatigue (<3%), vertigo (<3%), depression (<3%), malaise (<3%), somnolence (<3%)

Gastrointestinal: Nausea (3% to 9%), epigastric pain (3% to 9%), abdominal pain/cramps/distress (<3%), heartburn (3% to 9%), indigestion (3% to 9%), constipation (<3%), diarrhea (<3%), dyspepsia (3% to 9%)

Hematologic: Inhibition of platelet aggregation (3% to 9%)

Otic: Tinnitus (<3%)

<1%: Acute respiratory distress, agranulocytosis, allergic rhinitis, anaphylaxis, anemia, angioedema, anorexia, arrhythmias, aseptic meningitis, asthma, blurred vision, bone marrow suppression, bronchospasm, cholestatic jaundice, confusion, CHF, conjunctivitis, corneal opacities, cystitis, decreased hearing, depression, dilutional hyponatremia (I.V.), drowsiness, dry eyes, **dyspnea, epistaxis**, erythema multiforme, exfoliative dermatitis, fatigue, flatulence, gastritis, **GI bleeding/ulceration/perforation**, hallucinations, hemolytic anemia, hepatitis (including fatal cases), **hot flashes**, hyperkalemia, hypersensitivity reactions, **hypertension**, hypoglycemia (I.V.), interstitial nephritis, itching, leukopenia, nephrotic syndrome, oliguria, peripheral neuropathy, polydipsia, polyuria, proctitis, psychic disturbances, psychosis, rash, renal failure, retinal/macular disturbances, shock, somnolence, Stevens-Johnson syndrome, **stomatitis, tachycardia**, thrombocytopenia, toxic amblyopia, toxic epidermal necrolysis, urticaria

Drug Interactions Substrate of CYP2C8/9, 2C19; Inhibits CYP2C8/9, 2C19

Increased Effect/Toxicity: Indomethacin may increase serum potassium with potassium-sparing diuretics. Probenecid may increase indomethacin serum concentrations. Other NSAIDs may increase GI adverse effects. May increase nephrotoxicity of cyclosporine and increase renal adverse effects of ACE inhibitors. Indomethacin may increase serum concentrations of digoxin, methotrexate, lithium, and aminoglycosides (reported with I.V. use in neonates).

Decreased Effect: May decrease antihypertensive effects of beta-blockers, hydralazine, ACE inhibitors, and angiotensin II antagonists. Indomethacin may decrease the antihypertensive and diuretic effect of thiazides (hydrochlorothiazide, etc) and loop diuretics (furosemide, bumetanide).

Dietary/Ethanol/Herb Considerations

Ethanol: Avoid use; may enhance gastric mucosal irritation.

Food: Administer with food or milk to reduce GI upset; may cause bleeding, ulceration, or perforation. Food may decrease the rate but not the extent of absorption; may delay peak serum concentration. Avoid garlic, ginger, and green tea.

Herb/Nutraceutical: Avoid cat's claw, dong quai, evening primrose, feverfew, garlic, ginger, ginkgo biloba, ginseng, green tea, horse chestnut, and red clover due to additional antiplatelet activity. Avoid kava and valerian; may enhance benzodiazepine activity.

Pharmacodynamics/Kinetics
Onset of action: ~30 minutes
Duration: 4-6 hours
Absorption: Prompt and extensive
Distribution: V_d: 0.34-1.57 L/kg; crosses placenta; enters breast milk
Protein binding: 90%
Metabolism: Hepatic; significant enterohepatic recirculation
Half-life elimination: 4.5 hours; prolonged in neonates
Time to peak: Oral: ~3-4 hours
Excretion: Urine (primarily as glucuronide conjugates)
Pregnancy Risk Factor B/D (3rd trimester)
Generic Available Yes: Capsule, suspension

Indomethacin Sodium Trihydrate *see* Indomethacin *on page 719*

INF-alpha 2 *see* Interferon Alfa-2b *on page 727*

Infantaire [OTC] *see* Acetaminophen *on page 27*

Infants Tylenol® Cold [OTC] *see* Acetaminophen and Pseudoephedrine *on page 31*

Infants' Tylenol® Cold Plus Cough Concentrated Drops [OTC] *see* Acetaminophen, Dextromethorphan, and Pseudoephedrine *on page 35*

Infasurf® *see* Calfactant *on page 232*

INFeD® *see* Iron Dextran Complex *on page 743*

Inflamase® Forte *see* PrednisoLONE *on page 1110*

Inflamase® Mild *see* PrednisoLONE *on page 1110*

Infliximab (in FLIKS e mab)

U.S. Brand Names Remicade®
Canadian Brand Names Remicade®
Pharmacologic Category Antirheumatic, Disease Modifying; Gastrointestinal Agent, Miscellaneous; Monoclonal Antibody
Synonyms Infliximab, Recombinant
Use
Crohn's disease: Reduce the signs and symptoms of moderate to severe disease in patients who have an inadequate response to conventional therapy; reduce the number of draining enterocutaneous fistulas in fistulizing disease
Rheumatoid arthritis: Used with methotrexate in patients who have had an inadequate response to methotrexate alone; used with methotrexate to inhibit the progression of structural damage and improve physical function in patients with moderate to severe disease

Local Anesthetic/Vasoconstrictor Precautions No information available to require special precautions

Effects on Dental Treatment Upper respiratory tract infection (16% to 26%), cough (5% to 13%), sinusitis (5% to 13%), pharyngitis (9% to 11%), candidiasis (~5%), fever (8% to 10%)

Dosage I.V.: Adults:
Crohn's disease:
Moderately- to severely-active: 5 mg/kg as a single infusion over a minimum of 2 hours
Fistulizing: 5 mg/kg as an infusion over a minimum of 2 hours; dose repeated at 2- and 6 weeks after the initial infusion
Rheumatoid arthritis (in combination with methotrexate therapy): 3 mg/kg followed by an additional 3 mg/kg at 2- and 6 weeks after the first dose; then repeat every 8 weeks thereafter; doses have ranged from 3-10 mg/kg intravenous infusion repeated at 4-week intervals or 8-week intervals
Dosing adjustment in renal/hepatic impairment: No specific recommendations

Mechanism of Action Infliximab is a chimeric monoclonal antibody that binds to human tumor necrosis factor alpha (TNFα) receptor sites, thereby interfering with endogenous TNFα activity. Biological activities of TNFα include the induction of pro-inflammatory cytokines (interleukins), enhancement of leukocyte migration, activation of neutrophils and eosinophils, and the induction of acute phase reactants and tissue degrading enzymes. Animal models have shown TNFα expression causes polyarthritis, and infliximab can prevent disease as well as allow diseased joints to heal.

Other Adverse Effects Although profile is similar, frequency of effects may be different in specific populations (Crohn's disease vs rheumatoid arthritis).

>10%:
Central nervous system: Headache (22% to 23%), fatigue (8% to 11%)
Dermatologic: Rash (6% to 12%)
Gastrointestinal: Nausea (17%), diarrhea (3% to 13%), abdominal pain (10% to 12%)
Local: Infusion reactions (19%)
Miscellaneous: Development of antinuclear antibodies (34%); infections (32%)
Crohn's patients with fistulizing disease: Development of new abscess (12%, 8-16 weeks after the last infusion)

(Continued)

Infliximab *(Continued)*

2% to 10%:

Cardiovascular: Chest pain (5% to 6%, similar to placebo)

Central nervous system: Pain (8% to 9%), dizziness (8% to 10%, similar to placebo)

Dermatologic: Pruritus (5% to 6%)

Gastrointestinal: Vomiting (7% to 9%), dyspepsia (5% to 6%)

Genitourinary: Urinary tract infection (3% to 8%, similar to placebo)

Neuromuscular & skeletal: Arthralgia (5% to 6%), back pain (5% to 6%)

Respiratory: Bronchitis (6% to 7%), rhinitis (6% to 9%)

Miscellaneous: Development of antibodies to double-stranded DNA (9%)

<2%: Abscess, abdominal hernia, adult respiratory distress syndrome, ALT increased (mild, incidence increased with concomitant methotrexate therapy), anemia, **anxiety**, appendicitis, **arrhythmia**, arthritis, AST increased (mild, incidence increased with concomitant methotrexate therapy), atrioventricular block, azotemia, **bacterial infection**, basal cell carcinoma, biliary pain, bone fracture, bradycardia, brain infarction, breast cancer, cardiac arrest, cardiac failure, cellulitis, ceruminosis, cholecystitis, cholelithiasis, confusion, Crohn's disease, dehydration, delirium, depression, diaphragmatic hernia, dyspnea, dysuria, edema, encephalopathy, endometriosis, endophthalmitis, fungal infection, furunculosis, gastric ulcer, gastrointestinal hemorrhage, hemarthrosis, hepatitis cholestatic, herpes zoster, hydronephrosis, **hypertension, hypotension**, intervertebral disk herniation, inflammation, injection site inflammation, intestinal obstruction, intestinal perforation, intestinal stenosis, joint cyst, joint degeneration, kidney infarction, leukopenia, lymphangitis, lupus erythematosus syndrome, lymphoma, myalgia, myocardial ischemia, osteoarthritis, osteoporosis, peripheral ischemia, pleural effusion, pleurisy, pneumonia, pneumothorax, pulmonary edema, pulmonary embolism, pulmonary infiltration, renal calculus, renal failure, **respiratory insufficiency**, rheumatoid nodules, **palpitation**, pancreatic insufficiency, pancreatitis, peritonitis, proctalgia, pyelonephritis, rectal adenocarcinoma, sepsis, skin cancer, somnolence, splenic infarction, spondylolisthesis, spinal stenosis, splenomegaly, suicide attempt, diaphoresis increased, symphyseolysis, **syncope, tachycardia**, tendon disorder, tendon injury, thrombocytopenia, thrombophlebitis (deep), ulceration, upper motor neuron lesion, ureteral obstruction, weakness, weight loss, worsening rheumatoid arthritis

Postmarketing and/or case reports: Demyelinating disorders (eg, multiple sclerosis, optic neuritis); Guillain-Barré syndrome, interstitial fibrosis, interstitial pneumonitis, latent tuberculosis reactivation, neuropathy, worsening CHF

Drug Interactions Decreased toxicity of immunosuppressants; may decrease risk of infusion related reactions and development of anti-double-stranded DNA antibodies.

Pharmacodynamics/Kinetics

Onset of action: Crohn's disease: ~2 weeks

Half-life elimination: 8-9.5 days

Pregnancy Risk Factor B (manufacturer)

Generic Available No

Infliximab, Recombinant *see* Infliximab *on page 721*

Influenza Virus Vaccine (in floo EN za VYE rus vak SEEN)

Related Information

Immunizations (Vaccines) *on page 1612*

U.S. Brand Names FluShield®; Fluvirin®; Fluzone®

Canadian Brand Names Fluviral S/F®; Fluzone®; Vaxigrip®

Pharmacologic Category Vaccine

Synonyms Influenza Virus Vaccine (inactivated whole-virus); Influenza Virus Vaccine (purified split-virus); Influenza Virus Vaccine (purified surface antigen); Influenza Virus Vaccine (split-virus)

Use Provide active immunity to influenza virus strains contained in the vaccine; for high-risk persons, previous year vaccines should not be used to prevent present year influenza

Groups at Increased Risk for Influenza-Related Complications:

- Persons ≥65 years of age
- Residents of nursing homes and other chronic-care facilities that house persons of any age with chronic medical conditions
- Adults and children with chronic disorders of the pulmonary or cardiovascular systems, including children with asthma
- Adults and children who have required regular medical follow-up or hospitalization during the preceding year because of chronic metabolic diseases (including diabetes mellitus), renal dysfunction, hemoglobinopathies, or immunosuppression (including immunosuppression caused by medications)
- Children and adolescents (6 months to 18 years of age) who are receiving long-term aspirin therapy and therefore, may be at risk for developing Reye's syndrome after influenza

- Women who will be in the 2nd or 3rd trimester of pregnancy during the influenza season

Otherwise healthy children aged 6-23 months, healthy persons who may transmit influenza to those at risk, and others who are interested in immunization to influenza virus should receive the vaccine as long as supply is available.

Local Anesthetic/Vasoconstrictor Precautions No information available to require special precautions

Effects on Dental Treatment No significant effects or complications reported

Restrictions Influenza vaccines from previous seasons must not be used. Pharmacies will stock the formulations(s) standardized according to the USPHS. Federal law requires that the date of administration, the vaccine manufacturer, lot number of vaccine, and the administering person's name, title, and address be entered into the patient's permanent medical record.

Dosage Optimal time to receive vaccine is October-November; however, vaccination can continue into December and later as long as vaccine is available. I.M.:

FluShield®, Fluzone®:

Children 6-35 months: 0.25 mL (1 or 2 doses; see **Note**)

Children 3-8 years: 0.5 mL (1 or 2 doses; see **Note**)

Children ≥9 years and Adults: 0.5 mL (1 dose)

Fluvirin®:

Children 4-8 years: 0.5 mL (1 or 2 doses; see **Note**)

Children ≥9 years and Adults: 0.5 mL (1 dose)

Note: Previously unvaccinated children <9 years should receive 2 doses, given >1 month apart in order to achieve satisfactory antibody response.

Mechanism of Action Promotes immunity to influenza virus by inducing specific antibody production. Each year the formulation is standardized according to the U.S. Public Health Service. Preparations from previous seasons must not be used.

Other Adverse Effects All serious adverse reactions must be reported to the U.S. Department of Health and Human Services (DHHS) Vaccine Adverse Event Reporting System (VAERS) 1-800-822-7967.

Frequency not defined:

Central nervous system: Fever and malaise (may start within 6-12 hours and last 1-2 days; incidence equal to placebo in adults; occurs more frequently than placebo in children); GBS (previously reported with older vaccine formulations; relationship to current formulations not known, however, patients with history of GBS have a greater likelihood of developing GBS than those without)

Dermatology: Angioedema, urticaria

Local: Tenderness, redness, or induration at the site of injection (10% to 64%; May last up to 2 days)

Neuromuscular & skeletal: Myalgia (may start within 6-12 hours and last 1-2 days; incidence equal to placebo in adults; occurs more frequently than placebo in children)

Miscellaneous: Allergic or anaphylactoid reactions (most likely to residual egg protein; includes allergic asthma, angioedema, hives, systemic anaphylaxis)

Pharmacodynamics/Kinetics

Onset: Protective antibody levels achieved ~2 weeks after vaccination

Duration: Protective antibody levels persist approximately ≥6 months

Pregnancy Risk Factor C

Generic Available No

Selected Readings Centers for Disease Control, "Recommendations of the Advisory Committee on Immunization Practices (ACIP): General Recommendations on Immunization," *MMWR*, 1994, 43(RR-1):23.

Influenza Virus Vaccine (inactivated whole-virus) *see* Influenza Virus Vaccine *on page 722*

Influenza Virus Vaccine (purified split-virus) *see* Influenza Virus Vaccine *on page 722*

Influenza Virus Vaccine (purified surface antigen) *see* Influenza Virus Vaccine *on page 722*

Influenza Virus Vaccine (split-virus) *see* Influenza Virus Vaccine *on page 722*

Infumorph® *see* Morphine Sulfate *on page 931*

INH *see* Isoniazid *on page 748*

Innohep® *see* Tinzaparin *on page 1311*

INOmax® *see* Nitric Oxide *on page 979*

Inspra™ *see* Eplerenone *on page 502*

Insta-Glucose® [OTC] *see* Glucose (Instant) *on page 641*

Insulin Preparations (IN su lin prep a RAY shuns)

Related Information

Endocrine Disorders and Pregnancy *on page 1479*

U.S. Brand Names Humalog®; Humalog® Mix 75/25™; Humulin® 50/50; Humulin® 70/30; Humulin® L; Humulin® N; Humulin® R; Humulin® R (Concentrated) U-500; Humulin® U; Lantus®; Lente® Iletin® II; Novolin® 70/30; Novolin® L; Novolin® N; (Continued)

Insulin Preparations *(Continued)*

Novolin® R; NovoLog®; NovoLog® Mix 70/30; NPH Iletin® II; Regular Iletin® II; Velosulin® BR (Buffered)

Canadian Brand Names Humalog®; Humalog® Mix 25™; Humulin®; Iletin® II Pork; Novolin® ge; NovoRapid®

Mexican Brand Names Humulin 20/80®; Humulin 30/70®; Humulin L®; Humulin N®; Humulin R®; Insulina Lenta; Insulina NPH; Insulina Regular; Insulin Novolin 30/70®; Insulin Novolin L®; Insulin Novolin N®; Insulin Novolin R®

Pharmacologic Category Antidiabetic Agent, Insulin; Antidote

Use Treatment of type 1 diabetes mellitus (insulin dependent, IDDM); type 2 diabetes mellitus (noninsulin dependent, NIDDM) unresponsive to treatment with diet and/or oral hypoglycemics; adjunct to parenteral nutrition; hyperkalemia (regular insulin only; use with glucose to shift potassium into cells to lower serum potassium levels)

Local Anesthetic/Vasoconstrictor Precautions No information available to require special precautions

Effects on Dental Treatment Type 1 diabetics (insulin-dependent) should be appointed for dental treatment in the morning in order to minimize chance of stress-induced hypoglycemia.

Dosage Dose requires continuous medical supervision; may administer I.V. (regular), I.M., S.C.

Diabetes mellitus: The number and size of daily doses, time of administration, and diet and exercise require continuous medical supervision. In addition, specific formulations may require distinct administration procedures.

Lispro should be given within 15 minutes before or immediately after a meal

Aspart should be given immediately before a meal (within 5-10 minutes of the start of a meal)

Human regular insulin should be given within 30-60 minutes before a meal.

Intermediate-acting insulins may be administered 1-2 times/day.

Long-acting insulins may be administered once daily.

Insulin glargine (Lantus®) should be administered subcutaneously once daily at bedtime. Maintenance doses should be administered subcutaneously and sites should be rotated to prevent lipodystrophy.

Children and Adults: 0.5-1 unit/kg/day in divided doses

Adolescents (growth spurts): 0.8-1.2 units/kg/day in divided doses

Adjust dose to maintain premeal and bedtime blood glucose of 80-140 mg/dL (children <5 years: 100-200 mg/dL)

Insulin glargine (Lantus®):

Type 2 diabetes (patient not already on insulin): 10 units once daily, adjusted according to patient response (range in clinical study 2-100 units/day)

Patients already receiving insulin: In clinical studies, when changing to insulin glargine from once-daily NPH or Ultralente® insulin, the initial dose was not changed; when changing from twice-daily NPH to once-daily insulin glargine, the total daily dose was reduced by 20% and adjusted according to patient response

Hyperkalemia: Administer calcium gluconate and $NaHCO_3$ first then 50% dextrose at 0.5-1 mL/kg and insulin 1 unit for every 4-5 g dextrose given

Diabetic ketoacidosis: Children and Adults: Regular insulin: I.V. loading dose: 0.1 unit/kg, then maintenance continuous infusion: 0.1 unit/kg/hour (range: 0.05-0.2 units/kg/hour depending upon the rate of decrease of serum glucose - too rapid decrease of serum glucose may lead to cerebral edema).

Optimum rate of decrease (serum glucose): 80-100 mg/dL/hour

Note: Newly diagnosed patients with IDDM presenting in DKA and patients with blood sugars <800 mg/dL may be relatively "sensitive" to insulin and should receive loading and initial maintenance doses approximately $^1/_2$ of those indicated above.

Dosing adjustment in renal impairment (regular): Insulin requirements are reduced due to changes in insulin clearance or metabolism

Cl_{cr} 10-50 mL/minute: Administer at 75% of normal dose

Cl_{cr} <10 mL/minute: Administer at 25% to 50% of normal dose and monitor glucose closely

Hemodialysis: Because of a large molecular weight (6000 daltons), insulin is not significantly removed by either peritoneal or hemodialysis

Supplemental dose is unnecessary

Peritoneal dialysis: Supplemental dose is unnecessary

Continuous arteriovenous or venovenous hemofiltration effects: Supplemental dose is unnecessary

Mechanism of Action The principal hormone required for proper glucose utilization in normal metabolic processes; it is obtained from beef or pork pancreas or a biosynthetic process converting pork insulin to human insulin; insulins are categorized into 3 groups related to promptness, duration, and intensity of action

Other Adverse Effects Frequency not defined:

Cardiovascular: **Palpitation, tachycardia,** pallor

Central nervous system: Fatigue, mental confusion, loss of consciousness, headache, hypothermia

Dermatologic: Urticaria, redness
Endocrine & metabolic: Hypoglycemia
Gastrointestinal: Hunger, nausea, numbness of mouth
Local: Itching, edema, stinging, pain or warmth at injection site; atrophy or hypertrophy of S.C. fat tissue
Neuromuscular & skeletal: Muscle weakness, paresthesia, tremors
Ocular: Transient presbyopia or blurred vision
Miscellaneous: **Diaphoresis, anaphylaxis**

Drug Interactions Induces CYP1A2

Increased Effect/Toxicity:

Increased hypoglycemic effect of insulin with alcohol, alpha-blockers, anabolic steroids, beta-blockers (nonselective beta-blockers may delay recovery from hypoglycemic episodes and mask signs/symptoms of hypoglycemia; cardioselective beta-blocker agents may be alternatives), clofibrate, guanethidine, MAO inhibitors, pentamidine, phenylbutazone, salicylates, sulfinpyrazone, and tetracyclines.

Insulin increases the risk of hypoglycemia associated with oral hypoglycemic agents (including sulfonylureas, metformin, pioglitazone, rosiglitazone, and troglitazone).

Decreased Effect: Decreased hypoglycemic effect of insulin with corticosteroids, dextrothyroxine, diltiazem, dobutamine, epinephrine, niacin, oral contraceptives, thiazide diuretics, thyroid hormone, and smoking. Buffering agent in Velosulin® BR may alter the activity of other insulin products.

Dietary/Ethanol/Herb Considerations

Ethanol: Avoid use; may increase hypoglycemia.

Food: Patient must start eating within 5-10 minutes after insulin aspart injection (NovoLog®). Insulin shifts potassium from extracellular to intracellular space; decreases potassium serum concentration; monitor. Dietary modification based on ADA recommendations is part of therapy.

Herb/Nutraceutical: Use caution with black cohosh, chromium, garlic, gymnema, and horse chestnut; may increase hypoglycemia.

Pharmacodynamics/Kinetics

Onset of action and duration: Biosynthetic NPH human insulin shows a more rapid onset and shorter duration of action than corresponding porcine insulins; human insulin and purified porcine regular insulin are similarly efficacious following S.C. administration. The duration of action of highly purified porcine insulins is shorter than that of conventional insulin equivalents. Duration depends on type of preparation and route of administration as well as patient-related variables. In general, the larger the dose of insulin, the longer the duration of activity.

Absorption: Biosynthetic regular human insulin is absorbed from the S.C. injection site more rapidly than insulins of animal origin (60-90 minutes peak vs 120-150 minutes peak respectively) and lowers the initial blood glucose much faster. Human Ultralente® insulin is absorbed about twice as quickly as its bovine equivalent, and bioavailability is also improved. Human Lente® insulin preparations are also absorbed more quickly than their animal equivalents. Insulin glargine (Lantus®) is designed to form microprecipitates when injected subcutaneously. Small amounts of insulin glargine are then released over a 24-hour period, with no pronounced peak. Insulin glargine (Lantus®) for the treatment of type 1 diabetes (insulin dependent, IDDM) and type 2 diabetes mellitus (noninsulin dependent, NIDDM) in patients who require basal (long-acting) insulin.

Bioavailability: Medium-acting S.C. Lente®-type human insulins did not differ from the corresponding porcine insulins

Lispro (Humalog®):
Onset: 0.25 hours; Peak effect: 0.5-1.5 hours; Duration: 6-8 hours

Insulin aspart (NovoLog®):
Onset: 0.5 hours; Peak effect: 1-3 hours; Duration: 3-5 hours

Insulin, regular (Novolin® R):
Onset: 0.5-1 hours; Peak effect: 2-3 hours; Duration: 8-12 hours

Isophane insulin suspension (NPH) (Novolin® N):
Onset: 1-1.5 hours; Peak effect: 4-12 hours; Duration: 24 hours

Insulin zinc suspension (Lente®):
Onset: 1-2.5 hours; Peak effect: 8-12 hours; Duration: 18-24 hours

Isophane insulin suspension and regular insulin injection (Novolin® 70/30):
Onset: 0.5 hours; Peak effect: 2-12 hours; Duration: 24 hours

Extended insulin zinc suspension (Ultralente®):
Onset: 4-8 hours; Peak effect: 16-18 hours; Duration: >36 hours

Insulin glargine (Lantus®):
Duration: 24 hours

Pregnancy Risk Factor B; C (insulin glargine [Lantus®]; insulin aspart [NovoLog®])

Generic Available No

Comments The term "purified" refers to insulin preparations containing no more than 10 ppm proinsulin (purified and human insulins are less immunogenic).

Intal® *see* Cromolyn Sodium *on page 375*

Integrilin® *see* Eptifibatide *on page 507*

α-2-interferon *see* Interferon Alfa-2b *on page 727*

Interferon Alfa-2a (in ter FEER on AL fu-too ay)

Related Information

Systemic Viral Diseases *on page 1517*

U.S. Brand Names Roferon-A®

Canadian Brand Names Roferon-A®

Pharmacologic Category Interferon

Synonyms IFLrA; rIFN-A

Use

Patients >18 years of age: Hairy cell leukemia, AIDS-related Kaposi's sarcoma, chronic hepatitis C

Children and Adults: Chronic myelogenous leukemia (CML), Philadelphia chromosome positive, within 1 year of diagnosis (limited experience in children)

Unlabeled/Investigational Use Adjuvant therapy for malignant melanoma, AIDS-related thrombocytopenia, cutaneous ulcerations of Behçet's disease, brain tumors, metastatic ileal carcinoid tumors, cervical and colorectal cancers, genital warts, idiopathic mixed cryoglobulinemia, hemangioma, hepatitis D, hepatocellular carcinoma, idiopathic hypereosinophilic syndrome, mycosis fungoides, Sézary syndrome, low-grade non-Hodgkin's lymphoma, macular degeneration, multiple myeloma, renal cell carcinoma, basal and squamous cell skin cancer, essential thrombocythemia, cutaneous T-cell lymphoma

Local Anesthetic/Vasoconstrictor Precautions No information available to require special precautions

Effects on Dental Treatment

>10%: Significant xerostomia, metallic taste, hypertension (11%), chest pain (4% to 11%), taste change (13%), loss of taste, cough (27%), irritation of oropharynx (14%), flu-like syndrome (≤92%), diaphoresis (15%)

1% to 10%: Dyspnea (7.5%), epistaxis (4%), rhinitis (3%), palpitations (<3%), acute myocardial infarction (~1%), hypotension (6%), supraventricular tachyarrhythmias,

Dosage Refer to individual protocols.

Children (limited data):

Chronic myelogenous leukemia (CML): I.M.: 2.5-5 million units/m^2/day; **Note:** In juveniles, higher dosages (30 million units/m^2/day) have been associated with severe adverse events, including death

Adults:

Hairy cell leukemia: S.C., I.M.: 3 million units/day for 16-24 weeks, then 3 million units 3 times/week for up to 6-24 months

Chronic myelogenous leukemia (CML): S.C., I.M.: 9 million units/day, continue treatment until disease progression

AIDS-related Kaposi's sarcoma: S.C., I.M.: 36 million units/day for 10-12 weeks, then 36 million units 3 times/week; to minimize adverse reactions, can use escalating dose (3-, 9-, then 18 million units each day for 3 days, then 36 million units daily thereafter). If severe reactions occur, reduce dose by 50% or discontinue until reaction subsides.

Hepatitis C: S.C., I.M.: 3 million units 3 times/week for 12 months

Dosing adjustment in renal impairment: Not removed by hemodialysis

Dosing adjustment for toxicity: If severe adverse reactions occur, modify dosage (reduce dose by 50%) or temporarily discontinue treatment until reaction subsides.

Mechanism of Action Alpha interferons are a family of proteins, produced by nucleated cells, that have antiviral, antiproliferative, and immune-regulating activity. There are 16 known subtypes of alpha interferons. Interferons interact with cells through high affinity cell surface receptors. Following activation, multiple effects can be detected including induction of gene transcription. Inhibits cellular growth, alters the state of cellular differentiation, interferes with oncogene expression, alters cell surface antigen expression, increases phagocytic activity of macrophages, and augments cytotoxicity of lymphocytes for target cells

Other Adverse Effects A flu-like syndrome (fever, chills, tachycardia, malaise, myalgia, arthralgia, headache) occurs within 1-2 hours of administration; may last up to 24 hours and may be dose-limiting (symptoms in up to 92% of patients). For the listing below, the percentage of incidence noted generally corresponds to highest reported ranges. Incidence depends upon dosage and indication.

>10%:

Cardiovascular: Edema (11%)

Central nervous system: Psychiatric disturbances (including depression and suicidal behavior/ideation; reported incidence highly variable, generally >15%), fatigue (90%), headache (52%), dizziness (21%), irritability (15%), insomnia (14%), somnolence, lethargy, confusion, mental impairment, motor weakness (most frequently seen at high doses [>100 million units]; usually reverses within a few days), vertigo (19%), mental status changes (12%)

Dermatologic: Rash (usually maculopapular) on the trunk and extremities (7% to 18%), alopecia (19% to 22%), pruritus (13%), dry skin
Endocrine & metabolic: Hypocalcemia (10% to 51%), hyperglycemia (33% to 39%), elevation of transaminase levels (25% to 30%), elevation of alkaline phosphatase (48%)
Gastrointestinal: Anorexia (30% to 70%), abdominal cramps, abdominal pain, nausea (28% to 53%), vomiting (10% to 30%, usually mild), diarrhea (22% to 34%, may be severe)
Hematologic (often due to underlying disease): Myelosuppression; neutropenia (32% to 70%); thrombocytopenia (22% to 70%); anemia (24% to 65%; may be dose-limiting, usually seen only during the first 6 months of therapy)
Onset: 7-10 days
Nadir: 14 days, may be delayed 20-40 days in hairy cell leukemia
Recovery: 21 days
Hepatic: Elevation of AST (SGOT) (77% to 80%), LDH (47%), bilirubin (31%)
Local: Injection site reaction (29%)
Neuromuscular & skeletal: Weakness (may be severe at doses >20,000,000 units/day); arthralgia and myalgia (5% to 73%, usually during the first 72 hours of treatment); rigors
Renal: Proteinuria (15% to 25%)

1% to 10%:
Central nervous system: Confusion (10%), delirium
Dermatologic: Erythema (diffuse), urticaria
Endocrine & metabolic: Hyperphosphatemia (2%)
Gastrointestinal: Stomatitis, pancreatitis (<5%), flatulence, liver pain
Genitourinary: Impotence (6%), menstrual irregularities
Neuromuscular & skeletal: Leg cramps; peripheral neuropathy, paresthesias (7%), and numbness (4%) are more common in patients previously treated with vinca alkaloids or receiving concurrent vinblastine
Ocular: Conjunctivitis (4%)
Miscellaneous: Antibody production to interferon (10%)

<1%: Abdominal fullness, aplastic anemia, arthritis, autoimmune reaction with worsening of liver disease, **bronchospasm**, cardiomyopathy, **coagulopathy, coma, CHF, cutaneous eruptions**, decreased libido, decreased visual acuity, distal cyanosis, diffuse encephalopathy, dysphasia, eczema, EEG abnormalities, elevation of BUN/creatinine, hallucinations, hemolytic anemia, hypermotility, hypertriglyceridemia, hyponatremia (SIADH), hypo- and hyperthyroidism, mania, gait disturbance, **GI hemorrhage**, leukopenia, lupus erythematosus syndrome, nasal congestion, nephrotic syndrome, pneumonia, pneumonitis, presenile dementia, proteinuria, psychotic episodes, Raynaud's phenomenon, renal failure (acute), seborrhea, **seizures, stroke, syncope**, tachypnea, vasculitis

Drug Interactions Inhibits CYP1A2

Increased Effect/Toxicity: Cimetidine may augment the antitumor effects of interferon in melanoma. Theophylline clearance has been reported to be decreased in hepatitis patients receiving interferon. Vinblastine enhances interferon toxicity in several patients; increased incidence of paresthesia has also been noted. Interferons may increase the adverse/toxic effects of ACE inhibitors, specifically the development of granulocytopenia. Agranulocytosis has been reported with concurrent use of clozapine (case report). Interferons may increase the anticoagulant effects of warfarin, and interferons may increase serum levels of zidovudine.

Decreased Effect: Prednisone may decrease the therapeutic effects of interferon alpha. A decreased response to erythropoietin has been reported (case reports) in patients receiving interferons. Interferon alpha may decrease the serum concentrations of melphalan (may or may not decrease toxicity of melphalan).

Pharmacodynamics/Kinetics

Absorption: Filtered and absorbed at the renal tubule
Distribution: V_d: 0.223-0.748 L/kg
Metabolism: Primarily renal; filtered through glomeruli and undergoes rapid proteolytic degradation during tubular reabsorption
Bioavailability: I.M.: 83%; S.C.: 90%
Half-life elimination: I.V.: 3.7-8.5 hours (mean ~5 hours)
Time to peak, serum: I.M., S.C.: ~6-8 hours

Pregnancy Risk Factor C

Generic Available No

Interferon Alfa-2a (PEG Conjugate) *see* Peginterferon Alfa-2a *on page 1040*

Interferon Alfa-2b (in ter FEER on AL fu-too bee)

Related Information

Systemic Viral Diseases *on page 1517*

U.S. Brand Names Intron® A

Canadian Brand Names Intron® A

Pharmacologic Category Interferon

Synonyms INF-alpha 2; α-2-interferon; rLFN-α2

Use

Patients >1 year of age: Chronic hepatitis B

(Continued)

Interferon Alfa-2b *(Continued)*

Patients >18 years of age: Condyloma acuminata, chronic hepatitis C, hairy cell leukemia, malignant melanoma, AIDS-related Kaposi's sarcoma, follicular non-Hodgkin's lymphoma

Unlabeled/Investigational Use

Unlabeled: Treatment of AIDS-related thrombocytopenia, cutaneous ulcerations of Behçet's disease, carcinoid syndrome, cervical cancer, lymphomatoid granulomatosis, genital herpes, hepatitis D, chronic myelogenous leukemia (CML), non-Hodgkin's lymphomas (other than follicular lymphoma, see approved use), polycythemia vera, medullary thyroid carcinoma, multiple myeloma, renal cell carcinoma, basal and squamous cell skin cancers, essential thrombocytopenia, thrombocytopenic purpura

Investigational: West Nile virus

Local Anesthetic/Vasoconstrictor Precautions No information available to require special precautions

Effects on Dental Treatment

>10%: Xerostomia (1% to 28%), metallic taste, chest pain (2% to 28%), fever (34% to 94%), gingivitis (2% to 14%), taste change (2% to 24%), dyspnea (1% to 34%), cough (1% to 31%), pharyngitis (1% to 31%), flu-like symptoms (5% to 79%), hyperglycemia (33% to 39%), paresthesia (1% to 21%), diaphoresis (2% to 21%)

1% to 10%: Hypertension (9% in hepatitis C), anxiety (1% to 9%), nervousness (1% to 3%), nasal congestion (1% to 10%)

<5%: Angina, arrhythmia, atrial fibrillation, bradycardia, tachycardia, CHF, hypotension, pulmonary embolism, myocardial infarction, aphasia, Bell's palsy, coma, seizures, dysphonia, extrapyramidal disorder, flushing, hallucinations, manic reaction, migraine, neuropathy, paranoia, psychosis, stroke, syncope, tremor, diabetes mellitus, hyperglycemia, esophagitis, gastritis, GI hemorrhage, gingival hyperplasia, mucositis, stomatitis, loss of taste, asthma, bronchospasm, hypoventilation, pulmonary fibrosis, pneumonitis, respiratory insufficiency, acute hypersensitivity reactions, allergic reactions hemoptysis

Dosage Refer to individual protocols

Children 1-17 years: Chronic hepatitis B: S.C.: 3 million units/m^2 3 times/week for 1 week; then 6 million units/m^2 3 times/week; maximum: 10 million units 3 times/week; total duration of therapy 16-24 weeks

Adults:

Hairy cell leukemia: I.M., S.C.: 2 million units/m^2 3 times/week for 2-6 months

Lymphoma (follicular): S.C.: 5 million units 3 times/week for up to 18 months

Malignant melanoma: 20 million units/m^2 I.V. for 5 consecutive days per week for 4 weeks, then 10 million units/m^2 S.C. 3 times/week for 48 weeks

AIDS-related Kaposi's sarcoma: I.M., S.C.: 30 million units/m^2 3 times/week

Chronic hepatitis B: I.M., S.C.: 5 million units/day or 10 million units 3 times/week for 16 weeks

Chronic hepatitis C: I.M., S.C.: 3 million units 3 times/week for 16 weeks. In patients with normalization of ALT at 16 weeks, continue treatment for 18-24 months; consider discontinuation if normalization does not occur at 16 weeks. **Note:** May be used in combination therapy with ribavirin in previously untreated patients or in patients who relapse following alpha interferon therapy; refer to Interferon Alfa-2b and Ribavirin Combination Pack monograph.

Condyloma acuminata: Intralesionally: 1 million units/lesion (maximum: 5 lesions/treatment) 3 times/week (on alternate days) for 3 weeks. Use 1 million unit per 0.1 mL concentration.

Dosing adjustment in renal impairment: Not removed by peritoneal or hemodialysis

Dosing adjustment for toxicity:

Reduce dose by 50% if WBC <1500 cells/mm^3, granulocytes <750 cells/mm^3 (<1000 cells/mm^3 in children), or platelet count <50,000 cells/mm^3 (<100,000 cells/mm^3 in children)

Interrupt therapy if WBC <1200 cells/mm^3, granulocytes <500 cells/mm^3 (<750 cells/mm^3 in children), or platelet count <30,000 cells/mm^3 (<70,000 cells/mm^3 in children)

Mechanism of Action Alpha interferons are a family of proteins, produced by nucleated cells, that have antiviral, antiproliferative, and immune-regulating activity. There are 16 known subtypes of alpha interferons. Interferons interact with cells through high affinity cell surface receptors. Following activation, multiple effects can be detected including induction of gene transcription. Inhibits cellular growth, alters the state of cellular differentiation, interferes with oncogene expression, alters cell surface antigen expression, increases phagocytic activity of macrophages, and augments cytotoxicity of lymphocytes for target cells

Other Adverse Effects In a majority of patients, a flu-like syndrome (fever, chills, tachycardia, malaise, myalgia, headache), occurs within 1-2 hours of administration; may last up to 24 hours and may be dose-limiting.

>10%:

Central nervous system: Fatigue (8% to 96%), headache (21% to 62%), depression (4% to 40%), somnolence (1% to 33%), irritability (1% to 22%), paresthesia (1% to 21%; more common in patients previously treated with vinca alkaloids or receiving concurrent vinblastine), dizziness (7% to 23%), confusion (1% to 12%), malaise (3% to 14%), pain (3% to 15%), insomnia (1% to 12%), impaired concentration (1% to 14%; usually reverses within a few days), amnesia (1% to 14%), chills (45% to 54%)

Dermatologic: Alopecia (8% to 38%), rash (usually maculopapular) on the trunk and extremities (1% to 25%), pruritus (3% to 11%), dry skin (1% to 10%)

Endocrine & metabolic: Hypocalcemia (10% to 51%), amenorrhea (up to 12% in lymphoma)

Gastrointestinal: Anorexia (1% to 69%), nausea (19% to 66%), vomiting (2% to 32%, usually mild), diarrhea (2% to 45%, may be severe), abdominal pain (2% to 23%), constipation (1% to 14%)

Hematologic: Myelosuppression; neutropenia (30% to 66%); thrombocytopenia (5% to 15%); anemia (15% to 32%; may be dose-limiting, usually seen only during the first 6 months of therapy)

Onset: 7-10 days

Nadir: 14 days, may be delayed 20-40 days in hairy cell leukemia

Recovery: 21 days

Hepatic: Increased transaminases (increased SGOT in up to 63%), elevation of alkaline phosphatase (48%), right upper quadrant pain (15% in hepatitis C)

Local: Injection site reaction (1% to 20%)

Neuromuscular & skeletal: Weakness (5% to 63%) may be severe at doses >20,000,000 units/day; mild arthralgia and myalgia (5% to 75% - usually during the first 72 hours of treatment), rigors (2% to 42%), back pain (1% to 19%), musculoskeletal pain (1% to 21%), paresthesia (1% to 21%)

Renal: Urinary tract infection (up to 5% in hepatitis C)

Miscellaneous: Loss of smell

5% to 10%:

Central nervous system: Vertigo (up to 8% in lymphoma)

Dermatologic: Dermatitis (1% to 8%)

Endocrine & metabolic: Decreased libido (1% to 5%)

Gastrointestinal: Loose stools (1% to 21%), dyspepsia (2% to 8%)

Neuromuscular & skeletal: Hypoesthesia (1% to 10%)

<5% (Limited to important or life-threatening):

Cardiovascular: Vasculitis, cardiomegaly, cardiomyopathy, Raynaud's phenomenon, thrombosis

Central nervous system: Abnormal coordination, aggravated depression, aphasia, ataxia, suicidal ideation, suicide attempt

Dermatologic: Diffuse erythema, eczema, epidermal necrolysis, hirsutism, psoriasis, urticaria

Endocrine & metabolic: Hyperthyroidism, hypothyroidism, hypertriglyceridemia, goiter, pancreatitis

Gastrointestinal: Ascites, colitis, rectal hemorrhage

Genitourinary: Cystitis, incontinence, dysuria

Hematologic: Anemia, granulocytopenia, leukopenia, hemolytic anemia, thrombocytopenic purpura

Hepatic: Hyperbilirubinemia, jaundice, hepatic encephalopathy (rare), hepatic failure (rare), hepatotoxic reaction

Neuromuscular & skeletal: Arthritis, leg cramps, polyarteritis nodosa, tendonitis, rheumatoid arthritis, spondylitis, lupus erythematosus

Ocular: Abnormal vision, nystagmus

Renal: Proteinuria, hematuria, increased BUN, nephrotic syndrome, renal failure

Respiratory: Pleural effusion

Drug Interactions Inhibits CYP1A2

Increased Effect/Toxicity: Cimetidine may augment the antitumor effects of interferon in melanoma. Theophylline clearance has been reported to be decreased in hepatitis patients receiving interferon. Vinblastine enhances interferon toxicity in several patients; increased incidence of paresthesia has also been noted. Interferons may increase the adverse/toxic effects of ACE inhibitors, specifically the development of granulocytopenia. Agranulocytosis has been reported with concurrent use of clozapine (case report). Interferons may increase the anticoagulant effects of warfarin, and interferons may increase serum levels of zidovudine.

Pharmacodynamics/Kinetics

Distribution: V_d: 31 L; but has been noted to be much greater (370-720 L) in leukemia patients receiving continuous infusion IFN; IFN does not penetrate the CSF

Metabolism: Primarily renal

Bioavailability: I.M.: 83%; S.C.: 90%

Half-life elimination: I.M., I.V.: 2 hours; S.C.: 3 hours

Time to peak, serum: I.M., S.C.: ~3-12 hours

Pregnancy Risk Factor C

Generic Available No

Interferon Alfa-2b and Ribavirin

(in ter FEER on AL fu-too bee & rye bu VYE rin)

Related Information

Interferon Alfa-2b *on page 727*

Ribavirin *on page 1176*

U.S. Brand Names Rebetron®

Canadian Brand Names Rebetron®

Pharmacologic Category Antiviral Agent; Interferon

Synonyms Ribavirin and Interferon Alfa-2b Combination Pack

Use The combination therapy of oral ribavirin with interferon alfa-2b, recombinant (Intron® A) injection is indicated for the treatment of chronic hepatitis C in patients with compensated liver disease who have relapsed after alpha interferon therapy.

Local Anesthetic/Vasoconstrictor Precautions No information available to require special precautions

Effects on Dental Treatment

>10%: Xerostomia, metallic taste, dyspnea (19%), flu-like syndrome (14%)

1% to 10%: Chest pain (5%), taste perversion (7%), sinusitis (9%), nervousness (4%)

Dosage

Children: Chronic hepatitis C: **Note:** Safety and efficacy have not been established; dosing based on pharmacokinetic profile: Recommended dosage of combination therapy (Intron® A with Rebetrol®):

Intron® A: S.C.:

25-61 kg: 3 million int. units/m^2 3 times/week

>61 kg: Refer to adult dosing

Rebetrol® capsule: Oral:

25-36 kg: 400 mg/day (200 mg twice daily)

37-49 kg: 600 mg/day (200 mg in morning and 400 mg in evening)

50-61 kg: 800 mg/day (400 mg twice daily)

>61 kg: Refer to adult dosing

Adults: Chronic hepatitis C: Recommended dosage of combination therapy:

Intron® A: S.C.: 3 million int. units 3 times/week **and**

Rebetrol® capsule: Oral: Range: 1000-1200 mg in a divided daily (morning and evening) dose for 24 weeks

≤75 kg (165 pounds): 1000 mg/day (two 200 mg capsules in the morning and three 200 mg capsules in the evening)

>75 kg: 1200 mg/day (three 200 mg capsules in the morning and three 200 mg capsules in the evening)

Mechanism of Action

Interferon Alfa-2b: Alpha interferons are a family of proteins, produced by nucleated cells, that have antiviral, antiproliferative, and immune-regulating activity. There are 16 known subtypes of alpha interferons. Interferons interact with cells through high affinity cell surface receptors. Following activation, multiple effects can be detected including induction of gene transcription. Inhibits cellular growth, alters the state of cellular differentiation, interferes with oncogene expression, alters cell surface antigen expression, increases phagocytic activity of macrophages, and augments cytotoxicity of lymphocytes for target cells

Ribavirin: Inhibits replication of RNA and DNA viruses; inhibits influenza virus RNA polymerase activity and inhibits the initiation and elongation of RNA fragments resulting in inhibition of viral protein synthesis

Other Adverse Effects Specific to combination regimen in previously untreated hepatitis patients (see individual agents for additional adverse reactions reported with each agent during therapy for other diseases):

>10%

Central nervous system: Fatigue (68%), headache (63%), insomnia (39%), fever (37%), depression (32%), irritability (23%), dizziness (17%), impaired concentration (11%)

Dermatologic: Alopecia (28%), pruritus (21%), rash (20%)

Gastrointestinal: Nausea (38%), anorexia (27%), dyspepsia (14%), vomiting (11%)

Hematologic: Leukopenia, neutropenia (usually recovers within 4 weeks of treatment discontinuation), anemia

Hepatic: Hyperbilirubinemia (27% - only 0.9% >3.0 mg/dL)

Local: Injection site inflammation (13%)

Neuromuscular & skeletal: Myalgia (61%), rigors (40%), arthralgia (30%), musculoskeletal pain (20%)

1% to 10%:

Central nervous system: Emotional lability (7%)

Endocrine & metabolic: Thyroid abnormalities (hyper- or hypothyroidism), increased serum uric acid, hyperglycemia

Hematologic: Hemolytic anemia (10%), thrombocytopenia, anemia

Local: Injection site reaction (7%)

Neuromuscular & skeletal: Weakness (9%)

<1%: **Acute hypersensitivity reactions, anaphylaxis**, angioedema, aplastic anemia (very rare), **arrhythmia, bronchoconstriction**, cardiomyopathy, cotton wool spots, **diabetes**, hearing loss, hepatotoxic reactions, **hypotension, MI, pneumonia, pneumonitis**, retinal hemorrhages, retinal artery or vein obstruction, severe psychiatric reactions, suicidal behavior, suicidal ideation, tinnitus, urticaria; rare cases of autoimmune diseases including vasculitis, polyarteritis reaction, rheumatoid arthritis, lupus erythematosus, and Raynaud's phenomenon

Postmarketing and/or case reports: Hypertriglyceridemia, nephrotic syndrome, pancreatitis, **hallucinations**, renal failure, sarcoidosis

Drug Interactions

Increased Effect/Toxicity: Interferon alpha: Cimetidine may augment the antitumor effects of interferon in melanoma. Theophylline clearance has been reported to be decreased in hepatitis patients receiving interferon. Vinblastine enhances interferon toxicity in several patients; increased incidence of paresthesia has also been noted. Interferons may increase the adverse/toxic effects of ACE inhibitors, specifically the development of granulocytopenia. Agranulocytosis has been reported with concurrent use of clozapine (case report). Interferons may increase the anticoagulant effects of warfarin, and interferons may increase serum levels of zidovudine. Concomitant use of ribavirin and nucleoside analogues may increase the risk of developing lactic acidosis.

Decreased Effect:

Interferon alpha: Prednisone may decrease the therapeutic effects of interferon alpha. A decreased response to erythropoietin has been reported (case reports) in patients receiving interferons. Interferon alpha may decrease the serum concentrations of melphalan (may or may not decrease toxicity of melphalan). Thyroid dysfunction has been reported during treatment; monitor response to thyroid hormones.

Ribavirin: Decreased effect of zidovudine.

Pregnancy Risk Factor X

Generic Available No

Interferon Alfa-n3 (in ter FEER on AL fu-en three)

Related Information

Systemic Viral Diseases *on page 1517*

U.S. Brand Names Alferon® N

Canadian Brand Names Alferon® N

Pharmacologic Category Interferon

Use Patients ≥18 years of age: Intralesional treatment of refractory or recurring genital or venereal warts (condylomata acuminata)

Local Anesthetic/Vasoconstrictor Precautions No information available to require special precautions

Effects on Dental Treatment

>10%: Xerostomia, metallic taste

1% to 10%: Tongue hyperesthesia (1%), abnormal taste (1%), thirst (1%), rhinitis (2%), pharyngitis (1%), nosebleed (1%), increased diaphoresis (2%)

Dosage Adults: Inject 250,000 units (0.05 mL) in each wart twice weekly for a maximum of 8 weeks; therapy should not be repeated for at least 3 months after the initial 8-week course of therapy

Mechanism of Action Interferons interact with cells through high affinity cell surface receptors. Following activation, multiple effects can be detected including induction of gene transcription. Inhibits cellular growth, alters the state of cellular differentiation, interferes with oncogene expression, alters cell surface antigen expression, increases phagocytic activity of macrophages, and augments cytotoxicity of lymphocytes for target cells

Other Adverse Effects Specific to intralesional administration in patients with condylomata acuminata:

>10%:

Central nervous system: Fever (40%), headache (31%), chills (14%), fatigue (14%)

Hematologic: Decreased WBC (11%)

Neuromuscular & skeletal: Myalgia (45%)

Miscellaneous: Flu-like syndrome (30% headache, fever, and/or myalgia; abated with repeated dosing)

1% to 10%:

Central nervous system: Malaise (9%), dizziness (9%), depression (2%), insomnia (2%)

Dermatologic: Pruritus (2%)

Gastrointestinal: Nausea (45), vomiting (3%), dyspepsia (3%), diarrhea (2%)

Genitourinary: Groin lymph node swelling (1%)

Neuromuscular & skeletal: Arthralgia (5%), back pain (4%), cramps (1%), paresthesia (1%)

Ocular: Visual disturbance (1%)

Miscellaneous: Vasovagal reaction (2%)

<1%: Dysuria, **hot flashes**, impaired concentration, **nervousness**, photosensitivity

(Continued)

Interferon Alfa-n3 *(Continued)*

Rare adverse reactions reported with other alfa-interferons include depression, suicide, autoimmune and ophthalmic disorders.

Drug Interactions

Increased Effect/Toxicity: Interferons may increase the adverse/toxic effects of ACE inhibitors, specifically the development of granulocytopenia. Risk: Monitor A case report of agranulocytosis has been reported with concurrent use of clozapine. Case reports of decreased hematopoietic effect with erythropoietin. Interferon alpha may decrease the P450 isoenzyme metabolism of theophylline. Interferons may increase the anticoagulant effects of warfarin. Interferons may decrease the metabolism of zidovudine.

Decreased Effect: Interferon alpha may decrease the serum concentrations of melphalan; this may or may not decrease the potential toxicity of melphalan. Prednisone may decrease the therapeutic effects of Interferon alpha.

Pregnancy Risk Factor C

Generic Available No

Interferon Beta-1a (in ter FEER on BAY tu-wun ay)

U.S. Brand Names Avonex®; Rebif®

Canadian Brand Names Avonex®; Rebif®

Mexican Brand Names Betaferon®; Rebif®

Pharmacologic Category Interferon

Synonyms rIFN beta-1a

Use Treatment of relapsing forms of multiple sclerosis (MS)

Local Anesthetic/Vasoconstrictor Precautions No information available to require special precautions

Effects on Dental Treatment

>10%: Upper respiratory tract infection (31%), sinusitis (18%), rhinitis (15% to 17%), fever (23% to 28%), flu-like symptoms (61%; headache, fever, myalgia, weakness; may diminish with repeated dosing), infection (11%)

1% to 10%: Dyspnea (6%), xerostomia (5%), otitis media (6%)

Dosage Adults:

I.M. (Avonex®): 30 mcg once weekly

S.C. (Rebif®): Initial: 8.8 mcg 3 times/week, increasing over a 4-week period to the recommended dose of 44 mcg 3 times/week; doses should be separated by at least 48 hours

Mechanism of Action Interferon beta differs from naturally occurring human protein by a single amino acid substitution and the lack of carbohydrate side chains; alters the expression and response to surface antigens and can enhance immune cell activities. Properties of interferon beta that modify biologic responses are mediated by cell surface receptor interactions; mechanism in the treatment of MS is unknown.

Other Adverse Effects In a comparative study, the adverse effect profiles of Avonex® and Rebif® were noted to be similar; with the exception of three adverse events noted to occur more frequently in the Rebif® group: Transaminase elevations, local reactions, and reductions in white blood cell counts.

Highest reported frequency for either product;either from placebo-controlled trials or comparative studies (some effects reported for only one product):

>10%:

Central nervous system: Headache (30% to 70%), fever (23% to 28%), chills (21%), sleep disturbance (19%), dizziness (15%), depression (11% to 13%), insomnia (10% to 13%)

Gastrointestinal: Nausea (33%), abdominal pain (9% to 22%) diarrhea (16%), dyspepsia (11%)

Hematologic: Leukopenia (up to 36% in Rebif® patients), lymphadenopathy (12%)

Hepatic: Transaminases increased (up to 27% with Rebif®; hepatic dysfunction noted in <10%)

Local: Injection site disorders: A comparative trial noted events in 80% with Rebif® versus 24% with Avonex® (includes inflammation, pain, bruising, or site reaction)

Neuromuscular & skeletal: Myalgia (25% to 34%), back pain (23% to 25%), skeletal pain (15%), weakness (21%)

Ocular: Visual abnormalities (13%)

Respiratory: Upper respiratory tract infection (31%), sinusitis (18%), rhinitis (15% to 17%)

Miscellaneous; Flu-like symptoms (61%), infection (11%)

1% to 10%:

Cardiovascular: Chest pain (8%), syncope (4%), vasodilation (4%)

Central nervous system: Somnolence (5%), suicidal tendency (4%), malaise (5%), seizure (5%), ataxia (5%)

Dermatologic: Urticaria (5%), alopecia (4%), rash (7%)

Endocrine & metabolic: Thyroid abnormalities (up to 6% with Rebif®)

Gastrointestinal: Abdominal pain (9%), anorexia (7%), xerostomia (5%)
Genitourinary: Vaginitis (4%), ovarian cyst (3%), urinary frequency (7%), incontinence (4%)
Hematologic: Thrombocytopenia (8%), anemia (8%), eosinophilia (5%)
Hepatic: Hepatic function abnormalities (9%), hyperbilirubinemia (3%)
Neuromuscular & skeletal: Arthralgia (9%), muscle spasm (7%), rigors (13%)
Ocular: Dry eyes (3%)
Otic: Otitis media (6%), hearing decreased (3%)
Respiratory: Dyspnea (6%)
Miscellaneous: Herpesvirus infection (3%), hypersensitivity reaction (3%)

<1% (Limited to important or life-threatening): Amnesia, anaphylaxis, basal cell carcinoma, Bell's palsy, cardiac arrest, colitis, gastrointestinal hemorrhage, hypothyroidism, injection site necrosis, intestinal perforation, myasthenia, osteonecrosis, pharyngeal edema, photosensitivity, psychosis, pulmonary embolism, rash, sepsis, vaginal hemorrhage

Postmarketing and/or case reports: Arrhythmia, autoimmune disorders, erythema multiforme, hepatic failure, idiopathic thrombocytopenia, pancytopenia, Stevens-Johnson syndrome

Drug Interactions Increased Effect/Toxicity: Interferons may increase the adverse/toxic effects of ACE inhibitors, specifically the development of granulocytopenia. Agranulocytosis has been reported with concurrent use of clozapine (case report). Interferons may increase the anticoagulant effects of warfarin, and interferons may increase serum levels of zidovudine.

Pharmacodynamics/Kinetics Limited data due to small doses used
Half-life elimination: Avonex®: 10 hours; Rebif®: 69 hours
Time to peak, serum: Avonex® (I.M.): 3-15 hours; Rebif® (S.C.): 14 hours

Pregnancy Risk Factor C

Generic Available No

Interferon Beta-1b (in ter FEER on BAY tu-wun bee)

U.S. Brand Names Betaseron®

Canadian Brand Names Betaseron®

Mexican Brand Names Betaferon®

Pharmacologic Category Interferon

Synonyms rIFN beta-1b

Use Reduces the frequency of clinical exacerbations in ambulatory patients with relapsing-remitting multiple sclerosis (MS)

Local Anesthetic/Vasoconstrictor Precautions No information available to require special precautions

Effects on Dental Treatment

>10%: Headache (84%), fever (59%), anxiety (15%), migraine (12%), hypoglycemia (15%), sinusitis (36%), flu-like symptoms (76% headache, fever, chills, malaise, and/or myalgias), increased diaphoresis (23%),

1% to 10%: Edema (8%), palpitation (8%), hypertension (7%), tachycardia (6%), nervousness (8%), speech disorder (3%), seizure (2%), dyspnea (8%), laryngitis (6%)

Dosage S.C.:
Children <18 years: Use not recommended
Adults >18 years: 0.25 mg (8 million units) every other day

Mechanism of Action Interferon beta-1b differs from naturally occurring human protein by a single amino acid substitution and the lack of carbohydrate side chains; alters the expression and response to surface antigens and can enhance immune cell activities. Properties of interferon beta-1b that modify biologic responses are mediated by cell surface receptor interactions; mechanism in the treatment of MS is unknown.

Other Adverse Effects

>10%:
Central nervous system: Pain (52%), chills (46%), dizziness (35%), malaise (15%)
Endocrine & metabolic: Dysmenorrhea (18%), menstrual disorder (17%), metrorrhagia (15%)
Gastrointestinal: Diarrhea (35%), abdominal pain (32%), constipation (24%), vomiting (21%)
Hematologic: Lymphopenia (82%), neutropenia (18%), leukopenia (16%), lymphadenopathy (14%)
Hepatic: SGPT increased >5x baseline (19%), SGOT increased >5x baseline (4%)
Local: Injection site reaction (85%)
Neuromuscular & skeletal: Weakness (49%), myalgia (44%), hypertonia (26%), myasthenia (13%)
Ocular: Conjunctivitis (12%)

1% to 10%:
Cardiovascular: Peripheral vascular disorder (5%), hemorrhage (3%)

(Continued)

Interferon Beta-1b *(Continued)*

Central nervous system: Nervousness (8%), somnolence (6%), confusion (4%), speech disorder (3%), seizure (2%), suicide attempt (2%), hyperkinesias (2%), amnesia (2%)
Dermatologic: Alopecia (4%)
Endocrine & metabolic: Breast pain (7%), menorrhagia (6%), fibrocystic breast (3%), breast neoplasm (2%), goiter (2%)
Genitourinary: Pelvic pain (6%), cystitis (8%), urinary urgency (4%), weight gain (4%), weight loss (4%)
Hepatic: Bilirubin increased >2.5x baseline (6%), SGOT increased >5x baseline (4%)
Local: Injection site necrosis (5%)
Ocular: Abnormal vision (7%)
Renal: Proteinuria (5%)
Respiratory: Dyspnea (8%), laryngitis (6%)

<1% (Limited to important or life-threatening): **Anaphylactoid reaction,** anemia, apnea, **arrhythmia, asthma**, blindness, **cardiac arrest,** cardiomegaly, cerebral hemorrhage, cholecystitis, **coma, delirium, diabetes mellitus, diabetes insipidus**, erythema nodosum, **esophagitis**, ethanol intolerance, exfoliative dermatitis, **GI hemorrhage, hallucinations, heart failure**, hematemesis, hepatitis, hepatomegaly, hypercalcemia, **hyperglycemia, hypoglycemia**, hypothermia, hypothyroidism, manic reaction, **MI**, skin necrosis, pancreatitis, pericardial effusion, photosensitivity, psoriasis, psychosis, pulmonary embolism, rash (maculopapular and vesiculobullous), renal calculus, sepsis, **shock**, SIADH, **syncope**, thrombocytopenia, tremor, vaginal hemorrhage

Drug Interactions Increased Effect/Toxicity: Interferons may increase the adverse/toxic effects of ACE inhibitors, specifically the development of granulocytopenia. Risk: Monitor A case report of agranulocytosis has been reported with concurrent use of clozapine. Case reports of decreased hematopoietic effect with erythropoietin. Interferon alpha may decrease the P450 isoenzyme metabolism of theophylline. Interferons may increase the anticoagulant effects of warfarin. Interferons may decrease the metabolism of zidovudine.

Pharmacodynamics/Kinetics Limited data due to small doses used
Half-life elimination: 8 minutes to 4.3 hours
Time to peak, serum: 1-8 hours

Pregnancy Risk Factor C

Generic Available No

Interferon Gamma-1b (in ter FEER on GAM u-wun bee)

U.S. Brand Names Actimmune®

Canadian Brand Names Actimmune®

Pharmacologic Category Interferon

Use Reduce frequency and severity of serious infections associated with chronic granulomatous disease; delay time to disease progression in patients with severe, malignant osteopetrosis

Local Anesthetic/Vasoconstrictor Precautions No information available to require special precautions

Effects on Dental Treatment No significant effects or complications reported

Dosage If severe reactions occur, modify dose (50% reduction) or therapy should be discontinued until adverse reactions abate.
Chronic granulomatous disease: Children >1 year and Adults: S.C.:
BSA ≤0.5 m^2: 1.5 mcg/kg/dose 3 times/week
BSA >0.5 m^2: 50 mcg/m^2 (1 million int. units/m^2) 3 times/week

Severe, malignant osteopetrosis: Children >1 year: S.C.:
BSA ≤0.5 m^2: 1.5 mcg/kg/dose 3 times/week
BSA >0.5 m^2: 50 mcg/m^2 (1 million int. units/m^2) 3 times/week

Note: Previously expressed as 1.5 million units/m^2; 50 mcg is equivalent to 1 million int. units/m^2.

Other Adverse Effects Based on 50 mcg/m^2 dose administered 3 times weekly for chronic granulomatous disease:

>10%:
Central nervous system: Fever (52%), headache (33%), chills (14%), fatigue (14%)
Dermatologic: Rash (17%)
Gastrointestinal: Diarrhea (14%), vomiting (13%)
Local: Injection site erythema or tenderness (14%)

1% to 10%:
Central nervous system: Depression (3%)
Gastrointestinal: Nausea (10%), abdominal pain (8%)
Neuromuscular & skeletal: Myalgia (6%), arthralgia (2%), back pain (2%)

Drug Interactions Inhibits CYP1A2, 2E1
Increased Effect/Toxicity: Interferon gamma-1b may increase hepatic enzymes or enhance myelosuppression when taken with other myelosuppressive agents.

May decrease cytochrome P450 concentrations leading to increased serum concentrations of drugs metabolized by this pathway.

Dietary/Ethanol/Herb Considerations Herb/Nutraceutical: Dietary supplements containing aristolochic acid (found most often in Chinese medicines/herbal therapies) have been associated with cases of nephropathy and ESRD.

Pharmacodynamics/Kinetics

Absorption: I.M., S.C.: Slowly

Half-life elimination: I.V.: 38 minutes; I.M., S.C.: 3-6 hours

Time to peak, plasma: I.M.: 4 hours (1.5 ng/mL); S.C.: 7 hours (0.6 ng/mL)

Pregnancy Risk Factor C

Generic Available No

Comments More heat- and acid-labile than alfa interferons

Interleukin-1 Receptor antagonist *see* Anakinra *on page 108*

Interleukin-2 *see* Aldesleukin *on page 50*

Interleukin-11 *see* Oprelvekin *on page 1003*

Intralipid® *see* Fat Emulsion *on page 558*

Intravenous Fat Emulsion *see* Fat Emulsion *on page 558*

Intrifiban *see* Eptifibatide *on page 507*

Intron® A *see* Interferon Alfa-2b *on page 727*

Invanz® *see* Ertapenem *on page 511*

Inversine® *see* Mecamylamine *on page 846*

Invirase® *see* Saquinavir *on page 1207*

Iodex [OTC] *see* Iodine *on page 735*

Iodine (EYE oh dyne)

U.S. Brand Names Iodex [OTC]; Iodoflex™; Iodosorb®

Pharmacologic Category Topical Skin Product

Use Used topically as an antiseptic in the management of minor, superficial skin wounds and has been used to disinfect the skin preoperatively

Local Anesthetic/Vasoconstrictor Precautions No information available to require special precautions

Effects on Dental Treatment No significant effects or complications reported

Dosage Apply topically as necessary to affected areas of skin

Other Adverse Effects Frequency not defined:

Central nervous system: **Fever, headache**

Dermatologic: Skin rash, angioedema, urticaria, acne

Endocrine & metabolic: Hypothyroidism

Gastrointestinal: **Metallic taste**, diarrhea

Hematologic: Eosinophilia, hemorrhage (mucosal)

Neuromuscular & skeletal: Arthralgia

Ocular: Swelling of eyelids

Respiratory: Pulmonary edema

Miscellaneous: Lymph node enlargement

Drug Interactions Decreased Effect: Sodium thiosulfate inactivates iodine.

Pregnancy Risk Factor D

Generic Available Yes

Comments Solutions of sodium thiosulfate may be used to remove iodine stains from skin and clothing.

Iodine *see* Trace Metals *on page 1328*

Iodoflex™ *see* Iodine *on page 735*

Iodopen® *see* Trace Metals *on page 1328*

Iodoquinol (eye oh doe KWIN ole)

U.S. Brand Names Yodoxin®

Canadian Brand Names Diodoquin®

Pharmacologic Category Amebicide

Synonyms Diiodohydroxyquin

Use Treatment of acute and chronic intestinal amebiasis; asymptomatic cyst passers; *Blastocystis hominis* infections; ineffective for amebic hepatitis or hepatic abscess

Local Anesthetic/Vasoconstrictor Precautions No information available to require special precautions

Effects on Dental Treatment No significant effects or complications reported

Dosage Oral:

Children: 30-40 mg/kg/day (maximum: 650 mg/dose) in 3 divided doses for 20 days; not to exceed 1.95 g/day

Adults: 650 mg 3 times/day after meals for 20 days; not to exceed 1.95 g/day

Mechanism of Action Contact amebicide that works in the lumen of the intestine by an unknown mechanism

Other Adverse Effects Frequency not defined:

Central nervous system: Fever, chills, agitation, retrograde amnesia, headache

Dermatologic: Rash, urticaria, pruritus

(Continued)

Iodoquinol *(Continued)*

Endocrine & metabolic: Thyroid gland enlargement
Gastrointestinal: Diarrhea, nausea, vomiting, stomach pain, abdominal cramps
Neuromuscular & skeletal: Peripheral neuropathy, weakness
Ocular: Optic neuritis, optic atrophy, visual impairment
Miscellaneous: Itching of rectal area

Pharmacodynamics/Kinetics
Absorption: Poor and erratic
Metabolism: Hepatic
Excretion: Feces (high percentage)

Pregnancy Risk Factor C

Generic Available No

Iodoquinol and Hydrocortisone

(eye oh doe KWIN ole & hye droe KOR ti sone)

Related Information
Hydrocortisone *on page 688*
Iodoquinol *on page 735*

U.S. Brand Names Dermazene®; Vytone®

Pharmacologic Category Antifungal Agent, Topical; Corticosteroid, Topical

Synonyms Hydrocortisone and Iodoquinol

Use Treatment of eczema; infectious dermatitis; chronic eczematoid otitis externa; mycotic dermatoses

Local Anesthetic/Vasoconstrictor Precautions No information available to require special precautions

Effects on Dental Treatment >10%: Epistaxis, nervousness,

Dosage Apply 3-4 times/day

Other Adverse Effects

Based on iodoquinol component (frequency not defined):
- Central nervous system: Fever, chills, agitation, retrograde amnesia, headache
- Dermatologic: Rash, urticaria, pruritus
- Endocrine & metabolic: Thyroid gland enlargement
- Gastrointestinal: Diarrhea, nausea, vomiting, stomach pain, abdominal cramps
- Neuromuscular & skeletal: Peripheral neuropathy, weakness
- Ocular: Optic neuritis, optic atrophy, visual impairment
- Miscellaneous: Itching of rectal area

Based on hydrocortisone component:

>10%:
- Central nervous system: Insomnia
- Gastrointestinal: Increased appetite, indigestion

1% to 10%:
- Dermatologic: Hirsutism
- Endocrine & metabolic: Diabetes mellitus
- Neuromuscular & skeletal: Arthralgia
- Ocular: Cataracts

<1%: **Hypertension**, edema, euphoria, delirium, **headache, hallucinations, seizures**, mood swings, acne, dermatitis, skin atrophy, bruising, hyperpigmentation, hypokalemia, hyperglycemia, Cushing's syndrome, sodium and water retention, bone growth suppression, amenorrhea, peptic ulcer, abdominal distention, **ulcerative esophagitis**, pancreatitis, muscle wasting, hypersensitivity reactions, immunosuppression

Pregnancy Risk Factor C

Generic Available Yes

Iodosorb® *see* Iodine *on page 735*

Iohexol *see* Radiological/Contrast Media (Nonionic) *on page 1165*

Ionamin® *see* Phentermine *on page 1069*

Ionil® [OTC] *see* Salicylic Acid *on page 1204*

Ionil® Plus [OTC] *see* Salicylic Acid *on page 1204*

Iopamidol *see* Radiological/Contrast Media (Nonionic) *on page 1165*

Iopidine® *see* Apraclonidine *on page 118*

Iosat™ [OTC] *see* Potassium Iodide *on page 1101*

Ioversol *see* Radiological/Contrast Media (Nonionic) *on page 1165*

Ipecac Syrup

(IP e kak SIR up)

Pharmacologic Category Antidote

Use Treatment of acute oral drug overdosage and in certain poisonings

Local Anesthetic/Vasoconstrictor Precautions No information available to require special precautions

Effects on Dental Treatment No significant effects or complications reported

Dosage Oral:
Children:
6-12 months: 5-10 mL followed by 10-20 mL/kg of water; repeat dose one time if vomiting does not occur within 20 minutes
1-12 years: 15 mL followed by 10-20 mL/kg of water; repeat dose one time if vomiting does not occur within 20 minutes
If emesis does not occur within 30 minutes after second dose, ipecac must be removed from stomach by gastric lavage
Adults: 15-30 mL followed by 200-300 mL of water; repeat dose one time if vomiting does not occur within 20 minutes

Mechanism of Action Irritates the gastric mucosa and stimulates the medullary chemoreceptor trigger zone to induce vomiting

Other Adverse Effects Frequency not defined:
Cardiovascular: Cardiotoxicity
Central nervous system: Lethargy
Gastrointestinal: Protracted vomiting, diarrhea
Neuromuscular & skeletal: Myopathy

Drug Interactions
Increased Effect/Toxicity: Phenothiazines (chlorpromazine has been associated with serious dystonic reactions).
Decreased Effect: Activated charcoal decreases effect of ipecac syrup.

Dietary/Ethanol/Herb Considerations Food: Milk and carbonated beverages decrease effectiveness.

Pharmacodynamics/Kinetics
Onset of action: 15-30 minutes
Duration: 20-25 minutes; 60 minutes in some cases
Absorption: Significant amounts, mainly when it does not produce emesis
Excretion: Urine; emetine (alkaloid component) may be detected in urine 60 days after excess dose or chronic use

Pregnancy Risk Factor C

Generic Available Yes

I-Pentolate® *see* Cyclopentolate *on page 380*
IPM Wound Gel™ [OTC] *see* Sodium Hyaluronate *on page 1230*
IPOL® *see* Poliovirus Vaccine (Inactivated) *on page 1093*

Ipratropium (i pra TROE pee um)

Related Information
Ipratropium and Albuterol *on page 738*
Respiratory Diseases *on page 1476*

U.S. Brand Names Atrovent®

Canadian Brand Names Alti-Ipratropium; Apo®-Ipravent; Atrovent®; Gen-Ipratropium; Novo-Ipramide; Novo-Ipramide; Nu-Ipratropium; PMS-Ipratropium

Mexican Brand Names Atrovent®

Pharmacologic Category Anticholinergic Agent

Synonyms Ipratropium Bromide

Use Anticholinergic bronchodilator used in bronchospasm associated with COPD, bronchitis, and emphysema; symptomatic relief of rhinorrhea associated with the common cold and allergic and nonallergic rhinitis

Local Anesthetic/Vasoconstrictor Precautions No information available to require special precautions

Effects on Dental Treatment
Inhalation, aerosol and solution:
>10%: Xerostomia, changes in salivation
<10%: Upper respiratory infection (13%), bronchitis (15%)
1% to 10%: Palpitations (2%), nervousness (3%), dry mucous membranes, bronchospasm (2%), pharyngitis (3%), rhinitis (2%), sinusitis (5%), nasal congestion, dyspnea (10%), increased sputum (1%), flu-like symptoms
Nasal spray: Epistaxis (8%), nasal dryness (5%)

Dosage
Nebulization:
Infants and Children ≤12 years: 125-250 mcg 3 times/day
Children >12 years and Adults: 500 mcg (one unit-dose vial) 3-4 times/day with doses 6-8 hours apart

Oral inhalation: MDI:
Children 3-12 years: 1-2 inhalations 3 times/day, up to 6 inhalations/24 hours
Children >12 years and Adults: 2 inhalations 4 times/day, up to 12 inhalations/24 hours

Intranasal: Nasal spray:
Symptomatic relief of rhinorrhea associated with the common cold (safety and efficacy of use beyond 4 days in patients with the common cold have not been established):
Children 5-11 years: 0.06%: 2 sprays in each nostril 3 times/day

(Continued)

Ipratropium *(Continued)*

Children ≥5 years and Adults: 0.06%: 2 sprays in each nostril 3-4 times/day

Symptomatic relief of rhinorrhea associated with allergic/nonallergic rhinitis: Children ≥6 years and Adults: 0.03%: 2 sprays in each nostril 2-3 times/day

Mechanism of Action Blocks the action of acetylcholine at parasympathetic sites in bronchial smooth muscle causing bronchodilation

Other Adverse Effects

Inhalation, aerosol and solution:

1% to 10%:

Central nervous system: Dizziness (2%), fatigue, headache (6%), pain (4%)

Dermatologic: Rash (1%)

Gastrointestinal: Nausea, GI upset

Nasal spray: Nausea (2%)

<1%: Urticaria, **stomatitis, mucosal ulcers**, insomnia, tremor, constipation, hypersensitivity reactions, urinary retention, blurred vision

Drug Interactions Increased Effect/Toxicity: Increased therapeutic effect with albuterol. Increased toxicity with anticholinergics or drugs with anticholinergic properties and dronabinol.

Pharmacodynamics/Kinetics

Onset of action: Bronchodilation: 1-3 minutes

Peak effect: 1.5-2 hours

Duration: ≤4-6 hours

Absorption: Negligible

Distribution: Inhalation: 15% of dose reaches lower airways

Pregnancy Risk Factor B

Generic Available Yes: Solution for nebulization

Ipratropium and Albuterol (i pra TROE pee um & al BYOO ter ole)

Related Information

Albuterol *on page 48*

Ipratropium *on page 737*

U.S. Brand Names Combivent®; DuoNeb™

Canadian Brand Names Combivent®

Pharmacologic Category Bronchodilator

Synonyms Albuterol and Ipratropium

Use Treatment of COPD in those patients that are currently on a regular bronchodilator who continue to have bronchospasms and require a second bronchodilator

Local Anesthetic/Vasoconstrictor Precautions No information available to require special precautions

Effects on Dental Treatment

>10%: Xerostomia, increased diaphoresis, tachycardia, palpitations

<10%: Upper respiratory infection (13%), bronchitis (15%)

1% to 10%: Dry mucous membrane, nasal congestion, dyspnea (10%), increased sputum (1%), bronchospasm (2%), pharyngitis (3%), rhinitis (2%), sinusitis (5%), flu-like symptoms, nervousness (3%) flushing, hypertension, hypotension, nervousness, headache, unusual taste, cough

Dosage Adults:

Inhalation: 2 inhalations 4 times/day (maximum: 12 inhalations/24 hours)

Inhalation via nebulization: Initial: 3 mL every 6 hours (maximum: 3 mL every 4 hours)

Mechanism of Action See individual agents.

Other Adverse Effects

Based on ipratropium component:

Inhalation, aerosol and solution:

1% to 10%:

Cardiovascular: Palpitations (2%)

Central nervous system: Dizziness (2%), fatigue, headache (6%), pain (4%)

Dermatologic: Rash (1%)

Gastrointestinal: Nausea, GI upset

<1%: Urticaria, **stomatitis**, insomnia, **tremor, mucosal ulcers,** constipation, hypersensitivity reactions, urinary retention, blurred vision

Based on albuterol component:

>10%: Gastrointestinal: GI upset, nausea

1% to 10%:

Central nervous system: CNS stimulation, hyperactivity, insomnia, dizziness, lightheadedness, drowsiness,

Gastrointestinal: Heartburn, vomiting

Genitourinary: Dysuria

Neuromuscular & skeletal: Muscle cramping, tremor, weakness

<1%: **Chest pain**, unusual pallor, loss of appetite, paradoxical bronchospasm, hypokalemia

Pregnancy Risk Factor C

Generic Available No

Ipratropium Bromide *see* Ipratropium *on page 737*
I-Prin [OTC] *see* Ibuprofen *on page 703*
Iproveratril Hydrochloride *see* Verapamil *on page 1382*
IPV *see* Poliovirus Vaccine (Inactivated) *on page 1093*

Irbesartan (ir be SAR tan)

U.S. Brand Names Avapro®

Canadian Brand Names Avapro®

Mexican Brand Names Aprovel®; Avapro®

Pharmacologic Category Angiotensin II Receptor Blocker

Use Treatment of hypertension alone or in combination with other antihypertensives; treatment of diabetic nephropathy in patients with type 2 diabetes mellitus (noninsulin dependent, NIDDM) and hypertension

Local Anesthetic/Vasoconstrictor Precautions No information available to require special precautions

Effects on Dental Treatment >10%: Orthostatic hypotension (5%, diabetic nephropathy), upper respiratory infection (9%)

Dosage Oral:

Hypertension:

Children:

<6 years: Safety and efficacy have not been established.

≥6-12 years: Initial: 75 mg once daily; may be titrated to a maximum of 150 mg once daily

Children ≥13 years and Adults: 150 mg once daily; patients may be titrated to 300 mg once daily

Note: Starting dose in volume-depleted patients should be 75 mg

Nephropathy in patients with type 2 diabetes and hypertension: Adults: Target dose: 300 mg once daily

Dosing adjustment in renal impairment: None required in mild to severe impairment unless the patient is also volume depleted

Mechanism of Action Irbesartan is an angiotensin receptor antagonist. Angiotensin II acts as a vasoconstrictor. In addition to causing direct vasoconstriction, angiotensin II also stimulates the release of aldosterone. Once aldosterone is released, sodium as well as water are reabsorbed. The end result is an elevation in blood pressure. Irbesartan binds to the AT1 angiotensin II receptor. This binding prevents angiotensin II from binding to the receptor thereby blocking the vasoconstriction and the aldosterone secreting effects of angiotensin II.

Other Adverse Effects Percentage of incidence is reported for patients with hypertension (unless otherwise indicated):

>10%: Endocrine & metabolic: Hyperkalemia (19%, diabetic nephropathy)

1% to 10%:

Central nervous system: Fatigue (4%), dizziness (10%, diabetic nephropathy)

Gastrointestinal: Diarrhea (3%), dyspepsia (2%)

Respiratory: Cough (2.8% versus 2.7% in placebo)

>1% but frequency ≤ placebo: Abdominal pain, **anxiety, chest pain,** edema, **headache, influenza**, musculoskeletal pain, nausea, **nervousness, pharyngitis,** rash, **rhinitis, sinus abnormality, syncope, tachycardia,** urinary tract infection, vertigo, vomiting

<1% (Limited to important or life-threatening): Abdominal distension, abnormal urination, **angina, arrhythmia, arthritis, bronchitis**, bursitis, **cardiopulmonary arrest**, cerebrovascular accident, chest pain (noncardiac), chills, **congestion**, conjunctivitis, constipation, depression, dermatitis, dyspnea, ear infection, ear pain, ecchymosis, **epistaxis**, erythema, **facial edema, fever**, flatulence, **flushing, gastroenteritis**, gout, hearing abnormality, **heart failure, hypertension, hypertensive crisis, hypotension**, libido decreased, **MI**, muscle aches, muscle cramps, muscle weakness, numbness, **orthostatic hypotension**, paresthesia, prostate disorder, pruritus, pulmonary congestion, serum creatinine increased (0.7% versus 0.9% in placebo), sexual dysfunction, sleep disturbance, somnolence, TIA, tremor, upper extremity edema, vision disturbance, wheezing.

May be associated with worsening of renal function in patients dependent on renin-angiotensin-aldosterone system.

Postmarketing reports: Angioedema, jaundice, transaminases increased, urticaria

Drug Interactions Substrate of CYP2C8/9; Inhibits CYP2C8/9, 3A4

Increased Effect/Toxicity: Potassium salts/supplements, co-trimoxazole (high dose), ACE inhibitors, and potassium-sparing diuretics (amiloride, spironolactone, triamterene) may increase the risk of hyperkalemia.

Dietary/Ethanol/Herb Considerations

Ethanol: Avoid use; may increase risk of hypotension or dizziness.

Food: May be taken with food; avoid caffeine (eg, colas, chocolate), garlic, and licorice.

Herb/Nutraceutical: Avoid black cohosh, dong quai, and evening primrose due to estrogenic activity. Avoid ephedra, ginseng, and yohimbe; may worsen hypertension. Avoid garlic; may have increased antihypertensive effect. Avoid ginger due to positive inotropic effects; theoretically, may cause arrhythmia. Avoid hawthorn;

(Continued)

Irbesartan *(Continued)*

may lower peripheral vascular resistance resulting in additive decrease in BP. Avoid licorice.

Pharmacodynamics/Kinetics

Onset of action: Peak effect: 1-2 hours

Duration: >24 hours

Distribution: V_d: 53-93 L

Protein binding, plasma: 90%

Metabolism: Hepatic, primarily CYP2C9

Bioavailability: 60% to 80%

Half-life elimination: Terminal: 11-15 hours

Time to peak, serum: 1.5-2 hours

Excretion: Feces (80%); urine (20%)

Pregnancy Risk Factor C/D (2nd and 3rd trimesters)

Generic Available No

Irbesartan and Hydrochlorothiazide

(ir be SAR tan & hye droe klor oh THYE a zide)

Related Information

Hydrochlorothiazide *on page 675*

Irbesartan *on page 739*

U.S. Brand Names Avalide®

Canadian Brand Names Avalide®

Pharmacologic Category Antihypertensive Agent Combination

Synonyms Avapro® HCT; Hydrochlorothiazide and Irbesartan

Use Combination therapy for the management of hypertension

Local Anesthetic/Vasoconstrictor Precautions No information available to require special precautions

Effects on Dental Treatment No significant effects or complications reported

Dosage Dose must be individualized. A patient who is not controlled with either agent alone may be switched to the combination product. Mean effect increases with the dose of each component. The lowest dosage available is irbesartan 150 mg/hydrochlorothiazide 12.5 mg. Dose increases should be made not more frequently than every 2-4 weeks.

Mechanism of Action

Irbesartan: Irbesartan is an angiotensin receptor antagonist. Angiotensin II acts as a vasoconstrictor. In addition to causing direct vasoconstriction, angiotensin II also stimulates the release of aldosterone. Once aldosterone is released, sodium as well as water are reabsorbed. The end result is an elevation in blood pressure. Irbesartan binds to the AT1 angiotensin II receptor. This binding prevents angiotensin II from binding to the receptor thereby blocking the vasoconstriction and the aldosterone secreting effects of angiotensin II.

Hydrochlorothiazide: Inhibits sodium reabsorption in the distal tubules causing increased excretion of sodium and water as well as potassium and hydrogen ions

Pregnancy Risk Factor C/D (2nd and 3rd trimesters)

Generic Available No

Ircon® [OTC] *see* Iron Supplements *on page 745*

Irinotecan (eye rye no TEE kan)

U.S. Brand Names Camptosar®

Canadian Brand Names Camptosar®

Mexican Brand Names Camptosar®

Pharmacologic Category Antineoplastic Agent, Natural Source (Plant) Derivative

Synonyms Camptothecin-11; CPT-11

Use A component of first-line therapy in combination with 5-fluorouracil and leucovorin for the treatment of metastatic carcinoma of the colon or rectum; treatment of metastatic carcinoma of the colon or rectum which has recurred or progressed following fluorouracil-based therapy

Unlabeled/Investigational Use Treatment of cervical, gastric, pancreatic, breast, and lung (small cell and nonsmall cell) cancers; leukemia, lymphoma

Local Anesthetic/Vasoconstrictor Precautions No information available to require special precautions

Effects on Dental Treatment >10%: Vasodilation, diaphoresis, fever (45.4%), dyspnea (22%), coughing, rhinitis

Dosage It is recommended that new courses begin only after the granulocyte count recovers to ≥1500/mm^3, the platelet count recovers to ≥100,000/mm^3, and treatment-related diarrhea has fully resolved. Treatment should be delayed 1-2 weeks to allow for recovery from treatment-related toxicities. If the patient has not recovered after a 2-week delay, consideration should be given to discontinuing irinotecan. Courses may be repeated indefinitely as long as the patient continues to experience clinical benefit. Refer to individual protocols.

Adults: I.V.:

Single-agent therapy:

Weekly regimen: 125 mg/m^2 over 90 minutes on days 1, 8, 15, and 22, followed by a 2-week rest

Adjusted dose level -1: 100 mg/m^2

Adjusted dose level -2: 75 mg/m^2

Once-every-3-week regimen: 350 mg/m^2 over 90 minutes, once every 3 weeks

Adjusted dose level -1: 300 mg/m^2

Adjusted dose level -2: 250 mg/m^2

A reduction in the starting dose by one dose level may be considered for patients ≥65 years of age, prior pelvic/abdominal radiotherapy, performance status of 2, or increased bilirubin (dosing for patients with a bilirubin >2 mg/dL cannot be recommended based on lack of data per manufacturer). Depending on the patient's ability to tolerate therapy, doses should be adjusted in increments of 25-50 mg/m^2. Irinotecan doses may range 50-150 mg/m^2.

Combination therapy with 5-FU and leucovorin: Six-week (42-day) cycle (next cycle beginning on day 45):

125 mg/m^2 over 90 minutes on days 1, 8, 15, and 22; to be given in combination with bolus leucovorin and 5-FU (leucovorin administered immediately following irinotecan; 5-FU immediately following leucovorin)

Adjusted dose level -1: 100 mg/m^2

Adjusted dose level -2: 75 mg/m^2

180 mg/m^2 over 90 minutes on days 1, 15, and 22; to be given in combination with infusional leucovorin and bolus/infusion 5-FU (leucovorin administered immediately following irinotecan; 5-FU immediately following leucovorin)

Adjusted dose level -1: 150 mg/m^2

Adjusted dose level -2: 120 mg/m^2

Dosing adjustment in renal impairment: Not evaluated

Dosing adjustment in hepatic impairment:

AUC of irinotecan and SN-38 have been reported to be higher in patients with known hepatic tumor involvement. The manufacturer recommends that no change in dosage or administration be made for patients with liver metastases and normal hepatic function.

Combination Schedules: Recommended Dosage Modifications[1]

Toxicity NCI[2] Grade (Value)	During a Cycle of Therapy	At the Start of Subsequent Cycles of Therapy (After Adequate Recovery), Compared to the Starting Dose in the Previous Cycle[1]
No toxicity	Maintain dose level	Maintain dose level
Neutropenia		
1 (1500-1999/mm^3)	Maintain dose level	Maintain dose level
2 (1000-1499/mm^3)	↓ 1 dose level	Maintain dose level
3 (500-999/mm^3)	Omit dose until resolved to ≤ grade 2, then ↓ 1 dose level	↓ 1 dose level
4 (<500/mm^3)	Omit dose until resolved to ≤ grade 2, then ↓ 2 dose levels	↓ 2 dose levels
Neutropenic Fever (grade 4 neutropenia and ≥ grade 2 fever)	Omit dose until resolved, then ↓ 2 dose levels	
Other Hematologic Toxicities	Dose modifications for leukopenia or thrombocytopenia during a course of therapy and at the start of subsequent courses of therapy are also based on NCI toxicity criteria and are the same as recommended for neutropenia above.	
Diarrhea		
1 (2-3 stools/day > pretreatment)	Delay dose until resolved to baseline, then give same dose	Maintain dose level
2 (4-6 stools/day > pretreatment)	Omit dose until resolved to baseline, then ↓ 1 dose level	Maintain dose level
3 (7-9 stools/day > pretreatment)	Omit dose until resolved to baseline, then ↓ by 1 dose level	↓ 1 dose level
4 (≥10 stools/day > pretreatment)	Omit dose until resolved to baseline, then ↓ 2 dose levels	↓ 2 dose levels
Other Nonhematologic Toxicities[3]		
1	Maintain dose level	Maintain dose level
2	Omit dose until resolved to ≤ grade 1, then ↓ 1 dose level	Maintain dose level
3	Omit dose until resolved to ≤ grade 2, then ↓ 1 dose level	↓ 1 dose level
4	Omit dose until resolved to ≤ grade 2, then ↓ 2 dose levels	↓ 2 dose levels
Mucositis and/or stomatitis	Decrease only 5-FU, not irinotecan	Decrease only 5-FU, not irinotecan

[1]All dose modifications should be based on the worst preceding toxicity.

[2]National Cancer Institute Common Toxicity Criteria (version 1.0)

[3]Excludes alopecia, anorexia, asthenia

(Continued)

Irinotecan *(Continued)*

In patients with a combined history of prior pelvic/abdominal irradiation and modestly elevated total serum bilirubin levels (1.0-2.0 mg/dL) prior to treatment with irinotecan, there may be substantially increased likelihood of grade 3 or 4 neutropenia. Consideration may be given to starting irinotecan at a lower dose (eg, 100 mg/m^2) in such patients. Definite recommendations regarding the most appropriate starting dose in patients who have pretreatment total serum bilirubin elevations >2.0 mg/dL are unavailable, but it is likely that lower starting doses will need to be considered in such patients.

Dosing adjustment for toxicities: It is recommended that new courses begin only after the granulocyte count recovers to ≥1500/mm^3, the platelet counts recovers to ≥100,000/mm^3, and treatment-related diarrhea has fully resolved. Depending on the patient's ability to tolerate therapy, doses should be adjusted in increments of 25-50 mg/m^2. Irinotecan doses may range 50-150 mg/m^2. Treatment should be delayed 1-2 weeks to allow for recovery from treatment-related toxicities. If the patient has not recovered after a 2-week delay, consideration should be given to discontinuing irinotecan. See tables on previous page and below.

Single-Agent Schedule: Recommended Dosage Modifications[1]

Toxicity NCI Grade[2] (Value)	During a Cycle of Therapy	At the Start of Subsequent Cycles of Therapy (After Adequate Recovery), Compared to the Starting Dose in the Previous Cycle[1]	
	Weekly	Weekly	Once Every 3 Weeks
No toxicity	Maintain dose level	↑ 25 mg/m^2 up to a maximum dose of 150 mg/m^2	Maintain dose level
Neutropenia			
1 (1500-1999/mm^3)	Maintain dose level	Maintain dose level	Maintain dose level
2 (1000-1499/mm^3)	↓ 25 mg/m^2	Maintain dose level	Maintain dose level
3 (500-999/mm^3)	Omit dose until resolved to ≤ grade 2, then ↓ 25 mg/m^2	↓ 25 mg/m^2	↓ 50 mg/m^2
4 (<500/mm^3)	Omit dose until resolved to ≤ grade 2, then ↓ 50 mg/m^2	↓ 50 mg/m^2	↓ 50 mg/m^2
Neutropenic Fever (grade 4 neutropenia and ≥ grade 2 fever)	Omit dose until resolved, then ↓ 50 mg/m^2	↓ 50 mg/m^2	↓ 50 mg/m^2
Other Hematologic Toxicities	Dose modifications for leukopenia, thrombocytopenia, and anemia during a course of therapy and at the start of subsequent courses of therapy are also based on NCI toxicity criteria and are the same as recommended for neutropenia above.		
Diarrhea			
1 (2-3 stools/day > pretreatment)	Maintain dose level	Maintain dose level	Maintain dose level
2 (4-6 stools/day > pretreatment)	↓ 25 mg/m^2	Maintain dose level	Maintain dose level
3 (7-9 stools/day > pretreatment)	Omit dose until resolved to ≤ grade 2, then ↓ 25 mg/m^2	↓ 25 mg/m^2	↓ 50 mg/m^2
4 (≥10 stools/day > pretreatment)	Omit dose until resolved to ≤ grade 2, then ↓ 50 mg/m^2	↓ 50 mg/m^2	↓ 50 mg/m^2
Other Nonhematologic Toxicities[3]			
1	Maintain dose level	Maintain dose level	Maintain dose level
2	↓ 25 mg/m^2	↓ 25 mg/m^2	↓ 50 mg/m^2
3	Omit dose until resolved to ≤ grade 2, then ↓ 25 mg/m^2	↓ 25 mg/m^2	↓ 50 mg/m^2
4	Omit dose until resolved to ≤ grade 2, then ↓ 50 mg/m^2	↓ 50 mg/m^2	↓ 50 mg/m^2

[1]All dose modifications should be based on the worst preceding toxicity.

[2]National Cancer Institute Common Toxicity Criteria (version 1.0)

[3]Excludes alopecia, anorexia, asthenia

Mechanism of Action Irinotecan and its active metabolite (SN-38) bind reversibly to topoisomerase I and stabilize the cleavable complex so that religation of the cleaved DNA strand cannot occur. This results in the accumulation of cleavable complexes and single-strand DNA breaks. This interaction results in double-stranded DNA breaks and cell death consistent with S-phase cell cycle specificity.

Other Adverse Effects

>10%:

Central nervous system: Insomnia, dizziness

Dermatologic: Alopecia (60.5%), rash

Gastrointestinal: Irinotecan therapy may induce two different forms of diarrhea. Onset, symptoms, proposed mechanisms and treatment are different. Overall, 56.9% of patients treated experience abdominal pain and/or cramping during therapy. Anorexia, constipation, flatulence, stomatitis, and dyspepsia have also been reported.

Diarrhea: Dose-limiting toxicity with weekly dosing regimen

Early diarrhea (50.7% incidence, grade 3/4 8%) usually occurs during or within 24 hours of administration. May be accompanied by symptoms of cramping, vomiting, flushing, and diaphoresis. It is thought to be mediated by cholinergic effects which can be successfully managed with atropine.

Late diarrhea (87.8% incidence) usually occurs >24 hours after treatment. National Cancer Institute (NCI) grade 3 or 4 diarrhea (31%) occurs in 30.6% of patients. Late diarrhea generally occurs with a median of 11 days after therapy and lasts approximately 3 days. Patients experiencing grade 3 or 4 diarrhea were noted to have symptoms a total of 7 days. Correlated with irinotecan or SN-38 levels in plasma and bile. Due to the duration, dehydration and electrolyte imbalances are significant clinical concerns. Loperamide therapy is recommended. The incidence of grade 3 or 4 late diarrhea is significantly higher in patients ≥65 years of age; close monitoring and prompt initiation of high-dose loperamide therapy is prudent (refer to Warnings/Precautions).

Emetic potential: Moderately high (86.2% incidence, however, only 12.5% grade 3 or 4 vomiting)

Hematologic: Myelosuppressive: Dose-limiting toxicity with 3 week dosing regimen

Grade 1-4 neutropenia occurred in 53.9% of patients. Patients who had previously received pelvic or abdominal radiation therapy were noted to have a significantly increased incidence of grade 3 or 4 neutropenia. White blood cell count nadir is 15 days after administration and is more frequent than thrombocytopenia. Recovery is usually within 24-28 days and cumulative toxicity has not been observed.

WBC: Mild to severe

Platelets: Mild

Onset: 10 days

Nadir: 14-16 days

Recovery: 21-28 days

Neuromuscular & skeletal: Weakness (75.7%)

Respiratory: Decreased DLCO (in a few patients)

1% to 10%: **Irritant chemotherapy**; thrombophlebitis has been reported

<1%, postmarketing and/or case reports: **Anaphylactoid reaction, anaphylaxis, bleeding**, colitis, ileus, renal failure (acute), renal impairment; pulmonary toxicity (dyspnea, fever, reticulonodular infiltrates on chest x-ray)

Drug Interactions Substrate of **CYP2B6, 3A4**

Increased Effect/Toxicity: Hold diuretics during dosing due to potential risk of dehydration secondary to vomiting and/or diarrhea induced by irinotecan. Prophylactic dexamethasone as an antiemetic may enhance lymphocytopenia. Prochlorperazine may increase incidence of akathisia. Adverse reactions such as myelosuppression and diarrhea would be expected to be exacerbated by other antineoplastic agents.

Pharmacodynamics/Kinetics

Distribution: V_d: 33-150 L/m^2

Protein binding, plasma: Parent drug: 30% to 68%; SN-38 (active drug): 95%

Metabolism: Via intestinal mucosa, plasma, hepatic, and perhaps in some tumors; converted to SN-38 by carboxylesterase enzymes; undergoes glucuronidation, the metabolite having much less activity than SN-38. Enterohepatic recirculation results in a second peak in the concentration of SN-38. The lactones of both irinotecan and SN-38 undergo hydrolysis to inactive hydroxy acid forms.

Half-life elimination: Parent drug: Alpha: 0.2 hours, Beta: 2.5 hours, Gamma: 14.2 hours; SN-38: 3-23.9 hours.

Time to peak: SN-38: 30-minute infusion: ~1 hour

Excretion: Urine (~20% of dose) within 24 hours; SN-38 excretion in 24 hours accounted for 0.25% of administered dose

Pregnancy Risk Factor D

Generic Available No

Iron Dextran Complex (EYE ern DEKS tran KOM pleks)

U.S. Brand Names Dexferrum®; INFeD®

Canadian Brand Names Dexiron™; Infufer®

Mexican Brand Names Driken

Pharmacologic Category Iron Salt

Use Treatment of microcytic hypochromic anemia resulting from iron deficiency in patients in whom oral administration is infeasible or ineffective

Local Anesthetic/Vasoconstrictor Precautions No information available to require special precautions

Effects on Dental Treatment

>10%: Metallic taste, flushing, fever, headache, diaphoresis; may be delayed 24-48 hours after I.V. administration or 3-4 days after I.M. administration.

1% to 10%: Hypotension (1% to 2%)

(Continued)

Iron Dextran Complex *(Continued)*

Dosage I.M. (Z-track method should be used for I.M. injection), I.V.:

A 0.5 mL test dose (0.25 mL in infants) should be given prior to starting iron dextran therapy; total dose should be divided into a daily schedule for I.M., total dose may be given as a single continuous infusion

Iron-deficiency anemia: Dose (mL) = 0.0476 x LBW (kg) x (normal hemoglobin - observed hemoglobin) + (1 mL/5 kg of LBW to maximum of 14 mL for iron stores)

LBW = Lean Body Weight

Iron replacement therapy for blood loss: Replacement iron (mg) = blood loss (mL) x hematocrit

Maximum daily dose (can administer total dose at one time I.V.):
- Infants <5 kg: 25 mg iron (0.5 mL)
- Children:
  - 5-10 kg: 50 mg iron (1 mL)
  - 10-50 kg: 100 mg iron (2 mL)
- Adults >50 kg: 100 mg iron (2 mL)

Mechanism of Action The released iron, from the plasma, eventually replenishes the depleted iron stores in the bone marrow where it is incorporated into hemoglobin

Other Adverse Effects Diaphoresis, urticaria, arthralgia, fever, chills, dizziness, headache, and nausea may be delayed 24-48 hours after I.V. administration or 3-4 days after I.M. administration.

>10%:
- Central nervous system: Dizziness, pain
- Gastrointestinal: Nausea, vomiting
- Local: Staining of skin at the site of I.M. injection

1% to 10%:
- Dermatologic: Urticaria (1% to 2%), phlebitis (1% to 2%)
- Gastrointestinal: Diarrhea
- Genitourinary: Discoloration of urine

<1%: **Cardiovascular collapse**, leukocytosis, chills, arthralgia, **respiratory difficulty,** lymphadenopathy, **anaphylaxis, shock**

Anaphylactoid reactions: Respiratory difficulties and cardiovascular collapse have been reported and occur most frequently within the first several minutes of administration.

Drug Interactions Decreased Effect: Decreased effect with chloramphenicol.

Dietary/Ethanol/Herb Considerations Food: Diary products may decrease bioavailability.

Pharmacodynamics/Kinetics

Absorption:
- I.M.: 50% to 90% is promptly absorbed, balance is slowly absorbed over month
- I.V.: Uptake of iron by the reticuloendothelial system appears to be constant at about 10-20 mg/hour

Excretion: Urine and feces via reticuloendothelial system

Pregnancy Risk Factor C

Generic Available No

Comments 2 mL of undiluted iron dextran is the maximum recommended daily dose; epinephrine should be immediately available in the event of acute hypersensitivity reaction

Iron Sucrose (EYE ern SOO krose)

U.S. Brand Names Venofer®

Pharmacologic Category Iron Salt

Use Treatment of iron-deficiency anemia in patients undergoing chronic hemodialysis who are receiving supplemental erythropoietin therapy

Local Anesthetic/Vasoconstrictor Precautions No information available to require special precautions

Effects on Dental Treatment
- >10%: Hypotension (36%)
- >5%: Headache
- 1% to 5%: Chest pain, hypertension, fever, dyspnea, pneumonia, cough

Dosage Doses expressed in mg of **elemental** iron

I.V.: Adults: Iron-deficiency anemia: 100 mg (5 mL of iron sucrose injection) administered 1-3 times/week during dialysis, to a total dose of 1000 mg (10 doses); administer no more than 3 times/week; may continue to administer at lowest dose necessary to maintain target hemoglobin, hematocrit, and iron storage parameters

Test dose: Product labeling does not indicate need for a test dose in product-naive patients; test doses were administered in some clinical trials as 50 mg (2.5 mL) in 50 mL 0.9% NaCl administered over 3-10 minutes

Elderly: Insufficient data to identify differences between elderly and other adults; use caution

Mechanism of Action Iron sucrose is dissociated by the reticuloendothelial system into iron and sucrose. The released iron increases serum iron concentrations and is incorporated into hemoglobin.

Other Adverse Effects Fatal and life-threatening anaphylactoid reactions (characterized by anaphylactic shock, loss of consciousness, collapse, hypotension, dyspnea, or convulsion) have been reported; hypotension may be related to total dose or rate of administration.

>5%:
- Gastrointestinal: Nausea, vomiting, diarrhea
- Neuromuscular & skeletal: Leg cramps (23%)

1% to 5%:
- Cardiovascular: Hypervolemia
- Central nervous system: Malaise, dizziness
- Dermatologic: Pruritus
- Gastrointestinal: Abdominal pain
- Hepatic: Elevated enzymes
- Local: Application site reaction
- Neuromuscular & skeletal: Musculoskeletal pain, weakness

<1%, postmarketing, and/or case reports: **Anaphylactoid reactions, anaphylactic shock, collapse, convulsion, facial rash, loss of consciousness**, necrotizing enterocolitis (reported in premature infants, no causal relationship established), urticaria

Drug Interactions Decreased Effect: Chloramphenicol may diminish the therapeutic effects of iron sucrose injection. Iron sucrose injection may reduce the absorption of oral iron preparations.

Pharmacodynamics/Kinetics
- Distribution: V_{dss}: Healthy adults: 7.9 L
- Metabolism: Dissociated into iron and sucrose by the reticuloendothelial system
- Half-life elimination: Healthy adults: 6 hours
- Excretion: Healthy adults: Urine (5%) within 24 hours

Pregnancy Risk Factor B

Generic Available No

Iron Sulfate (Ferrous Sulfate) *see* Iron Supplements *on page 745*

Iron Supplements (EYE ern SUP le ments)

U.S. Brand Names Femiron® [OTC]; Feostat® [OTC]; Feratab® [OTC]; Fer-Gen-Sol [OTC]; Fergon® [OTC]; Fer-In-Sol® [OTC]; Fer-Iron® [OTC]; Ferretts [OTC]; Ferro-Sequels® [OTC]; Hemocyte® [OTC]; Ircon® [OTC]; Nephro-Fer® [OTC]; Slow FE® [OTC]

Canadian Brand Names Apo®-Ferrous Gluconate; Apo®-Ferrous Sulfate; Palafer®; PMS-Ferrous Sulfate

Mexican Brand Names Ferval® Ferroso; Hemobion® 200; Hemobion® 400; Orafer®

Pharmacologic Category Iron Salt; Mineral, Oral; Mineral, Parenteral

Synonyms Ferrous Fumarate; Ferrous Gluconate; Ferrous Salts; Ferrous Sulfate; $FeSO_4$ (Ferrous Sulfate); Iron Sulfate (Ferrous Sulfate)

Use Prevention and treatment of iron deficiency anemias; supplemental therapy for patients receiving epoetin alfa

Local Anesthetic/Vasoconstrictor Precautions No information available to require special precautions

Effects on Dental Treatment Do not prescribe tetracyclines simultaneously with iron since GI tract absorption of both tetracycline and iron may be inhibited. Liquid preparations may temporarily stain teeth.

Frequency not defined: GI irritation, epigastric pain, nausea

Dosage Multiple salt forms of iron exist; close attention must be paid to the salt form when ordering and administering iron; incorrect selection or substitution of one salt for another without proper dosage adjustment may result in serious over- or underdosing. See table.

Recommended Daily Allowance of Iron (dosage expressed as elemental iron)

Age	RDA (mg)
<5 months	5
5 months to 10 years	10
Male	
11-18 years	12
>18 years	10
Female	
11-50 years	15
>50 years	10

(Continued)

Iron Supplements *(Continued)*

Children:

Oral: Dose expressed in terms of **elemental** iron:

Premature neonates: 2-4 mg elemental iron/kg/day divided every 12-24 hours (maximum dose: 15 mg/day)

Infants and Children:

Severe iron deficiency anemia: 4-6 mg elemental iron/kg/day in 3 divided doses

Mild to moderate iron deficiency anemia: 3 mg elemental iron/kg/day in 1-2 divided doses

Prophylaxis: 1-2 mg elemental iron/kg/day up to a maximum of 15 mg elemental iron/day

Adults:

Oral (Dose expressed in terms of **elemental** iron):

Iron deficiency: 60-100 mg elemental iron twice daily up to 60 mg elemental iron 4 times/day, or 50 mg elemental iron (extended release) 1-2 times/day

Prophylaxis: 60-100 mg elemental iron/day (see table)

Elemental Iron Content of Iron Salts

Iron Salt	Elemental Iron Content (% of salt form)	Approximate Equivalent Doses (mg of iron salt)
Ferrous fumarate	33	197
Ferrous gluconate	11.6	560
Ferrous sulfate	20	324

Mechanism of Action Released from plasma and eventually replenishes depleted iron stores in bone marrow where it is incorporated into hemoglobin; allows the transportation of oxygen via hemoglobin

Other Adverse Effects Frequency not defined:

Gastrointestinal: Diarrhea, dark stools, constipation

Genitourinary: Discoloration of urine (black or dark)

Drug Interactions

Increased Effect/Toxicity: Concurrent administration ≥200 mg vitamin C per 30 mg elemental iron increases absorption of oral iron.

Decreased Effect: Absorption of oral preparation of iron and tetracyclines is decreased when both of these drugs are given together. Absorption of quinolones may be decreased due to formation of a ferric ion-quinolone complex. Concurrent administration of antacids and cimetidine may decrease iron absorption. Iron may decrease absorption of penicillamine, methyldopa, and levodopa when given at the same time. Response to iron therapy may be delayed in patients receiving chloramphenicol.

Dietary/Ethanol/Herb Considerations Food: Milk, cereals, dietary fiber, tea, coffee, or eggs decrease absorption of iron. Some products contain sulfites and/or tartrazine which may cause allergic reactions in susceptible individuals.

Pregnancy Risk Factor A

Dosage Forms Elemental iron listed in brackets:

Ferrous fumarate:

Tablet: 325 mg [106 mg]

Femiron®: 63 mg [20 mg]

Ferretts: 325 mg [106 mg]

Hemocyte®: 324 mg [106 mg]

Ircon®: 200 mg [66 mg]

Nephro-Fer®: 350 mg [115 mg]

Tablet, chewable (Feostat®): 100 mg [33 mg] [chocolate flavor]

Tablet, timed release (Ferro-Sequels®): 150 mg [50 mg] [with docusate sodium and sodium benzoate]

Ferrous gluconate:

Tablet: 300 mg [34 mg]; 325 mg [36 mg]

Fergon®: 240 mg [27 mg]

Ferrous sulfate:

Drops, oral: 75 mg/0.6 mL (50 mL) [15 mg/0.6 mL]

Fer-Gen-Sol: 75 mg/0.6 mL (50 mL) [15 mg/0.6 mL] [lemon-lime flavor]

Fer-In-Sol®: 75 mg/0.6 mL (50 mL) [15 mg/0.6 mL] [contains 0.2% alcohol and sodium bisulfite]

Elixir: 220 mg/5 mL (480 mL) [44 mg/5 mL] [contains alcohol]

Tablet: 324 mg [65 mg]; 325 mg [65 mg]

Feratab®: 300 mg [60 mg]

Tablet, exsiccated (Feosol®): 200 mg [65 mg]

Tablet, exsiccated, timed release (Slow FE®): 160 mg [50 mg]

Generic Available Yes

ISD *see* Isosorbide Dinitrate *on page 750*
ISDN *see* Isosorbide Dinitrate *on page 750*
ISG *see* Immune Globulin (Intramuscular) *on page 713*
ISMN *see* Isosorbide Mononitrate *on page 751*
Ismo® *see* Isosorbide Mononitrate *on page 751*
Isoamyl Nitrite *see* Amyl Nitrite *on page 107*
Isobamate *see* Carisoprodol *on page 251*

Isocarboxazid (eye soe kar BOKS a zid)

U.S. Brand Names Marplan®

Pharmacologic Category Antidepressant, Monoamine Oxidase Inhibitor

Use Symptomatic treatment of atypical, nonendogenous or neurotic depression

Local Anesthetic/Vasoconstrictor Precautions Attempts should be made to avoid use of vasoconstrictor due to possibility of hypertensive episodes with monoamine oxidase inhibitors

Effects on Dental Treatment

>10%: Orthostatic hypotension

1% to 10%: Xerostomia, tachycardia, nervousness

Avoid use as an analgesic due to toxic reactions with MAO inhibitors.

Dosage Adults: Oral: 10 mg 3 times/day; reduce to 10-20 mg/day in divided doses when condition improves

Mechanism of Action Thought to act by increasing endogenous concentrations of epinephrine, norepinephrine, dopamine, and serotonin through inhibition of the enzyme (monoamine oxidase) responsible for the breakdown of these neurotransmitters

Other Adverse Effects

>10%:
- Central nervous system: Drowsiness
- Endocrine & metabolic: Decreased sexual ability
- Neuromuscular & skeletal: Weakness, trembling
- Ocular: Blurred vision

1% to 10%:
- Cardiovascular: Peripheral edema
- Central nervous system: Chills
- Gastrointestinal: Diarrhea, anorexia, constipation

<1%: Hepatitis, leukopenia, parkinsonian syndrome

Drug Interactions

Increased Effect/Toxicity: In general, the combined use with TCAs, venlafaxine, trazodone, dexfenfluramine, sibutramine, lithium, meperidine, fenfluramine, dextromethorphan, and SSRIs should be avoided due to the potential for severe adverse reactions (serotonin syndrome, death). MAO inhibitors (including isocarboxazid) may inhibit the metabolism of barbiturates and prolong their effect. Isocarboxazid in combination with amphetamines, other stimulants (methylphenidate), levodopa, metaraminol, reserpine, and decongestants (pseudoephedrine) may result in severe hypertensive reactions. Foods (eg, cheese) and beverages (eg, ethanol) containing tyramine should be avoided; hypertensive crisis may result. Isocarboxazid may increase the pressor response of norepinephrine and may prolong neuromuscular blockade produced by succinylcholine. Tramadol may increase the risk of seizures and serotonin syndrome in patients receiving an MAO inhibitor. Isocarboxazid may produce additive hypoglycemic effect in patients receiving hypoglycemic agents and may produce delirium in patients receiving disulfiram.

Decreased Effect: MAO inhibitors may inhibit the antihypertensive response to guanadrel or guanethidine.

Dietary/Ethanol/Herb Considerations

Ethanol: Avoid use; may contain tyramine (eg, Chianti, hearty red wine, and beer).

Food: Avoid food/beverages high in tyramine (eg, avocadoes, bananas, broad bean pods, canned figs, cheese, chicken liver, pickled herring, raisins, sour cream, soy sauce, yeast extracts, yogurt, pods, meats prepared with tenderizers, and foods aged to improve flavor); may cause sudden and severe high BP.

Pregnancy Risk Factor C

Generic Available No

Isoetharine (eye soe ETH a reen)

Related Information

Respiratory Diseases *on page 1476*

Canadian Brand Names Beta-2®; Bronkometer®; Bronkosol®

Pharmacologic Category Adrenergic Agonist Agent; Sympathomimetic

Synonyms Isoetharine Hydrochloride; Isoetharine Mesylate

Use Bronchodilator in bronchial asthma and for reversible bronchospasm occurring with bronchitis and emphysema

Local Anesthetic/Vasoconstrictor Precautions Isoetharine is selective for beta-adrenergic receptors and not alpha receptors; therefore, there is no precaution in the use of vasoconstrictor

(Continued)

Isoetharine *(Continued)*

Effects on Dental Treatment 1% to 10%: Xerostomia

Dosage Treatments are not usually repeated more than every 4 hours, except in severe cases

Nebulizer: Children: 0.01 mL/kg; minimum dose 0.1 mL; maximum dose: 0.5 mL diluted in 2-3 mL normal saline

Mechanism of Action Relaxes bronchial smooth muscle by action on beta$_2$-receptors with very little effect on heart rate

Other Adverse Effects Frequency not defined:

Cardiovascular: **Tachycardia, hypertension, palpitations**

Central nervous system: Dizziness, lightheadedness, **headache, nervousness**, insomnia

Gastrointestinal: Nausea, vomiting

Neuromuscular & skeletal: Trembling, weakness

Respiratory: **Paradoxical bronchospasm**

Drug Interactions

Increased toxicity with other sympathomimetics (eg, epinephrine).

Decreased effect with beta-blockers.

Dietary/Ethanol/Herb Considerations Herb/Nutraceutical: Avoid ephedra, ginseng, and yohimbe; may cause CNS stimulation.

Pharmacodynamics/Kinetics

Onset of action: Peak effect: Inhalation: 5-15 minutes

Duration: 1-4 hours

Metabolism: Hepatic, pulmonary, and other tissues

Excretion: Urine (90% primarily as metabolites)

Pregnancy Risk Factor C

Generic Available Yes

Isoetharine Hydrochloride *see* Isoetharine *on page 747*

Isoetharine Mesylate *see* Isoetharine *on page 747*

Isometheptene, Acetaminophen, and Dichloralphenazone *see* Acetaminophen, Isometheptene, and Dichloralphenazone *on page 36*

Isometheptene, Dichloralphenazone, and Acetaminophen *see* Acetaminophen, Isometheptene, and Dichloralphenazone *on page 36*

Isoniazid (eye soe NYE a zid)

Related Information

Nonviral Infectious Diseases *on page 1493*

Tuberculosis *on page 1493*

U.S. Brand Names Nydrazid®

Canadian Brand Names Isotamine®; PMS-Isoniazid

Pharmacologic Category Antitubercular Agent

Synonyms INH; Isonicotinic Acid Hydrazide

Use Treatment of susceptible tuberculosis infections; prophylactically in those individuals exposed to tuberculosis

Local Anesthetic/Vasoconstrictor Precautions No information available to require special precautions

Effects on Dental Treatment 1% to 10%: Xerostomia

Dosage Recommendations often change due to resistant strains and newly developed information; consult *MMWR* for current CDC recommendations: **Oral** (injectable is available for patients who are unable to either take or absorb oral therapy): A four-drug regimen (isoniazid, rifampin, pyrazinamide, and either streptomycin or ethambutol) is preferred for the initial, empiric treatment of TB. When the drug susceptibility results are available, the regimen should be altered as appropriate.

Infants and Children:

Prophylaxis: 10 mg/kg/day in 1-2 divided doses (maximum: 300 mg/day) 6 months in patients who do not have HIV infection and 12 months in patients who have HIV infection

Treatment:

Daily therapy: 10-20 mg/kg/day in 1-2 divided doses (maximum: 300 mg/day)

Directly observed therapy (DOT): Twice weekly therapy: 20-40 mg/kg (maximum: 900 mg/day); 3 times/week therapy: 20-40 mg/kg (maximum: 900 mg)

Adults:

Prophylaxis: 300 mg/day for 6 months in patients who do not have HIV infection and 12 months in patients who have HIV infection

Treatment:

Daily therapy: 5 mg/kg/day given daily (usual dose: 300 mg/day); 10 mg/kg/day in 1-2 divided doses in patients with disseminated disease

Directly observed therapy (DOT): Twice weekly therapy: 15 mg/kg (maximum: 900 mg); 3 times/week therapy: 15 mg/kg (maximum: 900 mg)

Note: Concomitant administration of 6-50 mg/day pyridoxine is recommended in malnourished patients or those prone to neuropathy (eg, alcoholics, diabetics)

Hemodialysis: Dialyzable (50% to 100%)

Administer dose postdialysis

Peritoneal dialysis effects: Dose for Cl_{cr} <10 mL/minute

Continuous arteriovenous or venovenous hemofiltration: Dose for Cl_{cr} <10 mL/minute

Dosing adjustment in hepatic impairment: Should be reduced in severe hepatic disease

Mechanism of Action Unknown, but may include the inhibition of myocolic acid synthesis resulting in disruption of the bacterial cell wall

Other Adverse Effects

>10%:

Gastrointestinal: Loss of appetite, nausea, vomiting, stomach pain

Hepatic: Mild increased LFTs (10% to 20%)

Neuromuscular & skeletal: Weakness, peripheral neuropathy (dose-related incidence, 10% to 20% incidence with 10 mg/kg/day)

1% to 10%:

Central nervous system: Dizziness, slurred speech, lethargy

Hepatic: Progressive liver damage (increases with age; 2.3% in patients >50 years)

Neuromuscular & skeletal: Hyper-reflexia

<1%: **Fever, seizures**, mental depression, psychosis, rash, blood dyscrasias, arthralgia, blurred vision, loss of vision

Drug Interactions Substrate of **CYP2E1**; Inhibits CYP1A2, 2C8/9, 2C19, 2D6, 2E1, 3A4; Induces CYP2E1 (after discontinuation)

Increased effect/toxicity of oral anticoagulants, carbamazepines, cycloserine, hydantoins, and hepatically metabolized benzodiazepines. Reaction with disulfiram.

Decreased effect of isoniazid with aluminum salts.

Dietary/Ethanol/Herb Considerations

Ethanol: Avoid use; increases the risk of hepatitis and may contain tyramine.

Food may decrease serum concentration. Avoid foods with histamine or tyramine (eg, cheese, broad beans, dry sausage, salami, nonfresh meat, liver pate, soy bean, liquid and powdered protein supplements, wine). Isoniazid decreases folic acid absorption and alters pyridoxine metabolism.

Pharmacodynamics/Kinetics

Absorption: Rapid and complete; rate can be slowed with food

Distribution: All body tissues and fluids including CSF; crosses placenta; enters breast milk

Protein binding: 10% to 15%

Metabolism: Hepatic with decay rate determined genetically by acetylation phenotype

Half-life elimination: Fast acetylators: 30-100 minutes; Slow acetylators: 2-5 hours; may be prolonged with hepatic or severe renal impairment

Time to peak, serum: 1-2 hours

Excretion: Urine (75% to 95%); feces; saliva

Pregnancy Risk Factor C

Generic Available Yes

Isoniazid and Rifampin *see* Rifampin and Isoniazid *on page 1181*

Isoniazid, Rifampin, and Pyrazinamide *see* Rifampin, Isoniazid, and Pyrazinamide *on page 1182*

Isonicotinic Acid Hydrazide *see* Isoniazid *on page 748*

Isonipecaine Hydrochloride *see* Meperidine *on page 858*

Isoprenaline Hydrochloride *see* Isoproterenol *on page 749*

Isoproterenol (eye soe proe TER e nole)

Related Information

Cardiovascular Diseases *on page 1456*

U.S. Brand Names Isuprel®

Pharmacologic Category $Beta_1$/$Beta_2$ Agonist

Synonyms Isoprenaline Hydrochloride; Isoproterenol Hydrochloride; Isoproterenol Sulfate

Use Ventricular arrhythmias due to AV nodal block; hemodynamically compromised bradyarrhythmias or atropine- and dopamine-resistant bradyarrhythmias (when transcutaneous/venous pacing is not available); temporary use in third-degree AV block until pacemaker insertion

Unlabeled/Investigational Use Temporizing measure before transvenous pacing for torsade de pointes; diagnostic aid (vasovagal syncope)

Local Anesthetic/Vasoconstrictor Precautions Isoproterenol is selective for beta-adrenergic receptors and not alpha receptors; therefore, there is no precaution in the use of vasoconstrictor such as epinephrine

Effects on Dental Treatment >10%: Xerostomia, changes in salivation

Dosage I.V.: Cardiac arrhythmias:

Children: Initial: 0.1 mcg/kg/minute (usual effective dose 0.2-2 mcg/kg/minute)

Adults: Initial: 2 mcg/minute; titrate to patient response (2-10 mcg/minute)

(Continued)

Isoproterenol *(Continued)*

Mechanism of Action Stimulates $beta_1$- and $beta_2$-receptors resulting in relaxation of bronchial, GI, and uterine smooth muscle, increased heart rate and contractility, vasodilation of peripheral vasculature

Other Adverse Effects Frequency not defined:

Cardiovascular: Premature ventricular beats, bradycardia, hypertension, hypotension, chest pain, palpitations, tachycardia, ventricular arrhythmias, MI size increased

Central nervous system: **Headache, nervousness, restlessness**

Gastrointestinal: Nausea, vomiting

Respiratory: **Dyspnea**

Drug Interactions Increased Effect/Toxicity: Sympathomimetic agents may cause headaches and elevate blood pressure. General anesthetics may cause arrhythmias.

Dietary/Ethanol/Herb Considerations Herb/Nutraceutical: Avoid ephedra, ginseng, and yohimbe; may cause CNS stimulation.

Pharmacodynamics/Kinetics

Onset of action: Bronchodilation: I.V.: Immediate

Duration: I.V.: 10-15 minutes

Metabolism: Via conjugation in many tissues including hepatic and pulmonary

Half-life elimination: 2.5-5 minutes

Excretion: Urine (primarily as sulfate conjugates)

Pregnancy Risk Factor C

Generic Available Yes

Isoproterenol Hydrochloride *see* Isoproterenol *on page 749*

Isoproterenol Sulfate *see* Isoproterenol *on page 749*

Isoptin® SR *see* Verapamil *on page 1382*

Isopto® Atropine *see* Atropine *on page 144*

Isopto® Carbachol *see* Carbachol *on page 241*

Isopto® Carpine *see* Pilocarpine *on page 1080*

Isopto® Homatropine *see* Homatropine *on page 670*

Isopto® Hyoscine *see* Scopolamine *on page 1210*

Isopto® Tears [OTC] *see* Artificial Tears *on page 128*

Isopto® Tears [OTC] *see* Hydroxypropyl Methylcellulose *on page 696*

Isordil® *see* Isosorbide Dinitrate *on page 750*

Isosorbide Dinitrate (eye soe SOR bide dye NYE trate)

Related Information

Cardiovascular Diseases *on page 1456*

Isosorbide Mononitrate *on page 751*

U.S. Brand Names Dilatrate®-SR; Isordil®

Canadian Brand Names Apo®-ISDN; Cedocard®-SR; Coronex®; Novo-Sorbide; PMS-Isosorbide

Mexican Brand Names Isoket®; Isorbid®

Pharmacologic Category Vasodilator

Synonyms ISD; ISDN

Use Prevention and treatment of angina pectoris; CHF; to relieve pain, dysphagia, and spasm in esophageal spasm with GE reflux

Local Anesthetic/Vasoconstrictor Precautions No information available to require special precautions

Effects on Dental Treatment No significant effects or complications reported

Dosage Adults (elderly should be given lowest recommended daily doses initially and titrate upward): Oral:

Angina: 5-40 mg 4 times/day or 40 mg every 8-12 hours in sustained-release dosage form

Congestive heart failure:

Initial dose: 10 mg 3 times/day

Target dose: 40 mg 3 times/day

Maximum dose: 80 mg 3 times/day

Sublingual: 2.5-10 mg every 4-6 hours

Chewable tablet: 5-10 mg every 2-3 hours

Tolerance to nitrate effects develops with chronic exposure

Dose escalation does not overcome this effect. Short periods (14 hours) of nitrate withdrawal help minimize tolerance.

Hemodialysis: During hemodialysis, administer dose postdialysis or administer supplemental 10-20 mg dose

Peritoneal dialysis: Supplemental dose is unnecessary

Mechanism of Action Stimulation of intracellular cyclic-GMP results in vascular smooth muscle relaxation of both arterial and venous vasculature. Increased venous pooling decreases left ventricular pressure (preload) and arterial dilatation decreases arterial resistance (afterload). Therefore, this reduces cardiac oxygen demand by decreasing left ventricular pressure and systemic vascular resistance by dilating arteries. Additionally, coronary artery dilation improves collateral flow to ischemic regions; esophageal smooth muscle is relaxed via the same mechanism.

Other Adverse Effects The incidence of hypotension and adverse cardiovascular events may be increased when used in combination with sildenafil (Viagra®).

Frequency not defined:

Cardiovascular: Hypotension (infrequent), postural hypotension, crescendo angina (uncommon), rebound hypertension (uncommon), pallor, cardiovascular collapse, tachycardia, shock, flushing, peripheral edema

Central nervous system: Headache (most common), lightheadedness (related to blood pressure changes), syncope (uncommon), dizziness, restlessness

Gastrointestinal: Nausea, vomiting, bowel incontinence, **xerostomia**

Genitourinary: Urinary incontinence

Hematologic: Methemoglobinemia (rare, overdose)

Neuromuscular & skeletal: Weakness

Ocular: Blurred vision

Miscellaneous: **Cold sweat**

Drug Interactions Substrate of **CYP3A4**

Increased Effect/Toxicity: Combinations of sildenafil and nitrates has been associated with severe hypotensive reactions and death.

Dietary/Ethanol/Herb Considerations

Ethanol: Use with caution; may increase risk of hypotension.

Herb/Nutraceutical: Avoid hawthorn; may lower peripheral vascular resistance resulting in additive decrease in BP.

Pharmacodynamics/Kinetics

Onset of action: Sublingual tablet: 2-10 minutes; Chewable tablet: 3 minutes; Oral tablet: 45-60 minutes

Duration: Sublingual tablet: 1-2 hours; Chewable tablet: 0.5-2 hours; Oral tablet: 4-6 hours

Metabolism: Extensively hepatic to conjugated metabolites, including isosorbide 5-mononitrate (active) and 2-mononitrate (active)

Half-life elimination: Parent drug: 1-4 hours; Metabolite (5-mononitrate): 4 hours

Excretion: Urine and feces

Pregnancy Risk Factor C

Generic Available Yes: Tablet

Isosorbide Mononitrate (eye soe SOR bide mon oh NYE trate)

Related Information

Cardiovascular Diseases *on page 1456*

Isosorbide Dinitrate *on page 750*

U.S. Brand Names Imdur®; Ismo®; Monoket®

Canadian Brand Names Imdur®

Mexican Brand Names Elantan®; Imdur®; Mono Mack®

Pharmacologic Category Vasodilator

Synonyms ISMN

Use Long-acting metabolite of the vasodilator isosorbide dinitrate used for the prophylactic treatment of angina pectoris

Local Anesthetic/Vasoconstrictor Precautions No information available to require special precautions

Effects on Dental Treatment

>10%: Headache (19% to 38%)

Dosage Adults and Geriatrics (start with lowest recommended dose): Oral:

Regular tablet: 5-10 mg twice daily with the two doses given 7 hours apart (eg, 8 AM and 3 PM) to decrease tolerance development; then titrate to 10 mg twice daily in first 2-3 days.

Extended release tablet: Initial: 30-60 mg given in morning as a single dose; titrate upward as needed, giving at least 3 days between increases; maximum daily single dose: 240 mg

Tolerance to nitrate effects develops with chronic exposure. Dose escalation does not overcome this effect. Tolerance can only be overcome by short periods of nitrate absence from the body. Short periods (10-12 hours) of nitrate withdrawal help minimize tolerance. Recommended dosage regimens incorporate this interval. General recommendations are to take the last dose of short-acting agents no later than 7 PM; administer 2 times/day rather than 4 times/day. Administer sustained release tablet once daily in the morning.

Mechanism of Action Prevailing mechanism of action for nitroglycerin (and other nitrates) is systemic venodilation, decreasing preload as measured by pulmonary capillary wedge pressure and left ventricular end diastolic volume and pressure; the average reduction in left ventricular end diastolic volume is 25% at rest, with a corresponding increase in ejection fractions of 50% to 60%. This effect improves congestive symptoms in heart failure and improves the myocardial perfusion gradient in patients with coronary artery disease.

Other Adverse Effects The incidence of hypotension and adverse cardiovascular events may be increased when used in combination with sildenafil (Viagra®).

(Continued)

Isosorbide Mononitrate *(Continued)*

1% to 10%:

Central nervous system: Dizziness (3% to 5%)

Gastrointestinal: Nausea/vomiting (2% to 4%)

<1% (Limited to important or life-threatening): Angina pectoris, **arrhythmias, atrial fibrillation, hypotension, palpitations, postural hypotension, premature ventricular contractions, supraventricular tachycardia, syncope,** pruritus, rash, abdominal pain, diarrhea, dyspepsia, tenesmus, **tooth disorder**, vomiting, dysuria, impotence, urinary frequency, asthenia, blurred vision, **cold sweat,** diplopia, edema, malaise, neck stiffness, rigors, agitation, anxiety, confusion, dyscoordination, hypoesthesia, nightmares, **bronchitis, pneumonia, upper respiratory tract infection**, arthralgia, methemoglobinemia (rare, overdose)

Drug Interactions Substrate of **CYP3A4**

Increased Effect/Toxicity: Combinations of sildenafil and nitrates has been associated with severe hypotensive reactions and death. CYP3A4 inhibitors may increase hypotensive response.

Dietary/Ethanol/Herb Considerations

Ethanol: Use with caution; may increase risk of hypotension.

Herb/Nutraceutical: Avoid hawthorn; may lower peripheral vascular resistance resulting in additive decrease in BP.

Pharmacodynamics/Kinetics

Onset of action: 30-60 minutes

Absorption: Nearly complete and low intersubject variability in its pharmacokinetic parameters and plasma concentrations

Metabolism: Hepatic

Half-life elimination: Mononitrate: ~4 hours

Excretion: Urine and feces

Pregnancy Risk Factor C

Generic Available Yes

Isotretinoin (eye soe TRET i noyn)

U.S. Brand Names Accutane®; Amnesteen™

Canadian Brand Names Accutane®; Isotrex®

Mexican Brand Names Isotrex®; Roaccutan®

Pharmacologic Category Retinoic Acid Derivative

Synonyms 13-*cis*-Retinoic Acid

Use Treatment of severe recalcitrant nodular acne unresponsive to conventional therapy

Unlabeled/Investigational Use Investigational: Treatment of children with metastatic neuroblastoma or leukemia that does not respond to conventional therapy

Local Anesthetic/Vasoconstrictor Precautions No information available to require special precautions

Effects on Dental Treatment >10%: Xerostomia, changes in salivation

Restrictions Prescriptions for Accutane® may not be dispensed unless they are affixed with a yellow self-adhesive Accutane® qualification sticker filled out by the prescriber. Telephone, fax, or computer-generated prescriptions are no longer valid. Prescribers will be provided with Accutane® qualification stickers after they have read the details of the S.M.A.R.T. program and have signed and mailed to the manufacturer their agreement to participate. A half-day continuing education program is also available.

Prescriptions may not be written for more than a 1-month supply and must be dispensed with a patient education guide every month. Prescriptions for females must be filled within 7 days of the date noted on the yellow sticker; prescriptions filled after 7 days of the noted date are considered to be expired and cannot be honored. Audits of pharmacies will be conducted to monitor program compliance. Pharmacists may call the manufacturer to confirm the prescriber's authority to write for this medication, however, this is not mandatory.

Females of childbearing potential must receive oral and written information reviewing the hazards of therapy and the effects that isotretinoin can have on a fetus. All patients (male and female) must read and sign the informed consent material provided in the pregnancy prevention program. Therapy should not begin without two negative pregnancy tests. Two forms of contraception (a primary and secondary form as described in the pregnancy prevention program materials) must be used during treatment and limitations to their use must be explained.

Dosage Oral:

Children: Maintenance therapy for neuroblastoma (investigational): 100-250 mg/m²/day in 2 divided doses

Children and Adults: Severe recalcitrant nodular acne: 0.5-2 mg/kg/day in 2 divided doses (dosages as low as 0.05 mg/kg/day have been reported to be beneficial) for 15-20 weeks or until the total cyst count decreases by 70%, whichever is sooner. A second course of therapy may be initiated after a period of ≥2 months off therapy.

Dosing adjustment in hepatic impairment: Dose reductions empirically are recommended in hepatitis disease

Mechanism of Action Reduces sebaceous gland size and reduces sebum production; regulates cell proliferation and differentiation

Other Adverse Effects Frequency not defined:

Cardiovascular: Palpitation, tachycardia, vascular thrombotic disease, stroke, chest pain, syncope, flushing

Central nervous system: Edema, fatigue, pseudotumor cerebri, dizziness, drowsiness, **headache**, insomnia, lethargy, malaise, **nervousness, paresthesias, seizures, stroke**, suicidal ideation, suicide attempts, suicide, depression, **psychosis, aggressive or violent behavior**, emotional instability

Dermatologic: Cutaneous allergic reactions, purpura, acne fulminans, alopecia, bruising, cheilitis, nasal dryness, dry skin, epistaxis, eruptive xanthomas, fragility of skin, hair abnormalities, hirsutism, hyperpigmentation, hypopigmentation, peeling of palms, peeling of soles, photoallergic reactions, photosensitizing reactions, pruritus, rash, dystrophy, paronychia, **facial erythema**, seborrhea, eczema, increased sunburn susceptibility, urticaria, **abnormal wound healing**

Endocrine & metabolic: Increased triglycerides (25%), elevated blood glucose, increased HDL, increased cholesterol, abnormal menses

Gastrointestinal: Weight loss, inflammatory bowel disease, regional ileitis, pancreatitis, **bleeding and inflammation of the gums**, colitis, nausea, nonspecific gastrointestinal symptoms

Genitourinary: Nonspecific urogenital findings

Hematologic: Anemia, thrombocytopenia, neutropenia, agranulocytosis, pyogenic granuloma

Hepatic: Hepatitis

Neuromuscular & skeletal: Skeletal hyperostosis, calcification of tendons and ligaments, premature epiphyseal closure, arthralgia, CPK elevations, arthritis, tendonitis, bone abnormalities, weakness, back pain (29% in pediatric patients), rhabdomyolysis (rare), bone mineral density decreased

Ocular: Corneal opacities, decreased night vision, cataracts, color vision disorder, conjunctivitis, dry eyes, eyelid inflammation, keratitis, optic neuritis, photophobia, visual disturbances

Otic: Hearing impairment, tinnitus

Renal: Vasculitis, glomerulonephritis,

Respiratory: **Bronchospasms, respiratory infection**, voice alteration, Wegener's granulomatosis

Miscellaneous: **Allergic reactions, anaphylactic reactions, lymphadenopathy, infection, disseminated herpes simplex, diaphoresis**

Drug Interactions

Increased Effect/Toxicity: Increased toxicity: Corticosteroids may cause osteoporosis; interactive effect with isotretinoin unknown; use with caution. Phenytoin may cause osteomalacia; interactive effect with isotretinoin unknown; use with caution. Cases of pseudotumor cerebri have been reported in concurrent use with tetracycline; avoid combination.

Decreased Effect: Isotretinoin may increase clearance of carbamazepine resulting in reduced carbamazepine levels. Microdosed progesterone preparations ("minipills") may not be an adequate form of contraception.

Dietary/Ethanol/Herb Considerations

Ethanol: Avoid or limit use; may increase triglyceride levels if taken in excess.

Food: Administer with food; food or milk may increase bioavailability. Additional vitamin A supplements may lead to vitamin A toxicity (dry skin, irritation, arthralgias, myalgias, abdominal pain, hepatic changes); avoid use.

Herb/Nutraceutical: Avoid dong quai and St John's Wort; may cause photosensitization and decrease the effectiveness of oral contraceptives.

Pharmacodynamics/Kinetics

Distribution: Crosses placenta

Protein binding: 99% to 100%; primarily albumin

Metabolism: Hepatic via CYP2B6, 2C8, 2C9, 2D6, 3A4; forms metabolites; major metabolite: 4-oxo-isotretinoin (active)

Half-life elimination: Terminal: Parent drug: 21 hours; Metabolite: 21-24 hours

Time to peak, serum: 3-5 hours

Excretion: Urine and feces (equal amounts)

Pregnancy Risk Factor X

Generic Available No

Isovue® *see* Radiological/Contrast Media (Nonionic) *on page 1165*

Isoxsuprine (eye SOKS syoo preen)

U.S. Brand Names Vasodilan®

Pharmacologic Category Vasodilator

Synonyms Isoxsuprine Hydrochloride

Use Treatment of peripheral vascular diseases, such as arteriosclerosis obliterans and Raynaud's disease

Local Anesthetic/Vasoconstrictor Precautions No information available to require special precautions

(Continued)

Isoxsuprine *(Continued)*

Effects on Dental Treatment May enhance effects of other vasodilators.

Dosage Oral: Adults: 10-20 mg 3-4 times/day; start with lower dose in elderly due to potential hypotension

Mechanism of Action In studies on normal human subjects, isoxsuprine increases muscle blood flow, but skin blood flow is usually unaffected. Rather than increasing muscle blood flow by beta-receptor stimulation, isoxsuprine probably has a direct action on vascular smooth muscle. The generally accepted mechanism of action of isoxsuprine on the uterus is beta-adrenergic stimulation. Isoxsuprine was shown to inhibit prostaglandin synthetase at high serum concentrations, with low concentrations there was an increase in the P-G synthesis.

Other Adverse Effects Frequency not defined:

Cardiovascular: **Hypotension, tachycardia, chest pain**
Central nervous system: Dizziness
Dermatologic: Rash
Gastrointestinal: Nausea, vomiting
Neuromuscular & skeletal: Weakness

Drug Interactions Increased effects with other vasodilators/hypotensive agents.

Pharmacodynamics/Kinetics

Absorption: Nearly complete
Half-life elimination, serum: Mean: 1.25 hours
Time to peak, serum: ~1 hour

Pregnancy Risk Factor C

Generic Available Yes

Isoxsuprine Hydrochloride *see* Isoxsuprine *on page 753*

Isradipine (iz RA di peen)

Related Information

Calcium Channel Blockers and Gingival Hyperplasia *on page 1598*
Calcium Channel Blockers, Comparative Pharmacokinetics *on page 1600*
Cardiovascular Diseases *on page 1456*

U.S. Brand Names DynaCirc®; DynaCirc® CR

Canadian Brand Names DynaCirc®

Mexican Brand Names DynaCirc®; DynaCirc SRO®

Pharmacologic Category Calcium Channel Blocker

Use Treatment of hypertension

Local Anesthetic/Vasoconstrictor Precautions No information available to require special precautions

Effects on Dental Treatment 1% to 10%: Dyspnea (1% to 3%), palpitations (dose-related 1% to 5%), flushing (dose-related 1% to 9%), tachycardia (1% to 3%), chest pain (2% to 3%)

Dosage Oral: Adults: 2.5 mg twice daily; antihypertensive response occurs in 2-3 hours; maximal response in 2-4 weeks; increase dose at 2- to 4-week intervals at 2.5-5 mg increments; usual dose range: 5-20 mg/day. **Note:** Most patients show no improvement with doses >10 mg/day except adverse reaction rate increases

Mechanism of Action Inhibits calcium ion from entering the "slow channels" or select voltage-sensitive areas of vascular smooth muscle and myocardium during depolarization, producing a relaxation of coronary vascular smooth muscle and coronary vasodilation; increases myocardial oxygen delivery in patients with vasospastic angina

Other Adverse Effects

>10%: Central nervous system: Headache (dose-related 2% to 22%)

1% to 10%:

- Cardiovascular: Edema (dose-related 1% to 9%)
- Central nervous system: Dizziness (2% to 8%), fatigue (dose-related 1% to 9%)
- Dermatologic: Rash (1.5% to 2%)
- Gastrointestinal: Nausea (1% to 5%), abdominal discomfort (≤3%), vomiting (≤1%), diarrhea (≤3%)
- Renal: Urinary frequency (1% to 3%)

0.5% to 1% (Limited to important or life-threatening): Pruritus, urticaria, cramps of legs and feet, **cough, dyspnea, hypotension, atrial fibrillation, ventricular fibrillation, MI, heart failure,** abdominal discomfort, constipation, diarrhea, nocturia, drowsiness, insomnia, lethargy, **nervousness**, weakness, impotence, decreased libido, depression, **syncope, paresthesias, transient ischemic attack, stroke**, hyperhidrosis, visual disturbance, **xerostomia, gingival hyperplasia, throat discomfort**, leukopenia, elevated LFTs, numbness

Drug Interactions Substrate of **CYP3A4**

Increased Effect/Toxicity: Isradipine may increase cardiovascular adverse effects of beta-blockers. Isradipine may minimally increase cyclosporine levels. Azole antifungals (and potentially other inhibitors of CYP3A4) may increase levels of isradipine; avoid this combination.

Decreased Effect: NSAIDs (diclofenac) may decrease the antihypertensive response of isradipine. Isradipine may cause a decrease in lovastatin effect.

Rifampin may reduce blood levels and effects of isradipine due to enzyme induction (other enzyme inducers may share this effect).

Dietary/Ethanol/Herb Considerations

Ethanol: Avoid use; increases serum concentration and risk of hypotension.

Food may increase serum concentration and delay absorption but does not affect bioavailability. Avoid grapefruit products; grapefruit juice increases bioavailability and increases AUC 2-fold; half-life remains unchanged. Avoid caffeine, garlic, and licorice.

Herb/Nutraceutical: Avoid black cohosh, dong quai, an evening primrose due to estrogenic activity. Avoid ephedra, ginseng, and yohimbe; may worsen hypertension. Avoid garlic; may have increased antihypertensive effect. Avoid ginger due to positive inotropic effects; theoretically, may cause arrhythmia. Avoid hawthorn; may lower peripheral vascular resistance resulting in additive decrease in BP. Avoid licorice. Avoid St John's wort; may decrease serum concentration.

Pharmacodynamics/Kinetics

Duration: 8-16 hours
Absorption: 90% to 95%
Protein binding: 95%
Metabolism: Hepatic; extensive first-pass effect
Bioavailability: 15% to 24%
Half-life elimination: 8 hours
Time to peak, serum: 1-1.5 hours
Excretion: Urine (as metabolites)

Pregnancy Risk Factor C

Generic Available No

Selected Readings Westbrook P, Bednarczyk EM, Carlson M, et al, "Regression of Nifedipine-Induced Gingival Hyperplasia Following Switch to a Same Class Calcium Channel Blocker, Isradipine," *J Periodontol*, 1997, 68(7):645-50.

Isuprel® *see* Isoproterenol *on page 749*

Itch-X® [OTC] *see* Pramoxine *on page 1105*

Itraconazole (i tra KOE na zole)

Related Information

Oral Fungal Infections *on page 1542*

U.S. Brand Names Sporanox®

Canadian Brand Names Sporanox®

Mexican Brand Names Carexan®; Isox®; Itranax®; Sporanox®

Pharmacologic Category Antifungal Agent, Oral

Use

Dental: Treatment of susceptible fungal infections in immunocompromised and immunocompetent patients including blastomycosis and histoplasmosis; also has activity against *Aspergillus, Candida, Coccidioides, Cryptococcus, Sporothrix*, and chromomycosis

Medical: Treatment of susceptible fungal infections in immunocompromised and immunocompetent patients including blastomycosis and histoplasmosis; indicated for aspergillosis, and onychomycosis of the toenail; treatment of onychomycosis of the fingernail without concomitant toenail infection via a pulse-type dosing regimen; has activity against *Aspergillus, Candida, Coccidioides, Cryptococcus, Sporothrix*, tinea unguium

Useful in superficial mycoses including dermatophytoses (eg, tinea capitis), pityriasis versicolor, sebopsoriasis, vaginal and chronic mucocutaneous candidiases; systemic mycoses including candidiasis, meningeal and disseminated cryptococcal infections, paracoccidioidomycosis, coccidioidomycoses; miscellaneous mycoses such as sporotrichosis, chromomycosis, leishmaniasis, fungal keratitis, alternariosis, zygomycosis

Intravenous solution is indicated in the treatment of blastomycosis, histoplasmosis (nonmeningeal), and aspergillosis (in patients intolerant or refractory to amphotericin B therapy)

Local Anesthetic/Vasoconstrictor Precautions No information available to require special precautions

Effects on Dental Treatment Listed incidences are for higher doses appropriate for systemic fungal infections.

>10%: Nausea (11%)

1% to 5%: Hypertension (3%), headache (4%), fatigue (2% to 3%), malaise (1%), fever (3%), dizziness (2%), vomiting (5%)

Dosage Capsule: Absorption is best if taken with food, therefore, it is best to administer itraconazole after meals; Solution: Should be taken on an empty stomach. Absorption of both products is significantly increased when taken with a cola beverage.

Children: Efficacy and safety not established; a small number of patients 3-16 years of age have been treated with 100 mg/day for systemic fungal infections with no serious adverse effects reported

(Continued)

Itraconazole *(Continued)*

Adults:

Oral:

Blastomycosis/histoplasmosis: 200 mg once daily, if no obvious improvement or there is evidence of progressive fungal disease, increase the dose in 100 mg increments to a maximum of 400 mg/day; doses >200 mg/day are given in 2 divided doses; length of therapy varies from 1 day to >6 months depending on the condition and mycological response

Aspergillosis: 200-400 mg/day

Onychomycosis: 200 mg once daily for 12 consecutive weeks

Life-threatening infections: Loading dose: 200 mg 3 times/day (600 mg/day) should be given for the first 3 days of therapy

Oropharyngeal and esophageal candidiasis: Oral solution: 100-200 mg once daily

I.V.: 200 mg twice daily for 4 doses, followed by 200 mg daily

Dosing adjustment in renal impairment: None; injection not recommended in patients with Cl_{cr} <30 mL/minute

Hemodialysis: Not dialyzable

Dosing adjustment in hepatic impairment: May be necessary; specific guidelines unavailable. Risk-to-benefit evaluation should be undertaken in patients who develop liver function abnormalities during treatment.

Mechanism of Action Interferes with cytochrome P450 activity, decreasing ergosterol synthesis (principal sterol in fungal cell membrane) and inhibiting cell membrane formation

Other Adverse Effects Listed incidences are for higher doses appropriate for systemic fungal infections.

1% to 10%:

Cardiovascular: Edema (4%)

Dermatologic: Rash (9%), pruritus (3%)

Endocrine & metabolic: Decreased libido (1%), hypertriglyceridemia, hypokalemia (2%)

Gastrointestinal: Abdominal pain (2%), anorexia (1%), diarrhea (3%)

Hepatic: Abnormal LFTs (3%), hepatitis

Renal: Albuminuria (1%)

<1%: Adrenal suppression, constipation, **gastritis,** gynecomastia, impotence, **somnolence,** tinnitus

Postmarketing and/or case reports: **Allergic reactions** (urticaria, angioedema), alopecia, **anaphylaxis, arrhythmia, CHF, hepatic failure,** menstrual disorders, neutropenia, peripheral neuropathy, pulmonary edema, Stevens-Johnson syndrome

Contraindications Hypersensitivity to itraconazole, any component of the formulation, or to other azoles; concurrent administration with astemizole, cisapride, dofetilide, ergot derivatives, lovastatin, midazolam, pimozide, quinidine, or simvastatin; treatment of onychomycosis in patients with evidence of left ventricular dysfunction, CHF, or a history of CHF

Warnings/Precautions Rare cases of serious cardiovascular adverse events, including death, ventricular tachycardia and torsade de pointes have been observed due to increased cisapride concentrations induced by itraconazole. Not recommended for use in patients with active liver disease, elevated liver enzymes, or prior hepatotoxic reactions to other drugs. Itraconazole has been associated with rare cases of serious hepatotoxicity (including fatal cases and cases within the first week of treatment); treatment should be discontinued in patients who develop clinical symptoms or abnormal LFTs during itraconazole therapy except in cases where expected benefit exceeds risk. Use with caution in patients with left ventricular dysfunction or a history of CHF when itraconazole is being used for indications other than onychomycosis. Discontinue if signs or symptoms of CHF occur or neuropathy during treatment. Due to differences in bioavailability, oral capsules and oral solution **cannot** be used interchangeably.

Drug Interactions Substrate of **CYP3A4**; Inhibits **CYP3A4**

Benzodiazepines: Alprazolam, diazepam, temazepam, triazolam, and midazolam serum concentrations may be increased; consider a benzodiazepine not metabolized by CYP3A4 (such as lorazepam) or another antifungal that is metabolized by CYP3A4

Buspirone: Serum concentrations may be increased; monitor for sedation

Busulfan: Serum concentrations may be increased; avoid concurrent use

Calcium channel blockers: Serum concentrations may be increased (applies to those agents metabolized by CYP3A4, including felodipine, nifedipine, and verapamil); consider another agent instead of a calcium channel blocker, another antifungal, or reduce the dose of the calcium channel blocker; monitor blood pressure

Cisapride; Serum concentration is increased which may lead to malignant arrhythmias; concurrent use is contraindicated

Didanosine: May decrease absorption of itraconazole (due to buffering capacity of oral solution); applies only to oral solution formulation of didanosine

Docetaxel: Serum concentrations may be increased; avoid concurrent use
Dofetilide: Serum levels/toxicity may be increased; concurrent use is contraindicated.
Enzyme inducers: Rifampin decreases itraconazole's serum concentration to levels which are no longer effective; avoid concurrent use. Other inducers (barbiturates, carbamazepine, rifabutin) may share this effect.
Erythromycin (and clarithromycin): May increase serum concentrations of itraconazole.
H_2 blockers: May decrease itraconazole absorption. Itraconazole depends on gastric acidity for absorption. Avoid concurrent use.
HMG-CoA reductase inhibitors (except pravastatin and fluvastatin): Serum concentrations may be increased. The risk of myopathy/rhabdomyolysis may be increased. Switch to pravastatin/fluvastatin or suspend treatment during course of itraconazole therapy.
Immunosuppressants: Cyclosporine, sirolimus, and tacrolimus: Serum concentrations may be increased; monitor serum concentrations and renal function
Methylprednisolone: Serum concentrations may be increased; monitor
Nevirapine: May decrease serum concentrations of itraconazole; monitor
Oral contraceptives: Efficacy may be reduced by itraconazole (limited data); use barrier birth control method during concurrent use
Phenytoin: Serum concentrations may be increased; monitor phenytoin levels and adjust dose as needed.
Pimozide: Serum levels/toxicity may be increased; concurrent use is contraindicated.
Protease inhibitors: May increase serum concentrations of itraconazole. Includes amprenavir, indinavir, nelfinavir, ritonavir, and saquinavir; monitor
Proton pump inhibitors: May decrease itraconazole absorption. Itraconazole depends on gastric acidity for absorption. Avoid concurrent use (includes omeprazole, lansoprazole).
Quinidine: Serum levels may be increased. Concurrent use is contraindicated.
Trimetrexate: Serum concentrations may be increased; monitor
Warfarin: Anticoagulant effects may be increased; monitor INR and adjust warfarin's dose as needed
Vinca alkaloids: Serum concentrations may be increased; avoid concurrent use
Zolpidem: Serum levels may be increased; monitor

Dietary/Ethanol/Herb Considerations

Ethanol: Avoid use; disulfiram-like reaction may occur.
Food: Administer capsules with food; gastric acidity required for absorption. Administer solution on an empty stomach, if possible; time to peak concentration prolonged by food. Avoid grapefruit products. Absorption of both products is increased when administered with a cola beverage.
Herb/Nutraceutical: Avoid St John's wort; may decrease serum concentration.

Pharmacodynamics/Kinetics

Absorption: Requires gastric acidity; capsule better absorbed with food, solution better absorbed on empty stomach; hypochlorhydria has been reported in HIV-infected patients; therefore, oral absorption in these patients may be decreased
Distribution: V_d (average): 796 ± 185 L or 10 L/kg; highly lipophilic and tissue concentrations are higher than plasma concentrations. The highest concentrations: adipose, omentum, endometrium, cervical and vaginal mucus, and skin/nails. Aqueous fluids (eg, CSF and urine) contain negligible amounts.
Protein binding, plasma: 99.9%; metabolite hydroxy-itraconazole: 99.5%
Metabolism: Extensively hepatic into >30 metabolites including hydroxy-itraconazole (major metabolite); appears to have *in vitro* antifungal activity. Main metabolic pathway is oxidation; may undergo saturation metabolism with multiple dosing.
Bioavailability: 55%; Fasting: 40%; Postprandial: 100%
Half-life elimination: Oral: After single 200 mg dose: 21 ± 5 hours; 64 hours at steady-state; I.V.: steady-state: 35 hours; steady-state concentrations are achieved in 13 days with multiple administration of itraconazole 100-400 mg/day.
Excretion: Feces (~3% to 18%); urine (~0.03% as parent drug, 40% as metabolites)

Pregnancy Risk Factor C

Dosage Forms CAP: 100 mg. **INJ, solution:** 10 mg/mL (25 mL) [packaged in a kit containing sodium chloride 0.9% (50 mL); filtered infusion set (1)]. **SOLN, oral:** 100 mg/10 mL (150 mL)

Generic Available No

Iveegam EN *see* Immune Globulin (Intravenous) *on page 714*

Ivermectin (eye ver MEK tin)

U.S. Brand Names Stromectol®

Pharmacologic Category Anthelmintic

Use Treatment of the following infections: Strongyloidiasis of the intestinal tract due to the nematode parasite *Strongyloides stercoralis*. Onchocerciasis due to the nematode parasite *Onchocerca volvulus*. Ivermectin is only active against the

(Continued)

Ivermectin *(Continued)*

immature form of *Onchocerca volvulus*, and the intestinal forms of *Strongyloides stercoralis*. Ivermectin has been used for other parasitic infections including *Ascaris lumbricoides*, Bancroftian filariasis, *Brugia malayi*, scabies, *Enterobius vermicularis*, *Mansonella ozzardi*, *Trichuris trichiura*.

Local Anesthetic/Vasoconstrictor Precautions No information available to require special precautions

Effects on Dental Treatment No significant effects or complications reported

Dosage Oral: Children ≥15 kg and Adults:

Strongyloidiasis: 200 mcg/kg as a single dose; follow-up stool examinations

Onchocerciasis: 150 mcg/kg as a single dose; retreatment may be required every 3-12 months until the adult worms die

Mechanism of Action Ivermectin is a semisynthetic antihelminthic agent; it binds selectively and with strong affinity to glutamate-gated chloride ion channels which occur in invertebrate nerve and muscle cells. This leads to increased permeability of cell membranes to chloride ions then hyperpolarization of the nerve or muscle cell, and death of the parasite.

Other Adverse Effects Frequency not defined:

Cardiovascular: Hypotension, mild EKG changes, peripheral and facial edema, transient tachycardia

Central nervous system: Dizziness, **headache**, hyperthermia, insomnia, somnolence, vertigo

Dermatologic: Pruritus, rash, urticaria

Gastrointestinal: Abdominal pain, diarrhea, nausea, vomiting

Hematologic: Eosinophilia, leukopenia

Hepatic: ALT/AST increased

Neuromuscular & skeletal: Limbitis, myalgia, **tremor**, weakness

Ocular: Blurred vision, mild conjunctivitis, punctate opacity

Mazzotti reaction (with onchocerciasis): Edema, fever, lymphadenopathy, ocular damage, pruritus, rash

Drug Interactions Substrate of CYP3A4

Pharmacodynamics/Kinetics

Onset of action: Peak effect: 3-6 months

Absorption: Well absorbed

Distribution: Does not cross blood-brain barrier

Half-life elimination: 16-35 hours

Metabolism: Hepatic (>97%)

Excretion: Urine (<1%); remainder in feces

Pregnancy Risk Factor C

Generic Available No

IVIG *see* Immune Globulin (Intravenous) *on page 714*

IvyBlock® [OTC] *see* Bentoquatam *on page 168*

Japanese Encephalitis Virus Vaccine (Inactivated)

(jap a NEEZ en sef a LYE tis VYE rus vak SEEN, in ak ti VAY ted)

Related Information

Immunizations (Vaccines) *on page 1612*

U.S. Brand Names JE-VAX®

Canadian Brand Names JE-VAX®

Pharmacologic Category Vaccine

Use Active immunization against Japanese encephalitis for persons 1 year of age and older who plan to spend 1 month or more in endemic areas in Asia, especially persons traveling during the transmission season or visiting rural areas; consider vaccination for shorter trips to epidemic areas or extensive outdoor activities in rural endemic areas; elderly (>55 years of age) individuals should be considered for vaccination, since they have increased risk of developing symptomatic illness after infection; those planning travel to or residence in endemic areas should consult the Travel Advisory Service (Central Campus) for specific advice

Local Anesthetic/Vasoconstrictor Precautions No information available to require special precautions

Effects on Dental Treatment No significant effects or complications reported

Restrictions Japanese encephalitis vaccine is currently available only from the Centers for Disease Control. Contact Centers for Disease Control at (404) 639-6370 (Mon-Fri) or (404) 639-2888 (nights, weekends, or holidays). Federal law requires that the date of administration, the vaccine manufacturer, lot number of vaccine, and the administering person's name, title and address be entered into the patient's permanent medical record.

Dosage U.S. recommended primary immunization schedule:

Children 1-3 years: S.C.: Three 0.5 mL doses given on days 0, 7, and 30; abbreviated schedules should be used only when necessary due to time constraints

Children >3 years and Adults: S.C.: Three 1 mL doses given on days 0, 7, and 30. Give third dose on day 14 when time does not permit waiting; 2 doses a week apart produce immunity in about 80% of recipients; the longest regimen yields highest titers after 6 months.

Booster dose: Give after 2 years, or according to current recommendation

Note: Travel should not commence for at least 10 days after the last dose of vaccine, to allow adequate antibody formation and recognition of any delayed adverse reaction

Advise concurrent use of other means to reduce the risk of mosquito exposure when possible, including bed nets, insect repellents, protective clothing, avoidance of travel in endemic areas, and avoidance of outdoor activity during twilight and evening periods

Other Adverse Effects Report allergic or unusual adverse reactions to the Vaccine Adverse Event Reporting System (VAERS) 1-800-822-7967.

Frequency not defined:

Cardiovascular: Angioedema, hypotension

Central nervous system: Fever, headache, dizziness, malaise, chills, encephalopathy, seizure, encephalitis

Dermatologic: Rash, urticaria, itching (with or without accompanying rash) erythema multiforme, erythema nodosum

Gastrointestinal: Nausea, vomiting, abdominal pain

Local: Tenderness, redness, and swelling at injection site

Neuromuscular & skeletal: Myalgia, peripheral neuropathy, joint swelling

Respiratory: Dyspnea

Miscellaneous: Anaphylactic reaction (rare)

Pregnancy Risk Factor C

Generic Available No

JE-VAX® *see* Japanese Encephalitis Virus Vaccine (Inactivated) *on page 758*

K+8 *see* Potassium Supplements *on page 1102*

K+10 *see* Potassium Supplements *on page 1102*

Kadian® *see* Morphine Sulfate *on page 931*

Kala® [OTC] *see Lactobacillus acidophilus* and *Lactobacillus bulgaricus on page 772*

Kaletra™ *see* Lopinavir and Ritonavir *on page 820*

Kalmz [OTC] *see* Phosphorated Carbohydrate Solution *on page 1078*

Kanamycin (kan a MYE sin)

Related Information

Nonviral Infectious Diseases *on page 1493*

U.S. Brand Names Kantrex®

Canadian Brand Names Kantrex®

Mexican Brand Names Koptin®; Randikan

Pharmacologic Category Antibiotic, Aminoglycoside

Synonyms Kanamycin Sulfate

Use Treatment of serious infections caused by susceptible strains of *E. coli, Proteus species, Enterobacter aerogenes, Klebsiella pneumoniae, Serratia marcescens,* and *Acinetobacter* species; second-line treatment of *Mycobacterium tuberculosis*

Local Anesthetic/Vasoconstrictor Precautions No information available to require special precautions

Effects on Dental Treatment No significant effects or complications reported

Dosage Dosing should be based on ideal body weight; must be further diluted prior to I.V. infusion.

Infections:

I.M., I.V.:

Children: 15 mg/kg/day in divided doses every 8-12 hours; for I.V., use sufficient amount to infuse solution over 30-60

Adults: 5-7.5 mg/kg/dose in divided doses every 8-12 hours (<15 mg/kg/day); for I.V., dilute 500 mg in 100-200 mL of appropriate solution or 1 g in 200-400 mL

Intraperitoneal: After contamination in surgery: 500 mg dilute in 20 mL sterile distilled water

Irrigating solution: 0.25%; maximum 1.5 g/day (via all administration routes)

Solution for aerosol: 250 mg diluted in 3 mL normal saline 2-4 times/day

Dosing adjustment/interval in renal impairment:

Cl_{cr} 50-80 mL/minute: Administer 60% to 90% of dose or administer every 8-12 hours

Cl_{cr} 10-50 mL/minute: Administer 30% to 70% of dose or administer every 12 hours

Cl_{cr} <10 mL/minute: Administer 20% to 30% of dose or administer every 24-48 hours

Mechanism of Action Interferes with protein synthesis in bacterial cell by binding to ribosomal subunit

Other Adverse Effects Frequency not defined:

Cardiovascular: Edema

(Continued)

Kanamycin *(Continued)*

Central nervous system: Neurotoxicity, drowsiness, **headache,** pseudomotor cerebri
Dermatologic: Skin itching, redness, rash, photosensitivity, erythema
Gastrointestinal: Nausea, vomiting, diarrhea, malabsorption syndrome (with prolonged and high-dose therapy of hepatic coma), anorexia, weight loss, **increased salivation**, enterocolitis
Hematologic: Granulocytopenia, agranulocytosis, thrombocytopenia
Local: Burning, stinging
Neuromuscular & skeletal: Weakness, **tremors**, muscle cramps
Otic: Ototoxicity (auditory and vestibular)
Renal: Nephrotoxicity
Respiratory: **Dyspnea**

Drug Interactions Increased toxicity may occur with amphotericin B, cisplatin, loop diuretics, neuromuscular-blocking agents. Use with bisphosphonate derivatives may lead to hypocalcemia.

Pharmacodynamics/Kinetics
Distribution:
Relative diffusion from blood into CSF: Good only with inflammation (exceeds usual MICs)
CSF:blood level ratio: Normal meninges: Nil; Inflamed meninges: 43%
Half-life elimination: 2-4 hours; Anuria: 80 hours; End-stage renal disease: 40-96 hours
Time to peak, serum: I.M.: 1-2 hours (decreased in burn patients)
Excretion: Urine (entire amount)

Pregnancy Risk Factor D
Generic Available No

Kanamycin Sulfate *see* Kanamycin *on page 759*
Kantrex® *see* Kanamycin *on page 759*
Kaodene® NN [OTC] *see* Kaolin and Pectin *on page 760*

Kaolin and Pectin (KAY oh lin & PEK tin)

U.S. Brand Names Kaodene® NN [OTC]; Kao-Spen® [OTC]; Kapectolin® [OTC]
Pharmacologic Category Antidiarrheal
Synonyms Pectin and Kaolin
Use Treatment of uncomplicated diarrhea
Local Anesthetic/Vasoconstrictor Precautions No information available to require special precautions
Effects on Dental Treatment No significant effects or complications reported
Dosage Oral:
Children:
<6 years: Do not use
6-12 years: 30-60 mL after each loose stool
Adults: 60-120 mL after each loose stool
Other Adverse Effects Frequency not defined: Gastrointestinal: Constipation, fecal impaction
Drug Interactions Decreased Effect: May decrease absorption of many drugs, including chloroquine, atenolol, metoprolol, propranolol, diflunisal, isoniazid, penicillamine, clindamycin, digoxin (give kaolin/pectin 2 hours before or 4 hours after medication).
Pregnancy Risk Factor C
Generic Available Yes

Kaon-Cl-10® *see* Potassium Supplements *on page 1102*
Kaon-Cl® 20 *see* Potassium Supplements *on page 1102*
Kaopectate® [OTC] *see* Bismuth *on page 186*
Kaopectate® Advanced Formula [DSC] [OTC] *see* Attapulgite *on page 146*
Kaopectate® Extra Strength [OTC] *see* Bismuth *on page 186*
Kaopectate® Maximum Strength Caplets [DSC] [OTC] *see* Attapulgite *on page 146*
Kao-Spen® [OTC] *see* Kaolin and Pectin *on page 760*
Kapectolin® [OTC] *see* Kaolin and Pectin *on page 760*
Kapectolin PG® *see* Hyoscyamine, Atropine, Scopolamine, Kaolin, Pectin, and Opium *on page 701*
Kariva™ *see* Combination Hormonal Contraceptives *on page 368*
Kay Ciel® *see* Potassium Supplements *on page 1102*
K+ Care® *see* Potassium Supplements *on page 1102*
K+ Care® ET *see* Potassium Supplements *on page 1102*
KCl (Potassium Chloride) *see* Potassium Supplements *on page 1102*
K-Dur® 10 *see* Potassium Supplements *on page 1102*
K-Dur® 20 *see* Potassium Supplements *on page 1102*
Keflex® *see* Cephalexin *on page 285*

Keftab® *see* Cephalexin *on page 285*
Kefurox® [DSC] *see* Cefuroxime *on page 279*
Kefzol® [DSC] *see* Cefazolin *on page 263*
Kemadrin® *see* Procyclidine *on page 1125*
Kenalog® *see* Triamcinolone *on page 1341*
Kenalog-10® *see* Triamcinolone *on page 1341*
Kenalog-40® *see* Triamcinolone *on page 1341*
Kenalog® in Orabase® *see* Triamcinolone Acetonide Dental Paste *on page 1344*
Keoxifene Hydrochloride *see* Raloxifene *on page 1165*
Keppra® *see* Levetiracetam *on page 787*
Keralyt® [OTC] *see* Salicylic Acid *on page 1204*
Kerlone® *see* Betaxolol *on page 180*
Ketalar® *see* Ketamine *on page 761*

Ketamine (KEET a meen)

U.S. Brand Names Ketalar®

Canadian Brand Names Ketalar®

Mexican Brand Names Ketalin®

Pharmacologic Category General Anesthetic

Synonyms Ketamine Hydrochloride

Use Induction and maintenance of general anesthesia, especially when cardiovascular depression must be avoided (ie, hypotension, hypovolemia, cardiomyopathy, constrictive pericarditis); sedation; analgesia

Local Anesthetic/Vasoconstrictor Precautions No information available to require special precautions

Effects on Dental Treatment

>10%: Hypertension, tachycardia, hallucinations, tonic-clonic movements, tremors, increased salivation

1% to 10%: Bradycardia, hypotension, respiratory depression

Restrictions C-III

Dosage Used in combination with anticholinergic agents to decrease hypersalivation

Children:

Oral: 6-10 mg/kg for 1 dose (mixed in 0.2-0.3 mL/kg of cola or other beverage) given 30 minutes before the procedure

I.M.: 3-7 mg/kg

I.V.: Range: 0.5-2 mg/kg, use smaller doses (0.5-1 mg/kg) for sedation for minor procedures; usual induction dosage: 1-2 mg/kg

Continuous I.V. infusion: Sedation: 5-20 mcg/kg/minute

Adults:

I.M.: 3-8 mg/kg

I.V.: Range: 1-4.5 mg/kg; usual induction dosage: 1-2 mg/kg

Children and Adults: Maintenance: Supplemental doses of $1/3$ to $1/2$ of initial dose

Mechanism of Action Produces a cataleptic-like state in which the patient is dissociated from the surrounding environment by direct action on the cortex and limbic system; releases endogenous catecholamines (epinephrine, norepinephrine) which maintain blood pressure and heart rate; reduces polysynaptic spinal reflexes; increases cerebral metabolism and cerebral blood flow while producing a noncompetitive block of the neuronal postsynaptic NMDA receptor; lowers seizure threshold

Other Adverse Effects Produces emergence psychosis including auditory and visual hallucinations, restlessness, disorientation, vivid dreams, and irrational behavior in 15% to 30% of patients; pretreatment with a benzodiazepine reduces incidence of psychosis by >50%. Spontaneous involuntary movements, nystagmus, hypertonus, and vocalizations are also commonly seen.

>10%:

Cardiovascular: Increased cardiac output, paradoxical direct myocardial depression

Central nervous system: Increased intracranial pressure, vivid dreams

Miscellaneous: Emergence reactions, vocalization

1% to 10%:

Dermatologic: Pain at injection site, skin rash

Gastrointestinal: Anorexia, nausea, vomiting

Ocular: Diplopia, nystagmus

<1%: **Anaphylaxis, cardiac arrhythmias, cough reflex may be depressed, decreased bronchospasm**, fasciculations, **hypersalivation, increased airway resistance**, increased intraocular pressure, increased metabolic rate, increased skeletal muscle tone, **laryngospasm, myocardial depression**, respiratory depression or apnea with large doses or rapid infusions

Drug Interactions Substrate of **CYP2B6, 2C8/9, 3A4**

Increased Effect/Toxicity: Barbiturates, narcotics, hydroxyzine increase prolonged recovery; nondepolarizing neuromuscular blockers may increase effects. Muscle relaxants, thyroid hormones may increase blood pressure and heart rate. Halothane may decrease BP.

(Continued)

Ketamine *(Continued)*

Pharmacodynamics/Kinetics

Onset of action:

I.V.: General anesthesia: 1-2 minutes; Sedation: 1-2 minutes

I.M.: General anesthesia: 3-8 minutes

Duration: I.V.: 5-15 minutes; I.M.: 12-25 minutes

Metabolism: Hepatic via hydroxylation and N-demethylation; the metabolite norketamine is 25% as potent as parent compound

Half-life elimination: 11-17 minutes; Elimination: 2.5-3.1 hours

Excretion: Clearance: 18 mL/kg/minute

Pregnancy Risk Factor D

Generic Available Yes

Comments The analgesia outlasts the general anesthetic component. Bronchodilation is beneficial in asthmatic or COPD patients. Laryngeal reflexes may remain intact or may be obtunded. The direct myocardial depressant action of ketamine can be seen in stressed, catecholamine-deficient patients.

Ketamine Hydrochloride *see* Ketamine *on page 761*

Ketoconazole (kee toe KOE na zole)

Related Information

Oral Fungal Infections *on page 1542*

Respiratory Diseases *on page 1476*

U.S. Brand Names Nizoral®; Nizoral® A-D [OTC]

Canadian Brand Names Apo®-Ketoconazole; Ketoderm®; Nizoral®; Novo-Ketoconazole

Mexican Brand Names Akorazol®; Conazol®; Cremosan®; Fungoral®; Konaderm®; Mi-Ke-Son's®; Mycodib®; Nizoral®; Onofin-K®; Termizol®; Tiniazol®

Pharmacologic Category Antifungal Agent, Oral; Antifungal Agent, Topical

Use

Dental: Treatment of susceptible fungal infections, including candidiasis, oral thrush, chronic mucocutaneous candidiasis, blastomycosis, histoplasmosis

Medical: Topical treatment of tinea corporis, cruris, and versicolor; cutaneous candidiasis; seborrheic dermatitis; blastomycosis, histoplasmosis, paracoccidioidomycosis, coccidioidomycosis, chromomycosis, candiduria, and certain recalcitrant cutaneous dermatophytoses

Local Anesthetic/Vasoconstrictor Precautions No information available to require special precautions

Effects on Dental Treatment Nausea/vomiting (3% to 10%; oral form)

Dosage

Oral:

Children ≥2 years: 3.3-6.6 mg/kg/day as a single dose for 1-2 weeks for candidiasis, for at least 4 weeks in recalcitrant dermatophyte infections, and for up to 6 months for other systemic mycoses

Adults: 200-400 mg/day as a single daily dose for durations as stated above

Shampoo: Apply twice weekly for 4 weeks with at least 3 days between each shampoo

Topical: Rub gently into the affected area once daily to twice daily

Dosing adjustment in hepatic impairment: Consider dose reduction in severe liver disease

Hemodialysis: Not dialyzable (0% to 5%)

Mechanism of Action Alters the permeability of the cell wall by blocking fungal cytochrome P450; inhibits biosynthesis of triglycerides and phospholipids by fungi; inhibits several fungal enzymes that results in a build-up of toxic concentrations of hydrogen peroxide

Other Adverse Effects

Oral:

1% to 10%:

Dermatologic: Pruritus (2%)

Gastrointestinal: Abdominal pain (1%)

<1%: **Headache, dizziness, somnolence, fever,** chills, bulging fontanelles, depression, gynecomastia, diarrhea, impotence, thrombocytopenia, leukopenia, hemolytic anemia, hepatotoxicity, photophobia

Cream: Severe irritation, pruritus, stinging (~5%)

Shampoo: Increases in normal hair loss, irritation (<1%), abnormal hair texture, scalp pustules, mild dryness of skin, itching, oiliness/dryness of hair

Contraindications Hypersensitivity to ketoconazole or any component of the formulation; CNS fungal infections (due to poor CNS penetration); coadministration with ergot derivatives, astemizole, or cisapride is contraindicated due to risk of potentially fatal cardiac arrhythmias

Warnings/Precautions Use with caution in patients with impaired hepatic function; has been associated with hepatotoxicity, including some fatalities; perform periodic LFTs; high doses of ketoconazole may depress adrenocortical function.

Drug Interactions Substrate of **CYP3A4**; Inhibits CYP1A2, 2A6, 2B6, 2C8/9, 2C19, **3A4**

Benzodiazepines: Alprazolam, diazepam, temazepam, triazolam, and midazolam serum concentrations may be increased; consider a benzodiazepine not metabolized by CYP3A4 (such as lorazepam) or another antifungal that is metabolized by CYP3A4. Concurrent use is contraindicated.
Buspirone: Serum concentrations may be increased; monitor for sedation
Busulfan: Serum concentrations may be increased; avoid concurrent use
Calcium channel blockers: Serum concentrations may be increased (applies to those agents metabolized by CYP3A4, including felodipine, nifedipine, and verapamil); consider another agent instead of a calcium channel blocker, another antifungal, or reduce the dose of the calcium channel blocker; monitor blood pressure
Cisapride: Serum concentration is increased which may lead to malignant arrhythmias; concurrent use is contraindicated
Didanosine: May decrease absorption of ketoconazole (due to buffering capacity of oral solution); applies only to oral solution formulation of didanosine
Docetaxel: Serum concentrations may be increased; avoid concurrent use
Enzyme inducers: Rifampin decreases ketoconazole's serum concentration to levels which are no longer effective; avoid concurrent use. Other inducers (barbiturates, carbamazepine, rifabutin) may share this effect.
Erythromycin (and clarithromycin): May increase serum concentrations of ketoconazole.
H_2 blockers: May decrease ketoconazole absorption. Ketoconazole depends on gastric acidity for absorption. Avoid concurrent use.
HMG-CoA reductase inhibitors (except pravastatin and fluvastatin): Serum concentrations may be increased. The risk of myopathy/rhabdomyolysis may be increased. Switch to pravastatin/fluvastatin or suspend treatment during course of ketoconazole therapy.
Immunosuppressants: Cyclosporine, sirolimus, and tacrolimus: Serum concentrations may be increased; monitor serum concentrations and renal function
Methylprednisolone: Serum concentrations may be increased; monitor
Nevirapine: May decrease serum concentrations of ketoconazole; monitor
Oral contraceptives: Efficacy may be reduced by ketoconazole (limited data); use barrier birth control method during concurrent use
Phenytoin: Serum concentrations may be increased; monitor phenytoin levels and adjust dose as needed
Protease inhibitors: May increase serum concentrations of ketoconazole. Includes amprenavir, indinavir, nelfinavir, ritonavir, and saquinavir; monitor
Proton pump inhibitors: May decrease ketoconazole absorption. Ketoconazole depends on gastric acidity for absorption. Avoid concurrent use (includes omeprazole, lansoprazole).
Quinidine: Serum levels may be increased; monitor
Trimetrexate: Serum concentrations may be increased; monitor
Warfarin: Anticoagulant effects may be increased; monitor INR and adjust warfarin's dose as needed
Vinca alkaloids: Serum concentrations may be increased; avoid concurrent use
Zolpidem: Serum levels may be increased; monitor

Dietary/Ethanol/Herb Considerations
Ethanol: Avoid use; may cause disulfiram-like reaction.
Food may prolong peak serum concentration; administer with food or milk to reduce GI upset.
Herb/Nutraceutical: Avoid St John's wort; may decrease serum concentration.

Pharmacodynamics/Kinetics
Absorption: Oral: Rapid (~75%); Shampoo: None
Distribution: Well into inflamed joint fluid, saliva, bile, urine, breast milk, sebum, cerumen, feces, tendons, skin and soft tissues, and testes; crosses blood-brain barrier poorly; only negligible amounts reach CSF
Protein binding: 93% to 96%
Metabolism: Partially hepatic via CYP3A4 to inactive compounds
Bioavailability: Decreases as gastric pH increases
Half-life elimination: Biphasic: Initial: 2 hours; Terminal: 8 hours
Time to peak, serum: 1-2 hours
Excretion: Feces (57%); urine (13%)

Pregnancy Risk Factor C

Dosage Forms CRM, topical: 2% (15 g, 30 g, 60 g). **SHAMP, topical** (Nizoral® A-D): 1% (6 mL, 120 mL, 210 mL). **TAB** (Nizoral®): 200 mg

Generic Available Yes

Ketoprofen (kee toe PROE fen)

Related Information
Oral Pain *on page 1524*
Rheumatoid Arthritis, Osteoarthritis, and Osteoporosis *on page 1488*
Temporomandibular Dysfunction (TMD) *on page 1562*

U.S. Brand Names Orudis® [DSC]; Orudis® KT [OTC]; Oruvail®
(Continued)

Ketoprofen *(Continued)*

Canadian Brand Names Apo®-Keto; Apo®-Keto-E; Apo®-Keto SR; Novo-Keto; Novo-Keto-EC; Nu-Ketoprofen; Nu-Ketoprofen-E; Orudis® SR; Oruvail®; Rhodis™; Rhodis-EC™; Rhodis SR™

Mexican Brand Names Keduril®; K-Profen®; Orudis®; Profenid®; Profenid® 200; Profenid®-IM

Pharmacologic Category Nonsteroidal Anti-inflammatory Drug (NSAID)

Synonyms Orudis® [DSC]

Use

Dental: Management of pain and swelling

Medical: Acute and long-term treatment of rheumatoid arthritis and osteoarthritis; primary dysmenorrhea; mild to moderate pain

Local Anesthetic/Vasoconstrictor Precautions No information available to require special precautions

Effects on Dental Treatment NSAID formulations are known to reversibly decrease platelet aggregation via mechanisms different than observed with aspirin. The dentist should be aware of the potential of abnormal coagulation. Caution should also be exercised in the use of NSAIDs in patients already on anticoagulant therapy with drugs such as warfarin (Coumadin®).

>10%: Headache (11%)

1% to 9%: Nervousness, vomiting (>1%), nausea (3% to 9%), abdominal distress/cramping/pain (3% to 9%), stomatitis (>1%)

Dosage Oral:

Children 3 months to 14 years: Fever: 0.5-1 mg/kg every 6-8 hours

Children >12 years and Adults:

Mild to moderate pain: 25-50 mg every 6-8 hours up to a maximum of 300 mg/day

Rheumatoid arthritis or osteoarthritis: 50-75 mg 3-4 times/day up to a maximum of 300 mg/day

Mechanism of Action Inhibits prostaglandin synthesis by decreasing the activity of the enzyme, cyclooxygenase, which results in decreased formation of prostaglandin precursors

Other Adverse Effects

>10%: Gastrointestinal: Dyspepsia (11%)

1% to 10%:

Dermatologic: Rash, itching

Endocrine & metabolic: Fluid retention

Gastrointestinal: Diarrhea (3% to 9%), constipation (3% to 9%), flatulence (3% to 9%), anorexia (>1%)

Genitourinary: Urinary tract infection (>1%)

Otic: Tinnitus

<1%: **CHF, hypertension, arrhythmias, tachycardia, confusion, hallucinations,** mental depression, **drowsiness,** insomnia, aseptic meningitis, urticaria, erythema multiforme, toxic epidermal necrolysis, Stevens-Johnson syndrome, angioedema, polydipsia, **hot flashes, gastritis, GI ulceration,** cystitis, polyuria, agranulocytosis, anemia, hemolytic anemia, bone marrow suppression, leukopenia, thrombocytopenia, hepatitis, peripheral neuropathy, toxic amblyopia, **blurred vision,** conjunctivitis, dry eyes, decreased hearing, **acute renal failure, allergic rhinitis, dyspnea, epistaxis**

Contraindications Hypersensitivity to ketoprofen, any component of the formulation, or other NSAIDs/aspirin; pregnancy (3rd trimester)

Warnings/Precautions Use with caution in patients with CHF, hypertension, dehydration, decreased renal or hepatic function, history of GI disease (bleeding or ulcers), or those receiving anticoagulants. Elderly are at a high risk for adverse effects from NSAIDs. As many as 60% of elderly can develop peptic ulceration and/or hemorrhage asymptomatically.

Use lowest effective dose for shortest period possible. Use of NSAIDs can compromise existing renal function especially when Cl_{cr} is <30 mL/minute. CNS adverse effects such as confusion, agitation, and hallucination are generally seen in overdose or high-dose situations; however, elderly may demonstrate these adverse effects at lower doses than younger adults. Withhold for at least 4-6 half-lives prior to surgical or dental procedures. Safety and efficacy in pediatric patients have not been established (per manufacturer).

Drug Interactions Inhibits CYP2C8/9

ACE inhibitors: Antihypertensive effects may be decreased by concurrent therapy with NSAIDs; monitor blood pressure

Angiotensin II antagonists: Antihypertensive effects may be decreased by concurrent therapy with NSAIDs; monitor blood pressure

Anticoagulants (warfarin, heparin, LMWHs) in combination with NSAIDs can cause increased risk of bleeding.

Other antiplatelet drugs (ticlopidine, clopidogrel, aspirin, abciximab, dipyridamole, eptifibatide, tirofiban) can cause an increased risk of bleeding.

Corticosteroids may increase the risk of GI ulceration; avoid concurrent use.

Cyclosporine: NSAIDs may increase serum creatinine, potassium, blood pressure, and cyclosporine levels; monitor cyclosporine levels and renal function carefully

Gentamicin and amikacin serum concentrations are increased by indomethacin in premature infants. Results may apply to other aminoglycosides and NSAIDs.

Hydralazine's antihypertensive effect is decreased; avoid concurrent use

Lithium levels can be increased; avoid concurrent use if possible or monitor lithium levels and adjust dose. Sulindac may have the least effect. When NSAID is stopped, lithium will need adjustment again.

Loop diuretics efficacy (diuretic and antihypertensive effect) is reduced. Indomethacin reduces this efficacy, however, it may be anticipated with any NSAID.

Thiazides antihypertensive effects are decreased; avoid concurrent use

Verapamil plasma concentration is decreased by diclofenac; avoid concurrent use

Warfarin's INRs may be increased by piroxicam. Other NSAIDs may have the same effect depending on dose and duration. Monitor INR closely. Use the lowest dose of NSAIDs possible and for the briefest duration.

Dietary/Ethanol/Herb Considerations

Ethanol: Avoid use due to GI irritation.

Food: Administer with food or milk to reduce GI upset. Although food affects the bioavailability of ketoprofen, analgesic efficacy is not significantly diminished. Food slows rate of absorption resulting in delayed and reduced peak serum concentration.

Herb/Nutraceutical: Avoid kava and valerian; may enhance benzodiazepine activity.

Pharmacodynamics/Kinetics

Onset of action: Peak effect: 1-2 hours

Absorption: Almost complete

Metabolism: Hepatic

Half-life elimination: 1-4 hours

Time to peak, serum: 0.5-2 hours

Excretion: Urine (60% to 75% primarily as glucuronide conjugates)

Pregnancy Risk Factor B/D (3rd trimester)

Dosage Forms CAP (Orudis® [DSC]): 50 mg, 75 mg. **CAP, extended release** (Oruvail®): 100 mg, 150 mg, 200 mg. **TAB** (Orudis® KT): 12.5 mg

Generic Available Yes: Capsule

Selected Readings

Balevi B, "Ketorolac Versus Ibuprofen: A Simple Cost-Efficacy Comparison for Dental Use," *J Can Dent Assoc*, 1994, 60(1):31-2.

Brooks PM and Day RO, "Nonsteroidal Anti-inflammatory Drugs - Differences and Similarities," *N Engl J Med*, 1991, 324(24):1716-25.

Cooper SA, "Ketoprofen in Oral Surgery Pain: A Review," *J Clin Pharmacol*, 1988, 28(12 Suppl):S40-6.

Hersh EV, "The Efficacy and Safety of Ketoprofen in Postsurgical Dental Pain," *Compendium*, 1991, 12(4):234.

Ketorolac (KEE toe role ak)

Related Information

Rheumatoid Arthritis, Osteoarthritis, and Osteoporosis *on page 1488*

Temporomandibular Dysfunction (TMD) *on page 1562*

U.S. Brand Names Acular®; Acular® PF; Toradol®

Canadian Brand Names Acular®; Apo®-Ketorolac; Apo®-Ketorolac Injectable; Novo-Ketorolac; Toradol®; Toradol® IM

Mexican Brand Names Acularen®; Alidol®; Dolac®; Dolac Inyectable; Dolac Oral; Dolotor®; Findol®; Supradol®

Pharmacologic Category Nonsteroidal Anti-inflammatory Drug (NSAID)

Synonyms Ketorolac Tromethamine

Use

Dental and Medical: Oral, injection: Short-term (≤5 days) management of moderately-severe acute pain requiring analgesia at the opioid level

Note: First parenteral NSAID for analgesia; 30 mg I.M. provides analgesia comparable to 12 mg of morphine or 100 mg of meperidine.

Medical: Ophthalmic: Temporary relief of ocular itching due to seasonal allergic conjunctivitis; postoperative inflammation following cataract extraction; reduction of ocular pain and photophobia following incisional refractive surgery

Local Anesthetic/Vasoconstrictor Precautions No information available to require special precautions

Effects on Dental Treatment NSAID formulations are known to reversibly decrease platelet aggregation via mechanisms different than observed with aspirin. The dentist should be aware of the potential of abnormal coagulation. Caution should also be exercised in the use of NSAIDs in patients already on anticoagulant therapy with drugs such as warfarin (Coumadin®).

Systemic:

>10%: Headache (17%), GI pain (13%), nausea (12%)

>1% to 10%: Hypertension, dizziness (7%), drowsiness (6%), vomiting, stomatitis, diaphoresis, xerostomia (1% to 10%), injection site pain (2%)

Dosage Use of any formulation except ophthalmic solution in children <16 years of age is outside of product labeling.

(Continued)

Ketorolac *(Continued)*

Children 2-16 years: Dosing guidelines are not established; **do not exceed adult doses**

Single-dose treatment:

I.M., I.V.: 0.4-1 mg/kg as a single dose; **Note:** Limited information exists. Single I.V. doses of 0.5 mg/kg, 0.75 mg/kg, 0.9 mg/kg and 1 mg/kg have been studied in children 2-16 years of age for postoperative analgesia. One study (Maunuksela, 1992) used a titrating dose starting with 0.2 mg/kg up to a total of 0.5 mg/kg (median dose required: 0.4 mg/kg).

Oral: One study used 1 mg/kg as a single dose for analgesia in 30 children (mean ± SD age: 3 ± 2.5 years) undergoing bilateral myringotomy

Multiple-dose treatment: I.M., I.V., Oral: No pediatric studies exist; one report (Buck, 1994) of the clinical experience with ketorolac in 112 children, 6 months to 19 years of age (mean: 9 years), described usual I.V. maintenance doses of 0.5 mg/kg every 6 hours (mean dose: 0.52 mg/kg; range: 0.17-1 mg/kg)

Adults (pain relief usually begins within 10 minutes with parenteral forms): **Note: The maximum combined duration of treatment (for parenteral and oral) is 5 days**; do not increase dose or frequency; supplement with low dose opioids if needed for breakthrough pain. For patients <50 kg and/or ≥65 years of age, see Elderly dosing.

I.M.: 60 mg as a single dose or 30 mg every 6 hours (maximum daily dose: 120 mg)

I.V.: 30 mg as a single dose or 30 mg every 6 hours (maximum daily dose: 120 mg)

Oral: 20 mg, followed by 10 mg every 4-6 hours; do not exceed 40 mg/day; oral dosing is intended to be a continuation of I.M. or I.V. therapy only

Ophthalmic: Children ≥3 years and Adults:

Allergic conjunctivitis (relief of ocular itching): Instill 1 drop (0.25 mg) 4 times/day for seasonal allergic conjunctivitis

Inflammation following cataract extraction: Instill 1 drop (0.25 mg) to affected eye(s) 4 times/day beginning 24 hours after surgery; continue for 2 weeks

Pain and photophobia following incisional refractive surgery: Instill 1 drop (0.25 mg) 4 times/day to affected eye for up to 3 days

Elderly >65 years: Renal insufficiency or weight <50 kg: **Note:** Ketorolac has decreased clearance and increased halflife in the elderly. In addition, the elderly have reported increased incidence of GI bleeding, ulceration, and perforation. The maximum combined duration of treatment (for parenteral and oral) is 5 days.

I.M.: 30 mg as a single dose or 15 mg every 6 hours (maximum daily dose: 60 mg)

I.V.: 15 mg as a single dose or 15 mg every 6 hours (maximum daily dose: 60 mg)

Oral: 10 mg every 4-6 hours; do not exceed 40 mg/day; oral dosing is intended to be a continuation of I.M. or I.V. therapy only

Dosing adjustment in renal impairment: Do not use in patients with advanced renal impairment. Patients with moderately-elevated serum creatinine should use half the recommended dose, not to exceed 60 mg/day I.M./I.V.

Dosing adjustment in hepatic impairment: Use with caution, may cause elevation of liver enzymes

Mechanism of Action Inhibits prostaglandin synthesis by decreasing the activity of the enzyme, cyclooxygenase, which results in decreased formation of prostaglandin precursors

Other Adverse Effects

>10%:

Systemic: Gastrointestinal: Dyspepsia (12%)

Ophthalmic solution: Ocular: Transient burning/stinging (Acular®: 40%; Acular® PF: 20%)

>1% to 10%:

Systemic:

Cardiovascular: Edema (4%)

Dermatologic: Pruritus, purpura, rash

Gastrointestinal: Diarrhea (7%), constipation, flatulence, GI fullness

Ophthalmic solution: Ocular: Irritation, allergic reactions, superficial infection, superficial keratitis, iritis, inflammation

≤1%:

Systemic: Abnormal dreams, **abnormal taste, abnormal thinking, abnormal vision,** anemia, anorexia, appetite increased, **cough,** depression, **dyspnea**, eosinophilia, **epistaxis, euphoria, excessive thirst, extrapyramidal symptoms, fever, gastritis, hallucinations,** hearing loss, hematuria, hyperkinesis, inability to concentrate, increased urinary frequency, **infections,** insomnia, **nervousness,** oliguria, pallor, **palpitations, paresthesia,** polyuria, proteinuria, pulmonary edema, rectal bleeding, **rhinitis, stupor, syncope,** tinnitus, **tremors,** urinary retention, urticaria, vertigo, **weakness,** weight gain

Ophthalmic solution: Dry eyes, corneal infiltrates, corneal ulcer, headache

Postmarketing and/or case reports: Acute pancreatitis, **acute renal failure, anaphylactoid reaction, anaphylaxis,** aseptic meningitis, **asthma,** azotemia, **bronchospasm,** cholestatic jaundice, **convulsions,** exfoliative dermatitis, **flank**

pain, flushing, GI hemorrhage or perforation, hematuria, hemolytic uremic syndrome, hepatitis, hyperkalemia, **hypersensitivity reactions,** hyponatremia, **hypotension, laryngeal edema,** leukopenia, **liver failure,** maculopapular rash, melena, myalgia, nephritis, **peptic ulceration, psychosis,** Stevens-Johnson syndrome, thrombocytopenia, **tongue edema**, toxic epidermal necrolysis, urticaria, **wound hemorrhage (postoperative)**

Contraindications Hypersensitivity to ketorolac, aspirin, other NSAIDs, or any component of the formulation; patients who have developed nasal polyps, angioedema, or bronchospastic reactions to other NSAIDs; active or history of peptic ulcer disease; recent or history of GI bleeding or perforation; patients with advanced renal disease or risk of renal failure; labor and delivery; nursing mothers; prophylaxis before major surgery; suspected or confirmed cerebrovascular bleeding; hemorrhagic diathesis; concurrent ASA or other NSAIDs; epidural or intrathecal administration; concomitant probenecid; pregnancy (3rd trimester)

Warnings/Precautions

Systemic: Treatment should be started with I.V./I.M. administration then changed to oral only as a continuation of treatment. Total therapy is not to exceed 5 days. Should not be used for minor or chronic pain. Hypersensitivity reactions have occurred flowing the first dose of ketorolac injection, including patients without prior exposure to ketorolac, aspirin, or other NSAIDs. Use extra caution and reduce dosages in the elderly because it is cleared renally somewhat slower, and the elderly are also more sensitive to the renal effects of NSAIDs and have a greater risk of GI perforation and bleeding; use with caution in patients with CHF, hypertension, dehydration, decreased renal or hepatic function, or those receiving anticoagulants. May prolong bleeding time; do not use when hemostasis is critical. Patients should be euvolemic prior to treatment. Low doses of narcotics may be needed for breakthrough pain. Withhold for at least 4-6 half-lives prior to surgical or dental procedures.

Ophthalmic: May increase bleeding time associated with ocular surgery. Use with caution in patients with known bleeding tendencies or those receiving anticoagulants. Do not administer while wearing soft contact lenses. Safety and efficacy in pediatric patients <3 years of age have not been established.

Drug Interactions

ACE inhibitors: Antihypertensive effects may be decreased by concurrent therapy with NSAIDs; monitor blood pressure.

Angiotensin II antagonists: Antihypertensive effects may be decreased by concurrent therapy with NSAIDs; monitor blood pressure.

Anticoagulants: Increased risk of bleeding complications with concomitant use; monitor closely.

Antiepileptic drugs (carbamazepine, phenytoin): Sporadic cases of seizures have been reported with concomitant use.

Diuretics: May see decreased effect of diuretics.

Lithium: May increase lithium levels; monitor.

Methotrexate: Severe bone marrow suppression, aplastic anemia, and GI toxicity have been reported with concomitant NSAID therapy. Avoid use during moderate or high-dose methotrexate (increased and prolonged methotrexate levels). NSAID use during low-dose treatment of rheumatoid arthritis has not been fully evaluated; extreme caution is warranted.

Nondepolarizing muscle relaxants: Concomitant use has resulted in apnea.

NSAIDs, salicylates: Concomitant use increases NSAID-induced adverse effects; contraindicated.

Probenecid: Probenecid significantly decreases ketorolac clearance, increases ketorolac plasma levels, and doubles the half-life of ketorolac; concomitant use is contraindicated.

Psychoactive drugs (alprazolam, fluoxetine, thiothixene): Hallucinations have been reported with concomitant use.

Dietary/Ethanol/Herb Considerations

Ethanol: Avoid use; may enhance gastric mucosal irritation.

Food: Administer with food or milk to reduce GI upset. Food decreases rate of absorption but extent remains the same. Oral: High-fat meals may delay time to peak (by ~1 hour) and decrease peak concentrations. Avoid garlic, ginger, and green tea.

Herb/Nutraceutical: Avoid cat's claw, dong quai, evening primrose, feverfew, garlic, ginger, ginkgo biloba, ginseng, green tea, horse chestnut, and red clover due to additional antiplatelet activity. Avoid kava and valerian; may enhance benzodiazepine activity.

Pharmacodynamics/Kinetics

Onset of action: Analgesic: I.M.: ~10 minutes

Peak effect: Analgesic: 2-3 hours

Duration: Analgesic: 6-8 hours

Absorption: Oral: Well absorbed

Distribution: Poor penetration into CSF; crosses placenta; enters breast milk

Protein binding: 99%

Metabolism: Hepatic

Half-life elimination: 2-8 hours; prolonged 30% to 50% in elderly

(Continued)

Ketorolac *(Continued)*

Time to peak, serum: I.M.: 30-60 minutes
Excretion: Urine (61% as unchanged drug)

Pregnancy Risk Factor C/D (3rd trimester); ophthalmic: C

Dosage Forms INJ, solution: 15 mg/mL (1 mL); 30 mg/mL (1 mL, 2 mL). **SOLN, ophthalmic** (Acular®): 0.5% (3 mL, 5 mL, 10 mL). **SOLN, ophthalmic** [preservative free] (Acular® PF): 0.5% (0.4 mL). **TAB** (Toradol®): 10 mg

Generic Available Yes: Injection, tablet

Comments According to the manufacturer, ketorolac has been used inappropriately by physicians in the past. The drug had been prescribed to NSAID-sensitive patients, patients with GI bleeding, and for long-term use; a warning has been issued regarding increased incidence and severity of GI complications with increasing doses and duration of use. Labeling now includes the statement that ketorolac inhibits platelet function and is indicated for up to 5 days use only.

Selected Readings

Ahmad N, Grad HA, Haas DA, et al, "The Efficacy of Nonopioid Analgesics for Postoperative Dental Pain: A Meta-analysis," *Anesth Prog*, 1997, 44(4):119-26.

Balevi B, "Ketorolac Versus Ibuprofen: A Simple Cost-Efficacy Comparison for Dental Use," *J Can Dent Assoc*, 1994, 60(1):31-2.

Forbes JA, Butterworth GA, Burchfield WH, et al, "Evaluation of Ketorolac, Aspirin, and an Acetaminophen-Codeine Combination in Postoperative Oral Surgery Pain," *Pharmacotherapy*, 1990, 10(6 Pt 2): 77S-93S.

Forbes JA, Kehm CJ, Grodin CD, et al, "Evaluation of Ketorolac, Ibuprofen, Acetaminophen, and an Acetaminophen-Codeine Combination in Postoperative Oral Surgery Pain," *Pharmacotherapy*, 1990, 10(6 Pt 2):94S-105S.

Fricke JR Jr, Angelocci D, Fox K, et al, "Comparison of the Efficacy and Safety of Ketorolac and Meperidine in the Relief of Dental Pain," *J Clin Pharmacol*, 1992, 32(4):376-84.

Fricke J, Halladay SC, Bynum L, et al, "Pain Relief After Dental Impaction Surgery Using Ketorolac, Hydrocodone Plus Acetaminophen, or Placebo," *Clin Ther*, 1993, 15(3):500-9.

Pendeville PE, Van Boven MJ, Contreras V, et al, "Ketorolac Tromethamine for Postoperative Analgesia in Oral Surgery," *Acta Anaesthesiol Belg*, 1995, 46(1):25-30.

Swift JQ, Roszkowski MT, Alton T, "Effect of Intra-articular Versus Systemic Anti-inflammatory Drugs in a Rabbit Model of Temporomandibular Joint Inflammation," *J Oral Maxillofac Surg*, 1998, 56(11):1288-95 (discussion 1295-6).

Walton GM, Rood JP, Snowdon AT, et al, "Ketorolac and Diclofenac for Postoperative Pain Relief Following Oral Surgery," *Br J Oral Maxillofac Surg*, 1993, 31(3):158-60.

Wynn RL, "Ketorolac (Toradol®) for Dental Pain," *Gen Dent*, 1992, 40(6):476-9.

Ketorolac Tromethamine *see* Ketorolac *on page 765*

Ketotifen (kee toe TYE fen)

U.S. Brand Names Zaditor™

Canadian Brand Names Apo®-Ketotifen; Novo-Ketotifen; Zaditen®; Zaditor™

Mexican Brand Names Kasmal®; Ventisol®; Zaditen®

Pharmacologic Category Antihistamine, H_1 Blocker, Ophthalmic

Synonyms Ketotifen Fumarate

Use Temporary prevention of eye itching due to allergic conjunctivitis

Local Anesthetic/Vasoconstrictor Precautions No information available to require special precautions

Effects on Dental Treatment 1% to 10%: Pharyngitis, flu-like syndrome

Dosage Children ≥3 years and Adults: Ophthalmic: Instill 1 drop into the affected eye(s) twice daily, every 8-12 hours

Mechanism of Action Relatively selective, noncompetitive H_1-receptor antagonist and mast cell stabilizer, inhibiting the release of mediators from cells involved in hypersensitivity reactions

Other Adverse Effects 1% to 10%: Ocular: Allergic reactions, burning or stinging, conjunctivitis, discharge, dry eyes, eye pain, eyelid disorder, itching, keratitis, lacrimation disorder, mydriasis, photophobia, rash

Pharmacodynamics/Kinetics

Onset of action: Minutes
Duration: 8-12 hours
Absorption: Minimally systemic

Pregnancy Risk Factor C

Generic Available No

Ketotifen Fumarate *see* Ketotifen *on page 768*
Key-E® [OTC] *see* Vitamin E *on page 1393*
Key- E® Kaps [OTC] *see* Vitamin E *on page 1393*
KI *see* Potassium Iodide *on page 1101*
Kidkare Decongestant [OTC] *see* Pseudoephedrine *on page 1146*
Kineret™ *see* Anakinra *on page 108*
Kinevac® *see* Sincalide *on page 1225*
Klaron® *see* Sulfacetamide *on page 1249*
Klerist-D® [OTC] *see* Chlorpheniramine and Pseudoephedrine *on page 308*
Klonopin™ *see* Clonazepam *on page 350*
K-Lor™ *see* Potassium Supplements *on page 1102*
Klor-Con® *see* Potassium Supplements *on page 1102*

Klor-Con® 8 *see* Potassium Supplements *on page 1102*
Klor-Con® 10 *see* Potassium Supplements *on page 1102*
Klor-Con®/25 *see* Potassium Supplements *on page 1102*
Klor-Con®/EF *see* Potassium Supplements *on page 1102*
Klor-Con® M10 *see* Potassium Supplements *on page 1102*
Klor-Con® M20 *see* Potassium Supplements *on page 1102*
Klotrix® *see* Potassium Supplements *on page 1102*
K-Lyte® *see* Potassium Supplements *on page 1102*
K-Lyte/Cl® *see* Potassium Supplements *on page 1102*
K-Lyte/Cl® 50 *see* Potassium Supplements *on page 1102*
K-Lyte® DS *see* Potassium Supplements *on page 1102*
Koāte®-DVI *see* Antihemophilic Factor (Human) *on page 113*
Kodet SE [OTC] *see* Pseudoephedrine *on page 1146*
Kogenate® FS *see* Antihemophilic Factor (Recombinant) *on page 115*
Kolephrin® GG/DM [OTC] *see* Guaifenesin and Dextromethorphan *on page 651*
Konsyl® [OTC] *see* Psyllium *on page 1149*
Konsyl-D® [OTC] *see* Psyllium *on page 1149*
Konsyl® Easy Mix [OTC] *see* Psyllium *on page 1149*
Konsyl® Orange [OTC] *see* Psyllium *on page 1149*
K-Phos® MF *see* Phosphate Supplements *on page 1076*
K-Phos® Neutral *see* Phosphate Supplements *on page 1076*
K-Phos® No. 2 *see* Phosphate Supplements *on page 1076*
K-Phos® Original *see* Phosphate Supplements *on page 1076*
K-Phos® Original *see* Potassium Acid Phosphate *on page 1100*
K-Phos® Original *see* Potassium Supplements *on page 1102*
Kristalose™ *see* Lactulose *on page 772*
K-Tab® *see* Potassium Supplements *on page 1102*
Kutrase® *see* Pancreatin *on page 1030*
Ku-Zyme® *see* Pancreatin *on page 1030*
Ku-Zyme® HP *see* Pancrelipase *on page 1030*
Kwelcof® *see* Hydrocodone and Guaifenesin *on page 683*
Kytril® *see* Granisetron *on page 648*
***L*-3-Hydroxytyrosine** *see* Levodopa *on page 792*
L-749,345 *see* Ertapenem *on page 511*

Labetalol (la BET a lole)

Related Information

Cardiovascular Diseases *on page 1456*

U.S. Brand Names Normodyne®; Trandate®

Canadian Brand Names Apo®-Labetalol; Normodyne®; Trandate®

Mexican Brand Names Midotens

Pharmacologic Category Beta Blocker With Alpha-Blocking Activity

Synonyms Ibidomide Hydrochloride; Labetalol Hydrochloride

Use Treatment of mild to severe hypertension; I.V. for hypertensive emergencies

Local Anesthetic/Vasoconstrictor Precautions Use with caution; epinephrine has interacted with nonselective beta-blockers to result in initial hypertensive episode followed by bradycardia

Effects on Dental Treatment 1% to 10%: Nasal congestion (1% to 6%), dyspnea (2%), hypotension (1% to 5%), headache (2%), taste disorder (1%)

Noncardioselective beta-blockers enhance the pressor response to epinephrine, resulting in hypertension and bradycardia. Many nonsteroidal anti-inflammatory drugs such as ibuprofen and indomethacin can reduce the hypotensive effect of beta-blockers after 3 or more weeks of therapy with the NSAID. Short-term NSAID use (ie, 3 days) requires no special precautions in patients taking beta-blockers.

Dosage Due to limited documentation of its use, labetalol should be initiated cautiously in pediatric patients with careful dosage adjustment and blood pressure monitoring.

Children:

- Oral: Limited information regarding labetalol use in pediatric patients is currently available in literature. Some centers recommend initial oral doses of 4 mg/kg/day in 2 divided doses. Reported oral doses have started at 3 mg/kg/day and 20 mg/kg/day and have increased up to 40 mg/kg/day.
- I.V., intermittent bolus doses of 0.3-1 mg/kg/dose have been reported.
- For treatment of pediatric hypertensive emergencies, initial continuous infusions of 0.4-1 mg/kg/hour with a maximum of 3 mg/kg/hour have been used. Administration requires the use of an infusion pump.

Adults:

- Oral: Initial: 100 mg twice daily, may increase as needed every 2-3 days by 100 mg until desired response is obtained; usual dose: 200-400 mg twice daily; may require up to 2.4 g/day.

(Continued)

Labetalol *(Continued)*

I.V.: 20 mg (0.25 mg/kg for an 80 kg patient) IVP over 2 minutes; may administer 40-80 mg at 10-minute intervals, up to 300 mg total dose.

I.V. infusion: Initial: 2 mg/minute; titrate to response up to 300 mg total dose, if needed. Administration requires the use of an infusion pump.

I.V. infusion (500 mg/250 mL D_5W) rates:
- 1 mg/minute: 30 mL/hour
- 2 mg/minute: 60 mL/hour
- 3 mg/minute: 90 mL/hour
- 4 mg/minute: 120 mL/hour
- 5 mg/minute: 150 mL/hour
- 6 mg/minute: 180 mL/hour

Dialysis: Not removed by hemo- or peritoneal dialysis; supplemental dose is unnecessary.

Dosing adjustment in hepatic impairment: Reduction may be necessary

Mechanism of Action Blocks alpha-, $beta_1$-, and $beta_2$-adrenergic receptor sites; elevated renins are reduced

Other Adverse Effects

>10%:
- Central nervous system: Dizziness (1% to 16%)
- Gastrointestinal: Nausea (≤19%)

1% to 10%:
- Cardiovascular: Edema (≤2%), hypotension (I.V. ≤58%)
- Central nervous system: Fatigue (1% to 10%), paresthesia (1% to 5%), vertigo (2%), weakness (1%)
- Dermatologic: Rash (1%), scalp tingling (1% to 5%)
- Gastrointestinal: Vomiting (<1% to 3%), dyspepsia (1% to 4%)
- Genitourinary: Ejaculatory failure (≤5%), impotence (1% to 4%)
- Hepatic: Increased transaminases (4%)
- Miscellaneous: Abnormal vision (1%)

<1% (Limited to important or life-threatening): **Hypotension, syncope, bradycardia, heart block, fever**, diarrhea, drowsiness, **increased diaphoresis,** systemic lupus erythematosus, positive ANA, dry eyes, antimitochondrial antibodies, hepatic necrosis, hepatitis, cholestatic jaundice, muscle cramps, toxic myopathy, bronchospasm, Peyronie's disease, alopecia (reversible), micturition difficulty, urinary retention, hypersensitivity, urticaria, angioedema, pruritus, **anaphylactoid reaction**, Raynaud's syndrome, claudication, **CHF, ventricular arrhythmias (I.V.)**

Postmarketing and/or case reports: Fever, toxic myopathy, muscle cramps, systemic lupus erythematosus, diabetes insipidus

Other adverse reactions noted with beta-adrenergic blocking agents include mental depression, catatonia, disorientation, short-term memory loss, emotional lability, clouded sensorium, intensification of pre-existing AV block, laryngospasm, respiratory distress, agranulocytosis, thrombocytopenic purpura, nonthrombocytopenic purpura, mesenteric artery thrombosis, and ischemic colitis.

Drug Interactions Substrate of **CYP2D6**; Inhibits CYP2D6

Increased Effect/Toxicity: Inhibitors of CYP2D6 including quinidine, paroxetine, and propafenone are likely to increase blood levels of labetalol. Cimetidine increases the bioavailability of labetalol. Labetalol has additive hypotensive effects with other antihypertensive agents. Concurrent use with alpha-blockers (prazosin, terazosin) and beta-blockers increases the risk of orthostasis. Concurrent use with diltiazem, verapamil, or digoxin may increase the risk of bradycardia with beta-blocking agents. Halothane, enflurane, isoflurane, and potentially other inhalation anesthetics may cause synergistic hypotension. Beta-blockers may affect the action or levels of ethanol, disopyramide, nondepolarizing muscle relaxants, and theophylline although the effects are difficult to predict.

Decreased Effect: Decreased effect of beta-blockers with aluminum salts, barbiturates, calcium salts, cholestyramine, colestipol, NSAIDs, penicillins (ampicillin), rifampin, salicylates, and sulfinpyrazone due to decreased bioavailability and plasma levels. Beta-blockers may decrease the effect of sulfonylureas.

Dietary/Ethanol/Herb Considerations

Ethanol: Avoid or limit use; may increase risk of hypotension or dizziness.

Food: Administer with food; may increase serum concentration. Avoid caffeine, garlic, and licorice.

Herb/Nutraceutical: Avoid black cohosh, dong quai, and evening primrose due to estrogenic activity. Avoid ephedra, ginseng, and yohimbe; may worsen hypertension. Avoid garlic; may have increased antihypertensive effect. Avoid hawthorn; may lower peripheral vascular resistance resulting in decrease in BP. Avoid ginger due to positive inotropic effects; theoretically, may cause arrhythmia. Avoid licorice; causes sodium and water retention and increases potassium loss.

Pharmacodynamics/Kinetics

Onset of action: Oral: 20 minutes to 2 hours; I.V.: 2-5 minutes
- Peak effect: Oral: 1-4 hours; I.V.: 5-15 minutes

Duration: Oral: 8-24 hours (dose dependent); I.V.: 2-4 hours

Distribution: V_d: Adults: 3-16 L/kg; mean: <9.4 L/kg; moderately lipid soluble, therefore, can enter CNS; crosses placenta; small amounts enter breast milk
Protein binding: 50%
Metabolism: Hepatic, primarily via glucuronide conjugation; extensive first-pass effect
Bioavailability: Oral: 25%; increased with liver disease, elderly, and concurrent cimetidine
Half-life elimination: Normal renal function: 2.5-8 hours
Excretion: Urine (<5% as unchanged drug)
Clearance: Possibly decreased in neonates/infants

Pregnancy Risk Factor C (manufacturer); D (2nd and 3rd trimesters - expert analysis)

Generic Available Yes

Labetalol Hydrochloride *see* Labetalol *on page 769*
Lac-Hydrin® *see* Lactic Acid and Ammonium Hydroxide *on page 771*
LAClotion™ *see* Lactic Acid and Ammonium Hydroxide *on page 771*
Lacrisert® *see* Hydroxypropyl Cellulose *on page 695*
Lactaid® [OTC] *see* Lactase *on page 771*
Lactaid® Extra Strength [OTC] *see* Lactase *on page 771*
Lactaid® Ultra [OTC] *see* Lactase *on page 771*

Lactase (LAK tase)

U.S. Brand Names Lactaid® [OTC]; Lactaid® Extra Strength [OTC]; Lactaid® Ultra [OTC]; Lactrase® [OTC]

Canadian Brand Names Dairyaid®

Pharmacologic Category Enzyme

Use Help digest lactose in milk for patients with lactose intolerance

Local Anesthetic/Vasoconstrictor Precautions No information available to require special precautions

Effects on Dental Treatment No significant effects or complications reported

Dosage Oral:
Capsule: 1-2 capsules taken with milk or meal; pretreat milk with 1-2 capsules/quart of milk
Liquid: 5-15 drops/quart of milk
Tablet: 1-3 tablets with meals

Dietary/Ethanol/Herb Considerations Food: May be taken with meals

Generic Available No

Lactic Acid and Ammonium Hydroxide

(LAK tik AS id & a MOE nee um hye DROKS ide)

U.S. Brand Names AmLactin® [OTC]; Lac-Hydrin®; LAClotion™

Pharmacologic Category Topical Skin Product

Synonyms Ammonium Lactate

Use Treatment of moderate to severe xerosis and ichthyosis vulgaris

Local Anesthetic/Vasoconstrictor Precautions No information available to require special precautions

Effects on Dental Treatment No significant effects or complications reported

Dosage Children ≥2 years and Adults: Topical: Apply twice daily to affected area; rub in well

Mechanism of Action Exact mechanism of action unknown; lactic acid is a normal component in blood and tissues. When applied topically to the skin, acts as a humectant.

Other Adverse Effects Dermatologic:
>10%: Rash, including erythema and irritation (2% to 15%); burning/stinging (2% to 15%)
1% to 10%: Itching (5%), dry skin (2%)

Pharmacodynamics/Kinetics Absorption: 6%

Pregnancy Risk Factor B

Generic Available No

Lactic Acid and Sodium-PCA

(LAK tik AS id & SOW dee um-pee see ay)

U.S. Brand Names LactiCare® [OTC]; Lactinol®; Lactinol-E®

Pharmacologic Category Topical Skin Product

Synonyms Sodium-PCA and Lactic Acid

Use Lubricate and moisturize the skin counteracting dryness and itching

Local Anesthetic/Vasoconstrictor Precautions No information available to require special precautions

Effects on Dental Treatment No significant effects or complications reported

Dosage Topical: Apply as needed

Generic Available No

LactiCare® [OTC] *see* Lactic Acid and Sodium-PCA *on page 771*

LactiCare-HC® *see* Hydrocortisone *on page 688*

Lactinex® [OTC] *see Lactobacillus acidophilus* and *Lactobacillus bulgaricus on page 772*

Lactinol® *see* Lactic Acid and Sodium-PCA *on page 771*

Lactinol-E® *see* Lactic Acid and Sodium-PCA *on page 771*

Lactobacillus acidophilus *see Lactobacillus acidophilus* and *Lactobacillus bulgaricus on page 772*

Lactobacillus acidophilus and *Lactobacillus bulgaricus*

(lak toe ba SIL us a si DO fil us)

Related Information

Bifidobacterium bifidum / Lactobacillus acidophilus on page 1422

Oral Nonviral Soft Tissue Ulcerations or Erosions *on page 1549*

U.S. Brand Names Bacid® [OTC]; Kala® [OTC]; Lactinex® [OTC]; Megadophilus® [OTC]; MoreDophilus® [OTC]; Probiotica® [OTC]; Superdophilus® [OTC]

Canadian Brand Names Bacid®; Fermalac

Mexican Brand Names Lacteol® Fort; Sinuberase®

Pharmacologic Category Antidiarrheal

Synonyms *Lactobacillus acidophilus*

Use Treatment of uncomplicated diarrhea particularly that caused by antibiotic therapy; re-establish normal physiologic and bacterial flora of the intestinal tract

Local Anesthetic/Vasoconstrictor Precautions No information available to require special precautions

Effects on Dental Treatment No significant effects or complications reported

Dosage Children >2 years and Adults: Oral:

Capsules: 2 capsules 2-4 times/day

Granules: 1 packet added to or taken with cereal, food, milk, fruit juice, or water, 3-4 times/day

Powder: 1 teaspoonful daily with liquid

Tablet, chewable: 4 tablets 3-4 times/day; may follow each dose with a small amount of milk, fruit juice, or water

Probiotica®: 1 tablet/day; chew thoroughly before swallowing

Mechanism of Action Creates an environment unfavorable to potentially pathogenic fungi or bacteria through the production of lactic acid, and favors establishment of an aciduric flora, thereby suppressing the growth of pathogenic microorganisms; helps re-establish normal intestinal flora

Dietary/Ethanol/Herb Considerations Food: Granules or contents of capsules may be added to cereal, milk, or fruit juice.

Pharmacodynamics/Kinetics

Absorption: Oral: None

Distribution: Local, primarily colon

Excretion: Feces

Pregnancy Risk Factor Not available

Generic Available Yes

Lactoflavin *see* Riboflavin *on page 1178*

Lactrase® [OTC] *see* Lactase *on page 771*

Lactulose (LAK tyoo lose)

U.S. Brand Names Cholac®; Constilac®; Constulose®; Enulose®; Generlac; Kristalose™

Canadian Brand Names Acilac; Apo®-Lactulose; Laxilose; PMS-Lactulose

Mexican Brand Names Lactulax®; Regulact®

Pharmacologic Category Ammonium Detoxicant; Laxative, Miscellaneous

Use Adjunct in the prevention and treatment of portal-systemic encephalopathy; treatment of chronic constipation

Local Anesthetic/Vasoconstrictor Precautions No information available to require special precautions

Effects on Dental Treatment No significant effects or complications reported

Dosage Diarrhea may indicate overdosage and responds to dose reduction

Prevention of portal systemic encephalopathy (PSE): Oral:

Infants: 2.5-10 mL/day divided 3-4 times/day; adjust dosage to produce 2-3 stools/day

Older Children: Daily dose of 40-90 mL divided 3-4 times/day; if initial dose causes diarrhea, then reduce it immediately; adjust dosage to produce 2-3 stools/day

Constipation: Oral:

Children: 5 g/day (7.5 mL) after breakfast

Adults: 15-30 mL/day increased to 60 mL/day if necessary

Acute PSE: Adults:

Oral: 20-30 g (30-45 mL) every 1-2 hours to induce rapid laxation; adjust dosage daily to produce 2-3 soft stools; doses of 30-45 mL may be given hourly to cause rapid laxation, then reduce to recommended dose; usual daily dose: 60-100 g (90-150 mL) daily

Rectal administration: 200 g (300 mL) diluted with 700 mL of H_2O or NS; administer rectally via rectal balloon catheter and retain 30-60 minutes every 4-6 hours

Mechanism of Action The bacterial degradation of lactulose resulting in an acidic pH inhibits the diffusion of NH_3 into the blood by causing the conversion of NH_3 to NH_4+; also enhances the diffusion of NH_3 from the blood into the gut where conversion to NH_4+ occurs; produces an osmotic effect in the colon with resultant distention promoting peristalsis

Other Adverse Effects Frequency not defined: Gastrointestinal: Flatulence, diarrhea (excessive dose), abdominal discomfort, nausea, vomiting, cramping

Drug Interactions Decreased Effect: Oral neomycin, laxatives, antacids

Dietary/Ethanol/Herb Considerations Food: Administer oral form with food, milk, juice, water, or citrus-flavored carbonated beverages; contraindicated in patients on galactose-restricted diet. Fluids, fruit, and fiber may reduce constipation.

Pharmacodynamics/Kinetics

Absorption: Not appreciable

Metabolism: Via colonic flora to lactic acid and acetic acid; requires colonic flora for drug activation

Excretion: Primarily feces and urine (~3%)

Pregnancy Risk Factor B

Generic Available Yes

Ladakamycin *see* Azacitidine *on page 149*
L-AmB *see* Amphotericin B (Liposomal) *on page 101*
Lamictal® *see* Lamotrigine *on page 774*
Lamisil® *see* Terbinafine *on page 1277*
Lamisil® AT™ [OTC] *see* Terbinafine *on page 1277*

Lamivudine (la MI vyoo deen)

Related Information

HIV Infection and AIDS *on page 1482*

Zidovudine and Lamivudine *on page 1407*

U.S. Brand Names Epivir®; Epivir-HBV®

Canadian Brand Names Heptovir®; 3TC®

Mexican Brand Names Combivir®; 3TC®

Pharmacologic Category Antiretroviral Agent, Reverse Transcriptase Inhibitor (Nucleoside)

Synonyms 3TC

Use

Epivir®: Treatment of HIV infection when antiretroviral therapy is warranted; should always be used as part of a multidrug regimen (at least three antiretroviral agents)

Epivir-HBV®: Treatment of chronic hepatitis B associated with evidence of hepatitis B viral replication and active liver inflammation

Unlabeled/Investigational Use Prevention of HIV following needlesticks (with or without protease inhibitor)

Local Anesthetic/Vasoconstrictor Precautions No information available to require special precautions

Effects on Dental Treatment 1% to 10%: Fever, nasal signs/symptoms, cough

Dosage The formulation and dosage of Epivir-HBV® are not appropriate for patients infected with both HBV and HIV. Use with at least two other antiretroviral agents when treating HIV.

Oral:

Children 3 months to 16 years: HIV: 4 mg/kg twice daily (maximum: 150 mg twice daily)

Children 2-17 years: Treatment of hepatitis B (Epivir-HBV®): 3 mg/kg once daily (maximum: 100 mg/day)

Adolescents and Adults: Prevention of HIV following needlesticks (unlabeled use): 150 mg twice daily (with zidovudine with or without a protease inhibitor, depending on risk)

Adults:

HIV: 150 mg twice daily **or** 300 mg once daily; <50 kg: 2 mg/kg twice daily

Treatment of hepatitis B (Epivir-HBV®): 100 mg/day

Dosing interval in renal impairment in pediatric patients: Insufficient data; however, dose reduction should be considered.

Dosing interval in renal impairment in patients >16 years for HIV:

Cl_{cr} 30-49 mL/minute: Administer 150 mg once daily

Cl_{cr} 15-29 mL/minute: Administer 150 mg first dose, then 100 mg once daily

Cl_{cr} 5-14 mL/minute: Administer 150 mg first dose, then 50 mg once daily

Cl_{cr} <5 mL/minute: Administer 50 mg first dose, then 25 mg once daily

Dosing interval in renal impairment in adult patients with hepatitis B:

Cl_{cr} 30-49: Administer 100 mg first dose then 50 mg once daily

Cl_{cr} 15-29: Administer 100 mg first dose then 25 mg once daily

Cl_{cr} 5-14: Administer 35 mg first dose then 15 mg once daily

(Continued)

Lamivudine *(Continued)*

Cl_{cr} <5: Administer 35 mg first dose then 10 mg once daily

Dialysis: No data available

Mechanism of Action After lamivudine is triphosphorylated, the principle mode of action is inhibition of HIV reverse transcription via viral DNA chain termination; inhibits RNA- and DNA-dependent DNA polymerase activities of reverse transcriptase. The monophosphate form of lamivudine is incorporated into the viral DNA by hepatitis B virus polymerase, resulting in DNA chain termination.

Other Adverse Effects As reported in adults treated for HIV infection:

>10%:

Central nervous system: Headache, fatigue

Gastrointestinal: Nausea, diarrhea, vomiting, pancreatitis (range: 0.5% to 18%; higher percentage in pediatric patients)

Neuromuscular & skeletal: Peripheral neuropathy, paresthesia, musculoskeletal pain

1% to 10%:

Central nervous system: Dizziness, depression, chills, insomnia

Dermatologic: Rash

Gastrointestinal: Anorexia, abdominal pain, heartburn, elevated amylase

Hematologic: Neutropenia

Hepatic: Elevated AST, ALT

Neuromuscular & skeletal: Myalgia, arthralgia

<1%, postmarketing, and/or case reports: Alopecia, **anaphylaxis,** anemia, hepatomegaly, hyperbilirubinemia, hyperglycemia, increased CPK, lactic acidosis, lymphadenopathy, peripheral neuropathy, pruritus, red cell aplasia, rhabdomyolysis, splenomegaly, steatosis, stomatitis, thrombocytopenia, urticaria, weakness

Drug Interactions

Increased Effect/Toxicity: Zidovudine concentrations increase significantly (~39%) with lamivudine coadministration. Trimethoprim/sulfamethoxazole increases lamivudine's blood levels. Concomitant use of ribavirin and nucleoside analogues may increase the risk of developing lactic acidosis (includes adefovir, didanosine, lamivudine, stavudine, zalcitabine, zidovudine).

Decreased Effect: Zalcitabine and lamivudine may inhibit the intracellular phosphorylation of each other; concomitant use should be avoided.

Dietary/Ethanol/Herb Considerations Food: May be taken with food; decreases the rate of absorption and C_{max}; however there is no change in the systemic AUC.

Pharmacodynamics/Kinetics

Absorption: Rapid

Distribution: V_d: 1.3 L/kg

Protein binding, plasma: <36%

Metabolism: 5.6% to trans-sulfoxide metabolite

Bioavailability: Absolute; Cp_{max} decreased with food although AUC not significantly affected

Children: 66%

Adults: 87%

Half-life elimination: Children: 2 hours; Adults: 5-7 hours

Excretion: Primarily urine (as unchanged drug)

Pregnancy Risk Factor C

Generic Available No

Lamivudine, Abacavir, and Zidovudine *see* Abacavir, Lamivudine, and Zidovudine *on page 23*

Lamivudine and Zidovudine *see* Zidovudine and Lamivudine *on page 1407*

Lamotrigine (la MOE tri jeen)

U.S. Brand Names Lamictal®

Canadian Brand Names Lamictal®

Mexican Brand Names Lamictal®

Pharmacologic Category Anticonvulsant, Miscellaneous

Synonyms BW-430C; LTG

Use Adjunctive therapy in the treatment of generalized seizures of Lennox-Gastaut syndrome and partial seizures in adults and children ≥2 years of age; conversion to monotherapy in adults with partial seizures who are receiving treatment with a single enzyme-inducing antiepileptic drug

Unlabeled/Investigational Use Treatment of bipolar disorder

Local Anesthetic/Vasoconstrictor Precautions No information available to require special precautions

Effects on Dental Treatment Rhinitis (7% to 14%), anxiety (4%), seizure (3% to 4%), flu-like syndrome (7%), fever (2% to 6%)

Dosage Only whole tablets should be used for dosing, round calculated dose down to the nearest whole tablet: Oral:

Children 2-12 years: Lennox-Gastaut (adjunctive) or partial seizures (adjunctive):
Note: Children 2-6 years will likely require maintenance doses at the higher end of recommended range:
Patients receiving AED regimens containing valproic acid:
Weeks 1 and 2: 0.15 mg/kg/day in 1-2 divided doses; round dose down to the nearest whole tablet. For patients >6.7 kg and <14 kg, dosing should be 2 mg every other day.
Weeks 3 and 4: 0.3 mg/kg/day in 1-2 divided doses; round dose down to the nearest whole tablet; may use combinations of 2 mg and 5 mg tablets. For patients >6.7 kg and <14 kg, dosing should be 2 mg/day.
Maintenance dose: Titrate dose to effect; after week 4, increase dose every 1-2 weeks by a calculated increment; calculate increment as 0.3 mg/kg/day rounded down to the nearest whole tablet; add this amount to the previously administered daily dose; usual maintenance: 1-5 mg/kg/day in 1-2 divided doses; maximum: 200 mg/day given in 1-2 divided doses
Patients receiving enzyme-inducing AED regimens without valproic acid:
Weeks 1 and 2: 0.6 mg/kg/day in 2 divided doses; round dose down to the nearest whole tablet
Weeks 3 and 4: 1.2 mg/kg/day in 2 divided doses; round dose down to the nearest whole tablet
Maintenance dose: Titrate dose to effect; after week 4, increase dose every 1-2 weeks by a calculated increment; calculate increment as 1.2 mg/kg/day rounded down to the nearest whole tablet; add this amount to the previously administered daily dose; usual maintenance: 5-15 mg/kg/day in 2 divided doses; maximum: 400 mg/day
Children >12 years: Lennox-Gastaut (adjunctive) or partial seizures (adjunctive): Refer to Adults dosing
Children ≥16 years: Conversion from single enzyme-inducing AED regimen to monotherapy: Refer to Adults dosing

Adults:
Lennox-Gastaut (adjunctive) or treatment of partial seizures (adjunctive):
Patients receiving AED regimens containing valproic acid:
Initial dose: 25 mg every other day for 2 weeks, then 25 mg every day for 2 weeks
Maintenance dose: 100-400 mg/day in 1-2 divided doses (usual range 100-200 mg/day). Dose may be increased by 25-50 mg every day for 1-2 weeks in order to achieve maintenance dose.
Patients receiving enzyme-inducing AED regimens without valproic acid:
Initial dose: 50 mg/day for 2 weeks, then 100 mg in 2 doses for 2 weeks; thereafter, daily dose can be increased by 100 mg every 1-2 weeks to be given in 2 divided doses
Usual maintenance dose: 300-500 mg/day in 2 divided doses; doses as high as 700 mg/day have been reported
Partial seizures (monotherapy) conversion from single enzyme-inducing AED regimen: Initial dose: 50 mg/day for 2 weeks, then 100 mg in 2 doses for 2 weeks; thereafter, daily dose should be increased by 100 mg every 1-2 weeks to be given in 2 divided doses until reaching a dose of 500 mg/day. Concomitant enzyme inducing AED should then be withdrawn by 20% decrements each week over a 4-week period. Patients should be monitored for rash.
Bipolar disorder (unlabeled use): 25 mg/day for 2 weeks, followed by 50 mg/day for 2 weeks, followed by 100 mg/day for 1 week; thereafter, daily dosage may be increased by 100 mg/week, up to a maximum of 500 mg/day as clinically indicated
Discontinuing therapy: Children and Adults: Decrease dose by ~50% per week, over at least 2 weeks unless safety concerns require a more rapid withdrawal.

Dosage adjustment in renal impairment: Decreased dosage may be effective in patients with significant renal impairment; use with caution
Dosage adjustment in hepatic impairment:
Child-Pugh Grade B: Reduce initial, escalation, and maintenance doses by 50%
Child-Pugh Grade C: Reduce initial, escalation, and maintenance doses by 75%

Mechanism of Action A triazine derivative which inhibits release of glutamate (an excitatory amino acid) and inhibits voltage-sensitive sodium channels, which stabilizes neuronal membranes. Lamotrigine has weak inhibitory effect on the 5-HT$_3$ receptor; *in vitro* inhibits dihydrofolate reductase.

Other Adverse Effects Percentages reported in adults receiving adjunctive therapy:
>10%:
Central nervous system: Headache (29%), dizziness (38%), ataxia (22%), somnolence (14%)
Gastrointestinal: Nausea (19%)
Ocular: Diplopia (28%), blurred vision (16%)
Respiratory: Rhinitis (14%)
1% to 10%:
Central nervous system: Depression (4%), anxiety (4%), irritability (3%), confusion, speech disorder (3%), difficulty concentrating (2%), malaise, seizure (2%
(Continued)

Lamotrigine *(Continued)*

to 3%), incoordination (6%), insomnia (6%), pain, amnesia, hostility, memory decreased, nervousness, vertigo

Dermatologic: Hypersensitivity rash (10%; serious rash requiring hospitalization - adults 0.3%, children 0.8%), pruritus (3%)

Gastrointestinal: Abdominal pain (5%), vomiting (9%), diarrhea (6%), dyspepsia (5%), constipation (4%), anorexia (2%), tooth disorder (3%)

Genitourinary: Vaginitis (4%), dysmenorrhea (7%), amenorrhea (2%)

Neuromuscular & skeletal: Tremor (4%), arthralgia (2%), neck pain (2%)

Ocular: Nystagmus (2%)

Miscellaneous: Flu syndrome (7%), fever (6%)

<1% (Limited to important or life-threatening): Acne, acute renal failure, allergic reactions, alopecia, anemia, angina, angioedema, atrial fibrillation, back pain, bronchospasm, bruising, chills, depersonalization, dyspnea, dysarthria, dysphagia, eosinophilia, erythema multiforme, facial edema, GI hemorrhage, gingival hyperplasia, halitosis, hemorrhage, hepatitis, hot flashes, hypertension, impotence, leukopenia, maculopapular rash, malaise, mania, migraine, movement disorder, palpitations, paralysis, photosensitivity (rare), postural hypotension, rash, Stevens-Johnson syndrome, stroke, suicidal ideation, urticaria, vesiculobullous rash

Postmarketing and/or case reports: Agranulocytosis, aplastic anemia, apnea, disseminated intravascular coagulation (DIC), esophagitis, hemolytic anemia, hypersensitivity reactions (including rhabdomyolysis), immunosuppression (progressive), lupus-like reaction, multiorgan failure, neutropenia, pancreatitis, pancytopenia, Parkinson's disease exacerbation, red cell aplasia, tics, toxic epidermal necrolysis, vasculitis

Drug Interactions Effects on CYP not characterized, may act as inducer.

Increased Effect/Toxicity: Lamotrigine may increase the epoxide metabolite of carbamazepine resulting in toxicity. Valproic acid increases blood levels of lamotrigine. Toxicity has been reported following addition of sertraline (limited documentation).

Decreased Effect: Acetaminophen (chronic administration), carbamazepine, oral contraceptives (estrogens), phenytoin, phenobarbital may decrease concentrations of lamotrigine; dosage adjustments may be needed when adding or withdrawing agent; monitor

Dietary/Ethanol/Herb Considerations

Ethanol: Avoid use; may increase CNS depression.

Food: Administer with food to reduce GI upset; absorption unaffected. Fluids, fruit, and fiber may reduce constipation.

Herb/Nutraceutical: Avoid evening primrose; decreases seizure threshold. Avoid gotu kola, kava, SAMe, St John's wort, and valerian; may increase CNS depression.

Pharmacodynamics/Kinetics

Distribution: V_d: 1.1 L/kg

Protein binding: 55%

Metabolism: Hepatic and renal; metabolized by glucuronic acid conjugation to inactive metabolites

Bioavailability: 98%

Half-life elimination: Adults: 25-33 hours; Concomitant valproic acid therapy: 59-70 hours; Concomitant phenytoin or carbamazepine therapy: 13-14 hours

Time to peak, plasma: 1-4 hours

Excretion: Urine (94%, ~90% as glucuronide conjugates and ~10% unchanged); feces (2%)

Pregnancy Risk Factor C

Generic Available No

Lamprene® *see* Clofazimine *on page 346*

Lanacane® [OTC] *see* Benzocaine *on page 169*

Lanaphilic® [OTC] *see* Urea *on page 1365*

Lanolin, Cetyl Alcohol, Glycerin, Petrolatum, and Mineral Oil

(LAN oh lin, SEE til AL koe hol, GLIS er in, pe troe LAY tum, & MIN er al oyl)

U.S. Brand Names Lubriderm® [OTC]; Lubriderm® Fragrance Free [OTC]

Pharmacologic Category Topical Skin Product

Synonyms Mineral Oil, Petrolatum, Lanolin, Cetyl Alcohol, and Glycerin

Use Treatment of dry skin

Local Anesthetic/Vasoconstrictor Precautions No information available to require special precautions

Effects on Dental Treatment No significant effects or complications reported

Dosage Topical: Apply to skin as necessary

Other Adverse Effects 1% to 10%: Local irritation

Pregnancy Risk Factor C

Generic Available Yes

Lanolin, Coal Tar, and Mineral Oil *see* Coal Tar, Lanolin, and Mineral Oil *on page 360*

Lanolin, Mineral Oil, and Coal Tar *see* Coal Tar, Lanolin, and Mineral Oil *on page 360*

Lanoxicaps® *see* Digoxin *on page 441*

Lanoxin® *see* Digoxin *on page 441*

Lansoprazole (lan SOE pra zole)

Related Information

Gastrointestinal Disorders *on page 1474*

U.S. Brand Names Prevacid®

Canadian Brand Names Prevacid®

Mexican Brand Names Ilsatec®; Ogastro®; Ulpax®

Pharmacologic Category Proton Pump Inhibitor

Use Short-term treatment of active duodenal ulcers; maintenance treatment of healed duodenal ulcers; as part of a multidrug regimen for *H. pylori* eradication to reduce the risk of duodenal ulcer recurrence; short-term treatment of active benign gastric ulcer; treatment of NSAID-associated gastric ulcer; to reduce the risk of NSAID-associated gastric ulcer in patients with a history of gastric ulcer who require an NSAID; short-term treatment of symptomatic GERD; short-term treatment for all grades of erosive esophagitis; to maintain healing of erosive esophagitis; long-term treatment of pathological hypersecretory conditions, including Zollinger-Ellison syndrome

Local Anesthetic/Vasoconstrictor Precautions No information available to require special precautions

Effects on Dental Treatment No significant effects or complications reported

Dosage Oral:

Children 1-11 years: GERD, erosive esophagitis:

≤30 kg: 15 mg once daily

>30 kg: 30 mg once daily

Adults:

Duodenal ulcer: Short-term treatment: 15 mg once daily for 4 weeks; maintenance therapy: 15 mg once daily

Gastric ulcer: Short-term treatment: 30 mg once daily for up to 8 weeks

NSAID-associated gastric ulcer (healing): 30 mg once daily for 8 weeks; controlled studies did not extend past 8 weeks of therapy

NSAID-associated gastric ulcer (to reduce risk): Oral: 15 mg once daily for up to 12 weeks; controlled studies did not extend past 12 weeks of therapy

Symptomatic GERD: Short-term treatment: 15 mg once daily for up to 8 weeks

Erosive esophagitis: Short-term treatment: 30 mg once daily for up to 8 weeks; continued treatment for an additional 8 weeks may be considered for recurrence or for patients that do not heal after the first 8 weeks of therapy; maintenance therapy: 15 mg once daily

Hypersecretory conditions: Initial: 60 mg once daily; adjust dose based upon patient response and to reduce acid secretion to <10 mEq/hour (5 mEq/hour in patients with prior gastric surgery); doses of 90 mg twice daily have been used; administer doses >120 mg/day in divided doses

Helicobacter pylori eradication: Currently accepted recommendations (may differ from product labeling): Dose varies with regimen: 30 mg once daily or 60 mg/day in 2 divided doses; requires combination therapy with antibiotics

Dosing adjustment in hepatic impairment: Reduction required in severe impairment

Mechanism of Action A proton pump inhibitor which decreases acid secretion in gastric parietal cells

Other Adverse Effects

1% to 10%: Gastrointestinal: Abdominal pain (2%), diarrhea (4%, more likely at doses of 60 mg/day), constipation (1%), nausea (1%)

<1%: Abdomen enlarged, abnormal dreams, abnormal menses, abnormal stools, **abnormal vision,** acne, **agitation,** albuminuria, **allergic reaction,** alkaline phosphatase increased, ALT increased, alopecia, **amnesia,** anemia, **angina, anorexia, anxiety,** apathy, appetite increased, **arrhythmia,** AST increased, asthenia, arthralgia, **arthritis, asthma,** back pain, bezoar, bilirubinemia, **blurred vision, bradycardia,** breast enlargement, breast pain, breast tenderness, **bronchitis,** bone disorder, **candidiasis,** carcinoma, cardiospasm, cerebrovascular accident, cerebral infarction, **chest pain,** chills, cholelithiasis, cholesterol increased, cholesterol decreased, colitis, **confusion,** conjunctivitis, **contact dermatitis, convulsion, cough increased,** creatinine increased, deafness, **dehydration,** depersonalization, depression, **diabetes mellitus,** diplopia, **dizziness,** dry eyes, **xerostomia,** dry skin, dyspepsia, **dysphagia, dyspnea,** dysmenorrhea, dysuria, ear disorder, edema, electrolytes imbalance, emotional lability, enteritis, eosinophilia, **epistaxis, eructation, esophageal ulcer, esophagitis,** eye pain, fecal discoloration, **fever,** fixed eruption, flatulence, **flu-like syndrome,** fundic gland polyps, **gastric nodules, gastrin levels increased, gastritis, gastroenteritis, GI anomaly, GI disorder, GI hemorrhage,** GGTP increased, GGTP decreased, glucocorticoids increased, globulins increased, **glossitis,**

(Continued)

Lansoprazole *(Continued)*

glycosuria, goiter, gout, **gum hemorrhage,** gynocomastia, hair disorder, **halitosis, hallucinations,** hematemesis, hematuria, hemiplegia, hemolysis, hemoptysis, **hiccup, hostility aggravated, hyperglycemia,** hyperkinesia, hyperlipemia, hypertonia, hypesthesia, **hypoglycemia, hypertension, hypotension,** hypothyroidism, impotence, **infection,** insomnia, **joint disorder,** kidney calculus, kidney pain, **laryngeal neoplasia,** LDH increased, **leg cramps,** leukorrhea, libido decreased, libido increased, LFTs abnormal, **lymphadenopathy,** maculopapular rash, **malaise,** melena, menorrhagia, menstrual disorder, **migraine, moniliasis (oral), oral ulceration, musculoskeletal pain,** myalgia, **myasthenia, MI,** nail disorder, **neck pain, neck rigidity, nervousness, neurosis, otitis media, pain, palpitations, paresthesia,** parosmia, pelvic pain, penis disorder, peripheral edema, **pharyngitis,** photophobia, **platelet abnormalities,** pleural disorder, **pneumonia,** polyuria, pruritus, rash, RBC abnormal, rectal disorder, rectal hemorrhage, **respiratory disorder**, retinal degeneration, **rhinitis, increased salivation, shock, sinusitis,** skin carcinoma, sleep disorder, **somnolence, stomatitis**, stridor, **sweating, syncope**, synovitis, **tachycardia, loss of taste, abnormal taste**, tenesmus, testis disorder, **thirst**, thinking abnormality, tinnitus, **tremor, tongue disorder**, ulcerative colitis, **ulcerative stomatitis, upper respiratory inflammation, upper respiratory infection**, urethral pain, urinary frequency, urination impaired, urticaria, vaginitis, **vasodilation,** vertigo, **visual field defect, vomiting,** WBC abnormal, weight gain/loss

Postmarketing and/or case reports: Agranulocytosis, **anaphylactoid reaction, aplastic anemia, dizziness, hepatotoxicity,** leukopenia, neutropenia, pancytopenia, speech disorder, thrombocytopenia, thrombotic thrombocytopenic purpura, urinary retention

Drug Interactions Substrate of CYP2C8/9, **2C19, 3A4**; Inhibits CYP2C8/9, **2C19**, 2D6, 3A4; Induces CYP1A2

Decreased Effect: Lansoprazole may decrease blood levels/absorption of ketoconazole, itraconazole, ampicillin esters, iron salts, digoxin and other drugs dependent upon acid for absorption. Lansoprazole may decrease theophylline levels (slightly). Sucralfate delays and reduces lansoprazole absorption by 30%.

Dietary/Ethanol/Herb Considerations

Ethanol: Avoid use; may cause gastric mucosal irritation.

Food may decrease serum concentration by 50%; administer on an empty stomach. Intact granules from capsules may be mixed with the following and then swallowed immediately: 1 tablespoon of applesauce, Ensure® pudding, cottage cheese, yogurt, or strained pears; ~60 mL orange, apple, cranberry, grape, pineapple, prune, tomato, or V-8® juice

Note: Delayed release oral suspension granules should be mixed with 2 tablespoonfuls of water (30 mL); no other liquid should be used.

Pharmacodynamics/Kinetics

Duration: >1 day
Absorption: Rapid
Protein binding: 97%
Metabolism: Hepatic and in parietal cells to two inactive metabolites
Bioavailability: 80%; decreased 50% if given 30 minutes after food
Half-life elimination: 2 hours; Elderly: 2.9 hours; Hepatic impairment: ≤7 hours
Time to peak, plasma: 1.7 hours
Excretion: Feces (67%); urine (33%)

Pregnancy Risk Factor B

Generic Available No

Lantus® *see* Insulin Preparations *on page 723*
L-Arginine *see* Arginine *on page 121*
Lariam® *see* Mefloquine *on page 852*
Larodopa® *see* Levodopa *on page 792*
Lasix® *see* Furosemide *on page 622*
L-asparaginase *see* Asparaginase *on page 129*
Lassar's Zinc Paste *see* Zinc Oxide *on page 1409*

Latanoprost (la TAN oh prost)

U.S. Brand Names Xalatan®

Canadian Brand Names Xalatan®

Mexican Brand Names Xalatan®

Pharmacologic Category Ophthalmic Agent, Antiglaucoma; Prostaglandin, Ophthalmic

Use Reduction of elevated intraocular pressure in patients with open-angle glaucoma or ocular hypertension

Local Anesthetic/Vasoconstrictor Precautions No information available to require special precautions

Effects on Dental Treatment 1% to 10%: Upper respiratory tract infection, cold, flu, chest pain, angina pectoris

Dosage Adults: Ophthalmic: 1 drop (1.5 mcg) in the affected eye(s) once daily in the evening; do not exceed the once daily dosage because it has been shown that more frequent administration may decrease the IOP lowering effect

Note: A medication delivery device (Xal-Ease™) is available for use with Xalatan®.

Mechanism of Action Latanoprost is a prostaglandin F_2-alpha analog believed to reduce intraocular pressure by increasing the outflow of the aqueous humor

Other Adverse Effects

>10%: Ocular: Blurred vision, burning and stinging, conjunctival hyperemia, foreign body sensation, itching, increased pigmentation of the iris, and punctate epithelial keratopathy

1% to 10%:

Dermatologic: Rash, allergic skin reaction

Neuromuscular & skeletal: Myalgia, arthralgia, back pain

Ocular: Dry eye, excessive tearing, eye pain, lid crusting, lid edema, lid erythema, lid discomfort/pain, photophobia

<1%: Conjunctivitis, diplopia, discharge from the eye, retinal artery embolus, retinal detachment, vitreous hemorrhage from diabetic retinopathy

Postmarketing and/or case reports: Asthma, corneal edema, corneal erosion, dyspnea, eyelash change, eyelid skin darkening, herpes keratitis, iritis, keratitis, macular edema, toxic epidermal necrolysis, uveitis

Drug Interactions Decreased Effect: *In vitro* studies have shown that precipitation occurs when eye drops containing thimerosal are mixed with latanoprost. If such drugs are used, administer with an interval of at least 5 minutes between applications. May be used concomitantly with other topical ophthalmic drugs if administration is separated by at least 5 minutes.

Pharmacodynamics/Kinetics

Onset of action: 3-4 hours

Peak effect: Maximum: 8-12 hours

Absorption: Through the cornea where the isopropyl ester prodrug is hydrolyzed by esterases to the biologically active acid. Peak concentration is reached in 2 hours after topical administration in the aqueous humor.

Distribution: V_d: 0.16 L/kg

Metabolism: Primarily hepatic via fatty acid beta-oxidation

Half-life elimination: 17 minutes

Excretion: Urine (as metabolites)

Pregnancy Risk Factor C

Generic Available No

l-Bunolol Hydrochloride *see* Levobunolol *on page 789*

L-Carnitine *see* Levocarnitine *on page 791*

LCD *see* Coal Tar *on page 359*

LCR *see* VinCRIStine *on page 1387*

L-Deprenyl *see* Selegiline *on page 1213*

L-Dopa *see* Levodopa *on page 792*

Leflunomide (le FLU no mide)

Related Information

Rheumatoid Arthritis, Osteoarthritis, and Osteoporosis *on page 1488*

U.S. Brand Names Arava™

Canadian Brand Names Arava™

Pharmacologic Category Antirheumatic, Disease Modifying

Use Treatment of active rheumatoid arthritis to reduce signs and symptoms and to retard structural damage as evidenced by x-ray erosions and joint space narrowing

Local Anesthetic/Vasoconstrictor Precautions No information available to require special precautions

Effects on Dental Treatment

>10%: Respiratory tract infection (15%)

1% to 10%: Stomatitis (3%), gingivitis (3%), oral candidiasis, enlarged salivary gland, tooth disorder, xerostomia, abnormal taste, hypertension (10%), chest pain (2%), palpitation, tachycardia, vasodilation headache (7%), fever, migraine, herpes infection, bruising, bronchitis (7%), cough (3%), pharyngitis (3%), pneumonia (2%), rhinitis (2%), sinusitis (2%), asthma, dyspnea, epistaxis, infection (4%)

Dosage Oral:

Adults: Initial: 100 mg/day for 3 days, followed by 20 mg/day; dosage may be decreased to 10 mg/day in patients who have difficulty tolerating the 20 mg dose. Due to the long halflife of the active metabolite, plasma levels may require a prolonged period to decline after dosage reduction.

Elderly: Although hepatic function may decline with age, no specific dosage adjustment is recommended. Patients should be monitored closely for adverse effects which may require dosage adjustment.

Dosing adjustment in renal impairment: No specific recommendations; not studied The free fraction of MI is doubled in dialysis patients. Patients should be monitored closely for adverse effects requiring dosage adjustment.

Dosing adjustment in hepatic impairment: No specific recommendations

(Continued)

Leflunomide *(Continued)*

Since the liver is involved in metabolic activation and subsequent metabolism/elimination of leflunomide, patients with hepatic impairment should be monitored closely for adverse effects requiring dosage adjustment.

Guidelines for dosage adjustment or discontinuation based on the severity and persistence of ALT elevation secondary to leflunomide have been developed. For ALT elevations >2 times the upper limit of normal, dosage reduction to 10 mg/day may allow continued administration (consider increased monitoring frequency - ie, weekly). Cholestyramine 8 g 3 times/day for 1-3 days may be administered to decrease plasma levels. If elevations >2 times but ≤3 times the upper limit of normal persist, liver biopsy is recommended. If elevations >3 times the upper limit of normal persist despite cholestyramine administration and dosage reduction, leflunomide should be discontinued and drug elimination should be enhanced with additional cholestyramine as indicated.

Mechanism of Action Inhibits pyrimidine synthesis, resulting in antiproliferative and anti-inflammatory effects

Other Adverse Effects

>10%: Gastrointestinal: Diarrhea (17%)

1% to 10%:

Cardiovascular: Vasculitis, varicose vein, edema (peripheral)

Central nervous system: Dizziness (4%), pain (2%), malaise, depression, insomnia, sleep disorder

Dermatologic: Alopecia (10%), rash (10%), pruritus (4%), dry skin (2%), eczema (2%), acne, dermatitis, hair discoloration, hematoma, nail disorder, subcutaneous nodule, skin disorder/discoloration, skin ulcer

Endocrine & metabolic: Hypokalemia (1%), **diabetes mellitus, hyperglycemia**, hyperlipidemia, hyperthyroidism, menstrual disorder

Gastrointestinal: Nausea (9%), abdominal pain (5%), dyspepsia (5%), weight loss (4%), anorexia (3%), gastroenteritis (3%), vomiting (3%), cholelithiasis, colitis, constipation, esophagitis, flatulence, gastritis, melena

Genitourinary: Urinary tract infection (5%), albuminuria, cystitis, dysuria, hematuria, vaginal candidiasis, prostate disorder, urinary frequency

Hematologic: Anemia

Hepatic: Abnormal LFTs (5%)

Neuromuscular & skeletal: Back pain (5%), joint disorder (4%), weakness (3%), tenosynovitis (3%), synovitis (2%), arthralgia (1%), paresthesia (2%), muscle cramps (1%), **neck pain**, pelvic pain, increased CPK, arthrosis, bursitis, myalgia, bone necrosis, bone pain, tendon rupture, neuralgia, neuritis

Ocular: Blurred vision, cataract, conjunctivitis, eye disorder

Respiratory: Lung disorder

Miscellaneous: Accidental injury (5%), allergic reactions (2%), diaphoresis

<1%, postmarketing and/or case reports: Anaphylaxis, eosinophilia, hepatotoxicity, hepatic failure, leukopenia, pancytopenia, Stevens-Johnson syndrome, thrombocytopenia, toxic epidermal necrolysis, urticaria

Drug Interactions Inhibits CYP2C8/9

Increased Effect/Toxicity: Theoretically, concomitant use of drugs metabolized by this enzyme, including many NSAIDs, may result in increased serum concentrations and possible toxic effects. Coadministration with methotrexate increases the risk of hepatotoxicity. Leflunomide may also enhance the hepatotoxicity of other drugs. Tolbutamide free fraction may be increased. Rifampin may increase serum concentrations of leflunomide. Leflunomide has uricosuric activity and may enhance activity of other uricosuric agents.

Decreased Effect: Administration of cholestyramine and activated charcoal enhance the elimination of leflunomide's active metabolite.

Dietary/Ethanol/Herb Considerations Food: No interactions with food have been noted.

Pharmacodynamics/Kinetics

Distribution: V_d: 0.13 L/kg

Metabolism: Hepatic to A77 1726 (MI) which accounts for nearly all pharmacologic activity; further metabolism to multiple inactive metabolites; undergoes enterohepatic recirculation

Bioavailability: 80%

Half-life elimination: Mean: 14-15 days; enterohepatic recycling appears to contribute to the long half-life of this agent, since activated charcoal and cholestyramine substantially reduce plasma half-life

Time to peak: 6-12 hours

Excretion: Feces (48%); urine (43%)

Pregnancy Risk Factor X

Generic Available No

Legatrin PM® [OTC] *see* Acetaminophen and Diphenhydramine *on page 30*

Lente® Iletin® II *see* Insulin Preparations *on page 723*

Lepirudin (leh puh ROO din)

Related Information

Cardiovascular Diseases *on page 1456*

U.S. Brand Names Refludan®

Canadian Brand Names Refludan®

Pharmacologic Category Anticoagulant, Thrombin Inhibitor

Synonyms Lepirudin (rDNA); Recombinant Hirudin

Use Indicated for anticoagulation in patients with heparin-induced thrombocytopenia (HIT) and associated thromboembolic disease in order to prevent further thromboembolic complications

Unlabeled/Investigational Use Investigational: Prevention or reduction of ischemic complications associated with unstable angina

Local Anesthetic/Vasoconstrictor Precautions No information available to require special precautions

Effects on Dental Treatment

>10%: HIT patients: Bleeding from puncture sites (11%), hematoma (11%) heart failure (3%), ventricular fibrillation (1%), fever (7%), epistaxis (4%)

1% to 10%: Non-HIT patients: Bronchospasm/stridor/dyspnea/cough

Dosage Dosing is weight-based, however, patients weighing >110 kg should not receive doses greater than the recommended dose for a patient weighing 110 kg (44 mg bolus and initial maximal infusion rate of 16.5 mg/hour).

Adults:

Maximum dose: Do not exceed 0.21 mg/kg/hour unless an evaluation of coagulation abnormalities limiting response has been completed.

Heparin-induced thrombocytopenia: Bolus dose: 0.4 mg/kg IVP (over 15-20 seconds), followed by continuous infusion at 0.15 mg/kg/hour; bolus and infusion must be reduced in renal insufficiency

Concomitant use with thrombolytic therapy: Bolus dose: 0.2 mg/kg IVP (over 15-20 seconds), followed by continuous infusion at 0.1 mg/kg/hour

Dosing adjustments during infusions: Monitor first aPTT 4 hours after the start of the infusion. Subsequent determinations of aPTT should be obtained at least once daily during treatment. More frequent monitoring is recommended in renally impaired patients. Any aPTT ratio measurement out of range (1.5-2.5) should be confirmed prior to adjusting dose, unless a clinical need for immediate reaction exists. If the aPTT is below target range, increase infusion by 20%. If the aPTT is in excess of the target range, decrease infusion rate by 50%. A repeat aPTT should be obtained 4 hours after any dosing change.

Use in patients scheduled for switch to oral anticoagulants: Reduce lepirudin dose gradually to reach aPTT ratio just above 1.5 before starting warfarin therapy; as soon as INR reaches 2.0, lepirudin therapy should be discontinued.

Dosing adjustment in renal impairment: All patients with a creatinine clearance of <60 mL/minute or a serum creatinine of >1.5 mg/dL should receive a reduction in lepirudin dosage; there is only limited information on the therapeutic use of lepirudin in HIT patients with significant renal impairment; the following dosage recommendations are mainly based on single-dose studies in a small number of patients with renal impairment.

Initial: Bolus dose: 0.2 mg/kg IVP (over 15-20 seconds), followed by adjusted infusion based on renal function; refer to the following infusion rate adjustments based on creatinine clearance (mL/minute) and serum creatinine (mg/dL):

Lepirudin infusion rates in patients with renal impairment: See table.

Lepirudin Infusion Rates in Patients With Renal Impairment

Creatinine Clearance (mL/minute)	Serum Creatinine (mg/dL)	Adjusted Infusion Rate	
		% of Standard Initial Infusion Rate	mg/kg/hour
45-60	1.6-2.0	50%	0.075
30-44	2.1-3.0	30%	0.045
15-29	3.1-6.0	15%	0.0225
<15	>6.0	Avoid or STOP infusion	

Acute renal failure or hemodialysis: Infusion is to be avoided or stopped. Following the bolus dose, additional bolus doses of 0.1 mg/kg may be administered every other day (only if aPTT falls below lower therapeutic limit).

Mechanism of Action Lepirudin is a highly specific direct inhibitor of thrombin; lepirudin is a recombinant hirudin derived from yeast cells

Other Adverse Effects Hemorrhage may occur at virtually any site; risk is dependent on multiple variables.

HIT patients:

>10%: Hematologic: Anemia (12%)

(Continued)

Lepirudin *(Continued)*

1% to 10%:

Cardiovascular: Pericardial effusion (1%)

Dermatologic: Eczema (3%), maculopapular rash (4%)

Gastrointestinal: GI bleeding/rectal bleeding (5%)

Genitourinary: Vaginal bleeding (2%)

Hepatic: Increased transaminases (6%)

Renal: Hematuria (4%)

<1% (Limited to important or life-threatening): Hemoperitoneum, hemoptysis, liver bleeding, pulmonary bleeding, retroperitoneal bleeding, **mouth bleeding**, pruritus, urticaria, injection site reactions, thrombocytopenia

Non-HIT populations (including those receiving thrombolytics and/or contrast media): <1% (Limited to important or life-threatening): Angioedema, laryngeal edema, **tongue edema**, intracranial bleeding (0.6%), allergic reactions (unspecified), anaphylactoid reactions, anaphylaxis, thrombocytopenia

Drug Interactions Increased Effect/Toxicity: Thrombolytics may enhance anticoagulant properties of lepirudin on aPTT and can increase the risk of bleeding complications. Bleeding risk may also be increased by oral anticoagulants (warfarin) and platelet function inhibitors (NSAIDs, dipyridamole, ticlopidine, clopidogrel, IIb/IIIa antagonists, and aspirin).

Dietary/Ethanol/Herb Considerations

Food: Avoid garlic, ginger, and green tea.

Herb/Nutraceutical: Avoid cat's claw, dong quai, evening primrose, feverfew, garlic, ginger, ginkgo biloba, ginseng, green tea, horse chestnut, and red clover due to additional antiplatelet activity.

Pharmacodynamics/Kinetics

Distribution: Two-compartment model; confined to extracellular fluids.

Metabolism: Via release of amino acids via catabolic hydrolysis of parent drug

Half-life elimination: Initial: ~10 minutes: Terminal: Healthy volunteers: 1.3 hours; Marked renal impairment (Cl_{cr} <15 mL/minute and on hemodialysis): ≤2 days

Excretion: Urine (~48%, 35% as unchanged drug and unchanged drug fragments of parent drug); systemic clearance is proportional to glomerular filtration rate or creatinine clearance

Pregnancy Risk Factor B

Generic Available No

Lepirudin (rDNA) *see* Lepirudin *on page 781*

Lescol® *see* Fluvastatin *on page 603*

Lescol® XL *see* Fluvastatin *on page 603*

Lessina™ *see* Combination Hormonal Contraceptives *on page 368*

Letrozole (LET roe zole)

U.S. Brand Names Femara®

Canadian Brand Names Femara®

Pharmacologic Category Antineoplastic Agent, Aromatase Inhibitor

Use First-line treatment of hormone receptor positive or hormone receptor unknown, locally advanced, or metastatic breast cancer in postmenopausal women; treatment of advanced breast cancer in postmenopausal women with disease progression following antiestrogen therapy

Local Anesthetic/Vasoconstrictor Precautions No information available to require special precautions

Effects on Dental Treatment

>10%: Hot flashes (5% to 19%), dyspnea (7% to 18%), cough (5% to 13%), nausea (13% to 17%), headache (8% to 12%). pain (8% to 22%)

1% to 10%: Chest pain (3% to 8%), hypertension (5% to 8%), anxiety (<5%), flu (5% to 6%), dizziness (3% to 5%), somnolence (2% to 3%), vomiting (7%), flu (6%) weakness (4% to 6%)

<2%: Angina, hemorrhagic stroke, MI, thrombotic stroke

Dosage Oral (refer to individual protocols):

Children: Use not recommended

Adults: Breast cancer in postmenopausal women: 2.5 mg once daily without regard to meals; continue treatment until tumor progression is evident. Patients treated with letrozole do not require glucocorticoid or mineralocorticoid replacement therapy.

Dosing adjustment in renal impairment: None required if Cl_{cr} ≥10 mL/minute

Mechanism of Action Nonsteroidal, competitive inhibitor of the aromatase enzyme system which binds to the heme group of aromatase, a cytochrome P450 enzyme which catalyzes conversion of androgens to estrogens (specifically, androstenedione to estrone and testosterone to estradiol). This leads to inhibition of the enzyme and a significant reduction in plasma estrogen levels. Does not affect synthesis of adrenal or thyroid hormones, aldosterone, or androgens.

Other Adverse Effects

>10%:

Central nervous system: Fatigue (6% to 13%)

Neuromuscular & skeletal: Musculoskeletal pain, bone pain (22%), back pain (18%), arthralgia (8% to 16%)

2% to 10%:

Cardiovascular: Peripheral edema (5%)

Central nervous system: Insomnia (7%) depression (<5%), vertigo (<5%)

Dermatologic: Rash (4% to 5%), alopecia (<5%), pruritus (1% to 2%)

Endocrine & metabolic: Breast pain (7%), hypercholesterolemia (3%), hypercalcemia (<5%)

Gastrointestinal: Constipation (6% to 10%), diarrhea (5% to 8%), abdominal pain (5% to 6%), anorexia (3% to 5%), dyspepsia (3% to 4%), weight loss (7%), weight gain (2%)

<2%: Cardiac ischemia, coronary artery disease, hemiparesis, bilirubin increased, transaminases increased, lymphopenia, portal vein thrombosis, pulmonary embolism, thrombocytopenia, thrombophlebitis, thrombotic stroke, transient ischemic attack, vaginal bleeding, venous thrombosis

Drug Interactions Substrate of CYP2A6, 3A4; Inhibits CYP2A6, 2C19

Increased Effect/Toxicity: Inhibitors of this enzyme may, in theory, increase letrozole blood levels. Letrozole inhibits cytochrome P450 isoenzyme 2A6 and 2C19 *in vitro* and may increase blood levels of drugs metabolized by these enzymes. Specific drug interaction studies have not been reported.

Pharmacodynamics/Kinetics

Absorption: Well absorbed; not affected by food

Distribution: V_d: ~1.9 L/kg

Protein binding, plasma: Weak

Metabolism: Hepatic via CYP3A4 and CYP2A6 to an inactive carbinol metabolite

Half-life elimination: Terminal: ~2 days

Time to steady state, plasma: 2-6 weeks

Excretion: Urine (6% as unchanged drug, 75% as glucuronide carbinol metabolite)

Pregnancy Risk Factor D

Generic Available No

Leucovorin (loo koe VOR in)

Mexican Brand Names Dalisol; Flynoken A; Medsavorin

Pharmacologic Category Antidote; Vitamin, Water Soluble

Synonyms Calcium Leucovorin; Citrovorum Factor; Folinic Acid; 5-Formyl Tetrahydrofolate; Leucovorin Calcium

Use Antidote for folic acid antagonists (methotrexate >100 mg/m^2, trimethoprim, pyrimethamine); treatment of megaloblastic anemias when folate is deficient as in infancy, sprue, pregnancy, and nutritional deficiency when oral folate therapy is not possible; in combination with fluorouracil in the treatment of malignancy

Local Anesthetic/Vasoconstrictor Precautions No information available to require special precautions

Effects on Dental Treatment No significant effects or complications reported

Dosage Children and Adults:

Treatment of folic acid antagonist overdosage (eg, pyrimethamine or trimethoprim): Oral: 2-15 mg/day for 3 days or until blood counts are normal or 5 mg every 3 days; doses of 6 mg/day are needed for patients with platelet counts <100,000/mm^3

Folate-deficient megaloblastic anemia: I.M.: 1 mg/day

Megaloblastic anemia secondary to congenital deficiency of dihydrofolate reductase: I.M.: 3-6 mg/day

Rescue dose (rescue therapy should start within 24 hours of MTX therapy): I.V.: 10 mg/m^2 to start, then 10 mg/m^2 every 6 hours orally for 72 hours until serum MTX concentration is <10^{-8} molar; if serum creatinine 24 hours after methotrexate is elevated 50% or more above the pre-MTX serum creatinine **or** the serum MTX concentration is >5×10^{-6} molar (see graph on next page), increase dose to 100 mg/m^2/dose (preservative-free) every 3 hours until serum methotrexate level is <1×10^{-8} molar

Investigational: Post I.T. methotrexate: Oral, I.V.: 12 mg/m^2 as a single dose; post high-dose methotrexate: 100-1000 mg/m^2/dose until the serum methotrexate level is less than 1×10^{-7} molar

The drug should be given parenterally instead of orally in patients with GI toxicity, nausea, vomiting, and when individual doses are >25 mg

Mechanism of Action A reduced form of folic acid, but does not require a reduction reaction by an enzyme for activation, allows for purine and thymidine synthesis, a necessity for normal erythropoiesis; leucovorin supplies the necessary cofactor blocked by MTX, enters the cells via the same active transport system as MTX

Other Adverse Effects Frequency not defined:

Dermatologic: Rash, pruritus, erythema, urticaria

Hematologic: Thrombocytosis

Respiratory: **Wheezing**

Miscellaneous: **Anaphylactoid reactions**

Drug Interactions

Increased toxicity of fluorouracil

Decreased effect of sulfamethoxazole and trimethoprim against *Pneumocystis carinii* pneumonitis.

(Continued)

Leucovorin *(Continued)*

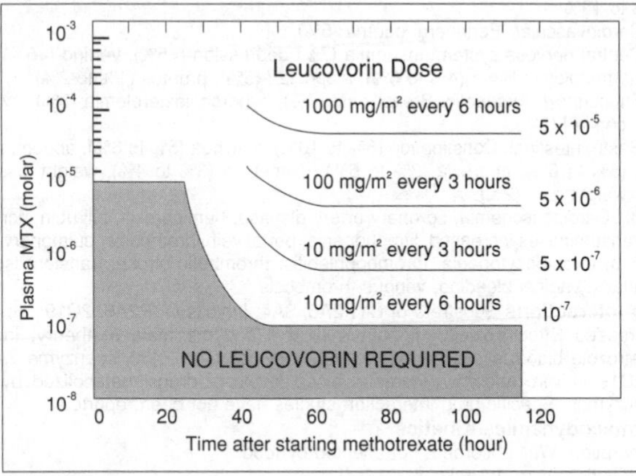

Dietary/Ethanol/Herb Considerations Food: Increase intake of foods high in folic acid if deficiency exists (meat proteins, bran, dried beans, asparagus, green leafy vegetables).

Pharmacodynamics/Kinetics

Onset of action: Oral: ~30 minutes; I.V.: ~5 minutes

Absorption: Oral, I.M.: Rapid and well absorbed

Metabolism: Intestinal mucosa and hepatically to 5-methyl-tetrahydrofolate (5MTHF; active)

Bioavailability: 31% (following 200 mg dose)

Half-life elimination: Leucovorin: 15 minutes; 5MTHF: 33-35 minutes

Excretion: Urine (80% to 90%); feces (5% to 8%)

Pregnancy Risk Factor C

Generic Available Yes

Leucovorin Calcium *see* Leucovorin *on page 783*

Leukeran® *see* Chlorambucil *on page 296*

Leukine® *see* Sargramostim *on page 1209*

Leuprolide (loo PROE lide)

U.S. Brand Names Eligard™; Lupron®; Lupron Depot®; Lupron Depot-Ped®; Viadur®

Canadian Brand Names Lupron®; Lupron® Depot®; Viadur®

Mexican Brand Names Lucrin; Lucrin Depot

Pharmacologic Category Antineoplastic Agent, Miscellaneous; Luteinizing Hormone-Releasing Hormone Analog

Synonyms Leuprolide Acetate; Leuprorelin; Leuprorelin Acetate

Use Palliative treatment of advanced prostate carcinoma; combination therapy with flutamide for treating metastatic prostatic carcinoma; management of endometriosis as initial treatment and/or treatment of recurrent symptoms; preoperative treatment of anemia caused by uterine leiomyomata (fibroids); central precocious puberty

Unlabeled/Investigational Use Treatment of infertility, benign prostatic hyperplasia (BPH), breast, ovarian, and endometrial cancer

Local Anesthetic/Vasoconstrictor Precautions No information available to require special precautions

Effects on Dental Treatment No significant effects or complications reported

Dosage

Children: Precocious puberty (consider discontinuing by age 11 for females and by age 12 for males):

- S.C. (Lupron®): 20-45 mcg/kg/day; titrate dose upward by 10 mcg/kg/day if down-regulation is not achieved
- I.M. (Lupron Depot-Ped®): 0.3 mg/kg/dose given every 28 days (minimum dose: 7.5 mg)
  - ≤25 kg: 7.5 mg
  - >25-37.5 kg: 11.25 mg
  - >37.5 kg: 15 mg
  - Titrate dose upward in 3.75 mg every 4 weeks if down-regulation is not achieved.

Adults:

Advanced prostatic carcinoma:

S.C.:

Eligard™: 7.5 mg monthly **or** 22.5 mg every 3 months

Lupron®: 1 mg/day
Viadur®: 65 mg implanted subcutaneously every 12 months
I.M.:
Lupron Depot®: 7.5 mg/dose given monthly (every 28-33 days) **or**
Lupron Depot-3®: 22.5 mg every 3 months **or**
Lupron Depot-4®: 30 mg every 4 months
Endometriosis: I.M.: Initial therapy may be with leuprolide alone or in combination with norethindrone; if retreatment for an additional 6 months is necessary, norethindrone should be used. Retreatment is not recommended for longer than one additional 6-month course.
Lupron Depot®: 3.75 mg/month for up to 6 months **or**
Lupron Depot-3®: 11.25 mg every 3 months for up to 2 doses (6 months total duration of treatment)
Uterine leiomyomata (fibroids): I.M. (in combination with iron):
Lupron Depot®: 3.75 mg/month for up to 3 months **or**
Lupron Depot-3®: 11.25 mg as a single injection

Mechanism of Action Potent inhibitor of gonadotropin secretion; continuous daily administration results in suppression of ovarian and testicular steroidogenesis due to decreased levels of LH and FSH with subsequent decrease in testosterone (male) and estrogen (female) levels

Other Adverse Effects
Children:
1% to 10%
Central nervous system: Pain (2%)
Dermatologic: Acne (2%), rash (2%), seborrhea (2%)
Genitourinary: Vaginitis (2%), vaginal bleeding (2%), vaginal discharge (2%)
Local: Injection site reaction (5%)
<1%: Alopecia, cervix disorder, dysphagia, emotional lability, **epistaxis, fever, gingivitis,** gynecomastia, **headache**, nausea, **nervousness,** peripheral edema, personality disorder, sexual maturity accelerated, skin striae, somnolence, **syncope**, urinary incontinence, **vasodilation**, vomiting, weight gain

Adults (frequency dependent upon formulation and indication):
Cardiovascular: Angina, atrial fibrillation, CHF, deep vein thrombosis, edema, hot flashes, hypertension, tachycardia
Central nervous system: Abnormal thinking, agitation, amnesia, confusion, convulsion, dementia, depression, dizziness, **fever, headache**, insomnia, pain, vertigo
Dermatologic: Alopecia, **bruising**, cellulitis
Endocrine & metabolic: Breast enlargement, breast tenderness, dehydration, hyperglycemia, hyperlipidemia, hyperphosphatemia, libido decreased, menstrual disorders, potassium decreased
Gastrointestinal: Anorexia, appetite increased, diarrhea, dysphagia, eructation, **GI hemorrhage, gingivitis, gum hemorrhage**, intestinal obstruction, peptic ulcer
Genitourinary: Balanitis, impotence, testicular atrophy, urinary disorder, vaginitis
Hematologic: Platelets decreased, PT prolonged, WBC increased
Hepatic: Hepatomegaly, LFTs abnormal
Local: Abscess, injection site reaction
Neuromuscular & skeletal: Leg cramps, myalgia, paresthesia, weakness
Renal: BUN increased
Respiratory: Allergic reaction, emphysema, hemoptysis, hypoxia, lung edema
Miscellaneous: **Body odor, flu-like syndrome**, neoplasm, voice alteration

Children and Adults: Postmarketing/case reports: **Anaphylactic reactions, asthmatic reactions,** bone density decreased, hypotension, induration at the injection site, peripheral neuropathy, photosensitivity, prostate pain, pulmonary embolism, rash, spinal fracture/paralysis, tenosynovitis-like symptoms, urticaria, WBC decreased

Pharmacodynamics/Kinetics
Onset of action: Following transient increase, testosterone suppression occurs in ~2-4 weeks of continued therapy
Distribution: Males: V_d: 27 L
Protein binding: 43% to 49%
Metabolism: Not well defined; forms smaller, inactive peptides and metabolites
Bioavailability: Oral: None; S.C.: 94%
Half-life elimination: 3 hours
Excretion: Urine (<5% as parent and major metabolite)

Pregnancy Risk Factor X

Generic Available Yes: Injection (solution)

Leuprolide Acetate *see* Leuprolide *on page 784*
Leuprorelin *see* Leuprolide *on page 784*
Leuprorelin Acetate *see* Leuprolide *on page 784*
Leurocristine *see* VinCRIStine *on page 1387*
Leustatin® *see* Cladribine *on page 336*

Levalbuterol (leve al BYOO ter ole)

U.S. Brand Names Xopenex®

Canadian Brand Names Xopenex®

Pharmacologic Category $Beta_2$ Agonist

Synonyms R-albuterol

Use Treatment or prevention of bronchospasm in adults and adolescents ≥6 years of age with reversible obstructive airway disease

Local Anesthetic/Vasoconstrictor Precautions No information available to require special precautions

Effects on Dental Treatment

>10%: Viral infection (7% to 12%), rhinitis (3% to 11%)

1% to 10%: Tachycardia (~3%), flu-like syndrome (1% to 4%), cough (1% to 4%), sinusitis (1% to 4%), nervousness (3% to 10%), tremor (≤7%), anxiety (≤3%), migraine (≤3%)

<2%: Abnormal EKG, asthma exacerbation, chest pain, diaphoresis, gastroenteritis, hypertension, hypotension, oropharyngeal dryness, paresthesia, syncope, wheezing

Dosage

Children 6-11 years: 0.31 mg 3 times/day via nebulization (maximum dose: 0.63 mg 3 times/day)

Children >12 years and Adults: Inhalation: 0.63 mg 3 times/day at intervals of 6-8 hours, via nebulization. Dosage may be increased to 1.25 mg 3 times/day with close monitoring for adverse effects. Most patients gain optimal benefit from regular use

Elderly: Only a small number of patients have been studied. Although greater sensitivity of some elderly patients cannot be ruled out, no overall differences in safety or effectiveness were observed. An initial dose of 0.63 mg should be used in all patients >65 years of age.

Mechanism of Action Relaxes bronchial smooth muscle by action on beta-2 receptors with little effect on heart rate

Other Adverse Effects Events reported include those ≥2% with incidence higher than placebo in patients ≥12 years of age.

>10%: Endocrine & metabolic: Increased serum glucose, decreased serum potassium

>2% to 10%:

Central nervous system: Dizziness (1% to 3%), pain (1% to 3%)

Gastrointestinal: Dyspepsia (1% to 3%)

Neuromuscular & skeletal: Leg cramps (≤3%)

Respiratory: Nasal edema (1% to 3%)

Miscellaneous: Accidental injury (≤3%)

<2%: Diarrhea, dyspepsia, chills, hypesthesia (hand), insomnia, itching eyes, lymphadenopathy, myalgia, nausea, immediate hypersensitivity reactions (angioedema, oropharyngeal edema, urticaria, rash, anaphylaxis)

Drug Interactions

Increased Effect/Toxicity: May add to effects of medications which deplete potassium (eg, loop or thiazide diuretics). Cardiac effects of levalbuterol may be potentiated in patients receiving MAO inhibitors, tricyclic antidepressants, sympathomimetics (eg, amphetamine, dobutamine), or inhaled anesthetics (eg, enflurane).

Decreased Effect: Beta-blockers (particularly nonselective agents) block the effect of levalbuterol. Digoxin levels may be decreased.

Pharmacodynamics/Kinetics

Onset of action: 10-17 minutes (measured as a 15% increase in FEV_1)

Peak effect: 1.5 hours

Duration: 5-6 hours (up to 8 hours in some patients)

Absorption: A portion of inhaled dose is absorbed to systemic circulation

Half-life elimination: 3.3-4 hours

Time to peak, serum: 0.2 hours

Pregnancy Risk Factor C

Generic Available No

Levamisole (lee VAM i sole)

U.S. Brand Names Ergamisol®

Canadian Brand Names Ergamisol®

Mexican Brand Names Decaris®

Pharmacologic Category Immune Modulator

Synonyms Levamisole Hydrochloride

Use Adjuvant treatment with fluorouracil in Dukes stage C colon cancer

Local Anesthetic/Vasoconstrictor Precautions No information available to require special precautions

Effects on Dental Treatment 1% to 10%: Fever, headache, nervousness, abnormal taste, stomatitis, rigors, paresthesia, infection

Dosage Oral:

Adults: Initial: 50 mg every 8 hours for 3 days, then 50 mg every 8 hours for 3 days every 2 weeks (fluorouracil is always given concomitantly)

Dosing adjustment in hepatic impairment: Specific guidelines unavailable

Mechanism of Action Clinically, combined therapy with levamisole and 5-fluorouracil has been effective in treating colon cancer patients, whereas demonstrable activity has been demonstrated. Due to the broad range of pharmacologic activities of levamisole, it has been suggested that the drug may act as a biochemical modulator (of fluorouracil, for example, in colon cancer), an effect entirely independent of immune modulation. Further studies are needed to evaluate the mechanisms of action of the drug in cancer patients.

Other Adverse Effects

>10%: Gastrointestinal: Nausea, diarrhea

1% to 10%:

Cardiovascular: Edema

Central nervous system: Fatigue, dizziness, somnolence, depression, insomnia

Dermatologic: Dermatitis, alopecia

Gastrointestinal: Anorexia, abdominal pain, constipation, vomiting

Hematologic: Leukopenia

Neuromuscular & skeletal: Arthralgia, myalgia

<1%: **Chest pain, anxiety**, pruritus, urticaria, flatulence, dyspepsia, thrombocytopenia, anemia, granulocytopenia, abnormal tearing, blurred vision, conjunctivitis, **epistaxis**, altered sense of smell, Stevens-Johnson syndrome

Drug Interactions Increased effect/toxicity of phenytoin.

Dietary/Ethanol/Herb Considerations Ethanol: Avoid use due to GI irritation and disulfiram-like reaction.

Pharmacodynamics/Kinetics

Absorption: Well absorbed

Metabolism: Hepatic (>70%)

Half-life elimination: 2-6 hours

Time to peak, serum: 1-2 hours

Excretion: Urine and feces within 48 hours

Pregnancy Risk Factor C

Generic Available No

Levamisole Hydrochloride *see* Levamisole *on page 786*

Levaquin® *see* Levofloxacin *on page 794*

Levarterenol Bitartrate *see* Norepinephrine *on page 985*

Levatol® *see* Penbutolol *on page 1045*

Levbid® *see* Hyoscyamine *on page 699*

Levetiracetam (lev e tir AS e tam)

U.S. Brand Names Keppra®

Canadian Brand Names Keppra®

Pharmacologic Category Anticonvulsant, Miscellaneous

Use Indicated as adjunctive therapy in the treatment of partial onset seizures in adults with epilepsy

Local Anesthetic/Vasoconstrictor Precautions No information available to require special precautions

Effects on Dental Treatment <10%: Anxiety, nervousness (4% vs 2% with placebo)

Dosage Oral:

Adults: Initial: 500 mg twice daily; additional dosing increments may be given (1000 mg/day additional every 2 weeks) to a maximum recommended daily dose of 3000 mg

Dosing adjustment in renal impairment:

Cl_{cr} >80 mL/minute: 500-1500 mg every 12 hours

Cl_{cr} 50-80 mL/minute: 500-1000 mg every 12 hours

Cl_{cr} 30-50 mL/minute: 250-750 mg every 12 hours

Cl_{cr} <30 mL/minute: 250-500 mg every 12 hours

End-stage renal disease patients using dialysis: 500-2000 mg every 24 hours

Mechanism of Action The precise mechanism by which levetiracetam exerts its antiepileptic effect is unknown and does not appear to derive from any interaction with known mechanisms involved in inhibitory and excitatory neurotransmission

Other Adverse Effects

>10%:

Central nervous system: Somnolence (15% vs 8% with placebo)

Neuromuscular & skeletal: Weakness (15% vs 9% with placebo)

<10%:

Central nervous system: Psychotic symptoms (1%), amnesia (2% vs 1% with placebo), ataxia (3% vs 1% with placebo), depression (4% vs 2% with placebo), dizziness (9% vs 4% with placebo), emotional lability (2%), vertigo (3% vs 1% with placebo), other behavioral symptoms (agitation, anger, aggression, irritability, hostility, apathy, depersonalization)

(Continued)

Levetiracetam *(Continued)*

Hematologic: Decreased erythrocyte counts (3%), decreased leukocytes (2% to 3%)

Neuromuscular & skeletal: Ataxia and other coordination difficulties (3% vs 2% with placebo), pain (7% vs 6% with placebo)

Ocular: Diplopia (2% vs 1% with placebo)

Postmarketing and/or case reports: Leukopenia, neutropenia, pancytopenia, thrombocytopenia

Drug Interactions No interaction was observed in pharmacokinetic trials with other anticonvulsants, including phenytoin, carbamazepine, valproic acid, phenobarbital, lamotrigine, gabapentin, and primidone.

Dietary/Ethanol/Herb Considerations

Ethanol: Avoid use; may increase CNS depression.

Food may delay but does not affect the extent of absorption.

Herb/Nutraceutical: Avoid gotu kola, kava, SAMe, St John's wort, and valerian; may increase CNS depression.

Pharmacodynamics/Kinetics

Onset of action: Peak effect: 1 hour

Absorption: Rapid and complete

Protein binding: <10%

Metabolism: Not extensive; primarily by enzymatic hydrolysis

Bioavailability: 100%

Half-life elimination: 6-8 hours

Excretion: Urine (66%)

Dialyzable: ~50% of pooled levetiracetam removed during standard 4-hour hemodialysis

Pregnancy Risk Factor C

Generic Available No

Levlen® *see* Combination Hormonal Contraceptives *on page 368*

Levlite™ *see* Combination Hormonal Contraceptives *on page 368*

Levobetaxolol (lee voe be TAX oh lol)

U.S. Brand Names Betaxon®

Canadian Brand Names Betaxon®

Pharmacologic Category Beta Blocker, Beta$_1$ Selective; Ophthalmic Agent, Antiglaucoma

Use Lowering of intraocular pressure in patients with chronic open-angle glaucoma or ocular hypertension

Local Anesthetic/Vasoconstrictor Precautions No information available to require special precautions

Effects on Dental Treatment Levobetaxolol is a cardioselective beta-blocker. Local anesthetic with vasoconstrictor can be safely used in patients medicated with levobetaxolol. Nonselective beta-blockers (ie, propranolol, nadolol) enhance the pressor response to epinephrine, resulting in hypertension and bradycardia; this has not been reported for levobetaxolol. Many nonsteroidal anti-inflammatory drugs such as ibuprofen and indomethacin can reduce the hypotensive effect of beta-blockers after 3 or more weeks of therapy with the NSAID. Short-term NSAID use (ie, 3 days) requires no special precautions in patients taking beta-blockers.

<2%: Tachycardia, bradycardia, hypertension, hypotension, headache, anxiety, abnormal taste, infection, bronchitis, dyspnea, pharyngitis, pneumonia, rhinitis, sinusitis, otitis media, dizziness

Dosage Adults: Ophthalmic: Instill 1 drop in affected eye(s) twice daily

Mechanism of Action Levobetaxolol is a cardioselective, beta$_1$-adrenergic receptor antagonist. It is the more active enantiomer of betaxolol. Reduces intraocular pressure by reducing the production of aqueous humor.

Other Adverse Effects

>10%: Ocular: Transient discomfort (11%)

2% to 10%: Ocular: Transient blurred vision (2%)

<2%:

Cardiovascular: Heart block

Central nervous system: Vertigo

Dermatologic: Alopecia, dermatitis, psoriasis

Endocrine & metabolic: **Diabetes**, hyperthyroidism, gout, hypercholesterolemia, hyperlipidemia

Gastrointestinal: Constipation, dyspepsia

Genitourinary: Cystitis

Neuromuscular & skeletal: Hypertonia, arthritis, tendonitis

Ocular: Cataracts, vitreous disorders

Otic: Ear pain, tinnitus

Miscellaneous: Breast abscess

Drug Interactions Increased Effect/Toxicity: Concurrent use of systemic beta-blockers, catecholamine-depleting agents (reserpine), antipsychotic agents may increase hypotension.

Pharmacodynamics/Kinetics
Onset of action: 30 minutes
Peak effect: 2 hours
Duration: 12 hours
Half-life elimination: 20 hours

Pregnancy Risk Factor C

Generic Available No

Levobunolol (lee voe BYOO noe lole)

U.S. Brand Names Betagan® Liquifilm®

Canadian Brand Names Apo®-Levobunolol; Betagan®; Novo-Levobunolol; Optho-Bunolol®; PMS-Levobunolol

Mexican Brand Names Betagan®

Pharmacologic Category Beta Blocker, Nonselective; Ophthalmic Agent, Antiglaucoma

Synonyms *l*-Bunolol Hydrochloride; Levobunolol Hydrochloride

Use To lower intraocular pressure in chronic open-angle glaucoma or ocular hypertension

Local Anesthetic/Vasoconstrictor Precautions No information available to require special precautions

Effects on Dental Treatment 1% to 10%: Bradycardia, arrhythmia, hypotension, bronchospasm, headache

Levobunolol is a nonselective beta-blocker and may enhance the pressor response to epinephrine, resulting in hypertension and bradycardia. Many nonsteroidal anti-inflammatory drugs such as ibuprofen and indomethacin can reduce the hypotensive effect of beta-blockers after 3 or more weeks of therapy with the NSAID. Short-term NSAID use (ie, 3 days) requires no special precautions in patients taking beta-blockers.

Dosage Adults: Ophthalmic: Instill 1 drop in the affected eye(s) 1-2 times/day

Mechanism of Action A nonselective beta-adrenergic blocking agent that lowers intraocular pressure by reducing aqueous humor production and possibly increases the outflow of aqueous humor

Other Adverse Effects
>10%: Ocular: Stinging/burning eyes
1% to 10%:
Central nervous system: Dizziness
Dermatologic: Alopecia, erythema
Local: Stinging, burning
Ocular: Blepharoconjunctivitis, conjunctivitis
<1%: Rash, itching, visual disturbances, keratitis, decreased visual acuity

Drug Interactions Increased Effect/Toxicity: Toxic effects may be increased with systemic beta-adrenergic blocking agents, ophthalmic epinephrine (increased blood pressure/loss of IOP effect), quinidine (sinus bradycardia), and verapamil (bradycardia and asystole have been reported).

Pharmacodynamics/Kinetics
Onset of action: ~1 hour
Peak effect: 2-6 hours
Duration: 1-7 days
Excretion: Not well defined

Pregnancy Risk Factor C

Generic Available Yes

Levobunolol Hydrochloride *see* Levobunolol *on page 789*

Levobupivacaine (LEE voe byoo PIV a kane)

Related Information
Oral Pain *on page 1524*

U.S. Brand Names Chirocaine®

Canadian Brand Names Chirocaine®

Pharmacologic Category Local Anesthetic

Use Production of local or regional anesthesia for surgery and obstetrics, and for postoperative pain management

Local Anesthetic/Vasoconstrictor Precautions No information available to require special precautions

Effects on Dental Treatment
>10%: Hypotension (20% to 31%), fever (7% to 17%),
1% to 10%: Abnormal EKG (3%), bradycardia (2%), tachycardia (2%), hypertension (1%), headache (5% to 7%), anxiety (1%), anesthesia (1%), rigors (3%), paresthesia (2%), cough (1%)

Dosage Adults: **Note:** Rapid injection of a large volume of local anesthetic solution should be avoided. Fractional (incremental) doses are recommended.
Guidelines (individual response varies): See table.

Maximum dosage: Epidural doses up to 375 mg have been administered incrementally to patients during a surgical procedure.

(Continued)

Levobupivacaine *(Continued)*

	Concentration	Volume	Dose	Motor Block
Surgical Anesthesia				
Epidural for surgery	0.5%-0.75%	10-20 mL	50-150 mg	Moderate to complete
Epidural - C-section	0.5%	20-30 mL	100-150 mg	Moderate to complete
Peripheral nerve	0.25%-0.5%	0.4 mL/kg (30 mL)	1-2 mg/kg (75-150 mg)	Moderate to complete
Ophthalmic	0.75%	5-15 mL	37.5-112.5 mg	Moderate to complete
Local infiltration	0.25%	60 mL	150 mg	Not applicable
Pain Management				
Labor analgesia (epidural bolus)	0.25%	10-20 mL	25-50 mg	Minimal to moderate
Postoperative pain (epidural infusion)	0.125%*-0.25%	4-10 mL/h	5-25 mg/h	Minimal to moderate

* 0.125%: Adjunct therapy with fentanyl or clonidine

Intraoperative block and postoperative pain: 695 mg in 24 hours
Postoperative epidural infusion over 24 hours: 570 mg
Single-fractionated injection for brachial plexus block: 300 mg

Mechanism of Action Levobupivacaine is the S-enantiomer of bupivacaine. It blocks both the initiation and transmission of nerve impulses by decreasing the neuronal membrane's permeability to sodium ions, which results in inhibition of depolarization with resultant blockade of conduction. Local anesthetics reversibly prevent generation and conduction of electrical impulses in neurons by decreasing the transient increase in permeability to sodium. The differential sensitivity generally depends on the size of the fiber; small fibers are more sensitive than larger fibers and require a longer period for recovery. Sensory pain fibers are usually blocked first, followed by fibers that transmit sensations of temperature, touch, and deep pressure. High concentrations block sympathetic somatic sensory and somatic motor fibers. The spread of anesthesia depends upon the distribution of the solution. This is primarily dependent on the site of administration and volume of drug injected.

Other Adverse Effects

>10%:

Central nervous system: Pain (postoperative) (7% to 18%)
Gastrointestinal: Nausea (12% to 21%), vomiting (8% to 14%)
Hematologic: Anemia (10% to 12%)

1% to 10%:

Central nervous system: Pain (4% to 8%), dizziness (5% to 6%), hypoesthesia (3%), somnolence (1%), hypothermia (2%)
Dermatologic: Pruritus (4% to 9%), purpura (1%)
Endocrine & metabolic: Breast pain (1% female)
Gastrointestinal: Constipation (3% to 7%), enlarged abdomen (3%), flatulence (2%), abdominal pain (2%), dyspepsia (2%), diarrhea (1%)
Genitourinary: Urinary incontinence (1%), urine flow decreased (1%), urinary tract infection (1%)
Hematologic: Leukocytosis (1%)
Neuromuscular & skeletal: Back pain (6%)
Ocular: Diplopia (3%)
Renal: Albuminuria (3%), hematuria (2%)
Miscellaneous: Fetal distress (5% to 10%), delayed delivery (6%), hemorrhage in pregnancy (2%), uterine abnormality (2%), increased wound drainage (1%)

<1%: Asthenia, edema, **postural hypotension**, hypokinesia, **involuntary muscle contraction, generalized spasm, tremor, syncope, arrhythmia, extrasystoles, atrial fibrillation, cardiac arrest**, ileus, elevated bilirubin, confusion, **apnea, bronchospasm, dyspnea, pulmonary edema, respiratory insufficiency, increased diaphoresis**, skin discoloration

Drug Interactions Substrate of CYP1A2, 3A4

Increased Effect/Toxicity: Although not specifically studied, inhibitors of CYP3A4 and CYP1A2 may increase levels/toxicity of levobupivacaine.

Dietary/Ethanol/Herb Considerations Herb/Nutraceutical: Avoid St John's wort; may decrease serum concentration.

Pharmacodynamics/Kinetics

Onset of action: Epidural: 10-14 minutes
Duration (dose dependent): 1-8 hours
Absorption: Dependent on route of administration and dose
Distribution: 67 L
Protein binding, plasma: >97%
Metabolism: Extensively hepatic via CYP3A4 and CYP1A2
Half-life elimination: 1.3 hours

Time to peak: Epidural: 30 minutes
Excretion: Urine (71%) and feces (24%) as metabolites

Pregnancy Risk Factor B

Generic Available No

Levocabastine (LEE voe kab as teen)

U.S. Brand Names Livostin®

Canadian Brand Names Livostin®

Mexican Brand Names Livostin®

Pharmacologic Category Antihistamine, H_1 Blocker, Ophthalmic

Synonyms Levocabastine Hydrochloride

Use Treatment of allergic conjunctivitis

Local Anesthetic/Vasoconstrictor Precautions No information available to require special precautions

Effects on Dental Treatment 1% to 10%: Xerostomia, headache, dyspnea

Dosage Children ≥12 years and Adults: Instill 1 drop in affected eye(s) 4 times/day for up to 2 weeks

Mechanism of Action Potent, selective histamine H_1-receptor antagonist for topical ophthalmic use

Other Adverse Effects

>10%: Local: Transient burning, stinging, discomfort

1% to 10%:

- Central nervous system: Somnolence, fatigue
- Dermatologic: Rash
- Ocular: Blurred vision, eye pain, somnolence, red eyes, eyelid edema

Pharmacodynamics/Kinetics Absorption: Topical: Systemic

Pregnancy Risk Factor C

Generic Available No

Levocabastine Hydrochloride *see* Levocabastine *on page 791*

Levocarnitine (lee voe KAR ni teen)

U.S. Brand Names Carnitor®

Canadian Brand Names Carnitor®

Mexican Brand Names Cardispan®

Pharmacologic Category Dietary Supplement

Synonyms L-Carnitine

Use Orphan drug:

Oral: Primary systemic carnitine deficiency; acute and chronic treatment of patients with an inborn error of metabolism which results in secondary carnitine deficiency

I.V.: Acute and chronic treatment of patients with an inborn error of metabolism which results in secondary carnitine deficiency; prevention and treatment of carnitine deficiency in patients with end-stage renal disease (ESRD) who are undergoing hemodialysis.

Local Anesthetic/Vasoconstrictor Precautions No information available to require special precautions

Effects on Dental Treatment

>10%: Hypertension (18% to 21%), fever (5% to 12%), paresthesia (3% to 12%),

1% to 10%: Allergic reaction (2% to 6%)

Dosage

Oral:

- Infants/Children: Initial: 50 mg/kg/day; titrate to 50-100 mg/kg/day in divided doses with a maximum dose of 3 g/day
- Adults: 990 mg (oral tablets) 2-3 times/day or 1-3 g/day (oral solution)

I.V.:

- Metabolic disorders: 50 mg/kg as a slow 2- to 3-minute I.V. bolus or by I.V. infusion
- Severe metabolic crisis:
  - A loading dose of 50 mg/kg over 2-3 minutes followed by an equivalent dose over the following 24 hours administered as every 3 hours or every 4 hours (never less than every 6 hours either by infusion or by intravenous injection)
  - All subsequent daily doses are recommended to be in the range of 50 mg/kg or as therapy may require (highest dose administered has been 300 mg/kg)
  - It is recommended that a plasma carnitine concentration be obtained prior to beginning parenteral therapy accompanied by weekly and monthly monitoring
- ESRD patients on hemodialysis:
  - Predialysis levocarnitine concentrations below normal (40-50 μmol/L): 10-20 mg/kg dry body weight as a slow 2- to 3-minute bolus after each dialysis session
  - Dosing adjustments should be guided by predialysis trough levocarnitine concentrations and downward dose adjustments (to 5 mg/kg after dialysis) may be made as early as every 3rd or 4th week of therapy

(Continued)

Levocarnitine *(Continued)*

Note: Safety and efficacy of oral carnitine have not been established in ESRD. Chronic administration of high oral doses to patients with severely compromised renal function or ESRD patients on dialysis may result in accumulation of metabolites.

Mechanism of Action Carnitine is a naturally occurring metabolic compound which functions as a carrier molecule for long-chain fatty acids within the mitochondria, facilitating energy production. Carnitine deficiency is associated with accumulation of excess acyl CoA esters and disruption of intermediary metabolism. Carnitine supplementation increases carnitine plasma concentrations. The effects on specific metabolic alterations have not been evaluated. ESRD patients on maintenance HD may have low plasma carnitine levels because of reduced intake of meat and dairy products, reduced renal synthesis, and dialytic losses. Certain clinical conditions (malaise, muscle weakness, cardiomyopathy and arrhythmias) in HD patients may be related to carnitine deficiency.

Other Adverse Effects Frequencies noted with I.V. therapy (hemodialysis patients):

Cardiovascular: Peripheral edema (3% to 6%)
Central nervous system: Dizziness (10% to 18%), depression (5% to 6%)
Endocrine & metabolic: Hypercalcemia (6% to 15%)
Gastrointestinal: Diarrhea (9% to 35%), abdominal pain (5% to 21%), vomiting (9% to 21%), nausea (5% to 12%)
Neuromuscular & skeletal: Weakness (9% to 12%)

Dietary/Ethanol/Herb Considerations Food: Tolerance may be improved by mixing the product with liquids or food and spacing doses evenly throughout the day with meals.

Pharmacodynamics/Kinetics

Metabolism: Hepatic (limited with moderate renal impairment), to trimethylamine (TMA) and trimethylamine N-oxide (TMAO)
Bioavailability: Tablet/solution: 15% to 16%
Half-life elimination: 17.4 hours
Time to peak: Tablet/solution: 3.3 hours
Excretion: Urine (4% to 9% as unchanged drug); metabolites also eliminated in urine

Pregnancy Risk Factor B

Generic Available Yes

Levodopa (lee voe DOE pa)

U.S. Brand Names Dopar®; Larodopa®

Canadian Brand Names Dopar®; Larodopa®

Pharmacologic Category Anti-Parkinson's Agent, Dopamine Agonist

Synonyms *L*-3-Hydroxytyrosine; *L*-Dopa

Use Treatment of Parkinson's disease

Unlabeled/Investigational Use Diagnostic agent for growth hormone deficiency

Local Anesthetic/Vasoconstrictor Precautions No information available to require special precautions

Effects on Dental Treatment 1% to 10%: Xerostomia

Dopaminergic therapy in Parkinson's disease (ie, treatment with levodopa) is associated with orthostatic hypotension. Patients medicated with levodopa should be carefully assisted from the chair and observed for signs of orthostatic hypotension.

Dosage Oral:

Children (administer as a single dose to evaluate growth hormone deficiency [unlabeled use]):
- 0.5 g/m^2 **or**
  - <30 lb: 125 mg
  - 30-70 lb: 250 mg
  - >70 lb: 500 mg

Adults: Parkinson's disease: 500-1000 mg/day in divided doses every 6-12 hours; increase by 100-750 mg/day every 3-7 days until response or total dose of 8000 mg is reached

A significant therapeutic response may not be obtained for 6 months

Mechanism of Action Increases dopamine levels in the brain, then stimulates dopaminergic receptors in the basal ganglia to improve the balance between cholinergic and dopaminergic activity

Other Adverse Effects Frequency not defined:

Cardiovascular: **Orthostatic hypotension, arrhythmias, chest pain, hypertension, syncope, palpitations**, phlebitis
Central nervous system: Dizziness, **anxiety**, confusion, nightmares, **headache, hallucinations**, on-off phenomenon, decreased mental acuity, memory impairment, **disorientation**, delusions, euphoria, **agitation**, somnolence, ataxia, insomnia, gait abnormalities, **nervousness, EPS, falling, psychosis**

Gastrointestinal: Anorexia, nausea, vomiting, constipation, **GI bleeding**, heartburn, duodenal ulcer, diarrhea, dyspepsia, **taste alterations, sialorrhea, increased salivation**

Genitourinary: Discoloration of urine, urinary frequency

Hematologic: Hemolytic anemia, agranulocytosis, thrombocytopenia, leukopenia, decreased hemoglobin and hematocrit, abnormalities in AST and ALT, LDH, bilirubin, BUN, Coombs' test

Neuromuscular & skeletal: Choreiform and involuntary movements, **paresthesia**, bone pain, shoulder pain, muscle cramps, weakness

Ocular: Blepharospasm

Renal: Difficult urination

Respiratory: **Dyspnea, cough**

Miscellaneous: **Hiccups**, discoloration of sweat

Drug Interactions

Increased Effect/Toxicity: Concurrent use of levodopa with nonselective MAO inhibitors may result in hypertensive reactions via an increased storage and release of dopamine, norepinephrine, or both. Use with carbidopa to minimize reactions if combination is necessary; otherwise avoid combination.

Decreased Effect: Antipsychotics, benzodiazepines, L-methionine, phenytoin, pyridoxine, spiramycin, and tacrine may inhibit the antiparkinsonian effects of levodopa; monitor for reduced effect. Antipsychotics may inhibit the antiparkinsonian effects of levodopa via dopamine receptor blockade. Use antipsychotics with low dopamine blockade (clozapine, olanzapine, quetiapine). High-protein diets may inhibit levodopa's efficacy; avoid high protein foods. Iron binds levodopa and reduces its bioavailability; separate doses of iron and levodopa.

Dietary/Ethanol/Herb Considerations

Ethanol: Avoid use due to CNS depression.

Food may decrease peak serum concentration; high protein diets (>2 g/kg) may decrease the efficacy of levodopa via competition with amino acids in crossing the blood-brain barrier. Avoid vitamin B_6 supplementation with dosages >200 mg/day.

Herb/Nutraceutical: Pyridoxine in doses >10-25 mg (for levodopa alone) or higher doses >200 mg/day (for levodopa/carbidopa) may decrease efficacy. Avoid gotu kola, kava, SAMe, St John's wort, and valerian; may increase CNS depression.

Pharmacodynamics/Kinetics

Duration: Variable, usually 6-12 hours

Absorption: May be reduced with a high-protein meal

Metabolism: Peripheral decarboxylation to dopamine; small amounts reach brain and are decarboxylated to active dopamine

Half-life elimination: 1.2-2.3 hours

Time to peak, serum: 1-2 hours

Excretion: Urine (80% as dopamine, norepinephrine, and homovanillic acid)

Pregnancy Risk Factor C

Generic Available No

Levodopa and Carbidopa (lee voe DOE pu & kar bi DOE pu)

Related Information

Carbidopa *on page 246*

Levodopa *on page 792*

U.S. Brand Names Sinemet®; Sinemet® CR

Canadian Brand Names Apo®-Levocarb; Endo®-Levodopa/Carbidopa; Novo-Levocarbidopa; Nu-Levocarb; Sinemet®; Sinemet® CR

Mexican Brand Names Racovel

Pharmacologic Category Anti-Parkinson's Agent, Dopamine Agonist

Synonyms Carbidopa and Levodopa

Use Idiopathic Parkinson's disease; postencephalitic parkinsonism; symptomatic parkinsonism

Unlabeled/Investigational Use Treatment of restless leg syndrome

Local Anesthetic/Vasoconstrictor Precautions No information available to require special precautions

Effects on Dental Treatment 1% to 10%: Xerostomia

Dopaminergic therapy in Parkinson's disease (ie, treatment with levodopa and carbidopa combination) is associated with orthostatic hypotension. Patients medicated with this drug combination should be carefully assisted from the chair and observed for signs of orthostatic hypotension.

Dosage Oral:

Adults: Initial: Carbidopa 25 mg/levodopa 100 mg 2-4 times/day, increase as necessary to a maximum of carbidopa 200 mg/levodopa 2000 mg per day

Restless leg syndrome (unlabeled use): Carbidopa 25 mg/levodopa 100 mg given 30-60 minutes before bedtime; may repeat dose once

Elderly: Initial: Carbidopa 25 mg/levodopa 100 mg twice daily, increase as necessary

Conversion from Sinemet® to Sinemet® CR (50/200): (Sinemet® [total daily dose

(Continued)

Levodopa and Carbidopa *(Continued)*

of levodopa] / Sinemet® CR):
300-400 mg / 1 tablet twice daily
500-600 mg / 1½ tablets twice daily or one 3 times/day
700-800 mg / 4 tablets in 3 or more divided doses
900-1000 mg / 5 tablets in 3 or more divided doses
Intervals between doses of Sinemet® CR should be 4-8 hours while awake

Mechanism of Action Parkinson's symptoms are due to a lack of striatal dopamine; levodopa circulates in the plasma to the blood-brain-barrier (BBB), where it crosses, to be converted by striatal enzymes to dopamine; carbidopa inhibits the peripheral plasma breakdown of levodopa by inhibiting its decarboxylation, and thereby increases available levodopa at the BBB

Other Adverse Effects Frequency not defined:

Cardiovascular: **Orthostatic hypotension, arrhythmias, chest pain, hypertension, syncope, palpitations**, phlebitis

Central nervous system: **Dizziness, anxiety**, confusion, nightmares, **headache, hallucinations**, on-off phenomenon, decreased mental acuity, memory impairment, **disorientation**, delusions, euphoria, **agitation**, somnolence, ataxia, insomnia, gait abnormalities, **nervousness, EPS, falling, psychosis**, peripheral neuropathy, **seizures** (causal relationship not established)

Dermatologic: Rash, alopecia, malignant melanoma, hypersensitivity (angioedema, urticaria, pruritus, bullous lesions, Henoch-Schönlein purpura)

Endocrine & metabolic: Increased libido

Gastrointestinal: Anorexia, nausea, vomiting, constipation, **GI bleeding**, duodenal ulcer, diarrhea, dyspepsia, **taste alterations, sialorrhea**, heartburn

Genitourinary: Discoloration of urine, urinary frequency

Hematologic: Hemolytic anemia, agranulocytosis, thrombocytopenia, leukopenia; decreased hemoglobin and hematocrit; abnormalities in AST and ALT, LDH, bilirubin, BUN, Coombs' test

Neuromuscular & skeletal: Choreiform and involuntary movements, **paresthesia**, bone pain, shoulder pain, muscle cramps, weakness

Ocular: Blepharospasm, oculogyric crises (may be associated with acute dystonic reactions)

Renal: Difficult urination

Respiratory: **Dyspnea, cough**

Miscellaneous: **Hiccups**, discoloration of sweat, diaphoresis (increased)

Drug Interactions

Increased Effect/Toxicity: Concurrent use of levodopa with nonselective MAO inhibitors may result in hypertensive reactions via an increased storage and release of dopamine, norepinephrine, or both. Use with carbidopa to minimize reactions if combination is necessary; otherwise avoid combination.

Decreased Effect: Antipsychotics, benzodiazepines, L-methionine, phenytoin, pyridoxine, spiramycin, and tacrine may inhibit the antiparkinsonian effects of levodopa; monitor for reduced effect. Antipsychotics may inhibit the antiparkinsonian effects of levodopa via dopamine receptor blockade. Use antipsychotics with low dopamine blockade (clozapine, olanzapine, quetiapine). High-protein diets may inhibit levodopa's efficacy; avoid high protein foods. Iron binds levodopa and reduces its bioavailability; separate doses of iron and levodopa.

Dietary/Ethanol/Herb Considerations

Ethanol: Avoid use due to CNS depression.

Food may decrease peak serum concentration; high protein diets (>2 g/kg) may decrease the efficacy of levodopa via competition with amino acids in crossing the blood-brain barrier. Avoid vitamin B_6 supplementation with dosages >200 mg/day.

Herb/Nutraceutical: Avoid kava; may decrease effects. Pyridoxine in doses >10-25 mg (for levodopa alone) or higher doses >200 mg/day (for levodopa/carbidopa) may decrease efficacy. Avoid gotu kola, SAMe, St John's wort, and valerian; may increase CNS depression.

Pharmacodynamics/Kinetics Duration: Variable, 6-12 hours; longer with sustained release forms

Pregnancy Risk Factor C

Generic Available Yes

Levo-Dromoran® *see* Levorphanol *on page 799*

Levofloxacin (lee voe FLOKS a sin)

Related Information

Sexually-Transmitted Diseases *on page 1502*
Tuberculosis *on page 1493*

U.S. Brand Names Levaquin®; Quixin™

Canadian Brand Names Levaquin®

Mexican Brand Names Elequine®; Tavanic®

Pharmacologic Category Antibiotic, Quinolone

Use

Systemic:

Acute bacterial exacerbation of chronic bronchitis due to *S. aureus, S. pneumoniae* (including penicillin-resistant strains), *H. influenzae, H. parainfluenzae,*or *M. catarrhalis*

Acute maxillary sinusitis due to *S. pneumoniae, H. influenzae,* or *M. catarrhalis*

Acute pyelonephritis caused by *E. coli*

Community-acquired pneumonia due to *S. aureus, S. pneumoniae* (including penicillin-resistant strains), *H. influenzae, H. parainfluenzae, M. catarrhalis, C. pneumoniae, L. pneumophila,* or *M. pneumoniae*

Nosocomial pneumonia due to methicillin-susceptible *S. aureus, Pseudomonas aeruginosa, Serratia marcescens, E. coli, K. pneumoniae, H. influenzae,* or *S. pneumoniae*

Skin or skin structure infections:

Complicated, due to methicillin-susceptible *S. aureus, Enterococcus faecalis, S. pyogenes,* or *Proteus mirabilis*

Uncomplicated, due to *S. aureus* or *S. pyogenes*

Urinary tract infections:

Complicated, due to gram-negative bacteria (*E. coli, Enterobacter cloacae, Klebsiella pneumoniae, Proteus mirabilis, Enterococcus faecalis,* or *Pseudomonas aeruginosa*)

Uncomplicated, due to *E. coli, K. pneumoniae,* or *S. saprophyticus*

Ophthalmic: Bacterial conjunctivitis due to *S. aureus, S. epidermidis, S. pneumoniae, Streptococcus* (groups C/F), *Streptococcus* (group G), Viridans group streptococci, *Corynebacterium* spp, *H. influenzae, Acinetobacter lwoffii,* or *Serratia marcescens*

Local Anesthetic/Vasoconstrictor Precautions No information available to require special precautions

Effects on Dental Treatment 1% to 10%: Fever, headache, pharyngitis, dizziness

Dosage

Adults: Oral, I.V. (infuse I.V. solution over 60 minutes):

Acute bacterial exacerbation of chronic bronchitis: 500 mg every 24 hours for at least 7 days

Nosocomial pneumonia: 750 mg every 24 hours for 7-14 days

Community-acquired pneumonia: 500 mg every 24 hours for 7-14 days

Acute maxillary sinusitis: 500 mg every 24 hours for 10-14 days

Uncomplicated skin infections: 500 mg every 24 hours for 7-10 days

Complicated skin infections: 750 mg every 24 hours for 7-14 days

Uncomplicated urinary tract infections: 250 mg once daily for 3 days

Complicated urinary tract infections, including acute pyelonephritis: 250 mg every 24 hours for 10 days

Children ≥1 year and Adults: Ophthalmic:

Treatment day 1 and day 2: Instill 1-2 drops into affected eye(s) every 2 hours while awake, up to 8 times/day

Treatment day 3 through day 7: Instill 1-2 drops into affected eye(s) every 4 hours while awake, up to 4 times/day

Dosing adjustment in renal impairment:

Chronic bronchitis, acute maxillary sinusitis, uncomplicated skin infection, community-acquired pneumonia:

Cl_{cr} 20-49 mL/minute: Administer 250 mg every 24 hours (initial: 500 mg)

Cl_{cr} 10-19 mL/minute: Administer 250 mg every 48 hours (initial: 500 mg)

Complicated UTI, acute pyelonephritis:

Cl_{cr} 20-49 mL/minute: No dosage adjustment required required

Cl_{cr} 10-19 mL/minute: Administer 250 mg every 48 hours

Uncomplicated UTI: No dosage adjustment required

Complicated skin infection or nosocomial pneumonia:

Cl_{cr} 20-49 mL/minute: Administer 750 mg every 48 hours mg

Cl_{cr} 10-19 mL/minute: Administer 500 mg every 48 hours (initial: 750 mg)

Hemodialysis/CAPD: 250 mg every 48 hours (initial: 500 mg for most infections; initial: 750 mg for complicated skin/soft tissue infections followed by 500 mg every 48 hours)

Mechanism of Action As the S (-) enantiomer of the fluoroquinolone, ofloxacin, levofloxacin, inhibits DNA-gyrase in susceptible organisms thereby inhibits relaxation of supercoiled DNA and promotes breakage of DNA strands. DNA gyrase (topoisomerase II), is an essential bacterial enzyme that maintains the superhelical structure of DNA and is required for DNA replication and transcription, DNA repair, recombination, and transposition.

Other Adverse Effects

1% to 10%:

Central nervous system: Insomnia

Gastrointestinal: Nausea, vomiting, diarrhea, constipation

Ocular (with ophthalmic solution use): Decreased vision (transient), foreign body sensation, transient ocular burning, ocular pain or discomfort, photophobia

(Continued)

Levofloxacin *(Continued)*

<1% (Limited to important or life-threatening):

Systemic: Acute renal failure; **allergic reaction (pneumonitis rash, pneumonitis, anaphylaxis); anaphylactoid reaction, arrhythmias (including ventricular tachycardia and torsade de pointes)**, arthralgia, **bradycardia, cardiac failure**, dysphonia, eosinophilia, erythema multiforme, granulocytopenia, hemolytic anemia, hepatic failure, hypertension, intracranial hypertension, jaundice, leukocytosis, leukopenia, leukorrhea, photosensitivity (<0.1%), pseudomembraneous colitis, pulmonary embolism, QT_c prolongation, seizures, Stevens-Johnson syndrome, **tachycardia**, tendon rupture, transaminases increased, thrombocytopenia, **tremor**

Ophthalmic solution: Allergic reaction, lid edema, ocular dryness, ocular itching

Drug Interactions Inhibits **CYP1A2**

Increased Effect/Toxicity: Quinolones may cause increased levels of azlocillin, cyclosporine, and caffeine/theophylline (effect of levofloxacin on theophylline metabolism appears limited). Azlocillin, cimetidine, loop diuretics (furosemide, torsemide), and probenecid increase quinolone levels (decreased renal secretion). An increased incidence of seizures may occur with foscarnet or NSAIDs. The hypoprothrombinemic effect of warfarin is enhanced by some quinolone antibiotics. QT_c-prolonging agents (including Class Ia and Class III antiarrhythmics, erythromycin, cisapride, antipsychotics, and cyclic antidepressants) should be avoided with levofloxacin. Levofloxacin does not alter warfarin levels, but may alter the gastrointestinal flora. Monitor INR closely during therapy. Concurrent use of corticosteroids may increase risk of tendon rupture.

Decreased Effect: Metal cations (magnesium, aluminum, iron, and zinc) bind quinolones in the gastrointestinal tract and inhibit absorption (by up to 98%). Due to electrolyte content, antacids, electrolyte supplements, sucralfate, quinapril, and some didanosine formulations should be avoided. Levofloxacin should be administered 2 hours before or 2 hours after these agents. Antineoplastic agents may decrease the absorption of quinolones.

Dietary/Ethanol/Herb Considerations Food: Administer on an empty stomach, if possible; food may decrease absorption if it contains divalent or trivalent cations.

Pharmacodynamics/Kinetics

Absorption: Rapid and complete

Distribution: V_d: 1.25 L/kg; CSF concentrations ~15% of serum levels; high concentrations are achieved in prostate and gynecological tissues, sinus, breast milk, and saliva

Protein binding: 50%

Metabolism: Minimally hepatic

Bioavailability: 100%

Half-life elimination: 6 hours

Time to peak, serum: 1 hour

Excretion: Primarily urine (as unchanged drug)

Pregnancy Risk Factor C

Generic Available No

Levomepromazine *see* Methotrimeprazine *on page 887*

Levomethadyl Acetate Hydrochloride

(lee voe METH a dil AS e tate hye droe KLOR ide)

U.S. Brand Names ORLAAM®

Pharmacologic Category Analgesic, Narcotic

Use Management of opiate dependence; should be reserved for use in treatment of opiate-addicted patients who fail to show an acceptable response to other adequate treatments for addiction

Local Anesthetic/Vasoconstrictor Precautions No information available to require special precautions

Effects on Dental Treatment

>10%: Flu-like syndrome

1% to 10%: CNS depression, sedation, headache, nervousness, euphoria, anxiety, hot flashes (males 2:1), xerostomia, nausea, vomiting, weakness, blurred vision

Restrictions C-II; must be dispensed in a designated clinic setting only

Dosage Adults: Oral: 20-40 mg at 48- or 72-hour intervals, with ranges of 10 mg to as high as 140 mg 3 times/week; adjust dose in increments of 5-10 mg (too rapid induction may lead to overdose); always dilute before administration and mix with diluent prior to dispensing

Mechanism of Action A synthetic opioid agonist with actions similar to morphine; principal actions are analgesia and sedation. Its clinical effects in the treatment of opiate abuse occur through two mechanisms: 1) cross-sensitivity for opiates of the morphine type, suppressing symptoms of withdrawal in opiate-dependent persons; 2) with chronic oral administration, can produce sufficient tolerance to block the subjective high of usual doses of parenterally administered opiates

Other Adverse Effects

>10%: Central nervous system: Malaise

1% to 10%:

Central nervous system: Chills, abnormal dreams, insomnia, hypesthesia

Gastrointestinal: Abdominal pain, constipation, diarrhea

Genitourinary: Urinary tract spasm, difficult ejaculation, impotence, decreased sex drive

Neuromuscular & skeletal: Arthralgia, back pain

Ocular: Miosis

<1%: Amenorrhea, amnesia, **angina, confusion**, hepatitis, **incoordination,** myalgia, **postural hypotension, seizures**, S-T segment increased, pyuria, tearing

Postmarketing and/or case reports: **Apnea**, breast enlargement, **cardiac arrest, chest pain, dyspnea, hallucinations, migraine, MI,** QT_c prolongation, **syncope, ventricular tachycardia; serious cardiac arrhythmias have been reported including torsade de pointes**

Drug Interactions Substrate of CYP2B6, **3A4**

Increased Effect/Toxicity: CNS depressants, including sedatives, tranquilizers, propoxyphene, antidepressants, benzodiazepines, and ethanol may result in serious overdose when used with levomethadyl. Enzyme inducers (carbamazepine, phenobarbital, rifampin, phenytoin) may enhance the metabolism of levomethadyl leading to an increase in levomethadyl peak effect (however, duration of action is shortened). Enzyme inhibitors such as erythromycin, cimetidine, and ketoconazole may increase the risk of arrhythmia (including torsade de pointes) or may increase the duration of action of levomethadyl. Concurrent use of QT_c-prolonging agents is contraindicated (includes class I and III antiarrhythmics, cisapride, erythromycin, select quinolones, mesoridazine, thioridazine, zonisamide). Concurrent use of MAO inhibitors is contraindicated (per manufacturer), or drugs with MAO-blocking activity (linezolid). Safety of selegiline (selective MAO type B inhibitor) not established.

Decreased Effect: Levomethadyl used in combination with naloxone, naltrexone, pentazocine, nalbuphine, butorphanol, and buprenorphine may result in withdrawal symptoms. The effect of meperidine may be decreased by levomethadyl. Enzyme inducers (carbamazepine, phenobarbital, rifampin, phenytoin) may shorten levomethadyl's duration of action. Enzyme inhibitors, such as erythromycin, cimetidine, and ketoconazole may slow the onset, lower the activity levomethadyl (may also increase duration of action).

Dietary/Ethanol/Herb Considerations

Ethanol: Avoid use; may increase CNS depression and lead to overdose.

Herb/Nutraceutical: Avoid gotu kola, kava, SAMe, St John's wort, and valerian; may increase CNS depression.

Pharmacodynamics/Kinetics

Protein binding: 80%

Metabolism: Hepatic to L-alpha-noracetylmethadol and L-alpha-dinoracetylmethadol (active metabolites)

Half-life elimination: 35-60 hours

Time to peak, serum: 1.5-6 hours

Excretion: Urine (as methadol and normethadol)

Pregnancy Risk Factor C

Generic Available No

Levonorgestrel (LEE voe nor jes trel)

Related Information

Endocrine Disorders and Pregnancy *on page 1479*

U.S. Brand Names Mirena®; Norplant® Implant [DSC]; Plan B®

Canadian Brand Names Mirena®; Norplant® Implant; Plan B™

Mexican Brand Names Microlut®

Pharmacologic Category Contraceptive

Synonyms LNg 20; Norplant® Implant [DSC]

Use Prevention of pregnancy

Local Anesthetic/Vasoconstrictor Precautions No information available to require special precautions

Effects on Dental Treatment Progestins may predispose the patient to gingival bleeding.

Intrauterine system: Migraine (<3%); >5%: Hypertension, headache, nervousness, CNS depression, upper respiratory tract infection, sinusitis

Oral tablets: Headache (17%), dizziness (11%), increased/prolonged bleeding (28%)

Dosage Adults:

Long-term prevention of pregnancy:

Subdermal capsules: Total administration doses (implanted): 216 mg in 6 capsules which should be implanted during the first 7 days of onset of menses subdermally in the upper arm; each Norplant® silastic capsule releases 80 mcg of levonorgestrel/day for 6-18 months, following which a rate of release of 25-30 mcg/day is maintained for ≤5 years; capsules should be removed by end of 5th year

(Continued)

Levonorgestrel *(Continued)*

Intrauterine system: To be inserted into uterine cavity; should be inserted within 7 days of onset of menstruation or immediately after 1st trimester abortion; releases 20 mcg levonorgestrel/day over 5 years. May be removed and replaced with a new unit at anytime during menstrual cycle; do not leave any one system in place for >5 years

Emergency contraception: Oral tablet: One 0.75 mg tablet as soon as possible within 72 hours of unprotected sexual intercourse; a second 0.75 mg tablet should be taken 12 hours after the first dose; may be used at any time during menstrual cycle

Elderly: Not intended for use in postmenopausal women

Dosing adjustment in renal/hepatic impairment: Safety and efficacy not established

Mechanism of Action Pregnancy may be prevented through several mechanisms: Thickening of cervical mucus, which inhibits sperm passage through the uterus and sperm survival; inhibition of ovulation, from a negative feedback mechanism on the hypothalamus, leading to reduced secretion of follicle stimulating hormone (FSH) and luteinizing hormone (LH); inhibition of implantation. Levonorgestrel is not effective once the implantation process has begun.

Other Adverse Effects

Intrauterine system:

>5%:

Dermatologic: Acne

Endocrine & metabolic: Breast pain, dysmenorrhea, decreased libido, abnormal Pap smear, amenorrhea (20% at 1 year), enlarged follicles (12%)

Gastrointestinal: Abdominal pain, nausea, weight gain

Genitourinary: Leukorrhea, vaginitis

Neuromuscular & skeletal: Back pain

<3% and postmarketing reports: Alopecia, anemia, cervicitis, dyspareunia, eczema, failed insertion, sepsis, vomiting

Oral tablets:

>10%:

Central nervous system: Fatigue (17%)

Endocrine & metabolic: Heavier menstrual bleeding (14%), lighter menstrual bleeding (12%), breast tenderness (11%)

Gastrointestinal: Nausea (23%), abdominal pain (18%),

1% to 10%: Gastrointestinal: Vomiting (6%), diarrhea (5%)

Subdermal capsules:

>10%: Endocrine & metabolic: Spotting (bleeding) (17%)

1% to 10%:

Endocrine & metabolic: Breast discharge (≥5%), menstrual irregularities

Gastrointestinal: Abdominal discomfort (≥5%)

Genitourinary: Cervicitis (≥5%), leukorrhea (≥5%), vaginitis (≥5%)

Local: Pain/itching at implant site (4%, usually transient)

Neuromuscular & skeletal: Musculoskeletal pain (≥5%)

Miscellaneous: Removal difficulties (6%); these may include multiple incisions, remaining capsule fragments, pain, multiple visits, deep placement, lengthy procedure

<1%, postmarketing, and/or case reports: Abscess, acne, adnexal enlargement, alopecia, **anxiety**, arm pain, blistering, breast cancer, bruising, cellulitis, change of appetite, congenital anomalies, depression, dermatitis, **dizziness**, DVT, dysmenorrhea, emotional lability, excessive scarring, fatigue, hirsutism, hypertrichosis, hyperpigmentation, idiopathic intracranial hypertension, induration, infection at implant site, mastalgia, **MI**, nausea, nerve injury, **nervousness**, numbness, phlebitis, pulmonary embolism, pruritus, rash, sloughing, **stroke**, superficial venous thrombosis, thrombotic thrombocytopenic purpura (TTP), tingling, ulcerations, urticaria, vomiting, weakness, weight gain

Drug Interactions Substrate of **CYP3A4**

Decreased Effect: Enzyme inducers: May increase the metabolism of levonorgestrel resulting in decreased effect; includes carbamazepine, phenobarbital, phenytoin, and rifampin; additional contraceptive measures may be needed with use of enzyme inducers or following their withdrawal

Dietary/Ethanol/Herb Considerations Herb/Nutraceutical: Avoid St John's wort; may decrease serum concentration.

Pharmacodynamics/Kinetics

Duration: Subdermal capsules and intrauterine system: Up to 5 years

Absorption: Rapid and complete

Protein binding: Highly bound to albumin and sex hormone-binding globulin

Metabolism: To inactive metabolites

Bioavailability: 100%

Half-life elimination: Oral tablet: ~24 hours

Excretion: Primarily urine

Pregnancy Risk Factor X

Generic Available No

Levophed® *see* Norepinephrine *on page 985*

Levora® *see* Combination Hormonal Contraceptives *on page 368*

Levorphanol (lee VOR fa nole)

U.S. Brand Names Levo-Dromoran®

Pharmacologic Category Analgesic, Narcotic

Synonyms Levorphanol Tartrate; Levorphan Tartrate

Use Relief of moderate to severe pain; also used parenterally for preoperative sedation and an adjunct to nitrous oxide/oxygen anesthesia; 2 mg levorphanol produces analgesia comparable to that produced by 10 mg of morphine

Local Anesthetic/Vasoconstrictor Precautions No information available to require special precautions

Effects on Dental Treatment ~10%: Xerostomia; normal salivary flow resumes upon discontinuation

Restrictions C-II

Dosage These are guidelines and do not represent the maximum doses that may be required in all patients. Doses should be titrated to pain relief/prevention.

Adults:

Acute pain (moderate to severe): Initial: Opiate-naive:

Oral: 2 mg every 6-8 hours as needed; patients with prior opiate exposure may require higher initial doses; usual dosage range: 2-4 mg every 6-8 hours as needed

I.M., S.C.: 1 mg every 6-8 hours as needed; patients with prior opiate exposure may require higher initial doses; usual dosage range: 1-2 mg every 6-8 hours as needed

Slow I.V.: Up to 1 mg/dose every 3-6 hours as needed; patients with prior opiate exposure may require higher initial doses

Chronic pain: Patients taking opioids chronically may become tolerant and require doses higher than the usual dosage range to maintain the desired effect. Tolerance can be managed by appropriate dose titration. There is no optimal or maximal dose for levorphanol in chronic pain. The appropriate dose is one that relieves pain throughout its dosing interval without causing unmanageable side effects.

Premedication: I.M., S.C.: 1-2 mg/dose 60-90 minutes prior to surgery; older or debilitated patients usually require less drug

Dosing adjustment in hepatic disease: Reduction necessary in liver disease

Mechanism of Action Levorphanol tartrate is a synthetic opioid agonist that is classified as a morphinan derivative. Opioids interact with stereospecific opioid receptors in various parts of the central nervous system and other tissues. Analgesic potency parallels the affinity for these binding sites. These drugs do not alter the threshold or responsiveness to pain, but the perception of pain.

Other Adverse Effects Frequency not defined:

Cardiovascular: Palpitations, hypotension, bradycardia, peripheral vasodilation, cardiac arrest, shock, tachycardia

Central nervous system: **CNS depression**, fatigue, drowsiness, **dizziness, nervousness, headache, restlessness**, anorexia, malaise, **confusion, coma, convulsion**, insomnia, amnesia, mental depression, **hallucinations, paradoxical CNS stimulation, intracranial pressure (increased)**

Dermatologic: Pruritus, urticaria, rash

Endocrine & metabolic: Antidiuretic hormone release

Gastrointestinal: Nausea, vomiting, dyspepsia, stomach cramps, constipation, abdominal pain, biliary tract spasm, paralytic ileus

Genitourinary: Decreased urination, urinary tract spasm, urinary retention

Local: Pain at injection site

Neuromuscular & skeletal: Weakness

Ocular: Miosis, diplopia

Respiratory: **Respiratory depression, apnea, hypoventilation**, cyanosis

Miscellaneous: Histamine release, physical and psychological dependence

Drug Interactions Increased Effect/Toxicity: CNS depression is enhanced with coadministration of other CNS depressants.

Dietary/Ethanol/Herb Considerations

Ethanol: Avoid use; may increase CNS depression.

Herb/Nutraceutical: Avoid gotu kola, kava, SAMe, St John's wort, and valerian; may increase CNS depression.

Pharmacodynamics/Kinetics

Onset of action: Oral: 10-60 minutes

Duration: 4-8 hours

Metabolism: Hepatic

Half-life elimination: 11-16 hours

Excretion: Urine (as inactive metabolite)

Pregnancy Risk Factor B/D (prolonged use or high doses at term)

Generic Available Yes: Tablet

Levorphanol Tartrate *see* Levorphanol *on page 799*

Levorphan Tartrate *see* Levorphanol *on page 799*

Levothroid® *see* Levothyroxine *on page 800*

Levothyroxine (lee voe thye ROKS een)

Related Information

Endocrine Disorders and Pregnancy *on page 1479*

U.S. Brand Names Levothroid®; Levoxyl®; Novothyrox; Synthroid®; Unithroid®

Canadian Brand Names Eltroxin®; Synthroid®

Mexican Brand Names Eutirox; Tiroidine

Pharmacologic Category Thyroid Product

Synonyms Levothyroxine Sodium; *L*-Thyroxine Sodium; T_4

Use Replacement or supplemental therapy in hypothyroidism; pituitary TSH suppression

Local Anesthetic/Vasoconstrictor Precautions No precautions with vasoconstrictor are necessary if patient is well controlled with levothyroxine

Effects on Dental Treatment No significant effects or complications reported

Dosage Doses should be adjusted based on clinical response and laboratory parameters.

Oral:

Children: Hypothyroidism:

Newborns: Initial: 10-15 mcg/kg/day. Lower doses of 25 mcg/day should be considered in newborns at risk for cardiac failure. Newborns with T_4 levels <5 mcg/dL should be started at 50 mcg/day. Adjust dose at 4- to 6-week intervals.

Infants and Children: Dose based on body weight and age as listed below. Children with severe or chronic hypothyroidism should be started at 25 mcg/day; adjust dose by 25 mcg every 2-4 weeks. In older children, hyperactivity may be decreased by starting with 1/4 of the recommended dose and increasing by 1/4 dose each week until the full replacement dose is reached. Refer to adult dosing once growth and puberty are complete.

0-3 months: 10-15 mcg/kg/day
3-6 months: 8-10 mcg/kg/day
6-12 months: 6-8 mcg/kg/day
1-5 years: 5-6 mcg/kg/day
6-12 years: 4-5 mcg/kg/day
>12 years: 2-3 mcg/kg/day

Adults:

Hypothyroidism: 1.7 mcg/kg/day in otherwise healthy adults <50 years old, children in whom growth and puberty are complete, and older adults who have been recently treated for hyperthyroidism or who have been hypothyroid for only a few months. Titrate dose every 6 weeks. Average starting dose ~100 mcg; usual doses are ≤200 mcg/day; doses ≥300 mcg/day are rare (consider poor compliance, malabsorption, and/or drug interactions). **Note:** For patients >50 years or patients with cardiac disease, refer to Elderly dosing.

Severe hypothyroidism: Initial: 12.5-25 mcg/day; adjust dose by 25 mcg/day every 2-4 weeks as appropriate; **Note:** Oral agents are not recommended for myxedema (see I.V. dosing).

Subclinical hypothyroidism (if treated): 1 mcg/kg/day

TSH suppression:

Well-differentiated thyroid cancer: Highly individualized; Doses >2 mcg/kg/day may be needed to suppress TSH to <0.1 mU/L.

Benign nodules and nontoxic multinodular goiter: Goal TSH suppression: 0.1-0.3 mU/L

Elderly: Hypothyroidism:

>50 years without cardiac disease **or** <50 years with cardiac disease: Initial: 25-50 mcg/day; adjust dose at 6- to 8-week intervals as needed

>50 years with cardiac disease: Initial: 12.5-25 mcg/day; adjust dose by 12.5-25 mcg increments at 4- to 6-week intervals

Note: Elderly patients may require <1 mcg/kg/day

I.M., I.V.: Children, Adults, Elderly: Hypothyroidism: 50% of the oral dose

I.V.:

Adults: Myxedema coma or stupor: 200-500 mcg, then 100-300 mcg the next day if necessary; smaller doses should be considered in patients with cardiovascular disease

Elderly: Myxedema coma: Refer to Adults dosing; lower doses may be needed

Mechanism of Action Exact mechanism of action is unknown; however, it is believed the thyroid hormone exerts its many metabolic effects through control of DNA transcription and protein synthesis; involved in normal metabolism, growth, and development; promotes gluconeogenesis, increases utilization and mobilization of glycogen stores, and stimulates protein synthesis, increases basal metabolic rate

Other Adverse Effects Frequency not defined:

Cardiovascular: **Angina, arrhythmias, hypertension, cardiac arrest, flushing, heart failure, MI, palpitations, increased pulse, tachycardia**

Central nervous system: **Anxiety, fatigue, fever, nervousness, seizures (rare), headache**, hyperactivity, emotional lability, insomnia, irritability, pseudotumor cerebri (children)

Dermatologic: Alopecia
Endocrine & metabolic: Fertility impaired, menstrual irregularities
Gastrointestinal: Abdominal cramps, appetite increased, diarrhea, vomiting, weight loss
Hepatic: LFTs increased
Neuromuscular & skeletal: Bone mineral density decreased, muscle weakness, tremors, slipped capital femoral epiphysis (children)
Respiratory: **Dyspnea**
Miscellaneous: **Diaphoresis**, heat intolerance, **hypersensitivity** to inactive ingredients (urticaria, pruritus, rash, flushing, angioedema, GI symptoms, fever, arthralgia, serum sickness, wheezing)

Drug Interactions CYP enzyme substrate (T_3 and T_4); thyroid hormone may alter metabolic activity of cytochrome P450 enzymes

Increased Effect/Toxicity: Levothyroxine may potentiate the hypoprothrombinemic effect of warfarin (and other oral anticoagulants). Tricyclic antidepressants (TCAs) coadministered with levothyroxine may increase potential for toxicity of both drugs. Coadministration with ketamine may lead to hypertension and tachycardia.

Decreased Effect: Some medications may decrease absorption of levothyroxine: Cholestyramine, colestipol (separate administration by at least 2 hours); aluminum- and magnesium-containing antacids, iron preparations, sucralfate, Kayexalate® (separate administration by at least 4 hours). Enzyme inducers (phenytoin, phenobarbital, carbamazepine, and rifampin/rifabutin) may decrease levothyroxine levels. Levothyroxine may decrease effect of oral sulfonylureas. Serum levels of digoxin and theophylline may be altered by thyroid function. Estrogens may decrease serum free-thyroxine concentrations.

Dietary/Ethanol/Herb Considerations Food: Administer tablets on an empty stomach; food may decrease oral absorption. Administration with enteral nutrition may cause reduced bioavailability and lower serum thyroxine levels leading to signs or symptoms of hypothyroidism. Limit intake of goitrogenic foods (eg, asparagus, cabbage, peas, turnip greens, broccoli, spinach, Brussels sprouts, lettuce, soybeans). Soybean flour (infant formula), walnuts, and dietary fiber may decrease absorption from the GI tract.

Pharmacodynamics/Kinetics

Onset of action: Therapeutic: Oral: 3-5 days; I.V. 6-8 hours
Peak effect: I.V.: ~24 hours
Absorption: Oral: Erratic (40% to 80%); decreases with age
Protein binding: >99%
Metabolism: Hepatic to triiodothyronine (active)
Time to peak, serum: 2-4 hours
Half-life elimination: Euthyroid: 6-7 days; Hypothyroid: 9-10 days; Hyperthyroid: 3-4 days
Excretion: Urine and feces; decreases with age

Pregnancy Risk Factor A

Generic Available Yes: Injection

Levothyroxine Sodium *see* Levothyroxine *on page 800*
Levoxyl® *see* Levothyroxine *on page 800*
Levsin® *see* Hyoscyamine *on page 699*
Levsinex® *see* Hyoscyamine *on page 699*
Levsin/SL® *see* Hyoscyamine *on page 699*
Levulan® Kerastick™ *see* Aminolevulinic Acid *on page 77*
Levulose, Dextrose and Phosphoric Acid *see* Phosphorated Carbohydrate Solution *on page 1078*
Lexapro™ *see* Escitalopram *on page 516*
Lexxel® *see* Enalapril and Felodipine *on page 494*
LFA-3/IgG(1) Fusion Protein, Human *see* Alefacept *on page 52*
***l*-Hyoscyamine Sulfate** *see* Hyoscyamine *on page 699*
Librax® *see* Clidinium and Chlordiazepoxide *on page 341*
Librium® *see* Chlordiazepoxide *on page 299*
LidaMantle® *see* Lidocaine *on page 801*
Lida-Mantle HC® *see* Lidocaine and Hydrocortisone *on page 805*
Lidex® *see* Fluocinonide *on page 585*
Lidex-E® *see* Fluocinonide *on page 585*

Lidocaine (LYE doe kane)

Related Information

Cardiovascular Diseases *on page 1456*
Management of Patients Undergoing Cancer Therapy *on page 1567*
Oral Pain *on page 1524*
Oral Viral Infections *on page 1545*

U.S. Brand Names Anestacon®; Band-Aid® Hurt-Free™ Antiseptic Wash [OTC]; Burnamycin [OTC]; Burn Jel [OTC]; Burn-O-Jel [OTC]; ELA-Max® [OTC]; ELA-Max® 5 [OTC]; LidaMantle®; Lidoderm®; Premjact® [OTC]; Solarcaine® Aloe (Continued)

Lidocaine *(Continued)*

Extra Burn Relief [OTC]; Topicaine® [OTC]; Xylocaine®; Xylocaine® MPF; Xylocaine® Viscous; Zilactin-L® [OTC]

Canadian Brand Names Lidodan™; Lidoderm®; Xylocaine®; Xylocard®; Zilactin®

Mexican Brand Names Pisacaina®; Uvega®; Xylocaina®

Pharmacologic Category Analgesic, Topical; Antiarrhythmic Agent, Class Ib; Local Anesthetic

Synonyms Lidocaine Hydrochloride; Lignocaine Hydrochloride

Use

Dental: Amide-type local anesthetic and topical local anesthetic

Patch: Production of mild topical anesthesia of accessible mucous membranes of the mouth prior to superficial dental procedures

Medical: Acute treatment of ventricular arrhythmias from MI, cardiac manipulation, digitalis intoxication; drug of choice for ventricular ectopy, ventricular tachycardia (VT), ventricular fibrillation (VF); for pulseless VT or VF preferably administer **after** defibrillation and epinephrine; control of premature ventricular contractions, wide-complex paroxysmal supraventricular tachycardia (PSVT); control of hemodynamically compromising PVCs; hemodynamically stable VT

ELA-Max® is a topical local anesthetic for use in laser, cosmetic, and outpatient surgeries; minor burns, cuts, and abrasions of the skin

Orphan drug (Lidoderm® Patch): Relief of allodynia (painful hypersensitivity) and chronic pain in postherpetic neuralgia

Local Anesthetic/Vasoconstrictor Precautions No information available to require special precautions

Effects on Dental Treatment Effects vary with route; many are dose-related (frequency not defined): Bradycardia, hypotension, heart block, arrhythmias, cardiovascular collapse, nausea, vomiting, taste disorder, blurred vision, dyspnea, respiratory depression or arrest, bronchospasm, allergic reaction, anaphylactoid reaction, lightheadedness, dizziness, tinnitus, blurred vision, vomiting, twitching, tremors, lethargy, coma, agitation, slurred speech, seizures, anxiety, euphoria, hallucinations, paresthesia, psychosis, contact dermatitis, heart block, cardiovascular collapse, asystole

Dosage

Topical: Apply to affected area as needed; maximum: 3 mg/kg/dose; do not repeat within 2 hours.

ELA-Max® cream: Apply 1/4 inch thick layer to intact skin. Leave on until adequate anesthetic effect is obtained. Remove cream and cleanse area before beginning procedure.

Injectable local anesthetic: Varies with procedure, degree of anesthesia needed, vascularity of tissue, duration of anesthesia required, and physical condition of patient; maximum: 4.5 mg/kg/dose; do not repeat within 2 hours.

Patch: Postherpetic neuralgia: Apply patch to most painful area. Up to 3 patches may be applied in a single application. Patch may remain in place for up to 12 hours in any 24-hour period.

Antiarrhythmic:

I.V.: 1-1.5 mg/kg bolus over 2-3 minutes; may repeat doses of 0.5-0.75 mg/kg in 5-10 minutes up to a total of 3 mg/kg; continuous infusion: 1-4 mg/minute

I.V. (2 g/250 mL D_5W) infusion rates (infusion pump should be used for I.V. infusion administration):

1 mg/minute: 7.5 mL/hour
2 mg/minute: 15 mL/hour
3 mg/minute: 22.5 mL/hour
4 mg/minute: 30 mL/hour

Ventricular fibrillation (after defibrillation and epinephrine): Initial: 1-1.5 mg/kg. Repeat 0.5-0.75 mg/kg bolus may be given 3-5 minutes after initial dose. Total dose should not exceed 200-300 mg during a 1-hour period or 3 mg/kg total dose. Follow with continuous infusion after return of perfusion.

Endotracheal: 2-2.5 times the I.V. dose (2-4 mg/kg diluted with NS to a total volume of 10 mL)

Dosing adjustment in renal impairment: Not dialyzable (0% to 5%) by hemo- or peritoneal dialysis; supplemental dose is unnecessary.

Dosing adjustment in hepatic impairment: Reduce dose in acute hepatitis and decompensated cirrhosis by 50%.

Mechanism of Action Class Ib antiarrhythmic; suppresses automaticity of conduction tissue, by increasing electrical stimulation threshold of ventricle, His-Purkinje system, and spontaneous depolarization of the ventricles during diastole by a direct action on the tissues; blocks both the initiation and conduction of nerve impulses by decreasing the neuronal membrane's permeability to sodium ions, which results in inhibition of depolarization with resultant blockade of conduction

Other Adverse Effects Effects vary with route; many are dose-related (frequency not always defined):

Cardiovascular: Sinus node supression, increased defibrillator threshold, vascular insufficiency (periarticular injections), arterial spasms

Central nervous system: Drowsiness postdose (usually a sign of high blood level)

Dermatologic: Itching, rash, edema of the skin

Local: Thrombophlebitis

Neuromuscular & skeletal: Transient radicular pain (subarachnoid administration; up to 1.9%)

Ocular: Diplopia

Following spinal anesthesia: Positional headache (3%), shivering (2%) nausea, peripheral nerve symptoms, respiratory inadequacy and double vision (<1%), hypotension, cauda equina syndrome

Postmarketing and/or case reports: **ARDS (inhalation), severe back pain,** methemoglobinemia, asystole

Contraindications Hypersensitivity to lidocaine or any component of the formulation; hypersensitivity to another local anesthetic of the amide type; Adam-Stokes syndrome; severe degrees of SA, AV, or intraventricular heart block (except in patients with a functioning artificial pacemaker)

Warnings/Precautions

Intravenous: Constant EKG monitoring is necessary during I.V. administration. Use cautiously in hepatic impairment, any degree of heart block, Wolff-Parkinson-White syndrome, CHF, marked hypoxia, severe respiratory depression, hypovolemia, history of malignant hyperthermia, or shock. Increased ventricular rate may be seen when administered to a patient with atrial fibrillation. Correct any underlying causes of ventricular arrhythmias. Monitor closely for signs and symptoms of CNS toxicity. The elderly may be prone to increased CNS and cardiovascular side effects. Reduce dose in hepatic dysfunction and CHF.

Injectable anesthetic: Follow appropriate administration techniques so as not to administer any intravascularly. Solutions containing antimicrobial preservatives should not be used for epidural or spinal anesthesia. Some solutions contain a bisulfite; avoid in patients who are allergic to bisulfite. Resuscitative equipment, medicine and oxygen should be available in case of emergency. Use products containing epinephrine cautiously in patients with significant vascular disease, compromised blood flow, or during or following general anesthesia (increased risk of arrhythmias). Adjust the dose for the elderly, pediatric, acutely ill, and debilitated patients.

Topical: ELA-Max® cream: Do not leave on large body areas for >2 hours. Observe young children closely to prevent accidental ingestion. Not for use ophthalmic use or for use on mucous membranes.

Drug Interactions Substrate of CYP1A2, 2A6, 2B6, 2C8/9, **2D6, 3A4**; Inhibits CYP1A2, 2D6

Cimetidine increases lidocaine blood levels; monitor levels or use an alternative H_2 antagonist.

Drugs which inhibit CYP3A4 may increase lidocaine blood levels.

Protease inhibitors like amprenavir and ritonavir may increase lidocaine blood levels.

Propranolol increases lidocaine blood levels.

Dietary/Ethanol/Herb Considerations

Food: Do not eat or drink for 1 hour following oral administration. Avoid grapefruit products; may increase serum concentration/toxicity.

Herb/Nutraceutical: Avoid St John's wort; may decrease serum concentration. Ginger has positive inotropic effects and theoretically could affect antiarrhythmic activity.

Pharmacodynamics/Kinetics

Onset of action: Single bolus dose: 45-90 seconds

Duration: 10-20 minutes

Distribution: V_d: 1.1-2.1 L/kg; alterable by many patient factors; decreased in CHF and liver disease; crosses blood-brain barrier

Protein binding: 60% to 80% to alpha$_1$ acid glycoprotein

Metabolism: 90% hepatic; active metabolites monoethylglycinexylidide (MEGX) and glycinexylidide (GX) can accumulate and may cause CNS toxicity

Half-life elimination: Biphasic: Prolonged with congestive heart failure, liver disease, shock, severe renal disease; Initial: 7-30 minutes; Terminal: Infants, premature: 3.2 hours, Adults: 1.5-2 hours

Pregnancy Risk Factor B (manufacturer); C (expert analysis)

Dosage Forms CRM, rectal (ELA-Max® 5): 5% (30 g). **CRM, topical** (ELA-Max®): 4% (5 g, 30 g). **CRM, topical**, as hydrochloride (LidaMantle®): 3% (30 g). **GEL, topical:** (Burn-O-Jel): 0.5% (90 g); (Topicaine®): 4% (1 g, 10 g, 30 g, 113 g). **GEL, topical**, as hydrochloride: 2% (30 g); (Burn Jel): 2% (3.5 g, 120 g); (Solarcaine® Aloe Extra Burn Relief): 0.5% (226 g). **INF** [premixed in D_5W]: 0.4% [4 mg/mL] (250 mL, 500 mL); 0.8% [8 mg/mL] (250 mL, 500 mL). **INJ, solution**: 0.5% [5 mg/mL] (50 mL); 1% [10 mg/mL] (5 mL, 20 mL, 30 mL, 50 mL); 1.5% [15 mg/mL] (20 mL); 2% [20 mg/mL] (2 mL, 5 mL, 20 mL, 30 mL, 50 mL); (Xylocaine®): 0.5% [5 mg/mL] (50 mL); 1% [10 mg/mL] (10 mL, 20 mL, 50 mL); 2% [20 mg/mL] (1.8 mL, 10 mL, 20 mL, 50 mL); 4% [40 mg/mL] (5 mL). **INJ, solution**, as hydrochloride [preservative free]: 0.5% [5 mg/mL] (50 mL); 1% [10 mg/mL] (2 mL, 5 mL, 30 mL); 1.5% [15 mg/mL] (20 mL); 2% [20 mg/mL] (5 mL, 10 mL); 4% [40 mg/mL] (5 mL); 10% [100 mg/mL] (10 mL); 20% [200 mg/mL] (10 mL); (Xylocaine® MPF): 0.5% [5 mg/mL] (50

(Continued)

Lidocaine *(Continued)*

mL); 1% [10 mg/mL] (2 mL, 5 mL, 10 mL, 20 mL, 30 mL); 1.5% [15 mg/mL] (10 mL, 20 mL); 2% [2 mg/mL] (2 mL, 5 mL, 10 mL); 4% [40 mg/mL] (5 mL). **INJ, solution** [premixed in $D_{7.5}W$; preservative free]: 5% (2 mL); (Xylocaine®-MPF): 1.5% (2 mL). **JELLY, topical:** (Anestacon®): 2% (15 mL, 240 mL); (Xylocaine®): 2% (5 mL, 10 mL, 20 mL, 30 mL). **LIQ, topical** (Zilactin®-L): 2.5% (7.5 mL). **OINT, topical:** 5% (37 g); (Xylocaine®): 2.5% (35 g) [OTC]; 5% (3.5 g, 35 g). **PATCH, transdermal** (Lidoderm®): 5% (30s). **SOLN, topical:** 2% [20 mg/mL] (15 mL, 240 mL); 4% [40 mg/mL] (50 mL); (Band-Aid® Hurt-Free™ Antiseptic Wash): 2% (180 mL); (Xylocaine®): 4% [40 mg/mL] (50 mL). **SOLN, viscous:** 2% [20 mg/mL] (20 mL, 100 mL); (Xylocaine® Viscous): 2% [20 mg/mL] (20 mL, 100 mL, 450 mL). **SPRAY, topical:** (Burnamycin): 0.5% (60 mL); (Premjact®): 9.6% (13 mL); (Solarcaine® Aloe Extra Burn Relief): 0.5% (127 g)

Generic Available Yes: Gel, injection, ointment, solution

Comments Lidocaine without epinephrine is not marketed as a dental 1.8 mL carpule, and as such, is not used as a dental local anesthetic.

Lidocaine and Epinephrine (LYE doe kane & ep i NEF rin)

Related Information

Epinephrine *on page 499*
Lidocaine *on page 801*
Oral Pain *on page 1524*

U.S. Brand Names Xylocaine® MPF With Epinephrine; Xylocaine® With Epinephrine

Canadian Brand Names Xylocaine® With Epinephrine

Mexican Brand Names Pisacaina; Uvega; Xylocaina

Pharmacologic Category Local Anesthetic, Dental; Local Anesthetic

Synonyms Epinephrine and Lidocaine

Use

Dental: Amide-type anesthetic used for local infiltration anesthesia; injection near nerve trunks to produce nerve block

Medical: Local infiltration anesthesia; AVS for nerve block

Local Anesthetic/Vasoconstrictor Precautions No information available to require special precautions

Effects on Dental Treatment It is common to misinterpret psychogenic responses to local anesthetic injection as an allergic reaction. Intraoral injections are perceived by many patients as a stressful procedure in dentistry. Common symptoms to this stress are diaphoresis, palpitations, hyperventilation, generalized pallor and a fainting feeling.

Degree of adverse effects in the CNS and cardiovascular system is directly related to the blood levels of lidocaine (frequency not defined; more likely to occur after systemic administration rather than infiltration): Bradycardia and reduction in cardiac output, nausea, vomiting

High blood levels: Anxiety, restlessness, disorientation, confusion, dizziness, tremors and seizures, followed by CNS depression resulting in somnolence, unconsciousness and possible respiratory arrest. In some cases, symptoms of CNS stimulation may be absent and the primary CNS effects are somnolence and unconsciousness.

Dosage Dosage varies with the anesthetic procedure, degree of anesthesia needed, vascularity of tissue, duration of anesthesia required, and physical condition of patient.

Dental anesthesia, infiltration, or conduction block:

Children <10 years: 20-30 mg (1-1.5 mL) of lidocaine hydrochloride as a 2% solution with epinephrine 1:100,000; maximum: 4-5 mg of lidocaine hydrochloride/kg of body weight or 100-150 mg as a single dose

Children >10 years and Adults: Do not exceed 6.6 mg/kg body weight or 300 mg of lidocaine hydrochloride and 3 mcg (0.003 mg) of epinephrine/kg of body

# of Cartridges (1.8 mL)	Lidocaine (2%) (mg)	Epinephrine 1:100,000 (mg)
1	36	0.018
2	72	0.036
3	108	0.054
4	144	0.072
5	180	0.090
6	216	0.108
7	252	0.126
8	288	0.144
9	324	0.162
10	360	0.180

weight or 0.2 mg epinephrine per dental appointment. The effective anesthetic dose varies with procedure, intensity of anesthesia needed, duration of anesthesia required, and physical condition of the patient. Always use the lowest effective dose along with careful aspiration.

The following numbers of dental carpules (1.8 mL) provide the indicated amounts of lidocaine hydrochloride 2% and epinephrine 1:100,000 (see table on previous page)

For most routine dental procedures, lidocaine hydrochloride 2% with epinephrine 1:100,000 is preferred. When a more pronounced hemostasis is required, a 1:50,000 epinephrine concentration should be used. The following numbers of dental carpules (1.8 mL) provide the indicated amounts of lidocaine hydrochloride 2% and epinephrine 1:50,000 (see table):

# of Cartridges (1.8 mL)	Lidocaine (2%) (mg)	Epinephrine 1:50,000 (mg)
1	36	0.036
2	72	0.072
3	108	0.108
4	144	0.144
5	180	0.180
6	216	0.216

Mechanism of Action Lidocaine blocks both the initiation and conduction of nerve impulses via decreased permeability of sodium ions; epinephrine increases the duration of action of lidocaine by causing vasoconstriction (via alpha effects) which slows the vascular absorption of lidocaine

Contraindications Hypersensitivity to local anesthetics of the amide type or any component of the formulation; myasthenia gravis; shock; cardiac conduction disease; also see individual agents

Warnings/Precautions Should be avoided in patients with uncontrolled hyperthyroidism. Should be used in minimal amounts in patients with significant cardiovascular problems (because of epinephrine component). Aspirate the syringe after tissue penetration and before injection to minimize chance of direct vascular injection.

Drug Interactions Lidocaine: Substrate of CYP1A2, 2A6, 2B6, 2C8/9, **2D6, 3A4**; Inhibits CYP1A2, 2D6

Epinephrine (and other direct alpha-agonists): Pressor response to I.V. epinephrine, norepinephrine, and phenylephrine may be enhanced in patients receiving TCAs (**Note:** Effect is unlikely with epinephrine or levonordefrin dosages typically administered as infiltration in combination with local anesthetics)

Pharmacodynamics/Kinetics

Onset of action: Peak effect: ~5 minutes

Duration: ~2 hours; dose and anesthetic procedure dependent

Pregnancy Risk Factor B

Breast-feeding Considerations Usual infiltration doses of lidocaine with epinephrine given to nursing mothers has not been shown to affect the health of the nursing infant.

Dosage Forms **INJ, solution**, with epinephrine 1:50,000 (Xylocaine® with Epinephrine): Lidocaine 2% [20 mg/mL] (1.8 mL). **INJ, solution**, with epinephrine 1:100,000: Lidocaine 1% [10 mg/mL] (20 mL, 30 mL, 50 mL); Lidocaine 2% (20 mL, 30 mL, 50 mL); (Xylocaine® with Epinephrine): Lidocaine 1% [10 mg/mL] (10 mL 20 mL, 50 mL); Lidocaine 2% (1.8 mL, 10 mL, 20 mL, 50 mL). **INJ, solution**, with epinephrine 1:200,000: Lidocaine 0.5% [5 mg/mL] (50 mL); (Xylocaine® with Epinephrine): Lidocaine 0.5% [5 mg/mL] (50 mL). **INJ, solution**, with epinephrine 1:200,000 [methylparaben free]: Lidocaine 1% [10 mg/mL] (30 mL); Lidocaine 1.5% (5 mL, 30 mL); Lidocaine 2% (20 mL); (Xylocaine® MPF with Epinephrine): Lidocaine 1% [10 mg/mL] (5 mL, 10 mL, 30 mL); 1.5% [15 mg/mL] (5 mL, 10 mL, 30 mL); Lidocaine 2% [20 mg/mL] (5 mL, 10 mL, 20 mL)

Generic Available Yes

Selected Readings

Ayoub ST and Coleman AE, "A Review of Local Anesthetics," *Gen Dent*, 1992, 40(4):285-7, 289-90.

Jastak JT and Yagiela JA, "Vasoconstrictors and Local Anesthesia: A Review and Rationale for Use," *J Am Dent Assoc*, 1983, 107(4):623-30.

MacKenzie TA and Young ER, "Local Anesthetic Update," *Anesth Prog*, 1993, 40(2):29-34.

Wynn RL, "Epinephrine Interactions With Beta-Blockers," *Gen Dent*, 1994, 42(1):16, 18.

Wynn RL, "Recent Research on Mechanisms of Local Anesthetics," *Gen Dent*, 1995, 43(4):316-8.

Yagiela JA, "Local Anesthetics," *Anesth Prog*, 1991, 38(4-5):128-41.

Lidocaine and Hydrocortisone

(LYE doe kane & hye droe KOR ti sone)

Related Information

Hydrocortisone *on page 688*

Lidocaine *on page 801*

U.S. Brand Names Lida-Mantle HC®

Pharmacologic Category Anesthetic/Corticosteroid

(Continued)

Lidocaine and Hydrocortisone *(Continued)*

Synonyms Hydrocortisone and Lidocaine

Use Topical anti-inflammatory and anesthetic for skin disorders

Local Anesthetic/Vasoconstrictor Precautions No information available to require special precautions

Effects on Dental Treatment No significant effects or complications reported

Dosage Topical: Apply 2-4 times/day

Pregnancy Risk Factor B (lidocaine); C (hydrocortisone)

Generic Available No

Lidocaine and Prilocaine (LYE doe kane & PRIL oh kane)

Related Information

Lidocaine *on page 801*

Prilocaine *on page 1114*

U.S. Brand Names EMLA®

Canadian Brand Names EMLA®

Pharmacologic Category Local Anesthetic, Dental; Local Anesthetic

Synonyms Prilocaine and Lidocaine

Use

Dental: Amide-type topical anesthetic for use on normal intact skin to provide local analgesia for minor procedures such as I.V. cannulation or venipuncture

Medical: Topical anesthetic for lumbar puncture, skin graft harvesting, superficial minor surgery of genital mucous membranes, and local anesthesia on normal skin; adjunct for local infiltration anesthesia in genital mucous membranes

Local Anesthetic/Vasoconstrictor Precautions No information available to require special precautions

Effects on Dental Treatment Frequency not defined: Hypotension, shock, bronchospasm, alteration in temperature sensation, hypersensitivity reactions, application site reactions (burning, stinging, edema)

Dosage Although the incidence of systemic adverse effects with EMLA® is very low, caution should be exercised, particularly when applying over large areas and leaving on for >2 hours. Dermal analgesia can be expected to increase for up to 3 hours under occlusive dressing and persist for 1-2 hours after removal of the cream. EMLA® should **not** be used in neonates with a gestation age <37 weeks nor in infants <12 months of age who are receiving treatment with methemoglobin-inducing agents. Children's dosing is based on age and weight. If a patient greater than 3 months old does not meet the minimum weight requirement, the maximum total dose should be restricted to the corresponding maximum based on patient weight.

Children (intact skin):

Age 0-3 months or <5 kg: Apply a maximum of 1 g over no more than 10 cm^2 of skin; leave on for no longer than 1 hour

Age 3 months to 12 months and >5 kg: Apply no more than a maximum 2 g total over no more than 20 cm^2 of skin; leave on for no longer than 4 hours

Age 1-6 years and >10 kg: Apply no more than a maximum of 10 g total over no more than 100 cm^2 of skin; leave on for no longer than 4 hours.

Age 7-12 years and >20 kg: Apply no more than a maximum 20 g total over no more than 200 cm^2 of skin; leave on for no longer than 4 hours.

Adults (intact skin):

EMLA® cream and EMLA® anesthetic disc: A thick layer of EMLA® cream is applied and covered with an occlusive dressing, or alternatively, an EMLA® anesthetic disc is applied.

Minor dermal procedures (eg, I.V. cannulation or venipuncture): Apply 2.5 g of cream (1/2 of the 5 g tube) over 20-25 cm of skin surface area, or 1 anesthetic disc (1 g over 10 cm^2) for at least 1 hour (In clinical trials, 2 sites were usually prepared in case there was a technical problem with cannulation or venipuncture at the first site.)

Major dermal procedures (eg, more painful dermatological procedures involving a larger skin area such as split thickness skin graft harvesting): Apply 2 g of cream per 10 cm^2 of skin and allow to remain in contact with the skin for at least 2 hours.

Adult male genital skin (eg, pretreatment prior to local anesthetic infiltration): Apply a thick layer of cream (1 g/10 cm^2) to the skin surface for 15 minutes. Local anesthetic infiltration should be performed immediately after removal of EMLA® cream.

Adult females: Genital mucous membranes: Minor procedures (eg, removal of condylomata acuminata, pretreatment for local anesthetic infiltration): Apply 5-10 g (thick layer) of cream for 5-10 minutes

Mechanism of Action Local anesthetic action occurs by stabilization of neuronal membranes and inhibiting the ionic fluxes required for the initiation and conduction of impulses

Other Adverse Effects Frequency not defined:

Dermatologic: Hyperpigmentation, erythema, itching, rash, burning, urticaria, angioedema

Genitourinary: Blistering of foreskin (rare)

Contraindications

Hypersensitivity to amide type anesthetic agents [ie, lidocaine, prilocaine, dibucaine, mepivacaine, bupivacaine, etidocaine]; hypersensitivity to any component of the formulation selected; application on mucous membranes or broken or inflamed skin; infants <1 month of age if gestational age is <37 weeks; infants <12 months of age receiving therapy with methemoglobin-inducing agents; children with congenital or idiopathic methemoglobinemia, or in children who are receiving medications associated with drug-induced methemoglobinemia [ie, acetaminophen (overdosage), benzocaine, chloroquine, dapsone, nitrofurantoin, nitroglycerin, nitroprusside, phenazopyridine, phenelzine, phenobarbital, phenytoin, quinine, sulfonamides]

Warnings/Precautions Use with caution in patients receiving class I antiarrhythmic drugs, since systemic absorption occurs and synergistic toxicity is possible. Although the incidence of systemic adverse reactions with EMLA® is very low, caution should be exercised, particularly when applying over large areas and leaving on for longer than 2 hours.

Drug Interactions Lidocaine: Substrate of CYP1A2, 2A6, 2B6, 2C8/9, **2D6, 3A4**; Inhibits CYP1A2, 2D6

Increased toxicity with drugs known to induce methemoglobinemia. Effects of Class I antiarrhythmic drugs (tocainide, mexiletine) are additive and potentially synergistic.

Pharmacodynamics/Kinetics

EMLA®:

Onset of action: 1 hour

Peak effect: 2-3 hours

Duration: 1-2 hours after removal

Absorption: Related to duration of application and area where applied

3-hour application: 3.6% lidocaine and 6.1% prilocaine

24-hour application: 16.2% lidocaine and 33.5% prilocaine

Pregnancy Risk Factor B

Breast-feeding Considerations Usual infiltration doses of lidocaine and prilocaine given to nursing mothers has not been shown to affect the health of the nursing infant.

Dosage Forms CRM, topical: Lidocaine 2.5% and prilocaine 2.5% (5 g, 30 g).

DISC, topical: 1 g (2s, 10s)

Generic Available No

Selected Readings

Broadman LM, Soliman IE, Hannallah RS, et al, "Analgesic Efficacy of Eutectic Mixture of Local Anesthetics (EMLA®) vs Intradermal Infiltration Prior to Venous Cannulation in Children," *Am J Anaesth*, 1987, 34:S56.

Halperin DL, Koren G, Attias D, et al, "Topical Skin Anesthesia for Venous Subcutaneous Drug Reservoir and Lumbar Puncture in Children," *Pediatrics*, 1989, 84(2):281-4.

Robieux I, Kumar R, Radhakrishnan S, et al, "Assessing Pain and Analgesia With a Lidocaine-Prilocaine Emulsion in Infants and Toddlers During Venipuncture," *J Pediatr*, 1991, 118(6):971-3.

Taddio A, Shennan AT, Stevens B, et al, "Safety of Lidocaine-Prilocaine Cream in the Treatment of Preterm Neonates," *J Pediatr*, 1995, 127(6):1002-5.

Vickers ER, Mazbani N, Gerzina TM, et al, "Pharmacokinetics of EMLA Cream 5% Application to Oral Mucosa," *Anesth Prog*, 1997, 44:32-7.

Lidocaine Hydrochloride *see* Lidocaine *on page 801*

Lidocaine (Transoral) (LYE doe kane trans OR al)

Related Information

Lidocaine *on page 801*

Oral Pain *on page 1524*

U.S. Brand Names DentiPatch®

Pharmacologic Category Local Anesthetic, Dental; Local Anesthetic, Transoral

Use Dental: Local anesthesia of the oral mucosa prior to oral injections and soft-tissue dental procedures

Local Anesthetic/Vasoconstrictor Precautions No information available to require special precautions

Effects on Dental Treatment No significant effects or complications reported

Dosage Apply one patch on selected area of oral mucosa.

According to the manufacturer, tips for applying lidocaine patch are the following:

Cotton roll isolation for all procedures except palatal application

Air dry with syringe on dental unit for 30 seconds

Apply patch to gingiva or mucosa

Apply firm finger pressure to patch for 30 seconds

Leave patch in place during scaling and root planing procedure; remove after 15 minutes. Patch should be removed after 5-10 minutes prior to giving injection.

Mechanism of Action Blocks both the initiation and conduction of nerve impulses by decreasing the neuronal membrane's permeability to sodium ions, which results in inhibition of depolarization with resultant blockade of conduction

Contraindications Hypersensitivity to lidocaine or any of component of the formulation

(Continued)

Lidocaine (Transoral) *(Continued)*

Pharmacodynamics/Kinetics

Onset of action: 2 minutes

Duration: Anesthesia: 40 minutes after 15-minute wear period

Dosage Forms PATCH: 23 mg/2 cm^2; 46.1 mg/2 cm^2 [50s, 100s]

Generic Available No

Comments Peak plasma levels were 10% of those seen following local infiltration anesthesia with 1.8 mL lidocaine and 1:100,000 epinephrine.

The manufacturer claims DentiPatch® is safe, with "negligible systemic absorption" of lidocaine. The agent is "clinically proven to prevent injection pain from 25-gauge needles that are inserted to the level of the bone." Data from controlled studies (235 patients) have shown no serious adverse effects with the application of lidocaine patch to the oral mucosa for 15 minutes.

Selected Readings

Hersh EV, Houpt MI, Cooper SA, et al, "Analgesic Efficacy and Safety of an Intraoral Lidocaine Patch," *J Am Dent Assoc*, 1996, 127(11):1626-34.

Houpt MI, Heins P, Lamster I, et al, "An Evaluation of Intraoral Lidocaine Patches in Reducing Needle-Insertion Pain," *Compend Contin Educ Dent*, 1997, 18(4):309-10, 312-4, 316.

"The Lidocaine Patch: A New Delivery System," *Biolog Ther Dent*, 1997, 13:17-22.

Lidoderm® *see* Lidocaine *on page 801*

Lignocaine Hydrochloride *see* Lidocaine *on page 801*

Limbitrol® *see* Amitriptyline and Chlordiazepoxide *on page 85*

Limbitrol® DS *see* Amitriptyline and Chlordiazepoxide *on page 85*

Lincocin® *see* Lincomycin *on page 808*

Lincomycin (lin koe MYE sin)

U.S. Brand Names Lincocin®

Canadian Brand Names Lincocin®

Mexican Brand Names Lincocin®; Princol®; Rimsalin®

Pharmacologic Category Antibiotic, Macrolide

Synonyms Lincomycin Hydrochloride

Use Treatment of susceptible bacterial infections, mainly those caused by streptococci and staphylococci resistant to other agents

Local Anesthetic/Vasoconstrictor Precautions No information available to require special precautions

Effects on Dental Treatment No significant effects or complications reported

Dosage

Children >1 month:

- Oral: 30-60 mg/kg/day in divided doses every 8 hours
- I.M.: 10 mg/kg every 8-12 hours
- I.V.: 10-20 mg/kg/day in divided doses every 8-12 hours

Adults:

- Oral: 500 mg every 6-8 hours
- I.M.: 600 mg every 12-24 hours
- I.V.: 600-1 g every 8-12 hours up to 8 g/day

Dosing interval in renal impairment:

- Cl_{cr} 10-50 mL/minute: Administer every 6-12 hours
- Cl_{cr} <10 mL/minute: Administer every 12 hours

Dosing adjustment in hepatic impairment: Reductions are indicated; specific guidelines unavailable

Mechanism of Action Lincosamide antibiotic which was isolated from a strain of *Streptomyces lincolnensis*; lincomycin, like clindamycin, inhibits bacterial protein synthesis by specifically binding on the 50S subunit and affecting the process of peptide chain initiation. Other macrolide antibiotics (erythromycin) also bind to the 50S subunit. Since only one molecule of antibiotic can bind to a single ribosome, the concomitant use of erythromycin and lincomycin is not recommended.

Other Adverse Effects Frequency not defined:

Central nervous system: Vertigo

Dermatologic: Vesiculobullous dermatitis (rare)

Gastrointestinal: Nausea, vomiting, diarrhea

Hematologic: Pancytopenia (rare)

Miscellaneous: Serum sickness (rare)

Drug Interactions

Increased effect/toxicity of neuromuscular blocking agents.

Decreased effect with erythromycin.

Dietary/Ethanol/Herb Considerations Food may decrease absorption.

Pharmacodynamics/Kinetics

Absorption: Oral: ~20% to 30%

Half-life elimination, serum: 2-11.5 hours

Time to peak, serum: Oral: 2-4 hours; I.M.: 1 hour

Pregnancy Risk Factor B

Generic Available No

Lincomycin Hydrochloride *see* Lincomycin *on page 808*

Lindane (LIN dane)

Canadian Brand Names Hexit™; PMS-Lindane

Mexican Brand Names Herklin; Herklin Shampoo®; Scabisan®; Scabisan Shampoo

Pharmacologic Category Antiparasitic Agent, Topical; Pediculocide; Scabicidal Agent

Synonyms Benzene Hexachloride; Gamma Benzene Hexachloride; Hexachlorocyclohexane

Use Treatment of scabies (*Sarcoptes scabiei*), *Pediculus capitis* (head lice), and *Pediculus pubis* (crab lice); FDA recommends reserving lindane as a second-line agent or with inadequate response to other therapies

Local Anesthetic/Vasoconstrictor Precautions No information available to require special precautions

Effects on Dental Treatment No significant effects or complications reported

Dosage Children and Adults: Topical:

Scabies: Apply a thin layer of lotion and massage it on skin from the neck to the toes (head to toe in infants). For adults, bathe and remove the drug after 8-12 hours; for children, wash off 6-8 hours after application (for infants, wash off 6 hours after application); repeat treatment in 7 days if lice or nits are still present

Pediculosis, capitis and pubis: 15-30 mL of shampoo is applied and lathered for 4-5 minutes; rinse hair thoroughly and comb with a fine tooth comb to remove nits; repeat treatment in 7 days if lice or nits are still present

Mechanism of Action Directly absorbed by parasites and ova through the exoskeleton; stimulates the nervous system resulting in seizures and death of parasitic arthropods

Other Adverse Effects <1% (Limited to important or life-threatening): Aplastic anemia, ataxia, burning and stinging, **arrhythmia**, contact dermatitis, **dizziness**, eczematous eruptions, **headache**, hematuria, hepatitis, nausea, pulmonary edema, **restlessness, seizures**, skin and adipose tissue may act as repositories, vomiting

Drug Interactions Increased Effect/Toxicity: Oil-based hair dressing may increase potential for toxicity of lindane.

Pharmacodynamics/Kinetics

Absorption: ≤13% systemically

Distribution: Stored in body fat; accumulates in brain; skin and adipose tissue may act as repositories

Metabolism: Hepatic

Half-life elimination: Children: 17-22 hours

Time to peak, serum: Children: 6 hours

Excretion: Urine and feces

Pregnancy Risk Factor B

Generic Available Yes

Linezolid (li NE zoe lid)

U.S. Brand Names Zyvox™

Canadian Brand Names Zyvoxam®

Pharmacologic Category Antibiotic, Oxazolidinone

Use Treatment of vancomycin-resistant *Enterococcus faecium* (VRE) infections, nosocomial pneumonia caused by *Staphylococcus aureus* including MRSA or *Streptococcus pneumoniae* (penicillin-susceptible strains only), complicated and uncomplicated skin and skin structure infections, and community-acquired pneumonia caused by susceptible gram-positive organisms.

Local Anesthetic/Vasoconstrictor Precautions Linezolid has mild monoamine oxidase inhibitor properties. The clinician is reminded that vasoconstrictors have the potential to interact with MAOIs to result in elevation of blood pressure. Caution is suggested.

Effects on Dental Treatment

>10%: Headache (≤11%)

1% to 10%: Hypertension (1% to 3%), fever (2%), nausea (3% to 10%), vomiting (1% to 4%)

≤2%: Oral moniliasis, taste alteration, tongue discoloration, dizziness (≤2%), fungal infections (≤2%)

Dosage

VRE infections: Oral, I.V.:

Infants (excluding preterm neonates <1 week) and Children ≤11 years: 10 mg/kg every 8 hours for 14-28 days

Children ≥12 years and Adults: 600 mg every 12 hours for 14-28 days

Nosocomial pneumonia, complicated skin and skin structure infections, community acquired pneumonia including concurrent bacteremia: Oral, I.V.:

Infants (excluding preterm neonates <1 week) and Children ≤11 years: 10 mg/kg every 8 hours for 10-14 days

Children ≥12 years and Adults: 600 mg every 12 hours for 10-14 days

Uncomplicated skin and skin structure infections: Oral:

Infants (excluding preterm neonates <1 week) and Children <5 years: 10 mg/kg every 8 hours for 10-14 days

(Continued)

Linezolid *(Continued)*

Children 5-11 years: 10 mg/kg every 12 hours for 10-14 days
Children ≥12-18 years: 600 mg every 12 hours for 10-14 days
Adults: 400 mg every 12 hours for 10-14 days

Mechanism of Action Inhibits bacterial protein synthesis by binding to bacterial 23S ribosomal RNA of the 50S subunit. This prevents the formation of a functional 70S initiation complex that is essential for the bacterial translation process. Linezolid is bacteriostatic against enterococci and staphylococci and bactericidal against most strains of streptococci.

Other Adverse Effects As reported in adults; frequency similar in pediatric patients:

1% to 10%:

Central nervous system: Insomnia (3%)
Dermatologic: Rash (2%)
Gastrointestinal: Diarrhea (3% to 11%), constipation (2%), pancreatitis
Genitourinary: Vaginal moniliasis (1% to 2%)
Hematologic: Thrombocytopenia (0.3% to 10%), anemia, leukopenia, neutropenia
Hepatic: Abnormal LFTs (0.4% to 1%)

<1%: *C. difficile*-related complications, increase in creatinine, dyspepsia, localized abdominal pain, pruritus

Postmarketing and/or case reports: Lactic acidosis, myelosuppression (including anemia, leukopenia, pancytopenia, and thrombocytopenia; may be more common in patients receiving linezolid for >2 weeks)

Drug Interactions Increased Effect/Toxicity: Linezolid is a reversible, nonselective inhibitor of MAO. Serotonergic agents (eg, TCAs, venlafaxine, trazodone, sibutramine, meperidine, dextromethorphan, and SSRIs) may cause a serotonin syndrome (eg, hyperpyrexia, cognitive dysfunction) when used concomitantly. Adrenergic agents (eg, phenylpropanolamine, pseudoephedrine, sympathomimetic agents, vasopressor or dopaminergic agents) may cause hypertension. Tramadol may increase the risk of seizures when used concurrently with linezolid. Myelosuppressive medications may increase risk of myelosuppression when used concurrently with linezolid.

Dietary/Ethanol/Herb Considerations

Ethanol: Avoid use; may contain tyramine (eg, wine) resulting in hypertensive crisis.

Food: May be taken with food; avoid caffeine (eg, colas, chocolate). Avoid food/beverages high in tyramine (eg, avocadoes, bananas, broad bean pods, canned figs, cheese, chicken liver, pickled herring, raisins, sour cream, soy sauce, yeast extracts, yogurt, pods, meats prepared with tenderizers, and foods aged to improve flavor); may cause sudden and severe high BP.

Pharmacodynamics/Kinetics

Absorption: Rapid and extensive
Distribution: V_{dss}: Adults: 40-50 L
Protein binding: Adults: 31%
Metabolism: Hepatic via oxidation of the morpholine ring, resulting in two inactive metabolites (aminoethoxyacetic acid, hydroxyethyl glycine); does not involve CYP
Bioavailability: 100%
Half-life elimination: Children ≥1 week (full-term) to 11 years: 1.5-3 hours; Adults: 4-5 hours
Time to peak: Adults: Oral: 1-2 hours
Excretion: Urine (30% as parent drug, 50% as metabolites); feces (9% as metabolites)
Nonrenal clearance: 65%; increased in children ≥1 week to 11 years

Pregnancy Risk Factor C

Generic Available No

Lioresal® *see* Baclofen *on page 158*

Liothyronine (lye oh THYE roe neen)

Related Information

Endocrine Disorders and Pregnancy *on page 1479*

U.S. Brand Names Cytomel®; Triostat®

Canadian Brand Names Cytomel®

Mexican Brand Names Triyotex®

Pharmacologic Category Thyroid Product

Synonyms Liothyronine Sodium; Sodium *L*-Triiodothyronine; T_3 Sodium

Use

Oral: Replacement or supplemental therapy in hypothyroidism; management of nontoxic goiter; a diagnostic aid

I.V.: Treatment of myxedema coma/precoma

Local Anesthetic/Vasoconstrictor Precautions No precautions with vasoconstrictor are necessary if patient is well controlled with liothyronine

Effects on Dental Treatment 1% to 10%: Arrhythmia (6%), tachycardia (3%), cardiopulmonary arrest (2%), hypotension (2%), MI (2%)

Dosage Doses should be adjusted based on clinical response and laboratory parameters.

Children: Congenital hypothyroidism: Oral: 5 mcg/day increase by 5 mcg every 3-4 days until the desired response is achieved. Usual maintenance dose: 20 mcg/day for infants, 50 mcg/day for children 1-3 years of age, and adult dose for children >3 years.

Adults:

Hypothyroidism: Oral: 25 mcg/day increase by increments of 12.5-25 mcg/day every 1-2 weeks to a maximum of 100 mcg/day; usual maintenance dose: 25-75 mcg/day.

Patients with cardiovascular disease: Refer to Elderly dosing.

T_3 suppression test: Oral: 75-100 mcg/day for 7 days; use lowest dose for elderly

Myxedema: Oral: Initial: 5 mcg/day; increase in increments of 5-10 mcg/day every 1-2 weeks. When 25 mcg/day is reached, dosage may be increased at intervals of 5-25 mcg/day every 1-2 weeks. Usual maintenance dose: 50-100 mcg/day.

Myxedema coma: I.V.: 25-50 mcg

Patients with known or suspected cardiovascular disease: 10-20 mcg

Note: Normally, at least 4 hours should be allowed between doses to adequately assess therapeutic response and no more than 12 hours should elapse between doses to avoid fluctuations in hormone levels. Oral therapy should be resumed as soon as the clinical situation has been stabilized and the patient is able to take oral medication. If levothyroxine rather than liothyronine sodium is used in initiating oral therapy, the physician should bear in mind that there is a delay of several days in the onset of levothyroxine activity and that I.V. therapy should be discontinued gradually.

Simple (nontoxic) goiter: Oral: Initial: 5 mcg/day; increase by 5-10 mcg every 1-2 weeks; after 25 mcg/day is reached, may increase dose by 12.5-25 mcg. Usual maintenance dose: 75 mcg/day

Elderly: Oral: 5 mcg/day; increase by 5 mcg/day every 2 weeks

Mechanism of Action Exact mechanism of action is unknown; however, it is believed the thyroid hormone exerts its many metabolic effects through control of DNA transcription and protein synthesis; involved in normal metabolism, growth, and development; promotes gluconeogenesis, increases utilization and mobilization of glycogen stores, and stimulates protein synthesis, increases basal metabolic rate

Other Adverse Effects <1%: Allergic skin reactions, **angina, CHF, fever, hypertension**, phlebitis, **twitching**

Drug Interactions

Increased Effect/Toxicity: Thyroid products may potentiate the hypoprothrombinemic effect of warfarin (and other oral anticoagulants). Tricyclic antidepressants (TCAs) may increase potential for toxicity of both drugs. Coadministration with ketamine may lead to hypertension and tachycardia.

Decreased Effect: Some medications may decrease absorption of liothyronine: Cholestyramine, colestipol (separate administration by at least 2 hours); aluminum- and magnesium-containing antacids, iron preparations, sucralfate, Kayexalate® (separate administration by at least 4 hours). Enzyme inducers (phenytoin, phenobarbital, carbamazepine, and rifampin/rifabutin) may decrease thyroid hormone levels. Thyroid hormone may decrease effect of oral sulfonylureas. Serum levels of digoxin and theophylline may be altered by thyroid function. Estrogens may decrease serum free-thyroxine concentrations.

Dietary/Ethanol/Herb Considerations Food: Limit intake of goitrogenic foods (asparagus, cabbage, peas, turnip greens, broccoli, spinach, Brussels sprouts, lettuce, soybeans).

Pharmacodynamics/Kinetics

Onset of action: 2-4 hours

Peak response: 2-3 days

Absorption: Oral: Well absorbed (95% in 4 hours)

Half-life elimination: 2.5 days

Excretion: Urine

Pregnancy Risk Factor A

Generic Available No

Liothyronine Sodium *see* Liothyronine *on page 810*

Liotrix (LYE oh triks)

Related Information

Endocrine Disorders and Pregnancy *on page 1479*

U.S. Brand Names Thyrolar®

Canadian Brand Names Thyrolar®

Pharmacologic Category Thyroid Product

Synonyms T_3/T_4 Liotrix

(Continued)

Liotrix *(Continued)*

Use Replacement or supplemental therapy in hypothyroidism (uniform mixture of T_4:T_3 in 4:1 ratio by weight); little advantage to this product exists and cost is not justified

Local Anesthetic/Vasoconstrictor Precautions No precautions with vasoconstrictor are necessary if patient is well controlled with liotrix

Effects on Dental Treatment Frequency not defined: Palpitations, cardiac arrhythmias, tachycardia, chest pain, nervousness, headache, fever, vomiting, tremors, dyspnea, diaphoresis

Dosage Oral:

Congenital hypothyroidism:

Children (dose of T_4 or levothyroxine/day):

0-6 months: 8-10 mcg/kg or 25-50 mcg/day

6-12 months: 6-8 mcg/kg or 50-75 mcg/day

1-5 years: 5-6 mcg/kg or 75-100 mcg/day

6-12 years: 4-5 mcg/kg or 100-150 mcg/day

>12 years: 2-3 mcg/kg or >150 mcg/day

Hypothyroidism (dose of thyroid equivalent):

Adults: 30 mg/day (15 mg/day if cardiovascular impairment), increasing by increments of 15 mg/day at 2- to 3-week intervals to a maximum of 180 mg/day (usual maintenance dose: 60-120 mg/day)

Elderly: Initial: 15 mg, adjust dose at 2- to 4-week intervals by increments of 15 mg

Mechanism of Action The primary active compound is T_3 (triiodothyronine), which may be converted from T_4 (thyroxine) and then circulates throughout the body to influence growth and maturation of various tissues. Liotrix is uniform mixture of synthetic T_4 and T_3 in 4:1 ratio; exact mechanism of action is unknown; however, it is believed the thyroid hormone exerts its many metabolic effects through control of DNA transcription and protein synthesis; involved in normal metabolism, growth, and development; promotes gluconeogenesis, increases utilization and mobilization of glycogen stores and stimulates protein synthesis, increases basal metabolic rate

Other Adverse Effects Frequency not defined:

Central nervous system: Insomnia, ataxia

Dermatologic: Alopecia

Endocrine & metabolic: Changes in menstrual cycle, weight loss, increased appetite

Gastrointestinal: Diarrhea, abdominal cramps, constipation

Neuromuscular & skeletal: Myalgia, hand tremors

Miscellaneous: Allergic skin reactions (rare)

Drug Interactions

Increased Effect/Toxicity: Thyroid products may potentiate the hypoprothrombinemic effect of warfarin (and other oral anticoagulants). Effect of warfarin may be dramatically increased when thyroid is added. However, the addition of warfarin in a patient previously receiving a stable dose of thyroid hormone does not require a significantly different dosing strategy. Tricyclic antidepressants (TCAs) may increase potential for toxicity of both drugs. Excessive thyroid replacement in patients receiving growth hormone may lead to accelerated epiphyseal closure; inadequate replacement interferes with growth response. Coadministration with ketamine may lead to hypertension and tachycardia.

Decreased Effect: Aluminum- and magnesium-containing antacids, iron preparations, sucralfate, cholestyramine, colestipol, and Kayexalate® may decrease absorption (separate administration by 8 hours). Enzyme inducers (phenytoin, phenobarbital, carbamazepine, and rifampin/rifabutin) may decrease thyroid hormone levels. Thyroid hormone may decrease effect of oral sulfonylureas. Dosage of thyroid hormone may need to be increased when SSRIs are added. Serum levels of digoxin and theophylline may be altered by thyroid function.

Pharmacodynamics/Kinetics

Absorption: 50% to 95%

Metabolism: Partially hepatic, renal, and in intestines

Half-life elimination: 6-7 days

Time to peak, serum: 12-48 hours

Excretion: Partially feces (as conjugated metabolites)

Pregnancy Risk Factor A

Generic Available No

Lipancreatin *see* Pancrelipase *on page 1030*

Lipitor® *see* Atorvastatin *on page 140*

Liposyn® III *see* Fat Emulsion *on page 558*

Lipram 4500 *see* Pancrelipase *on page 1030*

Lipram-CR *see* Pancrelipase *on page 1030*

Lipram-PN *see* Pancrelipase *on page 1030*

Lipram-UL *see* Pancrelipase *on page 1030*

Liquibid® *see* Guaifenesin *on page 650*

Liquibid® 1200 *see* Guaifenesin *on page 650*
Liquibid-D *see* Guaifenesin and Phenylephrine *on page 652*
Liqui-Char® [OTC] *see* Charcoal *on page 294*
Liquid Antidote *see* Charcoal *on page 294*
Liquifilm® Tears [OTC] *see* Artificial Tears *on page 128*
Liquiprin® for Children [OTC] *see* Acetaminophen *on page 27*

Lisinopril (lyse IN oh pril)

Related Information
Cardiovascular Diseases *on page 1456*

U.S. Brand Names Prinivil®; Zestril®

Canadian Brand Names Apo®-Lisinopril; Prinivil®; Zestril®

Mexican Brand Names Prinivil®; Zestril®

Pharmacologic Category Angiotensin-Converting Enzyme (ACE) Inhibitor

Use Treatment of hypertension, either alone or in combination with other antihypertensive agents; adjunctive therapy in treatment of CHF (afterload reduction); treatment of hemodynamically stable patients within 24 hours of acute MI, to improve survival; treatment of acute MI within 24 hours in hemodynamically stable patients to improve survival; treatment of left ventricular dysfunction after MI

Local Anesthetic/Vasoconstrictor Precautions No information available to require special precautions

Effects on Dental Treatment

>10%: Dizziness (5% to 12%), upper respiratory infection (2% to 12%)

1% to 9%: Orthostatic effects (1%), hypotension (1% to 4%), headache (4% to 6%), chest pain (3%), cough (4% to 9%), nausea (2%), vomiting (1%), fatigue (3%), weakness (1%)

Dosage Oral:

Hypertension:

Adults: Initial: 10 mg/day; increase doses 5-10 mg/day at 1- to 2-week intervals; maximum daily dose: 40 mg

Elderly: Initial: 2.5-5 mg/day; increase doses 2.5-5 mg/day at 1- to 2-week intervals; maximum daily dose: 40 mg

Patients taking diuretics should have them discontinued 2-3 days prior to initiating lisinopril if possible. Restart diuretic after blood pressure is stable if needed. If diuretic cannot be discontinued prior to therapy, begin with 5 mg with close supervision until stable blood pressure. In patients with hyponatremia (<130 mEq/L), start dose at 2.5 mg/day,

CHF: Adults: Initial: 5 mg; then increase by no more than 10 mg increments at intervals no less than 2 weeks to a maximum daily dose of 40 mg. Usual maintenance: 5-40 mg/day as a single dose. Patients should start/continue standard therapy, including diuretics, beta-blockers, and digoxin, as indicated.

Acute MI (within 24 hours in hemodynamically stable patients): Oral: 5 mg immediately, then 5 mg at 24 hours, 10 mg at 48 hours, and 10 mg every day thereafter for 6 weeks. Patients should continue to receive standard treatments such as thrombolytics, aspirin, and beta-blockers.

Dosing adjustment in renal impairment:

Cl_{cr} 10-50 mL/minute: Administer 50% to 75% of normal dose.

Cl_{cr} <10 mL/minute: Administer 25% to 50% of normal dose.

Hemodialysis: Dialyzable (50%)

Mechanism of Action Competitive inhibitor of angiotensin-converting enzyme (ACE); prevents conversion of angiotensin I to angiotensin II, a potent vasoconstrictor; results in lower levels of angiotensin II which causes an increase in plasma renin activity and a reduction in aldosterone secretion; a CNS mechanism may also be involved in hypotensive effect as angiotensin II increases adrenergic outflow from CNS; vasoactive kallikreins may be decreased in conversion to active hormones by ACE inhibitors, thus reducing blood pressure

Other Adverse Effects Includes data from hypertension and heart failure trials; higher ranges noted in CHF but frequency associated with placebo also increased in this population.

1% to 10%:

Dermatologic: Rash (1% to 2%)

Endocrine & metabolic: Hyperkalemia (2% to 5%)

Gastrointestinal: Diarrhea (3% to 4%), abdominal pain (2%)

Genitourinary: Impotence (1%)

Hematologic: Decreased hemoglobin (small)

Renal: Increased serum creatinine (often transient), increased BUN (2%); deterioration in renal function (in patients with bilateral renal artery stenosis or hypovolemia)

<1%: **Angioedema, anaphylactoid reactions**, edema, **cardiac arrest, MI**, cerebrovascular accident, pulmonary embolism, **arrhythmia, palpitation**, TIA, paroxysmal nocturnal dyspnea, **orthostatic hypotension**, peripheral edema, vasculitis, pancreatitis, jaundice (cholestatic), heartburn, GI cramps, constipation, flatulence, **xerostomia**, bone marrow suppression, neutropenia, thrombocytopenia, **diabetes mellitus**, weight gain/loss, **dehydration**, volume overload, gout,

(Continued)

Lisinopril *(Continued)*

arthritis, arthralgia, **stroke**, ataxia, **memory impairment, tremor**, peripheral neuropathy, **paresthesia, confusion**, insomnia, **somnolence, irritability, nervousness, bronchospasm**, infiltrates, **asthma**, pleural effusion, **bronchitis, wheezing, epistaxis, laryngitis, sinusitis, pharyngitis, rhinitis, rhinorrhea**, urticaria, alopecia, photosensitivity, pemphigus, erythema, **flushing, diaphoresis**, toxic epidermal necrolysis, Stevens-Johnson syndromes, vision loss, diplopia, **blurred vision,** tinnitus, photophobia, acute renal failure, oliguria, anuria, azotemia, renal dysfunction, dyspepsia, muscle cramps, decreased libido, vertigo, **nasal congestion**, increased transaminases, increased bilirubin, hyperkalemia, hyponatremia, hepatitis, systemic lupus erythematosus

Reported with ACE inhibitors: Elevated ESR; a syndrome which may include fever, myalgia, arthralgia, interstitial nephritis, vasculitis, rash, eosinophilia, positive ANA

Drug Interactions

Increased Effect/Toxicity:

Potassium supplements, co-trimoxazole (high dose), angiotensin II receptor antagonists (candesartan, losartan, irbesartan, etc), or potassium-sparing diuretics (amiloride, spironolactone, triamterene) may result in elevated serum potassium levels when combined with lisinopril. ACE inhibitor effects may be increased by phenothiazines or probenecid (increases levels of captopril). ACE inhibitors may increase serum concentrations/effects of digoxin, lithium, and sulfonlyureas.

Diuretics have additive hypotensive effects with ACE inhibitors, and hypovolemia increases the potential for adverse renal effects of ACE inhibitors. In patients with compromised renal function, coadministration with NSAIDs may result in further deterioration of renal function. Allopurinol and ACE inhibitors may cause a higher risk of hypersensitivity reaction when taken concurrently.

Decreased Effect: Aspirin (high dose) may reduce the therapeutic effects of ACE inhibitors; at low dosages this does not appear to be significant. Rifampin may decrease the effect of ACE inhibitors. Antacids may decrease the bioavailability of ACE inhibitors (may be more likely to occur with captopril); separate administration times by 1-2 hours. NSAIDs, specifically indomethacin, may reduce the hypotensive effects of ACE inhibitors. More likely to occur in low renin or volume dependent hypertensive patients.

Dietary/Ethanol/Herb Considerations

Ethanol: Avoid or limit use; may increase risk of hypotension or dizziness.

Food: May be taken with food; absorption unaffected. Avoid potassium supplements and salt substitutes containing potassium. Avoid caffeine, garlic, and licorice.

Herb/Nutraceutical: Avoid black cohosh, dong quai, and evening primrose due to estrogenic activity. Avoid ephedra, ginseng, and yohimbe; may worsen hypertension. Avoid garlic; may have increased antihypertensive effect. Avoid ginger due to positive inotropic effects; theoretically, may cause arrhythmia. Avoid hawthorn; may lower peripheral vascular resistance resulting in additive decrease in BP. Avoid licorice.

Pharmacodynamics/Kinetics

Onset of action: 1 hour

Peak effect: Hypotensive: Oral: ~6 hours

Duration: 24 hours

Absorption: Well absorbed; unaffected by food

Protein binding: 25%

Half-life elimination: 11-12 hours

Excretion: Primarily urine (as unchanged drug)

Pregnancy Risk Factor C/D (2nd and 3rd trimesters)

Generic Available Yes

Lisinopril and Hydrochlorothiazide

(lyse IN oh pril & hye droe klor oh THYE a zide)

Related Information

Cardiovascular Diseases *on page 1456*

Hydrochlorothiazide *on page 675*

Lisinopril *on page 813*

U.S. Brand Names Prinzide®; Zestoretic®

Canadian Brand Names Prinzide®; Zestoretic®

Pharmacologic Category Antihypertensive Agent Combination

Synonyms Hydrochlorothiazide and Lisinopril

Use Treatment of hypertension

Local Anesthetic/Vasoconstrictor Precautions No information available to require special precautions

Effects on Dental Treatment No significant effects or complications reported

Dosage Adults: Oral: Dosage is individualized; see each component for appropriate dosing suggestions; doses >80 mg/day lisinopril or >50 mg/day hydrochlorothiazide are not recommended.

Dietary/Ethanol/Herb Considerations Ethanol: Limit use; may increase risk of hypotension or dizziness.

Pregnancy Risk Factor C/D (2nd and 3rd trimesters)

Generic Available Yes

Lithium (LITH ee um)

U.S. Brand Names Eskalith®; Eskalith CR®; Lithobid®

Canadian Brand Names Apo®-Lithium; Carbolith™; Duralith®; Lithane™; PMS-Lithium Carbonate; PMS-Lithium Citrate

Mexican Brand Names Carbolit®; Lithellm® 300; Litheum®

Pharmacologic Category Lithium

Synonyms Lithium Carbonate; Lithium Citrate

Use Management of bipolar disorders; treatment of mania in individuals with bipolar disorder (maintenance treatment prevents or diminishes intensity of subsequent episodes)

Unlabeled/Investigational Use Potential augmenting agent for antidepressants; treatment of aggression, post-traumatic stress disorder, conduct disorders in children

Local Anesthetic/Vasoconstrictor Precautions No information available to require special precautions

Effects on Dental Treatment Avoid NSAIDs if analgesics are required since lithium toxicity has been reported with concomitant administration; acetaminophen products (ie, singly or with narcotics) are recommended.

Frequency not defined: Cardiac arrhythmias, hypotension, bradycardia, syncope, dizziness, blackout spells, seizures, sedation, restlessness, confusion, headache, stupor, coma, fatigue, lethargy, intellectual functioning, tics, slurred speech, hyperglycemia, diabetes insipidus, nausea, vomiting, xerostomia, metallic taste, salivary gland swelling, excessive salivation, tremor, muscle hyperirritability

Dosage Oral (monitor serum concentrations and clinical response [efficacy and toxicity] to determine proper dose):

Bipolar disorder:

- Children 6-12 years: 15-60 mg/kg/day in 3-4 divided doses; dose not to exceed usual adult dosage
- Adults: 900-2400 mg/day in 3-4 divided doses or 900-1800 mg/day (sustained release) in 2 divided doses
- Elderly: Initial dose: 300 mg once or twice daily; increase weekly in increments of 300 mg/day, monitoring levels; rarely need >900-1200 mg/day

Conduct disorder (unlabeled use): Children 6-12 years: 15-30 mg/kg/day in 3-4 divided doses; do not exceed usual adult dosage

Dosing adjustment in renal impairment:

- Cl_{cr} 10-50 mL/minute: Administer 50% to 75% of normal dose
- Cl_{cr} <10 mL/minute: Administer 25% to 50% of normal dose

Hemodialysis: Dialyzable (50% to 100%)

Mechanism of Action Alters cation transport across cell membrane in nerve and muscle cells and influences reuptake of serotonin and/or norepinephrine; second messenger systems involving the phosphatidylinositol cycle are inhibited; postsynaptic D2 receptor supersensitivity is inhibited

Other Adverse Effects Frequency not defined:

Cardiovascular: Sinus node dysfunction, flattened or inverted T waves (reversible), edema,

Central nervous system: Dystonia, pseudotumor cerebri, psychomotor retardation

Dermatologic: Dry hair, thinning hair, folliculitis, alopecia, exacerbation of psoriasis, rash

Endocrine & metabolic: Euthyroid goiter and/or hypothyroidism, hyperthyroidism

Gastrointestinal: Polydipsia, anorexia, diarrhea, weight gain

Genitourinary: Incontinence, polyuria, glycosuria, oliguria, albuminuria

Hematologic: Leukocytosis

Neuromuscular & skeletal: Ataxia, choreoathetoid movements, hyperactive deep tendon reflexes, myasthenia gravis (rare)

Ocular: Nystagmus, transient scotoma

Miscellaneous: Discoloration of fingers and toes

Drug Interactions

Increased Effect/Toxicity:

Concurrent use of lithium with carbamazepine, diltiazem, SSRIs (fluoxetine, fluvoxamine), haloperidol, methyldopa, metronidazole (rare), phenothiazines, phenytoin, TCAs, and verapamil may increase the risk for neurotoxicity. Lithium concentrations/toxicity may be increased by diuretics, NSAIDs (sulindac and aspirin may be exceptions), ACE inhibitors, angiotensin receptor antagonists (losartan), tetracyclines, or COX-2 inhibitors (celecoxib).

Lithium and MAO inhibitors should generally be avoided due to use reports of fatal malignant hyperpyrexia; risk with selective MAO type B inhibitors (selegiline) appears to be lower. Potassium iodide may enhance the hypothyroid effects of lithium. Combined use of lithium with tricyclic antidepressants or

(Continued)

Lithium *(Continued)*

sibutramine may increase the risk of serotonin syndrome; this combination is best avoided. Lithium may potentiate effect of neuromuscular blockers.

Decreased Effect: Combined use of lithium and chlorpromazine may lower serum concentrations of both drugs. Sodium bicarbonate and high sodium intake may reduce serum lithium concentrations via enhanced excretion. Lithium may blunt the pressor response to sympathomimetics (epinephrine, norepinephrine). Caffeine (xanthine derivatives) may lower lithium serum concentrations by increasing urinary lithium excretion (monitor).

Dietary/Ethanol/Herb Considerations Food may increase serum concentration. Limit caffeine.

Pharmacodynamics/Kinetics

Absorption: Rapid and complete

Distribution: V_d: Initial: 0.3-0.4 L/kg; V_{dss}: 0.7-1 L/kg; crosses placenta; enters breast milk at 35% to 50% the concentrations in serum; distribution is complete in 6-10 hours

Protein binding: Not protein bound

Metabolism: Not metabolized

Half-life elimination: 18-24 hours; can increase to more than 36 hours in elderly or with renal impairment

Time to peak, serum: Nonsustained release: ~0.5-2 hours

Excretion: Urine (90% to 98% as unchanged drug); sweat (4% to 5%); feces (1%)

Pregnancy Risk Factor D

Generic Available Yes

Lithium Carbonate *see* Lithium *on page 815*

Lithium Citrate *see* Lithium *on page 815*

Lithobid® *see* Lithium *on page 815*

Lithostat® *see* Acetohydroxamic Acid *on page 39*

Livostin® *see* Levocabastine *on page 791*

L-Lysine *see* Lysine *on page 832*

L-Lysine Hydrochloride *see* Lysine *on page 832*

LMD® *see* Dextran *on page 419*

LNg 20 *see* Levonorgestrel *on page 797*

LoCHOLEST® *see* Cholestyramine Resin *on page 318*

LoCHOLEST® Light *see* Cholestyramine Resin *on page 318*

Locoid® *see* Hydrocortisone *on page 688*

Locoid Lipocream® *see* Hydrocortisone *on page 688*

Lodine® *see* Etodolac *on page 547*

Lodine® XL *see* Etodolac *on page 547*

Lodosyn® *see* Carbidopa *on page 246*

Lodoxamide (loe DOKS a mide)

U.S. Brand Names Alomide®

Canadian Brand Names Alomide®

Pharmacologic Category Mast Cell Stabilizer

Synonyms Lodoxamide Tromethamine

Use Treatment of vernal keratoconjunctivitis, vernal conjunctivitis, and vernal keratitis

Local Anesthetic/Vasoconstrictor Precautions No information available to require special precautions

Effects on Dental Treatment 1% to 10%: Headache

Dosage Ophthalmic: Children ≥2 years and Adults: Instill 1-2 drops in eye(s) 4 times/day for up to 3 months

Mechanism of Action Mast cell stabilizer that inhibits the *in vivo* type I immediate hypersensitivity reaction to increase cutaneous vascular permeability associated with IgE and antigen-mediated reactions

Other Adverse Effects

>10%: Local: Transient burning, stinging, discomfort

1% to 10%: Ocular: Blurred vision, corneal erosion/ulcer, eye pain, corneal abrasion, blepharitis

<1%: **Dizziness, sneezing, nasal dryness, somnolence, nausea,** stomach discomfort, rash

Pharmacodynamics/Kinetics Absorption: Topical: Negligible

Pregnancy Risk Factor B

Generic Available No

Lodoxamide Tromethamine *see* Lodoxamide *on page 816*

Loestrin® *see* Combination Hormonal Contraceptives *on page 368*

Loestrin® Fe *see* Combination Hormonal Contraceptives *on page 368*

L-OHP *see* Oxaliplatin *on page 1008*

Lomefloxacin (loe me FLOKS a sin)

Related Information

Sexually-Transmitted Diseases *on page 1502*

U.S. Brand Names Maxaquin®

Mexican Brand Names Lomacin®; Maxaquin®

Pharmacologic Category Antibiotic, Quinolone

Synonyms Lomefloxacin Hydrochloride

Use Lower respiratory infections, acute bacterial exacerbation of chronic bronchitis, and urinary tract infections caused by *E. coli, K. pneumoniae, P. mirabilis, P. aeruginosa*; also has gram-positive activity including *S. pneumoniae* and some staphylococci; surgical prophylaxis (transrectal prostate biopsy or transurethral procedures)

Unlabeled/Investigational Use Treatment of skin infections, sexually-transmitted diseases

Local Anesthetic/Vasoconstrictor Precautions No information available to require special precautions

Effects on Dental Treatment 1% to 4%: Headache (3%), dizziness (2%), nausea (4%)

Dosage Oral: Adults:

Lower respiratory and urinary tract infections (UTI): 400 mg once daily for 10-14 days

Urinary tract infection (UTI) due to susceptible organisms:

- Females:
  - Uncomplicated cystitis caused by *Escherichia coli*: 400 mg once daily for 3 successive days
  - Uncomplicated cystitis caused by *Klebsiella pneumoniae, Proteus mirabilis*, or *Staphylococcus saprophyticus*: 400 mg once daily for 10 successive days
- Complicated UTI caused by *Escherichia coli, Klebsiella pneumoniae, Proteus mirabilis*, or *Pseudomonas aeruginosa*: 400 mg once daily for 14 successive days

Surgical prophylaxis: 400 mg 2-6 hours before surgery

Uncomplicated gonorrhea: 400 mg as a single dose

Elderly: No dosage adjustment with normal renal function

Dosing adjustment in renal impairment:

- Cl_{cr} 11-39 mL/minute: Loading dose: 400 mg, then 200 mg every day

Hemodialysis: Same as above

Mechanism of Action Inhibits DNA-gyrase in susceptible organisms thereby inhibits relaxation of supercoiled DNA and promotes breakage of DNA strands. DNA gyrase (topoisomerase II), is an essential bacterial enzyme that maintains the superhelical structure of DNA and is required for DNA replication and transcription, DNA repair, recombination, and transposition.

Other Adverse Effects

1% to 10%: Dermatologic: Photosensitivity (2%)

<1%: Abdominal pain, **abnormal taste, allergic reaction, angina pectoris**, anuria, **arrhythmia**, back pain, **bradycardia, cardiac failure, chest pain**, chills, **coma**, constipation, **convulsions, cough**, cyanosis, decreased heat tolerance, **increased diaphoresis, discoloration of tongue, dyspnea**, dysuria, earache, edema, **epistaxis**, extrasystoles, **facial edema, fatigue**, flatulence, **flu-like symptoms, flushing**, gout, hematuria, hyperkinesia, **hypertension, hypoglycemia, hypotension**, increased fibrinolysis, **leg cramps, malaise**, myalgia, **MI, paresthesia**, purpura, rash, **syncope, tachycardia, thirst**, thrombocytopenia, **tremor**, urinary disorders, vertigo, **vomiting, weakness, xerostomia**, tendon rupture and tendonitis

Drug Interactions Inhibits **CYP1A2**

Increased Effect/Toxicity: Quinolones can cause elevated levels of caffeine, warfarin, cyclosporine, and theophylline. Azlocillin, imipenem, cimetidine, loop diuretics, and probenecid may increase lomefloxacin serum levels. Increased CNS stimulation may occur with caffeine, theophylline, NSAIDs. Foscarnet has been associated with seizures in patients receiving quinolones. Concurrent use of corticosteroids may increase risk of tendon rupture.

Decreased Effect: Decreased absorption with antacids containing aluminum, magnesium, and/or calcium (by up to 98% if given at the same time). Antineoplastic agents may decrease quinolone absorption.

Dietary/Ethanol/Herb Considerations

Food: May be taken with food; may prolong peak serum concentration.

Herb/Nutraceutical: Avoid dong quai and St John's wort; may cause photosensitization.

Pharmacodynamics/Kinetics

Absorption: Well absorbed

Distribution: V_d: 2.4-3.5 L/kg; into bronchus, prostatic tissue, and urine

Protein binding: 20%

Half-life elimination: 5-7.5 hours

Excretion: Primarily urine (as unchanged drug)

Pregnancy Risk Factor C

Generic Available No

Lomefloxacin Hydrochloride *see* Lomefloxacin *on page 817*

Lomocot® *see* Diphenoxylate and Atropine *on page 453*

Lomotil® *see* Diphenoxylate and Atropine *on page 453*

Lomustine (loe MUS teen)

U.S. Brand Names CeeNU®

Canadian Brand Names CeeNU®

Mexican Brand Names CeeNU®

Pharmacologic Category Antineoplastic Agent, Alkylating Agent

Synonyms CCNU

Use Treatment of brain tumors and Hodgkin's disease, non-Hodgkin's lymphoma, melanoma, renal carcinoma, lung cancer, colon cancer

Local Anesthetic/Vasoconstrictor Precautions No information available to require special precautions

Effects on Dental Treatment No significant effects or complications reported

Dosage Oral (refer to individual protocols):

Children: 75-150 mg/m² as a single dose every 6 weeks; subsequent doses are readjusted after initial treatment according to platelet and leukocyte counts

Adults: 100-130 mg/m² as a single dose every 6 weeks; readjust after initial treatment according to platelet and leukocyte counts

With compromised marrow function: Initial dose: 100 mg/m² as a single dose every 6 weeks

Repeat courses should only be administered after adequate recovery: WBC >4000 and platelet counts >100,000

Subsequent dosing adjustment based on nadir:

Leukocytes 2000-2900/mm³, platelets 25,000-74,999/mm³: Administer 70% of prior dose

Leukocytes <2000/mm³, platelets <25,000/mm³: Administer 50% of prior dose

Dosing adjustment in renal impairment:

Cl_{cr} 10-50 mL/minute: Administer 75% of normal dose

Cl_{cr} <10 mL/minute: Administer 50% of normal dose

Hemodialysis: Supplemental dose is unnecessary

Peritoneal dialysis: Significant drug removal is unlikely based on physiochemical characteristics

Mechanism of Action Inhibits DNA and RNA synthesis via carbamylation of DNA polymerase, alkylation of DNA, and alteration of RNA, proteins, and enzymes

Other Adverse Effects

>10%:

Gastrointestinal: Nausea and vomiting (usually 3-6 hours after oral administration; administration of dose at bedtime, with an antiemetic, significantly reduces incidence and severity of nausea)

Hematologic: Myelosuppression (common, dose-limiting); may be cumulative and irreversible

Onset: 10-14 days

Nadir: Leukopenia: 6 weeks

Thrombocytopenia: 4 weeks

Recovery: 6-8 weeks

1% to 10%:

Dermatologic: Rash

Gastrointestinal: Anorexia, stomatitis, diarrhea

Genitourinary: Progressive azotemia, renal failure, decrease in kidney size

Hematologic: Anemia

Hepatic: Elevated liver enzymes, transient, reversible

<1%: Disorientation, lethargy, ataxia, dysarthria, alopecia, nephritis (associated with large cumulative doses), interstitial fibrosis and infiltrates (associated with cumulative doses >600-1000 mg, may be irreversible and fatal)

Drug Interactions Substrate of **CYP2D6**; Inhibits CYP2D6, 3A4

Increased Effect/Toxicity: Increased toxicity with cimetidine, reported to cause bone marrow depression or to potentiate the myelosuppressive effects of lomustine.

Decreased Effect: Decreased effect with phenobarbital, resulting in reduced efficacy of both drugs.

Dietary/Ethanol/Herb Considerations

Ethanol: Avoid use due to GI irritation.

Food: Administer with fluids on an empty stomach; no food or drink for 2 hours postdose to decrease nausea

Pharmacodynamics/Kinetics

Duration: Marrow recovery: ≤6 weeks

Absorption: Complete; appears in plasma within 3 minutes after administration

Distribution: Crosses blood-brain barrier to a greater degree than BCNU; CNS concentrations are equal to that of plasma

Protein binding: 50%

Metabolism: Rapidly hepatic via hydroxylation producing at least two active metabolites; enterohepatically recycled
Half-life elimination: Parent drug: 16-72 hours; Active metabolite: Terminal: 1.3-2 days
Time to peak, serum: Active metabolite: ~3 hours
Excretion: Urine; feces (<5%); expired air (<10%)

Pregnancy Risk Factor D
Generic Available No

Loniten® *see* Minoxidil *on page 917*
Lonox® *see* Diphenoxylate and Atropine *on page 453*
Lo/Ovral® *see* Combination Hormonal Contraceptives *on page 368*

Loperamide (loe PER a mide)

U.S. Brand Names Imodium® A-D [OTC]
Canadian Brand Names Apo®-Loperamide; Diarr-Eze; Imodium®; Loperacap; Novo-Loperamide; PMS-Loperamine; Rho®-Loperamine; Riva-Loperamine
Mexican Brand Names Acanol; Cryoperacid®; Pramidal®; Raxedin; Top-Dal®
Pharmacologic Category Antidiarrheal
Synonyms Loperamide Hydrochloride
Use Treatment of acute diarrhea and chronic diarrhea associated with inflammatory bowel disease; chronic functional diarrhea (idiopathic), chronic diarrhea caused by bowel resection or organic lesions; to decrease the volume of ileostomy discharge
Unlabeled/Investigational Use Treatment of traveler's diarrhea in combination with trimethoprim-sulfamethoxazole (co-trimoxazole) (3-day therapy)
Local Anesthetic/Vasoconstrictor Precautions No information available to require special precautions
Effects on Dental Treatment No significant effects or complications reported
Dosage Oral:

Children:
- Acute diarrhea: Initial doses (in first 24 hours):
  - 2-6 years: 1 mg 3 times/day
  - 6-8 years: 2 mg twice daily
  - 8-12 years: 2 mg 3 times/day
  - Maintenance: After initial dosing, 0.1 mg/kg doses after each loose stool, but not exceeding initial dosage
- Chronic diarrhea: 0.08-0.24 mg/kg/day divided 2-3 times/day, maximum: 2 mg/dose

Adults:
- Acute diarrhea: Initial: 4 mg (2 capsules), followed by 2 mg after each loose stool, up to 16 mg/day (8 capsules)
- Chronic diarrhea: Initial: Follow acute diarrhea; maintenance dose should be slowly titrated downward to minimum required to control symptoms (typically, 4-8 mg/day in divided doses)
- Traveler's diarrhea: Treat for no more than 2 days
  - 6-8 years: 1 mg after first loose stool followed by 1 mg after each subsequent stool; maximum dose: 4 mg/day
  - 9-11 years: 2 mg after first loose stool followed by 1 mg after each subsequent stool; maximum dose: 6 mg/day
  - 12 years to Adults: 4 mg after first loose stool followed by 2 mg after each subsequent stool; maximum dose: 8 mg/day

Mechanism of Action Acts directly on intestinal muscles to inhibit peristalsis and prolongs transit time enhancing fluid and electrolyte movement through intestinal mucosa; reduces fecal volume, increases viscosity, and diminishes fluid and electrolyte loss; demonstrates antisecretory activity; exhibits peripheral action
Other Adverse Effects Frequency not defined:
Cardiovascular: **Shock**
Central nervous system: **Dizziness, drowsiness, fatigue, sedation**
Dermatologic: Rash, toxic epidermal necrolysis
Gastrointestinal: Abdominal cramping, abdominal distention, constipation, nausea, paralytic ileus, vomiting, **xerostomia**
Miscellaneous: **Anaphylaxis**
Drug Interactions Increased Effect/Toxicity: Loperamide may potentiate the adverse effects of CNS depressants, phenothiazines, tricyclic antidepressants.
Pharmacodynamics/Kinetics
Onset of action: 0.5-1 hour
Absorption: <40%
Distribution: Low amounts enter breast milk
Protein binding: 97%
Metabolism: Hepatic (>50%) to inactive compounds
Half-life elimination: 7-14 hours
Excretion: Urine and feces (1% as metabolites, 30% to 40% as unchanged drug)
Pregnancy Risk Factor B
Generic Available Yes

Loperamide Hydrochloride *see* Loperamide *on page 819*

Lopid® *see* Gemfibrozil *on page 631*

Lopinavir *see* Lopinavir and Ritonavir *on page 820*

Lopinavir and Ritonavir (loe PIN a veer & rit ON uh veer)

U.S. Brand Names Kaletra™

Canadian Brand Names Kaletra™

Pharmacologic Category Antiretroviral Agent, Protease Inhibitor

Synonyms Lopinavir

Use Treatment of HIV infection in combination with other antiretroviral agents

Local Anesthetic/Vasoconstrictor Precautions No information available to require special precautions

Effects on Dental Treatment

1% to 10%: Headache (2% to 7%)

<2%: Chest pain, facial edema, hypertension, palpitations, agitation, anxiety, confusion, dizziness, facial paralysis, fever, migraine, nervousness, neuropathy, paresthesia, drowsiness, tremor, dehydration, xerostomia, dysphagia, esophagitis, gastritis, gastroenteritis, GI disorder, sialadenitis, stomatitis, abnormal taste, ulcerative stomatitis, bronchitis, dyspnea, rhinitis, sinusitis, diaphoresis, flu-like syndrome, viral infection, CNS depression, otitis media

Dosage Oral (take with food):

Children 6 months to 12 years: Dosage based on weight, presented based on mg of lopinavir (maximum dose: Lopinavir 400 mg/ritonavir 100 mg)

7-<15 kg: 12 mg/kg twice daily

15-40 kg: 10 mg/kg twice daily

>40 kg: Refer to adult dosing

Children >12 years and Adults: Lopinavir 400 mg/ritonavir 100 mg twice daily

Dosing adjustment when taken with efavirenz or nevirapine:

Children 6 months to 12 years:

7-<15 kg: 13 mg/kg twice daily

15-50 kg: 11 mg/kg twice daily

>50 kg: Refer to adult dosing

Children >12 years and Adults: Lopinavir 533 mg/ritonavir 133 mg twice daily

Elderly: Not studied; use with caution due to possible decreased hepatic, renal, and cardiac function

Dosing adjustment in renal impairment: Not studied; decrease in clearance not expected

Dosing comment in hepatic impairment: Plasma levels may be increased

Mechanism of Action A coformulation of lopinavir and ritonavir. The lopinavir component is the active inhibitor of HIV protease. Lopinavir inhibits HIV protease and renders the enzyme incapable of processing polyprotein precursor which leads to production of noninfectious immature HIV particles. The ritonavir component inhibits the CYP3A metabolism of lopinavir, allowing increased plasma levels of lopinavir.

Other Adverse Effects Protease inhibitors cause hyperglycemia and dyslipidemia (elevated cholesterol, triglycerides, and a redistribution of body fat centrally to cause "protease paunch," buffalo hump, facial atrophy, and breast enlargement).

>10%:

Endocrine & metabolic: Hypercholesterolemia (9% to 28%), triglycerides increased (9% to 28%)

Gastrointestinal: Diarrhea (16% to 24%), nausea (3% to 15%)

Hepatic: GGT increased (4% to 25%)

2% to 10%:

Central nervous system: Pain (≤2%), insomnia (1% to 2%)

Dermatologic: Rash (1% to 4%)

Endocrine & metabolic: Hyperglycemia (1% to 4%), hyperuricemia (up to 4%), sodium decreased (3% children), organic phosphorus decreased (up to 2%), amylase increased (2% to 10%)

Gastrointestinal: Abnormal stools (up to 6%), abdominal pain (2% to 4%), vomiting (2% to 5%), dyspepsia (0.5% to 2%)

Hematologic: Platelets decreased (4% children), neutrophils decreased (1% to 3%)

Hepatic: AST increased (2% to 9%), ALT increased (4% to 8%), bilirubin increased (children 3%)

Neuromuscular & skeletal: Weakness (4% to 7%)

<2%:

Cardiovascular: Deep vein thrombosis, edema, peripheral edema, vasculitis

Central nervous system: Abnormal dreams, abnormal thinking, amnesia, ataxia, chills, emotional lability, encephalopathy, malaise, peripheral neuritis,

Dermatologic: Acne, alopecia, benign neoplasm, dry skin, exfoliative dermatitis, furunculosis, maculopapular rash, nail disorder, pruritus, skin discoloration

Endocrine & metabolic: Cushing's syndrome, diabetes mellitus, glucose intolerance, gynecomastia, hypogonadism (male), hypothyroidism, lactic acidosis, libido decreased, weight gain

Gastrointestinal: Anorexia, constipation, dyspepsia, enterocolitis, eructation, fecal incontinence, flatulence, hemorrhagic colitis, increased appetite, pancreatitis, weight loss

Genitourinary: Abnormal ejaculation

Hematologic: Anemia, leukopenia, lymphadenopathy

Hepatic: Cholecystitis, hepatic dysfunction

Local: Thrombophlebitis

Neuromuscular & skeletal: Arthralgia, arthrosis, back pain, dyskinesia, hypertonia, myalgia

Ocular: Abnormal vision, eye disorder

Otic: Tinnitus

Renal: Kidney calculus, urine abnormality

Respiratory: Lung edema

Miscellaneous: Avitaminosis, obesity

Drug Interactions

Lopinavir: Substrate of 3A4

Ritonavir: Substrate of CYP1A2, 2B6, **2D6, 3A4**; Inhibits CYP2C8/9, 2C19, **2D6**, 2E1, **3A4**; Induces CYP1A2, 2C8/9, 3A4

Increased Effect/Toxicity:

Contraindicated drugs: Life-threatening arrhythmias may result from concurrent use of flecainide or propafenone. Concurrent use is contraindicated. Concurrent use of cisapride, pimozide, astemizole is also contraindicated. Some benzodiazepines (midazolam and triazolam) are contraindicated, due to the potential for increased response/respiratory depression. Concurrent use of ergot alkaloids is contraindicated, due to potential toxicity.

Serum levels of other antiarrhythmics, including amiodarone, bepridil, lidocaine (systemic), and quinidine may be increased with concurrent use. Serum levels of calcium channel blockers (including felodipine, nicardipine, and nifedipine), clarithromycin, immunosuppressants (cyclosporin, tacrolimus, sirolimus), HMG-CoA reductase inhibitors (lovastatin and simvastatin are not recommended, atorvastatin and cerivastatin should be used at lowest possible dose), itraconazole, ketoconazole, methadone, and rifabutin (decreased dose recommended) may be increased. Serum levels of protease inhibitors may be altered during concurrent therapy. Ritonavir may increase serum concentrations of amprenavir, indinavir, or saquinavir. Serum levels of sildenafil may be substantially increased (use caution at decreased dose of sildenafil, maximum of 25 mg in 48 hours). Warfarin serum levels may also be increased.

Delavirdine increases levels of lopinavir; dosing recommendations are not yet established.

Lopinavir/ritonavir solution contains alcohol, concurrent use with disulfiram or metronidazole should be avoided. May cause disulfiram-like reaction.

Decreased Effect: Carbamazepine, dexamethasone, phenobarbital, phenytoin, and rifampin may decrease levels of lopinavir. Non-nucleoside reverse transcriptase inhibitors: Efavirenz, nevirapine may decrease levels of lopinavir. To avoid incompatibility with didanosine, administer didanosine 1 hour before or 2 hours after lopinavir/ritonavir. Decreased levels of ethinyl estradiol may result from concurrent use. Lopinavir/ritonavir may decrease levels of abacavir, atovaquone, or zidovudine.

Dietary/Ethanol/Herb Considerations

Food: Administer with food.

Herb/Nutraceutical: Avoid St John's wort; may decrease serum concentration of protease inhibitors and lead to possible resistance.

Pharmacodynamics/Kinetics

Ritonavir: See Ritonavir monograph.

Lopinavir:

Protein binding: 98% to 99%

Metabolism: Hepatic via CYP3A; 13 metabolites identified

Half-life elimination: 5-6 hours

Excretion: Feces (83%, 20% as unchanged drug); urine (2%)

Pregnancy Risk Factor C

Generic Available No

Lopremone *see* Protirelin *on page 1144*

Lopressor® *see* Metoprolol *on page 901*

Loprox® *see* Ciclopirox *on page 322*

Lorabid® *see* Loracarbef *on page 821*

Loracarbef (lor u KAR bef)

U.S. Brand Names Lorabid®

Canadian Brand Names Lorabid™

Mexican Brand Names Carbac®; Lorabid®

Pharmacologic Category Antibiotic, Carbacephem

Use Infections caused by susceptible organisms involving the respiratory tract, acute otitis media, sinusitis, skin and skin structure, bone and joint, and urinary tract and gynecologic

(Continued)

Loracarbef *(Continued)*

Local Anesthetic/Vasoconstrictor Precautions No information available to require special precautions

Effects on Dental Treatment Headache (1% to 3%), somnolence (<2%), rhinitis (2% to 6%)

Dosage Oral:

Children:

Acute otitis media: 15 mg/kg twice daily for 10 days

Pharyngitis and impetigo: 7.5-15 mg/kg twice daily for 10 days

Adults:

Uncomplicated urinary tract infections: 200 mg once daily for 7 days

Skin and soft tissue: 200-400 mg every 12-24 hours

Uncomplicated pyelonephritis: 400 mg every 12 hours for 14 days

Upper/lower respiratory tract infection: 200-400 mg every 12-24 hours for 7-14 days

Dosing comments in renal impairment:

Cl_{cr} 10-49 mL/minute: 50% of usual dose at usual interval or usual dose given half as often

Cl_{cr} <10 mL/minute: Administer usual dose every 3-5 days

Hemodialysis: Doses should be administered after dialysis sessions

Mechanism of Action Inhibits bacterial cell wall synthesis by binding to one or more of the penicillin binding proteins (PBPs); inhibits the final transpeptidation step of peptidoglycan synthesis in bacterial cell walls, thus inhibiting cell wall biosynthesis. It is thought that beta-lactam antibiotics inactivate transpeptidase via acylation of the enzyme with cleavage of the CO-N bond of the beta-lactam ring. Upon exposure to beta-lactam antibiotics, bacteria eventually lyse due to ongoing activity of cell wall autolytic enzymes (autolysins and murein hydrolases) while cell wall assembly is arrested.

Other Adverse Effects

≥1%:

Dermatologic: Rash (1% to 3%)

Gastrointestinal: Diarrhea (4% to 6%), nausea (2%), vomiting (1% to 3%), anorexia (<2%), abdominal pain (1%)

Genitourinary: Vaginitis (1%)

<1%: **Anaphylaxis**, arthralgia, **candidiasis**, cholestasis, eosinophilia, hemolytic anemia, interstitial nephritis, jaundice, nephrotoxicity with transient elevations of BUN/creatinine, **nervousness**, neutropenia, positive Coombs' test, pruritus, pseudomembranous colitis, **seizures** (with high doses and renal dysfunction), serum sickness-like reaction, slightly increased AST/ALT, Stevens-Johnson syndrome, thrombocytopenia, urticaria

Drug Interactions Increased Effect/Toxicity: Loracarbef serum levels are increased with coadministered probenecid.

Dietary/Ethanol/Herb Considerations Food: Administer on an empty stomach at least 1 hour before or 2 hours after meal; food decreases and delays peak plasma concentration.

Pharmacodynamics/Kinetics

Absorption: Rapid

Half-life elimination: ~1 hour

Time to peak, serum: ~1 hour

Excretion: Clearance: Plasma: ~200-300 mL/minute

Pregnancy Risk Factor B

Generic Available No

Loratadine (lor AT a deen)

U.S. Brand Names Alavert™ [OTC]; Claritin® [OTC]

Canadian Brand Names Apo®-Loratadine; Claritin®; Claritin® Kids

Mexican Brand Names Clarityne®; Lertamine®; Lowadina; Sensibit®

Pharmacologic Category Antihistamine, Nonsedating

Use Relief of nasal and non-nasal symptoms of seasonal allergic rhinitis; treatment of chronic idiopathic urticaria

Local Anesthetic/Vasoconstrictor Precautions No information available to require special precautions

Effects on Dental Treatment

Adults:

>10%: Xerostomia (normal salivary flow resumes upon discontinuation), headache (12%)

1% to 10%: somnolence (8%),

Children: Nervousness (4% ages 6-12 years), wheezing (4% ages 6-12 years), viral infection (2% to 3% ages 2-5 years), upper respiratory infection (2% ages 6-12 years), epistaxis (2% to 3% ages 2-5 years), pharyngitis (2% to 3% ages 2-5 years), flu-like symptoms (2% to 3% ages 2-5 years)

Adults and Children: <2%: Agitation, altered taste, anxiety, bronchitis, bronchospasm, chest pain, confusion, coughing, increased diaphoresis, dizziness, dyspnea, flushing, gastritis, hemoptysis, hiccup, hypertension, hypotension, laryngitis, migraine, nasal dryness, palpitations, paresthesia, rigors, sinusitis, sneezing, supraventricular tachyarrhythmia, syncope, tachycardia, thirst, tremor

Dosage Oral: Seasonal allergic rhinitis, chronic idiopathic urticaria:

Children 2-5 years: 5 mg once daily

Children ≥6 years and Adults: 10 mg once daily

Elderly: Peak plasma levels are increased; elimination halflife is slightly increased; specific dosing adjustments are unavailable

Dosing adjustment in renal impairment: Cl_{cr} ≤30 mL/minute:

Children 2-5 years: 5 mg every other day

Children ≥6 years and Adults: 10 mg every other day

Dosing adjustment in hepatic impairment: Elimination halflife increases with severity of disease

Children 2-5 years: 5 mg every other day

Children ≥6 years and Adults: 10 mg every other day

Mechanism of Action Long-acting tricyclic antihistamine with selective peripheral histamine H_1-receptor antagonistic properties

Other Adverse Effects

Adults: Central nervous system: Fatigue (4%)

Children:

Central nervous system: Fatigue (3% ages 6-12 years, 2% to 3% ages 2-5 years), malaise (2% ages 6-12 years)

Dermatologic: Rash (2% to 3% ages 2-5 years)

Gastrointestinal: Abdominal pain (2% ages 6-12 years), stomatitis (2% to 3% ages 2-5 years)

Neuromuscular & skeletal: Hyperkinesia (3% ages 6-12 years)

Ocular: Conjunctivitis (2% ages 6-12 years)

Respiratory: Dysphonia (2% ages 6-12 years)

Adults and Children: <2%: Altered lacrimation, altered micturition, amnesia, angioneurotic edema, anorexia, appetite increased, arthralgia, back pain, blepharospasm, blurred vision, breast pain, constipation, depression, dermatitis, diarrhea, dry hair, dry skin, dysmenorrhea, dyspepsia, dysphonia, earache, eye pain, flatulence, hypertonia, hypoesthesia, impaired concentration, impotence, insomnia, irritability, leg cramps, libido decreased, loose stools, malaise, menorrhagia, myalgia, nausea, paroniria, photosensitivity, pruritus, purpura, tinnitus, urinary discoloration, urinary incontinence, urinary retention, urticaria, vaginitis, vertigo, vomiting, weakness, weight gain

Postmarketing and/or case reports: Abnormal hepatic function, alopecia, **anaphylaxis**, breast enlargement, erythema multiforme, hepatitis, hepatic necrosis, jaundice, peripheral edema, **seizures**, thrombocytopenia

Drug Interactions Substrate of CYP2D6, 3A4

Increased Effect/Toxicity: Increased plasma concentrations of loratadine and its active metabolite with ketoconazole and erythromycin, however, no change in QT_c interval was seen. Increased toxicity with procarbazine, other antihistamines, alcohol. Protease inhibitors (amprenavir, ritonavir, nelfinavir) may increase the serum levels of loratadine.

Dietary/Ethanol/Herb Considerations

Ethanol: Avoid use; although sedation is limited with loratadine, may increase risk of CNS depression.

Food increases bioavailability and delays peak serum concentration; administer on an empty stomach

Herb/Nutraceutical: Avoid St John's wort; may decrease serum concentration.

Pharmacodynamics/Kinetics

Onset of action: 1-3 hours

Peak effect: 8-12 hours

Duration: >24 hours

Absorption: Rapid

Distribution: Significant amounts enter breast milk

Metabolism: Extensively hepatic via CYP2D6 and 3A4 to active metabolite

Half-life elimination: 12-15 hours

Excretion: Urine (40%) and feces (40%) as metabolites

Pregnancy Risk Factor B

Generic Available No

Loratadine and Pseudoephedrine

(lor AT a deen & soo doe e FED rin)

Related Information

Loratadine *on page 822*

Oral Bacterial Infections *on page 1531*

Pseudoephedrine *on page 1146*

U.S. Brand Names Claritin-D® 12-Hour [OTC]; Claritin-D® 24-Hour [OTC]

Canadian Brand Names Chlor-Tripolon ND®; Claritin® Extra; Claritin® Liberator

Pharmacologic Category Antihistamine/Decongestant Combination

Synonyms Pseudoephedrine and Loratadine

Use Temporary relief of symptoms of seasonal allergic rhinitis and nasal congestion

(Continued)

Loratadine and Pseudoephedrine *(Continued)*

Local Anesthetic/Vasoconstrictor Precautions Use with caution since pseudoephedrine is a sympathomimetic amine which could interact with epinephrine to cause a pressor response

Effects on Dental Treatment

>10%: Xerostomia; normal salivary flow resumes upon discontinuation

1% to 10%: Tachycardia and palpitations (≤10%; use vasoconstrictor with caution), headache, dizziness (4%), slight to moderate drowsiness (6%), nervousness (3%), pharyngitis (5%), thickening of bronchial secretions, cough, diaphoresis

Dosage Oral:

Children ≥12 years and Adults:

Claritin-D® 12-Hour: 1 tablet every 12 hours

Claritin-D® 24-Hour: 1 tablet daily

Dosing adjustment in renal impairment:

Claritin-D® 12-Hour: 1 tablet daily

Claritin-D® 24-Hour: 1 tablet every other day

Other Adverse Effects

1% to 10%:

Central nervous system: Insomnia (5%), fatigue (3%)

Gastrointestinal: Weight gain, nausea (3%), diarrhea, abdominal pain, anorexia (2%)

Genitourinary: Dysuria, dysmenorrhea (2%)

Neuromuscular & skeletal: Arthralgia, weakness

<1%: Edema, **palpitations, hypertension, tachycardia, CNS depression, sedation**, paradoxical excitement, **convulsions, hallucinations**, angioedema, rash, photosensitivity, urinary retention, hepatitis, myalgia, **paresthesia, tremor**, blurred vision, **bronchospasm, epistaxis, dyspnea**

Pregnancy Risk Factor B

Generic Available No

Lorazepam (lor A ze pam)

Related Information

Patients Requiring Sedation *on page 1565*

Temporomandibular Dysfunction (TMD) *on page 1562*

U.S. Brand Names Ativan®; Lorazepam Intensol®

Canadian Brand Names Apo®-Lorazepam; Ativan®; Novo-Lorazepam®; Nu-Loraz; Riva-Lorazepam

Mexican Brand Names Ativan®; Sinestron®

Pharmacologic Category Benzodiazepine

Use

Oral: Management of anxiety disorders or short-term relief of the symptoms of anxiety or anxiety associated with depressive symptoms

I.V.: Status epilepticus, preanesthesia for desired amnesia, antiemetic adjunct

Unlabeled/Investigational Use Ethanol detoxification; treatment of insomnia, psychogenic catatonia, partial complex seizures

Local Anesthetic/Vasoconstrictor Precautions No information available to require special precautions

Effects on Dental Treatment

>10%: Xerostomia (normal salivary flow resumes upon discontinuation), sedation, respiratory depression

1% to 10%: Hypotension, nasal congestion, hyperventilation, apnea headache, depression, confusion, dizziness, akathisia, unsteadiness, disorientation

Restrictions C-IV

Dosage

Antiemetic:

Children 2-15 years: I.V.: 0.05 mg/kg (up to 2 mg/dose) prior to chemotherapy

Adults: Oral, I.V. (**Note:** May be administered sublingually; not a labeled route): 0.5-2 mg every 4-6 hours as needed

Anxiety and sedation:

Infants and Children: Oral, I.M., I.V.: Usual: 0.05 mg/kg/dose (range: 0.02-0.09 mg/kg) every 4-8 hours

I.V.: May use smaller doses (eg, 0.01-0.03 mg/kg) and repeat every 20 minutes, as needed to titrate to effect

Adults: Oral: 1-10 mg/day in 2-3 divided doses; usual dose: 2-6 mg/day in divided doses

Elderly: 0.5-4 mg/day; initial dose not to exceed 2 mg

Insomnia: Adults: Oral: 2-4 mg at bedtime

Preoperative: Adults:

I.M.: 0.05 mg/kg administered 2 hours before surgery (maximum: 4 mg/dose)

I.V.: 0.044 mg/kg 15-20 minutes before surgery (usual maximum: 2 mg/dose)

Operative amnesia: Adults: I.V.: Up to 0.05 mg/kg (maximum: 4 mg/dose)

Sedation (preprocedure): Infants and Children:

Oral, I.M., I.V.: Usual: 0.05 mg/kg (range: 0.02-0.09 mg/kg)

I.V.: May use smaller doses (eg, 0.01-0.03 mg/kg) and repeat every 20 minutes, as needed to titrate to effect

Status epilepticus: I.V.:

Infants and Children: 0.1 mg/kg slow I.V. over 2-5 minutes; do not exceed 4 mg/single dose; may repeat second dose of 0.05 mg/kg slow I.V. in 10-15 minutes if needed

Adolescents: 0.07 mg/kg slow I.V. over 2-5 minutes; maximum: 4 mg/dose; may repeat in 10-15 minutes

Adults: 4 mg/dose slow I.V. over 2-5 minutes; may repeat in 10-15 minutes; usual maximum dose: 8 mg

Rapid tranquilization of agitated patient (administer every 30-60 minutes):

Oral: 1-2 mg

I.M.: 0.5-1 mg

Average total dose for tranquilization: Oral, I.M.: 4-8 mg

Mechanism of Action Binds to stereospecific benzodiazepine receptors on the postsynaptic GABA neuron at several sites within the central nervous system, including the limbic system, reticular formation. Enhancement of the inhibitory effect of GABA on neuronal excitability results by increased neuronal membrane permeability to chloride ions. This shift in chloride ions results in hyperpolarization (a less excitable state) and stabilization.

Other Adverse Effects

1% to 10%:

Central nervous system: Amnesia

Dermatologic: Dermatitis, rash

Gastrointestinal: Weight gain/loss, nausea, changes in appetite

Neuromuscular & skeletal: Weakness

<1%: Blood dyscrasias, **increased salivation**, menstrual irregularities, physical and psychological dependence with prolonged use, reflex slowing, polyethylene glycol or propylene glycol poisoning (prolonged I.V. infusion)

Drug Interactions

Increased Effect/Toxicity: Ethanol and other CNS depressants may increase the CNS effects of lorazepam. Scopolamine in combination with parenteral lorazepam may increase the incidence of sedation, hallucinations, and irrational behavior. There are rare reports of significant respiratory depression, stupor, and/or hypotension with concomitant use of loxapine and lorazepam. Use caution if concomitant administration of loxapine and CNS drugs is required.

Decreased Effect: Oral contraceptives may increase the clearance of lorazepam. Lorazepam may decrease the antiparkinsonian efficacy of levodopa. Theophylline and other CNS stimulants may antagonize the sedative effects of lorazepam.

Dietary/Ethanol/Herb Considerations

Ethanol: Avoid use; may increase CNS depression.

Food: Avoid grapefruit products; may increase serum concentration/toxicity.

Herb/Nutraceutical: Avoid gotu kola, kava, SAMe, St John's wort, and valerian; may increase CNS depression. Melatonin may enhance activity of clonazepam; use cautiously.

Pharmacodynamics/Kinetics

Onset of action: Hypnosis: I.M.: 20-30 minutes; Sedation, anticonvulsant: I.V.: 5 minutes; oral: 0.5-1 hour

Duration: 6-8 hours

Absorption: Oral, I.M.: Prompt

Distribution:

V_d: Neonates: 0.76 L/kg, Adults: 1.3 L/kg; crosses placenta; enters breast milk

Protein binding: 85%; free fraction may be significantly higher in elderly

Metabolism: Hepatic to inactive compounds

Half-life elimination: Neonates: 40.2 hours; Older children: 10.5 hours; Adults: 12.9 hours; Elderly: 15.9 hours; End-stage renal disease: 32-70 hours

Excretion: Urine; feces (minimal)

Pregnancy Risk Factor D

Generic Available Yes

Lorazepam Intensol® *see* Lorazepam *on page 824*

Lorcet® 10/650 *see* Hydrocodone and Acetaminophen *on page 678*

Lorcet®-HD *see* Hydrocodone and Acetaminophen *on page 678*

Lorcet® Plus *see* Hydrocodone and Acetaminophen *on page 678*

Loroxide® [OTC] *see* Benzoyl Peroxide *on page 171*

Lortab® *see* Hydrocodone and Acetaminophen *on page 678*

Losartan (loe SAR tan)

Related Information

Cardiovascular Diseases *on page 1456*

U.S. Brand Names Cozaar®

Canadian Brand Names Cozaar®

Mexican Brand Names Cozaar®

Pharmacologic Category Angiotensin II Receptor Blocker

Synonyms DuP 753; Losartan Potassium; MK594

(Continued)

Losartan *(Continued)*

Use Treatment of hypertension; treatment of diabetic nephropathy in patients with type 2 diabetes mellitus (noninsulin dependent, NIDDM) and a history of hypertension

Local Anesthetic/Vasoconstrictor Precautions No information available to require special precautions

Effects on Dental Treatment

>10%: Chest pain (12% diabetic nephropathy), hypoglycemia (14% diabetic nephropathy) cough (11% diabetic nephropathy; 17% to 29% hypertension but similar to hydrochlorothiazide or placebo therapy)

1% to 10%: Hypotension (7% diabetic nephropathy), orthostatic hypotension (4% hypertension to 4% diabetic nephropathy), first-dose hypotension (dose-related: <1% with 50 mg, 2% with 100 mg), dizziness (4%), fever (4% diabetic nephropathy), bronchitis (10% diabetic nephropathy), upper respiratory infection (8%), nasal congestion (2%), sinusitis (1% hypertension to 6% diabetic nephropathy), infection (5% diabetic nephropathy), flu-like syndrome (10% diabetic nephropathy)

Dosage Oral: Adults:

Hypertension: The usual starting dose is 50 mg once daily. Can be administered once or twice daily with total daily doses ranging from 25-100 mg.

Usual initial doses in patients receiving diuretics or those with intravascular volume depletion: 25 mg

Nephropathy in patients with type 2 diabetes and hypertension: Initial: 50 mg once daily; can be increased to 100 mg once daily based on blood pressure response

Dosing adjustment in hepatic impairment: Reduce the initial dose to 25 mg/day; divide dosage intervals into two

Hemodialysis: Not removed

Mechanism of Action As a selective and competitive, nonpeptide angiotensin II receptor antagonist, losartan blocks the vasoconstrictor and aldosterone-secreting effects of angiotensin II; losartan interacts reversibly at the AT1 and AT2 receptors of many tissues and has slow dissociation kinetics; its affinity for the AT1 receptor is 1000 times greater than the AT2 receptor. Angiotensin II receptor antagonists may induce a more complete inhibition of the renin-angiotensin system than ACE inhibitors, they do not affect the response to bradykinin, and are less likely to be associated with nonrenin-angiotensin effects (eg, cough and angioedema). Losartan increases urinary flow rate and in addition to being natriuretic and kaliuretic, increases excretion of chloride, magnesium, uric acid, calcium, and phosphate.

Other Adverse Effects

>10%:

Central nervous system: Fatigue (14% diabetic nephropathy)

Gastrointestinal: Diarrhea (2% hypertension to 15% diabetic nephropathy)

Genitourinary: Urinary tract infection (13% diabetic nephropathy)

Hematologic: Anemia (14% diabetic nephropathy)

Neuromuscular & skeletal: Weakness (14% diabetic nephropathy), back pain (2% hypertension to 12% diabetic nephropathy)

1% to 10%:

Central nervous system: Hypoesthesia (5% diabetic nephropathy), insomnia (1%)

Dermatology: Cellulitis (7% diabetic nephropathy)

Endocrine: Hyperkalemia (<1% hypertension to 7% diabetic nephropathy)

Gastrointestinal: Gastritis (5% diabetic nephropathy), weight gain (4% diabetic nephropathy), dyspepsia (1% to 4%), abdominal pain (2%), nausea (2%)

Neuromuscular & skeletal: Muscular weakness (7% diabetic nephropathy), knee pain (5% diabetic nephropathy), leg pain (1% to 5%), muscle cramps (1%), myalgia (1%),

>1% but frequency ≤ placebo: Edema, abdominal pain, nausea, **headache, pharyngitis**

<1% (Limited to important or life-threatening): **Allergic reaction**, alopecia, **anaphylactic reactions**, anemia, angina, angioedema, anorexia, **anxiety**, arm pain, **arrhythmias**, arthralgia, arthritis, ataxia, AV block (second degree), bilirubin increased, blurred vision, **bradycardia, bronchitis**, BUN increased, **confusion**, conjunctivitis, constipation, CVA, **dental pain**, depression, dermatitis, **diaphoresis**, dry skin, **dyspnea**, ecchymosis, **epistaxis**, erythema, **facial edema, fever**, flatulence, **flushing**, gastritis, gout, hematocrit decreased, hemoglobin decreased, hepatitis, hip pain, hyperkalemia, hyponatremia, **hypotension**, impotence, joint swelling, libido decreased, memory impairment, **MI, migraine**, muscle weakness, **nervousness**, nocturia, **orthostatic effects, palpitations, paresthesia**, peripheral neuropathy, **pharyngitis**, photosensitivity, pruritus, rash, **rhinitis**, serum creatinine increased, sleep disorder, **somnolence, syncope, tachycardia, abnormal taste**, tinnitus, transaminases increased, **tremor**, urinary frequency, urticaria, **ventricular arrhythmias**, vertigo, visual acuity decreased, vomiting, **xerostomia**

Postmarketing and/or case reports: Acute psychosis with paranoid delusions, ageusia, anemia, dysgeusia, Henoch-Schönlein purpura, pancreatitis, maculopapular rash, vasculitis

Drug Interactions Substrate of **CYP2C8/9, 3A4**; Inhibits CYP1A2, 2C8/9, 2C19, 3A4

Increased Effect/Toxicity: Cimetidine may increase the absorption of losartan by 18% (clinical effect is unknown). Blood levels of losartan may be increased by inhibitors of CYP2C9 (amiodarone, fluoxetine, isoniazid, ritonavir, sulfonamides) and 3A4 (diltiazem, erythromycin, verapamil, ketoconazole, itraconazole). Potassium salts/supplements, co-trimoxazole (high dose), ACE inhibitors, and potassium-sparing diuretics (amiloride, spironolactone, triamterene) may increase the risk of hyperkalemia. Risk of lithium toxicity may be increased by losartan.

Decreased Effect: Phenobarbital (CYP3A4 and 2C8/9 inducer) caused a reduction of losartan in serum by 20%, clinical effect is unknown. Other enzyme inducers may affect serum concentrations of losartan. Rifampin may reduce antihypertensive efficacy of losartan. NSAIDs may decrease the efficacy of losartan.

Dietary/Ethanol/Herb Considerations

Ethanol: Avoid use; may increase risk of hypotension or dizziness.

Food: May be taken with food. Avoid caffeine, garlic, and licorice. Buttermilk, boiled milk, or yogurt may reduce diarrhea.

Herb/Nutraceutical: Avoid black cohosh, dong quai, and evening primrose due to estrogenic activity. Avoid ephedra, ginseng, and yohimbe; may worsen hypertension. Avoid garlic; may have increased antihypertensive effect. Avoid ginger due to positive inotropic effects; theoretically, may cause arrhythmia. Avoid hawthorn; may lower peripheral vascular resistance resulting in additive decrease in BP. Avoid St John's wort; may decrease serum concentration. Avoid licorice.

Pharmacodynamics/Kinetics

Onset of action: 6 hours

Distribution: V_d: Losartan: 34 L; E-3174: 12 L; does not cross blood brain barrier

Protein binding, plasma: High

Metabolism: Hepatic (14%) via CYP2C9 and 3A4 to active metabolite, E-3174 (40 times more potent than losartan); extensive first-pass effect

Bioavailability: 25% to 33%; AUC of E-3174 is four times greater than that of losartan

Half-life elimination: Losartan: 1.5-2 hours; E-3174: 6-9 hours

Time to peak, serum: Losartan: 1 hour; E-3174: 3-4 hours

Excretion: Feces (60%); urine (35%, 3% to 8% as unchanged drug, E-3174)

Clearance: Plasma: Losartan: 600 mL/minute; Active metabolite: 50 mL/minute

Pregnancy Risk Factor C/D (2nd and 3rd trimesters)

Generic Available No

Losartan and Hydrochlorothiazide

(loe SAR tan & hye droe klor oh THYE a zide)

Related Information

Hydrochlorothiazide *on page 675*

Losartan *on page 825*

U.S. Brand Names Hyzaar®

Canadian Brand Names Hyzaar®; Hyzaar® DS

Pharmacologic Category Antihypertensive Agent Combination

Synonyms Hydrochlorothiazide and Losartan

Use Treatment of hypertension

Local Anesthetic/Vasoconstrictor Precautions No information available to require special precautions

Effects on Dental Treatment No significant effects or complications reported

Dosage Adults: Oral: 1 tablet daily

Pregnancy Risk Factor C/D (2nd and 3rd trimesters)

Generic Available No

Losartan Potassium *see* Losartan *on page 825*

Lotemax® *see* Loteprednol *on page 827*

Lotensin® *see* Benazepril *on page 166*

Lotensin® HCT *see* Benazepril and Hydrochlorothiazide *on page 167*

Loteprednol (loe te PRED nol)

U.S. Brand Names Alrex®; Lotemax®

Canadian Brand Names Alrex®; Lotemax®

Pharmacologic Category Corticosteroid, Ophthalmic

Synonyms Loteprednol Etabonate

Use

Suspension, 0.2% (Alrex™): Temporary relief of signs and symptoms of seasonal allergic conjunctivitis

Suspension, 0.5% (Lotemax™): Inflammatory conditions (treatment of steroid-responsive inflammatory conditions of the palpebral and bulbar conjunctiva, cornea, and anterior segment of the globe such as allergic conjunctivitis, acne rosacea, superficial punctate keratitis, herpes zoster keratitis, iritis, cyclitis, selected infective conjunctivitis, when the inherent hazard of steroid use is accepted to obtain an advisable diminution in edema and inflammation) and treatment of postoperative inflammation following ocular surgery

(Continued)

Loteprednol *(Continued)*

Local Anesthetic/Vasoconstrictor Precautions No information available to require special precautions

Effects on Dental Treatment >10%: Rhinitis, pharyngitis, headache

Dosage Adults: Ophthalmic:

Suspension, 0.2% (Alrex™): Instill 1 drop into affected eye(s) 4 times/day

Suspension, 0.5% (Lotemax™):

Inflammatory conditions: Apply 1-2 drops into the conjunctival sac of the affected eye(s) 4 times/day. During the initial treatment within the first week, the dosing may be increased up to 1 drop every hour. Advise patients not to discontinue therapy prematurely. If signs and symptoms fail to improve after 2 days, re-evaluate the patient.

Postoperative inflammation: Apply 1-2 drops into the conjunctival sac of the operated eye(s) 4 times/day beginning 24 hours after surgery and continuing throughout the first 2 weeks of the postoperative period

Mechanism of Action Corticosteroids inhibit the inflammatory response including edema, capillary dilation, leukocyte migration, and scar formation. Loteprednol is highly lipid soluble and penetrates cells readily to induce the production of lipocortins. These proteins modulate the activity of prostaglandins and leukotrienes.

Other Adverse Effects

1% to 10%: Ocular: Abnormal vision/blurring, burning on instillation, chemosis, dry eyes, itching, injection, conjunctivitis/irritation, corneal abnormalities, eyelid erythema, papillae uveitis

<1%: Cataract formation, changes in visual acuity and/or field defects, global perforation in disease which thins cornea or sclera, increased intraocular pressure, secondary ocular infection

Pharmacodynamics/Kinetics Absorption: None

Pregnancy Risk Factor C

Generic Available No

Loteprednol Etabonate *see* Loteprednol *on page 827*

Lotrel® *see* Amlodipine and Benazepril *on page 89*

Lotrimin® *see* Clotrimazole *on page 356*

Lotrimin® AF [OTC] *see* Clotrimazole *on page 356*

Lotrimin® AF Powder/Spray [OTC] *see* Miconazole *on page 906*

Lotrimin® Ultra™ [OTC] *see* Butenafine *on page 217*

Lotrisone® *see* Betamethasone and Clotrimazole *on page 179*

Lotronex® *see* Alosetron *on page 60*

Lovastatin (LOE vu sta tin)

Related Information

Cardiovascular Diseases *on page 1456*

U.S. Brand Names Altocor™; Mevacor®

Canadian Brand Names Apo®-Lovastatin; Gen-Lovastatin; Mevacor®; ratio-Lovastatin

Mexican Brand Names Mevacor®

Pharmacologic Category Antilipemic Agent, HMG-CoA Reductase Inhibitor

Synonyms Mevinolin; Monacolin K

Use

Adjunct to dietary therapy to decrease elevated serum total and LDL-cholesterol concentrations in primary hypercholesterolemia

Primary prevention of coronary artery disease (patients without symptomatic disease with average to moderately elevated total and LDL-cholesterol and below average HDL-cholesterol); slow progression of coronary atherosclerosis in patients with coronary heart disease

Adjunct to dietary therapy in adolescent patients (10-17 years of age, females >1 year postmenarche) with heterozygous familial hypercholesterolemia having LDL >189 mg/dL, **or** LDL >160 mg/dL with positive family history of premature cardiovascular disease (CVD), **or** LDL >160 mg/dL with the presence of at least two other CVD risk factors

Local Anesthetic/Vasoconstrictor Precautions No information available to require special precautions

Effects on Dental Treatment Headache (2% to 3%), dizziness (0.5% to 1%)

Dosage Oral:

Adolescents 10-17 years: Immediate release tablet:

LDL reduction <20%: Initial: 10 mg/day with evening meal

LDL reduction ≥20%: Initial: 20 mg/day with evening meal

Usual range: 10-40 mg with evening meal, then adjust dose at 4-week intervals

Adults: Initial: 20 mg with evening meal, then adjust at 4-week intervals; maximum dose: 80 mg/day immediate release tablet **or** 60 mg/day extended release tablet; before initiation of therapy, patients should be placed on a standard cholesterol-lowering diet for 3-6 months and the diet should be continued during drug therapy. Patients receiving immunosuppressant drugs should start at 10 mg/day and not exceed 20 mg/day. Patients receiving concurrent therapy with fibrates should not exceed 20 mg lovastatin. Patients receiving amiodarone, niacin, or verapamil should not exceed 40 mg lovastatin daily.

Mechanism of Action Lovastatin acts by competitively inhibiting 3-hydroxyl-3-methylglutaryl-coenzyme A (HMG-CoA) reductase, the enzyme that catalyzes the rate-limiting step in cholesterol biosynthesis

Other Adverse Effects Percentages as reported with immediate release tablets (similar adverse reactions seen with extended release tablets):

>10%: Neuromuscular & skeletal: Increased CPK (>2x normal) (11%)

1% to 10%:

Dermatologic: Rash (0.8% to 1%)

Gastrointestinal: Abdominal pain (2% to 3%), constipation (2% to 4%), diarrhea (2% to 3%), dyspepsia (1% to 2%), flatulence (4% to 5%), nausea (2% to 3%)

Neuromuscular & skeletal: Myalgia (2% to 3%), weakness (1% to 2%), muscle cramps (0.6% to 1%)

Ocular: Blurred vision (0.8% to 1%)

<1% (Limited to important or life-threatening): **Chest pain, acid regurgitation, xerostomia, vomiting**, leg pain, arthralgia, insomnia, **paresthesia**, alopecia, pruritus, eye irritation, dermatomyositis

Additional class-related events or case reports (not necessarily reported with lovastatin therapy): Myopathy, increased CPK (>10x normal), rhabdomyolysis, renal failure (secondary to rhabdomyolysis), **alteration in taste**, impaired extraocular muscle movement, **facial paresis, tremor**, memory loss, vertigo, peripheral neuropathy, peripheral nerve palsy, **anxiety**, depression, psychic disturbance, **hypersensitivity reaction, angioedema, anaphylaxis**, systemic lupus erythematosus-like syndrome, polymyalgia rheumatica, vasculitis, purpura, thrombocytopenia, leukopenia, hemolytic anemia, positive ANA, increased ESR, eosinophilia, arthritis, urticaria, photosensitivity, **fever, flushing, dyspnea**, chills, malaise, rash, alopecia, pruritus, toxic epidermal necrolysis, erythema multiforme, Stevens-Johnson syndrome, pancreatitis, hepatitis, cholestatic jaundice, fatty liver, cirrhosis, fulminant hepatic necrosis, hepatoma, anorexia, vomiting, nodules, skin discoloration, **dryness of skin/mucous membranes**, nail changes, gynecomastia, decreased libido, erectile dysfunction, impotence, cataracts, ophthalmoplegia, elevated transaminases, increased alkaline phosphatase, increased GGT, hyperbilirubinemia, thyroid dysfunction

Drug Interactions Substrate of **CYP3A4**; Inhibits CYP2C8/9, 2D6

Increased Effect/Toxicity: Inhibitors of CYP3A4 (amiodarone, amprenavir, clarithromycin, cyclosporine, diltiazem, fluvoxamine, erythromycin, fluconazole, indinavir, itraconazole, ketoconazole, miconazole, nefazodone, nelfinavir, ritonavir, troleandomycin, and verapamil) increase lovastatin blood levels and may increase the risk of myopathy and rhabdomyolysis. Limit dose to ≤40 mg with amiodarone or verapamil. Suspend lovastatin therapy during concurrent clarithromycin, erythromycin, itraconazole, or ketoconazole therapy. Cyclosporine, clofibrate, fenofibrate, gemfibrozil, and niacin also may increase the risk of myopathy and rhabdomyolysis. Limit dose to ≤20 mg with concurrent gemfibrozil. The effect/toxicity of warfarin (elevated PT) and levothyroxine may be increased by lovastatin. Digoxin, norethindrone, and ethinyl estradiol levels may be increased. Effects are additive with other lipid-lowering therapies.

Decreased Effect: Cholestyramine taken with lovastatin reduces lovastatin absorption and effect.

Dietary/Ethanol/Herb Considerations

Ethanol: Avoid excessive consumption due to potential hepatic effects.

Administer with food; therapeutic effect may be decreased. Avoid grapefruit products; may increase serum concentration. Requires a standard cholesterol-lowering diet for 3-6 months prior to and during therapy.

Herb/Nutraceutical: Avoid St John's wort; may decrease serum concentration.

Pharmacodynamics/Kinetics

Onset of action: LDL-cholesterol reductions: 3 days

Absorption: 30%; increased with extended release tablets

Protein binding: 95%

Metabolism: Hepatic; extensive first-pass effect; hydrolyzed to B-hydroxy acid (active)

Bioavailability: Increased with extended release tablets

Half-life elimination: 1.1-1.7 hours

Time to peak, serum: 2-4 hours

Excretion: Feces (~80% to 85%); urine (10%)

Pregnancy Risk Factor X

Generic Available Yes: Immediate release tablet

Lovastatin and Niacin *see* Niacin and Lovastatin *on page 968*

Lovenox® *see* Enoxaparin *on page 495*

Low-Ogestrel® *see* Combination Hormonal Contraceptives *on page 368*

Loxapine (LOKS a peen)

U.S. Brand Names Loxitane®; Loxitane® C

Canadian Brand Names Apo®-Loxapine; Nu-Loxapine; PMS-Loxapine

(Continued)

Loxapine *(Continued)*

Pharmacologic Category Antipsychotic Agent, Dibenzoxazepine

Synonyms Loxapine Hydrochloride; Loxapine Succinate; Oxilapine Succinate

Use Management of psychotic disorders

Local Anesthetic/Vasoconstrictor Precautions Most pharmacology textbooks state that in presence of phenothiazines, systemic doses of epinephrine paradoxically decrease the blood pressure. This is the so called "epinephrine reversal" phenomenon. This has never been observed when epinephrine is given by infiltration as part of the anesthesia procedure.

Effects on Dental Treatment >10%: Xerostomia, changes in salivation

Significant hypotension may occur, especially when the drug is administered parenterally; orthostatic hypotension is due to alpha-receptor blockade, the elderly are at greater risk for orthostatic hypotension

Tardive dyskinesia: Prevalence rate may be 40% in elderly; development of the syndrome and the irreversible nature are proportional to duration and total cumulative dose over time. Extrapyramidal reactions are more common in elderly with up to 50% developing these reactions after 60 years of age; drug-induced **Parkinson's syndrome** occurs often; **Akathisia** is the most common extrapyramidal reaction in elderly.

Increased confusion, memory loss, psychotic behavior, and agitation frequently occur as a consequence of anticholinergic effects Antipsychotic associated sedation in nonpsychotic patients is extremely unpleasant due to feelings of depersonalization, derealization, and dysphoria

Dosage Oral:

Adults: 10 mg twice daily, increase dose until psychotic symptoms are controlled; usual dose range: 20-100 mg/day in divided doses 2-4 times/day; dosages >250 mg/day are not recommended

Elderly: 20-60 mg/day

Mechanism of Action Blocks postsynaptic mesolimbic D_1 and D_2 receptors in the brain, and also possesses serotonin 5-HT_2 blocking activity

Other Adverse Effects Frequency not defined:

Cardiovascular: **Orthostatic hypotension, tachycardia, arrhythmias,** abnormal T-waves with prolonged ventricular repolarization, **hypertension, hypotension, lightheadedness, syncope**

Central nervous system: **Drowsiness, extrapyramidal symptoms (dystonia, akathisia, pseudoparkinsonism, tardive dyskinesia, akinesia), dizziness, faintness,** ataxia, insomnia, **agitation, tension, seizures, slurred speech, confusion, headache,** neuroleptic malignant syndrome (NMS), altered central temperature regulation

Dermatologic: Rash, pruritus, photosensitivity, dermatitis, alopecia, seborrhea

Endocrine & metabolic: Enlargement of breasts, galactorrhea, amenorrhea, gynecomastia, menstrual irregularity

Gastrointestinal: Constipation, nausea, vomiting, weight gain/loss, adynamic ileus, polydipsia

Genitourinary: Urinary retention, sexual dysfunction

Hematologic: Agranulocytosis, leukopenia, thrombocytopenia

Neuromuscular & skeletal: Weakness

Ocular: Blurred vision

Respiratory: **Nasal congestion**

Drug Interactions

Increased Effect/Toxicity: Loxapine concentrations may be increased by chloroquine, propranolol, sulfadoxine-pyrimethamine. Loxapine may increased the effect and/or toxicity of antihypertensives, lithium, TCAs, CNS depressants (ethanol, narcotics), and trazodone. There are rare reports of significant respiratory depression, stupor, and/or hypotension with the concomitant use of loxapine and lorazepam. Use caution if the concomitant administration of loxapine and CNS drugs is required. Metoclopramide may increase risk of extrapyramidal symptoms (EPS).

Decreased Effect: Antipsychotics inhibit the activity of bromocriptine and levodopa. Benztropine (and other anticholinergics) may inhibit the therapeutic response to loxapine and excess anticholinergic effects may occur. Barbiturates and cigarette smoking may enhance the hepatic metabolism of loxapine. Loxapine and possibly other low potency antipsychotic may reverse the pressor effects of epinephrine.

Dietary/Ethanol/Herb Considerations

Ethanol: Avoid use; may increase CNS depression.

Herb/Nutraceutical: Avoid gotu kola, kava, SAMe, St John's wort, and valerian; may increase CNS depression.

Pharmacodynamics/Kinetics

Onset of action: Neuroleptic: Oral: 20-30 minutes

Peak effect: 1.5-3 hours

Duration: ~12 hours

Metabolism: Hepatic to glucuronide conjugates

Half-life elimination: Biphasic: Initial: 5 hours; Terminal: 12-19 hours

Excretion: Urine; feces (small amounts)

Pregnancy Risk Factor C

Generic Available Yes

Loxapine Hydrochloride *see* Loxapine *on page 829*
Loxapine Succinate *see* Loxapine *on page 829*
Loxitane® *see* Loxapine *on page 829*
Loxitane® C *see* Loxapine *on page 829*
Lozi-Flur™ *see* Fluoride *on page 586*
Lozol® *see* Indapamide *on page 716*
L-PAM *see* Melphalan *on page 855*
L-Sarcolysin *see* Melphalan *on page 855*
LTG *see* Lamotrigine *on page 774*
***L*-Thyroxine Sodium** *see* Levothyroxine *on page 800*
Lu-26-054 *see* Escitalopram *on page 516*
Lubriderm® [OTC] *see* Lanolin, Cetyl Alcohol, Glycerin, Petrolatum, and Mineral Oil *on page 776*
Lubriderm® Fragrance Free [OTC] *see* Lanolin, Cetyl Alcohol, Glycerin, Petrolatum, and Mineral Oil *on page 776*
Lufyllin® *see* Dyphylline *on page 485*
Lugol's Solution *see* Potassium Iodide *on page 1101*
Lumigan™ *see* Bimatoprost *on page 184*
Luminal® Sodium *see* Phenobarbital *on page 1066*
Lumitene™ *see* Beta-Carotene *on page 176*
Lunelle™ *see* Estradiol and Medroxyprogesterone *on page 523*
LupiCare™ Dandruff [OTC] *see* Salicylic Acid *on page 1204*
LupiCare™ II Psoriasis [OTC] *see* Salicylic Acid *on page 1204*
LupiCare™ Psoriasis [OTC] *see* Salicylic Acid *on page 1204*
Lupron® *see* Leuprolide *on page 784*
Lupron Depot® *see* Leuprolide *on page 784*
Lupron Depot-Ped® *see* Leuprolide *on page 784*
Luride® *see* Fluoride *on page 586*
Luride® Lozi-Tab® *see* Fluoride *on page 586*
Lustra® *see* Hydroquinone *on page 693*
Lustra-AF™ *see* Hydroquinone *on page 693*
Luvox® [DSC] *see* Fluvoxamine *on page 605*
Luxiq™ *see* Betamethasone *on page 177*
LY139603 *see* Atomoxetine *on page 139*
LY170053 *see* Olanzapine *on page 996*

Lymphocyte Immune Globulin (LIM foe syte i MYOON GLOB yoo lin)

U.S. Brand Names Atgam®

Canadian Brand Names Atgam®

Pharmacologic Category Immunosuppressant Agent

Synonyms Antithymocyte Globulin (Equine); Antithymocyte Immunoglobulin; ATG; Horse Antihuman Thymocyte Gamma Globulin

Use Prevention and treatment of acute renal and other solid organ allograft rejection; treatment of moderate to severe aplastic anemia in patients not considered suitable candidates for bone marrow transplantation; prevention of graft-versus-host disease following bone marrow transplantation

Local Anesthetic/Vasoconstrictor Precautions No information available to require special precautions

Effects on Dental Treatment

>10%: Fever, systemic infection

1% to 10%: stomatitis, GI bleeding hypotension, hypertension, tachycardia, chest pain, headache, dyspnea, sensitivity reactions (anaphylaxis may be indicated by hypotension, respiratory distress), serum sickness, viral infection

Dosage An intradermal skin test is recommended prior to administration of the initial dose of ATG; use 0.1 mL of a 1:1000 dilution of ATG in normal saline. A positive skin reaction consists of a wheal ≥10 mm in diameter. If a positive skin test occurs, the first infusion should be administered in a controlled environment with intensive life support immediately available. A systemic reaction precludes further administration of the drug. The absence of a reaction does **not** preclude the possibility of an immediate sensitivity reaction.

First dose: Premedicate with diphenhydramine 50 mg orally 30 minutes prior to and hydrocortisone 100 mg I.V. 15 minutes prior to infusion and acetaminophen 650 mg 2 hours after start of infusion

Children: I.V.:

Aplastic anemia protocol: 10-20 mg/kg/day for 8-14 days; then administer every other day for 7 more doses; addition doses may be given every other day for 21 total doses in 28 days

(Continued)

Lymphocyte Immune Globulin *(Continued)*

Renal allograft: 5-25 mg/kg/day

Adults: I.V.:

Aplastic anemia protocol: 10-20 mg/kg/day for 8-14 days, then administer every other day for 7 more doses

Renal allograft:

Rejection prophylaxis: 15 mg/kg/day for 14 days followed by 14 days of alternative day therapy at the same dose; the first dose should be administered within 24 hours before or after transplantation

Rejection treatment: 10-15 mg/kg/day for 14 days, then administer every other day for 10-14 days up to 21 doses in 28 days

Mechanism of Action May involve elimination of antigen-reactive T-lymphocytes (killer cells) in peripheral blood or alteration of T-cell function

Other Adverse Effects

>10%:

Central nervous system: Chills

Dermatologic: Rash

Hematologic: Leukopenia, thrombocytopenia

1% to 10%:

Cardiovascular: Edema

Central nervous system: Malaise, pain

Gastrointestinal: Diarrhea, nausea

Local: Edema or redness at injection site, thrombophlebitis

Neuromuscular & skeletal: Myalgia, back pain, arthralgia

Renal: Abnormal RFTs

<1%: **Seizures**, pruritus, urticaria, hemolysis, anemia, arthralgia, weakness, acute renal failure, lymphadenopathy

Pharmacodynamics/Kinetics

Distribution: Poorly into lymphoid tissues; binds to circulating lymphocytes, granulocytes, platelets, bone marrow cells

Half-life elimination, plasma: 1.5-12 days

Excretion: Urine (~1%)

Pregnancy Risk Factor C

Generic Available No

Lymphocyte Mitogenic Factor *see* Aldesleukin *on page 50*

Lysine (LYE seen)

U.S. Brand Names Lysinyl [OTC]

Pharmacologic Category Dietary Supplement

Synonyms L-Lysine; L-Lysine Hydrochloride

Use Improves utilization of vegetable proteins

Local Anesthetic/Vasoconstrictor Precautions No information available to require special precautions

Effects on Dental Treatment No significant effects or complications reported

Dosage Adults: Oral: 334-1500 mg/day

Pregnancy Risk Factor C

Generic Available Yes

Lysinyl [OTC] *see* Lysine *on page 832*

Lysodren® *see* Mitotane *on page 922*

Maalox® [OTC] *see* Aluminum Hydroxide and Magnesium Hydroxide *on page 69*

Maalox® Fast Release Liquid [OTC] *see* Aluminum Hydroxide, Magnesium Hydroxide, and Simethicone *on page 69*

Maalox® Max [OTC] *see* Aluminum Hydroxide, Magnesium Hydroxide, and Simethicone *on page 69*

Maalox® TC (Therapeutic Concentrate) [OTC] *see* Aluminum Hydroxide and Magnesium Hydroxide *on page 69*

Macrobid® *see* Nitrofurantoin *on page 980*

Macrodantin® *see* Nitrofurantoin *on page 980*

Mafenide (MA fe nide)

U.S. Brand Names Sulfamylon®

Pharmacologic Category Antibiotic, Topical

Synonyms Mafenide Acetate

Use Adjunct in the treatment of second- and third-degree burns to prevent septicemia caused by susceptible organisms such as *Pseudomonas aeruginosa*

Orphan drug: Prevention of graft loss of meshed autografts on excised burn wounds

Local Anesthetic/Vasoconstrictor Precautions No information available to require special precautions

Effects on Dental Treatment No significant effects or complications reported

Dosage Children and Adults: Topical: Apply once or twice daily with a sterile gloved hand; apply to a thickness of approximately 16 mm; the burned area should be covered with cream at all times

Mechanism of Action Interferes with bacterial folic acid synthesis through competitive inhibition of para-aminobenzoic acid

Other Adverse Effects Frequency not defined:

- Cardiovascular: **Facial edema**
- Central nervous system: Pain
- Dermatologic: Rash, erythema
- Endocrine & metabolic: Hyperchloremia, metabolic acidosis
- Hematologic: Porphyria, bone marrow suppression, hemolytic anemia, **bleeding**
- Local: Burning sensation, excoriation
- Respiratory: **Hyperventilation, tachypnea, dyspnea**
- Miscellaneous: **Hypersensitivity**

Pharmacodynamics/Kinetics

- Absorption: Diffuses through devascularized areas and is rapidly absorbed from burned surface
- Metabolism: To para-carboxybenzene sulfonamide, a carbonic anhydrase inhibitor
- Time to peak, serum: 2-4 hours
- Excretion: Urine (as metabolites)

Pregnancy Risk Factor C

Generic Available No

Mafenide Acetate *see* Mafenide *on page 832*

Magaldrate and Simethicone (MAG al drate & sye METH i kone)

Related Information

Simethicone *on page 1222*

U.S. Brand Names Riopan Plus® [OTC]; Riopan Plus® Double Strength [OTC]

Pharmacologic Category Antacid; Antiflatulent

Synonyms Simethicone and Magaldrate

Use Relief of hyperacidity associated with peptic ulcer, gastritis, peptic esophagitis and hiatal hernia which are accompanied by symptoms of gas

Local Anesthetic/Vasoconstrictor Precautions No information available to require special precautions

Effects on Dental Treatment No significant effects or complications reported

Dosage Adults: Oral: 540-1080 mg magaldrate between meals and at bedtime

Mechanism of Action Chemical entity known as hydroxy magnesium aluminate equivalent to magnesium oxide and aluminum oxide

Other Adverse Effects Frequency not defined:

Based on magaldrate component:

- Central nervous system: Encephalopathy
- Gastrointestinal: Constipation, chalky taste, stomach cramps, fecal impaction, diarrhea, nausea, vomiting, discoloration of feces (white speckles), rebound hyperacidity
- Endocrine & metabolic: Hypophosphatemia, hypermagnesemia, milk-alkali syndrome
- Neuromuscular & metabolic: Osteomalacia
- Miscellaneous: Aluminum intoxication

Pregnancy Risk Factor C

Generic Available Yes

Comments Unlike other magnesium containing antacids, Riopan® is safe to use in renal patients if used cautiously.

Mag Delay® [OTC] *see* Magnesium Chloride *on page 833*
Mag Delay® [OTC] *see* Magnesium Supplements *on page 837*
Mag G® [OTC] *see* Magnesium Supplements *on page 837*
Mag-Gel® 600 *see* Magnesium Supplements *on page 837*
Maginex™ [OTC] *see* Magnesium L-aspartate Hydrochloride *on page 836*
Maginex™ *see* Magnesium Supplements *on page 837*
Maginex™ DS [OTC] *see* Magnesium L-aspartate Hydrochloride *on page 836*
Maginex™ DS *see* Magnesium Supplements *on page 837*
Magnesia Magma *see* Magnesium Hydroxide *on page 835*
Magnesia Magma (Magnesium Hydroxide) *see* Magnesium Supplements *on page 837*
Magnesium Carbonate and Aluminum Hydroxide *see* Aluminum Hydroxide and Magnesium Carbonate *on page 68*

Magnesium Chloride (mag NEE zee um KLOR ide)

U.S. Brand Names Chloromag®; Mag Delay® [OTC]; Mag-SR® [OTC]; Slow-Mag® [OTC]

Pharmacologic Category Magnesium Salt

Use Correction or prevention of hypomagnesemia

(Continued)

Magnesium Chloride *(Continued)*

Local Anesthetic/Vasoconstrictor Precautions No information available to require special precautions

Effects on Dental Treatment 1% to 10%: CNS depression, drowsiness, flushing, respiratory paralysis

Magnesium products may prevent GI absorption of tetracyclines by forming a large ionized chelated molecule with the tetracyclines in the stomach. Tetracyclines should be given at least 1 hour before magnesium.

Dosage Dietary supplement:

Oral: Adults: 54-483 mg/day in divided doses; refer to product labeling. The recommended dietary allowance (RDA) of magnesium is 4.5 mg/kg which is a total daily allowance of 350-400 mg for adult men and 280-300 mg for adult women. During pregnancy the RDA is 300 mg and during lactation the RDA is 355 mg.

I.V. in TPN:

Children: 2-10 mEq/day

The usual recommended pediatric maintenance intake of magnesium ranges from 0.2-0.6 mEq/kg/day. The dose of magnesium may also be based on the caloric intake; on that basis, 3-10 mEq/day of magnesium are needed; maximum maintenance dose: 8-16 mEq/day

Adults: 8-24 mEq/day

Other Adverse Effects 1% to 10%:

Gastrointestinal: Diarrhea

Neuromuscular & skeletal: Blocked peripheral neuromuscular transmission, deep tendon reflexes

Pregnancy Risk Factor D

Generic Available Yes: Injection

Magnesium Chloride *see* Magnesium Supplements *on page 837*

Magnesium Citrate (mag NEE zee um SIT rate)

Canadian Brand Names Citro-Mag®

Pharmacologic Category Laxative, Saline; Magnesium Salt

Synonyms Citrate of Magnesia

Use Evacuation of bowel prior to certain surgical and diagnostic procedures or overdose situations

Local Anesthetic/Vasoconstrictor Precautions No information available to require special precautions

Effects on Dental Treatment 1% to 10%: Hypotension, respiratory depression

Magnesium products may prevent GI absorption of tetracyclines by forming a large ionized chelated molecule with the tetracyclines in the stomach. Tetracyclines should be given at least 1 hour before magnesium.

Dosage Cathartic: Oral:

Children:

<6 years: 0.5 mL/kg up to a maximum of 200 mL repeated every 4-6 hours until stools are clear

6-12 years: 100-150 mL

Children ≥12 years and Adults: ½ to 1 full bottle (120-300 mL)

Mechanism of Action Promotes bowel evacuation by causing osmotic retention of fluid which distends the colon with increased peristaltic activity

Other Adverse Effects 1% to 10%:

Endocrine & metabolic: Hypermagnesemia

Gastrointestinal: Abdominal cramps, diarrhea, gas formation

Dietary/Ethanol/Herb Considerations Food: Administer with water, fruit juice, or citrus-flavored carbonated beverage and chill before using. Magnesium content of 5 mL: 3.85-4.71 mEq

Pharmacodynamics/Kinetics

Absorption: Oral: 15% to 30%

Excretion: Urine

Pregnancy Risk Factor B

Generic Available Yes

Magnesium Citrate *see* Magnesium Supplements *on page 837*

Magnesium Gluconate (mag NEE zee um GLOO koe nate)

U.S. Brand Names Almora® [OTC], Mag G® [OTC]; Magonate® [OTC]; Magonate® Sport [OTC]; Magtrate® [OTC]

Pharmacologic Category Magnesium Salt

Use Dietary supplement for treatment of magnesium deficiencies

Local Anesthetic/Vasoconstrictor Precautions No information available to require special precautions

Effects on Dental Treatment Magnesium products may prevent GI absorption of tetracyclines by forming a large ionized chelated molecule with the tetracyclines in the stomach. Tetracyclines should be given at least 1 hour before magnesium.

Dosage The recommended dietary allowance (RDA) of magnesium is 4.5 mg/kg which is a total daily allowance of 350-400 mg for adult men and 280-300 mg for adult women. During pregnancy the RDA is 300 mg and during lactation the RDA is 355 mg.

Dietary supplement: Oral:
- Children: 3-6 mg/kg/day in divided doses 3-4 times/day; maximum: 400 mg/day
- Adults: 54-483 mg/day in divided doses; refer to product labeling

Dosing adjustment in renal impairment: Contraindicated in severe renal failure due to toxicity from accumulation
- Cl_{cr} <25 mL/minute: Monitor serum magnesium levels

Mechanism of Action Magnesium is important as a cofactor in many enzymatic reactions in the body involving protein synthesis and carbohydrate metabolism (at least 300 enzymatic reactions require magnesium). Actions on lipoprotein lipase have been found to be important in reducing serum cholesterol and on sodium/potassium ATPase in promoting polarization (ie, neuromuscular functioning).

Other Adverse Effects Frequency not defined: Gastrointestinal: Diarrhea (excessive dose)

Drug Interactions
- Increased Effect/Toxicity: Nondepolarizing neuromuscular blockers.
- Decreased Effect: Decreased absorption of aminoquinolones, digoxin, nitrofurantoin, penicillamine, and tetracyclines may occur with magnesium salts.

Pharmacodynamics/Kinetics Absorption: Oral: 15% to 30%

Generic Available Yes: Tablet

Comments Magnesium content of 500 mg: 27 mg

Magnesium Gluconate *see* Magnesium Supplements *on page 837*

Magnesium Hydroxide (mag NEE zee um hye DROKS ide)

U.S. Brand Names Phillips'® Milk of Magnesia [OTC]

Pharmacologic Category Antacid; Magnesium Salt

Synonyms Magnesia Magma; Milk of Magnesia; MOM

Use Short-term treatment of occasional constipation and symptoms of hyperacidity, magnesium replacement therapy

Local Anesthetic/Vasoconstrictor Precautions No information available to require special precautions

Effects on Dental Treatment Magnesium products may prevent GI absorption of tetracyclines by forming a large ionized chelated molecule with the tetracyclines in the stomach. Tetracyclines should be given at least 1 hour before magnesium.

Dosage Average daily intakes of dietary magnesium have declined in recent years due to processing of food. The latest estimate of the average American dietary intake was 349 mg/day.

Oral:
- Laxative:
  - Liquid:
    - Children
      - <2 years: 0.5 mL/kg/dose
      - 2-5 years: 5-15 mL/day (2.5-7.5 mL/day of liquid concentrate) or in divided doses
      - 6-12 years: 15-30 mL/day (7.5-15 mL/day of liquid concentrate) or in divided doses
    - Children ≥12 years and Adults: 30-60 mL/day (15-30 mL/day of liquid concentrate) or in divided doses
  - Tablet:
    - Children:
      - 2-5 years: 1-2 tablets before bedtime
      - 6-11 years: 3-4 tablets before bedtime
    - Children ≥12 years and Adults: 6-8 tablets before bedtime
- Antacid:
  - Liquid:
    - Children: 2.5-5 mL as needed up to 4 times/day
    - Adults: 5-15 mL (2.5-7.5 mL of liquid concentrate) as needed up to 4 times/day
  - Tablet:
    - Children 7-14 years: 1 tablet up to 4 times/day
    - Adults: 2-4 tablets up to 4 times/day

Dosing in renal impairment: Contraindicated in severe renal failure due to toxicity from accumulation
- Cl_{cr} <25 mL/minute: Monitor serum magnesium levels

Mechanism of Action Promotes bowel evacuation by causing osmotic retention of fluid which distends the colon with increased peristaltic activity; reacts with hydrochloric acid in stomach to form magnesium chloride

Other Adverse Effects Frequency not defined:
- Cardiovascular: **Hypotension**
- Endocrine & metabolic: Hypermagnesemia
- Gastrointestinal: Diarrhea, abdominal cramps
- Neuromuscular & skeletal: Muscle weakness

(Continued)

Magnesium Hydroxide *(Continued)*

Respiratory: **Respiratory depression**

Drug Interactions Decreased Effect: Absorption of tetracyclines, digoxin, iron salts, isoniazid, or quinolones may be decreased.

Dietary/Ethanol/Herb Considerations Food: Follow each dose with 8 oz water or citrus fruit juice.

Pharmacodynamics/Kinetics

Onset of action: Laxative: 4-8 hours

Excretion: Urine (up to 30% as absorbed magnesium ions); feces (as unabsorbed drug)

Pregnancy Risk Factor B

Generic Available Yes: Liquid

Magnesium Hydroxide *see* Magnesium Supplements *on page 837*

Magnesium Hydroxide, Aluminum Hydroxide, and Simethicone *see* Aluminum Hydroxide, Magnesium Hydroxide, and Simethicone *on page 69*

Magnesium Hydroxide and Aluminum Hydroxide *see* Aluminum Hydroxide and Magnesium Hydroxide *on page 69*

Magnesium Hydroxide and Mineral Oil

(mag NEE zee um hye DROKS ide & MIN er ol oyl)

Related Information

Magnesium Hydroxide *on page 835*

U.S. Brand Names Phillips' M-O® [OTC]

Pharmacologic Category Laxative

Synonyms MOM/Mineral Oil Emulsion

Use Short-term treatment of occasional constipation

Local Anesthetic/Vasoconstrictor Precautions No information available to require special precautions

Effects on Dental Treatment Magnesium products may prevent GI absorption of tetracyclines by forming a large ionized chelated molecule with the tetracyclines in the stomach. Tetracyclines should be given at least 1 hour before magnesium.

Dosage Oral:

Adults: 5-45 mL at bedtime

Product labeling:

Children 6-11 years: 5-15 mL at bedtime or upon rising

Children ≥12 years and Adults: 30-60 mL at bedtime or upon rising

Other Adverse Effects Frequency not defined:

Cardiovascular: **Hypotension**

Endocrine & metabolic: Hypermagnesemia

Gastrointestinal: Diarrhea, abdominal cramps

Neuromuscular & skeletal: Muscle weakness

Respiratory: **Respiratory depression**

Drug Interactions Decreased Effect: Absorption of tetracyclines, digoxin, iron salts, isoniazid, or quinolones may be decreased.

Pregnancy Risk Factor B

Generic Available No

Magnesium Hydroxide and Mineral Oil Emulsion *see* Magnesium Supplements *on page 837*

Magnesium Hydroxide, Famotidine, and Calcium Carbonate *see* Famotidine, Calcium Carbonate, and Magnesium Hydroxide *on page 557*

Magnesium L-aspartate Hydrochloride

(mag NEE zhum el as PAR tate hye droe KLOR ide)

U.S. Brand Names Maginex™ [OTC]; Maginex™ DS [OTC]

Pharmacologic Category Electrolyte Supplement, Oral

Synonyms MAH™

Use Dietary supplement

Local Anesthetic/Vasoconstrictor Precautions No information available to require special precautions

Effects on Dental Treatment Magnesium ions prevent GI absorption of tetracycline by forming a large, ionized, chelated molecule with the magnesium ion and tetracyclines in the stomach. Magnesium supplement should not be taken within 2-4 hours of oral tetracycline or other members of the tetracycline family.

Dosage Adults:

Recommended dietary allowance (RDA) of magnesium:

Male: 400-420 mg

Female: 310-320 mg

During pregnancy: 360 mg

During lactation: 320 mg

Dietary supplement: Oral: Magnesium-L-aspartate 1230 mg (magnesium 122 mg) up to 3 times/day

Dosing adjustment in renal impairment: Contraindicated in severe renal failure due to toxicity from accumulation

Other Adverse Effects Frequency not defined: Gastrointestinal: Diarrhea, loose stools

Dietary/Ethanol/Herb Considerations Food: Administer with food.

Magnesium L-aspartate Hydrochloride *see* Magnesium Supplements *on page 837*

Magnesium Oxide *see* Magnesium Supplements *on page 837*

Magnesium Salicylate (mag NEE zee um sa LIS i late)

Related Information

Rheumatoid Arthritis, Osteoarthritis, and Osteoporosis *on page 1488*

Temporomandibular Dysfunction (TMD) *on page 1562*

U.S. Brand Names Doan's® [OTC]; Doan's® Extra Strength [OTC]; Mobidin® [DSC]; Momentum® [OTC]

Mexican Brand Names Myoflex®

Pharmacologic Category Salicylate

Use Mild to moderate pain, fever, various inflammatory conditions

Local Anesthetic/Vasoconstrictor Precautions No information available to require special precautions

Effects on Dental Treatment NSAID formulations are known to reversibly decrease platelet aggregation via mechanisms different than observed with aspirin. The dentist should be aware of the potential of abnormal coagulation. Caution should also be exercised in the use of NSAIDs in patients already on anticoagulant therapy with drugs such as warfarin (Coumadin®).

Dosage Oral: Adults: 650 mg 4 times daily or 1090 mg 3 times daily; may increase to 3.6-4.8 mg/day in 3 or 4 divided doses

Drug Interactions Decreased Effect: May decrease absorption of aminoquinolones, digoxin, nitrofurantoin, penicillamine, and tetracyclines.

Generic Available Yes

Magnesium Sulfate *see* Magnesium Supplements *on page 837*

Magnesium Supplements (mag NEE zee um SUP le ments)

U.S. Brand Names Almora® [OTC]; Chloromag®; Mag Delay® [OTC]; Mag G® [OTC]; Mag-Gel® 600; Maginex™; Maginex™ DS; Magonate® [OTC]; Magonste® Sprot [OTC]; Mag-Ox 400® [OTC]; Mag-SR® [OTC]; Magtrate® [OTC]; Phillips'® Milk of Magnesia [OTC]; Phillips' M-O® [OTC]; Slow-Mag® [OTC]; Uro-Mag® [OTC]

Mexican Brand Names Leche De Magnesia Normex

Pharmacologic Category Electrolyte Supplement

Synonyms Citrate of Magnesia (Magnesium Citrate); Epsom Salts (Magnesium Sulfate); Magnesia Magma (Magnesium Hydroxide); Magnesium Chloride; Magnesium Citrate; Magnesium Gluconate; Magnesium Hydroxide; Magnesium Hydroxide and Mineral Oil Emulsion; Magnesium L-aspartate Hydrochloride; Magnesium Oxide; Magnesium Sulfate; Milk of Magnesia (Magnesium Hydroxide); MOM (Magnesium Hydroxide)

Use

Treatment and prevention of hypomagnesemia **(magnesium chloride, magnesium lactate, magnesium carbonate, magnesium sulfate, magnesium gluconate, and magnesium oxide)**

Treatment of hypertension **(magnesium sulfate)**

Treatment of encephalopathy and seizures associated with acute nephritis **(magnesium sulfate)**

Short-term treatment of constipation **(magnesium citrate, magnesium hydroxide, magnesium sulfate, and magnesium oxide)**

Treatment of hyperacidity symptoms **(magnesium hydroxide and magnesium oxide)**

Adjunctive treatment in moderate to severe acute asthma **(magnesium sulfate)**

Local Anesthetic/Vasoconstrictor Precautions No information available to require special precautions

Effects on Dental Treatment Magnesium products may prevent GI absorption of tetracyclines by forming a large, ionized, chelated molecule with the tetracyclines in the stomach, therefore, tetracyclines should be given at least 1 hour before magnesium-containing products.

Frequency not defined (related to serum level): Hypotension, weakness

>3 mg/dL: Depressed CNS, blocked peripheral neuromuscular transmission leading to anticonvulsant effects

>5 mg/dL: Flushing, somnolence

>12 mg/dL: Respiratory paralysis

Dosage Multiple salt forms of magnesium exist; close attention must be paid to the salt form when ordering and administering magnesium; incorrect selection or substitution of one salt for another without proper dosage adjustment may result in serious over- or underdosing. See table on next page.

Children: Note: Neonates: Avoid or use magnesium chloride injection with caution; avoid use of Magonate® solution (contains sodium benzoate and *in vitro* and animal

(Continued)

Magnesium Supplements *(Continued)*

Magnesium - Recommended Daily Allowance (RDA) (in terms of elemental magnesium)

Age	RDA (mg/day)
<5 months	40
5-12 months	60
1-3 years	80
4-6 years	120
7-10 years	170
Male	
11-14 years	270
15-18 years	400
>19 years	350
Female	
11-14 years	280
15-18 years	300
>19 years	280

studies have shown that benzoate, a metabolite of benzyl alcohol, displaces bilirubin from protein binding sites)

HYPOMAGNESEMIA:

Neonates: I.V.:

Magnesium sulfate: 25-50 mg/kg/dose (0.2-0.4 mEq/kg/dose) every 8-12 hours for 2-3 doses

Magnesium chloride: 0.2-0.4 mEq/kg/dose every 8-12 hours for 2-3 doses

Children:

I.M., I.V.:

Magnesium sulfate: 25-50 mg/kg/dose (0.2-0.4 mEq/kg/dose) every 4-6 hours for 3-4 doses; maximum single dose: 2000 mg (16 mEq)

Magnesium chloride: 0.2-0.4 mEq/kg/dose every 4-6 hours for 3-4 doses; maximum single dose 16 mEq

Oral:

Magnesium chloride, gluconate, lactate, carbonate, oxide, or sulfate salts: 10-20 mg/kg **elemental magnesium** per dose 4 times/day

DAILY MAINTENANCE MAGNESIUM: I.V.:

Magnesium sulfate or magnesium chloride:

Neonates, Infants, and Children ≤45 kg: 0.25-0.5 mEq/kg/day

Adolescents >45 kg: 0.2-0.5 mEq/kg/day or 3-10 mEq/1000 kcal/day (maximum 8-16 mEq/day)

MANAGEMENT OF SEIZURES AND HYPERTENSION: I.M., I.V.:

Magnesium sulfate: Children: 20-100 mg/kg/dose every 4-6 hours as needed; in severe cases doses as high as 200 mg/kg/dose have been used

BRONCHODILATION (adjunctive treatment in moderate to severe acute asthma; unlabeled use): I.V.:

Magnesium sulfate:

Children: 25 mg/kg/dose (maximum dose 2 g) as a single dose

Note: Literature evaluating magnesium sulfate's efficacy in the relief of bronchospasm has utilized single dosages in patient's with acute symptomatology who have received aerosol β-agonist therapy.

CATHARTIC: Oral:

Magnesium citrate (Citrate of magnesia):

<6 years: 2-4 mL/kg given once or in divided doses

6-12 years: 100-150 mL

≥12 years: 150-300 mL

Magnesium hydroxide (Milk of magnesia, MOM):

<2 years: 0.5 mL/kg/dose

2-5 years: 5-15 mL/day once or in divided doses

6-11 years: 15-30 mL/day once or in divided doses

≥12 years: 30-60 mL/day once or in divided doses

Magnesium hydroxide and mineral oil (Haley's M-O) (pediatric dosage to provide equivalent dosage of magnesium hydroxide):

<2 years: 0.6 mL/kg/dose
2-5 years: 6-18 mL/day once or in divided doses
6-11 years: 18-36 mL/day once or in divided doses
≥12 years: 30-45 mL once or in divided doses

Magnesium sulfate: Children: 0.25 g/kg/dose once or in divided doses

ANTACID Oral:

Magnesium hydroxide: Children: Liquid: 2.5-5 mL/dose, up to 4 times/day

Adults:

HYPOMAGNESEMIA:

Magnesium gluconate: Oral: 500-1000 mg 3 times/day

Magnesium sulfate:

I.M., I.V.: 1 g every 6 hours for 4 doses, or 250 mg/kg over a 4-hour period; for severe hypomagnesemia: 8-12 g/day in divided doses has been used

Oral: 3 g every 6 hours for 4 doses

DAILY MAINTENANCE MAGNESIUM: I.V.:

Magnesium sulfate or magnesium chloride: 0.2-0.5 mEq/kg/day or 3-10 mEq/1000 kcal/day (maximum 8-16 mEq/day)

MANAGEMENT OF SEIZURES AND HYPERTENSION: I.M., I.V.:

Magnesium sulfate: 1 g every 6 hours for 4 doses as needed

BRONCHODILATION (adjunctive treatment in moderate to severe acute asthma; unlabeled use): I.V.:

Magnesium sulfate: 2 g as a single dose

Note: Literature evaluating magnesium sulfate's efficacy in the relief of bronchospasm has utilized single dosages in patient's with acute symptomatology who have received aerosol β-agonist therapy.

CATHARTIC: Oral:

Magnesium citrate (Citrate of magnesia): 150-300 mL

Magnesium hydroxide (Milk of magnesia, MOM): 30-60 mL/day once or in divided doses

Magnesium hydroxide and mineral oil (Haley's M-O) (pediatric dosage to provide equivalent dosage of magnesium hydroxide) 30-45 mL once or in divided doses

Magnesium sulfate: 10-30 g

Magnesium oxide: Adults: 2-4 g at bedtime with full glass of water

ANTACID Oral:

Magnesium hydroxide:

Liquid: 5-15 mL/dose, up to 4 times/day
Liquid concentrate: 2.5-7.5 mL/dose, up to 4 times/day
Tablet: 622-1244 mg/dose, up to 4 times/day

Magnesium oxide: 140 mg 3-4 times/day or 400-840 mg/day

Dosing adjustment in renal impairment: Patients in severe renal failure should not receive magnesium due to toxicity from accumulation. Patients with a Cl_{cr} <25 mL/minute receiving magnesium should have serum magnesium levels monitored.

Mechanism of Action Important as a cofactor in many enzymatic reactions in the body; there are at least 300 enzymes which are dependent upon magnesium for normal functioning. Actions on lipoprotein lipase have been found to be important in reducing serum cholesterol. Magnesium is necessary for the maintaining of serum potassium and calcium levels due to its effect on the renal tubule. In the heart, magnesium acts as a calcium channel blocker. It also activates sodium potassium ATPase in the cell membrane to promote resting polarization and produce arrhythmias. Promotes bowel evacuation by causing osmotic retention of fluid which distends the colon and produces increased peristaltic activity when taken orally. To reduce stomach acidity, it reacts with hydrochloric acid in the stomach to form magnesium chloride.

Other Adverse Effects Frequency not defined (related to serum level):

>3 mg/dL: Depressed CNS, blocked peripheral neuromuscular transmission leading to anticonvulsant effects

>5 mg/dL: Depressed deep tendon reflexes, flushing, somnolence

>12 mg/dL: Respiratory paralysis, complete heart block

Endocrine & metabolic: Hypermagnesemia

Gastrointestinal: Diarrhea, abdominal cramps, gas formation

Drug Interactions

Increased Effect/Toxicity: If sufficient alkalinization of the urine by magnesium salts occurs, the excretion of salicylates is enhanced and the tubular reabsorption of quinidine is enhanced.

Decreased Effect: When given orally, may decrease the absorption of the following: H_2 antagonists, phenytoin, iron salts, penicillamine, tetracycline, ciprofloxacin, benzodiazepines, chloroquine, steroids, and glyburide. Systemic magnesium may enhance the effects of calcium channel blockers and neuromuscular blockers. May share additive CNS depressant effects with CNS depressants.

Dietary/Ethanol/Herb Considerations 1 g elemental magnesium = 83.3 mEq = 41.1 mmol

Pregnancy Risk Factor B

(Continued)

Magnesium Supplements *(Continued)*

Dosage Forms Elemental magnesium listed in brackets:

Magnesium chloride:

Injection, solution (Chloromag®): 200 mg/mL [1.97 mEq/mL] (50 mL)
Tablet, enteric coated (Slo-Mag®): 64 mg [contains elemental calcium 106 mg]
Tablet, extended release (Mag Delay®, May-SR®): 535 mg [64 mg]

Magnesium citrate:

Solution, oral: 290 mg/5 mL (300 mL) [cherry and lemon flavors]
Tablet: 100 mg

Magnesium gluconate:

Solution:
Magonate®: 1000 mg/5 mL (480 mL) [54 mg/5 mL] [contains sodium benzoate]
Magonate® Sport: 1000 mg/5 mL (30 mL) [54 mg/5 mL] [contains sodium benzoate; fruit flavor]
Tablet (Almora®, Mag G®, Magonate®, Magtrate®): 500 mg [27 mg]

Magnesium hydroxide:

Liquid, oral: 400 mg/5 mL (360 mL, 480 mL, 960 mL, 3780 mL)
Phillips'® Milk of Magnesia: 400 mg/5 mL (120 mL, 360 mL, 780 mL) [original, French vanilla, cherry, and mint flavors]
Liquid, oral concentrate: 800 mg/5 mL (100 mL, 400 mL)
Phillips'® Milk of Magnesia [concentrate]: 800 mg/5 mL (240 mL) [strawberry créme flavor]
Tablet, chewable (Phillips'® Milk of Magnesia): 311 mg [mint flavor]

Magnesium hydroxide and mineral oil: Suspension, oral: Magnesium hydroxide 300 mg and mineral oil 1.25 mL per 5 mL (360 mL, 780 mL) [original and mint flavors]

Magnesium L-aspartate hydrochloride:

Granules (Maginex™ DS): 1230 mg [10 mEq; 122 mg] [lemon flavor]
Tablet (Maginex™): 615 mg [5 mEq; 61 mg]

Magnesium oxide:

Capsule (Uro-Mag®): 140 mg [84 mg]
Tablet (Mag-Ox® 400): 400 mg [242 mg]

Magnesium sulfate:

Infusion [premixed in D_5W]: 10 mg/mL (100 mL); 20 mg/mL (500 mL, 1000 mL)
Infusion [premixed in water for injection]: 40 mg/mL (100 mL, 500 mL, 1000 mL); 80 mg/mL (50 mL)
Injection, solution: 125 mg/mL (8 mL); 500 mg/mL (2 mL, 5 mL, 10 mL, 20 mL, 50 mL)
Powder: Magnesium sulfate USP (480 g, 1810 g, 1920 g)

Generic Available Yes

Magnesium Trisilicate and Aluminum Hydroxide *see* Aluminum Hydroxide and Magnesium Trisilicate *on page 69*
Magonate® [OTC] *see* Magnesium Gluconate *on page 834*
Magonate® [OTC] *see* Magnesium Supplements *on page 837*
Magonate® Sport [OTC] *see* Magnesium Gluconate *on page 834*
Magonste® Sprot [OTC] *see* Magnesium Supplements *on page 837*
Mag-Ox 400® [OTC] *see* Magnesium Supplements *on page 837*
Mag-SR® [OTC] *see* Magnesium Chloride *on page 833*
Mag-SR® [OTC] *see* Magnesium Supplements *on page 837*
Magtrate® [OTC] *see* Magnesium Gluconate *on page 834*
Magtrate® [OTC] *see* Magnesium Supplements *on page 837*
MAH™ *see* Magnesium L-aspartate Hydrochloride *on page 836*
Malarone™ *see* Atovaquone and Proguanil *on page 143*
Mallamint® [OTC] *see* Calcium Supplements *on page 229*

Maltodextrin (mal toe DEK strin)

U.S. Brand Names Gelclair™; Multidex® [OTC]; OraRinse™ [OTC]

Pharmacologic Category Skin and Mucous Membrane Agent

Use

Dental: Oral: Management and relief of pain due to oral lesions (including mucositis/stomatitis), oral ulcers, or irritation; treatment of aphthous ulcers

Medical: Topical: Treatment of infected or noninfected wounds

Local Anesthetic/Vasoconstrictor Precautions No information available to require special precautions

Effects on Dental Treatment No significant effects or complications reported

Dosage Adults:

Oral: Management of pain due to oral lesions:

Gelclair™: Using contents of 1 reconstituted packet, rinse around mouth for ~1 minute, 3 times/day or more if needed; gargle and expectorate. May be used undiluted or with less dilution if adequate pain relief is not achieved.

OraRinse™: 1 tablespoonful, swish or gargle for ~1 minute, 4 times/day or more if needed

Topical: Wound dressing: Multidex®: After debridement and irrigation of wound, apply and cover with a nonadherent, nonocclusive dressing. May be applied to moist or dry, infected or noninfected wounds.

Mechanism of Action Forms a protective barrier over wound providing an environment which promotes tissue growth.

Contraindications Hypersensitivity to maltodextrin or any component of the formulation

Warnings/Precautions Oral: Avoid eating or drinking for 1 hour; products are not harmful if accidentally swallowed; notify healthcare provider if improvement is not seen within 7 days

Dietary/Ethanol/Herb Considerations Food: Avoid eating or drinking for 1 hour postadministration.

Dosage Forms **GEL, oral** [concentrate] (Gelclair™): 15 mL/packet (21s) [contains benzalkonium chloride and sodium benzoate]. **GEL, topical dressing** (Multidex®): (4 mL, 7 mL, 14 mL, 85 mL). **POWDER, for oral suspension** (OraRinse™): (19 g). **POWDER, topical dressing** (Multidex®): (6 g, 12 g, 25 g, 45 g)

Generic Available No

Comments

Gelclair™: Store at room temperature away from direct sunlight. Do not refrigerate. Gel may become darker or thicker over time; efficacy and safety are not affected if used prior to labeled expiration date. Mix contents of one packet with 40 mL of water. Stir and use at once. Product may be used undiluted if water is unavailable.

OraRinse™: Fill bottle with water to first arrow; shake vigorously until suspended; continue to fill to second arrow; shake well

Malt Soup Extract (molt soop EKS trakt)

U.S. Brand Names Maltsupex® [OTC]

Pharmacologic Category Laxative

Use Short-term treatment of constipation

Local Anesthetic/Vasoconstrictor Precautions No information available to require special precautions

Effects on Dental Treatment No significant effects or complications reported

Dosage Oral:

Infants >1 month:

- Breast-fed:
  - Liquid: 1-2 teaspoonfuls in 2-4 oz of water or fruit juice 1-2 times/day for 3-4 days
  - Powder: 4 g in 2-4 oz of water or fruit juice daily for 3-4 days
- Bottle-fed:
  - Liquid: ½ to 2 tablespoonfuls/day in formula for 3-4 days, then 1-2 teaspoonfuls/day
  - Powder: 8-16 g/day in formula for 3-4 days, then 4-8 g/day

Children:

- 2-6 years:
  - Liquid: 7.5 mL 1-2 times/day for 3-4 days
  - Powder: 8 g twice daily for 3-4 days
- 6-12 years:
  - Liquid: 15-30 mL 1-2 times/day for 3-4 days
  - Powder: Up to 16 g/day for 3-4 days

Children ≥12 years and Adults:

- Liquid: 30 mL twice daily for 3-4 days, then 15-30 mL at bedtime
- Powder: Up to 32 g twice daily for 3-4 days, then 16-32 g at bedtime
- Tablets: 4 tablets 4 times/day (maximum dose: 64 g/day)

Other Adverse Effects Frequency not defined: Gastrointestinal: Abdominal cramps, diarrhea, rectal obstruction

Generic Available No

Maltsupex® [OTC] *see* Malt Soup Extract *on page 841*
Mandelamine® *see* Methenamine *on page 879*
Mandol® [DSC] *see* Cefamandole *on page 263*
Mandrake *see* Podophyllum Resin *on page 1093*
Manganese *see* Trace Metals *on page 1328*
Mantoux *see* Tuberculin Tests *on page 1362*
Maolate® *see* Chlorphenesin *on page 306*
Mapap® [OTC] *see* Acetaminophen *on page 27*
Mapap® Children's [OTC] *see* Acetaminophen *on page 27*
Mapap® Extra Strength [OTC] *see* Acetaminophen *on page 27*
Mapap® Infants [OTC] *see* Acetaminophen *on page 27*

Maprotiline (ma PROE ti leen)

Canadian Brand Names Novo-Maprotiline

Mexican Brand Names Ludiomil®

Pharmacologic Category Antidepressant, Tetracyclic

(Continued)

Maprotiline *(Continued)*

Synonyms Maprotiline Hydrochloride

Use Treatment of depression and anxiety associated with depression

Unlabeled/Investigational Use Treatment of bulimia, duodenal ulcers, enuresis, urinary symptoms of multiple sclerosis (MS), pain, panic attacks, tension headaches, cocaine withdrawal symptoms

Local Anesthetic/Vasoconstrictor Precautions Although maprotiline is not a tricyclic antidepressant, it does block norepinephrine reuptake within CNS synapses as part of its mechanisms. It has been suggested that vasoconstrictor be administered with caution and to monitor vital signs in dental patients taking antidepressants that affect norepinephrine in this way, including maprotiline. Epinephrine, norepinephrine and levonordefrin have been shown to have an increased pressor response in combination with TCAs.

Effects on Dental Treatment

>10%: Xerostomia, changes in salivation, drowsiness

1% to 10%: Nervousness, anxiety, agitation, dizziness, headache, tremor

Long-term treatment with TCAs such as amoxapine increases the risk of caries by reducing salivation and salivary buffer capacity.

Dosage Oral:

Children 6-14 years: Depression/anxiety: 10 mg/day; increase to a maximum daily dose of 75 mg

Adults: Depression/anxiety: 75 mg/day to start, increase by 25 mg every 2 weeks up to 150-225 mg/day; given in 3 divided doses or in a single daily dose

Elderly: Depression/anxiety: Initial: 25 mg at bedtime, increase by 25 mg every 3 days for inpatients and weekly for outpatients if tolerated; usual maintenance dose: 50-75 mg/day, higher doses may be necessary in nonresponders

Mechanism of Action Traditionally believed to increase the synaptic concentration of norepinephrine in the central nervous system by inhibition of their reuptake by the presynaptic neuronal membrane. However, additional receptor effects have been found including desensitization of adenyl cyclase, down regulation of beta-adrenergic receptors, and down regulation of serotonin receptors.

Other Adverse Effects

1% to 10%:

Central nervous system: Insomnia, fatigue

Gastrointestinal: Constipation, nausea

Neuromuscular & skeletal: Weakness

Ocular: Blurred vision

<1%: Abdominal cramps, accommodation disturbances, **akathisia, arrhythmias**, ataxia, **bitter taste**, breast enlargement, **confusion**, decreased libido, delusions, **diaphoresis (excessive)**, diarrhea, **disorientation**, dysarthria, **dysphagia**, edema of testicles, **epigastric distress, EPS, exacerbation of psychosis, hallucinations, heart block, hyperglycemia, hypertension, hypomania, hypotension**, impotence, mania, motor hyperactivity, mydriasis, nightmares, numbness, **palpitations**, petechiae, photosensitivity, rash, **restlessness, seizures, syncope, tachycardia, tingling**, tinnitus, urinary retention, **vomiting**, weight gain/loss

Drug Interactions Substrate of **CYP2D6**

Increased Effect/Toxicity: Maprotiline may increase the effects of amphetamines, anticholinergics, other CNS depressants (sedatives, hypnotics, or ethanol), carbamazepine, tolazamide, chlorpropamide, and warfarin. When used with MAO inhibitors, hyperpyrexia, hypertension, tachycardia, confusion, seizures, and **deaths have been reported** (serotonin syndrome). The SSRIs (to varying degrees), cimetidine, fenfluramine, grapefruit juice, indinavir, methylphenidate, ritonavir, quinidine, diltiazem, valproate, and verapamil inhibit the metabolism of cyclic antidepressants and clinical toxicity may result. Use of lithium with a cyclic antidepressant may increase the risk for neurotoxicity. Phenothiazines may increase concentration of some cyclic antidepressants and cyclic antidepressants may increase the concentration of phenothiazines. Pressor response to I.V. epinephrine, norepinephrine, and phenylephrine may be enhanced in patients receiving cyclic antidepressants (**Note:** Effect is unlikely with epinephrine or levonordefrin dosages typically administered as infiltration in combination with local anesthetics). Combined use of beta-agonists or drugs which prolong QT_c (including quinidine, procainamide, disopyramide, cisapride, sparfloxacin, gatifloxacin, moxifloxacin) with cyclic antidepressants may predispose patients to cardiac arrhythmias.

Decreased Effect: Carbamazepine, phenobarbital, and rifampin may increase the metabolism of maprotiline resulting in a decreased effect. Maprotiline inhibits the antihypertensive response to bethanidine, clonidine, debrisoquin, guanadrel, guanethidine, guanabenz, or guanfacine. Cholestyramine and colestipol may bind cyclic antidepressants and reduce their absorption.

Dietary/Ethanol/Herb Considerations

Ethanol: Avoid use; may increase CNS depression.

Food: Avoid grapefruit products; may increase serum concentration/toxicity.

Herb/Nutraceutical: Avoid gotu kola, kava, SAMe, St John's wort, and valerian; may increase CNS depression.

Pharmacodynamics/Kinetics

Absorption: Slow

Protein binding: 88%

Metabolism: Hepatic to active and inactive compounds

Half-life elimination, serum: 27-58 hours (mean: 43 hours)

Time to peak, serum: Within 12 hours

Excretion: Urine (70%); feces (30%)

Pregnancy Risk Factor B

Generic Available Yes

Selected Readings

Boakes AJ, Laurence DR, Teoh PC, et al, "Interactions Between Sympathomimetic Amines and Antidepressant Agents in Man," *Br Med J*, 1973, 1(849):311-5.

Ganzber S, "Psychoactive Drugs," *ADA Guide to Dental Therapeutics,* 2nd edition, Chapter 21, Chicago, IL: ADA Publising, 2000, 382.

Jastak JT and Yagiela JA, "Vasoconstrictors and Local Anesthesia: A Review and Rationale for Use," *J Am Dent Assoc*, 1983, 107(4):623-30.

Mitchell JR, "Guanethidine and Related Agents. III Antagonism by Drugs Which Inhibit the Norepinephrine Pump in Man," *J Clin Invest*, 1970, 49(8):1596-604.

Rundegren J, van Dijken J, Mörnstad H, et al, "Oral Conditions in Patients Receiving Long-Term Treatment With Cyclic Antidepressant Drugs," *Swed Dent J*, 1985, 9(2):55-64.

Wynn RL, "New Antidepressant Medications," *Gen Dent*, 1997, 45(1):24-8.

Maprotiline Hydrochloride see Maprotiline *on page 841*

Marcaine® see Bupivacaine *on page 205*

Marcaine® Spinal see Bupivacaine *on page 205*

Marcaine® with Epinephrine see Bupivacaine and Epinephrine *on page 207*

Marcillin® see Ampicillin *on page 103*

Marezine® [OTC] see Cyclizine *on page 379*

Margesic® H see Hydrocodone and Acetaminophen *on page 678*

Marinol® see Dronabinol *on page 480*

Marplan® see Isocarboxazid *on page 747*

Matulane® see Procarbazine *on page 1122*

Mavik® see Trandolapril *on page 1331*

Maxair™ see Pirbuterol *on page 1090*

Maxair™ Autohaler™ see Pirbuterol *on page 1090*

Maxalt® see Rizatriptan *on page 1193*

Maxalt-MLT® see Rizatriptan *on page 1193*

Maxaquin® see Lomefloxacin *on page 817*

Maxidex® see Dexamethasone *on page 413*

Maxidone™ see Hydrocodone and Acetaminophen *on page 678*

Maxifed® see Guaifenesin and Pseudoephedrine *on page 652*

Maxifed® DM see Guaifenesin, Pseudoephedrine, and Dextromethorphan *on page 653*

Maxifed-G® see Guaifenesin and Pseudoephedrine *on page 652*

Maxiflor® see Diflorasone *on page 438*

Maxipime® see Cefepime *on page 267*

Maxitrol® see Neomycin, Polymyxin B, and Dexamethasone *on page 962*

Maxivate® see Betamethasone *on page 177*

Maxzide® see Hydrochlorothiazide and Triamterene *on page 677*

Maxzide®-25 see Hydrochlorothiazide and Triamterene *on page 677*

May Apple see Podophyllum Resin *on page 1093*

Mazanor® [DSC] see Mazindol *on page 843*

Mazindol (MAY zin dole)

U.S. Brand Names Mazanor® [DSC]; Sanorex® [DSC]

Canadian Brand Names Mazanor®; Sanorex®

Mexican Brand Names Diestet®; Solucaps®

Pharmacologic Category Anorexiant

Use Short-term adjunct in exogenous obesity

Local Anesthetic/Vasoconstrictor Precautions No information available to require special precautions

Effects on Dental Treatment >10%: Xerostomia, changes in salivation

Restrictions C-IV

Dosage Oral: Adults:

Initial: 1 mg once daily; adjust to patient response

Usual maintenance range: 2-3 mg/day in 1-3 divided doses

Note: Take 1 hour before meals to avoid GI discomfort

Mechanism of Action An isoindole with pharmacologic activity similar to amphetamine; produces CNS stimulation in humans and animals and appears to work primarily in the limbic system

Other Adverse Effects Frequency not defined:

Cardiovascular: **Palpitation, tachycardia**, edema

(Continued)

Mazindol *(Continued)*

Central nervous system: Insomnia, overstimulation, **dizziness**, dysphoria, **drowsiness, CNS depression, headache, restlessness**

Dermatologic: Rash, clamminess

Endocrine & metabolic: Changes in libido

Gastrointestinal: Nausea, constipation, vomiting, **unpleasant taste**, diarrhea, abdominal cramps

Genitourinary: Dysuria, polyuria, impotence

Neuromuscular & skeletal: **Tremor**, weakness

Ocular: Blurred vision, corneal opacities

Miscellaneous: **Diaphoresis (excessive)**

Drug Interactions

Increased Effect/Toxicity: Mazindol enhances the pressor effect of exogenous catecholamines (norepinephrine) and potential blood pressure increases in patients taking sympathomimetic medications.

Decreased Effect: Mazindol may decrease the hypotensive effect of guanethidine; monitor.

Dietary/Ethanol/Herb Considerations

Ethanol: Avoid use; may increase CNS depression.

Herb/Nutraceutical: Avoid gotu kola, kava, SAMe, St John's wort, and valerian; may increase CNS depression.

Pharmacodynamics/Kinetics

Half-life elimination: 33-55 hours

Excretion: Urine

Pregnancy Risk Factor C

Generic Available No

3M™ Cavilon™ Skin Cleanser [OTC] *see* Benzalkonium Chloride *on page 169*

MCH *see* Microfibrillar Collagen Hemostat *on page 907*

m-Cresyl Acetate (em-KREE sil AS e tate)

U.S. Brand Names Cresylate®

Pharmacologic Category Otic Agent, Anti-infective

Use Provides an acid medium; for external otitis infections caused by susceptible bacteria or fungus

Local Anesthetic/Vasoconstrictor Precautions No information available to require special precautions

Effects on Dental Treatment No significant effects or complications reported

Dosage Otic: Instill 2-4 drops as required

Generic Available No

MCT Oil® [OTC] *see* Medium Chain Triglycerides *on page 849*

MDL 73,147EF *see* Dolasetron *on page 465*

ME-500® *see* Methionine *on page 881*

Measles, Mumps, and Rubella Vaccines (Combined)

(MEE zels, mumpz & roo BEL a vak SEENS, kom BINED)

Related Information

Immunizations (Vaccines) *on page 1612*

U.S. Brand Names M-M-R® II

Canadian Brand Names M-M-R® II; Priorix™

Pharmacologic Category Vaccine, Live Virus

Synonyms MMR; Mumps, Measles and Rubella Vaccines, Combined; Rubella, Measles and Mumps Vaccines, Combined

Use Measles, mumps, and rubella prophylaxis

Local Anesthetic/Vasoconstrictor Precautions No information available to require special precautions

Effects on Dental Treatment No significant effects or complications reported

Restrictions Federal law requires that the date of administration, the vaccine manufacturer, lot number of vaccine, and the administering person's name, title and address be entered into the patient's permanent medical record.

Dosage S.C.:

Infants <12 months: If there is risk of exposure to measles, single-antigen measles vaccine should be administered at 6-11 months of age with a second dose (of MMR) at >12 months of age.

Children ≥12 months: 0.5 mL at 12 months and then repeated at 4-6 years of age. If the second dose was not received, the schedule should be completed by the 11- to 12-year old visit. Administer in outer aspect of the upper arm. Recommended age of primary immunization is 12-15 months; revaccination is recommended prior to elementary school.

Mechanism of Action As a live, attenuated vaccine, MMR vaccine offers active immunity to disease caused by the measles, mumps, and rubella viruses.

Other Adverse Effects All serious adverse reactions must be reported to the U.S. Department of Health and Human Services (DHHS) Vaccine Adverse Event Reporting System (VAERS) 1-800-822-7967.

Frequency not defined:

Cardiovascular: **Syncope,** vasculitis

Central nervous system: Ataxia, **dizziness**, febrile convulsions, **fever**, encephalitis, encephalopathy, Guillain-Barré syndrome, **headache, irritability,** malaise, measles inclusion body encephalitis, polyneuritis, polyneuropathy, **seizures,** subacute sclerosing panencephalitis

Dermatologic: Angioneurotic edema, erythema multiforme, purpura, rash, Stevens-Johnson syndrome, urticaria

Endocrine & metabolic: **Diabetes mellitus**

Gastrointestinal: Diarrhea, nausea, pancreatitis, **parotitis, sore throat, vomiting**

Genitourinary: Orchitis

Hematologic: Leukocytosis, thrombocytopenia

Local: Injection site reactions which include burning, induration, redness, stinging, swelling, tenderness, wheal and flare, vesiculation

Neuromuscular & skeletal: Arthralgia/arthritis (variable; highest rates in women, 12% to 26% versus children, up to 3%), myalgia, paresthesia

Ocular: Ocular palsies

Otic: **Otitis media**

Renal: Conjunctivitis, retinitis, optic neuritis, papillitis, retrobulbar neuritis

Respiratory: **Bronchospasm, cough, pneumonitis, rhinitis**

Miscellaneous: **Anaphylactoid reactions, anaphylaxis**, atypical measles, panniculitis, regional lymphadenopathy

Postmarketing and/or case reports: Aseptic meningitis (associated with Urabe strain of mumps vaccine)

Drug Interactions Decreased Effect: Immunosuppressant drugs (including high dose systemic corticosteroids) and/or immune globulin may decrease effect of vaccine; do not administer with vaccine. Effectiveness of MMR may be decreased if given within 30 days of varicella vaccine (effectiveness not decreased when administered simultaneously).

Pregnancy Risk Factor C

Generic Available No

Measles Virus Vaccine (Live) (MEE zels VYE rus vak SEEN, live)

Related Information

Immunizations (Vaccines) *on page 1612*

U.S. Brand Names Attenuvax®

Pharmacologic Category Vaccine, Live Virus

Synonyms More Attenuated Enders Strain; Rubeola Vaccine

Use Adults born before 1957 are generally considered to be immune. All those born in or after 1957 without documentation of live vaccine on or after first birthday, physician-diagnosed measles, or laboratory evidence of immunity should be vaccinated, ideally with two doses of vaccine separated by no less than 1 month. For those previously vaccinated with one dose of measles vaccine, revaccination is recommended for students entering colleges and other institutions of higher education, for healthcare workers at the time of employment, and for international travelers who visit endemic areas.

MMR is the vaccine of choice if recipients are likely to be susceptible to rubella and/or mumps as well as to measles. Persons vaccinated between 1963 and 1967 with a killed measles vaccine, followed by live vaccine within 3 months, or with a vaccine of unknown type should be revaccinated with live measles virus vaccine.

Local Anesthetic/Vasoconstrictor Precautions No information available to require special precautions

Effects on Dental Treatment

>10%: Fever (<100°F)

1% to 10%: Fever between 100°F and 103°F (usually between 5th and 12th days postvaccination)

Restrictions Federal law requires that the date of administration, the vaccine manufacturer, lot number of vaccine, and the administering person's name, title and address be entered into the patient's permanent medical record.

Dosage Children ≥15 months and Adults: S.C.: 0.5 mL in outer aspect of the upper arm, no routine boosters

Mechanism of Action Promotes active immunity to measles virus by inducing specific measles IgG and IgM antibodies.

Other Adverse Effects All serious adverse reactions must be reported to the U.S. Department of Health and Human Services (DHHS) Vaccine Adverse Event Reporting System (VAERS) 1-800-822-7967.

>10%:

Cardiovascular: Edema

Local: Burning or stinging, induration

(Continued)

Measles Virus Vaccine (Live) *(Continued)*

1% to 10%:

Dermatologic: Rash (rarely generalized)

<1%: Fatigue, **convulsions**, encephalitis, **confusion, severe headache, fever (>103°F - prolonged), palsies**, Guillain-Barré syndrome, ataxia, urticaria, itching, reddening of skin (especially around ears and eyes), erythema multiforme, **vomiting, sore throat**, diarrhea, thrombocytopenic purpura, diplopia, **stiff neck, dyspnea, cough, rhinitis**, lymphadenopathy, **coryza, allergic reactions**

Pregnancy Risk Factor X

Generic Available No

Comments Contains 25 mcg neomyciin per dose.

Mebaral® *see* Mephobarbital *on page 860*

Mebendazole (me BEN da zole)

U.S. Brand Names Vermox®

Canadian Brand Names Vermox®

Mexican Brand Names Helminzole; Mebensole; Revapol®; Soltric; Vermicol®; Vermidil®; Vermin®

Pharmacologic Category Anthelmintic

Use Treatment of pinworms (*Enterobius vermicularis*), whipworms (*Trichuris trichiura*), roundworms (*Ascaris lumbricoides*), and hookworms (*Ancylostoma duodenale*)

Local Anesthetic/Vasoconstrictor Precautions No information available to require special precautions

Effects on Dental Treatment No significant effects or complications reported

Dosage Children and Adults: Oral:

Pinworms: 100 mg as a single dose; may need to repeat after 2 weeks; treatment should include family members in close contact with patient

Whipworms, roundworms, hookworms: One tablet twice daily, morning and evening on 3 consecutive days; if patient is not cured within 3-4 weeks, a second course of treatment may be administered

Capillariasis: 200 mg twice daily for 20 days

Dosing adjustment in hepatic impairment: Reduction may be necessary in dysfunction

Hemodialysis: Not dialyzable (0% to 5%)

Mechanism of Action Selectively and irreversibly blocks glucose uptake and other nutrients in susceptible adult intestine-dwelling helminths

Other Adverse Effects Frequency not defined:

Cardiovascular: Angioedema

Central nervous system: **Fever, dizziness, headache, seizures**

Dermatologic: Rash, itching, alopecia (with high doses)

Gastrointestinal: Abdominal pain, diarrhea, nausea, **vomiting**

Hematologic: Neutropenia (sore throat, unusual fatigue)

Neuromuscular & skeletal: Unusual weakness

Drug Interactions Decreased Effect: Anticonvulsants such as carbamazepine and phenytoin may increase metabolism of mebendazole

Dietary/Ethanol/Herb Considerations Food may increase serum concentration.

Pharmacodynamics/Kinetics

Absorption: 2% to 10%

Distribution: To serum, cyst fluid, liver, omental fat, and pelvic, pulmonary, and hepatic cysts; highest concentrations found in liver; relatively high concentrations found in muscle-encysted *Trichinella spiralis* larvae; crosses placenta

Protein binding: 95%

Metabolism: Extensively hepatic

Half-life elimination: 1-11.5 hours

Time to peak, serum: 2-4 hours

Excretion: Primarily feces; urine (5% to 10%)

Pregnancy Risk Factor C

Generic Available Yes

Mecamylamine (mek a MIL a meen)

U.S. Brand Names Inversine®

Canadian Brand Names Inversine®

Pharmacologic Category Ganglionic Blocking Agent

Synonyms Mecamylamine Hydrochloride

Use Treatment of moderately severe to severe hypertension and in uncomplicated malignant hypertension

Unlabeled/Investigational Use Treatment of Tourette's syndrome

Local Anesthetic/Vasoconstrictor Precautions No information available to require special precautions

Effects on Dental Treatment >10%: Xerostomia

Dosage Oral:

Adults: 2.5 mg twice daily after meals for 2 days; increased by increments of 2.5 mg at intervals ≥2 days until desired blood pressure response is achieved; average daily dose: 25 mg (usually in 3 divided doses)

Reduce dosage of other antihypertensives when combined with mecamylamine with exception of thiazide diuretics which may be maintained at usual dose while decreasing mecamylamine by 50%

Dosing adjustment in renal impairment: Specific guidelines unavailable; use with caution

Mechanism of Action Mecamylamine is a ganglionic blocker. This agent inhibits acetylcholine at the autonomic ganglia, causing a decrease in blood pressure. Mecamylamine also blocks central nicotinic cholinergic receptors, which inhibits the effects of nicotine and may suppress the desire to smoke.

Other Adverse Effects Frequency not defined:

Cardiovascular: **Postural hypotension**

Central nervous system: **Drowsiness, convulsions, confusion**, mental depression

Endocrine & metabolic: Sexual ability decreased

Gastrointestinal: Loss of appetite, nausea, **vomiting**, bloating, frequent stools followed by severe constipation

Genitourinary: Dysuria

Neuromuscular & skeletal: **Uncontrolled movements of hands, arms, legs, or face; trembling**

Ocular: Blurred vision, enlarged pupils

Respiratory: **Dyspnea**

Drug Interactions Increased Effect/Toxicity: Sulfonamides and antibiotics that cause neuromuscular blockade may increase effect of mecamylamine. The action of mecamylamine may be increased by anesthesia, other antihypertensives, and alcohol.

Pregnancy Risk Factor C

Generic Available No

Mecamylamine Hydrochloride *see* Mecamylamine *on page 846*

Meclizine (MEK li zeen)

U.S. Brand Names Antivert®; Bonine® [OTC]; Dramamine® Less Drowsy Formula [OTC]

Canadian Brand Names Antivert®; Bonamine™; Bonine®

Pharmacologic Category Antiemetic; Antihistamine

Synonyms Meclizine Hydrochloride; Meclozine Hydrochloride

Use Prevention and treatment of symptoms of motion sickness; management of vertigo with diseases affecting the vestibular system

Local Anesthetic/Vasoconstrictor Precautions No information available to require special precautions

Effects on Dental Treatment

>10%: Slight to moderate drowsiness, thickening of bronchial secretions

≤10%: Significant xerostomia; normal salivary flow resumes upon discontinuation

1% to 10%: Headache, nervousness, dizziness, pharyngitis

Dosage Children >12 years and Adults: Oral:

Motion sickness: 12.5-25 mg 1 hour before travel, repeat dose every 12-24 hours if needed; doses up to 50 mg may be needed

Vertigo: 25-100 mg/day in divided doses

Mechanism of Action Has central anticholinergic action by blocking chemoreceptor trigger zone; decreases excitability of the middle ear labyrinth and blocks conduction in the middle ear vestibular-cerebellar pathways

Other Adverse Effects

1% to 10%:

Central nervous system: Fatigue

Gastrointestinal: Appetite increase, weight gain, nausea, diarrhea, abdominal pain

Neuromuscular & skeletal: Arthralgia

<1%: **Palpitations, hypotension**, depression, **sedation**, photosensitivity, rash, angioedema, urinary retention, hepatitis, myalgia, **tremor, paresthesia**, blurred vision, **bronchospasm, epistaxis**

Drug Interactions Increased toxicity with CNS depressants, neuroleptics, and anticholinergics.

Dietary/Ethanol/Herb Considerations

Ethanol: Avoid use; may increase CNS depression.

Herb/Nutraceutical: Avoid gotu kola, kava, SAMe, St John's wort, and valerian; may increase CNS depression.

Pharmacodynamics/Kinetics

Onset of action: ~1 hour

Duration: 8-24 hours

Metabolism: Hepatic

Half-life elimination: 6 hours

(Continued)

Meclizine *(Continued)*

Excretion: Urine (as metabolites); feces (as unchanged drug)

Pregnancy Risk Factor B

Generic Available Yes

Meclizine Hydrochloride *see* Meclizine *on page 847*

Meclofenamate (me kloe fen AM ate)

Related Information

Rheumatoid Arthritis, Osteoarthritis, and Osteoporosis *on page 1488*
Temporomandibular Dysfunction (TMD) *on page 1562*

Canadian Brand Names Meclomen®

Pharmacologic Category Nonsteroidal Anti-inflammatory Drug (NSAID)

Synonyms Meclofenamate Sodium

Use Treatment of inflammatory disorders, arthritis, mild to moderate pain, dysmenorrhea

Local Anesthetic/Vasoconstrictor Precautions No information available to require special precautions

Effects on Dental Treatment

>10%: Dizziness

1% to 10%: Headache, nervousness, vomiting

NSAID formulations are known to reversibly decrease platelet aggregation via mechanisms different than observed with aspirin. The dentist should be aware of the potential of abnormal coagulation. Caution should also be exercised in the use of NSAIDs in patients already on anticoagulant therapy with drugs such as warfarin (Coumadin®). Recovery of platelet function usually occurs 1-2 days after discontinuation of NSAIDs.

Dosage Children >14 years and Adults: Oral:

Mild to moderate pain: 50 mg every 4-6 hours, not to exceed 400 mg/day
Rheumatoid arthritis/osteoarthritis: 200-400 mg/day in 3-4 equal doses

Mechanism of Action Inhibits prostaglandin synthesis by decreasing the activity of the enzyme, cyclooxygenase, which results in decreased formation of prostaglandin precursors

Other Adverse Effects

>10%:
- Dermatologic: Rash
- Gastrointestinal: Abdominal cramps, heartburn, indigestion, nausea

1% to 10%:
- Dermatologic: Itching
- Endocrine & metabolic: Fluid retention
- Otic: Tinnitus

<1%: **CHF, hypertension, arrhythmia, tachycardia, confusion, hallucinations**, aseptic meningitis, mental depression, **drowsiness**, insomnia, urticaria, erythema multiforme, toxic epidermal necrolysis, Stevens-Johnson syndrome, angioedema, **polydipsia, hot flashes, gastritis, GI ulceration**, cystitis, polyuria, agranulocytosis, anemia, hemolytic anemia, bone marrow suppression, leukopenia, thrombocytopenia, hepatitis, peripheral neuropathy, toxic amblyopia, blurred vision, conjunctivitis, dry eyes, hearing loss, acute renal failure, **allergic rhinitis, dyspnea, epistaxis**

Drug Interactions

Increased Effect/Toxicity: Anticoagulants (warfarin, heparin, LMWHs) in combination with NSAIDs can cause increased risk of bleeding. Other antiplatelet drugs (ticlopidine, clopidogrel, aspirin, abciximab, dipyridamole, eptifibatide, tirofiban) can cause an increased risk of bleeding. NSAIDs may increase serum creatinine, potassium, blood pressure, and cyclosporine levels during concurrent therapy; monitor cyclosporine levels and renal function carefully. Lithium levels can be increased; avoid concurrent use if possible or monitor lithium levels and adjust dose. Sulindac may have the least effect. When NSAID is stopped, lithium will need adjustment again. Corticosteroids may increase the risk of GI ulceration; avoid concurrent use. Serum concentration/toxicity of methotrexate may be increased.

Decreased Effect: Antihypertensive effects of ACE-inhibitors, angiotensin antagonists, diuretics, and hydralazine may be decreased by concurrent therapy with NSAIDs; monitor blood pressure. Cholestyramine and colestipol reduce the bioavailability of diclofenac; separate administration times.

Dietary/Ethanol/Herb Considerations

Ethanol: Avoid use due to GI irritation.

Food: Administer with food or milk. Avoid excessive amounts of vitamin C and salicylate containing foods (eg, curry powder, prunes, raisins, tea, or licorice).

Herb/Nutraceutical: Avoid kava and valerian; may enhance benzodiazepine activity.

Pharmacodynamics/Kinetics

Duration: 2-4 hours
Distribution: Crosses placenta
Protein binding: 99%
Half-life elimination: 2-3.3 hours

Time to peak, serum: 0.5-1.5 hours
Excretion: Primarily urine and feces (as metabolites)

Pregnancy Risk Factor B/D (3rd trimester)

Generic Available Yes

Meclofenamate Sodium *see* Meclofenamate *on page 848*
Meclozine Hydrochloride *see* Meclizine *on page 847*
Medicinal Carbon *see* Charcoal *on page 294*
Medicinal Charcoal *see* Charcoal *on page 294*
Medicone® [OTC] *see* Phenylephrine *on page 1071*
Mediplast® [OTC] *see* Salicylic Acid *on page 1204*
Medi-Synal [OTC] *see* Acetaminophen and Pseudoephedrine *on page 31*

Medium Chain Triglycerides (mee DEE um chane trye GLIS er ides)

U.S. Brand Names MCT Oil® [OTC]

Canadian Brand Names MCT Oil®

Pharmacologic Category Dietary Supplement

Synonyms Triglycerides, Medium Chain

Use Dietary supplement for those who cannot digest long chain fats; malabsorption associated with disorders such as pancreatic insufficiency, bile salt deficiency, and bacterial overgrowth of the small bowel; induce ketosis as a prevention for seizures (akinetic, clonic, and petit mal)

Local Anesthetic/Vasoconstrictor Precautions No information available to require special precautions

Effects on Dental Treatment No significant effects or complications reported

Dosage Oral:

Infants: Initial: 0.5 mL every other feeding, then advance to every feeding, then increase in increments of 0.25-0.5 mL/feeding at intervals of 2-3 days as tolerated
Seizures: About 39 mL with each meal or 50% to 70% (800-1120 kcal) of total calories (1600 kcal) as the oil will induce ketosis necessary for seizure control
Cystic fibrosis: 3 tablespoons/day is tolerated without adverse symptoms by most children

Adults: 15 mL 3-4 times/day

Other Adverse Effects Frequency not defined:

Central nervous system: May result in **narcosis** and **coma** in cirrhotic patients due to high levels of medium chain fatty acids in the serum which then enter the cerebral spinal fluid; electroencephalogram effects include slowing of the alpha wave (can occur during infusion of fatty acids of 2-6 carbon lengths)

Endocrine & metabolic:
MCT therapy does not produce recognized metabolic side effects of any clinical importance, nor do they interfere with the metabolism of other food stuffs or with the absorption of drugs; when administered in the form of a mixed diet with carbohydrates and protein, there is no clinical evidence of **hyperketonemia**; hyperketonemia may occur in normal or diabetic subjects in the absence of carbohydrates; has been reported that MCT may increase hepatic free fatty acid synthesis and reduce ketone clearance
Fecal water, sodium and potassium excretion are decreased in patients with steatorrhea who are treated with MCT; enhanced calcium absorption has been demonstrated in patients with steatorrhea who are given MCT

Gastrointestinal: Nausea, occasional vomiting, gastritis and distention, diarrhea, and borborygmi are common adverse reactions occurring in about 10% of the patients receiving supplements or diets containing MCT; these symptoms may be related to rapid hydrolysis of MCT, high concentrations of free fatty acids in the stomach and small intestine, hyperosmolarity causing influx of large amounts of fluid, and lactose intolerance; abdominal cramps, nausea and vomiting occurred despite cautionary administration of MCT in small sips throughout meals, but subsided with continued administration

Dietary/Ethanol/Herb Considerations Food: Does not provide any essential fatty acids; only saturated fats are contained; supplementation with safflower, corn oil, or other polyunsaturated vegetable oil must be given to provide the patient with the essential fatty acids. The minimum daily requirement has not been established for oral intake, but 10-15 mL of safflower oil (60% to 70% linoleic acid) appears to be satisfactory. Contains 7.7 kcal/mL

Pregnancy Risk Factor C

Generic Available No

Medrol® *see* MethylPREDNISolone *on page 895*

MedroxyPROGESTERone (me DROKS ee proe JES te rone)

Related Information

Endocrine Disorders and Pregnancy *on page 1479*

U.S. Brand Names Depo-Provera®; Depo-Provera® Contraceptive; Provera®

Canadian Brand Names Alti-MPA; Depo-Prevera®; Gen-Medroxy; Novo-Medrone; Provera®

Mexican Brand Names Cycrin®; Depo-Provera®; Provera®

(Continued)

MedroxyPROGESTERone *(Continued)*

Pharmacologic Category Contraceptive; Progestin

Synonyms Acetoxymethylprogesterone; Medroxyprogesterone; Methylacetoxyprogesterone

Use Endometrial carcinoma or renal carcinoma as well as secondary amenorrhea or abnormal uterine bleeding due to hormonal imbalance; reduction of endometrial hyperplasia in postmenopausal women receiving 0.625 mg conjugated estrogens for 12-14 consecutive days per month; Depo-Provera® injection is used for the prevention of pregnancy

Unlabeled/Investigational Use Treatment of hypoventilation disorders, advanced breast cancer

Local Anesthetic/Vasoconstrictor Precautions No information available to require special precautions

Effects on Dental Treatment Progestins may predispose the patient to gingival bleeding.

Dosage

Adolescents and Adults: Oral:

Amenorrhea: 5-10 mg/day for 5-10 days or 2.5 mg/day

Abnormal uterine bleeding: 5-10 mg for 5-10 days starting on day 16 or 21 of cycle

Accompanying cyclic estrogen therapy, postmenopausal: 2.5-10 mg the last 10-13 days of estrogen dosing each month

Hypoventilation syndromes (unlabeled use): 20 mg 3 times/day

Adults:

I.M.:

Endometrial or renal carcinoma: 400-1000 mg/week

Contraception: 150 mg every 3 months

Dosing adjustment in hepatic impairment: Reduction required with alcoholic cirrhosis

Mechanism of Action Inhibits secretion of pituitary gonadotropins, which prevents follicular maturation and ovulation, stimulates growth of mammary tissue

Other Adverse Effects Frequency not defined:

Cardiovascular: Edema, embolism, central thrombosis

Central nervous system: Mental depression, insomnia, **somnolence, headache (rare), dizziness, fever**

Dermatologic: Melasma or chloasma, allergic rash with or without pruritus, acne, hirsutism, angioneurotic edema

Endocrine & metabolic: Breakthrough bleeding, spotting, changes in menstrual flow, amenorrhea, increased breast tenderness, changes in cervical erosion and secretions

Gastrointestinal: Weight gain/loss, anorexia, nausea

Hepatic: Cholestatic jaundice

Local: Pain at injection site, sterile abscess, thrombophlebitis

Neuromuscular & skeletal: Weakness

Respiratory: Pulmonary embolism

Miscellaneous: **Anaphylaxis**

Drug Interactions Substrate of **CYP3A4**; Induces CYP3A4

Decreased Effect: Aminoglutethimide may decrease effects by increasing hepatic metabolism.

Pharmacodynamics/Kinetics

Absorption: Oral: Well absorbed; I.M.: Slow

Protein binding: 90% primarily to albumin; not to sex-hormone-binding globulin

Metabolism: Oral: Hepatic via hydroxylated and conjugated

Bioavailability: 0.6% to 10%

Time to peak: Oral: 2-4 hours

Half-life elimination: Oral: 38-46 hours; I.M.: Acetate: 50 days

Excretion: Oral: Urine and feces

Pregnancy Risk Factor X

Generic Available Yes: Tablet

Medroxyprogesterone Acetate and Estradiol Cypionate *see* Estradiol and Medroxyprogesterone *on page 523*

Medroxyprogesterone and Estrogens (Conjugated) *see* Estrogens (Conjugated/Equine) and Medroxyprogesterone *on page 531*

Medrysone (ME dri sone)

U.S. Brand Names HMS Liquifilm®

Pharmacologic Category Corticosteroid, Ophthalmic

Use Treatment of allergic conjunctivitis, vernal conjunctivitis, episcleritis, ophthalmic epinephrine sensitivity reaction

Local Anesthetic/Vasoconstrictor Precautions No information available to require special precautions

Effects on Dental Treatment No significant effects or complications reported

Dosage Children ≥3 years and Adults: Ophthalmic: Instill 1 drop in conjunctival sac 2-4 times/day up to every 4 hours; may use every 1-2 hours during first 1-2 days

Mechanism of Action A synthetic corticosteroid; structurally related to progesterone; decreases inflammation by suppression of migration of polymorphonuclear leukocytes and reversal of increased capillary permeability

Other Adverse Effects Frequency not defined: Ocular: Acute anterior uveitis, allergic reactions, blurred vision (mild, temporary), burning, cataracts, conjunctivitis, corneal thinning, corneal ulcers, delayed wound healing, foreign body sensation, glaucoma, IOP increased, keratitis, mydriasis, optic nerve damage, ptosis, secondary ocular infection stinging, visual activity defects

Pharmacodynamics/Kinetics

Absorption: Through aqueous humor

Metabolism: Hepatic if absorbed

Excretion: Urine and feces

Pregnancy Risk Factor C

Generic Available No

Comments If no improvement after several days of treatment, discontinue medrysone and institute other therapy; duration of therapy: 3-4 days to several weeks dependent on type and severity of disease; taper dose to avoid disease exacerbation

Mefenamic Acid (me fe NAM ik AS id)

Related Information

Rheumatoid Arthritis, Osteoarthritis, and Osteoporosis *on page 1488*

Temporomandibular Dysfunction (TMD) *on page 1562*

U.S. Brand Names Ponstel®

Canadian Brand Names Apo®-Mefenamic; Nu-Mefenamic; PMS-Mefenamic Acid; Ponstan®; Ponstel®

Mexican Brand Names Ponstan®

Pharmacologic Category Nonsteroidal Anti-inflammatory Drug (NSAID)

Use Short-term relief of mild to moderate pain including primary dysmenorrhea

Local Anesthetic/Vasoconstrictor Precautions No information available to require special precautions

Effects on Dental Treatment 1% to 10%: Headache, nervousness, dizziness (3% to 9%), gastric or duodenal ulcer with bleeding or perforation (1% to 10%), gastritis (1% to 10%), vomiting (1% to 10%), bleeding (1% to 10%)

NSAID formulations are known to reversibly decrease platelet aggregation via mechanisms different than observed with aspirin. The dentist should be aware of the potential of abnormal coagulation. Caution should also be exercised in the use of NSAIDs in patients already on anticoagulant therapy with drugs such as warfarin (Coumadin®). Recovery of platelet function usually occurs 1-2 days after discontinuation of NSAIDs.

Dosage Oral:

Children >14 years and Adults: 500 mg to start then 250 mg every 4 hours as needed; maximum therapy: 1 week

Dosing comment in renal impairment: Use not recommended

Mechanism of Action Inhibits prostaglandin synthesis by decreasing the activity of the enzyme, cyclooxygenase, which results in decreased formation of prostaglandin precursors

Other Adverse Effects

1% to 10%:

- Dermatologic: Itching, rash
- Endocrine & metabolic: Fluid retention
- Gastrointestinal: Abdominal cramps, heartburn, indigestion, nausea (1% to 10%), diarrhea (1% to 10%), constipation (1% to 10%), abdominal distress/cramping/pain (1% to 10%), dyspepsia (1% to 10%), flatulence (1% to 10%)
- Hepatic: Elevated LFTs (1% to 10%)
- Otic: Tinnitus (1% to 10%)

<1%: **CHF, hypertension, arrhythmias, tachycardia, confusion, hallucinations**, aseptic meningitis, mental depression, **drowsiness**, insomnia, urticaria, erythema multiforme, toxic epidermal necrolysis, Stevens-Johnson syndrome, angioedema, **polydipsia, hot flashes, gastritis, GI ulceration**, cystitis, polyuria, agranulocytosis, anemia, hemolytic anemia, bone marrow suppression, leukopenia, thrombocytopenia, hepatitis, peripheral neuropathy, toxic amblyopia, blurred vision, conjunctivitis, dry eyes, hearing loss, acute renal failure, **dyspnea, allergic rhinitis, epistaxis, stomatitis**

Drug Interactions Substrate of CYP2C8/9; Inhibits CYP2C8/9

Increased Effect/Toxicity: Anticoagulants (warfarin, heparin, LMWHs) in combination with NSAIDs can cause increased risk of bleeding. Other antiplatelet drugs (ticlopidine, clopidogrel, aspirin, abciximab, dipyridamole, eptifibatide, tirofiban) can cause an increased risk of bleeding. NSAIDs may increase serum creatinine, potassium, blood pressure, and cyclosporine levels during concurrent therapy; monitor cyclosporine levels and renal function carefully. Lithium levels can be increased; avoid concurrent use if possible or monitor lithium levels and adjust

(Continued)

Mefenamic Acid *(Continued)*

dose. Sulindac may have the least effect. When NSAID is stopped, lithium will need adjustment again. Corticosteroids may increase the risk of GI ulceration; avoid concurrent use. Serum concentration/toxicity of methotrexate may be increased.

Decreased Effect: Antihypertensive effects of ACE-inhibitors, angiotensin antagonists, diuretics, and hydralazine may be decreased by concurrent therapy with NSAIDs; monitor blood pressure. Cholestyramine and colestipol reduce the bioavailability of diclofenac; separate administration times.

Dietary/Ethanol/Herb Considerations Ethanol: Avoid use due to GI irritation.

Pharmacodynamics/Kinetics

Onset of action: Peak effect: 2-4 hours

Duration: ≤6 hours

Protein binding: High

Metabolism: Conjugated hepatically

Half-life elimination: 3.5 hours

Excretion: Urine (50%) and feces as unchanged drug and metabolites

Pregnancy Risk Factor C/D (3rd trimester)

Generic Available No

Mefloquine (ME floe kwin)

U.S. Brand Names Lariam®

Canadian Brand Names Lariam®

Pharmacologic Category Antimalarial Agent

Synonyms Mefloquine Hydrochloride

Use Treatment of acute malarial infections and prevention of malaria

Local Anesthetic/Vasoconstrictor Precautions No information available to require special precautions

Effects on Dental Treatment 1% to 10%: Headache, fever, vomiting (3%), nausea

Dosage Oral (dose expressed as mg of mefloquine hydrochloride):

Children ≥6 months and >5 kg:

Malaria treatment: 20-25 mg/kg in 2 divided doses, taken 6-8 hours apart (maximum: 1250 mg) Take with food and an ample amount of water. If clinical improvement is not seen within 48-72 hours, an alternative therapy should be used for retreatment.

Malaria prophylaxis: 5 mg/kg/once weekly (maximum dose: 250 mg) starting 1 week before, arrival in endemic area, continuing weekly during travel and for 4 weeks after leaving endemic area. Take with food and an ample amount of water.

Adults:

Malaria treatment (mild to moderate infection): 5 tablets (1250 mg) as a single dose. Take with food and at least 8 oz of water. If clinical improvement is not seen within 48-72 hours, an alternative therapy should be used for retreatment.

Malaria prophylaxis: 1 tablet (250 mg) weekly starting 1 week before, arrival in endemic area, continuing weekly during travel and for 4 weeks after leaving endemic area. Take with food and at least 8 oz of water.

Dosage adjustment in hepatic impairment: Half-life may be prolonged and plasma levels may be higher.

Mechanism of Action Mefloquine is a quinoline-methanol compound structurally similar to quinine; mefloquine's effectiveness in the treatment and prophylaxis of malaria is due to the destruction of the asexual blood forms of the malarial pathogens that affect humans, *Plasmodium falciparum*, *P. vivax*, *P. malariae*, *P. ovale*

Other Adverse Effects

1% to 10%:

Central nervous system: Chills, fatigue

Dermatologic: Rash

Gastrointestinal: Appetite decreased, diarrhea, stomach pain

Neuromuscular & skeletal: Myalgia

Otic: Tinnitus

<1%: Alopecia, bradycardia, dizziness, emotional lability, extrasystoles, pruritus, seizures, syncope, weakness

Frequency not defined: Neuropsychiatric events

Postmarketing and/or case reports: Abnormal dreams, ataxia, aggressive behavior, agitation, anaphylaxis, anxiety, arthralgia, AV block, chest pain, conduction abnormalities (transient), confusion, convulsions, depression, diaphoresis (increased), dyspepsia, dyspnea, edema, encephalopathy, erythema multiforme, exanthema, hallucinations, hearing impairment, hypotension, insomnia, leukocytosis, malaise, mood changes, muscle cramps/weakness, palpitation, panic attacks, paranoia, paresthesia, psychosis, somnolence, Stevens-Johnson syndrome, suicidal ideation and behavior (causal relationship not established), tachycardia, thrombocytopenia, tremor, urticaria, vertigo, visual disturbances

Drug Interactions Substrate of **CYP3A4**; Inhibits CYP3A4

Increased Effect/Toxicity: Use caution with drugs that alter cardiac conduction; increased toxicity with chloroquine, quinine, and quinidine (hold treatment until at least 12 hours after these later drugs); increased toxicity with halofantrine (concurrent use is contraindicated)

Decreased Effect: Mefloquine may decrease the effect of valproic acid, carbamazepine, phenobarbital, and phenytoin.

Dietary/Ethanol/Herb Considerations Food: Administer with food and at least 8 oz water.

Pharmacodynamics/Kinetics

Absorption: Well absorbed

Distribution: V_d: 19 L/kg; blood, urine, CSF, tissues; enters breast milk

Protein binding: 98%

Metabolism: Extensively hepatic; forms metabolites

Bioavailability: Increased by food

Half-life elimination: 21-22 days

Time to peak, plasma: 6-24 hours (median: ~17 hours)

Excretion: Primarily bile and feces; urine (9% as unchanged drug, 4% as primary metabolite)

Pregnancy Risk Factor C

Generic Available Yes

Mefloquine Hydrochloride *see* Mefloquine *on page 852*

Mefoxin® *see* Cefoxitin *on page 272*

Megace® *see* Megestrol *on page 853*

Megadophilus® [OTC] *see Lactobacillus acidophilus* and *Lactobacillus bulgaricus on page 772*

Megestrol (me JES trole)

U.S. Brand Names Megace®

Canadian Brand Names Apo®-Megestrol; Lin-Megestrol; Megace®; Megace® OS; Nu-Megestrol

Pharmacologic Category Antineoplastic Agent, Miscellaneous; Progestin

Synonyms Megestrol Acetate

Use Palliative treatment of breast and endometrial carcinoma

Orphan drug: Treatment of anorexia, cachexia, or significant weight loss (≥10% baseline body weight); treatment of AIDS

Local Anesthetic/Vasoconstrictor Precautions No information available to require special precautions

Effects on Dental Treatment 1% to 10%: Hypertension (≤8%), CNS depression (≤6%), fever (2% to 6%), headache (≤10%), confusion (1% to 3%), convulsions (1% to 3%) hyperglycemia (≤6%), paresthesia (1% to 3%), dyspnea (1% to 3%), cough (1% to 3%)

Dosage Adults: Oral (refer to individual protocols):

Female:

Breast carcinoma: 40 mg 4 times/day

Endometrial: 40-320 mg/day in divided doses; use for 2 months to determine efficacy; maximum doses used have been up to 800 mg/day

Uterine bleeding: 40 mg 2-4 times/day

Male/Female: HIV-related cachexia: Initial dose: 800 mg/day; daily doses of 400 and 800 mg/day were found to be clinically effective

Dosing adjustment in renal impairment: Data unavailable; urinary excretion of megestrol acetate administered in doses of 4-90 mg ranged from 56% to 78% within 10 days

Hemodialysis: Megestrol acetate has not been tested for dialyzability; however, due to its low solubility, it is postulated that dialysis would not be an effective means of treating an overdose

Mechanism of Action A synthetic progestin with antiestrogenic properties which disrupt the estrogen receptor cycle. Megace® interferes with the normal estrogen cycle and results in a lower LH titer. May also have a direct effect on the endometrium. Megestrol is an antineoplastic progestin thought to act through an antileutenizing effect mediated via the pituitary.

Other Adverse Effects

Cardiovascular: Edema, cardiomyopathy

Central nervous system: Insomnia, pain (≤6%, similar to placebo)

Dermatologic: Allergic rash (2% to 12%) with or without pruritus, alopecia

Endocrine & metabolic: Breakthrough bleeding and amenorrhea, spotting, changes in menstrual flow, changes in cervical erosion and secretions, increased breast tenderness, changes in vaginal bleeding pattern, edema, fluid retention, **diabetes**, HPA axis suppression, adrenal insufficiency, Cushing's syndrome

Gastrointestinal: Weight gain (not attributed to edema or fluid retention), nausea (≤5%, less than placebo), vomiting, diarrhea (8% to 15%, similar to placebo), flatulence (≤10%), constipation (1% to 3%)

Genitourinary: Impotence (4% to 14%), decreased libido (≤5%)

Hepatic: Cholestatic jaundice, hepatotoxicity, hepatomegaly (1% to 3%)

Local: Thrombophlebitis

Neuromuscular & skeletal: Carpal tunnel syndrome, weakness

Respiratory: **Hyperpnea**

(Continued)

Megestrol *(Continued)*

Miscellaneous: **Diaphoresis**

Dietary/Ethanol/Herb Considerations Herb/Nutraceutical: Avoid black cohosh and dong quai in estrogen-dependent tumors.

Pharmacodynamics/Kinetics

Absorption: Well absorbed orally

Metabolism: Completely hepatic to free steroids and glucuronide conjugates

Time to peak, serum: 1-3 hours

Half-life elimination: 15-100 hours

Excretion: Urine (57% to 78% as steroid metabolites and inactive compound); feces (8% to 30%)

Pregnancy Risk Factor X

Generic Available Yes

Megestrol Acetate *see* Megestrol *on page 853*

Melanex® *see* Hydroquinone *on page 693*

Melfiat®: Obezine® *see* Phendimetrazine *on page 1064*

Mellaril® [DSC] *see* Thioridazine *on page 1298*

Meloxicam (mel OKS ee kam)

U.S. Brand Names MOBIC®

Canadian Brand Names MOBIC®; Mobicox®

Mexican Brand Names Masflex®; Mobicox®

Pharmacologic Category Nonsteroidal Anti-inflammatory Drug (NSAID)

Use Relief of signs and symptoms of osteoarthritis

Local Anesthetic/Vasoconstrictor Precautions No information available to require special precautions

Effects on Dental Treatment

1% to 10%: Upper respiratory infection (2% to 3%), pharyngitis (1% to 3%), flu-like symptoms (4% to 5%), falling (3%)

<2%: Taste perversion, ulcerative stomatitis, xerostomia

<2%: Allergic reaction, anaphylactic reaction, shock, hot flashes, syncope, angina, cardiac failure, hypertension, hypotension, myocardial infarction, seizures, paresthesia, tremor, xerostomia, duodenal ulcer, gastric ulcer, gastritis, gastroesophageal reflux, GI hemorrhage, intestinal perforation, duodenal perforation, gastric perforation, ulcerative stomatitis, arrhythmia, palpitations, tachycardia, dehydration, anxiety, confusion, nervousness, asthma, bronchospasm, dyspnea,

Dosage Oral:

Adult: Initial: 7.5 mg once daily; some patients may receive additional benefit from an increased dose of 15 mg once daily; maximum dose: 15 mg/day

Dosing adjustment in renal impairment: No specific recommendation for mild to moderate impairment; avoid use in significant impairment

Dosing adjustment in hepatic impairment: No specific adjustments; not studied in severe impairment

Elderly: No specific recommendations; increased concentrations may occur (particularly in females)

Mechanism of Action Inhibits prostaglandin synthesis by decreasing the activity of the enzyme, cyclooxygenase, which results in decreased formation of prostaglandin precursors

Other Adverse Effects

1% to 10%:

Cardiovascular: Edema (2% to 5%)

Central nervous system: Headache and dizziness (2% to 8%; less frequent than placebo in controlled trials)

Dermatologic: Rash (1% to 3%)

Gastrointestinal: Diarrhea (3% to 8%), dyspepsia (5%), nausea (4%), flatulence (3%), abdominal pain (2% to 3%)

<2%: Allergic reaction, anaphylactic reaction, shock, fatigue, hot flashes, malaise, syncope, weight changes, angina, cardiac failure, hypertension, hypotension, MI, vasculitis, seizures, paresthesia, tremor, vertigo, colitis, xerostomia, duodenal ulcer, gastric ulcer, gastritis, gastroesophageal reflux, gastrointestinal hemorrhage, hematemesis, intestinal perforation, melena, pancreatitis, duodenal perforation, gastric perforation, ulcerative stomatitis, arrhythmia, palpitations, tachycardia, agranulocytosis, leukopenia, purpura, thrombocytopenia, increased ALT, increased AST, hyperbilirubinemia, increased GGT, hepatitis, jaundice, hepatic failure, dehydration, abnormal dreams, anxiety, confusion, depression, nervousness, somnolence, asthma, bronchospasm, dyspnea, alopecia, angioedema, bullous eruption, erythema multiforme, photosensitivity reaction, pruritus, Stevens-Johnson syndrome, toxic epidermal necrolysis, urticaria, abnormal vision, conjunctivitis, tinnitus, albuminuria, increased BUN, increased creatinine, hematuria, interstitial nephritis, renal failure

Drug Interactions Substrate of CYP2C8/9, 3A4; Inhibits CYP2C8/9

Increased Effect/Toxicity: Anticoagulants (warfarin, heparin, LMWHs) in combination with NSAIDs can cause increased risk of bleeding. Antiplatelet drugs (ticlopidine, clopidogrel, aspirin, abciximab, dipyridamole, eptifibatide, tirofiban) can cause an increased risk of bleeding. Aspirin increases serum concentrations (AUC) of meloxicam (in addition to potential for additive adverse effects); concurrent use is not recommended. Corticosteroids may increase the risk of GI ulceration; avoid concurrent use. NSAIDs may increase serum creatinine, potassium, blood pressure, and cyclosporine levels; monitor cyclosporine levels and renal function carefully. Lithium levels can be increased; avoid concurrent use if possible or monitor lithium levels and adjust dose. When NSAID is stopped, lithium will need adjustment again. Serum concentration/toxicity of methotrexate may be increased. Warfarin INRs may be increased by meloxicam. Monitor INR closely, particularly during initiation or change in dose. May increase risk of bleeding. Use lowest possible dose for shortest duration possible.

Decreased Effect: Cholestyramine (and possibly colestipol) increases the clearance of meloxicam. Hydralazine's antihypertensive effect is decreased; avoid concurrent use. Loop diuretic efficacy (diuretic and antihypertensive effect) may be reduced by NSAIDs. Antihypertensive effects of thiazide diuretics are decreased; avoid concurrent use.

Dietary/Ethanol/Herb Considerations

Ethanol: Avoid use; may enhance gastric mucosal irritation.

Food: Administer with food or milk to reduce GI upset.

Pharmacodynamics/Kinetics

Distribution: 10 L

Protein binding: 99.4%

Metabolism: Hepatic via CYP2C9 and CYP3A4 (minor)

Bioavailability: 89%

Half-life elimination: 15-20 hours

Time to peak: 5-10 hours

Excretion: Urine and feces (as inactive metabolites)

Pregnancy Risk Factor C/D (3rd trimester)

Generic Available No

Melpaque HP® *see* Hydroquinone *on page 693*

Melphalan (MEL fa lan)

U.S. Brand Names Alkeran®

Canadian Brand Names Alkeran®

Mexican Brand Names Alkeran®

Pharmacologic Category Antineoplastic Agent, Alkylating Agent

Synonyms L-PAM; L-Sarcolysin; Phenylalanine Mustard

Use Palliative treatment of multiple myeloma and nonresectable epithelial ovarian carcinoma; neuroblastoma, rhabdomyosarcoma, breast cancer

Local Anesthetic/Vasoconstrictor Precautions No information available to require special precautions

Effects on Dental Treatment No significant effects or complications reported

Dosage Refer to individual protocols.

Oral: Dose should always be adjusted to patient response and weekly blood counts:

Children: 4-20 mg/m²/day for 1-21 days

Adults:

Multiple myeloma: 6 mg/day initially adjusted as indicated **or** 0.15 mg/kg/day for 7 days **or** 0.25 mg/kg/day for 4 days; repeat at 4- to 6-week intervals.

Ovarian carcinoma: 0.2 mg/kg/day for 5 days, repeat every 4-5 weeks.

I.V.:

Children:

Pediatric rhabdomyosarcoma: 10-35 mg/m²/dose every 21-28 days

High-dose melphalan with bone marrow transplantation for neuroblastoma: I.V.: 100-220 mg/m² as a single dose or divided into 2-5 daily doses. Infuse over 20-60 minutes.

Adults: Multiple myeloma: 16 mg/m² administered at 2-week intervals for 4 doses, then repeat monthly as per protocol for multiple myeloma.

Dosing adjustment in renal impairment:

Cl_{cr} 10-50 mL/minute: Administer at 75% of normal dose

Cl_{cr} <10 mL/minute: Administer at 50% of normal dose

or

BUN >30 mg/dL: Reduce dose by 50%

Serum creatinine >1.5 mg/dL: Reduce dose by 50%

Hemodialysis: Unknown

CAPD effects: Unknown

CAVH effects: Dose for GFR 10-50 mL/minute

Dosing adjustment in hepatic impairment: BUN >30 mg/dL: Reduce dose by 50%

Mechanism of Action Alkylating agent which is a derivative of mechlorethamine that inhibits DNA and RNA synthesis via formation of carbonium ions; cross-links strands of DNA

(Continued)

Melphalan *(Continued)*

Other Adverse Effects

>10%: Hematologic: Myelosuppressive: Leukopenia and thrombocytopenia are the most common effects of melphalan; irreversible bone marrow failure has been reported
- WBC: Moderate
- Platelets: Moderate
- Onset: 7 days
- Nadir: 8-10 days and 27-32 days
- Recovery: 42-50 days

1% to 10%:
- Cardiovascular: Vasculitis
- Dermatologic: Vesiculation of skin, alopecia, pruritus, rash
- Endocrine & metabolic: SIADH, sterility, amenorrhea
- Gastrointestinal: Nausea and vomiting (mild), stomatitis and diarrhea (infrequent)
- Genitourinary: Hemorrhagic cystitis, bladder irritation
- Hematologic: Anemia, agranulocytosis, hemolytic anemia
- Hepatic: Transaminases increased (hepatitis, jaundice have been reported)
- Respiratory: Pulmonary fibrosis, interstitial pneumonitis
- Miscellaneous: Hypersensitivity, secondary malignancy

Drug Interactions

Increased Effect/Toxicity: Cyclosporine: Risk of nephrotoxicity is increased by melphalan.

Decreased Effect: Cimetidine and other H_2 antagonists: The reduction in gastric pH has been reported to decrease bioavailability of melphalan by 30%.

Dietary/Ethanol/Herb Considerations

Ethanol: Avoid use due to GI irritation.

Food interferes with oral absorption.

Pharmacodynamics/Kinetics

Absorption: Oral: Variable and incomplete

Distribution: V_d: 0.5-0.6 L/kg throughout total body water

Bioavailability: Unpredictable, decreasing from 85% to 58% with repeated doses

Half-life elimination: Terminal: 1.5 hours

Time to peak, serum: ~2 hours

Excretion: Oral: Feces (20% to 50%); urine (10% to 30% as unchanged drug)

Pregnancy Risk Factor D

Generic Available No

Melquin-3® [OTC] *see* Hydroquinone *on page 693*

Melquin HP® *see* Hydroquinone *on page 693*

Menadol® [OTC] *see* Ibuprofen *on page 703*

Menest® *see* Estrogens (Esterified) *on page 533*

Meningococcal Polysaccharide Vaccine (Groups A, C, Y, and W-135)

(me NIN joe kok al pol i SAK a ride vak SEEN groops aye, see, why & dubl yoo won thur tee fyve)

Related Information

Immunizations (Vaccines) *on page 1612*

U.S. Brand Names Menomune®-A/C/Y/W-135

Pharmacologic Category Vaccine

Use

Immunization of persons ≥2 years of age in epidemic or endemic areas as might be determined in a population delineated by neighborhood, school, dormitory, or other reasonable boundary. The prevalent serogroup in such a situation should match a serogroup in the vaccine. Individuals at particular high-risk include persons with terminal component complement deficiencies and those with anatomic or functional asplenia.

Travelers visiting areas of a country that are recognized as having hyperendemic or epidemic meningococcal disease

Vaccinations should be considered for household or institutional contacts of persons with meningococcal disease as an adjunct to appropriate antibiotic chemoprophylaxis as well as medical and laboratory personnel at risk of exposure to meningococcal disease

Local Anesthetic/Vasoconstrictor Precautions No information available to require special precautions

Effects on Dental Treatment Headache (2% to 5%), fever (100°F to 106°F: 3%)

Restrictions Federal law requires that the date of administration, the vaccine manufacturer, lot number of vaccine, and the administering person's name, title and address be entered into the patient's permanent medical record.

Dosage One dose S.C. (0.5 mL); the need for booster is unknown; **Note:** Individuals who are sensitive to thimerosal should receive single-dose pack (reconstituted with 0.78 mL vial without preservative).

Mechanism of Action Induces the formation of bactericidal antibodies to meningococcal antigens; the presence of these antibodies is strongly correlated with immunity to meningococcal disease caused by *Neisseria meningitidis* groups A, C, Y and W-135.

Other Adverse Effects All serious adverse reactions must be reported to the U.S. Department of Health and Human Services (DHHS) Vaccine Adverse Event Reporting System (VAERS) 1-800-822-7967. Incidence of erythema, swelling, or tenderness may be higher in children.

>10%: Local: Tenderness (9% to 36% as reported in adults)

1% to 10%:

Central nervous system: Malaise (2%), chills (2%)

Local: Pain at injection site (2% to 3%), erythema (1% to 4%), induration (1% to 4%)

Pharmacodynamics/Kinetics

Onset of action: Antibody levels: 10-14 days

Duration: Antibodies against group A and C polysaccharides decline markedly (to prevaccination levels) over the first 3 years following a single dose of vaccine, especially in children <4 years of age

Pregnancy Risk Factor C

Generic Available No

Menomune®-A/C/Y/W-135 *see* Meningococcal Polysaccharide Vaccine (Groups A, C, Y, and W-135) *on page 856*

Menotropins (men oh TROE pins)

U.S. Brand Names Pergonal®; Repronex®

Canadian Brand Names Pergonal®

Mexican Brand Names HMG Massone®; Humegon®

Pharmacologic Category Gonadotropin; Ovulation Stimulator

Use Sequentially with hCG to induce ovulation and pregnancy in the infertile woman with functional anovulation or in patients who have previously received pituitary suppression; stimulation of multiple follicle development in ovulatory patients as part of an *in vitro* fertilization program; used with hCG in men to stimulate spermatogenesis in those with primary hypogonadotropic hypogonadism

Local Anesthetic/Vasoconstrictor Precautions No information available to require special precautions

Effects on Dental Treatment

1% to 10% (male): Erythrocytosis (dyspnea, dizziness, anorexia, syncope, epistaxis)

1% to 10% (female): Headache, vomiting, infection

Dosage Adults: I.M.:

Spermatogenesis (Male): Following pretreatment with hCG, 1 ampul 3 times/week and hCG 2000 units twice weekly until sperm is detected in the ejaculate (4-6 months) then may be increased to 2 ampuls of menotropins (150 units FSH/150 units LH) 3 times/week

Induction of ovulation (Female): 1 ampul/day (75 units of FSH and LH) for 9-12 days followed by 10,000 units hCG 1 day after the last dose; repeated at least twice at same level before increasing dosage to 2 ampuls (150 units FSH/150 units LH)

Repronex®: I.M., S.C.:

Infertile patients with oligo-anovulation: Initial: 150 int. units daily for the first 5 days of treatment. Adjustments should not be made more frequently than once every 2 days and should not exceed 75-150 int. units per adjustment. Maximum daily dose should not exceed 450 int. units and dosing beyond 12 days is not recommended. If patient's response to Repronex® is appropriate, hCG 5000-10,000 units should be given one day following the last dose of Repronex®. Hold dose if serum estradiol is >2000 pg/mL, if the ovaries are abnormally enlarged, or if abdominal pain occurs; the patient should also be advised to refrain from intercourse.

Assisted reproductive technologies: Initial (in patients who have received GnRH agonist or antagonist pituitary suppression): 225 int. units; adjustments in dose should not be made more frequently than once every 2 days and should not exceed more than 75-50 int. units per adjustment. The maximum daily doses of Repronex® given should not exceed 450 int. units and dosing beyond 12 days is not recommended. Once adequate follicular development is evident, hCG (5000-10,000 units) should be administered to induce final follicular maturation in preparation for oocyte retrieval. Withhold treatment when ovaries are abnormally enlarged on last day of therapy (to reduce chance of developing OHSS).

Mechanism of Action Actions occur as a result of both follicle stimulating hormone (FSH) effects and luteinizing hormone (LH) effects; menotropins stimulate the development and maturation of the ovarian follicle (FSH), cause ovulation (LH), and stimulate the development of the corpus luteum (LH); in males it stimulates spermatogenesis (LH)

Other Adverse Effects

Male:

>10%: Endocrine & metabolic: Gynecomastia

(Continued)

Menotropins *(Continued)*

Female:

1% to 10%:

Endocrine & metabolic: Breast tenderness

Gastrointestinal: Abdominal cramping, abdominal pain, diarrhea, enlarged abdomen, nausea

Genitourinary: Ectopic pregnancy, OHSS (% is dose-related), ovarian disease, vaginal hemorrhage

Local: Injection site edema/reaction

Miscellaneous: Pelvic pain

Frequency not defined:

Cardiovascular: **Stroke, tachycardia**, thrombosis (venous or arterial)

Central nervous system: **Dizziness**

Dermatologic: Angioedema, urticaria

Genitourinary: Adnexal torsion, hemoperitoneum, ovarian enlargement

Neuromuscular & skeletal: Limb necrosis

Respiratory: **Acute respiratory distress syndrome, atelectasis, dyspnea, embolism, laryngeal edema pulmonary infarction tachypnea**

Miscellaneous: **Allergic reactions, anaphylaxis**, rash

Drug Interactions Increased Effect/Toxicity: Clomiphene may decrease the amount of human menopausal gonadotropin (HMG) needed to induce ovulation (Gonadorelin, Factrel®); should not be used with drugs that stimulate ovulation.

Pharmacodynamics/Kinetics Excretion: Urine (~10% as unchanged drug)

Pregnancy Risk Factor X

Generic Available No

Mentax® *see* Butenafine *on page 217*

Mepenzolate (me PEN zoe late)

U.S. Brand Names Cantil®

Canadian Brand Names Cantil®

Pharmacologic Category Anticholinergic Agent; Antispasmodic Agent, Gastrointestinal

Synonyms Mepenzolate Bromide

Use Management of peptic ulcer disease; inhibit salivation and excessive secretions in respiratory tract preoperatively

Local Anesthetic/Vasoconstrictor Precautions No information available to require special precautions

Effects on Dental Treatment >10%: Xerostomia, dry throat

Dosage Adults: Oral: 25-50 mg 4 times/day with meals and at bedtime

Other Adverse Effects Frequency not defined:

Cardiovascular: **Palpitations, flushing**

Central nervous system: **Headache, nervousness, drowsiness, dizziness, confusion, fever**, CNS stimulation (large doses)

Dermatologic: Dry skin, urticaria

Gastrointestinal: Constipation, **dysphagia**, nausea, **vomiting**

Respiratory: **Nasal dryness**

Miscellaneous: Decreased diaphoresis, **hypersensitivity reactions, anaphylaxis**

Pregnancy Risk Factor C

Generic Available No

Mepenzolate Bromide *see* Mepenzolate *on page 858*

Meperidine (me PER i deen)

Related Information

Oral Pain *on page 1524*

U.S. Brand Names Demerol®; Meperitab®

Canadian Brand Names Demerol®

Pharmacologic Category Analgesic, Narcotic

Synonyms Isonipecaine Hydrochloride; Meperidine Hydrochloride; Pethidine Hydrochloride

Use

Dental: Adjunct in preoperative I.V. conscious sedation in patients undergoing dental surgery; alternate oral narcotic in patients allergic to codeine in treatment of moderate to moderate-severe pain

Medical: Management of moderate to severe pain; adjunct to anesthesia and preoperative sedation

Local Anesthetic/Vasoconstrictor Precautions No information available to require special precautions

Effects on Dental Treatment

1% to 10%: Xerostomia

Frequency not defined: Hypotension, fatigue, drowsiness, dizziness, nervousness, headache, restlessness, malaise, confusion, mental depression, hallucinations, paradoxical CNS stimulation, increased intracranial pressure, seizures (associated with metabolite accumulation), nausea, vomiting, cramps, biliary spasm, pain at injection site, weakness, dyspnea, histamine release, physical and psychological dependence

Restrictions C-II

Dosage These are guidelines and do not represent the maximum doses that may be required in all patients. Doses should be titrated to necessary analgesic effect. When changing route of administration, note that oral doses are about half as effective as parenteral dose. Oral route not recommended for chronic pain.

Children: Oral, I.M., I.V., S.C.: 1-1.5 mg/kg/dose every 3-4 hours as needed; 1-2 mg/kg as a single dose preoperative medication may be used; maximum 100 mg/dose

Adults: Oral, I.M., I.V.: S.C.: 50-150 mg/dose every 3-4 hours as needed

Elderly:

Oral: 50 mg every 4 hours

I.M.: 25 mg every 4 hours

Dosing adjustment in renal impairment: Avoid repeated administration in dysfunction:

Cl_{cr} 10-50 mL/minute: Administer at 75% of normal dose

Cl_{cr} <10 mL/minute: Administer at 50% of normal dose

Dosing adjustment/comments in hepatic impairment: Increased narcotic effect in cirrhosis; reduction in dose more important for oral than I.V. route

Mechanism of Action Binds to opiate receptors in the CNS, causing inhibition of ascending pain pathways, altering the perception of and response to pain; produces generalized CNS depression

Other Adverse Effects Frequency not defined:

Dermatologic: Rash, urticaria

Gastrointestinal: Constipation, anorexia, stomach cramps, paralytic ileus

Genitourinary: Ureteral spasms, decreased urination

Contraindications Hypersensitivity to meperidine or any component of the formulation; patients receiving MAO inhibitors presently or in the past 14 days; pregnancy (prolonged use or high doses near term)

Warnings/Precautions An opioid-containing analgesic regimen should be tailored to each patient's needs and based upon the type of pain being treated (acute versus chronic), the route of administration, degree of tolerance for opioids (naive versus chronic user), age, weight, and medical condition. The optimal analgesic dose varies widely among patients. Doses should be titrated to pain relief/prevention. Use for chronic pain management not recommended. Oral meperidine not recommended for acute pain management.

Use with caution in patients with pulmonary, hepatic, renal disorders, or increased intracranial pressure; use with caution in patients with renal failure or seizure disorders or those receiving high-dose meperidine; normeperidine (an active metabolite and CNS stimulant) may accumulate and precipitate twitches, tremors, or seizures; some preparations contain sulfites which may cause allergic reaction; not recommended as a drug of first choice for the treatment of chronic pain in the elderly due to the accumulation of normeperidine; for acute pain, its use should be limited to 1-2 doses; tolerance or drug dependence may result from extended use.

Drug Interactions

Increased Toxicity: May aggravate the adverse effects of isoniazid; MAO inhibitors, fluoxetine, and other serotonin uptake inhibitors greatly potentiate the effects of meperidine; acute opioid overdosage symptoms can be seen, including severe toxic reactions; CNS depressants, tricyclic antidepressants, phenothiazines may potentiate the effects of meperidine

Decreased Effect: Phenytoin may decrease the analgesic effects

Dietary/Ethanol/Herb Considerations

Ethanol: Avoid or limit use; may increase CNS depression.

Food: Glucose may cause hyperglycemia; monitor blood glucose concentrations.

Herb/Nutraceutical: Avoid gotu kola, kava, SAMe, St John's wort, and valerian; may increase CNS depression.

Pharmacodynamics/Kinetics

Onset of action: Analgesic: Oral, S.C., I.M.: 10-15 minutes; I.V.: ~5 minutes

Peak effect: Oral, S.C., I.M.: ~1 hour

Duration: Oral, S.C., I.M.: 2-4 hours

Distribution: Crosses placenta; enters breast milk

Protein binding: 65% to 75%

Metabolism: Hepatic; active metabolite (normeperidine)

Bioavailability: ~50% to 60%; increased with liver disease

Half-life elimination:

Parent drug: Terminal phase: Neonates: 23 hours (range: 12-39 hours); Adults: 2.5-4 hours, Liver disease: 7-11 hours

Normeperidine (active metabolite): 15-30 hours; can accumulate with high doses or with decreased renal function

Pregnancy Risk Factor B/D (prolonged use or high doses at term)

Dosage Forms INJ, solution [ampul]: 50 mg/mL (1.5 mL, 2 mL); [prefilled syringe]: 25 mg/mL (1 mL); 50 mg/mL (1 mL); 75 mg/mL (1 mL); 100 mg/mL (1 mL); [prefilled

(Continued)

Meperidine *(Continued)*

syringe for PCA pump]: 10 mg/mL (50 mL); [vial]: 50 mg/mL (1 mL, 30 mL); 100 mg/mL (20 mL). **SYR:** 50 mg/5 mL (5 mL, 500 mL); (Demerol®): 50 mg/5 mL (480 mL). **TAB** (Demerol®, Meperitab®): 50 mg, 100 mg

Generic Available Yes

Comments Meperidine is not to be used as the narcotic drug of first choice. It is recommended only to be used in codeine-allergic patients when a narcotic analgesic is indicated. Meperidine is not an anti-inflammatory agent. Meperidine, as with other narcotic analgesics, is recommended only for limited acute dosing (ie, 3 days or less); common adverse effects in the dental patient are nausea, sedation, and constipation. Meperidine has a significant addiction liability, especially when given long-term.

Meperidine and Promethazine (me PER i deen & proe METH a zeen)

Related Information

Meperidine *on page 858*

Promethazine *on page 1127*

Pharmacologic Category Analgesic Combination (Narcotic)

Synonyms Promethazine and Meperidine

Use Management of moderate to severe pain

Local Anesthetic/Vasoconstrictor Precautions No information available to require special precautions

Effects on Dental Treatment 1% to 10%: Xerostomia

Restrictions C-II

Dosage Adults: Oral: 1 capsule every 4-6 hours as needed

Other Adverse Effects Frequency not defined:

Based on meperidine component:

Cardiovascular: **Hypotension**

Central nervous system: Fatigue, **drowsiness, dizziness, nervousness, headache, restlessness, increased intracranial pressure, confusion, hallucinations**, mental depression, paradoxical CNS stimulation, malaise,

Dermatologic: Rash, urticaria

Gastrointestinal: Nausea, constipation, anorexia, stomach cramps, **biliary spasm, vomiting**

Genitourinary: Ureteral spasms, decreased urination, paralytic ileus

Local: Pain at injection site

Neuromuscular & skeletal: Weakness

Respiratory: **Dyspnea**

Miscellaneous: Histamine release, physical and psychological dependence

Based on promethazine component:

Cardiovascular: **Postural hypotension, tachycardia, dizziness**, nonspecific QT changes

Central nervous system: **Drowsiness, dystonias, akathisia, pseudoparkinsonism, tardive dyskinesia, neuroleptic malignant syndrome, seizures**

Dermatologic: Photosensitivity, dermatitis, skin pigmentation (slate gray)

Endocrine & metabolic: Lactation, breast engorgement, false-positive pregnancy test, amenorrhea, gynecomastia, hyper- or hypoglycemia

Gastrointestinal: Constipation, nausea

Genitourinary: Urinary retention, ejaculatory disorder, impotence

Hematologic: Agranulocytosis, eosinophilia, leukopenia, hemolytic anemia, aplastic anemia, thrombocytopenic purpura

Hepatic: Jaundice

Ocular: Blurred vision, corneal and lenticular changes, epithelial keratopathy, pigmentary retinopathy

Dietary/Ethanol/Herb Considerations

Ethanol: Avoid use; may increase CNS depression.

Herb/Nutraceutical: Avoid gotu kola, kava, SAMe, St John's wort, and valerian; may increase CNS depression.

Pregnancy Risk Factor B/D (prolonged use or high doses at term)

Generic Available Yes

Meperidine Hydrochloride *see* Meperidine *on page 858*

Meperitab® *see* Meperidine *on page 858*

Mephobarbital (me foe BAR bi tal)

U.S. Brand Names Mebaral®

Canadian Brand Names Mebaral®

Pharmacologic Category Barbiturate

Synonyms Methylphenobarbital

Use Sedative; treatment of grand mal and petit mal epilepsy

Local Anesthetic/Vasoconstrictor Precautions No information available to require special precautions

Effects on Dental Treatment >10%: Dizziness, lightheadedness, drowsiness, "hangover" effect

Restrictions C-IV

Dosage Oral:

Epilepsy:

Children: 6-12 mg/kg/day in 2-4 divided doses

Adults: 200-600 mg/day in 2-4 divided doses

Sedation:

Children:

<5 years: 16-32 mg 3-4 times/day

>5 years: 32-64 mg 3-4 times/day

Adults: 32-100 mg 3-4 times/day

Dosing adjustment in renal or hepatic impairment: Use with caution and reduce dosages

Mechanism of Action Increases seizure threshold in the motor cortex; depresses monosynaptic and polysynaptic transmission in the CNS

Other Adverse Effects 1% to 10%:

Central nervous system: **Confusion**, mental depression, unusual excitement, **nervousness, faint feeling, headache**, insomnia, nightmares

Gastrointestinal: Constipation, nausea, **vomiting**

Drug Interactions Substrate of CYP2B6, 2C8/9, **2C19**; Inhibits CYP2C19; Induces CYP2A6

Increased Effect/Toxicity: When combined with other CNS depressants, ethanol, narcotic analgesics, antidepressants, or benzodiazepines, additive respiratory and CNS depression may occur. Barbiturates may enhance the hepatotoxic potential of acetaminophen overdoses. Chloramphenicol, MAO inhibitors, valproic acid, and felbamate may inhibit barbiturate metabolism. Barbiturates may impair the absorption of griseofulvin, and may enhance the nephrotoxic effects of methoxyflurane. Concurrent use of phenobarbital with meperidine may result in increased CNS depression.

Decreased Effect: Barbiturates are hepatic enzyme inducers, and may increase the metabolism of antipsychotics, some beta-blockers (unlikely with atenolol and nadolol), calcium channel blockers, chloramphenicol, cimetidine, corticosteroids, cyclosporine, disopyramide, doxycycline, ethosuximide, felbamate, furosemide, griseofulvin, lamotrigine, phenytoin, propafenone, quinidine, tacrolimus, TCAs, and theophylline. Barbiturates may increase the metabolism of estrogens and reduce the efficacy of oral contraceptives; an alternative method of contraception should be considered. Barbiturates inhibit the hypoprothrombinemic effects of oral anticoagulants via increased metabolism. Barbiturates may enhance the metabolism of methadone resulting in methadone withdrawal.

Dietary/Ethanol/Herb Considerations Ethanol: Avoid use; increases effect/toxicity.

Pharmacodynamics/Kinetics

Onset of action: 20-60 minutes

Duration: 6-8 hours

Absorption: ~50%

Half-life elimination, serum: 34 hours

Pregnancy Risk Factor D

Generic Available No

Mephyton® *see* Phytonadione *on page 1079*

Mepivacaine (me PIV a kane)

U.S. Brand Names Carbocaine® [DSC]; Polocaine®; Polocaine® MPF

Canadian Brand Names Carbocaine®; Polocaine®

Pharmacologic Category Local Anesthetic

Synonyms Mepivacaine Hydrochloride

Use

Dental: Local anesthesia by nerve block, infiltration in dental procedures

Medical: Local anesthesia by nerve block; **not** for use in spinal anesthesia

Local Anesthetic/Vasoconstrictor Precautions No information available to require special precautions

Effects on Dental Treatment Degree of adverse effects in the CNS and cardiovascular system is directly related to blood levels of mepivacaine (frequency not defined; more likely to occur after systemic administration rather than infiltration): Bradycardia, cardiovascular collapse, hypotension, myocardial depression, ventricular arrhythmias, nausea, vomiting, respiratory arrest, anaphylactoid reactions, blurred vision, heart block, transient stinging or burning at injection site

High blood levels: Anxiety, restlessness, disorientation, confusion, dizziness, and seizures, followed by CNS depression resulting in somnolence, unconsciousness, and possible respiratory arrest.

In some cases, symptoms of CNS stimulation may be absent and the primary CNS effects are somnolence and unconsciousness.

Dosage Children and Adults: Injectable local anesthetic: Varies with procedure, degree of anesthesia needed, vascularity of tissue, duration of anesthesia required, and physical condition of patient

(Continued)

Mepivacaine *(Continued)*

Mechanism of Action Mepivacaine is an amino amide local anesthetic similar to lidocaine; like all local anesthetics, mepivacaine acts by preventing the generation and conduction of nerve impulses

Other Adverse Effects Frequency not defined (dependent on blood levels; more likely to occur after systemic administration rather than infiltration):

Cardiovascular: Edema, myocardial depression, angioneurotic edema

Dermatologic: Cutaneous lesions, urticaria

Otic: Tinnitus

Contraindications Hypersensitivity to mepivacaine, any component of the formulation, or other amide anesthetics; allergy to sodium bisulfate

Warnings/Precautions Use with caution in patients with cardiac disease, renal disease, and hyperthyroidism; convulsions due to systemic toxicity leading to cardiac arrest have been reported presumably due to intravascular injection

Pharmacodynamics/Kinetics

Onset of action: Epidural: 7-15 minutes

Duration: 2-2.5 hours; similar onset and duration following infiltration

Protein binding: 70% to 85%

Metabolism: Primarily hepatic via N-demethylation, hydroxylation, and glucuronidation

Half-life elimination: 1.9 hours

Excretion: Urine (95% as metabolites)

Pregnancy Risk Factor C

Dosage Forms INJ, solution (Carbocaine® [DSC]): 1% (30 mL, 50 mL); 2% (20 mL, 50 mL); (Polocaine®): 1% (50 mL); 2% (50 mL); (Polocaine® MPF): 1% (30 mL); 1.5% (30 mL); 3% (20 mL)

Generic Available No

Selected Readings Torres MJ, Garcia JJ, del Cano Moratinos AM, et al, "Fixed Drug Eruption Induced by Mepivacaine," *J Allergy Clin Immunol*, 1995, 96(1):130-1.

Mepivacaine and Levonordefrin

(me PIV a kane & lee voe nor DEF rin)

Related Information

Mepivacaine *on page 861*

Oral Pain *on page 1524*

U.S. Brand Names Carbocaine® 2% with Neo-Cobefrin®

Canadian Brand Names Polocaine® 2% and Levonordefrin 1:20,000

Pharmacologic Category Local Anesthetic, Dental; Local Anesthetic

Use Dental: Amide-type anesthetic used for local infiltration anesthesia; injection near nerve trunks to produce nerve block

Local Anesthetic/Vasoconstrictor Precautions No information available to require special precautions

Effects on Dental Treatment It is common to misinterpret psychogenic responses to local anesthetic injection as an allergic reaction. Intraoral injections are perceived by many patients as a stressful procedure in dentistry. Common symptoms to this stress are diaphoresis, palpitations, hyperventilation, generalized pallor and a fainting feeling. Patients may exhibit hypersensitivity to bisulfites contained in local anesthetic solution to prevent oxidation of levonordefrin. In general, patients reacting to bisulfites have a history of asthma and their airways are hyper-reactive to asthmatic syndrome.

Degree of adverse effects in the CNS and cardiovascular system is directly related to the blood levels of mepivacaine (frequency not defined; more likely to occur after systemic administration rather than infiltration): Bradycardia and reduction in cardiac output, nausea, vomiting, tremors, hypersensitivity reactions (extremely rare; may be manifest as dermatologic reactions and edema at injection site), asthmatic syndromes

High blood levels: Anxiety, restlessness, disorientation, confusion, dizziness, and seizures, followed by CNS depression resulting in somnolence, unconsciousness and possible respiratory arrest.

In some cases, symptoms of CNS stimulation may be absent and the primary CNS effects are somnolence and unconsciousness.

Dosage

Children <10 years: Maximum pediatric dosage must be carefully calculated on the basis of patient's weight but should not exceed 6.6 mg/kg of body weight or 180 mg of mepivacaine hydrochloride as a 2% solution with levonordefrin 1:20,000

Children >10 years and Adults:

Dental infiltration and nerve block, single site: 36 mg (1.8 mL) of mepivacaine hydrochloride as a 2% solution with levonordefrin 1:20,000

Entire oral cavity: 180 mg (9 mL) of mepivacaine hydrochloride as a 2% solution with levonordefrin 1:20,000; up to a maximum of 6.6 mg/kg of body weight but not to exceed 400 mg of mepivacaine hydrochloride per appointment. The effective anesthetic dose varies with procedure, intensity of anesthesia needed, duration of anesthesia required, and physical condition of the patient. Always use the lowest effective dose along with careful aspiration.

The following numbers of dental carpules (1.8 mL) provide the indicated amounts of mepivacaine hydrochloride 2% and levonordefrin 1:20,000 (see table).

# of Cartridges (1.8 mL)	Mepivacaine (2%) (mg)	Levonordefrin 1:20,000 (mg)
1	36	0.090
2	72	0.180
3	108	0.270
4	144	0.360
5	180	0.450
6	216	0.540
7	252	0.630
8	288	0.720
9	324	0.810
10	360	0.900

Mechanism of Action Local anesthetics bind selectively to the intracellular surface of sodium channels to block influx of sodium into the axon. As a result, depolarization necessary for action potential propagation and subsequent nerve function is prevented. The block at the sodium channel is reversible. When drug diffuses away from the axon, sodium channel function is restored and nerve propagation returns.

Levonordefrin prolongs the duration of the anesthetic actions of mepivacaine by causing vasoconstriction (alpha adrenergic receptor agonist) of the vasculature surrounding the nerve axons. This prevents the diffusion of mepivacaine away from the nerves resulting in a longer retention in the axon.

Contraindications Hypersensitivity to local anesthetics of the amide-type or any component of the formulation

Warnings/Precautions Should be avoided in patients with uncontrolled hyperthyroidism. Should be used in minimal amounts in patients with significant cardiovascular problems (because of levonordefrin component). Aspirate the syringe after tissue penetration and before injection to minimize chance of direct vascular injection.

Drug Interactions Increased Effect/Toxicity: Due to levonordefrin component, use with tricyclic antidepressants or MAO inhibitors could result in increased pressor response; use with nonselective beta-blockers (ie, propranolol) could result in serious hypertension and reflex bradycardia.

Pharmacodynamics/Kinetics

Duration: Upper jaw: 1-2.5 hours; Lower jaw: 2.5-5.5 hours

Infiltration: 50 minutes

Inferior alveolar block: 60-75 minutes

Pregnancy Risk Factor C

Breast-feeding Considerations Usual infiltration doses of mepivacaine with levonordefrin given to nursing mothers has not been shown to affect the health of the nursing infant.

Dosage Forms INJ: Mepivacaine hydrochloride 2% with levonordefrin 1:20,000 (1.8 mL) [dental cartridge]

Generic Available Yes

Selected Readings

Ayoub ST and Coleman AE, "A Review of Local Anesthetics," *Gen Dent*, 1992, 40(4):285-7, 289-90.

Jastak JT and Yagiela JA, "Vasoconstrictors and Local Anesthesia: A Review and Rationale for Use," *J Am Dent Assoc*, 1983, 107(4):623-30.

MacKenzie TA and Young ER, "Local Anesthetic Update," *Anesth Prog*, 1993, 40(2):29-34.

Wynn RL, "Epinephrine Interactions With Beta-Blockers," *Gen Dent*, 1994, 42(1):16, 18.

Wynn RL, "Recent Research on Mechanisms of Local Anesthetics," *Gen Dent*, 1995, 43(4):316-8.

Yagiela JA, "Local Anesthetics," *Anesth Prog*, 1991, 38(4-5):128-41.

Mepivacaine Dental Anesthetic

(me PIV a kane DEN tol an es THET ik)

Related Information

Mepivacaine *on page 861*

Oral Pain *on page 1524*

U.S. Brand Names Carbocaine® 3%

Canadian Brand Names Polocaine®

Pharmacologic Category Local Anesthetic, Dental; Local Anesthetic

Use Dental: Amide-type anesthetic used for local infiltration anesthesia; injection near nerve trunks to produce nerve block

Local Anesthetic/Vasoconstrictor Precautions No information available to require special precautions

Effects on Dental Treatment It is common to misinterpret psychogenic responses to local anesthetic injection as an allergic reaction. Intraoral injections are perceived by many patients as a stressful procedure in dentistry. Common symptoms to this

(Continued)

Mepivacaine Dental Anesthetic *(Continued)*

stress are diaphoresis, palpitations, hyperventilation, generalized pallor and a fainting feeling.

Degree of adverse effects in the CNS and cardiovascular system is directly related to the blood levels of mepivacaine.

Frequency not defined: Bradycardia and reduction in cardiac output, nausea, vomiting, tremors, asthmatic syndromes, hypersensitivity reactions (may manifest as dermatologic reactions and edema at injection site)

High blood levels: Anxiety, restlessness, disorientation, confusion, dizziness, tremors and seizures, followed by CNS depression resulting in somnolence, unconsciousness and possible respiratory arrest. In some cases, symptoms of CNS stimulation may be absent and the primary CNS effects are somnolence and unconsciousness.

Dosage

Children <10 years: Up to 5-6 mg/kg of body weight; maximum pediatric dosage must be carefully calculated on the basis of patient's weight but must not exceed 270 mg (9 mL) of the 3% solution

Children >10 years and Adults:

Dental anesthesia, single site in upper or lower jaw: 54 mg (1.8 mL) as a 3% solution

Infiltration and nerve block of entire oral cavity: 270 mg (9 mL) as a 3% solution; up to a maximum of 6.6 mg/kg of body weight but not to exceed 300 mg per appointment. Manufacturer's maximum recommended dose is not more than 400 mg to normal healthy adults. The effective anesthetic dose varies with procedure, intensity of anesthesia needed, duration of anesthesia required, and physical condition of the patient. Always use the lowest effective dose along with careful aspiration.

The following number of dental carpules (1.8 mL) provide the indicated amounts of mepivacaine dental anesthetic 3% (see table):

# of Cartridges (1.8 mL)	Mepivacaine (3%) (mg)
1	54
2	108
3	162
4	216
5	270
6	324
7	378
8	432

Mechanism of Action Local anesthetics bind selectively to the intracellular surface of sodium channels to block influx of sodium into the axon. As a result, depolarization necessary for action potential propagation and subsequent nerve function is prevented. The block at the sodium channel is reversible. When drug diffuses away from the axon, sodium channel function is restored and nerve propagation returns.

Other Adverse Effects related to the blood levels of mepivacaine. Hypersensitivity reactions may manifest as dermatologic reactions and edema at injection site.

Contraindications Hypersensitivity to local anesthetics of the amide type or any component of the formulation

Warnings/Precautions Aspirate the syringe after tissue penetration and before injection to minimize chance of direct vascular injection

Pharmacodynamics/Kinetics

Onset of action: Upper jaw: 30-120 seconds; Lower jaw: 1-4 minutes

Duration: Upper jaw: 20 minutes; Lower jaw: 40 minutes

Half-life elimination, serum: 1.9 hours

Pregnancy Risk Factor C

Breast-feeding Considerations Usual infiltration doses of mepivacaine dental anesthetic given to nursing mothers has not been shown to affect the health of the nursing infant.

Dosage Forms INJ: Mepivacaine hydrochloride 3% (1.8 mL) [dental cartridge]

Generic Available Yes

Selected Readings

Ayoub ST and Coleman AE, "A Review of Local Anesthetics," *Gen Dent*, 1992, 40(4):285-7, 289-90.

Wynn RL, "Recent Research on Mechanisms of Local Anesthetics," *Gen Dent*, 1995, 43(4):316-8.

Mepivacaine Hydrochloride *see* Mepivacaine *on page 861*

Meprobamate (me proe BA mate)

U.S. Brand Names Miltown®

Canadian Brand Names Novo-Mepro

Pharmacologic Category Antianxiety Agent, Miscellaneous

Use

Dental: Treatment of muscle spasm associated with acute temporomandibular joint pain; management of dental anxiety disorders

Medical: Management of anxiety disorders

Unlabeled/Investigational Use Treatment of muscle contraction/rigidity, headache, premenstrual tension, external sphincter spasticity, opisthotonos-associated with tetanus

Local Anesthetic/Vasoconstrictor Precautions No information available to require special precautions

Effects on Dental Treatment Frequency not defined: Syncope, palpitations, tachycardia, arrhythmia, drowsiness, dizziness, paradoxical excitement, confusion, slurred speech, headache, euphoria, paresthesia, overstimulation, vomiting, nausea, stomatitis, weakness, blurred vision, wheezing, dyspnea, bronchospasm, renal failure, ecchymosis

Restrictions C-IV

Dosage Guidelines from the CMS (Centers for Medicare and Medicaid Services), formerly known as HCFA, discourage use in residents of long-term care facilities.

Oral:

Children 6-12 years: Anxiety: 100-200 mg 2-3 times/day

Adults: Anxiety: 400 mg 3-4 times/day, up to 2400 mg/day

Dosing interval in renal impairment:

Cl_{cr} 10-50 mL/minute: Administer every 9-12 hours

Cl_{cr} <10 mL/minute: Administer every 12-18 hours

Hemodialysis: Moderately dialyzable (20% to 50%)

Dosing adjustment in hepatic impairment: Probably necessary in patients with liver disease

Mechanism of Action Affects the thalamus and limbic system; also appears to inhibit multineuronal spinal reflexes

Other Adverse Effects Frequency not defined:

Cardiovascular: Peripheral edema

Central nervous system: Ataxia, chills, vertigo

Dermatologic: Rashes, purpura, dermatitis, Stevens-Johnson syndrome, petechiae

Gastrointestinal: Diarrhea

Hematologic: Leukopenia, eosinophilia, agranulocytosis, aplastic anemia

Contraindications Hypersensitivity to meprobamate, related compounds (including carisoprodol), or any component of the formulation; acute intermittent porphyria; pre-existing CNS depression; narrow-angle glaucoma; severe uncontrolled pain; pregnancy

Warnings/Precautions Physical and psychological dependence and abuse may occur; abrupt cessation may precipitate withdrawal. Use with caution in patients with depression or suicidal tendencies, or in patients with a history of drug abuse. May cause CNS depression, which may impair physical or mental abilities. Patients must be cautioned about performing tasks which require mental alertness (ie, operating machinery or driving). Effects with other sedative drugs or ethanol may be potentiated. Not recommended in children <6 years of age; allergic reaction may occur in patients with history of dermatological condition (usually by fourth dose). Use with caution in patients with renal or hepatic impairment, or with a history of seizures. Use caution in the elderly as it may cause confusion, cognitive impairment, or excessive sedation.

Drug Interactions CNS depressants: Sedative effects may be additive with other CNS depressants; monitor for increased effect; includes barbiturates, benzodiazepines, narcotic analgesics, ethanol, and other sedative agents

Dietary/Ethanol/Herb Considerations

Ethanol: Avoid use; may increase CNS depression.

Herb/Nutraceutical: Avoid gotu kola, kava, SAMe, St John's wort, and valerian; may increase CNS depression.

Pharmacodynamics/Kinetics

Onset of action: Sedation: ~1 hour

Distribution: Crosses placenta; enters breast milk

Metabolism: Hepatic

Half-life elimination: 10 hours

Excretion: Urine (8% to 20% as unchanged drug); feces (10% as metabolites)

Pregnancy Risk Factor D

Breast-feeding Considerations Breast milk concentrations are higher than plasma; effects are unknown.

Dosage Forms TAB: 200 mg, 400 mg

Generic Available Yes

Meprobamate and Aspirin *see* Aspirin and Meprobamate *on page 136*

Mepron® *see* Atovaquone *on page 142*

Mequinol and Tretinoin (ME kwi nol & TRET i noyn)

U.S. Brand Names Solagé™

Canadian Brand Names Solagé™

(Continued)

Mequinol and Tretinoin *(Continued)*

Pharmacologic Category Retinoic Acid Derivative; Vitamin A Derivative; Vitamin, Topical

Use Treatment of solar lentigines; the efficacy of using Solagé™ daily for >24 weeks has not been established. The local cutaneous safety of Solagé™ in non-Caucasians has not been adequately established.

Local Anesthetic/Vasoconstrictor Precautions No information available to require special precautions

Effects on Dental Treatment No significant effects or complications reported

Dosage Solar lentigines: Topical: Apply twice daily to solar lentigines using the applicator tip while avoiding application to the surrounding skin. Separate application by at least 8 hours or as directed by physician.

Mechanism of Action Solar lentigines are localized, pigmented, macular lesions of the skin on areas of the body chronically exposed to the sun. Mequinol is a substrate for the enzyme tyrosinase and acts as a competitive inhibitor of the formation of melanin precursors. The mechanisms of depigmentation for both drugs is unknown.

Other Adverse Effects Dermatologic:

>10%: Erythema (49%), burning, stinging or tingling (26%), desquamation (14%), pruritus (12%),

1% to 10%: Skin irritation (5%), hypopigmentation (5%), halo hypopigmentation (7%), rash (3%), dry skin (3%), crusting (3%), vesicular bullae rash (2%), contact allergic reaction (1%)

Drug Interactions Tretinoin: Substrate of CYP2A6, 2B6, 2C8/9; Inhibits CYP2C8/9; Induces CYP2E1

Increased Effect/Toxicity: Avoid concurrent use of the following: Topical products with skin drying effects (eg, those containing alcohol, astringents, spices, or lime; medicated soaps or shampoos; permanent wave solutions; hair depilatories or waxes; and others); may increase skin irritation. Photosensitizing drugs (eg, thiazides, tetracyclines, fluoroquinolones, phenothiazines, sulfonamides) can further increase sun sensitivity.

Pharmacodynamics/Kinetics

Absorption: Percutaneous absorption was 4.4% of tretinoin when applied as 0.8 mL of Solagé™ to a 400 cm^2 area of the back

Time to peak: Mequinol: 2 hours

Pregnancy Risk Factor X

Generic Available No

Merbromin (mer BROE min)

U.S. Brand Names Mercurochrome®

Pharmacologic Category Topical Skin Product

Use Topical antiseptic

Local Anesthetic/Vasoconstrictor Precautions No information available to require special precautions

Effects on Dental Treatment No significant effects or complications reported

Dosage Apply freely, until injury has healed

Generic Available Yes

Mercaptopurine (mer kap toe PYOOR een)

U.S. Brand Names Purinethol®

Canadian Brand Names Purinethol®

Mexican Brand Names Purinethol®

Pharmacologic Category Antineoplastic Agent, Antimetabolite

Synonyms 6-Mercaptopurine; 6-MP

Use Maintenance therapy in acute lymphoblastic leukemia (ALL); other (less common) uses include chronic granulocytic leukemia, induction therapy in ALL, and treatment of non-Hodgkin's lymphomas

Local Anesthetic/Vasoconstrictor Precautions No information available to require special precautions

Effects on Dental Treatment 1% to 10%: Drug fever, nausea, vomiting, stomatitis, mucositis

Restrictions I.V. formulation is not commercially available in the U.S.

Dosage Oral (refer to individual protocols):

Children: Maintenance: 75 mg/m^2/day given once daily

Adults:

Induction: 2.5-5 mg/kg/day (100-200 mg)

Maintenance: 1.5-2.5 mg/kg/day **OR** 80-100 mg/m^2/day given once daily

Elderly: Due to renal decline with age, start with lower recommended doses for adults

Dosing adjustment in renal or hepatic impairment: Reduction required to avoid accumulation, specific guidelines unavailable.

Hemodialysis: Removed; supplemental dosing usually required

Mechanism of Action Purine antagonist which inhibits DNA and RNA synthesis; acts as false metabolite and is incorporated into DNA and RNA, eventually inhibiting their synthesis. 6-MP is substituted for hypoxanthine; must be metabolized to active nucleotides once inside the cell.

Other Adverse Effects

>10%:

Hematologic: Myelosuppression; leukopenia, thrombocytopenia, anemia
Onset: 7-10 days
Nadir: 14-16 days
Recovery: 21-28 days

Hepatic: Intrahepatic cholestasis and focal centralobular necrosis (40%), characterized by hyperbilirubinemia, increased alkaline phosphatase and AST, jaundice, ascites, encephalopathy; more common at doses >2.5 mg/kg/day. Usually occurs within 2 months of therapy but may occur within 1 week, or be delayed up to 8 years.

1% to 10%:

Dermatologic: Hyperpigmentation, rash
Endocrine & metabolic: Hyperuricemia
Gastrointestinal: Diarrhea, anorexia, stomach pain
Renal: Renal toxicity

<1%: Dry and scaling rash, **glossitis**, tarry stools, eosinophilia

Drug Interactions

Increased Effect/Toxicity: Allopurinol can cause increased levels of 6-MP by inhibition of xanthine oxidase. Decrease dose of 6-MP by 75% when both drugs are used concomitantly (seen only with oral 6-MP usage, not with I.V.); may potentiate effect of bone marrow suppression (reduce 6-MP to 25% of dose). Any agent which could potentially alter the metabolic function of the liver could produce higher drug levels and greater toxicities from either 6-MP or thioguanine (6-TG); doxorubicin produced synergistic liver toxicity with 6-MP in >50% of patients, which resolved with discontinuation of the 6-MP. Aminosalicylates (olsalazine, mesalamine, sulfasalazine) may inhibit TPMT, increasing toxicity/myelosuppression of mercaptopurine.

Decreased Effect: 6-MP inhibits the anticoagulation effect of warfarin by an unknown mechanism.

Pharmacodynamics/Kinetics

Absorption: Variable and incomplete (16% to 50%)
Distribution: V_d = total body water; CNS penetration is poor
Protein binding: 30%
Metabolism: Hepatic and in GI mucosa; hepatically via xanthine oxidase and methylation to sulfate conjugates, 6-thiouric acid, and other inactive compounds; first-pass effect
Half-life elimination (age dependent): Children: 21 minutes; Adults: 47 minutes
Time to peak, serum: ~2 hours
Excretion: Urine; following high (1 g/m^2) I.V. doses, 20% to 40% excreted unchanged; at lower doses renal elimination minor

Pregnancy Risk Factor D

Generic Available No

6-Mercaptopurine *see* Mercaptopurine *on page 866*
Mercapturic Acid *see* Acetylcysteine *on page 40*

Mercuric Oxide (mer KYOOR ik OKS ide)

Pharmacologic Category Antibiotic, Ophthalmic

Synonyms Yellow Mercuric Oxide

Use Treatment of irritation and minor infections of the eyelids

Local Anesthetic/Vasoconstrictor Precautions No information available to require special precautions

Effects on Dental Treatment No significant effects or complications reported

Dosage Apply small amount to inner surface of lower eyelid once or twice daily

Generic Available Yes

Mercurochrome® *see* Merbromin *on page 866*
Meridia® *see* Sibutramine *on page 1219*

Meropenem (mer oh PEN em)

U.S. Brand Names Merrem® I.V.

Canadian Brand Names Merrem®

Mexican Brand Names Merrem®

Pharmacologic Category Antibiotic, Carbapenem

Use Intra-abdominal infections (complicated appendicitis and peritonitis) caused by viridans group streptococci, *E. coli, K. pneumoniae, P. aeruginosa, B. fragilis, B. thetaiotaomicron*, and *Peptostreptococcus* sp; also indicated for bacterial meningitis in pediatric patients >3 months of age caused by *S. pneumoniae, H. influenzae*, and *N. meningitidis*; meropenem has also been used to treat soft tissue infections, febrile neutropenia, and urinary tract infections

(Continued)

Meropenem *(Continued)*

Local Anesthetic/Vasoconstrictor Precautions No information available to require special precautions

Effects on Dental Treatment 1% to 10%: Oral moniliasis (≤2%; pediatric patients), glossitis, headache (2%), vomiting (1% to 4%), apnea (1%), nausea (1% to 4%), sepsis (2%), septic shock (1%)

Dosage I.V.:

Neonates:

Preterm: 20 mg/kg/dose every 12 hours (may be increased to 40 mg/kg/dose if treating a highly resistant organism such as *Pseudomonas aeruginosa*)

Full-term (<3 months of age): 20 mg/kg/dose every 8 hours (may be increased to 40 mg/kg/dose if treating a highly resistant organism such as *Pseudomonas aeruginosa*)

Children >3 months (<50 kg):

Intra-abdominal infections: 20 mg/kg every 8 hours (maximum dose: 1 g every 8 hours)

Meningitis: 40 mg/kg every 8 hours (maximum dose: 2 g every 8 hours)

Children >50 kg:

Intra-abdominal infections: 1 g every 8 hours

Meningitis: 2 g every 8 hours

Adults: 1 g every 8 hours

Elderly: No differences in safety or efficacy have been reported. However, increased sensitivity may occur in some elderly patients; adjust dose based on renal function

Dosing adjustment in renal impairment: Adults:

Cl_{cr} 26-50 mL/minute: Administer 1 g every 12 hours

Cl_{cr} 10-25 mL/minute: Administer 500 mg every 12 hours

Cl_{cr} <10 mL/minute: Administer 500 mg every 24 hours

Dialysis: Meropenem and its metabolites are readily dialyzable

Continuous arteriovenous or venovenous hemodiafiltration effects: Dose as Cl_{cr} 10-50 mL/minute

Mechanism of Action Inhibits bacterial cell wall synthesis by binding to several of the penicillin-binding proteins, which in turn inhibit the final transpeptidation step of peptidoglycan synthesis in bacterial cell walls, thus inhibiting cell wall biosynthesis; bacteria eventually lyse due to ongoing activity of cell wall autolytic enzymes (autolysins and murein hydrolases) while cell wall assembly is arrested

Other Adverse Effects

1% to 10%:

Dermatologic: Rash (2% to 3%; includes diaper-area moniliasis in pediatrics), pruritus (1%)

Gastrointestinal: Diarrhea (4% to 5%), constipation (1%)

Local: Inflammation at the injection site (2%), phlebitis/thrombophlebitis (1%), injection site reaction (1%)

<1%: Abdominal enlargement, abdominal pain, agitation/delirium, anemia, anorexia, **anxiety, arrhythmias, asthma**, back pain, **chest pain**, chills, cholestatic jaundice/jaundice, **confusion, cough**, decreased platelets, decreased PT, depression, **diaphoresis, dizziness, dyspnea**, dyspepsia, dysuria, edema, eosinophilia, **epistaxis (0.2%), fever**, flatulence, **GI hemorrhage (0.5%), hallucinations, heart failure**, hemoperitoneum (0.2%), hepatic failure, **hypertension**, hypokalemia, **hypotension** ileus, increased BUN, increased creatinine, insomnia, intestinal obstruction, leukocytosis, melena (0.3%), **MI nervousness, paresthesia**, pelvic pain, pleural effusion, pulmonary edema, renal failure, **seizures**, skin ulcer, **somnolence, tachycardia**, thrombocytosis, urinary incontinence, urticaria, vaginal moniliasis, **weakness, whole body pain**

Postmarketing and/or case reports: Agranulocytosis, angioedema, erythema multiforme, leukopenia, neutropenia, Stevens-Johnson syndrome, toxic epidermal necrolysis

Drug Interactions

Increased Effect/Toxicity: Probenecid interferes with renal excretion of meropenem.

Decreased Effect: Serum concentrations of valproic acid may be reduced during meropenem therapy (potentially to subtherapeutic levels).

Dietary/Ethanol/Herb Considerations 1 g of meropenem contains 90.2 mg of sodium as sodium carbonate (3.92 mEq)

Pharmacodynamics/Kinetics

Distribution: V_d: Adults: ~0.3 L/kg, Children: 0.4-0.5 L/kg; penetrates well into most body fluids and tissues; CSF concentrations approximate those of the plasma

Protein binding: 2%

Metabolism: Hepatic; metabolized to open beta-lactam form (inactive)

Half-life elimination:

Normal renal function: 1-1.5 hours

Cl_{cr} 30-80 mL/minute: 1.9-3.3 hours

Cl_{cr} 2-30 mL/minute: 3.82-5.7 hours

Time to peak, tissue: 1 hour following infusion

Excretion: Urine (~25% as inactive metabolites)

Pregnancy Risk Factor B

Generic Available No

Selected Readings Wiseman LR, Wagstaff AJ, Brogden RN, et al, "Meropenem. A Review of Its Antibacterial Activity, Pharmacokinetic Properties, and Clinical Efficacy," *Drugs*, 1995, 50(1):73-101.

Merrem® I.V. *see* Meropenem *on page 867*

Mersol® [OTC] *see* Thimerosal *on page 1296*

Merthiolate® [OTC] *see* Thimerosal *on page 1296*

Meruvax® II *see* Rubella Virus Vaccine (Live) *on page 1202*

Mesalamine (me SAL a meen)

U.S. Brand Names Asacol®; Canasa™; Pentasa®; Rowasa®

Canadian Brand Names Asacol®; Mesasal®; Novo-5 ASA; Pentasa®; Quintasa®; Rowasa®; Salofalk®

Mexican Brand Names Salofalk®

Pharmacologic Category 5-Aminosalicylic Acid Derivative

Synonyms 5-Aminosalicylic Acid; 5-ASA; Fisalamine; Mesalazine

Use

Oral: Treatment and maintenance of remission of mildly to moderately active ulcerative colitis

Rectal: Treatment of active mild to moderate distal ulcerative colitis, proctosigmoiditis, or proctitis

Local Anesthetic/Vasoconstrictor Precautions No information available to require special precautions

Effects on Dental Treatment

>10%: Pharyngitis (11%)

1% to 10%: Chest pain (3%), dizziness (suppository: 3%), fever (enema: 3%; suppository: 1%), vomiting (5%), flu-like syndrome (3%; enema: 5%), diaphoresis (3%), cough (2%)

Dosage

Adults (usual course of therapy is 3-8 weeks):

Oral:

Treatment of ulcerative colitis:

Capsule: 1 g 4 times/day

Tablet: Initial: 800 mg (2 tablets) 3 times/day for 6 weeks

Maintenance of remission of ulcerative colitis:

Capsule: 1 g 4 times/day

Tablet: 1.6 g/day in divided doses

Rectal:

Retention enema: 60 mL (4 g) at bedtime, retained overnight, approximately 8 hours

Rectal suppository: Insert 1 suppository in rectum twice daily; retain suppositories for at least 1-3 hours to achieve maximum benefit

Canasa™: May increase to 3 times/day if inadequate response is seen after 2 weeks.

Note: Some patients may require rectal and oral therapy concurrently.

Elderly: See adult dosing; use with caution

Mechanism of Action Mesalamine (5-aminosalicylic acid) is the active component of sulfasalazine; the specific mechanism of action of mesalamine is unknown; however, it is thought that it modulates local chemical mediators of the inflammatory response, especially leukotrienes; action appears topical rather than systemic

Other Adverse Effects Effects vary depending upon dosage form (as reported with tablets, unless otherwise noted):

>10%:

Central nervous system: Pain (14%)

Gastrointestinal: Abdominal pain (18%; enema: 8%)

Genitourinary: Eructation (16%)

1% to 10%:

Cardiovascular: Peripheral edema (3%)

Central nervous system: Chills (3%), insomnia (2%), malaise (2%)

Dermatologic: Rash (6%; suppository: 1%), pruritus (3%; enema: 1%), acne (2%; suppository: 1%)

Gastrointestinal: Dyspepsia (6%), constipation (5%), colitis exacerbation (3%; suppository: 1%), nausea (capsule: 3%), flatulence (enema: 6%), hemorrhoids (enema: 1%), nausea and vomiting (capsule: 1%), rectal pain (enema: 1%; suppository: 2%)

Local: Pain on insertion of enema tip (enema: 1%)

Neuromuscular & skeletal: Back pain (7%; enema: 1%), arthralgia (5%), hypertonia (5%), myalgia (3%), arthritis (2%), leg/joint pain (enema: 2%),

Ocular: Conjunctivitis (2%)

<1%: Alopecia

Postmarketing and/or case reports: Agranulocytosis, alkaline phosphatase elevated, ALT elevated, anemia, anorexia, aplastic anemia, appetite increased, AST elevated, **asthma exacerbation**, bilirubin elevated, bloody diarrhea, blurred

(Continued)

Mesalamine *(Continued)*

vision, BUN elevated, **chest pain**, cholestatic jaundice, cholecystitis, confusion, depression, dry skin, dysuria, edema, emotional lability, eosinophilia, eosinophilic pneumonia, epididymitis, erythema nodosum, eye pain, **facial edema**, fibrosing alveolitis, gastritis, GGT elevated, gout, Guillain-Barré syndrome, hematuria, hepatitis, hepatocellular damage, hepatotoxicity, hyperesthesia, hypersensitivity pneumonitis, interstitial nephritis, interstitial pneumonia, jaundice, Kawasaki-like syndrome, LDH elevated, leukopenia, liver failure, liver necrosis, lupus-like syndrome, lymphadenopathy, menorrhagia, minimal change nephrotic syndrome, nephropathy, myocarditis, **neck pain, oral ulcers**, pancreatitis, pancytopenia, **perforated peptic ulcer**, pericarditis, peripheral neuropathy, pleuritis, psoriasis, pyoderma gangrenosum, serum creatinine elevated, **somnolence, abnormal taste**, thrombocytopenia, transverse myelitis, tinnitus, tremor, T-wave abnormalities, urinary urgency, urticaria, vertigo, **xerostomia**

Drug Interactions

Increased Effect/Toxicity: May increase risk of myelosuppression from azathioprine, mercaptopurine, and thioguanine.

Decreased digoxin bioavailability.

Dietary/Ethanol/Herb Considerations Food may decrease serum concentration with oral form. Boiled milk, buttermilk, or yogurt may reduce diarrhea.

Pharmacodynamics/Kinetics

Absorption: Rectal: Variable and dependent upon retention time, underlying GI disease, and colonic pH; Oral: Tablet: ~28%, Capsule: ~20% to 30%

Metabolism: Hepatic and via GI tract to acetyl-5-aminosalicylic acid

Half-life elimination: 5-ASA: 0.5-1.5 hours; acetyl-5-ASA: 5-10 hours

Time to peak, serum: 4-7 hours

Excretion: Urine (as metabolites); feces (<2%)

Pregnancy Risk Factor B

Generic Available No

Mesalazine *see* Mesalamine *on page 869*

Mesoridazine (mez oh RID a zeen)

U.S. Brand Names Serentil®

Canadian Brand Names Serentil®

Pharmacologic Category Antipsychotic Agent, Phenothiazine, Piperidine

Synonyms Mesoridazine Besylate

Use Management of schizophrenic patients who fail to respond adequately to treatment with other antipsychotic drugs, either because of insufficient effectiveness or the inability to achieve an effective dose due to intolerable adverse effects from these drugs

Unlabeled/Investigational Use Treatment of psychosis

Local Anesthetic/Vasoconstrictor Precautions No information available to require special precautions

Effects on Dental Treatment Frequency not defined: Hypotension, orthostatic hypotension, tachycardia, syncope, pseudoparkinsonism, akathisia, dystonias, tardive dyskinesia, dizziness, drowsiness, restlessness, slurred speech, impairment of temperature regulation, lowering of seizure threshold, nausea, vomiting, xerostomia, weakness, tremor, rigidity, nasal congestion

Dosage Concentrate may be diluted just prior to administration with distilled water, acidified tap water, orange or grape juice; do not prepare and store bulk dilutions

Adults: Schizophrenia/psychoses:

Oral: 25-50 mg 3 times/day; maximum: 100-400 mg/day

I.M.: Initial: 25 mg, repeat in 30-60 minutes as needed; optimal dosage range: 25-200 mg/day

Elderly: Behavioral symptoms associated with dementia:

Oral: Initial: 10 mg 1-2 times/day; if <10 mg/day is desired, consider administering 10 mg every other day (qod). Increase dose at 4- to 7-day intervals by 10-25 mg/day; increase dose intervals (bid, tid, etc) as necessary to control response or side effects. Maximum daily dose: 250 mg. Gradual increases (titration) may prevent some side effects or decrease their severity.

I.M.: Initial: 25 mg; repeat doses in 30-60 minutes if necessary. Dose range: 25-200 mg/day. Elderly usually require less than maximal daily dose.

Hemodialysis: Not dialyzable (0% to 5%)

Mechanism of Action Blockade of postsynaptic CNS dopamine$_2$ receptors in the mesolimbic and mesocortical areas

Other Adverse Effects Frequency not defined:

Cardiovascular: QT prolongation (dose dependent, up to 100% of patients at higher dosages), edema

Central nervous system: Ataxia, neuroleptic malignant syndrome (NMS)

Dermatologic: Increased sensitivity to sun, rash, itching, angioneurotic edema, dermatitis, discoloration of skin (blue-gray)

Endocrine & metabolic: Changes in menstrual cycle, changes in libido, gynecomastia, lactation, galactorrhea

Gastrointestinal: Constipation, stomach pain, weight gain

Genitourinary: Difficulty in urination, ejaculatory disturbances, impotence, enuresis, incontinence, priapism, urinary retention

Hematologic: Agranulocytosis, leukopenia, eosinophilia, thrombocytopenia, anemia, aplastic anemia

Hepatic: Cholestatic jaundice, hepatotoxicity

Ocular: Pigmentary retinopathy, photophobia, blurred vision, cornea and lens changes

Miscellaneous: Diaphoresis (decreased), lupus-like syndrome

Drug Interactions CYP1A2, 2D6, and 3A3/4 enzyme substrate; CYP2D6 enzyme inhibitor

Increased Effect/Toxicity: Use of mesoridazine with other agents known to prolong QT_c may increase the risk of malignant arrhythmias; concurrent use is contraindicated - includes type I and type III antiarrhythmics, TCAs, and some quinolone antibiotics (sparfloxacin, moxifloxacin, gatifloxacin). Mesoridazine may increase the effect and/or toxicity of antihypertensives, anticholinergics, lithium, CNS depressants (ethanol, narcotics), and trazodone. Metoclopramide may increase risk of extrapyramidal symptoms (EPS).

Decreased Effect: Mesoridazine may inhibit the activity of bromocriptine and levodopa. Benztropine (and other anticholinergics) may inhibit the therapeutic response to mesoridazine and excess anticholinergic effects may occur. Mesoridazine and possibly other low potency antipsychotic may reverse the pressor effects of epinephrine.

Dietary/Ethanol/Herb Considerations

Ethanol: Avoid use; may increase CNS depression.

Herb/Nutraceutical: Avoid gotu kola, kava, SAMe, St John's wort, and valerian; may increase CNS depression.

Pharmacodynamics/Kinetics

Duration: 4-6 hours

Absorption: Tablet: Erratic; Liquid: More dependable

Protein binding: 91% to 99%

Half-life elimination: 24-48 hours

Time to peak, serum: 2-4 hours; Steady-state serum: 4-7 days

Excretion: Urine

Pregnancy Risk Factor C

Generic Available No

Mesoridazine Besylate *see* Mesoridazine *on page 870*

Mestranol and Norethindrone (MES tra nole & nor eth IN drone)

Related Information

Endocrine Disorders and Pregnancy *on page 1479*

Norethindrone *on page 986*

U.S. Brand Names Necon® 1/50; Norinyl® 1+50; Ortho-Novum® 1/50

Canadian Brand Names Ortho-Novum® 1/50

Pharmacologic Category Contraceptive; Estrogen and Progestin Combination

Synonyms Norethindrone and Mestranol

Use Prevention of pregnancy

Unlabeled/Investigational Use Treatment of hypermenorrhea, endometriosis, female hypogonadism

Local Anesthetic/Vasoconstrictor Precautions No information available to require special precautions

Effects on Dental Treatment When prescribing antibiotics, patients must be advised to use additional methods of birth control when taking hormonal contraceptives.

Dosage Oral: Adults: Female: Contraception:

Schedule 1 (Sunday starter): Dose begins on first Sunday after onset of menstruation; if the menstrual period starts on Sunday, take first tablet that very same day. **With a Sunday start, an additional method of contraception should be used until after the first 7 days of consecutive administration.**

For 21-tablet package: Dosage is 1 tablet daily for 21 consecutive days, followed by 7 days off of the medication; a new course begins on the 8th day after the last tablet is taken.

For 28-tablet package: Dosage is 1 tablet daily without interruption.

Schedule 2 (Day 1 starter): Dose starts on first day of menstrual cycle taking 1 tablet daily.

For 21-tablet package: Dosage is 1 tablet daily for 21 consecutive days, followed by 7 days off of the medication; a new course begins on the 8th day after the last tablet is taken.

For 28-tablet package: Dosage is 1 tablet daily without interruption.

If all doses have been taken on schedule and one menstrual period is missed, continue dosing cycle. If two consecutive menstrual periods are missed, pregnancy test is required before new dosing cycle is started.

(Continued)

Mestranol and Norethindrone *(Continued)*

Missed doses **monophasic formulations** (refer to package insert for complete information):

One dose missed: Take as soon as remembered or take 2 tablets next day

Two consecutive doses missed in the first 2 weeks: Take 2 tablets as soon as remembered or 2 tablets next 2 days. **An additional method of contraception should be used for 7 days after missed dose.**

Two consecutive doses missed in week 3 or three consecutive doses missed at any time: **An additional method of contraception must be used for 7 days after a missed dose:**

Schedule 1 (Sunday starter): Continue dose of 1 tablet daily until Sunday, then discard the rest of the pack, and a new pack should be started that same day.

Schedule 2 (Day 1 starter): Current pack should be discarded, and a new pack should be started that same day.

Dosing adjustment in renal impairment: Specific guidelines unavailable; use with caution

Dosing adjustment in hepatic impairment: Contraindicated

Mechanism of Action Combination oral contraceptives inhibit ovulation via a negative feedback mechanism on the hypothalamus, which alters the normal pattern of gonadotropin secretion of a follicle-stimulating hormone (FSH) and luteinizing hormone by the anterior pituitary. The follicular phase FSH and midcycle surge of gonadotropins are inhibited. In addition, combination hormonal contraceptives produce alterations in the genital tract, including changes in the cervical mucus, rendering it unfavorable for sperm penetration even if ovulation occurs. Changes in the endometrium may also occur, producing an unfavorable environment for nidation. Combination hormonal contraceptive drugs may alter the tubal transport of the ova through the fallopian tubes. Progestational agents may also alter sperm fertility.

Other Adverse Effects Frequency not defined:

Cardiovascular: Arterial thromboembolism, cerebral hemorrhage, cerebral thrombosis, edema, hypertension, mesenteric thrombosis, MI

Central nervous system: Depression, dizziness, headache, migraine, nervousness, premenstrual syndrome, stroke

Dermatologic: Acne, erythema multiforme, erythema nodosum, hirsutism, loss of scalp hair, melasma (may persist), rash (allergic)

Endocrine & metabolic: Amenorrhea, breakthrough bleeding, breast enlargement, breast secretion, breast tenderness, carbohydrate intolerance, lactation decreased (postpartum), glucose tolerance decreased, libido changes, menstrual flow changes, sex hormone-binding globulins (SHBG) increased, spotting, temporary infertility (following discontinuation), thyroid-binding globulin increased, triglycerides increased

Gastrointestinal: Abdominal cramps, appetite changes, bloating, cholestasis, colitis, gallbladder disease, jaundice, nausea, vomiting, weight gain/loss

Genitourinary: Cervical erosion changes, cervical secretion changes, cystitis-like syndrome, vaginal candidiasis, vaginitis

Hematologic: Antithrombin III decreased, folate levels decreased, hemolytic uremic syndrome, norepinephrine induced platelet aggregability increased, porphyria, prothrombin increased; factors VII, VIII, IX, and X increased

Hepatic: Benign liver tumors, Budd-Chiari syndrome, cholestatic jaundice, hepatic adenomas

Local: Thrombophlebitis

Ocular: Cataracts, change in corneal curvature (steepening), contact lens intolerance, optic neuritis, retinal thrombosis

Renal: Impaired renal function

Respiratory: Pulmonary thromboembolism

Miscellaneous: Hemorrhagic eruption

Drug Interactions

Increased Effect/Toxicity: Acetaminophen and ascorbic acid may increase plasma levels of estrogen component. Atorvastatin and indinavir increase plasma levels of combination hormonal contraceptives. Combination hormonal contraceptives increase the plasma levels of alprazolam, chlordiazepoxide, cyclosporine, diazepam, prednisolone, selegiline, theophylline, tricyclic antidepressants. Combination hormonal contraceptives may increase (or decrease) the effects of coumarin derivatives.

Decreased Effect: Combination hormonal contraceptives may decrease plasma levels of acetaminophen, clofibric acid, lorazepam, morphine, oxazepam, salicylic acid, temazepam. Contraceptive effect decreased by acitretin, aminoglutethimide, amprenavir, anticonvulsants, griseofulvin, lopinavir, nelfinavir, nevirapine, penicillins (effect not consistent), rifampin, ritonavir, tetracyclines (effect not consistent) troglitazone. Combination hormonal contraceptives may decrease (or increase) the effects of coumarin derivatives.

Dietary/Ethanol/Herb Considerations

Food: CNS effects of caffeine may be enhanced. Avoid grapefruit products; grapefruit juice increases ethinyl estradiol concentrations and would be expected to increase progesterone serum concentration as well (clinical implications unclear).

Herb/Nutraceutical: Avoid black cohosh, dong quai, and evening primrose due to estrogenic activity. Avoid ginseng, red clover, and saw palmetto due to potential hormonal effect. Avoid St John's wort; may decrease the effectiveness of combination hormonal contraceptives by inducing hepatic enzymes.

Pharmacodynamics/Kinetics

Mestranol: Metabolism: Hepatic via demethylation to ethinyl estradiol

Norethindrone: See Norethindrone monograph and Ethinyl Estradiol monograph for additional information.

Pregnancy Risk Factor X

Generic Available Yes

Metacortandralone *see* PrednisoLONE *on page 1110*

Metadate® CD *see* Methylphenidate *on page 893*

Metadate™ ER *see* Methylphenidate *on page 893*

Metaglip™ *see* Glipizide and Metformin *on page 639*

Metamucil® [OTC] *see* Psyllium *on page 1149*

Metamucil® Smooth Texture [OTC] *see* Psyllium *on page 1149*

Metaproterenol (met a proe TER e nol)

Related Information

Respiratory Diseases *on page 1476*

U.S. Brand Names Alupent®

Pharmacologic Category $Beta_2$ Agonist

Synonyms Metaproterenol Sulfate; Orciprenaline Sulfate

Use Bronchodilator in reversible airway obstruction due to asthma or COPD; because of its delayed onset of action (1 hour) and prolonged effect (4 or more hours), this may not be the drug of choice for assessing response to a bronchodilator

Local Anesthetic/Vasoconstrictor Precautions No information available to require special precautions

Effects on Dental Treatment No significant effects or complications reported

Dosage

Oral:

Children:

<2 years: 0.4 mg/kg/dose given 3-4 times/day; in infants, the dose can be given every 8-12 hours

2-6 years: 1-2.6 mg/kg/day divided every 6 hours

6-9 years: 10 mg/dose 3-4 times/day

Children >9 years and Adults: 20 mg 3-4 times/day

Elderly: Initial: 10 mg 3-4 times/day, increasing as necessary up to 20 mg 3-4 times/day

Inhalation: Children >12 years and Adults: 2-3 inhalations every 3-4 hours, up to 12 inhalations in 24 hours

Nebulizer:

Infants and Children: 0.01-0.02 mL/kg of 5% solution; minimum dose: 0.1 mL; maximum dose: 0.3 mL diluted in 2-3 mL normal saline every 4-6 hours (may be given more frequently according to need)

Adolescents and Adults: 5-20 breaths of full strength 5% metaproterenol **or** 0.2 to 0.3 mL 5% metaproterenol in 2.5-3 mL normal saline until nebulized every 4-6 hours (can be given more frequently according to need)

Mechanism of Action Relaxes bronchial smooth muscle by action on $beta_2$-receptors with very little effect on heart rate

Other Adverse Effects

>10%:

Cardiovascular: Tachycardia (<17%)

Central nervous system: Nervousness (3% to 14%)

Neuromuscular & skeletal: Tremor (1% to 33%)

1% to 10%:

Cardiovascular: Palpitations (<4%)

Central nervous system: Headache (<4%), dizziness (1% to 4%), insomnia (2%)

Gastrointestinal: Nausea, vomiting, bad taste, heartburn (≥4%), xerostomia

Neuromuscular & skeletal: Trembling, muscle cramps, weakness (1%)

Respiratory: Coughing, pharyngitis (≤4%)

Miscellaneous: Diaphoresis (increased) (≤4%)

<1%: Paradoxical bronchospasm, hypertension, chest pain, angina, drowsiness, diarrhea, taste change

Drug Interactions

Increased Effect/Toxicity: Sympathomimetics, TCAs, MAO inhibitors taken with metaproterenol may result in toxicity. Inhaled ipratropium may increase duration of bronchodilation. Halothane may increase risk of malignant arrhythmias; avoid concurrent use.

Decreased Effect: Decreased effect of beta-blockers.

Pharmacodynamics/Kinetics

Onset of action: Bronchodilation: Oral: ~15 minutes; Inhalation: ~60 seconds

Peak effect: Oral: ~1 hour

(Continued)

Metaproterenol *(Continued)*

Duration: ~1-5 hours

Pregnancy Risk Factor C

Generic Available Yes; Excludes inhaler

Metaproterenol Sulfate *see* Metaproterenol *on page 873*

Metaxalone (me TAKS a lone)

U.S. Brand Names Skelaxin®

Canadian Brand Names Skelaxin®

Pharmacologic Category Skeletal Muscle Relaxant

Use Relief of discomfort associated with acute, painful musculoskeletal conditions

Local Anesthetic/Vasoconstrictor Precautions No information available to require special precautions

Effects on Dental Treatment No significant effects or complications reported

Dosage Children >12 years and Adults: Oral: 800 mg 3-4 times/day

Mechanism of Action Does not have a direct effect on skeletal muscle; most of its therapeutic effect comes from actions on the central nervous system

Other Adverse Effects Frequency not defined:

Central nervous system: Paradoxical stimulation, headache, drowsiness, dizziness, irritability

Dermatologic: Allergic dermatitis

Gastrointestinal: Nausea, vomiting, stomach cramps

Hematologic: Leukopenia, hemolytic anemia

Hepatic: Hepatotoxicity

Miscellaneous: Anaphylaxis

Drug Interactions Increased Effect/Toxicity: Additive effects with ethanol or CNS depressants

Dietary/Ethanol/Herb Considerations

Ethanol: Avoid use; may increase CNS depression.

Herb/Nutraceutical: Avoid gotu kola, kava, SAMe, St John's wort, and valerian; may increase CNS depression.

Pharmacodynamics/Kinetics

Onset of action: ~1 hour

Duration: ~4-6 hours

Metabolism: Hepatic

Bioavailability: Not established; food may increase

Half-life elimination: 9 hours

Time to peak: T_{max}: 3 hours

Excretion: Urine (as metabolites)

Pregnancy Risk Factor C

Generic Available No

Metformin (met FOR min)

Related Information

Endocrine Disorders and Pregnancy *on page 1479*

Glipizide and Metformin *on page 639*

Rosiglitazone and Metformin *on page 1200*

U.S. Brand Names Glucophage®; Glucophage® XR

Canadian Brand Names Alti-Metformin; Apo®-Metformin; Gen-Metformin; Glucophage®; Glycon; Novo-Metformin; Nu-Metformin; PMS-Metformin; Rho®-Metformin; Rhoxal-metformin FC

Mexican Brand Names Dabex®; Dimefor®; Glucophage®; Glucophage® Forte

Pharmacologic Category Antidiabetic Agent, Biguanide

Synonyms Metformin Hydrochloride

Use Management of type 2 diabetes mellitus (noninsulin dependent, NIDDM) as monotherapy when hyperglycemia cannot be managed on diet alone. May be used concomitantly with a sulfonylurea or insulin to improve glycemic control.

Unlabeled/Investigational Use Treatment of HIV lipodystrophy syndrome

Local Anesthetic/Vasoconstrictor Precautions No information available to require special precautions

Effects on Dental Treatment Metformin-dependent diabetics (noninsulin dependent, type 2) should be appointed for dental treatment in morning in order to minimize chance of stress-induced hypoglycemia.

Dosage Allow 1-2 weeks between dose titrations. Generally, clinically significant responses are not seen at doses <1500 mg daily; however, a lower recommended starting dose and gradual increased dosage is recommended to minimize GI symptoms.

Children 10-16 years: Management of type 2 diabetes mellitus: Oral: 500 mg tablets: Initial: 500 mg twice daily (give with the morning and evening meals); dosage increases should be made in increments of 1 tablet every week, given in divided doses, up to a maximum of 2000 mg/day

Adults: ≥17 years: Management of type 2 diabetes mellitus: Oral:

500 mg tablets: Initial: 500 mg twice daily (give with the morning and evening meals); dosage increases should be made in increments of 1 tablet every week, given in divided doses, up to a maximum of 2500 mg/day. Doses of up to 2000 mg/day may be given twice daily; if a dose of 2500 mg/day is required, it may be better tolerated 3 times/day (with meals).

850 mg tablets: Initial: 850 mg once daily (give with the morning meal); dosage increases should be made in increments of 1 tablet every **other** week, given in divided doses, up to a maximum of 2550 mg/day. Usual maintenance dose: 850 mg twice daily (with the morning and evening meals). Some patients may be given 850 mg 3 times/day (with meals).

Extended release tablets: Initial: 500 mg once daily (with the evening meal); dosage may be increased by 500 mg weekly; maximum dose: 2000 mg once daily. If glycemic control is not achieved at maximum dose, may divide dose to 1000 mg twice daily; if doses >2000 mg/day are needed, switch to regular release tablets and titrate to maximum dose of 2550 mg/day

Elderly: The initial and maintenance dosing should be conservative, due to the potential for decreased renal function. Generally, elderly patients should not be titrated to the maximum dose of metformin. Do not use in patients ≥80 years of age unless normal renal function has been established.

Transfer from other antidiabetic agents: No transition period is generally necessary except when transferring from chlorpropamide. When transferring from chlorpropamide, care should be exercised during the first 2 weeks because of the prolonged retention of chlorpropamide in the body, leading to overlapping drug effects and possible hypoglycemia.

Concomitant metformin and oral sulfonylurea therapy: If patients have not responded to 4 weeks of the maximum dose of metformin monotherapy, consider a gradual addition of an oral sulfonylurea, even if prior primary or secondary failure to a sulfonylurea has occurred. Continue metformin at the maximum dose.

Failed sulfonylurea therapy: Patients with prior failure on glyburide may be treated by gradual addition of metformin. Initiate with glyburide 20 mg and metformin 500 mg daily. Metformin dosage may be increased by 500 mg/day at weekly intervals, up to a maximum of 2500 mg/day (dosage of glyburide maintained at 20 mg/day).

Concomitant metformin and insulin therapy: Initial: 500 mg metformin once daily, continue current insulin dose; increase by 500 mg metformin weekly until adequate glycemic control is achieved

Maximum dose: 2500 mg metformin; 2000 mg metformin extended release

Decrease insulin dose 10% to 25% when FPG <120 mg/dL; monitor and make further adjustments as needed

Dosing adjustment in renal impairment: The plasma and blood halflife of metformin is prolonged and the renal clearance is decreased in proportion to the decrease in creatinine clearance. Metformin is contraindicated in the presence of renal dysfunction defined as a serum creatinine >1.5 mg/dL in males or >1.4 mg/dL in females or a creatinine clearance <60 mL/minute.

Dosing adjustment in hepatic impairment: Avoid metformin; liver disease is a risk factor for the development of lactic acidosis during metformin therapy.

Mechanism of Action Decreases hepatic glucose production, decreasing intestinal absorption of glucose and improves insulin sensitivity (increases peripheral glucose uptake and utilization)

Other Adverse Effects

>10%:

Gastrointestinal: Nausea/vomiting (6% to 25%), diarrhea (10% to 53%), flatulence (12%)

Neuromuscular & skeletal: Weakness (9%)

1% to 10%:

Cardiovascular: Chest discomfort, flushing, palpitation

Central nervous system: Headache (6%), chills, dizziness, lightheadedness

Dermatologic: Rash

Endocrine & metabolic: Hypoglycemia

Gastrointestinal: Indigestion (7%), abdominal discomfort (6%), abdominal distention, abnormal stools, constipation, dyspepsia/ heartburn, taste disorder

Neuromuscular & skeletal: Myalgia

Respiratory: Dyspnea, upper respiratory tract infection

Miscellaneous: Decreased vitamin B_{12} levels (7%), increased diaphoresis, flu-like syndrome, nail disorder

<1%: Megaloblastic anemia

Postmarketing and/or case reports: Lactic acidosis

Drug Interactions

Increased Effect/Toxicity: Furosemide and cimetidine may increase metformin blood levels. Cationic drugs (eg, amiloride, digoxin, morphine, procainamide, quinidine, quinine, ranitidine, triamterene, trimethoprim, and vancomycin) which are eliminated by renal tubular secretion have the potential to increase metformin levels by competing for common renal tubular transport systems.

Decreased Effect: Drugs which tend to produce hyperglycemia (eg, diuretics, corticosteroids, phenothiazines, thyroid products, estrogens, oral contraceptives,

(Continued)

Metformin *(Continued)*

phenytoin, nicotinic acid, sympathomimetics, calcium channel blocking drugs, isoniazid) may lead to a loss of glucose control.

Dietary/Ethanol/Herb Considerations

Ethanol: Avoid use; may increase risk of lactic acidosis and hypoglycemia.

Food: Administer with food to reduce GI upset; food decreases the extent and slightly delays the absorption. Dietary modification based on ADA recommendations is a part of therapy. Metformin may decrease absorption of vitamin B_{12} and/or folic acid; may require supplementation.

Herb/Nutraceutical: Black cohosh may enhance effects of antidiabetic agents. Use caution with chromium, garlic, gymnema, and horse chestnut; may cause hypoglycemia.

Pharmacodynamics/Kinetics

Onset of action: Within days; maximum effects up to 2 weeks

Distribution: V_d: 654 ± 358 L

Protein binding: 92% to 99%; Plasma: negligible

Bioavailability: Absolute: Fasting: 50% to 60%

Half-life elimination, plasma: 6.2 hours

Excretion: Urine (90% as unchanged drug)

Pregnancy Risk Factor B

Generic Available Yes: Regular release only

Metformin and Glipizide *see* Glipizide and Metformin *on page 639*

Metformin and Rosiglitazone *see* Rosiglitazone and Metformin *on page 1200*

Metformin Hydrochloride *see* Metformin *on page 874*

Metformin Hydrochloride and Rosiglitazone Maleate *see* Rosiglitazone and Metformin *on page 1200*

Methadone (METH a done)

U.S. Brand Names Dolophine®; Methadone Intensol™; Methadose®

Canadian Brand Names Dolophine®; Metadol™; Methadose®

Pharmacologic Category Analgesic, Narcotic

Synonyms Methadone Hydrochloride

Use Management of severe pain; detoxification and maintenance treatment of narcotic addiction (if used for detoxification and maintenance treatment of narcotic addiction, it must be part of an FDA-approved program)

Local Anesthetic/Vasoconstrictor Precautions No information available to require special precautions

Effects on Dental Treatment 1% to 10%: Significant xerostomia; normal salivary flow resumes upon discontinuation

Restrictions C-II

Dosage These are guidelines and do not represent the maximum doses that may be required in all patients. Methadone accumulates with repeated doses and dosage may need reduction after 3-5 days to prevent CNS depressant effects. Some patients may benefit from every 8-12 hour dosing interval for chronic pain management. Doses should be titrated to appropriate effects.

Children:

Pain (analgesia):

Oral, I.M., S.C.: 0.7 mg/kg/24 hours divided every 4-6 hours as needed or 0.1-0.2 mg/kg every 4-12 hours as needed; maximum: 10 mg/dose

I.V.: 0.1 mg/kg every 4 hours initially for 2-3 doses, then every 6-12 hours as needed; maximum: 10 mg/dose

Iatrogenic narcotic dependency: Oral: General guidelines: Initial: 0.05-0.1 mg/kg/dose every 6 hours; increase by 0.05 mg/kg/dose until withdrawal symptoms are controlled; after 24-48 hours, the dosing interval can be lengthened to every 12-24 hours; to taper dose, wean by 0.05 mg/kg/day; if withdrawal symptoms recur, taper at a slower rate

Adults:

Pain (analgesia):

Oral: Initial: 2.5-5 mg every 3-8 hours as needed; patients with prior opiate exposure may require higher initial doses; usual dosage range: 2.5-20 mg every 3-8 hours as needed

I.M., S.C.: 2.5-10 mg every 6-8 hours as needed; patients with prior opiate exposure may require higher initial doses

Detoxification: Oral: 15-40 mg/day

Maintenance treatment of opiate dependence: Oral: 20-120 mg/day

Dosing adjustment in renal impairment: Cl_{cr} <10 mL/minute: Administer at 50% to 75% of normal dose

Dosing adjustment/comments in hepatic disease: Avoid use in severe liver disease

Mechanism of Action Binds to opiate receptors in the CNS, causing inhibition of ascending pain pathways, altering the perception of and response to pain; produces generalized CNS depression

Other Adverse Effects Frequency not defined:

Cardiovascular: Bradycardia, peripheral vasodilation, cardiac arrest, syncope, faintness

Central nervous system: Euphoria, dysphoria, headache, insomnia, agitation, disorientation, drowsiness, dizziness, lightheadedness, sedation

Dermatologic: Pruritus, urticaria, rash

Endocrine & metabolic: Decreased libido

Gastrointestinal: Nausea, vomiting, constipation, anorexia, stomach cramps, biliary tract spasm

Genitourinary: Urinary retention or hesitancy, antidiuretic effect, impotence

Neuromuscular & skeletal: Weakness

Ocular: Miosis, visual disturbances

Respiratory: Respiratory depression, respiratory arrest

Miscellaneous: Physical and psychological dependence

Drug Interactions Substrate of CYP2C8/9, 2C19, 2D6, **3A4**; Inhibits **CYP2D6**, 3A4

Increased Effect/Toxicity: Fluconazole, itraconazole, and ketoconazole increase serum methadone concentrations via CYP3A4 inhibition; an increased narcotic effect may be experienced. Similar effects may be seen with ritonavir, nelfinavir, amiodarone, erythromycin, clarithromycin, diltiazem, verapamil, paroxetine, fluoxetine, and other inhibitors of CYP2D6 or CYP3A4.

Decreased Effect: Barbiturates, carbamazepine, nevirapine, phenytoin, primidone, rifampin and ritonavir may decrease serum methadone concentrations via enhanced hepatic metabolism; monitor for methadone withdrawal. Larger doses of methadone may be required.

Dietary/Ethanol/Herb Considerations

Ethanol: Avoid use; may increase CNS depression.

Food: Avoid grapefruit products. Oral dose for detoxification and maintenance may be administered in apple or grape juice.

Herb/Nutraceutical: Avoid gotu kola, kava, SAMe, and valerian; may increase CNS depression. Avoid St John's wort; may decrease serum concentration and increase CNS depression.

Pharmacodynamics/Kinetics

Onset of action: Oral: Analgesic: 0.5-1 hour; Parenteral: 10-20 minutes

Peak effect: Parenteral: 1-2 hours

Duration: Oral: 6-8 hours, increases to 22-48 hours with repeated doses

Distribution: Crosses placenta; enters breast milk

Protein binding: 80% to 85%

Metabolism: Hepatic via N-demethylation

Half-life elimination: 15-29 hours; may be prolonged with alkaline pH

Excretion: Urine (<10% as unchanged drug); increased with urine pH <6

Pregnancy Risk Factor B/D (prolonged use or high doses at term)

Generic Available Yes: Solution, tablet

Methadone Hydrochloride *see* Methadone *on page 876*

Methadone Intensol™ *see* Methadone *on page 876*

Methadose® *see* Methadone *on page 876*

Methaminodiazepoxide Hydrochloride *see* Chlordiazepoxide *on page 299*

Methamphetamine (meth am FET a meen)

U.S. Brand Names Desoxyn®

Canadian Brand Names Desoxyn®

Pharmacologic Category Stimulant

Synonyms Desoxyephedrine Hydrochloride; Methamphetamine Hydrochloride

Use Treatment of attention-deficit/hyperactivity disorder (ADHD); exogenous obesity (short-term adjunct)

Unlabeled/Investigational Use Treatment of narcolepsy

Local Anesthetic/Vasoconstrictor Precautions Use vasoconstriction with caution in patients taking methamphetamine. Amphetamines enhance the sympathomimetic response of epinephrine and norepinephrine leading to potential hypertension and cardiotoxicity.

Effects on Dental Treatment 1% to 10%: Xerostomia

Up to 10% of patients taking dextroamphetamines may present with hypertension. The use of local anesthetic without vasoconstrictor is recommended in these patients.

Restrictions C-II

Dosage Oral:

Children >6 years and Adults: ADHD: 2.5-5 mg 1-2 times/day; may increase by 5 mg increments at weekly intervals until optimum response is achieved, usually 20-25 mg/day

Children >12 years and Adults: Exogenous obesity: 5 mg 30 minutes before each meal; long-acting formulation: 10-15 mg in morning; treatment duration should not exceed a few weeks

Mechanism of Action A sympathomimetic amine related to ephedrine and amphetamine with CNS stimulant activity; peripheral actions include elevation of systolic

(Continued)

Methamphetamine *(Continued)*

and diastolic blood pressure and weak bronchodilator and respiratory stimulant action

Other Adverse Effects Frequency not defined:

Cardiovascular: Hypertension, tachycardia, palpitations

Central nervous system: Restlessness, headache, exacerbation of motor and phonic tics and Tourette's syndrome, dizziness, psychosis, dysphoria, overstimulation, euphoria, insomnia

Dermatologic: Rash, urticaria

Endocrine & metabolic: Change in libido

Gastrointestinal: Diarrhea, nausea, vomiting, stomach cramps, constipation, anorexia, weight loss, unpleasant taste

Genitourinary: Impotence

Neuromuscular & skeletal: Tremor

Miscellaneous: Suppression of growth in children, tolerance and withdrawal with prolonged use

Drug Interactions Substrate of **CYP2D6**

Increased Effect/Toxicity: Amphetamines may precipitate hypertensive crisis or serotonin syndrome in patients receiving MAO inhibitors (selegiline >10 mg/day, isocarboxazid, phenelzine, tranylcypromine, furazolidone). Serotonin syndrome has also been associated with combinations of amphetamines and SSRIs; these combinations should be avoided. TCAs may enhance the effects of amphetamines, potentially leading to hypertensive crisis. Large doses of antacids or urinary alkalinizers increase the half-life and duration of action of amphetamines. May precipitate arrhythmias in patients receiving general anesthetics. Inhibitors of CYP2D6 may increase the effects of amphetamines (includes amiodarone, cimetidine, delavirdine, fluoxetine, paroxetine, propafenone, quinidine, and ritonavir).

Decreased Effect: Amphetamines inhibit the antihypertensive response to guanethidine and guanadrel. Urinary acidifiers decrease the half-life and duration of action of amphetamines. Enzyme inducers (barbiturates, carbamazepine, phenytoin, and rifampin) may decrease serum concentrations of amphetamines.

Dietary/Ethanol/Herb Considerations

Ethanol: Avoid use; may cause CNS depression.

Food: Serum concentration may be altered if taken with acidic food, juices, or vitamin C; avoid caffeine.

Herb/Nutraceutical: Avoid ephedra, ginseng, and yohimbe; may cause hypertension or arrhythmias. Avoid gotu kola, kava, SAMe, St John's wort, and valerian; may increase CNS depression.

Pharmacodynamics/Kinetics

Absorption: Rapid from GI tract

Metabolism: Hepatic

Half-Life elimination: 4-5 hours

Excretion: Urine primarily (dependent on urine pH)

Pregnancy Risk Factor C

Generic Available No

Methamphetamine Hydrochloride *see* Methamphetamine *on page 877*

Methazolamide (meth a ZOE la mide)

U.S. Brand Names Neptazane® [DSC]

Canadian Brand Names Apo®-Methazolamide

Pharmacologic Category Carbonic Anhydrase Inhibitor; Diuretic, Carbonic Anhydrase Inhibitor; Ophthalmic Agent, Antiglaucoma

Use Adjunctive treatment of open-angle or secondary glaucoma; short-term therapy of narrow-angle glaucoma when delay of surgery is desired

Local Anesthetic/Vasoconstrictor Precautions No information available to require special precautions

Effects on Dental Treatment No significant effects or complications reported

Dosage Adults: Oral: 50-100 mg 2-3 times/day

Mechanism of Action Noncompetitive inhibition of the enzyme carbonic anhydrase; thought that carbonic anhydrase is located at the luminal border of cells of the proximal tubule. When the enzyme is inhibited, there is an increase in urine volume and a change to an alkaline pH with a subsequent decrease in the excretion of titratable acid and ammonia.

Other Adverse Effects Frequency not defined:

Central nervous system: Malaise, fever, mental depression, drowsiness, dizziness, nervousness, headache, confusion, seizures, fatigue, trembling, unsteadiness

Dermatologic: Urticaria, pruritus, photosensitivity, rash, Stevens-Johnson syndrome

Endocrine & metabolic: Hyperchloremic metabolic acidosis, hypokalemia, hyperglycemia

Gastrointestinal: Metallic taste, anorexia, nausea, vomiting, diarrhea, constipation, weight loss, GI irritation, xerostomia, black tarry stools

Genitourinary: Polyuria, crystalluria, hematuria, polyuria, renal calculi, impotence

Hematologic: Bone marrow depression, thrombocytopenia, thrombocytopenic purpura, hemolytic anemia, leukopenia, pancytopenia, agranulocytosis
Hepatic: Hepatic insufficiency
Neuromuscular & skeletal: Weakness, ataxia, paresthesias
Miscellaneous: Hypersensitivity

Drug Interactions

Increased Effect/Toxicity: Methazolamide may induce hypokalemia which would sensitize a patient to digitalis toxicity. Hypokalemia may be compounded with concurrent diuretic use or steroids. Methazolamide may increase the potential for salicylate toxicity. Primidone absorption may be delayed.

Decreased Effect: Increased lithium excretion and altered excretion of other drugs by alkalinization of the urine, such as amphetamines, quinidine, procainamide, methenamine, phenobarbital, and salicylates.

Pharmacodynamics/Kinetics

Onset of action: Slow in comparison with acetazolamide (2-4 hours)
Peak effect: 6-8 hours
Duration: 10-18 hours
Absorption: Slow
Distribution: Well into tissue
Protein binding: ~55%
Metabolism: Slowly from GI tract
Half-life elimination: ~14 hours
Excretion: Urine (~25% as unchanged drug)

Pregnancy Risk Factor C

Generic Available Yes

Methenamine (meth EN a meen)

U.S. Brand Names Hiprex®; Mandelamine®; Urex®

Canadian Brand Names Dehydral®; Hiprex®; Mandelamine®; Urasal®; Urex®

Pharmacologic Category Antibiotic, Miscellaneous

Synonyms Hexamethylenetetramine; Methenamine Hippurate; Methenamine Mandelate

Use Prophylaxis or suppression of recurrent urinary tract infections; urinary tract discomfort secondary to hypermotility

Local Anesthetic/Vasoconstrictor Precautions No information available to require special precautions

Effects on Dental Treatment No significant effects or complications reported

Dosage Oral:

Children:
<6 years: 0.25 g/30 lb 4 times/day
6-12 years:
Hippurate: 25-50 mg/kg/day divided every 12 hours or 0.5-1 g twice daily
Mandelate: 50-75 mg/kg/day divided every 6 hours or 0.5 g 4 times/day

Children >12 years and Adults:
Hippurate: 1 g twice daily
Mandelate: 1 g 4 times/day after meals and at bedtime

Dosing adjustment in renal impairment: Cl_{cr} <50 mL/minute: Avoid use

Mechanism of Action Methenamine is hydrolyzed to formaldehyde and ammonia in acidic urine; formaldehyde has nonspecific bactericidal action

Other Adverse Effects

1% to 10%:
Dermatologic: Rash (4%)
Gastrointestinal: Nausea, dyspepsia (4%)
Genitourinary: Dysuria (4%)

<1%: Bladder irritation, crystalluria (especially with large doses), increased AST/ALT (reversible, rare)

Drug Interactions

Increased Effect/Toxicity: Sulfonamides may precipitate in the urine.

Decreased Effect: Sodium bicarbonate and acetazolamide will decrease effect secondary to alkalinization of urine.

Dietary/Ethanol/Herb Considerations Food: Foods/diets which alkalinize urine pH >5.5 decrease therapeutic effect. Hiprex® contains tartrazine dye.

Pharmacodynamics/Kinetics

Absorption: Readily
Metabolism: Gastric juices: Hydrolyze 10% to 30% unless protected via enteric coating; Hepatic: ~10% to 25%
Half-life elimination: 3-6 hours
Excretion: Urine (~70% to 90% as unchanged drug) within 24 hours

Pregnancy Risk Factor C

Generic Available Yes

Methenamine Hippurate *see* Methenamine *on page 879*
Methenamine Mandelate *see* Methenamine *on page 879*

Methenamine, Sodium Biphosphate, Phenyl Salicylate, Methylene Blue, and Hyoscyamine

(meth EN a meen, SOW dee um bye FOS fate, fen nil sa LIS i late, METH i leen bloo, & hye oh SYE a meen)

Related Information

Hyoscyamine *on page 699*
Methenamine *on page 879*

U.S. Brand Names Urimar-T; Urimax®

Pharmacologic Category Antibiotic, Miscellaneous

Synonyms Hyoscyamine, Methenamine, Sodium Biphosphate, Phenyl Salicylate, and Methylene Blue; Methylene Blue, Methenamine, Sodium Biphosphate, Phenyl Salicylate, and Hyoscyamine; Phenyl Salicylate, Methenamine, Methylene Blue, Sodium Biphosphate, and Hyoscyamine; Sodium Biphosphate, Methenamine, Methylene Blue, Phenyl Salicylate, and Hyoscyamine

Use Treatment of symptoms of irritative voiding; relief of local symptoms associated with urinary tract infections; relief of urinary tract symptoms caused by diagnostic procedures

Local Anesthetic/Vasoconstrictor Precautions No information available to require special precautions

Effects on Dental Treatment No significant effects or complications reported

Dosage Oral:

Children >6 years: Dosage must be individualized
Adults: One tablet 4 times daily (followed by liberal fluid intake)

Other Adverse Effects Frequency not defined:

Cardiovascular: Tachycardia, flushing
Central nervous system: Dizziness
Gastrointestinal: Xerostomia, nausea, vomiting
Genitourinary: Urinary retention (acute), micturition difficulty, discoloration of urine (blue)
Ocular: Blurred vision
Respiratory: Dyspnea, shortness of breath

Pregnancy Risk Factor C

Generic Available No

Methergine® *see* Methylergonovine *on page 892*

Methimazole (meth IM a zole)

Related Information

Endocrine Disorders and Pregnancy *on page 1479*

U.S. Brand Names Tapazole®

Canadian Brand Names Tapazole®

Pharmacologic Category Antithyroid Agent

Synonyms Thiamazole

Use Palliative treatment of hyperthyroidism, return the hyperthyroid patient to a normal metabolic state prior to thyroidectomy, and to control thyrotoxic crisis that may accompany thyroidectomy. The use of antithyroid thioamides is as effective in elderly as they are in younger adults; however, the expense, potential adverse effects, and inconvenience (compliance, monitoring) make them undesirable. The use of radioiodine due to ease of administration and less concern for long-term side effects and reproduction problems (some older males) makes it a more appropriate therapy.

Local Anesthetic/Vasoconstrictor Precautions No information available to require special precautions

Effects on Dental Treatment No significant effects or complications reported

Dosage Oral: Administer in 3 equally divided doses at approximately 8-hour intervals

Children: Initial: 0.4 mg/kg/day in 3 divided doses; maintenance: 0.2 mg/kg/day in 3 divided doses up to 30 mg/24 hours maximum
Alternatively: Initial: 0.5-0.7 mg/kg/day **or** 15-20 mg/m²/day in 3 divided doses
Maintenance: ⅓ to ⅔ of the initial dose beginning when the patient is euthyroid
Maximum: 30 mg/24 hours

Adults: Initial: 15 mg/day for mild hyperthyroidism; 30-40 mg/day in moderately severe hyperthyroidism; 60 mg/day in severe hyperthyroidism; maintenance: 5-15 mg/day
Adjust dosage as required to achieve and maintain serum T_3, T_4, and TSH levels in the normal range. An elevated T_3 may be the sole indicator of inadequate treatment. An elevated TSH indicates excessive antithyroid treatment.

Mechanism of Action Inhibits the synthesis of thyroid hormones by blocking the oxidation of iodine in the thyroid gland, blocking iodine's ability to combine with tyrosine to form thyroxine and triiodothyronine (T_3), does not inactivate circulating T_4 and T_3

Other Adverse Effects Frequency not defined:

Cardiovascular: Edema

Central nervous system: Headache, vertigo, drowsiness, CNS stimulation, depression

Dermatologic: Skin rash, urticaria, pruritus, erythema nodosum, skin pigmentation, exfoliative dermatitis, alopecia

Endocrine & metabolic: Goiter

Gastrointestinal: Nausea, vomiting, stomach pain, abnormal taste, constipation, weight gain, salivary gland swelling

Hematologic: Leukopenia, agranulocytosis, granulocytopenia, thrombocytopenia, aplastic anemia, hypoprothrombinemia

Hepatic: Cholestatic jaundice, jaundice, hepatitis

Neuromuscular & skeletal: Arthralgia, paresthesia

Renal: Nephrotic syndrome

Miscellaneous: SLE-like syndrome

Drug Interactions Inhibits CYP1A2, 2A6, 2B6, 2C8/9, 2C19, 2D6, 2E1, 3A4

Increased Effect: Anticoagulant effect of warfarin may be increased. Dosage of some drugs (including beta-blockers, digoxin, and theophylline) require adjustment during treatment of hyperthyroidism.

Increased toxicity with lithium or potassium iodide.

Pharmacodynamics/Kinetics

Onset of action: Antithyroid: Oral: 12-18 hours

Duration: 36-72 hours

Distribution: Concentrated in thyroid gland; crosses placenta; enters breast milk (1:1)

Protein binding, plasma: None

Metabolism: Hepatic

Bioavailability: 80% to 95%

Half-life elimination: 4-13 hours

Excretion: Urine (80%)

Pregnancy Risk Factor D

Generic Available Yes

Methionine (me THYE oh neen)

U.S. Brand Names ME-500®; Pedameth®

Pharmacologic Category Dietary Supplement

Use Treatment of diaper rash and control of odor, dermatitis and ulceration caused by ammoniacal urine

Local Anesthetic/Vasoconstrictor Precautions No information available to require special precautions

Effects on Dental Treatment No significant effects or complications reported

Dosage Oral:

Children: Control of diaper rash: 75 mg in formula or other liquid 3-4 times/day for 3-5 days

Adults:

Control of odor in incontinent adults: 200-400 mg 3-4 times/day

Dietary supplement: 500 mg/day

Generic Available Yes

Methitest® *see* MethylTESTOSTERone *on page 897*

Methocarbamol (meth oh KAR ba mole)

Related Information

Temporomandibular Dysfunction (TMD) *on page 1562*

U.S. Brand Names Robaxin®

Canadian Brand Names Robaxin®

Pharmacologic Category Skeletal Muscle Relaxant

Use

Dental: Treatment of muscle spasm associated with acute temporomandibular joint pain (ie, TMD)

Medical: Treatment of muscle spasm associated with acute painful musculoskeletal conditions; supportive therapy in tetanus

Local Anesthetic/Vasoconstrictor Precautions No information available to require special precautions

Effects on Dental Treatment Frequency not defined: Facial flushing, bradycardia, hypotension, drowsiness, dizziness, lightheadedness, syncope, convulsions, headache, fever, nausea, vomiting, metallic taste, blurred vision, nasal congestion, allergic manifestations, anaphylactic reaction, allergic dermatitis, pain at injection site

Dosage

Children: Recommended **only** for use in tetanus: I.V.: 15 mg/kg/dose or 500 mg/m^2/dose, may repeat every 6 hours if needed; maximum dose: 1.8 g/m^2/day for 3 days only

Adults: **Muscle spasm:**

Oral: 1.5 g 4 times/day for 2-3 days, then decrease to 4-4.5 g/day in 3-6 divided doses

I.M., I.V.: 1 g every 8 hours if oral not possible

(Continued)

Methocarbamol *(Continued)*

Dosing comments in renal impairment: Do not administer parenteral formulation to patients with renal dysfunction.

Mechanism of Action Causes skeletal muscle relaxation by reducing the transmission of impulses from the spinal cord to skeletal muscle

Other Adverse Effects Frequency not defined:

Central nervous system: Vertigo
Dermatologic: urticaria, pruritus, rash
Hematologic: Leukopenia
Local: Thrombophlebitis
Ocular: Nystagmus, diplopia, conjunctivitis
Renal: Renal impairment

Contraindications Hypersensitivity to methocarbamol or any component of the formulation; renal impairment

Warnings/Precautions Rate of injection should not exceed 3 mL/minute; solution is hypertonic; avoid extravasation; use with caution in patients with a history of seizures

Drug Interactions Increased effect/toxicity with CNS depressants; pyridostigmine (a single case of worsening myasthenia has been reported following methocarbamol administration)

Dietary/Ethanol/Herb Considerations

Ethanol: Avoid use; may increase CNS depression.
Food: Tablets may be crushed and mixed with food or liquid.
Herb/Nutraceutical: Avoid gotu kola, kava, SAme, St John's wort, and valerian; may increase CNS depression.

Pharmacodynamics/Kinetics

Onset of action: Muscle relaxation: Oral: ~30 minutes
Metabolism: Hepatic
Half-life elimination: 1-2 hours
Time to peak, serum: ~2 hours
Excretion: Urine (as metabolites)

Pregnancy Risk Factor C

Dosage Forms INJ, solution: 100 mg/mL (10 mL). **TAB:** 500 mg, 750 mg

Generic Available Yes: Tablet

Methohexital (meth oh HEKS i tal)

U.S. Brand Names Brevital® Sodium

Canadian Brand Names Brevital®

Pharmacologic Category Barbiturate

Synonyms Methohexital Sodium

Use

Dental: Induction and maintenance of general anesthesia for short procedures

Medical: Pediatric patients (>1 month of age): Rectal or intramuscular induction of anesthesia prior to the use of other general anesthetic agents; adjunct to subpotent inhalational anesthetic agents for short surgical procedures; for short surgical, diagnostic, or therapeutic procedures associated with minimal painful stimuli

Local Anesthetic/Vasoconstrictor Precautions No information available to require special precautions

Effects on Dental Treatment Frequency not defined: Hypotension, seizures, headache, nausea, vomiting, tremor, twitching, rigidity, involuntary muscle movement, apnea, respiratory depression, laryngospasm, coughing, hiccups, pain on I.M. injection, peripheral vascular collapse

Restrictions C-IV

Dosage Doses must be titrated to effect.

Children 3-12 years:
I.M.: Preop: 5-10 mg/kg/dose
I.V.: Induction: 1-2 mg/kg/dose
Rectal: Preop/induction: 20-35 mg/kg/dose; usual 25 mg/kg/dose; administer as 10% aqueous solution

Adults: I.V.: Induction: 50-120 mg to start; 20-40 mg every 4-7 minutes

Dosing adjustment/comments in hepatic impairment: Lower dosage and monitor closely

Mechanism of Action Ultra short-acting I.V. barbiturate anesthetic

Other Adverse Effects Frequency not defined:

Gastrointestinal: Cramping, diarrhea, rectal bleeding, abdominal pain
Hematologic: Hemolytic anemia, thrombophlebitis
Hepatic: Elevated transaminases
Neuromuscular & skeletal: Radial nerve palsy

Contraindications Hypersensitivity to methohexital or any component of the formulation; porphyria

Warnings/Precautions Use with extreme caution in patients with liver impairment, asthma, cardiovascular instability

Drug Interactions

Acetaminophen: Barbiturates may enhance the hepatotoxic potential of acetaminophen overdoses

Antiarrhythmics: Barbiturates may increase the metabolism of antiarrhythmics, decreasing their clinical effect; includes disopyramide, propafenone, and quinidine

Anticonvulsants: Barbiturates may increase the metabolism of anticonvulsants; includes ethosuximide, felbamate (possibly), lamotrigine, phenytoin, tiagabine, topiramate, and zonisamide; does not appear to affect gabapentin or levetiracetam

Antineoplastics: Limited evidence suggests that enzyme-inducing anticonvulsant therapy may reduce the effectiveness of some chemotherapy regimens (specifically in ALL); teniposide and methotrexate may be cleared more rapidly in these patients

Antipsychotics: Barbiturates may enhance the metabolism (decrease the efficacy) of antipsychotics; monitor for altered response; dose adjustment may be needed

Beta-blockers: Metabolism of beta-blockers may be increased and clinical effect decreased; atenolol and nadolol are unlikely to interact given their renal elimination

Calcium channel blockers: Barbiturates may enhance the metabolism of calcium channel blockers, decreasing their clinical effect

Chloramphenicol: Barbiturates may increase the metabolism of chloramphenicol and chloramphenicol may inhibit barbiturate metabolism; monitor for altered response

Cimetidine: Barbiturates may enhance the metabolism of cimetidine, decreasing its clinical effect

CNS depressants: Sedative effects and/or respiratory depression with barbiturates may be additive with other CNS depressants; monitor for increased effect; includes ethanol, sedatives, antidepressants, narcotic analgesics, and benzodiazepines

Corticosteroids: Barbiturates may enhance the metabolism of corticosteroids, decreasing their clinical effect

Cyclosporine: Levels may be decreased by barbiturates; monitor

Doxycycline: Barbiturates may enhance the metabolism of doxycycline, decreasing its clinical effect; higher dosages may be required

Estrogens: Barbiturates may increase the metabolism of estrogens and reduce their efficacy

Felbamate may inhibit the metabolism of barbiturates and barbiturates may increase the metabolism of felbamate

Griseofulvin: Barbiturates may impair the absorption of griseofulvin, and griseofulvin metabolism may be increased by barbiturates, decreasing clinical effect

Guanfacine: Effect may be decreased by barbiturates

Immunosuppressants: Barbiturates may enhance the metabolism of immunosuppressants, decreasing its clinical effect; includes both cyclosporine and tacrolimus

Loop diuretics: Metabolism may be increased and clinical effects decreased; established for furosemide, effect with other loop diuretics not established

MAO inhibitors: Metabolism of barbiturates may be inhibited, increasing clinical effect or toxicity of the barbiturates

Methadone: Barbiturates may enhance the metabolism of methadone resulting in methadone withdrawal

Methoxyflurane: Barbiturates may enhance the nephrotoxic effects of methoxyflurane

Oral contraceptives: Barbiturates may enhance the metabolism of oral contraceptives, decreasing their clinical effect; an alternative method of contraception should be considered

Theophylline: Barbiturates may increase metabolism of theophylline derivatives and decrease their clinical effect

Tricyclic antidepressants: Barbiturates may increase metabolism of tricyclic antidepressants and decrease their clinical effect; sedative effects may be additive

Valproic acid: Metabolism of barbiturates may be inhibited by valproic acid; monitor for excessive sedation; a dose reduction may be needed

Warfarin: Barbiturates inhibit the hypoprothrombinemic effects of oral anticoagulants via increased metabolism; this combination should generally be avoided

Dietary/Ethanol/Herb Considerations Food: Do not administer if patient has food in stomach due to danger of vomiting during anesthesia.

Pharmacodynamics/Kinetics

Onset of action: I.V.: Immediately

Duration: Single dose: 10-20 minutes

Pregnancy Risk Factor C

Dosage Forms INJ, powder for reconstitution: 500 mg, 2.5 g, 5 g

Generic Available No

Selected Readings Dionne RA, Yagiela JA, Moore PA, et al, "Comparing Efficacy and Safety of Four Intravenous Sedation Regimens in Dental Outpatients," *Am Dent Assoc*, 2001, 132(6):740-51.

Methohexital Sodium *see* Methohexital *on page 882*

Methotrexate (meth oh TREKS ate)

Related Information

Rheumatoid Arthritis, Osteoarthritis, and Osteoporosis *on page 1488*

U.S. Brand Names Rheumatrex®; Trexall™

Canadian Brand Names Apo®-Methotrexate; ratio-Methotrexate

Mexican Brand Names Ledertrexate®; Texate®; Trixilem®

Pharmacologic Category Antineoplastic Agent, Antimetabolite

Synonyms Amethopterin; Methotrexate Sodium; MTX

Use Treatment of trophoblastic neoplasms; leukemias; psoriasis; rheumatoid arthritis (RA), including polyarticular-course juvenile rheumatoid arthritis (JRA); breast, head and neck, and lung carcinomas; osteosarcoma; sarcomas; carcinoma of gastric, esophagus, testes; lymphomas; mycosis fungoides (cutaneous T-cell lymphoma)

Local Anesthetic/Vasoconstrictor Precautions No information available to require special precautions

Effects on Dental Treatment >10%: Ulcerative stomatitis, nausea, vomiting, gingivitis, pharyngitis, glossitis, blurred vision, mucositis (dose dependent; appears 3-7 days post-therapy and resolves within 2 weeks)

Dosage Refer to individual protocols. May be administered orally, I.M., intra-arterially, intrathecally, or I.V.

Leucovorin may be administered concomitantly or within 24 hours of methotrexate - refer to for details

Children:

Dermatomyositis: Oral: 15-20 mg/m²/week as a single dose once weekly or 0.3-1 mg/kg/dose once weekly

Juvenile rheumatoid arthritis: Oral, I.M.: Recommended starting dose: 10 mg/m² once weekly (at higher doses, GI side effects may be decreased with I.M. administration); 5-15 mg/m²/week as a single dose **or** as 3 divided doses given 12 hours apart

Antineoplastic dosage range:

Oral, I.M.: 7.5-30 mg/m²/week **or** every 2 weeks

I.V.: 10-18,000 mg/m² bolus dosing **or** continuous infusion over 6-42 hours

For dosing schedules, see table:

Methotrexate Dosing Schedules

Dose	Route	Frequency
Conventional		
15-20 mg/m²	P.O.	Twice weekly
30-50 mg/m²	P.O., I.V.	Weekly
15 mg/day for 5 days	P.O., I.M.	Every 2-3 weeks
Intermediate		
50-150 mg/m²	I.V. push	Every 2-3 weeks
240 mg/m²*	I.V. infusion	Every 4-7 days
0.5-1 g/m²*	I.V. infusion	Every 2-3 weeks
High		
1-12 g/m²*	I.V. infusion	Every 1-3 weeks

*Followed with leucovorin rescue - refer to Leucovorin monograph for details.

Pediatric solid tumors (high-dose): I.V.:

<12 years: 12 g/m² (dosage range: 12-18 g)

≥12 years: 8 g/m² (maximum: 18 g)

Acute lymphocytic leukemia (intermediate-dose): I.V.: Loading: 100 mg/m² over 1 hour, followed by a 35-hour infusion of 900 mg/m²/day

Meningeal leukemia: I.T.: 10-15 mg/m² (maximum dose: 15 mg) **or**

≤3 months: 3 mg/dose

4-11 months: 6 mg/dose

1 year: 8 mg/dose

2 years: 10 mg/dose

≥3 years: 12 mg/dose

I.T. doses are prepared with preservative-free MTX only. Hydrocortisone may be added to the I.T. preparation; total volume should range from 3-6 mL. Doses should be repeated at 2- to 5-day intervals until CSF counts return to normal followed by a dose once weekly for 2 weeks then monthly thereafter.

Adults: I.V.: Range is wide from 30-40 mg/m²/week to 100-12,000 mg/m² with leucovorin rescue

Doses **not** requiring leucovorin rescue range from 30-40 mg/m² I.V. or I.M. repeated weekly, or oral regimens of 10 mg/m² twice weekly

High-dose MTX is considered to be >100 mg/m² and can be as high as 1500-7500 mg/m². These doses require leucovorin rescue. Patients receiving doses ≥1000 mg/m^2 should have their urine alkalinized with bicarbonate or Bicitra® prior to and following MTX therapy.

Trophoblastic neoplasms: Oral, I.M.: 15-30 mg/day for 5 days; repeat in 7 days for 3-5 courses

Head and neck cancer: Oral, I.M., I.V.: 25-50 mg/m^2 once weekly

Mycosis fungoides (cutaneous T-cell lymphoma): Oral, I.M.: Initial (early stages): 5-50 mg once weekly; dose reduction/cessation should be guided by response and hematologic monitoring. In patients with poor response to weekly therapy, MTX has also been given twice weekly in doses ranging from 15-37.5 mg.

Rheumatoid arthritis: Oral: 7.5 mg once weekly **OR** 2.5 mg every 12 hours for 3 doses/week generally; not to exceed 20 mg/week

Bone marrow suppression is increased at dosages >20 mg/week; absorption and GI effects may be improved with I.M. administration at higher end of dosage range

Psoriasis: Oral: 2.5-5 mg/dose every 12 hours for 3 doses given weekly **or** Oral, I.M.: 10-25 mg/dose given once weekly

Ectopic pregnancy: I.M./I.V.: 50 mg/m^2 single-dose without leucovorin rescue

Elderly: Rheumatoid arthritis/psoriasis: Oral: Initial: 5 mg once weekly; if nausea occurs, split dose to 2.5 mg every 12 hours for the day of administration; dose may be increased to 7.5 mg/week based on response, not to exceed 20 mg/week

Dosing adjustment in renal impairment:

Cl_{cr} 61-80 mL/minute: Reduce dose to 75% of usual dose

Cl_{cr} 51-60 mL/minute: Reduce dose to 70% of usual dose

Cl_{cr} 10-50 mL/minute: Reduce dose to 30% to 50% of usual dose

Cl_{cr} <10 mL/minute: Avoid use

Hemodialysis: Not dialyzable (0% to 5%); supplemental dose is unnecessary

Peritoneal dialysis: Supplemental dose is unnecessary

Dosing adjustment in hepatic impairment:

Bilirubin 3.1-5 mg/dL **or** AST >180 units: Administer 75% of usual dose

Bilirubin >5 mg/dL: Do not use

Mechanism of Action An antimetabolite that inhibits DNA synthesis and cell reproduction in malignant cells

Cytotoxicity is determined by both drug concentration and duration of cell exposure; extracellular drug concentrations of 1 x 10^{-8} M are required to inhibit thymidylate synthesis; reduced folates are able to rescue cells and reverse MTX toxicity if given within 40 hours of the MTX dose

Folates must be in the reduced form (FH_4) to be active

Folates are activated by dihydrofolate reductase (DHFR)

DHFR is inhibited by MTX (by binding irreversibly), causing an increase in the intracellular dihydrofolate pool (the inactive cofactor) and inhibition of both purine and thymidylate synthesis (TS)

MTX enters the cell through an energy-dependent and temperature-dependent process which is mediated by an intramembrane protein; this carrier mechanism is also used by naturally occurring reduced folates, including folinic acid (leucovorin), making this a competitive process

At high drug concentrations (>20 μM), MTX enters the cell by a second mechanism which is not shared by reduced folates; the process may be passive diffusion or a specific, saturable process, and provides a rationale for high-dose MTX

A small fraction of MTX is converted intracellularly to polyglutamates, which leads to a prolonged inhibition of DHFR

The MOA in the treatment of rheumatoid arthritis is unknown, but may affect immune function

In psoriasis, methotrexate is thought to target rapidly proliferating epithelial cells in the skin

Other Adverse Effects

>10%:

Cardiovascular: Vasculitis

Central nervous system (with I.T. administration only):

Arachnoiditis: Acute reaction manifested as severe headache, nuchal rigidity, vomiting, and fever; may be alleviated by reducing the dose

Subacute toxicity: 10% of patients treated with 12-15 mg/m^2 of I.T. MTX may develop this in the second or third week of therapy; consists of motor paralysis of extremities, cranial nerve palsy, seizures, or coma. This has also been seen in pediatric cases receiving very high-dose I.V. MTX (when enough MTX can get across into the CSF).

Demyelinating encephalopathy: Seen months or years after receiving MTX; usually in association with cranial irradiation or other systemic chemotherapy

Dermatologic: Reddening of skin

Endocrine & metabolic: Hyperuricemia, defective oogenesis or spermatogenesis

Gastrointestinal: Diarrhea, anorexia, intestinal perforation

Emetic potential:

<100 mg: Moderately low (10% to 30%)

≥100 mg or <250 mg: Moderate (30% to 60%)

≥250 mg: Moderately high (60% to 90%)

(Continued)

Methotrexate *(Continued)*

Hematologic: Leukopenia, thrombocytopenia
Renal: Renal failure, azotemia, nephropathy
Respiratory: Pharyngitis

1% to 10%:

Central nervous system: Dizziness, malaise, encephalopathy, seizures, fever, chills
Dermatologic: Alopecia, rash, photosensitivity, depigmentation or hyperpigmentation of skin
Endocrine & metabolic: Diabetes
Genitourinary: Cystitis
Hematologic: Hemorrhage
Myelosuppressive: This is the primary dose-limiting factor (along with mucositis) of MTX; occurs about 5-7 days after MTX therapy, and should resolve within 2 weeks
WBC: Mild
Platelets: Moderate
Onset: 7 days
Nadir: 10 days
Recovery: 21 days
Hepatic: Cirrhosis and portal fibrosis have been associated with chronic MTX therapy; acute elevation of liver enzymes are common after high-dose MTX, and usually resolve within 10 days.
Neuromuscular & skeletal: Arthralgia
Renal: Renal dysfunction: Manifested by an abrupt rise in serum creatinine and BUN and a fall in urine output; more common with high-dose MTX, and may be due to precipitation of the drug. The best treatment is prevention: Aggressively hydrate with 3 L/m^2/day starting 12 hours before therapy and continue for 24-36 hours; alkalinize the urine by adding 50 mEq of bicarbonate to each liter of fluid; keep urine flow over 100 mL/hour and urine pH >7.
Respiratory: Pneumonitis: Associated with fever, cough, and interstitial pulmonary infiltrates; treatment is to withhold MTX during the acute reaction; interstitial pneumonitis has been reported to occur with an incidence of 1% in patients with RA (dose 7.5-15 mg/week)

<1% (Limited to important or life-threatening): Anaphylaxis, decreased resistance to infection, osteonecrosis and soft tissue necrosis (with radiotherapy), plaque erosions (psoriasis)

Drug Interactions Involvement with CYP isoenzymes not defined; may act as inhibitor of some isoenzymes.

Increased Effect/Toxicity:

Live virus vaccines → vaccinia infections.
Vincristine: Inhibits MTX efflux from the cell, leading to increased and prolonged MTX levels in the cell; the dose of VCR needed to produce this effect is not achieved clinically.
Organic acids: Salicylates, sulfonamides, probenecid, and high doses of penicillins compete with MTX for transport and reduce renal tubular secretion. Salicylates and sulfonamides may also displace MTX from plasma proteins, increasing MTX levels.
Ara-C: Increased formation of the Ara-C nucleotide can occur when MTX precedes Ara-C, thus promoting the action of Ara-C.
Cyclosporine: CSA and MTX interfere with each other's renal elimination, which may result in increased toxicity.
Nonsteroidal anti-inflammatory drugs (NSAIDs): Severe bone marrow suppression, aplastic anemia, and GI toxicity have been reported with concomitant therapy. Should not be used during moderate or high-dose methotrexate due to increased and prolonged methotrexate levels (may increase toxicity). NSAID use during treatment of rheumatoid arthritis has not been fully explored, but continuation of prior regimen has been allowed in some circumstances, with cautious monitoring.
Patients receiving concomitant therapy with methotrexate and other potential hepatotoxins (eg, azathioprine, retinoids, sulfasalazine) should be closely monitored for possible increased risk of hepatotoxicity.

Decreased Effect: Corticosteroids have been reported to decrease methotrexate entry into leukemia cells. Administration should be separated by 12 hours. Dexamethasone has been reported to not affect methotrexate entry. May decrease phenytoin and 5-FU activity.

Dietary/Ethanol/Herb Considerations

Ethanol: Avoid use; may be associated with increased liver injury.
Food: May decrease peak serum concentration. Milk-rich foods may decrease absorption. Folate may decrease MTX response; avoid intake of extra dietary folic acid.
Herb/Nutraceutical: Avoid echinacea due to immunostimulant properties.

Pharmacodynamics/Kinetics

Onset of action: Antirheumatic: 3-6 weeks; additional improvement may continue longer than 12 weeks

Absorption: Oral: Rapid; well absorbed at low doses (<30 mg/m²), incomplete after large doses; I.M. injection: Complete

Distribution: Penetrates slowly into 3rd space fluids (eg, pleural effusions, ascites), exits slowly from these compartments (slower than from plasma); crosses placenta; small amounts enter breast milk; does not achieve therapeutic concentrations in CSF; must be given intrathecally if given for CNS prophylaxis or treatment; sustained concentrations retained in kidney and liver

Protein binding: 50%

Metabolism: <10%; degraded by intestinal flora to DAMPA by carboxypeptidase; hepatic aldehyde oxidase converts MTX to 7-OH MTX; polyglutamates are produced intracellularly and are just as potent as MTX; their production is dose- and duration-dependent and they are slowly eliminated by the cell once formed

Half-life elimination: Low dose: 3-10 hours; High dose: 8-12 hours

Time to peak, serum: Oral: 1-2 hours; Parenteral: 30-60 minutes

Excretion: Urine (44% to 100%); feces (small amounts)

Pregnancy Risk Factor D

Generic Available Yes

Methotrexate Sodium *see* Methotrexate *on page 884*

Methotrimeprazine (meth oh trye MEP ra zeen)

Canadian Brand Names Apo®-Methoprazine; Novo-Meprazine; Nozinan®

Mexican Brand Names Levocina®; Sinogan®

Pharmacologic Category Analgesic, Non-narcotic

Synonyms Levomepromazine; Methotrimeprazine Hydrochloride

Use Relief of moderate to severe pain in nonambulatory patients; for analgesia and sedation when respiratory depression is to be avoided, as in obstetrics; preanesthetic for producing sedation, somnolence and relief of apprehension and anxiety

Local Anesthetic/Vasoconstrictor Precautions No information available to require special precautions

Effects on Dental Treatment Anticholinergic side effects can cause a reduction of saliva production or secretion, contributing to discomfort and dental disease (ie, caries, oral candidiasis and periodontal disease); phenothiazines can cause extrapyramidal reactions which may appear as muscle twitching or increased motor activity of the face, neck or head.

Dosage Adults: I.M.:

Sedation analgesia: 10-20 mg every 4-6 hours as needed

Preoperative medication: 2-20 mg, 45 minutes to 3 hours before surgery

Postoperative analgesia: 2.5-7.5 mg every 4-6 hours is suggested as necessary since residual effects of anesthetic may be present

Pre- and postoperative hypotension: I.M.: 5-10 mg

Dosing adjustment in renal/hepatic impairment: Use with caution; specific guidelines unavailable

Mechanism of Action Methotrimeprazine is a phenothiazine with sites of action thought to be in the thalamus, hypothalamus, reticular and limbic systems, producing suppression of sensory impulses. This results with sedation, an elevated pain threshold, and induction of amnesia. The analgesic effect of methotrimeprazine is comparable to meperidine and morphine without the respiratory suppression. This agent also has antihistamine, anticholinergic, and antiepinephrine effects.

Other Adverse Effects

>10%:

- Cardiovascular: Hypotension, orthostatic hypotension
- Central nervous system: Pseudoparkinsonism, akathisia, dystonias, dizziness
- Gastrointestinal: Constipation
- Neuromuscular & skeletal: Tardive dyskinesia
- Ocular: Pigmentary retinopathy
- Respiratory: Nasal congestion
- Miscellaneous: Decreased diaphoresis

1% to 10%:

- Central nervous system: Dizziness
- Dermatologic: Increased sensitivity to sun, skin rash
- Endocrine & metabolic: Changes in menstrual cycle, ejaculatory disturbances, changes in libido, pain in breasts
- Gastrointestinal: Weight gain, nausea, vomiting, stomach pain
- Genitourinary: Dysuria
- Neuromuscular & skeletal: Trembling of fingers

Pharmacodynamics/Kinetics

Onset of action: Peak effect: 20-40 minutes

Duration: 4 hours

Half-life elimination, serum: 20 hours

Time to peak, serum: 0.5-1.5 hours

Pregnancy Risk Factor C

Generic Available No

Methotrimeprazine Hydrochloride *see* Methotrimeprazine *on page 887*

Methoxsalen (meth OKS a len)

U.S. Brand Names 8-MOP®; Oxsoralen®; Oxsoralen-Ultra®; Uvadex®

Canadian Brand Names 8-MOP®; Oxsoralen™; Oxsoralen-Ultra™; Ultramop™; Uvadex®

Mexican Brand Names Dermox®; Meladinina®; Oxsoralen®

Pharmacologic Category Psoralen

Synonyms Methoxypsoralen; 8-Methoxypsoralen; 8-MOP

Use

Oral: Symptomatic control of severe, recalcitrant disabling psoriasis, not responsive to other therapy when the diagnosis has been supported by biopsy. Administer only in conjunction with a schedule of controlled doses of long wave ultraviolet (UV) radiation; also used with long wave ultraviolet (UV) radiation for repigmentation of idiopathic vitiligo.

Topical: Repigmenting agent in vitiligo, used in conjunction with controlled doses of UVA or sunlight

Orphan drug (Uvadex®): Palliative treatment of skin manifestations of cutaneous T-cell lymphoma

Local Anesthetic/Vasoconstrictor Precautions No information available to require special precautions

Effects on Dental Treatment No significant effects or complications reported

Dosage

Children >12 years and Adults: Vitiligo:

Oral: 20 mg 2-4 hours before exposure to UVA light or sunlight; limit exposure to 15-40 minutes based on skin basic color and exposure

Topical: Apply lotion 1-2 hours before exposure to UVA light, no more than once weekly

Adults: Oral: Psoriasis: 10-70 mg $1^1/_2$-2 hours before exposure to UVA light, 2-3 times at least 48 hours apart; dosage is based upon patient's body weight and skin type

<30 kg: 10 mg
30-50 kg: 20 mg
51-65 kg: 30 mg
66-80 kg: 40 mg
81-90 kg: 50 mg
91-115 kg: 60 mg
>115 kg: 70 mg

Uvadex® sterile solution is used in conjunction with UVAR® Photopheresis System (consult user's guide): Treatment schedule: Two consecutive days every 4 weeks for a minimum of seven treatment cycles

Mechanism of Action Bonds covalently to pyrimidine bases in DNA, inhibits the synthesis of DNA, and suppresses cell division. The augmented sunburn reaction involves excitation of the methoxsalen molecule by radiation in the long-wave ultraviolet light (UVA), resulting in transference of energy to the methoxsalen molecule producing an excited state ("triplet electronic state"). The molecule, in this "triplet state", then reacts with cutaneous DNA.

Other Adverse Effects Frequency not always defined.

Cardiovascular: Severe edema, hypotension

Central nervous system: Nervousness, vertigo, depression

Dermatologic: Painful blistering, burning, and peeling of skin; pruritus (10%), freckling, hypopigmentation, rash, cheilitis, erythema, itching

Gastrointestinal: Nausea (10%)

Neuromuscular & skeletal: Loss of muscle coordination

Drug Interactions Substrate of CYP2A6; Inhibits **CYP1A2, 2A6**, 2C8/9, 2C19, 2D6, 2E1, 3A4

Increased Effect/Toxicity: Concomitant therapy with other photosensitizing agents such as anthralin, coal tar, griseofulvin, phenothiazines, nalidixic acid, sulfanilamides, tetracyclines, and thiazide diuretics.

Dietary/Ethanol/Herb Considerations Food may increase serum concentration. Avoid furocoumarin-containing foods (eg, limes, figs, parsley, celery, cloves, lemon, mustard, carrots).

Pharmacodynamics/Kinetics

Metabolism: Hepatic

Bioavailability: May be less with capsule than with gelcap

Time to peak, serum: Oral: 2-4 hours

Excretion: Urine (>90% as metabolites)

Pregnancy Risk Factor C

Generic Available No

Methoxypsoralen *see* Methoxsalen *on page 888*

8-Methoxypsoralen *see* Methoxsalen *on page 888*

Methscopolamine (meth skoe POL a meen)

U.S. Brand Names Pamine®

Canadian Brand Names Pamine®

Pharmacologic Category Anticholinergic Agent

Synonyms Methscopolamine Bromide

Use Adjunctive therapy in the treatment of peptic ulcer

Local Anesthetic/Vasoconstrictor Precautions No information available to require special precautions

Effects on Dental Treatment >10%: Xerostomia, changes in salivation, dry throat and nose

Anticholinergic side effects can cause a reduction of saliva production or secretion, contributing to discomfort and dental disease (ie, caries, oral candidiasis and periodontal disease).

Dosage Adults: Oral: 2.5 mg 30 minutes before meals or food and 2.5-5 mg at bedtime

Mechanism of Action Methscopolamine is a peripheral anticholinergic agent that does not cross the blood-brain barrier and provides a peripheral blockade of muscarinic receptors. This agent reduces the volume and the total acid content of gastric secretions, inhibits salivation, and reduces gastrointestinal motility.

Other Adverse Effects Frequency not defined:

Cardiovascular: Palpitations

Central nervous system: Headache, flushing, nervousness, drowsiness, dizziness, confusion, fever, CNS stimulation may be produced with large doses

Dermatologic: Dry skin, urticaria

Gastrointestinal: Constipation, dysphagia, nausea, vomiting

Miscellaneous: Decreased diaphoresis, hypersensitivity reactions, anaphylaxis

Pregnancy Risk Factor C

Generic Available No

Methscopolamine Bromide *see* Methscopolamine *on page 888*

Methsuximide (meth SUKS i mide)

U.S. Brand Names Celontin®

Canadian Brand Names Celontin®

Pharmacologic Category Anticonvulsant, Succinimide

Use Control of absence (petit mal) seizures that are refractory to other drugs

Unlabeled/Investigational Use Treatment of partial complex (psychomotor) seizures

Local Anesthetic/Vasoconstrictor Precautions No information available to require special precautions

Effects on Dental Treatment No significant effects or complications reported

Dosage Oral:

Children: Anticonvulsant: Initial: 10-15 mg/kg/day in 3-4 divided doses; increase weekly up to maximum of 30 mg/kg/day

Adults: Anticonvulsant: 300 mg/day for the first week; may increase by 300 mg/day at weekly intervals up to 1.2 g/day in 2-4 divided doses/day

Mechanism of Action Increases the seizure threshold and suppresses paroxysmal spike-and-wave pattern in absence seizures; depresses nerve transmission in the motor cortex

Other Adverse Effects Frequency not defined:

Cardiovascular: Hyperemia

Central nervous system: Ataxia, dizziness, drowsiness, headache, aggressiveness, mental depression, irritability, nervousness, insomnia, confusion, psychosis, suicidal behavior, auditory hallucinations

Dermatologic: Stevens-Johnson syndrome, rash, urticaria, pruritus

Gastrointestinal: Anorexia, nausea, vomiting, weight loss, diarrhea, epigastric and abdominal pain, constipation

Genitourinary: Proteinuria, hematuria (microscopic); cases of blood dyscrasias have been reported with succinimides

Hematologic: Leukopenia, pancytopenia, eosinophilia, monocytosis

Neuromuscular & skeletal: Cases of systemic lupus erythematosus have been reported

Ocular: Blurred vision, photophobia, peripheral edema

Drug Interactions Substrate of **CYP2C19**; Inhibits CYP2C19

Increased Effect/Toxicity: Sedative effects and/or respiratory depression may be additive with CNS depressants; includes ethanol, benzodiazepines, barbiturates, narcotic analgesics, and other sedative agents. Methsuximide may increase phenobarbital and/or phenytoin concentration.

Dietary/Ethanol/Herb Considerations

Ethanol: Avoid use; may enhance sedative effects and/or respiratory depression.

Herb/Nutraceutical: Avoid gotu kola, kava, SAMe, St John's wort, and valerian; may increase CNS depression.

Pharmacodynamics/Kinetics

Metabolism: Hepatic; rapidly demethylated to N-desmethylmethsuximide (active metabolite)

Half-life elimination: 2-4 hours

Time to peak, serum: Within 1-3 hours

Excretion: Urine (<1% as unchanged drug)

Pregnancy Risk Factor C

Generic Available No

Methyclothiazide (meth i kloe THYE a zide)

Related Information

Cardiovascular Diseases *on page 1456*

U.S. Brand Names Aquatensen®; Enduron®

Canadian Brand Names Aquatensen®; Enduron®

Pharmacologic Category Diuretic, Thiazide

Use Management of mild to moderate hypertension; treatment of edema in CHF and nephrotic syndrome

Local Anesthetic/Vasoconstrictor Precautions No information available to require special precautions

Effects on Dental Treatment No significant effects or complications reported

Dosage Adults: Oral:

Edema: 2.5-10 mg/day

Hypertension: 2.5-5 mg/day; may add another antihypertensive if 5 mg is not adequate after a trial of 8-12 weeks of therapy

Mechanism of Action Inhibits sodium reabsorption in the distal tubules causing increased excretion of sodium and water, as well as, potassium and hydrogen ions

Other Adverse Effects

1% to 10%:

Cardiovascular: Orthostatic hypotension

Dermatologic: Photosensitivity

Endocrine & metabolic: Hypokalemia

Gastrointestinal: Anorexia, epigastric distress

<1% (Limited to important or life-threatening): Agranulocytosis, aplastic anemia, cutaneous vasculitis, erythema multiforme, hemolytic anemia, hepatic function impairment, hypercalcemia, leukopenia, necrotizing angiitis, pancreatitis, respiratory distress, Stevens-Johnson syndrome, thrombocytopenia, vasculitis

Drug Interactions

Increased effect of methyclothiazide with furosemide and other loop diuretics. Increased hypotension and/or renal adverse effects of ACE inhibitors may result in aggressively diuresed patients. Beta-blockers increase hyperglycemic effects of thiazides in Type 2 diabetes mellitus. Cyclosporine and thiazides can increase the risk of gout or renal toxicity. Digoxin toxicity can be exacerbated if a thiazide induces hypokalemia or hypomagnesemia. Lithium toxicity can occur with thiazides due to reduced renal excretion of lithium. Thiazides may prolong the duration of action with neuromuscular blocking agents.

Decreased effect of oral hypoglycemics. Decreased absorption of thiazides with cholestyramine and colestipol. NSAIDs can decrease the efficacy of thiazides, reducing the diuretic and antihypertensive effects.

Dietary/Ethanol/Herb Considerations

Ethanol: Avoid use; may increase risk of hypotension or dizziness.

Food: Avoid caffeine, garlic, and licorice.

Herb/Nutraceutical: Avoid black cohosh, dong quai, and evening primrose due to estrogenic activity; dong quai may also cause photosensitization. Avoid ephedra, ginseng, and yohimbe; may worsen hypertension. Avoid garlic; may have increased antihypertensive effect. Avoid ginger due to positive inotropic effects; theoretically, may cause arrhythmia. Avoid hawthorn; may lower peripheral vascular resistance causing additional decrease in BP. Avoid licorice. Avoid St John's wort; may cause photosensitization.

Pharmacodynamics/Kinetics

Onset of action: Diuresis: 2 hours

Peak effect: 6 hours

Duration: ~1 day

Distribution: Crosses placenta; enters breast milk

Excretion: Urine (as unchanged drug)

Pregnancy Risk Factor B

Generic Available Yes

Methyclothiazide and Deserpidine

(meth i kloe THYE a zide & de SER pi deen)

U.S. Brand Names Enduronyl®; Enduronyl® Forte

Canadian Brand Names Enduronyl®; Enduronyl® Forte

Pharmacologic Category Antihypertensive Agent Combination

Synonyms Deserpidine and Methyclothiazide

Use Management of mild to moderately severe hypertension

Local Anesthetic/Vasoconstrictor Precautions No information available to require special precautions

Effects on Dental Treatment No significant effects or complications reported

Dosage Oral: Individualized, normally 1-4 tablets/day

Pregnancy Risk Factor C
Generic Available No

Methylacetoxyprogesterone *see* MedroxyPROGESTERone *on page 849*

Methylcellulose (meth il SEL yoo lose)

U.S. Brand Names Citrucel® [OTC]; FiberEase™ [OTC]
Pharmacologic Category Laxative
Use Adjunct in treatment of constipation
Local Anesthetic/Vasoconstrictor Precautions No information available to require special precautions
Effects on Dental Treatment No significant effects or complications reported
Dosage Oral:
Children 6-12 years:
Citrucel® caplet: 1 caplet up to 6 times/day; follow each dose with 8 oz of water
Citrucel® powder: Half the adult dose in 4 oz of cold water, 1-3 times/day
Children ≥12 years and Adults:
Citrucel® caplet: 2-4 caplets 1-3 times/day; follow each dose with 8 oz of water
Citrucel® powder: 1 heaping tablespoon (19 g) in 8 oz of cold water, 1-3 times/day
FiberEase™: 2 tablespoonfuls mixed in 7 oz of water, 1-3 times/day
Dietary/Ethanol/Herb Considerations Citrucel® powder (regular orange flavor): Each dose contains sodium 3 mg, potassium 105 mg, and 60 calories from sucrose
Pregnancy Risk Factor C
Generic Available No

Methyldopa (meth il DOE pu)

Related Information
Cardiovascular Diseases *on page 1456*
Canadian Brand Names Apo®-Methyldopa; Nu-Medopa
Mexican Brand Names Aldomet®
Pharmacologic Category Alpha-Adrenergic Inhibitor
Synonyms Methyldopate Hydrochloride
Use Management of moderate to severe hypertension
Local Anesthetic/Vasoconstrictor Precautions No information available to require special precautions
Effects on Dental Treatment 1% to 10%: Xerostomia
Anticholinergic side effects can cause a reduction of saliva production or secretion, contributing to discomfort and dental disease (ie, caries, oral candidiasis and periodontal disease).
Dosage
Children:
Oral: Initial: 10 mg/kg/day in 2-4 divided doses; increase every 2 days as needed to maximum dose of 65 mg/kg/day; do not exceed 3 g/day.
I.V.: 5-10 mg/kg/dose every 6-8 hours up to a total dose of 65 mg/kg/24 hours or 3 g/24 hours
Adults:
Oral: Initial: 250 mg 2-3 times/day; increase every 2 days as needed; usual dose 1-1.5 g/day in 2-4 divided doses; maximum dose: 3 g/day.
I.V.: 250-500 mg every 6-8 hours; maximum dose: 1 g every 6 hours
Dosing interval in renal impairment:
Cl_{cr} >50 mL/minute: Administer every 8 hours.
Cl_{cr} 10-50 mL/minute: Administer every 8-12 hours.
Cl_{cr} <10 mL/minute: Administer every 12-24 hours.
Hemodialysis: Slightly dialyzable (5% to 20%)
Mechanism of Action Stimulation of central alpha-adrenergic receptors by a false transmitter that results in a decreased sympathetic outflow to the heart, kidneys, and peripheral vasculature
Other Adverse Effects
>10%: Cardiovascular: Peripheral edema
1% to 10%:
Central nervous system: Drug fever, mental depression, anxiety, nightmares, drowsiness, headache
<1% (Limited to important or life-threatening): Orthostatic hypotension, bradycardia (sinus), sodium retention, sexual dysfunction, gynecomastia, hyperprolactinemia, thrombocytopenia, hemolytic anemia, positive Coombs' test, leukopenia, transient leukopenia or granulocytopenia, cholestasis or hepatitis and heptocellular injury, increased liver enzymes, jaundice, cirrhosis, dyspnea, SLE-like syndrome
Drug Interactions
Increased Effect/Toxicity: Beta-blockers, MAO inhibitors, phenothiazines, and sympathomimetics (including epinephrine) may result in hypertension (sometimes severe) when combined with methyldopa. Methyldopa may increase lithium serum levels resulting in lithium toxicity. Levodopa may cause enhanced blood pressure lowering; methyldopa may also potentiate the effect of levodopa. Tolbutamide, haloperidol, and anesthetics effects/toxicity are increased with methyldopa.
(Continued)

Methyldopa *(Continued)*

Decreased Effect: Iron supplements can interact and cause a significant **increase** in blood pressure. Ferrous sulfate and ferrous gluconate decrease bioavailability. Barbiturates and TCAs may reduce response to methyldopa.

Dietary/Ethanol/Herb Considerations

Ethanol: Avoid use; may increase risk of hypotension or dizziness.

Food: Avoid caffeine, garlic, and licorice.

Herb/Nutraceutical: Avoid black cohosh, dong quai, and evening primrose due to estrogenic activity. Avoid ephedra, ginseng, and yohimbe; may worsen hypertension. Avoid garlic; may have increased antihypertensive effect. Avoid ginger due to positive inotropic effects; theoretically, may cause arrhythmia. Avoid gotu kola, kava, SAMe, St John's wort, and valerian; may increase CNS depression. Avoid hawthorn; may lower peripheral vascular resistance resulting in additive decrease in BP. Avoid licorice.

Pharmacodynamics/Kinetics

Onset of action: Peak effect: Hypotensive: Oral/parenteral: 3-6 hours

Duration: 12-24 hours

Distribution: Crosses placenta; enters breast milk

Protein binding: <15%

Metabolism: Intestinal and hepatic

Half-life elimination: 75-80 minutes; End-stage renal disease: 6-16 hours

Excretion: Urine (85% as metabolites) within 24 hours

Pregnancy Risk Factor B

Generic Available Yes

Methyldopa and Chlorothiazide *see* Chlorothiazide and Methyldopa *on page 305*

Methyldopa and Hydrochlorothiazide

(meth il DOE pu & hye droe klore oh THYE a zide)

Related Information

Hydrochlorothiazide *on page 675*

U.S. Brand Names Aldoril®; Aldoril® D

Canadian Brand Names Apo®-Methazide

Pharmacologic Category Antihypertensive Agent Combination

Synonyms Hydrochlorothiazide and Methyldopa

Use Management of moderate to severe hypertension

Local Anesthetic/Vasoconstrictor Precautions No information available to require special precautions

Effects on Dental Treatment Anticholinergic side effects can cause a reduction of saliva production or secretion, contributing to discomfort and dental disease (ie, caries, oral candidiasis and periodontal disease).

Dosage Oral: Dosage titrated on individual components, then switch to combination product; no more than methyldopa 3 g/day and/or hydrochlorothiazide 50 mg/day; maintain initial dose for first 48 hours, then decrease or increase at intervals of not less than 2 days until an adequate response is achieved

Methyldopa 250 mg and hydrochlorothiazide 15 mg: 2-3 times/day

Methyldopa 250 mg and hydrochlorothiazide 25 mg: Twice daily

Methyldopa 500 mg and hydrochlorothiazide 30 mg: Once daily

Other Adverse Effects See individual agents.

Pregnancy Risk Factor C

Generic Available Yes

Methyldopate Hydrochloride *see* Methyldopa *on page 891*

Methylene Blue, Methenamine, Sodium Biphosphate, Phenyl Salicylate, and Hyoscyamine *see* Methenamine, Sodium Biphosphate, Phenyl Salicylate, Methylene Blue, and Hyoscyamine *on page 880*

Methylergometrine Maleate *see* Methylergonovine *on page 892*

Methylergonovine (meth il er goe NOE veen)

U.S. Brand Names Methergine®

Canadian Brand Names Methergine®

Pharmacologic Category Ergot Derivative

Synonyms Methylergometrine Maleate; Methylergonovine Maleate

Use Prevention and treatment of postpartum and postabortion hemorrhage caused by uterine atony or subinvolution

Local Anesthetic/Vasoconstrictor Precautions No information available to require special precautions

Effects on Dental Treatment No significant effects or complications reported

Dosage Adults:

Oral: 0.2 mg 3-4 times/day for 2-7 days

I.M.: 0.2 mg after delivery of anterior shoulder, after delivery of placenta, or during puerperium; may be repeated as required at intervals of 2-4 hours

I.V.: Same dose as I.M., but should not be routinely administered I.V. because of possibility of inducing sudden hypertension and cerebrovascular accident

Mechanism of Action Similar smooth muscle actions as seen with ergotamine; however, it affects primarily uterine smooth muscles producing sustained contractions and thereby shortens the third stage of labor

Other Adverse Effects Frequency not defined:

Cardiovascular: Hypertension, temporary chest pain, palpitations
Central nervous system: Hallucinations, dizziness, seizures, headache
Endocrine & metabolic: Water intoxication
Gastrointestinal: Nausea, vomiting, diarrhea, foul taste
Local: Thrombophlebitis
Neuromuscular & skeletal: Leg cramps
Otic: Tinnitus
Renal: Hematuria
Respiratory: Dyspnea, nasal congestion
Miscellaneous: Diaphoresis

Drug Interactions Substrate of **CYP3A4**

Increased effect with antifungals (azole derivatives); CYP3A4 inhibitors (eg, amiodarone, cimetidine, erythromycin, ritonavir); macrolide antibiotics; protease inhibitors; MAO inhibitors; beta blockers (vasoconstriction); sumatriptan (vasospasm); vasoconstrictors. Methylergonovine may increase the effects of sibutramine and other serotonin agonists (serotonin syndrome).

Decreased effect with antipsychotics, metoclopramide/

Pharmacodynamics/Kinetics

Onset of action: Oxytocic: Oral: 5-10 minutes; I.M.: 2-5 minutes; I.V.: Immediately
Duration: Oral: ~3 hours; I.M.: ~3 hours; I.V.: 45 minutes
Absorption: Rapid
Distribution: Rapid; primarily to plasma and extracellular fluid following I.V. administration; tissues
Metabolism: Hepatic
Half-life elimination: Biphasic: Initial: 1-5 minutes; Terminal: 0.5-2 hours
Time to peak, serum: 0.5-3 hours
Excretion: Urine and feces

Pregnancy Risk Factor C

Generic Available No

Methylergonovine Maleate *see* Methylergonovine *on page 892*
Methylin™ *see* Methylphenidate *on page 893*
Methylin™ ER *see* Methylphenidate *on page 893*
Methylmorphine *see* Codeine *on page 361*

Methylphenidate (meth il FEN i date)

U.S. Brand Names Concerta®; Metadate® CD; Metadate™ ER; Methylin™; Methylin™ ER; Ritalin®; Ritalin® LA; Ritalin-SR®

Canadian Brand Names PMS-Methylphenidate; Riphenidate; Ritalin®; Ritalin® SR

Mexican Brand Names Ritalin®

Pharmacologic Category Central Nervous System Stimulant

Synonyms Methylphenidate Hydrochloride

Use Treatment of attention-deficit/hyperactivity disorder (ADHD); symptomatic management of narcolepsy

Unlabeled/Investigational Use Treatment of depression (especially elderly or medically ill)

Local Anesthetic/Vasoconstrictor Precautions No information available to require special precautions

Effects on Dental Treatment Up to 10% of patients taking dextroamphetamines or amphetamine-like drugs may present with hypertension. The use of local anesthetic without vasoconstrictor is recommended in these patients.

Restrictions C-II

Dosage Oral (discontinue periodically to re-evaluate or if no improvement occurs within 1 month):

Children ≥6 years: ADHD: Initial: 0.3 mg/kg/dose or 2.5-5 mg/dose given before breakfast and lunch; increase by 0.1 mg/kg/dose or by 5-10 mg/day at weekly intervals; usual dose: 0.5-1 mg/kg/day; maximum dose: 2 mg/kg/day or 90 mg/day

Extended release products:

- Metadate™ ER, Methylin™ ER, Ritalin® SR: Duration of action is 8 hours. May be given in place of regular tablets, once the daily dose is titrated using the regular tablets and the titrated 8-hour dosage corresponds to sustained release tablet size.
- Metadate® CD, Ritalin® LA: Initial: 20 mg once daily; may be adjusted in 10-20 mg increments at weekly intervals; maximum: 60 mg/day
- Concerta™: Duration of action is 12 hours:
  - Children not currently taking methylphenidate:
    - Initial: 18 mg once daily in the morning
    - Adjustment: May increase to maximum of 54 mg/day in increments of 18 mg/day; dose may be adjusted at weekly intervals

(Continued)

Methylphenidate *(Continued)*

Children currently taking methylphenidate: **Note:** Dosing based on current regimen and clinical judgment; suggested dosing listed below:

Patients taking methylphenidate 5 mg 2-3 times/day or 20 mg/day sustained release formulation: Initial dose: 18 mg once every morning (maximum: 54 mg/day)

Patients taking methylphenidate 10 mg 2-3 times/day or 40 mg/day sustained release formulation: Initial dose: 36 mg once every morning (maximum: 54 mg/day)

Patients taking methylphenidate 15 mg 2-3 times/day or 60 mg/day sustained release formulation: Initial dose: 54 mg once every morning (maximum: 54 mg/day)

Note: A 27 mg dosage strength is available for situations in which a dosage between 18 mg and 36 mg is desired.

Adults:

Narcolepsy: 10 mg 2-3 times/day, up to 60 mg/day

Depression (unlabeled use): Initial: 2.5 mg every morning before 9 AM; dosage may be increased by 2.5-5 mg every 2-3 days as tolerated to a maximum of 20 mg/day; may be divided (ie, 7 AM and 12 noon), but should not be given after noon; do not use sustained release product

Mechanism of Action Mild CNS stimulant; blocks the reuptake mechanism of dopaminergic neurons; appears to stimulate the cerebral cortex and subcortical structures similar to amphetamines

Other Adverse Effects Frequency not defined:

Cardiovascular: Angina, cardiac arrhythmias, cerebral arteritis, cerebral occlusion, hypertension, hypotension, palpitations, pulse increase/decrease, tachycardia

Central nervous system: Depression, dizziness, drowsiness, fever, headache, insomnia, nervousness, neuroleptic malignant syndrome (NMS), Tourette's syndrome, toxic psychosis

Dermatologic: Erythema multiforme, exfoliative dermatitis, hair loss, rash, urticaria

Endocrine & metabolic: Growth retardation

Gastrointestinal: Abdominal pain, anorexia, nausea, vomiting, weight loss

Hematologic: Anemia, leukopenia, thrombocytopenic purpura

Hepatic: Abnormal LFTs, hepatic coma, transaminase elevation

Neuromuscular & skeletal: Arthralgia, dyskinesia

Ocular: Blurred vision

Renal: Necrotizing vasculitis

Respiratory: Cough increased, pharyngitis, sinusitis, upper respiratory tract infection

Miscellaneous: Hypersensitivity reactions

Drug Interactions Substrate of **CYP2D6**; Inhibits CYP2D6

Increased Effect/Toxicity: Methylphenidate may cause hypertensive effects when used in combination with MAO inhibitors or drugs with MAO-inhibiting activity (linezolid). Risk may be less with selegiline (MAO type B selective at low doses); it is best to avoid this combination. NMS has been reported in a patient receiving methylphenidate and venlafaxine. Methylphenidate may increase levels of phenytoin, phenobarbital, TCAs, and warfarin. Increased toxicity with clonidine and sibutramine.

Decreased Effect: Effectiveness of antihypertensive agents may be decreased. Carbamazepine may decrease the effect of methylphenidate.

Dietary/Ethanol/Herb Considerations

Ethanol: Avoid use; may cause CNS depression.

Food may increase oral absorption; administer 30-45 minutes before meals. Concerta™ is not affected by food and may be taken with meals. Metadate® CD should be taken before breakfast; food delays early peak and high-fat meals increase C_{max} and AUC. Metadate™ ER should be taken before breakfast and lunch.

Herb/Nutraceutical: Avoid ephedra, ginseng, and yohimbe; may cause hypertension or arrhythmias. Avoid gotu kola, kava, SAMe, St John's wort, and valerian; may increase CNS depression.

Pharmacodynamics/Kinetics

Onset of action: Peak effect:

Immediate release tablet: Cerebral stimulation: ~2 hours

Extended release capsule (Metadate® CD): Biphasic; initial peak similar to immediate release product, followed by second rising portion (corresponding to extended release portion)

Sustained release tablet: 4-7 hours

Osmotic release tablet (Concerta®): Initial: 1-2 hours

Duration: Immediate release tablet: 3-6 hours; Sustained release tablet: 8 hours

Absorption: Readily

Metabolism: Hepatic via de-esterification to active metabolite

Half-life elimination: 2-4 hours

Time to peak: C_{max}: 6-8 hours

Excretion: Urine (90% as metabolites and unchanged drug)

Pregnancy Risk Factor C

Generic Available Yes: Tablet

Methylphenidate Hydrochloride *see* Methylphenidate *on page 893*

Methylphenobarbital *see* Mephobarbital *on page 860*

Methylphenyl Isoxazolyl Penicillin *see* Oxacillin *on page 1007*

Methylphytyl Napthoquinone *see* Phytonadione *on page 1079*

MethylPREDNISolone (meth il pred NIS oh lone)

Related Information

Respiratory Diseases *on page 1476*

U.S. Brand Names A-Methapred®; Depo-Medrol®; Medrol®; Solu-Medrol®

Canadian Brand Names Depo-Medrol®; Medrol®; Solu-Medrol®

Mexican Brand Names Cryosolona

Pharmacologic Category Corticosteroid, Systemic

Synonyms 6-α-Methylprednisolone; Methylprednisolone Acetate; Methylprednisolone Sodium Succinate

Use

Dental: Treatment of a variety of oral diseases of allergic, inflammatory, or autoimmune origin

Medical: Anti-inflammatory or immunosuppressant agent in the treatment of a variety of diseases including those of hematologic, allergic, inflammatory, neoplastic, and autoimmune origin; prevention and treatment of graft-versus-host disease following allogeneic bone marrow transplantation

Unlabeled/Investigational Use Treatment of fibrosing-alveolitis phase of adult respiratory distress syndrome (ARDS)

Local Anesthetic/Vasoconstrictor Precautions No information available to require special precautions

Effects on Dental Treatment Frequency not defined: Hypertension, arrhythmias, nervousness, seizures, psychoses, headache, delirium, hallucinations, euphoria, skin atrophy, bruising, diabetes mellitus, hyperglycemia, peptic ulcer, nausea, vomiting, ulcerative esophagitis, weakness, increased fractures, infections, hypersensitivity reactions, intractable hiccups, pseudotumor cerebri, mood swings, osteoporosis

Dosage Dosing should be based on the lesser of ideal body weight or actual body weight. **Only sodium succinate may be given I.V.;** methylprednisolone sodium succinate is highly soluble and has a rapid effect by I.M. and I.V. routes. Methylprednisolone acetate has a low solubility and has a sustained I.M. effect.

Children:

Anti-inflammatory or immunosuppressive: Oral, I.M., I.V. (sodium succinate): 0.5-1.7 mg/kg/day **or** 5-25 mg/m²/day in divided doses every 6-12 hours; "Pulse" therapy: 15-30 mg/kg/dose over ≥30 minutes given once daily for 3 days

Status asthmaticus: I.V. (sodium succinate): Loading dose: 2 mg/kg/dose, then 0.5-1 mg/kg/dose every 6 hours for up to 5 days

Acute spinal cord injury: I.V. (sodium succinate): 30 mg/kg over 15 minutes, followed in 45 minutes by a continuous infusion of 5.4 mg/kg/hour for 23 hours

Lupus nephritis: I.V. (sodium succinate): 30 mg/kg over ≥30 minutes every other day for 6 doses

Adults:

Anti-inflammatory or immunosuppressive:

Oral: 2-60 mg/day in 1-4 divided doses to start, followed by gradual reduction in dosage to the lowest possible level consistent with maintaining an adequate clinical response.

I.M. (sodium succinate): 10-80 mg/day once daily

I.M. (acetate): 10-80 mg every 1-2 weeks

I.V. (sodium succinate): 10-40 mg over a period of several minutes and repeated I.V. or I.M. at intervals depending on clinical response; when high dosages are needed, give 30 mg/kg over a period ≥30 minutes and may be repeated every 4-6 hours for 48 hours.

Acute spinal cord injury: I.V. (sodium succinate): 30 mg/kg over 15 minutes, followed in 45 minutes by a continuous infusion of 5.4 mg/kg/hour for 23 hours

Status asthmaticus: I.V. (sodium succinate): Loading dose: 2 mg/kg/dose, then 0.5-1 mg/kg/dose every 6 hours for up to 5 days

High-dose therapy for acute spinal cord injury: I.V. bolus: 30 mg/kg over 15 minutes, followed 45 minutes later by an infusion of 5.4 mg/kg/hour for 23 hours

Lupus nephritis: High-dose "pulse" therapy: I.V. (sodium succinate): 1 g/day for 3 days

Aplastic anemia: I.V. (sodium succinate): 1 mg/kg/day or 40 mg/day (whichever dose is higher), for 4 days. After 4 days, change to oral and continue until day 10 or until symptoms of serum sickness resolve, then rapidly reduce over approximately 2 weeks.

Pneumocystis pneumonia in AIDs patients: I.V.: 40-60 mg every 6 hours for 7-10 days

Intra-articular (acetate): Administer every 1-5 weeks.

Large joints: 20-80 mg

(Continued)

MethylPREDNISolone *(Continued)*

Small joints: 4-10 mg
Intralesional (acetate): 20-60 mg every 1-5 weeks

Mechanism of Action In a tissue-specific manner, corticosteroids regulate gene expression subsequent to binding specific intracellular receptors and translocation into the nucleus. Corticosteroids exert a wide array of physiologic effects including modulation of carbohydrate, protein, and lipid metabolism and maintenance of fluid and electrolyte homeostasis. Moreover cardiovascular, immunologic, musculoskeletal, endocrine, and neurologic physiology are influenced by corticosteroids. Decreases inflammation by suppression of migration of polymorphonuclear leukocytes and reversal of increased capillary permeability.

Other Adverse Effects Frequency not defined:

Cardiovascular: Edema
Central nervous system: Insomnia, vertigo
Dermatologic: Hirsutism, acne, hyperpigmentation
Endocrine & metabolic: Adrenal suppression, hyperlipidemia, Cushing's syndrome, pituitary-adrenal axis suppression, growth suppression, glucose intolerance, hypokalemia, alkalosis, amenorrhea, sodium and water retention
Gastrointestinal: Increased appetite, indigestion, abdominal distention, pancreatitis
Hematologic: Transient leukocytosis
Neuromuscular & skeletal: Arthralgia
Ocular: Cataracts, glaucoma
Miscellaneous: Avascular necrosis, secondary malignancy

Contraindications Hypersensitivity to methylprednisolone or any component of the formulation; viral, fungal, or tubercular skin lesions; administration of live virus vaccines; serious infections, except septic shock or tuberculous meningitis. Methylprednisolone formulations containing benzyl alcohol preservative are contraindicated in infants.

Warnings/Precautions Use with caution in patients with hyperthyroidism, cirrhosis, nonspecific ulcerative colitis, hypertension, osteoporosis, thromboembolic tendencies, CHF, convulsive disorders, myasthenia gravis, thrombophlebitis, peptic ulcer, diabetes, glaucoma, cataracts, or tuberculosis. Use caution in hepatic impairment. Because of the risk of adverse effects, systemic corticosteroids should be used cautiously in the elderly, in the smallest possible dose, and for the shortest possible time

Acute adrenal insufficiency may occur with abrupt withdrawal after long-term therapy or with stress; young pediatric patients may be more susceptible to adrenal axis suppression from topical therapy

Drug Interactions Substrate of CYP3A4; Inhibits CYP3A4

Increased Toxicity:

Skin test antigens, immunizations decrease response and increase potential infections
Methylprednisolone may increase circulating glucose levels and may need adjustments of insulin or oral hypoglycemics

Decreased Effect:

Phenytoin, phenobarbital, rifampin increase clearance of methylprednisolone
Potassium depleting diuretics enhance potassium depletion

Dietary/Ethanol/Herb Considerations

Ethanol: Avoid use; may increase gastric mucosal irritation.
Food: Administer after meals or with food or milk. Methylprednisolone interferes with calcium absorption; requires diet rich in pyridoxine, vitamin C, vitamin D, folate, calcium, phosphorus, and protein. Limit caffeine.
Herb/Nutraceutical: Avoid cat's claw and echinacea due to immunostimulant properties. Avoid St John's wort; may decrease serum concentration.

Pharmacodynamics/Kinetics

Onset of action: Peak effect (route dependent): Oral: 1-2 hours; I.M.: 4-8 days; Intra-articular: 1 week; methylprednisolone sodium succinate is highly soluble and has a rapid effect by I.M. and I.V. routes
Duration (route dependent): Oral: 30-36 hours; I.M.: 1-4 weeks; Intra-articular: 1-5 weeks; methylprednisolone acetate has a low solubility and has a sustained I.M. effect
Distribution: V_d: 0.7-1.5 L/kg
Half-life elimination: 3-3.5 hours; reduced in obese
Excretion: Clearance: Reduced in obese

Pregnancy Risk Factor C

Dosage Forms **INJ, powder for reconstitution, as sodium succinate:** 40 mg, 125 mg, 500 mg; (A-Methapred®): 40 mg, 125 mg, 500 mg, 1000 mg; (Solu-Medrol®): 40 mg, 125 mg, 500 mg, 1 g, 2 g; (Solu-Medrol®): 500 mg, 1 g. **INJ, suspension, as acetate** (Depo-Medrol®): 20 mg/mL (5 mL); 40 mg/mL (5 mL); 80 mg/mL (5 mL). **INJ, suspension, as acetate** [single-dose vial] (Depo-Medrol®): 40 mg/mL (1 mL); 80 mg/mL (1 mL). **TAB:** 4 mg; (Medrol®): 2 mg, 4 mg, 8 mg, 16 mg, 32 mg. **TAB** [dose-pack]: 4 mg (21s)

Generic Available Yes

6-α-Methylprednisolone *see* MethylPREDNISolone *on page 895*

Methylprednisolone Acetate *see* MethylPREDNISolone *on page 895*
Methylprednisolone Sodium Succinate *see* MethylPREDNISolone *on page 895*
4-Methylpyrazole *see* Fomepizole *on page 609*
Methylrosaniline Chloride *see* Gentian Violet *on page 636*

MethylTESTOSTERone (meth il tes TOS te rone)

U.S. Brand Names Android®; Methitest®; Testred®; Virilon®

Pharmacologic Category Androgen

Use
Male: Hypogonadism; delayed puberty; impotence and climacteric symptoms
Female: Palliative treatment of metastatic breast cancer

Local Anesthetic/Vasoconstrictor Precautions No information available to require special precautions

Effects on Dental Treatment Frequency not defined: Headache, anxiety, GI irritation, nausea, vomiting, hypersensitivity reactions

Restrictions C-III

Dosage Adults (buccal absorption produces twice the androgenic activity of oral tablets):
Male:
- Hypogonadism, male climacteric and impotence: Oral: 10-40 mg/day
- Androgen deficiency:
  - Oral: 10-50 mg/day
  - Buccal: 5-25 mg/day
- Postpubertal cryptorchidism: Oral: 30 mg/day

Female:
- Breast pain/engorgement:
  - Oral: 80 mg/day for 3-5 days
  - Buccal: 40 mg/day for 3-5 days
- Breast cancer:
  - Oral: 50-200 mg/day
  - Buccal: 25-100 mg/day

Mechanism of Action Stimulates receptors in organs and tissues to promote growth and development of male sex organs and maintains secondary sex characteristics in androgen-deficient males

Other Adverse Effects Frequency not defined:
Male: Virilism, priapism, prostatic hyperplasia, prostatic carcinoma, impotence, testicular atrophy, gynecomastia
Female: Virilism, menstrual problems (amenorrhea), breast soreness, hirsutism (increase in pubic hair growth) atrophy
Cardiovascular: Edema
Central nervous system: Depression
Dermatologic: Acne, "male pattern" baldness, seborrhea
Endocrine & metabolic: Hypercalcemia, hypercholesterolemia
Hematologic: Leukopenia, polycythemia
Hepatic: Hepatic dysfunction, hepatic necrosis, cholestatic hepatitis

Drug Interactions
Increased effect of oral anticoagulants and hypoglycemic agents.
Increased toxicity may occur with cyclosporine; avoid concurrent use.
Decreased effect or oral anticoagulants.

Pharmacodynamics/Kinetics
Metabolism: Hepatic
Excretion: Urine

Pregnancy Risk Factor X

Generic Available No

Methysergide (meth i SER jide)

U.S. Brand Names Sansert® [DSC]

Canadian Brand Names Sansert®

Pharmacologic Category Ergot Derivative

Synonyms Methysergide Maleate; Sansert® [DSC]

Use Prophylaxis of vascular headache

Local Anesthetic/Vasoconstrictor Precautions No information available to require special precautions

Effects on Dental Treatment No significant effects or complications reported

Dosage Adults: Oral: 4-8 mg/day with meals; if no improvement is noted after 3 weeks, drug is unlikely to be beneficial; must not be given continuously for longer than 6 months, and a drug-free interval of 3-4 weeks must follow each 6-month course

Mechanism of Action Ergotamine congener, however, actions appear to differ; methysergide has minimal ergotamine-like oxytocic or vasoconstrictive properties, and has significantly greater serotonin-like properties

Other Adverse Effects Frequency not defined:
Cardiovascular: Postural hypotension, peripheral ischemia, peripheral edema, tachycardia, bradycardia, edema
(Continued)

Methysergide *(Continued)*

Central nervous system: Insomnia, drowsiness, euphoria, dizziness, seizures, fever
Dermatologic: Rash, telangiectasia, flushing
Endocrine & metabolic: Weight gain
Gastrointestinal: Nausea, vomiting, abdominal pain, diarrhea, heartburn
Hematologic: Neutropenia, eosinophilia, thrombocytopenia
Neuromuscular & skeletal: Weakness, myalgia, arthralgia
Note: Fibrotic complications: Retroperitoneal, pleuropulmonary, cardiac (aortic root, aortic valve, mitral valve) fibrosis, and Peyronie's disease have been reported.

Drug Interactions Substrate of **CYP3A4**

Increased effect with antifungals (azole derivatives); CYP3A4 inhibitors (eg, amiodarone, cimetidine, erythromycin, ritonavir); macrolide antibiotics; protease inhibitors; MAO inhibitors; sumatriptan (vasospasm). Methysergide may increase the effects of sibutramine and other serotonin agonists (serotonin syndrome).

Dietary/Ethanol/Herb Considerations Food: Administer with food.

Pharmacodynamics/Kinetics

Metabolism: Hepatic to methylergonovine and glucuronide metabolite
Half-life elimination: ~10 hours

Pregnancy Risk Factor X

Generic Available No

Methysergide Maleate *see* Methysergide *on page 897*

Metipranolol (met i PRAN oh lol)

U.S. Brand Names OptiPranolol®

Canadian Brand Names OptiPranolol®

Pharmacologic Category Beta Blocker, Nonselective; Ophthalmic Agent, Antiglaucoma

Synonyms Metipranolol Hydrochloride

Use Agent for lowering intraocular pressure in patients with chronic open-angle glaucoma

Local Anesthetic/Vasoconstrictor Precautions No information available to require special precautions

Effects on Dental Treatment Metipranolol is a nonselective beta-blocker and may enhance the pressor response to epinephrine, resulting in hypertension and bradycardia. Many nonsteroidal anti-inflammatory drugs such as ibuprofen and indomethacin can reduce the hypotensive effect of beta-blockers after 3 or more weeks of therapy with the NSAID. Short-term NSAID use (ie, 3 days) requires no special precautions in patients taking beta-blockers.

Dosage Ophthalmic: Adults: Instill 1 drop in the affected eye(s) twice daily

Mechanism of Action Beta-adrenoceptor-blocking agent; lacks intrinsic sympathomimetic activity and membrane-stabilizing effects and possesses only slight local anesthetic activity; mechanism of action of metipranolol in reducing intraocular pressure appears to be via reduced production of aqueous humor. This effect may be related to a reduction in blood flow to the iris root-ciliary body. It remains unclear if the reduction in intraocular pressure observed with beta-blockers is actually secondary to beta-adrenoceptor blockade.

Other Adverse Effects

>10%: Ocular: Mild ocular stinging and discomfort, eye irritation
1% to 10%: Ocular: Blurred vision, browache
<1%: Bradycardia, AV block, CHF, erythema, weakness, conjunctivitis, blepharitis, tearing, itching eyes, keratitis, photophobia, decreased corneal sensitivity, bronchospasm

Pharmacodynamics/Kinetics

Onset of action: ≤30 minutes
Peak effect: Maximum: ~2 hours
Duration: Intraocular pressure reduction: Up to 24 hours
Metabolism: Rapid and complete to deacetyl metipranolol, an active metabolite
Half-life elimination: ~3 hours

Pregnancy Risk Factor C

Generic Available Yes

Metipranolol Hydrochloride *see* Metipranolol *on page 898*

Metoclopramide (met oh kloe PRA mide)

Related Information

Endocrine Disorders and Pregnancy *on page 1479*

U.S. Brand Names Reglan®

Canadian Brand Names Apo®-Metoclop; Nu-Metoclopramide

Mexican Brand Names Carnotprim®; Carnotprim Primperan®; Carnotprim Primperan® Retard; Clorimet®; Meclomid®; Plasil®; Pramotil

Pharmacologic Category Gastrointestinal Agent, Prokinetic

Use Prevention and/or treatment of nausea and vomiting associated with chemotherapy, radiation therapy, or postsurgery; symptomatic treatment of diabetic gastric stasis; gastroesophageal reflux; facilitation of intubation of the small intestine

Local Anesthetic/Vasoconstrictor Precautions No information available to require special precautions

Effects on Dental Treatment 1% to 10%: Xerostomia

Dosage

Children:

Gastroesophageal reflux: Oral: 0.1-0.2 mg/kg/dose up to 4 times/day; efficacy of continuing metoclopramide beyond 12 weeks in reflux has not been determined; total daily dose should not exceed 0.5 mg/kg/day

Gastrointestinal hypomotility (gastroparesis): Oral, I.M., I.V.: 0.1 mg/kg/dose up to 4 times/day, not to exceed 0.5 mg/kg/day

Antiemetic (chemotherapy-induced emesis): I.V.: 1-2 mg/kg 30 minutes before chemotherapy and every 2-4 hours

Facilitate intubation: I.V.:

<6 years: 0.1 mg/kg

6-14 years: 2.5-5 mg

Adults:

Gastroesophageal reflux: Oral: 10-15 mg/dose up to 4 times/day 30 minutes before meals or food and at bedtime; single doses of 20 mg are occasionally needed for provoking situations; efficacy of continuing metoclopramide beyond 12 weeks in reflux has not been determined

Gastrointestinal hypomotility (gastroparesis):

Oral: 10 mg 30 minutes before each meal and at bedtime for 2-8 weeks

I.V. (for severe symptoms): 10 mg over 1-2 minutes; 10 days of I.V. therapy may be necessary for best response

Antiemetic (chemotherapy-induced emesis): I.V.: 1-2 mg/kg 30 minutes before chemotherapy and every 2-4 hours to every 4-6 hours (and usually given with diphenhydramine 25-50 mg I.V./oral)

Postoperative nausea and vomiting: I.M.: 10 mg near end of surgery; 20 mg doses may be used

Facilitate intubation: I.V.: 10 mg

Elderly:

Gastroesophageal reflux: Oral: 5 mg 4 times/day (30 minutes before meals and at bedtime); increase dose to 10 mg 4 times/day if no response at lower dose

Gastrointestinal hypomotility:

Oral: Initial: 5 mg 30 minutes before meals and at bedtime for 2-8 weeks; increase if necessary to 10 mg doses

I.V.: Initiate at 5 mg over 1-2 minutes; increase to 10 mg if necessary

Postoperative nausea and vomiting: I.M.: 5 mg near end of surgery; may repeat dose if necessary

Dosing adjustment in renal impairment:

Cl_{cr} 10-40 mL/minute: Administer at 50% of normal dose

Cl_{cr} <10 mL/minute: Administer at 25% of normal dose

Hemodialysis: Not dialyzable (0% to 5%); supplemental dose is unnecessary

Mechanism of Action Blocks dopamine receptors in chemoreceptor trigger zone of the CNS; enhances the response to acetylcholine of tissue in upper GI tract causing enhanced motility and accelerated gastric emptying without stimulating gastric, biliary, or pancreatic secretions

Other Adverse Effects Adverse reactions are more common/severe at dosages used for prophylaxis of chemotherapy-induced emesis.

>10%:

Central nervous system: Restlessness, drowsiness, extrapyramidal symptoms (high-dose, up to 34%)

Gastrointestinal: Diarrhea (may be dose-limiting)

Neuromuscular & skeletal: Weakness

1% to 10%:

Central nervous system: Insomnia, depression

Dermatologic: Rash

Endocrine & metabolic: Breast tenderness, prolactin stimulation

Gastrointestinal: Nausea

<1%: Agitation, agranulocytosis, allergic reaction, anxiety, AV block, bradycardia, CHF, constipation, fatigue, fluid retention, gynecomastia, hepatotoxicity, hypertension or hypotension, hyperprolactinemia, jaundice, methemoglobinemia, neuroleptic malignant syndrome (NMS), neutropenia, sulfhemoglobinemia, tachycardia, tardive dyskinesia

Drug Interactions Substrate of CYP1A2, 2D6; Inhibits CYP2D6

Increased Effect/Toxicity: Opiate analgesics may increase CNS depression. Metoclopramide may increase extrapyramidal symptoms (EPS) or risk when used concurrently with antipsychotic agents.

Decreased Effect: Anticholinergic agents antagonize metoclopramide's actions.

Dietary/Ethanol/Herb Considerations

Ethanol: Avoid use; may lead to increased CNS depression.

Herb/Nutraceutical: Avoid gotu kola, kava, SAMe, St John's wort, and valerian; may increase CNS depression.

(Continued)

Metoclopramide *(Continued)*

Pharmacodynamics/Kinetics

Onset of action: Oral: 0.5-1 hour; I.V.: 1-3 minutes

Duration: Therapeutic: 1-2 hours, regardless of route

Distribution: V_d: 2-4 L/kg; Crosses placenta; enters breast milk

Protein binding: 30% to 40%, primarily to α_1-acid glycoprotein

Half-life elimination: Normal renal function: 4-7 hours (may be dose dependent)

Time to peak, serum: Oral: 1-3 hours; I.M.: 2-3 hours; I.V.: Within 5 minutes; Rectal: 1-8 hours

Excretion: Urine (70% to 85%, ~19% as unchanged drug); feces (2% to 3%)

Pregnancy Risk Factor B

Generic Available Yes

Metolazone (me TOLE a zone)

Related Information

Cardiovascular Diseases *on page 1456*

U.S. Brand Names Mykrox®; Zaroxolyn®

Canadian Brand Names Mykrox®; Zaroxolyn®

Pharmacologic Category Diuretic, Thiazide-Related

Use Management of mild to moderate hypertension; treatment of edema in CHF and nephrotic syndrome, impaired renal function

Local Anesthetic/Vasoconstrictor Precautions No information available to require special precautions

Effects on Dental Treatment No significant effects or complications reported

Dosage Adults: Oral:

Edema: 5-20 mg/dose every 24 hours

Hypertension: 2.5-5 mg/dose every 24 hours

Hypertension (Mykrox®): 0.5 mg/day; if response is not adequate, increase dose to maximum of 1 mg/day

Dialysis: Not dialyzable (0% to 5%) via hemo- or peritoneal dialysis; supplemental dose is unnecessary

Mechanism of Action Inhibits sodium reabsorption in the distal tubules causing increased excretion of sodium and water, as well as, potassium and hydrogen ions

Other Adverse Effects

>10%: Central nervous system: Dizziness

1% to 10%:

Cardiovascular: Orthostatic hypotension, palpitations, chest pain, cold extremities (rapidly acting), edema (rapidly acting), venous thrombosis (slow acting), syncope (slow acting)

Central nervous system: Headache, fatigue, lethargy, malaise, lassitude, anxiety, depression, nervousness, "weird" feeling (rapidly acting), chills (slow acting)

Dermatologic: Rash, pruritus, dry skin (rapidly acting)

Endocrine & metabolic: Hypokalemia, impotence, reduced libido, excessive volume depletion (slow acting), hemoconcentration (slow acting), acute gouty attach (slow acting), weakness

Gastrointestinal: Nausea, vomiting, abdominal pain, cramping, bloating, diarrhea or constipation, xerostomia

Genitourinary: Nocturia

Neuromuscular & skeletal: Muscle cramps, spasm

Ocular: Eye itching (rapidly acting)

Otic: Tinnitus (rapidly acting)

Respiratory: Cough (rapidly acting), epistaxis (rapidly acting), sinus congestion (rapidly acting), sore throat (rapidly acting),

<1% (Limited to important or life-threatening): Agranulocytosis, aplastic anemia, glycosuria, hepatitis, hypercalcemia, hyperglycemia, leukopenia, pancreatitis, purpura, Stevens-Johnson syndrome, thrombocytopenia, toxic epidermal necrolysis

Drug Interactions

Increased Effect/Toxicity: Increased diuretic effect of metolazone with furosemide and other loop diuretics. Increased hypotension and/or renal adverse effects of ACE inhibitors may result in aggressively diuresed patients. Cyclosporine and thiazide-type diuretics can increase the risk of gout or renal toxicity. Digoxin toxicity can be exacerbated if a diuretic induces hypokalemia or hypomagnesemia. Lithium toxicity can occur with thiazide-type diuretics due to reduced renal excretion of lithium. Thiazide-type diuretics may prolong the duration of action of neuromuscular blocking agents.

Decreased Effect: Decreased absorption of metolazone with cholestyramine and colestipol. NSAIDs can decrease the efficacy of thiazide-type diuretics, reducing the diuretic and antihypertensive effects.

Dietary/Ethanol/Herb Considerations

Ethanol: Avoid use; may increase risk of hypotension or dizziness.

Food: Administer after breakfast. May require potassium supplementation; include bananas and oranges in diet. Fluids, fruit, and fiber may reduce constipation. Avoid caffeine, garlic, and licorice.

Herb/Nutraceutical: Avoid black cohosh, dong quai, and evening primrose due to estrogenic activity; dong quai may also cause photosensitization. Avoid ephedra, ginseng, and yohimbe; may worsen hypertension. Avoid escin (from the horse chestnut seed); may have additive diuretic effects. Avoid garlic; may have increased antihypertensive effect. Avoid hawthorn; may lower peripheral vascular resistance and cause more BP reductions. Avoid licorice. Avoid St John's wort; may cause photosensitization.

Pharmacodynamics/Kinetics

Onset of action: Diuresis: ~60 minutes

Duration: 12-24 hours

Absorption: Incomplete

Distribution: Crosses placenta; enters breast milk

Protein binding: 95%

Metabolism: Undergoes enterohepatic recirculation

Bioavailability: Mykrox® reportedly has highest

Half-life elimination (renal function dependent): 6-20 hours

Excretion: Urine (80% to 95%)

Pregnancy Risk Factor B (manufacturer); D (expert analysis)

Generic Available No

Metoprolol (me toe PROE lole)

Related Information

Cardiovascular Diseases *on page 1456*

U.S. Brand Names Lopressor®; Toprol-XL®

Canadian Brand Names Apo®-Metoprolol; Betaloc®; Betaloc® Durules®; Lopressor®; Novo-Metoprolol; Nu-Metop; PMS-Metoprolol; Toprol-XL®

Mexican Brand Names Kenaprol; Lopresor®; Proken M®; Prolaken®; Ritmolol®; Selectadril®; Seloken®; Selopres

Pharmacologic Category Beta Blocker, $Beta_1$ Selective

Synonyms Metoprolol Tartrate

Use Treatment of hypertension and angina pectoris; prevention of MI, atrial fibrillation, flutter, symptomatic treatment of hypertrophic subaortic stenosis; to reduce mortality/hospitalization in patients with CHF (stable NYHA Class II or III) in patients already receiving ACE inhibitors, diuretics, and/or digoxin (sustained-release only)

Unlabeled/Investigational Use Treatment of ventricular arrhythmias, atrial ectopy, essential tremor, aggressive behavior; prophylaxis of migraine headaches

Local Anesthetic/Vasoconstrictor Precautions No information available to require special precautions

Effects on Dental Treatment Metoprolol is a cardioselective beta-blocker. Local anesthetic with vasoconstrictor can be safely used in patients medicated with metoprolol. Nonselective beta-blockers (ie, propranolol, nadolol) enhance the pressor response to epinephrine, resulting in hypertension and bradycardia; this has not been reported for metoprolol. Many nonsteroidal anti-inflammatory drugs such as ibuprofen and indomethacin can reduce the hypotensive effect of beta-blockers after 3 or more weeks of therapy with the NSAID. Short-term NSAID use (ie, 3 days) requires no special precautions in patients taking beta-blockers.

Dosage

Children: Oral: 1-5 mg/kg/24 hours divided twice daily; allow 3 days between dose adjustments

Adults:

Hypertension, angina, SVT, MI prophylaxis: Oral: 100-450 mg/day in 2-3 divided doses, begin with 50 mg twice daily and increase doses at weekly intervals to desired effect

Extended release: Same daily dose administered as a single dose

I.V.: Hypertension: Has been given in dosages 1.25-5 mg every 6-12 hours in patients unable to take oral medications

CHF: Oral (extended release): Initial: 25 mg once daily (reduce to 12.5 mg once daily in NYHA class higher than class II); may double dosage every 2 weeks as tolerated, up to 200 mg/day

Myocardial infarction (acute): I.V.: 5 mg every 2 minutes for 3 doses in early treatment of MI; thereafter give 50 mg orally every 6 hours 15 minutes after last I.V. dose and continue for 48 hours; then administer a maintenance dose of 100 mg twice daily.

Elderly: Oral: Initial: 25 mg/day; usual range: 25-300 mg/day

Extended release: 25-50 mg/day initially as a single dose; increase at 1- to 2-week intervals.

Hemodialysis: Administer dose posthemodialysis or administer 50 mg supplemental dose; supplemental dose is unnecessary following peritoneal dialysis

Dosing adjustment in hepatic disease: Reduction probably necessary

Mechanism of Action Selective inhibitor of $beta_1$-adrenergic receptors; competitively blocks $beta_1$-receptors, with little or no effect on $beta_2$-receptors at doses <100 mg; does not exhibit any membrane stabilizing or intrinsic sympathomimetic activity

(Continued)

Metoprolol *(Continued)*

Other Adverse Effects

>10%:

Central nervous system: Drowsiness, insomnia

Endocrine & metabolic: Decreased sexual ability

1% to 10%:

Cardiovascular: Bradycardia, palpitations, edema, CHF, reduced peripheral circulation

Central nervous system: Mental depression

Gastrointestinal: Diarrhea or constipation, nausea, vomiting, stomach discomfort

Respiratory: Bronchospasm

Miscellaneous: Cold extremities

<1% (Limited to important or life-threatening): Arrhythmias, arthralgia, chest pain, confusion (especially in the elderly), depression, dyspnea, hallucinations, headache, hepatic dysfunction, hepatitis, jaundice, leukopenia, nervousness, orthostatic hypotension, thrombocytopenia

Drug Interactions Substrate of CYP2C19, **2D6**; Inhibits CYP2D6

Increased Effect/Toxicity: Metoprolol may increase the effects of other drugs which slow AV conduction (digoxin, verapamil, diltiazem), alpha-blockers (prazosin, terazosin), and alpha-adrenergic stimulants (epinephrine, phenylephrine). Metoprolol may mask the tachycardia from hypoglycemia caused by insulin and oral hypoglycemics. In patients receiving concurrent therapy, the risk of hypertensive crisis is increased when either clonidine or the beta-blocker is withdrawn. Reserpine has been shown to enhance the effect of beta-blockers. Beta-blockers may increase the action or levels of ethanol, disopyramide, nondepolarizing muscle relaxants, and theophylline although the effects are difficult to predict.

Decreased Effect: Decreased effect of beta-blockers with aluminum salts, barbiturates, calcium salts, cholestyramine, colestipol, NSAIDs, penicillins (ampicillin), rifampin, salicylates, and sulfinpyrazone due to decreased bioavailability and plasma levels. Beta-blockers may decrease the effect of sulfonylureas.

Dietary/Ethanol/Herb Considerations

Ethanol: Limit use; may increase risk of hypotension or dizziness.

Food increases absorption and may increase serum concentration. Avoid caffeine, garlic, and licorice.

Herb/Nutraceutical: Avoid black cohosh, dong quai, and evening primrose due to estrogenic activity. Avoid ephedra, ginseng, and yohimbe; may worsen hypertension. Avoid garlic; may have increased antihypertensive effect. Avoid ginger due to positive inotropic effects; theoretically, may cause arrhythmia. Avoid hawthorn; may lower peripheral vascular resistance resulting in additive decrease in BP. Avoid licorice.

Pharmacodynamics/Kinetics

Onset of action: Peak effect: Antihypertensive: Oral: 1.5-4 hours

Duration: 10-20 hours

Absorption: 95%

Protein binding: 8%

Metabolism: Extensively hepatic; significant first-pass effect

Bioavailability: Oral: 40% to 50%

Half-life elimination: 3-4 hours; End-stage renal disease: 2.5-4.5 hours

Excretion: Urine (3% to 10% as unchanged drug)

Pregnancy Risk Factor C (manufacturer); D (2nd and 3rd trimesters - expert analysis)

Generic Available Yes: Injection, tablet (nonextended release)

Selected Readings

Foster CA and Aston SJ, "Propranolol-Epinephrine Interaction: A Potential Disaster," *Plast Reconstr Surg*, 1983, 72(1):74-8.

Wong DG, Spence JD, Lamki L, et al, "Effect of Nonsteroidal Anti-inflammatory Drugs on Control of Hypertension of Beta-Blockers and Diuretics," *Lancet*, 1986, 1(8488):997-1001.

Wynn RL, "Dental Nonsteroidal Anti-inflammatory Drugs and Prostaglandin-Based Drug Interactions, Part Two," *Gen Dent*, 1992, 40(2):104, 106, 108.

Wynn RL, "Epinephrine Interactions With Beta-Blockers," *Gen Dent*, 1994, 42(1):16, 18.

Metoprolol Tartrate *see* Metoprolol *on page 901*

Metrizamide *see* Radiological/Contrast Media (Nonionic) *on page 1165*

MetroCream® *see* Metronidazole *on page 902*

MetroGel® *see* Metronidazole *on page 902*

MetroGel-Vaginal® *see* Metronidazole *on page 902*

MetroLotion® *see* Metronidazole *on page 902*

Metronidazole (me troe NI du zole)

Related Information

Antibiotic Prophylaxis, Preprocedural Guidelines for Dental Patients *on page 1507*

Gastrointestinal Disorders *on page 1474*

Oral Bacterial Infections *on page 1531*

Oral Nonviral Soft Tissue Ulcerations or Erosions *on page 1549*

Periodontal Diseases *on page 1540*

Sexually-Transmitted Diseases *on page 1502*

U.S. Brand Names Flagyl®; Flagyl ER®; MetroCream®; MetroGel®; MetroGel-Vaginal®; MetroLotion®; Noritate™

Canadian Brand Names Apo®-Metronidazole; Flagyl®; Florazole® ER; MetroCream™; Metrogel®; Nidagel™; Noritate®; Novo-Nidazol

Mexican Brand Names Ameblin®; Flagenase®; Flagyl®; Fresenizol®; MetroGel®; Milezzol; Nidrozol®; Otrozol; Selegil®; Servizol®; Vatrix-S; Vertisal®

Pharmacologic Category Amebicide; Antibiotic, Topical; Antibiotic, Miscellaneous; Antiprotozoal

Synonyms Metronidazole Hydrochloride

Use

Dental: Treatment of oral soft tissue infections due to anaerobic bacteria including all anaerobic cocci, anaerobic gram-negative bacilli (*Bacteroides*), and gram-positive spore-forming bacilli (*Clostridium*). Useful as single agent or in combination with amoxicillin, Augmentin®, or ciprofloxacin in the treatment of periodontitis associated with the presence of *Actinobacillus actinomycetemcomitans*, (AA).

Medical: Treatment of susceptible anaerobic bacterial and protozoal infections in the following conditions: Amebiasis, symptomatic and asymptomatic trichomoniasis; skin and skin structure infections; CNS infections; intra-abdominal infections (as part of combination regimen); systemic anaerobic infections; treatment of antibiotic-associated pseudomembranous colitis (AAPC), bacterial vaginosis; as part of a multidrug regimen for *H. pylori* eradication to reduce the risk of duodenal ulcer recurrence; also used in Crohn's disease and hepatic encephalopathy

Orphan drug (MetroGel® Topical): Treatment of acne rosacea

Local Anesthetic/Vasoconstrictor Precautions No information available to require special precautions

Effects on Dental Treatment

Systemic: >10%: Dizziness, headache, nausea (12%), vomiting (12%)

Vaginal: 1% to 10%: Altered taste, xerostomia, furry tongue, nausea, vomiting

Dosage

Infants and Children:

Amebiasis: Oral: 35-50 mg/kg/day in divided doses every 8 hours for 10 days

Trichomoniasis: Oral: 15-30 mg/kg/day in divided doses every 8 hours for 7 days

Anaerobic infections:

Oral: 15-35 mg/kg/day in divided doses every 8 hours

I.V.: 30 mg/kg/day in divided doses every 6 hours

Clostridium difficile (antibiotic-associated colitis): Oral: 20 mg/kg/day divided every 6 hours

Maximum dose: 2 g/day

Adults:

Amebiasis: Oral: 500-750 mg every 8 hours for 5-10 days

Trichomoniasis: Oral: 250 mg every 8 hours for 7 days or 2 g as a single dose

Anaerobic infections: Oral, I.V.: 500 mg every 6-8 hours, not to exceed 4 g/day

Antibiotic-associated pseudomembranous colitis: Oral: 250-500 mg 3-4 times/day for 10-14 days

Helicobacter pylori eradication: 250 mg with meals and at bedtime for 14 days; requires combination therapy with at least one other antibiotic and an acid-suppressing agent (proton pump inhibitor or H_2 blocker)

Vaginosis: 1 applicatorful (~37.5 mg metronidazole) intravaginally once or twice daily for 5 days; apply once in morning and evening if using twice daily, if daily, use at bedtime

Elderly: Use lower end of dosing recommendations for adults, do not administer as a single dose

Topical (acne rosacea therapy): Apply and rub a thin film twice daily, morning and evening, to entire affected areas after washing. Significant therapeutic results should be noticed within 3 weeks. Clinical studies have demonstrated continuing improvement through 9 weeks of therapy.

Dosing adjustment in renal impairment: Cl_{cr} <10 mL/minute: Administer 50% of dose or every 12 hours

Hemodialysis: Extensively removed by hemodialysis and peritoneal dialysis (50% to 100%); administer dose posthemodialysis

Peritoneal dialysis: Dose as for Cl_{cr} <10 mL/minute

Continuous arteriovenous or venovenous hemofiltration: Administer usual dose

Dosing adjustment/comments in hepatic impairment: Unchanged in mild disease; reduce dosage in severe disease

Mechanism of Action Reduced to a product which interacts with DNA to cause a loss of helical DNA structure and strand breakage resulting in inhibition of protein synthesis and cell death in susceptible organisms

Other Adverse Effects

Systemic:

>10%:

Gastrointestinal (12%): Diarrhea, loss of appetite

(Continued)

Metronidazole *(Continued)*

<1%: Ataxia, **seizures, disulfiram-type reaction with ethanol,** dark urine, pancreatitis, vaginal candidiasis, leukopenia, thrombophlebitis, neuropathy, **hypersensitivity, xerostomia, metallic taste, furry tongue, change in taste sensation**

Topical:

1% to 10%:

Dermatologic: Dry skin, redness (or other signs of skin irritation not present before therapy), stinging or burning of skin

Ocular: Watering of eyes

Vaginal:

>10%: Genitourinary: *Candida* cervicitis or vaginitis

1% to 10%:

Central nervous system: Diarrhea, anorexia

Genitourinary: Burning or irritation of penis of sexual partner; burning or increased frequency of urination, vulvitis, dark urine

Contraindications Hypersensitivity to metronidazole or any component of the formulation; pregnancy (1st trimester - found to be carcinogenic in rats)

Warnings/Precautions Use with caution in patients with liver impairment due to potential accumulation, blood dyscrasias; history of seizures, CHF, or other sodium retaining states; reduce dosage in patients with severe liver impairment, CNS disease, and severe renal failure (Cl_{cr} <10 mL/minute); if *H. pylori* is not eradicated in patients being treated with metronidazole in a regimen, it should be assumed that metronidazole-resistance has occurred and it should not again be used; seizures and neuropathies have been reported especially with increased doses and chronic treatment; if this occurs, discontinue therapy

Drug Interactions Inhibits CYP2C8/9, 3A4

Increased Effect: May inhibit metabolism of cisapride, causing potential arrhythmias; avoid concurrent use. May increase lithium levels/toxicity; monitor. Cimetidine may increase metronidazole levels. Phenytoin, phenobarbital may increase metabolism of metronidazole, potentially decreasing its effect. Increased P-T prolongation with warfarin.

Dietary/Ethanol/Herb Considerations

Ethanol: Avoid alcohol-containing drugs or food during therapy and for 72 hours following discontinuation; metronidazole inhibits ethanol's usual metabolism and may cause disulfiram-like reaction (flushing, headache, nausea, vomiting, sweating or tachycardia).

Food: Administer oral forms with food to reduce GI upset; peak antibiotic serum concentration is lowered and delayed by food, but total drug absorption is not affected.

Pharmacodynamics/Kinetics

Absorption: Oral: Well absorbed; Topical: Concentrations achieved systemically after application of 1 g topically are 10 times less than those obtained after a 250 mg oral dose

Distribution: To saliva, bile, seminal fluid, breast milk, bone, liver, and liver abscesses, lung and vaginal secretions; crosses placenta and blood-brain barrier CSF:blood level ratio: Normal meninges: 16% to 43%; Inflamed meninges: 100%

Protein binding: <20%

Metabolism: Hepatic (30% to 60%)

Half-life elimination: Neonates: 25-75 hours; Others: 6-8 hours, prolonged with hepatic impairment; End-stage renal disease: 21 hours

Time to peak, serum: Oral: Immediate release: 1-2 hours

Excretion: Urine (20% to 40% as unchanged drug); feces (6% to 15%)

Pregnancy Risk Factor B (may be contraindicated in 1st trimester)

Breast-feeding Considerations It is suggested to stop breast-feeding for 12-24 hours following single dose therapy to allow excretion of dose.

Dosage Forms CAP (Flagyl®): 375 mg. **CRM, topical** (MetroCream®): 0.75% (45 g); (Noritate™): 1% (30 g). **GEL, topical** (MetroGel®): 0.75% [7.5 mg/mL] (30 g, 45 g). **GEL, vaginal** (MetroGel-Vaginal®): 0.75% (70 g). **INF** [premixed iso-osmotic sodium chloride solution]: 500 mg (100 mL). **INJ, powder for reconstitution** (Flagyl®): 500 mg. **LOTION** (MetroLotion®): 0.75% (60 mL). **TAB** (Flagyl®): 250 mg, 500 mg. **TAB, extended release** (Flagyl® ER): 750 mg

Generic Available Yes: Infusion and tablet only

Selected Readings

Eisenberg L, Suchow R, Coles RS, et al, "The Effects of Metronidazole Administration on Clinical and Microbiologic Parameters of Periodontal Disease," *Clin Prev Dent*, 1991, 13(1):28-34.

Jenkins WM, MacFarlane TW, Gilmour WH, et al, "Systemic Metronidazole in the Treatment of Periodontitis," *J Clin Periodontol*, 1989, 16(7):433-50.

Loesche WJ, Giordano JR, Hujoel P, et al, "Metronidazole in Periodontitis: Reduced Need for Surgery," *J Clin Periodontol*, 1992, 19(2):103-12.

Loesche WJ, Schmidt E, Smith BA, et al, "Effects of Metronidazole on Periodontal Treatment Needs," *J Periodontol*, 1991, 62(4):247-57.

Soder PO, Frithiof L, Wikner S, et al, "The Effect of Systemic Metronidazole After Nonsurgical Treatment in Moderate and Advanced Periodontitis in Young Adults," *J Periodontol*, 1990, 61(5):281-8.

Wynn RL, Bergman SA, Meiller TF, et al, "Antibiotics in Treating Oral-Facial Infections of Odontogenic Origin: An Update", *Gen Dent*, 2001, 49(3):238-40, 242, 244 passim.

Metronidazole, Bismuth Subsalicylate, and Tetracycline *see* Bismuth, Metronidazole, and Tetracycline *on page 187*

Metronidazole Hydrochloride *see* Metronidazole *on page 902*

Metronidazole, Tetracycline, and Bismuth Subsalicylate *see* Bismuth, Metronidazole, and Tetracycline *on page 187*

Metyrosine (me TYE roe seen)

U.S. Brand Names Demser®

Canadian Brand Names Demser®

Pharmacologic Category Tyrosine Hydroxylase Inhibitor

Synonyms AMPT; OGMT

Use Short-term management of pheochromocytoma before surgery, long-term management when surgery is contraindicated or when chronic malignant pheochromocytoma exists

Local Anesthetic/Vasoconstrictor Precautions No information available to require special precautions

Effects on Dental Treatment

>10%: Drowsiness, extrapyramidal symptoms

1% to 10%: Nausea, vomiting, xerostomia

Dosage Oral:

Children >12 years and Adults: Initial: 250 mg 4 times/day, increased by 250-500 mg/day up to 4 g/day; maintenance: 2-3 g/day in 4 divided doses; for preoperative preparation, administer optimum effective dosage for 5-7 days

Dosing adjustment in renal impairment: Consider adjustment

Mechanism of Action Blocks the rate-limiting step in the biosynthetic pathway of catecholamines. It is a tyrosine hydroxylase inhibitor, blocking the conversion of tyrosine to dihydroxyphenylalanine. This inhibition results in decreased levels of endogenous catecholamines. Catecholamine biosynthesis is reduced by 35% to 80% in patients treated with metyrosine 1-4 g/day.

Other Adverse Effects

>10%: Gastrointestinal: Diarrhea

1% to 10%:

Endocrine & metabolic: Galactorrhea, edema of the breasts

Genitourinary: Impotence

<1%: **Lower extremity edema,** depression, **hallucinations, disorientation, parkinsonism,** urticaria, urinary problems, anemia, eosinophilia, hematuria, hyperstimulation (after withdrawal)

Drug Interactions Increased Toxicity: Phenothiazines, haloperidol may potentiate EPS.

Dietary/Ethanol/Herb Considerations

Ethanol: Avoid use due to additive CNS effect.

Herb/Nutraceutical: Avoid gotu kola, kava, SAMe, St John's wort, and valerian; may increase CNS depression.

Pharmacodynamics/Kinetics

Half-life elimination: 7.2 hours

Excretion: Primarily urine (as unchanged drug)

Pregnancy Risk Factor C

Generic Available No

Mevacor® *see* Lovastatin *on page 828*

Mevinolin *see* Lovastatin *on page 828*

Mexiletine (MEKS i le teen)

Related Information

Cardiovascular Diseases *on page 1456*

U.S. Brand Names Mexitil®

Canadian Brand Names Novo-Mexiletine

Pharmacologic Category Antiarrhythmic Agent, Class Ib

Use Management of serious ventricular arrhythmias; suppression of PVCs

Unlabeled/Investigational Use Treatment of diabetic neuropathy

Local Anesthetic/Vasoconstrictor Precautions No information available to require special precautions

Effects on Dental Treatment 1% to 10%: Xerostomia

Dosage Oral: Oral: Initial: 200 mg every 8 hours (may load with 400 mg if necessary); adjust dose every 2-3 days; usual dose: 200-300 mg every 8 hours; maximum dose: 1.2 g/day (some patients respond to every 12-hour dosing). When switching from another antiarrhythmic, initiate a 200 mg dose 6-12 hours after stopping former agents, 3-6 hours after stopping procainamide.

Dosing adjustment in hepatic impairment: Reduce to 25% to 30% of usual dose

Mechanism of Action Class IB antiarrhythmic, structurally related to lidocaine, which inhibits inward sodium current, decreases rate of rise of phase 0, increases effective refractory period/action potential duration ratio

(Continued)

Mexiletine *(Continued)*

Other Adverse Effects

>10%:

Central nervous system: Lightheadedness (11% to 25%), dizziness (20% to 25%), nervousness (5% to 10%), incoordination (10%)

Gastrointestinal: GI distress (41%), nausea/vomiting (40%)

Neuromuscular & skeletal: Trembling, unsteady gait, tremor (13%), ataxia (10% to 20%)

1% to 10%:

Cardiovascular: Chest pain (3% to 8%), premature ventricular contractions (1% to 2%), palpitations (4% to 8%), angina (2%), proarrhythmic (10% to 15% in patients with malignant arrhythmias)

Central nervous system: Confusion, headache, insomnia (5% to 7%), depression (2%)

Dermatologic: Rash (4%)

Gastrointestinal: Constipation or diarrhea (4% to 5%), abdominal pain (1%)

Neuromuscular & skeletal: Weakness (5%), numbness of fingers or toes (2% to 4%), paresthesias (2%), arthralgias (1%)

Ocular: Blurred vision (5% to 7%), nystagmus (6%)

Otic: Tinnitus (2% to 3%)

Respiratory: Dyspnea (3%)

<1% (Limited to important or life-threatening): Leukopenia, agranulocytosis, thrombocytopenia, positive antinuclear antibody, SLE syndrome, increased LFTs, diplopia, syncope, edema, hot flashes, hypertension, short-term memory loss, psychological changes, psychosis, convulsion, diaphoresis, urinary hesitancy, urinary retention, malaise, impotence, decreased libido, pharyngitis, dysphagia, esophageal ulceration, upper GI bleeding, increased transaminases, hepatitis, hepatic necrosis, exfoliative dermatitis, Stevens-Johnson syndrome, CHF (patients with pre-existing ventricular dysfunction), diaphoresis, salivary changes, alopecia, pancreatitis (rare), myelofibrosis (patients with pre-existing myeloid abnormalities), hypotension, sinus arrest, AV block, conduction disturbances, cardiogenic shock, torsade de pointes, hallucinations, seizures, peptic ulcer, drug-induced lupus-like syndrome

Postmarketing and/or case reports: Pulmonary fibrosis, urticaria

Drug Interactions Substrate of **CYP1A2, 2D6**; Inhibits CYP1A2

Increased Effect/Toxicity: Mexiletine and caffeine or theophylline may result in elevated levels of theophylline and caffeine. Quinidine, fluvoxamine, and urinary alkalinizers (antacids, sodium bicarbonate, acetazolamide) may increase mexiletine blood levels.

Decreased Effect: Decreased mexiletine plasma levels when used with phenobarbital, phenytoin, rifampin, cimetidine, or other hepatic enzyme inducers. Urinary acidifying agents may decrease mexiletine levels.

Dietary/Ethanol/Herb Considerations

Food: Administer with food; may decrease the rate but not the extent of oral absorption. Diets which affect urine pH can increase or decrease excretion of mexiletine; avoid dietary changes that alter urine pH.

Herb/Nutraceutical: Ginger has positive inotropic effects and theoretically could affect antiarrhythmic activity.

Pharmacodynamics/Kinetics

Absorption: Elderly have a slightly slower rate, but extent of absorption is the same as young adults

Distribution: V_d: 5-7 L/kg

Protein binding: 50% to 70%

Metabolism: Hepatic; low first-pass effect

Half-life elimination: Adults: 10-14 hours (average: elderly: 14.4 hours, younger adults: 12 hours); prolonged with hepatic impairment or heart failure

Time to peak: 2-3 hours

Excretion: Urine (10% to 15% as unchanged drug); urinary acidification increases excretion, alkalinization decreases excretion

Pregnancy Risk Factor C

Generic Available Yes

Mexitil® *see* Mexiletine *on page 905*

MG217 Sal-Acid® [OTC] *see* Salicylic Acid *on page 1204*

Miacalcin® *see* Calcitonin *on page 222*

Micaderm® [OTC] *see* Miconazole *on page 906*

Micanol® *see* Anthralin *on page 111*

Micardis® *see* Telmisartan *on page 1269*

Micardis® HCT *see* Telmisartan and Hydrochlorothiazide *on page 1270*

Micatin® [OTC] *see* Miconazole *on page 906*

Miconazole (mi KON a zole)

U.S. Brand Names Aloe Vesta® 2-n-1 Antifungal [OTC]; Baza® Antifungal [OTC]; Carrington Antifungal [OTC]; Femizol-M™ [OTC]; Fungoid® Tincture [OTC];

Lotrimin® AF Powder/Spray [OTC]; Micaderm® [OTC]; Micatin® [OTC]; Micro-Guard® [OTC]; Mitrazol™ [OTC]; Monistat® 1 Combination Pack [OTC]; Monistat® 3 [OTC]; Monistat® 7 [OTC]; Monistat-Derm®; Triple Care® Antifungal [OTC]; Zeasorb®-AF [OTC]

Canadian Brand Names Dermazole; Micatin®; Micozole; Monistat®; Monistat®-3

Mexican Brand Names Aloid®; Daktarin®; Dermifun®; Fungiquim; Gyno-Daktarin; Gyno-Daktarin V; Lotrimin AF®; Neomicol®

Pharmacologic Category Antifungal Agent, Topical; Antifungal Agent, Vaginal

Synonyms Miconazole Nitrate

Use Treatment of vulvovaginal candidiasis and a variety of skin and mucous membrane fungal infections

Local Anesthetic/Vasoconstrictor Precautions No information available to require special precautions

Effects on Dental Treatment No significant effects or complications reported

Dosage

Topical: Children and Adults: **Note:** Not for OTC use in children <2 years:

Tinea pedis and tinea corporis: Apply twice daily for 4 weeks

Tinea cruris: Apply twice daily for 2 weeks

Vaginal: Adults: Vulvovaginal candidiasis:

Cream, 2%: Insert 1 applicatorful at bedtime for 7 days

Cream, 4%: Insert 1 applicatorful at bedtime for 3 days

Suppository, 100 mg: Insert 1 suppository at bedtime for 7 days

Suppository, 200 mg: Insert 1 suppository at bedtime for 3 days

Suppository, 1200 mg: Insert 1 suppository at bedtime (a one-time dose)

Note: Many products are available as a combination pack, with a suppository for vaginal instillation and cream to relieve external symptoms.

Mechanism of Action Inhibits biosynthesis of ergosterol, damaging the fungal cell wall membrane, which increases permeability causing leaking of nutrients

Other Adverse Effects Frequency not defined:

Topical: Allergic contact dermatitis, burning, maceration

Vaginal: Abdominal cramps, burning, irritation, itching

Drug Interactions Substrate of **CYP3A4**; Inhibits CYP2A6, 2C8/9, 2E1, 3A4

Increased Effect/Toxicity:

The majority of reported drug interactions were observed following intravenous miconazole administration. Although systemic absorption following topical and/or vaginal administration is low, potential interactions due to CYP isoenzyme inhibition may occur (rarely). This may be particularly true in situations where topical absorption may be increased (ie, inflamed tissue).

Miconazole coadministered with warfarin has increased the anticoagulant effect of warfarin (including reports associated with vaginal miconazole therapy of as little as 3 days). Phenytoin levels may be increased. Miconazole may inhibit the metabolism of oral sulfonylureas. Concurrent administration of cisapride is contraindicated due to an increased risk of cardiotoxicity.

Decreased Effect: Amphotericin B may decrease antifungal effect of both agents.

Dietary/Ethanol/Herb Considerations Herb/Nutraceutical: Avoid St John's wort; may decrease serum concentration.

Pharmacodynamics/Kinetics

Absorption: Topical: Negligible

Distribution: Widely to body tissues; penetrates well into inflamed joints, vitreous humor of eye, and peritoneal cavity, but poorly into saliva and sputum; crosses blood-brain barrier but only to a small extent

Protein binding: 91% to 93%

Metabolism: Hepatic

Half-life elimination: Multiphasic: Initial: 40 minutes; Secondary: 126 minutes; Terminal: 24 hours

Excretion: Feces (~50%); urine (<1% as unchanged drug)

Pregnancy Risk Factor C

Generic Available Yes

Miconazole Nitrate *see* Miconazole *on page 906*

MICRhoGAM® *see* Rh_o(D) Immune Globulin *on page 1175*

Microfibrillar Collagen Hemostat

(mye kro FI bri lar KOL la jen HEE moe stat)

U.S. Brand Names Avitene®; Helistat®

Pharmacologic Category Hemostatic Agent

Synonyms Collagen; MCH

Use Dental and Medical: Adjunct to hemostasis when control of bleeding by ligature is ineffective or impractical

Local Anesthetic/Vasoconstrictor Precautions No information available to require special precautions

Effects on Dental Treatment Frequency not defined: Potentiation of infection, allergic reaction, adhesion formation, foreign body reaction

Dosage Apply dry directly to source of bleeding.

(Continued)

Microfibrillar Collagen Hemostat *(Continued)*

Mechanism of Action Microfibrillar collagen hemostat is an absorbable topical hemostatic agent prepared from purified bovine corium collagen and shredded into fibrils. Physically, microfibrillar collagen hemostat yields a large surface area. Chemically, it is collagen with hydrochloric acid noncovalently bound to some of the available amino groups in the collagen molecules. When in contact with a bleeding surface, microfibrillar collagen hemostat attracts platelets which adhere to its fibrils and undergo the release phenomenon. This triggers aggregation of the platelets into thrombi in the interstices of the fibrous mass, initiating the formation of a physiologic platelet plug.

Contraindications Hypersensitivity to any component of the formulation; closure of skin incisions, contaminated wounds

Warnings/Precautions Fragments of MCH may pass through filters of blood scavenging systems, avoid reintroduction of blood from operative sites treated with MCH; after several minutes remove excess material

Pharmacodynamics/Kinetics Absorption: By animal tissue in 3 months

Pregnancy Risk Factor C

Dosage Forms SPONGE (Avitene®): 2 cm x 6.25 cm x 7 mm (12s); 8 cm x 6.25 cm x 1 cm (6s); 8 cm x 12.5 cm x 1 cm (6s); 8 cm x 12.5 cm x 3 mm (6s); 8 cm x 25 cm x1 cm (6s); (Helisat®): 0.5 inch x 1 inch x 7 mm (18s)

Generic Available No

MicrogestinTM Fe *see* Combination Hormonal Contraceptives *on page 368*
Micro-Guard® [OTC] *see* Miconazole *on page 906*
microK® *see* Potassium Supplements *on page 1102*
microK® 10 *see* Potassium Supplements *on page 1102*
Micronase® *see* GlyBURIDE *on page 642*
microNefrin® *see* Epinephrine (Racemic) *on page 500*
Micronor® *see* Norethindrone *on page 986*
MicrozideTM *see* Hydrochlorothiazide *on page 675*
Midamor® *see* Amiloride *on page 75*

Midazolam (MID ay zoe lam)

U.S. Brand Names Versed® [DSC]

Canadian Brand Names Apo®-Midazolam

Mexican Brand Names Dormicum®

Pharmacologic Category Benzodiazepine

Synonyms Midazolam Hydrochloride; Versed® [DSC]

Use

Dental: Sedation component in I.V. conscious sedation in oral surgery patients; syrup formulation is used for children to help alleviate anxiety before a dental procedure

Medical: Preoperative sedation; conscious sedation prior to diagnostic or radiographic procedures; ICU sedation (continuous infusion); intravenous anesthesia (induction/maintenance)

Unlabeled/Investigational Use Treatment of anxiety, status epilepticus

Local Anesthetic/Vasoconstrictor Precautions No information available to require special precautions

Effects on Dental Treatment

Children:

>10%: Apnea (3%)

1% to 3%: Hypotension (3%), seizure-like activity (1%), paradoxical reaction (2%), hiccups (1%)

Adults: 1% to 10%: Drowsiness (1%), hiccups (4%), oversedation, headache (1%), nausea (3%), cough (1%), physical and psychological dependence, vomiting (3%), pain and local reactions at injection site (4% I.M., 5% I.V.; severity less than diazepam)

Restrictions C-IV

Dosage Dosage needs to be individualized based on the patient's age, underlying diseases, and concurrent medications. Decrease dose (by ~30%) if narcotics or other CNS depressants are administered concomitantly. Children <6 years may require higher doses and closer monitoring than older children; calculate dose on ideal body weight. **Personnel and equipment needed for standard respiratory resuscitation should be immediately available during administration.**

Children: Conscious sedation for procedures or preoperative sedation:

Oral: 0.25-0.5 mg/kg as a single dose preprocedure, up to a maximum of 20 mg; administer 30-45 minutes prior to procedure. Children <6 years and uncooperative patients may require as much as 1 mg/kg as a single dose; 0.25 mg/kg may suffice for children 6-16 years of age.

Intranasal (not an approved route): 0.2 mg/kg (up to 0.4 mg/kg in some studies), to a maximum of 15 mg; may be administered 30-45 minutes prior to procedure

I.M.: 0.1-0.15 mg/kg 30-60 minutes before surgery or procedure; range 0.05-0.15 mg/kg; doses up to 0.5 mg/kg have been used in more anxious patients; maximum total dose: 10 mg

I.V.:

Infants <6 months: Limited information is available in nonintubated infants; dosing recommendations not clear; infants <6 months are at higher risk for airway obstruction and hypoventilation; titrate dose in small increments to desired effect; monitor carefully

Infants 6 months to Children 5 years: Initial: 0.05-0.1 mg/kg; titrate dose carefully; total dose of 0.6 mg/kg may be required; usual maximum total dose: 6 mg

Children 6-12 years: Initial: 0.025-0.05 mg/kg; titrate dose carefully; total doses of 0.4 mg/kg may be required; usual maximum total dose: 10 mg

Children 12-16 years: Dose as adults; usual maximum total dose: 10 mg

Conscious sedation during mechanical ventilation: Children: Loading dose: 0.05-0.2 mg/kg, followed by initial continuous infusion: 0.06-0.12 mg/kg/hour (1-2 mcg/kg/minute); titrate to the desired effect; usual range: 0.4-6 mcg/kg/minute

Status epilepticus refractory to standard therapy (unlabeled use): Infants >2 months and Children: Loading dose: 0.15 mg/kg followed by a continuous infusion of 1 mcg/kg/minute; titrate dose upward every 5 minutes until clinical seizure activity is controlled; mean infusion rate required in 24 children was 2.3 mcg/kg/minute with a range of 1-18 mcg/kg/minute

Adults:

Preoperative sedation:

I.M.: 0.07-0.08 mg/kg 30-60 minutes prior to surgery/procedure; usual dose: 5 mg; **Note:** Reduce dose in patients with COPD, high-risk patients, patients ≥60 years of age, and patients receiving other narcotics or CNS depressants

I.V.: 0.02-0.04 mg/kg; repeat every 5 minutes as needed to desired effect or up to 0.1-0.2 mg/kg

Intranasal (not an approved route): 0.2 mg/kg (up to 0.4 mg/kg in some studies); administer 30-45 minutes prior to surgery/procedure

Conscious sedation: I.V.: Initial: 0.5-2 mg slow I.V. over at least 2 minutes; slowly titrate to effect by repeating doses every 2-3 minutes if needed; usual total dose: 2.5-5 mg; use decreased doses in elderly

Healthy Adults <60 years: Some patients respond to doses as low as 1 mg; no more than 2.5 mg should be administered over a period of 2 minutes. Additional doses of midazolam may be administered after a 2-minute waiting period and evaluation of sedation after each dose increment. A total dose >5 mg is generally not needed. If narcotics or other CNS depressants are administered concomitantly, the midazolam dose should be reduced by 30%.

Anesthesia: I.V.:

Induction:

0.3-0.35 mg/kg (up to 0.6 mg/kg in resistant cases)

Premedicated patients: 0.15-0.35 mg/kg

Maintenance: 0.05-0.3 mg/kg as needed, or continuous infusion 0.25-1.5 mcg/kg/minute

Sedation in mechanically-ventilated patients: I.V. continuous infusion: 100 mg in 250 mL D_5W or NS (if patient is fluid-restricted, may concentrate up to a maximum of 0.5 mg/mL); initial dose: 0.01-0.05 mg/kg (~0.5-4 mg for a typical adult) initially and either repeated at 10-15 minute intervals until adequate sedation is achieved or continuous infusion rates of 0.02-0.1 mg/kg/hour (1-7 mg/hour) and titrate to reach desired level of sedation

Elderly: I.V.: Conscious sedation: Initial: 0.5 mg slow I.V.; give no more than 1.5 mg in a 2-minute period; if additional titration is needed, give no more than 1 mg over 2 minutes, waiting another 2 or more minutes to evaluate sedative effect; a total dose of >3.5 mg is rarely necessary

Dosing adjustment in renal impairment:

Hemodialysis: Supplemental dose is unnecessary

Peritoneal dialysis: Significant drug removal is unlikely based on physiochemical characteristics

Mechanism of Action Binds to stereospecific benzodiazepine receptors on the postsynaptic GABA neuron at several sites within the central nervous system, including the limbic system, reticular formation. Enhancement of the inhibitory effect of GABA on neuronal excitability results by increased neuronal membrane permeability to chloride ions. This shift in chloride ions results in hyperpolarization (a less excitable state) and stabilization.

Other Adverse Effects

1% to 10%: Ocular: Nystagmus (1% children)

<1%: **Acid taste, agitation, amnesia, bigeminy, bradycardia, bronchospasm, confusion, dyspnea, emergence delirium, euphoria, excessive salivation, hallucinations, hyperventilation, laryngospasm**, PVC, rash, **tachycardia, wheezing**

Contraindications Hypersensitivity to midazolam or any component of the formulation, including benzyl alcohol (cross-sensitivity with other benzodiazepines may

(Continued)

Midazolam *(Continued)*

exist); parenteral form is not for intrathecal or epidural injection; narrow-angle glaucoma; pregnancy

Warnings/Precautions May cause severe respiratory depression, respiratory arrest, or apnea. Use with extreme caution, particularly in noncritical care settings. Appropriate resuscitative equipment and qualified personnel must be available for administration and monitoring. Initial dosing must be cautiously titrated and individualized, particularly in elderly or debilitated patients, patients with hepatic impairment (including alcoholics), or in renal impairment, particularly if other CNS depressants (including opiates) are used concurrently. Initial doses in elderly or debilitated patients should not exceed 2.5 mg. Use with caution in patients with respiratory disease or impaired gag reflex. Use during upper airway procedures may increase risk of hypoventilation. Prolonged responses have been noted following extended administration by continuous infusion (possibly due to metabolite accumulation) or in the presence of drugs which inhibit midazolam metabolism.

May cause hypotension - hemodynamic events are more common in pediatric patients or patients with hemodynamic instability. Hypotension and/or respiratory depression may occur more frequently in patients who have received narcotic analgesics. Use with caution in obese patients, chronic renal failure, and CHF. Parenteral form contains benzyl alcohol - avoid rapid injection in neonates or prolonged infusions. Does not protect against increases in heart rate or blood pressure during intubation. Should not be used in shock, coma, or acute alcohol intoxication. Avoid intra-arterial administration or extravasation of parenteral formulation.

Causes CNS depression (dose-related) resulting in sedation, dizziness, confusion, or ataxia which may impair physical and mental capabilities. Patients must be cautioned about performing tasks which require mental alertness (ie, operating machinery or driving). A minimum of 1 day should elapse after midazolam administration before attempting these tasks. Use with caution in patients receiving other CNS depressants or psychoactive agents. Effects with other sedative drugs or ethanol may be potentiated. Benzodiazepines have been associated with falls and traumatic injury and should be used with extreme caution in patients who are at risk of these events (especially the elderly).

Midazolam causes anterograde amnesia. Paradoxical reactions, including hyperactive or aggressive behavior have been reported with benzodiazepines, particularly in adolescent/pediatric or psychiatric patients. Does not have analgesic, antidepressant, or antipsychotic properties.

Benzodiazepines have been associated with dependence and acute withdrawal symptoms on discontinuation or reduction in dose. Acute withdrawal, including seizures, may be precipitated after administration of flumazenil to patients receiving long-term benzodiazepine therapy.

Drug Interactions Substrate of CYP2B6, **3A4**; Inhibits CYP2C8/9, 3A4

CNS depressants: Sedative effects and/or respiratory depression may be additive with CNS depressants; includes ethanol, barbiturates, narcotic analgesics, and other sedative agents; monitor for increased effect. **If narcotics or other CNS depressants are administered concomitantly, the midazolam dose should be reduced by 30% if <65 years of age, or by at least 50% if >65 years of age.**

CYP3A4 inhibitors: Serum level and/or toxicity of some benzodiazepines may be increased; inhibitors include amiodarone, cimetidine, clarithromycin, erythromycin, delavirdine, diltiazem, dirithromycin, disulfiram, fluoxetine, fluvoxamine, grapefruit juice, indinavir, itraconazole, ketoconazole, nefazodone, nevirapine, propoxyphene, quinupristin-dalfopristin, ritonavir, saquinavir, verapamil, zafirlukast, zileuton; monitor for altered benzodiazepine response. **Use is contraindicated with amprenavir and ritonavir.**

Enzyme inducers: Metabolism of some benzodiazepines may be increased, decreasing their therapeutic effect; consider using an alternative sedative/hypnotic agent; potential inducers include phenobarbital, phenytoin, carbamazepine, rifampin, and rifabutin

Levodopa: Therapeutic effects may be diminished in some patients following the addition of a benzodiazepine; limited/inconsistent data

Oral contraceptives: May decrease the clearance of some benzodiazepines (those which undergo oxidative metabolism); monitor for increased benzodiazepine effect

Saquinavir: A 56% reduction in clearance and a doubling of midazolam's half-life were seen with concurrent administration with saquinavir.

Theophylline: May partially antagonize some of the effects of benzodiazepines; monitor for decreased response; may require higher doses for sedation

Dietary/Ethanol/Herb Considerations

Ethanol: Avoid use; may increase CNS depression.

Food: Grapefruit products may increase serum concentration of midazolam; avoid concurrent use with oral form.

Herb/Nutraceutical: Avoid gotu kola, kava, SAMe, and valerian; may increase CNS depression. Avoid St John's wort; may decrease serum concentration and increase CNS depression. Melatonin may enhance activity of clonazepam; use cautiously.

Pharmacodynamics/Kinetics

Onset of action: I.M.: Sedation: ~15 minutes; I.V.: 1-5 minutes

Peak effect: I.M.: 0.5-1 hour

Duration: I.M.: Up to 6 hours; Mean: 2 hours

Absorption: Oral: Rapid

Distribution: V_d: 0.8-2.5 L/kg; increased with congestive heart failure (CHF) and chronic renal failure

Protein binding: 95%

Metabolism: Extensively hepatic via CYP3A4

Bioavailability: Mean: 45%

Half-life elimination: 1-4 hours; prolonged with cirrhosis, congestive heart failure, obesity, and elderly

Excretion: Urine (as glucuronide conjugated metabolites); feces (~2% to 10%)

Pregnancy Risk Factor D

Dosage Forms INJ, solution (Versed® [DSC]): 1 mg/mL (2 mL, 5 mL, 10 mL); 5 mg/mL (1 mL, 2 mL, 5 mL, 10 mL). **INJ, solution** [preservative free]: 1 mg/mL (2 mL, 5 mL); 5 mg/mL (1 mL, 2 mL). **SYR** (Versed® [DSC]): 2 mg/mL (118 mL)

Generic Available Yes: Injection

Selected Readings Dionne RA, Yagiela JA, Moore PA, et al, "Comparing Efficacy and Safety of Four Intravenous Sedation Regimens in Dental Outpatients," *Am Dent Assoc*, 2001, 132(6):740-51.

Midazolam Hydrochloride *see* Midazolam *on page 908*

Midodrine (MI doe dreen)

U.S. Brand Names ProAmatine®

Canadian Brand Names Amatine®

Pharmacologic Category Alpha$_1$ Agonist

Synonyms Midodrine Hydrochloride

Use Orphan drug: Treatment of symptomatic orthostatic hypotension

Unlabeled/Investigational Use Investigational: Management of urinary incontinence

Local Anesthetic/Vasoconstrictor Precautions No information available to require special precautions

Effects on Dental Treatment

>10%: Paresthesia (18.3%), xerostomia (>10%)

1% to 10%: Supine hypertension (7%), facial flushing, confusion, anxiety, dizziness, nausea, pain (5%)

Dosage Oral:

Adults: 10 mg 3 times/day during daytime hours (every 3-4 hours) when patient is upright (maximum: 40 mg/day)

Dosing adjustment in renal impairment: 2.5 mg 3 times/day, gradually increasing as tolerated

Mechanism of Action Midodrine forms an active metabolite, desglymidodrine, that is an alpha$_1$-agonist. This agent increases arteriolar and venous tone resulting in a rise in standing, sitting, and supine systolic and diastolic blood pressure in patients with orthostatic hypotension. See table.

Causes of Orthostatic Hypotension

Primary Autonomic Causes
Pure autonomic failure (Bradbury-Eggleston syndrome, idiopathic orthostatic hypotension)
Autonomic failure with multiple system atrophy (Shy-Drager syndrome)
Familial dysautonomia (Riley-Day syndrome)
Dopamine beta-hydroxylase deficiency
Secondary Autonomic Causes
Chronic alcoholism
Parkinson's disease
Diabetes mellitus
Porphyria
Amyloidosis
Various carcinomas
Vitamin B_1 or B_{12} deficiency
Nonautonomic Causes
Hypovolemia (such as associated with hemorrhage, burns, or hemodialysis) and dehydration
Diminished homeostatic regulation (such as associated with aging, pregnancy, fever, or prolonged best rest)
Medications (eg, antihypertensives, insulin, tricyclic antidepressants)

(Continued)

Midodrine *(Continued)*

Other Adverse Effects

>10%:

Dermatologic: Piloerection (13%), pruritus (12%)

Genitourinary: Urinary urgency, retention, or polyuria, dysuria (up to 13%)

1% to 10%:

Central nervous system: Chills (5%)

Dermatologic: Rash, dry skin (2%)

Gastrointestinal: Abdominal pain

<1%: **Headache,** insomnia, flatulence, **leg cramps, visual changes**

Drug Interactions Increased Effect/Toxicity: Concomitant fludrocortisone results in hypernatremia or an increase in intraocular pressure and glaucoma. Bradycardia may be accentuated with concomitant administration of cardiac glycosides, psychotherapeutics, and beta-blockers. Alpha agonists may increase the pressure effects and alpha antagonists may negate the effects of midodrine.

Pharmacodynamics/Kinetics

Onset of action: ~1 hour

Duration: 2-3 hours

Absorption: Rapid

Distribution: V_d (desglymidodrine): <1.6 L/kg; poorly across membrane (eg, blood brain barrier)

Protein binding: Minimal

Metabolism: Hepatic; rapid deglycination to desglymidodrine occurs in many tissues and plasma

Bioavailability: Absolute: 93%

Half-life elimination: Active drug: ~3-4 hours; Prodrug: 25 minutes

Time to peak, serum: Active drug: 1-2 hours; Prodrug: 30 minutes

Excretion: Urine (2% to 4%)

Clearance: Desglymidodrine: 385 mL/minute (predominantly by renal secretion)

Pregnancy Risk Factor C

Generic Available No

Midodrine Hydrochloride *see* Midodrine *on page 911*

Midol® Maximum Strength Cramp Formula [OTC] *see* Ibuprofen *on page 703*

Midrin® *see* Acetaminophen, Isometheptene, and Dichloralphenazone *on page 36*

Mifeprex® *see* Mifepristone *on page 912*

Mifepristone (mi fe PRIS tone)

U.S. Brand Names Mifeprex®

Pharmacologic Category Abortifacient; Antineoplastic Agent, Hormone Antagonist; Antiprogestin

Synonyms RU-486; RU-38486

Use Medical termination of intrauterine pregnancy, through day 49 of pregnancy. Patients may need treatment with misoprostol and possibly surgery to complete therapy

Unlabeled/Investigational Use Treatment of unresectable meningioma, breast and ovarian cancers, adrenal cortical carcinoma

Local Anesthetic/Vasoconstrictor Precautions No information available to require special precautions

Effects on Dental Treatment

>10%: Headache (2% to 31%), dizziness (1% to 12%), nausea (43% to 61%), vomiting (18% to 26%),

1% to 4%: Syncope (1%), fatigue (10%), fever (4%), anxiety (2%), fainting (2%), rigors (3%), leg pain (2%), weakness (2%), sinusitis (2%), viral infection (4%)

Restrictions There are currently no clinical trials with mifepristone in oncology open in the U.S.; investigators wishing to obtain the agent for use in oncology patients must apply for a patient-specific IND from the FDA. Mifepristone will be supplied only to licensed physicians who sign and return a "Prescriber's Agreement." Distribution of mifepristone will be subject to specific requirements imposed by the distributor. Mifepristone will **not** be available to the public through licensed pharmacies.

Dosage Oral:

Adults: Termination of pregnancy: Treatment consists of three office visits by the patient; the patient must read medication guide and sign patient agreement prior to treatment:

Day 1: 600 mg (three 200 mg tablets) taken as a single dose under physician supervision

Day 3: Patient must return to the healthcare provider 2 days following administration of mifepristone; if termination of pregnancy cannot be confirmed using ultrasound or clinical examination: 400 mcg (two 200 mcg tablets) of misoprostol; patient may need treatment for cramps or GI symptoms at this time

Day 14: Patient must return to the healthcare provider ~14 days after administration of mifepristone; confirm complete termination of pregnancy by ultrasound or clinical exam. Surgical termination is recommended to manage treatment failures.

Dosing adjustment for elderly or in renal/hepatic impairment: Safety and efficacy not established; use with caution due to CYP3A4 metabolism

Unlabeled use: Refer to individual protocols; dose used in meningioma is usually 200 mg/day, continued based on toxicity and response

Mechanism of Action Mifepristone, a synthetic steroid, competitively binds to the intracellular progesterone receptor, blocking the effects of progesterone. When used for the termination of pregnancy, this leads to contraction-inducing activity in the myometrium. In the absence of progesterone, mifepristone acts as a partial progesterone agonist. Mifepristone also has weak antiglucocorticoid and antiandrogenic properties; it blocks the feedback effect of cortisol on corticotropin secretion.

Other Adverse Effects Vaginal bleeding and uterine cramping are expected to occur when this medication is used to terminate a pregnancy; 90% of women using this medication for this purpose also report adverse reactions

>10%:
- Gastrointestinal: Abdominal pain (cramping) (96%), diarrhea (12% to 20%)
- Genitourinary: Uterine cramping (83%)

1% to 10%:
- Central nervous system: Insomnia (3%)
- Gastrointestinal: Dyspepsia (3%)
- Genitourinary: Uterine hemorrhage (5%), vaginitis (3%), pelvic pain (2%)
- Hematologic: Decreased hemoglobin >2 g/dL (6%), anemia (2%), leukorrhea (2%)
- Neuromuscular & skeletal: Back pain (9%)

<1%: Significant SGOT, SGPT, alkaline phosphatase, and GT changes have been reported (rarely)

Postmarketing and/or case reports: **MI**, ruptured ectopic pregnancy, **bacterial infection**

In trials for unresectable meningioma, the most common adverse effects included fatigue, hot flashes, gynecomastia or breast tenderness, hair thinning, and rash. In premenopausal women, vaginal bleeding may be seen shortly after beginning therapy and cessation of menses is common. Thyroiditis and effects related to antiglucocorticoid activity have also been noted.

Drug Interactions Substrate of CYP3A4; Inhibits CYP2D6, 3A4

Increased Effect/Toxicity: There are no reported interactions. It might be anticipated that the effects of one or both agents would be minimized if mifepristone were administered concurrently with a progestin (exogenous). During concurrent use of CYP3A4 inhibitors, serum level and/or toxicity of mifepristone may be increased; inhibitors include amiodarone, cimetidine, clarithromycin, erythromycin, delavirdine, diltiazem, dirithromycin, disulfiram, fluoxetine, fluvoxamine, grapefruit juice, indinavir, itraconazole, ketoconazole, nefazodone, nevirapine, propoxyphene, quinupristin-dalfopristin, ritonavir, saquinavir, verapamil, zafirlukast, zileuton; monitor for altered response

Decreased Effect: Enzyme inducers may increase the metabolism of mifepristone resulting in decreased effect; includes carbamazepine, dexamethasone, phenobarbital, phenytoin, and rifampin. St John's wort may induce mifepristone metabolism, leading to decreased levels.

Dietary/Ethanol/Herb Considerations Food: Avoid grapefruit products; may inhibit metabolism leading to increased serum concentration.

Pharmacodynamics/Kinetics

Protein binding: 98% to albumin and α_1-acid glycoprotein

Metabolism: Hepatic via CYP3A4 to three metabolites (may possess some antiprogestin and antiglucocorticoid activity)

Bioavailability: 69%

Half-life elimination: Terminal: 18 hours following a slower phase where 50% eliminated between 12-72 hours

Time to peak: 90 minutes

Excretion: Feces (83%); urine (9%)

Pregnancy Risk Factor X

Generic Available No

Miglitol (MIG li tol)

Related Information

Endocrine Disorders and Pregnancy *on page 1479*

U.S. Brand Names Glyset®

Canadian Brand Names Glyset®

Pharmacologic Category Antidiabetic Agent, Alpha-Glucosidase Inhibitor

Use Type 2 diabetes mellitus (noninsulin-dependent, NIDDM):

Monotherapy adjunct to diet to improve glycemic control in patients with type 2 diabetes mellitus (noninsulin-dependent, NIDDM) whose hyperglycemia cannot be managed with diet alone

(Continued)

Miglitol *(Continued)*

Combination therapy with a sulfonylurea when diet plus either miglitol or a sulfonylurea alone do not result in adequate glycemic control. The effect of miglitol to enhance glycemic control is additive to that of sulfonylureas when used in combination.

Local Anesthetic/Vasoconstrictor Precautions No information available to require special precautions

Effects on Dental Treatment No significant effects or complications reported

Dosage Oral:

Adults: 25 mg 3 times/day with the first bite of food at each meal; the dose may be increased to 50 mg 3 times/day after 4-8 weeks; maximum recommended dose: 100 mg 3 times/day

Dosing adjustment in renal impairment: Primarily excreted by the kidneys; little information in Cl_{cr} <25 mL/minute

Mechanism of Action In contrast to sulfonylureas, miglitol does not enhance insulin secretion; the antihyperglycemic action of miglitol results from a reversible inhibition of membrane-bound intestinal alpha-glucosidases which hydrolyze oligosaccharides and disaccharides to glucose and other monosaccharides in the brush border of the small intestine; in diabetic patients, this enzyme inhibition results in delayed glucose absorption and lowering of postprandial hyperglycemia

Other Adverse Effects

>10%: Gastrointestinal: Flatulence (42%), diarrhea (29%), abdominal pain (12%)

1% to 10%: Dermatologic: Rash

Drug Interactions Decreased Effect: Miglitol may decrease the absorption and bioavailability of digoxin, propranolol, and ranitidine. Digestive enzymes (amylase, pancreatin, charcoal) may reduce the effect of miglitol and should **not** be taken concomitantly.

Pharmacodynamics/Kinetics

Absorption: Saturable at high doses: 25 mg dose: Completely absorbed; 100 mg dose: 50% to 70% absorbed

Distribution: V_d: 0.18 L/kg

Protein binding: <4%

Metabolism: None

Half-life elimination: ~2 hours

Time to peak: 2-3 hours

Excretion: Urine (as unchanged drug)

Pregnancy Risk Factor B

Generic Available No

Migranal® *see* Dihydroergotamine *on page 445*

Migratine® *see* Acetaminophen, Isometheptene, and Dichloralphenazone *on page 36*

Milk of Magnesia *see* Magnesium Hydroxide *on page 835*

Milk of Magnesia (Magnesium Hydroxide) *see* Magnesium Supplements *on page 837*

Milophene® *see* ClomiPHENE *on page 348*

Milrinone (MIL ri none)

U.S. Brand Names Primacor®

Canadian Brand Names Primacor®

Pharmacologic Category Phosphodiesterase Enzyme Inhibitor

Synonyms Milrinone Lactate

Use Short-term I.V. therapy of CHF; calcium antagonist intoxication

Local Anesthetic/Vasoconstrictor Precautions No information available to require special precautions

Effects on Dental Treatment 1% to 10%: Arrhythmias, hypotension, headache

Dosage I.V.:

Adults: Loading dose: 50 mcg/kg administered over 10 minutes followed by a maintenance dose titrated according to the hemodynamic and clinical response; see following table:

Maintenance Dosage	Dose Rate (mcg/kg/min)	Total Dose (mg/kg/24 h)
Minimum	0.375	0.59
Standard	0.500	0.77
Maximum	0.750	1.13

Dosing adjustment in renal impairment:

Cl_{cr} 50 mL/minute/1.73 m^2: Administer 0.43 mcg/kg/minute.
Cl_{cr} 40 mL/minute/1.73 m^2: Administer 0.38 mcg/kg/minute.
Cl_{cr} 30 mL/minute/1.73 m^2: Administer 0.33 mcg/kg/minute.
Cl_{cr} 20 mL/minute/1.73 m^2: Administer 0.28 mcg/kg/minute.
Cl_{cr} 10 mL/minute/1.73 m^2: Administer 0.23 mcg/kg/minute.
Cl_{cr} 5 mL/minute/1.73 m^2: Administer 0.2 mcg/kg/minute.

Mechanism of Action Phosphodiesterase inhibitor resulting in vasodilation

Other Adverse Effects <1% (Limited to important or life-threatening): **Atrial fibrillation, chest pain,** hypokalemia, LFT abnormalities, **MI,** thrombocytopenia, **ventricular fibrillation**

Pharmacodynamics/Kinetics

Onset of action: I.V.: 5-15 minutes

Serum level: I.V.: Following a 125 mcg/kg dose, peak plasma concentrations ~1000 ng/mL were observed at 2 minutes postinjection, decreasing to <100 ng/mL in 2 hours

Drug concentration levels:

Therapeutic:

Serum levels of 166 ng/mL, achieved during I.V. infusions of 0.25-1 mcg/kg/minute, were associated with sustained hemodynamic benefit in severe congestive heart failure patients over a 24-hour period

Maximum beneficial effects on cardiac output and pulmonary capillary wedge pressure following I.V. infusion have been associated with plasma milrinone concentrations of 150-250 ng/mL

Toxic: Serum concentrations >250-300 ng/mL have been associated with marked reductions in mean arterial pressure and tachycardia; however, more studies are required to determine the toxic serum levels for milrinone

Distribution: V_{dss}: 0.32 L/kg; Severe congestive heart failure (CHF): V_d: 0.33-0.47 L/kg; not significantly bound to tissues; excretion in breast milk unknown

Protein binding, plasma: ~70%

Metabolism: Hepatic (12%)

Half-life elimination: I.V.: 136 minutes in patients with CHF; patients with severe CHF have a more prolonged half-life, with values ranging from 1.7-2.7 hours. Patients with CHF have a reduction in the systemic clearance of milrinone, resulting in a prolonged elimination half-life. Alternatively, one study reported that 1 month of therapy with milrinone did not change the pharmacokinetic parameters for patients with CHF despite improvement in cardiac function.

Excretion: I.V.: Urine (85% as unchanged drug) within 24 hours; active tubular secretion is a major elimination pathway for milrinone

Clearance: I.V. bolus: 25.9 ± 5.7 L/hour (0.37 L/hour/kg); Severe congestive heart failure: 0.11-0.13 L/hour/kg. The reduction in clearance may be a result of reduced renal function. Creatinine clearance values were ½ those reported for healthy adults in patients with severe congestive heart failure (52 vs 119 mL/minute).

Pregnancy Risk Factor C

Generic Available Yes: Injection

Milrinone Lactate *see* Milrinone *on page 914*

Miltown® *see* Meprobamate *on page 864*

Mineral Oil, Coal Tar, and Lanolin *see* Coal Tar, Lanolin, and Mineral Oil *on page 360*

Mineral Oil, Lanolin, and Coal Tar *see* Coal Tar, Lanolin, and Mineral Oil *on page 360*

Mineral Oil, Petrolatum, Lanolin, Cetyl Alcohol, and Glycerin *see* Lanolin, Cetyl Alcohol, Glycerin, Petrolatum, and Mineral Oil *on page 776*

Minidyne® [OTC] *see* Povidone-Iodine *on page 1104*

Minipress® *see* Prazosin *on page 1108*

Minitran™ *see* Nitroglycerin *on page 981*

Minizide® *see* Prazosin and Polythiazide *on page 1109*

Minocin® *see* Minocycline *on page 915*

Minocycline (mi noe SYE kleen)

U.S. Brand Names Dynacin®; Minocin®

Canadian Brand Names Alti-Minocycline; Apo®-Minocycline; Gen-Minocycline; Minocin®; Novo-Minocycline; PMS-Minocycline; Rhoxal-minocycline

Mexican Brand Names Minocin®

Pharmacologic Category Antibiotic, Tetracycline Derivative

Synonyms Minocycline Hydrochloride; Vectrin® [DSC]

Use

Dental: Treatment of periodontitis associated with presence of *Actinobacillus actinomycetemcomitans* (AA); as adjunctive therapy in recurrent aphthous ulcers

Medical: Treatment of susceptible bacterial infections of both gram-negative and gram-positive organisms; treatment of anthrax (inhalation, cutaneous, and GI); acne, meningococcal carrier state

Local Anesthetic/Vasoconstrictor Precautions No information available to require special precautions

Effects on Dental Treatment Opportunistic "superinfection" with *Candida albicans*; tetracyclines are not recommended for use during pregnancy or in children ≤8 years of age since they have been reported to cause enamel hypoplasia and permanent teeth discoloration. The use of tetracycline's should only be used in these patients if other agents are contraindicated or alternative antimicrobials will not eradicate the organism. Long-term use associated with oral candidiasis.

(Continued)

Minocycline *(Continued)*

>10%: Discoloration of teeth (children)

1% to 10%: Lightheadedness, nausea

Dosage

Children >8 years: Oral, I.V.: Initial: 4 mg/kg followed by 2 mg/kg/dose every 12 hours

Adults:

Infection: Oral, I.V.: 200 mg stat, 100 mg every 12 hours not to exceed 400 mg/24 hours

Acne: Oral: 50 mg 1-3 times/day

Hemodialysis: Not dialyzable (0% to 5%)

Mechanism of Action Inhibits bacterial protein synthesis by binding with the 30S and possibly the 50S ribosomal subunit(s) of susceptible bacteria; cell wall synthesis is not affected

Other Adverse Effects

1% to 10%:

Central nervous system: Vertigo

Dermatologic: Photosensitivity

Gastrointestinal: Diarrhea

<1%: Abdominal cramps, acute renal failure, **anaphylaxis,** angioedema, anorexia, azotemia, **diabetes insipidus,** eosinophilia, erythema multiforme, **esophagitis,** exfoliative dermatitis, hemolytic anemia, hepatitis, **hepatic failure,** neutropenia, **paresthesia,** pericarditis, pigmentation of nails, pruritus, **pseudotumor cerebri** (eg, blurred vision, bulging fontanels in infants, headache, increased intracranial pressure), rash, Stevens-Johnson syndrome, **superinfections,** thrombocytopenia, thyroid dysfunction (extremely rare), tinnitus, urticaria, **vomiting**

Contraindications Hypersensitivity to minocycline, other tetracyclines, or any component of the formulation; pregnancy

Warnings/Precautions Avoid use during tooth development (children ≤8 years of age) unless other drugs are not likely to be effective or are contraindicated. May be associated with increases in BUN secondary to antianabolic effects. Avoid in renal insufficiency (associated with hepatotoxicity). CNS effects (lightheadedness, vertigo) may occur, potentially affecting a patient's ability to drive or operate heavy machinery. Has been associated (rarely) with pseudotumor cerebri. May cause photosensitivity.

Drug Interactions

Calcium-, magnesium-, or aluminum-containing antacids, oral contraceptives, iron, zinc, sodium bicarbonate, penicillins, cimetidine: May decrease absorption of tetracyclines

Although no clinical evidence exists, tetracyclines may bind with bismuth or calcium carbonate, an excipient in bismuth subsalicylate, during treatment for *H. pylori.*

Digoxin: Tetracyclines may rarely increase digoxin serum levels.

Methoxyflurane anesthesia when concurrent with tetracyclines may cause fatal nephrotoxicity.

Oral contraceptives: Anecdotal reports suggesting decreased contraceptive efficacy with tetracyclines have been refuted by more rigorous scientific and clinical data.

Warfarin: Hypoprothrombinemic response may be increased with tetracyclines; monitor INR closely during initiation or discontinuation.

Dietary/Ethanol/Herb Considerations Herb/Nutraceutical: Avoid dong quai and St John's wort; may cause photosensitization.

Pharmacodynamics/Kinetics

Absorption: Well absorbed

Distribution: Majority deposits for extended periods in fat; crosses placenta; enters breast milk

Protein binding: 70% to 75%

Half-life elimination: 15 hours

Excretion: Urine

Pregnancy Risk Factor D

Breast-feeding Considerations Although tetracyclines are excreted in limited amounts, the potential for staining of unerupted teeth has led some experts to recommend against breast-feeding. The AAP identified tetracyclines as "compatible" with breast-feeding.

Dosage Forms CAP: 50 mg, 75 mg, 100 mg; (Dynacin®): 50 mg, 75 mg, 100 mg. **CAP, pellet-filled** (Minocin®): 50 mg, 100 mg. **INJ, powder for reconstitution** (Minocin®): 100 mg

Generic Available Yes

Minocycline Hydrochloride *see* Minocycline *on page 915*

Minocycline Hydrochloride Periodontal Microspheres

(mi noe SYE kleen hye droe KLORe ide per ee oh DON tol MYE kroe sfeerz)

Related Information

Minocycline *on page 915*

U.S. Brand Names Arestin™

Pharmacologic Category Antibiotic, Tetracycline Derivative

Use Dental: Adjunct to scaling and root planing procedures for reduction of pocket depth in patients with adult periodontitis. May be used as part of a periodontal maintenance program which includes good oral hygiene, scaling, and root planing.

Local Anesthetic/Vasoconstrictor Precautions No information available to require special precautions

Effects on Dental Treatment Patients should avoid the following postadministration: Eating hard, crunchy, or sticky foods for 1 week; brushing for a 12-hour period; touching treated areas; use of interproximal cleaning devices for 10 days

Frequency not defined: Headache, pain, periodontitis, tooth disorder, dental caries, dental pain, gingivitis, stomatitis, oral ulceration, dyspepsia, dental infection, mucous membrane disorder, pharyngitis, infection, flu syndrome

Dosage Arestin™ is a variable dose product; dependent upon the size, shape, and number of pockets being treated. Administration of Arestin™ does not require local anesthesia. Professional subgingival administration is accomplished by inserting the unit-dose cartridge to the base of the periodontal pocket and then pressing the thumb ring in the handle mechanism to expel the powder while gradually withdrawing the tip from the base of the pocket. The handle mechanism should be sterilized between patients. Arestin™ does not have to be removed (it is bioresorbable) nor is an adhesive dressing required.

Mechanism of Action Minocycline, a member of the tetracycline class of antibiotics, has a broad spectrum of activity. It is bacteriostatic and exerts its antimicrobial activity by inhibiting protein synthesis.

Contraindications Known hypersensitivity to minocycline, tetracyclines, or any component of the formulation; pregnancy

Warnings/Precautions The use of the tetracycline class during tooth development (last half of pregnancy, infancy, and childhood to 8 years of age) may cause permanent discoloration of the teeth (yellow-gray brown). This adverse reaction is more common during long-term use of the drugs, but has been observed following repeated short-term courses. Enamel hypoplasia has also been reported. Tetracycline drugs, therefore, should not be used in this age group, or in pregnant or nursing women, unless the potential benefits are considered to outweigh the potential risks. Results of animal studies indicate that tetracyclines cross the placenta, are found in fetal tissues, and can have toxic effects on the developing fetus (often related to retardation of skeletal development). Evidence of embryotoxicity has also been noted in animals treated early in pregnancy. If any tetracyclines are used during pregnancy, or if the patient becomes pregnant while taking this drug, the patient should be apprised of the potential hazard to the fetus. Photosensitivity manifested by an exaggerated sunburn reaction has been observed in some individuals taking tetracyclines. Patients apt to be exposed to direct sunlight or ultraviolet light should be advised that this reaction can occur with tetracycline drugs, and treatment should be discontinued at the first evidence of skin erythema.

The use of Arestin™ in an acutely abscessed periodontal pocket has not been studied and is not recommended. While no overgrowth by opportunistic microorganisms, such as yeast, were noted during clinical studies, as with other antimicrobials, the use of Arestin™ may result in overgrowth of nonsusceptible microorganisms including fungi. The effects of treatment for >6 months have not been studied. Arestin™ should be used with caution in patients having a history of predisposition to oral candidiasis. The safety and effectiveness of Arestin™ have not been established for the treatment of periodontitis in patients with coexistent oral candidiasis. Arestin™ has not been clinically tested in immunocompromised patients (such as those immunocompromised by diabetes, chemotherapy, radiation therapy, or infection with HIV). If superinfection is suspected, appropriate measures should be taken. Arestin™ has not been clinically tested for use in the regeneration of alveolar bone, either in preparation for or in conjunction with the placement of endosseous (dental) implants or in the treatment of failing implants.

Pregnancy Risk Factor D

Dosage Forms **POWDER**, dry [microspheres] (Arestin™): 1 mg/unit-dose cartridge [12/tray]

Generic Available No

Minoxidil (mi NOKS i dil)

Related Information

Cardiovascular Diseases *on page 1456*

U.S. Brand Names Loniten®; Rogaine® Extra Strength for Men [OTC]; Rogaine® for Men [OTC]; Rogaine® for Women [OTC]

Canadian Brand Names Apo®-Gain; Minox; Rogaine®

Mexican Brand Names Regaine®

Pharmacologic Category Topical Skin Product; Vasodilator

Use Management of severe hypertension (usually in combination with a diuretic and beta-blocker); treatment (topical formulation) of alopecia androgenetica in males and females

Local Anesthetic/Vasoconstrictor Precautions No information available to require special precautions

(Continued)

Minoxidil *(Continued)*

Effects on Dental Treatment No significant effects or complications reported

Dosage

Children <12 years: Hypertension: Oral: Initial: 0.1-0.2 mg/kg once daily; maximum: 5 mg/day; increase gradually every 3 days; usual dosage: 0.25-1 mg/kg/day in 1-2 divided doses; maximum: 50 mg/day

Children >12 years and Adults: Hypertension: Oral: Initial: 5 mg once daily, increase gradually every 3 days; usual dose: 10-40 mg/day in 1-2 divided doses; maximum: 100 mg/day

Adults: Alopecia: Topical: Apply twice daily; 4 months of therapy may be necessary for hair growth.

Elderly: Initial: 2.5 mg once daily; increase gradually.

Note: Dosing adjustment is needed when added to concomitant therapy.

Dialysis: Supplemental dose is unnecessary via hemo- or peritoneal dialysis.

Mechanism of Action Produces vasodilation by directly relaxing arteriolar smooth muscle, with little effect on veins; effects may be mediated by cyclic AMP; stimulation of hair growth is secondary to vasodilation, increased cutaneous blood flow and stimulation of resting hair follicles

Other Adverse Effects

Oral: Incidence of reactions not always reported.

Cardiovascular: Peripheral edema (7%), sodium and water retention, CHF, tachycardia, angina pectoris, pericardial effusion with or without tamponade, pericarditis, EKG changes (T-wave changes, 60%), rebound hypertension (in children after a gradual withdrawal)

Central nervous system: Headache (rare), fatigue

Dermatologic: Hypertrichosis (common, 80%), transient pruritus, changes in pigmentation (rare), serosanguineous bullae (rare), rash (rare), Stevens-Johnson syndrome

Endocrine & metabolic: Breast tenderness (rare, <1%), gynecomastia (rare), polymenorrhea (rare)

Gastrointestinal: Weight gain, nausea (rare), vomiting

Hematologic: Intermittent claudication (rare), thrombocytopenia (rare), decreased hematocrit (hemodilution), decreased hemoglobin (hemodilution), decreased erythrocyte count (hemodilution), leukopenia (rare)

Hepatic: Increased alkaline phosphatase

Renal: Transient increase in serum BUN and creatinine

Respiratory: Pulmonary edema

Topical: Incidence of adverse events is not always reported.

Cardiovascular: Increased left ventricular end-diastolic volume, increased cardiac output, increased left ventricular mass, dizziness, tachycardia, edema, transient chest pain, palpitation, increase or decrease in blood pressure, increase or decrease in pulse rate (1.5%, placebo 1.6%)

Central nervous system: Headache, dizziness, weakness, taste alterations, faintness, lightheadedness (3.4%, placebo 3.5%), vertigo (1.2%, placebo 1.2%), anxiety (rare), mental depression (rare), fatigue (rare 0.4%, placebo 1%)

Dermatologic: Local irritation, dryness, erythema, allergic contact dermatitis (7.4%, placebo 5.4%), pruritus, scaling/flaking, eczema, seborrhea, papular rash, folliculitis, local erythema, flushing, exacerbation of hair loss, alopecia, hypertrichosis, increased hair growth outside the area of application (face, beard, eyebrows, ear, arm)

Endocrine & metabolic: Menstrual changes, breast symptoms (0.5%, placebo 0.5%)

Gastrointestinal: Diarrhea, nausea, vomiting (4.3%, placebo 6.6%), weight gain (1.2%, placebo 1.3%)

Genitourinary: Urinary tract infections (rare), renal calculi (rare), urethritis (rare), prostatitis (rare), epididymitis (rare), impotence (rare)

Hematologic: Lymphadenopathy, thrombocytopenia, anemia (0.3%, placebo 0.6%)

Neuromuscular & skeletal: Fractures, back pain, retrosternal chest pain of muscular origin, tendonitis (2.6%, placebo 2.2%)

Ocular: Conjunctivitis, visual disturbances, decreased visual acuity

Respiratory: Bronchitis, upper respiratory infections, sinusitis (7.2%, placebo 8.6%)

Drug Interactions Increased Effect/Toxicity: Concurrent use of guanethidine can cause severe orthostasis; avoid concurrent use - discontinue 1-3 weeks prior to initiating minoxidil. Effects of other antihypertensives may be additive with minoxidil.

Dietary/Ethanol/Herb Considerations

Food: Avoid licorice

Herb/Nutraceutical: Avoid licorice; causes sodium and water retention and increases potassium loss.

Pharmacodynamics/Kinetics

Onset of action: Hypotensive: Oral: ~30 minutes

Peak effect: 2-8 hours

Duration: 2-5 days

Protein binding: None

Metabolism: 88%, primarily via glucuronidation
Bioavailability: Oral: 90%
Half-life elimination: Adults: 3.5-4.2 hours
Excretion: Urine (12% as unchanged drug)

Pregnancy Risk Factor C

Generic Available Yes

Mintezol® *see* Thiabendazole *on page 1294*
Miochol-E® *see* Acetylcholine *on page 39*
Miostat® *see* Carbachol *on page 241*
Miradon® *see* Anisindione *on page 110*
MiraLax™ *see* Polyethylene Glycol-Electrolyte Solution *on page 1094*
Mirapex® *see* Pramipexole *on page 1105*
Miraphen PSE *see* Guaifenesin and Pseudoephedrine *on page 652*
Mircette® *see* Combination Hormonal Contraceptives *on page 368*
Mirena® *see* Levonorgestrel *on page 797*

Mirtazapine (mir TAZ a peen)

U.S. Brand Names Remeron®; Remeron SolTab®

Canadian Brand Names Remeron®

Mexican Brand Names Remeron®

Pharmacologic Category Antidepressant, Alpha-2 Antagonist

Use Treatment of depression

Local Anesthetic/Vasoconstrictor Precautions Although mirtazapine is not a tricyclic antidepressant, it does block norepinephrine reuptake within CNS synapses as part of its mechanisms. It has been suggested that vasoconstrictor be administered with caution and to monitor vital signs in dental patients taking antidepressants that affect norepinephrine in this way, including mirtazapine.

Effects on Dental Treatment ≤25%: Significant xerostomia

Dosage Oral:

Children: Safety and efficacy not established

Treatment of depression: Adults: Initial: 15 mg nightly, titrate up to 15-45 mg/day with dose increases made no more frequently than every 1-2 weeks; there is an inverse relationship between dose and sedation

Elderly: Decreased clearance seen (40% males, 10% females); no specific adjustments recommended by manufacturer

Dosing adjustment in renal impairment:
- Cl_{cr} 11-39 mL/minute: 30% decreased clearance
- Cl_{cr} <10 mL/minute: 50% decreased clearance

Dosing adjustment in hepatic impairment: Clearance decreased by 30%

Mechanism of Action Mirtazapine is a tetracyclic antidepressant that works by its central presynaptic alpha$_2$-adrenergic antagonist effects, which results in increased release of norepinephrine and serotonin. It is also a potent antagonist of 5-HT_2 and 5-HT_3 serotonin receptors and H1 histamine receptors and a moderate peripheral alpha$_1$-adrenergic and muscarinic antagonist; it does not inhibit the reuptake of norepinephrine or serotonin.

Other Adverse Effects

>10%:
- Central nervous system: Somnolence (54%)
- Endocrine & metabolic: Cholesterol increased
- Gastrointestinal: Constipation (13%), appetite increased (17%), weight gain (12%; weight gain of >7% reported in 8% of adults, ≤49% of pediatric patients)

1% to 10%:
- Cardiovascular: Hypertension, vasodilatation, peripheral edema (2%), edema (1%)
- Central nervous system: Dizziness (7%), abnormal dreams (4%), abnormal thoughts (3%), confusion (2%), malaise
- Endocrine & metabolic: Triglycerides increased
- Gastrointestinal: Vomiting, anorexia, abdominal pain
- Genitourinary: Urinary frequency (2%)
- Neuromuscular & skeletal: Myalgia (2%), back pain (2%), arthralgias, tremor (2%), weakness (8%)
- Respiratory: Dyspnea (1%)
- Miscellaneous: Flu-like symptoms (5%), thirst

<1%: Abdomen enlarged, abnormal ejaculation, accommodation abnormality, acne, agitation, agranulocytosis, akathisia, alopecia, amenorrhea, amnesia, anemia, angina pectoris, anxiety, apathy, aphasia, **aphthous stomatitis**, arthrosis, arthritis, asphyxia, asthma, ataxia, atrial arrhythmia, bigeminy, blepharitis, bone pain, bradycardia, breast engorgement, breast enlargement, breast pain, bronchitis, bursitis, cardiomegaly, cellulitis, cerebral ischemia, chest pain, chills, cholecystitis, cirrhosis, colitis, conjunctivitis, coordination abnormal, cough, cystitis, deafness, dehydration, delirium, delusions, dementia, depersonalization, depression, diabetes mellitus, diplopia, drug dependence, dry skin, dysarthria, dyskinesia, dysmenorrhea, dystonia, dysuria, ear pain, emotional lability, epistaxis, eructation, euphoria, exfoliative dermatitis, extrapyramidal syndrome,

(Continued)

Mirtazapine *(Continued)*

eye pain, facial edema, fever, fracture, gastritis, gastroenteritis, glaucoma, **glossitis**, goiter, gout, grand mal seizure, **gum hemorrhage**, hallucinations, hematuria, herpes simplex, herpes zoster, hiccup, hostility, hypokinesia, hyperacusis, hyperkinesias, hypesthesia, hypotension, hypothyroidism, hypotonia, impotence, increased salivation, intestinal obstruction, keratoconjunctivitis, kidney calculus, lacrimation disorder, laryngitis, left heart failure, leukopenia, leukorrhea, libido increased, LFTs abnormal, lymphadenopathy, lymphocytosis, manic reaction, menorrhagia, metrorrhagia, migraine, MI, myoclonus, myositis, nausea, neck pain, neck rigidity, neurosis, nystagmus, oral moniliasis, osteoporosis, otitis media, pancreatitis, pancytopenia, paralysis, paranoid reaction, paresthesia, parosmia, petechia, phlebitis, photosensitivity reaction, pneumonia, pneumothorax, polyuria, pruritus, psychotic depression, pulmonary embolus, rash, reflexes increased, salivary gland enlargement, seborrhea, sinusitis, skin hypertrophy, skin ulcer, stomatitis, stupor, syncope, **loss of taste**, tendon rupture, tenosynovitis, thrombocytopenia, tongue discoloration, tongue edema, twitching, ulcer, ulcerative stomatitis, urethritis, urinary incontinence, urinary retention, urinary tract infection, urinary urgency, urticaria, vaginitis, vascular headache, ventricular extrasystoles, vertigo, weight loss, withdrawal syndrome

Postmarketing and/or case reports: Torsade de pointes (1 case reported)

Drug Interactions Substrate of **CYP1A2**, 2C8/9, **2D6, 3A4**; Inhibits CYP1A2, 3A4

Increased sedative effect seen with CNS depressants, CYP inhibitors, linezolid, MAO inhibitors, selegiline, and sibutramine.

Decreased effect seen with clonidine, CYP inducers.

Dietary/Ethanol/Herb Considerations

Avoid ethanol; may increase CNS depression.

Herb/Nutraceutical: Avoid kava, SAMe, and valerian; may increase CNS depression. Avoid St John's wort; may decrease serum concentration and increase CNS depression.

Pharmacodynamics/Kinetics

Protein binding: 85%

Metabolism: Extensively hepatic via CYP1A2, 2C9, 2D6, 3A4 and via demethylation and hydroxylation

Bioavailability: 50%

Half-life elimination: 20-40 hours; hampered with renal or hepatic impairment

Time to peak, serum: 2 hours

Excretion: Urine (75%) and feces (15%) as metabolites

Pregnancy Risk Factor C

Generic Available Yes: Tablet

Selected Readings Ganzber S, "Psychoactive Drugs," *ADA Guide to Dental Therapeutics,* 2nd edition, Chapter 21, Chicago, IL: ADA Publishing, 2000, 382.

Misoprostol (mye soe PROST ole)

U.S. Brand Names Cytotec®

Canadian Brand Names Apo®-Misoprostol; Cytotec®; Novo-Misoprostol

Mexican Brand Names Cytotec®

Pharmacologic Category Prostaglandin

Use Prevention of NSAID-induced gastric ulcers; medical termination of pregnancy of ≤49 days (in conjunction with mifepristone)

Unlabeled/Investigational Use Cervical ripening and labor induction; treatment of NSAID-induced nephropathy, fat malabsorption in cystic fibrosis

Local Anesthetic/Vasoconstrictor Precautions No information available to require special precautions

Effects on Dental Treatment No significant effects or complications reported

Dosage

Oral:

Children 8-16 years: Fat absorption in cystic fibrosis (unlabeled use): 100 mcg 4 times/day

Adults:

Prevention of NSAID-induced gastric ulcers: 200 mcg 4 times/day with food; if not tolerated, may decrease dose to 100 mcg 4 times/day with food or 200 mcg twice daily with food; last dose of the day should be taken at bedtime

Medical termination of pregnancy: Refer to Mifepristone monograph.

Intravaginal: Adults: Labor induction or cervical ripening (unlabeled use): 25 mcg (1/4 of 100 mcg tablet); may repeat at intervals no more frequent than every 3-6 hours. Do not use in patients with previous cesarean delivery or prior major uterine surgery.

Mechanism of Action Misoprostol is a synthetic prostaglandin E_1 analog that replaces the protective prostaglandins consumed with prostaglandin-inhibiting therapies (eg, NSAIDs); has been shown to induce uterine contractions

Other Adverse Effects

>10%: Gastrointestinal: Diarrhea, abdominal pain

1% to 10%:

Central nervous system: Headache

Gastrointestinal: Constipation, flatulence, nausea, dyspepsia, vomiting

<1%: Uterine stimulation, vaginal bleeding

Postmarketing and/or case reports: Abnormal taste, abnormal vision, alkaline phosphatase increased, alopecia, anaphylaxis, anemia, amylase increase, anxiety, appetite changes, arrhythmia, arthralgia, back pain, breast pain, bronchospasm, cardiac enzymes increased, chest pain, confusion, deafness, depression, dermatitis, diaphoresis, drowsiness, dysphagia, dyspnea, earache, edema, epistaxis, ESR increased, fetal or infant death (when used during pregnancy), fever, GI bleeding, GI inflammation, gingivitis, glycosuria, gout, hypertension, hypotension, impotence, loss of libido, muscle cramps, myalgia, neuropathy, neurosis, nitrogen increased, pallor, phlebitis, purpura, rash, reflux, rigors, stiffness, syncope, thirst, thrombocytopenia, tinnitus, uterine rupture, weakness, weight changes

Drug Interactions Decreased Effect: Antacids may diminish absorption (not clinically significant).

Dietary/Ethanol/Herb Considerations Food: Administration with food may reduce diarrhea; food may decrease peak serum concentration (not clinically significant).

Pharmacodynamics/Kinetics

Absorption: Rapid

Metabolism: Hepatic; rapidly de-esterified to misoprostol acid (active)

Half-life elimination: Metabolite: 20-40 minutes

Time to peak, serum: Active metabolite: Fasting: 15-30 minutes

Excretion: Urine (64% to 73%) and feces (15%) within 24 hours

Pregnancy Risk Factor X

Generic Available Yes

Misoprostol and Diclofenac *see* Diclofenac and Misoprostol *on page 431*

Mitomycin (mye toe MYE sin)

U.S. Brand Names Mitozytrex™; Mutamycin®

Canadian Brand Names Mutamycin®

Mexican Brand Names Mitocin®

Pharmacologic Category Antineoplastic Agent, Antibiotic

Synonyms Mitomycin-C; MTC

Use Therapy of disseminated adenocarcinoma of stomach or pancreas in combination with other approved chemotherapeutic agents; bladder cancer, colorectal cancer

Unlabeled/Investigational Use Prevention of excess scarring in glaucoma filtration procedures in patients at high risk of bleb failure

Local Anesthetic/Vasoconstrictor Precautions No information available to require special precautions

Effects on Dental Treatment No significant effects or complications reported

Dosage Refer to individual protocols. Children and Adults:

Single agent therapy: I.V.: 20 mg/m^2 every 6-8 weeks

Combination therapy: I.V.: 10 mg/m^2 every 6-8 weeks

Mitozytrex™: I.V.: 15 mg/m^2 every 6-8 weeks

Bladder carcinoma: Intravesicular instillation (unapproved route): 20-40 mg/dose (1 mg/mL in sterile aqueous solution) instilled into the bladder for 3 hours repeated up to 3 times/week for up to 20 procedures per course

Glaucoma surgery (unlabeled use): Dosages and techniques vary; 0.2-0.5 mg may be applied to a pledget (using a 0.2-0.5 mg/mL solution), and placed in contact with the surgical wound for 2-5 minutes; other protocols have been reported

Dosing adjustment in renal impairment: Varying approaches to dosing adjustments have been published; consult individual protocols.

Cl_{cr} <10 mL/minute: Administer 75% of normal dose

Note: The manufacturers state that products should not be given to patients with serum creatinine >1.7 mg/dL. Mitozytrex™ should not be used if Cl_{cr} <30 mL/minute.

Hemodialysis: Unknown

CAPD effects: Unknown

CAVH effects: Unknown

Dosing adjustment in hepatic impairment: Specific recommendations unavailable

Mechanism of Action Isolated from *Streptomyces caespitosus*; acts primarily as an alkylating agent and produces DNA cross-linking (primarily with guanine and cytosine pairs); cell-cycle nonspecific; inhibits DNA and RNA synthesis by alkylation and cross-linking the strands of DNA

Other Adverse Effects

>10%:

Cardiovascular: Congestive heart failure (3% to 15%) (doses >30 mg/m^2)

Central nervous system: Fever (14%)

Dermatologic: Alopecia, nail banding/discoloration

Gastrointestinal: Nausea, vomiting and anorexia (14%)

Hematologic: Anemia (19% to 24%); myelosuppression, common, dose-limiting, delayed

Onset: 3 weeks

(Continued)

Mitomycin *(Continued)*

Nadir: 4-6 weeks
Recovery: 6-8 weeks
1% to 10%:
Dermatologic: Rash
Gastrointestinal: Stomatitis
Neuromuscular: Paresthesias
Renal: Creatinine increased (2%)
Respiratory: Interstitial pneumonitis, infiltrates, dyspnea, cough (7%)
<1%: Malaise, pruritus, extravasation reactions, hemolytic uremic syndrome, renal failure, bladder fibrosis/contraction (intravesical administration)

Drug Interactions Increased Effect/Toxicity: *Vinca* alkaloids or doxorubicin may enhance cardiac toxicity when coadministered with mitomycin.

Dietary/Ethanol/Herb Considerations Herb/Nutraceutical: Avoid black cohosh and dong quai in estrogen-dependent tumors.

Pharmacodynamics/Kinetics

Distribution: V_d: 22 L/m^2; high drug concentrations found in kidney, tongue, muscle, heart, and lung tissue; probably not distributed into the CNS
Metabolism: Hepatic
Half-life elimination: 23-78 minutes; Terminal: 50 minutes
Excretion: Mitomycin: Urine (<10% as unchanged drug), with elevated serum concentrations; HPβCD: Urine (93% as unchanged drug)

Pregnancy Risk Factor D

Generic Available Yes

Mitomycin-C *see* Mitomycin *on page 921*

Mitotane (MYE toe tane)

U.S. Brand Names Lysodren®

Canadian Brand Names Lysodren®

Pharmacologic Category Antineoplastic Agent, Miscellaneous

Synonyms o,p′-DDD

Use Treatment of adrenocortical carcinoma

Unlabeled/Investigational Use Treatment of Cushing's syndrome

Local Anesthetic/Vasoconstrictor Precautions No information available to require special precautions

Effects on Dental Treatment No significant effects or complications reported

Dosage Oral:

Children: 0.1-0.5 mg/kg or 1-2 g/day in divided doses increasing gradually to a maximum of 5-7 g/day
Adults: Start at 1-6 g/day in divided doses, then increase incrementally to 8-10 g/day in 3-4 divided doses; dose is changed on basis of side effect with aim of giving as high a dose as tolerated; maximum daily dose: 18 g
Dosing adjustment in hepatic impairment: May require reduction

Mechanism of Action Causes adrenal cortical atrophy; drug affects mitochondria in adrenal cortical cells and decreases production of cortisol; also alters the peripheral metabolism of steroids

Other Adverse Effects The following reactions are reversible:

Central nervous system: CNS depression (32%), dizziness (15%), headache (5%), confusion (3%)
Dermatologic: Skin rash (12%)
Gastrointestinal: Anorexia (24%), nausea (39%), vomiting (37%), diarrhea (13%)
Neuromuscular & skeletal: Muscle tremor (3%), weakness (12%)

Drug Interactions

Increased Effect/Toxicity: CNS depressants taken with mitotane may enhance CNS depression.
Decreased Effect: Mitotane may enhance the clearance of barbiturates and warfarin by induction of the hepatic microsomal enzyme system resulting in a decreased effect. Coadministration of spironolactone has resulted in negation of mitotane's effect. Mitotane may increase clearance of phenytoin by microsomal enzyme stimulation.

Dietary/Ethanol/Herb Considerations

Ethanol: Avoid use; may increase CNS depression.
Herb/Nutraceutical: Avoid gotu kola, kava, SAMe, St John's wort, and valerian; may increase CNS depression.

Pharmacodynamics/Kinetics

Absorption: Oral: ~35% to 40%
Distribution: Stored mainly in fat tissue but is found in all body tissues
Metabolism: Hepatic and other tissues
Half-life elimination: 18-159 days
Time to peak, serum: 3-5 hours
Excretion: Urine and feces (as metabolites)

Pregnancy Risk Factor C

Generic Available No

Mitoxantrone (mye toe ZAN trone)

U.S. Brand Names Novantrone®

Canadian Brand Names Novantrone®

Mexican Brand Names Misostol; Mitroxone® [inj.]; Novantrone®

Pharmacologic Category Antineoplastic Agent, Antibiotic

Synonyms DHAD; Mitoxantrone Hydrochloride

Use Treatment of acute nonlymphocytic leukemia (ANLL) in adults in combination with other agents; very active against various leukemias, lymphoma, and breast cancer; moderately active against pediatric sarcoma; treatment of secondary (chronic) progressive, progressive relapsing, or worsening relapsing-remitting multiple sclerosis; treatment of pain related to advanced hormone-refractory prostate cancer (in combination with corticosteroids)

Local Anesthetic/Vasoconstrictor Precautions No information available to require special precautions

Effects on Dental Treatment No significant effects or complications reported

Dosage Refer to individual protocols. I.V. (dilute in D_5W or NS):

ANLL leukemias:

Children ≤2 years: 0.4 mg/kg/day once daily for 3-5 days

Children >2 years and Adults: 12 mg/m²/day once daily for 3 days; acute leukemia in relapse: 8-12 mg/m²/day once daily for 4-5 days

Solid tumors:

Children: 18-20 mg/m² every 3-4 weeks **OR** 5-8 mg/m² every week

Adults: 12-14 mg/m² every 3-4 weeks **OR** 2-4 mg/m²/day for 5 days every 4 weeks

Maximum total dose: 80-120 mg/m² in patients with predisposing factor and <160 mg in patients with no predisposing factor

Hormone-refractory prostate cancer: Adults: 12-14 mg/m² over 5-15 minutes via intravenous infusion every 21 days

Multiple sclerosis: Adults: 12 mg/m² over 5-15 minutes via intravenous infusion every 3 months; do **not** use if LVEF <50% (or following significant reduction); cumulative lifetime dose should not exceed ≥140 mg/m²

Elderly: Clearance is decreased; use with caution

Dosing adjustment in renal impairment: Safety and efficacy not established

Hemodialysis: Supplemental dose is unnecessary

Peritoneal dialysis: Supplemental dose is unnecessary

Dosing adjustment in hepatic impairment: Official recommendations not established; not indicated for patients with MS who are hepatically impaired. Use with caution when used to treat other indications.

Moderate dysfunction (bilirubin 1.5-3 mg/dL): Some clinicians recommend a 50% dosage reduction

Severe dysfunction (bilirubin >3.0 mg/dL) have a lower total body clearance and may require a dosage adjustment to 8 mg/m²; some clinicians recommend a dosage reduction to 25% of dose

Dose modifications based on degree of leukopenia or thrombocytopenia: See table.

Granulocyte Count Nadir (cells/mm²)	Platelet Count Nadir (cells/mm²)	Total Bilirubin (mg/dL)	Dose Adjustment
>2000	>150,000	<1.5	Increase by 1 mg/m²
1000-2000	75,000-150,000	<1.5	Maintain same dose
<1000	<75,000	1.5-3	Decrease by 1 mg/m²

Mechanism of Action Analogue of the anthracyclines, but different in mechanism of action, cardiac toxicity, and potential for tissue necrosis; mitoxantrone does intercalate DNA; binds to nucleic acids and inhibits DNA and RNA synthesis by template disordering and steric obstruction; replication is decreased by binding to DNA topoisomerase II (enzyme responsible for DNA helix supercoiling); active throughout entire cell cycle; does not appear to produce free radicals

Other Adverse Effects Reported with any indication; incidence varies based on treatment/dose

>10%:

Cardiovascular: Abnormal EKG, arrhythmia (3% to 18%), edema, nail bed changes

Central nervous system: Fatigue, fever, headache (6% to 13%)

Dermatologic: Alopecia (20% to 61%)

Endocrine & metabolic: Amenorrhea, menstrual disorder

Gastrointestinal: Abdominal pain, anorexia, nausea (29% to 76%), constipation, diarrhea (16% to 47%), GI bleeding, mucositis (10% to 29%), stomatitis, vomiting, weight gain/loss

Genitourinary: Abnormal urine, urinary tract infection

Hematologic: Decreased hemoglobin, leukopenia, lymphopenia, petechiae/bruising; myelosuppressive effects of chemotherapy:

WBC: Mild

Platelets: Mild

(Continued)

Mitoxantrone *(Continued)*

Onset: 7-10 days
Nadir: 14 days
Recovery: 21 days

Hepatic: Increased GGT
Neuromuscular & skeletal: Weakness (24%)
Respiratory: Cough, dyspnea, upper respiratory tract infection
Miscellaneous: Fungal infections, infection, sepsis

1% to 10%:

Cardiovascular: CHF, ischemia, decreased LVEF (≤5%)
Central nervous system: Chills, anxiety, depression, seizures
Dermatologic: Skin infection
Endocrine & metabolic: Hypocalcemia, hypokalemia, hyponatremia, hyperglycemia
Gastrointestinal: Dyspepsia, aphthosis
Genitourinary: Impotence, proteinuria, renal failure, sterility
Hematologic: Anemia, granulocytopenia, hemorrhage
Hepatic: Jaundice, increased SGOT, increased SGPT
Neuromuscular & skeletal: Back pain, myalgia, arthralgia
Ocular: Blurred vision, conjunctivitis
Renal: Hematuria
Respiratory: Pneumonia, rhinitis, sinusitis
Miscellaneous: Systemic infection, sweats, development of secondary leukemia (~1% to 2%)

<1% or frequency not defined: Acute leukemia, allergic reaction, anaphylactoid reactions, anaphylaxis, EKG changes, hypotension, extravasation and phlebitis at the infusion site, interstitial pneumonitis (has occurred during combination chemotherapy), irritant chemotherapy with blue skin discoloration, rash, tachycardia

Drug Interactions Inhibits CYP3A4

Decreased Effect: Impaired immune response to vaccines; possible infection postadministration (patients receiving immunosuppressants)

Dietary/Ethanol/Herb Considerations Herb/Nutraceutical: Avoid black cohosh and dong quai in estrogen-dependent tumors.

Pharmacodynamics/Kinetics

Absorption: Oral: Poor
Distribution: V_d: 14 L/kg; distributes into pleural fluid, kidney, thyroid, liver, heart, and red blood cells
Protein binding: >95%, 76% to albumin
Metabolism: Hepatic; pathway not determined
Half-life elimination: Terminal: 23-215 hours; may be prolonged with hepatic impairment
Excretion: Urine (6% to 11%) and feces as unchanged drug and metabolites

Pregnancy Risk Factor D

Generic Available No

Mitoxantrone Hydrochloride *see* Mitoxantrone *on page 923*
Mitozytrex™ *see* Mitomycin *on page 921*
Mitrazol™ [OTC] *see* Miconazole *on page 906*
Mitrolan® Chewable Tablet [OTC] *see* Calcium Polycarbophil *on page 228*
MK383 *see* Tirofiban *on page 1313*
MK462 *see* Rizatriptan *on page 1193*
MK594 *see* Losartan *on page 825*
MK-0826 *see* Ertapenem *on page 511*
MMR *see* Measles, Mumps, and Rubella Vaccines (Combined) *on page 844*
M-M-R® II *see* Measles, Mumps, and Rubella Vaccines (Combined) *on page 844*
Moban® *see* Molindone *on page 927*
MOBIC® *see* Meloxicam *on page 854*
Mobidin® [DSC] *see* Magnesium Salicylate *on page 837*
Mobisyl® [OTC] *see* Triethanolamine Salicylate *on page 1348*

Modafinil (moe DAF i nil)

U.S. Brand Names Provigil®

Canadian Brand Names Alertec®; Provigil®

Pharmacologic Category Stimulant

Use Improve wakefulness in patients with excessive daytime sleepiness associated with narcolepsy

Unlabeled/Investigational Use Treatment of attention-deficit/hyperactivity disorder (ADHD), fatigue in MS and other disorders

Local Anesthetic/Vasoconstrictor Precautions No information available to require special precautions

Effects on Dental Treatment Xerostomia (5%), oral ulceration and gingivitis (1%)

Restrictions C-IV

Dosage Oral:

Children: ADHD (unlabeled use): 50-100 mg once daily

Adults:

ADHD (unlabeled use): 100-300 mg once daily

Narcolepsy: Initial: 200 mg as a single daily dose in the morning

Doses of 400 mg/day, given as a single dose, have been well tolerated, but there is no consistent evidence that this dose confers additional benefit

Elderly: Elimination of modafinil and its metabolites may be reduced as a consequence of aging and as a result, lower doses should be considered.

Dosing adjustment in renal impairment: Safety and efficacy in severe impairment not established

Dosing adjustment in hepatic impairment: Reduce dose to one-half of that recommended for patients with normal liver function

Mechanism of Action The exact mechanism of action is unclear, it does not appear to alter the release of dopamine or norepinephrine, it may exert its stimulant effects by decreasing GABA-mediated neurotransmission, although this theory has not yet been fully evaluated; several studies also suggest that an intact central alpha-adrenergic system is required for modafinil's activity; the drug increases high-frequency alpha waves while decreasing both delta and theta wave activity, and these effects are consistent with generalized increases in mental alertness

Other Adverse Effects Limited to reports equal to or greater than placebo-related events.

<10%:

Cardiovascular: Chest pain (2%), hypertension (2%), hypotension (2%), vasodilation (1%), arrhythmia (1%), syncope (1%)

Central nervous system: Headache (50%, compared to 40% with placebo), nervousness (8%), dizziness (5%), depression (4%), anxiety (4%), cataplexy (3%), insomnia (3%), chills (2%), fever (1%), confusion (1%), amnesia (1%), emotional lability (1%), ataxia (1%)

Dermatologic: Dry skin (1%)

Endocrine & metabolic: Hyperglycemia (1%), albuminuria (1%)

Gastrointestinal: Diarrhea (8%), nausea (13%, compared to 4% with placebo), anorexia (5%), vomiting (1%)

Genitourinary: Abnormal urine (1%), urinary retention (1%), ejaculatory disturbance (1%)

Hematologic: Eosinophilia (1%)

Hepatic: Abnormal LFTs (3%)

Neuromuscular & skeletal: Paresthesias (3%), dyskinesia (2%), neck pain (2%), hypertonia (2%), neck rigidity (1%), joint disorder (1%), tremor (1%)

Ocular: Amblyopia (2%), abnormal vision (2%)

Respiratory: Pharyngitis (6%), rhinitis (11%, compared to 8% with placebo), lung disorder (4%), dyspnea (2%), asthma (1%), epistaxis (1%)

Drug Interactions Substrate of **CYP3A4**; Inhibits CYP2C8/9, 2C19; Induces CYP1A2, 2B6, 3A4

Increased Effect/Toxicity: Modafinil may increase levels of diazepam, mephenytoin, phenytoin, propranolol, and warfarin. In populations deficient in the CYP2D6 isoenzyme, where CYP2C19 acts as a secondary metabolic pathway, concentrations of tricyclic antidepressants and selective serotonin reuptake inhibitors may be increased during coadministration.

Decreased Effect: Modafinil may decrease serum concentrations of oral contraceptives, cyclosporine, and to a lesser degree, theophylline. Agents that induce CYP3A4, including phenobarbital, carbamazepine, and rifampin may result in decreased modafinil levels. There is also evidence to suggest that modafinil may induce its own metabolism.

Pharmacodynamics/Kinetics Modafinil is a racemic compound (10% *d*-isomer and 90% *l*-isomer at steady state) whose enantiomers have different pharmacokinetics

Distribution: V_d: 0.9 L/kg

Protein binding: 60%, primarily to albumin

Metabolism: Hepatic; multiple pathways including CYP3A4

Half-life elimination: Effective half-life: 15 hours; Steady-state: 2-4 days

Time to peak, serum: 2-4 hours

Excretion: Urine (as metabolites, <10% as unchanged drug)

Pregnancy Risk Factor C

Generic Available No

Modane® Bulk [OTC] *see* Psyllium *on page 1149*

Modane Tablets® [OTC] *see* Bisacodyl *on page 186*

Modicon® *see* Combination Hormonal Contraceptives *on page 368*

Modified Dakin's Solution *see* Sodium Hypochlorite Solution *on page 1231*

Modified Shohl's Solution *see* Sodium Citrate and Citric Acid *on page 1230*

Moducal® [OTC] *see* Glucose Polymers *on page 641*

Moduretic® *see* Amiloride and Hydrochlorothiazide *on page 76*

Moexipril (mo EKS i pril)

Related Information

Cardiovascular Diseases *on page 1456*

Moexipril and Hydrochlorothiazide *on page 927*

U.S. Brand Names Univasc®

Pharmacologic Category Angiotensin-Converting Enzyme (ACE) Inhibitor

Synonyms Moexipril Hydrochloride

Use Treatment of hypertension, alone or in combination with thiazide diuretics; treatment of left ventricular dysfunction after MI

Local Anesthetic/Vasoconstrictor Precautions No information available to require special precautions

Effects on Dental Treatment No significant effects or complications reported

Dosage Oral:

Adults: Initial: 7.5 mg once daily (in patients **not** receiving diuretics), 1 hour prior to a meal **or** 3.75 mg once daily (when combined with thiazide diuretics); maintenance dose: 7.5-30 mg/day in 1 or 2 divided doses 1 hour before meals

Dosing adjustment in renal impairment: Cl_{cr} ≤40 mL/minute: Patients may be cautiously placed on 3.75 mg once daily, then upwardly titrated to a maximum of 15 mg/day.

Mechanism of Action Competitive inhibitor of angiotensin-converting enzyme (ACE); prevents conversion of angiotensin I to angiotensin II, a potent vasoconstrictor; results in lower levels of angiotensin II which causes an increase in plasma renin activity and a reduction in aldosterone secretion

Other Adverse Effects

1% to 10%:

Cardiovascular: Hypotension, peripheral edema

Central nervous system: Headache, dizziness, fatigue

Dermatologic: Rash, alopecia, flushing, rash

Endocrine & metabolic: Hyperkalemia, hyponatremia

Gastrointestinal: Diarrhea, nausea, heartburn

Genitourinary: Polyuria

Neuromuscular & skeletal: Myalgia

Renal: Reversible increases in creatinine or BUN

Respiratory: Cough, pharyngitis, upper respiratory infection, sinusitis

<1% (Limited to important or life-threatening): Alopecia, chest pain, MI, palpitations, arrhythmias, syncope, cerebrovascular accident, orthostatic hypotension, hypercholesterolemia, anemia, elevated LFTs, hepatitis, oliguria, proteinuria, bronchospasm, dyspnea, eosinophilic pneumonitis

Drug Interactions

Increased Effect/Toxicity:

Potassium supplements, co-trimoxazole (high dose), angiotensin II receptor antagonists (candesartan, losartan, irbesartan, etc), or potassium-sparing diuretics (amiloride, spironolactone, triamterene) may result in elevated serum potassium levels when combined with moexipril. ACE inhibitor effects may be increased by probenecid (increases levels of captopril). ACE inhibitors may increase serum concentrations/effects of digoxin, lithium, and sulfonlyureas.

Diuretics have additive hypotensive effects with ACE inhibitors, and hypovolemia increases the potential for adverse renal effects of ACE inhibitors. In patients with compromised renal function, coadministration with NSAIDs may result in further deterioration of renal function. Allopurinol and ACE inhibitors may cause a higher risk of hypersensitivity reaction when taken concurrently.

Decreased Effect: Aspirin (high dose) may reduce the therapeutic effects of ACE inhibitors; at low dosages this does not appear to be significant. Rifampin may decrease the effect of ACE inhibitors. Antacids may decrease the bioavailability of ACE inhibitors (may be more likely to occur with captopril); separate administration times by 1-2 hours. NSAIDs, specifically indomethacin, may reduce the hypotensive effects of ACE inhibitors. More likely to occur in low renin or volume dependent hypertensive patients.

Dietary/Ethanol/Herb Considerations

Ethanol: Avoid use; may increase risk of hypotension or dizziness.

Food: Administer on an empty stomach; food may delay and reduce peak serum concentration. Avoid caffeine, garlic, and licorice.

Herb/Nutraceutical: Avoid black cohosh, dong quai, and evening primrose due to estrogenic activity. Avoid ephedra, ginseng, and yohimbe; may worsen hypertension. Avoid garlic; may have increased antihypertensive effect. Avoid ginger due to positive inotropic effects; theoretically, may cause arrhythmia. Avoid hawthorn; may decrease peripheral vascular resistance and cause additive decrease in BP. Avoid licorice.

Pharmacodynamics/Kinetics

Onset of action: Peak effect: 1-2 hours

Duration: >24 hours

Distribution: V_d (moexiprilat): 180 L

Protein binding, plasma: Moexipril: 90%; Moexiprilat: 50% to 70%

Metabolism: Parent drug: Hepatic and via GI tract to moexiprilat, 1000 times more potent than parent
Bioavailability: Moexiprilat: 13%; reduced with food (AUC decreased by ~40%)
Half-life elimination: Moexipril: 1 hour; Moexiprilat: 2-9 hours
Time to peak: 1.5 hours
Excretion: Feces (50%)

Pregnancy Risk Factor C/D (2nd and 3rd trimesters)

Generic Available No

Moexipril and Hydrochlorothiazide

(mo EKS i pril & hye droe klor oh THYE a zide)

Related Information

Hydrochlorothiazide *on page 675*
Moexipril *on page 926*

U.S. Brand Names Uniretic®

Canadian Brand Names Uniretic™

Pharmacologic Category Antihypertensive Agent Combination

Synonyms Hydrochlorothiazide and Moexipril

Use Combination therapy for hypertension, however, not indicated for initial treatment of hypertension; replacement therapy in patients receiving separate dosage forms (for patient convenience); when monotherapy with one component fails to achieve desired antihypertensive effect, or when dose-limiting adverse effects limit upward titration of monotherapy

Local Anesthetic/Vasoconstrictor Precautions No information available to require special precautions

Effects on Dental Treatment No significant effects or complications reported

Dosage Adults: Oral: 7.5-30 mg of moexipril, taken either in a single or divided dose one hour before meals; hydrochlorothiazide dose should be ≤50 mg/day

Mechanism of Action See individual agents.

Other Adverse Effects See individual agents.

Dietary/Ethanol/Herb Considerations Ethanol: Limit use; may increase risk of hypotension or dizziness.

Pregnancy Risk Factor C/D (2nd and 3rd trimesters)

Generic Available No

Moexipril Hydrochloride *see* Moexipril *on page 926*
Moi-Stir® [OTC] *see* Saliva Substitute *on page 1205*
Moisture® Eyes [OTC] *see* Artificial Tears *on page 128*
Moisture® Eyes PM [OTC] *see* Artificial Tears *on page 128*

Molindone

(moe LIN done)

U.S. Brand Names Moban®

Canadian Brand Names Moban®

Pharmacologic Category Antipsychotic Agent, Dihydoindoline

Synonyms Molindone Hydrochloride

Use Management of schizophrenia

Unlabeled/Investigational Use Management of psychotic disorders

Local Anesthetic/Vasoconstrictor Precautions No information available to require special precautions

Effects on Dental Treatment >10%: Xerostomia, changes in salivation

Anticholinergic side effects can cause a reduction of saliva production or secretion, contributing to discomfort and dental disease (ie, caries, oral candidiasis and periodontal disease). Molindone can cause extrapyramidal reactions which may appear as muscle twitching or increased motor activity of the face, neck or head.

Dosage Oral:

Children: Schizophrenia/psychoses:
3-5 years: 1-2.5 mg/day in 4 divided doses
5-12 years: 0.5-1 mg/kg/day in 4 divided doses

Adults: Schizophrenia/psychoses: 50-75 mg/day increase at 3- to 4-day intervals up to 225 mg/day

Elderly: Behavioral symptoms associated with dementia: Initial: 5-10 mg 1-2 times/day; increase at 4- to 7-day intervals by 5-10 mg/day; increase dosing intervals (bid, tid, etc) as necessary to control response or side effects.

Mechanism of Action Mechanism of action mimics that of chlorpromazine; however, it produces more extrapyramidal symptoms and less sedation than chlorpromazine

Other Adverse Effects Frequency not defined:

Cardiovascular: Orthostatic hypotension, tachycardia, arrhythmias

Central nervous system: Extrapyramidal reactions (akathisia, pseudoparkinsonism, dystonia, tardive dyskinesia), mental depression, altered central temperature regulation, sedation, drowsiness, restlessness, anxiety, hyperactivity, euphoria, seizures, neuroleptic malignant syndrome (NMS)

Dermatologic: Pruritus, rash, photosensitivity

(Continued)

Molindone *(Continued)*

Endocrine & metabolic: Change in menstrual periods, edema of breasts, amenorrhea, galactorrhea, gynecomastia

Gastrointestinal: Constipation, nausea, weight gain (minimal compared to other antipsychotics), weight loss, **increased salivation**

Genitourinary: Urinary retention, priapism

Hematologic: Leukopenia, leukocytosis

Ocular: Blurred vision, retinal pigmentation

Miscellaneous: Diaphoresis (decreased)

Drug Interactions CYP2D6 enzyme substrate

Increased Effect/Toxicity: Molindone concentrations may be increased by chloroquine, propranolol, sulfadoxine-pyrimethamine. Molindone may increase the effect and/or toxicity of antihypertensives, lithium, TCAs, CNS depressants (ethanol, narcotics), and trazodone. Metoclopramide may increase risk of extrapyramidal symptoms (EPS).

Decreased Effect: Antipsychotics inhibit the activity of bromocriptine and levodopa. Benztropine (and other anticholinergics) may inhibit the therapeutic response to molindone and excess anticholinergic effects may occur. Barbiturates and cigarette smoking may enhance the hepatic metabolism of molindone. Molindone and possibly other low potency antipsychotic may reverse the pressor effects of epinephrine.

Dietary/Ethanol/Herb Considerations

Ethanol: Avoid use; may increase CNS depression.

Herb/Nutraceutical: Avoid gotu kola, kava, SAMe, St John's wort, and valerian; may increase CNS depression.

Pharmacodynamics/Kinetics

Metabolism: Hepatic

Half-life elimination: 1.5 hours

Time to peak, serum: ~1.5 hours

Excretion: Urine and feces (90%) within 24 hours

Pregnancy Risk Factor C

Generic Available No

Molindone Hydrochloride *see* Molindone *on page 927*

Mollifene® Ear Wax Removing Formula [OTC] *see* Carbamide Peroxide *on page 244*

Molybdenum *see* Trace Metals *on page 1328*

Molypen® *see* Trace Metals *on page 1328*

MOM *see* Magnesium Hydroxide *on page 835*

Momentum® [OTC] *see* Magnesium Salicylate *on page 837*

Mometasone Furoate (moe MET a sone FYOOR oh ate)

Related Information

Respiratory Diseases *on page 1476*

U.S. Brand Names Elocon®; Nasonex®

Canadian Brand Names Elocom®; Nasonex®

Pharmacologic Category Corticosteroid, Nasal; Corticosteroid, Topical

Use Relief of the inflammatory and pruritic manifestations of corticosteroid-responsive dermatoses (medium potency topical corticosteroid); treatment of nasal symptoms of seasonal and perennial allergic rhinitis in adults and children ≥2 years of age; prevention of nasal symptoms associated with seasonal allergic rhinitis in children ≥12 years of age and adults

Local Anesthetic/Vasoconstrictor Precautions No information available to require special precautions

Effects on Dental Treatment Nasal:

>10%: Headache (17% to 26%), pharyngitis (10% to 12%), cough (7% to 13%), epistaxis (8% to 11%), viral infection (8% to 14%),

1% to 10%: Chest pain, vomiting (1% to 5%), nausea, upper respiratory tract infection (5% to 6%), sinusitis (4% to 5%), asthma, bronchitis, rhinitis, wheezing, flu-like symptoms, otitis media

Dosage

Nasal spray:

Children 2-11 years: 1 spray (50 mcg) in each nostril daily

Children ≥12 years and Adults: 2 sprays (100 mcg) in each nostril daily; when used for the prevention of allergic rhinitis, treatment should begin 2-4 weeks prior to pollen season

Topical: Apply sparingly, do not use occlusive dressings. Therapy should be discontinued when control is achieved; if no improvement is seen in 2 weeks, reassessment of diagnosis may be necessary.

Cream, ointment: Children ≥2 years and Adults: Apply a thin film to affected area once daily; do not use in pediatric patients for longer than 3 weeks

Lotion: Children ≥12 years and Adults: Apply a few drops to affected area once daily

Mechanism of Action May depress the formation, release, and activity of endogenous chemical mediators of inflammation (kinins, histamine, liposomal enzymes, prostaglandins). Leukocytes and macrophages may have to be present for the initiation of responses mediated by the above substances. Inhibits the margination and subsequent cell migration to the area of injury, and also reverses the dilatation and increased vessel permeability in the area resulting in decreased access of cells to the sites of injury.

Other Adverse Effects

Nasal:

1% to 10%:

Endocrine & metabolic: Dysmenorrhea (1% to 5%)

Gastrointestinal: Diarrhea, dyspepsia

Neuromuscular & skeletal: Musculoskeletal pain (1% to 5%), arthralgia, myalgia

Ocular: Conjunctivitis

Otic: Earache

Respiratory: Nasal irritation

<1%: **Nasal ulcers, oral candidiasis**

Postmarketing and/or case reports: **Anaphylaxis**, angioedema, **nasal septal perforation**

Topical:

1% to 10%: Dermatologic: Bacterial skin infection, burning, furunculosis, pruritus, skin atrophy, tingling/stinging

<1%: Folliculitis, glucocorticoid levels decreased (pediatric patients), moniliasis, paresthesia, skin depigmentation, skin atrophy

Postmarketing and/or case reports: Rosacea

Cataract formation, reduction in growth velocity, and HPA axis suppression have been reported with other corticosteroids

Drug Interactions Substrate of CYP3A4

Pharmacodynamics/Kinetics

Absorption:

Nasal: Mometasone furoate monohydrate: Undetectable in plasma

Ointment: 0.7%; increased by occlusive dressings

Protein binding: Mometasone furoate: 98% to 99%

Metabolism: Mometasone furoate: Hepatic via CYP3A4; forms metabolite

Half-life elimination: I.V.: 5.8 hours

Excretion: Bile, urine

Pregnancy Risk Factor C

Generic Available Yes: Ointment

MOM (Magnesium Hydroxide) *see* Magnesium Supplements *on page 837*

MOM/Mineral Oil Emulsion *see* Magnesium Hydroxide and Mineral Oil *on page 836*

Monacolin K *see* Lovastatin *on page 828*

Monarc® M *see* Antihemophilic Factor (Human) *on page 113*

Monistat® 1 Combination Pack [OTC] *see* Miconazole *on page 906*

Monistat® 3 [OTC] *see* Miconazole *on page 906*

Monistat® 7 [OTC] *see* Miconazole *on page 906*

Monistat-Derm® *see* Miconazole *on page 906*

Monobenzone (mon oh BEN zone)

U.S. Brand Names Benoquin®

Pharmacologic Category Topical Skin Product

Use Final depigmentation in extensive vitiligo

Local Anesthetic/Vasoconstrictor Precautions No information available to require special precautions

Effects on Dental Treatment No significant effects or complications reported

Dosage Adults: Topical: Apply 2-3 times daily

Other Adverse Effects 1% to 10%: Irritation, burning sensation, dermatitis

Pregnancy Risk Factor C

Generic Available No

Monocid® [DSC] *see* Cefonicid *on page 269*

Monoclate-P® *see* Antihemophilic Factor (Human) *on page 113*

Monoclonal Antibody *see* Muromonab-CD3 *on page 938*

Monodox® *see* Doxycycline *on page 476*

Monoethanolamine *see* Ethanolamine Oleate *on page 540*

Mono-Gesic® *see* Salsalate *on page 1206*

Monoket® *see* Isosorbide Mononitrate *on page 751*

Monopril® *see* Fosinopril *on page 616*

Monopril-HCT® *see* Fosinopril and Hydrochlorothiazide *on page 617*

Montelukast (mon te LOO kast)

Related Information

Respiratory Diseases *on page 1476*

(Continued)

Montelukast *(Continued)*

U.S. Brand Names Singulair®

Canadian Brand Names Singulair®

Mexican Brand Names Singulair®

Pharmacologic Category Leukotriene Receptor Antagonist

Synonyms Montelukast Sodium

Use Prophylaxis and chronic treatment of asthma in adults and children ≥1 year of age; relief of symptoms of seasonal allergic rhinitis in adults and children ≥2 years of age

Local Anesthetic/Vasoconstrictor Precautions No information available to require special precautions

Effects on Dental Treatment No significant effects or complications reported

Restrictions Singulair® oral granules received FDA approval July, 2002. A formal marketing date has not been announced.

Dosage Oral:

Children:

<1 year: Safety and efficacy have not been established

12-23 months: Asthma: 4 mg (oral granules) once daily, taken in the evening

2-5 years: Asthma or seasonal allergic rhinitis: 4 mg (chewable tablet or oral granules) once daily, taken in the evening

6-14 years: Asthma or seasonal allergic rhinitis: Chew one 5 mg chewable tablet/day, taken in the evening

Children ≥15 years and Adults: Asthma or seasonal allergic rhinitis: 10 mg/day, taken in the evening

Mechanism of Action Selective leukotriene receptor antagonist that inhibits the cysteinyl leukotriene receptor. Cysteinyl leukotrienes and leukotriene receptor occupation have been correlated with the pathophysiology of asthma, including airway edema, smooth muscle contraction, and altered cellular activity associated with the inflammatory process, which contribute to the signs and symptoms of asthma.

Other Adverse Effects (As reported in adults with asthma)

>10%: Central nervous system: Headache (18%)

1% to 10%:

Central nervous system: Dizziness (2%), fatigue (2%), fever (2%)

Dermatologic: Rash (2%)

Gastrointestinal: Dyspepsia (2%), dental pain (2%), gastroenteritis (2%), abdominal pain (3%)

Neuromuscular & skeletal: Weakness (2%)

Respiratory: Cough (3%), nasal congestion (2%)

Miscellaneous: Flu-like symptoms (4%), trauma (1%)

Postmarketing and/or case reports: Agitation, anaphylaxis, angioedema, bleeding tendency, bruising, diarrhea, dream abnormalities, drowsiness, edema, eosinophilia, erythema nodosum, hallucinations, hepatic eosinophilic infiltration (rare), insomnia, irritability, muscle cramps, myalgia, nausea, palpitations, pancreatitis, pruritus, restlessness, seizures, urticaria, vasculitis, vomiting

Drug Interactions Substrate of **CYP2C8/9, 3A4**; Inhibits CYP2C8/9

Decreased Effect: Phenobarbital decreases montelukast area under the curve by 40%. Clinical significance is uncertain. Rifampin may increase the metabolism of montelukast similar to phenobarbital. No dosage adjustment is recommended when taking phenobarbital with montelukast.

Dietary/Ethanol/Herb Considerations Herb/Nutraceutical: Avoid St John's wort; may decrease serum concentration.

Pharmacodynamics/Kinetics

Duration: >24 hours

Absorption: Rapid

Distribution: V_d: 8-11 L

Protein binding, plasma: >99%

Metabolism: Extensively hepatic via CYP3A4 and 2C8/9

Bioavailability: Tablet: 10 mg: Mean: 64%; 5 mg: 63% to 73%

Half-life elimination, plasma: Mean: 2.7-5.5 hours

Time to peak, serum: Tablet: 10 mg: 3-4 hours; 5 mg: 2-2.5 hours; 4 mg: 2 hours

Excretion: Feces (86%); urine (<0.2%)

Pregnancy Risk Factor B

Generic Available No

Montelukast Sodium *see* Montelukast *on page 929*

Monurol™ *see* Fosfomycin *on page 615*

8-MOP® *see* Methoxsalen *on page 888*

More Attenuated Enders Strain *see* Measles Virus Vaccine (Live) *on page 845*

MoreDophilus® [OTC] *see Lactobacillus acidophilus* and *Lactobacillus bulgaricus on page 772*

Moricizine (mor I siz een)

Related Information

Cardiovascular Diseases *on page 1456*

U.S. Brand Names Ethmozine®

Canadian Brand Names Ethmozine®

Pharmacologic Category Antiarrhythmic Agent, Class I

Synonyms Moricizine Hydrochloride

Use Treatment of ventricular tachycardia and life-threatening ventricular arrhythmias

Unlabeled/Investigational Use Treatment of PVCs, complete and nonsustained ventricular tachycardia, atrial arrhythmias

Local Anesthetic/Vasoconstrictor Precautions No information available to require special precautions

Effects on Dental Treatment No significant effects or complications reported

Dosage Oral:

Adults: 200-300 mg every 8 hours, adjust dosage at 150 mg/day at 3-day intervals.

Recommendations for transferring patients from other antiarrhythmic agents to Ethmozine®: See table.

Moricizine

Transferred From	Start Ethmozine®
Encainide, propafenone, tocainide, or mexiletine	8-12 hours after last dose
Flecainide	12-24 hours after last dose
Procainamide	3-6 hours after last dose
Quinidine, disopyramide	6-12 hours after last dose

Dosing interval in renal or hepatic impairment: Start at 600 mg/day or less.

Mechanism of Action Class I antiarrhythmic agent; reduces the fast inward current carried by sodium ions, shortens Phase I and Phase II repolarization, resulting in decreased action potential duration and effective refractory period

Other Adverse Effects

>10%: Central nervous system: Dizziness

1% to 10%:

Cardiovascular: Proarrhythmia, palpitations, cardiac death, EKG abnormalities, CHF

Central nervous system: Headache, fatigue, insomnia

Endocrine & metabolic: Decreased libido

Gastrointestinal: Nausea, diarrhea, ileus

Ocular: Blurred vision, periorbital edema

Respiratory: Dyspnea

<1% (Limited to important or life-threatening): Ventricular tachycardia, cardiac chest pain, hypotension or hypertension, syncope, supraventricular arrhythmias, MI, apnea

Drug Interactions Substrate of **CYP3A4**; Induces CYP1A2, 3A4

Increased Effect/Toxicity: Moricizine levels may be increased by cimetidine and diltiazem. Digoxin may result in additive prolongation of the PR interval when combined with moricizine (but not rate of second- and third-degree AV block). Drugs which may prolong QT interval (including cisapride, erythromycin, phenothiazines, cyclic antidepressants, and some quinolones) are contraindicated with type Ia antiarrhythmics. Moricizine has some type Ia activity, and caution should be used.

Decreased Effect: Moricizine may decrease levels of theophylline (50%) and diltiazem.

Dietary/Ethanol/Herb Considerations

Food: May decrease peak serum concentration; administer on an empty stomach.

Herb/Nutraceutical: Ginger has positive inotropic effects and theoretically could affect antiarrhythmic activity.

Pharmacodynamics/Kinetics

Protein binding, plasma: 95%

Metabolism: Significant first-pass effect; some enterohepatic recycling

Bioavailability: 38%

Half-life elimination: Healthy volunteers: 3-4 hours; Cardiac disease: 6-13 hours

Excretion: Feces (56%); urine (39%)

Pregnancy Risk Factor B

Generic Available No

Moricizine Hydrochloride *see* Moricizine *on page 931*

Morphine Sulfate (MOR feen SUL fate)

Related Information

Dental Office Emergencies *on page 1582*

Oxymorphone *on page 1024*

U.S. Brand Names Astramorph/PF™; Avinza™; Duramorph®; Infumorph®; Kadian®; MS Contin®; MSIR®; Oramorph SR®; RMS®; Roxanol®; Roxanol 100®; Roxanol®-T

(Continued)

Morphine Sulfate *(Continued)*

Canadian Brand Names Kadian®; M-Eslon®; Morphine HP®; Morphine LP® Epidural; M.O.S.-Sulfate®; MS Contin®; MS-IR®; ratio-Morphine SR; Statex®

Mexican Brand Names Analfin®; Duralmor L.P.®; Graten®; Kapanol®; MST Continus®

Pharmacologic Category Analgesic, Narcotic

Synonyms MS

Use Relief of moderate to severe acute and chronic pain; relief of pain of MI; relief of dyspnea of acute left ventricular failure and pulmonary edema; preanesthetic medication

Orphan drug (Infumorph™): Used in microinfusion devices for intraspinal administration in treatment of intractable chronic pain

Local Anesthetic/Vasoconstrictor Precautions No information available to require special precautions

Effects on Dental Treatment Xerostomia (78%)

Anticholinergic side effects can cause a reduction of saliva production or secretion, contributing to discomfort and dental disease (ie, caries, oral candidiasis and periodontal disease).

Restrictions C-II

Dosage These are guidelines and do not represent the maximum doses that may be required in all patients. Doses should be titrated to pain relief/prevention.

Children >6 months and <50 kg: Acute pain (moderate to severe):
- Oral (prompt release): 0.15-0.3 mg/kg every 3-4 hours as needed
- I.M.: 0.1 mg/kg every 3-4 hours as needed
- I.V.: 0.05-0.1 mg/kg every 3-4 hours as needed
- I.V. infusion: Range: 10-30 mcg/kg/hour

Adolescents >12 years: Sedation/analgesia for procedures: I.V.: 3-4 mg and repeat in 5 minutes if necessary

Adults: Acute pain (moderate to severe):
- Oral: Prompt release formulations: Opiate-naive: Initial: 10 mg every 3-4 hours as needed; patients with prior opiate exposure may require higher initial doses: usual dosage range: 10-30 mg every 3-4 hours as needed
- Oral: Controlled-, extended-, or sustained-release formulations: **Note:** A patient's morphine requirement should be established using prompt-release formulations. Conversion to long-acting products may be considered when chronic, continuous treatment is required. Higher dosages should be reserved for use only in opioid-tolerant patients.
  - Capsules, extended release (Avinza™): Daily dose administered once daily (for best results, administer at same time each day)
  - Capsules, sustained release (Kadian®): Daily dose administered once daily or in 2 divided doses daily (every 12 hours)
  - Tablets, controlled release (MS Contin®), sustained release (Oramorph SR®), or extended release: Daily dose divided and administered every 8 or every 12 hours
- I.V.: Initial: Opiate-naive: 2.5-5 mg every 3-4 hours; patients with prior opiate exposure may require higher initial doses. **Note:** Repeated doses (up to every 5 minutes if needed) in small increments (eg, 1-4 mg) may be preferred to larger and less frequent doses.
- I.V., S.C. continuous infusion: 0.8-10 mg/hour; may increase depending on pain relief/adverse effects: usual range: up to 80 mg/hour although higher doses may be required
  - Mechanically-ventilated patients (based on 70 kg patient): 0.7-10 mg every 1-2 hours as needed; infusion: 5-35 mg/hour
  - Patient-controlled analgesia (PCA): (Opiate-naive: Consider lower end of dosing range):
    - Usual concentration: 1 mg/mL
    - Demand dose: Usual: 1 mg; range: 0.5-2.5 mg
    - Lockout interval: 5-10 minutes
- Epidural: **Note:** Administer with extreme caution and in reduced dosage to geriatric or debilitated patients.
  - Bolus dose: 1-6 mg
  - Infusion rate: 0.1-1 mg/hour
  - Maximum dose: 10 mg/24 hours
- Intrathecal (IT): One-tenth of epidural dose; **Note:** Administer with extreme caution and in reduced dosage to geriatric or debilitated patients.
  - Opiate-naive: 0.2-1 mg/dose (may provide adequate relief for 24 hours); repeat doses **not** recommended except to establish initial IT dose.
- I.M., S.C.: **Note:** Repeated S.C. administration causes local tissue irritation, pain, and induration.
  - Initial: Opiate-naive: 5-10 mg every 3-4 hours as needed; patients with prior opiate exposure may require higher initial doses; usual dosage range: 5-20 mg every 3-4 hours as needed
- Rectal: 10-20 mg every 3- 4 hours

Chronic pain: Patients taking opioids chronically may become tolerant and require doses higher than the usual dosage range to maintain the desired effect. Tolerance can be managed by appropriate dose titration. There is no optimal or maximal dose for morphine in chronic pain. The appropriate dose is one that relieves pain throughout its dosing interval without causing unmanageable side effects.

Elderly or debilitated patients: Use with caution; may require dose reduction

Dosage adjustment in renal impairment:

Cl_{cr} 10-50 mL/minute: Administer at 75% of normal dose

Cl_{cr} <10 mL/minute: Administer at 50% of normal dose

Dosage adjustment in hepatic disease: Unchanged in mild liver disease; substantial extrahepatic metabolism may occur; excessive sedation may occur in cirrhosis

Mechanism of Action Binds to opiate receptors in the CNS, causing inhibition of ascending pain pathways, altering the perception of and response to pain; produces generalized CNS depression

Other Adverse Effects Percentages are based on a study in 19 chronic cancer pain patients (*J Pain Symptom Manage*, 1995, 10:416-22). Chronic use of various opioids in cancer pain is accompanied by similar adverse reactions; individual patient differences are unpredictable, and percentage may differ in acute pain (surgical) treatment.

>10%:

Cardiovascular: Palpitations, hypotension, bradycardia

Central nervous system: Drowsiness (48%, tolerance usually develops to drowsiness with regular dosing for 1-2 weeks); dizziness (20%); confusion

Dermatologic: Pruritus (may be secondary to histamine release)

Gastrointestinal: Nausea (28%, tolerance usually develops to nausea and vomiting with chronic use); vomiting (9%); constipation (40%, tolerance develops very slowly if at all)

Genitourinary: Urinary retention (16%)

Local: Pain at injection site

Neuromuscular & skeletal: Weakness

Miscellaneous: Histamine release

1% to 10%:

Central nervous system: Restlessness, headache, false feeling of well being

Gastrointestinal: Anorexia, GI irritation, paralytic ileus

Genitourinary: Decreased urination

Neuromuscular & skeletal: Trembling

Ocular: Vision problems

Respiratory: Respiratory depression, dyspnea

<1%: Anaphylaxis, intestinal obstruction, peripheral vasodilation, insomnia, mental depression, hallucinations, paradoxical CNS stimulation, increased intracranial pressure, biliary tract spasm, urinary tract spasm, muscle rigidity, miosis, increased LFTs

Frequency not defined:

Cardiovascular: Flushing

Central nervous system: CNS depression, sedation

Endocrine & metabolic: Antidiuretic hormone release

Miscellaneous: Diaphoresis, physical and psychological dependence

Drug Interactions Substrate of CYP2D6

Increased Effect/Toxicity: CNS depressants (phenothiazines, tranquilizers, anxiolytics, sedatives, hypnotics, or alcohol), tricyclic antidepressants may potentiate the effects of morphine and other opiate agonists. Dextroamphetamine may enhance the analgesic effect of morphine and other opiate agonists. Concurrent use of MAO inhibitors and meperidine has been associated with significant adverse effects. Use caution with morphine. Some manufacturers recommend avoiding use within 14 days of MAO inhibitors.

Decreased Effect: Diuretic effects may be decreased (due to antidiuretic hormone release).

Dietary/Ethanol/Herb Considerations

Ethanol: Avoid use; may increase CNS depression.

Food: Administer consistently in regard to meals; may administer with food to reduce GI upset. Food may increase bioavailability of oral solution (ie, a report of 34% increase in morphine AUC when morphine oral solution followed a high-fat meal). The bioavailability of Oramorph SR™ does not appear to be affected by food.

Herb/Nutraceutical: Avoid kava, gotu kola, St John's wort, and valerian; may increase CNS depression.

Pharmacodynamics/Kinetics

Onset of action: Oral: 1 hour; I.V.: 5-10 minutes

Duration: Pain relief (not sustained/controlled/extended release forms): 4 hours

Absorption: Variable

Distribution: Binds to opioid receptors in the CNS and periphery (eg, GI tract)

Metabolism: Hepatic via conjugation with glucuronic acid to morphine-3-glucuronide (inactive), morphine-6-glucuronide (active), and in lesser

(Continued)

Morphine Sulfate *(Continued)*

amounts, morphine-3-6-diglucuronide; other minor metabolites include normorphine (active) and the 3-ethereal sulfate

Bioavailability: Oral: 17% to 33% (first-pass effect limits oral bioavailability; oral:parenteral effectiveness reportedly varies from 1:6 in opioid naive patients to 1:3 with chronic use)

Half-life elimination: Adults: 2-4 hours (not sustained/controlled/extended release forms)

Excretion: Urine (primarily as morphine-3-glucuronide, ~2% to 12% excreted unchanged); feces (~7% to 10%). It has been suggested that accumulation of morphine-6-glucuronide might cause toxicity with renal insufficiency. All of the metabolites (ie, morphine-3-glucuronide, morphine-6-glucuronide, and normorphine) have been suggested as possible causes of neurotoxicity (eg, myoclonus).

Pregnancy Risk Factor B/D (prolonged use or high doses at term)

Generic Available Yes: Excludes capsule, controlled release tablet, sustained release tablet

Morrhuate Sodium (MOR yoo ate SOW dee um)

U.S. Brand Names Scleromate™

Pharmacologic Category Sclerosing Agent

Use Treatment of small, uncomplicated varicose veins of the lower extremities

Local Anesthetic/Vasoconstrictor Precautions No information available to require special precautions

Effects on Dental Treatment No significant effects or complications reported

Dosage Adults: I.V.: 50-250 mg, repeated at 5- to 7-day intervals (50-100 mg for small veins, 150-250 mg for large veins)

Mechanism of Action Both varicose veins and esophageal varices are treated by the thrombotic action of morrhuate sodium. By causing inflammation of the vein's intima, a thrombus is formed. Occlusion secondary to the fibrous tissue and the thrombus results in the obliteration of the vein.

Other Adverse Effects Frequency not defined:

Cardiovascular: Thrombosis, valvular incompetency, vascular collapse
Central nervous system: Drowsiness, headache, dizziness
Dermatologic: Urticaria
Gastrointestinal: Nausea, vomiting
Local: Burning at the site of injection, severe extravasation effects
Neuromuscular & skeletal: Weakness
Respiratory: Asthma
Miscellaneous: Anaphylaxis, hypersensitivity reactions

Pharmacodynamics/Kinetics

Onset of action: ~5 minutes
Absorption: Most stays at site of injection
Distribution: Esophageal varices treatment: ~20% of dose to lungs

Pregnancy Risk Factor C

Generic Available No

Mosco® Corn and Callus Remover [OTC] *see* Salicylic Acid *on page 1204*
Motofen® *see* Difenoxin and Atropine *on page 437*
Motrin® *see* Ibuprofen *on page 703*
Motrin® Children's [OTC] *see* Ibuprofen *on page 703*
Motrin® Cold, Children's [OTC] *see* Pseudoephedrine and Ibuprofen *on page 1148*
Motrin® IB [OTC] *see* Ibuprofen *on page 703*
Motrin® Infants' [OTC] *see* Ibuprofen *on page 703*
Motrin® Junior Strength [OTC] *see* Ibuprofen *on page 703*
Motrin® Migraine Pain [OTC] *see* Ibuprofen *on page 703*
Motrin® Sinus Headache [OTC] *see* Pseudoephedrine and Ibuprofen *on page 1148*
Mouthkote® [OTC] *see* Saliva Substitute *on page 1205*

Mouthwash (Antiseptic) (MOWTH wosh an ti SEP tik)

Related Information

Antiplaque Agents *on page 1554*
Dentin Hypersensitivity, High Caries Index, and Xerostomia *on page 1553*
Oral Bacterial Infections *on page 1531*
Oral Nonviral Soft Tissue Ulcerations or Erosions *on page 1549*
Oral Rinse Products *on page 1634*
Periodontal Diseases *on page 1540*

Pharmacologic Category Antimicrobial Mouth Rinse; Antiplaque Agent

Use Used exclusively in dental applications (help prevent and reduce plaque and gingivitis; bad breath)

Local Anesthetic/Vasoconstrictor Precautions No information available to require special precautions

Effects on Dental Treatment No significant effects or complications reported

Dosage Rinse full strength for 30 seconds with 20 mL (2/3 fluid ounce or 4 teaspoonfuls) morning and night

Comments Active ingredients:

Listerine® Antiseptic: Thymol 0.064%, eucalyptus 0.092%, methyl salicylate 0.060%, menthol 0.042%, alcohol 26.9%, water, benzoic acid, poloxamer 407, sodium benzoate, caramel

Fresh Burst Listerine® Antiseptic: Thymol 0.064%, eucalyptus 0.092%, methyl salicylate 0.060%, menthol 0.042%, alcohol 26.9%, water, benzoic acid, poloxamer 407, sodium benzoate, flavoring, sodium, saccharin, sodium citrate, citric acid, D&C yellow #10, FD&C green #3

Cool Mint Listerine® Antiseptic: Thymol 0.064%, eucalyptus 0.092%, methyl salicylate 0.060%, menthol 0.042%, alcohol 26.9%, water, benzoic acid, poloxamer 407, sodium benzoate, flavoring, sodium, saccharin, sodium citrate, citric acid, FD&C green #3

The following information is endorsed on the label of the Listerine® products by the Council on Scientific Affairs, American Dental Association: "Listerine® Antiseptic has been shown to help prevent and reduce supragingival plaque accumulation and gingivitis when used in a conscientiously applied program of oral hygiene and regular professional care. Its effect on periodontitis has not been determined."

Moxifloxacin (moks i FLOKS a sin)

Related Information

Oral Bacterial Infections *on page 1531*
Respiratory Diseases *on page 1476*

U.S. Brand Names Avelox®; Avelox® I.V.

Canadian Brand Names Avelox®

Pharmacologic Category Antibiotic, Quinolone

Synonyms Moxifloxacin Hydrochloride

Use Treatment of mild to moderate community-acquired pneumonia, acute bacterial exacerbation of chronic bronchitis, acute bacterial sinusitis, uncomplicated skin infections

Local Anesthetic/Vasoconstrictor Precautions No information available to require special precautions

Effects on Dental Treatment No significant effects or complications reported

Dosage Oral, I.V.:

Adults:

Acute bacterial sinusitis: 400 mg every 24 hours for 10 days

Chronic bronchitis, acute bacterial exacerbation: 400 mg every 24 hours for 5 days

Note: Avelox® ABC Pack™ (Avelox® Bronchitis Course) contains five tablets of 400 mg each.

Community-acquired pneumonia: 400 mg every 24 hours for 7-14 days

Uncomplicated skin infections: 400 mg every 24 hours for 7 days

Dosing adjustment in hepatic impairment: None required in mild to moderate insufficiency (Child-Pugh Class A and B); use not recommended in severe insufficiency

Mechanism of Action Moxifloxacin is a DNA gyrase inhibitor, and also inhibits topoisomerase IV. DNA gyrase (topoisomerase II) is an essential bacterial enzyme that maintains the superhelical structure of DNA. DNA gyrase is required for DNA replication and transcription, DNA repair, recombination, and transposition; inhibition is bactericidal.

Other Adverse Effects

3% to 10%:

Central nervous system: Dizziness (3%)

Gastrointestinal: Nausea (7%), diarrhea (6%)

0.1% to 3%:

Cardiovascular: Chest pain, hypertension, palpitation, peripheral edema, QT prolongation, tachycardia

Central nervous system: Anxiety, chills, confusion, headache, insomnia, nervousness, pain, somnolence, tremor, vertigo

Dermatologic: Dry skin, pruritus, rash (maculopapular, purpuric, pustular)

Endocrine & metabolic: Serum chloride increased (≥2%), serum ionized calcium increased (≥2%), serum glucose decreased (≥2%)

Gastrointestinal: Abdominal pain, amylase increased, amylase decreased (≥2%), anorexia, constipation, xerostomia, dyspepsia, flatulence, glossitis, lactic dehydrogenase increased, stomatitis, abnormal taste, vomiting

Hematologic: Eosinophilia, leukopenia, PT decreased, thrombocythemia, thrombocytopenia

Increased serum levels of the following (≥2%): MCH, neutrophils, PT ratio, WBC

Decreased serum levels of the following (≥2%): Basophils, eosinophils, hemoglobin, PT ratio, RBC, neutrophils

Hepatic: Bilirubin decreased (≥2%), cholestatic jaundice, GGTP increased, LFTs abnormal

Local: Injection site reaction

(Continued)

Moxifloxacin *(Continued)*

Neuromuscular & skeletal: Arthralgia, back pain, leg pain, myalgia, paresthesia, malaise, weakness
Renal: Serum albumin increased (≥2%)
Respiratory: Dyspnea, pharyngitis, pneumonia, rhinitis, sinusitis, PO_2 increased (≥2%)
Miscellaneous: Allergic reaction, infection, moniliasis, diaphoresis

<0.1%, postmarketing, and/or case reports: Abnormal dreams, agitation, amblyopia, amnesia, anaphylactic reaction, anaphylactic shock, anemia, aphasia, arthritis, asthma, atrial fibrillation, *C. difficile*-positive diarrhea, convulsions, depersonalization, depression, dysphagia, EKG abnormalities, emotional lability, face edema, gastritis, hallucinations, hyperglycemia, hyperlipidemia, hypertonia, hyperuricemia, hypesthesia, hypotension, incoordination, jaundice, kidney function abnormalities, parosmia, pelvic pain, PT increased, sleep disorder, speech disorder, supraventricular tachycardia, loss of taste, tendon disorder, thinking abnormal, thromboplastin decreased, tinnitus, tongue discoloration, urticaria, ventricular tachycardia, vision abnormalities

Drug Interactions

Increased Effect/Toxicity: Drugs which prolong QT interval (including Class Ia and Class III antiarrhythmics, erythromycin, cisapride, antipsychotics, and cyclic antidepressants) are contraindicated with moxifloxacin. Cimetidine and probenecid increase quinolone levels. An increased incidence of seizures may occur with foscarnet or NSAIDs. Serum levels of some quinolones are increased by loop diuretic administration. Digoxin levels may be increased in some patients by quinolones. The hypoprothrombinemic effect of warfarin is enhanced by some quinolone antibiotics. Monitoring of the INR during concurrent therapy is recommended by the manufacturer. Concurrent use of corticosteroids may increase risk of tendon rupture.

Decreased Effect: Metal cations (magnesium, aluminum, iron, and zinc) bind quinolones in the gastrointestinal tract and inhibit absorption (by up to 98%). Antacids, multivitamins with minerals, sucralfate, and some didanosine formulations should be avoided. Moxifloxacin should be administered 4 hours before or 8 hours (a minimum of 2 hours before and 2 hours after) after these agents. Antineoplastic agents may decrease the absorption of quinolones.

Dietary/Ethanol/Herb Considerations

Food: May be taken with food; absorption unaffected by high-fat meal or yogurt. Avoid iron, zinc, or multivitamins with minerals 4 hours before or 8 hours after administration.

Herb/Nutraceutical: Avoid dong quai and St John's wort; may cause photosensitization.

Pharmacodynamics/Kinetics

Absorption: Well absorbed; not affected by high fat meal or yogurt
Distribution: V_d: 1.7 to 2.7 L/kg; tissue concentrations often exceed plasma concentrations in respiratory tissues, alveolar macrophages, and sinus tissues
Protein binding: 50%
Metabolism: Hepatic via glucuronide (14%) and sulfate (38%) conjugation
Bioavailability: 90%
Half-life elimination: Oral: 12 hours; I.V.: 15 hours
Excretion: Feces (25%) and urine (20%) as unchanged drug; sulfate conjugates in feces, glucuronide conjugates in urine

Pregnancy Risk Factor C

Generic Available No

Moxifloxacin Hydrochloride *see* Moxifloxacin *on page 935*
Moxilin® *see* Amoxicillin *on page 93*
4-MP *see* Fomepizole *on page 609*
6-MP *see* Mercaptopurine *on page 866*
MPA and Estrogens (Conjugated) *see* Estrogens (Conjugated/Equine) and Medroxyprogesterone *on page 531*
MS *see* Morphine Sulfate *on page 931*
MS Contin® *see* Morphine Sulfate *on page 931*
MSIR® *see* Morphine Sulfate *on page 931*
MTC *see* Mitomycin *on page 921*
M.T.E.-4® *see* Trace Metals *on page 1328*
M.T.E.-5® *see* Trace Metals *on page 1328*
M.T.E.-6® *see* Trace Metals *on page 1328*
M.T.E.-7® *see* Trace Metals *on page 1328*
MTX *see* Methotrexate *on page 884*
Mucinex™ [OTC] *see* Guaifenesin *on page 650*
Mucomyst® *see* Acetylcysteine *on page 40*
Mucosil™ *see* Acetylcysteine *on page 40*
Multidex® [OTC] *see* Maltodextrin *on page 840*
Multiple Vitamins *see* Vitamins (Multiple/Oral) *on page 1394*

Multitest CMI® *see* Skin Test Antigens (Multiple) *on page 1227*
Multitrace™-4 *see* Trace Metals *on page 1328*
Multitrace™-4 Neonatal *see* Trace Metals *on page 1328*
Multitrace™-4 Pediatric *see* Trace Metals *on page 1328*
Multitrace™-5 *see* Trace Metals *on page 1328*
Mumps, Measles and Rubella Vaccines, Combined *see* Measles, Mumps, and Rubella Vaccines (Combined) *on page 844*
Mumpsvax® *see* Mumps Virus Vaccine (Live/Attenuated) *on page 937*

Mumps Virus Vaccine (Live/Attenuated)

(mumpz VYE rus vak SEEN, lyve, a ten YOO ay ted)

Related Information

Immunizations (Vaccines) *on page 1612*

U.S. Brand Names Mumpsvax®

Canadian Brand Names Mumpsvax®

Pharmacologic Category Vaccine

Use Mumps prophylaxis by promoting active immunity

Note: Trivalent measles-mumps-rubella (MMR) vaccine is the preferred agent for most children and many adults; persons born prior to 1957 are generally considered immune and need not be vaccinated

Local Anesthetic/Vasoconstrictor Precautions No information available to require special precautions

Effects on Dental Treatment No significant effects or complications reported

Restrictions Federal law requires that the date of administration, the vaccine manufacturer, lot number of vaccine, and the administering person's name, title and address be entered into the patient's permanent medical record.

Dosage Children ≥15 months and Adults: 0.5 mL S.C. in outer aspect of the upper arm, no booster

Mechanism of Action Promotes active immunity to mumps virus by inducing specific antibodies.

Other Adverse Effects All serious adverse reactions must be reported to the U.S. Department of Health and Human Services (DHHS) Vaccine Adverse Event Reporting System (VAERS) 1-800-822-7967.

>10%: Local: Burning or stinging at injection site

1% to 10%:

Central nervous system: Fever (≤100°F)
Dermatologic: Rash
Endocrine & metabolic: Parotitis

<1%: Convulsions, confusion, severe or continuing headache, fever (>103°F), orchitis in postpubescent and adult males, thrombocytopenia, purpura, anaphylactic reactions

Pregnancy Risk Factor X

Generic Available No

Mupirocin

(myoo PEER oh sin)

U.S. Brand Names Bactroban®; Bactroban® Nasal

Canadian Brand Names Bactroban®

Mexican Brand Names Bactroban®; Mupiban

Pharmacologic Category Antibiotic, Topical

Synonyms Mupirocin Calcium; Pseudomonic Acid A

Use

Intranasal: Eradication of nasal colonization with MRSA in adult patients and healthcare workers

Topical treatment of impetigo due to *Staphylococcus aureus*, beta-hemolytic *Streptococcus*, and *S. pyogenes*

Unlabeled/Investigational Use Intranasal: Surgical prophylaxis to prevent wound infections

Local Anesthetic/Vasoconstrictor Precautions No information available to require special precautions

Effects on Dental Treatment No significant effects or complications reported

Dosage

Children ≥12 years and Adults: Intranasal: Approximately one-half of the ointment from the single-use tube should be applied into one nostril and the other half into the other nostril twice daily for 5 days

Children ≥3 months and Adults: Topical: Apply small amount to affected area 2-5 times/day for 5-14 days

Mechanism of Action Binds to bacterial isoleucyl transfer-RNA synthetase resulting in the inhibition of protein and RNA synthesis

Other Adverse Effects Frequency not defined:

Central nervous system: Dizziness, headache
Dermatologic: Pruritus, rash, erythema, dry skin, cellulitis, dermatitis
Gastrointestinal: Nausea, abnormal taste
Local: Burning, stinging, tenderness, edema, pain

(Continued)

Mupirocin *(Continued)*

Respiratory: Rhinitis, upper respiratory tract infection, pharyngitis, cough

Pharmacodynamics/Kinetics

Absorption: Topical: Penetrates outer layers of skin; systemic absorption minimal through intact skin

Protein binding: 95%

Metabolism: Skin: 3% to monic acid

Half-life elimination: 17-36 minutes

Excretion: Urine

Pregnancy Risk Factor B

Generic Available No

Mupirocin Calcium *see* Mupirocin *on page 937*

Murine® Ear Drops [OTC] *see* Carbamide Peroxide *on page 244*

Murine® Tears [OTC] *see* Artificial Tears *on page 128*

Murine® Tears Plus [OTC] *see* Tetrahydrozoline *on page 1288*

Muro 128® [OTC] *see* Sodium Chloride *on page 1229*

Murocel® [OTC] *see* Artificial Tears *on page 128*

Murocoll-2® *see* Phenylephrine and Scopolamine *on page 1072*

Muromonab-CD3 (myoor oh MOE nab-see dee three)

U.S. Brand Names Orthoclone OKT® 3

Canadian Brand Names Orthoclone OKT® 3

Mexican Brand Names Orthoclone OKT3®

Pharmacologic Category Immunosuppressant Agent

Synonyms Monoclonal Antibody; OKT3

Use Treatment of acute allograft rejection in renal transplant patients; treatment of acute hepatic, kidney, and pancreas rejection episodes resistant to conventional treatment. Acute graft-versus-host disease following bone marrow transplantation resistant to conventional treatment.

Local Anesthetic/Vasoconstrictor Precautions No information available to require special precautions

Effects on Dental Treatment No significant effects or complications reported

Dosage I.V. (refer to individual protocols):

Children <30 kg: 2.5 mg/day once daily for 7-14 days

Children >30 kg: 5 mg/day once daily for 7-14 days

OR

Children <12 years: 0.1 mg/kg/day once daily for 10-14 days

Children ≥12 years and Adults: 5 mg/day once daily for 10-14 days

Hemodialysis: Molecular size of OKT3 is 150,000 daltons; not dialyzed by most standard dialyzers; however, may be dialyzed by high flux dialysis; OKT3 will be removed by plasmapheresis; administer following dialysis treatments

Peritoneal dialysis: Significant drug removal is unlikely based on physiochemical characteristics

Mechanism of Action Reverses graft rejection by binding to T cells and interfering with their function by binding T-cell receptor-associated CD3 glycoprotein

Other Adverse Effects

>10%:

"First-dose" (cytokine release) effects: Onset: 1-3 hours after the dose; duration: 12-16 hours. Severity is mild to life-threatening. Signs and symptoms include fever, chilling, dyspnea, wheezing, chest pain, chest tightness, nausea, vomiting, and diarrhea. Hypervolemic pulmonary edema, nephrotoxicity, meningitis, and encephalopathy are possible. Reactions tend to decrease with repeated doses.

Cardiovascular: Tachycardia (including ventricular)

Central nervous system: Dizziness, faintness

Gastrointestinal: Diarrhea, nausea, vomiting

Hematologic: Transient lymphopenia

Neuromuscular & skeletal: Trembling

Respiratory: Dyspnea

1% to 10%:

Central nervous system: Headache

Neuromuscular & skeletal: Stiff neck

Ocular: Photophobia

Respiratory: Pulmonary edema

<1%: Hypertension, hypotension, chest pain, tightness, aseptic meningitis, seizures, fatigue, confusion, coma, hallucinations, pyrexia, pruritus, rash, arthralgia, tremor, increased BUN and creatinine, dyspnea, wheezing. Sensitivity reactions: Anaphylactic-type reactions, flu-like symptoms (ie, fever, chills), infection, pancytopenia, secondary lymphoproliferative disorder or lymphoma, thrombosis of major vessels in renal allograft.

Drug Interactions

Increased Effect/Toxicity: Recommend decreasing dose of prednisone to 0.5 mg/kg, azathioprine to 0.5 mg/kg (approximate 50% decrease in dose), and discontinuing cyclosporine while patient is receiving OKT3.

Decreased Effect: Decreased effect with immunosuppressive drugs.

Pharmacodynamics/Kinetics

Duration: 7 days after discontinuation

Time to peak: Steady-state: Trough: 3-14 days

Pregnancy Risk Factor C

Generic Available No

Comments Recommend decreasing dose of prednisone to 0.5 mg/kg, azathioprine to 0.5 mg/kg (approximate 50% decrease in dose), and discontinuing cyclosporine while patient is receiving OKT3

Muse® Pellet *see* Alprostadil *on page 63*

Mutamycin® *see* Mitomycin *on page 921*

Myambutol® *see* Ethambutol *on page 539*

Mycelex® *see* Clotrimazole *on page 356*

Mycelex®-3 [OTC] *see* Butoconazole *on page 218*

Mycelex®-3 *see* Clotrimazole *on page 356*

Mycelex®-7 [OTC] *see* Clotrimazole *on page 356*

Mycelex® Twin Pack [OTC] *see* Clotrimazole *on page 356*

Myciguent [OTC] *see* Neomycin *on page 961*

Mycinettes® [OTC] *see* Benzocaine *on page 169*

Mycitracin® [OTC] *see* Bacitracin, Neomycin, and Polymyxin B *on page 157*

Mycobutin® *see* Rifabutin *on page 1179*

Mycolog®-II *see* Nystatin and Triamcinolone *on page 992*

Myco-Nail [OTC] *see* Triacetin *on page 1340*

Mycophenolate (mye koe FEN oh late)

U.S. Brand Names CellCept®

Canadian Brand Names CellCept®

Pharmacologic Category Immunosuppressant Agent

Synonyms Mycophenolate Mofetil

Use Prophylaxis of organ rejection concomitantly with cyclosporine and corticosteroids in patients receiving allogenic renal, cardiac, or hepatic transplants. Intravenous formulation is an alternative dosage form to oral capsules, suspension, and tablets.

Unlabeled/Investigational Use Treatment of rejection in liver transplant patients unable to tolerate tacrolimus or cyclosporine due to neurotoxicity, mild rejection in heart transplant patients, moderate-severe psoriasis

Local Anesthetic/Vasoconstrictor Precautions No information available to require special precautions

Effects on Dental Treatment No significant effects or complications reported

Dosage

Children: Renal transplant: Oral:

Suspension: 600 mg/m²/dose twice daily; maximum dose: 1 g twice daily

Alternatively, may use solid dosage forms according to BSA as follows:

BSA 1.25-1.5 m²: 750 mg capsule twice daily

BSA >1.5 m²: 1 g capsule or tablet twice daily

Adults: The initial dose should be given as soon as possible following transplantation; intravenous solution may be given until the oral medication can be tolerated (up to 14 days)

Renal transplant:

Oral: 1 g twice daily. Although a dose of 1.5 g twice daily was used in clinical trials and shown to be effective, no efficacy advantage was established. Patients receiving 2 g/day demonstrated an overall better safety profile than patients receiving 3 g/day. Doses >2 g/day are not recommended in these patients because of the possibility for enhanced immunosuppression as well as toxicities.

I.V.: 1 g twice daily

Cardiac transplantation:

Oral: 1.5 g twice daily

I.V.: 1.5 g twice daily

Hepatic transplantation:

Oral: 1.5 g twice daily

I.V.: 1 g twice daily

Elderly: Use caution due to possibility of increased hepatic, renal or cardiac dysfunction; may be increased risk of certain infections, GI hemorrhage, and pulmonary edema, compared to younger patients

Dosing adjustment in renal impairment:

Renal transplant: GFR <25 mL/minute in patients outside the immediate post-transplant period: Doses of >1 g administered twice daily should be avoided; patients should also be carefully observed; no dose adjustments are

(Continued)

Mycophenolate *(Continued)*

needed in renal transplant patients experiencing delayed graft function postoperatively

Cardiac or liver transplant: No data available; mycophenolate may be used in cardiac or hepatic transplant patients with severe chronic renal impairment if the potential benefit outweighs the potential risk

Hemodialysis: Not removed; supplemental dose is unnecessary

Peritoneal dialysis: Supplemental dose is unnecessary

Dosing adjustment in hepatic impairment: None required in severe hepatic parenchymal disease; unknown in hepatic disease with other etiologies

Dosing adjustment for toxicity (neutropenia): ANC <1.3 x $10^3/\mu L$: Dosing should be interrupted or the dose reduced, appropriate diagnostic tests performed and patients managed appropriately

Mechanism of Action Inhibition of purine synthesis of human lymphocytes and proliferation of human lymphocytes

Other Adverse Effects As reported in adults following oral dosing of mycophenolate alone in renal, cardiac, and hepatic allograft rejection studies. In general, lower doses used in renal rejection patients had less adverse effects than higher doses. Rates of adverse effects were similar for each indication, except for those unique to the specific organ involved. The type of adverse effects observed in pediatric patients was similar to those seen in adults; abdominal pain, anemia, diarrhea, fever, hypertension, infection, pharyngitis, respiratory tract infection, sepsis, and vomiting were seen in higher proportion; lymphoproliferative disorder was the only type of malignancy observed.

>10%:

Cardiovascular: Hypertension (28% to 77%), peripheral edema (27% to 64%), hypotension (18% to 32%), edema (12% to 28%), cardiovascular disorder (26%), chest pain (13% to 26%), tachycardia (20% to 22%), arrhythmia (19%), bradycardia (17%), hypervolemia (17%), pericardial effusion (16%), heart failure (12%)

Central nervous system: Pain (31% to 76%), headache (16% to 54%), fever (21% to 52%), insomnia (9% to 52%), tremor (11% to 34%), anxiety (19% to 28%), dizziness (6% to 28%), depression (16% to 17%), confusion (13% to 17%), agitation (13%), chills (11%), somnolence (11%), nervousness (10% to 11%)

Dermatologic: Rash (18% to 22%), pruritus (14%), skin disorder (12%), diaphoresis (11%), acne (10% to 12%)

Endocrine & metabolic: Hyperglycemia (9% to 47%), hypercholesterolemia (8% to 41%), hypomagnesemia (18% to 39%), hypokalemia (10% to 37%), hypocalcemia (30%), elevated LDH (23%), hyperkalemia (9% to 22%), elevated AST (17%), elevated ALT (16%), hyperuricemia (16%), hypophosphatemia (12% to 16%), acidosis (14%), hypoproteinemia (13%), hyponatremia (11%)

Gastrointestinal: Abdominal pain (25% to 62%), nausea (20% to 54%), diarrhea (31% to 51%), constipation (18% to 41%), vomiting (12% to 34%), anorexia (25%), dyspepsia (13% to 22%), abdominal enlargement (19%), weight gain (16%), flatulence (13% to 14%), oral moniliasis (10% to 12%), nausea and vomiting (10% to 11%)

Genitourinary: Urinary tract infection (13% to 37%), urinary tract disorder

Hematologic: Leukopenia (23% to 46%), anemia (26% to 43%), leukocytosis (7% to 40%), thrombocytopenia (8% to 38%), hypochromic anemia (7% to 25%), ecchymosis (17%)

Hepatic: Abnormal LFTs (25%), ascites (24%), bilirubinemia (14% to 18%), cholangitis (14%), hepatitis (13%), cholestatic jaundice (12%)

Neuromuscular & skeletal: Back pain (12% to 47%), weakness (14% to 43%), paresthesia (15% to 21%), leg cramps (17%), hypertonia (16%), myasthenia (12%), myalgia (12%)

Ocular: Amblyopia (15%)

Renal: Elevated creatinine (20% to 40%), elevated BUN (10% to 35%), abnormal kidney function (22% to 27%), oliguria (14% to 17%), hematuria (12% to 14%), kidney tubular necrosis (6% to 10%)

Respiratory: Respiratory infection (16% to 37%), dyspnea (15% to 37%), pleural effusion (17% to 34%), increased cough (13% to 31%), lung disorder (22% to 30%), sinusitis (11% to 26%), rhinitis (19%), pharyngitis (9% to 18%), pneumonia (11% to 14%), atelectasis (13%), asthma (11%), bronchitis

Miscellaneous: Infection (18% to 27%), sepsis (18% to 27%), herpes simplex (10% to 21%), accidental injury (11% to 19%), mucocutaneous *Candida* (15% to 18%), CMV viremia/syndrome (12% to 14%), hernia (12%), CMV tissue invasive disease (6% to 11%), herpes zoster cutaneous disease (6% to 11%)

1% to 10%:

Cardiovascular: I.V.: Thrombosis (4%)

Dermatologic: Nonmelanoma skin carcinomas (2% to 4%)

Endocrine & metabolic: Hypoglycemia (10%)

Hematologic: Severe neutropenia (2% to 4%), lymphoproliferative disease/lymphoma (0.4% to 1%)

Local: I.V.: Phlebitis (4%)

Miscellaneous: Abnormal healing (10%), peritonitis (10%), fatal sepsis (2% to 5%), *Aspergillus/Mucor* (<4%), *Candida* fungemia/disseminated disease (<4%), *Candida* tissue invasive disease (<4%), *Candida* urinary tract infection (<4%), cryptococcosis (<4%), herpes zoster visceral disease (<4%), *Pneumocystis carinii* (<4%), malignancy (0.7% to 2%)

<1% or postmarketing experience: Colitis, infectious endocarditis, interstitial lung disorders, meningitis, pancreatitis, pulmonary fibrosis (rare, fatalities reported)

Drug Interactions

Increased Effect/Toxicity: Acyclovir and ganciclovir levels may increase due to competition for tubular secretion of these drugs. Probenecid may increase mycophenolate levels due to inhibition of tubular secretion. High doses of salicylates may increase free fraction of mycophenolic acid. Azathioprine's bone marrow suppression may be potentiated; do not administer together.

Decreased Effect: Antacids decrease serum levels (C_{max} and AUC); **do not administer together**. Cholestyramine resin decreases serum levels; **do not administer together**. Avoid use of live vaccines; vaccinations may be less effective. During concurrent use of oral contraceptives, progesterone levels are not significantly affected, however, effect on estrogen component varies; an additional form of contraception should be used.

Dietary/Ethanol/Herb Considerations

Food decreases C_{max} of MPA by 40% but the extent of absorption is not changed. Oral forms should be taken on an empty stomach; may be administered with food in stable renal transplant patients, if necessary.

Herb/Nutraceutical: Avoid cat's claw and echinacea due to immunostimulant properties.

Pharmacodynamics/Kinetics

Onset of action: Peak effect: Correlation of toxicity or efficacy is still being developed, however, one study indicated that 12-hour AUCs >40 mcg/mL/hour were correlated with efficacy and decreased episodes of rejection

Absorption: AUC values for MPA are lower in the early post-transplant period versus later (>3 months) post-transplant period. The extent of absorption in pediatrics is similar to that seen in adults, although there was wide variability reported.

Distribution: Oral: 4 L/kg; I.V.: 3.6 L/kg

Protein binding: MPA: 97%, MPAG 82%

Metabolism: Hepatic and via GI tract; hydrolyzed to mycophenolic acid (MPA; active metabolite); enterohepatic recirculation of MPA may occur; MPA is glucuronidated to MPAG (inactive metabolite)

Bioavailability: Oral: 94%

Half-life elimination: Oral: 17 hours; I.V.: 18 hours

Excretion: MPAG: Urine and feces; MPA: Urine (87% as inactive MPAG)

Pregnancy Risk Factor C (manufacturer)

Generic Available No

Mycophenolate Mofetil *see* Mycophenolate *on page 939*

Mycostatin® *see* Nystatin *on page 992*

Mydfrin® *see* Phenylephrine *on page 1071*

Mydriacyl® *see* Tropicamide *on page 1360*

Mykrox® *see* Metolazone *on page 900*

Mylanta® Extra Strength Liquid [OTC] *see* Aluminum Hydroxide, Magnesium Hydroxide, and Simethicone *on page 69*

Mylanta® Gas [OTC] *see* Simethicone *on page 1222*

Mylanta® Gas Maximum Strength [OTC] *see* Simethicone *on page 1222*

Mylanta® Liquid [OTC] *see* Aluminum Hydroxide, Magnesium Hydroxide, and Simethicone *on page 69*

Myleran® *see* Busulfan *on page 212*

Mylicon® Infants [OTC] *see* Simethicone *on page 1222*

Mylocel™ *see* Hydroxyurea *on page 696*

Mylotarg® *see* Gemtuzumab Ozogamicin *on page 632*

Myobloc® *see* Botulinum Toxin Type B *on page 195*

Myoflex® [OTC] *see* Triethanolamine Salicylate *on page 1348*

Mysoline® *see* Primidone *on page 1118*

Mytelase® *see* Ambenonium *on page 72*

Mytrex® *see* Nystatin and Triamcinolone *on page 992*

Mytussin® AC *see* Guaifenesin and Codeine *on page 650*

Mytussin® DAC *see* Guaifenesin, Pseudoephedrine, and Codeine *on page 653*

Mytussin® DM [OTC] *see* Guaifenesin and Dextromethorphan *on page 651*

Nabi-HB® *see* Hepatitis B Immune Globulin *on page 666*

Nabumetone (na BYOO me tone)

Related Information

Rheumatoid Arthritis, Osteoarthritis, and Osteoporosis *on page 1488*

Temporomandibular Dysfunction (TMD) *on page 1562*

(Continued)

Nabumetone *(Continued)*

U.S. Brand Names Relafen®

Canadian Brand Names Apo®-Nabumetone; Gen-Nabumetone; Relafen™; Rhoxal-nabumetone

Mexican Brand Names Relifex®

Pharmacologic Category Nonsteroidal Anti-inflammatory Drug (NSAID)

Use Management of osteoarthritis and rheumatoid arthritis

Unlabeled/Investigational Use Treatment of sunburn, mild to moderate pain

Local Anesthetic/Vasoconstrictor Precautions No information available to require special precautions

Effects on Dental Treatment 1% to 10%: Xerostomia

NSAID formulations are known to reversibly decrease platelet aggregation via mechanisms different than observed with aspirin. The dentist should be aware of the potential of abnormal coagulation. Caution should also be exercised in the use of NSAIDs in patients already on anticoagulant therapy with drugs such as warfarin (Coumadin®).

Dosage Oral:

Adults: 1000 mg/day; an additional 500-1000 mg may be needed in some patients to obtain more symptomatic relief; may be administered once or twice daily

Dosing adjustment in renal impairment: None; adverse effects from accumulation of inactive metabolites (excreted renally) have not been studied and should be considered

Mechanism of Action Nabumetone is a nonacidic NSAID that is rapidly metabolized after absorption to a major active metabolite, 6-methoxy-2-naphthylacetic acid. As found with previous NSAIDs, nabumetone's active metabolite inhibits the cyclooxygenase enzyme which is indirectly responsible for the production of inflammation and pain during arthritis by way of enhancing the production of endoperoxides and prostaglandins E_2 and I_2 (prostacyclin). The active metabolite of nabumetone is felt to be the compound primarily responsible for therapeutic effect. Comparatively, the parent drug is a poor inhibitor of prostaglandin synthesis.

Other Adverse Effects

>10%:

Central nervous system: Dizziness

Dermatologic: Rash

Gastrointestinal: Abdominal cramps, abdominal pain (12%), diarrhea (14%), dyspepsia (13%), heartburn, indigestion, nausea

1% to 10%:

Central nervous system: Headache, nervousness

Dermatologic: Itching

Endocrine & metabolic: Fluid retention

Gastrointestinal: Vomiting

Otic: Tinnitus

<1%: Abnormal vision, acne, agitation, albuminuria, alopecia, anemia, angina, angioneurotic edema, anorexia, anxiety, arrhythmia, asthma, azotemia, bullous eruptions, cholestatic jaundice, confusion, depression, duodenal ulcer, dysphagia, dyspnea, fever, gallstones, gastric ulcer, gastroenteritis, gingivitis, GI bleeding, granulocytopenia, hyperglycemia, hypertension, hyperuricemia, hypokalemia, impotence, leukopenia, liver function abnormalities, malaise, melena, MI, nephrolithiasis, nightmares, pancreatitis, paresthesia, photosensitivity, pseudoporphyria cutanea tarda, syncope, thrombocytopenia, thrombophlebitis, tremor, urticaria, vasculitis, vertigo, weakness

Postmarketing and/or case reports: Anaphylactoid reaction, anaphylaxis, CHF, eosinophilic pneumonia, erythema multiforme, hepatic failure, hepatitis, hypersensitivity pneumonitis, interstitial nephritis, interstitial pneumonitis, nephrotic syndrome, renal failure, Stevens-Johnson syndrome, toxic epidermal necrolysis

Drug Interactions

Increased Effect/Toxicity: NSAIDs may increase digoxin, methotrexate, and lithium serum concentrations. The renal adverse effects of ACE inhibitors may be potentiated by NSAIDs. Potential for bleeding may be increased with anticoagulants or antiplatelet agents. Concurrent use of corticosteroids may increase the risk of GI ulceration.

Decreased Effect: NSAIDs may decrease the effect of some antihypertensive agents, including ACE inhibitors, angiotensin receptor antagonists, and hydralazine. The efficacy of diuretics (loop and/or thiazide) may be decreased.

Dietary/Ethanol/Herb Considerations

Ethanol: Avoid use; may enhance gastric mucosal irritation.

Food: Administer with food or milk to reduce GI upset; may increase peak serum concentration. Avoid garlic, ginger, or green tea.

Herb/Nutraceutical: Avoid cat's claw, dong quai, evening primrose, feverfew, garlic, ginger, ginkgo biloba, ginseng, green tea, horse chestnut, and red clover due to additional antiplatelet activity.

Pharmacodynamics/Kinetics

Onset of action: Several days

Distribution: Diffusion occurs readily into synovial fluid

Protein binding: >99%

Metabolism: Prodrug, rapidly metabolized to an active metabolite (6-methoxy-2-naphthylacetic acid); extensive first-pass effect

Half-life elimination: Major metabolite: 24 hours

Time to peak, serum: Metabolite: Oral: 3-6 hours; Synovial fluid: 4-12 hours

Excretion: Urine (80%) and feces (10%) with little as unchanged drug

Pregnancy Risk Factor C/D (3rd trimester)

Generic Available Yes

NAC *see* Acetylcysteine *on page 40*

***N*-Acetylcysteine** *see* Acetylcysteine *on page 40*

***N*-Acetyl-L-cysteine** *see* Acetylcysteine *on page 40*

N-Acetyl-P-Aminophenol *see* Acetaminophen *on page 27*

NaCl *see* Sodium Chloride *on page 1229*

Nadolol (nay DOE lole)

Related Information

Cardiovascular Diseases *on page 1456*

U.S. Brand Names Corgard®

Canadian Brand Names Alti-Nadolol; Apo®-Nadol; Corgard®; Novo-Nadolol

Pharmacologic Category Beta Blocker, Nonselective

Use Treatment of hypertension and angina pectoris; prophylaxis of migraine headaches

Local Anesthetic/Vasoconstrictor Precautions Use with caution; epinephrine has interacted with nonselective beta-blockers to result in initial hypertensive episode followed by bradycardia

Effects on Dental Treatment Nadolol is a nonselective beta-blocker and may enhance the pressor response to epinephrine, resulting in hypertension and bradycardia. Many nonsteroidal anti-inflammatory drugs such as ibuprofen and indomethacin can reduce the hypotensive effect of beta-blockers after 3 or more weeks of therapy with the NSAID. Short-term NSAID use (ie, 3 days) requires no special precautions in patients taking beta-blockers.

Dosage Oral:

Adults: Initial: 40 mg/day, increase dosage gradually by 40-80 mg increments at 3- to 7-day intervals until optimum clinical response is obtained with profound slowing of heart rate; doses up to 160-240 mg/day in angina and 240-320 mg/day in hypertension may be necessary.

Elderly: Initial: 20 mg/day; increase doses by 20 mg increments at 3- to 7-day intervals; usual dosage range: 20-240 mg/day.

Dosing adjustment in renal impairment:

Cl_{cr} 31-40 mL/minute: Administer every 24-36 hours or administer 50% of normal dose.

Cl_{cr} 10-30 mL/minute: Administer every 24-48 hours or administer 50% of normal dose.

Cl_{cr} <10 mL/minute: Administer every 40-60 hours or administer 25% of normal dose.

Hemodialysis: Moderately dialyzable (20% to 50%); administer dose postdialysis or administer 40 mg supplemental dose.

Peritoneal dialysis: Supplemental dose is unnecessary.

Dosing adjustment in hepatic disease: Reduction probably necessary.

Mechanism of Action Competitively blocks response to beta$_1$- and beta$_2$-adrenergic stimulation; does not exhibit any membrane stabilizing or intrinsic sympathomimetic activity

Other Adverse Effects

>10%:

Central nervous system: Drowsiness, insomnia

Endocrine & metabolic: Decreased sexual ability

1% to 10%:

Cardiovascular: Bradycardia, palpitations, edema, CHF, reduced peripheral circulation

Central nervous system: Mental depression

Gastrointestinal: Diarrhea or constipation, nausea, vomiting, stomach discomfort

Respiratory: Bronchospasm

Miscellaneous: Cold extremities

<1% (Limited to important or life-threatening): Chest pain, arrhythmias, orthostatic hypotension, nervousness, headache, depression, hallucinations, confusion (especially in the elderly), thrombocytopenia, leukopenia, dyspnea

Drug Interactions

Increased Effect/Toxicity: The heart rate lowering effects of nadolol are additive with other drugs which slow AV conduction (digoxin, verapamil, diltiazem). Concurrent use of alpha-blockers (prazosin, terazosin) with beta-blockers may increase risk of orthostasis. Nadolol may mask the tachycardia from hypoglycemia caused by insulin and oral hypoglycemics. In patients receiving concurrent therapy, the risk of hypertensive crisis is increased when either clonidine or the beta-blocker is withdrawn. Reserpine has been shown to enhance the effect of

(Continued)

Nadolol *(Continued)*

beta-blockers. Avoid using with alpha-adrenergic stimulants (phenylephrine, epinephrine, etc) which may have exaggerated hypertensive responses. Beta-blockers may affect the action or levels of ethanol, disopyramide, nondepolarizing muscle relaxants, and theophylline although the effects are difficult to predict. The vasoconstrictive effects of ergot alkaloids may be enhanced.

Decreased Effect: Decreased effect of beta-blockers with aluminum salts, barbiturates, calcium salts, cholestyramine, colestipol, NSAIDs, penicillins (ampicillin), rifampin, salicylates, and sulfinpyrazone due to decreased bioavailability and plasma levels. Beta-blockers may decrease the effect of sulfonylureas (possibly hyperglycemia). Nonselective beta-blockers blunt the effect of beta-2 adrenergic agonists (albuterol).

Dietary/Ethanol/Herb Considerations

Ethanol: Limit use; may increase risk of hypotension or dizziness.

Food: May be taken with food; avoid caffeine, garlic, ginger, and licorice.

Herb/Nutraceutical: Avoid black cohosh, dong quai, and evening primrose due to estrogenic activity. Avoid ephedra, ginseng, and yohimbe; may worsen hypertension. Avoid garlic (may have increased antihypertensive effect). Avoid ginger; may have positive inotropic effects. Avoid hawthorn; may decrease peripheral vascular resistance and cause BP to decrease more than expected. Avoid licorice; causes sodium and water retention and increases potassium loss.

Pharmacodynamics/Kinetics

Duration: 17-24 hours

Absorption: 30% to 40%

Distribution: Concentration in human breast milk is 4.6 times higher than serum

Protein binding: 28%

Half-life elimination: Adults: 10-24 hours; prolonged with renal impairment; End-stage renal disease: 45 hours

Time to peak, serum: 2-4 hours

Excretion: Urine (as unchanged drug)

Pregnancy Risk Factor C

Generic Available Yes

Selected Readings

Foster CA and Aston SJ, "Propranolol-Epinephrine Interaction: A Potential Disaster," *Plast Reconstr Surg*, 1983, 72(1):74-8.

Wong DG, Spence JD, Lamki L, et al, "Effect of Nonsteroidal Anti-inflammatory Drugs on Control of Hypertension of Beta-Blockers and Diuretics," *Lancet*, 1986, 1(8488):997-1001.

Wynn RL, "Dental Nonsteroidal Anti-inflammatory Drugs and Prostaglandin-Based Drug Interactions, Part Two," *Gen Dent*, 1992, 40(2):104, 106, 108.

Wynn RL, "Epinephrine Interactions With Beta-Blockers," *Gen Dent*, 1994, 42(1):16, 18.

Nafarelin (NAF a re lin)

U.S. Brand Names Synarel®

Canadian Brand Names Synarel®

Mexican Brand Names Synarel®

Pharmacologic Category Hormone, Posterior Pituitary; Luteinizing Hormone-Releasing Hormone Analog

Synonyms Nafarelin Acetate

Use Treatment of endometriosis, including pain and reduction of lesions; treatment of central precocious puberty (gonadotropin-dependent precocious puberty) in children of both sexes

Local Anesthetic/Vasoconstrictor Precautions No information available to require special precautions

Effects on Dental Treatment No significant effects or complications reported

Dosage

Endometriosis: Adults: Female: 1 spray (200 mcg) in 1 nostril each morning and the other nostril each evening starting on days 2-4 of menstrual cycle for 6 months

Central precocious puberty: Children: Males/Females: 2 sprays (400 mcg) into each nostril in the morning 2 sprays (400 mcg) into each nostril in the evening. If inadequate suppression, may increase dose to 3 sprays (600 mcg) into alternating nostrils 3 times/day.

Mechanism of Action Potent synthetic decapeptide analogue of gonadotropin-releasing hormone (GnRH; LHRH) which is approximately 200 times more potent than GnRH in terms of pituitary release of luteinizing hormone (LH) and follicle-stimulating hormone (FSH). Effects on the pituitary gland and sex hormones are dependent upon its length of administration. After acute administration, an initial stimulation of the release of LH and FSH from the pituitary is observed; an increase in androgens and estrogens subsequently follows. Continued administration of nafarelin, however, suppresses gonadotrope responsiveness to endogenous GnRH resulting in reduced secretion of LH and FSH and, secondarily, decreased ovarian and testicular steroid production.

Other Adverse Effects

>10%:

Central nervous system: Headache, emotional lability

Dermatologic: Acne

Endocrine & metabolic: Hot flashes, decreased libido, decreased breast size
Genitourinary: Vaginal dryness
Neuromuscular & skeletal: Myalgia
Respiratory: Nasal irritation

1% to 10%:

Cardiovascular: Edema, chest pain
Central nervous system: Insomnia
Dermatologic: Urticaria, rash, pruritus, seborrhea
Respiratory: Dyspnea

<1%: Increased libido, weight loss

Pharmacodynamics/Kinetics

Protein binding, plasma: 80%
Time to peak, serum: 10-45 minutes

Pregnancy Risk Factor X

Generic Available No

Nafarelin Acetate *see* Nafarelin *on page 944*

Nafcillin (naf SIL in)

Canadian Brand Names Nallpen®; Unipen®

Pharmacologic Category Antibiotic, Penicillin

Synonyms Ethoxynaphthamido Penicillin Sodium; Nafcillin Sodium; Nallpen [DSC]; Sodium Nafcillin

Use Treatment of infections such as osteomyelitis, septicemia, endocarditis, and CNS infections caused by susceptible strains of staphylococci species

Local Anesthetic/Vasoconstrictor Precautions No information available to require special precautions

Effects on Dental Treatment Prolonged use of penicillins may lead to the development of oral candidiasis.

Dosage

Neonates:

<2000 g, <7 days: 50 mg/kg/day divided every 12 hours
<2000 g, >7 days: 75 mg/kg/day divided every 8 hours
>2000 g, <7 days: 50 mg/kg/day divided every 8 hours
>2000 g, >7 days: 75 mg/kg/day divided every 6 hours

Children:

I.M.: 25 mg/kg twice daily
I.V.:

Mild to moderate infections: 50-100 mg/kg/day in divided doses every 6 hours
Severe infections: 100-200 mg/kg/day in divided doses every 4-6 hours

Maximum dose: 12 g/day

Adults:

I.M.: 500 mg every 4-6 hours
I.V.: 500-2000 mg every 4-6 hours

Dosing adjustment in renal/hepatic impairment: In patients with both hepatic and renal impairment, modification of dosage may be necessary; no data available.

Dialysis: Not dialyzable (0% to 5%) via hemodialysis; supplemental dosage unnecessary with hemo- or peritoneal dialysis or continuous arteriovenous or venovenous hemofiltration

Mechanism of Action Interferes with bacterial cell wall synthesis during active multiplication, causing cell wall death and resultant bactericidal activity against susceptible bacteria

Other Adverse Effects Frequency not defined:

Central nervous system: Pain, fever
Dermatologic: Rash
Gastrointestinal: Nausea, diarrhea
Hematologic: Agranulocytosis, bone marrow depression, neutropenia
Local: Pain, swelling, inflammation, phlebitis, skin sloughing, and thrombophlebitis at the injection site; oxacillin (less likely to cause phlebitis) is often preferred in pediatric patients
Renal: Interstitial nephritis (acute)
Miscellaneous: Hypersensitivity reactions

Drug Interactions Induces **CYP3A4**

Increased Effect/Toxicity: Probenecid may cause an increase in nafcillin levels.

Decreased Effect: Chloramphenicol may decrease nafcillin efficacy. If taken concomitantly with warfarin, nafcillin may inhibit the anticoagulant response to warfarin. This effect may persist for up to 30 days after nafcillin has been discontinued. Subtherapeutic cyclosporine levels may result when taken concomitantly with nafcillin. Although anecdotal reports suggest oral contraceptive efficacy could be reduced by penicillins, this has been refuted by more rigorous scientific and clinical data.

Dietary/Ethanol/Herb Considerations Food: Administer on an empty stomach; food may decrease serum concentration.

(Continued)

Nafcillin *(Continued)*

Pharmacodynamics/Kinetics

Distribution: Widely distributed; CSF penetration is poor but enhanced by meningeal inflammation; crosses placenta

Protein binding: 70% to 90%

Metabolism: Primarily hepatic; undergoes enterohepatic recirculation

Half-life elimination:

Neonates: <3 weeks: 2.2-5.5 hours; 4-9 weeks: 1.2-2.3 hours

Children 3 months to 14 years: 0.75-1.9 hours

Adults: 30 minutes to 1.5 hours with normal renal and hepatic function

Time to peak, serum: I.M.: 30-60 minutes

Excretion: Primarily feces; urine (10% to 30% as unchanged drug)

Pregnancy Risk Factor B

Generic Available Yes

Nafcillin Sodium *see* Nafcillin *on page 945*

Naftifine (NAF ti feen)

Related Information

Oral Fungal Infections *on page 1542*

U.S. Brand Names Naftin®

Pharmacologic Category Antifungal Agent, Topical

Synonyms Naftifine Hydrochloride

Use Topical treatment of tinea cruris (jock itch), tinea corporis (ringworm), and tinea pedis (athlete's foot)

Local Anesthetic/Vasoconstrictor Precautions No information available to require special precautions

Effects on Dental Treatment No significant effects or complications reported

Dosage Adults: Topical: Apply cream once daily and gel twice daily (morning and evening) for up to 4 weeks

Mechanism of Action Synthetic, broad-spectrum antifungal agent in the allylamine class; appears to have both fungistatic and fungicidal activity. Exhibits antifungal activity by selectively inhibiting the enzyme squalene epoxidase in a dose-dependent manner which results in the primary sterol, ergosterol, within the fungal membrane not being synthesized.

Other Adverse Effects

>10%: Local: Burning, stinging

1% to 10%:

Dermatologic: Erythema, itching

Local: Dryness, irritation

Pharmacodynamics/Kinetics

Absorption: Systemic: Cream: 6%; Gel: ≤4%

Half-life elimination: 2-3 days

Excretion: Urine and feces (as metabolites)

Pregnancy Risk Factor B

Generic Available No

Naftifine Hydrochloride *see* Naftifine *on page 946*

Naftin® *see* Naftifine *on page 946*

$NaHCO_3$ *see* Sodium Bicarbonate *on page 1227*

Nalbuphine (NAL byoo feen)

U.S. Brand Names Nubain®

Canadian Brand Names Nubain®

Mexican Brand Names Bufigen®; Nalcryn®; Nubain®

Pharmacologic Category Analgesic, Narcotic

Synonyms Nalbuphine Hydrochloride

Use Relief of moderate to severe pain; preoperative analgesia, postoperative and surgical anesthesia, and obstetrical analgesia during labor and delivery

Local Anesthetic/Vasoconstrictor Precautions No information available to require special precautions

Effects on Dental Treatment Anticholinergic side effects can cause a reduction of saliva production or secretion, contributing to discomfort and dental disease (ie, caries, oral candidiasis and periodontal disease).

Dosage I.M., I.V., S.C.:

Children 10 months to 14 years: Premedication: 0.2 mg/kg; maximum: 20 mg/dose

Adults: 10 mg/70 kg every 3-6 hours; maximum single dose: 20 mg; maximum daily dose: 160 mg

Dosing adjustment in hepatic impairment: Use with caution and reduce dose

Mechanism of Action Binds to opiate receptors in the CNS, causing inhibition of ascending pain pathways, altering the perception of and response to pain; produces generalized CNS depression

Other Adverse Effects

>10%:

Central nervous system: Fatigue, drowsiness

Miscellaneous: Histamine release

1% to 10%:

Cardiovascular: Hypotension

Central nervous system: Headache, nightmares, dizziness

Gastrointestinal: Anorexia, nausea, vomiting, xerostomia

Local: Pain at injection site

Neuromuscular & skeletal: Weakness

<1% (Limited to important or life-threatening): Bradycardia, dyspnea, hypertension, narcotic withdrawal, pulmonary edema, tachycardia

Drug Interactions Increased Effect/Toxicity: Barbiturate anesthetics may increase CNS depression.

Dietary/Ethanol/Herb Considerations

Ethanol: Avoid use; may increase CNS depression.

Herb/Nutraceutical: Avoid gotu kola, kava, SAMe, St John's wort, and valerian; may increase CNS depression.

Pharmacodynamics/Kinetics

Onset of action: Peak effect: I.M.: 30 minutes; I.V.: 1-3 minutes

Metabolism: Hepatic

Half-life elimination: 3.5-5 hours

Excretion: Feces; urine (~7% as metabolites)

Pregnancy Risk Factor B/D (prolonged use or high doses at term)

Generic Available Yes

Nalbuphine Hydrochloride *see* Nalbuphine *on page 946*

Nalfon® *see* Fenoprofen *on page 563*

Nalidixic Acid (nal i DIKS ik AS id)

U.S. Brand Names NegGram®

Canadian Brand Names NegGram®

Pharmacologic Category Antibiotic, Quinolone

Synonyms Nalidixinic Acid

Use Treatment of urinary tract infections

Local Anesthetic/Vasoconstrictor Precautions No information available to require special precautions

Effects on Dental Treatment No significant effects or complications reported

Dosage Oral:

Children 3 months to 12 years: 55 mg/kg/day divided every 6 hours; suppressive therapy is 33 mg/kg/day divided every 6 hours

Adults: 1 g 4 times/day for 2 weeks; then suppressive therapy of 500 mg 4 times/day

Dosing comments in renal impairment: Cl_{cr} <50 mL/minute: Avoid use

Mechanism of Action Inhibits DNA polymerization in late stages of chromosomal replication

Other Adverse Effects

Central nervous system: Dizziness, drowsiness, headache, increased intracranial pressure, malaise, vertigo, confusion, toxic psychosis, convulsions, fever, chills

Dermatologic: Rash, urticaria, photosensitivity reactions

Endocrine & metabolic: Metabolic acidosis

Gastrointestinal: Nausea, vomiting

Hematologic: Leukopenia, thrombocytopenia

Hepatic: Hepatotoxicity

Ocular: Visual disturbances

Miscellaneous: Quinolones have been associated with tendonitis and tendon rupture

Drug Interactions Inhibits **CYP1A2**

Increased Effect/Toxicity: Nalidixic acid increases the levels/effect of cyclosporine, caffeine, theophylline, and warfarin. The CNS-stimulating effect of some quinolones may be enhanced by NSAIDs, and foscarnet has been associated with an increased risk of seizures with some quinolones. Serum levels of some quinolones are increased by loop diuretics, probenecid, and cimetidine (and possibly other H_2-blockers) due to altered renal elimination. This effect may be more important for quinolones with high percentage of renal elimination than with nalidixic acid. Concurrent use of corticosteroids may increase risk of tendon rupture.

Decreased Effect: Enteral feedings may decrease plasma concentrations of nalidixic acid probably by >30% inhibition of absorption. Aluminum/magnesium products, didanosine, quinapril, and sucralfate may decrease absorption of nalidixic acid by ≥90% if administered concurrently. (Administer nalidixic acid at least 4 hours and preferably 6 hours after the dose of these agents.) Calcium, iron, zinc, and multivitamins with minerals products may decrease absorption of nalidixic acid significantly if administered concurrently. (Administer nalidixic acid 2

(Continued)

Nalidixic Acid *(Continued)*

hours before dose or at least 2 hours after the dose of these agents). Antineoplastic agents may decrease quinolone absorption.

Dietary/Ethanol/Herb Considerations Administer with food to reduce GI upset.

Pharmacodynamics/Kinetics

Distribution: Achieves significant antibacterial concentrations only in the urinary tract; crosses placenta; enters breast milk

Protein binding: 90%

Metabolism: Partially hepatic

Half-life elimination: 6-7 hours; significantly prolonged with renal impairment

Time to peak, serum: 1-2 hours

Excretion: Urine (as unchanged drug, 80% as metabolites); feces (small amounts)

Pregnancy Risk Factor B

Generic Available No

Nalidixinic Acid *see* Nalidixic Acid *on page 947*

Nallpen [DSC] *see* Nafcillin *on page 945*

***N*-allylnoroxymorphine Hydrochloride** *see* Naloxone *on page 949*

Nalmefene (NAL me feen)

U.S. Brand Names Revex®

Pharmacologic Category Antidote

Synonyms Nalmefene Hydrochloride

Use Complete or partial reversal of opioid drug effects, including respiratory depression induced by natural or synthetic opioids; reversal of postoperative opioid depression; management of known or suspected opioid overdose

Local Anesthetic/Vasoconstrictor Precautions No information available to require special precautions

Effects on Dental Treatment No significant effects or complications reported

Dosage

Reversal of postoperative opioid depression: Blue labeled product (100 mcg/mL): Titrate to reverse the undesired effects of opioids; initial dose for nonopioid dependent patients: 0.25 mcg/kg followed by 0.25 mcg/kg incremental doses at 2- to 5-minute intervals; after a total dose >1 mcg/kg, further therapeutic response is unlikely

Management of known/suspected opioid overdose: Green labeled product (1000 mcg/mL): Initial dose: 0.5 mg/70 kg; may repeat with 1 mg/70 kg in 2-5 minutes; further increase beyond a total dose of 1.5 mg/70 kg will not likely result in improved response and may result in cardiovascular stress and precipitated withdrawal syndrome. (If opioid dependency is suspected, administer a challenge dose of 0.1 mg/70 kg; if no withdrawal symptoms are observed in 2 minutes, the recommended doses can be administered.)

Note: If recurrence of respiratory depression is noted, dose may again be titrated to clinical effect using incremental doses.

Note: If I.V. access is lost or not readily obtainable, a single S.C. or I.M. dose of 1 mg may be effective in 5-15 minutes.

Dosing adjustment in renal or hepatic impairment: Not necessary with single uses, however, slow administration (over 60 seconds) of incremental doses is recommended to minimize hypertension and dizziness

Mechanism of Action As a 6-methylene analog of naltrexone, nalmefene acts as a competitive antagonist at opioid receptor sites, preventing or reversing the respiratory depression, sedation, and hypotension induced by opiates; no pharmacologic activity of its own (eg, opioid agonist activity) has been demonstrated

Other Adverse Effects

>10%: Gastrointestinal: Nausea

1% to 10%:

Cardiovascular: Tachycardia, hypertension, hypotension, vasodilation

Central nervous system: Fever, dizziness, headache, chills

Gastrointestinal: Vomiting

Miscellaneous: Postoperative pain

<1%: Agitation, arrhythmia, bradycardia, confusion, depression, diarrhea, myoclonus, nervousness, pharyngitis, pruritus, somnolence, tremor, urinary retention, xerostomia

Drug Interactions Increased Effect/Toxicity: Potential increased risk of seizures may exist with use of flumazenil and nalmefene coadministration.

Pharmacodynamics/Kinetics

Onset of action: I.M., S.C.: 5-15 minutes

Distribution: V_d: 8.6 L/kg; rapid

Protein binding: 45%

Metabolism: Hepatic via glucuronide conjugation to metabolites with little or no activity

Bioavailability: I.M., I.V., S.C.: 100%

Half-life elimination: 10.8 hours

Time to peak, serum: I.M.: 2.3 hours; I.V.: <2 minutes; S.C.: 1.5 hours

Excretion: Feces (17%); urine (<5% as unchanged drug)
Clearance: 0.8 L/hour/kg

Pregnancy Risk Factor B

Generic Available No

Comments Nalmefene is supplied in two concentrations 100 mcg/mL has a blue label, 1000 mcg/mL has a green label. Proper steps should be used to prevent use of the incorrect dosage strength. The duration of action of nalmefene is as long as most opioid analgesics; may cause acute withdrawal symptoms in individuals who have some degree of tolerance to and dependence on opioids. The goal of treatment in the postoperative setting is to achieve reversal of excessive opioid effects without inducing a complete reversal and acute pain. If opioid dependence is suspected, nalmefene should only be used in opioid overdose if the likelihood of overdose is high based on history or the clinical presentation of respiratory depression with concurrent pupillary constriction is present.

Nalmefene Hydrochloride *see* Nalmefene *on page 948*

Naloxone (nal OKS one)

Related Information

Dental Office Emergencies *on page 1582*

U.S. Brand Names Narcan®

Canadian Brand Names Narcan®

Mexican Brand Names Narcanti®

Pharmacologic Category Antidote

Synonyms *N*-allylnoroxymorphine Hydrochloride; Naloxone Hydrochloride

Use

Dental: Reverse overdose effects of the two narcotic agents, fentanyl and meperidine, used in the technique of I.V. conscious sedation

Medical:

Complete or partial reversal of opioid depression, including respiratory depression, induced by natural and synthetic opioids (including propoxyphene, methadone, and certain mixed agonist-antagonist analgesics, such as nalbuphine, pentazocine, and butorphanol):

Diagnosis of suspected opioid tolerance or acute opioid overdose

Adjunctive agent to increase BP in the management of septic shock

Unlabeled/Investigational Use Treatment of PCP and toxic ethanol ingestion

Local Anesthetic/Vasoconstrictor Precautions No information available to require special precautions

Effects on Dental Treatment Frequency not defined: Hypertension, hypotension, tachycardia, ventricular arrhythmias, cardiac arrest, irritability, anxiety, narcotic withdrawal, restlessness, seizures, nausea, vomiting, tremors, dyspnea, runny nose, sneezing, diaphoresis

Dosage I.M., I.V. (preferred), intratracheal, S.C.:

Postanesthesia narcotic reversal: Infants and Children: 0.01 mg/kg; may repeat every 2-3 minutes, as needed based on response

Opiate intoxication:

Children:

Birth (including premature infants) to 5 years or <20 kg: 0.1 mg/kg; repeat every 2-3 minutes if needed; may need to repeat doses every 20-60 minutes

>5 years or ≥20 kg: 2 mg/dose; if no response, repeat every 2-3 minutes; may need to repeat doses every 20-60 minutes

Children and Adults: Continuous infusion: I.V.: If continuous infusion is required, calculate dosage/hour based on effective intermittent dose used and duration of adequate response seen, titrate dose 0.04-0.16 mg/kg/hour for 2-5 days in children, adult dose typically 0.25-6.25 mg/hour (short-term infusions as high as 2.4 mg/kg/hour have been tolerated in adults during treatment for septic shock); alternatively, continuous infusion utilizes $^2/_3$ of the initial naloxone bolus on an hourly basis; add 10 times this dose to each liter of D_5W and infuse at a rate of 100 mL/hour; $^1/_2$ of the initial bolus dose should be readministered 15 minutes after initiation of the continuous infusion to prevent a drop in naloxone levels; increase infusion rate as needed to assure adequate ventilation

Narcotic overdose: Adults: I.V.: 0.4-2 mg every 2-3 minutes as needed; may need to repeat doses every 20-60 minutes, if no response is observed after 10 mg, question the diagnosis. **Note:** Use 0.1-0.2 mg increments in patients who are opioid dependent and in postoperative patients to avoid large cardiovascular changes.

Mechanism of Action Pure opioid antagonist that competes and displaces narcotics at opioid receptor sites

Other Adverse Effects Frequency not defined:

Gastrointestinal: Diarrhea

Respiratory: Pulmonary edema

Contraindications Hypersensitivity to naloxone or any component of the formulation

Warnings/Precautions Due to an association between naloxone and acute pulmonary edema, use with caution in patients with cardiovascular disease or in

(Continued)

Naloxone *(Continued)*

patients receiving medications with potential adverse cardiovascular effects (eg, hypotension, pulmonary edema or arrhythmias). Excessive dosages should be avoided after use of opiates in surgery. Abrupt postoperative reversal may result in nausea, vomiting, sweating, tachycardia, hypertension, seizures, and other cardiovascular events (including pulmonary edema and arrhythmias). May precipitate withdrawal symptoms in patients addicted to opiates, including pain, hypertension, sweating, agitation, irritability; in neonates: shrill cry, failure to feed. Recurrence of respiratory depression is possible if the opioid involved is long-acting; observe patients until there is no reasonable risk of recurrent respiratory depression.

Drug Interactions Narcotic analgesics: Decreased effect of narcotic analgesics; may precipitate acute withdrawal reaction in physically dependent patients

Pharmacodynamics/Kinetics

Onset of action: Endotracheal, I.M., S.C.: 2-5 minutes; I.V.: ~2 minutes

Duration: 20-60 minutes; since shorter than that of most opioids, repeated doses are usually needed

Distribution: Crosses placenta

Metabolism: Primarily hepatic via glucuronidation

Half-life elimination: Neonates: 1.2-3 hours; Adults: 1-1.5 hours

Excretion: Urine (as metabolites)

Pregnancy Risk Factor C

Breast-feeding Considerations No data reported. Since naloxone is used for opiate reversal the concern should be on opiate drug levels in a breast-feeding mother and transfer to the infant rather than naloxone exposure. The safest approach would be **not** to breast-feed.

Dosage Forms INJ, neonatal solution: 0.02 mg/mL (2 mL). **INJ, solution:** 0.4 mg/mL (1 mL, 2 mL, 10 mL); 1 mg/mL (2 mL, 10 mL)

Generic Available Yes

Naloxone Hydrochloride *see* Naloxone *on page 949*

Naltrexone (nal TREKS one)

U.S. Brand Names ReVia®

Canadian Brand Names ReVia®

Pharmacologic Category Antidote

Synonyms Naltrexone Hydrochloride

Use Treatment of ethanol dependence; blockade of the effects of exogenously administered opioids

Local Anesthetic/Vasoconstrictor Precautions No information available to require special precautions

Effects on Dental Treatment No significant effects or complications reported

Dosage Do not give until patient is opioid-free for 7-10 days as determined by urine analysis.

Adults: Oral: 25 mg; if no withdrawal signs within 1 hour give another 25 mg; maintenance regimen is flexible, variable and individualized (50 mg/day to 100-150 mg 3 times/week for 12 weeks); up to 800 mg/day has been tolerated in adults without an adverse effect

Dosing cautions in renal/hepatic impairment: Use with caution; an increase in naltrexone AUC of approximately five- and tenfold in patients with compensated or decompensated liver cirrhosis respectively, compared with normal liver function has been reported.

Mechanism of Action Naltrexone (a pure opioid antagonist) is a cyclopropyl derivative of oxymorphone similar in structure to naloxone and nalorphine (a morphine derivative); it acts as a competitive antagonist at opioid receptor sites

Other Adverse Effects

>10%:

Central nervous system: Insomnia, nervousness, headache, low energy

Gastrointestinal: Abdominal cramping, nausea, vomiting

Neuromuscular & skeletal: Arthralgia

1% to 10%:

Central nervous system: Increased energy, feeling down, irritability, dizziness, anxiety, somnolence

Dermatologic: Rash

Endocrine & metabolic: Polydipsia

Gastrointestinal: Diarrhea, constipation

Genitourinary: Delayed ejaculation, impotency

<1%: Bad dreams, blurred vision, confusion, depression, disorientation, edema, fatigue, hallucinations, increased blood pressure, itching, rhinorrhea, narcotic withdrawal, nasal congestion, nightmares, palpitations, paranoia, restlessness, sneezing, suicide attempts, tachycardia

Drug Interactions

Increased Effect/Toxicity: Lethargy and somnolence have been reported with the combination of naltrexone and thioridazine.

Decreased Effect: Naltrexone decreases effects of opioid-containing products.

Dietary/Ethanol/Herb Considerations
Ethanol: Avoid use; may increase CNS depression.
Herb/Nutraceutical: Avoid gotu kola, kava, SAMe, St John's wort, and valerian; may increase CNS depression.

Pharmacodynamics/Kinetics
Duration: 50 mg: 24 hours; 100 mg: 48 hours; 150 mg: 72 hours
Absorption: Almost complete
Distribution: V_d: 19 L/kg; widely throughout the body but considerable interindividual variation exists
Protein binding: 21%
Metabolism: Extensive first-pass effect to 6-β-naltrexol
Half-life elimination: 4 hours; 6-β-naltrexol: 13 hours
Time to peak, serum: ~60 minutes
Excretion: Primarily urine (as metabolites and unchanged drug)

Pregnancy Risk Factor C

Generic Available Yes

Naltrexone Hydrochloride *see* Naltrexone *on page 950*

Nandrolone (NAN droe lone)

U.S. Brand Names Deca-Durabolin® [DSC]

Canadian Brand Names Deca-Durabolin®; Durabolin®

Mexican Brand Names Deca-Durabolin®

Pharmacologic Category Androgen

Synonyms Deca-Durabolin® [DSC]; Nandrolone Decanoate; Nandrolone Phenpropionate

Use Control of metastatic breast cancer; management of anemia of renal insufficiency

Local Anesthetic/Vasoconstrictor Precautions No information available to require special precautions

Effects on Dental Treatment No significant effects or complications reported

Restrictions C-III

Dosage Deep I.M. (into gluteal muscle):
Children 2-13 years (decanoate): 25-50 mg every 3-4 weeks
Adults:
Male:
Breast cancer (phenpropionate): 50-100 mg/week
Anemia of renal insufficiency (decanoate): 100-200 mg/week
Female: 50-100 mg/week
Breast cancer (phenpropionate): 50-100 mg/week
Anemia of renal insufficiency (decanoate): 50-100 mg/week

Mechanism of Action Promotes tissue-building processes, increases production of erythropoietin, causes protein anabolism; increases hemoglobin and red blood cell volume

Other Adverse Effects

Male:
Postpubertal:
>10%:
Dermatologic: Acne
Endocrine & metabolic: Gynecomastia
Genitourinary: Bladder irritability, priapism
1% to 10%:
Central nervous system: Insomnia, chills
Endocrine & metabolic: Decreased libido, hepatic dysfunction
Gastrointestinal: Nausea, diarrhea
Genitourinary: Prostatic hyperplasia (elderly)
Hematologic: Iron-deficiency anemia, suppression of clotting factors
<1%: Hepatic necrosis, hepatocellular carcinoma
Prepubertal:
>10%:
Dermatologic: Acne
Endocrine & metabolic: Virilism
1% to 10%:
Central nervous system: Chills, insomnia
Dermatologic: Hyperpigmentation
Gastrointestinal: Diarrhea, nausea
Hematologic: Iron deficiency anemia, suppression of clotting
<1%: Hepatocellular carcinoma, necrosis

Female:
>10%: Endocrine & metabolic: Virilism
1% to 10%:
Central nervous system: Chills, insomnia
Endocrine & metabolic: Hypercalcemia
Gastrointestinal: Nausea, diarrhea
Hematologic: Iron deficiency anemia, suppression of clotting factors

(Continued)

Nandrolone *(Continued)*

Hepatic: Hepatic dysfunction

<1%: Hepatic necrosis, hepatocellular carcinoma

Drug Interactions Increased Effect/Toxicity: Nandrolone may increase the effect of oral anticoagulants, insulin, oral hypoglycemic agents, adrenal steroids, or ACTH when taken together.

Pharmacodynamics/Kinetics

Onset of action: 3-6 months

Duration: Up to 30 days

Absorption: I.M.: 77%

Metabolism: Hepatic

Excretion: Urine

Pregnancy Risk Factor X

Generic Available Yes

Nandrolone Decanoate *see* Nandrolone *on page 951*

Nandrolone Phenpropionate *see* Nandrolone *on page 951*

Naphazoline (naf AZ oh leen)

U.S. Brand Names AK-Con™; Albalon®; Allersol®; Clear Eyes® [OTC]; Clear Eyes® ACR [OTC]; Naphcon® [OTC]; Privine® [OTC]; VasoClear® [OTC]

Canadian Brand Names Naphcon Forte®; Vasocon®

Mexican Brand Names Afazol Grin®

Pharmacologic Category Alpha$_1$ Agonist; Ophthalmic Agent, Vasoconstrictor

Synonyms Naphazoline Hydrochloride

Use Topical ocular vasoconstrictor; will temporarily relieve congestion, itching, and minor irritation, and to control hyperemia in patients with superficial corneal vascularity; treatment of nasal congestion; adjunct for sinusitis

Local Anesthetic/Vasoconstrictor Precautions No information available to require special precautions

Effects on Dental Treatment No significant effects or complications reported

Dosage Use in children <6 years of age not recommended due to CNS depression (especially in infants).

Nasal:

Children:

6-12 years: 1 spray of 0.05% into each nostril every 6 hours if necessary; therapy should not exceed 3-5 days

Children >12 years and Adults: 0.05%, instill 1-2 drops or sprays every 6 hours if needed; therapy should not exceed 3-5 days

Ophthalmic: Children >6 years and Adults: Instill 1-2 drops into conjunctival sac of affected eye(s) every 3-4 hours; therapy generally should not exceed 3-4 days

Mechanism of Action Stimulates alpha-adrenergic receptors in the arterioles of the conjunctiva and the nasal mucosa to produce vasoconstriction

Other Adverse Effects Frequency not defined:

Cardiovascular: Systemic cardiovascular stimulation

Central nervous system: Dizziness, headache, nervousness

Gastrointestinal: Nausea

Local: Transient stinging, nasal mucosa irritation, dryness, rebound congestion

Ocular: Mydriasis, increased intraocular pressure, blurring of vision

Respiratory: Sneezing

Pharmacodynamics/Kinetics

Onset of action: Decongestant: Topical: ~10 minutes

Duration: 2-6 hours

Pregnancy Risk Factor C

Generic Available Yes: Ophthalmic solution

Naphazoline and Antazoline (naf AZ oh leen & an TAZ oh leen)

Related Information

Naphazoline *on page 952*

U.S. Brand Names Vasocon-A® [OTC]

Canadian Brand Names Albalon®-A Liquifilm; Vasocon-A®

Pharmacologic Category Ophthalmic Agent, Vasoconstrictor

Synonyms Antazoline and Naphazoline

Use Topical ocular congestion, irritation, and itching

Local Anesthetic/Vasoconstrictor Precautions No information available to require special precautions

Effects on Dental Treatment No significant effects or complications reported

Dosage Ophthalmic: 1-2 drops every 3-4 hours; discontinue if patient experiences ocular pain, visual changes, ocular redness or irritation, or if condition worsens or persists for >72 hours.

Other Adverse Effects Frequency not defined:

Cardiovascular: Systemic cardiovascular stimulation, hypertension

Central nervous system: Nervousness, dizziness, headache

Gastrointestinal: Nausea
Local: Transient stinging
Neuromuscular & skeletal: Weakness
Ocular: Mydriasis, increased intraocular pressure, blurring of vision
Respiratory: Nasal mucosa irritation, dryness, rebound congestion
Miscellaneous: Diaphoresis

Pregnancy Risk Factor C

Generic Available No

Naphazoline and Pheniramine (naf AZ oh leen & fen NIR a meen)

Related Information

Naphazoline *on page 952*

U.S. Brand Names Naphcon-A® [OTC]; Opcon-A® [OTC]; Visine-A™ [OTC]

Canadian Brand Names Naphcon®-A

Pharmacologic Category Ophthalmic Agent, Vasoconstrictor

Synonyms Pheniramine and Naphazoline

Use Topical ocular vasoconstrictor

Local Anesthetic/Vasoconstrictor Precautions No information available to require special precautions

Effects on Dental Treatment No significant effects or complications reported

Dosage Ophthalmic: 1-2 drops every 3-4 hours

Other Adverse Effects 1% to 10%:

Ocular: Pupillary dilation, increase in intraocular pressure
Systemic effects due to absorption:
Cardiovascular: Hypertension, cardiac irregularities
Endocrine & metabolic: Hyperglycemia

Pregnancy Risk Factor C

Generic Available Yes

Naphazoline Hydrochloride *see* Naphazoline *on page 952*
Naphcon® [OTC] *see* Naphazoline *on page 952*
Naphcon-A® [OTC] *see* Naphazoline and Pheniramine *on page 953*
Naprelan® *see* Naproxen *on page 953*
Naprosyn® *see* Naproxen *on page 953*

Naproxen (na PROKS en)

Related Information

Oral Pain *on page 1524*
Rheumatoid Arthritis, Osteoarthritis, and Osteoporosis *on page 1488*
Temporomandibular Dysfunction (TMD) *on page 1562*

U.S. Brand Names Aleve® [OTC]; Anaprox®; Anaprox® DS; EC-Naprosyn®; Naprelan®; Naprosyn®

Canadian Brand Names Anaprox®; Anaprox® DS; Apo®-Napro-Na; Apo®-Napro-Na DS; Apo®-Naproxen; Apo®-Naproxen SR; Gen-Naproxen EC; Naprosyn®; Naxen®; Novo-Naproc EC; Novo-Naprox; Novo-Naprox Sodium; Novo-Naprox Sodium DS; Novo-Naprox SR; Nu-Naprox; Riva-Naproxen

Mexican Brand Names Artron®; Atiflan; Atiquim®; Dafloxen®; Faraxen; Flanax®; Flexen; Flogen®; Fuxen®; Naprodil®; Naxen®; Naxil; Neonaxil®; Nixal®; Novaxen®; Pactens®; Pronaxil®; Supradol®; Tandax®; Velsay

Pharmacologic Category Nonsteroidal Anti-inflammatory Drug (NSAID)

Synonyms Naproxen Sodium

Use

Dental: Management of pain and swelling

Medical: Management of inflammatory disease and rheumatoid disorders (including juvenile rheumatoid arthritis); acute gout; mild to moderate pain; dysmenorrhea; fever, migraine headache

Local Anesthetic/Vasoconstrictor Precautions No information available to require special precautions

Effects on Dental Treatment NSAID formulations are known to reversibly decrease platelet aggregation via mechanisms different than observed with aspirin. The dentist should be aware of the potential of abnormal coagulation. Caution should also be exercised in the use of NSAIDs in patients already on anticoagulant therapy with drugs such as warfarin (Coumadin®).

>10%: Headache (11%)

1% to 10%: Nervousness, malaise (<3%), somnolence (3% to 9%), nausea (3% to 9%), GI bleeding/ulcers/perforation, stomatitis (<3%), dyspnea (3% to 9%), abdominal distress/cramps/pain (3% to 9%), ecchymosis (3% to 9%)

Dosage Oral:

Children >2 years:
Fever: 2.5-10 mg/kg/dose; maximum: 10 mg/kg/day
Juvenile arthritis: 10 mg/kg/day in 2 divided doses

(Continued)

Naproxen *(Continued)*

Adults:

Rheumatoid arthritis, osteoarthritis, and ankylosing spondylitis: 500-1000 mg/day in 2 divided doses; may increase to 1.5 g/day of naproxen base for limited time period

Mild to moderate pain or dysmenorrhea: Initial: 500 mg, then 250 mg every 6-8 hours; maximum: 1250 mg/day naproxen base

Dosing adjustment in hepatic impairment: Reduce dose to 50%

Mechanism of Action Inhibits prostaglandin synthesis by decreasing the activity of the enzyme, cyclooxygenase, which results in decreased formation of prostaglandin precursors

Other Adverse Effects

1% to 10%:

Dermatologic: Itching, pruritus, rash

Endocrine & metabolic: Fluid retention (3% to 9%)

Gastrointestinal: Abdominal discomfort, constipation (3% to 9%), indigestion, diarrhea (<3%), dyspepsia (<3%), heartburn (<3%)

Hematologic: Hemolysis (3% to 9%)

Otic: Tinnitus (3% to 9%)

<1%: **Acute renal failure,** agranulocytosis, **allergic rhinitis,** anemia, angioedema, **arrhythmias,** aseptic meningitis, **blurred vision,** bone marrow suppression, **bronchospasm, confusion, CHF,** conjunctivitis, cystitis, decreased hearing, **drowsiness,** dry eyes, edema, **epistaxis,** erythema, **fatigue, gastritis, hallucinations,** hemolytic anemia, hepatitis, **hot flashes, hypertension, inhibition of platelet aggregation,** insomnia, leukopenia, mental depression, multiforme, peripheral neuropathy, polydipsia, polyuria, **prolonged bleeding time, renal dysfunction,** Stevens-Johnson syndrome, **tachycardia,** thrombocytopenia, toxic amblyopia, toxic epidermal necrolysis, urticaria, **vomiting**

Contraindications Hypersensitivity to naproxen, aspirin, other NSAIDs, or any component of the formulation; pregnancy (3rd trimester)

Warnings/Precautions Use with caution in patients with GI disease (bleeding or ulcers), cardiovascular disease (CHF, hypertension), dehydration, renal or hepatic impairment, and patients receiving anticoagulants; perform ophthalmologic evaluation for those who develop eye complaints during therapy (blurred vision, diminished vision, changes in color vision, retinal changes); NSAIDs may mask signs/symptoms of infections; photosensitivity reported. Elderly are at a high risk for adverse effects (including GI and CNS adverse effects) from NSAIDs. As many as 60% of elderly can develop peptic ulceration and/or hemorrhage asymptomatically. Use lowest effective dose for shortest period possible. Use of NSAIDs can compromise existing renal function especially when Cl_{cr} is <30 mL/minute. Withhold for at least 4-6 half-lives prior to surgical or dental procedures.

Drug Interactions Substrate of CYP1A2, 2C8/9

ACE inhibitors: Antihypertensive effects may be decreased by concurrent therapy with NSAIDs; monitor blood pressure.

Angiotensin II antagonists: Antihypertensive effects may be decreased by concurrent therapy with NSAIDs; monitor blood pressure.

Anticoagulants (warfarin, heparin, LMWHs) in combination with NSAIDs can cause increased risk of bleeding.

Antiplatelet drugs (ticlopidine, clopidogrel, aspirin, abciximab, dipyridamole, eptifibatide, tirofiban) can cause an increased risk of bleeding.

Corticosteroids may increase the risk of GI ulceration; avoid concurrent use.

Cyclosporine: NSAIDs may increase serum creatinine, potassium, blood pressure, and cyclosporine levels; monitor cyclosporine levels and renal function carefully.

Hydralazine's antihypertensive effect is decreased; avoid concurrent use.

Lithium levels can be increased; avoid concurrent use if possible or monitor lithium levels and adjust dose. Sulindac may have the least effect. When NSAID is stopped, lithium will need adjustment again.

Loop diuretics efficacy (diuretic and antihypertensive effect) is reduced. Indomethacin reduces this efficacy, however, it may be anticipated with any NSAID.

Methotrexate: Severe bone marrow suppression, aplastic anemia, and GI toxicity have been reported with concomitant NSAID therapy. Avoid use during moderate or high-dose methotrexate (increased and prolonged methotrexate levels). NSAID use during low-dose treatment of rheumatoid arthritis has not been fully evaluated; extreme caution is warranted.

Thiazides antihypertensive effects are decreased; avoid concurrent use.

Warfarin's INRs may be increased by naproxen. Other NSAIDs may have the same effect depending on dose and duration. Monitor INR closely. Use the lowest dose of NSAIDs possible and for the briefest duration.

Dietary/Ethanol/Herb Considerations

Ethanol: Avoid or limit use; may enhance gastric mucosal irritation.

Food may decrease absorption. Administer with food or milk to reduce GI upset; may cause bleeding, perforation, and ulceration. Avoid garlic, ginger, and green tea.

Herb/Nutraceutical: Avoid cat's claw, dong quai, evening primrose, feverfew, garlic, ginger, ginkgo biloba, ginseng, green tea, horse chestnut, and red clover due to additional antiplatelet activity. Avoid kava and valerian; may enhance benzodiazepine activity.

Pharmacodynamics/Kinetics

Onset of action: Analgesic: 1 hour; Anti-inflammatory: ~2 weeks
Peak effect: Anti-inflammatory: 2-4 weeks
Duration: Analgesic: ≤7 hours; Anti-inflammatory: ≤12 hours
Absorption: Almost 100%
Protein binding: >90%; increased free fraction in elderly
Half-life elimination: Normal renal function: 12-15 hours; End-stage renal disease: Unchanged
Time to peak, serum: 1-2 hours
Excretion: Urine (95%)

Pregnancy Risk Factor B/D (3rd trimester)

Dosage Forms CAPLET (Aleve®): 220 mg. **GELCAP** (Aleve®): 220 mg. **SUSP, oral** (Naprosyn®): 125 mg/5 mL (480 mL). **TAB:** 220 mg, 275 mg, 550 mg; (Aleve®): 220 mg; (Anaprox®): 275 mg; (Anaprox® DS): 550 mg; (Naprosyn®): 250 mg, 375 mg, 500 mg. **TAB, controlled release**: 550 mg; (Naprelan®): 421.5 mg, 550 mg. **TAB, delayed release** (EC-Naprosyn®): 375 mg, 500 mg

Generic Available Yes

Comments The sodium salt of naproxen provides better effects because of better oral absorption; the sodium salt also provides a faster onset and a longer duration of action. Naproxen: Naprosyn®; naproxen sodium: Anaprox®; 275 mg of Anaprox® equivalent to 250 mg of Naprosyn®

Selected Readings

Ahmad N, Grad HA, Haas DA, et al, "The Efficacy of Nonopioid Analgesics for Postoperative Dental Pain: A Meta-Analysis," *Anesth Prog*, 1997, 44(4):119-26.

Brooks PM and Day RO, "Nonsteroidal Anti-inflammatory Drugs - Differences and Similarities," *N Engl J Med*, 1991, 324(24):1716-25.

Dionne R, "Additive Analgesia Without Opioid Side Effects," *Compend Contin Educ Dent*, 2000, 21(7):572-4, 576-7.

Dionne RA and Berthold CW, "Therapeutic Uses of Nonsteroidal Anti-Inflammatory Drugs in Dentistry," *Crit Rev Oral Biol Med*, 2001, 12(4):315-30.

Forbes JA, Keller CK, Smith JW, et al, "Analgesic Effect of Naproxen Sodium, Codeine, a Naproxen-Codeine Combination and Aspirin on the Postoperative Pain of Oral Surgery," *Pharmacotherapy*, 1986, 6(5):211-8.

Nguyen AM, Graham DY, Gage T, et al, "Nonsteroidal Anti-Inflammatory Drug Use in Dentistry: Gastrointestinal Implications," *Gen Dent*, 1999, 47(6):590-6.

Naproxen Sodium *see* Naproxen *on page 953*

Naqua® *see* Trichlormethiazide *on page 1347*

Naratriptan (NAR a trip tan)

U.S. Brand Names Amerge®

Canadian Brand Names Amerge®

Mexican Brand Names Naramig®

Pharmacologic Category Serotonin 5-HT_{1D} Receptor Agonist

Synonyms Naratriptan Hydrochloride

Use Treatment of acute migraine headache with or without aura

Local Anesthetic/Vasoconstrictor Precautions No information available to require special precautions

Effects on Dental Treatment No significant effects or complications reported

Dosage Oral:

Adults: 1-2.5 mg at the onset of headache; it is recommended to use the lowest possible dose to minimize adverse effects. If headache returns or does not fully resolve, the dose may be repeated after 4 hours; do not exceed 5 mg in 24 hours.
Elderly: Use not recommended
Dosing in renal impairment:
Cl_{cr}: 18-39 mL/minute: Initial: 1 mg; do not exceed 2.5 mg in 24 hours
Cl_{cr}: <15 mL/minute: Do not use
Dosing in hepatic impairment: Contraindicated in patients with severe liver failure; maximum dose: 2.5 mg in 24 hours for patients with mild or moderate liver failure; recommended starting dose: 1 mg

Mechanism of Action The therapeutic effect for migraine is due to serotonin agonist activity

Other Adverse Effects

1% to 10%:
Central nervous system: Dizziness, drowsiness, malaise/fatigue
Gastrointestinal: Nausea, vomiting
Neuromuscular & skeletal: Paresthesias
Miscellaneous: Pain or pressure in throat or neck

<1% (Limited to important or life-threatening): Coronary artery vasospasm, transient myocardial ischemia, MI, ventricular tachycardia, ventricular fibrillation, palpitations, hypertension, EKG changes (PR prolongation, QT_c prolongation, premature ventricular contractions, atrial flutter, or atrial fibrillation) hypotension, heart murmurs, bradycardia, hyperlipidemia, hypercholesterolemia, hypothyroidism, hyperglycemia, glycosuria, ketonuria, eye hemorrhage, abnormal LFTs, abnormal bilirubin tests, convulsions, allergic reaction, panic, hallucinations

(Continued)

Naratriptan *(Continued)*

Drug Interactions

Increased Effect/Toxicity: Ergot-containing drugs (dihydroergotamine or methysergide) may cause vasospastic reactions when taken with naratriptan. Avoid concomitant use with ergots; separate dose of naratriptan and ergots by at least 24 hours. Oral contraceptives taken with naratriptan reduced the clearance of naratriptan ~30% which may contribute to adverse effects. Selective serotonin reuptake inhibitors (SSRIs) (eg, fluoxetine, fluvoxamine, paroxetine, sertraline) may cause lack of coordination, hyper-reflexia, or weakness and should be avoided when taking naratriptan.

Decreased Effect: Smoking increases the clearance of naratriptan.

Dietary/Ethanol/Herb Considerations Ethanol: Avoid use; may cause or worsen headaches.

Pharmacodynamics/Kinetics

Onset of action: 30 minutes
Absorption: Well absorbed
Protein binding, plasma: 28% to 31%
Metabolism: Hepatic via CYP
Bioavailability: 70%
Time to peak: 2-3 hours
Excretion: Urine

Pregnancy Risk Factor C

Generic Available No

Naratriptan Hydrochloride *see* Naratriptan *on page 955*
Narcan® *see* Naloxone *on page 949*
Nardil® *see* Phenelzine *on page 1065*
Naropin® *see* Ropivacaine *on page 1198*
Nasacort® *see* Triamcinolone *on page 1341*
Nasacort® AQ *see* Triamcinolone *on page 1341*
NāSal™ [OTC] *see* Sodium Chloride *on page 1229*
Nasalcrom® [OTC] *see* Cromolyn Sodium *on page 375*
Nasalide® *see* Flunisolide *on page 582*
Nasal Moist® [OTC] *see* Sodium Chloride *on page 1229*
Nasarel® *see* Flunisolide *on page 582*
Nascobal® *see* Cyanocobalamin *on page 377*
Nasonex® *see* Mometasone Furoate *on page 928*
Natacyn® *see* Natamycin *on page 956*

Natamycin (na ta MYE sin)

U.S. Brand Names Natacyn®

Canadian Brand Names Natacyn®

Pharmacologic Category Antifungal Agent, Ophthalmic

Synonyms Pimaricin

Use Treatment of blepharitis, conjunctivitis, and keratitis caused by susceptible fungi (*Aspergillus, Candida*), *Cephalosporium, Curvularia, Fusarium, Penicillium, Microsporum, Epidermophyton, Blastomyces dermatitidis, Coccidioides immitis, Cryptococcus neoformans, Histoplasma capsulatum, Sporothrix schenckii*, and *Trichomonas vaginalis*

Local Anesthetic/Vasoconstrictor Precautions No information available to require special precautions

Effects on Dental Treatment No significant effects or complications reported

Dosage Adults: Ophthalmic: Instill 1 drop in conjunctival sac every 1-2 hours, after 3-4 days reduce to one drop 6-8 times/day; usual course of therapy is 2-3 weeks.

Mechanism of Action Increases cell membrane permeability in susceptible fungi

Other Adverse Effects Frequency not defined: Ocular: Blurred vision, photophobia, eye pain, eye irritation not present before therapy

Drug Interactions Increased Effect/Toxicity: Topical corticosteroids (concomitant use contraindicated).

Pharmacodynamics/Kinetics

Absorption: Ophthalmic: Systemic, <2%
Distribution: Adheres to cornea, retained in conjunctival fornices

Pregnancy Risk Factor C

Generic Available No

Natrecor® *see* Nesiritide *on page 964*
Natriuretic Peptide *see* Nesiritide *on page 964*
Natural Lung Surfactant *see* Beractant *on page 176*
Nature's Tears® [OTC] *see* Artificial Tears *on page 128*
Nature-Throid® NT *see* Thyroid *on page 1303*
Naturetin® *see* Bendroflumethiazide *on page 168*
Nausetrol® [OTC] *see* Phosphorated Carbohydrate Solution *on page 1078*

Navane® *see* Thiothixene *on page 1301*
Navelbine® *see* Vinorelbine *on page 1389*
Na-Zone® [OTC] *see* Sodium Chloride *on page 1229*
n-Docosanol *see* Docosanol *on page 463*
Nebcin® *see* Tobramycin *on page 1315*
NebuPent® *see* Pentamidine *on page 1052*
Necon® 0.5/35 *see* Combination Hormonal Contraceptives *on page 368*
Necon® 1/35 *see* Combination Hormonal Contraceptives *on page 368*
Necon® 1/50 *see* Mestranol and Norethindrone *on page 871*
Necon® 7/7/7 *see* Combination Hormonal Contraceptives *on page 368*
Necon® 10/11 *see* Combination Hormonal Contraceptives *on page 368*

Nedocromil (ne doe KROE mil)

Related Information

Respiratory Diseases *on page 1476*

U.S. Brand Names Alocril™; Tilade®

Canadian Brand Names Alocril™; Tilade®

Pharmacologic Category Mast Cell Stabilizer

Synonyms Nedocromil Sodium

Use

Aerosol: Maintenance therapy in patients with mild to moderate bronchial asthma
Ophthalmic: Treatment of itching associated with allergic conjunctivitis

Local Anesthetic/Vasoconstrictor Precautions No information available to require special precautions

Effects on Dental Treatment No significant effects or complications reported

Dosage

Inhalation: Children >6 years and Adults: 2 inhalations 4 times/day; may reduce dosage to 2-3 times/day once desired clinical response to initial dose is observed
Ophthalmic: 1-2 drops in each eye twice daily

Mechanism of Action Inhibits the activation of and mediator release from a variety of inflammatory cell types associated with asthma including eosinophils, neutrophils, macrophages, mast cells, monocytes, and platelets; it inhibits the release of histamine, leukotrienes, and slow-reacting substance of anaphylaxis; it inhibits the development of early and late bronchoconstriction responses to inhaled antigen

Other Adverse Effects

Inhalation aerosol:

>10%: Gastrointestinal: Unpleasant taste
1% to 10%:
Cardiovascular: Chest pain
Central nervous system: Dizziness, dysphonia, headache, fatigue
Dermatologic: Rash
Gastrointestinal: Nausea, vomiting, dyspepsia, diarrhea, abdominal pain, xerostomia, unpleasant taste
Hepatic: Increased ALT
Neuromuscular & skeletal: Arthritis, tremor
Respiratory: Cough, pharyngitis, rhinitis, bronchitis, upper respiratory infection, bronchospasm, increased sputum production

Ophthalmic solution:

>10%:
Central nervous system: Headache (40%)
Gastrointestinal: Unpleasant taste
Ocular: Burning, irritation, stinging
Respiratory: Nasal congestion
1% to 10%:
Ocular: Conjunctivitis, eye redness, photophobia
Respiratory: Asthma, rhinitis

Pharmacodynamics/Kinetics

Duration: Therapeutic effect: 2 hours
Protein binding, plasma: 89%
Bioavailability: 7% to 9%
Half-life elimination: 1.5-2 hours
Excretion: Urine (as unchanged drug)

Pregnancy Risk Factor B

Generic Available No

Comments Not a bronchodilator; should not be used for reversal of acute bronchospasm; no known therapeutic systemic activity when inhaled

Nedocromil Sodium *see* Nedocromil *on page 957*

Nefazodone (nef AY zoe done)

U.S. Brand Names Serzone®

Canadian Brand Names Apo®-Nefazodone; Lin-Nefazodone; Serzone-5HT$_2$®

Pharmacologic Category Antidepressant, Serotonin Reuptake Inhibitor/Antagonist

(Continued)

Nefazodone *(Continued)*

Synonyms Nefazodone Hydrochloride

Use Treatment of depression

Unlabeled/Investigational Use Treatment of post-traumatic stress disorder

Local Anesthetic/Vasoconstrictor Precautions Although nefazodone is not a tricyclic antidepressant, it does block norepinephrine reuptake within CNS synapses as part of its mechanisms. It has been suggested that vasoconstrictor be administered with caution and to monitor vital signs in dental patients taking antidepressants that affect norepinephrine in this way, including nefazodone.

Effects on Dental Treatment >10%: Significant xerostomia; normal salivary flow resumes upon discontinuation

Dosage Oral:

Children and Adolescents: Depression: Target dose: 300-400 mg/day (mean: 3.4 mg/kg)

Adults: Depression: 200 mg/day, administered in 2 divided doses initially, with a range of 300-600 mg/day in 2 divided doses thereafter

Mechanism of Action Inhibits neuronal reuptake of serotonin and norepinephrine; also blocks 5-HT_2 and $alpha_1$ receptors; has no significant affinity for $alpha_2$, beta-adrenergic, 5-HT_{1A}, cholinergic, dopaminergic, or benzodiazepine receptors

Other Adverse Effects

>10%:

Central nervous system: Headache, drowsiness, insomnia, agitation, dizziness

Gastrointestinal: Nausea, constipation

Neuromuscular & skeletal: Weakness

1% to 10%:

Cardiovascular: Bradycardia, hypotension, peripheral edema, postural hypotension, vasodilation

Central nervous system: Chills, fever, incoordination, lightheadedness, confusion, memory impairment, abnormal dreams, decreased concentration, ataxia, psychomotor retardation, tremor

Dermatologic: Pruritus, rash

Endocrine & metabolic: Breast pain, impotence, libido decreased

Gastrointestinal: Gastroenteritis, vomiting, dyspepsia, diarrhea, increased appetite, thirst, **abnormal taste**

Genitourinary: Urinary frequency, urinary retention

Hematologic: Hematocrit decreased

Neuromuscular & skeletal: Arthralgia, hypertonia, paresthesia, neck rigidity, tremor

Ocular: Blurred vision (9%), abnormal vision (7%), eye pain, visual field defect

Otic: Tinnitus

Respiratory: Bronchitis, cough, dyspnea, pharyngitis

Miscellaneous: Flu syndrome, infection

<1%: Abdomen enlarged, abnormal gait, accommodation abnormality, acne, allergic reaction, alopecia, ALT increased, amenorrhea, anemia, angina pectoris, anorgasmia, apathy, arthritis, AST increased, asthma, attention decreased, AV block, breast enlargement, bruising, bursitis, cellulitis, cerebrovascular accident, colitis, CHF, conjunctivitis, cystitis, deafness, depersonalization, derealization, diplopia, dry eyes, dry skin, dehydration, dysarthria, ear pain, eczema, ejaculation abnormal, epistaxis, eructation, esophagitis, euphoria, **facial edema, gastritis, gingivitis**, glaucoma, gout, halitosis, hallucinations, hangover effect, hematuria, hemorrhage, hernia, hiccup, hostility, hyperacusis, hypercholesteremia, hyperesthesia, hyperkinesia, hypertension, hyperventilation, hypoglycemia, hypotonia, keratoconjunctivitis, kidney calculus, lactic dehydrogenase increased, **laryngitis**, leukopenia, libido increased, LFTs abnormal, lymphadenopathy, maculopapular rash, malaise, menorrhagia, metrorrhagia, **oral ulceration**, muscle stiffness, myoclonus, mydriasis, neuralgia, neuroleptic malignant syndrome, night blindness, nocturia, oliguria, **oral moniliasis**, pallor, paranoid reaction, pelvic pain, periodontal abscess, **peptic ulcer**, photophobia, photosensitivity, pneumonia, polyuria, ptosis, rectal hemorrhage, salivation increased, stomatitis, suicide attempt, suicidal thoughts, suicide, **syncope, tachycardia, loss of taste**, tendonitis, contracture, tenosynovitis, abnormal thinking, **twitching**, ulcerative colitis, urticaria, enlarged uterine fibroids, uterine hemorrhage, urinary incontinence, urinary urgency, ventricular extrasystoles, vaginal hemorrhage, varicose vein, vertigo, vesiculobullous rash, voice alteration, weight loss, **yawn**

Postmarketing and/or case reports: Angioedema, convulsions, galactorrhea, grand mal seizures, gynocomastia, hepatic failure, hepatic necrosis, hepatitis, hyponatremia, priapism, prolactin increased, rhabdomyolysis (with lovastatin/simvastatin), serotonin syndrome, Stevens-Johnson syndrome, thrombocytopenia

Drug Interactions Substrate of **CYP2D6, 3A4**; Inhibits CYP1A2, 2B6, 2D6, **3A4**

Increased Effect/Toxicity:

CYP3A4 substrates: Serum concentrations of drugs metabolized by CYP3A4 may be elevated by nefazodone; cisapride, pimozide, HMG-CoA reductase inhibitors (lovastatin, simvastatin), and triazolam are contraindicated.

Nefazodone may increase the serum levels/effects of antiarrhythmics (amiodarone, lidocaine, propafenone, quinidine), some antipsychotics (clozapine, haloperidol, mesoridazine, quetiapine, and risperidone), some benzodiazepines (triazolam is contraindicated; decrease alprazolam dose by 50%), buspirone (limit buspirone dose to <2.5 mg/day), calcium channel blockers, cyclosporine, digoxin, donepezil, methadone, oral contraceptives, protease inhibitors (ritonavir, saquinavir), sibutramine, sildenafil, tacrolimus, tricyclic antidepressants, vinca alkaloids, and zolpidem.

CYP3A4 inhibitors: Serum level and/or toxicity of nefazodone may be increased; inhibitors include amiodarone, cimetidine, clarithromycin, erythromycin, delavirdine, diltiazem, dirithromycin, disulfiram, fluoxetine, fluvoxamine, grapefruit juice, indinavir, itraconazole, ketoconazole, metronidazole, nevirapine, propoxyphene, quinupristin-dalfopristin, ritonavir, saquinavir, verapamil, zafirlukast, zileuton

MAO inhibitors: Concurrent use may lead to serotonin syndrome; avoid concurrent use or use within 14 days (includes phenelzine, isocarboxazid, and linezolid). Selegiline may increase the risk of serotonin syndrome, particularly at higher doses (>10 mg/day, where selectivity for MAO type B is decreased).

Theoretically, concurrent use of buspirone, meperidine, serotonin agonists (sumatriptan, rizatriptan), SSRIs, and venlafaxine may result in serotonin syndrome.

Decreased Effect: Carbamazepine may reduce serum concentrations of nefazodone - concurrent administration should be avoided.

Dietary/Ethanol/Herb Considerations

Ethanol: Avoid use; may increase CNS depression.

Food may decrease bioavailability and delay absorption. Grapefruit products may increase serum concentration and/or toxicity.

Herb/Nutraceutical: Avoid kava, SAMe, St John's wort, tryptophan, and valerian; may increase risk of serotonin syndrome and/or excessive sedation. Melatonin may enhance activity of clonazepam; use cautiously.

Pharmacodynamics/Kinetics

Onset of action: Therapeutic: Up to 6 weeks

Metabolism: Hepatic to three active metabolites: Triazoledione, hydroxynefazodone, and m-chlorophenylpiperazine (mCPP)

Bioavailability: 20% (variable)

Half-life elimination: Parent drug: 2-4 hours; active metabolites persist longer

Time to peak, serum: 1 hour, prolonged in presence of food

Excretion: Primarily urine (as metabolites); feces

Pregnancy Risk Factor C

Generic Available No

Selected Readings Ganzber S, "Psychoactive Drugs," *ADA Guide to Dental Therapeutics,* 2nd edition, Chapter 21, Chicago, IL: ADA Publishing, 2000, 382.

Nefazodone Hydrochloride *see* Nefazodone *on page 957*

NegGram® *see* Nalidixic Acid *on page 947*

Nelfinavir (nel FIN a veer)

Related Information

HIV Infection and AIDS *on page 1482*

Oral Viral Infections *on page 1545*

Tuberculosis *on page 1493*

U.S. Brand Names Viracept®

Canadian Brand Names Viracept®

Pharmacologic Category Antiretroviral Agent, Protease Inhibitor

Use In combination with other antiretroviral therapy in the treatment of HIV infection

Local Anesthetic/Vasoconstrictor Precautions No information available to require special precautions

Effects on Dental Treatment <1%: Mouth ulcers

Dosage Oral:

Children 2-13 years (labeled dose): 20-30 mg/kg 3 times/day with a meal or light snack; if tablets are unable to be taken, use oral powder in small amount of water, milk, formula, or dietary supplements; do not use acidic food/juice or store for >6 hours

Note: Clinically, dosages as high as 45 mg/kg every 8 hours are used; twice-daily dosages of 50-55 mg/kg are under investigation in older children (>6 years)

Adults: 750 mg 3 times/day with meals or 1250 mg twice daily with meals in combination with other antiretroviral therapies

Note: Dosing adjustments for nelfinavir when administered in combination with ritonavir: Nelfinavir 500-750 mg twice daily plus ritonavir 400 mg twice daily

Dosing adjustment in hepatic impairment: Use with caution; eliminated predominantly by the liver

Mechanism of Action Inhibits the HIV-1 protease; inhibition of the viral protease prevents cleavage of the gag-pol polyprotein resulting in the production of immature, noninfectious virus

(Continued)

Nelfinavir *(Continued)*

Other Adverse Effects Protease inhibitors cause dyslipidemia which includes elevated cholesterol and triglycerides and a redistribution of body fat centrally to cause "protease paunch", buffalo hump, facial atrophy, and breast enlargement. These agents also cause hyperglycemia.

>10%: Gastrointestinal: Diarrhea (19%)

1% to 10%:

Central nervous system: Impaired concentration
Dermatologic: Rash
Gastrointestinal: Nausea, flatulence, abdominal pain
Neuromuscular & skeletal: Weakness

<1%: Anxiety, depression, dizziness, emotional lability, hyperkinesia, insomnia, migraine, seizures, sleep disorder, somnolence, suicide ideation, fever, headache, malaise, dermatitis, pruritus, urticaria, increased LFTs, hyperlipemia, hyperuricemia, hypoglycemia, anorexia, dyspepsia, epigastric pain, oral ulceration, GI bleeding, pancreatitis, vomiting, kidney calculus, sexual dysfunction, anemia, leukopenia, thrombocytopenia, hepatitis, arthralgia, arthritis, cramps, myalgia, myasthenia, myopathy, paresthesia, back pain, dyspnea, pharyngitis, rhinitis, sinusitis, diaphoresis, allergy, redistribution of body fat, jaundice, metabolic acidosis

Drug Interactions Substrate of CYP2C8/9, **2C19**, 2D6, **3A4**; Inhibits CYP1A2, 2B6, 2C8/9, 2C19, 2D6, **3A4**

Increased Effect/Toxicity: Nelfinavir inhibits the metabolism of cisapride, astemizole, amiodarone, quinidine, lovastatin, simvastatin - should not be administered concurrently due to risk of life-threatening cardiac arrhythmias. Concentrations of atorvastatin and cerivastatin may be increased by nelfinavir. Do not administer with ergot alkaloids. Rifabutin plasma levels (AUC) are increased when coadministered with nelfinavir (decrease rifabutin dose by 50%). Nelfinavir increases levels of ketoconazole and indinavir. An increase in midazolam and triazolam serum levels may occur resulting in significant oversedation when administered with nelfinavir. Indinavir and ritonavir may increase nelfinavir plasma concentrations resulting in potential increases in side effects (the safety of these combinations have not been established). Concentrations of nelfinavir may be doubled during therapy with delavirdine. Sildenafil serum concentration may be substantially increased (do not exceed single doses of 25 mg in 48 hours).

Decreased Effect: Rifampin decreases nelfinavir's blood levels (AUC decreased by ~82%); the two drugs should not be administered concurrently. Serum levels of ethinyl estradiol and norethindrone (including many oral contraceptives) may decrease significantly with administration of nelfinavir. Patients should use alternative methods of contraceptives during nelfinavir therapy. Phenobarbital, phenytoin, and carbamazepine may decrease serum levels and consequently effectiveness of nelfinavir. Delavirdine concentrations may be decreased by up to 50% during nelfinavir treatment. Nelfinavir's effectiveness may be decreased with concomitant nevirapine use.

Dietary/Ethanol/Herb Considerations

Food: Administer with food to increase absorption; food increases plasma concentration time curve (AUC) by 2- to 3-fold. Do not administer with acidic or citric food/fluids (eg, apple juice, applesauce, orange juice); combination may have a bitter taste. Mix powder in a small amount of water, milk, formula, soy milk, soy formula, or dietary supplement.

Herb/Nutraceutical: Avoid St John's wort; may decrease serum concentration.

Pharmacodynamics/Kinetics

Absorption: Food increases plasma concentration-time curve (AUC) by two- to threefold

Distribution: V_d: 2-7 L/kg

Protein binding: 98%

Metabolism: Hepatic via CYP3A4; major metabolite has activity comparable to parent drug

Half-life elimination: 3.5-5 hours

Time to peak, serum: 2-4 hours

Excretion: Feces (98% to 99%, 78% as metabolites, 22% as unchanged drug); urine (1% to 2%)

Pregnancy Risk Factor B

Generic Available No

Nembutal® *see* Pentobarbital *on page 1055*
Neo-Calglucon® [OTC] *see* Calcium Glubionate *on page 225*
Neo-Calglucon® [OTC] *see* Calcium Supplements *on page 229*
NeoCeuticals™ Acne Spot Treatment [OTC] *see* Salicylic Acid *on page 1204*
NeoDecadron® *see* Neomycin and Dexamethasone *on page 961*
Neo-Fradin™ *see* Neomycin *on page 961*
Neoloid® [OTC] *see* Castor Oil *on page 259*

Neomycin (nee oh MYE sin)

Related Information

Neomycin and Polymyxin B *on page 962*
Neomycin, Polymyxin B, and Dexamethasone *on page 962*
Neomycin, Polymyxin B, and Prednisolone *on page 963*

U.S. Brand Names Myciguent [OTC]; Neo-Fradin™; Neo-Rx

Pharmacologic Category Ammonium Detoxicant; Antibiotic, Aminoglycoside; Antibiotic, Topical

Synonyms Neomycin Sulfate

Use Orally to prepare GI tract for surgery; topically to treat minor skin infections; treatment of diarrhea caused by *E. coli*; adjunct in the treatment of hepatic encephalopathy

Local Anesthetic/Vasoconstrictor Precautions No information available to require special precautions

Effects on Dental Treatment No significant effects or complications reported

Dosage

Children: Oral:

Preoperative intestinal antisepsis: 90 mg/kg/day divided every 4 hours for 2 days; or 25 mg/kg at 1 PM, 2 PM, and 11 PM on the day preceding surgery as an adjunct to mechanical cleansing of the intestine and in combination with erythromycin base

Hepatic coma: 50-100 mg/kg/day in divided doses every 6-8 hours or 2.5-7 g/m^2/day divided every 4-6 hours for 5-6 days not to exceed 12 g/day

Children and Adults: Topical: Apply ointment 1-4 times/day; topical solutions containing 0.1% to 1% neomycin have been used for irrigation

Adults: Oral:

Preoperative intestinal antisepsis: 1 g each hour for 4 doses then 1 g every 4 hours for 5 doses; or 1 g at 1 PM, 2 PM, and 11 PM on day preceding surgery as an adjunct to mechanical cleansing of the bowel and oral erythromycin; or 6 g/day divided every 4 hours for 2-3 days

Hepatic coma: 500-2000 mg every 6-8 hours or 4-12 g/day divided every 4-6 hours for 5-6 days

Chronic hepatic insufficiency: 4 g/day for an indefinite period

Mechanism of Action Interferes with bacterial protein synthesis by binding to 30S ribosomal subunits

Other Adverse Effects

Oral:

>10%: Gastrointestinal: Nausea, diarrhea, vomiting, irritation or soreness of the mouth or rectal area

<1% (Limited to important or life-threatening): Dyspnea, eosinophilia, nephrotoxicity, neurotoxicity, ototoxicity (auditory), ototoxicity (vestibular)

Topical: >10%: Dermatologic: Contact dermatitis

Drug Interactions

Increased Effect/Toxicity: Oral neomycin may potentiate the effects of oral anticoagulants. Neomycin may increase the adverse effects with other neurotoxic, ototoxic, or nephrotoxic drugs.

Decreased Effect: May decrease GI absorption of digoxin and methotrexate.

Pharmacodynamics/Kinetics

Absorption: Oral, percutaneous: Poor (3%)
Distribution: V_d: 0.36 L/kg
Metabolism: Slightly hepatic
Half-life elimination (age and renal function dependent): 3 hours
Time to peak, serum: Oral: 1-4 hours; I.M.: ~2 hours
Excretion: Feces (97% of oral dose as unchanged drug); urine (30% to 50% of absorbed drug as unchanged drug)

Pregnancy Risk Factor C

Generic Available Yes

Neomycin and Dexamethasone

(nee oh MYE sin & deks a METH a sone)

Related Information

Dexamethasone *on page 413*

U.S. Brand Names NeoDecadron®

Pharmacologic Category Antibiotic/Corticosteroid, Ophthalmic

Synonyms Dexamethasone and Neomycin

Use Treatment of steroid responsive inflammatory conditions of the palpebral and bulbar conjunctiva, lid, cornea, and anterior segment of the globe

Local Anesthetic/Vasoconstrictor Precautions No information available to require special precautions

Effects on Dental Treatment No significant effects or complications reported

Dosage Ophthalmic: Instill 1-2 drops in eye(s) every 3-4 hours

Other Adverse Effects <1%: Burning, local irritation or transient stinging; epithelial punctate keratitis, increased intraocular pressure, mydriasis, ptosis, and possible corneal or scleral malacia can occur

(Continued)

Neomycin and Dexamethasone *(Continued)*

Pregnancy Risk Factor C

Generic Available No

Neomycin and Polymyxin B (nee oh MYE sin & pol i MIKS in bee)

Related Information

Neomycin *on page 961*

Polymyxin B *on page 1095*

U.S. Brand Names Neosporin® G.U. Irrigant

Canadian Brand Names Cortimyxin®; Neosporin® Irrigating Solution

Pharmacologic Category Antibiotic, Topical

Synonyms Polymyxin B and Neomycin

Use Short-term as a continuous irrigant or rinse in the urinary bladder to prevent bacteriuria and gram-negative rod septicemia associated with the use of indwelling catheters; to help prevent infection in minor cuts, scrapes, and burns

Local Anesthetic/Vasoconstrictor Precautions No information available to require special precautions

Effects on Dental Treatment No significant effects or complications reported

Dosage Children and Adults: Bladder irrigation: **Not for injection**; add 1 mL irrigant to 1 liter isotonic saline solution and connect container to the inflow of lumen of 3-way catheter. Continuous irrigant or rinse in the urinary bladder for up to a maximum of 10 days with administration rate adjusted to patient's urine output; usually no more than 1 L of irrigant is used per day.

Mechanism of Action See individual agents.

Other Adverse Effects Frequency not defined:

Dermatologic: Contact dermatitis, erythema, rash, urticaria

Genitourinary: Bladder irritation

Local: Burning

Neuromuscular & skeletal: Neuromuscular blockade

Otic: Ototoxicity

Renal: Nephrotoxicity

Pharmacodynamics/Kinetics Absorption: Topical: Not absorbed following application to intact skin; absorbed through denuded or abraded skin, peritoneum, wounds, or ulcers

Pregnancy Risk Factor C/D (for G.U. irrigant)

Generic Available No

Neomycin, Bacitracin, and Polymyxin B *see* Bacitracin, Neomycin, and Polymyxin B *on page 157*

Neomycin, Bacitracin, Polymyxin B, and Hydrocortisone *see* Bacitracin, Neomycin, Polymyxin B, and Hydrocortisone *on page 158*

Neomycin, Colistin, and Hydrocortisone *see* Colistin, Neomycin, and Hydrocortisone *on page 367*

Neomycin, Polymyxin B, and Dexamethasone

(nee oh MYE sin, pol i MIKS in bee, & deks a METH a sone)

Related Information

Dexamethasone *on page 413*

Neomycin *on page 961*

Polymyxin B *on page 1095*

U.S. Brand Names AK-Trol®; Dexacidin®; Dexacine™; Maxitrol®

Canadian Brand Names Dioptrol®; Maxitrol®

Pharmacologic Category Antibiotic/Corticosteroid, Ophthalmic

Synonyms Dexamethasone, Neomycin, and Polymyxin B; Polymyxin B, Neomycin, and Dexamethasone

Use Steroid-responsive inflammatory ocular conditions in which a corticosteroid is indicated and where bacterial infection or a risk of bacterial infection exists

Local Anesthetic/Vasoconstrictor Precautions No information available to require special precautions

Effects on Dental Treatment No significant effects or complications reported

Dosage Children and Adults: Ophthalmic:

Ointment: Place a small amount (~½") in the affected eye 3-4 times/day or apply at bedtime as an adjunct with drops

Suspension: Instill 1-2 drops into affected eye(s) every 3-4 hours; in severe disease, drops may be used hourly and tapered to discontinuation

Mechanism of Action See individual agents.

Other Adverse Effects Frequency not defined: Ocular: Cutaneous sensitization, eye pain, development of glaucoma, cataract, increased intraocular pressure, optic nerve damage

Pregnancy Risk Factor C

Generic Available Yes

Neomycin, Polymyxin B, and Gramicidin

(nee oh MYE sin, pol i MIKS in bee, & gram i SYE din)

Related Information

Neomycin *on page 961*

U.S. Brand Names Neosporin® Ophthalmic Solution

Canadian Brand Names Neosporin®; Optimyxin Plus®

Mexican Brand Names Neosporin® Oftalmico

Pharmacologic Category Antibiotic, Ophthalmic

Synonyms Gramicidin, Neomycin, and Polymyxin B; Polymyxin B, Neomycin, and Gramicidin

Use Treatment of superficial ocular infection

Local Anesthetic/Vasoconstrictor Precautions No information available to require special precautions

Effects on Dental Treatment No significant effects or complications reported

Dosage Children and Adults: Ophthalmic: Instill 1-2 drops 4-6 times/day or more frequently as required for severe infections

Mechanism of Action Interferes with bacterial protein synthesis by binding to 30S ribosomal subunits; binds to phospholipids, alters permeability, and damages the bacterial cytoplasmic membrane permitting leakage of intracellular constituents

Other Adverse Effects Frequency not defined: Ocular: Transient irritation, burning, stinging, itching, inflammation, angioneurotic edema, urticaria, vesicular and maculopapular dermatitis

Pregnancy Risk Factor C

Generic Available Yes

Neomycin, Polymyxin B, and Hydrocortisone

(nee oh MYE sin, pol i MIKS in bee, & hye droe KOR ti sone)

Related Information

Hydrocortisone *on page 688*

Neomycin *on page 961*

U.S. Brand Names AntibiOtic® Ear; Cortisporin® Cream; Cortisporin® Ophthalmic; Cortisporin® Otic; PediOtic®

Canadian Brand Names Cortimyxin®; Cortisporin®

Pharmacologic Category Antibiotic/Corticosteroid, Ophthalmic; Antibiotic/Corticosteroid, Otic; Topical Skin Product

Synonyms Hydrocortisone, Neomycin, and Polymyxin B; Polymyxin B, Neomycin, and Hydrocortisone

Use Steroid-responsive inflammatory condition for which a corticosteroid is indicated and where bacterial infection or a risk of bacterial infection exists

Local Anesthetic/Vasoconstrictor Precautions No information available to require special precautions

Effects on Dental Treatment No significant effects or complications reported

Dosage Duration of use should be limited to 10 days unless otherwise directed by the physician

Otic solution is used **only** for swimmer's ear (infections of external auditory canal)

Otic:

- Children: Instill 3 drops into affected ear 3-4 times/day
- Adults: Instill 4 drops 3-4 times/day; otic suspension is the preferred otic preparation

Children and Adults:

- Ophthalmic: Drops: Instill 1-2 drops 2-4 times/day, or more frequently as required for severe infections; in acute infections, instill 1-2 drops every 15-30 minutes gradually reducing the frequency of administration as the infection is controlled
- Topical: Apply a thin layer 1-4 times/day. Therapy should be discontinued when control is achieved; if no improvement is seen, reassessment of diagnosis may be necessary.

Mechanism of Action See individual agents.

Other Adverse Effects Frequency not defined:

Dermatologic: Contact dermatitis, erythema, rash, urticaria

Local: Burning, itching, swelling, pain, stinging

Ocular: Intraocular pressure increased, glaucoma, cataracts, conjunctival erythema, transient irritation, burning, stinging, itching, inflammation, angioneurotic edema, urticaria, vesicular and maculopapular dermatitis

Otic: Ototoxicity

Miscellaneous: Hypersensitivity, sensitization to neomycin, secondary infections

Pregnancy Risk Factor C

Generic Available Yes

Neomycin, Polymyxin B, and Prednisolone

(nee oh MYE sin, pol i MIKS in bee, & pred NIS oh lone)

Related Information

Neomycin *on page 961*

Polymyxin B *on page 1095*

PrednisoLONE *on page 1110*

(Continued)

Neomycin, Polymyxin B, and Prednisolone *(Continued)*

U.S. Brand Names Poly-Pred®

Pharmacologic Category Antibiotic/Corticosteroid, Ophthalmic

Synonyms Polymyxin B, Neomycin, and Prednisolone; Prednisolone, Neomycin, and Polymyxin B

Use Steroid-responsive inflammatory ocular condition in which bacterial infection or a risk of bacterial ocular infection exists

Local Anesthetic/Vasoconstrictor Precautions No information available to require special precautions

Effects on Dental Treatment No significant effects or complications reported

Dosage Children and Adults: Ophthalmic: Instill 1-2 drops every 3-4 hours; acute infections may require every 30-minute instillation initially with frequency of administration reduced as the infection is brought under control. To treat the lids: Instill 1-2 drops every 3-4 hours, close the eye and rub the excess on the lids and lid margins.

Mechanism of Action See individual agents.

Other Adverse Effects Frequency not defined:

Dermatologic: Cutaneous sensitization, skin rash, delayed wound healing

Ocular: Increased intraocular pressure, glaucoma, optic nerve damage, cataracts, conjunctival sensitization, transient irritation, burning, stinging, itching, inflammation, angioneurotic edema, urticaria, vesicular and maculopapular dermatitis

Pregnancy Risk Factor C

Generic Available No

Neomycin Sulfate *see* Neomycin *on page 961*

Neonatal Trace Metals *see* Trace Metals *on page 1328*

Neoral® *see* CycloSPORINE *on page 383*

Neo-Rx *see* Neomycin *on page 961*

Neosar® *see* Cyclophosphamide *on page 381*

Neosporin® G.U. Irrigant *see* Neomycin and Polymyxin B *on page 962*

Neosporin® Ophthalmic Ointment *see* Bacitracin, Neomycin, and Polymyxin B *on page 157*

Neosporin® Ophthalmic Solution *see* Neomycin, Polymyxin B, and Gramicidin *on page 963*

Neosporin® Topical [OTC] *see* Bacitracin, Neomycin, and Polymyxin B *on page 157*

NeoStrata AHA [OTC] *see* Hydroquinone *on page 693*

Neo-Synephrine® 12 Hour [OTC] *see* Oxymetazoline *on page 1022*

Neo-Synephrine® 12 Hour Extra Moisturizing [OTC] *see* Oxymetazoline *on page 1022*

Neo-Synephrine® Extra Strength [OTC] *see* Phenylephrine *on page 1071*

Neo-Synephrine® Mild [OTC] *see* Phenylephrine *on page 1071*

Neo-Synephrine® Ophthalmic *see* Phenylephrine *on page 1071*

Neo-Synephrine® Regular Strength [OTC] *see* Phenylephrine *on page 1071*

Neotrace-4® *see* Trace Metals *on page 1328*

Nephro-Calci® [OTC] *see* Calcium Supplements *on page 229*

Nephrocaps® *see* Vitamin B Complex, Vitamin C, and Folic Acid *on page 1393*

Nephro-Fer® [OTC] *see* Iron Supplements *on page 745*

Neptazane® [DSC] *see* Methazolamide *on page 878*

Nesacaine® *see* Chloroprocaine *on page 302*

Nesacaine®-MPF *see* Chloroprocaine *on page 302*

Nesiritide (ni SIR i tide)

U.S. Brand Names Natrecor®

Pharmacologic Category Natriuretic Peptide, B-type, Human; Vasodilator

Synonyms B-type Natriuretic Peptide (Human); hBNP; Natriuretic Peptide

Use Treatment of acutely decompensated CHF (CHF) in patients with dyspnea at rest or with minimal activity

Local Anesthetic/Vasoconstrictor Precautions No information available to require special precautions

Effects on Dental Treatment No significant effects or complications reported

Dosage I.V.:

Adults: Initial: 2 mcg/kg (bolus); followed by continuous infusion at 0.01 mcg/kg/minute; **Note:** Should not be initiated at a dosage higher than initial recommended dose. At intervals of ≥3 hours, the dosage may be increased by 0.005 mcg/kg/minute (preceded by a bolus of 1 mcg/kg), up to a maximum of 0.03 mcg/kg/minute. Increases beyond the initial infusion rate should be limited to selected patients and accompanied by hemodynamic monitoring.

Patients experiencing hypotension during the infusion: Infusion should be interrupted. May attempt to restart at a lower dose (reduce initial infusion dose by 30% and omit bolus).

Mechanism of Action Binds to guanylate cyclase receptor on vascular smooth muscle and endothelial cells, increasing intracellular cyclic GMP, resulting in smooth muscle cell relaxation. Has been shown to produce dose-dependent reductions in pulmonary capillary wedge pressure (PCWP) and systemic arterial pressure.

Other Adverse Effects Note: Frequencies cited below were recorded in VMAC trial at dosages similar to approved labeling. Higher frequencies have been observed in trials using higher dosages of nesiritide.

>10%:

Cardiovascular: Hypotension (total: 11%; symptomatic: 4% at recommended dose, up to 17% at higher doses)

Renal: Increased serum creatinine (28% with >0.5 mg/dL increase over baseline)

1% to 10%:

Cardiovascular: Ventricular tachycardia (3%)*, ventricular extrasystoles (3%)*, angina (2%)*, bradycardia (1%), tachycardia, atrial fibrillation, AV node conduction abnormalities

Central nervous system: Headache (8%)*, dizziness (3%)*, insomnia (2%), anxiety (3%), fever, confusion, paresthesia, somnolence, tremor

Dermatologic: Pruritus, rash

Gastrointestinal: Nausea (4%)*, abdominal pain (1%)*, vomiting (1%)*

Hematologic: Anemia

Local: Injection site reaction

Neuromuscular & skeletal: Back pain (4%), leg cramps

Ocular: Amblyopia

Respiratory: Cough (increased), hemoptysis, apnea

Miscellaneous: Increased diaphoresis

*Frequency less than or equal to placebo or other standard therapy

Drug Interactions Increased Effect/Toxicity: An increased frequency of symptomatic hypotension was observed with concurrent administration of ACE inhibitors. Other hypotensive agents are likely to have additive effects on hypotension. In patients receiving diuretic therapy leading to depletion of intravascular volume, the risk of hypotension and/or renal impairment may be increased. Nesiritide should be avoided in patients with low filling pressures.

Pharmacodynamics/Kinetics

Onset of action: 15 minutes (60% of 3-hour effect achieved)

Duration: >60 minutes (up to several hours) for systolic blood pressure; hemodynamic effects persist longer than serum half-life would predict

Distribution: V_{ss}: 0.19 L/kg

Metabolism: Proteolytic cleavage by vascular endopeptidases and proteolysis following receptor binding and cellular internalization

Half-life elimination: Initial (distribution) 2 minutes; Terminal: 18 minutes

Time to peak: 1 hour

Excretion: Urine

Pregnancy Risk Factor C

Generic Available No

Neulasta™ *see* Pegfilgrastim *on page 1040*
Neumega® *see* Oprelvekin *on page 1003*
Neupogen® *see* Filgrastim *on page 571*
Neurontin® *see* Gabapentin *on page 624*
Neut® *see* Sodium Bicarbonate *on page 1227*
NeutraCare® *see* Fluoride *on page 586*
NeutraGard® [OTC] *see* Fluoride *on page 586*
Neutra-Phos® [OTC] *see* Phosphate Supplements *on page 1076*
Neutra-Phos®-K [OTC] *see* Phosphate Supplements *on page 1076*
Neutrexin® *see* Trimetrexate Glucuronate *on page 1354*
Neutrogena® Acne Mask [OTC] *see* Benzoyl Peroxide *on page 171*
Neutrogena® Acne Wash [OTC] *see* Salicylic Acid *on page 1204*
Neutrogena® Body Clear™ [OTC] *see* Salicylic Acid *on page 1204*
Neutrogena® Clear Pore [OTC] *see* Salicylic Acid *on page 1204*
Neutrogena® Clear Pore Shine Control [OTC] *see* Salicylic Acid *on page 1204*
Neutrogena® Healthy Scalp [OTC] *see* Salicylic Acid *on page 1204*
Neutrogena® Maximum Strength T/Sal® [OTC] *see* Salicylic Acid *on page 1204*
Neutrogena® On The Spot® Acne Patch [OTC] *see* Salicylic Acid *on page 1204*
Neutrogena® On The Spot® Acne Treatment [OTC] *see* Benzoyl Peroxide *on page 171*
Neutrogena® T/Derm *see* Coal Tar *on page 359*
Neutrogena® T/Sal [OTC] *see* Coal Tar and Salicylic Acid *on page 359*

Nevirapine (ne VYE ra peen)

Related Information

HIV Infection and AIDS *on page 1482*
Tuberculosis *on page 1493*

(Continued)

Nevirapine *(Continued)*

U.S. Brand Names Viramune®

Canadian Brand Names Viramune®

Mexican Brand Names Viramune®

Pharmacologic Category Antiretroviral Agent, Reverse Transcriptase Inhibitor (Non-nucleoside)

Use In combination therapy with other antiretroviral agents for the treatment of HIV-1 in adults

Local Anesthetic/Vasoconstrictor Precautions No information available to require special precautions

Effects on Dental Treatment Ulcerative stomatitis (4%)

Dosage Oral:

Children 2 months to <8 years: Initial: 4 mg/kg/dose once daily for 14 days; increase dose to every 12 hours if no rash or other adverse effects occur; maintenance dose: 7 mg/kg/dose every 12 hours; maximum dose: 200 mg/dose every 12 hours

Children ≥8 years: Initial: 4 mg/kg/dose once daily for 14 days; increase dose to 4 mg/kg/dose every 12 hours if no rash or other adverse effects occur; maximum dose: 200 mg/dose every 12 hours

Note: Alternative pediatric dosing (unlabeled): 120-200 mg/m^2 every 12 hours; this dosing has been proposed due to the fact that dosing based on mg/kg may result in an abrupt decrease in dose at the 8th birthday, which may be inappropriate.

Adults: Initial: 200 mg once daily for 14 days; maintenance: 200 mg twice daily (in combination with an additional antiretroviral agent)

Note: If therapy is interrupted for >7 days, restart with initial dose for 14 days

Mechanism of Action As a non-nucleoside reverse transcriptase inhibitor, nevirapine has activity against HIV-1 by binding to reverse transcriptase. It consequently blocks the RNA-dependent and DNA-dependent DNA polymerase activities including HIV-1 replication. It does not require intracellular phosphorylation for antiviral activity.

Other Adverse Effects

>10%:

Central nervous system: Headache (11%), fever (8% to 11%)

Dermatologic: Rash (15% to 20%)

Gastrointestinal: Diarrhea (15% to 20%)

Hematologic: Neutropenia (10% to 11%)

1% to 10%:

Gastrointestinal: Nausea, abdominal pain (2%)

Hematologic: Anemia

Hepatic: Hepatitis, increased LFTs (2% to 4%)

Neuromuscular & skeletal: Peripheral neuropathy, paresthesia (2%), myalgia

<1%: Thrombocytopenia, Stevens-Johnson syndrome, hepatotoxicity, hepatic necrosis, cholestatic hepatitis, hepatic failure

Hypersensitivity (frequency not defined): Symptoms of severe hypersensitivity/dermatologic reactions may include: Severe rash (or rash with fever), blisters, **oral lesions, facial edema, muscle or joint aches**, general malaise, hepatitis, eosinophilia, granulocytopenia, conjunctivitis, lymphadenopathy, or renal dysfunction. Nevirapine should be permanently discontinued.

Drug Interactions Substrate of CYP2B6, 2D6, **3A4**; Inhibits CYP1A2, 2D6, 3A4; Induces **CYP2B6, 3A4**

Increased Effect/Toxicity: Cimetidine, itraconazole, ketoconazole, and some macrolide antibiotics may increase nevirapine plasma concentrations. Increased toxicity when used concomitantly with protease inhibitors or oral contraceptives. Ketoconazole should NOT be coadministered. Concurrent administration of prednisone for the initial 14 days of nevirapine therapy was associated with an increased incidence and severity of rash.

Decreased Effect: Rifampin and rifabutin may decrease nevirapine concentrations due to induction of CYP3A; since nevirapine may decrease concentrations of protease inhibitors (eg, indinavir, saquinavir), they should not be administered concomitantly or doses should be increased. Nevirapine may decrease the effectiveness of oral contraceptives - suggest alternate method of birth control. Nevirapine also decreases the effect of ketoconazole and methadone. Nevirapine may decrease serum concentrations of some protease inhibitors (AUC of indinavir and saquinavir may be decreased - no effect noted with ritonavir), specific dosage adjustments have not been recommended (no adjustment recommended for ritonavir).

Dietary/Ethanol/Herb Considerations Herb/Nutraceutical: Avoid St John's wort; may decrease serum concentration.

Pharmacodynamics/Kinetics

Absorption: >90%

Distribution: Widely; V_d: 1.2-1.4 L/kg; crosses placenta; enters breast milk; CSF penetration approximates 50% of plasma

Protein binding, plasma: 50% to 60%

Metabolism: Extensively hepatic via CYP3A4 (hydroxylation to inactive compounds); may undergo enterohepatic recycling

Half-life elimination: Decreases over 2- to 4-week time with chronic dosing due to autoinduction (ie, half-life = 45 hours initially and decreases to 23 hours)

Time to peak, serum: 2-4 hours

Excretion: Urine (as metabolites, <3% as unchanged drug)

Pregnancy Risk Factor C

Generic Available No

Nexium® *see* Esomeprazole *on page 519*

Niacin (NYE a sin)

Related Information

Cardiovascular Diseases *on page 1456*

U.S. Brand Names Niacor®; Niaspan®; Nicotinex [OTC]; Slo-Niacin® [OTC]

Canadian Brand Names Niaspan®

Mexican Brand Names Hipocol®; Pepevit®

Pharmacologic Category Antilipemic Agent, Miscellaneous; Vitamin, Water Soluble

Synonyms Nicotinic Acid; Vitamin B_3

Use Adjunctive treatment of dyslipidemias (alone or with lovastatin or bile acid sequestrant); peripheral vascular disease and circulatory disorders; treatment of pellagra; dietary supplement

Local Anesthetic/Vasoconstrictor Precautions No information available to require special precautions

Effects on Dental Treatment No significant effects or complications reported

Dosage

Children: Oral:
- Pellagra: 50-100 mg/dose 3 times/day
- Recommended daily allowances:
  - 0-0.5 years: 5 mg/day
  - 0.5-1 year: 6 mg/day
  - 1-3 years: 9 mg/day
  - 4-6 years: 12 mg/day
  - 7-10 years: 13 mg/day

Children and Adolescents: Recommended daily allowances:
- Male:
  - 11-14 years: 17 mg/day
  - 15-18 years: 20 mg/day
  - 19-24 years: 19 mg/day
- Female: 11-24 years: 15 mg/day

Adults: Oral:
- Recommended daily allowances:
  - Male: 25-50 years: 19 mg/day; >51 years: 15 mg/day
  - Female: 25-50 years: 15 mg/day; >51 years: 13 mg/day
- Hyperlipidemia: Usual target dose: 1.5-6 g/day in 3 divided doses with or after meals using a dosage titration schedule; extended release: 375 mg to 2 g once daily at bedtime
  - Regular release formulation (Niacor®): Initial: 250 mg once daily (with evening meal); increase frequency and/or dose every 4-7 days to desired response or first-level therapeutic dose (1.5-2 g/day in 2-3 divided doses); after 2 months, may increase at 2- to 4-week intervals to 3 g/day in 3 divided doses
  - Extended release formulation (Niaspan®): 500 mg at bedtime for 4 weeks, then 1 g at bedtime for 4 weeks; adjust dose to response and tolerance; can increase to a maximum of 2 g/day, but only at 500 mg/day at 4-week intervals
  - With lovastatin: Maximum lovastatin dose: 40 mg/day
- Pellagra: 50-100 mg 3-4 times/day, maximum: 500 mg/day
- Niacin deficiency: 10-20 mg/day, maximum: 100 mg/day

Dosing adjustment in renal impairment: Use with caution

Dosing adjustment in hepatic impairment: Not recommended for use in significant or unexplained dysfunction

Dosage adjustment for toxicity: Transaminases rise to 3 times ULN: Discontinue therapy.

Mechanism of Action Component of two coenzymes which is necessary for tissue respiration, lipid metabolism, and glycogenolysis; inhibits the synthesis of very low density lipoproteins

Other Adverse Effects Frequency not defined:

Cardiovascular: Arrhythmias, atrial fibrillation, edema, flushing, hypotension, orthostasis, palpitations, syncope (rare), tachycardia

Central nervous system: Chills, dizziness, insomnia, migraine

Dermatologic: Acanthosis nigricans, dry skin, hyperpigmentation, maculopapular rash, pruritus, rash, urticaria,

Endocrine & metabolic: Glucose tolerance decreased, gout, phosphorous levels decreased, uric acid level increased

Gastrointestinal: Abdominal pain, nausea, peptic ulcers, vomiting

(Continued)

Niacin *(Continued)*

Hepatic: Hepatic necrosis (rare), jaundice, liver enzymes elevated
Neuromuscular & skeletal: Myalgia, myopathy (with concurrent HMG-CoA reductase inhibitor), rhabdomyolysis (with concurrent HMG-CoA reductase inhibitor; rare), weakness
Ocular: Cystoid macular edema, toxic amblyopia
Respiratory: Dyspnea
Miscellaneous: Diaphoresis

Drug Interactions

Increased Effect/Toxicity: Use with adrenergic blocking agents may result in additive vasodilating effect and postural hypotension.

Decreased Effect: The effect of oral hypoglycemics may be decreased by niacin. Niacin may inhibit uricosuric effects of sulfinpyrazone and probenecid. Aspirin (or other NSAIDs) decreases niacin-induced flushing. Bile acid sequestrants decrease the absorption of niacin.

Dietary/Ethanol/Herb Considerations Food: Administer with food; low-fat meal if treating hyperlipidemia. Avoid hot drinks around the time of niacin dose.

Pharmacodynamics/Kinetics

Absorption: Rapid and extensive
Distribution: Mainly to hepatic, renal, and adipose tissue
Metabolism: Extensive first-pass effects; converted to nicotinamide (dose dependent); niacinamide (30%) hepatically metabolized
Half-life elimination: 45 minutes
Time to peak, serum: Immediate release formulation: ~45 minutes; extended release formulation: 4-5 hours
Excretion: Urine (unchanged drug and metabolites); with larger doses, greater percentage as unchanged drug

Pregnancy Risk Factor A/C (dose exceeding RDA recommendation)
Generic Available Yes

Niacinamide (nye a SIN a mide)

Pharmacologic Category Vitamin, Water Soluble
Synonyms Nicotinamide; Vitamin B_3
Use Prophylaxis and treatment of pellagra
Local Anesthetic/Vasoconstrictor Precautions No information available to require special precautions
Effects on Dental Treatment No significant effects or complications reported
Dosage Oral:

Children: Pellagra: 100-300 mg/day in divided doses
Adults: 50 mg 3-10 times/day
Pellagra: 300-500 mg/day
Recommended daily allowance: 13-19 mg/day

Mechanism of Action Used by the body as a source of niacin; is a component of two coenzymes which is necessary for tissue respiration, lipid metabolism, and glycogenolysis; inhibits the synthesis of very low density lipoproteins; does not have hypolipidemia or vasodilating effects

Other Adverse Effects Frequency not defined:

Cardiovascular: Tachycardia
Dermatologic: Increased sebaceous gland activity, rash
Gastrointestinal: Bloating, flatulence, nausea
Neuromuscular & skeletal: Paresthesia in extremities
Ocular: Blurred vision
Respiratory: Wheezing

Pharmacodynamics/Kinetics

Absorption: Rapid
Metabolism: Hepatic
Half-life elimination: 45 minutes
Time to peak, serum: 20-70 minutes
Excretion: Urine

Pregnancy Risk Factor A/C (dose exceeding RDA recommendation)
Generic Available Yes

Niacin and Lovastatin (NYE a sin & LOE va sta tin)

Related Information

Lovastatin *on page 828*
Niacin *on page 967*

U.S. Brand Names Advicor™
Pharmacologic Category Antilipemic Agent, HMG-CoA Reductase Inhibitor; Antilipemic Agent, Miscellaneous
Synonyms Lovastatin and Niacin
Use Treatment of primary hypercholesterolemia (heterozygous familial and nonfamilial) and mixed dyslipidemia (Fredrickson types IIa and IIb) in patients previously treated with either agent alone (patients who require further lowering of triglycerides or increase in HDL-cholesterol from addition of niacin or further

lowering of LDL-cholesterol from addition of lovastatin). Combination product; not intended for initial treatment.

Local Anesthetic/Vasoconstrictor Precautions No information available to require special precautions

Effects on Dental Treatment No significant effects or complications reported

Dosage Dosage forms are a fixed combination of niacin and lovastatin.

Oral: Adults: Lowest dose: Niacin 500 mg/lovastatin 20 mg; may increase by not more than 500 mg (niacin) at 4-week intervals (maximum dose: Niacin 2000 mg/lovastatin 40 mg daily); should be taken at bedtime with a low-fat snack

Not for use as initial therapy of dyslipidemias. May be substituted for equivalent dose of Niaspan®, however, manufacturer does not recommend direct substitution with other niacin products.

Mechanism of Action Lovastatin acts by competitively inhibiting 3-hydroxyl-3-methylglutaryl-coenzyme A (HMG-CoA) reductase, the enzyme that catalyzes the rate-limiting step in cholesterol biosynthesis. Niacin is a component of two coenzymes which is necessary for tissue respiration, lipid metabolism, and glycogenolysis; inhibits the synthesis of very low density lipoproteins.

Other Adverse Effects

>10%: Cardiovascular: Flushing

1% to 10%:

Central nervous system: Headache (9%), pain (8%)

Dermatologic: Pruritus (7%), rash (5%)

Endocrine & metabolic: Hyperglycemia (4%)

Gastrointestinal: Nausea (7%), diarrhea (6%), abdominal pain (4%), dyspepsia (3%), vomiting (3%)

Neuromuscular & skeletal: Back pain (5%), weakness (5%), myalgia (3%)

Miscellaneous: Flu-like syndrome (6%)

Other uncommon adverse reactions reported with niacin and/or lovastatin include: Alkaline phosphatase increased, alopecia, anaphylaxis, angioedema, anemia, anorexia, anxiety, arthritis, cataracts, chills, cholestatic jaundice, cirrhosis, CPK increased (>10x normal), depression, dryness of skin/mucous membranes, dyspnea, eosinophilia, erectile dysfunction, erythema multiforme, ESR increased, facial paresis, fatty liver, fever, flushing, GGT increased, gout, gynecomastia, hemolytic anemia, hepatitis, hepatic necrosis (fulminant), hepatoma, hyperbilirubinemia, hypersensitivity reaction, hypotension, impotence, impaired extraocular muscle movement, leukopenia, libido decreased, memory loss, malaise, myopathy, nail changes, nodules, ophthalmoplegia, pancreatitis, paresthesia, peptic ulcer, peripheral nerve palsy, peripheral neuropathy, photosensitivity, polymyalgia rheumatica, pruritus, psychic disturbance, positive ANA, purpura, rhabdomyolysis, rash, renal failure, skin discoloration, Stevens-Johnson syndrome, syncope, systemic lupus erythematosus-like syndrome, taste alteration, thrombocytopenia, thyroid dysfunction, toxic epidermal necrolysis, transaminases elevated, tremor, urticaria, vasculitis, vertigo, vomiting

Dietary/Ethanol/Herb Considerations

Ethanol: Limit use; large amounts may increase risk of liver damage.

Administer with a low-fat snack at bedtime; food may decrease lovastatin absorption. Avoid grapefruit products; may increase lovastatin serum concentration. Requires a standard cholesterol-lowering diet 6 months prior to and during therapy.

Herb/Nutraceutical: Avoid St John's wort; may decrease serum concentration.

Pregnancy Risk Factor X

Generic Available No

Niacor® *see* Niacin *on page 967*

Niaspan® *see* Niacin *on page 967*

NiCARdipine (nye KAR de peen)

Related Information

Calcium Channel Blockers and Gingival Hyperplasia *on page 1598*

Calcium Channel Blockers, Comparative Pharmacokinetics *on page 1600*

Cardiovascular Diseases *on page 1456*

U.S. Brand Names Cardene®; Cardene® I.V.; Cardene® SR

Mexican Brand Names Ridene®

Pharmacologic Category Calcium Channel Blocker

Synonyms Nicardipine Hydrochloride

Use Chronic stable angina (immediate-release product only); management of essential hypertension (immediate and sustained release; parenteral only for short time that oral treatment is not feasible)

Unlabeled/Investigational Use Treatment of CHF

Local Anesthetic/Vasoconstrictor Precautions No information available to require special precautions

Effects on Dental Treatment 1% to 10%: Xerostomia

Other drugs of this class can cause gingival hyperplasia (ie, nifedipine). The first case of nicardipine-induced gingival hyperplasia has been reported in a child taking 40-50 mg daily for 20 months.

(Continued)

NiCARdipine *(Continued)*

Dosage The total daily dose of immediate-release product may not automatically be equivalent to the daily sustained-release dose; use caution in converting.

Adults:

Oral:

Immediate release: Initial: 20 mg 3 times/day; usual: 20-40 mg 3 times/day (allow 3 days between dose increases)

Sustained release: Initial: 30 mg twice daily, titrate up to 60 mg twice daily

I.V. (dilute to 0.1 mg/mL): Initial: 5 mg/hour increased by 2.5 mg/hour every 15 minutes to a maximum of 15 mg/hour

Dosing adjustment in renal impairment: Titrate dose beginning with 20 mg 3 times/day (immediate release) or 30 mg twice daily (sustained release).

Dosing adjustment in hepatic impairment: Starting dose: 20 mg twice daily (immediate release) with titration.

Equivalent oral vs I.V. infusion doses:

20 mg every 8 hours oral, equivalent to 0.5 mg/hour I.V. infusion

30 mg every 8 hours oral, equivalent to 1.2 mg/hour I.V. infusion

40 mg every 8 hours oral, equivalent to 2.2 mg/hour I.V. infusion

Mechanism of Action Inhibits calcium ion from entering the "slow channels" or select voltage-sensitive areas of vascular smooth muscle and myocardium during depolarization, producing a relaxation of coronary vascular smooth muscle and coronary vasodilation; increases myocardial oxygen delivery in patients with vasospastic angina

Other Adverse Effects

1% to 10%:

Cardiovascular: Flushing (6% to 10%), palpitations (3% to 4%), tachycardia (1% to 4%), peripheral edema (dose-related 7% to 8%), increased angina (dose-related 6%), hypotension (I.V. 6%), orthostasis (I.V. 1%)

Central nervous system: Headache (6% to 15%), dizziness (4% to 7%), somnolence (4% to 6%), paresthesia (1%)

Dermatologic: Rash (1%)

Gastrointestinal: Nausea (2% to 5%)

Genitourinary: Polyuria (1%)

Local: Injection site reaction (I.V. 1%)

Neuromuscular & skeletal: Weakness (4% to 6%), myalgia (1%)

Miscellaneous: Diaphoresis

<1% (Limited to important or life-threatening): Abnormal EKG, insomnia, malaise, abnormal dreams, vomiting, constipation, nocturia, tremor, nervousness, malaise, dyspnea, syncope, sustained tachycardia, injection site pain (I.V.), hypokalemia, intracranial hemorrhage, dyspnea

Case report: Parotitis

Drug Interactions Substrate of CYP1A2, 2C8/9, 2D6, 2E1, **3A4**; Inhibits CYP2C8/9, 2C19, 2D6, 3A4

Increased Effect/Toxicity: H_2 blockers (cimetidine) may increase the bioavailability of nicardipine. Serum concentrations/toxicity of nicardipine may be increased by inhibitors of CYP3A4, including amprenavir, cimetidine, ciprofloxacin, clarithromycin, clozapine, diltiazem, disulfiram, digoxin, erythromycin, ethanol, fluconazole, fluoxetine, fluvoxamine, grapefruit juice, isoniazid, itraconazole, ketoconazole, labetalol, levodopa, loxapine, metoprolol, metronidazole, miconazole, nefazodone, nelfinavir, omeprazole, phenytoin, propranolol, rifabutin, rifampin, ritonavir, troleandomycin, valproic acid, and verapamil. Calcium may reduce the calcium channel blocker's effects, particularly hypotension. Cyclosporine levels (and possibly tacrolimus) may be increased by nicardipine. May increase effect of vecuronium (reduce dose 25%) and increase serum levels of metoprolol.

Decreased Effect: Rifampin (and potentially other enzyme inducers) increase the metabolism of calcium channel blockers.

Dietary/Ethanol/Herb Considerations

Ethanol: Avoid use; may increase CNS depression.

Food may decrease average serum concentration. Avoid grapefruit products; may increase serum concentration. Avoid caffeine, garlic, and licorice.

Herb/Nutraceutical: Avoid black cohosh, dong quai, and evening primrose due to estrogenic activity. Avoid ephedra, ginseng, and yohimbe; may worsen hypertension. Avoid garlic; may have increased antihypertensive effect. Avoid ginger due to positive inotropic effects; theoretically, may cause arrhythmia. Avoid gotu kola, kava, SAMe, and valerian; may increase CNS depression. Avoid hawthorn; may lower peripheral vascular resistance resulting in additive decrease in BP. Avoid licorice. Avoid St John's wort; may decrease serum concentration and increase CNS depression.

Pharmacodynamics/Kinetics

Onset of action: Oral: 1-2 hours; I.V.: 10 minutes; Hypotension: ~20 minutes

Duration: 2-6 hours

Absorption: Oral: ~100%

Protein binding: 95%

Metabolism: Hepatic; extensive first-pass effect
Bioavailability: 35%
Half-life elimination: 2-4 hours
Time to peak, serum: 20-120 minutes
Excretion: Urine (as metabolites)

Pregnancy Risk Factor C

Generic Available Yes: Capsule

Selected Readings Pascual-Castroviejo I and Pascual Pascual SI, "Nicardipine-Induced Gingival Hyperplasia," *Neurologia*, 1997, 12(1):37-9.

Nicardipine Hydrochloride *see* NiCARdipine *on page 969*
NicoDerm® CQ® [OTC] *see* Nicotine *on page 971*
Nicorette® [OTC] *see* Nicotine *on page 971*
Nicotinamide *see* Niacinamide *on page 968*

Nicotine (nik oh TEEN)

Related Information

Chemical Dependency and Smoking Cessation *on page 1574*

U.S. Brand Names Commit™ [OTC]; NicoDerm® CQ® [OTC]; Nicorette® [OTC]; Nicotrol® Inhaler; Nicotrol® NS; Nicotrol® Patch [OTC]

Canadian Brand Names Habitrol®; Nicoderm®; Nicorette®; Nicorette® Plus; Nicotrol®

Mexican Brand Names Nicolan; Nicotinell TTS®

Pharmacologic Category Smoking Cessation Aid

Use Dental and Medical: Treatment to aid smoking cessation for the relief of nicotine withdrawal symptoms (including nicotine craving)

Unlabeled/Investigational Use Transdermal: Management of ulcerative colitis

Local Anesthetic/Vasoconstrictor Precautions No information available to require special precautions

Effects on Dental Treatment

Chewing gum form:

- >10%: Excessive salivation, mouth/throat soreness, jaw muscle ache, hiccups, tachycardia, headache (mild), vomiting, belching, nausea
- 1% to 10%: Xerostomia, dizziness, nervousness, GI distress, hoarseness, hiccups, muscle pain

Transdermal:

- >10%: Rhinitis, cough, pharyngitis, sinusitis
- 1% to 10%: Chest pain, anxiety, dizziness, somnolence, xerostomia, nausea

Dosage

Smoking deterrent: Patients should be advised to completely stop smoking upon initiation of therapy.

Gum: Chew 1 piece of gum when urge to smoke, up to 30 pieces/day; most patients require 10-12 pieces of gum/day

Inhaler: Usually 6-16 cartridges per day; best effect was achieved by frequent continuous puffing (20 minutes); recommended duration of treatment is 3 months, after which patients may be weaned from the inhaler by gradual reduction of the daily dose over 6-12 weeks

Lozenge: Patients who smoke their first cigarette within 30 minutes of waking should use the 4 mg strength; otherwise the 2 mg strength is recommended.

Weeks 1-6: One lozenge every 1-2 hours
Weeks 7-9: One lozenge every 2-4 hours
Weeks 10-12: One lozenge every 4-8 hours

Note: Use at least 9 lozenges/day during first 6 weeks to improve chances of quitting; do not use more than one lozenge at a time (maximum: 5 lozenges every 6 hours, 20 lozenges/day)

Transdermal patch: Apply new patch every 24 hours to nonhairy, clean, dry skin on the upper body or upper outer arm; each patch should be applied to a different site. **Note:** Adjustment may be required during initial treatment (move to higher dose if experiencing withdrawal symptoms; lower dose if side effects are experienced).

Habitrol®, NicoDerm CQ®:

Patients smoking ≥10 cigarettes/day: Begin with **step 1** (21 mg/day) for 4-6 weeks, followed by **step 2** (14 mg/day) for 2 weeks; finish with **step 3** (7 mg/day) for 2 weeks

Patients smoking <10 cigarettes/day: Begin with **step 2** (14 mg/day) for 6 weeks, followed by **step 3** (7 mg/day) for 2 weeks

Note: Initial starting dose for patients <100 pounds, history of cardiovascular disease: 14 mg/day for 4-6 weeks, followed by 7 mg/day for 2-4 weeks

Note: Patients receiving >600 mg/day of cimetidine: Decrease to the next lower patch size

Nicotrol®: One patch daily for 6 weeks

Note: Benefits of use of nicotine transdermal patches beyond 3 months have not been demonstrated.

(Continued)

Nicotine *(Continued)*

Spray: 1-2 sprays/hour; do not exceed more than 5 doses (10 sprays) per hour; each dose (2 sprays) contains 1 mg of nicotine. **Warning:** A dose of 40 mg can cause fatalities.

Ulcerative colitis (unlabeled use): Transdermal: Titrated to 22-25 mg/day

Mechanism of Action Nicotine is one of two naturally-occurring alkaloids which exhibit their primary effects via autonomic ganglia stimulation. The other alkaloid is lobeline which has many actions similar to those of nicotine but is less potent. Nicotine is a potent ganglionic and central nervous system stimulant, the actions of which are mediated via nicotine-specific receptors. Biphasic actions are observed depending upon the dose administered. The main effect of nicotine in small doses is stimulation of all autonomic ganglia; with larger doses, initial stimulation is followed by blockade of transmission. Biphasic effects are also evident in the adrenal medulla; discharge of catecholamines occurs with small doses, whereas prevention of catecholamines release is seen with higher doses as a response to splanchnic nerve stimulation. Stimulation of the central nervous system (CNS) is characterized by tremors and respiratory excitation. However, convulsions may occur with higher doses, along with respiratory failure secondary to both central paralysis and peripheral blockade to respiratory muscles.

Other Adverse Effects

Chewing gum/lozenge:

- >10%: Gastrointestinal: Indigestion, increased appetite
- 1% to 10%:
  - Central nervous system: Insomnia
  - Endocrine & metabolic: Dysmenorrhea
- <1%: **Atrial fibrillation**, erythema, hypersensitivity reactions, itching

Transdermal systems:

- >10%:
  - Central nervous system: Insomnia, abnormal dreams
  - Dermatologic: Pruritus, erythema
  - Local: Application site reaction
- 1% to 10%:
  - Central nervous system: Dysphoria, difficulty concentrating
  - Dermatologic: Rash
  - Gastrointestinal: Diarrhea, dyspepsia, constipation, anorexia, abdominal pain
  - Neuromuscular & skeletal: Arthralgia, myalgia
- <1%: **Atrial fibrillation, hypersensitivity reactions, itching, tremor, nervousness, abnormal taste**

Contraindications Hypersensitivity to nicotine or any component of the formulation; patients who are smoking during the postmyocardial infarction period; patients with life-threatening arrhythmias, or severe or worsening angina pectoris; active temporomandibular joint disease (gum); pregnancy; not for use in nonsmokers

Warnings/Precautions The risk versus the benefits must be weighed for each of these groups: patients with CAD, serious cardiac arrhythmias, vasospastic disease. Use caution in patients with hyperthyroidism, pheochromocytoma, or insulin-dependent diabetes. Use with caution in oropharyngeal inflammation and in patients with history of esophagitis, peptic ulcer, coronary artery disease, vasospastic disease, angina, hypertension, hyperthyroidism, pheochromocytoma, diabetes, severe renal dysfunction, and hepatic dysfunction. The inhaler should be used with caution in patients with bronchospastic disease (other forms of nicotine replacement may be preferred). Safety and efficacy have not been established in pediatric patients. Cautious use of topical nicotine in patients with certain skin diseases. Hypersensitivity to the topical products can occur. Dental problems may be worsened by chewing the gum. Urge patients to stop smoking completely when initiating therapy.

Drug Interactions Substrate of CYP1A2, 2A6, 2B6, 2C8/9, 2C19, 2D6, 2E1, 3A4; Inhibits CYP2A6

Adenosine: Nicotine increases the hemodynamic and AV blocking effects of adenosine; monitor

Bupropion: Monitor for treatment-emergent hypertension in patients treated with the combination of nicotine patch and bupropion

Cimetidine; May increases nicotine concentrations; therefore, may decrease amount of gum or patches needed

Dietary/Ethanol/Herb Considerations Food: Lozenge: Acidic foods/beverages decrease absorption of nicotine. Each lozenge contains phenylalanine 3.4 mg.

Pharmacodynamics/Kinetics

Onset of action: Intranasal: More closely approximate the time course of plasma nicotine levels observed after cigarette smoking than other dosage forms

Duration: Transdermal: 24 hours

Absorption: Transdermal: Slow

Metabolism: Hepatic, primarily to cotinine ($^1/_5$ as active)

Half-life elimination: 4 hours

Time to peak, serum: Transdermal: 8-9 hours

Excretion: Urine

Clearance: Renal: pH dependent

Pregnancy Risk Factor D (transdermal); X (chewing gum)

Dosage Forms GUM, chewing, as polacrilex (Nicorette®): 2 mg/square (48s, 108s, 168s); 4 mg/square (48s, 108s, 168s). **LOZ, as polacrilex** (Commit™): 2 mg, 4 mg. **Oral inhalation system** (Nicotrol® Inhaler): 10 mg cartridge (42s). **PATCH, transdermal:** 7 mg/24 hours (7s, 30s); 14 mg/24 hours (7s, 14s, 30s); 21 mg/24 hours (7s, 14s, 30s); Kit (Step 1): 21 mg/24 hours (28s); (Step 2): 14 mg/24 hours (14s); (Step 3): 7 mg/24 hours (14s); (NicoDerm® CQ®) [clear patch]: 7 mg/24 hours (14s); 14 mg/24 hours (14s); 21 mg/24 hours (14s); (NicoDerm® CQ®) [tan patch]: 7 mg/24 hours (14s); 14 mg/24 hours (14s); 21 mg/24 hours (7s, 14s); (Nicotrol®): 15 mg/16 hours (7s). **SPRAY, intranasal** (Nicotrol® NS): 10 mg/mL (10 mL)

Generic Available Yes: Transdermal patch and gum

Comments At least 10 reported studies have documented the effectiveness of nicotine patches in smoking cessation. Approximately 45% of treated patients quit smoking after 6 weeks of patch therapy. Control patients given placebo patches accounted for about a 20% success rate. At 52 weeks, approximately 1/2 of the 45% 6-week successful patients continued to abstain. Control placebo patients accounted for an approximate 11% success rate after 52 weeks.

Selected Readings

Christen AG and Christen JA, "The Prescription of Transdermal Nicotine Patches for Tobacco-Using Dental Patients: Current Status in Indiana," *J Indiana Dent Assoc*, 1992, 71(6):12-8.

Li Wan Po A, "Transdermal Nicotine in Smoking Cessation. A Meta-analysis," *Eur J Clin Pharmacol*, 1993, 45(6):519-28.

Stafne EE, "The Nicotine Transdermal Patch: Use in the Dental Office Tobacco Cessation Program," *Northwest Dent*, 1994, 73(3):19-22.

Transdermal Nicotine Study Group, "Transdermal Nicotine for Smoking Cessation. Six-Month Results from Two Multicenter Controlled Clinical Trials," *JAMA*, 1991, 266(22):3133-8.

Westman EC, Levin ED, and Rose JE, "The Nicotine Patch in Smoking Cessation," *Arch Intern Med*, 1993, 153(16):1917-23.

Wynn RL, "Nicotine Patches in Smoking Cessation," *AGD Impact*, 1994, 22:14.

Nicotinex [OTC] *see* Niacin *on page 967*

Nicotinic Acid *see* Niacin *on page 967*

Nicotrol® Inhaler *see* Nicotine *on page 971*

Nicotrol® NS *see* Nicotine *on page 971*

Nicotrol® Patch [OTC] *see* Nicotine *on page 971*

Nifedical™ XL *see* NIFEdipine *on page 973*

NIFEdipine (nye FED i peen)

Related Information

Calcium Channel Blockers and Gingival Hyperplasia *on page 1598*

Calcium Channel Blockers, Comparative Pharmacokinetics *on page 1600*

Cardiovascular Diseases *on page 1456*

U.S. Brand Names Adalat® CC; Nifedical™ XL; Procardia®; Procardia XL®

Canadian Brand Names Adalat® XL®; Apo®-Nifed; Apo®-Nifed PA; Novo-Nifedin; Nu-Nifed; Procardia®

Mexican Brand Names Adalat®; Adalat® Oros; Adalat® Retard; Corogal; Corotrend®; Corotrend Retard; Dilafed; Nifedipres®; Noviken-N

Pharmacologic Category Calcium Channel Blocker

Use Angina and hypertension (sustained release only), pulmonary hypertension

Local Anesthetic/Vasoconstrictor Precautions No information available to require special precautions

Effects on Dental Treatment Nifedipine has been reported to cause 10% incidence of gingival hyperplasia; effects from 30-100 mg/day have appeared after 1-9 months. Discontinuance results in complete disappearance or marked regression of symptoms; symptoms will reappear upon remedication. Marked regression occurs after 1 week and complete disappearance of symptoms has occurred within 15 days. If a gingivectomy is performed and use of the drug is continued or resumed, hyperplasia usually will recur. The success of the gingivectomy usually requires that the medication be discontinued or that a switch to a noncalcium channel blocker be made. If for some reason nifedipine cannot be discontinued, hyperplasia has not recurred after gingivectomy when extensive plaque control was performed. If nifedipine is changed to another class of cardiovascular agent, the gingival hyperplasia will probably regress and resolve. Switching to another calcium channel blocker may result in continued hyperplasia.

>10%: Flushing (10% to 25%), Dizziness/lightheadedness/giddiness (10% to 27%), headache (10% to 23%), nausea/heartburn (10% to 11%), weakness (10% to 12%)

≥1% to 10%: Palpitations (≤2% to 7%), transient hypotension (dose-related 5%), CHF (2%), nervousness (≤2% to 7%), shakiness (≤2%), jitteriness (≤2%), difficulties in balance (≤2%), fever (≤2%), muscle cramps/tremor (≤2% to 8%), inflammation (≤2%), joint stiffness (≤2%), blurred vision (≤2%), cough/wheezing (6%), nasal congestion/sore throat (≤2% to 6%), chest congestion (≤2%), dyspnea (≤2%), diaphoresis (≤2%)

Dosage Oral:

Children: Hypertrophic cardiomyopathy: 0.6-0.9 mg/kg/24 hours in 3-4 divided doses

(Continued)

NIFEdipine *(Continued)*

Adolescents and Adults: (**Note:** When switching from immediate release to sustained release formulations, total daily dose will start the same)

Initial: 30 mg once daily as sustained release formulation, or if indicated, 10 mg 3 times/day as capsules

Usual dose: 10-30 mg 3 times/day as capsules or 30-60 mg once daily as sustained release

Maximum dose: 120-180 mg/day

Increase sustained release at 7- to 14-day intervals

Hemodialysis: Supplemental dose unnecessary.

Peritoneal dialysis effects: Supplemental dose unnecessary.

Dosing adjustment in hepatic impairment: Reduce oral dose by 50% to 60% in patients with cirrhosis.

Mechanism of Action Inhibits calcium ion from entering the "slow channels" or select voltage-sensitive areas of vascular smooth muscle and myocardium during depolarization, producing a relaxation of coronary vascular smooth muscle and coronary vasodilation; increases myocardial oxygen delivery in patients with vasospastic angina

Other Adverse Effects

>10%:

Cardiovascular: Peripheral edema (dose-related 7% to 10%; up to 50%)

≥1% to 10%:

Central nervous system: Sleep disturbances (≤2%), chills (≤2%)

Dermatologic: Dermatitis (≤2%), pruritus (≤2%), urticaria (≤2%)

Endocrine & metabolic: Sexual difficulties (≤2%)

Gastrointestinal: Diarrhea (≤2%), constipation (≤2%), cramps (≤2%), flatulence (≤2%)

<1% (Limited to important or life-threatening): **Syncope,** erythromelalgia, thrombocytopenia, anemia, leukopenia, purpura, allergic hepatitis, angioedema, **gingival hyperplasia,** depression, **paranoid syndrome, transient blindness,** tinnitus, nocturia, polyuria, arthritis with positive ANA, exfoliative dermatitis, gynecomastia, myalgia, **memory dysfunction, fever,** bezoars (sustained-release preparations), **reflux, myoclonus, angina,** ischemia

Postmarketing and/or case reports: Phototoxicity, EPS, aplastic anemia, agranulocytosis, purpura, Stevens-Johnson syndrome, cerebral ischemia, parotitis, dysgeusia, dysosmia, nocturnal enuresis, erythema multiforme

Reported with use of sublingual short-acting nifedipine: Cerebrovascular ischemia, **syncope,** heart block, **stroke, sinus arrest, severe hypotension, acute MI,** EKG changes, and fetal distress

Drug Interactions Substrate of CYP2D6, **3A4**; Inhibits CYP1A2, 2C8/9, 2D6, 3A4

Increased Effect/Toxicity: H_2-blockers may increase bioavailability and serum concentrations of nifedipine. Serum concentrations/toxicity of nifedipine may be increased by inhibitors of CYP3A4, including amprenavir, cimetidine, ciprofloxacin, clarithromycin, clozapine, diltiazem, disulfiram, digoxin, erythromycin, ethanol, fluconazole, fluoxetine, fluvoxamine, grapefruit juice, isoniazid, itraconazole, ketoconazole, labetalol, levodopa, loxapine, metoprolol, metronidazole, miconazole, nefazodone, nelfinavir, omeprazole, phenytoin, rifabutin, rifampin, ritonavir, troleandomycin, valproic acid, and verapamil. Nifedipine may increase serum levels of digoxin, phenytoin, theophylline, and vincristine.

Decreased Effect: Phenobarbital and nifedipine may decrease nifedipine levels. Quinidine and nifedipine may decrease quinidine serum levels. Rifampin and nifedipine may decrease nifedipine serum levels. Calcium may reduce the hypotension from of calcium channel blockers.

Dietary/Ethanol/Herb Considerations

Ethanol: Avoid use; may increase serum concentration; watch for greater hypotensive effect; may increase CNS depression.

Food may decrease serum concentration and rate but not extent of absorption of Procardia XL®. Avoid grapefruit products; may increase therapeutic and vasodilator effects, including severe hypotension and myocardial ischemia. Avoid caffeine, garlic, and licorice.

Herb/Nutraceutical: Avoid black cohosh, dong quai, and evening primrose due to estrogenic activity. Avoid ephedra, ginseng, and yohimbe; may worsen hypertension. Avoid garlic; may have increased antihypertensive effect. Avoid ginger due to positive inotropic effects; theoretically, may cause arrhythmia. Avoid gotu kola, kava, SAMe, and valerian; may increase CNS depression. Avoid hawthorn; may decrease peripheral vascular resistance. Avoid licorice. Avoid St John's wort; may decrease serum concentration and increase CNS depression.

Pharmacodynamics/Kinetics

Onset of action: ~20 minutes

Protein binding (concentration dependent): 92% to 98%

Metabolism: Hepatic to inactive metabolites

Bioavailability: Capsules: 45% to 75%; Sustained release: 65% to 86%

Half-life elimination: Adults: Healthy: 2-5 hours, Cirrhosis: 7 hours; Elderly: 6.7 hours

Excretion: Urine

Pregnancy Risk Factor C
Generic Available Yes
Selected Readings

Deen-Duggins L, Fry HR, Clay JR, et al, "Nifedipine-Associated Gingival Overgrowth: A Survey of the Literature and Report of Four Cases," *Quintessence Int*, 1996, 27(3):163-70.

Desai P and Silver JG, "Drug-Induced Gingival Enlargements," *J Can Dent Assoc*, 1998, 64(4):263-8.

Harel-Raviv M, Eckler M, Lalani K, et al, "Nifedipine-Induced Gingival Hyperplasia. A Comprehensive Review and Analysis," *Oral Surg Oral Med Oral Pathol Oral Radiol Endod*, 1995, 79(6):715-22.

Lederman D, Lumerman H, Reuben S, et al, "Gingival Hyperplasia Associated With Nifedipine Therapy," *Oral Surg Oral Med Oral Pathol*, 1984, 57(6):620-2.

Lucas RM, Howell LP, and Wall BA, "Nifedipine-Induced Gingival Hyperplasia: A Histochemical and Ultrastructural Study," *J Periodontol*, 1985, 56(4):211-5.

Nery EB, Edson RG, Lee KK, et al, "Prevalence of Nifedipine-Induced Gingival Hyperplasia," *J Periodontol*, 1995, 66(7):572-8.

Nishikawa SJ, Tada H, Hamasaki A, et al, "Nifedipine-Induced Gingival Hyperplasia: A Clinical and In Vitro Study," *J Periodontol*, 1991, 62(1):30-5.

Pilloni A, Camargo PM, Carere M, et al, "Surgical Treatment of Cyclosporine A- and Nifedipine-Induced Gingival Enlargement: Gingivectomy Versus Periodontal Flap," *J Periodontol*, 1998, 69(7):791-7.

Saito K, Mori S, Iwakura M, et al, "Immunohistochemical Localization of Transforming Growth Factor Beta, Basic Fibroblast Growth Factor and Heparin Sulphate Glycosaminoglycan in Gingival Hyperplasia Induced by Nifedipine and Phenytoin," *J Periodontal Res*, 1996, 31(8):545-5.

Silverstein LH, Koch JP, Lefkove MD, et al, "Nifedipine-Induced Gingival Enlargement Around Dental Implants: A Clinical Report," *J Oral Implantol*, 1995, 21(2):116-20.

Westbrook P, Bednarczyk EM, Carlson M, et al, "Regression of Nifedipine-Induced Gingival Hyperplasia Following Switch to a Same Class Calcium Channel Blocker, Isradipine," *J Periodontol*, 1997, 68(7):645-50.

Wynn RL, "Calcium Channel Blockers and Gingival Hyperplasia," *Gen Dent*, 1991, 39(4):240-3.

Wynn RL, "Update on Calcium Channel Blocker-Induced Gingival Hyperplasia," *Gen Dent*, 1995, 43(3):218-22.

Niferex® [OTC] *see* Polysaccharide-Iron Complex *on page 1096*

Niferex® 150 [OTC] *see* Polysaccharide-Iron Complex *on page 1096*

Nilandron® *see* Nilutamide *on page 975*

Nilutamide (ni Loo tu mide)

U.S. Brand Names Nilandron®

Canadian Brand Names Anandron®

Pharmacologic Category Antineoplastic Agent, Antiandrogen

Use Treatment of metastatic prostate cancer

Local Anesthetic/Vasoconstrictor Precautions No information available to require special precautions

Effects on Dental Treatment No significant effects or complications reported

Dosage Refer to individual protocols.

Adults: Oral: 300 mg daily for 30 days starting the same day or day after surgical castration, then 150 mg/day

Mechanism of Action Nonsteroidal antiandrogen that inhibits androgen uptake or inhibits binding of androgen in target tissues

Other Adverse Effects

>10%:

- Central nervous system: Headache, insomnia
- Endocrine & metabolic: Hot flashes (30% to 67%), gynecomastia (10%)
- Gastrointestinal: Nausea (mild - 10% to 32%), abdominal pain (10%), constipation, anorexia
- Genitourinary: Testicular atrophy (16%), libido decreased
- Hepatic: Transient elevation in serum transaminases (8% to 13%)
- Ocular: Impaired dark adaptation (13% to 57%), usually reversible with dose reduction, may require discontinuation of the drug in 1% to 2% of patients
- Respiratory: Dyspnea (11%)

1% to 10%:

- Cardiovascular: Chest pain, edema, heart failure, hypertension, syncope
- Central nervous system: Dizziness, drowsiness, malaise, hypesthesia, depression
- Dermatologic: Pruritus, alopecia, dry skin, rash
- Endocrine & metabolic: Disulfiram-like reaction (hot flashes, rashes) (5%); Flu-like syndrome, fever
- Gastrointestinal: Vomiting, diarrhea, dyspepsia, GI hemorrhage, melena, weight loss, xerostomia
- Genitourinary: Hematuria, nocturia
- Hematologic: Anemia
- Hepatic: Hepatitis (1%)
- Neuromuscular & skeletal: Arthritis, paresthesia
- Ocular: Chromatopsia (9%), abnormal vision (6% to 7%), cataracts, photophobia
- Respiratory: Interstitial pneumonitis (2% - typically exertional dyspnea, cough, chest pain, and fever; most often occurring within the first 3 months of treatment); rhinitis
- Miscellaneous: Diaphoresis

<1%: Aplastic anemia

Dietary/Ethanol/Herb Considerations

Ethanol: Avoid use; up to 5% of patients may experience a systemic reaction (flushing, hypotension, malaise).

(Continued)

Nilutamide *(Continued)*

Herb/Nutraceutical: Avoid St John's wort; may decrease serum concentration.

Pharmacodynamics/Kinetics

Absorption: Rapid and complete

Protein binding: 72% to 85%

Metabolism: Hepatic, forms active metabolites

Half-life elimination: Terminal: 23-87 hours; Metabolites: 35-137 hours

Excretion: Urine (up to 78% at 120 hours; <1% as unchanged drug); feces (1% to 7%)

Pregnancy Risk Factor C

Generic Available No

Nimodipine (nye MOE di peen)

Related Information

Calcium Channel Blockers and Gingival Hyperplasia *on page 1598*

Calcium Channel Blockers, Comparative Pharmacokinetics *on page 1600*

Cardiovascular Diseases *on page 1456*

U.S. Brand Names Nimotop®

Canadian Brand Names Nimotop®

Mexican Brand Names Nimotop®

Pharmacologic Category Calcium Channel Blocker

Use Spasm following subarachnoid hemorrhage from ruptured intracranial aneurysms regardless of the patients neurological condition postictus (Hunt and Hess grades I-V)

Local Anesthetic/Vasoconstrictor Precautions No information available to require special precautions

Effects on Dental Treatment Other drugs of this class can cause gingival hyperplasia (ie, nifedipine) but there have been no reports for nimodipine.

Dosage Oral:

Adults: 60 mg every 4 hours for 21 days, start therapy within 96 hours after subarachnoid hemorrhage.

Dialysis: Not removed by hemo- or peritoneal dialysis; supplemental dose is unnecessary.

Dosing adjustment in hepatic impairment: Reduce to 30 mg every 4 hours in liver failure

Mechanism of Action Nimodipine shares the pharmacology of other calcium channel blockers; animal studies indicate that nimodipine has a greater effect on cerebral arterials than other arterials; this increased specificity may be due to the drug's increased lipophilicity and cerebral distribution as compared to nifedipine; inhibits calcium ion from entering the "slow channels" or select voltage sensitive areas of vascular smooth muscle and myocardium during depolarization

Other Adverse Effects

1% to 10%:

Cardiovascular: Reductions in systemic blood pressure (1% to 8%)

Central nervous system: Headache (1% to 4%)

Dermatologic: Rash (1% to 2%)

Gastrointestinal: Diarrhea (2% to 4%), abdominal discomfort (2%)

≤1% (Limited to important or life-threatening): Edema (≤1%), EKG abnormalities (≤1%), tachycardia (≤1%), bradycardia (≤1%), depression (≤1%), acne (≤1%), nausea (≤1%), hemorrhage, hepatitis, muscle cramps/pain (≤1%), dyspnea (≤1%). itching, GI hemorrhage, thrombocytopenia, anemia, palpitations, vomiting, flushing, diaphoresis, wheezing, lightheadedness, dizziness, rebound vasospasm, jaundice, hypertension, hematoma, neurological deterioration, CHF, hyponatremia, disseminated intravascular coagulation, deep vein thrombosis

Case report: Disseminated intravascular coagulation (DIC)

Drug Interactions Substrate of **CYP3A4**

Increased Effect/Toxicity: Calcium channel blockers and nimodipine may result in enhanced cardiovascular effects of other calcium channel blockers. Cimetidine, omeprazole, and valproic acid may increase serum nimodipine levels. The effects of antihypertensive agents may be increased by nimodipine. Azole antifungals (itraconazole, ketoconazole, fluconazole), erythromycin, protease inhibitors (amprenavir, nelfinavir, ritonavir) and other inhibitors of cytochrome P450 isoenzyme 3A4 may inhibit calcium channel blocker metabolism.

Decreased Effect: Rifampin (and potentially other enzyme inducers) increase the metabolism of calcium channel blockers.

Dietary/Ethanol/Herb Considerations

Ethanol: Avoid use; may increase risk of hypotension or dizziness.

Food: Avoid grapefruit products; bioavailability increases 1.5-fold when taken concurrently. Avoid caffeine, garlic, and licorice.

Herb/Nutraceutical: Avoid black cohosh, dong quai, and evening primrose due to estrogenic activity. Avoid ephedra, ginseng, and yohimbe; may worsen hypertension. Avoid garlic; may have increased antihypertensive effect. Avoid ginger due to positive inotropic effects; theoretically, may cause arrhythmia. Avoid hawthorn;

may lower peripheral vascular resistance causing additional decrease in BP. Avoid licorice. Avoid St John's wort; may decrease serum concentration.

Pharmacodynamics/Kinetics

Protein binding: >95%

Metabolism: Extensively hepatic

Bioavailability: 13%

Half-life elimination: 3 hours; prolonged with renal impairment

Time to peak, serum: ~1 hour

Excretion: Urine (50%) and feces (32%) within 4 days

Pregnancy Risk Factor C

Generic Available No

Nimotop® *see* Nimodipine *on page 976*

Nipent® *see* Pentostatin *on page 1057*

Nisoldipine (NYE sole di peen)

Related Information

Calcium Channel Blockers, Comparative Pharmacokinetics *on page 1600*

Cardiovascular Diseases *on page 1456*

U.S. Brand Names Sular®

Mexican Brand Names Sular®; Syscor®

Pharmacologic Category Calcium Channel Blocker

Use Management of hypertension, alone or in combination with other antihypertensive agents

Local Anesthetic/Vasoconstrictor Precautions No information available to require special precautions

Effects on Dental Treatment 1% to 10%: Xerostomia

Dosage Adults: Oral: Initial: 20 mg once daily, then increase by 10 mg/week (or longer intervals) to attain adequate control of blood pressure; doses >60 mg once daily are not recommended. A starting dose not exceeding 10 mg/day is recommended for the elderly and those with hepatic impairment.

Mechanism of Action As a dihydropyridine calcium channel blocker, structurally similar to nifedipine, nisoldipine impedes the movement of calcium ions into vascular smooth muscle and cardiac muscle. Dihydropyridines are potent vasodilators and are not as likely to suppress cardiac contractility and slow cardiac conduction as other calcium antagonists such as verapamil and diltiazem; nisoldipine is 5-10 times as potent a vasodilator as nifedipine.

Other Adverse Effects

>10%:

Cardiovascular: Peripheral edema (dose-related 7% to 29%)

Central nervous system: Headache (22%)

1% to 10%:

Cardiovascular: Chest pain (2%), palpitations (3%), vasodilation (4%)

Central nervous system: Dizziness (3% to 10%)

Dermatologic: Rash (2%)

Gastrointestinal: Nausea (2%)

Respiratory: Pharyngitis (5%), sinusitis (3%), dyspnea (3%), cough (5%)

<1% (Limited to important or life-threatening): Cellulite, chills, facial edema, fever, flu syndrome, malaise, atria fibrillation, CVA, CHF, first-degree AV block, hypertension, angina, pulmonary edema, jugular venous distention, migraine, MI, postural hypertension, ventricular extrasystoles, supraventricular tachycardia, syncope, systolic ejection murmur, T-wave abnormalities on EKG (flattening, inversion, nonspecific changes), venous insufficiency, abnormal LFTs, anorexia, colitis, diarrhea, dyspepsia, dysphagia, flatulence, gastritis, gastrointestinal hemorrhage, **glossitis, gingival hyperplasia**, hepatomegaly, increased appetite, melena, oral ulceration, diabetes mellitus, thyroiditis, anemia, ecchymoses, leukopenia, petechiae, gout, hypokalemia, increased serum creatine kinase, increased nonprotein nitrogen, weight gain, weight loss, arthralgia, arthritis, leg cramps, myalgia, myasthenia, myositis, tenosynovitis, abnormal dreams, abnormal thinking and confusion, amnesia, anxiety, ataxia, cerebral ischemia, decreased libido, depression, hypesthesia, hypertonia, insomnia, nervousness, paresthesia, somnolence, tremor, vertigo, asthma, dyspnea, end inspiratory wheeze and fine rales, epistaxis, increased cough, laryngitis, pharyngitis, pleural effusions, rhinitis, sinusitis, acne, alopecia, dry skin, exfoliative dermatitis, fungal dermatitis, herpes simplex, herpes zoster, maculopapular rash, pruritus, pustular rash, skin discoloration, skin ulcer, diaphoresis, urticaria, abnormal vision, amblyopia, blepharitis, conjunctivitis, ear pain, glaucoma, itchy eyes, keratoconjunctivitis, otitis media, retinal detachment, tinnitus, watery eyes, abnormal taste, temporary unilateral loss of vision, vitreous floater, watery eyes, dysuria, hematuria, impotence, nocturia, urinary frequency, increased BUN and serum creatinine, vaginal hemorrhage, vaginitis, gynecomastia

Case report: Cholestatic jaundice

Drug Interactions Substrate of **CYP3A4**; Inhibits CYP1A2, 3A4

Increased Effect/Toxicity: H_2-antagonists or omeprazole may cause an increase in the serum concentrations of nisoldipine. Digoxin and nisoldipine may increase

(Continued)

Nisoldipine *(Continued)*

digoxin effect. Azole antifungals (itraconazole, ketoconazole, fluconazole), erythromycin, and other inhibitors of cytochrome P450 isoenzyme 3A4 may inhibit calcium channel blocker metabolism. Calcium may reduce the calcium channel blocker's effects, particularly hypotension.

Decreased Effect: Rifampin, phenytoin, and potentially other enzyme inducers decrease the levels of nisoldipine. Calcium may decrease the hypotension from calcium channel blockers.

Dietary/Ethanol/Herb Considerations

Ethanol: Avoid use; may increase risk of hypotension or dizziness.

Food: Bioavailability may be increased if taken with high-lipid foods or grapefruit products; avoid grapefruit products before and after administration. Avoid caffeine, garlic, and licorice.

Herb/Nutraceutical: Avoid black cohosh, dong quai, and evening primrose due to estrogenic activity. Avoid ephedra, ginseng, and yohimbe; may worsen hypertension. Avoid garlic; may have increased antihypertensive effect. Avoid ginger due to positive inotropic effects; theoretically, may cause arrhythmia. Avoid hawthorn; may decrease peripheral vascular resistance. Avoid licorice. Avoid St John's wort; may decrease serum concentration.

Pharmacodynamics/Kinetics

Duration: >24 hours

Absorption: Well absorbed

Metabolism: Extensively hepatic to inactive metabolites; first-pass effect

Bioavailability: 5%

Half-life elimination: 7-12 hours

Time to peak: 6-12 hours

Excretion: Urine

Pregnancy Risk Factor C

Generic Available No

Nitalapram *see* Citalopram *on page 334*

Nitazoxanide (nye ta ZOKS a nide)

U.S. Brand Names Alinia™

Pharmacologic Category Antiprotozoal

Synonyms NTZ

Use Treatment of diarrhea caused by *Cryptosporidium parvum* and *Giardia lamblia* in pediatric patients 1-11 years of age

Local Anesthetic/Vasoconstrictor Precautions No information available to require special precautions

Effects on Dental Treatment No significant effects or complications reported

Dosage Oral: Diarrhea: Children:

12-47 months: 100 mg every 12 hours for 3 days

4-11 years: 200 mg every 12 hours for 3 days

Dosing adjustment in renal/hepatic impairment: Specific recommendations unavailable; use with caution

Mechanism of Action Nitazoxanide is rapidly metabolized to the active metabolite tizoxanide *in vivo.* Activity may be due to interference with the pyruvate:ferredoxin oxidoreductase (PFOR) enzyme-dependent electron transfer reaction which is essential to anaerobic metabolism. *In vitro*, nitazoxanide and tizoxanide inhibit the growth of sporozoites and oocysts of *Cryptosporidium parvum* and trophozoites of *Giardia lamblia.*

Other Adverse Effects Rates of adverse effects were similar to those reported with placebo.

1% to 10%:

Central nervous system: Headache (1%)

Gastrointestinal: Abdominal pain (8%), diarrhea (2%), vomiting (1%)

<1%: ALT increased, anorexia, appetite increased, creatinine increased, diaphoresis, dizziness, eye discoloration (pale yellow), fever, flatulence, infection, malaise, nausea, pruritus, rhinitis, salivary glands enlarged, urine discoloration

Dietary/Ethanol/Herb Considerations Food: Should be taken with food; contains sucrose 1.48 g/5 mL.

Pharmacodynamics/Kinetics

Protein binding: Tizoxanide: >99%

Metabolism: Hepatic, to an active metabolite, tizoxanide. Tizoxanide undergoes conjugation to form tizoxanide glucuronide. Nitazoxanide is not detectable in the serum following oral administration.

Time to peak, plasma: Tizoxanide and tizoxanide glucuronide: 1-4 hours

Excretion: Tizoxanide: Urine, bile, and feces; Tizoxanide glucuronide: Urine and bile

Pregnancy Risk Factor B

Generic Available No

Nitisinone (ni TIS i known)

U.S. Brand Names Orfadin®

Pharmacologic Category 4-Hydroxyphenylpyruvate Dioxygenase Inhibitor

Use Treatment of hereditary tyrosinemia type 1 (HT-1); to be used with dietary restriction of tyrosine and phenylalanine

Local Anesthetic/Vasoconstrictor Precautions No information available to require special precautions

Effects on Dental Treatment No significant effects or complications reported

Restrictions Distributed by Rare Disease Therapeutics, Inc (contact 615-399-0700)

Dosage Must be used in conjunction with a low protein diet restricted in tyrosine and phenylalanine.

Oral:

Children and Adults: Initial: 1 mg/kg/day in divided doses, given in the morning and evening, 1 hour before meals; doses do not need to be divided evenly

Infants may require maximal dose once liver function has improved.

Dose adjustment: If biochemical parameters (see Monitoring Parameters) are not normalized within in 1-month period, dose may be increased to 1.5 mg/kg/day (maximum dose: 2 mg/kg/day).

Mechanism of Action In patients with HT-1, tyrosine metabolism is interrupted due to a lack of the enzyme (fumarylacetoacetate hydrolase) needed in the last step of tyrosine degradation. Toxic metabolites of tyrosine accumulate and cause liver and kidney toxicity. Nitisinone competitively inhibits 4-hydroxyphenyl-pyruvate dioxygenase, an enzyme needed earlier in the tyrosine degradation pathway, and therefore prevents the build-up of the damaging metabolites.

Other Adverse Effects

1% to 10%:

Dermatologic: Alopecia (1%), dry skin (1%), exfoliative dermatitis (1%), maculopapular rash (1%), pruritus (1%)

Hematologic: Thrombocytopenia (3%), leukopenia (3%), porphyria (1%), epistaxis (1%)

Hepatic: Hepatic neoplasm (8%), hepatic failure (7%)

Ocular: Conjunctivitis (2%), corneal opacity (2%), keratitis (2%), photophobia (2%), cataracts (1%), blepharitis (1%), eye pain (1%)

<1%: Abdominal pain, amenorrhea, brain tumor, bronchitis, cyanosis, dehydration, diarrhea, enanthema, encephalopathy, gastritis, gastroenteritis, gastrointestinal hemorrhage, headache, hepatic dysfunction, hepatomegaly, hyperkinesias, infection, liver enzyme elevation, melena, nervousness, otitis, pathologic fracture, respiratory insufficiency, seizures, septicemia, somnolence, thirst, tooth discoloration

Dietary/Ethanol/Herb Considerations Food: Effect unknown; administer 1 hour prior to meal. Tyrosine toxicity can occur without proper dietary restriction of tyrosine and phenylalanine.

Pharmacodynamics/Kinetics Limited pharmacokinetic studies in children or HT-1 patients.

Bioavailability: Animal studies: >90%

Half-life elimination: Terminal: Male: Healthy: 54 hours

Time to peak: 3 hours

Excretion (animal studies): Urine

Pregnancy Risk Factor C

Generic Available No

Nitrek® *see* Nitroglycerin *on page 981*

Nitric Oxide (NYE trik OKS ide)

U.S. Brand Names INOmax®

Canadian Brand Names INOmax®

Pharmacologic Category Vasodilator, Pulmonary

Use Treatment of term and near-term (>34 weeks) neonates with hypoxic respiratory failure associated with pulmonary hypertension; used concurrently with ventilatory support and other agents

Unlabeled/Investigational Use Treatment of adult respiratory distress syndrome (ARDS)

Local Anesthetic/Vasoconstrictor Precautions No information available to require special precautions

Effects on Dental Treatment No significant effects or complications reported

Dosage Neonates (up to 14 days old): 20 ppm. Treatment should be maintained up to 14 days or until the underlying oxygen desaturation has resolved and the neonate is ready to be weaned from therapy. In the CINRGI trial, patients whose oxygenation improved had their dose reduced to 5 ppm at the end of 4 hours of treatment. Doses above 20 ppm should not be used because of the risk of methemoglobinemia and elevated NO_2.

Mechanism of Action In neonates with persistent pulmonary hypertension, nitric oxide improves oxygenation. Nitric oxide relaxes vascular smooth muscle by binding to the heme moiety of cytosolic guanylate cyclase, activating guanylate

(Continued)

Nitric Oxide *(Continued)*

cyclase and increasing intracellular levels of cyclic guanosine 3',5'-monophosphate, which leads to vasodilation. When inhaled, pulmonary vasodilation occurs and an increase in the partial pressure of arterial oxygen results. Dilation of pulmonary vessels in well ventilated lung areas redistributes blood flow away from lung areas where ventilation/perfusion ratios are poor.

Other Adverse Effects

>10%:
- Cardiovascular: Hypotension (13%)
- Miscellaneous: Withdrawal syndrome (12%)

1% to 10%:
- Dermatologic: Cellulitis (5%)
- Endocrine & metabolic: Hyperglycemia (8%)
- Genitourinary: Hematuria (8%)
- Respiratory: Stridor (5%)
- Miscellaneous: Sepsis (7%), infection (6%)

Atelectasis occurred in 9% of patients receiving placebo and in 9% of those receiving inhaled nitric oxide.

Pharmacodynamics/Kinetics

Absorption: Systemic after inhalation

Metabolism: Nitric oxide combines with hemoglobin that is 60% to 100% oxygenated. Nitric oxide combines with oxyhemoglobin to produce methemoglobin and nitrate. Within the pulmonary system, nitric oxide can combine with oxygen and water to produce nitrogen dioxide and nitrite respectively, which interact with oxyhemoglobin to then produce methemoglobin and nitrate. At 80 ppm the methemoglobin percent is ~5% after 8 hours of administration. Methemoglobin levels >7% were attained only in patients receiving 80 ppm.

Excretion: Urine (as nitrate)
- Clearance: Nitrate: At a rate approaching the glomerular filtration rate

Pregnancy Risk Factor C

Generic Available No

Nitro-Bid® *see* Nitroglycerin *on page 981*

Nitro-Dur® *see* Nitroglycerin *on page 981*

Nitrofurantoin (nye troe fyoor AN toin)

U.S. Brand Names Furadantin®; Macrobid®; Macrodantin®

Canadian Brand Names Apo®-Nitrofurantoin; MacroBID®; Macrodantin®; Novo-Furantoin

Mexican Brand Names Furadantina; Macrodantina®

Pharmacologic Category Antibiotic, Miscellaneous

Use Prevention and treatment of urinary tract infections caused by susceptible gram-negative and some gram-positive organisms; *Pseudomonas*, *Serratia*, and most species of *Proteus* are generally resistant to nitrofurantoin

Local Anesthetic/Vasoconstrictor Precautions No information available to require special precautions

Effects on Dental Treatment No significant effects or complications reported

Dosage Oral:

Children >1 month: 5-7 mg/kg/day in divided doses every 6 hours; maximum: 400 mg/day
- Chronic therapy: 1-2 mg/kg/day in divided doses every 12-24 hours; maximum dose: 100 mg/day

Adults: 50-100 mg/dose every 6 hours
- Macrocrystal/monohydrate: 100 mg twice daily
- Prophylaxis or chronic therapy: 50-100 mg/dose at bedtime

Dosing adjustment in renal impairment: Cl_{cr} <50 mL/minute: Avoid use

Avoid use in hemo and peritoneal dialysis and continuous arteriovenous or venovenous hemofiltration

Mechanism of Action Inhibits several bacterial enzyme systems including acetyl coenzyme A interfering with metabolism and possibly cell wall synthesis

Other Adverse Effects Frequency not defined:
- Cardiovascular: Chest pains
- Central nervous system: Chills, dizziness, drowsiness, fatigue, fever, headache
- Dermatologic: Exfoliative dermatitis, itching, rash
- Gastrointestinal: *C. difficile*-colitis, diarrhea, loss of appetite/vomiting/nausea (most common), sore throat, stomach upset
- Hematologic: Hemolytic anemia
- Hepatic: Hepatitis, increased LFTs
- Neuromuscular & skeletal: Arthralgia, numbness, paresthesia, weakness
- Respiratory: Cough, dyspnea, pneumonitis, pulmonary fibrosis
- Miscellaneous: Hypersensitivity, lupus-like syndrome

Drug Interactions

Increased Effect/Toxicity: Probenecid decreases renal excretion of nitrofurantoin.

Decreased Effect: Antacids decrease absorption of nitrofurantoin.

Dietary/Ethanol/Herb Considerations

Ethanol: Avoid use; may increase CNS depression.

Food may increase serum concentration.

Herb/Nutraceutical: Avoid gotu kola, kava, SAMe, St John's wort, and valerian; may increase CNS depression.

Pharmacodynamics/Kinetics

Absorption: Well absorbed; macrocrystalline form absorbed more slowly due to slower dissolution (causes less GI distress)

Distribution: V_d: 0.8 L/kg; crosses placenta; enters breast milk

Protein binding: ~40%

Metabolism: Body tissues (except plasma) metabolize 60% of drug to inactive metabolites

Bioavailability: Increased with food

Half-life elimination: 20-60 minutes; prolonged with renal impairment

Excretion: Urine (40%) and feces (small amounts) as metabolites and unchanged drug

Pregnancy Risk Factor B

Generic Available Yes: Capsule, macrocrystal

Nitrogard® *see* Nitroglycerin *on page 981*

Nitroglycerin (nye troe GLI ser in)

Related Information

Cardiovascular Diseases *on page 1456*

Dental Office Emergencies *on page 1582*

U.S. Brand Names Deponit® [DSC]; Minitran™; Nitrek®; Nitro-Bid®; Nitro-Dur®; Nitrogard®; Nitrol®; Nitrolingual®; NitroQuick®; Nitrostat®; Nitro-Tab®; NitroTime®

Canadian Brand Names Gen-Nitro; Minitran™; Nitro-Dur®; Nitrol®; Nitrostat™; Rho-Nitro; Transderm-Nitro®

Mexican Brand Names Anglix®; Cardinit®; Minitran®; Nitradisc®; Nitroderm TTS®; Nitro-Dur®

Pharmacologic Category Vasodilator

Synonyms Deponit® [DSC]; Glyceryl Trinitrate; Nitroglycerol; NTG

Use Treatment of angina pectoris; I.V. for CHF (especially when associated with acute MI); pulmonary hypertension; hypertensive emergencies occurring perioperatively (especially during cardiovascular surgery)

Local Anesthetic/Vasoconstrictor Precautions No information available to require special precautions

Effects on Dental Treatment No significant effects or complications reported

Dosage Note: Hemodynamic and antianginal tolerance often develop within 24-48 hours of continuous nitrate administration

Children: Pulmonary hypertension: Continuous infusion: Start 0.25-0.5 mcg/kg/minute and titrate by 1 mcg/kg/minute at 20- to 60-minute intervals to desired effect; usual dose: 1-3 mcg/kg/minute; maximum: 5 mcg/kg/minute

Adults:

Buccal: Initial: 1 mg every 3-5 hours while awake (3 times/day); titrate dosage upward if angina occurs with tablet in place

Oral: 2.5-9 mg 2-4 times/day (up to 26 mg 4 times/day)

I.V.: 5 mcg/minute, increase by 5 mcg/minute every 3-5 minutes to 20 mcg/minute; if no response at 20 mcg/minute increase by 10 mcg/minute every 3-5 minutes, up to 200 mcg/minute

Ointment: ½" upon rising and ½" 6 hours later; the dose may be doubled and even doubled again as needed

Patch, transdermal: Initial: 0.2-0.4 mg/hour, titrate to doses of 0.4-0.8 mg/hour; tolerance is minimized by using a patch-on period of 12-14 hours and patch-off period of 10-12 hours

Sublingual: 0.2-0.6 mg every 5 minutes for maximum of 3 doses in 15 minutes; may also use prophylactically 5-10 minutes prior to activities which may provoke an attack

Translingual: 1-2 sprays into mouth under tongue every 3-5 minutes for maximum of 3 doses in 15 minutes, may also be used 5-10 minutes prior to activities which may provoke an attack prophylactically

Hemodialysis: Supplemental dose is unnecessary

Peritoneal dialysis: Supplemental dose is unnecessary

May need to use nitrate-free interval (10-12 hours/day) to avoid tolerance development; gradually decrease dose in patients receiving NTG for prolonged period to avoid withdrawal reaction

Elderly: In general, dose selection should be cautious, usually starting at the low end of the dosing range

Mechanism of Action Reduces cardiac oxygen demand by decreasing left ventricular pressure and systemic vascular resistance; dilates coronary arteries and improves collateral flow to ischemic regions

Other Adverse Effects

Spray or patch:

>10%: Central nervous system: Headache (patch 63%, spray 50%)

(Continued)

Nitroglycerin *(Continued)*

1% to 10%:

Cardiovascular: Hypotension (patch 4%), increased angina (patch 2%)

Central nervous system: Lightheadedness (patch 6%), syncope (patch 4%)

<1% (Limited to important or life-threatening): Allergic reactions, application site irritation (patch), rash, dizziness, weakness, restlessness, pallor, perspiration, collapse, exfoliative dermatitis, vertigo, palpitations, methemoglobinemia (rare, overdose)

Topical, sublingual, intravenous: Frequency not defined:

Cardiovascular: Hypotension (infrequent), postural hypotension, crescendo angina (uncommon), rebound hypertension (uncommon), pallor, cardiovascular collapse, tachycardia, shock, flushing, peripheral edema

Central nervous system: Headache (most common), lightheadedness (related to blood pressure changes), syncope (uncommon), dizziness, restlessness

Gastrointestinal: Nausea, vomiting, bowel incontinence, xerostomia

Genitourinary: Urinary incontinence

Hematologic: Methemoglobinemia (rare, overdose)

Neuromuscular & skeletal: Weakness

Ocular: Blurred vision

Miscellaneous: Cold sweat

The incidence of hypotension and adverse cardiovascular events may be increased when used in combination with sildenafil (Viagra®).

Drug Interactions

Increased Effect/Toxicity: Has been associated with severe reactions and death when sildenafil is given concurrently with nitrites. Ethanol can cause hypotension when nitrates are taken 1 hour or more after ethanol ingestion.

Decreased Effect: I.V. nitroglycerin may antagonize the anticoagulant effect of heparin (possibly only at high nitroglycerin dosages); monitor closely. May need to decrease heparin dosage when nitroglycerin is discontinued. Alteplase (tissue plasminogen activator) has a lesser effect when used with I.V. nitroglycerin; avoid concurrent use. Ergot alkaloids may cause an increase in blood pressure and decrease in antianginal effects; avoid concurrent use.

Dietary/Ethanol/Herb Considerations

Ethanol: Avoid use; may cause hypotension within 1 hour of coadministration.

Food: Avoid caffeine (eg, colas, chocolate), garlic, and licorice.

Herb/Nutraceutical: Avoid black cohosh, dong quai, and evening primrose due to estrogenic activity. Avoid ephedra, ginseng, and yohimbe; may cause arrhythmias or hypertension. Avoid garlic; may have increased antihypertensive effect. Avoid ginger due to positive inotropic effects; theoretically, may cause arrhythmia. Avoid hawthorn; may decrease peripheral vascular resistance and cause additional decrease in BP. Avoid licorice.

Pharmacodynamics/Kinetics

Onset of action: Sublingual tablet: 1-3 minutes; Translingual spray: 2 minutes; Buccal tablet: 2-5 minutes; Sustained release: 20-45 minutes; Topical: 15-60 minutes; Transdermal: 40-60 minutes; I.V. drip: Immediate

Peak effect: Sublingual tablet: 4-8 minutes; Translingual spray: 4-10 minutes; Buccal tablet: 4-10 minutes; Sustained release: 45-120 minutes; Topical: 30-120 minutes; Transdermal: 60-180 minutes; I.V. drip: Immediate

Duration: Sublingual tablet: 30-60 minutes; Translingual spray: 30-60 minutes; Buccal tablet: 2 hours; Sustained release: 4-8 hours; Topical: 2-12 hours; Transdermal: 18-24 hours; I.V. drip: 3-5 minutes

Protein binding: 60%

Metabolism: Extensive first-pass effect

Half-life elimination: 1-4 minutes

Excretion: Urine (as inactive metabolites)

Pregnancy Risk Factor C

Generic Available Yes: Capsule, injection, patch, tablet

Nitroglycerol *see* Nitroglycerin *on page 981*

Nitrol® *see* Nitroglycerin *on page 981*

Nitrolingual® *see* Nitroglycerin *on page 981*

Nitropress® *see* Nitroprusside *on page 982*

Nitroprusside (nye troe PRUS ide)

U.S. Brand Names Nitropress®

Canadian Brand Names Nipride®

Pharmacologic Category Vasodilator

Synonyms Nitroprusside Sodium; Sodium Nitroferricyanide; Sodium Nitroprusside

Use Management of hypertensive crises; CHF; used for controlled hypotension to reduce bleeding during surgery

Local Anesthetic/Vasoconstrictor Precautions No information available to require special precautions

Effects on Dental Treatment No significant effects or complications reported

Dosage Administration requires the use of an infusion pump. Average dose: 5 mcg/kg/minute.

Children: Pulmonary hypertension: I.V.: Initial: 1 mcg/kg/minute by continuous I.V. infusion; increase in increments of 1 mcg/kg/minute at intervals of 20-60 minutes; titrating to the desired response; usual dose: 3 mcg/kg/minute, rarely need >4 mcg/kg/minute; maximum: 5 mcg/kg/minute.

Adults: I.V. Initial: 0.3-0.5 mcg/kg/minute; increase in increments of 0.5 mcg/kg/minute, titrating to the desired hemodynamic effect or the appearance of headache or nausea; usual dose: 3 mcg/kg/minute; rarely need >4 mcg/kg/minute; maximum: 10 mcg/kg/minute. When administered by prolonged infusion faster than 2 mcg/kg/minute, cyanide is generated faster than an unaided patient can handle.

Mechanism of Action Causes peripheral vasodilation by direct action on venous and arteriolar smooth muscle, thus reducing peripheral resistance; will increase cardiac output by decreasing afterload; reduces aortal and left ventricular impedance

Other Adverse Effects 1% to 10%:

Cardiovascular: Excessive hypotensive response, palpitations, substernal distress
Central nervous system: Disorientation, psychosis, headache, restlessness
Endocrine & metabolic: Thyroid suppression
Gastrointestinal: Nausea, vomiting
Neuromuscular & skeletal: Weakness, muscle spasm
Otic: Tinnitus
Respiratory: Hypoxia
Miscellaneous: Diaphoresis, thiocyanate toxicity

Pharmacodynamics/Kinetics

Onset of action: BP reduction <2 minutes
Duration: 1-10 minutes
Metabolism: Nitroprusside is converted to cyanide ions in the bloodstream; decomposes to prussic acid which in the presence of sulfur donor is converted to thiocyanate (hepatic and renal rhodanase systems)
Half-life elimination: Parent drug: <10 minutes; Thiocyanate: 2.7-7 days
Excretion: Urine (as thiocyanate)

Pregnancy Risk Factor C

Generic Available Yes: Solution

Nitroprusside Sodium *see* Nitroprusside *on page 982*
NitroQuick® *see* Nitroglycerin *on page 981*
Nitrostat® *see* Nitroglycerin *on page 981*
Nitro-Tab® *see* Nitroglycerin *on page 981*
NitroTime® *see* Nitroglycerin *on page 981*

Nitrous Oxide (NYE trus OKS ide)

Related Information

Patients Requiring Sedation *on page 1565*

Pharmacologic Category Dental Gases; General Anesthetic

Use

Dental: To induce sedation and analgesia in anxious dental patients

Medical: Produces sedation and analgesia; principal adjunct to inhalation and intravenous general anesthesia

Local Anesthetic/Vasoconstrictor Precautions No information available to require special precautions

Effects on Dental Treatment No significant effects or complications reported

Dosage Children and Adults:

Sedation and analgesia for dental procedure: Concentrations of 25% to 50% nitrous oxide with oxygen

Sedation and analgesia for surgical procedure: Concentrations of 25% to 50% nitrous oxide with oxygen. For general anesthesia, concentrations of 40% to 70% via mask or endotracheal tube. Minimal alveolar concentration (MAC), which can be considered the ED_{50} of inhalational anesthetics, is 105%; therefore delivery in a hyperbaric chamber is necessary to use as a complete anesthetic. When administered at 70%, reduces the MAC of other anesthetics by half.

Mechanism of Action General CNS depressant action; may act similarly as inhalant general anesthetics by stabilizing axonal membranes to partially inhibit action potentials leading to sedation; may partially act on opiate receptor systems to cause mild analgesia; central sympathetic stimulating action supports blood pressure, systemic vascular resistance, and cardiac output; it does not depress carbon dioxide drive to breath. Nitrous oxide increases cerebral blood flow and intracranial pressure while decreasing hepatic and renal blood flow; has analgesic action similar to morphine.

Other Adverse Effects Methionine synthase, a vitamin B_{12} dependent enzyme, is inactivated following prolonged administration of nitrous oxide, and the subsequent interference with DNA synthesis prevents production of both leukocytes and red blood cells by bone marrow **(does not occur within the time frame of clinical use).**

(Continued)

Nitrous Oxide *(Continued)*

Contraindications Hypersensitivity to nitrous oxide or any component of the formulation; nitrous oxide should not be administered without oxygen; should not be given to patients after a full meal

Warnings/Precautions Nausea and vomiting occurs postoperatively in ~15% of patients. Prolonged use may produce bone marrow suppression and/or neurologic dysfunction. Oxygen should be briefly administered during emergence from prolonged anesthesia with nitrous oxide to prevent diffusion hypoxia. Patients with vitamin B_{12} deficiency (pernicious anemia) and those with other nutritional deficiencies (alcoholics) are at increased risk of developing neurologic disease and bone marrow suppression with exposure to nitrous oxide. May be addictive.

Pharmacodynamics/Kinetics
Onset of action: Inhalation: 2-5 minutes
Absorption: Rapid via lungs; blood/gas partition coefficient is 0.47
Metabolism: Body: <0.004%
Excretion: Primarily exhaled gases; skin (minimal amounts)

Pregnancy Risk Factor No data reported

Dosage Forms Supplied in blue cylinders

Generic Available Yes

Comments An increased risk of renal and hepatic diseases and peripheral neuropathy similar to that of vitamin B_{12} deficiency have been reported in dental personnel who work in areas where nitrous oxide is frequently used without an enclosed gas scavenging system. Female dental personnel who were exposed to unscavenged nitrous oxide for more than 5 hours/week were significantly less fertile than women who were not exposed, or who were exposed to lower levels of scavenged or unscavenged nitrous oxide. Fertility was measured by the number of menstrual cycles, without use of contraception, required to become pregnant. Women who were exposed to nitrous oxide for more than 5 hours/week were only 41% as likely as unexposed women to conceive during each monthly cycle.

Nix® [OTC] *see* Permethrin *on page 1062*

Nizatidine (ni ZA ti deen)

Related Information
Gastrointestinal Disorders *on page 1474*

U.S. Brand Names Axid®; Axid® AR [OTC]

Canadian Brand Names Apo®-Nizatidine; Axid®; Novo-Nizatidine; PMS-Nizatidine

Mexican Brand Names Axid®

Pharmacologic Category Histamine H_2 Antagonist

Use Treatment and maintenance of duodenal ulcer; treatment of benign gastric ulcer; treatment of gastroesophageal reflux disease (GERD); OTC tablet used for the prevention of meal-induced heartburn, acid indigestion, and sour stomach

Unlabeled/Investigational Use Part of a multidrug regimen for *H. pylori* eradication to reduce the risk of duodenal ulcer recurrence

Local Anesthetic/Vasoconstrictor Precautions No information available to require special precautions

Effects on Dental Treatment
>10%: Headache (16%)
1% to 10%: Dizziness, somnolence, nervousness, anxiety, nausea, vomiting, xerostomia

Dosage Adults: Oral:
Active duodenal ulcer:
Treatment: 300 mg at bedtime or 150 mg twice daily
Maintenance: 150 mg/day
Gastric ulcer: 150 mg twice daily or 300 mg at bedtime
GERD: 150 mg twice daily
Meal-induced heartburn, acid indigestion, and sour stomach: 75 mg tablet [OTC] twice daily, 30 to 60 minutes prior to consuming food or beverages
Helicobacter pylori eradication (unlabeled use): 150 mg twice daily; requires combination therapy
Dosing adjustment in renal impairment:
Cl_{cr} 50-80 mL/minute: Administer 75% of normal dose
Cl_{cr} 10-50 mL/minute: Administer 50% of normal dose or 150 mg/day for active treatment and 150 mg every other day for maintenance treatment
Cl_{cr} <10 mL/minute: Administer 25% of normal dose or 150 mg every other day for treatment and 150 mg every 3 days for maintenance treatment

Mechanism of Action Nizatidine is an H_2-receptor antagonist. In healthy volunteers, nizatidine has been effective in suppressing gastric acid secretion induced by pentagastrin infusion or food. Nizatidine reduces gastric acid secretion by 30% to 78%. This compares with a 60% reduction by cimetidine. Nizatidine 100 mg is reported to provide equivalent acid suppression as cimetidine 300 mg.

Other Adverse Effects
1% to 10%:
Central nervous system: Insomnia
Dermatologic: Rash, pruritus

Gastrointestinal: Abdominal pain, constipation, diarrhea, flatulence, heartburn, anorexia

<1% (Limited to important or life-threatening): **Ventricular tachycardia,** anemia, eosinophilia, thrombocytopenic purpura, elevated AST or ALT, elevated alkaline phosphatase, hepatitis, jaundice, **bronchospasm, laryngeal edema**

Drug Interactions

Decreased Effect: May decrease the absorption of itraconazole or ketoconazole.

Dietary/Ethanol/Herb Considerations Ethanol: Avoid use; may cause gastric mucosal irritation.

Pharmacodynamics/Kinetics

Distribution: V_d: 0.8-1.5 L/kg

Protein binding: 35% to α_1-acid glycoprotein

Metabolism: Partially hepatic

Bioavailability: >70%

Half-life elimination: 1-2 hours; prolonged with renal impairment

Time to peak, plasma: 0.5-3.0 hours

Excretion: Urine (~60% as unchanged drug); feces (<6%)

Pregnancy Risk Factor C

Generic Available Yes: Capsule

Nizoral® *see* Ketoconazole *on page 762*

Nizoral® A-D [OTC] *see* Ketoconazole *on page 762*

N-Methylhydrazine *see* Procarbazine *on page 1122*

Nolahist® [OTC] *see* Phenindamine *on page 1066*

Nolvadex® *see* Tamoxifen *on page 1264*

Nonoxynol 9 (non OKS i nole nine)

U.S. Brand Names Advantage-S™ [OTC]; Aqua Lube Plus [OTC]; Conceptrol® [OTC]; Delfen® [OTC]; Emko® [OTC]; Encare® [OTC]; Gynol II® [OTC]; Semicid® [OTC]; Shur-Seal® [OTC]; VCF™ [OTC]

Canadian Brand Names Advantage 24™

Pharmacologic Category Spermicide

Use Spermatocide in contraception

Local Anesthetic/Vasoconstrictor Precautions No information available to require special precautions

Effects on Dental Treatment No significant effects or complications reported

Dosage Insert into vagina at least 10 minutes before intercourse (but not longer than 1 hour); refer to specific product labeling

Other Adverse Effects Frequency not defined: Genitourinary: Irritation of mucous membranes (including vaginal/urethral)

Pregnancy Risk Factor C

Generic Available No

No Pain-HP® [OTC] *see* Capsaicin *on page 238*

Noradrenaline *see* Norepinephrine *on page 985*

Noradrenaline Acid Tartrate *see* Norepinephrine *on page 985*

Norco® *see* Hydrocodone and Acetaminophen *on page 678*

Nordeoxyguanosine *see* Ganciclovir *on page 626*

Nordette® *see* Combination Hormonal Contraceptives *on page 368*

Norditropin® *see* Human Growth Hormone *on page 671*

Norditropin® Cartridges *see* Human Growth Hormone *on page 671*

Norepinephrine (nor ep i NEF rin)

U.S. Brand Names Levophed®

Canadian Brand Names Levophed®

Pharmacologic Category Alpha/Beta Agonist

Synonyms Levarterenol Bitartrate; Noradrenaline; Noradrenaline Acid Tartrate; Norepinephrine Bitartrate

Use Treatment of shock which persists after adequate fluid volume replacement

Local Anesthetic/Vasoconstrictor Precautions No information available to require special precautions

Effects on Dental Treatment No significant effects or complications reported

Dosage Administration requires the use of an infusion pump!

Note: Norepinephrine dosage is stated in terms of norepinephrine base and intravenous formulation is norepinephrine bitartrate

Norepinephrine bitartrate 2 mg = Norepinephrine base 1 mg

Continuous I.V. infusion:

Children: Initial: 0.05-0.1 mcg/kg/minute; titrate to desired effect; maximum dose: 1-2 mcg/kg/minute

Adults: Initial: 0.5-1 mcg/minute and titrate to desired response; 8-30 mcg/minute is usual range; range used in clinical trials: 0.01-3 mcg/kg/minute; ACLS dosage range: 0.5-30 mcg/minute

Mechanism of Action Stimulates $beta_1$-adrenergic receptors and alpha-adrenergic receptors causing increased contractility and heart rate as well as vasoconstriction, (Continued)

Norepinephrine *(Continued)*

thereby increasing systemic blood pressure and coronary blood flow; clinically alpha effects (vasoconstriction) are greater than beta effects (inotropic and chronotropic effects)

Other Adverse Effects Frequency not defined:

Cardiovascular: Bradycardia, arrhythmias, peripheral (digital) ischemia
Central nervous system: Headache (transient), anxiety
Local: Skin necrosis (with extravasation)
Respiratory: Dyspnea, respiratory difficulty

Drug Interactions

Increased Effect/Toxicity: The effects of norepinephrine may be increased by tricyclic antidepressants, MAO inhibitors, antihistamines (diphenhydramine, tripelennamine), beta-blockers (nonselective), guanethidine, ergot alkaloids, reserpine, and methyldopa. Atropine sulfate may block the reflex bradycardia caused by norepinephrine and enhances the vasopressor response.

Decreased Effect: Alpha-blockers may blunt response to norepinephrine.

Pharmacodynamics/Kinetics

Onset of action: I.V.: Very rapid-acting
Duration: Limited
Metabolism: Via catechol-o-methyltransferase (COMT) and monoamine oxidase (MAO)
Excretion: Urine (84% to 96% as inactive metabolites)

Pregnancy Risk Factor C

Generic Available No

Selected Readings Martin C, Papazian L, Perrin G, et al, "Norepinephrine or Dopamine for the Treatment of Hyperdynamic Septic Shock?" *Chest*, 1993, 103(6):1826-31.

Norepinephrine Bitartrate *see* Norepinephrine *on page 985*

Norethindrone (nor eth IN drone)

Related Information

Endocrine Disorders and Pregnancy *on page 1479*

U.S. Brand Names Aygestin®; Camila™; Errin™; Micronor®; Nor-QD®

Canadian Brand Names Micronor®; Norlutate®

Mexican Brand Names Syngestal

Pharmacologic Category Contraceptive; Progestin

Synonyms Norethindrone Acetate; Norethisterone

Use Treatment of amenorrhea; abnormal uterine bleeding; endometriosis, oral contraceptive; **higher rate of failure with progestin only contraceptives**

Local Anesthetic/Vasoconstrictor Precautions No information available to require special precautions

Effects on Dental Treatment Until we know more about the mechanism of interaction, caution is required in prescribing antibiotics to female dental patients taking progestin-only hormonal contraceptives.

Dosage Oral: Adolescents and Adults: Female:

Contraception: Progesterone only: Norethindrone 0.35 mg every day of the year starting on first day of menstruation; if one dose is missed, discontinue and use an alternative method of contraception

Amenorrhea and abnormal uterine bleeding:

Norethindrone: 5-20 mg/day for 5-10 days during the second half of the menstrual cycle

Acetate salt: 2.5-10 mg/day for 5-10 days during the second half of the menstrual cycle

Endometriosis:

Norethindrone: 10 mg/day for 2 weeks; increase at increments of 5 mg/day every 2 weeks until 30 mg/day; continue for 6-9 months or until breakthrough bleeding demands temporary termination

Acetate salt: 5 mg/day for 14 days; increase at increments of 2.5 mg/day every 2 weeks up to 15 mg/day; continue for 6-9 months or until breakthrough bleeding demands temporary termination

Mechanism of Action Inhibits secretion of pituitary gonadotropin (LH) which prevents follicular maturation and ovulation

Other Adverse Effects

>10%:

Cardiovascular: Edema
Endocrine & metabolic: Breakthrough bleeding, spotting, changes in menstrual flow, amenorrhea
Gastrointestinal: Anorexia
Local: Pain at injection site
Neuromuscular & skeletal: Weakness

1% to 10%:

Cardiovascular: Edema
Central nervous system: Mental depression, fever, insomnia

Dermatologic: Melasma or chloasma, allergic rash with or without pruritus
Endocrine & metabolic: Increased breast tenderness
Gastrointestinal: Weight gain/loss
Genitourinary: Changes in cervical erosion and secretions
Hepatic: Cholestatic jaundice

Drug Interactions Substrate of **CYP3A4**; Induces CYP2C19

Decreased Effect: Rifampin (potentially other enzyme inducers) and nelfinavir decrease the pharmacologic effect of norethindrone.

Dietary/Ethanol/Herb Considerations

Food: Limit caffeine.

Herb/Nutraceutical: High-dose vitamin C (1 g/day) may increase adverse effects. Avoid St John's wort.

Pharmacodynamics/Kinetics

Absorption: Oral, transdermal: Rapidly absorbed
Distribution: V_d: 2-4 L/kg
Protein binding: 61% to albumin; 36% to sex-hormone-binding globulin (SHBG); SHBG capacity affected by plasma ethinyl estradiol levels
Metabolism: Oral: Hepatic via reduction and conjugation; first-pass effect
Bioavailability: 64%
Half-life elimination: 5-14 hours
Time to peak: 1-2 hours
Excretion: Primarily urine (as metabolites)

Pregnancy Risk Factor X

Generic Available Yes

Norethindrone Acetate *see* Norethindrone *on page 986*
Norethindrone and Estradiol *see* Estradiol and Norethindrone *on page 525*
Norethindrone and Mestranol *see* Mestranol and Norethindrone *on page 871*
Norethisterone *see* Norethindrone *on page 986*
Norflex™ *see* Orphenadrine *on page 1005*

Norfloxacin (nor FLOKS a sin)

Related Information

Sexually-Transmitted Diseases *on page 1502*

U.S. Brand Names Noroxin®

Canadian Brand Names Apo®-Norflox; Norfloxacine®; Novo-Norfloxacin; PMS-Norfloxacin; Riva-Norfloxacin

Mexican Brand Names Difoxacil®; Floxacin®; Noroxin®; Oranor®

Pharmacologic Category Antibiotic, Quinolone

Use Uncomplicated urinary tract infections and cystitis caused by susceptible gram-negative and gram-positive bacteria; sexually-transmitted disease (eg, uncomplicated urethral and cervical gonorrhea) caused by *N. gonorrhoeae*; prostatitis due to *E. coli*

Local Anesthetic/Vasoconstrictor Precautions No information available to require special precautions

Effects on Dental Treatment No significant effects or complications reported

Dosage Oral: Adults:

Urinary tract infections: 400 mg twice daily for 3-21 days depending on severity of infection or organism sensitivity; maximum: 800 mg/day

Uncomplicated gonorrhea: 800 mg as a single dose (CDC recommends as an alternative regimen to ciprofloxacin or ofloxacin)

Prostatitis: 400 mg every 12 hours for 4 weeks

Dosing interval in renal impairment: Cl_{cr} 10-30 mL/minute: Urinary tract infections: Administer 400 mg every 24 hours

Mechanism of Action Norfloxacin is a DNA gyrase inhibitor. DNA gyrase is an essential bacterial enzyme that maintains the superhelical structure of DNA. DNA gyrase is required for DNA replication and transcription, DNA repair, recombination, and transposition; bactericidal

Other Adverse Effects

1% to 10%:

Central nervous system: Headache (3%), dizziness (3%)
Gastrointestinal: Nausea (4%)
Neuromuscular & skeletal: Weakness (1%)

<1%, postmarketing, and/or case reports: Abdominal pain, acute renal failure, anaphylactoid reactions, angioedema, anorexia, anxiety, arthralgia, arthritis, ataxia, back pain, bitter taste, cholestatic jaundice, confusion, constipation, depression, diarrhea, diplopia, dysgeusia, dyspepsia, dyspnea, erythema multiforme, erythema, exacerbation of myasthenia gravis, exfoliative dermatitis, fever, flatulence, GI bleeding, Guillain-Barré syndrome, heartburn, hemolytic anemia (sometimes associated with G6PD deficiency), hepatitis, hyperhidrosis, increased serum creatinine/BUN, increased transaminases, insomnia, jaundice, leukopenia, loose stools, myalgia, myoclonus, neutropenia, pancreatitis, paresthesias, peripheral neuropathy, photosensitivity, pruritus, pseudomembraneous colitis, psychotic

(Continued)

Norfloxacin *(Continued)*

reactions, rash, seizures, somnolence, Stevens-Johnson syndrome, thrombocytopenia, tinnitus, toxic epidermal necrolysis, transient hearing loss, tremor, urticaria, vasculitis, vomiting, weakness, xerostomia; quinolones have been associated with tendonitis and tendon rupture

Drug Interactions Inhibits **CYP1A2**, 3A4

Increased Effect/Toxicity: Quinolones cause increased levels of caffeine, warfarin, cyclosporine, and theophylline. Cimetidine and probenecid may increase norfloxacin serum levels. Concurrent use of corticosteroids may increase risk of tendon rupture.

Decreased Effect: Decreased absorption with antacids containing aluminum, magnesium, and/or calcium (by up to 98% if given at the same time); decreased serum levels of fluoroquinolones by antineoplastics; nitrofurantoin may antagonize effects of norfloxacin; phenytoin serum levels may be decreased by fluoroquinolones; didanosine (chewable/buffered or pediatric powder) may decrease quinolone absorption

Dietary/Ethanol/Herb Considerations

Food: Dairy products may decrease average peak serum concentration. Administer oral forms on an empty stomach.

Herb/Nutraceutical: Avoid dong quai and St John's wort; may cause photosensitization.

Pharmacodynamics/Kinetics

Absorption: Oral: Rapid, up to 40%

Distribution: Crosses placenta; small amounts enter breast milk

Protein binding: 15%

Metabolism: Hepatic

Half-life elimination: 3-4 hours; Renal impairment (Cl_{cr} ≤30 mL/minute): 6.5 hours; Elderly: 4 hours

Time to peak, serum: 1-2 hours

Excretion: Urine (26% to 36%); feces (30%)

Pregnancy Risk Factor C

Generic Available No

Norgesic™ *see* Orphenadrine, Aspirin, and Caffeine *on page 1005*

Norgesic™ Forte *see* Orphenadrine, Aspirin, and Caffeine *on page 1005*

Norgestimate and Estradiol *see* Estradiol and Norgestimate *on page 526*

Norgestrel (nor JES trel)

Related Information

Endocrine Disorders and Pregnancy *on page 1479*

U.S. Brand Names Ovrette®

Canadian Brand Names Ovrette®

Pharmacologic Category Contraceptive

Use Prevention of pregnancy; **progestin only products have higher risk of failure in contraceptive use**

Local Anesthetic/Vasoconstrictor Precautions No information available to require special precautions

Effects on Dental Treatment Until we know more about the mechanism of interaction, caution is required in prescribing antibiotics to female dental patients taking progestin-only hormonal contraceptives.

Dosage Oral: Administer daily, starting the first day of menstruation, take 1 tablet at the same time each day, every day of the year. If one dose is missed, take as soon as remembered, then next tablet at regular time; if two doses are missed, take 1 tablet as soon as it is remembered, followed by an additional dose that same day at the usual time. When one or two doses are missed, additional contraceptive measures should be used until 14 consecutive tablets have been taken. If three doses are missed, discontinue norgestrel and use an additional form of birth control until menses or pregnancy is ruled out.

Mechanism of Action Inhibits secretion of pituitary gonadotropin (LH) which prevents follicular maturation and ovulation

Other Adverse Effects Frequency not defined:

Cardiovascular: Embolism, cerebral thrombosis, edema

Central nervous system: Mental depression, fever, insomnia

Dermatologic: Melasma or chloasma, allergic rash with or without pruritus

Endocrine & metabolic: Breakthrough bleeding, spotting, changes in menstrual flow, amenorrhea, changes in cervical erosion and secretions, increased breast tenderness

Gastrointestinal: Weight gain/loss, anorexia

Hepatic: Cholestatic jaundice

Local: Thrombophlebitis

Neuromuscular & skeletal: Weakness

Drug Interactions Substrate of **CYP3A4**

Increased Effect/Toxicity: Oral contraceptives may increase toxicity of acetaminophen, anticoagulants, benzodiazepines, caffeine, corticosteroids, metoprolol, theophylline, and tricyclic antidepressants.

Decreased Effect: Azole antifungals (ketoconazole, itraconazole, fluconazole), barbiturates, hydantoins (phenytoin), carbamazepine, and rifampin decrease oral contraceptive efficacy due to increased metabolism. Antibiotics (penicillins, tetracyclines, griseofulvin) may decrease efficacy of oral contraceptives.

Dietary/Ethanol/Herb Considerations

Food: CNS effects of caffeine may be enhanced.

Herb/Nutraceutical: Avoid St John's wort; may decrease serum concentration. Avoid black cohosh, dong quai, and evening primrose due to estrogenic activity. Avoid ginseng, red clover, and saw palmetto due to potential hormonal effect.

Pharmacodynamics/Kinetics

Absorption: Oral: Well absorbed

Protein binding: >97% to sex-hormone-binding globulin

Metabolism: Primarily hepatic via reduction and conjugation

Half-life elimination: ~20 hours

Excretion: Urine (as metabolites)

Pregnancy Risk Factor X

Generic Available No

Norinyl® 1+35 *see* Combination Hormonal Contraceptives *on page 368*

Norinyl® 1+50 *see* Mestranol and Norethindrone *on page 871*

Noritate™ *see* Metronidazole *on page 902*

Normal Saline *see* Sodium Chloride *on page 1229*

Normodyne® *see* Labetalol *on page 769*

Noroxin® *see* Norfloxacin *on page 987*

Norpace® *see* Disopyramide *on page 458*

Norpace® CR *see* Disopyramide *on page 458*

Norplant® Implant [DSC] *see* Levonorgestrel *on page 797*

Norpramin® *see* Desipramine *on page 408*

Nor-QD® *see* Norethindrone *on page 986*

Nortrel™ *see* Combination Hormonal Contraceptives *on page 368*

Nortrel™ 7/7/7 *see* Combination Hormonal Contraceptives *on page 368*

Nortriptyline (nor TRIP ti leen)

U.S. Brand Names Aventyl® HCl; Pamelor®

Canadian Brand Names Alti-Nortriptyline; Apo®-Nortriptyline; Aventyl®; Gen-Nortriptyline; Norventyl; Novo-Nortriptyline; Nu-Nortriptyline; PMS-Nortriptyline

Pharmacologic Category Antidepressant, Tricyclic (Secondary Amine)

Synonyms Nortriptyline Hydrochloride

Use Treatment of symptoms of depression

Unlabeled/Investigational Use Treatment of chronic pain, anxiety disorders, enuresis, attention-deficit/hyperactivity disorder (ADHD)

Local Anesthetic/Vasoconstrictor Precautions Use with caution; epinephrine, norepinephrine and levonordefrin have been shown to have an increased pressor response in combination with TCAs

Effects on Dental Treatment >10%: Xerostomia

Long-term treatment with TCAs such as nortriptyline increases the risk of caries by reducing salivation and salivary buffer capacity.

Dosage Oral:

Nocturnal enuresis:

Children:

6-7 years (20-25 kg): 10 mg/day

8-11 years (25-35 kg): 10-20 mg/day

>11 years (35-54 kg): 25-35 mg/day

Depression or ADHD (unlabeled use):

Children 6-12 years: 1-3 mg/kg/day or 10-20 mg/day in 3-4 divided doses

Adolescents: 30-100 mg/day in divided doses

Depression:

Adults: 25 mg 3-4 times/day up to 150 mg/day

Elderly (**Note:** Nortriptyline is one of the best tolerated TCAs in the elderly)

Initial: 10-25 mg at bedtime

Dosage can be increased by 25 mg every 3 days for inpatients and weekly for outpatients if tolerated

Usual maintenance dose: 75 mg as a single bedtime dose or 2 divided doses; however, lower or higher doses may be required to stay within the therapeutic window

Dosing adjustment in hepatic impairment: Lower doses and slower titration dependent on individualization of dosage is recommended

Mechanism of Action Traditionally believed to increase the synaptic concentration of serotonin and/or norepinephrine in the central nervous system by inhibition of their reuptake by the presynaptic neuronal membrane. However, additional receptor effects have been found including desensitization of adenyl cyclase, down

(Continued)

Nortriptyline *(Continued)*

regulation of beta-adrenergic receptors, and down regulation of serotonin receptors.

Other Adverse Effects Frequency not defined:

Cardiovascular: Postural hypotension, arrhythmias, hypertension, heart block, tachycardia, palpitations, MI

Central nervous system: Confusion, delirium, hallucinations, restlessness, insomnia, disorientation, delusions, anxiety, agitation, panic, nightmares, hypomania, exacerbation of psychosis, incoordination, ataxia, extrapyramidal symptoms, seizures

Dermatologic: Alopecia, photosensitivity, rash, petechiae, urticaria, itching

Endocrine & metabolic: Sexual dysfunction, gynecomastia, breast enlargement, galactorrhea, increase or decrease in libido, increase in blood sugar, SIADH

Gastrointestinal: Constipation, vomiting, anorexia, diarrhea, abdominal cramps, black tongue, nausea, unpleasant taste, weight gain/loss

Genitourinary: Urinary retention, delayed micturition, impotence, testicular edema

Hematologic: Rarely agranulocytosis, eosinophilia, purpura, thrombocytopenia

Hepatic: Increased liver enzymes, cholestatic jaundice

Neuromuscular & skeletal: Tremor, numbness, tingling, paresthesias, peripheral neuropathy

Ocular: Blurred vision, eye pain, disturbances in accommodation, mydriasis

Otic: Tinnitus

Miscellaneous: Diaphoresis (excessive), allergic reactions

Drug Interactions Substrate of CYP1A2, 2C19, **2D6**, 3A4; Inhibits CYP2D6, 2E1

Increased Effect/Toxicity: Nortriptyline increases the effects of amphetamines, anticholinergics, other CNS depressants (sedatives, hypnotics, ethanol), chlorpropamide, tolazamide, and warfarin. When used with MAO inhibitors, hyperpyrexia, hypertension, tachycardia, confusion, seizures, and **deaths have been reported** (serotonin syndrome). Serotonin syndrome has also been reported with ritonavir (rare). The SSRIs (to varying degrees), cimetidine, grapefruit juice, indinavir, methylphenidate, ritonavir, quinidine, diltiazem, and verapamil inhibit the metabolism of TCAs and clinical toxicity may result. Use of lithium with a TCA may increase the risk for neurotoxicity. Phenothiazines may increase concentration of some TCAs and TCAs may increase concentration of phenothiazines. Pressor response to I.V. epinephrine, norepinephrine, and phenylephrine may be enhanced in patients receiving TCAs (**Note:** Effect is unlikely with epinephrine or levonordefrin dosages typically administered as infiltration in combination with local anesthetics). Combined use of beta-agonists or drugs which prolong QT_c (including quinidine, procainamide, disopyramide, cisapride, sparfloxacin, gatifloxacin, moxifloxacin) with TCAs may predispose patients to cardiac arrhythmias. Use with altretamine may cause orthostatic hypotension.

Decreased Effect: Carbamazepine, phenobarbital, and rifampin may increase the metabolism of nortriptyline resulting in decreased effect of nortriptyline. Nortriptyline inhibits the antihypertensive response to bethanidine, clonidine, debrisoquin, guanadrel, guanethidine, guanabenz, or guanfacine. Cholestyramine and colestipol may bind TCAs and reduce their absorption; monitor for altered response.

Dietary/Ethanol/Herb Considerations

Ethanol: Avoid use; may increase CNS depression.

Food: Avoid grapefruit products; may inhibit the metabolism of some TCAs and clinical toxicity may result.

Herb/Nutraceutical: Avoid gotu kola, kava, SAMe, St John's wort, tryptophan, and valerian; may increase risk of serotonin syndrome and/or excessive sedation.

Pharmacodynamics/Kinetics

Onset of action: Therapeutic: 1-3 weeks

Distribution: V_d: 21 L/kg

Protein binding: 93% to 95%

Metabolism: Primarily hepatic; extensive first-pass effect

Half-life elimination: 28-31 hours

Time to peak, serum: 7-8.5 hours

Excretion: Urine (as metabolites and small amounts of unchanged drug); feces (small amounts)

Pregnancy Risk Factor D

Generic Available Yes

Selected Readings

Friedlander AH, Mahler ME, "Major Depressive Disorder. Psychopathology, Medical Management, and Dental Implications," *J Am Dent Assoc*, 201, 132(5):629-38.

Ganzberg S, "Psychoactive Drugs," *ADA Guide to Dental Therapeutics*, 2nd ed, Chicago, IL: ADA Publishing, a Division of ADA Business Enterprises, Inc, 2000, 376-405.

Jastak JT and Yagiela JA, "Vasoconstrictors and Local Anesthesia: A Review and Rationale for Use," *J Am Dent Assoc*, 1983, 107(4):623-30.

Mitchell JR, "Guanethidine and Related Agents. III Antagonism by Drugs Which Inhibit the Norepinephrine Pump in Man," *J Clin Invest*, 1970, 49(8):1596-604.

Rundegren J, van Dijken J, Mörnstad H, et al, "Oral Conditions in Patients Receiving Long-Term Treatment With Cyclic Antidepressant Drugs," *Swed Dent J*, 1985, 9(2):55-64.

Yagiela JA, "Adverse Drug Interactions in Dental Practice: Interactions Associated With Vasoconstrictors. Part V of a Series," *J Am Dent Assoc*, 1999, 130(5):701-9.

Nortriptyline Hydrochloride *see* Nortriptyline *on page 989*
Norvasc® *see* Amlodipine *on page 87*
Norvir® *see* Ritonavir *on page 1188*
Nostril® [OTC] *see* Phenylephrine *on page 1071*
Nōstrilla® [OTC] *see* Oxymetazoline *on page 1022*
Novantrone® *see* Mitoxantrone *on page 923*
Novarel™ *see* Chorionic Gonadotropin (Human) *on page 320*
Novocain® *see* Procaine *on page 1121*
Novolin® 70/30 *see* Insulin Preparations *on page 723*
Novolin® L *see* Insulin Preparations *on page 723*
Novolin® N *see* Insulin Preparations *on page 723*
Novolin® R *see* Insulin Preparations *on page 723*
NovoLog® *see* Insulin Preparations *on page 723*
NovoLog® Mix 70/30 *see* Insulin Preparations *on page 723*
Novo-Seven® *see* Factor VIIa (Recombinant) *on page 554*
Novothyrox *see* Levothyroxine *on page 800*
NPH Iletin® II *see* Insulin Preparations *on page 723*
NSC-3053 *see* Dactinomycin *on page 393*
NSC-3088 *see* Chlorambucil *on page 296*
NSC-13875 *see* Altretamine *on page 66*
NSC-26271 *see* Cyclophosphamide *on page 381*
NSC-102816 *see* Azacitidine *on page 149*
NSC-106977 (*Erwinia*) *see* Asparaginase *on page 129*
NSC-109229 (*E. coli*) *see* Asparaginase *on page 129*
NSC-123127 *see* DOXOrubicin *on page 473*
NSC-125066 *see* Bleomycin *on page 190*
NSC-373364 *see* Aldesleukin *on page 50*
NTG *see* Nitroglycerin *on page 981*
NTZ *see* Nitazoxanide *on page 978*
Nubain® *see* Nalbuphine *on page 946*
Nucofed® Expectorant *see* Guaifenesin, Pseudoephedrine, and Codeine *on page 653*
Nucofed® Pediatric Expectorant *see* Guaifenesin, Pseudoephedrine, and Codeine *on page 653*
Nucotuss® *see* Guaifenesin, Pseudoephedrine, and Codeine *on page 653*
Nu-Iron® 150 [OTC] *see* Polysaccharide-Iron Complex *on page 1096*
NuLev™ *see* Hyoscyamine *on page 699*
Nullo® [OTC] *see* Chlorophyll *on page 302*
NuLytely® *see* Polyethylene Glycol-Electrolyte Solution *on page 1094*
Numorphan® *see* Oxymorphone *on page 1024*
Nupercainal® [OTC] *see* Dibucaine *on page 427*
Nupercainal® Hydrocortisone Cream [OTC] *see* Hydrocortisone *on page 688*
Nuquin HP® *see* Hydroquinone *on page 693*
Nu-Tears® [OTC] *see* Artificial Tears *on page 128*
Nu-Tears® II [OTC] *see* Artificial Tears *on page 128*
Nutracort® *see* Hydrocortisone *on page 688*
Nutraplus® [OTC] *see* Urea *on page 1365*
Nutropin® *see* Human Growth Hormone *on page 671*
Nutropin AQ® *see* Human Growth Hormone *on page 671*
Nutropin Depot® *see* Human Growth Hormone *on page 671*
NuvaRing® *see* Combination Hormonal Contraceptives *on page 368*
Nydrazid® *see* Isoniazid *on page 748*

Nylidrin (NYE li drin)

U.S. Brand Names Arlidin®

Canadian Brand Names Arlidin®

Pharmacologic Category Vasodilator, Peripheral

Use Considered "possibly effective" for increasing blood supply to treat peripheral disease (arteriosclerosis obliterans, diabetic vascular disease, nocturnal leg cramps, Raynaud's disease, frost bite, ischemic ulcer, thrombophlebitis) and circulatory disturbances of the inner ear (cochlear ischemia, macular or ampullar ischemia, etc)

Local Anesthetic/Vasoconstrictor Precautions No information available to require special precautions

Effects on Dental Treatment No significant effects or complications reported

Dosage Adults: Oral: 3-12 mg 3-4 times/day

Mechanism of Action Nylidrin is a peripheral vasodilator; this results from direct relaxation of vascular smooth muscle and beta agonist action. Nylidrin does not (Continued)

Nylidrin *(Continued)*

appear to affect cutaneous blood flow; it reportedly increases heart rate and cardiac output; cutaneous blood flow is not enhanced to any appreciable extent.

Other Adverse Effects

1% to 10%:

Central nervous system: Nervousness

Neuromuscular & skeletal: Trembling

<1%: Dizziness, nausea, palpitations, postural hypotension, vomiting, weakness

Pregnancy Risk Factor C

Nystatin (nye STAT in)

Related Information

Management of Patients Undergoing Cancer Therapy *on page 1567*
Oral Fungal Infections *on page 1542*
Sexually-Transmitted Diseases *on page 1502*

U.S. Brand Names Bio-Statin®; Mycostatin®; Nystat-Rx®; Nystop®; Pedi-Dri®

Canadian Brand Names Candistatin®; Mycostatin®; Nilstat; Nyaderm; PMS-Nystatin

Mexican Brand Names Micostatin®; Nistaquim

Pharmacologic Category Antifungal Agent, Oral Nonabsorbed; Antifungal Agent, Topical; Antifungal Agent, Vaginal

Use Dental: Treatment of susceptible cutaneous, mucocutaneous, and oral cavity fungal infections normally caused by the *Candida* species

Local Anesthetic/Vasoconstrictor Precautions No information available to require special precautions

Effects on Dental Treatment

1% to 10%: Vomiting, nausea

Frequency not defined: Contact dermatitis

Dosage

Oral candidiasis:

Suspension (swish and swallow orally):

Premature infants: 100,000 units 4 times/day

Infants: 200,000 units 4 times/day or 100,000 units to each side of mouth 4 times/day

Children and Adults: 400,000-600,000 units 4 times/day

Troche: Children and Adults: 200,000-400,000 units 4-5 times/day

Powder for compounding: Children and Adults: 1/8 teaspoon (500,000 units) to equal approximately 1/2 cup of water; give 4 times/day

Mucocutaneous infections: Children and Adults: Topical: Apply 2-3 times/day to affected areas; very moist topical lesions are treated best with powder

Intestinal infections: Adults: Oral: 500,000-1,000,000 units every 8 hours

Vaginal infections: Adults: Vaginal tablets: Insert 1 tablet/day at bedtime for 2 weeks

Mechanism of Action Binds to sterols in fungal cell membrane, changing the cell wall permeability allowing for leakage of cellular contents

Other Adverse Effects

1% to 10%: Gastrointestinal: Diarrhea, stomach pain

<1%: **Hypersensitivity reactions**

Frequency not defined: Dermatologic: Stevens-Johnson syndrome

Contraindications Hypersensitivity to nystatin or any component of the formulation

Dietary/Ethanol/Herb Considerations Do not permit patient to eat or drink for 10 minutes after oral dosing.

Pharmacodynamics/Kinetics

Onset of action: Symptomatic relief from candidiasis: 24-72 hours

Absorption: Topical: None through mucous membranes or intact skin; Oral: Poorly absorbed

Excretion: Feces (as unchanged drug)

Pregnancy Risk Factor B/C (oral)

Dosage Forms CAP (Bio-Statin®): 500,000 units, 1 million units. **CRM, topical:** 100,000 units/g (15 g, 30 g); (Mycostatin®): 100,000 units/g (30 g). **LOZ** (Mycostatin®): 200,000 units. **OINT, topical:** 100,000 units/g (15 g, 30 g). **POWDER, for prescription compounding**: 50 million units (10 g), 150 million units (30 g), 500 million units (100 g), 2 billion units (400 g); (Nystat-Rx®): 50 million units (10 g), 150 million units (30 g), 500 million units (100 g), 1 billion units (190 g), 2 billion units (350 g). **POWDER, topical** (Mycostatin®, Nystop®): 100,000 units/g (15 g); (Pedi-Dri®): 100,000 units/g (56.7 g). **SUSP, oral:** 100,000 units/mL (5 mL, 60 mL, 480 mL); (Mycostatin®): 100,000 units/mL (60 mL, 480 mL). **TAB** (Mycostatin®): 500,000 units. **TAB, vaginal:** 100,000 units (15s).

Generic Available Yes: Cream, ointment, suspension, tablet

Nystatin and Triamcinolone (nye STAT in & trye am SIN oh lone)

Related Information

Nystatin *on page 992*
Oral Fungal Infections *on page 1542*

Triamcinolone *on page 1341*

U.S. Brand Names Mycolog®-II; Mytrex®

Pharmacologic Category Antifungal Agent, Topical; Corticosteroid, Topical

Synonyms Triamcinolone and Nystatin

Use Treatment of cutaneous candidiasis

Local Anesthetic/Vasoconstrictor Precautions No information available to require special precautions

Effects on Dental Treatment No significant effects or complications reported

Dosage Children and Adults: Topical: Apply sparingly 2-4 times/day. Therapy should be discontinued when control is achieved; if no improvement is seen, reassessment of diagnosis may be necessary.

Mechanism of Action Nystatin is an antifungal agent that binds to sterols in fungal cell membrane, changing the cell wall permeability allowing for leakage of cellular contents. Triamcinolone is a synthetic corticosteroid; it decreases inflammation by suppression of migration of polymorphonuclear leukocytes and reversal of increased capillary permeability. It suppresses the immune system reducing activity and volume of the lymphatic system. It suppresses adrenal function at high doses.

Other Adverse Effects 1% to 10%:

Dermatologic: Dryness, folliculitis, hypertrichosis, acne, hypopigmentation, allergic dermatitis, maceration of the skin, skin atrophy

Local: Burning, itching, irritation

Miscellaneous: Increased incidence of secondary infection

Pregnancy Risk Factor C

Generic Available Yes

Nystat-Rx® *see* Nystatin *on page 992*

Nystop® *see* Nystatin *on page 992*

Nytol® [OTC] *see* DiphenhydrAMINE *on page 451*

Nytol® Maximum Strength [OTC] *see* DiphenhydrAMINE *on page 451*

Occlusal®-HP [OTC] *see* Salicylic Acid *on page 1204*

Ocean® [OTC] *see* Sodium Chloride *on page 1229*

OCL® [DSC] *see* Polyethylene Glycol-Electrolyte Solution *on page 1094*

Octreotide (ok TREE oh tide)

U.S. Brand Names Sandostatin®; Sandostatin LAR®

Canadian Brand Names Sandostatin®; Sandostatin LAR®

Mexican Brand Names Sandostatina®

Pharmacologic Category Antidiarrheal; Somatostatin Analog

Synonyms Octreotide Acetate

Use Control of symptoms in patients with metastatic carcinoid and vasoactive intestinal peptide-secreting tumors (VIPomas); pancreatic tumors, gastrinoma, secretory diarrhea, acromegaly

Unlabeled/Investigational Use Treatment of AIDS-associated secretory diarrhea, breast cancer, cryptosporidiosis, Cushing's syndrome, insulinomas, small bowel fistulas, postgastrectomy dumping syndrome, chemotherapy-induced diarrhea, graft-versus-host disease (GVHD) induced diarrhea, Zollinger-Ellison syndrome, congenital hyperinsulinism; control bleeding of esophageal varices

Local Anesthetic/Vasoconstrictor Precautions No information available to require special precautions

Effects on Dental Treatment No significant effects or complications reported

Dosage

Infants and Children:

Diarrhea: I.V., S.C.: Doses of 1-10 mcg/kg every 12 hours have been used in children beginning at the low end of the range and increasing by 0.3 mcg/kg/dose at 3-day intervals. Suppression of growth hormone (animal data) is of concern when used as long-term therapy.

Congenital hyperinsulinism (unlabeled): S.C.: Doses of 3-40 mcg/kg/day have been used

Adults: S.C.: Initial: 50 mcg 1-2 times/day and titrate dose based on patient tolerance and response

Carcinoid: 100-600 mcg/day in 2-4 divided doses

VIPomas: 200-300 mcg/day in 2-4 divided doses

Diarrhea: Initial: I.V.: 50-100 mcg every 8 hours; increase by 100 mcg/dose at 48-hour intervals; maximum dose: 500 mcg every 8 hours

Esophageal varices bleeding: I.V. bolus: 25-50 mcg followed by continuous I.V. infusion of 25-50 mcg/hour

Acromegaly: Initial: S.C.: 50 mcg 3 times/day; titrate to achieve growth hormone levels <5 ng/mL or IGF-I (somatomedin C) levels <1.9 U/mL in males and <2.2 U/mL in females; usual effective dose 100 mcg 3 times/day; range 300-1500 mcg/day

Note: Should be withdrawn yearly for a 4-week interval in patients who have received irradiation. Resume if levels increase and signs/symptoms recur.

Acromegaly, carcinoid tumors, and VIPomas (depot injection): Patients must be stabilized on subcutaneous octreotide for at least 2 weeks before switching to

(Continued)

Octreotide *(Continued)*

the long-acting depot: Upon switch: 20 mg I.M. intragluteally every 4 weeks for 2-3 months, then the dose may be modified based upon response

Dosing adjustment for acromegaly: After 3 months of depot injections the dosage may be continued or modified as follows:

GH ≤2.5 ng/mL, IGF-1 is normal, symptoms controlled: Maintain octreotide LAR® at 20 mg I.M. every 4 weeks

GH >2.5 ng/mL, IGF-1 is elevated, and/or symptoms uncontrolled: Increase octreotide LAR® to 30 mg I.M. every 4 weeks

GH ≤1 ng/mL, IGF-1 is normal, symptoms controlled: Reduce octreotide LAR® to 10 mg I.M. every 4 weeks

Dosages >40 mg are not recommended

Dosing adjustment for carcinoid tumors and VIPomas: After 2 months of depot injections the dosage may be continued or modified as follows:

Increase to 30 mg I.M. every 4 weeks if symptoms are inadequately controlled

Decrease to 10 mg I.M. every 4 weeks, for a trial period, if initially responsive to 20 mg dose

Dosage >30 mg is not recommended

Mechanism of Action Mimics natural somatostatin by inhibiting serotonin release, and the secretion of gastrin, VIP, insulin, glucagon, secretin, motilin, and pancreatic polypeptide. Decreases growth hormone and IGF-1 in acromegaly.

Other Adverse Effects

>10%:

Cardiovascular: Sinus bradycardia (19% to 25%)

Endocrine & metabolic: Hyperglycemia (15% acromegaly, 27% carcinoid)

Gastrointestinal: Diarrhea (36% to 58% acromegaly), abdominal pain (30% to 44% acromegaly), flatulence (13% to 26% acromegaly), constipation (9% to 19% acromegaly), nausea (10% to 30%)

1% to 10%:

Cardiovascular: Flushing, edema, conduction abnormalities (9% to 10%), arrhythmias (3% to 9%)

Central nervous system: Fatigue, headache, dizziness, vertigo, anorexia, depression

Endocrine & metabolic: Hypoglycemia (2% acromegaly, 4% carcinoid), hyperglycemia (1%), hypothyroidism, galactorrhea

Gastrointestinal: Nausea, vomiting, diarrhea, constipation, abdominal pain, cramping, discomfort, fat malabsorption, loose stools, flatulence, tenesmus

Hepatic: Jaundice, hepatitis, increase LFTs, cholelithiasis has occurred, presumably by altering fat absorption and decreasing the motility of the gallbladder

Local: Pain at injection site (dose-related)

Neuromuscular & skeletal: Weakness

<1%: Chest pain, hypertensive reaction, anxiety, fever, hyperesthesia, alopecia, wheal/erythema, rash, thrombophlebitis, leg cramps, Bell's palsy, muscle cramping, burning eyes, throat discomfort, rhinorrhea, dyspnea, gallstones

Drug Interactions CYP2D6 (high dose) and 3A enzyme inhibitor

Increased Effect/Toxicity: Octreotide may increase the effect of insulin or sulfonylurea agents which may result in hypoglycemia.

Decreased Effect: Octreotide may lower cyclosporine serum levels (case report of a transplant rejection due to reduction of serum cyclosporine levels). Codeine effect may be reduced.

Dietary/Ethanol/Herb Considerations Administer injections between meals to reduce GI effects.

Pharmacodynamics/Kinetics

Duration: S.C.: 6-12 hours

Absorption: S.C.: Rapid

Distribution: V_d: 14 L

Protein binding: 65% to lipoproteins

Metabolism: Extensively hepatic

Bioavailability: S.C.: 100%

Half-life elimination: 60-110 minutes

Excretion: Urine (32%)

Pregnancy Risk Factor B

Generic Available No

Octreotide Acetate *see* Octreotide *on page 993*

Ocu-Chlor® *see* Chloramphenicol *on page 297*

OcuClear® [OTC] [DSC] *see* Oxymetazoline *on page 1022*

OcuCoat® [OTC] *see* Artificial Tears *on page 128*

OcuCoat® PF [OTC] *see* Artificial Tears *on page 128*

Ocufen® *see* Flurbiprofen *on page 596*

Ocuflox® *see* Ofloxacin *on page 995*

Ocupress® Ophthalmic *see* Carteolol *on page 254*

Ocusulf-10 *see* Sulfacetamide *on page 1249*

Ofloxacin (oh FLOKS a sin)

Related Information

Nonviral Infectious Diseases *on page 1493*
Sexually-Transmitted Diseases *on page 1502*
Tuberculosis *on page 1493*

U.S. Brand Names Floxin®; Ocuflox®

Canadian Brand Names Apo®-Oflox; Floxin®; Ocuflox®

Mexican Brand Names Bactocin®; Floxil®; Floxstat®; Ocuflox®

Pharmacologic Category Antibiotic, Quinolone

Use Quinolone antibiotic for skin and skin structure, lower respiratory, and urinary tract infections and sexually-transmitted diseases. Active against many gram-positive and gram-negative aerobic bacteria.

Ophthalmic: Treatment of superficial ocular infections involving the conjunctiva or cornea due to strains of susceptible organisms

Otic: Otitis externa, chronic suppurative otitis media (patients >12 years of age); acute otitis media

Local Anesthetic/Vasoconstrictor Precautions No information available to require special precautions

Effects on Dental Treatment No significant effects or complications reported

Dosage

Oral, I.V.: Adults:

- Lower respiratory tract infection: 400 mg every 12 hours for 10 days
- Epididymitis (gonorrhea): 300 mg twice daily for 10 days
- Cervicitis due to *C. trachomatis* and/or *N. gonorrhoeae*: 300 mg every 12 hours for 7 days
- Skin/skin structure: 400 mg every 12 hours for 10 days
- Urinary tract infection: 200-400 mg every 12 hours for 3-10 days
- Prostatitis: 300 mg every 12 hours for 6 weeks

Ophthalmic: Children >1 year and Adults:

- Conjunctivitis: Instill 1-2 drops in affected eye(s) every 2-4 hours for the first 2 days, then use 4 times/day for an additional 5 days
- Corneal ulcer: Instill 1-2 drops every 30 minutes while awake and every 4-6 hours after retiring for the first 2 days; beginning on day 3, instill 1-2 drops every hour while awake for 4-6 additional days; thereafter, 1-2 drops 4 times/day until clinical cure.

Otic:

- Children 1-12 years: Otitis externa or acute otitis media with tympanostomy tubes: Instill 5 drops into affected ear(s) twice daily for 10 days
- Children >12 years and Adults:
  - Chronic otitis media with perforated tympanic membranes: Otic: 10 drops into affected ear twice daily for 14 days
  - Chronic suppurative otitis media: Instill 10 drops into affected ear(s) twice daily for 14 days
  - Otitis externa: Instill 10 drops into affected ear(s) twice daily for 10 days

Dosing adjustment/interval in renal impairment: Adults: I.V., Oral:

- Cl_{cr} 10-50 mL/minute: Administer 200-400 mg every 24 hours
- Cl_{cr} <10 mL/minute: Administer 100-200 mg every 24 hours

Continuous arteriovenous or venovenous hemodiafiltration effects: Administer 300 mg every 24 hours

Mechanism of Action Ofloxacin is a DNA gyrase inhibitor. DNA gyrase is an essential bacterial enzyme that maintains the superhelical structure of DNA. DNA gyrase is required for DNA replication and transcription, DNA repair, recombination, and transposition; bactericidal

Other Adverse Effects

Ophthalmic:

- >10%: Ocular: Burning or other discomfort of the eye, crusting or crystals in corner of eye
- 1% to 10%:
  - Gastrointestinal: Bad taste instillation
  - Ocular: Foreign body sensation, conjunctival hyperemia, itching of eye, ocular or facial edema, redness, stinging, photophobia
- <1% (Limited to important or life-threatening): Dizziness, nausea

Otic: Local reactions (3%), earache (1%), tinnitus, otorrhagia

Systemic:

- 1% to 10%:
  - Cardiovascular: Chest pain (1% to 3%)
  - Central nervous system: Headache (1% to 9%), insomnia (3% to 7%), dizziness (1% to 5%), fatigue (1% to 3%), somnolence (1% to 3%), sleep disorders, nervousness (1% to 3%), pyrexia (1% to 3%), pain
  - Dermatologic: Rash/pruritus (1% to 3%)
  - Gastrointestinal: Diarrhea (1% to 4%), vomiting (1% to 3%), GI distress, cramps, abdominal cramps (1% to 3%), flatulence (1% to 3%), abnormal taste (1% to 3%), xerostomia (1% to 3%), decreased appetite, nausea (3% to 10%)
  - Genitourinary: Vaginitis (1% to 3%), external genital pruritus in women

(Continued)

Ofloxacin *(Continued)*

Local: Pain at injection site

Ocular: Superinfection (ophthalmic), photophobia, lacrimation, dry eyes, stinging, visual disturbances (1% to 3%)

Miscellaneous: Trunk pain

<1% (Limited to important or life-threatening): Seizure, syncope, vasculitis, edema, hypertension, palpitations, vasodilation, anxiety, cognitive change, depression, dream abnormality, euphoria, hallucinations, vertigo, chills, malaise, extremity pain, weight loss, paresthesia, Stevens-Johnson syndrome, Tourette's syndrome, weakness, photophobia, photosensitivity, interstitial nephritis, vasculitis, hepatitis, decreased hearing acuity, tinnitus, cough, thirst; quinolones have been associated with tendonitis and tendon rupture

Drug Interactions Inhibits CYP1A2

Increased Effect/Toxicity: Quinolones can cause increased caffeine, warfarin, cyclosporine, and theophylline levels (unlikely to occur with ofloxacin). Azlocillin, cimetidine, and probenecid may increase ofloxacin serum levels. Foscarnet and NSAIDs have been associated with an increased risk of seizures with some quinolones. Serum levels of some quinolones are increased by loop diuretic administration. The hypoprothrombinemic effect of warfarin is enhanced by some quinolone antibiotics. Ofloxacin does not alter warfarin levels, but may alter the gastrointestinal flora which may increase warfarin's effect. Concurrent use of corticosteroids may increase risk of tendon rupture.

Decreased Effect: Metal cations (magnesium, aluminum, iron, and zinc) bind quinolones in the gastrointestinal tract and inhibit absorption (as much as 98%). Antacids, electrolyte supplements, sucralfate, quinapril, and some didanosine formulations should be avoided. Ofloxacin should be administered 4 hours before or 8 hours after these agents. Antineoplastic agents may decrease the absorption of quinolones.

Dietary/Ethanol/Herb Considerations

Food may decrease average peak serum concentration by 20%.

Herb/Nutraceutical: Avoid dong quai and St John's wort; may cause photosensitization.

Pharmacodynamics/Kinetics

Absorption: Well absorbed; food causes only minor alterations

Distribution: V_d: 2.4-3.5 L/kg

Protein binding: 20%

Half-life elimination: 5-7.5 hours; prolonged with renal impairment

Excretion: Primarily urine (as unchanged drug)

Pregnancy Risk Factor C

Generic Available No

Ogen® *see* Estropipate *on page 536*

Ogestrel® *see* Combination Hormonal Contraceptives *on page 368*

OGMT *see* Metyrosine *on page 905*

OKT3 *see* Muromonab-CD3 *on page 938*

Olanzapine (oh LAN za peen)

U.S. Brand Names Zyprexa®; Zyprexa® Zydis®

Canadian Brand Names Zyprexa®; Zyprexa® Zydis®

Mexican Brand Names Zyprexa®

Pharmacologic Category Antipsychotic Agent, Thienobenzodiazepine

Synonyms LY170053

Use Treatment of the manifestations of schizophrenia; short-term treatment of acute mania episodes associated with bipolar mania

Unlabeled/Investigational Use Treatment of psychotic symptoms

Local Anesthetic/Vasoconstrictor Precautions No information available to require special precautions

Effects on Dental Treatment No significant effects or complications reported

Dosage Oral:

Children: Schizophrenia/bipolar disorder: Initial: 2.5 mg/day; titrate as necessary to 20 mg/day (0.12-0.29 mg/kg/day)

Adults:

Schizophrenia: Usual starting dose: 5-10 mg once daily; increase to 10 mg once daily within 5-7 days, thereafter adjust by 5-10 mg/day at 1-week intervals, up to a maximum of 20 mg/day; doses of 30-50 mg/day have been used; typical dosage range: 10-30 mg/day

Bipolar mania: Usual starting dose: 10-15 mg once daily; increase by 5 mg/day at intervals of not less than 24 hours; maximum dose: 20 mg/day

Elderly: Schizophrenia: Usual starting dose: 2.5 mg/day, increase as clinically indicated and monitor blood pressure; typical dosage range: 2.5-10 mg/day

Dialysis: Not removed

Mechanism of Action Olanzapine is a thienobenzodiazepine neuroleptic; thought to work by antagonizing dopamine and serotonin activities. It is a selective monoaminergic antagonist with high affinity binding to serotonin 5-HT_{2A} and 5-HT_{2C}, dopamine D_{1-4}, muscarinic M_{1-5}, histamine H_1- and $alpha_1$-adrenergic receptor sites. Olanzapine binds weakly to GABA-A, BZD, and beta-adrenergic receptors.

Other Adverse Effects

>10%: Central nervous system: Headache, somnolence, insomnia, agitation, nervousness, hostility, dizziness

1% to 10%:

Cardiovascular: Postural hypotension, tachycardia, hypotension, peripheral edema

Central nervous system: Dystonic reactions, parkinsonian events, amnesia, euphoria, stuttering, akathisia, anxiety, personality changes, fever

Dermatologic: Rash

Gastrointestinal: Xerostomia, constipation, abdominal pain, weight gain, increased appetite

Genitourinary: Premenstrual syndrome

Neuromuscular & skeletal: Arthralgia, neck rigidity, twitching, hypertonia, tremor

Ocular: Amblyopia

Respiratory: Rhinitis, cough, pharyngitis

<1%: Agranulocytosis, diabetes mellitus, hyperglycemia, neuroleptic malignant syndrome, neutropenia, priapism, seizures, tardive dyskinesia

Drug Interactions Substrate of CYP1A2, 2D6; Inhibits CYP1A2, 2C8/9, 2C19, 2D6, 3A4

Increased Effect/Toxicity: Olanzapine levels may be increased by CYP1A2 inhibitors such as cimetidine and fluvoxamine. Sedations from olanzapine is increased with ethanol or other CNS depressants. The risk of hypotension and orthostatic hypotension from olanzapine is increased by concurrent antihypertensives. Metoclopramide may increase risk of extrapyramidal symptoms (EPS).

Decreased Effect: Olanzapine levels may be decreased by cytochrome P450 enzyme inducers such as rifampin, omeprazole, and carbamazepine (also cigarette smoking). Olanzapine may antagonize the effects of levodopa and dopamine agonists.

Dietary/Ethanol/Herb Considerations

Ethanol: Avoid use; may increase CNS depression and enhance orthostatic hypotension.

Herb/Nutraceutical: Avoid dong quai; may cause photosensitization. Avoid gotu kola, kava, SAMe, and valerian; may increase CNS depression. Avoid St John's wort; may cause photosensitization and increase CNS depression.

Pharmacodynamics/Kinetics

Absorption: Well absorbed; not affected by food; tablets and orally-disintegrating tablets are bioequivalent

Distribution: V_d: Extensive, 1000 L

Protein binding, plasma: 93% bound to albumin and $alpha_1$-glycoprotein

Metabolism: Highly metabolized via direct glucuronidation and cytochrome P450 mediated oxidation (CYP1A2, CYP2D6)

Half-life elimination: 21-54 hours; ~1.5 times greater in elderly

Time to peak: ~6 hours

Excretion: 40% removed via first pass metabolism; urine (57%, 7% as unchanged drug); feces (30%)

Clearance: 40% increase in olanzapine clearance in smokers

Pregnancy Risk Factor C

Generic Available No

Oleovitamin A *see* Vitamin A *on page 1390*

Oleum Ricini *see* Castor Oil *on page 259*

Olmesartan (ole me SAR tan)

U.S. Brand Names Benicar™

Pharmacologic Category Angiotensin II Receptor Blocker

Synonyms Olmesartan Medoxomil

Use Treatment of hypertension with or without concurrent use of other antihypertensive agents

Local Anesthetic/Vasoconstrictor Precautions No information available to require special precautions

Effects on Dental Treatment No significant effects or complications reported

Dosage Oral: Adults: Initial: Usual starting dose is 20 mg once daily; if initial response is inadequate, may be increased to 40 mg once daily after 2 weeks. May administer with other antihypertensive agents if blood pressure inadequately controlled with olmesartan. Consider lower starting dose in patients with possible depletion of intravascular volume (eg, patients receiving diuretics).

Mechanism of Action As a selective and competitive, nonpeptide angiotensin II receptor antagonist, olmesartan blocks the vasoconstrictor and aldosterone-secreting effects of angiotensin II; olmesartan interacts reversibly at the AT1 and AT2 receptors of many tissues and has slow dissociation kinetics; its affinity for

(Continued)

Olmesartan *(Continued)*

the AT1 receptor is 12,500 times greater than the AT2 receptor. Angiotensin II receptor antagonists may induce a more complete inhibition of the renin-angiotensin system than ACE inhibitors, they do not affect the response to bradykinin, and are less likely to be associated with nonrenin-angiotensin effects (eg, cough and angioedema). Olmesartan increases urinary flow rate and, in addition to being natriuretic and kaliuretic, increases excretion of chloride, magnesium, uric acid, calcium, and phosphate.

Other Adverse Effects

1% to 10%:

Central nervous system: Dizziness (3%), headache

Endocrine & metabolic: Hyperglycemia, hypertriglyceridemia

Gastrointestinal: Diarrhea

Neuromuscular & skeletal: Back pain, CPK increased

Renal: Hematuria

Respiratory: Bronchitis, pharyngitis, rhinitis, sinusitis, upper respiratory tract infection

Miscellaneous: Flu-like syndrome

<1%: Abdominal pain, arthralgia, arthritis, bilirubin increased, chest pain, dyspepsia, facial edema, fatigue, gastroenteritis, hypercholesterolemia, hyperlipidemia, hyperuricemia, insomnia, liver enzymes increased, myalgia, nausea, pain, peripheral edema, rash, skeletal pain, tachycardia, urinary tract infection, vertigo

Drug Interactions

Increased Effect/Toxicity: The risk of hyperkalemia may be increased during concomitant use with potassium-sparing diuretics, potassium supplements, and trimethoprim; may increase risk of lithium toxicity.

Decreased Effect: NSAIDs may decrease the efficacy of olmesartan.

Dietary/Ethanol/Herb Considerations

Ethanol: Avoid use; may increase risk of hypotension or dizziness.

Food does not affect bioavailability. Boiled milk, buttermilk, or yogurt may reduce diarrhea. Avoid caffeine, garlic, and licorice.

Herb/Nutraceutical: Avoid black cohosh, dong quai, and evening primrose due to estrogenic activity. Avoid ephedra, ginseng, and yohimbe; may worsen hypertension. Avoid garlic; may have increased antihypertensive effect. Avoid ginger due to positive inotropic effects; theoretically, may cause arrhythmia. Avoid hawthorn; may lower peripheral vascular resistance causing additional decrease in BP. Avoid licorice.

Pharmacodynamics/Kinetics

Distribution: 17 L; does not cross the blood-brain barrier (animal studies)

Protein binding: 99%

Metabolism: Olmesartan medoxomil is hydrolyzed in the GI tract to active olmesartan. No further metabolism occurs.

Bioavailability: 26%

Half-life elimination: Terminal: 13 hours

Time to peak: 1-2 hours

Excretion: All as unchanged drug: Feces (50% to 65%); urine (35% to 50%)

Pregnancy Risk Factor C/D (2nd and 3rd trimesters)

Generic Available No

Olmesartan Medoxomil *see* Olmesartan *on page 997*

Olopatadine (oh LOP ah tah deen)

U.S. Brand Names Patanol®

Canadian Brand Names Patanol®

Pharmacologic Category Antihistamine; Ophthalmic Agent, Miscellaneous

Use Treatment of the signs and symptoms of allergic conjunctivitis

Local Anesthetic/Vasoconstrictor Precautions No information available to require special precautions

Effects on Dental Treatment No significant effects or complications reported

Dosage Adults: Ophthalmic: 1 to 2 drops in affected eye(s) twice daily every 6 to 8 hours; results from an environmental study demonstrated that olopatadine was effective when dosed twice daily for up to 6 weeks

Other Adverse Effects

>5%: Central nervous system: Headache (7%)

<5%:

Central nervous system: Weakness, cold syndrome

Gastrointestinal: Taste perversion

Ocular: Burning, stinging, dry eyes, foreign body sensation, hyperemia, keratitis, eyelid edema, itching

Respiratory: Pharyngitis, rhinitis, sinusitis

Pregnancy Risk Factor C

Generic Available No

Olsalazine (ole SAL a zeen)

U.S. Brand Names Dipentum®

Canadian Brand Names Dipentum®

Pharmacologic Category 5-Aminosalicylic Acid Derivative

Synonyms Olsalazine Sodium

Use Maintenance of remission of ulcerative colitis in patients intolerant to sulfasalazine

Local Anesthetic/Vasoconstrictor Precautions No information available to require special precautions

Effects on Dental Treatment No significant effects or complications reported

Dosage Adults: Oral: 1 g/day in 2 divided doses

Mechanism of Action The mechanism of action appears to be topical rather than systemic

Other Adverse Effects

>10%: Gastrointestinal: Diarrhea, cramps, abdominal pain

1% to 10%:

- Central nervous system: Headache, fatigue, depression
- Dermatologic: Rash, itching
- Gastrointestinal: Nausea, heartburn, bloating, anorexia
- Neuromuscular & skeletal: Arthralgia

<1% (Limited to important or life-threatening): Blood dyscrasias, hepatitis, jaundice, cholestatic jaundice, cirrhosis, hepatic necrosis, and Kawasaki-like syndrome

Drug Interactions Increased Effect/Toxicity: Olsalazine has been reported to increase the prothrombin time in patients taking warfarin. Olsalazine may increase the risk of myelosuppression with azathioprine, mesalamine, or sulfasalazine.

Pharmacodynamics/Kinetics

Absorption: <3%; very little intact olsalazine is systemically absorbed

Protein binding, plasma: >99%

Metabolism: Primarily via colonic bacteria to active drug, 5-aminosalicylic acid

Half-life elimination: 56 minutes

Time to peak: ~1 hour

Excretion: Primarily feces

Pregnancy Risk Factor C

Generic Available No

Olsalazine Sodium *see* Olsalazine *on page 999*

Olux® *see* Clobetasol *on page 345*

Omeprazole (oh ME pray zole)

Related Information

Gastrointestinal Disorders *on page 1474*

U.S. Brand Names Prilosec®

Canadian Brand Names Losec®

Mexican Brand Names Inhibitron®; Losec®; Olexin®; Osiren®; Ozoken; Prazidec®; Prazolit®; Ulsen®

Pharmacologic Category Proton Pump Inhibitor

Use Short-term (4-8 weeks) treatment of active duodenal ulcer disease or active benign gastric ulcer; treatment of heartburn and other symptoms associated with gastroesophageal reflux disease (GERD); short-term (4-8 weeks) treatment of endoscopically-diagnosed erosive esophagitis; maintenance healing of erosive esophagitis; long-term treatment of pathological hypersecretory conditions; as part of a multidrug regimen for *H. pylori* eradication to reduce the risk of duodenal ulcer recurrence

Unlabeled/Investigational Use Treatment and prophylaxis of NSAID-induced ulcers

Local Anesthetic/Vasoconstrictor Precautions No information available to require special precautions

Effects on Dental Treatment No significant effects or complications reported

Dosage Oral:

Children ≥2 years: GERD or other acid-related disorders:

- <20 kg: 10 mg once daily
- ≥20 kg: 20 mg once daily

Adults:

- Active duodenal ulcer: 20 mg/day for 4-8 weeks
- Gastric ulcers: 40 mg/day for 4-8 weeks
- Symptomatic GERD: 20 mg/day for up to 4 weeks
- Erosive esophagitis: 20 mg/day for 4-8 weeks
- *Helicobacter pylori* eradication: Dose varies with regimen: 20 mg once daily **or** 40 mg/day as single dose or in 2 divided doses; requires combination therapy with antibiotics
- Pathological hypersecretory conditions: Initial: 60 mg once daily; doses up to 120 mg 3 times/day have been administered; administer daily doses >80 mg in divided doses

(Continued)

Omeprazole *(Continued)*

Mechanism of Action Suppresses gastric acid secretion by inhibiting the parietal cell H+/K+ ATP pump

Other Adverse Effects

1% to 10%:

Central nervous system: Headache (7%), dizziness (2%)

Dermatologic: Rash (2%)

Gastrointestinal: Diarrhea (3%), abdominal pain (2%), nausea (2%), vomiting (2%), constipation (1%), abnormal taste (<1% to 15%)

Neuromuscular & skeletal: Weakness (1%), back pain (1%)

Respiratory: Upper respiratory infection (2%), cough (1%)

<1%: Abdominal swelling, abnormal dreams, aggression, agranulocytosis, alopecia, anemia, angina, angioedema, anorexia, anxiety, apathy, atrophic gastritis, benign gastric polyps, bradycardia, jaundice, confusion, depression, diaphoresis, xerostomia, dry skin, elevated serum creatinine, elevated serum transaminases, toxic epidermal necrolysis, epistaxis, erythema multiforme, esophageal candidiasis, fatigue, fecal discoloration, fever, flatulence, glycosuria, gynecomastia, hallucinations, hematuria, hemifacial dysesthesia, hemolytic anemia, hepatic encephalopathy, hepatic failure hepatic necrosis, hypertension, hypoglycemia, hyponatremia, increased serum alkaline, insomnia, interstitial nephritis, irritable colon, joint pain, leg pain, leukocytosis, liver disease (hepatocellular, cholestatic, mixed), malaise, microscopic pyuria, mucosal atrophy (tongue), muscle cramps, muscle weakness, myalgia, nervousness, neutropenia, pain, palpitation, pancreatitis, pancytopenia, paresthesia, peripheral edema, pharyngeal pain, phosphatase, proteinuria, pruritus, psychic disturbance, skin inflammation, somnolence, Stevens-Johnson syndrome, tachycardia, testicular pain, thrombocytopenia, tinnitus, tremor, urinary frequency, urinary tract infection, urticaria, vertigo, weight gain

Drug Interactions Substrate of CYP2A6, 2C8/9, **2C19**, 2D6, 3A4; Inhibits CYP2C8/9, **2C19**, 2D6, **3A4**; Induces CYP1A2

Increased Effect/Toxicity: Omeprazole may increase the half-life of diazepam, digoxin, phenytoin, warfarin, and other drugs metabolized by the liver. Voriconazole may significantly increase serum levels of omeprazole (for omeprazole dosages >40 mg/day, reduce omeprazole dose by 50%). Serum levels of other proton pump inhibitors may also be increased.

Decreased Effect: The clinical effect of ketoconazole, itraconazole, and other drugs dependent upon acid for absorption is reduced; voriconazole not affected. Theophylline clearance is increased slightly.

Dietary/Ethanol/Herb Considerations

Ethanol: Avoid use; may cause gastric mucosal irritation.

Food delays absorption. Capsule may be opened and contents added to applesauce.

Herb/Nutraceutical: Avoid St John's wort; may decrease serum concentration.

Pharmacodynamics/Kinetics

Onset of action: Antisecretory: ~1 hour

Peak effect: 2 hours

Duration: 72 hours

Protein binding: 95%

Metabolism: Extensively hepatic

Half-life elimination: 0.5-1 hour

Excretion: Urine (77% as metabolites, very small amount as unchanged drug)

Pregnancy Risk Factor C

Generic Available Yes

Omnicef® *see* Cefdinir *on page 265*

Omnipaque® *see* Radiological/Contrast Media (Nonionic) *on page 1165*

Oncaspar® *see* Pegaspargase *on page 1039*

Oncovin® [DSC] *see* VinCRIStine *on page 1387*

Ondansetron (on DAN se tron)

U.S. Brand Names Zofran®; Zofran® ODT

Canadian Brand Names Zofran®; Zofran® ODT

Mexican Brand Names Zofran®

Pharmacologic Category Selective 5-HT_3 Receptor Antagonist

Synonyms Ondansetron Hydrochloride

Use Prevention of nausea and vomiting associated with moderately to highly emetogenic cancer chemotherapy; radiotherapy in patients receiving total body irradiation or fractions to the abdomen; postoperatively, when nausea and vomiting should be avoided

Unlabeled/Investigational Use Treatment of early-onset alcoholism

Local Anesthetic/Vasoconstrictor Precautions No information available to require special precautions

Effects on Dental Treatment 1% to 10%: Xerostomia

Dosage

Children:

I.V.:

Chemotherapy-induced emesis: 4-18 years: 0.15 mg/kg/dose administered 30 minutes prior to chemotherapy, 4 and 8 hours after the first dose

Postoperative nausea and vomiting: 2-12 years:

≤40 kg: 0.1 mg/kg

>40 kg: 4 mg

Oral: Chemotherapy-induced emesis of moderately-emetogenic agents:

4-11 years: 4 mg 30 minutes before chemotherapy; repeat 4 and 8 hours after initial dose, then 4 mg every 8 hours for 1-2 days after chemotherapy completed

≥12 years: Refer to adult dosing.

Adults:

I.V.: Chemotherapy-induced emesis: Administer either three 0.15 mg/kg doses or a single 32 mg dose:

Three-dose regimen: Initial dose is given 30 minutes prior to chemotherapy with subsequent doses administered 4 and 8 hours after the first dose

Single-dose regimen: 32 mg is infused over 15 minutes beginning 30 minutes before the start of emetogenic chemotherapy

I.M., I.V.: Postoperative nausea and vomiting: 4 mg as a single dose approximately 30 minutes before the end of anesthesia, or as treatment if vomiting occurs after surgery

Oral:

Chemotherapy-induced emesis:

Highly-emetogenic agents/single-day therapy: 24 mg given 30 minutes prior to the start of therapy

Moderately-emetogenic agents: 8 mg every 8 hours for 2 doses beginning 30 minutes before chemotherapy, then 8 mg every 12 hours for 1-2 days after chemotherapy completed

Total body irradiation: 8 mg 1-2 hours before each fraction of radiotherapy administered each day

Single high-dose fraction radiotherapy to abdomen: 8 mg 1-2 hours before irradiation, then 8 mg every 8 hours after first dose for 1-2 days after completion of radiotherapy

Daily fractionated radiotherapy to abdomen: 8 mg 1-2 hours before irradiation, then 8 mg every 8 hours after first dose for each day of radiotherapy

Postoperative nausea and vomiting: 16 mg given 1 hour prior to induction of anesthesia

Dosing adjustment in hepatic impairment: Maximum daily dose: 8 mg in patients with severe liver disease (Child-Pugh score ≥10)

Mechanism of Action Selective 5-HT_3-receptor antagonist, blocking serotonin, both peripherally on vagal nerve terminals and centrally in the chemoreceptor trigger zone

Other Adverse Effects

>10%:

Cardiovascular: Malaise/fatigue (9% to 13%)

Central nervous system: Headache (9% to 27%)

1% to 10%:

Central nervous system: Drowsiness (8%), fever (2% to 8%), dizziness (4% to 7%), anxiety (6%), cold sensation (2%)

Dermatologic: Pruritus (2% to 5%), rash (1%)

Gastrointestinal: Constipation (6% to 9%), diarrhea (3% to 7%)

Genitourinary: Gynecological disorder (7%), urinary retention (5%)

Hepatic: Increased ALT/AST (1% to 2%)

Local: Injection site reaction (4%)

Neuromuscular & skeletal: Paresthesia (2%)

Respiratory: Hypoxia (9%)

<1%: Anaphylaxis, angina, bronchospasm, EKG changes, extrapyramidal symptoms, grand mal seizures, hypokalemia, tachycardia, vascular occlusive events

Postmarketing and/or case reports: Angioedema, cardiopulmonary arrest, dystonic reactions, flushing, hiccups, hypersensitivity reactions, hypotension, laryngeal edema, laryngospasm, oculogyric crisis, shock, dyspnea, stridor, urticaria

Drug Interactions Substrate of CYP1A2, 2C8/9, 2D6, 2E1, **3A4**; Inhibits CYP1A2, 2C8/9, 2D6

Increased Effect/Toxicity: Increased toxicity: CYP1A2, 2D6, 2E1, and 3A4 enzyme inhibitors (eg, cimetidine, allopurinol, and disulfiram) may change the clearance of ondansetron; monitor

Decreased Effect: Decreased effect: CYP1A2, 2D6, 2E1, and 3A4 enzyme inducers (eg, barbiturates, carbamazepine, rifampin, phenytoin, and phenylbutazone) may change the clearance of ondansetron; monitor

Dietary/Ethanol/Herb Considerations

Food increases the extent of absorption; C_{max} and T_{max} do not change much.

Herb/Nutraceutical: Avoid St John's wort; may decrease serum concentration.

(Continued)

Ondansetron *(Continued)*

Pharmacodynamics/Kinetics

Onset of action: ~30 minutes

Distribution: V_d: 2.2-2.5 L/kg

Protein binding, plasma: 70% to 76%

Metabolism: Extensively hepatic via hydroxylation, followed by glucuronide or sulfate conjugation; CYP1A2, CYP2D6, and CYP3A4 substrate; some demethylation occurs

Bioavailability: Oral: 56% to 71%; Rectal: 58% to 74%

Half-life elimination: Children <15 years: 2-3 hours; Adults: 3-6 hours

Time to peak: Oral: ~2 hours

Excretion: Urine (44% to 60% as metabolites, 5% to 10% as unchanged drug); feces (~25%)

Pregnancy Risk Factor B

Generic Available No

Ondansetron Hydrochloride *see* Ondansetron *on page 1000*

One-A-Day® 50 Plus Formula [OTC] *see* Vitamins (Multiple/Oral) *on page 1394*

One-A-Day® Active Formula [OTC] *see* Vitamins (Multiple/Oral) *on page 1394*

One-A -Day® Essential Formula [OTC] *see* Vitamins (Multiple/Oral) *on page 1394*

One-A-Day® Maximum Formula [OTC] *see* Vitamins (Multiple/Oral) *on page 1394*

One-A- Day® Men's Formula [OTC] *see* Vitamins (Multiple/Oral) *on page 1394*

One-A-Day® Today [OTC] *see* Vitamins (Multiple/Oral) *on page 1394*

One-A-Day® Women's Formula [OTC] *see* Vitamins (Multiple/Oral) *on page 1394*

ONTAK® *see* Denileukin Diftitox *on page 407*

Onxol™ *see* Paclitaxel *on page 1026*

Ony-Clear [OTC] *see* Benzalkonium Chloride *on page 169*

OPC13013 *see* Cilostazol *on page 325*

OPC-14597 *see* Aripiprazole *on page 122*

OP-CCK *see* Sincalide *on page 1225*

Opcon-A® [OTC] *see* Naphazoline and Pheniramine *on page 953*

o,p′-DDD *see* Mitotane *on page 922*

Operand® [OTC] *see* Povidone-Iodine *on page 1104*

Ophthetic® *see* Proparacaine *on page 1132*

Opium and Belladonna *see* Belladonna and Opium *on page 164*

Opium Tincture (OH pee um TING chur)

Pharmacologic Category Analgesic, Narcotic; Antidiarrheal

Synonyms DTO; Opium Tincture, Deodorized

Use Treatment of diarrhea or relief of pain

Local Anesthetic/Vasoconstrictor Precautions No information available to require special precautions

Effects on Dental Treatment No significant effects or complications reported

Restrictions C-II

Dosage Oral:

Children:

Diarrhea: 0.005-0.01 mL/kg/dose every 3-4 hours for a maximum of 6 doses/24 hours

Analgesia: 0.01-0.02 mL/kg/dose every 3-4 hours

Adults:

Diarrhea: 0.3-1 mL/dose every 2-6 hours to maximum of 6 mL/24 hours

Analgesia: 0.6-1.5 mL/dose every 3-4 hours

Mechanism of Action Contains many narcotic alkaloids including morphine; its mechanism for gastric motility inhibition is primarily due to this morphine content; it results in a decrease in digestive secretions, an increase in GI muscle tone, and therefore a reduction in GI propulsion

Other Adverse Effects Frequency not defined:

Cardiovascular: Palpitations, hypotension, bradycardia, peripheral vasodilation,

Central nervous system: Drowsiness, dizziness, restlessness, headache, malaise, CNS depression, increased intracranial pressure, insomnia, mental depression

Gastrointestinal: Nausea, vomiting, constipation, anorexia, stomach cramps, biliary tract spasm

Genitourinary: Decreased urination, urinary tract spasm

Neuromuscular & skeletal: Weakness

Ocular: Miosis

Respiratory: Respiratory depression

Miscellaneous: Histamine release, physical and psychological dependence

Drug Interactions Increased Effect/Toxicity: Opium tincture and CNS depressants, MAO inhibitors, tricyclic antidepressants may potentiate the effects of opiate agonists (eg, codeine, morphine, etc). Dextroamphetamine may enhance the analgesic effect of opiate agonists.

Dietary/Ethanol/Herb Considerations
Ethanol: Avoid use; may increase CNS depression.
Herb/Nutraceutical: Avoid gotu kola, kava, SAMe, St John's wort, and valerian; may increase CNS depression.

Pharmacodynamics/Kinetics
Duration: 4-5 hours
Absorption: Variable
Metabolism: Hepatic
Excretion: Urine

Pregnancy Risk Factor B/D (prolonged use or high doses at term)
Generic Available Yes

Opium Tincture, Deodorized *see* Opium Tincture *on page 1002*

Oprelvekin (oh PREL ve kin)

U.S. Brand Names Neumega®
Pharmacologic Category Biological Response Modulator; Human Growth Factor
Synonyms IL-11; Interleukin-11; Recombinant Human Interleukin-11; Recombinant Interleukin-11; rhIL-11; rIL-11
Use Prevention of severe thrombocytopenia and the reduction of the need for platelet transfusions following myelosuppressive chemotherapy in patients with nonmyeloid malignancies who are at high risk of severe thrombocytopenia.
Local Anesthetic/Vasoconstrictor Precautions No information available to require special precautions
Effects on Dental Treatment No significant effects or complications reported
Dosage S.C.:
Children: 75-100 mcg/kg once daily for 10-21 days (until postnadir platelet count ≥50,000 cells/μL)
Note: The manufacturer states that, until efficacy/toxicity parameters are established, the use of oprelvekin in pediatric patients (particularly those <12 years of age) should be restricted to use in controlled clinical trials.
Adults: 50 mcg/kg once daily for 10-21 days (until postnadir platelet count ≥50,000 cells/μL)
Mechanism of Action Oprelvekin stimulates multiple stages of megakaryocytopoiesis and thrombopoiesis, resulting in proliferation of megakaryocyte progenitors and megakaryocyte maturation
Other Adverse Effects
>10%:
Cardiovascular: Tachycardia (19% to 30%), palpitations (14% to 24%), atrial arrhythmias (12%), peripheral edema (60% to 75%)
Central nervous system: Headache (41%), dizziness (38%), insomnia (33%), fatigue (30%), fever (36%)
Dermatologic: Rash (25%)
Endocrine & metabolic: Fluid retention
Gastrointestinal: Nausea (50% to 77%), vomiting, anorexia
Hematologic: Anemia (100%), probably a dilutional phenomena; appears within 3 days of initiation of therapy, resolves in about 2 weeks after cessation of oprelvekin
Neuromuscular & skeletal: Arthralgia, myalgias
Ocular: Papilledema: (frequency estimated to be up to 33% in pediatric patients, 1.5% in adults)
Respiratory: Dyspnea (48%), pleural effusions (10%)
1% to 10%:
Cardiovascular: Syncope (6% to 13%)
Gastrointestinal: Weight gain (5%)

Pharmacodynamics/Kinetics
Metabolism: Uncertain
Half-life elimination: Terminal: 5-8 hours
Time to peak, serum: 1-6 hours
Excretion: Urine (primarily as metabolites)

Pregnancy Risk Factor C
Generic Available No

Opticaine® *see* Tetracaine *on page 1284*
Opticrom® *see* Cromolyn Sodium *on page 375*
Opticyl® *see* Tropicamide *on page 1360*
Optigene® 3 [OTC] *see* Tetrahydrozoline *on page 1288*
Optimine® *see* Azatadine *on page 149*
OptiPranolol® *see* Metipranolol *on page 898*
Optiray® *see* Radiological/Contrast Media (Nonionic) *on page 1165*
Optivar™ *see* Azelastine *on page 151*
Orabase®-B [OTC] *see* Benzocaine *on page 169*
Orabase® With Benzocaine [OTC] *see* Benzocaine, Gelatin, Pectin, and Sodium Carboxymethylcellulose *on page 171*
Oracit® *see* Sodium Citrate and Citric Acid *on page 1230*

Orajel® [OTC] *see* Benzocaine *on page 169*
Orajel® Baby [OTC] *see* Benzocaine *on page 169*
Orajel® Baby Nighttime [OTC] *see* Benzocaine *on page 169*
Orajel® Maximum Strength [OTC] *see* Benzocaine *on page 169*
Orajel® Perioseptic® [OTC] *see* Carbamide Peroxide *on page 244*
Oramorph SR® *see* Morphine Sulfate *on page 931*
Oranyl [OTC] *see* Pseudoephedrine *on page 1146*
Orap® *see* Pimozide *on page 1083*
Orapred® *see* PrednisoLONE *on page 1110*
OraRinse™ [OTC] *see* Maltodextrin *on page 840*
Orasol® [OTC] *see* Benzocaine *on page 169*
Orciprenaline Sulfate *see* Metaproterenol *on page 873*
Oretic® *see* Hydrochlorothiazide *on page 675*
Orfadin® *see* Nitisinone *on page 979*
Organidin® NR *see* Guaifenesin *on page 650*
Orgaran® [DSC] *see* Danaparoid *on page 395*
Orinase Diagnostic® [DSC] *see* TOLBUTamide *on page 1319*
ORLAAM® *see* Levomethadyl Acetate Hydrochloride *on page 796*

Orlistat (OR li stat)

U.S. Brand Names Xenical®

Canadian Brand Names Xenical®

Mexican Brand Names Xenical®

Pharmacologic Category Lipase Inhibitor

Use Management of obesity, including weight loss and weight management when used in conjunction with a reduced-calorie diet; reduce the risk of weight regain after prior weight loss; indicated for obese patients with an initial body mass index (BMI) ≥30 kg/m^2 or ≥27 kg/m^2 in the presence of other risk factors

Local Anesthetic/Vasoconstrictor Precautions No information available to require special precautions

Effects on Dental Treatment No significant effects or complications reported

Dosage Oral: Adults: 120 mg 3 times/day with each main meal containing fat (during or up to 1 hour after the meal); omit dose if meal is occasionally missed or contains no fat. **Note:** A once-daily multivitamin containing the fat-soluble vitamins (A, D, E, and K) should be administered at least 2 hours prior to orlistat.

Mechanism of Action Orlistat is a reversible inhibitor of lipases; it exerts its therapeutic activity in the lumen of the stomach and small intestine by forming a covalent bond with the active serine residue site of gastric and pancreatic lipases; the inactivated enzymes are thus unavailable to hydrolyze dietary fat in the form of triglycerides into absorbable free fatty acids and monoglycerides; as undigested triglycerides are not absorbed, the resulting caloric deficit may have a positive effect on weight control; systemic absorption of the drug is therefore not needed for activity; at the recommended therapeutic dose of 120 mg 3 times/day, orlistat inhibits dietary fat absorption by approximately 30%

Other Adverse Effects

>10%

- Central nervous system: Headache (31%)
- Gastrointestinal: Oily spotting (27%), abdominal pain/discomfort (26%), flatus with discharge (24%), fatty/oily stool (20%), fecal urgency (22%), oily evacuation (12%), increased defecation (11%)
- Neuromuscular & skeletal: Back pain (14%)
- Respiratory: Upper respiratory infection (38%)

1% to 10%

- Central nervous system: Fatigue (7%), anxiety (5%), sleep disorder (4%)
- Dermatologic: Dry skin (2%)
- Endocrine & metabolic: Menstrual irregularities (10%)
- Gastrointestinal: Fecal incontinence (8%), nausea (8%), infectious diarrhea (5%), rectal pain/discomfort (5%), vomiting (4%)
- Neuromuscular & skeletal: Arthritis (5%), myalgia (4%)
- Otic: Otitis (4%)

<1%: Allergic reactions, anaphylaxis, angioedema, pruritus, rash, urticaria

Drug Interactions Decreased Effect: Vitamin K absorption may be decreased when taken with orlistat. Coadministration with cyclosporine may decrease plasma levels of cyclosporine.

Pregnancy Risk Factor B

Generic Available No

Ornex® [OTC] *see* Acetaminophen and Pseudoephedrine *on page 31*
Ornex® Maximum Strength [OTC] *see* Acetaminophen and Pseudoephedrine *on page 31*

Orphenadrine (or FEN a dreen)

Related Information

Temporomandibular Dysfunction (TMD) *on page 1562*

U.S. Brand Names Norflex™

Canadian Brand Names Norflex™; Orphenace®; Rhoxal-orphendrine

Pharmacologic Category Anti-Parkinson's Agent, Anticholinergic; Skeletal Muscle Relaxant

Synonyms Orphenadrine Citrate

Use Treatment of muscle spasm associated with acute painful musculoskeletal conditions; supportive therapy in tetanus

Local Anesthetic/Vasoconstrictor Precautions No information available to require special precautions

Effects on Dental Treatment The peripheral anticholinergic effects of orphenadrine may decrease or inhibit salivary flow; normal salivation will return with cessation of drug therapy.

Dosage Adults:

Oral: 100 mg twice daily

I.M., I.V.: 60 mg every 12 hours

Mechanism of Action Indirect skeletal muscle relaxant thought to work by central atropine-like effects; has some euphorigenic and analgesic properties

Other Adverse Effects

>10%:

- Central nervous system: Drowsiness, dizziness
- Ocular: Blurred vision

1% to 10%:

- Cardiovascular: Flushing of face, tachycardia, syncope
- Dermatologic: Rash
- Gastrointestinal: Nausea, vomiting, constipation
- Genitourinary: Decreased urination
- Neuromuscular & skeletal: Weakness
- Ocular: Nystagmus, increased intraocular pressure
- Respiratory: Nasal congestion

<1%: Hallucinations, aplastic anemia

Drug Interactions Substrate of CYP1A2, 2B6, 2D6, 3A4; Inhibits CYP1A2, 2A6, 2B6, 2C8/9, 2C19, 2D6, 2E1, **3A4**

Increased Effect/Toxicity: Orphenadrine may increase potential for anticholinergic adverse effects of anticholinergic agents; includes drugs with high anticholinergic activity (diphenhydramine, TCAs, phenothiazines). Sedative effects of may be additive in concurrent use of orphenadrine and CNS depressants (monitor). Effects of levodopa may be decreased by orphenadrine. Monitor.

Dietary/Ethanol/Herb Considerations

Ethanol: Avoid use; may increase CNS depression.

Herb/Nutraceutical: Avoid gotu kola, kava, SAMe, and valerian; may increase CNS depression. Avoid St John's wort; may decrease serum concentration and increase CNS depression.

Pharmacodynamics/Kinetics

Onset of effect: Peak effect: Oral: 2-4 hours

Duration: 4-6 hours

Protein binding: 20%

Metabolism: Extensively hepatic

Half-life elimination: 14-16 hours

Excretion: Primarily urine (8% as unchanged drug)

Pregnancy Risk Factor C

Generic Available Yes

Orphenadrine, Aspirin, and Caffeine

(or FEN a dreen, AS pir in, & KAF een)

Related Information

Aspirin *on page 131*

Orphenadrine *on page 1005*

U.S. Brand Names Norgesic™; Norgesic™ Forte; Orphengesic; Orphengesic Forte

Canadian Brand Names Norgesic™; Norgesic™ Forte

Pharmacologic Category Skeletal Muscle Relaxant

Synonyms Aspirin, Orphenadrine, and Caffeine; Caffeine, Orphenadrine, and Aspirin

Use Relief of discomfort associated with skeletal muscular conditions

Local Anesthetic/Vasoconstrictor Precautions No information available to require special precautions

Effects on Dental Treatment The peripheral anticholinergic effects of orphenadrine may decrease or inhibit salivary flow; normal salivation will return with cessation of drug therapy.

Dosage Oral: 1-2 tablets 3-4 times/day

(Continued)

Orphenadrine, Aspirin, and Caffeine *(Continued)*

Dietary/Ethanol/Herb Considerations

Ethanol: Avoid use; may increase CNS depression and enhance gastric mucosal irritation.

Herb/Nutraceutical: Avoid gotu kola, kava, SAMe, St John's wort, and valerian; may increase CNS depression.

Pregnancy Risk Factor D

Generic Available Yes

Orphenadrine Citrate *see* Orphenadrine *on page 1005*
Orphengesic *see* Orphenadrine, Aspirin, and Caffeine *on page 1005*
Orphengesic Forte *see* Orphenadrine, Aspirin, and Caffeine *on page 1005*
Ortho-Cept® *see* Combination Hormonal Contraceptives *on page 368*
Orthoclone OKT® 3 *see* Muromonab-CD3 *on page 938*
Ortho-Cyclen® Lo *see* Combination Hormonal Contraceptives *on page 368*
Ortho-Est® *see* Estropipate *on page 536*
Ortho Evra™ *see* Combination Hormonal Contraceptives *on page 368*
Ortho-Novum® *see* Combination Hormonal Contraceptives *on page 368*
Ortho-Novum® 1/50 *see* Mestranol and Norethindrone *on page 871*
Ortho-Prefest® *see* Estradiol and Norgestimate *on page 526*
Ortho Sprintec™ *see* Combination Hormonal Contraceptives *on page 368*
Orudis® [DSC] *see* Ketoprofen *on page 763*
Orudis® KT [OTC] *see* Ketoprofen *on page 763*
Oruvail® *see* Ketoprofen *on page 763*
Os-Cal® 500 [OTC] *see* Calcium Supplements *on page 229*

Oseltamivir (o sel TAM i veer)

Related Information

Systemic Viral Diseases *on page 1517*

U.S. Brand Names Tamiflu®

Canadian Brand Names Tamiflu®

Pharmacologic Category Antiviral Agent; Neuraminidase Inhibitor

Synonyms Oseltamivir Phosphate

Use Treatment of uncomplicated acute illness due to influenza (A or B) infection in adults and children >1 year of age who have been symptomatic for no more than 2 days; prophylaxis against influenza (A or B) infection in adults and adolescents ≥13 years of age

Local Anesthetic/Vasoconstrictor Precautions No information available to require special precautions

Effects on Dental Treatment Single doses of 1000 mg have resulted in nausea and vomiting.

Dosage Oral:

Treatment: Initiate treatment within 2 days of onset of symptoms; duration of treatment: 5 days:

Children: 1-12 years:

≤15 kg: 30 mg twice daily

>15 kg - ≤23 kg: 45 mg twice daily

>23 kg - ≤40 kg: 60 mg twice daily

>40 kg: 75 mg twice daily

Adolescents and Adults: 75 mg twice daily

Prophylaxis: Adolescents and Adults: 75 mg once daily for at least 7 days; treatment should begin within 2 days of contact with an infected individual. During community outbreaks, dosing is 75 mg once daily. May be used for up to 6 weeks; duration of protection lasts for length of dosing period

Elderly: No adjustments required

Dosing adjustment in renal impairment:

Cl_{cr} 10-30 mL/minute:

Treatment: Reduce dose to 75 mg once daily for 5 days

Prophylaxis: 75 mg every other day

Cl_{cr} <10 mL/minute: Has not been studied

Dosing adjustment in hepatic impairment: Not evaluated

Mechanism of Action Oseltamivir, a prodrug, is hydrolyzed to the active form, oseltamivir carboxylate. It is thought to inhibit influenza virus neuraminidase, with the possibility of alteration of virus particle aggregation and release. In clinical studies of the influenza virus, 1.3% of post-treatment isolates had decreased neuraminidase susceptibility to oseltamivir carboxylate.

Other Adverse Effects

As seen with **treatment** doses: 1% to 10%:

Central nervous system: Insomnia (adults 1%), vertigo (adults 1%)

Gastrointestinal: Nausea (adults 10%), vomiting (adults 9%, children 15%), abdominal pain (children 5%)

Ocular: Conjunctivitis (children 1%)

Otic: Ear disorder (children 2%)

Respiratory: Epistaxis (children 3%)

Similar adverse effects were seen in **prophylactic** use, however, the incidence was generally less. The following reactions were seen more commonly with prophylactic use: Headache (20%), fatigue (8%), diarrhea (3%)

<1% and case reports (any indication): Aggravation of diabetes, anemia, arrhythmia, confusion, hepatitis, humerus fracture, peritonsillar abscess, pneumonia, pseudomembranous colitis, pyrexia, rash, seizure, transaminases increased, toxic epidermal necrolysis, unstable angina, swelling of face or tongue

Drug Interactions Increased Effect/Toxicity: Cimetidine and amoxicillin have no effect on plasma concentrations. Probenecid increases oseltamivir carboxylate serum concentration by twofold. Dosage adjustments are not required.

Dietary/Ethanol/Herb Considerations Food: Administer with food to reduce GI upset.

Pharmacodynamics/Kinetics

Absorption: Well absorbed

Distribution: V_d: 23-26 L (oseltamivir carboxylate)

Protein binding, plasma: Oseltamivir carboxylate: 3%; Oseltamivir: 42%

Metabolism: Hepatic (90%) to oseltamivir carboxylate; neither the parent drug nor active metabolite has any effect on CYP

Bioavailability: 75% reaches systemic circulation in active form

Half-life elimination: Oseltamivir carboxylate: 6-10 hours; similar in geriatrics (68-78 years)

Time to peak: C_{max}: Oseltamivir: 65 ng/mL; Oseltamivir carboxylate: 348 ng/mL

Excretion: Urine (as carboxylate metabolite)

Pregnancy Risk Factor C

Generic Available No

Oseltamivir Phosphate *see* Oseltamivir *on page 1006*

Osmoglyn® *see* Glycerin *on page 644*

Otic Domeboro® *see* Aluminum Acetate and Acetic Acid *on page 67*

Otrivin® [OTC] [DSC] *see* Xylometazoline *on page 1401*

Otrivin® Pediatric [OTC] [DSC] *see* Xylometazoline *on page 1401*

Ovace™ *see* Sulfacetamide *on page 1249*

Ovcon® *see* Combination Hormonal Contraceptives *on page 368*

Ovidrel® *see* Chorionic Gonadotropin (Recombinant) *on page 321*

Ovral® *see* Combination Hormonal Contraceptives *on page 368*

Ovrette® *see* Norgestrel *on page 988*

Oxacillin (oks u SIL in)

Pharmacologic Category Antibiotic, Penicillin

Synonyms Methylphenyl Isoxazolyl Penicillin; Oxacillin Sodium

Use Treatment of infections such as osteomyelitis, septicemia, endocarditis, and CNS infections caused by susceptible strains of *Staphylococcus*

Local Anesthetic/Vasoconstrictor Precautions No information available to require special precautions

Effects on Dental Treatment Prolonged use of penicillins may lead to development of oral candidiasis.

Dosage I.M., I.V.:

Neonates:

Postnatal age <7 days:

<2000 g: 25 mg/kg/dose every 12 hours

>2000 g: 25 mg/kg/dose every 8 hours

Postnatal age >7 days:

<1200 g: 25 mg/kg/dose every 12 hours

1200-2000 g: 30 mg/kg/dose every 8 hours

>2000 g: 37.5 mg/kg/dose every 6 hours

Infants and Children: 150-200 mg/kg/day in divided doses every 6 hours; maximum dose: 12 g/day

Adults: 250 mg to 2 g/dose every 4-6 hours

Dosing adjustment in renal impairment: Cl_{cr} <10 mL/minute: Use lower range of the usual dosage

Hemodialysis: Not dialyzable (0% to 5%)

Mechanism of Action Inhibits bacterial cell wall synthesis by binding to one or more of the penicillin binding proteins (PBPs); which in turn inhibits the final transpeptidation step of peptidoglycan synthesis in bacterial cell walls, thus inhibiting cell wall biosynthesis. Bacteria eventually lyse due to ongoing activity of cell wall autolytic enzymes (autolysins and murein hydrolases) while cell wall assembly is arrested.

Other Adverse Effects Frequency not defined:

Central nervous system: Fever

Dermatologic: Rash

Gastrointestinal: Nausea, diarrhea, vomiting

Hematologic: Eosinophilia, leukopenia, neutropenia, thrombocytopenia, agranulocytosis

(Continued)

Oxacillin *(Continued)*

Hepatic: Hepatotoxicity, AST increased
Renal: Acute interstitial nephritis, hematuria
Miscellaneous: Serum sickness-like reactions

Drug Interactions

Increased Effect/Toxicity: Probenecid increases penicillin levels. Penicillins and anticoagulants may increase the effect of anticoagulants.

Decreased Effect: Although anecdotal reports suggest oral contraceptive efficacy could be reduced by penicillins, this has been refuted by more rigorous scientific and clinical data.

Dietary/Ethanol/Herb Considerations Food may decrease serum concentration.

Pharmacodynamics/Kinetics

Distribution: Into bile, synovial and pleural fluids, bronchial secretions, peritoneal, and pericardial fluids; crosses placenta; enters breast milk; penetrates the blood-brain barrier only when meninges are inflamed
Protein binding: ~94%
Metabolism: Hepatic to active metabolites
Half-life elimination: Children 1 week to 2 years: 0.9-1.8 hours; Adults: 23-60 minutes; prolonged in neonates and with renal impairment
Time to peak, serum: I.M.: 30-60 minutes
Excretion: Urine and feces (small amounts as unchanged drug and metabolites)

Pregnancy Risk Factor B

Generic Available Yes

Oxacillin Sodium *see* Oxacillin *on page 1007*

Oxaliplatin (ox AL i pla tin)

U.S. Brand Names Eloxatin™

Pharmacologic Category Antineoplastic Agent, Alkylating Agent

Synonyms Diaminocyclohexane Oxalatoplatinum; L-OHP

Use Treatment of metastatic colon or rectal carcinoma, in combination with fluorouracil (5-FU) and leucovorin, in patients whose disease has recurred or progressed during or within 6 months of completing therapy with 5-FU/leucovorin and irinotecan

Unlabeled/Investigational Use Orphan drug: Treatment of ovarian cancer

Local Anesthetic/Vasoconstrictor Precautions No information available to require special precautions

Effects on Dental Treatment No significant effects or complications reported

Dosage Dosed in combination with 5-FU/leucovorin on Day 1 of a 2-day treatment protocol that is repeated on a 2-week cycle; premedication with antiemetics is recommended.

Adults: I.V.:
Day 1: 85 mg/m^2 oxaliplatin infused over 2 hours (administered simultaneously with leucovorin via a Y-line), followed by a 5-FU bolus and 22-hour infusion of 5-FU
Day 2: Leucovorin and 5-FU administered as on Day 1.

Elderly: No dosing adjustment recommended

Dosing adjustment for toxicity: Prolongation of oxaliplatin infusion time from 2 hours to 6 hours may reduce some acute toxicities.
Persistent grade 2 neuropathy: Consider reducing dose to 65 mg/m^2
Persistent grade 3 neuropathy: Consider discontinuing therapy
Patients recovering from grade 3/4 GI or hematologic toxicity: Consider reduced dose (65 mg/m^2)

Dosing adjustment in renal impairment: Use with caution; specific guidelines not established

Mechanism of Action Oxaliplatin is an alkylating agent. Following intracellular hydrolysis of the "leaving group," the platinum compound binds to DNA, RNA, or proteins. Oxaliplatin is thought to be noncross-resistant with cisplatin and carboplatin on the basis of lack of recognition of oxaliplatin/DNA adducts by DNA repair systems.

Other Adverse Effects Based on clinical trial data using oxaliplatin alone. Some adverse effects may be increased when therapy is combined with 5-FU/leucovorin.

>10%:
Central nervous system: Fatigue (61%), fever (25%), pain (14%), headache (13%), insomnia (11%)
Gastrointestinal: Nausea (64%), diarrhea (46%), vomiting (37%), abdominal pain (31%), constipation (31%), anorexia (20%), stomatitis (14%)
Hematologic: Anemia (64%), thrombocytopenia (30%), leukopenia (13%)
Hepatic: SGOT increased (54%), SGPT increased (36%); total bilirubin increased (13%)
Neuromuscular & skeletal: Neuropathy, peripheral (acute 65%, persistent 43%), back pain (11%)
Respiratory: Dyspnea (13%), coughing (11%)

1% to 10%:
Cardiovascular: Edema (10%), chest pain (5%), flushing (3%), thromboembolism (2%)

Central nervous system: Rigors (9%), dizziness (7%), hand-foot syndrome (1%)
Dermatologic: Rash (5%), alopecia (3%)
Endocrine & metabolic: Dehydration (5%), hypokalemia (3%)
Gastrointestinal: Dyspepsia (7%), abnormal taste (5%), flatulence (3%), mucositis (2%), gastroesophageal reflux (1%)
Genitourinary: Dysuria (1%)
Hematologic: Neutropenia (7%)
Local: Injection site reaction (9%)
Neuromuscular & skeletal: Arthralgia (7%)
Ocular: Abnormal lacrimation (1%)
Renal: Serum creatinine increased (10%)
Respiratory: URI (7%), rhinitis (6%), epistaxis (2%), pharyngitis (2%)
Miscellaneous: Allergic reactions (3%), hiccup (2%)

Postmarketing and/or case reports: Anaphylactic shock, angioedema, cranial nerve palsies, deep tendon reflex loss, deafness, decreased visual acuity, dysarthria, fasciculations, hemolytic uremia syndrome, ileus, immuno-allergic thrombocytopenia, interstitial lung diseases, intestinal obstruction, Lhermittes' sign, metabolic acidosis, optic neuritis, pancreatitis, pulmonary fibrosis, visual field disturbance

Drug Interactions Increased Effect/Toxicity: Taxane derivatives may increase oxaliplatin toxicity if administered before the platin as a sequential infusion; nephrotoxic agents (aminoglycosides) may increase oxaliplatin toxicity

Pharmacodynamics/Kinetics

Distribution: 400 L
Protein binding: >90% primarily albumin and gamma globulin (irreversible binding to platinum)
Metabolism: Nonenzymatic (rapid and extensive), forms active and inactive derivatives
Half-life elimination: 391 hours; Distribution: 0.4-16.8 hours
Excretion: Primarily urine

Pregnancy Risk Factor D

Generic Available No

Oxandrin® *see* Oxandrolone *on page 1009*

Oxandrolone (oks AN droe lone)

U.S. Brand Names Oxandrin®

Pharmacologic Category Androgen

Use Adjunctive therapy to promote weight gain after weight loss following extensive surgery, chronic infections, or severe trauma, and in some patients who, without definite pathophysiologic reasons, fail to gain or to maintain normal weight

Local Anesthetic/Vasoconstrictor Precautions No information available to require special precautions

Effects on Dental Treatment No significant effects or complications reported

Restrictions C-III

Dosage

Children: Total daily dose: ≤0.1 mg/kg **or** ≤0.045 mg/lb

Adults: 2.5 mg 2-4 times/day; however, since the response of individuals to anabolic steroids varies, a daily dose of as little as 2.5 mg or as much as 20 mg may be required to achieve the desired response. A course of therapy of 2-4 weeks is usually adequate. This may be repeated intermittently as needed.

Dosing adjustment in renal impairment: Use with caution due to propensity to cause edema and water retention

Dosing adjustment in hepatic impairment: Use with caution; no specific recommendations

Mechanism of Action Synthetic testosterone derivative with similar androgenic and anabolic actions

Other Adverse Effects

Male:

Postpubertal:

>10%:
Dermatologic: Acne
Endocrine & metabolic: Gynecomastia
Genitourinary: Bladder irritability, priapism

1% to 10%:
Central nervous system: Insomnia, chills
Endocrine & metabolic: Decreased libido, hepatic dysfunction
Gastrointestinal: Nausea, diarrhea
Genitourinary: Prostatic hyperplasia (elderly)
Hematologic: Iron-deficiency anemia, suppression of clotting factors

<1%: Hepatic necrosis, hepatocellular carcinoma

Prepubertal:

>10%:
Dermatologic: Acne
Endocrine & metabolic: Virilism

1% to 10%:
Central nervous system: Chills, insomnia,

(Continued)

Oxandrolone *(Continued)*

Dermatologic: Hyperpigmentation
Gastrointestinal: Diarrhea, nausea
Hematologic: Iron deficiency anemia, suppression of clotting factors
<1%: Hepatic necrosis, hepatocellular carcinoma

Female:
>10%: Endocrine & metabolic: Virilism
1% to 10%:
Central nervous system: Chills, insomnia
Endocrine & metabolic: Hypercalcemia
Gastrointestinal: Nausea, diarrhea
Hematologic: Iron deficiency anemia, suppression of clotting factors
Hepatic: Hepatic dysfunction
<1%: Hepatic necrosis, hepatocellular carcinoma

Drug Interactions Increased Effect/Toxicity: ACTH, adrenal steroids may increase risk of edema and acne. Stanozolol enhances the hypoprothrombinemic effects of oral anticoagulants, and enhances the hypoglycemic effects of insulin and sulfonylureas (oral hypoglycemics).

Pharmacodynamics/Kinetics
Onset of action: 1 month
Absorption: High
Distribution: V_d: 0.578 L/kg
Protein binding, plasma: 94% to 97%
Metabolism: Hepatic
Excretion: Urine (60%); feces (3%)

Pregnancy Risk Factor X

Generic Available No

Oxaprozin (oks a PROE zin)

Related Information
Rheumatoid Arthritis, Osteoarthritis, and Osteoporosis *on page 1488*
Temporomandibular Dysfunction (TMD) *on page 1562*

U.S. Brand Names Daypro®

Canadian Brand Names Apo®-Oxaprozin; Daypro®; Rhoxal-oxaprozin

Pharmacologic Category Nonsteroidal Anti-inflammatory Drug (NSAID)

Use Acute and long-term use in the management of signs and symptoms of osteoarthritis and rheumatoid arthritis; juvenile rheumatoid arthritis

Local Anesthetic/Vasoconstrictor Precautions No information available to require special precautions

Effects on Dental Treatment NSAID formulations are known to reversibly decrease platelet aggregation via mechanisms different than observed with aspirin. The dentist should be aware of the potential of abnormal coagulation. Caution should also be exercised in the use of NSAIDs in patients already on anticoagulant therapy with drugs such as warfarin (Coumadin®).

Dosage Oral (individualize dosage to lowest effective dose to minimize adverse effects):
Children 6-16 years: Juvenile rheumatoid arthritis:
22-31 kg: 600 mg once daily
32-54 kg: 900 mg once daily
≥55 kg: 1200 mg once daily
Adults:
Osteoarthritis: 1200 mg once daily; patients should be titrated to lowest dose possible; patients with low body weight should start with 600 mg daily
Rheumatoid arthritis: 1200 mg once daily; a one-time loading dose of up to 1800 mg/day or 26 mg/kg (whichever is lower) may be given
Maximum daily dose: 1800 mg or 26 mg/kg (whichever is lower) in divided doses
Dosing adjustment in renal impairment: 600 mg once daily; dose may be increased to 1200 mg with close monitoring
Dosing adjustment in hepatic impairment: Use caution in severe dysfunction

Mechanism of Action Inhibits prostaglandin synthesis by decreasing the activity of the enzyme, cyclooxygenase, which results in decreased formation of prostaglandin precursors

Other Adverse Effects
1% to 10%:
Cardiovascular: Edema
Central nervous system: Confusion, depression, dizziness, headache, sedation, sleep disturbance, somnolence
Dermatologic: Pruritus, rash
Gastrointestinal: Abdominal distress, abdominal pain, anorexia, constipation, diarrhea, flatulence, gastrointestinal ulcer, gross bleeding with perforation, heartburn, nausea, vomiting
Hematologic: Anemia, bleeding time increased
Hepatic: Liver enzyme elevation
Otic: Tinnitus

Renal: Dysuria, renal function abnormal, urinary frequency

<1% (effects reported with oxaprozin or other NSAIDs): Acute interstitial nephritis, acute renal failure, agranulocytosis, alopecia, anaphylaxis, angioedema, anxiety, asthma, blurred vision, bruising, CHF, conjunctivitis, cystitis, dream abnormalities, drowsiness, dyspnea, eosinophilia, erythema multiforme, esophagitis, exfoliative dermatitis, fever, gastritis, GI bleeding, glossitis, hearing decreased, hematemesis, hematuria, hemorrhoidal bleeding, hepatitis, hypersensitivity reaction, hypertension, infection, insomnia, jaundice, leukopenia, liver function abnormalities, malaise, melena, menstrual flow increased/decreased, nephrotic syndrome, nervousness, oliguria, palpitations, pancreatitis, pancytopenia, paresthesia, peptic ulcer, photosensitivity, pneumonia, polyuria, proteinuria, pseudoporphyria, pulmonary infections, purpura, rectal bleeding, renal insufficiency, respiratory depression, sepsis, serum sickness, sinusitis, Stevens-Johnson syndrome, stomatitis, syncope, tachycardia,taste alteration, thrombocytopenia, toxic epidermal necrolysis, tremors, upper respiratory tract infections, vertigo, weakness, weight changes, xerostomia

Drug Interactions CYP2C9 enzyme inhibitor

Increased Effect/Toxicity: Oxaprozin may increase cyclosporine, digoxin, lithium, and methotrexate serum concentrations. The renal adverse effects of ACE inhibitors may be potentiated by NSAIDs. Corticosteroids may increase the risk of GI ulceration. The risk of bleeding with anticoagulants (warfarin, antiplatelet agents, low molecular weight heparins) may be increased.

Decreased Effect: Oxaprozin may decrease the effect of some antihypertensive agents (including ACE inhibitors and angiotensin antagonists) and diuretics.

Dietary/Ethanol/Herb Considerations

Ethanol: Avoid use; may enhance gastric mucosal irritation.

Food: Avoid garlic, ginger, and green tea.

Herb/Nutraceutical: Avoid cat's claw, dong quai, evening primrose, feverfew, garlic, ginger, ginkgo biloba, ginseng, green tea, horse chestnut, and red clover due to additional antiplatelet activity. Avoid kava and valerian; may enhance benzodiazepine activity.

Pharmacodynamics/Kinetics

Absorption: Almost complete

Protein binding: >99%

Metabolism: Hepatic via oxidation and glucuronidation; no active metabolites

Half-life elimination: 40-50 hours

Time to peak: 2-4 hours

Excretion: Urine (5% unchanged, 65% as metabolites); feces (35% as metabolites)

Pregnancy Risk Factor C/D (3rd trimester)

Generic Available No

Oxazepam (oks A ze pam)

Related Information

Patients Requiring Sedation *on page 1565*

U.S. Brand Names Serax®

Canadian Brand Names Apo®-Oxazepam; Novoxapram®; Oxpram®; PMS-Oxazepam

Pharmacologic Category Benzodiazepine

Use Treatment of anxiety; management of ethanol withdrawal

Unlabeled/Investigational Use Anticonvulsant in management of simple partial seizures; hypnotic

Local Anesthetic/Vasoconstrictor Precautions No information available to require special precautions

Effects on Dental Treatment >10%: Xerostomia; normal salivary flow resumes upon discontinuation

Restrictions C-IV

Dosage Oral:

Children: Anxiety: 1 mg/kg/day has been administered

Adults:

Anxiety: 10-30 mg 3-4 times/day

Ethanol withdrawal: 15-30 mg 3-4 times/day

Hypnotic: 15-30 mg

Elderly: Oral: Anxiety: 10 mg 2-3 times/day; increase gradually as needed to a total of 30-45 mg/day. Dose titration should be slow to evaluate sensitivity.

Hemodialysis: Not dialyzable (0% to 5%)

Mechanism of Action Binds to stereospecific benzodiazepine receptors on the postsynaptic GABA neuron at several sites within the central nervous system, including the limbic system, reticular formation. Enhancement of the inhibitory effect of GABA on neuronal excitability results by increased neuronal membrane permeability to chloride ions. This shift in chloride ions results in hyperpolarization (a less excitable state) and stabilization.

Other Adverse Effects Frequency not defined:

Cardiovascular: Syncope (rare), edema

(Continued)

Oxazepam *(Continued)*

Central nervous system: Drowsiness, ataxia, dizziness, vertigo, memory impairment, headache, paradoxical reactions (excitement, stimulation of effect), lethargy, amnesia, euphoria
Dermatologic: Rash
Endocrine & metabolic: Decreased libido, menstrual irregularities
Genitourinary: Incontinence
Hematologic: Leukopenia, blood dyscrasias
Hepatic: Jaundice
Neuromuscular & skeletal: Dysarthria, tremor, reflex slowing
Ocular: Blurred vision, diplopia
Miscellaneous: Drug dependence

Drug Interactions

Increased Effect/Toxicity: Ethanol and other CNS depressants may increase the CNS effects of oxazepam. Oxazepam may decrease the antiparkinsonian efficacy of levodopa. Flumazenil may cause seizures if administered following long-term benzodiazepine treatment.

Decreased Effect: Oral contraceptives may increase the clearance of oxazepam. Theophylline and other CNS stimulants may antagonize the sedative effects of oxazepam. Phenytoin may increase the clearance of oxazepam.

Dietary/Ethanol/Herb Considerations

Ethanol: Avoid use; may increase CNS depression.
Food: Fluids, fruit, and fiber may reduce constipation.
Herb/Nutraceutical: Avoid gotu kola, kava, SAMe, St John's wort, and valerian; may increase CNS depression.

Pharmacodynamics/Kinetics

Absorption: Almost complete
Protein binding: 86% to 99%
Metabolism: Hepatic to inactive compounds (primarily as glucuronides)
Half-life elimination: 2.8-5.7 hours
Time to peak, serum: 2-4 hours
Excretion: Urine (as unchanged drug (50%) and metabolites)

Pregnancy Risk Factor D

Generic Available Yes: Capsule

Oxcarbazepine (ox kar BAZ e peen)

U.S. Brand Names Trileptal®

Canadian Brand Names Trileptal®

Mexican Brand Names Trileptal®

Pharmacologic Category Anticonvulsant, Miscellaneous

Synonyms GP 47680

Use Monotherapy or adjunctive therapy in the treatment of partial seizures in adults with epilepsy; adjunctive therapy in the treatment of partial seizures in children (4-16 years of age) with epilepsy

Unlabeled/Investigational Use Antimanic

Local Anesthetic/Vasoconstrictor Precautions No information available to require special precautions

Effects on Dental Treatment No significant effects or complications reported

Dosage Oral:

Children:

Adjunctive therapy: 8-10 mg/kg/day, not to exceed 600 mg/day, given in 2 divided daily doses. Maintenance dose should be achieved over 2 weeks, and is dependent upon patient weight, according to the following:
20-29 kg: 900 mg/day in 2 divided doses
29.1-39 kg: 1200 mg/day in 2 divided doses
>39 kg: 1800 mg/day in 2 divided doses

Adults:

Adjunctive therapy: Initial: 300 mg twice daily; dose may be increased by as much as 600 mg/day at weekly intervals; recommended daily dose: 1200 mg/day in 2 divided doses. Although daily doses >1200 mg/day demonstrated greater efficacy, most patients were unable to tolerate 2400 mg/day (due to CNS effects).

Conversion to monotherapy: Oxcarbazepine 600 mg/day in twice daily divided doses while simultaneously initiating the reduction of the dose of the concomitant antiepileptic drug. The concomitant dosage should be withdrawn over 3-6 weeks, while the maximum dose of oxcarbazepine should be reached in about 2-4 weeks. Recommended daily dose: 2400 mg/day.

Initiation of monotherapy: Oxcarbazepine should be initiated at a dose of 600 mg/day in twice daily divided doses; doses may be titrated upward by 300 mg/day every third day to a final dose of 1200 mg/day given in 2 daily divided doses

Dosing adjustment in renal impairment: Initiate at one-half the usual starting dose (300 mg/day) and increase slowly to achieve the desired clinical response

Mechanism of Action Pharmacological activity results from both oxcarbazepine and its monohydroxy metabolite (MHD). Precise mechanism of anticonvulsant effect has not been defined. Oxcarbazepine and MHD block voltage sensitive sodium channels, stabilizing hyperexcited neuronal membranes, inhibiting repetitive firing, and decreasing the propagation of synaptic impulses. These actions are believed to prevent the spread of seizures. Oxcarbazepine and MHD also increase potassium conductance and modulate the activity of high-voltage activated calcium channels.

Other Adverse Effects As reported in adults with doses of up to 2400 mg/day (includes patients on monotherapy, adjunctive therapy, and those not previously on AEDs); incidence in children was similar:

>10%:

- Central nervous system: Dizziness (22% to 49%), somnolence (20% to 36%), headache (13% to 32%, placebo 23%), ataxia (5% to 31%), fatigue (12% to 15%), vertigo (6% to 15%)
- Gastrointestinal: Vomiting (7% to 36%), nausea (15% to 29%), abdominal pain (10% to 13%)
- Neuromuscular & skeletal: Abnormal gait (5% to 17%), tremor (3% to 16%)
- Ocular: Diplopia (14% to 40%), nystagmus (7% to 26%), abnormal vision (4% to 14%)

1% to 10%:

- Cardiovascular: Hypotension (1% to 2%), leg edema (1% to 2%, placebo 1%)
- Central nervous system: Nervousness (2% to 5%, placebo 1% to 2%), amnesia (4%), abnormal thinking (2% to 4%), insomnia (2% to 4%), speech disorder (1% to 3%), EEG abnormalities (2%), abnormal feelings (1% to 2%), agitation (1% to 2%, placebo 1%), confusion (1% to 2%, placebo 1%)
- Dermatologic: Rash (4%), acne (1% to 2%)
- Endocrine & metabolic: Hyponatremia (1% to 3%, placebo 1%)
- Gastrointestinal: Diarrhea (5% to 7%), dyspepsia (5% to 6%), constipation (2% to 6%, placebo 0% to 4%), gastritis (1% to 2%, placebo 1%), weight gain (1% to 2%, placebo 1%)
- Neuromuscular & skeletal: Weakness (3% to 6%, placebo 5%), back pain (4%), falling down (4%), abnormal coordination (1% to 4%, placebo 1% to 2%), dysmetria (1% to 3%), sprains/strains (2%), muscle weakness (1% to 2%)
- Ocular: Abnormal accommodation (2%)
- Respiratory: Upper respiratory tract infection (7%), rhinitis (2% to 5%, placebo 4%), chest infection (4%), epistaxis (4%), sinusitis (4%)

Postmarketing and/or case reports: Aggressive reaction, alopecia, amnesia, angioedema, anguish, anxiety, apathy, aphasia, appetite increased, asthma, arthralgia, aura, biliary pain, blood in stool, bradycardia, bruising, cardiac failure, cataract, cerebral hemorrhage, chest pain, cholelithiasis, colitis, conjunctival hemorrhage, consciousness decreased, contact dermatitis, convulsions aggravated, delirium, delusion, xerostomia, duodenal ulcer, dysphagia, dysphonia, dyspnea, dystonia, dysuria, eczema, emotional lability, enteritis, eructation, erythema multiforme, erythematosus rash, esophagitis, eosinophilia, euphoria, eye edema, extrapyramidal disorder, facial rash, feeling drunk, fever, flatulence, flushing, folliculitis, gastric ulcer, genital pruritus, GGT increased, gingival bleeding, gum hyperplasia, heat rash, hematuria, hemianopia, hemiplegia, hematemesis, hemorrhoids, hiccups, hot flashes, hyperglycemia, hyperkinesia, hyper-reflexia, hypersensitivity reaction, hypertonia, hypertension, hypocalcemia, hypochondrium pain, hypoesthesia, hypoglycemia, hypokalemia, hypokinesia, hyporeflexia, hypotonia, hysteria, intermenstrual bleeding, laryngismus, leukopenia, leukorrhea, libido decreased/increased, liver enzymes elevated, lymphadenopathy, maculopapular rash, malaise, manic reaction, migraine, menorrhagia, micturition frequency, muscle contractions (involuntary), mydriasis, neuralgia, oculogyric crisis, otitis externa, palpitation, panic disorder, paralysis, paroniria, personality disorder, photophobia, photosensitivity reaction, pleurisy, postural hypotension, priapism, psoriasis, purpura, psychosis, ptosis, rectal hemorrhage, renal calculus, renal pain, retching, rigors, scotoma, sialoadenitis, serum transaminase increased, Stevens-Johnson syndrome, stupor, syncope, systemic lupus erythematosus, tachycardia, abnormal taste, tetany, thrombocytopenia, tinnitus, toxic epidermal necrolysis, ulcerative stomatitis, urinary tract pain, urticaria, vitiligo, weight loss, xerophthalmia

Drug Interactions Inhibits CYP2C19; Induces **CYP3A4**

Increased Effect/Toxicity: Serum concentrations of phenytoin and phenobarbital are increased by oxcarbazepine.

Decreased Effect: Oxcarbazine serum concentrations may be reduced by carbamazepine, phenytoin, phenobarbital, valproic acid and verapamil (decreases levels of active oxcarbazepine metabolite). Oxcarbazepine reduces the serum concentrations of felodipine (similar effects may be anticipated with other dihydropyridines), oral contraceptives (use alternative contraceptive measures), and verapamil.

Dietary/Ethanol/Herb Considerations

Ethanol: Avoid use; may increase CNS depression.

Food: May be taken with food

Herb/Nutraceutical: Avoid evening primrose (decreases seizure threshold). Avoid gotu kola, kava, SAMe, and valerian; may increase CNS depression. Avoid St John's wort; may decrease serum concentration and increase CNS depression.

(Continued)

Oxcarbazepine *(Continued)*

Pharmacodynamics/Kinetics

Absorption: Complete; food has no affect on rate or extent

Distribution: MHD: V_d: 49 L

Protein binding, serum: MHD: 40%

Metabolism: Hepatic to 10-monohydroxy metabolite (active); MHD which is further conjugated to DHD (inactive)

Bioavailability: Decreased in children <8 years; increased in elderly >60 years

Half-life elimination: Parent drug: 2 hours; MHD: 9 hours; Cl_{cr} 30 mL/minute: 19 hours

Time to peak, serum: 4.5 hours (3-13 hours)

Excretion: Urine (95%, <1% as unchanged oxcarbazepine, 27% as unchanged MHD, 49% as MHD glucuronides); feces (<4%)

Pregnancy Risk Factor C

Generic Available No

Oxiconazole (oks i KON u zole)

Related Information

Oral Fungal Infections *on page 1542*

U.S. Brand Names Oxistat®

Canadian Brand Names Oxistat®; Oxizole®

Mexican Brand Names Gyno-Myfungar®; Myfungar®; Oxistat®

Pharmacologic Category Antifungal Agent, Topical

Synonyms Oxiconazole Nitrate

Use Treatment of tinea pedis (athlete's foot), tinea cruris (jock itch), and tinea corporis (ringworm)

Local Anesthetic/Vasoconstrictor Precautions No information available to require special precautions

Effects on Dental Treatment No significant effects or complications reported

Dosage Children and Adults: Topical: Apply once to twice daily to affected areas for 2 weeks (tinea corporis/tinea cruris) to 1 month (tinea pedis)

Mechanism of Action The cytoplasmic membrane integrity of fungi is destroyed by oxiconazole which exerts a fungicidal activity through inhibition of ergosterol synthesis. Effective for treatment of tinea pedis, tinea cruris, and tinea corporis. Active against *Trichophyton rubrum, Trichophyton mentagrophytes, Trichophyton violaceum, Microsporum canis, Microsporum audouini, Microsporum gypseum, Epidermophyton floccosum, Candida albicans*, and *Malassezia furfur*.

Other Adverse Effects 1% to 10%:

Dermatologic: Itching, erythema

Local: Transient burning, local irritation, stinging, dryness

Pharmacodynamics/Kinetics

Absorption: In each layer of the dermis; very little systemically after one topical dose

Distribution: To each layer of the dermis; enters breast milk

Excretion: Urine (<0.3%)

Pregnancy Risk Factor B

Generic Available No

Oxiconazole Nitrate *see* Oxiconazole *on page 1014*

Oxilapine Succinate *see* Loxapine *on page 829*

Oxipor® VHC [OTC] *see* Coal Tar *on page 359*

Oxistat® *see* Oxiconazole *on page 1014*

Oxpentifylline *see* Pentoxifylline *on page 1058*

Oxprenolol (ox PREN oh lole)

Canadian Brand Names Slow-Trasicor®; Trasicor®

Pharmacologic Category Antihypertensive; Beta-adrenergic Blocker, Noncardioselective

Synonyms Oxprenolol Hydrochloride

Use Treatment of mild or moderate hypertension

Unlabeled/Investigational Use Treatment of nonsevere hypertension in pregnancy (second-line agent)

Local Anesthetic/Vasoconstrictor Precautions No information available to require special precautions

Effects on Dental Treatment Nonselective beta-blockers may enhance the pressor response to epinephrine, resulting in hypertension and bradycardia. Many nonsteroidal anti-inflammatory drugs such as ibuprofen and indomethacin can reduce the hypotensive effect of beta-blockers after 3 or more weeks of therapy with the NSAID. Short-term NSAID use (ie, 3 days) requires no special precautions in patients taking beta-blockers.

Dosage Oral: Adults:

Initial: 20 mg 3 times/day (regular-release formulation); increase by 60 mg/day (in 3 divided doses) at 1-2 week intervals until adequate control is obtained

Maintenance: 120-320 mg/day; do not exceed 480 mg; may switch to slow-release formulation once-daily dosing at this time

Mechanism of Action Oxprenolol has a competitive ability to antagonize catecholamine-induced tachycardia at the beta-receptor sites in the heart, thus decreasing cardiac output, inhibits of renin release by the kidneys, and inhibits the vasomotor centers.

Other Adverse Effects Frequency not defined:

Cardiovascular: Congestive heart failure, pulmonary edema, cardiac enlargement, postural hypotension, severe bradycardia, lengthening of PR interval, second- and third-degree AV block, sinus arrest, palpitations, chest pain; peripheral vascular disorders, Raynaud's phenomenon, claudication, hot flashes

Central nervous system: Vertigo, syncope, lightheadedness, headache, dizziness, anxiety, mental depression, nervousness, irritability, hallucinations, sleep disturbances, nightmares, insomnia, weakness, sedation, vivid dreams, slurred speech

Dermatological: Dry skin, rash, pruritus

Endocrine & metabolic: Decreased libido, impotence, weight gain; elevated transaminases, alkaline phosphatase, and bilirubin; hypoglycemia

Gastrointestinal: Diarrhea, constipation, flatulence, heartburn, anorexia, nausea, vomiting, abdominal pain, xerostomia

Hematological: Thrombocytopenia, leukopenia

Neuromuscular & skeletal: Paresthesia

Ocular: Keratoconjunctivitis, dry eyes, itching eyes, blurred vision

Otic: Tinnitus

Renal: Elevated BUN

Respiratory: Dyspnea, wheezing, bronchospasm, nasal congestion, status asthmaticus

Miscellaneous: Diaphoresis, exertional tiredness

Drug Interactions Inhibits CYP2D6

Increased Effect/Toxicity:

Antiarrhythmic agents (quinidine, amiodarone) may be potentiated by oxprenolol. Concomitant use of I.V. calcium channel blockers with AV-blocking potential (eg, diltiazem and verapamil) may lead to severe hypotension, cardiac arrhythmias, and cardiac arrest. Catecholamine-depleting drugs (reserpine, guanethidine) may produce any excessive reduction of sympathetic activity, leading to severe bradycardia and hypotension. Ergot alkaloids may cause deterioration in peripheral blood flow, leading to peripheral ischemia. Inhalational anesthetics may cause cardiodepressant effects in patients receiving oxprenolol. Oxprenolol may potentiate hypoglycemic effects of insulin and hypoglycemic agents. Concomitant use of MAO inhibitors may produce any excessive reduction of sympathetic activity. CNS depressants (opiate analgesics, antihistamines, ethanol, and psychoactive drugs) may potentiate CNS depressant effects of oxprenolol.

Decreased Effect: Concomitant use of NSAIDs (indomethacin) may decrease antihypertensive effect of oxprenolol. Concomitant use of sympathomimetic agents (eg, epinephrine) may cause hypertensive reactions.

Dietary/Ethanol/Herb Considerations

Ethanol: Avoid use; may increase CNS depression.

Herb/Nutraceutical: Avoid black cohosh, dong quai, and evening primrose due to estrogenic activity. Avoid ephedra, ginseng, and yohimbe; may worsen hypertension. Avoid gotu kola, kava, SAMe, St John's wort, and valerian; may increase CNS depression.

Pharmacodynamics/Kinetics

Duration of beta-blocking effects: Immediate-release tablet: 8-12 hours; Slow-release tablet: Up to 24 hours

Absorption: 20% to 70%

Distribution: 1.3 L/kg

Protein binding: 80%

Metabolism: Hepatic first-pass effect

Half-life elimination: 1.3-1.5 hours

Time to peak, serum: Immediate-release tablet: 0.5-1.5 hours; Slow-release tablet: 2-4 hours

Excretion: Urine (as inactive metabolites, <5% as unchanged drug); major metabolite is glucuronide

Pregnancy Risk Factor Not assigned (similar agents rated C/D)

Generic Available No

Oxprenolol Hydrochloride *see* Oxprenolol *on page 1014*

Oxsoralen® *see* Methoxsalen *on page 888*

Oxsoralen-Ultra® *see* Methoxsalen *on page 888*

Oxy 10® Balanced Medicated Face Wash [OTC] *see* Benzoyl Peroxide *on page 171*

Oxy Balance® [OTC] *see* Salicylic Acid *on page 1204*

Oxy® Balance Deep Pore [OTC] *see* Salicylic Acid *on page 1204*

Oxybutynin (oks i BYOO ti nin)

U.S. Brand Names Ditropan®; Ditropan® XL; Oxytrol™

Canadian Brand Names Ditropan®; Ditropan® XL; Gen-Oxybutynin; Novo-Oxybutynin; Nu-Oxybutyn; PMS-Oxybutynin

Mexican Brand Names Tavor®

Pharmacologic Category Antispasmodic Agent, Urinary

Synonyms Oxybutynin Chloride

Use Antispasmodic for neurogenic bladder (urgency, frequency, urge incontinence) and uninhibited bladder

Local Anesthetic/Vasoconstrictor Precautions No information available to require special precautions

Effects on Dental Treatment >10%: Xerostomia, changes in salivation

Prolonged use may decrease or inhibit salivary flow; normal salivation resumes upon discontinuation

Dosage

Oral:

Children:

1-5 years (unlabeled use): 0.2 mg/kg/dose 2-4 times/day

>5 years: 5 mg twice daily, up to 5 mg 3-4 times/day maximum

Adults: 5 mg 2-3 times/day up to 5 mg 4 times/day maximum

Extended release: Initial: 5 mg once daily, may increase in 5-10 mg increments; maximum: 30 mg daily

Elderly: 2.5-5 mg twice daily; increase by 2.5 mg increments every 1-2 days

Transdermal: Adults: Apply one 3.9 mg/day patch twice weekly (every 3-4 days)

Note: Should be discontinued periodically to determine whether the patient can manage without the drug and to minimize resistance to the drug.

Mechanism of Action Direct antispasmodic effect on smooth muscle, also inhibits the action of acetylcholine on smooth muscle (exhibits 1/5 the anticholinergic activity of atropine, but is 4-10 times the antispasmodic activity); does not block effects at skeletal muscle or at autonomic ganglia; increases bladder capacity, decreases uninhibited contractions, and delays desire to void; therefore, decreases urgency and frequency

Other Adverse Effects

Oral: Frequency not defined:

Cardiovascular: Tachycardia, palpitations, vasodilation

Central nervous system: Drowsiness, dizziness, insomnia, fever, headache, hallucinations, restlessness

Dermatologic: Rash

Endocrine & metabolic: Flow of breast milk decreased, impotence

Gastrointestinal: Xerostomia, constipation, nausea, vomiting

Genitourinary: Urinary hesitancy or retention

Neuromuscular & skeletal: Weakness

Ocular: Blurred vision, mydriatic effect, amblyopia, cycloplegia, intraocular pressure increased, lacrimation decreased

Miscellaneous: Diaphoresis (decreased), allergic reaction

Transdermal:

>10%: Local: Application site reaction (17%), pruritus (14%)

1% to 10%:

Gastrointestinal: Xerostomia (4% to 10%), diarrhea (3%), constipation (3%)

Genitourinary: Dysuria (2%)

Local: Erythema (6% to 8%), vesicles (3%), rash (3%)

Ocular: Vision changes (3%)

Drug Interactions Substrate of CYP3A4; Inhibits CYP2D6, 3A4

Increased Effect/Toxicity: Additive sedation with CNS depressants and ethanol. Additive anticholinergic effects with antihistamines and anticholinergic agents. Effects of CYP2D6 substrates may be increased by concurrent therapy with beta-blockers, many phenothiazines, and tricyclic antidepressants. CYP3A4 inhibitors may increase effects of oxybutynin during concurrent therapy; inhibitors include amiodarone, ciprofloxacin, clarithromycin, diltiazem, erythromycin, itraconazole, ketoconazole, protease inhibitors, and verapamil.

Dietary/Ethanol/Herb Considerations

Ethanol: Avoid use; may increase CNS depression.

Oral formulations should be taken on an empty stomach with water.

Herb/Nutraceutical: Avoid gotu kola, kava, SAMe, St John's wort, and valerian; may increase CNS depression.

Pharmacodynamics/Kinetics

Onset of action: Oral: 30-60 minutes

Peak effect: 3-6 hours

Duration: 6-10 hours

Absorption: Rapid and well absorbed; Transdermal: High

Distribution: V_d: 193 L

Metabolism: Hepatic via CYP3A4; Oral: High first-pass metabolism; I.V.: Forms active metabolites

Half-life elimination: I.V.: ~2 hours (parent drug), 7-8 hours (metabolites)

Time to peak, serum: Oral: ~60 minutes; Transdermal: 24-48 hours
Excretion: Urine

Pregnancy Risk Factor B

Generic Available Yes: Excludes extended release formulation or transdermal patch

Oxybutynin Chloride *see* Oxybutynin *on page 1016*

Oxycel® *see* Cellulose (Oxidized) *on page 284*

Oxychlorosene (oks i KLOR oh seen)

U.S. Brand Names Clorpactin® WCS-90 [OTC]

Pharmacologic Category Antibiotic, Topical

Synonyms Oxychlorosene Sodium

Use Treatment of localized infections

Local Anesthetic/Vasoconstrictor Precautions No information available to require special precautions

Effects on Dental Treatment No significant effects or complications reported

Dosage Topical (0.1% to 0.5% solutions): Powder must be diluted with sterile water or isotonic saline; apply by irrigation, instillation, spray, soaks, or wet compresses

Generic Available No

Oxychlorosene Sodium *see* Oxychlorosene *on page 1017*

Oxycodone (oks i KOE done)

Related Information

Oral Pain *on page 1524*
Oxycodone and Aspirin *on page 1020*

U.S. Brand Names OxyContin®; Oxydose™; OxyFast®; OxyIR®; Percolone® [DSC]; Roxicodone™; Roxicodone™ Intensol™

Canadian Brand Names OxyContin®; Oxy.IR®; Supeudol®

Mexican Brand Names OxyContin®

Pharmacologic Category Analgesic, Narcotic

Synonyms Dihydrohydroxycodeinone; Oxycodone Hydrochloride; Percolone® [DSC]

Use

Dental: Treatment of postoperative pain

Medical: Around-the-clock management of moderate to severe pain when an analgesic is needed for an extended period of time.

OxyContin® is not intended for use as an "as needed" analgesic or for immediately-postoperative pain management; should be used postoperatively only if the patient has received it prior to surgery or if severe, persistent pain is anticipated.

Local Anesthetic/Vasoconstrictor Precautions No information available to require special precautions

Effects on Dental Treatment

>10%: Hypotension, drowsiness, dizziness, vomiting, fatigue, nausea, weakness

1% to 10%: Xerostomia, nervousness, headache, restlessness, confusion, biliary spasm, dyspnea, malaise, pain at injection site

Restrictions C-II

Dosage Oral:

- Immediate release:
  - Children:
    - 6-12 years: 1.25 mg every 6 hours as needed
    - >12 years: 2.5 mg every 6 hours as needed
  - Adults: 5 mg every 6 hours as needed
- Controlled release: Adults:
  - Opioid naive (not currently on opioid): 10 mg every 12 hours
  - Currently on opioid/ASA or acetaminophen or NSAID combination:
    - 1-5 tablets: 10-20 mg every 12 hours
    - 6-9 tablets: 20-30 mg every 12 hours
    - 10-12 tablets: 30-40 mg every 12 hours
    - May continue the nonopioid as a separate drug.
  - Currently on opioids: Use standard conversion chart to convert daily dose to oxycodone equivalent. Divide daily dose in 2 (for every 12-hour dosing) and round down to nearest dosage form.
- Dosing adjustment in hepatic impairment: Reduce dosage in patients with severe liver disease

Mechanism of Action Binds to opiate receptors in the CNS, causing inhibition of ascending pain pathways, altering the perception of and response to pain; produces generalized CNS depression

Other Adverse Effects Deaths due to overdose have been reported due to misuse/abuse after crushing the sustained release tablets.

1% to 10%:

Gastrointestinal: Anorexia, stomach cramps, constipation
Genitourinary: Ureteral spasms, decreased urination

(Continued)

Oxycodone *(Continued)*

<1%: Mental depression, **hallucinations, paradoxical CNS stimulation, increased intracranial pressure**, skin rash, urticaria, paralytic ileus, **histamine release, physical and psychological dependence**

Contraindications Hypersensitivity to oxycodone or any component of the formulation; significant respiratory depression; hypercarbia; acute or severe bronchial asthma; OxyContin® is also contraindicated in paralytic ileus (known or suspected); pregnancy (prolonged use or high doses at term)

Warnings/Precautions Use with caution in patients with hypersensitivity reactions to other phenanthrene derivative opioid agonists (morphine, hydrocodone, hydromorphone, levorphanol, oxycodone, oxymorphone), respiratory diseases including asthma, emphysema, or COPD. Use with caution in pancreatitis or biliary tract disease, acute alcoholism (including delirium tremens), adrenocortical insufficiency, CNS depression/coma, kyphoscoliosis (or other skeletal disorder which may alter respiratory function), hypothyroidism (including myxedema), prostatic hyperplasia, urethral stricture, and toxic psychosis.

Use with caution in the elderly, debilitated, severe hepatic or renal function. Hemodynamic effects (hypotension, orthostasis) may be exaggerated in patients with hypovolemia, concurrent vasodilating drugs, or in patients with head injury. Respiratory depressant effects and capacity to elevate CSF pressure may be exaggerated in presence of head injury, other intracranial lesion, or pre-existing intracranial pressure. Tolerance or drug dependence may result from extended use. Healthcare provider should be alert to problems of abuse, misuse, and diversion. Do **not** crush controlled-release tablets. Some preparations contain sulfites which may cause allergic reactions. OxyContin® 80 mg and 160 mg strengths are for use only in opioid-tolerant patients requiring high daily dosages >160 mg (80 mg formulation) or >320 mg (160 mg formulation).

Drug Interactions Substrate of **CYP2D6**

Increased Toxicity: CNS depressants, MAO inhibitors, general anesthetics, and tricyclic antidepressants may potentiate the effects of opiate agonists; dextroamphetamine may enhance the analgesic effect of opiate agonists

Dietary/Ethanol/Herb Considerations

Ethanol: Avoid use; may cause CNS depression.

Herb/Nutraceutical: Avoid gotu kola, kava, SAMe, St John's wort, and valerian; may increase CNS depression.

Pharmacodynamics/Kinetics

Onset of action: Pain relief: 10-15 minutes
  Peak effect: 0.5-1 hour
Duration: 3-6 hours; Controlled release: ≤12 hours
Metabolism: Hepatic
Half-life elimination: 2-3 hours
Excretion: Urine

Pregnancy Risk Factor B/D (prolonged use or high doses at term)

Dosage Forms CAP, immediate release (OxyIR®): 5 mg. **SOLN, oral** (Roxicodone™): 5 mg/mL (5 mL, 500 mL). **SOLN, oral concentrate**: (Oxydose™, OxyFast®, Roxicodone Intensol®: 20 mg/mL (30 mL). **TAB:** (Percolone® [DSC]): 5 mg; (Roxicodone™): 5 mg, 15 mg, 30 mg. **TAB, controlled release** (OxyContin®): 10 mg, 20 mg, 40 mg, 80 mg, 160 mg

Generic Available Yes

Comments Prophylactic use of a laxative should be considered; oxycodone, as with other narcotic analgesics, is recommended only for limited acute dosing (ie, 3 days or less). The most common adverse effect is nausea, followed by sedation and constipation. Oxycodone has an addictive liability, especially when given long-term.

Selected Readings Wynn RL, "Narcotic Analgesics for Dental Pain: Available Products, Strengths, and Formulations," *Gen Dent*, 2001, 49(2)126-36.

Oxycodone and Acetaminophen

(oks i KOE done & a seet a MIN oh fen)

Related Information

Acetaminophen *on page 27*
Oral Pain *on page 1524*
Oxycodone *on page 1017*

U.S. Brand Names Endocet®; Percocet® 2.5/325; Percocet® 5/325; Percocet® 7.5/325; Percocet® 7.5/500; Percocet® 10/325; Percocet® 10/650; Roxicet®; Roxicet® 5/500; Tylox®

Canadian Brand Names Endocet®; Oxycocet®; Percocet®; Percocet®-Demi

Pharmacologic Category Analgesic, Narcotic

Synonyms Acetaminophen and Oxycodone

Use

Dental: Treatment of postoperative pain

Medical: Management of moderate to severe pain

Local Anesthetic/Vasoconstrictor Precautions No information available to require special precautions

Effects on Dental Treatment The most common adverse effects are nausea and sedation.

1% to 10%: Xerostomia

Frequency not defined: Dizziness, lightheadedness, sedation, euphoria, allergic reaction, nausea, vomiting, respiratory failure

Restrictions C-II

Dosage Doses should be given every 4-6 hours as needed and titrated to appropriate analgesic effects. Initial dose is based on the **oxycodone** content; however, the maximum daily dose is based on the **acetaminophen** content.

Oral:

Children: Maximum acetaminophen dose: Children <45 kg: 90 mg/kg/day; children >45 kg: 4 g/day

Mild to moderate pain: Initial dose, **based on oxycodone content:** 0.05-0.1 mg/kg/dose

Severe pain: Initial dose, **based on oxycodone content:** 0.3 mg/kg/dose

Adults:

Mild to moderate pain: Initial dose, **based on oxycodone content:** 5 mg

Severe pain: Initial dose, **based on oxycodone content:** 15-30 mg. Do not exceed acetaminophen 4 g/day.

Elderly: Doses should be titrated to appropriate analgesic effects: Initial dose, **based on oxycodone content:** 2.5-5 mg every 6 hours. Do not exceed acetaminophen 4 g/day.

Dosing adjustment in hepatic impairment: Dose should be reduced in patients with severe liver disease.

Mechanism of Action

Oxycodone, as with other narcotic (opiate) analgesics, blocks pain perception in the cerebral cortex by binding to specific receptor molecules (opiate receptors) within the neuronal membranes of synapses. This binding results in a decreased synaptic chemical transmission throughout the CNS thus inhibiting the flow of pain sensations into the higher centers. Mu and kappa are the two subtypes of the opiate receptor which oxycodone binds to to cause analgesia.

Acetaminophen inhibits the synthesis of prostaglandins in the CNS and peripherally blocks pain impulse generation; produces antipyresis from inhibition of hypothalamic heat-regulating center

Other Adverse Effects Frequency not defined:

Central nervous system: Dysphoria

Dermatologic: Pruritus, skin rash

Gastrointestinal: Constipation

Contraindications Hypersensitivity to oxycodone, acetaminophen, or any component of the formulation; severe respiratory depression (in absence of resuscitative equipment or ventilatory support); pregnancy (prolonged periods or high doses at term)

Warnings/Precautions Use with caution in patients with hypersensitivity reactions to other phenanthrene-derivative opioid agonists (morphine, codeine, hydrocodone, hydromorphone, levorphanol, oxymorphone); respiratory diseases including asthma, emphysema, COPD, or severe liver or renal insufficiency, hypothyroidism, Addison's disease, prostatic hypertrophy, or urethral stricture; some preparations contain sulfites which may cause allergic reactions; may be habit-forming

Use with caution in patients with head injury and increased intracranial pressure (respiratory depressant effects increased and may also elevate CSF pressure). May mask diagnosis or clinical course in patients with acute abdominal conditions.

Enhanced analgesia has been seen in elderly patients on therapeutic doses of narcotics; duration of action may be increased in the elderly; the elderly may be particularly susceptible to the CNS depressant and constipating effects of narcotics

Dietary/Ethanol/Herb Considerations

Ethanol: Avoid use; may increase CNS depression. Excessive intake may increase the risk of acetaminophen-induced hepatotoxicity.

Herb/Nutraceutical: Avoid gotu kola, kava, SAMe, St John's wort, and valerian; may increase CNS depression.

Pregnancy Risk Factor C/D (prolonged periods or high doses at term)

Breast-feeding Considerations

Oxycodone: Excreted in breast milk. If occasional doses are used during breast-feeding, monitor infant for sedation, GI effects and changes in feeding pattern.

Acetaminophen: May be taken while breast-feeding

Dosage Forms CAP (Tylox®): Oxycodone 5 mg and acetaminophen 500 mg. **CAPLET** (Roxicet® 5/500): Oxycodone 5 mg and acetaminophen 500 mg. **SOLN, oral** (Roxicet®): Oxycodone 5 mg and acetaminophen 325 mg per 5 mL (5 mL, 500 mL). **TAB:** Oxycodone hydrochloride 5 mg and acetaminophen 325 mg; oxycodone hydrochloride 7.5 mg and acetaminophen 500 mg; oxycodone hydrochloride 10 mg and acetaminophen 650 mg; (Endocet®, Percocet® 5/325): Oxycodone 5 mg and acetaminophen 325 mg; (Percocet® 2.5/325): Oxycodone 2.5 mg and acetaminophen 325 mg; (Percocet® 7.5/325): Oxycodone 7.5 mg and acetaminophen 325

(Continued)

Oxycodone and Acetaminophen *(Continued)*

mg; (Percocet® 7.5/500): Oxycodone 7.5 mg and acetaminophen 500 mg; (Percocet® 10/325): Oxycodone 10 mg and acetaminophen 325 mg; (Percocet® 10/650): Oxycodone 10 mg and acetaminophen 650 mg; (Roxicet®): Oxycodone 5 mg and acetaminophen 325 mg

Generic Available Yes

Comments Oxycodone, as with other narcotic analgesics, is recommended only for limited acute dosing (ie, 3 days or less). Oxycodone has an addictive liability, especially when given long-term. The acetaminophen component requires use with caution in patients with alcoholic liver disease.

Acetaminophen: A study by Hylek, et al, suggested that the combination of acetaminophen with warfarin (Coumadin®) may cause enhanced anticoagulation. The following recommendations have been made by Hylek, et al, and supported by an editorial in *JAMA* by Bell.

Dose and duration of acetaminophen should be as low as possible, individualized and monitored

For patients who reported taking the equivalent of at least 4 regular strength (325 mg) tablets for longer than a week, the odds of having an INR >6.0 were increased 10-fold above those not taking acetaminophen. Risk decreased with lower intakes of acetaminophen reaching a background level of risk at a dose of 6 or fewer 325 mg tablets per week.

Selected Readings

Bell WR, "Acetaminophen and Warfarin: Undesirable Synergy," *JAMA*, 1998, 279(9):702-3.

Botting RM, "Mechanism of Action of Acetaminophen: Is There a Cyclooxygenase 3?," *Clin Infect Dis*, 2000, Suppl 5:S202-10.

Cooper SA, Precheur H, Rauch D, et al, "Evaluation of Oxycodone and Acetaminophen in Treatment of Postoperative Pain," *Oral Surg Oral Med Oral Pathol*, 1980, 50(6):496-501.

Dart RC, Kuffner EK, and Rumack BH, "Treatment of Pain or Fever with Paracetamol (Acetaminophen) in the Alcoholic Patient: A Systematic Review," *Am J Ther*, 2000, 7(2):123-34.

Dionne RA, "New Approaches to Preventing and Treating Postoperative Pain," *J Am Dent Assoc*, 1992, 123(6):26-34.

Gobetti JP, "Controlling Dental Pain," *J Am Dent Assoc*, 1992, 123(6):47-52.

Grant JA and Weiler JM, "A Report of a Rare Immediate Reaction After Ingestion of Acetaminophen," *Ann Allergy Asthma Immunol*, 2001, 87(3):227-9.

Hylek EM, Heiman H, Skates SJ, et al, "Acetaminophen and Other Risk Factors for Excessive Warfarin Anticoagulation 1998," *JAMA*, 1998, 279(9):702-3.

Kwan D, Bartle WR, and Walker SE, "The Effects of Acetaminophen on Pharmacokinetics and Pharmacodynamics of Warfarin," *J Clin Pharmacol*, 1999, 39(1):68-75.

McClain CJ, Price S, Barve S, et al, "Acetaminophen Hepatotoxicity: An Update," *Curr Gastroenterol Rep*, 1999, 1(1):42-9.

Shek KL, Chan LN, and Nutescu E, "Warfarin-Acetaminophen Drug Interaction Revisited," *Pharmacotherapy*, 1999, 19(10):1153-8.

Tanaka E, Yamazaki K, and Misawa S, "Update: The Clinical Importance of Acetaminophen Hepatotoxicity in Nonalcoholic and Alcoholic Subjects," *J Clin Pharm Ther*, 2000, 25(5):325-32.

Wynn RL, "Narcotic Analgesics for Dental Pain: Available Products, Strengths, and Formulations," *Gen Dent*, 2001, 49(2):126-8, 130, 132 passim.

Oxycodone and Aspirin (oks i KOE done & AS pir in)

Related Information

Aspirin *on page 131*
Oral Pain *on page 1524*
Oxycodone *on page 1017*

U.S. Brand Names Endodan®; Percodan®; Percodan®-Demi [DSC]

Canadian Brand Names Endodan®; Oxycodan®; Percodan®; Percodan®-Demi

Pharmacologic Category Analgesic, Narcotic

Synonyms Aspirin and Oxycodone; Percodan®-Demi [DSC]

Use

Dental: Treatment of postoperative pain

Medical: Relief of pain

Local Anesthetic/Vasoconstrictor Precautions No information available to require special precautions

Effects on Dental Treatment May have anticoagulant effects which may affect bleeding time. The elderly are a high-risk population for adverse effects from NSAIDs. As much as 60% of elderly patients with GI complications from NSAIDs can develop peptic ulceration and/or hemorrhage asymptomatically. Concomitant disease and drug use contribute to the risk of GI adverse effects. Enhanced analgesia has been seen with therapeutic doses of narcotics; duration of action may be increased. Elderly may also be particularly susceptible to the CNS depressant effects of narcotics.

>10%: Hypotension, drowsiness, dizziness, vomiting, nausea, fatigue, weakness

1% to 10%: Xerostomia, nervousness, headache, restlessness, confusion, GI ulceration, biliary spasm, dyspnea, anaphylactic shock, malaise

Restrictions C-II

Dosage Oral (based on oxycodone combined salts):

Children: 0.05-0.15 mg/kg/dose every 4-6 hours as needed; maximum: 5 mg/dose (1 tablet Percodan® or 2 tablets Percodan®-Demi/dose)

Adults: Percodan®: 1 tablet every 6 hours as needed for pain or Percodan®-Demi: 1-2 tablets every 6 hours as needed for pain

Dosing adjustment in hepatic impairment: Dose should be reduced in patients with severe liver disease

Mechanism of Action

Oxycodone, as with other narcotic (opiate) analgesics, blocks pain perception in the cerebral cortex by binding to specific receptor molecules (opiate receptors) within the neuronal membranes of synapses. This binding results in a decreased synaptic chemical transmission throughout the CNS thus inhibiting the flow of pain sensations into the higher centers. Mu and kappa are the two subtypes of the opiate receptor which oxycodone binds to to cause analgesia.

Aspirin inhibits prostaglandin synthesis by decreasing the activity of the enzyme, cyclooxygenase, which results in decreased formation of prostaglandin precursors, acts on the hypothalamic heat-regulating center to reduce fever, blocks thromboxane synthetase action which prevents formation of the platelet-aggregating substance thromboxane A_2

Other Adverse Effects

>10%: Gastrointestinal: Heartburn, stomach pains, dyspepsia

1% to 10%:

- Dermatologic: Rash
- Gastrointestinal: Anorexia, stomach cramps, constipation
- Genitourinary: Ureteral spasms, decreased urination
- Hematologic: Hemolytic anemia
- Local: Pain at injection site

<1%: Mental depression, **hallucinations, paradoxical CNS stimulation, increased intracranial pressure**, insomnia, **jitters,** rash, urticaria, paralytic ileus, occult bleeding, **prolongation of bleeding time**, leukopenia, thrombocytopenia, iron-deficiency anemia, hepatotoxicity, **impaired renal function, bronchospasm, physical and psychological dependence, histamine release**

Contraindications Hypersensitivity to oxycodone, aspirin, or any component of the formulation; severe respiratory depression; pregnancy

Warnings/Precautions Use with caution in patients with hypersensitivity to other phenanthrene derivative opioid agonists (morphine, codeine, hydrocodone, hydromorphone, oxymorphone, levorphanol); children and teenagers should not be given aspirin products if chickenpox or flu symptoms are present; aspirin use has been associated with Reye's syndrome; severe liver or renal insufficiency, pre-existing CNS and depression

Use with caution in patients with platelet and bleeding disorders, renal dysfunction, erosive gastritis, or peptic ulcer disease, previous nonreaction does not guarantee future safe taking of medication; use with caution in impaired hepatic function; do not use aspirin in children <16 years of age for chickenpox or flu symptoms due to the association with Reye's syndrome. Avoid aspirin, if possible, for 1 week prior to dental or surgical procedures due to possibility of postoperative bleeding.

Enhanced analgesia has been seen in elderly patients on therapeutic doses of narcotics; duration of action may be increased in the elderly; the elderly may be particularly susceptible to the CNS depressant and constipating effects of narcotics. Use lowest effective dose for shortest period possible. Consider renal function decline with age. Use with caution in patients with history of asthma.

Dietary/Ethanol/Herb Considerations

Ethanol: Avoid use; may increase CNS depression and enhance gastric mucosal irritation.

Food: May be taken with food

Herb/Nutraceutical: Avoid gotu kola, kava, SAMe, St John's wort, and valerian; may increase CNS depression.

Pregnancy Risk Factor D

Breast-feeding Considerations

Aspirin: Caution is suggested due to potential adverse effects in nursing infants.

Oxycodone: No data reported.

Dosage Forms TAB: Oxycodone 4.5 mg, oxycodone 0.38 mg, and aspirin 325 mg; (Endodan®, Percodan®): Oxycodone 4.5 mg, oxycodone 0.38 mg, and aspirin 325 mg; (Percodan®-Demi [DSC]): Oxycodone 2.25 mg, oxycodone 0.19 mg, and aspirin 325 mg

Generic Available Yes

Comments Oxycodone, as with other narcotic analgesics, is recommended only for limited acute dosing (ie, 3 days or less). Oxycodone has an addictive liability, especially when given long-term.

Selected Readings

Dionne RA, "New Approaches to Preventing and Treating Postoperative Pain," *J Am Dent Assoc*, 1992, 123(6):26-34.

Gobetti JP, "Controlling Dental Pain," *J Am Dent Assoc*, 1992, 123(6):47-52.

Wynn RL, "Narcotic Analgesics for Dental Pain: Available Products, Strengths, and Formulations," *Gen Dent*, 2001, 49(2):126-8, 130, 132 passim.

Oxycodone Hydrochloride *see* Oxycodone *on page 1017*

OxyContin® *see* Oxycodone *on page 1017*

Oxydose™ *see* Oxycodone *on page 1017*

OxyFast® *see* Oxycodone *on page 1017*

Oxygen (OKS i jen)

Related Information

Dental Office Emergencies *on page 1582*

Pharmacologic Category Dental Gases

Use

Dental: Administered as a supplement with nitrous oxide to ensure adequate ventilation during sedation; a resuscitative agent for medical emergencies in dental office

Medical: Treatment of various clinical disorders, both respiratory and nonrespiratory; relief of arterial hypoxia and secondary complications; treatment of pulmonary hypertension, polycythemia secondary to hypoxemia, chronic disease states complicated by anemia, cancer, migraine headaches, coronary artery disease, seizure disorders, sickle-cell crisis and sleep apnea

Local Anesthetic/Vasoconstrictor Precautions No information available to require special precautions

Effects on Dental Treatment No significant effects or complications reported

Dosage Children and Adults: Average rate of 2 L/minute

Mechanism of Action Increased oxygen in tidal volume and oxygenation of tissues at molecular level

Contraindications No data reported

Warnings/Precautions Oxygen-induced hypoventilation is the greatest potential hazard of oxygen therapy. In patients with severe COPD, the respiratory drive results from hypoxic stimulation of the carotid chemoreceptors. If this hypoxic drive is diminished by excessive oxygen therapy, hypoventilation may occur and further carbon dioxide retention with possible cessation of ventilation.

Pregnancy Risk Factor No data reported

Dosage Forms GAS, liquid for: Large reservoir holding 75-100 lb liquid oxygen in compressed-gas system [high-pressure tank in sizes "H" (6900 L of oxygen), "E" (622 L of oxygen), "D" (356 L of oxygen)]

Generic Available Yes

OxyIR® *see* Oxycodone *on page 1017*

Oxymetazoline (oks i met AZ oh leen)

Related Information

Oral Bacterial Infections *on page 1531*

U.S. Brand Names Afrin® [OTC]; Afrin® Extra Moisturizing [OTC]; Afrin® Original [OTC]; Afrin® Severe Congestion [OTC]; Afrin® Sinus [OTC]; Duramist® Plus [OTC]; Duration® [OTC]; Genasal [OTC]; Neo-Synephrine® 12 Hour [OTC]; Neo-Synephrine® 12 Hour Extra Moisturizing [OTC]; Nōstrilla® [OTC]; OcuClear® [OTC] [DSC]; Twice-A-Day® [OTC]; Vicks Sinex® 12 Hour Ultrafine Mist [OTC]; Visine® L.R. [OTC]; 4-Way® Long Acting [OTC]

Canadian Brand Names Claritin® Allergic Decongestant; Dristan® Long Lasting Nasal; Drixoral® Nasal

Mexican Brand Names Afrin®; Iliadin®; Ocuclear®; Oxylin®; Visine A.D.®

Pharmacologic Category Adrenergic Agonist Agent; Vasoconstrictor

Synonyms Oxymetazoline Hydrochloride

Use

Dental: Symptomatic relief of nasal mucosal congestion

Medical:

Adjunctive therapy of middle ear infections, associated with acute or chronic rhinitis, the common cold, sinusitis, hay fever, or other allergies

Ophthalmic: Relief of redness of eye due to minor eye irritations

Local Anesthetic/Vasoconstrictor Precautions No information available to require special precautions

Effects on Dental Treatment

>10%: Nasal dryness, sneezing, transient nasal burning and stinging

1% to 10%: Hypertension, palpitations, rebound congestion (with prolonged use)

Dosage

Intranasal (therapy should not exceed 3-5 days):

Children 2-5 years: 0.025% solution: Instill 2-3 drops in each nostril twice daily

Children ≥6 years and Adults: 0.05% solution: Instill 2-3 drops or 2-3 sprays into each nostril twice daily

Ophthalmic: Children >6 years and Adults: 0.025% solution: Instill 1-2 drops in affected eye(s) every 6 hours as needed or as directed by healthcare provider

Mechanism of Action Stimulates alpha-adrenergic receptors in the arterioles of the nasal mucosa to produce vasoconstriction

Contraindications Hypersensitivity to oxymetazoline or any component of the formulation

Warnings/Precautions Rebound congestion may occur with extended use (>3 days); use with caution in the presence of hypertension, diabetes, hyperthyroidism, heart disease, coronary artery disease, cerebral arteriosclerosis, or long-standing bronchial asthma

Drug Interactions Increased toxicity with MAO inhibitors

Pharmacodynamics/Kinetics
Onset of action: Intranasal: 5-10 minutes
Duration: 5-6 hours

Pregnancy Risk Factor C

Dosage Forms SOLN, intranasal spray: 0.05% (15 mL, 30 mL); (Afrin®, Afrin® Extra Moisturizing, Afrin® Severe Congestion, Afrin® Sinus, Duramist® Plus, Neo-Synephrine® 12 Hour, Nōstrilla®, Vicks Sinex® 12 Hour Ultrafine Mist, 4-Way® Long Acting Nasal, Neo-Synephrine® 12 Hour Extra Moisturizing, Nōstrilla®): 0.05% (15 mL); (Afrin® Original): 0.05% (15 mL, 30 mL, 45 mL); (Duration®): 0.05% (30 mL); (Genasal): 0.05% (15 mL, 30 mL); **SOLN, ophthalmic** (OcuClear® [DSC], Visine® L.R.): 0.025% (15 mL, 30 mL)

Generic Available Yes

Oxymetazoline Hydrochloride *see* Oxymetazoline *on page 1022*

Oxymetholone (oks i METH oh lone)

U.S. Brand Names Anadrol®

Pharmacologic Category Anabolic Steroid

Use Anemias caused by the administration of myelotoxic drugs

Local Anesthetic/Vasoconstrictor Precautions No information available to require special precautions

Effects on Dental Treatment No significant effects or complications reported

Restrictions C-III

Dosage Oral:

Adults: Erythropoietic effects: 1-5 mg/kg/day in one daily dose; usual effective dose: 1-2 mg/kg/day; give for a minimum trial of 3-6 months because response may be delayed

Dosing adjustment in hepatic impairment: Use with caution due to hepatotoxic potential; contraindicated in severe impairment

Mechanism of Action Stimulates receptors in organs and tissues to promote growth and development of male sex organs and maintains secondary sex characteristics in androgen-deficient males

Other Adverse Effects

Male:

Postpubertal:
- >10%:
  - Dermatologic: Acne
  - Endocrine & metabolic: Gynecomastia
  - Genitourinary: Bladder irritability, priapism
- 1% to 10%:
  - Central nervous system: Insomnia, chills
  - Endocrine & metabolic: Decreased libido
  - Gastrointestinal: Nausea, diarrhea
  - Genitourinary: Prostatic hyperplasia (elderly)
  - Hematologic: Iron-deficiency anemia, suppression of clotting factors
  - Hepatic: Hepatic dysfunction
- <1%: Hepatic necrosis, hepatocellular carcinoma

Prepubertal:
- >10%:
  - Dermatologic: Acne
  - Endocrine & metabolic: Virilism
- 1% to 10%:
  - Central nervous system: Chills, insomnia
  - Dermatologic: Hyperpigmentation
  - Gastrointestinal: Diarrhea, nausea
  - Hematologic: Iron-deficiency anemia, suppression of clotting factors
- <1%: Hepatic necrosis, hepatocellular carcinoma

Female:
- >10%: Endocrine & metabolic: Virilism
- 1% to 10%:
  - Central nervous system: Chills, insomnia
  - Endocrine & metabolic: Hypercalcemia
  - Gastrointestinal: Nausea, diarrhea
  - Hematologic: Iron-deficiency anemia, suppression of clotting factors
  - Hepatic: Hepatic dysfunction
- <1%: Hepatic necrosis, hepatocellular carcinoma

Drug Interactions Increased Effect/Toxicity: Oxymetholone may increase prothrombin times in patients receiving warfarin, leading to toxicity. Insulin effects may be enhanced, leading to hypoglycemia.

Pharmacodynamics/Kinetics
Onset of action: 2-6 months
Half-life elimination: 9 hours
Excretion: Urine (20% to 25%)

Pregnancy Risk Factor X

Generic Available No

Oxymorphone (oks i MOR fone)

U.S. Brand Names Numorphan®

Canadian Brand Names Numorphan®

Pharmacologic Category Analgesic, Narcotic

Synonyms Oxymorphone Hydrochloride

Use Management of moderate to severe pain and preoperatively as a sedative and a supplement to anesthesia

Local Anesthetic/Vasoconstrictor Precautions No information available to require special precautions

Effects on Dental Treatment Anticholinergic side effects can cause a reduction of saliva production or secretion, contributing to discomfort and dental disease (ie, caries, oral candidiasis and periodontal disease).

Restrictions C-II

Dosage More frequent dosing may be required.

Adults:

- I.M., S.C.: 0.5 mg initially, 1-1.5 mg every 4-6 hours as needed
- I.V.: 0.5 mg initially
- Rectal: 5 mg every 4-6 hours

Mechanism of Action Oxymorphone hydrochloride (Numorphan®) is a potent narcotic analgesic with uses similar to those of morphine. The drug is a semisynthetic derivative of morphine (phenanthrene derivative) and is closely related to hydromorphone chemically (Dilaudid®).

Other Adverse Effects

>10%:

- Cardiovascular: Hypotension
- Central nervous system: Fatigue, drowsiness, dizziness
- Gastrointestinal: Nausea, vomiting, constipation
- Neuromuscular & skeletal: Weakness
- Miscellaneous: Histamine release

1% to 10%:

- Central nervous system: Nervousness, headache, restlessness, malaise, confusion
- Gastrointestinal: Anorexia, stomach cramps, xerostomia, biliary spasm
- Genitourinary: Decreased urination, ureteral spasms
- Local: Pain at injection site
- Respiratory: Dyspnea

<1%: Mental depression, hallucinations, paradoxical CNS stimulation, increased intracranial pressure, rash, urticaria, paralytic ileus, histamine release, physical and psychological dependence

Drug Interactions

Increased Effect/Toxicity: Increased effect/toxicity with CNS depressants (phenothiazines, tranquilizers, anxiolytics, sedatives, hypnotics, alcohol), tricyclic antidepressants, and dextroamphetamine.

Decreased Effect: Decreased effect with phenothiazines.

Dietary/Ethanol/Herb Considerations

Ethanol: Avoid use; may increase CNS depression.

Herb/Nutraceutical: Avoid gotu kola, kava, SAMe, St John's wort, and valerian; may increase CNS depression.

Pharmacodynamics/Kinetics

Onset of action: Analgesic: I.V., I.M., S.C.: 5-10 minutes; Rectal: 15-30 minutes

Duration: Analgesic: Parenteral, rectal: 3-4 hours

Metabolism: Hepatic via glucuronidation

Excretion: Urine

Pregnancy Risk Factor B/D (prolonged use or high doses at term)

Generic Available No

Oxymorphone Hydrochloride *see* Oxymorphone *on page 1024*

Oxytetracycline (oks i tet ra SYE kleen)

U.S. Brand Names Terramycin® I.M.

Canadian Brand Names Terramycin®

Mexican Brand Names Oxitraklin®; Terramicina®

Pharmacologic Category Antibiotic, Tetracycline Derivative

Synonyms Oxytetracycline Hydrochloride

Use Treatment of susceptible bacterial infections; both gram-positive and gram-negative, as well as, *Rickettsia* and *Mycoplasma* organisms

Local Anesthetic/Vasoconstrictor Precautions No information available to require special precautions

Effects on Dental Treatment Tetracyclines are not recommended for use during pregnancy or in children ≤8 years of age since they have been reported to cause enamel hypoplasia and permanent teeth discoloration. Tetracyclines should only be used in these patients if other agents are contraindicated or alternative antimicrobials will not eradicate the organism. Long-term use associated with oral candidiasis.

Dosage I.M.:
Children >8 years: 15-25 mg/kg/day (maximum: 250 mg/dose) in divided doses every 8-12 hours
Adults: 250 mg every 24 hours or 300 mg/day divided every 8-12 hours
Dosing interval in renal impairment: Cl_{cr} <10 mL/minute: Administer every 24 hours or avoid use if possible
Dosing adjustment in hepatic impairment: Avoid in severe liver disease

Mechanism of Action Inhibits bacterial protein synthesis by binding with the 30S and possibly the 50S ribosomal subunit(s) of susceptible bacteria, cell wall synthesis is not affected

Other Adverse Effects Frequency not defined; also refer to Tetracycline monograph
Cardiovascular: Pericarditis
Central nervous system: Bulging fontanels (infants), intracranial hypertension (adults)
Dermatologic: Angioneurotic edema, erythematous rash, exfoliative dermatitis (uncommon), maculopapular rash, photosensitivity, urticaria
Gastrointestinal: Anogenital inflammatory lesions, diarrhea, dysphagia, enamel hyperplasia, enterocolitis, glossitis, nausea, tooth discoloration, vomiting
Hematologic: Anemia, eosinophilia, neutropenia, thrombocytopenia
Local: Irritation
Renal: BUN increased
Miscellaneous: Anaphylactoid purpura, anaphylaxis, hypersensitivity reaction, SLE exacerbation

Drug Interactions
Increased Effect/Toxicity: Oral anticoagulant (warfarin) effects may be increased.
Decreased Effect: Barbiturates, phenytoin, and carbamazepine decrease serum levels of tetracyclines. Although anecdotal reports suggest oral contraceptive efficacy could be reduced by tetracyclines, this has been refuted by more rigorous scientific and clinical data.

Dietary/Ethanol/Herb Considerations Food: Dairy products may decrease serum concentration.

Pharmacodynamics/Kinetics
Absorption: Poor
Distribution: Crosses placenta
Metabolism: Hepatic (small amounts)
Half-life elimination: 8.5-9.6 hours; prolonged with renal impairment
Excretion: Urine; feces

Pregnancy Risk Factor D

Generic Available No

Oxytetracycline and Hydrocortisone

(oks i tet ra SYE kleen & hye droe KOR ti sone)

Related Information
Hydrocortisone *on page 688*
Oxytetracycline *on page 1024*

U.S. Brand Names Terra-Cortril® [DSC]

Pharmacologic Category Antibiotic/Corticosteroid, Ophthalmic

Synonyms Hydrocortisone and Oxytetracycline; Terra-Cortril® [DSC]

Use Treatment of susceptible ophthalmic bacterial infections with associated swelling

Local Anesthetic/Vasoconstrictor Precautions No information available to require special precautions

Effects on Dental Treatment No significant effects or complications reported

Dosage Ophthalmic: Adults: Instill 1-2 drops in eye(s) every 3-4 hours

Pregnancy Risk Factor C

Generic Available No

Oxytetracycline and Polymyxin B

(oks i tet ra SYE kleen & pol i MIKS in bee)

Related Information
Oxytetracycline *on page 1024*
Polymyxin B *on page 1095*

U.S. Brand Names Terramycin® w/Polymyxin B Ophthalmic

Pharmacologic Category Antibiotic, Ophthalmic; Antibiotic, Otic

Synonyms Polymyxin B and Oxytetracycline

Use Treatment of superficial ocular infections involving the conjunctiva and/or cornea

Local Anesthetic/Vasoconstrictor Precautions No information available to require special precautions

Effects on Dental Treatment No significant effects or complications reported

Dosage Topical: Apply 1/2" of ointment onto the lower lid of affected eye 2-4 times/day

Pregnancy Risk Factor D

Generic Available No

Oxytetracycline Hydrochloride *see* Oxytetracycline *on page 1024*

Oxytocin (oks i TOE sin)

U.S. Brand Names Pitocin®

Canadian Brand Names Pitocin®; Syntocinon®

Mexican Brand Names Oxitopisa; Syntocinon®; Xitocin; Xitocin®

Pharmacologic Category Oxytocic Agent

Synonyms Pit

Use Induces labor at term; controls postpartum bleeding

Local Anesthetic/Vasoconstrictor Precautions No information available to require special precautions

Effects on Dental Treatment No significant effects or complications reported

Dosage I.V. administration requires the use of an infusion pump. Adults:

Induction of labor: I.V.: 0.001-0.002 units/minute; increase by 0.001-0.002 units every 15-30 minutes until contraction pattern has been established; maximum dose should not exceed 20 milliunits/minute

Postpartum bleeding:

I.M.: Total dose of 10 units after delivery

I.V.: 10-40 units by I.V. infusion in 1000 mL of intravenous fluid at a rate sufficient to control uterine atony

Mechanism of Action Produces the rhythmic uterine contractions characteristic to delivery

Other Adverse Effects

Fetal: <1%: Bradycardia, arrhythmias, intracranial hemorrhage, brain damage, neonatal jaundice, hypoxia, death

Maternal: <1%: Arrhythmias, premature ventricular contractions, hypotension, tachycardia, seizures, coma, SIADH with hyponatremia, nausea, vomiting, pelvic hematoma, postpartum hemorrhage, increased uterine motility, fatal afibrinogenemia, increased blood loss, death, anaphylactic reactions

Pharmacodynamics/Kinetics

Onset of action: Uterine contractions: I.V.: ~1 minute

Duration: <30 minutes

Metabolism: Rapidly hepatic and via plasma (by oxytocinase) and to a smaller degree the mammary gland

Half-life elimination: 1-5 minutes

Excretion: Urine

Pregnancy Risk Factor X

Generic Available Yes

Oxytrol™ *see* Oxybutynin *on page 1016*

Oyst-Cal 500 [OTC] *see* Calcium Supplements *on page 229*

Oystercal® 500 *see* Calcium Supplements *on page 229*

P-071 *see* Cetirizine *on page 289*

Pacerone® *see* Amiodarone *on page 80*

Paclitaxel (PAK li taks il)

U.S. Brand Names Onxol™; Taxol®

Canadian Brand Names Taxol®

Mexican Brand Names Bris Taxol®; Praxel®

Pharmacologic Category Antineoplastic Agent, Natural Source (Plant) Derivative

Use Treatment of advanced carcinoma of the ovary in combination with cisplatin; treatment of metastatic carcinoma of the ovary after failure of first-line or subsequent chemotherapy; adjuvant treatment of node-positive breast cancer administered sequentially to standard doxorubicin-containing chemotherapy; treatment of metastatic breast cancer after failure of combination chemotherapy or relapse within 6 months of adjuvant chemotherapy; treatment of nonsmall cell lung cancer; second-line treatment of AIDS-related Kaposi's sarcoma

Local Anesthetic/Vasoconstrictor Precautions No information available to require special precautions

Effects on Dental Treatment No significant effects or complications reported

Dosage Premedication with dexamethasone (20 mg orally or I.V. at 12 and 6 hours **or** 14 and 7 hours before the dose), diphenhydramine (50 mg I.V. 30-60 minutes prior to the dose), and cimetidine, famotidine or ranitidine (I.V. 30-60 minutes prior to the dose) is recommended

Adults: I.V.: Refer to individual protocols

Ovarian carcinoma:

First-line therapy: 175 mg/m^2 over 3 hours every 3 weeks

or 135 mg/m^2 over 24 hours every 3 weeks

After failure of first-line therapy: 135-175 mg/m^2 over 3 hours every 3 weeks (doses up to 350 mg/m^2 have been studied, but are not generally recommended)

or 50-80 mg/m^2 over 1-3 hours weekly

or 1.4-4 mg/m^2/day continuous infusion for 14 days every 4 weeks

Metastatic breast cancer:

Adjuvant treatment of node-positive breast cancer: 175 mg/m^2 over 3 hours every 3 weeks for 4 courses

Metastatic or recurrent disease: 175 mg/m² over 3 hours every 3 weeks
Nonsmall cell lung carcinoma: 135 mg/m² over 24 hours, followed by cisplatin 75 mg/m²; repeat every 3 weeks
AIDS-related Kaposi's sarcoma: 135 mg/m² over 3 hours every 3 weeks **or** 100 mg/m² over 3 hours every 2 weeks

Dosage modification for toxicity (solid tumors, including ovary, breast, and lung carcinoma): Courses of paclitaxel should not be repeated until the neutrophil count is ≥1500 cells/mm³ and the platelet count is ≥100,000 cells/mm³; reduce dosage by 20% for patients experiencing severe peripheral neuropathy or severe neutropenia (neutrophil <500 cells/mm³ for a week or longer)

Dosage modification for immunosuppression in advanced HIV disease: Paclitaxel should not be given to patients with HIV if the baseline or subsequent neutrophil count is <1000 cells/mm³. Additional modifications include: Reduce dosage of dexamethasone in premedication to 10 mg orally; reduce dosage by 20% in patients experiencing severe peripheral neuropathy or severe neutropenia (neutrophil <500 cells/mm³ for a week or longer); initiate concurrent hematopoietic growth factor (G-CSF) as clinically indicated

Hemodialysis: Significant drug removal is unlikely based on physiochemical characteristics

Peritoneal dialysis: Significant drug removal is unlikely based on physiochemical characteristics

Dosing adjustment in hepatic impairment:
Total bilirubin ≤1.5 mg/dL and AST >2 times normal limits: Total dose <135 mg/m²
Total bilirubin 1.6-3.0 mg/dL: Total dose ≤75 mg/m²
Total bilirubin ≥3.1 mg/dL: Total dose ≤50 mg/m²

Mechanism of Action Paclitaxel exerts its effects on microtubules and their protein subunits, tubulin dimers. Microtubules serve as facilitators of intracellular transport and maintain the integrity and function of cells. Paclitaxel promotes microtubule assembly by enhancing the action of tubulin dimers, stabilizing existing microtubules, and inhibiting their disassembly. Maintaining microtubule assembly inhibits mitosis and cell death. The G_2- and M-phases of the cell cycle are affected. In addition, the drug can distort mitotic spindles, resulting in the breakage of chromosomes.

Other Adverse Effects

>10%:
Allergic: Appear to be primarily nonimmunologically mediated release of histamine and other vasoactive substances; almost always seen within the first hour of an infusion (~75% occur within 10 minutes of starting the infusion); incidence is significantly reduced by premedication
Cardiovascular: Bradycardia (transient, 25%)
Hematologic: Myelosuppression, leukopenia, neutropenia (6% to 21%), thrombocytopenia
Onset: 8-11 days
Nadir: 15-21 days
Recovery: 21 days
Dermatologic: Alopecia (87%), venous erythema, tenderness, discomfort, phlebitis (2%)
Neurotoxicity: Sensory and/or autonomic neuropathy (numbness, tingling, burning pain), myopathy or myopathic effects (25% to 55%), and central nervous system toxicity. May be cumulative and dose-limiting.
Gastrointestinal: Severe, potentially dose-limiting mucositis, stomatitis (15%), most common at doses >390 mg/m²
Hepatic: Mild increases in liver enzymes
Neuromuscular & skeletal: Arthralgia, myalgia

1% to 10%:
Cardiovascular: Myocardial infarction
Gastrointestinal: Mild nausea and vomiting (5% to 6%), diarrhea (5% to 6%)
Hematologic: Anemia

<1%: Ataxia, atrial fibrillation, enterocolitis, hepatic encephalopathy, intestinal obstruction, interstitial pneumonia, necrotic changes and ulceration following extravasation, neuroencephalopathy, ototoxicity (tinnitus and hearing loss), pancreatitis, paralytic ileus, pruritus, pulmonary fibrosis, radiation recall, radiation pneumonitis, rash, seizures, Stevens-Johnson syndrome, toxic epidermal necrolysis, visual disturbances (scintillating scotomata)

Drug Interactions Substrate of **CYP2C8/9, 3A4**; Induces CYP3A4

Increased Effect/Toxicity: In Phase I trials, myelosuppression was more profound when given after cisplatin than with alternative sequence. Pharmacokinetic data demonstrates a decrease in clearance of ~33% when administered following cisplatin. Possibility of an inhibition of metabolism in patients treated with ketoconazole. When administered as sequential infusions, observational studies indicate a potential for increased toxicity when platinum derivatives (carboplatin, cisplatin) are administered before taxane derivatives (docetaxel, paclitaxel).

Decreased Effect: Paclitaxel metabolism is dependent on cytochrome P450 isoenzymes. Inducers of these enzymes may decrease the effect of paclitaxel.

(Continued)

Paclitaxel *(Continued)*

Dietary/Ethanol/Herb Considerations Herb/Nutraceutical: Avoid black cohosh, dong quai, and evening primrose in estrogen-dependent tumors. Avoid gotu kola, kava, SAMe, St John's wort, and valerian; may increase CNS depression.

Pharmacodynamics/Kinetics

Distribution: V_{dss}: 42-162 L/m^2, indicating extensive extravascular distribution and/or tissue binding; initial rapid decline represents distribution to the peripheral compartment and significant elimination of the drug; later phase is due to a relatively slow efflux of paclitaxel from the peripheral compartment

Protein binding: 89% to 98%

Metabolism: Hepatic in animals; evidence suggests similar in humans

Half-life elimination: Mean: Terminal: 5.3-17.4 hours

Excretion: Urine (as unchanged drug); 1.3% to 12.6%

Clearance: Mean: Total body: After 1- and 6-hour infusions: 5.8-16.3 L/hour/m^2; After 24-hour infusions: 14.2-17.2 L/hour/m^2

Pregnancy Risk Factor D

Generic Available Yes

Pain-A-Lay® [OTC] *see* Phenol *on page 1068*

Palgic®-D *see* Carbinoxamine and Pseudoephedrine *on page 247*

Palgic®-DS *see* Carbinoxamine and Pseudoephedrine *on page 247*

Palivizumab (pah li VIZ yoo mab)

U.S. Brand Names Synagis®

Canadian Brand Names Synagis®

Pharmacologic Category Monoclonal Antibody

Use Prevention of serious lower respiratory tract disease caused by respiratory syncytial virus (RSV) in infants and children <2 years of age at high risk of RSV disease

Local Anesthetic/Vasoconstrictor Precautions No information available to require special precautions

Effects on Dental Treatment No significant effects or complications reported

Dosage I.M.: Infants and Children: 15 mg/kg of body weight, monthly throughout RSV season (First dose administered prior to commencement of RSV season)

Mechanism of Action Exhibits neutralizing and fusion-inhibitory activity against RSV; these activities inhibit RSV replication in laboratory and clinical studies

Other Adverse Effects Incidence similar between the palivizumab and placebo groups.

>1%:

- Central nervous system: Nervousness, fever
- Dermatologic: Fungal dermatitis, eczema, seborrhea, rash
- Gastrointestinal: Diarrhea, vomiting, gastroenteritis
- Hematologic: Anemia
- Hepatic: ALT increase, abnormal LFTs
- Local: Injection site reaction, erythema, induration
- Ocular: Conjunctivitis
- Otic: Otitis media
- Respiratory: Cough, wheezing, bronchiolitis, pneumonia, bronchitis, asthma, croup, dyspnea, sinusitis, apnea, upper respiratory infection, rhinitis
- Miscellaneous: Oral moniliasis, failure to thrive, viral infection, flu syndrome

Postmarketing and/or case reports: Hypersensitivity reactions, anaphylaxis (very rare)

Pharmacodynamics/Kinetics

Half-life elimination: Children <24 months: 20 days; Adults: 18 days

Time to peak, serum: 48 hours

Pregnancy Risk Factor C

Generic Available No

Selected Readings

Johnson S, Oliver C, Prince GA, et al, "Development of a Humanized Monoclonal Antibody (MEDI-493) With Potent *In Vitro* and *In Vivo* Activity Against Respiratory Syncytial Virus," *J Infect Dis*, 1997, 176(5):1215-24.

Subramanian KN, Weisman, LE, Rhodes T, et al, "Safety, Tolerance and Pharmacokinetics of a Humanized Monoclonal Antibody to Respiratory Syncytial Virus in Premature Infants With Bronchopulmonary Dysplasia. MEDI-493 Study Group," *Pediatr Infect Dis J*, 1998, 17(2):110-5.

Welliver RC, "Respiratory Syncytial Virus Immunoglobulin and Monoclonal Antibodies in the Prevention and Treatment of Respiratory Syncytial Virus Infection," *Semin Perinatol*, 1998, 22(1):87-95.

Palmer's® Skin Success Acne [OTC] *see* Benzoyl Peroxide *on page 171*

Palmer's Skin Success Acne Cleanser [OTC] *see* Salicylic Acid *on page 1204*

Palmer's® Skin Success Fade Cream™ [OTC] *see* Hydroquinone *on page 693*

Palmitate-A® [OTC] *see* Vitamin A *on page 1390*

PALS® [OTC] *see* Chlorophyll *on page 302*

Pamelor® *see* Nortriptyline *on page 989*

Pamidronate (pa mi DROE nate)

U.S. Brand Names Aredia®

Canadian Brand Names Aredia®

Pharmacologic Category Antidote; Bisphosphonate Derivative

Synonyms Pamidronate Disodium

Use Treatment of hypercalcemia associated with malignancy; treatment of osteolytic bone lesions associated with multiple myeloma or metastatic breast cancer; moderate to severe Paget's disease of bone

Local Anesthetic/Vasoconstrictor Precautions No information available to require special precautions

Effects on Dental Treatment No significant effects or complications reported

Dosage Drug must be diluted properly before administration and infused intravenously slowly. Due to risk of nephrotoxicity, doses should not exceed 90 mg.

I.V.: Adults:

Hypercalcemia of malignancy:

Moderate cancer-related hypercalcemia (corrected serum calcium: 12-13.5 mg/dL): 60-90 mg, as a single dose, given as a slow infusion over 2-24 hours; dose should be diluted in 1000 mL 0.45% NaCl, 0.9% NaCl, or D_5W

Severe cancer-related hypercalcemia (corrected serum calcium: >13.5 mg/dL): 90 mg, as a single dose, as a slow infusion over 2-24 hours; dose should be diluted in 1000 mL 0.45% NaCl, 0.9% NaCl, or D_5W

A period of 7 days should elapse before the use of second course; repeat infusions every 2-3 weeks have been suggested, however, could be administered every 2-3 months according to the degree and of severity of hypercalcemia and/or the type of malignancy.

Note: Some investigators have suggested a lack of a dose-response relationship. Courses of pamidronate for hypercalcemia may be repeated at varying intervals, depending on the duration of normocalcemia (median 2-3 weeks), but the manufacturer recommends a minimum interval between courses of 7 days. Oral etidronate at a dose of 20 mg/kg/day has been used to maintain the calcium lowering effect following I.V. bisphosphonates, although it is of limited effectiveness.

Osteolytic bone lesions with multiple myeloma: 90 mg in 500 mL D_5W, 0.45% NaCl or 0.9% NaCl administered over 4 hours on a monthly basis

Osteolytic bone lesions with metastatic breast cancer: 90 mg in 250 mL D_5W, 0.45% NaCl or 0.9% NaCl administered over 2 hours, repeated every 3-4 weeks

Paget's disease: 30 mg in 500 mL 0.45% NaCl, 0.9% NaCl or D_5W administered over 4 hours for 3 consecutive days

Dosing adjustment in renal impairment: Use not recommended in severe impairment (patients with bone metastases)

Renal toxicity: In patients with bone metastases, treatment should be withheld in patients who experience deterioration in renal function (increase of serum creatinine ≥0.5 mg/dL in patients with normal baseline or ≥1.0 mg/dL in patients with abnormal baseline). Resumption of therapy may be considered when serum creatinine returns to within 10% of baseline.

Mechanism of Action A biphosphonate which inhibits bone resorption via actions on osteoclasts or on osteoclast precursors. Does not appear to produce any significant effects on renal tubular calcium handling and is poorly absorbed following oral administration (high oral doses have been reported effective); therefore, I.V. therapy is preferred.

Other Adverse Effects As reported with hypercalcemia of malignancy; percentage of adverse effect varies upon dose and duration of infusion.

>10%:

Central nervous system: Fever (18% to 26%), fatigue (12%)

Endocrine & metabolic: Hypophosphatemia (9% to 18%), hypokalemia (4% to 18%), hypomagnesemia (4% to 12%), hypocalcemia (1% to 12%)

Gastrointestinal: Nausea (up to 18%), anorexia (1% to 12%)

Local: Infusion site reaction (up to 18%)

1% to 10%:

Cardiovascular: Atrial fibrillation (up to 6%), hypertension (up to 6%), syncope (up to 6%), tachycardia (up to 6%), atrial flutter (up to 1%), cardiac failure (up to 1%)

Central nervous system: Somnolence (1% to 6%), psychosis (up to 4%), insomnia (up to 1%)

Endocrine & metabolic: Hypothyroidism (6%)

Gastrointestinal: Constipation (4% to 6%), stomatitis (up to 1%)

Hematologic: Leukopenia (up to 4%), neutropenia (up to 1%), thrombocytopenia (up to 1%)

Neuromuscular & skeletal: Myalgia (up to 1%)

Renal: Uremia (up to 4%)

Respiratory: Rales (up to 6%), rhinitis (up to 6%), upper respiratory tract infection (up to 3%)

<1%: Iritis, episcleritis, scleritis, uveitis

(Continued)

Pamidronate *(Continued)*

Postmarketing and/or case reports: Allergic reaction, anaphylactic shock, angioedema, hypotension

Pharmacodynamics/Kinetics

Onset of action: 24-48 hours

Peak effect: Maximum: 5-7 days

Absorption: Poor; pharmacokinetic studies lacking

Metabolism: Not metabolized

Half-life elimination: 21-35 hours; Bone: Terminal: ~300 days

Excretion: Biphasic; urine (~50% as unchanged drug) within 120 hours

Pregnancy Risk Factor D

Generic Available Yes

Pamidronate Disodium *see* Pamidronate *on page 1029*

Pamine® *see* Methscopolamine *on page 888*

p-Aminoclonidine *see* Apraclonidine *on page 118*

Pan-2400™ [OTC] *see* Pancreatin *on page 1030*

Pancof®-XP *see* Hydrocodone, Pseudoephedrine, and Guaifenesin *on page 687*

Pancrease® *see* Pancrelipase *on page 1030*

Pancrease® MT *see* Pancrelipase *on page 1030*

Pancreatin (PAN kree a tin)

U.S. Brand Names Hi-Vegi-Lip® [OTC]; Kutrase®; Ku-Zyme®; Pan-2400™ [OTC]; Pancreatin 4X [OTC]; Pancreatin 8X [OTC]; Veg-Pancreatin 4X [OTC]

Mexican Brand Names Creon®; Optifree®; Pancrease®; Selecto®

Pharmacologic Category Enzyme

Use Relief of functional indigestion due to enzyme deficiency or imbalance

Local Anesthetic/Vasoconstrictor Precautions No information available to require special precautions

Effects on Dental Treatment No significant effects or complications reported

Dosage Oral: Adults: Actual dose varies with condition of patient and is usually given with each meal or snack.

Ku-Zyme®: 1-2 capsules with each meal or snack

Kutrase®: 1 capsule with each meal or snack

Mechanism of Action An enzyme supplement, not a replacement, which contains a combination of lipase, amylase and protease; enhances the digestion of proteins, starch and fat in the stomach and intestines; on a weight basis, pancreatin has $^1/_{12}$ the lipolytic activity of pancrelipase.

Other Adverse Effects Frequency not defined:

Gastrointestinal: Loose stools (decrease dose)

Respiratory: Mucous membrane irritation or precipitation of asthma attack (due to inhalation of airborne powder)

Dietary/Ethanol/Herb Considerations Food: Administer with food; capsules may be opened and sprinkled on soft food.

Pregnancy Risk Factor C

Generic Available Yes

Pancreatin 4X [OTC] *see* Pancreatin *on page 1030*

Pancreatin 8X [OTC] *see* Pancreatin *on page 1030*

Pancrecarb MS® *see* Pancrelipase *on page 1030*

Pancrelipase (pan kre LI payz)

U.S. Brand Names Creon®; Ku-Zyme® HP; Lipram 4500; Lipram-CR; Lipram-PN; Lipram-UL; Pancrease®; Pancrease® MT; Pancrecarb MS®; Pangestyme™ CN; Pangestyme™ EC; Pangestyme™ MT; Pangestyme™ UL; Ultrase®; Ultrase® MT; Viokase®

Canadian Brand Names Cotazym®; Creon® 5; Creon® 10; Creon® 20; Creon® 25; Pancrease®; Pancrease® MT; Ultrase®; Ultrase® MT; Viokase®

Pharmacologic Category Enzyme

Synonyms Lipancreatin; Zymase® [DSC]

Use Replacement therapy in symptomatic treatment of malabsorption syndrome caused by pancreatic insufficiency

Unlabeled/Investigational Use Treatment of occluded feeding tubes

Local Anesthetic/Vasoconstrictor Precautions No information available to require special precautions

Effects on Dental Treatment No significant effects or complications reported

Dosage Oral:

Powder: Actual dose depends on the condition being treated and the digestive requirements of the patient

Children <1 year: Start with $^1/_8$ teaspoonful with feedings

Adults: 0.7 g ($^1/_4$ teaspoonful) with meals

Capsules/tablets: The following dosage recommendations are only an approximation for initial dosages. The actual dosage will depend on the condition being treated and the digestive requirements of the individual patient. Adjust dose based on body weight and stool fat content. Total daily dose reflects ~3 meals/day and 2-3 snacks/day, with half the mealtime dose given with a snack. Older patients may need less units/kg due to increased weight, but decreased ingestion of fat/kg. Maximum dose: 2500 units of lipase/kg/meal (10,000 units of lipase/kg/day)

Children:

<1 year: 2000 units of lipase with meals

1-6 years: 4000-8000 units of lipase with meals and 4000 units with snacks

7-12 years: 4000-12,000 units of lipase with meals and snacks

Adults: 4000-48,000 units of lipase with meals and with snacks

Occluded feeding tubes: One tablet of Viokase® crushed with one 325 mg tablet of sodium bicarbonate (to activate the Viokase®) in 5 mL of water can be instilled into the nasogastric tube and clamped for 5 minutes; then, flushed with 50 mL of tap water

Mechanism of Action Pancrelipase is a natural product harvested from the hog pancreas. It contains a combination of lipase, amylase, and protease. Products are formulated to dissolve in the more basic pH of the duodenum so that they may act locally to break down fats, protein, and starch.

Other Adverse Effects Frequency not defined; occurrence of events may be dose-related.

Central nervous system: Pain

Dermatologic: Rash

Endocrine & metabolic: Hyperuricemia

Gastrointestinal: Nausea, cramps, constipation, diarrhea, perianal irritation/inflammation (large doses), irritation of the mouth, abdominal pain, intestinal obstruction, vomiting, flatulence, melena, weight loss, fibrotic strictures, greasy stools

Ocular: Lacrimation

Renal: Hyperuricosuria

Respiratory: Sneezing, dyspnea, bronchospasm

Miscellaneous: Allergic reactions

Dietary/Ethanol/Herb Considerations Food: Administer with food. Delayed-release capsules containing enteric coated microspheres or microtablets may also be opened and the contents sprinkled on soft food with a low pH such as applesauce or gelatin; apricot, banana, or sweet potato baby food; or baby formula; avoid placing contents of opened capsules on alkaline food with pH >5.5 (eg, dairy products). May impair absorption of oral iron and folic acid. Requires high-calorie diet, appropriate for age and clinical status.

Pharmacodynamics/Kinetics

Absorption: None; acts locally in GI tract

Excretion: Feces

Pregnancy Risk Factor B/C (product specific)

Generic Available Yes

Comments Concomitant administration of conventional pancreatin enzymes with an H_2-receptor antagonist has been used to decrease the inactivation of enzyme activity.

Pandel® *see* Hydrocortisone *on page 688*

Pangestyme™ CN *see* Pancrelipase *on page 1030*

Pangestyme™ EC *see* Pancrelipase *on page 1030*

Pangestyme™ MT *see* Pancrelipase *on page 1030*

Pangestyme™ UL *see* Pancrelipase *on page 1030*

Panglobulin® *see* Immune Globulin (Intravenous) *on page 714*

Panhematin® *see* Hemin *on page 661*

PanMist®-DM *see* Guaifenesin, Pseudoephedrine, and Dextromethorphan *on page 653*

PanMist® Jr. *see* Guaifenesin and Pseudoephedrine *on page 652*

PanMist® LA *see* Guaifenesin and Pseudoephedrine *on page 652*

PanMist® S *see* Guaifenesin and Pseudoephedrine *on page 652*

PanOxyl® *see* Benzoyl Peroxide *on page 171*

PanOxyl®-AQ *see* Benzoyl Peroxide *on page 171*

PanOxyl® Bar [OTC] *see* Benzoyl Peroxide *on page 171*

Panretin® *see* Alitretinoin *on page 57*

Panthoderm® [OTC] *see* Dexpanthenol *on page 418*

Pantoprazole (pan TOE pray zole)

Related Information

Gastrointestinal Disorders *on page 1474*

U.S. Brand Names Protonix®

Canadian Brand Names Panto™ IV; Pantoloc™; Protonix®

Mexican Brand Names Pantozol®; Zurcal®

Pharmacologic Category Proton Pump Inhibitor

Use

Oral: Treatment and maintenance of healing of erosive esophagitis associated with GERD; reduction in relapse rates of daytime and nighttime heartburn symptoms

(Continued)

Pantoprazole *(Continued)*

in GERD; hypersecretory disorders associated with Zollinger-Ellison syndrome or other neoplastic disorders

I.V.: As an alternative to oral therapy in patients unable to continue oral pantoprazole; hypersecretory disorders associated with Zollinger-Ellison syndrome or other neoplastic disorders

Unlabeled/Investigational Use Treatment of peptic ulcer disease, active ulcer bleeding with parenterally-administered pantoprazole; adjunct treatment with antibiotics for *Helicobacter pylori* eradication

Local Anesthetic/Vasoconstrictor Precautions No information available to require special precautions

Effects on Dental Treatment No significant effects or complications reported

Dosage Adults:

Oral:

Erosive esophagitis associated with GERD:

Treatment: 40 mg once daily for up to 8 weeks; an additional 8 weeks may be used in patients who have not healed after an 8-week course

Maintenance of healing: 40 mg once daily

Note: Lower doses (20 mg once daily) have been used successfully in mild GERD treatment and maintenance of healing

Hypersecretory disorders (including Zollinger-Ellison): Initial: 40 mg twice daily; adjust dose based on patient needs; doses up to 240 mg/day have been administered

I.V.:

Erosive esophagitis associated with GERD: 40 mg once daily (infused over 15 minutes) for 7-10 days

Helicobacter pylori eradication (unlabeled use): Doses up to 40 mg twice daily have been used as part of combination therapy

Hypersecretory disorders: 80 mg twice daily; adjust dose based on acid output measurements; 160-240 mg/day in divided doses has been used for a limited period (up to 7 days)

Hemodialysis: Not removed

Mechanism of Action Suppresses gastric acid secretin by inhibiting the parietal cell H^+/K^+ ATP pump

Other Adverse Effects

1% to 10%:

Cardiovascular: Chest pain (I.V. ≤6%)

Central nervous system: Pain, migraine, anxiety, dizziness, headache (I.V. >1%)

Dermatologic: Rash (I.V. 6%), pruritus (I.V. 4%)

Endocrine & metabolic: Hyperglycemia (1%), hyperlipidemia

Gastrointestinal: Diarrhea (4%), constipation, dyspepsia, gastroenteritis, nausea, rectal disorder, vomiting, abdominal pain (I.V. 12%)

Genitourinary: Urinary frequency, urinary tract infection

Hepatic: Liver function test abnormality, increased SGPT

Local: Injection site pain (>1%)

Neuromuscular & skeletal: Weakness, back pain, neck pain, arthralgia, hypertonia

Respiratory: Bronchitis, increased cough, dyspnea, pharyngitis, rhinitis, sinusitis, upper respiratory tract infection

Miscellaneous: Flu syndrome, infection

<1%: Abnormal vision, acne, albuminuria, allergic reaction, alopecia, amblyopia, anemia, angina pectoris, anorexia, aphthous stomatitis, arrhythmia, arthritis, asthma, balanitis, bone pain, breast pain, bursitis, cataract, cholecystitis, cholelithiasis, cholestatic jaundice, colitis, confusion, CHF, contact dermatitis, convulsion, cystitis, deafness, decreased reflexes, decreased libido, dehydration, depression, diabetes mellitus, diplopia, xerostomia, dry skin, duodenitis, dysarthria, dysmenorrhea, dysphagia, dysuria, ear pain, ecchymosis, eczema, EKG abnormality, eosinophilia, epididymitis, epistaxis, extraocular palsy, fever, fungal dermatitis, gastrointestinal carcinoma, gastrointestinal hemorrhage, gastrointestinal moniliasis, generalized edema, gingivitis, glaucoma, glossitis, glycosuria, goiter, gout, halitosis, hallucinations, hematuria, hemorrhage, hepatitis, herpes simplex, herpes zoster, hypercholesterolemia, hyperkinesia, hypertension, hyperuricemia, hypotension, impaired urination, impotence, increased alkaline phosphatase, increased appetite, increased creatinine, increased transaminases, kidney calculus, kidney pain, laryngitis, leg cramps, leukocytosis, leukopenia, lichenoid dermatitis, maculopapular rash, oral ulceration, myalgia, myocardial ischemia, neck rigidity, neoplasm, nervousness, neuralgia, neuritis, nocturia, oral moniliasis, otitis externa, pain, palpitation, paresthesia, pneumonia, pyelonephritis, rectal hemorrhage, retinal vascular disorder, scrotal edema, skin ulcer, somnolence, stomach ulcer, stomatitis, diaphoresis, syncope, tachycardia, abnormal taste, tenosynovitis, thrombocytopenia, thrombosis, tongue discoloration, tremor, urethritis, urticaria, thrombophlebitis (I.V.), vaginitis, vasodilation, vertigo, voice alteration

Postmarketing and/or case reports: Anaphylaxis, angioedema, anterior ischemic optic neuropathy, blurred vision, erythema multiforme, hepatic failure, hypokinesia, pancytopenia, rhabdomyolysis, increased salivation, speech disorder, Stevens-Johnson syndrome, pancreatitis, tinnitus, toxic epidermal necrolysis

Drug Interactions Substrate of **CYP2C19**, 3A4; Induces CYP1A2, 3A4

Decreased Effect: Drugs (eg, itraconazole, ketoconazole, and other azole antifungals, ampicillin esters, iron salts) where absorption is determined by an acidic gastric pH, may have decreased absorption when used concurrently. Monitor for change in effectiveness.

Dietary/Ethanol/Herb Considerations

Ethanol: Avoid use; may cause gastric mucosal irritation.

Food: Oral form may be taken with food.

Pharmacodynamics/Kinetics

Absorption: Well absorbed

Distribution: V_d: 11-24 L

Protein binding: 98%, primarily to albumin

Metabolism: Extensively hepatic; CYP2C19 (demethylation), CYP3A4; no evidence that metabolites have pharmacologic activity

Bioavailability: 77%

Half-life elimination: 1 hour

Time to peak: Oral: 2.5 hours

Excretion: Urine (71%); feces (18%)

Pregnancy Risk Factor B

Generic Available No

Pantothenic Acid (pan toe THEN ik AS id)

Pharmacologic Category Vitamin, Water Soluble

Synonyms Calcium Pantothenate; Vitamin B_5

Use Pantothenic acid deficiency

Local Anesthetic/Vasoconstrictor Precautions No information available to require special precautions

Effects on Dental Treatment No significant effects or complications reported

Dosage Adults: Oral: Recommended daily dose 4-7 mg/day

Pregnancy Risk Factor A/C (dose exceeding RDA recommendation)

Generic Available Yes

Pantothenyl Alcohol *see* Dexpanthenol *on page 418*

Papaverine (pa PAV er een)

U.S. Brand Names Para-Time S.R.®

Pharmacologic Category Vasodilator

Synonyms Papaverine Hydrochloride; Pavabid® [DSC]

Use Oral: Relief of peripheral and cerebral ischemia associated with arterial spasm and myocardial ischemia complicated by arrhythmias

Unlabeled/Investigational Use Investigational: Parenteral: Treatment of various vascular spasms associated with muscle spasms as in myocardial infarction, angina, peripheral and pulmonary embolism, peripheral vascular disease, angiospastic states, and visceral spasm (ureteral, biliary, and GI colic); testing for impotence

Local Anesthetic/Vasoconstrictor Precautions No information available to require special precautions

Effects on Dental Treatment No significant effects or complications reported

Dosage

I.M., I.V.:

Children: 6 mg/kg/day in 4 divided doses

Adults: 30-65 mg (rarely up to 120 mg); may repeat every 3 hours

Oral, sustained release: Adults: 150-300 mg every 12 hours; in difficult cases: 150 mg every 8 hours

Mechanism of Action Smooth muscle spasmolytic producing a generalized smooth muscle relaxation including: vasodilatation, gastrointestinal sphincter relaxation, bronchiolar muscle relaxation, and potentially a depressed myocardium (with large doses); muscle relaxation may occur due to inhibition or cyclic nucleotide phosphodiesterase, increasing cyclic AMP; muscle relaxation is unrelated to nerve innervation; papaverine increases cerebral blood flow in normal subjects; oxygen uptake is unaltered

Other Adverse Effects Frequency not defined:

Cardiovascular: Arrhythmias (with rapid I.V. use), flushing of the face, mild hypertension, tachycardias

Central nervous system: Drowsiness, headache, lethargy, sedation, vertigo

Gastrointestinal: Abdominal distress, anorexia, constipation, diarrhea, nausea

Hepatic: Chronic hepatitis, hepatic hypersensitivity

Respiratory: Apnea (with rapid I.V. use)

Drug Interactions CYP2D6 enzyme substrate

Decreased Effect: Papaverine decreases the effects of levodopa.

(Continued)

Papaverine *(Continued)*

Dietary/Ethanol/Herb Considerations

Ethanol: Avoid use; may increase CNS depression.

Herb/Nutraceutical: Avoid gotu kola, kava, SAMe, St John's wort, and valerian; may increase CNS depression.

Pharmacodynamics/Kinetics

Onset of action: Oral: Rapid
Protein binding: 90%
Metabolism: Rapidly hepatic
Half-life elimination: 0.5-1.5 hours
Excretion: Primarily urine (as metabolites)

Pregnancy Risk Factor C

Generic Available Yes

Papaverine Hydrochloride *see* Papaverine *on page 1033*
Para-Aminosalicylate Sodium *see* Aminosalicylic Acid *on page 79*
Paracetamol *see* Acetaminophen *on page 27*
Parafon Forte® DSC *see* Chlorzoxazone *on page 316*
Paraplatin® *see* Carboplatin *on page 248*
Parathyroid Hormone (1-34) *see* Teriparatide *on page 1280*
Para-Time S.R.® *see* Papaverine *on page 1033*

Paregoric (par e GOR ik)

Pharmacologic Category Analgesic, Narcotic

Synonyms Camphorated Tincture of Opium

Use Treatment of diarrhea or relief of pain; neonatal opiate withdrawal

Local Anesthetic/Vasoconstrictor Precautions No information available to require special precautions

Effects on Dental Treatment No significant effects or complications reported

Restrictions C-III

Dosage Oral:

Neonatal opiate withdrawal: 3-6 drops every 3-6 hours as needed, or initially 0.2 mL every 3 hours; increase dosage by approximately 0.05 mL every 3 hours until withdrawal symptoms are controlled; it is rare to exceed 0.7 mL/dose. Stabilize withdrawal symptoms for 3-5 days, then gradually decrease dosage over a 2- to 4-week period.

Children: 0.25-0.5 mL/kg 1-4 times/day

Adults: 5-10 mL 1-4 times/day

Mechanism of Action Increases smooth muscle tone in GI tract, decreases motility and peristalsis, diminishes digestive secretions

Other Adverse Effects Frequency not defined:

Cardiovascular: Hypotension, peripheral vasodilation

Central nervous system: Drowsiness, dizziness, insomnia, CNS depression, mental depression, increased intracranial pressure, restlessness, headache, malaise

Gastrointestinal: Constipation, anorexia, stomach cramps, nausea, vomiting, biliary tract spasm

Genitourinary: Ureteral spasms, decreased urination, urinary tract spasm

Hepatic: Increased LFTs

Neuromuscular & skeletal: Weakness

Ocular: Miosis

Respiratory: Respiratory depression

Miscellaneous: Physical and psychological dependence, histamine release

Drug Interactions Increased Effect/Toxicity: Increased effect/toxicity with CNS depressants (eg, alcohol, narcotics, benzodiazepines, tricyclic antidepressants, MAO inhibitors, phenothiazine).

Dietary/Ethanol/Herb Considerations

Ethanol: Avoid use; may increase CNS depression.

Herb/Nutraceutical: Avoid gotu kola, kava, SAMe, St John's wort, and valerian; may increase CNS depression.

Pharmacodynamics/Kinetics In terms of opium:

Metabolism: Hepatic

Excretion: Urine (primarily as morphine glucuronide conjugates and unchanged drug - morphine, codeine, papaverine, etc)

Pregnancy Risk Factor B/D (prolonged use or high doses)

Generic Available Yes

Paremyd® *see* Hydroxyamphetamine and Tropicamide *on page 694*

Paricalcitol (par e KAL si tol)

U.S. Brand Names Zemplar™

Canadian Brand Names Zemplar™

Pharmacologic Category Vitamin D Analog

Use Prevention and treatment of secondary hyperparathyroidism associated with chronic renal failure. Has been evaluated only in hemodialysis patients.

Local Anesthetic/Vasoconstrictor Precautions No information available to require special precautions

Effects on Dental Treatment No significant effects or complications reported

Dosage Adults: I.V.: 0.04-0.1 mcg/kg (2.8-7 mcg) given as a bolus dose no more frequently than every other day at any time during dialysis; doses as high as 0.24 mcg/kg (16.8 mcg) have been administered safely; usually start with 0.04 mcg/kg 3 times/week by I.V. bolus, increased by 0.04 mcg/kg every 2 weeks; the dose of paricalcitol should be adjusted based on serum PTH levels, as follows:

- Same or increasing serum PTH level: Increase paricalcitol dose
- Serum PTH level decreased by <30%: Increase paricalcitol dose
- Serum PTH level decreased by >30% and <60%: Maintain paricalcitol dose
- Serum PTH level decrease by >60%: Decrease paricalcitol dose
- Serum PTH level 1.5-3 times upper limit of normal: Maintain paricalcitol dose

Mechanism of Action Synthetic vitamin D analog which has been shown to reduce PTH serum concentrations

Other Adverse Effects The three most frequently reported events in clinical studies were nausea, vomiting, and edema, which are commonly seen in hemodialysis patients.

>10%: Gastrointestinal: Nausea (13%)

1% to 10%:
- Cardiovascular: Palpitations, peripheral edema (7%)
- Central nervous system: Chills, malaise, fever, lightheadedness (5%)
- Gastrointestinal: Vomiting (8%), GI bleeding (5%), xerostomia (3%)
- Respiratory: Pneumonia (5%)
- Miscellaneous: Flu-like symptoms, sepsis

Drug Interactions Increased Effect/Toxicity: Phosphate or vitamin D-related compounds should not be taken concurrently. Digitalis toxicity is potentiated by hypercalcemia.

Dietary/Ethanol/Herb Considerations Avoid other phosphate or vitamin D supplements or related compounds.

Pharmacodynamics/Kinetics

Protein binding: >99%

Excretion: Feces (74%) in healthy subjects; urine (16%); 51% to 59% as metabolites

Pregnancy Risk Factor C

Generic Available No

Paripriazole *see* Rabeprazole *on page 1162*

Parlodel® *see* Bromocriptine *on page 199*

Parnate® *see* Tranylcypromine *on page 1334*

Paromomycin (par oh moe MYE sin)

U.S. Brand Names Humatin®

Canadian Brand Names Humatin®

Pharmacologic Category Amebicide

Synonyms Paromomycin Sulfate

Use Treatment of acute and chronic intestinal amebiasis; preoperatively to suppress intestinal flora; tapeworm infestations; treatment of *Cryptosporidium*

Local Anesthetic/Vasoconstrictor Precautions No information available to require special precautions

Effects on Dental Treatment No significant effects or complications reported

Dosage Oral:

Intestinal amebiasis: Children and Adults: 25-35 mg/kg/day in 3 divided doses for 5-10 days

Dientamoeba fragilis: Children and Adults: 25-30 mg/kg/day in 3 divided doses for 7 days

Cryptosporidium: Adults with AIDS: 1.5-2.25 g/day in 3-6 divided doses for 10-14 days (occasionally courses of up to 4-8 weeks may be needed)

Tapeworm (fish, dog, bovine, porcine):
- Children: 11 mg/kg every 15 minutes for 4 doses
- Adults: 1 g every 15 minutes for 4 doses

Hepatic coma: Adults: 4 g/day in 2-4 divided doses for 5-6 days

Dwarf tapeworm: Children and Adults: 45 mg/kg/dose every day for 5-7 days

Mechanism of Action Acts directly on ameba; has antibacterial activity against normal and pathogenic organisms in the GI tract; interferes with bacterial protein synthesis by binding to 30S ribosomal subunits

Other Adverse Effects

1% to 10%: Gastrointestinal: Diarrhea, abdominal cramps, nausea, vomiting, heartburn

<1%: Headache, vertigo, exanthema, rash, pruritus, steatorrhea, secondary enterocolitis, eosinophilia, ototoxicity

Dietary/Ethanol/Herb Considerations Food: May cause malabsorption of xylose, sucrose, and fats.

(Continued)

Paromomycin *(Continued)*

Pharmacodynamics/Kinetics

Absorption: None

Excretion: Feces (100% as unchanged drug)

Pregnancy Risk Factor C

Generic Available Yes

Paromomycin Sulfate *see* Paromomycin *on page 1035*

Paroxetine (pa ROKS e teen)

U.S. Brand Names Paxil®; Paxil® CR™

Canadian Brand Names Paxil®; Paxil® CR™

Mexican Brand Names Aropax®; Paxil®

Pharmacologic Category Antidepressant, Selective Serotonin Reuptake Inhibitor

Use Treatment of depression in adults; treatment of panic disorder with or without agoraphobia; obsessive-compulsive disorder (OCD) in adults; social anxiety disorder (social phobia); generalized anxiety disorder (GAD); post-traumatic stress disorder (PTSD)

Paxil® CR™: Treatment of depression; treatment of panic disorder

Unlabeled/Investigational Use Treatment of eating disorders, impulse control disorders, self-injurious behavior, premenstrual disorders, vasomotor symptoms of menopause, depression and obsessive-compulsive disorder (OCD) in children

Local Anesthetic/Vasoconstrictor Precautions Although caution should be used in patients taking tricyclic antidepressants, no interactions have been reported with vasoconstrictor and paroxetine, a nontricyclic antidepressant which acts to increase serotonin

Effects on Dental Treatment

Problems with SSRI-induced bruxism have been reported and may preclude their use; clinicians attempting to evaluate any patient with bruxism or involuntary muscle movement, who is simultaneously being treated with an SSRI drug, should be aware of the potential association.

Prolonged use may decrease or inhibit salivary flow; normal salivation resumes upon discontinuation.

>10%: Xerostomia, changes in salivation

>10%: Headache, somnolence, dizziness, nausea, weakness, diaphoresis

1% to 10%: Palpitations, vasodilation, postural hypotension, nervousness, anxiety, yawning, vomiting, abnormal taste, tremors, paresthesia

Dosage Oral:

Children:

- Depression (unlabeled use): Initial: 10 mg/day and adjusted upward on an individual basis to 20 mg/day
- OCD (unlabeled use): Initial: 10 mg/day and titrate up as necessary to 60 mg/day
- Self-injurious behavior (unlabeled use): 20 mg/day

Adults:

- Depression: Initial: 20 mg once daily, preferably in the morning; increase if needed by 10 mg/day increments at intervals of at least 1 week; maximum dose: 50 mg/day
  - Paxil® CR™: Initial: 25 mg once daily; increase if needed by 12.5 mg/day increments at intervals of at least 1 week; maximum dose: 62.5 mg/day
- GAD: Initial: 20 mg once daily, preferably in the morning; doses of 20-50 mg/day were used in clinical trials, however, no greater benefit was seen with doses >20 mg. If dose is increased, adjust in increments of 10 mg/day at 1-week intervals.
- OCD: Initial: 20 mg once daily, preferably in the morning; increase if needed by 10 mg/day increments at intervals of at least 1 week; recommended dose: 40 mg/day; range: 20-60 mg/day; maximum dose: 60 mg/day
- Panic disorder: Initial: 10 mg once daily, preferably in the morning; increase if needed by 10 mg/day increments at intervals of at least 1 week; recommended dose: 40 mg/day; range: 10-60 mg/day; maximum dose: 60 mg/day
  - Paxil® CR™: Initial: 12 mg once daily; increase if needed by 12.5 mg/day at intervals of at least 1 week; maximum dose: 75 mg/day
- PTSD: Initial: 20 mg once daily, preferably in the morning; increase if needed by 10 mg/day increments at intervals of at least 1 week; range: 20-50 mg
- Social anxiety disorder: Initial: 20 mg once daily, preferably in the morning; recommended dose: 20 mg/day; range: 20-60 mg/day; doses >20 mg may not have additional benefit

Elderly: Initial: 10 mg/day; increase if needed by 10 mg/day increments at intervals of at least 1 week; maximum dose: 40 mg/day

- Paxil® CR™; Initial: 12.5 mg/day; increase if needed by 12.5 mg/day increments at intervals of at least 1 week; maximum dose: 50 mg/day

Note: Upon discontinuation of paroxetine therapy, gradually taper dose (taper-phase regimen used in PTSD/GAD clinical trials involved an incremental decrease in the daily dose by 10 mg/day at weekly intervals; when 20 mg/day dose was reached, this dose was continued for 1 week before treatment was stopped).

Dosing adjustment in severe renal/hepatic impairment: Adults: Initial: 10 mg/day; increase if needed by 10 mg/day increments at intervals of at least 1 week; maximum dose: 40 mg/day

Paxil® CR™: Initial: 12.5 mg/day; increase if needed by 12.5 mg/day increments at intervals of at least 1 week; maximum dose: 50 mg/day

Mechanism of Action Paroxetine is a selective serotonin reuptake inhibitor, chemically unrelated to tricyclic, tetracyclic, or other antidepressants; presumably, the inhibition of serotonin reuptake from brain synapse stimulated serotonin activity in the brain

Other Adverse Effects

>10%:

Central nervous system: Insomnia

Gastrointestinal: Constipation, diarrhea

Genitourinary: Ejaculatory disturbances

1% to 10%:

Central nervous system: Abnormal dreams

Dermatologic: Rash

Endocrine & metabolic: Decreased libido, delayed ejaculation

Gastrointestinal: Anorexia, flatulence, dyspepsia, weight gain

Genitourinary: Urinary frequency, impotence

Neuromuscular & skeletal: Myopathy, myalgia

<1%: Acne, akinesia, alopecia, amenorrhea, **anaphylactoid reaction,** anemia, angioedema, **arthritis, asthma, atrial fibrillation, bradycardia, bruxism**, bundle branch block, colitis, **dysphasia, EPS, ear pain,** erythema multiforme, exfoliative dermatitis, eye pain, **hypotension,** leukopenia, **mania, migraine, myasthenia, thirst**

Postmarketing and/or case reports: Acute renal failure, allergic alveolitis, **anaphylaxis,** aplastic anemia, agranulocytosis, bone marrow aplasia, eclampsia, Guillain-Barré syndrome, hemolytic anemia, hepatic necrosis, **laryngismus,** neuroleptic malignant syndrome, optic neuritis, pancreatitis, pancytopenia, porphyria, priapism, **pulmonary hypertension, seizures (including status epilepticus), serotonin syndrome,** SIADH, thrombocytopenia, **torsade de pointes,** toxic epidermal necrolysis, **ventricular fibrillation, ventricular tachycardia, withdrawal reactions** (dizziness; sensory disturbances - eg, paresthesias such as electric shock sensations; agitation; anxiety; nausea; diaphoresis - particularly following abrupt withdrawal)

Drug Interactions Substrate of **CYP2D6**; Inhibits CYP1A2, **2B6**, 2C8/9, 2C19, **2D6**, 3A4

Increased Effect/Toxicity:

MAO inhibitors: Paroxetine should not be used with nonselective MAO inhibitors (phenelzine, isocarboxazid) or other drugs with MAO inhibition (linezolid); fatal reactions have been reported. Wait 5 weeks after stopping fluoxetine before starting a nonselective MAO inhibitor and 2 weeks after stopping an MAO inhibitor before starting paroxetine. Concurrent selegiline has been associated with mania, hypertension, or serotonin syndrome (risk may be reduced relative to nonselective MAO inhibitors).

Phenothiazines: Paroxetine may inhibit the metabolism of thioridazine or mesoridazine, resulting in increased plasma levels and increasing the risk of QT_c interval prolongation. This may lead to serious ventricular arrhythmias, such as torsade de pointes-type arrhythmias and sudden death. Do not use together. Wait at least 5 weeks after discontinuing paroxetine prior to starting thioridazine.

Combined used of SSRIs and amphetamines, buspirone, meperidine, nefazodone, serotonin agonists (such as sumatriptan), sibutramine, other SSRIs, sympathomimetics, ritonavir, tramadol, and venlafaxine may increase the risk of serotonin syndrome. Paroxetine may increase serum levels/effects of benzodiazepines (alprazolam and diazepam), carbamazepine, carvedilol, clozapine, cyclosporine (and possibly tacrolimus), dextromethorphan, digoxin, haloperidol, HMG-CoA reductase inhibitors (lovastatin and simvastatin - increasing the risk of rhabdomyolysis), phenytoin, propafenone, theophylline, trazodone, tricyclic antidepressants, and valproic acid. Concurrent lithium may increase risk of nephrotoxicity. Risk of hyponatremia may increase with concurrent use of loop diuretics (bumetanide, furosemide, torsemide). Paroxetine may increase the hypoprothrombinemic response to warfarin.

Combined use of sumatriptan (and other serotonin agonists) may result in toxicity; weakness, hyper-reflexia, and incoordination have been observed with sumatriptan and SSRIs. In addition, concurrent use may theoretically increase the risk of serotonin syndrome; includes sumatriptan, naratriptan, rizatriptan, and zolmitriptan.

Decreased Effect: Cyproheptadine, a serotonin antagonist, may inhibit the effects of serotonin reuptake inhibitors (paroxetine).

(Continued)

Paroxetine *(Continued)*

Dietary/Ethanol/Herb Considerations

Ethanol: Although ethanol may not cause much CNS depression here, depressed patients should avoid/limit intake.

Food: May be taken with food; increases peak concentration, but bioavailability is not significantly altered. Avoid caffeine.

Herb/Nutraceutical: Avoid kava, SAMe, St John's wort, and valerian; may increase CNS depression. Avoid melatonin; may cause acute psychosis. Avoid tryptophan; may cause serotonin syndrome.

Pharmacodynamics/Kinetics

Protein binding: 93% to 95%

Metabolism: Extensively hepatic via CYP

Half-life elimination: 21 hours

Time to peak: 5.2 hours

Excretion: Feces and urine (as metabolites)

Pregnancy Risk Factor C

Generic Available No

Selected Readings Gerber PE and Lynd LD, "Selective Serotonin Reuptake Inhibitor-Induced Movement Disorders," *Ann Pharmacother*, 1998, 32(6):692-8.

PAS *see* Aminosalicylic Acid *on page 79*

Paser® *see* Aminosalicylic Acid *on page 79*

Patanol® *see* Olopatadine *on page 998*

Pavabid® [DSC] *see* Papaverine *on page 1033*

Paxil® *see* Paroxetine *on page 1036*

Paxil® CR™ *see* Paroxetine *on page 1036*

PBZ® *see* Tripelennamine *on page 1356*

PBZ-SR® *see* Tripelennamine *on page 1356*

PCA *see* Procainamide *on page 1119*

PCE® *see* Erythromycin *on page 512*

PCV7 *see* Pneumococcal Conjugate Vaccine (7-Valent) *on page 1091*

Pectin and Kaolin *see* Kaolin and Pectin *on page 760*

Pedameth® *see* Methionine *on page 881*

PediaCare® Decongestant Infants [OTC] *see* Pseudoephedrine *on page 1146*

Pediacare® Decongestant Plus Cough [OTC] *see* Pseudoephedrine and Dextromethorphan *on page 1147*

Pediacare® Long Acting Cough Plus Cold [OTC] *see* Pseudoephedrine and Dextromethorphan *on page 1147*

Pediacof® *see* Chlorpheniramine, Phenylephrine, Codeine, and Potassium Iodide *on page 311*

Pediaflor® *see* Fluoride *on page 586*

Pediamist® [OTC] *see* Sodium Chloride *on page 1229*

Pediapred® *see* PrednisoLONE *on page 1110*

Pediarix™ *see* Diphtheria, Tetanus Toxoids, Acellular Pertussis, Hepatitis B (Recombinant), and Poliovirus (Inactivated) Vaccine *on page 454*

Pediazole® *see* Erythromycin and Sulfisoxazole *on page 516*

Pedi-Boro® [OTC] *see* Aluminum Sulfate and Calcium Acetate *on page 70*

Pedi-Dri® *see* Nystatin *on page 992*

PediOtic® *see* Neomycin, Polymyxin B, and Hydrocortisone *on page 963*

Pedisilk® [OTC] *see* Salicylic Acid *on page 1204*

Pedituss® *see* Chlorpheniramine, Phenylephrine, Codeine, and Potassium Iodide *on page 311*

Pedtrace-4® *see* Trace Metals *on page 1328*

PedvaxHIB® *see* *Haemophilus* b Conjugate Vaccine *on page 656*

Pegademase Bovine (peg A de mase BOE vine)

U.S. Brand Names Adagen®

Canadian Brand Names Adagen®

Pharmacologic Category Enzyme

Use Orphan drug: Enzyme replacement therapy for adenosine deaminase (ADA) deficiency in patients with severe combined immunodeficiency disease (SCID) who can not benefit from bone marrow transplant; not a cure for SCID, unlike bone marrow transplants, injections must be used the rest of the child's life, therefore is not really an alternative

Local Anesthetic/Vasoconstrictor Precautions No information available to require special precautions

Effects on Dental Treatment No significant effects or complications reported

Dosage Children: I.M.: Dose given every 7 days, 10 units/kg the first dose, 15 units/kg the second dose, and 20 units/kg the third dose; maintenance dose: 20 units/kg/week is recommended depending on patient's ADA level; maximum single dose: 30 units/kg

Mechanism of Action Adenosine deaminase is an enzyme that catalyzes the deamination of both adenosine and deoxyadenosine. Hereditary lack of adenosine deaminase activity results in severe combined immunodeficiency disease, a fatal disorder of infancy characterized by profound defects of both cellular and humoral immunity. It is estimated that 25% of patients with the autosomal recessive form of severe combined immunodeficiency lack adenosine deaminase.

Other Adverse Effects <1%: Headache, pain at injection site

Pharmacodynamics/Kinetics

Absorption: Rapid

Half-life elimination: 48-72 hours

Time to peak: Plasma adenosine deaminase activity: 2-3 weeks

Pregnancy Risk Factor C

Generic Available No

Peganone® *see* Ethotoin *on page 544*

Pegaspargase (peg AS par jase)

U.S. Brand Names Oncaspar®

Pharmacologic Category Antineoplastic Agent, Miscellaneous

Synonyms PEG-L-asparaginase

Use Treatment of acute lymphocytic leukemia, blast crisis of chronic lymphocytic leukemia (CLL), salvage therapy of non-Hodgkin's lymphoma; may be used in some patients who have had hypersensitivity reactions to *E. coli* asparaginase

Local Anesthetic/Vasoconstrictor Precautions No information available to require special precautions

Effects on Dental Treatment No significant effects or complications reported

Dosage Refer to individual protocols; dose must be individualized based upon clinical response and tolerance of the patient

I.M. administration is **preferred** over I.V. administration; I.M. administration may decrease the incidence of hepatotoxicity, coagulopathy, and GI and renal disorders

Children: I.M., I.V.:

Body surface area <0.6 m^2: 82.5 international units/kg every 14 days

Body surface area ≥0.6 m^2: 2500 international units/m^2 every 14 days

Adults: I.M., I.V.: 2500 international units/m^2 every 14 days

Hemodialysis: Significant drug removal is unlikely based on physiochemical characteristics

Peritoneal dialysis: Significant drug removal is unlikely based on physiochemical characteristics

Mechanism of Action Pegaspargase is a modified version of the enzyme L-asparaginase; the L-asparaginase used in the manufacture of pegaspargase is derived from *Escherichia coli*

Some malignant cells (ie, lymphoblastic leukemia cells and those of lymphocyte derivation) must acquire the amino acid asparagine from surrounding fluid such as blood, whereas normal cells can synthesize their own asparagine. Asparaginase is an enzyme that deaminates asparagine to aspartic acid and ammonia in the plasma and extracellular fluid and therefore deprives tumor cells of the amino acid for protein synthesis.

Other Adverse Effects In general, pegaspargase toxicities tend to be less frequent and appear somewhat later than comparable toxicities of asparaginase. Intramuscular rather than intravenous injection may decrease the incidence of coagulopathy; GI, hepatic, and renal toxicity.

>10%:

Cardiovascular: Edema

Central nervous system: Fatigue, disorientation (10%)

Gastrointestinal: Nausea, vomiting (50% to 60%), generally mild to moderate, but may be severe and protracted in some patients; anorexia (33%); abdominal pain (38%); diarrhea (28%); increased serum lipase and amylase

Hematologic: Hypofibrinogenemia and depression of clotting factors V and VII, variable decreases in factors VII and IX, severe protein C deficiency and decrease in antithrombin III - overt bleeding is uncommon, but may be dose-limiting, or fatal in some patients

Neuromuscular & skeletal: Weakness (33%)

Miscellaneous: Acute allergic reactions, including fever, rash, urticaria, arthralgia, hypotension, angioedema, bronchospasm, anaphylaxis (10% to 30%) - dose-limiting in some patients

1% to 10%:

Cardiovascular: Hypotension, tachycardia, thrombosis

Dermatologic: Urticaria, erythema, lip edema

Endocrine & metabolic: Hyperglycemia (3%)

Gastrointestinal: Acute pancreatitis (1%)

<1%: Agitation, bronchospasm, coma, convulsions, depression, dyspnea, hallucinations, paresthesias, parkinsonian symptoms (tremor, increased muscle tone), seizures, somnolence; transient elevations of transaminases, bilirubin, and alkaline phosphatase

(Continued)

Pegaspargase *(Continued)*

Mild to moderate myelosuppression, leukopenia, anemia, thrombocytopenia; onset: 7 days; nadir: 14 days; recovery: 21 days

Drug Interactions

Increased Effect/Toxicity: Decreased metabolism of cyclophosphamide. Increased hepatotoxicity of mercaptopurine. Imbalances in coagulation factors have been noted with the use of pegaspargase and aspirin, dipyridamole, heparin, warfarin, or NSAIDs; use with caution. An increased toxicity has been noticed when asparaginase is administered with vincristine (neuropathy) and prednisone (hyperglycemia).

Decreased Effect: Asparaginase terminates methotrexate action by inhibition of protein synthesis and prevention of cell entry into the S Phase.

Pharmacodynamics/Kinetics

Duration: Asparaginase was measurable for at least 15 days following initial treatment with pegaspargase

Distribution: V_d: 4-5 L/kg; 70% to 80% of plasma volume; does not penetrate the CSF

Metabolism: Systemically degraded

Half-life elimination: 5.73 days; unaffected by age, renal or hepatic function

Excretion: Urine (trace amounts)

Pregnancy Risk Factor C

Generic Available No

Pegasys® *see* Peginterferon Alfa-2a *on page 1040*

Pegfilgrastim (peg fil GRA stim)

U.S. Brand Names Neulasta™

Pharmacologic Category Colony Stimulating Factor

Synonyms G-CSF (PEG Conjugate); Granulocyte Colony Stimulating Factor (PEG Conjugate)

Use Decrease the incidence of infection, by stimulation of granulocyte production, in patients with nonmyeloid malignancies receiving myelosuppressive therapy associated with a significant risk of febrile neutropenia

Local Anesthetic/Vasoconstrictor Precautions No information available to require special precautions

Effects on Dental Treatment No significant effects or complications reported

Dosage S.C.: Adolescents >45 kg and Adults: 6 mg once per chemotherapy cycle; do not administer in the period between 14 days before and 24 hours after administration of cytotoxic chemotherapy; do not use in patients infants, children and smaller adolescents weighing <45 kg

Mechanism of Action Stimulates the production, maturation, and activation of neutrophils, pegfilgrastim activates neutrophils to increase both their migration and cytotoxicity. Pegfilgrastim has a prolonged duration of effect relative to filgrastim and a reduced renal clearance.

Other Adverse Effects

>10%

Neuromuscular & skeletal: Bone pain (medullary, 26%)

Hepatic: Increased LDH (19%)

1% to 10%

Endocrine & metabolic: Uric acid increased (8%)

Hepatic: Alkaline phosphatase increased (9%)

<1%: Leukocytosis, hypoxia. **Note**: Rare adverse reactions reported for filgrastim include adult respiratory distress syndrome, allergic reactions (including urticaria, rash or anaphylaxis), sickle cell crisis (in patients with sickle cell disease), and splenic rupture (following use for peripheral blood progenitor cell [PBPC] mobilization). Cytopenias resulting from an antibody response to exogenous growth factors have been reported on rare occasions in patients treated with other recombinant growth factors.

Drug Interactions Increased Effect/Toxicity: Lithium may potentiate release of neutrophils.

Pharmacodynamics/Kinetics Half-life elimination: S.C.: 15-80 hours

Pregnancy Risk Factor C

Generic Available No

Peginterferon Alfa-2a (peg in ter FEER on AL fu-too ay)

U.S. Brand Names Pegasys®

Pharmacologic Category Interferon

Synonyms Interferon Alfa-2a (PEG Conjugate); Pegylated Interferon Alfa-2a

Use Treatment of chronic hepatitis C, alone or in combination with ribavirin, in patients with compensated liver disease

Local Anesthetic/Vasoconstrictor Precautions No information available to require special precautions

Effects on Dental Treatment No significant effects or complications reported

Dosage S.C.: Adults: Chronic hepatitis C:

Monotherapy: 180 mcg once weekly for 48 weeks

Combination therapy with ribavirin: Recommended dosage: 180 mcg once/week with ribavirin (Copegus™)

Note: Duration of therapy based on genotype:

Genotype 1,4: Treat for 48 weeks

Genotype 2,3: Treat for 24 weeks

Dose modification:

For moderate to severe adverse reactions: Initial: 135 mcg/week; may need decreased to 90 mcg/week in some cases

Based on hematologic parameters:

ANC <750/mm³: 135 mcg/week

ANC <500/mm³: Suspend therapy until >1000/mm³, then restart at 90 mcg/week and monitor

Platelet count <50,000/mm³: 90 mcg/week

Platelet count <25,000/mm³: Discontinue therapy

Depression (severity based on DSM-IV criteria):

Mild depression: No dosage adjustment required; evaluate once weekly by visit/phone call. If depression remains stable, continue weekly visits. If depression improves, resume normal visit schedule

Moderate depression: Decrease interferon dose to 90-135 mcg once/week; evaluate once weekly with an office visit at least every other week. If depression remains stable, consider psychiatric evaluation and continue with reduced dosing. If symptoms improve and remain stable for 4 weeks, resume normal visit schedule; continue reduced dosing or return to normal dose.

Severe depression: Discontinue interferon permanently. Obtain immediate psychiatric consultation. Discontinue ribavirin if using concurrently.

Dosing adjustment in renal impairment: End-stage renal disease requiring hemodialysis: 135 mcg/week; monitor for toxicity

Dosing adjustment in hepatic impairment: ALT progressively rising above baseline: Decrease dose to 135 mcg/week. If ALT continues to rise or is accompanied by increased bilirubin or hepatic decompensation, discontinue therapy immediately.

Mechanism of Action Alpha interferons are a family of proteins, produced by nucleated cells, that have antiviral, antiproliferative, and immune-regulating activity. There are 16 known subtypes of alpha interferons. Interferons interact with cells through high affinity cell surface receptors. Following activation, multiple effects can be detected including induction of gene transcription. Inhibits cellular growth, alters the state of cellular differentiation, interferes with oncogene expression, alters cell surface antigen expression, increases phagocytic activity of macrophages, and augments cytotoxicity of lymphocytes for target cells.

Other Adverse Effects Note: Percentages indicated as "with ribavirin" are those which have been seen with peginterferon alfa-2b/ribavirin combination therapy.

>10%:

Central nervous system: Headache (54%), fatigue (50%), pyrexia (36%), insomnia (19%; 30% with ribavirin), depression (1% to 18%), dizziness (16%), irritability (13%), irritability/anxiety/nervousness (33% with ribavirin), pain (11%)

Dermatologic: Alopecia (23%), pruritus (12%; 19% with ribavirin), dermatitis (16% with ribavirin)

Gastrointestinal: Nausea (5% to 23%), anorexia (17%; 24% with ribavirin), diarrhea (16%), abdominal pain (15%)

Hematologic: Neutropenia (21%), lymphopenia (14% with ribavirin), anemia (11% with ribavirin)

Local: Injection site reaction (22%)

Neuromuscular & skeletal: Myalgia (37%), rigors (32%), arthralgia (28%)

Respiratory: Dyspnea (13% with ribavirin)

1% to 10%:

Central nervous system: Concentration impaired (8%), anxiety (6%), memory impaired (5%)

Dermatologic: Dermatitis (8%), rash (5%), eczema (5% with ribavirin)

Endocrine & metabolic: Hypothyroidism (4%), hyperthyroidism (1%)

Gastrointestinal: Xerostomia (6%), vomiting (5%)

Hematologic: Thrombocytopenia (5%), platelets decreased <50,000/mm³ (5%)

Neuromuscular & skeletal: Back pain (9%), weakness (5%)

Miscellaneous: Diaphoresis (6%)

≤1%, postmarketing, and/or case reports: Arrhythmia, autoimmune disorders, bronchiolitis obliterans, cerebral hemorrhage, chest pain, cholangitis, coma, cotton wool spots, diabetes mellitus, dyspnea, endocarditis, fatty liver, hemoglobin decreased, hematocrit decreased, hepatic dysfunction, hypersensitivity reactions, hypertension, interstitial pneumonitis, MI, myositis, optic neuritis, papilledema, pancreatitis (with ribavirin), peptic ulcer, peripheral neuropathy, pneumonia, pulmonary embolism, pulmonary infiltrates, retinal hemorrhage, retinopathy, sarcoidosis, substance overdose, suicidal ideation, suicide, supraventricular arrhythmias, vision decreased/loss

Drug Interactions Inhibits CYP1A2

Increased Effect/Toxicity: Interferons may increase the risk of neutropenia when used with ACE inhibitors; fluorouracil concentrations doubled with interferon

(Continued)

Peginterferon Alfa-2a *(Continued)*

alpha-2b; interferon alpha may decrease the metabolism of theophylline and zidovudine; interferons may increase the anticoagulant effects of warfarin

Decreased Effect: Prednisone may decrease the therapeutic effects of interferon alpha; interferon alpha may decrease the serum concentrations of melphalan

Dietary/Ethanol/Herb Considerations Ethanol: Avoid use in patients with hepatitis C virus.

Pharmacodynamics/Kinetics

Half-life elimination: Terminal: 80 hours; increased with renal dysfunction

Time to peak, serum: 72-96 hours

Pregnancy Risk Factor C

Generic Available No

Peginterferon Alfa-2b (peg in ter FEER on AL fu-too bee)

Related Information

Systemic Viral Diseases *on page 1517*

U.S. Brand Names PEG-Intron®

Canadian Brand Names PEG-Intron®

Pharmacologic Category Interferon

Use Treatment of chronic hepatitis C (as monotherapy or in combination with ribavirin) in adult patients who have never received interferon alpha and have compensated liver disease

Local Anesthetic/Vasoconstrictor Precautions No information available to require special precautions

Effects on Dental Treatment No significant effects or complications reported

Restrictions Patients must have an Access Assurance ID number (obtained by calling Schering-Plough at 1-888-437-2608). Pharmacists should receive the ID number from the patient, and must obtain an order authorization number from the manufacturer prior to placing an order with their wholesaler (effective October 22, 2001). The patient's authorization number will be retained throughout therapy. This number may be inactivated if the patient fails to fill the prescription over any 60-day period, and access will no longer be assured by the manufacturer.

Dosage S.C.:

Children: Safety and efficacy not established

Adults: Chronic hepatitis C: Administer dose once weekly; **Note:** Usual duration is for 1 year; after 24 weeks of treatment, if serum HCV RNA is not below the limit of detection of the assay, consider discontinuation:

Monotherapy: Initial:

- ≤45 kg: 40 mcg
- 46-56 kg: 50 mcg
- 57-72 kg: 64 mcg
- 73-88 kg: 80 mcg
- 89-106 kg: 96 mcg
- 107-136 kg: 120 mcg
- 137-160 kg: 150 mcg

Combination therapy with ribavirin (400 mg twice daily): Initial: 1.5 mcg/kg/week

- <40 kg: 50 mcg
- 40-50 kg: 64 mcg
- 51-60 kg: 80 mcg
- 61-75 kg: 96 mcg
- 76-85 kg: 120 mcg
- >85 kg: 150 mcg

Elderly: No specific recommendations; assessment of renal function is critical

Dosing adjustment if serious adverse event occurs: Depression (severity based upon DSM-IV criteria):

Mild depression: No dosage adjustment required; evaluate once weekly by visit/phone call. If depression remains stable, continue weekly visits. If depression improves, resume normal visit schedule.

Moderate depression: Decrease interferon dose by 50%; evaluate once weekly with an office visit at least every other week. If depression remains stable, consider psychiatric evaluation and continue with reduced dosing. If symptoms improve and remain stable for 4 weeks, resume normal visit schedule; continue reduced dosing or return to normal dose.

Severe depression: Discontinue interferon and ribavirin permanently. Obtain immediate psychiatric consultation.

Dosing adjustment in renal impairment: Monitor for signs and symptoms of toxicity and if toxicity occurs then adjust dose. Do not use patients with Cl_{cr} <50 mL/minute. Patients were excluded from the clinical trials if serum creatinine >1.5 times the upper limits of normal.

Dosing adjustment in hepatic impairment: Contraindicated in decompensated liver disease

Dosing adjustment in hematologic toxicity:

Hemoglobin:

Hemoglobin <10 g/dL: Continue current peginterferon alfa-2b dose; decrease ribavirin dose by 200 mg/day.

Hemoglobin <8.5 g/dL: Permanently discontinue peginterferon alfa-2b and ribavirin.

Hemoglobin decrease >2 g/dL in any 4-week period and stable cardiac disease: Decrease peginterferon alfa-2b dose by half; decrease ribavirin dose by 200 mg per day. Hemoglobin <12 g/dL after ribavirin dose is decreased: Permanently discontinue both peginterferon alfa-2b and ribavirin.

White blood cells:

WBC <1.5 x 10^9/L: Decrease peginterferon alfa-2b dose by half.

WBC <1.0 x 10^9/L: Permanently discontinue peginterferon alfa-2b and ribavirin.

Neutrophils:

Neutrophils <0.75 x 10^9/L: Decrease peginterferon alfa-2b dose by half.

Neutrophils <0.5 x 10^9/L: Permanently discontinue peginterferon alfa-2b and ribavirin.

Platelets:

Platelet count <80 x 10^9 /L: Decrease peginterferon alfa-2b dose by half.

Platelet count <50 x 10^9/L: Permanently discontinue peginterferon alfa-2b and ribavirin.

Mechanism of Action Alpha interferons are a family of proteins, produced by nucleated cells, that have antiviral, antiproliferative, and immune-regulating activity. There are 16 known subtypes of alpha interferons. Interferons interact with cells through high affinity cell surface receptors. Following activation, multiple effects can be detected including induction of gene transcription. Inhibits cellular growth, alters the state of cellular differentiation, interferes with oncogene expression, alters cell surface antigen expression, increases phagocytic activity of macrophages, and augments cytotoxicity of lymphocytes for target cells.

Other Adverse Effects

>10% :

Central nervous system: Headache (56%), fatigue (52%), depression (16% to 29%), anxiety/emotional liability/irritability (28%), insomnia (23%), fever (22%), dizziness (12%), impaired concentration (5% to 12%), pain (12%)

Dermatologic: Alopecia (22%), pruritus (12%), dry skin (11%)

Gastrointestinal: Nausea (26%), anorexia (20%), diarrhea (18%), abdominal pain (15%), weight loss (11%)

Local: Injection site inflammation/reaction (47%),

Neuromuscular & skeletal: Musculoskeletal pain (56%), myalgia (38% to 42%), rigors (23% to 45%)

Respiratory: Epistaxis (14%), nasopharyngitis (11%)

Miscellaneous: Flu-like syndrome (46%), viral infection (11%)

>1% to 10%:

Cardiovascular: Flushing (6%)

Central nervous system: Malaise (8%)

Dermatologic: Rash (6%), dermatitis (7%)

Endocrine & metabolic: Hypothyroidism (5%)

Gastrointestinal: Vomiting (7%), dyspepsia (6%), abnormal taste

Hematologic: Neutropenia, thrombocytopenia

Hepatic: Transient increase in transaminases (10%), hepatomegaly (6%)

Local: Injection site pain (2%)

Neuromuscular & skeletal: Hypertonia (5%)

Respiratory: Pharyngitis (10%), sinusitis (7%), cough (6%)

Miscellaneous: Diaphoresis (6%)

≤1%: Abscess, aggressive behavior, anaphylaxis, anemia, angioedema, aplastic anemia, arrhythmias, autoimmune disorder (eg, thyroiditis, thrombocytopenia, rheumatoid arthritis, interstitial nephritis, systemic lupus erythematosus, psoriasis) or exacerbation of disorder, bronchoconstriction, cardiomyopathy, cotton wool spots, diabetes mellitus, drug addiction relapse, drug overdose, dyspnea, facial oculomotor nerve palsy, hallucinations, hemorrhagic colitis, homicidal ideation, hyperglycemia, hypersensitivity reactions, hyperthyroidism, hypotension, loss of consciousness, MI, nerve palsy, neutralizing antibodies, pancreatitis, severe neutropenia (<0.5 x 10^9/L), severe thrombocytopenia (<50,000/mm^3), pneumonia, pneumonitis, polyneuropathy, retinopathy, optic neuritis, hearing impairment, psychosis, pulmonary infiltrates, retinal artery or vein obstruction, retinal hemorrhage, retinal ischemia, severe depression, suicidal behavior, suicidal ideation, supraventricular arrhythmias, tachycardia, transient ischemic attack, ulcerative colitis, urticaria

Drug Interactions Inhibits CYP1A2

Increased Effect/Toxicity: ACE inhibitors, clozapine, erythropoietin may increase risk of bone marrow suppression. Fluorouracil, theophylline, zidovudine concentrations may increase. Warfarin's anticoagulant effect may increase.

Decreased Effect: Melphalan concentrations may decrease. Prednisone may decrease effects of interferon alpha.

(Continued)

Peginterferon Alfa-2b *(Continued)*

Dietary/Ethanol/Herb Considerations Ethanol: Avoid use in patients with hepatitis C virus.

Pharmacodynamics/Kinetics

Bioavailability: Increases with chronic dosing

Half-life elimination: 40 hours

Time to peak: 15-44 hours

Excretion: Urine (30%)

Pregnancy Risk Factor C (manufacturer) as monotherapy; X in combination with ribavirin

Generic Available No

PEG-Intron® *see* Peginterferon Alfa-2b *on page 1042*

PEG-L-asparaginase *see* Pegaspargase *on page 1039*

Pegylated Interferon Alfa-2a *see* Peginterferon Alfa-2a *on page 1040*

PemADD® *see* Pemoline *on page 1044*

PemADD® CT *see* Pemoline *on page 1044*

Pemirolast (pe MIR oh last)

U.S. Brand Names Alamast™

Canadian Brand Names Alamast™

Pharmacologic Category Mast Cell Stabilizer; Ophthalmic Agent, Miscellaneous

Use Prevention of itching of the eye due to allergic conjunctivitis

Local Anesthetic/Vasoconstrictor Precautions No information available to require special precautions

Effects on Dental Treatment No significant effects or complications reported

Dosage Children >3 years and Adults: 1-2 drops instilled in affected eye(s) 4 times/day

Mechanism of Action Mast cell stabilizer that inhibits the *in vivo* type I immediate hypersensitivity reaction; in addition, inhibits chemotaxis of eosinophils into the ocular tissue and blocks their release of mediators; also reported to prevent calcium influx into mast cells following antigen stimulation

Other Adverse Effects

>10%:

- Central nervous system: Headache (10% to 25%)
- Respiratory: Rhinitis (10% to 25%)
- Miscellaneous: Cold/flu symptoms (10% to 25%)

<5%:

- Central nervous system: Fever
- Endocrine & metabolic: Dysmenorrhea
- Neuromuscular & skeletal: Back pain
- Ocular: Burning eyes, dry eyes, foreign body sensation, ocular discomfort
- Respiratory: Bronchitis, cough, sinusitis, sneezing/nasal congestion

Pharmacodynamics/Kinetics

Onset of action: A few days

Peak effect: 4 weeks

Absorption: Systemic

Half-life elimination: 4.5 hours

Excretion: Urine (10% to 15%)

Pregnancy Risk Factor C

Generic Available No

Pemoline (PEM oh leen)

U.S. Brand Names Cylert®; PemADD®; PemADD® CT

Pharmacologic Category Stimulant

Synonyms Phenylisohydantoin; PIO

Use Treatment of attention-deficit/hyperactivity disorder (ADHD) (not first-line)

Unlabeled/Investigational Use Treatment of narcolepsy

Local Anesthetic/Vasoconstrictor Precautions Pemoline has minimal sympathomimetic effects; there are no precautions in using vasoconstrictors

Effects on Dental Treatment No significant effects or complications reported

Restrictions C-IV

Dosage Oral:

Children ≥6 years: Initial: 37.5 mg given once daily in the morning, increase by 18.75 mg/day at weekly intervals; usual effective dose range: 56.25-75 mg/day; maximum: 112.5 mg/day; dosage range: 0.5-3 mg/kg/24 hours; significant benefit may not be evident until third or fourth week of administration

Dosing adjustment in renal impairment: Cl_{cr} <50 mL/minute: Avoid use

Mechanism of Action Blocks the reuptake mechanism of dopaminergic neurons, appears to act at the cerebral cortex and subcortical structures; CNS and respiratory stimulant with weak sympathomimetic effects; actions may be mediated via increase in CNS dopamine

Other Adverse Effects Frequency not defined:

Central nervous system: Insomnia, dizziness, drowsiness, mental depression, increased irritability, seizures, precipitation of Tourette's syndrome, hallucinations, headache, movement disorders

Dermatologic: Rash

Endocrine & metabolic: Suppression of growth in children

Gastrointestinal: Anorexia, weight loss, stomach pain, nausea

Hematologic: Aplastic anemia

Hepatic: Increased liver enzyme (usually reversible upon discontinuation), hepatitis, jaundice, hepatic failure

Drug Interactions

Increased Effect/Toxicity: Use caution when pemoline is used with other CNS-acting medications.

Decreased Effect: Pemoline in combination with antiepileptic medications may decrease seizure threshold.

Dietary/Ethanol/Herb Considerations

Ethanol: Avoid use; may increase CNS depression.

Herb/Nutraceutical: Avoid gotu kola, kava, SAMe, St John's wort, and valerian; may increase CNS depression.

Pharmacodynamics/Kinetics

Onset of action: Peak effect: 4 hours

Duration: 8 hours

Protein binding: 50%

Metabolism: Partially hepatic

Half-life elimination: Children: 7-8.6 hours; Adults: 12 hours

Time to peak, serum: 2-4 hours

Excretion: Urine; feces (negligible amounts)

Pregnancy Risk Factor B

Generic Available Yes

Penbutolol (pen BYOO toe lole)

Related Information

Cardiovascular Diseases *on page 1456*

U.S. Brand Names Levatol®

Canadian Brand Names Levatol®

Pharmacologic Category Beta Blocker With Intrinsic Sympathomimetic Activity

Synonyms Penbutolol Sulfate

Use Treatment of mild to moderate arterial hypertension

Local Anesthetic/Vasoconstrictor Precautions No information available to require special precautions

Effects on Dental Treatment 1% to 10%: Xerostomia

Penbutolol is a nonselective beta-blocker and may enhance the pressor response to epinephrine, resulting in hypertension and bradycardia. Many nonsteroidal anti-inflammatory drugs such as ibuprofen and indomethacin can reduce the hypotensive effect of beta-blockers after 3 or more weeks of therapy with the NSAID. Short-term NSAID use (ie, 3 days) requires no special precautions in patients taking beta-blockers.

Dosage Adults: Oral: Initial: 20 mg once daily, full effect of a 20 or 40 mg dose is seen by the end of a 2-week period, doses of 40-80 mg have been tolerated but have shown little additional antihypertensive effects

Mechanism of Action Blocks both $beta_1$- and $beta_2$-receptors and has mild intrinsic sympathomimetic activity; has negative inotropic and chronotropic effects and can significantly slow AV nodal conduction

Other Adverse Effects

1% to 10%:

Cardiovascular: Congestive heart failure, arrhythmia

Central nervous system: Mental depression, headache, dizziness, fatigue

Gastrointestinal: Nausea, diarrhea, dyspepsia

Neuromuscular & skeletal: Arthralgia

<1% (Limited to important or life-threatening): AV block, bradycardia, bronchospasm, cold extremities, confusion, cough, edema, hypoglycemia, hypotension, insomnia, lethargy, ischemic colitis, mesenteric arterial thrombosis, nightmares, purpura, Raynaud's phenomena, thrombocytopenia

Drug Interactions

Increased Effect/Toxicity: The heart rate lowering effects of propranolol are beta-blockers are additive with other drugs which slow AV conduction (digoxin, verapamil, diltiazem). Concurrent use of beta-blockers may increase the effects of alpha-blockers (prazosin, terazosin), alpha-adrenergic stimulants (epinephrine, phenylephrine), and the vasoconstrictive effects of ergot alkaloids. Beta-blockers may mask the tachycardia from hypoglycemia caused by insulin and oral hypoglycemics. In patients receiving concurrent therapy, the risk of hypertensive crisis is increased when either clonidine or the beta-blocker is withdrawn. Beta-blockers may increase the action or levels of ethanol, disopyramide, nondepolarizing muscle relaxants, and theophylline although the effects are difficult to predict.

(Continued)

Penbutolol *(Continued)*

Beta-blocker effects may be enhanced by oral contraceptives, flecainide, haloperidol (hypotensive effects), H_2-antagonists (cimetidine, possibly ranitidine), hydralazine, loop diuretics, possibly MAO inhibitors, phenothiazines, propafenone, quinidine (in extensive metabolizers), ciprofloxacin, thyroid hormones (when hypothyroid patient is converted to euthyroid state). Beta-blockers may increase the effect/toxicity of flecainide, haloperidol (hypotensive effects), hydralazine, phenothiazines, acetaminophen, anticoagulants (warfarin), and benzodiazepines.

Decreased Effect: Aluminum salts, barbiturates, calcium salts, cholestyramine, colestipol, NSAIDs, penicillins (ampicillin), rifampin, salicylates, and sulfinpyrazone decrease effect of beta-blockers due to decreased bioavailability and plasma levels. Beta-blockers may decrease the effect of sulfonylureas. Nonselective beta-blockers blunt the response to beta-2 adrenergic agonists (albuterol).

Dietary/Ethanol/Herb Considerations Ethanol: Avoid use; penbutolol may increase the action or levels of ethanol.

Pharmacodynamics/Kinetics

Absorption: ~100%

Protein binding: 80% to 98%

Metabolism: Extensively hepatic (oxidation and conjugation)

Bioavailability: ~100%

Half-life elimination: 5 hours

Excretion: Urine

Pregnancy Risk Factor C (manufacturer); D (2nd and 3rd trimester - expert analysis)

Generic Available No

Selected Readings

Foster CA and Aston SJ, "Propranolol-Epinephrine Interaction: A Potential Disaster," *Plast Reconstr Surg*, 1983, 72(1):74-8.

Wong DG, Spence JD, Lamki L, et al, "Effect of Nonsteroidal Anti-inflammatory Drugs on Control of Hypertension of Beta-Blockers and Diuretics," *Lancet*, 1986, 1(8488):997-1001.

Wynn RL, "Dental Nonsteroidal Anti-inflammatory Drugs and Prostaglandin-Based Drug Interactions, Part Two," *Gen Dent*, 1992, 40(2):104, 106, 108.

Wynn RL, "Epinephrine Interactions With Beta-Blockers," *Gen Dent*, 1994, 42(1):16, 18.

Penbutolol Sulfate *see* Penbutolol *on page 1045*

Penciclovir (pen SYE kloe veer)

Related Information

Oral Viral Infections *on page 1545*

Systemic Viral Diseases *on page 1517*

U.S. Brand Names Denavir®

Pharmacologic Category Antiviral Agent

Use Topical treatment of herpes simplex labialis (cold sores); potentially used for Epstein-Barr virus infections

Local Anesthetic/Vasoconstrictor Precautions No information available to require special precautions

Effects on Dental Treatment Headache (5.3%)

Dosage Apply cream at the first sign or symptom of cold sore (eg, tingling, swelling); apply every 2 hours during waking hours for 4 days

Mechanism of Action In cells infected with HSV-1 or HSV-2, viral thymidine kinase phosphorylates penciclovir to a monophosphate form which, in turn, is converted to penciclovir triphosphate by cellular kinases. Penciclovir triphosphate inhibits HSV polymerase competitively with deoxyguanosine triphosphate. Consequently, herpes viral DNA synthesis and, therefore, replication are selectively inhibited

Other Adverse Effects

>10%: Dermatologic: Mild erythema (50%)

<1%: Local anesthesia (0.9%)

Pharmacodynamics/Kinetics Absorption: Topical: None

Pregnancy Risk Factor B

Generic Available No

Penicillamine (pen i SIL a meen)

U.S. Brand Names Cuprimine®; Depen®

Canadian Brand Names Cuprimine®; Depen®

Mexican Brand Names Adalken®; Sufortan®; Sufortanon®

Pharmacologic Category Chelating Agent

Synonyms D-3-Mercaptovaline; β,β-Dimethylcysteine; D-Penicillamine

Use Treatment of Wilson's disease, cystinuria, adjunct in the treatment of rheumatoid arthritis; lead, mercury, copper, and possibly gold poisoning. (**Note:** Oral DMSA is preferable for lead or mercury poisoning); primary biliary cirrhosis; as adjunctive therapy following initial treatment with calcium EDTA or BAL

Local Anesthetic/Vasoconstrictor Precautions No information available to require special precautions

Effects on Dental Treatment No significant effects or complications reported

Dosage Oral:

Rheumatoid arthritis:

Children: Initial: 3 mg/kg/day (≤250 mg/day) for 3 months, then 6 mg/kg/day (≤500 mg/day) in divided doses twice daily for 3 months to a maximum of 10 mg/kg/day in 3-4 divided doses

Adults: 125-250 mg/day, may increase dose at 1- to 3-month intervals up to 1-1.5 g/day

Wilson's disease (doses titrated to maintain urinary copper excretion >1 mg/day):

Infants <6 months: 250 mg/dose once daily

Children <12 years: 250 mg/dose 2-3 times/day

Adults: 250 mg 4 times/day

Cystinuria:

Children: 30 mg/kg/day in 4 divided doses

Adults: 1-4 g/day in divided doses every 6 hours

Lead poisoning (continue until blood lead level is <60 µg/dL): Children and Adults: 25-35 mg/kg/d, administered in 3-4 divided doses; initiating treatment at 25% of this dose and gradually increasing to the full dose over 2-3 weeks may minimize adverse reactions

Primary biliary cirrhosis: 250 mg/day to start, increase by 250 mg every 2 weeks up to a maintenance dose of 1 g/day, usually given 250 mg 4 times/day

Arsenic poisoning: Children: 100 mg/kg/day in divided doses every 6 hours for 5 days; maximum: 1 g/day

Dosing adjustment in renal impairment: Cl_{cr} <50 mL/minute: Avoid use

Mechanism of Action Chelates with lead, copper, mercury and other heavy metals to form stable, soluble complexes that are excreted in urine; depresses circulating IgM rheumatoid factor, depresses T-cell but not B-cell activity; combines with cystine to form a compound which is more soluble, thus cystine calculi are prevented

Other Adverse Effects

>10%:

Dermatologic: Rash, urticaria, itching (44% to 50%)

Gastrointestinal: Hypogeusia (25% to 33%)

Neuromuscular & skeletal: Arthralgia

1% to 10%:

Cardiovascular: Edema of the face, feet, or lower legs

Central nervous system: Fever, chills

Gastrointestinal: Weight gain, sore throat

Genitourinary: Bloody or cloudy urine

Hematologic: Aplastic or hemolytic anemia, leukopenia (2%), thrombocytopenia (4%)

Miscellaneous: White spots on lips or mouth, positive ANA

<1%: Allergic reactions, anorexia, cholestatic jaundice, coughing, fatigue, hepatitis, increased friability of the skin, iron deficiency, lymphadenopathy, myasthenia gravis syndrome, nausea, nephrotic syndrome, pancreatitis, pemphigus, optic neuritis, SLE-like syndrome, spitting of blood, tinnitus, toxic epidermal necrolysis, vomiting, weakness, wheezing

Drug Interactions

Increased Effect/Toxicity: Increased effect or toxicity of gold, antimalarials, immunosuppressants, and phenylbutazone (hematologic, renal toxicity).

Decreased Effect: Decreased effect of penicillamine when taken with iron and zinc salts, antacids (magnesium, calcium, aluminum), and food. Digoxin levels may be decreased when taken with penicillamine.

Dietary/Ethanol/Herb Considerations

Ethanol: Avoid or limit use.

Food: Administer on an empty stomach if possible; food may decrease serum concentration. Do not administer with milk; may mix contents of capsule with fruit juice or chilled pureed fruit. Iron and zinc may decrease drug action. Increase dietary intake of pyridoxine. For Wilson's disease, decrease dietary copper and avoid broccoli, chocolate, liver, molasses, mushrooms, nuts, raisins, and shellfish. For lead poisoning, decrease dietary calcium.

Pharmacodynamics/Kinetics

Absorption: 40% to 70%

Protein binding: 80% to albumin

Metabolism: Hepatic (small amounts)

Half-life elimination: 1.7-3.2 hours

Time to peak, serum: ~2 hours

Excretion: Urine (30% to 60% as unchanged drug)

Pregnancy Risk Factor D

Generic Available No

Selected Readings Rosa FW, "Teratogen Update. Penicillamine," *Teratology*, 1986, 33(1):127-31.

Penicillin G Benzathine (pen i SIL in jee BENZ a theen)

Related Information

Nonviral Infectious Diseases *on page 1493*

(Continued)

Penicillin G Benzathine *(Continued)*

Sexually-Transmitted Diseases *on page 1502*

U.S. Brand Names Bicillin® L-A; Permapen® Isoject®

Mexican Brand Names Bencelin®; Benzanil®; Benzetacil®; Benzilfan

Pharmacologic Category Antibiotic, Penicillin

Synonyms Benzathine Benzylpenicillin; Benzathine Penicillin G; Benzylpenicillin Benzathine

Use Active against some gram-positive organisms, few gram-negative organisms such as *Neisseria gonorrhoeae*, and some anaerobes and spirochetes; used in the treatment of syphilis; used only for the treatment of mild to moderately severe infections caused by organisms susceptible to low concentrations of penicillin G or for prophylaxis of infections caused by these organisms

Local Anesthetic/Vasoconstrictor Precautions No information available to require special precautions

Effects on Dental Treatment No significant effects or complications reported

Dosage I.M.: Administer undiluted injection; higher doses result in more sustained rather than higher levels. Use a penicillin G benzathine-penicillin G procaine combination to achieve early peak levels in acute infections.

Infants and Children:
- Group A streptococcal upper respiratory infection: 25,000-50,000 units/kg as a single dose; maximum: 1.2 million units
- Prophylaxis of recurrent rheumatic fever: 25,000-50,000 units/kg every 3-4 weeks; maximum: 1.2 million units/dose
- Early syphilis: 50,000 units/kg as a single injection; maximum: 2.4 million units
- Syphilis of more than 1-year duration: 50,000 units/kg every week for 3 doses; maximum: 2.4 million units/dose

Adults:
- Group A streptococcal upper respiratory infection: 1.2 million units as a single dose
- Prophylaxis of recurrent rheumatic fever: 1.2 million units every 3-4 weeks or 600,000 units twice monthly
- Early syphilis: 2.4 million units as a single dose in 2 injection sites
- Syphilis of more than 1-year duration: 2.4 million units in 2 injection sites once weekly for 3 doses
- Not indicated as single drug therapy for neurosyphilis, but may be given 1 time/week for 3 weeks following I.V. treatment; refer to Penicillin G Parenteral/Aqueous monograph for dosing

Mechanism of Action Interferes with bacterial cell wall synthesis during active multiplication, causing cell wall death and resultant bactericidal activity against susceptible bacteria

Other Adverse Effects Frequency not defined:
- Central nervous system: Convulsions, confusion, drowsiness, myoclonus, fever
- Dermatologic: Rash
- Endocrine & metabolic: Electrolyte imbalance
- Hematologic: Positive Coombs' reaction, hemolytic anemia
- Local: Pain, thrombophlebitis
- Renal: Acute interstitial nephritis
- Miscellaneous: Anaphylaxis, hypersensitivity reactions, Jarisch-Herxheimer reaction

Drug Interactions
- Increased Effect/Toxicity: Probenecid increases penicillin levels. Aminoglycosides may lead to synergistic efficacy.
- Decreased Effect: Tetracyclines may decrease penicillin effectiveness. Although anecdotal reports suggest oral contraceptive efficacy could be reduced by penicillins, this has been refuted by more rigorous scientific and clinical data.

Pharmacodynamics/Kinetics
- Duration: 1-4 weeks (dose dependent); larger doses result in more sustained levels
- Absorption: I.M.: Slow
- Time to peak, serum: 12-24 hours

Pregnancy Risk Factor B

Generic Available No

Penicillin G Benzathine and Penicillin G Procaine

(pen i SIL in jee BENZ a theen & pen i SIL in jee PROE kane)

U.S. Brand Names Bicillin® C-R; Bicillin® C-R 900/300

Pharmacologic Category Antibiotic, Penicillin

Synonyms Penicillin G Benzathine and Procaine; Penicillin G Procaine and Benzathine Combined; Penicillin G Procaine and Penicillin G Benzathine

Use May be used in specific situations in the treatment of streptococcal infections

Local Anesthetic/Vasoconstrictor Precautions No information available to require special precautions

Effects on Dental Treatment No significant effects or complications reported

Dosage I.M.:
Children:
<30 lb: 600,000 units in a single dose
30-60 lb: 900,000 units to 1.2 million units in a single dose
Children >60 lb and Adults: 2.4 million units in a single dose

Mechanism of Action Inhibits bacterial cell wall synthesis by binding to one or more of the penicillin binding proteins (PBPs); which in turn inhibits the final transpeptidation step of peptidoglycan synthesis in bacterial cell walls, thus inhibiting cell wall biosynthesis. Bacteria eventually lyse due to ongoing activity of cell wall autolytic enzymes (autolysins and murein hydrolases) while cell wall assembly is arrested.

Other Adverse Effects Frequency not defined:
Central nervous system: CNS toxicity (convulsions, confusion, drowsiness, myoclonus)
Hematologic: Positive Coombs' reaction, hemolytic anemia
Renal: Interstitial nephritis
Miscellaneous: Hypersensitivity reactions, Jarisch-Herxheimer reaction

Drug Interactions
Increased Effect/Toxicity: Probenecid increases penicillin levels. Aminoglycosides may lead to synergistic efficacy. Warfarin effects may be increased.
Decreased Effect: Tetracyclines may decrease penicillin effectiveness. Although anecdotal reports suggest oral contraceptive efficacy could be reduced by penicillins, this has been refuted by more rigorous scientific and clinical data.

Pregnancy Risk Factor B

Generic Available No

Penicillin G Benzathine and Procaine *see* Penicillin G Benzathine and Penicillin G Procaine *on page 1048*

Penicillin G (Parenteral/Aqueous)

(pen i SIL in jee, pa REN ter ol, AY kwee us)

Related Information
Nonviral Infectious Diseases *on page 1493*

U.S. Brand Names Pfizerpen®

Canadian Brand Names Pfizerpen®

Mexican Brand Names Benzanil; Lentopenil

Pharmacologic Category Antibiotic, Penicillin

Synonyms Benzylpenicillin Potassium; Benzylpenicillin Sodium; Crystalline Penicillin; Penicillin G Potassium; Penicillin G Sodium

Use Active against some gram-positive organisms, generally not *Staphylococcus aureus*; some gram-negative organisms such as *Neisseria gonorrhoeae*, and some anaerobes and spirochetes

Local Anesthetic/Vasoconstrictor Precautions No information available to require special precautions

Effects on Dental Treatment No significant effects or complications reported

Dosage I.M., I.V.:
Infants:
<7 days, <2000 g: 50,000 units/kg/day in divided doses every 12 hours
<7 days, >2000 g: 50,000 units/kg/day in divided doses every 8 hours
>7 days, <2000 g: 75,000 units/kg/day in divided doses every 8 hours
>7 days, >2000 g: 100,000 units/kg/day in divided doses every 6 hours
Infants and Children (sodium salt is preferred in children): 100,000-250,000 units/kg/day in divided doses every 4 hours
Severe infections: Up to 400,000 units/kg/day in divided doses every 4 hours; maximum dose: 24 million units/day
Congenital syphilis:
Newborns: 50,000 units/kg/day I.V. every 8-12 hours for 10-14 days
Infants: 50,000 units/kg every 4-6 hours for 10-14 days
Disseminated gonococcal infections or gonococcus ophthalmia (if organism proven sensitive): 100,000 units/kg/day in 2 equal doses (4 equal doses/day for infants >1 week)
Gonococcal meningitis: 150,000 units/kg in 2 equal doses (4 doses/day for infants >1 week)
Adults: 2-24 million units/day in divided doses every 4 hours depending on sensitivity of the organism and severity of the infection
Neurosyphilis: 18-24 million units/day in divided doses every 3-4 hours for 10-14 days
Dosing interval in renal impairment:
Cl_{cr} 30-50 mL/minute: Administer every 6 hours
Cl_{cr} 10-30 mL/minute: Administer every 8 hours
Cl_{cr} <10 mL/minute: Administer every 12 hours
Hemodialysis: Moderately dialyzable (20% to 50%)
Continuous arteriovenous or venovenous hemodiafiltration effects: Dose as for Cl_{cr} 10-50 mL/minute

(Continued)

Penicillin G (Parenteral/Aqueous) *(Continued)*

Mechanism of Action Interferes with bacterial cell wall synthesis during active multiplication, causing cell wall death and resultant bactericidal activity against susceptible bacteria

Other Adverse Effects Frequency not defined:

Central nervous system: Convulsions, confusion, drowsiness, myoclonus, fever
Dermatologic: Rash
Endocrine & metabolic: Electrolyte imbalance
Hematologic: Positive Coombs' reaction, hemolytic anemia
Local: Thrombophlebitis
Renal: Acute interstitial nephritis
Miscellaneous: Anaphylaxis, hypersensitivity reactions, Jarisch-Herxheimer reaction

Drug Interactions

Increased Effect/Toxicity: Probenecid increases penicillin levels. Aminoglycosides may lead to synergistic efficacy.

Decreased Effect: Tetracyclines may decrease penicillin effectiveness. Although anecdotal reports suggest oral contraceptive efficacy could be reduced by penicillins, this has been refuted by more rigorous scientific and clinical data.

Pharmacodynamics/Kinetics

Distribution: Poor penetration across blood-brain barrier, despite inflamed meninges; crosses placenta; enters breast milk

Relative diffusion from blood into CSF: Good only with inflammation (exceeds usual MICs)

CSF:blood level ratio: Normal meninges: <1%; Inflamed meninges: 3% to 5%

Protein binding: 65%
Metabolism: Hepatic (30%) to penicilloic acid
Half-life elimination:

Neonates: <6 days old: 3.2-3.4 hours; 7-13 days old: 1.2-2.2 hours; >14 days old: 0.9-1.9 hours
Children and Adults: Normal renal function: 20-50 minutes
End-stage renal disease: 3.3-5.1 hours

Time to peak, serum: I.M.: ~30 minutes; I.V. ~1 hour
Excretion: Urine

Pregnancy Risk Factor B

Generic Available Yes

Penicillin G Potassium *see* Penicillin G (Parenteral/Aqueous) *on page 1049*

Penicillin G Procaine (pen i SIL in jee PROE kane)

Related Information

Sexually-Transmitted Diseases *on page 1502*

Canadian Brand Names Pfizerpen-AS®; Wycillin®

Mexican Brand Names Penicil; Penipot; Penprocilina

Pharmacologic Category Antibiotic, Penicillin

Synonyms APPG; Aqueous Procaine Penicillin G; Procaine Benzylpenicillin; Procaine Penicillin G

Use Moderately severe infections due to *Treponema pallidum* and other penicillin G-sensitive microorganisms that are susceptible to low, but prolonged serum penicillin concentrations; anthrax due to *Bacillus anthracis* (postexposure) to reduce the incidence or progression of disease following exposure to aerolized *Bacillus anthracis*

Local Anesthetic/Vasoconstrictor Precautions No information available to require special precautions

Effects on Dental Treatment No significant effects or complications reported

Dosage I.M.:

Children: 25,000-50,000 units/kg/day in divided doses 1-2 times/day; not to exceed 4.8 million units/24 hours

Anthrax, inhalational (postexposure prophylaxis): 25,000 units/kg every 12 hours (maximum: 1,200,000 units every 12 hours); see "Note" in Adults dosing

Congenital syphilis: 50,000 units/kg/day for 10-14 days

Adults: 0.6-4.8 million units/day in divided doses every 12-24 hours

Anthrax:

Inhalational (postexposure prophylaxis): 1,200,000 units every 12 hours

Note: Overall treatment duration should be 60 days. Available safety data suggest continued administration of penicillin G procaine for longer than 2 weeks may incur additional risk for adverse reactions. Clinicians may consider switching to effective alternative treatment for completion of therapy beyond 2 weeks.

Cutaneous (treatment): 600,000-1,200,000 units/day; alternative therapy is recommended in severe cutaneous or other forms of anthrax infection

Endocarditis caused by susceptible viridans *Streptococcus* (when used in conjunction with an aminoglycoside): 1.2 million units every 6 hours for 2-4 weeks

Neurosyphilis: I.M.: 2-4 million units/day with 500 mg probenecid by mouth 4 times/day for 10-14 days; **penicillin G aqueous I.V. is the preferred agent**

Hemodialysis: Moderately dialyzable (20% to 50%)

Mechanism of Action Inhibits bacterial cell wall synthesis by binding to one or more of the penicillin binding proteins (PBPs); which in turn inhibits the final transpeptidation step of peptidoglycan synthesis in bacterial cell walls, thus inhibiting cell wall biosynthesis. Bacteria eventually lyse due to ongoing activity of cell wall autolytic enzymes (autolysins and murein hydrolases) while cell wall assembly is arrested.

Other Adverse Effects Frequency not defined:

Cardiovascular: Myocardial depression, vasodilation, conduction disturbances

Central nervous system: Confusion, drowsiness, myoclonus, CNS stimulation, seizures

Hematologic: Positive Coombs' reaction, hemolytic anemia, neutropenia

Local: Pain at injection site, thrombophlebitis, sterile abscess at injection site

Renal: Interstitial nephritis

Miscellaneous: Pseudoanaphylactic reactions, hypersensitivity reactions, Jarisch-Herxheimer reaction, serum sickness

Drug Interactions

Increased Effect/Toxicity: Probenecid increases penicillin levels. Aminoglycosides may lead to synergistic efficacy.

Decreased Effect: Tetracyclines may decrease penicillin effectiveness. Although anecdotal reports suggest oral contraceptive efficacy could be reduced by penicillins, this has been refuted by more rigorous scientific and clinical data.

Pharmacodynamics/Kinetics

Duration: Therapeutic: 15-24 hours

Absorption: I.M.: Slow

Distribution: Penetration across the blood-brain barrier is poor, despite inflamed meninges; enters breast milk

Protein binding: 65%

Metabolism: ~30% hepatically inactivated

Time to peak, serum: 1-4 hours

Excretion: Urine (60% to 90% as unchanged drug)

Clearance: Renal: Delayed in neonates, young infants, and with impaired renal function

Pregnancy Risk Factor B

Generic Available Yes

Penicillin G Procaine and Benzathine Combined *see* Penicillin G Benzathine and Penicillin G Procaine *on page 1048*

Penicillin G Procaine and Penicillin G Benzathine *see* Penicillin G Benzathine and Penicillin G Procaine *on page 1048*

Penicillin G Sodium *see* Penicillin G (Parenteral/Aqueous) *on page 1049*

Penicillin V Potassium (pen i SIL in vee poe TASS ee um)

Related Information

Antibiotic Prophylaxis, Preprocedural Guidelines for Dental Patients *on page 1507*

Oral Bacterial Infections *on page 1531*

Oral Viral Infections *on page 1545*

U.S. Brand Names Veetids®

Canadian Brand Names Apo®-Pen VK; Nadopen-V®; Novo-Pen-VK®; Nu-Pen-VK®; PVF® K

Mexican Brand Names Anapenil; Pen-Vi-K

Pharmacologic Category Antibiotic, Penicillin

Synonyms Pen VK; Phenoxymethyl Penicillin

Use

Dental: Antibiotic of first choice in treating common orofacial infections caused by aerobic gram-positive cocci and anaerobes. These orofacial infections include cellulitis, periapical abscess, periodontal abscess, acute suppurative pulpitis, oronasal fistula, pericoronitis, osteitis, osteomyelitis, postsurgical and post-traumatic infection. It is **no longer recommended for dental procedure prophylaxis.**

Medical: Treatment of moderate to severe susceptible bacterial infections involving the respiratory tract, otitis media, sinusitis, skin, and urinary tract; prophylaxis in rheumatic fever

Local Anesthetic/Vasoconstrictor Precautions No information available to require special precautions

Effects on Dental Treatment >10%: Vomiting, nausea, oral candidiasis (prolonged use)

Dosage Oral:

Systemic infections:

Children <12 years: 25-50 mg/kg/day in divided doses every 6-8 hours; maximum dose: 3 g/day

Children ≥12 years and Adults: 125-500 mg every 6-8 hours

(Continued)

Penicillin V Potassium *(Continued)*

Prophylaxis of pneumococcal infections:
- Children <5 years: 125 mg twice daily
- Children ≥5 years and Adults: 250 mg twice daily

Prophylaxis of recurrent rheumatic fever:
- Children <5 years: 125 mg twice daily
- Children ≥5 years and Adults: 250 mg twice daily

Dosing interval in renal impairment: Cl_{cr} <10 mL/minute: Administer 250 mg every 6 hours

Mechanism of Action Inhibits bacterial cell wall synthesis by binding to one or more of the penicillin binding proteins (PBPs); which in turn inhibits the final transpeptidation step of peptidoglycan synthesis in bacterial cell walls, thus inhibiting cell wall biosynthesis. Bacteria eventually lyse due to ongoing activity of cell wall autolytic enzymes (autolysins and murein hydrolases) while cell wall assembly is arrested.

Other Adverse Effects

>10%: Gastrointestinal: Mild diarrhea

<1%: **Convulsions, fever**, hemolytic anemia, positive Coombs' reaction, acute interstitial nephritis, **hypersensitivity reactions, anaphylaxis**

Contraindications Hypersensitivity to penicillin or any component of the formulation

Warnings/Precautions Use with caution in patients with severe renal impairment (modify dosage), history of seizures, or hypersensitivity to cephalosporins

Drug Interactions

Aminoglycosides: May be synergistic against selected organisms

Oral contraceptives: Anecdotal reports suggesting decreased contraceptive efficacy with penicillins have been refuted by more rigorous scientific and clinical data.

Probenecid, disulfiram: May increase penicillin levels

Tetracyclines: May decrease penicillin effectiveness

Warfarin: Effects of warfarin may be increased

Dietary/Ethanol/Herb Considerations Food decreases drug absorption rate and serum concentration.

Pharmacodynamics/Kinetics

Absorption: 60% to 73%

Distribution: Enters breast milk

Protein binding, plasma: 80%

Half-life elimination: 30 minutes; prolonged with renal impairment

Time to peak, serum: 0.5-1 hour

Excretion: Urine (as unchanged drug and metabolites)

Pregnancy Risk Factor B

Breast-feeding Considerations No data reported; however, other penicillins may be taken while breast-feeding.

Dosage Forms 250 mg = 400,000 units

POWDER, oral solution: 125 mg/5 mL (80 mL, 100 mL, 150 mL, 200 mL); 250 mg/5 mL (80 mL, 100 mL, 150 mL, 200 mL). **TAB:** 250 mg, 500 mg

Generic Available Yes

Selected Readings

Wynn RL and Bergman SA, "Antibiotics and Their Use in the Treatment of Orofacial Infections, Part I," *Gen Dent*, 1994, 42(5):398, 400, 402.

Wynn RL and Bergman SA, "Antibiotics and Their Use in the Treatment of Orofacial Infections, Part II," *Gen Dent*, 1994, 42(6):498-502.

Wynn RL, Bergman SA, Meiller TF, et al, "Antibiotics in Treating Oral-Facial Infections of Odontogenic Origin: An Update", *Gen Dent*, 2001, 49(3):238-40, 242, 244 passim.

Penicilloyl-polylysine *see* Benzylpenicilloyl-polylysine *on page 174*

Penlac™ *see* Ciclopirox *on page 322*

Pentam-300® *see* Pentamidine *on page 1052*

Pentamidine (pen TAM i deen)

U.S. Brand Names NebuPent®; Pentam-300®

Canadian Brand Names Pentacarinat®

Mexican Brand Names Pentacarinat®

Pharmacologic Category Antibiotic, Miscellaneous

Synonyms Pentamidine Isethionate

Use Treatment and prevention of pneumonia caused by *Pneumocystis carinii*; treatment of trypanosomiasis and visceral leishmaniasis

Local Anesthetic/Vasoconstrictor Precautions No information available to require special precautions

Effects on Dental Treatment No significant effects or complications reported

Dosage

Children:

Treatment: I.M., I.V. (I.V. preferred): 4 mg/kg/day once daily for 10-14 days

Prevention:

I.M., I.V.: 4 mg/kg monthly or every 2 weeks

Inhalation (aerosolized pentamidine in children ≥5 years): 300 mg/dose given every 3-4 weeks via Respirgard® II inhaler (8 mg/kg dose has also been used in children <5 years)

Treatment of trypanosomiasis: I.V.: 4 mg/kg/day once daily for 10 days

Adults:

Treatment: I.M., I.V. (I.V. preferred): 4 mg/kg/day once daily for 14-21 days

Prevention: Inhalation: 300 mg every 4 weeks via Respirgard® II nebulizer

Dialysis: Not removed by hemo or peritoneal dialysis or continuous arteriovenous or venovenous hemofiltration; supplemental dosage is unnecessary

Dosing adjustment in renal impairment: Adults: I.V.:

Cl_{cr} 10-50 mL/minute: Administer 4 mg/kg every 24-36 hours

Cl_{cr} <10 mL/minute: Administer 4 mg/kg every 48 hours

Mechanism of Action Interferes with RNA/DNA, phospholipids and protein synthesis, through inhibition of oxidative phosphorylation and/or interference with incorporation of nucleotides and nucleic acids into RNA and DNA, in protozoa

Other Adverse Effects Injection (I); Aerosol (A)

>10%:

Cardiovascular: Chest pain (A - 10% to 23%)

Central nervous system: Fatigue (A - 50% to 70%); dizziness (A - 31% to 47%)

Dermatologic: Rash (31% to 47%)

Endocrine & metabolic: Hyperkalemia

Gastrointestinal: Anorexia (A - 50% to 70%), nausea (A - 10% to 23%)

Local: Local reactions at injection site

Renal: Increased creatinine (I - 23%)

Respiratory: Wheezing (A - 10% to 23%), dyspnea (A - 50% to 70%), coughing (A - 31% to 47%), pharyngitis (10% to 23%)

1% to 10%:

Cardiovascular: Hypotension (I - 4%)

Central nervous system: Confusion/hallucinations (1% to 2%), headache (A - 1% to 5%)

Dermatologic: Rash (I - 3.3%)

Endocrine & metabolic: Hypoglycemia <25 mg/dL (I - 2.4%)

Gastrointestinal: Nausea/anorexia (I - 6%), diarrhea (A - 1% to 5%), vomiting

Hematologic: Severe leukopenia (I - 2.8%), thrombocytopenia <20,000/mm^3 (I - 1.7%), anemia (A - 1% to 5%)

Hepatic: Increased LFTs (I - 8.7%)

<1%: Hypotension <60 mm Hg systolic (I - 0.9%), tachycardia, arrhythmias, dizziness (I), fever, fatigue (I), hyperglycemia or hypoglycemia, hypocalcemia, pancreatitis, megaloblastic anemia, granulocytopenia, leukopenia, renal insufficiency, extrapulmonary pneumocystosis, irritation of the airway, pneumothorax, Jarisch-Herxheimer-like reaction, mild renal or hepatic injury

Drug Interactions Substrate of **CYP2C19**; Inhibits CYP2D6

Increased Effect/Toxicity: Pentamidine may potentiate the effect of other drugs which prolong QT interval (cisapride, astemizole, sparfloxacin, gatifloxacin, moxifloxacin, and type Ia and type III antiarrhythmics).

Dietary/Ethanol/Herb Considerations

Ethanol: Avoid use; may increase CNS depression or aggravate hypoglycemia.

Herb/Nutraceutical: Avoid gotu kola, kava, SAMe, St John's wort, and valerian; may increase CNS depression.

Pharmacodynamics/Kinetics

Absorption: I.M.: Well absorbed; Inhalation: Limited systemic absorption

Half-life elimination: Terminal: 6.4-9.4 hours; may be prolonged with severe renal impairment

Excretion: Urine (33% to 66% as unchanged drug)

Pregnancy Risk Factor C

Generic Available Yes: Injection

Pentamidine Isethionate *see* Pentamidine *on page 1052*

Pentasa® *see* Mesalamine *on page 869*

Pentaspan® *see* Pentastarch *on page 1053*

Pentastarch (PEN ta starch)

U.S. Brand Names Pentaspan®

Canadian Brand Names Pentaspan®

Mexican Brand Names Pentaspan®

Pharmacologic Category Blood Modifiers

Use Orphan drug: Adjunct in leukapheresis to improve harvesting and increase yield of leukocytes by centrifugal means

Local Anesthetic/Vasoconstrictor Precautions No information available to require special precautions

Effects on Dental Treatment No significant effects or complications reported

Dosage 250-700 mL to which citrate anticoagulant has been added is administered by adding to the input line of the centrifugation apparatus at a ratio of 1:8-1:13 to venous whole blood

Generic Available No

Pentazocine (pen TAZ oh seen)

U.S. Brand Names Talwin®; Talwin® NX

Canadian Brand Names Talwin®

Pharmacologic Category Analgesic, Narcotic

Synonyms Pentazocine Hydrochloride; Pentazocine Lactate

Use Relief of moderate to severe pain; has also been used as a sedative prior to surgery and as a supplement to surgical anesthesia

Local Anesthetic/Vasoconstrictor Precautions No information available to require special precautions

Effects on Dental Treatment No significant effects or complications reported

Restrictions C-IV

Dosage

Children: I.M., S.C.:
- 5-8 years: 15 mg
- 8-14 years: 30 mg

Children >12 years and Adults: Oral: 50 mg every 3-4 hours; may increase to 100 mg/dose if needed, but should not exceed 600 mg/day

Adults:
- I.M., S.C.: 30-60 mg every 3-4 hours, not to exceed total daily dose of 360 mg
- I.V.: 30 mg every 3-4 hours

Elderly: Dosing should be started at the lower end of range; population may be more sensitive to analgesic and sedating effects; assessment of renal function is critical

Dosing adjustment in renal impairment:
- Cl_{cr} 10-50 mL/minute: Administer 75% of normal dose
- Cl_{cr} <10 mL/minute: Administer 50% of normal dose

Dosing adjustment in hepatic impairment: Reduce dose or avoid use in liver disease

Mechanism of Action Binds to opiate receptors in the CNS, causing inhibition of ascending pain pathways, altering the perception of and response to pain; produces generalized CNS depression; partial agonist-antagonist

Other Adverse Effects Frequency not defined:

Cardiovascular: Hypotension, palpitations, peripheral vasodilation

Central nervous system: Malaise, headache, restlessness, nightmares, insomnia, CNS depression, sedation, hallucinations, confusion, disorientation, dizziness, euphoria, drowsiness

Dermatologic: Rash, pruritus

Gastrointestinal: Nausea, vomiting, xerostomia, constipation, anorexia, diarrhea, GI irritation, biliary tract spasm

Genitourinary: Urinary tract spasm

Local: Tissue damage and irritation with I.M./S.C. use

Neuromuscular & skeletal: Weakness

Ocular: Blurred vision, miosis

Respiratory: Dyspnea, respiratory depression (rare)

Miscellaneous: Histamine release, physical and psychological dependence

Drug Interactions CYP2D6 enzyme substrate

Increased Effect/Toxicity: Increased effect/toxicity with tripelennamine (can be lethal), CNS depressants (eg, phenothiazines, tranquilizers, anxiolytics, sedatives, hypnotics, alcohol).

Decreased Effect: May potentiate or reduce analgesic effect of opiate agonist (eg, morphine) depending on patients tolerance to opiates; can precipitate withdrawal in narcotic addicts.

Dietary/Ethanol/Herb Considerations

Ethanol: Avoid use; may increase CNS depression.

Herb/Nutraceutical: Avoid gotu kola, kava, SAMe, St John's wort, and valerian; may increase CNS depression.

Pharmacodynamics/Kinetics

Onset of action: Oral, I.M., S.C.: 15-30 minutes; I.V.: 2-3 minutes

Duration: Oral: 4-5 hours; Parenteral: 2-3 hours

Protein binding: 60%

Metabolism: Hepatic via oxidative and glucuronide conjugation pathways; extensive first-pass effect

Bioavailability: Oral: ~20%; increased to 60% to 70% with cirrhosis

Half-life elimination: 2-3 hours; prolonged with hepatic impairment

Excretion: Urine (small amounts as unchanged drug)

Pregnancy Risk Factor B/D (prolonged use or high doses at term)

Generic Available Yes: Tablet

Pentazocine Combinations (pen TAZ oh seen kom bi NAY shuns)

Related Information

Acetaminophen *on page 27*
Aspirin *on page 131*
Pentazocine *on page 1054*

U.S. Brand Names Talacen®

Pharmacologic Category Analgesic Combination (Narcotic)

Use Relief of moderate to severe pain; sedative prior to surgery; supplement to surgical anesthesia

Local Anesthetic/Vasoconstrictor Precautions No information available to require special precautions

Effects on Dental Treatment No significant effects or complications reported

Dosage Adults: Oral: 2 tablets 3-4 times/day

Other Adverse Effects Abrupt discontinuation after sustained use (generally >10 days) may cause withdrawal symptoms.

Frequency not defined:

Cardiovascular: Tachycardia or bradycardia, hypertension or hypotension

Central nervous system: Nervousness, headache, restlessness, malaise, dizziness, fatigue, drowsiness, false sense of well-being, convulsions, increased intracranial pressure

Dermatologic: Rash, urticaria, erythema multiforme, Stevens-Johnson syndrome

Gastrointestinal: Nausea, vomiting, xerostomia, biliary spasm, constipation

Genitourinary: Ureteral spasms, decreased urination

Local: Pain at injection site

Neuromuscular & skeletal: Weakness

Ocular: Blurred vision

Respiratory: Dyspnea

Miscellaneous: Histamine release

Dietary/Ethanol/Herb Considerations

Ethanol: Avoid use; may increase CNS depression.

Herb/Nutraceutical: Avoid gotu kola, kava, SAMe, St John's wort, and valerian; may increase CNS depression.

Pregnancy Risk Factor D/C (Talacen®)

Generic Available No

Pentazocine Hydrochloride *see* Pentazocine *on page 1054*

Pentazocine Lactate *see* Pentazocine *on page 1054*

Pentobarbital (pen toe BAR bi tal)

U.S. Brand Names Nembutal®

Canadian Brand Names Nembutal® Sodium

Pharmacologic Category Anticonvulsant, Barbiturate; Barbiturate

Synonyms Pentobarbital Sodium

Use Sedative/hypnotic; preanesthetic; high-dose barbiturate coma for treatment of increased intracranial pressure or status epilepticus unresponsive to other therapy

Unlabeled/Investigational Use Tolerance test during withdrawal of sedative hypnotics

Local Anesthetic/Vasoconstrictor Precautions No information available to require special precautions

Effects on Dental Treatment No significant effects or complications reported

Restrictions C-II (capsules, injection); C-III (suppositories)

Dosage

Children:

Sedative: Oral: 2-6 mg/kg/day divided in 3 doses; maximum: 100 mg/day

Hypnotic: I.M.: 2-6 mg/kg; maximum: 100 mg/dose

Sedative/hypnotic: Rectal:

2 months to 1 year (10-20 lb): 30 mg

1-4 years (20-40 lb): 30-60 mg

5-12 years (40-80 lb): 60 mg

12-14 years (80-110 lb): 60-120 mg

or

<4 years: 3-6 mg/kg/dose

>4 years: 1.5-3 mg/kg/dose

Preoperative/preprocedure sedation: ≥6 months:

Note: Limited information is available for infants <6 months of age.

Oral, I.M., rectal: 2-6 mg/kg; maximum: 100 mg/dose

I.V.: 1-3 mg/kg to a maximum of 100 mg until asleep

Conscious sedation prior to a procedure: Children 5-12 years: I.V.: 2 mg/kg 5-10 minutes before procedures, may repeat one time

Adolescents: Conscious sedation: Oral, I.V.: 100 mg prior to a procedure

Children and Adults: Barbiturate coma in head injury patients: I.V.: Loading dose: 5-10 mg/kg given slowly over 1-2 hours; monitor blood pressure and respiratory rate; Maintenance infusion: Initial: 1 mg/kg/hour; may increase to 2-3 mg/kg/hour; maintain burst suppression on EEG

Status epilepticus: I.V.: **Note**: Intubation required; monitor hemodynamics

Children: Loading dose: 5-15 mg/kg given slowly over 1-2 hours; maintenance infusion: 0.5-5 mg/kg/hour

Adults: Loading dose: 2-15 mg/kg given slowly over 1-2 hours; maintenance infusion: 0.5-3 mg/kg/hour

(Continued)

Pentobarbital *(Continued)*

Adults:

Hypnotic:

Oral: 100-200 mg at bedtime or 20 mg 3-4 times/day for daytime sedation

I.M.: 150-200 mg

I.V.: Initial: 100 mg, may repeat every 1-3 minutes up to 200-500 mg total dose

Rectal: 120-200 mg at bedtime

Preoperative sedation: I.M.: 150-200 mg

Tolerance testing (unlabeled use): 200 mg every 2 hours until signs of intoxication are exhibited at any time during the 2 hours after the dose; maximum dose: 1000 mg

Dosing adjustment in hepatic impairment: Reduction required in severe dysfunction

Mechanism of Action Short-acting barbiturate with sedative, hypnotic, and anticonvulsant properties. Barbiturates depress the sensory cortex, decrease motor activity, alter cerebellar function, and produce drowsiness, sedation, and hypnosis. In high doses, barbiturates exhibit anticonvulsant activity; barbiturates produce dose-dependent respiratory depression.

Other Adverse Effects Frequency not defined:

Cardiovascular: Bradycardia, hypotension, syncope

Central nervous system: Drowsiness, lethargy, CNS excitation or depression, impaired judgment, "hangover" effect, confusion, somnolence, agitation, hyperkinesia, ataxia, nervousness, headache, insomnia, nightmares, hallucinations, anxiety, dizziness

Dermatologic: Rash, exfoliative dermatitis, Stevens-Johnson syndrome

Gastrointestinal: Nausea, vomiting, constipation

Hematologic: Agranulocytosis, thrombocytopenia, megaloblastic anemia

Local: Pain at injection site, thrombophlebitis with I.V. use

Renal: Oliguria

Respiratory: Laryngospasm, respiratory depression, apnea (especially with rapid I.V. use), hypoventilation, apnea

Miscellaneous: Gangrene with inadvertent intra-arterial injection

Drug Interactions Induces **CYP2A6, 3A4**

Increased Effect/Toxicity: When combined with other CNS depressants, ethanol, narcotic analgesics, antidepressants, or benzodiazepines, additive respiratory and CNS depression may occur. Chronic use of barbiturates may enhance the hepatotoxic potential of acetaminophen overdoses. Chloramphenicol, MAO inhibitors, valproic acid, and felbamate may inhibit barbiturate metabolism. Barbiturates may impair the absorption of griseofulvin, and may enhance the nephrotoxic effects of methoxyflurane.

Decreased Effect: Barbiturates such as pentobarbital are hepatic enzyme inducers, and (only with chronic use) may increase the metabolism of antipsychotics, some beta-blockers (unlikely with atenolol and nadolol), calcium channel blockers, chloramphenicol, cimetidine, corticosteroids, cyclosporine, disopyramide, doxycycline, ethosuximide, felbamate, furosemide, griseofulvin, lamotrigine, phenytoin, propafenone, quinidine, tacrolimus, TCAs, and theophylline. Barbiturates may increase the metabolism of estrogens and reduce the efficacy of oral contraceptives; an alternative method of contraception should be considered. Barbiturates inhibit the hypoprothrombinemic effects of oral anticoagulants via increased metabolism. Barbiturates may enhance the metabolism of methadone resulting in methadone withdrawal.

Dietary/Ethanol/Herb Considerations

Ethanol: Avoid use; may increase CNS depression.

Food may decrease the rate but not the extent of oral absorption.

Herb/Nutraceutical: Avoid gotu kola, kava, SAMe, St John's wort, and valerian; may increase CNS depression.

Pharmacodynamics/Kinetics

Onset of action: Oral, rectal: 15-60 minutes; I.M.: 10-15 minutes; I.V.: ~1 minute

Duration: Oral, rectal: 1-4 hours; I.V.: 15 minutes

Distribution: V_d: Children: 0.8 L/kg; Adults: 1 L/kg

Protein binding: 35% to 55%

Metabolism: Extensively hepatic via hydroxylation and oxidation pathways

Half-life elimination: Terminal: Children: 25 hours; Adults: Healthy: 22 hours (range: 35-50 hours)

Excretion: Urine (<1% as unchanged drug)

Pregnancy Risk Factor D

Generic Available No

Pentobarbital Sodium *see* Pentobarbital *on page 1055*

Pentosan Polysulfate Sodium

(PEN toe san pol i SUL fate SOW dee um)

U.S. Brand Names Elmiron®

Canadian Brand Names Elmiron™

Pharmacologic Category Analgesic, Urinary

Synonyms PPS

Use Orphan drug: Relief of bladder pain or discomfort due to interstitial cystitis

Local Anesthetic/Vasoconstrictor Precautions No information available to require special precautions

Effects on Dental Treatment 1% to 10%: Headache (3%), dizziness (1%), nausea

Dosage Adults: Oral: 100 mg 3 times/day taken with water 1 hour before or 2 hours after meals

Patients should be evaluated at 3 months and may be continued an additional 3 months if there has been no improvement and if there are no therapy-limiting side effects. **The risks and benefits of continued use beyond 6 months in patients who have not responded is not yet known.**

Mechanism of Action Although pentosan polysulfate sodium is a low-molecular weight heparinoid, it is not known whether these properties play a role in its mechanism of action in treating interstitial cystitis; the drug appears to adhere to the bladder wall mucosa where it may act as a buffer to protect the tissues from irritating substances in the urine.

Other Adverse Effects

1% to 10%:

Central nervous system: Depression (2%)
Dermatologic: Alopecia, rash, pruritus
Gastrointestinal: Diarrhea, dyspepsia, abdominal pain
Hepatic: Liver function test abnormalities (1%)

<1%: **Allergic reactions,** amblyopia, anemia, anorexia, **bruising,** colitis, conjunctivitis, constipation, **dyspnea, epistaxis, esophagitis,** flatulence, **gastritis, gum bleeding, oral ulceration, increased partial thromboplastin time,** insomnia, leukopenia, optic neuritis, pharyngitis, photosensitivity, prolonged PT, pruritus, retinal hemorrhage, **rhinitis**, thrombocytopenia, tinnitus, urticaria, **vomiting**

Drug Interactions Increased Effect/Toxicity: Although there is no information about potential drug interactions, it is expected that pentosan polysulfate sodium would have at least additive anticoagulant effects when administered with anticoagulant drugs such as warfarin or heparin, and possible similar effects when administered with aspirin or thrombolytics.

Pharmacodynamics/Kinetics

Absorption: ~3%
Metabolism: Hepatic and via spleen
Half-life elimination: 4.8 hours
Excretion: Urine (3% as unchanged drug)

Pregnancy Risk Factor B

Generic Available No

Pentostatin (PEN toe stat in)

U.S. Brand Names Nipent®

Canadian Brand Names Nipent®

Pharmacologic Category Antineoplastic Agent, Antibiotic

Synonyms DCF; Deoxycoformycin; 2′-deoxycoformycin

Use Treatment of adult patients with alpha-interferon-refractory hairy cell leukemia; non-Hodgkin's lymphoma, cutaneous T-cell lymphoma

Local Anesthetic/Vasoconstrictor Precautions No information available to require special precautions

Effects on Dental Treatment 1% to 20%: Dyspnea, pneumonia, bronchitis, pharyngitis, rhinitis, epistaxis, sinusitis (3% to 7%), chest pain, arrhythmia

Dosage Refractory hairy cell leukemia: Adults (refer to individual protocols): 4 mg/m^2 every other week; I.V. bolus over ≥3-5 minutes in D_5W or NS at concentrations ≥2 mg/mL

Dosing interval in renal impairment:

Cl_{cr} <60 mL/minute: Use extreme caution
Cl_{cr} 50-60 mL/minute: 2 mg/m^2/dose

Mechanism of Action Pentostatin is a purine antimetabolite that inhibits adenosine deaminase, preventing the deamination of adenosine to inosine. Accumulation of deoxyadenosine (dAdo) and deoxyadenosine 5′-triphosphate (dATP) results in a reduction of purine metabolism and DNA synthesis and cell death.

Other Adverse Effects

>10%:

Central nervous system: Fever, chills, infection (57%), severe, life-threatening (35%); headache, lethargy, seizures, coma (10% to 15%), potentially dose-limiting, uncommon at doses 4 mg/m^2
Dermatologic: Skin rashes (25% to 30%), alopecia (10%)
Gastrointestinal: Mild to moderate nausea, vomiting (60%), controlled with non-5-HT_3 antagonist antiemetics; stomatitis, diarrhea (13%), anorexia
Genitourinary: Acute renal failure (35%)
Hematologic: Thrombocytopenia (50%), dose-limiting in 25% of patients; anemia (40% to 45%), neutropenia, mild to moderate, not dose-limiting (11%)
Nadir: 7 days
Recovery: 10-14 days

(Continued)

Pentostatin *(Continued)*

Hepatic: Mild to moderate increases in transaminase levels (30%), usually transient; hepatitis (19%), usually reversible

Respiratory: Pulmonary edema (15%; may be exacerbated by fludarabine)

1% to 10%:

Cardiovascular: Peripheral edema

Central nervous system: Opportunistic infections (8%); anxiety, confusion, depression, dizziness, insomnia, nervousness, somnolence, myalgias, malaise

Dermatologic: Dry skin, eczema, pruritus

Gastrointestinal: Constipation, flatulence, weight loss

Neuromuscular & skeletal: Paresthesia, weakness

Ocular: Moderate to severe keratoconjunctivitis, abnormal vision, eye pain

Otic: Ear pain

<1%: Dysuria, hematuria, hypersensitivity reactions, increased BUN, thrombophlebitis

Drug Interactions Increased toxicity with vidarabine, fludarabine, and allopurinol.

Pharmacodynamics/Kinetics

Distribution: I.V.: V_d: 36.1 L (20.1 L/m^2); rapidly to body tissues

Half-life elimination: Distribution half-life: 30-85 minutes; Terminal: 5-15 hours

Excretion: Urine (~50% to 96%) within 24 hours (30% to 90% as unchanged drug)

Pregnancy Risk Factor D

Generic Available No

Pentothal® *see* Thiopental *on page 1297*

Pentoxifylline (pen toks I fi leen)

U.S. Brand Names Pentoxil®; Trental®

Canadian Brand Names Albert® Pentoxifylline; Apo®-Pentoxifylline SR; Nu-Pentoxifylline SR; ratio-Pentoxifylline; Trental®

Mexican Brand Names Fixoten®; Kentadin®; Peridane®; Sufisal®; Trental®; Vasofyl®

Pharmacologic Category Blood Viscosity Reducer Agent

Synonyms Oxpentifylline

Use Treatment of intermittent claudication on the basis of chronic occlusive arterial disease of the limbs; may improve function and symptoms, but not intended to replace more definitive therapy

Unlabeled/Investigational Use AIDS patients with increased TNF, CVA, cerebrovascular diseases, diabetic atherosclerosis, diabetic neuropathy, gangrene, hemodialysis shunt thrombosis, vascular impotence, cerebral malaria, septic shock, sickle cell syndromes, and vasculitis

Local Anesthetic/Vasoconstrictor Precautions No information available to require special precautions

Effects on Dental Treatment No significant effects or complications reported

Dosage Adults: Oral: 400 mg 3 times/day with meals; may reduce to 400 mg twice daily if GI or CNS side effects occur

Mechanism of Action Mechanism of action remains unclear; is thought to reduce blood viscosity and improve blood flow by altering the rheology of red blood cells

Other Adverse Effects

1% to 10%:

Central nervous system: Dizziness, headache

Gastrointestinal: Dyspepsia, nausea, vomiting

<1%; Angioedema, arrhythmias, chest pain, cholecystitis, congestion, dyspnea, hallucinations, hepatitis, jaundice, rash, tremor

Drug Interactions Inhibits CYP1A2

Increased Effect/Toxicity: Pentoxifylline levels may be increased with cimetidine and other H_2 antagonists. May increase anticoagulation with warfarin. Pentoxifylline may increase the serum levels of theophylline.

Decreased Effect: Blood pressure changes (decreases) have been observed with the addition of pentoxifylline therapy in patients receiving antihypertensives.

Dietary/Ethanol/Herb Considerations

Food: Administer with food to reduce GI upset; may decrease peak serum concentration and rate but not extent of absorption.

Herb/Nutraceutical: Avoid garlic and ginkgo biloba; may have additive neurostatic effect. Avoid ginger; may inhibit platelet aggregation resulting in additive hemostatic effects. Avoid horse chestnut; may increase bleeding risk due to antiplatelet effects.

Pharmacodynamics/Kinetics

Absorption: Well absorbed

Metabolism: Hepatic and via erythrocytes; extensive first-pass effect

Half-life elimination: Parent drug: 24-48 minutes; Metabolites: 60-96 minutes

Time to peak, serum: 2-4 hours

Excretion: Primarily urine

Pregnancy Risk Factor C

Generic Available Yes

Pentoxil® *see* Pentoxifylline *on page 1058*
Pentrax® [OTC] *see* Coal Tar *on page 359*
Pen VK *see* Penicillin V Potassium *on page 1051*
Pepcid® *see* Famotidine *on page 556*
Pepcid® AC [OTC] *see* Famotidine *on page 556*
Pepcid® Complete [OTC] *see* Famotidine, Calcium Carbonate, and Magnesium Hydroxide *on page 557*
Pepto-Bismol® [OTC] *see* Bismuth *on page 186*
Pepto-Bismol® Maximum Strength [OTC] *see* Bismuth *on page 186*
Percocet® 2.5/325 *see* Oxycodone and Acetaminophen *on page 1018*
Percocet® 5/325 *see* Oxycodone and Acetaminophen *on page 1018*
Percocet® 7.5/325 *see* Oxycodone and Acetaminophen *on page 1018*
Percocet® 7.5/500 *see* Oxycodone and Acetaminophen *on page 1018*
Percocet® 10/325 *see* Oxycodone and Acetaminophen *on page 1018*
Percocet® 10/650 *see* Oxycodone and Acetaminophen *on page 1018*
Percodan® *see* Oxycodone and Aspirin *on page 1020*
Percodan®-Demi [DSC] *see* Oxycodone and Aspirin *on page 1020*
Percogesic® [OTC] *see* Acetaminophen and Phenyltoloxamine *on page 31*
Percolone® [DSC] *see* Oxycodone *on page 1017*
Perdiem® Fiber Therapy [OTC] *see* Psyllium *on page 1149*

Pergolide (PER go lide)

U.S. Brand Names Permax®

Canadian Brand Names Permax®

Mexican Brand Names Permax®

Pharmacologic Category Anti-Parkinson's Agent, Dopamine Agonist; Ergot Derivative

Synonyms Pergolide Mesylate

Use Adjunctive treatment to levodopa/carbidopa in the management of Parkinson's disease

Unlabeled/Investigational Use Treatment of Tourette's disorder, chronic motor or vocal tic disorders

Local Anesthetic/Vasoconstrictor Precautions No information available to require special precautions

Effects on Dental Treatment 1% to 10%: Xerostomia; normal salivary flow resumes upon discontinuation

Prolonged use may decrease or inhibit salivary flow, contributing to discomfort and dental disease (ie, oral candidiasis and periodontal disease).

Dosage When adding pergolide to levodopa/carbidopa, the dose of the latter can usually and should be decreased. Patients no longer responsive to bromocriptine may benefit by being switched to pergolide. Oral:

Children and Adolescents: Tourette's disorder, chronic motor or vocal disorder (unlabeled uses): Up to 300 mcg/day

Adults: Parkinson's disease: Start with 0.05 mg/day for 2 days, then increase dosage by 0.1 or 0.15 mg/day every 3 days over next 12 days, increase dose by 0.25 mg/day every 3 days until optimal therapeutic dose is achieved, up to 5 mg/day maximum; usual dosage range: 2-3 mg/day in 3 divided doses

Mechanism of Action Pergolide is a semisynthetic ergot alkaloid similar to bromocriptine but stated to be more potent (10-1000 times) and longer-acting; it is a centrally-active dopamine agonist stimulating both D_1 and D_2 receptors. Pergolide is believed to exert its therapeutic effect by directly stimulating postsynaptic dopamine receptors in the nigrostriatal system.

Other Adverse Effects

>10%:

Central nervous system: Dizziness (19%), hallucinations (14%), dystonia (12%), somnolence (10%), confusion (10%)

Gastrointestinal: Nausea (24%), constipation (11%)

Neuromuscular & skeletal: Dyskinesia (62%)

Respiratory: Rhinitis (12%)

1% to 10%:

Cardiovascular: Hypotension or postural hypotension (10%), peripheral edema (7%), chest pain (4%), vasodilation (3%), palpitation (2%), syncope (2%), arrhythmias (1%), hypertension (2%), MI (1%)

Central nervous system: Insomnia (8%), pain (7%), anxiety (6%), psychosis (2%), EPS (2%), incoordination (2%), chills (1%)

Dermatologic: Rash (3%)

Gastrointestinal: Diarrhea (6%), dyspepsia (6%), abdominal pain (6%), anorexia (5%), xerostomia (4%), vomiting (3%), dysphagia (1%), nausea (1%)

Hematologic: Anemia (1%)

Neuromuscular & skeletal: Myalgia (1%), neuralgia (1%)

Ocular: Abnormal vision (6%), diplopia (2%)

Respiratory: Dyspnea (5%), epistaxis (2%)

Miscellaneous: Flu syndrome (3%), hiccups (1%)

(Continued)

Pergolide *(Continued)*

<1% (Limited to important or life-threatening): A-V block, facial paralysis, intestinal obstruction, intracranial hypertension, laryngeal edema, neuritis, pancreatitis, pericarditis, pericardial effusion, pleural effusion, pleural fibrosis, pleuritis, pneumothorax, retroperitoneal fibrosis, vasculitis

Postmarketing and/or case reports: Neuroleptic malignant syndrome (NMS; associated with rapid discontinuation), valvular fibrosis

Drug Interactions Substrate of **CYP3A4**; Inhibits **CYP2D6**, 3A4

Increased Effect/Toxicity: Effects of pergolide may be increased by antifungals (azole derivatives); CYP3A4 inhibitors (eg, amiodarone, cimetidine, erythromycin, ritonavir); macrolide antibiotics; levodopa (hallucinations); protease inhibitors; MAO inhibitors. Pergolide may increase the effects of CYP2D6 substrates (eg, TCAs, fluoxetine, fluvoxamine, risperidone); sibutramine; and other serotonin agonists (serotonin syndrome).

Decreased Effect: Effects of pergolide may be diminished by antipsychotics, metoclopramide.

Dietary/Ethanol/Herb Considerations

Ethanol: Avoid use; may cause CNS depression.

Herb/Nutraceutical: Avoid gotu kola, kava, SAMe, St John's wort, and valerian; may increase CNS depression.

Pharmacodynamics/Kinetics

Absorption: Well absorbed

Protein binding, plasma: 90%

Metabolism: Extensively hepatic

Half-life elimination: 27 hours

Excretion: Urine (~50%); feces (50%)

Pregnancy Risk Factor B

Generic Available Yes

Pergolide Mesylate *see* Pergolide *on page 1059*
Pergonal® *see* Menotropins *on page 857*
Periactin® *see* Cyproheptadine *on page 387*
Peri-Colace® [OTC] *see* Docusate and Casanthranol *on page 464*
Peridex® *see* Chlorhexidine Gluconate *on page 300*

Perindopril Erbumine (per IN doe pril er BYOO meen)

U.S. Brand Names Aceon®

Canadian Brand Names Coversyl®

Mexican Brand Names Coversyl®

Pharmacologic Category Angiotensin-Converting Enzyme (ACE) Inhibitor

Use Treatment of stage I or II hypertension and CHF; treatment of left ventricular dysfunction after MI

Local Anesthetic/Vasoconstrictor Precautions No information available to require special precautions

Effects on Dental Treatment No significant effects or complications reported

Dosage Adults: Oral:

CHF: 4 mg once daily

Hypertension: Initial: 4 mg/day but may be titrated to response; usual range: 4-8 mg/day, maximum: 16 mg/day

Elderly: Dose reduction of 50% is recommended due to bioavailability and lower renal clearance

Dosing adjustment in renal impairment:

Cl_{cr} >60 mL/minute: Administer 4 mg/day.

Cl_{cr} 30-60 mL/minute: Administer 2 mg/day.

Cl_{cr} 15-29 mL/minute: Administer 2 mg every other day.

Cl_{cr} <15 mL/minute: Administer 2 mg on the day of dialysis.

Hemodialysis: Perindopril and its metabolites are dialyzable

Mechanism of Action Competitive inhibitor of angiotensin-converting enzyme (ACE); prevents conversion of angiotensin I to angiotensin II, a potent vasoconstrictor; results in lower levels of angiotensin II which, in turn, causes an increase in plasma renin activity and a reduction in aldosterone secretion

Other Adverse Effects

>10% Central nervous system: Headache (23%)

1% to 10%:

Cardiovascular: edema (4%), chest pain (2%)

Central nervous system: Dizziness (8%), sleep disorders (3%), depression (2%), fever (2%), weakness (8%), nervousness (1%)

Dermatologic: Rash (2%)

Endocrine & metabolic: Hyperkalemia (1%), increased triglycerides (1%)

Gastrointestinal: Nausea (2%), diarrhea (4%), vomiting (2%), dyspepsia (2%), abdominal pain (3%), flatulence (1%)

Genitourinary: Sexual dysfunction (male: 1%)

Hepatic: Increased ALT (2%)

Neuromuscular & skeletal: Back pain (6%), upper extremity pain (3%), lower extremity pain (5%), paresthesia (2%), joint pain (1%), myalgia (1%), arthritis (1%)

Renal: Proteinuria (2%)

Respiratory: Cough (incidence is higher in women, 3:1) (12%), sinusitis (5%), rhinitis (5%), pharyngitis (3%)

Otic: Tinnitus (2%)

Miscellaneous: Viral infection (3%)

Note: Some reactions occurred at an incidence >1% but ≤ placebo.

<1% (Limited to important or life-threatening): Amnesia, anaphylaxis, angioedema (0.1%), anxiety, arthralgia, bronchitis, bruising, cerebral vascular accident (0.2%), chills, conduction abnormalities, conjunctivitis, constipation, decreased uric acid, diaphoresis, dry skin, dyspnea, earache, epistaxis, erythema, facial edema, flank pain, gastroenteritis, gout, hematoma, hematuria, hyperglycemia, hypokalemia, hypotension, increased alkaline phosphatase, increased appetite, increased AST, increased serum creatinine, malaise, migraine, MI, nephrolithiasis, orthostatic hypotension, pain, pruritus, psychosocial disorder, pulmonary fibrosis (<0.1%), purpura (0.1%), rhinorrhea, sneezing, syncope, tinea, urinary frequency, urinary retention, vaginitis, vasodilation, ventricular extrasystole, vertigo, xerostomia

Additional adverse effects associated with with **ACE inhibitors** include agranulocytosis (especially in patients with renal impairment or collagen vascular disease), neutropenia, decreases in creatinine clearance in some elderly hypertensive patients or those with chronic renal failure, and worsening of renal function in patients with bilateral renal artery stenosis or hypovolemic patients (diuretic therapy). In addition, a syndrome which may include fever, myalgia, arthralgia, interstitial nephritis, vasculitis, rash, eosinophilia and positive ANA, and elevated ESR has been reported with ACE inhibitors.

Drug Interactions

Increased Effect/Toxicity: Coadministration of the following drugs may result in elevated serum potassium levels: Potassium supplements, sulfamethoxazole and trimethoprim (high dose), angiotensin II receptor antagonists (candesartan, losartan, irbesartan, etc), or potassium-sparing diuretics (amiloride, spironolactone, triamterene). ACE inhibitor effects may be increased by phenothiazines or probenecid (increases levels of captopril). ACE inhibitors may increase serum concentrations/effects of digoxin, lithium, and sulfonlyureas. Diuretics have additive hypotensive effects with ACE inhibitors, and hypovolemia increases the potential for adverse renal effects of ACE inhibitors. In patients with compromised renal function, coadministration with NSAIDs may result in further deterioration of renal function. Allopurinol and ACE inhibitors may cause a higher risk of hypersensitivity reaction when taken concurrently.

Decreased Effect: Aspirin (high dose) may reduce the therapeutic effects of ACE inhibitors; at low dosages this does not appear to be significant. Rifampin may decrease the effect of ACE inhibitors. Antacids may decrease the bioavailability of ACE inhibitors (may be more likely to occur with captopril); separate administration times by 1-2 hours. NSAIDs, specifically indomethacin, may reduce the hypotensive effects of ACE inhibitors. More likely to occur in low renin or volume dependent hypertensive patients.

Dietary/Ethanol/Herb Considerations

Ethanol: Avoid use; may increase risk of hypotension or dizziness.

Food may lower active metabolite concentrations. Avoid caffeine (eg, colas, chocolate), garlic, and licorice.

Herb/Nutraceutical: Avoid black cohosh, dong quai, and evening primrose due to estrogenic activity. Avoid ephedra, ginseng, and yohimbe; may worsen hypertension. Avoid garlic; may have increased antihypertensive effect. Avoid ginger due to positive inotropic effects; theoretically, may cause arrhythmia. Avoid hawthorn; may lower peripheral vascular resistance resulting in additive decrease in BP. Avoid licorice.

Pharmacodynamics/Kinetics

Onset of action: Peak effect: 1-2 hours

Distribution: Small amounts enter breast milk

Protein binding: Perindopril: 60%; Perindoprilat: 10% to 20%

Metabolism: Hepatically hydrolyzed to active metabolite, perindoprilat (~17% to 20% of a dose) and other inactive metabolites

Bioavailability: Perindopril: 65% to 95%

Half-life elimination: Parent drug: 1.5-3 hours; Metabolite: Effective: 3-10 hours, Terminal: 30-120 hours

Time to peak: Chronic therapy: Perindopril: 1 hour; Perindoprilat: 3-4 hours (maximum perindoprilat serum levels are 2-3 times higher and T_{max} is shorter following chronic therapy); CHF: Perindoprilat: 6 hours

Excretion: Urine (75%, 10% as unchanged drug)

Pregnancy Risk Factor D (especially 2nd and 3rd trimesters)

Generic Available No

PerioChip® *see* Chlorhexidine Gluconate *on page 300*

PerioGard® *see* Chlorhexidine Gluconate *on page 300*

Periostat® *see* Doxycycline Subantimicrobial *on page 480*

Permapen® Isoject® *see* Penicillin G Benzathine *on page 1047*

Permax® *see* Pergolide *on page 1059*

Permethrin (per METH rin)

U.S. Brand Names A200® Lice [OTC]; Acticin®; Elimite®; Nix® [OTC]; Rid® Spray [OTC]

Canadian Brand Names Kwellada-P™; Nix®

Mexican Brand Names Novo-Herklin 2000®

Pharmacologic Category Antiparasitic Agent, Topical; Scabicidal Agent

Use Single-application treatment of infestation with *Pediculus humanus capitis* (head louse) and its nits or *Sarcoptes scabiei* (scabies); indicated for prophylactic use during epidemics of lice

Local Anesthetic/Vasoconstrictor Precautions No information available to require special precautions

Effects on Dental Treatment No significant effects or complications reported

Dosage Topical:

Head lice: Children >2 months and Adults: After hair has been washed with shampoo, rinsed with water, and towel dried, apply a sufficient volume of topical liquid (lotion or cream rinse) to saturate the hair and scalp. Leave on hair for 10 minutes before rinsing off with water; remove remaining nits; may repeat in 1 week if lice or nits still present.

Scabies: Apply cream from head to toe; leave on for 8-14 hours before washing off with water; for infants, also apply on the hairline, neck, scalp, temple, and forehead; may reapply in 1 week if live mites appear

Permethrin 5% cream was shown to be safe and effective when applied to an infant <1 month of age with neonatal scabies; time of application was limited to 6 hours before rinsing with soap and water

Mechanism of Action Inhibits sodium ion influx through nerve cell membrane channels in parasites resulting in delayed repolarization and thus paralysis and death of the pest

Other Adverse Effects 1% to 10%:

Dermatologic: Pruritus, erythema, rash of the scalp

Local: Burning, stinging, tingling, numbness or scalp discomfort, edema

Pharmacodynamics/Kinetics

Absorption: <2%

Metabolism: Hepatic via ester hydrolysis to inactive metabolites

Excretion: Urine

Pregnancy Risk Factor B

Generic Available Yes: Excludes spray

Perphenazine (per FEN a zeen)

U.S. Brand Names Trilafon® [DSC]

Canadian Brand Names Apo®-Perphenazine; Trilafon®

Mexican Brand Names Leptopsique®

Pharmacologic Category Antipsychotic Agent, Phenothiazine, Piperazine

Use Treatment of severe schizophrenia; nausea and vomiting

Unlabeled/Investigational Use Treatment of ethanol withdrawal symptoms, dementia in elderly, Tourette's syndrome, Huntington's chorea, spasmodic torticollis, Reye's syndrome, psychosis

Local Anesthetic/Vasoconstrictor Precautions Most pharmacology textbooks state that in presence of phenothiazines, systemic doses of epinephrine paradoxically decrease the blood pressure. This is the so called "epinephrine reversal" phenomenon. This has never been observed when epinephrine is given by infiltration as part of the anesthesia procedure.

Effects on Dental Treatment

Significant hypotension may occur, especially when the drug is administered parenterally; orthostatic hypotension is due to alpha-receptor blockade, the elderly are at greater risk for orthostatic hypotension.

Tardive dyskinesia: Prevalence rate may be 40% in elderly; development of the syndrome and the irreversible nature are proportional to duration and total cumulative dose over time. Extrapyramidal reactions are more common in elderly with up to 50% developing these reactions after 60 years of age; drug-induced **Parkinson's syndrome** occurs often; **Akathisia** is the most common extrapyramidal reaction in elderly.

Increased confusion, memory loss, psychotic behavior, and agitation frequently occur as a consequence of anticholinergic effects. Antipsychotic associated sedation in nonpsychotic patients is extremely unpleasant due to feelings of depersonalization, derealization, and dysphoria

Dosage

Children:

Schizophrenia/psychoses:

Oral:

1-6 years: 4-6 mg/day in divided doses

6-12 years: 6 mg/day in divided doses
>12 years: 4-16 mg 2-4 times/day
I.M.: 5 mg every 6 hours
Nausea/vomiting: I.M.: 5 mg every 6 hours

Adults:
Schizophrenia/psychoses:
Oral: 4-16 mg 2-4 times/day not to exceed 64 mg/day
I.M.: 5 mg every 6 hours up to 15 mg/day in ambulatory patients and 30 mg/day in hospitalized patients
Nausea/vomiting:
Oral: 8-16 mg/day in divided doses up to 24 mg/day
I.M.: 5-10 mg every 6 hours as necessary up to 15 mg/day in ambulatory patients and 30 mg/day in hospitalized patients
I.V. (severe): 1 mg at 1- to 2-minute intervals up to a total of 5 mg

Elderly: Behavioral symptoms associated with dementia: Oral: Initial: 2-4 mg 1-2 times/day; increase at 4- to 7-day intervals by 2-4 mg/day. Increase dose intervals (bid, tid, etc) as necessary to control behavior response or side effects. Maximum daily dose: 32 mg; gradual increase (titration) and bedtime administration may prevent some side effects or decrease their severity.

Hemodialysis: Not dialyzable (0% to 5%)

Dosing adjustment in hepatic impairment: Consider reductions; specific guidelines unavailable

Mechanism of Action Blocks postsynaptic mesolimbic dopaminergic receptors in the brain; exhibits alpha-adrenergic blocking effect and depresses the release of hypothalamic and hypophyseal hormones

Other Adverse Effects Frequency not defined:

Cardiovascular: Hypotension, orthostatic hypotension, hypertension, tachycardia, bradycardia, dizziness, cardiac arrest

Central nervous system: Extrapyramidal symptoms (pseudoparkinsonism, akathisia, dystonias, tardive dyskinesia), dizziness, cerebral edema, seizures, headache, drowsiness, paradoxical excitement, restlessness, hyperactivity, insomnia, neuroleptic malignant syndrome (NMS), impairment of temperature regulation

Dermatologic: Increased sensitivity to sun, rash, discoloration of skin (blue-gray)

Endocrine & metabolic: Hypoglycemia, hyperglycemia, galactorrhea, lactation, breast enlargement, gynecomastia, menstrual irregularity, amenorrhea, SIADH, changes in libido

Gastrointestinal: Constipation, weight gain, vomiting, stomach pain, nausea, xerostomia, salivation, diarrhea, anorexia, ileus

Genitourinary: Difficulty in urination, ejaculatory disturbances, incontinence, polyuria, ejaculating dysfunction, priapism

Hematologic: Agranulocytosis, leukopenia, eosinophilia, hemolytic anemia, thrombocytopenic purpura, pancytopenia

Hepatic: Cholestatic jaundice, hepatotoxicity

Neuromuscular & skeletal: Tremor

Ocular: Pigmentary retinopathy, blurred vision, cornea and lens changes

Respiratory: Nasal congestion

Miscellaneous: Diaphoresis

Drug Interactions Substrate of CYP1A2, 2C8/9, 2C19, **2D6**, 3A4; Inhibits CYP1A2, **2D6**

Increased Effect/Toxicity: Effects on CNS depression may be additive when perphenazine is combined with CNS depressants (narcotic analgesics, ethanol, barbiturates, cyclic antidepressants, antihistamines, or sedative-hypnotics). Perphenazine may increase the effects/toxicity of anticholinergics, antihypertensives, lithium (rare neurotoxicity), trazodone, or valproic acid. Concurrent use with TCA may produce increased toxicity or altered therapeutic response. Chloroquine and propranolol may increase perphenazine concentrations. Hypotension may occur when perphenazine is combined with epinephrine. May increase the risk of arrhythmia when combined with antiarrhythmics, cisapride, pimozide, sparfloxacin, or other drugs which prolong QT interval. Metoclopramide may increase risk of extrapyramidal symptoms (EPS). Drugs which inhibit CYP2D6 may increase serum concentrations of perphenazine (includes amiodarone, cimetidine, delavirdine, fluoxetine, paroxetine, propafenone, quinidine, ritonavir, and sertraline).

Decreased Effect: Phenothiazines inhibit the ability of bromocriptine to lower serum prolactin concentrations. Benztropine (and other anticholinergics) may inhibit the therapeutic response to perphenazine and excess anticholinergic effects may occur. Cigarette smoking and barbiturates may enhance the hepatic metabolism of chlorpromazine. Antihypertensive effects of guanethidine and guanadrel may be inhibited by perphenazine. Perphenazine may inhibit the antiparkinsonian effect of levodopa. Perphenazine and possibly other low potency antipsychotics may reverse the pressor effects of epinephrine.

Dietary/Ethanol/Herb Considerations

Ethanol: Avoid use; may increase CNS depression

(Continued)

Perphenazine *(Continued)*

Food: Oral concentration may be diluted with water, milk, or citrus juice; do not dilute with coffee, tea, or liquids containing apple juice. Avoid caffeine. Fluids, fruit, and fiber may reduce constipation.

Herb/Nutraceutical: Avoid gotu kola, kava, SAMe, St John's wort, and valerian; may increase CNS depression.

Pharmacodynamics/Kinetics

Absorption: Oral: Well absorbed

Distribution: Crosses placenta

Metabolism: Extensively hepatic to metabolites via sulfoxidation, hydroxylation, dealkylation, and glucuronidation

Half-life elimination: Perphenazine: 9-12 hours; 7-hydroxyperphenazine: 11.3 hours

Time to peak, serum: Perphenazine: 1-3 hours; 7-hydroxyperphenazine: 2-4 hours

Excretion: Urine and feces

Pregnancy Risk Factor C

Generic Available Yes

Perphenazine and Amitriptyline *see* Amitriptyline and Perphenazine *on page 85*

Persantine® *see* Dipyridamole *on page 456*

Pertussin® DM [OTC] *see* Dextromethorphan *on page 423*

Pethidine Hydrochloride *see* Meperidine *on page 858*

PFA *see* Foscarnet *on page 613*

Pfizerpen® *see* Penicillin G (Parenteral/Aqueous) *on page 1049*

PGE_1 *see* Alprostadil *on page 63*

PGE_2 *see* Dinoprostone *on page 450*

PGI_2 *see* Epoprostenol *on page 505*

PGX *see* Epoprostenol *on page 505*

Phanasin [OTC] *see* Guaifenesin *on page 650*

Pharmaflur® *see* Fluoride *on page 586*

Pharmaflur® 1.1 *see* Fluoride *on page 586*

Phazyme® Quick Dissolve [OTC] *see* Simethicone *on page 1222*

Phazyme® Ultra Strength [OTC] *see* Simethicone *on page 1222*

Phenaphen® With Codeine *see* Acetaminophen and Codeine *on page 29*

Phenazopyridine (fen az oh PEER i deen)

U.S. Brand Names Azo-Gesic® [OTC]; Azo-Standard® [OTC]; Prodium® [OTC]; Pyridium®; ReAzo [OTC]; Uristat® [OTC]; UTI Relief® [OTC]

Canadian Brand Names Phenazo™; Pyridium®

Mexican Brand Names Azo Wintomylon; Madel; Urovalidin

Pharmacologic Category Analgesic, Urinary

Synonyms Phenazopyridine Hydrochloride; Phenylazo Diamino Pyridine Hydrochloride

Use Symptomatic relief of urinary burning, itching, frequency and urgency in association with urinary tract infection or following urologic procedures

Local Anesthetic/Vasoconstrictor Precautions No information available to require special precautions

Effects on Dental Treatment No significant effects or complications reported

Dosage Oral:

Children: 12 mg/kg/day in 3 divided doses administered after meals for 2 days

Adults: 100-200 mg 3 times/day after meals for 2 days when used concomitantly with an antibacterial agent

Dosing interval in renal impairment:

Cl_{cr} 50-80 mL/minute: Administer every 8-16 hours

Cl_{cr} <50 mL/minute: Avoid use

Mechanism of Action An azo dye which exerts local anesthetic or analgesic action on urinary tract mucosa through an unknown mechanism

Other Adverse Effects

1% to 10%:

Central nervous system: Headache, dizziness

Gastrointestinal: Stomach cramps

<1%: Acute renal failure, methemoglobinemia, hemolytic anemia, hepatitis, rash, skin pigmentation, vertigo

Pharmacodynamics/Kinetics

Metabolism: Hepatic and via other tissues

Excretion: Urine (65% as unchanged drug)

Pregnancy Risk Factor B

Generic Available Yes

Phenazopyridine Hydrochloride *see* Phenazopyridine *on page 1064*

Phendimetrazine (fen dye ME tra zeen)

U.S. Brand Names Bontril PDM®; Bontril® Slow-Release; Melfiat®: Obezine®; Prelu-2®

Canadian Brand Names Bontril®; Plegine®; Statobex®

Pharmacologic Category Anorexiant

Synonyms Phendimetrazine Tartrate

Use Appetite suppressant during the first few weeks of dieting to help establish new eating habits; its effectiveness lasts only for short periods (3-12 weeks)

Local Anesthetic/Vasoconstrictor Precautions Use vasoconstrictor with caution in patients taking phendimetrazine. Phendimetrazine can enhance the sympathomimetic response to epinephrine leading to potential hypertension and cardiotoxicity.

Effects on Dental Treatment Patients taking phendimetrazine may present with hypertension; monitor BP.

Restrictions C-III

Dosage Adults: Oral:

Regular capsule or tablet: 35 mg 2 or 3 times daily, 1 hour before meals

Sustained release: 105 mg once daily in the morning before breakfast

Other Adverse Effects Frequency not defined:

Cardiovascular: Hypertension, tachycardia, arrhythmias

Central nervous system: Euphoria, nervousness, insomnia, confusion, mental depression, restlessness, headache

Dermatologic: Alopecia

Endocrine & metabolic: Changes in libido

Gastrointestinal: Nausea, vomiting, constipation, diarrhea, abdominal cramps

Genitourinary: Dysuria

Hematologic: Blood dyscrasias

Neuromuscular & skeletal: Tremor, myalgia

Ocular: Blurred vision

Renal: Polyuria

Respiratory: Dyspnea

Miscellaneous: Diaphoresis (increased)

Generic Available Yes

Phendimetrazine Tartrate *see* Phendimetrazine *on page 1064*

Phenelzine (FEN el zeen)

U.S. Brand Names Nardil®

Canadian Brand Names Nardil®

Pharmacologic Category Antidepressant, Monoamine Oxidase Inhibitor

Synonyms Phenelzine Sulfate

Use Symptomatic treatment of atypical, nonendogenous, or neurotic depression

Unlabeled/Investigational Use Treatment of selective mutism

Local Anesthetic/Vasoconstrictor Precautions Attempts should be made to avoid use of vasoconstrictor due to possibility of hypertensive episodes with monoamine oxidase inhibitors

Effects on Dental Treatment >10%: Orthostatic hypotension, xerostomia, changes in salivation

Avoid use as an analgesic due to toxic reactions with MAO inhibitors.

Dosage Oral:

Children: Selective mutism (unlabeled use): 30-60 mg/day

Adults: Depression: 15 mg 3 times/day; may increase to 60-90 mg/day during early phase of treatment, then reduce dose for maintenance therapy slowly after maximum benefit is obtained; takes 2-4 weeks for a significant response to occur

Elderly: Depression: Initial: 7.5 mg/day; increase by 7.5-15 mg/day every 3-4 days as tolerated; usual therapeutic dose: 15-60 mg/day in 3-4 divided doses

Mechanism of Action Thought to act by increasing endogenous concentrations of norepinephrine, dopamine, and serotonin through inhibition of the enzyme (monoamine oxidase) responsible for the breakdown of these neurotransmitters

Other Adverse Effects Frequency not defined:

Cardiovascular: Orthostatic hypotension, edema

Central nervous system: Dizziness, headache, drowsiness, sleep disturbances, fatigue, hyper-reflexia, twitching, ataxia, mania

Dermatologic: Rash, pruritus

Endocrine & metabolic: Decreased sexual ability (anorgasmia, ejaculatory disturbances, impotence), hypernatremia, hypermetabolic syndrome

Gastrointestinal: Constipation, weight gain

Genitourinary: Urinary retention

Hematologic: Leukopenia

Hepatic: Hepatitis

Neuromuscular & skeletal: Weakness, tremor, myoclonus

Ocular: Blurred vision, glaucoma

Miscellaneous: Diaphoresis

Drug Interactions

Increased Effect/Toxicity: In general, the combined use of phenelzine with TCAs, venlafaxine, trazodone, dexfenfluramine, sibutramine, lithium, meperidine, fenfluramine, dextromethorphan, and SSRIs should be avoided due to the potential for severe adverse reactions (serotonin syndrome, death). MAO inhibitors

(Continued)

Phenelzine *(Continued)*

(including phenelzine) may inhibit the metabolism of barbiturates and prolong their effect. Phenelzine in combination with amphetamines, other stimulants (methylphenidate), levodopa, metaraminol, reserpine, and decongestants (pseudoephedrine) may result in severe hypertensive reactions. Foods (eg, cheese) and beverages (eg, ethanol) containing tyramine should be avoided; hypertensive crisis may result. Phenelzine may increase the pressor response of norepinephrine and may prolong neuromuscular blockade produced by succinylcholine. Tramadol may increase the risk of seizures and serotonin syndrome in patients receiving an MAO inhibitor. Phenelzine may produce additive hypoglycemic effect in patients receiving hypoglycemic agents and may produce delirium in patients receiving disulfiram.

Decreased Effect: Phenelzine (and other MAO inhibitors) inhibits the antihypertensive response to guanadrel or guanethidine.

Dietary/Ethanol/Herb Considerations

Ethanol: Avoid beverages containing tyramine (eg, wine); may induce a severe hypertensive response.

Food: Avoid food/beverages high in tyramine (eg, avocadoes, bananas, broad bean pods, canned figs, cheese, chicken liver, pickled herring, raisins, sour cream, soy sauce, yeast extracts, yogurt, pods, meats prepared with tenderizers, and foods aged to improve flavor); may cause sudden and severe high BP. Avoid foods containing tryptophan, dopamine, chocolate, or caffeine.

Pharmacodynamics/Kinetics

Onset of action: Therapeutic: 2-4 weeks

Duration: May continue to have a therapeutic effect and interactions 2 weeks after discontinuing therapy

Absorption: Well absorbed

Excretion: Urine (primarily as metabolites and unchanged drug)

Pregnancy Risk Factor C

Generic Available No

Phenelzine Sulfate *see* Phenelzine *on page 1065*

Phenergan® With Codeine *see* Promethazine and Codeine *on page 1129*

Phenindamine (fen IN dah meen)

U.S. Brand Names Nolahist® [OTC]

Canadian Brand Names Nolahist®

Pharmacologic Category Antihistamine

Synonyms Phenindamine Tartrate

Use Treatment of perennial and seasonal allergic rhinitis and chronic urticaria

Local Anesthetic/Vasoconstrictor Precautions No information available to require special precautions

Effects on Dental Treatment No significant effects or complications reported

Dosage Oral:

Children <6 years: As directed by physician

Children 6 to <12 years: 12.5 mg every 4-6 hours, up to 75 mg/24 hours

Adults: 25 mg every 4-6 hours, up to 150 mg/24 hours

Generic Available No

Phenindamine Tartrate *see* Phenindamine *on page 1066*

Pheniramine and Naphazoline *see* Naphazoline and Pheniramine *on page 953*

Phenobarbital (fee noe BAR bi tal)

U.S. Brand Names Luminal® Sodium

Mexican Brand Names Alepsal

Pharmacologic Category Anticonvulsant, Barbiturate; Barbiturate

Synonyms Phenobarbital Sodium; Phenobarbitone; Phenylethylmalonylurea

Use Management of generalized tonic-clonic (grand mal) and partial seizures; sedative

Unlabeled/Investigational Use Treatment of febrile seizures in children, neonatal seizures, management of sedative/hypnotic withdrawal; treatment and prophylaxis of neonatal hyperbilirubinemia and lowering of bilirubin in chronic cholestasis

Local Anesthetic/Vasoconstrictor Precautions No information available to require special precautions

Effects on Dental Treatment No significant effects or complications reported

Restrictions C-IV

Dosage

Children:

- Sedation: Oral: 2 mg/kg 3 times/day
- Hypnotic: I.M., I.V., S.C.: 3-5 mg/kg at bedtime
- Preoperative sedation: Oral, I.M., I.V.: 1-3 mg/kg 1-1.5 hours before procedure

Adults:

- Sedation: Oral, I.M.: 30-120 mg/day in 2-3 divided doses
- Hypnotic: Oral, I.M., I.V., S.C.: 100-320 mg at bedtime
- Preoperative sedation: I.M.: 100-200 mg 1-1.5 hours before procedure

Anticonvulsant: Status epilepticus: **Loading dose:** I.V.:

Infants and Children: 10-20 mg/kg in a single or divided dose; in select patients may administer additional 5 mg/kg/dose every 15-30 minutes until seizure is controlled or a total dose of 40 mg/kg is reached

Adults: 300-800 mg initially followed by 120-240 mg/dose at 20-minute intervals until seizures are controlled or a total dose of 1-2 g

Anticonvulsant maintenance dose: Oral, I.V.:

Infants: 5-8 mg/kg/day in 1-2 divided doses

Children:

1-5 years: 6-8 mg/kg/day in 1-2 divided doses

5-12 years: 4-6 mg/kg/day in 1-2 divided doses

Children >12 years and Adults: 1-3 mg/kg/day in divided doses or 50-100 mg 2-3 times/day

Sedative/hypnotic withdrawal (unlabeled use): Initial daily requirement is determined by substituting phenobarbital 30 mg for every 100 mg pentobarbital used during tolerance testing; then daily requirement is decreased by 10% of initial dose

Dosing interval in renal impairment: Cl_{cr} <10 mL/minute: Administer every 12-16 hours

Hemodialysis: Moderately dialyzable (20% to 50%)

Dosing adjustment in hepatic impairment: Increased side effects may occur in severe impairment; monitor plasma levels and adjust dose accordingly

Mechanism of Action Short-acting barbiturate with sedative, hypnotic, and anticonvulsant properties. Barbiturates depress the sensory cortex, decrease motor activity, alter cerebellar function, and produce drowsiness, sedation, and hypnosis. In high doses, barbiturates exhibit anticonvulsant activity; barbiturates produce dose-dependent respiratory depression.

Other Adverse Effects Frequency not defined:

Cardiovascular: Bradycardia, hypotension, syncope

Central nervous system: Drowsiness, lethargy, CNS excitation or depression, impaired judgment, "hangover" effect, confusion, somnolence, agitation, hyperkinesia, ataxia, nervousness, headache, insomnia, nightmares, hallucinations, anxiety, dizziness

Dermatologic: Rash, exfoliative dermatitis, Stevens-Johnson syndrome

Gastrointestinal: Nausea, vomiting, constipation

Hematologic: Agranulocytosis, thrombocytopenia, megaloblastic anemia

Local: Pain at injection site, thrombophlebitis with I.V. use

Renal: Oliguria

Respiratory: Laryngospasm, respiratory depression, apnea (especially with rapid I.V. use), hypoventilation

Miscellaneous: Gangrene with inadvertent intra-arterial injection

Drug Interactions Substrate of CYP2C8/9, **2C19**, 2E1; Induces **CYP1A2, 2A6, 2B6, 2C8/9, 3A4**

Increased Effect/Toxicity: When combined with other CNS depressants, ethanol, narcotic analgesics, antidepressants, or benzodiazepines, additive respiratory and CNS depression may occur. Barbiturates may enhance the hepatotoxic potential of acetaminophen overdoses. Chloramphenicol, MAO inhibitors, valproic acid, and felbamate may inhibit barbiturate metabolism. Barbiturates may impair the absorption of griseofulvin, and may enhance the nephrotoxic effects of methoxyflurane. Concurrent use of phenobarbital with meperidine may result in increased CNS depression. Concurrent use of phenobarbital with primidone may result in elevated phenobarbital serum concentrations.

Decreased Effect: Barbiturates are hepatic enzyme inducers, and may increase the metabolism of antipsychotics, some beta-blockers (unlikely with atenolol and nadolol), calcium channel blockers, chloramphenicol, cimetidine, corticosteroids, cyclosporine, disopyramide, doxycycline, ethosuximide, felbamate, furosemide, griseofulvin, lamotrigine, phenytoin, propafenone, quinidine, tacrolimus, TCAs, and theophylline. Barbiturates may increase the metabolism of estrogens and reduce the efficacy of oral contraceptives; an alternative method of contraception should be considered. Barbiturates inhibit the hypoprothrombinemic effects of oral anticoagulants via increased metabolism. Barbiturates may enhance the metabolism of methadone resulting in methadone withdrawal.

Dietary/Ethanol/Herb Considerations

Ethanol: Avoid use; may increase CNS depression.

Food: Requires diet rich in vitamin D; may require calcium supplementation. May reduce effects of caffeine. Avoid grapefruit products; may increase serum concentration.

Herb/Nutraceutical: Avoid evening primrose; decreases seizure threshold. Avoid gotu kola, kava, SAMe, St John's wort, and valerian; may increase CNS depression.

Pharmacodynamics/Kinetics

Onset of action: Oral: Hypnosis: 20-60 minutes; I.V.: ~5 minutes

Peak effect: I.V.: ~30 minutes

Duration: Oral: 6-10 hours; I.V.: 4-10 hours

Absorption: Oral: 70% to 90%

(Continued)

Phenobarbital *(Continued)*

Protein binding: 20% to 45%; decreased in neonates
Metabolism: Hepatic via hydroxylation and glucuronide conjugation
Half-life elimination: Neonates: 45-500 hours; Infants: 20-133 hours; Children: 37-73 hours; Adults: 53-140 hours
Time to peak, serum: Oral: 1-6 hours
Excretion: Urine (20% to 50% as unchanged drug)

Pregnancy Risk Factor D

Generic Available Yes

Phenobarbital, Belladonna, and Ergotamine Tartrate *see* Belladonna, Phenobarbital, and Ergotamine *on page 165*

Phenobarbital, Hyoscyamine, Atropine, and Scopolamine *see* Hyoscyamine, Atropine, Scopolamine, and Phenobarbital *on page 700*

Phenobarbital Sodium *see* Phenobarbital *on page 1066*

Phenobarbitone *see* Phenobarbital *on page 1066*

Phenol (FEE nol)

Related Information

Mouth Pain, Cold Sore, and Canker Sore Products *on page 1630*

U.S. Brand Names Cēpastat® [OTC]; Cēpastat® Extra Strength [OTC]; Chloraseptic® Gargle [OTC]; Chloraseptic® Mouth Pain Spray [OTC]; Chloraseptic® Rinse [OTC]; Chloraseptic® Spray [OTC]; Chloraseptic® Spray for Kids [OTC]; Pain-A-Lay® [OTC]; Ulcerease® [OTC]

Canadian Brand Names P & S™ Liquid Phenol

Pharmacologic Category Pharmaceutical Aid

Synonyms Carbolic Acid

Use Relief of sore throat pain, mouth, gum, and throat irritations; neurologic pain, rectal prolapse, hemorrhoids, hydrocele

Local Anesthetic/Vasoconstrictor Precautions No information available to require special precautions

Effects on Dental Treatment No significant effects or complications reported

Dosage

Allow to dissolve slowly in mouth; may be repeated every 2 hours as needed
For each neurolysis procedure: 0.5-2 mL (up to 7.5 mL may be needed)

Other Adverse Effects Frequency not defined:

In overdose situation:

Cardiovascular: Hypotension, cardiovascular collapse, tachycardia, atrial and ventricular arrhythmias, edema
Central nervous system: slurred speech, CNS depression, agitation, confusion, seizures, coma
Dermatologic: White, red, or brown skin discoloration
Gastrointestinal: Nausea, vomiting, oral burns, GI ulceration, GI bleeding
Genitourinary: Urine discoloration (green)
Hematologic: Hemorrhage
Local: Irritation, burns
Renal: Nephritis
Respiratory: Bronchospasm/wheezing, coughing, dyspnea, pneumonia, pulmonary

When used for spinal neurolysis/motor point blocks:

Cardiovascular: Dysrhythmias
Central nervous system: Headache, hyperesthesia, dysesthesia
Gastrointestinal: Bowel incontinence
Genitourinary: Urinary incontinence
Local: Tissue necrosis, pain at injection site
Neuromuscular & skeletal: Motor weakness, nerve damage
Respiratory: Pleural irritation

Pregnancy Risk Factor C

Generic Available Yes: Oral spray

Phenol and Camphor *see* Camphor and Phenol *on page 232*

Phenoptic® *see* Phenylephrine *on page 1071*

Phenoxybenzamine (fen oks ee BEN za meen)

U.S. Brand Names Dibenzyline®

Canadian Brand Names Dibenzyline®

Pharmacologic Category Alpha$_1$ Blocker

Synonyms Phenoxybenzamine Hydrochloride

Use Symptomatic management of pheochromocytoma; treatment of hypertensive crisis caused by sympathomimetic amines

Unlabeled/Investigational Use Treatment of micturition problems associated with neurogenic bladder, functional outlet obstruction, and partial prostate obstruction

Local Anesthetic/Vasoconstrictor Precautions No information available to require special precautions

Effects on Dental Treatment No significant effects or complications reported

Dosage Oral:

Children: Initial: 0.2 mg/kg (maximum: 10 mg) once daily, increase by 0.2 mg/kg increments; usual maintenance dose: 0.4-1.2 mg/kg/day every 6-8 hours, higher doses may be necessary

Adults: Initial: 10 mg twice daily, increase by 10 mg every other day until optimum dose is achieved; usual range: 20-40 mg 2-3 times/day

Mechanism of Action Produces long-lasting noncompetitive alpha-adrenergic blockade of postganglionic synapses in exocrine glands and smooth muscle; relaxes urethra and increases opening of the bladder

Other Adverse Effects Frequency not defined:

Cardiovascular: Postural hypotension, tachycardia, syncope, shock

Central nervous system: Lethargy, headache, confusion, fatigue

Gastrointestinal: Vomiting, nausea, diarrhea, xerostomia

Genitourinary: Inhibition of ejaculation

Neuromuscular & skeletal: Weakness

Ocular: Miosis

Respiratory: Nasal congestion

Drug Interactions

Increased Effect/Toxicity: Beta-blockers may result in increased toxicity (hypotension, tachycardia).

Decreased Effect: Alpha adrenergic agonists decrease the effect of phenoxybenzamine.

Dietary/Ethanol/Herb Considerations Ethanol: Avoid use.

Pharmacodynamics/Kinetics

Onset of action: ~2 hours

Peak effect: 4-6 hours

Duration: ≥4 days

Half-life elimination: 24 hours

Excretion: Primarily urine and feces

Pregnancy Risk Factor C

Generic Available No

Phenoxybenzamine Hydrochloride *see* Phenoxybenzamine *on page 1068*

Phenoxymethyl Penicillin *see* Penicillin V Potassium *on page 1051*

Phentermine (FEN ter meen)

U.S. Brand Names Adipex-P®; Ionamin®

Canadian Brand Names Ionamin®

Mexican Brand Names Ifa Reduccing "S"®

Pharmacologic Category Anorexiant

Synonyms Phentermine Hydrochloride

Use Short-term adjunct in a regimen of weight reduction based on exercise, behavioral modification, and caloric reduction in the management of exogenous obesity for patients with an initial body mass index ≥30 kg/m^2 or ≥27 kg/m^2 in the presence of other risk factors (diabetes, hypertension)

Local Anesthetic/Vasoconstrictor Precautions Use vasoconstriction with caution in patients taking phentermine. Amphetamines enhance the sympathomimetic response of epinephrine and norepinephrine leading to potential hypertension and cardiotoxicity.

Effects on Dental Treatment Up to 10% of patients may present with hypertension. The use of local anesthetic without vasoconstrictor is recommended in these patients.

Restrictions C-IV

Dosage Oral: Adults: Obesity: 8 mg 3 times/day 30 minutes before meals or food or 15-37.5 mg/day before breakfast or 10-14 hours before retiring

Mechanism of Action Phentermine is structurally similar to dextroamphetamine and is comparable to dextroamphetamine as an appetite suppressant, but is generally associated with a lower incidence and severity of CNS side effects. Phentermine, like other anorexiants, stimulates the hypothalamus to result in decreased appetite; anorexiant effects are most likely mediated via norepinephrine and dopamine metabolism. However, other CNS effects or metabolic effects may be involved.

Other Adverse Effects Frequency not defined:

Cardiovascular: Palpitations, tachycardia, primary pulmonary hypertension and/or regurgitant cardiac valvular disease

Central nervous system: Euphoria, insomnia, overstimulation, dizziness, dysphoria, headache, restlessness, psychosis

Dermatologic: Urticaria

Endocrine & metabolic: Changes in libido, impotence

Gastrointestinal: Nausea, constipation, diarrhea, **xerostomia, unpleasant taste**

Hematologic: Blood dyscrasias

Neuromuscular & skeletal: Tremor

Ocular: Blurred vision

(Continued)

Phentermine *(Continued)*

Drug Interactions

Increased Effect/Toxicity: Dosage of hypoglycemic agents may need to be adjusted when phentermine is used in a diabetic receiving a special diet. Concurrent use of MAO inhibitors and drugs with MAO activity (furazolidone, linezolid) may be associated with hypertensive episodes. Concurrent use of SSRIs may be associated with a risk of serotonin syndrome.

Decreased Effect: Phentermine may decrease the effect of antihypertensive medications The efficacy of anorexiants may be decreased by antipsychotics; in addition, amphetamines or related compounds may induce an increase in psychotic symptoms in some patients. Amphetamines (and related compounds) inhibit the antihypertensive response to guanethidine; probably also may occur with guanadrel.

Pharmacodynamics/Kinetics

Duration: Resin produces more prolonged clinical effects

Absorption: Well absorbed; resin absorbed slower

Half-life elimination: 20 hours

Excretion: Primarily urine (as unchanged drug)

Pregnancy Risk Factor C

Generic Available Yes

Comments Many diet physicians have prescribed fenfluramine ("fen") and phentermine ("phen"). When taken together the combination is known as "fen-phen". The diet drug dexfenfluramine (Redux®) is chemically similar to fenfluramine (Pondimin®) and was also used in combination with phentermine called "Redux-phen". While each of the three drugs alone had approval from the FDA for sale in the treatment of obesity, neither combination had an official approval. The use of the combinations in the treatment of obesity was considered an "off-label" use. Reports in medical literature have been accumulating for some years about significant side effects associated with fenfluramine and dexfenfluramine. In 1997, the manufacturers, at the urging of the FDA, agreed to voluntarily withdraw the drugs from the market. The action was based on findings from physicians who evaluated patients taking fenfluramine and dexfenfluramine with echocardiograms. The findings indicated that approximately 30% of patients had abnormal echocardiograms, even though they had no symptoms. This was a much higher than expected percentage of abnormal test results. This conclusion was based on a sample of 291 patients examined by five different physicians. Under normal conditions, fewer than 1% of patients would be expected to show signs of heart valve disease. The findings suggested that fenfluramine and dexfenfluramine were the likely cause of heart valve problems of the type that promoted FDA's earlier warnings concerning "fen-phen". The earlier warning included the following: The mitral valve and other valves in the heart are damaged by a strange white coating and allow blood to flow back, causing heart muscle damage. In several cases, valve replacement surgery has been done. As a rule, the person must, thereafter for life, be on a blood thinner to prevent clots from the mechanical valve. This type of valve damage had only been seen before in persons who were exposed to large amounts of serotonin. The fenfluramine increases the availability of serotonin.

Phentermine Hydrochloride *see* Phentermine *on page 1069*

Phentolamine (fen TOLE a meen)

Canadian Brand Names Regitine®; Rogitine®

Mexican Brand Names Z-Max®

Pharmacologic Category Alpha$_1$ Blocker

Synonyms Phentolamine Mesylate

Use Diagnosis of pheochromocytoma and treatment of hypertension associated with pheochromocytoma or other caused by excess sympathomimetic amines; as treatment of dermal necrosis after extravasation of drugs with alpha-adrenergic effects (norepinephrine, dopamine, epinephrine, dobutamine)

Local Anesthetic/Vasoconstrictor Precautions Although the alpha-adrenergic blocking effects could antagonize epinephrine, there is no information available to require special precautions

Effects on Dental Treatment No significant effects or complications reported

Dosage

Treatment of alpha-adrenergic drug extravasation: S.C.:

Children: 0.1-0.2 mg/kg diluted in 10 mL 0.9% sodium chloride infiltrated into area of extravasation within 12 hours

Adults: Infiltrate area with small amount of solution made by diluting 5-10 mg in 10 mL 0.9% sodium chloride within 12 hours of extravasation; do not exceed 0.1-0.2 mg/kg or 5 mg total

If dose is effective, normal skin color should return to the blanched area within 1 hour

Diagnosis of pheochromocytoma: I.M., I.V.:

Children: 0.05-0.1 mg/kg/dose, maximum single dose: 5 mg

Adults: 5 mg

Surgery for pheochromocytoma: Hypertension: I.M., I.V.:

Children: 0.05-0.1 mg/kg/dose given 1-2 hours before procedure; repeat as needed every 2-4 hours until hypertension is controlled; maximum single dose: 5 mg

Adults: 5 mg given 1-2 hours before procedure and repeated as needed every 2-4 hours

Hypertensive crisis: Adults: 5-20 mg

Mechanism of Action Competitively blocks alpha-adrenergic receptors to produce brief antagonism of circulating epinephrine and norepinephrine to reduce hypertension caused by alpha effects of these catecholamines; also has a positive inotropic and chronotropic effect on the heart

Other Adverse Effects Frequency not defined:

Cardiovascular: Hypotension, tachycardia, arrhythmia, flushing, orthostatic hypotension

Central nervous system: Weakness, dizziness

Gastrointestinal: Nausea, vomiting, diarrhea

Respiratory: Nasal congestion

Case report: Pulmonary hypertension

Drug Interactions Decreased effect of phentolamine with epinephrine and ephedrine.

Dietary/Ethanol/Herb Considerations Ethanol: Avoid use; increases toxicity.

Pharmacodynamics/Kinetics

Onset of action: I.M.: 15-20 minutes; I.V.: Immediate

Duration: I.M.: 30-45 minutes; I.V.: 15-30 minutes

Metabolism: Hepatic

Half-life elimination: 19 minutes

Excretion: Urine (10% as unchanged drug)

Pregnancy Risk Factor C

Generic Available Yes

Phentolamine Mesylate *see* Phentolamine *on page 1070*

Phenylalanine Mustard *see* Melphalan *on page 855*

Phenylazo Diamino Pyridine Hydrochloride *see* Phenazopyridine *on page 1064*

Phenylephrine (fen il EF rin)

Related Information

Guaifenesin and Phenylephrine *on page 652*

U.S. Brand Names AK-Dilate®; AK-Nefrin®; Formulation R™ [OTC]; Medicone® [OTC]; Mydfrin®; Neo-Synephrine® Extra Strength [OTC]; Neo-Synephrine® Mild [OTC]; Neo-Synephrine® Ophthalmic; Neo-Synephrine® Regular Strength [OTC]; Nostril® [OTC]; Phenoptic®; Prefrin™ [DSC]; Relief® [OTC]; Vicks® Sinex® Nasal Spray [OTC]; Vicks® Sinex® UltraFine Mist [OTC]

Canadian Brand Names Dionephrine®; Mydfrin®; Neo-Synephrine®

Pharmacologic Category Alpha/Beta Agonist; Ophthalmic Agent, Antiglaucoma; Ophthalmic Agent, Mydriatic

Synonyms Phenylephrine Hydrochloride

Use Treatment of hypotension, vascular failure in shock; as a vasoconstrictor in regional analgesia; symptomatic relief of nasal and nasopharyngeal mucosal congestion; as a mydriatic in ophthalmic procedures and treatment of wide-angle glaucoma; supraventricular tachycardia

Local Anesthetic/Vasoconstrictor Precautions Use with caution since phenylephrine is a sympathomimetic amine which could interact with epinephrine to cause a pressor response

Effects on Dental Treatment ≤10%: Tachycardia, palpitations, xerostomia; use vasoconstrictor with caution

Dosage

Ophthalmic procedures:

Infants <1 year: Instill 1 drop of 2.5% 15-30 minutes before procedures

Children and Adults: Instill 1 drop of 2.5% or 10% solution, may repeat in 10-60 minutes as needed

Nasal decongestant (therapy should not exceed 3 continuous days):

Children:

2-6 years: Instill 1 drop every 2-4 hours of 0.125% solution as needed

6-12 years: Instill 1-2 sprays or instill 1-2 drops every 4 hours of 0.25% solution as needed

Children >12 years and Adults: Instill 1-2 sprays or instill 1-2 drops every 4 hours of 0.25% to 0.5% solution as needed; 1% solution may be used in adult in cases of extreme nasal congestion; do not use nasal solutions more than 3 days

Hypotension/shock:

Children:

I.M., S.C.: 0.1 mg/kg/dose every 1-2 hours as needed (maximum: 5 mg)

I.V. bolus: 5-20 mcg/kg/dose every 10-15 minutes as needed

I.V. infusion: 0.1-0.5 mcg/kg/minute

(Continued)

Phenylephrine *(Continued)*

Adults:

I.M., S.C.: 2-5 mg/dose every 1-2 hours as needed (initial dose should not exceed 5 mg)

I.V. bolus: 0.1-0.5 mg/dose every 10-15 minutes as needed (initial dose should not exceed 0.5 mg)

I.V. infusion: 10 mg in 250 mL D_5W or NS (1:25,000 dilution) (40 mcg/mL); start at 100-180 mcg/minute (2-5 mL/minute; 50-90 drops/minute) initially; when blood pressure is stabilized, maintenance rate: 40-60 mcg/minute (20-30 drops/minute); rates up to 360 mcg/minute have been reported; dosing range: 0.4-9.1 mcg/kg/minute

Note: Concentrations up to 100-500 mg in 250 mL have been used.

Paroxysmal supraventricular tachycardia: I.V.:

Children: 5-10 mcg/kg/dose over 20-30 seconds

Adults: 0.25-0.5 mg/dose over 20-30 seconds

Mechanism of Action Potent, direct-acting alpha-adrenergic stimulator with weak beta-adrenergic activity; causes vasoconstriction of the arterioles of the nasal mucosa and conjunctiva; activates the dilator muscle of the pupil to cause contraction; produces vasoconstriction of arterioles in the body; produces systemic arterial vasoconstriction

Other Adverse Effects Frequency not defined:

Cardiovascular: Reflex bradycardia, excitability, restlessness, arrhythmias (rare), precordial pain or discomfort, pallor, hypertension, severe peripheral and visceral vasoconstriction, decreased cardiac output

Central nervous system: Headache, anxiety, weakness, dizziness, tremor, paresthesia, restlessness

Endocrine & metabolic: Metabolic acidosis

Local: Extravasation which may lead to necrosis and sloughing of surrounding tissue, blanching of skin

Neuromuscular & skeletal: Pilomotor response, weakness

Renal: Decreased renal perfusion, reduced urine output, reduced urine output

Respiratory: Respiratory distress

Drug Interactions

Increased Effect/Toxicity: Phenylephrine, taken with sympathomimetics, may induce tachycardia or arrhythmias. If taken with MAO inhibitors or oxytocic agents, actions may be potentiated.

Decreased Effect: Alpha- and beta-adrenergic blocking agents may have a decreased effect if taken with phenylephrine.

Dietary/Ethanol/Herb Considerations Herb/Nutraceutical: Avoid ephedra, ginseng, and yohimbe; may cause CNS stimulation.

Pharmacodynamics/Kinetics

Onset of action: I.M., S.C.: 10-15 minutes; I.V.: Immediate

Duration: I.M.: 0.5-2 hours; I.V.: 15-30 minutes; S.C.: 1 hour

Metabolism: Hepatically and via intestinal monoamine oxidase to phenolic conjugates

Half-life elimination: 2.5 hours; prolonged after long-term infusion

Excretion: Urine (90%)

Pregnancy Risk Factor C

Generic Available Yes: Excludes nasal drops and spray

Phenylephrine and Chlorpheniramine *see* Chlorpheniramine and Phenylephrine *on page 308*

Phenylephrine and Cyclopentolate *see* Cyclopentolate and Phenylephrine *on page 381*

Phenylephrine and Guaifenesin *see* Guaifenesin and Phenylephrine *on page 652*

Phenylephrine and Promethazine *see* Promethazine and Phenylephrine *on page 1129*

Phenylephrine and Scopolamine (fen il EF rin & skoe POL a meen)

Related Information

Phenylephrine *on page 1071*

Scopolamine *on page 1210*

U.S. Brand Names Murocoll-2®

Pharmacologic Category Anticholinergic/Adrenergic Agonist

Synonyms Scopolamine and Phenylephrine

Use Mydriasis, cycloplegia, and to break posterior synechiae in iritis

Local Anesthetic/Vasoconstrictor Precautions Use with caution since phenylephrine is a sympathomimetic amine which could interact with epinephrine to cause a pressor response

Effects on Dental Treatment This form of phenylephrine will have no effect on dental treatment when given as eye drops.

Dosage Ophthalmic: Instill 1-2 drops into eye(s); repeat in 5 minutes

Pregnancy Risk Factor C

Generic Available No

Phenylephrine and Zinc Sulfate (fen il EF rin & zingk SUL fate)

Related Information

Phenylephrine *on page 1071*

U.S. Brand Names Zincfrin® [OTC]

Canadian Brand Names Zincfrin®

Pharmacologic Category Adrenergic Agonist Agent

Synonyms Zinc Sulfate and Phenylephrine

Use Soothe, moisturize, and remove redness due to minor eye irritation

Local Anesthetic/Vasoconstrictor Precautions No information available to require special precautions

Effects on Dental Treatment No significant effects or complications reported

Dosage Ophthalmic: Instill 1-2 drops in eye(s) 2-4 times/day as needed

Generic Available No

Phenylephrine Hydrochloride *see* Phenylephrine *on page 1071*

Phenylephrine, Hydrocodone, Chlorpheniramine, Acetaminophen, and Caffeine *see* Hydrocodone, Chlorpheniramine, Phenylephrine, Acetaminophen, and Caffeine *on page 686*

Phenylephrine, Promethazine, and Codeine *see* Promethazine, Phenylephrine, and Codeine *on page 1130*

Phenylethylmalonylurea *see* Phenobarbital *on page 1066*

Phenylgesic® [OTC] *see* Acetaminophen and Phenyltoloxamine *on page 31*

Phenylisohydantoin *see* Pemoline *on page 1044*

Phenyl Salicylate, Methenamine, Methylene Blue, Sodium Biphosphate, and Hyoscyamine *see* Methenamine, Sodium Biphosphate, Phenyl Salicylate, Methylene Blue, and Hyoscyamine *on page 880*

Phenyltoloxamine and Acetaminophen *see* Acetaminophen and Phenyltoloxamine *on page 31*

Phenytek™ *see* Phenytoin *on page 1073*

Phenytoin (FEN i toyn)

Related Information

Cardiovascular Diseases *on page 1456*

Fosphenytoin *on page 618*

U.S. Brand Names Dilantin®; Phenytek™

Canadian Brand Names Dilantin®

Mexican Brand Names Epamin®; Fenidantoin®; Fenitron®; Hidantoina®

Pharmacologic Category Antiarrhythmic Agent, Class Ib; Anticonvulsant, Hydantoin

Synonyms Diphenylhydantoin; DPH; Phenytoin Sodium; Phenytoin Sodium, Extended; Phenytoin Sodium, Prompt

Use Management of generalized tonic-clonic (grand mal), complex partial seizures; prevention of seizures following head trauma/neurosurgery

Unlabeled/Investigational Use Treatment of ventricular arrhythmias (including those associated with digitalis intoxication, prolonged QT interval, and surgical repair of congenital heart diseases in children), epidermolysis bullosa

Local Anesthetic/Vasoconstrictor Precautions No information available to require special precautions

Effects on Dental Treatment Gingival hyperplasia is a common problem observed during the first 6 months of phenytoin therapy appearing as gingivitis or gum inflammation. To minimize severity and growth rate of gingival tissue begin a program of professional cleaning and patient plaque control within 10 days of starting anticonvulsant therapy.

Dosage

Status epilepticus: I.V.:

- Infants and Children: Loading dose: 15-20 mg/kg in a single or divided dose; maintenance dose: Initial: 5 mg/kg/day in 2 divided doses; usual doses:
  - 6 months to 3 years: 8-10 mg/kg/day
  - 4-6 years: 7.5-9 mg/kg/day
  - 7-9 years: 7-8 mg/kg/day
  - 10-16 years: 6-7 mg/kg/day, some patients may require every 8 hours dosing
- Adults: Loading dose: Manufacturer recommends 10-15 mg/kg, however, 15-25 mg/kg has been used clinically; maintenance dose: 300 mg/day or 5-6 mg/kg/day in 3 divided doses or 1-2 divided doses using extended release

Anticonvulsant: Children and Adults: Oral:

- Loading dose: 15-20 mg/kg; based on phenytoin serum concentrations and recent dosing history; administer oral loading dose in 3 divided doses given every 2-4 hours to decrease GI adverse effects and to ensure complete oral absorption; maintenance dose: same as I.V.
- Neurosurgery (prophylactic): 100-200 mg at approximately 4-hour intervals during surgery and during the immediate postoperative period

Dosing adjustment in renal/hepatic impairment: Usual dosing safe in mild liver disease; clearance may be substantially reduced in cirrhosis and plasma level

(Continued)

Phenytoin *(Continued)*

monitoring with dose adjustment advisable. Free phenytoin levels should be monitored closely.

Mechanism of Action Stabilizes neuronal membranes and decreases seizure activity by increasing efflux or decreasing influx of sodium ions across cell membranes in the motor cortex during generation of nerve impulses; prolongs effective refractory period and suppresses ventricular pacemaker automaticity, shortens action potential in the heart

Other Adverse Effects I.V. effects: Hypotension, bradycardia, cardiac arrhythmias, cardiovascular collapse (especially with rapid I.V. use), venous irritation and pain, thrombophlebitis

Effects not related to plasma phenytoin concentrations: Hypertrichosis, gingival hypertrophy, thickening of facial features, carbohydrate intolerance, folic acid deficiency, peripheral neuropathy, vitamin D deficiency, osteomalacia, systemic lupus erythematosus

Concentration-related effects: Nystagmus, blurred vision, diplopia, ataxia, slurred speech, dizziness, drowsiness, lethargy, coma, rash, fever, nausea, vomiting, gum tenderness, confusion, mood changes, folic acid depletion, osteomalacia, hyperglycemia

Related to elevated concentrations:

>20 mcg/mL: Far lateral nystagmus

>30 mcg/mL: 45° lateral gaze nystagmus and ataxia

>40 mcg/mL: Decreased mentation

>100 mcg/mL: Death

Cardiovascular: Hypotension, bradycardia, cardiac arrhythmias, cardiovascular collapse

Central nervous system: Psychiatric changes, slurred speech, dizziness, drowsiness, headache, insomnia

Dermatologic: Rash

Gastrointestinal: Constipation, nausea, vomiting, **enlargement of lips**

Hematologic: Leukopenia, thrombocytopenia, agranulocytosis

Hepatic: Hepatitis

Local: Thrombophlebitis

Neuromuscular & skeletal: Tremor, peripheral neuropathy, paresthesia

Ocular: Diplopia, nystagmus, blurred vision

Rarely seen effects: SLE-like syndrome, lymphadenopathy, hepatitis, Stevens-Johnson syndrome, blood dyscrasias, dyskinesias, pseudolymphoma, lymphoma, venous irritation and pain, coarsening of facial features, hypertrichosis

Drug Interactions Substrate of **CYP2C8/9, 2C19**, 3A4; Induces **CYP2B6, 2C8/9, 2C19, 3A4**

Increased Effect/Toxicity: Phenytoin serum concentrations may be increased by isoniazid, chloramphenicol, ticlopidine, or fluconazole. In addition, trimethoprim, sulfamethoxazole, valproic acid, sulfamethizole, sulfaphenazole, nifedipine, omeprazole, phenylbutazone, phenobarbital, amiodarone, chloramphenicol, cimetidine, ciprofloxacin, disulfiram, enoxacin, norfloxacin, felbamate, fluconazole, fluoxetine, influenza vaccine, isoniazid, and metronidazole inhibit the metabolism of phenytoin resulting in increased serum phenytoin concentrations. Valproic acid may increase, decrease, or have no effect on phenytoin serum concentrations. Phenytoin may increase the effect of dopamine (enhanced hypotension), warfarin (transiently enhanced anticoagulation), or increase the rate of conversion of primidone to phenobarbital resulting in increased phenobarbital serum concentrations. Phenytoin may enhance the hepatotoxic potential of acetaminophen. Concurrent use of acetazolamide and phenytoin may result in an increased risk of osteomalacia. Concurrent use of phenytoin and lithium has resulted in lithium intoxication. Phenytoin enhances the conversion of primidone to phenobarbital resulting in elevated phenobarbital serum concentrations. Valproic acid and sulfisoxazole may displace phenytoin from binding sites, transiently increasing phenytoin free levels.

Decreased Effect: The blood levels of phenytoin may be decreased by carbamazepine, rifampin, amiodarone, cisplatin, disulfiram, vinblastine, bleomycin, folic acid, phenobarbital, ethanol (chronic), pyridoxine, vigabatrin, and theophylline. Sucralfate and continuous NG feedings may decrease absorption of phenytoin. Phenytoin induces hepatic enzymes, and may decrease the effect of oral contraceptives, itraconazole, mebendazole, methadone, oral midazolam, valproic acid, cyclosporine, theophylline, doxycycline, quinidine, mexiletine, disopyramide. Phenytoin also may increase the metabolism of alprazolam, amiodarone, bromfenac, carbamazepine, clozapine, cyclosporine, diazepam, disopyramide, doxycycline, felbamate, furosemide, itraconazole, lamotrigine, mebendazole, meperidine, methadone, metyrapone, mexiletine, midazolam, oral contraceptives, quetiapine, quinidine, tacrolimus, teniposide, theophylline, thyroid hormones, triazolam, and valproic acid resulting in decreased levels/effect. Phenytoin may inhibit the anti-Parkinson effect of levodopa. Long-term concurrent use of phenytoin may inhibit hypoprothrombinemic response to warfarin. Phenytoin may reduce the effectiveness of some nondepolarizing neuromuscular blocking agents.

Dietary/Ethanol/Herb Considerations

Ethanol: Avoid or limit use; acute use inhibits metabolism (watch for sedation) and chronic use stimulates metabolism of phenytoin.

Food: Administer with food to reduce GI upset; may alter serum concentration. Tube feedings decrease bioavailability; do not administer 2 hours before to 2 hours after phenytoin administration. Enteral feedings can decrease phenytoin oral absorption by up to 80%; be consistent in administration of enteral feedings throughout therapy. Caffeine's effects are decreased. Hypocalcemia has been reported in patients taking prolonged high-dose therapy with an anticonvulsant. May require vitamin D supplementation to prevent hypocalcemia. May decrease mucosal uptake of folic acid; may require prophylactic doses of folic acid and cyanocobalamin (folate supplementation may increase seizures in some patients).

Herb/Nutraceutical: Avoid evening primrose; decreases seizure threshold. Avoid gotu kola, kava, SAMe, St John's wort, and valerian; may increase CNS depression.

Pharmacodynamics/Kinetics

Onset of action: I.V.: ~0.5-1 hour

Absorption: Oral: Slow

Distribution: V_d:

- Neonates: Premature: 1-1.2 L/kg; Full-term: 0.8-0.9 L/kg
- Infants: 0.7-0.8 L/kg
- Children: 0.7 L/kg
- Adults: 0.6-0.7 L/kg

Protein binding:

- Neonates: ≥80% (≤20% free)
- Infants: ≥85% (≤15% free)
- Adults: 90% to 95%
- Others: Decreased protein binding
  - **Disease states resulting in a decrease in serum albumin concentration**: Burns, hepatic cirrhosis, nephrotic syndrome, pregnancy, cystic fibrosis
  - **Disease states resulting in an apparent decrease in affinity of phenytoin for serum albumin**: Renal failure, jaundice (severe), other drugs (displacers), hyperbilirubinemia (total bilirubin >15 mg/dL), Cl_{cr} <25 mL/minute (unbound fraction is increased two- to threefold in uremia)

Metabolism: Follows dose-dependent capacity-limited (Michaelis-Menten) pharmacokinetics with increased V_{max} in infants >6 months of age and children versus adults; major metabolite (via oxidation), HPPA, undergoes enterohepatic recirculation

Bioavailability: Form dependent

Half-life elimination: Oral: 22 hours (range: 7-42 hours)

Time to peak, serum (form dependent): Oral: Extended-release capsule: 4-12 hours; Immediate release preparation: 2-3 hours

Excretion: Urine (<5% as unchanged drug); as glucuronides

- Clearance: Highly variable, dependent upon intrinsic hepatic function and dose administered; increased clearance and decreased serum concentrations with febrile illness

Pregnancy Risk Factor D

Generic Available Yes: Excludes chewable tablet, extended release capsule

Selected Readings

Dooley G and Vasan N, "Dilantin® Hyperplasia: A Review of the Literature," *J N Z Soc Periodontol*, 1989, 68:19-22.

Iacopino AM, Doxey D, Cutler CW, et al, "Phenytoin and Cyclosporine A Specifically Regulate Macrophage Phenotype and Expression of Platelet-Derived Growth Factor and Interleukin-1 *In Vitro* and *In Vivo*: Possible Molecular Mechanism of Drug-Induced Gingival Hyperplasia," *J Periodontol*, 1997, 68(1):73-83.

Pihlstrom BL, "Prevention and Treatment of Dilantin®-Associated Gingival Enlargement," *Compendium*, 1990, 14:S506-10.

Saito K, Mori S, Iwakura M, et al, "Immunohistochemical Localization of Transforming Growth Factor Beta, Basic Fibroblast Growth Factor and Heparin Sulphate Glycosaminoglycan in Gingival Hyperplasia Induced by Nifedipine and Phenytoin," *J Periodontal Res*, 1996, 31(8):545-5.

Zhou LX, Pihlstrom B, Hardwick JP, et al, "Metabolism of Phenytoin by the Gingiva of Normal Humans: The Possible Role of Reactive Metabolites of Phenytoin in the Initiation of Gingival Hyperplasia," *Clin Pharmacol Ther*, 1996, 60(2):191-8.

Phenytoin Sodium *see* Phenytoin *on page 1073*

Phenytoin Sodium, Extended *see* Phenytoin *on page 1073*

Phenytoin Sodium, Prompt *see* Phenytoin *on page 1073*

Phillips'® Milk of Magnesia [OTC] *see* Magnesium Hydroxide *on page 835*

Phillips'® Milk of Magnesia [OTC] *see* Magnesium Supplements *on page 837*

Phillips' M-O® [OTC] *see* Magnesium Hydroxide and Mineral Oil *on page 836*

Phillips' M-O® [OTC] *see* Magnesium Supplements *on page 837*

Phillips'® Stool Softener Laxative [OTC] *see* Docusate *on page 463*

pHisoHex® *see* Hexachlorophene *on page 669*

Phos-Flur® *see* Fluoride *on page 586*

Phos-Flur® Rinse [OTC] *see* Fluoride *on page 586*
PhosLo® *see* Calcium Supplements *on page 229*

Phosphate Supplements (FOS fate SUP le ments)

U.S. Brand Names Fleet® Enema [OTC]; Fleet® Phospho®-Soda [OTC]; K-Phos® MF; K-Phos® Neutral; K-Phos® No. 2; K-Phos® Original; Neutra-Phos® [OTC]; Neutra-Phos®-K [OTC]; Uro-KP-Neutral®; Visicol™

Pharmacologic Category Cathartic; Electrolyte Supplement, Oral; Electrolyte Supplement, Parenteral; Laxative, Bowel Evacuant

Synonyms Potassium Acid Phosphate; Potassium Phosphate; Potassium Phosphate and Sodium Phosphate; Sodium Phosphate

Use Treatment and prevention of hypophosphatemia; short-term treatment of constipation (oral/rectal); evacuation of the colon for rectal and bowel exams; source of phosphate in large volume I.V. fluids and parenteral nutrition; urinary acidifier (potassium acid phosphate) for reduction in formation of calcium stones

Local Anesthetic/Vasoconstrictor Precautions No information available to require special precautions

Effects on Dental Treatment Frequency not defined:

Potassium salt form: arrhythmias, heart block, cardiac arrest

Hypotension, confusion, seizures, dizziness, headache, nausea, vomiting, mucosal bleeding, superficial mucosal ulcerations paresthesia, bone and joint pain, weakness, muscle cramps

Dosage Phosphate supplements are either sodium or potassium salt forms. Consider the contribution of these electrolytes also when determining appropriate phosphate replacement.

I.V. doses should be incorporated into the patient's maintenance I.V. fluids; intermittent I.V. infusion should be reserved for severe depletion situations; requires continuous cardiac monitoring (for potassium salts). It is difficult to determine total body phosphorus deficit, the following dosages are empiric guidelines: **Note:** Doses listed as mmol of **phosphate**:

Children:

Hypophosphatemia: Intermittent I.V. infusion:
- Low dose: 0.08 mmol/kg over 6 hours; use if recent losses and uncomplicated
- Intermediate dose: 0.16-0.24 mmol/kg over 4-6 hours; use if serum phosphorus level 0.5-1 mg/dL
- High dose: 0.36 mmol/kg over 6 hours; use if serum phosphorus <0.5 mg/dL
- Maintenance:
  - I.V.: 0.5-1.5 mmol/kg/day
  - Oral: 2-3 mmol/kg/day in divided doses

Laxative: Oral

Neutra-Phos®, Neutra-Phos®-K, or Uro-KP-Neutral®:
- Children <4 years: 1 capsule or packet (250 mg phosphorus/8 mmol) 4 times/day; dilute as instructed
- Children >4 years: 1-2 capsules or packets (250-500 mg phosphorus/8-16 mmol) 4 times/day; dilute as instructed

Fleet® Phospho®-Soda:® Oral:
- Children 5-9 years: 5-10 mL as a single dose
- Children 10-12 years: 10-20 mL as a single dose
- Children ≥12 years: 20-45 mL as a single dose

Enema: (not for use in children <2 years of age; tips are latex free):

Fleet® Enema:
- Children 2-4 years: One-half contents of one 2.25 oz pediatric enema
- Children 5-12 years: Contents of one 2.25 oz pediatric enema, may repeat
- Children ≥12 years: Contents of one 4.5 oz enema as a single dose, may repeat

Adults:

Hypophosphatemia: Intermittent I.V. infusion: Varying dosages: 0.15-0.3 mmol/kg/dose over 12 hours; may repeat as needed to achieve desired serum level **or** 15 mmol/dose over 2 hours; use if serum phosphorus <2 mg/dL **or**
- Low dose: 0.16 mmol/kg over 4-6 hours; use if serum phosphorus level 2.3-3 mg/dL
- Intermediate dose: 0.32 mmol/kg over 4-6 hours; use if serum phosphorus level 1.6-2.2 mg/dL
- High dose: 0.64 mmol/kg over 8-12 hours; use if serum phosphorus <1.5 mg/dL

Maintenance:
- I.V.: 50-70 mmol/day
- Oral: 50-150 mmol/day in divided doses

Laxative: Oral:
- 1-2 capsules or packets (250-500 mg phosphorus/8-16 mmol) 4 times/day; dilute as instructed
- Fleet® Phospho®-Soda:® 20-45 mL as a single dose

Enema (tips are latex free): Administer contents of one 4.5 oz enema as a single dose; may repeat

Note: Correct electrolyte abnormalities before treatment; inadequate fluid intake may lead to excessive fluid loss and hypovolemia. May cause colonic mucosal aphthous ulcerations; use with caution in patients with an acute exacerbation of chronic inflammatory bowel disease (absorption may be enhanced), debilitated patients, and those with a colostomy.

Bowel cleansing prior to colonoscopy (Visicol™): Oral: A total of 40 tablets divided as follows:

Evening before colonoscopy: 3 tablets every 15 minutes for 6 doses, then 2 additional tablets in 15 minutes (total of 20 tablets)

3-5 hours prior to colonoscopy: 3 tablets every 15 minutes for 6 doses, then 2 additional tablets in 15 minutes (total of 20 tablets)

Note: Each dose should be taken with a minimum of 8 oz. of clear liquids. Do not repeat treatment within 7 days. Do not use additional agents, especially sodium phosphate products.

Urinary acidification: Oral (K-Phos® Original): 2 tablets 4 times/day

Mechanism of Action Participates in bone deposition, calcium metabolism, utilization of B complex vitamins, and acts as a buffer in acid-base equilibrium; as a laxative, it exerts osmotic effect in the small intestine by drawing water into the lumen of the gut, producing distension, promoting peristalsis, and evacuation of the bowel.

Other Adverse Effects Frequency not defined:

Cardiovascular: Edema

Central nervous system: Tetany, calcium phosphate precipitation

Endocrine & metabolic: Hyperphosphatemia, hyperkalemia **(potassium salt form)**, hypocalcemia, hypernatremia **(sodium salt form)**

Gastrointestinal: Diarrhea, flatulence (oral form), abdominal bloating, abdominal pain

Local: Phlebitis (parenteral forms)

Neuromuscular & skeletal: Arthralgia

Renal: Acute renal failure

Case reports: Tablet: **Atrial fibrillation (following severe vomiting)**

Drug Interactions

Increased Effect/Toxicity: Do not use with other phosphate-containing products, fatalities reported. Potassium-containing preparations should be used with caution in patients receiving ACE-inhibitors, salt substitutes, or potassium-sparing diuretics.

Decreased Effect: Oral phosphate preparations may reduce absorption of some medications due to rapid intestinal peristalsis; do not administer with sucralfate, iron supplements, or antacids which contain aluminum, calcium, or magnesium (may result in binding of the phosphate and reduced absorption).

Dietary/Ethanol/Herb Considerations Food: Avoid coadministration with foods containing oxalates (ie, berries, nuts, chocolate, beans, celery, tomato) or phytates (ie, bran, whole wheat).

Pregnancy Risk Factor C

Dosage Forms

Enema: Monobasic sodium phosphate 19 g and dibasic sodium phosphate 7 g per 118 mL delivered dose (135 mL)

Fleet® Enema: Monobasic sodium phosphate 19 g and dibasic sodium phosphate 7 g per 118 mL delivered dose (135 mL)

Fleet® Enema for Children: Monobasic sodium phosphate 9.5 g and dibasic sodium phosphate 3.5 g per 59 mL delivered dose (68 mL)

Injection: solution, as potassium phosphate: Phosphate 3 mmol and potassium 4.4 mEq per mL (5 mL, 15 mL, 50 mL)

Injection, solution, as sodium phosphate [preservative free]: Phosphate 3 mmol and sodium 4 mEq per mL (5 mL, 15 mL, 50 mL)

Powder:

Neutra-Phos®: Phosphorus 250 mg [8 mmol], potassium 278 mg [7.125 mEq], and sodium 164 mg [7.125 mEq] per packet (100s)

Neutra-Phos®-K: Elemental phosphorus 250 mg [8 mmol] and potassium 556 mg [14.25 mEq] per packet (100s) [sodium free]

Solution, oral (Fleet® Phospho®-Soda): Phosphate 4 mmol and sodium 4.82 mEq per mL (45 mL, 90 mL) [equivalent to monobasic sodium phosphate monohydrate 2.4 g and dibasic sodium phosphate heptahydrate 0.9 g per 5 mL; ginger-lemon flavor or unflavored]

Tablet:

K-Phos® MF: Phosphorus 125.6 mg [4 mmol], potassium 44.5 mg [1.1 mEq], and sodium 67 mg [2.9 mEq]

K-Phos® Neutral: Phosphorus 250 mg [8 mmol], potassium 45 mg [1.1 mEq], and sodium 298 mg [13 mEq] per tablet

K-Phos® No. 2: Phosphorus 250 mg [8 mmol], potassium 88 mg [2.3 mEq], and sodium 134 mg [5.8 mEq]

K-Phos® Original: Phosphorus 114 mg [3.7 mmol] and potassium 144 mg [3.7 mEq] per tablet [sodium free]

Uro-KP-Neutral®: Phosphorus 258 mg [8 mmol], potassium 49.4 mg [1.27 mEq], and sodium 262.4 mg [10.9 mEq]

(Continued)

Phosphate Supplements *(Continued)*

Visicol™: Sodium phosphate monobasic monohydrate 1.102 g and sodium phosphate dibasic anhydrous 0.398 g [1.5 g total sodium phosphate per tablet]

Generic Available Yes

Phospholine Iodide® *see* Echothiophate Iodide *on page 485*

Phosphonoformate *see* Foscarnet *on page 613*

Phosphonoformic Acid *see* Foscarnet *on page 613*

Phosphorated Carbohydrate Solution

(FOS for ate ed kar boe HYE drate soe LOO shun)

U.S. Brand Names Emetrol® [OTC]; Especol® [OTC]; Kalmz [OTC]; Nausetrol® [OTC]

Pharmacologic Category Antiemetic

Synonyms Dextrose, Levulose and Phosphoric Acid; Levulose, Dextrose and Phosphoric Acid; Phosphoric Acid, Levulose and Dextrose

Use Relief of nausea associated with upset stomach that occurs with intestinal flu, food indiscretions, and emotional upsets

Unlabeled/Investigational Use Relief of nausea associated with pregnancy

Local Anesthetic/Vasoconstrictor Precautions No information available to require special precautions

Effects on Dental Treatment No significant effects or complications reported

Dosage Oral:

Motion sickness and vomiting due to drug therapy: 5 mL doses for young children; 15 mL doses for older children and adults

Nausea associated with pregnancy (unlabeled use): 15-30 mL on arising; repeat every 3 hours or when nausea threatens

Regurgitation in infants: 5 or 10 mL, 10-15 minutes before each feeding; in refractory cases: 10-15 mL, 30 minutes before each feeding

Vomiting due to psychogenic factors:

Children: 5-10 mL; repeat dose every 15 minutes until distress subsides; do not take for more than 1 hour

Adults: 15-30 mL; repeat dose every 15 minutes until distress subsides; do not take for more than 1 hour

Other Adverse Effects 1% to 10%: Gastrointestinal: Abdominal pain, diarrhea

Generic Available Yes

Phosphoric Acid, Levulose and Dextrose *see* Phosphorated Carbohydrate Solution *on page 1078*

Photofrin® *see* Porfimer *on page 1098*

p-Hydroxyampicillin *see* Amoxicillin *on page 93*

Phylloquinone *see* Phytonadione *on page 1079*

Physostigmine

(fye zoe STIG meen)

Canadian Brand Names Eserine®; Isopto® Eserine

Pharmacologic Category Acetylcholinesterase Inhibitor; Ophthalmic Agent, Antiglaucoma

Synonyms Eserine Salicylate; Physostigmine Salicylate; Physostigmine Sulfate

Use Reverse toxic CNS effects caused by anticholinergic drugs; used as miotic in treatment of glaucoma

Local Anesthetic/Vasoconstrictor Precautions No information available to require special precautions

Effects on Dental Treatment No significant effects or complications reported

Dosage

Children: Anticholinergic drug overdose: Reserve for life-threatening situations only: I.V.: 0.01-0.03 mg/kg/dose (maximum: 0.5 mg/minute); may repeat after 5-10 minutes to a maximum total dose of 2 mg or until response occurs or adverse cholinergic effects occur

Adults: Anticholinergic drug overdose:

I.M., I.V., S.C.: 0.5-2 mg to start, repeat every 20 minutes until response occurs or adverse effect occurs

Repeat 1-4 mg every 30-60 minutes as life-threatening signs (arrhythmias, seizures, deep coma) recur; maximum I.V. rate: 1 mg/minute

Ophthalmic: Ointment: Instill a small quantity to lower fornix up to 3 times/day

Mechanism of Action Inhibits destruction of acetylcholine by acetylcholinesterase which facilitates transmission of impulses across myoneural junction and prolongs the central and peripheral effects of acetylcholine

Other Adverse Effects Frequency not defined:

Ophthalmic:

Central nervous system: Headache, browache

Dermatologic: Burning, redness

Ocular: Lacrimation, marked miosis, blurred vision, eye pain

Miscellaneous: Diaphoresis

Systemic:

Cardiovascular: Palpitations, bradycardia

Central nervous system: Restlessness, nervousness, hallucinations, seizures

Gastrointestinal: Nausea, salivation, diarrhea, stomach pains

Genitourinary: Frequent urge to urinate

Neuromuscular & skeletal: Muscle twitching

Ocular: Lacrimation, miosis

Respiratory: Dyspnea, bronchospasm, respiratory paralysis, pulmonary edema

Miscellaneous: Diaphoresis

Drug Interactions

Increased Effect: Succinylcholine may increase neuromuscular blockade with systemic administration.

Increased toxicity with bethanechol, methacholine.

Pharmacodynamics/Kinetics

Onset of action: Ophthalmic: ~2 minutes; Parenteral: ~5 minutes

Duration: Ophthalmic: 12-48 hours; Parenteral: 0.5-5 hours

Absorption: I.M., ophthalmic, S.C.: Readily absorbed

Distribution: Crosses blood-brain barrier readily and reverses both central and peripheral anticholinergic effects

Metabolism: Hepatic and via hydrolysis by cholinesterases

Half-life elimination: 15-40 minutes

Pregnancy Risk Factor C

Generic Available Yes

Physostigmine Salicylate *see* Physostigmine *on page 1078*

Physostigmine Sulfate *see* Physostigmine *on page 1078*

Phytomenadione *see* Phytonadione *on page 1079*

Phytonadione (fye toe na DYE one)

U.S. Brand Names AquaMEPHYTON®; Mephyton®

Canadian Brand Names AquaMEPHYTON®; Konakion; Mephyton®

Mexican Brand Names Konakion®

Pharmacologic Category Vitamin, Fat Soluble

Synonyms Methylphytyl Napthoquinone; Phylloquinone; Phytomenadione; Vitamin K_1

Use Prevention and treatment of hypoprothrombinemia caused by drug-induced or anticoagulant-induced vitamin K deficiency, hemorrhagic disease of the newborn; phytonadione is more effective and is preferred to other vitamin K preparations in the presence of impending hemorrhage; oral absorption depends on the presence of bile salts

Local Anesthetic/Vasoconstrictor Precautions No information available to require special precautions

Effects on Dental Treatment No significant effects or complications reported

Dosage S.C. is the preferred (per manufacturer) parenteral route; I.V. route should be restricted for emergency use only

- Minimum daily requirement: Not well established
  - Infants: 1-5 mcg/kg/day
  - Adults: 0.03 mcg/kg/day
- Hemorrhagic disease of the newborn:
  - Prophylaxis: I.M.: 0.5-1 mg within 1 hour of birth
  - Treatment: I.M., S.C.: 1-2 mg/dose/day
- Oral anticoagulant overdose:
  - Infants and Children:
    - No bleeding, rapid reversal needed, patient **will require** further oral anticoagulant therapy: S.C., I.V.: 0.5-2 mg
    - No bleeding, rapid reversal needed, patient **will not require** further oral anticoagulant therapy: S.C., I.V.: 2-5 mg
    - Significant bleeding, not life-threatening: S.C., I.V.: 0.5-2 mg
    - Significant bleeding, life-threatening: I.V.: 5 mg over 10-20 minutes
  - Adults: Oral, I.V., S.C.: 1-10 mg/dose depending on degree of INR elevation
    - Serious bleeding or major overdose: 10 mg I.V. (slow infusion); may repeat every 12 hours (have required doses up to 25 mg)
- Vitamin K deficiency: Due to drugs, malabsorption, or decreased synthesis of vitamin K
  - Infants and Children:
    - Oral: 2.5-5 mg/24 hours
    - I.M., I.V., S.C.: 1-2 mg/dose as a single dose
  - Adults:
    - Oral: 5-25 mg/24 hours
    - I.M., I.V., S.C.: 10 mg

Mechanism of Action Promotes liver synthesis of clotting factors (II, VII, IX, X); however, the exact mechanism as to this stimulation is unknown. Menadiol is a water soluble form of vitamin K; phytonadione has a more rapid and prolonged effect than menadione; menadiol sodium diphosphate (K_4) is half as potent as menadione (K_3).

(Continued)

Phytonadione *(Continued)*

Other Adverse Effects <1%: Abnormal taste, anaphylaxis, cyanosis, diaphoresis, dizziness (rarely), dyspnea, GI upset (oral), hemolysis in neonates and in patients with G6PD deficiency, hypersensitivity reactions, hypotension (rarely), pain, tenderness at injection site, transient flushing reaction

Drug Interactions Decreased Effect: The anticoagulant effects of warfarin, dicumarol, anisindione are reversed by phytonadione.

Pharmacodynamics/Kinetics

Onset of action: Increased coagulation factors: Oral: 6-12 hours; Parenteral: 1-2 hours; prothrombin may become normal after 12-14 hours

Absorption: Oral: From intestines in presence of bile

Metabolism: Rapidly hepatic

Excretion: Urine and feces

Pregnancy Risk Factor C

Generic Available Yes: Injection

Pilocar® *see* Pilocarpine *on page 1080*

Pilocarpine (pye loe KAR peen)

Related Information

Management of Patients Undergoing Cancer Therapy *on page 1567*

U.S. Brand Names Isopto® Carpine; Pilocar®; Pilopine HS®; Piloptic®; Salagen®

Canadian Brand Names Diocarpine; Isopto® Carpine; Pilopine HS®; Salagen®

Mexican Brand Names Pilo Grin®; Pilogrin

Pharmacologic Category Cholinergic Agonist; Ophthalmic Agent, Antiglaucoma; Ophthalmic Agent, Miotic

Synonyms Pilocarpine Hydrochloride; Pilocarpine Nitrate

Use

Ophthalmic: Management of chronic simple glaucoma, chronic and acute angle-closure glaucoma

Oral: Symptomatic treatment of xerostomia caused by salivary gland hypofunction resulting from radiotherapy for cancer of the head and neck or Sjögren's syndrome

Unlabeled/Investigational Use Counter effects of cycloplegics

Local Anesthetic/Vasoconstrictor Precautions No information available to require special precautions

Effects on Dental Treatment No significant effects or complications reported

Dosage Adults:

Ophthalmic:

Glaucoma:

Solution: Instill 1-2 drops up to 6 times/day; adjust the concentration and frequency as required to control elevated intraocular pressure

Gel: Instill 0.5" ribbon into lower conjunctival sac once daily at bedtime

Ocular systems: Systems are labeled in terms of mean rate of release of pilocarpine over 7 days; begin with 20 mcg/hour at night and adjust based on response

To counteract the mydriatic effects of sympathomimetic agents (unlabeled use):

Solution: Instill 1 drop of a 1% solution in the affected eye

Oral: Xerostomia:

Following head and neck cancer: 5 mg 3 times/day, titration up to 10 mg 3 times/day may be considered for patients who have not responded adequately; do not exceed 2 tablets/dose

Sjögren's syndrome: 5 mg 4 times/day

Dosing adjustment in hepatic impairment: Oral: Patients with moderate impairment: 5 mg 2 times/day regardless of indication; adjust dose based on response and tolerability. Do not use with severe impairment (Child-Pugh score 10-15).

Mechanism of Action Directly stimulates cholinergic receptors in the eye causing miosis (by contraction of the iris sphincter), loss of accommodation (by constriction of ciliary muscle), and lowering of intraocular pressure (with decreased resistance to aqueous humor outflow)

Other Adverse Effects

Ophthalmic: Frequency not defined:

Cardiovascular: Hypertension, tachycardia

Dermatologic: Diaphoresis

Gastrointestinal: Diarrhea, nausea, salivation, vomiting

Ocular: Burning, ciliary spasm, conjunctival vascular congestion, corneal granularity (gel 10%), lacrimation, lens opacity, myopia, retinal detachment, supraorbital or temporal headache, visual acuity decreased

Respiratory: Bronchial spasm, pulmonary edema

Oral (frequency varies by indication and dose):

>10%:

Cardiovascular: Flushing (8% to 13%)

Central nervous system: Chills (3% to 15%), dizziness (5% to 12%), headache (11%)

Dermatologic: Diaphoresis (29% to 68%)
Gastrointestinal: Nausea (6% to 15%)
Genitourinary: Urinary frequency (9% to 12%)
Neuromuscular & skeletal: Weakness (2% to 12%)
Respiratory: Rhinitis (5% to 14%)

1% to 10%:
Cardiovascular: Edema (<1% to 5%), facial edema, hypertension (3%), palpitation, tachycardia
Central nervous system: Pain (4%), fever, somnolence
Dermatologic: Pruritus, rash
Gastrointestinal: Diarrhea (4% to 7%), dyspepsia (7%), vomiting (3% to 4%), constipation, flatulence, glossitis, salivation increased, stomatitis, abnormal taste
Genitourinary: Vaginitis, urinary incontinence
Neuromuscular & skeletal: Myalgias, tremor
Ocular: Lacrimation (6%), amblyopia (4%), abnormal vision, blurred vision, conjunctivitis,
Otic: Tinnitus
Respiratory: Cough increased, dysphagia, epistaxis, sinusitis
Miscellaneous: Allergic reaction, voice alteration

<1%: Abnormal dreams, abnormal thinking, alopecia, angina pectoris, anorexia, anxiety, aphasia, appetite increased, arrhythmia, arthralgia, arthritis, bilirubinemia, body odor, bone disorder, bradycardia, breast pain, bronchitis, cataract, cholelithiasis, colitis, confusion, contact dermatitis, cyst, deafness, depression, dry eyes, xerostomia, dry skin, dyspnea, dysuria, ear pain, EKG abnormality, eczema, emotional lability, eructation, erythema nodosum, esophagitis, exfoliative dermatitis, eye hemorrhage, eye pain, gastritis, gastroenteritis, gastrointestinal disorder, gingivitis, glaucoma, hematuria, hepatitis, herpes simplex, hiccup, hyperkinesias, hypesthesia, hypoglycemia, hypotension, hypothermia, insomnia, intracranial hemorrhage, laryngismus, laryngitis, leg cramps, leukopenia, LFTs abnormal, lymphadenopathy, mastitis, melena, menorrhagia, metrorrhagia, migraine, moniliasis, myasthenia, MI, neck pain, photosensitivity reaction, nervousness, ovarian disorder, pancreatitis, paresthesias, parotid gland enlargement, peripheral edema, platelet abnormality, pneumonia, pyuria, salivary gland enlargement, salpingitis, seborrhea, skin ulcer, speech disorder, sputum increased, stridor, syncope, loss of taste, tendon disorder, tenosynovitis, thrombocythemia, thrombocytopenia, thrombosis, tongue disorder, twitching, urethral pain, urinary impairment, urinary urgency, vaginal hemorrhage, vaginal moniliasis, vesiculobullous rash, WBC abnormality, yawning

Drug Interactions Inhibits CYP2A6, 2E1, 3A4

Increased Effect/Toxicity: Concurrent use with beta-blockers may cause conduction disturbances.

Decreased Effect: May decrease effects of anticholinergic drugs (atropine, ipratropium).

Dietary/Ethanol/Herb Considerations Food: Avoid administering oral formulation with high-fat meal; fat decreases the rate of absorption, maximum concentration and increases the time it takes to reach maximum concentration.

Pharmacodynamics/Kinetics

Onset of action:
Ophthalmic: Miosis: 10-30 minutes; Intraocular pressure reduction: 1 hour
Oral: 20 minutes

Duration:
Ophthalmic: Miosis: 4-8 hours; Intraocular pressure reduction: 4-12 hours
Oral: 3-5 hours

Half-life elimination: Oral: 0.76-1.35 hours; increased with hepatic impairment

Excretion: Urine

Pregnancy Risk Factor C

Generic Available Yes: Hydrochloride solution

Pilocarpine (Dental) (pye loe KAR peen)

Related Information

Dentin Hypersensitivity, High Caries Index, and Xerostomia *on page 1553*
Pilocarpine *on page 1080*

U.S. Brand Names Salagen®

Canadian Brand Names Salagen®

Pharmacologic Category Cholinergic Agonist; Salivary Stimulant

Use Dental: Treatment of xerostomia caused by radiation therapy in patients with head and neck cancer and from Sjögren's syndrome

Local Anesthetic/Vasoconstrictor Precautions No information available to require special precautions

Effects on Dental Treatment

>10%: Sweating, increased salivation (therapeutic effect)

1% to 10%: Flushing, hypertension, tachycardia, headache, tremors, nausea, vomiting, epistaxis, rhinitis, weakness, dysphagia

Dosage Minimum 90-day therapy for optimum effects

(Continued)

Pilocarpine (Dental) *(Continued)*

Adults: 1-2 tablets 3-4 times/day not to exceed 30 mg/day

Mechanism of Action Stimulates the muscarinic-type acetylcholine receptors in the salivary glands within the parasympathetic division of the autonomic nervous system to cause an increase in serous-type saliva

Other Adverse Effects Systemic: 1% to 10%:

Cardiovascular: Edema

Central nervous system: Chills

Gastrointestinal: Heartburn

Genitourinary: Polyuria

Ocular: Amblyopia

Respiratory: Voice change

Contraindications Hypersensitivity to pilocarpine or any component of the formulation; uncontrolled asthma, angle-closure glaucoma, severe hepatic impairment

Warnings/Precautions Use caution with cardiovascular disease; patients may have difficulty compensating for transient changes in hemodynamics or rhythm induced by pilocarpine. Use caution with controlled asthma, chronic bronchitis or COPD; may increase airway resistance, bronchial smooth muscle tone, and bronchial secretions. Use caution with cholelithiasis, biliary tract disease, nephrolithiasis; adjust dose with moderate hepatic impairment.

Drug Interactions Increased Effect/Toxicity: Concurrent use with anticholinergics may cause antagonism of pilocarpine's cholinergic effect; medications with cholinergic actions may result in additive cholinergic effects. Beta-adrenergic receptor blocking drugs when used with pilocarpine may increase the possibility of myocardial conduction disturbances.

Pharmacodynamics/Kinetics

Onset of action: 20 minutes after single dose

Duration: 3-5 hours

Halflife, elimination: 0.76 hours

Time to peak: 1.25 hours

Dosage Forms TAB (Salagen®): 5 mg

Generic Available No

Comments Pilocarpine may have potential as a salivary stimulant in individuals suffering from xerostomia induced by antidepressants and other medications. At the present time however, the FDA has not approved pilocarpine for use in drug-induced xerostomia (clinical studies required). In an attempt to discern the efficacy of pilocarpine as a salivary stimulant in patients suffering from Sjögren's syndrome (SS), Rhodus and Schuh studied 9 patients with SS given daily doses of pilocarpine over a 6-week period. A dose of 5 mg daily produced a significant overall increase in both whole unstimulated salivary flow and parotid stimulated salivary flow. These results support the use of pilocarpine to increase salivary flow in patients with SS.

Selected Readings

Davies AN and Singer J, "A Comparison of Artificial Saliva and Pilocarpine in Radiation-Induced Xerostomia," *J Laryngol Otol*, 1994, 108(8):663-5.

Fox PC, "Management of Dry Mouth," *Dent Clin North Am*, 1997, 41(4):863-75.

Fox PC, Atkinson JC, Macynski AA, et al, " Pilocarpine Treatment of Salivary Gland Hypofunction and Dry Mouth (Xerostomia)," *Arch Intern Med*, 1991, 151(6):1149-52.

Garg AK and Malo M, "Manifestations and Treatment of Xerostomia and Associated Oral Effects Secondary to Head and Neck Radiation Therapy," *J Am Dent Assoc*, 1997, 128(8):1128-33.

Johnson JT, Ferretti GA, Nethery WJ, et al, "Oral Pilocarpine for Postirradiation Xerostomia in Patients With Head and Neck Cancer," *N Engl J Med*, 1993, 329(6):390-5.

Nagler RM and Laufer D, "Protection Against Irradiation-Induced Damage to Salivary Glands by Adrenergic Agonist Administration," *Int J Radiat Oncol Biol Phys*, 1998, 40(2):477-81.

Nelson JD, Friedlaender M, Yeatts RP, et al, "Oral Pilocarpine for Symptomatic Relief of Keratoconjunctivitis Sicca in Patients With Sjögren's Syndrome. The MGI PHARMA Sjögren's Syndrome Study Group," *Adv Exp Med Biol*, 1998, 438:979-83.

Rhodus NL and Schuh MJ, "Effects of Pilocarpine on Salivary Flow in Patients With Sjögren's Syndrome," *Oral Surg Oral Med Oral Pathol*, 1991, 72(5):545-9.

Rieke JW, Hafermann MD, Johnson JT, et al, "Oral Pilocarpine for Radiation-Induced Xerostomia: Integrated Efficacy and Safety Results From Two Prospective Randomized Clinical Trials," *Int J Radiat Oncol Biol Phys*, 1995, 31(3):661-9.

Rousseau P, "Pilocarpine in Radiation-Induced Xerostomia," *Am J Hosp Palliat Care*, 1995, 12(2):38-9.

Schuller DE, Stevens P, Clausen KP, et al, "Treatment of Radiation Side Effects With Pilocarpine," *J Surg Oncol*, 1989, 42(4):272-6.

Singhal S, Mehta J, Rattenbury H, et al, "Oral Pilocarpine Hydrochloride for the Treatment of Refractory Xerostomia Associated With Chronic Graft-Versus-Host Disease," *Blood*, 1995, 85(4):1147-8.

Valdez IH, Wolff A, Atkinson JC, et al, "Use of Pilocarpine During Head and Neck Radiation Therapy to Reduce Xerostomia Salivary Dysfunction," *Cancer*, 1993, 71(5):1848-51.

Wiseman LR and Faulds D, "Oral Pilocarpine: A Review of Its Pharmacological Properties and Clinical Potential in Xerostomia," *Drugs*, 1995, 49(1):143-55.

Wynn RL, "Oral Pilocarpine (Salagen®) - A Recently Approved Salivary Stimulant," *Gen Dent*, 1996, 44(1):26,29-30.

Zimmerman RP, Mark RJ, Tran LM, et al, "Concomitant Pilocarpine During Head and Neck Irradiation Is Associated With Decreased Post-Treatment Xerostomia," *Int J Radiat Oncol Biol Phys*, 1997, 37(3):571-5.

Pilocarpine Hydrochloride *see* Pilocarpine *on page 1080*

Pilocarpine Nitrate *see* Pilocarpine *on page 1080*

Pilopine HS® *see* Pilocarpine *on page 1080*

Piloptic® *see* Pilocarpine *on page 1080*

Pima® *see* Potassium Iodide *on page 1101*

Pimaricin *see* Natamycin *on page 956*

Pimecrolimus (pim e KROE li mus)

U.S. Brand Names Elidel®

Pharmacologic Category Immunosuppressant Agent; Topical Skin Product

Use Short-term and intermittent long-term treatment of mild to moderate atopic dermatitis in patients not responsive to conventional therapy or when conventional therapy is not appropriate

Local Anesthetic/Vasoconstrictor Precautions No information available to require special precautions

Effects on Dental Treatment 1% to 10%: Ear infection (0.6% to 6%), nasal congestion (0.6% to 3%)

Dosage Children ≥2 years and Adults: Topical: Apply thin layer to affected area twice daily; rub in gently and completely. **Note:** Continue as long as signs and symptoms persist; discontinue if resolution occurs; re-evaluate if symptoms persist >6 weeks.

Mechanism of Action Penetrates inflamed epidermis to inhibit T cell activation by blocking transcription of proinflammatory cytokine genes such as interleukin-2, interferon gamma (Th1-type), interleukin-4, and interleukin-10 (Th2-type). Blocks catalytic function of calcineurin. Prevents release of inflammatory cytokines and mediators from mast cells *in vitro* after stimulation by antigen/IgE.

Other Adverse Effects

>10% :

- Central nervous system: Headache (7% to 25%), pyrexia (1% to 13%)
- Local: Burning at application site (2% to 26%)
- Respiratory: Nasopharyngitis (8% to 27%), cough (2% to 16%), upper respiratory tract infection (4% to 19%), bronchitis (0.4% to 11%)
- Miscellaneous: Influenza (3% to 13%)

1% to 10%:

- Dermatologic: Skin papilloma (warts) (up to 3%), molluscum contagiosum (0.7% to 2%), herpes simplex dermatitis (up to 2%)
- Gastrointestinal: Diarrhea (0.6% to 8%), constipation (up to 4%)
- Local: Irritation at application site (0.4% to 6%), erythema at application site (0.4% to 2%), pruritus at application site (0.6% to 6%)
- Ocular: Eye infection (up to 1%)
- Respiratory: Pharyngitis (0.7% to 8%), sinusitis (0.6% to 3%)
- Miscellaneous: Viral infection (up to 7%), herpes simplex infections (0.4% to 4%), tonsillitis (0.4% to 6%)

Adverse events ≤ placebo: Abdominal pain, acne, arthralgias, asthma exacerbation, back pain, bacterial infection, conjunctivitis, dyspnea, dysmenorrhea, earache, epistaxis, folliculitis, hypersensitivity, impetigo, nausea, otitis media, pharyngitis (streptococcal), pneumonia, rhinorrhea, rhinitis, sinus congestion, skin infection, sore throat, Staphylococcal infection, toothache, urticaria, vomiting, wheezing

<1%: Eczema herpeticum, lymphadenopathy

Drug Interactions Substrate of CYP3A4

Increased Effect/Toxicity: CYP3A inhibitors may increase pimecrolimus levels in patients where increased absorption expected.

Pharmacodynamics/Kinetics Absorption: Poor when applied to 13% to 62% body surface area for up to a year

Pregnancy Risk Factor C

Generic Available No

Pimozide (PI moe zide)

U.S. Brand Names Orap®

Canadian Brand Names Orap®

Pharmacologic Category Antipsychotic Agent, Diphenylbutylperidine

Use Suppression of severe motor and phonic tics in patients with Tourette's disorder who have failed to respond satisfactorily to standard treatment

Unlabeled/Investigational Use Treatment of psychosis, delusions focused on physical symptoms (ie, preoccupation with parasitic infestation), Huntington's chorea

Local Anesthetic/Vasoconstrictor Precautions No information available to require special precautions

Effects on Dental Treatment Tourette's disorder: Xerostomia (25%), increased salivation (14%), taste disturbance (5%)

Dosage Oral:

Children ≤12 years: Tourette's disorder: Initial: 1-2 mg/day in divided doses; usual range: 2-4 mg/day; do not exceed 10 mg/day (0.2 mg/kg/day)

Children >12 years and Adults: Tourette's disorder: Initial: 1-2 mg/day in divided doses, then increase dosage as needed every other day; range is usually 7-16 mg/day, maximum dose: 20 mg/day or 0.3 mg/kg/day should not be exceeded.

(Continued)

Pimozide *(Continued)*

Note: Sudden unexpected deaths have occurred in patients taking doses >10 mg. Therefore, dosages exceeding 10 mg/day are generally not recommended.

Dosing adjustment in hepatic impairment: Reduction required in liver disease

Mechanism of Action A potent centrally-acting dopamine-receptor antagonist resulting in its characteristic neuroleptic effects

Other Adverse Effects

Frequencies >1% reported in adults (limited data) and/or children with Tourette's disorder:

Cardiovascular: Abnormal EKG (3%)

Central nervous system: Somnolence (up to 28% in children), sedation (14%), akathisia (8%), drowsiness (7%), hyperkinesias (6%), insomnia (2%), depression (2%), headache (1%), nervousness (1% to 8%)

Dermatologic: Rash (8%)

Gastrointestinal: Constipation (20%), diarrhea (5%), thirst (5%), appetite increased (5%), dysphagia (3%)

Genitourinary: Impotence (15%)

Neuromuscular & skeletal: Weakness (22%), muscle tightness (15%), rigidity (10%), myalgia (3%), torticollis (3%), tremor (3%)

Ocular: Visual disturbance (6% to 20%), accommodation decreased (20%)

Miscellaneous: Speech disorder (10%)

Frequency not established (reported in disorders other than Tourette's disorder): Anorexia, blood dyscrasias, breast edema, chest pain, diaphoresis, dizziness, excitement; extrapyramidal symptoms (akathisia, akinesia, dystonia, pseudoparkinsonism, tardive dyskinesia); facial edema, gingival hyperplasia (case report), hypertension, hyponatremia, hypotension, jaundice, libido decreased, nausea, neuroleptic malignant syndrome, orthostatic hypotension, palpitations, periorbital edema, postural hypotension, QT_c prolongation, seizure, tachycardia, ventricular arrhythmias, vomiting, weight gain/loss

Drug Interactions Substrate of **CYP1A2, 3A4**; Inhibits **CYP2D6**, 3A4

Increased Effect/Toxicity: Concurrent use with QT_c-prolonging agents is contraindicated including Class Ia and Class III antiarrhythmics, arsenic trioxide, chlorpromazine, dolasetron, droperidol, halofantrine, levomethadyl, mefloquine, pentamidine, probucol, tacrolimus, ziprasidone, mesoridazine, thioridazine, tricyclic antidepressants, and some quinolone antibiotics (sparfloxacin, moxifloxacin, and gatifloxacin). Pimozide levels/toxicity may be increased by CYP3A4 inhibitors including macrolide antibiotics (clarithromycin, erythromycin, dirithromycin, troleandomycin), azole antifungals (fluconazole, itraconazole), protease inhibitors (amprenavir, nelfinavir, ritonavir), nefazodone, and zileuton; may predispose to life-threatening arrhythmias (use is contraindicated). Chloroquine, propranolol, and sulfadoxine-pyrimethamine also may increase pimozide concentrations. Concurrent use with TCA may produce increased toxicity or altered therapeutic response. Pimozide plus lithium may (rarely) produce neurotoxicity. Pimozide and CNS depressants (ethanol, narcotics) may produce additive CNS depressant effects. Pimozide with fluoxetine has been associated with the development of bradycardia (case report). Metoclopramide may increase risk of extrapyramidal symptoms (EPS).

Decreased Effect: Barbiturates and carbamazepine may increase the metabolism of pimozide, lowering its serum levels. Benztropine (and other anticholinergics) may inhibit the therapeutic response to pimozide. Antipsychotics such as pimozide inhibit the ability of bromocriptine to lower serum prolactin concentrations. The antihypertensive effects of guanethidine and guanadrel may be inhibited by pimozide. Pimozide may inhibit the antiparkinsonian effect of levodopa. Pimozide (and possibly other low potency antipsychotics) may reverse the pressor effects of epinephrine.

Dietary/Ethanol/Herb Considerations

Ethanol: Avoid use; may increase CNS depression.

Food: Avoid grapefruit products; may increase serum concentration.

Herb/Nutraceutical: Avoid gotu kola, kava, SAMe, and valerian; may increase CNS depression. Avoid St John's wort; may decrease serum concentration and increase CNS depression.

Pharmacodynamics/Kinetics

Absorption: 50%

Protein binding: 99%

Metabolism: Hepatic; significant first-pass effect

Half-life elimination: 50 hours

Time to peak, serum: 6-8 hours

Excretion: Urine

Pregnancy Risk Factor C

Generic Available No

Selected Readings "Pimozide (Orap) Contraindicated With Clarithromycin (Biaxin®) and Other Macrolide Antibiotics," *FDA Medical Bulletin*, October 1996, 26(3).

Pindolol (PIN doe lole)

Related Information

Cardiovascular Diseases *on page 1456*

Canadian Brand Names Apo®-Pindol; Gen-Pindolol; Novo-Pindol; Nu-Pindol; PMS-Pindolol; Visken®

Pharmacologic Category Beta Blocker With Intrinsic Sympathomimetic Activity

Use Management of hypertension

Unlabeled/Investigational Use Potential augmenting agent for antidepressants; treatment of ventricular arrhythmias/tachycardia, antipsychotic-induced akathisia, situational anxiety, aggressive behavior associated with dementia

Local Anesthetic/Vasoconstrictor Precautions Use with caution; epinephrine has interacted with nonselective beta-blockers to result in initial hypertensive episode followed by bradycardia

Effects on Dental Treatment Pindolol is a nonselective beta-blocker and may enhance the pressor response to epinephrine, resulting in hypertension and bradycardia. Many nonsteroidal anti-inflammatory drugs such as ibuprofen and indomethacin can reduce the hypotensive effect of beta-blockers after 3 or more weeks of therapy with the NSAID. Short-term NSAID use (ie, 3 days) requires no special precautions in patients taking beta-blockers.

Dosage Oral:

Adults:

Hypertension: Initial: 5 mg twice daily, increase as necessary by 10 mg/day every 3-4 weeks; maximum daily dose: 60 mg

Antidepressant augmentation: 2.5 mg 3 times/day

Elderly: Initial: 5 mg once daily, increase as necessary by 5 mg/day every 3-4 weeks

Dosing adjustment in renal/hepatic impairment: Reduction required in severe impairment

Mechanism of Action Blocks both $beta_1$- and $beta_2$-receptors and has mild intrinsic sympathomimetic activity; pindolol has negative inotropic and chronotropic effects and can significantly slow AV nodal conduction. Augmentive action of antidepressants thought to be mediated via a serotonin 1A autoreceptor antagonism.

Other Adverse Effects

1% to 10%:

Cardiovascular: Chest pain (3%), edema (6%)

Central nervous system: Nightmares/vivid dreams (5%), dizziness (9%), insomnia (10%), fatigue (8%), nervousness (7%), anxiety (<2%)

Dermatologic: Rash, itching (4%)

Gastrointestinal: Nausea (5%), abdominal discomfort (4%)

Neuromuscular & skeletal: Weakness (4%), paresthesia (3%), arthralgia (7%), muscle pain (10%)

Respiratory: Dyspnea (5%)

<1%: Bradycardia, CHF, claudication, confusion, dry eyes, hallucinations, hypotension, impotence, mental depression, palpitations, thrombocytopenia, wheezing

Drug Interactions Substrate of **CYP2D6**; Inhibits CYP2D6

Increased Effect/Toxicity: Pindolol may increase the effects of other drugs which slow AV conduction (digoxin, verapamil, diltiazem), alpha-blockers (prazosin, terazosin), and alpha-adrenergic stimulants (epinephrine, phenylephrine). Pindolol may mask the tachycardia from hypoglycemia caused by insulin and oral hypoglycemics. In patients receiving concurrent therapy, the risk of hypertensive crisis is increased when either clonidine or the beta-blocker is withdrawn. Reserpine has been shown to enhance the effect of beta-blockers. Beta-blockers may increase the action or levels of ethanol, disopyramide, nondepolarizing muscle relaxants, and theophylline although the effects are difficult to predict.

Decreased Effect: Decreased levels/effect of pindolol with aluminum salts, barbiturates, calcium salts, cholestyramine, colestipol, NSAIDs, penicillins (ampicillin), rifampin, salicylates, and sulfinpyrazone due to decreased bioavailability and plasma levels. Beta-blockers may decrease the effect of sulfonylureas (possibly hyperglycemia). Nonselective beta-blockers blunt the effect of beta-2 adrenergic agonists (albuterol).

Dietary/Ethanol/Herb Considerations

Ethanol: Limit use; may increase risk of hypotension or dizziness.

Herb/Nutraceutical: Avoid black cohosh, dong quai, and evening primrose due to estrogenic activity. Avoid ephedra, ginseng, and yohimbe; may worsen hypertension.

Pharmacodynamics/Kinetics

Absorption: Rapid, 50% to 95%

Protein binding: 50%

Metabolism: Hepatic (60% to 65%) to conjugates

Half-life elimination: 2.5-4 hours; prolonged with renal impairment, age, and cirrhosis

Time to peak, serum: 1-2 hours

Excretion: Urine (35% to 50% as unchanged drug)

Pregnancy Risk Factor B

(Continued)

Pindolol *(Continued)*

Generic Available Yes

Selected Readings

Foster CA and Aston SJ, "Propranolol-Epinephrine Interaction: A Potential Disaster," *Plast Reconstr Surg*, 1983, 72(1):74-8.
Wong DG, Spence JD, Lamki L, et al, "Effect of Nonsteroidal Anti-inflammatory Drugs on Control of Hypertension of Beta-Blockers and Diuretics," *Lancet*, 1986, 1(8488):997-1001.
Wynn RL, "Dental Nonsteroidal Anti-inflammatory Drugs and Prostaglandin-Based Drug Interactions, Part Two," *Gen Dent*, 1992, 40(2):104, 106, 108.
Wynn RL, "Epinephrine Interactions With Beta-Blockers," *Gen Dent*, 1994, 42(1):16, 18.

Pink Bismuth *see* Bismuth *on page 186*
Pin-X® [OTC] *see* Pyrantel Pamoate *on page 1150*
PIO *see* Pemoline *on page 1044*

Pioglitazone (pye oh GLI tu zone)

U.S. Brand Names Actos®

Canadian Brand Names Actos®

Pharmacologic Category Antidiabetic Agent, Thiazolidinedione

Use

Type 2 diabetes mellitus (noninsulin dependent, NIDDM), monotherapy: Adjunct to diet and exercise, to improve glycemic control

Type 2 diabetes mellitus (noninsulin dependent, NIDDM), combination therapy with sulfonylurea, metformin, or insulin: When diet, exercise, and a single agent alone does not result in adequate glycemic control

Local Anesthetic/Vasoconstrictor Precautions No information available to require special precautions

Effects on Dental Treatment Pioglitazone-dependent diabetics should be appointed for dental treatment in morning in order to minimize chance of stress-induced hypoglycemia.

Dosage Adults: Oral:

Monotherapy: Initial: 15-30 mg once daily; if response is inadequate, the dosage may be increased in increments up to 45 mg once daily; maximum recommended dose: 45 mg once daily

Combination therapy:

With sulfonylureas: Initial: 15-30 mg once daily; dose of sulfonylurea should be reduced if the patient reports hypoglycemia

With metformin: Initial: 15-30 mg once daily; it is unlikely that the dose of metformin will need to be reduced due to hypoglycemia

With insulin: Initial: 15-30 mg once daily; dose of insulin should be reduced by 10% to 25% if the patient reports hypoglycemia or if the plasma glucose falls to <100 mg/dL. Doses >30 mg/day have not been evaluated in combination regimens.

A 1-week washout period is recommended in patients with normal liver enzymes who are changed from troglitazone to pioglitazone therapy.

Dosing adjustment in hepatic impairment: Clearance is significantly lower; do not initiate in active liver disease or if patient exhibits increased transaminases (>2.5 times the upper limit of normal) at baseline

Mechanism of Action Thiazolidinedione antidiabetic agent that lowers blood glucose by improving target cell response to insulin, without increasing pancreatic insulin secretion. It has a mechanism of action that is dependent on the presence of insulin for activity. Pioglitazone is a potent and selective agonist for peroxisome proliferator-activated receptor-gamma (PPARgamma). Activation of nuclear PPAR-gamma receptors influences the production of a number of gene products involved in glucose and lipid metabolism.

Other Adverse Effects

>10%:

Endocrine & metabolic: Decreased serum triglycerides, increased HDL-cholesterol

Gastrointestinal: Weight gain

Respiratory: Upper respiratory tract infection (13%)

1% to 10%:

Cardiovascular: Edema (5%) (in combination trials with sulfonylureas or insulin, the incidence of edema was as high as 15%)

Central nervous system: Headache (9%), fatigue (4%)

Endocrine & metabolic: Aggravation of diabetes mellitus (5%), hypoglycemia (range 2% to 15% when used in combination with sulfonylureas or insulin)

Hematologic; Anemia (1%)

Neuromuscular & skeletal: Myalgia (5%)

Respiratory: Sinusitis (6%), pharyngitis (5%)

<1%: Elevated CPK, elevated transaminases

Postmarketing and/or case reports: Congestive heart failure, hepatic failure (very rare), hepatitis

Drug Interactions Substrate of **CYP2C8/9, 3A4**; Inhibits CYP2C8/9, 2C19; Induces CYP3A4

Increased Effect/Toxicity: Ketoconazole (*in vitro*) inhibits metabolism of pioglitazone. Other inhibitors of CYP3A4, including itraconazole, are likely to decrease pioglitazone metabolism. Patients receiving inhibitors of CYP3A4 should have their glycemic control evaluated more frequently.

Decreased Effect: Effects of oral contraceptives may be decreased, based on data from a related compound. This has not been specifically evaluated for pioglitazone. CYP3A4 inducers may decrease the therapeutic effect of pioglitazone.

Dietary/Ethanol/Herb Considerations

Ethanol: Use with caution; may increase risk of hypoglycemia.

Food: May be taken with food; delays peak concentrations but the extent of absorption is not affected. Management of type 2 diabetes mellitus (noninsulin dependent, NIDDM) should include diet control.

Herb/Nutraceutical: Use caution with chromium, garlic, and gymnema; may cause hypoglycemia. Avoid St John's wort; may decrease serum concentration.

Pharmacodynamics/Kinetics

Onset of action: Delayed

Peak effect: Glucose control: Several weeks

Distribution: V_{ss} (apparent): 0.63 L/kg

Protein binding: 99.8%

Metabolism: Hepatic (99%) via CYP2C8/9 and 3A4 to both active and inactive metabolites

Half-life elimination: Parent drug: 3-7 hours; Total: 16-24 hours

Time to peak: ~2 hours

Excretion: Urine (15% to 30%) and feces as metabolites

Pregnancy Risk Factor C

Generic Available No

Piperacillin (pi PER a sil in)

U.S. Brand Names Pipracil®

Canadian Brand Names Pipracil®

Pharmacologic Category Antibiotic, Penicillin

Synonyms Piperacillin Sodium

Use Treatment of susceptible infections such as septicemia, acute and chronic respiratory tract infections, skin and soft tissue infections, and urinary tract infections due to susceptible strains of *Pseudomonas*, *Proteus*, and *Escherichia coli* and *Enterobacter*; active against some streptococci and some anaerobic bacteria; febrile neutropenia (as part of combination regimen)

Local Anesthetic/Vasoconstrictor Precautions No information available to require special precautions

Effects on Dental Treatment Prolonged use of penicillins may lead to development of oral candidiasis.

Dosage

Neonates: 100 mg/kg every 12 hours

Infants and Children: I.M., I.V.: 200-300 mg/kg/day in divided doses every 4-6 hours

Higher doses have been used in cystic fibrosis: 350-500 mg/kg/day in divided doses every 4-6 hours

Adults: I.M., I.V.:

Moderate infections (urinary tract infections): 2-3 g/dose every 6-12 hours; maximum: 2 g I.M./site

Serious infections: 3-4 g/dose every 4-6 hours; maximum: 24 g/24 hours

Uncomplicated gonorrhea: 2 g I.M. in a single dose accompanied by 1 g probenecid 30 minutes prior to injection

Dosing adjustment in renal impairment: Adults: I.V.:

Cl_{cr} 20-40 mL/minute: Administer 3-4 g every 8 hours

Cl_{cr} <20 mL/minute: Administer 3-4 g every 12 hours

Moderately dialyzable (20% to 50%)

Continuous arteriovenous or venovenous hemodiafiltration effects: Dose as for Cl_{cr} 10-50 mL/minute

Mechanism of Action Inhibits bacterial cell wall synthesis by binding to one or more of the penicillin binding proteins (PBPs); which in turn inhibits the final transpeptidation step of peptidoglycan synthesis in bacterial cell walls, thus inhibiting cell wall biosynthesis. Bacteria eventually lyse due to ongoing activity of cell wall autolytic enzymes (autolysins and murein hydrolases) while cell wall assembly is arrested.

Other Adverse Effects Frequency not defined:

Central nervous system: Confusion, convulsions, drowsiness, fever, Jarisch-Herxheimer reaction

Dermatologic: Rash

Endocrine & metabolic: Electrolyte imbalance

Hematologic: Abnormal platelet aggregation and prolonged PT (high doses), hemolytic anemia, Coombs' reaction (positive)

Local: Thrombophlebitis

Neuromuscular & skeletal: Myoclonus

Renal: Acute interstitial nephritis

Miscellaneous: Anaphylaxis, hypersensitivity reactions

(Continued)

Piperacillin *(Continued)*

Drug Interactions

Increased Effect/Toxicity: Probenecid may increase penicillin levels. Neuromuscular blockers may increase duration of blockade.

Decreased Effect: Tetracyclines may decrease penicillin effectiveness. High concentrations of piperacillin may cause physical inactivation of aminoglycosides and lead to potential toxicity in patients with mild-moderate renal dysfunction. Although anecdotal reports suggest oral contraceptive efficacy could be reduced by penicillins, this has been refuted by more rigorous scientific and clinical data.

Pharmacodynamics/Kinetics

Absorption: I.M.: 70% to 80%

Distribution: Crosses placenta; low concentrations enter breast milk

Protein binding: 22%

Half-life elimination (dose dependent; prolonged with moderately severe renal or hepatic impairment):

Neonates: 1-5 days old: 3.6 hours; >6 days old: 2.1-2.7 hours

Children: 1-6 months: 0.79 hour; 6 months to 12 years: 0.39-0.5 hour

Adults: 36-80 minutes

Time to peak, serum: I.M.: 30-50 minutes

Excretion: Primarily urine; partially feces

Pregnancy Risk Factor B

Generic Available No

Piperacillin and Tazobactam Sodium

(pi PER a sil in & ta zoe BAK tam SOW dee um)

Related Information

Piperacillin *on page 1087*

U.S. Brand Names Zosyn®

Canadian Brand Names Tacozin®

Pharmacologic Category Antibiotic, Penicillin

Synonyms Piperacillin Sodium and Tazobactam Sodium

Use Treatment of infections of lower respiratory tract, urinary tract, skin and skin structures, gynecologic, bone and joint infections, and septicemia caused by susceptible organisms. Tazobactam expands activity of piperacillin to include beta-lactamase producing strains of *S. aureus*, *H. influenzae*, *Bacteroides*, and other gram-negative bacteria.

Local Anesthetic/Vasoconstrictor Precautions No information available to require special precautions

Effects on Dental Treatment Prolonged use of penicillins may lead to development of oral candidiasis.

Dosage

Children <12 years: Use not recommended due to lack of data

Children >12 years and Adults:

Severe infections: I.V.: Piperacillin/tazobactam 4/0.5 g every 8 hours or 3/0.375 g every 6 hours

Moderate infections: I.M.: Piperacillin/tazobactam 2/0.25 g every 6-8 hours; treatment should be continued for ≥7-10 days depending on severity of disease (**Note:** I.M. route not FDA-approved)

Dosing interval in renal impairment:

Cl_{cr} 20-40 mL/minute: Administer 2/0.25 g every 6 hours

Cl_{cr} <20 mL/minute: Administer 2/0.25 g every 8 hours

Hemodialysis: Administer 2/0.25 g every 8 hours with an additional dose of 0.75 g after each dialysis

Continuous arteriovenous or venovenous hemodiafiltration effects: Dose as for Cl_{cr} 10-50 mL/minute

Mechanism of Action Inhibits bacterial cell wall synthesis by binding to one or more of the penicillin binding proteins (PBPs); which in turn inhibits the final transpeptidation step of peptidoglycan synthesis in bacterial cell walls, thus inhibiting cell wall biosynthesis. Bacteria eventually lyse due to ongoing activity of cell wall autolytic enzymes (autolysins and murein hydrolases) while cell wall assembly is arrested. Tazobactam inhibits many beta-lactamases, including staphylococcal penicillinase and Richmond and Sykes types II, III, IV, and V, including extended spectrum enzymes; it has only limited activity against class I beta-lactamases other than class Ic types.

Other Adverse Effects

>10%: Gastrointestinal: Diarrhea (11%)

1% to 10%:

Cardiovascular: Hypertension (2%)

Central nervous system: Insomnia (7%), headache (7% to 8%), agitation (2%), fever (2%), dizziness (1%)

Dermatologic: Rash (4%), pruritus (3%)

Gastrointestinal: Constipation (7% to 8%), nausea (7%), vomiting/dyspepsia (3%)

Respiratory: Rhinitis/dyspnea (~1%)

Miscellaneous: Serum sickness-like reaction

<1%: Bronchospasm, cholestatic jaundice, *Clostridium difficile* colitis, confusion, edema, erythema multiforme, hemolytic anemia, hepatitis, hepatotoxicity, hypotension, interstitial nephritis, leukopenia, pseudomembranous colitis, seizures, Stevens-Johnson syndrome, thrombocytopenia

Several laboratory abnormalities have rarely been associated with piperacillin/tazobactam including reversible eosinophilia, and neutropenia (associated most often with prolonged therapy), positive direct Coombs' test, prolonged PT and aPTT, transient elevations of LFT, increases in creatinine

Drug Interactions

Increased Effect/Toxicity: Probenecid may increase penicillin levels. Neuromuscular blockers may increase duration of blockade.

Decreased Effect: Tetracyclines may decrease penicillin effectiveness. Aminoglycosides may cause physical inactivation of aminoglycosides in the presence of high concentrations of piperacillin and potential toxicity in patients with mild-moderate renal dysfunction. Although anecdotal reports suggest oral contraceptive efficacy could be reduced by penicillins, this has been refuted by more rigorous scientific and clinical data.

Pharmacodynamics/Kinetics Both AUC and peak concentrations are dose proportional; hepatic impairment does not affect kinetics

Distribution: Well into lungs, intestinal mucosa, skin, muscle, uterus, ovary, prostate, gallbladder, and bile; penetration into CSF is low in subject with noninflamed meninges

Protein binding: Piperacillin: ~26% to 33%; Tazobactam: 31% to 32%

Metabolism: Piperacillin: 6% to 9%; Tazobactam: ~26%

Half-life elimination: Piperacillin: 1 hour; Metabolite: 1-1.5 hours; Tazobactam: 0.7-0.9 hour

Excretion: Both piperacillin and tazobactam are directly proportional to renal function

Piperacillin: Urine (50% to 70%); feces (10% to 20%)

Tazobactam: Urine (26% as inactive metabolite) within 24 hours

Pregnancy Risk Factor B

Generic Available No

Piperacillin Sodium *see* Piperacillin *on page 1087*

Piperacillin Sodium and Tazobactam Sodium *see* Piperacillin and Tazobactam Sodium *on page 1088*

Piperazine (PI per a zeen)

Canadian Brand Names Entacyl®

Mexican Brand Names Desparasil®

Pharmacologic Category Anthelmintic

Synonyms Piperazine Citrate

Use Treatment of pinworm and roundworm infections (used as an alternative to first-line agents, mebendazole, or pyrantel pamoate)

Local Anesthetic/Vasoconstrictor Precautions No information available to require special precautions

Effects on Dental Treatment No significant effects or complications reported

Dosage Oral:

Pinworms: Children and Adults: 65 mg/kg/day (not to exceed 2.5 g/day) as a single daily dose for 7 days; in severe infections, repeat course after a 1-week interval

Roundworms:

Children: 75 mg/kg/day as a single daily dose for 2 days; maximum: 3.5 g/day

Adults: 3.5 g/day for 2 days (in severe infections, repeat course, after a 1-week interval)

Mechanism of Action Causes muscle paralysis of the roundworm by blocking the effects of acetylcholine at the neuromuscular junction

Other Adverse Effects <1%: Bronchospasms, diarrhea, dizziness, EEG changes, headache, hemolytic anemia, hypersensitivity reactions, nausea, seizures, vertigo, visual impairment, vomiting, weakness

Drug Interactions Decreased Effect: Pyrantel pamoate (antagonistic mode of action)

Pharmacodynamics/Kinetics

Absorption: Well absorbed

Time to peak, serum: 1 hour

Excretion: Urine (as unchanged drug and metabolites)

Pregnancy Risk Factor B

Generic Available Yes

Piperazine Citrate *see* Piperazine *on page 1089*

Piperazine Estrone Sulfate *see* Estropipate *on page 536*

Piperonyl Butoxide and Pyrethrins *see* Pyrethrins and Piperonyl Butoxide *on page 1151*

Pipracil® *see* Piperacillin *on page 1087*

Pirbuterol (peer BYOO ter ole)

Related Information

Respiratory Diseases *on page 1476*

U.S. Brand Names Maxair™; Maxair™ Autohaler™

Pharmacologic Category $Beta_2$ Agonist

Synonyms Pirbuterol Acetate

Use Prevention and treatment of reversible bronchospasm including asthma

Local Anesthetic/Vasoconstrictor Precautions No information available to require special precautions

Effects on Dental Treatment 1% to 10%: Xerostomia

Dosage Children ≥12 years and Adults: 2 inhalations every 4-6 hours for prevention; two inhalations at an interval of at least 1-3 minutes, followed by a third inhalation in treatment of bronchospasm, not to exceed 12 inhalations/day

Mechanism of Action Pirbuterol is a $beta_2$-adrenergic agonist with a similar structure to albuterol, specifically a pyridine ring has been substituted for the benzene ring in albuterol. The increased $beta_2$ selectivity of pirbuterol results from the substitution of a tertiary butyl group on the nitrogen of the side chain, which additionally imparts resistance of pirbuterol to degradation by monoamine oxidase and provides a lengthened duration of action in comparison to the less selective previous beta-agonist agents.

Other Adverse Effects

>10%:
- Central nervous system: Nervousness (7%)
- Neuromuscular & skeletal: Trembling (6%)

1% to 10%:
- Cardiovascular: Palpitations (2%), tachycardia (1%)
- Central nervous system: Headache (2%), dizziness (1%)
- Gastrointestinal: Nausea (2%)
- Respiratory: Cough (1%)

<1%: Abdominal pain/cramps, alopecia, anxiety, bruising, chest pain, confusion, depression, diarrhea, edema, flushing, glossitis, hyperkinesia, hypotension, insomnia, pruritus, rash, skipped beats, smell/taste changes, sore throat, stomatitis, syncope, vomiting, weakness, numbness in extremities, weight gain

Drug Interactions

Increased toxicity with other beta agonists, MAO inhibitors, and TCAs.

Decreased effect with beta-blockers.

Pharmacodynamics/Kinetics

Onset of action: Peak effect: Therapeutic: Oral: 2-3 hours with peak serum concentration of 6.2-9.8 mcg/L; Inhalation: 0.5-1 hour

Half-life elimination: 2-3 hours

Metabolism: Hepatic

Excretion: Urine (10% as unchanged drug)

Pregnancy Risk Factor C

Generic Available No

Pirbuterol Acetate *see* Pirbuterol *on page 1090*

Piroxicam (peer OKS i kam)

Related Information

Rheumatoid Arthritis, Osteoarthritis, and Osteoporosis *on page 1488*

Temporomandibular Dysfunction (TMD) *on page 1562*

U.S. Brand Names Feldene®

Canadian Brand Names Apo®-Piroxicam; Feldene™; Gen-Piroxicam; Novo-Pirocam®; Nu-Pirox; Pexicam®

Mexican Brand Names Androxicam®; Artinor®; Artyflam; Brexicam®; Citoken® Dixonal®; Dolzycam®; Facicam®; Feldene®; Flogosan®; Osteral®; Oxicanol®; Piroxan®; Piroxen; Rogal®

Pharmacologic Category Nonsteroidal Anti-inflammatory Drug (NSAID)

Use Management of inflammatory disorders; symptomatic treatment of acute and chronic rheumatoid arthritis, osteoarthritis, and ankylosing spondylitis; also used to treat sunburn

Local Anesthetic/Vasoconstrictor Precautions No information available to require special precautions

Effects on Dental Treatment NSAID formulations are known to reversibly decrease platelet aggregation via mechanisms different than observed with aspirin. The dentist should be aware of the potential of abnormal coagulation. Caution should also be exercised in the use of NSAIDs in patients already on anticoagulant therapy with drugs such as warfarin (Coumadin®).

Dosage Oral:

Children: 0.2-0.3 mg/kg/day once daily; maximum dose: 15 mg/day

Adults: 10-20 mg/day once daily; although associated with increase in GI adverse effects, doses >20 mg/day have been used (ie, 30-40 mg/day)

Dosing adjustment in hepatic impairment: Reduction required

Mechanism of Action Inhibits prostaglandin synthesis, acts on the hypothalamus heat-regulating center to reduce fever, blocks prostaglandin synthetase action which prevents formation of the platelet-aggregating substance thromboxane A_2; decreases pain receptor sensitivity. Other proposed mechanisms of action for salicylate anti-inflammatory action are lysosomal stabilization, kinin and leukotriene production, alteration of chemotactic factors, and inhibition of neutrophil activation. This latter mechanism may be the most significant pharmacologic action to reduce inflammation.

Other Adverse Effects

>10%:
- Central nervous system: Dizziness
- Dermatologic: Rash
- Gastrointestinal: Abdominal cramps, heartburn, indigestion, nausea

1% to 10%:
- Central nervous system: Headache, nervousness
- Dermatologic: Itching
- Endocrine & metabolic: Fluid retention
- Gastrointestinal: Vomiting
- Otic: Tinnitus

<1%: Acute renal failure, agranulocytosis, allergic rhinitis, anemia, angioedema, arrhythmias, aseptic meningitis, blurred vision, bone marrow suppression, confusion, CHF, conjunctivitis, cystitis, decreased hearing, drowsiness, dry eyes, dyspnea, epistaxis, erythema multiforme, gastritis, GI ulceration, hallucinations, hemolytic anemia, hepatitis, hot flashes, hypertension, insomnia, leukopenia, mental depression, peripheral neuropathy, polydipsia, polyuria, Stevens-Johnson syndrome, tachycardia, thrombocytopenia, toxic amblyopia, toxic epidermal necrolysis, urticaria

Drug Interactions Substrate of CYP2C8/9

Increased effect/toxicity of lithium, warfarin, and methotrexate (controversial).

Decreased effect of diuretics, beta-blockers. Decreased effect with aspirin, antacids, and cholestyramine.

Dietary/Ethanol/Herb Considerations

Ethanol: Avoid use; may enhance gastric mucosal irritation.

Food: Administer with food to reduce GI upset; food may delay onset of action.

Herb/Nutraceutical: Avoid cat's claw, dong quai, evening primrose, feverfew, garlic, ginkgo biloba, ginseng, green tea, horse chestnut, and red clover due to additional antiplatelet activity. Avoid kava and valerian; may enhance benzodiazepine activity.

Pharmacodynamics/Kinetics

Onset of action: Analgesic: ~1 hour
- Peak effect: 3-5 hours

Protein binding: 99%

Metabolism: Hepatic

Half-life elimination: 45-50 hours

Excretion: Primarily urine and feces (small amounts) as unchanged drug (5%) and metabolites

Pregnancy Risk Factor B/D (3rd trimester or near term)

Generic Available Yes

***p*-Isobutylhydratropic Acid** *see* Ibuprofen *on page 703*

Pit *see* Oxytocin *on page 1026*

Pitocin® *see* Oxytocin *on page 1026*

Pitressin® *see* Vasopressin *on page 1379*

Pix Carbonis *see* Coal Tar *on page 359*

Plan B® *see* Levonorgestrel *on page 797*

Plantago Seed *see* Psyllium *on page 1149*

Plantain Seed *see* Psyllium *on page 1149*

Plaquenil® *see* Hydroxychloroquine *on page 694*

Platinol® *see* Cisplatin *on page 332*

Platinol®-AQ *see* Cisplatin *on page 332*

Plavix® *see* Clopidogrel *on page 353*

Plendil® *see* Felodipine *on page 560*

Pletal® *see* Cilostazol *on page 325*

PMPA *see* Tenofovir *on page 1275*

Pneumococcal 7-Valent Conjugate Vaccine *see* Pneumococcal Conjugate Vaccine (7-Valent) *on page 1091*

Pneumococcal Conjugate Vaccine (7-Valent)

(noo moe KOK ul KON joo get vak SEEN, seven vay lent)

Related Information

Immunizations (Vaccines) *on page 1612*

U.S. Brand Names Prevnar®

Canadian Brand Names Prevnar®

Pharmacologic Category Vaccine

(Continued)

Pneumococcal Conjugate Vaccine (7-Valent) *(Continued)*

Synonyms Diphtheria CRM_{197} Protein; PCV7; Pneumococcal 7-Valent Conjugate Vaccine

Use Immunization of infants and toddlers against *Streptococcus pneumoniae* infection caused by serotypes included in the vaccine

Advisory Committee on Immunization Practices (ACIP) guidelines also recommend PCV7 for use in:

All children ≥23 months

Children ages 24-59 months with: Sickle cell disease (including other sickle cell hemoglobinopathies, asplenia, splenic dysfunction), HIV infection, immunocompromising conditions (congenital immunodeficiencies, renal failure, nephrotic syndrome, diseases associated with immunosuppressive or radiation therapy, solid organ transplant), chronic illnesses (cardiac disease, cerebrospinal fluid leaks, diabetes mellitus, pulmonary disease excluding asthma unless on high dose corticosteroids); cochlear implants

Consider use in all children 24-59 months with priority given to:

Children 24-35 months

Children 24-59 months who are of Alaska native, American Indian, or African-American descent

Children 24-59 months who attend group day care centers

Local Anesthetic/Vasoconstrictor Precautions No information available to require special precautions

Effects on Dental Treatment No significant effects or complications reported

Restrictions Federal law requires that the date of administration, the vaccine manufacturer, lot number of vaccine, and the administering person's name, title and address be entered into the patient's permanent medical record.

Dosage I.M.:

Infants: 2-6 months: 0.5 mL at approximately 2-month intervals for 3 consecutive doses, followed by a fourth dose of 0.5 mL at 12-15 months of age; first dose may be given as young as 6 weeks of age, but is typically given at 2 months of age. In case of a moderate shortage of vaccine, defer the fourth dose until shortage is resolved; in case of a severe shortage of vaccine, defer third and fourth doses until shortage is resolved.

Previously Unvaccinated Infants and Children:

7-11 months: 0.5 mL for a total of 3 doses; 2 doses at least 4 weeks apart, followed by a third dose after the 1-year birthday (12-15 months), separated from the second dose by at least 2 months. In case of a severe shortage of vaccine, defer the third dose until shortage is resolved.

12-23 months: 0.5 mL for a total of 2 doses, separated by at least 2 months. In case of a severe shortage of vaccine, defer the second dose until shortage is resolved.

24-59 months:

Healthy Children: 0.5 mL as a single dose. In case of a severe shortage of vaccine, defer dosing until shortage is resolved.

Children with sickle cell disease, asplenia, HIV infection, chronic illness or immunocompromising conditions (not including bone marrow transplants - results pending; use PPV23 [pneumococcal polysaccharide vaccine, polyvalent] at 12- and 24-months until studies are complete): 0.5 mL for a total of 2 doses, separated by 2 months

Previously Vaccinated Children with a lapse in vaccine administration:

7-11 months: Previously received 1 or 2 doses PCV7: 0.5 mL dose at 7-11 months of age, followed by a second dose ≥2 months later at 12-15 months of age

12-23 months:

Previously received 1 dose before 12 months of age: 0.5 mL dose, followed by a second dose ≥2 months later

Previously received 2 doses before age 12 months: 0.5 mL dose ≥2 months after the most recent dose

24-59 months: Any incomplete schedule: 0.5 mL as a single dose; **Note:** Patients with chronic diseases or immunosuppressing conditions should receive 2 doses ≥2 months apart

Mechanism of Action Contains saccharides of capsular antigens of serotypes 4, 6B, 9V, 18C, 19F, and 23F, individually conjugated to CRM197 protein

Other Adverse Effects All serious adverse reactions must be reported to the U.S. Department of Health and Human Services (DHHS) Vaccine Adverse Event Reporting System (VAERS) 1-800-822-7967.

>10%:

Central nervous system: Fever, irritability, drowsiness, restlessness

Dermatologic: Erythema

Gastrointestinal: Decreased appetite, vomiting, diarrhea

Local: Induration, tenderness, nodule

1% to 10%: Dermatologic: Rash (0.5% to 1.4%)

Pregnancy Risk Factor C

Generic Available No

Pneumotussin® *see* Hydrocodone and Guaifenesin *on page 683*

Podocon-25® *see* Podophyllum Resin *on page 1093*

Podofilox (po do FIL oks)

U.S. Brand Names Condylox®

Canadian Brand Names Condyline™; Wartec®

Pharmacologic Category Keratolytic Agent; Topical Skin Product

Use Treatment of external genital warts

Local Anesthetic/Vasoconstrictor Precautions No information available to require special precautions

Effects on Dental Treatment No significant effects or complications reported

Dosage Topical: Adults: Apply twice daily (morning and evening) for 3 consecutive days, then withhold use for 4 consecutive days; this cycle may be repeated up to 4 times until there is no visible wart tissue

Pregnancy Risk Factor C

Generic Available Yes: Topical solution

Podophyllin *see* Podophyllum Resin *on page 1093*

Podophyllum Resin (po DOF fil um REZ in)

U.S. Brand Names Podocon-25®

Canadian Brand Names Podofilm®

Pharmacologic Category Keratolytic Agent

Synonyms Mandrake; May Apple; Podophyllin

Use Topical treatment of benign growths including external genital and perianal warts, papillomas, fibroids; compound benzoin tincture generally is used as the medium for topical application

Local Anesthetic/Vasoconstrictor Precautions No information available to require special precautions

Effects on Dental Treatment No significant effects or complications reported

Dosage Topical:

- Children and Adults: 10% to 25% solution in compound benzoin tincture; apply drug to dry surface, use 1 drop at a time allowing drying between drops until area is covered; total volume should be limited to <0.5 mL per treatment session
- Condylomata acuminatum: 25% solution is applied daily; use a 10% solution when applied to or near mucous membranes
- Verrucae: 25% solution is applied 3-5 times/day directly to the wart

Mechanism of Action Directly affects epithelial cell metabolism by arresting mitosis through binding to a protein subunit of spindle microtubules (tubulin)

Other Adverse Effects

- 1% to 10%:
  - Dermatologic: Pruritus
  - Gastrointestinal: Nausea, vomiting, abdominal pain, diarrhea
- <1%: Confusion, lethargy, hallucinations, leukopenia, thrombocytopenia, hepatotoxicity, peripheral neuropathy, renal failure

Pregnancy Risk Factor X

Generic Available No

Polaramine® [DSC] *see* Dexchlorpheniramine *on page 416*

Poliovirus Vaccine (Inactivated)

(POE lee oh VYE rus vak SEEN, in ak ti VAY ted)

Related Information

- Diphtheria, Tetanus Toxoids, Acellular Pertussis, Hepatitis B (Recombinant), and Poliovirus (Inactivated) Vaccine *on page 454*
- Immunizations (Vaccines) *on page 1612*

U.S. Brand Names IPOL®

Canadian Brand Names IPOL™

Pharmacologic Category Vaccine

Synonyms Enhanced-potency Inactivated Poliovirus Vaccine; IPV; Salk Vaccine

Use

As the global eradication of poliomyelitis continues, the risk for importation of wild-type poliovirus into the United States decreases dramatically. To eliminate the risk for vaccine-associated paralytic poliomyelitis (VAPP), an all-IPV schedule is recommended for routine childhood vaccination in the United States. All children should receive four doses of IPV (at age 2 months, age 4 months, between ages 6-18 months, and between ages 4-6 years). Oral poliovirus vaccine (OPV), if available, may be used only for the following special circumstances:

- Mass vaccination campaigns to control outbreaks of paralytic polio
- Unvaccinated children who will be traveling within 4 weeks to areas where polio is endemic or epidemic
- Children of parents who do not accept the recommended number of vaccine injections; these children may receive OPV only for the third or fourth dose or both. In this situation, healthcare providers should administer OPV only after discussing the risk for VAPP with parents or caregivers.

(Continued)

Poliovirus Vaccine (Inactivated) *(Continued)*

OPV supplies are expected to be very limited in the United States after inventories are depleted. ACIP reaffirms its support for the global eradication initiative and use of OPV as the vaccine of choice to eradicate polio where it is endemic.

Local Anesthetic/Vasoconstrictor Precautions No information available to require special precautions

Effects on Dental Treatment No significant effects or complications reported

Restrictions Federal law requires that the date of administration, the vaccine manufacturer, lot number of vaccine, and the administering person's name, title, and address be entered into the patient's permanent medical record.

Dosage S.C.: **Enhanced-potency inactivated poliovirus vaccine (E-IPV) is preferred for primary vaccination of adults**, two doses S.C. 4-8 weeks apart, a third dose 6-12 months after the second. For adults with a completed primary series and for whom a booster is indicated, either OPV or E-IPV can be given (E-IPV preferred). If immediate protection is needed, either OPV or E-IPV is recommended.

Other Adverse Effects All serious adverse reactions must be reported to the U.S. Department of Health and Human Services (DHHS) Vaccine Adverse Event Reporting System (VAERS) 1-800-822-7967.

1% to 10%:

Central nervous system: Fever (>101.3°F)

Dermatologic: Rash

Local: Tenderness or pain at injection site

<1%: Crying, decreased appetite, dyspnea, erythema, fatigue, fussiness, Guillain-Barré, reddening of skin, sleepiness, weakness

Pregnancy Risk Factor C

Generic Available No

Polocaine® *see* Mepivacaine *on page 861*

Polocaine® MPF *see* Mepivacaine *on page 861*

Polycitra® *see* Citric Acid, Sodium Citrate, and Potassium Citrate *on page 335*

Polycitra®-K *see* Potassium Citrate and Citric Acid *on page 1101*

Polycose® [OTC] *see* Glucose Polymers *on page 641*

Polyethylene Glycol-Electrolyte Solution

(pol ee ETH i leen GLYE kol-ee LEK troe lyte soe LOO shun)

U.S. Brand Names Colyte®; GoLYTELY®; MiraLax™; NuLytely®; OCL® [DSC]

Canadian Brand Names Colyte™; Klean-Prep®; Klean-Prep®; Lyteprep™; PegLyte®; Peglyte™

Pharmacologic Category Cathartic; Laxative, Bowel Evacuant

Synonyms Electrolyte Lavage Solution

Use Bowel cleansing prior to GI examination or following toxic ingestion (electrolyte containing solutions only); treatment of occasional constipation (MiraLax™)

Local Anesthetic/Vasoconstrictor Precautions No information available to require special precautions

Effects on Dental Treatment No significant effects or complications reported

Dosage

Oral:

Children ≥6 months: Bowel cleansing prior to GI exam (solutions with electrolytes only): 25-40 mL/kg/hour for 4-10 hours (until rectal effluent is clear). Ideally, patients should fast for ~3-4 hours prior to administration; absolutely no solid food for at least 2 hours before the solution is given. The solution may be given via nasogastric tube to patients who are unwilling or unable to drink the solution. Patients <2 years should be monitored closely.

Adults:

Bowel cleansing prior to GI exam (solutions with electrolytes only): 240 mL (8 oz) every 10 minutes, until 4 L are consumed or the rectal effluent is clear; rapid drinking of each portion is preferred to drinking small amounts continuously. Ideally, patients should fast for ~3-4 hours prior to administration; absolutely no solid food for at least 2 hours before the solution is given. The solution may be given via nasogastric tube to patients who are unwilling or unable to drink the solution.

Occasional constipation (MiraLax™): 17 g of powder (~1 heaping tablespoon) dissolved in 8 oz of water; once daily; do not use for >2 weeks.

Nasogastric tube:

Children ≥6 months: Bowel cleansing prior to GI exam (solutions with electrolytes only): 25 mL/kg/hour until rectal effluent is clear. Ideally, patients should fast for ~3-4 hours prior to administration; absolutely no solid food for at least 2 hours before the solution is given.

Adults: Bowel cleansing prior to GI exam (solutions with electrolytes only): 20-30 mL/minute (1.2-1.8 L/hour); the first bowel movement should occur ~1 hour after the start of administration. Ideally, patients should fast for ~3-4 hours prior to administration; absolutely no solid food for at least 2 hours before the solution is given.

Mechanism of Action Induces catharsis by strong electrolyte and osmotic effects

Other Adverse Effects Frequency not defined:

Dermatologic: Dermatitis, rash, urticaria

Gastrointestinal: Nausea, abdominal fullness, bloating, abdominal cramps, vomiting, anal irritation, diarrhea, flatulence

Postmarketing and/or case reports: Upper GI bleeding, Mallory-Weiss tear, esophageal perforation, asystole, dyspnea (acute), pulmonary edema, vomiting with aspiration of PEG, anaphylaxis; dehydration and hypokalemia have been reported in children

Drug Interactions Decreased Effect: Oral medications should not be administered within 1 hour of start of therapy.

Dietary/Ethanol/Herb Considerations Food: For bowel cleansing prior to GI exam, the patient should fast for ~3-4 hours prior to administration, but in no case should solid food be given for at least 2 hours before the solution is given. Do not add flavorings as additional ingredients before use

Pharmacodynamics/Kinetics Onset of effect: Oral: Bowel cleansing: ~1-2 hours; Constipation: 48-96 hours

Pregnancy Risk Factor C

Generic Available No

Polygam® S/D *see* Immune Globulin (Intravenous) *on page 714*

Polymyxin B (pol i MIKS in bee)

Related Information

Neomycin and Polymyxin B *on page 962*

Neomycin, Polymyxin B, and Dexamethasone *on page 962*

Neomycin, Polymyxin B, and Prednisolone *on page 963*

U.S. Brand Names Poly-Rx

Pharmacologic Category Antibiotic, Irrigation; Antibiotic, Miscellaneous

Synonyms Polymyxin B Sulfate

Use Treatment of acute infections caused by susceptible strains of *Pseudomonas aeruginosa*; used occasionally for gut decontamination; parenteral use of polymyxin B has mainly been replaced by less toxic antibiotics, reserved for life-threatening infections caused by organisms resistant to the preferred drugs (eg, pseudomonal meningitis - intrathecal administration)

Local Anesthetic/Vasoconstrictor Precautions No information available to require special precautions

Effects on Dental Treatment No significant effects or complications reported

Dosage

Otic (in combination with other drugs): 1-2 drops, 3-4 times/day; should be used sparingly to avoid accumulation of excess debris

Infants <2 years:

I.M.: Up to 40,000 units/kg/day divided every 6 hours (not routinely recommended due to pain at injection sites)

I.V.: Up to 40,000 units/kg/day divided every 12 hours

Intrathecal: 20,000 units/day for 3-4 days, then 25,000 units every other day for at least 2 weeks after CSF cultures are negative and CSF (glucose) has returned to within normal limits

Children ≥2 years and Adults:

I.M.: 25,000-30,000 units/kg/day divided every 4-6 hours (not routinely recommended due to pain at injection sites)

I.V.: 15,000-25,000 units/kg/day divided every 12 hours

Intrathecal: 50,000 units/day for 3-4 days, then every other day for at least 2 weeks after CSF cultures are negative and CSF (glucose) has returned to within normal limits

Total daily dose should not exceed 2,000,000 units/day

Bladder irrigation: Continuous irrigant or rinse in the urinary bladder for up to 10 days using 20 mg (equal to 200,000 units) added to 1 L of normal saline; usually no more than 1 L of irrigant is used per day unless urine flow rate is high; administration rate is adjusted to patient's urine output

Topical irrigation or topical solution: 500,000 units/L of normal saline; topical irrigation should not exceed 2 million units/day in adults

Gut sterilization: Oral: 15,000-25,000 units/kg/day in divided doses every 6 hours

Clostridium difficile enteritis: Oral: 25,000 units every 6 hours for 10 days

Ophthalmic: A concentration of 0.1% to 0.25% is administered as 1-3 drops every hour, then increasing the interval as response indicates to 1-2 drops 4-6 times/day

Dosing adjustment in renal impairment:

Cl_{cr} 20-50 mL/minute: Administer 75% to 100% of normal dose every 12 hours

Cl_{cr} 5-20 mL/minute: Administer 50% of normal dose every 12 hours

Cl_{cr} <5 mL/minute: Administer 15% of normal dose every 12 hours

Mechanism of Action Binds to phospholipids, alters permeability, and damages the bacterial cytoplasmic membrane permitting leakage of intracellular constituents

Other Adverse Effects Frequency not defined:

Cardiovascular: Facial flushing

(Continued)

Polymyxin B *(Continued)*

Central nervous system: Neurotoxicity (irritability, drowsiness, ataxia, perioral paresthesia, numbness of the extremities, and blurring of vision); dizziness, drug fever, meningeal irritation with intrathecal administration
Dermatologic: Urticarial rash
Endocrine & metabolic: Hypocalcemia, hyponatremia, hypokalemia, hypochloremia
Local: Pain at injection site
Neuromuscular & skeletal: Neuromuscular blockade, weakness
Renal: Nephrotoxicity
Respiratory: Respiratory arrest
Miscellaneous: Anaphylactoid reaction

Drug Interactions Increased Effect/Toxicity: Increased/prolonged effect of neuromuscular blocking agents.

Pharmacodynamics/Kinetics

Absorption: Well absorbed from peritoneum; minimal from GI tract (except in neonates) from mucous membranes or intact skin
Distribution: Minimal into CSF; does not cross placenta
Half-life elimination: 4.5-6 hours; prolonged with renal impairment
Time to peak, serum: I.M.: ~2 hours
Excretion: Urine (>60% primarily as unchanged drug)

Pregnancy Risk Factor B (per expert opinion)

Generic Available Yes

Polymyxin B and Bacitracin *see* Bacitracin and Polymyxin B *on page 157*

Polymyxin B and Neomycin *see* Neomycin and Polymyxin B *on page 962*

Polymyxin B and Oxytetracycline *see* Oxytetracycline and Polymyxin B *on page 1025*

Polymyxin B and Trimethoprim *see* Trimethoprim and Polymyxin B *on page 1353*

Polymyxin B, Bacitracin, and Neomycin *see* Bacitracin, Neomycin, and Polymyxin B *on page 157*

Polymyxin B, Bacitracin, Neomycin, and Hydrocortisone *see* Bacitracin, Neomycin, Polymyxin B, and Hydrocortisone *on page 158*

Polymyxin B, Chloramphenicol, and Hydrocortisone *see* Chloramphenicol, Polymyxin B, and Hydrocortisone *on page 299*

Polymyxin B, Hydrocortisone, and Chloramphenicol *see* Chloramphenicol, Polymyxin B, and Hydrocortisone *on page 299*

Polymyxin B, Neomycin, and Dexamethasone *see* Neomycin, Polymyxin B, and Dexamethasone *on page 962*

Polymyxin B, Neomycin, and Gramicidin *see* Neomycin, Polymyxin B, and Gramicidin *on page 963*

Polymyxin B, Neomycin, and Hydrocortisone *see* Neomycin, Polymyxin B, and Hydrocortisone *on page 963*

Polymyxin B, Neomycin, and Prednisolone *see* Neomycin, Polymyxin B, and Prednisolone *on page 963*

Polymyxin B Sulfate *see* Polymyxin B *on page 1095*

Poly-Pred® *see* Neomycin, Polymyxin B, and Prednisolone *on page 963*

Poly-Rx *see* Polymyxin B *on page 1095*

Polysaccharide-Iron Complex (pol i SAK a ride-EYE ern KOM pleks)

U.S. Brand Names Fe-Tinic™ 150 [OTC]; Hytinic® [OTC]; Niferex® [OTC]; Niferex® 150 [OTC]; Nu-Iron® 150 [OTC]

Pharmacologic Category Iron Salt

Use Prevention and treatment of iron-deficiency anemias

Local Anesthetic/Vasoconstrictor Precautions No information available to require special precautions

Effects on Dental Treatment No significant effects or complications reported

Dosage

Children ≥6 years: Tablets/elixir: 50-100 mg/day; may be given in divided doses
Adults:
  Tablets/elixir: 50-100 mg twice daily
  Capsules: 150-300 mg/day

Other Adverse Effects

>10%: Gastrointestinal: Stomach cramping, constipation, nausea, vomiting, dark stools, GI irritation, epigastric pain, nausea
1% to 10%:
  Gastrointestinal: Heartburn, diarrhea
  Genitourinary: Discolored urine
  Miscellaneous: Staining of teeth
<1%: Contact irritation

Pregnancy Risk Factor A

Generic Available Yes: Capsule

Comments 100% elemental iron

Polysporin® Ophthalmic *see* Bacitracin and Polymyxin B *on page 157*

Polysporin® Topical [OTC] *see* Bacitracin and Polymyxin B *on page 157*

Polytar® [OTC] *see* Coal Tar *on page 359*

Polythiazide (pol i THYE a zide)

Related Information

Cardiovascular Diseases *on page 1456*

U.S. Brand Names Renese®

Pharmacologic Category Diuretic, Thiazide

Use Adjunctive therapy in treatment of edema and hypertension

Local Anesthetic/Vasoconstrictor Precautions No information available to require special precautions

Effects on Dental Treatment No significant effects or complications reported

Dosage Adults: Oral:

Edema: 1-4 mg/day

Hypertension: 2-4 mg/day

Mechanism of Action The diuretic mechanism of action of the thiazides is primarily inhibition of sodium, chloride, and water reabsorption in the renal distal tubules, thereby producing diuresis with a resultant reduction in plasma volume. The antihypertensive mechanism of action of the thiazides is unknown. It is known that doses of thiazides produce greater reductions in blood pressure than equivalent diuretic doses of loop diuretics (eg, furosemide). There has been speculation that the thiazides may have some influence on vascular tone mediated through sodium depletion, but this remains to be proven.

Other Adverse Effects

1% to 10%: Hypokalemia

<1% (Limited to important or life-threatening): Anorexia, blood dyscrasias (rarely), drowsiness, hepatitis, hypotension; fluid and electrolyte imbalances (hypercalcemia, hypocalcemia, hypomagnesemia, hyponatremia); hyperglycemia, nausea, pancreatitis, photosensitivity, polyuria, prerenal azotemia, rash, uremia, vomiting

Drug Interactions

Increased Effect/Toxicity: Increased effect of thiazides with furosemide and other loop diuretics. Increased hypotension and/or renal adverse effects of ACE inhibitors may result in aggressively diuresed patients. Beta-blockers increase hyperglycemic effects of thiazides in type 2 diabetes mellitus. Cyclosporine and thiazides can increase the risk of gout or renal toxicity. Digoxin toxicity can be exacerbated if a thiazide induces hypokalemia or hypomagnesemia. Lithium toxicity can occur with thiazides due to reduced renal excretion of lithium. Thiazides may prolong the duration of action with neuromuscular blocking agents.

Decreased Effect: Effects of oral hypoglycemics may be decreased. Decreased absorption of hydrochlorothiazide with cholestyramine and colestipol. NSAIDs can decrease the efficacy of thiazides, reducing the diuretic and antihypertensive effects.

Pharmacodynamics/Kinetics

Onset of action: Diuresis: ~2 hours

Duration: 24-48 hours

Pregnancy Risk Factor D

Generic Available No

Polythiazide and Prazosin *see* Prazosin and Polythiazide *on page 1109*

Polytrim® *see* Trimethoprim and Polymyxin B *on page 1353*

Polyvinyl Alcohol *see* Artificial Tears *on page 128*

Ponstel® *see* Mefenamic Acid *on page 851*

Pontocaine® *see* Tetracaine *on page 1284*

Pontocaine® With Dextrose *see* Tetracaine and Dextrose *on page 1285*

Poractant Alfa (por AKT ent AL fu)

U.S. Brand Names Curosurf®

Canadian Brand Names Curosurf®

Pharmacologic Category Lung Surfactant

Use Orphan drug: Treatment and prevention of respiratory distress syndrome (RDS) in premature infants

Local Anesthetic/Vasoconstrictor Precautions No information available to require special precautions

Effects on Dental Treatment No significant effects or complications reported

Dosage Intratracheal use **only**: Premature infant with RDS: Initial dose is 2.5 mL/kg of birth weight. Up to 2 subsequent doses of 1.25 mL/kg birth weight can be administered at 12-hour intervals if needed in infants who continue to require mechanical ventilation and supplemental oxygen.

Mechanism of Action Endogenous pulmonary surfactant reduces surface tension at the air-liquid interface of the alveoli during ventilation and stabilizes the alveoli against collapse at resting transpulmonary pressures. A deficiency of pulmonary surfactant in preterm infants results in respiratory distress syndrome characterized by poor lung expansion, inadequate gas exchange, and atelectasis. Poractant

(Continued)

Poractant Alfa *(Continued)*

alpha compensates for the surfactant deficiency and restores surface activity to the infant's lungs. It reduces mortality and pneumothoraces associated with RDS.

Other Adverse Effects Frequency not defined:

Cardiovascular: Bradycardia, hypotension

Gastrointestinal: Endotracheal tube blockage

Respiratory: Oxygen desaturation

Pharmacodynamics/Kinetics Information limited to animal models. No human information about pharmacokinetics exists.

Generic Available No

Porfimer (POR fi mer)

U.S. Brand Names Photofrin®

Canadian Brand Names Photofrin®

Pharmacologic Category Antineoplastic Agent, Miscellaneous

Synonyms CL184116; Dihematoporphyrin Ether; Porfimer Sodium

Use Orphan drug: Photodynamic therapy (PDT) with porfimer for palliation of patients with completely obstructing esophageal cancer, or of patients with partially obstructing esophageal cancer who cannot be satisfactorily treated with Nd:YAG laser therapy; completely- or partially-obstructing endobronchial nonsmall cell lung cancer; microinvasive endobronchial nonsmall cell lung cancer

Local Anesthetic/Vasoconstrictor Precautions No information available to require special precautions

Effects on Dental Treatment No significant effects or complications reported

Dosage I.V. (refer to individual protocols):

Children: Safety and efficacy have not been established

Adults: I.V.: 2 mg/kg over 3-5 minutes

Photodynamic therapy is a two-stage process requiring administration of both drug and light. The first stage of PDT is the I.V. injection of porfimer. Illumination with laser light 40-50 hours following the injection with porfimer constitutes the second stage of therapy. A second laser light application may be given 90-120 hours after injection, preceded by gentle debridement of residual tumor.

Patients may receive a second course of PDT a minimum of 30 days after the initial therapy; up to three courses of PDT (each separated by a minimum of 30 days) can be given. Before each course of treatment, evaluate patients for the presence of a tracheoesophageal or bronchoesophageal fistula.

Mechanism of Action Photosensitizing agent used in the photodynamic therapy (PDT) of tumors: cytotoxic and antitumor actions of porfimer are light and oxygen dependent. Cellular damage caused by porfimer PDT is a consequence of the propagation of radical reactions.

Other Adverse Effects

>10%:

Cardiovascular: Atrial fibrillation, chest pain

Central nervous system: Fever, pain, insomnia

Dermatologic: Photosensitivity reaction (minor reactions may occur in up to 100%)

Gastrointestinal: Abdominal pain, constipation, dysphagia, nausea, vomiting

Hematologic: Anemia

Neuromuscular & skeletal: Back pain

Respiratory: Dyspnea, pharyngitis, pleural effusion, pneumonia, respiratory insufficiency

1% to 10%:

Cardiovascular: Hypertension, hypotension, edema, cardiac failure, tachycardia, chest pain (substernal)

Central nervous system: Anxiety, confusion

Dermatologic: Increased hair growth, skin discoloration, skin wrinkles, skin nodules, increased skin fragility

Endocrine & metabolic: Dehydration

Gastrointestinal: Diarrhea, dyspepsia, eructation, esophageal edema, esophageal tumor bleeding, esophageal stricture, esophagitis, hematemesis, melena, weight loss, anorexia

Genitourinary: Urinary tract infection

Neuromuscular & skeletal: Weakness

Respiratory: Coughing, tracheoesophageal fistula

Miscellaneous: Moniliasis, surgical complication

Drug Interactions

Increased Effect/Toxicity: Concomitant administration of other photosensitizing agents (eg, tetracyclines, sulfonamides, phenothiazines, sulfonylureas, thiazide diuretics, griseofulvin) could increase the photosensitivity reaction.

Decreased Effect: Compounds that quench active oxygen species or scavenge radicals (eg, dimethyl sulfoxide, beta-carotene, ethanol, mannitol) would be expected to decrease photodynamic therapy (PDT) activity. Allopurinol, calcium channel blockers, and some prostaglandin synthesis inhibitors could interfere with porfimer. Drugs that decrease clotting, vasoconstriction, or platelet aggregation could decrease the efficacy of PDT. Glucocorticoid hormones may decrease the efficacy of the treatment.

Dietary/Ethanol/Herb Considerations Ethanol: Avoid use; may decrease photodynamic therapy (PDT) activity.

Pharmacodynamics/Kinetics

Distribution: V_{dss}: 0.49 L/kg
Protein binding, plasma: 90%
Half-life elimination: 250 hours
Time to peak, serum: ~2 hours
Excretion: Clearance: Plasma: Total: 0.051 mL/minute/kg

Pregnancy Risk Factor C

Generic Available No

Porfimer Sodium *see* Porfimer *on page 1098*

Portia™ *see* Combination Hormonal Contraceptives *on page 368*

Post Peel Healing Balm [OTC] *see* Hydrocortisone *on page 688*

Posture® [OTC] *see* Calcium Phosphate (Tribasic) *on page 227*

Posture® [OTC] *see* Calcium Supplements *on page 229*

Potassium Acetate (poe TASS ee um AS e tate)

Pharmacologic Category Electrolyte Supplement, Parenteral

Use Potassium deficiency; to avoid chloride when high concentration of potassium is needed, source of bicarbonate

Local Anesthetic/Vasoconstrictor Precautions No information available to require special precautions

Effects on Dental Treatment No significant effects or complications reported

Dosage I.V. doses should be incorporated into the patient's maintenance I.V. fluids, intermittent I.V. potassium administration should be reserved for severe depletion situations and requires EKG monitoring; doses listed as mEq of potassium

Treatment of hypokalemia: I.V.:
- Children: 2-5 mEq/kg/day
- Adults: 40-100 mEq/day

I.V. intermittent infusion (must be diluted prior to administration):
- Children: 0.5-1 mEq/kg/dose (maximum: 30 mEq/dose) to infuse at 0.3-0.5 mEq/kg/hour (maximum: 1 mEq/kg/hour)
- Adults: 5-10 mEq/dose (maximum: 40 mEq/dose) to infuse over 2-3 hours (maximum: 40 mEq over 1 hour)

Note: Continuous cardiac monitor recommended for rates >0.5 mEq/hour

Potassium dosage/rate of infusion guidelines:
- Serum potassium >2.5 mEq/L: Maximum infusion rate: 10 mEq/hour; maximum concentration: 40 mEq/L; maximum 24-hour dose: 200 mEq
- Serum potassium <2.5 mEq/L: Maximum infusion rate: 40 mEq/hour; maximum concentration: 80 mEq/L; maximum 24-hour dose: 400 mEq

Mechanism of Action Potassium is the major cation of intracellular fluid and is essential for the conduction of nerve impulses in heart, brain, and skeletal muscle; contraction of cardiac, skeletal and smooth muscles; maintenance of normal renal function, acid-base balance, carbohydrate metabolism, and gastric secretion

Other Adverse Effects

1% to 10%:
- Cardiovascular: Bradycardia
- Endocrine & metabolic: Hyperkalemia
- Neuromuscular & skeletal: Weakness
- Respiratory: Dyspnea
- Local: Local tissue necrosis with extravasation

<1%: Abdominal pain, alkalosis, chest pain, mental confusion, paralysis, paresthesia, phlebitis, throat pain

Drug Interactions Increased Effect/Toxicity: Potassium-sparing diuretics, salt substitutes, and ACE inhibitors

Pharmacodynamics/Kinetics

Distribution: Enters cells via active transport from extracellular fluid
Excretion: Primarily urine; skin and feces (small amounts); most intestinal potassium reabsorbed

Pregnancy Risk Factor C

Generic Available Yes

Comments 1 mEq of acetate is equivalent to the alkalinizing effect of 1 mEq of bicarbonate.

Potassium Acetate *see* Potassium Supplements *on page 1102*

Potassium Acetate, Potassium Bicarbonate, and Potassium Citrate *see* Potassium Supplements *on page 1102*

Potassium Acid Phosphate *see* Phosphate Supplements *on page 1076*

Potassium Acid Phosphate (poe TASS ee um AS id FOS fate)

U.S. Brand Names K-Phos® Original

Pharmacologic Category Urinary Acidifying Agent

Use Acidifies urine and lowers urinary calcium concentration; reduces odor and rash caused by ammoniacal urine; increases the antibacterial activity of methenamine

Local Anesthetic/Vasoconstrictor Precautions No information available to require special precautions

Effects on Dental Treatment No significant effects or complications reported

Dosage Adults: Oral: 1000 mg dissolved in 6-8 oz of water 4 times/day with meals and at bedtime; for best results, soak tablets in water for 2-5 minutes, then stir and swallow

Mechanism of Action The principal intracellular cation; involved in transmission of nerve impulses, muscle contractions, enzyme activity, and glucose utilization

Other Adverse Effects

>10%: Gastrointestinal: Diarrhea, nausea, stomach pain, flatulence, vomiting

1% to 10%:

- Cardiovascular: Bradycardia
- Endocrine & metabolic: Hyperkalemia
- Local: Local tissue necrosis with extravasation
- Neuromuscular & skeletal: Weakness
- Respiratory: Dyspnea

<1%: Abdominal pain, alkalosis, arrhythmia, arthralgia, bone pain, chest pain, decreased urine output, dyspnea, edema, weight gain, hyperphosphatemia, hypocalcemia, mental confusion, pain of extremities, paralysis, paresthesia, phlebitis, tetany, thirst, throat pain, weakness of extremities

Drug Interactions

Increased Effect/Toxicity: Potassium-sparing diuretics, salt substitutes, salicylates, and ACE inhibitors

Decreased Effect: Antacids containing magnesium, calcium or aluminum (bind phosphate and decreased its absorption)

Pharmacodynamics/Kinetics

Absorption: Well absorbed from upper GI tract

Distribution: Enters cells via active transport from extracellular fluid

Excretion: Primarily urine; skin and feces (small amounts); most intestinal potassium reabsorbed

Pregnancy Risk Factor C

Generic Available No

Potassium Acid Phosphate *see* Potassium Supplements *on page 1102*

Potassium Bicarbonate *see* Potassium Supplements *on page 1102*

Potassium Bicarbonate and Potassium Chloride *see* Potassium Supplements *on page 1102*

Potassium Bicarbonate and Potassium Citrate *see* Potassium Supplements *on page 1102*

Potassium Chloride *see* Potassium Supplements *on page 1102*

Potassium Citrate (poe TASS ee um SIT rate)

U.S. Brand Names Urocit®-K

Canadian Brand Names K-Lyte®; Polycitra®

Pharmacologic Category Alkalinizing Agent

Use Prevention of uric acid nephrolithiasis; prevention of calcium renal stones in patients with hypocitraturia; urinary alkalinizer when sodium citrate is contraindicated

Local Anesthetic/Vasoconstrictor Precautions No information available to require special precautions

Effects on Dental Treatment No significant effects or complications reported

Dosage Adults: Oral: 10-20 mEq 3 times/day with meals up to 100 mEq/day

Other Adverse Effects

>10%: Gastrointestinal: Diarrhea, nausea, stomach pain, flatulence, vomiting (oral)

1% to 10%:

- Cardiovascular: Bradycardia
- Endocrine & metabolic: Hyperkalemia, metabolic alkalosis in patients with severe renal failure
- Neuromuscular & skeletal: Weakness
- Respiratory: Dyspnea

<1% (Limited to important or life-threatening): Arrhythmias, chest pain, heart block, hypotension

Drug Interactions Increased Effect/Toxicity: Concurrent administration with potassium-containing medications, potassium-sparing diuretics, ACE inhibitors, or cardiac glycosides could lead to toxicity.

Pharmacodynamics/Kinetics Metabolism: Hepatic to bicarbonate

Pregnancy Risk Factor Not available

Generic Available No

Comments Parenteral K_3PO_4 contains 3 mmol of phosphorous/mL and 4.4 mEq of potassium/mL. If ordering by phosphorous content, use mmol instead of mEq since the mEq value for phosphorous varies with the pH of the solution due to valence changes of the phosphorus ion. (1 mmol of phosphorous = 31 mg)

Potassium Citrate *see* Potassium Supplements *on page 1102*

Potassium Citrate and Citric Acid

(poe TASS ee um SIT rate & SI trik AS id)

Related Information

Potassium Citrate *on page 1100*

U.S. Brand Names Cytra-K; Polycitra®-K

Pharmacologic Category Alkalinizing Agent

Synonyms Citric Acid and Potassium Citrate

Use Treatment of metabolic acidosis; alkalinizing agent in conditions where long-term maintenance of an alkaline urine is desirable

Local Anesthetic/Vasoconstrictor Precautions No information available to require special precautions

Effects on Dental Treatment No significant effects or complications reported

Dosage Oral:

Mild to moderate hypocitraturia: 10 mEq 3 times/day with meals

Severe hypocitraturia: Initial: 20 mEq 3 times/day or 15 mEq 4 times/day with meals or within 30 minutes after meals; do not exceed 100 mEq/day

Other Adverse Effects

>10%: Gastrointestinal: Diarrhea, nausea, stomach pain, flatulence, vomiting (oral)

1% to 10%:

- Cardiovascular: Bradycardia
- Endocrine & metabolic: Hyperkalemia, metabolic alkalosis in patients with severe renal failure
- Neuromuscular & skeletal: Weakness
- Respiratory: Dyspnea

<1% (Limited to important or life-threatening): Chest pain, arrhythmias, heart block, hypotension

Drug Interactions Increased Effect/Toxicity: Concurrent administration with potassium-containing medications, potassium-sparing diuretics, ACE inhibitors, or cardiac glycosides could lead to toxicity.

Dietary/Ethanol/Herb Considerations Potassium citrate 3.4 mmol/5 mL and citric acid 1.6 mmol/5 mL = total of 5.0 mmol/5 mL citrate content

Pharmacodynamics/Kinetics Metabolism: To potassium bicarbonate; citric acid is metabolized to CO_2 and H_2O

Pregnancy Risk Factor A

Generic Available No

Potassium Citrate, Citric Acid, and Sodium Citrate *see* Citric Acid, Sodium Citrate, and Potassium Citrate *on page 335*

Potassium Citrate Mixture and Sodium Citrate *see* Citric Acid, Sodium Citrate, and Potassium Citrate *on page 335*

Potassium Gluconate *see* Potassium Supplements *on page 1102*

Potassium Iodide (poe TASS ee um EYE oh dide)

Related Information

Endocrine Disorders and Pregnancy *on page 1479*

U.S. Brand Names Iosat™ [OTC]; Pima®; SSKI®

Pharmacologic Category Antithyroid Agent; Expectorant

Synonyms KI; Lugol's Solution; Strong Iodine Solution

Use Expectorant for the symptomatic treatment of chronic pulmonary diseases complicated by mucous; reduce thyroid vascularity prior to thyroidectomy and management of thyrotoxic crisis; block thyroidal uptake of radioactive isotopes of iodine in a radiation emergency or other exposure to radioactive iodine

Unlabeled/Investigational Use Treatment of lymphocutaneous and cutaneous sporotrichosis

Local Anesthetic/Vasoconstrictor Precautions No information available to require special precautions

Effects on Dental Treatment No significant effects or complications reported

Dosage Oral:

Adults: RDA: 150 mcg (iodide)

Expectorant:

- Children (Pima®):
  - <3 years: 162 mg 3 times day
  - >3 years: 325 mg 3 times/day
- Adults:
  - Pima®: 325-650 mg 3 times/day
  - SSKI®: 300-600 mg 3-4 times/day

(Continued)

Potassium Iodide *(Continued)*

Preoperative thyroidectomy: Children and Adults: 50-250 mg (1-5 drops SSKI®) 3 times/day **or** 0.1-0.3 mL (3-5 drops) of strong iodine (Lugol's solution) 3 times/day; administer for 10 days before surgery

Radiation protectant to radioactive isotopes of iodine (Pima®):

Children:

Infants up to 1 year: 65 mg once daily for 10 days; start 24 hours prior to exposure

>1 year: 130 mg once daily for 10 days; start 24 hours prior to exposure

Adults: 195 mg once daily for 10 days; start 24 hours prior to exposure

To reduce risk of thyroid cancer following nuclear accident (dosing should continue until risk of exposure has passed or other measures are implemented):

Children (see adult dose for children >68 kg):

Infants <1 month: 16 mg once daily

1 month to 3 years: 32 mg once daily

3-18 years: 65 mg once daily

Children >68 kg and Adults (including pregnant/lactating women): 130 mg once daily

Thyrotoxic crisis:

Infants <1 year: 150-250 mg (3-5 drops SSKI®) 3 times/day

Children and Adults: 300-500 mg (6-10 drops SSKI®) 3 times/day or 1 mL strong iodine (Lugol's solution) 3 times/day

Sporotrichosis (cutaneous, lymphocutaneous): Adults: Oral: Initial: 5 drops (SSKI®) 3 times/day; increase to 40-50 drops (SSKI®) 3 times/day as tolerated for 3-6 months

Mechanism of Action Reduces viscosity of mucus by increasing respiratory tract secretions; inhibits secretion of thyroid hormone, fosters colloid accumulation in thyroid follicles

Other Adverse Effects Frequency not defined:

Cardiovascular: Irregular heart beat

Central nervous system: Confusion, tiredness, fever

Dermatologic: Skin rash

Endocrine & metabolic: Goiter, salivary gland swelling/tenderness, thyroid adenoma, swelling of neck/throat, myxedema, lymph node swelling

Gastrointestinal: Diarrhea, gastrointestinal bleeding, metallic taste, nausea, stomach pain, stomach upset, vomiting

Neuromuscular & skeletal: Numbness, tingling, weakness

Miscellaneous: Chronic iodine poisoning (with prolonged treatment/high doses); iodism, hypersensitivity reactions (angioedema, cutaneous and mucosal hemorrhage, serum sickness-like symptoms)

Drug Interactions Increased Effect/Toxicity: Lithium may cause additive hypothyroid effects; ACE-inhibitors, potassium-sparing diuretics, and potassium/potassium-containing products may lead to hyperkalemia, cardiac arrhythmias, or cardiac arrest

Dietary/Ethanol/Herb Considerations Food: Administer with food to reduce GI upset.

Pharmacodynamics/Kinetics

Onset of action: 24-48 hours

Peak effect: 10-15 days after continuous therapy

Duration: May persist for up to 6 weeks

Excretion: Clearance: Euthyroid patient: Renal: 2 times that of thyroid

Pregnancy Risk Factor D

Generic Available Yes

Potassium Phosphate *see* Phosphate Supplements *on page 1076*

Potassium Phosphate and Sodium Phosphate *see* Phosphate Supplements *on page 1076*

Potassium Supplements (poe TASS ee um SUP le ments)

U.S. Brand Names Effer-K™; Glu-K® [OTC]; K+8; K+10; Kaon-Cl-10®; Kaon-Cl® 20; Kay Ciel®; K+ Care®; K+ Care® ET; K-Dur® 10; K-Dur® 20; K-Lor™; Klor-Con®; Klor-Con® 8; Klor-Con® 10; Klor-Con®/25; Klor-Con®/EF; Klor-Con® M10; Klor-Con® M20; Klotrix®; K-Lyte®; K-Lyte/Cl®; K-Lyte/Cl® 50; K-Lyte® DS; K-Phos® Original; K-Tab®; microK®; microK® 10; Rum-K®; Tri-K®; Urocit®-K

Mexican Brand Names Celek® 20; Clor-K-Zaf®; Cloruro® De Potasio Kaliolite®

Pharmacologic Category Electrolyte Supplement; Electrolyte Supplement, Oral; Electrolyte Supplement, Parenteral

Synonyms KCl (Potassium Chloride); Potassium Acetate; Potassium Acetate, Potassium Bicarbonate, and Potassium Citrate; Potassium Acid Phosphate; Potassium Bicarbonate; Potassium Bicarbonate and Potassium Chloride; Potassium Bicarbonate and Potassium Citrate; Potassium Chloride; Potassium Citrate; Potassium Gluconate

Use Potassium deficiency; treatment or prevention of hypokalemia

Local Anesthetic/Vasoconstrictor Precautions No information available to require special precautions

Effects on Dental Treatment Frequency not defined (usually dependent on rate of elimination or serum concentration): Confusion, weakness, dyspnea, paresthesia, flaccid paralysis

Oral: Nausea, vomiting GI lesions

Dosage Injections should be administered only in patients with adequate urine flow; must be diluted before I.V. use and infused slowly. I.V. doses should be incorporated into the patient's maintenance I.V. fluids; intermittent I.V. potassium administration should be reserved for severe depletion situations and requires EKG monitoring. Doses listed as mEq of **potassium**. When using microencapsulated or wax matrix formulations, use no more than 20 mEq as a single dose.

Do not use in patients with severe tissue trauma. Solid oral dosage forms are contraindicated in patients in whom there is a structural, pathological, and/or pharmacologic cause for delay or arrest in passage through the GI tract. Oral liquid preparation should be used in patients with esophageal compression or delayed gastric emptying time.

Children:

Normal daily requirement: Oral, I.V.:
- Neonates and Infants: 2-6 mEq/kg/day
- Children: 2-3 mEq/kg/day

Prevention of hypokalemia during diuretic therapy: Oral:
- Neonates, Infants, and Children: 1-2 mEq/kg/day in 1-2 divided doses

Treatment of hypokalemia: Oral, I.V.: Neonates, Infants, and Children: 2-5 mEq/kg/day in divided doses

Treatment of hypokalemia: I.V. intermittent infusion (must be diluted prior to administration): Neonates, Infants, and Children: 0.5-1 mEq/kg/dose (maximum dose: 30 mEq) to infuse at 0.3-0.5 mEq/kg/hour (maximum dose: 1 mEq/kg/hour)

Adults:

Normal daily requirement: Oral, I.V.: 40-80 mEq/day

Prevention of hypokalemia during diuretic therapy: Oral: 20-40 mEq/day in 1-2 divided doses

Treatment of hypokalemia: Oral, I.V.: 40-100 mEq/day in divided doses

Treatment of hypokalemia: I.V. intermittent infusion (must be diluted prior to administration): 10-20 mEq/dose (maximum dose: 40 mEq/dose) to infuse over 2-3 hours (maximum dose: 40 mEq over 1 hour)

Mechanism of Action The major cation of intracellular fluid, it is essential for the conduction of nerve impulses in heart, brain, and skeletal muscle; contraction of cardiac, skeletal, and smooth muscles; maintenance of normal renal function, acid-base balance (acetate form), carbohydrate metabolism, and gastric secretion.

Other Adverse Effects Usually dependent on rate of elimination or serum concentration; frequency not defined:

Cardiovascular (with rapid I.V. administration or at high serum concentrations): Arrhythmias and cardiac arrest, heart block, hypotension, bradycardia, chest pain

Endocrine & metabolic: Hyperkalemia, metabolic alkalosis (acetate salt)

Gastrointestinal: Oral: Diarrhea, abdominal pain, flatulence

Local: Pain at the site of injection, phlebitis, tissue necrosis with extravasation

Drug Interactions Increased Effect/Toxicity: Potassium-sparing diuretics, salt substitutes, ACE inhibitors such as captopril and enalapril may result in increased serum potassium.

Dietary/Ethanol/Herb Considerations Some oral products contain tartrazine which may cause allergic reactions in susceptible individuals.

Pregnancy Risk Factor C

Dosage Forms

Potassium acetate: Injection, solution: 2 mEq/mL (20 mL, 50 mL, 100 mL); 4 mEq/mL (50 mL)

Potassium acetate, potassium bicarbonate, and potassium citrate: Solution, oral: Potassium 45 mEq/15 mL (480 mL) [from potassium acetate 1500 mg, potassium bicarbonate 1500 mg, and potassium citrate 1500 mg per 15 mL]

Potassium acid phosphate: Tablet [scored]: 500 mg [phosphorus 114 mg and potassium 144 mg (3.7 mEq) per tablet; sodium free]

Potassium bicarbonate: Tablet for oral solution, effervescent: Potassium 25 mEq

Potassium bicarbonate and potassium chloride:

Tablet for oral solution, effervescent:
- K-Lyte/Cl®: Potassium chloride 25 mEq [potassium chloride 1.5 g and potassium bicarbonate 0.5 g; citrus or fruit punch flavor]
- K-Lyte/Cl® 50: Potassium chloride 50 mEq [potassium chloride 2.24 g and potassium bicarbonate 2 g; citrus or fruit punch flavor]

Potassium bicarbonate and potassium citrate:

Tablet, effervescent: Potassium 25 mEq
- Effer-K™: Potassium 25 mEq
- Klor-Con®/EF: Potassium 25 mEq [orange flavor]
- K-Lyte®: Potassium 25 mEq [lime or orange flavor]
- K-Lyte® DS: Potassium 50 mEq [lime or orange flavor]

Potassium chloride:

Capsule, extended release: 10 mEq [800 mg]

(Continued)

Potassium Supplements *(Continued)*

microK® [microencapsulated]: 8 mEq [600 mg]
microK® 10 [microencapsulated]: 10 mEq [800 mg]
Infusion [premixed in D_5W]: 20 mEq (1000 mL); 30 mEq (1000 mL); 40 mEq (1000 mL)
Infusion [premixed in D_5W and LR]: 20 mEq (1000 mL); 30 mEq (1000 mL)
Infusion [premixed in D_5W and 1/4NS]: 10 mEq (500 mL, 1000 mL); 20 mEq (1000 mL); 30 mEq (1000 mL); 40 mEq (1000 mL)
Infusion [premixed in D_5W and 1/2NS]: 20 mEq (1000 mL); 40 mEq (1000 mL)
Infusion [premixed in D_5 and NS]: 20 mEq (1000 mL); 40 mEq (1000 mL)
Infusion [premixed in D_5W and sodium chloride 0.3%]: 10 mEq (500 mL); 20 mEq (1000 mL)
Infusion [premixed in NS]: 20 mEq (1000 mL); 40 mEq (1000 mL)
Infusion [premixed in SWFI]: 10 mEq (50 mL, 100 mL); 20 mEq (50 mL, 100 mL); 30 mEq (100 mL); 40 mEq (100 mL)
Injection, solution [concentrate]: 2 mEq/mL (5 mL, 10 mL, 15 mL, 20 mL, 250 mL)
Powder, for oral solution: 20 mEq/packet (30s, 100s, 1000s)
K+ Care: 20 mEq/packet (30s) [fruit or orange flavor]
K-Lor®: 20 mEq/packet (30s, 100s)
Kay Ciel® 10%: 20 mEq/packet (30s, 100s) [sugar free]
Klor-Con®: 20 mEq/packet (30s, 100s) [sugar free]
Klor-Con®/25: 25 mEq/packet (30s, 100s) [sugar free]
Solution, oral: 20 mEq/15 mL (480 mL); 40 mEq/15 mL (480 mL)
Kaon-Cl 20: 40 mEq/15 mL (480 ml) [sugar free; contains alcohol; cherry flavor]
Kay Ciel®: 10%: 20 mEq/15 mL (120 mL, 480 mL) [sugar free; contains alcohol]
Rum-K: 20 mEq/10 mL (480 mL) [alcohol free, sugar free; butter/rum flavor]
Tablet, extended release: 8 mEq [600 mg]; 10 mEq [800 mg]; 20 mEq [1500 mg]
K+8: 8 mEq [600 mg]
K+10: 10 mEq [800 mg]
K-Dur® 10 [microencapsulated]: 10 mEq [800 mg]
K-Dur® 20 [microencapsulated]: 20 mEq [1500 mg; scored]
K-Tab®: 10 mEq [800 mg]
Kaon-Cl® 10 [film coated]: 10 mEq [800 mg
Klor-Con® 8: 8 mEq [600 mg; wax matrix]
Klor-Con® 10: 10 mEq [800 mg; wax matrix]
Klor-Con® M10 [microencapsulated]: 10 mEq [800 mg]
Klor-Con® M20 [microencapsulated]: 20 mEq [1500 mg; scored]
Tablet, slow release:
Klotrix® [film coated]: 10 mEq [800 mg; wax matrix]
Potassium citrate: Tablet: 540 mg [5 mEq]; 1080 mg [10 mEq]
Potassium gluconate:
Tablet: 500 mg, 610 mg
Glu-K®: 486 mg
Tablet, timed release: 595 mg

Generic Available Yes

Povidone-Iodine (POE vi done EYE oh dyne)

Related Information
Animal and Human Bites Guidelines *on page 1580*
Management of Patients Undergoing Cancer Therapy *on page 1567*

U.S. Brand Names ACU-dyne® [OTC]; Betadine® [OTC]; Betadine® Ophthalmic; Minidyne® [OTC]; Operand® [OTC]; Summer's Eve® Medicated Douche [OTC]; Vagi-Gard® [OTC]

Canadian Brand Names Betadine®; Proviodine

Mexican Brand Names Isodine®; Yodine®

Pharmacologic Category Antibiotic, Ophthalmic; Antibiotic, Topical; Antibiotic, Vaginal; Topical Skin Product

Use External antiseptic with broad microbicidal spectrum against bacteria, fungi, viruses, protozoa, and yeasts

Local Anesthetic/Vasoconstrictor Precautions No information available to require special precautions

Effects on Dental Treatment No significant effects or complications reported

Dosage
Shampoo: Apply 2 teaspoons to hair and scalp, lather and rinse; repeat application 2 times/week until improvement is noted, then shampoo weekly
Topical: Apply as needed for treatment and prevention of susceptible microbial infections

Mechanism of Action Povidone-iodine is known to be a powerful broad spectrum germicidal agent effective against a wide range of bacteria, viruses, fungi, protozoa, and spores.

Other Adverse Effects
1% to 10%:
Dermatologic: Rash, pruritus
Local: Local edema

<1%: Systemic absorption in extensive burns causing iododerma, metabolic acidosis, renal impairment

Pharmacodynamics/Kinetics Absorption: Topical: Healthy volunteers: Little systemic absorption; Vaginal: Rapid, serum concentrations of total iodine and inorganic iodide are increased significantly

Pregnancy Risk Factor D

Generic Available Yes

PPD *see* Tuberculin Tests *on page 1362*

PPL *see* Benzylpenicilloyl-polylysine *on page 174*

PPS *see* Pentosan Polysulfate Sodium *on page 1056*

Pramipexole (pra mi PEKS ole)

U.S. Brand Names Mirapex®

Canadian Brand Names Mirapex®

Pharmacologic Category Anti-Parkinson's Agent, Dopamine Agonist

Use Treatment of the signs and symptoms of idiopathic Parkinson's disease

Unlabeled/Investigational Use Treatment of depression

Local Anesthetic/Vasoconstrictor Precautions No information available to require special precautions

Effects on Dental Treatment No significant effects or complications reported

Dosage Adults: Oral: Initial: 0.375 mg/day given in 3 divided doses, increase gradually by 0.125 mg/dose every 5-7 days; range: 1.5-4.5 mg/day

Mechanism of Action Pramipexole is a nonergot dopamine agonist with specificity for the D_2 subfamily dopamine receptor, and has also been shown to bind to D_3 and D_4 receptors. By binding to these receptors, it is thought that pramipexole can stimulate dopamine activity on the nerves of the striatum and substantia nigra.

Other Adverse Effects

>10%:

Cardiovascular: Postural hypotension

Central nervous system: Asthenia, dizziness, somnolence, insomnia, hallucinations, abnormal dreams

Gastrointestinal: Nausea, constipation

Neuromuscular & skeletal: Weakness, dyskinesia, EPS

1% to 10%:

Cardiovascular: Edema, postural hypotension, syncope, tachycardia, chest pain

Central nervous system: Malaise, confusion, amnesia, dystonias, akathisia, thinking abnormalities, myoclonus, hyperesthesia, gait abnormalities, hypertonia, paranoia

Endocrine & metabolic: Decreased libido

Gastrointestinal: Anorexia, weight loss, xerostomia

Genitourinary: Urinary frequency (up to 6%), impotence

Neuromuscular & skeletal: Muscle twitching, leg cramps, arthritis, bursitis

Ocular: Vision abnormalities (3%)

Respiratory: Dyspnea, rhinitis

<1%: Liver transaminases increased

Frequency not defined, dose-related: Falling asleep during activities of daily living

Drug Interactions

Increased Effect/Toxicity: Cimetidine in combination with pramipexole produced a 50% increase in AUC and a 40% increase in half-life. Drugs secreted by the cationic transport system (diltiazem, triamterene, verapamil, quinidine, quinine, ranitidine) decrease the clearance of pramipexole by ~20%.

Decreased Effect: Dopamine antagonists (antipsychotics, metoclopramide) may decrease the efficiency of pramipexole.

Dietary/Ethanol/Herb Considerations

Ethanol: Avoid use; may increase CNS depression.

Food does not affect the extent of drug absorption, although the time to maximal plasma concentration is delayed by 1 hour when taken with a meal.

Herb/Nutraceutical: Avoid kava, SAMe, St John's wort, tryptophan, and valerian; may increase risk of serotonin syndrome and/or excessive sedation.

Pharmacodynamics/Kinetics

Protein binding: 15%

Bioavailability: 90%

Half-life elimination: ~8 hours; Elderly: 12-14 hours

Time to peak, serum: ~2 hours

Excretion: Urine (90% as unchanged drug)

Pregnancy Risk Factor C

Generic Available No

Pramosone® *see* Pramoxine and Hydrocortisone *on page 1106*

Pramoxine (pra MOKS een)

U.S. Brand Names Anusol® Ointment [OTC]; Itch-X® [OTC]; Prax® [OTC]; ProctoFoam® NS [OTC]; Tronolane® [OTC]

Pharmacologic Category Local Anesthetic

(Continued)

Pramoxine *(Continued)*

Synonyms Pramoxine Hydrochloride

Use Temporary relief of pain and itching associated with anogenital pruritus or irritation; dermatosis, minor burns, or hemorrhoids

Local Anesthetic/Vasoconstrictor Precautions No information available to require special precautions

Effects on Dental Treatment No significant effects or complications reported

Dosage Adults: Topical: Apply as directed, usually every 3-4 hours to affected area (maximum adult dose: 200 mg)

Mechanism of Action Pramoxine, like other anesthetics, decreases the neuronal membrane's permeability to sodium ions; both initiation and conduction of nerve impulses are blocked, thus depolarization of the neuron is inhibited

Other Adverse Effects

1% to 10%:

Dermatologic: Angioedema

Local: Contact dermatitis, burning, stinging

<1%: Edema, methemoglobinemia in infants, urethritis, urticaria, tenderness

Pharmacodynamics/Kinetics

Onset of action: Therapeutic: 2-5 minutes

Peak effect: 3-5 minutes

Duration: Several days

Pregnancy Risk Factor C

Generic Available No

Pramoxine and Hydrocortisone

(pra MOKS een & hye droe KOR ti sone)

Related Information

Hydrocortisone *on page 688*

Pramoxine *on page 1105*

U.S. Brand Names Analpram-HC®; Enzone®; Epifoam®; Pramosone®; ProctoFoam®-HC; Zone-A®; Zone-A Forte®

Canadian Brand Names Pramox® HC; Proctofoam™-HC

Pharmacologic Category Anesthetic/Corticosteroid

Synonyms Hydrocortisone and Pramoxine

Use Treatment of severe anorectal or perianal swelling

Local Anesthetic/Vasoconstrictor Precautions No information available to require special precautions

Effects on Dental Treatment No significant effects or complications reported

Dosage Apply to affected areas 3-4 times/day

Pregnancy Risk Factor C

Generic Available No

Pramoxine Hydrochloride *see* Pramoxine *on page 1105*

Prandin® *see* Repaglinide *on page 1172*

Pravachol® *see* Pravastatin *on page 1106*

Pravastatin (PRA va stat in)

Related Information

Cardiovascular Diseases *on page 1456*

U.S. Brand Names Pravachol®

Canadian Brand Names Apo®-Pravastatin; Lin-Pravastatin; Novo-Pravastatin; Pravachol®

Mexican Brand Names Pravacol®

Pharmacologic Category Antilipemic Agent, HMG-CoA Reductase Inhibitor

Synonyms Pravastatin Sodium

Use Use with dietary therapy for the following:

Primary prevention of coronary events: In hypercholesterolemic patients without established coronary heart disease to reduce cardiovascular morbidity (MI, coronary revascularization procedures) and mortality.

Secondary prevention of cardiovascular events in patients with established coronary heart disease: To slow the progression of coronary atherosclerosis; to reduce cardiovascular morbidity (MI, coronary vascular procedures) and to reduce mortality; to reduce the risk of stroke and transient ischemic attacks

Hyperlipidemias: Reduce elevations in total cholesterol, LDL-C, apolipoprotein B, and triglycerides (elevations of 1 or more components are present in Fredrickson type IIa, IIb, III, and IV hyperlipidemias)

Heterozygous familial hypercholesterolemia (HeFH): In pediatric patients, 8-18 years of age, with HeFH having ≥190 mg/dL **or** LDL ≥160 mg/dL with positive family history of premature cardiovascular disease (CVD) or 2 or more CVD risk factors in the pediatric patient

Local Anesthetic/Vasoconstrictor Precautions No information available to require special precautions

Effects on Dental Treatment No effects of complications reported

Dosage Doses should be individualized according to the baseline LDL-cholesterol levels, the recommended goal of therapy, and patient response. Adjustments should be made at intervals of 4 weeks or more; doses may need adjusted based on concomitant medications.

Oral:

Children: HeFH:

8-13 years: 20 mg/day

14-18 years: 40 mg/day

Dosing adjustment for pravastatin based on concomitant immunosuppressants (ie, cyclosporine): Refer to Adults dosing section

Adults: Hyperlipidemias, primary prevention of coronary events, secondary prevention of cardiovascular events: Initial: 40 mg once daily; titrate dosage to response; usual range: 10-80 mg; (maximum dose: 80 mg once daily)

Dosing adjustment for pravastatin based on concomitant immunosuppressants (ie, cyclosporine): Initial: 10 mg/day, titrate with caution (maximum dose: 20 mg/day)

Elderly: No specific recommendations; clearance is reduced resulting in an increase in AUC between 25% to 50% but substantial accumulation is not expected.

Dosing adjustment in renal/hepatic impairment: Initial: 10 mg/day

Mechanism of Action Pravastatin is a competitive inhibitor of 3-hydroxy-3-methylglutaryl coenzyme A (HMG-CoA) reductase, which is the rate-limiting enzyme involved in *de novo* cholesterol synthesis.

Other Adverse Effects As reported in short-term trials; safety and tolerability with long-term use were similar to placebo

1% to 10%:

Cardiovascular: Chest pain (4%)

Central nervous system: Headache (2% to 6%), fatigue (4%), dizziness (1% to 3%)

Dermatologic: Rash (4%)

Gastrointestinal: Nausea/vomiting (7%), diarrhea (6%), heartburn (3%)

Hepatic: Increased transaminases (>3x normal on two occasions - 1%)

Neuromuscular & skeletal: Myalgia (2%)

Respiratory: Cough (3%)

Miscellaneous: Influenza (2%)

<1%: Allergy, alopecia, appetite decreased, dermatitis, dry skin, edema, fever, flushing, insomnia, lens opacity, libido change, memory impairment, muscle weakness, neuropathy, paresthesia, pruritus, sexual dysfunction, abnormal taste, tremor, urticaria, vertigo

Postmarketing and/or case reports: Anaphylaxis, cholestatic jaundice, cirrhosis, cranial nerve dysfunction, dermatomyositis, erythema multiforme, ESR increase, fulminant hepatic necrosis, gynecomastia, hemolytic anemia, hepatitis, hepatoma, lupus erythematosus-like syndrome, myopathy, pancreatitis, peripheral nerve palsy, polymyalgia rheumatica, positive ANA, purpura, rhabdomyolysis, Stevens-Johnson syndrome, vasculitis

Additional class-related events or case reports (not necessarily reported with pravastatin therapy): Angioedema, cataracts, depression, dyspnea, eosinophilia, erectile dysfunction, facial paresis, hypersensitivity reaction, impaired extraocular muscle movement, impotence, leukopenia, malaise, memory loss, ophthalmoplegia, paresthesia, peripheral neuropathy, photosensitivity, psychic disturbance, skin discoloration, thrombocytopenia, thyroid dysfunction, toxic epidermal necrolysis, transaminases increased, vomiting

Drug Interactions Substrate of CYP3A4; Inhibits CYP2C8/9, 2D6, 3A4

Increased Effect/Toxicity: Clofibrate, fenofibrate, gemfibrozil, and niacin may increase the risk of myopathy and rhabdomyolysis. Imidazole antifungals (itraconazole, ketoconazole), P-glycoprotein inhibitors may increase pravastatin concentrations.

Decreased Effect: Concurrent administration of cholestyramine or colestipol can decrease pravastatin absorption.

Dietary/Ethanol/Herb Considerations

Ethanol: Large amounts may increase risk of liver damage.

Food: May be taken with food; requires a standard cholesterol-lowering diet for 3-6 months prior to and during therapy.

Herb/Nutraceutical: Avoid St John's wort; may decrease serum concentration.

Pharmacodynamics/Kinetics

Onset of action: Several days

Peak effect: 4 weeks

Absorption: Poor

Protein binding: 50%

Metabolism: Hepatic to at least two metabolites

Bioavailability: 17%

Half-life elimination: ~2-3 hours

Time to peak, serum: 1-1.5 hours

Excretion: Urine (≤20%, 8% as unchanged drug)

Pregnancy Risk Factor X

Generic Available No

Pravastatin Sodium *see* Pravastatin *on page 1106*

Prax® [OTC] *see* Pramoxine *on page 1105*

Praziquantel (pray zi KWON tel)

U.S. Brand Names Biltricide®

Canadian Brand Names Biltricide®

Mexican Brand Names Cesol®; Cisticid®; Tecprazin

Pharmacologic Category Anthelmintic

Use All stages of schistosomiasis caused by all *Schistosoma* species pathogenic to humans; clonorchiasis and opisthorchiasis

Unlabeled/Investigational Use Treatment of cysticercosis, flukes, and many intestinal tapeworms

Local Anesthetic/Vasoconstrictor Precautions No information available to require special precautions

Effects on Dental Treatment No significant effects or complications reported

Dosage Children >4 years and Adults: Oral:

Schistosomiasis: 20 mg/kg/dose 2-3 times/day for 1 day at 4- to 6-hour intervals
Flukes: 25 mg/kg/dose every 8 hours for 1-2 days
Cysticercosis: 50 mg/kg/day divided every 8 hours for 14 days
Tapeworms: 10-20 mg/kg as a single dose (25 mg/kg for *Hymenolepis nana*)
Clonorchiasis/opisthorchiasis: 3 doses of 25 mg/kg as a 1-day treatment

Mechanism of Action Increases the cell permeability to calcium in schistosomes, causing strong contractions and paralysis of worm musculature leading to detachment of suckers from the blood vessel walls and to dislodgment

Other Adverse Effects

1% to 10%:

Central nervous system: Dizziness, drowsiness, headache, malaise, CSF reaction syndrome in patients being treated for neurocysticercosis
Gastrointestinal: Abdominal pain, loss of appetite, nausea, vomiting
Miscellaneous: Diaphoresis

<1%: Diarrhea, fever, itching, rash, urticaria

Drug Interactions Inhibits CYP2D6

Pharmacodynamics/Kinetics

Absorption: Oral: ~80%
Distribution: CSF concentration is 14% to 20% of plasma concentration; enters breast milk
Protein binding: ~80%
Metabolism: Extensive first-pass effect
Half-life elimination: Parent drug: 0.8-1.5 hours; Metabolites: 4.5 hours
Time to peak, serum: 1-3 hours
Excretion: Urine (99% as metabolites)

Pregnancy Risk Factor B

Generic Available No

Prazosin (PRA zoe sin)

Related Information

Cardiovascular Diseases *on page 1456*

U.S. Brand Names Minipress®

Canadian Brand Names Apo®-Prazo; Minipress™; Novo-Prazin; Nu-Prazo

Mexican Brand Names Minipres®; Sinozzard®

Pharmacologic Category Alpha$_1$ Blocker

Synonyms Furazosin; Prazosin Hydrochloride

Use Treatment of hypertension

Unlabeled/Investigational Use Treatment of benign prostatic hyperplasia (BPH), Raynaud's syndrome

Local Anesthetic/Vasoconstrictor Precautions No information available to require special precautions

Effects on Dental Treatment ≤10%: Significant xerostomia

Significant orthostatic hypotension a possibility; monitor patient when getting out of dental chair.

Dosage Oral:

Children: Initial: 5 mcg/kg/dose (to assess hypotensive effects); usual dosing interval: every 6 hours; increase dosage gradually up to maximum of 25 mcg/kg/dose every 6 hours

Adults:

Hypertension: Initial: 1 mg/dose 2-3 times/day; usual maintenance dose: 3-15 mg/day in divided doses 2-4 times/day; maximum daily dose: 20 mg
Hypertensive urgency: 10-20 mg once, may repeat in 30 minutes
Raynaud's (unlabeled use): 0.5-3 mg twice daily
Benign prostatic hyperplasia (unlabeled use): 2 mg twice daily

Mechanism of Action Competitively inhibits postsynaptic alpha-adrenergic receptors which results in vasodilation of veins and arterioles and a decrease in total peripheral resistance and blood pressure

Other Adverse Effects

>10%: Central nervous system: Dizziness (10%)

1% to 10%:

Cardiovascular: Palpitations (5%), edema, orthostatic hypotension, syncope (1%)

Central nervous system: Headache (8%), drowsiness (8%), weakness (7%), vertigo, depression, nervousness

Dermatologic: Rash (1% to 4%)

Endocrine & metabolic: Decreased energy (7%)

Gastrointestinal: Nausea (5%), vomiting, diarrhea, constipation

Genitourinary: Urinary frequency (1% to 5%)

Ocular: Blurred vision, reddened sclera

Respiratory: Dyspnea, epistaxis, nasal congestion

<1% (Limited to important or life-threatening): Abdominal discomfort, alopecia, angina, bradycardia, cataracts (both development and disappearance have been reported), hallucinations, impotence, incontinence, lichen planus, liver function abnormalities, MI, narcolepsy (worsened), pancreatitis, paresthesia, pigmentary mottling and serous retinopathy, priapism, pruritus, tachycardia, tinnitus

Postmarketing and/or case reports: Allergic reaction, cataplexy, enuresis, eye pain, gynecomastia, leukopenia, systemic lupus erythematosus, urticaria, vasculitis

Drug Interactions

Increased Effect/Toxicity: Prazosin's hypotensive effect may be increased with beta-blockers, diuretics, ACE inhibitors, calcium channel blockers, and other antihypertensive medications. Concurrent use with tricyclic antidepressants (TCAs) and low-potency antipsychotics may increase risk of orthostasis.

Decreased Effect: Decreased antihypertensive effect if taken with NSAIDs.

Dietary/Ethanol/Herb Considerations

Ethanol: Avoid use; may increase vasodilation.

Food has variable effects on absorption. Avoid caffeine (eg, colas, chocolate), garlic, and licorice.

Herb/Nutraceutical: Avoid black cohosh, dong quai, and evening primrose due to estrogenic activity. Avoid ephedra, ginseng, and yohimbe; may worsen hypertension. Avoid garlic; may have increased antihypertensive effect. Avoid ginger due to positive inotropic effects; theoretically, may cause arrhythmia. Avoid hawthorn; may lower peripheral vascular resistance causing additional decrease in BP. Avoid licorice. Avoid saw palmetto due to limited experience with this combination.

Pharmacodynamics/Kinetics

Onset of action: BP reduction: ~2 hours

Maximum decrease: 2-4 hours

Duration: 10-24 hours

Distribution: Hypertensive adults: V_d: 0.5 L/kg

Protein binding: 92% to 97%

Metabolism: Extensively hepatic

Bioavailability: 43% to 82%

Half-life elimination: 2-4 hours; prolonged with congestive heart failure

Excretion: Urine (6% to 10% as unchanged drug)

Pregnancy Risk Factor C

Generic Available Yes

Prazosin and Polythiazide (PRA zoe sin & pol i THYE a zide)

Related Information

Polythiazide *on page 1097*

Prazosin *on page 1108*

U.S. Brand Names Minizide®

Pharmacologic Category Antihypertensive Agent Combination

Synonyms Polythiazide and Prazosin

Use Management of mild to moderate hypertension

Local Anesthetic/Vasoconstrictor Precautions No information available to require special precautions

Effects on Dental Treatment ≤10%: Significant xerostomia

Significant orthostatic hypotension a possibility; monitor patient when getting out of dental chair.

Dosage Adults: Oral: 1 capsule 2-3 times/day

Pregnancy Risk Factor C

Generic Available No

Prazosin Hydrochloride *see* Prazosin *on page 1108*

Precedex™ *see* Dexmedetomidine *on page 416*

Precose® *see* Acarbose *on page 24*

Pred Forte® *see* PrednisoLONE *on page 1110*

Pred-G® *see* Prednisolone and Gentamicin *on page 1112*

Pred Mild® *see* PrednisoLONE *on page 1110*

Prednicarbate (PRED ni kar bate)

U.S. Brand Names Dermatop®

Canadian Brand Names Dermatop®

Pharmacologic Category Corticosteroid, Topical

Use Relief of the inflammatory and pruritic manifestations of corticosteroid-responsive dermatoses (medium potency topical corticosteroid)

Local Anesthetic/Vasoconstrictor Precautions No information available to require special precautions

Effects on Dental Treatment No significant effects or complications reported

Dosage Adults: Topical: Apply a thin film to affected area twice daily. Therapy should be discontinued when control is achieved; if no improvement is seen, reassessment of diagnosis may be necessary.

Mechanism of Action Topical corticosteroids have anti-inflammatory, antipruritic, vasoconstrictive, and antiproliferative actions

Other Adverse Effects

1% to 10%: Dermatologic: Skin atrophy, shininess, thinness, mild telangiectasia

<1%: Pruritus, edema, urticaria, burning, allergic contact dermatitis and rash, folliculitis, acneiform eruptions, hypopigmentation, perioral dermatitis, secondary infection, striae, miliaria, paresthesia

Pregnancy Risk Factor C

Generic Available No

PrednisoLONE (pred NIS oh lone)

Related Information

Neomycin, Polymyxin B, and Prednisolone *on page 963*
PredniSONE *on page 1112*
Respiratory Diseases *on page 1476*

U.S. Brand Names AK-Pred®; Econopred®; Econopred® Plus; Inflamase® Forte; Inflamase® Mild; Orapred®; Pediapred®; Pred Forte®; Pred Mild®; Prelone®

Canadian Brand Names Diopred®; Hydeltra T.B.A.®; Inflamase® Forte; Inflamase® Mild; Novo-Prednisolone®; Ophtho-Tate®; Ophtho-tate®; Pediapred®; Pred Forte®; Pred Mild®

Mexican Brand Names Fisopred®; Sophipren Ofteno

Pharmacologic Category Corticosteroid, Ophthalmic; Corticosteroid, Systemic

Synonyms Deltahydrocortisone; Metacortandralone; Prednisolone Acetate; Prednisolone Acetate, Ophthalmic; Prednisolone Sodium Phosphate; Prednisolone Sodium Phosphate, Ophthalmic

Use

Dental: Treatment of a variety of oral diseases of allergic, inflammatory, or autoimmune origin

Medical: Treatment of palpebral and bulbar conjunctivitis; corneal injury from chemical, radiation, thermal burns, or foreign body penetration; endocrine disorders, rheumatic disorders, collagen diseases, dermatologic diseases, allergic states, ophthalmic diseases, respiratory diseases, hematologic disorders, neoplastic diseases, edematous states, and GI diseases; useful in patients with inability to activate prednisone (liver disease)

Local Anesthetic/Vasoconstrictor Precautions No information available to require special precautions

Effects on Dental Treatment

>10%: Nervousness

1% to 10%: Epistaxis, diabetes mellitus

Dosage Dose depends upon condition being treated and response of patient; dosage for infants and children should be based on severity of the disease and response of the patient rather than on strict adherence to dosage indicated by age, weight, or body surface area. Consider alternate day therapy for long-term therapy. Discontinuation of long-term therapy requires gradual withdrawal by tapering the dose.

Children: Oral:
- Acute asthma: 1-2 mg/kg/day in divided doses 1-2 times/day for 3-5 days
- Anti-inflammatory or immunosuppressive dose: 0.1-2 mg/kg/day in divided doses 1-4 times/day
- Nephrotic syndrome:
  - Initial (first 3 episodes): 2 mg/kg/day **or** 60 mg/m^2/day (maximum: 80 mg/day) in divided doses 3-4 times/day until urine is protein free for 3 consecutive days (maximum: 28 days); followed by 1-1.5 mg/kg/dose **or** 40 mg/m^2/dose given every other day for 4 weeks
  - Maintenance (long-term maintenance dose for frequent relapses): 0.5-1 mg/kg/dose given every other day for 3-6 months

Adults: Oral:
- Usual range: 5-60 mg/day
- Multiple sclerosis: 200 mg/day for 1 week followed by 80 mg every other day for 1 month
- Rheumatoid arthritis: Initial: 5-7.5 mg/day; adjust dose as necessary

Elderly: Use lowest effective dose

Dosing adjustment in hyperthyroidism: Prednisolone dose may need to be increased to achieve adequate therapeutic effects

Hemodialysis: Slightly dialyzable (5% to 20%); administer dose posthemodialysis

Peritoneal dialysis: Supplemental dose is unnecessary

Ophthalmic suspension/solution: Children and Adults: Instill 1-2 drops into conjunctival sac every hour during day, every 2 hours at night until favorable response is obtained, then use 1 drop every 4 hours

Mechanism of Action Decreases inflammation by suppression of migration of polymorphonuclear leukocytes and reversal of increased capillary permeability; suppresses the immune system by reducing activity and volume of the lymphatic system

Other Adverse Effects

>10%:

Central nervous system: Insomnia

Gastrointestinal: Increased appetite, indigestion

1% to 10%:

Dermatologic: Hirsutism

Neuromuscular & skeletal: Arthralgia

Ocular: Cataracts, glaucoma

<1%: Abdominal distention, edema, **hypertension**, vertigo, **seizures, psychoses, pseudotumor cerebri, headache, mood swings, delirium, hallucinations, euphoria,** acne, **skin atrophy, bruising**, hyperpigmentation, Cushing's syndrome, pituitary-adrenal axis suppression, growth suppression, glucose intolerance, hypokalemia, alkalosis, amenorrhea, sodium and water retention, **hyperglycemia, peptic ulcer, nausea, vomiting, ulcerative esophagitis**, pancreatitis, **muscle weakness, osteoporosis, increased fractures, muscle wasting, hypersensitivity reactions**

Contraindications Hypersensitivity to prednisolone or any component of the formulation; acute superficial herpes simplex keratitis; systemic fungal infections; varicella

Warnings/Precautions Use with caution in patients with hyperthyroidism, cirrhosis, nonspecific ulcerative colitis, hypertension, osteoporosis, thromboembolic tendencies, CHF, convulsive disorders, myasthenia gravis, thrombophlebitis, peptic ulcer, diabetes; acute adrenal insufficiency may occur with abrupt withdrawal after long-term therapy or with stress; young pediatric patients may be more susceptible to adrenal axis suppression from topical therapy. Because of the risk of adverse effects, systemic corticosteroids should be used cautiously in the elderly, in the smallest possible dose, and for the shortest possible time.

Drug Interactions Substrate of CYP3A4; Inhibits CYP3A4

Decreased effect of salicylates, vaccines, and toxoids. Barbiturates, phenytoin, rifampin decrease corticosteroid effectiveness.

Dietary/Ethanol/Herb Considerations

Ethanol: Avoid use; may increase gastric mucosal irritation.

Food: Administer with food or milk to reduce GI upset. Prednisolone interferes with calcium absorption; increase intake of calcium, folate, phosphorus, pyridoxine, vitamin C, and vitamin D. Limit caffeine.

Herb/Nutraceutical: Avoid cat's claw and echinacea due to immunostimulant properties. Avoid St John's wort; may decrease serum concentration.

Pharmacodynamics/Kinetics

Duration: 18-36 hours

Protein binding (concentration dependent): 65% to 91%

Metabolism: Primarily hepatic, but also metabolized in most tissues, to inactive compounds

Half-life elimination: 3.6 hours; End-stage renal disease: 3-5 hours

Excretion: Primarily urine (as glucuronides, sulfates, and unconjugated metabolites)

Pregnancy Risk Factor C

Dosage Forms **SOLN, ophthalmic, as sodium phosphate:** 1% (5 mL, 10 mL, 15 mL); (AK-Pred®): 1% (5 mL, 15 mL); (Inflamase® Forte): 1% (5 mL, 10 mL, 15 mL); (Inflamase® Mild): 0.125% (5 mL, 10 mL). **SOLN, oral, as sodium phosphate:** Prednisolone base 5 mg/5 mL (120 mL); (Orapred®): 20 mg/5 mL (240 mL); (Pediapred®): 6.7 mg/5 mL (120 mL). **SUSP, ophthalmic, as acetate:** 1% (5 mL, 10 mL, 15 mL); (Econopred®): 0.125% (5 mL, 10 mL); (Econopred® Plus): 1% (5 mL, 10 mL); (Pred Forte®): 1% (1 mL, 5 mL, 10 mL, 15 mL); (Pred Mild®): 0.12% (5 mL, 10 mL). **SYRUP, as base:** 5 mg/5 mL (120 mL), 15 mg/5 mL (240 mL, 480 mL); (Prelone®): 5 mg/5 mL (120 mL), 15 mg/5 mL (240 mL, 480 mL). **TAB, as base:** 5 mg

Generic Available Yes

Prednisolone Acetate *see* PrednisoLONE *on page 1110*

Prednisolone Acetate, Ophthalmic *see* PrednisoLONE *on page 1110*

Prednisolone and Chloramphenicol *see* Chloramphenicol and Prednisolone *on page 299*

Prednisolone and Gentamicin (pred NIS oh lone & jen tu MYE sin)

Related Information

PrednisoLONE *on page 1110*

U.S. Brand Names Pred-G®

Pharmacologic Category Antibiotic/Corticosteroid, Ophthalmic

Synonyms Gentamicin and Prednisolone

Use Treatment of steroid responsive inflammatory conditions and superficial ocular infections due to strains of microorganisms susceptible to gentamicin such as *Staphylococcus, E. coli, H. influenzae, Klebsiella, Neisseria, Pseudomonas, Proteus,* and *Serratia* species

Local Anesthetic/Vasoconstrictor Precautions No information available to require special precautions

Effects on Dental Treatment Frequency not defined: Delayed wound healing, secondary infection

Dosage Children and Adults: Ophthalmic: 1 drop 2-4 times/day; during the initial 24-48 hours, the dosing frequency may be increased if necessary

Other Adverse Effects Frequency not defined:

Local: Burning, stinging

Ocular: Intraocular pressure increased, glaucoma, superficial punctate keratitis, optic nerve damage (infrequent), posterior subcapsular cataract formation

Pregnancy Risk Factor C

Generic Available No

Prednisolone and Sulfacetamide *see* Sulfacetamide and Prednisolone *on page 1250*

Prednisolone, Neomycin, and Polymyxin B *see* Neomycin, Polymyxin B, and Prednisolone *on page 963*

Prednisolone Sodium Phosphate *see* PrednisoLONE *on page 1110*

Prednisolone Sodium Phosphate, Ophthalmic *see* PrednisoLONE *on page 1110*

PredniSONE (PRED ni sone)

Related Information

Oral Nonviral Soft Tissue Ulcerations or Erosions *on page 1549*

PrednisoLONE *on page 1110*

Respiratory Diseases *on page 1476*

Rheumatoid Arthritis, Osteoarthritis, and Osteoporosis *on page 1488*

U.S. Brand Names Deltasone®; Prednisone Intensol™; Sterapred®; Sterapred® DS

Canadian Brand Names Apo®-Prednisone; Winpred™

Mexican Brand Names Meticorten®; Prednidib®

Pharmacologic Category Corticosteroid, Systemic

Synonyms Deltacortisone; Deltadehydrocortisone

Use

Dental: Treatment of a variety of oral diseases of allergic, inflammatory, or autoimmune origin

Medical: Treatment of a variety of diseases including adrenocortical insufficiency, hypercalcemia, rheumatic, and collagen disorders; dermatologic, ocular, respiratory, GI, and neoplastic diseases; organ transplantation and a variety of diseases including those of hematologic, allergic, inflammatory, and autoimmune in origin

Unlabeled/Investigational Use Investigational: Prevention of postherpetic neuralgia and relief of acute pain in the early stages

Local Anesthetic/Vasoconstrictor Precautions No information available to require special precautions

Effects on Dental Treatment

>10%: Nervousness

1% to 10%: Diabetes mellitus, epistaxis, hyperglycemia

Dosage Dose depends upon condition being treated and response of patient; dosage for infants and children should be based on severity of the disease and response of the patient rather than on strict adherence to dosage indicated by age, weight, or body surface area. Consider alternate day therapy for long-term therapy. Discontinuation of long-term therapy requires gradual withdrawal by tapering the dose. Not available in injectable form, prednisolone must be used.

Oral:

Children:

Anti-inflammatory or immunosuppressive dose: 0.05-2 mg/kg/day divided 1-4 times/day

Acute asthma: 1-2 mg/kg/day in divided doses 1-2 times/day for 3-5 days

Alternatively (for 3- to 5-day "burst"):

<1 year: 10 mg every 12 hours

1-4 years: 20 mg every 12 hours

5-13 years: 30 mg every 12 hours

>13 years: 40 mg every 12 hours

Asthma long-term therapy (alternative dosing by age):

<1 year: 10 mg every other day

1-4 years: 20 mg every other day

5-13 years: 30 mg every other day
>13 years: 40 mg every other day
Nephrotic syndrome:
Initial (first 3 episodes): 2 mg/kg/day **or** 60 mg/m²/day (maximum: 80 mg/day) in divided doses 3-4 times/day until urine is protein free for 3 consecutive days (maximum: 28 days); followed by 1-1.5 mg/kg/dose **or** 40 mg/m²/dose given every other day for 4 weeks
Maintenance dose (long-term maintenance dose for frequent relapses): 0.5-1 mg/kg/dose given every other day for 3-6 months
Children and Adults: Physiologic replacement: 4-5 mg/m²/day
Children ≥5 years and Adults: Asthma:
Moderate persistent: Inhaled corticosteroid (medium dose) or inhaled corticosteroid (low-medium dose) with a long-acting bronchodilator
Severe persistent: Inhaled corticosteroid (high dose) and corticosteroid tablets or syrup long term: 2 mg/kg/day, generally not to exceed 60 mg/day
Adults:
Immunosuppression/chemotherapy adjunct: Range: 5-60 mg/day in divided doses 1-4 times/day
Allergic reaction (contact dermatitis):
Day 1: 30 mg divided as 10 mg before breakfast, 5 mg at lunch, 5 mg at dinner, 10 mg at bedtime
Day 2: 5 mg at breakfast, 5 mg at lunch, 5 mg at dinner, 10 mg at bedtime
Day 3: 5 mg 4 times/day (with meals and at bedtime)
Day 4: 5 mg 3 times/day (breakfast, lunch, bedtime)
Day 5: 5 mg 2 times/day (breakfast, bedtime)
Day 6: 5 mg before breakfast
Pneumocystis carinii pneumonia (PCP):
40 mg twice daily for 5 days **followed by**
40 mg once daily for 5 days **followed by**
20 mg once daily for 11 days or until antimicrobial regimen is completed
Thyrotoxicosis: Oral: 60 mg/day
Chemotherapy (refer to individual protocols): Oral: Range: 20 mg/day to 100 mg/m²/day
Rheumatoid arthritis: Oral: Use lowest possible daily dose (often ≤7.5 mg/day)
Idiopathic thrombocytopenia purpura (ITP): Oral: 60 mg daily for 4-6 weeks, gradually tapered over several weeks
Systemic lupus erythematosus (SLE): Oral:
Acute: 1-2 mg/kg/day in 2-3 divided doses
Maintenance: Reduce to lowest possible dose, usually <1 mg/kg/day as single dose (morning)
Elderly: Use the lowest effective dose
Dosing adjustment in hepatic impairment: Prednisone is inactive and must be metabolized by the liver to prednisolone. This conversion may be impaired in patients with liver disease, however, prednisolone levels are observed to be higher in patients with severe liver failure than in normal patients. Therefore, compensation for the inadequate conversion of prednisone to prednisolone occurs.
Dosing adjustment in hyperthyroidism: Prednisone dose may need to be increased to achieve adequate therapeutic effects
Hemodialysis: Supplemental dose is unnecessary
Peritoneal dialysis: Supplemental dose is unnecessary

Mechanism of Action Decreases inflammation by suppression of migration of polymorphonuclear leukocytes and reversal of increased capillary permeability; suppresses the immune system by reducing activity and volume of the lymphatic system; suppresses adrenal function at high doses. Antitumor effects may be related to inhibition of glucose transport, phosphorylation, or induction of cell death in immature lymphocytes. Antiemetic effects are thought to occur due to blockade of cerebral innervation of the emetic center via inhibition of prostaglandin synthesis.

Other Adverse Effects
>10%:
Central nervous system: Insomnia
Gastrointestinal: Increased appetite, indigestion
1% to 10%:
Dermatologic: Hirsutism
Endocrine & metabolic: Glucose intolerance
Neuromuscular & skeletal: Arthralgia
Ocular: Cataracts, glaucoma
<1%: Abdominal distention, edema, **hypertension**, vertigo, **seizures, psychoses, pseudotumor cerebri, headache, mood swings, delirium, hallucinations, euphoria,** acne, **skin atrophy, bruising**, hyperpigmentation, Cushing's syndrome, pituitary-adrenal axis suppression, growth suppression, glucose intolerance, hypokalemia, alkalosis, amenorrhea, sodium and water retention, **hyperglycemia, peptic ulcer, nausea, vomiting, ulcerative esophagitis**, pancreatitis, **muscle weakness, osteoporosis, increased fractures, muscle wasting, hypersensitivity reactions**
(Continued)

PredniSONE *(Continued)*

Contraindications Hypersensitivity to prednisone or any component of the formulation; serious infections, except tuberculous meningitis; systemic fungal infections; varicella

Warnings/Precautions Withdraw therapy with gradual tapering of dose, may retard bone growth. Use with caution in patients with hypothyroidism, cirrhosis, CHF, ulcerative colitis, thromboembolic disorders, and patients at increased risk for peptic ulcer disease. Corticosteroids should be used with caution in patients with diabetes, hypertension, osteoporosis, glaucoma, cataracts, or tuberculosis. Use caution in hepatic impairment. Because of the risk of adverse effects, systemic corticosteroids should be used cautiously in the elderly, in the smallest possible dose, and for the shortest possible time.

Drug Interactions Substrate of CYP3A4; Induces CYP2C19, 3A4

Increased Effect/Toxicity: NSAIDs: Concurrent use of prednisone may increase the risk of GI ulceration.

Decreased effect of salicylates, vaccines, and toxoids. Barbiturates, phenytoin, and rifampin decrease corticosteroid effectiveness.

Dietary/Ethanol/Herb Considerations

Ethanol: Avoid use; may increase gastric mucosal irritation.

Food: Administer after meals or with food or milk. Prednisone interferes with calcium absorption; increase dietary intake of pyridoxine, vitamin C, vitamin D, folate, calcium, and phosphorus. Limit caffeine.

Herb/Nutraceutical: Avoid cat's claw and echinacea due to immunostimulant properties. Avoid St John's wort; may decrease serum concentration.

Pharmacodynamics/Kinetics

Protein binding (concentration dependent): 65% to 91%

Metabolism: Hepatically converted from prednisone (inactive) to prednisolone (active); may be impaired with hepatic dysfunction

Half-life elimination: Normal renal function: 2.5-3.5 hours

See Prednisolone monograph for complete information.

Pregnancy Risk Factor B

Breast-feeding Considerations Crosses into breast milk. No data on clinical effects on the infant. AAP considers **compatible** with breast-feeding.

Dosage Forms SOLN, oral: 1 mg/mL (5 mL, 120 mL, 500 mL). **SOLN, oral concentrate** (Prednisone Intensol™): 5 mg/mL (30 mL). **TAB:** 1 mg, 2.5 mg, 5 mg, 10 mg, 20 mg, 50 mg; (Deltasone®): 2.5 mg, 10 mg, 20 mg, 50 mg; (Sterapred®): 5 mg; (Sterapred® DS): 10 mg

Generic Available Yes

Prednisone Intensol™ *see* PredniSONE *on page 1112*

Prefrin™ [DSC] *see* Phenylephrine *on page 1071*

Pregnenedione *see* Progesterone *on page 1125*

Pregnyl® *see* Chorionic Gonadotropin (Human) *on page 320*

Prelone® *see* PrednisoLONE *on page 1110*

Prelu-2® *see* Phendimetrazine *on page 1064*

Premarin® *see* Estrogens (Conjugated/Equine) *on page 529*

Premjact® [OTC] *see* Lidocaine *on page 801*

Premphase® *see* Estrogens (Conjugated/Equine) and Medroxyprogesterone *on page 531*

Prempro™ *see* Estrogens (Conjugated/Equine) and Medroxyprogesterone *on page 531*

Preparation H® Hydrocortisone [OTC] *see* Hydrocortisone *on page 688*

Pre-Pen® *see* Benzylpenicilloyl-polylysine *on page 174*

Prepidil® *see* Dinoprostone *on page 450*

Pretz-D® [OTC] *see* Ephedrine *on page 499*

Pretz® Irrigation [OTC] *see* Sodium Chloride *on page 1229*

Prevacid® *see* Lansoprazole *on page 777*

Prevalite® *see* Cholestyramine Resin *on page 318*

PREVEN® *see* Combination Hormonal Contraceptives *on page 368*

PreviDent® *see* Fluoride *on page 586*

PreviDent® 5000 Plus™ *see* Fluoride *on page 586*

Prevnar® *see* Pneumococcal Conjugate Vaccine (7-Valent) *on page 1091*

Priftin® *see* Rifapentine *on page 1182*

Prilocaine (PRIL oh kane)

Related Information

Oral Pain *on page 1524*

U.S. Brand Names Citanest® Plain

Canadian Brand Names Citanest® Forte; Citanest® Plain

Mexican Brand Names Citanest Octapressin®

Pharmacologic Category Local Anesthetic, Dental; Local Anesthetic

Use Dental: Amide-type anesthetic used for local infiltration anesthesia; injection near nerve trunks to produce nerve block

Local Anesthetic/Vasoconstrictor Precautions No information available to require special precautions

Effects on Dental Treatment It is common to misinterpret psychogenic responses to local anesthetic injection as an allergic reaction. Intraoral injections are perceived by many patients as a stressful procedure in dentistry. Common symptoms to this stress are diaphoresis, palpitations, hyperventilation, generalized pallor and a fainting feeling.

Degree of adverse effects in the CNS and cardiovascular system is directly related to blood levels of prilocaine (frequency not defined; more likely to occur after systemic administration rather than infiltration): Bradycardia and reduction in cardiac output, hypersensitivity reactions (may be manifest as dermatologic reactions and edema at injection site), asthmatic syndromes

High blood levels: Anxiety, restlessness, disorientation, confusion, dizziness, tremors, and seizures, followed by CNS depression, resulting in somnolence, unconsciousness and possible respiratory arrest; nausea and vomiting

In some cases, symptoms of CNS stimulation may be absent and the primary CNS effects are somnolence and unconsciousness.

Dosage

Children <10 years: Doses >40 mg (1 mL) as a 4% solution per procedure rarely needed

Children >10 years and Adults: Dental anesthesia, infiltration, or conduction block: Initial: 40-80 mg (1-2 mL) as a 4% solution; up to a maximum of 400 mg (10 mL) as a 4% solution within a 2-hour period. Manufacturer's maximum recommended dose is not more than 600 mg to normal healthy adults. The effective anesthetic dose varies with procedure, intensity of anesthesia needed, duration of anesthesia required and physical condition of the patient. Always use the lowest effective dose along with careful aspiration.

The following numbers of dental carpules (1.8 mL) provide the indicated amounts of prilocaine hydrochloride 4% (see table).

# of Cartridges (1.8 mL)	Prilocaine HCl 4% (mg)
1	72
2	144
3	216
4	288
5	360
6	432
7	504
8	576

Mechanism of Action Local anesthetics bind selectively to the intracellular surface of sodium channels to block influx of sodium into the axon. As a result, depolarization necessary for action potential propagation and subsequent nerve function is prevented. The block at the sodium channel is reversible. When drug diffuses away from the axon, sodium channel function is restored and nerve propagation returns.

Contraindications Hypersensitivity to local anesthetics of the amide type or any component of the formulation

Warnings/Precautions Aspirate the syringe after tissue penetration and before injection to minimize chance of direct vascular injection

Pharmacodynamics/Kinetics

Onset of action: Infiltration: ~2 minutes; Inferior alveolar nerve block: ~3 minutes

Duration: Infiltration: Complete anesthesia for procedures lasting 20 minutes; Inferior alveolar nerve block: ~2.5 hours

Distribution: V_d: 0.7-4.4 L/kg; crosses blood-brain barrier

Protein binding: 55%

Metabolism: Hepatic and renal

Half-life elimination: 10-150 minutes; prolonged with hepatic or renal impairment

Pregnancy Risk Factor B

Breast-feeding Considerations Usual infiltration doses of prilocaine given to nursing mothers has not been shown to affect the health of the nursing infant.

Dosage Forms INJ, solution [prefilled cartridge]: Prilocaine 4% (1.8 mL)

Generic Available No

Selected Readings

Jastak JT and Yagiela JA, "Vasoconstrictors and Local Anesthesia: A Review and Rationale for Use," *J Am Dent Assoc*, 1983, 107(4):623-30.

MacKenzie TA and Young ER, "Local Anesthetic Update," *Anesth Prog*, 1993, 40(2):29-34.

Wynn RL, "Epinephrine Interactions With Beta-Blockers," *Gen Dent*, 1994, 42(1):16, 18.

Yagiela JA, "Local Anesthetics," *Anesth Prog*, 1991, 38(4-5):128-41.

Prilocaine and Epinephrine (PRIL oh kane & ep i NEF rin)

Related Information

Oral Pain *on page 1524*

Prilocaine *on page 1114*

U.S. Brand Names Citanest® Forte

Pharmacologic Category Local Anesthetic, Dental; Local Anesthetic

Use Dental: Amide-type anesthetic used for local infiltration anesthesia; injection near nerve trunks to produce nerve block

Local Anesthetic/Vasoconstrictor Precautions No information available to require special precautions

Effects on Dental Treatment It is common to misinterpret psychogenic responses to local anesthetic injection as an allergic reaction. Intraoral injections are perceived by many patients as a stressful procedure in dentistry. Common symptoms to this stress are diaphoresis, palpitations, hyperventilation, generalized pallor and a fainting feeling. Patients may exhibit hypersensitivity to bisulfites contained in local anesthetic solution to prevent oxidation of epinephrine. In general, patients reacting to bisulfites have a history of asthma and their airways are hyper-reactive to asthmatic syndrome.

Degree of adverse effects in the CNS and cardiovascular system is directly related to blood levels of prilocaine (frequency not defined; more likely to occur after systemic administration rather than infiltration): Bradycardia and reduction in cardiac output, hypersensitivity reactions (extremely rare; may be manifest as dermatologic reactions and edema at injection site), asthmatic syndromes

High blood levels: Anxiety, restlessness, disorientation, confusion, dizziness, tremors, and seizures, followed by CNS depression, resulting in somnolence, unconsciousness and possible respiratory arrest; nausea and vomiting

In some cases, symptoms of CNS stimulation may be absent and the primary CNS effects are somnolence and unconsciousness.

Dosage

Children <10 years: Doses >40 mg (1 mL) of prilocaine hydrochloride as a 4% solution with epinephrine 1:200,000 are rarely needed

Children >10 years and Adults: Dental anesthesia, infiltration, or conduction block: Initial: 40-80 mg (1-2 mL) of prilocaine hydrochloride as a 4% solution with epinephrine 1:200,000; up to a maximum of 400 mg (10 mL) of prilocaine hydrochloride within a 2-hour period. The effective anesthetic dose varies with procedure, intensity of anesthesia needed, duration of anesthesia required, and physical condition of the patient. Always use the lowest effective dose along with careful aspiration.

The following numbers of dental carpules (1.8 mL) provide the indicated amounts of prilocaine hydrochloride 4% and epinephrine 1:200,000 (see table).

Prilocaine and Epinephrine

# of Cartridges	Mg Prilocaine (4%)	Mg Vasoconstrictor (Epinephrine 1:200,000)
1	72	0.009
2	144	0.018
3	216	0.027
4	288	0.036
5	360	0.045
6	432	0.054
7	504	0.063
8	576	0.072

Mechanism of Action Local anesthetics bind selectively to the intracellular surface of sodium channels to block influx of sodium into the axon. As a result, depolarization necessary for action potential propagation and subsequent nerve function is prevented. The block at the sodium channel is reversible. When drug diffuses away from the axon, sodium channel function is restored and nerve propagation returns.

Epinephrine prolongs the duration of the anesthetic actions of prilocaine by causing vasoconstriction (alpha adrenergic receptor agonist) of the vasculature surrounding the nerve axons. This prevents the diffusion of prilocaine away from the nerves resulting in a longer retention in the axon.

Contraindications Hypersensitivity to local anesthetics of the amide-type or any component of the formulation

Warnings/Precautions Should be avoided in patients with uncontrolled hyperthyroidism. Should be used in minimal amounts in patients with significant cardiovascular problems (because of epinephrine component). Aspirate the syringe after tissue penetration and before injection to minimize chance of direct vascular injection

Drug Interactions

MAO inhibitors: Administration of local anesthetic solutions containing epinephrine may produce severe, prolonged hypertension

Beta-blockers, nonselective (ie, propranolol): Concurrent use could result in serious hypertension and reflex bradycardia

Tricyclic antidepressants: Pressor response to I.V. epinephrine, norepinephrine, and phenylephrine may be enhanced in patients receiving TCAs (**Note:** Effect is unlikely with epinephrine or levonordefrin dosages typically administered as infiltration in combination with local anesthetics)

Pharmacodynamics/Kinetics

Onset of action: Infiltration: <2 minutes; Inferior alveolar nerve block: <3 minutes

Duration: Infiltration: 2.25 hours; Inferior alveolar nerve block: 3 hours

Pregnancy Risk Factor C

Breast-feeding Considerations Usual infiltration doses of prilocaine with epinephrine given to nursing mothers has not been shown to affect the health of the nursing infant.

Dosage Forms INJ: Prilocaine hydrochloride 4% with epinephrine 1:200,000 (1.8 mL) [cartridge, 100/box]

Generic Available No

Selected Readings

Ayoub ST and Coleman AE, "A Review of Local Anesthetics," *Gen Dent*, 1992, 40(4):285-7, 289-90.

Blanton PL and Roda RS, "The Anatomy of Local Anesthesia," *J Calif Dent Assoc*, 1995, 23(4):55-65.

Jastak JT and Yagiela JA, "Vasoconstrictors and Local Anesthesia: A Review and Rationale for Use," *J Am Dent Assoc*, 1983, 107(4):623-30.

MacKenzie TA and Young ER, "Local Anesthetic Update," *Anesth Prog*, 1993, 40(2):29-34.

Wynn RL, "Epinephrine Interactions With Beta-Blockers," *Gen Dent*, 1994, 42(1):16, 18.

Yagiela JA, "Local Anesthetics," *Anesth Prog*, 1991, 38(4-5):128-41.

Yagiela JA, "Vasoconstrictor Agents for Local Anesthesia," *Anesth Prog*, 1995, 42(3-4):116-20.

Prilocaine and Lidocaine *see* Lidocaine and Prilocaine *on page 806*

Prilosec® *see* Omeprazole *on page 999*

Primaclone *see* Primidone *on page 1118*

Primacor® *see* Milrinone *on page 914*

Primaquine (PRIM a kween)

Pharmacologic Category Aminoquinoline (Antimalarial)

Synonyms Primaquine Phosphate; Prymaccone

Use Provides radical cure of *P. vivax* or *P. ovale* malaria after a clinical attack has been confirmed by blood smear or serologic titer and postexposure prophylaxis

Local Anesthetic/Vasoconstrictor Precautions No information available to require special precautions

Effects on Dental Treatment No significant effects or complications reported

Dosage Oral:

Children: 0.3 mg base/kg/day once daily for 14 days (not to exceed 15 mg/day) or 0.9 mg base/kg once weekly for 8 weeks not to exceed 45 mg base/week

Adults: 15 mg/day (base) once daily for 14 days or 45 mg base once weekly for 8 weeks

CDC treatment recommendations: Begin therapy during last 2 weeks of, or following a course of, suppression with chloroquine or a comparable drug

Mechanism of Action Eliminates the primary tissue exoerythrocytic forms of *P. falciparum*; disrupts mitochondria and binds to DNA

Other Adverse Effects

>10%:

Gastrointestinal: Abdominal pain, nausea, vomiting

Hematologic: Hemolytic anemia in G6PD deficiency

1% to 10%: Hematologic: Methemoglobinemia in NADH-methemoglobin reductase-deficient individuals

<1%: Agranulocytosis, arrhythmias, headache, interference with visual accommodation, leukopenia, leukocytosis, pruritus

Drug Interactions Substrate of **CYP3A4**; Inhibits CYP2D6, 3A4; Induces CYP1A2

Increased effect/toxicity with quinacrine.

Dietary/Ethanol/Herb Considerations Ethanol: Avoid use due to GI irritation.

Pharmacodynamics/Kinetics

Absorption: Well absorbed

Metabolism: Hepatic to carboxyprimaquine (active)

Half-life elimination: 3.7-9.6 hours

Time to peak, serum: 1-2 hours

Excretion: Urine (small amounts as unchanged drug)

Pregnancy Risk Factor C

Generic Available Yes

Primaquine Phosphate *see* Primaquine *on page 1117*

Primaxin® *see* Imipenem and Cilastatin *on page 709*

Primidone (PRI mi done)

U.S. Brand Names Mysoline®

Canadian Brand Names Apo®-Primidone; Mysoline®

Mexican Brand Names Mysoline®

Pharmacologic Category Anticonvulsant, Miscellaneous; Barbiturate

Synonyms Desoxyphenobarbital; Primaclone

Use Management of grand mal, psychomotor, and focal seizures

Unlabeled/Investigational Use Treatment of benign familial tremor (essential tremor)

Local Anesthetic/Vasoconstrictor Precautions No information available to require special precautions

Effects on Dental Treatment No significant effects or complications reported

Dosage Oral:

Children <8 years: Initial: 50-125 mg/day given at bedtime; increase by 50-125 mg/day increments every 3-7 days; usual dose: 10-25 mg/kg/day in divided doses 3-4 times/day

Children ≥8 years and Adults: Initial: 125-250 mg/day at bedtime; increase by 125-250 mg/day every 3-7 days; usual dose: 750-1500 mg/day in divided doses 3-4 times/day with maximum dosage of 2 g/day

Dosing interval in renal impairment:

Cl_{cr} 50-80 mL/minute: Administer every 8 hours

Cl_{cr} 10-50 mL/minute: Administer every 8-12 hours

Cl_{cr} <10 mL/minute: Administer every 12-24 hours

Hemodialysis: Moderately dialyzable (20% to 50%); administer dose postdialysis or administer supplemental 30% dose

Mechanism of Action Decreases neuron excitability, raises seizure threshold similar to phenobarbital; primidone has two active metabolites, phenobarbital and phenylethylmalonamide (PEMA); PEMA may enhance the activity of phenobarbital

Other Adverse Effects Frequency not defined:

Central nervous system: Drowsiness, vertigo, ataxia, lethargy, behavior change, fatigue, hyperirritability

Dermatologic: Rash

Gastrointestinal: Nausea, vomiting, anorexia

Genitourinary: Impotence

Hematologic: Agranulocytopenia, agranulocytosis, anemia

Ocular: Diplopia, nystagmus

Drug Interactions Metabolized to phenobarbital; Induces **CYP1A2, 2B6, 2C8/9, 3A4**

Increased Effect/Toxicity: Central nervous system depression (and possible respiratory depression) may be increased when combined with other CNS depressants, benzodiazepines, valproic acid, chloramphenicol, or antidepressants. MAO inhibitors may prolong the effect of primidone.

Decreased Effect: Primidone may induce the hepatic metabolism of many drugs due to enzyme induction, and may reduce the efficacy of beta-blockers, chloramphenicol, cimetidine, clozapine, corticosteroids, cyclosporine, disopyramide, doxycycline, ethosuximide, furosemide, griseofulvin, haloperidol, lamotrigine, methadone, nifedipine, oral contraceptives, phenothiazine, phenytoin, propafenone, quinidine, tacrolimus, TCAs, theophylline, warfarin, and verapamil.

Dietary/Ethanol/Herb Considerations

Ethanol: Avoid use; may increase CNS depression

Food: Protein-deficient diets increase duration of action of primidone.

Herb/Nutraceutical: Avoid kava, gotu kola, St John's wort, and valerian; may increase CNS depression.

Pharmacodynamics/Kinetics

Distribution: Adults: V_d: 2-3 L/kg

Protein binding: 99%

Metabolism: Hepatic to phenobarbital (active) and phenylethylmalonamide (PEMA)

Bioavailability: 60% to 80%

Half-life elimination (age dependent): Primidone: 10-12 hours; PEMA: 16 hours; Phenobarbital: 52-118 hours

Time to peak, serum: ~4 hours

Excretion: Urine (15% to 25% as unchanged drug and active metabolites)

Pregnancy Risk Factor D

Generic Available Yes

Primsol® *see* Trimethoprim *on page 1352*

Principen® *see* Ampicillin *on page 103*

Prinivil® *see* Lisinopril *on page 813*

Prinzide® *see* Lisinopril and Hydrochlorothiazide *on page 814*

Pristinamycin *see* Quinupristin and Dalfopristin *on page 1161*

Privine® [OTC] *see* Naphazoline *on page 952*

ProAmatine® *see* Midodrine *on page 911*

Probenecid (proe BEN e sid)

Related Information

Sexually-Transmitted Diseases *on page 1502*

Canadian Brand Names Benuryl™

Mexican Brand Names Benecid®; Benecid Probenecida Valdecasas

Pharmacologic Category Uricosuric Agent

Synonyms Benemid [DSC]

Use Prevention of gouty arthritis; hyperuricemia; prolongation of beta-lactam effect (ie, serum levels)

Local Anesthetic/Vasoconstrictor Precautions No information available to require special precautions

Effects on Dental Treatment No significant effects or complications reported

Dosage Oral:

Children:

<2 years: Use not recommended

2-14 years: Prolong penicillin serum levels: 25 mg/kg starting dose, then 40 mg/kg/day given 4 times/day

Gonorrhea: <45 kg: 25 mg/kg x 1 (maximum: 1 g/dose) 30 minutes before penicillin, ampicillin or amoxicillin

Adults:

Hyperuricemia with gout: 250 mg twice daily for one week; increase to 250-500 mg/day; may increase by 500 mg/month, if needed, to maximum of 2-3 g/day (dosages may be increased by 500 mg every 6 months if serum urate concentrations are controlled)

Prolong penicillin serum levels: 500 mg 4 times/day

Gonorrhea: 1 g 30 minutes before penicillin, ampicillin, procaine, or amoxicillin

Pelvic inflammatory disease: Cefoxitin 2 g I.M. plus probenecid 1 g orally as a single dose

Neurosyphilis: Aqueous procaine penicillin 2.4 million units/day I.M. plus probenecid 500 mg 4 times/day for 10-14 days

Dosing comment in renal impairment: Cl_{cr} <50 mL/minute: Avoid use

Mechanism of Action Competitively inhibits the reabsorption of uric acid at the proximal convoluted tubule, thereby promoting its excretion and reducing serum uric acid levels; increases plasma levels of weak organic acids (penicillins, cephalosporins, or other beta-lactam antibiotics) by competitively inhibiting their renal tubular secretion

Other Adverse Effects Frequency not defined:

Cardiovascular: Flushing of face

Central nervous system: Headache, dizziness

Dermatologic: Rash, itching

Gastrointestinal: Anorexia, nausea, vomiting, sore gums

Genitourinary: Painful urination

Hematologic: Aplastic anemia, hemolytic anemia, leukopenia

Hepatic: Hepatic necrosis

Neuromuscular & skeletal: Gouty arthritis (acute)

Renal: Renal calculi, nephrotic syndrome, urate nephropathy

Miscellaneous: Anaphylaxis

Drug Interactions Inhibits CYP2C19

Increased Effect/Toxicity: Increases methotrexate toxic potential. Probenecid increases the serum concentrations of quinolones and beta-lactams such as penicillins and cephalosporins. Also increases levels/toxicity of acyclovir, diflunisal, ketorolac, thiopental, benzodiazepines, dapsone, fluoroquinolones, methotrexate, NSAIDs, sulfonylureas, zidovudine.

Decreased Effect: Salicylates (high-dose) may decrease uricosuria. Decreased urinary levels of nitrofurantoin may decrease efficacy.

Pharmacodynamics/Kinetics

Onset of action: Effect on penicillin levels: 2 hours

Absorption: Rapid and complete

Metabolism: Hepatic

Half-life elimination (dose dependent): Normal renal function: 6-12 hours

Time to peak, serum: 2-4 hours

Excretion: Urine

Pregnancy Risk Factor B

Generic Available Yes

Probenecid and Colchicine *see* Colchicine and Probenecid *on page 364*

Probiotica® [OTC] *see Lactobacillus acidophilus* and *Lactobacillus bulgaricus on page 772*

Procainamide (proe kane A mide)

Related Information

Cardiovascular Diseases *on page 1456*

U.S. Brand Names Procanbid®; Pronestyl®; Pronestyl-SR®

Canadian Brand Names Apo®-Procainamide; Procan® SR; Pronestyl®-SR

Pharmacologic Category Antiarrhythmic Agent, Class Ia

(Continued)

Procainamide *(Continued)*

Synonyms PCA; Procainamide Hydrochloride; Procaine Amide Hydrochloride

Use Treatment of ventricular tachycardia (VT), premature ventricular contractions, paroxysmal atrial tachycardia (PSVT), and atrial fibrillation (AF); prevent recurrence of ventricular tachycardia, paroxysmal supraventricular tachycardia, atrial fibrillation or flutter

Unlabeled/Investigational Use ACLS guidelines: Treatment of intermittent/recurrent VF or pulseless VT not responsive to earlier interventions, monomorphic VT (EF >40%, no CHF), polymorphic VT with normal baseline QT interval, wide complex tachycardia of unknown type (EF >40%, no CHF, patient stable), refractory paroxysmal SVT, atrial fibrillation or flutter (EF >40%, no CHF) including pre-excitation syndrome

Local Anesthetic/Vasoconstrictor Precautions No information available to require special precautions

Effects on Dental Treatment No significant effects or complications reported

Dosage Must be titrated to patient's response

Children:

Oral: 15-50 mg/kg/24 hours divided every 3-6 hours

I.M.: 50 mg/kg/24 hours divided into doses of $^1/_8$ to $^1/_4$ every 3-6 hours in divided doses until oral therapy is possible

I.V. (infusion requires use of an infusion pump):

Load: 3-6 mg/kg/dose over 5 minutes not to exceed 100 mg/dose; may repeat every 5-10 minutes to maximum of 15 mg/kg/load

Maintenance as continuous I.V. infusion: 20-80 mcg/kg/minute; maximum: 2 g/24 hours

Adults:

Oral: 250-500 mg/dose every 3-6 hours or 500 mg to 1 g every 6 hours sustained release; usual dose: 50 mg/kg/24 hours; maximum: 4 g/24 hours (**Note:** Twice daily dosing approved for Procanbid®)

I.M.: 0.5-1 g every 4-8 hours until oral therapy is possible

I.V. (infusion requires use of an infusion pump): Loading dose: 15-18 mg/kg administered as slow infusion over 25-30 minutes or 100-200 mg/dose repeated every 5 minutes as needed to a total dose of 1 g; maintenance dose: 1-4 mg/minute by continuous infusion

Infusion rate: **2 g/250 mL** D_5W/NS (I.V. infusion requires use of an infusion pump):

1 mg/minute: 7.5 mL/hour
2 mg/minute: 15 mL/hour
3 mg/minute: 22.5 mL/hour
4 mg/minute: 30 mL/hour
5 mg/minute: 37.5 mL/hour
6 mg/minute: 45 mL/hour

Intermittent/recurrent VF or pulseless VT:

Initial: 20-30 mg/minute (maximum: 50 mg/minute if necessary), up to a total of 17 mg/kg. ACLS guidelines: I.V.: Infuse 20 mg/minute until arrhythmia is controlled, hypotension occurs, QRS complex widens by 50% of its original width, or total of 17 mg/kg is given.

Note: Reduce to 12 mg/kg in setting of cardiac or renal dysfunction

I.V. maintenance infusion: 1-4 mg/minute; monitor levels and do not exceed 3 mg/minute for >24 hours in adults with renal failure.

Dosing interval in renal impairment:

Cl_{cr} 10-50 mL/minute: Administer every 6-12 hours.

Cl_{cr} <10 mL/minute: Administer every 8-24 hours.

Dialysis:

Procainamide: Moderately hemodialyzable (20% to 50%): 200 mg supplemental dose posthemodialysis is recommended.

N-acetylprocainamide: Not dialyzable (0% to 5%)

Procainamide/N-acetylprocainamide: Not peritoneal dialyzable (0% to 5%)

Procainamide/N-acetylprocainamide: Replace by blood level during continuous arteriovenous or venovenous hemofiltration

Dosing adjustment in hepatic impairment: Reduce dose by 50%.

Mechanism of Action Decreases myocardial excitability and conduction velocity and may depress myocardial contractility, by increasing the electrical stimulation threshold of ventricle, His-Purkinje system and through direct cardiac effects

Other Adverse Effects

>1%:

Cardiovascular: Hypotension (I.V. up to 5%)

Dermatologic: Rash

Gastrointestinal: Diarrhea (3% to 4%), nausea, vomiting, taste disorder, GI complaints (3% to 4%)

<1% (Limited to important or life-threatening): New or worsened arrhythmias (proarrhythmic effect), tachycardia, QT prolongation (excessive), second-degree heart block, torsade de pointes, ventricular arrhythmias, depressed myocardial contractility, paradoxical increase in ventricular rate in atrial fibrillation/flutter, dizziness, lightheadedness, confusion, hallucinations, mental depression, disorientation,

fever, drug fever, rash, urticaria, pruritus, angioneurotic edema, flushing, maculopapular rash, hemolytic anemia, agranulocytosis, neutropenia, thrombocytopenia (0.5%), positive Coombs' test, bone marrow suppression, hypoplastic anemia, leukopenia, pancytopenia, aplastic anemia, elevated transaminases, increased alkaline phosphatase, hyperbilirubinemia, hepatic failure,granulomatous hepatitis, intrahepatic cholestasis, arthralgia, myalgia (<0.5%), worsening of myasthenia gravis, neuromuscular blockade, weakness, peripheral/polyneuropathy, myopathy, pleural effusion, SLE-like syndrome (increased incidence with long-term therapy: arthralgia, pleural pain, abdominal pain, arthralgia, pleural effusion, pericarditis, fever, chills, myalgia, rash); positive ANA

Postmarketing and/or case reports: Pancreatitis, pseudo-obstruction, tremor, mania, myocarditis, vasculitis, psychosis, cerebellar ataxia, demyelinating polyradiculoneuropathy, respiratory failure due to myopathy, pulmonary embolism, myopathy

Drug Interactions Substrate of **CYP2D6**

Increased Effect/Toxicity:

Amiodarone, cimetidine, ofloxacin (and potentially other renally eliminated quinolones), ranitidine, and trimethoprim increase procainamide and NAPA blood levels; consider reducing procainamide dosage by 25% with concurrent use. Cisapride and procainamide may increase the risk of malignant arrhythmia; concurrent use is contraindicated. Procainamide may potentiate effects of neuromuscular blocking agents.

Drugs which may prolong the QT interval include amiodarone, amitriptyline, astemizole, bepridil, cisapride, disopyramide, erythromycin, haloperidol, imipramine, pimozide, quinidine, sotalol, mesoridazine, thioridazine, and some quinolone antibiotics (sparfloxacin, gatifloxacin, moxifloxacin); concurrent use may result in additional prolongation of the QT interval.

Dietary/Ethanol/Herb Considerations

Ethanol: Avoid use; acute consumption decreases serum concentration.

Food: Administer on an empty stomach.

Herb/Nutraceutical: Avoid ephedra; may worsen arrhythmia.

Pharmacodynamics/Kinetics

Onset of action: I.M. 10-30 minutes

Distribution: V_d: Children: 2.2 L/kg; Adults: 2 L/kg; Congestive heart failure or shock: Decreased V_d

Protein binding: 15% to 20%

Metabolism: Hepatic via acetylation to produce N-acetyl procainamide (NAPA) (active metabolite)

Bioavailability: Oral: 75% to 95%

Half-life elimination:

Procainamide (hepatic acetylator, phenotype, cardiac and renal function dependent):

Children: 1.7 hours; Adults: 2.5-4.7 hours; Anephric: 11 hours

NAPA (dependent upon renal function):

Children: 6 hours; Adults: 6-8 hours; Anephric: 42 hours

Time to peak, serum: Capsule: 45 minutes to 2.5 hours; I.M.: 15-60 minutes

Excretion: Urine (25% as NAPA)

Pregnancy Risk Factor C

Generic Available Yes: Excludes tablet

Procainamide Hydrochloride *see* Procainamide *on page 1119*

Procaine (PROE kane)

U.S. Brand Names Novocain®

Canadian Brand Names Novocain®

Pharmacologic Category Local Anesthetic

Synonyms Procaine Hydrochloride

Use Produces spinal anesthesia and epidural and peripheral nerve block by injection and infiltration methods

Local Anesthetic/Vasoconstrictor Precautions No information available to require special precautions

Effects on Dental Treatment This is no longer a useful anesthetic in dentistry due to high incidence of allergic reactions.

Dosage Dose varies with procedure, desired depth, and duration of anesthesia, desired muscle relaxation, vascularity of tissues, physical condition, and age of patient

Mechanism of Action Blocks both the initiation and conduction of nerve impulses by decreasing the neuronal membrane's permeability to sodium ions, which results in inhibition of depolarization with resultant blockade of conduction

Other Adverse Effects

1% to 10%: Local: Burning sensation at site of injection, tissue irritation, pain at injection site

<1%: Anaphylactoid reaction, aseptic meningitis resulting in paralysis can occur, chills, CNS stimulation followed by CNS depression, discoloration of skin, miosis, nausea, tinnitus, vomiting

(Continued)

Procaine *(Continued)*

Drug Interactions Decreased effect of sulfonamides with the PABA metabolite of procaine, chloroprocaine, and tetracaine.

Note: Decreased/increased effect of vasopressors, ergot alkaloids, and MAO inhibitors on blood pressure when using anesthetic solutions with a vasoconstrictor.

Pharmacodynamics/Kinetics

Onset of action: 2-5 minutes

Duration (patient, type of block, concentration, and method of anesthesia dependent); 0.5-1.5 hours

Metabolism: Rapidly hydrolyzed by plasma enzymes to para-aminobenzoic acid and diethylaminoethanol (80% conjugated before elimination)

Half-life elimination: 7.7 minutes

Excretion: Urine (as metabolites and some unchanged drug)

Pregnancy Risk Factor C

Generic Available Yes

Procaine Amide Hydrochloride *see* Procainamide *on page 1119*

Procaine Benzylpenicillin *see* Penicillin G Procaine *on page 1050*

Procaine Hydrochloride *see* Procaine *on page 1121*

Procaine Penicillin G *see* Penicillin G Procaine *on page 1050*

Procanbid® *see* Procainamide *on page 1119*

Procarbazine (proe KAR ba zeen)

U.S. Brand Names Matulane®

Canadian Brand Names Matulane®; Natulan®

Mexican Brand Names Natulan®

Pharmacologic Category Antineoplastic Agent, Alkylating Agent

Synonyms Benzmethyzin; N-Methylhydrazine; Procarbazine Hydrochloride

Use Treatment of Hodgkin's disease; other uses include non-Hodgkin's lymphoma, brain tumors, melanoma, lung cancer, multiple myeloma

Local Anesthetic/Vasoconstrictor Precautions No information available to require special precautions

Effects on Dental Treatment No significant effects or complications reported

Dosage Refer to individual protocols. Dose based on patient's ideal weight if the patient is obese or has abnormal fluid retention. Oral:

Children:

BMT aplastic anemia conditioning regimen: 12.5 mg/kg/dose every other day for 4 doses

Hodgkin's disease: MOPP/IC-MOPP regimens: 100 mg/m^2/day for 14 days and repeated every 4 weeks

Neuroblastoma and medulloblastoma: Doses as high as 100-200 mg/m^2/day once daily have been used

Adults: Initial: 2-4 mg/kg/day in single or divided doses for 7 days then increase dose to 4-6 mg/kg/day until response is obtained or leukocyte count decreased <4000/mm^3 or the platelet count decreased <100,000/mm^3; maintenance: 1-2 mg/kg/day

In MOPP, 100 mg/m^2/day on days 1-14 of a 28-day cycle

Dosing in renal/hepatic impairment: Use with caution, may result in increased toxicity

Mechanism of Action Mechanism of action is not clear, methylating of nucleic acids; inhibits DNA, RNA, and protein synthesis; may damage DNA directly and suppresses mitosis; metabolic activation required by host

Other Adverse Effects Frequency not defined:

Central nervous system: Reports of neurotoxicity with procarbazine generally originate from early usage with single agent oral (continuous) or I.V. dosing; CNS depression is commonly reported to be additive with other CNS depressants

Hematologic: Myelosuppression, hemolysis in patients with G6PD deficiency

Gastrointestinal: Nausea and vomiting (60% to 90%); increasing the dose in a stepwise fashion over several days may minimize this

Genitourinary: Reproductive dysfunction >10% (in animals, hormone treatment has prevented azoospermia)

Respiratory: Pulmonary toxicity (<1%); the most commonly reported pulmonary toxicity is a hypersensitivity pneumonitis which responds to steroids and discontinuation of the drug. At least one report of persistent pulmonary fibrosis has been reported, however, a higher incidence (18%) of pulmonary toxicity (fibrosis) was reported when procarbazine was given prior to BCNU (BCNU alone does cause pulmonary fibrosis).

Miscellaneous: Second malignancies (cumulative incidence 2% to 15% reported with MOPP combination therapy)

Drug Interactions Increased Effect/Toxicity: Sympathomimetic amines (epinephrine and amphetamines) and antidepressants (tricyclics) should be used cautiously with procarbazine. Barbiturates, narcotics, phenothiazines, and other CNS depressants can cause somnolence, ataxia, and other symptoms of CNS depression.

Dietary/Ethanol/Herb Considerations

Avoid ethanol and ethanol-containing products due to disulfiram-like reaction (headache, respiratory difficulties, nausea, vomiting, sweating, thirst, hypotension, and flushing).

Food: Avoid tyramine-containing foods (eg, cheese); hypertensive crisis (life-threatening), intracranial bleeding, and headache have been reported.

Pharmacodynamics/Kinetics

Absorption: Rapid and complete

Distribution: Crosses blood-brain barrier; distributes into CSF

Metabolism: Hepatic and renal

Half-life elimination: 1 hour

Excretion: Urine and respiratory tract (<5% as unchanged drug, 70% as metabolites)

Pregnancy Risk Factor D

Generic Available No

Procarbazine Hydrochloride *see* Procarbazine *on page 1122*

Procardia® *see* NIFEdipine *on page 973*

Procardia XL® *see* NIFEdipine *on page 973*

Procetofene *see* Fenofibrate *on page 561*

Prochieve™ *see* Progesterone *on page 1125*

Prochlorperazine (proe klor PER a zeen)

U.S. Brand Names Compazine®; Compro™

Canadian Brand Names Apo®-Prochlorperazine; Compazine®; Nu-Prochlor; Stemetil®

Pharmacologic Category Antipsychotic Agent, Phenothiazine, Piperazine

Synonyms Prochlorperazine Edisylate; Prochlorperazine Maleate

Use Management of nausea and vomiting; psychosis; anxiety

Unlabeled/Investigational Use Treatment of dementia behavior

Local Anesthetic/Vasoconstrictor Precautions Most pharmacology textbooks state that in presence of phenothiazines, systemic doses of epinephrine paradoxically decrease the blood pressure. This is the so called "epinephrine reversal" phenomenon. This has never been observed when epinephrine is given by infiltration as part of the anesthesia procedure.

Effects on Dental Treatment >10%: Xerostomia, changes in salivation

Significant hypotension may occur especially when the drug is administered parenterally; orthostatic hypotension is due to alpha-receptor blockade, the elderly are at greater risk for orthostatic hypotension.

Tardive dyskinesia: Prevalence rate may be 40% in elderly; development of the syndrome and the irreversible nature are proportional to duration and total cumulative dose over time. Extrapyramidal reactions are more common in elderly with up to 50% developing these reactions after 60 years of age; drug-induced **Parkinson's syndrome** occurs often; **Akathisia** is the most common extrapyramidal reaction in elderly.

Increased confusion, memory loss, psychotic behavior, and agitation frequently occur as a consequence of anticholinergic effects. Antipsychotic associated sedation in nonpsychotic patients is extremely unpleasant due to feelings of depersonalization, derealization, and dysphoria.

Dosage Use not recommended in children <10 kg or <2 years of age.

Antiemetic: Children:

Oral, rectal:

>10 kg: 0.4 mg/kg/24 hours in 3-4 divided doses; **or**

9-14 kg: 2.5 mg every 12-24 hours as needed; maximum: 7.5 mg/day

14-18 kg: 2.5 mg every 8-12 hours as needed; maximum: 10 mg/day

18-39 kg: 2.5 mg every 8 hours or 5 mg every 12 hours as needed; maximum: 15 mg/day

I.M.: 0.1-0.15 mg/kg/dose; usual: 0.13 mg/kg/dose; change to oral as soon as possible

Antiemetic: Adults:

Oral:

Tablet: 5-10 mg 3-4 times/day; usual maximum: 40 mg/day

Capsule, sustained action: 15 mg upon arising or 10 mg every 12 hours

I.M.: 5-10 mg every 3-4 hours; usual maximum: 40 mg/day

I.V.: 2.5-10 mg; maximum 10 mg/dose or 40 mg/day; may repeat dose every 3-4 hours as needed

Rectal: 25 mg twice daily

Surgical nausea/vomiting: Adults:

I.M.: 5-10 mg 1-2 hours before induction; may repeat once if necessary

I.V.: 5-10 mg 15-30 minutes before induction; may repeat once if necessary

Antipsychotic:

Children 2-12 years:

Oral, rectal: 2.5 mg 2-3 times/day; increase dosage as needed to maximum daily dose of 20 mg for 2-5 years and 25 mg for 6-12 years

I.M.: 0.13 mg/kg/dose; change to oral as soon as possible

(Continued)

Prochlorperazine *(Continued)*

Adults:

Oral: 5-10 mg 3-4 times/day; doses up to 150 mg/day may be required in some patients for treatment of severe disturbances

I.M.: 10-20 mg every 4-6 hours may be required in some patients for treatment of severe disturbances; change to oral as soon as possible

Nonpsychotic anxiety: Oral: Adults: Usual dose: 15-20 mg/day in divided doses; do not give doses >20 mg/day or for longer than 12 weeks

Elderly: Behavioral symptoms associated with dementia: Initial: 2.5-5 mg 1-2 times/day; increase dose at 4- to 7-day intervals by 2.5-5 mg/day; increase dosing intervals (twice daily, 3 times/day, etc) as necessary to control response or side effects; maximum daily dose should probably not exceed 75 mg; gradual increases (titration) may prevent some side effects or decrease their severity

Hemodialysis: Not dialyzable (0% to 5%)

Mechanism of Action Blocks postsynaptic mesolimbic dopaminergic D_1 and D_2 receptors in the brain, including the medullary chemoreceptor trigger zone; exhibits a strong alpha-adrenergic and anticholinergic blocking effect and depresses the release of hypothalamic and hypophyseal hormones; believed to depress the reticular activating system, thus affecting basal metabolism, body temperature, wakefulness, vasomotor tone and emesis

Other Adverse Effects Frequency not defined:

Cardiovascular: Hypotension, orthostatic hypotension, hypertension, tachycardia, bradycardia, dizziness, cardiac arrest

Central nervous system: Extrapyramidal symptoms (pseudoparkinsonism, akathisia, dystonias, tardive dyskinesia), dizziness, cerebral edema, seizures, headache, drowsiness, paradoxical excitement, restlessness, hyperactivity, insomnia, neuroleptic malignant syndrome (NMS), impairment of temperature regulation

Dermatologic: Increased sensitivity to sun, rash, discoloration of skin (blue-gray)

Endocrine & metabolic: Hypoglycemia, hyperglycemia, galactorrhea, lactation, breast enlargement, gynecomastia, menstrual irregularity, amenorrhea, SIADH, changes in libido

Gastrointestinal: Constipation, weight gain, vomiting, stomach pain, nausea, diarrhea, anorexia, ileus, **increased salivation**

Genitourinary: Difficulty in urination, ejaculatory disturbances, incontinence, polyuria, ejaculating dysfunction, priapism

Hematologic: Agranulocytosis, leukopenia, eosinophilia, hemolytic anemia, thrombocytopenic purpura, pancytopenia

Hepatic: Cholestatic jaundice, hepatotoxicity

Neuromuscular & skeletal: Tremor

Ocular: Pigmentary retinopathy, blurred vision, cornea and lens changes

Respiratory: Nasal congestion

Miscellaneous: Diaphoresis

Drug Interactions Possible CYP2D6 enzyme substrate

Increased Effect/Toxicity: Chloroquine, propranolol, and sulfadoxine-pyrimethamine may increase prochlorperazine concentrations. Concurrent use with TCA may produce increased toxicity or altered therapeutic response. Prochlorperazine plus lithium may rarely produce neurotoxicity. Prochlorperazine may produce additive CNS depressant effects with CNS depressants (ethanol, narcotics). Metoclopramide may increase risk of extrapyramidal symptoms (EPS).

Decreased Effect: Barbiturates and carbamazepine may increase the metabolism of prochlorperazine, lowering its serum levels. Benztropine (and other anticholinergics) may inhibit the therapeutic response to prochlorperazine. Antipsychotics such as prochlorperazine inhibit the ability of bromocriptine to lower serum prolactin concentrations. The antihypertensive effects of guanethidine and guanadrel may be inhibited by prochlorperazine. Prochlorperazine may inhibit the antiparkinsonian effect of levodopa. Prochlorperazine (and possibly other low potency antipsychotics) may reverse the pressor effects of epinephrine.

Dietary/Ethanol/Herb Considerations

Ethanol: Avoid use; may increase CNS depression.

Food: May be taken with food; increase intake of riboflavin and limit caffeine.

Herb/Nutraceutical: Avoid dong quai; may cause photosensitization. Avoid gotu kola, kava, SAMe, and valerian; may increase CNS depression. Avoid St John's wort; may cause photosensitization and increase CNS depression.

Pharmacodynamics/Kinetics

Onset of action: Oral: 30-40 minutes; I.M.: 10-20 minutes; Rectal: ~60 minutes

Duration: I.M., oral extended-release: 12 hours; Rectal, immediate release: 3-4 hours

Distribution: V_d: 1400-1548 L; crosses placenta; enters breast milk

Metabolism: Primarily hepatic; N-desmethyl prochlorperazine (major active metabolite)

Bioavailability: Oral: 12.5%

Half-life elimination: Oral: 3-5 hours; I.V.: ~7 hours

Pregnancy Risk Factor C

Generic Available Yes: Injection, tablet, suppository

Prochlorperazine Edisylate *see* Prochlorperazine *on page 1123*
Prochlorperazine Maleate *see* Prochlorperazine *on page 1123*
Procrit® *see* Epoetin Alfa *on page 503*
Proctocort® *see* Hydrocortisone *on page 688*
ProctoCream® HC *see* Hydrocortisone *on page 688*
Proctofene *see* Fenofibrate *on page 561*
ProctoFoam®-HC *see* Pramoxine and Hydrocortisone *on page 1106*
ProctoFoam® NS [OTC] *see* Pramoxine *on page 1105*
Proctosol-HC® *see* Hydrocortisone *on page 688*

Procyclidine (proe SYE kli deen)

U.S. Brand Names Kemadrin®

Canadian Brand Names PMS-Procyclidine; Procyclid™

Pharmacologic Category Anticholinergic Agent; Anti-Parkinson's Agent, Anticholinergic

Synonyms Procyclidine Hydrochloride

Use Relieves symptoms of parkinsonian syndrome and drug-induced extrapyramidal symptoms

Local Anesthetic/Vasoconstrictor Precautions No information available to require special precautions

Effects on Dental Treatment >10%: Xerostomia, dry throat and nose

Prolonged use of antidyskinetics may decrease or inhibit salivary flow, contributing to discomfort and dental disease (ie, caries, oral candidiasis, and periodontal disease).

Dosage Oral:

Adults: 2.5 mg 3 times/day after meals; if tolerated, gradually increase dose, maximum of 20 mg/day if necessary

Dosing adjustment in hepatic impairment: Decrease dose to a twice daily dosing regimen

Mechanism of Action Thought to act by blocking excess acetylcholine at cerebral synapses; many of its effects are due to its pharmacologic similarities with atropine; it exerts an antispasmodic effect on smooth muscle, is a potent mydriatic; inhibits salivation

Other Adverse Effects Frequency not defined:

Cardiovascular: Tachycardia, palpitations

Central nervous system: Confusion, drowsiness, headache, loss of memory, fatigue, ataxia, giddiness, lightheadedness

Dermatologic: Dry skin, increased sensitivity to light, rash

Gastrointestinal: Constipation, nausea, vomiting, epigastric distress

Genitourinary: Difficult urination

Neuromuscular & skeletal: Weakness

Ocular: Increased intraocular pain, blurred vision, mydriasis

Miscellaneous: Diaphoresis (decreased)

Drug Interactions

Increased Effect/Toxicity: Central and/or peripheral anticholinergic syndrome can occur when administered with amantadine, rimantadine, narcotic analgesics, phenothiazines and other antipsychotics (especially with high anticholinergic activity), tricyclic antidepressants, quinidine and some other antiarrhythmics, and antihistamines.

Decreased Effect: May increase gastric degradation of levodopa and decrease the amount of levodopa absorbed by delaying gastric emptying; the opposite may be true for digoxin. Therapeutic effects of cholinergic agents (tacrine, donepezil) and neuroleptics may be antagonized.

Dietary/Ethanol/Herb Considerations

Ethanol: Avoid use; may increase CNS depression.

Food: Limit caffeine.

Herb/Nutraceutical: Avoid dong quai; may cause photosensitization. Avoid gotu kola, kava, SAMe, and valerian; may increase CNS depression. Avoid St John's wort; may cause photosensitization and increase CNS depression.

Pharmacodynamics/Kinetics

Onset of action: 30-40 minutes

Duration: 4-6 hours

Pregnancy Risk Factor C

Generic Available No

Procyclidine Hydrochloride *see* Procyclidine *on page 1125*
Prodium® [OTC] *see* Phenazopyridine *on page 1064*
Profasi® *see* Chorionic Gonadotropin (Human) *on page 320*
Profilnine® SD *see* Factor IX Complex (Human) *on page 553*
Progestasert® *see* Progesterone *on page 1125*

Progesterone (proe JES ter one)

U.S. Brand Names Crinone®; Prochieve™; Progestasert®; Prometrium®

Canadian Brand Names Crinone®; Prometrium®

(Continued)

Progesterone *(Continued)*

Mexican Brand Names Crinone®; Crinone® V; Utrogestan

Pharmacologic Category Progestin

Synonyms Pregnenedione; Progestin

Use

Oral: Prevention of endometrial hyperplasia in nonhysterectomized, postmenopausal women who are receiving conjugated estrogen tablets; secondary amenorrhea

I.M.: Amenorrhea; abnormal uterine bleeding due to hormonal imbalance

Intrauterine device (IUD): Contraception in women who have had at least one child, are in a stable and mutually-monogamous relationship, and have no history of pelvic inflammatory disease; amenorrhea; functional uterine bleeding

Intravaginal gel: Part of assisted reproductive technology (ART) for infertile women with progesterone deficiency; secondary amenorrhea

Local Anesthetic/Vasoconstrictor Precautions No information available to require special precautions

Effects on Dental Treatment Progestins may predispose the patient to gingival bleeding.

Dosage

I.M.: Adults: Female:

Amenorrhea: 5-10 mg/day for 6-8 consecutive days

Functional uterine bleeding: 5-10 mg/day for 6 doses

IUD: Adults: Female: Contraception: Insert a single system into the uterine cavity; contraceptive effectiveness is retained for 1 year and system must be replaced 1 year after insertion

Oral: Adults: Female:

Prevention of endometrial hyperplasia (in postmenopausal women with a uterus who are receiving daily conjugated estrogen tablets): 200 mg as a single daily dose every evening for 12 days sequentially per 28-day cycle

Amenorrhea: 400 mg every evening for 10 days

Intravaginal gel: Adults: Female:

ART in women who require progesterone supplementation: 90 mg (8% gel) once daily; if pregnancy occurs, may continue treatment for up to 10-12 weeks

ART in women with partial or complete ovarian failure: 90 mg (8% gel) intravaginally twice daily; if pregnancy occurs, may continue up to 10-12 weeks

Secondary amenorrhea: 45 mg (4% gel) intravaginally every other day for up to 6 doses; women who fail to respond may be increased to 90 mg (8% gel) every other day for up to 6 doses

Mechanism of Action Natural steroid hormone that induces secretory changes in the endometrium, promotes mammary gland development, relaxes uterine smooth muscle, blocks follicular maturation and ovulation, and maintains pregnancy

Other Adverse Effects

Intrauterine device:

Cardiovascular: Bradycardia and syncope (secondary to insertion)

Central nervous system: Pain

Endocrine & metabolic: Amenorrhea, delayed menses, dysmenorrhea, ectopic pregnancy, endometritis, pregnancy, septic abortion, prolonged menstrual flow, spontaneous abortion, spotting

Genitourinary: Cervical erosion, dyspareunia, leukorrhea, pelvic infection, tubal damage, tubo-ovarian abscess, vaginitis

Hematologic: Anemia

Local: Embedment or fragmentation of the IUD, perforation of uterus and cervix

Neuromuscular & skeletal: Backache

Miscellaneous: Abscess formation and erosion of adjacent area, abdominal adhesions, complete or partial IUD expulsion, congenital anomalies, cramping, cystic masses in the pelvis, death, difficult removal, fetal damage, hormonal imbalance, intestinal penetration, intestinal obstruction, local inflammatory reaction, loss of fertility, peritonitis, septicemia

Injection (I.M.):

Cardiovascular: Edema

Central nervous system: Depression, fever, insomnia, somnolence

Dermatologic: Acne, allergic rash (rare), alopecia, hirsutism, pruritus, rash, urticaria

Endocrine & metabolic: Amenorrhea, breakthrough bleeding, breast tenderness, galactorrhea, menstrual flow changes, spotting

Gastrointestinal: Nausea, weight gain, weight loss

Genitourinary: Cervical erosion changes, cervical secretion changes

Hepatic: Cholestatic jaundice

Local: Pain at the injection site

Miscellaneous: Anaphylactoid reactions

Oral capsule:

>10%:

Central nervous system: Dizziness (16%)

Endocrine & metabolic: Breast pain (11%)

5% to 10%:

Central nervous system: Headache (10%), fatigue (7%), emotional lability (6%), irritability (5%)

Gastrointestinal: Abdominal pain (10%), abdominal distention (6%)

Neuromuscular & skeletal: Musculoskeletal pain (6%)

Respiratory: Upper respiratory tract infection (5%)

Miscellaneous: Viral infection (7%)

<5%: Dry mouth, accidental injury, chest pain, fever, hypertension, confusion, somnolence, speech disorder, constipation, dyspepsia, gastroenteritis, hemorrhagic rectum, hiatus hernia, vomiting, earache, palpitation, edema, arthritis, leg cramps, hypertonia, muscle disorder, myalgia, angina pectoris, anxiety, impaired concentration, insomnia, personality disorder, leukorrhea, uterine fibroid, vaginal dryness, fungal vaginitis, vaginitis, abscess, herpes simplex, bronchitis, nasal congestion, pharyngitis, pneumonitis, sinusitis, acne, verruca, urinary tract infection, abnormal vision, lymphadenopathy

Postmarketing and/or case reports: Hepatitis (reversible), elevated transaminases, syncope, hypotension

Drug Interactions Substrate of CYP1A2, 2A6, 2C8/9, **2C19**, 2D6, **3A4**; Inhibits CYP2C8/9, 2C19

Increased Effect/Toxicity: Ketoconazole may increase the bioavailability of progesterone. Progesterone may increase concentrations of estrogenic compounds during concurrent therapy with conjugated estrogens.

Decreased Effect: Aminoglutethimide may decrease effect by increasing hepatic metabolism.

Dietary/Ethanol/Herb Considerations

Food increases oral bioavailability.

Herb/Nutraceutical: Avoid St John's wort; may decrease serum concentration.

Pharmacodynamics/Kinetics

Duration: 24 hours

Protein binding: 96% to 99%

Metabolism: Hepatic

Half-life elimination: 5 minutes

Time to peak: Oral: 1.5-2.3 hours

Excretion: Urine (50% to 60%); feces (~10%)

Pregnancy Risk Factor B (Prometrium®, per manufacturer); none established for gel (Crinone®), injection (contraindicated), or intrauterine device (contraindicated)

Generic Available Yes: Injection

Progestin *see* Progesterone *on page 1125*

Proglycem® *see* Diazoxide *on page 427*

Prograf® *see* Tacrolimus *on page 1261*

Proguanil and Atovaquone *see* Atovaquone and Proguanil *on page 143*

ProHance® *see* Radiological/Contrast Media (Nonionic) *on page 1165*

Prolastin® *see* Alpha$_1$-Proteinase Inhibitor *on page 61*

Proleukin® *see* Aldesleukin *on page 50*

Prolex-D *see* Guaifenesin and Phenylephrine *on page 652*

Prolixin® *see* Fluphenazine *on page 593*

Prolixin Decanoate® *see* Fluphenazine *on page 593*

Prolixin Enanthate® [DSC] *see* Fluphenazine *on page 593*

Proloprim® *see* Trimethoprim *on page 1352*

Promethazine (proe METH a zeen)

Canadian Brand Names Phenergan®

Pharmacologic Category Antiemetic

Synonyms Promethazine Hydrochloride

Use Symptomatic treatment of various allergic conditions; antiemetic; motion sickness; sedative; analgesic adjunct for control of postoperative pain; anesthetic adjunct

Local Anesthetic/Vasoconstrictor Precautions Most pharmacology textbooks state that in presence of phenothiazines, systemic doses of epinephrine paradoxically decrease the blood pressure. This is the so called "epinephrine reversal" phenomenon. This has never been observed when epinephrine is given by infiltration as part of the anesthesia procedure.

Effects on Dental Treatment 1% to 10%: Xerostomia

Significant hypotension may occur, especially when the drug is administered parenterally; orthostatic hypotension is due to alpha-receptor blockade, the elderly are at greater risk for orthostatic hypotension.

Tardive dyskinesia: Prevalence rate may be 40% in elderly; development of the syndrome and the irreversible nature are proportional to duration and total cumulative dose over time. Extrapyramidal reactions are more common in elderly with up to 50% developing these reactions after 60 years of age; drug-induced **Parkinson's syndrome** occurs often; **akathisia** is the most common extrapyramidal reaction in elderly.

(Continued)

Promethazine *(Continued)*

Increased confusion, memory loss, psychotic behavior, and agitation frequently occur as a consequence of anticholinergic effects. Antipsychotic associated sedation in nonpsychotic patients is extremely unpleasant due to feelings of depersonalization, derealization, and dysphoria.

Dosage

Children:

Antihistamine: Oral, rectal: 0.1 mg/kg/dose every 6 hours during the day and 0.5 mg/kg/dose at bedtime as needed

Antiemetic: Oral, I.M., I.V., rectal: 0.25-1 mg/kg 4-6 times/day as needed

Motion sickness: Oral, rectal: 0.5 mg/kg/dose 30 minutes to 1 hour before departure, then every 12 hours as needed

Sedation: Oral, I.M., I.V., rectal: 0.5-1 mg/kg/dose every 6 hours as needed

Adults:

Antihistamine (including allergic reactions to blood or plasma):

Oral, rectal: 12.5 mg 3 times/day and 25 mg at bedtime

I.M., I.V.: 25 mg, may repeat in 2 hours when necessary; switch to oral route as soon as feasible

Antiemetic: Oral, I.M., I.V., rectal: 12.5-25 mg every 4 hours as needed

Motion sickness: Oral, rectal: 25 mg 30-60 minutes before departure, then every 12 hours as needed

Sedation: Oral, I.M., I.V., rectal: 25-50 mg/dose

Hemodialysis: Not dialyzable (0% to 5%)

Mechanism of Action Blocks postsynaptic mesolimbic dopaminergic receptors in the brain; exhibits a strong alpha-adrenergic blocking effect and depresses the release of hypothalamic and hypophyseal hormones; competes with histamine for the H_1-receptor; reduces stimuli to the brainstem reticular system

Other Adverse Effects Frequency not defined:

Cardiovascular: Postural hypotension, tachycardia, dizziness, nonspecific QT changes

Central nervous system: Drowsiness, dystonias, akathisia, pseudoparkinsonism, tardive dyskinesia, neuroleptic malignant syndrome, seizures

Dermatologic: Photosensitivity, dermatitis, skin pigmentation (slate gray)

Endocrine & metabolic: Lactation, breast engorgement, false-positive pregnancy test, amenorrhea, gynecomastia, hyper- or hypoglycemia

Gastrointestinal: Constipation, nausea

Genitourinary: Urinary retention, ejaculatory disorder, impotence

Hematologic: Agranulocytosis, eosinophilia, leukopenia, hemolytic anemia, aplastic anemia, thrombocytopenic purpura

Hepatic: Jaundice

Ocular: Blurred vision, corneal and lenticular changes, epithelial keratopathy, pigmentary retinopathy

Drug Interactions Substrate of **CYP2B6, 2D6**; Inhibits CYP2D6

Increased Effect/Toxicity: Chloroquine, propranolol, and sulfadoxine-pyrimethamine also may increase promethazine concentrations. Concurrent use with TCA may produce increased toxicity or altered therapeutic response. Promethazine plus lithium may rarely produce neurotoxicity. Concurrent use of promethazine and CNS depressants (ethanol, narcotics) may produce additive depressant effects.

Decreased Effect: Barbiturates and carbamazepine may increase the metabolism of promethazine, lowering its serum levels. Benztropine (and other anticholinergics) may inhibit the therapeutic response to promethazine. Promethazine may inhibit the ability of bromocriptine to lower serum prolactin concentrations. The antihypertensive effects of guanethidine and guanadrel may be inhibited by promethazine. Promethazine may inhibit the antiparkinsonian effect of levodopa. Promethazine (and possibly other low potency antipsychotics) may reverse the pressor effects of epinephrine.

Dietary/Ethanol/Herb Considerations

Ethanol: Avoid use; may increase CNS depression.

Food: May be taken with food; increase intake of riboflavin.

Herb/Nutraceutical: Avoid gotu kola, kava, SAMe, St John's wort, and valerian; may increase CNS depression.

Pharmacodynamics/Kinetics

Onset of action: I.M.: ~20 minutes; I.V.: 3-5 minutes

Peak effect: C_{max}: 9.04 mg/mL (suppository); 19.3 mg/mL (syrup)

Duration: 2-6 hours

Absorption:

I.M.: Bioavailability may be greater than with oral or rectal administration

Oral: Rapid and complete; large first pass effect limits systemic bioavailability

Distribution: V_d: 171 L

Protein binding: 93%

Metabolism: Hepatic; primarily oxidation

Time to maximum serum concentration: 4.4 hours (syrup); 6.7-8.6 hours (suppositories)

Excretion: Primarily urine and feces (as inactive metabolites)

Pregnancy Risk Factor C

Generic Available Yes

Promethazine and Codeine (proe METH a zeen & KOE deen)

Related Information

Codeine *on page 361*

Promethazine *on page 1127*

U.S. Brand Names Phenergan® With Codeine

Pharmacologic Category Antihistamine/Antitussive

Synonyms Codeine and Promethazine

Use Temporary relief of coughs and upper respiratory symptoms associated with allergy or the common cold

Local Anesthetic/Vasoconstrictor Precautions No information available to require special precautions

Effects on Dental Treatment Although promethazine is a phenothiazine derivative, extrapyramidal reactions or tardive dyskinesias are not seen with the use of this drug.

Restrictions C-V

Dosage Oral (in terms of codeine):

Children: 1-1.5 mg/kg/day every 4 hours as needed; maximum: 30 mg/day **or**

2-6 years: 1.25-2.5 mL every 4-6 hours or 2.5-5 mg/dose every 4-6 hours as needed; maximum: 30 mg codeine/day

6-12 years: 2.5-5 mL every 4-6 hours as needed or 5-10 mg/dose every 4-6 hours as needed; maximum: 60 mg codeine/day

Adults: 10-20 mg/dose every 4-6 hours as needed; maximum: 120 mg codeine/day; or 5-10 mL every 4-6 hours as needed

Dietary/Ethanol/Herb Considerations

Ethanol: Avoid use; may increase CNS depression.

Herb/Nutraceutical: Avoid gotu kola, kava, SAMe, St John's wort, and valerian; may increase CNS depression.

Pregnancy Risk Factor C

Generic Available Yes

Promethazine and Dextromethorphan

(proe METH a zeen & deks troe meth OR fan)

Related Information

Dextromethorphan *on page 423*

Promethazine *on page 1127*

Canadian Brand Names Promatussin® DM

Pharmacologic Category Antihistamine/Antitussive

Synonyms Dextromethorphan and Promethazine

Use Temporary relief of coughs and upper respiratory symptoms associated with allergy or the common cold

Local Anesthetic/Vasoconstrictor Precautions No information available to require special precautions

Effects on Dental Treatment Although promethazine is a phenothiazine derivative, extrapyramidal reactions or tardive dyskinesias are not seen with the use of this drug.

Dosage Oral:

Children:

2-6 years: 1.25-2.5 mL every 4-6 hours up to 10 mL in 24 hours

6-12 years: 2.5-5 mL every 4-6 hours up to 20 mL in 24 hours

Adults: 5 mL every 4-6 hours up to 30 mL in 24 hours

Dietary/Ethanol/Herb Considerations

Ethanol: Avoid use; may increase CNS depression.

Herb/Nutraceutical: Avoid gotu kola, kava, SAMe, St John's wort, and valerian; may increase CNS depression.

Pregnancy Risk Factor C

Generic Available Yes

Promethazine and Meperidine *see* Meperidine and Promethazine *on page 860*

Promethazine and Phenylephrine

(proe METH a zeen & fen il EF rin)

Related Information

Phenylephrine *on page 1071*

Promethazine *on page 1127*

Pharmacologic Category Antihistamine/Decongestant Combination

Synonyms Phenylephrine and Promethazine

Use Temporary relief of upper respiratory symptoms associated with allergy or the common cold

Local Anesthetic/Vasoconstrictor Precautions

Phenylephrine: Use with caution since phenylephrine is a sympathomimetic amine which could interact with epinephrine to cause a pressor response

Promethazine: No information available to require special precautions

(Continued)

Promethazine and Phenylephrine *(Continued)*

Effects on Dental Treatment Phenylephrine: ≤10%: Tachycardia, palpitations, xerostomia; use vasoconstrictor with caution

Although promethazine is a phenothiazine derivative, extrapyramidal reactions or tardive dyskinesias are not seen with the use of this drug.

Dosage Oral:

Children:

2-6 years: 1.25 mL every 4-6 hours, not to exceed 7.5 mL in 24 hours

6-12 years: 2.5 mL every 4-6 hours, not to exceed 15 mL in 24 hours

Children >12 years and Adults: 5 mL every 4-6 hours, not to exceed 30 mL in 24 hours

Dietary/Ethanol/Herb Considerations

Ethanol: Avoid use; may increase CNS depression.

Herb/Nutraceutical: Avoid gotu kola, kava, SAMe, St John's wort, and valerian; may increase CNS depression.

Pregnancy Risk Factor C

Generic Available Yes

Promethazine Hydrochloride *see* Promethazine *on page 1127*

Promethazine, Phenylephrine, and Codeine

(proe METH a zeen, fen il EF rin, & KOE deen)

Related Information

Codeine *on page 361*
Phenylephrine *on page 1071*
Promethazine *on page 1127*

Pharmacologic Category Antihistamine/Decongestant/Antitussive

Synonyms Codeine, Promethazine, and Phenylephrine; Phenylephrine, Promethazine, and Codeine

Use Temporary relief of coughs and upper respiratory symptoms including nasal congestion

Local Anesthetic/Vasoconstrictor Precautions

Phenylephrine: Use with caution since phenylephrine is a sympathomimetic amine which could interact with epinephrine to cause a pressor response

Promethazine: No information available to require special precautions

Effects on Dental Treatment Phenylephrine: ≤10%: Tachycardia, palpitations, xerostomia; use vasoconstrictor with caution

Although promethazine is a phenothiazine derivative, extrapyramidal reactions or tardive dyskinesias are not seen with the use of this drug.

Restrictions C-V

Dosage Oral:

Children (expressed in terms of codeine dosage): 1-1.5 mg/kg/day every 4 hours, maximum: 30 mg/day **or**

<2 years: Use not recommended

2-6 years:

Weight 25 lb: 1.25-2.5 mL every 4-6 hours, not to exceed 6 mL/24 hours

Weight 30 lb: 1.25-2.5 mL every 4-6 hours, not to exceed 7 mL/24 hours

Weight 35 lb: 1.25-2.5 mL every 4-6 hours, not to exceed 8 mL/24 hours

Weight 40 lb: 1.25-2.5 mL every 4-6 hours, not to exceed 9 mL/24 hours

6 to <12 years: 2.5-5 mL every 4-6 hours, not to exceed 15 mL/24 hours

Adults: 5 mL every 4-6 hours, not to exceed 30 mL/24 hours

Dietary/Ethanol/Herb Considerations

Ethanol: Avoid use; may increase CNS depression.

Herb/Nutraceutical: Avoid gotu kola, kava, SAMe, St John's wort, and valerian; may increase CNS depression.

Pregnancy Risk Factor C

Generic Available Yes

Prometrium® *see* Progesterone *on page 1125*

Promit® *see* Dextran 1 *on page 420*

Pronap-100® *see* Propoxyphene and Acetaminophen *on page 1136*

Pronestyl® *see* Procainamide *on page 1119*

Pronestyl-SR® *see* Procainamide *on page 1119*

Pronto® [OTC] *see* Pyrethrins and Piperonyl Butoxide *on page 1151*

Propafenone (proe pu FEEN one)

Related Information

Cardiovascular Diseases *on page 1456*

U.S. Brand Names Rythmol®

Canadian Brand Names Apo®-Propafenone; Rythmol®

Mexican Brand Names Nistaken®; Norfenon®

Pharmacologic Category Antiarrhythmic Agent, Class Ic

Synonyms Propafenone Hydrochloride

Use Life-threatening ventricular arrhythmias

Unlabeled/Investigational Use Treatment of supraventricular tachycardias, including those patients with Wolff-Parkinson-White syndrome

Local Anesthetic/Vasoconstrictor Precautions No information available to require special precautions

Effects on Dental Treatment >10%: Significant xerostomia; normal salivary flow resumes upon discontinuation

Dosage Oral:

Adults: 150 mg every 8 hours, increase at 3- to 4-day intervals up to 300 mg every 8 hours. **Note:** Patients who exhibit significant widening of QRS complex or second- or third-degree AV block may need dose reduction.

Dosing adjustment in hepatic impairment: Reduction required

Mechanism of Action Propafenone is a class 1c antiarrhythmic agent which possesses local anesthetic properties, blocks the fast inward sodium current, and slows the rate of increase of the action potential. Prolongs conduction and refractoriness in all areas of the myocardium, with a slightly more pronounced effect on intraventricular conduction; it prolongs effective refractory period, reduces spontaneous automaticity and exhibits some beta-blockade activity.

Other Adverse Effects

1% to 10%:

Cardiovascular: New or worsened arrhythmias (proarrhythmic effect) (2% to 10%), angina (2% to 5%), CHF (1% to 4%), ventricular tachycardia (1% to 3%), palpitations (1% to 3%), AV block (first-degree) (1% to 3%), syncope (1% to 2%), increased QRS interval (1% to 2%), chest pain (1% to 2%), PVCs (1% to 2%), bradycardia (1% to 2%), edema (≤1%), bundle branch block (≤1%), atrial fibrillation (1%), hypotension (≤1%), intraventricular conduction delay (0% to 1%)

Central nervous system: Dizziness (4% to 15%), fatigue (2% to 6%), headache (2% to 5%), weakness (1% to 2%), ataxia (≤2%), insomnia (≤2%), anxiety (1% to 2%), drowsiness (1%)

Dermatologic: Rash (1% to 3%)

Gastrointestinal: Nausea/vomiting (2% to 11%), unusual taste (3% to 23%), constipation (2% to 7%), dyspepsia (1% to 3%), diarrhea (1% to 3%), anorexia (1% to 2%), abdominal pain (1% to 2%), flatulence (≤1%)

Neuromuscular & skeletal: Tremor (≤1%), arthralgia (≤1%)

Ocular: Blurred vision (1% to 6%)

Respiratory: Dyspnea (2% to 5%)

Miscellaneous: Diaphoresis (1%)

<1% (Limited to important or life-threatening): Agranulocytosis, leukopenia, thrombocytopenia, purpura, granulocytopenia, anemia, increased bleeding time, hepatitis (0.03%), increased serum transaminases (0.2%), prolonged PR interval, sinus node dysfunction, cholestasis (0.1%), gastroenteritis, positive ANA titers (0.7%), lupus erythematosus, AV block (second or third degree), AV dissociation, cardiac arrest, flushing, sinus arrest, abnormal speech, abnormal dreams, abnormal vision, apnea, coma, confusion, depression, memory loss, paresthesia, numbness, psychosis, seizures (0.3%), tinnitus, abnormal smell sensation, vertigo, alopecia, eye irritation, SIADH, hyponatremia, impotence, hyperglycemia, kidney failure, muscle cramps, muscle weakness, nephrotic syndrome, pain, pruritus, CHF, renal failure, nephrotic syndrome

Postmarketing and/or case reports: Peripheral neuropathy, mania, amnesia

Drug Interactions Substrate of CYP1A2, **2D6**, 3A4; Inhibits CYP1A2, 2D6

Increased Effect/Toxicity: Amprenavir, cimetidine, metoprolol, propranolol, quinidine, and ritonavir may increase propafenone levels; concurrent use is contraindicated. Digoxin (reduce dose by 25%), cyclosporine, local anesthetics, theophylline, and warfarin blood levels are increased by propafenone.

Decreased Effect: Enzyme inducers (phenobarbital, phenytoin, rifabutin, rifampin) may decrease propafenone blood levels.

Dietary/Ethanol/Herb Considerations

Ethanol: Avoid use; may increase risk of hypotension or dizziness.

Food may be increase serum concentration. Avoid caffeine (eg, colas, chocolate), garlic, and licorice.

Herb/Nutraceutical: Avoid black cohosh, dong quai, and evening primrose due to estrogenic activity. Avoid ephedra, ginseng, and yohimbe; may worsen arrhythmia. Avoid garlic; may have increased antihypertensive effect. Avoid ginger due to positive inotropic effects; theoretically, may cause arrhythmia. Avoid hawthorn; may lower peripheral vascular resistance causing additional decrease in BP. Avoid licorice. Avoid St John's wort; may decrease serum concentration.

Pharmacodynamics/Kinetics

Absorption: Well absorbed

Metabolism: Hepatic; two genetically determined metabolism groups exist: fast or slow metabolizers; 10% of Caucasians are slow metabolizers; exhibits nonlinear pharmacokinetics; when dose is increased from 300-900 mg/day, serum concentrations increase tenfold; this nonlinearity is thought to be due to saturable first-pass effect

Bioavailability: 150 mg: 3.4%; 300 mg: 10.6%

(Continued)

Propafenone *(Continued)*

Half-life elimination: Single dose (100-300 mg): 2-8 hours; Chronic dosing: 10-32 hours

Time to peak: 150 mg dose: 2 hours, 300 mg dose: 3 hours

Pregnancy Risk Factor C

Generic Available Yes

Propafenone Hydrochloride *see* Propafenone *on page 1130*

Propantheline (proe PAN the leen)

Canadian Brand Names Propanthel™

Pharmacologic Category Anticholinergic Agent

Synonyms Propantheline Bromide

Use

Dental: Induce dry field (xerostomia) in oral cavity

Medical: Adjunctive treatment of peptic ulcer, irritable bowel syndrome (IBS), pancreatitis, ureteral and urinary bladder spasm; reduce duodenal motility during diagnostic radiologic procedures

Local Anesthetic/Vasoconstrictor Precautions No information available to require special precautions

Effects on Dental Treatment >10%: Significant xerostomia (therapeutic effect), dry throat, nasal dryness, dysphagia

Dosage Oral:

Preprocedure to induce xerostomia: Adults: 15-30 mg as a single dose 1 hour before procedure

Antisecretory:

Children: 1-2 mg/kg/day in 3-4 divided doses

Adults: 15 mg 3 times/day before meals or food and 30 mg at bedtime

Elderly: 7.5 mg 3 times/day before meals and at bedtime

Antispasmodic:

Children: 2-3 mg/kg/day in divided doses every 4-6 hours and at bedtime

Adults: 15 mg 3 times/day before meals or food and 30 mg at bedtime

Mechanism of Action Competitively blocks the action of acetylcholine at postganglionic parasympathetic receptor sites

Other Adverse Effects Frequency not defined:

Dermatologic: Dry skin

Gastrointestinal: Constipation

Miscellaneous: Diaphoresis (decreased)

Contraindications Hypersensitivity to propantheline or any component of the formulation; ulcerative colitis, toxic megacolon, obstructive disease of the GI or urinary tract; narrow-angle glaucoma; myasthenia gravis

Warnings/Precautions Use with caution in patients with hyperthyroidism, hepatic, cardiac, or renal disease, hypertension, GI infections, or other endocrine diseases.

Drug Interactions

Decreased effect with antacids (decreased absorption); decreased effect of sustained release dosage forms (decreased absorption)

Increased effect/toxicity with anticholinergics, disopyramide, narcotic analgesics, bretylium, type I antiarrhythmics, antihistamines, phenothiazines, TCAs, corticosteroids (increased IOP), CNS depressants (sedation), adenosine, amiodarone, beta-blockers, amoxapine

Dietary/Ethanol/Herb Considerations Food: Administer 30 minutes before meals to ensure peak effect occurs at the proper time.

Pharmacodynamics/Kinetics

Onset of action: 30-45 minutes

Duration: 4-6 hours

Half-life elimination, serum: Average: 1.6 hours

Pregnancy Risk Factor C

Breast-feeding Considerations No data reported; however, atropine may be taken while breast-feeding.

Dosage Forms TAB: 15 mg

Generic Available Yes

Propantheline Bromide *see* Propantheline *on page 1132*

Propa pH [OTC] *see* Salicylic Acid *on page 1204*

Proparacaine (proe PAR a kane)

U.S. Brand Names Alcaine®; Ophthetic®

Canadian Brand Names Alcaine®; Diocaine®

Pharmacologic Category Local Anesthetic, Ophthalmic

Synonyms Proparacaine Hydrochloride; Proxymetacaine

Use Anesthesia for tonometry, gonioscopy; suture removal from cornea; removal of corneal foreign body; cataract extraction, glaucoma surgery; short operative procedure involving the cornea and conjunctiva

Local Anesthetic/Vasoconstrictor Precautions No information available to require special precautions

Effects on Dental Treatment No significant effects or complications reported

Dosage Children and Adults:

Ophthalmic surgery: Instill 1 drop of 0.5% solution in eye every 5-10 minutes for 5-7 doses

Tonometry, gonioscopy, suture removal: Instill 1-2 drops of 0.5% solution in eye just prior to procedure

Mechanism of Action Prevents initiation and transmission of impulse at the nerve cell membrane by decreasing ion permeability through stabilizing

Other Adverse Effects

1% to 10%: Local: Burning, stinging, redness

<1%: Allergic contact dermatitis, arrhythmias, blurred vision, CNS depression, conjunctival congestion and hemorrhage, corneal opacification, diaphoresis (increased), epithelium, erosion of the corneal iritis, irritation, keratitis, lacrimation, sensitization

Drug Interactions Increased Effect/Toxicity: Effects of phenylephrine and tropicamide (ophthalmics) are increased

Pharmacodynamics/Kinetics

Onset of action: ~20 seconds

Duration: 15-20 minutes

Pregnancy Risk Factor C

Generic Available Yes

Proparacaine and Fluorescein (proe PAR a kane & FLORE e seen)

Related Information

Proparacaine *on page 1132*

U.S. Brand Names Flucaine®; Fluoracaine®

Pharmacologic Category Diagnostic Agent; Local Anesthetic

Use Anesthesia for tonometry, gonioscopy; suture removal from cornea; removal of corneal foreign body; cataract extraction, glaucoma surgery

Local Anesthetic/Vasoconstrictor Precautions No information available to require special precautions

Effects on Dental Treatment No significant effects or complications reported

Dosage

Ophthalmic surgery: Children and Adults: Instill 1 drop in each eye every 5-10 minutes for 5-7 doses

Tonometry, gonioscopy, suture removal: Adults: Instill 1-2 drops in each eye just prior to procedure

Mechanism of Action Prevents initiation and transmission of impulse at the nerve cell membrane by decreasing ion permeability through stabilizing

Other Adverse Effects

1% to 10%: Local: Burning, stinging of eye

<1%: Allergic contact dermatitis, irritation, sensitization, erosion of the corneal epithelium, conjunctival congestion and hemorrhage, keratitis, iritis, corneal opacification

Pharmacodynamics/Kinetics

Onset of action: ~20 seconds

Duration: 15-20 minutes

Pregnancy Risk Factor C

Generic Available Yes

Proparacaine Hydrochloride *see* Proparacaine *on page 1132*

Propecia® *see* Finasteride *on page 572*

Propine® *see* Dipivefrin *on page 455*

Proplex® T *see* Factor IX Complex (Human) *on page 553*

Propofol (PROE po fole)

U.S. Brand Names Diprivan®

Canadian Brand Names Diprivan®

Mexican Brand Names Diprivan®; Fresofol®; Recofol®

Pharmacologic Category General Anesthetic

Use Induction of anesthesia for inpatient or outpatient surgery in patients ≥3 years of age; maintenance of anesthesia for inpatient or outpatient surgery in patients >2 months of age; in adults, for the induction and maintenance of monitored anesthesia care sedation during diagnostic procedures; may be used (for patients >18 years of age who are intubated and mechanically ventilated) as an alternative to benzodiazepines for the treatment of agitation in the intensive care unit

Unlabeled/Investigational Use Postoperative antiemetic; treatment of refractory delirium tremens

Local Anesthetic/Vasoconstrictor Precautions No information available to require special precautions

Effects on Dental Treatment No significant effects or complications reported

Dosage Dosage must be individualized based on total body weight and titrated to the desired clinical effect; wait at least 3-5 minutes between dosage adjustments to

(Continued)

Propofol *(Continued)*

clinically assess drug effects; smaller doses are required when used with narcotics; the following are general dosing guidelines:

General anesthesia:

Induction: I.V.:

Children 3-16 years, ASA I or II: 2.5-3.5 mg/kg over 20-30 seconds; use a lower dose for children ASA III or IV

Adults, ASA I or II, <55 years: 2-2.5 mg/kg (~40 mg every 10 seconds until onset of induction)

Elderly, debilitated, hypovolemic, or ASA III or IV: 1-1.5 mg/kg (~20 mg every 10 seconds until onset of induction)

Cardiac anesthesia: 0.5-1.5 mg/kg (~20 mg every 10 seconds until onset of induction)

Neurosurgical patients: 1-2 mg/kg (~20 mg every 10 seconds until onset of induction)

Maintenance: I.V. infusion:

Children 2 months to 16 years, ASA I or II: Initial: 200-300 mcg/kg/minute; decrease dose after 30 minutes if clinical signs of light anesthesia are absent; usual infusion rate: 125-150 mcg/kg/minute (range: 125-300 mcg/kg/minute; 7.5-18 mg/kg/hour); children ≤5 years may require larger infusion rates compared to older children

Adults, ASA I or II, <55 years: Initial: 150-200 mcg/kg/minute for 10-15 minutes; decrease by 30% to 50% during first 30 minutes of maintenance; usual infusion rate: 100-200 mcg/kg/minute (6-12 mg/kg/hour)

Elderly, debilitated, hypovolemic, ASA III or IV: 50-100 mcg/kg/minute (3-6 mg/kg/ hour)

Cardiac anesthesia:

Low-dose propofol with primary opioid: 50-100 mcg/kg/minute (see manufacturer's labeling)

Primary propofol with secondary opioid: 100-150 mcg/kg/minute

Neurosurgical patients: 100-200 mcg/kg/minute (6-12 mg/kg/hour)

Maintenance: I.V. intermittent bolus: Adults, ASA I or II, <55 years: 20-50 mg increments as needed

Monitored anesthesia care sedation:

Initiation:

Adults, ASA I or II, <55 years: Slow I.V. infusion: 100-150 mcg/kg/minute for 3-5 minutes **or** slow injection: 0.5 mg/kg over 3-5 minutes

Elderly, debilitated, neurosurgical, or ASA III or IV patients: Use similar doses to healthy adults; avoid rapid I.V. boluses

Maintenance:

Adults, ASA I or II, <55 years: I.V. infusion using variable rates (preferred over intermittent boluses): 25-75 mcg/kg/minute **or** incremental bolus doses: 10 mg or 20 mg

Elderly, debilitated, neurosurgical, or ASA III or IV patients: Use 80% of healthy adult dose; **do not** use rapid bolus doses (single or repeated)

ICU sedation in intubated mechanically-ventilated patients: Avoid rapid bolus injection; individualize dose and titrate to response

Adults: Continuous infusion: Initial: 0.3 mg/kg/hour; increase by 0.3-0.6 mg/kg/hour every 5-10 minutes until desired sedation level is achieved; usual maintenance: 0.3-3 mg/kg/hour or higher; reduce dose by 80% in elderly, debilitated, and ASA III or IV patients; reduce dose after adequate sedation established and adjust to response (ie, evaluate frequently to use minimum dose for sedation). Some clinicians recommend daily interruption of infusion to perform clinical evaluation.

Mechanism of Action Propofol is a hindered phenolic compound with intravenous general anesthetic properties. The drug is unrelated to any of the currently used barbiturate, opioid, benzodiazepine, arylcyclohexylamine, or imidazole intravenous anesthetic agents.

Other Adverse Effects

>10%:

Cardiovascular: Hypotension (3% to 26% adults, 17% children)

Central nervous system: Movement (17% children)

Local: Injection site burning, stinging, or pain (adults 18%, children 10%)

Respiratory: Apnea, lasting 30-60 seconds (24% adults, 10% children); Apnea, lasting >60 seconds (12% adults, 5% children)

3% to 10%:

Cardiovascular: Hypertension (8% children)

Central nervous system: Movement (adults)

Dermatologic: Pruritus (adults), rash

Endocrine & metabolic: Hyperlipidemia

Respiratory: Respiratory acidosis during weaning

1% to 3%:

Cardiovascular: Arrhythmia, bradycardia, decreased cardiac output, tachycardia

Dermatologic: Pruritus (children)

<1%: Agitation; amblyopia; anaphylaxis; anaphylactoid reaction; anticholinergic syndrome; bigeminy; chills; cough; dizziness; delirium; discoloration (green) of urine, hair, or nailbeds; dystonia; EKG abnormal; extremity pain; fever; flushing; hemorrhage; hypersalivation; hypertonia; hypomagnesemia; hypoxia; laryngospasm; leukocytosis; lung function decreased; myalgia; nausea; paresthesia; perinatal disorder; phlebitis; premature atrial contractions; premature ventricular contractions; somnolence; syncope; thrombosis; urine cloudy; vision abnormality; wheezing

Postmarketing and/or case reports: Asystole, cardiac arrest, perioperative myoclonia (rarely including convulsions and opisthotonos), postoperative pancreatitis, postoperative unconsciousness with or without increase in muscle tone, pulmonary edema, rhabdomyolysis, increased serum triglycerides; infusion site reactions include pain, swelling, blisters and/or tissue necrosis following accidental extravasation

Drug Interactions Substrate of CYP1A2, 2A6, **2B6, 2C8/9**, 2C19, 2D6, 2E1, 3A4; Inhibits CYP1A2, 2C8/9, 2D6, 2E1, 3A4

Increased Toxicity: Propofol may potentiate the neuromuscular blockade of vecuronium. Additive CNS depression and respiratory depression may necessitate dosage reduction when used with anesthetics, benzodiazepines, opiates, ethanol, narcotics, phenothiazines.

Dietary/Ethanol/Herb Considerations

Ethanol: Avoid use; may cause additive CNS and respiratory depression.

Food: EDTA, an ingredient of propofol emulsion, may lead to decreased zinc levels in patients on prolonged therapy (>5 days) or those predisposed to deficiency (burns, diarrhea, and/or major sepsis). Propofol is formulated in an oil-in-water emulsion. If patient is on parenteral nutrition, may require adjustment in the amount of lipid infused. Propofol emulsion contains 1.1 kcal/mL.

Herb/Nutraceutical: Avoid gotu kola, kava, SAMe, St John's wort, and valerian; may increase CNS depression.

Pharmacodynamics/Kinetics

Onset of action: Anesthetic: Bolus infusion (dose dependent): 9-51 seconds (average 30 seconds)

Duration (dose and rate dependent): 3-10 minutes

Distribution: V_d: 2-10 L/kg; highly lipophilic

Protein binding: 97% to 99%

Metabolism: Hepatic to water-soluble sulfate and glucuronide conjugates

Half-life elimination: Biphasic: Initial: 40 minutes; Terminal: 4-7 hours (up to 1-3 days)

Excretion: Urine (~88% as metabolites, 40% as glucuronide metabolite); feces (<2%)

Clearance: 20-30 mL/kg/minute; total body clearance exceeds liver blood flow

Pregnancy Risk Factor B

Generic Available Yes

Comments Formulated into an emulsion containing 10% w/v soybean oil, 1.2% w/v purified egg phosphatide, and 2.25% w/v glycerol; this emulsion vehicle is chemically similar to 10% Intralipid®

Injection contains EDTA as a preservative

Propoxyphene (proe POKS i feen)

U.S. Brand Names Darvon®; Darvon-N®

Canadian Brand Names Darvon-N®; 642® Tablet

Pharmacologic Category Analgesic, Narcotic

Synonyms Dextropropoxyphene; Propoxyphene Hydrochloride; Propoxyphene Napsylate

Use Management of mild to moderate pain

Local Anesthetic/Vasoconstrictor Precautions No information available to require special precautions

Effects on Dental Treatment 1% to 10%: Xerostomia

Restrictions C-IV

Dosage Oral:

Children: Doses for children are not well established; doses of the hydrochloride of 2-3 mg/kg/d divided every 6 hours have been used

Adults:

Hydrochloride: 65 mg every 3-4 hours as needed for pain; maximum: 390 mg/day

Napsylate: 100 mg every 4 hours as needed for pain; maximum: 600 mg/day

Dosing comments in renal impairment: Cl_{cr} <10 mL/minute: Avoid use

Hemodialysis: Not dialyzable (0% to 5%)

Dosing adjustment in hepatic impairment: Reduction required

Mechanism of Action Propoxyphene is a weak narcotic analgesic which acts through binding to opiate receptors to inhibit ascending pain pathways. Propoxyphene, as with other narcotic (opiate) analgesics, blocks pain perception in the cerebral cortex by binding to specific receptor molecules (opiate receptors) within the neuronal membranes of synapses. This binding results in a decreased synaptic

(Continued)

Propoxyphene *(Continued)*

chemical transmission throughout the CNS thus inhibiting the flow of pain sensations into the higher centers. Mu and kappa are the two subtypes of the opiate receptor which propoxyphene binds to to cause analgesia.

Other Adverse Effects Frequency not defined:

Cardiovascular: Hypotension, bundle branch block

Central nervous system: Dizziness, lightheadedness, sedation, paradoxical excitement and insomnia, fatigue, drowsiness, mental depression, hallucinations, paradoxical CNS stimulation, increased intracranial pressure, nervousness, headache, restlessness, malaise, confusion

Dermatologic: Rash, urticaria

Endocrine & metabolic: May decrease glucose, urinary 17-OHCS

Gastrointestinal: Anorexia, stomach cramps, biliary spasm, nausea, vomiting, constipation, paralytic ileus

Genitourinary: Decreased urination, ureteral spasms

Neuromuscular & skeletal: Weakness

Hepatic: Increased liver enzymes (may increase LFTs)

Respiratory: Dyspnea

Miscellaneous: Psychologic and physical dependence with prolonged use, histamine release

Drug Interactions Inhibits CYP2C8/9, 2D6, 3A4

Increased Effect/Toxicity: CNS depressants (phenothiazines, tranquilizers, anxiolytics, sedatives, hypnotics, or alcohol) may potentiate pharmacologic effects. Propoxyphene may inhibit the metabolism and increase the serum concentrations of carbamazepine, phenobarbital, MAO inhibitors, tricyclic antidepressants, and warfarin.

Decreased Effect: Decreased effect with cigarette smoking.

Dietary/Ethanol/Herb Considerations

Ethanol: Avoid or limit use; may increase CNS depression.

Food: Administer on an empty stomach if possible; food may decrease rate of absorption but slightly increase bioavailability.

Herb/Nutraceutical: Avoid gotu kola, kava, SAMe, St John's wort, and valerian; may increase CNS depression.

Pharmacodynamics/Kinetics

Onset of action: 0.5-1 hour

Duration: 4-6 hours

Metabolism: Hepatic to active metabolite (norpropoxyphene) and inactive metabolites; first-pass effect

Bioavailability: 30% to 70%

Half-life elimination: Adults: Parent drug: 8-24 hours (mean: ~15 hours); Norpropoxyphene: 34 hours

Excretion: Urine (20% to 25%)

Pregnancy Risk Factor C/D (prolonged use)

Generic Available Yes: Capsule

Propoxyphene and Acetaminophen

(proe POKS i feen & a seet a MIN oh fen)

Related Information

Acetaminophen *on page 27*

Propoxyphene *on page 1135*

U.S. Brand Names Darvocet-N® 50; Darvocet-N® 100; Pronap-100®

Canadian Brand Names Darvocet-N® 50; Darvocet-N® 100

Pharmacologic Category Analgesic Combination (Narcotic)

Synonyms Propoxyphene Hydrochloride and Acetaminophen; Propoxyphene Napsylate and Acetaminophen

Use

Dental: Treatment of postoperative pain

Medical: Management of mild to moderate pain

Local Anesthetic/Vasoconstrictor Precautions No information available to require special precautions

Effects on Dental Treatment Frequency not defined: Based on propoxyphene component: Hypotension, dizziness, lightheadedness, sedation, fatigue, drowsiness, hallucinations, paradoxical CNS stimulation, increased intracranial pressure, nervousness, headache, restlessness, malaise, confusion, xerostomia, biliary spasm, nausea, vomiting, weakness, dyspnea, psychologic and physical dependence (prolonged use), histamine release

Restrictions C-IV

Dosage Dosage of acetaminophen should not exceed 4 g/day (6 tablets of Darvocet-N® 100); less in patients with ethanol use due to increased CNS depression.

Adults: Oral:

Darvocet-N®: 1-2 tablets every 4 hours as needed; maximum: 600 mg propoxyphene napsylate/day

Darvocet-N® 100: 1 tablet every 4 hours as needed; maximum: 600 mg propoxyphene napsylate/day

Mechanism of Action

Propoxyphene is a weak narcotic analgesic which acts through binding to opiate receptors to inhibit ascending pain pathways

Propoxyphene, as with other narcotic (opiate) analgesics, blocks pain perception in the cerebral cortex by binding to specific receptor molecules (opiate receptors) within the neuronal membranes of synapses. This binding results in a decreased synaptic chemical transmission throughout the CNS thus inhibiting the flow of pain sensations into the higher centers. Mu and kappa are the two subtypes of the opiate receptor which propoxyphene binds to to cause analgesia.

Acetaminophen inhibits the synthesis of prostaglandins in the CNS and peripherally blocks pain impulse generation; produces antipyresis from inhibition of hypothalamic heat-regulating center

Other Adverse Effects Frequency not defined:

Based on propoxyphene component:

- Central nervous system: Mental depression,
- Dermatologic: Rash, urticaria
- Endocrine & metabolic: May decrease glucose, urinary 17-OHCS
- Gastrointestinal: Anorexia, stomach cramps constipation, paralytic ileus
- Genitourinary: Decreased urination, ureteral spasms
- Hepatic: Increased liver enzymes (may increase LFTs)

Based on acetaminophen component: May increase chloride, bilirubin, uric acid, glucose, ammonia, alkaline phosphatase; may decrease sodium, bicarbonate, calcium

<1%: Rash, **nausea, vomiting**, blood dyscrasias (neutropenia, pancytopenia, leukopenia), anemia, analgesic nephropathy, nephrotoxicity (chronic overdose), **hypersensitivity reactions (rare)**

Contraindications Hypersensitivity to propoxyphene, acetaminophen, or any component of the formulation; patients with known G6PD deficiency

Warnings/Precautions When given in excessive doses, either alone or in combination with other CNS depressants, propoxyphene is a major cause of drug-related deaths; do not exceed recommended dosage; give with caution in patients dependent on opiates, substitution may result in acute opiate withdrawal symptoms

Dietary/Ethanol/Herb Considerations Food: Administer on an empty stomach; glucose may cause hyperglycemia (monitor blood glucose concentrations).

Based on **propoxyphene** component:

- Ethanol: Avoid or limit use; may increase CNS depression.
- Food may decrease rate of absorption, but slightly increase bioavailability.

Based on **acetaminophen** component:

- Ethanol: Excessive intake may increase the risk of acetaminophen-induced hepatotoxicity; avoid use or limit to <3 drinks/day.
- Food may slightly delay absorption of extended-release preparations; rate of absorption may be decreased when given with food high in carbohydrates.
- Herb/Nutraceutical: Avoid St John's wort; may decrease serum concentration.

Pregnancy Risk Factor C

Dosage Forms TAB: Propoxyphene hydrochloride 65 mg and acetaminophen 650 mg, propoxyphene napsylate 100 mg, and acetaminophen 650 mg; (Darvocet-N® 50): Propoxyphene napsylate 50 mg and acetaminophen 325 mg; (Darvocet-N® 100, Pronap-100®): Propoxyphene napsylate 100 mg and acetaminophen 650 mg

Generic Available Yes

Comments Propoxyphene is a narcotic analgesic and shares many properties including addiction liability. The acetaminophen component requires use with caution in patients with alcoholic liver disease.

Selected Readings

Botting RM, "Mechanism of Action of Acetaminophen: Is There a Cyclooxygenase 3?," *Clin Infect Dis*, 2000, Suppl 5:S202-10.

Dart RC, Kuffner EK, and Rumack BH, "Treatment of Pain or Fever with Paracetamol (Acetaminophen) in the Alcoholic Patient: A Systematic Review," *Am J Ther*, 2000, 7(2):123-34.

Grant JA and Weiler JM, "A Report of a Rare Immediate Reaction After Ingestion of Acetaminophen," *Ann Allergy Asthma Immunol*, 2001, 87(3):227-9.

Kwan D, Bartle WR, and Walker SE, "The Effects of Acetaminophen on Pharmacokinetics and Pharmacodynamics of Warfarin," *J Clin Pharmacol*, 1999, 39(1):68-75.

McClain CJ, Price S, Barve S, et al, "Acetaminophen Hepatotoxicity: An Update," *Curr Gastroenterol Rep*, 1999, 1(1):42-9.

Shek KL, Chan LN, and Nutescu E, "Warfarin-Acetaminophen Drug Interaction Revisited," *Pharmacotherapy*, 1999, 19(10):1153-8.

Tanaka E, Yamazaki K, and Misawa S, "Update: The Clinical Importance of Acetaminophen Hepatotoxicity in Nonalcoholic and Alcoholic Subjects," *J Clin Pharm Ther*, 2000, 25(5):325-32.

Propoxyphene and Aspirin (proe POKS i feen & AS pir in)

Related Information

Aspirin *on page 131*

Propoxyphene *on page 1135*

U.S. Brand Names Darvon® Compound-65 Pulvules®

Pharmacologic Category Analgesic Combination (Narcotic)

(Continued)

Propoxyphene and Aspirin *(Continued)*

Synonyms Propoxyphene Hydrochloride and Aspirin; Propoxyphene Napsylate and Aspirin

Use

Dental: Treatment of postoperative pain

Medical: Management of mild to moderate pain

Local Anesthetic/Vasoconstrictor Precautions No information available to require special precautions

Effects on Dental Treatment As with all drugs which may affect hemostasis, bleeding is associated with aspirin. Hemorrhage may occur at virtually any site; risk is dependent on multiple variables including dosage, concurrent use of multiple agents which alter hemostasis, and patient susceptibility. Many adverse effects of aspirin are dose-related, and are rare at low dosages. Other serious reactions are idiosyncratic, related to allergy or individual sensitivity.

Elderly are a high-risk population for adverse effects from nonsteroidal anti-inflammatory agents. As much as 60% of elderly patients with GI complications from NSAIDs can develop peptic ulceration and/or hemorrhage asymptomatically. Concomitant disease and drug use contribute to the risk of GI adverse effects. Use lowest effective dose for shortest period possible. Consider renal function decline with age.

Frequency not always defined:

Based on propoxyphene component: Hypotension, dizziness, lightheadedness, sedation, fatigue, drowsiness, hallucinations, paradoxical CNS stimulation, increased intracranial pressure, nervousness, headache, restlessness, malaise, confusion, xerostomia, biliary spasm, nausea, vomiting, weakness, dyspnea, psychologic and physical dependence (prolonged use), histamine release

Based on aspirin component: Hypotension, tachycardia, dysrhythmias, fatigue, nervousness, agitation, confusion, dizziness, headache, lethargy, coma, dehydration, hypoglycemia (children), hyperglycemia, nausea, vomiting, epigastric discomfort, GI ulceration (6% to 31%), gastric erosions, gastric erythema, duodenal ulcers, increased PT, coagulopathy, weakness, asthma, bronchospasm, dyspnea, laryngeal edema, hyperpnea, tachypnea, respiratory alkalosis, anaphylaxis, esophageal stricture, esophagitis with esophageal ulcer, esophageal hematoma, oral mucosal ulcers (aspirin-containing chewing gum), delirium, rhinosinusitis

Restrictions C-IV

Dosage Oral:

Children: Use not recommended

Adults: 1-2 capsules every 4 hours as needed

Mechanism of Action

Propoxyphene is a weak narcotic analgesic which acts through binding to opiate receptors to inhibit ascending pain pathways

Propoxyphene, as with other narcotic (opiate) analgesics, blocks pain perception in the cerebral cortex by binding to specific receptor molecules (opiate receptors) within the neuronal membranes of synapses. This binding results in a decreased synaptic chemical transmission throughout the CNS thus inhibiting the flow of pain sensations into the higher centers. Mu and kappa are the two subtypes of the opiate receptor to which propoxyphene binds to cause analgesia.

Aspirin inhibits prostaglandin synthesis by decreasing the activity of the enzyme, cyclooxygenase, which results in decreased formation of prostaglandin precursors, acts on the hypothalamic heat-regulating center to reduce fever, blocks thromboxane synthetase action which prevents formation of the platelet-aggregating substance thromboxane A_2

Other Adverse Effects Frequency not defined:

Based on propoxyphene component:

- Central nervous system: Mental depression
- Dermatologic: Rash, urticaria
- Endocrine & metabolic: May decrease glucose, urinary 17-OHCS
- Gastrointestinal: Anorexia, stomach cramps, constipation, paralytic ileus
- Genitourinary: Decreased urination, ureteral spasms
- Hepatic: Increased liver enzymes (may increase LFTs)

Based on aspirin component:

- Cardiovascular: Edema
- Central nervous system: Insomnia, cerebral edema, hyperthermia
- Dermatologic: Rash, angioedema, urticaria
- Endocrine & metabolic: Acidosis, hyperkalemia, hypernatremia (buffered forms)
- Gastrointestinal: Dyspepsia, heartburn, stomach pains
- Hematologic: Anemia, disseminated intravascular coagulation, thrombocytopenia, hemolytic anemia, iron-deficiency anemia
- Hepatic: Hepatotoxicity, increased transaminases, hepatitis (reversible)
- Neuromuscular & skeletal: Rhabdomyolysis, acetabular bone destruction (OA)
- Otic: Hearing loss, tinnitus

Renal: Interstitial nephritis, papillary necrosis, proteinuria, renal impairment, renal failure (including cases caused by rhabdomyolysis), increased BUN, increased serum creatinine

Respiratory: Noncardiogenic pulmonary edema

Miscellaneous: Prolonged pregnancy and labor, stillbirths, low birth weight, peripartum bleeding, Reye's syndrome

Case reports: Colonic ulceration, coronary artery spasm, **conduction defect and atrial fibrillation (toxicity),** ischemic brain infarction, colitis, rectal stenosis (suppository), cholestatic jaundice, **periorbital edema**

Contraindications Hypersensitivity to propoxyphene, aspirin, or any component of the formulation

Warnings/Precautions When given in excessive doses, either alone or in combination with other CNS depressants, propoxyphene is a major cause of drug-related deaths. Do not exceed recommended dosage. Due to aspirin component, do not use in children <16 years of age for chickenpox or flu symptoms before a physician is consulted about Reye's syndrome. Avoid use in active peptic ulcer disease. Use with caution in patients with platelet and bleeding disorders, renal dysfunction, erosive gastritis. Previous nonreaction does not guarantee future safe taking of medication. Use with caution in impaired hepatic function and patients with history of asthma. Avoid aspirin-containing products, if possible, for 1 week prior to dental or surgical procedures due to possibility of postoperative bleeding.

Dietary/Ethanol/Herb Considerations

Ethanol: Avoid use; may increase CNS depression and enhance gastric mucosal irritation.

Herb/Nutraceutical: Avoid gotu kola, kava, SAMe, St John's wort, and valerian; may increase CNS depression.

Pregnancy Risk Factor D

Breast-feeding Considerations

Propoxyphene: May be taken while breast-feeding.

Aspirin: Use cautiously due to potential adverse effects in nursing infants.

Dosage Forms CAP (Darvon® Compound-65, PC-Cap®): Propoxyphene 65 mg and aspirin 389 mg with caffeine 32.4 mg

Generic Available No

Comments Propoxyphene is a narcotic analgesic and shares many properties including addiction liability. The aspirin component could have anticoagulant effects and could possibly affect bleeding times.

Propoxyphene Hydrochloride *see* Propoxyphene *on page 1135*

Propoxyphene Hydrochloride and Acetaminophen *see* Propoxyphene and Acetaminophen *on page 1136*

Propoxyphene Hydrochloride and Aspirin *see* Propoxyphene and Aspirin *on page 1137*

Propoxyphene Napsylate *see* Propoxyphene *on page 1135*

Propoxyphene Napsylate and Acetaminophen *see* Propoxyphene and Acetaminophen *on page 1136*

Propoxyphene Napsylate and Aspirin *see* Propoxyphene and Aspirin *on page 1137*

Propranolol (proe PRAN oh lole)

Related Information

Cardiovascular Diseases *on page 1456*

Endocrine Disorders and Pregnancy *on page 1479*

U.S. Brand Names Inderal®; Inderal® LA; Propranolol Intensol™

Canadian Brand Names Apo®-Propranolol; Inderal®; Inderal®-LA; Nu-Propranolol

Mexican Brand Names Inderalici; PMS-Propranolol®

Pharmacologic Category Antiarrhythmic Agent, Class II; Beta Blocker, Nonselective

Synonyms Propranolol Hydrochloride

Use Management of hypertension; angina pectoris; pheochromocytoma; essential tremor; tetralogy of Fallot cyanotic spells; arrhythmias (such as atrial fibrillation and flutter, AV nodal re-entrant tachycardias, and catecholamine-induced arrhythmias); prevention of MI; migraine headache; symptomatic treatment of hypertrophic subaortic stenosis

Unlabeled/Investigational Use Treatment of tremor due to Parkinson's disease, ethanol withdrawal symptoms, aggressive behavior, antipsychotic-induced akathisia, anxiety, schizophrenia, acute panic; prevention of bleeding esophageal varices, gastric bleeding in portal hypertension

Local Anesthetic/Vasoconstrictor Precautions Use with caution; epinephrine has interacted with nonselective beta-blockers to result in initial hypertensive episode followed by bradycardia

Effects on Dental Treatment Propranolol is a nonselective beta-blocker and may enhance the pressor response to epinephrine, resulting in hypertension and bradycardia. Many nonsteroidal anti-inflammatory drugs such as ibuprofen and indomethacin can reduce the hypotensive effect of beta-blockers after 3 or more weeks

(Continued)

Propranolol *(Continued)*

of therapy with the NSAID. Short-term NSAID use (ie, 3 days) requires no special precautions in patients taking beta-blockers.

Dosage

Tachyarrhythmias:

Oral:

Children: Initial: 0.5-1 mg/kg/day in divided doses every 6-8 hours; titrate dosage upward every 3-7 days; usual dose: 2-4 mg/kg/day; higher doses may be needed; do not exceed 16 mg/kg/day or 60 mg/day

Adults: 10-30 mg/dose every 6-8 hours

Elderly: Initial: 10 mg twice daily; increase dosage every 3-7 days; usual dosage range: 10-320 mg given in 2 divided doses

I.V.:

Children: 0.01-0.1 mg/kg slow IVP over 10 minutes; maximum dose: 1 mg

Adults: 1 mg/dose slow IVP; repeat every 5 minutes up to a total of 5 mg

Hypertension: Oral:

Children: Initial: 0.5-1 mg/kg/day in divided doses every 6-12 hours; increase gradually every 3-7 days; maximum: 2 mg/kg/24 hours

Adults: Initial: 40 mg twice daily; increase dosage every 3-7 days; usual dose: ≤320 mg divided in 2-3 doses/day; maximum daily dose: 640 mg

Long-acting formulation: Initial: 80 mg once daily; usual maintenance: 120-160 mg once daily; maximum daily dose: 640 mg

Migraine headache prophylaxis: Oral:

Children: 0.6-1.5 mg/kg/day **or**

≤35 kg: 10-20 mg 3 times/day

>35 kg: 20-40 mg 3 times/day

Adults: Initial: 80 mg/day divided every 6-8 hours; increase by 20-40 mg/dose every 3-4 weeks to a maximum of 160-240 mg/day given in divided doses every 6-8 hours; if satisfactory response not achieved within 6 weeks of starting therapy, drug should be withdrawn gradually over several weeks

Long-acting formulation: Initial: 80 mg once daily; effective dose range: 160-240 mg once daily

Tetralogy spells: Children:

Oral: 1-2 mg/kg/day every 6 hours as needed, may increase by 1 mg/kg/day to a maximum of 5 mg/kg/day, or if refractory may increase slowly to a maximum of 10-15 mg/kg/day

I.V.: 0.15-0.25 mg/kg/dose slow IVP; may repeat in 15 minutes

Thyrotoxicosis:

Adolescents and Adults: Oral: 10-40 mg/dose every 6 hours

Adults: I.V.: 1-3 mg/dose slow IVP as a single dose

Adults: Oral:

Akathisia: 30-120 mg/day in 2-3 divided doses

Angina: 80-320 mg/day in doses divided 2-4 times/day

Long-acting formulation: Initial: 80 mg once daily; maximum dose: 320 mg once daily

Essential tremor: 20-40 mg twice daily initially; maintenance doses: usually 120-320 mg/day

Hypertrophic subaortic stenosis: 20-40 mg 3-4 times/day

Long-acting formulation: 80-160 mg once daily

Myocardial infarction prophylaxis: 180-240 mg/day in 3-4 divided doses

Pheochromocytoma: 30-60 mg/day in divided doses

Dosing adjustment in renal impairment:

Cl_{cr} 31-40 mL/minute: Administer every 24-36 hours or administer 50% of normal dose

Cl_{cr} 10-30 mL/minute: Administer every 24-48 hours or administer 50% of normal dose

Cl_{cr} <10 mL/minute: Administer every 40-60 hours or administer 25% of normal dose

Hemodialysis: Not dialyzable (0% to 5%); supplemental dose is unnecessary

Peritoneal dialysis: Supplemental dose is unnecessary

Dosing adjustment in hepatic disease: Marked slowing of heart rate may occur in cirrhosis with conventional doses; low initial dose and regular heart rate monitoring

Mechanism of Action Nonselective beta-adrenergic blocker (class II antiarrhythmic); competitively blocks response to $beta_1$- and $beta_2$-adrenergic stimulation which results in decreases in heart rate, myocardial contractility, blood pressure, and myocardial oxygen demand

Other Adverse Effects Frequency not defined:

Cardiovascular: Bradycardia, CHF, reduced peripheral circulation, chest pain, hypotension, impaired myocardial contractility, worsening of AV conduction disturbance, cardiogenic shock, Raynaud's syndrome, mesenteric thrombosis (rare)

Central nervous system: Mental depression, lightheadedness, amnesia, emotional lability, confusion, hallucinations, dizziness, insomnia, fatigue, vivid dreams, lethargy, cold extremities, vertigo, syncope, cognitive dysfunction, psychosis, hypersomnolence

Dermatologic: Rash, alopecia, exfoliative dermatitis, psoriasiform eruptions, eczematous eruptions, hyperkeratosis, nail changes, pruritus, urticaria, ulcerative lichenoid, contact dermatitis

Endocrine & metabolic: Hypoglycemia, hyperglycemia, hyperlipidemia, hyperkalemia

Gastrointestinal: Diarrhea, nausea, vomiting, stomach discomfort, constipation, anorexia

Genitourinary: Impotence, proteinuria (rare), oliguria (rare), interstitial nephritis (rare), Peyronie's disease

Hematologic: Agranulocytosis, thrombocytopenia, thrombocytopenic purpura

Neuromuscular & skeletal: Weakness, carpal tunnel syndrome (rare), paresthesias, myotonus, polyarthritis, arthropathy

Respiratory: Wheezing, pharyngitis, bronchospasm, pulmonary edema

Ocular: Hyperemia of the conjunctiva, decreased tear production, decreased visual acuity, mydriasis

Miscellaneous: Lupus-like syndrome (rare)

Drug Interactions Substrate of **CYP1A2, 2C19, 2D6**, 3A4; Inhibits CYP1A2, 2D6

Increased Effect/Toxicity: The heart rate lowering effects of propranolol are additive with other drugs which slow AV conduction (digoxin, verapamil, diltiazem). Reserpine increases the effects of propranolol. Concurrent use of propranolol may increase the effects of alpha-blockers (prazosin, terazosin), alpha-adrenergic stimulants (epinephrine, phenylephrine), and the vasoconstrictive effects of ergot alkaloids. Propranolol may mask the tachycardia from hypoglycemia caused by insulin and oral hypoglycemics. In patients receiving concurrent therapy, the risk of hypertensive crisis is increased when either clonidine or the beta-blocker is withdrawn. Beta-blockers may increase the action or levels of ethanol, disopyramide, nondepolarizing muscle relaxants, and theophylline although the effects are difficult to predict. Beta-blocker effects may be enhanced by oral contraceptives, flecainide, haloperidol (hypotensive effects), H_2-antagonists (cimetidine, possibly ranitidine), hydralazine, loop diuretics, possibly MAO inhibitors, phenothiazines, propafenone, quinidine (in extensive metabolizers), ciprofloxacin, thyroid hormones (when hypothyroid patient is converted to euthyroid state). Beta-blockers may increase the effect/toxicity of flecainide, haloperidol (hypotensive effects), hydralazine, phenothiazines, acetaminophen, anticoagulants (warfarin), and benzodiazepines.

Decreased Effect: Aluminum salts, barbiturates, calcium salts, cholestyramine, colestipol, NSAIDs, penicillins (ampicillin), rifampin, salicylates, and sulfinpyrazone decrease effect of beta-blockers due to decreased bioavailability and plasma levels. Beta-blockers may decrease the effect of sulfonylureas. Ascorbic acid decreases propranolol Cp_{max} and AUC and increases the T_{max} significantly resulting in a greater decrease in the reduction of heart rate, possibly due to decreased absorption and first pass metabolism (n=5). Nefazodone decreased peak plasma levels and AUC of propranolol and increases time to reach steady-state; monitoring of clinical response is recommended. Nonselective beta-blockers blunt the response to beta-2 adrenergic agonists (albuterol).

Dietary/Ethanol/Herb Considerations

Ethanol: Avoid or limit use; may increase risk of hypotension or dizziness.

Food may increase serum concentration; protein-rich foods may increase bioavailability. A change in diet from high carbohydrate/low protein to low carbohydrate/high protein may result in increased oral clearance. Avoid caffeine (eg, colas, chocolate), garlic, and licorice.

Herb/Nutraceutical: Avoid black cohosh, dong quai, and evening primrose due to estrogenic activity. Avoid ephedra, ginseng, and yohimbe; may worsen hypertension or arrhythmia. Avoid garlic; may have increased antihypertensive effect. Avoid ginger due to positive inotropic effects; theoretically, may cause arrhythmia. Avoid hawthorn; may lower peripheral vascular resistance causing additional decrease in BP. Avoid licorice; causes sodium and water retention and increases potassium loss.

Pharmacodynamics/Kinetics

Onset of action: Beta-blockade: Oral: 1-2 hours

Duration: ~6 hours

Distribution: V_d: 3.9 L/kg in adults; crosses placenta; small amounts enter breast milk

Protein binding: Newborns: 68%; Adults: 93%

Metabolism: Hepatic to active and inactive compounds; extensive first-pass effect

Bioavailability: 30% to 40%; may be increased in Down syndrome

Half-life elimination: Neonates and Infants: Possible increased half-life; Children: 3.9-6.4 hours; Adults: 4-6 hours

Excretion: Urine (96% to 99%)

Pregnancy Risk Factor C (manufacturer); D (2nd and 3rd trimesters - expert analysis)

(Continued)

Propranolol *(Continued)*

Generic Available Yes: Excludes capsule

Selected Readings

Foster CA and Aston SJ, "Propranolol-Epinephrine Interaction: A Potential Disaster," *Plast Reconstr Surg*, 1983, 72(1):74-8.

Wong DG, Spence JD, Lamki L, et al, "Effect of Nonsteroidal Anti-inflammatory Drugs on Control of Hypertension of Beta-Blockers and Diuretics," *Lancet*, 1986, 1(8488):997-1001.

Wynn RL, "Dental Nonsteroidal Anti-inflammatory Drugs and Prostaglandin-Based Drug Interactions, Part Two," *Gen Dent*, 1992, 40(2):104, 106, 108.

Wynn RL, "Epinephrine Interactions With Beta-Blockers," *Gen Dent*, 1994, 42(1):16, 18.

Propranolol and Hydrochlorothiazide

(proe PRAN oh lole & hye droe klor oh THYE a zide)

Related Information

Hydrochlorothiazide *on page 675*

Propranolol *on page 1139*

U.S. Brand Names Inderide®

Pharmacologic Category Antihypertensive Agent Combination

Synonyms Hydrochlorothiazide and Propranolol

Use Management of hypertension

Local Anesthetic/Vasoconstrictor Precautions Use with caution; epinephrine has interacted with nonselective beta-blockers to result in initial hypertensive episode followed by bradycardia

Effects on Dental Treatment Noncardioselective beta-blockers (ie, propranolol, nadolol) enhance the pressor response to epinephrine, resulting in hypertension and bradycardia. Many nonsteroidal anti-inflammatory drugs such as ibuprofen and indomethacin can reduce the hypotensive effect of beta-blockers after 3 or more weeks of therapy with the NSAID. Short-term NSAID use (ie, 3 days) requires no special precautions in patients taking beta-blockers.

Dosage Oral: Adults: Hypertension: Dose is individualized; typical dosages of **hydrochlorothiazide**: 12.5-50 mg/day; initial dose of **propranolol**: 80 mg/day

Daily dose of tablet form should be divided into 2 daily doses; may be used to maximum dosage of up to 160 mg of propranolol; higher dosages would result in higher than optimal thiazide dosages.

Long acting capsules may be given once daily.

Other Adverse Effects See individual agents.

Dietary/Ethanol/Herb Considerations Ethanol: Limit use; may increase risk of hypotension or dizziness.

Pregnancy Risk Factor C

Generic Available Yes

Propranolol Hydrochloride *see* Propranolol *on page 1139*

Propranolol Intensol™ *see* Propranolol *on page 1139*

Propulsid® *see* Cisapride *on page 332*

Propylene Glycol Diacetate, Acetic Acid, and Hydrocortisone *see* Acetic Acid, Propylene Glycol Diacetate, and Hydrocortisone *on page 38*

Propylene Glycol Diacetate, Hydrocortisone, and Acetic Acid *see* Acetic Acid, Propylene Glycol Diacetate, and Hydrocortisone *on page 38*

Propylhexedrine

(proe pil HEKS e dreen)

U.S. Brand Names Benzedrex® [OTC]

Pharmacologic Category Adrenergic Agonist Agent

Use Topical nasal decongestant

Local Anesthetic/Vasoconstrictor Precautions No information available to require special precautions

Effects on Dental Treatment No significant effects or complications reported

Dosage Inhale through each nostril while blocking the other

Generic Available No

Comments Drug has been extracted from inhaler and injected I.V. as an amphetamine substitute

2-Propylpentanoic Acid *see* Valproic Acid and Derivatives *on page 1371*

Propylthiouracil

(proe pil thye oh YOOR a sil)

Related Information

Endocrine Disorders and Pregnancy *on page 1479*

Canadian Brand Names Propyl-Thyracil®

Pharmacologic Category Antithyroid Agent

Synonyms PTU

Use Palliative treatment of hyperthyroidism as an adjunct to ameliorate hyperthyroidism in preparation for surgical treatment or radioactive iodine therapy; management of thyrotoxic crisis

Local Anesthetic/Vasoconstrictor Precautions No information available to require special precautions

Effects on Dental Treatment No significant effects or complications reported

Dosage Administer in 3 equally divided doses at approximately 8-hour intervals. Adjust dosage to maintain T_3, T_4, and TSH levels in normal range; elevated T_3 may be sole indicator of inadequate treatment. Elevated TSH indicates excessive antithyroid treatment.

Oral:

Children: Initial: 5-7 mg/kg/day **or** 150-200 mg/m²/day in divided doses every 8 hours

or

6-10 years: 50-150 mg/day

>10 years: 150-300 mg/day

Maintenance: Determined by patient response **or** ⅓ to ⅔ of the initial dose in divided doses every 8-12 hours. This usually begins after 2 months on an effective initial dose.

Adults: Initial: 300 mg/day in divided doses every 8 hours. In patients with severe hyperthyroidism, very large goiters, or both, the initial dosage is usually 450 mg/day; an occasional patient will require 600-900 mg/day; maintenance: 100-150 mg/day in divided doses every 8-12 hours

Elderly: Initial: 150-300 mg/day

Withdrawal of therapy: Therapy should be withdrawn gradually with evaluation of the patient every 4-6 weeks for the first 3 months then every 3 months for the first year after discontinuation of therapy to detect any reoccurrence of a hyperthyroid state.

Mechanism of Action Inhibits the synthesis of thyroid hormones by blocking the oxidation of iodine in the thyroid gland; blocks synthesis of thyroxine and triiodothyronine

Other Adverse Effects Frequency not defined:

Cardiovascular: Edema, cutaneous vasculitis, leukocytoclastic vasculitis, ANCA-positive vasculitis

Central nervous system: Fever, drowsiness, vertigo, headache, drug fever, dizziness, neuritis

Dermatologic: Skin rash, urticaria, pruritus, exfoliative dermatitis, alopecia, erythema nodosum

Endocrine & metabolic: Goiter, weight gain, swollen salivary glands

Gastrointestinal: Nausea, vomiting, loss of taste, stomach pain, constipation

Hematologic: Leukopenia, agranulocytosis, thrombocytopenia, bleeding, aplastic anemia

Hepatic: Cholestatic jaundice, hepatitis

Neuromuscular & skeletal: Arthralgia, paresthesia

Renal: Nephritis, glomerulonephritis, acute renal failure

Respiratory: Interstitial pneumonitis, alveolar hemorrhage

Miscellaneous: SLE-like syndrome

Drug Interactions

Increased Effect/Toxicity: Propylthiouracil may increase the anticoagulant activity of warfarin.

Decreased Effect: Oral anticoagulant activity is increased only until metabolic effect stabilizes. Anticoagulants may be potentiated by antivitamin K effect of propylthiouracil. Correction of hyperthyroidism may alter disposition of beta-blockers, digoxin, and theophylline, necessitating a dose reduction of these agents.

Dietary/Ethanol/Herb Considerations Food may alter serum concentration; administer with consistency in regard to meals.

Pharmacodynamics/Kinetics

Onset of action: Therapeutic: 24-36 hours

Peak effect: Remission: 4 months of continued therapy

Duration: 2-3 hours

Distribution: Concentrated in the thyroid gland

Protein binding: 75% to 80%

Metabolism: Hepatic

Bioavailability: 80% to 95%

Half-life elimination: 1.5-5 hours; End-stage renal disease: 8.5 hours

Time to peak, serum: ~1 hour

Excretion: Urine (35%)

Pregnancy Risk Factor D

Generic Available Yes

2-Propylvaleric Acid *see* Valproic Acid and Derivatives *on page 1371*

Proscar® *see* Finasteride *on page 572*

ProSom® *see* Estazolam *on page 521*

Prostacyclin *see* Epoprostenol *on page 505*

Prostaglandin E_1 *see* Alprostadil *on page 63*

Prostaglandin E_2 *see* Dinoprostone *on page 450*

Prostin E_2® *see* Dinoprostone *on page 450*

Prostin VR Pediatric® *see* Alprostadil *on page 63*

Protamine Sulfate (PROE ta meen SUL fate)

Pharmacologic Category Antidote

Use Treatment of heparin overdosage; neutralize heparin during surgery or dialysis procedures

Local Anesthetic/Vasoconstrictor Precautions No information available to require special precautions

Effects on Dental Treatment No significant effects or complications reported

Dosage Protamine dosage is determined by the dosage of heparin; 1 mg of protamine neutralizes 90 USP units of heparin (lung) and 115 USP units of heparin (intestinal); maximum dose: 50 mg

In the situation of heparin overdosage, since blood heparin concentrations decrease rapidly **after** administration, adjust the protamine dosage depending upon the duration of time since heparin administration as follows: See table.

Time Elapsed	Dose of Protamine (mg) to Neutralize 100 units of Heparin
Immediate	1-1.5
30-60 min	0.5-0.75
>2 h	0.25-0.375

If heparin administered by deep S.C. injection, use 1-1.5 mg protamine per 100 units heparin; this may be done by a portion of the dose (eg, 25-50 mg) given slowly I.V. followed by the remaining portion as a continuous infusion over 8-16 hours (the expected absorption time of the S.C. heparin dose)

Mechanism of Action Combines with strongly acidic heparin to form a stable complex (salt) neutralizing the anticoagulant activity of both drugs

Other Adverse Effects Frequency not defined:

Cardiovascular: Sudden fall in blood pressure, bradycardia, flushing, hypotension
Central nervous system: Lassitude
Gastrointestinal: Nausea, vomiting
Hematologic: Hemorrhage
Respiratory: Dyspnea, pulmonary hypertension
Miscellaneous: Hypersensitivity reactions

Pharmacodynamics/Kinetics Onset of action: I.V.: Heparin neutralization: ~5 minutes

Pregnancy Risk Factor C

Generic Available Yes

Comments Heparin rebound associated with anticoagulation and bleeding has been reported to occur occasionally; symptoms typically occur 8-9 hours after protamine administration, but may occur as long as 18 hours later

Protein C (Activated), Human, Recombinant *see* Drotrecogin Alfa *on page 483*

Prothrombin Complex Concentrate *see* Factor IX Complex (Human) *on page 553*

Protirelin (proe TYE re lin)

U.S. Brand Names Thyrel® TRH

Canadian Brand Names Relefact® TRH

Pharmacologic Category Diagnostic Agent

Synonyms Lopremone; Thyrotropin Releasing Hormone; TRH

Use Adjunct in the diagnostic assessment of thyroid function, and an adjunct to other diagnostic procedures in patients with pituitary or hypothalamic dysfunction; also causes release of prolactin from the pituitary and is used to detect defective control of prolactin secretion

Local Anesthetic/Vasoconstrictor Precautions No information available to require special precautions

Effects on Dental Treatment >10%: Xerostomia

Dosage I.V.:

Infants and Children <6 years: Experience limited, but doses of 7 mcg/kg have been administered
Children 6-16 years: 7 mcg/kg to a maximum dose of 500 mcg
Adults: 500 mcg (range 200-500 mcg)

Mechanism of Action Increase release of thyroid stimulating hormone from the anterior pituitary

Other Adverse Effects

>10%:
Central nervous system: Headache, lightheadedness
Dermatologic: Flushing of face
Gastrointestinal: Nausea
Genitourinary: Urge to urinate

1% to 10%:
Central nervous system: Anxiety
Endocrine & metabolic: Breast enlargement and leaking in lactating women
Gastrointestinal: Bad taste in mouth, abdominal discomfort

Neuromuscular & skeletal: Tingling
Miscellaneous: Diaphoresis

Drug Interactions Decreased Effect: Aspirin, levodopa, thyroid hormones, adrenocorticoid drugs

Pharmacodynamics/Kinetics
Onset of action: Peak effect: TSH: 20-30 minutes
Duration: TSH returns to baseline after ~3 hours
Half-life elimination, serum: Mean plasma: 5 minutes

Pregnancy Risk Factor C

Generic Available No

Protonix® *see* Pantoprazole *on page 1031*

Protopic® *see* Tacrolimus *on page 1261*

Protriptyline (proe TRIP ti leen)

U.S. Brand Names Vivactil®

Pharmacologic Category Antidepressant, Tricyclic (Secondary Amine)

Synonyms Protriptyline Hydrochloride

Use Treatment of depression

Local Anesthetic/Vasoconstrictor Precautions No information available to require special precautions

Effects on Dental Treatment >10%: Xerostomia, changes in salivation

Long-term treatment with TCAs such as protriptyline increases the risk of caries by reducing salivation and salivary buffer capacity.

Dosage Oral:
Adolescents: 15-20 mg/day
Adults: 15-60 mg in 3-4 divided doses
Elderly: 15-20 mg/day

Mechanism of Action Increases the synaptic concentration of serotonin and/or norepinephrine in the central nervous system by inhibition of their reuptake by the presynaptic neuronal membrane

Other Adverse Effects Frequency not defined:
Cardiovascular: Arrhythmias, hypotension, MI, stroke, heart block, hypertension, tachycardia, palpitations
Central nervous system: Dizziness, drowsiness, headache, confusion, delirium, hallucinations, restlessness, insomnia, nightmares, fatigue, delusions, anxiety, agitation, hypomania, exacerbation of psychosis, panic, seizures, incoordination, ataxia, EPS
Dermatologic: Alopecia, photosensitivity, rash, petechiae, urticaria, itching
Endocrine & metabolic: Breast enlargement, galactorrhea, SIADH, gynecomastia, increased or decreased libido
Gastrointestinal: Constipation, unpleasant taste, weight gain/loss, increased appetite, nausea, diarrhea, heartburn, vomiting, anorexia, **trouble with gums, decreased lower esophageal sphincter tone (may cause GE reflux)**
Genitourinary: Difficult urination, impotence, testicular edema
Hematologic: Agranulocytosis, leukopenia, eosinophilia, thrombocytopenia, purpura
Hepatic: Cholestatic jaundice, increased liver enzymes
Neuromuscular & skeletal: Fine muscle tremors, weakness, tremor, numbness, tingling
Ocular: Blurred vision, eye pain, increased intraocular pressure
Otic: Tinnitus
Miscellaneous: Diaphoresis (excessive), allergic reactions

Drug Interactions CYP2D6 enzyme substrate

Increased Effect/Toxicity: Protriptyline increases the effects of amphetamines, anticholinergics, other CNS depressants (sedatives, hypnotics, or ethanol), chlorpropamide, tolazamide, and warfarin. When used with MAO inhibitors, hyperpyrexia, hypertension, tachycardia, confusion, seizures, and **deaths have been reported** (serotonin syndrome). The SSRIs (to varying degrees), cimetidine, grapefruit juice, indinavir, methylphenidate, ritonavir, quinidine, diltiazem, and verapamil inhibit the metabolism of TCAs and clinical toxicity may result. Use of lithium with a TCA may increase the risk for neurotoxicity. Phenothiazines may increase concentration of some TCAs and TCAs may increase concentration of phenothiazines. Pressor response to I.V. epinephrine, norepinephrine, and phenylephrine may be enhanced in patients receiving TCAs (**Note:** Effect is unlikely with epinephrine or levonordefrin dosages typically administered as infiltration in combination with local anesthetics). Combined use of beta-agonists or drugs which prolong QT_c (including quinidine, procainamide, disopyramide, cisapride, sparfloxacin, gatifloxacin, moxifloxacin) with TCAs may predispose patients to cardiac arrhythmias.

Decreased Effect: Carbamazepine, phenobarbital, and rifampin may increase the metabolism of protriptyline, decreasing its effects. Protriptyline inhibits the antihypertensive response to bethanidine, clonidine, debrisoquin, guanadrel, guanethidine, guanabenz, guanfacine. Cimetidine and methylphenidate may decrease the

(Continued)

Protriptyline *(Continued)*

metabolism of protriptyline. Cholestyramine and colestipol may bind TCAs and reduce their absorption.

Dietary/Ethanol/Herb Considerations

Ethanol: Avoid use; may increase CNS depression.

Food: Avoid grapefruit products; may inhibit the metabolism of some TCAs and clinical toxicity may result.

Herb/Nutraceutical: Avoid kava, SAMe, St John's wort, tryptophan, and valerian; may increase risk of serotonin syndrome and/or excessive sedation.

Pharmacodynamics/Kinetics

Distribution: Crosses placenta

Protein binding: 92%

Metabolism: Extensively hepatic via N-oxidation, hydroxylation, and glucuronidation; first-pass effect (10% to 25%)

Half-life elimination: 54-92 hours (average: 74 hours)

Time to peak, serum: 24-30 hours

Excretion: Urine

Pregnancy Risk Factor C

Generic Available No

Selected Readings

Friedlander AH, Mahler ME, "Major Depressive Disorder. Psychopathology, Medical Management, and Dental Implications," *J Am Dent Assoc*, 201, 132(5):629-38.

Ganzberg S, "Psychoactive Drugs," *ADA Guide to Dental Therapeutics*, 2nd ed, Chicago, IL: ADA Publishing, a Division of ADA Business Enterprises, Inc, 2000, 376-405.

Jastak JT and Yagiela JA, "Vasoconstrictors and Local Anesthesia: A Review and Rationale for Use," *J Am Dent Assoc*, 1983, 107(4):623-30.

Mitchell JR, "Guanethidine and Related Agents. III Antagonism by Drugs Which Inhibit the Norepinephrine Pump in Man," *J Clin Invest*, 1970, 49(8):1596-604.

Rundegren J, van Dijken J, Mörnstad H, et al, "Oral Conditions in Patients Receiving Long-Term Treatment With Cyclic Antidepressant Drugs," *Swed Dent J*, 1985, 9(2):55-64.

Yagiela JA, "Adverse Drug Interactions in Dental Practice: Interactions Associated With Vasoconstrictors. Part V of a Series," *J Am Dent Assoc*, 1999, 130(5):701-9.

Protriptyline Hydrochloride *see* Protriptyline *on page 1145*

Protropin® *see* Human Growth Hormone *on page 671*

Proventil® *see* Albuterol *on page 48*

Proventil® HFA *see* Albuterol *on page 48*

Proventil® Repetabs® *see* Albuterol *on page 48*

Provera® *see* MedroxyPROGESTERone *on page 849*

Provigil® *see* Modafinil *on page 924*

Provisc® *see* Sodium Hyaluronate *on page 1230*

Proxigel® Oral [OTC] *see* Carbamide Peroxide *on page 244*

Proxymetacaine *see* Proparacaine *on page 1132*

Prozac® *see* Fluoxetine *on page 589*

Prozac® Weekly™ *see* Fluoxetine *on page 589*

PRP-D *see Haemophilus* b Conjugate Vaccine *on page 656*

Prudoxin™ *see* Doxepin *on page 471*

Prymaccone *see* Primaquine *on page 1117*

Pseudoephedrine (soo doe e FED rin)

Related Information

Diphenhydramine and Pseudoephedrine *on page 453*

Guaifenesin, Pseudoephedrine, and Dextromethorphan *on page 653*

Oral Bacterial Infections *on page 1531*

U.S. Brand Names Biofed [OTC]; Decofed® [OTC]; Dimetapp® 12-Hour Non-Drowsy Extentabs® [OTC]; Dimetapp® Decongestant [OTC]; Genaphed® [OTC]; Kidkare Decongestant [OTC]; Kodet SE [OTC]; Oranyl [OTC]; PediaCare® Decongestant Infants [OTC]; Silfedrine Children's [OTC]; Sudafed® [OTC]; Sudafed® 12 Hour [OTC]; Sudafed® 24 Hour [OTC]; Sudafed® Children's [OTC]; Sudodrin [OTC]; Triaminic® Allergy Congestion [OTC]

Canadian Brand Names Balminil® Decongestant; Contac® Cold 12 Hour Relief Non Drowsy; Drixoral® ND; Eltor®; PMS-Pseudoephedrine; Pseudofrin; Robidrine®; Sudafed® Decongestant; Triaminic® Allergy Congestion

Mexican Brand Names Lertamine-D®; Sudafed®

Pharmacologic Category Alpha/Beta Agonist

Synonyms *d*-Isoephedrine Hydrochloride; Pseudoephedrine Hydrochloride; Pseudoephedrine Sulfate

Use Temporary symptomatic relief of nasal congestion due to common cold, upper respiratory allergies, and sinusitis; also promotes nasal or sinus drainage

Local Anesthetic/Vasoconstrictor Precautions Use with caution since pseudoephedrine is a sympathomimetic amine which could interact with epinephrine to cause a pressor response

Effects on Dental Treatment ≤10%: Tachycardia, palpitations, xerostomia; use vasoconstrictor with caution

Dosage Oral:
Children:
<2 years: 4 mg/kg/day in divided doses every 6 hours
2-5 years: 15 mg every 6 hours; maximum: 60 mg/24 hours
6-12 years: 30 mg every 6 hours; maximum: 120 mg/24 hours
Adults: 30-60 mg every 4-6 hours, sustained release: 120 mg every 12 hours; maximum: 240 mg/24 hours
Dosing adjustment in renal impairment: Reduction required

Mechanism of Action Directly stimulates alpha-adrenergic receptors of respiratory mucosa causing vasoconstriction; directly stimulates beta-adrenergic receptors causing bronchial relaxation, increased heart rate and contractility

Other Adverse Effects Frequency not defined:
Cardiovascular: Arrhythmias
Central nervous system: Nervousness, transient stimulation, insomnia, excitability, dizziness, drowsiness, convulsions, hallucinations, headache
Gastrointestinal: Nausea, vomiting
Genitourinary: Dysuria
Neuromuscular & skeletal: Weakness, tremor
Respiratory: Dyspnea
Miscellaneous: Diaphoresis

Drug Interactions
Increased Effect/Toxicity: MAO inhibitors may increase blood pressure effects of pseudoephedrine. Sympathomimetic agents may increase toxicity.
Decreased Effect: Decreased effect of methyldopa, reserpine.

Dietary/Ethanol/Herb Considerations
Ethanol: Avoid use, may increase CNS depression.
Food: Administer with water or milk; food may delay onset of action.
Herb/Nutraceutical: Avoid ephedra, ginseng, and yohimbe; may cause hypertension. Avoid gotu kola, kava, SAMe, St John's wort, and valerian; may increase CNS depression.

Pharmacodynamics/Kinetics
Onset of action: Decongestant: Oral: 15-30 minutes
Duration: Immediate release tablet: 4-6 hours; Extended release: ≤12 hours
Absorption: Rapid
Metabolism: Partially hepatic
Half-life elimination: 9-16 hours
Excretion: Urine (70% to 90% as unchanged drug, 1% to 6% as active norpseudoephedrine); dependent on urine pH and flow rate; alkaline urine decreases renal elimination of pseudoephedrine

Pregnancy Risk Factor C

Generic Available Yes: Tablet, syrup

Pseudoephedrine, Acetaminophen, and Chlorpheniramine *see* Acetaminophen, Chlorpheniramine, and Pseudoephedrine *on page 35*

Pseudoephedrine, Acetaminophen, and Dextromethorphan *see* Acetaminophen, Dextromethorphan, and Pseudoephedrine *on page 35*

Pseudoephedrine and Acetaminophen *see* Acetaminophen and Pseudoephedrine *on page 31*

Pseudoephedrine and Acrivastine *see* Acrivastine and Pseudoephedrine *on page 41*

Pseudoephedrine and Azatadine *see* Azatadine and Pseudoephedrine *on page 150*

Pseudoephedrine and Brompheniramine *see* Brompheniramine and Pseudoephedrine *on page 201*

Pseudoephedrine and Carbinoxamine *see* Carbinoxamine and Pseudoephedrine *on page 247*

Pseudoephedrine and Chlorpheniramine *see* Chlorpheniramine and Pseudoephedrine *on page 308*

Pseudoephedrine and Dexbrompheniramine *see* Dexbrompheniramine and Pseudoephedrine *on page 415*

Pseudoephedrine and Dextromethorphan

(soo doe e FED rin & deks troe meth OR fan)

Related Information
Dextromethorphan *on page 423*
Pseudoephedrine *on page 1146*

U.S. Brand Names Children's Sudafed® Cough & Cold [OTC]; Pediacare® Decongestant Plus Cough [OTC]; Pediacare® Long Acting Cough Plus Cold [OTC]; Robitussin® Maximum Strength Cough & Cold [OTC]; Robitussin® Pediatric Cough & Cold [OTC]; Vicks® 44D Cough & Head Congestion [OTC]

Canadian Brand Names Balminil DM D; Benylin® DM-D; Koffex DM-D; Novahistex® DM Decongestant; Novahistine® DM Decongestant; Robitussin® Childrens Cough & Cold

Pharmacologic Category Antitussive/Decongestant

Synonyms Dextromethorphan and Pseudoephedrine

(Continued)

Pseudoephedrine and Dextromethorphan *(Continued)*

Use Temporary symptomatic relief of nasal congestion due to common cold, upper respiratory allergies, and sinusitis; also promotes nasal or sinus drainage; symptomatic relief of coughs caused by minor viral upper respiratory tract infections or inhaled irritants; most effective for a chronic nonproductive cough

Local Anesthetic/Vasoconstrictor Precautions Use with caution since pseudoephedrine is a sympathomimetic amine which could interact with epinephrine to cause a pressor response

Effects on Dental Treatment ≤10%: Tachycardia, palpitations, xerostomia; use vasoconstrictor with caution

Dosage Oral:

Children: Dose should be based on pseudoephedrine component

Adults: 5-10 mL every 6 hours

Other Adverse Effects Frequency not defined:

Based on **pseudoephedrine** component:

Cardiovascular: Arrhythmias

Central nervous system: Nervousness, transient stimulation, insomnia, excitability, dizziness, drowsiness, convulsions, hallucinations, headache

Gastrointestinal: Nausea, vomiting

Genitourinary: Dysuria

Neuromuscular & skeletal: Weakness, tremor

Respiratory: Dyspnea

Miscellaneous: Diaphoresis

Based on **dextromethorphan** component: Abdominal discomfort coma, constipation, dizziness, drowsiness, GI upset, nausea, respiratory depression

Generic Available Yes: Liquid

Pseudoephedrine and Diphenhydramine *see* Diphenhydramine and Pseudoephedrine *on page 453*

Pseudoephedrine and Fexofenadine *see* Fexofenadine and Pseudoephedrine *on page 570*

Pseudoephedrine and Guaifenesin *see* Guaifenesin and Pseudoephedrine *on page 652*

Pseudoephedrine and Ibuprofen

(soo doe e FED rin & eye byoo PROE fen)

Related Information

Ibuprofen *on page 703*

Pseudoephedrine *on page 1146*

U.S. Brand Names Advil® Cold, Children's [OTC]; Advil® Cold & Sinus [OTC]; Dristan® Sinus [OTC]; Motrin® Cold, Children's [OTC]; Motrin® Sinus Headache [OTC]

Canadian Brand Names Advil® Cold & Sinus; Dristan® Sinus; Sudafed® Sinus Advance

Pharmacologic Category Decongestant/Analgesic

Synonyms Ibuprofen and Pseudoephedrine

Use For temporary relief of cold, sinus and flu symptoms (including nasal congestion, headache, sore throat, minor body aches and pains, and fever)

Local Anesthetic/Vasoconstrictor Precautions Use with caution since pseudoephedrine is a sympathomimetic amine which could interact with epinephrine to cause a pressor response

Effects on Dental Treatment ≤10%: Tachycardia, palpitations, xerostomia; use vasoconstrictor with caution

Dosage OTC labeling: Oral:

Children: Ibuprofen 100 mg and pseudoephedrine 15 mg per 5 mL: May repeat dose every 6 hours (maximum: 4 doses/24 hours); dose should be based on weight when possible. Contact healthcare provider if symptoms have not improved within 3 days (2 days if treating sore throat accompanied by fever).

2-5 years or 11 to <22 kg (24-47 pounds): 5 mL

6-11 years or 22-43 kg (48-95 pounds): 10 mL

Children ≥12 years and Adults: Ibuprofen 200 mg and pseudoephedrine 30 mg per tablet: One tablet every 4-6 hours as needed; may increase to 2 tablets if necessary (maximum: 6 tablets/24 hours). Contact healthcare provider if symptoms have not improved within 7 days when treating cold symptoms or within 3 days when treating fever.

Dietary/Ethanol/Herb Considerations Ethanol: Avoid use; may enhance gastric mucosal irritation.

Generic Available No

Pseudoephedrine and Loratadine *see* Loratadine and Pseudoephedrine *on page 823*

Pseudoephedrine and Triprolidine *see* Triprolidine and Pseudoephedrine *on page 1356*

Pseudoephedrine, Carbinoxamine, and Dextromethorphan *see* Carbinoxamine, Pseudoephedrine, and Dextromethorphan *on page 247*

Pseudoephedrine, Chlorpheniramine, and Acetaminophen *see* Acetaminophen, Chlorpheniramine, and Pseudoephedrine *on page 35*

Pseudoephedrine, Dextromethorphan, and Acetaminophen *see* Acetaminophen, Dextromethorphan, and Pseudoephedrine *on page 35*

Pseudoephedrine, Dextromethorphan, and Carbinoxamine *see* Carbinoxamine, Pseudoephedrine, and Dextromethorphan *on page 247*

Pseudoephedrine, Dextromethorphan, and Guaifenesin *see* Guaifenesin, Pseudoephedrine, and Dextromethorphan *on page 653*

Pseudoephedrine, Guaifenesin, and Codeine *see* Guaifenesin, Pseudoephedrine, and Codeine *on page 653*

Pseudoephedrine Hydrochloride *see* Pseudoephedrine *on page 1146*

Pseudoephedrine Hydrochloride and Cetirizine Hydrochloride *see* Cetirizine and Pseudoephedrine *on page 290*

Pseudoephedrine, Hydrocodone, and Guaifenesin *see* Hydrocodone, Pseudoephedrine, and Guaifenesin *on page 687*

Pseudoephedrine Sulfate *see* Pseudoephedrine *on page 1146*

Pseudoephedrine, Triprolidine, and Codeine Pseudoephedrine, Codeine, and Triprolidine *see* Triprolidine, Pseudoephedrine, and Codeine *on page 1357*

Pseudo-Gest Plus® [OTC] *see* Chlorpheniramine and Pseudoephedrine *on page 308*

Pseudo GG TR *see* Guaifenesin and Pseudoephedrine *on page 652*

Pseudomonic Acid A *see* Mupirocin *on page 937*

Pseudovent™, Pseudovent™-Ped *see* Guaifenesin and Pseudoephedrine *on page 652*

Psorcon® *see* Diflorasone *on page 438*

Psorcon® e™ *see* Diflorasone *on page 438*

psoriGel® [OTC] *see* Coal Tar *on page 359*

P & S Plus® [OTC] *see* Coal Tar and Salicylic Acid *on page 359*

Psyllium (SIL i yum)

U.S. Brand Names Fiberall®; Genfiber® [OTC]; Hydrocil® [OTC]; Konsyl® [OTC]; Konsyl-D® [OTC]; Konsyl® Easy Mix [OTC]; Konsyl® Orange [OTC]; Metamucil® [OTC]; Metamucil® Smooth Texture [OTC]; Modane® Bulk [OTC]; Perdiem® Fiber Therapy [OTC]; Reguloid® [OTC]; Serutan® [OTC]

Canadian Brand Names Metamucil®; Novo-Mucilax

Pharmacologic Category Antidiarrheal; Laxative, Bulk-Producing

Synonyms Plantago Seed; Plantain Seed; Psyllium Hydrophilic Mucilloid

Use Treatment of chronic atonic or spastic constipation and in constipation associated with rectal disorders; management of irritable bowel syndrome

Local Anesthetic/Vasoconstrictor Precautions No information available to require special precautions

Effects on Dental Treatment No significant effects or complications reported

Dosage Oral (administer at least 2 hours before or after other drugs):

Children 6-11 years: Approximately 1/2 adult dosage

Children ≥12 years and Adults: Take 1 dose up to 3 times/day; all doses should be followed with 8 oz of water or liquid

- Capsule: 4 capsules/dose (range: 2-6); swallow capsules one at a time
- Powder: 1 rounded tablespoonful/dose (1 teaspoonful/dose for many sugar free or select concentrated products) mixed in 8 oz liquid
- Tablet: 1 tablet/dose
- Wafer: 2 wafers/dose

Mechanism of Action Adsorbs water in the intestine to form a viscous liquid which promotes peristalsis and reduces transit time

Other Adverse Effects Frequency not defined:

Gastrointestinal: Esophageal or bowel obstruction, diarrhea, constipation, abdominal cramps

Respiratory: Bronchospasm

Miscellaneous: Anaphylaxis upon inhalation in susceptible individuals, rhinoconjunctivitis

Drug Interactions Decreased effect of warfarin, digitalis, potassium-sparing diuretics, salicylates, tetracyclines, and nitrofurantoin when coadministered; separate administration times to reduce potential for interaction.

Dietary/Ethanol/Herb Considerations Food: Some products contain aspartame, dextrose, or sucrose; check individual product information for nutritional information.

Pharmacodynamics/Kinetics

Onset of action: 12-24 hours

- Peak effect: 2-3 days

Absorption: None; small amounts of grain extracts present in the preparation have been reportedly absorbed following colonic hydrolysis

Pregnancy Risk Factor B

Generic Available Yes: Powder

Psyllium Hydrophilic Mucilloid *see* Psyllium *on page 1149*

P.T.E.-4® *see* Trace Metals *on page 1328*
P.T.E.-5® *see* Trace Metals *on page 1328*
Pteroylglutamic Acid *see* Folic Acid *on page 606*
PTU *see* Propylthiouracil *on page 1142*
Pulmicort Respules™ *see* Budesonide *on page 202*
Pulmicort Turbuhaler® *see* Budesonide *on page 202*
Pulmozyme® *see* Dornase Alfa *on page 467*
Puralube® Tears [OTC] *see* Artificial Tears *on page 128*
Purge® [OTC] *see* Castor Oil *on page 259*
Purinethol® *see* Mercaptopurine *on page 866*

Pyrantel Pamoate (pi RAN tel PAM oh ate)

U.S. Brand Names Pin-X® [OTC]; Reese's® Pinworm Medicine [OTC]

Canadian Brand Names Combantrin™

Mexican Brand Names Combantrin®

Pharmacologic Category Anthelmintic

Use Treatment of pinworms (*Enterobius vermicularis*), whipworms (*Trichuris trichiura*), roundworms (*Ascaris lumbricoides*), and hookworms (*Ancylostoma duodenale*)

Local Anesthetic/Vasoconstrictor Precautions No information available to require special precautions

Effects on Dental Treatment No significant effects or complications reported

Dosage Children and Adults (purgation is not required prior to use): Oral:

Roundworm, pinworm, or trichostrongyliasis: 11 mg/kg administered as a single dose; maximum dose: 1 g. (**Note:** For pinworm infection, dosage should be repeated in 2 weeks and all family members should be treated).

Hookworm: 11 mg/kg administered once daily for 3 days

Mechanism of Action Causes the release of acetylcholine and inhibits cholinesterase; acts as a depolarizing neuromuscular blocker, paralyzing the helminths

Other Adverse Effects Frequency not defined:

Central nervous system: Dizziness, drowsiness, insomnia, headache
Dermatologic: Rash
Gastrointestinal: Anorexia, nausea, vomiting, abdominal cramps, diarrhea, tenesmus
Hepatic: Elevated liver enzymes
Neuromuscular & skeletal: Weakness

Drug Interactions Decreased effect with piperazine

Pharmacodynamics/Kinetics

Absorption: Oral: Poor
Metabolism: Partially hepatic
Time to peak, serum: 1-3 hours
Excretion: Feces (50% as unchanged drug); urine (7% as unchanged drug)

Pregnancy Risk Factor C

Generic Available No

Comments Purgation is not required prior to use

Pyrazinamide (peer a ZIN u mide)

Related Information

Nonviral Infectious Diseases *on page 1493*
Tuberculosis *on page 1493*

Canadian Brand Names Tebrazid™

Mexican Brand Names Braccoprial®

Pharmacologic Category Antitubercular Agent

Synonyms Pyrazinoic Acid Amide

Use Adjunctive treatment of tuberculosis in combination with other antituberculosis agents in combination with rifampin or rifabutin for prevention of tuberculosis (as an alternative to isoniazid monotherapy)

Local Anesthetic/Vasoconstrictor Precautions No information available to require special precautions

Effects on Dental Treatment No significant effects or complications reported

Dosage Oral (calculate dose on ideal body weight rather than total body weight):

Note: A four-drug regimen (isoniazid, rifampin, pyrazinamide, and either streptomycin or ethambutol) is preferred for the initial, empiric treatment of TB. When the drug susceptibility results are available, the regimen should be altered as appropriate.

Children and Adults:
- Daily therapy: 15-30 mg/kg/day (maximum: 2 g/day)
- Directly observed therapy (DOT):
  - Twice weekly: 50-70 mg/kg (maximum: 4 g)
  - Three times/week: 50-70 mg/kg (maximum: 3 g)
- Prevention of tuberculosis (in combination with rifampin or rifabutin): 15-30 mg/kg/day for 2 months

Elderly: Start with a lower daily dose (15 mg/kg) and increase as tolerated

Dosing adjustment in renal impairment: Cl_{cr} <50 mL/minute: Avoid use or reduce dose to 12-20 mg/kg/day

Dosing adjustment in hepatic impairment: Reduction required

Mechanism of Action Converted to pyrazinoic acid in susceptible strains of *Mycobacterium* which lowers the pH of the environment; exact mechanism of action has not been elucidated

Other Adverse Effects

1% to 10%:

Central nervous system: Malaise

Gastrointestinal: Nausea, vomiting, anorexia

Neuromuscular & skeletal: Arthralgia, myalgia

<1%: Fever, rash, itching, acne, photosensitivity, gout, dysuria, porphyria, thrombocytopenia, hepatotoxicity, interstitial nephritis

Drug Interactions Increased Effect/Toxicity: Combination therapy with rifampin and pyrazinamide has been associated with severe and fatal hepatotoxic reactions.

Pharmacodynamics/Kinetics Bacteriostatic or bactericidal depending on drug's concentration at infection site

Absorption: Well absorbed

Distribution: Widely into body tissues and fluids including liver, lung, and CSF

Relative diffusion from blood into CSF: Adequate with or without inflammation (exceeds usual MICs)

CSF:blood level ratio: Inflamed meninges: 100%

Protein binding: 50%

Metabolism: Hepatic

Half-life elimination: 9-10 hours

Time to peak, serum: Within 2 hours

Excretion: Urine (4% as unchanged drug)

Pregnancy Risk Factor C

Generic Available Yes

Pyrazinamide, Rifampin, and Isoniazid *see* Rifampin, Isoniazid, and Pyrazinamide *on page 1182*

Pyrazinoic Acid Amide *see* Pyrazinamide *on page 1150*

Pyrethrins and Piperonyl Butoxide

(pye RE thrins & pi PER oh nil byoo TOKS ide)

U.S. Brand Names A-200® Maximum Strength [OTC]; Pronto® [OTC]; Pyrinyl Plus® [OTC]; RID® Maximum Strength [OTC]; Tisit® [OTC]; Tisit® Blue Gel [OTC]

Canadian Brand Names Pronto® Lice Control; R & C™ II; R & C™ Shampoo/Conditioner; RID® Mousse

Pharmacologic Category Antiparasitic Agent, Topical; Pediculocide; Shampoo, Pediculocide

Synonyms Piperonyl Butoxide and Pyrethrins

Use Treatment of *Pediculus humanus* infestations (head lice, body lice, pubic lice and their eggs)

Local Anesthetic/Vasoconstrictor Precautions No information available to require special precautions

Effects on Dental Treatment No effects or complications reported

Dosage Application of pyrethrins: Topical:

Apply enough solution to completely wet infested area, including hair

Allow to remain on area for 10 minutes

Wash and rinse with large amounts of warm water

Use fine-toothed comb to remove lice and eggs from hair

Shampoo hair to restore body and luster

Treatment may be repeated if necessary once in a 24-hour period

Repeat treatment in 7-10 days to kill newly hatched lice

Mechanism of Action Pyrethrins are derived from flowers that belong to the chrysanthemum family. The mechanism of action on the neuronal membranes of lice is similar to that of DDT. Piperonyl butoxide is usually added to pyrethrin to enhance the product's activity by decreasing the metabolism of pyrethrins in arthropods.

Other Adverse Effects Frequency not defined.

Dermatologic: Pruritus

Local: Burning, stinging, irritation with repeat use

Pharmacodynamics/Kinetics

Onset of action: ~30 minutes

Absorption: Minimal

Metabolism: Via ester hydrolysis and hydroxylation

Pregnancy Risk Factor C

Generic Available Yes: Shampoo

Pyridium® *see* Phenazopyridine *on page 1064*

Pyridoxine (peer i DOKS een)

U.S. Brand Names Aminoxin® [OTC]

Mexican Brand Names Benadon

Pharmacologic Category Vitamin, Water Soluble

Synonyms Pyridoxine Hydrochloride; Vitamin B_6

Use Prevention and treatment of vitamin B_6 deficiency, pyridoxine-dependent seizures in infants; adjunct to treatment of acute toxicity from isoniazid, cycloserine, or hydralazine overdose

Local Anesthetic/Vasoconstrictor Precautions No information available to require special precautions

Effects on Dental Treatment No significant effects or complications reported

Dosage

Recommended daily allowance (RDA):
- Children:
  - 1-3 years: 0.9 mg
  - 4-6 years: 1.3 mg
  - 7-10 years: 1.6 mg
- Adults:
  - Male: 1.7-2.0 mg
  - Female: 1.4-1.6 mg

Pyridoxine-dependent Infants:
- Oral: 2-100 mg/day
- I.M., I.V., S.C.: 10-100 mg

Dietary deficiency: Oral:
- Children: 5-25 mg/24 hours for 3 weeks, then 1.5-2.5 mg/day in multiple vitamin product
- Adults: 10-20 mg/day for 3 weeks

Drug-induced neuritis (eg, isoniazid, hydralazine, penicillamine, cycloserine): Oral:
- Children:
  - Treatment: 10-50 mg/24 hours
  - Prophylaxis: 1-2 mg/kg/24 hours
- Adults:
  - Treatment: 100-200 mg/24 hours
  - Prophylaxis: 25-100 mg/24 hours

Treatment of seizures and/or coma from acute isoniazid toxicity, a dose of pyridoxine hydrochloride equal to the amount of INH ingested can be given I.M./I.V. in divided doses together with other anticonvulsants; if the amount INH ingested is not known, administer 5 g I.V. pyridoxine

Treatment of acute hydralazine toxicity, a pyridoxine dose of 25 mg/kg in divided doses I.M./I.V. has been used

Mechanism of Action Precursor to pyridoxal, which functions in the metabolism of proteins, carbohydrates, and fats; pyridoxal also aids in the release of liver and muscle-stored glycogen and in the synthesis of GABA (within the central nervous system) and heme

Other Adverse Effects Frequency not defined:
- Central nervous system: Headache, seizures (following very large I.V. doses), sensory neuropathy
- Endocrine & metabolic: Decreased serum folic acid secretions
- Gastrointestinal: Nausea
- Hepatic: Increased AST
- Neuromuscular & skeletal: Paresthesia
- Miscellaneous: Allergic reactions

Drug Interactions Decreased Effect: Pyridoxine may decrease serum levels of levodopa, phenobarbital, and phenytoin (patients taking levodopa without carbidopa should avoid supplemental vitamin B_6 >5 mg per day, which includes multivitamin preparations).

Pharmacodynamics/Kinetics
- Absorption: Enteral, parenteral: Well absorbed
- Metabolism: Via 4-pyridoxic acid (active form) and other metabolites
- Half-life elimination: 15-20 days
- Excretion: Urine

Pregnancy Risk Factor A/C (dose exceeding RDA recommendation)

Generic Available Yes

Pyridoxine, Folic Acid, and Cyanocobalamin *see* Folic Acid, Cyanocobalamin, and Pyridoxine *on page 607*

Pyridoxine Hydrochloride *see* Pyridoxine *on page 1152*

Pyrimethamine (peer i METH a meen)

U.S. Brand Names Daraprim®

Canadian Brand Names Daraprim®

Mexican Brand Names Daraprim®

Pharmacologic Category Antimalarial Agent

Use Prophylaxis of malaria due to susceptible strains of plasmodia; used in conjunction with quinine and sulfadiazine for the treatment of uncomplicated attacks of chloroquine-resistant *P. falciparum* malaria; used in conjunction with fast-acting schizonticide to initiate transmission control and suppression cure; synergistic combination with sulfonamide in treatment of toxoplasmosis

Local Anesthetic/Vasoconstrictor Precautions No information available to require special precautions

Effects on Dental Treatment Atrophic glossitis has been reported.

Dosage

Malaria chemoprophylaxis (for areas where chloroquine-resistant *P. falciparum* exists): Begin prophylaxis 2 weeks before entering endemic area:
- Children: 0.5 mg/kg once weekly; not to exceed 25 mg/dose
  or
- Children:
  - <4 years: 6.25 mg once weekly
  - 4-10 years: 12.5 mg once weekly
- Children >10 years and Adults: 25 mg once weekly
- Dosage should be continued for all age groups for at least 6-10 weeks after leaving endemic areas

Chloroquine-resistant *P. falciparum* malaria (when used in conjunction with quinine and sulfadiazine):
- Children:
  - <10 kg: 6.25 mg/day once daily for 3 days
  - 10-20 kg: 12.5 mg/day once daily for 3 days
  - 20-40 kg: 25 mg/day once daily for 3 days
- Adults: 25 mg twice daily for 3 days

Toxoplasmosis:
- Infants for congenital toxoplasmosis: Oral: 1 mg/kg once daily for 6 months with sulfadiazine then every other month with sulfa, alternating with spiramycin.
- Children: Loading dose: 2 mg/kg/day divided into 2 equal daily doses for 1-3 days (maximum: 100 mg/day) followed by 1 mg/kg/day divided into 2 doses for 4 weeks; maximum: 25 mg/day
  - With sulfadiazine or trisulfapyrimidines: 2 mg/kg/day divided every 12 hours for 3 days followed by 1 mg/kg/day once daily or divided twice daily for 4 weeks given with trisulfapyrimidines or sulfadiazine
- Adults: 50-75 mg/day together with 1-4 g of a sulfonamide for 1-3 weeks depending on patient's tolerance and response, then reduce dose by 50% and continue for 4-5 weeks **or** 25-50 mg/day for 3-4 weeks

Prophylaxis for first episode of *Toxoplasma gondii*:
- Children ≥1 month of age: 1 mg/kg/day once daily with dapsone, plus oral folinic acid 5 mg every 3 days
- Adolescents and Adults: 50 mg once weekly with dapsone, plus oral folinic acid 25 mg once weekly

Prophylaxis to prevent recurrence of *Toxoplasma gondii:*
- Children ≥1 month of age: 1 mg/kg/day once daily given with sulfadiazine or clindamycin, plus oral folinic acid 5 mg every 3 days
- Adolescents and Adults: 25-50 mg once daily in combination with sulfadiazine or clindamycin, plus oral folinic acid 10-25 mg daily **or** with atovaquone, plus oral folinic acid 10 mg daily

Mechanism of Action Inhibits parasitic dihydrofolate reductase, resulting in inhibition of vital tetrahydrofolic acid synthesis

Other Adverse Effects Frequency not defined:
- Cardiovascular: Arrhythmias (large doses)
- Central nervous system: Depression, fever, insomnia, lightheadedness, malaise, seizures
- Dermatologic: Abnormal skin pigmentation, dermatitis, erythema multiforme, rash, Stevens-Johnson syndrome
- Gastrointestinal: Anorexia, abdominal cramps, vomiting, diarrhea, xerostomia, atrophic glossitis
- Hematologic: Megaloblastic anemia, leukopenia, pancytopenia, thrombocytopenia, pulmonary eosinophilia
- Miscellaneous: Anaphylaxis

Drug Interactions Inhibits CYP2D6
- Increased effect with sulfonamides (synergy), methotrexate, and TMP/SMZ.
- Decreased Effect: Pyrimethamine effectiveness is decreased by acid.

Pharmacodynamics/Kinetics
- Onset of action: ~1 hour
- Absorption: Well absorbed
- Distribution: Widely, mainly in blood cells, kidneys, lungs, liver, and spleen; crosses into CSF; crosses placenta; enters breast milk
- Protein binding: 80% to 87%
- Metabolism: Hepatic
- Half-life elimination: 80-95 hours
- Time to peak, serum: 1.5-8 hours
- Excretion: Urine (20% to 30% as unchanged drug)

Pregnancy Risk Factor C

Generic Available No

Pyrimethamine and Sulfadoxine *see* Sulfadoxine and Pyrimethamine *on page 1252*

Pyrinyl Plus® [OTC] *see* Pyrethrins and Piperonyl Butoxide *on page 1151*

Pyrithione Zinc (peer i THYE one zingk)

U.S. Brand Names DHS™ Zinc [OTC]; Head & Shoulders® Classic Clean [OTC]; Head & Shoulders® Classic Clean 2-In-1 [OTC]; Head & Shoulders® Dry Scalp Care [OTC]; Head & Shoulders® Extra Fullness [OTC]; Head & Shoulders® Refresh [OTC]; Head & Shoulders® Smooth & Silky 2-In-1 [OTC]; Zincon® [OTC]; ZNP® Bar [OTC]

Mexican Brand Names ZNP Shampoo®

Pharmacologic Category Topical Skin Product

Use Relieves the itching, irritation and scalp flaking associated with dandruff and/or seborrheal dermatitis of the scalp

Local Anesthetic/Vasoconstrictor Precautions No information available to require special precautions

Effects on Dental Treatment No significant effects or complications reported

Dosage Shampoo hair twice weekly, wet hair, apply to scalp and massage vigorously, rinse and repeat

Generic Available No

Quaternium-18 Bentonite *see* Bentoquatam *on page 168*

Quazepam (KWAY ze pam)

U.S. Brand Names Doral®

Canadian Brand Names Doral®

Pharmacologic Category Benzodiazepine

Use Treatment of insomnia

Local Anesthetic/Vasoconstrictor Precautions No information available to require special precautions

Effects on Dental Treatment >10%: Xerostomia; normal salivary flow resumes upon discontinuation

Restrictions C-IV

Dosage Adults: Oral: Initial: 15 mg at bedtime, in some patients the dose may be reduced to 7.5 mg after a few nights

Elderly: Dosing should be cautious; begin at lower end of dosing range (ie, 7.5 mg)

Dosing adjustment in hepatic impairment: Reduction may be necessary

Mechanism of Action Binds to stereospecific benzodiazepine receptors on the postsynaptic GABA neuron at several sites within the central nervous system, including the limbic system, reticular formation. Enhancement of the inhibitory effect of GABA on neuronal excitability results by increased neuronal membrane permeability to chloride ions. This shift in chloride ions results in hyperpolarization (a less excitable state) and stabilization.

Other Adverse Effects Frequency not defined:

Cardiovascular: Palpitations

Central nervous system: Drowsiness, fatigue, ataxia, memory impairment, anxiety, depression, headache, confusion, nervousness, dizziness, incoordination, hypo- and hyperkinesia, agitation, euphoria, paranoid reaction, nightmares, abnormal thinking

Dermatologic: Dermatitis, pruritus, rash

Endocrine & metabolic: Decreased libido, menstrual irregularities

Gastrointestinal: Constipation, diarrhea, dyspepsia, anorexia, abnormal taste perception, nausea, vomiting, increased or decreased appetite, abdominal pain

Genitourinary: Impotence, incontinence

Hematologic: Blood dyscrasias

Neuromuscular & skeletal: Dysarthria, rigidity, tremor, muscle cramps, reflex slowing

Ocular: Blurred vision

Miscellaneous: Drug dependence

Drug Interactions Substrate of CYP3A4

Increased Effect/Toxicity: Serum levels and/or toxicity of quazepam may be increased by cimetidine, ciprofloxacin, clarithromycin, clozapine, CNS depressants, diltiazem, disulfiram, digoxin, erythromycin, ethanol, fluconazole, fluoxetine, fluvoxamine, grapefruit juice, isoniazid, itraconazole, ketoconazole, labetalol, levodopa, loxapine, metoprolol, metronidazole, miconazole, nefazodone, omeprazole, phenytoin, rifabutin, rifampin, troleandomycin, valproic acid, and verapamil.

Decreased Effect: Carbamazepine, rifampin, rifabutin may enhance the metabolism of quazepam and decrease its therapeutic effect.

Dietary/Ethanol/Herb Considerations

Ethanol: Avoid use; may increase CNS depression.

Food: Avoid grapefruit products; may increase serum concentration/toxicity.

Herb/Nutraceutical: Avoid gotu kola, kava, SAMe, St John's wort, and valerian; may increase CNS depression.

Pharmacodynamics/Kinetics

Absorption: Rapid

Protein binding: 95%

Half-life elimination, serum: Parent drug: 25-41 hours; Active metabolite: 40-114 hours

Pregnancy Risk Factor X

Generic Available No

Questran® *see* Cholestyramine Resin *on page 318*

Questran® Light *see* Cholestyramine Resin *on page 318*

Quetiapine (kwe TYE a peen)

U.S. Brand Names Seroquel®

Canadian Brand Names Seroquel®

Mexican Brand Names Seroquel®

Pharmacologic Category Antipsychotic Agent, Dibenzothiazepine

Synonyms Quetiapine Fumarate

Use Treatment of schizophrenia

Unlabeled/Investigational Use Treatment of mania, bipolar disorder (children and adults), autism, psychosis in children

Local Anesthetic/Vasoconstrictor Precautions No information available to require special precautions

Effects on Dental Treatment No significant effects or complications reported

Dosage Oral:

Children and Adolescents:

Autism (unlabeled use): 100-350 mg/day (1.6-5.2 mg/kg/day)

Psychosis and mania (unlabeled use): Initial: 25 mg twice daily; titrate as necessary to 450 mg/day

Adults: Schizophrenia/psychoses: Initial: 25 mg twice daily; increase in increments of 25-50 mg 2-3 times/day on the second and third day, if tolerated, to a target dose of 300-400 mg in 2-3 divided doses by day 4. Make further adjustments as needed at intervals of at least 2 days in adjustments of 25-50 mg twice daily. Usual maintenance range: 300-800 mg/day

Elderly: 50-200 mg/day; 40% lower mean oral clearance in adults >65 years of age; higher plasma levels expected

Dosing comments in hepatic insufficiency: Adjustment may be required; 30% lower mean oral clearance of quetiapine than normal subjects; higher plasma levels expected in hepatically impaired subjects

Mechanism of Action Mechanism of action of quetiapine, as with other antipsychotic drugs, is unknown. However, it has been proposed that this drug's antipsychotic activity is mediated through a combination of dopamine type 2 (D_2) and serotonin type 2 (5-HT_2) antagonism. However, it is an antagonist at multiple neurotransmitter receptors in the brain: serotonin 5-HT_{1A} and 5-HT_2, dopamine D_1 and D_2, histamine H_1, and adrenergic alpha$_1$- and alpha$_2$-receptors; but appears to have no appreciable affinity at cholinergic muscarinic and benzodiazepine receptors.

Antagonism at receptors other than dopamine and 5-HT_2 with similar receptor affinities may explain some of the other effects of quetiapine. The drug's antagonism of histamine H_1-receptors may explain the somnolence observed with it. The drug's antagonism of adrenergic alpha$_1$-receptors may explain the orthostatic hypotension observed with it.

Other Adverse Effects

>10%:

Central nervous system: Headache, somnolence

Gastrointestinal: Weight gain

1% to 10%:

Cardiovascular: Postural hypotension, tachycardia, palpitations

Central nervous system: Dizziness

Dermatologic: Rash

Gastrointestinal: Abdominal pain, constipation, xerostomia, dyspepsia, anorexia

Hematologic: Leukopenia

Neuromuscular & skeletal: Dysarthria, back pain, weakness

Respiratory: Rhinitis, pharyngitis, cough, dyspnea

Miscellaneous: Diaphoresis

<1%: Abnormal dreams, anemia, bradycardia, diabetes mellitus, elevated alkaline phosphatase, elevated GGT, epistaxis, hyperglycemia, hyperlipidemia, hypothyroidism, increased appetite, increased salivation, involuntary movements, leukocytosis, QT prolongation, rash, tardive dyskinesia, vertigo

Drug Interactions Substrate of CYP2D6, **3A4**

Increased Effect/Toxicity: Quetiapine reduces the metabolism of lorazepam (by 20%). The effects of other centrally-acting drugs, sedatives, or ethanol may be potentiated by quetiapine. Quetiapine may enhance the effects of antihypertensive agents. Although data is not yet available, caution is advised with inhibitors of CYP3A4 (eg, ketoconazole, erythromycin), which may increase levels of

(Continued)

Quetiapine *(Continued)*

quetiapine. Cimetidine increases blood levels of quetiapine (quetiapine's clearance is reduced by by 20%). Metoclopramide may increase risk of extrapyramidal symptoms (EPS).

Decreased Effect: The metabolism of quetiapine may be increased when administered with enzyme-inducing drugs (phenytoin, rifampin, barbiturates, carbamazepine). Thioridazine increases quetiapine's clearance (by 65%).

Dietary/Ethanol/Herb Considerations

Ethanol: Avoid use; may cause excessive impairment in cognition/motor function.

Food: May be taken with food; in healthy volunteers, administration with food resulted in an increase in the peak serum concentration and AUC (each by ~15%) compared to the fasting state.

Herb/Nutraceutical: Avoid gotu kola, kava, SAMe, and valerian; may increase CNS depression. Avoid St John's wort; may decrease serum concentration and increase CNS depression.

Pharmacodynamics/Kinetics

Absorption: Accumulation is predictable upon multiple dosing

Distribution: V_{dss}: ~2 days; unlikely to interfere with the metabolism of drugs dependent on CYP

Protein binding, plasma: 83%

Metabolism: Primarily hepatic; both metabolites are pharmacologically inactive

Bioavailability: 100%

Half-life elimination: Mean: Terminal: ~6 hours

Time to peak, plasma: 1.5 hours

Excretion: Urine (73% as metabolites, <1% as unchanged drug); feces (20%)

Pregnancy Risk Factor C

Generic Available No

Quetiapine Fumarate *see* Quetiapine *on page 1155*

Quibron® *see* Theophylline and Guaifenesin *on page 1293*

Quibron®-T *see* Theophylline *on page 1291*

Quibron®-T/SR *see* Theophylline *on page 1291*

Quinaglute® Dura-Tabs® *see* Quinidine *on page 1158*

Quinalbarbitone Sodium *see* Secobarbital *on page 1212*

Quinapril (KWIN a pril)

Related Information

Cardiovascular Diseases *on page 1456*

U.S. Brand Names Accupril®

Canadian Brand Names Accupril™

Mexican Brand Names Acupril®

Pharmacologic Category Angiotensin-Converting Enzyme (ACE) Inhibitor

Synonyms Quinapril Hydrochloride

Use Management of hypertension; treatment of CHF

Unlabeled/Investigational Use Treatment of left ventricular dysfunction after myocardial infarction

Local Anesthetic/Vasoconstrictor Precautions No information available to require special precautions

Effects on Dental Treatment No significant effects or complications reported

Dosage

Adults: Oral:

Hypertension: Initial: 10-20 mg once daily, adjust according to blood pressure response at peak and trough blood levels; initial dose may be reduced to 5 mg in patients receiving diuretic therapy if the diuretic is continued (normal dosage range is 20-80 mg/day for hypertension)

Congestive heart failure or post-MI: Initial: 5 mg once daily, titrated at weekly intervals to 20-40 mg daily in 2 divided doses

Elderly: Initial: 2.5-5 mg/day; increase dosage at increments of 2.5-5 mg at 1- to 2-week intervals.

Dosing adjustment in renal impairment: Lower initial doses should be used; after initial dose (if tolerated), administer initial dose twice daily; may be increased at weekly intervals to optimal response:

Hypertension: Initial:

Cl_{cr} >60 mL/minute: Administer 10 mg/day

Cl_{cr} 30-60 mL/minute: Administer 5 mg/day

Cl_{cr} 10-30 mL/minute: Administer 2.5 mg/day

Congestive heart failure: Initial:

Cl_{cr} >30 mL/minute: Administer 5 mg/day

Cl_{cr} 10-30 mL/minute: Administer 2.5 mg/day

Dosing comments in hepatic impairment: In patients with alcoholic cirrhosis, hydrolysis of quinapril to quinaprilat is impaired; however, the subsequent elimination of quinaprilat is unaltered.

Mechanism of Action Competitive inhibitor of angiotensin-converting enzyme (ACE); prevents conversion of angiotensin I to angiotensin II, a potent vasoconstrictor; results in lower levels of angiotensin II which causes an increase in plasma renin activity and a reduction in aldosterone secretion; a CNS mechanism may also be involved in hypotensive effect as angiotensin II increases adrenergic outflow from CNS; vasoactive kallikreins may be decreased in conversion to active hormones by ACE inhibitors, thus reducing blood pressure

Other Adverse Effects Note: Frequency ranges include data from hypertension and heart failure trials. Higher rates of adverse reactions have generally been noted in patients with CHF. However, the frequency of adverse effects associated with placebo is also increased in this population.

1% to 10%:

Cardiovascular: Hypotension (3%), chest pain (2%), first-dose hypotension (up to 3%)

Central nervous system: Dizziness (4% to 8%), headache (2% to 6%), fatigue (3%)

Dermatologic: Rash (1%)

Endocrine & metabolic: Hyperkalemia (2%)

Gastrointestinal: Vomiting/nausea (1% to 2%), diarrhea (2%)

Neuromuscular & skeletal: Myalgias (2% to 5%), back pain (1%)

Renal: Increased BUN/serum creatinine (2%, transient elevations may occur with a higher frequency), worsening of renal function (in patients with bilateral renal artery stenosis or hypovolemia)

Respiratory: Upper respiratory symptoms, cough (2% to 4%; up to 13% in some studies), dyspnea (2%)

<1% (Limited to important or life-threatening): Angioedema, arthralgia, edema, back pain, malaise, viral infection, palpitation, vasodilation, tachycardia, heart failure, hyperkalemia, MI, cerebrovascular accident, hypertensive crisis, angina, orthostatic hypotension, arrhythmia, shock, hemolytic anemia, xerostomia, constipation, gastrointestinal hemorrhage, pancreatitis, abnormal LFTs, somnolence, vertigo, syncope, nervousness, depression, insomnia, paresthesia, alopecia, increased diaphoresis, pemphigus, pruritus, exfoliative dermatitis, photosensitivity, dermatopolymyositis, impotence, acute renal failure, eosinophilic pneumonitis, amblyopia, pharyngitis, agranulocytosis, hepatitis, thrombocytopenia

A syndrome which may include fever, myalgia, arthralgia, interstitial nephritis, vasculitis, rash, eosinophilia and positive ANA, and elevated ESR has been reported with ACE inhibitors. In addition, pancreatitis, hepatic necrosis, neutropenia, and/or agranulocytosis (particularly in patients with collagen-vascular disease or renal impairment) have been associated with many ACE inhibitors.

Drug Interactions

Increased Effect/Toxicity:

The following drugs may result in elevated serum potassium levels when combined with quinapril: Potassium supplements, sulfamethoxazole and trimethoprim (high dose), angiotensin II receptor antagonists (candesartan, losartan, irbesartan, etc), or potassium-sparing diuretics (amiloride, spironolactone, triamterene)

ACE inhibitor effects may be increased by phenothiazines or probenecid (increases levels of captopril). ACE inhibitors may increase serum concentrations/effects of digoxin, lithium, and sulfonlyureas. Diuretics have additive hypotensive effects with ACE inhibitors, and hypovolemia increases the potential for adverse renal effects of ACE inhibitors. In patients with compromised renal function, coadministration with NSAIDs may result in further deterioration of renal function. Allopurinol and ACE inhibitors may cause a higher risk of hypersensitivity reaction when taken concurrently.

Decreased Effect: Quinapril may reduce the absorption of quinolones and tetracycline antibiotics. Aspirin (high dose) may reduce the therapeutic effects of ACE inhibitors; at low dosages this does not appear to be significant. Rifampin may decrease the effect of ACE inhibitors. Antacids may decrease the bioavailability of ACE inhibitors (may be more likely to occur with captopril); separate administration times by 1-2 hours. NSAIDs, specifically indomethacin, may reduce the hypotensive effects of ACE inhibitors.

Dietary/Ethanol/Herb Considerations

Ethanol: Avoid use; may increase risk of hypotension or dizziness.

Food: Administer on an empty stomach; avoid caffeine (eg, colas, chocolate), garlic, and licorice.

Herb/Nutraceutical: Avoid black cohosh, dong quai, and evening primrose due to estrogenic activity. Avoid ephedra, ginseng, and yohimbe; may worsen hypertension. Avoid garlic; may have increased antihypertensive effect. Avoid ginger due to positive inotropic effects; theoretically, may cause arrhythmia. Avoid hawthorn; may lower peripheral vascular resistance causing additional decrease in BP.

Pharmacodynamics/Kinetics

Onset of action: 1 hour

Duration: 24 hours

Absorption: Quinapril: ≥60%

Protein binding: Quinapril: 97%; Quinaprilat: 97%

(Continued)

Quinapril *(Continued)*

Metabolism: Rapidly hydrolyzed to quinaprilat, the active metabolite
Half-life elimination: Quinapril: 0.8 hours; Quinaprilat: 3 hours; increases as Cl_{cr} decreases
Time to peak, serum: Quinapril: 1 hour; Quinaprilat: ~2 hours
Excretion: Urine (50% to 60% primarily as quinaprilat)

Pregnancy Risk Factor C/D (2nd and 3rd trimesters)

Generic Available No

Quinapril and Hydrochlorothiazide

(KWIN a pril & hye droe klor oh THYE a zide)

Related Information

Hydrochlorothiazide *on page 675*
Quinapril *on page 1156*

U.S. Brand Names Accuretic™

Canadian Brand Names Accuretic™

Pharmacologic Category Angiotensin-Converting Enzyme (ACE) Inhibitor; Antihypertensive; Diuretic, Thiazide

Synonyms Hydrochlorothiazide and Quinapril

Use Treatment of hypertension (not for initial therapy)

Local Anesthetic/Vasoconstrictor Precautions No information available to require special precautions

Effects on Dental Treatment No significant effects or complications reported

Dosage Oral:

Children: Safety and efficacy not established.
Adults: Initial:
- Patients who have failed quinapril monotherapy:
  - Quinapril 10 mg/hydrochlorothiazide 12.5 mg **or**
  - Quinapril 20 mg/hydrochlorothiazide 12.5 mg once daily
- Patients with adequate blood pressure control on hydrochlorothiazide 25 mg/day, but significant potassium loss:
  - Quinapril 10 mg/hydrochlorothiazide 12.5 mg **or**
  - Quinapril 20 mg/hydrochlorothiazide 12.5 mg once daily
- **Note:** Clinical trials of quinapril/hydrochlorothiazide combinations used quinapril doses of 2.5-40 mg/day and hydrochlorothiazide doses of 6.25-25 mg/day.

Dosing adjustment in renal impairment: Cl_{cr} <30 mL/minute/1.73 m^2 or serum creatinine ≤3 mg/dL: Use not recommended.

Other Adverse Effects

1% to 10%:
- Central nervous system: Dizziness (5%), somnolence (1%)
- Neuromuscular & skeletal: Weakness (1%)
- Renal: Serum creatinine increase (3%), blood urea nitrogen increase (4%)
- Respiratory: Cough (3%), bronchitis (1%)

<1%: Acute renal failure, agranulocytosis, alopecia, angina pectoris, arrhythmia, arthralgia, calcium increase (serum), cerebrovascular accident, cholesterol increase (serum), diaphoresis increased, dyspnea, erythema multiforme, exfoliative dermatitis, gastrointestinal hemorrhage, glucose increase (serum), heart failure, hypercalcemia, hyperkalemia, hypertensive crisis, impotence, LFTs abnormalities, magnesium increase (serum), malaise, MI, nervousness, orthostatic hypotension, palpitation, pancreatitis, paresthesia, pemphigus, photosensitivity, pruritus, sinusitis, tachycardia, uric acid increase (serum), thrombocytopenia, triglyceride increase (serum), vertigo, xerostomia

Postmarketing and/or case reports: Abnormal gait, abnormal vision, albuminuria, amnesia, anemia, arthritis, ascites, asthma, bradycardia, cellulitis, cholestatic jaundice, cor pulmonale, deep thrombosis, diarrhea, esophagitis, generalized edema, hematuria, hemiplegia, hepatitis, kidney function abnormality, maculopapular rash, meningism, myopathy, myositis, nephrosis, paralysis, petechiae, pneumonia, pyuria, shock, urticaria, vasculitis, weight loss

Dietary/Ethanol/Herb Considerations Food: May be taken with food

Pregnancy Risk Factor C (1st trimester)/D (2nd and 3rd trimesters)

Generic Available No

Quinapril Hydrochloride *see* Quinapril *on page 1156*
Quinidex® Extentabs® *see* Quinidine *on page 1158*

Quinidine (KWIN i deen)

Related Information

Cardiovascular Diseases *on page 1456*

U.S. Brand Names Quinaglute® Dura-Tabs®; Quinidex® Extentabs®

Canadian Brand Names Apo®-Quin-G; Apo®-Quinidine; BioQuin® Durules™; Novo-Quinidin; Quinate®

Mexican Brand Names Quini Durules®

Pharmacologic Category Antiarrhythmic Agent, Class Ia

Synonyms Quinidine Gluconate; Quinidine Polygalacturonate; Quinidine Sulfate

Use Prophylaxis after cardioversion of atrial fibrillation and/or flutter to maintain normal sinus rhythm; prevent recurrence of paroxysmal supraventricular tachycardia, paroxysmal AV junctional rhythm, paroxysmal ventricular tachycardia, paroxysmal atrial fibrillation, and atrial or ventricular premature contractions; has activity against *Plasmodium falciparum* malaria

Local Anesthetic/Vasoconstrictor Precautions No information available to require special precautions

Effects on Dental Treatment When taken over a long period of time, the anticholinergic side effects from quinidine can cause a reduction of saliva production or secretion contributing to discomfort and dental disease (ie, caries, oral candidiasis and periodontal disease).

Dosage Dosage expressed in terms of the salt: 267 mg of quinidine gluconate = 200 mg of quinidine sulfate.

Children: Test dose for idiosyncratic reaction (sulfate, oral or gluconate, I.M.): 2 mg/kg or 60 mg/m^2

Oral (quinidine sulfate): 15-60 mg/kg/day in 4-5 divided doses or 6 mg/kg every 4-6 hours; usual 30 mg/kg/day or 900 mg/m^2/day given in 5 daily doses

I.V. **not** recommended (quinidine gluconate): 2-10 mg/kg/dose given at a rate ≤10 mg/minute every 3-6 hours as needed

Adults: Test dose: Oral, I.M.: 200 mg administered several hours before full dosage (to determine possibility of idiosyncratic reaction)

Oral (for malaria):

Sulfate: 100-600 mg/dose every 4-6 hours; begin at 200 mg/dose and titrate to desired effect (maximum daily dose: 3-4 g)

Gluconate: 324-972 mg every 8-12 hours

I.M.: 400 mg/dose every 2-6 hours; initial dose: 600 mg (gluconate)

I.V.: 200-400 mg/dose diluted and given at a rate ≤10 mg/minute; may require as much as 500-750 mg

Dosing adjustment in renal impairment: Cl_{cr} <10 mL/minute: Administer 75% of normal dose.

Hemodialysis: Slightly hemodialyzable (5% to 20%); 200 mg supplemental dose posthemodialysis is recommended.

Peritoneal dialysis: Not dialyzable (0% to 5%)

Dosing adjustment/comments in hepatic impairment: Larger loading dose may be indicated, reduce maintenance doses by 50% and monitor serum levels closely.

Mechanism of Action Class 1a antiarrhythmic agent; depresses phase O of the action potential; decreases myocardial excitability and conduction velocity, and myocardial contractility by decreasing sodium influx during depolarization and potassium efflux in repolarization; also reduces calcium transport across cell membrane

Other Adverse Effects

Frequency not defined: Hypotension, syncope

>10%:

Cardiovascular: QT_c prolongation (modest prolongation is common, however, excessive prolongation is rare and indicates toxicity)

Central nervous system: Lightheadedness (15%)

Gastrointestinal: Diarrhea (35%), upper GI distress, bitter taste, diarrhea, anorexia, nausea, vomiting, stomach cramping (22%)

1% to 10%:

Cardiovascular: Angina (6%), palpitation (7%), new or worsened arrhythmias (proarrhythmic effect)

Central nervous system: Syncope (1% to 8%), headache (7%), fatigue (7%), weakness (5%), sleep disturbance (3%), tremor (2%), nervousness (2%), incoordination (1%)

Dermatologic: Rash (5%)

Ocular: Blurred vision

Otic: Tinnitus

Respiratory: Wheezing

<1% (Limited to important or life-threatening): Tachycardia, QT_c prolongation (excessive), torsade de pointes, heart block, ventricular fibrillation, ventricular tachycardia, paradoxical increase in ventricular rate during atrial fibrillation/flutter, exacerbated bradycardia (in sick sinus syndrome), vascular collapse, confusion, delirium, vertigo, impaired hearing, respiratory depression, pneumonitis, bronchospasm, fever, urticaria, flushing, exfoliative rash, psoriaform rash, pruritus, lymphadenopathy, hemolytic anemia, vasculitis, thrombocytopenic purpura, thrombocytopenia, pancytopenia, uveitis, angioedema, agranulocytosis, sicca syndrome, arthralgia, myalgia, increased CPK, drug-induced lupus-like syndrome, cerebral hypoperfusion (possibly resulting in ataxia, apprehension and seizures), acute psychotic reactions, depression, hallucinations, mydriasis, disturbed color perception, night blindness, scotoma, optic neuritis, visual field loss, photosensitivity, abnormal pigmentation, granulomatous hepatitis, hepatotoxic reaction (rare), eczematous dermatitis, livedo reticularis

Postmarketing and/or case reports: Melanin pigmentation of the hard palate, esophagitis, nephropathy, cholestasis, pneumonitis, lichen planus

(Continued)

Quinidine *(Continued)*

Note: Cinchonism, a syndrome which may include tinnitus, high-frequency hearing loss, deafness, vertigo, blurred vision, diplopia, photophobia, headache, confusion, and delirium has been associated with quinidine use. Usually associated with chronic toxicity, this syndrome has also been described after brief exposure to a moderate dose in sensitive patients. Vomiting and diarrhea may also occur as isolated reactions to therapeutic quinidine levels.

Drug Interactions Substrate of CYP2C8/9, 2E1, **3A4**; Inhibits CYP2C8/9, **2D6**, 3A4

Increased Effect/Toxicity:

Quinidine potentiates nondepolarizing and depolarizing muscle relaxants. Quinidine may increase plasma concentration of digoxin; closely monitor digoxin concentrations. Digoxin dosage may need to be reduced (by 50%) when quinidine is initiated; new steady-state digoxin plasma concentrations occur in 5-7 days. When combined with quinidine, amiloride may cause prolonged ventricular conduction leading to arrhythmias. Urinary alkalinizers (antacids, sodium bicarbonate, acetazolamide) increase quinidine blood levels. Warfarin effects may be increased by quinidine.

Amprenavir, amiodarone, cimetidine, clarithromycin, diltiazem, erythromycin, itraconazole, ketoconazole, nelfinavir, ritonavir, troleandomycin, and verapamil (as well as other inhibitors of cytochrome P450 isoenzyme 3A4 may increase quinidine blood levels). Quinidine may increase blood levels of metoprolol mexiletine, nifedipine, propafenone, propranolol, and timolol.

Effects may be additive with drugs which prolong the QT interval, including amiodarone, amitriptyline, astemizole, bepridil, cisapride (use is contraindicated), disopyramide, erythromycin, haloperidol, imipramine, pimozide, procainamide, sotalol, thioridazine, and some quinolones (sparfloxacin, gatifloxacin, moxifloxacin - concurrent use is contraindicated).

Decreased Effect: Analgesic efficacy of codeine may be reduced. Enzyme inducers (aminoglutethimide, carbamazepine, phenobarbital, phenytoin, primidone, rifabutin, rifampin) may decrease quinidine blood levels.

Dietary/Ethanol/Herb Considerations

Food may increase serum concentration; has a variable effect on absorption of sustained release formulation. Avoid grapefruit products; may decrease absorption. Excessive intake of fruit juices or vitamin C may decrease urine pH resulting in increased clearance and decreased serum concentration. Alkaline foods may increase serum concentration. Buttermilk, boiled milk, or yogurt may reduce diarrhea. Dietary salt may alter the rate and extent of absorption; decreased salt intake may lead to increased quinidine serum concentration; avoid changes in dietary salt intake. Avoid caffeine (eg, colas, chocolate), garlic, and licorice.

Herb/Nutraceutical: Avoid black cohosh, dong quai, and evening primrose due to estrogenic activity. Avoid ephedra, ginseng, and yohimbe; may worsen arrhythmia. Avoid garlic; may have increased antihypertensive effect. Avoid ginger due to positive inotropic effects; theoretically, may cause arrhythmia. Avoid hawthorn; may lower peripheral vascular resistance causing additional decrease in BP. Avoid licorice. Avoid St John's wort; may decrease serum concentration.

Pharmacodynamics/Kinetics

Distribution: V_d: Adults: 2-3.5 L/kg, decreased with congestive heart failure, malaria; increased with cirrhosis; crosses placenta; enters breast milk

Protein binding:

Newborns: 60% to 70%; decreased protein binding with cyanotic congenital heart disease, cirrhosis, or acute myocardial infarction

Adults: 80% to 90%

Metabolism: Extensively hepatic (50% to 90%) to inactive compounds

Bioavailability: Sulfate: 80%; Gluconate: 70%

Half-life elimination, plasma: Children: 2.5-6.7 hours; Adults: 6-8 hours; prolonged with elderly, cirrhosis, and congestive heart failure

Excretion: Urine (15% to 25% as unchanged drug)

Pregnancy Risk Factor C

Generic Available Yes

Quinidine Gluconate *see* Quinidine *on page 1158*

Quinidine Polygalacturonate *see* Quinidine *on page 1158*

Quinidine Sulfate *see* Quinidine *on page 1158*

Quinine (KWYE nine)

Canadian Brand Names Quinine-Odan™

Pharmacologic Category Antimalarial Agent

Synonyms Quinine Sulfate

Use In conjunction with other antimalarial agents, suppression or treatment of chloroquine-resistant *P. falciparum* malaria; treatment of *Babesia microti* infection in conjunction with clindamycin

Unlabeled/Investigational Use Prevention and treatment of nocturnal recumbency leg muscle cramps

Local Anesthetic/Vasoconstrictor Precautions No information available to require special precautions

Effects on Dental Treatment No significant effects or complications reported

Dosage Oral:

Children:

Treatment of chloroquine-resistant malaria: 25-30 mg/kg/day in divided doses every 8 hours for 3-7 days with tetracycline (consider risk versus benefit in children <8 years of age)

Babesiosis: 25 mg/kg/day divided every 8 hours for 7 days

Adults:

Treatment of chloroquine-resistant malaria: 650 mg every 8 hours for 3-7 days with tetracycline

Suppression of malaria: 325 mg twice daily and continued for 6 weeks after exposure

Babesiosis: 650 mg every 6-8 hours for 7 days

Leg cramps: 200-300 mg at bedtime

Dosing adjustment in renal impairment:

Cl_{cr} 10-50 mL/minute: Administer every 8-12 hours or 75% of normal dose

Cl_{cr} <10 mL/minute: Administer every 24 hours or 30% to 50% of normal dose

Dialysis: Not removed

Peritoneal dialysis: Dose as for Cl_{cr} <10 mL/minute

Continuous arteriovenous or venovenous hemodiafiltration effects: Dose for Cl_{cr} 10-50 mL/minute

Mechanism of Action Depresses oxygen uptake and carbohydrate metabolism; intercalates into DNA, disrupting the parasite's replication and transcription; affects calcium distribution within muscle fibers and decreases the excitability of the motor end-plate region; cardiovascular effects similar to quinidine

Other Adverse Effects

Frequency not defined:

Central nervous system: Severe headache

Gastrointestinal: Nausea, vomiting, diarrhea

Ocular: Blurred vision

Otic: Tinnitus

Miscellaneous: Cinchonism (risk of cinchonism is directly related to dose and duration of therapy)

<1%: Flushing of the skin, anginal symptoms, fever, rash, pruritus, hypoglycemia, epigastric pain, hemolysis in G6PD deficiency, thrombocytopenia, hepatitis, nightblindness, diplopia, optic atrophy, impaired hearing, hypersensitivity reactions

Drug Interactions Substrate of CYP1A2, 2C19, 3A4; Inhibits CYP2C8/9, **2D6**, 3A4

Increased Effect/Toxicity: Beta-blockers + quinine may increase bradycardia. Quinine may enhance warfarin anticoagulant effect. Quinine potentiates nondepolarizing and depolarizing muscle relaxants. Quinine may increase plasma concentration of digoxin. Closely monitor digoxin concentrations. Digoxin dosage may need to be reduced (by one-half) when quinine is initiated. New steady-state digoxin plasma concentrations occur in 5-7 days. Verapamil, amiodarone, alkalinizing agents, and cimetidine may increase quinine serum concentrations.

Decreased Effect: Phenobarbital, phenytoin, and rifampin may decrease quinine serum concentrations.

Dietary/Ethanol/Herb Considerations

Food: Administer with food to reduce GI upset.

Herb/Nutraceutical: Avoid St John's wort; may decrease serum concentration.

Pharmacodynamics/Kinetics

Absorption: Readily, mainly from upper small intestine

Protein binding: 70% to 95%

Metabolism: Primarily hepatic

Half-life elimination: Children: 6-12 hours; Adults: 8-14 hours

Time to peak, serum: 1-3 hours

Excretion: Feces and saliva; urine (<5% as unchanged drug)

Pregnancy Risk Factor X

Generic Available Yes

Quinine Sulfate *see* Quinine *on page 1160*

Quinol *see* Hydroquinone *on page 693*

Quinupristin and Dalfopristin (kwi NYOO pris tin & dal FOE pris tin)

U.S. Brand Names Synercid®

Canadian Brand Names Synercid®

Pharmacologic Category Antibiotic, Streptogramin

Synonyms Pristinamycin; RP59500

Use Treatment of serious or life-threatening infections associated with vancomycin-resistant *Enterococcus faecium* bacteremia; treatment of complicated skin and skin structure infections caused by methcillin-susceptible *Staphylococcus aureus* or *Streptococcus pyogenes*

(Continued)

Quinupristin and Dalfopristin *(Continued)*

Has been studied in the treatment of a variety of infections caused by *Enterococcus faecium* (not *E. fecalis*) including vancomycin-resistant strains. May also be effective in the treatment of serious infections caused by *Staphylococcus* species including those resistant to methicillin.

Local Anesthetic/Vasoconstrictor Precautions No information available to require special precautions

Effects on Dental Treatment No significant effects or complications reported

Dosage I.V.:

Children (limited information): Dosages similar to adult dosing have been used in the treatment of complicated skin/soft tissue infections and infections caused by vancomycin-resistant *Enterococcus faecium*

CNS shunt infection due to vancomycin-resistant *Enterococcus faecium*: 7.5 mg/kg/dose every 8 hours; concurrent intrathecal doses of 1-2 mg/day have been administered for up to 68 days

Adults:

Vancomycin-resistant *Enterococcus faecium:* 7.5 mg/kg every 8 hours

Complicated skin and skin structure infection: 7.5 mg/kg every 12 hours

Mechanism of Action Quinupristin/dalfopristin inhibits bacterial protein synthesis by binding to different sites on the 50S bacterial ribosomal subunit thereby inhibiting protein synthesis

Other Adverse Effects

>10%:

Hepatic: Hyperbilirubinemia (3% to 35%)

Local: Inflammation at infusion site (38% to 42%), local pain (40% to 44%), local edema (17% to 18%), infusion site reaction (12% to 13%)

1% to 10%:

Central nervous system: Pain (2% to 3%), headache (2%)

Dermatologic: Pruritus (2%), rash (3%)

Endocrine & metabolic: Hyperglycemia (1%)

Gastrointestinal: Nausea (3% to 5%), diarrhea (3%), vomiting (3% to 4%)

Hematologic: Anemia (3%)

Hepatic: Increased LDH (3%), increased GGT (2%)

Local: Thrombophlebitis (2%)

Neuromuscular & skeletal: Arthralgia (<1% to 8%), myalgia (<1% to 5%), Increased CPK (2%)

<1%: Abdominal pain, allergic reaction, anaphylactoid reaction, anxiety, apnea, arrhythmia, bone pain, cardiac arrest, chest pain, coagulation disorder, confusion, constipation, dizziness, dysautonomia, dyspepsia, dyspnea, encephalopathy, fever, gastrointestinal hemorrhage, gout, hematuria, hemolysis, hemolytic anemia, hepatitis, hyperkalemia, hypertonia, hypoglycemia, hyponatremia, hypotension, hypoventilation, hypovolemia, increased BUN, increased serum creatinine, increased transaminases, infection, insomnia, leg cramps, maculopapular rash, mesenteric artery occlusion, myasthenia, neck rigidity, neuropathy, oral candidiasis, palpitation, pancreatitis, pancytopenia, paraplegia, paresthesia, pericarditis, peripheral edema, phlebitis, pleural effusion, pseudomembranous colitis, respiratory distress, seizures, shock, skin ulcer, stomatitis, diaphoresis, syncope, thrombocytopenia, tremor, urticaria, vaginitis, vasodilation

Drug Interactions Quinupristin: Inhibits CYP3A4

Increased Effect/Toxicity: Astemizole and cisapride (which may prolong QT_c interval and lead to arrhythmias) should be avoided. The metabolism of midazolam and nifedipine have been demonstrated to be inhibited *in vitro.* An increase in cyclosporine levels has been documented in patients receiving concomitant therapy. Other medications metabolized by CYP3A4, including protease inhibitors, non-nucleoside reverse transcriptase inhibitors, benzodiazepines, calcium channel blockers, some HMG-CoA reductase inhibitors, immunosuppressive agents, corticosteroids, carbamazepine, quinidine, lidocaine, and disopyramide are predicted to have increased plasma concentrations during concurrent dosing.

Pharmacodynamics/Kinetics

Distribution: Quinupristin: 0.45 L/kg; Dalfopristin: 0.24 L/kg

Protein binding: Moderate

Metabolism: To active metabolites via nonenzymatic reactions

Half-life elimination: Quinupristin: 0.85 hour; Dalfopristin: 0.7 hour (mean elimination half-lives, including metabolites: 3 and 1 hours, respectively)

Excretion: Feces (75% to 77% as unchanged drug and metabolites); urine (15% to 19%)

Pregnancy Risk Factor B

Generic Available No

Quixin™ *see* Levofloxacin *on page 794*

QVAR™ *see* Beclomethasone *on page 163*

Rabeprazole (ra BE pray zole)

U.S. Brand Names Aciphex®

Canadian Brand Names Aciphex®; Pariet®

Mexican Brand Names Pariet®

Pharmacologic Category Proton Pump Inhibitor

Synonyms Pariprazole

Use Short-term (4-8 weeks) treatment and maintenance of erosive or ulcerative gastroesophageal reflux disease (GERD); symptomatic GERD; short-term (up to 4 weeks) treatment of duodenal ulcers; long-term treatment of pathological hypersecretory conditions, including Zollinger-Ellison syndrome; *H. pylori* eradication (in combination with amoxicillin and clarithromycin)

Unlabeled/Investigational Use Maintenance of duodenal ulcer

Local Anesthetic/Vasoconstrictor Precautions No information available to require special precautions

Effects on Dental Treatment No significant effects or complications reported

Dosage Oral: Adults >18 years and Elderly:

GERD: 20 mg once daily for 4-8 weeks; maintenance: 20 mg once daily

Duodenal ulcer: 20 mg/day after breakfast for 4 weeks

H. pylori eradication: 20 mg twice daily for 7 days; to be administered with amoxicillin 1000 mg and clarithromycin 500 mg, also given twice daily for 7 days. **Note:** All three medications should be given together with morning and evening meals.

Hypersecretory conditions: 60 mg once daily; dose may need to be adjusted as necessary. Doses as high as 100 mg once daily and 60 mg twice daily have been used.

Dosing adjustment in hepatic impairment: None required for mild to moderate; use caution in severe impairment

Mechanism of Action Potent proton pump inhibitor; suppresses gastric acid secretion by inhibiting the parietal cell H+/K+ ATP pump

Other Adverse Effects

1% to 10%: Central nervous system: Headache

<1%: Abdomen enlarged (rare), abdominal pain, abnormal dreams, abnormal stools, abnormal vision, agitation (rare), allergic reaction, alopecia, amblyopia, amnesia (rare), anemia, angina pectoris, anorexia, anxiety, apnea (rare), appetite increased, arthritis, arthrosis, asthma, bloody diarrhea (rare), blurred vision (rare), bone pain, bradycardia (rare), breast enlargement, bundle branch block, bursitis, cataract, chest pain substernal, chills, cholangitis (rare), cholecystitis, cholelithiasis, colitis, confusion (rare), constipation, convulsions, corneal opacity (rare), cystitis, deafness, deafness (rare), dehydration, depression, diaphoresis, diarrhea, diplopia (rare), dizziness, dry eyes, xerostomia, dry skin (rare), duodenitis (rare), dysmenorrhea, dyspepsia, dysphagia, dyspnea, dysuria, ecchymosis, edema, electrocardiogram abnormal, epistaxis, eructation, esophagitis, extrapyramidal syndrome (rare), eye pain (rare), facial edema (rare), fever, flatulence, gastroenteritis, gastrointestinal hemorrhage (rare), gingivitis, glaucoma, glossitis, gout, hangover effect (rare), hematuria (rare), hepatic encephalopathy (rare), hepatitis (rare), hepatoma (rare), herpes zoster (rare), hiccups, hyperkinesia (rare), hypertension, hyperthyroidism, hypertonia, hyperventilation, hypochromic anemia, hypothyroidism, hypoventilation (rare), impotence (rare), insomnia, kidney calculus, laryngitis, leg cramps, leukorrhea (rare), libido decreased, liver fatty deposit (rare), lymphadenopathy, malaise, melena, menorrhagia (rare), metrorrhagia, MI, migraine, oral ulceration, myalgia, nausea, neck rigidity, nervousness, neuralgia, neuropathy, orchitis (rare), otitis media, palpitation, pancreatitis, paresthesia, peripheral edema, photosensitivity reaction, polyuria, proctitis, pruritus, psoriasis (rare), pulmonary embolus (rare), rash, rectal hemorrhage, retinal degeneration (rare), salivary gland enlargement (rare), sinus bradycardia, skin discoloration (rare), somnolence, stomatitis, strabismus (rare), supraventricular tachycardia (rare), syncope, tachycardia, thirst (rare), tinnitus, tremor, twitching (rare), urinary frequency, urinary incontinence (rare), urticaria, vertigo, vomiting, weakness, weight gain/loss

Postmarketing and/or case reports: Sudden death, coma, hyperammonemia, jaundice, rhabdomyolysis, disorientation, delirium, anaphylaxis, angioedema, bullous and other drug eruptions of the skin, interstitial pneumonia, TSH elevations; in most instances, the relationship to rabeprazole sodium was unclear. In addition, agranulocytosis, hemolytic anemia, leukopenia, pancytopenia, and thrombocytopenia have been reported.

Drug Interactions Substrate of **CYP2C19, 3A4**; Inhibits CYP2C19, 3A4

Increased Effect/Toxicity: Rabeprazole (in extremely high concentrations) may increase serum levels of digoxin and cyclosporine. Rabeprazole may increase INR and PT when used with warfarin; monitor.

Decreased Effect: Rabeprazole may decrease bioavailability of ketoconazole or itraconazole.

Dietary/Ethanol/Herb Considerations Ethanol: Avoid use; may cause gastric mucosal irritation.

Pharmacodynamics/Kinetics

Onset of action: 1 hour

Duration: 24 hours

Absorption: Oral: Well absorbed within 1 hour

Distribution: 96.3%

Protein binding, serum: 94.8% to 97.5%

(Continued)

Rabeprazole *(Continued)*

Metabolism: Hepatic via CYP3A and 2C19 to inactive metabolites
Bioavailability: Oral: 52%
Half-life elimination (dose dependent): 0.85-2 hours
Time to peak, plasma: 2-5 hours
Excretion: Urine (90% primarily as thioether carboxylic acid); remainder in feces

Pregnancy Risk Factor B

Generic Available No

Rabies Immune Globulin (Human)

(RAY beez i MYOON GLOB yoo lin, HYOO min)

Related Information

Animal and Human Bites Guidelines *on page 1580*
Immunizations (Vaccines) *on page 1612*

U.S. Brand Names BayRab®; Imogam®

Canadian Brand Names BayRab™; Imogam® Rabies Pasteurized

Pharmacologic Category Immune Globulin

Synonyms RIG

Use Part of postexposure prophylaxis of persons with rabies exposure who lack a history of pre-exposure or postexposure prophylaxis with rabies vaccine or a recently documented neutralizing antibody response to previous rabies vaccination; although it is preferable to administer RIG with the first dose of vaccine, it can be given up to 8 days after vaccination

Local Anesthetic/Vasoconstrictor Precautions No information available to require special precautions

Effects on Dental Treatment No significant effects or complications reported

Restrictions Federal law requires that the date of administration, the vaccine manufacturer, lot number of vaccine, and the administering person's name, title and address be entered into the patient's permanent medical record.

Dosage Children and Adults: I.M.: 20 units/kg in a single dose (RIG should always be administered as part of rabies vaccine (HDCV)) regimen (as soon as possible after the first dose of vaccine, up to 8 days); infiltrate 1/2 of the dose locally around the wound; administer the remainder I.M.

Note: Persons known to have an adequate titer or who have been completely immunized with rabies vaccine should not receive RIG, only booster doses of HDCV

Mechanism of Action Rabies immune globulin is a solution of globulins dried from the plasma or serum of selected adult human donors who have been immunized with rabies vaccine and have developed high titers of rabies antibody. It generally contains 10% to 18% of protein of which not less than 80% is monomeric immunoglobulin G.

Other Adverse Effects

1% to 10%:

Central nervous system: Fever (mild)
Local: Soreness at injection site

<1%: Urticaria, angioedema, stiffness, soreness of muscles, anaphylactic shock

Pregnancy Risk Factor C

Generic Available No

Rabies Virus Vaccine (RAY beez VYE rus vak SEEN)

Related Information

Animal and Human Bites Guidelines *on page 1580*
Immunizations (Vaccines) *on page 1612*

U.S. Brand Names Imovax® Rabies

Canadian Brand Names Imovax® Rabies

Pharmacologic Category Vaccine

Synonyms HDCV; Human Diploid Cell Cultures Rabies Vaccine

Use Pre-exposure immunization: Vaccinate persons with greater than usual risk due to occupation or avocation including veterinarians, rangers, animal handlers, certain laboratory workers, and persons living in or visiting countries for longer than 1 month where rabies is a constant threat.

Postexposure prophylaxis: If a bite from a carrier animal is unprovoked, if it is not captured and rabies is present in that species and area, administer rabies immune globulin (RIG) and the vaccine as indicated

Local Anesthetic/Vasoconstrictor Precautions No information available to require special precautions

Effects on Dental Treatment No significant effects or complications reported

Restrictions Federal law requires that the date of administration, the vaccine manufacturer, lot number of vaccine, and the administering person's name, title and address be entered into the patient's permanent medical record.

Dosage

Pre-exposure prophylaxis: 1 mL I.M. on days 0, 7, and 21 to 28. **Note:** Prolonging the interval between doses does not interfere with immunity achieved after the concluding dose of the basic series.

Postexposure prophylaxis: All postexposure treatment should begin with immediate cleansing of the wound with soap and water

Persons not previously immunized as above: Rabies immune globulin 20 units/kg body weight, half infiltrated at bite site if possible, remainder I.M.; and 5 doses of rabies vaccine, 1 mL I.M., one each on days 0, 3, 7, 14, 28

Persons who have previously received postexposure prophylaxis with rabies vaccine, received a recommended I.M. pre-exposure series of rabies vaccine or have a previously documented rabies antibody titer considered adequate: 1 mL of either vaccine I.M. only on days 0 and 3; do not administer RIG

Booster (for occupational or other continuing risk): 1 mL I.M. every 2-5 years or based on antibody titers

Mechanism of Action Rabies vaccine is an inactivated virus vaccine which promotes immunity by inducing an active immune response. The production of specific antibodies requires about 7-10 days to develop. Rabies immune globulin or antirabies serum, equine (ARS) is given in conjunction with rabies vaccine to provide immune protection until an antibody response can occur.

Other Adverse Effects Mild systemic reactions occur at an incidence of ~8% to 10% with RVA and 20% with HDCV. **All serious adverse reactions must be reported to the U.S. Department of Health and Human Services (DHHS) Vaccine Adverse Event Reporting System (VAERS) 1-800-822-7967.**

Cardiovascular: Edema

Central nervous system: Dizziness, malaise, encephalomyelitis, transverse myelitis, fever, pain, headache, neuroparalytic reactions

Dermatologic: Itching, erythema

Gastrointestinal: Nausea, abdominal pain

Local: Local discomfort, pain at injection site

Neuromuscular & skeletal: Myalgia

Note: Serum sickness reaction is much less frequent with RVA (<1%) vs the HDCV (6%).

Pharmacodynamics/Kinetics

Onset of action: I.M.: Rabies antibody: ~7-10 days

Peak effect: ~30-60 days

Duration: ≥1 year

Pregnancy Risk Factor C

Generic Available No

Radiological/Contrast Media (Nonionic)

(ray deo LO jik ul/KON trast MEE diu non eye ON ik)

U.S. Brand Names Amipaque®; Isovue®; Omnipaque®; Optiray®; ProHance®

Pharmacologic Category Radiopaque Agents

Synonyms Gadoteridol; Iohexol; Iopamidol; Ioversol; Metrizamide

Use Enhance visualization of structures during radiologic procedures

Local Anesthetic/Vasoconstrictor Precautions No information available to require special precautions

Effects on Dental Treatment

1.4%: Taste perversion

<1%: Xerostomia, edematous and/or itching tongue, gingivitis

Generic Available Yes

rAHF *see* Antihemophilic Factor (Recombinant) *on page 115*

R-albuterol *see* Levalbuterol *on page 786*

Raloxifene (ral OKS i feen)

Related Information

Endocrine Disorders and Pregnancy *on page 1479*

U.S. Brand Names Evista®

Canadian Brand Names Evista®

Mexican Brand Names Evista®

Pharmacologic Category Selective Estrogen Receptor Modulator (SERM)

Synonyms Keoxifene Hydrochloride; Raloxifene Hydrochloride

Use Prevention and treatment of osteoporosis in postmenopausal women

Local Anesthetic/Vasoconstrictor Precautions No information available to require special precautions

Effects on Dental Treatment No significant effects or complications reported

Dosage Adults: Female: Oral: 60 mg/day which may be administered any time of the day without regard to meals

Mechanism of Action A selective estrogen receptor modulator, meaning that it affects some of the same receptors that estrogen does, but not all, and in some instances, it antagonizes or blocks estrogen; it acts like estrogen to prevent bone loss and improve lipid profiles (decreases total and LDL-cholesterol but does not

(Continued)

Raloxifene *(Continued)*

raise triglycerides), but it has the potential to block some estrogen effects such as those that lead to breast cancer and uterine cancer

Other Adverse Effects Note: Has been associated with increased risk of thromboembolism (DVT, PE) and superficial thrombophlebitis; risk is similar to reported risk of HRT

≥2%:
- Cardiovascular: Chest pain
- Central nervous system: Migraine, depression, insomnia, fever
- Dermatologic: Rash
- Endocrine & metabolic: Hot flashes
- Gastrointestinal: Nausea, dyspepsia, vomiting, flatulence, gastroenteritis, weight gain
- Genitourinary: Vaginitis, urinary tract infection, cystitis, leukorrhea
- Neuromuscular & skeletal: Leg cramps, arthralgia, myalgia, arthritis
- Respiratory: Sinusitis, pharyngitis, cough, pneumonia, laryngitis
- Miscellaneous: Infection, flu syndrome, diaphoresis

<1%: Hypertriglyceridemia (in women with a history of increased triglycerides in response to oral estrogens)

Postmarketing and/or case reports: Retinal vein occlusion

Drug Interactions

Increased Effect/Toxicity: May interact with highly protein-bound drugs, increasing effects of either agent; use caution with highly protein-bound drugs, warfarin, clofibrate, indomethacin, naproxen, ibuprofen, diazepam, phenytoin, or tamoxifen.

Decreased Effect: Ampicillin and cholestyramine reduce raloxifene absorption/blood levels.

Dietary/Ethanol/Herb Considerations Ethanol: Avoid use; may increase risk of osteoporosis.

Pharmacodynamics/Kinetics
- Onset of action: 8 weeks
- Absorption: ~60%
- Distribution: 2348 L/kg
- Protein binding: >95% to albumin and α-glycoprotein
- Metabolism: Extensive first-pass effect
- Bioavailability: ~2%
- Half-life elimination: 27.7-32.5 hours
- Excretion: Primarily feces; urine (0.2%)

Pregnancy Risk Factor X

Generic Available No

Raloxifene Hydrochloride *see* Raloxifene *on page 1165*

Ramipril (ra MI pril)

Related Information

Cardiovascular Diseases *on page 1456*

U.S. Brand Names Altace®

Canadian Brand Names Altace®

Mexican Brand Names Ramace®; Tritace®

Pharmacologic Category Angiotensin-Converting Enzyme (ACE) Inhibitor

Use Treatment of hypertension, alone or in combination with thiazide diuretics; treatment of CHF; treatment of left ventricular dysfunction after MI; to reduce risk of heart attack, stroke, and death in patients at increased risk for these problems

Local Anesthetic/Vasoconstrictor Precautions No information available to require special precautions

Effects on Dental Treatment No significant effects or complications reported

Dosage Adults: Oral:

Hypertension: 2.5-5 mg once daily, maximum: 20 mg/day

Reduction in risk of MI, stroke, and death from cardiovascular causes: Initial: 2.5 mg once daily for 1 week, then 5 mg once daily for the next 3 weeks, then increase as tolerated to 10 mg once daily (may be given as divided dose)

Heart failure postmyocardial infarction: Initial: 2.5 mg twice daily titrated upward, if possible, to 5 mg twice daily.

Note: The dose of any concomitant diuretic should be reduced. If the diuretic cannot be discontinued, initiate therapy with 1.25 mg. After the initial dose, the patient should be monitored carefully until blood pressure has stabilized.

Dosing adjustment in renal impairment:
- Cl_{cr} <40 mL/minute: Administer 25% of normal dose.
- Renal failure and hypertension: Administer 1.25 mg once daily, titrated upward as possible.
- Renal failure and heart failure: Administer 1.25 mg once daily, increasing to 1.25 mg twice daily up to 2.5 mg twice daily as tolerated.

Mechanism of Action Ramipril is an ACE inhibitor which prevents the formation of angiotensin II from angiotensin I and exhibits pharmacologic effects that are similar to captopril. Ramipril must undergo enzymatic saponification by esterases in the liver to its biologically active metabolite, ramiprilat. The pharmacodynamic effects of ramipril result from the high-affinity, competitive, reversible binding of ramiprilat to angiotensin-converting enzyme thus preventing the formation of the potent vasoconstrictor angiotensin II. This isomerized enzyme-inhibitor complex has a slow rate of dissociation, which results in high potency and a long duration of action; a CNS mechanism may also be involved in the hypotensive effect as angiotensin II increases adrenergic outflow from CNS; vasoactive kallikreins may be decreased in conversion to active hormones by ACE inhibitors, thus reducing blood pressure

Other Adverse Effects Note: Frequency ranges include data from hypertension and heart failure trials. Higher rates of adverse reactions have generally been noted in patients with CHF. However, the frequency of adverse effects associated with placebo is also increased in this population.

>10%: Respiratory: Cough (increased) (7% to 12%)

1% to 10%:

Cardiovascular: Hypotension (11%), angina (3%), postural hypotension (2%), syncope (2%)

Central nervous system: Headache (1% to 5%), dizziness (2% to 4%), fatigue (2%), vertigo (2%)

Endocrine & metabolic: Hyperkalemia (1% to 10%)

Gastrointestinal: Nausea/vomiting (1% to 2%)

Neuromuscular & skeletal: Chest pain (noncardiac) (1%)

Renal: Renal dysfunction (1%), elevation in serum creatinine (1% to 2%), increased BUN (<1% to 3%); transient elevations of creatinine and/or BUN may occur more frequently

Respiratory: Cough (estimated 1% to 10%)

<1%: Agranulocytosis, abdominal pain, amnesia, anaphylactoid reaction, angina, angioedema, anorexia, anxiety, arrhythmia, arthralgia, arthritis, bone marrow depression, cerebrovascular events, constipation, convulsions, decreased hematocrit, decreased hemoglobin, depression, diarrhea, dyspepsia, dysphagia, dyspnea, edema, elevated transaminase levels, eosinophilia, epistaxis, erythema multiforme, gastroenteritis, hearing loss, hemolytic anemia, hepatitis, hypersensitivity reactions (fever, rash, urticaria), hyponatremia, impotence, increased diaphoresis, increased salivation, insomnia, malaise, myalgia, MI, nervousness, neuralgia, neuropathy, onycholysis, palpitation, pancreatitis, pancytopenia, paresthesia, pemphigoid, pemphigus, photosensitivity, proteinuria, purpura, somnolence, Stevens-Johnson syndrome, symptomatic hypotension, syncope, abnormal taste, thrombocytopenia, tinnitus, toxic epidermal necrolysis, tremor, vertigo, vision disturbances, weight gain, xerostomia

Postmarketing and/or case reports: Agitation

Worsening of renal function may occur in patients with bilateral renal artery stenosis or in hypovolemia. In addition, a syndrome which may include fever, myalgia, arthralgia, interstitial nephritis, vasculitis, rash, eosinophilia and positive ANA, and elevated ESR has been reported with ACE inhibitors. Risk of pancreatitis and agranulocytosis may be increased in patients with collagen vascular disease or renal impairment.

Drug Interactions

Increased Effect/Toxicity: Potassium supplements, co-trimoxazole (high dose), angiotensin II receptor antagonists (candesartan, losartan, irbesartan, etc), or potassium-sparing diuretics (amiloride, spironolactone, triamterene) may result in elevated serum potassium levels when combined with ramipril. ACE inhibitor effects may be increased by phenothiazines or probenecid (increases levels of captopril). ACE inhibitors may increase serum concentrations/effects of digoxin, lithium, and sulfonlyureas.

Diuretics have additive hypotensive effects with ACE inhibitors, and hypovolemia increases the potential for adverse renal effects of ACE inhibitors. In patients with compromised renal function, coadministration with NSAIDs may result in further deterioration of renal function. Allopurinol and ACE inhibitors may cause a higher risk of hypersensitivity reaction when taken concurrently.

Decreased Effect: Aspirin (high dose) may reduce the therapeutic effects of ACE inhibitors; at low dosages this does not appear to be significant. Rifampin may decrease the effect of ACE inhibitors. Antacids may decrease the bioavailability of ACE inhibitors (may be more likely to occur with captopril); separate administration times by 1-2 hours. NSAIDs, specifically indomethacin, may reduce the hypotensive effects of ACE inhibitors. More likely to occur in low renin or volume dependent hypertensive patients.

Dietary/Ethanol/Herb Considerations

Ethanol: Avoid use; may increase risk of hypotension or dizziness.

Food: Avoid caffeine (eg, colas, chocolate), garlic, and licorice.

Herb/Nutraceutical: Avoid black cohosh, dong quai, and evening primrose due to estrogenic activity. Avoid ephedra, ginseng, and yohimbe; may worsen hypertension. Avoid garlic; may have increased antihypertensive effect. Avoid ginger due to positive inotropic effects; theoretically, may cause arrhythmia. Avoid hawthorn; may lower peripheral vascular resistance causing additional decrease in BP.

Pharmacodynamics/Kinetics

Onset of action: 1-2 hours

(Continued)

Ramipril *(Continued)*

Duration: 24 hours
Absorption: Well absorbed (50% to 60%)
Distribution: Plasma levels decline in a triphasic fashion; rapid decline is a distribution phase to peripheral compartment, plasma protein and tissue ACE (half-life 2-4 hours); 2nd phase is an apparent elimination phase representing the clearance of free ramiprilat (half-life: 9-18 hours); and final phase is the terminal elimination phase representing the equilibrium phase between tissue binding and dissociation
Metabolism: Hepatic to the active form, ramiprilat
Half-life elimination: Ramiprilat: Effective: 13-17 hours; Terminal: >50 hours
Time to peak, serum: ~1 hour
Excretion: Urine (60%) and feces (40%) as parent drug and metabolites

Pregnancy Risk Factor C/D (2nd and 3rd trimesters)

Generic Available No

Ranitidine (ra NI ti deen)

Related Information

Gastrointestinal Disorders *on page 1474*

U.S. Brand Names Zantac®; Zantac® 75 [OTC]

Canadian Brand Names Alti-Ranitidine; Apo®-Ranitidine; Gen-Ranidine; Novo-Ranidine; Nu-Ranit; PMS-Ranitidine; Rhoxal-ranitidine; Zantac®; Zantac 75®

Mexican Brand Names Acloral®; Alter H2®; Alvidina®; Anistal®; Azanplus®; Azantac®; Cauteridol®; Credaxol®; Galidrin®; Gastrec; Microtid; Neugal®; Ranifur®; Ranisen®; Raudil®; Serviradine®; Ulcedin®; Ulsaven®; Ultran®

Pharmacologic Category Histamine H_2 Antagonist

Synonyms Ranitidine Hydrochloride

Use

Zantac®: Short-term and maintenance therapy of duodenal ulcer, gastric ulcer, gastroesophageal reflux, active benign ulcer, erosive esophagitis, and pathological hypersecretory conditions; as part of a multidrug regimen for *H. pylori* eradication to reduce the risk of duodenal ulcer recurrence

Zantac® 75 [OTC]: Relief of heartburn, acid indigestion, and sour stomach

Unlabeled/Investigational Use Treatment of recurrent postoperative ulcer, upper GI bleeding, prevention of acid-aspiration pneumonitis during surgery; prevention of stress-induced ulcers

Local Anesthetic/Vasoconstrictor Precautions No information available to require special precautions

Effects on Dental Treatment No significant effects or complications reported

Dosage

Children 1 month to 16 years:
- Duodenal and gastric ulcer:
  - Oral:
    - Treatment: 2-4 mg/kg/day divided twice daily; maximum treatment dose: 300 mg/day
    - Maintenance: 2-4 mg/kg once daily; maximum maintenance dose: 150 mg/day
  - I.V.: 2-4 mg/kg/day divided every 6-8 hours; maximum: 150 mg/day
- GERD and erosive esophagitis:
  - Oral: 5-10 mg/kg/day divided twice daily; maximum: GERD: 300 mg/day, erosive esophagitis: 600 mg/day
  - I.V.: 2-4 mg/kg/day divided every 6-8 hours; maximum: 150 mg/day **or as an alternative**
    - Continuous infusion: Initial: 1 mg/kg/dose for one dose followed by infusion of 0.08-0.17 mg/kg/hour or 2-4 mg/kg/day

Children ≥12 years: Prevention of heartburn: Oral: Zantac® 75 [OTC]: 75 mg 30-60 minutes before eating food or drinking beverages which cause heartburn; maximum: 150 mg/24 hours; do not use for more than 14 days

Adults:
- Duodenal ulcer: Oral: Treatment: 150 mg twice daily, or 300 mg once daily after the evening meal or at bedtime; maintenance: 150 mg once daily at bedtime
- *Helicobacter pylori* eradication: 150 mg twice daily; requires combination therapy
- Pathological hypersecretory conditions:
  - Oral: 150 mg twice daily; adjust dose or frequency as clinically indicated; doses of up to 6 g/day have been used
  - I.V.: Continuous infusion for Zollinger-Ellison: 1 mg/kg/hour; measure gastric acid output at 4 hours, if >10 mEq or if patient is symptomatic, increase dose in increments of 0.5 mg/kg/hour; doses of up to 2.5 mg/kg/hour have been used
- Gastric ulcer, benign: Oral: 150 mg twice daily; maintenance: 150 mg once daily at bedtime
- Erosive esophagitis: Oral: Treatment: 150 mg 4 times/day; maintenance: 150 mg twice daily

Prevention of heartburn: Oral: Zantac® 75 [OTC]: 75 mg 30-60 minutes before eating food or drinking beverages which cause heartburn; maximum: 150 mg in 24 hours; do not use for more than 14 days

Patients not able to take oral medication:

I.M.: 50 mg every 6-8 hours

I.V.: Intermittent bolus or infusion: 50 mg every 6-8 hours

Continuous I.V. infusion: 6.25 mg/hour

Elderly: Ulcer healing rates and incidence of adverse effects are similar in the elderly, when compared to younger patients; dosing adjustments unnecessary based on age alone

Dosing adjustment in renal impairment: Adults: Cl_{cr} <50 mL/minute:

Oral: 150 mg every 24 hours; adjust dose cautiously if needed

I.V.: 50 mg every 18-24 hours; adjust dose cautiously if needed

Hemodialysis: Adjust dosing schedule so that dose coincides with the end of hemodialysis

Dosing adjustment in hepatic impairment: None; monitor for minor changes in ranitidine halflife, distribution, clearance, and bioavailability

Mechanism of Action Competitive inhibition of histamine at H_2-receptors of the gastric parietal cells, which inhibits gastric acid secretion, gastric volume, and hydrogen ion concentration are reduced. Does not affect pepsin secretion, pentagastrin-stimulated intrinsic factor secretion, or serum gastrin.

Other Adverse Effects Frequency not defined:

Cardiovascular: Atrioventricular block, bradycardia, premature ventricular beats, tachycardia, vasculitis

Central nervous system: Agitation, dizziness, depression, hallucinations, headache, insomnia, malaise, mental confusion, somnolence, vertigo

Dermatologic: Alopecia, erythema multiforme, rash

Endocrine & metabolic: Gynocomastia, impotence, increased prolactin levels, loss of libido

Gastrointestinal: Abdominal discomfort/pain, constipation, diarrhea, nausea, pancreatitis, vomiting

Hematologic: Acquired hemolytic anemia, agranulocytosis, aplastic anemia, granulocytopenia, leukopenia, pancytopenia, thrombocytopenia

Hepatic: Hepatic failure, hepatitis

Local: Transient pain, burning or itching at the injection site

Neuromuscular & skeletal: Arthralgia, involuntary motor disturbance, myalgia

Ocular: Blurred vision

Renal: Increased serum creatinine

Miscellaneous: Anaphylaxis, angioneurotic edema, hypersensitivity reactions

Drug Interactions Substrate of CYP1A2, 2C19, 2D6; Inhibits CYP1A2, 2D6

Increased effect/toxicity of cyclosporine (increased serum creatinine), gentamicin (neuromuscular blockade), glipizide, glyburide, midazolam (increased concentrations), metoprolol, pentoxifylline, phenytoin, quinidine, and triazolam.

Decreased Effect: Variable effects on warfarin. Antacids may decrease absorption of ranitidine. Ketoconazole and itraconazole absorptions are decreased. May produce altered serum levels of procainamide and ferrous sulfate. Decreased effect of nondepolarizing muscle relaxants, cefpodoxime, cyanocobalamin (decreased absorption), diazepam, and oxaprozin.

Decreased toxicity of atropine.

Dietary/Ethanol/Herb Considerations

Ethanol: Avoid use; may cause gastric mucosal irritation.

Food does not interfere with absorption.

Pharmacodynamics/Kinetics

Absorption: Oral: 50%

Distribution: Normal renal function: V_d: 1.7 L/kg; Cl_{cr} 25-35 mL/minute: 1.76 L/kg minimally penetrates the blood-brain barrier; enters breast milk

Protein binding: 15%

Metabolism: Hepatic to N-oxide, S-oxide, and N-desmethyl metabolites

Bioavailability: Oral: 48%

Half-life elimination:

Oral: Normal renal function: 2.5-3 hours; Cl_{cr} 25-35 mL/minute: 4.8 hours

I.V.: Normal renal function: 2-2.5 hours

Time to peak, serum: Oral: 2-3 hours; I.M.: ≤15 minutes

Excretion: Urine: Oral: 30%, I.V.: 70% (as unchanged drug); feces (as metabolites)

Pregnancy Risk Factor B

Generic Available Yes; Excludes effervescent granules and tablets, injection

Ranitidine Hydrochloride *see* Ranitidine *on page 1168*

Rapamune® *see* Sirolimus *on page 1225*

Rasburicase (ras BYOOR i kayz)

U.S. Brand Names Elitek™

Pharmacologic Category Enzyme; Enzyme, Urate-Oxidase (Recombinant)

(Continued)

Rasburicase *(Continued)*

Use Initial management of uric acid levels in pediatric patients with leukemia, lymphoma, and solid tumor malignancies receiving anticancer therapy expected to result in tumor lysis and elevation of plasma uric acid

Local Anesthetic/Vasoconstrictor Precautions No information available to require special precautions

Effects on Dental Treatment No significant effects or complications reported

Dosage I.V.: Children: Management of uric acid levels: 0.15 mg/kg or 0.2 mg/kg once daily for 5 days; begin chemotherapy 4-24 hours after the first dose

Note: Adults and Elderly: Refer to pediatric dosing; insufficient data collected in adult/geriatric patients to determine response to treatment

Mechanism of Action Rasburicase is a recombinant urate-oxidase enzyme, which converts uric acid to allantoin (an inactive and soluble metabolite of uric acid); it does not inhibit the formation of uric acid.

Other Adverse Effects As reported in patients receiving rasburicase with antitumor therapy versus active-control:

>10%:

Central nervous system: Fever (5% to 46%), headache (26%)

Dermatologic: Rash (13%)

Gastrointestinal: Vomiting (50%), nausea (27%), abdominal pain (20%), constipation (20%), mucositis (2% to 15%), diarrhea (≤1% to 20%)

1% to 10%:

Hematologic: Neutropenia with fever (4%), neutropenia (2%)

Respiratory: Respiratory distress (3%)

Miscellaneous: Sepsis (3%)

<1%: Acute renal failure, anaphylaxis, arrhythmia, cardiac arrest, cardiac failure, cellulitis, cerebrovascular disorder, chest pain, convulsions, cyanosis, dehydration, hemolysis, hemorrhage, hot flashes, ileus, infection, intestinal obstruction, methemoglobinemia, MI, pancytopenia, paresthesia, pneumonia, pulmonary edema, pulmonary hypertension, retinal hemorrhage, rigors, thrombosis, thrombophlebitis

Pharmacodynamics/Kinetics

Distribution: Pediatric patients: 110-127 mL/kg

Half-life elimination: Pediatric patients: 18 hours

Pregnancy Risk Factor C

Generic Available No

Rauwolfia Serpentina (rah WOOL fee u ser pen TEEN u)

Pharmacologic Category Rauwolfia Alkaloid

Synonyms Whole Root Rauwolfia

Use Mild essential hypertension; relief of agitated psychotic states

Local Anesthetic/Vasoconstrictor Precautions No information available to require special precautions

Effects on Dental Treatment No significant effects or complications reported

Dosage Adults: Oral: 200-400 mg/day in 2 divided doses

Other Adverse Effects Frequency not defined:

Cardiovascular: Hypotension, tachycardia, flushing

Central nervous system: Drowsiness, fatigue, CNS depression, coma, parkinsonism, hypothermia

Endocrine & metabolic: Sodium and water retention, gynecomastia, galactorrhea

Gastrointestinal: Abdominal cramps, nausea, vomiting, gastric acid secretion (increased), xerostomia, diarrhea

Ocular: Miosis, conjunctival flushing

Respiratory: Nasal congestion

Drug Interactions Increased Effect/Toxicity: Effects may be additive with other antihypertensives. May increase effect of CNS depressants.

Pregnancy Risk Factor C

Generic Available Yes

Rea-Lo® [OTC] *see* Urea *on page 1365*

ReAzo [OTC] *see* Phenazopyridine *on page 1064*

Rebetol® *see* Ribavirin *on page 1176*

Rebetron® *see* Interferon Alfa-2b and Ribavirin *on page 730*

Rebif® *see* Interferon Beta-1a *on page 732*

Recombinant Hirudin *see* Lepirudin *on page 781*

Recombinant Human Deoxyribonuclease *see* Dornase Alfa *on page 467*

Recombinant Human Follicle Stimulating Hormone *see* Follitropins *on page 607*

Recombinant Human Interleukin-11 *see* Oprelvekin *on page 1003*

Recombinant Human Parathyroid Hormone (1-34) *see* Teriparatide *on page 1280*

Recombinant Human Platelet-Derived Growth Factor B *see* Becaplermin *on page 162*

Recombinant Interleukin-11 *see* Oprelvekin *on page 1003*
Recombinant Plasminogen Activator *see* Reteplase *on page 1174*
Recombinate™ *see* Antihemophilic Factor (Recombinant) *on page 115*
Recombivax HB® *see* Hepatitis B Vaccine *on page 666*
Redutemp® [OTC] *see* Acetaminophen *on page 27*
Reese's® Pinworm Medicine [OTC] *see* Pyrantel Pamoate *on page 1150*
ReFacto® *see* Antihemophilic Factor (Recombinant) *on page 115*
Refludan® *see* Lepirudin *on page 781*
Refresh® [OTC] *see* Artificial Tears *on page 128*
Refresh® Plus [OTC] *see* Artificial Tears *on page 128*
Refresh® Tears [OTC] *see* Artificial Tears *on page 128*
Reglan® *see* Metoclopramide *on page 898*
Regranex® *see* Becaplermin *on page 162*
Regular Iletin® II *see* Insulin Preparations *on page 723*
Reguloid® [OTC] *see* Psyllium *on page 1149*
Relafen® *see* Nabumetone *on page 941*
Relenza® *see* Zanamivir *on page 1405*
Relief® [OTC] *see* Phenylephrine *on page 1071*
Relpax® *see* Eletriptan *on page 490*
Remeron® *see* Mirtazapine *on page 919*
Remeron SolTab® *see* Mirtazapine *on page 919*
Remicade® *see* Infliximab *on page 721*

Remifentanil (rem i FEN ta nil)

U.S. Brand Names Ultiva®
Canadian Brand Names Ultiva®
Mexican Brand Names Ultiva®
Pharmacologic Category Analgesic, Narcotic
Synonyms GI87084B
Use Analgesic for use during general anesthesia for continued analgesia in children ≥2 years of age and adults
Unlabeled/Investigational Use Management of pain in mechanically-ventilated patients
Local Anesthetic/Vasoconstrictor Precautions No information available to require special precautions
Effects on Dental Treatment No significant effects or complications reported
Restrictions C-II
Dosage I.V. continuous infusion:

- Children ≥2 years: Per kg doses are the same as for adult patients
- Adults:
  - Induction: 0.5-1 mcg/kg/minute
  - Maintenance:
    - With nitrous oxide (66%): 0.4 mcg/kg/minute (range: 0.1-2 mcg/kg/minute)
    - With isoflurane: 0.25 mcg/kg/minute (range: 0.05-2 mcg/kg/minute)
    - With propofol: 0.25 mcg/kg/minute (range: 0.05-2 mcg/kg/minute)
  - Continuation as an analgesic in immediate postoperative period: 0.1 mcg/kg/minute (range: 0.025-0.2 mcg/kg/minute)
  - Mechanically-ventilated patients: Acute pain (moderate to severe) (unlabeled use): 0.6-15 mcg/kg/hour
- Elderly: Doses should be decreased by ½ and titrated due to increased sensitivity to effects.

Mechanism of Action Binds with stereospecific mu-opioid receptors at many sites within the CNS, increases pain threshold, alters pain reception, inhibits ascending pain pathways
Other Adverse Effects

- >10%: Gastrointestinal: Nausea, vomiting
- 1% to 10%:
  - Cardiovascular: Hypotension, bradycardia, tachycardia, hypertension
  - Central nervous system: Dizziness, headache, agitation, fever
  - Dermatologic: Pruritus
  - Ocular: Visual disturbances
  - Respiratory: Respiratory depression, apnea, hypoxia
  - Miscellaneous: Shivering, postoperative pain

Drug Interactions Increased Effect/Toxicity: Additive effects with other CNS depressants.
Pharmacodynamics/Kinetics

- Onset of action: I.V.: 1-3 minutes
- Protein binding: 92%
- Metabolism: Rapid via blood and tissue esterases
- Half-life elimination (dose dependent): 10 minutes
- Excretion: Urine

Pregnancy Risk Factor C
Generic Available No

Remodulin™ *see* Treprostinil *on page 1337*

Renacidin® *see* Citric Acid Bladder Mixture *on page 335*

Renagel® *see* Sevelamer *on page 1218*

Renese® *see* Polythiazide *on page 1097*

Renova® *see* Tretinoin (Topical) *on page 1340*

Rentamine® [OTC] *see* Chlorpheniramine, Ephedrine, Phenylephrine, and Carbetapentane *on page 309*

ReoPro® *see* Abciximab *on page 23*

Repaglinide (re PAG li nide)

Related Information

Endocrine Disorders and Pregnancy *on page 1479*

U.S. Brand Names Prandin®

Canadian Brand Names GlucoNorm®; Prandin®

Pharmacologic Category Antidiabetic Agent, Miscellaneous

Use Management of type 2 diabetes mellitus (noninsulin dependent, NIDDM)

An adjunct to diet and exercise to lower the blood glucose in patients with type 2 diabetes mellitus whose hyperglycemia cannot be controlled satisfactorily by diet and exercise alone

In combination with metformin or thiazolidinediones to lower blood glucose in patients whose hyperglycemia cannot be controlled by exercise, diet and either agent alone

Local Anesthetic/Vasoconstrictor Precautions No information available to require special precautions

Effects on Dental Treatment No significant effects or complications reported

Dosage Adults: Oral: Should be taken within 15 minutes of the meal, but time may vary from immediately preceding the meal to as long as 30 minutes before the meal

Initial: For patients not previously treated or whose Hb A_{1c} is <8%, the starting dose is 0.5 mg. For patients previously treated with blood glucose-lowering agents whose Hb A_{1c} is ≥8%, the initial dose is 1 or 2 mg before each meal.

Dose adjustment: Determine dosing adjustments by blood glucose response, usually fasting blood glucose. Double the preprandial dose up to 4 mg until satisfactory blood glucose response is achieved. At least 1 week should elapse to assess response after each dose adjustment.

Dose range: 0.5-4 mg taken with meals. Repaglinide may be dosed preprandial 2, 3 or 4 times/day in response to changes in the patient's meal pattern. Maximum recommended daily dose: 16 mg.

Patients receiving other oral hypoglycemic agents: When repaglinide is used to replace therapy with other oral hypoglycemic agents, it may be started the day after the final dose is given. Observe patients carefully for hypoglycemia because of potential overlapping of drug effects. When transferred from longer halflife sulfonylureas (eg, chlorpropamide), close monitoring may be indicated for up to ≥1 week.

Combination therapy: If repaglinide monotherapy does not result in adequate glycemic control, metformin or a thiazolidinedione may be added. Or, if metformin or thiazolidinedione therapy does not provide adequate control, repaglinide may be added. The starting dose and dose adjustments for combination therapy are the same as repaglinide monotherapy. Carefully adjust the dose of each drug to determine the minimal dose required to achieve the desired pharmacologic effect. Failure to do so could result in an increase in the incidence of hypoglycemic episodes. Use appropriate monitoring of FPG and Hb A_{1c} measurements to ensure that the patient is not subjected to excessive drug exposure or increased probability of secondary drug failure. If glucose is not achieved after a suitable trial of combination therapy, consider discontinuing these drugs and using insulin.

Dosing adjustment in renal impairment:

Cl_{cr} 40-80 mL/minute (mild to moderate renal dysfunction): Initial dosage adjustment does not appear to be necessary.

Cl_{cr} 20-40 mL/minute: Initiate 0.5 mg with meals; titrate carefully.

Dosing adjustment in hepatic impairment: Use conservative initial and maintenance doses. Use longer intervals between dosage adjustments.

Mechanism of Action Nonsulfonylurea hypoglycemic agent of the meglitinide class (the nonsulfonylurea moiety of glyburide) used in the management of type 2 diabetes mellitus; stimulates insulin release from the pancreatic beta cells

Other Adverse Effects

>10%:

Central nervous system: Headache (9% to 11%)

Endocrine & metabolic: Hypoglycemia (16% to 31%)

Respiratory: Upper respiratory tract infection (10% to 16%)

1% to 10%:

Cardiovascular: Chest pain (2% to 3%)

Gastrointestinal: Nausea (3% to 5%), heartburn (2% to 4%), vomiting (2% to 3%) constipation (2% to 3%), diarrhea (4% to 5%), tooth disorder (<1% to 2%)
Genitourinary: Urinary tract infection (2% to 3%)
Neuromuscular & skeletal: Arthralgia (3% to 6%), back pain (5% to 6%), paresthesia (2% to 3%)
Respiratory: Sinusitis (3% to 6%), rhinitis (3% to 7%), bronchitis (2% to 6%)
Miscellaneous: Allergy (1% to 2%)

<1%: Anaphylactoid reaction, leukopenia, LFTs increased, thrombocytopenia

Postmarketing and/or case reports: Alopecia, hemolytic anemia, hepatic dysfunction (severe), pancreatitis, Stevens-Johnson syndrome

Drug Interactions Substrate of CYP2C8/9, **3A4**

Increased Effect/Toxicity: Agents that inhibit CYP3A4 (eg, ketoconazole, miconazole, erythromycin, clarithromycin) may increase repaglinide concentrations. The effect of repaglinide may be potentiated when given concomitantly with other highly protein-bound drugs (ie, phenylbutazone, oral anticoagulants, hydantoins, salicylates, NSAIDs, sulfonamides). Concurrent use of other hypoglycemic agents may increase risk of hypoglycemia.

Decreased Effect: Drugs which induce cytochrome P450 isoenzyme 3A4 may increase metabolism of repaglinide (phenytoin, rifampin, barbiturates, carbamazepine). Certain drugs (thiazides, diuretics, corticosteroids, phenothiazines, thyroid products, estrogens, oral contraceptives, phenytoin, nicotinic acid, sympathomimetics, calcium channel blockers, isoniazid) tend to produce hyperglycemia and may lead to loss of glycemic control.

Dietary/Ethanol/Herb Considerations

Ethanol: Avoid use; may increase risk of hypoglycemia.

Food: Administer 15-30 minutes before meals; food decreases the AUC of repaglinide. Dietary modification based on ADA recommendations is a part of therapy. Avoid garlic.

Herb/Nutraceutical: Avoid black cohosh; may enhance effects of antidiabetic agents. Avoid chromium, garlic, gymnema, and horse chestnut; may cause hypoglycemia. Avoid St John's wort; may decrease serum concentration.

Pharmacodynamics/Kinetics

Onset of action: Single dose: Increased insulin levels: ~15-60 minutes
Duration: 4-6 hours
Absorption: Rapid and complete
Distribution: V_d: 31 L
Protein binding, plasma: >98%
Metabolism: Hepatic via CYP3A4 isoenzyme and glucuronidation to inactive metabolites
Bioavailability: Mean absolute: ~56%
Half-life elimination: 1 hour
Time to peak, plasma: ~1 hour
Excretion: Within 96 hours: Feces (~90%, <2% as parent drug); Urine (~8%)

Pregnancy Risk Factor C

Generic Available No

Comments Known as GlucoNorm® in Canada, NovoNorm™ elsewhere

Repan® *see* Butalbital, Acetaminophen, and Caffeine *on page 214*
Repronex® *see* Menotropins *on page 857*
Requip® *see* Ropinirole *on page 1196*
Rescriptor® *see* Delavirdine *on page 405*

Reserpine (re SER peen)

Related Information

Cardiovascular Diseases *on page 1456*

Pharmacologic Category Rauwolfia Alkaloid

Use Management of mild to moderate hypertension

Unlabeled/Investigational Use Management of tardive dyskinesia, schizophrenia

Local Anesthetic/Vasoconstrictor Precautions No information available to require special precautions

Effects on Dental Treatment >10%: Xerostomia, changes in salivation

Dosage

Oral:

Children: Hypertension: 0.01-0.02 mg/kg/24 hours divided every 12 hours; maximum dose: 0.25 mg/day (not recommended in children)

Adults:

Hypertension (may take 3 weeks for full effect): 0.1-0.25 mg/day in 1-2 doses; initial: 0.5 mg/day for 1-2 weeks; maintenance: reduce to 0.1-0.25 mg/day;

Tardive dyskinesia/schizophrenia: Initial: 0.5 mg/day; usual range: 0.1-1 mg

Elderly: Initial: 0.05 mg once daily, increasing by 0.05 mg every week as necessary

Dosing adjustment in renal impairment: Cl_{cr} <10 mL/minute: Avoid use

Dialysis: Not removed by hemo or peritoneal dialysis; supplemental dose is unnecessary

(Continued)

Reserpine *(Continued)*

Mechanism of Action Reduces blood pressure via depletion of sympathetic biogenic amines (norepinephrine and dopamine); this also commonly results in sedative effects

Other Adverse Effects Frequency not defined:

Cardiovascular: Peripheral edema, arrhythmias, bradycardia, chest pain, PVC, hypotension

Central nervous system: Dizziness, headache, nightmares, nervousness, drowsiness, fatigue, mental depression, parkinsonism, dull sensorium, syncope, paradoxical anxiety

Dermatologic: Rash, pruritus, flushing of skin

Gastrointestinal: Anorexia, diarrhea, nausea, vomiting, weight gain, increased gastric acid secretion, **increased salivation**

Genitourinary: Impotence, decreased libido

Hematologic: Thrombocytopenia purpura

Ocular: Blurred vision

Respiratory: Nasal congestion, dyspnea, epistaxis

Drug Interactions

Increased Effect/Toxicity: Reserpine may cause hypertensive reactions in patients receiving an MAO inhibitor; use an alternative antihypertensive. Reserpine may increase the effect of beta-blockers. May increase effects of CNS depressants and/or ethanol. May increase the effects/toxicity of levodopa, quinidine, procainamide, and digitalis glycosides.

Decreased Effect: Tricyclic antidepressants may increase antihypertensive effect.

Dietary/Ethanol/Herb Considerations

Ethanol: Avoid use; may increase CNS depression.

Food: Avoid caffeine (eg, colas, chocolate), garlic, and licorice.

Herb/Nutraceutical: Avoid black cohosh, dong quai, and evening primrose due to estrogenic activity. Avoid ephedra, ginseng, and yohimbe; may worsen hypertension. Avoid garlic; may have increased antihypertensive effect. Avoid ginger due to positive inotropic effects; theoretically, may cause arrhythmia. Avoid gotu kola, kava, SAMe, St John's wort, and valerian; may increase CNS depression. Avoid hawthorn; may lower peripheral vascular resistance causing additional decrease in BP. Avoid licorice.

Pharmacodynamics/Kinetics

Onset of action: Antihypertensive: 3-6 days

Duration: 2-6 weeks

Absorption: ~40%

Distribution: Crosses placenta; enters breast milk

Protein binding: 96%

Metabolism: Extensively hepatic (>90%)

Half-life elimination: 50-100 hours

Excretion: Feces (30% to 60%); urine (10%)

Pregnancy Risk Factor C

Generic Available Yes

Reserpine and Chlorothiazide *see* Chlorothiazide and Reserpine *on page 306*

Reserpine, Hydralazine, and Hydrochlorothiazide *see* Hydralazine, Hydrochlorothiazide, and Reserpine *on page 675*

Respa-1st® *see* Guaifenesin and Pseudoephedrine *on page 652*

Respa® DM *see* Guaifenesin and Dextromethorphan *on page 651*

Respa-GF® *see* Guaifenesin *on page 650*

Respaire®-60 SR *see* Guaifenesin and Pseudoephedrine *on page 652*

Respaire®-120 SR *see* Guaifenesin and Pseudoephedrine *on page 652*

Restasis™ *see* CycloSPORINE *on page 383*

Restoril® *see* Temazepam *on page 1271*

Retavase® *see* Reteplase *on page 1174*

Reteplase (RE te playz)

U.S. Brand Names Retavase®

Canadian Brand Names Retavase®

Pharmacologic Category Thrombolytic Agent

Synonyms Recombinant Plasminogen Activator; r-PA

Use Management of acute MI (AMI); improvement of ventricular function; reduction of the incidence of CHF and the reduction of mortality following AMI

Local Anesthetic/Vasoconstrictor Precautions No information available to require special precautions

Effects on Dental Treatment No significant effects or complications reported

Dosage

Children: Use not recommended

Adults: 10 units I.V. over 2 minutes, followed by a second dose 30 minutes later of 10 units I.V. over 2 minutes

Withhold second dose if serious bleeding or anaphylaxis occurs

Mechanism of Action Reteplase is a nonglycosylated form of tPA produced by recombinant DNA technology using *E. coli*; it initiates local fibrinolysis by binding to fibrin in a thrombus (clot) and converts entrapped plasminogen to plasmin

Other Adverse Effects Bleeding is the most frequent adverse effect associated with reteplase. Heparin and aspirin have been administered concurrently with reteplase in clinical trials. The incidence of adverse events is a reflection of these combined therapies, and are comparable with comparison thrombolytics.

>10%: Local: Injection site bleeding (4.6% to 48.6%)

1% to 10%:
- Gastrointestinal: Bleeding (1.8% to 9.0%)
- Genitourinary: Bleeding (0.9% to 9.5%)
- Hematologic: Anemia (0.9% to 2.6%)

<1% (Limited to important or life-threatening): Intracranial hemorrhage (0.8%), allergic/anaphylactoid reactions, cholesterol embolization

Other adverse effects noted are frequently associated with MI (and therefore may or may not be attributable to Retavase®) and include arrhythmias, hypotension, cardiogenic shock, pulmonary edema, cardiac arrest, reinfarction, pericarditis, tamponade, thrombosis, and embolism.

Drug Interactions

Increased Effect/Toxicity: The risk of bleeding associated with reteplase may be increased by oral anticoagulants (warfarin), heparin, low molecular weight heparins, and drugs which affect platelet function (eg, NSAIDs, dipyridamole, ticlopidine, clopidogrel, IIb/IIIa antagonists). Concurrent use with aspirin and heparin may increase the risk of bleeding; however, aspirin and heparin were used concomitantly with reteplase in the majority of patients in clinical studies.

Decreased Effect: Aminocaproic acid (antifibrinolytic agent) may decrease effectiveness of thrombolytic agents.

Pharmacodynamics/Kinetics

Onset of action: Thrombolysis: 30-90 minutes

Half-life elimination: 13-16 minutes

Excretion: Feces and urine

Clearance: Plasma: 250-450 mL/minute

Pregnancy Risk Factor C

Generic Available No

Retin-A® *see* Tretinoin (Topical) *on page 1340*
Retin-A® Micro *see* Tretinoin (Topical) *on page 1340*
Retinoic Acid *see* Tretinoin (Topical) *on page 1340*
Retrovir® *see* Zidovudine *on page 1406*
Revex® *see* Nalmefene *on page 948*
Rēv-Eyes™ *see* Dapiprazole *on page 399*
ReVia® *see* Naltrexone *on page 950*
rFSH-alpha *see* Follitropins *on page 607*
rFSH-beta *see* Follitropins *on page 607*
rFVIIa *see* Factor VIIa (Recombinant) *on page 554*
R-Gel® [OTC] *see* Capsaicin *on page 238*
R-Gene® *see* Arginine *on page 121*
rGM-CSF *see* Sargramostim *on page 1209*
r-hCG *see* Chorionic Gonadotropin (Recombinant) *on page 321*
Rheumatrex® *see* Methotrexate *on page 884*
rhFSH-alpha *see* Follitropins *on page 607*
rhFSH-beta *see* Follitropins *on page 607*
rhIL-11 *see* Oprelvekin *on page 1003*
Rhinatate® *see* Chlorpheniramine, Pyrilamine, and Phenylephrine *on page 312*
Rhinocort® [DSC] *see* Budesonide *on page 202*
Rhinocort® Aqua™ *see* Budesonide *on page 202*
Rhinosyn® [OTC] *see* Chlorpheniramine and Pseudoephedrine *on page 308*
Rhinosyn-PD® [OTC] *see* Chlorpheniramine and Pseudoephedrine *on page 308*

Rh_o(D) Immune Globulin (ar aych oh, dee, i MYOON GLOB yoo lin)

Related Information

Immunizations (Vaccines) *on page 1612*

U.S. Brand Names BayRho-D® Full-Dose; BayRho-D® Mini-Dose; MICRhoGAM®; RhoGAM®; WinRho SDF®

Canadian Brand Names BayRho-D® Full-Dose

Pharmacologic Category Immune Globulin

Use Prevention of isoimmunization in Rh-negative individuals exposed to Rh-positive blood during delivery of an Rh-positive infant, as a result of an abortion, following amniocentesis or abdominal trauma, or following a transfusion accident; prevention of hemolytic disease of the newborn if there is a subsequent pregnancy with an Rh-positive fetus

(Continued)

Rh_o(D) Immune Globulin *(Continued)*

Local Anesthetic/Vasoconstrictor Precautions No information available to require special precautions

Effects on Dental Treatment No significant effects or complications reported

Restrictions Federal law requires that the date of administration, the vaccine manufacturer, lot number of vaccine, and the administering person's name, title and address be entered into the patient's permanent medical record.

Dosage Adults (administered I.M. to mothers **not** to infant) I.M.:

Obstetrical usage: 1 vial (300 mcg) prevents maternal sensitization if fetal packed red blood cell volume that has entered the circulation is <15 mL; if it is more, give additional vials. The number of vials = RBC volume of the calculated fetomaternal hemorrhage divided by 15 mL

Postpartum prophylaxis: 300 mcg within 72 hours of delivery

Antepartum prophylaxis: 300 mcg at approximately 26-28 weeks gestation; followed by 300 mcg within 72 hours of delivery if infant is Rh-positive

Following miscarriage, abortion, or termination of ectopic pregnancy at up to 13 weeks of gestation: 50 mcg ideally within 3 hours, but may be given up to 72 hours after; if pregnancy has been terminated at 13 or more weeks of gestation, administer 300 mcg

Mechanism of Action

Rh suppression: Suppresses the immune response and antibody formation of Rh_o(D) negative individuals to Rh_o(D) positive red blood cells.

ITP: Coats the patients Rh_o(D) positive red blood cells with antibody, so that as they are cleared by the spleen, the spleens ability to clear antibody-coated cells is saturated, sparing the platelets.

Other Adverse Effects Frequency not defined:

Cardiovascular: Hypotension, pallor, vasodilation

Central nervous system: Chills, dizziness, fever, headache, somnolence

Dermatologic: Pruritus, rash

Gastrointestinal: Abdominal pain, diarrhea

Hematologic: Hemoglobin decreased (patients with ITP), intravascular hemolysis (patients with ITP)

Local: Injection site reaction: Discomfort, induration, mild pain, redness, swelling

Neuromuscular & skeletal: Back pain, hyperkinesia, myalgia, weakness

Miscellaneous: Anaphylaxis, diaphoresis, LDH increased

Drug Interactions Decreased Effect: Rh_o(D) immune globulin may interfere with the response of live vaccines; vaccines should not be administered within 3 months after Rh_o(D)

Pharmacodynamics/Kinetics

Onset of platelet increase: ITP: 1-3 days

Duration: Suppression of Rh isoimmunization: ~12 weeks; Treatment of ITP: 3-4 weeks

Distribution: V_d: I.M.: 8.59 L

Half-life elimination: 21-30 days

Time to peak, plasma: I.M.: 5-10 days

Pregnancy Risk Factor C

Generic Available No

RhoGAM® *see* Rh_o(D) Immune Globulin *on page 1175*

rhPTH(1-34) *see* Teriparatide *on page 1280*

HuEPO-α *see* Epoetin Alfa *on page 503*

Ribavirin (rye bu VYE rin)

Related Information

Systemic Viral Diseases *on page 1517*

U.S. Brand Names Copegus™; Rebetol®; Virazole®

Canadian Brand Names Virazole™

Mexican Brand Names Vilona®; Vilona Pediatrica; Virazide®

Pharmacologic Category Antiviral Agent

Synonyms RTCA; Tribavirin

Use

Inhalation: Treatment of patients with respiratory syncytial virus (RSV) infections; may also be used in other viral infections including influenza A and B and adenovirus; specially indicated for treatment of severe lower respiratory tract RSV infections in patients with an underlying compromising condition (prematurity, bronchopulmonary dysplasia and other chronic lung conditions, congenital heart disease, immunodeficiency, immunosuppression), and recent transplant recipients

Oral capsule:

In combination with interferon alfa-2b (Intron® A) injection for the treatment of chronic hepatitis C in patients with compensated liver disease who have relapsed after alpha interferon therapy or were previously untreated with alpha interferons

In combination with peginterferon alfa-2b (PEG-Intron™) injection for the treatment of chronic hepatitis C in patients with compensated liver disease who were previously untreated with alpha interferons

Oral tablet: In combination with peginterferon alfa-2a (Pegasys®) injection for the treatment of chronic hepatitis C in patients with compensated liver disease who were previously untreated with alpha interferons

Unlabeled/Investigational Use Treatment of West Nile virus, hemorrhagic fever virus infections with renal syndrome (ie, Lassa, Venezuelan, Korean hemorrhagic fever, Sabia, Argentian hemorrhagic fever, Bolivian hemorrhagic fever, Junin, Machupa)

Local Anesthetic/Vasoconstrictor Precautions No information available to require special precautions

Effects on Dental Treatment No significant effects or complications reported

Dosage

Aerosol inhalation: Infants and children: Use with Viratek® small particle aerosol generator (SPAG-2) at a concentration of 20 mg/mL (6 g reconstituted with 300 mL of sterile water without preservatives). Continuous aerosol administration: 12-18 hours/day for 3 days, up to 7 days in length

Oral capsule:

Children: Chronic hepatitis C (in combination with interferon alfa-2b): **Note:** Safety and efficacy have not been established; dosing based on pharmacokinetic profile:

25-36 kg: 400 mg/day (200 mg twice daily)

37-49 kg: 600 mg/day (200 mg in morning and 400 mg in evening)

50-61 kg: 800 mg/day (400 mg twice daily)

>61 kg: Refer to adult dosing

Note: Also refer to Interferon Alfa-2b/Ribavirin combination pack monograph.

Adults:

Chronic hepatitis C (in combination with interferon alfa-2b):

≤75 kg: 400 mg in the morning, then 600 mg in the evening

>75 kg: 600 mg in the morning, then 600 mg in the evening

Note: If HCV-RNA is undetectable at 24 weeks, duration of therapy is 48 weeks. In patients who relapse following interferon therapy, duration of dual therapy is 24 weeks.

Note: Also refer to Interferon Alfa-2b/Ribavirin combination pack monograph.

Chronic hepatitis C (in combination with peginterferon alfa-2b): 400 mg twice daily; duration of therapy is 1 year; after 24 weeks of treatment, if serum HCV-RNA is not below the limit of detection of the assay, consider discontinuation.

Oral tablet: Adults:

Chronic hepatitis C, genotype 1,4 (in combination with peginterferon alfa-2a):

<75kg: 1000 mg/day in 2 divided doses for 48 weeks

≥75kg: 1200 mg/day in 2 divided doses for 48 weeks

Chronic hepatitis C, genotype 2,3 (in combination with peginterferon alfa-2a): 800 mg/day in 2 divided doses for 24 weeks

Note: Also refer to Peginterferon Alfa-2a monograph.

Dosing adjustment in renal impairment: Cl_{cr} <50 mL/minute: Oral route is contraindicated

Dosing adjustment for toxicity: Oral: Capsule, tablet:

Patient **without** cardiac history:

Hemoglobin <10 g/dL: Decrease dose to 600 mg/day

Hemoglobin <8.5 g/dL: Permanently discontinue treatment

Patient **with** cardiac history:

Hemoglobin has ≥2 g/dL decrease during any 4-week period of treatment: Decrease dose to 600 mg/day

Hemoglobin <12 g/dL after 4 weeks of reduced dose: Permanently discontinue treatment

Mechanism of Action Inhibits replication of RNA and DNA viruses; inhibits influenza virus RNA polymerase activity and inhibits the initiation and elongation of RNA fragments resulting in inhibition of viral protein synthesis

Other Adverse Effects

Inhalation:

1% to 10%:

Central nervous system: Fatigue, headache, insomnia

Gastrointestinal: Nausea, anorexia

Hematologic: Anemia

<1% Hypotension, cardiac arrest, digitalis toxicity, conjunctivitis, mild bronchospasm, worsening of respiratory function, apnea

Note: Incidence of adverse effects (approximate) in healthcare workers: Headache (51%); conjunctivitis (32%); rhinitis, nausea, rash, dizziness, pharyngitis, and lacrimation (10% to 20%)

(Continued)

Ribavirin *(Continued)*

Oral (all adverse reactions are documented while receiving combination therapy with interferon alpha-2b):

>10%:

Central nervous system: Dizziness (17% to 26%), headache (63% to 66%)*, fatigue (60% to 70%)*, fever (32% to 41%)*, insomnia (26% to 39%), irritability (23% to 32%), depression (23% to 36%)*, emotional lability (7% to 12%)*, impaired concentration (10% to 14%)*

Dermatologic: Alopecia (27% to 32%), rash (20% to 28%), pruritus (13% to 21%)

Gastrointestinal: Nausea (38% to 47%), anorexia (21% to 27%), dyspepsia (14% to 16%), vomiting (9% to 12%)*

Hematologic: Decreased hemoglobin (25% to 36%), decreased WBC, absolute neutrophil count <0.5 x 10^9/L (5% to 11%), thrombocytopenia (6% to 14%), hyperbilirubinemia (24% to 34%), hemolysis

Neuromuscular & skeletal: Myalgia (61% to 64%)*, arthralgia (29% to 33%)*, musculoskeletal pain (20% to 28%), rigors (40% to 43%)

Respiratory: Dyspnea (17% to 19%), sinusitis (9% to 12%)*, nasal congestion

Miscellaneous: Flu-like syndrome (13% to 18%)*

*Similar to interferon alone

1% to 10%:

Cardiovascular: Chest pain (5% to 9%)*

Central nervous system: Nervousness (~5%)*

Gastrointestinal: Taste perversion (6% to 8%)

Hematologic: Hemolytic anemia (~10%)

Neuromuscular & skeletal: Weakness (9% to 10%)

*Similar to interferon alone

<1%: Diabetes mellitus, gout, pancreatitis, pulmonary dysfunction, suicidal ideation, thyroid function test abnormalities

Postmarketing and/or case reports: Hearing disorder, vertigo, sarcoidosis

Drug Interactions

Increased Effect/Toxicity: Concomitant use of ribavirin and nucleoside analogues may increase the risk of developing lactic acidosis (includes adefovir, didanosine, lamivudine, stavudine, zalcitabine, zidovudine). Concurrent use with didanosine has been noted to increase the risk of pancreatitis and/or peripheral neuropathy in addition to lactic acidosis. Suspend therapy of signs/symptoms of toxicity are present.

Decreased effect of zidovudine.

Dietary/Ethanol/Herb Considerations Food: Administer consistently in regard to food. High-fat meal (54 g fat) increases the AUC and C_{max} by 70% with oral form.

Pharmacodynamics/Kinetics

Absorption: Inhalation: Systemic; dependent upon respiratory factors and method of drug delivery; maximal absorption occurs with the use of aerosol generator via endotracheal tube; highest concentrations in respiratory tract and erythrocytes

Distribution: Oral capsule: Single dose: V_d 2825 L; distribution significantly prolonged in the erythrocyte (16-40 days), which can be used as a marker for intracellular metabolism

Protein binding: Oral: None

Metabolism: Hepatically and intracellularly (forms active metabolites); may be necessary for drug action

Bioavailability: Oral: 64%

Half-life elimination, plasma:

Children: Inhalation: 6.5-11 hours

Adults: Oral capsule, single dose: 24 hours in healthy adults, 44 hours with chronic hepatitis C infection (increases to ~298 hours at steady state)

Time to peak, serum: Inhalation: At end of inhalation period; Oral capsule: Multiple doses: 3 hours

Excretion: Inhalation: Urine (40% as unchanged drug and metabolites); Oral capsule: Urine (61%), feces (12%)

Pregnancy Risk Factor X

Generic Available No

Comments RSV season is usually December to April; viral shedding period for RSV is usually 3-8 days.

Ribavirin and Interferon Alfa-2b Combination Pack *see* Interferon Alfa-2b and Ribavirin *on page 730*

Riboflavin (RYE boe flay vin)

Pharmacologic Category Vitamin, Water Soluble

Synonyms Lactoflavin; Vitamin B_2; Vitamin G

Use Dental and Medical: Prevention of riboflavin deficiency; treatment of ariboflavinosis

Local Anesthetic/Vasoconstrictor Precautions No information available to require special precautions

Effects on Dental Treatment No significant effects or complications reported

Dosage Oral:
Riboflavin deficiency:
Children: 2.5-10 mg/day in divided doses
Adults: 5-30 mg/day in divided doses
Recommended daily allowance:
Children: 0.4-1.8 mg
Adults: 1.2-1.7 mg

Mechanism of Action Component of flavoprotein enzymes that work together, which are necessary for normal tissue respiration; also needed for activation of pyridoxine and conversion of tryptophan to niacin

Other Adverse Effects Frequency not defined: Genitourinary: Discoloration of urine (yellow-orange)

Warnings/Precautions Riboflavin deficiency often occurs in the presence of other B vitamin deficiencies

Drug Interactions Decreased effect with probenecid due to decreased absorption.

Pharmacodynamics/Kinetics
Absorption: Readily via GI tract, however, food increases extent; decreased with hepatitis, cirrhosis, or biliary obstruction
Metabolism: None
Half-life elimination: Biologic: 66-84 minutes
Excretion: Urine (9%) as unchanged drug

Pregnancy Risk Factor A/C (dose exceeding RDA recommendation)

Dosage Forms CAP: 100 mg. **TAB:** 25 mg, 50 mg, 100 mg

Generic Available Yes

Ridaura® *see* Auranofin *on page 147*

RID® Maximum Strength [OTC] *see* Pyrethrins and Piperonyl Butoxide *on page 1151*

Rid® Spray [OTC] *see* Permethrin *on page 1062*

Rifabutin (rif a BYOO tin)

Related Information
Nonviral Infectious Diseases *on page 1493*
Systemic Viral Diseases *on page 1517*

U.S. Brand Names Mycobutin®

Canadian Brand Names Mycobutin®

Pharmacologic Category Antibiotic, Miscellaneous; Antitubercular Agent

Synonyms Ansamycin

Use Prevention of disseminated *Mycobacterium avium* complex (MAC) in patients with advanced HIV infection; also utilized in multiple drug regimens for treatment of MAC

Local Anesthetic/Vasoconstrictor Precautions No information available to require special precautions

Effects on Dental Treatment No significant effects or complications reported

Dosage Oral:
Children >1 year:
Treatment: Patients not receiving NNRTIs or protease inhibitors:
Initial phase (2 weeks to 2 months): 10-20 mg/kg daily (maximum: 300 mg).
Second phase: 10-20 mg/kg daily (maximum: 300 mg) or twice weekly
Prophylaxis: 5 mg/kg daily; higher dosages have been used in limited trials
Adults:
Treatment:
Patients not receiving NNRTIs or protease inhibitors:
Initial phase: 5 mg/kg daily (maximum: 300 mg)
Second phase: 5 mg/kg daily or twice weekly
Patients receiving nelfinavir, amprenavir, indinavir: Reduce dose to 150 mg/day; no change in dose if administered twice weekly
Prophylaxis: 300 mg once daily (alone or in combination with azithromycin)
Dosing adjustment in renal impairment: Cl_{cr} <30 mL/minute: Reduce dose by 50%

Mechanism of Action Inhibits DNA-dependent RNA polymerase at the beta subunit which prevents chain initiation

Other Adverse Effects
>10%:
Dermatologic: Rash (11%)
Genitourinary: Discoloration of urine (30%)
Hematologic: Neutropenia (25%), leukopenia (17%)
1% to 10%:
Central nervous system: Headache (3%)
Gastrointestinal: Vomiting/nausea (3%), abdominal pain (4%), diarrhea (3%), anorexia (2%), flatulence (2%), eructation (3%)
Hematologic: Anemia, thrombocytopenia (5%)
Hepatic: Increased AST/ALT (7% to 9%)
Neuromuscular & skeletal: Myalgia
<1%: Chest pain, fever, insomnia, dyspepsia, dyspnea, abnormal taste, uveitis

Drug Interactions Substrate of **CYP1A2, 3A4**; Induces **CYP3A4**
(Continued)

Rifabutin *(Continued)*

Increased Effect/Toxicity: Concentrations of rifabutin are increased by indinavir (reduce rifabutin to 50% of standard dose) and ritonavir (reduce rifabutin dose to 150 mg every other day). Fluconazole increases rifabutin concentrations.

Decreased Effect: Rifabutin may decreased plasma concentrations (due to induction of liver enzymes) of verapamil, methadone, digoxin, cyclosporine, corticosteroids, oral anticoagulants, theophylline, barbiturates, chloramphenicol, itraconazole, ketoconazole, oral contraceptives, quinidine, protease inhibitors (indinavir, nelfinavir, ritonavir, saquinavir), non-nucleoside reverse transcriptase inhibitors, halothane, and clarithromycin.

Dietary/Ethanol/Herb Considerations Food: High-fat meal may decrease the rate but not the extent of absorption.

Pharmacodynamics/Kinetics

Absorption: Readily, 53%

Distribution: V_d: 9.32 L/kg; distributes to body tissues including the lungs, liver, spleen, eyes, and kidneys

Protein binding: 85%

Metabolism: To active and inactive metabolites

Bioavailability: Absolute: HIV: 20%

Half-life elimination: Terminal: 45 hours (range: 16-69 hours)

Time to peak, serum: 2-4 hours

Excretion: Urine (10% as unchanged drug, 53% as metabolites); feces (10% as unchanged drug, 30% as metabolites)

Pregnancy Risk Factor B

Generic Available No

Rifadin® *see* Rifampin *on page 1180*

Rifamate® *see* Rifampin and Isoniazid *on page 1181*

Rifampicin *see* Rifampin *on page 1180*

Rifampin (RIF am pin)

Related Information

Nonviral Infectious Diseases *on page 1493*

Rifapentine *on page 1182*

Tuberculosis *on page 1493*

U.S. Brand Names Rifadin®; Rimactane®

Canadian Brand Names Rifadin®; Rofact™

Mexican Brand Names Pestarin®; Rifadin®; Rimactan®

Pharmacologic Category Antibiotic, Miscellaneous; Antitubercular Agent

Synonyms Rifampicin

Use Management of active tuberculosis in combination with other agents; eliminate meningococci from asymptomatic carriers; prophylaxis of *Haemophilus influenzae* type b infection; used in combination with other anti-infectives in the treatment of staphylococcal infections; *Legionella* pneumonia

Local Anesthetic/Vasoconstrictor Precautions No information available to require special precautions

Effects on Dental Treatment No significant effects or complications reported

Dosage Oral (I.V. infusion dose is the same as for the oral route):

Tuberculosis therapy: Note: A four-drug regimen (isoniazid, rifampin, pyrazinamide, and either streptomycin or ethambutol) is preferred for the initial, empiric treatment of TB. When the drug susceptibility results are available, the regimen should be altered as appropriate.

Infants and Children <12 years:

Daily therapy: 10-20 mg/kg/day usually as a single dose (maximum: 600 mg/day)

Directly observed therapy (DOT): Twice weekly: 10-20 mg/kg (maximum: 600 mg); 3 times/week: 10-20 mg/kg (maximum: 600 mg)

Adults:

Daily therapy: 10 mg/kg/day (maximum: 600 mg/day)

Directly observed therapy (DOT): Twice weekly: 10 mg/kg (maximum: 600 mg); 3 times/week: 10 mg/kg (maximum: 600 mg)

Tuberculosis prevention: As an alternative to isoniazid:

Children: 10-20 mg/kg/day (maximum: 600 mg/day)

Adults: 10 mg/kg/day (maximum: 600 mg/day) for 2 months in combination with pyrazinamide

H. influenzae prophylaxis:

Infants and Children: 20 mg/kg/day every 24 hours for 4 days, not to exceed 600 mg/dose

Adults: 600 mg every 24 hours for 4 days

Leprosy: Adults:

Multibacillary: 600 mg once monthly for 24 months in combination with ofloxacin and minocycline

Paucibacillary: 600 mg once monthly for 6 months in combination with dapsone

Single lesion: 600 mg as a single dose in combination with ofloxacin 400 mg and minocycline 100 mg

Meningococcal meningitis prophylaxis:

Infants <1 month: 10 mg/kg/day in divided doses every 12 hours for 2 days

Infants ≥1 month and Children: 20 mg/kg/day in divided doses every 12 hours for 2 days

Adults: 600 mg every 12 hours for 2 days

Nasal carriers of *Staphylococcus aureus*:

Children: 15 mg/kg/day divided every 12 hours for 5-10 days in combination with other antibiotics

Adults: 600 mg/day for 5-10 days in combination with other antibiotics

Synergy for *Staphylococcus aureus* infections: Adults: 300-600 mg twice daily with other antibiotics

Dosing adjustment in hepatic impairment: Reduction may be necessary to reduce hepatotoxicity

Hemodialysis or peritoneal dialysis: Plasma rifampin concentrations are not significantly affected by hemodialysis or peritoneal dialysis.

Mechanism of Action Inhibits bacterial RNA synthesis by binding to the beta subunit of DNA-dependent RNA polymerase, blocking RNA transcription

Other Adverse Effects

Frequency not defined:

Cardiovascular: Flushing, edema

Central nervous system: Headache, drowsiness, dizziness, confusion, numbness, behavioral changes, ataxia

Dermatologic: Pruritus, urticaria, pemphigoid reaction

Hematologic: Eosinophilia, leukopenia, hemolysis, hemolytic anemia, thrombocytopenia (especially with high-dose therapy)

Hepatic: Hepatitis (rare)

Neuromuscular & skeletal: Myalgia, weakness, osteomalacia

Ocular: Visual changes, exudative conjunctivitis

1% to 10%:

Dermatologic: Rash (1% to 5%)

Gastrointestinal (1% to 2%): Epigastric distress, anorexia, nausea, vomiting, diarrhea, cramps, pseudomembranous colitis, pancreatitis

Hepatic: Increased LFTs (up to 14%)

Drug Interactions Substrate of **CYP2A6, 2C8/9, 3A4**; Induces **CYP1A2, 2A6, 2B6, 2C8/9, 2C19, 3A4**

Increased Effect/Toxicity: Rifampin levels may be increased when given with co-trimoxazole, probenecid, or ritonavir. Rifampin given with halothane or isoniazid increases the potential for hepatotoxicity. Combination therapy with rifampin and pyrazinamide has been associated with severe and fatal hepatotoxic reactions.

Decreased Effect: Rifampin induces liver enzymes which may decrease the plasma concentration of calcium channel blockers (verapamil, diltiazem, nifedipine), methadone, digoxin, cyclosporine, corticosteroids, haloperidol, oral anticoagulants, theophylline, barbiturates, chloramphenicol, imidazole antifungals (ketoconazole), oral contraceptives, acetaminophen, benzodiazepines, hydantoins, sulfa drugs, enalapril, beta-blockers, clofibrate, dapsone, antiarrhythmics (disopyramide, mexiletine, quinidine, tocainide), doxycycline, fluoroquinolones, levothyroxine, nortriptyline, tacrolimus, zidovudine, protease inhibitors (ie, amprenavir), and non-nucleoside reverse transcriptase inhibitors.

Dietary/Ethanol/Herb Considerations

Ethanol: Avoid use; may increase risk of hepatotoxicity.

Food may decrease serum concentration; administer on an empty stomach.

Herb/Nutraceutical: Avoid St John's wort; may decrease serum concentration.

Pharmacodynamics/Kinetics

Duration: ≤24 hours

Absorption: Oral: Well absorbed; food may delay or slightly reduce peak

Distribution: Highly lipophilic; crosses blood-brain barrier well

Relative diffusion from blood into CSF: Adequate with or without inflammation (exceeds usual MICs)

CSF:blood level ratio: Inflamed meninges: 25%

Protein binding: 80%

Metabolism: Hepatic; undergoes enterohepatic recirculation

Half-life elimination: 3-4 hours; prolonged with hepatic impairment; End-stage renal disease: 1.8-11 hours

Time to peak, serum: Oral: 2-4 hours

Excretion: Feces (60% to 65%) and urine (~30%) as unchanged drug

Pregnancy Risk Factor C

Generic Available Yes

Rifampin and Isoniazid (RIF am pin & eye soe NYE a zid)

Related Information

Isoniazid *on page 748*

Rifampin *on page 1180*

U.S. Brand Names Rifamate®

Canadian Brand Names Rifamate®

(Continued)

Rifampin and Isoniazid *(Continued)*

Pharmacologic Category Antibiotic, Miscellaneous

Synonyms Isoniazid and Rifampin

Use Management of active tuberculosis; see individual agents for additional information

Local Anesthetic/Vasoconstrictor Precautions No information available to require special precautions

Effects on Dental Treatment No significant effects or complications reported

Dosage Oral: 2 capsules/day

Dietary/Ethanol/Herb Considerations

Ethanol: Avoid use; may increase risk of hepatotoxicity.

Food may decrease serum concentration. Clinically severe elevated blood pressure may occur if taken with tyramine-containing foods. Isoniazid decreases folic acid absorption and alters pyridoxine metabolism.

Pregnancy Risk Factor C

Generic Available No

Rifampin, Isoniazid, and Pyrazinamide

(RIF am pin, eye soe NYE a zid, & peer a ZIN a mide)

Related Information

Isoniazid *on page 748*
Pyrazinamide *on page 1150*
Rifampin *on page 1180*

U.S. Brand Names Rifater®

Canadian Brand Names Rifater™

Pharmacologic Category Antibiotic, Miscellaneous

Synonyms Isoniazid, Rifampin, and Pyrazinamide; Pyrazinamide, Rifampin, and Isoniazid

Use Management of active tuberculosis; see individual agents for additional information

Local Anesthetic/Vasoconstrictor Precautions No information available to require special precautions

Effects on Dental Treatment No significant effects or complications reported

Dosage Adults: Oral: Patients weighing:

≤44 kg: 4 tablets
45-54 kg: 5 tablets
≥55 kg: 6 tablets
Doses should be administered in a single daily dose

Other Adverse Effects See individual agents.

Drug Interactions

Increased Effect/Toxicity: Increased effect/toxicity: Combination therapy with rifampin and pyrazinamide has been associated with severe and fatal hepatotoxic reactions.

Based on **rifampin** component: Rifampin levels may be increased when given with co-trimoxazole, probenecid, or ritonavir. Rifampin given with halothane or isoniazid increases the potential for hepatotoxicity.

Dietary/Ethanol/Herb Considerations

Ethanol: Avoid use; increases the risk of hepatitis.

Food may decrease serum concentration; administer on an empty stomach. Clinically severe elevated blood pressure may occur if taken with tyramine-containing foods. Isoniazid alters pyridoxine metabolism and decreases folic acid absorption.

Pregnancy Risk Factor C

Generic Available No

Rifapentine (RIF a pen teen)

Related Information

Rifampin *on page 1180*

U.S. Brand Names Priftin®

Canadian Brand Names Priftin®

Pharmacologic Category Antitubercular Agent

Use Treatment of pulmonary tuberculosis; rifapentine must always be used in conjunction with at least one other antituberculosis drug to which the isolate is susceptible; it may also be necessary to add a third agent (either streptomycin or ethambutol) until susceptibility is known.

Local Anesthetic/Vasoconstrictor Precautions No information available to require special precautions

Effects on Dental Treatment No significant effects or complications reported

Dosage

Children: Data available

Adults: **Rifapentine should not be used alone**; initial phase should include a 3- to 4-drug regimen

Intensive phase of short-term therapy: 600 mg (four 150 mg tablets) given weekly (every 72 hours); following the intensive phase, treatment should continue with rifapentine 600 mg once weekly for 4 months in combination with INH or appropriate agent for susceptible organisms

Dosing adjustment in renal/hepatic impairment: Data unavailable

Mechanism of Action Inhibits DNA-dependent RNA polymerase in susceptible strains of *Mycobacterium tuberculosis* (but not in mammalian cells). Rifapentine is bactericidal against both intracellular and extracellular MTB organisms. MTB resistant to other rifamycins including rifampin are likely to be resistant to rifapentine. Cross-resistance does not appear between rifapentine and other nonrifamycin antimycobacterial agents.

Other Adverse Effects

>10%: Endocrine & metabolic: Hyperuricemia (most likely due to pyrazinamide from initiation phase combination therapy)

1% to 10%:

- Cardiovascular: Hypertension
- Central nervous system: Headache, dizziness
- Dermatologic: Rash, pruritus, acne
- Gastrointestinal: Anorexia, nausea, vomiting, dyspepsia, diarrhea
- Hematologic: Neutropenia, lymphopenia, anemia, leukopenia, thrombocytosis
- Hepatic: Increased ALT/AST
- Neuromuscular & skeletal: Arthralgia, pain
- Renal: Pyuria, proteinuria, hematuria, urinary casts
- Respiratory: Hemoptysis

<1%: Peripheral edema, aggressive reaction, fatigue, urticaria, skin discoloration, hyperkalemia, hypovolemia, increased alkaline phosphatase, increased LDH, constipation, esophagitis, gastritis, pancreatitis, thrombocytopenia, neutrophilia, leukocytosis, purpura, hematoma, bilirubinemia, hepatitis, gout, arthrosis

Postmarketing and/or case reports: Rifampin has been associated with exacerbation of porphyria. Rifapentine is assumed to share this potential.

Drug Interactions Induces **CYP2C8/9, 3A4**

Decreased Effect:

Rifapentine may increase the metabolism of coadministered drugs that are metabolized by these enzymes. Enzymes are induced within 4 days after the first dose and returned to baseline 14 days after discontinuation of rifapentine. The magnitude of enzyme induction is dose and frequency dependent.

Rifampin has been shown to accelerate the metabolism and may reduce activity of the following drugs (therefore, rifapentine may also do the same): Phenytoin, disopyramide, mexiletine, quinidine, tocainide, chloramphenicol, clarithromycin, dapsone, doxycycline, fluoroquinolones, warfarin, fluconazole, itraconazole, ketoconazole, barbiturates, benzodiazepines, beta-blockers, diltiazem, nifedipine, verapamil, corticosteroids, cardiac glycoside preparations, clofibrate, oral or other systemic hormonal contraceptives, haloperidol, HIV protease inhibitors, sulfonylureas, cyclosporine, tacrolimus, levothyroxine, methadone, progestins, quinine, delavirdine, zidovudine, sildenafil, theophylline, amitriptyline, and nortriptyline.

Rifapentine should be used with extreme caution, if at all, in patients who are also taking protease inhibitors.

Patients using oral or other systemic hormonal contraceptives should be advised to change to nonhormonal methods of birth control when receiving concomitant rifapentine.

Dietary/Ethanol/Herb Considerations Food increases AUC and maximum serum concentration by 43% and 44%, respectively, as compared to fasting conditions.

Pharmacodynamics/Kinetics

Absorption: Food increases AUC and C_{max} by 43% and 44% respectively.

Distribution: V_d: ~70.2 L; rifapentine and metabolite accumulate in human monocyte-derived macrophages with intracellular/extracellular ratios of 24:1 and 7:1 respectively

Protein binding: Rifapentine and 25-desacetyl metabolite: 97.7% and 93.2%, primarily to albumin

Metabolism: Hepatic; hydrolyzed by an esterase and esterase enzyme to form the active metabolite 25-desacetyl rifapentine

Bioavailability: ~70%

Half-life elimination: Rifapentine: 14-17 hours; 25-desacetyl rifapentine: 13 hours

Time to peak, serum: 5-6 hours

Excretion: Urine (17% primarily as metabolites)

Pregnancy Risk Factor C

Generic Available No

Rifater® *see* Rifampin, Isoniazid, and Pyrazinamide *on page 1182*

rIFN-A *see* Interferon Alfa-2a *on page 726*

rIFN beta-1a *see* Interferon Beta-1a *on page 732*

rIFN beta-1b *see* Interferon Beta-1b *on page 733*

RIG *see* Rabies Immune Globulin (Human) *on page 1164*

rIL-11 *see* Oprelvekin *on page 1003*

Rilutek® *see* Riluzole *on page 1184*

Riluzole (RIL yoo zole)

U.S. Brand Names Rilutek®

Canadian Brand Names Rilutek®

Mexican Brand Names Rilutek®

Pharmacologic Category Glutamate Inhibitor

Synonyms 2-Amino-6-Trifluoromethoxy-benzothiazole; RP54274

Use Orphan drug: Treatment of amyotrophic lateral sclerosis (ALS); riluzole can extend survival or time to tracheostomy

Local Anesthetic/Vasoconstrictor Precautions No information available to require special precautions

Effects on Dental Treatment No significant effects or complications reported

Dosage Adults: Oral: 50 mg every 12 hours; no increased benefit can be expected from higher daily doses, but adverse events are increased

Dosing adjustment in smoking: Cigarette smoking is known to induce CYP1A2; patients who smoke cigarettes would be expected to eliminate riluzole faster. There is no information, however, on the effect of, or need for, dosage adjustment in these patients.

Dosing adjustment in special populations: Females and Japanese patients may possess a lower metabolic capacity to eliminate riluzole compared with male and Caucasian subjects, respectively

Dosing adjustment in renal impairment: Use with caution

Dosing adjustment in hepatic impairment: Use with caution in patients with current evidence or history of abnormal liver function indicated by significant abnormalities in serum transaminase, bilirubin or GGT levels. Baseline elevations of several LFTs (especially elevated bilirubin) should preclude use of riluzole.

Mechanism of Action Inhibitory effect on glutamate release, inactivation of voltage-dependent sodium channels; and ability to interfere with intracellular events that follow transmitter binding at excitatory amino acid receptors

Other Adverse Effects

>10%:
- Gastrointestinal: Nausea (10% to 21%)
- Neuromuscular & skeletal: Weakness (15% to 20%)
- Respiratory: Decreased lung function (10% to 16%)

1% to 10%:
- Cardiovascular: Hypertension, tachycardia, postural hypotension, edema
- Central nervous system: headache, dizziness, somnolence, insomnia, malaise, depression, vertigo, agitation, tremor, circumoral paresthesia
- Dermatologic: Pruritus, eczema, alopecia
- Gastrointestinal: Abdominal pain, diarrhea, anorexia, dyspepsia, vomiting, stomatitis
- Neuromuscular & skeletal: Arthralgia, back pain
- Respiratory: Rhinitis, increased cough
- Miscellaneous: Aggravation reaction

<1% (Limited to important or life-threatening): Seizures, neutropenia, exfoliative dermatitis

Drug Interactions Substrate of **CYP1A2**

Increased Effect/Toxicity: Inhibitors of CYP1A2 (eg, caffeine, theophylline, amitriptyline, quinolones) could decrease the rate of riluzole elimination resulting in accumulation of riluzole.

Decreased Effect: Drugs that induce CYP1A2 (eg, cigarette smoke, charbroiled food, rifampin, omeprazole) could increase the rate of riluzole elimination.

Dietary/Ethanol/Herb Considerations

Ethanol: Avoid use due to CNS depression.

Food: High-fat meals decrease absorption, AUC by 20%, and peak blood concentration by 45%.

Herb/Nutraceutical: Avoid gotu kola, kava, SAMe, St John's wort, and valerian; may increase CNS depression.

Pharmacodynamics/Kinetics

Absorption: 90%; high fat meal decreases AUC by 20%, peak blood levels by 45%

Protein binding, plasma: 96%, primarily to albumin and lipoproteins

Metabolism: Extensively hepatic to six major and a number of minor metabolites via CYP1A2 dependent hydroxylation and glucuronidation

Bioavailability: Oral: Absolute: 50%

Half-life elimination: 12 hours

Excretion: Urine (90%; 85% as metabolites, 2% as unchanged drug) and feces (5%) within 7 days

Pregnancy Risk Factor C

Generic Available No

Rimactane® *see* Rifampin *on page 1180*

Rimantadine (ri MAN ta deen)

Related Information

Systemic Viral Diseases *on page 1517*

U.S. Brand Names Flumadine®

Canadian Brand Names Flumadine®

Pharmacologic Category Antiviral Agent

Synonyms Rimantadine Hydrochloride

Use Prophylaxis (adults and children >1 year of age) and treatment (adults) of influenza A viral infection

Local Anesthetic/Vasoconstrictor Precautions No information available to require special precautions

Effects on Dental Treatment 1% to 10%: Xerostomia

Dosage Oral:

Prophylaxis:

- Children <10 years: 5 mg/kg once daily; maximum: 150 mg
- Children >10 years and Adults: 100 mg twice daily; decrease to 100 mg/day in elderly or in patients with severe hepatic or renal impairment (Cl_{cr} ≤10 mL/minute)

Treatment: Adults: 100 mg twice daily; decrease to 100 mg/day in elderly or in patients with severe hepatic or renal impairment (Cl_{cr} ≤10 mL/minute)

Mechanism of Action Exerts its inhibitory effect on three antigenic subtypes of influenza A virus (H1N1, H2N2, H3N2) early in the viral replicative cycle, possibly inhibiting the uncoating process; it has no activity against influenza B virus and is two- to eightfold more active than amantadine

Other Adverse Effects 1% to 10%:

Cardiovascular: Orthostatic hypotension, edema

Central nervous system: Dizziness (2%), confusion, headache (1%), insomnia (2%), difficulty in concentrating, anxiety (1%), restlessness, irritability, hallucinations; incidence of CNS side effects may be less than that associated with amantadine

Gastrointestinal: Nausea (3%), vomiting (2%), abdominal pain (1%), anorexia (2%)

Genitourinary: Urinary retention

Drug Interactions

Increased Effect/Toxicity: Cimetidine increases blood levels/toxicity of rimantadine.

Decreased Effect: Acetaminophen may cause a small reduction in AUC and peak concentration of rimantadine. Peak plasma and AUC concentrations of rimantadine are slightly reduced by aspirin.

Dietary/Ethanol/Herb Considerations

Ethanol: Avoid use; may increase CNS depression.

Food: Administer with food to reduce GI upset; food does not affect rate or extent of absorption.

Herb/Nutraceutical: Avoid gotu kola, kava, SAMe, St John's wort, and valerian; may increase CNS depression.

Pharmacodynamics/Kinetics

Onset of action: Antiviral activity: No data exist establishing a correlation between plasma concentration and antiviral effect

Absorption: Tablet and syrup formulations are equally absorbed

Metabolism: Extensively hepatic

Half-life elimination: 25.4 hours; prolonged in elderly

Time to peak: 6 hours

Excretion: Urine (<25% as unchanged drug)

Clearance: Hemodialysis does not contribute to clearance

Pregnancy Risk Factor C

Generic Available Yes: Tablet

Rimantadine Hydrochloride *see* Rimantadine *on page 1185*

Rimexolone (ri MEKS oh lone)

U.S. Brand Names Vexol®

Canadian Brand Names Vexol®

Pharmacologic Category Corticosteroid, Ophthalmic

Use Treatment of inflammation after ocular surgery and the treatment of anterior uveitis

Local Anesthetic/Vasoconstrictor Precautions No information available to require special precautions

Effects on Dental Treatment No significant effects or complications reported

Dosage Adults: Ophthalmic: Instill 1 drop in conjunctival sac 2-4 times/day up to every 4 hours; may use every 1-2 hours during first 1-2 days

Mechanism of Action Decreases inflammation by suppression of migration of polymorphonuclear leukocytes and reversal of increased capillary permeability

Other Adverse Effects

1% to 10%: Ocular: Temporary mild blurred vision

(Continued)

Rimexolone *(Continued)*

<1%: Stinging, burning eyes, corneal thinning, increased intraocular pressure, glaucoma, damage to the optic nerve, defects in visual activity, cataracts, secondary ocular infection

Pharmacodynamics/Kinetics

Absorption: Through aqueous humor

Metabolism: Hepatic for any amount of drug absorbed

Excretion: Urine and feces

Pregnancy Risk Factor C

Generic Available No

Riopan Plus® [OTC] *see* Magaldrate and Simethicone *on page 833*

Riopan Plus® Double Strength [OTC] *see* Magaldrate and Simethicone *on page 833*

Risedronate (ris ED roe nate)

Related Information

Rheumatoid Arthritis, Osteoarthritis, and Osteoporosis *on page 1488*

U.S. Brand Names Actonel®

Canadian Brand Names Actonel®

Pharmacologic Category Bisphosphonate Derivative

Synonyms Risedronate Sodium

Use Paget's disease of the bone; treatment and prevention of glucocorticoid-induced osteoporosis; treatment and prevention of osteoporosis in postmenopausal women

Local Anesthetic/Vasoconstrictor Precautions No information available to require special precautions

Effects on Dental Treatment No significant effects or complications reported

Dosage Oral (should be taken at least 30 minutes before the first food or drink of the day other than water):

Adults (patients should receive supplemental calcium and vitamin D if dietary intake is inadequate):

Paget's disease of bone: 30 mg once daily for 2 months

Retreatment may be considered (following post-treatment observation of at least 2 months) if relapse occurs, or if treatment fails to normalize serum alkaline phosphatase. For retreatment, the dose and duration of therapy are the same as for initial treatment. No data are available on more than one course of retreatment.

Osteoporosis (postmenopausal) prevention and treatment: 5 mg once daily; efficacy for use longer than 1 year has not been established; **alternatively,** a dose of 35 mg once weekly has been demonstrated to be effective

Osteoporosis (glucocorticoid-induced) prevention and treatment: 5 mg once daily

Elderly: No dosage adjustment required in $Cl_{cr} \geq 30$ mL/minute.

Dosing adjustment in renal impairment: $Cl_{cr} < 30$ mL/minute: Use not recommended

Mechanism of Action A bisphosphonate which inhibits bone resorption via actions on osteoclasts or on osteoclast precursors; decreases the rate of bone resorption direction, leading to an indirect decrease in bone formation

Other Adverse Effects

Seen in patients taking 30 mg/day for Paget's disease:

>10%:

Central nervous system: Headache (18%)

Dermatologic: Rash (11%)

Gastrointestinal: Diarrhea (20%), abdominal pain (11%)

Neuromuscular & skeletal: Arthralgia (33%)

Miscellaneous: Flu-like syndrome (10%)

1% to 10%:

Cardiovascular: Peripheral edema (8%)

Central nervous system: Chest pain (7%), dizziness (7%)

Gastrointestinal: Nausea (10%), constipation (7%), belching (3%), colitis (3%, placebo 3%)

Neuromuscular & skeletal: Weakness (5%), bone pain (5%, placebo 5%), leg cramps (3%, placebo 3%), myasthenia (3%)

Ocular: Amblyopia (3%, placebo 3%), dry eye (3%)

Otic: Tinnitus (3%, placebo 3%)

Respiratory: Sinusitis (5%), bronchitis (3%, placebo 5%) <1%: Acute iritis

Miscellaneous: Neoplasm (3%)

Seen in patient taking 5 mg/day for osteoporosis (events similar to those seen with placebo)

>10%:

Central nervous system: Pain (14%)

Gastrointestinal: Abdominal pain (12%), diarrhea (11%), nausea (11%)

Genitourinary: Urinary tract infection (11%)

Neuromuscular & skeletal: Back pain (26%), arthralgia (24%)

1% to 10%:
Cardiovascular: Hypertension (10%), chest pain (5%), cardiovascular disorder (2%), angina (2%)
Central nervous system: Depression (7%), dizziness (6%), insomnia (5%), anxiety (4%), vertigo (3%)
Dermatologic: Rash (8%), bruising (4%), pruritus (3%), skin carcinoma (2%)
Gastrointestinal: Flatulence (5), gastritis (2%), gastrointestinal disorder (2%), rectal disorder (2%), tooth disorder (2%)
Genitourinary: Cystitis (4%)
Hematologic: Anemia (2%)
Neuromuscular & skeletal: Joint disorder (7%), myalgia (7%), neck pain (5%), asthenia (5%), bone pain (5%), bone disorder (4%), neuralgia (4%), leg cramps (4%), bursitis (3%), tendon disorder (3%), hypertonia (2%), paresthesia (2%)
Ocular: Cataract (6%), conjunctivitis (3%)
Otic: Otitis media (2%)
Respiratory: Pharyngitis (6%), rhinitis (6%), dyspnea (4%), pneumonia (3%)
Miscellaneous: Neoplasm(3%), hernia (3%)
<1%: Duodenitis, glossitis, abnormal LFTs, iritis

Drug Interactions Decreased Effect: Calcium supplements and antacids interfere with absorption of risedronate (take at a different time of the day than risedronate).

Dietary/Ethanol/Herb Considerations
Ethanol: Avoid use; may increase risk of osteoporosis.
Food may reduce absorption (similar to other bisphosphonates); administer ≥30 minutes before the first food or drink of the day other than water. Mean oral bioavailability is decreased when given with food.
Calcium supplements interfere with absorption of risedronate (take at a different time of the day than risedronate).

Pharmacodynamics/Kinetics
Onset of action: May require weeks
Absorption: Rapid
Distribution: V_d: 6.3 L/kg
Protein binding: ~24%
Metabolism: None
Bioavailability: Poor, ~0.54% to 0.75%
Half-life elimination: Terminal: 480 hours
Excretion: Urine (up to 80%); feces (as unabsorbed drug)

Pregnancy Risk Factor C

Generic Available No

Risedronate Sodium *see* Risedronate *on page 1186*

Risperdal® *see* Risperidone *on page 1187*

Risperdal Consta™ [Investigational] *see* Risperidone *on page 1187*

Risperidone (ris PER i done)

U.S. Brand Names Risperdal®; Risperdal Consta™ [Investigational]

Canadian Brand Names Risperdal®

Mexican Brand Names Risperdal®

Pharmacologic Category Antipsychotic Agent, Benzisoxazole

Use Management of psychotic disorders (eg, schizophrenia)

Unlabeled/Investigational Use Treatment of behavioral symptoms associated with dementia in elderly, bipolar disorder, mania, Tourette's disorder, pervasive developmental disorder, autism in children and adolescents

Local Anesthetic/Vasoconstrictor Precautions No information available to require special precautions

Effects on Dental Treatment 1% to 10%: Significant xerostomia and orthostatic hypotension; resolves upon discontinuation

Dosage
Oral:
Children and Adolescents:
Pervasive developmental disorder (unlabeled use): Initial: 0.25 mg twice daily; titrate up 0.25 mg/day every 5-7 days; optimal dose range: 0.75-3 mg/day
Autism (unlabeled use): Initial: 0.25 mg at bedtime; titrate to 1 mg/day (0.1 mg/kg/day)
Schizophrenia: Initial: 0.5 mg twice daily; titrate as necessary up to 2-6 mg/day
Bipolar disorder (unlabeled use): Initial: 0.5 mg; titrate to 0.5-3 mg/day
Tourette's disorder (unlabeled use): Initial: 0.5 mg; titrate to 2-4 mg/day
Adults: Recommended starting dose: 0.5-1 mg twice daily; slowly increase to the optimum range of 3-6 mg/day; may be given as a single daily dose once maintenance dose is achieved; daily dosages >10 mg does not appear to confer any additional benefit, and the incidence of extrapyramidal symptoms is higher than with lower doses
Elderly: A starting dose of 0.25-1 mg in 1-2 divided doses, and titration should progress slowly. Additional monitoring of renal function and orthostatic blood pressure may be warranted. If once-a-day dosing in the elderly or debilitated

(Continued)

Risperidone *(Continued)*

patient is considered, a twice daily regimen should be used to titrate to the target dose, and this dose should be maintained for 2-3 days prior to attempts to switch to a once-daily regimen.

I.M.: Adults: Risperdal Consta™ (currently investigational, not commercially available): 25 mg every 2 weeks; some patients may benefit from larger doses; maximum dose not to exceed 50 mg every 2 weeks

Note: Oral risperidone (or other antipsychotic) should be administered with the initial injection of Risperdal Consta™ and continued for 3 weeks to maintain adequate therapeutic plasma concentrations prior to main release phase of risperidone from injection site.

Dosing adjustment in renal/hepatic impairment: Starting dose of 0.25-0.5 mg twice daily is advisable

Mechanism of Action Risperidone is a benzisoxazole derivative, mixed serotonin-dopamine antagonist; binds to 5-HT_2-receptors in the CNS and in the periphery with a very high affinity; binds to dopamine-D_2 receptors with less affinity. The binding affinity to the dopamine-D_2 receptor is 20 times lower than the 5-HT_2 affinity. The addition of serotonin antagonism to dopamine antagonism (classic neuroleptic mechanism) is thought to improve negative symptoms of psychoses and reduce the incidence of extrapyramidal side effects. Alpha$_1$, alpha$_2$ adrenergic, and histaminergic receptors are also antagonized with high affinity. Risperidone has low to moderate affinity for 5-HT_{1C}, 5-HT_{1D}, and 5-HT_{1A} receptors, weak affinity for D_1 and no affinity for muscarinics or beta$_1$ and beta$_2$ receptors

Other Adverse Effects

>10%: Central nervous system: Insomnia, agitation, anxiety, headache

1% to 10%:

Cardiovascular: Tachycardia, hypotension

Central nervous system: Sedation, dizziness, restlessness, extrapyramidal symptoms (dose dependent), dystonic reactions, pseudoparkinson, tardive dyskinesia, neuroleptic malignant syndrome, altered central temperature regulation

Dermatologic: Photosensitivity (rare), rash, dry skin

Endocrine & metabolic: Amenorrhea, galactorrhea, gynecomastia, sexual dysfunction

Gastrointestinal: Constipation, GI upset, dyspepsia, vomiting, abdominal pain, nausea, anorexia, weight gain

Genitourinary: Polyuria

Ocular: Abnormal vision

Respiratory: Rhinitis, coughing, sinusitis, pharyngitis, dyspnea

<1%: Diabetes mellitus, hyperglycemia

Frequency not defined: Gastrointestinal: Dysphagia, esophageal dysmotility

Drug Interactions Substrate of **CYP2D6**, 3A4; Inhibits CYP2D6, 3A4

Increased Effect/Toxicity: Risperidone may enhance the hypotensive effects of antihypertensive agents. Clozapine decreases clearance of risperidone. Metoclopramide may increase risk of extrapyramidal symptoms (EPS).

Decreased Effect: Risperidone may antagonize effects of levodopa. Carbamazepine decreases risperidone serum concentrations.

Dietary/Ethanol/Herb Considerations

Ethanol: Avoid use; may increase CNS depression.

Food: Avoid grapefruit products; may increase serum concentration. Dilute solution with water, milk, or orange juice; do not dilute with beverages containing tannin, or pectinate (eg, colas, tea). Avoid caffeine.

Herb/Nutraceutical: Avoid gotu kola, kava, SAMe, St John's wort, and valerian; may increase CNS depression.

Pharmacodynamics/Kinetics

Absorption: Rapid and well absorbed; food does not affect rate or extent

Protein binding, plasma: Risperidone 90%; 9-hydroxyrisperidone: 77%

Metabolism: Extensively hepatic via CYP2D6 to 9-hydroxyrisperidone (equi-effective with risperidone); *N*-dealkylation is a second minor pathway

Bioavailability: Tablet: 70%; Solution: 74.5%

Half-life elimination: 20 hours (risperidone and its active metabolite 9-hydroxyrisperidone)

Time to peak, plasma: Risperidone: Within 1 hour; 9-hydroxyrisperidone: Extensive metabolizers: 3 hours; Poor metabolizers: 17 hours

Excretion: Urine (70%); feces (15%)

Pregnancy Risk Factor C

Generic Available No

Ritalin® *see* Methylphenidate *on page 893*

Ritalin® LA *see* Methylphenidate *on page 893*

Ritalin-SR® *see* Methylphenidate *on page 893*

Ritonavir (rye TON a veer)

Related Information

HIV Infection and AIDS *on page 1482*

Tuberculosis *on page 1493*

U.S. Brand Names Norvir®

Canadian Brand Names Norvir®; Norvir® SEC

Mexican Brand Names Norvir®

Pharmacologic Category Antiretroviral Agent, Protease Inhibitor

Use Treatment of HIV infection; should always be used as part of a multidrug regimen (at least 3 antiretroviral agents)

Local Anesthetic/Vasoconstrictor Precautions No information available to require special precautions

Effects on Dental Treatment 1% to 10%: Xerostomia

Dosage Oral:

Children ≥2 years: 250 mg/m^2 twice daily; titrate dose upward to 400 mg/m^2 twice daily (maximum: 600 mg twice daily)

Adults: 600 mg twice daily; dose escalation tends to avoid nausea that many patients experience upon initiation of full dosing. Escalate the dose as follows: 300 mg twice daily for 1 day, 400 mg twice daily for 2 days, 500 mg twice daily for 1 day, then 600 mg twice daily. Ritonavir may be better tolerated when used in combination with other antiretrovirals by initiating the drug alone and subsequently adding the second agent within 2 weeks.

Note: Dosing adjustments for ritonavir when administered in combination therapy:

Amprenavir: Adjustments necessary for each agent:

Amprenavir 1200 mg with ritonavir 200 mg once daily **or**

Amprenavir 600 mg with ritonavir 100 mg twice daily

Amprenavir plus efavirenz (3-drug regimen): Amprenavir 1200 mg twice daily plus ritonavir 200 mg twice daily plus efavirenz at standard dose

Indinavir: Adjustments necessary for both agents:

Indinavir 800 mg twice daily plus ritonavir 100-200 mg twice daily **or**

Indinavir 400 mg twice daily plus ritonavir 400 mg twice daily

Nelfinavir or saquinavir: Ritonavir 400 mg twice daily

Dosing adjustment in hepatic impairment: None required in mild impairment; insufficient data in moderate-severe impairment; caution advised with severe impairment

Mechanism of Action Ritonavir inhibits HIV protease and renders the enzyme incapable of processing of polyprotein precursor which leads to production of noninfectious immature HIV particles

Other Adverse Effects Protease inhibitors cause dyslipidemia which includes elevated cholesterol and triglycerides and a redistribution of body fat centrally to cause "protease paunch," buffalo hump, facial atrophy, and breast enlargement. These agents also cause hyperglycemia.

>10%:

Endocrine & metabolic: Increased triglycerides

Gastrointestinal: Diarrhea, nausea, vomiting, abnormal taste

Hematologic: Anemia, decreased WBCs

Hepatic: Increased GGT

Neuromuscular & skeletal: Weakness

1% to 10%:

Cardiovascular: Vasodilation

Central nervous system: Fever, headache, malaise, dizziness, insomnia, somnolence, thinking abnormally

Dermatologic: Rash

Endocrine & metabolic: Hyperlipidemia, increased uric acid, increased glucose

Gastrointestinal: Abdominal pain, anorexia, constipation, dyspepsia, flatulence, local throat irritation

Hematologic: Neutropenia, eosinophilia, neutrophilia, prolonged PT, leukocytosis

Hepatic: Increased LFTs

Neuromuscular & skeletal: Increased CPK, myalgia, paresthesia

Respiratory: Pharyngitis

Miscellaneous: Diaphoresis, increased potassium, increased calcium

Drug Interactions Substrate of CYP1A2, 2B6, **2D6, 3A4**; Inhibits CYP2C8/9, 2C19, **2D6**, 2E1, **3A4**; Induces CYP1A2, 2C8/9, 3A4

Increased Effect/Toxicity: Concurrent use of amiodarone, bepridil, cisapride, flecainide, pimozide, propafenone, and quinidine is contraindicated. Serum concentrations/toxicity of many benzodiazepines may be increased; midazolam and triazolam are contraindicated. Concurrent use of ergot alkaloids (dihydroergotamine, ergotamine, ergonovine, methylergonovine) with ritonavir is also contraindicated (may cause vasospasm and peripheral ischemia). HMG-CoA reductase inhibitors serum concentrations may be increased by ritonavir, increasing the risk of myopathy/rhabdomyolysis; lovastatin and simvastatin are contraindicated; fluvastatin and pravastatin may be safer alternatives. Serum concentrations of meperidine's neuroexcitatory metabolite (normeperidine) are increased by ritonavir, which may increase the risk of CNS toxicity/seizures. Rifabutin and rifabutin metabolite serum concentrations may be increased by ritonavir; reduce rifabutin dose to 150 mg every other day. Sildenafil serum concentrations may be increased by ritonavir; when used concurrently, do not exceed a maximum sildenafil dose of 25 mg in a 48-hour period. Saquinavir's serum concentrations

(Continued)

Ritonavir *(Continued)*

are increased by ritonavir; the dosage of both agents should be reduced to 400 mg twice daily. Concurrent therapy with amprenavir may result in increased serum concentrations: dosage adjustment is recommended. Metronidazole or disulfiram may cause disulfiram reaction (oral solution contains 43% ethanol).

Ritonavir may also increase the serum concentrations of the following drugs (dose decrease may be needed): Benzodiazepines, beta-blockers (metoprolol, timolol), bupropion, calcium channel blockers (diltiazem, nifedipine, verapamil), carbamazepine, clarithromycin, clonazepam, clorazepate, clozapine, cyclosporin, dexamethasone, disopyramide, dronabinol, ethosuximide, fluoxetine (and other SSRIs), indinavir, ketoconazole, lidocaine, methamphetamine, mexiletine, nefazodone, perphenazine, prednisone, propoxyphene, piroxicam, quinine, risperidone, tacrolimus, tramadol, thioridazine, tricyclic antidepressants (including desipramine), and zolpidem. Serum concentrations of rifabutin may be increased by ritonavir; dosage adjustment required.

Decreased Effect: The administration of didanosine (buffered formulation) should be separated from ritonavir by 2.5 hours to limit interaction with ritonavir. Concurrent use of rifampin, rifabutin, dexamethasone, and many anticonvulsants may lower serum concentration of ritonavir. Ritonavir may reduce the concentration of ethinyl estradiol which may result in loss of contraception (including combination products). Theophylline concentrations may be reduced in concurrent therapy. Levels of didanosine and zidovudine may be decreased by ritonavir, however, no dosage adjustment is necessary. In addition, ritonavir may decrease the serum concentrations of the following drugs: Atovaquone, divalproex, lamotrigine, methadone, phenytoin, warfarin.

Dietary/Ethanol/Herb Considerations

Ethanol: Oral solution contains 43% ethanol by volume.

Food: Administer with food; enhances absorption. Liquid forms may be mixed with chocolate milk or nutritional supplement to mask unpleasant taste. Buttermilk, boiled milk, or yogurt may reduce diarrhea.

Herb/Nutraceutical: Avoid St John's wort; may decrease serum concentration.

Pharmacodynamics/Kinetics

Absorption: Variable, with or without food

Distribution: High concentrations in serum and lymph nodes

Protein binding: 98% to 99%

Metabolism: Hepatic; five metabolites, low concentration of an active metabolite achieved in plasma (oxidative); see Drug Interactions

Half-life elimination: 3-5 hours

Excretion: Urine (negligible amounts)

Pregnancy Risk Factor B

Generic Available No

Selected Readings Ouellet D, Hsu A, Granneman GR, et al, "Pharmacokinetic Interaction Between Ritonavir and Clarithromycin," *Clin Pharmacol Ther*, 1998, 64(4):355-62.

Rituxan® *see* Rituximab *on page 1190*

Rituximab (ri TUK si mab)

U.S. Brand Names Rituxan®

Canadian Brand Names Rituxan®

Mexican Brand Names Mabthera®

Pharmacologic Category Antineoplastic Agent, Monoclonal Antibody

Synonyms C2B8

Use Treatment of patients with relapsed or refractory low-grade or follicular, CD20 positive, B-cell non-Hodgkin's lymphoma; treatment (as part of combination therapy with radiolabeled ibritumomab) of patients with relapsed or refractory low-grade, follicular, or transformed B-cell non-Hodgkin's lymphoma (including rituximab refractory follicular non-Hodgkin's lymphoma)

Local Anesthetic/Vasoconstrictor Precautions No information available to require special precautions

Effects on Dental Treatment No significant effects or complications reported

Dosage Adults: I.V. (refer to individual protocols): **Do not administer I.V. push or bolus** (hypersensitivity reactions may occur). Consider premedication (consisting of acetaminophen and diphenhydramine) before each infusion of rituximab. Premedication may attenuate infusion-related events. Because transient hypotension may occur during infusion, give consideration to withholding antihypertensive medications 12 hours prior to rituximab infusion.

I.V. infusion: 375 mg/m^2 once weekly for 4 doses (days 1, 8, 15, and 22).

As part of combination therapy with ibritumomab (Zevalin™ therapeutic regimen): Two infusions of rituximab are completed, separated by 7-9 days (corresponding to two infusions of ibritumomab with differing radiolabels).

Rituximab dose (also see Ibritumomab monograph):

Step 1: 250 mg/m^2 at an initial rate of 50 mg/hour. If hypersensitivity or infusion-related events do not occur, increase infusion in increments of 50 mg/

hour every 30 minutes, to a maximum of 400 mg/hour. Infusions should be temporarily slowed or interrupted if hypersensitivity or infusion related events occur. The infusion may be resumed at ½ the previous rate upon improvement of symptoms.

Step 2: 250 mg/m^2 at an initial rate of 100 mg/hour (50 mg/hour if infusion-related events occurred with the first infusion). If hypersensitivity or infusion-related events do not occur, increase infusion in increments of 100 mg/hour every 30 minutes, to a maximum of 400 mg/hour, as tolerated.

Mechanism of Action Rituximab is a monoclonal antibody directed against the CD20 antigen on B-lymphocytes. CD20 regulates cell cycle initiation; and, possibly, functions as a calcium channel. Rituximab binds to the antigen on the cell surface, activating complement-dependent cytotoxicity; and to human Fc receptors, mediating cell killing through an antibody-dependent cellular toxicity. The CD20 antigen is also expressed on >90% of B-cell non-Hodgkin's lymphomas (NHL) but is not found on hematopoietic stem cells, pro-B cells, normal plasma cells, or other normal tissues.

Other Adverse Effects

>10%:

Central nervous system: Headache, fever, chills

Gastrointestinal: Nausea

Hematologic: Leukopenia

Neuromuscular & skeletal: Asthenia

Miscellaneous: Angioedema

Immunologic: Rituximab-induced B-cell depletion occurred in 70% to 80% of patients and was associated with decreased serum immunoglobulins in a minority of patients. The incidence of infections does not appear to be increased. During the treatment period, 50 patients in the pivotal trial developed infectious events, including six grade 3 events (there were no grade 4 events. The six serious events were not associated with neutropenia).

Infusion-related: An infusion-related symptom complex consisting of fever and chills/rigors occurred in the majority of patients during the first rituximab infusion. Other frequent infusion-related symptoms included nausea, urticaria, fatigue, headache, pruritus, bronchospasm, dyspnea, sensation of tongue or throat swelling (angioedema), rhinitis, vomiting, hypotension, flushing, and pain at disease sites. These reactions generally occurred within 30 minutes to 2 hours of beginning the first infusion, and resolved with slowing or interruption of the infusion and with supportive care (I.V. saline, diphenhydramine, and acetaminophen). The incidence of infusion related events decreased from 80% during the first to ~40% with subsequent infusions. Mild to moderate hypotension requiring interruption of rituximab infusion, with or without the administration of I.V. saline, occurred in 10%. Isolated occurrences of severe reactions requiring epinephrine have been reported in patients receiving rituximab for other indicators. Angioedema was reported in 13% and was serious in one patient.

1% to 10%:

Cardiovascular: Hypotension

Central nervous system: Myalgia, dizziness

Dermatologic: Pruritus, rash, urticaria

Gastrointestinal: Vomiting, abdominal pain

Hematologic: Thrombocytopenia, neutropenia; during the treatment period (up to 30 days following the last dose), the following occurred: Severe thrombocytopenia, severe neutropenia, and severe anemia

Respiratory: Bronchospasm occurred in 8%; 25% of these patients were treated with bronchodilators; rhinitis

Miscellaneous: Throat irritation

<1%:

Four patients developed arrhythmias during rituximab infusion. One of the four discontinued treatment based on ventricular tachycardia and supraventricular tachycardias. The other three patients experienced trigeminy and irregular pulses and did not require discontinuation of therapy. Angina was reported during infusion and MI occurred 4 days postinfusion in one subject with a history of MI.

A single occurrence of transient aplastic anemia (pure red-cell aplasia) and two occurrences of hemolytic anemia were reported.

Note: The following adverse events were reported more frequently in retreated patients: Asthenia, throat irritation, flushing, tachycardia, anorexia, leukopenia, thrombocytopenia, anemia, peripheral edema, dizziness, depression, respiratory symptoms, night sweats, pruritus.

Pharmacodynamics/Kinetics

Duration: Detectable in serum 3-6 months after completion of treatment; B-cell recovery begins ~6 months following completion of treatment; median B-cell levels return to normal by 12 months following completion of treatment

Absorption: I.V.: Immediate and results in a rapid and sustained depletion of circulating and tissue-based B cells

(Continued)

Rituximab *(Continued)*

Half-life elimination:

>100 mg/m^2: 4.4 days (range 1.6-10.5 days)

375 mg/m^2: 50 hours (following first dose) to 174 hours (following fourth dose)

Excretion: Uncertain; may undergo phagocytosis and catabolism in the reticuloendothelial system (RES)

Pregnancy Risk Factor C

Generic Available No

Rivastigmine (ri va STIG meen)

U.S. Brand Names Exelon®

Canadian Brand Names Exelon®

Mexican Brand Names Exelon®

Pharmacologic Category Acetylcholinesterase Inhibitor (Central)

Synonyms ENA 713; SDZ ENA 713

Use Mild to moderate dementia from Alzheimer's disease

Local Anesthetic/Vasoconstrictor Precautions No information available to require special precautions

Effects on Dental Treatment No significant effects or complications reported

Dosage Oral:

Adults: Mild to moderate Alzheimer's dementia: Initial: 1.5 mg twice daily to start; if dose is tolerated for at least 2 weeks then it may be increased to 3 mg twice daily; increases to 4.5 mg twice daily and 6 mg twice daily should only be attempted after at least 2 weeks at the previous dose; maximum dose: 6 mg twice daily. If adverse events such as nausea, vomiting, abdominal pain, or loss of appetite occur, the patient should be instructed to discontinue treatment for several doses then restart at the same or next lower dosage level; antiemetics have been used to control GI symptoms. If treatment is interrupted for longer than several days, restart the treatment at the lowest dose and titrate as previously described.

Elderly: Clearance is significantly lower in patients >60 years of age, but dosage adjustments are not recommended. Titrate dose to individual's tolerance.

Dosing adjustment in renal impairment: Titrate to individual's tolerance

Dosing adjustment in hepatic impairment: Clearance is significantly reduced in mild to moderately impairment; use lowest possible dose and titrate according to individual's tolerance (consider waiting >2 weeks between dosage adjustments)

Mechanism of Action A deficiency of cortical acetylcholine is thought to account for some of the symptoms of Alzheimer's disease; rivastigmine increases acetylcholine in the central nervous system through reversible inhibition of its hydrolysis by cholinesterase

Other Adverse Effects

>10%:

Central nervous system: Dizziness (21%), headache (17%)

Gastrointestinal: Nausea (47%), vomiting (31%), diarrhea (19%), anorexia (17%), abdominal pain (13%)

2% to 10%:

Cardiovascular: Syncope (3%), hypertension (3%)

Central nervous system: Fatigue (9%), insomnia (9%), confusion (8%), depression (6%), anxiety (5%), malaise (5%), somnolence (5%), hallucinations (4%), aggressiveness (3%)

Gastrointestinal: Dyspepsia (9%), constipation (5%), flatulence (4%), weight loss (3%), eructation (2%)

Genitourinary: Urinary tract infection (7%)

Neuromuscular & skeletal: Weakness (6%), tremor (4%)

Respiratory: Rhinitis (4%)

Miscellaneous: Increased diaphoresis (4%), flu-like syndrome (3%)

>2% (but frequency equal to placebo): Chest pain, peripheral edema, vertigo, back pain, arthralgia, pain, bone fracture, agitation, nervousness, delusion, paranoid reaction, upper respiratory tract infections, infection, coughing, pharyngitis, bronchitis, rash, urinary incontinence.

<2% (Limited to important or life-threatening symptoms; reactions may be at a similar frequency to placebo): Fever, edema, allergy, periorbital or facial edema, hypothermia, hypotension, postural hypotension, cardiac failure, ataxia, convulsions, apraxia, aphasia, dysphonia, hyperkinesia, hypertonia, hypokinesia, migraine, neuralgia, peripheral neuropathy, hypothyroidism, peptic ulcer, gastroesophageal reflux, GI hemorrhage, intestinal obstruction, pancreatitis, colitis, atrial fibrillation, bradycardia, AV block, bundle branch block, sick sinus syndrome, cardiac arrest, supraventricular tachycardia, tachycardia, abnormal hepatic function, cholecystitis, dehydration, arthritis, angina pectoris, MI, epistaxis, hematoma, thrombocytopenia, purpura, delirium, emotional lability, psychosis, anemia, bronchospasm, apnea, rashes (maculopapular, eczema, bullous, exfoliative, psoriaform, erythematous), urticaria, acute renal failure, peripheral ischemia, pulmonary embolism, thrombosis, thrombophlebitis, intracranial hemorrhage, conjunctival hemorrhage, diplopia, glaucoma, lymphadenopathy, leukocytosis.

Postmarketing and/or case reports: Stevens-Johnson syndrome, severe vomiting with esophageal rupture (following inappropriate reinitiation of dose)

Drug Interactions

Increased Effect/Toxicity: Beta-blockers without ISA activity may increase risk of bradycardia. Calcium channel blockers (diltiazem or verapamil) may increase risk of bradycardia. Cholinergic agonists effects may be increased with rivastigmine. Cigarette use increases the clearance of rivastigmine by 23%. Depolarizing neuromuscular blocking agents effects may be increased with rivastigmine. Digoxin may increase risk of bradycardia.

Decreased Effect: Anticholinergic agents effects may be reduced with rivastigmine.

Dietary/Ethanol/Herb Considerations

Ethanol: Avoid use due to risk of sedation; may increase GI irritation.

Food delays absorption by 90 minutes, lowers C_{max} by 30% and increases AUC by 30%.

Herb/Nutraceutical: Avoid gotu kola, kava, SAMe, St John's wort, and valerian; may increase CNS depression.

Pharmacodynamics/Kinetics

Absorption: Fasting: Rapid and complete within 1 hour

Distribution: V_d: 1.8-2.7 L/kg

Protein binding: 40%

Metabolism: Extensively via cholinesterase-mediated hydrolysis in the brain; metabolite undergoes N-demethylation and/or sulfate conjugation hepatically; CYP minimally involved; linear kinetics at 3 mg twice daily, but nonlinear at higher doses

Bioavailability: 40%

Half-life elimination: 1.5 hours

Time to peak: 1 hour

Excretion: Urine (97% as metabolites); feces (0.4%)

Pregnancy Risk Factor B

Generic Available No

Rizatriptan (rye za TRIP tan)

U.S. Brand Names Maxalt®; Maxalt-MLT®

Canadian Brand Names Maxalt™; Maxalt RPD™

Mexican Brand Names Maxalt®

Pharmacologic Category Serotonin 5-HT_{1D} Receptor Agonist

Synonyms MK462

Use Acute treatment of migraine with or without aura

Local Anesthetic/Vasoconstrictor Precautions No information available to require special precautions

Effects on Dental Treatment 1% to 10%: BP increase, chest pain (5%), palpitations, dizziness, drowsiness, fatigue (13% to 30%; dose-related), flushing, hot flashes, nausea, xerostomia (<5%), dyspnea

Dosage Note: In patients with risk factors for coronary artery disease, following adequate evaluation to establish the absence of coronary artery disease, the initial dose should be administered in a setting where response may be evaluated (physician's office or similarly staffed setting). EKG monitoring may be considered.

Oral: 5-10 mg, repeat after 2 hours if significant relief is not attained; maximum: 30 mg in a 24-hour period (use 5 mg dose in patients receiving propranolol with a maximum of 15 mg in 24 hours)

Note: For orally-disintegrating tablets (Maxalt-MLT™): Patient should be instructed to place tablet on tongue and allow to dissolve. Dissolved tablet will be swallowed with saliva.

Mechanism of Action Selective agonist for serotonin (5-HT_{1D} receptor) in cranial arteries to cause vasoconstriction and reduce sterile inflammation associated with antidromic neuronal transmission correlating with relief of migraine

Other Adverse Effects

1% to 10%:

Endocrine & metabolic: Mild increase in growth hormone

Gastrointestinal: Abdominal pain

<1%: Akinesia, **angina, arrhythmia,** arthralgia, **blurred vision,** bradykinesia, decreased mental activity, **diaphoresis,** diarrhea, dry eyes, eye pain, **facial edema, bradycardia,** chills, **hangover, heat sensitivity muscle weakness,** myalgia, **nasopharyngeal irritation, neck pain/stiffness, neurological/psychiatric abnormalities, pharyngitis,** polyuria, pruritus, **syncope, tachycardia,** tinnitus

Postmarketing and/or case reports: Angioedema, dysgeusia, myocardial ischemia, **MI, stroke,** toxic epidermal necrolysis, **wheezing**

Drug Interactions Increased Effect/Toxicity: Use within 24 hours of another selective 5-HT_1 antagonist or ergot-containing drug should be avoided due to possible additive vasoconstriction. Use with propranolol increased plasma concentration of rizatriptan by 70%. Rarely, concurrent use with SSRIs results in weakness and incoordination; monitor closely. MAO inhibitors and nonselective MAO inhibitors increase concentration of rizatriptan.

Dietary/Ethanol/Herb Considerations Food delays absorption.

(Continued)

Rizatriptan *(Continued)*

Pharmacodynamics/Kinetics

Onset of action: ~30 minutes
Duration: 14-16 hours
Protein binding: 14%
Metabolism: Via monoamine oxidase-A; first-pass effect
Bioavailability: 40% to 50%
Half-life elimination: 2-3 hours
Time to peak: 1-1.5 hours
Excretion: Urine (82%, 8% to 16% as unchanged drug); feces (12%)

Pregnancy Risk Factor C

Generic Available No

rLFN-α2 *see* Interferon Alfa-2b *on page 727*
RMS® *see* Morphine Sulfate *on page 931*
RO5-420 *see* Flunitrazepam *on page 583*
Robafen® AC *see* Guaifenesin and Codeine *on page 650*
Robaxin® *see* Methocarbamol *on page 881*
Robinul® *see* Glycopyrrolate *on page 645*
Robinul® Forte *see* Glycopyrrolate *on page 645*
Robitussin® [OTC] *see* Guaifenesin *on page 650*
Robitussin® A-C [DSC] *see* Guaifenesin and Codeine *on page 650*
Robitussin® CF [OTC] *see* Guaifenesin, Pseudoephedrine, and Dextromethorphan *on page 653*
Robitussin® Cold and Congestion [OTC] *see* Guaifenesin, Pseudoephedrine, and Dextromethorphan *on page 653*
Robitussin® Cough and Cold Infant [OTC] *see* Guaifenesin, Pseudoephedrine, and Dextromethorphan *on page 653*
Robitussin®-DAC [DSC] *see* Guaifenesin, Pseudoephedrine, and Codeine *on page 653*
Robitussin® DM [OTC] *see* Guaifenesin and Dextromethorphan *on page 651*
Robitussin® Maximum Strength Cough [OTC] *see* Dextromethorphan *on page 423*
Robitussin® Maximum Strength Cough & Cold [OTC] *see* Pseudoephedrine and Dextromethorphan *on page 1147*
Robitussin-PE® [OTC] *see* Guaifenesin and Pseudoephedrine *on page 652*
Robitussin® Pediatric Cough [OTC] *see* Dextromethorphan *on page 423*
Robitussin® Pediatric Cough & Cold [OTC] *see* Pseudoephedrine and Dextromethorphan *on page 1147*
Robitussin® Severe Congestion [OTC] *see* Guaifenesin and Pseudoephedrine *on page 652*
Robitussin® Sugar Free Cough [OTC] *see* Guaifenesin and Dextromethorphan *on page 651*
Rocaltrol® *see* Calcitriol *on page 223*
Rocephin® *see* Ceftriaxone *on page 278*

Rofecoxib (roe fe COX ib)

Related Information

Oral Pain *on page 1524*
Rheumatoid Arthritis, Osteoarthritis, and Osteoporosis *on page 1488*

U.S. Brand Names Vioxx®

Canadian Brand Names Vioxx®

Pharmacologic Category Nonsteroidal Anti-inflammatory Drug (NSAID), COX-2 Selective

Use

Dental and Medical: Management of acute pain in adults

Medical: Relief of the signs and symptoms of osteoarthritis; treatment of primary dysmenorrhea; relief of signs and symptoms of rheumatoid arthritis in adults

Local Anesthetic/Vasoconstrictor Precautions No information available to require special precautions

Effects on Dental Treatment

2% to 10%: Hypertension (≤10%), headache (5%), dizziness (3%), nausea (5%), epigastric discomfort (4%), dry socket (post-dental extraction alveolitis 2%), upper respiratory infection (9%), bronchitis (2%), sinusitis (3%), flu-like syndrome (3%), weakness (2%)

≤2%: Chest pain, atrial fibrillation, bradycardia, arrhythmia, palpitations, tachycardia, anxiety, CNS depression, migraine, paresthesia, somnolence, fever, GI reflux, xerostomia, esophagitis, gastritis, gastroenteritis, oral ulceration, dental caries, aphthous stomatitis, hematoma, asthma, cough, dyspnea, pneumonia, respiratory infection, pulmonary congestion, rhinitis, epistaxis, laryngitis, dry throat, pharyngitis, tonsillitis, allergy, fungal infection, syncope, viral syndrome, herpes simplex, increased diaphoresis, otic pain, otitis media, muscle spasm, sciatica, joint pain, swelling, muscle cramps, blurred vision, contact dermatitis

Dosage Adult: Oral:

Acute pain or management of dysmenorrhea: 50 mg once daily as needed (use for longer than 5 days has not been studied)

Osteoarthritis: 12.5 mg once daily; may be increased to a maximum of 25 mg once daily

Rheumatoid arthritis: 25 mg once daily

Elderly: No specific adjustment is recommended; use the lowest recommended dose. AUC may be increased by 34%, compared to younger subjects.

Dosing comment in renal impairment: Use in advanced renal disease is not recommended

Dosing adjustment in hepatic impairment: No specific recommendations; AUC may be increased by 69%

Mechanism of Action Inhibits prostaglandin synthesis by decreasing the activity of the enzyme, cyclooxygenase-2 (COX-2), which results in decreased formation of prostaglandin precursors. Rofecoxib does not inhibit cyclooxygenase-1 (COX-1) at therapeutic concentrations.

Other Adverse Effects

2% to 7%:

- Cardiovascular: Peripheral edema (4%)
- Gastrointestinal: Diarrhea (7%), heartburn (4%), dyspepsia (4%), abdominal pain (3%)
- Genitourinary: Urinary tract infection (3%)
- Neuromuscular & skeletal: Back pain (3%)

≤2%:

- Cardiovascular: Upper extremity edema, venous insufficiency, fluid retention
- Central nervous system: Decreased mental acuity, hypesthesia, insomnia, neuropathy, vertigo
- Dermatologic: Alopecia, atopic dermatitis, basal cell carcinoma, pruritus, rash, erythema, urticaria, dry skin
- Endocrine & metabolic: Weight gain, hypercholesteremia
- Gastrointestinal: Abdominal distension, abdominal tenderness, constipation, flatulence, hematochezia, hemorrhoids
- Genitourinary: Breast mass, cystitis, dysuria, menopausal disorder, nocturia, urinary retention, vaginitis, pelvic pain
- Neuromuscular & skeletal: Arthralgia, bursitis, cartilage trauma, myalgia, tendonitis, traumatic arthropathy, fracture (wrist)
- Ocular: Conjunctivitis
- Otic: Tinnitus
- Respiratory: Diaphragmatic hernia
- Miscellaneous: Insect bite reaction

<0.1% (Limited to important or life-threatening): **CHF, stroke**, deep venous thrombosis, **MI, pulmonary embolism, unstable angina, transient ischemic attack**, colitis, colonic neoplasm, cholecystitis, **duodenal ulcer, duodenal perforation, GI bleeding or perforation**, intestinal obstruction, pancreatitis, lymphoma, breast cancer, prostatic cancer, urolithiasis, **anaphylactoid reaction**, angioedema, aseptic meningitis, **hallucinations**

Contraindications Hypersensitivity to rofecoxib or any component of the formulation, aspirin, or other NSAIDs; pregnancy (3rd trimester)

Warnings/Precautions Gastrointestinal irritation, ulceration, bleeding, and perforation may occur with NSAIDs (rofecoxib has been associated with rates of these events which are lower than naproxen, a nonselective NSAID). Use with caution in patients with a history of GI disease (bleeding or ulcers), decreased renal function, hepatic disease, CHF, hypertension, or asthma. Edema, GI irritation, and/or hypertension occur at an increased frequency with chronic use of 50 mg/day. Use with caution in patients with ischemic heart disease; antiplatelet therapies should be considered (rofecoxib is not a substitute for antiplatelet agents). Anaphylactoid reactions may occur, even with no prior exposure to rofecoxib.

Drug Interactions Substrate of CYP2C8/9; Inhibits **CYP1A2**; Induces CYP3A4

ACE inhibitors: Antihypertensive effects may be reduced by rofecoxib.

Aspirin: Rofecoxib may be used with low-dose aspirin, however, rates of gastrointestinal bleeding may be increased with coadministration.

Cimetidine increases AUC of rofecoxib by 23%.

Diuretics: Thiazide diuretics, loop diuretics: Effects may be diminished by rofecoxib.

Lithium: Serum concentrations/toxicity may be increased by rofecoxib; monitor.

Methotrexate: Severe bone marrow suppression, aplastic anemia, and GI toxicity have been reported with concomitant NSAID therapy. Selective COX-2 inhibitors appear to have a lower risk of this toxicity, however, caution is warranted.

Rifampin reduces the serum concentration of rofecoxib by ~50%.

Theophylline: Serum concentrations may be increased during therapy with rofecoxib; monitor.

Warfarin: Rofecoxib may increase the INR in patients receiving warfarin and may increase the risk of bleeding complications. However, rofecoxib does not appear to inhibit platelet aggregation.

Dietary/Ethanol/Herb Considerations

Ethanol: Avoid use; may increase gastric mucosal irritation.

(Continued)

Rofecoxib *(Continued)*

Food: May be taken with food; time to peak concentrations are delayed when taken with a high-fat meal, but peak concentration and AUC are unchanged.

Pharmacodynamics/Kinetics

Onset of action: 45 minutes

Duration: Up to >24 hours

Distribution: V_{dss} (apparent): 86-91 L

Protein binding: 87%

Metabolism: Hepatic (99%); minor metabolism via CYP2C8/9 isoenzyme

Half-life elimination: 17 hours

Time to peak: 2-3 hours

Excretion: Urine (as metabolites, <1% as unchanged drug)

Pregnancy Risk Factor C/D (3rd trimester)

Breast-feeding Considerations In animal studies, rofecoxib has been found to be excreted in milk. It is not known whether rofecoxib is excreted in human milk. Because many drugs are excreted in milk, and the potential for serious adverse reactions exists, a decision should be made whether to discontinue nursing or discontinue the drug, taking into account the importance of the drug to the mother.

Dosage Forms SUSP, oral: 12.5 mg/5 mL (150 mL); 25 mg/5 mL (150 mL). **TAB:** 12.5 mg, 25 mg, 50 mg

Generic Available No

Selected Readings

Bombardier C, Laine L, Reicin A, et al, "Comparison of Upper Gastrointestinal Toxicity of Rofecoxib and Naproxen in Patients With Rheumatoid Arthritis. VIGOR Study Group," *N Engl J Med*, 2000, 343(21):1520-8.

Change DJ, Fricke JR, Bird SR, et al, "Rofecoxib Versus Codeine/Acetaminophen in Postoperative Dental Pain: A Double-Blind, Randomized, Placebo- and Active Comparator-Controlled Clinical Trial," *Clin Ther*, 2001, 23(9):1446-55.

Ehrich EW, Dallob A, De Lepeleire I, et al, "Characterization of Rofecoxib as a Cyclo-oxygenase-2 Isoform Inhibitor and Demonstration of Analgesia in the Dental Pain Model," *Clin Pharmacol Ther*, 1999, 65(3):336-47.

Greenberg HE, Gottesdiener K, Huntington M, et al, "A New Cyclo-oxygenase-2 Inhibitor, Rofecoxib (Vioxx®), Did Not Alter the Antiplatelet Effects of Low-Dose Aspirin in Healthy Volunteers," *J Clin Pharmacol*, 2000, 40(12 Pt 2):1509-15.

Hawkey CJ, Jackson L, Harper SE, et al, "Review Article: The Gastrointestinal Safety Profile of Rofecoxib, a Highly Selective Inhibitor of Cyclo-oxygenase-2 in Humans," *Aliment Pharmacol Ther*, 2001, 15(1):1-9.

Malmstrom K, Daniels S, Kotey P, et al, "Comparison of Rofecoxib and Celecoxib, two Cyclooxygenase-2 Inhibitors, in Postoperative Dental Pain: A Randomized Placebo- and Active-Comparator-Controlled Clinical Trial," *Clin Ther*, 1999, 21(10):1653-63.

Moore PA and Hersh EV, "Celecoxib and Rofecoxib. The Role of COX-2 Inhibitors in Dental Practice," *J Am Dent Assoc*, 2001, 132(4):451-6.

Morrison BW, Christensen S, Yuan W, et al, "Analgesic Efficacy of the Cyclo-oxygenase-2-Specific Inhibitor Rofecoxib in Postdental Surgery Pain: A Randomized, Controlled Trial," *Clin Ther*, 1999, 21(6):943-53.

Mullican WS and Lacy JR, "Tramadol/Acetaminophen Combination Tablets and Codeine/Acetaminophen Combination Capsules for the Management of Chronic Pain: A Comparative Trial," *Clin Ther*, 2001, 23(9):1429-45.

Wynn RL, "The New COX-2 Inhibitors: Rofecoxib (Vioxx®) and Celecoxib (Celebrex™)," *Gen Dent*, 2000, 48(1):16-20.

Wynn RL, "NSAIDS and Cardiovascular Effects, Celecoxib for Dental Pain, and a New Analgesic - Tramadol with Acetaminophen," *Gen Dent*, 2002, 50(3):218-222.

Roferon-A® *see* Interferon Alfa-2a *on page 726*

Rogaine® Extra Strength for Men [OTC] *see* Minoxidil *on page 917*

Rogaine® for Men [OTC] *see* Minoxidil *on page 917*

Rogaine® for Women [OTC] *see* Minoxidil *on page 917*

Rohypnol *see* Flunitrazepam *on page 583*

Rolaids® Calcium Rich [OTC] *see* Calcium Supplements *on page 229*

Rolatuss® Plain *see* Chlorpheniramine and Phenylephrine *on page 308*

Romazicon® *see* Flumazenil *on page 581*

Romilar® AC *see* Guaifenesin and Codeine *on page 650*

Romycin® *see* Erythromycin *on page 512*

Rondec®-DM Drops *see* Carbinoxamine, Pseudoephedrine, and Dextromethorphan *on page 247*

Rondec® Drops *see* Carbinoxamine and Pseudoephedrine *on page 247*

Rondec® Syrup *see* Brompheniramine and Pseudoephedrine *on page 201*

Rondec® Tablets *see* Carbinoxamine and Pseudoephedrine *on page 247*

Rondec-TR® *see* Carbinoxamine and Pseudoephedrine *on page 247*

Ropinirole (roe PIN i role)

U.S. Brand Names Requip®

Canadian Brand Names ReQuip™

Pharmacologic Category Anti-Parkinson's Agent, Dopamine Agonist

Synonyms Ropinirole Hydrochloride

Use Treatment of idiopathic Parkinson's disease; in patients with early Parkinson's disease who were not receiving concomitant levodopa therapy as well as in patients with advanced disease on concomitant levodopa

Local Anesthetic/Vasoconstrictor Precautions No information available to require special precautions

Effects on Dental Treatment Xerostomia (5%), increased salivation (2%)

Dosage Adults: Oral: The dosage should be increased to achieve a maximum therapeutic effect, balanced against the principal side effects of nausea, dizziness, somnolence and dyskinesia

Recommended starting dose is 0.25 mg 3 times/day; based on individual patient response, the dosage should be titrated with weekly increments as described below:

- •Week 1: 0.25 mg 3 times/day; total daily dose: 0.75 mg
- •Week 2: 0.5 mg 3 times/day; total daily dose: 1.5 mg
- •Week 3: 0.75 mg 3 times/day; total daily dose: 2.25 mg
- •Week 4: 1 mg 3 times/day; total daily dose: 3 mg

After week 4, if necessary, daily dosage may be increased by 1.5 mg per day on a weekly basis up to a dose of 9 mg/day, and then by up to 3 mg/day weekly to a total of 24 mg/day

Removal by hemodialysis is unlikely.

Mechanism of Action Ropinirole has a high relative *in vitro* specificity and full intrinsic activity at the D_2 and D_3 dopamine receptor subtypes, binding with higher affinity to D_3 than to D_2 or D_4 receptor subtypes; relevance of D_3 receptor binding in Parkinson's disease is unknown. Ropinirole has moderate *in vitro* affinity for opioid receptors. Ropinirole and its metabolites have negligible *in vitro* affinity for dopamine D_1, 5-HT_1, 5-HT_2, benzodiazepine, GABA, muscarinic, $alpha_1$-, $alpha_2$-, and beta-adrenoreceptors. Although precise mechanism of action of ropinirole is unknown, it is believed to be due to stimulation of postsynaptic dopamine D_2-type receptors within the caudate-putamen in the brain. Ropinirole caused decreases in systolic and diastolic blood pressure at doses >0.25 mg. The mechanism of ropinirole-induced postural hypotension is believed to be due to D_2-mediated blunting of the noradrenergic response to standing and subsequent decrease in peripheral vascular resistance.

Other Adverse Effects

Early Parkinson's disease (without levodopa):

>10%:

Cardiovascular: Syncope (12%)

Central nervous system: Dizziness (40%), somnolence (40%), fatigue (11%)

Gastrointestinal: Nausea (60%), vomiting (12%)

Miscellaneous: Viral infection (11%)

1% to 10%:

Cardiovascular: Dependent/leg edema (6% to 7%), orthostasis (6%), hypertension (5%), chest pain (4%), flushing (3%), palpitations (3%), peripheral ischemia (3%), hypotension (2%), tachycardia (2%),

Central nervous system: Pain (8%), confusion (5%), hallucinations (5%, dose-related), hypoesthesia (4%), amnesia (3%), malaise (3%), vertigo (2%), yawning (3%)

Gastrointestinal: Constipation (>5%), dyspepsia (10%), abdominal pain (6%), anorexia (4%), flatulence (3%)

Genitourinary: Urinary tract infection (5%), impotence (3%)

Hepatic: Elevated alkaline phosphatase (3%)

Neuromuscular & skeletal: Weakness (6%)

Ocular: Abnormal vision (6%), xerophthalmia (2%)

Respiratory: Pharyngitis (6%), rhinitis (4%), sinusitis (4%), dyspnea (3%)

Miscellaneous: Diaphoresis (increased) (6%)

Advanced Parkinson's disease (with levodopa):

>10%:

Central nervous system: Dizziness (26%), somnolence (20%), headache (17%)

Gastrointestinal: Nausea (30%)

Neuromuscular & skeletal: Dyskinesias (34%)

1% to 10%:

Cardiovascular: Syncope (3%), hypotension (2%)

Central nervous system: Hallucinations (10%, dose-related), aggravated parkinsonism, confusion (9%), pain (5%), paresis (3%), amnesia (5%), anxiety (6%), abnormal dreaming (3%), insomnia

Gastrointestinal: Abdominal pain (9%), vomiting (7%), constipation (6%), diarrhea (5%), dysphagia (2%), flatulence (2%), weight loss (2%)

Genitourinary: Urinary tract infections

Hematologic: Anemia (2%)

Neuromuscular & skeletal: Falls (10%), arthralgia (7%), tremor (6%), hypokinesia (5%), paresthesia (5%), arthritis (3%)

Respiratory: Upper respiratory tract infection (9%), dyspnea (3%)

Miscellaneous: Injury, increased diaphoresis (7%), viral infection, increased drug level (7%)

Other adverse effects (all phase 2/3 trials):

1% to 10%:

Central nervous system: Neuralgia (>1%)

Renal: Elevated BUN (>1%)

(Continued)

Ropinirole *(Continued)*

<1% (Limited to important or life-threatening): Abnormal coordination, acidosis, agitation, angina, aphasia, asthma, bradycardia, bundle branch block, cardiac arrest, cardiac failure, cholecystitis, choreoathetosis, coma, delirium, delusion, dementia, diabetes mellitus, dysphonia, eosinophilia, extrapyramidal symptoms, gangrene, gastrointestinal hemorrhage, gastrointestinal ulceration, glaucoma, goiter, gynecomastia, hyperbilirubinemia, hyperkalemia, hyperthyroidism, hypoglycemia, hyponatremia, hypothyroidism, leukopenia, lymphopenia, limb embolism, manic reaction, pancreatitis, paralysis, paranoid reaction, peripheral neuropathy, photosensitivity, pleural effusion, pulmonary edema, pulmonary embolism, rash, renal calculus, renal failure (acute), seizures, sepsis, SIADH, stomatitis, stupor, suicide attempt, tachycardia, thrombocytopenia, thrombosis, tinnitus, torticollis, urticaria, ventricular tachycardia

Drug Interactions Substrate of **CYP1A2**, 3A4; Inhibits CYP1A2, **2D6**

Increased Effect/Toxicity: Inhibitors of CYP1A2 inhibitors may increase serum concentrations of ropinirole; inhibitors include cimetidine, ciprofloxacin, erythromycin, fluvoxamine, isoniazid, ritonavir, and zileuton. Estrogens may also reduce the metabolism of ropinirole; dosage adjustments may be needed.

Decreased Effect: Antipsychotics, enzyme inducers (barbiturates, carbamazepine, phenytoin, rifampin, rifabutin), cigarette smoking, and metoclopramide may reduce the effect or serum concentrations of ropinirole.

Dietary/Ethanol/Herb Considerations

Ethanol: Avoid use; may increase CNS depression.

May be taken with food

Herb/Nutraceutical: Avoid gotu kola, kava, SAMe, St John's wort, and valerian; may increase CNS depression.

Pharmacodynamics/Kinetics

Absorption: Not affected by food

Distribution: V_d: 525 L

Metabolism: Extensively hepatic via CYP1A2 to inactive metabolites; first-pass effect

Bioavailability: Absolute: 55%

Half-life elimination: ~6 hours

Time to peak: ~1-2 hours; T_{max} increased by 2.5 hours when drug taken with food

Excretion: Clearance: Reduced by 30% in patients >65 years of age

Pregnancy Risk Factor C

Generic Available No

Ropinirole Hydrochloride *see* Ropinirole *on page 1196*

Ropivacaine (roe PIV a kane)

Related Information

Oral Pain *on page 1524*

U.S. Brand Names Naropin®

Canadian Brand Names Naropin®

Mexican Brand Names Naropin®

Pharmacologic Category Local Anesthetic

Synonyms Ropivacaine Hydrochloride

Use Local anesthetic (injectable) for use in surgery, postoperative pain management, and obstetrical procedures when local or regional anesthesia is needed. It can be administered via local infiltration, epidural block and epidural infusion, or intermittent bolus.

Local Anesthetic/Vasoconstrictor Precautions No information available to require special precautions

Effects on Dental Treatment No significant effects or complications reported

Dosage Dose varies with procedure, onset and depth of anesthesia desired, vascularity of tissues, duration of anesthesia, and condition of patient: Adults:

- Surgical anesthesia:
  - Lumbar epidural: 15-30 mL of 0.5% to 1% solution
  - Lumbar epidural block for cesarean section:
    - 20-30 mL dose of 0.5% solution
    - 15-20 mL dose of 0.75% solution
  - Thoracic epidural block: 5-15 mL dose of 0.5% to 0.75% solution
  - Major nerve block:
    - 35-50 mL dose of 0.5% solution (175-250 mg)
    - 10-40 mL dose of 0.75% solution (75-300 mg)
  - Field block: 1-40 mL dose of 0.5% solution (5-200 mg)
- Labor pain management: Lumbar epidural: Initial: 10-20 mL 0.2% solution; continuous infusion dose: 6-14 mL/hour of 0.2% solution with incremental injections of 10-15 mL/hour of 0.2% solution
- Postoperative pain management:
  - Lumbar or thoracic epidural: Continuous infusion dose: 6-14 mL/hour of 0.2% solution

Infiltration/minor nerve block:
1-100 mL dose of 0.2% solution
1-40 mL dose of 0.5% solution

Mechanism of Action Blocks both the initiation and conduction of nerve impulses by decreasing the neuronal membrane's permeability to sodium ions, which results in inhibition of depolarization with resultant blockade of conduction

Other Adverse Effects

>5% (dose and route related):
- Cardiovascular: Hypotension, bradycardia
- Central nervous system: Headache
- Dermatologic: Pruritus
- Gastrointestinal: Nausea, vomiting
- Neuromuscular & skeletal: Back pain, paresthesia
- Miscellaneous: Shivering

1% to 5% (dose-related):
- Cardiovascular: Hypertension, tachycardia
- Central nervous system: Dizziness, anxiety, lightheadedness
- Endocrine & metabolic: Hypokalemia
- Neuromuscular & skeletal: Hypoesthesia, rigors, circumoral paresthesia
- Otic: Tinnitus
- Respiratory: Dyspnea

<1% (Limited to important or life-threatening): Angioedema, apnea (usually associated with epidural block in head/neck region), bronchospasm, cardiac arrest, cardiovascular collapse, hallucinations, hyperthermia, myocardial depression, rash, seizures, syncope, tinnitus, ventricular arrhythmia

Drug Interactions Substrate of CYP1A2, 2B6, 2D6, 3A4

Increased Effect/Toxicity: Other local anesthetics or agents structurally related to the amide-type anesthetics. Increased toxicity possible (but not yet reported) with drugs that decrease cytochrome P450 1A enzyme function. SSRIs may increase ropivacaine levels.

Pharmacodynamics/Kinetics

Onset of action: Anesthesia (route dependent): 3-15 minutes
Duration (dose and route dependent): 3-15 hours
Metabolism: Hepatic
Half-life elimination: Epidural: 5-7 hours; I.V.: 2.4 hours
Excretion: Urine (86% as metabolites)

Pregnancy Risk Factor B

Generic Available No

Comments Not available with vasoconstrictor (epinephrine) and not available in dental (1.8 mL) carpules

Ropivacaine Hydrochloride *see* Ropivacaine *on page 1198*

Rosiglitazone (roh si GLI ta zone)

Related Information

Rosiglitazone and Metformin *on page 1200*

U.S. Brand Names Avandia®

Canadian Brand Names Avandia®

Pharmacologic Category Antidiabetic Agent, Thiazolidinedione

Use Type 2 diabetes mellitus (noninsulin dependent, NIDDM):

Monotherapy: Improve glycemic control as an adjunct to diet and exercise

Combination therapy: In combination with metformin or a sulfonylurea when diet, exercise, and metformin or a sulfonylurea alone do not result in adequate glycemic control; **or** when diet, exercise, and rosiglitazone alone do not result in adequate glycemic control

Local Anesthetic/Vasoconstrictor Precautions No information available to require special precautions

Effects on Dental Treatment Rosiglitazone-dependent diabetics should be appointed for dental treatment in morning in order to minimize chance of stress-induced hypoglycemia.

Dosage Oral:

Adults: Initial: 4 mg daily as a single daily dose or in divided doses twice daily. If response is inadequate after 12 weeks of treatment, the dosage may be increased to 8 mg daily as a single daily dose or in divided doses twice daily. In clinical trials, the 4 mg twice-daily regimen resulted in the greatest reduction in fasting plasma glucose and Hb A_{1c}. (**Note:** Doses >4 mg in combination with sulfonylureas have not been evaluated in clinical trials.)

Dosage comment in hepatic impairment: Clearance is significantly lower in hepatic impairment. Therapy should not be initiated if the patient exhibits active liver disease of increased transaminases (>2.5 times the upper limit of normal) at baseline.

Mechanism of Action Thiazolidinedione antidiabetic agent that lowers blood glucose by improving target cell response to insulin, without increasing pancreatic insulin secretion. It has a mechanism of action that is dependent on the presence of insulin for activity.

(Continued)

Rosiglitazone *(Continued)*

Other Adverse Effects Rare cases of hepatocellular injury have been reported in men in their 60s within 2-3 weeks after initiation of rosiglitazone therapy. LFTs in these patients revealed severe hepatocellular injury which responded with rapid improvement of liver function and resolution of symptoms upon discontinuation of rosiglitazone. Patients were also receiving other potentially hepatotoxic medications (*Ann Intern Med*, 2000, 132:121-4; 132:164-6).

>10%: Endocrine & metabolic: Weight gain, increase in total cholesterol, increased LDL-cholesterol, increased HDL-cholesterol

1% to 10%:

Cardiovascular: Edema (5%)
Central nervous system: Headache (6%), fatigue (4%)
Endocrine & metabolic: Hyperglycemia (4%), hypoglycemia (1% to 2%)
Gastrointestinal: Diarrhea (2%)
Hematologic: Anemia (2%)
Neuromuscular & skeletal: Back pain (4%)
Respiratory: Upper respiratory tract infection (10%), sinusitis (3%)
Miscellaneous: Injury (8%)

<1%, postmarketing and/or case reports: CHF (or exacerbation), elevated transaminases, hepatic failure, hepatitis, increased bilirubin, pulmonary edema, weight gain (rapid, excessive; due to fluid accumulation)

Drug Interactions Substrate of **CYP2C8/9**; Inhibits CYP2C8/9

Increased Effect/Toxicity: When rosiglitazone was coadministered with glyburide, metformin, digoxin, warfarin, ethanol, or ranitidine, no significant pharmacokinetic alterations were observed.

Dietary/Ethanol/Herb Considerations

Ethanol: Avoid use; may cause hypoglycemia.

Food: May be taken with food; lowers peak concentration by 28% (not clinically significant). Requires diet management.

Herb/Nutraceutical: Avoid black cohosh; may enhance effects of antidiabetic agents. Avoid chromium, garlic, gymnema, and horse chestnut; may cause hypoglycemia.

Pharmacodynamics/Kinetics

Onset of action: Delayed; Maximum effect: Up to 12 weeks
Distribution: V_{dss} (apparent): 17.6 L
Protein binding: 99.8%
Metabolism: Hepatic (99%) via CYP2C8; minor metabolism via CYP2C9
Bioavailability: 99%
Half-life elimination: 3.15-3.59 hours
Time to peak: 1 hour
Excretion: Urine (64%) and feces (23%) as metabolites

Pregnancy Risk Factor C

Generic Available No

Rosiglitazone and Metformin (roh si GLI ta zone & met FOR min)

Related Information

Metformin *on page 874*
Rosiglitazone *on page 1199*

U.S. Brand Names Avandamet™

Pharmacologic Category Antidiabetic Agent, Biguanide; Antidiabetic Agent, Thiazolidinedione

Synonyms Metformin and Rosiglitazone; Metformin Hydrochloride and Rosiglitazone Maleate; Rosiglitazone Maleate and Metformin Hydrochloride

Use Management of type 2 diabetes mellitus (noninsulin dependent, NIDDM) in patients who are already treated with the combination of rosiglitazone and metformin, or who are not adequately controlled on metformin alone. Used as an adjunct to diet and exercise to lower the blood glucose when hyperglycemia cannot be controlled satisfactorily by diet and exercise alone

Local Anesthetic/Vasoconstrictor Precautions No information available to require special precautions

Effects on Dental Treatment Dependent diabetics (noninsulin dependent, type 2) should be appointed in the morning in order to minimize chance of stress-induced hypoglycemia.

Dosage Oral:

Adults: Type 2 diabetes mellitus: Initial dose should be based on current dose of rosiglitazone and/or metformin; daily dose should be divided and given with meals

Patients inadequately controlled on **metformin alone**: Initial dose: Rosiglitazone 4 mg/day plus current dose of metformin

Patients inadequately controlled on **rosiglitazone alone**: Initial dose: Metformin 1000 mg/day plus current dose of rosiglitazone

Note: When switching from combination rosiglitazone and metformin as separate tablets: Use current dose

Dose adjustment: Doses may be increased as increments of rosiglitazone 4 mg and/or metformin 500 mg, up to the maximum dose; doses should be titrated gradually.

After a change in the metformin dosage, titration can be done after 1-2 weeks

After a change in the rosiglitazone dosage, titration can be done after 8-12 weeks

Maximum dose: Rosiglitazone 8 mg/metformin 2000 mg daily

Elderly: The initial and maintenance dosing should be conservative, due to the potential for decreased renal function (monitor). Generally, elderly patients should not be titrated to the maximum; do not use in patients ≥80 years unless normal renal function has been established.

Dosing adjustment in renal impairment: Do not use with serum creatinine ≥1.5 mg/dL in males; ≥1.4 mg/dL in females; or abnormal clearance

Dosing adjustment in hepatic impairment: Do not use with active liver disease or ALT >2.5 times the upper limit of normal

Mechanism of Action Rosiglitazone is a thiazolidinedione antidiabetic agent that lowers blood glucose by improving target cell response to insulin, without increasing pancreatic insulin secretion. It has a mechanism of action that is dependent on the presence of insulin for activity. Metformin decreases hepatic glucose production, decreasing intestinal absorption of glucose, and improves insulin sensitivity (increases peripheral glucose uptake and utilization).

Other Adverse Effects Also see individual agents. Percentages of adverse effects as reported with the combination product.

>10%:

Gastrointestinal: Diarrhea (13%)

Respiratory: Upper respiratory tract infection (16%)

1% to 10%:

Cardiovascular: Edema (4%)

Central nervous system: Headache (7%), fatigue (6%)

Endocrine & metabolic: Hypoglycemia (3%), hyperglycemia (2%)

Hematologic: Anemia (7%)

Neuromuscular & skeletal: Arthralgia (5%), back pain (5%)

Respiratory: Sinusitis (6%)

Miscellaneous: Viral infection (5%)

Dietary/Ethanol/Herb Considerations

Ethanol: Avoid use.

Food: Administer with food. Dietary modification based on ADA recommendations is a part of therapy. Monitor for signs and symptoms of vitamin B_{12} and folic acid deficiency; supplementation may be required.

Pregnancy Risk Factor C

Generic Available No

Rosiglitazone Maleate and Metformin Hydrochloride *see* Rosiglitazone and Metformin *on page 1200*

Rosuvastatin (roe SOO va sta tin)

Canadian Brand Names Crestor®

Pharmacologic Category Antilipemic Agent, HMG-CoA Reductase Inhibitor

Synonyms Rosuvastatin Calcium

Use Used with dietary therapy for hyperlipidemias to reduce elevations in total cholesterol (TC), LDL-C, apolipoprotein B, TC:HDL-C ratio, and triglycerides (TG) in patients with primary hypercholesterolemia (Fredrickson type IIa or IIb hyperlipidemias); treatment of homozygous familial hypercholesterolemia

Local Anesthetic/Vasoconstrictor Precautions No information available to require special precautions

Effects on Dental Treatment 1% to 10%: Dizziness, nausea, weakness

Dosage Adults: Oral: Initial: 10 mg once daily (20 mg in patients with severe hypercholesterolemia); after 2 weeks, may be increased to 20 mg once daily. Maximum dose: 40 mg once daily; in patients receiving gemfibrozil, limit maximum dose to 20 mg.

Dosage adjustment in renal impairment:

Cl_{cr} <30 mL/minute/1.73 m^2: Do not exceed 10 mg once daily.

Dosage adjustment in hepatic impairment:

Moderate to severe: Do not exceed 20 mg once daily.

Mechanism of Action Inhibitor of 3-hydroxy-3-methylglutaryl coenzyme A (HMG-CoA) reductase, the rate-limiting enzyme in cholesterol synthesis (reduces the production of mevalonic acid from HMG-CoA); this then results in a compensatory increase in the expression of LDL receptors on hepatocyte membranes and a stimulation of LDL catabolism

Other Adverse Effects

1% to 10%:

Gastrointestinal: Constipation

Neuromuscular & skeletal: Myalgia

(Continued)

Rosuvastatin *(Continued)*

<1% (Limited to important or life-threatening): Myopathy, rhabdomyolysis (rare, high doses), renal impairment (rare, high doses), transaminase increases (dose-related)

Reported with other HMG-CoA reductase inhibitors: **Hypersensitivity syndrome (eg, anaphylaxis**, angioedema, arthralgia, erythema multiforme, eosinophilia, hemolytic anemia, lupus syndrome, photosensitivity, polymyalgia rheumatica, positive ANA, purpura, Stevens-Johnson syndrome, toxic epidermal necrolysis, urticaria, or vasculitis)

Drug Interactions Substrate of CYP2C9, 3A4

Increased Effect/Toxicity: Cyclosporine may increase serum concentrations of rosuvastatin (up to 10-fold); concurrent use is contraindicated. Serum concentrations of rosuvastatin may be increased (doubled) during concurrent administration of gemfibrozil; limit initial dose to 10 mg/day and limit maximum dose to 20 mg/day. Clofibrate or fenofibrate may increase the risk of myopathy and rhabdomyolysis with HMG-CoA reductase inhibitors (not established with rosuvastatin), and the effects on lipids may be additive. The anticoagulant effects of warfarin may be increased by rosuvastatin (monitor).

Decreased Effect: Plasma concentrations of rosuvastatin may be decreased when given with magnesium/aluminum hydroxide-containing antacids (reported with atorvastatin and pravastatin); clinical efficacy is not altered, no dosage adjustment is necessary. Cholestyramine and colestipol (bile acid sequestrants) may reduce absorption of several HMG-CoA reductase inhibitors; separate administration times by at least 4 hours; cholesterol-lowering effects are additive.

Dietary/Ethanol/Herb Considerations

Ethanol: Avoid excessive consumption due to potential hepatic effects.

Food: May be taken with food

Pharmacodynamics/Kinetics

Onset: Within 1 week; maximal at 4 weeks

Distribution: V_d: 134 L

Protein binding: 90%

Metabolism: Hepatic (10%), via CYP2C9 (1 active metabolite identified)

Bioavailability: 20% (high first-pass extraction by liver)

Half-life elimination: 19 hours

Time to peak, plasma: 3-5 hours

Excretion: Feces (90%), primarily as unchanged drug

Pregnancy Risk Factor X

Generic Available No

Rosuvastatin Calcium *see* Rosuvastatin *on page 1201*

Rowasa® *see* Mesalamine *on page 869*

Roxanol® *see* Morphine Sulfate *on page 931*

Roxanol 100® *see* Morphine Sulfate *on page 931*

Roxanol®-T *see* Morphine Sulfate *on page 931*

Roxicet® *see* Oxycodone and Acetaminophen *on page 1018*

Roxicet® 5/500 *see* Oxycodone and Acetaminophen *on page 1018*

Roxicodone™ *see* Oxycodone *on page 1017*

Roxicodone™ Intensol™ *see* Oxycodone *on page 1017*

RP54274 *see* Riluzole *on page 1184*

RP59500 *see* Quinupristin and Dalfopristin *on page 1161*

r-PA *see* Reteplase *on page 1174*

rPDGF-BB *see* Becaplermin *on page 162*

R-Tannamine® *see* Chlorpheniramine, Pyrilamine, and Phenylephrine *on page 312*

R-Tannate® *see* Chlorpheniramine, Pyrilamine, and Phenylephrine *on page 312*

RTCA *see* Ribavirin *on page 1176*

RU-486 *see* Mifepristone *on page 912*

RU-38486 *see* Mifepristone *on page 912*

Rubella, Measles and Mumps Vaccines, Combined *see* Measles, Mumps, and Rubella Vaccines (Combined) *on page 844*

Rubella Virus Vaccine (Live) (roo BEL u VYE rus vak SEEN, lyve)

Related Information

Immunizations (Vaccines) *on page 1612*

U.S. Brand Names Meruvax® II

Pharmacologic Category Vaccine

Synonyms German Measles Vaccine

Use Selective active immunization against rubella; vaccination is routinely recommended for persons from 12 months of age to puberty. All adults, both male and female, lacking documentation of live vaccine on or after first birthday, or laboratory evidence of immunity (particularly women of childbearing age and young adults who work in or congregate in hospitals, colleges, and on military bases) should be vaccinated. Susceptible travelers should be vaccinated.

Note: Trivalent measles - mumps - rubella (MMR) vaccine is the preferred immunizing agent for most children and many adults.

Local Anesthetic/Vasoconstrictor Precautions No information available to require special precautions

Effects on Dental Treatment No significant effects or complications reported

Restrictions Federal law requires that the date of administration, the vaccine manufacturer, lot number of vaccine, and the administering person's name, title and address be entered into the patient's permanent medical record.

Dosage Children ≥12 months and Adults: S.C.: 0.5 mL in outer aspect of upper arm; children vaccinated before 12 months of age should be revaccinated. Recommended age for primary immunization is 12-15 months; revaccination with MMR-II is recommended prior to elementary school.

Mechanism of Action Rubella vaccine is a live attenuated vaccine that contains the Wistar Institute RA 27/3 strain, which is adapted to and propagated in human diploid cell culture. Promotes active immunity by inducing rubella hemagglutination-inhibiting antibodies.

Other Adverse Effects All serious adverse reactions must be reported to the U.S. Department of Health and Human Services (DHHS) Vaccine Adverse Event Reporting System (VAERS) 1-800-822-7967.

Frequency not defined:

Cardiovascular: Syncope, vasculitis

Central nervous system: Dizziness, encephalitis, fever, Guillain-Barré syndrome, headache, irritability, malaise, polyneuritis, polyneuropathy

Dermatologic: Angioneurotic edema, erythema multiforme, purpura, rash, Stevens-Johnson syndrome, urticaria

Gastrointestinal: Diarrhea, nausea, sore throat, vomiting

Hematologic: Leukocytosis, thrombocytopenia

Local: Injection site reactions which include burning, induration, pain, redness, stinging, wheal and flare

Neuromuscular & skeletal: Arthralgia/arthritis (variable; highest rates in women, 12% to 26% versus children, up to 3%), myalgia, paresthesia

Ocular: Conjunctivitis, optic neuritis, papillitis, retrobulbar neuritis

Otic: Nerve deafness, **otitis media**

Respiratory: Bronchial spasm, cough, rhinitis

Miscellaneous: Anaphylactoid reactions, anaphylaxis, regional lymphadenopathy

Drug Interactions Decreased Effect: Immunosuppressant drugs (including high-dose systemic corticosteroids), immune globulin, whole blood, or plasma may decrease effect of vaccine; do not administer with vaccine. Effectiveness may be decreased if given within 30 days of varicella vaccine (effectiveness not decreased when administered simultaneously).

Pharmacodynamics/Kinetics Onset of action: Antibodies to vaccine: 2-4 weeks

Pregnancy Risk Factor C

Generic Available No

Comments Federal law requires that the date of administration, the vaccine manufacturer, lot number of vaccine, and the administering person's name, title and address be entered into the patient's permanent record

Rubeola Vaccine *see* Measles Virus Vaccine (Live) *on page 845*

Rubex® *see* DOXOrubicin *on page 473*

Rubidomycin Hydrochloride *see* DAUNOrubicin Hydrochloride *on page 402*

Rum-K® *see* Potassium Supplements *on page 1102*

Ru-Tuss® *see* Chlorpheniramine and Phenylephrine *on page 308*

Ryna® [OTC] *see* Chlorpheniramine and Pseudoephedrine *on page 308*

Ryna-C® *see* Chlorpheniramine, Pseudoephedrine, and Codeine *on page 311*

Rynatan® Pediatric Suspension *see* Chlorpheniramine, Pyrilamine, and Phenylephrine *on page 312*

Rynatan® Tablet *see* Azatadine and Pseudoephedrine *on page 150*

Rynatuss® [OTC] *see* Chlorpheniramine, Ephedrine, Phenylephrine, and Carbetapentane *on page 309*

Rynatuss® Pediatric Suspension [OTC] *see* Chlorpheniramine, Ephedrine, Phenylephrine, and Carbetapentane *on page 309*

Rythmol® *see* Propafenone *on page 1130*

S-2® *see* Epinephrine (Racemic) *on page 500*

Sacrosidase (sak RO si dayz)

U.S. Brand Names Sucraid®

Canadian Brand Names Sucraid®

Pharmacologic Category Enzyme, Gastrointestinal

Use Orphan drug: Oral replacement therapy in sucrase deficiency, as seen in congenital sucrase-isomaltase deficiency (CSID)

Local Anesthetic/Vasoconstrictor Precautions No information available to require special precautions

Effects on Dental Treatment No significant effects or complications reported

(Continued)

Sacrosidase *(Continued)*

Dosage Oral:

Infants ≥5 months and Children <15 kg: 8500 int. units (1 mL) per meal or snack

Children >15 kg and Adults: 17,000 int. units (2 mL) per meal or snack

Doses should be diluted with 2-4 oz of water, milk, or formula with each meal or snack. Approximately one-half of the dose may be taken before, and the remainder of a dose taken at the completion of each meal or snack.

Mechanism of Action Sacrosidase is a naturally-occurring gastrointestinal enzyme which breaks down the disaccharide sucrose to its monosaccharide components. Hydrolysis is necessary to allow absorption of these nutrients.

Other Adverse Effects

1% to 10%: Gastrointestinal: Abdominal pain, vomiting, nausea, diarrhea, constipation

<1%: Bronchospasm, dehydration, headache, hypersensitivity reaction, insomnia, nervousness

Dietary/Ethanol/Herb Considerations Food: May be inactivated or denatured if administered with fruit juice or warm/hot food or liquids. Since isomaltase deficiency is not addressed by supplementation of sacrosidase, adherence to a low-starch diet may be required.

Pharmacodynamics/Kinetics

Absorption: Amino acids

Metabolism: GI tract to individual amino acids

Pregnancy Risk Factor C

Generic Available No

Comments Oral solution contains 50% glycerol

Safe Tussin® 30 [OTC] *see* Guaifenesin and Dextromethorphan *on page 651*
Saizen® *see* Human Growth Hormone *on page 671*
SalAc® [OTC] *see* Salicylic Acid *on page 1204*
Sal-Acid® [OTC] *see* Salicylic Acid *on page 1204*
Salactic® [OTC] *see* Salicylic Acid *on page 1204*
Salagen® *see* Pilocarpine *on page 1080*
Salagen® *see* Pilocarpine (Dental) *on page 1081*
Salbutamol *see* Albuterol *on page 48*
Salflex® *see* Salsalate *on page 1206*
Salicylazosulfapyridine *see* Sulfasalazine *on page 1254*

Salicylic Acid (sal i SIL ik AS id)

U.S. Brand Names Compound W® [OTC]; Compound W® One Step Wart Remover [OTC]; DHS™ Sal [OTC]; Dr. Scholl's® Callus Remover [OTC]; Dr. Scholl's® Clear Away [OTC]; DuoFilm® [OTC]; DuoPlant® [DSC] [OTC]; Freezone® [OTC]; Fung-O® [OTC]; Gordofilm® [OTC]; Hydrisalic™ [OTC]; Ionil® [OTC]; Ionil® Plus [OTC]; Keralyt® [OTC]; LupiCare™ Dandruff [OTC]; LupiCare™ II Psoriasis [OTC]; LupiCare™ Psoriasis [OTC]; Mediplast® [OTC]; MG217 Sal-Acid® [OTC]; Mosco® Corn and Callus Remover [OTC]; NeoCeuticals™ Acne Spot Treatment [OTC]; Neutrogena® Acne Wash [OTC]; Neutrogena® Body Clear™ [OTC]; Neutrogena® Clear Pore [OTC]; Neutrogena® Clear Pore Shine Control [OTC]; Neutrogena® Healthy Scalp [OTC]; Neutrogena® Maximum Strength T/Sal® [OTC]; Neutrogena® On The Spot® Acne Patch [OTC]; Occlusal®-HP [OTC]; Oxy Balance® [OTC]; Oxy® Balance Deep Pore [OTC]; Palmer's Skin Success Acne Cleanser [OTC]; Pedisilk® [OTC]; Propa pH [OTC]; SalAc® [OTC]; Sal-Acid® [OTC]; Salactic® [OTC]; Sal-Plant® [OTC]; Stri-dex® [OTC]; Stri-dex® Body Focus [OTC]; Stri-dex® Facewipes To Go™ [OTC]; Stri-dex® Maximum Strength [OTC]; Tinamed® [OTC]; Tiseb® [OTC]; Trans-Ver-Sal® [OTC]; Wart-Off® Maximum Strength [OTC]; Zapzyt® Acne Wash [OTC]; Zapzyt® Pore Treatment [OTC]

Canadian Brand Names Duofilm®; Duoforte® 27; Occlusal™; Occlusal™-HP; Sebcur®; Soluver®; Soluver® Plus; Trans-Plantar®; Trans-Ver-Sal®

Mexican Brand Names DuoPlant®; Ionil®; Ionil Plus®; Trans-Ver-Sal®

Pharmacologic Category Keratolytic Agent

Use Topically for its keratolytic effect in controlling seborrheic dermatitis or psoriasis of body and scalp, dandruff, and other scaling dermatoses; also used to remove warts, corns, and calluses; acne

Local Anesthetic/Vasoconstrictor Precautions No information available to require special precautions

Effects on Dental Treatment No significant effects or complications reported

Dosage Children and Adults (consult specific product labeling for use in children <12 years):

Acne:

Cream, cloth, foam, or liquid cleansers (2%): Use to cleanse skin once or twice daily. Massage gently into skin, work into lather and rinse thoroughly. Cloths should be wet with water prior to using and disposed of (not flushed) after use.

Gel (0.5% or 2%): Apply small amount to face in the morning or evening; if peeling occurs, may be used every other day. Some products may be labeled for OTC use up to 3 or 4 times per day. Apply to clean, dry skin.

Pads (0.5% or 2%): Use pad to cover affected area with thin layer of salicylic acid one to three times a day. Apply to clean, dry skin. Do not leave pad on skin.

Patch (2%): At bedtime, after washing face, allow skin to dry at least 5 minutes. Apply patch directly over pimple being treated. Remove in the morning.

Shower/bath gels or soap (2%): Use once daily in shower or bath to massage over skin prone to acne. Rinse well.

Callus, corns, or warts:

Gel or liquid (17%): Apply to each wart and allow to dry. May repeat once or twice daily, up to 12 weeks. Apply to clean dry area.

Gel (6%): Apply to affected area once daily, generally used at night and rinsed off in the morning.

Plaster or transdermal patch (40%): Apply directly over affected area, leave in place for 48 hours. Some products may be cut to fit area or secured with adhesive strips. May repeat procedure for up to 12 weeks. Apply to clean, dry skin

Transdermal patch (15%): Apply directly over affected area at bedtime, leave in place overnight and remove in the morning. Patch should be trimmed to cover affected area. May repeat daily for up to 12 weeks.

Dandruff, psoriasis, or seborrheic dermatitis:

Cream (2.5%): Apply to affected area 3-4 times daily. Apply to clean, dry skin. Some products may be left in place overnight.

Ointment (3%): Apply to scales or plaques on skin up to 4 times per day (not for scalp or face)

Shampoo (1.8% to 3%): Massage into wet hair or affected area; leave in place for several minutes; rinse thoroughly. Labeled for OTC use 2-3 times a week, or as directed by healthcare provider. Some products may be left in place overnight.

Mechanism of Action Produces desquamation of hyperkeratotic epithelium via dissolution of the intercellular cement which causes the cornified tissue to swell, soften, macerate, and desquamate. Salicylic acid is keratolytic at concentrations of 3% to 6%; it becomes destructive to tissue at concentrations >6%. Concentrations of 6% to 60% are used to remove corns and warts and in the treatment of psoriasis and other hyperkeratotic disorders.

Other Adverse Effects Frequency not defined:

Central nervous system: Dizziness, mental confusion, headache

Local: Burning and irritation at site of exposure on normal tissue, peeling, scaling

Otic: Tinnitus

Respiratory: Hyperventilation

Pharmacodynamics/Kinetics

Absorption: Percutaneous; systemic toxicity unlikely with normal use

Time to peak, serum: Within 5 hours of application with occlusion

Pregnancy Risk Factor C

Generic Available Yes: Gel, soap

Salicylic Acid and Coal Tar *see* Coal Tar and Salicylic Acid *on page 359*

Salicylsalicylic Acid *see* Salsalate *on page 1206*

SalineX® [OTC] *see* Sodium Chloride *on page 1229*

Salivart® [OTC] *see* Saliva Substitute *on page 1205*

Saliva Substitute (sa LYE vu SUB sti toot)

Related Information

Management of Patients Undergoing Cancer Therapy *on page 1567*

U.S. Brand Names Entertainer's Secret® [OTC]; Moi-Stir® [OTC]; Mouthkote® [OTC]; Salivart® [OTC]; Saliva Substitute™ [OTC]; Salix® [OTC]

Pharmacologic Category Gastrointestinal Agent, Miscellaneous

Use Relief of dry mouth and throat in xerostomia

Local Anesthetic/Vasoconstrictor Precautions No information available to require special precautions

Effects on Dental Treatment No significant effects or complications reported

Dosage Use as needed

Generic Available No

Salix® [OTC] *see* Saliva Substitute *on page 1205*

Salk Vaccine *see* Poliovirus Vaccine (Inactivated) *on page 1093*

Salmeterol (sal ME te role)

Related Information

Fluticasone and Salmeterol *on page 601*

Respiratory Diseases *on page 1476*

U.S. Brand Names Serevent®; Serevent® Diskus®

Canadian Brand Names Serevent®

Mexican Brand Names Serevent®; Zamtirel

Pharmacologic Category $Beta_2$ Agonist

Synonyms Salmeterol Xinafoate

Use Maintenance treatment of asthma and in prevention of bronchospasm (inhalation aerosol in patients >12 years of age; inhalation powder in patients ≥4 years of

(Continued)

Salmeterol *(Continued)*

age) with reversible obstructive airway disease, including patients with symptoms of nocturnal asthma, who require regular treatment with inhaled, short-acting beta$_2$ agonists; prevention of exercise-induced bronchospasm; maintenance treatment of bronchospasm associated with COPD

Local Anesthetic/Vasoconstrictor Precautions No information available to require special precautions

Effects on Dental Treatment No significant effects or complications reported

Dosage

Note: Do **not** use spacer with inhalation powder

Asthma, maintenance and prevention:
- Inhalation, aerosol: Children ≥12 years and Adults: 42 mcg (2 puffs) twice daily (12 hours apart)
- Inhalation, powder (Serevent® Diskus®): Children ≥4 years and Adults: One inhalation (50 mcg) twice daily

Exercise-induced asthma, prevention:
- Inhalation, aerosol: Children ≥12 years and Adults: 42 mcg (2 puffs) 30-60 minutes prior to exercise; additional doses should not be used for 12 hours
- Inhalation, powder (Serevent® Diskus®): Children ≥4 years and Adults: One inhalation (50 mcg) at least 30 minutes prior to exercise; additional doses should not be used for 12 hours

COPD (maintenance treatment of associated bronchospasm):
- Inhalation, aerosol: Adults: 42 micrograms (2 puffs) twice daily (morning and evening, 12 hours apart)
- Inhalation, powder (Serevent® Diskus®): Adults: One inhalation (50 mcg) twice daily, ~12 hours apart

Mechanism of Action Relaxes bronchial smooth muscle by selective action on beta$_2$-receptors with little effect on heart rate; because salmeterol acts locally in the lung, therapeutic effect is not predicted by plasma levels

Other Adverse Effects

>10%:
- Central nervous system: Headache
- Respiratory: Pharyngitis

1% to 10%:
- Cardiovascular: Tachycardia, palpitations, elevation or depression of blood pressure, cardiac arrhythmias
- Central nervous system: Nervousness, CNS stimulation, hyperactivity, insomnia, malaise, dizziness
- Gastrointestinal: GI upset, diarrhea, nausea
- Neuromuscular & skeletal: Tremors (may be more common in the elderly), myalgias, back pain, arthralgia
- Respiratory: Upper respiratory infection, cough, bronchitis

<1% (Limited to important or life-threatening): Immediate hypersensitivity reactions (rash, urticaria, bronchospasm), paradoxical bronchospasms, laryngeal spasm, arrhythmias, atrial fibrillation

Postmarketing and/or case reports: Oropharyngeal irritation, hypertension

Drug Interactions CYP3A3/4 enzyme substrate

Increased Toxicity (cardiovascular): MAO inhibitors, tricyclic antidepressants
- Increased Effect: Inhaled corticosteroids: The addition of salmeterol has been demonstrated to improve response to inhaled corticosteroids (as compared to increasing steroid dosage).

Decreased Effect: Beta-adrenergic blockers (eg, propranolol)

Pharmacodynamics/Kinetics

Onset of action: 5-20 minutes (average 10 minutes)
- Peak effect: 2-4 hours

Duration: 12 hours
Protein binding: 94% to 98%
Metabolism: Hepatically hydroxylated
Half-life elimination: 3-4 hours

Pregnancy Risk Factor C

Generic Available No

Salmeterol and Fluticasone *see* Fluticasone and Salmeterol *on page 601*

Salmeterol Xinafoate *see* Salmeterol *on page 1205*

Sal-Plant® [OTC] *see* Salicylic Acid *on page 1204*

Salsalate (SAL sa late)

Related Information

Rheumatoid Arthritis, Osteoarthritis, and Osteoporosis *on page 1488*
Temporomandibular Dysfunction (TMD) *on page 1562*

U.S. Brand Names Amigesic®; Disalcid® [DSC]; Mono-Gesic®; Salflex®

Canadian Brand Names Amigesic®; Salflex®

Pharmacologic Category Salicylate

Synonyms Disalcid® [DSC]; Disalicylic Acid; Salicylsalicylic Acid

Use Treatment of minor pain or fever; arthritis

Local Anesthetic/Vasoconstrictor Precautions No information available to require special precautions

Effects on Dental Treatment NSAID formulations are known to reversibly decrease platelet aggregation via mechanisms different than observed with aspirin. The dentist should be aware of the potential of abnormal coagulation. Caution should also be exercised in the use of NSAIDs in patients already on anticoagulant therapy with drugs such as warfarin (Coumadin®).

Dosage Oral:

Adults: 3 g/day in 2-3 divided doses

Dosing comments in renal impairment: End-stage renal disease with hemodialysis: 750 mg twice daily with an additional 500 mg after dialysis

Mechanism of Action Inhibits prostaglandin synthesis, acts on the hypothalamus heat-regulating center to reduce fever, blocks prostaglandin synthetase action which prevents formation of the platelet-aggregating substance thromboxane A_2

Other Adverse Effects

>10%: Gastrointestinal: Nausea, heartburn, stomach pains, dyspepsia

1% to 10%:

- Central nervous system: Fatigue
- Dermatologic: Rash
- Gastrointestinal: Gastrointestinal ulceration
- Hematologic: Hemolytic anemia
- Neuromuscular & skeletal: Weakness
- Respiratory: Dyspnea
- Miscellaneous: Anaphylactic shock

<1%: Insomnia, nervousness, jitters, leukopenia, thrombocytopenia, iron-deficiency anemia, does not appear to inhibit platelet aggregation, occult bleeding, hepatotoxicity, impaired renal function, bronchospasm

Drug Interactions

Increased Effect/Toxicity: Increased effect/toxicity of oral anticoagulants, hypoglycemics, and methotrexate.

Decreased Effect: Decreased effect with urinary alkalinizers, antacids, and corticosteroids. Decreased effect of uricosurics and spironolactone.

Dietary/Ethanol/Herb Considerations

Ethanol: Avoid use; may enhance gastric mucosal irritation.

Food: Administer with food or milk to reduce GI upset; food may delay peak serum concentration. Avoid garlic, ginger, and green tea.

Herb/Nutraceutical: Avoid cat's claw, dong quai, evening primrose, feverfew, garlic, ginger, ginkgo biloba, ginseng, green tea, horse chestnut, and red clover due to additional antiplatelet activity.

Pharmacodynamics/Kinetics

Onset of action: Therapeutic: 3-4 days of continuous dosing

Absorption: Complete from small intestine

Metabolism: Hepatically hydrolyzed to two moles of salicylic acid (active)

Half-life elimination: 7-8 hours

Excretion: Primarily urine

Pregnancy Risk Factor C/D (3rd trimester)

Generic Available Yes

Salt *see* Sodium Chloride *on page 1229*

Sal-Tropine™ *see* Atropine Sulfate Dental Tablets *on page 145*

Sandimmune® *see* CycloSPORINE *on page 383*

Sandostatin® *see* Octreotide *on page 993*

Sandostatin LAR® *see* Octreotide *on page 993*

Sani-Supp® [OTC] *see* Glycerin *on page 644*

Sanorex® [DSC] *see* Mazindol *on page 843*

Sansert® [DSC] *see* Methysergide *on page 897*

Santyl® *see* Collagenase *on page 367*

Saquinavir (sa KWIN a veer)

Related Information

HIV Infection and AIDS *on page 1482*

Tuberculosis *on page 1493*

U.S. Brand Names Fortovase®; Invirase®

Canadian Brand Names Fortovase™; Invirase®

Mexican Brand Names Invirase®

Pharmacologic Category Antiretroviral Agent, Protease Inhibitor

Synonyms Saquinavir Mesylate

Use Treatment of HIV infection in selected patients; used in combination with at least two other antiretroviral agents

Local Anesthetic/Vasoconstrictor Precautions No information available to require special precautions

Effects on Dental Treatment No significant effects or complications reported

(Continued)

Saquinavir *(Continued)*

Dosage Oral:

Children and Adolescents <16 years: Safety and efficacy have not been established; dosages of 33-50 mg/kg/dose 3 times/day are under study

Adults: **Note:** Fortovase® and Invirase® are not bioequivalent and should not be used interchangeably; only Fortovase® should be used to initiate therapy:

Fortovase®: Six 200 mg capsules (1200 mg) 3 times/day within 2 hours after a meal in combination with a nucleoside analog

Invirase®: Three 200 mg capsules (600 mg) 3 times/day within 2 hours after a full meal in combination with a nucleoside analog

Note: Dosing adjustment of either Fortovase® or Invirase® in combination with ritonavir: 400 mg twice daily

Note: Dosing adjustments of Fortovase® when administered in combination therapy:

Delavirdine: Fortovase® 800 mg 3 times/day

Lopinavir and ritonavir (Kaletra™): Fortovase® 800 mg twice daily

Nelfinavir: Fortovase® 800 mg 3 times/day or 1200 mg twice daily

Elderly: Clinical studies did not include sufficient numbers of patients ≥65 years of age; use caution due to increased frequency of organ dysfunction

Mechanism of Action As an inhibitor of HIV protease, saquinavir prevents the cleavage of viral polyprotein precursors which are needed to generate functional proteins in and maturation of HIV-infected cells

Other Adverse Effects Protease inhibitors cause dyslipidemia which includes elevated cholesterol and triglycerides and a redistribution of body fat centrally to cause "protease paunch", buffalo hump, facial atrophy, and breast enlargement. These agents also cause hyperglycemia.

1% to 10%:

Dermatologic: Rash

Endocrine & metabolic: Hyperglycemia

Gastrointestinal: Diarrhea, abdominal discomfort, nausea, abdominal pain, buccal mucosa ulceration

Neuromuscular & skeletal: Paresthesia, weakness, increased CPK

<1%: Headache, confusion, seizures, ataxia, pain, Stevens-Johnson syndrome, hypoglycemia, hyper- and hypokalemia, low serum amylase, upper quadrant abdominal pain, acute myeloblastic leukemia, hemolytic anemia, thrombocytopenia, jaundice, ascites, bullous skin eruption, polyarthritis, portal hypertension, exacerbation of chronic liver disease, elevated LFTs, altered AST/ALT, bilirubin, hemoglobin, thrombophlebitis

Drug Interactions Substrate of CYP2D6, **3A4**; Inhibits CYP2C8/9, 2C19, 2D6, **3A4**

Increased Effect:

Ketoconazole significantly increases plasma levels and AUC of saquinavir; as a known, although not potent inhibitor of the cytochrome P450 system, saquinavir may decrease the metabolism of astemizole, as well as cisapride and ergot derivatives (and result in rare but serious effects including cardiac arrhythmias); other drugs which may have increased adverse effects if coadministered with saquinavir include benzodiazepines (midazolam and triazolam), calcium channel blockers, clindamycin, dapsone, ergot alkaloids, and quinidine. Both clarithromycin and saquinavir levels/effects may be increased with coadministration. Delavirdine may increase concentration; ritonavir may increase AUC >17-fold; concurrent administration of nelfinavir results in increase in nelfinavir (18%) and saquinavir (mean: 392%).

Saquinavir increased serum concentrations of simvastatin, lovastatin, and atorvastatin; risk of myopathy/rhabdomyolysis may be increased. Use cautiously with HMG-CoA reductase inhibitors. Avoid use with simvastatin and lovastatin. Use caution with atorvastatin and cerivastatin (fluvastatin and pravastatin are not metabolized by CYP3A4).

Sildenafil serum concentrations are increased in concurrent therapy (limit sildenafil dosage to 25 mg).

Decreased Effect: Nevirapine, rifabutin, rifampin, phenobarbital, phenytoin, dexamethasone, and carbamazepine may decrease saquinavir concentrations. Saquinavir may decrease delavirdine concentrations.

Dietary/Ethanol/Herb Considerations

Food: Administer within 2 hours of a meal; a high-fat meal maximizes bioavailability. Avoid grapefruit products; may increase serum concentration.

Herb/Nutraceutical: Avoid St John's wort; may decrease serum concentration.

Pharmacodynamics/Kinetics

Absorption: Poor; increased with high fat meal; Fortovase® has improved absorption over Invirase®

Distribution: V_d: 700 L; does not distribute into CSF

Protein binding, plasma: ~98%

Metabolism: Extensively hepatic via CYP3A4; extensive first-pass effect

Bioavailability: Invirase®: ~4%; Fortovase®: 12% to 15%

Excretion: Feces (81% to 88%), urine (1% to 3%) within 5 days

Pregnancy Risk Factor B

Generic Available No

Saquinavir Mesylate *see* Saquinavir *on page 1207*
Sarafem™ *see* Fluoxetine *on page 589*

Sargramostim (sar GRAM oh stim)

U.S. Brand Names Leukine®
Canadian Brand Names Leukine™
Mexican Brand Names Leucomax®
Pharmacologic Category Colony Stimulating Factor
Synonyms GM-CSF; Granulocyte-Macrophage Colony Stimulating Factor; rGM-CSF

Use

Myeloid reconstitution after autologous bone marrow transplantation: Non-Hodgkin's lymphoma (NHL), acute lymphoblastic leukemia (ALL), Hodgkin's lymphoma, metastatic breast cancer

Myeloid reconstitution after allogeneic bone marrow transplantation

Peripheral stem cell transplantation: Metastatic breast cancer, non-Hodgkin's lymphoma, Hodgkin's lymphoma, multiple myeloma

Orphan drug:

Acute myelogenous leukemia (AML) following induction chemotherapy in older adults to shorten time to neutrophil recovery and to reduce the incidence of severe and life-threatening infections and infections resulting in death

Bone marrow transplant (allogeneic or autologous) failure or engraftment delay

Safety and efficacy of GM-CSF given simultaneously with cytotoxic chemotherapy have not been established. Concurrent treatment may increase myelosuppression.

Local Anesthetic/Vasoconstrictor Precautions No information available to require special precautions

Effects on Dental Treatment No significant effects or complications reported

Dosage

Children and Adults: I.V. infusion over ≥2 hours or S.C.

Existing clinical data suggest that starting GM-CSF between 24 and 72 hours subsequent to chemotherapy may provide optimal neutrophil recover; continue therapy until the occurrence of an absolute neutrophil count of 10,000/μL after the neutrophil nadir

The available data suggest that rounding the dose to the nearest vial size may enhance patient convenience and reduce costs without clinical detriment

Myeloid reconstitution after peripheral stem cell, allogeneic or autologous bone marrow transplant: I.V.: 250 mcg/m^2/day for 21 days to begin 2-4 hours after the marrow infusion on day 0 of autologous bone marrow transplant or ≥24 hours after chemotherapy or 12 hours after last dose of radiotherapy

If a severe adverse reaction occurs, reduce or temporarily discontinue the dose until the reaction abates

If blast cells appear or progression of the underlying disease occurs, disrupt treatment

Interrupt or reduce the dose by half if ANC is >20,000 cells/mm^3

Patients should not receive sargramostim until the postmarrow infusion ANC is <500 cells/mm^3

Neutrophil recovery following chemotherapy in AML: I.V.: 250 mcg/m^2/day over a 4-hour period starting approximately day 11 or 4 days following the completion of induction chemotherapy, if day 10 bone marrow is hypoblastic with <5% blasts

If a second cycle of chemotherapy is necessary, administer ~4 days after the completion of chemotherapy if the bone marrow is hypoblastic with <5% blasts

Continue sargramostim until ANC is >1500 cells/mm^3 for consecutive days or a maximum of 42 days

Discontinue sargramostim immediately if leukemic regrowth occurs

If a severe adverse reaction occurs, reduce the dose by 50% or temporarily discontinue the dose until the reaction abates

Mobilization of peripheral blood progenitor cells: I.V.: 250 mcg/m^2/day over 24 hours or S.C. once daily

Continue the same dose through the period of PBPC collection

The optimal schedule for PBPC collection has not been established (usually begun by day 5 and performed daily until protocol specified targets are achieved)

If WBC >50,000 cells/mm^3, reduce the dose by 50%

If adequate numbers of progenitor cells are not collected, consider other mobilization therapy

Postperipheral blood progenitor cell transplantation: I.V.: 250 mcg/m^2/day over 24 hours or S.C. once daily beginning immediately following infusion of progenitor cells and continuing until ANC is >1500 for 3 consecutive days is attained

BMT failure or engraftment delay: I.V.: 250 mcg/m^2/day for 14 days as a 2-hour infusion

(Continued)

Sargramostim *(Continued)*

The dose can be repeated after 7 days off therapy if engraftment has not occurred

If engraftment still has not occurred, a third course of 500 mcg/m²/day for 14 days may be tried after another 7 days off therapy; if there is still no improvement, it is unlikely that further dose escalation will be beneficial

If a severe adverse reaction occurs, reduce or temporarily discontinue the dose until the reaction abates

If blast cells appear or disease progression occurs, discontinue treatment

Mechanism of Action Stimulates proliferation, differentiation and functional activity of neutrophils, eosinophils, monocytes, and macrophages, as indicated: See table.

Comparative Effects — G-CSF vs. GM-CSF

Proliferation/Differentiation	G-CSF (Filgrastim)	GM-CSF (Sargramostim)
Neutrophils	Yes	Yes
Eosinophils	No	Yes
Macrophages	No	Yes
Neutrophil migration	Enhanced	Inhibited

Other Adverse Effects

>10%:

Cardiovascular: Hypotension, tachycardia, flushing, and syncope may occur with the first dose of a cycle ("first-dose effect"); peripheral edema (11%)

Central nervous system: Headache (26%)

Dermatologic: Rash, alopecia

Endocrine & metabolic: Polydypsia

Gastrointestinal: Diarrhea (52% to 89%), stomatitis, mucositis

Local: Local reactions at the injection site (~50%)

Neuromuscular & skeletal: Myalgia (18%), arthralgia (21%), bone pain

Renal: Increased serum creatinine (14%)

Respiratory: Dyspnea (28%)

1% to 10%:

Cardiovascular: Transient supraventricular arrhythmias; chest pain; capillary leak syndrome; pericardial effusion (4%)

Central nervous system: Headache

Gastrointestinal: Nausea, vomiting

Hematologic: Leukocytosis, thrombocytopenia

Neuromuscular & skeletal: Weakness

Respiratory: Cough; pleural effusion (1%)

<1%: Anaphylaxis, anorexia, constipation, fever, lethargy, malaise, pericarditis, rigors, sore throat, thrombophlebitis

Postmarketing and/or case reports: Arrhythmia, eosinophilia, thrombosis

Drug Interactions Increased Effect/Toxicity: Lithium, corticosteroids may potentiate myeloproliferative effects.

Pharmacodynamics/Kinetics

Onset of action: Increase in WBC: 7-14 days

Duration: WBCs return to baseline within 1 week of discontinuing drug

Half-life elimination: 2 hours

Time to peak, serum: S.C.: 1-2 hours

Pregnancy Risk Factor C

Generic Available No

Comments Reimbursement Hotline (Leukine®): 1-800-321-4669

Sarnol®-HC [OTC] *see* Hydrocortisone *on page 688*

S-Citalopram *see* Escitalopram *on page 516*

Scleromate™ *see* Morrhuate Sodium *on page 934*

Scopace™ *see* Scopolamine *on page 1210*

Scopolamine (skoe POL a meen)

U.S. Brand Names Isopto® Hyoscine; Scopace™; Transderm Scōp®

Canadian Brand Names Transderm-V®

Pharmacologic Category Anticholinergic Agent

Synonyms Hyoscine; Scopolamine Hydrobromide

Use Preoperative medication to produce amnesia and decrease salivary and respiratory secretions; to produce cycloplegia and mydriasis; treatment of iridocyclitis; prevention of motion sickness; prevention of nausea/vomiting associated with anesthesia or opiate analgesia (patch); symptomatic treatment of postencephalitic parkinsonism and paralysis agitans (oral); inhibits excessive motility and hypertonus of the GI tract in such conditions as the irritable colon syndrome, mild dysentery, diverticulitis, pylorospasm, and cardiospasm

Local Anesthetic/Vasoconstrictor Precautions No information available to require special precautions

Effects on Dental Treatment >10%: Significant xerostomia, dry throat (transdermal); normal salivary flow resumes upon discontinuation

Dosage

Preoperatively:

Children: I.M., S.C.: 6 mcg/kg/dose (maximum: 0.3 mg/dose) or 0.2 mg/m^2 may be repeated every 6-8 hours **or** alternatively:

4-7 months: 0.1 mg

7 months to 3 years: 0.15 mg

3-8 years: 0.2 mg

8-12 years: 0.3 mg

Adults:

I.M., I.V., S.C.: 0.3-0.65 mg; may be repeated every 4-6 hours

Transdermal patch: Apply 2.5 cm^2 patch to hairless area behind ear the night before surgery or 1 hour prior to cesarean section (the patch should be applied no sooner than 1 hour before surgery for best results and removed 24 hours after surgery)

Motion sickness: Transdermal: Children >12 years and Adults: Apply 1 disc behind the ear at least 4 hours prior to exposure and every 3 days as needed; effective if applied as soon as 2-3 hours before anticipated need, best if 12 hours before

Ophthalmic:

Refraction:

Children: Instill 1 drop of 0.25% to eye(s) twice daily for 2 days before procedure

Adults: Instill 1-2 drops of 0.25% to eye(s) 1 hour before procedure

Iridocyclitis:

Children: Instill 1 drop of 0.25% to eye(s) up to 3 times/day

Adults: Instill 1-2 drops of 0.25% to eye(s) up to 4 times/day

Oral: Parkinsonism, spasticity, motion sickness: 0.4-0.8 mg as a range; the dosage may be cautiously increased in parkinsonism and spastic states.

Mechanism of Action Blocks the action of acetylcholine at parasympathetic sites in smooth muscle, secretory glands and the CNS; increases cardiac output, dries secretions, antagonizes histamine and serotonin

Other Adverse Effects Frequency not defined:

Ophthalmic (systemic adverse effects have been reported):

Cardiovascular: Vascular congestion, edema

Central nervous system: Drowsiness

Dermatologic: Eczematoid dermatitis

Ocular: Blurred vision, photophobia, local irritation, increased intraocular pressure, follicular conjunctivitis, exudate

Respiratory: Congestion

Systemic:

Cardiovascular: Orthostatic hypotension, ventricular fibrillation, tachycardia, palpitations

Central nervous system: Confusion, drowsiness, headache, loss of memory, ataxia, fatigue

Dermatologic: Dry skin, increased sensitivity to light, rash

Endocrine & metabolic: Decreased flow of breast milk

Gastrointestinal: Constipation, dysphagia, bloated feeling, nausea, vomiting

Genitourinary: Dysuria

Local: Irritation at injection site

Neuromuscular & skeletal: Weakness

Ocular: Increased intraocular pain, blurred vision

Respiratory: Dry nose, diaphoresis (decreased)

Postmarketing and/or case reports: Restlessness, hallucinations

Drug Interactions

Increased Effect/Toxicity: Additive adverse effects with other anticholinergic agents.

Decreased Effect: Decreased effect of acetaminophen, levodopa, ketoconazole, digoxin, riboflavin, and potassium chloride in wax matrix preparations.

Dietary/Ethanol/Herb Considerations

Ethanol: Avoid use; may increase CNS depression.

Food: Fluids, fruit, and fiber may reduce constipation.

Herb/Nutraceutical: Avoid gotu kola, kava, SAMe, St John's wort, and valerian; may increase CNS depression.

Pharmacodynamics/Kinetics

Onset of action: Oral, I.M.: 0.5-1 hour; I.V.: 10 minutes

Peak effect: 20-60 minutes; may take 3-7 days for full recovery; transdermal: 24 hours

Duration: Oral, I.M.: 4-6 hours; I.V.: 2 hours

Absorption: Well absorbed from all routes

Protein binding, plasma: Reversible

Metabolism: Hepatic

Excretion: Urine

Pregnancy Risk Factor C

Generic Available Yes

Scopolamine and Phenylephrine *see* Phenylephrine and Scopolamine *on page 1072*

Scopolamine Hydrobromide *see* Scopolamine *on page 1210*

Scopolamine, Hyoscyamine, Atropine, and Phenobarbital *see* Hyoscyamine, Atropine, Scopolamine, and Phenobarbital *on page 700*

Scot-Tussin DM® Cough Chasers [OTC] *see* Dextromethorphan *on page 423*

Scot-Tussin® Sugar Free Expectorant [OTC] *see* Guaifenesin *on page 650*

SDZ ENA 713 *see* Rivastigmine *on page 1192*

SeaMist® [OTC] *see* Sodium Chloride *on page 1229*

Seba-Gel™ *see* Benzoyl Peroxide *on page 171*

Secobarbital (see koe BAR bi tol)

U.S. Brand Names Seconal®

Pharmacologic Category Barbiturate

Synonyms Quinalbarbitone Sodium; Secobarbital Sodium

Use Preanesthetic agent; short-term treatment of insomnia

Local Anesthetic/Vasoconstrictor Precautions No information available to require special precautions

Effects on Dental Treatment No significant effects or complications reported

Restrictions C-II

Dosage Oral:

Children:

Preoperative sedation: 2-6 mg/kg (maximum dose: 100 mg/dose) 1-2 hours before procedure

Sedation: 6 mg/kg/day divided every 8 hours

Adults:

Hypnotic: Usual: 100 mg/dose at bedtime; range 100-200 mg/dose

Preoperative sedation: 100-300 mg 1-2 hours before procedure

Mechanism of Action Depresses CNS activity by binding to barbiturate site at GABA-receptor complex enhancing GABA activity, depressing reticular activity system; higher doses may be gabamimetic

Other Adverse Effects Frequency not defined:

Cardiovascular: Hypotension

Central nervous system: Dizziness, lightheadedness, "hangover" effect, drowsiness, CNS depression, fever, confusion, mental depression, unusual excitement, nervousness, faint feeling, headache, insomnia, nightmares, hallucinations

Dermatologic: Exfoliative dermatitis, rash, Stevens-Johnson syndrome

Gastrointestinal: Nausea, vomiting, constipation

Hematologic: Agranulocytosis, megaloblastic anemia, thrombocytopenia, thrombophlebitis, urticaria apnea

Local: Pain at injection site

Respiratory: Respiratory depression, laryngospasm

Drug Interactions Induces **CYP2A6, 2C8/9**

Increased Effect/Toxicity: Increased toxicity when combined with other CNS depressants, antidepressants, benzodiazepines, chloramphenicol, or valproic acid; respiratory and CNS depression may be additive. MAO inhibitors may prolong the effect of secobarbital. Barbiturates may enhance the hepatotoxic potential of acetaminophen (due to an increased formation of toxic metabolites). Chloramphenicol may inhibit the metabolism of barbiturates.

Decreased Effect: Barbiturates, such as secobarbital, are hepatic enzyme inducers, and may increase the metabolism of antipsychotics, some beta-blockers (unlikely with atenolol and nadolol), calcium channel blockers, chloramphenicol, cimetidine, corticosteroids, cyclosporine, disopyramide, doxycycline, ethosuximide, felbamate, furosemide, griseofulvin, lamotrigine, phenytoin, propafenone, quinidine, tacrolimus, TCAs, and theophylline. Barbiturates may increase the metabolism of estrogens and reduce the efficacy of oral contraceptives; an alternative method of contraception should be considered. Barbiturates inhibit the hypoprothrombinemic effects of oral anticoagulants via increased metabolism. Barbiturates may enhance the metabolism of methadone resulting in methadone withdrawal.

Dietary/Ethanol/Herb Considerations

Ethanol: Avoid use; may increase CNS depression.

Herb/Nutraceutical: Avoid gotu kola, kava, SAMe, St John's wort, and valerian; may increase CNS depression.

Pharmacodynamics/Kinetics

Onset of hypnosis: 15-30 minutes

Duration: 3-4 hours with 100 mg dose

Distribution: 1.5 L/kg; crosses the placenta; appears in breast milk

Protein binding: 45% to 60%

Metabolism: Hepatic, by microsomal enzyme system

Half-life elimination: 15-40 hours, mean: 28 hours

Time to peak, serum: Within 2-4 hours

Excretion: Urine (as inactive metabolites, small amounts as unchanged drug)

Pregnancy Risk Factor D

Generic Available No

Secobarbital and Amobarbital *see* Amobarbital and Secobarbital *on page 91*

Secobarbital Sodium *see* Secobarbital *on page 1212*

Seconal® *see* Secobarbital *on page 1212*

SecreFlo™ *see* Secretin *on page 1213*

Secretin (SEE kre tin)

U.S. Brand Names SecreFlo™

Pharmacologic Category Diagnostic Agent

Use Secretin-stimulation testing to aid in diagnosis of pancreatic exocrine dysfunction; diagnosis of gastrinoma (Zollinger-Ellison syndrome); facilitation of ERCP visualization

Unlabeled/Investigational Use Diagnosis of some hepatobiliary disease such as obstructive jaundice

Local Anesthetic/Vasoconstrictor Precautions No information available to require special precautions

Effects on Dental Treatment No significant effects or complications reported

Restrictions In the U.S., no secretin product has been available, except for research protocols, since 1999.

Dosage I.V.: Adults: **Note:** A test dose of 0.2 mcg (0.1 mL) is injected to test for possible allergy. Dosing may be completed if no reaction occurs after 1 minute.

Diagnosis of pancreatic dysfunction, facilitation of ERCP: 0.2 mcg/kg over 1 minute

Diagnosis of gastrinoma: 0.4 mcg/kg over 1 minute

Mechanism of Action SecreFlo™ is a synthetic formulation of the porcine hormone secretin. This hormone is normally secreted by duodenal mucosa and upper jejunal mucosa which increases the volume and bicarbonate content of pancreatic juice; stimulates the flow of hepatic bile with a high bicarbonate concentration; stimulates gastrin release in patients with Zollinger-Ellison syndrome.

Other Adverse Effects

1% to 10%: Gastrointestinal: Abdominal discomfort (1%), nausea (1%)

<1%: Abdominal cramping, allergic reactions, bloating, bradycardia, diarrhea, fever, hypersensitivity reaction, hypotension, syncope, respiratory distress (transient), vomiting

Drug Interactions Decreased Effect: The response to secretin stimulation may be blunted by drugs with high anticholinergic activity such as tricyclic antidepressants, phenothiazines, and antihistamines as well as anticholinergic agents (ie, atropine, benztropine, biperiden).

Pharmacodynamics/Kinetics

Peak output of pancreatic secretions: ~30 minutes

Duration: At least 2 hours

Half-life elimination: 27 minutes

Pregnancy Risk Factor C

Generic Available No

Sectral® *see* Acebutolol *on page 25*

Selegiline (se LEJ i leen)

U.S. Brand Names Eldepryl®

Canadian Brand Names Apo®-Selegiline; Eldepryl®; Gen-Selegiline; Novo-Selegiline; Nu-Selegiline

Mexican Brand Names Niar®

Pharmacologic Category Antidepressant, Monoamine Oxidase Inhibitor; Anti-Parkinson's Agent, MAO Type B Inhibitor

Synonyms Deprenyl; L-Deprenyl; Selegiline Hydrochloride

Use Adjunct in the management of parkinsonian patients in which levodopa/carbidopa therapy is deteriorating

Unlabeled/Investigational Use Treatment of early Parkinson's disease, attention-deficit/hyperactivity disorder (ADHD), negative symptoms of schizophrenia, extrapyramidal symptoms, depression, Alzheimer's disease (studies have shown some improvement in behavioral and cognitive performance)

Local Anesthetic/Vasoconstrictor Precautions Selegiline in doses of 10 mg a day or less does not inhibit type-A MAO. Therefore, there are no precautions with the use of vasoconstrictors.

Effects on Dental Treatment >10%: Xerostomia, changes in salivation

Anticholinergic side effects can cause a reduction of saliva production or secretion, contributing to discomfort and dental disease (ie, caries, oral candidiasis and periodontal disease).

Dosage Oral:

Children and Adolescents: ADHD (unlabeled use): 5-15 mg/day

Adults: Parkinson's disease: 5 mg twice daily with breakfast and lunch or 10 mg in the morning

Elderly: Parkinson's disease: Initial: 5 mg in the morning, may increase to a total of 10 mg/day

(Continued)

Selegiline *(Continued)*

Mechanism of Action Potent monoamine oxidase (MAO) type-B inhibitor; MAO type B plays a major role in the metabolism of dopamine; selegiline may also increase dopaminergic activity by interfering with dopamine reuptake at the synapse

Other Adverse Effects Frequency not defined:

Cardiovascular: Orthostatic hypotension, hypertension, arrhythmias, palpitations, angina, tachycardia, peripheral edema, bradycardia, syncope

Central nervous system: Hallucinations, dizziness, confusion, anxiety, depression, drowsiness, behavior/mood changes, dreams/nightmares, fatigue, delusions

Dermatologic: Rash, photosensitivity

Gastrointestinal: Nausea, vomiting, constipation, weight loss, anorexia, diarrhea, heartburn

Genitourinary: Nocturia, prostatic hyperplasia, urinary retention, sexual dysfunction

Neuromuscular & skeletal: Tremor, chorea, loss of balance, restlessness, bradykinesia

Ocular: Blepharospasm, blurred vision

Miscellaneous: Diaphoresis (increased)

Drug Interactions Substrate of CYP1A2, 2A6, **2B6, 2C8/9**, 2D6, 3A4; Inhibits CYP1A2, 2A6, 2C8/9, 2C19, 2D6, 2E1, 3A4

Increased Effect/Toxicity: Concurrent use of selegiline (high dose) in combination with amphetamines, methylphenidate, dextromethorphan, fenfluramine, meperidine, nefazodone, sibutramine, tramadol, trazodone, tricyclic antidepressants, and venlafaxine may result in serotonin syndrome; these combinations are best avoided. Concurrent use of selegiline with an SSRI may result in mania or hypertension; it is generally best to avoid these combinations. Selegiline (>10 mg/day) in combination with tyramine (cheese, ethanol) may increase the pressor response; avoid high tyramine-containing foods in patients receiving >10 mg/day of selegiline. The toxicity of levodopa (hypertension), lithium (hyperpyrexia), and reserpine may be increased by MAO inhibitors.

Dietary/Ethanol/Herb Considerations

Ethanol: Avoid use; may contain tyramine (eg, Chianti, hearty red wine, and beer).

Food: Avoid food/beverages high in tyramine (eg, avocadoes, bananas, broad bean pods, canned figs, cheese, chicken liver, pickled herring, raisins, sour cream, soy sauce, yeast extracts, yogurt, pods, meats prepared with tenderizers, and foods aged to improve flavor); may cause sudden and severe high BP (risk increases with doses of selegiline (>10 mg/day) but generally not a problem). Avoid caffeine; even small amounts may produce irregular heartbeat or high blood pressure and can interact with this medication for up to 2 weeks after stopping its use.

Herb/Nutraceutical: Avoid ephedra, ginseng, and yohimbe; may cause arrhythmia. Avoid kava, SAMe, St John's wort, tryptophan, and valerian; may increase risk of serotonin syndrome and/or excessive sedation.

Pharmacodynamics/Kinetics

Onset of action: Therapeutic: Within 1 hour

Duration: 24-72 hours

Half-life elimination: Steady state: 10 hours

Metabolism: Hepatic to amphetamine and methamphetamine

Pregnancy Risk Factor C

Generic Available Yes

Selegiline Hydrochloride *see* Selegiline *on page 1213*

Selenium (se LEE nee um)

U.S. Brand Names Selepen®

Pharmacologic Category Trace Element, Parenteral

Synonyms Selenium Sulfide

Use Trace metal supplement

Local Anesthetic/Vasoconstrictor Precautions No information available to require special precautions

Effects on Dental Treatment No significant effects or complications reported

Dosage I.V. in TPN solutions:

Children: 3 mcg/kg/day

Adults:

- Metabolically stable: 20-40 mcg/day
- Deficiency from prolonged TPN support: 100 mcg/day for 24 and 21 days

Mechanism of Action Part of glutathione peroxidase which protects cell components from oxidative damage due to peroxidases produced in cellular metabolism

Other Adverse Effects Frequency not defined:

Central nervous system: Lethargy

Dermatologic: Alopecia or hair discoloration

Gastrointestinal: Vomiting following long-term use on damaged skin; abdominal pain, garlic breath

Local: Irritation

Neuromuscular & skeletal: Tremor

Miscellaneous: Diaphoresis

Pharmacodynamics/Kinetics Excretion: Urine, feces, lungs, skin

Pregnancy Risk Factor C

Generic Available Yes

Selenium *see* Trace Metals *on page 1328*

Selenium Sulfide *see* Selenium *on page 1214*

Selepen® *see* Selenium *on page 1214*

Selepen® *see* Trace Metals *on page 1328*

Semicid® [OTC] *see* Nonoxynol 9 *on page 985*

Semprex®-D *see* Acrivastine and Pseudoephedrine *on page 41*

Senexon® [OTC] *see* Senna *on page 1215*

Senna (SEN nu)

U.S. Brand Names Agoral® Maximum Strength Laxative [OTC]; Evac-U-Gen [OTC]; ex-lax® [OTC]; ex-lax® Maximum Strength [OTC]; Fletcher's® Castoria® [OTC]; Senexon® [OTC]; Senna-Gen® [OTC]; Sennatural™ [OTC]; Senokot® [OTC]; Senokot® Children's [OTC]; SenokotXTRA® [OTC]; X-Prep® [OTC]

Pharmacologic Category Laxative, Stimulant

Synonyms *C. angustifolia*; *Cassia acutifolia*; Senna Alexandria

Use Short-term treatment of constipation; evacuate the colon for bowel or rectal examinations

Local Anesthetic/Vasoconstrictor Precautions No information available to require special precautions

Effects on Dental Treatment Frequency not defined: Nausea, vomiting

Dosage Oral:

Bowel evacuation: OTC labeling: Children ≥12 years and Adults: Usual dose: Sennosides 130 mg (X-Prep® 75 mL) between 2-4 PM the afternoon of the day prior to procedure

Constipation: OTC ranges:

Children :

2-6 years:

Sennosides: Initial: 3.75 mg once daily (maximum: 15 mg/day, divided twice daily)

Senna concentrate: 33.3 mg/mL: 5-10 mL up to twice daily

6-12 years:

Sennosides: Initial: 8.6 mg once daily (maximum: 50 mg/day, divided twice daily)

Senna concentrate: 33.3 mg/mL: 10-30 mL up to twice daily

Children ≥12 years and Adults: Sennosides 15 mg once daily (maximum: 70-100 mg/day, divided twice daily)

Elderly: Consider half the initial dose in older, debilitated patients.

Mechanism of Action Hydrolyzed by bacteria in the colon thus releasing active sennosides; active metabolite (aglycone) acts as a local irritant on the colon, stimulates Auerbach's plexus to produce peristalsis; contains up to 3% anthraquinone glycosides

Other Adverse Effects Frequency not defined: Gastrointestinal: Diarrhea, abdominal cramps

Generic Available Yes: Tablet

Senna Alexandria *see* Senna *on page 1215*

Senna-Gen® [OTC] *see* Senna *on page 1215*

Sennatural™ [OTC] *see* Senna *on page 1215*

Senokot® [OTC] *see* Senna *on page 1215*

Senokot® Children's [OTC] *see* Senna *on page 1215*

SenokotXTRA® [OTC] *see* Senna *on page 1215*

Sensorcaine® *see* Bupivacaine *on page 205*

Sensorcaine®-MPF *see* Bupivacaine *on page 205*

Septocaine™ *see* Articaine Hydrochloride and Epinephrine (U.S.) *on page 125*

Septra® *see* Sulfamethoxazole and Trimethoprim *on page 1253*

Septra® DS *see* Sulfamethoxazole and Trimethoprim *on page 1253*

Serax® *see* Oxazepam *on page 1011*

Serentil® *see* Mesoridazine *on page 870*

Serevent® *see* Salmeterol *on page 1205*

Serevent® Diskus® *see* Salmeterol *on page 1205*

Sermorelin Acetate (ser moe REL in AS e tate)

U.S. Brand Names Geref® [DSC]; Geref® Diagnostic

Mexican Brand Names Geref®

Pharmacologic Category Diagnostic Agent; Growth Hormone

Use

Geref® Diagnostic: For evaluation of the ability of the pituitary gland to secrete growth hormone (GH)

(Continued)

Sermorelin Acetate *(Continued)*

Geref® injection: Treatment of idiopathic growth hormone deficiency in children

Orphan drug: Sermorelin has been designated an orphan product for AIDS-associated catabolism or weight loss, and as an adjunct to gonadotropin on ovulation induction.

Local Anesthetic/Vasoconstrictor Precautions No information available to require special precautions

Effects on Dental Treatment No significant effects or complications reported

Dosage

Children: Treatment of idiopathic growth hormone deficiency: S.C.: 30 mcg/kg at bedtime; discontinue when epiphyses are fused

Children and Adults: Diagnostic: I.V.: 1 mcg/kg as a single dose in the morning following an overnight fast

Note: Response to diagnostic test may be decreased in patients >40 years

Other Adverse Effects Frequency not defined:

Cardiovascular: Tightness in the chest
Central nervous system: Headache, dizziness, hyperactivity, somnolence
Dermatologic: Transient flushing of the face, urticaria
Gastrointestinal: Dysphagia, nausea, vomiting
Local: Pain, redness, and/or swelling at the injection site

Contraindications Hypersensitivity to sermorelin acetate, mannitol, or any component of the formulation

Drug Interactions The test should not be conducted in the presence of drugs that directly affect the pituitary secretion of somatotropin. These include preparations that contain or release somatostatin, insulin, glucocorticoids, or cyclooxygenase inhibitors such as ASA or indomethacin. Somatotropin levels may be transiently elevated by clonidine, levodopa, and insulin-induced hypoglycemia. Response to sermorelin may be blunted in patients who are receiving muscarinic antagonists (atropine) or who are hypothyroid or being treated with antithyroid medications such as propylthiouracil. Obesity, hyperglycemia, and elevated plasma fatty acids generally are associated with subnormal GH responses to sermorelin. Exogenous growth hormone therapy should be discontinued at least 1 week before administering the test.

Pharmacodynamics/Kinetics Onset of action: Peak response: Diagnostic: Children 30 ± 27 minutes; Adults: 35 ± 29 minutes

Pregnancy Risk Factor C

Dosage Forms INJ, powder for reconstitution (Geref® [DSC]): 0.5 mg, 1 mg; (Geref® Diagnostic): 50 mcg

Generic Available No

Seromycin® Pulvules® *see* CycloSERINE *on page 383*
Serophene® *see* ClomiPHENE *on page 348*
Seroquel® *see* Quetiapine *on page 1155*
Serostim® *see* Human Growth Hormone *on page 671*

Sertraline (SER tra leen)

U.S. Brand Names Zoloft®

Canadian Brand Names Apo®-Sertraline; Gen-Sertraline; Novo-Sertraline; ratio-Sertraline; Rhoxal-sertraline; Zoloft™

Mexican Brand Names Altruline®

Pharmacologic Category Antidepressant, Selective Serotonin Reuptake Inhibitor

Synonyms Sertraline Hydrochloride

Use Treatment of major depression, obsessive-compulsive disorder (OCD), panic disorder, post-traumatic stress disorder (PTSD), premenstrual dysphoric disorder (PMDD), social anxiety disorder

Unlabeled/Investigational Use Treatment of eating, anxiety, or impulse control disorders

Local Anesthetic/Vasoconstrictor Precautions Although caution should be used in patients taking tricyclic antidepressants, no interactions have been reported with vasoconstrictor and sertraline, a nontricyclic antidepressant which acts to increase serotonin

Effects on Dental Treatment

>10%: Somnolence, dizziness, headache, fatigue, xerostomia, nausea,

1% to 10%: Palpitations, agitation, anxiety, nervousness, vomiting, tremors, paresthesia, abnormal vision, increased diaphoresis

Dosage Oral:

Children and Adolescents: Depression/OCD:

6-12 years: Initial: 25 mg once daily
13-17 years: Initial: 50 mg once daily

Note: May increase by 50 mg/day increments at intervals of not less than 1 week if tolerated to 100 mg/day; additional increases may be necessary; maximum: 200 mg/day. If somnolence is noted, give at bedtime.

Adults:

Depression/OCD: Oral: Initial: 50 mg/day (see "Note" above)

Panic disorder, PTSD, social anxiety disorder: Initial: 25 mg once daily; increase to 50 mg once daily after 1 week (see "Note" above)

PMDD: 50 mg/day either daily throughout menstrual cycle **or** limited to the luteal phase of menstrual cycle, depending on physician assessment. Patients not responding to 50 mg/day may benefit from dose increases (50 mg increments per menstrual cycle) up to 150 mg/day when dosing throughout menstrual cycle **or** up to 100 mg day when dosing during luteal phase only. If a 100 mg/day dose has been established with luteal phase dosing, a 50 mg/day titration step for 3 days should be utilized at the beginning of each luteal phase dosing period.

Elderly: Depression/OCD: Start treatment with 25 mg/day in the morning and increase by 25 mg/day increments every 2-3 days if tolerated to 50-100 mg/day; additional increases may be necessary; maximum dose: 200 mg/day

Dosing adjustment in renal impairment: Multiple-dose pharmacokinetics are unaffected

Hemodialysis: Not removed

Dosing adjustment in hepatic impairment: Use lower dose or less frequent dosing; extensively metabolized by the liver

Mechanism of Action Antidepressant with selective inhibitory effects on presynaptic serotonin (5-HT) reuptake and only very weak effects on norepinephrine and dopamine neuronal uptake. *In vitro* studies demonstrate no significant affinity for adrenergic, cholinergic, GABA, dopaminergic, histaminergic, serotonergic, or benzodiazepine receptors.

Other Adverse Effects

>10%:

- Central nervous system: Insomnia
- Gastrointestinal: Diarrhea
- Genitourinary: Ejaculatory disturbances

1% to 10%:

- Dermatologic: Rash
- Endocrine & metabolic: Libido decreased
- Gastrointestinal: Constipation, anorexia, dyspepsia, flatulence, weight gain
- Genitourinary: Micturition disorders
- Ocular: Visual difficulty
- Otic: Tinnitus

Postmarketing and/or case reports: Abdominal pain, acute renal failure, agranulocytosis, allergic reaction, anaphylactoid reaction, angioedema, aplastic anemia, atrial arrhythmias, AV block, bilirubin increased, blindness, bradycardia, cataract, dystonia, extrapyramidal symptoms, galactorrhea, gum hyperplasia, gynecomastia, hallucinations, hepatic failure, hepatitis, hepatomegaly, hyperglycemia, hyperprolactinemia, hypothyroidism, jaundice, leukopenia, lupus-like syndrome, neuroleptic malignant syndrome, oculogyric crisis, serotonin syndrome, SIADH, Stevens-Johnson syndrome (and other severe dermatologic reactions), optic neuritis, pancreatitis (rare), photosensitivity, priapism, psychosis, PT/INR increased, pulmonary hypertension, QT_c prolongation, serum sickness, thrombocytopenia, transaminases increased, vasculitis, ventricular tachycardia (including torsade de pointes)

Drug Interactions Substrate of **CYP2B6, 2C8/9, 2C19**, 2D6, **3A4**; Inhibits CYP1A2, **2B6**, 2C8/9, **2C19**, 2D6, 3A4

Increased Effect/Toxicity:

MAO inhibitors: Sertraline should not be used with nonselective MAO inhibitors (phenelzine, isocarboxazid) or other drugs with MAO inhibition (linezolid); fatal reactions have been reported. Wait 5 weeks after stopping sertraline before starting a nonselective MAO inhibitor and 2 weeks after stopping an MAO inhibitor before starting sertraline. Concurrent selegiline has been associated with mania, hypertension, or serotonin syndrome (risk may be reduced relative to nonselective MAO inhibitors). Sertraline may increase serum concentrations of pimozide; concurrent use is contraindicated.

Combined used of SSRIs and amphetamines, buspirone, meperidine, nefazodone, serotonin agonists (such as sumatriptan), sibutramine, other SSRIs, sympathomimetics, ritonavir, tramadol, and venlafaxine may increase the risk of serotonin syndrome. Sertraline may increase serum levels/effects of benzodiazepines (alprazolam and diazepam), carbamazepine, carvedilol, clozapine, cyclosporine (and possibly tacrolimus), dextromethorphan, digoxin, haloperidol, HMG-CoA reductase inhibitors (lovastatin and simvastatin - increasing the risk of rhabdomyolysis, despite sertraline's weak inhibition), phenytoin, propafenone, trazodone, tricyclic antidepressants, and valproic acid. Concurrent lithium may increase risk of nephrotoxicity. Risk of hyponatremia may increase with concurrent use of loop diuretics (bumetanide, furosemide, torsemide). Sertraline may increase the hypoprothrombinemic response to warfarin.

Combined use of sumatriptan (and other serotonin agonists) may result in toxicity; weakness, hyper-reflexia, and incoordination have been observed with sumatriptan and SSRIs. In addition, concurrent use may theoretically increase the risk of serotonin syndrome; includes sumatriptan, naratriptan, rizatriptan, and zolmitriptan.

(Continued)

Sertraline *(Continued)*

Phenothiazines: CYP3A4 inhibitors (including sertraline) may inhibit the metabolism of thioridazine or mesoridazine, resulting in increased plasma levels and increasing the risk of QT_c interval prolongation. This may lead to serious ventricular arrhythmias, such as torsade de pointes-type arrhythmias and sudden death. Do not use together. Wait at least 5 weeks after discontinuing sertraline prior to starting thioridazine.

Decreased Effect: Sertraline may decrease the metabolism of tolbutamide; monitor for changes in glucose control.

Dietary/Ethanol/Herb Considerations

Ethanol: Avoid use; may increase CNS depression.

Food may increase average peak serum concentration.

Herb/Nutraceutical: Avoid gotu kola, kava, SAMe, St John's wort, and valerian; may increase CNS depression. Avoid melatonin; may cause acute psychosis. Avoid tryptophan; may cause serotonin syndrome. Avoid St John's wort; a number of case reports of serotonin syndrome have occurred as a result of concurrent use (eg, hypertension, hyperthermia, myoclonus, and mental status changes).

Pharmacodynamics/Kinetics

Absorption: Slow

Protein binding: High

Metabolism: Hepatic; extensive first-pass metabolism

Bioavailability: 88%

Half-life elimination: Parent drug: 26 hours; Metabolite N-desmethylsertraline: 66 hours (range: 62-104 hours)

Time to peak, plasma: 4.5-8.4 hours

Excretion: Urine and feces

Pregnancy Risk Factor C

Generic Available No

Comments Problems with SSRI-induced bruxism have been reported and may preclude their use; clinicians attempting to evaluate any patient with bruxism or involuntary muscle movement, who is simultaneously being treated with an SSRI drug, should be aware of the potential association.

Selected Readings Gerber PE and Lynd LD, "Selective Serotonin Reuptake Inhibitor-Induced Movement Disorders," *Ann Pharmacother*, 1998, 32(6):692-8.

Sertraline Hydrochloride *see* Sertraline *on page 1216*

Serutan® [OTC] *see* Psyllium *on page 1149*

Serzone® *see* Nefazodone *on page 957*

Sevelamer (se VEL u mer)

U.S. Brand Names Renagel®

Canadian Brand Names Renagel®

Pharmacologic Category Phosphate Binder

Synonyms Sevelamer Hydrochloride

Use Reduction of serum phosphorous in patients with end-stage renal disease

Local Anesthetic/Vasoconstrictor Precautions No information available to require special precautions

Effects on Dental Treatment No significant effects or complications reported

Dosage Adults: Oral: Patients not taking a phosphate binder: 800-1600 mg 3 times/day with meals; the initial dose may be based on serum phosphorous:

(Phosphorous: Initial Dose:)

- >6.0 mg/dL and <7.5 mg/dL: 800 mg 3 times/day
- ≥7.5 mg/dL and <9.0 mg/dL: 1200-1600 mg 3 times/day
- ≥9.0 mg/dL: 1600 mg 3 times/day

Dosage should be adjusted based on serum phosphorous concentration, with a goal of lowering to <6.0 mg/dL; maximum daily dose studied was equivalent to 30 capsules/day

Mechanism of Action Sevelamer (a polymeric compound) binds phosphate within the intestinal lumen, limiting absorption and decreasing serum phosphate concentrations without altering calcium, aluminum, or bicarbonate concentrations

Other Adverse Effects

>10%:

- Cardiovascular: Hypotension (11%), thrombosis (10%)
- Central nervous system: Headache (10%)
- Endocrine & metabolic: Decreased absorption of vitamins D, E, K and folic acid
- Gastrointestinal: Diarrhea (16%), dyspepsia (5% to 11%), vomiting (12%)
- Neuromuscular & skeletal: Pain (13%)
- Miscellaneous: Infection (15%)

1% to 10%:

- Cardiovascular: Hypertension (9%)
- Gastrointestinal: Nausea (7%), flatulence (4%), diarrhea (4%), constipation (2%)
- Respiratory: Cough (4%)

Drug Interactions Decreased Effect: Sevelamer may bind to some drugs in the gastrointestinal tract and decrease their absorption. When changes in absorption of oral medications may have significant clinical consequences (such as antiarrhythmic and antiseizure medications), these medications should be taken at least 1 hour before or 3 hours after a dose of sevelamer.

Dietary/Ethanol/Herb Considerations Administer with meals.

Pharmacodynamics/Kinetics

Absorption: None

Excretion: Feces

Pregnancy Risk Factor C

Generic Available No

Sevelamer Hydrochloride *see* Sevelamer *on page 1218*

Shur-Seal® [OTC] *see* Nonoxynol 9 *on page 985*

Sibutramine (si BYOO tra meen)

U.S. Brand Names Meridia®

Canadian Brand Names Meridia®

Mexican Brand Names Raductil®; Reductil®

Pharmacologic Category Anorexiant

Synonyms Sibutramine Hydrochloride Monohydrate

Use Management of obesity, including weight loss and maintenance of weight loss, and should be used in conjunction with a reduced calorie diet

Local Anesthetic/Vasoconstrictor Precautions No information available to require special precautions

Effects on Dental Treatment No significant effects or complications reported

Restrictions C-IV; recommended only for obese patients with a body mass index ≥30 kg/m² or ≥27 kg/m² in the presence of other risk factors such as hypertension, diabetes, and/or dyslipidemia

Dosage Adults ≥16 years: Initial: 10 mg once daily; after 4 weeks may titrate up to 15 mg once daily as needed and tolerated (may be used for up to 2 years, per manufacturer labeling)

Mechanism of Action Sibutramine blocks the neuronal uptake of norepinephrine and, to a lesser extent, serotonin and dopamine

Other Adverse Effects

>10%

Central nervous system: Headache, insomnia

Gastrointestinal: Anorexia, xerostomia, constipation

Respiratory: Rhinitis

1% to 10%

Cardiovascular: Tachycardia, vasodilation, hypertension, palpitations, chest pain, edema

Central nervous system: Migraine, dizziness, nervousness, anxiety, depression, somnolence, CNS stimulation, emotional liability

Dermatologic: Rash

Endocrine & metabolic: Dysmenorrhea

Gastrointestinal: Increased appetite, nausea, dyspepsia, gastritis, vomiting, abnormal taste, abdominal pain

Neuromuscular & skeletal: Weakness, arthralgia, back pain

Respiratory: Pharyngitis, sinusitis, cough, laryngitis

Miscellaneous: Diaphoresis, flu-like syndrome, allergic reactions, thirst

Postmarketing and/or case reports (frequency not defined; limited to important or life-threatening): Anaphylactic shock, anaphylactoid reaction, angina, arrhythmia, atrial fibrillation, CHF, cardiac arrest, syncope, torsade de pointes, transient ischemic attack, stroke, ventricular dysrhythmias, cholecystitis, cholelithiasis, GI hemorrhage, intestinal obstruction, goiter, hyperthyroidism, hypothyroidism, mania, serotonin syndrome, vascular headache, alopecia, increased intraocular pressure, photosensitivity, impotence

Drug Interactions Substrate of **CYP3A4**

Increased Effect/Toxicity: Serotonergic agents such as buspirone, selective serotonin reuptake inhibitors (eg, citalopram, fluoxetine, fluvoxamine, paroxetine, sertraline), sumatriptan (and similar serotonin agonists), dihydroergotamine, lithium, tryptophan, some opioid/analgesics (eg, meperidine, tramadol), and venlafaxine, when combined with sibutramine may result in serotonin syndrome. Dextromethorphan, MAO inhibitors and other drugs that can raise the blood pressure (eg decongestants, centrally-acting weight loss products, amphetamines, and amphetamine-like compounds) can increase the possibility of sibutramine-associated cardiovascular complications. Sibutramine may increase serum levels of tricyclic antidepressants. Theoretically, inhibitors of CYP3A4 (including ketoconazole, itraconazole, erythromycin) may increase sibutramine levels.

Decreased Effect: Inducers of CYP3A4 (including phenytoin, phenobarbital, carbamazepine, and rifampin) theoretically may reduce sibutramine serum concentrations.

Dietary/Ethanol/Herb Considerations

Ethanol: Avoid or limit use

(Continued)

Sibutramine *(Continued)*

Food: Administer with food to reduce GI upset. Most effective as an appetite suppressant when combined with a low calorie diet and behavior modification counseling. Avoid grapefruit products; may reduce metabolism and increase serum concentration.

Herb/Nutraceutical: Avoid St John's wort; may decrease serum concentration and increase risk for serotonin syndrome. Avoid tryptophan; may cause serotonin syndrome.

Pharmacodynamics/Kinetics

Absorption: Rapid

Protein binding, plasma: 94% to 97%

Metabolism: Hepatic; undergoes first-pass metabolism via CYP3A4

Time to peak: Within 3-4 hours

Excretion: Primarily urine (77%); feces

Pregnancy Risk Factor C

Generic Available No

Comments The mechanism of action is thought to be different from the "fen" drugs. Sibutramine works to suppress the appetite by inhibiting the reuptake of norepinephrine and serotonin. Unlike dexfenfluramine and fenfluramine, it is not a serotonin releaser. Sibutramine is closer chemically to the widely used antidepressants such as fluoxetine (Prozac®). The FDA approved sibutramine over the objections of its own advisory panel, who called the drug too risky. FDA reported that the drug causes blood pressure to increase, generally by a small amount, though in some patients the increases were higher. It is now recommended that patients taking sibutramine have their blood pressure evaluated regularly.

Selected Readings Wynn RL, "Sibutramine (Meridia) - Dental Considerations for a New Weight Control Drug," *Gen Dent*, 1998, 46(4):332-5.

Sibutramine Hydrochloride Monohydrate *see* Sibutramine *on page 1219*

Siladryl® Allergy [OTC] *see* DiphenhydrAMINE *on page 451*

Silafed® [OTC] *see* Triprolidine and Pseudoephedrine *on page 1356*

Silapap® Children's [OTC] *see* Acetaminophen *on page 27*

Silapap® Infants [OTC] *see* Acetaminophen *on page 27*

Sildenafil (sil DEN a fil)

U.S. Brand Names Viagra®

Canadian Brand Names Viagra®

Mexican Brand Names Viagra®

Pharmacologic Category Phosphodiesterase Enzyme Inhibitor

Synonyms UK 92480

Use Treatment of erectile dysfunction

Unlabeled/Investigational Use Treatment of psychotropic-induced sexual dysfunction

Local Anesthetic/Vasoconstrictor Precautions No information available to require special precautions

Effects on Dental Treatment No significant effects or complications reported

Dosage Oral:

Adults: 50 mg once daily (as needed); may be taken anywhere from 30 minutes to 4 hours before sexual activity. Based on effectiveness and tolerance, the dose may be increased to a maximum recommended dose of 100 mg or decreased to 25 mg.

Dosing adjustment for elderly (>65 years of age), hepatic impairment (cirrhosis), severe renal impairment (creatinine clearance <30 mL/minute), or concomitant use of potent cytochrome P450 3A4 inhibitors (erythromycin, ketoconazole, itraconazole, ritonavir, amprenavir): Higher plasma levels have been associated which may result in increase in efficacy and adverse effects and a starting dose of 25 mg should be considered

Mechanism of Action Does not directly cause penile erections, but affects the response to sexual stimulation. The physiologic mechanism of erection of the penis involves release of nitric oxide (NO) in the corpus cavernosum during sexual stimulation. NO then activates the enzyme guanylate cyclase, which results in increased levels of cyclic guanosine monophosphate (cGMP), producing smooth muscle relaxation and inflow of blood to the corpus cavernosum. Sildenafil enhances the effect of NO by inhibiting phosphodiesterase type 5 (PDE5), which is responsible for degradation of cGMP in the corpus cavernosum; when sexual stimulation causes local release of NO, inhibition of PDE5 by sildenafil causes increased levels of cGMP in the corpus cavernosum, resulting in smooth muscle relaxation and inflow of blood to the corpus cavernosum; at recommended doses, it has no effect in the absence of sexual stimulation.

Other Adverse Effects

>10%: Central nervous system: Headache

Note: Dyspepsia and abnormal vision (color changes, blurred or increased sensitivity to light) occurred at an incidence of >10% with doses of 100 mg.

1% to 10%:
- Cardiovascular: Flushing
- Central nervous system: Dizziness
- Dermatologic: Rash
- Genitourinary: Urinary tract infection
- Ophthalmic: Abnormal vision (color changes, blurred or increased sensitivity to light)
- Respiratory: Nasal congestion

<2% (Limited to important of life-threatening): Allergic reaction, angina pectoris anorgasmia, asthma, AV block, cardiac arrest, cardiomyopathy, cataract, cerebral thrombosis, colitis, dyspnea, edema, exfoliative dermatitis, eye hemorrhage, gout, heart failure, hyperglycemia, hypotension, migraine, myocardial ischemia, neuralgia, photosensitivity, postural hypotension, priapism, rectal hemorrhage, seizures, shock, syncope, vertigo

Warnings/Precautions There is a degree of cardiac risk associated with sexual activity; therefore, physicians may wish to consider the cardiovascular status of their patients prior to initiating any treatment for erectile dysfunction. Agents for the treatment of erectile dysfunction should be used with caution in patients with anatomical deformation of the penis (angulation, cavernosal fibrosis, or Peyronie's disease), or in patients who have conditions which may predispose them to priapism (sickle cell anemia, multiple myeloma, leukemia).

The safety and efficacy of sildenafil with other treatments for erectile dysfunction have not been studied and are, therefore, not recommended as combination therapy.

A minority of patients with retinitis pigmentosa have generic disorders of retinal phosphodiesterases. There is no safety information on the administration of sildenafil to these patients and sildenafil should be administered with caution.

Drug Interactions Substrate of CYP2C8/9, **3A4**; Inhibits CYP1A2, 2C8/9, 2C19, 2D6, 2E1, 3A4

Increased Effect/Toxicity: Sildenafil potentiates the hypotensive effects of nitrates (amyl nitrate, isosorbide dinitrate, isosorbide mononitrate, nitroglycerin); severe reactions have occurred and concurrent use is contraindicated. Concomitant use of alpha-blockers (doxazosin) may lead to symptomatic hypotension in some patients (sildenafil in doses >25 mg should not be given within 4 hours of administering an alpha-blocker). Sildenafil may potentiate the effect of other antihypertensives. Serum concentrations/toxicity of sildenafil may be increased by inhibitors of CYP3A4, including amprenavir, cimetidine, ciprofloxacin, clarithromycin, clozapine, diltiazem, disulfiram, digoxin, erythromycin, ethanol, fluconazole, fluoxetine, fluvoxamine, grapefruit juice, ritonavir, isoniazid, itraconazole, ketoconazole, labetalol, levodopa, loxapine, metoprolol, metronidazole, miconazole, nefazodone, nelfinavir, omeprazole, phenytoin, rifabutin, rifampin, ritonavir, troleandomycin, valproic acid, and verapamil. Sildenafil may potentiate bleeding in patients receiving heparin. A reduction in sildenafil's dose is recommended when used with ritonavir or indinavir (no more than 25 mg/dose; no more than 25 mg in 48 hours).

Decreased Effect: Enzyme inducers (including phenytoin, carbamazepine, phenobarbital, rifampin) may decrease the serum concentration and efficacy of sildenafil.

Dietary/Ethanol/Herb Considerations

Ethanol: Avoid use; may increase serum concentration.

Food: High fat meal reduces amount and rate of absorption. Avoid grapefruit products; may increase serum concentration/toxicity.

Herb/Nutraceutical: Avoid St John's wort; may decrease serum concentration.

Pharmacodynamics/Kinetics

Onset of action: ~60 minutes
Duration: 2-4 hours
Absorption: Rapid
Protein binding, plasma: ~96%
Metabolism: Hepatic via CYP3A4 (major) and CYP2C9 (minor route)
Bioavailability: 40%
Half-life elimination: 4 hours
Time to peak: 30-120 minutes
Excretion: Feces (80%); urine (13%)

Pregnancy Risk Factor B

Generic Available No

Silexin® [OTC] *see* Guaifenesin and Dextromethorphan *on page 651*

Silfedrine Children's [OTC] *see* Pseudoephedrine *on page 1146*

Silphen® [OTC] *see* DiphenhydrAMINE *on page 451*

Silphen DM® [OTC] *see* Dextromethorphan *on page 423*

Silvadene® *see* Silver Sulfadiazine *on page 1222*

Silver Nitrate (SIL ver NYE trate)

Pharmacologic Category Antibiotic, Ophthalmic; Antibiotic, Topical; Cauterizing Agent, Topical; Topical Skin Product, Antibacterial

(Continued)

Silver Nitrate *(Continued)*

Synonyms $AgNO_3$

Use Cauterization of wounds and sluggish ulcers, removal of granulation tissue and warts, aseptic prophylaxis of burns

Local Anesthetic/Vasoconstrictor Precautions No information available to require special precautions

Effects on Dental Treatment No significant effects or complications reported

Dosage Children and Adults:

Sticks: Apply to mucous membranes and other moist skin surfaces only on area to be treated 2-3 times/week for 2-3 weeks

Topical solution: Apply a cotton applicator dipped in solution on the affected area 2-3 times/week for 2-3 weeks

Mechanism of Action Free silver ions precipitate bacterial proteins by combining with chloride in tissue forming silver chloride; coagulates cellular protein to form an eschar; silver ions or salts or colloidal silver preparations can inhibit the growth of both gram-positive and gram-negative bacteria. This germicidal action is attributed to the precipitation of bacterial proteins by liberated silver ions. Silver nitrate coagulates cellular protein to form an eschar, and this mode of action is the postulated mechanism for control of benign hematuria, rhinitis, and recurrent pneumothorax.

Other Adverse Effects Frequency not defined:

Dermatologic: Burning and skin irritation, staining of the skin

Endocrine & metabolic: Hyponatremia

Hematologic: Methemoglobinemia

Pharmacodynamics/Kinetics

Absorption: Because silver ions readily combine with protein, there is minimal GI and cutaneous absorption of the 0.5% and 1% preparations

Excretion: Highest amounts of silver noted on autopsy have been in kidneys, excretion in urine is minimal

Pregnancy Risk Factor C

Generic Available Yes

Silver Sulfadiazine (SIL ver sul fa DYE a zeen)

U.S. Brand Names Silvadene®; SSD®; SSD® AF; Thermazene®

Canadian Brand Names Dermazin™; Flamazine®; SSD™

Pharmacologic Category Antibiotic, Topical

Use Prevention and treatment of infection in second and third degree burns

Local Anesthetic/Vasoconstrictor Precautions No information available to require special precautions

Effects on Dental Treatment No significant effects or complications reported

Dosage Children and Adults: Topical: Apply once or twice daily with a sterile-gloved hand; apply to a thickness of $^1/_{16}$"; burned area should be covered with cream at all times

Mechanism of Action Acts upon the bacterial cell wall and cell membrane. Bactericidal for many gram-negative and gram-positive bacteria and is effective against yeast. Active against *Pseudomonas aeruginosa, Pseudomonas maltophilia, Enterobacter* species, *Klebsiella* species, *Serratia* species, *Escherichia coli, Proteus mirabilis, Morganella morganii, Providencia rettgeri, Proteus vulgaris, Providencia* species, *Citrobacter* species, *Acinetobacter calcoaceticus, Staphylococcus aureus, Staphylococcus epidermidis, Enterococcus* species, *Candida albicans, Corynebacterium diphtheriae,* and *Clostridium perfringens*

Other Adverse Effects Frequency not defined:

Dermatologic: Itching, rash, erythema multiforme, discoloration of skin, photosensitivity

Hematologic: Hemolytic anemia, leukopenia, agranulocytosis, aplastic anemia

Hepatic: Hepatitis

Renal: Interstitial nephritis

Miscellaneous: Allergic reactions may be related to sulfa component

Drug Interactions Decreased Effect: Topical proteolytic enzymes are inactivated by silver sulfadiazine.

Pharmacodynamics/Kinetics

Absorption: Significant percutaneous absorption of silver sulfadiazine can occur especially when applied to extensive burns

Half-life elimination: 10 hours; prolonged with renal impairment

Time to peak, serum: 3-11 days of continuous therapy

Excretion: Urine (~50% as unchanged drug)

Pregnancy Risk Factor B

Generic Available Yes

Simethicone (sye METH i kone)

U.S. Brand Names Alka-Seltzer® Gas Relief [OTC]; Baby Gasz [OTC]; Flatulex® [OTC]; Gas-X® [OTC]; Gas-X® Extra Strength [OTC]; Genasyme® [OTC]; Mylanta® Gas [OTC]; Mylanta® Gas Maximum Strength [OTC]; Mylicon® Infants [OTC]; Phazyme® Quick Dissolve [OTC]; Phazyme® Ultra Strength [OTC]

Canadian Brand Names Ovol®; Phazyme™

Pharmacologic Category Antiflatulent

Synonyms Activated Dimethicone; Activated Methylpolysiloxane

Use Relieves flatulence and functional gastric bloating, and postoperative gas pains

Local Anesthetic/Vasoconstrictor Precautions No information available to require special precautions

Effects on Dental Treatment No significant effects or complications reported

Dosage Oral:

Infants: 20 mg 4 times/day

Children <12 years: 40 mg 4 times/day

Children >12 years and Adults: 40-120 mg after meals and at bedtime as needed, not to exceed 500 mg/day

Mechanism of Action Decreases the surface tension of gas bubbles thereby disperses and prevents gas pockets in the GI system

Other Adverse Effects No data reported

Dietary/Ethanol/Herb Considerations Food: Avoid carbonated beverages and gas-forming foods.

Pregnancy Risk Factor C

Generic Available Yes: Tablet, suspension

Simethicone, Aluminum Hydroxide, and Magnesium Hydroxide *see* Aluminum Hydroxide, Magnesium Hydroxide, and Simethicone *on page 69*

Simethicone and Calcium Carbonate *see* Calcium Carbonate and Simethicone *on page 224*

Simethicone and Magaldrate *see* Magaldrate and Simethicone *on page 833*

Simply Cough™ [OTC] *see* Dextromethorphan *on page 423*

Simply Saline™ [OTC] *see* Sodium Chloride *on page 1229*

Simulect® *see* Basiliximab *on page 160*

Simvastatin (SIM va stat in)

Related Information

Cardiovascular Diseases *on page 1456*

U.S. Brand Names Zocor®

Canadian Brand Names Zocor®

Mexican Brand Names Zocor®

Pharmacologic Category Antilipemic Agent, HMG-CoA Reductase Inhibitor

Use Used with dietary therapy for the following:

Secondary prevention of cardiovascular events in hypercholesterolemic patients with established coronary heart disease: To reduce cardiovascular morbidity (MI, coronary revascularization procedures) and mortality; to reduce the risk of stroke and transient ischemic attacks

Hyperlipidemias: To reduce elevations in total cholesterol, LDL-C, apolipoprotein B, and triglycerides in patients with primary hypercholesterolemia (elevations of 1 or more components are present in Fredrickson type IIa, IIb, III, and IV hyperlipidemias); treatment of homozygous familial hypercholesterolemia

Heterozygous familial hypercholesterolemia (HeFH): In adolescent patients (10-17 years of age, females >1 year postmenarche) with HeFH having LDL-C ≥190 mg/dL **or** LDL ≥160 mg/dL with positive family history of premature cardiovascular disease (CVD), or 2 or more CVD risk factors in the adolescent patient

Local Anesthetic/Vasoconstrictor Precautions No information available to require special precautions

Effects on Dental Treatment No significant effects or complications reported

Dosage Doses should be individualized according to the baseline LDL-cholesterol levels, the recommended goal of therapy, and the patient's response. Adjustments should be made at intervals of 4 weeks or more; doses may need adjusted based on concomitant medications.

Oral:

Children 10-17 years (females >1 year postmenarche): HeFH: 10 mg once daily in the evening; range: 10-40 mg/day (maximum: 40 mg/day)

Dosing adjustment for simvastatin with concomitant cyclosporine, fibrates, niacin, amiodarone, or verapamil: Refer to drug-specific dosing in Adults dosing section

Adults:

Homozygous familial hypercholesterolemia: 40 mg once daily in the evening **or** 80 mg/day (given as 20 mg, 20 mg, and 40 mg evening dose)

Prevention of cardiovascular events, hyperlipidemias: 20 mg once daily in the evening; range: 5-80 mg/day

Patients requiring only moderate reduction of LDL-cholesterol may be started at 10 mg once daily

Patients requiring reduction of >45% in low-density lipoprotein (LDL) cholesterol may be started at 40 mg once daily in the evening

Dosing adjustment with concomitant medications:

Cyclosporine: Initial: 5 mg simvastatin, should **not** exceed 10 mg/day

Fibrates or niacin: Simvastatin dose should **not** exceed 10 mg/day

(Continued)

Simvastatin *(Continued)*

Amiodarone or verapamil: Simvastatin dose should **not** exceed 20 mg/day

Dosing adjustment in renal impairment: Because simvastatin does not undergo significant renal excretion, modification of dose should not be necessary in patients with mild to moderate renal insufficiency.

Severe renal impairment: Cl_{cr} <10 mL/minute: Initial: 5 mg/day with close monitoring.

Mechanism of Action Simvastatin is a methylated derivative of lovastatin that acts by competitively inhibiting 3-hydroxy-3-methylglutaryl-coenzyme A (HMG-CoA) reductase, the enzyme that catalyzes the rate-limiting step in cholesterol biosynthesis

Other Adverse Effects

1% to 10%:

Gastrointestinal: Constipation (2%), dyspepsia (1%), flatulence (2%)

Neuromuscular & skeletal: CPK elevation (>3x normal on one or more occasions - 5%)

Respiratory: Upper respiratory infection (2%)

<1%: Thrombocytopenia, dizziness, headache, vertigo, weakness, fatigue, insomnia, nausea, diarrhea, abdominal pain

Postmarketing and/or case reports: Hypotension, depression, dermatomyositis, lichen planus, photosensitivity

Additional class-related events or case reports (not necessarily reported with simvastatin therapy): Alopecia, alteration in taste, anaphylaxis, angioedema, anorexia, anxiety, arthritis, cataracts, chills, cholestatic jaundice, cirrhosis, decreased libido, depression, dermatomyositis, dryness of skin/mucous membranes, dyspnea, elevated transaminases, eosinophilia, erectile dysfunction/impotence, erythema multiforme, facial paresis, fatty liver, fever, flushing, fulminant hepatic necrosis, gynecomastia, hemolytic anemia, hepatitis, hepatoma, hyperbilirubinemia, hypersensitivity reaction, impaired extraocular muscle movement, increased alkaline phosphatase, increased CPK (>10x normal), increased ESR, increased GGT, leukopenia, malaise, memory loss, myopathy, nail changes, nodules, ophthalmoplegia, pancreatitis, paresthesia, peripheral nerve palsy, peripheral neuropathy, photosensitivity, polymyalgia rheumatica, positive ANA, pruritus, psychic disturbance, purpura, rash, renal failure (secondary to rhabdomyolysis), rhabdomyolysis, skin discoloration, Stevens-Johnson syndrome, systemic lupus erythematosus-like syndrome, thrombocytopenia, thyroid dysfunction, toxic epidermal necrolysis, tremor, urticaria, vasculitis, vertigo, vomiting

Drug Interactions Substrate of **CYP3A4**; Inhibits CYP2C8/9, 2D6

Increased Effect/Toxicity: Risk of myopathy/rhabdomyolysis may be increased by concurrent use of lipid-lowering agents which may cause rhabdomyolysis (gemfibrozil, fibric acid derivatives, or niacin at doses ≥1 g/day), or during concurrent use of potent CYP3A4 inhibitors (including amiodarone, clarithromycin, cyclosporine, danazol, diltiazem, erythromycin, fluconazole, itraconazole, ketoconazole, nefazodone, verapamil or protease inhibitors such as indinavir, nelfinavir, ritonavir or saquinavir). In large quantities (ie, >1 quart/day), grapefruit juice may also increase simvastatin serum concentrations, increasing the risk of rhabdomyolysis. In general, concurrent use with CYP3A4 inhibitors is not recommended; manufacturer recommends limiting simvastatin dose to 20 mg/day when used with amiodarone or verapamil, and 10 mg/day when used with cyclosporine, gemfibrozil, or fibric acid derivatives. The anticoagulant effect of warfarin may be increased by simvastatin. Cholesterol-lowering effects are additive with bile-acid sequestrants (colestipol and cholestyramine).

Decreased Effect: When taken within 1 before or up to 2 hours after cholestyramine, a decrease in absorption of simvastatin can occur.

Dietary/Ethanol/Herb Considerations

Ethanol: Avoid excessive consumption due to potential hepatic effects.

Food: Avoid grapefruit products; may inhibit metabolism and increase serum concentration.

Herb/Nutraceutical: Avoid St John's wort; may decrease serum concentration.

Pharmacodynamics/Kinetics

Onset of action: >3 days

Peak effect: 2 weeks

Absorption: 85%

Protein binding: ~95%

Metabolism: Hepatic via CYP3A4; extensive first-pass effect

Bioavailability: <5%

Half-life elimination: Unknown

Time to peak: 1.3-2.4 hours

Excretion: Feces (60%); urine (13%)

Pregnancy Risk Factor X

Generic Available No

Sincalide (SIN ka lide)

U.S. Brand Names Kinevac®

Pharmacologic Category Diagnostic Agent

Synonyms C8-CCK; OP-CCK

Use Postevacuation cholecystography; gallbladder bile sampling; stimulate pancreatic secretion for analysis

Local Anesthetic/Vasoconstrictor Precautions No information available to require special precautions

Effects on Dental Treatment No significant effects or complications reported

Dosage Adults: I.V.:

Contraction of gallbladder: 0.02 mcg/kg over 30 seconds to 1 minute, may repeat in 15 minutes a 0.04 mcg/kg dose

Pancreatic function: 0.02 mcg/kg over 30 minutes administered after secretin

Mechanism of Action Stimulates contraction of the gallbladder and simultaneous relaxation of the sphincter of Oddi, inhibits gastric emptying, and increases intestinal motility. Graded doses have been shown to produce graded decreases in small intestinal transit time, thought to be mediated by acetylcholine.

Other Adverse Effects 1% to 10%:

Cardiovascular: Flushing

Central nervous system: Dizziness

Gastrointestinal: Nausea, abdominal pain, urge to defecate

Pharmacodynamics/Kinetics

Onset of action: Contraction of the gallbladder: ~5-15 minutes

Duration: ~1 hour

Pregnancy Risk Factor B

Generic Available No

Sinemet® *see* Levodopa and Carbidopa *on page 793*

Sinemet® CR *see* Levodopa and Carbidopa *on page 793*

Sinequan® *see* Doxepin *on page 471*

Singulair® *see* Montelukast *on page 929*

Sinus-Relief® [OTC] *see* Acetaminophen and Pseudoephedrine *on page 31*

Sinutab® Sinus Allergy Maximum Strength [OTC] *see* Acetaminophen, Chlorpheniramine, and Pseudoephedrine *on page 35*

Sinutab® Sinus Maximum Strength Without Drowsiness [OTC] *see* Acetaminophen and Pseudoephedrine *on page 31*

Sirdalud® *see* Tizanidine *on page 1314*

Sirolimus (sir OH li mus)

U.S. Brand Names Rapamune®

Canadian Brand Names Rapamune®

Pharmacologic Category Immunosuppressant Agent

Use Prophylaxis of organ rejection in patients receiving renal transplants, in combination with cyclosporine and corticosteroids

Unlabeled/Investigational Use Investigational: Immunosuppression in other forms of solid organ transplantation

Local Anesthetic/Vasoconstrictor Precautions No information available to require special precautions

Effects on Dental Treatment 3% to 20%: Otitis media

Dosage Oral:

Children ≥13 years or Adults <40 kg: Loading dose: 3 mg/m² (day 1); followed by a maintenance of 1 mg/m²/day.

Adults ≥40 kg: Loading dose: For *de novo* transplant recipients, a loading dose of 3 times the daily maintenance dose should be administered on day 1 of dosing. Maintenance dose: 2 mg/day. Doses should be taken 4 hours after cyclosporine, and should be taken consistently either with or without food.

Dosing adjustment in hepatic impairment: Reduce maintenance dose by approximately 33%; loading dose is unchanged.

Mechanism of Action Sirolimus inhibits T-lymphocyte activation and proliferation in response to antigenic and cytokine stimulation. Its mechanism differs from other immunosuppressants. It inhibits acute rejection of allografts and prolongs graft survival.

Other Adverse Effects Incidence of many adverse effects is dose-related.

>20%:

- Cardiovascular: Hypertension (39% to 49%), peripheral edema (54% to 64%), edema (16% to 24%), chest pain (16% to 24%)
- Central nervous system: Fever (23% to 34%), headache (23% to 34%), pain (24% to 33%), insomnia (13% to 22%)
- Dermatologic: Acne (20% to 31%)
- Endocrine & metabolic: Hypercholesterolemia (38% to 46%), hypophosphatemia (15% to 23%), hyperlipidemia (38% to 57%), hypokalemia (11% to 21%)

(Continued)

Sirolimus *(Continued)*

Gastrointestinal: Abdominal pain (28% to 36%), nausea (25% to 36%), vomiting (19% to 25%), diarrhea (25% to 42%), constipation (28% to 38%), dyspepsia (17% to 25%), weight gain (8% to 21%)

Genitourinary: Urinary tract infection (20% to 33%)

Hematologic: Anemia (23% to 37%), thrombocytopenia (13% to 40%)

Neuromuscular & skeletal: Arthralgia (25% to 31%), weakness (22% to 40%), back pain (16% to 26%), tremor (21% to 31%)

Renal: Increased serum creatinine (35% to 40%)

Respiratory: Dyspnea (22% to 30%), upper respiratory infection (20% to 26%), pharyngitis (16% to 21%)

3% to 20%:

Cardiovascular: Atrial fibrillation, CHF, hypervolemia, hypotension, palpitation, peripheral vascular disorder, postural hypotension, syncope, tachycardia, thrombosis, vasodilation

Central nervous system: Chills, malaise, anxiety, confusion, depression, dizziness, emotional lability, hypesthesia, hypotonia, insomnia, neuropathy, somnolence

Dermatologic: Dermatitis (fungal), hirsutism, pruritus, skin hypertrophy, dermal ulcer, ecchymosis, cellulitis, rash (10% to 20%)

Endocrine & metabolic: Cushing's syndrome, diabetes mellitus, glycosuria, acidosis, dehydration, hypercalcemia, hyperglycemia, hyperphosphatemia, hypocalcemia, hypoglycemia, hypomagnesemia, hyponatremia, hyperkalemia (12% to 17%)

Gastrointestinal: Enlarged abdomen, anorexia, dysphagia, eructation, esophagitis, flatulence, gastritis, gastroenteritis, gingivitis, gingival hyperplasia, ileus, mouth ulceration, oral moniliasis, stomatitis, weight loss

Genitourinary: Pelvic pain, scrotal edema, testis disorder, impotence

Hematologic: Leukocytosis, polycythemia, TTP, hemolytic-uremic syndrome, hemorrhage, leukopenia (9% to 15%)

Hepatic: Abnormal LFTs, increased alkaline phosphatase, increased LDH, increased transaminases, ascites

Local: Thrombophlebitis

Neuromuscular & skeletal: Increased CPK, arthrosis, bone necrosis, leg cramps, myalgia, osteoporosis, tetany, hypertonia, paresthesia

Ocular: Abnormal vision, cataract, conjunctivitis

Otic: Ear pain, deafness, otitis media, tinnitus

Renal: Increased BUN, albuminuria, bladder pain, dysuria, hematuria, hydronephrosis, kidney pain, tubular necrosis, nocturia, oliguria, pyuria, nephropathy (toxic), urinary frequency, urinary incontinence, urinary retention

Respiratory: Asthma, atelectasis, bronchitis, cough, epistaxis, hypoxia, lung edema, pleural effusion, pneumonia, rhinitis, sinusitis

Miscellaneous: Abscess, facial edema, flu-like syndrome, hernia, infection, lymphadenopathy, lymphocele, peritonitis, sepsis, diaphoresis

Postmarketing and/or case reports: Interstitial lung disease (pneumonitis, pulmonary fibrosis, and bronchiolitis obliterans organizing pneumonia) with no identified infectious etiology; fascial dehiscence; hepatic necrosis; pancytopenia; anastomotic disruption. In liver transplant patients (not an approved use), an increase in hepatic artery thrombosis and graft failure were noted in clinical trials. In lung transplant patients (not an approved use), bronchial anastomotic dehiscence have been reported.

Drug Interactions Substrate of **CYP3A4**; Inhibits CYP3A4

Increased Effect/Toxicity: Cyclosporine increases sirolimus concentrations during concurrent therapy, and cyclosporine levels may be increased. Diltiazem, ketoconazole, voriconazole, and rifampin increase serum concentrations of sirolimus. Avoid potent CYP3A4 inhibitors (ketoconazole, voriconazole). Other inhibitors of CYP3A4 (eg, calcium channel blockers, antifungal agents, macrolide antibiotics, gastrointestinal prokinetic agents, HIV-protease inhibitors) are likely to increase sirolimus concentrations.

Decreased Effect: Inducers of CYP3A4 (eg, rifampin, phenobarbital, carbamazepine, rifabutin, phenytoin) are likely to decrease serum concentrations of sirolimus.

Dietary/Ethanol/Herb Considerations

Food: Administer with food to reduce GI upset; high-fat meals decrease peak concentration but increase AUC by 35%. Administer with consistency in regard to food to minimize variability. Never mix solution with anything but water or orange juice. Avoid grapefruit products; may decrease clearance.

Herb/Nutraceutical: Avoid cat's claw and echinacea due to immunostimulant properties. Ginkgo biloba has been reported to protect the liver. Avoid St John's wort; may decrease serum concentration.

Pharmacodynamics/Kinetics

Absorption: Rapid

Distribution: 12 L/kg (± 7.52 L/kg)

Protein binding: 92%, primarily to albumin

Metabolism: Extensively hepatic via CYP3A4 and P-glycoprotein

Bioavailability: 14%
Half-life elimination: Mean: 62 hours
Time to peak: 1-3 hours
Excretion: Feces (91%); urine (2.2%)

Pregnancy Risk Factor C

Generic Available No

SK *see* Streptokinase *on page 1243*
SK and F 104864 *see* Topotecan *on page 1325*
Skelaxin® *see* Metaxalone *on page 874*
Skelid® *see* Tiludronate *on page 1309*
SKF 104864 *see* Topotecan *on page 1325*
SKF 104864-A *see* Topotecan *on page 1325*

Skin Test Antigens (Multiple) (skin test AN ti jenz, MUL ti pul)

U.S. Brand Names Multitest CMI®

Canadian Brand Names Multitest® CMI

Pharmacologic Category Diagnostic Agent

Use Detection of nonresponsiveness to antigens by means of delayed hypersensitivity skin testing

Local Anesthetic/Vasoconstrictor Precautions No information available to require special precautions

Effects on Dental Treatment No significant effects or complications reported

Dosage For percutaneous administration:

Test Head No. 1 = Tetanus toxoid antigen
Test Head No. 2 = Diphtheria toxoid antigen
Test Head No. 3 = *Streptococcus* antigen
Test Head No. 4 = Tuberculin, old
Test Head No. 5 = Glycerin negative control
Test Head No. 6 = *Candida* antigen
Test Head No. 7 = *Trichophyton* antigen
Test Head No. 8 = *Proteus* antigen

Select only test sites that permit sufficient surface area and subcutaneous tissue to allow adequate penetration of all eight points, avoid hairy areas. Press loaded unit into the skin with sufficient pressure to puncture the skin and allow adequate penetration of all points, maintain firm contact for at least 5 seconds, during application the device should not be "rocked" back and forth and side to side without removing any of the test heads from the skin sites.

If adequate pressure is applied it will be possible to observe:

1. The puncture marks of the nine tines on each of the eight test heads
2. An imprint of the circular platform surrounding each test head
3. Residual antigen and glycerin at each of the eight sites

If any of the above three criteria are not fully followed, the test results may not be reliable.

Reading should be done in good light, read the test sites at both 24 and 48 hours, the largest reaction recorded from the two readings at each test site should be used. If two readings are not possible, a single 48 hour is recommended. A positive reaction from any of the seven delayed hypersensitivity skin test antigens is **induration ≥2 mm** providing there is no induration at the negative control site. The size of the induration reactions with this test may be smaller than those obtained with other intradermal procedures.

Other Adverse Effects 1% to 10%: Local: Irritation

Pregnancy Risk Factor C

Generic Available No

Sleepinal® [OTC] *see* DiphenhydrAMINE *on page 451*
Slo-Niacin® [OTC] *see* Niacin *on page 967*
Slow FE® [OTC] *see* Iron Supplements *on page 745*
Slow-Mag® [OTC] *see* Magnesium Chloride *on page 833*
Slow-Mag® [OTC] *see* Magnesium Supplements *on page 837*
Smelling Salts *see* Ammonia Spirit (Aromatic) *on page 89*
SMZ-TMP *see* Sulfamethoxazole and Trimethoprim *on page 1253*
Sodium 4-Hydroxybutyrate *see* Sodium Oxybate *on page 1231*
Sodium Acid Carbonate *see* Sodium Bicarbonate *on page 1227*
Sodium Benzoate and Caffeine *see* Caffeine and Sodium Benzoate *on page 221*

Sodium Bicarbonate (SOW dee um bye KAR bun ate)

U.S. Brand Names Brioschi® [OTC]; Neut®

Pharmacologic Category Alkalinizing Agent; Antacid; Electrolyte Supplement, Oral; Electrolyte Supplement, Parenteral

Synonyms Baking Soda; $NaHCO_3$; Sodium Acid Carbonate; Sodium Hydrogen Carbonate

(Continued)

Sodium Bicarbonate *(Continued)*

Use Management of metabolic acidosis; gastric hyperacidity; as an alkalinization agent for the urine; treatment of hyperkalemia; management of overdose of certain drugs, including tricyclic antidepressants and aspirin

Local Anesthetic/Vasoconstrictor Precautions No information available to require special precautions

Effects on Dental Treatment No significant effects or complications reported

Dosage

Cardiac arrest: **Routine use of $NaHCO_3$ is not recommended and should be given only after adequate alveolar ventilation has been established and effective cardiac compressions are provided**

Infants and Children: I.V.: 0.5-1 mEq/kg/dose repeated every 10 minutes or as indicated by arterial blood gases; rate of infusion should not exceed 10 mEq/minute; neonates and children <2 years of age should receive 4.2% (0.5 mEq/mL) solution

Adults: I.V.: Initial: 1 mEq/kg/dose one time; maintenance: 0.5 mEq/kg/dose every 10 minutes or as indicated by arterial blood gases

Metabolic acidosis: Dosage should be based on the following formula if blood gases and pH measurements are available:

Infants and Children:

HCO_3^-(mEq) = 0.3 x weight (kg) x base deficit (mEq/L) **or**

HCO_3^-(mEq) = 0.5 x weight (kg) x [24 - serum HCO_3^- (mEq/L)]

Adults:

HCO_3^-(mEq) = 0.2 x weight (kg) x base deficit (mEq/L) **or**

HCO_3^-(mEq) = 0.5 x weight (kg) x [24 - serum HCO_3^- (mEq/L)]

If acid-base status is unavailable: Dose for older Children and Adults: 2-5 mEq/kg I.V. infusion over 4-8 hours; subsequent doses should be based on patient's acid-base status

Chronic renal failure: Oral: Initiate when plasma HCO_3^- <15 mEq/L

Children: 1-3 mEq/kg/day

Adults: Start with 20-36 mEq/day in divided doses, titrate to bicarbonate level of 18-20 mEq/L

Hyperkalemia: Adults: I.V.: 1 mEq/kg over 5 minutes

Renal tubular acidosis: Oral:

Distal:

Children: 2-3 mEq/kg/day

Adults: 0.5-2 mEq/kg/day in 4-5 divided doses

Proximal: Children: Initial: 5-10 mEq/kg/day; maintenance: Increase as required to maintain serum bicarbonate in the normal range

Urine alkalinization: Oral:

Children: 1-10 mEq (84-840 mg)/kg/day in divided doses every 4-6 hours; dose should be titrated to desired urinary pH

Adults: Initial: 48 mEq (4 g), then 12-24 mEq (1-2 g) every 4 hours; dose should be titrated to desired urinary pH; doses up to 16 g/day (200 mEq) in patients <60 years and 8 g (100 mEq) in patients >60 years

Antacid: Adults: Oral: 325 mg to 2 g 1-4 times/day

Mechanism of Action Dissociates to provide bicarbonate ion which neutralizes hydrogen ion concentration and raises blood and urinary pH

Other Adverse Effects Frequency not defined:

Cardiovascular: Cerebral hemorrhage, CHF (aggravated), edema

Central nervous system: Tetany

Gastrointestinal: Belching

Endocrine & metabolic: Hypernatremia, hyperosmolality, hypocalcemia, hypokalemia, increased affinity of hemoglobin for oxygen-reduced pH in myocardial tissue necrosis when extravasated, intracranial acidosis, metabolic alkalosis, milk-alkali syndrome (especially with renal dysfunction)

Gastrointestinal: Flatulence (with oral), gastric distension

Respiratory: Pulmonary edema

Drug Interactions

Increased Effect/Toxicity: Increased toxicity/levels of amphetamines, ephedrine, pseudoephedrine, flecainide, quinidine, and quinine due to urinary alkalinization.

Decreased Effect: Decreased effect/levels of lithium, chlorpropamide, and salicylates due to urinary alkalinization.

Dietary/Ethanol/Herb Considerations Food: Administer 1-3 hours after meals. Concurrent doses with iron may decrease iron absorption.

Pharmacodynamics/Kinetics

Onset of action: Oral: Rapid; I.V.: 15 minutes

Duration: Oral: 8-10 minutes; I.V.: 1-2 hours

Absorption: Oral: Well absorbed

Excretion: Urine (<1%)

Pregnancy Risk Factor C

Generic Available Yes

Sodium Biphosphate, Methenamine, Methylene Blue, Phenyl Salicylate, and Hyoscyamine *see* Methenamine, Sodium Biphosphate, Phenyl Salicylate, Methylene Blue, and Hyoscyamine *on page 880*

Sodium Cellulose Phosphate *see* Cellulose Sodium Phosphate *on page 284*

Sodium Chloride (SOW dee um KLOR ide)

U.S. Brand Names Altamist [OTC]; Ayr® Baby Saline [OTC]; Ayr® Saline [OTC]; Ayr® Saline Mist [OTC]; Breathe Right® Saline [OTC]; Broncho Saline® [OTC]; Entsol® [OTC]; Muro 128® [OTC]; NāSal™ [OTC]; Nasal Moist® [OTC]; Na-Zone® [OTC]; Ocean® [OTC]; Pediamist® [OTC]; Pretz® Irrigation [OTC]; SalineX® [OTC]; SeaMist® [OTC]; Simply Saline™ [OTC]; Wound Wash Saline™ [OTC]

Pharmacologic Category Electrolyte Supplement, Oral; Electrolyte Supplement, Parenteral; Lubricant, Ocular; Sodium Salt

Synonyms NaCl; Normal Saline; Salt

Use

Parenteral: Restores sodium ion in patients with restricted oral intake (especially hyponatremia states or low salt syndrome). In general, parenteral saline uses:

Bacteriostatic sodium chloride: Dilution or dissolving drugs for I.M., I.V., or S.C. injections

Concentrated sodium chloride: Additive for parenteral fluid therapy

Hypertonic sodium chloride: For severe hyponatremia and hypochloremia

Hypotonic sodium chloride: Hydrating solution

Normal saline: Restores water/sodium losses

Pharmaceutical aid/diluent for infusion of compatible drug additives

Ophthalmic: Reduces corneal edema

Oral: Restores sodium losses

Inhalation: Restores moisture to pulmonary system; loosens and thins congestion caused by colds or allergies; diluent for bronchodilator solutions that require dilution before inhalation

Intranasal: Restores moisture to nasal membranes

Irrigation: Wound cleansing, irrigation, and flushing

Local Anesthetic/Vasoconstrictor Precautions No information available to require special precautions

Effects on Dental Treatment No significant effects or complications reported

Dosage

Children: I.V.: Hypertonic solutions (>0.9%) should only be used for the initial treatment of acute serious symptomatic hyponatremia; maintenance: 3-4 mEq/kg/day; maximum: 100-150 mEq/day; dosage varies widely depending on clinical condition

Replacement: Determined by laboratory determinations mEq

Sodium deficiency (mEq/kg) = [% dehydration (L/kg)/100 x 70 (mEq/L)] + [0.6 (L/kg) x (140 - serum sodium) (mEq/L)]

Children ≥2 years and Adults:

Intranasal: 2-3 sprays in each nostril as needed

Irrigation: Spray affected area

Children and Adults: Inhalation: Bronchodilator diluent: 1-3 sprays (1-3 mL) to dilute bronchodilator solution in nebulizer prior to administration

Adults:

GU irrigant: 1-3 L/day by intermittent irrigation

Heat cramps: Oral: 0.5-1 g with full glass of water, up to 4.8 g/day

Replacement I.V.: Determined by laboratory determinations mEq

Sodium deficiency (mEq/kg) = [% dehydration (L/kg)/100 x 70 (mEq/L)] + [0.6 (L/kg) x (140 - serum sodium) (mEq/L)]

To correct acute, serious hyponatremia: mEq sodium = [desired sodium (mEq/L) - actual sodium (mEq/L)] x [0.6 x wt (kg)]; for acute correction use 125 mEq/L as the desired serum sodium; acutely correct serum sodium in 5 mEq/L/dose

Approximate Deficits of Water and Electrolytes in Moderately Severe Dehydration*

Condition	Water (mL/kg)	Sodium (mEq/kg)
Fasting and thirsting	100-120	5-7
Diarrhea		
isonatremic	100-120	8-10
hypernatremic	100-120	2-4
hyponatremic	100-120	10-12
Pyloric stenosis	100-120	8-10
Diabetic acidosis	100-120	9-10

*A **negative** deficit indicates total body **excess** prior to treatment.

Adapted from Behrman RE, Kleigman RM, Nelson WE, et al, eds, *Nelson Textbook of Pediatrics*, 14th ed, WB Saunders Co, 1992.

(Continued)

Sodium Chloride *(Continued)*

increments; more gradual correction in increments of 10 mEq/L/day is indicated in the asymptomatic patient

Chloride maintenance electrolyte requirement in parenteral nutrition: 2-4 mEq/kg/24 hours or 25-40 mEq/1000 kcals/24 hours; maximum: 100-150 mEq/24 hours

Sodium maintenance electrolyte requirement in parenteral nutrition: 3-4 mEq/kg/24 hours or 25-40 mEq/1000 kcals/24 hours; maximum: 100-150 mEq/24 hours.

Ophthalmic:

Ointment: Apply once daily or more often

Solution: Instill 1-2 drops into affected eye(s) every 3-4 hours

Mechanism of Action Principal extracellular cation; functions in fluid and electrolyte balance, osmotic pressure control, and water distribution

Other Adverse Effects Frequency not defined:

Cardiovascular: Congestive conditions

Endocrine & metabolic: Extravasation, hypervolemia, hypernatremia, dilution of serum electrolytes, overhydration, hypokalemia

Local: Thrombosis, phlebitis, extravasation

Respiratory: Pulmonary edema

Drug Interactions Decreased Effect: Lithium serum concentrations may be decreased.

Pharmacodynamics/Kinetics

Absorption: Oral, I.V.: Rapid

Distribution: Widely distributed

Excretion: Primarily urine; also sweat, tears, saliva

Pregnancy Risk Factor C

Generic Available Yes

Sodium Citrate and Citric Acid

(SOW dee um SIT rate & SI trik AS id)

U.S. Brand Names Bicitra®; Cytra-2; Oracit®

Canadian Brand Names PMS-Dicitrate™

Pharmacologic Category Alkalinizing Agent

Synonyms Modified Shohl's Solution

Use Treatment of metabolic acidosis; alkalinizing agent in conditions where long-term maintenance of an alkaline urine is desirable

Local Anesthetic/Vasoconstrictor Precautions No information available to require special precautions

Effects on Dental Treatment No significant effects or complications reported

Dosage Oral: Systemic alkalization:

Infants and Children: 2-3 mEq/kg/day in divided doses 3-4 times/day **or** 5-15 mL with water after meals and at bedtime

Adults: 10-30 mL with water after meals and at bedtime

Other Adverse Effects Frequency not defined:

Central nervous system: Tetany

Endocrine & metabolic: Metabolic alkalosis, hyperkalemia

Gastrointestinal: Diarrhea, nausea, vomiting

Drug Interactions

Increased Effect/Toxicity: Increased toxicity/levels of amphetamines, ephedrine, pseudoephedrine, flecainide, quinidine, and quinine due to urinary alkalinization.

Decreased Effect: Decreased effect/levels of lithium, chlorpropamide, and salicylates due to urinary alkalinization.

Dietary/Ethanol/Herb Considerations Food: Administer after meals to avoid laxative effect.

Pharmacodynamics/Kinetics

Metabolism: Oxidized to sodium bicarbonate

Excretion: Urine (<5% as sodium citrate)

Pregnancy Risk Factor Not established

Generic Available Yes

Sodium Citrate and Potassium Citrate Mixture *see* Citric Acid, Sodium Citrate, and Potassium Citrate *on page 335*

Sodium Citrate, Citric Acid, and Potassium Citrate *see* Citric Acid, Sodium Citrate, and Potassium Citrate *on page 335*

Sodium Edetate *see* Edetate Disodium *on page 488*

Sodium Etidronate *see* Etidronate Disodium *on page 546*

Sodium Ferric Gluconate *see* Ferric Gluconate *on page 568*

Sodium Fluoride *see* Fluoride *on page 586*

Sodium Hyaluronate

(SOW dee um hye al yoor ON ate)

U.S. Brand Names Biolon™; Healon®; Healon®5; Healon GV®; Hyalgan®; IPM Wound Gel™ [OTC]; Provisc®; Supartz™; Vitrax®

Canadian Brand Names Biolon™; Cystistat®; Eyestil; Healon®; Healon® GV; Suplasyn®

Mexican Brand Names Biolon®; Healon®

Pharmacologic Category Ophthalmic Agent, Viscoelastic; Skin and Mucous Membrane Agent

Synonyms Hyaluronic Acid

Use

Intra-articular injection (Hyalgan®): Treatment of pain in osteoarthritis in knee in patients who have failed nonpharmacologic treatment and simple analgesics

Ophthalmic: Surgical aid in cataract extraction, intraocular implantation, corneal transplant, glaucoma filtration, and retinal attachment surgery

Topical: Management of skin ulcers and wounds

Local Anesthetic/Vasoconstrictor Precautions No information available to require special precautions

Effects on Dental Treatment No significant effects or complications reported

Dosage Adults:

Intra-articular:

Hyalgen®: Inject 20 mg (2 mL) once weekly for 5 weeks; some patients may benefit with a total of 3 injections

Supartz™: Inject 25 mg (2.5 mL) once weekly for 5 weeks

Ophthalmic: Depends upon procedure (slowly introduce a sufficient quantity into eye)

Topical: Apply to clean dry ulcer or wound, and cover with nonstick dressing; repeat daily. Discontinue if wound size increase after 3-4 applications.

Mechanism of Action Functions as a tissue lubricant and is thought to play an important role in modulating the interactions between adjacent tissues. Sodium hyaluronate is a polysaccharide which is distributed widely in the extracellular matrix of connective tissue in man. (Vitreous and aqueous humor of the eye, synovial fluid, skin, and umbilical cord.) Sodium hyaluronate forms a viscoelastic solution in water (at physiological pH and ionic strength) which makes it suitable for aqueous and vitreous humor in ophthalmic surgery.

Other Adverse Effects Frequency not defined:

Central nervous system: Headache

Dermatologic: Itching

Local: Injection site: Bruising, pain, rash

Ocular: Postoperative inflammatory reactions (iritis, hypopyon), corneal edema, corneal decompensation, transient postoperative increase in IOP

Postmarketing and/or case reports: Anaphylaxis, allergic reactions, hypotensive crisis

Pharmacodynamics/Kinetics

Distribution: Intravitreous injection: Diffusion occurs slowly

Excretion: Ophthalmic: Via Canal of Schlemm

Pregnancy Risk Factor C

Generic Available No

Sodium Hyaluronate-Chrondroitin Sulfate *see* Chondroitin Sulfate and Sodium Hyaluronate *on page 320*

Sodium Hydrogen Carbonate *see* Sodium Bicarbonate *on page 1227*

Sodium Hypochlorite Solution

(SOW dee um hye poe KLORE ite soe LOO shun)

U.S. Brand Names Dakin's Solution

Pharmacologic Category Disinfectant, Antibacterial, Topical

Synonyms Dakin's Solution; Modified Dakin's Solution

Use Treatment of athlete's foot (0.5%); wound irrigation (0.5%); disinfection of utensils and equipment (5%)

Local Anesthetic/Vasoconstrictor Precautions No information available to require special precautions

Effects on Dental Treatment No significant effects or complications reported

Dosage Topical irrigation

Other Adverse Effects Frequency not defined:

Dermatologic: Irritating to skin

Hematologic: Dissolves blood clots, delays clotting

Pregnancy Risk Factor C

Generic Available No

Sodium *L*-Triiodothyronine *see* Liothyronine *on page 810*

Sodium Nafcillin *see* Nafcillin *on page 945*

Sodium Nitroferricyanide *see* Nitroprusside *on page 982*

Sodium Nitroprusside *see* Nitroprusside *on page 982*

Sodium Oxybate

(SOW dee um oks i BATE)

U.S. Brand Names Xyrem®

Pharmacologic Category Central Nervous System Depressant

(Continued)

Sodium Oxybate *(Continued)*

Synonyms Gamma Hydroxybutyric Acid; GHB; 4-Hydroxybutyrate; Sodium 4-Hydroxybutyrate

Use Orphan drug: Treatment of cataplexy in patients with narcolepsy

Local Anesthetic/Vasoconstrictor Precautions No information available to require special precautions

Effects on Dental Treatment

>10%: Dizziness (23% to 34%), headache (9% to 31%), pain (9% to 20%), somnolence (12% to 15%), confusion (9% to 14%), diaphoresis (3% to 11%), nausea (6% to 34%), vomiting (6% to 11%), pharyngitis (11%), infection (7% to 15%)

1% to 10%: Hypertension (6%), amnesia (3% to 6%), anxiety (3% to 6%), abnormal thinking (3% to 6%), agitation, convulsion, stupor, tremor

Restrictions C-I (illicit use); C-III (medical use)

Sodium oxybate oral solution will be available only to prescribers enrolled in the Xyrem® Success Program℠ and dispensed to the patient through the designated centralized pharmacy. Prior to dispensing the first prescription, prescribers will be sent educational materials to be reviewed with the patient and enrollment forms for the postmarketing surveillance program. Patients must be seen at least every 3 months; prescriptions can be written for a maximum of 3 months (the first prescription may only be written for a 1-month supply).

Dosage Oral:

Children ≥16 years and Adults: Treatment of cataplexy in patients with narcolepsy: Initial: 4.5 g/day, in 2 equal doses; first dose to be given at bedtime after the patient is in bed, and second dose to be given 2.5-4 hours later. Dose may be increased or adjusted in 2-week intervals; average dose: 6-9 g/day (maximum: 9 g/day)

Elderly: Not studied in patients >65 years

Dosing adjustment in renal impairment: None; consider sodium content

Dosing adjustment in hepatic impairment: Decrease starting dose to half and titrate doses carefully in patients with liver dysfunction. Elimination halflife significantly longer in patients with Child's class C liver dysfunction.

Mechanism of Action The exact mechanism for the efficacy of sodium oxybate the treatment of cataplexy in patients with narcolepsy is not known.

Other Adverse Effects

>10%:

Central nervous system: Sleep disorder (6% to 14%)

Genitourinary: Urinary incontinence (5% to 14%, usually nocturnal)

1% to 10%:

Cardiovascular: Edema

Central nervous system: Dream abnormality (3% to 9%), sleepwalking (7%), depression (6%), insomnia (5%), ataxia, chills

Dermatologic: Acne, alopecia, rash

Endocrine & metabolic: Dysmenorrhea (3% to 6%)

Gastrointestinal: Dyspepsia (6% to 9%), diarrhea (6% to 8%), abdominal pain (6%), anorexia, constipation, weight gain

Hepatic: Alkaline phosphatase increased, hypercholesteremia, hypocalcemia

Neuromuscular & skeletal: Hypesthesia (6%), myasthenia (3% to 6%), arthritis, leg cramps, myalgia

Ocular: Amblyopia (6%)

Otic: Tinnitus (6%)

Renal: Albuminuria, cystitis, hematuria, metrorrhagia, urinary frequency

<1%: Abdomen enlarged, akathisia, ALT/AST increased, anemia, apathy, apnea, bilirubinemia, **bruising, coma**, contact dermatitis, creatinine increased, **dehydration**, depersonalization, **epistaxis**, euphoria, hangover, **hiccup**, hyperuricemia, **hyperglycemia**, hypernatremia, hypertonia, leukocytosis, decreased libido, lymphadenopathy, **oral ulceration**, myoclonus, **neck rigidity**, neuralgia, **paralysis**, polycythemia, positive ANA test, **stomatitis, suicidal behavior/thoughts, syncope, loss of taste, thirst**, urinary urgency, urticaria

Drug Interactions Increased effect/toxicity with CNS depressants; concomitant use is contraindicated.

Dietary/Ethanol/Herb Considerations

Ethanol: Avoid use; increases CNS depression.

Food: High-fat meal decreases bioavailability, delays absorption, and decreases peak serum level. Administer on an empty stomach; separate last meal (or food) and first dose by several hours; try to take at similar time each day. Contains sodium 0.5 g per 3 g dose or 1.6 g per 9 g dose.

Herb/Nutraceutical: Avoid any products that may cause CNS depression (eg, kava kava, St John's wort, or valerian).

Pharmacodynamics/Kinetics

Absorption: Rapid

Distribution: 190-384 mL/kg

Protein binding: <1%

Metabolism: Primarily via the Krebs cycle to form water and carbon dioxide; secondarily via beta oxidation; significant first-pass effect; no active metabolites; metabolic pathways are saturable

Bioavailability: 25%

Half-life elimination: 30-60 minutes

Time to peak: 30-75 minutes

Excretion: Primarily pulmonary (as carbon dioxide); urine (<5% unchanged drug)

Pregnancy Risk Factor B

Generic Available No

Comments Sodium oxybate is a known substance of abuse. When used illegally, it has been referred to as a "date-rape drug". The dentist should be aware of patients showing signs of CNS depression, as with all other drugs in this class.

Sodium PAS *see* Aminosalicylic Acid *on page 79*

Sodium-PCA and Lactic Acid *see* Lactic Acid and Sodium-PCA *on page 771*

Sodium Phenylbutyrate (SOW dee um fen il BYOO ti rate)

U.S. Brand Names Buphenyl®

Pharmacologic Category Urea Cycle Disorder (UCD) Treatment Agent

Synonyms Ammonapse

Use Orphan drug: Adjunctive therapy in the chronic management of urea cycle disorder involving deficiencies of carbamoylphosphate synthetase, ornithine transcarbamylase, or argininosuccinic acid synthetase

Local Anesthetic/Vasoconstrictor Precautions No information available to require special precautions

Effects on Dental Treatment No significant effects or complications reported

Dosage Oral:

Powder: Patients weighing <20 kg: 450-600 mg/kg/day or 9.9-13 g/m²/day, administered in equally divided amounts with each meal or feeding, four to six times daily; safety and efficacy of doses >20 g/day has not been established

Tablet: Children >20 kg and Adults: 450-600 mg/kg/day or 9.9-13 g/m²/day, administered in equally divided amounts with each meal; safety and efficacy of doses >20 g/day have not been established

Mechanism of Action Sodium phenylbutyrate is a prodrug that, when given orally, is rapidly converted to phenylacetate, which is in turn conjugated with glutamine to form the active compound phenylacetylglutamine; phenylacetylglutamine serves as a substitute for urea and is excreted in the urine whereby it carries with it 2 moles of nitrogen per mole of phenylacetylglutamine and can thereby assist in the clearance of nitrogenous waste in patients with urea cycle disorders

Other Adverse Effects

>10%: Endocrine & metabolic: Amenorrhea, menstrual dysfunction

1% to 10%:

Gastrointestinal: Anorexia, abnormal taste

Miscellaneous: Offensive body odor

Pregnancy Risk Factor C

Generic Available No

Sodium Phosphate *see* Phosphate Supplements *on page 1076*

Sodium Sulfacetamide *see* Sulfacetamide *on page 1249*

Sodium Thiosulfate (SOW dee um thye oh SUL fate)

U.S. Brand Names Versiclear™

Pharmacologic Category Antidote

Use

Parenteral: Used alone or with sodium nitrite or amyl nitrite in cyanide poisoning or arsenic poisoning; reduce the risk of nephrotoxicity associated with cisplatin therapy

Topical: Treatment of tinea versicolor

Local Anesthetic/Vasoconstrictor Precautions No information available to require special precautions

Effects on Dental Treatment No significant effects or complications reported

Dosage

Cyanide and nitroprusside antidote: I.V.:

Children <25 kg: 50 mg/kg after receiving 4.5-10 mg/kg sodium nitrite; a half dose of each may be repeated if necessary

Children >25 kg and Adults: 12.5 g after 300 mg of sodium nitrite; a half dose of each may be repeated if necessary

Cyanide poisoning: I.V.: Dose should be based on determination as with nitrite, at rate of 2.5-5 mL/minute to maximum of 50 mL.

Variation of sodium nitrate and sodium thiosulfate dose, based on hemoglobin concentration*: See table on next page.

Cisplatin rescue should be given before or during cisplatin administration: I.V. infusion (in sterile water): 12 g/m² over 6 hours or 9 g/m² I.V. push followed by 1.2 g/m² continuous infusion for 6 hours

(Continued)

Sodium Thiosulfate *(Continued)*

Variation of Sodium Nitrite and Sodium Thiosulfate Dose With Hemoglobin Concentration*

Hemoglobin (g/dL)	Initial Dose Sodium Nitrite (mg/kg)	Initial Dose Sodium Nitrite 3% (mL/kg)	Initial Dose Sodium Thiosulfate 25% (mL/kg)
7	5.8	0.19	0.95
8	6.6	0.22	1.10
9	7.5	0.25	1.25
10	8.3	0.27	1.35
11	9.1	0.30	1.50
12	10.0	0.33	1.65
13	10.8	0.36	1.80
14	11.6	0.39	1.95

*Adapted from Berlin DM Jr, "The Treatment of Cyanide Poisoning in Children," *Pediatrics*, 1970, 46:793.

Arsenic poisoning: I.V.: 1 mL first day, 2 mL second day, 3 mL third day, 4 mL fourth day, 5 mL on alternate days thereafter

Children and Adults: Topical: 20% to 25% solution: Apply a thin layer to affected areas twice daily

Mechanism of Action

Cyanide toxicity: Increases the rate of detoxification of cyanide by the enzyme rhodanese by providing an extra sulfur

Cisplatin toxicity: Complexes with cisplatin to form a compound that is nontoxic to either normal or cancerous cells

Other Adverse Effects 1% to 10%:

Cardiovascular: Hypotension

Central nervous system: Coma, CNS depression secondary to thiocyanate intoxication, psychosis, confusion

Dermatologic: Contact dermatitis, local irritation

Neuromuscular & skeletal: Weakness

Otic: Tinnitus

Pharmacodynamics/Kinetics

Absorption: Oral: Poor

Distribution: Extracellular fluid

Half-life elimination: 0.65 hour

Excretion: Urine (28.5% as unchanged drug)

Pregnancy Risk Factor C

Generic Available Yes: Injection

Comments White, odorless crystals or powder with a salty taste; normal body burden: 1.5 mg/kg

Solagé™ *see* Mequinol and Tretinoin *on page 865*

Solaquin® [OTC] *see* Hydroquinone *on page 693*

Solaquin Forte® *see* Hydroquinone *on page 693*

Solaraze™ *see* Diclofenac *on page 429*

Solarcaine® [OTC] *see* Benzocaine *on page 169*

Solarcaine® Aloe Extra Burn Relief [OTC] *see* Lidocaine *on page 801*

Solganal® *see* Aurothioglucose *on page 148*

Solu-Cortef® *see* Hydrocortisone *on page 688*

Solu-Medrol® *see* MethylPREDNISolone *on page 895*

Solurex® *see* Dexamethasone *on page 413*

Solurex L.A.® *see* Dexamethasone *on page 413*

Soma® *see* Carisoprodol *on page 251*

Soma® Compound *see* Carisoprodol and Aspirin *on page 252*

Soma® Compound w/Codeine *see* Carisoprodol, Aspirin, and Codeine *on page 252*

Somatrem *see* Human Growth Hormone *on page 671*

Somatropin *see* Human Growth Hormone *on page 671*

Sominex® [OTC] *see* DiphenhydrAMINE *on page 451*

Sominex® Maximum Strength [OTC] *see* DiphenhydrAMINE *on page 451*

Sonata® *see* Zaleplon *on page 1404*

Sorbitol (SOR bi tole)

Pharmacologic Category Genitourinary Irrigant; Laxative, Miscellaneous

Use Genitourinary irrigant in transurethral prostatic resection or other transurethral resection or other transurethral surgical procedures; diuretic; humectant; sweetening agent; hyperosmotic laxative; facilitate the passage of sodium polystyrene sulfonate through the intestinal tract

Local Anesthetic/Vasoconstrictor Precautions No information available to require special precautions

Effects on Dental Treatment No significant effects or complications reported

Dosage Hyperosmotic laxative (as single dose, at infrequent intervals):

Children 2-11 years:

Oral: 2 mL/kg (as 70% solution)

Rectal enema: 30-60 mL as 25% to 30% solution

Children >12 years and Adults:

Oral: 30-150 mL (as 70% solution)

Rectal enema: 120 mL as 25% to 30% solution

Adjunct to sodium polystyrene sulfonate: 15 mL as 70% solution orally until diarrhea occurs (10-20 mL/2 hours) or 20-100 mL as an oral vehicle for the sodium polystyrene sulfonate resin

When administered with charcoal:

Oral:

Children: 4.3 mL/kg of 35% sorbitol with 1 g/kg of activated charcoal

Adults: 4.3 mL/kg of 70% sorbitol with 1 g/kg of activated charcoal every 4 hours until first stool containing charcoal is passed

Topical: 3% to 3.3% as transurethral surgical procedure irrigation

Mechanism of Action A polyalcoholic sugar with osmotic cathartic actions

Other Adverse Effects Frequency not defined:

Cardiovascular: Edema

Endocrine & metabolic: Fluid and electrolyte losses, lactic acidosis

Gastrointestinal: Diarrhea, nausea, vomiting, abdominal discomfort, xerostomia

Pharmacodynamics/Kinetics

Onset of action: 0.25-1 hour

Absorption: Oral, rectal: Poor

Metabolism: Primarily hepatic to fructose

Generic Available Yes

Sorine® *see* Sotalol *on page 1235*

Sotalol (SOE tu lole)

Related Information

Cardiovascular Diseases *on page 1456*

U.S. Brand Names Betapace®; Betapace AF®; Sorine®

Canadian Brand Names Alti-Sotalol; Apo®-Sotalol; Betapace AF™; Gen-Sotalol; Lin-Sotalol; Novo-Sotalol; Nu-Sotalol; PMS-Sotalol; Rho®-Sotalol; Sotacor®

Pharmacologic Category Antiarrhythmic Agent, Class II; Antiarrhythmic Agent, Class III; Beta Blocker, Nonselective

Synonyms Sotalol Hydrochloride

Use Treatment of documented ventricular arrhythmias (ie, sustained ventricular tachycardia), that in the judgment of the physician are life-threatening; maintenance of normal sinus rhythm in patients with symptomatic atrial fibrillation and atrial flutter who are currently in sinus rhythm. Manufacturer states substitutions should not be made for Betapace AF® since Betapace AF® is distributed with a patient package insert specific for atrial fibrillation/flutter.

Local Anesthetic/Vasoconstrictor Precautions Use with caution; epinephrine has interacted with nonselective beta-blockers to result in initial hypertensive episode followed by bradycardia

Effects on Dental Treatment Sotalol is a nonselective beta-blocker and may enhance the pressor response to epinephrine, resulting in hypertension and bradycardia. Many nonsteroidal anti-inflammatory drugs such as ibuprofen and indomethacin can reduce the hypotensive effect of beta-blockers after 3 or more weeks of therapy with the NSAID. Short-term NSAID use (ie, 3 days) requires no special precautions in patients taking beta-blockers.

Dosage Sotalol should be initiated and doses increased in a hospital with facilities for cardiac rhythm monitoring and assessment. Proarrhythmic events can occur after initiation of therapy and with each upward dosage adjustment.

Children: Oral: The safety and efficacy of sotalol in children have not been established

Note: Dosing per manufacturer, based on pediatric pharmacokinetic data; wait at least 36 hours between dosage adjustments to allow monitoring of QT intervals

≤2 years: Dosage should be adjusted (decreased) by plotting of the child's age on a logarithmic scale; see graph or refer to manufacturer's package labeling.

>2 years: Initial: 90 mg/m²/day in 3 divided doses; may be incrementally increased to a maximum of 180 mg/m²/day

Adults: Oral:

Ventricular arrhythmias (Betapace®, Sorine®):

Initial: 80 mg twice daily

Dose may be increased gradually to 240-320 mg/day; allow 3 days between dosing increments in order to attain steady-state plasma concentrations and to allow monitoring of QT intervals

Most patients respond to a total daily dose of 160-320 mg/day in 2-3 divided doses.

(Continued)

Sotalol *(Continued)*

Sotalol Age Factor Nomogram for Patients ≤2 Years of Age

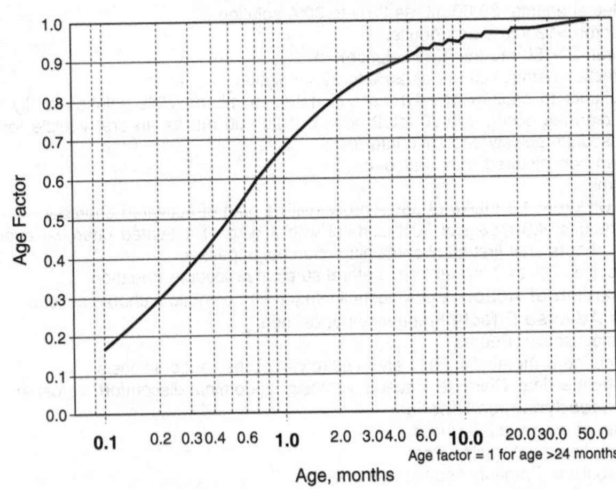

Adapted from U.S. Food and Drug Administration. http://www.fda.gov/cder/foi/label/2001/2115s3lbl.PDF

Some patients, with life-threatening refractory ventricular arrhythmias, may require doses as high as 480-640 mg/day; however, these doses should only be prescribed when the potential benefit outweighs the increased of adverse events.

Atrial fibrillation or atrial flutter (Betapace AF®): Initial: 80 mg twice daily

If the initial dose does not reduce the frequency of relapses of atrial fibrillation/flutter and is tolerated without excessive QT prolongation (not >520 msec) after 3 days, the dose may be increased to 120 mg twice daily. This may be further increased to 160 mg twice daily if response is inadequate and QT prolongation is not excessive.

Elderly: Age does not significantly alter the pharmacokinetics of sotalol, but impaired renal function in elderly patients can increase the terminal halflife, resulting in increased drug accumulation

Dosing adjustment in renal impairment:

Children: Safety and efficacy not established.

Adults: Impaired renal function can increase the terminal halflife, resulting in increased drug accumulation. Sotalol (Betapace AF®) is contraindicated per the manufacturer for treatment of atrial fibrillation/flutter in patients with a Cl_{cr} <40 mL/minute.

Ventricular arrhythmias (Betapace®, Sorine®):

Cl_{cr} >60 mL/minute: Administer every 12 hours
Cl_{cr} 30-60 mL/minute: Administer every 24 hours
Cl_{cr} 10-30 mL/minute: Administer every 36-48 hours
Cl_{cr} <10 mL/minute: Individualize dose

Atrial fibrillation/flutter (Betapace AF®):

Cl_{cr} >60 mL/minute: Administer every 12 hours
Cl_{cr} 40-60 mL/minute: Administer every 24 hours
Cl_{cr} <40 mL/minute: Use is contraindicated

Dialysis: Hemodialysis would be expected to reduce sotalol plasma concentrations because sotalol is not bound to plasma proteins and does not undergo extensive metabolism; administer dose postdialysis or administer supplemental 80 mg dose; peritoneal dialysis does not remove sotalol; supplemental dose is unnecessary

Mechanism of Action

Beta-blocker which contains both beta-adrenoreceptor-blocking (Vaughan Williams Class II) and cardiac action potential duration prolongation (Vaughan Williams Class III) properties

Class II effects: Increased sinus cycle length, slowed heart rate, decreased AV nodal conduction, and increased AV nodal refractoriness

Class III effects: Prolongation of the atrial and ventricular monophasic action potentials, and effective refractory prolongation of atrial muscle, ventricular muscle, and atrioventricular accessory pathways in both the antegrade and retrograde directions

Sotalol is a racemic mixture of *d*- and *l*-sotalol; both isomers have similar Class III antiarrhythmic effects while the *l*-isomer is responsible for virtually all of the beta-blocking activity

Sotalol has both $beta_1$- and $beta_2$-receptor blocking activity

The beta-blocking effect of sotalol is a noncardioselective [half maximal at about 80 mg/day and maximal at doses of 320-640 mg/day]. Significant beta-blockade occurs at oral doses as low as 25 mg/day.

The Class III effects are seen only at oral doses ≥160 mg/day

Other Adverse Effects

>10%:

- Cardiovascular: Bradycardia (16%), chest pain (16%), palpitations (14%)
- Central nervous system: Fatigue (20%), dizziness (20%), lightheadedness (12%)
- Neuromuscular & skeletal: Weakness (13%)
- Respiratory: Dyspnea (21%)

1% to 10%:

- Cardiovascular: Congestive heart failure (5%), peripheral vascular disorders (3%), edema (8%), abnormal EKG (7%), hypotension (6%), proarrhythmia (5%), syncope (5%)
- Central nervous system: Mental confusion (6%), anxiety (4%), headache (8%), sleep problems (8%), depression (4%)
- Dermatologic: Itching/rash (5%)
- Endocrine & metabolic: Decreased sexual ability (3%)
- Gastrointestinal: Diarrhea (7%), nausea/vomiting (10%), stomach discomfort (3% to 6%), flatulence (2%)
- Genitourinary: Impotence (2%)
- Hematologic: Bleeding (2%)
- Neuromuscular & skeletal: Paresthesia (4%), extremity pain (7%), back pain (3%)
- Ocular: Visual problems (5%)
- Respiratory: Upper respiratory problems (5% to 8%), asthma (2%)

<1% (Limited to important or life-threatening): Raynaud's phenomenon, red crusted skin, skin necrosis after extravasation, phlebitis, diaphoresis, cold extremities, increased serum transaminases, emotional lability, clouded sensorium, incoordination, vertigo, paralysis, thrombocytopenia, eosinophilia, leukopenia, photosensitivity reaction, fever, pulmonary edema, hyperlipidemia, myalgia, pruritus, alopecia, xerostomia

Postmarketing and/or case reports: Leukocytoclastic vasculitis, retroperitoneal fibrosis, bronchiolitis obliterans with organized pneumonia

Drug Interactions

Increased Effect/Toxicity: Increased effect/toxicity of beta-blockers with calcium blockers since there may be additive effects on AV conduction or ventricular function. Sotalol in combination with amiodarone. Other agents which prolong QT interval, including Class I antiarrhythmic agents, bepridil, cisapride (use is contraindicated), erythromycin, haloperidol, pimozide, phenothiazines, tricyclic antidepressants, specific quinolones (sparfloxacin, gatifloxacin, moxifloxacin), or astemizole may increase the effect of sotalol on the prolongation of QT interval. When used concurrently with clonidine, sotalol may increase the risk of rebound hypertension after or during withdrawal of either agent. Beta-blocker and catecholamine depleting agents (reserpine or guanethidine) may result in additive hypotension or bradycardia. Beta-blockers may increase the action or levels of ethanol, nondepolarizing muscle relaxants, and theophylline although the effects are difficult to predict.

Decreased Effect: Decreased effect of sotalol may occur with aluminum-magnesium antacids (if taken within 2 hours), aluminum salts, barbiturates, calcium salts, cholestyramine, colestipol, NSAIDs, penicillins (ampicillin), rifampin, salicylates, and sulfinpyrazone due to decreased bioavailability and plasma levels. Beta-blockers may decrease the effect of sulfonylureas. Beta-agonists such as albuterol, terbutaline may have less of a therapeutic effect when administered concomitantly.

Dietary/Ethanol/Herb Considerations

Ethanol: Limit use; may increase risk of hypotension or dizziness.

Food: Administer on an empty stomach; food decreases absorption 20% to 30%. Fluids, fruit, and fiber may reduce constipation. Avoid caffeine (eg, colas, chocolate), garlic, and licorice.

Herb/Nutraceutical: Avoid black cohosh, dong quai, and evening primrose due to estrogenic activity. Avoid ephedra, ginseng, and yohimbe; may worsen arrhythmia. Avoid garlic; may have increased antihypertensive effect. Avoid ginger due to positive inotropic effects; theoretically, may cause arrhythmia. Avoid hawthorn; may have cardiac electrophysiology effects like class III antiarrhythmics. Avoid licorice.

Pharmacodynamics/Kinetics

Onset of action: Rapid, 1-2 hours

Peak effect: 2.5-4 hours

Duration: 8-16 hours

Absorption: Decreased 20% to 30% by meals compared to fasting

(Continued)

Sotalol *(Continued)*

Distribution: Low lipid solubility; enters milk of laboratory animals and is reported to be present in human milk
Protein binding: None
Metabolism: None
Bioavailability: 90% to 100%
Half-life elimination: 12 hours; Children: 9.5 hours; terminal half-life decreases with age <2 years (may by ≥1 week in neonates)
Excretion: Urine (as unchanged drug)

Pregnancy Risk Factor B

Generic Available Yes: Betapace®, Sorine®

Selected Readings

Foster CA and Aston SJ, "Propranolol-Epinephrine Interaction: A Potential Disaster," *Plast Reconstr Surg*, 1983, 72(1):74-8.
Wong DG, Spence JD, Lamki L, et al, "Effect of Nonsteroidal Anti-inflammatory Drugs on Control of Hypertension of Beta-Blockers and Diuretics," *Lancet*, 1986, 1(8488):997-1001.
Wynn RL, "Dental Nonsteroidal Anti-inflammatory Drugs and Prostaglandin-Based Drug Interactions, Part Two," *Gen Dent*, 1992, 40(2):104, 106, 108.
Wynn RL, "Epinephrine Interactions With Beta-Blockers," *Gen Dent*, 1994, 42(1):16, 18.

Sotalol Hydrochloride *see* Sotalol *on page 1235*
Spacol *see* Hyoscyamine *on page 699*
Spacol T/S *see* Hyoscyamine *on page 699*

Sparfloxacin (spar FLOKS a sin)

U.S. Brand Names Zagam®

Pharmacologic Category Antibiotic, Quinolone

Use Treatment of adults with community-acquired pneumonia caused by *C. pneumoniae, H. influenzae, H. parainfluenzae, M. catarrhalis, M. pneumoniae* or *S. pneumoniae*; treatment of acute bacterial exacerbations of chronic bronchitis caused by *C. pneumoniae, E. cloacae, H. influenzae, H. parainfluenzae, K. pneumoniae, M. catarrhalis, S. aureus* or *S. pneumoniae*

Local Anesthetic/Vasoconstrictor Precautions No information available to require special precautions

Effects on Dental Treatment No significant effects or complications reported

Dosage Adults: Oral:
Loading dose: 2 tablets (400 mg) on day 1
Maintenance: 1 tablet (200 mg) daily for 10 days total therapy (total 11 tablets)
Dosing adjustment in renal impairment: Cl_{cr} <50 mL/minute: Administer 400 mg on day 1, then 200 mg every 48 hours for a total of 9 days of therapy (total 6 tablets)

Mechanism of Action Inhibits DNA-gyrase in susceptible organisms; inhibits relaxation of supercoiled DNA and promotes breakage of double-stranded DNA

Other Adverse Effects
1% to 10%:
Cardiovascular: QT_c interval prolongation (1.3%)
Central nervous system: Insomnia, dizziness, headache, agitation, sleep disorders, anxiety, delirium
Dermatologic: Photosensitivity reaction, pruritus, vasodilatation
Gastrointestinal: Diarrhea, dyspepsia, nausea, abdominal pain, vomiting, flatulence, abnormal taste, xerostomia
Hematologic: Leukopenia, eosinophilia, anemia
Hepatic: Increased LFTs
<1% (Limited to important or life-threatening): Arrhythmias, angina pectoris, atrial fibrillation, atrial flutter, complete AV block, postural hypotension, migraine, ecchymosis, exfoliative dermatitis, angioedema, asthma, dyspnea; quinolones have been associated with tendonitis and tendon rupture

Drug Interactions Inhibits **CYP1A2**
Increased Effect/Toxicity: Quinolones cause increased levels of caffeine, warfarin, cyclosporine, and theophylline (although one study indicates that sparfloxacin may not affect theophylline metabolism). Cimetidine, and probenecid increase quinolone levels. An increased incidence of seizures may occur with foscarnet and NSAIDs. Sparfloxacin does not appear to alter warfarin levels, but warfarin effect may be increased due possible effects on gastrointestinal flora. Concurrent use of corticosteroids may increase risk of tendon rupture.
Decreased Effect: Decreased absorption with antacids containing aluminum, didanosine (chewable/buffered tablets or pediatric powder for oral solution), magnesium, zinc, iron and/or calcium (by up to 98% if given at the same time). Phenytoin serum levels may be reduced by quinolones. Antineoplastic agents may also decrease serum levels of fluoroquinolones.

Dietary/Ethanol/Herb Considerations Herb/Nutraceutical: Avoid dong quai and St John's wort; may cause photosensitization.

Pharmacodynamics/Kinetics
Absorption: Unaffected by food or milk; reduced ~50% by concurrent administration of aluminum- and magnesium-containing antacids
Distribution: Widely throughout the body
Metabolism: Hepatic, but does not utilize CYP

Half-life elimination: Mean terminal: 20 hours (range: 16-30 hours)
Time to peak, serum: 3-5 hours
Excretion: Urine (~10% as unchanged drug) and feces (equal amounts)

Pregnancy Risk Factor C

Generic Available No

Spectazole® *see* Econazole *on page 486*

Spectinomycin (spek ti noe MYE sin)

Related Information

Nonviral Infectious Diseases *on page 1493*
Sexually-Transmitted Diseases *on page 1502*

U.S. Brand Names Trobicin®

Mexican Brand Names Trobicin®

Pharmacologic Category Antibiotic, Miscellaneous

Synonyms Spectinomycin Hydrochloride

Use Treatment of uncomplicated gonorrhea

Local Anesthetic/Vasoconstrictor Precautions No information available to require special precautions

Effects on Dental Treatment No significant effects or complications reported

Dosage I.M.:

Children:
<45 kg: 40 mg/kg/dose 1 time (ceftriaxone preferred)
≥45 kg: Refer to adult dosing.

Children >8 years who are allergic to PCNS/cephalosporins may be treated with oral tetracycline

Adults:
Uncomplicated urethral, cervical, pharyngeal, or rectal gonorrhea: 2 g deep I.M. or 4 g where antibiotic resistance is prevalent 1 time; 4 g (10 mL) dose should be given as two 5 mL injections, followed by adequate chlamydial treatment (doxycycline 100 mg twice daily for 7 days)
Disseminated gonococcal infection: 2 g every 12 hours

Hemodialysis: 50% removed by hemodialysis

Mechanism of Action A bacteriostatic antibiotic that selectively binds to the 30s subunits of ribosomes, and thereby inhibiting bacterial protein synthesis

Other Adverse Effects <1%: Chills, dizziness, headache, nausea, pain at injection site, pruritus, rash, urticaria, vomiting

Pharmacodynamics/Kinetics

Duration: Up to 8 hours
Absorption: I.M.: Rapid and almost complete
Distribution: Concentrates in urine; does not distribute well into the saliva
Half-life elimination: 1.7 hours
Time to peak: ~1 hour
Excretion: Urine (70% to 100% as unchanged drug)

Pregnancy Risk Factor B

Generic Available No

Spectinomycin Hydrochloride *see* Spectinomycin *on page 1239*

Spectracef™ *see* Cefditoren *on page 265*

Spectrocin Plus® [OTC] *see* Bacitracin, Neomycin, Polymyxin B, and Lidocaine *on page 158*

Spiramycin (speer a MYE sin)

Canadian Brand Names Rovamycine®

Pharmacologic Category Antibiotic, Macrolide

Use Treatment of infections of the respiratory tract, buccal cavity, skin and soft tissues due to susceptible organisms. *N. gonorrhoeae*: as an alternate choice of treatment for gonorrhea in patients allergic to the penicillins. Before treatment of gonorrhea, the possibility of concomitant infection due to *T. pallidum* should be excluded.

Unlabeled/Investigational Use Treatment of *Toxoplasma gondii* to prevent transmission from mother to fetus

Local Anesthetic/Vasoconstrictor Precautions No information available to require special precautions

Effects on Dental Treatment No significant effects or complications reported

Dosage Oral:

Children: Dosage by body weight; usual dosage 150,000 int. units/kg; expressed as the number of 750,000 int. unit (Rovamycine® "250") capsules per day. Daily dose should be administered in 2-3 divided doses.
15 kg = 3 capsules per day
20 kg = 4 capsules per day
30 kg = 6 capsules per day
Note: In severe infections, dosage may be increased by 50%.

(Continued)

Spiramycin *(Continued)*

Adults:

Mild to moderate infections: 6,000,000 to 9,000,000 int. units (4-6 capsules of Rovamycine® "500" per day) in 2 divided doses

Severe infections: 12,000,000 to 15,000,000 int. units (8-10 capsules of Rovamycine® "500" per day) in 2 divided doses

Gonorrhea: 12,000,000 to 13,500,000 int. units (8-9 capsules of Rovamycine® "500") as a single dose

Mechanism of Action Inhibits growth of susceptible organisms; mechanism not established.

Other Adverse Effects Frequency not defined:

Central nervous system: Paresthesia (rare)

Dermatologic: Rash, urticaria, pruritus, angioedema (rare)

Gastrointestinal: Nausea, vomiting, diarrhea, pseudomembranous colitis (rare)

Hepatic: Transaminases increased

Miscellaneous: Anaphylactic shock (rare)

Note: Rare adverse reactions associated with other macrolide antibiotics include life-threatening ventricular arrhythmias, prolongation of QT_c, and neuromuscular blockade.

Drug Interactions Substrate of **CYP3A4**

Decreased Effect: Reported to decrease carbidopa absorption and decrease levodopa concentrations.

Dietary/Ethanol/Herb Considerations Food: Administer with food to reduce GI upset.

Pregnancy Risk Factor Not assigned (other macrolides rated B); C per expert analysis

Generic Available No

Spironolactone (speer on oh LAK tone)

Related Information

Cardiovascular Diseases *on page 1456*

U.S. Brand Names Aldactone®

Canadian Brand Names Aldactone®; Novo-Spiroton

Mexican Brand Names Aldactone®

Pharmacologic Category Diuretic, Potassium Sparing

Use Management of edema associated with excessive aldosterone excretion; hypertension; primary hyperaldosteronism; hypokalemia; treatment of hirsutism; cirrhosis of liver accompanied by edema or ascites. The benefits of spironolactone were additive to the benefits of ACE inhibition in patients with severe CHF (further reducing mortality by 30% over 2 years) in RALES - a large controlled clinical trial.

Local Anesthetic/Vasoconstrictor Precautions No information available to require special precautions

Effects on Dental Treatment No significant effects or complications reported

Dosage To reduce delay in onset of effect, a loading dose of 2 or 3 times the daily dose may be administered on the first day of therapy. Oral:

Neonates: Diuretic: 1-3 mg/kg/day divided every 12-24 hours

Children:

Diuretic, hypertension: 1.5-3.5 mg/kg/day **or** 60 mg/m²/day in divided doses every 6-24 hours

Diagnosis of primary aldosteronism: 125-375 mg/m²/day in divided doses

Vaso-occlusive disease: 7.5 mg/kg/day in divided doses twice daily (not FDA approved)

Adults:

Edema, hypertension, hypokalemia: 25-200 mg/day in 1-2 divided doses

Diagnosis of primary aldosteronism: 100-400 mg/day in 1-2 divided doses

Hirsutism in women: 50-200 mg/day in 1-2 divided doses

CHF, severe (with ACE inhibitor and a loop diuretic ± digoxin): 25 mg/day, increased or reduced depending on individual response and evidence of hyperkalemia

Elderly: Initial: 25-50 mg/day in 1-2 divided doses, increasing by 25-50 mg every 5 days as needed.

Dosing interval in renal impairment:

Cl_{cr} 10-50 mL/minute: Administer every 12-24 hours.

Cl_{cr} <10 mL/minute: Avoid use.

Mechanism of Action Competes with aldosterone for receptor sites in the distal renal tubules, increasing sodium chloride and water excretion while conserving potassium and hydrogen ions; may block the effect of aldosterone on arteriolar smooth muscle as well

Other Adverse Effects Incidence of adverse events is not always reported. (Mean daily dose: 26 mg)

Cardiovascular: Edema (2%, placebo 2%)

Central nervous system: Disorders (23%, placebo 21%) which may include drowsiness, lethargy, headache, mental confusion, drug fever, ataxia, fatigue

Dermatologic: Maculopapular, erythematous cutaneous eruptions, urticaria, hirsutism, eosinophilia

Endocrine & metabolic: Gynecomastia (men 9%; placebo 1%), breast pain (men 2%; placebo 0.1%), serious hyperkalemia (2%, placebo 1%), hyponatremia, dehydration, hyperchloremic metabolic acidosis in decompensated hepatic cirrhosis, inability to achieve or maintain an erection, irregular menses, amenorrhea, postmenopausal bleeding

Gastrointestinal: Disorders (29%, placebo 29%) which may include anorexia, nausea, cramping, diarrhea, gastric bleeding, ulceration, gastritis, vomiting

Genitourinary: Disorders (12%, placebo 11%)

Hematologic: Agranulocytosis

Hepatic: Cholestatic/hepatocellular toxicity

Renal: Increased BUN concentration

Respiratory: Disorders (32%, placebo 34%)

Miscellaneous: Deepening of the voice, anaphylactic reaction, breast cancer

Drug Interactions

Increased Effect/Toxicity: Concurrent use of spironolactone with other potassium-sparing diuretics, potassium supplements, angiotensin-receptor antagonists, co-trimoxazole (high dose), and ACE inhibitors can increase the risk of hyperkalemia, especially in patients with renal impairment. Cholestyramine can cause hyperchloremic acidosis in cirrhotic patients; avoid concurrent use.

Decreased Effect: The effects of digoxin (loss of positive inotropic effect) and mitotane may be reduced by spironolactone. Salicylates and NSAIDs (indomethacin) may decrease the natriuretic effect of spironolactone.

Dietary/Ethanol/Herb Considerations

Food: Administer with food or milk to increase absorption. Avoid salt substitutes or low-salt milk; diuretic does not cause potassium loss and ingestion of these products may result in additional potassium. Avoid licorice; glycyrrhizic acid has aldosterone properties and may antagonize effects.

Herb/Nutraceutical: Avoid hawthorn; may decrease peripheral vascular resistance and cause additive decrease in BP. Avoid licorice due to mineralocorticoid activity.

Pharmacodynamics/Kinetics

Protein binding: 91% to 98%

Metabolism: Hepatic to multiple metabolites, including canrenone (active)

Half-life elimination: 78-84 minutes

Time to peak, serum: 1-3 hours (primarily as the active metabolite)

Excretion: Urine and feces

Pregnancy Risk Factor C/D in pregnancy-induced hypertension (per expert analysis)

Generic Available Yes

Spironolactone and Hydrochlorothiazide *see* Hydrochlorothiazide and Spironolactone *on page 677*

Sporanox® *see* Itraconazole *on page 755*

Sportscreme® [OTC] *see* Triethanolamine Salicylate *on page 1348*

SSD® *see* Silver Sulfadiazine *on page 1222*

SSD® AF *see* Silver Sulfadiazine *on page 1222*

SSKI® *see* Potassium Iodide *on page 1101*

Stadol® *see* Butorphanol *on page 218*

Stadol® NS *see* Butorphanol *on page 218*

Stagesic® *see* Hydrocodone and Acetaminophen *on page 678*

Stan-gard® *see* Fluoride *on page 586*

Stannous Fluoride *see* Fluoride *on page 586*

Stanozolol (stan OH zoe lole)

U.S. Brand Names Winstrol®

Pharmacologic Category Anabolic Steroid

Use Prophylactic use against hereditary angioedema

Local Anesthetic/Vasoconstrictor Precautions No information available to require special precautions

Effects on Dental Treatment No significant effects or complications reported

Restrictions C-III

Dosage

Children: Acute attacks:

<6 years: 1 mg/day

6-12 years: 2 mg/day

Adults: Oral: Initial: 2 mg 3 times/day, may then reduce to a maintenance dose of 2 mg/day or 2 mg every other day after 1-3 months

Dosing adjustment in hepatic impairment: Use not recommended in severe dysfunction

Mechanism of Action Synthetic testosterone derivative with similar androgenic and anabolic actions

(Continued)

Stanozolol *(Continued)*

Other Adverse Effects

Male:

Postpubertal:

>10%:

Dermatologic: Acne

Endocrine & metabolic: Gynecomastia

Genitourinary: Bladder irritability, priapism

1% to 10%:

Central nervous system: Insomnia, chills

Endocrine & metabolic: Decreased libido, hepatic dysfunction

Gastrointestinal: Nausea, diarrhea

Genitourinary: Prostatic hyperplasia (elderly)

Hematologic: Iron-deficiency anemia, suppression of clotting factors

<1%: Hepatic necrosis, hepatocellular carcinoma

Prepubertal:

>10%:

Dermatologic: Acne

Endocrine & metabolic: Virilism

1% to 10%:

Central nervous system: Chills, insomnia, factors

Dermatologic: Hyperpigmentation

Gastrointestinal: Diarrhea, nausea

Hematologic: Iron deficiency anemia, suppression of clotting

<1%: Hepatic necrosis, hepatocellular carcinoma

Female:

>10%: Endocrine & metabolic: Virilism

1% to 10%:

Central nervous system: Chills, insomnia

Endocrine & metabolic: Hypercalcemia

Gastrointestinal: Nausea, diarrhea

Hematologic: Iron deficiency anemia, suppression of clotting factors

Hepatic: Hepatic dysfunction

<1%: Hepatic necrosis, hepatocellular carcinoma

Drug Interactions Increased Effect/Toxicity: ACTH, adrenal steroids may increase risk of edema and acne. Stanozolol enhances the hypoprothrombinemic effects of oral anticoagulants and enhances the hypoglycemic effects of insulin and sulfonylureas (oral hypoglycemics).

Pharmacodynamics/Kinetics

Metabolism: Hepatic

Excretion: Urine (90%); feces (6%)

Pregnancy Risk Factor X

Generic Available No

Staticin® *see* Erythromycin *on page 512*

Stat Touch 2 [OTC] [DSC] *see* Chlorhexidine Gluconate *on page 300*

Stavudine (STAV yoo deen)

Related Information

HIV Infection and AIDS *on page 1482*

U.S. Brand Names Zerit®

Canadian Brand Names Zerit®

Mexican Brand Names Zerit®

Pharmacologic Category Antiretroviral Agent, Reverse Transcriptase Inhibitor (Nucleoside)

Synonyms d4T

Use Treatment of adults with HIV infection in combination with other antiretroviral agents

Local Anesthetic/Vasoconstrictor Precautions No information available to require special precautions

Effects on Dental Treatment No significant effects or complications reported

Dosage Oral:

Newborns (Birth to 13 days): 0.5 mg/kg every 12 hours

Children:

>14 days and <30 kg: 1 mg/kg every 12 hours

≥30 kg: 30 mg every 12 hours

Adults:

≥60 kg: 40 mg every 12 hours

<60 kg: 30 mg every 12 hours

Dose may be cut in half if symptoms of peripheral neuropathy occur

Elderly: Monitor closely for signs and symptoms of peripheral neuropathy; dosage should be carefully adjusted to renal function

Dosing adjustment in renal impairment:
- Cl_{cr} >50 mL/minute:
  - ≥60 kg: 40 mg every 12 hours
  - <60 kg: 30 mg every 12 hours
- Cl_{cr} 26-50 mL/minute:
  - ≥60 kg: 20 mg every 12 hours
  - <60 kg: 15 mg every 12 hours
- Hemodialysis:
  - ≥60 kg: 20 mg every 24 hours
  - <60 kg: 15 mg every 24 hours

Mechanism of Action Stavudine is a thymidine analog which interferes with HIV viral DNA dependent DNA polymerase resulting in inhibition of viral replication; nucleoside reverse transcriptase inhibitor

Other Adverse Effects All adverse reactions reported below were similar to comparative agent, zidovudine, except for peripheral neuropathy, which was greater for stavudine.

>10%:
- Central nervous system: Headache, chills/fever, malaise, insomnia, anxiety, depression, pain
- Dermatologic: Rash
- Gastrointestinal: Nausea, vomiting, diarrhea, pancreatitis, abdominal pain
- Neuromuscular & skeletal: Peripheral neuropathy (15% to 21%)

1% to 10%:
- Hematologic: Neutropenia, thrombocytopenia
- Hepatic: Increased hepatic transaminases, increased bilirubin
- Neuromuscular & skeletal: Myalgia, back pain, weakness

Postmarketing and/or case reports: Allergic reaction, anemia, anorexia, hepatomegaly, hepatic failure, hepatic steatosis, insomnia, lactic acidosis, leukopenia, motor weakness (severe), pancreatitis, redistribution/accumulation of body fat

Drug Interactions

Increased Effect/Toxicity: Drugs associated with peripheral neuropathy (chloramphenicol, cisplatin, dapsone, ethionamide, gold, hydralazine, iodoquinol, isoniazid, lithium, metronidazole, nitrofurantoin, pentamidine, phenytoin, ribavirin, vincristine) may increase risk for stavudine peripheral neuropathy. Risk of neuropathy, pancreatitis, or lactic acidosis and severe hepatomegaly is increased with concurrent use of didanosine and hydroxyurea. Concomitant use of ribavirin and nucleoside analogues may increase the risk of developing lactic acidosis (includes adefovir, didanosine, lamivudine, stavudine, zalcitabine, zidovudine).

Decreased Effect: Stavudine may decrease the activity of zidovudine (based on *in vitro* data).

Pharmacodynamics/Kinetics
- Distribution: V_d: 0.5 L/kg
- Bioavailability: 86.4%
- Half-life elimination: 1-1.6 hours
- Time to peak, serum: 1 hour
- Excretion: Urine (40%)

Pregnancy Risk Factor C

Generic Available No

Stelazine® *see* Trifluoperazine *on page 1349*
Sterapred® *see* PredniSONE *on page 1112*
Sterapred® DS *see* PredniSONE *on page 1112*
Stilbestrol *see* Diethylstilbestrol *on page 437*
Stimate™ *see* Desmopressin *on page 410*
St. Joseph® Pain Reliever [OTC] *see* Aspirin *on page 131*
Stop® *see* Fluoride *on page 586*
Strattera™ *see* Atomoxetine *on page 139*
Streptase® *see* Streptokinase *on page 1243*

Streptokinase (strep toe KYE nase)

Related Information

Cardiovascular Diseases *on page 1456*

U.S. Brand Names Streptase®

Canadian Brand Names Streptase®

Mexican Brand Names Streptase®

Pharmacologic Category Thrombolytic Agent

Synonyms SK

Use Thrombolytic agent used in treatment of recent severe or massive deep vein thrombosis, pulmonary emboli, MI, and occluded arteriovenous cannulas

Local Anesthetic/Vasoconstrictor Precautions No information available to require special precautions

Effects on Dental Treatment No significant effects or complications reported

(Continued)

Streptokinase *(Continued)*

Dosage I.V.:

Children: Safety and efficacy not established; limited studies have used 3500-4000 units/kg over 30 minutes followed by 1000-1500 units/kg/hour.

Clotted catheter: I.V.: **Note:** Not recommended due to possibility of allergic reactions with repeated doses: 10,000-25,000 units diluted in NS to a final volume equivalent to catheter volume; instill into catheter and leave in place for 1 hour, then aspirate contents out of catheter and flush catheter with normal saline.

Adults: Antibodies to streptokinase remain for at least 3-6 months after initial dose:

Administration requires the use of an infusion pump.

An intradermal skin test of 100 units has been suggested to predict allergic response to streptokinase. If a positive reaction is not seen after 15-20 minutes, a therapeutic dose may be administered.

Guidelines for acute MI (AMI): 1.5 million units over 60 minutes

Administration:

Dilute two 750,000 unit vials of streptokinase with 5 mL dextrose 5% in water (D_5W) each, gently swirl to dissolve.

Add this dose of the 1.5 million units to 150 mL D_5W.

This should be infused over 60 minutes; an in-line filter ≥0.45 micron should be used.

Monitor for the first few hours for signs of anaphylaxis or allergic reaction. **Infusion should be slowed if blood pressure falls by 25 mm Hg or terminated if asthmatic symptoms appear**.

Following completion of streptokinase, initiate heparin, if directed, when aPTT returns to less than 2 times the upper limit of control; do not use a bolus, but initiate infusion adjusted to a target aPTT of 1.5-2 times the upper limit of control. If prolonged (>48 hours) heparin is required, infusion may be switched to subcutaneous therapy.

Guidelines for acute pulmonary embolism (APE): 3 million unit dose over 24 hours

Administration:

Dilute four 750,000 unit vials of streptokinase with 5 mL dextrose 5% in water (D_5W) each, gently swirl to dissolve.

Add this dose of 3 million units to 250 mL D_5W, an in-line filter ≥0.45 micron should be used.

Administer 250,000 units (23 mL) over 30 minutes followed by 100,000 units/hour (9 mL/hour) for 24 hours.

Monitor for the first few hours for signs of anaphylaxis or allergic reaction. **Infusion should be slowed if blood pressure is lowered by 25 mm Hg or if asthmatic symptoms appear**.

Begin heparin 1000 units/hour about 3-4 hours after completion of streptokinase infusion or when PTT is <100 seconds.

Monitor PT, PTT, and fibrinogen levels during therapy.

Thromboses: 250,000 units to start, then 100,000 units/hour for 24-72 hours depending on location.

Cannula occlusion: 250,000 units into cannula, clamp for 2 hours, then aspirate contents and flush with normal saline; use not recommended

Mechanism of Action Activates the conversion of plasminogen to plasmin by forming a complex, exposing plasminogen-activating site, and cleaving a peptide bond that converts plasminogen to plasmin; plasmin degrades fibrin, fibrinogen and other procoagulant proteins into soluble fragments; effective both outside and within the formed thrombus/embolus

Other Adverse Effects As with all drugs which may affect hemostasis, bleeding is the major adverse effect associated with streptokinase. Hemorrhage may occur at virtually any site. Risk is dependent on multiple variables, including the dosage administered, concurrent use of multiple agents which alter hemostasis, and patient predisposition (including hypertension). Rapid lysis of coronary artery thrombi by thrombolytic agents may be associated with reperfusion-related atrial and/or ventricular arrhythmias.

>10%:

Cardiovascular: Hypotension

Local: Injection site bleeding

1% to 10%:

Central nervous system: Fever (1% to 4%)

Dermatologic: Bruising, rash, pruritus

Gastrointestinal: Gastrointestinal hemorrhage, nausea, vomiting

Genitourinary: Genitourinary hemorrhage

Hematologic: Anemia

Neuromuscular & skeletal: Muscle pain

Ocular: Eye hemorrhage, periorbital edema

Respiratory: Bronchospasm, epistaxis

Miscellaneous: Diaphoresis

<1%: Intracranial hemorrhage, retroperitoneal hemorrhage, pericardial hemorrhage, gingival hemorrhage, epistaxis, allergic reactions, anaphylaxis, anaphylactic shock, angioneurotic edema, anaphylactoid reactions, laryngeal edema,

urticaria, back pain (during infusion), elevated transaminases, respiratory depression, morbilliform, erysipelas-like rash, hemarthrosis

Postmarketing and/or case reports: Guillain-Barré syndrome, Parsonage-Turner syndrome, splenic rupture, acute tubular necrosis, cholesterol embolization, ARDS

Additional cardiovascular events associated with use in MI: AV block, cardiogenic shock, heart failure, cardiac arrest, recurrent ischemia/infarction, myocardial rupture, electromechanical dissociation, pericardial effusion, pericarditis, mitral regurgitation, cardiac tamponade, thromboembolism, pulmonary edema, asystole, ventricular tachycardia

Drug Interactions

Increased Effect/Toxicity: The risk of bleeding with streptokinase is increased by oral anticoagulants (warfarin), heparin, low molecular weight heparins, and drugs which affect platelet function (eg, NSAIDs, dipyridamole, ticlopidine, clopidogrel, IIb/IIIa antagonists). Although concurrent use with aspirin and heparin may increase the risk of bleeding. Aspirin and heparin were used concomitantly with streptokinase in the majority of patients in clinical studies of MI.

Decreased Effect: Antifibrinolytic agents (aminocaproic acid) may decrease effectiveness to thrombolytic agents.

Dietary/Ethanol/Herb Considerations

Food: Avoid garlic, ginger, and green tea.

Herb/Nutraceutical: Avoid cat's claw, dong quai, evening primrose, feverfew, garlic, ginkgo biloba, ginger, ginseng, green tea, horse chestnut, and red clover due to additional antiplatelet activity.

Pharmacodynamics/Kinetics

Onset of action: Activation of plasminogen occurs almost immediately

Duration: Fibrinolytic effect: Several hours; Anticoagulant effect: 12-24 hours

Half-life elimination: 83 minutes

Excretion: By circulating antibodies and the reticuloendothelial system

Pregnancy Risk Factor C

Generic Available No

Streptomycin (strep toe MYE sin)

Related Information

Nonviral Infectious Diseases *on page 1493*

Tuberculosis *on page 1493*

Pharmacologic Category Antibiotic, Aminoglycoside; Antitubercular Agent

Synonyms Streptomycin Sulfate

Use Part of combination therapy of active tuberculosis; used in combination with other agents for treatment of streptococcal or enterococcal endocarditis, mycobacterial infections, plague, tularemia, and brucellosis

Local Anesthetic/Vasoconstrictor Precautions No information available to require special precautions

Effects on Dental Treatment No significant effects or complications reported

Dosage

Children:

Tuberculosis:

Daily therapy: 20-40 mg/kg/day (maximum: 1 g/day)

Directly observed therapy (DOT): Twice weekly: 20-40 mg/kg (maximum: 1 g)

DOT: 3 times/week: 25-30 mg/kg (maximum: 1 g)

Adults:

Tuberculosis:

Daily therapy: 15 mg/kg/day (maximum: 1 g)

Directly observed therapy (DOT): Twice weekly: 25-30 mg/kg (maximum: 1.5 g)

DOT: 3 times/week: 25-30 mg/kg (maximum: 1 g)

Enterococcal endocarditis: 1 g every 12 hours for 2 weeks, 500 mg every 12 hours for 4 weeks in combination with penicillin

Streptococcal endocarditis: 1 g every 12 hours for 1 week, 500 mg every 12 hours for 1 week

Tularemia: 1-2 g/day in divided doses for 7-10 days or until patient is afebrile for 5-7 days

Plague: 2-4 g/day in divided doses until the patient is afebrile for at least 3 days

Elderly: 10 mg/kg/day, not to exceed 750 mg/day; dosing interval should be adjusted for renal function; some authors suggest not to give more than 5 days/week or give as 20-25 mg/kg/dose twice weekly

Dosing interval in renal impairment:

Cl_{cr} 10-50 mL/minute: Administer every 24-72 hours

Cl_{cr} <10 mL/minute: Administer every 72-96 hours

Removed by hemo and peritoneal dialysis: Administer dose postdialysis

Mechanism of Action Inhibits bacterial protein synthesis by binding directly to the 30S ribosomal subunits causing faulty peptide sequence to form in the protein chain

Other Adverse Effects Frequency not defined:

Cardiovascular: Hypotension

(Continued)

Streptomycin *(Continued)*

Central nervous system: Neurotoxicity, drowsiness, headache, drug fever, paresthesia
Dermatologic: Skin rash
Gastrointestinal: Nausea, vomiting
Hematologic: Eosinophilia, anemia
Neuromuscular & skeletal: Arthralgia, weakness, tremor
Otic: Ototoxicity (auditory and vestibular)
Renal: Nephrotoxicity
Respiratory: Difficulty in breathing

Drug Interactions Increased effect with depolarizing and nondepolarizing neuromuscular blocking agents. Concurrent use with amphotericin or loop diuretics may increase nephrotoxicity.

Pharmacodynamics/Kinetics
Absorption: I.M.: Well absorbed
Distribution: To extracellular fluid including serum, abscesses, ascitic, pericardial, pleural, synovial, lymphatic, and peritoneal fluids; crosses placenta; small amounts enter breast milk
Protein binding: 34%
Half-life elimination: Newborns: 4-10 hours; Adults: 2-4.7 hours, prolonged with renal impairment
Time to peak: Within 1 hour
Excretion: Urine (90% as unchanged drug); feces, saliva, sweat, and tears (<1%)

Pregnancy Risk Factor D

Generic Available Yes

Streptomycin Sulfate *see* Streptomycin *on page 1245*

Streptozocin (strep toe ZOE sin)

U.S. Brand Names Zanosar®

Canadian Brand Names Zanosar®

Pharmacologic Category Antineoplastic Agent, Alkylating Agent

Use Treatment of metastatic islet cell carcinoma of the pancreas, carcinoid tumor and syndrome, Hodgkin's disease, palliative treatment of colorectal cancer

Local Anesthetic/Vasoconstrictor Precautions No information available to require special precautions

Effects on Dental Treatment No significant effects or complications reported

Dosage I.V. (refer to individual protocols):
Children and Adults:
Single agent therapy: 1-1.5 g/m^2 weekly for 6 weeks followed by a 4-week observation period
Combination therapy: 0.5-1 g/m^2 for 5 consecutive days followed by a 4- to 6-week observation period
Dosing adjustment in renal impairment:
Cl_{cr} 10-50 mL/minute: Administer 75% of dose
Cl_{cr} <10 mL/minute: Administer 50% of dose
Hemodialysis and CAPD/CAVH effects: Data unavailable
Dosing adjustment in hepatic impairment: Reduction required in severe liver disease

Mechanism of Action Interferes with the normal function of DNA by alkylation and cross-linking the strands of DNA, and by possible protein modification

Other Adverse Effects
>10%:
Gastrointestinal: Nausea and vomiting in all patients usually 1-4 hours after infusion; diarrhea in 10% of patients; increased LFTs and hypoalbuminemia
Emetic potential: High (>90%)
Time course of nausea/vomiting: Onset 1-3 hours; Duration: 1-12 hours
Renal: Renal dysfunction occurs in 65% of patients; proteinuria, decreased Cl_{cr}, increased BUN, hypophosphatemia, and renal tubular acidosis; use caution with patients on other nephrotoxic agents; nephrotoxicity (25% to 75% of patients)
1% to 10%:
Endocrine & metabolic: Hypoglycemia: Seen in 6% of patients; may be prevented with the administration of nicotinamide
Gastrointestinal: Diarrhea
Local: Pain at injection site
<1%: Confusion, lethargy, depression, leukopenia, thrombocytopenia, liver dysfunction, secondary malignancy
Myelosuppressive:
WBC: Mild
Platelets: Mild
Onset: 7 days
Nadir: 14 days
Recovery: 21 days

Drug Interactions

Increased Effect/Toxicity: Doxorubicin prolongs half-life and thus prolonged leukopenia and thrombocytopenia.

Decreased Effect: Phenytoin results in negation of streptozocin cytotoxicity.

Pharmacodynamics/Kinetics

Duration: Disappears from serum in 4 hours

Distribution: Concentrates in liver, intestine, pancreas, and kidney

Metabolism: Rapidly hepatic

Half-life elimination: 35-40 minutes

Excretion: Urine (60% to 70% as metabolites); exhaled gases (5%); feces (1%)

Pregnancy Risk Factor C

Generic Available No

Stri-dex® [OTC] *see* Salicylic Acid *on page 1204*

Stri-dex® Body Focus [OTC] *see* Salicylic Acid *on page 1204*

Stri-dex® Facewipes To Go™ [OTC] *see* Salicylic Acid *on page 1204*

Stri-dex® Maximum Strength [OTC] *see* Salicylic Acid *on page 1204*

Stromectol® *see* Ivermectin *on page 757*

Strong Iodine Solution *see* Potassium Iodide *on page 1101*

Sublimaze® *see* Fentanyl *on page 565*

Subutex® *see* Buprenorphine *on page 208*

Sucraid® *see* Sacrosidase *on page 1203*

Sucralfate (soo KRAL fate)

Related Information

Management of Patients Undergoing Cancer Therapy *on page 1567*

U.S. Brand Names Carafate®

Canadian Brand Names Apo®-Sucralate; Novo-Sucralate; Nu-Sucralate; PMS-Sucralate; Sulcrate®; Sulcrate® Suspension Plus

Mexican Brand Names Antepsin

Pharmacologic Category Gastrointestinal Agent, Miscellaneous

Synonyms Aluminum Sucrose Sulfate, Basic

Use Short-term management of duodenal ulcers; maintenance of duodenal ulcers

Unlabeled/Investigational Use Treatment of gastric ulcers, GERD, esophagitis; NSAID-induced mucosal damage; prevention of stress ulcers; postsclerotherapy for esophageal variceal bleeding

Suspension: May be used topically for treatment of stomatitis due to cancer chemotherapy and other causes of esophageal and gastric erosions (eg, GERD, esophagitis)

Local Anesthetic/Vasoconstrictor Precautions No information available to require special precautions

Effects on Dental Treatment No significant effects or complications reported

Dosage Oral:

Children: Dose not established, doses of 40-80 mg/kg/day divided every 6 hours have been used

Stomatitis (unlabeled use): 2.5-5 mL (1 g/10 mL suspension), swish and spit or swish and swallow 4 times/day

Adults:

Stress ulcer prophylaxis: 1 g 4 times/day

Stress ulcer treatment: 1 g every 4 hours

Duodenal ulcer:

Treatment: 1 g 4 times/day on an empty stomach and at bedtime for 4-8 weeks, or alternatively 2 g twice daily; treatment is recommended for 4-8 weeks in adults, the elderly may require 12 weeks

Maintenance: Prophylaxis: 1 g twice daily

Stomatitis (unlabeled use): 1 g/10 mL suspension, swish and spit or swish and swallow 4 times/day

Dosage comment in renal impairment: Aluminum salt is minimally absorbed (<5%), however, may accumulate in renal failure

Mechanism of Action Forms a complex by binding with positively charged proteins in exudates, forming a viscous paste-like, adhesive substance. This selectively forms a protective coating that protects the lining against peptic acid, pepsin, and bile salts.

Other Adverse Effects

1% to 10%: Gastrointestinal: Constipation

<1%: Back pain, bezoar formation, diarrhea, dizziness, gastric discomfort; hypersensitivity (pruritus, urticaria, angioedema); indigestion, insomnia, nausea, pruritus, rash, sleepiness, vertigo, vomiting, xerostomia

Drug Interactions Decreased Effect: Sucralfate may alter the absorption of digoxin, phenytoin (hydantoins), warfarin, ketoconazole, quinidine, quinolones, tetracycline, theophylline. Because of the potential for sucralfate to alter the absorption of some drugs; separate administration (take other medications at least 2 hours before sucralfate). The potential for decreased absorption should be considered when alterations in bioavailability are believed to be critical.

(Continued)

Sucralfate *(Continued)*

Dietary/Ethanol/Herb Considerations

Ethanol: Avoid or limit use; may enhance gastric mucosal irritation.

Food: Sucralfate may interfere with absorption of vitamin A, vitamin D, vitamin E, and vitamin K.

Pharmacodynamics/Kinetics

Onset of action: Paste formation and ulcer adhesion: 1-2 hours

Duration: Up to 6 hours

Absorption: Oral: <5%

Distribution: Acts locally at ulcer sites; unbound in GI tract to aluminum and sucrose octasulfate

Metabolism: None

Excretion: Urine (small amounts as unchanged compounds)

Pregnancy Risk Factor B

Generic Available Yes

Sucrets® Original [OTC] *see* Hexylresorcinol *on page 670*

Sudafed® [OTC] *see* Pseudoephedrine *on page 1146*

Sudafed® 12 Hour [OTC] *see* Pseudoephedrine *on page 1146*

Sudafed® 24 Hour [OTC] *see* Pseudoephedrine *on page 1146*

Sudafed® Children's [OTC] *see* Pseudoephedrine *on page 1146*

Sudafed® Cold & Allergy [OTC] *see* Chlorpheniramine and Pseudoephedrine *on page 308*

Sudafed® Cold and Sinus [OTC] *see* Acetaminophen and Pseudoephedrine *on page 31*

Sudafed® Severe Cold [OTC] *see* Acetaminophen, Dextromethorphan, and Pseudoephedrine *on page 35*

Sudafed® Sinus Headache [OTC] *see* Acetaminophen and Pseudoephedrine *on page 31*

Sudodrin [OTC] *see* Pseudoephedrine *on page 1146*

Sufenta® *see* Sufentanil *on page 1248*

Sufentanil (soo FEN tu nil)

U.S. Brand Names Sufenta®

Canadian Brand Names Sufenta®

Pharmacologic Category Analgesic, Narcotic; General Anesthetic

Synonyms Sufentanil Citrate

Use Analgesic supplement in maintenance of balanced general anesthesia

Local Anesthetic/Vasoconstrictor Precautions No information available to require special precautions

Effects on Dental Treatment No significant effects or complications reported

Restrictions C-II

Dosage

Children 2-12 years: 10-25 mcg/kg (10-15 mcg/kg most common dose) with 100% O_2, maintenance: up to 1-2 mcg/kg total dose

Adults: Dose should be based on body weight. **Note:** In obese patients (ie, >20% above ideal body weight), use lean body weight to determine dosage.

- 1-2 mcg/kg with N_2O/O_2 for endotracheal intubation; maintenance: 10-25 mcg as needed
- 2-8 mcg/kg with N_2O/O_2 more complicated major surgical procedures; maintenance: 10-50 mcg as needed
- 8-30 mcg/kg with 100% O_2 and muscle relaxant produces sleep; at doses ≥8 mcg/kg maintains a deep level of anesthesia; maintenance: 10-50 mcg as needed

Mechanism of Action Binds to opioid receptors throughout the CNS. Once receptor binding occurs, effects are exerted by opening K+ channels and inhibiting Ca++ channels. These mechanisms increase pain threshold, alter pain perception, inhibit ascending pain pathways; short-acting narcotic

Other Adverse Effects

>10%:

- Cardiovascular: Bradycardia, hypotension
- Central nervous system: Somnolence
- Gastrointestinal: Nausea, vomiting
- Respiratory: Respiratory depression

1% to 10%:

- Cardiovascular: Cardiac arrhythmias, orthostatic hypotension
- Central nervous system: CNS depression, confusion
- Gastrointestinal: Biliary spasm
- Ocular: Blurred vision

<1%: Bronchospasm, circulatory depression; cold, clammy skin; convulsions, dizziness, dysesthesia, itching, laryngospasm, mental depression, paradoxical CNS excitation or delirium, physical and psychological dependence with prolonged use, skin rash, urinary tract spasm, urticaria

Drug Interactions Substrate of **CYP3A4**

Increased effct/toxicity with CNS depressants or beta-blockers. May increase response to neuromuscular blocking agents.

Pharmacodynamics/Kinetics

Onset of action: 1-3 minutes

Duration: Dose dependent

Metabolism: Primarily hepatic

Pregnancy Risk Factor C

Generic Available Yes

Sufentanil Citrate *see* Sufentanil *on page 1248*

Sular® *see* Nisoldipine *on page 977*

Sulbactam and Ampicillin *see* Ampicillin and Sulbactam *on page 104*

Sulconazole (sul KON u zole)

U.S. Brand Names Exelderm®

Canadian Brand Names Exelderm®

Pharmacologic Category Antifungal Agent, Topical

Synonyms Sulconazole Nitrate

Use Treatment of superficial fungal infections of the skin, including tinea cruris (jock itch), tinea corporis (ringworm), tinea versicolor, and possibly tinea pedis (athlete's foot, cream only)

Local Anesthetic/Vasoconstrictor Precautions No information available to require special precautions

Effects on Dental Treatment No significant effects or complications reported

Dosage Adults: Topical: Apply a small amount to the affected area and gently massage once or twice daily for 3 weeks (tinea cruris, tinea corporis, tinea versicolor) to 4 weeks (tinea pedis).

Mechanism of Action Substituted imidazole derivative which inhibits metabolic reactions necessary for the synthesis of ergosterol, an essential membrane component. The end result is usually fungistatic; however, sulconazole may act as a fungicide in *Candida albicans* and parapsilosis during certain growth phases.

Other Adverse Effects 1% to 10%:

Dermatologic: Itching

Local: Burning, stinging, redness

Pharmacodynamics/Kinetics

Absorption: Topical: ~8.7% percutaneously

Excretion: Primarily urine

Pregnancy Risk Factor C

Generic Available No

Sulconazole Nitrate *see* Sulconazole *on page 1249*

Sulf-10® *see* Sulfacetamide *on page 1249*

Sulfabenzamide, Sulfacetamide, and Sulfathiazole

(sul fu BENZ u mide, sul fu SEE tu mide, & sul fu THYE u zole)

Related Information

Sulfacetamide *on page 1249*

U.S. Brand Names V.V.S.®

Pharmacologic Category Antibiotic, Vaginal

Synonyms Triple Sulfa

Use Treatment of *Haemophilus vaginalis* vaginitis

Local Anesthetic/Vasoconstrictor Precautions No information available to require special precautions

Effects on Dental Treatment No significant effects or complications reported

Dosage Intravaginal: Adults: Female: Cream: Insert one applicatorful into vagina twice daily for 4-6 days; dosage may then be decreased to ½ to ¼ of an applicatorful twice daily

Mechanism of Action Interferes with microbial folic acid synthesis and growth via inhibition of para-aminobenzoic acid metabolism

Other Adverse Effects Frequency not defined:

Dermatologic: Pruritus, urticaria, Stevens-Johnson syndrome

Local: Local irritation

Miscellaneous: Allergic reactions

Pharmacodynamics/Kinetics

Absorption: Absorption from vagina is variable and unreliable

Metabolism: Primarily via acetylation

Excretion: Urine

Pregnancy Risk Factor C (avoid if near term)

Generic Available Yes

Sulfacetamide (sul fu SEE tu mide)

U.S. Brand Names AK-Sulf®; Bleph®-10; Carmol® Scalp; Klaron®; Ocusulf-10; Ovace™; Sulf-10®

Canadian Brand Names Cetamide™; Diosulf™; Sodium Sulamyd®

(Continued)

Sulfacetamide *(Continued)*

Mexican Brand Names Ceta Sulfa®

Pharmacologic Category Antibiotic, Ophthalmic; Antibiotic, Sulfonamide Derivative

Synonyms Sodium Sulfacetamide; Sulfacetamide Sodium

Use Treatment and prophylaxis of conjunctivitis due to susceptible organisms; corneal ulcers; adjunctive treatment with systemic sulfonamides for therapy of trachoma; topical application in scaling dermatosis (seborrheic); bacterial infections of the skin

Local Anesthetic/Vasoconstrictor Precautions No information available to require special precautions

Effects on Dental Treatment No significant effects or complications reported

Dosage

Children >2 months and Adults: Ophthalmic:

Ointment: Apply to lower conjunctival sac 1-4 times/day and at bedtime

Solution: Instill 1-3 drops several times daily up to every 2-3 hours in lower conjunctival sac during waking hours and less frequently at night

Children >12 years and Adults: Topical:

Seborrheic dermatitis: Apply at bedtime and allow to remain overnight; in severe cases, may apply twice daily

Secondary cutaneous bacterial infections: Apply 2-4 times/day until infection clears

Mechanism of Action Interferes with bacterial growth by inhibiting bacterial folic acid synthesis through competitive antagonism of PABA

Other Adverse Effects

1% to 10%: Local: Irritation, stinging, burning

<1%: Headache, Stevens-Johnson syndrome, exfoliative dermatitis, toxic epidermal necrolysis, blurred vision, browache, hypersensitivity reactions

Drug Interactions Decreased Effect: Silver containing products are incompatible with sulfacetamide solutions.

Pharmacodynamics/Kinetics

Half-life elimination: 7-13 hours

Excretion: When absorbed, primarily urine (as unchanged drug)

Pregnancy Risk Factor C

Generic Available Yes: Ointment, solution

Sulfacetamide and Fluorometholone

(sul fu SEE tu mide & flore oh METH oh lone)

Related Information

Fluorometholone *on page 587*

Sulfacetamide *on page 1249*

U.S. Brand Names FML-S®

Pharmacologic Category Antibiotic/Corticosteroid, Ophthalmic

Synonyms Fluorometholone and Sulfacetamide

Use Steroid-responsive inflammatory ocular conditions where infection is present or there is a risk of infection

Local Anesthetic/Vasoconstrictor Precautions No information available to require special precautions

Effects on Dental Treatment No significant effects or complications reported

Dosage Children >2 months and Adults: Ophthalmic: Instill 1-3 drops every 2-3 hours while awake

Pregnancy Risk Factor C

Generic Available No

Sulfacetamide and Prednisolone

(sul fu SEE tu mide & pred NIS oh lone)

Related Information

PrednisoLONE *on page 1110*

Sulfacetamide *on page 1249*

U.S. Brand Names Blephamide®; Vasocidin®

Canadian Brand Names Blephamide®; Dioptimyd®; Vasocidin®

Pharmacologic Category Antibiotic/Corticosteroid, Ophthalmic

Synonyms Prednisolone and Sulfacetamide; Sulfacetamide Sodium and Prednisolone

Use Steroid-responsive inflammatory ocular conditions where infection is present or there is a risk of infection; ophthalmic suspension may be used as an otic preparation

Local Anesthetic/Vasoconstrictor Precautions No information available to require special precautions

Effects on Dental Treatment No significant effects or complications reported

Dosage Children >2 months and Adults: Ophthalmic:

Ointment: Apply to lower conjunctival sac 1-4 times/day

Solution: Instill 1-3 drops every 2-3 hours while awake

Mechanism of Action Interferes with bacterial growth by inhibiting bacterial folic acid synthesis through competitive antagonism of PABA; decreases inflammation by suppression of migration of polymorphonuclear leukocytes and reversal of increased capillary permeability; suppresses the immune system by reducing activity and volume of the lymphatic system

Other Adverse Effects

1% to 10%: Local: Burning, stinging

<1%: Cataracts, Cushing's syndrome, fractures, glaucoma, growth suppression, headache, muscle weakness, nausea, osteoporosis, peptic ulcer, pituitary-adrenal axis suppression, pseudotumor cerebri, psychoses, seizures, skin atrophy, Stevens-Johnson syndrome, vertigo, vomiting

Pregnancy Risk Factor C

Generic Available Yes: Suspension

Sulfacetamide Sodium *see* Sulfacetamide *on page 1249*

Sulfacetamide Sodium and Prednisolone *see* Sulfacetamide and Prednisolone *on page 1250*

SulfaDIAZINE (sul fu DYE a zeen)

Pharmacologic Category Antibiotic, Sulfonamide Derivative

Use Treatment of urinary tract infections and nocardiosis, rheumatic fever prophylaxis; adjunctive treatment in toxoplasmosis; uncomplicated attack of malaria

Local Anesthetic/Vasoconstrictor Precautions No information available to require special precautions

Effects on Dental Treatment No significant effects or complications reported

Dosage Oral:

Asymptomatic meningococcal carriers:
- Infants 1-12 months: 500 mg once daily for 2 days
- Children 1-12 years: 500 mg twice daily for 2 days
- Adults: 1 g twice daily for 2 days

Congenital toxoplasmosis:
- Newborns and Children <2 months: 100 mg/kg/day divided every 6 hours in conjunction with pyrimethamine 1 mg/kg/day once daily and supplemental folinic acid 5 mg every 3 days for 6 months
- Children >2 months: 25-50 mg/kg/dose 4 times/day

Nocardiosis: 4-8 g/day for a minimum of 6 weeks

Toxoplasmosis:
- Children >2 months: Loading dose: 75 mg/kg; maintenance dose: 120-150 mg/kg/day, maximum dose: 6 g/day; divided every 4-6 hours in conjunction with pyrimethamine 2 mg/kg/day divided every 12 hours for 3 days followed by 1 mg/kg/day once daily with supplemental folinic acid
- Adults: 2-6 g/day in divided doses every 6 hours in conjunction with pyrimethamine 50-75 mg/day and with supplemental folinic acid

Prevention of recurrent attacks of rheumatic fever:
- >30 kg: 1 g/day
- <30 kg: 0.5 g/day

Mechanism of Action Interferes with bacterial growth by inhibiting bacterial folic acid synthesis through competitive antagonism of PABA

Other Adverse Effects Frequency not defined:

Central nervous system: Fever, dizziness, headache

Dermatologic: Lyell's syndrome, Stevens-Johnson syndrome, itching, rash, photosensitivity

Endocrine & metabolic: Thyroid function disturbance

Gastrointestinal: Anorexia, nausea, vomiting, diarrhea

Genitourinary: Crystalluria

Hematologic: Granulocytopenia, leukopenia, thrombocytopenia, aplastic anemia, hemolytic anemia

Hepatic: Hepatitis, jaundice

Renal: Hematuria, acute nephropathy, interstitial nephritis

Miscellaneous: Serum sickness-like reactions

Drug Interactions Substrate of **CYP2C8/9**, 2E1, 3A4; Inhibits CYP2C8/9

Increased effect of oral anticoagulants and oral hypoglycemic agents.

Decreased effect with PABA or PABA metabolites of drugs (eg, procaine, proparacaine, tetracaine, sunblock).

Dietary/Ethanol/Herb Considerations

Food: Avoid large quantities of vitamin C or acidifying agents (cranberry juice) to prevent crystalluria.

Herb/Nutraceutical: Avoid dong quai and St John's wort; may cause photosensitization.

Pharmacodynamics/Kinetics

Absorption: Well absorbed

Distribution: Throughout body tissues and fluids including pleural, peritoneal, synovial, and ocular fluids; throughout total body water; readily diffused into CSF; enters breast milk

Metabolism: Via N-acetylation

Half-life elimination: 10 hours

(Continued)

SulfaDIAZINE *(Continued)*

Time to peak: Within 3-6 hours

Excretion: Urine (43% to 60% as unchanged drug, 15% to 40% as metabolites)

Pregnancy Risk Factor B/D (at term)

Generic Available Yes

Sulfadoxine and Pyrimethamine

(sul fu DOKS een & peer i METH u meen)

Related Information

Pyrimethamine *on page 1152*

U.S. Brand Names Fansidar®

Pharmacologic Category Antimalarial Agent

Synonyms Pyrimethamine and Sulfadoxine

Use Treatment of *Plasmodium falciparum* malaria in patients in whom chloroquine resistance is suspected; malaria prophylaxis for travelers to areas where chloroquine-resistant malaria is endemic

Local Anesthetic/Vasoconstrictor Precautions No information available to require special precautions

Effects on Dental Treatment No significant effects or complications reported

Dosage Children and Adults: Oral:

Treatment of acute attack of malaria: A single dose of the following number of Fansidar® tablets is used in sequence with quinine or alone:

2-11 months: 1/4 tablet
1-3 years: 1/2 tablet
4-8 years: 1 tablet
9-14 years: 2 tablets
>14 years: 3 tablets

Malaria prophylaxis: A single dose should be carried for self-treatment in the event of febrile illness when medical attention is not immediately available:

2-11 months: 1/4 tablet
1-3 years: 1/2 tablet
4-8 years: 1 tablet
9-14 years: 2 tablets
>14 years and Adults: 3 tablets

Mechanism of Action Sulfadoxine interferes with bacterial folic acid synthesis and growth via competitive inhibition of para-aminiobenzoic acid; pyrimethamine inhibits microbial dihydrofolate reductase, resulting in inhibition of tetrahydrofolic acid synthesis

Other Adverse Effects Frequency not defined:

Central nervous system: Ataxia, seizures, headache

Dermatologic: Photosensitivity, Stevens-Johnson syndrome, erythema multiforme, toxic epidermal necrolysis, rash

Endocrine & metabolic: Thyroid function dysfunction

Gastrointestinal: Atrophic glossitis, vomiting, gastritis, anorexia, glossitis

Genitourinary: Crystalluria

Hematologic: Megaloblastic anemia, leukopenia, thrombocytopenia, pancytopenia

Hepatic: Hepatic necrosis, hepatitis

Neuromuscular & skeletal: Tremors

Respiratory: Respiratory failure

Miscellaneous: Hypersensitivity

Drug Interactions Pyrimethamine: Inhibits CYP2D6

Increased Effect/Toxicity: Hydantoin (phenytoin) levels may be increased. Effect of oral hypoglycemics (rare, but severe) may occur. Combination with methenamine may result in crystalluria; avoid use. May increase methotrexate-induced bone marrow suppression. NSAIDs and salicylates may increase sulfonamide concentrations. Effect of warfarin may be increased.

Decreased Effect: Cyclosporine concentrations may be decreased; monitor levels and renal function. PABA (para-aminobenzoic acid - may be found in some vitamin supplements): interferes with the antibacterial activity of sulfonamides; avoid concurrent use. Pyrimethamine effectiveness decreased by acid.

Pharmacodynamics/Kinetics

Absorption: Well absorbed

Distribution: Sulfadoxine: Well distributed like other sulfonamides; Pyrimethamine: Widely distributed, mainly in blood cells, kidneys, lungs, liver, and spleen

Metabolism: Pyrimethamine: Hepatic; Sulfadoxine: None

Half-life elimination: Pyrimethamine: 80-95 hours; Sulfadoxine: 5-8 days

Time to peak, serum: 2-8 hours

Excretion: Urine (as unchanged drug and several unidentified metabolites)

Pregnancy Risk Factor C/D (at term)

Generic Available No

Sulfamethoxazole and Trimethoprim

(sul fa meth OKS a zole & trye METH oh prim)

Related Information

Animal and Human Bites Guidelines *on page 1580*

Trimethoprim *on page 1352*

U.S. Brand Names Bactrim™; Bactrim™ DS; Septra®; Septra® DS

Canadian Brand Names Apo®-Sulfatrim; Novo-Trimel; Novo-Trimel D.S.; Nu-Cotrimox®; Septra®; Septra® DS; Septra® Injection

Mexican Brand Names Anitrim; Bactelan; Batrizol; Ectaprim®; Ectaprim®-F; Enterobacticel; Esteprim; Isobac; Kelfiprim; Metoxiprim; Syraprim; Tribakin; Trimesuxol; Trimetoger; Trimetox; Trimzol

Pharmacologic Category Antibiotic, Sulfonamide Derivative; Antibiotic, Miscellaneous

Synonyms Co-Trimoxazole; SMZ-TMP; TMP-SMZ; Trimethoprim and Sulfamethoxazole

Use

Oral treatment of urinary tract infections due to *E. coli*, *Klebsiella* and *Enterobacter* sp, *M. morganii*, *P. mirabilis* and *P. vulgaris*; acute otitis media in children and acute exacerbations of chronic bronchitis in adults due to susceptible strains of *H. influenzae* or *S. pneumoniae*; prophylaxis of *Pneumocystis carinii* pneumonitis (PCP), traveler's diarrhea due to enterotoxigenic *E. coli* or *Cyclospora*

I.V. treatment or severe or complicated infections when oral therapy is not feasible, for documented PCP, empiric treatment of PCP in immune compromised patients; treatment of documented or suspected shigellosis, typhoid fever, *Nocardia asteroides* infection, or other infections caused by susceptible bacteria

Unlabeled/Investigational Use Treatment of cholera and salmonella-type infections and nocardiosis, chronic prostatitis; prophylaxis in neutropenic patients with *P. carinii* infections, in leukemics, and in patients following renal transplantation, to decrease incidence of gram-negative rod infections

Local Anesthetic/Vasoconstrictor Precautions No information available to require special precautions

Effects on Dental Treatment Frequency not defined (GI effects most common): Confusion, hallucinations, seizures, fever, hyperglycemia, nausea, vomiting, stomatitis, cough, dyspnea, serum sickness

Dosage Dosage recommendations are based on the trimethoprim component

Children >2 months:

- Mild to moderate infections: Oral, I.V.: 8 mg TMP/kg/day in divided doses every 12 hours
- Serious infection/*Pneumocystis*: I.V.: 20 mg TMP/kg/day in divided doses every 6 hours
- Urinary tract infection prophylaxis: Oral: 2 mg TMP/kg/dose daily
- Prophylaxis of *Pneumocystis*: Oral, I.V.: 10 mg TMP/kg/day or 150 mg TMP/m^2/day in divided doses every 12 hours for 3 days/week; dose should not exceed 320 mg trimethoprim and 1600 mg sulfamethoxazole 3 days/week
- Cholera: Oral, I.V.: 5 mg TMP/kg twice daily for 3 days
- *Cyclospora:* Oral, I.V.: 5 mg TMP/kg twice daily for 7 days

Adults:

- Urinary tract infection/chronic bronchitis: Oral: 1 double strength tablet every 12 hours for 10-14 days
- Sepsis: I.V.: 20 TMP/kg/day divided every 6 hours
- *Pneumocystis carinii*:
  - Prophylaxis: Oral: 1 double strength tablet daily or 3 times/week
  - Treatment: Oral, I.V.: 15-20 mg TMP/kg/day in 3-4 divided doses
- Cholera: Oral, I.V.: 160 mg TMP twice daily for 3 days
- *Cyclospora:* Oral, I.V.: 160 mg TMP twice daily for 7 days
- *Nocardia:* Oral, I.V.: 640 mg TMP/day in divided doses for several months (duration is controversial; an average of 7 months has been reported)

Dosing adjustment in renal impairment: Adults:

I.V.:

- Cl_{cr} 15-30 mL/minute: Administer 2.5-5 mg/kg every 12 hours
- Cl_{cr} <15 mL/minute: Administer 2.5-5 mg/kg every 24 hours

Oral:

- Cl_{cr} 15-30 mL/minute: Administer 1 double strength tablet every 24 hours or 1 single strength tablet every 12 hours
- Cl_{cr} <15 mL/minute: Use not recommended

Mechanism of Action Sulfamethoxazole interferes with bacterial folic acid synthesis and growth via inhibition of dihydrofolic acid formation from para-aminobenzoic acid; trimethoprim inhibits dihydrofolic acid reduction to tetrahydrofolate resulting in sequential inhibition of enzymes of the folic acid pathway

Other Adverse Effects Rare life-threatening reactions reported including severe dermatologic reactions and hepatotoxic reactions. Most other reactions listed are rare, however, frequency cannot be accurately estimated.

Cardiovascular: Allergic myocarditis

(Continued)

Sulfamethoxazole and Trimethoprim *(Continued)*

Central nervous system: Depression, aseptic meningitis, peripheral neuritis, ataxia, kernicterus (in neonates)

Dermatologic: Rashes, pruritus, urticaria, photosensitivity; rare reactions include erythema multiforme, Stevens-Johnson syndrome, toxic epidermal necrolysis, exfoliative dermatitis, and Henoch-Schönlein purpura

Endocrine & metabolic: Hyperkalemia (generally at high dosages)

Gastrointestinal: Anorexia, diarrhea, pseudomembranous colitis, pancreatitis

Hematologic: Thrombocytopenia, megaloblastic anemia, granulocytopenia, eosinophilia, pancytopenia, aplastic anemia, methemoglobinemia, hemolysis (with G6PD deficiency), agranulocytosis

Hepatic: Elevated serum transaminases, hepatotoxicity (including hepatitis, cholestasis, and hepatic necrosis), hyperbilirubinemia

Neuromuscular & skeletal: Arthralgia, myalgia, rhabdomyolysis

Renal: Interstitial nephritis, crystalluria, renal failure, nephrotoxicity (in association with cyclosporine), diuresis

Respiratory: Pulmonary infiltrates

Miscellaneous: Angioedema, periarteritis nodosa (rare), systemic lupus erythematosus (rare)

Drug Interactions

Sulfamethoxazole: Substrate of **CYP2C8/9**, 3A4; Inhibits CYP2C8/9

Trimethoprim: Substrate of **CYP2C8/9, 3A4**; Inhibits CYP2C8/9

Increased Effect/Toxicity: May increase effect of sulfonylureas and oral anticoagulants (warfarin). May displace highly protein-bound drugs like methotrexate, phenytoin, or cyclosporine causing increased free serum concentrations, leading to increased toxicity of these agents (may also compete for renal excretion of methotrexate). May enhance nephrotoxicity of cyclosporine and increase digoxin concentrations.

Decreased effect of cyclosporines and tricyclic antidepressants. Procaine and indomethacin may cause decreased effect of sulfamethoxazole and trimethoprim.

Dietary/Ethanol/Herb Considerations

Food: Administer on an empty stomach.

Herb/Nutraceutical: Avoid dong quai and St John's wort; may cause photosensitization.

Pregnancy Risk Factor C/D (at term - expert analysis)

Generic Available Yes

Sulfamylon® *see* Mafenide *on page 832*

Sulfasalazine (sul fa SAL a zeen)

U.S. Brand Names Azulfidine®; Azulfidine® EN-tabs®

Canadian Brand Names Alti-Sulfasalazine; Salazopyrin®; Salazopyrin En-Tabs®

Pharmacologic Category 5-Aminosalicylic Acid Derivative

Synonyms Salicylazosulfapyridine

Use Management of ulcerative colitis; enteric coated tablets are also used for rheumatoid arthritis (including juvenile rheumatoid arthritis) in patients who inadequately respond to analgesics and NSAIDs

Unlabeled/Investigational Use Treatment of ankylosing spondylitis, collagenous colitis, Crohn's disease, psoriasis, psoriatic arthritis, juvenile chronic arthritis

Local Anesthetic/Vasoconstrictor Precautions No information available to require special precautions

Effects on Dental Treatment No significant effects or complications reported

Dosage Oral:

Children ≥2 years: Ulcerative colitis: Initial: 40-60 mg/kg/day in 3-6 divided doses; maintenance dose: 20-30 mg/kg/day in 4 divided doses

Children ≥6 years: Juvenile rheumatoid arthritis: Enteric coated tablet: 30-50 mg/kg/day in 2 divided doses; Initial: Begin with 1/4 to 1/3 of expected maintenance dose; increase weekly; maximum: 2 g/day typically

Adults:

Ulcerative colitis: Initial: 1 g 3-4 times/day, 2 g/day maintenance in divided doses; may initiate therapy with 0.5-1 g/day

Rheumatoid arthritis: Enteric coated tablet: Initial: 0.5-1 g/day; increase weekly to maintenance dose of 2 g/day in 2 divided doses; maximum: 3 g/day (if response to 2 g/day is inadequate after 12 weeks of treatment)

Dosing interval in renal impairment:

Cl_{cr} 10-30 mL/minute: Administer twice daily

Cl_{cr} <10 mL/minute: Administer once daily

Dosing adjustment in hepatic impairment: Avoid use

Mechanism of Action Acts locally in the colon to decrease the inflammatory response and systemically interferes with secretion by inhibiting prostaglandin synthesis

Other Adverse Effects

>10%:

Central nervous system: Headache (33%)

Dermatologic: Photosensitivity

Gastrointestinal: Anorexia, nausea, vomiting, diarrhea (33%), gastric distress
Genitourinary: Reversible oligospermia (33%)

<3%:
Dermatologic: Urticaria/pruritus (<3%)
Hematologic: Hemolytic anemia (<3%), Heinz body anemia (<3%)

<0.1%: Alopecia, anaphylaxis, aplastic anemia, ataxia, convulsions, crystalluria, depression, drowsiness, epidermal necrolysis, exfoliative dermatitis, granulocytopenia, hallucinations, hearing loss, hematuria, hepatitis, insomnia, interstitial nephritis, jaundice, leukopenia, Lyell's syndrome, myelodysplastic syndrome, nephropathy (acute), neutropenic enterocolitis, pancreatitis, peripheral neuropathy, photosensitization, rhabdomyolysis, serum sickness-like reactions, skin discoloration, Stevens-Johnson syndrome, thrombocytopenia, thyroid function disturbance, tinnitus, urine discoloration, vasculitis, vertigo

Additional events reported with sulfonamides and/or 5-ASA derivatives: Cholestatic jaundice, eosinophilia pneumonitis, erythema multiforme, fibrosing alveolitis, hepatic necrosis, Kawasaki-like syndrome, SLE-like syndrome, pericarditis, seizures, transverse myelitis

Drug Interactions

Increased Effect/Toxicity: May increase hydantoin levels. Effects of thiopental, oral hypoglycemics, and oral anticoagulants may be increased. Sulfasalazine may increase the risk of myelosuppression with azathioprine, mercaptopurine, or thioguanine (due to TPMT inhibition); may also increase the toxicity of methotrexate. Risk of thrombocytopenia may be increased with thiazide diuretics. Concurrent methenamine may increase risk of crystalluria.

Decreased effect with iron, digoxin, and PABA or PABA-metabolites of drugs (eg, procaine, proparacaine, tetracaine).

Dietary/Ethanol/Herb Considerations

Food may impair folate absorption.

Herb/Nutraceutical: Avoid dong quai and St John's wort; may cause photosensitization.

Pharmacodynamics/Kinetics

Absorption: 10% to 15% as unchanged drug from small intestine

Distribution: Small amounts enter feces and breast milk

Metabolism: Via colonic intestinal flora to sulfapyridine and 5-aminosalicylic acid (5-ASA); following absorption, sulfapyridine undergoes N-acetylation and ring hydroxylation while 5-ASA undergoes N-acetylation

Half-life elimination: 5.7-10 hours

Excretion: Primarily urine (as unchanged drug, components, and acetylated metabolites)

Pregnancy Risk Factor B/D (at term)

Generic Available Yes: Tablet; excludes delayed release

Sulfinpyrazone (sul fin PEER a zone)

Canadian Brand Names Apo®-Sulfinpyrazone; Nu-Sulfinpyrazone

Pharmacologic Category Uricosuric Agent

Use Treatment of chronic gouty arthritis and intermittent gouty arthritis

Unlabeled/Investigational Use Decrease incidence of sudden death postmyocardial infarction

Local Anesthetic/Vasoconstrictor Precautions No information available to require special precautions

Effects on Dental Treatment No significant effects or complications reported

Dosage Oral:

Adults: 100-200 mg twice daily; maximum daily dose: 800 mg

Dosing adjustment in renal impairment: Cl_{cr} <50 mL/minute: Avoid use

Mechanism of Action Acts by increasing the urinary excretion of uric acid, thereby decreasing blood urate levels; this effect is therapeutically useful in treating patients with acute intermittent gout, chronic tophaceous gout, and acts to promote resorption of tophi; also has antithrombic and platelet inhibitory effects

Other Adverse Effects Frequency not defined:

Cardiovascular: Flushing
Central nervous system: Dizziness, headache
Dermatologic: Dermatitis, rash
Gastrointestinal (most frequent adverse effects): Nausea, vomiting, stomach pain
Genitourinary: Polyuria
Hematologic: Anemia, leukopenia, increased bleeding time (decreased platelet aggregation)
Hepatic: Hepatic necrosis
Renal: Nephrotic syndrome, uric acid stones

Drug Interactions Substrate of **CYP2C8/9**, 3A4; Inhibits CYP2C8/9; Induces CYP3A4

Increased effect of oral hypoglycemics and anticoagulants.

Increased effect/toxicity: Risk of acetaminophen hepatotoxicity is increased, while therapeutic effects may be reduced.

Decreased effect of theophylline, verapamil. Decreased uricosuric activity with salicylates, niacins.

(Continued)

Sulfinpyrazone *(Continued)*

Dietary/Ethanol/Herb Considerations Herb/Nutraceutical: Avoid dong quai and St John's wort; may cause photosensitization.

Pharmacodynamics/Kinetics
Absorption: Rapid and complete
Metabolism: Hepatic to two active metabolites
Half-life elimination: 2.7-6 hours
Time to peak, serum: 1.6 hours
Excretion: Urine (22% to 50% as unchanged drug)

Pregnancy Risk Factor C/D (near term - expert analysis)

Generic Available Yes

SulfiSOXAZOLE (sul fi SOKS a zole)

U.S. Brand Names Gantrisin®

Canadian Brand Names Novo-Soxazole®; Sulfizole®

Pharmacologic Category Antibiotic, Sulfonamide Derivative

Synonyms Sulfisoxazole Acetyl; Sulphafurazole

Use Treatment of urinary tract infections, otitis media, *Chlamydia*; nocardiosis; treatment of acute pelvic inflammatory disease in prepubertal children; often used in combination with trimethoprim

Local Anesthetic/Vasoconstrictor Precautions No information available to require special precautions

Effects on Dental Treatment No significant effects or complications reported

Dosage Oral:
Children >2 months: Initial: 75 mg/kg, followed by 120-150 mg/kg/day in divided doses every 4-6 hours; not to exceed 6 g/day
Adults: Initial: 2-4 g, then 4-8 g/day in divided doses every 4-6 hours
Dosing interval in renal impairment:
Cl_{cr} 10-50 mL/minute: Administer every 8-12 hours
Cl_{cr} <10 mL/minute: Administer every 12-24 hours
Hemodialysis: >50% removed

Mechanism of Action Interferes with bacterial growth by inhibiting bacterial folic acid synthesis through competitive antagonism of PABA

Other Adverse Effects Frequency not defined:
Cardiovascular: Vasculitis
Central nervous system: Fever, dizziness, headache
Dermatologic: Itching, rash, photosensitivity, Lyell's syndrome, Stevens-Johnson syndrome
Endocrine & metabolic: Thyroid function disturbance
Gastrointestinal: Anorexia, nausea, vomiting, diarrhea
Genitourinary: Crystalluria, hematuria,
Hematologic: Granulocytopenia, leukopenia, thrombocytopenia, aplastic anemia, hemolytic anemia
Hepatic: Jaundice, hepatitis
Renal: Interstitial nephritis
Miscellaneous: Serum sickness-like reactions

Drug Interactions Substrate of **CYP2C8/9**; Inhibits CYP2C8/9
Increased effect of oral anticoagulants, methotrexate, and oral hypoglycemic agents. May increase phenytoin levels. Risk of adverse reactions (thrombocytopenia purpura) may be increased by thiazide.
Decreased effect with PABA or PABA-metabolites of drugs (eg, procaine, proparacaine, tetracaine), thiopental. May decrease cyclosporine levels.

Dietary/Ethanol/Herb Considerations
Food interferes with folate absorption.
Herb/Nutraceutical: Avoid dong quai and St John's wort; may cause photosensitization.

Pharmacodynamics/Kinetics
Absorption: Sulfisoxazole acetyl is hydrolyzed in GI tract to sulfisoxazole which is readily absorbed
Distribution: Crosses placenta; enters breast milk
CSF:blood level ratio: Normal meninges: 50% to 80%; Inflamed meninges: 80+%
Protein binding: 85% to 88%
Metabolism: Hepatic via acetylation and glucuronide conjugation to inactive compounds
Half-life elimination: 4-7 hours; prolonged with renal impairment
Time to peak, serum: 2-3 hours
Excretion: Urine (95%, 40% to 60% as unchanged drug) within 24 hours

Pregnancy Risk Factor B/D (near term)

Generic Available Yes: Tablet

Sulfisoxazole Acetyl *see* SulfiSOXAZOLE *on page 1256*

Sulfisoxazole and Erythromycin *see* Erythromycin and Sulfisoxazole *on page 516*

Sulfonated Phenolics in Aqueous Solution

(sul fo NATE ed fe NOL iks in AY kwee us soe LOO shun)

U.S. Brand Names Debacterol®

Pharmacologic Category Aphthous Ulcer Treatment Agent

Use Dental: Therapeutic cauterization in the treatment of oral mucosal lesions (aphthous stomatitis, gingivitis, moderate to severe periodontitis)

Local Anesthetic/Vasoconstrictor Precautions No effects or complications reported

Effects on Dental Treatment In most patients, a stinging sensation will be felt immediately. Ulcer pain should subside almost immediately after rinsing.

Restrictions Currently available only by direct distribution to healthcare providers from the manufacturer. Contact Northern Research Laboratories at (888)884-4675.

Dosage One application per ulcer is usually sufficient. If the ulcer pain returns shortly after rinsing, additional applications may be applied as part of the same treatment session until the ulcer remains pain-free after rinsing. It is not recommended that more than one treatment be applied to each ulcer. Prior to application/treatment, the ulcerated mucosal area should be thoroughly dried with a cotton-tipped applicator or similar method. After drying, dip a cotton-tipped applicator into the solution and apply directly to the ulcerated area (most patients experience a brief stinging sensation immediately) and hold the applicator in contact with the ulcer for at least 5-10 seconds. The patient should then thoroughly rinse out the mouth with water and spit out the rinse water. The stinging sensation and ulcer pain will subside almost immediately after the rinse, larger ulcers may require 1-2 minutes for relief. If excess irritation occurs during use, a rinse with sodium bicarbonate (baking soda) solution will neutralize the reaction (use 0.5 teaspoon in 120 mL water).

Mechanism of Action Semiviscous, chemical cautery agent which provides controlled, focal debridement and sterilization of necrotic tissues; relieving pain, sealing damaged tissue, and providing local antiseptic action

Contraindications For external use only

Warnings/Precautions Prolonged use of Debacterol® on normal tissue should be avoided. If ingested, do not induce vomiting; immediately dilute with milk or water and get medical help or contact a Poison Control Center. If eye exposure occurs, immediately remove contact lenses, irrigate eyes for at least 15 minutes with lukewarm water, and contact a physician. Safety and efficacy in children <12 years have not been established.

Pregnancy Risk Factor C

Breast-feeding Considerations Unknown if excreted in breast milk; use with caution

Dosage Forms SOLN, topical [for oral mucosa] (Debacterol®): Sulfonated phenolics 22% and sulfuric acid 30% (1 mL)

Generic Available No

Selected Readings Rhodus NL and Bereuter J, "An Evaluation of a Chemical Cautery Agent and an Anti-inflammatory Ointment for the Treatment of Recurrent Aphthous Stomatitis: A Pilot Study," *Quintessence Int*, 1998, 29(12):769-73.

Sulindac (sul IN dak)

Related Information

Rheumatoid Arthritis, Osteoarthritis, and Osteoporosis *on page 1488*

Temporomandibular Dysfunction (TMD) *on page 1562*

U.S. Brand Names Clinoril®

Canadian Brand Names Apo®-Sulin; Novo-Sundac; Nu-Sundac

Mexican Brand Names Clinoril®; Copal®; Kenalin®

Pharmacologic Category Nonsteroidal Anti-inflammatory Drug (NSAID)

Use Management of inflammatory disease, rheumatoid disorders, acute gouty arthritis; structurally similar to indomethacin but acts like aspirin; safest NSAID for use in mild renal impairment

Local Anesthetic/Vasoconstrictor Precautions No information available to require special precautions

Effects on Dental Treatment NSAID formulations are known to reversibly decrease platelet aggregation via mechanisms different than observed with aspirin. The dentist should be aware of the potential of abnormal coagulation. Caution should also be exercised in the use of NSAIDs in patients already on anticoagulant therapy with drugs such as warfarin (Coumadin®).

Dosage Maximum therapeutic response may not be realized for up to 3 weeks

Oral:

- Children: Dose not established
- Adults: 150-200 mg twice daily or 300-400 mg once daily; not to exceed 400 mg/day
- Dosing adjustment in hepatic impairment: Reduction required

Mechanism of Action Inhibits prostaglandin synthesis by decreasing the activity of the enzyme, cyclooxygenase, which results in decreased formation of prostaglandin precursors

(Continued)

Sulindac *(Continued)*

Other Adverse Effects

1% to 10%:

Cardiovascular: Edema

Central nervous system: Dizziness, headache, nervousness

Dermatologic: Pruritus, rash

Gastrointestinal: GI pain, heartburn, nausea, vomiting, diarrhea, constipation, flatulence, anorexia, abdominal cramps

Otic: Tinnitus

<1% (Limited to important or life-threatening): Congestive heart failure, hypertension, palpitation, arrhythmia, convulsions, aseptic meningitis, erythema multiforme, toxic epidermal necrolysis, Stevens-Johnson syndrome, exfoliative dermatitis, anaphylaxis, angioneurotic edema, peptic ulcer, GI bleeding, GI perforation, agranulocytosis, aplastic anemia, hemolytic anemia, bone marrow depression, leukopenia, thrombocytopenia, neutropenia, increased PT, abnormal LFTs, pancreatitis, jaundice, hepatitis, hepatic failure, proteinuria, crystalluria, renal impairment, renal failure, nephrotic syndrome, interstitial nephritis, bronchial spasm, dyspnea, depression, psychosis, hypersensitivity reaction

Drug Interactions CYP2C9 enzyme inhibitor

Increased toxicity of digoxin, anticoagulants, methotrexate, lithium, aminoglycosides antibiotics (reported in neonates), cyclosporine (increased nephrotoxicity), and potassium-sparing diuretics (hyperkalemia). Increased toxicity with probenecid, NSAIDs.

Decreased effect of diuretics, beta-blockers, hydralazine, and captopril.

Dietary/Ethanol/Herb Considerations

Ethanol: Avoid use; may enhance gastric mucosal irritation.

Food: Administer with food or milk to reduce GI upset; may decrease therapeutic effect and rate but not extent of oral absorption. Avoid garlic, ginger, and green tea.

Herb/Nutraceutical: Avoid cat's claw, dong quai, evening primrose, feverfew, garlic, ginger, ginkgo biloba, ginseng, green tea, horse chestnut, and red clover due to additional antiplatelet activity. Avoid kava and valerian; may enhance benzodiazepine activity.

Pharmacodynamics/Kinetics

Onset of action: Analgesic: ~1 hour

Duration: 12-24 hours

Absorption: 90%

Metabolism: Hepatic; prodrug requiring metabolic activation to sulfide metabolite (active) for therapeutic effects and to sulfone metabolites (inactive)

Half-life elimination: Parent drug: 7 hours; Active metabolite: 18 hours

Excretion: Urine (50%); feces (25%)

Pregnancy Risk Factor B/D (3rd trimester)

Generic Available Yes

Sulphafurazole *see* SulfiSOXAZOLE *on page 1256*

Sumatriptan (SOO ma trip tan)

U.S. Brand Names Imitrex®

Canadian Brand Names Imitrex®

Mexican Brand Names Imigran®

Pharmacologic Category Serotonin 5-HT_{1D} Receptor Agonist

Synonyms Sumatriptan Succinate

Use Acute treatment of migraine with or without aura

Sumatriptan injection: Acute treatment of cluster headache episodes

Local Anesthetic/Vasoconstrictor Precautions No information available to require special precautions

Effects on Dental Treatment No significant effects or complications reported

Dosage Adults:

Oral: A single dose of 25 mg, 50 mg, or 100 mg (taken with fluids). If a satisfactory response has not been obtained at 2 hours, a second dose may be administered. Results from clinical trials show that initial doses of 50 mg and 100 mg are more effective than doses of 25 mg, and that 100 mg doses do not provide a greater effect than 50 mg and may have increased incidence of side effects. Although doses of up to 300 mg/day have been studied, the total daily dose should not exceed 200 mg. The safety of treating an average of >4 headaches in a 30-day period have not been established.

Intranasal: A single dose of 5 mg, 10 mg, or 20 mg administered in one nostril. A 10 mg dose may be achieved by administering a single 5 mg dose in each nostril. If headache returns, the dose may be repeated once after 2 hours, not to exceed a total daily dose of 40 mg. The safety of treating an average of >4 headaches in a 30-day period has not been established.

S.C.: 6 mg; a second injection may be administered at least 1 hour after the initial dose, but not more than 2 injections in a 24-hour period. If side effects are dose-limiting, lower doses may be used.

Elderly: Use of tablet is not recommended; use of nasal spray has not been studied; pharmacokinetics of injection are similar to healthy patients

Dosing adjustment in hepatic impairment: Contraindicated in severe impairment. Bioavailability of oral form is increased; do not exceed single doses of 50 mg. The nasal spray has not been studied in patients with hepatic impairment, however, because the spray does not undergo first-pass metabolism, levels would not be expected to alter.

Mechanism of Action Selective agonist for serotonin (5-HT_{1D} receptor) in cranial arteries to cause vasoconstriction and reduces sterile inflammation associated with antidromic neuronal transmission correlating with relief of migraine

Other Adverse Effects

>10%:

Central nervous system: Dizziness (injection 12%), warm/hot sensation (injection 11%)

Gastrointestinal: Bad taste (nasal spray 13% to 24%), nausea (nasal spray 11% to 13%), vomiting (nasal spray 11% to 13%)

Local: Injection: Pain at the injection site (59%)

Neuromuscular & skeletal: Tingling (injection 13%)

1% to 10%:

Cardiovascular: Chest pain/tightness/heaviness/pressure (injection 2% to 3%, tablet 1% to 2%)

Central nervous system: Burning (injection 7%), dizziness (nasal spray 1% to 2%, tablet >1%), feeling of heaviness (injection 7%), flushing (injection 7%), pressure sensation (injection 7%), feeling of tightness (injection 5%), numbness (injection 5%), drowsiness (injection 3%, tablet >1%), malaise/fatigue (tablet 2% to 3%, injection 1%), feeling strange (injection 2%), headache (injection 2%, tablet >1%), tight feeling in head (injection 2%), nonspecified pain (tablet 1% to 2%, placebo 1%), vertigo (tablet <1% to 2%, nasal spray 1% to 2%), migraine (tablet >1%), sleepiness (tablet >1%), cold sensation (injection 1%), anxiety (injection 1%)

Gastrointestinal: Nausea (tablet >1%), vomiting (tablet >1%), **xerostomia** (tablet >1%), abdominal discomfort (injection 1%), dysphagia (injection 1%)

Neuromuscular & skeletal: Neck, throat, and jaw pain/tightness/pressure (injection 2% to 5%, tablet 2% to 3%), mouth/tongue discomfort (injection 5%), paresthesia (tablet 3% to 5%), weakness (injection 5%), myalgia (injection 2%), muscle cramps (injection 1%)

Ocular: Vision alterations (injection 1%)

Respiratory: Nasal disorder/discomfort (nasal spray 2% to 4%, injection 2%), throat discomfort (injection 3%, nasal spray 1% to 2%)

Miscellaneous: Warm/cold sensation (tablet 2% to 3%, placebo 2%), nonspecified pressure/tightness/heaviness (tablet 1% to 3%, placebo 2%), diaphoresis (injection 2%)

<1%: Postmarketing and uncontrolled studies (limited to important or life-threatening): Abdominal aortic aneurysm, abdominal discomfort, abnormal menstrual cycle, abnormal/elevated LFTs, accommodation disorders, acute renal failure, agitation, anaphylactoid reaction, anaphylaxis, anemia, angioneurotic edema, arrhythmia, atrial fibrillation, bronchospasm, cerebral ischemia, cerebrovascular accident, convulsions, deafness, death, decreased appetite, dental pain, diarrhea, dyspeptic symptoms, dysphagia, dystonic reaction, EKG changes, fluid disturbances (including retention), flushing, gastrointestinal pain, hallucinations, heart block, hematuria, hemolytic anemia, hiccoughs, hypersensitivity reactions, increased intracranial pressure, increased TSH, intestinal obstruction, ischemic colitis, joint ache, muscle stiffness, nose/throat hemorrhage, numbness of tongue, optic neuropathy (ischemic), pancytopenia, paresthesia, phlebitis, photosensitivity, Prinzmetal's angina, pruritus, psychomotor disorders, pulmonary embolism, rash, Raynaud syndrome, sensation changes, shock, subarachnoid hemorrhage, swallowing disorders, syncope, thrombocytopenia, thrombophlebitis, thrombosis, transient myocardial ischemia, vasculitis, vision loss, xerostomia

Drug Interactions Increased toxicity with ergot-containing drugs, avoid use, wait 24 hours from last ergot containing drug (dihydroergotamine, or methysergide) before administering sumatriptan. MAO inhibitors decrease clearance of sumatriptan increasing the risk of systemic sumatriptan toxic effects. Sumatriptan may enhance CNS toxic effects when taken with selective serotonin reuptake inhibitors (SSRIs) like fluoxetine, fluvoxamine, paroxetine, or sertraline.

Dietary/Ethanol/Herb Considerations Ethanol: Avoid use; may cause or worsen headaches.

Pharmacodynamics/Kinetics

Onset of action: ~30 minutes

Distribution: V_d: 2.4 L/kg

Protein binding: 14% to 21%

Bioavailability: S.C.: 97% ± 16% of that following I.V. injection

Half-life elimination: Injection, tablet: 2.5 hours; Nasal spray: 2 hours

Time to peak, serum: 5-20 minutes

(Continued)

Sumatriptan *(Continued)*

Excretion:

Injection: Urine (38% as indole acetic acid metabolite, 22% as unchanged drug)

Nasal spray: Urine (42% as indole acetic acid metabolite, 3% as unchanged drug)

Tablet: Urine (60% as indole acetic acid metabolite, 3% as unchanged drug); feces (40%)

Pregnancy Risk Factor C

Generic Available No

Sumatriptan Succinate *see* Sumatriptan *on page 1258*

Summer's Eve® Medicated Douche [OTC] *see* Povidone-Iodine *on page 1104*

Summer's Eve® SpecialCare™ Medicated Anti-Itch Cream [OTC] *see* Hydrocortisone *on page 688*

Sumycin® *see* Tetracycline *on page 1286*

Supartz™ *see* Sodium Hyaluronate *on page 1230*

Superdophilus® [OTC] *see Lactobacillus acidophilus* and *Lactobacillus bulgaricus on page 772*

Suprax® [DSC] *see* Cefixime *on page 268*

Surbex-T® Filmtabs® [OTC] *see* Vitamin B Complex and Vitamin C *on page 1392*

Surbex® With C Filmtabs® [OTC] *see* Vitamin B Complex and Vitamin C *on page 1392*

Sureprin 81™ [OTC] *see* Aspirin *on page 131*

Surfak® [OTC] *see* Docusate *on page 463*

Surgicel® *see* Cellulose (Oxidized) *on page 284*

Surgicel® Absorbable Hemostat *see* Cellulose (Oxidized/Regenerated) *on page 284*

Surmontil® *see* Trimipramine *on page 1354*

Survanta® *see* Beractant *on page 176*

Sus-Phrine® (Dental) *see* Epinephrine *on page 499*

Sustiva® *see* Efavirenz *on page 488*

Su-Tuss®-HD *see* Hydrocodone, Pseudoephedrine, and Guaifenesin *on page 687*

Sween Cream® [OTC] *see* Vitamin A and Vitamin D *on page 1392*

Symax SL *see* Hyoscyamine *on page 699*

Symax SR *see* Hyoscyamine *on page 699*

Symmetrel® *see* Amantadine *on page 70*

Synacthen *see* Cosyntropin *on page 374*

Synagis® *see* Palivizumab *on page 1028*

Synalar® *see* Fluocinolone *on page 584*

Synalgos®-DC *see* Dihydrocodeine, Aspirin, and Caffeine *on page 444*

Synarel® *see* Nafarelin *on page 944*

Synercid® *see* Quinupristin and Dalfopristin *on page 1161*

Synthetic Lung Surfactant *see* Colfosceril Palmitate *on page 366*

Synthroid® *see* Levothyroxine *on page 800*

T_3 Sodium *see* Liothyronine *on page 810*

T_3/T_4 Liotrix *see* Liotrix *on page 811*

T_4 *see* Levothyroxine *on page 800*

T-20 *see* Enfuvirtide *on page 495*

Tac™-3 [DSC] *see* Triamcinolone *on page 1341*

Tacrine (TAK reen)

U.S. Brand Names Cognex®

Pharmacologic Category Acetylcholinesterase Inhibitor (Central)

Synonyms Tacrine Hydrochloride; Tetrahydroaminoacrine; THA

Use Treatment of mild to moderate dementia of the Alzheimer's type

Local Anesthetic/Vasoconstrictor Precautions No information available to require special precautions

Effects on Dental Treatment No significant effects or complications reported

Dosage Adults: Initial: 10 mg 4 times/day; may increase by 40 mg/day adjusted every 6 weeks; maximum: 160 mg/day; best administered separate from meal times.

Dose adjustment based upon transaminase elevations:

ALT ≤3 x ULN*: Continue titration

ALT >3 to ≤5 x ULN*: Decrease dose by 40 mg/day, resume when ALT returns to normal

ALT >5 x ULN*: Stop treatment, may rechallenge upon return of ALT to normal

*ULN = upper limit of normal

Patients with clinical jaundice confirmed by elevated total bilirubin (>3 mg/dL) should not be rechallenged with tacrine

Mechanism of Action Centrally-acting cholinesterase inhibitor. It elevates acetylcholine in cerebral cortex by slowing the degradation of acetylcholine.

Other Adverse Effects

>10%:

Central nervous system: Headache, dizziness
Gastrointestinal: Nausea, vomiting, diarrhea
Miscellaneous: Elevated transaminases

1% to 10%:

Cardiovascular: Flushing
Central nervous system: Confusion, ataxia, insomnia, somnolence, depression, anxiety, fatigue
Dermatologic: Rash
Gastrointestinal: Dyspepsia, anorexia, abdominal pain, flatulence, constipation, weight loss
Neuromuscular & skeletal: Myalgia, tremor
Respiratory: Rhinitis

Drug Interactions Substrate of **CYP1A2**; Inhibits CYP1A2

Increased Effect/Toxicity: Tacrine in combination with other cholinergic agents (eg, ambenonium, edrophonium, neostigmine, pyridostigmine, bethanechol), will likely produce additive cholinergic effects. Tacrine in combination with beta-blockers may produce additive bradycardia. Tacrine may increase the levels/effect of succinylcholine and theophylline. in elevated plasma levels. Fluvoxamine, enoxacin, and cimetidine increase tacrine concentrations via enzyme inhibition (CYP1A2).

Decreased Effect: Enzyme inducers and cigarette smoking may reduce tacrine plasma levels via enzyme induction (CYP1A2). Tacrine may worsen Parkinson's disease and inhibit the effects of levodopa. Tacrine may antagonize the therapeutic effect of anticholinergic agents (benztropine, trihexphenidyl).

Dietary/Ethanol/Herb Considerations Food decreases bioavailability.

Pharmacodynamics/Kinetics

Absorption: Oral: Rapid
Distribution: V_d: Mean: 349 L; reduced by food
Protein binding, plasma: 55%
Metabolism: Extensively by CYP450 to multiple metabolites; first pass effect
Bioavailability: Absolute: 17%
Half-life elimination, serum: 2-4 hours; Steady-state: 24-36 hours
Time to peak, plasma: 1-2 hours

Pregnancy Risk Factor C

Generic Available No

Tacrine Hydrochloride *see* Tacrine *on page 1260*

Tacrolimus (ta KROE li mus)

U.S. Brand Names Prograf®; Protopic®

Canadian Brand Names Prograf®; Protopic®

Mexican Brand Names Prograf®

Pharmacologic Category Immunosuppressant Agent; Topical Skin Product

Synonyms FK506

Use

Oral/injection: Potent immunosuppressive drug used in liver or kidney transplant recipients

Topical: Moderate to severe atopic dermatitis in patients not responsive to conventional therapy or when conventional therapy is not appropriate

Unlabeled/Investigational Use Potent immunosuppressive drug for recipients of heart, lung, small bowel, peripheral stem cell/bone marrow transplantations

Local Anesthetic/Vasoconstrictor Precautions No information available to require special precautions

Effects on Dental Treatment 3% to 15%: Otitis media

Dosage

Children:

Liver transplant: Patients without pre-existing renal or hepatic dysfunction have required and tolerated higher doses than adults to achieve similar blood concentrations. It is recommended that therapy be initiated at high end of the recommended adult I.V. and oral dosing ranges; dosage adjustments may be required.

Oral: Initial dose: 0.15-0.20 mg/kg/day in 2 divided doses, given every 12 hours; begin oral dose no sooner than 6 hours post-transplant; adjunctive therapy with corticosteroids is recommended; if switching from I.V. to oral, the oral dose should be started 8-12 hours after stopping the infusion

Typical whole blood trough concentrations: Months 1-12: 5-20 ng/mL

I.V.: **Note:** I.V. route should only be used in patients not able to take oral medications, anaphylaxis has been reported. Initial dose: 0.03-0.05 mg/kg/day as a continuous infusion; begin no sooner than 6 hours post-transplant; adjunctive therapy with corticosteroids is recommended; continue only until oral medication can be tolerated

(Continued)

Tacrolimus *(Continued)*

Children ≥2 years: Moderate to severe atopic dermatitis: Topical: Apply 0.03% ointment to affected area twice daily; rub in gently and completely; continue applications for 1 week after symptoms have cleared

Adults:

Kidney transplant:

Oral: Initial dose: 0.2 mg/kg/day in 2 divided doses, given every 12 hours; initial dose may be given within 24 hours of transplant, but should be delayed until renal function has recovered; African-American patients may require larger doses to maintain trough concentration

Typical whole blood trough concentrations: Months 1-3: 7- 20 ng/mL; months 4-12: 5-15 ng/mL

I.V.: **Note:** I.V. route should only be used in patients not able to take oral medications, anaphylaxis has been reported. Initial dose: 0.03-0.05 mg/kg/day as a continuous infusion; begin no sooner than 6 hours post-transplant, starting at lower end of the dosage range; adjunctive therapy with corticosteroids is recommended; continue only until oral medication can be tolerated

Liver transplant:

Oral: Initial dose: 0.1-0.15 mg/kg/day in 2 divided doses, given every 12 hours; begin oral dose no sooner than 6 hours post-transplant; adjunctive therapy with corticosteroids is recommended; if switching from I.V. to oral, the oral dose should be started 8-12 hours after stopping the infusion

Typical whole blood trough concentrations: Months 1-12: 5-20 ng/mL

I.V.: **Note:** I.V. route should only be used in patients not able to take oral medications, anaphylaxis has been reported. Initial dose: 0.03-0.05 mg/kg/day as a continuous infusion; begin no sooner than 6 hours post-transplant starting at lower end of the dosage range; adjunctive therapy with corticosteroids is recommended; continue only until oral medication can be tolerated

Prevention of graft-vs-host disease: I.V.: 0.03 mg/kg/day as continuous infusion

Moderate to severe atopic dermatitis: Topical: Apply 0.03% or 0.1% ointment to affected area twice daily; rub in gently and completely; continue applications for 1 week after symptoms have cleared

Dosing adjustment in renal impairment: Evidence suggests that lower doses should be used; patients should receive doses at the lowest value of the recommended I.V. and oral dosing ranges; further reductions in dose below these ranges may be required.

Tacrolimus therapy should usually be delayed up to 48 hours or longer in patients with postoperative oliguria

Hemodialysis: Not removed by hemodialysis; supplemental dose is unnecessary

Peritoneal dialysis: Significant drug removal is unlikely based on physiochemical characteristics

Dosing adjustment in hepatic impairment: Use of tacrolimus in liver transplant recipients experiencing post-transplant hepatic impairment may be associated with increased risk of developing renal insufficiency related to high whole blood levels of tacrolimus. The presence of moderate-to-severe hepatic dysfunction (serum bilirubin >2 mg/dL) appears to affect the metabolism of FK506. The halflife of the drug was prolonged and the clearance reduced after I.V. administration. The bioavailability of FK506 was also increased after oral administration. The higher plasma concentrations as determined by ELISA, in patients with severe hepatic dysfunction are probably due to the accumulation of FK506 metabolites of lower activity. These patients should be monitored closely and dosage adjustments should be considered. Some evidence indicates that lower doses could be used in these patients.

Mechanism of Action Suppresses cellular immunity (inhibits T-lymphocyte activation), possibly by binding to an intracellular protein, FKBP-12

Other Adverse Effects

Oral, I.V.:

≥15%

Cardiovascular: Chest pain, hypertension

Central nervous system: Dizziness, headache, insomnia, tremor (headache and tremor are associated with high whole blood concentrations and may respond to decreased dosage)

Dermatologic: Pruritus, rash

Endocrine & metabolic: Diabetes mellitus, hyperglycemia, hyperkalemia, hyperlipemia, hypomagnesemia, hypophosphatemia

Gastrointestinal: Abdominal pain, constipation, diarrhea, dyspepsia, nausea, vomiting

Genitourinary: Urinary tract infection

Hematologic: Anemia, leukocytosis, thrombocytopenia

Hepatic: Ascites

Neuromuscular & skeletal: Arthralgia, back pain, weakness, paresthesia

Renal: Abnormal kidney function, increased creatinine, oliguria, urinary tract infection, increased BUN

Respiratory: Atelectasis, dyspnea, increased cough

3% to 15%:

Cardiovascular: Abnormal EKG, angina pectoris, deep thrombophlebitis, hemorrhage, hypotension, hypervolemia, generalized edema, peripheral vascular disorder, phlebitis, postural hypotension, tachycardia, thrombosis, vasodilation

Central nervous system: Abnormal dreams, abnormal thinking, agitation, amnesia, anxiety, chills, confusion, depression, emotional lability, encephalopathy, hallucinations, nervousness, psychosis, somnolence

Dermatologic: Acne, alopecia, cellulitis, exfoliative dermatitis, fungal dermatitis, hirsutism, increased diaphoresis, photosensitivity reaction, skin discoloration, skin disorder, skin ulcer

Endocrine & metabolic: Acidosis, alkalosis, Cushing's syndrome, decreased bicarbonate, decreased serum iron, diabetes mellitus, hypercalcemia, hypercholesterolemia, hyperphosphatemia, hypoproteinemia, increased alkaline phosphatase, increase LDH

Gastrointestinal: Anorexia, cramps, dysphagia, enlarged abdomen, esophagitis, flatulence, gastritis, GI perforation/hemorrhage, ileus, increased appetite, oral moniliasis, rectal disorder, stomatitis, weight gain

Genitourinary: Urinary frequency, urinary incontinence, vaginitis, cystitis, dysuria

Hematologic: Bruising, coagulation disorder, decreased prothrombin, hypochromic anemia, leukopenia, polycythemia

Hepatic: Abnormal LFTs, bilirubinemia, cholangitis, cholestatic jaundice, hepatitis, increased ALT, increased AST, increased GGT, jaundice, liver damage

Neuromuscular & skeletal: Hypertonia, incoordination, joint disorder, leg cramps, myalgia, myasthenia, myoclonus, neuropathy, osteoporosis

Ocular: Abnormal vision, amblyopia

Otic: Ear pain, tinnitus

Renal: Albuminuria

Respiratory: Asthma, bronchitis, lung disorder, pharyngitis, pneumonia, pneumothorax, pulmonary edema, respiratory disorder, rhinitis, sinusitis, voice alteration

Miscellaneous: Abscess, abnormal healing, allergic reaction, flu-like syndrome, generalized spasm, hernia, herpes simplex, peritonitis, sepsis

Postmarketing and/or case reports: Acute renal failure, anaphylaxis, coma, deafness, delirium, hearing loss, hemolytic-uremic syndrome, leukoencephalopathy, lymphoproliferative disorder (related to EBV), myocardial hypertrophy (associated with ventricular dysfunction), pancreatitis, seizures, Stevens-Johnson syndrome, thrombocytopenic purpura, torsade de pointes

Topical (as reported in children and adults, unless otherwise noted):

>10%:

Central nervous system: Headache (5% to 20%), fever (1% to 21%)

Dermatologic: Skin burning (43% to 58%), pruritus (41% to 46%), erythema (12% to 28%)

Respiratory: Increased cough (18% children)

Miscellaneous: Flu-like syndrome (23% to 28%), allergic reaction (4% to 12%)

1% to 10%:

Cardiovascular: Peripheral edema (3% to 4% adults)

Central nervous system: Hyperesthesia (3% to 7% adults), pain (1% to 2%)

Dermatologic: Skin tingling (2% to 8%), acne (4% to 7% adults), folliculitis (2% to 6%), urticaria (1% to 6%), rash (2% to 5%), pustular rash (2% to 4%), vesiculobullous rash (4% children), contact dermatitis (3% to 4%), cyst (1% to 3% adults), eczema herpeticum (1% to 2%), fungal dermatitis (1% to 2% adults), sunburn (1% to 2% adults), dry skin (1% children)

Endocrine & metabolic: Dysmenorrhea (4% women)

Gastrointestinal: Diarrhea (3% to 5%), dyspepsia (1% to 4% adults), abdominal pain (3% children), vomiting (1% adults), gastroenteritis (adults 2%), nausea (1% children)

Neuromuscular & skeletal: Myalgia (2% to 3% adults), weakness (2% to 3% adults), back pain (2% adults)

Ocular: Conjunctivitis (2% adults)

Otic: Otitis media (12% children)

Respiratory: Rhinitis (6% children), sinusitis (2% to 4% adults), bronchitis (2% adults), pneumonia (1% adults)

Miscellaneous: Ethanol intolerance (3% to 7% adults), varicella/herpes zoster (1% to 5%), lymphadenopathy (3% children)

≥1%: Alopecia, increased ALT, increased AST, anaphylactoid reaction, angina pectoris, angioedema, anorexia, anxiety, arrhythmia, arthralgia, arthritis, bilirubinemia, breast pain, cellulitis, cerebrovascular accident, cheilitis, chills, constipation, increased creatinine, dehydration, depression, dizziness, dyspnea, ear pain, ecchymosis, edema, epistaxis, exacerbation of untreated area, eye pain, furunculosis, gastritis, hernia, hyperglycemia, hypertension, hypoglycemia, hypoxia, laryngitis, leukocytosis, leukopenia, abnormal LFTs, lymphadenopathy (0.8%), malaise, migraine, neck pain, neuritis, palpitations, paresthesia, peripheral vascular disorder, photosensitivity reaction, skin discoloration, diaphoresis, abnormal taste, unintended pregnancy, vaginal moniliasis, vasodilation, vertigo

(Continued)

Tacrolimus *(Continued)*

Drug Interactions Substrate of **CYP3A4**; Inhibits CYP3A4

Increased Effect/Toxicity: Amphotericin B and other nephrotoxic antibiotics have the potential to increase tacrolimus-associated nephrotoxicity. Agents which may increase tacrolimus plasma concentrations resulting in toxicity are erythromycin, clarithromycin, clotrimazole, fluconazole, itraconazole, ketoconazole, diltiazem, nicardipine, verapamil, bromocriptine, cimetidine, cisapride, danazol, metoclopramide, methylprednisolone, and cyclosporine (synergistic immunosuppression). Voriconazole may increase tacrolimus serum concentrations; decrease tacrolimus dosage by 66% when initiating voriconazole.

Decreased Effect: Antacids impair tacrolimus absorption; separate administration by at least 2 hours. Agents which may decrease tacrolimus plasma concentrations and reduce the therapeutic effect include rifampin, rifabutin, phenytoin, phenobarbital, and carbamazepine.

Dietary/Ethanol/Herb Considerations

Food: Administer capsules on an empty stomach, 30 minutes before or after meal; food decreases rate and extent of absorption. High-fat meals have most pronounced effect (35% decrease in AUC, 77% decrease in C_{max}). Avoid grapefruit products; may increase serum concentration/toxicity. Be consistent with timing and composition of meals if GI intolerance occurs (per manufacturer).

Herb/Nutraceutical: Avoid St John's wort; may decrease serum concentration.

Pharmacodynamics/Kinetics

Absorption: Better in resected patients with a closed stoma; unlike cyclosporine, clamping of the T-tube in liver transplant patients does not alter trough concentrations or AUC

Oral: Incomplete and variable; food within 15 minutes of administration decreases absorption (27%)

Topical: Serum concentrations range from undetectable to 20 ng/mL (<5 ng/mL in majority of adult patients studied)

Protein binding: 99%

Metabolism: Extensively hepatic via CYP3A4 to eight possible metabolites (major metabolite, 31-demethyl tacrolimus, shows same activity as tacrolimus *in vitro*)

Bioavailability: Oral: Adults: 7% to 28%, Children: 10% to 52%; Topical: <0.5%; Absolute: Unknown

Half-life elimination: Variable, 21-61 hours in healthy volunteers

Time to peak: 0.5-4 hours

Excretion: Feces (~92%); feces/urine (<1% as unchanged drug)

Pregnancy Risk Factor C

Generic Available No

Tagamet® *see* Cimetidine *on page 326*

Tagamet® HB 200 [OTC] *see* Cimetidine *on page 326*

Talacen® *see* Pentazocine Combinations *on page 1054*

Talwin® *see* Pentazocine *on page 1054*

Talwin® NX *see* Pentazocine *on page 1054*

Tambocor™ *see* Flecainide *on page 574*

Tamiflu® *see* Oseltamivir *on page 1006*

Tamoxifen (ta MOKS i fen)

U.S. Brand Names Nolvadex®

Canadian Brand Names Apo®-Tamox; Gen-Tamoxifen; Nolvadex®; Nolvadex®-D; Novo-Tamoxifen; PMS-Tamoxifen; Tamofen®

Mexican Brand Names Bilem; Cryoxifeno; Nolvadex®; Tamoxan; Taxus®; Tecnofen®

Pharmacologic Category Antineoplastic Agent, Estrogen Receptor Antagonist

Synonyms Tamoxifen Citrate

Use Palliative or adjunctive treatment of advanced breast cancer; reduce the incidence of breast cancer in women at high risk (at least 35 years of age with 5-year predicted risk ≥1.67% calculated by Gail Model); reduce risk of invasive breast cancer in women with ductal carcinoma *in situ* (DCIS); metastatic male breast cancer

Unlabeled/Investigational Use Treatment of mastalgia, gynecomastia, pancreatic carcinoma, precocious puberty in females (secondary to McCune-Albright syndrome); induction of ovulation

Local Anesthetic/Vasoconstrictor Precautions No information available to require special precautions

Effects on Dental Treatment No significant effects or complications reported

Dosage Oral (refer to individual protocols):

Children: Female: Precocious puberty and McCune-Albright syndrome (unlabeled use): A dose of 20 mg/day has been reported in patients 2-10 years of age; safety and efficacy have not been established for treatment of longer than 1 year duration

Adults:

Breast cancer:

Metastatic (males and females) or adjuvant therapy (females): 20-40 mg/day; dosages >20 mg/day in divided doses; 20 mg/day is most common

Prevention (high-risk females): 20 mg/day for 5 years

DCIS (females): 20 mg once daily for 5 years

Note: Higher dosages (up to 700 mg/day) have been investigated for use in modulation of multidrug resistance (MDR), but are not routinely used in clinical practice

Induction of ovulation (unlabeled use): 5-40 mg twice daily for 4 days

Mechanism of Action Competitively binds to estrogen receptors on tumors and other tissue targets, producing a nuclear complex that decreases DNA synthesis and inhibits estrogen effects; nonsteroidal agent with potent antiestrogenic properties which compete with estrogen for binding sites in breast and other tissues; cells accumulate in the G_0 and G_1 phases; therefore, tamoxifen is cytostatic rather than cytocidal.

Other Adverse Effects Note: Differences in the frequency of some adverse events may be related to use for a specific indication.

Frequency not defined: Depression, dizziness, headache, hypercalcemia, lightheadedness, peripheral edema, pruritus vulvae, abnormal taste, vaginal dryness

>10%:

Cardiovascular: Fluid retention (32%)

Central nervous system: Mood changes (up to 12%; may include depression)

Dermatologic: Skin changes (19%)

Endocrine & metabolic: Hot flashes (64% to 80%), weight loss (23%)

Gastrointestinal: Nausea (26%)

Genitourinary: Vaginal bleeding (up to 23%), vaginal discharge (30% to 55%), menstrual irregularities (25%)

Neuromuscular & skeletal: Bone pain, tumor pain, and local disease flare (including increase in lesion size and erythema) during treatment of metastatic breast cancer (generally resolves with continuation)

1% to 10%:

Dermatologic: Alopecia (<1% to 5%)

Gastrointestinal: Constipation (up to 4%)

Hematologic: Thrombocytopenia (<1% to 2%)

Hepatic: SGOT increased (2%), serum bilirubin increased (2%)

Renal: Serum creatinine increased (up to 2%)

Miscellaneous: Infection/sepsis (up to 6%), allergic reaction (up to 3%)

<1% (Limited to important or life-threatening): Angioedema, bullous pemphigoid, deep vein thrombosis, erythema multiforme, hypersensitivity reactions, hypertriglyceridemia, interstitial pneumonitis, pancreatitis, phlebitis, pulmonary embolism, rash, retinopathy (optic disc swelling, retinal hemorrhage, visual impairment associated with doses >200 mg/day), Stevens-Johnson syndrome

Warnings/Precautions The Food and Drug Administration (FDA) and AstraZeneca have added a black box warning to the Nolvadex (tamoxifen) product labeling, concerning its use in women taking this medication to reduce the risk of developing breast cancer. This would include women at high risk for cancer and women with ductal carcinoma in situ (DCIS).

Serious and life-threatening events (including stroke, pulmonary emboli, and uterine malignancy) have occurred at an incidence greater than placebo during use for cancer risk reduction; these events are rare, but require consideration in risk:benefit evaluation. Use with caution in patients with leukopenia, thrombocytopenia, or hyperlipidemias; ovulation may be induced; decreased visual acuity, retinopathy, corneal changes, and increased incidence of cataracts have been reported; hypercalcemia in patients with bone metastasis; hepatocellular carcinomas have been reported in some studies, relationship to treatment is unclear. Endometrial hyperplasia and polyps have occurred. Increased risk of uterine or endometrial cancer; monitor.

Drug Interactions Substrate of CYP2A6, 2B6, **2C8/9, 2D6**, 2E1, **3A4**; Inhibits CYP2B6, 2C8/9, 3A4

Increased Effect/Toxicity: Allopurinol and tamoxifen results in exacerbation of allopurinol-induced hepatotoxicity. Cyclosporine serum levels may be increased when taken with tamoxifen. Bromocriptine may increase serum levels of tamoxifen. Concomitant use of warfarin is contraindicated when used for risk reduction; results in significant enhancement of the anticoagulant effects of warfarin.

Decreased Effect: CYP3A4 inducers may decrease serum levels of tamoxifen. Letrozole serum levels may be reduced by tamoxifen.

Dietary/Ethanol/Herb Considerations Herb/Nutraceutical: Avoid black cohosh and dong quai in estrogen-dependent tumors.

Pharmacodynamics/Kinetics

Absorption: Well absorbed

Distribution: High concentrations found in uterus, endometrial and breast tissue

Protein binding: 99%

Metabolism: Hepatic (via CYP3A4) to major metabolites, desmethyltamoxifen and 4-hydroxytamoxifen; undergoes enterohepatic recirculation

(Continued)

Tamoxifen *(Continued)*

Half-life elimination: Distribution: 7-14 hours; Elimination: 5-7 days; Metabolites: 14 days
Time to peak, serum: 5 hours
Excretion: Feces (26% to 51%); urine (9% to 13%)

Pregnancy Risk Factor D
Generic Available Yes

Tamoxifen Citrate *see* Tamoxifen *on page 1264*

Tamsulosin (tam SOO loe sin)

U.S. Brand Names Flomax®
Canadian Brand Names Flomax®
Mexican Brand Names Secotex®
Pharmacologic Category Alpha$_1$ Blocker
Synonyms Tamsulosin Hydrochloride
Use Treatment of signs and symptoms of benign prostatic hyperplasia (BPH)

Local Anesthetic/Vasoconstrictor Precautions No information available to require special precautions

Effects on Dental Treatment No significant effects or complications reported

Dosage Oral: Adults: 0.4 mg once daily approximately 30 minutes after the same meal each day

Mechanism of Action An antagonist of alpha$_{1A}$ adrenoreceptors in the prostate. Three subtypes identified: alpha$_{1A}$, alpha$_{1B}$, alpha$_{1D}$ have distribution that differs between human organs and tissue. Approximately 70% of the alpha$_1$-receptors in human prostate are of alpha$_{1A}$ subtype. The symptoms associated with benign prostatic hyperplasia (BPH) are related to bladder outlet obstruction, which is comprised of two underlying components: static and dynamic. Static is related to an increase in prostate size, partially caused by a proliferation of smooth muscle cells in the prostatic stroma. Severity of BPH symptoms and the degree of urethral obstruction do not correlate well with the size of the prostate. Dynamic is a function of an increase in smooth muscle tone in the prostate and bladder neck leading to constriction of the bladder outlet. Smooth muscle tone is mediated by the sympathetic nervous stimulation of alpha$_1$ adrenoreceptors, which are abundant in the prostate, prostatic capsule, prostatic urethra, and bladder neck. Blockade of these adrenoreceptors can cause smooth muscles in the bladder neck and prostate to relax, resulting in an improvement in urine flow rate and a reduction in symptoms of BPH.

Other Adverse Effects

Orthostatic hypotension (by testing criteria): First-dose orthostatic hypotension at 4 hours postdose has been observed in 7% of patients following a 0.4 mg dose as compared to 3% in a placebo group. Overall, at least one positive test was observed in 16% of patients receiving 0.4 mg and 19% of patients receiving the 0.8 mg dose as compared to 11% in a placebo group. **Percentages correspond to the 0.4 mg and 0.8 mg doses, respectively.**

>10%:
- Central nervous system: Headache (19% to 21%), dizziness (15% to 17%)
- Genitourinary: Abnormal ejaculation (8% to 18%)
- Respiratory: Rhinitis (13% to 18%)

1% to 10%:
- Cardiovascular: Chest pain (~4%)
- Central nervous system: Weakness (8% to 9%), somnolence (3% to 4%), insomnia (1% to 2%)
- Endocrine & metabolic: Decreased libido (1% to 2%)
- Gastrointestinal: Diarrhea (4% to 6%), nausea (3% to 4%), stomach discomfort (2% to 3%), bitter taste (2% to 3%)
- Neuromuscular & skeletal: Back pain (7% to 8%)
- Ocular: Amblyopia (0.2% to 2%)
- Respiratory: Pharyngitis (6% to 5%), cough (3% to 5%), sinusitis (2% to 4%)
- Miscellaneous: Infection (9% to 11%), tooth disorder (1% to 2%)

<1% (Limited to important or life-threatening): Orthostasis (symptomatic) (0.2% to 0.4%), syncope (0.2% to 0.4%), vertigo (0.6% to 1%)

Postmarketing and/or case reports: Allergic reactions (rash, angioedema, pruritus, urticaria) priapism; constipation, elevated transaminases, palpitations, vomiting

Drug Interactions Substrate of **CYP2D6, 3A4**

Increased Effect/Toxicity: Metabolized by cytochrome P450 isoenzymes. Profile of involved isoenzymes has not been established. Concurrent cimetidine therapy increased AUC of tamsulosin by 44%. Use with caution in patients receiving concurrent warfarin therapy (may increase anticoagulant effect). Do not use in combination with other alpha-blocking drugs.

Decreased Effect: Metabolism by cytochrome P450 isoenzymes may, in theory, be influenced by enzyme-inducing agents, resulting in decreased effects.

Dietary/Ethanol/Herb Considerations

Food: The time to peak (T_{max}) is reached in 4-5 hours under fasting conditions and 6-7 hours with food. Fasting conditions result in a 30% increase in bioavailability and 40% to 70% increase in peak concentration (C_{max}) compared to fed conditions.

Herb/Nutraceutical: Avoid saw palmetto due to limited experience with this combination.

Pharmacodynamics/Kinetics

Absorption: >90%

Protein binding: 94% to 99%, primarily to alpha$_1$ acid glycoprotein (AAG); not affected by amitriptyline, diclofenac, glyburide, simvastatin plus simvastatin-hydroxy acid metabolite, warfarin, diazepam, propranolol, trichlormethiazide, or chlormadinone, nor does tamsulosin effect extent of binding of these drugs

Metabolism: Hepatic via CYP; metabolites undergo extensive conjugation to glucuronide or sulfate

Bioavailability: Fasting: 30% increase

Steady-state: By the fifth day of once daily dosing

Half-life elimination: Healthy volunteers: 9-13 hours; Target population: 14-15 hours

Time to peak: C_{max}: Fasting: 40% to 70% increase; T_{max}: Fasting: 4-5 hours; With food: 6-7 hours

Excretion: Urine (<10% as unchanged drug)

Pregnancy Risk Factor B

Generic Available No

Tamsulosin Hydrochloride *see* Tamsulosin *on page 1266*

Tannic-12 *see* Carbetapentane and Chlorpheniramine *on page 245*

Tannic-12 S *see* Carbetapentane and Chlorpheniramine *on page 245*

Tanoral® *see* Chlorpheniramine, Pyrilamine, and Phenylephrine *on page 312*

Tao® *see* Troleandomycin *on page 1359*

Tapazole® *see* Methimazole *on page 880*

Targretin® *see* Bexarotene *on page 182*

Tarka® *see* Trandolapril and Verapamil *on page 1332*

Tasmar® *see* Tolcapone *on page 1320*

Tavist® *see* Clemastine *on page 340*

Tavist®-1 [OTC] *see* Clemastine *on page 340*

Taxol® *see* Paclitaxel *on page 1026*

Taxotere® *see* Docetaxel *on page 461*

Tazarotene (taz AR oh teen)

U.S. Brand Names Avage™; Tazorac®

Canadian Brand Names Tazorac®

Pharmacologic Category Keratolytic Agent

Use Topical treatment of facial acne vulgaris; topical treatment of stable plaque psoriasis of up to 20% body surface area involvement; mitigation (palliation) of facial skin wrinkling, facial mottled hyper/hypopigmentation, and benign facial lentigines

Local Anesthetic/Vasoconstrictor Precautions No information available to require special precautions

Effects on Dental Treatment No significant effects or complications reported

Dosage Topical: **Note:** In patients experiencing excessive pruritus, burning, skin redness, or peeling, discontinue until integrity of the skin is restored, or reduce dosing to an interval the patient is able to tolerate.

Children ≥12 years and Adults:

Acne: Tazorac® cream/gel 0.1%: Cleanse the face gently. After the skin is dry, apply a thin film of tazarotene (2 mg/cm^2) once daily, in the evening, to the skin where the acne lesions appear; use enough to cover the entire affected area

Psoriasis: Tazorac® gel 0.05% or 0.1%: Apply once daily, in the evening, to psoriatic lesions using enough (2 mg/cm^2) to cover only the lesion with a thin film to no more than 20% of body surface area. If a bath or shower is taken prior to application, dry the skin before applying. Unaffected skin may be more susceptible to irritation, avoid application to these areas.

Children ≥17 years and Adults: Palliation of fine facial wrinkles, facial mottled hyper/hypopigmentation, benign facial lentigines: Avage™: Apply a pea-sized amount once daily to clean dry face at bedtime; lightly cover entire face including eyelids if desired. Emollients or moisturizers may be applied before or after; if applied before tazarotene, ensure cream or lotion has absorbed into the skin and has dried completely.

Adults: Psoriasis: Tazorac® cream 0.05% or 0.1%: Apply once daily, in the evening, to psoriatic lesions using enough (2 mg/cm^2) to cover only the lesion with a thin film to no more than 20% of body surface area. If a bath or shower is taken prior to application, dry the skin before applying. Unaffected skin may be more susceptible to irritation, avoid application to these areas.

(Continued)

Tazarotene *(Continued)*

Elderly: No differences in safety or efficacy were seen when administered to patients >65 years of age; may experience increased sensitivity

Mechanism of Action Synthetic, acetylenic retinoid which modulates differentiation and proliferation of epithelial tissue and exerts some degree of anti-inflammatory and immunological activity

Other Adverse Effects Percentage of incidence varies with formulation and/or strength:

>10%: Dermatologic: Burning/stinging, desquamation, dry skin, erythema, pruritus, skin pain, worsening of psoriasis

1% to 10%: Dermatologic: Contact dermatitis, discoloration, fissuring, hypertriglyceridemia, inflammation, irritation, localized bleeding, rash

Frequency not defined:

Dermatologic: Photosensitization

Neuromuscular & skeletal: Peripheral neuropathy

Drug Interactions Increased toxicity may occur with sulfur, benzoyl peroxide, salicylic acid, resorcinol, or any product with strong drying effects (including alcohol-containing compounds) due to increased drying actions. May augment phototoxicity of sensitizing medications (thiazides, tetracyclines, fluoroquinolones, phenothiazines, sulfonamides).

Pharmacodynamics/Kinetics

Duration: Therapeutic: Psoriasis: Effects have been observed for up to 3 months after a 3-month course of topical treatment

Absorption: Minimal following cutaneous application (≤6% of dose)

Distribution: Retained in skin for prolonged periods after topical application.

Protein binding: >99%

Metabolism: Prodrug, rapidly metabolized via esterases to an active metabolite (tazarotenic acid) following topical application and systemic absorption; tazarotenic acid undergoes further hepatic metabolism

Half-life elimination: 18 hours

Excretion: Urine and feces (as metabolites)

Pregnancy Risk Factor X

Generic Available No

Tazicef® *see* Ceftazidime *on page 275*

Tazidime® *see* Ceftazidime *on page 275*

Tazorac® *see* Tazarotene *on page 1267*

3TC *see* Lamivudine *on page 773*

3TC, Abacavir, and Zidovudine *see* Abacavir, Lamivudine, and Zidovudine *on page 23*

T-Cell Growth Factor *see* Aldesleukin *on page 50*

TCGF *see* Aldesleukin *on page 50*

TCN *see* Tetracycline *on page 1286*

TDF *see* Tenofovir *on page 1275*

Teargen® [OTC] *see* Artificial Tears *on page 128*

Teargen® II [OTC] *see* Artificial Tears *on page 128*

Tearisol® [OTC] *see* Artificial Tears *on page 128*

Tearisol® [OTC] *see* Hydroxypropyl Methylcellulose *on page 696*

Tears Again® [OTC] *see* Artificial Tears *on page 128*

Tears Naturale® [OTC] *see* Artificial Tears *on page 128*

Tears Naturale® Free [OTC] *see* Artificial Tears *on page 128*

Tears Naturale® II [OTC] *see* Artificial Tears *on page 128*

Tears Plus® [OTC] *see* Artificial Tears *on page 128*

Tears Renewed® [OTC] *see* Artificial Tears *on page 128*

Tegaserod (teg a SER od)

U.S. Brand Names Zelnorm™

Canadian Brand Names Zelnorm™

Pharmacologic Category Serotonin 5-HT_4 Receptor Agonist

Synonyms HTF919; Tegaserod Maleate

Use Short-term treatment of constipation-predominate irritable bowel syndrome (IBS) in women

Local Anesthetic/Vasoconstrictor Precautions No information available to require special precautions

Effects on Dental Treatment No significant effects or complications reported

Dosage Oral:

Adults: Female: IBS with constipation: 6 mg twice daily, before meals, for 4-6 weeks; may consider continuing treatment for an additional 4-6 weeks in patients who respond initially.

Elderly: No dosing adjustment recommended

Dosing adjustment in renal impairment: C_{max} and AUC of the inactive metabolite are increased with renal impairment.

Severe impairment: Use is contraindicated

Dosing adjustment in hepatic impairment: C_{max} and AUC of tegaserod are increased with hepatic impairment.

Mild impairment: Use with caution; no recommendations available

Moderate to severe impairment: Contraindicated

Mechanism of Action Tegaserod is a partial neuronal 5-HT_4 receptor agonist. Its action at the receptor site leads to stimulation of the peristaltic reflex and intestinal secretion, and moderation of visceral sensitivity.

Other Adverse Effects

>10%:

Central nervous system: Headache (15%)

Gastrointestinal: Abdominal pain (12%)

1% to 10%:

Central nervous system: Dizziness (4%), migraine (2%)

Gastrointestinal: Diarrhea (9%), nausea (8%), flatulence (6%)

Neuromuscular & skeletal: Back pain (5%), arthropathy (2%), leg pain (1%)

<1%: Albuminuria, angina pectoris, appendicitis, appetite increased, arrhythmia, asthma, breast carcinoma, bundle branch block, cholecystitis, concentration impaired, CPK increased, cramps, depression, diaphoresis, emotional lability, eructation, facial edema, fecal incontinence, flushing, hypotension, irritable colon, menorrhagia, micturition, miscarriage, ovarian cyst, pain, polyuria, pruritus, renal pain, serum bilirubin increased, SGOT increased, SGPT increased, sleep disorder, subileus, suicide attempt, supraventricular tachycardia, syncope, tenesmus, vertigo

Postmarketing and/or case reports: Bile duct stone, cholecystitis with elevated transaminases, sphincter of Oddi spasm (suspected)

Dietary/Ethanol/Herb Considerations Food: Administer on an empty stomach, 30 minutes before meals; bioavailability is decreased by 40% to 65% and C_{max} is decreased by 20% to 40% when taken with food. T_{max} is prolonged from 1 hour up to 2 hours when taken following a meal, but decreased to 0.7 hours when taken 30 minutes before a meal.

Pharmacodynamics/Kinetics

Distribution: V_d: 368 ± 223 L

Protein binding: 98% primarily to α_1-acid glycoprotein

Metabolism: GI: Hydrolysis in the stomach; Hepatic: Oxidation, conjugation, and glucuronidation; metabolite (negligible activity); significant first-pass effect

Bioavailability: Fasting: 10%

Half-life elimination: I.V.: 11 ± 5 hours

Time to peak: 1 hour

Excretion: Feces (~66% as unchanged drug); urine (~33% as metabolites)

Pregnancy Risk Factor B

Generic Available No

Tegaserod Maleate *see* Tegaserod *on page 1268*

Tegretol® *see* Carbamazepine *on page 241*

Tegretol®-XR *see* Carbamazepine *on page 241*

Tegrin® Dandruff Shampoo [OTC] *see* Coal Tar *on page 359*

Telmisartan (tel mi SAR tan)

U.S. Brand Names Micardis®

Canadian Brand Names Micardis®

Pharmacologic Category Angiotensin II Receptor Blocker

Use Treatment of hypertension; may be used alone or in combination with other antihypertensive agents

Local Anesthetic/Vasoconstrictor Precautions No information available to require special precautions

Effects on Dental Treatment No significant effects or complications reported

Dosage Oral:

Adults: Initial: 40 mg once daily; usual maintenance dose range: 20-80 mg/day. Patients with volume depletion should be initiated on the lower dosage with close supervision.

Dosing adjustment in hepatic impairment: Supervise closely

Mechanism of Action Angiotensin II acts as a vasoconstrictor. In addition to causing direct vasoconstriction, angiotensin II also stimulates the release of aldosterone. Once aldosterone is released, sodium as well as water are reabsorbed. The end result is an elevation in blood pressure. Telmisartan is a nonpeptide AT1 angiotensin II receptor antagonist. This binding prevents angiotensin II from binding to the receptor thereby blocking the vasoconstriction and the aldosterone secreting effects of angiotensin II.

Other Adverse Effects May be associated with worsening of renal function in patients dependent on renin-angiotensin-aldosterone system.

1% to 10%:

Cardiovascular: Hypertension (1%), chest pain (1%), peripheral edema (1%)

Central nervous system: Headache (1%), dizziness (1%), pain (1%), fatigue (1%)

(Continued)

Telmisartan *(Continued)*

Gastrointestinal: Diarrhea (3%), dyspepsia (1%), nausea (1%), abdominal pain (1%)

Genitourinary: Urinary tract infection (1%)

Neuromuscular & skeletal: Back pain (3%), myalgia (1%)

Respiratory: Upper respiratory infection (7%), sinusitis (3%), pharyngitis (1%), cough (2%)

Miscellaneous: Flu-like syndrome (1%)

<1% (Limited to important or life-threatening): Angioedema, allergic reaction, elevated liver enzymes, decrease in hemoglobin, increased serum creatinine and BUN, impotence, diaphoresis, flushing, fever, malaise, palpitations, angina, tachycardia, abnormal EKG, insomnia, anxiety, nervousness, migraine, vertigo, depression, somnolence, paresthesia, involuntary muscle contractions, constipation, flatulence, xerostomia, hemorrhoids, gastroenteritis, enteritis, reflux, toothache, gout, hypercholesterolemia, diabetes mellitus, arthritis, arthralgia, leg cramps, fungal infection, abscess, otitis media, asthma, dyspnea, bronchitis, rhinitis, epistaxis, dermatitis, eczema, pruritus, rash, frequent urination, cystitis, abnormal vision, conjunctivitis, tinnitus, earache, cerebrovascular disorder

Drug Interactions Inhibits CYP2C19

Increased Effect/Toxicity: Telmisartan may increase serum digoxin concentrations. Potassium salts/supplements, co-trimoxazole (high dose), ACE inhibitors, and potassium-sparing diuretics (amiloride, spironolactone, triamterene) may increase the risk of hyperkalemia with telmisartan.

Decreased Effect: Telmisartan decreased the trough concentrations of warfarin during concurrent therapy, however, INR was not changed.

Dietary/Ethanol/Herb Considerations

Ethanol: Avoid use; may increase risk of hypotension or dizziness.

Food: May be taken with food; avoid caffeine (eg, colas, chocolate), garlic, and licorice.

Herb/Nutraceutical: Avoid black cohosh, dong quai, and evening primrose due to estrogenic activity. Avoid ephedra, ginseng, and yohimbe; may worsen hypertension. Avoid garlic; may have increased antihypertensive effect. Avoid ginger due to positive inotropic effects; theoretically, may cause arrhythmia. Avoid hawthorn; may decrease peripheral vascular resistance causing additional decrease in BP. Avoid licorice.

Pharmacodynamics/Kinetics Orally active, not a prodrug

Onset of action: 1-2 hours

Peak effect: 0.5-1 hours

Duration: Up to 24 hours

Protein binding: >99.5%

Metabolism: Hepatic via conjugation to inactive metabolites; not metabolized via CYP

Bioavailability (dose dependent): 42% to 58%

Half-life elimination: Terminal: 24 hours

Excretion: Feces (97%)

Clearance: Total body: 800 mL/minute

Pregnancy Risk Factor C (1st trimester); D (2nd and 3rd trimesters)

Generic Available No

Telmisartan and HCTZ *see* Telmisartan and Hydrochlorothiazide *on page 1270*

Telmisartan and Hydrochlorothiazide

(tel mi SAR tan & hye droe klor oh THYE a zide)

Related Information

Hydrochlorothiazide *on page 675*

Telmisartan *on page 1269*

U.S. Brand Names Micardis® HCT

Canadian Brand Names Micardis® Plus

Pharmacologic Category Angiotensin II Receptor Blocker Combination; Antihypertensive Agent Combination

Synonyms HCTZ and Telmisartan; Hydrochlorothiazide and Telmisartan; Telmisartan and HCTZ

Use Treatment of hypertension; combination product should not be used for initial therapy

Local Anesthetic/Vasoconstrictor Precautions No information available to require special precautions

Effects on Dental Treatment No significant effects or complications reported

Dosage Adults: Oral:

Replacement therapy: Combination product can be substituted for individual titrated agents. Initiation of combination therapy when monotherapy has failed to achieve desired effects:

Patients currently on telmisartan: Initial dose if blood pressure is not currently controlled on monotherapy of 80 mg telmisartan: Telmisartan 80 mg/hydrochlorothiazide 12.5 mg once daily; may titrate up to telmisartan 160 mg/hydrochlorothiazide 25 mg if needed

Patients currently on HCTZ: Initial dose if blood pressure is not currently controlled on monotherapy of 25 mg once daily, or is controlled and experiencing hypokalemia: Telmisartan 80 mg/hydrochlorothiazide 12.5 mg once daily; may titrate up to telmisartan 160 mg/hydrochlorothiazide 25 mg if blood pressure remains uncontrolled after 2-4 weeks of therapy

Dosing adjustment in renal impairment:

Cl_{cr} >30 mL/minute: Usual recommended dose

Cl_{cr} <30 mL/minute: Use not recommended

Dosing adjustment in hepatic impairment: Initial: telmisartan 40 mg/hydrochlorothiazide 12.5 mg; contraindicated in severe impairment

Elderly: No dosing adjustment based on age; monitor renal and hepatic function

Mechanism of Action

Telmisartan: Telmisartan is an angiotensin receptor antagonist. Angiotensin II acts as a vasoconstrictor. In addition to causing direct vasoconstriction, angiotensin II also stimulates the release of aldosterone. Once aldosterone is released, sodium as well as water are reabsorbed. The end result is an elevation in blood pressure. Telmisartan binds to the AT1 angiotensin II receptor. This binding prevents angiotensin II from binding to the receptor thereby blocking the vasoconstriction and the aldosterone secreting effects of angiotensin II.

Hydrochlorothiazide: Inhibits sodium reabsorption in the distal tubules causing increased excretion of sodium and water as well as potassium and hydrogen ions

Other Adverse Effects The following reactions have been reported with the combination product; see individual agents for additional adverse reactions that may be expected from each agent.

2% to 10%:

Central nervous system: Dizziness (5%)

Gastrointestinal: Diarrhea (3%), nausea (2%)

Renal: Elevated BUN (3%)

Respiratory: Upper respiratory tract infection (8%), sinusitis (4%)

Miscellaneous: Flu-like syndrome (2%)

<2%: Abdominal pain, back pain, bilirubin increased, bronchitis, dyspepsia, hematocrit decreased, hemoglobin decreased, hypokalemia, liver enzymes increased, pharyngitis, postural hypotension, rash, serum creatinine increased, tachycardia, vomiting

Dietary/Ethanol/Herb Considerations

Ethanol: Avoid use; may potentiate orthostatic hypotension.

Food: May be taken with food

Pregnancy Risk Factor C (1st trimester); D (2nd and 3rd trimesters)

Generic Available No

Selected Readings Conlin P, Moore T, Swartz S, et al, "Effect of Indomethacin on Blood Pressure Lowering by Captopril and Losartan in Hypertensive Patients," *Hypertension*, 2000, 36(3):461-5.

Temazepam (te MAZ e pam)

U.S. Brand Names Restoril®

Canadian Brand Names Apo®-Temazepam; Gen-Temazepam; Novo-Temazepam; Nu-Temazepam; PMS-Temazepam; Restoril®

Pharmacologic Category Benzodiazepine

Use Short-term treatment of insomnia

Unlabeled/Investigational Use Treatment of anxiety; adjunct in treatment of depression; management of panic attacks

Local Anesthetic/Vasoconstrictor Precautions No information available to require special precautions

Effects on Dental Treatment >10%: Significant xerostomia; normal salivary flow resumes upon discontinuation

Restrictions C-IV

Dosage Oral:

Adults: 15-30 mg at bedtime

Elderly or debilitated patients: 15 mg

Mechanism of Action Binds to stereospecific benzodiazepine receptors on the postsynaptic GABA neuron at several sites within the central nervous system, including the limbic system, reticular formation. Enhancement of the inhibitory effect of GABA on neuronal excitability results by increased neuronal membrane permeability to chloride ions. This shift in chloride ions results in hyperpolarization (a less excitable state) and stabilization.

Other Adverse Effects

1% to 10%:

Central nervous system: Confusion, dizziness, drowsiness, fatigue, anxiety, headache, lethargy, hangover, euphoria, vertigo

Dermatologic: Rash

Endocrine & metabolic: Decreased libido

Gastrointestinal: Diarrhea

Neuromuscular & skeletal: Dysarthria, weakness

Ocular: Blurred vision

Miscellaneous: Diaphoresis

(Continued)

Temazepam *(Continued)*

<1%: Amnesia, anorexia, ataxia, back pain, blood dyscrasias, drug dependence, increased dreaming, menstrual irregularities, palpitations, paradoxical reactions, reflex slowing, tremor, vomiting

Drug Interactions Substrate of CYP2B6, 2C8/9, 2C19, 3A4

Increased Effect/Toxicity: Temazepam potentiates the CNS depressant effects of narcotic analgesics, barbiturates, phenothiazines, ethanol, antihistamines, MAO inhibitors, sedative-hypnotics, and cyclic antidepressants. Serum levels of temazepam may be increased by inhibitors of CYP3A4, including cimetidine, ciprofloxacin, clarithromycin, clozapine, diltiazem, disulfiram, digoxin, erythromycin, ethanol, fluconazole, fluoxetine, fluvoxamine, grapefruit juice, isoniazid, itraconazole, ketoconazole, labetalol, levodopa, loxapine, metoprolol, metronidazole, miconazole, nefazodone, omeprazole, phenytoin, rifabutin, rifampin, troleandomycin, valproic acid, and verapamil.

Decreased Effect: Oral contraceptives may increase the clearance of temazepam. Temazepam may decrease the antiparkinsonian efficacy of levodopa. Theophylline and other CNS stimulants may antagonize the sedative effects of temazepam. Carbamazepine, rifampin, rifabutin may enhance the metabolism of temazepam and decrease its therapeutic effect.

Dietary/Ethanol/Herb Considerations

Ethanol: Avoid use; may increase CNS depression.

Food: Administration with food reduces GI upset; avoid grapefruit products; may increase serum concentration.

Herb/Nutraceutical: Avoid gotu kola, kava, SAMe, and valerian; may increase CNS depression. Avoid St John's wort; may decrease serum concentration and increase CNS depression. Melatonin may increase benzodiazepine binding at receptor sites causing enhancement of activity of clonazepam; use cautiously.

Pharmacodynamics/Kinetics

Distribution: V_d: 1.4 L/kg

Protein binding: 96%

Metabolism: Hepatic

Half-life elimination: 9.5-12.4 hours

Time to peak, serum: 2-3 hours

Excretion: Urine (80% to 90% as inactive metabolites)

Pregnancy Risk Factor X

Generic Available Yes

Temodar® *see* Temozolomide *on page 1272*

Temovate® *see* Clobetasol *on page 345*

Temovate E® *see* Clobetasol *on page 345*

Temozolomide (te mo ZOLE oh mide)

U.S. Brand Names Temodar®

Canadian Brand Names Temodal™; Tomedar®

Pharmacologic Category Antineoplastic Agent, Alkylating Agent

Use Treatment of adult patients with refractory (first relapse) anaplastic astrocytoma who have experienced disease progression on nitrosourea and procarbazine

Unlabeled/Investigational Use Treatment of glioma, first relapse/advanced metastatic malignant melanoma

Local Anesthetic/Vasoconstrictor Precautions No information available to require special precautions

Effects on Dental Treatment No significant effects or complications reported

Dosage Therapy can be continued until disease progression. Treatment could be continued for a maximum of 2 years in the clinical trial, but the optimum duration of therapy is not known. Refer to individual protocols.

Dosage is adjusted according to nadir neutrophil and platelet counts of previous cycle and counts at the time of the next cycle Measure day 22 ANC and platelets. Measure day 29 ANC and platelets. Based on lowest counts at either day 22 or day 29:

On day 22 or day 29, if ANC <1000/µL or the platelet count is <50,000/µL, postpone therapy until ANC >1500/µL and platelet count >100,000/µL. Reduce dose by 50 mg/m² for subsequent cycle.

If ANC 1000-1500/µL or platelets 50,000-100,000/µL, postpone therapy until ANC >1500/µL and platelet count >100,000/µL; maintain initial dose.

If ANC >1500/µL (on day 22 and day 29) and platelet count >100,000/µL, increase dose to, or maintain dose at 200 mg/m²/day for 5 for subsequent cycle.

Usual dose: Oral: 150-200 mg/m²/day for 5 days; repeat every 28 days.

Elderly: Patients ≥70 years of age had a higher incidence of grade 4 neutropenia and thrombocytopenia in the first cycle of therapy than patients <70 years of age

Dosing adjustment in renal impairment: No guidelines exist; use with caution in severe impairment (Cl_{cr} <39 mL/minute)

Dosing adjustment in hepatic impairment: Use with caution in severe impairment

Mechanism of Action Like DTIC, temozolomide is converted to the active alkylating metabolite MTIC. Unlike DTIC, however, this conversion is spontaneous, nonenzymatic, and occurs under physiologic conditions in all tissues to which the drug distributes.

Other Adverse Effects

>10%:

Cardiovascular: Peripheral edema (11%)

Central nervous system: Headache (41%), fatigue (34%), convulsions (23%), hemiparesis (29%), dizziness (19%), fever (11%), coordination abnormality (11%), amnesia (10%), insomnia (10%), somnolence. In the case of CNS malignancies, it is difficult to distinguish the relative contributions of temozolomide and progressive disease to CNS symptoms.

Gastrointestinal: Nausea (53%), vomiting (42%), constipation (33%), diarrhea (16%)

Hematologic: Neutropenia (grade 3-4, 14%), thrombocytopenia (grade 3-4 19%)

Neuromuscular & skeletal: Weakness (13%)

1% to 10%:

Central nervous system: Ataxia (8%), confusion (5%), anxiety (7%), depression (6%)

Dermatologic: Rash (8%), pruritus (8%)

Endocrine & metabolic: Hypercorticism (8%), breast pain (6%), weight gain (5%)

Gastrointestinal: Dysphagia (7%), abdominal pain (9%), anorexia (9%)

Genitourinary: Increased micturition frequency (6%)

Hematologic: Anemia (8%; grade 3-4, 4%)

Neuromuscular & skeletal: Paresthesia (9%), back pain (8%), myalgia (5%)

Ocular: Diplopia (5%), vision abnormality (5%)

Respiratory: Pharyngitis (8%), sinusitis (6%), cough (5%)

<1%: Allergic reactions, anaphylaxis, erythema multiforme

Drug Interactions Decreased Effect: Although valproic acid reduces the clearance of temozolomide by 5%, the clinical significance of this is unknown.

Dietary/Ethanol/Herb Considerations Food reduces rate and extent of absorption; incidence of nausea/vomiting is decreased when taken on an empty stomach.

Pharmacodynamics/Kinetics

Distribution: V_d: Parent drug: 0.4 L/kg

Protein binding: 15%

Metabolism: Prodrug, hydrolyzed to the active form, MTIC; MTIC is eventually eliminated as CO_2 and 5-aminoimidazole-4-carboxamide (AIC), a natural constituent in urine

Bioavailability: 100%

Half-life elimination: Mean: Parent drug: 1.8 hours

Time to peak: Empty stomach: 1 hour

Excretion: Urine (5% to 7% of total)

Pregnancy Risk Factor D

Generic Available No

Tenecteplase (ten EK te playz)

U.S. Brand Names TNKase™

Canadian Brand Names TNKase™

Pharmacologic Category Thrombolytic Agent

Use Thrombolytic agent used in the management of acute MI for the lysis of thrombi in the coronary vasculature to restore perfusion and reduce mortality.

Local Anesthetic/Vasoconstrictor Precautions No information available to require special precautions

Effects on Dental Treatment No significant effects or complications reported

Dosage I.V.:

Adult: Recommended total dose should not exceed 50 mg and is based on patient's weight; administer as a bolus over 5 seconds

If patient's weight:

<60 kg, dose: 30 mg

≥60 to <70 kg, dose: 35 mg

≥70 to <80 kg, dose: 40 mg

≥80 to <90 kg, dose: 45 mg

≥90 kg, dose: 50 mg

All patients received 150-325 mg of aspirin as soon as possible and then daily. Intravenous heparin was initiated as soon as possible and aPTT was maintained between 50-70 seconds.

Elderly: Although dosage adjustments are not recommended, the elderly have a higher incidence of morbidity and mortality with the use of tenecteplase. The 30-day mortality in the ASSENT-2 trial was 2.5% for patients <65 years, 8.5% for patients 65-74 years, and 16.2% for patients ≥75 years. The intracranial hemorrhage rate was 0.4% for patients <65, 1.6 % for patients 65-74 years, and 1.7 % for patients ≥75. The risks and benefits of use should be weighted carefully in the elderly.

Dosing adjustment in renal impairment: No formal recommendations

Dosing adjustment in hepatic impairment: Severe hepatic failure is a relative contraindication; no recommendations for mild to moderate

(Continued)

Tenecteplase *(Continued)*

Mechanism of Action Initiates fibrinolysis by binding to fibrin and converting plasminogen to plasmin.

Other Adverse Effects As with all drugs which may affect hemostasis, bleeding is the major adverse effect associated with tenecteplase. Hemorrhage may occur at virtually any site. Risk is dependent on multiple variables, including the dosage administered, concurrent use of multiple agents which alter hemostasis, and patient predisposition. Rapid lysis of coronary artery thrombi by thrombolytic agents may be associated with reperfusion-related arterial and/or ventricular arrhythmias. The incidence of stroke and bleeding increase in patients >65 years.

>10%:

Hematologic: Bleeding (22% minor: ASSENT-2 trial)
Local: Hematoma (12% minor)

1% to 10%:

Central nervous system: Stroke (2%)
Gastrointestinal: GI hemorrhage (1% major, 2% minor), epistaxis (2% minor)
Genitourinary: GU bleeding (4% minor)
Hematologic: Bleeding (5% major: ASSENT-2 trial)
Local: Bleeding at catheter puncture site (4% minor), hematoma (2% major)
Respiratory: Pharyngeal bleeding (3% minor)

<1%: Intracranial hemorrhage (0.9%), retroperitoneal bleeding, respiratory tract bleeding, anaphylaxis, angioedema, laryngeal edema, rash, urticaria, cholesterol embolism (clinical features may include livedo reticularis, "purple toe" syndrome, acute renal failure, gangrenous digits, hypertension, pancreatitis, MI, cerebral infarction, spinal cord infarction, retinal artery occlusion, bowel infarction, rhabdomyolysis), GU bleeding (<1% major), bleeding at catheter puncture site (<1% major)

Additional cardiovascular events associated with use in MI: Cardiogenic shock, arrhythmias, AV block, pulmonary edema, heart failure, cardiac arrest, recurrent myocardial ischemia, myocardial reinfarction, myocardial rupture, cardiac tamponade, pericarditis, pericardial effusion, mitral regurgitation, thrombosis, embolism, electromechanical dissociation, hypotension, fever, nausea, vomiting

Drug Interactions

Increased Effect/Toxicity: Drugs which affect platelet function (eg, NSAIDs, dipyridamole, ticlopidine, clopidogrel, IIb/IIIa antagonists) may potentiate the risk of hemorrhage; use with caution. Use with aspirin and heparin may increase bleeding. However, aspirin and heparin were used concomitantly with tenecteplase in the majority of patients in clinical studies. Risk of bleeding may be increased during concurrent therapy with arfarin or oral anticoagulants.

Decreased Effect: Aminocaproic acid (antifibrinolytic agent) may decrease effectiveness.

Pharmacodynamics/Kinetics

Distribution: V_d is weight related and approximates plasma volume
Metabolism: Primarily hepatic
Half-life elimination: 90-130 minutes
Excretion: Clearance: Plasma: 99-119 mL/minute

Pregnancy Risk Factor C

Generic Available No

Tenex® *see* Guanfacine *on page 655*

Teniposide (ten i POE side)

U.S. Brand Names Vumon

Canadian Brand Names Vumon®

Mexican Brand Names Vumon®

Pharmacologic Category Antineoplastic Agent, Miscellaneous

Synonyms EPT; VM-26

Use Treatment of acute lymphocytic leukemia, small cell lung cancer

Local Anesthetic/Vasoconstrictor Precautions No information available to require special precautions

Effects on Dental Treatment No significant effects or complications reported

Dosage I.V.:

Children: 130 mg/m²/week, increasing to 150 mg/m² after 3 weeks and up to 180 mg/m² after 6 weeks

Acute lymphoblastic leukemia (ALL): 165 mg/m² twice weekly for 8-9 doses **or** 250 mg/m² weekly for 4-8 weeks

Adults: 50-180 mg/m² once or twice weekly for 4-6 weeks or 20-60 mg/m²/day for 5 days

Small cell lung cancer: 80-90 mg/m²/day for 5 days every 4-6 weeks

Dosing adjustment in renal/hepatic impairment: Data insufficient; adjustments may be necessary in significant impairment

Dosing adjustment in Down syndrome patients: Reduce initial dosing; administer the first course at half the usual dose. Patients with both Down syndrome and leukemia may be especially sensitive to myelosuppressive chemotherapy.

Mechanism of Action Teniposide does not inhibit microtubular assembly; it has been shown to delay transit of cells through the S phase and arrest cells in late S or early G_2 phase. Teniposide is a topoisomerase II inhibitor, and appears to cause DNA strand breaks by inhibition of strand-passing and DNA ligase action.

Other Adverse Effects

>10%:

Gastrointestinal: Mucositis (75%); diarrhea, nausea, vomiting (20% to 30%); anorexia

Hematologic: Myelosuppression, leukopenia, neutropenia (95%), thrombocytopenia (65% to 80%), anemia

Onset: 5-7 days

Nadir: 7-10 days

Recovery: 21-28 days

1% to 10%:

Cardiovascular: Hypotension (2%), associated with rapid (<30 minutes) infusions

Dermatologic: Alopecia (9%), rash (3%)

Miscellaneous: Anaphylactoid reactions (5%) (fever, rash, hypertension, hypotension, dyspnea, bronchospasm), usually seen with rapid (<30 minutes) infusions

<1%: Lethargy, peripheral neuropathies, somnolence

Drug Interactions Substrate of **CYP3A4**; Inhibits CYP2C8/9, 3A4

Increased Effect/Toxicity: Alteration of methotrexate (MTX) transport has been found as a slow efflux of MTX and its polyglutamated form out of the cell, leading to intercellular accumulation of MTX. Sodium salicylate, sulfamethizole, and tolbutamide displace teniposide from protein-binding sites which could cause substantial increases in free drug levels, resulting in potentiation of toxicity. Concurrent use of vincristine may increase the incidence of peripheral neuropathy.

Decreased Effect: Barbiturates, phenytoin (and other CYP3A4 inducers) may decrease teniposide efficacy.

Dietary/Ethanol/Herb Considerations Herb/Nutraceutical: Avoid St John's wort; may decrease serum concentration.

Pharmacodynamics/Kinetics

Distribution: V_d: 0.28 L/kg; Adults: 8-44 L; Children: 3-11 L; mainly into liver, kidneys, small intestine, and adrenals; crosses blood-brain barrier to a limited extent

Protein binding: 99.4%

Metabolism: Extensively hepatic

Half-life elimination: 5 hours

Excretion: Urine (44%, 21% as unchanged drug); feces (≤10%)

Pregnancy Risk Factor D

Generic Available No

Tenofovir (te NOE fo veer)

Related Information

HIV Infection and AIDS *on page 1482*

U.S. Brand Names Viread™

Pharmacologic Category Antiretroviral Agent, Reverse Transcriptase Inhibitor (Nucleotide)

Synonyms PMPA; TDF; Tenofovir Disoproxil Fumarate

Use Management of HIV infections in combination with at least two other antiretroviral agents

Local Anesthetic/Vasoconstrictor Precautions No information available to require special precautions

Effects on Dental Treatment No significant effects or complications reported

Dosage Oral:

Adults: HIV infection: 300 mg once daily

Dosing adjustment in renal impairment: Avoid use in Cl_{cr} <60 mL/minute; guidelines unavailable

Mechanism of Action Tenofovir disoproxil fumarate (TDF) is an analog of adenosine 5'-monophosphate; it interferes with the HIV viral RNA dependent DNA polymerase resulting in inhibition of viral replication. TDF is first converted intracellularly by hydrolysis to tenofovir and subsequently phosphorylated to the active tenofovir diphosphate; nucleotide reverse transcriptase inhibitor.

Other Adverse Effects Clinical trials involved addition to prior antiretroviral therapy. Frequencies listed are treatment-emergent adverse effects noted at higher frequency than in the placebo group.

>10%: Gastrointestinal: Nausea (11%)

1% to 10%:

Endocrine & metabolic: Glycosuria (3%, frequency equal to placebo); other metabolic effects (hyperglycemia, hypertriglyceridemia) noted at frequencies less than placebo

Gastrointestinal: Diarrhea (9%), vomiting (5%), flatulence (4%), abdominal pain (3%, frequency equal to placebo), anorexia (3%)

Hematologic: Neutropenia (1%, frequency equal to placebo)

Hepatic: Increased transaminases (2% to 4%)

(Continued)

Tenofovir *(Continued)*

Neuromuscular & skeletal: Weakness (8%, frequency equal to placebo)

Postmarketing and/or case reports: Dizziness, dyspnea, Fanconi syndrome, hypophosphatemia, lactic acidosis, pancreatitis, rash, renal failure, serum creatinine increased, weakness

Note: Uncommon, but significant adverse reactions reported with other reverse transcriptase inhibitors include pancreatitis, peripheral neuropathy, and myopathy.

Drug Interactions Inhibits CYP1A2

Increased Effect/Toxicity: Concurrent use has been noted to increase serum concentrations/exposure to didanosine and its metabolites, potentially increasing the risk of didanosine toxicity (pancreatitis, peripheral neuropathy, or lactic acidosis); use caution and monitor closely; suspend therapy if signs/symptoms of toxicity are present. Drugs which may compete for renal tubule secretion (including acyclovir, cidofovir, ganciclovir, valacyclovir, valganciclovir) may increase the serum concentrations of tenofovir. Drugs causing nephrotoxicity may reduce elimination of tenofovir. Lopinavir/ritonavir may increase serum concentrations of tenofovir.

Decreased Effect: Serum levels of lopinavir and/or ritonavir may be decreased by tenofovir.

Dietary/Ethanol/Herb Considerations Food: Administer with food to increase absorption; fatty meals may increase the bioavailability.

Pharmacodynamics/Kinetics

Distribution: 1.2-1.3 L/kg

Protein binding: 7% to serum proteins

Metabolism: Tenofovir disoproxil fumarate (TDF) is converted intracellularly by hydrolysis (by nonCYP enzymes) to tenofovir, then phosphorylated to the active tenofovir diphosphate

Bioavailability: 25% (fasting); increases ~40% with high-fat meal

Time to peak, serum: Fasting: 1 hour; With food: 2 hours

Excretion: Urine (70% to 80%) via filtration and active secretion, primarily as unchanged tenofovir

Pregnancy Risk Factor B

Generic Available No

Tenofovir Disoproxil Fumarate *see* Tenofovir *on page 1275*

Tenoretic® *see* Atenolol and Chlorthalidone *on page 138*

Tenormin® *see* Atenolol *on page 137*

Tenuate® *see* Diethylpropion *on page 436*

Tenuate® Dospan® *see* Diethylpropion *on page 436*

Tequin® *see* Gatifloxacin *on page 628*

Terazol® 3 *see* Terconazole *on page 1279*

Terazol® 7 *see* Terconazole *on page 1279*

Terazosin (ter AY zoe sin)

Related Information

Cardiovascular Diseases *on page 1456*

U.S. Brand Names Hytrin®

Canadian Brand Names Alti-Terazosin; Apo®-Terazosin; Hytrin®; Novo-Terazosin; Nu-Terazosin; PMS-Terazosin

Mexican Brand Names Adecur®; Hytrin®

Pharmacologic Category $Alpha_1$ Blocker

Use Management of mild to moderate hypertension; alone or in combination with other agents such as diuretics or beta-blockers; benign prostate hyperplasia (BPH)

Local Anesthetic/Vasoconstrictor Precautions No information available to require special precautions

Effects on Dental Treatment ≤10%: Xerostomia

Dosage Oral: Adults:

Hypertension: Initial: 1 mg at bedtime; slowly increase dose to achieve desired blood pressure, up to 20 mg/day; usual dose: 1-5 mg/day

Dosage reduction may be needed when adding a diuretic or other antihypertensive agent; if drug is discontinued for greater than several days, consider beginning with initial dose and retitrate as needed; dosage may be given on a twice daily regimen if response is diminished at 24 hours and hypotensive is observed at 2-4 hours following a dose

Benign prostatic hyperplasia: Initial: 1 mg at bedtime, increasing as needed; most patients require 10 mg day; if no response after 4-6 weeks of 10 mg/day, may increase to 20 mg/day

Mechanism of Action $Alpha_1$-specific blocking agent with minimal $alpha_2$ effects; this allows peripheral postsynaptic blockade, with the resultant decrease in arterial tone, while preserving the negative feedback loop which is mediated by the peripheral presynaptic $alpha_2$-receptors; terazosin relaxes the smooth muscle of the bladder neck, thus reducing bladder outlet obstruction

Other Adverse Effects Asthenia, postural hypotension, dizziness, somnolence, nasal congestion/rhinitis, and impotence were the only events noted in clinical trials to occur at a frequency significantly greater than placebo ($p < 0.05$).

>10%: Central nervous system: Dizziness, headache, muscle weakness

1% to 10%:

Cardiovascular: Edema, palpitations, chest pain, peripheral edema (3%), orthostatic hypotension (3% to 4%), tachycardia

Central nervous system: Fatigue, nervousness, drowsiness

Genitourinary: Urinary incontinence

Ocular: Blurred vision

Respiratory: Dyspnea, nasal congestion

<1% (Limited to important or life-threatening): Sexual dysfunction, syncope (0.8%)

Postmarketing and/or case reports: Allergic reactions, anaphylaxis, atrial fibrillation, priapism, thrombocytopenia

Drug Interactions

Increased Effect/Toxicity: Terazosin's hypotensive effect is increased with beta-blockers, diuretics, ACE inhibitors, calcium channel blockers, and other antihypertensive medications.

Decreased Effect: Decreased antihypertensive response with NSAIDs. Alpha-blockers reduce the response to pressor agents (norepinephrine).

Dietary/Ethanol/Herb Considerations

Ethanol: Use with caution; may increase risk of hypotension or dizziness.

Food: May be taken with food; avoid caffeine (eg, colas, chocolate), garlic, and licorice.

Herb/Nutraceutical: Avoid black cohosh, dong quai, and evening primrose due to estrogenic activity. Avoid ephedra, ginseng, and yohimbe; may worsen hypertension. Avoid garlic; may have increased antihypertensive effect. Avoid ginger due to positive inotropic effects; theoretically, may cause arrhythmia. Avoid hawthorn; may lower peripheral vascular resistance causing additional decrease in BP. Avoid licorice and saw palmetto.

Pharmacodynamics/Kinetics

Onset of action: 1-2 hours

Absorption: Rapid

Protein binding: 90% to 95%

Metabolism: Extensively hepatic

Half-life elimination: 9.2-12 hours

Time to peak, serum: ~1 hour

Excretion: Feces (60%); urine (40%)

Pregnancy Risk Factor C

Generic Available Yes

Terbinafine (TER bin a feen)

U.S. Brand Names Lamisil®; Lamisil® AT™ [OTC]

Canadian Brand Names Apo®-Terbinafine; Gen-Terbinafine; Lamisil®; Novo-Terbinafine; PMS-Terbinafine

Mexican Brand Names Lamisil®

Pharmacologic Category Antifungal Agent, Oral; Antifungal Agent, Topical

Synonyms Terbinafine Hydrochloride

Use Active against most strains of *Trichophyton mentagrophytes*, *Trichophyton rubrum*; may be effective for infections of *Microsporum gypseum* and *M. nanum*, *Trichophyton verrucosum*, *Epidermophyton floccosum*, *Candida albicans*, and *Scopulariopsis brevicaulis*

Oral: Treatment of onychomycosis of the toenail or fingernail due to susceptible dermatophytes

Topical: Antifungal for the treatment of tinea pedis (athlete's foot), tinea cruris (jock itch), and tinea corporis (ringworm) [OTC/prescription formulations]; tinea versicolor [prescription formulations]

Unlabeled/Investigational Use Topical: Treatment of cutaneous candidiasis and pityriasis versicolor

Local Anesthetic/Vasoconstrictor Precautions No information available to require special precautions

Effects on Dental Treatment No significant effects or complications reported

Dosage

Children ≥12 years and Adults:

Topical cream, solution:

Athlete's foot (tinea pedis): Apply to affected area twice daily for at least 1 week, not to exceed 4 weeks [OTC/prescription formulations]

Ringworm (tinea corporis) and jock itch (tinea cruris): Apply cream to affected area once or twice daily for at least 1 week, not to exceed 4 weeks; apply solution once daily for 7 days [OTC formulations]

Adults:

Oral:

Superficial mycoses: Fingernail: 250 mg/day for up to 6 weeks; toenail: 250 mg/day for 12 weeks; doses may be given in two divided doses

(Continued)

Terbinafine *(Continued)*

Systemic mycosis: 250-500 mg/day for up to 16 months

Topical solution: Tinea versicolor: Apply to affected area twice daily for 1 week [prescription formulation]

Dosing adjustment in renal impairment: Oral: Specific guidelines not available; dose reduction in significant renal insufficiency (GFR <50 mL/minute) recommended

Dosing adjustment in hepatic impairment: Clearance decreased by ~50% with hepatic cirrhosis

Mechanism of Action Synthetic alkylamine derivative which inhibits squalene epoxidase, a key enzyme in sterol biosynthesis in fungi. This results in a deficiency in ergosterol within the fungal cell wall and results in fungal cell death.

Other Adverse Effects

Oral:

1% to 10%:

Central nervous system: Headache, dizziness, vertigo

Dermatologic: Rash, pruritus, and alopecia with oral therapy

Gastrointestinal: Nausea, diarrhea, dyspepsia, abdominal pain, appetite decrease, abnormal taste

Hematologic: Lymphocytopenia

Hepatic: Liver enzyme elevations

Ocular: Visual disturbance

Miscellaneous: Allergic reaction

<1%, postmarketing and/or case reports: Agranulocytosis, allergic reactions, anaphylaxis, hepatic failure, neutropenia, Stevens-Johnson syndrome, abnormal taste (with prolonged recovery and weight loss), thrombocytopenia, toxic epidermal necrolysis; changes in ocular lens and retina have been reported (clinical significance unknown)

Topical: 1% to 10%:

Dermatologic: Pruritus, contact dermatitis, irritation, burning, dryness

Local: Irritation, stinging

Drug Interactions Substrate of **CYP3A4**; Inhibits CYP2D6; Induces CYP3A4

Increased Effect/Toxicity: Terbinafine clearance is decreased by cimetidine (33%); caffeine clearance is decreased by terbinafine (19%); effects of drugs metabolized by CYP2D6 (including beta-blockers, SSRIs, MAO inhibitors, tricyclic antidepressants) may be increased; warfarin effects may be increased

Decreased Effect: Cyclosporine clearance is increased (~15%) with concomitant terbinafine; rifampin increases terbinafine clearance (100%); rifampin increases the metabolism of terbinafine (decreases serum concentration)

Pharmacodynamics/Kinetics

Absorption: Topical: Limited (<5%); Oral: >70%

Distribution: V_d: 2000 L; distributed to sebum and skin predominantly

Protein binding, plasma: >99%

Metabolism: Hepatic; no active metabolites; first-pass effect; little effect on CYP

Bioavailability: Oral: 40%

Half-life elimination:

Topical: 22-26 hours

Oral: Terminal half-life: 200-400 hours; very slow release of drug from skin and adipose tissues occurs

Time to peak, plasma: 1-2 hours

Excretion: Urine (70% to 75%)

Pregnancy Risk Factor B

Generic Available No

Selected Readings

Abdel-Rahman SM and Nahata MC, "Oral Terbinafine: A New Antifungal Agent," *Ann Pharmacother*, 1997, 31(4):445-56.

Amichai B and Grunwald MH, "Adverse Drug Reactions of the New Oral Antifungal Agents - Terbinafine, Fluconazole, and Itraconazole," *Int J Dermatol*, 1998, 37(6):410-5.

Angello JT, Voytovich RM, and Jan SA, "A Cost/Efficacy Analysis of Oral Antifungals Indicated for the Treatment of Onychomycosis: Griseofulvin, Itraconazole, and Terbinafine," *Am J Manag Care*, 1997, 3(3):443-50.

De Backer M, De Vroey C, Lesaffre E, et al, "Twelve Weeks of Continuous Oral Therapy for Toenail Onychomycosis Caused by Dermatophytes: A Double-Blind Comparative Trial of Terbinafine 250 mg/day Versus Itraconazole 200 mg/day," *J Am Acad Dermatol*, 1998, 38(5 Pt 3):S57-63.

Dwyer CM, White MI, and Sinclair TS, "Cholestatic Jaundice Due to Terbinafine," *Br J Dermatol*, 1997, 136(6):976-7.

Gupta AK and Shear NH, "Terbinafine: An Update," *J Am Acad Dermatol*, 1997, 37(6):979-88.

Gupta AK, Sibbald RG, Knowles SR, et al, "Terbinafine Therapy May Be Associated With the Development of Psoriasis De Novo or Its Exacerbation: Four Case Reports and a Review of Drug Induced Psoriasis," *J Am Acad Dermatol*, 1997, 36(5 Part 2):858-62.

Jones TC, "Overview of the Use of Terbinafine in Children," *Br J Dermatol*, 1995, 132(5):683-9.

Trepanier EF and Amsden GW, "Current Issues in Onchomycosis," *Ann Pharmacother*, 1998, 32(2):204-14.

Terbinafine Hydrochloride *see* Terbinafine *on page 1277*

Terbutaline (ter BYOO ta leen)

Related Information

Respiratory Diseases *on page 1476*

U.S. Brand Names Brethine®
Canadian Brand Names Bricanyl® [DSC]
Mexican Brand Names Bricanyl®; Taziken®
Pharmacologic Category Beta$_2$ Agonist
Synonyms Brethaire® [DSC]; Bricanyl® [DSC]
Use Bronchodilator in reversible airway obstruction and bronchial asthma; tocolytic agent
Unlabeled/Investigational Use Tocolytic agent for management of preterm labor
Local Anesthetic/Vasoconstrictor Precautions No information available to require special precautions
Effects on Dental Treatment 1% to 10%: Xerostomia
Dosage

Children <12 years: Bronchoconstriction:
- Oral: Initial: 0.05 mg/kg/dose 3 times/day, increased gradually as required; maximum: 0.15 mg/kg/dose 3-4 times/day or a total of 5 mg/24 hours
- S.C.: 0.005-0.01 mg/kg/dose to a maximum of 0.3 mg/dose every 15-20 minutes for 3 doses

Children >12 years and Adults: Bronchoconstriction:
- Oral:
  - 12-15 years: 2.5 mg every 6 hours 3 times/day; not to exceed 7.5 mg in 24 hours
  - >15 years: 5 mg/dose every 6 hours 3 times/day; if side effects occur, reduce dose to 2.5 mg every 6 hours; not to exceed 15 mg in 24 hours
- S.C.: 0.25 mg/dose repeated in 15-30 minutes for one time only; a total dose of 0.5 mg should not be exceeded within a 4-hour period inhalations

Adults: Premature labor (tocolysis; unlabeled use):
- Acute: I.V. 2.5-10 mcg/minute; increased gradually every 10-20 minutes; effective maximum dosages from 17.5-30 mcg/minute have been used with caution. Duration of infusion is at least 12 hours.
- Maintenance: Oral: 2.5-10 mg every 4-6 hours for as long as necessary to prolong pregnancy depending on patient tolerance

Dosing adjustment in renal impairment:
- Cl_{cr} 10-50 mL/minute: Administer at 50% of normal dose
- Cl_{cr} <10 mL/minute: Avoid use

Mechanism of Action Relaxes bronchial smooth muscle by action on beta$_2$-receptors with less effect on heart rate
Other Adverse Effects

>10%:
- Central nervous system: Nervousness, restlessness
- Neuromuscular & skeletal: Trembling

1% to 10%:
- Cardiovascular: Tachycardia, hypertension
- Central nervous system: Dizziness, drowsiness, headache, insomnia
- Gastrointestinal: Nausea, vomiting, bad taste in mouth
- Neuromuscular & skeletal: Muscle cramps, weakness
- Miscellaneous: Diaphoresis

<1%: Chest pain, arrhythmias, paradoxical bronchospasm

Drug Interactions

Increased toxicity with MAO inhibitors and TCAs.
Decreased effect with beta-blockers.

Dietary/Ethanol/Herb Considerations Herb/Nutraceutical: Avoid ephedra, ginseng, and yohimbe; may cause CNS stimulation.
Pharmacodynamics/Kinetics

Onset of action: Oral: 30-45 minutes; S.C.: 6-15 minutes
Protein binding: 25%
Metabolism: Hepatic to inactive sulfate conjugates
Bioavailability: S.C. doses are more bioavailable than oral
Half-life elimination: 11-16 hours
Excretion: Urine

Pregnancy Risk Factor B
Generic Available Yes: Tablet

Terconazole (ter KONE a zole)

U.S. Brand Names Terazol® 3; Terazol® 7
Canadian Brand Names Terazol®
Mexican Brand Names Fungistat®; Fungistat Dual
Pharmacologic Category Antifungal Agent, Vaginal
Synonyms Triaconazole
Use Local treatment of vulvovaginal candidiasis
Local Anesthetic/Vasoconstrictor Precautions No information available to require special precautions
Effects on Dental Treatment No significant effects or complications reported

(Continued)

Terconazole *(Continued)*

Dosage Adults: Female:

Terazol® 3 vaginal cream: Insert 1 applicatorful intravaginally at bedtime for 3 consecutive days

Terazol® 7 vaginal cream: Insert 1 applicatorful intravaginally at bedtime for 7 consecutive days

Terazol® 3 vaginal suppository: Insert 1 suppository intravaginally at bedtime for 3 consecutive days

Mechanism of Action Triazole ketal antifungal agent; involves inhibition of fungal cytochrome P450. Specifically, terconazole inhibits cytochrome P450-dependent 14-alpha-demethylase which results in accumulation of membrane disturbing 14-alpha-demethylsterols and ergosterol depletion.

Other Adverse Effects

1% to 10%:

Central nervous system; Fever, chills

Gastrointestinal: Abdominal pain

Genitourinary: Vulvar/vaginal burning, dysmenorrhea

<1% (Limited to important or life-threatening): Vulvar itching, soreness, edema, or discharge; polyuria; burning or itching of penis of sexual partner; flu-like syndrome

Pharmacodynamics/Kinetics Absorption: Extent of systemic absorption after vaginal administration may be dependent on presence of a uterus; 5% to 8% in women who had a hysterectomy versus 12% to 16% in nonhysterectomy women

Pregnancy Risk Factor C

Generic Available No

Teriparatide (ter i PAR a tide)

U.S. Brand Names Forteo™

Pharmacologic Category Parathyroid Hormone Analog

Synonyms Parathyroid Hormone (1-34); Recombinant Human Parathyroid Hormone (1-34); rhPTH(1-34)

Use Treatment of osteoporosis in postmenopausal women at high risk of fracture; treatment of primary or hypogonadal osteoporosis in men at high risk of fracture

Local Anesthetic/Vasoconstrictor Precautions No information available to require special precautions

Effects on Dental Treatment No significant effects or complications reported

Dosage S.C.:

Adults: 20 mcg once daily; **Note:** Initial administration should occur under circumstances in which the patient may sit or lie down, in the event of orthostasis.

Dosing adjustment in renal impairment: None; bioavailability and halflife increase with Cl_{cr} <30 mL/minute.

Mechanism of Action Teriparatide is a recombinant formulation of endogenous parathyroid hormone (PTH), containing a 34-amino-acid sequence which is identical to the N-terminal portion of this hormone. The pharmacologic activity of teriparatide is similar to the physiologic activity of PTH, stimulating osteoblast function, increasing gastrointestinal calcium absorption, increasing renal tubular reabsorption of calcium. Treatment with teriparatide increases bone mineral density, bone mass, and strength. In postmenopausal women, it has been shown to decrease osteoporosis-related fractures.

Other Adverse Effects 1% to 10%:

Cardiovascular: Chest pain (3%), syncope (3%)

Central nervous system: Dizziness (8%), depression (4%), vertigo (4%)

Dermatologic: Rash (5%)

Endocrine & metabolic: Hypercalcemia (transient increases noted 4-6 hours post-dose in 11% of women and 6% of men)

Gastrointestinal: Nausea (9%), dyspepsia (5%), vomiting (3%), tooth disorder (2%)

Genitourinary: Hyperuricemia (3%)

Neuromuscular & skeletal: Arthralgia (10%), weakness (9%), leg cramps (3%)

Respiratory: Rhinitis (10%), pharyngitis (6%), dyspnea (4%), pneumonia (4%)

Miscellaneous: Antibodies to teriparatide (3% of women in long-term treatment; hypersensitivity reactions or decreased efficacy were not associated in preclinical trials)

Drug Interactions Increased Effect/Toxicity: Digitalis serum concentrations are not affected, however, transient hypercalcemia may increase risk of digitalis toxicity (case reports).

Dietary/Ethanol/Herb Considerations

Ethanol: Avoid use; may increase risk of osteoporosis.

Herb/Nutraceutical: Ensure adequate calcium and vitamin D intake.

Pharmacodynamics/Kinetics

Distribution: V_d: 0.12 L/kg

Metabolism: Hepatic (nonspecific proteolysis)

Bioavailability: 95%

Half-life elimination: Serum: I.V.: 5 minutes; S.C.: 1 hour

Excretion: Urine (as metabolites)

Pregnancy Risk Factor C

Generic Available No

Terpin Hydrate and Codeine (TER pin HYE drate & KOE deen)

Related Information

Codeine *on page 361*

Pharmacologic Category Expectorant

Synonyms ETH and C

Use Symptomatic relief of cough

Local Anesthetic/Vasoconstrictor Precautions No information available to require special precautions

Effects on Dental Treatment No significant effects or complications reported

Restrictions C-V

Dosage Based on codeine content

Adults: 10-20 mg/dose every 4-6 hours as needed

Children (not recommended): 1-1.5 mg/kg/24 hours divided every 4 hours; maximum: 30 mg/24 hours

2-6 years: 1.25-2.5 mL every 4-6 hours as needed

6-12 years: 2.5-5 mL every 4-6 hours as needed

Other Adverse Effects Frequency not defined:

Central nervous system: Drowsiness

Gastrointestinal: Nausea, vomiting

Pharmacodynamics/Kinetics See Codeine monograph.

Pregnancy Risk Factor C

Generic Available Yes

Terra-Cortril® [DSC] *see* Oxytetracycline and Hydrocortisone *on page 1025*

Terramycin® I.M. *see* Oxytetracycline *on page 1024*

Terramycin® w/Polymyxin B Ophthalmic *see* Oxytetracycline and Polymyxin B *on page 1025*

Teslac® *see* Testolactone *on page 1281*

TESPA *see* Thiotepa *on page 1300*

Tessalon® *see* Benzonatate *on page 171*

Testim™ *see* Testosterone *on page 1281*

Testoderm® *see* Testosterone *on page 1281*

Testoderm® TTS [DSC] *see* Testosterone *on page 1281*

Testoderm® with Adhesive *see* Testosterone *on page 1281*

Testolactone (tes toe LAK tone)

U.S. Brand Names Teslac®

Canadian Brand Names Teslac®

Pharmacologic Category Androgen

Use Palliative treatment of advanced disseminated breast carcinoma

Local Anesthetic/Vasoconstrictor Precautions No information available to require special precautions

Effects on Dental Treatment No significant effects or complications reported

Restrictions C-III

Dosage Adults: Female: Oral: 250 mg 4 times/day for at least 3 months; desired response may take as long as 3 months

Mechanism of Action Testolactone is a synthetic testosterone derivative without significant androgen activity. The drug inhibits steroid aromatase activity, thereby blocking the production of estradiol and estrone from androgen precursors such as testosterone and androstenedione. Unfortunately, the enzymatic block provided by testolactone is transient and is usually limited to a period of 3 months.

Other Adverse Effects 1% to 10%:

Cardiovascular: Edema

Dermatologic: Maculopapular rash

Endocrine & metabolic: Hypercalcemia

Gastrointestinal: Anorexia, diarrhea, nausea, edema of the tongue

Neuromuscular & skeletal: Paresthesias, peripheral neuropathies

Drug Interactions Increased effects of oral anticoagulants.

Pharmacodynamics/Kinetics

Absorption: Well absorbed

Metabolism: Hepatic

Excretion: Urine

Pregnancy Risk Factor C

Generic Available No

Testopel® *see* Testosterone *on page 1281*

Testosterone (tes TOS ter one)

U.S. Brand Names Androderm®; AndroGel®; Delatestryl®; Depo®-Testosterone; Testim™; Testoderm®; Testoderm® TTS [DSC]; Testoderm® with Adhesive; Testopel®

(Continued)

Testosterone *(Continued)*

Canadian Brand Names Andriol®; Androderm®; AndroGel®; Andropository; Delatestryl®; Depotest® 100; Everone® 200; Testoderm®; Virilon® IM

Pharmacologic Category Androgen

Synonyms Aqueous Testosterone; Testosterone Cypionate; Testosterone Enanthate; Testosterone Propionate

Use

Injection: Androgen replacement therapy in the treatment of delayed male puberty; male hypogonadism (primary or hypogonadotropic); inoperable female breast cancer (enanthate only)

Pellet: Androgen replacement therapy in the treatment of delayed male puberty; male hypogonadism (primary or hypogonadotropic)

Topical: Male hypogonadism (primary or hypogonadotropic)

Local Anesthetic/Vasoconstrictor Precautions No information available to require special precautions

Effects on Dental Treatment No significant effects or complications reported

Restrictions C-III

Dosage

Adolescents: I.M.:

Male hypogonadism:

Initiation of pubertal growth: 40-50 mg/m^2/dose (cypionate or enanthate ester) monthly until the growth rate falls to prepubertal levels

Terminal growth phase: 100 mg/m^2/dose (cypionate or enanthate ester) monthly until growth ceases

Maintenance virilizing dose: 100 mg/m^2/dose (cypionate or enanthate ester) twice monthly

Delayed male puberty: 40-50 mg/m^2/dose monthly (cypionate or enanthate ester) for 6 months

Adolescents and Adults: Pellet (for subcutaneous implantation): Delayed male puberty, male hypogonadism: 150-450 mg every 3-6 months

Adults:

I.M.:

Female: Inoperable breast cancer: Testosterone enanthate: 200-400 mg every 2-4 weeks

Male: Long-acting formulations: Testosterone enanthate (in oil)/testosterone cypionate (in oil):

Hypogonadism: 50-400 mg every 2-4 weeks

Delayed puberty: 50-200 mg every 2-4 weeks for a limited duration

Transdermal: Primary male hypogonadism **or** hypogonadotropic hypogonadism:

Testoderm®: Apply 6 mg patch daily to scrotum (if scrotum is inadequate, use a 4 mg daily system)

Androderm®: Apply two systems nightly to clean, dry area on the back, abdomen, upper arms, or thighs for 24 hours for a total of 5 mg day

AndroGel®, Testim™: 5 g (to deliver 50 mg of testosterone with 5 mg systemically absorbed) applied once daily (preferably in the morning) to clean, dry, intact skin of the shoulder and upper arms. AndroGel® may also be applied to the abdomen. Dosage may be increased to a maximum of 10 g (100 mg). Upon opening the packet(s), the entire contents should be squeezed into the palm of the hand and immediately applied to the application site(s). Application sites should be allowed to dry for a few minutes prior to dressing. Hands should be washed with soap and water after application. **Do not apply testosterone gel to the genitals**.

Dosing adjustment in hepatic impairment: Reduction required

Mechanism of Action Principal endogenous androgen responsible for promoting the growth and development of the male sex organs and maintaining secondary sex characteristics in androgen-deficient males

Other Adverse Effects Frequency not defined:

Cardiovascular: Flushing, edema

Central nervous system: Excitation, aggressive behavior, sleeplessness, anxiety, mental depression, headache

Dermatologic: Hirsutism (increase in pubic hair growth), acne

Endocrine & metabolic: Menstrual problems (amenorrhea), virilism, breast soreness, gynecomastia, hypercalcemia, hypoglycemia

Gastrointestinal: Nausea, vomiting, GI irritation

Genitourinary: Prostatic hyperplasia, prostatic carcinoma, impotence, testicular atrophy, epididymitis, priapism, bladder irritability

Hepatic: Hepatic dysfunction, cholestatic hepatitis, hepatic necrosis

Hematologic: Leukopenia, polycythemia, suppression of clotting factors

Miscellaneous: Hypersensitivity reactions

Drug Interactions Substrate of CYP2B6, 2C8/9, 2C19, 3A4; Inhibits CYP3A4

Increased Effect/Toxicity: Warfarin and testosterone: Effects of oral anticoagulants may be enhanced. Testosterone may increase levels of oxyphenbutazone. May enhance fluid retention from corticosteroids.

Dietary/Ethanol/Herb Considerations Herb/Nutraceutical: Avoid St John's wort; may decrease serum concentration.

Pharmacodynamics/Kinetics

Duration (route and ester dependent): I.M.: Cypionate and enanthate esters have longest duration, ≤2-4 weeks

Absorption: Transdermal gel: ~10% of dose

Distribution: Crosses placenta; enters breast milk

Protein binding: 98% to transcortin and albumin

Metabolism: Hepatic; forms metabolites

Half-life elimination: 10-100 minutes

Excretion: Urine (90%); feces (6%)

Pregnancy Risk Factor X

Generic Available No

Testosterone and Estradiol *see* Estradiol and Testosterone *on page 527*

Testosterone Cypionate *see* Testosterone *on page 1281*

Testosterone Enanthate *see* Testosterone *on page 1281*

Testosterone Propionate *see* Testosterone *on page 1281*

Testred® *see* MethylTESTOSTERone *on page 897*

Tetanus Immune Globulin (Human)

(TET a nus i MYOON GLOB yoo lin HYOO min)

Related Information

Animal and Human Bites Guidelines *on page 1580*

U.S. Brand Names BayTet™

Canadian Brand Names BayTet™

Pharmacologic Category Immune Globulin

Synonyms TIG

Use Passive immunization against tetanus; tetanus immune globulin is preferred over tetanus antitoxin for treatment of active tetanus; part of the management of an unclean, wound in a person whose history of previous receipt of tetanus toxoid is unknown or who has received less than three doses of tetanus toxoid; elderly may require TIG more often than younger patients with tetanus infection due to declining antibody titers with age

Local Anesthetic/Vasoconstrictor Precautions No information available to require special precautions

Effects on Dental Treatment No significant effects or complications reported

Dosage I.M.:

Prophylaxis of tetanus:

Children: 4 units/kg; some recommend administering 250 units to small children

Adults: 250 units

Treatment of tetanus:

Children: 500-3000 units; some should infiltrate locally around the wound

Adults: 3000-6000 units

Mechanism of Action Passive immunity toward tetanus

Other Adverse Effects

>10%: Local: Pain, tenderness, erythema at injection site

1% to 10%:

Central nervous system: Fever (mild)

Dermatologic: Urticaria, angioedema

Neuromuscular & skeletal: Muscle stiffness

Miscellaneous: Anaphylaxis reaction

<1%: Sensitization to repeated injections

Pharmacodynamics/Kinetics Absorption: Well absorbed

Pregnancy Risk Factor C

Generic Available No

Tetanus Toxoid (Adsorbed) (TET a nus TOKS oyd, ad ZORBD)

Related Information

Diphtheria, Tetanus Toxoids, Acellular Pertussis, Hepatitis B (Recombinant), and Poliovirus (Inactivated) Vaccine *on page 454*

Pharmacologic Category Toxoid

Use Selective induction of active immunity against tetanus in selected patients. **Note:** Tetanus and diphtheria toxoids for adult use (Td) is the preferred immunizing agent for most adults and for children after their seventh birthday. Young children should receive trivalent DTwP or DTaP (diphtheria/tetanus/pertussis - whole cell or acellular), as part of their childhood immunization program, unless pertussis is contraindicated, then TD is warranted.

Local Anesthetic/Vasoconstrictor Precautions No information available to require special precautions

Effects on Dental Treatment No significant effects or complications reported

Restrictions Federal law requires that the date of administration, the vaccine manufacturer, lot number of vaccine, and the administering person's name, title and address be entered into the patient's permanent medical record.

(Continued)

Tetanus Toxoid (Adsorbed) *(Continued)*

Dosage Adults: I.M.:

Primary immunization: 0.5 mL; repeat 0.5 mL at 4-8 weeks after first dose and at 6-12 months after second dose

Routine booster doses are recommended only every 5-10 years

Mechanism of Action Tetanus toxoid preparations contain the toxin produced by virulent tetanus bacilli (detoxified growth products of *Clostridium tetani*). The toxin has been modified by treatment with formaldehyde so that it has lost toxicity but still retains ability to act as antigen and produce active immunity; the aluminum salt, a mineral adjuvant, delays the rate of absorption and prolongs and enhances its properties; duration ~10 years.

Other Adverse Effects

>10%: Local: Induration/redness at injection site

1% to 10%:

Central nervous system: Chills, fever

Local: Sterile abscess at injection site

Miscellaneous: Allergic reaction

<1%: Fever >103°F, malaise, neurological disturbances, blistering at injection site, Arthus-type hypersensitivity reactions

Pharmacodynamics/Kinetics Duration: Primary immunization: ~10 years

Pregnancy Risk Factor C

Generic Available No

Tetanus Toxoid (Fluid) (TET a nus TOKS oyd FLOO id)

Related Information

Diphtheria, Tetanus Toxoids, Acellular Pertussis, Hepatitis B (Recombinant), and Poliovirus (Inactivated) Vaccine *on page 454*

Pharmacologic Category Toxoid

Synonyms Tetanus Toxoid Plain

Use Detection of delayed hypersensitivity and assessment of cell-mediated immunity; active immunization against tetanus in the rare adult or child who is allergic to the aluminum adjuvant (a product containing adsorbed tetanus toxoid is preferred)

Local Anesthetic/Vasoconstrictor Precautions No information available to require special precautions

Effects on Dental Treatment No significant effects or complications reported

Restrictions Federal law requires that the date of administration, the vaccine manufacturer, lot number of vaccine, and the administering person's name, title and address be entered into the patient's permanent medical record.

Dosage

Anergy testing: Intradermal: 0.1 mL

Primary immunization (**Note:** Td, TD, DTaP/DTwP are recommended): Adults: Inject 3 doses of 0.5 mL I.M. or S.C. at 4- to 8-week intervals; administer fourth dose 6-12 months after third dose

Booster doses: I.M., S.C.: 0.5 mL every 10 years

Mechanism of Action Tetanus toxoid preparations contain the toxin produced by virulent tetanus bacilli (detoxified growth products of *Clostridium tetani*). The toxin has been modified by treatment with formaldehyde so that is has lost toxicity but still retains ability to act as antigen and produce active immunity.

Other Adverse Effects Frequency not defined: Very hypersensitive persons may develop a local reaction at the injection site; urticaria, anaphylactic reactions, shock and death are possible.

Pregnancy Risk Factor C

Generic Available No

Tetanus Toxoid Plain *see* Tetanus Toxoid (Fluid) *on page 1284*

Tetracaine (TET ra kane)

Related Information

Mouth Pain, Cold Sore, and Canker Sore Products *on page 1630*

Oral Nonviral Soft Tissue Ulcerations or Erosions *on page 1549*

Oral Pain *on page 1524*

U.S. Brand Names AK-T-Caine™; Cēpacol Viractin® [OTC]; Opticaine®; Pontocaine®

Canadian Brand Names Ametop™; Pontocaine®

Pharmacologic Category Local Anesthetic, Dental; Local Anesthetic

Synonyms Amethocaine Hydrochloride; Tetracaine Hydrochloride

Use

Dental: Ester-type local anesthetic; applied topically to throat for various diagnostic procedures and on cold sores and fever blisters for pain; **~10 times more potent than procaine (Novocain®)**

Medical: Spinal anesthesia; local anesthesia in the eye and on nose or throat for various diagnostic and examination purposes; topical analgesic

Local Anesthetic/Vasoconstrictor Precautions No information available to require special precautions

Effects on Dental Treatment Frequency not defined: Injection: Cardiac arrest, hypotension, convulsions, dizziness, drowsiness, nervousness, unconsciousness, nausea, vomiting, tremors, blurred vision, respiratory arrest, allergic reaction

Dosage

Children ≥2 years and Adults: **Topical gel** [OTC]: Cold sores and fever blisters: Apply to affected area up to 3-4 times/day for up to 7 days

Adults:

Topical mucous membranes (2% solution): Apply as needed; dose should not exceed 20 mg

Ophthalmic solution (not for prolonged use): Instill 1-2 drops

Spinal anesthesia:

High, medium, low, and saddle blocks: 0.2% to 0.3% solution

Prolonged (2-3 hours): 1% solution

Subarachnoid injection: 5-20 mg

Saddle block: 2-5 mg; a 1% solution should be diluted with equal volume of CSF before administration

Mechanism of Action Ester local anesthetic blocks both the initiation and conduction of nerve impulses by decreasing the neuronal membrane's permeability to sodium ions, which results in inhibition of depolarization with resultant blockade of conduction

Other Adverse Effects Frequency not defined:

Injection:

Central nervous system: Chills

Ocular: Pupil constriction

Otic: Tinnitus

Ophthalmic: Ocular: Chemosis, lacrimation, photophobia, transient stinging

With chronic use: Corneal erosions, corneal healing retardation, corneal opacification (permanent), corneal scarring, keratitis (severe)

Contraindications Hypersensitivity to tetracaine or any component of the formulation; ophthalmic secondary bacterial infection; liver disease; CNS disease or meningitis (if used for epidural or spinal anesthesia); myasthenia gravis

Warnings/Precautions Ophthalmic preparations may delay wound healing; use with caution in patients with cardiac disease and hyperthyroidism

Drug Interactions Decreased effect: Aminosalicylic acid, sulfonamides effects may be antagonized

Pharmacodynamics/Kinetics

Onset of action: Anesthetic: Ophthalmic: ~60 seconds; Topical or spinal injection: 3-8 minutes after applied to mucous membranes or when saddle block administered for spinal anesthesia

Metabolism: Hepatic; detoxified by plasma esterases to aminobenzoic acid

Excretion: Urine

Pregnancy Risk Factor C

Dosage Forms Gel (Cēpacol Viractin®): 2% (7.1 g). **INJ, solution** (Pontocaine®): 1% [10 mg/mL] (2 mL). **INJ, solution** [premixed in dextrose 6%] (Pontocaine®): 0.3% [3 mg/mL] (5 mL). **INJ, powder for reconstitution** (Pontocaine®): 20 mg. **SOLN, ophthalmic:** 0.5% [5 mg/mL] (15 mL); (AK-T-Caine™, Opticaine®): 0.5% (15 mL); (Pontocaine®): 0.5% (15 mL, 59 mL). **SOLN, topical** (Pontocaine®): 2% [20 mg/mL] (30 mL, 118 mL)

Generic Available Yes: Ophthalmic solution

Tetracaine and Dextrose (TET ra kane & DEKS trose)

Related Information

Oral Pain *on page 1524*

Tetracaine *on page 1284*

U.S. Brand Names Pontocaine® With Dextrose

Pharmacologic Category Local Anesthetic

Synonyms Dextrose and Tetracaine

Use Spinal anesthesia (saddle block)

Local Anesthetic/Vasoconstrictor Precautions No information available to require special precautions

Effects on Dental Treatment No significant effects or complications reported

Dosage Dose varies with procedure, depth of anesthesia, duration desired and physical condition of patient

Pharmacodynamics/Kinetics See Tetracaine monograph.

Pregnancy Risk Factor C

Generic Available Yes

Tetracaine Hydrochloride *see* Tetracaine *on page 1284*

Tetracaine Hydrochloride, Benzocaine Butyl Aminobenzoate, and Benzalkonium Chloride *see* Benzocaine, Butyl Aminobenzoate, Tetracaine, and Benzalkonium Chloride *on page 170*

Tetracosactide *see* Cosyntropin *on page 374*

Tetracycline (tet ra SYE kleen)

Related Information

Gastrointestinal Disorders *on page 1474*
Oral Bacterial Infections *on page 1531*
Oral Nonviral Soft Tissue Ulcerations or Erosions *on page 1549*
Periodontal Diseases *on page 1540*
Sexually-Transmitted Diseases *on page 1502*

U.S. Brand Names Sumycin®; Wesmycin®

Canadian Brand Names Apo®-Tetra; Novo-Tetra; Nu-Tetra

Mexican Brand Names Acromicina; Ambotetra; Quimocyclar; Terranumonyl; Tetra-Atlantis®; Zorbenal-G

Pharmacologic Category Antibiotic, Ophthalmic; Antibiotic, Tetracycline Derivative; Antibiotic, Topical

Synonyms Achromycin® [DSC]; TCN; Tetracycline Hydrochloride

Use

Dental: Treatment of periodontitis associated with presence of *Actinobacillus actinomycetemcomitans* (AA); adjunctive therapy for recurrent aphthous ulcers

Medical: Treatment of susceptible bacterial infections (both gram-positive and gram-negative organisms) and infections due to *Mycoplasma*, *Chlamydia*, and *Rickettsia*; treatment of acne, exacerbations of chronic bronchitis, gonorrhea and syphilis in patients allergic to penicillin; part of a multidrug regimen for *H. pylori* eradication to reduce the risk of duodenal ulcer recurrence

Local Anesthetic/Vasoconstrictor Precautions No information available to require special precautions

Effects on Dental Treatment Opportunistic "superinfection" with *Candida albicans*; tetracyclines are not recommended for use during pregnancy or in children ≤8 years of age since they have been reported to cause enamel hypoplasia and permanent teeth discoloration. The use of tetracyclines should only be used in these patients if other agents are contraindicated or alternative antimicrobials will not eradicate the organism. Long-term use associated with oral candidiasis.

Frequency not defined: Intracranial pressure increased, paresthesia, diabetes insipidus syndrome, discoloration of teeth and enamel hypoplasia (young children), nausea, vomiting, esophagitis, antibiotic-associated pseudomembranous colitis, staphylococcal enterocolitis, superinfections, anaphylaxis, hypersensitivity reactions, candidal superinfection, acute renal failure, renal damage

Dosage

Children >8 years: **Oral:** 25-50 mg/kg/day in divided doses every 6 hours

Children >8 years and Adults:

- **Topical:** Apply to affected areas 1-4 times/day
- Ophthalmic:
  - Ointment: Instill every 2-12 hours
  - Suspension: Instill 1-2 drops 2-4 times/day or more often as needed

Adults: **Oral:** 250-500 mg/dose every 6 hours until improvement (usually ≥10 days)

- *Helicobacter pylori* eradication: 500 mg 2-4 times/day depending on regimen; requires combination therapy with at least one other antibiotic and an acid-suppressing agent (proton pump inhibitor or H_2 blocker)

Dosing interval in renal impairment:

- Cl_{cr} 50-80 mL/minute: Administer every 8-12 hours
- Cl_{cr} 10-50 mL/minute: Administer every 12-24 hours
- Cl_{cr} <10 mL/minute: Administer every 24 hours

Dialysis: Slightly dialyzable (5% to 20%) via hemo- and peritoneal dialysis or via continuous arteriovenous or venovenous hemofiltration; no supplemental dosage necessary

Dosing adjustment in hepatic impairment: Avoid use or maximum dose is 1 g/day

Mechanism of Action Inhibits bacterial protein synthesis by binding with the 30S and possibly the 50S ribosomal subunit(s) of susceptible bacteria; may also cause alterations in the cytoplasmic membrane

Other Adverse Effects Frequency not defined:

Cardiovascular: Pericarditis
Central nervous system: Pseudotumor cerebri
Dermatologic: Photosensitivity, pruritus, pigmentation of nails, exfoliative dermatitis
Gastrointestinal: Diarrhea, anorexia, abdominal cramps, pancreatitis
Hematologic: Thrombophlebitis
Hepatic: Hepatotoxicity
Renal: Azotemia

Contraindications Hypersensitivity to tetracycline or any component of the formulation; do not administer to children ≤8 years of age; pregnancy

Warnings/Precautions Use of tetracyclines during tooth development may cause permanent discoloration of the teeth and enamel, hypoplasia and retardation of skeletal development and bone growth with risk being the greatest for children <4 years and those receiving high doses; use with caution in patients with renal or hepatic impairment (eg, elderly); dosage modification required in patients with renal impairment since it may increase BUN as an antianabolic agent; pseudotumor cerebri has been reported with tetracycline use (usually resolves with discontinuation); outdated drug can cause nephropathy; superinfection possible; use protective measure to avoid photosensitivity

Drug Interactions Substrate of **CYP3A4**; Inhibits CYP3A4

Decreased effect: Calcium-, magnesium-, or aluminum-containing antacids, iron, zinc, sodium bicarbonate, penicillins, cimetidine may decrease tetracycline absorption

Although no clinical evidence exists, may bind with bismuth or calcium carbonate, an excipient in bismuth subsalicylate, during treatment for *H. pylori*

Digoxin: Tetracyclines may rarely increase digoxin serum levels.

Methoxyflurane anesthesia when concurrent with tetracycline may cause fatal nephrotoxicity.

Oral contraceptives: Anecdotal reports suggesting decreased contraceptive efficacy with tetracyclines have been refuted by more rigorous scientific and clinical data.

Warfarin with tetracyclines may result in increased anticoagulation.

Dietary/Ethanol/Herb Considerations

Food: Administer on an empty stomach, 1 hour before or 2 hours after meals; food decreases absorption. Avoid dairy products and iron supplements within 3 hours of administration; tetracycline decreases absorption of magnesium, zinc, calcium, iron, and amino acids.

Herb/Nutraceutical: Avoid dong quai and St John's wort; may cause additional photosensitization.

Pharmacodynamics/Kinetics

Absorption: Oral: 75%

Distribution: Small amount appears in bile

Relative diffusion from blood into CSF: Good only with inflammation (exceeds usual MICs)

CSF:blood level ratio: Inflamed meninges: 25%

Protein binding: ~65%

Half-life elimination: Normal renal function: 8-11 hours; End-stage renal disease: 57-108 hours

Time to peak, serum: Oral: 2-4 hours

Excretion: Urine (60% as unchanged drug); feces (as active form)

Pregnancy Risk Factor D

Breast-feeding Considerations Negligible absorption by infant; potential to stain infants' unerupted teeth

Dosage Forms CAP: 250 mg, 500 mg; (Wesmycin®): 250 mg. **SUSP, oral** (Sumycin®): 125 mg/5 mL (480 mL). **TAB** (Sumycin®): 250 mg, 500 mg

Generic Available Yes: Capsule

Selected Readings

Gordon JM and Walker CB, "Current Status of Systemic Antibiotic Usage in Destructive Periodontal Disease," *J Periodontol*, 1993, 64(8 Suppl): 760-71.

Rams TE and Slots J, "Antibiotics in Periodontal Therapy: An Update," *Compendium*, 1992, 13(12):1130, 1132, 1134.

Seymour RA and Heasman PA, "Tetracyclines in the Management of Periodontal Diseases. A Review," *J Clin Periodontol*, 1995, 22(1):22-35.

Seymour RA and Heasman PA, "Pharmacological Control of Periodontal Disease. II. Antimicrobial Agents," *J Dent*, 1995, 23(1):5-14

Tetracycline, Bismuth Subsalicylate, and Metronidazole *see* Bismuth, Metronidazole, and Tetracycline *on page 187*

Tetracycline Hydrochloride *see* Tetracycline *on page 1286*

Tetracycline, Metronidazole, and Bismuth Subsalicylate *see* Bismuth, Metronidazole, and Tetracycline *on page 187*

Tetracycline Periodontal Fibers

(tet ru SYE kleen per ee oh DON tol FYE berz)

Related Information

Tetracycline *on page 1286*

U.S. Brand Names Actisite®

Pharmacologic Category Antibacterial, Dental

Use Dental: Treatment of adult periodontitis; as an adjunct to scaling and root planing for the reduction of pocket depth and bleeding on probing in selected patients with adult periodontitis

Local Anesthetic/Vasoconstrictor Precautions No information available to require special precautions

Effects on Dental Treatment 1% to 10%: Gingival inflammation, mouth pain, glossitis, candidiasis, staining of tongue, local erythema following removal, discomfort from fiber placement

Dosage

Children: Has not been established

Adults: Insert fiber to fill the periodontal pocket; each fiber contains 12.7 mg of tetracycline in 23 cm (9 inches) and provides continuous release of drug for 10 days; fibers are to be secured in pocket with cyanoacrylate adhesive and left in place for 10 days

(Continued)

Tetracycline Periodontal Fibers *(Continued)*

Mechanism of Action Tetracycline is an antibiotic which inhibits growth of susceptible microorganisms. Tetracycline binds primarily to the 30S subunits of bacterial ribosomes, and appears to prevent access of aminoacyl tRNA to the acceptor site on the mRNA-ribosome complex. The fiber releases tetracycline into the periodontal site at a rate of 2 mcg/cm/hour.

Contraindications Hypersensitivity to tetracyclines or any component of the formulation

Warnings/Precautions Use of tetracyclines is not recommended during pregnancy because of interference with fetal bone and dental development

Dietary/Ethanol/Herb Considerations

Food: Avoid dairy products and iron supplements within 3 hours of use; tetracycline decreases absorption of magnesium, zinc, calcium, iron, and amino acids.

Herb/Nutraceutical: Avoid dong quai and St John's wort; may cause additional photosensitization.

Pharmacodynamics/Kinetics

The fiber releases tetracycline at a rate of 2 mcg/cm/hour

Tissue fluid concentrations:

Gingival fluid: ~1590 mcg/mL of tetracycline per site over 10 days

Plasma: During fiber treatment of up to 11 teeth, the tetracycline plasma concentration was below any detectable levels (<0.1 mcg/mL)

Oral: 500 mg of tetracycline produces a peak plasma level of 3-4 mcg/mL

Saliva: ~50.7 mcg/mL of tetracycline immediately after fiber treatment of 9 teeth

Pregnancy Risk Factor C

Dosage Forms FIBER: 23 cm (9") in length [12.7 mg of tetracycline hydrochloride per fiber]

Generic Available No

Comments A number of different facultative and obligate anaerobic bacteria have been found to be causative factors in periodontal disease. These include *Actinobacillus actinomycetemcomitans* (AA), *Fusobacterium nucleatum*, and *Porphyromonas gingivalis*. These bacteria are sensitive to tetracyclines at similar concentrations as those released from the tetracycline-impregnated fibers. Placement of tetracycline periodontal fibers into gingival pockets decreases inflammation, edema, pocket depth, and bleeding upon probing.

Selected Readings

Baer PN, "Actisite (Tetracycline Hydrochloride Periodontal Fiber): A Critique," *Periodontal Clin Investig*, 1994, 16(2):5-7.

Greenstein G, "Treating Periodontal Diseases With Tetracycline-Impregnated Fibers: Data and Controversies," *Compend Contin Educ Dent*, 1995, 16(5)448-55.

Kerry G, "Tetracycline-Loaded Fibers as Adjunctive Treatment in Periodontal Disease," *J Am Dent Assoc*, 1994, 125(9):1199-203.

Michalowicz BS, Pihlstrom BL, Drisko CL, et al, "Evaluation of Periodontal Treatments Using Controlled-Release Tetracycline Fibers: Maintenance Response," *J Periodontol*, 1995, 66(8):708-15.

Mombelli A, Lehmann B, Tonetti M, et al, "Clinical Response to Local Delivery of Tetracycline in Relation to Overall and Local Periodontal Conditions," *J Clin Periodontol*, 1997, 24(7):470-77.

Vandekerckhove BN, Quirynen M, and van Steenberghe D, "The Use of Tetracycline-Containing Controlled-Release Fibers in the Treatment of Refractory Periodontitis," *J Periodontol*, 1997, 68(4):353-61.

Tetrahydroaminoacrine *see* Tacrine *on page 1260*

Tetrahydrocannabinol *see* Dronabinol *on page 480*

Tetrahydrozoline (tet ra hye DROZ a leen)

U.S. Brand Names Eye-Sine™ [OTC]; Geneye® [OTC]; Murine® Tears Plus [OTC]; Optigene® 3 [OTC]; Tyzine®; Tyzine® Pediatric; Visine® Advanced Relief [OTC]; Visine® Original [OTC]

Mexican Brand Names Visine®

Pharmacologic Category Adrenergic Agonist Agent; Ophthalmic Agent, Vasoconstrictor

Synonyms Tetrahydrozoline Hydrochloride; Tetryzoline

Use Symptomatic relief of nasal congestion and conjunctival congestion

Local Anesthetic/Vasoconstrictor Precautions No information available to require special precautions

Effects on Dental Treatment No significant effects or complications reported

Dosage

Nasal congestion: Intranasal:

Children 2-6 years: Instill 2-3 drops of 0.05% solution every 4-6 hours as needed, no more frequent than every 3 hours

Children >6 years and Adults: Instill 2-4 drops or 3-4 sprays of 0.1% solution every 3-4 hours as needed, no more frequent than every 3 hours

Conjunctival congestion: Ophthalmic: Adults: Instill 1-2 drops in each eye 2-4 times/day

Mechanism of Action Stimulates alpha-adrenergic receptors in the arterioles of the conjunctiva and the nasal mucosa to produce vasoconstriction

Other Adverse Effects

>10%:

Local: Transient stinging

Respiratory: Sneezing

1% to 10%:

Cardiovascular: Tachycardia, palpitations, hypertension, heart rate

Central nervous system: Headache

Neuromuscular & skeletal: Tremor

Ocular: Blurred vision

Pharmacodynamics/Kinetics

Onset of action: Decongestant: Intranasal: 4-8 hours

Duration: Ophthalmic vasoconstriction: 2-3 hours

Pregnancy Risk Factor C

Generic Available Yes: Ophthalmic solution

Tetrahydrozoline Hydrochloride *see* Tetrahydrozoline *on page 1288*

Tetryzoline *see* Tetrahydrozoline *on page 1288*

Teveten® *see* Eprosartan *on page 506*

Texacort® *see* Hydrocortisone *on page 688*

TG *see* Thioguanine *on page 1296*

6-TG *see* Thioguanine *on page 1296*

T/Gel® [OTC] *see* Coal Tar *on page 359*

THA *see* Tacrine *on page 1260*

Thalidomide (tha LI doe mide)

Related Information

HIV Infection and AIDS *on page 1482*

Oral Nonviral Soft Tissue Ulcerations or Erosions *on page 1549*

U.S. Brand Names Thalomid®

Canadian Brand Names Thalomid®

Pharmacologic Category Immunosuppressant Agent

Use Treatment and maintenance of cutaneous manifestations of erythema nodosum leprosum

Orphan drug: Treatment of Crohn's disease

Unlabeled/Investigational Use Treatment or prevention of graft-versus-host reactions after bone marrow transplantation; AIDS-related aphthous stomatitis; Langerhans cell histiocytosis, Behçet's syndrome; hypnotic agent; also may be effective in rheumatoid arthritis, discoid lupus erythematosus, and erythema multiforme; useful in type 2 lepra reactions, but not type 1; renal cell carcinoma, multiple myeloma, myeloma, Waldenström's macroglobulinemia

Local Anesthetic/Vasoconstrictor Precautions No information available to require special precautions

Effects on Dental Treatment 1% to 10%: Oral moniliasis (6.3% to 11.1% of HIV-seropositive patients), toothache, xerostomia (8.3% to 9.4%), aphthous stomatitis

Restrictions Thalidomide is approved for marketing only under a special distribution program. This program, called the "System for Thalidomide Education and Prescribing Safety" (STEPS™), has been approved by the FDA. Prescribing and dispensing of thalidomide is restricted to prescribers and pharmacists registered with the program. Prior to dispensing, an authorization number must be obtained (1-888-423-5436) from Celgene (write authorization number on prescription). No more than a 4-week supply should be dispensed. Blister packs should be dispensed intact (do not repackage capsules). Prescriptions must be filled within 7 days.

Dosage Oral:

Cutaneous ENL:

Initiate dosing at 100-300 mg/day taken once daily at bedtime with water (at least 1 hour after evening meal)

Patients weighing <50 kg: Initiate at lower end of the dosing range

Severe cutaneous reaction or previously requiring high dose may be initiated at 400 mg/day; doses may be divided, but taken 1 hour after meals

Dosing should continue until active reaction subsides (usually at least 2 weeks), then tapered in 50 mg decrements every 2-4 weeks

Patients who flare during tapering or with a history or requiring prolonged maintenance should be maintained on the minimum dosage necessary to control the reaction. Efforts to taper should be repeated every 3-6 months, in increments of 50 mg every 2-4 weeks.

Behçet's syndrome (unlabeled use): 100-400 mg/day

Graft-vs-host reactions (unlabeled use): 100-1600 mg/day; usual initial dose: 200 mg 4 times/day for use up to 700 days

AIDS-related aphthous stomatitis (unlabeled use): 200 mg twice daily for 5 days, then 200 mg/day for up to 8 weeks

Discoid lupus erythematosus (unlabeled use): 100-400 mg/day; maintenance dose: 25-50 mg

Mechanism of Action A derivative of glutethimide; mode of action for immunosuppression is unclear; inhibition of neutrophil chemotaxis and decreased monocyte

(Continued)

Thalidomide *(Continued)*

phagocytosis may occur; may cause 50% to 80% reduction of tumor necrosis factor - alpha

Other Adverse Effects

Controlled clinical trials: ENL:

>10%:

Central nervous system: Somnolence (37.5%), headache (12.5%)

Dermatologic: Rash (20.8%)

1% to 10%:

Cardiovascular: Peripheral edema

Central nervous system: Dizziness (4.2%), vertigo (8.3%), chills, malaise (8.3%)

Dermatologic: Dermatitis (fungal) (4.2%), nail disorder (4.2%), pruritus (8.3%), rash (maculopapular) (4.2%)

Gastrointestinal (4.2%): Constipation, diarrhea, nausea, abdominal pain

Genitourinary: Impotence (8.2%)

Neuromuscular & skeletal: Asthenia (8.3%), pain (8.3%), back pain (4.2%), neck pain (4.2%), neck rigidity (4.2%), tremor (4.2%)

Respiratory (4.2%): Pharyngitis, rhinitis, sinusitis

HIV-seropositive:

General: An increased viral load has been noted in patients treated with thalidomide. This is of uncertain clinical significance - see monitoring

>10%:

Central nervous system: Somnolence (36% to 37%), dizziness (18.7% to 19.4%), fever (19.4% to 21.9%), headache (16.7% to 18.7%)

Dermatologic: Rash (25%), maculopapular rash (16.7% to 18.7%), acne (3.1% to 11.1%)

Gastrointestinal: AST increase (2.8% to 12.5%), diarrhea (11.1% to 18.7%), nausea (≤12.5%)

Hematologic: Leukopenia (16.7% to 25%), anemia (5.6% to 12.5%)

Neuromuscular & skeletal: Paresthesia (5.6% to 15.6%), weakness (5.6% to 21.9%)

Miscellaneous: Diaphoresis (≤12.5%), lymphadenopathy (5.6% to 12.5%)

1% to 10%:

Cardiovascular: Peripheral edema (3.1% to 8.3%)

Central nervous system: Nervousness (2.8% to 9.4%), insomnia (≤9.4%), agitation (≤9.4%), chills (≤9.4%)

Dermatologic: Dermatitis (fungal) (5.6% to 9.4%), nail disorder (≤3.1%), pruritus (2.8% to 6.3%)

Gastrointestinal: Anorexia (2.8% to 9.4%), constipation (2.8% to 9.4%), flatulence (8.3% to 9.4%), multiple abnormalities LFTs (≤9.4%), abdominal pain (2.8% to 3.1%)

Neuromuscular & skeletal: Back pain (≤5%), pain (≤3.1%)

Respiratory: Pharyngitis (6.3% to 8.3%), sinusitis (3.1% to 8.3%)

Miscellaneous: Accidental injury (≤5.6%), infection (6.3% to 8.3%)

Literature reports of other adverse reactions (Limited to important or life-threatening): Acute renal failure, bradycardia, CML, dyspnea, erythema nodosum, Hodgkin's disease, hypersensitivity, hyperthyroidism, lymphopenia, myxedema, orthostatic hypotension, pancytopenia, photosensitivity, Raynaud's syndrome, seizures, Stevens-Johnson syndrome, suicide attempt, toxic epidermal necrolysis

Drug Interactions Increased Effect/Toxicity: Other medications known to cause peripheral neuropathy should be used with caution in patients receiving thalidomide; thalidomide may enhance the sedative activity of other drugs such as ethanol, barbiturates, reserpine, and chlorpromazine

Dietary/Ethanol/Herb Considerations

Ethanol: Avoid use; may increase sedation.

Food: Administer at least 1 hour after evening meal. Fluids, fruit, and fiber may reduce constipation. Buttermilk, boiled milk, or yogurt may reduce diarrhea.

Herb/Nutraceutical: Avoid cat's claw due to immunostimulant properties. Avoid gotu kola, kava, SAMe, St John's wort, and valerian; may increase CNS depression.

Pharmacodynamics/Kinetics

Distribution: V_d: 120 L

Metabolism: Hepatic

Half-life elimination: 8.7 hours

Time to peak, plasma: 2-6 hours

Pregnancy Risk Factor X

Generic Available No

Selected Readings Jacobson JM, Greenspan JS, Spritzler J, et al, "Thalidomide for the Treatment of Oral Aphthous Ulcers in Patients With Human Immunodeficiency Virus Infection. National Institute of Allergy and Infectious Diseases AIDS Clinical Trials Group," *N Engl J Med*, 1997, 336(21):1487-93.

Thalitone® *see* Chlorthalidone *on page 315*

Thalomid® *see* Thalidomide *on page 1289*

THAM® *see* Tromethamine *on page 1360*

THC *see* Dronabinol *on page 480*

Theo-24® *see* Theophylline *on page 1291*

Theochron® *see* Theophylline *on page 1291*

Theolair™ *see* Theophylline *on page 1291*

Theolair-SR® [DSC] *see* Theophylline *on page 1291*

Theolate *see* Theophylline and Guaifenesin *on page 1293*

Theophylline (thee OF i lin)

Related Information

Aminophylline *on page 78*

Respiratory Diseases *on page 1476*

U.S. Brand Names Elixophyllin®; Quibron®-T; Quibron®-T/SR; Theo-24®; Theochron®; Theolair™; Theolair-SR® [DSC]; T-Phyl®; Uniphyl®

Canadian Brand Names Apo®-Theo LA; Novo-Theophyl SR; PMS-Theophylline; Pulmophylline; Quibron®-T/SR; ratio-Theo-Bronc; Theochron® SR; Theo-Dur®; Theolair™; Uniphyl® SRT

Mexican Brand Names Slo-Bid®; Teolong®; Uni-Dur®

Pharmacologic Category Theophylline Derivative

Synonyms Theophylline Anhydrous

Use Treatment of symptoms and reversible airway obstruction due to chronic asthma, chronic bronchitis, or COPD

Local Anesthetic/Vasoconstrictor Precautions No information available to require special precautions

Effects on Dental Treatment Prescribe erythromycin products with caution to patients taking theophylline products. Erythromycin will delay the normal metabolic inactivation of theophyllines leading to increased blood levels; this has resulted in nausea, vomiting, and CNS restlessness. Azithromycin does not cause these effects in combination with theophylline products.

Dosage Use ideal body weight for obese patients

I.V.: Initial: Maintenance infusion rates:

Children:

6 weeks to 6 months: 0.5 mg/kg/hour

6 months to 1 year: 0.6-0.7 mg/kg/hour

Children >1 year and Adults:

Acute bronchospasm: See table on next page.

Approximate I.V. maintenance dosages are based upon continuous infusions; bolus dosing (often used in children <6 months of age) may be determined by multiplying the hourly infusion rate by 24 hours and dividing by the desired number of doses/day. See the following:

Maintenance dose for acute symptoms: See table below.

Dosage should be adjusted according to serum level measurements during the first 12- to 24-hour period. See table on next page.

Maintenance Dose for Acute Symptoms

Population Group	Oral Theophylline (mg/kg/day)	I.V. Aminophylline
Premature infant or newborn - 6 wk (for apnea/bradycardia)	4	5 mg/kg/day
6 wk - 6 mo	10	12 mg/kg/day or continuous I.V. infusion*
Infants 6 mo - 1 y	12-18	15 mg/kg/day or continuous I.V. infusion*
Children 1-9 y	20-24	1 mg/kg/h
Children 9-12 y, and adolescent daily smokers of cigarettes or marijuana, and otherwise healthy adult smokers <50 y	16	0.9 mg/kg/h
Adolescents 12-16 y (nonsmokers)	13	0.7 mg/kg/h
Otherwise healthy nonsmoking adults (including elderly patients)	10 (not to exceed 900 mg/day)	0.5 mg/kg/h
Cardiac decompensation, cor pulmonale and/or liver dysfunction	5 (not to exceed 400 mg/day)	0.25 mg/kg/h

*For continuous I.V. infusion divide total daily dose by 24 = mg/kg/h.

(Continued)

Approximate I.V. Theophylline Dosage for Treatment of Acute Bronchospasm

Group	Dosage for Next 12 h*	Dosage After 12 h*
Infants 6 wk - 6 mo	0.5 mg/kg/h	
Children 6 mo - 1 y	0.6-0.7 mg/kg/h	
Children 1-9 y	0.95 mg/kg/h (1.2 mg/kg/h)	0.79 mg/kg/h (1 mg/kg/h)
Children 9-16 y and young adult smokers	0.79 mg/kg/h (1 mg/kg/h)	0.63 mg/kg/h (0.8 mg/kg/h)
Healthy, nonsmoking adults	0.55 mg/kg/h (0.7 mg/kg/h)	0.39 mg/kg/h (0.5 mg/kg/h)
Older patients and patients with cor pulmonale	0.47 mg/kg/h (0.6 mg/kg/h)	0.24 mg/kg/h (0.3 mg/kg/h)
Patients with congestive heart failure or liver failure	0.39 mg/kg/h (0.5 mg/kg/h)	0.08-0.16 mg/kg/h (0.1-0.2 mg/kg/h)

*Equivalent hydrous aminophylline dosage indicated in parentheses.

Dosage Adjustment After Serum Theophylline Measurement

Serum Theophylline		Guidelines
Within normal limits	10-20 mcg/mL	Maintain dosage if tolerated. Recheck serum theophylline concentration at 6- to 12-month intervals.*
Too high	20-25 mcg/mL	Decrease doses by about 10%. Recheck serum theophylline concentration after 3 days and then at 6- to 12-month intervals.*
	25-30 mcg/mL	Skip next dose and decrease subsequent doses by about 25%. Recheck serum theophylline.
	>30 mcg/mL	Skip next 2 doses and decrease subsequent doses by 50%. Recheck serum theophylline.
Too low	7.5-10 mcg/mL	Increase dose by about 25%.† Recheck serum theophylline concentration after 3 days and then at 6- to 12-month intervals.*
	5-7.5 mcg/mL	Increase dose by about 25% to the nearest dose increment† and recheck serum theophylline for guidance in further dosage adjustment (another increase will probably be needed, but this provides a safety check).

*Finer adjustments in dosage may be needed for some patients.

†Dividing the daily dose into 3 doses administered at 8-hour intervals may be indicated if symptoms occur repeatedly at the end of a dosing interval.

From Weinberger M and Hendeles L, "Practical Guide to UsingTheophylline," *J Resp Dis*, 1981,2:12-27.

Oral Theophylline Dosage for Bronchial Asthma*

Age	Initial 3 Days	Second 3 Days	Steady-State Maintenance
<1 y	0.2 x (age in weeks) + 5		0.3 x (age in weeks) + 8
1-9 y	16 up to a maximum of 400 mg/24 h	20	22
9-12 y	16 up to a maximum of 400 mg/24 h	16 up to a maximum of 600 mg/24 h	20 up to a maximum of 800 mg/24 h
12-16 y	16 up to a maximum of 400 mg/24 h	16 up to a maximum of 600 mg/24 h	18 up to a maximum of 900 mg/24 h
Adults	400 mg/24 h	600 mg/24 h	900 mg/24 h

*Dose in mg/kg/24 hours of theophylline.

Oral theophylline: Initial dosage recommendation: Loading dose (to achieve a serum level of about 10 mcg/mL; loading doses should be given using a rapidly absorbed oral product **not** a sustained release product):

If no theophylline has been administered in the previous 24 hours: 4-6 mg/kg theophylline

If theophylline has been administered in the previous 24 hours: administer 1/2 loading dose or 2-3 mg/kg theophylline can be given in emergencies when serum levels are unavailable

On the average, for every 1 mg/kg theophylline given, blood levels will rise 2 mcg/mL

Ideally, defer the loading dose if a serum theophylline concentration can be obtained rapidly. However, if this is not possible, exercise clinical judgment. If the patient is not experiencing theophylline toxicity, this is unlikely to result in dangerous adverse effects.

Oral theophylline dosage for bronchial asthma (by age): See previous table.

Increasing dose: The dosage may be increased in approximately 25% increments at 2- to 3-day intervals so long as the drug is tolerated or until the maximum dose is reached

Maintenance dose: In children and healthy adults, a slow-release product can be used; the total daily dose can be divided every 8-12 hours

Mechanism of Action Causes bronchodilatation, diuresis, CNS and cardiac stimulation, and gastric acid secretion by blocking phosphodiesterase which increases tissue concentrations of cyclic adenine monophosphate (cAMP) which in turn promotes catecholamine stimulation of lipolysis, glycogenolysis, and gluconeogenesis and induces release of epinephrine from adrenal medulla cells

Other Adverse Effects

Adverse reactions/theophylline serum level: (Adverse effects do not necessarily occur according to serum levels. Arrhythmia and seizure can occur without seeing the other adverse effects).

15-25 mcg/mL: GI upset, diarrhea, nausea/vomiting, abdominal pain, nervousness, headache, insomnia, agitation, dizziness, muscle cramp, tremor

25-35 mcg/mL: Tachycardia, occasional PVC

>35 mcg/mL: Ventricular tachycardia, frequent PVC, seizure

Uncommon at serum theophylline concentrations ≤20 mcg/mL

1% to 10%:

Cardiovascular: Tachycardia

Central nervous system: Nervousness, restlessness

Gastrointestinal: Nausea, vomiting

<1% (Limited to important or life-threatening): Insomnia, irritability, seizures, tremor

Drug Interactions Substrate of **CYP1A2**, 2C8/9, 2D6, **2E1**, **3A4**; Inhibits CYP1A2

Increased Effect/Toxicity: Changes in diet may affect the elimination of theophylline. The following may increase serum theophylline levels: propranolol, allopurinol (>600 mg/day), erythromycin, cimetidine, troleandomycin, ciprofloxacin (other quinolone antibiotics), oral contraceptives, beta-blockers, calcium channel blockers, corticosteroids, disulfiram, ephedrine, influenza virus vaccine, interferon, macrolides, mexiletine, thiabendazole, thyroid hormones, carbamazepine, isoniazid, and loop diuretics. Other inhibitors of cytochrome P450 1A2 may increase theophylline levels.

Decreased Effect: Changes in diet may affect the elimination of theophylline. Charcoal-broiled foods may increase elimination, reducing half-life by 50%. The following factors decrease theophylline serum levels: Smoking (cigarettes, marijuana), high protein/low carbohydrate diet, charcoal, phenytoin, phenobarbital, carbamazepine, rifampin, ritonavir, I.V. isoproterenol, aminoglutethimide, barbiturates, hydantoins, ketoconazole, sulfinpyrazone, isoniazid, loop diuretics, and sympathomimetics.

Dietary/Ethanol/Herb Considerations Food does not appreciably affect the absorption of liquid, fast-release products, and most sustained-release products, but may induce a sudden release (dose-dumping) of once-daily sustained-release products resulting in an increase in serum concentration and potential toxicity. Avoid excessive amounts of caffeine, carbohydrates, and protein; limit charcoal-broiled foods.

Pharmacodynamics/Kinetics

Onset of action: I.V.: <30 minutes

Absorption: Oral (formulation dependent): ≤100%

Protein binding: 40%, primarily to albumin

Metabolism: Hepatic

Half-life elimination (age, liver and cardiac function, lung disease, and smoking history dependent): Highly variable

Excretion: Urine

Pregnancy Risk Factor C

Generic Available Yes: Elixir, extended release tablet, infusion, oral solution

Theophylline and Guaifenesin (thee OF i lin & gwye FEN e sin)

Related Information

Guaifenesin *on page 650*

(Continued)

Theophylline and Guaifenesin *(Continued)*

Theophylline *on page 1291*

U.S. Brand Names Elixophyllin-GG®; Quibron®; Theolate

Pharmacologic Category Theophylline Derivative

Synonyms Guaifenesin and Theophylline

Use Symptomatic treatment of bronchospasm associated with bronchial asthma, chronic bronchitis, and pulmonary emphysema

Local Anesthetic/Vasoconstrictor Precautions No information available to require special precautions

Effects on Dental Treatment Prescribe erythromycin products with caution to patients taking theophylline products. Erythromycin will delay the normal metabolic inactivation of theophyllines leading to increased blood levels; this has resulted in nausea, vomiting, and CNS restlessness.

Dosage Adults: Oral: 16 mg/kg/day or 400 mg theophylline/day, in divided doses, every 6-8 hours

Dietary/Ethanol/Herb Considerations Food does not appreciably affect the absorption of liquid, fast-release products and most sustained-release products, but may induce a sudden release (dose-dumping) of once-daily sustained-release products resulting in an increase in serum concentration and potential toxicity. Avoid excessive amounts of caffeine, carbohydrates, and protein; limit charcoal-broiled foods.

Pregnancy Risk Factor C

Generic Available No

Theophylline Anhydrous *see* Theophylline *on page 1291*

Theophylline Ethylenediamine *see* Aminophylline *on page 78*

Theracort® [OTC] *see* Hydrocortisone *on page 688*

TheraCys® *see* BCG Vaccine *on page 161*

Thera-Flu® Flu and Cold *see* Acetaminophen, Chlorpheniramine, and Pseudoephedrine *on page 35*

Thera-Flu® Non-Drowsy Flu, Cold and Cough [OTC] *see* Acetaminophen, Dextromethorphan, and Pseudoephedrine *on page 35*

Thera-Flur-N® *see* Fluoride *on page 586*

Theragran® Heart Right™ [OTC] *see* Vitamins (Multiple/Oral) *on page 1394*

Theragran-M® Advanced Formula [OTC] *see* Vitamins (Multiple/Oral) *on page 1394*

Theramycin Z® *see* Erythromycin *on page 512*

Therapeutic Multivitamins *see* Vitamins (Multiple/Oral) *on page 1394*

Thermazene® *see* Silver Sulfadiazine *on page 1222*

Thiabendazole (thye a BEN da zole)

U.S. Brand Names Mintezol®

Pharmacologic Category Anthelmintic

Synonyms Tiabendazole

Use Treatment of strongyloidiasis, cutaneous larva migrans, visceral larva migrans, dracunculiasis, trichinosis, and mixed helminthic infections

Local Anesthetic/Vasoconstrictor Precautions No information available to require special precautions

Effects on Dental Treatment No significant effects or complications reported

Dosage Purgation is not required prior to use; drinking of fruit juice aids in expulsion of worms by removing the mucous to which the intestinal tapeworms attach themselves.

Children and Adults: Oral: 50 mg/kg/day divided every 12 hours (if >68 kg: 1.5 g/dose); maximum dose: 3 g/day

Treatment duration:

- Strongyloidiasis, ascariasis, uncinariasis, trichuriasis: For 2 consecutive days
- Cutaneous larva migrans: For 2-5 consecutive days
- Visceral larva migrans: For 5-7 consecutive days
- Trichinosis: For 2-4 consecutive days
- Dracunculosis: 50-75 mg/kg/day divided every 12 hours for 3 days

Dosing comments in renal/hepatic impairment: Use with caution

Mechanism of Action Inhibits helminth-specific mitochondrial fumarate reductase

Other Adverse Effects Frequency not defined:

Central nervous system: Seizures, hallucinations, delirium, dizziness, drowsiness, headache, chills

Dermatologic: Rash, Stevens-Johnson syndrome, pruritus, angioedema

Endocrine & metabolic: Hyperglycemia

Gastrointestinal: Anorexia, diarrhea, nausea, vomiting, drying of mucous membranes, abdominal pain

Genitourinary: Malodor of urine, hematuria, crystalluria, enuresis

Hematologic: Leukopenia

Hepatic: Jaundice, cholestasis, hepatic failure, hepatotoxicity

Neuromuscular & skeletal: Numbness, incoordination

Ocular: Visual changes, dry eyes, Sicca syndrome
Otic: Tinnitus
Renal: Nephrotoxicity
Miscellaneous: Anaphylaxis, hypersensitivity reactions, lymphadenopathy

Drug Interactions Substrate of CYP1A2
Increased effects of theophylline and other xanthines.

Pharmacodynamics/Kinetics
Absorption: Rapid and well absorbed
Metabolism: Rapidly hepatic
Half-life elimination: 1.2 hours
Time to peak, plasma: Oral suspension: Within 1-2 hours
Excretion: Urine (87%) and feces (5%) primarily as conjugated metabolites

Pregnancy Risk Factor C

Generic Available No

Thiamazole *see* Methimazole *on page 880*
Thiamilate® [OTC] *see* Thiamine *on page 1295*

Thiamine (THYE a min)

U.S. Brand Names Thiamilate® [OTC]

Canadian Brand Names Betaxin®

Mexican Brand Names Benerva®

Pharmacologic Category Vitamin, Water Soluble

Synonyms Aneurine Hydrochloride; Thiamine Hydrochloride; Thiaminium Chloride Hydrochloride; Vitamin B_1

Use Treatment of thiamine deficiency including beriberi, Wernicke's encephalopathy syndrome, and peripheral neuritis associated with pellagra, alcoholic patients with altered sensorium; various genetic metabolic disorders

Local Anesthetic/Vasoconstrictor Precautions No information available to require special precautions

Effects on Dental Treatment No significant effects or complications reported

Dosage
Recommended daily allowance:
- <6 months: 0.3 mg
- 6 months to 1 year: 0.4 mg
- 1-3 years: 0.7 mg
- 4-6 years: 0.9 mg
- 7-10 years: 1 mg
- 11-14 years: 1.1-1.3 mg
- >14 years: 1-1.5 mg

Thiamine deficiency (beriberi):
- Children: 10-25 mg/dose I.M. or I.V. daily (if critically ill), or 10-50 mg/dose orally every day for 2 weeks, then 5-10 mg/dose orally daily for 1 month
- Adults: 5-30 mg/dose I.M. or I.V. 3 times/day (if critically ill); then orally 5-30 mg/day in single or divided doses 3 times/day for 1 month

Wernicke's encephalopathy: Adults: Initial: 100 mg I.V., then 50-100 mg/day I.M. or I.V. until consuming a regular, balanced diet

Dietary supplement (depends on caloric or carbohydrate content of the diet):
- Infants: 0.3-0.5 mg/day
- Children: 0.5-1 mg/day
- Adults: 1-2 mg/day

Note: The above doses can be found in multivitamin preparations

Metabolic disorders: Oral: Adults: 10-20 mg/day (dosages up to 4 g/day in divided doses have been used)

Mechanism of Action An essential coenzyme in carbohydrate metabolism by combining with adenosine triphosphate to form thiamine pyrophosphate

Other Adverse Effects <1%: Cardiovascular collapse and death, warmth, rash, angioedema, paresthesia

Dietary/Ethanol/Herb Considerations Food: High carbohydrate diets may increase thiamine requirement.

Pharmacodynamics/Kinetics
Absorption: Oral: Adequate; I.M.: Rapid and complete
Excretion: Urine (as unchanged drug and as pyrimidine after body storage sites become saturated)

Pregnancy Risk Factor A/C (dose exceeding RDA recommendation)

Generic Available Yes

Thiamine Hydrochloride *see* Thiamine *on page 1295*
Thiaminium Chloride Hydrochloride *see* Thiamine *on page 1295*

Thiethylperazine (thye eth il PER a zeen)

U.S. Brand Names Torecan®

Canadian Brand Names Torecan®

Mexican Brand Names Torecan®

Pharmacologic Category Antiemetic

(Continued)

Thiethylperazine *(Continued)*

Synonyms Thiethylperazine Maleate

Use Relief of nausea and vomiting

Unlabeled/Investigational Use Treatment of vertigo

Local Anesthetic/Vasoconstrictor Precautions No information available to require special precautions

Effects on Dental Treatment >10%: Xerostomia, changes in salivation

Dosage Children >12 years and Adults:

Oral, I.M., rectal: 10 mg 1-3 times/day as needed

I.V. and S.C. routes of administration are not recommended

Hemodialysis: Not dialyzable (0% to 5%)

Dosing comments in hepatic impairment: Use with caution

Mechanism of Action Blocks postsynaptic mesolimbic dopaminergic receptors in the brain; exhibits a strong alpha-adrenergic blocking effect and depresses the release of hypothalamic and hypophyseal hormones; acts directly on chemoreceptor trigger zone and vomiting center

Other Adverse Effects

>10%:

- Central nervous system: Drowsiness, dizziness
- Respiratory: Dry nose

1% to 10%:

- Cardiovascular: Tachycardia, orthostatic hypotension
- Central nervous system: Confusion, convulsions, extrapyramidal symptoms, tardive dyskinesia, fever, headache
- Hematologic: Agranulocytosis
- Hepatic: Cholestatic jaundice
- Otic: Tinnitus

Drug Interactions Increased effect with CNS depressants (eg, anesthetics, opiates, tranquilizers, alcohol), lithium, atropine, epinephrine, MAO inhibitors, and TCAs.

Dietary/Ethanol/Herb Considerations

Ethanol: Avoid use; may increase CNS depression.

Herb/Nutraceutical: Avoid gotu kola, kava, SAMe, St John's wort, and valerian; may increase CNS depression.

Pharmacodynamics/Kinetics

Onset of action: Antiemetic: ~30 minutes

Duration: ~4 hours

Pregnancy Risk Factor X

Generic Available No

Thiethylperazine Maleate *see* Thiethylperazine *on page 1295*

Thimerosal (thye MER oh sal)

U.S. Brand Names Mersol® [OTC]; Merthiolate® [OTC]

Pharmacologic Category Antibiotic, Topical

Use Organomercurial antiseptic with sustained bacteriostatic and fungistatic activity

Local Anesthetic/Vasoconstrictor Precautions No information available to require special precautions

Effects on Dental Treatment No significant effects or complications reported

Dosage Apply 1-3 times/day

Generic Available Yes

Thioguanine (thye oh GWAH neen)

Canadian Brand Names Lanvis®

Pharmacologic Category Antineoplastic Agent, Antimetabolite

Synonyms 2-Amino-6-Mercaptopurine; TG; 6-TG; 6-Thioguanine; Tioguanine

Use Remission induction, consolidation, and maintenance therapy of acute myelogenous (nonlymphocytic) leukemia; treatment of chronic myelogenous leukemia and granulocytic leukemia

Local Anesthetic/Vasoconstrictor Precautions No information available to require special precautions

Effects on Dental Treatment No significant effects or complications reported

Dosage Total daily dose can be given at one time; offers little advantage over mercaptopurine; is sometimes ordered as 6-thioguanine, with 6 being part of the drug name and not a unit or strength

Oral (refer to individual protocols):

- Infants and Children <3 years: Combination drug therapy for acute nonlymphocytic leukemia: 3.3 mg/kg/day in divided doses twice daily for 4 days
- Children and Adults: 2-3 mg/kg/day calculated to nearest 20 mg or 75-200 mg/m^2/day in 1-2 divided doses for 5-7 days or until remission is attained

Dosing adjustment in renal/hepatic impairment: Reduction required

Mechanism of Action Purine analog that is incorporated into DNA and RNA resulting in the blockage of synthesis and metabolism of purine nucleotides

Other Adverse Effects
>10%:
Hematologic: Myelosuppressive:
WBC: Moderate
Platelets: Moderate
Onset: 7-10 days
Nadir: 14 days
Recovery: 21 days
1% to 10%:
Dermatologic: Skin rash
Endocrine & metabolic: Hyperuricemia
Gastrointestinal: Mild nausea or vomiting, anorexia, stomatitis, diarrhea
Emetic potential: Low (<10%)
Neuromuscular & skeletal: Unsteady gait
<1%: Neurotoxicity, photosensitivity, hepatitis, jaundice, veno-occlusive hepatic disease

Drug Interactions Increased Effect/Toxicity: Allopurinol can be used in full doses with 6-TG unlike 6-MP. Use with busulfan may cause hepatotoxicity and esophageal varices. Aminosalicylates (olsalazine, mesalamine, sulfasalazine) may inhibit TPMT, increasing toxicity/myelosuppression of thioguanine.

Dietary/Ethanol/Herb Considerations Food: Administer between meals to enhance absorption.

Pharmacodynamics/Kinetics
Absorption: 30%
Distribution: Crosses placenta
Metabolism: Rapidly and extensively hepatic to 2-amino-6-methylthioguanine (active) and inactive compounds
Half-life elimination: Terminal: 11 hours
Time to peak, serum: Within 8 hours
Excretion: Urine

Pregnancy Risk Factor D

Generic Available Yes

6-Thioguanine *see* Thioguanine *on page 1296*
Thiola® *see* Tiopronin *on page 1313*

Thiopental (thye oh PEN tal)

U.S. Brand Names Pentothal®

Canadian Brand Names Pentothal®

Mexican Brand Names Pentothal Sodico®; Sodipental®

Pharmacologic Category Anticonvulsant, Barbiturate; Barbiturate; General Anesthetic

Synonyms Thiopental Sodium

Use Induction of anesthesia; adjunct for intubation in head injury patients; control of convulsive states; treatment of elevated intracranial pressure

Local Anesthetic/Vasoconstrictor Precautions No information available to require special precautions

Effects on Dental Treatment No significant effects or complications reported

Restrictions C-III

Dosage Accumulation may occur with chronic dosing due to lipid solubility; prolonged recovery may result from redistribution of thiopental from fat stores
I.V.:
Induction anesthesia:
Infants: 5-8 mg/kg
Children 1-12 years: 5-6 mg/kg
Adults: 3-5 mg/kg
Maintenance anesthesia:
Children: 1 mg/kg as needed
Adults: 25-100 mg as needed
Increased intracranial pressure: Children and Adults: 1.5-5 mg/kg/dose; repeat as needed to control intracranial pressure
Seizures:
Children: 2-3 mg/kg/dose; repeat as needed
Adults: 75-250 mg/dose; repeat as needed

Rectal administration (patient should be NPO for no less than 3 hours prior to administration):
Suggested initial doses of thiopental rectal suspension are:
<3 months: 15 mg/kg/dose
>3 months: 25 mg/kg/dose
Note: The age of a premature infant should be adjusted to reflect the age that the infant would have been if full-term (eg, an infant, now age 4 months, who was 2 months premature should be considered to be a 2-month old infant).
Doses should be rounded downward to the nearest 50 mg increment to allow for accurate measurement of the dose

(Continued)

Thiopental *(Continued)*

Inactive or debilitated patients and patients recently medicated with other sedatives (eg, chloral hydrate, meperidine, chlorpromazine, and promethazine), may require smaller doses than usual

If the patient is not sedated within 15-20 minutes, a single repeat dose of thiopental can be given. The single repeat doses are:

<3 months: <7.5 mg/kg/dose

>3 months: 15 mg/kg/dose

Children weighing >34 kg should not receive >1 g as a total dose (initial plus repeat doses)

Adults weighing >90 kg should not receive >3 g as a total dose (initial plus repeat doses)

Neither adults nor children should receive more than one course of thiopental rectal suspension (initial dose plus repeat dose) per 24-hour period

Dosing adjustment in renal impairment: Cl_{cr} <10 mL/minute: Administer at 75% of normal dose

Mechanism of Action Short-acting barbiturate with sedative, hypnotic, and anticonvulsant properties. Barbiturates depress the sensory cortex, decrease motor activity, alter cerebellar function, and produce drowsiness, sedation, and hypnosis. In high doses, barbiturates exhibit anticonvulsant activity; barbiturates produce dose-dependent respiratory depression.

Other Adverse Effects Frequency not defined:

Cardiovascular: Bradycardia, hypotension, syncope

Central nervous system: Drowsiness, lethargy, CNS excitation or depression, impaired judgment, "hangover" effect, confusion, somnolence, agitation, hyperkinesia, ataxia, nervousness, headache, insomnia, nightmares, hallucinations, anxiety, dizziness, shivering

Dermatologic: Rash, exfoliative dermatitis, Stevens-Johnson syndrome

Gastrointestinal: Nausea, vomiting, constipation

Hematologic: Agranulocytosis, thrombocytopenia, megaloblastic anemia, immune hemolytic anemia (rare)

Local: Pain at injection site, thrombophlebitis with I.V. use

Renal: Oliguria

Respiratory: Laryngospasm, respiratory depression, apnea (especially with rapid I.V. use), hypoventilation, apnea, sneezing, coughing, bronchospasm

Miscellaneous: Gangrene with inadvertent intra-arterial injection, anaphylaxis, anaphylactic reactions

Drug Interactions Increased Effect/Toxicity: In chronic use, barbiturates are potent inducers of CYP isoenzymes resulting in multiple interactions with medication groups. When used for limited periods, thiopental is not likely to interact via this mechanism. Sedative effects and/or respiratory depression with barbiturates may be additive with other CNS depressants; includes ethanol, sedatives, antidepressants, narcotic analgesics, and benzodiazepines. Felbamate may inhibit the metabolism of barbiturates and barbiturates may increase the metabolism of felbamate. Barbiturates may enhance the nephrotoxic effects of methoxyflurane

Dietary/Ethanol/Herb Considerations

Ethanol: Avoid use; may increase CNS and respiratory depression.

Herb/Nutraceutical: Avoid gotu kola, kava, SAMe, St John's wort, and valerian; may increase CNS depression.

Pharmacodynamics/Kinetics

Onset of action: Anesthetic: I.V.: 30-60 seconds

Duration: 5-30 minutes

Distribution: V_d: 1.4 L/kg

Protein binding: 72% to 86%

Metabolism: Hepatic, primarily to inactive metabolites but pentobarbital is also formed

Half-life elimination: 3-11.5 hours; decreased in children

Pregnancy Risk Factor C

Generic Available Yes

Thiopental Sodium *see* Thiopental *on page 1297*

Thiophosphoramide *see* Thiotepa *on page 1300*

Thioplex® *see* Thiotepa *on page 1300*

Thioridazine (thye oh RID a zeen)

U.S. Brand Names Mellaril® [DSC]; Thioridazine Intensol™

Canadian Brand Names Apo®-Thioridazine; Mellaril®

Mexican Brand Names Melleril®

Pharmacologic Category Antipsychotic Agent, Phenothiazine, Piperidine

Synonyms Thioridazine Hydrochloride

Use Management of schizophrenic patients who fail to respond adequately to treatment with other antipsychotic drugs, either because of insufficient effectiveness or the inability to achieve an effective dose due to intolerable adverse effects from those medications

Unlabeled/Investigational Use Treatment of psychosis

Local Anesthetic/Vasoconstrictor Precautions Most pharmacology textbooks state that in the presence of phenothiazines, systemic doses of epinephrine paradoxically decrease the blood pressure. This is the so called "epinephrine reversal" phenomenon. This has never been observed when epinephrine is given by infiltration as part of the anesthesia procedure.

Effects on Dental Treatment >10%: Xerostomia, changes in salivation

Significant hypotension may occur, especially when the drug is administered parenterally; orthostatic hypotension is due to alpha-receptor blockade, the elderly are at greater risk for orthostatic hypotension.

Tardive dyskinesia; Prevalence rate may be 40% in elderly; development of the syndrome and the irreversible nature are proportional to duration and total cumulative dose over time. Extrapyramidal reactions are more common in elderly with up to 50% developing these reactions after 60 years of age; drug-induced **Parkinson's syndrome** occurs often; **Akathisia** is the most common extrapyramidal reaction in elderly.

Increased confusion, memory loss, psychotic behavior, and agitation frequently occur as a consequence of anticholinergic effects. Antipsychotic associated sedation in nonpsychotic patients is extremely unpleasant due to feelings of depersonalization, derealization, and dysphoria.

Dosage Oral:

Children >2-12 years: Range: 0.5-3 mg/kg/day in 2-3 divided doses; usual: 1 mg/kg/day; maximum: 3 mg/kg/day

Behavior problems: Initial: 10 mg 2-3 times/day, increase gradually

Severe psychoses: Initial: 25 mg 2-3 times/day, increase gradually

Children >12 years and Adults:

Schizophrenia/psychoses: Initial: 50-100 mg 3 times/day with gradual increments as needed and tolerated; maximum: 800 mg/day in 2-4 divided doses; if >65 years, initial dose: 10 mg 3 times/day

Depressive disorders/dementia: Initial: 25 mg 3 times/day; maintenance dose: 20-200 mg/day

Elderly: Behavioral symptoms associated with dementia: Oral: Initial: 10-25 mg 1-2 times/day; increase at 4- to 7-day intervals by 10-25 mg/day; increase dose intervals (qd, bid, etc) as necessary to control response or side effects. Maximum daily dose: 400 mg; gradual increases (titration) may prevent some side effects or decrease their severity.

Hemodialysis: Not dialyzable (0% to 5%)

Mechanism of Action Blocks postsynaptic mesolimbic dopaminergic receptors in the brain; exhibits a strong alpha-adrenergic blocking effect and depresses the release of hypothalamic and hypophyseal hormones

Other Adverse Effects Frequency not defined:

Cardiovascular: Hypotension, orthostatic hypotension, peripheral edema, EKG changes

Central nervous system: EPS (pseudoparkinsonism, akathisia, dystonias, tardive dyskinesia), dizziness, drowsiness, neuroleptic malignant syndrome (NMS), impairment of temperature regulation, lowering of seizures threshold, seizure

Dermatologic: Increased sensitivity to sun, rash, discoloration of skin (blue-gray)

Endocrine & metabolic: Changes in menstrual cycle, changes in libido, breast pain, galactorrhea, amenorrhea

Gastrointestinal: Constipation, weight gain, nausea, vomiting, stomach pain, nausea, vomiting, diarrhea

Genitourinary: Difficulty in urination, ejaculatory disturbances, urinary retention, priapism

Hematologic: Agranulocytosis, leukopenia

Hepatic: Cholestatic jaundice, hepatotoxicity

Neuromuscular & skeletal: Tremor

Ocular: Pigmentary retinopathy, blurred vision, cornea and lens changes

Respiratory: Nasal congestion

Drug Interactions Substrate of CYP2C19, **2D6**; Inhibits CYP1A2, **2D6**, 2E1

Increased Effect/Toxicity: Concurrent use of phenothiazines with an antihypertensive may produce additive hypotensive effects (particularly orthostasis). Concurrent use of beta-blockers may increase the risk of arrhythmia; propranolol and pindolol are **contraindicated.** Phenothiazines inhibit the ability of bromocriptine to lower serum prolactin concentrations. Serum concentrations of carvedilol or valproic acid may be increased by phenothiazines. The sedative effects of CNS depressants or ethanol may be additive with phenothiazines. Phenothiazines and trazodone may produce additive hypotensive effects Concurrent use of phenothiazines and tricyclic antidepressants may produce increased toxicity or altered therapeutic response. Metoclopramide may increase risk of extrapyramidal symptoms (EPS). Effects on QT_c interval may be additive with phenothiazines, increasing the risk of malignant arrhythmias; includes type Ia antiarrhythmics, TCAs, and some quinolone antibiotics (sparfloxacin, moxifloxacin and gatifloxacin). **These agents are contraindicated with thioridazine.** Potassium depleting agents may increase the risk of serious arrhythmias with thioridazine (includes many diuretics, aminoglycosides, and amphotericin). Metabolism of

(Continued)

Thioridazine *(Continued)*

phenothiazines may be decreased with CYP2D6 inhibitors, increasing clinical effect or toxicity. Inhibitors include amiodarone, cimetidine, delavirdine, fluoxetine, paroxetine, propafenone, quinidine, and ritonavir; monitor for increased effect/toxicity. **Thioridazine is contraindicated with inhibitors of this enzyme, including fluoxetine and paroxetine.** Inhibitors of CYP1A2, including cimetidine, ciprofloxacin, fluvoxamine, isoniazid, ritonavir, and zileuton may also decrease thioridazine metabolism. **Concurrent use with fluvoxamine is contraindicated.** Phenothiazines may produce neurotoxicity with lithium; this is a rare effect. Rare cases of respiratory paralysis have been reported with concurrent use of phenothiazines and polypeptide antibiotics. Naltrexone in combination with thioridazine has been reported to cause lethargy and somnolence. Phenylpropanolamine has been reported to result in cardiac arrhythmias when combined with thioridazine.

Decreased Effect: Aluminum salts may decrease the absorption of phenothiazines. The efficacy of amphetamines may be diminished by antipsychotics; in addition, amphetamines may increase psychotic symptoms; avoid concurrent use. Anticholinergics may inhibit the therapeutic response to phenothiazines and excess anticholinergic effects may occur (includes benztropine, trihexyphenidyl, biperiden, and drugs with significant anticholinergic activity). Chlorpromazine (and possibly other low potency antipsychotics) may diminish the pressor effects of epinephrine. The antihypertensive effects of guanethidine or guanadrel may be inhibited by phenothiazines. Phenothiazines may inhibit the antiparkinsonian effect of levodopa. Enzyme inducers may enhance the hepatic metabolism of phenothiazines; larger doses may be required; includes rifampin, rifabutin, barbiturates, phenytoin, and cigarette smoking.

Dietary/Ethanol/Herb Considerations

Ethanol: Avoid use; may increase CNS depression.

Herb/Nutraceutical: Avoid dong quai; may cause photosensitization. Avoid gotu kola, kava, SAMe, and valerian; may increase CNS depression. Avoid St John's wort; may cause photosensitization and increase CNS depression.

Pharmacodynamics/Kinetics

Duration: 4-5 days

Half-life elimination: 21-25 hours

Time to peak, serum: ~1 hour

Pregnancy Risk Factor C

Generic Available Yes

Thioridazine Hydrochloride *see* Thioridazine *on page 1298*

Thioridazine Intensol™ *see* Thioridazine *on page 1298*

Thiotepa (thye oh TEP a)

U.S. Brand Names Thioplex®

Pharmacologic Category Antineoplastic Agent, Alkylating Agent

Synonyms TESPA; Thiophosphoramide; Triethylenethiophosphoramide; TSPA

Use Treatment of superficial tumors of the bladder; palliative treatment of adenocarcinoma of breast or ovary; lymphomas and sarcomas; controlling intracavitary effusions caused by metastatic tumors; I.T. use: CNS leukemia/lymphoma, CNS metastases

Local Anesthetic/Vasoconstrictor Precautions No information available to require special precautions

Effects on Dental Treatment No significant effects or complications reported

Dosage Refer to individual protocols; dosing must be based on the clinical and hematologic response of the patient

Children: Sarcomas: I.V.: 25-65 mg/m^2 as a single dose every 21 days

Adults:

- I.M., I.V., S.C.: 30-60 mg/m^2 once per week
- I.V. doses of 0.3-0.4 mg/kg by rapid I.V. administration every 1-4 weeks, or 0.2 mg/kg or 6-8 mg/m^2/day for 4-5 days every 2-4 weeks
- High-dose therapy for bone marrow transplant: I.V.: 500 mg/m^2; up to 900 mg/m^2
- I.M. doses of 15-30 mg in various schedules have been given
- Intracavitary: 0.6-0.8 mg/kg
- Intrapericardial dose: Usually 15-30 mg
- Dosing comments/adjustment in renal impairment: Use with extreme caution; may require reduction. Less than 3% of alkylating species are detected in the urine in 24 hours.
- Intrathecal: Doses of 1-10 mg/m^2 administered 1-2 times/week in concentrations of 1 mg/mL diluted with preservative-free sterile water for injection
- Intravesical: Used for treatment of carcinoma of the bladder; patients should be dehydrated for 8-12 hours prior to treatment; instill 60 mg (in 30-60 mL of NS) into the bladder and retain for a minimum of 2 hours. Patient should be positioned every 15 minutes for maximal area exposure. Instillations usually once a week for 4 weeks. Monitor for bone marrow suppression.

Intratumor: Use a 22-gauge needle to inject thiotepa directly into the tumor. Initial dose: 0.6-0.8 mg/kg (diluted to 10 mg/mL) are used every 1-4 weeks; maintenance dose: 0.07-0.8 mg/kg are administered at 1- to 4-week intervals

Ophthalmic: 0.05% solution in LR has been instilled into the eye every 3 hours for 6-8 weeks for the prevention of pterygium recurrence

Mechanism of Action Alkylating agent that reacts with DNA phosphate groups to produce cross-linking of DNA strands leading to inhibition of DNA, RNA, and protein synthesis; mechanism of action has not been explored as thoroughly as the other alkylating agents, it is presumed that the aziridine rings open and react as nitrogen mustard; reactivity is enhanced at a lower pH

Other Adverse Effects

>10%:

Hematopoietic: Dose-limiting toxicity which is dose-related and cumulative; moderate to severe leukopenia and severe thrombocytopenia have occurred. Anemia and pancytopenia may become fatal, so careful hematologic monitoring is required; intravesical administration may cause bone marrow suppression as well.

Hematologic: Myelosuppressive:

WBC: Moderate

Platelets: Severe

Onset: 7-10 days

Nadir: 14 days

Recovery: 28 days

Local: Pain at injection site

1% to 10%:

Central nervous system: Dizziness, fever, headache

Dermatologic: Alopecia, rash, pruritus, hyperpigmentation with high-dose therapy

Endocrine & metabolic: Hyperuricemia

Gastrointestinal: Anorexia, nausea and vomiting rarely occur

Emetic potential: Low (<10%)

Genitourinary: Hemorrhagic cystitis

Renal: Hematuria

Miscellaneous: Tightness of the throat, allergic reactions

<1%: Stomatitis, anaphylaxis; like other alkylating agents, this drug is carcinogenic

Drug Interactions Inhibits CYP2B6

Increased Effect/Toxicity: Other alkylating agents or irradiation used concomitantly with thiotepa intensifies toxicity rather than enhancing therapeutic response. Prolonged muscular paralysis and respiratory depression may occur when neuromuscular blocking agents are administered. Succinylcholine and other neuromuscular blocking agents' action can be prolonged due to thiotepa inhibiting plasma pseudocholinesterase.

Dietary/Ethanol/Herb Considerations

Ethanol: Avoid use due to GI irritation.

Herb/Nutraceutical: Avoid black cohosh and dong quai in estrogen-dependent tumors.

Pharmacodynamics/Kinetics

Absorption: Intracavitary instillation: Unreliable (10% to 100%) through bladder mucosa; I.M.: variable

Metabolism: Extensively hepatic

Half-life elimination: Terminal (dose-dependent clearance): 109 minutes

Excretion: Urine (as metabolites and unchanged drug)

Pregnancy Risk Factor D

Generic Available Yes

Thiothixene (thye oh THIKS een)

U.S. Brand Names Navane®

Canadian Brand Names Navane®

Pharmacologic Category Antipsychotic Agent, Thioxanthene Derivative

Synonyms Tiotixene

Use Management of schizophrenia

Unlabeled/Investigational Use Treatment of psychotic disorders

Local Anesthetic/Vasoconstrictor Precautions Most pharmacology textbooks state that in presence of phenothiazines, systemic doses of epinephrine paradoxically decrease the blood pressure. This is the so called "epinephrine reversal" phenomenon. This has never been observed when epinephrine is given by infiltration as part of the anesthesia procedure.

Effects on Dental Treatment

Significant hypotension may occur, especially when the drug is administered parenterally; orthostatic hypotension is due to alpha-receptor blockade, the elderly are at greater risk for orthostatic hypotension.

Tardive dyskinesia: Prevalence rate may be 40% in elderly; development of the syndrome and the irreversible nature are proportional to duration and total cumulative dose over time. Extrapyramidal reactions are more common in elderly with up to 50% developing these reactions after 60 years of age; drug-induced

(Continued)

Thiothixene *(Continued)*

Parkinson's syndrome occurs often; **Akathisia** is the most common extrapyramidal reaction in elderly.

Increased confusion, memory loss, psychotic behavior, and agitation frequently occur as a consequence of anticholinergic effects. Antipsychotic associated sedation in nonpsychotic patients is extremely unpleasant due to feelings of depersonalization, derealization, and dysphoria.

Dosage

Children <12 years (unlabeled): Schizophrenia/psychoses: Oral: 0.25 mg/kg/24 hours in divided doses (dose not well established; use not recommended)

Children >12 years and Adults: Mild to moderate psychosis:

Oral: 2 mg 3 times/day, up to 20-30 mg/day; more severe psychosis: Initial: 5 mg 2 times/day, may increase gradually, if necessary; maximum: 60 mg/day

I.M.: 4 mg 2-4 times/day, increase dose gradually; usual: 16-20 mg/day; maximum: 30 mg/day; change to oral dose as soon as able

Rapid tranquilization of the agitated patient (administered every 30-60 minutes):

Oral: 5-10 mg

I.M.: 10-20 mg

Average total dose for tranquilization: 15-30 mg

Hemodialysis: Not dialyzable (0% to 5%)

Mechanism of Action Elicits antipsychotic activity by postsynaptic blockade of CNS dopamine receptors resulting in inhibition of dopamine-mediated effects; also has alpha-adrenergic blocking activity

Other Adverse Effects Frequency not defined:

Cardiovascular: Hypotension, tachycardia, syncope, nonspecific EKG changes

Central nervous system: Extrapyramidal symptoms (pseudoparkinsonism, akathisia, dystonias, lightheadedness, tardive dyskinesia), dizziness, drowsiness, restlessness, agitation, insomnia

Dermatologic: Discoloration of skin (blue-gray), rash, pruritus, urticaria, photosensitivity

Endocrine & metabolic: Changes in menstrual cycle, changes in libido, breast pain, galactorrhea, lactation, amenorrhea, gynecomastia, hyperglycemia, hypoglycemia

Gastrointestinal: Weight gain, nausea, vomiting, stomach pain, constipation, xerostomia, increased salivation

Genitourinary: Difficulty in urination, ejaculatory disturbances, impotence

Hematologic: Leukopenia, leukocytes

Neuromuscular & skeletal: Tremors

Ocular: Pigmentary retinopathy, blurred vision

Respiratory: Nasal congestion

Miscellaneous: Diaphoresis

Drug Interactions Substrate of **CYP1A2**; Inhibits CYP2D6

Increased Effect/Toxicity: Thiothixene and CNS depressants (ethanol, narcotics) may produce additive CNS depressant effects. Thiothixene may increase the effect/toxicity of antihypertensives, benztropine (and other anticholinergic agents), lithium, trazodone, and TCAs. Thiothixene's concentrations may be increased by chloroquine, sulfadoxine-pyrimethamine, and propranolol. Metoclopramide may increase risk of extrapyramidal symptoms (EPS).

Decreased Effect: Thiothixene inhibits the activity of guanadrel, guanethidine, levodopa, and bromocriptine. Benztropine (and other anticholinergics) may inhibit the therapeutic response to thiothixene. Barbiturates and cigarette smoking may enhance the hepatic metabolism of thiothixene. Thiothixene and low potency antipsychotics may reverse the pressor effects of epinephrine.

Dietary/Ethanol/Herb Considerations

Ethanol: Avoid use; may increase CNS depression.

Herb/Nutraceutical: Avoid gotu kola, kava, SAMe, St John's wort, and valerian; may increase CNS depression.

Pharmacodynamics/Kinetics

Metabolism: Extensively hepatic

Half-life elimination: >24 hours with chronic use

Pregnancy Risk Factor C

Generic Available Yes

Thorazine® *see* ChlorproMAZINE *on page 312*

Thrombate III™ *see* Antithrombin III *on page 117*

Thrombin-JMI® *see* Thrombin (Topical) *on page 1302*

Thrombin (Topical) (THROM bin, TOP i kal)

U.S. Brand Names Thrombin-JMI®; Thrombogen®

Canadian Brand Names Thrombostat™

Pharmacologic Category Hemostatic Agent

Use Dental and Medical: Hemostasis whenever minor bleeding from capillaries and small venules is accessible

Local Anesthetic/Vasoconstrictor Precautions No information available to require special precautions

Effects on Dental Treatment 1% to 10%: Fever, allergic-type reaction

Dosage Use 1000-2000 units/mL of solution where bleeding is profuse; apply powder directly to the site of bleeding or on oozing surfaces; use 100 units/mL for bleeding from skin or mucosal surfaces

Mechanism of Action Catalyzes the conversion of fibrinogen to fibrin

Contraindications Hypersensitivity to thrombin or any component of the formulation

Warnings/Precautions Do not inject, for topical use only

Pregnancy Risk Factor C

Dosage Forms POWDER for reconstitution, topical: (Thrombin-JMI®): 1000 units, 5000 units, 10,000 units, 20,000 units, 50,000 units; (Thrombin-JMI® Spray Kit): 5000 unit, 10,000 units, 20,000 units; (Thrombin-JMI® Syringe Spray Kit): 10,000 units, 20,000 units; (Thrombogen®): 5000 units, 20,000 units; (Thrombogen® Spray Kit): 10,000 units, 20,000 units

Generic Available No

Comments Topical thrombin is not to be used in conjunction with oxidized cellulose.

Thrombogen® *see* Thrombin (Topical) *on page 1302*

Thymocyte Stimulating Factor *see* Aldesleukin *on page 50*

Thyrel® TRH *see* Protirelin *on page 1144*

Thyrogen® *see* Thyrotropin Alpha *on page 1304*

Thyroid (THYE royd)

Related Information

Endocrine Disorders and Pregnancy *on page 1479*

U.S. Brand Names Armour® Thyroid; Nature-Throid® NT; Westhroid®

Pharmacologic Category Thyroid Product

Synonyms Desiccated Thyroid; Thyroid Extract; Thyroid USP

Use Replacement or supplemental therapy in hypothyroidism; pituitary TSH suppressants (thyroid nodules, thyroiditis, multinodular goiter, thyroid cancer), thyrotoxicosis, diagnostic suppression tests

Local Anesthetic/Vasoconstrictor Precautions No precautions with vasoconstrictor are necessary if patient is well controlled with thyroid preparations

Effects on Dental Treatment No significant effects or complications reported

Dosage Oral:

Children: See table.

Recommended Pediatric Dosage for Congenital Hypothyroidism

Age	Daily Dose (mg)	Daily Dose/kg (mg)
0-6 mo	15-30	4.8-6
6-12 mo	30-45	3.6-4.8
1-5 y	45-60	3-3.6
6-12 y	60-90	2.4-3
>12 y	>90	1.2-1.8

Adults: Initial: 15-30 mg; increase with 15 mg increments every 2-4 weeks; use 15 mg in patients with cardiovascular disease or myxedema. Maintenance dose: Usually 60-120 mg/day; monitor TSH and clinical symptoms.

Thyroid cancer: Requires larger amounts than replacement therapy

Mechanism of Action The primary active compound is T_3 (triiodothyronine), which may be converted from T_4 (thyroxine) and then circulates throughout the body to influence growth and maturation of various tissues; exact mechanism of action is unknown; however, it is believed the thyroid hormone exerts its many metabolic effects through control of DNA transcription and protein synthesis; involved in normal metabolism, growth, and development; promotes gluconeogenesis, increases utilization and mobilization of glycogen stores and stimulates protein synthesis, increases basal metabolic rate

Other Adverse Effects <1%: Abdominal cramps, alopecia, ataxia, cardiac arrhythmias, changes in menstrual cycle, chest pain, constipation, diaphoresis, diarrhea, dyspnea, excessive bone loss with overtreatment (excess thyroid replacement), fever, hand tremors, headache, heat intolerance, increased appetite, insomnia, myalgia, nervousness, palpitations, tachycardia, tremor, vomiting, weight loss

Drug Interactions

Increased Effect/Toxicity: Thyroid may potentiate the hypoprothrombinemic effect of oral anticoagulants. Tricyclic antidepressants (TAD) coadministered with thyroid hormone may increase potential for toxicity of both drugs.

Decreased Effect: Thyroid hormones increase the therapeutic need for oral hypoglycemics or insulin. Cholestyramine can bind thyroid and reduce its absorption. Phenytoin may decrease thyroxine serum levels. Thyroid hormone may decrease effect of oral sulfonylureas.

(Continued)

Thyroid *(Continued)*

Pharmacodynamics/Kinetics

Absorption: T_4: 48% to 79%; T_3: 95%; desiccated thyroid contains thyroxine, liothyronine, and iodine (primarily bound)

Metabolism: Thyroxine: Largely converted to liothyronine

Half-life elimination, serum: Liothyronine: 1-2 days; Thyroxine: 6-7 days

Pregnancy Risk Factor A

Generic Available Yes

Thyroid Extract *see* Thyroid *on page 1303*

Thyroid USP *see* Thyroid *on page 1303*

Thyrolar® *see* Liotrix *on page 811*

Thyrotropin Alpha (thye roe TROE pin AL fu)

U.S. Brand Names Thyrogen®

Canadian Brand Names Thyrogen®

Pharmacologic Category Diagnostic Agent

Synonyms Human Thyroid Stimulating Hormone; TSH

Use As an adjunctive diagnostic tool for serum thyroglobulin (Tg) testing with or without radioiodine imaging in the follow-up of patients with well-differentiated thyroid cancer

Potential clinical use:

1. Patients with an undetectable Tg on thyroid hormone suppressive therapy to exclude the diagnosis of residual or recurrent thyroid cancer
2. Patients requiring serum Tg testing and radioiodine imaging who are unwilling to undergo thyroid hormone withdrawal testing and whose treating physician believes that use of a less sensitive test is justified
3. Patients who are either unable to mount an adequate endogenous TSH response to thyroid hormone withdrawal or in whom withdrawal is medically contraindicated

Local Anesthetic/Vasoconstrictor Precautions No information available to require special precautions

Effects on Dental Treatment No significant effects or complications reported

Dosage Children >16 years and Adults: I.M.: 0.9 mg every 24 hours for 2 doses or every 72 hours for 3 doses

For radioiodine imaging, radioiodine administration should be given 24 hours following the final Thyrogen® injection. Scanning should be performed 48 hours after radioiodine administration (72 hours after the final injection of Thyrogen®).

For serum testing, serum Tg should be obtained 72 hours after final injection.

Mechanism of Action An exogenous source of human TSH that offers an additional diagnostic tool in the follow-up of patients with a history of well-differentiated thyroid cancer. Binding of thyrotropin alpha to TSH receptors on normal thyroid epithelial cells or on well-differentiated thyroid cancer tissue stimulates iodine uptake and organification and synthesis and secretion of thyroglobulin, triiodothyronine, and thyroxine.

Other Adverse Effects 1% to 10%:

Central nervous system: Headache, chills, fever, dizziness

Gastrointestinal: Nausea, vomiting

Neuromuscular & skeletal: Weakness, paresthesia

Miscellaneous: Flu-like syndrome

Pharmacodynamics/Kinetics

Half-life elimination: 25 ± 10 hours

Time to peak: Mean: 3-24 hours after injection

Pregnancy Risk Factor C

Generic Available No

Thyrotropin Releasing Hormone *see* Protirelin *on page 1144*

Tiabendazole *see* Thiabendazole *on page 1294*

Tiagabine (tye AG i been)

U.S. Brand Names Gabitril®

Canadian Brand Names Gabitril®

Pharmacologic Category Anticonvulsant, Miscellaneous

Synonyms Tiagabine Hydrochloride

Use Adjunctive therapy in adults and children ≥12 years of age in the treatment of partial seizures

Unlabeled/Investigational Use Treatment of bipolar disorder

Local Anesthetic/Vasoconstrictor Precautions No information available to require special precautions

Effects on Dental Treatment No significant effects or complications reported

Dosage Oral (administer with food):

Children 12-18 years: 4 mg once daily for 1 week; may increase to 8 mg daily in 2 divided doses for 1 week; then may increase by 4-8 mg weekly to response or up to 32 mg daily in 2-4 divided doses

Adults: 4 mg once daily for 1 week; may increase by 4-8 mg weekly to response or up to 56 mg daily in 2-4 divided doses

Mechanism of Action The exact mechanism by which tiagabine exerts antiseizure activity is not definitively known; however, *in vitro* experiments demonstrate that it enhances the activity of gamma aminobutyric acid (GABA), the major neuroinhibitory transmitter in the nervous system; it is thought that binding to the GABA uptake carrier inhibits the uptake of GABA into presynaptic neurons, allowing an increased amount of GABA to be available to postsynaptic neurons; based on *in vitro* studies, tiagabine does not inhibit the uptake of dopamine, norepinephrine, serotonin, glutamate, or choline

Other Adverse Effects

>10%:

Central nervous system: Dizziness, somnolence
Gastrointestinal: Nausea
Neuromuscular & skeletal: Weakness

1% to 10%:

Central nervous system: Nervousness, difficulty with concentration, insomnia, ataxia, confusion, speech disorder, depression, emotional lability, abnormal gait, hostility
Dermatologic: Rash, pruritus
Gastrointestinal: Diarrhea, vomiting, increased appetite
Neuromuscular & skeletal: Tremor, paresthesia
Ocular: Nystagmus
Otic: Hearing impairment
Respiratory: Pharyngitis, cough

Drug Interactions Substrate of **3A4**

Increased Effect/Toxicity: Valproate increased free tiagabine concentrations by 40%.

Decreased Effect: Primidone, phenobarbital, phenytoin, and carbamazepine increase tiagabine clearance by 60%.

Dietary/Ethanol/Herb Considerations

Ethanol: Avoid use; may increase CNS depression.

Food reduces the rate but not extent of absorption. Avoid grapefruit products; may increase serum plasma concentration.

Herb/Nutraceutical: Avoid gotu kola, kava, SAMe, and valerian; may increase CNS depression. Avoid St John's wort; may decrease serum concentration and increase CNS depression.

Pharmacodynamics/Kinetics

Absorption: Rapid (within 1 hour); prolonged with food
Protein binding: 96%, primarily to albumin and α_1-acid glycoprotein
Metabolism: Hepatic via CYP (primarily 3A4)
Bioavailability: Oral: Absolute: 90%
Half-life elimination: 6.7 hours
Time to peak, plasma: 45 minutes
Excretion: Feces (63%) and urine (25%, 2% as unchanged drug); primarily as metabolites

Pregnancy Risk Factor C

Generic Available No

Selected Readings Patsalos PN and Sander JW, "Newer Antiepileptic Drugs: Towards an Improved Risk-Benefit Ratio," *Drug Saf*, 1994, 11(1):37-67.

Tiagabine Hydrochloride *see* Tiagabine *on page 1304*
Tiazac® *see* Diltiazem *on page 447*
Ticar® *see* Ticarcillin *on page 1305*

Ticarcillin (tye kar SIL in)

U.S. Brand Names Ticar®

Mexican Brand Names Timentin®

Pharmacologic Category Antibiotic, Penicillin

Synonyms Ticarcillin Disodium

Use Treatment of susceptible infections such as septicemia, acute and chronic respiratory tract infections, skin and soft tissue infections, and urinary tract infections due to susceptible strains of *Pseudomonas*, and other gram-negative bacteria

Local Anesthetic/Vasoconstrictor Precautions No information available to require special precautions

Effects on Dental Treatment Prolonged use of penicillins may lead to development of oral candidiasis.

Dosage Ticarcillin is generally given I.V., I.M. injection is only for the treatment of uncomplicated urinary tract infections and dose should not exceed 2 g/injection when administered I.M.

Neonates: I.M., I.V.:

Postnatal age <7 days:
<2000 g: 75 mg/kg/dose every 12 hours
>2000 g: 75 mg/kg/dose every 8 hours

(Continued)

Ticarcillin *(Continued)*

Postnatal age >7 days:
<1200 g: 75 mg/kg/dose every 12 hours
1200-2000 g: 75 mg/kg/dose every 8 hours
>2000 g: 75 mg/kg/dose every 6 hours
Infants and Children:
Systemic infections: I.V.: 200-300 mg/kg/day in divided doses every 4-6 hours
Urinary tract infections: I.M., I.V.: 50-100 mg/kg/day in divided doses every 6-8 hours
Maximum dose: 24 g/day
Adults: I.M., I.V.: 1-4 g every 4-6 hours, usual dose: 3 g I.V. every 4-6 hours
Dosing adjustment in renal impairment: Adults:
Cl_{cr} 30-60 mL/minute: 2 g every 4 hours or 3 g every 8 hours
Cl_{cr} 10-30 mL/minute: 2 g every 8 hours or 3 g every 12 hours
Cl_{cr} <10 mL/minute: 2 g every 12 hours
Moderately dialyzable (20% to 50%)
Continuous arteriovenous or venovenous hemodiafiltration effects: Dose as for Cl_{cr} 10-50 mL/minute

Mechanism of Action Inhibits bacterial cell wall synthesis by binding to one or more of the penicillin binding proteins (PBPs); which in turn inhibits the final transpeptidation step of peptidoglycan synthesis in bacterial cell walls, thus inhibiting cell wall biosynthesis. Bacteria eventually lyse due to ongoing activity of cell wall autolytic enzymes (autolysins and murein hydrolases) while cell wall assembly is arrested.

Other Adverse Effects Frequency not defined:
Central nervous system: Confusion, convulsions, drowsiness, fever, Jarisch-Herxheimer reaction
Dermatologic: Rash
Endocrine & metabolic: Electrolyte imbalance
Gastrointestinal: *Clostridium difficile* colitis
Hematologic: Bleeding, eosinophilia, hemolytic anemia, leukopenia, neutropenia, positive Coombs' reaction, thrombocytopenia
Hepatic: Hepatotoxicity, jaundice
Local: Thrombophlebitis
Neuromuscular & skeletal: Myoclonus
Renal: Interstitial nephritis (acute)
Miscellaneous: Anaphylaxis, hypersensitivity reactions

Drug Interactions
Increased Effect/Toxicity: Probenecid may increase penicillin levels. Neuromuscular blockers may have an increased duration of action (neuromuscular blockade).
Decreased Effect: Tetracyclines may decrease penicillin effectiveness. Aminoglycosides may cause physical inactivation of aminoglycosides in the presence of high concentrations of ticarcillin and potential toxicity in patients with mild-moderate renal dysfunction. Although anecdotal reports suggest oral contraceptive efficacy could be reduced by penicillins, this has been refuted by more rigorous scientific and clinical data.

Pharmacodynamics/Kinetics
Absorption: I.M.: 86%
Distribution: Blister fluid, lymph tissue, and gallbladder; low concentrations into CSF increasing with inflamed meninges, otherwise widely distributed; crosses placenta; enters breast milk (low concentrations)
Protein binding: 45% to 65%
Half-life elimination:
Neonates: <1 week old: 3.5-5.6 hours; 1-8 weeks old: 1.3-2.2 hours
Children 5-13 years: 0.9 hour
Adults: 66-72 minutes; prolonged with renal and/or hepatic impairment
Time to peak, serum: I.M.: 30-75 minutes
Excretion: Almost entirely urine (as unchanged drug and metabolites); feces (3.5%)

Pregnancy Risk Factor B
Generic Available No

Ticarcillin and Clavulanate Potassium

(tye kar SIL in & klav yoo LAN ate poe TASS ee um)

Related Information
Ticarcillin *on page 1305*

U.S. Brand Names Timentin®
Canadian Brand Names Timentin®
Pharmacologic Category Antibiotic, Penicillin
Synonyms Ticarcillin and Clavulanic Acid
Use Treatment of infections of lower respiratory tract, urinary tract, skin and skin structures, bone and joint, and septicemia caused by susceptible organisms. Clavulanate expands activity of ticarcillin to include beta-lactamase producing strains of

S. aureus, H. influenzae, Bacteroides species, and some other gram-negative bacilli

Local Anesthetic/Vasoconstrictor Precautions No information available to require special precautions

Effects on Dental Treatment Prolonged use of penicillins may lead to development of oral candidiasis.

Dosage I.V.:

Children and Adults <60 kg: 200-300 mg of ticarcillin component/kg/day in divided doses every 4-6 hours

Children >60 kg and Adults: 3.1 g (ticarcillin 3 g plus clavulanic acid 0.1 g) every 4-6 hours; maximum: 24 g/day

Urinary tract infections: 3.1 g every 6-8 hours

Dosing adjustment in renal impairment:

Cl_{cr} 30-60 mL/minute: Administer 2 g every 4 hours or 3.1 g every 8 hours

Cl_{cr} 10-30 mL/minute: Administer 2 g every 8 hours or 3.1 g every 12 hours

Cl_{cr} <10 mL/minute: Administer 2 g every 12 hours

Moderately dialyzable (20% to 50%)

Continuous arteriovenous or venovenous hemodiafiltration effects: Dose as for Cl_{cr} 10-50 mL/minute

Peritoneal dialysis: 3.1 g every 12 hours

Hemodialysis: 2 g every 12 hours; supplemented with 3.1 g after each dialysis

Dosing adjustment in hepatic dysfunction: Cl_{cr} <10 mL/minute: 2 g every 24 hours

Mechanism of Action Inhibits bacterial cell wall synthesis by binding to one or more of the penicillin binding proteins (PBPs); which in turn inhibits the final transpeptidation step of peptidoglycan synthesis in bacterial cell walls, thus inhibiting cell wall biosynthesis. Bacteria eventually lyse due to ongoing activity of cell wall autolytic enzymes (autolysins and murein hydrolases) while cell wall assembly is arrested.

Other Adverse Effects Frequency not defined:

Central nervous system: Confusion, convulsions, drowsiness, fever, Jarisch-Herxheimer reaction

Dermatologic: Rash, erythema multiforme, toxic epidermal necrolysis, Stevens-Johnson syndrome

Endocrine & metabolic: Electrolyte imbalance

Gastrointestinal: *Clostridium difficile* colitis

Hematologic: Bleeding, hemolytic anemia, leukopenia, neutropenia, positive Coombs' reaction, thrombocytopenia

Hepatic: Hepatotoxicity, jaundice

Local: Thrombophlebitis

Neuromuscular & skeletal: Myoclonus

Renal: Interstitial nephritis (acute)

Miscellaneous: Anaphylaxis, hypersensitivity reactions

Drug Interactions

Increased Effect/Toxicity: Probenecid may increase penicillin levels. Neuromuscular blockers may have an increased duration of action (neuromuscular blockade).

Decreased Effect: Tetracyclines may decrease penicillin effectiveness. Aminoglycosides may cause physical inactivation of aminoglycosides in the presence of high concentrations of ticarcillin and potential toxicity in patients with mild-moderate renal dysfunction. Although anecdotal reports suggest oral contraceptive efficacy could be reduced by penicillins, this has been refuted by more rigorous scientific and clinical data.

Pharmacodynamics/Kinetics

Ticarcillin: See Ticarcillin monograph.

Clavulanic acid:

Protein binding: 9% to 30%

Metabolism: Hepatic

Half-life elimination: 66-90 minutes

Excretion: Urine (45% as unchanged drug)

Clearance: Does not affect clearance of ticarcillin

Pregnancy Risk Factor B

Generic Available No

Ticarcillin and Clavulanic Acid *see* Ticarcillin and Clavulanate Potassium *on page 1306*

Ticarcillin Disodium *see* Ticarcillin *on page 1305*

TICE® BCG *see* BCG Vaccine *on page 161*

Ticlid® *see* Ticlopidine *on page 1307*

Ticlopidine (tye KLOE pi deen)

Related Information

Cardiovascular Diseases *on page 1456*

U.S. Brand Names Ticlid®

Canadian Brand Names Alti-Ticlopidine; Apo®-Ticlopidine; Gen-Ticlopidine; Nu-Ticlopidine; PMS-Ticlopidine; Rhoxal-ticlopidine; Ticlid®

(Continued)

Ticlopidine *(Continued)*

Mexican Brand Names Ticlid®

Pharmacologic Category Antiplatelet Agent

Synonyms Ticlopidine Hydrochloride

Use Platelet aggregation inhibitor that reduces the risk of thrombotic stroke in patients who have had a stroke or stroke precursors. **Note:** Due to its association with life-threatening hematologic disorders, ticlopidine should be reserved for patients who are intolerant to aspirin, or who have failed aspirin therapy. Adjunctive therapy (with aspirin) following successful coronary stent implantation to reduce the incidence of subacute stent thrombosis.

Unlabeled/Investigational Use Treatment of diabetic microangiopathy, ischemic heart disease;prevention of postoperative DVT; reduction of graft loss following renal transplant; protection of aortocoronary bypass grafts,

Local Anesthetic/Vasoconstrictor Precautions No information available to require special precautions

Effects on Dental Treatment No significant effects or complications reported; if a patient is to undergo elective surgery and an antiplatelet effect is not desired, ticlopidine should be discontinued at least 7 days prior to surgery.

Dosage Oral: Adults:

Stroke prevention: 250 mg twice daily with food

Coronary artery stenting (initiate after successful implantation): 250 mg twice daily with food (in combination with antiplatelet doses of aspirin) for up to 30 days

Mechanism of Action Ticlopidine is an inhibitor of platelet function with a mechanism which is different from other antiplatelet drugs. The drug significantly increases bleeding time. This effect may not be solely related to ticlopidine's effect on platelets. The prolongation of the bleeding time caused by ticlopidine is further increased by the addition of aspirin in *ex vivo* experiments. Although many metabolites of ticlopidine have been found, none have been shown to account for *in vivo* activity.

Other Adverse Effects As with all drugs which may affect hemostasis, bleeding is associated with ticlopidine. Hemorrhage may occur at virtually any site. Risk is dependent on multiple variables, including the use of multiple agents which alter hemostasis and patient susceptibility.

>10%:

Endocrine & metabolic: Increased total cholesterol (increases of ~8% to 10% within 1 month of therapy)

Gastrointestinal: Diarrhea (13%)

1% to 10%:

Central nervous system: Dizziness (1%)

Dermatologic: Rash (5%), purpura (2%), pruritus (1%)

Gastrointestinal: Nausea (7%), dyspepsia (7%), gastrointestinal pain (4%), vomiting (2%), flatulence (2%), anorexia (1%)

Hematologic: Neutropenia (2%)

Hepatic: Abnormal LFTs (1%)

<1% (Limited to important or life-threatening): Thrombotic thrombocytopenic purpura (TTP), thrombocytopenia (immune), agranulocytosis, eosinophilia, pancytopenia, thrombocytosis, anaphylaxis, bone marrow suppression, gastrointestinal bleeding, ecchymosis, epistaxis, hematuria, menorrhagia, conjunctival bleeding, intracranial bleeding (rare), urticaria, exfoliative dermatitis, Stevens-Johnson syndrome, erythema multiforme, maculopapular rash, erythema nodosum, headache, weakness, pain, tinnitus, hemolytic anemia, aplastic anemia, hepatitis, jaundice, hepatic necrosis, peptic ulcer, renal failure, nephrotic syndrome, hyponatremia, vasculitis, sepsis, pneumonitis (allergic), angioedema, positive ANA, systemic lupus erythematosus, peripheral neuropathy, serum sickness, arthropathy, myositis

Postmarketing and/or case reports: Chronic diarrhea, increase in serum creatinine, bronchiolitis obliterans-organized pneumonia

Drug Interactions Substrate of **CYP3A4**; Inhibits **CYP1A2, 2C8/9, 2C19**, 2D6

Increased Effect/Toxicity: Ticlopidine may increase effect/toxicity of aspirin, anticoagulants, theophylline, and NSAIDs. Cimetidine may increase ticlopidine blood levels. Phenytoin blood levels may be increased by ticlopidine (case reports).

Decreased Effect: Decreased effect of ticlopidine with antacids (decreased absorption). Ticlopidine may decrease the effect of digoxin, cyclosporine.

Dietary/Ethanol/Herb Considerations

Food may increase bioavailability 20%; high-fat meals increase absorption.

Herb/Nutraceutical: Avoid cat's claw, dong quai, evening primrose, feverfew, garlic, ginkgo biloba, ginger, ginseng, green tea, horse chestnut, and red clover due to additional antiplatelet activity.

Pharmacodynamics/Kinetics

Onset of action: ~6 hours

Peak effect: 3-5 days; serum levels do not correlate with clinical antiplatelet activity

Metabolism: Extensively hepatic; has at least one active metabolite

Half-life elimination: 24 hours

Pregnancy Risk Factor B

Generic Available Yes

Ticlopidine Hydrochloride *see* Ticlopidine *on page 1307*

TIG *see* Tetanus Immune Globulin (Human) *on page 1283*

Tigan® *see* Trimethobenzamide *on page 1352*

Tikosyn™ *see* Dofetilide *on page 464*

Tilade® *see* Nedocromil *on page 957*

Tiludronate (tye LOO droe nate)

U.S. Brand Names Skelid®

Pharmacologic Category Bisphosphonate Derivative

Synonyms Tiludronate Disodium

Use Treatment of Paget's disease of the bone in patients who have a level of serum alkaline phosphatase (SAP) at least twice the upper limit of normal, or who are symptomatic, or who are at risk for future complications of their disease

Local Anesthetic/Vasoconstrictor Precautions No information available to require special precautions

Effects on Dental Treatment No significant effects or complications reported

Dosage Oral (should be taken with 6-8 oz of plain water and not taken within 2 hours of food):

Adults: 400 mg (2 tablets of tiludronic acid) daily for a period of 3 months; allow an interval of 3 months to assess response

Dosing adjustment in renal impairment: Cl_{cr} <30 mL/minute: Use not recommended

Mechanism of Action Inhibition of normal and abnormal bone resorption. Inhibits osteoclasts through at least two mechanisms: disruption of the cytoskeletal ring structure, possibly by inhibition of protein-tyrosine-phosphatase, thus leading to the detachment of osteoclasts from the bone surface area and the inhibition of the osteoclast proton pump.

Other Adverse Effects The following events occurred >2% and at a frequency > placebo:

1% to 10%:

Cardiovascular: Chest pain (3%), edema (3%)

Central nervous system: Dizziness (4%), paresthesia (4%)

Dermatologic: Rash (3%), skin disorder (3%)

Gastrointestinal: Nausea (9%), diarrhea (9%), heartburn (5%), vomiting (4%), flatulence (3%)

Neuromuscular & skeletal: Arthrosis (3%)

Ocular: cataract (3%), conjunctivitis (3%), glaucoma (3%)

Respiratory: Rhinitis (5%), sinusitis (5%), coughing (3%), pharyngitis (3%)

<1% (Limited to important or life-threatening): Stevens-Johnson syndrome

Drug Interactions

Increased Effect/Toxicity: Administration of indomethacin increases bioavailability of tiludronate two- to fourfold.

Decreased Effect: Concurrent administration of calcium salts, aluminum- or magnesium-containing antacids, and aspirin markedly decrease absorption/bioavailability (by 50% to 60%) of tiludronate if given within 2 hours of a dose.

Dietary/Ethanol/Herb Considerations Food: In single-dose studies, the bioavailability of tiludronate was reduced by 90% when an oral dose was administered with, or 2 hours after, a standard breakfast compared to the same dose administered after an overnight fast and 4 hours before a standard breakfast.

Pharmacodynamics/Kinetics

Onset of action: Delayed, may require several weeks

Absorption: Rapid

Distribution: Widely to bone and soft tissue

Protein binding: 90%, primarily to albumin

Metabolism: Little, if any

Bioavailability: 6%; reduced by food

Half-life elimination: Healthy volunteers: 50 hours; Pagetic patients: 150 hours

Time to peak, plasma: ~2 hours

Excretion: Urine (60% as unchanged drug) within 13 days

Pregnancy Risk Factor C

Generic Available No

Tiludronate Disodium *see* Tiludronate *on page 1309*

Timentin® *see* Ticarcillin and Clavulanate Potassium *on page 1306*

Timolol (TYE moe lole)

Related Information

Cardiovascular Diseases *on page 1456*

U.S. Brand Names Betimol®; Blocadren®; Timoptic®; Timoptic® OcuDose®; Timoptic-XE®

Canadian Brand Names Alti-Timolol; Apo®-Timol; Apo®-Timop; Gen-Timolol; Nu-Timolol; Phoxal-timolol; PMS-Timolol; Tim-AK; Timoptic®; Timoptic-XE®

Mexican Brand Names Imot Ofteno; Shemol®; Timoptol®; Timoptol® XE

(Continued)

Timolol *(Continued)*

Pharmacologic Category Beta Blocker, Nonselective; Ophthalmic Agent, Antiglaucoma

Synonyms Timolol Hemihydrate; Timolol Maleate

Use Ophthalmic dosage form used in treatment of elevated intraocular pressure such as glaucoma or ocular hypertension; oral dosage form used for treatment of hypertension and angina, to reduce mortality following MI, and for prophylaxis of migraine

Local Anesthetic/Vasoconstrictor Precautions No information available to require special precautions

Effects on Dental Treatment Timolol is a nonselective beta-blocker and may enhance the pressor response to epinephrine, resulting in hypertension and bradycardia. Many nonsteroidal anti-inflammatory drugs such as ibuprofen and indomethacin can reduce the hypotensive effect of beta-blockers after 3 or more weeks of therapy with the NSAID. Short-term NSAID use (ie, 3 days) requires no special precautions in patients taking beta-blockers.

Dosage

Children and Adults: Ophthalmic:

Solution: Initial: 0.25% solution, instill 1 drop twice daily; increase to 0.5% solution if response not adequate; decrease to 1 drop/day if controlled; do not exceed 1 drop twice daily of 0.5% solution

Gel-forming solution (Timoptic-XE®): Instill 1 drop (either 0.25% or 0.5%) once daily

Adults: Oral:

Hypertension: Initial: 10 mg twice daily, increase gradually every 7 days, usual dosage: 20-40 mg/day in 2 divided doses; maximum: 60 mg/day

Prevention of MI: 10 mg twice daily initiated within 1-4 weeks after infarction

Migraine headache: Initial: 10 mg twice daily, increase to maximum of 30 mg/day

Mechanism of Action Blocks both $beta_1$- and $beta_2$-adrenergic receptors, reduces intraocular pressure by reducing aqueous humor production or possibly outflow; reduces blood pressure by blocking adrenergic receptors and decreasing sympathetic outflow, produces a negative chronotropic and inotropic activity through an unknown mechanism

Other Adverse Effects

Ophthalmic:

>10%: Ocular: Conjunctival hyperemia

1% to 10%: Ocular: Anisocoria, corneal punctate keratitis, keratitis, corneal staining, decreased corneal sensitivity, eye pain, vision disturbances

<1%: Systemic allergic reaction (anaphylaxis, angioedema, rash, urticaria)

Systemic:

>10%:

Central nervous system: Drowsiness, insomnia

Endocrine & metabolic: Decreased sexual ability

1% to 10%:

Cardiovascular: Bradycardia, palpitations, edema, CHF, reduced peripheral circulation

Central nervous system: Mental depression

Gastrointestinal: Diarrhea or constipation, nausea, vomiting, stomach discomfort

Respiratory: Bronchospasm

Miscellaneous: Cold extremities

<1% (Limited to important or life-threatening): Anaphylaxis, angioedema, arrhythmias, chest pain, confusion (especially in the elderly), depression, dyspnea, hallucinations, headache, leukopenia, memory loss, nervousness, nightmares, orthostatic hypotension, psoriasis, rash, Raynaud's phenomenon, retroperitoneal fibrosis, thrombocytopenia, urticaria

Drug Interactions Substrate of **CYP2D6**; Inhibits CYP2D6

Increased Effect/Toxicity: The heart rate lowering effects of timolol are additive with other drugs which slow AV conduction (digoxin, verapamil, diltiazem). Reserpine increases the effects of timolol. Concurrent use of timolol may increase the effects of alpha-blockers (prazosin, terazosin), alpha-adrenergic stimulants (epinephrine, phenylephrine), and the vasoconstrictive effects of ergot alkaloids. Timolol may mask the tachycardia from hypoglycemia caused by insulin and oral hypoglycemics. In patients receiving concurrent therapy, the risk of hypertensive crisis is increased when either clonidine or the beta-blocker is withdrawn. Beta-blockers may increase the action or levels of ethanol, disopyramide, nondepolarizing muscle relaxants, and theophylline although the effects are difficult to predict.

Decreased effect of timolol with aluminum salts, barbiturates, calcium salts, cholestyramine, colestipol, NSAIDs, penicillins (ampicillin), rifampin, salicylates, and sulfinpyrazone due to decreased bioavailability and plasma levels. Beta-blockers may decrease the effect of sulfonylureas. Beta-blockers may affect the action or levels of ethanol, disopyramide, nondepolarizing muscle relaxants, and theophylline, although the effects are difficult to predict.

Dietary/Ethanol/Herb Considerations

Ethanol: Limit use; may increase risk of hypotension or dizziness.

Food: Administer oral formulation with food at the same time each day.

Pharmacodynamics/Kinetics

Onset of action: Hypotensive: Oral: 15-45 minutes

Peak effect: 0.5-2.5 hours

Duration: ~4 hours; Ophthalmic: Intraocular: 24 hours

Protein binding: 60%

Metabolism: Extensively hepatic; extensive first-pass effect

Half-life elimination: 2-2.7 hours; prolonged with renal impairment

Excretion: Urine (15% to 20% as unchanged drug)

Pregnancy Risk Factor C (manufacturer); D (2nd and 3rd trimesters - expert analysis)

Generic Available Yes; Excludes hemihydrate and preservative free maleate ophthalmic solutions

Selected Readings

Foster CA and Aston SJ, "Propranolol-Epinephrine Interaction: A Potential Disaster," *Plast Reconstr Surg*, 1983, 72(1):74-8.

Wong DG, Spence JD, Lamki L, et al, "Effect of Nonsteroidal Anti-inflammatory Drugs on Control of Hypertension of Beta-Blockers and Diuretics," *Lancet*, 1986, 1(8488):997-1001.

Wynn RL, "Dental Nonsteroidal Anti-inflammatory Drugs and Prostaglandin-Based Drug Interactions, Part Two," *Gen Dent*, 1992, 40(2):104, 106, 108.

Wynn RL, "Epinephrine Interactions With Beta-Blockers," *Gen Dent*, 1994, 42(1):16, 18.

Timolol Hemihydrate *see* Timolol *on page 1309*

Timolol Maleate *see* Timolol *on page 1309*

Timoptic® *see* Timolol *on page 1309*

Timoptic® OcuDose® *see* Timolol *on page 1309*

Timoptic-XE® *see* Timolol *on page 1309*

Tinactin® Antifungal [OTC] *see* Tolnaftate *on page 1322*

Tinactin® Antifungal Jock Itch [OTC] *see* Tolnaftate *on page 1322*

Tinaderm [OTC] *see* Tolnaftate *on page 1322*

Tinamed® [OTC] *see* Salicylic Acid *on page 1204*

TinBen® [OTC] *see* Benzoin *on page 171*

Tine Test *see* Tuberculin Tests *on page 1362*

Ting® [OTC] *see* Tolnaftate *on page 1322*

Tinzaparin (tin ZA pa rin)

U.S. Brand Names Innohep®

Canadian Brand Names Innohep®

Pharmacologic Category Low Molecular Weight Heparin

Synonyms Tinzaparin Sodium

Use Treatment of acute symptomatic deep vein thrombosis, with or without pulmonary embolism, in conjunction with warfarin sodium

Local Anesthetic/Vasoconstrictor Precautions No information available to require special precautions

Effects on Dental Treatment

No significant effects or complications reported

Patients undergoing treatment with low molecular weight heparins have an increased risk of hemorrhage during surgery.

Dosage S.C.:

Adults: 175 anti-Xa int. units/kg of body weight once daily. Warfarin sodium should be started when appropriate. Administer tinzaparin for at least 6 days and until patient is adequately anticoagulated with warfarin.

Note: To calculate the volume of solution to administer per dose: Volume to be administered (mL) = patient weight (kg) x 0.00875 mL/kg (may be rounded off to the nearest 0.05 mL)

Elderly: No significant differences in safety or response were seen when used in patients ≥65 years of age. However, increased sensitivity to tinzaparin in elderly patients may be possible due to a decline in renal function.

Dosing adjustment in renal impairment: Clearance decreased 24% in severe impairment; use with caution.

Dosing adjustment in hepatic impairment: No specific recommendations

Mechanism of Action Standard heparin consists of components with molecular weights ranging from 4000-30,000 daltons with a mean of 16,000 daltons. Heparin acts as an anticoagulant by enhancing the inhibition rate of clotting proteases by antithrombin III, impairing normal hemostasis and inhibition of factor Xa. Low molecular weight heparins have a small effect on the activated partial thromboplastin time and strongly inhibit factor Xa. The primary inhibitory activity of tinzaparin is through antithrombin. Tinzaparin is derived from porcine heparin that undergoes controlled enzymatic depolymerization. The average molecular weight of tinzaparin ranges between 5500 and 7500 daltons which is distributed as (<10%) 2000 daltons (60% to 72%) 2000-8000 daltons, and (22% to 36%) >8000 daltons. The antifactor Xa activity is approximately 100 int. units/mg.

Other Adverse Effects As with all anticoagulants, bleeding is the major adverse effect of tinzaparin. Hemorrhage may occur at virtually any site. Risk is dependent on multiple variables.

(Continued)

Tinzaparin *(Continued)*

>10%:
Hepatic: Increased ALT (13%)
Local: Injection site hematoma (16%)

1% to 10%:
Cardiovascular: Angina pectoris, chest pain (2%), hypertension, hypotension, tachycardia
Central nervous system: Confusion, dizziness, fever (2%), headache (2%), insomnia, pain (2%)
Dermatologic: Bullous eruption, pruritus, rash (1%), skin disorder
Gastrointestinal: Constipation (1%), dyspepsia, flatulence, nausea (2%), nonspecified gastrointestinal disorder, vomiting (1%)
Genitourinary: Dysuria, urinary retention, urinary tract infection (4%)
Hematologic: Anemia, hematoma, hemorrhage (2%), thrombocytopenia (1%)
Hepatic: Increased AST (9%)
Local: Deep vein thrombosis, injection site hematoma
Neuromuscular & skeletal: Back pain (2%)
Renal: Hematuria (1%)
Respiratory: Dyspnea (1%), epistaxis (2%), pneumonia, pulmonary embolism (2%), respiratory disorder
Miscellaneous: Impaired healing, infection, unclassified reactions

<1%: Abdominal pain, diarrhea, major bleeding

Additional serious adverse reactions reported in clinical trials and postmarketing experience: Abscess, acute febrile reaction, agranulocytosis, allergic purpura, allergic reaction, angioedema, anorectal bleeding, cardiac arrhythmia, cellulitis, cerebral hemorrhage, cholestatic hepatitis, coronary thrombosis, dependent edema, epidermal necrolysis, erythematous gastrointestinal hemorrhage, granulocytopenia, hemarthrosis, hematemesis, hemoptysis, injection site bleeding, intracranial hemorrhage, ischemic necrosis, melena, MI, necrosis, neoplasm, ocular hemorrhage, pancytopenia, peripheral ischemia, priapism, purpura, rash, retroperitoneal/intra-abdominal bleeding, severe thrombocytopenia, skin necrosis, spinal epidural hematoma, Stevens-Johnson syndrome, thromboembolism, urticaria, vaginal hemorrhage, wound hematoma

Postmarketing and/or case reports: The following adverse effects have been reported in infants of women receiving tinzaparin during pregnancy (relationship has not been established): Cleft palate (one report), optic nerve hypoplasia (one report), trisomy 21 (one report), fetal death/miscarriage, fetal distress, neonatal hypotonia, cutis aplasia of the scalp

Drug Interactions
Increased Effect/Toxicity: Drugs which affect platelet function (eg, aspirin, NSAIDs, dipyridamole, ticlopidine, clopidogrel, sulfinpyrazone, dextran) may potentiate the risk of hemorrhage. Thrombolytic agents increase the risk of hemorrhage. Risk of bleeding may be increased during concurrent therapy with warfarin. Tinzaparin is commonly continued during the initiation of warfarin therapy to assure anticoagulation and to protect against possible transient hypercoagulability.

Pharmacodynamics/Kinetics
Onset of action: 2-3 hours
Distribution: 3-5 L
Half-life elimination: 3-4 hours
Metabolism: Partially metabolized by desulphation and depolymerization
Bioavailability: 87%
Time to peak: 4-5 hours
Excretion: Urine

Pregnancy Risk Factor B

Generic Available No

Tinzaparin Sodium *see* Tinzaparin *on page 1311*

Tioconazole (tye oh KONE a zole)

U.S. Brand Names 1-Day™ [OTC]; Vagistat®-1 [OTC]

Pharmacologic Category Antifungal Agent, Vaginal

Use Local treatment of vulvovaginal candidiasis

Local Anesthetic/Vasoconstrictor Precautions No information available to require special precautions

Effects on Dental Treatment No significant effects or complications reported

Dosage Adults: Vaginal: Insert 1 applicatorful in vagina, just prior to bedtime, as a single dose

Mechanism of Action A 1-substituted imidazole derivative with a broad antifungal spectrum against a wide variety of dermatophytes and yeasts, including *Trichophyton mentagrophytes*, *T. rubrum*, *T. erinacei*, *T. tonsurans*, *Microsporum canis*, *Microsporum gypseum*, and *Candida albicans*. Both agents appear to be similarly effective against *Epidermophyton floccosum*.

Other Adverse Effects Frequency not defined:
Central nervous system: Headache
Gastrointestinal: Abdominal pain

Dermatologic: Burning, desquamation

Genitourinary: Discharge, dyspareunia, dysuria, irritation, itching, nocturia, vaginal pain, vaginitis, vulvar swelling

Pharmacodynamics/Kinetics

Onset of action: Some improvement: Within 24 hours; Complete relief: Within 7 days

Absorption: Intravaginal: Systemic (small amounts)

Distribution: Vaginal fluid: 24-72 hours

Excretion: Urine and feces

Pregnancy Risk Factor C

Generic Available No

Tioguanine *see* Thioguanine *on page 1296*

Tiopronin (tye oh PROE nin)

U.S. Brand Names Thiola®

Canadian Brand Names Thiola™

Pharmacologic Category Urinary Tract Product

Use Prevention of kidney stone (cystine) formation in patients with severe homozygous cystinuric who have urinary cystine >500 mg/day who are resistant to treatment with high fluid intake, alkali, and diet modification, or who have had adverse reactions to penicillamine

Local Anesthetic/Vasoconstrictor Precautions No information available to require special precautions

Effects on Dental Treatment No significant effects or complications reported

Dosage Adults: Initial dose is 800 mg/day, average dose is 1000 mg/day

Pregnancy Risk Factor C

Generic Available No

Tiotixene *see* Thiothixene *on page 1301*

Tirofiban (tye roe FYE ban)

Related Information

Cardiovascular Diseases *on page 1456*

U.S. Brand Names Aggrastat®

Canadian Brand Names Aggrastat®

Mexican Brand Names Agrastat®

Pharmacologic Category Antiplatelet Agent, Glycoprotein IIb/IIIa Inhibitor

Synonyms MK383; Tirofiban Hydrochloride

Use In combination with heparin, is indicated for the treatment of acute coronary syndrome, including patients who are to be managed medically and those undergoing PTCA or atherectomy. In this setting, it has been shown to decrease the rate of a combined endpoint of death, new MI or refractory ischemia/repeat cardiac procedure.

Local Anesthetic/Vasoconstrictor Precautions No information available to require special precautions

Effects on Dental Treatment No significant effects or complications reported

Tirofiban Dosing
(Using 50 mcg/mL Concentration)

Patient Weight (kg)	Patients With Normal Renal Function		Patients With Renal Dysfunction	
	30-Min Loading Infusion Rate (mL/h)	Maintenance Infusion Rate (mL/h)	30-Min Loading Infusion Rate (mL/h)	Maintenance Infusion Rate (mL/h)
30-37	16	4	8	2
38-45	20	5	10	3
46-54	24	6	12	3
55-62	28	7	14	4
63-70	32	8	16	4
71-79	36	9	18	5
80-87	40	10	20	5
88-95	44	11	22	6
96-104	48	12	24	6
105-112	52	13	26	7
113-120	56	14	28	7
121-128	60	15	30	8
128-137	64	16	32	8
138-145	68	17	34	9
146-153	72	18	36	9

(Continued)

Tirofiban *(Continued)*

Dosage I.V.:

Adults: Initial rate of 0.4 mcg/kg/minute for 30 minutes and then continued at 0.1 mcg/kg/minute; dosing should be continued through angiography and for 12-24 hours after angioplasty or atherectomy. See table on previous page.

Dosing adjustment in severe renal impairment: Cl_{cr} <30 mL/minute: Reduce dose to 50% of normal rate.

Mechanism of Action A reversible antagonist of fibrinogen binding to the GP IIb/IIIa receptor, the major platelet surface receptor involved in platelet aggregation. When administered intravenously, it inhibits *ex vivo* platelet aggregation in a dose- and concentration-dependent manner. When given according to the recommended regimen, >90% inhibition is attained by the end of the 30-minute infusion. Platelet aggregation inhibition is reversible following cessation of the infusion.

Other Adverse Effects Bleeding is the major drug-related adverse effect. Patients received background treatment with aspirin and heparin. Major bleeding was reported in 1.4% to 2.2%; minor bleeding in 10.5% to 12%; transfusion was required in 4% to 4.3%.

>1% (nonbleeding adverse events):

- Cardiovascular: Bradycardia (4%), coronary artery dissection (5%), edema (2%)
- Central nervous system: Dizziness (3%), fever (>1%), headache (>1%), vasovagal reaction (2%)
- Gastrointestinal: Nausea (>1%)
- Genitourinary: Pelvic pain (6%)
- Hematologic: Thrombocytopenia: <90,000/mm^3 (1.5%), <50,000/mm^3 (0.3%)
- Neuromuscular & skeletal: Leg pain (3%)
- Miscellaneous: Diaphoresis (2%)

<1% (Limited to important or life-threatening): Intracranial bleeding (up to 0.1%), GI bleeding (0.1% to 0.2%), retroperitoneal bleeding (up to 0.6%), GU bleeding (up to 0.1%), hemopericardium, hives, pulmonary alveolar hemorrhage, rash, anaphylaxis (case reports), severe (<10,000/mm^3) thrombocytopenia (rare), spinal-epidural hematoma, urticaria

Drug Interactions

Increased Effect/Toxicity: Use of tirofiban with aspirin and heparin is associated with an increase in bleeding over aspirin and heparin alone; however, efficacy of tirofiban is improved. Risk of bleeding is increased when used with thrombolytics, oral anticoagulants, NSAIDs, dipyridamole, ticlopidine, and clopidogrel. Avoid concomitant use of other IIb/IIIa antagonists. Cephalosporins which contain the MTT side chain may theoretically increase the risk of hemorrhage.

Decreased Effect: Levothyroxine and omeprazole decrease tirofiban levels; however, the clinical significance of this interaction remains to be demonstrated.

Pharmacodynamics/Kinetics

Distribution: 35% unbound

Metabolism: Minimally hepatic

Half-life elimination: 2 hours

Excretion: Urine (65%) and feces (25%) primarily as unchanged drug

Clearance: Elderly: Reduced by 19% to 26%

Pregnancy Risk Factor B

Generic Available No

Tirofiban Hydrochloride *see* Tirofiban *on page 1313*

Tiseb® [OTC] *see* Salicylic Acid *on page 1204*

Tisit® [OTC] *see* Pyrethrins and Piperonyl Butoxide *on page 1151*

Tisit® Blue Gel [OTC] *see* Pyrethrins and Piperonyl Butoxide *on page 1151*

Tisseel® VH *see* Fibrin Sealant Kit *on page 570*

Titralac® Plus Liquid [OTC] *see* Calcium Carbonate and Simethicone *on page 224*

Tizanidine (tye ZAN i deen)

U.S. Brand Names Zanaflex®

Canadian Brand Names Zanaflex®

Mexican Brand Names Sirdalud®

Pharmacologic Category $Alpha_2$-Adrenergic Agonist

Synonyms Sirdalud®

Use Skeletal muscle relaxant used for treatment of muscle spasticity

Unlabeled/Investigational Use Treatment of tension headaches, low back pain, trigeminal neuralgia

Local Anesthetic/Vasoconstrictor Precautions No information available to require special precautions

Effects on Dental Treatment >10%: Significant xerostomia; normal salivary flow resumes upon discontinuation

Dosage

Adults: 2-4 mg 3 times/day

Usual initial dose: 4 mg, may increase by 2-4 mg as needed for satisfactory reduction of muscle tone every 6-8 hours to a maximum of three doses in any 24 hour period

Maximum dose: 36 mg/day

Dosing adjustment in renal/hepatic impairment: May require reduction or less frequent dosing

Mechanism of Action An alpha$_2$-adrenergic agonist agent which decreases excitatory input to alpha motor neurons; an imidazole derivative chemically-related to clonidine, which acts as a centrally acting muscle relaxant with alpha$_2$-adrenergic agonist properties; acts on the level of the spinal cord

Other Adverse Effects

>10%:

Cardiovascular: Hypotension

Central nervous system: Sedation, daytime drowsiness, somnolence

1% to 10%:

Cardiovascular: Bradycardia, syncope

Central nervous system: Fatigue, dizziness, anxiety, nervousness, insomnia

Dermatologic: Pruritus, skin rash

Gastrointestinal: Nausea, vomiting, dyspepsia, constipation, diarrhea

Hepatic: Elevation of liver enzymes

Neuromuscular & skeletal: Muscle weakness, tremor

<1%: Palpitations, ventricular extrasystoles, psychotic-like symptoms, visual hallucinations, delusions, hepatic failure

Drug Interactions

Increased effect: Oral contraceptives

Increased toxicity: Additive hypotensive effects may be seen with diuretics, other alpha adrenergic agonists, or antihypertensives; CNS depression with alcohol, baclofen or other CNS depressants

Dietary/Ethanol/Herb Considerations

Ethanol: Avoid use; may increase CNS depression.

Food increases maximum concentration of tizanidine by 33% and reduces the time to peak serum concentration by 40 minutes; extent of absorption is unchanged.

Herb/Nutraceutical: Avoid gotu kola, kava, SAMe, St John's wort, and valerian; may increase CNS depression.

Pharmacodynamics/Kinetics

Duration: 3-6 hours

Bioavailability: 40%

Half-life elimination: 2.5 hours

Time to peak, serum: 1-5 hours

Pregnancy Risk Factor C

Generic Available Yes

TMP *see* Trimethoprim *on page 1352*

TMP-SMZ *see* Sulfamethoxazole and Trimethoprim *on page 1253*

TNKase™ *see* Tenecteplase *on page 1273*

TOBI® *see* Tobramycin *on page 1315*

TobraDex® *see* Tobramycin and Dexamethasone *on page 1317*

Tobramycin (toe bra MYE sin)

U.S. Brand Names AKTob®; Nebcin®; TOBI®; Tobrex®

Canadian Brand Names Nebcin®; PMS-Tobramycin; TOBI®; Tobrex®; Tomycine™

Mexican Brand Names Tobra; Tobrex®; Trazil®; Trazil Ofteno/Ungena

Pharmacologic Category Antibiotic, Aminoglycoside; Antibiotic, Ophthalmic

Synonyms Tobramycin Sulfate

Use Treatment of documented or suspected infections caused by susceptible gram-negative bacilli including *Pseudomonas aeruginosa*; topically used to treat superficial ophthalmic infections caused by susceptible bacteria. Tobramycin solution for inhalation is indicated for the management of cystic fibrosis patients (>6 years of age) with *Pseudomonas aeruginosa*.

Local Anesthetic/Vasoconstrictor Precautions No information available to require special precautions

Effects on Dental Treatment No significant effects or complications reported

Dosage Individualization is critical because of the low therapeutic index. Use of ideal body weight (IBW) for determining the mg/kg/dose appears to be more accurate than dosing on the basis of total body weight (TBW). In morbid obesity, dosage requirement may best be estimated using a dosing weight of IBW + 0.4 (TBW - IBW). Initial and periodic peak and trough plasma drug levels should be determined, particularly in critically ill patients with serious infections or in disease states known to significantly alter aminoglycoside pharmacokinetics (eg, cystic fibrosis, burns, or major surgery). Two to three serum level measurements should be obtained after the initial dose to measure the halflife in order to determine the frequency of subsequent doses.

Once daily dosing: Higher peak serum drug concentration to MIC ratios, demonstrated aminoglycoside postantibiotic effect, decreased renal cortex drug uptake,

(Continued)

Tobramycin *(Continued)*

and improved cost-time efficiency are supportive reasons for the use of once daily dosing regimens for aminoglycosides. Current research indicates these regimens to be as effective for non-life-threatening infections, with no higher incidence of nephrotoxicity, than those requiring multiple daily doses. Doses are determined by calculating the entire day's dose via usual multiple dose calculation techniques and administering this quantity as a single dose. Doses are then adjusted to maintain mean serum concentrations above the MIC(s) of the causative organism(s). (Example: 2.5-5 mg/kg as a single dose; expected Cp_{max}: 10-20 mcg/mL and Cp_{min}: <1 mcg/mL). Further research is needed for universal recommendation in all patient populations and gram-negative disease; exceptions may include those with known high clearance (eg, children, patients with cystic fibrosis, or burns who may require shorter dosage intervals) and patients with renal function impairment for whom longer than conventional dosage intervals are usually required. Some clinicians suggest a daily dose of 4-7 mg/kg for all patients with normal renal function. This dose is at least as efficacious with similar, if not less, toxicity than conventional dosing.

Infants and Children <5 years: I.M., I.V.: 2.5 mg/kg/dose every 8 hours

Children >5 years: 1.5-2.5 mg/kg/dose every 8 hours

Note: Some patients may require larger or more frequent doses if serum levels document the need (ie, cystic fibrosis or febrile granulocytopenic patients).

Adults: I.M., I.V.:
- Severe life-threatening infections: 2-2.5 mg/kg/dose
- Urinary tract infection: 1.5 mg/kg/dose
- Synergy (for gram-positive infections): 1 mg/kg/dose

Children and Adults: Ophthalmic: Instill 1-2 drops of solution every 4 hours; apply ointment 2-3 times/day; for severe infections apply ointment every 3-4 hours, or solution 2 drops every 30-60 minutes initially, then reduce to less frequent intervals

Inhalation:
- Standard aerosolized tobramycin:
  - Children: 40-80 mg 2-3 times/day
  - Adults: 60-80 mg 3 times/day
- High-dose regimen: Children ≥6 years and Adults: 300 mg every 12 hours (do not administer doses less than 6 hours apart); administer in repeated cycles of 28 days on drug followed by 28 days off drug

Dosing interval in renal impairment:
- Cl_{cr} ≥60 mL/minute: Administer every 8 hours
- Cl_{cr} 40-60 mL/minute: Administer every 12 hours
- Cl_{cr} 20-40 mL/minute: Administer every 24 hours
- Cl_{cr} 10-20 mL/minute: Administer every 48 hours
- Cl_{cr} <10 mL/minute: Administer every 72 hours

Hemodialysis: Dialyzable; 30% removal of aminoglycosides occurs during 4 hours of HD - administer dose after dialysis and follow levels

Continuous arteriovenous or venovenous hemofiltration: Dose as for Cl_{cr} of 10-40 mL/minute and follow levels
- Administration in CAPD fluid:
  - Gram-negative infection: 4-8 mg/L (4-8 mcg/mL) of CAPD fluid
  - Gram-positive infection (ie, synergy): 3-4 mg/L (3-4 mcg/mL) of CAPD fluid
- Administration IVPB/I.M.: Dose as for Cl_{cr} <10 mL/minute and follow levels

Dosing adjustment in hepatic impairment: Monitor plasma concentrations

Mechanism of Action Interferes with bacterial protein synthesis by binding to 30S and 50S ribosomal subunits resulting in a defective bacterial cell membrane

Other Adverse Effects

1% to 10%:
- Neuromuscular & skeletal: Neurotoxicity (neuromuscular blockade)
- Otic: Ototoxicity (auditory and vestibular)
- Renal: Nephrotoxicity

<1%: Hypotension, drug fever, headache, drowsiness, rash, nausea, vomiting, eosinophilia, anemia, paresthesia, tremor, arthralgia, weakness, lacrimation, itching eyes, edema of the eyelid, keratitis, dyspnea

Drug Interactions Increased Effect/Toxicity: Increased antimicrobial effect of tobramycin with extended spectrum penicillins (synergistic). Neuromuscular blockers may have an increased duration of action (neuromuscular blockade). Amphotericin B, cephalosporins, and loop diuretics may increase the risk of nephrotoxicity.

Dietary/Ethanol/Herb Considerations Food: May require supplementation of calcium, magnesium, and potassium

Pharmacodynamics/Kinetics

Absorption: I.M.: Rapid and complete

Distribution: V_d: 0.2-0.3 L/kg; Pediatrics: 0.2-0.7 L/kg; to extracellular fluid including serum, abscesses, ascitic, pericardial, pleural, synovial, lymphatic, and peritoneal fluids; crosses placenta; poor penetration into CSF, eye, bone, prostate

Protein binding: <30%

Half-life elimination:

Neonates: ≤1200 g: 11 hours; >1200 g: 2-9 hours

Adults: 2-3 hours; directly dependent upon glomerular filtration rate

Adults with impaired renal function: 5-70 hours

Time to peak, serum: I.M.: 30-60 minutes; I.V.: ~30 minutes

Excretion: Normal renal function: Urine (~90% to 95%) within 24 hours

Pregnancy Risk Factor C

Generic Available Yes; Excludes ophthalmic ointment, powder for injection, solution for nebulization

Tobramycin and Dexamethasone

(toe bra MYE sin & deks a METH a sone)

Related Information

Dexamethasone *on page 413*

Tobramycin *on page 1315*

U.S. Brand Names TobraDex®

Canadian Brand Names Tobradex®

Pharmacologic Category Antibiotic/Corticosteroid, Ophthalmic

Synonyms Dexamethasone and Tobramycin

Use Treatment of external ocular infection caused by susceptible gram-negative bacteria and steroid responsive inflammatory conditions of the palpebral and bulbar conjunctiva, lid, cornea, and anterior segment of the globe

Local Anesthetic/Vasoconstrictor Precautions No information available to require special precautions

Effects on Dental Treatment No significant effects or complications reported

Dosage Children and Adults: Ophthalmic: Instill 1-2 drops of solution every 4 hours; apply ointment 2-3 times/day; for severe infections apply ointment every 3-4 hours, or solution 2 drops every 30-60 minutes initially, then reduce to less frequent intervals

Mechanism of Action Refer to individual monographs for Dexamethasone and Tobramycin

Other Adverse Effects Frequency not defined:

Dermatologic: Allergic contact dermatitis, delayed wound healing

Ocular: Lacrimation, itching, edema of eyelid, keratitis, increased intraocular pressure, glaucoma, cataract formation

Dietary/Ethanol/Herb Considerations Based on tobramycin component:

Food: May require supplementation of calcium, magnesium, and potassium

Pharmacodynamics/Kinetics

Absorption: Into aqueous humor

Time to peak, serum: 1-2 hours in the cornea and aqueous humor

Pregnancy Risk Factor B

Generic Available No

Tobramycin Sulfate *see* Tobramycin *on page 1315*

Tobrex® *see* Tobramycin *on page 1315*

Tocainide (toe KAY nide)

Related Information

Cardiovascular Diseases *on page 1456*

U.S. Brand Names Tonocard®

Canadian Brand Names Tonocard®

Pharmacologic Category Antiarrhythmic Agent, Class Ib

Synonyms Tocainide Hydrochloride

Use Suppression and prevention of symptomatic life-threatening ventricular arrhythmias

Unlabeled/Investigational Use Treatment of trigeminal neuralgia

Local Anesthetic/Vasoconstrictor Precautions No information available to require special precautions

Effects on Dental Treatment No significant effects or complications reported

Dosage Oral:

Adults: 1200-1800 mg/day in 3 divided doses, up to 2400 mg/day

Dosing adjustment in renal impairment: Cl_{cr} <30 mL/minute: Administer 50% of normal dose or 600 mg once daily.

Hemodialysis: Moderately dialyzable (20% to 50%)

Dosing adjustment in hepatic impairment: Maximum daily dose: 1200 mg

Mechanism of Action Class 1B antiarrhythmic agent; suppresses automaticity of conduction tissue, by increasing electrical stimulation threshold of ventricle, His-Purkinje system, and spontaneous depolarization of the ventricles during diastole by a direct action on the tissues; blocks both the initiation and conduction of nerve impulses by decreasing the neuronal membrane's permeability to sodium ions, which results in inhibition of depolarization with resultant blockade of conduction

(Continued)

Tocainide *(Continued)*

Other Adverse Effects

>10%:

Central nervous system: Dizziness (8% to 15%)

Gastrointestinal: Nausea (14% to 15%)

1% to 10%:

Cardiovascular: Tachycardia (3%), bradycardia/angina/palpitations (0.5% to 1.8%), hypotension (3%)

Central nervous system: Nervousness (0.5% to 1.5%), confusion (2% to 3%), headache (4.6%), anxiety, incoordination, giddiness, vertigo

Dermatologic: Rash (0.5% to 8.4%)

Gastrointestinal: Vomiting (4.5%), diarrhea (4% to 5%), anorexia (1% to 2%), loss of taste

Neuromuscular & skeletal: Paresthesia (3.5% to 9%), tremor (dose-related: 2.9% to 8.4%), ataxia (dose-related: 2.9% to 8.4%), hot and cold sensations

Ocular: Blurred vision (~1.5%), nystagmus (1%)

<1% (Limited to important or life-threatening): Hypersensitivity reactions, increased ANA, sinoatrial block, syncope, vasovagal episodes, diaphoresis, edema, fever, chills, cinchonism, asthenia, malaise, AV block, hypertension, increased QRS duration, prolonged QT interval, right bundle branch block, cardiomegaly, angina, pulmonary embolism, sinus arrest, vasculitis, orthostatic hypotension, pericarditis, hepatitis, jaundice, abnormal LFTs, pancreatitis, abdominal pain, constipation, dysphagia, dyspepsia, stomatitis, xerostomia, muscle cramps, neck pain, depression, psychosis, psychic disturbances, agitation, decreased mental acuity, dysarthria, impaired memory, slurred speech, sleep disturbance, insomnia, local anesthesia, myasthenia gravis, convulsions, coma, pneumonia, interstitial pneumonitis, fibrosing alveolitis, pulmonary fibrosis, dyspnea, hiccup, yawning, pulmonary edema, respiratory arrest, urticaria, alopecia, pallor, pruritus, erythema multiforme, exfoliative dermatitis, Stevens-Johnson syndrome, diplopia, earache, abnormal taste, urinary retention, polyuria, hallucinations, delirium

Postmarketing and/or case reports: Pericarditis, immune complex glomerulonephritis, granulomatous hepatitis

Note: Rare, potentially severe hematologic reactions, have occurred (generally within the first 12 weeks of therapy). These may include agranulocytosis, bone marrow depression, aplastic anemia, hypoplastic anemia, hemolytic anemia, anemia, leukopenia, neutropenia, thrombocytopenia, and eosinophilia.

Drug Interactions Inhibits CYP1A2

Increased Effect/Toxicity: Tocainide may increase serum levels of caffeine and theophylline.

Decreased Effect: Decreased tocainide plasma levels with cimetidine, phenobarbital, phenytoin, rifampin, and other hepatic enzyme inducers.

Dietary/Ethanol/Herb Considerations

Food: Administer with food.

Herb/Nutraceutical: Ginger has positive inotropic effects and theoretically could affect antiarrhythmia activity.

Pharmacodynamics/Kinetics

Absorption: Oral: 99% to 100%

Distribution: V_d: 1.62-3.2 L/kg

Protein binding: 10% to 20%

Metabolism: Hepatic to inactive metabolites; negligible first-pass effect

Half-life elimination: 11-14 hours; Renal and hepatic impairment: 23-27 hours

Time to peak, serum: 30-160 minutes

Excretion: Urine (40% to 50% as unchanged drug)

Pregnancy Risk Factor C

Generic Available No

Tocainide Hydrochloride *see* Tocainide *on page 1317*

Tofranil® *see* Imipramine *on page 711*

Tofranil-PM® *see* Imipramine *on page 711*

TOLAZamide (tole AZ a mide)

Related Information

Endocrine Disorders and Pregnancy *on page 1479*

U.S. Brand Names Tolinase®

Canadian Brand Names Tolinase®

Pharmacologic Category Antidiabetic Agent, Sulfonylurea

Use Adjunct to diet for the management of mild to moderately severe, stable, type 2 diabetes mellitus (noninsulin dependent, NIDDM)

Local Anesthetic/Vasoconstrictor Precautions No information available to require special precautions

Effects on Dental Treatment Use salicylates with caution in patients taking tolazamide due to potential increased hypoglycemia; NSAIDs such as ibuprofen and naproxen may be safely used. Tolazamide-dependent diabetics (noninsulin dependent, type 2) should be appointed for dental treatment in morning in order to minimize chance of stress-induced hypoglycemia.

Dosage Oral (doses >1000 mg/day normally do not improve diabetic control):

Adults:

Initial: 100-250 mg/day with breakfast or the first main meal of the day

Fasting blood sugar <200 mg/dL: 100 mg/day

Fasting blood sugar >200 mg/dL: 250 mg/day

Patient is malnourished, underweight, elderly, or not eating properly: 100 mg/day

Adjust dose in increments of 100-250 mg/day at weekly intervals to response. If >500 mg/day is required, give in divided doses twice daily; maximum daily dose: 1 g (doses >1 g/day are not likely to improve control)

Conversion from insulin → tolazamide

10 units day = 100 mg/day

20-40 units/day = 250 mg/day

>40 units/day = 250 mg/day and 50% of insulin dose

Doses >500 mg/day should be given in 2 divided doses

Dosing adjustment in renal impairment: Conservative initial and maintenance doses are recommended because tolazamide is metabolized to active metabolites, which are eliminated in the urine

Dosing adjustment in hepatic impairment: Conservative initial and maintenance doses and careful monitoring of blood glucose are recommended.

Mechanism of Action Stimulates insulin release from the pancreatic beta cells; reduces glucose output from the liver; insulin sensitivity is increased at peripheral target sites

Other Adverse Effects Frequency not defined:

Central nervous system: Headache, dizziness

Dermatologic: Rash, urticaria, photosensitivity

Endocrine & metabolic: Hypoglycemia, SIADH

Gastrointestinal: Anorexia, nausea, vomiting, diarrhea, constipation, heartburn, epigastric fullness

Hematologic: Aplastic anemia, hemolytic anemia, bone marrow suppression, thrombocytopenia, agranulocytosis

Hepatic: Cholestatic jaundice

Renal: Diuretic effect

Drug Interactions

Increased Effect/Toxicity: Salicylates, anticoagulants, H_2 antagonists, TCAs, MAO inhibitors, beta-blockers, and thiazides may increase effect of sulfonylureas.

Decreased Effect: Many drugs, including corticosteroids, beta-blockers, and thiazides may alter response to oral hypoglycemics.

Dietary/Ethanol/Herb Considerations

Ethanol: Avoid use; may increase risk of hypoglycemia and cause disulfiram-like reaction.

Food: Avoid garlic; may increase blood insulin concentration.

Herb/Nutraceutical: Avoid black cohosh; may enhance effects of antidiabetic agents. Avoid chromium, garlic, and horse chestnut; may cause hypoglycemia.

Pharmacodynamics/Kinetics

Onset of action: 4-6 hours

Duration: 10-24 hours

Protein binding: >98%

Metabolism: Extensively hepatic to one active and three inactive metabolites

Half-life elimination: 7 hours

Excretion: Urine

Pregnancy Risk Factor D

Generic Available Yes

TOLBUTamide (tole BYOO ta mide)

Related Information

Endocrine Disorders and Pregnancy *on page 1479*

U.S. Brand Names Orinase Diagnostic® [DSC]; Tol-Tab®

Canadian Brand Names Apo®-Tolbutamide

Mexican Brand Names Artosin; Diaval®; Rastinon®

Pharmacologic Category Antidiabetic Agent, Sulfonylurea

Synonyms Tolbutamide Sodium

Use Adjunct to diet for the management of mild to moderately severe, stable, type 2 diabetes mellitus (noninsulin dependent, NIDDM)

Local Anesthetic/Vasoconstrictor Precautions No information available to require special precautions

Effects on Dental Treatment Use salicylates with caution in patients taking tolazamide due to potential increased hypoglycemia; NSAIDs such as ibuprofen and naproxen may be safely used. Tolbutamide-dependent diabetics (noninsulin dependent, type 2) should be appointed for dental treatment in morning in order to minimize chance of stress-induced hypoglycemia.

Dosage Divided doses may improve GI tolerance.

(Continued)

TOLBUTamide *(Continued)*

Adults:

Oral: Initial: 1-2 g/day as a single dose in the morning or in divided doses throughout the day. Total doses may be taken in the morning; however, divided doses may allow increased GI tolerance. Maintenance dose: 0.25-3 g/day; however, a maintenance dose >2 g/day is seldom required.

I.V. bolus: 1 g over 2-3 minutes

Elderly: Oral: Initial: 250 mg 1-3 times/day; usual: 500-2000 mg; maximum: 3 g/day

Hemodialysis: Not dialyzable (0% to 5%)

Dosing adjustment in hepatic impairment: Reduction may be required

Mechanism of Action Stimulates insulin release from the pancreatic beta cells; reduces glucose output from the liver; insulin sensitivity is increased at peripheral target sites, suppression of glucagon may also contribute

Other Adverse Effects Frequency not defined:

Cardiovascular: Venospasm

Central nervous system: Headache, dizziness

Dermatologic: Skin rash, urticaria, photosensitivity

Endocrine & metabolic: Hypoglycemia, SIADH

Gastrointestinal: Constipation, diarrhea, heartburn, anorexia, epigastric fullness, taste alteration

Hematologic: Aplastic anemia, hemolytic anemia, bone marrow suppression, thrombocytopenia, leukopenia, agranulocytosis

Hepatic: Cholestatic jaundice

Local: Thrombophlebitis

Otic: Tinnitus

Miscellaneous: Hypersensitivity reaction, disulfiram-like reactions

Drug Interactions Substrate of **CYP2C8/9**, 2C19; Inhibits CYP2C8/9

Increased Effect/Toxicity: A number of drugs increase the effect of first-generation sulfonylureas (tolbutamide) including salicylates, chloramphenicol, anticoagulants, H_2 antagonists, tricyclic antidepressants, MAO inhibitors, beta-blockers, and thiazide diuretics.

Decreased Effect: Drugs with increase glucose (corticosteroids, thiazides) may decrease the effect of tolbutamide.

Dietary/Ethanol/Herb Considerations

Ethanol: Avoid use; may increase risk of hypoglycemia.

Herb/Nutraceutical: Avoid chromium, garlic and gymnema; may cause hypoglycemia.

Pharmacodynamics/Kinetics

Onset of action: Peak effect: Hypoglycemic action: Oral: 1-3 hours; I.V.: 30 minutes

Duration: Oral: 6-24 hours; I.V.: 3 hours

Absorption: Oral: Rapid

Distribution: V_d: 6-10 L; increased with decreased albumin concentrations

Protein binding: 95% to 97%, primarily to albumin

Metabolism: Hepatic to hydroxymethyltolbutamide (mildly active) and carboxytolbutamide (inactive); metabolism does not appear to be affected by age

Half-life elimination: Plasma: 4-25 hours; Elimination: 4-9 hours

Time to peak, serum: 3-5 hours

Excretion: Urine (<2% as unchanged drug, primarily as metabolites)

Pregnancy Risk Factor D

Generic Available Yes: Tablet

Tolbutamide Sodium *see* TOLBUTamide *on page 1319*

Tolcapone (TOLE ka pone)

U.S. Brand Names Tasmar®

Mexican Brand Names Tasmar®

Pharmacologic Category Anti-Parkinson's Agent, COMT Inhibitor

Use Adjunct to levodopa and carbidopa for the treatment of signs and symptoms of idiopathic Parkinson's disease

Local Anesthetic/Vasoconstrictor Precautions No information available to require special precautions

Effects on Dental Treatment Dopaminergic therapy in Parkinson's disease (ie, treatment with levodopa) is associated with orthostatic hypotension. Tolcapone enhances levodopa bioavailability and may increase the occurrence of hypotension/syncope in the dental patient. The patient should be carefully assisted from the chair and observed for signs of orthostatic hypotension.

Dosage Adults: Oral: Initial: 100-200 mg 3 times/day; levodopa therapy may need to be decreased upon initiation of tolcapone

Mechanism of Action Tolcapone is a selective and reversible inhibitor of catechol-o-methyltransferase (COMT)

Other Adverse Effects

>10%:

Cardiovascular: Orthostatic hypotension

Central nervous system: Sleep disorder, excessive dreaming, somnolence, headache

Gastrointestinal: Nausea, diarrhea, anorexia
Neuromuscular & skeletal: Dyskinesia, dystonia, muscle cramps

1% to 10%:

Central nervous system: Hallucinations, fatigue, loss of balance, hyperkinesia
Gastrointestinal: Vomiting, constipation, xerostomia, abdominal pain, flatulence, dyspepsia
Genitourinary: Urine discoloration
Neuromuscular & skeletal: Paresthesia, stiffness
Miscellaneous: Diaphoresis (increased)

Drug Interactions Inhibits CYP2C8/9

Increased Effect/Toxicity: Tolcapone may increase the effect/levels of methyldopa, dobutamine, apomorphine, and isoproterenol due to inhibition of catechol-O-methyl transferase enzymes (COMT).

Dietary/Ethanol/Herb Considerations

Ethanol: Avoid use; may increase CNS depression.
Food decreases bioavailability by 10% to 20% if ingested within 1 hour before or 2 hours after the dose.
Herb/Nutraceutical: Avoid gotu kola, kava, SAMe, St John's wort, valerian; may increase CNS depression.

Pharmacodynamics/Kinetics

Absorption: Rapid
Protein binding: >99.0%
Metabolism: Glucuronidation
Bioavailability: 65%
Half-life elimination: 2-3 hours
Time to peak: ~2 hours
Excretion: Urine and feces (40%)

Pregnancy Risk Factor C

Generic Available No

Tolectin® *see* Tolmetin *on page 1321*
Tolectin® DS *see* Tolmetin *on page 1321*
Tolinase® *see* TOLAZamide *on page 1318*

Tolmetin (TOLE met in)

Related Information

Rheumatoid Arthritis, Osteoarthritis, and Osteoporosis *on page 1488*
Temporomandibular Dysfunction (TMD) *on page 1562*

U.S. Brand Names Tolectin®; Tolectin® DS

Canadian Brand Names Tolectin®

Mexican Brand Names Tolectin®

Pharmacologic Category Nonsteroidal Anti-inflammatory Drug (NSAID)

Synonyms Tolmetin Sodium

Use Treatment of rheumatoid arthritis and osteoarthritis, juvenile rheumatoid arthritis

Local Anesthetic/Vasoconstrictor Precautions No information available to require special precautions

Effects on Dental Treatment NSAID formulations are known to reversibly decrease platelet aggregation via mechanisms different than observed with aspirin. The dentist should be aware of the potential of abnormal coagulation. Caution should also be exercised in the use of NSAIDs in patients already on anticoagulant therapy with drugs such as warfarin (Coumadin®).

Dosage Oral:

Children ≥2 years:

Anti-inflammatory: Initial: 20 mg/kg/day in 3 divided doses, then 15-30 mg/kg/day in 3 divided doses
Analgesic: 5-7 mg/kg/dose every 6-8 hours

Adults: 400 mg 3 times/day; usual dose: 600 mg to 1.8 g/day; maximum: 2 g/day

Mechanism of Action Inhibits prostaglandin synthesis by decreasing the activity of the enzyme, cyclooxygenase, which results in decreased formation of prostaglandin precursors

Other Adverse Effects

1% to 10%:

Cardiovascular: Chest pain, hypertension, edema
Central nervous system: Headache, dizziness, drowsiness, depression
Dermatologic: Skin irritation
Endocrine & metabolic: Weight gain/loss
Gastrointestinal: Heartburn, abdominal pain, diarrhea, flatulence, vomiting, constipation, gastritis, peptic ulcer, nausea
Genitourinary: Urinary Tract Infection
Hematologic: Elevated BUN, transient decreases in hemoglobin/hematocrit
Ocular: Visual disturbances
Otic: Tinnitus

<1%: Congestive heart failure, hypertension, arrhythmias, tachycardia, confusion, hallucinations, aseptic meningitis, mental depression, drowsiness, insomnia, urticaria, erythema multiforme, toxic epidermal necrolysis, Stevens-Johnson

(Continued)

Tolmetin *(Continued)*

syndrome, angioedema, polydipsia, hot flashes, gastritis, GI ulceration, cystitis, polyuria, agranulocytosis, anemia, hemolytic anemia, bone marrow suppression, leukopenia, thrombocytopenia, hepatitis, peripheral neuropathy, toxic amblyopia, blurred vision, conjunctivitis, dry eyes, decreased hearing, acute renal failure, allergic rhinitis, dyspnea, bronchospasm, epistaxis

Drug Interactions

Increased toxicity of digoxin, methotrexate, cyclosporine, lithium, insulin, sulfonylureas, potassium-sparing diuretics, and aspirin.

Decreased effect with aspirin. Decreased effect of thiazides and furosemide.

Dietary/Ethanol/Herb Considerations

Ethanol: Avoid use; may enhance gastric mucosal irritation.

Food: Administer with food or milk to reduce GI upset; may decrease serum concentration. Avoid garlic, ginger, and green tea.

Herb/Nutraceutical: Avoid cat's claw, dong quai, evening primrose, feverfew, garlic, ginger, ginkgo biloba, ginseng, green tea, horse chestnut, and red clover due to additional antiplatelet activity. Avoid kava and valerian; may enhance benzodiazepine activity.

Pharmacodynamics/Kinetics

Onset of action: Analgesic: 1-2 hours; Anti-inflammatory: Days to weeks

Absorption: Well absorbed

Bioavailability: Reduced 16% with food or milk

Half-life elimination: Biphasic: Rapid: 1-2 hours; Slow: 5 hours

Time to peak, serum: 30-60 minutes

Excretion: Urine (as inactive metabolites or conjugates) within 24 hours

Pregnancy Risk Factor C/D (3rd trimester or at term)

Generic Available Yes

Tolmetin Sodium *see* Tolmetin *on page 1321*

Tolnaftate (tole NAF tate)

U.S. Brand Names Absorbine Jr.® Antifungal [OTC]; Aftate® Antifungal [OTC]; Fungi-Guard [OTC]; Tinactin® Antifungal [OTC]; Tinactin® Antifungal Jock Itch [OTC]; Tinaderm [OTC]; Ting® [OTC]

Canadian Brand Names Pitrex

Mexican Brand Names Tinaderm®

Pharmacologic Category Antifungal Agent, Topical

Use Treatment of tinea pedis, tinea cruris, and tinea corporis fungal infections

Local Anesthetic/Vasoconstrictor Precautions No information available to require special precautions

Effects on Dental Treatment No significant effects or complications reported

Dosage Children ≥2 years and Adults: Topical: Wash and dry affected area; spray aerosol or apply 1-3 drops of solution or a small amount of cream, gel, or powder and rub into the affected areas 2 times/day (may use for up to 4 weeks for tinea pedis or tinea corporis, and up to 2 weeks for tinea cruris)

Mechanism of Action Distorts the hyphae and stunts mycelial growth in susceptible fungi

Other Adverse Effects Frequency not defined:

Dermatologic: Pruritus, contact dermatitis

Local: Irritation, stinging

Pharmacodynamics/Kinetics Onset of action: 24-72 hours

Pregnancy Risk Factor C

Generic Available Yes: Cream, powder, solution

Tol-Tab® *see* TOLBUTamide *on page 1319*

Tolterodine (tole TER oh dine)

U.S. Brand Names Detrol®; Detrol® LA

Canadian Brand Names Detrol®; Unidet®

Mexican Brand Names Detrusitol®

Pharmacologic Category Anticholinergic Agent

Synonyms Tolterodine Tartrate

Use Treatment of patients with an overactive bladder with symptoms of urinary frequency, urgency, or urge incontinence

Local Anesthetic/Vasoconstrictor Precautions No information available to require special precautions

Effects on Dental Treatment The anticholinergic effects of tolterodine are selective for the urinary bladder rather than salivary glands; xerostomia should not be significant.

Dosage

Children: Safety and efficacy in pediatric patients have not been established

Adults: Treatment of overactive bladder: Oral:

Immediate release tablet: 2 mg twice daily; the dose may be lowered to 1 mg twice daily based on individual response and tolerability

Dosing adjustment in patients concurrently taking CYP3A4 inhibitors: 1 mg twice daily

Extended release capsule: 4 mg once a day; dose may be lowered to 2 mg daily based on individual response and tolerability

Dosing adjustment in patients concurrently taking CYP3A4 inhibitors: 2 mg daily

Elderly: Safety and efficacy in patients >64 years was found to be similar to that in younger patients; no dosage adjustment is needed based on age

Dosing adjustment in renal impairment: Use with caution (studies conducted in patients with Cl_{cr} 10-30 mL/minute):

Immediate release tablet: 1 mg twice daily

Extended release capsule: 2 mg daily

Dosing adjustment in hepatic impairment:

Immediate release tablet: 1 mg twice daily

Extended release capsule: 2 mg daily

Mechanism of Action Tolterodine is a competitive antagonist of muscarinic receptors. In animal models, tolterodine demonstrates selectivity for urinary bladder receptors over salivary receptors. Urinary bladder contraction is mediated by muscarinic receptors. Tolterodine increases residual urine volume and decreases detrusor muscle pressure.

Other Adverse Effects As reported with immediate release tablet, unless otherwise specified

>10%: Gastrointestinal: Dry mouth (35%; extended release capsules 23%)

1% to 10%:

Cardiovascular: Chest pain (2%)

Central nervous system: Headache (7%; extended release capsules 6%), somnolence (3%; extended release capsules 3%), fatigue (4%; extended release capsules 2%), dizziness (5%; extended release capsules 2%), anxiety (extended release capsules 1%)

Dermatologic: Dry skin (1%)

Gastrointestinal: Abdominal pain (5%; extended release capsules 4%), constipation (7%; extended release capsules 6%), dyspepsia (4%; extended release capsules 3%), diarrhea (4%), weight gain (1%)

Genitourinary: Dysuria (2%; extended release capsules 1%)

Neuromuscular & skeletal: Arthralgia (2%)

Ocular: Abnormal vision (2%; extended release capsules 1%), dry eyes (3%; extended release capsules 3%)

Respiratory: Bronchitis (2%), sinusitis (extended release capsules 2%)

Postmarketing and/or case reports: Anaphylactoid reactions, tachycardia, peripheral edema

Drug Interactions Substrate of CYP2C8/9, 2C19, **2D6, 3A4**

Increased Effect/Toxicity:

Serum levels and/or toxicity of tolterodine may be increased by drugs which inhibit CYP2D6; effect was seen with fluoxetine. Inhibitors include amiodarone, cimetidine, delavirdine, paroxetine, propafenone, quinidine, and ritonavir. No dosage adjustment was needed in patients coadministered tolterodine and fluoxetine.

Serum level and/or toxicity of tolterodine may be increased by drugs which inhibit CYP3A4, particularly in patients who are poor metabolizers via CYP2D6; effect was seen with ketoconazole. Other inhibitors include amiodarone, cimetidine, clarithromycin, cyclosporine, erythromycin, delavirdine, diltiazem, dirithromycin, disulfiram, fluoxetine, fluvoxamine, grapefruit juice, indinavir, itraconazole, nefazodone, nevirapine, propoxyphene, quinupristin-dalfopristin, ritonavir, saquinavir, verapamil, vinblastine, zafirlukast, zileuton.

Dietary/Ethanol/Herb Considerations

Food increases bioavailability (~53%) of tablets, but not extended release capsules. Avoid grapefruit products; may increase serum concentration/toxicity (unlikely secondary to high oral bioavailability).

Herb/Nutraceutical: Avoid St John's wort; may decrease serum concentration.

Pharmacodynamics/Kinetics

Absorption: Immediate release tablet: Rapid

Distribution: I.V.: V_d: 113 ± 27 L

Protein binding: Highly bound to $alpha_1$-acid glycoprotein

Metabolism: Extensively hepatic, primarily via CYP2D6 (some metabolites share activity) and 3A4 usually (minor pathway). In patients with a genetic deficiency of CYP2D6, metabolism via 3A4 predominates. Forms three active metabolites.

Bioavailability: Immediate release tablet: 77%; increased with food

Half-life elimination:

Immediate release tablet: Extensive metabolizers: ~2 hours; Poor metabolizers: ~10 hours

Extended release capsule: Extensive metabolizers: ~7 hours; Poor metabolizers: ~18 hours

Time to peak: Immediate release tablet: 1-2 hours; Extended release tablet: 2-6 hours

(Continued)

Tolterodine *(Continued)*

Excretion: Urine (77% as unchanged drug, 5% to 14% as metabolites, <1% as metabolites in poor metabolizers); feces (17%, <1% as unchanged drug, <2.5% in poor metabolizers)

Pregnancy Risk Factor C

Generic Available No

Tolterodine Tartrate *see* Tolterodine *on page 1322*
Tolu-Sed® DM [OTC] *see* Guaifenesin and Dextromethorphan *on page 651*
Tomoxetine *see* Atomoxetine *on page 139*
Tonocard® *see* Tocainide *on page 1317*
Topamax® *see* Topiramate *on page 1324*
Topicaine® [OTC] *see* Lidocaine *on page 801*
Topicort® *see* Desoximetasone *on page 412*
Topicort®-LP *see* Desoximetasone *on page 412*

Topiramate (toe PYE ra mate)

U.S. Brand Names Topamax®

Canadian Brand Names Topamax®

Mexican Brand Names Topamax®

Pharmacologic Category Anticonvulsant, Miscellaneous

Use In adults and pediatric patients (ages 2-16 years), adjunctive therapy for partial onset seizures and adjunctive therapy of primary generalized tonic-clonic seizures; treatment of seizures associated with Lennox-Gastaut syndrome in patients ≥2 years of age

Unlabeled/Investigational Use Treatment of bipolar disorder, infantile spasms, neuropathic pain, migraine or cluster headaches

Local Anesthetic/Vasoconstrictor Precautions No information available to require special precautions

Effects on Dental Treatment 1% to 10%: Gingivitis, xerostomia

Dosage Oral:

Children 2-16 years: Partial seizures (adjunctive therapy), primary generalized tonic-clonic seizures (adjunctive therapy), or seizure associated with Lennox-Gastaut syndrome: Initial dose titration should begin at 25 mg (or less, based on a range of 1-3 mg/kg/day) nightly for the first week; dosage may be increased in increments of 1-3 mg/kg/day (administered in 2 divided doses) at 1- or 2-week intervals to a total daily dose of 5-9 mg/kg/day.

Adults:

Partial onset seizures (adjunctive therapy), primary generalized tonic-clonic seizures (adjunctive therapy): Initial: 25-50 mg/day; titrate in increments of 25-50 mg per week until an effective daily dose is reached; the daily dose may be increased by 25 mg at weekly intervals for the first 4 weeks; thereafter, the daily dose may be increased by 25-50 mg weekly to an effective daily dose (usually at least 400 mg); usual maximum dose: 1600 mg/day

Note: A more rapid titration schedule has been previously recommended (ie, 50 mg/week), and may be attempted in some clinical situations; however, this may reduce the patient's ability to tolerate topiramate.

Migraine, cluster headache (unlabeled uses): Initial: 25 mg/day, titrated at weekly intervals in 25 mg increments, up to 200 mg/day

Dosing adjustment in renal impairment: Cl_{cr} <70 mL/minute: Administer 50% dose and titrate more slowly

Hemodialysis: Supplemental dose may be needed during hemodialysis

Dosing adjustment in hepatic impairment: Clearance may be reduced

Mechanism of Action Mechanism is not fully understood, it is thought to decrease seizure frequency by blocking sodium channels in neurons, enhancing GABA activity and by blocking glutamate activity

Other Adverse Effects

>10%:

Central nervous system: Dizziness, ataxia, somnolence, psychomotor slowing, nervousness, memory difficulties, speech problems, fatigue
Gastrointestinal: Nausea
Neuromuscular & skeletal: Paresthesia, tremor
Ocular: Nystagmus, diplopia, abnormal vision
Respiratory: Upper respiratory infections

1% to 10%:

Cardiovascular: Chest pain, edema
Central nervous system: Language problems, abnormal coordination, confusion, depression, difficulty concentrating, hypoesthesia
Endocrine & metabolic: Hot flashes
Gastrointestinal: Dyspepsia, abdominal pain, anorexia, constipation, weight loss
Neuromuscular & skeletal: Myalgia, weakness, back pain, leg pain, rigors
Otic: Decreased hearing
Renal: Nephrolithiasis
Respiratory: Pharyngitis, sinusitis, epistaxis

Miscellaneous: Flu-like symptoms

<1%: Apraxia, AV block, bone marrow depression, delirium, dyskinesia, encephalopathy, eosinophilia, granulocytopenia, manic reaction, neuropathy, pancytopenia, paranoid reaction, photosensitivity, psychosis, renal calculus, suicidal behavior, tinnitus

Postmarketing and/or case reports: Hepatic failure, hepatitis, pancreatitis, renal tubular acidosis, syndrome of acute myopia/secondary angle-closure glaucoma

Drug Interactions Inhibits CYP2C19; Induces CYP3A4

Increased Effect/Toxicity: Concomitant administration with other CNS depressants will increase its sedative effects. Coadministration with other carbonic anhydrase inhibitors may increase the chance of nephrolithiasis. Topiramate may increase phenytoin concentration by 25%.

Decreased Effect: Phenytoin can decrease topiramate levels by as much as 48%, carbamazepine reduces it by 40%, and valproic acid reduces topiramate by 14%. Digoxin levels and ethinyl estradiol blood levels are decreased when coadministered with topiramate. Topiramate may decrease valproic acid concentration by 11%.

Dietary/Ethanol/Herb Considerations

Ethanol: Avoid use; may increase CNS depression.

Food: May be taken with food

Herb/Nutraceutical: Avoid evening primrose; decreases seizure threshold. Avoid gotu kola, kava, SAMe, St John's wort, and valerian; may increase CNS depression.

Pharmacodynamics/Kinetics

Absorption: Good; unaffected by food

Protein binding: 13% to 17%

Metabolism: Minimally hepatic via hydroxylation, hydrolysis, glucuronidation

Bioavailability: 80%

Half-life elimination: Mean: Adults: 21 hours; shorter in pediatric patients; clearance is 50% higher in pediatric patients

Time to peak, serum: ~2-4 hours

Excretion: Urine (~70% as unchanged drug)

Dialyzable: ~30%

Pregnancy Risk Factor C

Generic Available No

TOPO *see* Topotecan *on page 1325*

Toposar® *see* Etoposide *on page 549*

Topotecan (toe poe TEE kan)

U.S. Brand Names Hycamtin®

Canadian Brand Names Hycamtin™

Pharmacologic Category Antineoplastic Agent, Natural Source (Plant) Derivative

Synonyms Hycamptamine; SK and F 104864; SKF 104864; SKF 104864-A; TOPO; Topotecan Hydrochloride; TPT

Use Treatment of metastatic carcinoma of the ovary after failure of initial or subsequent chemotherapy; second-line treatment of small cell lung cancer

Unlabeled/Investigational Use Investigational: Treatment of nonsmall cell lung cancer, sarcoma (pediatrics)

Local Anesthetic/Vasoconstrictor Precautions No information available to require special precautions

Effects on Dental Treatment No significant effects or complications reported

Dosage Adults: Refer to individual protocols.

Metastatic ovarian cancer and small cell lung cancer: IVPB: 1.5 mg/m²/day for 5 days; repeated every 21 days (neutrophil count should be >1500/mm³ and platelet count should be >100,000/mm³)

Dosing adjustment for hematological effects: If neutrophil count <1500/mm³, reduce dose by 0.25 mg/m²/day for 5 days for next cycle

Dosing adjustment in renal impairment:

- Cl_{cr} 20-39 mL/minute: Administer 50% of normal dose
- Cl_{cr} <20 mL/minute: Do not use; insufficient data

Hemodialysis: Supplemental dose is unnecessary

Dosing adjustment in hepatic impairment: Bilirubin 1.5-10 mg/dL: None

Mechanism of Action Inhibits topoisomerase I (an enzyme which relaxes torsionally strained-coiled duplex DNA) to prevent DNA replication and translocation; topotecan acts in S phase

Other Adverse Effects

>10%:

Central nervous system: Headache

Dermatologic: Alopecia (reversible)

Gastrointestinal: Nausea, vomiting, diarrhea

Emetic potential: Moderately low (10% to 30%)

(Continued)

Topotecan *(Continued)*

Hematologic: Myelosuppressive: Principle dose-limiting toxicity; white blood cell count nadir is 8-11 days after administration and is more frequent than thrombocytopenia (at lower doses); recover is usually within 21 days and cumulative toxicity has not been noted.

WBC: Mild to severe
Platelets: Mild (at low doses)
Nadir: 8-11 days
Recovery: 14-21 days

1% to 10%:

Neuromuscular & skeletal: Paresthesia
Respiratory: Dyspnea

<1%: Mild erythema and bruising

Drug Interactions Increased Effect/Toxicity: Concurrent administration of TPT and G-CSF in clinical trials results in severe myelosuppression. Concurrent *in vitro* exposure to TPT and the topoisomerase II inhibitor etoposide results in no altered effect; sequential exposure results in potentiation. Concurrent exposure to TPT and 5-azacytidine results in potentiation both *in vitro* and *in vivo*. Myelosuppression was more severe when given in combination with cisplatin.

Dietary/Ethanol/Herb Considerations Ethanol: Avoid use due to GI irritation.

Pharmacodynamics/Kinetics

Absorption: Oral: ~30%
Distribution: V_{dss} of the lactone is high (mean: 87.3 L/mm^2; range: 25.6-186 L/mm^2), suggesting wide distribution and/or tissue sequestering
Protein binding: 35%
Metabolism: Undergoes a rapid, pH-dependent opening of the lactone ring to yield a relatively inactive hydroxy acid in plasma
Half-life elimination: 3 hours
Excretion: Urine (30%) within 24 hours

Pregnancy Risk Factor D

Generic Available No

Topotecan Hydrochloride *see* Topotecan *on page 1325*
Toprol-XL® *see* Metoprolol *on page 901*
Toradol® *see* Ketorolac *on page 765*
Torecan® *see* Thiethylperazine *on page 1295*

Toremifene (TORE em i feen)

U.S. Brand Names Fareston®

Canadian Brand Names Fareston®

Mexican Brand Names Fareston®

Pharmacologic Category Antineoplastic Agent, Estrogen Receptor Antagonist

Synonyms FC1157a; Toremifene Citrate

Use Treatment of metastatic breast cancer in postmenopausal women with estrogen-receptor (ER) positive or ER unknown tumors

Local Anesthetic/Vasoconstrictor Precautions No information available to require special precautions

Effects on Dental Treatment No significant effects or complications reported

Dosage Refer to individual protocols.

Adults: Oral: 60 mg once daily, generally continued until disease progression is observed

Dosing adjustment in hepatic impairment: Specific guidelines unavailable; extensively metabolized in the liver

Mechanism of Action Nonsteroidal, triphenylethylene derivative. Competitively binds to estrogen receptors on tumors and other tissue targets, producing a nuclear complex that decreases DNA synthesis and inhibits estrogen effects. Nonsteroidal agent with potent antiestrogenic properties which compete with estrogen for binding sites in breast and other tissues; cells accumulate in the G_0 and G_1 phases; therefore, tamoxifen is cytostatic rather than cytocidal.

Other Adverse Effects

>10%:

Endocrine & metabolic: Vaginal discharge, hot flashes
Gastrointestinal: Nausea, vomiting
Miscellaneous: Diaphoresis

1% to 10%:

Cardiovascular: Thromboembolism: Tamoxifen has been associated with the occurrence of venous thrombosis and pulmonary embolism; arterial thrombosis has also been described in a few case reports; cardiac failure, MI, edema
Central nervous system: Dizziness
Endocrine & metabolic: Hypercalcemia may occur in patients with bone metastases; galactorrhea and vitamin deficiency, menstrual irregularities
Genitourinary: Vaginal bleeding or discharge, endometriosis, priapism, possible endometrial cancer

Ocular: Ophthalmologic effects (visual acuity changes, cataracts, or retinopathy), corneal opacities, dry eyes

Drug Interactions Substrate of CYP1A2, **3A4**

Increased Effect/Toxicity: Enzyme inhibitors (such as ketoconazole or erythromycin) may increase blood levels of toremifene. Concurrent therapy with warfarin results in significant enhancement of anticoagulant effects; has been speculated that a ↓ in antitumor effect of tamoxifen may also occur due to alterations in the percentage of active tamoxifen metabolites.

Decreased Effect: Phenobarbital, phenytoin, and carbamazepine increase the rate of toremifene metabolism and lower blood levels.

Pharmacodynamics/Kinetics

Absorption: Well absorbed

Distribution: V_d: 580 L

Protein binding, plasma: >99.5%, primarily to albumin

Metabolism: Extensively hepatic, principally by CYP3A4 to N-demethyltoremifene, which is also antiestrogenic but with weak *in vivo* antitumor potency

Half-life elimination: ~5 days

Time to peak, serum: ~3 hours

Excretion: Primarily feces; urine (10%) during a 1-week period

Pregnancy Risk Factor D

Generic Available No

Selected Readings

Gams R, "Phase III Trials of Toremifene vs Tamoxifen," *Oncology*, 1997, 11(5 Suppl 4): 23-8.

Hamm JT, "Phase I and II Studies of Toremifene," *Oncology*, 1997, 11(5 Suppl 4):19-22.

Holli K, "Evolving Role of Toremifene in the Adjuvant Setting," *Oncology*, 1997, 11(5 Suppl 4):48-51.

Kangas L, "Review of the Pharmacological Properties of Toremifene," *J Steroid Biochem*, 1990, 36(3):191-5.

Pyrhönen S, Valavaara R, Modig H, et al, "Comparison of Toremifene and Tamoxifen in Postmenopausal Patients With Advanced Breast Cancer: A Randomized Double-Blind, the "Nordic" Phase III Study," *Br J Cancer*, 1997, 76(2):270-7.

Williams GM and Jeffrey AM, "Safety Assessment of Tamoxifen and Toremifene," *Oncology*, 1997, 11(5 Suppl 4):41-7.

Toremifene Citrate *see* Toremifene *on page 1326*

Tornalate® [DSC] *see* Bitolterol *on page 189*

Torsemide (TOR se mide)

Related Information

Cardiovascular Diseases *on page 1456*

U.S. Brand Names Demadex®

Pharmacologic Category Diuretic, Loop

Use Management of edema associated with CHF and hepatic or renal disease; used alone or in combination with antihypertensives in treatment of hypertension; I.V. form is indicated when rapid onset is desired

Local Anesthetic/Vasoconstrictor Precautions No information available to require special precautions

Effects on Dental Treatment No significant effects or complications reported

Dosage Adults: Oral, I.V.:

Congestive heart failure: 10-20 mg once daily; may increase gradually for chronic treatment by doubling dose until the diuretic response is apparent (for acute treatment, I.V. dose may be repeated every 2 hours with double the dose as needed)

Chronic renal failure: 20 mg once daily; increase as described above

Hepatic cirrhosis: 5-10 mg once daily with an aldosterone antagonist or a potassium-sparing diuretic; increase as described above

Hypertension: 5 mg once daily; increase to 10 mg after 4-6 weeks if an adequate hypotensive response is not apparent; if still not effective, an additional antihypertensive agent may be added

Mechanism of Action Inhibits reabsorption of sodium and chloride in the ascending loop of Henle and distal renal tubule, interfering with the chloride-binding cotransport system, thus causing increased excretion of water, sodium, chloride, magnesium, and calcium; does not alter GFR, renal plasma flow, or acid-base balance

Other Adverse Effects

1% to 10%:

Cardiovascular: Edema (1.1%), EKG abnormality (2%), chest pain (1.2%)

Central nervous system: Headache (7.3%), dizziness (3.2%), insomnia (1.2%), nervousness (1%)

Endocrine & metabolic: Hyperglycemia, hyperuricemia, hypokalemia

Gastrointestinal: Diarrhea (2%), constipation (1.8%), nausea (1.8%), dyspepsia (1.6%), sore throat (1.6%)

Genitourinary: Excessive urination (6.7%)

Neuromuscular & skeletal: Weakness (2%), arthralgia (1.8%), myalgia (1.6%)

Respiratory: Rhinitis (2.8%), cough increase (2%)

<1% (Limited to important or life-threatening): Syncope, atrial fibrillation, hypotension, ventricular tachycardia, shunt thrombosis, hypovolemia, GI hemorrhage, rash, rectal bleeding, angioedema, hypernatremia

(Continued)

Torsemide *(Continued)*

Drug Interactions Substrate of **CYP2C8/9**; Inhibits CYP2C19

Increased Effect/Toxicity:

Torsemide-induced hypokalemia may predispose to digoxin toxicity and may increase the risk of arrhythmia with drugs which may prolong QT interval, including type Ia and type III antiarrhythmic agents, cisapride, and some quinolones (sparfloxacin, gatifloxacin, and moxifloxacin). The risk of toxicity from lithium and salicylates (high dose) may be increased by loop diuretics. Hypotensive effects and/or adverse renal effects of ACE inhibitors and NSAIDs are potentiated by bumetanide-induced hypovolemia. The effects of peripheral adrenergic-blocking drugs or ganglionic blockers may be increased by bumetanide.

Torsemide may increase the risk of ototoxicity with other ototoxic agents (aminoglycosides, cis-platinum), especially in patients with renal dysfunction. Synergistic diuretic effects occur with thiazide-type diuretics. Diuretics tend to be synergistic with other antihypertensive agents, and hypotension may occur.

Decreased Effect: Torsemide efficacy may be decreased with NSAIDs. Torsemide action may be reduced with probenecid. Diuretic action may be impaired in patients with cirrhosis and ascites if used with salicylates. Glucose tolerance may be decreased when used with sulfonylureas.

Dietary/Ethanol/Herb Considerations

Ethanol: Avoid use; may increase risk of hypotension or dizziness.

Food: May be taken with food or milk; increase intake of potassium-rich foods (eg, bananas and citrus fruits). Fluids, fruit, and fiber may reduce constipation. Avoid caffeine (eg, colas, chocolate), garlic, and licorice.

Herb/Nutraceutical: Avoid black cohosh, dong quai, and evening primrose due to estrogenic activity. Avoid ephedra, ginseng, and yohimbe; may worsen hypertension. Avoid garlic; may have increased antihypertensive effect. Avoid ginger due to positive inotropic effects; theoretically, may cause arrhythmia. Avoid hawthorn; may lower peripheral vascular resistance resulting in additive decrease in BP. Avoid licorice.

Pharmacodynamics/Kinetics

Onset of action: Diuresis: 30-60 minutes

Peak effect: 1-4 hours

Duration: ~6 hours

Absorption: Oral: Rapid

Protein binding, plasma: ~97% to 99%

Metabolism: Hepatic (80%) via CYP

Bioavailability: 80% to 90%

Half-life elimination: 2-4; Cirrhosis: 7-8 hours

Excretion: Urine (20% as unchanged drug)

Pregnancy Risk Factor B

Generic Available Yes: Tablet

Touro™ Allergy *see* Brompheniramine and Pseudoephedrine *on page 201*

Touro™ CC *see* Guaifenesin, Pseudoephedrine, and Dextromethorphan *on page 653*

Touro® DM *see* Guaifenesin and Dextromethorphan *on page 651*

Touro Ex® *see* Guaifenesin *on page 650*

Touro LA® *see* Guaifenesin and Pseudoephedrine *on page 652*

tPA *see* Alteplase *on page 65*

T-Phyl® *see* Theophylline *on page 1291*

TPT *see* Topotecan *on page 1325*

Trace Metals (trase MET als)

U.S. Brand Names Iodopen®; Molypen®; M.T.E.-4®; M.T.E.-5®; M.T.E.-6®; M.T.E.-7®; Multitrace™-4; Multitrace™-4 Neonatal; Multitrace™-4 Pediatric; Multitrace™-5; Neotrace-4®; Pedtrace-4®; P.T.E.-4®; P.T.E.-5®; Selepen®

Pharmacologic Category Trace Element, Parenteral

Synonyms Chromium; Copper; Iodine; Manganese; Molybdenum; Neonatal Trace Metals; Selenium; Zinc

Use Prevention and correction of trace metal deficiencies

Local Anesthetic/Vasoconstrictor Precautions No information available to require special precautions

Effects on Dental Treatment No significant effects or complications reported

Dosage Recommended daily parenteral dosage: See table on next page.

Dietary/Ethanol/Herb Considerations Food: Administration with bran products, protein, and phytates decreases absorption of oral zinc.

Pregnancy Risk Factor C

Generic Available Yes

Comments Persistent diarrhea or excessive GI fluid losses from ostomy sites may grossly increase zinc losses

Recommended Daily Parenteral Dosage

	Infants	Children	Adults
Chromium[1]	0.2 mcg/kg	0.2 mcg/kg (max: 5 mcg)	10-15 mcg
Copper[2]	20 mcg/kg	20 mcg/kg (max: 300 mcg)	0.5-1.5 mg
Manganese[2,3]	1 mcg/kg	1 mcg/kg (max: 50 mcg)	150-800 mcg
Molybdenum[1,4]	0.25 mcg/kg	0.25 mcg/kg (max: 5 mcg)	20-120 mcg
Selenium[1,4]	2 mcg/kg	2 mcg/kg (max: 30 mcg)	20-40 mcg
Zinc			
preterm	400 mcg/kg	50 mcg/kg (max: 5 mg)	2.5-4 mg
term <3 mo	250 mcg/kg		
term >3 mo	100 mcg/kg		

[1]Omit in patients with renal dysfunction.
[2]Omit in patients with obstructive jaundice.
[3]Current available commercial products are not in appropriate ratios to maintain this recommendation — doses of up to 10 mcg/kg have been used.
[4]Indicated for use in long-term parenteral nutrition patients.

Tracleer™ *see* Bosentan *on page 192*

Tramadol (TRA ma dole)

U.S. Brand Names Ultram®

Canadian Brand Names Ultram®

Mexican Brand Names Nobligan®; Prontofort®; Tradol®

Pharmacologic Category Analgesic, Non-narcotic

Synonyms Tramadol Hydrochloride

Use Dental and Medical: Relief of moderate to moderately severe pain

Local Anesthetic/Vasoconstrictor Precautions No information available to require special precautions

Effects on Dental Treatment

>10%: Xerostomia, changes in salivation, dizziness, headache, somnolence, nausea

1% to 10%: Vasodilation, agitation, anxiety, confusion, nervousness, hallucinations, tremor, vomiting, diaphoresis, euphoria, incoordination, malaise, visual disturbance, hypertonia, spasticity, weakness

Dosage Oral:

Adults: Moderate to severe chronic pain: 50-100 mg every 4-6 hours, not to exceed 400 mg/day

For patients not requiring rapid onset of effect, tolerability may be improved by starting dose at 25 mg/day and titrating dose by 25 mg every 3 days, until reaching 25 mg 4 times/day. Dose may then be increased by 50 mg every 3 days as tolerated, to reach dose of 50 mg 4 times/day.

Elderly: >75 years: 50-100 mg every 4-6 hours (not to exceed 300 mg/day); see dosing adjustments for renal and hepatic impairment

Dosing adjustment in renal impairment: Cl_{cr} <30 mL/minute: Administer 50-100 mg dose every 12 hours (maximum: 200 mg/day)

Dosing adjustment in hepatic impairment: Cirrhosis: Recommended dose: 50 mg every 12 hours

Mechanism of Action Binds to μ-opiate receptors in the CNS causing inhibition of ascending pain pathways, altering the perception of and response to pain; also inhibits the reuptake of norepinephrine and serotonin, which also modifies the ascending pain pathway

Other Adverse Effects Incidence may increase over time.

>10%:

Central nervous system: Vertigo

Gastrointestinal: Constipation

1% to 10%:

Central nervous system: Emotional lability, sleep disorder

Dermatologic: Pruritus, rash

Endocrine & metabolic: Menopausal symptoms

Gastrointestinal: Abdominal pain, anorexia, diarrhea, dyspepsia, flatulence

Genitourinary: Urinary frequency, urinary retention

Ocular: Miosis

<1%: **Abnormal gait, allergic reaction, amnesia, anaphylactoid reactions, anaphylaxis**, angioedema, **bronchospasm, cognitive dysfunction, concentration difficulty, death**, depression, **dyspnea**, dysuria, **hallucinations**, menstrual disorder, **orthostatic hypotension, paresthesia, seizure, serotonin syndrome, suicidal tendency, syncope, abnormal taste, tachycardia**,

(Continued)

Tramadol *(Continued)*

Stevens-Johnson syndrome, toxic epidermal necrolysis, **tremor**, urticaria, vesicles, weight loss

Postmarketing and/or case reports: **Abnormal EKG**, cataracts, creatinine increased, deafness, **GI bleeding**, hemoglobin decreased, hepatitis, **hypertension, hypotension**, liver enzymes elevated, liver failure, **migraine, speech disorders, stomatitis, palpitations**, proteinuria, pulmonary edema, pulmonary embolism, myocardial ischemia, tinnitus

Contraindications Hypersensitivity to tramadol, opioids, or any component of the formulation; opioid-dependent patients; acute intoxication with alcohol, hypnotics, centrally-acting analgesics, opioids, or psychotropic drugs

Warnings/Precautions Should be used only with extreme caution in patients receiving MAO inhibitors. May cause CNS depression and/or respiratory depression, particularly when combined with other CNS depressants. Use with caution and reduce dosage when administered to patients receiving other CNS depressants. An increased risk of seizures may occur in patients receiving serotonin reuptake inhibitors (SSRIs or anorectics), tricyclic antidepressants, other cyclic compounds (including cyclobenzaprine, promethazine), neuroleptics, MAO inhibitors, or drugs which may lower seizure threshold. Patients with a history of seizures, or with a risk of seizures (head trauma, metabolic disorders, CNS infection, or malignancy, or during ethanol/drug withdrawal) are also at increased risk.

Elderly patients and patients with chronic respiratory disorders may be at greater risk of adverse events. Use with caution in patients with increased intracranial pressure or head injury. Use tramadol with caution and reduce dosage in patients with liver disease or renal dysfunction and in patients with myxedema, hypothyroidism, or hypoadrenalism. Not recommended during pregnancy or in nursing mothers. Tolerance or drug dependence may result from extended use; abrupt discontinuation should be avoided. Safety and efficacy in pediatric patients have not been established.

Drug Interactions Substrate of **CYP2D6**, 3A4

Amphetamines: May increase the risk of seizures with tramadol.

Carbamazepine: Decreases half-life of tramadol by 33% to 50%.

CYP2D6 inhibitors: May increase tramadol serum concentrations.

Digoxin: Rare reports of digoxin toxicity with concomitant tramadol use.

Linezolid: May be associated with increased risk of seizures (due to MAO inhibition)

MAO inhibitors: May increases the risk of seizures.

Naloxone: May increase the risk of seizures (if administered in tramadol overdose)

Neuroleptic agents: May increase the risk of tramadol-associated seizures and may have additive CNS depressant effects.

Opioids: May increase the risk of seizures, and may have additive CNS depressant effects.

Quinidine: May increase the tramadol serum concentrations.

Selegiline: An increased risk of seizures has been associated with MAO inhibitors. It is not clear if drugs with selective MAO type B inhibition are safer than nonselective agents.

SSRIs: May increase the risk of seizures with tramadol. Includes citalopram, fluoxetine, paroxetine, sertraline.

Tricyclic antidepressants: May increase the risk of seizures.

Warfarin: Concomitant use may lead to an elevation of prothrombin times; monitor.

Dietary/Ethanol/Herb Considerations

Ethanol: Avoid use; may increase CNS depression.

Food: May be taken with food; absorption unaffected. Fluids, fruit, and fiber may reduce constipation.

Herb/Nutraceutical: Avoid gotu kola, kava, SAMe, St John's wort, and valerian; may increase CNS depression.

Pharmacodynamics/Kinetics

Onset of action: ~1 hour

Duration of action: 9 hours

Absorption: Rapid and complete

Distribution: V_d: 2.5-3 L/kg

Protein binding, plasma: 20%

Metabolism: Extensively hepatic via demethylation, glucuronidation, and sulfation; has pharmacologically active metabolite formed by CYP2D6

Bioavailability: 75%

Half-life elimination: Tramadol: ~6 hours; Active metabolite: 7 hours; prolonged in elderly, hepatic or renal impairment

Time to peak: 2 hours

Excretion: Urine (as metabolites)

Pregnancy Risk Factor C

Breast-feeding Considerations Not recommended for postdelivery analgesia in nursing mothers.

Dosage Forms TAB: 50 mg

Generic Available Yes

Comments Literature reports suggest that the efficacy of tramadol in oral surgery pain is equivalent to the combination of aspirin and codeine. One study (Olson et al 1990) showed acetaminophen and dextropropoxyphene combination to be superior to tramadol and another study showed tramadol to be superior to acetaminophen and dextropropoxyphene combination. Tramadol appears to be at least equal to if not better than codeine alone. Seizures have been reported with the use of tramadol.

Selected Readings

Collins M, Young I, Sweeney P, et al, "The Effect of Tramadol on Dento-Alveolar Surgical Pain," *Br J Oral Maxillofac Surg*, 1997, 35(1):54-8.

Kahn LH, Alderfer RJ, and Graham DJ, "Seizures Reported With Tramadol," *JAMA*, 1997, 278(20):1661.

Lewis KS and Han NH, "Tramadol: A New Centrally Acting Analgesic," *Am J Health Syst Pharm*, 1997, 54(6):643-52.

Sunshine A, "New Clinical Experience With Tramadol," *Drugs*, 1994, 47(Suppl 1):8-18.

Sunshine A, Olson NZ, Zighelboim I, et al, "Analgesic Oral Efficacy of Tramadol Hydrochloride in Postoperative Pain," *Clin Pharmacol Ther*, 1992; 51(6):740-6.

Wynn RL, "Tramadol (Ultram) - A New Kind of Analgesic," *Gen Dent*, 1996, 44(3):216-8,220.

Tramadol Hydrochloride *see* Tramadol *on page 1329*

Tramadol Hydrochloride and Acetaminophen *see* Acetaminophen and Tramadol *on page 32*

Trandate® *see* Labetalol *on page 769*

Trandolapril (tran DOE la pril)

U.S. Brand Names Mavik®

Canadian Brand Names Mavik™

Mexican Brand Names Gopten®

Pharmacologic Category Angiotensin-Converting Enzyme (ACE) Inhibitor

Use Management of hypertension alone or in combination with other antihypertensive agents; treatment of left ventricular dysfunction after MI

Unlabeled/Investigational Use As a class, ACE inhibitors are recommended in the treatment of systolic CHF

Local Anesthetic/Vasoconstrictor Precautions No information available to require special precautions

Effects on Dental Treatment No significant effects or complications reported

Dosage Adults: Oral:

Hypertension: Initial dose in patients not receiving a diuretic: 1 mg/day (2 mg/day in black patients). Adjust dosage according to the blood pressure response. Make dosage adjustments at intervals of ≥1 week. Most patients have required dosages of 2-4 mg/day. There is a little experience with doses >8 mg/day. Patients inadequately treated with once daily dosing at 4 mg may be treated with twice daily dosing. If blood pressure is not adequately controlled with trandolapril monotherapy, a diuretic may be added.

Heart failure postmyocardial infarction or left ventricular dysfunction postmyocardial infarction: Initial: 1 mg/day; titrate patients (as tolerated) towards the target dose of 4 mg/day. If a 4 mg dose is not tolerated, patients can continue therapy with the greatest tolerated dose.

Dosing adjustment in renal impairment: Cl_{cr} ≤30 mL/minute: Recommended starting dose: 0.5 mg/day.

Dosing adjustment in hepatic impairment: Cirrhosis: Recommended starting dose: 0.5 mg/day.

Mechanism of Action Trandolapril is an ACE inhibitor which prevents the formation of angiotensin II from angiotensin I. Trandolapril must undergo enzymatic hydrolysis, mainly in liver, to its biologically active metabolite, trandolaprilat. A CNS mechanism may also be involved in the hypotensive effect as angiotensin II increases adrenergic outflow from the CNS. Vasoactive kallikrein's may be decreased in conversion to active hormones by ACE inhibitors, thus, reducing blood pressure.

Other Adverse Effects Note: Frequency ranges include data from hypertension and heart failure trials. Higher rates of adverse reactions have generally been noted in patients with CHF. However, the frequency of adverse effects associated with placebo is also increased in this population.

>1%:

Cardiovascular: Hypotension (<1% to 11%), bradycardia (<1% to 4.7%), intermittent claudication (3.8%), stroke (3.3%)

Central nervous system: Dizziness (1.3% to 23%), syncope (5.9%), asthenia (3.3%)

Endocrine & metabolic: Elevated uric acid (15%), hyperkalemia (5.3%), hypocalcemia (4.7%)

Gastrointestinal: Dyspepsia (6.4%), gastritis (4.2%)

Neuromuscular & skeletal: Myalgia (4.7%)

Renal: Elevated BUN (9%), elevated serum creatinine (1.1% to 4.7%) Respiratory: Cough (1.9% to 35%)

<1% (Limited to important or life-threatening): Chest pain, AV block (first-degree), edema, flushing, palpitations, drowsiness, insomnia, paresthesia, vertigo, pruritus, rash, pemphigus, epistaxis, pharyngitis, upper respiratory tract infection,

(Continued)

Trandolapril *(Continued)*

anxiety, impotence, decreased libido, abdominal distension, abdominal pain, constipation, dyspepsia, diarrhea, vomiting, pancreatitis, leukopenia, neutropenia, thrombocytopenia, increased serum creatinine, increased ALT, muscle pain, gout, dyspnea, angioedema, laryngeal edema, symptomatic hypotension, transaminase elevation, increased bilirubin. Worsening of renal function may occur in patients with bilateral renal artery stenosis or in hypovolemic patients. In addition, a syndrome which may include fever, myalgia, arthralgia, interstitial nephritis, vasculitis, rash, eosinophilia and positive ANA, and elevated ESR has been reported with ACE inhibitors.

Drug Interactions

Increased Effect/Toxicity: Potassium supplements, co-trimoxazole (high dose), angiotensin II receptor antagonists (candesartan, losartan, irbesartan, etc), or potassium-sparing diuretics (amiloride, spironolactone, triamterene) may result in elevated serum potassium levels when combined with trandolapril. ACE inhibitor effects may be increased by phenothiazines or probenecid (increases levels of captopril). ACE inhibitors may increase serum concentrations/effects of digoxin, lithium, and sulfonlyureas.

Diuretics have additive hypotensive effects with ACE inhibitors, and hypovolemia increases the potential for adverse renal effects of ACE inhibitors. In patients with compromised renal function, coadministration with NSAIDs may result in further deterioration of renal function. Allopurinol and ACE inhibitors may cause a higher risk of hypersensitivity reaction when taken concurrently.

Decreased Effect: Aspirin (high dose) may reduce the therapeutic effects of ACE inhibitors; at low dosages this does not appear to be significant. Rifampin may decrease the effect of ACE inhibitors. Antacids may decrease the bioavailability of ACE inhibitors (may be more likely to occur with captopril); separate administration times by 1-2 hours. NSAIDs, specifically indomethacin, may reduce the hypotensive effects of ACE inhibitors. More likely to occur in low renin or volume dependent hypertensive patients.

Dietary/Ethanol/Herb Considerations

Ethanol: Avoid use; may increase risk of hypotension or dizziness.

Food: Avoid caffeine (eg, colas, chocolate), garlic, and licorice.

Herb/Nutraceutical: Avoid black cohosh, dong quai, and evening primrose due to estrogenic activity. Avoid ephedra, ginseng, and yohimbe; may worsen hypertension. Avoid garlic; may have increased antihypertensive effect. Avoid ginger due to positive inotropic effects; theoretically, may cause arrhythmia. Avoid hawthorn; may lower peripheral vascular resistance causing additional decrease in BP. Avoid licorice.

Pharmacodynamics/Kinetics

Onset of action: 1-2 hours

Peak effect: Reduction in blood pressure: 6 hours

Duration: Prolonged; 72 hours after single dose

Absorption: Rapid

Distribution: Trandolaprilat (active metabolite) is very lipophilic in comparison to other ACE inhibitors

Protein binding: 80%

Metabolism: Hepatically hydrolyzed to active metabolite, trandolaprilat

Half-life elimination:

Trandolapril: 6 hours; Trandolaprilat: Effective: 10 hours, Terminal: 24 hours

Elimination: As metabolites in urine;

Time to peak: Parent: 1 hour; Active metabolite trandolaprilat: 4-10 hours

Excretion: Urine (as metabolites)

Clearance: Reduce dose in renal failure; creatinine clearances ≤30 mL/minute result in accumulation of active metabolite

Pregnancy Risk Factor C/D (2nd and 3rd trimesters)

Generic Available No

Selected Readings

Bevan EG, McInnes GT, Aldigier JC, et al, "Effect of Renal Function on the Pharmacokinetics and Pharmacodynamics of Trandolapril," *Br J Clin Pharmacol*, 1993, 35(2):128-35.

Conen H and Brunner HR, "Pharmacologic Profile of Trandolapril, A New Angiotensin-Converting Enzyme Inhibitor," *Am J Heart*, 1993, 125(5 Pt 2):1524-31.

Zannad F, "Trandolapril. How Does It Differ From Other Angiotensin-Converting Enzyme Inhibitors?" *Drugs*, 1993, 46(Suppl 2):172-81.

Trandolapril and Verapamil (tran DOE la pril & ver AP a mil)

Related Information

Trandolapril *on page 1331*

Verapamil *on page 1382*

U.S. Brand Names Tarka®

Canadian Brand Names Tarka®

Pharmacologic Category Antihypertensive Agent Combination

Synonyms Verapamil and Trandolapril

Use Combination drug for the treatment of hypertension, however, not indicated for initial treatment of hypertension; replacement therapy in patients receiving separate dosage forms (for patient convenience); when monotherapy with one component fails to achieve desired antihypertensive effect, or when dose-limiting adverse effects limit upward titration of monotherapy

Local Anesthetic/Vasoconstrictor Precautions No information available to require special precautions

Effects on Dental Treatment No significant effects or complications reported

Dosage Dose is individualized

Dietary/Ethanol/Herb Considerations Based on verapamil component:

Ethanol: Avoid use; may increase risk of hypotension or dizziness.

Food: Avoid caffeine (eg, colas, chocolate), garlic, and licorice.

Herb/Nutraceutical: Avoid black cohosh, dong quai, and evening primrose due to estrogenic activity. Avoid ephedra, ginseng, and yohimbe; may worsen hypertension. Avoid garlic; may have increased antihypertensive effect. Avoid ginger due to positive inotropic effects; theoretically, may cause arrhythmia. Avoid hawthorn; may lower peripheral vascular resistance causing additional decrease in BP. Avoid licorice.

Pregnancy Risk Factor C/D (2nd and 3rd trimesters)

Generic Available No

Tranexamic Acid (tran eks AM ik AS id)

U.S. Brand Names Cyklokapron®

Canadian Brand Names Cyklokapron®

Pharmacologic Category Antihemophilic Agent

Use Short-term use (2-8 days) in hemophilia patients during and following tooth extraction to reduce or prevent hemorrhage

Unlabeled/Investigational Use Alternative to aminocaproic acid for subarachnoid hemorrhage

Local Anesthetic/Vasoconstrictor Precautions No information available to require special precautions

Effects on Dental Treatment No significant effects or complications reported

Dosage Children and Adults: I.V.: 10 mg/kg immediately before surgery, then 25 mg/kg/dose orally 3-4 times/day for 2-8 days

Alternatively:

Oral: 25 mg/kg 3-4 times/day beginning 1 day prior to surgery

I.V.: 10 mg/kg 3-4 times/day in patients who are unable to take oral

Dosing adjustment in renal impairment:

Cl_{cr} 50-80 mL/minute: Administer 50% of normal dose or 10 mg/kg twice daily I.V. or 15 mg/kg twice daily orally

Cl_{cr} 10-50 mL/minute: Administer 25% of normal dose or 10 mg/kg/day I.V. or 15 mg/kg/day orally

Cl_{cr} <10 mL/minute: Administer 10% of normal dose or 10 mg/kg/dose every 48 hours I.V. or 15 mg/kg/dose every 48 hours orally

Mechanism of Action Forms a reversible complex that displaces plasminogen from fibrin resulting in inhibition of fibrinolysis; it also inhibits the proteolytic activity of plasmin

Other Adverse Effects

>10%: Gastrointestinal: Nausea, diarrhea, vomiting

1% to 10%:

Cardiovascular: Hypotension, thrombosis

Ocular: Blurred vision

<1%: Unusual menstrual discomfort

Postmarketing and/or case reports: Deep venous thrombosis (DVT), pulmonary embolus (PE), renal cortical necrosis, retinal artery obstruction, retinal vein obstruction, ureteral obstruction

Drug Interactions Increased Effect/Toxicity: Chlorpromazine may increase cerebral vasospasm and ischemia. Coadministrations of Factor IX complex or anti-inhibitor coagulant concentrates may increase risk of thrombosis.

Pharmacodynamics/Kinetics

Half-life elimination: 2-10 hours

Excretion: Urine (>90% as unchanged drug)

Pregnancy Risk Factor B

Generic Available No

Comments Antifibrinolytic drugs are useful for the control of bleeding after dental extractions in patients with hemophilia because the oral mucosa and saliva are rich in plasminogen activators. In a clinical trial, tranexamic acid reduced recurrent bleeding and the amount of clotting-factor-replacement therapy needed. In adults, the oral dose was 20-25 mg/kg tranexamic acid every 8 hours until the dental sockets were completely healed. Mouthwashes containing tranexamic acid are effective for preventing oral bleeding in patients with hemophilia and in patients requiring dental extraction while receiving long-term oral anticoagulant therapy.

Immediately before dental extraction in hemophilic patients, administer 10 mg/kg tranexamic acid I.V. together with replacement therapy. Following surgery, a dose of 25 mg/kg may be given orally 3-4 times/day for 2-8 days.

(Continued)

Tranexamic Acid *(Continued)*

Selected Readings

Mannucci PM, "Hemostatic Drugs," *N Eng J Med*, 1998, 339(4):245-53.

Sindet-Pedersen S, "Distribution of Tranexamic Acid to Plasma and Saliva After Oral Administration and Mouth Rinsing: A Pharmacokinetic Study," *J Clin Pharmacol*, 1987, 27(12):1005-8.

Sindet-Pedersen S, Ramstron G, Bernvil S, et al, "Hemostatic Effect of Tranexamic Acid Mouthwash in Anticoagulant-Treated Patients Undergoing Oral Surgery," *N Engl J Med*, 1989, 320(13):840-3.

Transamine Sulphate *see* Tranylcypromine *on page 1334*

Transderm Scōp® *see* Scopolamine *on page 1210*

***trans*-Retinoic Acid** *see* Tretinoin (Topical) *on page 1340*

Trans-Ver-Sal® [OTC] *see* Salicylic Acid *on page 1204*

Tranxene® *see* Clorazepate *on page 355*

Tranylcypromine (tran il SIP roe meen)

U.S. Brand Names Parnate®

Canadian Brand Names Parnate®

Pharmacologic Category Antidepressant, Monoamine Oxidase Inhibitor

Synonyms Transamine Sulphate; Tranylcypromine Sulfate

Use Treatment of major depressive episode without melancholia

Unlabeled/Investigational Use Treatment of post-traumatic stress disorder

Local Anesthetic/Vasoconstrictor Precautions Attempts should be made to avoid use of vasoconstrictor due to possibility of hypertensive episodes with monoamine oxidase inhibitors

Effects on Dental Treatment >10%: Orthostatic hypotension

Avoid use as an analgesic due to toxic reactions with MAO inhibitors.

Dosage Oral:

Adults: 10 mg twice daily, increase by 10 mg increments at 1- to 3-week intervals; maximum: 60 mg/day

Dosing comments in hepatic impairment: Use with care and monitor plasma levels and patient response closely

Mechanism of Action Thought to act by increasing endogenous concentrations of epinephrine, norepinephrine, dopamine and serotonin through inhibition of the enzyme (monoamine oxidase) responsible for the breakdown of these neurotransmitters

Other Adverse Effects Frequency not defined:

Cardiovascular: Edema

Central nervous system: Dizziness, headache, drowsiness, sleep disturbances, fatigue, hyper-reflexia, twitching, ataxia, mania, akinesia, confusion, disorientation, memory loss

Dermatologic: Rash, pruritus, urticaria, localized scleroderma, cystic acne (flare), alopecia

Endocrine & metabolic: Sexual dysfunction (anorgasmia, ejaculatory disturbances, impotence), hypernatremia, hypermetabolic syndrome, SIADH

Gastrointestinal: **Xerostomia**, constipation, weight gain

Genitourinary: Urinary retention, incontinence

Hematologic: Leukopenia, agranulocytosis

Hepatic: Hepatitis

Neuromuscular & skeletal: Weakness, tremor, myoclonus

Ocular: Blurred vision, glaucoma

Miscellaneous: Diaphoresis

Drug Interactions Inhibits CYP1A2, **2A6**, 2C8/9, 2C19, 2D6, 2E1, 3A4

Increased Effect/Toxicity: In general, the combined use of tranylcypromine with TCAs, venlafaxine, trazodone, dexfenfluramine, sibutramine, lithium, meperidine, fenfluramine, dextromethorphan, and SSRIs should be avoided due to the potential for severe adverse reactions (serotonin syndrome, death). Tranylcypromine in combination with amphetamines, other stimulants (methylphenidate), levodopa, metaraminol, buspirone, bupropion, reserpine, and decongestants (pseudoephedrine) may result in severe hypertensive reactions. MAO inhibitors (including tranylcypromine) may inhibit the metabolism of barbiturates and prolong their effect. Foods (eg, cheese) and beverages (eg, ethanol) containing tyramine should be avoided; hypertensive crisis may result. Tranylcypromine may increase the pressor response of norepinephrine and may prolong neuromuscular blockade produced by succinylcholine. Tramadol may increase the risk of seizures and serotonin syndrome in patients receiving an MAO inhibitor. Tranylcypromine may produce additive hypoglycemic effect in patients receiving hypoglycemic agents and may produce delirium in patients receiving disulfiram. Tryptophan combined use with an MAO inhibitor has been reported to cause disorientation, confusion, anxiety, delirium, agitation, hypomanic signs, ataxia, and myoclonus; concurrent use is contraindicated.

Decreased Effect: Tranylcypromine inhibits the antihypertensive response to guanadrel or guanethidine.

Dietary/Ethanol/Herb Considerations

Ethanol: Avoid use; many contain tyramine (eg, wine).

Food: Avoid food/beverages high in tyramine (eg, avocadoes, bananas, broad bean pods, canned figs, cheese, chicken liver, pickled herring, raisins, sour cream, soy sauce, yeast extracts, yogurt, pods, meats prepared with tenderizers, and foods aged to improve flavor); may cause sudden and severe high BP. Avoid foods containing tryptophan or dopamine, chocolate or caffeine. Boiled milk, buttermilk, or yogurt may reduce diarrhea. Fluids, fruit, and fiber may reduce constipation. Avoid caffeine.

Herb/Nutraceutical: Avoid ephedra, ginseng, and yohimbe; may cause hypertension. Avoid ginkgo biloba (may lead to MAO inhibitor toxicity), SAMe, St John's wort, and valerian.

Pharmacodynamics/Kinetics

Onset of action: Therapeutic: 2-3 weeks continued dosing

Half-life elimination: 90-190 minutes

Time to peak, serum: ~2 hours

Excretion: Urine

Pregnancy Risk Factor C

Generic Available No

Tranylcypromine Sulfate *see* Tranylcypromine *on page 1334*

Trastuzumab (tras TU zoo mab)

U.S. Brand Names Herceptin®

Canadian Brand Names Herceptin®

Pharmacologic Category Monoclonal Antibody

Use

Single agent for the treatment of patients with metastatic breast cancer whose tumors overexpress the HER-2/*neu* protein and who have received one or more chemotherapy regimens for their metastatic disease

Combination therapy with paclitaxel for the treatment of patients with metastatic breast cancer whose tumors overexpress the HER-2/*neu* protein and who have not received chemotherapy for their metastatic disease

Note: HER-2/*neu* protein overexpression or amplification has been noted in ovarian, gastric, colorectal, endometrial, lung, bladder, prostate, and salivary gland tumors. It is not yet known whether trastuzumab may be effective in these other carcinomas which overexpress HER-2/*neu* protein.

Local Anesthetic/Vasoconstrictor Precautions No information available to require special precautions

Effects on Dental Treatment No significant effects or complications reported

Dosage I.V. infusion:

Adults:

Initial loading dose: 4 mg/kg intravenous infusion over 90 minutes

Maintenance dose: 2 mg/kg intravenous infusion over 90 minutes (can be administered over 30 minutes if prior infusions are well tolerated) weekly until disease progression

Dosing adjustment in renal impairment: Data suggest that the disposition of trastuzumab is not altered based on age or serum creatinine (up to 2 mg/dL); however, no formal interaction studies have been performed

Dosing adjustment in hepatic impairment: Data unavailable

Mechanism of Action Trastuzumab is a monoclonal antibody which binds to the extracellular domain of the human epidermal growth factor receptor 2 protein (HER2); it mediates antibody-dependent cellular cytotoxicity against cells which overproduce HER2

Other Adverse Effects

>10%:

Central nervous system: Pain (47%), fever (36%), chills (32%), headache (26%)

Dermatologic: Rash (18%)

Gastrointestinal: Nausea (33%), diarrhea (25%), vomiting (23%), abdominal pain (22%), anorexia (14%)

Neuromuscular & skeletal: Weakness (42%), back pain (22%)

Respiratory: Cough (26%), dyspnea (22%), rhinitis (14%), pharyngitis (12%)

Miscellaneous: Infection (20%)

1% to 10%:

Cardiovascular: Peripheral edema (10%), CHF (7%), tachycardia (5%)

Central nervous system: Insomnia (14%), dizziness (13%), paresthesia (9%), depression (6%), peripheral neuritis (2%), neuropathy (1%)

Dermatologic: Herpes simplex (2%), acne (2%)

Gastrointestinal: Nausea and vomiting (8%)

Genitourinary: Urinary tract infection (5%)

Hematologic: Anemia (4%), leukopenia (3%)

Neuromuscular & skeletal: Bone pain (7%), arthralgia (6%)

Respiratory: Sinusitis (9%)

Miscellaneous: Flu syndrome (10%), accidental injury (6%), allergic reaction (3%)

<1%: **Adult respiratory distress syndrome (ARDS)**, amblyopia, anaphylaxis, anaphylactoid reaction, angioedema, **arrhythmia, bronchospasm, cardiac arrest**, cellulitis, coagulopathy, colitis, deafness, **esophageal ulcer**, ascites, gastroenteritis, hematemesis, hemorrhage, hemorrhagic cystitis, hepatic failure,

(Continued)

Trastuzumab *(Continued)*

hepatitis, hydrocephalus, hydronephrosis, hypotension, hypothyroidism, ileus, intestinal obstruction, leukemia (acute), lymphangitis, pancreatitis, pancytopenia, pericardial effusion, pyelonephritis, radiation injury, renal failure, **respiratory distress**, severe infusion reaction, shock, syncope, stomatitis, vascular thrombosis

Drug Interactions Increased Effect/Toxicity: Paclitaxel may result in a decrease in clearance of trastuzumab, increasing serum concentrations.

Pharmacodynamics/Kinetics

Distribution: V_d: 44 mL/kg

Half-life elimination: Mean: 5.8 days (range: 1-32 days)

Pregnancy Risk Factor B

Generic Available No

Trasylol® *see* Aprotinin *on page 119*

Travatan® *see* Travoprost *on page 1336*

Travoprost (TRA voe prost)

U.S. Brand Names Travatan®

Canadian Brand Names Travatan®

Mexican Brand Names Travatan®

Pharmacologic Category Prostaglandin, Ophthalmic

Use Reduction of elevated intraocular pressure in patients with open-angle glaucoma or ocular hypertension who are intolerant of the other IOP-lowering medications or insufficiently responsive (failed to achieve target IOP determined after multiple measurements over time) to another IOP-lowering medication

Local Anesthetic/Vasoconstrictor Precautions No information available to require special precautions

Effects on Dental Treatment No significant effects or complications reported

Dosage Ophthalmic: Adults: Glaucoma (open angle) or ocular hypertension: Instill 1 drop into affected eye(s) once daily in the evening; do not exceed once-daily dosing (may decrease IOP-lowering effect). If used with other topical ophthalmic agents, separate administration by at least 5 minutes.

Mechanism of Action A selective FP prostanoid receptor agonist which lowers intraocular pressure by increasing outflow

Other Adverse Effects

>10%: Ocular: Hyperemia (35% to 50%)

5% to 10%: Ocular: Decreased visual acuity, eye discomfort, foreign body sensation, pain, pruritus

1% to 5%:

Cardiovascular: Angina pectoris, bradycardia, hypotension, hypertension

Central nervous system: Depression, pain, anxiety, headache

Endocrine & metabolic: Hypercholesterolemia

Gastrointestinal: Dyspepsia

Genitourinary: Prostate disorder, urinary incontinence

Neuromuscular & skeletal: Arthritis, back pain, chest pain

Ocular (1% to 4%): Abnormal vision, blepharitis, blurred vision, conjunctivitis, dry eye, iris discoloration, keratitis, lid margin crusting, photophobia, subconjunctival hemorrhage, cataract, tearing, periorbital skin discoloration (darkening), eyelash darkening, eyelash growth increased

Respiratory: Bronchitis, sinusitis

Postmarketing and/or case reports: Bacterial keratitis (due to solution contamination)

Pharmacodynamics/Kinetics

Onset of action: ~2 hours

Peak effect: 12 hours

Duration: Plasma levels decrease to <10 pg/mL within 1 hour

Absorption: Absorbed via cornea

Metabolism: Hydrolyzed by esterases in the cornea to active free acid; systemically; the free acid is metabolized to inactive metabolites

Pregnancy Risk Factor C

Generic Available No

Trazodone (TRAZ oh done)

U.S. Brand Names Desyrel®

Canadian Brand Names Alti-Trazodone; Apo®-Trazodone; Apo®-Trazodone D; Desyrel®; Gen-Trazodone; Novo-Trazodone; Nu-Trazodone; PMS-Trazodone

Pharmacologic Category Antidepressant, Serotonin Reuptake Inhibitor/Antagonist

Synonyms Trazodone Hydrochloride

Use Treatment of depression

Unlabeled/Investigational Use Potential augmenting agent for antidepressants; hypnotic

Local Anesthetic/Vasoconstrictor Precautions No information available to require special precautions

Effects on Dental Treatment >10%: Xerostomia (especially in the elderly; may contribute to periodontal diseases and oral discomfort)

Trazodone elicits anticholinergic effects; much less frequent than with tricyclic antidepressants.

Dosage Oral: Therapeutic effects may take up to 6 weeks to occur; therapy is normally maintained for 6-12 months after optimum response is reached to prevent recurrence of depression

Children 6-12 years: Depression: Initial: 1.5-2 mg/kg/day in divided doses; increase gradually every 3-4 days as needed; maximum: 6 mg/kg/day in 3 divided doses

Adolescents: Depression: Initial: 25-50 mg/day; increase to 100-150 mg/day in divided doses

Adults:

Depression: Initial: 150 mg/day in 3 divided doses (may increase by 50 mg/day every 3-7 days); maximum: 600 mg/day

Sedation/hypnotic (unlabeled use): 25-50 mg at bedtime (often in combination with daytime SSRIs); may increase up to 200 mg at bedtime

Elderly: 25-50 mg at bedtime with 25-50 mg/day dose increase every 3 days for inpatients and weekly for outpatients, if tolerated; usual dose: 75-150 mg/day

Mechanism of Action Inhibits reuptake of serotonin, causes adrenoreceptor subsensitivity, and induces significant changes in 5-HT presynaptic receptor adrenoreceptors. Trazodone also significantly blocks histamine (H_1) and alpha$_1$-adrenergic receptors.

Other Adverse Effects

>10%:

Central nervous system: Dizziness, headache, sedation

Gastrointestinal: Nausea

1% to 10%:

Cardiovascular: Syncope, hypertension, hypotension, edema

Central nervous system: Confusion, decreased concentration, fatigue, incoordination

Gastrointestinal: Diarrhea, constipation, weight gain/loss

Neuromuscular & skeletal: Tremor, myalgia

Ocular: Blurred vision

Respiratory: Nasal congestion

<1%: Agitation, bradycardia, extrapyramidal symptoms, hepatitis, priapism, rash, seizures, tachycardia, urinary retention

Drug Interactions Substrate of CYP2D6, **3A4**; Inhibits CYP2D6

Increased Effect/Toxicity: Trazodone, in combination with other serotonergic agents (buspirone, MAO inhibitors), may produce additive serotonergic effects, including serotonin syndrome. Trazodone, in combination with other psychotropics (low potency antipsychotics), may result in additional hypotension. Trazodone, in combination with ethanol, may result in additive sedation and impairment of motor skills. Fluoxetine may inhibit the metabolism of trazodone resulting in elevated plasma levels.

Decreased Effect: Trazodone inhibits the hypotensive response to clonidine.

Dietary/Ethanol/Herb Considerations

Ethanol: Avoid use; may increase CNS depression.

Food may increase time to peak serum concentration up to 2.5 hours.

Herb/Nutraceutical: Avoid gotu kola, kava, SAMe, St John's wort, tryptophan, and valerian; may increase risk of serotonin syndrome and/or excessive sedation.

Pharmacodynamics/Kinetics

Onset of action: Therapeutic: 1-3 weeks

Protein binding: 85% to 95%

Metabolism: Hepatic

Half-life elimination: 7-8 hours, two compartment kinetics

Time to peak, serum: 30-100 minutes; delayed with food (up to 2.5 hours)

Excretion: Primarily urine; secondarily feces

Pregnancy Risk Factor C

Generic Available Yes

Trazodone Hydrochloride *see* Trazodone *on page 1336*

Trecator®-SC *see* Ethionamide *on page 542*

Trelstar™ Depot *see* Triptorelin *on page 1358*

Trelstar™ LA *see* Triptorelin *on page 1358*

Trental® *see* Pentoxifylline *on page 1058*

Treprostinil (tre PROST in il)

U.S. Brand Names Remodulin™

Pharmacologic Category Vasodilator

Synonyms Treprostinil Sodium

Use Treatment of pulmonary arterial hypertension (PAH) in patients with NYHA Class II-IV symptoms to decrease exercise-associated symptoms

(Continued)

Treprostinil *(Continued)*

Local Anesthetic/Vasoconstrictor Precautions No information available to require special precautions

Effects on Dental Treatment No significant effects or complications reported

Dosage S.C. infusion:

Adults: PAH: Initial: 1.25 ng/kg/minute continuous; if dose cannot be tolerated, reduce to 0.625 ng/kg/minute. Increase at rate not >1.25 ng/kg/minute per week for first 4 weeks, and not >2.5 ng/kg/minute per week for remainder of therapy. Limited experience with doses >40 ng/kg/minute.

Note: Dose must be carefully and individually titrated (symptom improvement with minimal adverse effects).

Elderly: Limited experience; use caution

Dosing adjustment in renal impairment: No specific recommendations; use with caution.

Dosing adjustment in hepatic impairment:

Mild to moderate: Initial: 0.625 ng/kg/minute; increase with caution.

Severe: No data available.

Mechanism of Action Treprostinil is a direct dilator of both pulmonary and systemic arterial vascular beds; also inhibits platelet aggregation.

Other Adverse Effects

>10%:

Cardiovascular: Vasodilation (11%)

Central nervous system: Headache (27%)

Dermatologic: Rash (14%)

Gastrointestinal: Diarrhea (25%), nausea (22%)

Local: Infusion site pain (85%), infusion site reaction (83%)

Miscellaneous: Jaw pain (13%)

1% to 10%:

Cardiovascular: Edema (9%), hypotension (4%)

Central nervous system: Dizziness (9%)

Dermatologic: Pruritus (8%)

Drug Interactions Increased Effect/Toxicity: Concomitant use of treprostinil with other agents that inhibit platelet aggregation (eg, NSAIDs, ASA, antiplatelet agents) or promote anticoagulation (eg, warfarin) may increase the risk of bleeding.

Pharmacodynamics/Kinetics

Absorption: S.C.: Rapidly and completely

Distribution: 14 L/70 kg lean body weight

Protein binding: 91%

Metabolism: Hepatic (enzymes unknown); forms metabolites

Bioavailability: 100%

Half-life elimination: Terminal: 2-4 hours

Excretion: Urine (4% as unchanged drug; 64% as metabolites); feces (13%)

Pregnancy Risk Factor B

Generic Available No

Treprostinil Sodium *see* Treprostinil *on page 1337*

Tretinoin *see* Tretinoin (Oral) *on page 1338*

Tretinoin *see* Tretinoin (Topical) *on page 1340*

Tretinoin, Fluocinolone Acetonide, and Hydroquinone *see* Fluocinolone, Hydroquinone, and Tretinoin *on page 585*

Tretinoin (Oral) (TRET i noin, ORE ul)

U.S. Brand Names Vesanoid®

Canadian Brand Names Vesanoid®

Pharmacologic Category Antineoplastic Agent, Miscellaneous

Synonyms All-*trans*-Retinoic Acid; Tretinoin

Use Acute promyelocytic leukemia (APL): Induction of remission in patients with APL, French American British (FAB) classification M3 (including the M3 variant), characterized by the presence of the t(15;17) translocation or the presence of the PML/RARα gene who are refractory to or who have relapsed from anthracycline chemotherapy, or for whom anthracycline-based chemotherapy is contraindicated. Tretinoin is for the induction of remission only. All patients should receive an accepted form of remission consolidation or maintenance therapy for APL after completion of induction therapy with tretinoin.

Local Anesthetic/Vasoconstrictor Precautions No information available to require special precautions

Effects on Dental Treatment >10%: Xerostomia

Dosage Oral:

Children: There are limited clinical data on the pediatric use of tretinoin. Of 15 pediatric patients (age range: 1-16 years) treated with tretinoin, the incidence of complete remission was 67%. Safety and efficacy in pediatric patients <1 year of age have not been established. Some pediatric patients experience severe headache and pseudotumor cerebri, requiring analgesic treatment and lumbar puncture for relief. Increased caution is recommended. Consider dose reduction in children experiencing serious or intolerable toxicity; however, the efficacy and safety of tretinoin at doses <45 mg/m^2/day have not been evaluated.

Adults: 45 mg/m^2/day administered as two evenly divided doses until complete remission is documented. Discontinue therapy 30 days after achievement of complete remission or after 90 days of treatment, whichever occurs first. If after initiation of treatment the presence of the t(15;17) translocation is not confirmed by cytogenetics or by polymerase chain reaction studies and the patient has not responded to tretinoin, consider alternative therapy.

Note: Tretinoin is for the induction of remission only. Optimal consolidation or maintenance regimens have not been determined. All patients should therefore receive a standard consolidation or maintenance chemotherapy regimen for APL after induction therapy with tretinoin unless otherwise contraindicated.

Mechanism of Action Retinoid that induces maturation of acute promyelocytic leukemia (APL) cells in cultures; induces cytodifferentiation and decreased proliferation of APL cells

Other Adverse Effects Virtually all patients experience some drug-related toxicity, especially headache, fever, weakness and fatigue. These adverse effects are seldom permanent or irreversible nor do they usually require therapy interruption

>10%:

Cardiovascular: Arrhythmias, flushing, hypotension, hypertension, peripheral edema, chest discomfort, edema

Central nervous system: Dizziness, anxiety, insomnia, depression, confusion, malaise, pain

Dermatologic: Burning, redness, cheilitis, inflammation of lips, dry skin, pruritus, photosensitivity

Endocrine & metabolic: Increased serum concentration of triglycerides

Gastrointestinal: GI hemorrhage, abdominal pain, other GI disorders, diarrhea, constipation, dyspepsia, abdominal distention, weight gain/loss

Hematologic: Hemorrhage, disseminated intravascular coagulation

Local: Phlebitis, injection site reactions

Neuromuscular & skeletal: Bone pain, arthralgia, myalgia, paresthesia

Ocular: Itching of eye

Renal: Renal insufficiency

Respiratory: Upper respiratory tract disorders, dyspnea, respiratory insufficiency, pleural effusion, pneumonia, rales, expiratory wheezing, nasal dryness

Miscellaneous: Infections, shivering

1% to 10%:

Cardiovascular: Cardiac failure, cardiac arrest, MI, enlarged heart, heart murmur, ischemia, stroke, myocarditis, pericarditis, pulmonary hypertension, secondary cardiomyopathy, cerebral hemorrhage, pallor

Central nervous system: Intracranial hypertension, agitation, hallucination, agnosia, aphasia, cerebellar edema, cerebellar disorders, convulsions, coma, CNS depression, encephalopathy, hypotaxia, no light reflex, neurologic reaction, spinal cord disorder, unconsciousness, dementia, forgetfulness, somnolence, slow speech, hypothermia

Dermatologic: Skin peeling on hands or soles of feet, rash, cellulitis

Endocrine & metabolic: Fluid imbalance, acidosis

Gastrointestinal: Hepatosplenomegaly, ulcer

Genitourinary: Dysuria, polyuria, enlarged prostate

Hepatic: Ascites, hepatitis

Neuromuscular & skeletal: Tremor, leg weakness, hyporeflexia, dysarthria, facial paralysis, hemiplegia, flank pain, asterixis, abnormal gait

Ocular: Dry eyes, photophobia

Renal: Acute renal failure, renal tubular necrosis

Respiratory: Lower respiratory tract disorders, pulmonary infiltration, bronchial asthma, pulmonary/larynx edema, unspecified pulmonary disease

Miscellaneous: Face edema, lymph disorders

<1%: Mood changes, pseudomotor cerebri, alopecia, hyperuricemia, anorexia, nausea, vomiting, inflammatory bowel syndrome, **bleeding gums**, increase in erythrocyte sedimentation rate, decrease in hemoglobin and hematocrit, conjunctivitis, corneal opacities, optic neuritis, cataracts

Drug Interactions Substrate of CYP2A6, 2B6, 2C8/9; Inhibits CYP2C8/9; Induces CYP2E1

Increased Effect/Toxicity: Ketoconazole increases the mean plasma AUC of tretinoin. Other drugs which inhibit CYP3A4 would be expected to increase tretinoin concentrations, potentially increasing toxicity.

Dietary/Ethanol/Herb Considerations

Ethanol: Avoid use; may increase CNS depression.

Food has been shown to enhance absorption of retinoids. Avoid additional vitamin A supplementation; may lead to vitamin A toxicity.

Herb/Nutraceutical: Avoid dong quai; may cause photosensitization. Avoid Avoid gotu kola, kava, SAMe, St John's wort, and valerian; may increase CNS depression. St John's wort; may decrease serum concentration and cause photosensitization.

(Continued)

Tretinoin (Oral) *(Continued)*

Pharmacodynamics/Kinetics

Protein binding: >95%

Metabolism: Hepatic via CYP; primary metabolite: 4-oxo-all-*trans*- retinoic acid

Half-life elimination: Terminal: Parent drug: 0.5-2 hours

Time to peak, serum: 1-2 hours

Excretion: Urine (63%); feces (30%)

Pregnancy Risk Factor D

Generic Available No

Tretinoin (Topical) (TRET i noyn, TOP i kal)

U.S. Brand Names Altinac™; Avita®; Renova®; Retin-A®; Retin-A® Micro

Canadian Brand Names Rejuva-A®; Retin-A®; Retin-A® Micro; Retinova®

Mexican Brand Names Stieva-A®; Stieva-A® 0.025%

Pharmacologic Category Retinoic Acid Derivative

Synonyms Retinoic Acid; *trans*-Retinoic Acid; Tretinoin; Vitamin A Acid

Use Treatment of acne vulgaris; photodamaged skin; palliation of fine wrinkles, mottled hyperpigmentation, and tactile roughness of facial skin as part of a comprehensive skin care and sun avoidance program

Unlabeled/Investigational Use Treatment of some skin cancers

Local Anesthetic/Vasoconstrictor Precautions No information available to require special precautions

Effects on Dental Treatment No significant effects or complications reported

Dosage Topical:

Children >12 years and Adults: Acne vulgaris: Begin therapy with a weaker formulation of tretinoin (0.025% cream, 0.04% microsphere gel, or 0.01% gel) and increase the concentration as tolerated; apply once daily to acne lesions before retiring or on alternate days; if stinging or irritation develop, decrease frequency of application

Adults ≥18: Palliation of fine wrinkles, mottled hyperpigmentation, and tactile roughness of facial skin: Pea-sized amount of the 0.02% or 0.05% emollient cream applied to entire face once daily in the evening

Elderly: Use of the 0.02% emollient cream in patients 65-71 years of age showed similar improvement in fine wrinkles as seen in patients <65 years. Safety and efficacy of the 0.02% cream have not been established in patients >71 years of age. Safety and efficacy of the 0.05% cream have not been established in patients >50 years of age.

Mechanism of Action Keratinocytes in the sebaceous follicle become less adherent which allows for easy removal; inhibits microcomedone formation and eliminates lesions already present

Other Adverse Effects

>10%: Dermatologic: Excessive dryness, erythema, scaling of the skin, pruritus

1% to 10%:

Dermatologic: Hyperpigmentation or hypopigmentation, photosensitivity, initial acne flare-up

Local: Edema, blistering, stinging

Drug Interactions Substrate of CYP2A6, 2B6, 2C8/9; Inhibits CYP2C8/9; Induces CYP2E1

Increased Effect/Toxicity: Topical application of sulfur, benzoyl peroxide, salicylic acid, resorcinol, or any product with strong drying effects potentiates adverse reactions with tretinoin. Photosensitizing medications (thiazides, tetracyclines, fluoroquinolones, phenothiazines, sulfonamides) augment phototoxicity and should not be used when treating palliation of fine wrinkles, mottled hyperpigmentation, and tactile roughness of facial skin.

Dietary/Ethanol/Herb Considerations

Food: Avoid excessive intake of vitamin A (cod liver oil, halibut fish oil).

Herb/Nutraceutical: Avoid dong quai and St John's wort; may cause photosensitization.

Pharmacodynamics/Kinetics

Absorption: Minimal

Metabolism: Hepatic for the small amount absorbed

Excretion: Urine and feces

Pregnancy Risk Factor C

Generic Available Yes: Cream, gel

Trexall™ *see* Methotrexate *on page 884*

TRH *see* Protirelin *on page 1144*

Triacetin (trye a SEE tin)

U.S. Brand Names Myco-Nail [OTC]

Pharmacologic Category Antifungal Agent, Topical

Synonyms Glycerol Triacetate

Use Fungistat for athlete's foot and other superficial fungal infections

Local Anesthetic/Vasoconstrictor Precautions No information available to require special precautions

Effects on Dental Treatment No significant effects or complications reported

Dosage Apply twice daily, cleanse areas with dilute alcohol or mild soap and water before application; continue treatment for 7 days after symptoms have disappeared

Generic Available No

Triacetyloleandomycin *see* Troleandomycin *on page 1359*

Triacin-C® [DSC] *see* Triprolidine, Pseudoephedrine, and Codeine *on page 1357*

Triaconazole *see* Terconazole *on page 1279*

Triamcinolone (trye am SIN oh lone)

Related Information

Oral Nonviral Soft Tissue Ulcerations or Erosions *on page 1549*
Respiratory Diseases *on page 1476*
Triamcinolone Acetonide Dental Paste *on page 1344*

U.S. Brand Names Aristocort®; Aristocort® A; Aristocort® Forte; Aristospan®; Azmacort®; Kenalog®; Kenalog-10®; Kenalog-40®; Nasacort®; Nasacort® AQ; Tac™-3 [DSC]; Triderm®; Tri-Nasal®

Canadian Brand Names Aristocort®; Aristospan®; Azmacort®; Kenalog®; Kenalog® in Orabase; Nasacort® AQ; Oracort; Triaderm; Trinasal®

Mexican Brand Names Kenacort®; Ledercort; Triamsicort®; Zamacort®

Pharmacologic Category Corticosteroid, Adrenal; Corticosteroid, Inhalant (Oral); Corticosteroid, Nasal; Corticosteroid, Systemic; Corticosteroid, Topical

Synonyms Triamcinolone Acetonide, Aerosol; Triamcinolone Acetonide, Parenteral; Triamcinolone Diacetate, Oral; Triamcinolone Diacetate, Parenteral; Triamcinolone Hexacetonide; Triamcinolone, Oral

Use

Dental

Inhalation: Control of bronchial asthma and related bronchospastic conditions

Intranasal: Management of seasonal and perennial allergic rhinitis in patients ≥12 years of age

Oral, topical: Adjunctive treatment and temporary relief of symptoms associated with oral inflammatory lesions and ulcerative lesions resulting from trauma

Systemic: Treatment of allergic states and respiratory diseases

Medical:

Systemic: Treatment of adrenocortical insufficiency, rheumatic disorders, systemic lupus erythematosus, and other diseases requiring anti-inflammatory or immunosuppressive effects

Topical: Treatment of inflammatory dermatoses responsive to steroids

Local Anesthetic/Vasoconstrictor Precautions No information available to require special precautions

Effects on Dental Treatment Frequency not defined:

Systemic: CHF, hypertension, convulsions, fever, headache, increased intracranial pressure, bruising, thin/fragile skin, impaired wound healing, diabetes mellitus (manifestations of latent disease), nausea, [oral *Monilia* (oral inhaler), peptic ulcer, ulcerative esophagitis, decreased muscle mass, weakness, pathologic fracture of long bones, vertebral compression fractures, cough increased (nasal spray), epistaxis (nasal inhaler/spray), pharyngitis (nasal spray/oral inhaler), sinusitis (oral inhaler), anaphylaxis, increased diaphoresis

Topical: Allergic contact dermatitis, skin infection (secondary), perioral dermatitis, atrophy of oral mucosa, burning, irritation

Dosage The lowest possible dose should be used to control the condition; when dose reduction is possible, the dose should be reduced gradually. Parenteral dose

Triamcinolone Dosing

<table>
<tr><th></th><th>Acetonide</th><th>Diacetate</th><th>Hexacetonide</th></tr>
<tr><td>Intrasynovial</td><td>2.5-40 mg</td><td>5-40 mg</td><td></td></tr>
<tr><td>Intralesional</td><td rowspan="2">1-30 mg</td><td rowspan="2">5-48 mg (max: 12.5 mg/site; 25 mg/lesion; 75 mg/wk)</td><td rowspan="2">≤0.5 mg/sq inch affected area</td></tr>
<tr><td>Sublesional</td></tr>
<tr><td>Systemic I.M.</td><td>2.5-60 mg/dose
Children 6-12 years: 40 mg
Children >12 years and Adults: 60 mg</td><td>3-48 mg/day
40 mg/wk (average)</td><td></td></tr>
<tr><td>Intra-articular</td><td>2.5-40 mg</td><td>5-40 mg</td><td>2-20 mg</td></tr>
<tr><td>large joints</td><td>5-15 mg</td><td>25 mg</td><td>10-20 mg</td></tr>
<tr><td>small joints</td><td>2.5-5 mg</td><td>2-5 mg</td><td>2-6 mg</td></tr>
<tr><td>Tendon sheaths</td><td rowspan="2">2.5-10 mg</td><td rowspan="3"></td><td rowspan="3"></td></tr>
<tr><td>Intrabursal</td></tr>
<tr><td>Intradermal</td><td>1 mg/site</td></tr>
</table>

(Continued)

Triamcinolone *(Continued)*

is usually 1/3 to 1/2 the oral dose given every 12 hours. In life-threatening situations, parenteral doses larger than the oral dose may be needed.

Injection: See table on previous page.

Intranasal: Perennial allergic rhinitis, seasonal allergic rhinitis:

Nasal spray:

Children 6-11 years: 110 mcg/day as 1 spray in each nostril once daily.

Children ≥12 years and Adults: 220 mcg/day as 2 sprays in each nostril once daily

Nasal inhaler:

Children 6-11 years: Initial: 220 mcg/day as 2 sprays in each nostril once daily

Children ≥12 years and Adults: Initial: 220 mcg/day as 2 sprays in each nostril once daily; may increase dose to 440 mcg/day (given once daily or divided and given 2 or 4 times/day)

Oral: Adults:

Acute rheumatic carditis: Initial: 20-60 mg/day; reduce dose during maintenance therapy

Acute seasonal or perennial allergic rhinitis: 8-12 mg/day

Adrenocortical insufficiency: Range 4-12 mg/day

Bronchial asthma: 8-16 mg/day

Dermatological disorders, contact/atopic dermatitis: Initial: 8-16 mg/day

Ophthalmic disorders: 12-40 mg/day

Rheumatic disorders: Range: 8-16 mg/day

SLE: Initial: 20-32 mg/day, some patients may need initial doses ≥48 mg; reduce dose during maintenance therapy

Oral inhalation: Asthma:

Children 6-12 years: 100-200 mcg 3-4 times/day **or** 200-400 mcg twice daily; maximum dose: 1200 mg/day

Children >12 years and Adults: 200 mcg 3-4 times/day **or** 400 mcg twice daily; maximum dose: 1600 mcg/day

Oral topical: Oral inflammatory lesions/ulcers: Press a small dab (about 1/4 inch) to the lesion until a thin film develops. A larger quantity may be required for coverage of some lesions. For optimal results use only enough to coat the lesion with a thin film; do not rub in.

Topical:

Cream, Ointment: Apply thin film to affected areas 2-4 times/day

Spray: Apply to affected area 3-4 times/day

Mechanism of Action Decreases inflammation by suppression of migration of polymorphonuclear leukocytes and reversal of increased capillary permeability; suppresses the immune system by reducing activity and volume of the lymphatic system; suppresses adrenal function at high doses

Other Adverse Effects Frequency not defined:

Systemic:

Central nervous system: Vertigo

Dermatologic: Facial erythema, petechiae, photosensitivity, rash

Endocrine & metabolic: Adrenocortical/pituitary unresponsiveness (particularly during stress), decreased carbohydrate tolerance, cushingoid state, fluid retention, growth suppression (children), hypokalemic alkalosis, menstrual irregularities, negative nitrogen balance, potassium loss, sodium retention

Gastrointestinal: Abdominal distention, diarrhea, dyspepsia, pancreatitis, weight gain

Local: Skin atrophy (at the injection site)

Neuromuscular & skeletal: Femoral/humeral head aseptic necrosis, steroid myopathy

Ocular: Cataracts, intraocular pressure increased, exophthalmos, glaucoma

Miscellaneous: Suppression to skin tests

Topical: Dermatologic: Itching, dryness, folliculitis, hypertrichosis, acneiform eruptions, hypopigmentation, skin maceration, striae, miliaria, skin atrophy

Contraindications Hypersensitivity to triamcinolone or any component of the formulation; systemic fungal infections; serious infections (except septic shock or tuberculous meningitis); primary treatment of status asthmaticus; fungal, viral, or bacterial infections of the mouth or throat (oral topical formulation)

Warnings/Precautions May cause suppression of hypothalamic-pituitary-adrenal (HPA) axis, particularly in younger children or in patients receiving high doses for prolonged periods. Particular care is required when patients are transferred from systemic corticosteroids to inhaled products due to possible adrenal insufficiency or withdrawal from steroids, including an increase in allergic symptoms. Patients receiving 20 mg per day of prednisone (or equivalent) may be most susceptible. Fatalities have occurred due to adrenal insufficiency in asthmatic patients during and after transfer from systemic corticosteroids to aerosol steroids; aerosol steroids do **not** provide the systemic steroid needed to treat patients having trauma, surgery, or infections. Withdrawal and discontinuation of the corticosteroid should be done slowly and carefully

Use with caution in patients with hypothyroidism, cirrhosis, nonspecific ulcerative colitis and patients at increased risk for peptic ulcer disease. Corticosteroids should be used with caution in patients with diabetes, hypertension, osteoporosis, glaucoma, cataracts, or tuberculosis. Use caution in hepatic impairment. Do not use occlusive dressings on weeping or exudative lesions and general caution with occlusive dressings should be observed; discontinue if skin irritation or contact dermatitis should occur; do not use in patients with decreased skin circulation; avoid the use of high potency steroids on the face.

Because of the risk of adverse effects, systemic corticosteroids should be used cautiously in the elderly, in the smallest possible dose, and for the shortest possible time. Azmacort® (metered dose inhaler) comes with its own spacer device attached and may be easier to use in older patients.

Controlled clinical studies have shown that orally-inhaled and intranasal corticosteroids may cause a reduction in growth velocity in pediatric patients. (In studies of orally-inhaled corticosteroids, the mean reduction in growth velocity was approximately 1 centimeter per year [range 0.3-1.8 cm per year] and appears to be related to dose and duration of exposure.) The growth of pediatric patients receiving inhaled corticosteroids, should be monitored routinely (eg, via stadiometry). To minimize the systemic effects of orally-inhaled and intranasal corticosteroids, each patient should be titrated to the lowest effective dose.

May suppress the immune system, patients may be more susceptible to infection. Use with caution in patients with systemic infections or ocular herpes simplex. Avoid exposure to chickenpox and measles.

Oral topical: Discontinue if local irritation or sensitization should develop. If significant regeneration or repair of oral tissues has not occurred in seven days, re-evaluation of the etiology of the oral lesion is advised.

Drug Interactions

Increased Effect: Salmeterol: The addition of salmeterol has been demonstrated to improve response to inhaled corticosteroids (as compared to increasing steroid dosage).

Increased Toxicity: Salicylates may increase risk of GI ulceration

Decreased Effect: Barbiturates, phenytoin, rifampin increase metabolism of triamcinolone; vaccine and toxoid effects may be reduced

Dietary/Ethanol/Herb Considerations

Ethanol: Avoid use; may enhance gastric mucosal irritation.

Food: Administer with food to reduce GI upset; food interferes with calcium absorption.

Herb/Nutraceutical: Avoid cat's claw and echinacea due to immunostimulant properties.

Pharmacodynamics/Kinetics

Duration: Oral: 8-12 hours

Absorption: Topical: Systemic

Time to peak: I.M.: 8-10 hours

Half-life elimination: Biologic: 18-36 hours

Pregnancy Risk Factor C

Breast-feeding Considerations It is not known if triamcinolone is excreted in breast milk, however, other corticosteroids are excreted. Prednisone and prednisolone are excreted in breast milk; the AAP considers them to be "usually compatible" with breast-feeding. Hypertension was reported in a nursing infant when a topical corticosteroid was applied to the nipples of the mother.

Dosage Forms **AERO, for nasal inhalation, as acetonide** (Nasacort®): 55 mcg/inhalation (10 g). **AERO, for nasal inhalation, as acetonide** [spray] (Nasacort® AQ): 55 mcg/inhalation (16.5 g); (Tri-Nasal®): 50 mcg/inhalation (15 mL). **AERO, for oral inhalation, as acetonide** (Azmacort®): 100 mcg per actuation (20 g). **AERO, topical, as acetonide** (Kenalog®): 0.2 mg/2-second spray (63 g). **CRM, as acetonide:** 0.025% (15 g, 80 g); 0.1% (15 g, 30 g, 80 g, 454 g, 2270 g); 0.5% (15 g); (Aristocort® A): 0.025% (15 g, 60 g); 0.1% (15 g, 60 g); 0.5% (15 g); (Kenalog®): 0.1% (15 g, 60 g, 80 g); 0.5% (20 g); (Triderm®): 0.1% (30 g, 85 g). **INJ, suspension, as acetonide** (Kenalog-10®): 10 mg/mL (5 mL) [not for I.V. or I.M. use]; (Kenalog-40®): 40 mg/mL (1 mL, 5 mL, 10 mL) [not for I.V. or intradermal use]; (Tac™-3 [DSC]): 3 mg/mL (5 mL). **INJ, suspension, as diacetate** (Aristocort®): 25 mg/mL (5 mL) [not for I.V. use]; (Aristocort® Forte): 40 mg/mL (1 mL, 5mL) [not for I.V. use]. **INJ, suspension, as hexacetonide** (Aristospan®): 5 mg/mL (5 mL); 20 mg/mL (1 mL, 5 mL) [not for I.V. use]. **LOTION, as acetonide:** 0.025% (60 mL); 0.1% (60 mL). **OINT, topical, as acetonide:** 0.025% (80 g); 0.1% (15 g, 80 g); (Aristocort® A, Kenalog®): 0.1% (15 g, 60 g). **TAB** (Aristocort®): 4 mg

Generic Available Yes: Cream, lotion, ointment

Comments Triamcinolone 16 mg is equivalent to cortisone 100 mg (no mineralocorticoid activity).

Triamcinolone Acetonide, Aerosol *see* Triamcinolone *on page 1341*

Triamcinolone Acetonide Dental Paste

(trye am SIN oh lone a SEE toe nide DEN tal paste)

Related Information

Triamcinolone *on page 1341*

U.S. Brand Names Kenalog® in Orabase®

Canadian Brand Names Oracort®

Pharmacologic Category Anti-inflammatory Agent; Corticosteroid, Topical

Use

Dental: For adjunctive treatment and for the temporary relief of symptoms associated with oral inflammatory and ulcerative lesions, resulting from trauma

Medical: Treatment of localized inflammation responsive to steroids

Local Anesthetic/Vasoconstrictor Precautions No information available to require special precautions

Effects on Dental Treatment Frequency not defined: Local irritation

Dosage Oral, topical: Press a small dab (about 1/4 inch) to the lesion until a thin film develops. A larger quantity may be required for coverage of some lesions. For optimal results use only enough to coat the lesion with a thin film.

Mechanism of Action Decreases inflammation by suppression of migration of polymorphonuclear leukocytes and reversal of increased capillary permeability; suppresses the immune system by reducing activity and volume of the lymphatic system; suppresses adrenal function at high doses

Contraindications Hypersensitivity to triamcinolone or any component of the formulation; contraindicated in the presence of fungal, viral, or bacterial infections of the mouth or throat

Warnings/Precautions Patients with tuberculosis, peptic ulcer or diabetes mellitus should not be treated with any corticosteroid preparation without the advice of the patient's physician. Normal immune responses of the oral tissues are depressed in patients receiving topical corticosteroid therapy. Virulent strains of oral microorganisms may multiply without producing the usual warning symptoms of oral infections. The small amount of steroid released from the topical preparation makes systemic effects very unlikely. If local irritation or sensitization should develop, the preparation should be discontinued. If significant regeneration or repair of oral tissues has not occurred in seven days, re-evaluation of the etiology of the oral lesion is advised.

Dietary/Ethanol/Herb Considerations Herb/Nutraceutical: Avoid cat's claw and echinacea due to immunostimulant properties.

Pharmacodynamics/Kinetics

Absorption: Systemic

Half-life elimination, serum: Biological: 18-36 hours

Pregnancy Risk Factor C

Dosage Forms PASTE, oral, topical [tube]: 5 g [each g provides 1 mg (0.1%) triamcinolone in emollient paste containing gelatin, pectin, and carboxymethylcellulose sodium with a polyethylene and mineral oil gel base]

Generic Available Yes

Comments When applying to tissues, attempts to spread this preparation may result in a granular, gritty sensation and cause it to crumble. This preparation should be applied at bedtime to permit steroid contact with the lesion throughout the night.

Triamcinolone Acetonide, Parenteral *see* Triamcinolone *on page 1341*

Triamcinolone and Nystatin *see* Nystatin and Triamcinolone *on page 992*

Triamcinolone Diacetate, Oral *see* Triamcinolone *on page 1341*

Triamcinolone Diacetate, Parenteral *see* Triamcinolone *on page 1341*

Triamcinolone Hexacetonide *see* Triamcinolone *on page 1341*

Triamcinolone, Oral *see* Triamcinolone *on page 1341*

Triaminic® Allergy Congestion [OTC] *see* Pseudoephedrine *on page 1146*

Triaminic® Sore Throat Formula [OTC] *see* Acetaminophen, Dextromethorphan, and Pseudoephedrine *on page 35*

Triamterene

(trye AM ter een)

Related Information

Cardiovascular Diseases *on page 1456*

U.S. Brand Names Dyrenium®

Pharmacologic Category Diuretic, Potassium Sparing

Use Alone or in combination with other diuretics in treatment of edema and hypertension; decreases potassium excretion caused by kaliuretic diuretics

Local Anesthetic/Vasoconstrictor Precautions No information available to require special precautions

Effects on Dental Treatment No significant effects or complications reported

Dosage Oral:

Adults: 100-300 mg/day in 1-2 divided doses; maximum dose: 300 mg/day

Dosing comment in renal impairment: Cl_{cr} <10 mL/minute: Avoid use.

Dosing adjustment in hepatic impairment: Reduction recommended in cirrhosis.

Mechanism of Action Interferes with potassium/sodium exchange (active transport) in the distal tubule, cortical collecting tubule and collecting duct by inhibiting sodium, potassium-ATPase; decreases calcium excretion; increases magnesium loss

Other Adverse Effects

1% to 10%:

Cardiovascular: Hypotension, edema, CHF, bradycardia

Central nervous system: Dizziness, headache, fatigue

Gastrointestinal: Constipation, nausea

Respiratory: Dyspnea

<1% (Limited to important or life-threatening): Inability to achieve or maintain an erection, agranulocytosis, thrombocytopenia

Drug Interactions Increased Effect/Toxicity: ACE inhibitors or spironolactone can cause hyperkalemia, especially in patients with renal impairment, potassium-rich diets, or on other drugs causing hyperkalemia; avoid concurrent use or monitor closely. Potassium supplements may further increase potassium retention and cause hyperkalemia; avoid concurrent use.

Dietary/Ethanol/Herb Considerations Food: May be taken with food; avoid salt substitutes and low-salt milk; diuretic does not cause potassium loss and ingestion of these products may result in additional potassium.

Pharmacodynamics/Kinetics

Onset of action: Diuresis: 2-4 hours

Duration: 7-9 hours

Absorption: Unreliable

Pregnancy Risk Factor B (manufacturer); D (expert analysis)

Generic Available No

Triamterene and Hydrochlorothiazide *see* Hydrochlorothiazide and Triamterene *on page 677*

Triavil® *see* Amitriptyline and Perphenazine *on page 85*

Triaz® *see* Benzoyl Peroxide *on page 171*

Triaz® Cleanser *see* Benzoyl Peroxide *on page 171*

Triazolam (trye AY zoe lam)

Related Information

Patients Requiring Sedation *on page 1565*

U.S. Brand Names Halcion®

Canadian Brand Names Apo®-Triazo; Gen-Triazolam; Halcion®

Mexican Brand Names Halcion®

Pharmacologic Category Benzodiazepine

Use

Dental: Oral premedication before dental procedures

Medical: Short-term treatment of insomnia

Local Anesthetic/Vasoconstrictor Precautions No information available to require special precautions

Effects on Dental Treatment

>10%: Drowsiness, anteriograde amnesia

1% to 10%: Headache, dizziness, nervousness, lightheadedness, nausea, vomiting

Restrictions C-IV

Dosage Oral:

Children <18 years: Dosage not established

Adults:

Hypnotic: 0.125-0.25 mg at bedtime

Sedation for dental procedure: 0.25 mg taken the evening before oral surgery; or 0.25 mg 1 hour before procedure

Dosing adjustment/comments in hepatic impairment: Reduce dose or avoid use in cirrhosis

Mechanism of Action Binds to stereospecific benzodiazepine receptors on the postsynaptic GABA neuron at several sites within the central nervous system, including the limbic system, reticular formation. Enhancement of the inhibitory effect of GABA on neuronal excitability results by increased neuronal membrane permeability to chloride ions. This shift in chloride ions results in hyperpolarization (a less excitable state) and stabilization.

Other Adverse Effects

1% to 10%: Central nervous system: Ataxia

<1%: **Cramps, confusion, CNS depression, euphoria, fatigue, memory impairment, pain, tachycardia, visual disturbance**

Contraindications Hypersensitivity to triazolam or any component of the formulation (cross-sensitivity with other benzodiazepines may exist); concurrent therapy with CYP3A4 inhibitors (including ketoconazole, itraconazole, and nefazodone); pregnancy

Warnings/Precautions Should be used only after evaluation of potential causes of sleep disturbance. Failure of sleep disturbance to resolve after 7-10 days may indicate psychiatric or medical illness. A worsening of insomnia or the emergence

(Continued)

Triazolam *(Continued)*

of new abnormalities of thought or behavior may represent unrecognized psychiatric or medical illness and requires immediate and careful evaluation.

An increase in daytime anxiety may occur after as few as 10 days of continuous use, which may be related to withdrawal reaction in some patients. Anterograde amnesia may occur at a higher rate with triazolam than with other benzodiazepines. Use with caution in elderly or debilitated patients, patients with hepatic disease (including alcoholics), or renal impairment. Use with caution in patients with respiratory disease or impaired gag reflex. Avoid use in patients with sleep apnea.

Causes CNS depression (dose-related) resulting in sedation, dizziness, confusion, or ataxia which may impair physical and mental capabilities. Patients must be cautioned about performing tasks which require mental alertness (ie, operating machinery or driving). Use with caution in patients receiving other CNS depressants or psychoactive agents. Effects with other sedative drugs or ethanol may be potentiated. Benzodiazepines have been associated with falls and traumatic injury and should be used with extreme caution in patients who are at risk of these events (especially the elderly).

Use caution in patients with depression, particularly if suicidal risk may be present. Use with caution in patients with a history of drug dependence. Benzodiazepines have been associated with dependence and acute withdrawal symptoms on discontinuation or reduction in dose. Acute withdrawal, including seizures, may be precipitated after administration of flumazenil to patients receiving long-term benzodiazepine therapy.

Paradoxical reactions, including hyperactive or aggressive behavior have been reported with benzodiazepines, particularly in adolescent/pediatric or psychiatric patients. Does not have analgesic, antidepressant, or antipsychotic properties.

Drug Interactions Substrate of **CYP3A4**; Inhibits CYP2C8/9

CNS depressants: Sedative effects and/or respiratory depression may be additive with CNS depressants; includes ethanol, barbiturates, narcotic analgesics, and other sedative agents; monitor for increased effect

CYP3A4 inhibitors: Serum level and/or toxicity of some benzodiazepines may be increased; inhibitors include amiodarone, cimetidine, clarithromycin, erythromycin, delavirdine, diltiazem, dirithromycin, disulfiram, fluoxetine, fluvoxamine, grapefruit juice, indinavir, itraconazole, ketoconazole, nefazodone, nevirapine, propoxyphene, quinupristin-dalfopristin, ritonavir, saquinavir, verapamil, zafirlukast, zileuton; monitor for altered benzodiazepine response

Enzyme inducers: Metabolism of some benzodiazepines may be increased, decreasing their therapeutic effect; consider using an alternative sedative/hypnotic agent; potential inducers include phenobarbital, phenytoin, carbamazepine, rifampin, and rifabutin

Levodopa: Therapeutic effects may be diminished in some patients following the addition of a benzodiazepine; limited/inconsistent data

Oral contraceptives: May decrease the clearance of some benzodiazepines (those which undergo oxidative metabolism); monitor for increased benzodiazepine effect

Theophylline: May partially antagonize some of the effects of benzodiazepines; monitor for decreased response; may require higher doses for sedation

Dietary/Ethanol/Herb Considerations

Ethanol: Avoid use; may increase CNS depression.

Food may decrease the rate of absorption. Avoid grapefruit products; may increase serum concentration.

Herb/Nutraceutical: Avoid gotu kola, kava, SAMe, and valerian; may increase CNS depression. Avoid St John's wort; may decrease serum concentration and increase CNS depression. Melatonin may increase benzodiazepine binding at receptor sites causing enhancement of activity of triazolam; use cautiously.

Pharmacodynamics/Kinetics

Onset of action: Hypnotic: 15-30 minutes

Duration: 6-7 hours

Distribution: V_d: 0.8-1.8 L/kg

Protein binding: 89%

Metabolism: Extensively hepatic

Half-life elimination: 1.7-5 hours

Excretion: Urine as unchanged drug and metabolites

Pregnancy Risk Factor X

Dosage Forms TAB: 0.125 mg, 0.25 mg

Generic Available Yes

Comments Triazolam (0.25 mg) 1 hour prior to dental procedure has been used as an oral pre-op sedative

Selected Readings

Berthold CW, Dionne RA, and Corey SE, "Comparison of Sublingually and Orally Administered Triazolam for Premedication Before Oral Surgery," *Oral Surg Oral Med Oral Pathol Oral Radiol Endod*, 1997, 84(2):119-24.

Berthold CW, Schneider A, and Dionne RA, "Using Triazolam to Reduce Dental Anxiety," *J Am Dent Assoc*, 1993, 124(11):58-64.

Kaufman E, Hargreaves KM, and Dionne RA, "Comparison of Oral Triazolam and Nitrous Oxide With Placebo and Intravenous Diazepam for Outpatient Premedication," *Oral Surg Oral Med Oral Pathol*, 1993, 75(2):156-64.
Kurzrock M, "Triazolam and Dental Anxiety," *J Am Dent Assoc*, 1994, 125(4):358, 360.
Lieblich SE and Horswell B, "Attenuation of Anxiety in Ambulatory Oral Surgery Patients With Oral Triazolam," *J Oral Maxillofac Surg*, 1991, 49(8):792-7.
Milgrom P, Quarnstrom FC, Longley A, et al, "The Efficacy and Memory Effects of Oral Triazolam Premedication in Highly Anxious Dental Patients," *Anesth Prog*, 1994, 41(3):70-6.

Tribavirin *see* Ribavirin *on page 1176*

Tricalcium Phosphate *see* Calcium Phosphate (Tribasic) *on page 227*

Tri-Chlor® *see* Trichloroacetic Acid *on page 1347*

Trichlormethiazide (trye klor meth EYE a zide)

Related Information
Cardiovascular Diseases *on page 1456*

U.S. Brand Names Naqua®

Canadian Brand Names Metahydrin®; Metatensin®; Naqua®; Trichlorex®

Pharmacologic Category Diuretic, Thiazide

Use Management of mild to moderate hypertension; treatment of edema in CHF and nephrotic syndrome

Local Anesthetic/Vasoconstrictor Precautions No information available to require special precautions

Effects on Dental Treatment No significant effects or complications reported

Dosage Oral:
Adults: 1-4 mg/day; initially doses may be given twice daily.
Dosing adjustment in renal impairment: Reduction required

Mechanism of Action The diuretic mechanism of action of the thiazides is primarily inhibition of sodium, chloride, and water reabsorption in the renal distal tubules, thereby producing diuresis with a resultant reduction in plasma volume. The antihypertensive mechanism of action of the thiazides is unknown. It is known that doses of thiazides produce greater reduction in blood pressure than equivalent diuretic doses of loop diuretics. There has been speculation that the thiazides may have some influence on vascular tone mediated through sodium depletion, but this remains to be proven.

Other Adverse Effects
1% to 10%:
Endocrine & metabolic: Hypokalemia
Respiratory: Dyspnea (<5%)
<1% (Limited to important or life-threatening): Hypotension, photosensitivity, lichenoid dermatitis; fluid and electrolyte imbalances (hypercalcemia, hypocalcemia, hypomagnesemia, hyponatremia); hyperglycemia, rarely blood dyscrasias, pancreatitis, prerenal azotemia

Drug Interactions
Increased effect of thiazides with furosemide and other loop diuretics. Increased hypotension and/or renal adverse effects of ACE inhibitors may result in aggressively diuresed patients. Beta-blockers increase hyperglycemic effects of thiazides in type 2 diabetes mellitus. Cyclosporine and thiazides can increase the risk of gout or renal toxicity. Digoxin toxicity can be exacerbated if a thiazide induces hypokalemia or hypomagnesemia. Lithium toxicity can occur with thiazides due to reduced renal excretion of lithium. Thiazides may prolong the duration of action with neuromuscular blocking agents.
Decreased effect of oral hypoglycemics. Decreased absorption of thiazides with cholestyramine and colestipol. NSAIDs can decrease the efficacy of thiazides, reducing the diuretic and antihypertensive effects.

Pharmacodynamics/Kinetics
Onset of action: Diuresis: ~2 hours
Peak effect: 4 hours
Duration: 12-24 hours

Pregnancy Risk Factor D

Generic Available Yes

Trichloroacetaldehyde Monohydrate *see* Chloral Hydrate *on page 295*

Trichloroacetic Acid (trye klor oh a SEE tik AS id)

U.S. Brand Names Tri-Chlor®

Pharmacologic Category Keratolytic Agent

Use Debride callous tissue

Local Anesthetic/Vasoconstrictor Precautions No information available to require special precautions

Effects on Dental Treatment No significant effects or complications reported

Dosage Topical: Apply to verruca, cover with bandage for 5-6 days, remove verruca, reapply as needed

Generic Available Yes

Trichloromonofluoromethane and Dichlorodifluoromethane *see* Dichlorodifluoromethane and Trichloromonofluoromethane *on page 428*

Triclosan and Fluoride (trye KLOE san & FLOR ide)

Related Information

Fluoride *on page 586*

Periodontal Diseases *on page 1540*

U.S. Brand Names Colgate Total® Toothpaste

Pharmacologic Category Antibacterial, Dental; Mineral (Oral/Topical)

Synonyms Fluoride and Triclosan (Dental)

Use Used exclusively in dental applications (anticavity, antigingivitis, antiplaque toothpaste)

Local Anesthetic/Vasoconstrictor Precautions No information available to require special precautions

Effects on Dental Treatment No significant effects or complications reported

Dosage Brush teeth thoroughly after each meal or at least twice daily

Mechanism of Action Triclosan is an antibacterial agent which helps to prevent gingivitis with regular use. Fluoride promotes remineralization of decalcified enamel, inhibits the cariogenic microbial process in dental plaque, and increases tooth resistance to acid dissolution

Other Adverse Effects No data reported

Pregnancy Risk Factor No data reported

Comments It has been shown that stannous fluoride and triclosan when formulated into a toothpaste vehicle provide plaque inhibitory effects. To provide a longer retention time of the triclosan in plaque, a polymer has been added to the toothpaste vehicle. The polymer is known as PVM/MA which stands for polyvinylmethyl ether/maleic acid copolymer, and is listed as an inactive ingredient (PVM/MA Copolymer) on the manufacturer's label. Studies have reported that the retention of triclosan in plaque (exceeding the minimal inhibitory concentration) after polymer application was 14 hours after brushing. Ongoing studies are evaluating the effects of triclosan/copolymer on alveolar bone loss. Rosling et al. have reported that the daily use of Colgate Total® reduced (1) the frequency of deep periodontal pockets and (2) the number of sites that exhibited additional probing attachment and bone loss.

Selected Readings

Binney A, Addy M, Owens J, et al, "A Comparison of Triclosan and Stannous Fluoride Toothpastes for Inhibition of Plaque Regrowth. A Crossover Study Designed to Access Carry Over," *J Clin Periodontol*, 1997, 24(3):166-70.

Ellwood RP, Worthington HV, Blinkhorn AS, et al, "Effect of a Triclosan/Copolymer Dentifrice on the Incidence of Periodontal Attachment Loss in Adolescents," *J Clin Periodontol*, 1998, 25(5):363-7.

Mandel ID, "The New Toothpastes," *J Calif Dent Assoc*, 1998, 26(3):186-90.

Rosling B, Wannfors B, Volpe AR, et a, "The Use of a Triclosan/Copolymer Dentifrice May Retard the Progression of Periodontitis," *J Clin Periodontol*, 1997, 24(12):873-80.

TriCor® *see* Fenofibrate *on page 561*

Tricosal® *see* Choline Magnesium Trisalicylate *on page 319*

Tri-Cyclen® *see* Combination Hormonal Contraceptives *on page 368*

Triderm® *see* Triamcinolone *on page 1341*

Tridesilon® *see* Desonide *on page 412*

Tridione® *see* Trimethadione *on page 1351*

Triethanolamine Polypeptide Oleate-Condensate

(trye eth a NOLE a meen pol i PEP tide OH lee ate-KON den sate)

U.S. Brand Names Cerumenex®

Canadian Brand Names Cerumenex®

Pharmacologic Category Otic Agent, Cerumenolytic

Use Removal of ear wax (cerumen)

Local Anesthetic/Vasoconstrictor Precautions No information available to require special precautions

Effects on Dental Treatment No significant effects or complications reported

Dosage Children and Adults: Otic: Fill ear canal, insert cotton plug; allow to remain 15-30 minutes; flush ear with lukewarm water as a single treatment; if a second application is needed for unusually hard impactions, repeat the procedure

Mechanism of Action Emulsifies and disperses accumulated cerumen

Other Adverse Effects <1%: Mild erythema and pruritus, severe eczematoid reactions, localized dermatitis

Pharmacodynamics/Kinetics Onset of action: Slight disintegration of very hard ear wax by 24 hours

Pregnancy Risk Factor C

Generic Available No

Triethanolamine Salicylate (trye eth u NOLE u meen su LIS i late)

U.S. Brand Names Mobisyl® [OTC]; Myoflex® [OTC]; Sportscreme® [OTC]

Canadian Brand Names Antiphlogistine Rub A-535 No Odour; Myoflex®

Pharmacologic Category Analgesic, Topical; Salicylate; Topical Skin Product

Use Relief of pain of muscular aches, rheumatism, neuralgia, sprains, arthritis on intact skin

Local Anesthetic/Vasoconstrictor Precautions No information available to require special precautions

Effects on Dental Treatment No significant effects or complications reported

Dosage Topical: Apply to area as needed

Other Adverse Effects 1% to 10%:

Central nervous system: Confusion, drowsiness
Gastrointestinal: Nausea, vomiting, diarrhea
Respiratory: Hyperventilation

Generic Available Yes

Triethylenethiophosphoramide *see* Thiotepa *on page 1300*

Trifluoperazine (trye floo oh PER a zeen)

U.S. Brand Names Stelazine®

Canadian Brand Names Apo®-Trifluoperazine; Novo-Trifluzine; PMS-Trifluoperazine; Terfluzine

Mexican Brand Names Flupazine®; Stelazine®

Pharmacologic Category Antipsychotic Agent, Phenothiazine, Piperazine

Synonyms Trifluoperazine Hydrochloride

Use Treatment of schizophrenia

Unlabeled/Investigational Use Management of psychotic disorders

Local Anesthetic/Vasoconstrictor Precautions Most pharmacology textbooks state that in presence of phenothiazines, systemic doses of epinephrine paradoxically decrease the blood pressure. This is the so called "epinephrine reversal" phenomenon. This has never been observed when epinephrine is given by infiltration as part of the anesthesia procedure.

Effects on Dental Treatment

Significant hypotension may occur, especially when the drug is administered parenterally; orthostatic hypotension is due to alpha-receptor blockade, the elderly are at greater risk for orthostatic hypotension.

Tardive dyskinesia: Prevalence rate may be 40% in elderly; development of the syndrome and the irreversible nature are proportional to duration and total cumulative dose over time. Extrapyramidal reactions are more common in elderly with up to 50% developing these reactions after 60 years of age; drug-induced **Parkinson's syndrome** occurs often; **Akathisia** is the most common extrapyramidal reaction in elderly.

Increased confusion, memory loss, psychotic behavior, and agitation frequently occur as a consequence of anticholinergic effects; may be confused with original neurotic symptoms. Antipsychotic-associated sedation in nonpsychotic patients is extremely unpleasant due to feelings of depersonalization, derealization, and dysphoria.

Dosage

Children 6-12 years: Schizophrenia/psychoses:

- Oral: Hospitalized or well-supervised patients: Initial: 1 mg 1-2 times/day, gradually increase until symptoms are controlled or adverse effects become troublesome; maximum: 15 mg/day
- I.M.: 1 mg twice daily

Adults:

- Schizophrenia/psychoses:
  - Outpatients: Oral: 1-2 mg twice daily
  - Hospitalized or well-supervised patients: Initial: 2-5 mg twice daily with optimum response in the 15-20 mg/day range; do not exceed 40 mg/day
  - I.M.: 1-2 mg every 4-6 hours as needed up to 10 mg/24 hours maximum
- Nonpsychotic anxiety: Oral: 1-2 mg twice daily; maximum: 6 mg/day; therapy for anxiety should not exceed 12 weeks; do not exceed 6 mg/day for longer than 12 weeks when treating anxiety; agitation, jitteriness, or insomnia may be confused with original neurotic or psychotic symptoms

Elderly:

- Schizophrenia/psychoses:
  - Oral: Dose selection should start at the low end of the dosage range and titration must be gradual.
  - I.M.: Initial: 1 mg every 4-6 hours; increase at 1 mg increments; do not exceed 6 mg/day
- Behavioral symptoms associated with dementia behavior: Oral: Initial: 0.5-1 mg 1-2 times/day; increase dose at 4- to 7-day intervals by 0.5-1 mg/day; increase dosing intervals (bid, tid, etc) as necessary to control response or side effects. Maximum daily dose: 40 mg. Gradual increases (titration) may prevent some side effects or decrease their severity.

Hemodialysis: Not dialyzable (0% to 5%)

Mechanism of Action Blocks postsynaptic mesolimbic dopaminergic receptors in the brain; exhibits alpha-adrenergic blocking effect and depresses the release of hypothalamic and hypophyseal hormones

Other Adverse Effects Frequency not defined:

Cardiovascular: Hypotension, orthostatic hypotension, cardiac arrest

(Continued)

Trifluoperazine *(Continued)*

Central nervous system: Extrapyramidal symptoms (pseudoparkinsonism, akathisia, dystonias, tardive dyskinesia), dizziness, headache, neuroleptic malignant syndrome (NMS), impairment of temperature regulation, lowering of seizures threshold

Dermatologic: Increased sensitivity to sun, rash, discoloration of skin (blue-gray)

Endocrine & metabolic: Changes in menstrual cycle, changes in libido, breast pain, hyperglycemia, hypoglycemia, gynecomastia, lactation, galactorrhea

Gastrointestinal: Constipation, weight gain, nausea, vomiting, stomach pain, xerostomia

Genitourinary: Difficulty in urination, ejaculatory disturbances, urinary retention, priapism

Hematologic: Agranulocytosis, leukopenia, pancytopenia, thrombocytopenic purpura, eosinophilia, hemolytic anemia, aplastic anemia

Hepatic: Cholestatic jaundice, hepatotoxicity

Neuromuscular & skeletal: Tremor

Ocular: Pigmentary retinopathy, cornea and lens changes

Respiratory: Nasal congestion

Drug Interactions Substrate of **CYP1A2**

Increased Effect/Toxicity: Trifluoperazine's effects on CNS depression may be additive when trifluoperazine is combined with CNS depressants (narcotic analgesics, ethanol, barbiturates, cyclic antidepressants, antihistamines, or sedative-hypnotics). Trifluoperazine may increase the effects/toxicity of anticholinergics, antihypertensives, lithium (rare neurotoxicity), trazodone, or valproic acid. Concurrent use with TCA may produce increased toxicity or altered therapeutic response. Chloroquine and propranolol may increase trifluoperazine concentrations. Hypotension may occur when trifluoperazine is combined with epinephrine. May increase the risk of arrhythmia when combined with antiarrhythmics, cisapride, pimozide, sparfloxacin, or other drugs which prolong QT interval. Metoclopramide may increase risk of extrapyramidal symptoms (EPS).

Decreased Effect: Phenothiazines inhibit the effects of levodopa, guanadrel, guanethidine, and bromocriptine. Benztropine (and other anticholinergics) may inhibit the therapeutic response to trifluoperazine and excess anticholinergic effects may occur. Cigarette smoking and barbiturates may enhance the hepatic metabolism of trifluoperazine. Trifluoperazine and possibly other low potency antipsychotics may reverse the pressor effects of epinephrine.

Dietary/Ethanol/Herb Considerations

Ethanol: Avoid use; may increase CNS depression.

Food: Administer with food to decrease GI upset.

Herb/Nutraceutical: Avoid dong quai; may cause photosensitization. Avoid gotu kola, kava, SAMe, and valerian; may increase CNS depression. Avoid St John's wort; may cause photosensitization and increase CNS depression.

Pharmacodynamics/Kinetics

Metabolism: Extensively hepatic

Half-life elimination: >24 hours with chronic use

Pregnancy Risk Factor C

Generic Available Yes: Tablet

Trifluoperazine Hydrochloride *see* Trifluoperazine *on page 1349*

Trifluorothymidine *see* Trifluridine *on page 1350*

Trifluridine (trye FLORE i deen)

Related Information

Systemic Viral Diseases *on page 1517*

U.S. Brand Names Viroptic®

Canadian Brand Names Viroptic®

Pharmacologic Category Antiviral Agent, Ophthalmic

Synonyms F_3T; Trifluorothymidine

Use Treatment of primary keratoconjunctivitis and recurrent epithelial keratitis caused by herpes simplex virus types I and II

Local Anesthetic/Vasoconstrictor Precautions No information available to require special precautions

Effects on Dental Treatment No significant effects or complications reported

Dosage Adults: Instill 1 drop into affected eye every 2 hours while awake, to a maximum of 9 drops/day, until re-epithelialization of corneal ulcer occurs; then use 1 drop every 4 hours for another 7 days; do **not** exceed 21 days of treatment; if improvement has not taken place in 7-14 days, consider another form of therapy

Mechanism of Action Interferes with viral replication by incorporating into viral DNA in place of thymidine, inhibiting thymidylate synthetase resulting in the formation of defective proteins

Other Adverse Effects

1% to 10%: Local: Burning, stinging

<1%: Hyperemia, palpebral edema, epithelial keratopathy, keratitis, stromal edema, increased intraocular pressure, hypersensitivity reactions

Pharmacodynamics/Kinetics Absorption: Ophthalmic: Systemic absorption negligible, corneal penetration adequate

Pregnancy Risk Factor C

Generic Available Yes

Triglycerides, Medium Chain *see* Medium Chain Triglycerides *on page 849*

Trihexyphenidyl (trye heks ee FEN i dil)

Canadian Brand Names Apo®-Trihex

Mexican Brand Names Hipokinon®

Pharmacologic Category Anticholinergic Agent; Anti-Parkinson's Agent, Anticholinergic

Synonyms Benzhexol Hydrochloride; Trihexyphenidyl Hydrochloride

Use Adjunctive treatment of Parkinson's disease; treatment of drug-induced extrapyramidal symptoms

Local Anesthetic/Vasoconstrictor Precautions No information available to require special precautions

Effects on Dental Treatment Prolonged xerostomia may contribute to discomfort and dental disease (ie, caries, periodontal disease, and oral candidiasis).

>10%: Xerostomia, dry throat; normal salivary flow resumes upon discontinuation

Frequency not defined (dose-related): Tachycardia, confusion, agitation, euphoria, drowsiness, headache, dizziness, nervousness, delusions, hallucinations, paranoia, nausea, vomiting, weakness, blurred vision, nasal dryness

Dosage Adults: Oral: Initial: 1-2 mg/day, increase by 2 mg increments at intervals of 3-5 days; usual dose: 5-15 mg/day in 3-4 divided doses

Mechanism of Action Exerts a direct inhibitory effect on the parasympathetic nervous system. It also has a relaxing effect on smooth musculature; exerted both directly on the muscle itself and indirectly through parasympathetic nervous system (inhibitory effect)

Other Adverse Effects Frequency not defined (dose-related):

Dermatologic: Dry skin, increased sensitivity to light, rash

Gastrointestinal: Constipation, ileus, parotitis

Genitourinary: Urinary retention

Ocular: Mydriasis, increase in intraocular pressure, glaucoma

Miscellaneous: Diaphoresis (decreased)

Drug Interactions

Increased Effect/Toxicity: Central and/or peripheral anticholinergic syndrome can occur when administered with amantadine, rimantadine, narcotic analgesics, phenothiazines and other antipsychotics (especially with high anticholinergic activity), tricyclic antidepressants, quinidine and some other antiarrhythmics, and antihistamines.

Decreased Effect: May increase gastric degradation of levodopa and decrease the amount of levodopa absorbed by delaying gastric emptying; the opposite may be true for digoxin. Therapeutic effects of cholinergic agents (tacrine, donepezil) and neuroleptics may be antagonized.

Dietary/Ethanol/Herb Considerations

Ethanol: Avoid use; may increase CNS depression.

Herb/Nutraceutical: Avoid gotu kola, kava, SAMe, St John's wort, and valerian; may increase CNS depression.

Pharmacodynamics/Kinetics

Onset of action: Peak effect: ~1 hour

Half-life elimination: 3.3-4.1 hours

Time to peak, serum: 1-1.5 hours

Excretion: Primarily urine

Pregnancy Risk Factor C

Generic Available Yes

Trihexyphenidyl Hydrochloride *see* Trihexyphenidyl *on page 1351*

Tri-K® *see* Potassium Supplements *on page 1102*

Trilafon® [DSC] *see* Perphenazine *on page 1062*

Trileptal® *see* Oxcarbazepine *on page 1012*

Tri-Levlen® *see* Combination Hormonal Contraceptives *on page 368*

Trilisate® *see* Choline Magnesium Trisalicylate *on page 319*

Tri-Luma™ *see* Fluocinolone, Hydroquinone, and Tretinoin *on page 585*

Tri-Luma *see* Furazolidone *on page 622*

Trimethadione (trye meth a DYE one)

U.S. Brand Names Tridione®

Pharmacologic Category Anticonvulsant, Oxazolidinedione

Synonyms Troxidone

Use Control absence (petit mal) seizures refractory to other drugs

Local Anesthetic/Vasoconstrictor Precautions No information available to require special precautions

Effects on Dental Treatment No significant effects or complications reported

(Continued)

Trimethadione *(Continued)*

Dosage Oral:

Children: Seizure disorders: Initial: 25-50 mg/kg/24 hours in 3-4 equally divided doses every 6-8 hours

Adults: Seizure disorders: Initial: 900 mg/day in 3-4 equally divided doses, increase by 300 mg/day at weekly intervals until therapeutic results or toxic symptoms appear

Dosing interval in renal impairment:

Cl_{cr} 10-50 mL/minute: Administer every 8-12 hours

Cl_{cr} <10 mL/minute: Administer every 12-24 hours

Mechanism of Action An oxazolidinedione with anticonvulsant sedative properties; elevates the cortical and basal seizure thresholds, and reduces the synaptic response to low frequency impulses

Other Adverse Effects Frequency not defined:

Central nervous system: Drowsiness, hiccups

Dermatologic: Alopecia, exfoliative dermatitis, rash

Endocrine & metabolic: Porphyria

Gastrointestinal: Anorexia, vomiting, stomach upset, abdominal pain, weight loss

Hematologic: Aplastic anemia, agranulocytosis, thrombocytopenia,

Hepatic: Hepatitis, jaundice

Neuromuscular & skeletal: Myasthenia gravis-like syndrome

Ocular: Diplopia, photophobia, hemeralopia, nystagmus, scotomata

Renal: Nephrosis, proteinuria

Miscellaneous: Lupus

Drug Interactions Substrate of CYP2C8/9, 2C19, **2E1**, 3A4

Pregnancy Risk Factor D

Generic Available No

Trimethobenzamide (trye meth oh BEN za mide)

U.S. Brand Names Tigan®

Canadian Brand Names Tigan®

Pharmacologic Category Anticholinergic Agent; Antiemetic

Synonyms Trimethobenzamide Hydrochloride

Use Treatment of postoperative nausea and vomiting; nausea associated with gastroenteritis

Local Anesthetic/Vasoconstrictor Precautions No information available to require special precautions

Effects on Dental Treatment No significant effects or complications reported

Dosage Rectal use is contraindicated in neonates and premature infants

Children:

Rectal: <14 kg: 100 mg 3-4 times/day

Oral, rectal: 14-40 kg: 100-200 mg 3-4 times/day

Adults:

Oral: 250-300 mg 3-4 times/day

I.M., rectal: 200 mg 3-4 times/day

Mechanism of Action Acts centrally to inhibit the medullary chemoreceptor trigger zone

Other Adverse Effects Frequency not defined:

Cardiovascular: Hypotension

Central nervous system: Coma, depression, disorientation, dizziness, drowsiness, EPS, headache, opisthotonos, Parkinson-like syndrome, seizures

Hematologic: Blood dyscrasias

Hepatic: Jaundice

Neuromuscular & skeletal: Muscle cramps

Ocular: Blurred vision

Miscellaneous: Hypersensitivity reactions

Dietary/Ethanol/Herb Considerations Ethanol: Avoid concomitant use

Pharmacodynamics/Kinetics

Onset of action: Antiemetic: Oral: 10-40 minutes; I.M.: 15-35 minutes

Duration: 3-4 hours

Absorption: Rectal: ~60%

Bioavailability: Oral: 100%

Half-life elimination: 7-9 hours

Time to peak: Oral: 45 minutes; I.M.: 30 minutes

Excretion: Urine (30% to 50%)

Pregnancy Risk Factor C

Generic Available Yes: Injection

Trimethobenzamide Hydrochloride *see* Trimethobenzamide *on page 1352*

Trimethoprim (trye METH oh prim)

U.S. Brand Names Primsol®; Proloprim®

Canadian Brand Names Apo®-Trimethoprim; Proloprim®

Mexican Brand Names Bactilen®; Bactiver®; Bactrim®; Bactropin®; Bateral®; Batrizol®; Dibaprim®; Ectaprim®; Esteprim®; Maxtrim®; Metoxiprim®; Septrin®; Servitrim®; Tribakin®; Trimetoger®; Trimetox®; Trimexazol®; Trimexole-F®

Pharmacologic Category Antibiotic, Miscellaneous

Synonyms TMP

Use Treatment of urinary tract infections due to susceptible strains of *E. coli*, *P. mirabilis*, *K. pneumoniae*, *Enterobacter* sp and coagulase-negative *Staphylococcus* including *S. saprophyticus*; acute otitis media in children; acute exacerbations of chronic bronchitis in adults; in combination with other agents for treatment of toxoplasmosis, *Pneumocystis carinii*; treatment of superficial ocular infections involving the conjunctiva and cornea

Local Anesthetic/Vasoconstrictor Precautions No information available to require special precautions

Effects on Dental Treatment No significant effects or complications reported

Dosage Oral:

Children: 4 mg/kg/day in divided doses every 12 hours

Adults: 100 mg every 12 hours or 200 mg every 24 hours; in the treatment of *Pneumocystis carinii* pneumonia; dose may be as high as 15-20 mg/kg/day in 3-4 divided doses

Dosing interval in renal impairment:

Cl_{cr} 15-30 mL/minute: Administer 100 mg every 18 hours or 50 mg every 12 hours

Cl_{cr} <15 mL/minute: Administer 100 mg every 24 hours or avoid use

Hemodialysis: Moderately dialyzable (20% to 50%)

Mechanism of Action Inhibits folic acid reduction to tetrahydrofolate, and thereby inhibits microbial growth

Other Adverse Effects Frequency not defined:

Central nervous system: Aseptic meningitis (rare), fever

Dermatologic: Maculopapular rash (3% to 7% at 200 mg/day; incidence higher with larger daily doses), erythema multiforme (rare), exfoliative dermatitis (rare), pruritus (common), phototoxic skin eruptions, Stevens-Johnson syndrome (rare), toxic epidermal necrolysis (rare)

Endocrine & metabolic: Hyperkalemia, hyponatremia

Gastrointestinal: Epigastric distress, glossitis, nausea, vomiting

Hematologic: Leukopenia, megaloblastic anemia, methemoglobinemia, neutropenia, thrombocytopenia

Hepatic: Liver enzyme elevation, cholestatic jaundice (rare)

Renal: BUN and creatinine increased

Miscellaneous: Anaphylaxis, hypersensitivity reactions

Drug Interactions Substrate of **CYP2C8/9, 3A4**; Inhibits CYP2C8/9

Increased effect/toxicity/levels of phenytoin. Concurrent use with ACE inhibitors increases risk of hyperkalemia. Increased myelosuppression with methotrexate. May increase levels of digoxin. Concurrent use with dapsone may increase levels of dapsone and trimethoprim. Concurrent use with procainamide may increase levels of procainamide and trimethoprim.

Dietary/Ethanol/Herb Considerations Food: Administer with food or milk. May require folic acid supplementation.

Pharmacodynamics/Kinetics

Absorption: Readily and extensive

Distribution: Widely into body tissues and fluids (middle ear, prostate, bile, aqueous humor, CSF); crosses placenta; enters breast milk

Protein binding: 42% to 46%

Metabolism: Partially hepatic

Half-life elimination: 8-14 hours; prolonged with renal impairment

Time to peak, serum: 1-4 hours

Excretion: Urine (60% to 80%) as unchanged drug

Pregnancy Risk Factor C

Generic Available Yes: Tablet

Trimethoprim and Polymyxin B

(trye METH oh prim & pol i MIKS in bee)

Related Information

Polymyxin B *on page 1095*

U.S. Brand Names Polytrim®

Canadian Brand Names PMS-Polytrimethoprim; Polytrim™

Pharmacologic Category Antibiotic, Ophthalmic

Synonyms Polymyxin B and Trimethoprim

Use Treatment of surface ocular bacterial conjunctivitis and blepharoconjunctivitis

Local Anesthetic/Vasoconstrictor Precautions No information available to require special precautions

Effects on Dental Treatment No significant effects or complications reported

Dosage Instill 1-2 drops in eye(s) every 4-6 hours

Elderly: No overall differences observed between elderly and other adults

Other Adverse Effects 1% to 10%: Local: Burning, stinging, itching, increased redness

(Continued)

Trimethoprim and Polymyxin B *(Continued)*

Dietary/Ethanol/Herb Considerations Based on trimethoprim component:

Food: Administer with food or milk. Trimethoprim may cause folic acid deficiency requiring supplementation.

Pregnancy Risk Factor C

Generic Available Yes

Trimethoprim and Sulfamethoxazole *see* Sulfamethoxazole and Trimethoprim *on page 1253*

Trimetrexate Glucuronate (tri me TREKS ate gloo KYOOR oh nate)

U.S. Brand Names Neutrexin®

Pharmacologic Category Antineoplastic Agent, Miscellaneous

Use Alternative therapy for the treatment of moderate-to-severe *Pneumocystis carinii* pneumonia (PCP) in immunocompromised patients, including patients with acquired immunodeficiency syndrome (AIDS), who are intolerant of, or are refractory to, co-trimoxazole therapy or for whom co-trimoxazole and pentamidine are contraindicated. **Concurrent folinic acid (leucovorin) must always be administered.**

Local Anesthetic/Vasoconstrictor Precautions No information available to require special precautions

Effects on Dental Treatment No significant effects or complications reported

Dosage I.V.:

Adults: 45 mg/m² once daily for 21 days; concurrent leucovorin 20 mg/m² every 6 hours must be administered daily (oral or I.V.) during treatment and for 72 hours past the last dose of trimetrexate glucuronate (for a total of 24 days)

Alternative dosing based on weight:

<50 kg:Trimetrexate glucuronate 1.5 mg/kg/day; leucovorin 0.6 mg/kg 4 times/day

50-80 kg:Trimetrexate glucuronate 1.2 mg/kg/day; leucovorin 0.5 mg/kg/4 times/day

>80 kg: Trimetrexate glucuronate 1 mg/kg/day; leucovorin 0.5 mg/kg/4 times/day

Note: Oral doses of leucovorin should be rounded up to the next higher 25 mg increment.

Dosing adjustment in hepatic impairment: No specific recommendations

Mechanism of Action Exerts an antimicrobial effect through potent inhibition of the enzyme dihydrofolate reductase (DHFR)

Other Adverse Effects

>10%:

Hematologic: Neutropenia

Hepatic: LFTs increased

1% to 10%:

Central nervous system: Seizures, fever

Dermatologic: Rash

Gastrointestinal: Stomatitis, nausea, vomiting

Hematologic: Thrombocytopenia, anemia

Neuromuscular & skeletal: Peripheral neuropathy

Renal: Increased serum creatinine

Miscellaneous: Flu-like illness, hypersensitivity reactions, anaphylactoid reactions

Drug Interactions Metabolized by cytochrome isoenzyme, possibly CYP3A3/4

Increased Effect/Toxicity: Cimetidine, clotrimazole, and ketoconazole may decrease trimetrexate metabolism, resulting in increased serum levels. Trimetrexate may increase toxicity (infections) of live virus vaccines.

Pharmacodynamics/Kinetics

Distribution: V_d: 0.62 L/kg

Metabolism: Extensively hepatic

Half-life elimination: 15-17 hours

Pregnancy Risk Factor D

Generic Available No

Trimipramine (trye MI pra meen)

U.S. Brand Names Surmontil®

Canadian Brand Names Apo®-Trimip; Novo-Tripramine; Nu-Trimipramine; Rhotrimine®; Surmontil®

Pharmacologic Category Antidepressant, Tricyclic (Tertiary Amine)

Synonyms Trimipramine Maleate

Use Treatment of depression

Local Anesthetic/Vasoconstrictor Precautions Use with caution; epinephrine, norepinephrine and levonordefrin have been shown to have an increased pressor response in combination with TCAs

Effects on Dental Treatment >10%: Xerostomia

Long-term treatment with TCAs such as trimipramine increases the risk of caries by reducing salivation and salivary buffer capacity.

Dosage Oral:

Adults: 50-150 mg/day as a single bedtime dose up to a maximum of 200 mg/day outpatient and 300 mg/day inpatient

Elderly: Adequate studies have not been done in the elderly. In general, dosing should be cautious, starting at the lower end of dosing range.

Mechanism of Action Increases the synaptic concentration of serotonin and/or norepinephrine in the central nervous system by inhibition of their reuptake by the presynaptic neuronal membrane

Other Adverse Effects Frequency not defined:

Cardiovascular: Arrhythmias, hypotension, hypertension, tachycardia, palpitations, heart block, stroke, MI

Central nervous system: Headache, exacerbation of psychosis, confusion, delirium, hallucinations, nervousness, restlessness, delusions, agitation, insomnia, nightmares, anxiety, seizures, drowsiness

Dermatologic: Photosensitivity, rash, petechiae, itching

Endocrine & metabolic: Sexual dysfunction, breast enlargement, galactorrhea, SIADH

Gastrointestinal: Constipation, increased appetite, nausea, unpleasant taste, weight gain, diarrhea, heartburn, vomiting, anorexia, **trouble with gums, decreased lower esophageal sphincter tone (may cause GE reflux)**

Genitourinary: Difficult urination, urinary retention, testicular edema

Hematologic: Agranulocytosis, eosinophilia, purpura, thrombocytopenia

Hepatic: Cholestatic jaundice, increased liver enzymes

Neuromuscular & skeletal: Tremors, numbness, tingling, paresthesia, incoordination, ataxia, peripheral neuropathy, extrapyramidal symptoms

Ocular: Blurred vision, eye pain, disturbances in accommodation, mydriasis, increased intraocular pressure

Otic: Tinnitus

Miscellaneous: Allergic reactions

Drug Interactions Substrate of **CYP2C19, 2D6, 3A4**

Increased Effect/Toxicity: Trimipramine increases the effects of amphetamines, anticholinergics, other CNS depressants (sedatives, hypnotics, or ethanol), chlorpropamide, tolazamide, and warfarin. When used with MAO inhibitors, hyperpyrexia, hypertension, tachycardia, confusion, seizures, and **deaths have been reported** (serotonin syndrome). Serotonin syndrome has also been reported with ritonavir (rare). The SSRIs (to varying degrees), cimetidine, grapefruit juice, indinavir, methylphenidate, ritonavir, quinidine, diltiazem, and verapamil inhibit the metabolism of TCAs and clinical toxicity may result. Use of lithium with a TCA may increase the risk for neurotoxicity. Phenothiazines may increase concentration of some TCAs and TCAs may increase concentration of phenothiazines. Pressor response to I.V. epinephrine, norepinephrine, and phenylephrine may be enhanced in patients receiving TCAs (**Note:** Effect is unlikely with epinephrine or levonordefrin dosages typically administered as infiltration in combination with local anesthetics). Combined use of beta-agonists or drugs which prolong QT_c (including quinidine, procainamide, disopyramide, cisapride, sparfloxacin, gatifloxacin, moxifloxacin) with TCAs may predispose patients to cardiac arrhythmias.

Decreased Effect: Carbamazepine, phenobarbital, and rifampin may increase the metabolism of trimipramine resulting in decreased effect of trimipramine. Trimipramine inhibits the antihypertensive response to bethanidine, clonidine, debrisoquin, guanadrel, guanethidine, guanabenz, and guanfacine. Cholestyramine and colestipol may bind TCAs and reduce their absorption; monitor for altered response.

Dietary/Ethanol/Herb Considerations

Ethanol: Avoid use; may increase CNS depression.

Food: Avoid grapefruit products; may inhibit the metabolism of some TCAs and clinical toxicity may result.

Herb/Nutraceutical: Avoid kava, SAMe, St John's wort, tryptophan, and valerian; may increase risk of serotonin syndrome and/or excessive sedation.

Pharmacodynamics/Kinetics

Distribution: V_d: 17-48 L/kg

Protein binding: 95%; free drug: 3% to 7%

Metabolism: Hepatic; significant first-pass effect

Bioavailability: 18% to 63%

Half-life elimination: 16-40 hours

Excretion: Urine

Pregnancy Risk Factor C

Generic Available No

Selected Readings

Friedlander AH, Mahler ME, "Major Depressive Disorder. Psychopathology, Medical Management, and Dental Implications," *J Am Dent Assoc*, 201, 132(5):629-38.

Ganzberg S, "Psychoactive Drugs," *ADA Guide to Dental Therapeutics*, 2nd ed, Chicago, IL: ADA Publishing, a Division of ADA Business Enterprises, Inc, 2000, 376-405.

Yagiela JA, "Adverse Drug Interactions in Dental Practice: Interactions Associated With Vasoconstrictors. Part V of a Series," *J Am Dent Assoc*, 1999, 130(5):701-9.

Trimipramine Maleate *see* Trimipramine *on page 1354*

Trimox® *see* Amoxicillin *on page 93*
Trinalin® *see* Azatadine and Pseudoephedrine *on page 150*
Tri-Nasal® *see* Triamcinolone *on page 1341*
Tri-Norinyl® *see* Combination Hormonal Contraceptives *on page 368*
Triostat® *see* Liothyronine *on page 810*
Triotann® *see* Chlorpheniramine, Pyrilamine, and Phenylephrine *on page 312*

Tripelennamine (tri pel EN a meen)

U.S. Brand Names PBZ®; PBZ-SR®

Pharmacologic Category Antihistamine

Synonyms Tripelennamine Citrate; Tripelennamine Hydrochloride

Use Perennial and seasonal allergic rhinitis and other allergic symptoms including urticaria

Local Anesthetic/Vasoconstrictor Precautions No information available to require special precautions

Effects on Dental Treatment >10%: Xerostomia, changes in salivation

Chronic use of antihistamines will inhibit salivary flow, particularly in elderly patients; this may contribute to periodontal disease and oral discomfort.

Dosage Oral:

Infants and Children: 5 mg/kg/day in 4-6 divided doses, up to 300 mg/day maximum

Adults: 25-50 mg every 4-6 hours, extended release tablets 100 mg morning and evening up to 100 mg every 8 hours

Mechanism of Action Competes with histamine for H_1-receptor sites on effector cells in the gastrointestinal tract, blood vessels, and respiratory tract

Other Adverse Effects

>10%:

- Central nervous system: Slight to moderate drowsiness
- Respiratory: Thickening of bronchial secretions

1% to 10%:

- Central nervous system: Headache, fatigue, nervousness, dizziness
- Gastrointestinal: Appetite increase, weight gain, nausea, diarrhea, abdominal pain
- Neuromuscular & skeletal: Arthralgia
- Respiratory: Pharyngitis

<1%: Edema, palpitations, hypotension, depression, sedation, paradoxical excitement, insomnia, angioedema, photosensitivity, rash, urinary retention, hepatitis, myalgia, paresthesia, tremor, blurred vision, bronchospasm, epistaxis

Drug Interactions Inhibits CYP2D6

Increased effect/toxicity with CNS depressants, and MAO inhibitors.

Dietary/Ethanol/Herb Considerations

Ethanol: Avoid use; increases CNS depression.

Herb/Nutraceutical: Avoid gotu kola, kava, SAMe, St John's wort, and valerian; may increase CNS depression.

Pharmacodynamics/Kinetics

Onset of action: Antihistaminic: 15-30 minutes

Duration: 4-6 hours (up to 8 hours with PBZ-SR®)

Metabolism: Almost completely hepatic

Excretion: Urine

Pregnancy Risk Factor B

Generic Available Yes

Tripelennamine Citrate *see* Tripelennamine *on page 1356*
Tripelennamine Hydrochloride *see* Tripelennamine *on page 1356*
Triphasil® *see* Combination Hormonal Contraceptives *on page 368*
Triple Antibiotic® *see* Bacitracin, Neomycin, and Polymyxin B *on page 157*
Triple Care® Antifungal [OTC] *see* Miconazole *on page 906*
Triple Sulfa *see* Sulfabenzamide, Sulfacetamide, and Sulfathiazole *on page 1249*

Triprolidine and Pseudoephedrine

(trye PROE li deen & soo doe e FED rin)

Related Information

Pseudoephedrine *on page 1146*

U.S. Brand Names Actifed® Cold and Allergy [OTC]; Allerfrim® [OTC]; Allerphed® [OTC]; Aphedrid™ [OTC]; Aprodine® [OTC]; Genac® [OTC]; Silafed® [OTC]; Tri-Sudo® [OTC]; Uni-Fed® [OTC]

Canadian Brand Names Actifed®

Pharmacologic Category Alpha/Beta Agonist; Antihistamine

Synonyms Pseudoephedrine and Triprolidine

Use Temporary relief of nasal congestion, decongest sinus openings, running nose, sneezing, itching of nose or throat and itchy, watery eyes due to common cold, hay fever, or other upper respiratory allergies

Local Anesthetic/Vasoconstrictor Precautions Use with caution since pseudoephedrine is a sympathomimetic amine which could interact with epinephrine to cause a pressor response

Effects on Dental Treatment Chronic use of antihistamines will inhibit salivary flow, particularly in elderly patients; this may contribute to periodontal disease and oral discomfort.

Dosage Oral:

Children:

Syrup:

4 months to 2 years: 1.25 mL 3-4 times/day

2-4 years: 2.5 mL 3-4 times/day

4-6 years: 3.75 mL 3-4 times/day

6-12 years: 5 mL every 4-6 hours; do not exceed 4 doses in 24 hours

Tablet: ½ every 4-6 hours; do not exceed 4 doses in 24 hours

Children >12 years and Adults:

Syrup: 10 mL every 4-6 hours; do not exceed 4 doses in 24 hours

Tablet: 1 every 4-6 hours; do not exceed 4 doses in 24 hours

Mechanism of Action Refer to Pseudoephedrine monograph

Triprolidine is a member of the propylamine (alkylamine) chemical class of H_1-antagonist antihistamines. As such, it is considered to be relatively less sedating than traditional antihistamines of the ethanolamine, phenothiazine, and ethylenediamine classes of antihistamines. Triprolidine has a shorter half-life and duration of action than most of the other alkylamine antihistamines. Like all H_1-antagonist antihistamines, the mechanism of action of triprolidine is believed to involve competitive blockade of H_1-receptor sites resulting in the inability of histamine to combine with its receptor sites and exert its usual effects on target cells. Antihistamines do not interrupt any effects of histamine which have already occurred. Therefore, these agents are used more successfully in the prevention rather than the treatment of histamine-induced reactions.

Other Adverse Effects Frequency not defined:

Cardiovascular: Tachycardia

Central nervous system: Drowsiness, nervousness, insomnia, transient stimulation, headache, fatigue, dizziness

Respiratory: Thickening of bronchial secretions, pharyngitis

Gastrointestinal: Appetite increase, weight gain, nausea, diarrhea, abdominal pain, xerostomia

Genitourinary: Dysuria

Neuromuscular & skeletal: Arthralgia, weakness

Miscellaneous: Diaphoresis

Drug Interactions Triprolidine: Inhibits CYP2D6

Increased toxicity with MAO inhibitors or drugs with MAO inhibiting activity such as linezolid or furazolidone (hypertensive crisis). May increase toxicity of sympathomimetics, CNS depressants, and alcohol.

Decreased effect of guanethidine, reserpine, methyldopa.

Dietary/Ethanol/Herb Considerations

Ethanol: Avoid use; may increase CNS depression.

Herb/Nutraceutical: Avoid gotu kola, kava, SAMe, St John's wort, and valerian; may increase CNS depression.

Pharmacodynamics/Kinetics See Pseudoephedrine monograph.

Pregnancy Risk Factor C

Generic Available Yes

Triprolidine, Codeine, and Pseudoephedrine *see* Triprolidine, Pseudoephedrine, and Codeine *on page 1357*

Triprolidine, Pseudoephedrine, and Codeine

(trye PROE li deen, soo doe e FED rin, & KOE deen)

Related Information

Codeine *on page 361*

Pseudoephedrine *on page 1146*

U.S. Brand Names Triacin-C® [DSC]

Canadian Brand Names CoActifed®

Pharmacologic Category Antihistamine/Decongestant/Antitussive

Synonyms Codeine, Pseudoephedrine, and Triprolidine; Pseudoephedrine, Triprolidine, and Codeine Pseudoephedrine, Codeine, and Triprolidine; Triprolidine, Codeine, and Pseudoephedrine; Triprolidine, Pseudoephedrine, and Codeine, Triprolidine, and Pseudoephedrine

Use Symptomatic relief of upper respiratory symptoms and cough

Local Anesthetic/Vasoconstrictor Precautions Use with caution since pseudoephedrine is a sympathomimetic amine which could interact with epinephrine to cause a pressor response

Effects on Dental Treatment ≤10%: Tachycardia, palpitations, xerostomia; use vasoconstrictor with caution

Restrictions C-V

Dosage Oral:

Children:

2-6 years: 2.5 mL 4 times/day

7-12 years: 5 mL 4 times/day

(Continued)

Triprolidine, Pseudoephedrine, and Codeine *(Continued)*

Children >12 years and Adults: 10 mL 4 times/day

Dietary/Ethanol/Herb Considerations

Ethanol: Avoid use; may increase CNS depression.

Herb/Nutraceutical: Avoid gotu kola, kava, SAMe, St John's wort, and valerian; may increase CNS depression.

Pharmacodynamics/Kinetics See Pseudoephedrine and Codeine monographs.

Pregnancy Risk Factor C

Generic Available No

Triprolidine, Pseudoephedrine, and Codeine, Triprolidine, and Pseudoephedrine *see* Triprolidine, Pseudoephedrine, and Codeine *on page 1357*

TripTone® [OTC] *see* DimenhyDRINATE *on page 449*

Triptorelin (trip toe REL in)

U.S. Brand Names Trelstar™ Depot; Trelstar™ LA

Canadian Brand Names Trelstar™ Depot

Pharmacologic Category Luteinizing Hormone-Releasing Hormone Analog

Synonyms Triptorelin Pamoate

Use Palliative treatment of advanced prostate cancer as an alternative to orchiectomy or estrogen administration

Local Anesthetic/Vasoconstrictor Precautions No information available to require special precautions

Effects on Dental Treatment No significant effects or complications reported

Dosage I.M.: Adults: Prostate cancer:

Trelstar™ Depot: 3.75 mg once every 28 days

Trelstar™ LA: 11.25 mg once every 84 days

Dosing comment in renal/hepatic impairment: Two- to fourfold higher exposure than young healthy males; clinical consequences of this increase are unknown

Mechanism of Action Causes suppression of ovarian and testicular steroidogenesis due to decreased levels of LH and FSH with subsequent decrease in testosterone (male) and estrogen (female) levels. After chronic and continuous administration, usually 2-4 weeks after initiation, a sustained decrease in LH and FSH secretion occurs.

Other Adverse Effects As reported with Trelstar™ Depot and Trelstar™ LA; frequency of effect may vary by product:

>10%:

- Endocrine & metabolic: Hot flashes (59% to 73%), glucose increased, hemoglobin decreased, RBC count decreased
- Hepatic: Alkaline phosphatase increased, ALT increased, AST increased
- Neuromuscular & skeletal: Skeletal pain (12% to 13%)
- Renal: BUN increased

1% to 10%:

- Cardiovascular: Leg edema (6%), hypertension (4%), chest pain (2%), peripheral edema (1%)
- Central nervous system: Headache (5% to 7%), dizziness (1% to 3%), pain (2% to 3%), emotional lability (1%), fatigue (2%), insomnia (2%)
- Dermatologic: Rash (2%), pruritus (1%)
- Endocrine & metabolic: Alkaline phosphatase increased (2%), breast pain (2%), gynocomastia (2%), libido decreased (2%)
- Gastrointestinal: Nausea (3%), anorexia (2%), constipation (2%), dyspepsia (2%), vomiting (2%), abdominal pain (1%), diarrhea (1%)
- Genitourinary: Dysuria (5%), impotence (2% to 7%), urinary retention (1%), urinary tract infection (1%)
- Hematologic: Anemia (1%)
- Local: Injection site pain (4%)
- Neuromuscular & skeletal: Leg pain (2% to 5%), back pain (3%), arthralgia (2%), leg cramps (2%), myalgia (1%), weakness (1%)
- Ocular: Conjunctivitis (1%), eye pain (1%)
- Respiratory: Cough (2%), dyspnea (1%), pharyngitis (1%)

Postmarketing and/or case reports: Anaphylaxis, angioedema, hypersensitivity reactions, spinal cord compression, renal dysfunction

Drug Interactions Hyperprolactinemic drugs (dopamine antagonists such as antipsychotics, and metoclopramide) are contraindicated.

Pharmacodynamics/Kinetics

Absorption: Oral: Not active

Distribution: V_d: 30-33 L

Protein binding: None

Metabolism: Unknown; unlikely to involve CYP; no known metabolites

Half-life elimination: 2.8 ± 1.2 hours

- Moderate to severe renal impairment: 6.5-7.7 hours
- Hepatic impairment: 7.6 hours

Time to peak: 1-3 hours

Excretion: Urine (42% as intact peptide); hepatic

Pregnancy Risk Factor X
Generic Available No

Triptorelin Pamoate *see* Triptorelin *on page 1358*
Tris Buffer *see* Tromethamine *on page 1360*
Tris(hydroxymethyl)aminomethane *see* Tromethamine *on page 1360*
Tri-Sudo® [OTC] *see* Triprolidine and Pseudoephedrine *on page 1356*
Tri-Tannate® *see* Chlorpheniramine, Pyrilamine, and Phenylephrine *on page 312*
Tri-Tannate Plus® [OTC] *see* Chlorpheniramine, Ephedrine, Phenylephrine, and Carbetapentane *on page 309*
Trivagizole 3™ *see* Clotrimazole *on page 356*
Trivora® *see* Combination Hormonal Contraceptives *on page 368*
Trizivir® *see* Abacavir, Lamivudine, and Zidovudine *on page 23*
Trobicin® *see* Spectinomycin *on page 1239*
Trocaine® [OTC] *see* Benzocaine *on page 169*

Troleandomycin (troe lee an doe MYE sin)

U.S. Brand Names Tao®
Pharmacologic Category Antibiotic, Macrolide
Synonyms Triacetyloleandomycin
Use Antibiotic with spectrum of activity similar to erythromycin

Orphan drug: Adjunct in the treatment of corticosteroid-dependent asthma due to its steroid-sparing properties

Local Anesthetic/Vasoconstrictor Precautions No information available to require special precautions

Effects on Dental Treatment No significant effects or complications reported

Dosage Oral:

Children 7-13 years: 25-40 mg/kg/day divided every 6 hours (125-250 mg every 6 hours)

Adjunct in corticosteroid-dependent asthma: 14 mg/kg/day in divided doses every 6-12 hours not to exceed 250 mg every 6 hours; dose is tapered to once daily then alternate day dosing

Adults: 250-500 mg 4 times/day (around-the-clock every 6 hours)

Mechanism of Action Decreases methylprednisolone clearance from a linear first order decline to a nonlinear decline in plasma concentration. Troleandomycin also has an undefined action independent of its effects on steroid elimination. Inhibits RNA-dependent protein synthesis at the chain elongation step; binds to the 50S ribosomal subunit resulting in blockage of transpeptidation.

Other Adverse Effects Frequency not defined:

Gastrointestinal: Abdominal cramping and discomfort (dose-related), nausea, vomiting, diarrhea, rectal burning

Dermatologic: Urticaria, rashes

Hepatic: Cholestatic jaundice

Drug Interactions Substrate of **CYP3A4**; Inhibits **CYP3A4**

Increased Effect/Toxicity:

Avoid concomitant use of the following with troleandomycin due to increased risk of malignant arrhythmias: Astemizole, cisapride, gatifloxacin, moxifloxacin, pimozide, sparfloxacin, thioridazine. Other agents that prolong the QT_c interval, including type Ia (eg, quinidine) and type III antiarrhythmic agents, and selected antipsychotic agents (eg, mesoridazine, thioridazine) should be used with extreme caution.

Troleandomycin may increase the serum concentrations (and possibly the toxicity) of the following agents: Alfentanil (and possibly other narcotic analgesics), benzodiazepines (alprazolam, diazepam, midazolam, triazolam), buspirone, calcium channel blockers, dihydropyridine (felodipine), carbamazepine, cilostazol, clozapine, colchicine, cyclosporine, digoxin, disopyramide, ergot alkaloids (eg, bromocriptine), HMG-CoA reductase inhibitors (except fluvastatin, pravastatin), loratadine, methylprednisolone, rifabutin, tacrolimus, theophylline, sildenafil, valproate, vinblastine, vincristine, zopiclone.

The effects of neuromuscular-blocking agents and warfarin have been potentiated by troleandomycin. Troleandomycin serum concentrations may be increased by amprenavir (and possibly other protease inhibitors).

Decreased Effect: Troleandomycin may decrease the serum concentrations of zafirlukast. Troleandomycin may antagonize the therapeutic effects of clindamycin and lincomycin.

Dietary/Ethanol/Herb Considerations Food delays but has no effect on the extent of absorption.

Pharmacodynamics/Kinetics

Time to peak, serum: ~2 hours

Excretion: Urine (10% to 25% as active drug); feces

Pregnancy Risk Factor C
Generic Available No

Tromethamine (troe METH a meen)

U.S. Brand Names THAM®

Pharmacologic Category Alkalinizing Agent

Synonyms Tris Buffer; Tris(hydroxymethyl)aminomethane

Use Correction of metabolic acidosis associated with cardiac bypass surgery or cardiac arrest; to correct excess acidity of stored blood that is preserved with acid citrate dextrose; to prime the pump-oxygenator during cardiac bypass surgery; indicated in infants needing alkalinization after receiving maximum sodium bicarbonate (8-10 mEq/kg/24 hours); (advantage of THAM® is that it alkalinizes without increasing pCO_2 and sodium)

Local Anesthetic/Vasoconstrictor Precautions No information available to require special precautions

Effects on Dental Treatment No significant effects or complications reported

Dosage

Neonates and Infants: Metabolic acidosis associated with RDS: Initial: Approximately 1 mL/kg for each pH unit below 7.4; additional doses determined by changes in PaO_2, pH, and pCO_2; **Note:** Although THAM® solution does not raise pCO_2 when treating metabolic acidosis with concurrent respiratory acidosis, bicarbonate may be preferred because the osmotic effects of THAM® are greater.

Adults: Dose depends on buffer base deficit; when deficit is known: tromethamine (mL of 0.3 M solution) = body weight (kg) x base deficit (mEq/L); when base deficit is not known: 3-6 mL/kg/dose I.V. (1-2 mEq/kg/dose)

Metabolic acidosis with cardiac arrest:

I.V.: 3.5-6 mL/kg (1-2 mEq/kg/dose) into large peripheral vein; 500-1000 mL if needed in adults

I.V. continuous drip: Infuse slowly by syringe pump over 3-6 hours

Acidosis associated with cardiac bypass surgery: Average dose: 9 mL/kg (2.7 mEq/kg); 500 mL is adequate for most adults; maximum dose: 500 mg/kg in ≤1 hour

Excess acidity of acid citrate dextrose priming blood: 14-70 mL of 0.3 molar solution added to each 500 mL of blood

Dosing comments in renal impairment: Use with caution and monitor for hyperkalemia and EKG

Mechanism of Action Acts as a proton acceptor, which combines with hydrogen ions to form bicarbonate buffer, to correct acidosis

Other Adverse Effects

1% to 10%:

Cardiovascular: Venospasm

Local: Tissue irritation, necrosis with extravasation

<1%: Apnea, respiratory depression, hyperosmolality of serum, hyperkalemia, hypoglycemia (transient), increased blood coagulation time, liver cell destruction from direct contact with THAM®; infusion via low-lying umbilical venous catheters has been associated with hepatocellular necrosis

Pharmacodynamics/Kinetics

Absorption: 30% of dose is not ionized

Excretion: Urine (>75%) within 3 hours

Pregnancy Risk Factor C

Generic Available No

Comments 1 mM = 120 mg = 3.3 mL = 1 mEq of THAM®

Tronolane® [OTC] *see* Pramoxine *on page 1105*

Tropicacyl® *see* Tropicamide *on page 1360*

Tropicamide (troe PIK a mide)

U.S. Brand Names Mydriacyl®; Opticyl®; Tropicacyl®

Canadian Brand Names Diotrope®; Mydriacyl®

Pharmacologic Category Ophthalmic Agent, Mydriatic

Synonyms Bistropamide

Use Short-acting mydriatic used in diagnostic procedures; as well as preoperatively and postoperatively; treatment of some cases of acute iritis, iridocyclitis, and keratitis

Local Anesthetic/Vasoconstrictor Precautions No information available to require special precautions

Effects on Dental Treatment No significant effects or complications reported

Dosage Ophthalmic: Children and Adults (individuals with heavily pigmented eyes may require larger doses):

Cycloplegia: Instill 1-2 drops (1%); may repeat in 5 minutes

Exam must be performed within 30 minutes after the repeat dose; if the patient is not examined within 20-30 minutes, instill an additional drop

Mydriasis: Instill 1-2 drops (0.5%) 15-20 minutes before exam; may repeat every 30 minutes as needed

Mechanism of Action Prevents the sphincter muscle of the iris and the muscle of the ciliary body from responding to cholinergic stimulation

Other Adverse Effects Frequency not defined:

Cardiovascular: Tachycardia, vascular congestion, edema

Central nervous system: Parasympathetic stimulations, drowsiness, headache

Dermatologic: Eczematoid dermatitis

Gastrointestinal: Xerostomia

Local: Transient stinging

Ocular: Blurred vision, photophobia with or without corneal staining, increased intraocular pressure, follicular conjunctivitis

Pharmacodynamics/Kinetics

Onset of action: Mydriasis: ~20-40 minutes; Cycloplegia: ~30 minutes

Duration: Mydriasis: ~6-7 hours; Cycloplegia: <6 hours

Pregnancy Risk Factor C

Generic Available Yes

Tropicamide and Hydroxyamphetamine *see* Hydroxyamphetamine and Tropicamide *on page 694*

Trovafloxacin/Alatrofloxacin

(TROE vu floks u sin/a lat roe FLOKS u sin)

U.S. Brand Names Trovan®

Mexican Brand Names Trovan®

Pharmacologic Category Antibiotic, Quinolone

Synonyms Alatrofloxacin Mesylate; CP-99,219-27

Use Should be used only in life- or limb-threatening infections

Treatment of nosocomial pneumonia, community-acquired pneumonia, complicated intra-abdominal infections, gynecologic/pelvic infections, complicated skin and skin structure infections

Local Anesthetic/Vasoconstrictor Precautions No information available to require special precautions

Effects on Dental Treatment No significant effects or complications reported

Dosage Adults:

Nosocomial pneumonia: I.V.: 300 mg single dose followed by 200 mg/day orally for a total duration of 10-14 days

Community-acquired pneumonia: Oral, I.V.: 200 mg/day for 7-14 days

Complicated intra-abdominal infections, including postsurgical infections/gynecologic and pelvic infections: I.V.: 300 mg as a single dose followed by 200 mg/day orally for a total duration of 7-14 days

Skin and skin structure infections, complicated, including diabetic foot infections: Oral, I.V.: 200 mg/day for 10-14 days

Hemodialysis: Not sufficiently removed

Dosing adjustment in hepatic impairment:

Mild to moderate cirrhosis:

Initial dose for normal hepatic function: 300 mg I.V.; 200 mg I.V. or oral; 100 mg oral

Reduced dose: 200 mg I.V.; 100 mg I.V. or oral; 100 mg oral

Mechanism of Action Inhibits DNA-gyrase in susceptible organisms; inhibits relaxation of supercoiled DNA and promotes breakage of double-stranded DNA

Other Adverse Effects Note: Fatalities have occurred in patients developing hepatic necrosis.

1% to 10% (range reported in clinical trials):

Central nervous system: Dizziness (2% to 11%), lightheadedness (<1% to 4%), headache (1% to 5%)

Dermatologic: Rash (<1% to 2%), pruritus (<1% to 2%)

Gastrointestinal: Nausea (4% to 8%), abdominal pain (<1% to 1%), vomiting, diarrhea

Genitourinary: Vaginitis (<1% to 1%)

Hepatic: Increased LFTs

Local: Injection site reaction, pain, or inflammation

<1%: Phototoxicity, convulsions, dyskinesia, pseudomembranous colitis, allergic/anaphylactoid reaction, tendonitis, bronchospasm, interstitial nephritis, anaphylaxis, hepatic necrosis, pancreatitis, Stevens-Johnson syndrome; quinolones have been associated with tendon rupture

Drug Interactions

Increased Effect/Toxicity: Concurrent use of corticosteroids may increase risk of tendon rupture.

Decreased Effect: Coadministration with antacids containing aluminum or magnesium, citric acid/sodium citrate, sucralfate, and iron markedly reduces absorption of trovafloxacin. Separate oral administration by at least 2 hours. Coadministration of intravenous morphine also reduces absorption. Separate I.V. morphine by 2 hours (when trovafloxacin is taken in fasting state) or 4 hours (when taken with food). Do not administer multivalent cations (eg, calcium, magnesium) through the same intravenous line.

Dietary/Ethanol/Herb Considerations

Food: Avoid dairy products; may decrease absorption of oral form. Enteral feedings may also limit absorption.

(Continued)

Trovafloxacin/Alatrofloxacin *(Continued)*

Herb/Nutraceutical: Avoid dong quai and St John's wort; may cause photosensitization.

Pharmacodynamics/Kinetics

Distribution: Concentration in most tissues greater than plasma or serum
Protein binding: 76%
Metabolism: Hepatic conjugation; glucuronidation 13%, acetylation 9%
Bioavailability: 88%
Half-life elimination: 9-12 hours
Time to peak, serum: Oral: Within 2 hours
Excretion: Feces (43% as unchanged drug); urine (6% as unchanged drug)

Pregnancy Risk Factor C

Generic Available No

Comments *In vitro* trovafloxacin was more active than sparfloxacin, ofloxacin, ciprofloxacin, ceftriaxone, erythromycin and vancomycin against *S. pneumoniae.* It was also more active against penicillin-resistant strains than ceftriaxone, erythromycin or vancomycin. Trovafloxacin is very effective in bronchitis and pneumonia. It has good activity against resistant organisms, and penetration of the cerebral spinal fluid giving potential in the treatment of CNS infections.

Trovan® *see* Trovafloxacin/Alatrofloxacin *on page 1361*
Troxidone *see* Trimethadione *on page 1351*
Truphylline® *see* Aminophylline *on page 78*
Trusopt® *see* Dorzolamide *on page 468*

Trypsin, Balsam Peru, and Castor Oil

(TRIP sin, BOL sum pe ROO, & KAS ter oyl)

U.S. Brand Names Granulex®

Pharmacologic Category Protectant, Topical

Use Treatment of decubitus ulcers, varicose ulcers, debridement of eschar, dehiscent wounds and sunburn

Local Anesthetic/Vasoconstrictor Precautions No information available to require special precautions

Effects on Dental Treatment No significant effects or complications reported

Dosage Topical: Apply a minimum of twice daily or as often as necessary

Generic Available Yes

TSH *see* Thyrotropin Alpha *on page 1304*
TSPA *see* Thiotepa *on page 1300*
TST *see* Tuberculin Tests *on page 1362*
T-Stat® *see* Erythromycin *on page 512*
Tuberculin Skin Test *see* Tuberculin Tests *on page 1362*

Tuberculin Tests (too BER kyoo lin tests)

U.S. Brand Names Aplisol®; Tubersol®

Pharmacologic Category Diagnostic Agent

Synonyms Mantoux; PPD; Tine Test; TST; Tuberculin Skin Test

Use Skin test in diagnosis of tuberculosis, cell-mediated immunodeficiencies

Local Anesthetic/Vasoconstrictor Precautions No information available to require special precautions

Effects on Dental Treatment No significant effects or complications reported

Restrictions Whenever administered, a record should be made of the administration technique (Mantoux method, disposable multiple-puncture device), tuberculin used (OT or PPD), manufacturer and lot number of tuberculin used, date of administration, date of test reading, and the size of the reaction in millimeters (mm).

Dosage Children and Adults: Intradermal: 0.1 mL about 4" below elbow; use 1/4" to 1/2" or 26- or 27-gauge needle; significant reactions are ≥5 mm in diameter

Interpretation of induration of tuberculin skin test injections: Positive: ≥10 mm; inconclusive: 5-9 mm; negative: <5 mm

Interpretation of induration of Tine test injections: Positive: >2 mm and vesiculation present; inconclusive: <2 mm (give patient Mantoux test of 5 TU/0.1 mL - base decisions on results of Mantoux test); negative: <2 mm or erythema of any size (no need for retesting unless person is a contact of a patient with tuberculosis or there is clinical evidence suggestive of the disease)

Mechanism of Action Tuberculosis results in individuals becoming sensitized to certain antigenic components of the *M. tuberculosis* organism. Culture extracts called tuberculins are contained in tuberculin skin test preparations. Upon intracutaneous injection of these culture extracts, a classic delayed (cellular) hypersensitivity reaction occurs. This reaction is characteristic of a delayed course (peak occurs >24 hours after injection, induration of the skin secondary to cell infiltration, and occasional vesiculation and necrosis). Delayed hypersensitivity reactions to tuberculin may indicate infection with a variety of nontuberculosis mycobacteria, or vaccination with the live attenuated mycobacterial strain of *M. bovis* vaccine, BCG, in addition to previous natural infection with *M. tuberculosis*.

Other Adverse Effects Frequency not defined:
Dermatologic: Ulceration, necrosis, vesiculation
Local: Pain at injection site

Pharmacodynamics/Kinetics
Onset of action: Delayed hypersensitivity reactions: 5-6 hours
Peak effect: 48-72 hours
Duration: Reactions subside over a few days

Pregnancy Risk Factor C

Generic Available No

Tubersol® *see* Tuberculin Tests *on page 1362*
Tuinal® *see* Amobarbital and Secobarbital *on page 91*
Tums® [OTC] *see* Calcium Supplements *on page 229*
Tums® E-X Extra Strength Tablet [OTC] *see* Calcium Supplements *on page 229*
Tums® Ultra® [OTC] *see* Calcium Supplements *on page 229*
Tussend® Expectorant *see* Hydrocodone, Pseudoephedrine, and Guaifenesin *on page 687*
Tussi-12® *see* Carbetapentane and Chlorpheniramine *on page 245*
Tussi-12 S™ *see* Carbetapentane and Chlorpheniramine *on page 245*
Tussigon® *see* Hydrocodone and Homatropine *on page 684*
Tussionex® *see* Hydrocodone and Chlorpheniramine *on page 682*
Tussi-Organidin® DM NR *see* Guaifenesin and Dextromethorphan *on page 651*
Tussi-Organidin® NR *see* Guaifenesin and Codeine *on page 650*
Tussi-Organidin® S-NR *see* Guaifenesin and Codeine *on page 650*
Tusstat® *see* DiphenhydrAMINE *on page 451*
Twice-A-Day® [OTC] *see* Oxymetazoline *on page 1022*
Twilite® [OTC] *see* DiphenhydrAMINE *on page 451*
Twinrix® *see* Hepatitis A (Inactivated) and Hepatitis B (Recombinant) Vaccine *on page 664*
Tylenol® [OTC] *see* Acetaminophen *on page 27*
Tylenol® Allergy Sinus [OTC] *see* Acetaminophen, Chlorpheniramine, and Pseudoephedrine *on page 35*
Tylenol® Arthritis Pain [OTC] *see* Acetaminophen *on page 27*
Tylenol® Children's [OTC] *see* Acetaminophen *on page 27*
Tylenol® Cold Non-Drowsy [OTC] *see* Acetaminophen, Dextromethorphan, and Pseudoephedrine *on page 35*
Tylenol® Extra Strength [OTC] *see* Acetaminophen *on page 27*
Tylenol® Flu Non-Drowsy Maximum Strength [OTC] *see* Acetaminophen, Dextromethorphan, and Pseudoephedrine *on page 35*
Tylenol® Infants [OTC] *see* Acetaminophen *on page 27*
Tylenol® Junior Strength [OTC] *see* Acetaminophen *on page 27*
Tylenol® PM Extra Strength [OTC] *see* Acetaminophen and Diphenhydramine *on page 30*
Tylenol® Severe Allergy [OTC] *see* Acetaminophen and Diphenhydramine *on page 30*
Tylenol® Sinus Non-Drowsy [OTC] *see* Acetaminophen and Pseudoephedrine *on page 31*
Tylenol® Sore Throat [OTC] *see* Acetaminophen *on page 27*
Tylenol® With Codeine *see* Acetaminophen and Codeine *on page 29*
Tylox® *see* Oxycodone and Acetaminophen *on page 1018*
Typhim Vi® *see* Typhoid Vaccine *on page 1363*

Typhoid Vaccine (TYE foyd vak SEEN)

Related Information
Immunizations (Vaccines) *on page 1612*

U.S. Brand Names Typhim Vi®; Vivotif Berna®

Canadian Brand Names Vivotif Berna®

Pharmacologic Category Vaccine

Synonyms Typhoid Vaccine Live Oral Ty21a

Use Typhoid vaccine: Live, attenuated Ty21a typhoid vaccine should not be administered to immunocompromised persons, including those known to be infected with HIV. Parenteral inactivated vaccine is a theoretically safer alternative for this group.
Parenteral: Promotes active immunity to typhoid fever for patients intimately exposed to a typhoid carrier or foreign travel to a typhoid fever endemic area
Oral: For immunization of children >6 years of age and adults who expect intimate exposure of or household contact with typhoid fever, travelers to areas of world with risk of exposure to typhoid fever, and workers in microbiology laboratories with expected frequent contact with *S. typhi*

Local Anesthetic/Vasoconstrictor Precautions No information available to require special precautions

Effects on Dental Treatment No significant effects or complications reported

(Continued)

Typhoid Vaccine *(Continued)*

Restrictions Federal law requires that the date of administration, the vaccine manufacturer, lot number of vaccine, and the administering person's name, title and address be entered into the patient's permanent medical record.

Dosage

S.C. (AKD and H-P):

Children 6 months to 10 years: 0.25 mL; repeat in ≥4 weeks (total immunization is 2 doses)

Children >10 years and Adults: 0.5 mL; repeat dose in ≥4 weeks (total immunization is 2 doses)

Booster: 0.25 mL every 3 years for children 6 months to 10 years and 0.5 mL every 3 years for children >10 years and adults

Oral: Adults:

Primary immunization: 1 capsule on alternate days (day 1, 3, 5, and 7)

Booster immunization: Repeat full course of primary immunization every 5 years

Mechanism of Action Virulent strains of *Salmonella typhi* cause disease by penetrating the intestinal mucosa and entering the systemic circulation via the lymphatic vasculature. One possible mechanism of conferring immunity may be the provocation of a local immune response in the intestinal tract induced by oral ingesting of a live strain with subsequent aborted infection. The ability of *Salmonella typhi* to produce clinical disease (and to elicit an immune response) is dependent on the bacteria having a complete lipopolysaccharide. The live attenuate Ty21a strain lacks the enzyme UDP-4-galactose epimerase so that lipopolysaccharide is only synthesized under conditions that induce bacterial autolysis. Thus, the strain remains avirulent despite the production of sufficient lipopolysaccharide to evoke a protective immune response. Despite low levels of lipopolysaccharide synthesis, cells lyse before gaining a virulent phenotype due to the intracellular accumulation of metabolic intermediates.

Other Adverse Effects All serious adverse reactions must be reported to the U.S. Department of Health and Human Services (DHHS) Vaccine Adverse Event Reporting System (VAERS) 1-800-822-7967.

Oral:

1% to 10%:

Central nervous system: Headache, fever

Dermatologic: Rash

Gastrointestinal: Abdominal discomfort, stomach cramps, diarrhea, nausea, vomiting

<1%: Anaphylactic reaction

Injection:

>10%:

Central nervous system: Headache (13% to 20%), fever (3% to 11%), malaise (4% to 24%)

Dermatologic: Local tenderness (13% to 98%), induration (5% to 15%), pain at injection site (7% to 41%)

1% to 10%:

Central nervous system: Fever ≥100°F (2%)

Gastrointestinal: Nausea (2% to 8%), diarrhea (3% to 4%), vomiting (2%)

Local: Erythema at injection site (4% to 5%)

Neuromuscular & skeletal: Myalgia (3% to 7%)

<1%: Hypotension, allergic reactions

Pharmacodynamics/Kinetics

Onset of action: Immunity to *Salmonella typhi*: Oral: ~1 week

Duration: Immunity: Oral: ~5 years; Parenteral: ~3 years

Pregnancy Risk Factor C

Generic Available No

Typhoid Vaccine Live Oral Ty21a *see* Typhoid Vaccine *on page 1363*

Tyzine® *see* Tetrahydrozoline *on page 1288*

Tyzine® Pediatric *see* Tetrahydrozoline *on page 1288*

U-90152S *see* Delavirdine *on page 405*

UCB-P071 *see* Cetirizine *on page 289*

UK 92480 *see* Sildenafil *on page 1220*

UK109496 *see* Voriconazole *on page 1395*

Ulcerease® [OTC] *see* Phenol *on page 1068*

Ultiva® *see* Remifentanil *on page 1171*

Ultracet™ *see* Acetaminophen and Tramadol *on page 32*

Ultram® *see* Tramadol *on page 1329*

Ultra Mide® *see* Urea *on page 1365*

Ultrase® *see* Pancrelipase *on page 1030*

Ultrase® MT *see* Pancrelipase *on page 1030*

Ultra Tears® [OTC] *see* Artificial Tears *on page 128*

Ultravate® *see* Halobetasol *on page 658*

Unasyn® *see* Ampicillin and Sulbactam *on page 104*

Undecylenic Acid and Derivatives

(un de sil EN ik AS id & du RIV u tivz)

U.S. Brand Names Fungi-Nail® [OTC]

Pharmacologic Category Antifungal Agent, Topical

Synonyms Zinc Undecylenate

Use Treatment of athlete's foot (tinea pedis); ringworm (except nails and scalp)

Local Anesthetic/Vasoconstrictor Precautions No information available to require special precautions

Effects on Dental Treatment No significant effects or complications reported

Dosage Children and Adults: Topical: Apply twice daily to affected area for 4 weeks; apply to clean, dry area

Other Adverse Effects 1% to 10%: Dermatologic: Skin irritation, sensitization

Generic Available No

Uni-Fed® [OTC] *see* Triprolidine and Pseudoephedrine *on page 1356*

Uniphyl® *see* Theophylline *on page 1291*

Uniretic® *see* Moexipril and Hydrochlorothiazide *on page 927*

Unisom® Maximum Strength SleepGels® [OTC] *see* DiphenhydrAMINE *on page 451*

Unithroid® *see* Levothyroxine *on page 800*

Univasc® *see* Moexipril *on page 926*

Unna's Boot *see* Zinc Gelatin *on page 1409*

Unna's Paste *see* Zinc Gelatin *on page 1409*

Urea (yoor EE u)

U.S. Brand Names Amino-Cerv™; Aquacare® [OTC]; Aquaphilic® With Carbamide [OTC]; Carmol® 10 [OTC]; Carmol® 20 [OTC]; Carmol® 40; Carmol® Deep Cleaning; Gormel® [OTC]; Lanaphilic® [OTC]; Nutraplus® [OTC]; Rea-Lo® [OTC]; Ultra Mide®; Ureacin® [OTC]; Ureaphil® [DSC]; Vanamide™

Canadian Brand Names UltraMide 25™; Uremol®; Urisec®

Mexican Brand Names Derma Keri®; Dermoplast®

Pharmacologic Category Diuretic, Osmotic; Keratolytic Agent; Topical Skin Product

Synonyms Carbamide

Use

Injection: Reduces intracranial pressure (ICP) and intraocular pressure (IOP)

Vaginal: Treatment of cervicitis

Topical: Keratolytic agent to soften nails or skin; moisturizer for dry, rough skin [OTC]

Local Anesthetic/Vasoconstrictor Precautions No information available to require special precautions

Effects on Dental Treatment No significant effects or complications reported

Dosage

Reduction of intracranial or intraocular pressure: I.V. slow infusion:

- Children:
  - <2 years: 0.1-0.5 g/kg
  - >2 years: 0.5-1.5 g/kg
- Adults: 1-1.5 g/kg slow infusion (1-2½ hours); maximum: 120 g/24 hours
- Elderly: Start at low end of dosing range; use caution due to greater frequency of renal, hepatic, and cardiac dysfunction

Hyperkeratotic conditions, dry skin: Adults: Topical: Apply 1-3 times/day

Cervicitis: Adults: Vaginal: Insert 1 applicatorful in vagina at bedtime for 2-4 weeks

Mechanism of Action Injection: Elevates plasma osmolality by inhibiting tubular reabsorption of water, thus enhancing the flow of water into extracellular fluid

Other Adverse Effects Frequency not defined:

Injection:

- Central nervous system: **Headache**
- Endocrine & metabolic: Electrolyte imbalance
- Gastrointestinal: **Nausea, vomiting**
- Local: Tissue necrosis from extravasation of I.V. preparation

Topical: Local: Transient stinging, local irritation

Drug Interactions Decreased Effect: Urea increases lithium excretion

Pharmacodynamics/Kinetics Injection:

Onset of action: Therapeutic: Maximum: 1-2 hours

Duration: 3-6 hours (diuresis can continue for up to 10 hours)

Half-life elimination: 1 hour

Excretion: Urine (as unchanged drug)

Pregnancy Risk Factor C

Generic Available No

Urea and Hydrocortisone (yoor EE u & hye droe KORE ti zone)

Related Information

Hydrocortisone *on page 688*

Urea *on page 1365*

(Continued)

Urea and Hydrocortisone *(Continued)*

U.S. Brand Names Carmol-HC®

Canadian Brand Names Ti-U-Lac® H; Uremol® HC

Pharmacologic Category Corticosteroid, Topical

Synonyms Hydrocortisone and Urea

Use Inflammation of corticosteroid-responsive dermatoses

Local Anesthetic/Vasoconstrictor Precautions No information available to require special precautions

Effects on Dental Treatment No significant effects or complications reported

Dosage Apply thin film and rub in well 1-4 times/day. Therapy should be discontinued when control is achieved; if no improvement is seen, reassessment of diagnosis may be necessary.

Pregnancy Risk Factor C

Generic Available No

Ureacin® [OTC] *see* Urea *on page 1365*

Urea Peroxide *see* Carbamide Peroxide *on page 244*

Ureaphil® [DSC] *see* Urea *on page 1365*

Urecholine® *see* Bethanechol *on page 181*

Urex® *see* Methenamine *on page 879*

Urimar-T *see* Methenamine, Sodium Biphosphate, Phenyl Salicylate, Methylene Blue, and Hyoscyamine *on page 880*

Urimax® *see* Methenamine, Sodium Biphosphate, Phenyl Salicylate, Methylene Blue, and Hyoscyamine *on page 880*

Urispas® *see* Flavoxate *on page 573*

Uristat® [OTC] *see* Phenazopyridine *on page 1064*

Urocit®-K *see* Potassium Citrate *on page 1100*

Urocit®-K *see* Potassium Supplements *on page 1102*

Urofollitropin *see* Follitropins *on page 607*

Uro-KP-Neutral® *see* Phosphate Supplements *on page 1076*

Uro-Mag® [OTC] *see* Magnesium Supplements *on page 837*

Urso® *see* Ursodiol *on page 1366*

Ursodeoxycholic Acid *see* Ursodiol *on page 1366*

Ursodiol (ER soe dye ole)

U.S. Brand Names Actigall®; Urso®

Canadian Brand Names Urso®

Mexican Brand Names Ursofalk®

Pharmacologic Category Gallstone Dissolution Agent

Synonyms Ursodeoxycholic Acid

Use Actigall®: Gallbladder stone dissolution; prevention of gallstones in obese patients experiencing rapid weight loss; Urso®: Primary biliary cirrhosis

Unlabeled/Investigational Use Liver transplantation

Local Anesthetic/Vasoconstrictor Precautions No information available to require special precautions

Effects on Dental Treatment No significant effects or complications reported

Dosage Adults: Oral:

Gallstone dissolution: 8-10 mg/kg/day in 2-3 divided doses; use beyond 24 months is not established; obtain ultrasound images at 6-month intervals for the first year of therapy; 30% of patients have stone recurrence after dissolution

Gallstone prevention: 300 mg twice daily

Primary biliary cirrhosis: 13-15 mg/kg/day in 4 divided doses (with food)

Mechanism of Action Decreases the cholesterol content of bile and bile stones by reducing the secretion of cholesterol from the liver and the fractional reabsorption of cholesterol by the intestines. Mechanism of action in primary biliary cirrhosis is not clearly defined.

Other Adverse Effects

>10%:

Central nervous system: Headache (up to 25%), dizziness (up to 17%)

Gastrointestinal: In treatment of primary biliary cirrhosis: Constipation (up to 26%)

1% to 10%:

Dermatologic: Rash (<1% to 3%), alopecia (<1% to 5%)

Gastrointestinal:

In gallstone dissolution: Most GI events (diarrhea, nausea, vomiting) are similar to placebo and attributable to gallstone disease.

In treatment of primary biliary cirrhosis: Diarrhea (1%)

Hematologic: Leukopenia (3%)

Miscellaneous: Allergy (5%)

<1%: Abdominal pain, biliary pain, fatigue, metallic taste, nausea, pruritus, vomiting

In treatment of primary biliary cirrhosis: Constipation, dyspepsia, headache

Drug Interactions Decreased Effect: Decreased effect with aluminum-containing antacids, cholestyramine, colestipol, clofibrate, and oral contraceptives (estrogens).

Dietary/Ethanol/Herb Considerations Food: Administer Urso® with food.

Pharmacodynamics/Kinetics

Metabolism: Undergoes extensive enterohepatic recycling; following hepatic conjugation and biliary secretion, the drug is hydrolyzed to active ursodiol, where it is recycled or transformed to lithocholic acid by colonic microbial flora

Half-life elimination: 100 hours

Excretion: Feces

Pregnancy Risk Factor B

Generic Available Yes: Capsule

UTI Relief® [OTC] *see* Phenazopyridine *on page 1064*

Uvadex® *see* Methoxsalen *on page 888*

Vagifem® *see* Estradiol *on page 521*

Vagi-Gard® [OTC] *see* Povidone-Iodine *on page 1104*

Vagistat®-1 [OTC] *see* Tioconazole *on page 1312*

Valacyclovir (val ay SYE kloe veer)

Related Information

Acyclovir *on page 42*

Sexually-Transmitted Diseases *on page 1502*

Systemic Viral Diseases *on page 1517*

U.S. Brand Names Valtrex®

Canadian Brand Names Valtrex®

Pharmacologic Category Antiviral Agent, Oral

Synonyms Valacyclovir Hydrochloride

Use Treatment of herpes zoster (shingles) in immunocompetent patients; episodic treatment or prophylaxis of recurrent genital herpes in immunocompetent patients; for first episode genital herpes; treatment of herpes labialis (cold sores)

Local Anesthetic/Vasoconstrictor Precautions No information available to require special precautions

Effects on Dental Treatment

>10%: Headache (14% to 35%), nausea (6% to 15%)

1% to 7%: Dizziness (2% to 4%), CNS depression (≤7%), vomiting (≤6%)

Dosage Oral:

Adolescents ≥12 years and Adults: **Herpes labialis (cold sores):** 2 g twice daily for 1 day (separate doses by ~12 hours)

Adults:

- Herpes zoster (shingles): 1 g 3 times/day for 7 days
- Genital herpes:
  - Initial episode: 1 g 2 times/day for 10 days
  - Episodic treatment: 500 mg twice daily for 3 days
  - Prophylaxis: 500-1000 mg once daily

Dosing interval in renal impairment:

- Herpes zoster: Adults:
  - Cl_{cr} 30-49 mL/minute: 1 g every 12 hours
  - Cl_{cr} 10-29 mL/minute: 1 g every 24 hours
  - Cl_{cr} <10 mL/minute: 500 mg every 24 hours
- Genital herpes: Adults:
  - Initial episode:
    - Cl_{cr} 10-29 mL/minute: 1 g every 24 hours
    - Cl_{cr} <10 mL/minute: 500 mg every 24 hours
  - Episodic treatment: Cl_{cr} <10-29 mL/minute: 500 mg every 24 hours
  - Prophylaxis: Cl_{cr} <10-29 mL/minute:
    - For usual dose of 1 g every 24 hours, decrease dose to 500 mg every 24 hours
    - For usual dose of 500 mg every 24 hours, decrease dose to 500 mg every 48 hours
- **Herpes labialis:** Adolescents ≥12 years and Adults:
  - Cl_{cr} 30-49 mL/minute: 1 g every 12 hours for 2 doses
  - Cl_{cr} 10-29 mL/minute: 500 mg every 12 hours for 2 doses
  - Cl_{cr} <10 mL/minute: 500 mg as a single dose

Hemodialysis: Dialyzable (~33% removed during 4-hour session); administer dose postdialysis

Chronic ambulatory peritoneal dialysis/continuous arteriovenous hemofiltration dialysis: Pharmacokinetic parameters are similar to those in patients with ESRD; supplemental dose not needed following dialysis

Mechanism of Action Valacyclovir is rapidly and nearly completely converted to acyclovir by intestinal and hepatic metabolism. Acyclovir is converted to acyclovir monophosphate by virus-specific thymidine kinase then further converted to acyclovir triphosphate by other cellular enzymes. Acyclovir triphosphate inhibits DNA synthesis and viral replication by competing with deoxyguanosine triphosphate for viral DNA polymerase and being incorporated into viral DNA.

Other Adverse Effects

>10%: Gastrointestinal: Abdominal pain (2% to 11%)

(Continued)

Valacyclovir *(Continued)*

1% to 8%:
Endocrine: Dysmenorrhea (≤1% to 8%)
Hematologic: Leukopenia (≤1%), thrombocytopenia (≤1%)
Hepatic: AST increased (1% to 4%)
Neuromuscular & skeletal: Arthralgia (≤1 to 6%)
<1%: Anemia
Postmarketing and/or case reports: **Acute hypersensitivity reactions, agitation, anaphylaxis,** aplastic anemia, **auditory amd visual hallucinations,** creatinine increased, **coma, confusion, consciousness decreased,** diarrhea, encephalopathy, **facial edema,** erythema multiforme, hepatitis, **hypertension, mania,** photosensitivity reaction, **psychosis,** rash, renal failure, **tachycardia,** thrombotic thrombocytopenic purpura/hemolytic uremic syndrome, **visual disturbances**

Warnings/Precautions Thrombotic thrombocytopenic purpura/hemolytic uremic syndrome has occurred in immunocompromised patients (at doses of 8 g/day); use caution and adjust the dose in elderly patients or those with renal insufficiency and in patients receiving concurrent nephrotoxic agents; treatment should begin as soon as possible after the first signs and symptoms (within 72 hours of onset of first diagnosis or within 24 hours of onset of recurrent episodes); safety and efficacy in children have not been established, except in adolescents for the treatment of herpes labialis

Drug Interactions
Increased Effect/Toxicity: Valacyclovir and acyclovir have increased CNS side effects with zidovudine and probenecid.
Decreased Effect: Cimetidine and/or probenecid has decreased the rate but not the extent of valacyclovir conversion to acyclovir leading to decreased effectiveness of valacyclovir.

Dietary/Ethanol/Herb Considerations Food: May be taken with food

Pharmacodynamics/Kinetics
Absorption: Rapid
Distribution: Acyclovir is widely distributed throughout the body including brain, kidney, lungs, liver, spleen, muscle, uterus, vagina, and CSF
Protein binding: 13.5% to 17.9%
Metabolism: Hepatic; valacyclovir is rapidly and nearly completely converted to acyclovir and L-valine by first-pass effect; acyclovir is hepatically metabolized to a very small extent by aldehyde oxidase and by alcohol and aldehyde dehydrogenase (inactive metabolites)
Bioavailability: ~55% once converted to acyclovir
Half-life elimination: Normal renal function: Adults: Acyclovir: 2.5-3.3 hours, Valacyclovir: ~30 minutes; End-stage renal disease: Acyclovir: 14-20 hours
Excretion: Urine: Acyclovir: 88%, Valacyclovir: 46%; feces: Valacyclovir: 47%

Pregnancy Risk Factor B

Generic Available No

Valacyclovir Hydrochloride *see* Valacyclovir *on page 1367*
Valcyte™ *see* Valganciclovir *on page 1370*

Valdecoxib (val de KOKS ib)

U.S. Brand Names Bextra®

Pharmacologic Category Nonsteroidal Anti-inflammatory Drug (NSAID), COX-2 Selective

Use
Dental (unlabeled): Treatment of postoperative pain
Medical: Relief of signs and symptoms of osteoarthritis and adult rheumatoid arthritis; treatment of primary dysmenorrhea

Local Anesthetic/Vasoconstrictor Precautions No information available to require special precautions

Effects on Dental Treatment
2% to 9%: Hypertension (2%), headache (5% to 9%), dizziness (3%), nausea (6% to 7%), upper respiratory tract infection (6% to 7%), sinusitis (2% to 3%), flu-like symptoms (2%)
<2%: Allergy, aneurysm, angina, anxiety, arrhythmia, atrial fibrillation, bradycardia, bronchitis, bronchospasm, chest pain, CHF, convulsion, cough, diabetes mellitus, duodenal ulcer, duodenitis, dyspnea, EKG abnormality, epistaxis, eructation, esophageal perforation, esophagitis, facial edema, fever, gastric ulcer, gastritis, gastroenteritis, gastroesophageal reflux, GI bleeding, halitosis, hot flashes, hyperglycemia, hypertension exacerbation, hypertensive encephalopathy, hypotension, laryngitis, migraine, myocardial infarction, neck stiffness, nervousness, palpitations, paresthesia, periorbital swelling, pharyngitis, pneumonia, rhinitis, somnolence, stomatitis, increased sweating, syncope, tachycardia, abnormal taste, thirst, twitching, tremors, unstable angina, hemorrhage, ventricular fibrillation, vomiting, earache, xerostomia, bruising, dysphagia, blurred vision, dermatitis (contact and fungal), fatigue, emphysema, hematoma, hypocalcemia, lymphadenopathy, lymphangitis, lymphopenia, malaise, osteoporosis, pain, weakness, anaphylaxis, anorexia, heart block, dysphagia

Dosage Oral: Adults:

Osteoarthritis and rheumatoid arthritis: 10 mg once daily; **Note:** No additional benefits seen with 20 mg/day

Primary dysmenorrhea: 20 mg twice daily as needed

Dosing adjustment in renal/hepatic impairment: Use not recommended in advanced disease

Mechanism of Action Inhibits prostaglandin synthesis by decreasing the activity of the enzyme, cyclooxygenase-2 (COX-2), which results in decreased formation of prostaglandin precursors. Does not affect platelet function.

Other Adverse Effects

2% to 10%:

Cardiovascular: Peripheral edema (2% to 3%)

Dermatologic: Rash (1% to 2%)

Gastrointestinal: Dyspepsia (8% to 9%), abdominal pain (7% to 8%), diarrhea (5% to 6%), flatulence (3% to 4%), abdominal fullness (2%)

Neuromuscular & skeletal: Back pain (2% to 3%), myalgia (2%)

Otic: Tinnitus

<2%: Acne, albuminuria, alkaline phosphatase increased, ALT increased, alopecia, amenorrhea, anemia, aortic stenosis, appetite increased, arthralgia, AST increased, breast neoplasm, BUN increased, cardiomyopathy, carotid stenosis, cataracts, cellulitis, cervical dysplasia, chills, colitis, conjunctivitis, constipation, coronary thrombosis, CPK increased, creatinine increased, cystitis, depression exacerbation, diverticulosis, dry skin, dysmenorrhea, dysuria, eczema, edema, eosinophilia, eye pain, fecal incontinence, glycosuria, goiter, gout, heart murmur, hemangioma, hematemesis, hematuria, hematochezia, hemorrhoids, hepatitis, hypercholesterolemia, hyperkalemia, hyperlipemia, hyperparathyroidism, hypertonia, hyperuricemia, hypoesthesia, hypokalemia, intermittent claudication, impotence, insomnia, keratitis, LDH increased, leukopenia, leukocytosis, leukorrhea, lipoma, LFTs increased, mastitis, melena, menorrhagia, menstrual bloating, micturition frequency increased, mitral insufficiency, morbid dreaming, myocardial ischemia, neuralgia, neuropathy, ovarian cyst (malignant), pericarditis, photosensitivity, pleurisy, pruritus, pyuria, rash erythematous, rash maculopapular, rash psoriaform, skin hypertrophy, skin ulceration, stool frequency increased, synovitis, tendonitis, tenesmus, thrombocytopenia, thrombophlebitis, urinary incontinence, urinary tract infection, urticaria, vaginal hemorrhage, varicose vein, vertigo, weight gain/loss, xerophthalmia, hiatal hernia

Postmarketing and/or case reports: Angioedema, erythema multiforme, exfoliative dermatitis, Stevens-Johnson syndrome, toxic epidermal necrolysis

Contraindications Hypersensitivity to valdecoxib, sulfonamides, or any component of the formulation; patients who have experienced asthma, urticaria, or allergic-type reactions to aspirin or NSAIDs; pregnancy (3rd trimester)

Warnings/Precautions Anaphylactic/anaphylactoid reactions may occur, even with no prior exposure to valdecoxib. Serious dermatologic reactions have been reported; discontinue in any patients who develop rash or any signs of hypersensitivity. Use with caution in patients with decreased renal function, hepatic disease, CHF, hypertension, dehydration, or asthma. Use caution in patients with known or suspected deficiency of cytochrome P450 isoenzyme 2C9. Use in patients with severe hepatic impairment (Child-Pugh Class C) is not recommended. Safety and efficacy have not been established for patients <18 years of age.

GI irritation, ulceration, bleeding, and perforation may occur with NSAIDs (it is unclear whether valdecoxib is associated with rates of these events which are similar to nonselective NSAIDs). Use with caution in patients with a history of GI disease (bleeding or ulcers) or risk factor for GI bleeding, use lowest dose for shortest time possible.

Drug Interactions Substrate of CYP2C8/9, 3A4; Inhibits CYP2C8/9, 2C19

ACE inhibitors: Antihypertensive effects may be decreased by concurrent therapy with NSAIDs; monitor blood pressure.

Angiotensin II antagonists: Antihypertensive effects may be decreased by concurrent therapy with NSAIDs; monitor blood pressure.

Anticoagulants (warfarin, heparin, LMWHs): In combination with NSAIDs, can cause increased risk of bleeding.

Antiplatelet drugs (ticlopidine, clopidogrel, aspirin, abciximab, dipyridamole, eptifibatide, tirofiban): Can cause an increased risk of bleeding.

Corticosteroids: May increase the risk of GI ulceration; avoid concurrent use

Cyclosporine: NSAIDs may increase serum creatinine, potassium, blood pressure, and cyclosporine levels; monitor cyclosporine levels and renal function carefully.

CYP2C8/9 inhibitors: May increase valdecoxib levels. Use caution with concurrent use; inhibitors include amiodarone, cimetidine, fluconazole, fluoxetine, isoniazid, metronidazole, omeprazole, valproic acid.

CYP3A4 inhibitors: May increase valdecoxib levels. Use caution with concurrent use; inhibitors include amiodarone, cimetidine, clarithromycin, erythromycin, delavirdine, diltiazem, disulfiram, fluoxetine, fluvoxamine, grapefruit juice, nefazodone, nevirapine, propoxyphene, quinupristin-dalfopristin, verapamil, zafirlukast, zileuton

Hydralazine: Antihypertensive effect is decreased; avoid concurrent use

(Continued)

Valdecoxib *(Continued)*

Lithium levels can be increased; avoid concurrent use if possible or monitor lithium levels and adjust dose. Sulindac may have the least effect. When NSAID is stopped, lithium will need adjustment again.

Loop diuretics: Diuretic and antihypertensive efficacy is reduced. May be anticipated with any NSAID.

Methotrexate: Severe bone marrow suppression, aplastic anemia, and GI toxicity have been reported with concomitant NSAID therapy. Selective COX-2 inhibitors appear to have a lower risk of this toxicity, however, caution is warranted.

Thiazides: Diuretic efficacy is reduced.

Warfarin: Valdecoxib (40 mg twice daily) caused a significant increase in plasma warfarin exposure (12% R-warfarin, 15% S-warfarin). May increase the anticoagulant effects of warfarin. Monitor INR closely.

Dietary/Ethanol/Herb Considerations

Ethanol: Avoid use; may enhance gastric mucosal irritation.

Food: May be taken with food; high-fat meal delays time to peak by 1-2 hours. Avoid garlic, ginger, and green tea.

Herb/Nutraceutical: Avoid cat's claw, dong quai, evening primrose, feverfew, garlic, ginger, ginkgo biloba, ginseng, green tea, horse chestnut, and red clover due to additional antiplatelet activity.

Pharmacodynamics/Kinetics

Onset of action: Dysmenorrhea: 60 minutes

Distribution: V_d: 86 L

Protein binding: 98%

Metabolism: Extensively hepatic via CYP3A4 and 2C9; glucuronidation

Bioavailability: 83%

Half-life elimination: 8-11 hours

Time to peak: 2.25-3 hours

Excretion: Primarily urine (as metabolites)

Pregnancy Risk Factor C/D (3rd trimester)

Dosage Forms TAB: 10 mg, 20 mg

Generic Available No

Valganciclovir (val gan SYE kloe veer)

Related Information

Ganciclovir *on page 626*

U.S. Brand Names Valcyte™

Canadian Brand Names Valcyte™

Pharmacologic Category Antiviral Agent

Synonyms Valganciclovir Hydrochloride

Use Treatment of cytomegalovirus (CMV) retinitis in patients with acquired immunodeficiency syndrome (AIDS)

Unlabeled/Investigational Use Treatment and prophylaxis of CMV in patients undergoing transplantation

Local Anesthetic/Vasoconstrictor Precautions No information available to require special precautions

Effects on Dental Treatment No significant effects or complications reported

Dosage Oral: Adults:

CMV retinitis:

Induction: 900 mg twice daily for 21 days (with food)

Maintenance: Following induction treatment, or for patients with inactive CMV retinitis who require maintenance therapy: Recommended dose: 900 mg once daily (with food)

CMV prophylaxis/treatment in transplantation (unlabeled use): Various regimens (ranging from full dose to "maintenance dosing") have been used in patients with a variety of organ transplants for CMV prophylaxis based on CMV serologic status.

Dosage adjustment in renal impairment:

Induction dose (for 21 days):

Cl_{cr} 40-59 mL/minute: 450 mg twice daily

Cl_{cr} 25-39 mL/minute: 450 mg once daily

Cl_{cr} 10-24 mL/minute: 450 mg every 2 days

Maintenance dose:

Cl_{cr} 40-59 mL/minute: 450 mg once daily

Cl_{cr} 25-39 mL/minute: 450 mg every 2 days

Cl_{cr} 10-24 mL/minute: 450 mg twice weekly

Note: Valganciclovir is not recommended in patients receiving hemodialysis. For patients on hemodialysis (Cl_{cr} <10 mL/minute), it is recommended that ganciclovir be used (dose adjusted as specified for ganciclovir).

Mechanism of Action Valganciclovir is rapidly converted to ganciclovir in the body. The bioavailability of ganciclovir from valganciclovir is increased tenfold compared to the oral ganciclovir. A dose of 900 mg achieved systemic exposure of ganciclovir comparable to that achieved with the recommended doses of intravenous ganciclovir of 5 mg/kg. Ganciclovir is phosphorylated to a substrate which competitively inhibits the binding of deoxyguanosine triphosphate to DNA polymerase resulting in inhibition of viral DNA synthesis.

Other Adverse Effects

>10%:

Central nervous system: Fever (31%), headache (9% to 22%), insomnia (16%)
Gastrointestinal: Diarrhea (16% to 41%), nausea (8% to 30%), vomiting (21%), abdominal pain (15%)
Hematologic: Granulocytopenia (11% to 27%), anemia (8% to 26%)
Ocular: Retinal detachment (15%)

1% to 10%:

Central nervous system: Peripheral neuropathy (9%), paresthesia (8%), seizures (<5%), psychosis, hallucinations (<5%), confusion (<5%), agitation (<5%)
Hematologic: Thrombocytopenia (8%), pancytopenia (<5%), bone marrow depression (<5%), aplastic anemia (<5%), bleeding (potentially life-threatening due to thrombocytopenia <5%)
Renal: Decreased renal function (<5%)
Miscellaneous: Local and systemic infections, including sepsis (<5%); allergic reaction (<5%)

<1%: Valganciclovir is expected to share the toxicities which may occur at a low incidence or due to idiosyncratic reactions which have been associated with ganciclovir

Drug Interactions

Increased Effect/Toxicity: Reported for ganciclovir: Immunosuppressive agents may increase hematologic toxicity of ganciclovir. Imipenem/cilastatin may increase seizure potential. Oral ganciclovir increases blood levels of zidovudine, although zidovudine decreases steady-state levels of ganciclovir. Since both drugs have the potential to cause neutropenia and anemia, some patients may not tolerate concomitant therapy with these drugs at full dosage. Didanosine levels are increased with concurrent ganciclovir. Other nephrotoxic drugs (eg, amphotericin and cyclosporine) may have additive nephrotoxicity with ganciclovir.

Decreased Effect: Reported for ganciclovir: A decrease in blood levels of ganciclovir AUC may occur when used with didanosine.

Dietary/Ethanol/Herb Considerations Food: Administer with food; a high-fat meal increased AUC by 30%.

Pharmacodynamics/Kinetics

Absorption: Well absorbed; high-fat meal increases AUC by 30%
Distribution: Ganciclovir: V_d: 15.26 L/1.73 m^2; widely to all tissues including CSF and ocular tissue
Protein binding: 1% to 2%
Metabolism: Converted to ganciclovir by intestinal mucosal cells and hepatocytes
Bioavailability: With food: 60%
Half-life elimination: Ganciclovir: 4.08 hours; prolonged with renal impairment; Severe renal impairment: Up to 68 hours
Excretion: Urine (primarily as ganciclovir)

Pregnancy Risk Factor C

Generic Available No

Valganciclovir Hydrochloride *see* Valganciclovir *on page 1370*
Valium® *see* Diazepam *on page 424*
Valorin [OTC] *see* Acetaminophen *on page 27*
Valorin Extra [OTC] *see* Acetaminophen *on page 27*
Valproate Semisodium *see* Valproic Acid and Derivatives *on page 1371*
Valproate Sodium *see* Valproic Acid and Derivatives *on page 1371*
Valproic Acid *see* Valproic Acid and Derivatives *on page 1371*

Valproic Acid and Derivatives

(val PROE ik AS id & dah RIV ah tives)

U.S. Brand Names Depacon®; Depakene®; Depakote® Delayed Release; Depakote® ER; Depakote® Sprinkle®

Canadian Brand Names Alti-Divalproex; Apo®-Divalproex; Depakene®; Epival® ER; Epival® I.V.; Gen-Divalproex; Novo-Divalproex; Nu-Divalproex; PMS-Valproic Acid; PMS-Valproic Acid E.C.; Rhoxal-valproic

Mexican Brand Names Atemperator-S®; Cryoval®; Depakene®; Epival®; Leptilan®; Valprosid®

Pharmacologic Category Anticonvulsant, Miscellaneous

Synonyms Dipropylacetic Acid; Divalproex Sodium; DPA; 2-Propylpentanoic Acid; 2-Propylvaleric Acid; Valproate Semisodium; Valproate Sodium; Valproic Acid

Use Monotherapy and adjunctive therapy in the treatment of patients with complex partial seizures; monotherapy and adjunctive therapy of simple and complex absence seizures; adjunctive therapy patients with multiple seizure types that include absence seizures

Mania associated with bipolar disorder (Depakote®)

Migraine prophylaxis (Depakote®, Depakote® ER)

Unlabeled/Investigational Use Treatment of behavior disorders in Alzheimer's disease

(Continued)

Valproic Acid and Derivatives *(Continued)*

Local Anesthetic/Vasoconstrictor Precautions No information available to require special precautions

Effects on Dental Treatment 1% to 10%: Otitis media

Dosage

Seizures:

Children >10 years and Adults:

Oral: Initial: 10-15 mg/kg/day in 1-3 divided doses; increase by 5-10 mg/kg/day at weekly intervals until therapeutic levels are achieved; maintenance: 30-60 mg/kg/day. Adult usual dose: 1000-2500 mg/day. **Note:** Regular release and delayed release formulations are usually given in 2-4 divided doses/day, extended release formulation (Depakote® ER) is usually given once daily. Conversion to Depakote® ER from a stable dose of Depakote® may require an increase in the total daily dose between 8% and 20% to maintain similar serum concentrations.

Children receiving more than one anticonvulsant (ie, polytherapy) may require doses up to 100 mg/kg/day in 3-4 divided doses

I.V.: Administer as a 60-minute infusion (≤20 mg/minute) with the same frequency as oral products; switch patient to oral products as soon as possible. Rapid infusions have been given: ≤15 mg/kg over 5-10 minutes. (1.5-3 mg/kg/minute).

Rectal (unlabeled): Dilute syrup 1:1 with water for use as a retention enema; loading dose: 17-20 mg/kg one time; maintenance: 10-15 mg/kg/dose every 8 hours

Mania: Adults: Oral: 750 mg/day in divided doses; dose should be adjusted as rapidly as possible to desired clinical effect; a loading dose of 20 mg/kg may be used; maximum recommended dosage: 60 mg/kg/day

Migraine prophylaxis: Adults: Oral:

Extended release tablets: 500 mg once daily for 7 days, then increase to 1000 mg once daily; adjust dose based on patient response; usual dosage range 500-1000 mg/day

Delayed release tablets: 250 mg twice daily; adjust dose based on patient response, up to 1000 mg/day

Elderly: Elimination is decreased; studies of patients with dementia show a high incidence of somnolence. In some patients, this was associated with weight loss. Starting doses should be lower and increases should be slow, with careful monitoring of nutritional intake and dehydration. Safety and efficacy for use in patients >65 years have not been studied for migraine prophylaxis.

Dosing adjustment in renal impairment: A 27% reduction in clearance of unbound valproate is seen in patients with Cl_{cr} <10 mL/minute. Hemodialysis reduces valproate concentrations by 20%, therefore no dose adjustment is needed in patients with renal failure. Protein binding is reduced, monitoring only total valproate concentrations may be misleading.

Dosing adjustment/comments in hepatic impairment: Reduction required; clearance is decreased. Hepatic disease is also associated with increased albumin concentrations and 2- to 2.6-fold increase in the unbound fraction. Free concentrations of valproate may be elevated while total concentrations appear normal.

Mechanism of Action Causes increased availability of gamma-aminobutyric acid (GABA), an inhibitory neurotransmitter, to brain neurons or may enhance the action of GABA or mimic its action at postsynaptic receptor sites

Other Adverse Effects Reported when used as monotherapy for complex partial seizures:

>10%:

Central nervous system: Somnolence (18% to 30%), dizziness (13% to 18%), insomnia (9% to 15%), nervousness (7% to 11%)

Dermatologic: Alopecia (13% to 24%)

Gastrointestinal: Nausea (26% to 34%), diarrhea (19% to 23%), vomiting (15% to 23%), abdominal pain (9% to 12%), dyspepsia (10% to 11%), anorexia (4% to 11%)

Hematologic: Thrombocytopenia (1% to 24%)

Neuromuscular & skeletal: Tremor (19% to 57%), weakness (10% to 21%)

Respiratory: Respiratory tract infection (13% to 20%), pharyngitis (2% to 8%), dyspnea (1% to 5%)

1% to 10%

Cardiovascular: Hypertension, palpitation, peripheral edema (3% to 8%), tachycardia, chest pain

Central nervous system: Amnesia (4% to 7%), abnormal dreams, anxiety, confusion, depression (4% to 5%), malaise, personality disorder

Dermatologic: Bruising (4% to 5%), dry skin, petechia, pruritus, rash

Endocrine & metabolic: Amenorrhea, dysmenorrhea

Gastrointestinal: Eructation, flatulence, hematemesis, increased appetite, pancreatitis, periodontal abscess, abnormal taste, weight gain (4% to 9%)

Genitourinary: Urinary frequency, urinary incontinence, vaginitis

Hepatic: Increased AST and ALT

Neuromuscular & skeletal: Abnormal gait, arthralgia, back pain, hypertonia, incoordination, leg cramps, myalgia, myasthenia, paresthesia, twitching
Ocular: Amblyopia/blurred vision (4% to 8%), abnormal vision, nystagmus (1% to 7%)
Otic: Deafness, tinnitus (1% to 7%)
Respiratory: Epistaxis, increased cough, pneumonia, sinusitis

Additional adverse effects: Frequency not defined:
Cardiovascular: Bradycardia
Central nervous system: Aggression, ataxia, behavioral deterioration, cerebral atrophy (reversible), dementia, emotional upset, encephalopathy (rare), fever, hallucinations, headache, hostility, hyperactivity, hypesthesia, incoordination, Parkinsonism, psychosis, vertigo
Dermatologic: Cutaneous vasculitis, erythema multiforme, photosensitivity, Stevens-Johnson syndrome, toxic epidermal necrolysis (rare)
Endocrine & metabolic: Breast enlargement, galactorrhea, hyperammonemia, hyponatremia, inappropriate ADH secretion, irregular menses, parotid gland swelling, polycystic ovary disease (rare), abnormal thyroid function tests
Genitourinary: Enuresis, urinary tract infection
Hematologic: Anemia, aplastic anemia, bone marrow suppression, eosinophilia, hematoma formation, hemorrhage, hypofibrinogenemia, intermittent porphyria, leukopenia, lymphocytosis, macrocytosis, pancytopenia
Hepatic: Bilirubin increased, hyperammonemic encephalopathy (in patients with UCD)
Neuromuscular & skeletal: Asterixis, bone pain, dysarthria
Ocular: Diplopia, "spots before the eyes"
Renal: Fanconi-like syndrome (rare, in children)
Miscellaneous: Anaphylaxis, decreased carnitine, hyperglycinemia, lupus

Postmarketing and/or case reports: Life-threatening pancreatitis (2 cases out of 2416 patients), occurring at the start of therapy or following years of use, has been reported in adults and children. Some cases have been hemorrhagic with rapid progression of initial symptoms to death. Cases have also been reported upon rechallenge.

Drug Interactions For valproic acid: Substrate of CYP2A6, 2B6, 2C8/9, 2C19, 2E1; Inhibits CYP2C8/9, 2C19, 2D6, 3A4; Induces CYP2A6

Increased Effect/Toxicity: Absence seizures have been reported in patients receiving VPA and clonazepam. Valproic acid may increase, decrease, or have no effect on carbamazepine and phenytoin levels. Valproic acid may increase serum concentrations of carbamazepine - epoxide (active metabolite). Valproic acid may increase serum concentrations of diazepam, lamotrigine, nimodipine, and phenobarbital, and tricyclic antidepressants. Chlorpromazine (and possibly other phenothiazines), macrolide antibiotics (clarithromycin, erythromycin, troleandomycin), felbamate, and isoniazid may inhibit the metabolism of valproic acid. Aspirin or other salicylates may displace valproic acid from protein-binding sites, leading to acute toxicity. CYP2C18/19 inhibitors may increase serum concentrations of valproic acid (ie, cimetidine, felbamate, fluoxetine, and fluvoxamine).

Decreased Effect: Valproic acid may displace clozapine from protein binding site resulting in decreased clozapine serum concentrations. Carbamazepine, lamotrigine, and phenytoin may induce the metabolism of valproic acid. Cholestyramine (and possibly colestipol) may bind valproic acid in GI tract, decreasing absorption. Acyclovir may reduce valproic acid levels. Mefloquine may decrease serum concentration of valproic acid.

Dietary/Ethanol/Herb Considerations

Ethanol: Avoid use; may increase CNS depression.

Food: Administer with food or milk to reduce GI upset. Food may decrease serum concentration; delays but does not affect the extent of absorption. Milk has no effect on absorption. Coated particles of divalproex sodium may be mixed with semisolid food (eg, applesauce or pudding). Do not mix oral solution with carbonated beverages; generates valproic acid and may cause mouth and throat irritation.

Herb/Nutraceutical: Avoid evening primrose; decreases seizure threshold. Avoid gotu kola, kava, SAMe, St John's wort, and valerian; may increase CNS depression.

Pharmacodynamics/Kinetics

Distribution: Total valproate: 11 L/1.73 m^2; free valproate 92 L/1.73 m^2
Protein binding (dose dependent): 80% to 90%
Metabolism: Extensively hepatic via glucuronide conjugation and mitochondrial beta-oxidation. The relationship between dose and total valproate concentration is nonlinear; concentration does not increase proportionally with the dose, but increases to a lesser extent due to saturable plasma protein binding. The kinetics of unbound drug are linear.
Bioavailability: Extended release: 90% of I.V. dose and 81% to 90% of delayed release dose
Half-life elimination: (increased in neonates and with liver disease): Children: 4-14 hours; Adults: 9-16 hours
Time to peak, serum: 1-4 hours; Divalproex (enteric coated): 3-5 hours

(Continued)

Valproic Acid and Derivatives *(Continued)*

Excretion: Urine (30% to 50% as glucuronide conjugate, 3% as unchanged drug)

Pregnancy Risk Factor D

Generic Available Yes (valproic acid)

Selected Readings Redington K, Wells C, and Petito F, "Erythromycin and Valproic Acid Interaction," *Ann Intern Med*, 1992, 116(10):877-8.

Valrubicin (val roo BYE sin)

U.S. Brand Names Valstar®

Canadian Brand Names Valstar®; Valtaxin®

Pharmacologic Category Antineoplastic Agent, Anthracycline

Use Intravesical therapy of BCG-refractory carcinoma *in situ* of the urinary bladder

Local Anesthetic/Vasoconstrictor Precautions No information available to require special precautions

Effects on Dental Treatment No significant effects or complications reported

Dosage Intravesical:

Adults: 800 mg once weekly for 6 weeks

Dosing adjustment in renal/hepatic impairment: No specific recommendations

Mechanism of Action Blocks function of DNA topoisomerase II; inhibits DNA synthesis, causes extensive chromosomal damage, and arrests cell development

Other Adverse Effects

>10%: Genitourinary: Frequency (61%), dysuria (56%), urgency (57%), bladder spasm (31%), hematuria (29%), bladder pain (28%), urinary incontinence (22%), cystitis (15%), urinary tract infection (15%)

1% to 10%:

Cardiovascular: Chest pain (2%), vasodilation (2%), peripheral edema (1%)

Central nervous system: Headache (4%), malaise (4%), dizziness (3%), fever (2%)

Dermatologic: Rash (3%)

Endocrine & metabolic: Hyperglycemia (1%)

Gastrointestinal: Abdominal pain (5%), nausea (5%), diarrhea (3%), vomiting (2%), flatulence (1%)

Genitourinary: Nocturia (7%), burning symptoms (5%), urinary retention (4%), urethral pain (3%), pelvic pain (1%), hematuria (microscopic) (3%)

Hematologic: Anemia (2%)

Neuromuscular & skeletal: Weakness (4%), back pain (3%), myalgia (1%)

Respiratory: Pneumonia (1%)

<1%: Tenesmus, pruritus, abnormal taste, skin irritation, decreased urine flow, urethritis

Pharmacodynamics/Kinetics

Absorption: Well absorbed into bladder tissue, negligible systemic absorption. Trauma to mucosa may increase absorption, and perforation greatly increases absorption with significant systemic myelotoxicity.

Metabolism: Negligible after intravesical instillation and 2 hour retention

Excretion: Urine when expelled from urinary bladder (98.6% as intact drug; 0.4% as *N*-trifluoroacetyladriamycin)

Pregnancy Risk Factor C

Generic Available No

Valsartan (val SAR tan)

U.S. Brand Names Diovan®

Canadian Brand Names Diovan®

Mexican Brand Names Diovan®

Pharmacologic Category Angiotensin II Receptor Blocker

Use Alone or in combination with other antihypertensive agents in treating essential hypertension; treatment of heart failure (NYHA Class II-IV) in patients intolerant to angiotensin converting enzyme (ACE) inhibitors

Local Anesthetic/Vasoconstrictor Precautions No information available to require special precautions

Effects on Dental Treatment No significant effects or complications reported

Dosage Adults: Oral:

Hypertension: Initial: 80 mg or 160 mg once daily (in patients who are not volume depleted); majority of effect within 2 weeks, maximal effects in 4-6 weeks; dose may be increased to achieve desired effect; maximum recommended dose: 320 mg/day

Heart failure: Initial: 40 mg twice daily; titrate dose to 80-160 mg twice daily, as tolerated; maximum daily dose: 320 mg. **Note:** Do not use with ACE inhibitors and beta blockers.

Dosing adjustment in renal impairment: None required if Cl_{cr} >10 mL/minute.

Dosing adjustment in hepatic impairment: Mild - moderate: ≤80 mg/day

Dialysis: Not significantly removed

Mechanism of Action As a prodrug, valsartan produces direct antagonism of the angiotensin II (AT2) receptors, unlike the ACE inhibitors. It displaces angiotensin II from the AT1 receptor and produces its blood pressure lowering effects by antagonizing AT1-induced vasoconstriction, aldosterone release, catecholamine release, arginine vasopressin release, water intake, and hypertrophic responses. This action results in more efficient blockade of the cardiovascular effects of angiotensin II and fewer side effects than the ACE inhibitors.

Other Adverse Effects

Hypertension: Similar incidence to placebo; independent of race, age, and gender.

>1%:

Central nervous system: Dizziness (2% to 8%), fatigue (2%)
Endocrine & metabolic: Serum potassium increased (4.4%)
Gastrointestinal: Abdominal pain (2%)
Hematologic: Neutropenia (1.9%)
Respiratory: Cough (2.6% versus 1.5% in placebo)
Miscellaneous: Viral infection (3%)

>1% but frequency ≤ placebo: Headache, upper respiratory infection, cough, diarrhea, rhinitis, sinusitis, nausea, pharyngitis, edema, arthralgia

Heart failure:

>10%: Central nervous system: Dizziness (17%)

1% to 10%:

Cardiovascular: Hypotension (7%), postural hypotension (2%)
Central nervous system: Fatigue (3%)
Endocrine & metabolic: Hyperkalemia (2%)
Gastrointestinal: Diarrhea (5%)
Neuromuscular & skeletal: Arthralgia (3%), back pain (3%)
Renal: Creatinine elevated >50% (4%)

All indications:

<1%: Allergic reactions, anemia, angioedema, anorexia, anxiety, asthenia, back pain, chest pain, constipation, creatinine increased (0.8% in hypertensive patients), dyspepsia, dyspnea, flatulence, hematocrit/hemoglobin decreased, impotence, insomnia, muscle cramps, myalgia, orthostatic effects, palpitations, paresthesia, pruritus, rash, serum transaminases increased, somnolence, syncope, vertigo, vomiting, xerostomia. May be associated with worsening of renal function in patients dependent on renin-angiotensin-aldosterone system.

Postmarketing and/or case reports: Angioedema, hepatitis, impaired renal function, hyperkalemia (hypertensive patients), alopecia

Drug Interactions Inhibits CYP2C8/9

Increased Effect/Toxicity: Valsartan blood levels may be increased by cimetidine and monoxidine; clinical effect is unknown. Concurrent use of potassium salts/supplements, co-trimoxazole (high dose), ACE inhibitors, and potassium-sparing diuretics (amiloride, spironolactone, triamterene) may increase the risk of hyperkalemia.

Decreased Effect: Phenobarbital, ketoconazole, troleandomycin, sulfaphenazole

Dietary/Ethanol/Herb Considerations

Ethanol: Avoid use; may increase risk of dizziness or hypotension.

Food decreases rate (50%) and extent of absorption by 40%. Avoid caffeine (eg, colas, chocolate), garlic, and licorice.

Herb/Nutraceutical: Avoid black cohosh, dong quai, and evening primrose due to estrogenic activity. Avoid ephedra, ginseng, and yohimbe; may worsen hypertension. Avoid garlic; may have increased antihypertensive effect. Avoid ginger due to positive inotropic effects; theoretically, may cause arrhythmia. Avoid hawthorn; may lower peripheral vascular resistance causing additional decrease in BP. Avoid licorice.

Pharmacodynamics/Kinetics

Onset of action: Peak antihypertensive effect: 2-4 weeks
Distribution: V_d: 17 L (adults)
Protein binding: 95%, primarily albumin
Metabolism: To inactive metabolite
Bioavailability: 25% (range 10% to 35%)
Half-life elimination: 6 hours
Time to peak, serum: 2-4 hours
Excretion: Feces (83%) and urine (13%) as unchanged drug

Pregnancy Risk Factor C/D (2nd and 3rd trimesters)

Generic Available No

Valsartan and Hydrochlorothiazide

(val SAR tan & hye droe klor oh THYE a zide)

Related Information

Hydrochlorothiazide *on page 675*
Valsartan *on page 1374*

U.S. Brand Names Diovan HCT®

Canadian Brand Names Diovan HCT®

Pharmacologic Category Antihypertensive Agent Combination

Synonyms Hydrochlorothiazide and Valsartan

Use Treatment of hypertension (not indicated for initial therapy)

(Continued)

Valsartan and Hydrochlorothiazide *(Continued)*

Local Anesthetic/Vasoconstrictor Precautions No information available to require special precautions

Effects on Dental Treatment No significant effects or complications reported

Dosage Adults: Oral: Dose is individualized

Other Adverse Effects See individual agents.

Dietary/Ethanol/Herb Considerations Based on valsartan component:

Ethanol: Avoid use; may increase risk of dizziness or hypotension.

Food decreases rate (50%) and extent of absorption by 40%. Avoid caffeine (eg, colas, chocolate), garlic, and licorice.

Herb/Nutraceutical: Avoid black cohosh, dong quai, and evening primrose due to estrogenic activity. Avoid ephedra, ginseng, and yohimbe; may worsen hypertension. Avoid garlic; may have increased antihypertensive effect. Avoid ginger due to positive inotropic effects; theoretically, may cause arrhythmia. Avoid hawthorn; may lower peripheral vascular resistance causing additional decrease in BP. Avoid licorice.

Pregnancy Risk Factor C (1st trimester); D (2nd and 3rd trimester)

Generic Available No

Valstar® *see* Valrubicin *on page 1374*

Valtrex® *see* Valacyclovir *on page 1367*

Vanamide™ *see* Urea *on page 1365*

Vanatrip® *see* Amitriptyline *on page 83*

Vancenase® AQ 84 mcg [DSC] *see* Beclomethasone *on page 163*

Vancenase® Pockethaler® [DSC] *see* Beclomethasone *on page 163*

Vanceril® [DSC] *see* Beclomethasone *on page 163*

Vancocin® *see* Vancomycin *on page 1376*

Vancomycin (van koe MYE sin)

Related Information

Cardiovascular Diseases *on page 1456*

U.S. Brand Names Vancocin®

Canadian Brand Names Vancocin®

Mexican Brand Names Balcoran; Vancocin®; Vanmicina®

Pharmacologic Category Antibiotic, Miscellaneous

Synonyms Vancomycin Hydrochloride

Use Dental and Medical: Treatment of infections due to documented or suspected methicillin-resistant *S. aureus* or beta-lactam resistant coagulase negative *Staphylococcus* and serious or life-threatening infections (ie, endocarditis, meningitis) due to documented or suspected staphylococcal or streptococcal infections in patients who are allergic to penicillins and/or cephalosporins; empiric therapy of infections associated with gram-positive organisms; used orally for staphylococcal enterocolitis or for antibiotic-associated pseudomembranous colitis produced by *C. difficile*

Local Anesthetic/Vasoconstrictor Precautions No information available to require special precautions

Effects on Dental Treatment The "red man syndrome" characterized by skin rash and hypotension is not an allergic reaction but rather is associated with too rapid infusion of the drug. To alleviate or prevent the reaction, infuse vancomycin at a rate of ≥30 minutes for each 500 mg of drug being administered (eg, 1 g over ≥60 minutes); 1.5 g over ≥90 minutes.

>10%:

- Oral form: Bitter taste, nausea, vomiting
- Parenteral form: Hypotension, flushing

1% to 10%: Drug fever

Dosage Initial dosage recommendation: I.V.:

Neonates:

- Postnatal age ≤7 days:
  - <1200 g: 15 mg/kg/dose every 24 hours
  - 1200-2000 g: 10 mg/kg/dose every 12 hours
  - >2000 g: 15 mg/kg/dose every 12 hours
- Postnatal age >7 days:
  - <1200 g: 15 mg/kg/dose every 24 hours
  - ≥1200 g: 10 mg/kg/dose divided every 8 hours

Infants >1 month and Children:

40 mg/kg/day in divided doses every 6 hours

Prophylaxis for bacterial endocarditis:

Dental, oral, or upper respiratory tract surgery: 20 mg/kg 1 hour prior to the procedure

GI/GU procedure: 20 mg/kg plus gentamicin 2 mg/kg 1 hour prior to surgery

Infants >1 month and Children with staphylococcal central nervous system infection: 60 mg/kg/day in divided doses every 6 hours

Adults:

With normal renal function: 1 g **or** 10-15 mg/kg/dose every 12 hours

Prophylaxis for bacterial endocarditis:

Dental, oral, or upper respiratory tract surgery: 1 g 1 hour before surgery

GI/GU procedure: 1 g plus 1.5 mg/kg gentamicin 1 hour prior to surgery

Dosing interval in renal impairment (vancomycin levels should be monitored in patients with any renal impairment:

Cl_{cr} >60 mL/minute: Start with 1 g or 10-15 mg/kg/dose every 12 hours

Cl_{cr} 40-60 mL/minute: Start with 1 g or 10-15 mg/kg/dose every 24 hours

Cl_{cr} <40 mL/minute: Will need longer intervals; determine by serum concentration monitoring

Hemodialysis: Not dialyzable (0% to 5%); generally not removed; exception minimal-moderate removal by some of the newer high-flux filters; dose may need to be administered more frequently; monitor serum concentrations

Continuous ambulatory peritoneal dialysis (CAPD): Not significantly removed; administration via CAPD fluid: 15-30 mg/L (15-30 mcg/mL) of CAPD fluid

Continuous arteriovenous hemofiltration: Dose as for Cl_{cr} 10-40 mL/minute

Antibiotic lock technique (for catheter infections): 2 mg/mL in SWI/NS or D_5W; instill 3-5 mL into catheter port as a flush solution instead of heparin lock (**Note:** Do not mix with any other solutions)

Intrathecal: Vancomycin is available as a powder for injection and may be diluted to 1-5 mg/mL concentration in preservative-free 0.9% sodium chloride for administration into the CSF

Neonates: 5-10 mg/day

Children: 5-20 mg/day

Adults: Up to 20 mg/day

Oral: Pseudomembranous colitis produced by *C. difficile*:

Neonates: 10 mg/kg/day in divided doses

Children: 40 mg/kg/day in divided doses, added to fluids

Adults: 125 mg 4 times/day for 10 days

Mechanism of Action Inhibits bacterial cell wall synthesis by blocking glycopeptide polymerization through binding tightly to D-alanyl-D-alanine portion of cell wall precursor

Other Adverse Effects

Oral:

1% to 10%:

Central nervous system: Chills

Hematologic: Eosinophilia

<1%: Vasculitis, thrombocytopenia, ototoxicity, renal failure, interstitial nephritis

Parenteral:

>10%: Dermatologic: Erythematous rash on face and upper body (red neck or red man syndrome - infusion rate related)

1% to 10%:

Central nervous system: Chills

Dermatologic: Rash

Hematologic: Eosinophilia, reversible neutropenia

<1%: Vasculitis, Stevens-Johnson syndrome, ototoxicity (especially with large doses), thrombocytopenia, renal failure (especially with renal dysfunction or pre-existing hearing loss)

Contraindications Hypersensitivity to vancomycin or any component of the formulation; avoid in patients with previous severe hearing loss

Warnings/Precautions Use with caution in patients with renal impairment or those receiving other nephrotoxic or ototoxic drugs; dosage modification required in patients with impaired renal function (especially elderly)

Drug Interactions Increased Toxicity: Anesthetic agents; other ototoxic or nephrotoxic agents

Dietary/Ethanol/Herb Considerations Food: Administer oral form with food to reduce GI upset.

Pharmacodynamics/Kinetics

Absorption: Oral: Poor; I.M.: Erratic; Intraperitoneal: ~38%

Distribution: Widely in body tissues and fluids. except for CSF

Relative diffusion from blood into CSF: Good only with inflammation (exceeds usual MICs)

CSF:blood level ratio: Normal meninges: Nil; Inflamed meninges: 20% to 30%

Protein binding: 10% to 50%

Half-life elimination: Biphasic: Terminal:

Newborns: 6-10 hours

Infants and Children 3 months to 4 years: 4 hours

Children >3 years: 2.2-3 hours

Adults: 5-11 hours; significantly prolonged with renal impairment

End-stage renal disease: 200-250 hours

Time to peak, serum: I.V.: 45-65 minutes

Excretion: I.V.: Urine (80% to 90% as unchanged drug); Oral: Primarily feces

Pregnancy Risk Factor C

Breast-feeding Considerations Vancomycin is excreted in breast milk but is poorly absorbed from the gastrointestinal tract. Therefore, systemic absorption

(Continued)

Vancomycin *(Continued)*

would not be expected. Theoretically, vancomycin in the GI tract may affect the normal bowel flora in the infant, resulting in diarrhea.

Dosage Forms CAP (Vancocin®): 125 mg, 250 mg. **INF** [premixed in iso-osmotic dextrose]: 500 mg (100 mL); 1 g (200 mL). **INJ, powder for reconstitution:** 500 mg, 1 g, 5 g, 10 g; (Vancocin® [DSC]): 500 mg, 1 g, 10 g. **POWDER, oral solution** (Vancocin®): 1 g, 10 g

Generic Available Yes: Injection

Vancomycin Hydrochloride *see* Vancomycin *on page 1376*

Vaniqa™ *see* Eflornithine *on page 489*

Vanoxide-HC® *see* Benzoyl Peroxide and Hydrocortisone *on page 172*

Vanquish® Extra Strength Pain Reliever [OTC] *see* Acetaminophen, Aspirin, and Caffeine *on page 34*

Van R Gingibraid® *see* Epinephrine (Racemic) and Aluminum Potassium Sulfate *on page 501*

Vantin® *see* Cefpodoxime *on page 273*

Vaponefrin® *see* Epinephrine (Racemic) *on page 500*

VAQTA® *see* Hepatitis A Vaccine *on page 665*

Varicella-Zoster Immune Globulin (Human)

(var i SEL u- ZOS ter i MYOON GLOB yoo lin HYOO min)

Related Information

Immunizations (Vaccines) *on page 1612*

Pharmacologic Category Immune Globulin

Synonyms VZIG

Use Passive immunization of susceptible immunodeficient patients after exposure to varicella; most effective if begun within 96 hours of exposure; there is no evidence VZIG modifies established varicella-zoster infections.

Restrict administration to those patients meeting the following criteria:

Neoplastic disease (eg, leukemia or lymphoma)

Congenital or acquired immunodeficiency

Immunosuppressive therapy with steroids, antimetabolites or other immunosuppressive treatment regimens

Newborn of mother who had onset of chickenpox within 5 days before delivery or within 48 hours after delivery

Premature (≥28 weeks gestation) whose mother has no history of chickenpox

Premature (<28 weeks gestation or ≤1000 g VZIG) regardless of maternal history

One of the following types of exposure to chickenpox or zoster patient(s) may warrant administration:

Continuous household contact

Playmate contact (>1 hour play indoors)

Hospital contact (in same 2-4 bedroom or adjacent beds in a large ward or prolonged face-to-face contact with an infectious staff member or patient)

Susceptible to varicella-zoster

Age <15 years; administer to immunocompromised adolescents and adults and to other older patients on an individual basis

An acceptable alternative to VZIG prophylaxis is to treat varicella, if it occurs, with high-dose I.V. acyclovir

Age is the most important risk factor for reactivation of varicella zoster; persons <50 years of age have incidence of 2.5 cases per 1000, whereas those 60-79 have 6.5 cases per 1000 and those >80 years have 10 cases per 1000

Local Anesthetic/Vasoconstrictor Precautions No information available to require special precautions

Effects on Dental Treatment No significant effects or complications reported

Dosage High risk susceptible patients who are exposed again more than 3 weeks after a prior dose of VZIG should receive another full dose; there is no evidence VZIG modifies established varicella-zoster infections.

I.M.: Administer by deep injection in the gluteal muscle or in another large muscle mass. Inject 125 units/10 kg (22 lb); maximum dose: 625 units (5 vials); minimum dose: 125 units; do not administer fractional doses. Do not inject I.V.
VZIG dose based on weight: See table.

VZIG Dose Based on Weight

Weight of Patient		Dose	
kg	**lb**	**Units**	**No. of Vials**
0-10	0-22	125	1
10.1-20	22.1-44	250	2
20.1-30	44.1-66	375	3
30.1-40	66.1-88	500	4
>40	>88	625	5

Mechanism of Action The exact mechanism has not been clarified but the antibodies in varicella-zoster immune globulin most likely neutralize the varicella-zoster virus and prevent its pathological actions

Other Adverse Effects

1% to 10%: Local: Discomfort at the site of injection (pain, redness, edema)

<1%: Malaise, headache, rash, angioedema, GI symptoms, respiratory symptom, anaphylactic shock

Pregnancy Risk Factor C

Generic Available No

Comments Should be administered within 96 hours of exposure

Vascor® *see* Bepridil *on page 174*

Vaseretic® *see* Enalapril and Hydrochlorothiazide *on page 494*

Vasocidin® *see* Sulfacetamide and Prednisolone *on page 1250*

VasoClear® [OTC] *see* Naphazoline *on page 952*

Vasocon-A® [OTC] *see* Naphazoline and Antazoline *on page 952*

Vasodilan® *see* Isoxsuprine *on page 753*

Vasopressin (vay zoe PRES in)

U.S. Brand Names Pitressin®

Canadian Brand Names Pressyn®

Pharmacologic Category Antidiuretic Hormone Analog; Hormone, Posterior Pituitary

Synonyms ADH; Antidiuretic Hormone; 8-Arginine Vasopressin; Vasopressin Tannate

Use Treatment of diabetes insipidus; prevention and treatment of postoperative abdominal distention; differential diagnosis of diabetes insipidus

Unlabeled/Investigational Use Adjunct in the treatment of GI hemorrhage and esophageal varices; treatment of pulseless ventricular tachycardia (VT)/ventricular fibrillation (VF), vasodilatory shock (septic shock)

Local Anesthetic/Vasoconstrictor Precautions No information available to require special precautions

Effects on Dental Treatment No significant effects or complications reported

Dosage

Diabetes insipidus (highly variable dosage; titrated based on serum and urine sodium and osmolality in addition to fluid balance and urine output):

I.M., S.C.:

Children: 2.5-10 units 2-4 times/day as needed

Adults: 5-10 units 2-4 times/day as needed (dosage range 5-60 units/day)

Continuous I.V. infusion: Children and Adults: 0.5 milliunit/kg/hour (0.0005 unit/kg/hour); double dosage as needed every 30 minutes to a maximum of 0.01 unit/kg/hour

Intranasal: Administer on cotton pledget, as nasal spray, or by dropper

Abdominal distention: Adults: I.M.: 5 mg stat, 10 mg every 3-4 hours

GI hemorrhage (unlabeled use): I.V. infusion: Dilute in NS or D_5W to 0.1-1 unit/mL

Children: Initial: 0.002-0.005 units/kg/minute; titrate dose as needed; maximum: 0.01 unit/kg/minute; continue at same dosage (if bleeding stops) for 12 hours, then taper off over 24-48 hours

Adults: Initial: 0.2-0.4 unit/minute, then titrate dose as needed, if bleeding stops; continue at same dose for 12 hours, taper off over 24-48 hours

Pulseless VT/VF (ACLS protocol): I.V.: 40 int. units (as a single dose only); if no I.V. access, administer 40 int. units diluted with NS (to a total volume of 10 mL) endotracheally

Vasodilatory shock/septic shock (unlabeled use): Adults: I.V.: Vasopressin has been used in doses of 0.01-0.1 units/minute for the treatment of septic shock. Doses >0.05 units/minute may have more cardiovascular side effects. Most case reports have used 0.04 units/minute continuous infusion as a fixed dose.

Dosing adjustment in hepatic impairment: Some patients respond to much lower doses with cirrhosis

Mechanism of Action Increases cyclic adenosine monophosphate (cAMP) which increases water permeability at the renal tubule resulting in decreased urine volume and increased osmolality; causes peristalsis by directly stimulating the smooth muscle in the GI tract

Other Adverse Effects Frequency not defined:

Cardiovascular: Increased blood pressure, arrhythmias, venous thrombosis, vasoconstriction (with higher doses), angina, MI

Central nervous system: Pounding in the head, fever, vertigo

Dermatologic: Urticaria, circumoral pallor

Gastrointestinal: Flatulence, abdominal cramps, nausea, vomiting

Genitourinary: Uterine contraction

Neuromuscular & skeletal: Tremor

Respiratory: Bronchial constriction

Miscellaneous: Diaphoresis

(Continued)

Vasopressin *(Continued)*

Drug Interactions

Increased Effect/Toxicity: Chlorpropamide, urea, clofibrate, carbamazepine, and fludrocortisone potentiate antidiuretic response.

Decreased Effect: Lithium, epinephrine, demeclocycline, heparin, and ethanol block antidiuretic activity to varying degrees.

Dietary/Ethanol/Herb Considerations Ethanol: Avoid use due to effects on ADH.

Pharmacodynamics/Kinetics

Onset of action: Nasal: 1 hour

Duration: Nasal: 3-8 hours; I.M., S.C.: 2-8 hours

Metabolism: Nasal/Parenteral: Hepatic, renal

Half-life elimination: Nasal: 15 minutes; Parenteral: 10-20 minutes

Excretion: Nasal: Urine; S.C.: Urine (5% as unchanged drug) after 4 hours

Pregnancy Risk Factor C

Generic Available No

Vasopressin Tannate *see* Vasopressin *on page 1379*

Vasotec® *see* Enalapril *on page 492*

Vasotec® I.V. *see* Enalapril *on page 492*

VCF™ [OTC] *see* Nonoxynol 9 *on page 985*

VCR *see* VinCRIStine *on page 1387*

V-Dec-M® *see* Guaifenesin and Pseudoephedrine *on page 652*

Vectrin® [DSC] *see* Minocycline *on page 915*

Veetids® *see* Penicillin V Potassium *on page 1051*

Veg-Pancreatin 4X [OTC] *see* Pancreatin *on page 1030*

Velban® [DSC] *see* VinBLAStine *on page 1386*

Velosef® *see* Cephradine *on page 288*

Velosulin® BR (Buffered) *see* Insulin Preparations *on page 723*

Venlafaxine (VEN la faks een)

U.S. Brand Names Effexor®; Effexor® XR

Canadian Brand Names Effexor®; Effexor® XR

Mexican Brand Names Efexor®

Pharmacologic Category Antidepressant, Serotonin/Norepinephrine Reuptake Inhibitor

Use Treatment of depression, generalized anxiety disorder (GAD), social anxiety disorder

Unlabeled/Investigational Use Treatment of obsessive-compulsive disorder (OCD), chronic fatigue syndrome, hot flashes, neuropathic pain, attention-deficit/hyperactivity disorder (ADHD) and autism in children

Local Anesthetic/Vasoconstrictor Precautions Although venlafaxine is not a tricyclic antidepressant, it does block norepinephrine reuptake within CNS synapses as part of its mechanisms. It has been suggested that vasoconstrictor be administered with caution and to monitor vital signs in dental patients taking antidepressants that affect norepinephrine in this way. This is particularly important in patients taking venlafaxine, which has been noted to produce a sustained increase in diastolic blood pressure and heart rate as a side effect.

Effects on Dental Treatment Significant xerostomia (22%); may contribute to oral discomfort, especially in the elderly

Dosage Oral:

Children and Adolescents:

ADHD (unlabeled use): Initial: 12.5 mg/day

Children <40 kg: Increase by 12.5 mg/week to maximum of 50 mg/day in 2 divided doses

Children ≥40 kg: Increase by 25 mg/week to maximum of 75 mg/day in 3 divided doses.

Mean dose: 60 mg or 1.4 mg/kg administered in 2-3 divided doses

Autism (unlabeled use): Initial: 12.5 mg/day; adjust to 6.25-50 mg/day

Adults:

Depression: Immediate-release tablets: 75 mg/day, administered in 2 or 3 divided doses, taken with food; dose may be increased in 75 mg/day increments at intervals of at least 4 days, up to 225-375 mg/day

Depression, GAD, social anxiety disorder: Extended-release capsules: 75 mg once daily taken with food; for some new patients, it may be desirable to start at 37.5 mg/day for 4-7 days before increasing to 75 mg once daily; dose may be increased by up to 75 mg/day increments every 4 days as tolerated, up to a maximum of 225 mg/day

Note: When discontinuing this medication after more than 1 week of treatment, it is generally recommended that the dose be tapered. If venlafaxine is used for 6 weeks or longer, the dose should be tapered over 2 weeks when discontinuing its use.

Dosing adjustment in renal impairment: Cl_{cr} 10-70 mL/minute: Decrease dose by 25%; decrease total daily dose by 50% if dialysis patients; dialysis patients should receive dosing after completion of dialysis

Dosing adjustment in moderate hepatic impairment: Reduce total daily dosage by 50%

Mechanism of Action Venlafaxine and its active metabolite o-desmethylvenlafaxine (ODV) are potent inhibitors of neuronal serotonin and norepinephrine reuptake and weak inhibitors of dopamine reuptake

Other Adverse Effects

≥10%:

Central nervous system: Headache (25%), somnolence (23%), dizziness (19%), insomnia (18%), nervousness (13%)

Gastrointestinal: Nausea (37%), constipation (15%), anorexia (11%)

Genitourinary: Abnormal ejaculation/orgasm (12%)

Neuromuscular & skeletal: Weakness (12%)

Miscellaneous: Diaphoresis (12%)

1% to 10%:

Cardiovascular: Vasodilation (4%), hypertension (dose-related; 3% in patients receiving <100 mg/day, up to 13% in patients receiving >300 mg/day), tachycardia (2%), chest pain (2%), postural hypotension (1%)

Central nervous system: Anxiety (6%), abnormal dreams (4%), yawning (3%), agitation (2%), confusion (2%), abnormal thinking (2%), depersonalization (1%), depression (1%)

Dermatologic: Rash (3%), pruritus (1%)

Endocrine & metabolic: Decreased libido

Gastrointestinal: Diarrhea (8%), vomiting (6%), dyspepsia (5%), flatulence (3%), abnormal taste (2%), weight loss (1%)

Genitourinary: Impotence (6%), urinary frequency (3%), impaired urination (2%), orgasm disturbance (2%), urinary retention (1%)

Neuromuscular & skeletal: Tremor (5%), hypertonia (3%), paresthesia (3%), twitching (1%)

Ocular: Blurred vision (6%), mydriasis (2%)

Otic: Tinnitus (2%)

Miscellaneous: Infection (6%), chills (3%), trauma (2%)

<1%, postmarketing and/or case reports (limited to important or life-threatening): Abnormal vision, agranulocytosis, akathisia, anaphylaxis, aplastic anemia, asthma, bronchitis, catatonia, delirium, dyspnea, emotional lability, epidermal necrolysis, erythema multiforme, erythema nodosum, exfoliative dermatitis, extrapyramidal symptoms, hallucinations, hemorrhage (including ophthalmic and gastrointestinal), hepatic failure, hepatic necrosis, hirsutism, increased transaminases/GGT, manic reaction (0.5%), metrorrhagia, pancreatitis, prostatitis, psychosis, rash (maculopapular, pustular, or vesiculobullous), seizure, serotonin syndrome, SIADH, Stevens-Johnson syndrome, tardive dyskinesia, torticollis, vaginitis, vertigo

Drug Interactions Substrate of CYP2C8/9, 2C19, **2D6, 3A4**; Inhibits CYP2B6, 2D6, 3A4

Increased Effect/Toxicity: Concurrent use of MAO inhibitors (phenelzine, isocarboxazid), or drugs with MAO inhibitor activity (linezolid) may result in serotonin syndrome; should not be used within 2 weeks of each other. Selegiline may have a lower risk of this effect, particularly at low dosages, due to selectivity for MAO type B. In addition, concurrent use of buspirone, lithium, meperidine, nefazodone, selegiline, serotonin agonists (sumatriptan, naratriptan), sibutramine, SSRIs, trazodone, or tricyclic antidepressants may increase the risk of serotonin syndrome. Serum levels of haloperidol may be increased by venlafaxine. Inhibitors of CYP2D6 or CYP3A4 may increase the serum levels and/or toxicity of venlafaxine.

Decreased Effect: Serum levels of indinavir may be reduced be venlafaxine (AUC reduced by 28%) - clinical significance not determined. Enzyme inducers (carbamazepine, phenytoin, phenobarbital) may reduce the serum concentrations of venlafaxine.

Dietary/Ethanol/Herb Considerations

Ethanol: Avoid use; may increase CNS depression.

Food: Administer with food. Avoid caffeine and grapefruit products. Extended release capsule: Contents may be sprinkled on a spoonful of applesauce and swallowed immediately without chewing; followed with a glass of water to ensure complete swallowing of the pellets.

Herb/Nutraceutical: Avoid gotu kola, kava, SAMe, St John's wort, tryptophan, and valerian; may increase risk of serotonin syndrome and/or excessive sedation. Avoid melatonin; may cause acute psychosis.

Pharmacodynamics/Kinetics

Absorption: Oral: 92% to 100%; food has no significant effect on the absorption of venlafaxine or formation of the active metabolite O-desmethylvenlafaxine (ODV)

Distribution: At steady state: Venlafaxine 7.5 ± 3.7 L/kg, ODV 5.7 ± 1.8 L/Kg

Protein binding: Bound to human plasma protein: Venlafaxine 27%, ODV 30%

(Continued)

Venlafaxine *(Continued)*

Metabolism: Hepatic via CYP2D6 to active metabolite, O-desmethylvenlafaxine (ODV); other metabolites include N-desmethylvenlafaxine and N,O-didesmethylvenlafaxine

Bioavailability: Absolute: ~45%

Half-life elimination: Venlafaxine: 3-7 hours; ODV: 9-13 hours; Steady-state, plasma: Venlafaxine/ODV: Within 3 days of multiple dose therapy; prolonged with cirrhosis (Adults: Venlafaxine: ~30%, ODV: ~60%) and with dialysis (Adults: Venlafaxine: ~180%, ODV: ~142%)

Time to peak:

- Immediate release: Venlafaxine: 2 hours, ODV: 3 hours
- Extended release: Venlafaxine: 5.5 hours, ODV: 9 hours

Excretion: Urine (~87%, 5% as unchanged drug, 29% as unconjugated ODV, 26% as conjugated ODV, 27% as minor metabolites) within 48 hours

Clearance at steady state: Venlafaxine: 1.3 ± 0.6 L/hour/kg, ODV: 0.4 ± 0.2 L/hour/kg

- Clearance decreased with:
  - Cirrhosis: Adults: Venlafaxine: ~50%, ODV: ~30%
  - Severe cirrhosis: Adults: Venlafaxine: ~90%
  - Renal impairment (Cl_{cr} 10-70 mL/minute): Adults: Venlafaxine: ~24%
  - Dialysis: Adults: Venlafaxine: ~57%, ODV: ~56%; due to large volume of distribution, a significant amount of drug is not likely to be removed.

Pregnancy Risk Factor C

Generic Available No

Selected Readings Ganzber S, "Psychoactive Drugs," *ADA Guide to Dental Therapeutics,* 2nd edition, Chapter 21, Chicago, IL: ADA Publising, 2000, 381.

Venofer® *see* Iron Sucrose *on page 744*

Venoglobulin®-S *see* Immune Globulin (Intravenous) *on page 714*

Ventolin® *see* Albuterol *on page 48*

Ventolin® HFA *see* Albuterol *on page 48*

VePesid® *see* Etoposide *on page 549*

Verapamil (ver AP a mil)

Related Information

Calcium Channel Blockers and Gingival Hyperplasia *on page 1598*

Calcium Channel Blockers, Comparative Pharmacokinetics *on page 1600*

Cardiovascular Diseases *on page 1456*

U.S. Brand Names Calan®; Calan® SR; Covera-HS®; Isoptin® SR; Verelan®; Verelan® PM

Canadian Brand Names Alti-Verapamil; Apo®-Verap; Calan®; Chronovera®; Covera®; Gen-Verapamil; Gen-Verapamil SR; Isoptin®; Isoptin® I.V.; Isoptin® SR; Novo-Veramil; Novo-Veramil SR; Nu-Verap; Tarka®

Mexican Brand Names Cronovera®; Dilacoran®; Dilacoran HTA; Dilacoran Retard; Veraken; Verdilac

Pharmacologic Category Antiarrhythmic Agent, Class IV; Calcium Channel Blocker

Synonyms Iproveratril Hydrochloride; Verapamil Hydrochloride

Use Orally for treatment of angina pectoris (vasospastic, chronic stable, unstable) and hypertension; I.V. for supraventricular tachyarrhythmias (PSVT, atrial fibrillation, atrial flutter)

Unlabeled/Investigational Use Treatment of migraine headaches, hypertrophic cardiomyopathy, bipolar disorder (manic manifestations)

Local Anesthetic/Vasoconstrictor Precautions No information available to require special precautions

Effects on Dental Treatment Gingival hyperplasia (19%)

Calcium channel blockers (CCB) have been reported to cause gingival hyperplasia (GH). Verapamil induced GH has appeared 11 months or more after subjects took daily doses of 240-360 mg. The severity of hyperplastic syndrome does not seem to be dose-dependent. Gingivectomy is only successful if CCB therapy is discontinued. GH regresses markedly 1 week after CCB discontinuance with all symptoms resolving in 2 months. If a patient must continue CCB therapy, begin a program of professional cleaning and patient plaque control to minimize severity and growth rate of gingival tissue.

Dosage

- Children: SVT:
  - I.V.:
    - <1 year: 0.1-0.2 mg/kg over 2 minutes; repeat every 30 minutes as needed
    - 1-15 years: 0.1-0.3 mg/kg over 2 minutes; maximum: 5 mg/dose, may repeat dose in 15 minutes if adequate response not achieved; maximum for second dose: 10 mg/dose
  - Oral (dose not well established):
    - 1-5 years: 4-8 mg/kg/day in 3 divided doses **or** 40-80 mg every 8 hours

>5 years: 80 mg every 6-8 hours

Adults:

SVT: I.V.: 2.5-5 mg (over 2 minutes); second dose of 5-10 mg (~0.15 mg/kg) may be given 15-30 minutes after the initial dose if patient tolerates, but does not respond to initial dose; maximum total dose: 20 mg

Angina: Oral: Initial dose: 80-120 mg 3 times/day (elderly or small stature: 40 mg 3 times/day); range: 240-480 mg/day in 3-4 divided doses

Hypertension: Oral: 80 mg 3 times/day or 240 mg/day (sustained release); range: 240-480 mg/day; 120 mg/day in the elderly or small patients (no evidence of additional benefit in doses >360 mg/day).

Note: One time per day dosing is recommended at bedtime with Covera-HS®.

Dosing adjustment in renal impairment: Cl_{cr} <10 mL/minute: Administer at 50% to 75% of normal dose.

Dialysis: Not dialyzable (0% to 5 %) via hemo- or peritoneal dialysis; supplemental dose is unnecessary.

Dosing adjustment in hepatic impairment: Reduce dose in cirrhosis, reduce dose to 20% to 50% of normal and monitor EKG.

Mechanism of Action Inhibits calcium ion from entering the "slow channels" or select voltage-sensitive areas of vascular smooth muscle and myocardium during depolarization; produces a relaxation of coronary vascular smooth muscle and coronary vasodilation; increases myocardial oxygen delivery in patients with vasospastic angina; slows automaticity and conduction of AV node.

Other Adverse Effects

1% to 10%:

Cardiovascular: Bradycardia (1.4% oral, 1.2% I.V.); first-, second-, or third-degree AV block (1.2% oral, unknown I.V.); CHF (1.8% oral); hypotension (2.5% oral, 3% I.V.); peripheral edema (1.9% oral), symptomatic hypotension (1.5% I.V.); severe tachycardia (1% I.V.)

Central nervous system: Dizziness (3.3% oral, 1.2% I.V.), fatigue (1.7% oral), headache (2.2% oral, 1.2% I.V.)

Dermatologic: Rash (1.2% oral)

Gastrointestinal: Constipation (12% up to 42% in clinical trials), nausea (2.7% oral, 0.9% I.V.)

Respiratory: Dyspnea (1.4% oral)

Oral: <1% (Limited to important or life-threatening): Angina, atrioventricular dissociation, chest pain, claudication, MI, palpitations, purpura (vasculitis), syncope, diarrhea, xerostomia, gastrointestinal distress, gingival hyperplasia, ecchymosis, bruising, cerebrovascular accident, confusion, equilibrium disorders, insomnia, muscle cramps, paresthesia, psychotic symptoms, shakiness, somnolence, arthralgia, rash, exanthema, hair loss, hyperkeratosis, macules, diaphoresis, urticaria, Stevens-Johnson syndrome, erythema multiforme, blurred vision, tinnitus, gynecomastia, galactorrhea/hyperprolactinemia, increased urination, spotty menstruation, impotence, flushing, abdominal discomfort

I.V.: <1% (Limited to important or life-threatening): Bronchi/laryngeal spasm, itching, urticaria, emotional depression, rotary nystagmus, sleepiness, vertigo, muscle fatigue, diaphoresis, respiratory failure, myoclonus

Postmarketing and/or case reports: Stevens-Johnson syndrome, erythema multiforme, exfoliative dermatitis, EPS, gynecomastia, eosinophilia, ventricular fibrillation, asystole, electrical mechanical dissociation, shock, myoclonus, Parkinsonian syndrome, GI obstruction, pulmonary edema, respiratory failure, hair color change

Drug Interactions Substrate of CYP1A2, 2B6, 2C8/9, 2C18, 2E1, **3A4**; Inhibits CYP1A2, 2C8/9, 2D6, **3A4**

Increased Effect/Toxicity: Use of verapamil with amiodarone, beta-blockers, or flecainide may lead to bradycardia and decreased cardiac output. Aspirin and concurrent verapamil use may increase bleeding times. Azole antifungals, cimetidine, erythromycin may inhibit verapamil metabolism, increasing serum concentrations/effect of verapamil. Lithium neurotoxicity may result when verapamil is added. Effect of nondepolarizing neuromuscular blocker is prolonged by verapamil. Cisapride and astemizole levels may be increased by verapamil, potentially resulting in life-threatening arrhythmias; avoid concurrent use. Serum concentrations of the following drugs may be increased by verapamil: Alfentanil, buspirone, carbamazepine, cyclosporine, digoxin, doxorubicin, ethanol, HMG-CoA reductase inhibitors (atorvastatin, cerivastatin, lovastatin, simvastatin), midazolam, prazosin, quinidine, tacrolimus, and theophylline.

Decreased Effect: Rifampin or phenobarbital may decrease verapamil serum concentrations by increased hepatic metabolism. Lithium levels may be decreased by verapamil. Nafcillin decreases plasma concentration of verapamil.

Dietary/Ethanol/Herb Considerations

Ethanol: Avoid or limit use; effects may be increased by verapamil.

Food: Administer sustained release product with food or milk; may sprinkle contents of capsule onto food. Avoid grapefruit products; may increase serum concentration. Fluids, fruit, and fiber may reduce constipation. Buttermilk, boiled milk, or yogurt may reduce diarrhea. Avoid caffeine (eg, colas, chocolate), garlic, and licorice.

(Continued)

Verapamil *(Continued)*

Herb/Nutraceutical: Avoid black cohosh, dong quai, and evening primrose due to estrogenic activity. Avoid ephedra, ginseng, and yohimbe; may worsen arrhythmia or hypertension. Avoid garlic; may have increased antihypertensive effect. Avoid ginger due to positive inotropic effects; theoretically, may cause arrhythmia. Avoid hawthorn; may lower peripheral vascular resistance and enhance reductions in BP. Avoid licorice. Avoid St John's wort; may decrease serum concentration.

Pharmacodynamics/Kinetics

Onset of action: Peak effect: Oral: Immediate release: 2 hours; I.V.: 1-5 minutes

Duration: Oral: Immediate release tablets: 6-8 hours; I.V.: 10-20 minutes

Protein binding: 90%

Metabolism: Hepatic via multiple CYP isoenzymes; extensive first-pass effect

Bioavailability: Oral: 20% to 30%

Half-life elimination: Infants: 4.4-6.9 hours; Adults: Single dose: 2-8 hours, Multiple doses: Up to 12 hours; prolonged with hepatic cirrhosis

Excretion: Urine (70%, 3% to 4% as unchanged drug); feces (16%)

Pregnancy Risk Factor C

Generic Available Yes

Selected Readings Wynn RL, "Update on Calcium Channel Blocker Induced Gingival Hyperplasia," *Gen Dent*, 1995, 43(3):218-22.

Verapamil and Trandolapril *see* Trandolapril and Verapamil *on page 1332*

Verapamil Hydrochloride *see* Verapamil *on page 1382*

Verelan® *see* Verapamil *on page 1382*

Verelan® PM *see* Verapamil *on page 1382*

Vermox® *see* Mebendazole *on page 846*

Verr-Canth™ *see* Cantharidin *on page 234*

Versacaps® *see* Guaifenesin and Pseudoephedrine *on page 652*

Versed® [DSC] *see* Midazolam *on page 908*

Versiclear™ *see* Sodium Thiosulfate *on page 1233*

Vesanoid® *see* Tretinoin (Oral) *on page 1338*

Vexol® *see* Rimexolone *on page 1185*

VFEND® *see* Voriconazole *on page 1395*

Viadur® *see* Leuprolide *on page 784*

Viagra® *see* Sildenafil *on page 1220*

Vibramycin® *see* Doxycycline *on page 476*

Vibra-Tabs® *see* Doxycycline *on page 476*

Vicks® 44® Cough Relief [OTC] *see* Dextromethorphan *on page 423*

Vicks® 44D Cough & Head Congestion [OTC] *see* Pseudoephedrine and Dextromethorphan *on page 1147*

Vicks® 44E [OTC] *see* Guaifenesin and Dextromethorphan *on page 651*

Vicks® DayQuil® Cold and Flu Non-Drowsy [OTC] *see* Acetaminophen, Dextromethorphan, and Pseudoephedrine *on page 35*

Vicks® Pediatric Formula 44E [OTC] *see* Guaifenesin and Dextromethorphan *on page 651*

Vicks Sinex® 12 Hour Ultrafine Mist [OTC] *see* Oxymetazoline *on page 1022*

Vicks® Sinex® Nasal Spray [OTC] *see* Phenylephrine *on page 1071*

Vicks® Sinex® UltraFine Mist [OTC] *see* Phenylephrine *on page 1071*

Vicodin® *see* Hydrocodone and Acetaminophen *on page 678*

Vicodin® ES *see* Hydrocodone and Acetaminophen *on page 678*

Vicodin® HP *see* Hydrocodone and Acetaminophen *on page 678*

Vicodin Tuss® *see* Hydrocodone and Guaifenesin *on page 683*

Vicon Forte® *see* Vitamins (Multiple/Oral) *on page 1394*

Vicon Plus® [OTC] *see* Vitamins (Multiple/Oral) *on page 1394*

Vicoprofen® *see* Hydrocodone and Ibuprofen *on page 684*

Vidarabine (vye DAIR u been)

Related Information

Oral Viral Infections *on page 1545*

Systemic Viral Diseases *on page 1517*

U.S. Brand Names Vira-A® [DSC]

Mexican Brand Names Adena a Ungena

Pharmacologic Category Antiviral Agent, Ophthalmic

Synonyms Adenine Arabinoside; Ara-A; Arabinofuranosyladenine; Vidarabine Monohydrate; Vira-A® [DSC]

Use Treatment of acute keratoconjunctivitis and epithelial keratitis due to herpes simplex virus type 1 and 2; superficial keratitis caused by herpes simplex virus

Local Anesthetic/Vasoconstrictor Precautions No information available to require special precautions

Effects on Dental Treatment No significant effects or complications reported

Dosage Children and Adults: Ophthalmic: Keratoconjunctivitis: Instill 1/2" of ointment in lower conjunctival sac 5 times/day every 3 hours while awake until complete re-epithelialization has occurred, then twice daily for an additional 7 days

Mechanism of Action Inhibits viral DNA synthesis by blocking DNA polymerase

Other Adverse Effects Frequency not defined: Ocular: Burning eyes, lacrimation, keratitis, photophobia, foreign body sensation, uveitis

Drug Interactions Increased Effect/Toxicity: Allopurinol (may increase vidarabine levels).

Pregnancy Risk Factor C

Generic Available No

Vidarabine Monohydrate *see* Vidarabine *on page 1384*

Vi-Daylin® + Iron Liquid [OTC] *see* Vitamins (Multiple/Oral) *on page 1394*

Vi-Daylin® Liquid [OTC] *see* Vitamins (Multiple/Oral) *on page 1394*

Videx® *see* Didanosine *on page 434*

Videx® EC *see* Didanosine *on page 434*

Vigabatrin (vye GA ba trin)

Canadian Brand Names Sabril®

Pharmacologic Category Anticonvulsant, Miscellaneous

Use Active management of partial or secondary generalized seizures not controlled by usual treatments; treatment of infantile spasms

Unlabeled/Investigational Use Treatment of spasticity, tardive dyskinesias

Local Anesthetic/Vasoconstrictor Precautions No information available to require special precautions

Effects on Dental Treatment No significant effects or complications reported

Dosage Oral:

Children: **Note:** Administer daily dose in 2 divided doses, especially in the higher dosage ranges:

Adjunctive treatment of seizures: Initial: 40 mg/kg/day; maintenance dosages based on patient weight:

10-15 kg: 0.5-1 g/day

16-30 kg: 1-1.5 g/day

31-50 kg: 1.5-3 g/day

>50 kg: 2-3 g/day

Infantile spasms: 50-100 mg/kg/day, depending on severity of symptoms; higher doses (up to 150 mg/kg/day) have been used in some cases.

Adults: Adjunctive treatment of seizures: Initial: 1 g/day (severe manifestations may require 2 g/day); dose may be given as a single daily dose or divided into 2 equal doses. Increase daily dose by 0.5 g based on response and tolerability. Optimal dose range: 2-3 g/day (maximum dose: 3 g/day)

Elderly: Initiate at low end of dosage range; monitor closely for sedation and confusion

Dosing adjustment in renal impairment: Cl_{cr} <60 mL/minute: Initiate at lower dosage; monitor closely for sedation and confusion

Mechanism of Action Irreversibly inhibits gamma-aminobutyric acid transaminase (GABA-T), increasing the levels of the inhibitory compound gamma amino butyric acid (GABA) within the brain. Duration of effect is dependent upon rate of GABA-T resynthesis.

Other Adverse Effects

>10%

Central nervous system: Fatigue (27%), headache (26%), drowsiness (22%), dizziness (19%), depression (13%), tremor (11%), agitation (11%). **Note:** In pediatric use, hyperactivity (hyperkinesia, agitation, excitation, or restlessness) was reported in 11% of patients.

Endocrine & metabolic: Weight gain (12%)

Ophthalmic: Visual field defects (33%), abnormal vision (11%)

1% to 10%

Cardiovascular: Edema (dependent), chest pain

Central nervous system: Amnesia, confusion, paresthesia, impaired concentration, insomnia, anxiety, emotional lability, abnormal thinking, speech disorder, vertigo, aggression, nervousness, personality disorder

Dermatologic: Rash (5%, similar to placebo), skin disorder

Endocrine & metabolic: Increased appetite, dysmenorrhea, menstrual disorder

Gastrointestinal: Nausea, diarrhea, abdominal pain, constipation, vomiting

Genitourinary: Urinary tract infection

Hematologic: Purpura

Neuromuscular & skeletal: Ataxia, arthralgia, back pain, abnormal coordination, abnormal gait, weakness, hyporeflexia, arthrosis

Ophthalmologic: Nystagmus, diplopia, eye pain

Otic: Ear pain

Respiratory: Throat irritation, nasal congestion, upper respiratory tract infection, sinusitis

<1% (Limited to important or life-threatening): Bilateral optic disc pallor, optic/retinal atrophy, and rare optic neuritis have been reported (usually in first year of

(Continued)

Vigabatrin *(Continued)*

therapy). Additional rare reactions include hallucinations, hypomania, mania, psychosis, suicidal behavior, angioedema, hypersensitivity, urticaria, and stupor.

Drug Interactions Decreased Effect: Serum concentrations of phenytoin and phenobarbital may be decreased by vigabatrin.

Dietary/Ethanol/Herb Considerations

Ethanol: Avoid use; may increase CNS depression.

Food: Administer with food to reduce GI upset; small, frequent meals, chewing gum, or sucking lozenges may reduce nausea and vomiting. Fluids, fruit, and fiber may reduce constipation.

Herb/Nutraceutical: Avoid evening primrose; decreases seizure threshold. Avoid gotu kola, kava, SAMe, St John's wort, and valerian; may increase CNS depression.

Pharmacodynamics/Kinetics

Duration (rate of GABA-T resynthesis dependent): Variable (not strictly correlated to serum concentrations)

Absorption: Rapid

Metabolism: Minimal

Half-life elimination: 5-8 hours; Elderly: Up to 13 hours

Time to peak: 2 hours

Excretion: Urine (70%, as unchanged drug)

Pregnancy Risk Factor Not assigned; contraindicated per manufacturer

Generic Available No

VinBLAStine (vin BLAS teen)

U.S. Brand Names Velban® [DSC]

Canadian Brand Names Velban®

Mexican Brand Names Lemblastine®

Pharmacologic Category Antineoplastic Agent, Natural Source (Plant) Derivative

Synonyms Velban® [DSC]; Vinblastine Sulfate; Vincaleukoblastine; VLB

Use Treatment of Hodgkin's and non-Hodgkin's lymphoma, testicular, lung, head and neck, breast, and renal carcinomas, Mycosis fungoides, Kaposi's sarcoma, histiocytosis, choriocarcinoma, and idiopathic thrombocytopenic purpura

Local Anesthetic/Vasoconstrictor Precautions No information available to require special precautions

Effects on Dental Treatment No significant effects or complications reported

Dosage Refer to individual protocols. Varies depending upon clinical and hematological response. Give at intervals of at least 14 days and only after leukocyte count has returned to at least 4000/mm^3; maintenance therapy should be titrated according to leukocyte count. Dosage should be reduced in patients with recent exposure to radiation therapy or chemotherapy; single doses in these patients should not exceed 5.5 mg/m^2.

Children and Adults: I.V.: 4-20 mg/m^2 (0.1-0.5 mg/kg) every 7-10 days **or** 5-day continuous infusion of 1.5-2 mg/m^2/day **or** 0.1-0.5 mg/kg/week

Dosing adjustment in hepatic impairment:

- Serum bilirubin 1.5-3.0 mg/dL or AST 60-180 units: Administer 50% of normal dose
- Serum bilirubin 3.0-5.0 mg/dL: Administer 25% of dose
- Serum bilirubin >5.0 mg/dL or AST >180 units: Omit dose

Mechanism of Action VLB binds to tubulin and inhibits microtubule formation, therefore, arresting the cell at metaphase by disrupting the formation of the mitotic spindle; it is specific for the M and S phases; binds to microtubular protein of the mitotic spindle causing metaphase arrest

Other Adverse Effects

>10%:

Dermatologic: Alopecia

Gastrointestinal: Nausea and vomiting are most common and are easily controlled with standard antiemetics; constipation, diarrhea (less common), stomatitis, abdominal cramps, anorexia, metallic taste

Emetic potential: Moderate (30% to 60%)

Hematologic: May cause severe bone marrow suppression and is the dose-limiting toxicity of VLB (unlike vincristine); severe granulocytopenia and thrombocytopenia may occur following the administration of VLB and nadir 5-10 days after treatment

Myelosuppressive:

- WBC: Moderate - severe
- Platelets: Moderate - severe
- Onset: 4-7 days
- Nadir: 5-10 days
- Recovery: 17 days

1% to 10%:

Cardiovascular: Hypertension, Raynaud's phenomenon

Central nervous system: Depression, malaise, headache, seizures

Dermatologic: Rash, photosensitivity, dermatitis

Endocrine & metabolic: Hyperuricemia

Extravasation: VLB is a vesicant and can cause tissue irritation and necrosis if infiltrated; if extravasation occurs, follow institutional policy, which may include hyaluronidase and hot compresses

Vesicant chemotherapy

Gastrointestinal: Paralytic ileus, stomatitis

Genitourinary: Urinary retention

Neuromuscular & skeletal: Jaw pain, myalgia, paresthesia

Respiratory: Bronchospasm

<1%: VLB rarely produces neurotoxicity at clinical doses; however, neurotoxicity may be seen, especially at high doses; if it occurs, symptoms are similar to VCR toxicity (ie, peripheral neuropathy, loss of deep tendon reflexes, headache, weakness, urinary retention, and GI symptoms, tachycardia, orthostatic hypotension, convulsions); hemorrhagic colitis

Drug Interactions Substrate of CYP2D6, **3A4**; Inhibits CYP2D6, 3A4

Increased Effect/Toxicity: Vinblastine levels may be increased when given with drugs that inhibit cytochrome P450 3A enzyme substrate. Previous or simultaneous use with mitomycin-C has resulted in acute shortness of breath and severe bronchospasm within minutes or several hours after *Vinca* alkaloid injection and may occur up to 2 weeks after the dose of mitomycin. Mitomycin-C in combination with administration of VLB may cause acute shortness of breath and severe bronchospasm, onset may be within minutes or several hours after VLB injection.

Decreased Effect: Phenytoin plasma levels may be reduced with concomitant combination chemotherapy with vinblastine. Alpha-interferon enhances interferon toxicity; phenytoin may ↓ plasma levels.

Dietary/Ethanol/Herb Considerations Herb/Nutraceutical: Avoid black cohosh and dong quai in estrogen-dependent tumors. Avoid St John's wort; may decrease serum concentration.

Pharmacodynamics/Kinetics

Distribution: V_d: 27.3 L/kg; binds extensively to tissues; does not penetrate CNS or other fatty tissues; distributes to liver

Protein binding: 99%

Metabolism: Hepatic to active metabolite

Half-life elimination: Biphasic: Initial: 0.164 hours; Terminal: 25 hours

Excretion: Feces (95%); urine (<1% as unchanged drug)

Pregnancy Risk Factor D

Generic Available Yes

Vinblastine Sulfate *see* VinBLAStine *on page 1386*

Vincaleukoblastine *see* VinBLAStine *on page 1386*

Vincasar PFS® *see* VinCRIStine *on page 1387*

VinCRIStine (vin KRIS teen)

U.S. Brand Names Oncovin® [DSC]; Vincasar PFS®

Canadian Brand Names Oncovin®; Vincasar® PFS™

Mexican Brand Names Citomid®; Vintec®

Pharmacologic Category Antineoplastic Agent, Natural Source (Plant) Derivative

Synonyms LCR; Leurocristine; Oncovin® [DSC]; VCR; Vincristine Sulfate

Use Treatment of leukemias, Hodgkin's disease, non-Hodgkin's lymphomas, Wilms' tumor, neuroblastoma, rhabdomyosarcoma

Local Anesthetic/Vasoconstrictor Precautions No information available to require special precautions

Effects on Dental Treatment No significant effects or complications reported

Dosage I.V.: Refer to individual protocols as dosages vary with protocol used; adjustments are made depending upon clinical and hematological response and upon adverse reactions

Children ≤10 kg or BSA <1 m^2: Initial therapy: 0.05 mg/kg once weekly then titrate dose; maximum single dose: 2 mg

Children >10 kg or BSA ≥1 m^2: 1-2 mg/m^2, may repeat once weekly for 3-6 weeks; maximum single dose: 2 mg

Neuroblastoma: I.V. continuous infusion with doxorubicin: 1 mg/m^2/day for 72 hours

Adults: 0.4-1.4 mg/m^2 (up to 2 mg maximum in most patients); may repeat every week

Dosing adjustment in hepatic impairment:

Serum bilirubin 1.5-3.0 mg/dL or AST 60-180 units: Administer 50% of normal dose

Serum bilirubin 3.0-5.0 mg/dL: Administer 25% of dose

Serum bilirubin >5.0 mg/dL or AST >180 units: Omit dose

The average total dose per course of treatment should be around 2-2.5 mg; some recommend capping the dose at 2 mg maximum to reduce toxicity; however, it is felt that this measure can reduce the efficacy of the drug

Mechanism of Action Binds to microtubular protein of the mitotic spindle causing metaphase arrest; cell-cycle phase specific in the M and S phases

(Continued)

VinCRIStine *(Continued)*

Other Adverse Effects

>10%:

Dermatologic: Alopecia occurs in 20% to 70% of patients

Extravasation: VCR is a vesicant and can cause tissue irritation and necrosis if infiltrated; if extravasation occurs, follow institutional policy, which may include hyaluronidase and hot compresses

Vesicant chemotherapy

1% to 10%:

Cardiovascular: Orthostatic hypotension or hypertension, hypertension, hypotension

Central nervous system: Motor difficulties, seizures, headache, CNS depression, cranial nerve paralysis, fever

Dermatologic: Rash

Endocrine & metabolic: Hyperuricemia

SIADH: Rarely occurs, but may be related to the neurologic toxicity; may cause symptomatic hyponatremia with seizures; the increase in serum ADH concentration usually subsides within 2-3 days after onset

Gastrointestinal: Constipation and possible paralytic ileus secondary to neurologic toxicity; oral ulceration, abdominal cramps, anorexia, metallic taste, bloating, nausea, vomiting, weight loss, diarrhea

Emetic potential: Low (<10%)

Local: Phlebitis

Neurologic: Alterations in mental status such as depression, confusion, or insomnia; constipation, paralytic ileus, and urinary tract disturbances may occur. All patients should be on a prophylactic bowel management regimen. Cranial nerve palsies, headaches, jaw pain, optic atrophy with blindness have been reported. Intrathecal administration of VCR has uniformly caused death; VCR should **never** be administered by this route. Neurologic effects of VCR may be additive with those of other neurotoxic agents and spinal cord irradiation.

Neuromuscular & skeletal: Jaw pain, leg pain, myalgia, cramping, numbness, weakness

Peripheral neuropathy: Frequently the dose-limiting toxicity of VCR. Most frequent in patients >40 years of age; occurs usually after an average of 3 weekly doses, but may occur after just one dose. Manifested as loss of the deep tendon reflexes in the lower extremities, numbness, tingling, pain, paresthesias of the fingers and toes (stocking glove sensation), and "foot drop" or "wrist drop"

Ocular: Photophobia

<1%: Stomatitis

Myelosuppressive: Occasionally mild leukopenia and thrombocytopenia may occur

WBC: Rare

Platelets: Rare

Onset: 7 days

Nadir: 10 days

Recovery: 21 days

Drug Interactions Substrate of **CYP3A4**; Inhibits CYP3A4

Increased Effect/Toxicity: Vincristine levels may be increased when given with drugs that inhibit cytochrome P450 3A enzyme (itraconazole has been shown to increase onset and severity of neuromuscular adverse effects of vincristine). Digoxin plasma levels and renal excretion may decrease with combination chemotherapy including vincristine. Vincristine should be given 12-24 hours before asparaginase to minimize toxicity (may decrease the hepatic clearance of vincristine). Acute pulmonary reactions may occur with mitomycin-C. Previous or simultaneous use with mitomycin-C has resulted in acute shortness of breath and severe bronchospasm within minutes or several hours after *Vinca* alkaloid injection and may occur up to 2 weeks after the dose of mitomycin.

Decreased Effect: Digoxin and phenytoin levels may decrease with combination chemotherapy.

Dietary/Ethanol/Herb Considerations Herb/Nutraceutical: Avoid St John's wort; may decrease serum concentration.

Pharmacodynamics/Kinetics

Absorption: Oral: Poor

Distribution: Poor penetration into CSF; rapidly removed from bloodstream and tightly bound to tissues; penetrates blood-brain barrier poorly

Protein binding: 75%

Metabolism: Extensively hepatic

Half-life elimination: Terminal: 24 hours

Excretion: Feces (~80%); urine (<1% as unchanged drug)

Pregnancy Risk Factor D

Generic Available Yes

Vincristine Sulfate *see* VinCRIStine *on page 1387*

Vinorelbine (vi NOR el been)

U.S. Brand Names Navelbine®

Canadian Brand Names Navelbine®

Mexican Brand Names Navelbine®

Pharmacologic Category Antineoplastic Agent, Natural Source (Plant) Derivative

Synonyms Vinorelbine Tartrate

Use Treatment of nonsmall cell lung cancer (as a single agent or in combination with cisplatin)

Unlabeled/Investigational Use Treatment of breast cancer, ovarian carcinoma (cisplatin-resistant), Hodgkin's disease

Local Anesthetic/Vasoconstrictor Precautions No information available to require special precautions

Effects on Dental Treatment No significant effects or complications reported

Dosage Refer to individual protocols; varies depending upon clinical and hematological response

Adults: I.V.:

Single-agent therapy: 30 mg/m² every 7 days

Combination therapy with cisplatin: 25 mg/m² every 7 days (with cisplatin 100 mg/m² every 4 weeks); **Alternatively:** 30 mg/m² in combination with cisplatin 120 mg/m² on days 1 and 29, then every 6 weeks

Dosing adjustment in hematological toxicity: Granulocyte counts should be ≥1000 cells/mm³ prior to the administration of vinorelbine. Adjustments in the dosage of vinorelbine should be based on granulocyte counts obtained on the day of treatment as follows:

Granulocytes ≥1500 cells/mm³ on day of treatment: Administer 100% of starting dose

Granulocytes 1000-1499 cells/mm³ on day of treatment: Administer 50% of starting dose

Granulocytes <1000 cells/mm³ on day of treatment: Do not administer. Repeat granulocyte count in one week; if 3 consecutive doses are held because granulocyte count is <1000 cells/mm³, discontinue vinorelbine

For patients who, during treatment, have experienced fever and/or sepsis while granulocytopenic or had 2 consecutive weekly doses held due to granulocytopenia, subsequent doses of vinorelbine should be:

75% of starting dose for granulocytes ≥1500 cells/mm³

37.5% of starting dose for granulocytes 1000-1499 cells/mm³

Dosing adjustment in renal impairment: None; if moderate or severe neurotoxicity develops, discontinue therapy

Dosing adjustment in hepatic impairment: Use with caution; in patients who develop hyperbilirubinemia during treatment with vinorelbine, the dose should be adjusted for total bilirubin as follows:

Serum bilirubin ≤2 mg/dL: Administer 100% of starting dose

Serum bilirubin 2.1-3 mg/dL: Administer 50% of starting dose

Serum bilirubin >3 mg/dL: Administer 25% of starting dose

Dosing adjustment in patients with concurrent hematologic toxicity and hepatic impairment: Administer the lower doses determined from the above recommendations

Mechanism of Action Semisynthetic vinca alkaloid which binds to tubulin and inhibits microtubule formation, therefore, arresting the cell at metaphase by disrupting the formation of the mitotic spindle; it is specific for the M and S phases; binds to microtubular protein of the mitotic spindle causing metaphase arrest

Other Adverse Effects

>10%:

Central nervous system: Fatigue (27%)

Dermatologic: Alopecia (12%)

Gastrointestinal: Nausea (44%, severe <2%) and vomiting (20%) are most common and are easily controlled with standard antiemetics; constipation (35%), diarrhea (17%)

Emetic potential: Moderate (30% to 60%)

Hematologic: May cause severe bone marrow suppression and is the dose-limiting toxicity of vinorelbine; severe granulocytopenia (90%) may occur following the administration of vinorelbine; leukopenia (92%), anemia (83%)

Myelosuppressive:

WBC: Moderate - severe

Onset: 4-7 days

Nadir: 7-10 days

Recovery: 14-21 days

Hepatic: Elevated SGOT (67%), elevated total bilirubin (13%)

Local: Injection site reaction (28%), injection site pain (16%)

Neuromuscular & skeletal: Weakness (36%), peripheral neuropathy (20% to 25%)

1% to 10%:

Cardiovascular: Chest pain (5%)

Gastrointestinal: Paralytic ileus (1%)

(Continued)

Vinorelbine *(Continued)*

Hematologic: Thrombocytopenia (5%)

Local: Extravasation: Vesicant and can cause tissue irritation and necrosis if infiltrated; if extravasation occurs, follow institutional policy, which may include hyaluronidase and hot compresses; phlebitis (7%)

Vesicant chemotherapy

Neuromuscular & skeletal: Mild to moderate peripheral neuropathy manifested by paresthesia and hyperesthesia, loss of deep tendon reflexes (<5%); myalgia (<5%), arthralgia (<5%), jaw pain (<5%)

Respiratory: Dyspnea (3% to 7%)

<1%: Hemorrhagic cystitis, severe peripheral neuropathy (generally reversible), syndrome of inappropriate ADH secretion

Postmarketing and/or case reports: Angioedema, headache, DVT, flushing, hypertension, hypotension, vasodilation, tachycardia, hyponatremia, abdominal pain, dysphagia, esophagitis, mucositis, back pain, gait instability, muscle weakness, anaphylaxis, tumor pain, pancreatitis, pneumonia, pulmonary edema, pulmonary embolus, radiation recall (dermatitis, esophagitis)

Drug Interactions Substrate of CYP2D6, **3A4**; Inhibits CYP2D6, 3A4

Increased Effect/Toxicity: Previous or simultaneous use with mitomycin-C has resulted in acute shortness of breath and severe bronchospasm within minutes or several hours after *Vinca* alkaloid injection and may occur up to 2 weeks after the dose of mitomycin.

Cisplatin: Incidence of granulocytopenia is significantly higher than with single-agent vinorelbine.

Dietary/Ethanol/Herb Considerations Herb/Nutraceutical: Avoid St John's wort; may decrease serum concentration.

Pharmacodynamics/Kinetics

Absorption: Unreliable; must be given I.V.

Distribution: V_d: 25.4-40.1 L/kg; binds extensively to human platelets and lymphocytes (79.6% to 91.2%)

Protein binding: 80% to 90%

Metabolism: Extensively hepatic to two metabolites, deacetylvinorelbine (active) and vinorelbine N-oxide

Bioavailability: Oral: 26% to 45%

Half-life elimination: Triphasic: Terminal: 27.7-43.6 hours

Excretion: Feces (46%); urine (18%)

Clearance: Plasma: Mean: 0.97-1.26 L/hour/kg

Pregnancy Risk Factor D

Generic Available Yes

Vinorelbine Tartrate *see* Vinorelbine *on page 1389*

Viokase® *see* Pancrelipase *on page 1030*

Viosterol *see* Ergocalciferol *on page 508*

Vioxx® *see* Rofecoxib *on page 1194*

Vira-A® [DSC] *see* Vidarabine *on page 1384*

Viracept® *see* Nelfinavir *on page 959*

Viramune® *see* Nevirapine *on page 965*

Virazole® *see* Ribavirin *on page 1176*

Viread™ *see* Tenofovir *on page 1275*

Virilon® *see* MethylTESTOSTERone *on page 897*

Viroptic® *see* Trifluridine *on page 1350*

Viscoat® *see* Chondroitin Sulfate and Sodium Hyaluronate *on page 320*

Visicol™ *see* Phosphate Supplements *on page 1076*

Visine-A™ [OTC] *see* Naphazoline and Pheniramine *on page 953*

Visine® Advanced Relief [OTC] *see* Tetrahydrozoline *on page 1288*

Visine® L.R. [OTC] *see* Oxymetazoline *on page 1022*

Visine® Original [OTC] *see* Tetrahydrozoline *on page 1288*

Vistaril® *see* HydrOXYzine *on page 697*

Vistide® *see* Cidofovir *on page 323*

Vita-C® [OTC] *see* Ascorbic Acid *on page 128*

Vitacon Forte *see* Vitamins (Multiple/Oral) *on page 1394*

Vitamin A (VYE tu min ay)

U.S. Brand Names Aquasol A®; Palmitate-A® [OTC]

Mexican Brand Names Arovit; A-Vicon; A-Vitex

Pharmacologic Category Vitamin, Fat Soluble

Synonyms Oleovitamin A

Use Treatment and prevention of vitamin A deficiency; parenteral (I.M.) route is indicated when oral administration is not feasible or when absorption is insufficient (malabsorption syndrome)

Local Anesthetic/Vasoconstrictor Precautions No information available to require special precautions

Effects on Dental Treatment No significant effects or complications reported

Dosage

RDA:

<1 year: 375 mcg
1-3 years: 400 mcg
4-6 years: 500 mcg*
7-10 years: 700 mcg*
>10 years: 800-1000 mcg*
Male: 1000 mcg
Female: 800 mcg
* mcg retinol equivalent (0.3 mcg retinol = 1 unit vitamin A)

Vitamin A supplementation in measles (recommendation of the World Health Organization): Children: Oral: Administer as a single dose; repeat the next day and at 4 weeks for children with ophthalmologic evidence of vitamin A deficiency:

6 months to 1 year: 100,000 units
>1 year: 200,000 units

Note: Use of vitamin A in measles is recommended only for patients 6 months to 2 years of age hospitalized with measles and its complications **or** patients >6 months of age who have any of the following risk factors and who are not already receiving vitamin A: immunodeficiency, ophthalmologic evidence of vitamin A deficiency including night blindness, Bitot's spots or evidence of xerophthalmia, impaired intestinal absorption, moderate to severe malnutrition including that associated with eating disorders, or recent immigration from areas where high mortality rates from measles have been observed

Note: Monitor patients closely; dosages >25,000 units/kg have been associated with toxicity

Severe deficiency with xerophthalmia: Oral:

Children 1-8 years: 5000-10,000 units/kg/day for 5 days or until recovery occurs
Children >8 years and Adults: 500,000 units/day for 3 days, then 50,000 units/day for 14 days, then 10,000-20,000 units/day for 2 months

Deficiency (without corneal changes): Oral:

Infants <1 year: 100,000 units every 4-6 months
Children 1-8 years: 200,000 units every 4-6 months
Children >8 years and Adults: 100,000 units/day for 3 days then 50,000 units/day for 14 days

Deficiency: I.M.: **Note:** I.M. route is indicated when oral administration is not feasible or when absorption is insufficient (malabsorption syndrome):

Infants: 7500-15,000 units/day for 10 days
Children 1-8 years: 17,500-35,000 units/day for 10 days
Children >8 years and Adults: 100,000 units/day for 3 days, followed by 50,000 units/day for 2 weeks

Note: Follow-up therapy with an oral therapeutic multivitamin (containing additional vitamin A) is recommended:

Low Birth Weight Infants: Additional vitamin A is recommended, however, no dosage amount has been established
Children ≤8 years: 5000-10,000 units/day
Children >8 years and Adults: 10,000-20,000 units/day

Malabsorption syndrome (prophylaxis): Children >8 years and Adults: Oral: 10,000-50,000 units/day of water miscible product

Dietary supplement: Oral:

Infants up to 6 months: 1500 units/day
Children:

6 months to 3 years: 1500-2000 units/day
4-6 years: 2500 units/day
7-10 years: 3300-3500 units/day

Children >10 years and Adults: 4000-5000 units/day

Mechanism of Action Needed for bone development, growth, visual adaptation to darkness, testicular and ovarian function, and as a cofactor in many biochemical processes

Other Adverse Effects 1% to 10%:

Central nervous system: Irritability, vertigo, lethargy, malaise, fever, headache
Dermatologic: Drying or cracking of skin
Endocrine & metabolic: Hypercalcemia
Gastrointestinal: Weight loss
Ocular: Visual changes
Miscellaneous: Hypervitaminosis A

Drug Interactions

Increased Effect/Toxicity: Retinoids may have additive adverse effects.

Decreased Effect: Cholestyramine resin decreases absorption of vitamin A. Neomycin and mineral oil may also interfere with vitamin A absorption.

Pharmacodynamics/Kinetics

Absorption: Vitamin A in dosages **not** exceeding physiologic replacement is well absorbed after oral administration; water miscible preparations are absorbed more rapidly than oil preparations; large oral doses, conditions of fat malabsorption, low protein intake, or hepatic or pancreatic disease reduces oral absorption

(Continued)

Vitamin A *(Continued)*

Distribution: Large amounts concentrate for storage in the liver; enters breast milk
Metabolism: Conjugated with glucuronide; undergoes enterohepatic recirculation
Excretion: Feces

Pregnancy Risk Factor A/X (dose exceeding RDA recommendation)

Dosage Forms CAP [softgel]: 10,000 units, 25,000 units. **INJ, solution** (Aquasol A®): 50,000 units/mL (2 mL). **TAB** (Palmitate-A®): 5000 units, 15,000 units

Generic Available Yes: Capsule

Vitamin A Acid *see* Tretinoin (Topical) *on page 1340*

Vitamin A and Vitamin D (VYE ta min aye & VYE ta min dee)

U.S. Brand Names A and D® Ointment [OTC]; Baza® Clear [OTC]; Clocream [OTC]; Sween Cream® [OTC]

Pharmacologic Category Topical Skin Product

Synonyms Cod Liver Oil

Use Temporary relief of discomfort due to chapped skin, diaper rash, minor burns, abrasions, as well as irritations associated with ostomy skin care

Local Anesthetic/Vasoconstrictor Precautions No information available to require special precautions

Effects on Dental Treatment No significant effects or complications reported

Dosage Topical: Apply locally with gentle massage as needed

Other Adverse Effects Frequency not defined: Local: Irritation

Pregnancy Risk Factor B

Dosage Forms CAP: Vitamin A 1250 int. units and vitamin D 135 int. units; Vitamin A 5000 int. units and vitamin D 400 int. units; Vitamin A 10,000 int. units and vitamin D 400 int. units; Vitamin A 25,000 int. units and vitamin D 400 int. units. **CRM** (Sween Cream®): 14 g, 57 g, 142 g, 255 g. **OINT:** 5 g, 60 g, 120 g, 454 g; (A and D® Ointment): 45 g, 120 g, 454 g; (Baza® Clear): 15 g, 50 g, 150 g, 240 g; (Clocream): 30 g

Generic Available Yes: Capsule, ointment

Vitamin B_1 *see* Thiamine *on page 1295*
Vitamin B_2 *see* Riboflavin *on page 1178*
Vitamin B_3 *see* Niacin *on page 967*
Vitamin B_3 *see* Niacinamide *on page 968*
Vitamin B_5 *see* Pantothenic Acid *on page 1033*
Vitamin B_6 *see* Pyridoxine *on page 1152*
Vitamin B_{12} *see* Cyanocobalamin *on page 377*
Vitamin B_{12} *see* Hydroxocobalamin *on page 693*

Vitamin B Complex (VYE tu min bee KOM pleks)

Related Information

Vitamin B Complex Combination Products *on page 1640*

U.S. Brand Names Apatate® [OTC]; Gevrabon® [OTC]

Canadian Brand Names Penta/3B®; Vita 3B

Pharmacologic Category Vitamin, Water Soluble

Use Supportive nutritional supplementation in conditions in which water-soluble vitamins are required like GI disorders, chronic alcoholism, pregnancy, severe burns, and recovery from surgery

Local Anesthetic/Vasoconstrictor Precautions No information available to require special precautions

Effects on Dental Treatment No significant effects or complications reported

Dosage Dosage is usually 1 tablet or capsule/day; please refer to product labeling

Generic Available Yes

Vitamin B Complex and Vitamin C

(VYE tu min bee KOM pleks & VYE tu min see)

Related Information

Vitamin B Complex Combination Products *on page 1640*

U.S. Brand Names Allbee® With C [OTC]; Surbex-T® Filmtabs® [OTC]; Surbex® With C Filmtabs® [OTC]

Canadian Brand Names Penta/3B®+C; Vita 3B+C

Pharmacologic Category Vitamin, Water Soluble

Use Supportive nutritional supplementation in conditions in which water-soluble vitamins are required like GI disorders, chronic alcoholism, pregnancy, severe burns, and recovery from surgery

Local Anesthetic/Vasoconstrictor Precautions No information available to require special precautions

Effects on Dental Treatment No significant effects or complications reported

Dosage Adults: Oral: 1 every day

Generic Available Yes

Vitamin B Complex, Vitamin C, and Folic Acid

(VYE tu min bee KOM pleks, VYE tu min see, & FOE lik AS id)

Related Information

Vitamin B Complex Combination Products *on page 1640*

U.S. Brand Names Nephrocaps®

Pharmacologic Category Vitamin, Water Soluble

Use Supportive nutritional supplementation in conditions in which water-soluble vitamins are required like GI disorders, chronic alcoholism, pregnancy, severe burns, and recovery from surgery

Local Anesthetic/Vasoconstrictor Precautions No information available to require special precautions

Effects on Dental Treatment No significant effects or complications reported

Dosage Adults: Oral: 1 every day

Generic Available Yes

Vitamin C *see* Ascorbic Acid *on page 128*

Vitamin D_2 *see* Ergocalciferol *on page 508*

Vitamin E (VYE tu min ee)

U.S. Brand Names Aqua Gem E® [OTC]; Aquasol E® [OTC]; E-Gems® [OTC]; Key-E® [OTC]; Key- E® Kaps [OTC]

Pharmacologic Category Vitamin, Fat Soluble

Synonyms *d*-Alpha Tocopherol; *dl*-Alpha Tocopherol

Use Dental and Medical: Prevention and treatment of hemolytic anemia secondary to vitamin E deficiency; dietary supplement

Unlabeled/Investigational Use To reduce the risk of bronchopulmonary dysplasia or retrolental fibroplasia in infants exposed to high concentrations of oxygen; prevention and treatment of tardive dyskinesia and Alzheimer's disease

Local Anesthetic/Vasoconstrictor Precautions No information available to require special precautions

Effects on Dental Treatment No significant effects or complications reported

Dosage One unit of vitamin E = 1 mg *dl*-alpha-tocopherol acetate. Oral:

Recommended daily allowance (RDA):
- Premature infants ≤3 months: 17 mg (25 units)
- Infants:
  - ≤6 months: 3 mg (4.5 units)
  - 7-12 months: 4 mg (6 units)
- Children:
  - 1-3 years: 6 mg (9 units); upper limit of intake should not exceed 200 mg/day
  - 4-8 years: 7 mg (10.5 units); upper limit of intake should not exceed 300 mg/day
  - 9-13 years: 11 mg (16.5 units); upper limit of intake should not exceed 600 mg/day
  - 14-18 years: 15 mg (22.5 units); upper limit of intake should not exceed 800 mg/day
- Adults: 15 mg (22.5 units); upper limit of intake should not exceed 1000 mg/day
- Pregnant female:
  - ≤18 years: 15 mg (22.5 units); upper level of intake should not exceed 800 mg/day
  - 19-50 years: 15 mg (22.5 units); upper level of intake should not exceed 1000 mg/day
- Lactating female:
  - ≤18 years: 19 mg (28.5 units); upper level of intake should not exceed 800 mg/day
  - 19-50 years: 19 mg (28.5 units); upper level of intake should not exceed 1000 mg/day

Vitamin E deficiency:
- Children (with malabsorption syndrome): 1 unit/kg/day of water miscible vitamin E (to raise plasma tocopherol concentrations to the normal range within 2 months and to maintain normal plasma concentrations)
- Adults: 60-75 units/day

Prevention of vitamin E deficiency: Adults: 30 units/day

Prevention of retinopathy of prematurity or BPD secondary to O_2 therapy (AAP considers this use investigational and routine use is not recommended):
- Retinopathy prophylaxis: 15-30 units/kg/day to maintain plasma levels between 1.5-2 µg/mL (may need as high as 100 units/kg/day)

Cystic fibrosis, beta-thalassemia, sickle cell anemia may require higher daily maintenance doses:
- Children:
  - Cystic fibrosis: 100-400 units/day
  - Beta-thalassemia: 750 units/day
- Adults:
  - Sickle cell: 450 units/day
  - Alzheimer's disease: 1000 units twice daily

(Continued)

Vitamin E *(Continued)*

Tardive dyskinesia: 1600 units/day

Mechanism of Action Prevents oxidation of vitamin A and C; protects polyunsaturated fatty acids in membranes from attack by free radicals and protects red blood cells against hemolysis

Other Adverse Effects <1%: **Blurred vision, contact dermatitis (topical form),** diarrhea, **fatigue,** gonadal dysfunction, **headache**, intestinal cramps, **nausea, weakness**

Contraindications Hypersensitivity to vitamin E or any component of the formulation; I.V. route

Warnings/Precautions May induce vitamin K deficiency; necrotizing enterocolitis has been associated with oral administration of large dosages (eg, >200 units/day) of a hyperosmolar vitamin E preparation in low birth weight infants

Drug Interactions

Cholestyramine (and colestipol): May reduce absorption of vitamin E

Iron: Vitamin E may impair the hematologic response to iron in children with iron-deficiency anemia; monitor

Orlistat: May reduce absorption of vitamin E

Warfarin: Vitamin E may alter the effect of vitamin K actions on clotting factors resulting in an increase hypoprothrombinemic response to warfarin; monitor

Pharmacodynamics/Kinetics

Absorption: Oral: Depends on presence of bile; reduced in conditions of malabsorption, in low birth weight premature infants, and as dosage increases; water miscible preparations are better absorbed than oil preparations

Distribution: To all body tissues, especially adipose tissue, where it is stored

Metabolism: Hepatic to glucuronides

Excretion: Feces

Pregnancy Risk Factor A/C (dose exceeding RDA recommendation)

Dosage Forms CAP: 100 units, 200 units, 400 units, 500 units, 600 units, 1000 units; (Aqua Gem E®, Key-E Kaps®): 200 units, 400 units; (E-Gems®): 30 units, 100 units, 600 units, 800 units, 1000 units, 1200 units. **CRM:** 100 units/g (60 g); (Key-E®): 30 units/g (60 g, 120 g, 480 g). **Oil:** 100 units/0.25 mL (60 mL); 1150 units/0.25 mL (30 mL, 60 mL, 120 mL); (E-Gem®): 100 units/10 drops (15 mL, 60 mL). **OINT, topical** (Key-E®): 30 units/g (60 g, 120 g, 480 g). **POWDER** (Key-E®): 700 units/dose (15 g, 75 g, 1000 g). **SOLN, oral drops** (Aquasol E®): 15 units/0.3 mL (12 mL, 30 mL). **SUPP** (Key-E®): 30 units (12s, 24s). **SPRAY** (Key-E®): 30 units/3 seconds (105 g). **TAB:** 100 units, 200 units, 400 units, 500 units, 800 units; (Key-E®): 100 units, 200 units, 400 units

Generic Available Yes

Vitamin G *see* Riboflavin *on page 1178*

Vitamin K_1 *see* Phytonadione *on page 1079*

Vitamins (Multiple/Oral) (VYE tu minz, MUL ti pul, ORE ul)

U.S. Brand Names Centrum® [OTC]; Centrum® Performance™ [OTC]; Centrum® Silver® [OTC]; Geritol® Tonic [OTC]; Iberet® [OTC]; Iberet®-500 [OTC]; Iberet-Folic-500®; One-A-Day® 50 Plus Formula [OTC]; One-A-Day® Active Formula [OTC]; One-A -Day® Essential Formula [OTC]; One-A-Day® Maximum Formula [OTC]; One-A- Day® Men's Formula [OTC]; One-A-Day® Today [OTC]; One-A-Day® Women's Formula [OTC]; Theragran® Heart Right™ [OTC]; Theragran-M® Advanced Formula [OTC]; Vicon Forte®; Vicon Plus® [OTC]; Vi-Daylin® + Iron Liquid [OTC]; Vi-Daylin® Liquid [OTC]; Vitacon Forte

Mexican Brand Names Clanda®; Complan; Suplena; Vi-Syneral

Pharmacologic Category Vitamin

Synonyms Multiple Vitamins; Therapeutic Multivitamins; Vitamins, Multiple (Oral); Vitamins, Multiple (Therapeutic); Vitamins, Multiple With Iron

Use Prevention/treatment of vitamin and mineral deficiencies; labeled for OTC use as a dietary supplement

Local Anesthetic/Vasoconstrictor Precautions No information available to require special precautions

Effects on Dental Treatment No significant effects or complications reported

Dosage Oral: Adults: Daily dose of adult preparations varies by product. Generally, 1 tablet or capsule or 5-15 mL of liquid per day. Consult package labeling. Prescription doses may be higher for burn or cystic fibrosis patients.

Other Adverse Effects 1% to 10%: Hypervitaminosis (refer to individual entries)

Contraindications Hypersensitivity to any component of the formulation; pre-existing hypervitaminosis

Warnings/Precautions RDA values are not requirements, but are recommended daily intakes of certain essential nutrients; use with caution in patients with severe renal or hepatic dysfunction or failure. Adult preparations may contain amounts of ethanol or iron which should not be used in children.

Dietary/Ethanol/Herb Considerations Food: Iron absorption is inhibited by eggs and milk. May administer with food to decrease stomach upset.

Pregnancy Risk Factor A (at RDA recommended dose)

Dosage Forms See Adult Multivitamin Products on page 1637 of the Appendix.
Generic Available Yes

Vitamins, Multiple (Therapeutic) *see* Vitamins (Multiple/Oral) *on page 1394*
Vitamins, Multiple With Iron *see* Vitamins (Multiple/Oral) *on page 1394*
Vitelle™ Irospan® [OTC] *see* Ferrous Sulfate and Ascorbic Acid *on page 569*
Vitrasert® *see* Ganciclovir *on page 626*
Vitravene™ *see* Fomivirsen *on page 611*
Vitrax® *see* Sodium Hyaluronate *on page 1230*
Vitussin *see* Hydrocodone and Guaifenesin *on page 683*
Vivactil® *see* Protriptyline *on page 1145*
Viva-Drops® [OTC] *see* Artificial Tears *on page 128*
Vivelle® *see* Estradiol *on page 521*
Vivelle-Dot® *see* Estradiol *on page 521*
Vivotif Berna® *see* Typhoid Vaccine *on page 1363*
VLB *see* VinBLAStine *on page 1386*
VM-26 *see* Teniposide *on page 1274*
Volmax® *see* Albuterol *on page 48*
Voltaren® *see* Diclofenac *on page 429*
Voltaren Ophthalmic® *see* Diclofenac *on page 429*
Voltaren®-XR *see* Diclofenac *on page 429*

Voriconazole (vor i KOE na zole)

U.S. Brand Names VFEND®
Pharmacologic Category Antifungal Agent, Oral; Antifungal Agent, Parenteral
Synonyms UK109496
Use Dental and Medical: Treatment of invasive aspergillosis and serious fungal infections caused by *Scedosporium apiospermum* and *Fusarium* spp (including *Fusarium solanae*) in patients intolerant of, or refractory to, other therapy
Local Anesthetic/Vasoconstrictor Precautions No information available to require special precautions
Effects on Dental Treatment
>10%: Visual changes (~30%; photophobia, color changes, increased or decreased visual acuity, blurred vision)
1% to 10%: Tachycardia (3%), hypertension (2%), hypotension (2%), vasodilation (2%), fever (6%), headache (3%), hallucinations (3%), dizziness (1%), nausea (6%), vomiting (5%), xerostomia (1%)

Dosage
Children <12 years: No data available
Children ≥12 years and Adults: I.V.: Initial: Loading dose: 6 mg/kg every 12 hours for 2 doses; followed by maintenance dose of 4 mg/kg every 12 hours
Conversion to oral dosing:
Patients >40 kg: 200 mg every 12 hours
Patients ≤40 kg: 100 mg every 12 hours
Note: Dosage may be increased by 100 mg/dose in patients who fail to respond adequately (50 mg/dose in patients ≤40 kg)
Dosing adjustment in patients unable to tolerate treatment:
I.V.: Dose may be reduced to 3 mg/kg every 12 hours
Oral: Dose may be reduced in 50 mg increments to a minimum dosage of 200 mg every 12 hours in patients weighing >40 kg (100 mg every 12 hours in patients ≤40 kg)
Dosing adjustment in patients receiving concomitant phenytoin:
I.V.: Increase maintenance dosage to 5 mg/kg every 12 hours
Oral: Increase dose from 200 mg to 400 mg every 12 hours in patients >40 kg (100 mg to 200 mg every 12 hours in patients ≤40 kg)
Dosing adjustment in renal impairment: In patients with Cl_{cr} <50 mL/minute, accumulation of the intravenous vehicle (SBECD) occurs. After initial loading dose, oral voriconazole should be administered to these patients, unless an assessment of the benefit:risk to the patient justifies the use of I.V. voriconazole. Monitor serum creatinine and change to oral voriconazole therapy when possible.
Dosing adjustment in hepatic impairment:
Mild to moderate hepatic dysfunction (Child-Pugh Class A and B): Following standard loading dose, reduce maintenance dosage by 50%
Severe hepatic impairment: Should only be used if benefit outweighs risk; monitor closely for toxicity

Mechanism of Action Interferes with fungal cytochrome P450 activity, decreasing ergosterol synthesis (principal sterol in fungal cell membrane) and inhibiting fungal cell membrane formation.
Other Adverse Effects Reported from all trials, including immunocompromised patients (cause:effect relationship not established for many reactions):
1% to 10%:
Cardiovascular: Peripheral edema (1%)
Central nervous system: Chills (4%)
(Continued)

Voriconazole *(Continued)*

Gastrointestinal: Diarrhea (1%), abdominal pain (2%)

Hematologic: Thrombocytopenia (1%)

Hepatic: Alkaline phosphatase increased (4%), serum transaminases increased (2%), AST increased (2%), ALT increased (2%), cholestatic jaundice (1%)

Renal: Acute renal failure (1%)

<1% (Limited to important or life-threatening): Acute tubular necrosis, adrenal cortical insufficiency, agranulocytosis, **allergic reaction, anaphylactoid reaction**, anemia (aplastic), anemia (macrocytic, megaloblastic, or microcytic), angioedema, aplastic anemia, ataxia, **atrial arrhythmia, atrial fibrillation**, AV block, **bigeminy,** bone marrow depression, bone necrosis, **bradycardia**, brain edema, bundle branch block, **cardiac arrest**, cerebral hemorrhage, cholecystitis, cholelithiasis, color blindness, **coma, CHF, convulsion, delirium, dementia**, depersonalization, depression, DIC, discoid lupus erythematosus, **duodenal ulcer perforation, dyspnea**, encephalopathy, enlarged liver, enlarged spleen, eosinophilia, erythema multiforme, exfoliative dermatitis, **extrapyramidal symptoms**, fixed drug eruption, **GI hemorrhage, grand mal seizure**, Guillain-Barré syndrome, hematemesis, hemolytic anemia, hepatic coma, hepatic failure, hepatitis, intestinal perforation, intracranial hypertension, leukopenia, lung edema, **myasthenia, MI**, neuropathy, night blindness, optic atrophy, optic neuritis, pancreatitis, pancytopenia, papilledema, **paresthesia**, photosensitivity, **psychosis**, pulmonary embolus, QT interval prolongation, **respiratory distress syndrome, sepsis,** Stevens-Johnson syndrome, **suicidal ideation, supraventricular tachycardia, syncope**, thrombotic thrombocytopenic purpura, toxic epidermal necrolysis, **ventricular arrhythmia, ventricular fibrillation, ventricular tachycardia (including possible torsade de pointes)**, vertigo, **visual field defect**

Contraindications Hypersensitivity to voriconazole or any component of the formulation (cross-reaction with other azole antifungal agents may occur but has not been established, use caution); coadministration of CYP3A4 substrates which may lead to QT_c prolongation (cisapride, pimozide, or quinidine); coadministration with barbiturates (long acting), carbamazepine, ergot alkaloids, rifampin, rifabutin, and sirolimus; pregnancy (unless risk:benefit justifies use)

Warnings/Precautions Visual changes are commonly associated with treatment, including blurred vision, changes in visual acuity, color changes, and photophobia. Patients should be warned to avoid tasks which depend on vision, including operating machinery or driving. Changes are reversible on discontinuation following brief exposure/treatment regimens (≤28 days); reversibility following long-term administration has not been evaluated.

Serious hepatic reactions (including hepatitis, cholestasis, and fulminant hepatic failure) have occurred during treatment, primarily in patients with serious concomitant medical conditions, including hematological malignancy. However, hepatotoxicity has occurred in patients with no identifiable risk factors. Use caution in patients with pre-existing hepatic impairment (dose adjustment required).

Voriconazole tablets contain lactose; avoid administration in hereditary galactose intolerance, Lapp lactase deficiency, or glucose-galactose malabsorption. Avoid/limit use of intravenous formulation in patients with renal impairment; intravenous formulation contains excipient sulfobutyl ether beta-cyclodextrin (SBECD), which may accumulate in renal insufficiency. Infusion-related reactions may occur with intravenous dosing. Consider discontinuation of infusion if reaction is severe.

Avoid use in pregnancy, unless an evaluation of the potential benefit justifies possible risk to the fetus. Safety and efficacy have not been established in children <12 years of age.

Drug Interactions Substrate of **CYP2C8/9, 2C19**, 3A4; Inhibits CYP2C8/9, 2C19, 3A4

Benzodiazepines (metabolized by oxidation): Alprazolam, diazepam, temazepam, triazolam, and midazolam serum concentrations/toxicity may be increased.

Buspirone: Serum concentrations may be increased; monitor for sedation.

Busulfan: Serum concentrations may be increased; avoid concurrent use.

Calcium channel blockers: Serum concentrations may be increased (applies to those agents metabolized by CYP3A4, including felodipine, nifedipine, and verapamil).

Cisapride: Serum concentrations may be increased which may lead to malignant arrhythmias; concurrent use is contraindicated.

Docetaxel: Serum concentrations may be increased; avoid concurrent use.

Dofetilide: Serum levels/toxicity may be increased; avoid concurrent use.

Enzyme inducers: Rifampin decreases voriconazole's serum concentration to levels which are no longer effective; concurrent use is contraindicated. Other inducers (barbiturates, carbamazepine, rifabutin) may share this effect. Rifabutin serum levels are increased by voriconazole; concurrent use is contraindicated.

Ergot alkaloids: Serum levels may be increased by voriconazole, leading to ergot toxicity; concurrent use is contraindicated.

Erythromycin (and clarithromycin): Although voriconazole is a substrate for CYP3A4, no significant increase in serum levels was noted during concurrent erythromycin, likely reflecting a limited role in voriconazole metabolism.

H_2 antagonists: Changes in gastric acidity do not appear to significantly affect voriconazole absorption.

HMG-CoA reductase inhibitors (except pravastatin and fluvastatin): Serum concentrations may be increased. The risk of myopathy/rhabdomyolysis may be increased. Switch to pravastatin/fluvastatin or monitor for development of myopathy.

Immunosuppressants (cyclosporine, sirolimus, and tacrolimus): Serum concentrations may be increased; monitor serum concentrations and renal function. Concurrent use of sirolimus is contraindicated. Decrease cyclosporine dosage by 50% when initiating voriconazole, decreased tacrolimus dosage by 66% when initiating voriconazole.

Methylprednisolone: Serum concentrations may be increased; monitor.

NNRTIs: Effects on serum concentrations may be difficult to predict. Serum levels of voriconazole may be increased by efavirenz or delavirdine. Serum levels may be decreased by efavirenz or nevirapine. Monitor closely for efficacy/toxicity.

Phenytoin: Serum concentrations of voriconazole may be decreased; adjust dose of voriconazole; monitor phenytoin levels and adjust dose as needed.

Pimozide: Serum levels/toxicity may be increased; concurrent use is contraindicated.

Protease inhibitors: Indinavir did not appear to alter voriconazole serum concentrations during concurrent treatment. Other protease inhibitors may result in increased voriconazole concentrations.

Proton pump inhibitors: Changes in gastric acidity do not appear to significantly affect voriconazole absorption. However, voriconazole may significantly increase serum levels of omeprazole. For omeprazole dosages >40 mg/day, reduce omeprazole dosage by 50%. Serum levels of other proton pump inhibitors may also be increased.

Quinidine: Serum levels may be increased; concurrent use is contraindicated.

Sulfonylureas: Serum levels may be increased by voriconazole, potentially leading to hypoglycemia; monitor.

Trimetrexate: Serum concentrations may be increased; monitor.

Warfarin: Anticoagulant effects may be increased; monitor INR.

Vinca alkaloids: Serum concentrations may be increased; consider reduced dosage of vinca alkaloid.

Zolpidem: Serum levels may be increased; monitor.

Dietary/Ethanol/Herb Considerations

Food may decrease absorption; should be taken 1 hour before or 1 hour after a meal. Avoid grapefruit products; may increase voriconazole serum levels.

Herb/Nutraceutical: Avoid St John's wort; may decrease serum concentration.

Pharmacodynamics/Kinetics

Absorption: Well absorbed after oral administration

Distribution: V_d: 4.6 L/kg

Protein binding: 58%

Metabolism: Hepatic, via CYP2C19 (major pathway) and CYP2C9 and CYP3A4 (less significant); saturable (may demonstrate nonlinearity)

Bioavailability: 96%

Half-life elimination (dose dependent): Variable

Time to peak: 1-2 hours

Excretion: Urine (as inactive metabolites)

Pregnancy Risk Factor D

Breast-feeding Considerations Excretion in breast milk has not been investigated; avoid breast-feeding until additional data are available.

Dosage Forms INJ, powder for reconstitution: 200 mg. **TAB:** 50 mg, 200 mg

Generic Available No

VōSol® HC *see* Acetic Acid, Propylene Glycol Diacetate, and Hydrocortisone *on page 38*

VoSpire ER™ *see* Albuterol *on page 48*

VP-16 *see* Etoposide *on page 549*

VP-16-213 *see* Etoposide *on page 549*

Vumon *see* Teniposide *on page 1274*

V.V.S.® *see* Sulfabenzamide, Sulfacetamide, and Sulfathiazole *on page 1249*

Vytone® *see* Iodoquinol and Hydrocortisone *on page 736*

VZIG *see* Varicella-Zoster Immune Globulin (Human) *on page 1378*

Warfarin (WAR far in)

Related Information

Cardiovascular Diseases *on page 1456*

Dicumarol *on page 433*

U.S. Brand Names Coumadin®

Canadian Brand Names Apo®-Warfarin; Coumadin®; Gen-Warfarin; Taro-Warfarin

Mexican Brand Names Dimantil

(Continued)

Warfarin *(Continued)*

Pharmacologic Category Anticoagulant, Coumarin Derivative

Synonyms Warfarin Sodium

Use Prophylaxis and treatment of venous thrombosis, pulmonary embolism and thromboembolic disorders; atrial fibrillation with risk of embolism and as an adjunct in the prophylaxis of systemic embolism after MI

Unlabeled/Investigational Use Prevention of recurrent transient ischemic attacks and to reduce risk of recurrent myocardial infarction

Local Anesthetic/Vasoconstrictor Precautions No information available to require special precautions

Effects on Dental Treatment Signs of warfarin overdose may first appear as bleeding from gingival tissue; consultation with prescribing physician is advisable prior to surgery to determine temporary dose reduction or withdrawal of medication.

Dosage

Oral:

Infants and Children: 0.05-0.34 mg/kg/day; infants <12 months of age may require doses at or near the high end of this range; consistent anticoagulation may be difficult to maintain in children <5 years of age

Adults: Initial dosing must be individualized based upon patient's end organ function, concurrent therapy, and risk of bleeding; ACCP recommendation: 5 mg/day for 2-5 days, then adjust dose according to results of PT; usual maintenance dose ranges from 2-10 mg/day (selected sensitive patients may require less; resistant patients may require higher dosages).

Note: Lower starting doses may be required for patients with hepatic impairment, poor nutrition, CHF, elderly, or a high risk of bleeding. Higher initial doses may be reasonable in selected patients (ie, receiving enzyme-inducing agents and with low risk of bleeding).

I.V. (administer as a slow bolus injection): 2-5 mg/day

Dosing comment in hepatic disease: Monitor effect at usual doses; the response to oral anticoagulants may be markedly enhanced in obstructive jaundice (due to reduced vitamin K absorption) and also in hepatitis and cirrhosis (due to decreased production of vitamin K-dependent clotting factors); prothrombin index should be closely monitored

Mechanism of Action Interferes with hepatic synthesis of vitamin K-dependent coagulation factors (II, VII, IX, X)

Other Adverse Effects As with all anticoagulants, bleeding is the major adverse effect of warfarin. Hemorrhage may occur at virtually any site. Risk is dependent on multiple variables, including the intensity of anticoagulation and patient susceptibility.

Additional adverse effects are often related to idiosyncratic reactions, and the frequency cannot be accurately estimated.

Cardiovascular: Vasculitis, edema, hemorrhagic shock

Central nervous system: Fever, lethargy, malaise, asthenia, pain, headache, dizziness, stroke

Dermatologic: Rash, dermatitis, bullous eruptions, urticaria, pruritus, alopecia

Gastrointestinal: Anorexia, nausea, vomiting, stomach cramps, abdominal pain, diarrhea, flatulence, gastrointestinal bleeding, abnormal taste, oral ulceration

Genitourinary: Priapism, hematuria

Hematologic: Hemorrhage, leukopenia, unrecognized bleeding sites (eg, colon cancer) may be uncovered by anticoagulation, retroperitoneal hematoma, agranulocytosis

Hepatic: Increased transaminases, hepatic injury, jaundice,

Neuromuscular & skeletal: Paresthesia, osteoporosis

Respiratory: Hemoptysis, epistaxis, pulmonary hemorrhage, tracheobronchial calcification

Miscellaneous: Hypersensitivity/allergic reactions

Skin necrosis/gangrene, due to paradoxical local thrombosis, is a known but rare risk of warfarin therapy. Its onset is usually within the first few days of therapy and is frequently localized to the limbs, breast or penis. The risk of this effect is increased in patients with protein C or S deficiency.

"Purple toes syndrome," caused by cholesterol microembolization, also occurs rarely. Typically, this occurs after several weeks of therapy, and may present as a dark, purplish, mottled discoloration of the plantar and lateral surfaces. Other manifestations of cholesterol microembolization may include rash, livedo reticularis, rash, gangrene, abrupt and intense pain in lower extremities, abdominal, flank, or back pain, hematuria, renal insufficiency, hypertension, cerebral ischemia, spinal cord infarction, or other symptom of vascular compromise.

Warnings/Precautions Use care in the selection of patients appropriate for this treatment. Ensure patient cooperation especially from the alcoholic, illicit drug user, demented, or psychotic patient. Use with caution in trauma, acute infection (antibiotics and fever may alter affects), renal insufficiency, prolonged dietary insufficiencies (vitamin K deficiency), moderate-severe hypertension, polycythemia vera, vasculitis, open wound, active TB, history of PUD, anaphylactic disorders, indwelling catheters, severe diabetes, thyroid disease, severe renal disease, and menstruating and postpartum women. Use with caution in protein C deficiency.

Hemorrhage is the most serious risk of therapy. Patient must be instructed to report bleeding, accidents, or falls. Patient must also report any new or discontinued medications, herbal or alternative products used, significant changes in smoking or dietary habits. Necrosis or gangrene of the skin and other tissues can occur (rarely) due to early hypercoagulability. "Purple toes syndrome," due to cholesterol microembolization, may rarely occur (often after several weeks of therapy). Women may be at risk of developing ovarian hemorrhage at the time of ovulation. The elderly may be more sensitive to anticoagulant therapy.

Drug Interactions Substrate of CYP1A2, **2C8/9**, 2C19, 3A4; Inhibits CYP2C8/9, 2C19

Enhanced Anticoagulant Effects

Decrease Vitamin K	Displace Anticoagulant	Inhibit Metabolism	Other
Oral antibiotics: Can ↑/↓ INR Check INR 3 days after a patient begins antibiotics to see the INR value and adjust the warfarin dose accordingly	Chloral hydrate	Allopurinol	Acetaminophen
	Clofibrate	Amiodarone	Anabolic steroids
	Diazoxide	Azole antifungals	Clarithromycin
	Ethacrynic acid	Capecitabine	Clofibrate
	Miconazole (including intravaginal use)	Chloramphenicol	Danazol
		Chlorpropamide	Erythromycin
		Cimetidine	Gemfibrozil
	Nalidixic acid	Ciprofloxacin	Glucagon
	Phenylbutazone	Co-trimoxazole	Influenza vaccine
	Salicylates	Disulfiram	Propranolol
	Sulfonamides	Ethanol (acute ingestion)[1]	Propylthiouracil
	Sulfonylureas	Flutamide	Ranitidine
		Isoniazid	SSRIs
		Metronidazole	Sulindac
		Norfloxacin	Tetracycline
		Ofloxacin	Thyroid drugs
		Omperazole	Vitamin E (≥400 int. units)
		Phenylbutazone	
		Phenytoin	
		Propafenone	
		Propoxyphene	
		Protease inhibitors	
		Quinidine	
		"Statins"[2]	
		Sulfinpyrazone	
		Sulfonamides	
		Tamoxifen	
		Tolbutamide	
		Zafirlukast	
		Zileuton	

[1]The hypoprothrombinemic effect of oral anticoagulants has been reported to be both increased and decreased during chronic and excessive alcohol ingestion. Data are insufficient to predict the direction of this interaction in alcoholic patients.

[2]Particularly lovastatin and fluvastatin; others (atorvastatin, pravastatin) rarely associated with increased PT.

Decreased Anticoagulant Effects

Induction of Enzymes		Increased Procoagulant Factors	Decreased Drug Absorption	Other
Barbiturates	Nafcillin	Estrogens	Aluminum hydroxide	Ethchlorvynol
Carbamazepine	Phenytoin	Oral contraceptives	Cholestyramine*	Griseofulvin
Glutethimide	Rifampin	Vitamin K (including nutritional supplements)	Colestipol*	Spironolactone†
Griseofulvin				Sucralfate

Decreased anticoagulant effect may occur when these drugs are administered with oral anticoagulants.

*Cholestyramine and colestipol may increase the anticoagulant effect by binding vitamin K in the gut; yet, the decreased drug absorption appears to be of more concern.

†Diuretic-induced hemoconcentration with subsequent concentration of clotting factors has been reported to decrease the effects of oral anticoagulants.

Increased Bleeding Tendency

Inhibit Platelet Aggregation	Inhibit Procoagulant Factors	Ulcerogenic Drugs
Cephalosporins Dipyridamole Indomethacin Oxyphenbutazone Penicillin, parenteral Phenylbutazone Salicylates Sulfinpyrazone	Antimetabolites Quinidine Quinine Salicylates	Adrenal corticosteroids Indomethacin Oxyphenbutazone Phenylbutazone Potassium products Salicylates

Use of these agents with oral anticoagulants may increase the chances of hemorrhage.

Dietary/Ethanol/Herb Considerations

Ethanol: Avoid use; hypoprothrombinemic effect of oral anticoagulants reported to be both increased and decreased during chronic and excessive alcohol ingestion. Data insufficient to predict direction of interaction in alcoholics.

Food: Anticoagulant effects may be decreased if taken with foods rich in vitamin K (eg, beef liver, pork liver, green tea and leafy green vegetables) Do not alter diet during therapy; a balanced diet with a consistent intake of 70-140 mcg/day of vitamin K is essential. Avoid large amounts of alfalfa, asparagus, broccoli, Brussels sprouts, cabbage, cauliflower, green teas, kale, lettuce, spinach, turnip greens, and watercress. Vitamin E may increase effect. Many enteral products contain large amounts o vitamin K. Avoid garlic, ginger, and green tea.

Herb/Nutraceutical: Avoid alfalfa; contains large amounts of vitamin. Avoid cat's claw, dong quai, evening primrose, feverfew, garlic, ginkgo biloba, ginger, ginseng, green tea, horse chestnut, and red clover due to additional antiplatelet activity. Avoid coenzyme Q_{10}; may decrease response to warfarin. Avoid St John's wort; may decrease serum concentration.

Pharmacodynamics/Kinetics

Onset of action: Anticoagulation: Oral: 36-72 hours

Peak effect: Full therapeutic effect: 5-7 days; INR may increase in 36-72 hours

Duration: 2-5 days

Absorption: Oral: Rapid

Metabolism: Hepatic

Half-life elimination: 20-60 hours; Mean: 40 hours; highly variable among individuals

Pregnancy Risk Factor D

Generic Available Yes: Tablet

Warfarin Sodium *see* Warfarin *on page 1397*
Wart-Off® Maximum Strength [OTC] *see* Salicylic Acid *on page 1204*
4-Way® Long Acting [OTC] *see* Oxymetazoline *on page 1022*
WelChol™ *see* Colesevelam *on page 365*
Wellbutrin® *see* BuPROPion *on page 209*
Wellbutrin SR® *see* BuPROPion *on page 209*
Wesmycin® *see* Tetracycline *on page 1286*
Westcort® *see* Hydrocortisone *on page 688*
Westhroid® *see* Thyroid *on page 1303*
Whole Root Rauwolfia *see* Rauwolfia Serpentina *on page 1170*
Wigraine® *see* Ergotamine *on page 510*
WinRho SDF® *see* Rh_o(D) Immune Globulin *on page 1175*
Winstrol® *see* Stanozolol *on page 1241*
Wound Wash Saline™ [OTC] *see* Sodium Chloride *on page 1229*
WR-139013 *see* Chlorambucil *on page 296*
Wytensin® [DSC] *see* Guanabenz *on page 654*
Xalatan® *see* Latanoprost *on page 778*
Xanax® *see* Alprazolam *on page 61*
Xanax XR® *see* Alprazolam *on page 61*
Xeloda® *see* Capecitabine *on page 235*
Xenical® *see* Orlistat *on page 1004*
Xigris® *see* Drotrecogin Alfa *on page 483*
Xopenex® *see* Levalbuterol *on page 786*
X-Prep® [OTC] *see* Senna *on page 1215*

X-Seb™ T [OTC] *see* Coal Tar and Salicylic Acid *on page 359*

Xylocaine® *see* Lidocaine *on page 801*

Xylocaine® MPF *see* Lidocaine *on page 801*

Xylocaine® MPF With Epinephrine *see* Lidocaine and Epinephrine *on page 804*

Xylocaine® Viscous *see* Lidocaine *on page 801*

Xylocaine® With Epinephrine *see* Lidocaine and Epinephrine *on page 804*

Xylometazoline (zye loe met AZ oh leen)

U.S. Brand Names Otrivin® [OTC] [DSC]; Otrivin® Pediatric [OTC] [DSC]

Canadian Brand Names Decongest

Pharmacologic Category Vasoconstrictor, Nasal

Synonyms Otrivin® [OTC] [DSC]; Otrivin® Pediatric [OTC] [DSC]; Xylometazoline Hydrochloride

Use Symptomatic relief of nasal and nasopharyngeal mucosal congestion

Local Anesthetic/Vasoconstrictor Precautions No information available to require special precautions

Effects on Dental Treatment No significant effects or complications reported

Dosage

Children 2-12 years: Instill 2-3 drops (0.05%) in each nostril every 8-10 hours

Children >12 years and Adults: Instill 2-3 drops or sprays (0.1%) in each nostril every 8-10 hours

Mechanism of Action Stimulates alpha-adrenergic receptors in the arterioles of the conjunctiva and the nasal mucosa to produce vasoconstriction

Other Adverse Effects Frequency not defined:

Cardiovascular: Palpitations

Central nervous system: Drowsiness, dizziness, seizures, headache

Ocular: Blurred vision, ocular irritation, photophobia

Miscellaneous: Diaphoresis

Pharmacodynamics/Kinetics

Onset of action: Intranasal: Local vasoconstriction: 5-10 minutes

Duration: 5-6 hours

Pregnancy Risk Factor C

Generic Available No

Xylometazoline Hydrochloride *see* Xylometazoline *on page 1401*

Xyrem® *see* Sodium Oxybate *on page 1231*

Y-90 Zevalin *see* Ibritumomab *on page 702*

Yasmin® *see* Combination Hormonal Contraceptives *on page 368*

Yellow Mercuric Oxide *see* Mercuric Oxide *on page 867*

Yocon® *see* Yohimbine *on page 1401*

Yodoxin® *see* Iodoquinol *on page 735*

Yohimbine (yo HIM byne)

Related Information

Yohimbe *on page 1451*

U.S. Brand Names Aphrodyne®; Yocon®

Canadian Brand Names PMS-Yohimbine; Yocon®

Pharmacologic Category Impotency Agent

Synonyms Yohimbine Hydrochloride

Use No FDA sanctioned indications

Unlabeled/Investigational Use Treatment of SSRI-induced sexual dysfunction, impotence; weight loss; sympathicolytic and mydriatic; aphrodisiac

Local Anesthetic/Vasoconstrictor Precautions No information available to require special precautions

Effects on Dental Treatment No significant effects or complications reported

Dosage Adults: Oral:

Male erectile impotence: 5.4 mg tablet 3 times/day have been used. If side effects occur, reduce to $\frac{1}{2}$ tablet (2.7 mg) 3 times/day followed by gradual increases to 1 tablet 3 times/day. Results of therapy >10 weeks are not known.

Orthostatic hypotension: Doses of 12.5 mg/day have been utilized; however, more research is necessary

Mechanism of Action Derived from the bark of the yohimbe tree (*Corynanthe yohimbe*), this indole alkaloid produces a presynaptic alpha$_2$-adrenergic blockade. Peripheral autonomic effect is to increase cholinergic and decrease adrenergic activity; yohimbine exerts a stimulating effect on the mood and a mild antidiuretic effect.

Other Adverse Effects Frequency not defined:

Cardiovascular: Tachycardia, hypertension, hypotension (orthostatic), flushing

Central nervous system: Anxiety, mania, hallucinations, irritability, dizziness, psychosis, insomnia, headache, panic attacks

Gastrointestinal: Nausea, vomiting, anorexia, salivation

Neuromuscular & skeletal: Tremors

Miscellaneous: Antidiuretic action, diaphoresis

(Continued)

Yohimbine *(Continued)*

Drug Interactions Substrate of CYP2D6; Inhibits CYP2D6

Increased Effect/Toxicity: Caution with other CNS acting drugs. When used in combination with CYP3A4 inhibitors, serum level and/or toxicity of yohimbine may be increased; inhibitors include amiodarone, cimetidine, clarithromycin, erythromycin, delavirdine, diltiazem, dirithromycin, disulfiram, fluoxetine, fluvoxamine, grapefruit juice, indinavir, itraconazole, ketoconazole, metronidazole, nefazodone, nevirapine, propoxyphene, quinupristin-dalfopristin, ritonavir, saquinavir, verapamil, zafirlukast, zileuton; monitor for altered response. MAO inhibitors or drugs with MAO inhibition (linezolid, furazolidone) theoretically may increase toxicity or adverse effects

Dietary/Ethanol/Herb Considerations Food: Avoid grapefruit products may; increase serum concentration/toxicity.

Pharmacodynamics/Kinetics

Duration of action: Usually 3-4 hours, but may last 36 hours

Absorption: 33%

Distribution: V_d: 0.3-3 L/kg

Half-life elimination: 0.6 hour

Generic Available Yes

Comments Also a street drug of abuse that can be smoked; has a bitter taste. Dissociative state may resemble phencyclidine intoxication.

Yohimbine Hydrochloride *see* Yohimbine *on page 1401*

Zaditor™ *see* Ketotifen *on page 768*

Zafirlukast (za FIR loo kast)

Related Information

Respiratory Diseases *on page 1476*

U.S. Brand Names Accolate®

Canadian Brand Names Accolate®

Mexican Brand Names Accolate®

Pharmacologic Category Leukotriene Receptor Antagonist

Synonyms ICI 204, 219

Use Prophylaxis and chronic treatment of asthma in adults and children ≥5 years of age

Local Anesthetic/Vasoconstrictor Precautions No information available to require special precautions

Effects on Dental Treatment No significant effects or complications reported

Dosage Oral:

Children <5 years: Safety and effectiveness have not been established

Children 5-11 years: 10 mg twice daily

Children ≥12 years and Adults: 20 mg twice daily

Elderly: The mean dose (mg/kg) normalized AUC and C_{max} increase and plasma clearance decreases with increasing age. In patients >65 years of age, there is a two- to threefold greater C_{max} and AUC compared to younger adults.

Dosing adjustment in hepatic impairment: 50% to 60% greater C_{max} and AUC compared to normal subjects

Mechanism of Action Zafirlukast is a selectively and competitive leukotriene-receptor antagonist (LTRA) of leukotriene D4 and E4 (LTD4 and LTE4), components of slow-reacting substance of anaphylaxis (SRSA). Cysteinyl leukotriene production and receptor occupation have been correlated with the pathophysiology of asthma, including airway edema, smooth muscle constriction and altered cellular activity associated with the inflammatory process, which contribute to the signs and symptoms of asthma.

Other Adverse Effects

>10%: Central nervous system: Headache (12.9%)

1% to 10%:

- Central nervous system: Dizziness, pain, fever
- Gastrointestinal: Nausea, diarrhea, abdominal pain, vomiting, dyspepsia
- Hepatic: SGPT elevation
- Neuromuscular & skeletal: Back pain, myalgia, weakness

<1%: Postmarketing and/or case reports: Symptomatic hepatitis, hepatic failure, hyperbilirubinemia, systemic eosinophilia with clinical features of Churg-Strauss syndrome (rare), hypersensitivity reactions (urticaria, angioedema, rash), agranulocytosis, bleeding, bruising, edema, arthralgia

Drug Interactions Substrate of **CYP2C8/9**; Inhibits CYP1A2, 2C8/9, 2C19, 2D6, 3A4

Increased Effect/Toxicity: Zafirlukast concentrations are increased by aspirin. Warfarin effect may be increased with zafirlukast. Zafirlukast may increase theophylline levels.

Decreased Effect: Zafirlukast concentrations may be reduced by erythromycin.

Dietary/Ethanol/Herb Considerations Food decreases bioavailability by 40%.

Pharmacodynamics/Kinetics

Protein binding: >99%, primarily to albumin

Metabolism: Extensively hepatic via CYP2C9
Bioavailability: Reduced 40% with food
Half-life elimination: 10 hours
Time to peak, serum: 3 hours
Excretion: Urine (10%); feces

Pregnancy Risk Factor B

Generic Available No

Zagam® *see* Sparfloxacin *on page 1238*

Zalcitabine (zal SITE a been)

Related Information
HIV Infection and AIDS *on page 1482*

U.S. Brand Names Hivid®

Canadian Brand Names Hivid®

Mexican Brand Names Hivid®

Pharmacologic Category Antiretroviral Agent, Reverse Transcriptase Inhibitor (Nucleoside)

Synonyms ddC; Dideoxycytidine

Use In combination with at least two other antiretrovirals in the treatment of patients with HIV infection; it is not recommended that zalcitabine be given in combination with didanosine, stavudine, or lamivudine due to overlapping toxicities, virologic interactions, or lack of clinical data

Local Anesthetic/Vasoconstrictor Precautions No information available to require special precautions

Effects on Dental Treatment >10%: Oral ulcerations

Dosage Oral:
Neonates: Dose unknown
Infants and Children <13 years: Safety and efficacy have not been established; suggested usual dose: 0.01 mg/kg every 8 hours; range: 0.005-0.01 mg/kg every 8 hours
Adolescents and Adults: 0.75 mg 3 times/day
Dosing adjustment in renal impairment: Adults:
Cl_{cr} 10-40 mL/minute: 0.75 mg every 12 hours
Cl_{cr} <10 mL/minute: 0.75 mg every 24 hours
Moderately dialyzable (20% to 50%)

Mechanism of Action Purine nucleoside analogue, zalcitabine or 2′,3′-dideoxycytidine (ddC) is converted to active metabolite ddCTP; lack the presence of the 3′-hydroxyl group necessary for phosphodiester linkages during DNA replication. As a result viral replication is prematurely terminated. ddCTP acts as a competitor for binding sites on the HIV-RNA dependent DNA polymerase (reverse transcriptase) to further contribute to inhibition of viral replication.

Other Adverse Effects
>10%:
Central nervous system: Fever (5% to 17%), malaise (2% to 13%)
Neuromuscular & skeletal: Peripheral neuropathy (28%)

1% to 10%:
Central nervous system: Headache (2%), dizziness (1%), fatigue (4%), seizures (1.3%)
Dermatologic: Rash (2% to 11%), pruritus (3% to 5%)
Endocrine & metabolic: Hypoglycemia (2% to 6%), hyponatremia (4%), hyperglycemia (1% to 6%)
Gastrointestinal: Nausea (3%), dysphagia (1% to 4%), anorexia (4%), abdominal pain (3% to 8%), vomiting (1% to 3%), diarrhea (<1% to 10%), weight loss, increased amylase (3% to 8%)
Hematologic: Anemia (occurs as early as 2-4 weeks), granulocytopenia (usually after 6-8 weeks)
Hepatic: Abnormal hepatic function (9%), hyperbilirubinemia (2% to 5%)
Neuromuscular & skeletal: Myalgia (1% to 6%), foot pain
Respiratory: Pharyngitis (2%), cough (6%), nasal discharge (4%)

<1% (Limited to important or life-threatening): Atrial fibrillation, chest pain, constipation, edema, epistaxis, heart racing, hepatic failure, hepatitis, hepatomegaly, hypersensitivity (including anaphylaxis), hypertension, hypocalcemia, jaundice, lactic acidosis, myositis, night sweats, pain, palpitations, pancreatitis, redistribution/accumulation of body fat, syncope, tachycardia, weakness

Drug Interactions
Increased Effect/Toxicity: Amphotericin, foscarnet, and aminoglycosides may potentiate the risk of developing peripheral neuropathy or other toxicities associated with zalcitabine by interfering with the renal elimination of zalcitabine. Other drugs associated with peripheral neuropathy include chloramphenicol, cisplatin, dapsone, disulfiram, ethionamide, glutethimide, gold, hydralazine, iodoquinol, isoniazid, metronidazole, nitrofurantoin, phenytoin, ribavirin, and vincristine. Concomitant use with zalcitabine may increase risk of peripheral neuropathy.
(Continued)

Zalcitabine *(Continued)*

Concomitant use of zalcitabine with didanosine is not recommended. Concomitant use of ribavirin and nucleoside analogues may increase the risk of developing lactic acidosis (includes adefovir, didanosine, lamivudine, stavudine, zalcitabine, zidovudine).

Decreased Effect: It is not recommended that zalcitabine be given in combination with didanosine, stavudine, or lamivudine due to overlapping toxicities, virologic interactions, or lack of clinical data. Doxorubicin and lamivudine have been shown *in vitro* to decrease zalcitabine phosphorylation. Magnesium/aluminum-containing antacids and metoclopramide may decrease the absorption of zalcitabine.

Dietary/Ethanol/Herb Considerations Food decreases peak plasma concentration by 39%; may decrease extent and rate of absorption.

Pharmacodynamics/Kinetics

Absorption: Well, but variable; decreased 39% with food

Distribution: Minimal data available; variable CSF penetration

Protein binding: <4%

Metabolism: Intracellularly to active triphosphorylated agent

Bioavailability: >80%

Half-life elimination: 2.9 hours; Renal impairment: ≤8.5 hours

Excretion: Urine (>70% as unchanged drug)

Pregnancy Risk Factor C

Generic Available No

Zaleplon (ZAL e plon)

U.S. Brand Names Sonata®

Canadian Brand Names Sonata®; Starnoc®

Pharmacologic Category Hypnotic, Nonbenzodiazepine

Use Short-term (7-10 days) treatment of insomnia (has been demonstrated to be effective for up to 5 weeks in controlled trial)

Local Anesthetic/Vasoconstrictor Precautions No information available to require special precautions

Effects on Dental Treatment No significant effects or complications reported

Restrictions C-IV

Dosage Oral:

Adults: 10 mg at bedtime (range: 5-20 mg); has been used for up to 5 weeks of treatment in controlled trial setting

Elderly: 5 mg at bedtime

Dosing adjustment in renal impairment: None for mild to moderate; use in severe renal impairment not adequately studied

Dosing adjustment in hepatic impairment: Mild to moderate impairment: 5 mg; use not recommended in severe impairment

Mechanism of Action Zaleplon is unrelated to benzodiazepines, barbiturates, or other hypnotics. However, it interacts with the benzodiazepine GABA receptor complex. Nonclinical studies have shown that it binds selectively to the brain omega-1 receptor situated on the alpha subunit of the GABA-A receptor complex.

Other Adverse Effects

1% to 10%:

- Cardiovascular: Peripheral edema, chest pain
- Central nervous system: Amnesia, anxiety, depersonalization, dizziness, hallucinations, hypesthesia, somnolence, vertigo, malaise, depression, lightheadedness, impaired coordination, fever, migraine
- Dermatologic: Photosensitivity reaction, rash, pruritus
- Gastrointestinal: Abdominal pain, anorexia, colitis, dyspepsia, nausea, constipation, xerostomia
- Genitourinary: Dysmenorrhea
- Neuromuscular & skeletal: Paresthesia, tremor, myalgia, weakness, back pain, arthralgia
- Ocular: Abnormal vision, eye pain
- Otic: Hyperacusis
- Miscellaneous: Parosmia

1% (Limited to important or life-threatening): Alopecia, angina, ataxia, bundle branch block, dysarthria, dystonia, eosinophilia, facial paralysis, glaucoma, intestinal obstruction, paresthesia, pericardial effusion, ptosis, pulmonary embolus, syncope, urinary retention, ventricular tachycardia

Drug Interactions Substrate of CYP3A4

Increased Effect/Toxicity: Zaleplon potentiates the CNS effects of CNS depressants, including alcohol, imipramine, and thioridazine. Cimetidine increases concentrations of zaleplon. Avoid concurrent use or use 5 mg zaleplon as starting dose in patient receiving cimetidine.

Decreased Effect: CYP3A4 inducers (eg, phenytoin, carbamazepine, phenobarbital) could lead to ineffectiveness of zaleplon.

Dietary/Ethanol/Herb Considerations

Ethanol: Avoid use; may increase CNS depression

Food: High fat meal prolongs absorption, delays t_{max} by 2 hours, and reduces C_{max} by 35%.

Herb/Nutraceutical: Avoid gotu kola, kava, SAMe, and valerian; may increase CNS depression. Avoid St John's wort; may decrease serum concentration and increase CNS depression.

Pharmacodynamics/Kinetics

Onset of action: Rapid

Peak effect: ~1 hour

Duration: 6-8 hours

Absorption: Rapid and almost complete

Distribution: V_d: 1.4 L/kg

Protein binding: 60% ± 15%

Metabolism: Extensive, primarily via aldehyde oxidase to form 5-oxo-zaleplon and to a lesser extent by CYP3A4 to desethylzaleplon; all metabolites are pharmacologically inactive

Bioavailability: 30%

Half-life elimination: 1 hour

Time to peak, serum: 1 hour

Excretion: Urine (primarily metabolites, <1% as unchanged drug)

Clearance: Plasma: Oral: 3 L/hour/kg

Pregnancy Risk Factor C

Generic Available No

Zanaflex® *see* Tizanidine *on page 1314*

Zanamivir (za NA mi veer)

Related Information

Systemic Viral Diseases *on page 1517*

U.S. Brand Names Relenza®

Canadian Brand Names Relenza®

Pharmacologic Category Antiviral Agent; Neuraminidase Inhibitor

Use Treatment of uncomplicated acute illness due to influenza virus in adults and children ≥7 years of age. Treatment should only be initiated in patients who have been symptomatic for no more than 2 days.

Unlabeled/Investigational Use Investigational: Prophylaxis against influenza A/B infections

Local Anesthetic/Vasoconstrictor Precautions No information available to require special precautions

Effects on Dental Treatment No significant effects or complications reported

Dosage Children ≥7 years and Adults: 2 inhalations (10 mg total) twice daily for 5 days. Two doses should be taken on the first day of dosing, regardless of interval, while doses should be spaced by approximately 12 hours on subsequent days.

Prophylaxis (investigational use): 2 inhalations (10 mg) once daily for duration of exposure period (6 weeks has been used in clinical trial)

Mechanism of Action Zanamivir inhibits influenza virus neuraminidase enzymes, potentially altering virus particle aggregation and release.

Other Adverse Effects Most adverse reactions occurred at a frequency which was equal to the control (lactose vehicle).

>1.5%:

Central nervous system: Headache (2%), dizziness (2%)

Gastrointestinal: Nausea (3%), diarrhea (3% adults, 2% children), vomiting (1% adults, 2% children)

Respiratory: Sinusitis (3%), bronchitis (2%), cough (2%), other nasal signs and symptoms (2%), infection (ear, nose, and throat; 2% adults, 5% children)

<1.5%: Malaise, fatigue, fever, abdominal pain, myalgia, arthralgia, and urticaria

In addition, the following adverse reactions have been reported during postmarketing use: Allergic or allergic-like reaction (including oropharyngeal edema), arrhythmias, syncope, seizures, bronchospasm, dyspnea, facial edema, rash (including serious cutaneous reactions)

Pharmacodynamics/Kinetics

Absorption: Inhalation: 4% to 17%

Protein binding, plasma: <10%

Metabolism: None

Half-life elimination, serum: 2.5-5.1 hours

Excretion: Urine (as unchanged drug)

Pregnancy Risk Factor C

Generic Available No

Zanosar® *see* Streptozocin *on page 1246*

Zantac® *see* Ranitidine *on page 1168*

Zantac® 75 [OTC] *see* Ranitidine *on page 1168*

Zapzyt® [OTC] *see* Benzoyl Peroxide *on page 171*

Zapzyt® Acne Wash [OTC] *see* Salicylic Acid *on page 1204*

Zapzyt® Pore Treatment [OTC] *see* Salicylic Acid *on page 1204*

Zarontin® *see* Ethosuximide *on page 543*

Zaroxolyn® *see* Metolazone *on page 900*
ZDV *see* Zidovudine *on page 1406*
ZDV, Abacavir, and Lamivudine *see* Abacavir, Lamivudine, and Zidovudine *on page 23*
Zeasorb®-AF [OTC] *see* Miconazole *on page 906*
Zebeta® *see* Bisoprolol *on page 188*
Zelnorm™ *see* Tegaserod *on page 1268*
Zemplar™ *see* Paricalcitol *on page 1034*
Zenapax® *see* Daclizumab *on page 392*
Zephiran® [OTC] *see* Benzalkonium Chloride *on page 169*
Zephrex® *see* Guaifenesin and Pseudoephedrine *on page 652*
Zephrex LA® *see* Guaifenesin and Pseudoephedrine *on page 652*
Zerit® *see* Stavudine *on page 1242*
Zestoretic® *see* Lisinopril and Hydrochlorothiazide *on page 814*
Zestril® *see* Lisinopril *on page 813*
Zetar® [OTC] *see* Coal Tar *on page 359*
Zetia™ *see* Ezetimibe *on page 553*
Zevalin™ *see* Ibritumomab *on page 702*
Ziac® *see* Bisoprolol and Hydrochlorothiazide *on page 189*
Ziagen® *see* Abacavir *on page 22*

Zidovudine (zye DOE vyoo deen)

Related Information

HIV Infection and AIDS *on page 1482*
Systemic Viral Diseases *on page 1517*
Zidovudine and Lamivudine *on page 1407*

U.S. Brand Names Retrovir®

Canadian Brand Names Apo®-Zidovudine; AZT™; Novo-AZT; Retrovir®

Mexican Brand Names Combivir®; Dipedyne; Isadol®; Kenamil; Retrovir AZT®

Pharmacologic Category Antiretroviral Agent, Reverse Transcriptase Inhibitor (Nucleoside)

Synonyms Azidothymidine; AZT; Compound S; ZDV

Use Management of patients with HIV infections in combination with at least two other antiretroviral agents; for prevention of maternal/fetal HIV transmission as monotherapy

Unlabeled/Investigational Use Postexposure prophylaxis for HIV exposure as part of a multidrug regimen

Local Anesthetic/Vasoconstrictor Precautions No information available to require special precautions

Effects on Dental Treatment No significant effects or complications reported

Dosage Patients should receive I.V. therapy only until oral therapy can be administered.

Prevention of maternal-fetal HIV transmission:
- Neonatal: Oral: 2 mg/kg/dose every 6 hours for 6 weeks beginning 6-12 hours after birth; infants unable to receive oral dosing may receive 1.5 mg/kg I.V. infused over 30 minutes every 6 hours
- Maternal (may delay treatment until after 10-12 weeks gestation): Oral (per HIV/ATIS 2001 guidelines): 200 mg 3 times/day or 300 mg twice daily until start of labor
  - During labor and delivery, administer zidovudine I.V. at 2 mg/kg over 1 hour followed by a continuous I.V. infusion of 1 mg/kg/hour until the umbilical cord is clamped

Children 3 months to 12 years for HIV infection:
- Oral: 160 mg/m²/dose every 8 hours; dosage range: 90 mg/m²/dose to 180 mg/m²/dose every 6-8 hours; some Working Group members use a dose of 180 mg/m² every 12 hours when using in drug combinations with other antiretroviral compounds, but data on this dosing in children is limited
- I.V. continuous infusion: 20 mg/m²/hour
- I.V. intermittent infusion: 120 mg/m²/dose every 6 hours

Adults:
- Oral: 300 mg twice daily or 200 mg 3 times/day
- I.V.: 1-2 mg/kg/dose (infused over 1 hour) administered every 4 hours around-the-clock (6 doses/day)
- Prevention of HIV following needlesticks: 200 mg 3 times/day plus lamivudine 150 mg twice daily; a protease inhibitor (eg, indinavir) may be added for high risk exposures; begin therapy within 2 hours of exposure if possible

Dosing adjustment in renal impairment: Cl_{cr} <10 mL/minute: May require minor adjustment

Hemodialysis: At least partially removed by hemo- and peritoneal dialysis; administer dose after hemodialysis or administer 100 mg supplemental dose; during CAPD, dose as for Cl_{cr} <10 mL/minute

Continuous arteriovenous or venovenous hemodiafiltration effects: Administer 100 mg every 8 hours

Dosing adjustment in hepatic impairment: Reduce dose by 50% or double dosing interval in patients with cirrhosis

Mechanism of Action Zidovudine is a thymidine analog which interferes with the HIV viral RNA dependent DNA polymerase resulting in inhibition of viral replication; nucleoside reverse transcriptase inhibitor

Other Adverse Effects

>10%:

Central nervous system: Severe headache (42%), fever (16%)

Dermatologic: Rash (17%)

Gastrointestinal: Nausea (46% to 61%), anorexia (11%), diarrhea (17%), pain (20%), vomiting (6% to 25%)

Hematologic: Anemia (23% in children), leukopenia, granulocytopenia (39% in children)

Neuromuscular & skeletal: Weakness (19%)

1% to 10%:

Central nervous system: Malaise (8%), dizziness (6%), insomnia (5%), somnolence (8%)

Dermatologic: Hyperpigmentation of nails (bluish-brown)

Gastrointestinal: Dyspepsia (5%)

Hematologic: Changes in platelet count

Neuromuscular & skeletal: Paresthesia (6%)

<1%, postmarketing and/or case reports: Amblyopia, anxiety, aplastic anemia, back pain, cardiomyopathy, chest pain, confusion, constipation, cough, CPK increased, depression, diaphoresis, dizziness, dysphagia, dyspnea, flatulence, flu-like syndrome, generalized pain, gynecomastia, hearing loss, hemolytic anemia, hepatitis, hepatomegaly with steatosis, jaundice, lactic acidosis, LDH increased, leukopenia, loss of mental acuity, lymphadenopathy, macular edema, mania, mouth ulcer, muscle spasm, myopathy and myositis with pathological changes (similar to that produced by HIV disease), oral mucosal pigmentation, pancreatitis, pancytopenia with marrow hypoplasia, paresthesia, photophobia, pruritus, pure red cell aplasia, rash, rhabdomyolysis, rhinitis, seizures, sensitization reactions (including anaphylaxis and angioedema), sinusitis, skin and nail pigmentation changes, somnolence, Stevens-Johnson syndrome, syncope, taste perversion, toxic epidermal necrolysis, tremor, urinary frequency, urinary hesitancy, urticaria, vasculitis, vertigo

Drug Interactions Substrate of CYP2A6, 2C8/9, 2C19, 3A4

Increased Effect/Toxicity: Coadministration of zidovudine with drugs that are nephrotoxic (amphotericin B), cytotoxic (flucytosine, vincristine, vinblastine, doxorubicin, interferon), inhibit glucuronidation or excretion (acetaminophen, cimetidine, indomethacin, lorazepam, probenecid, aspirin), or interfere with RBC/WBC number or function (acyclovir, ganciclovir, pentamidine, dapsone). Clarithromycin may increase blood levels of zidovudine (although total body exposure was unaffected, peak plasma concentrations were increased). Valproic acid significantly increases zidovudine's blood levels (believed due to inhibition first pass metabolism). Concomitant use of ribavirin and nucleoside analogues may increase the risk of developing lactic acidosis (includes adefovir, didanosine, lamivudine, stavudine, zalcitabine, zidovudine).

Decreased Effect: *In vitro* evidence suggests zidovudine's antiretroviral activity may be antagonized by doxorubicin, ribavirin, and/or stavudine; avoid concurrent use.

Dietary/Ethanol/Herb Considerations Food may decrease serum concentration; administration with a fatty meal decreases AUC and peak plasma concentration.

Pharmacodynamics/Kinetics

Absorption: Oral: 66% to 70%

Distribution: Significant penetration into the CSF; crosses placenta

Relative diffusion from blood into CSF: Adequate with or without inflammation (exceeds usual MICs)

CSF:blood level ratio: Normal meninges: ~60%

Protein binding: 25% to 38%

Metabolism: Hepatic via glucuronidation to inactive metabolites; extensive first-pass effect

Half-life elimination: Terminal: 60 minutes

Time to peak, serum: 30-90 minutes

Excretion:

Oral: Urine (72% to 74% as metabolites, 14% to 18% as unchanged drug)

I.V.: Urine (45% to 60% as metabolites, 18% to 29% as unchanged drug)

Pregnancy Risk Factor C

Generic Available No

Zidovudine, Abacavir, and Lamivudine *see* Abacavir, Lamivudine, and Zidovudine *on page 23*

Zidovudine and Lamivudine (zye DOE vyoo deen & la MI vyoo deen)

Related Information

HIV Infection and AIDS *on page 1482*

(Continued)

Zidovudine and Lamivudine *(Continued)*

Lamivudine *on page 773*
Zidovudine *on page 1406*

U.S. Brand Names Combivir®

Canadian Brand Names Combivir®

Pharmacologic Category Antiretroviral Agent, Reverse Transcriptase Inhibitor (Nucleoside)

Synonyms AZT + 3TC; Lamivudine and Zidovudine

Use Treatment of HIV infection when therapy is warranted based on clinical and/or immunological evidence of disease progression. Combivir® given twice daily, provides an alternative regimen to lamivudine 150 mg twice daily plus zidovudine 600 mg/day in divided doses; this drug form reduces capsule/tablet intake for these two drugs to 2 per day instead of up to 8.

Local Anesthetic/Vasoconstrictor Precautions No information available to require special precautions

Effects on Dental Treatment No significant effects or complications reported

Dosage Children >12 years and Adults: Oral: One tablet twice daily

Mechanism of Action The combination of zidovudine and lamivudine are believed to act synergistically to inhibit reverse transcriptase via DNA chain termination after incorporation of the nucleoside analogue as well as to delay the emergence of mutations conferring resistance

Other Adverse Effects See individual agents.

Dietary/Ethanol/Herb Considerations Food may decrease serum concentration.

Pregnancy Risk Factor C

Generic Available No

Zilactin®-B [OTC] *see* Benzocaine *on page 169*

Zilactin® Baby [OTC] *see* Benzocaine *on page 169*

Zilactin-L® [OTC] *see* Lidocaine *on page 801*

Zileuton (zye LOO ton)

Related Information

Respiratory Diseases *on page 1476*

U.S. Brand Names Zyflo™

Pharmacologic Category 5-Lipoxygenase Inhibitor

Use Prophylaxis and chronic treatment of asthma in children ≥12 years of age and adults

Local Anesthetic/Vasoconstrictor Precautions No information available to require special precautions

Effects on Dental Treatment No significant effects or complications reported

Dosage Oral:

Children ≥12 years of age and Adults: 600 mg 4 times/day with meals and at bedtime

Elderly: Zileuton pharmacokinetics were similar in healthy elderly subjects (>65 years) compared with healthy younger adults (18-40 years)

Dosing adjustment in renal impairment: None (even during dialysis)

Dosing adjustment in hepatic impairment: Contraindicated in active liver disease

Mechanism of Action Specific inhibitor of 5-lipoxygenase and thus inhibits leukotriene (LTB1, LTC1, LTD1 and LTE1) formation. Leukotrienes are substances that induce numerous biological effects including augmentation of neutrophil and eosinophil migration, neutrophil and monocyte aggregation, leukocyte adhesion, increased capillary permeability and smooth muscle contraction.

Other Adverse Effects

>10%:
- Central nervous system: Headache (25%)
- Hepatic: ALT elevation (12%)

1% to 10%:
- Cardiovascular: Chest pain
- Central nervous system: Pain, dizziness, fever, insomnia, malaise, nervousness, somnolence
- Gastrointestinal: Dyspepsia, nausea, abdominal pain, constipation, flatulence
- Hematologic: Low white blood cell count
- Neuromuscular & skeletal: Myalgia, arthralgia, weakness
- Ocular: Conjunctivitis

<1% (Limited to important or life-threatening): Rash, urticaria

Drug Interactions Substrate of CYP1A2, 2C8/9, 3A4; Inhibits CYP1A2

Increased Effect/Toxicity: Zileuton increases concentrations/effects of of beta-blockers (propranolol), theophylline, and warfarin. Potentially, it may increase levels of many drugs, including cisapride, due to inhibition of CYP3A4.

Dietary/Ethanol/Herb Considerations

Ethanol: Avoid use; may increase CNS depression.

Herb/Nutraceutical: Avoid gotu kola, kava, SAMe, and valerian; may increase CNS depression. Avoid St John's wort; may decrease serum concentration and increase CNS depression.

Pharmacodynamics/Kinetics
Absorption: Rapid
Distribution: 1.2 L/kg
Protein binding: 93%
Metabolism: Several metabolites in plasma and urine; metabolized by CYP1A2, 2C9, and 3A4
Bioavailability: Unknown
Half-life elimination: 2.5 hours
Time to peak, serum: 1.7 hours
Excretion: Urine (~95% primarily as metabolites); feces (~2%)
Pregnancy Risk Factor C
Generic Available No

Zinacef® *see* Cefuroxime *on page 279*

Zinc *see* Trace Metals *on page 1328*

Zinc Acetate *see* Zinc Supplements *on page 1410*

Zinc Chloride (zingk KLOR ide)

Pharmacologic Category Trace Element
Use Cofactor for replacement therapy to different enzymes helps maintain normal growth rates, normal skin hydration and senses of taste and smell
Local Anesthetic/Vasoconstrictor Precautions No information available to require special precautions
Effects on Dental Treatment No significant effects or complications reported
Dosage Clinical response may not occur for up to 6-8 weeks
Supplemental to I.V. solutions:
Premature Infants <1500 g, up to 3 kg: 300 mcg/kg/day
Full-term Infants and Children ≤5 years: 100 mcg/kg/day
Adults:
Stable with fluid loss from small bowel: 12.2 mg zinc/liter TPN or 17.1 mg zinc/kg (added to 1000 mL I.V. fluids) of stool or ileostomy output
Metabolically stable: 2.5-4 mg/day, add 2 mg/day for acute catabolic states
Other Adverse Effects <1%: Hypotension, indigestion, jaundice, leukopenia, nausea, neutropenia, pulmonary edema, vomiting
Pregnancy Risk Factor C
Generic Available Yes
Comments Clinical response may not occur for up to 6-8 weeks

Zincfrin® [OTC] *see* Phenylephrine and Zinc Sulfate *on page 1073*

Zinc Gelatin (zingk JEL ah tin)

U.S. Brand Names Gelucast®
Pharmacologic Category Topical Skin Product
Synonyms Dome Paste Bandage; Unna's Boot; Unna's Paste; Zinc Gelatin Boot
Use As a protectant and to support varicosities and similar lesions of the lower limbs
Local Anesthetic/Vasoconstrictor Precautions No information available to require special precautions
Effects on Dental Treatment No significant effects or complications reported
Dosage Apply externally as an occlusive boot
Other Adverse Effects 1% to 10%: Local: Irritation
Generic Available Yes

Zinc Gelatin Boot *see* Zinc Gelatin *on page 1409*

Zincon® [OTC] *see* Pyrithione Zinc *on page 1154*

Zinc Oxide (zingk OKS ide)

U.S. Brand Names Ammens® Medicated Deodorant [OTC]; Balmex® [OTC]; Boudreaux's® Butt Paste [OTC]; Critic-Aid Skin Care® [OTC]; Desitin® [OTC]; Desitin® Creamy [OTC]
Canadian Brand Names Zincofax®
Pharmacologic Category Topical Skin Product
Synonyms Base Ointment; Lassar's Zinc Paste
Use Protective coating for mild skin irritations and abrasions, soothing and protective ointment to promote healing of chapped skin, diaper rash
Local Anesthetic/Vasoconstrictor Precautions No information available to require special precautions
Effects on Dental Treatment No significant effects or complications reported
Dosage Infants, Children, and Adults: Topical: Apply as required for affected areas several times daily
Mechanism of Action Mild astringent with weak antiseptic properties
Other Adverse Effects 1% to 10%: Local: Skin sensitivity, irritation
Generic Available Yes: Ointment

Zinc Sulfate *see* Zinc Supplements *on page 1410*

Zinc Sulfate and Phenylephrine *see* Phenylephrine and Zinc Sulfate *on page 1073*

Zinc Supplements (zingk SUP le ments)

Pharmacologic Category Electrolyte Supplement; Mineral, Oral; Mineral, Parenteral; Trace Element

Synonyms Zinc Acetate; Zinc Sulfate

Use Cofactor for replacement therapy to different enzymes helps maintain normal growth rates, normal skin hydration and senses of taste and smell; zinc supplement (oral and parenteral); may improve wound healing in those who are deficient. May be useful to promote wound healing in patients with pressure sores.

Local Anesthetic/Vasoconstrictor Precautions No information available to require special precautions

Effects on Dental Treatment No significant effects or complications reported

Dosage Clinical response may not occur for up to 6-8 weeks

RDA: Oral:

Birth to 6 months: 3 mg elemental zinc/day
6-12 months: 5 mg elemental zinc/day
1-10 years: 10 mg elemental zinc/day (44 mg zinc sulfate)
≥11 years: 15 mg elemental zinc/day (65 mg zinc sulfate)

Zinc deficiency: Zinc sulfate: Oral:

Infants and Children: 0.5-1 mg elemental zinc/kg/day divided 1-3 times/day; somewhat larger quantities may be needed if there is impaired intestinal absorption or an excessive loss of zinc

Adults: 110-220 mg zinc sulfate (25-50 mg elemental zinc)/dose 3 times/day

Zinc supplements:

Parenteral: TPN: I.V. infusion (chloride or sulfate): Supplemental to I.V. solutions (clinical response may not occur for up to 6-8 weeks):

Premature Infants <1500 g, up to 3 kg: 300 mcg/kg/day
Full-term Infants and Children ≤5 years: 100 mcg/kg/day

or

Premature Infants: 400 mcg/kg/day
Term <3 months: 250 mcg/kg/day
Term >3 months: 100 mcg/kg/day
Children: 50 mcg/kg/day
Adults:

Stable with fluid loss from small bowel: 12.2 mg zinc/liter TPN or 17.1 mg zinc/kg (added to 1000 mL I.V. fluids) of stool or ileostomy output

Metabolically stable: 2.5-4 mg/day, add 2 mg/day for acute catabolic states

Mechanism of Action Provides for normal growth and tissue repair, is a cofactor for >70 enzymes; ophthalmic astringent and weak antiseptic due to precipitation of protein and clearing mucus from outer surface of the eye

Dietary/Ethanol/Herb Considerations Food: Administer with food to reduce GI upset; avoid foods high in calcium or phosphorus. Caffeine and dairy products may decrease serum concentration.

Zinc Undecylenate *see* Undecylenic Acid and Derivatives *on page 1365*
Zinecard® *see* Dexrazoxane *on page 419*
Zithromax® *see* Azithromycin *on page 153*
ZNP® Bar [OTC] *see* Pyrithione Zinc *on page 1154*
Zocor® *see* Simvastatin *on page 1223*
Zofran® *see* Ondansetron *on page 1000*
Zofran® ODT *see* Ondansetron *on page 1000*
Zoladex® *see* Goserelin *on page 647*
Zoledronate *see* Zoledronic Acid *on page 1410*

Zoledronic Acid (ZOE le dron ik AS id)

U.S. Brand Names Zometa®

Canadian Brand Names Zometa®

Mexican Brand Names Zometa®

Pharmacologic Category Bisphosphonate Derivative

Synonyms CGP-42446; Zoledronate

Use Treatment of hypercalcemia of malignancy, multiple myeloma, and bone metastases of solid tumors in conjunction with standard antineoplastic therapy

Local Anesthetic/Vasoconstrictor Precautions No information to require special precautions

Effects on Dental Treatment No significant effects or complications reported

Dosage I.V.: Adults:

Hypercalcemia of malignancy (albumin-corrected serum calcium ≥12 mg/dL): 4 mg (maximum) given as a single dose infused over **no less than 15 minutes**; patients should be adequately hydrated prior to treatment (restoring urine output to ~2 L/day). Monitor serum calcium and wait at least 7 days before considering retreatment. Dosing adjustment may be needed in patients with decreased renal function following treatment.

Multiple myeloma or metastatic bone lesions from solid tumors: 4 mg given over 15 minutes every 3-4 weeks; duration of treatment ranges from 9-15 months

Note: Patients should receive a daily calcium supplement and multivitamin containing vitamin D

Dosing adjustment in renal impairment: Specific guidelines unavailable

Patients with hypercalcemia of malignancy and pretreatment serum creatinine ≥4.5 mg/dL were excluded from clinical trials.

Patients with bone metastases and pretreatment serum creatinine >3 mg/dL were excluded from clinical trials.

Dosing adjustment in hepatic impairment: Specific guidelines unavailable.

Dosing adjustment for toxicity:

Hypercalcemia of malignancy: Evidence of renal deterioration: Evaluate risk versus benefit.

Bone metastases: Evidence of renal deterioration: Discontinue further dosing until renal function returns to baseline: renal deterioration defined as follows:

Normal baseline creatinine: Increase of 0.5 mg/dL

Abnormal baseline creatinine: Increase of 1 mg/dL

Mechanism of Action A bisphosphonate which inhibits bone resorption via actions on osteoclasts or on osteoclast precursors; inhibits osteoclastic activity and skeletal calcium release induced by tumors.

Other Adverse Effects

>10%:

Cardiovascular: Leg edema (up to 19%)

Central nervous system: Fever (30% to 44%), headache (18%), insomnia (15%), anxiety (9% to 14%), dizziness (14%), agitation (13%)

Dermatologic: Alopecia (11%)

Endocrine & metabolic: Hypophosphatemia (13%), hypokalemia (12%), dehydration (up to 12%)

Gastrointestinal: Diarrhea (17% to 22%), abdominal pain (12% to 16%)

Genitourinary: Urinary tract infection (11% to 14%)

Hematologic: Anemia (22% to 29%), neutropenia (11%)

Neuromuscular & skeletal: Myalgia (21%), paresthesias (18%), arthralgia (18%) skeletal pain (12%)

Respiratory: Dyspnea (22%), coughing (12% to 19%)

1% to 10%:

Cardiovascular: Hypotension (10%), chest pain

Central nervous system: Hypoesthesia (10%)

Dermatologic: Dermatitis (10%)

Endocrine & metabolic: Hypomagnesemia (up to 10%), hypocalcemia, hypophosphatemia (9%), hypermagnesemia (Grade 3: 2%)

Gastrointestinal: Anorexia (9%), mucositis, dysphagia

Genitourinary: Urinary tract infection (14%)

Hematologic: Thrombocytopenia, pancytopenia

Neuromuscular & skeletal: Arthralgia, rigors (10%)

Renal: Serum creatinine increased

Respiratory: Pleural effusion , upper respiratory tract infection (8%)

<1%: Conjunctivitis, flu-like symptoms, injection site reactions, pruritus, rash

Symptoms of hypercalcemia include polyuria, nephrolithiasis, anorexia, nausea, vomiting, constipation, weakness, fatigue, confusion, stupor, and coma. These may not be drug-related adverse events, but related to the underlying metabolic condition.

Drug Interactions Increased Effect/Toxicity: Aminoglycosides may also lower serum calcium levels; loop diuretics increase risk of hypocalcemia; thalidomide increases renal toxicity

Pharmacodynamics/Kinetics

Onset of action: Maximum effect may not been seen for 7 days

Distribution: Binds to bone

Protein binding: ~22%

Half-life elimination: Triphasic; Terminal: 167 hours

Excretion: Urine (44% ± 18% as unchanged drug) within 24 hours; feces (<3%)

Pregnancy Risk Factor D

Generic Available No

Zolmitriptan (zohl mi TRIP tan)

U.S. Brand Names Zomig®; Zomig-ZMT™

Canadian Brand Names Zomig®; Zomig® Rapimelt

Mexican Brand Names Zomig®

Pharmacologic Category Serotonin 5-HT_{1D} Receptor Agonist

Synonyms 311C90

Use Acute treatment of migraine with or without auras

Local Anesthetic/Vasoconstrictor Precautions No information available to require special precautions

Effects on Dental Treatment No significant effects or complications reported

Dosage Oral:

Children: Safety and efficacy have not been established

(Continued)

Zolmitriptan *(Continued)*

Adults: Migraine:

Tablet: Initial: ≤2.5 mg at the onset of migraine headache; may break 2.5 mg tablet in half

Orally-disintegrating tablet: Initial: 2.5 mg at the onset of migraine headache

Note: Use the lowest possible dose to minimize adverse events. If the headache returns, the dose may be repeated after 2 hours; do not exceed 10 mg within a 24-hour period. Controlled trials have not established the effectiveness of a second dose if the initial one was ineffective

Elderly: No dosage adjustment needed but elderly patients are more likely to have underlying cardiovascular disease and should have careful evaluation of cardiovascular system before prescribing.

Dosing adjustment in renal impairment: None; 25% reduction in clearance in patients with severe renal impairment (Cl_{cr} 5-25 mL/minute)

Dosing adjustment in hepatic impairment: Use doses <2.5 mg; patients with moderate-severe impairment may have decreased clearance; significant elevation in blood pressure was observed in some patients

Mechanism of Action Selective agonist for serotonin (5-HT_{1B} and 5-HT_{1D} receptors) in cranial arteries to cause vasoconstriction and reduce sterile inflammation associated with antidromic neuronal transmission correlating with relief of migraine

Other Adverse Effects

1% to 10%:

Cardiovascular: Chest pain (2% to 4%), palpitations (up to 2%)

Central nervous system: Dizziness (6% to 10%), somnolence (5% to 8%), pain (2% to 3%), vertigo (≤2%)

Gastrointestinal: Nausea (4% to 9%), xerostomia (3% to 5%), dyspepsia (1% to 3%), dysphagia (≤2%)

Neuromuscular & skeletal: Paresthesia (5% to 9%), weakness (3% to 9%), warm/cold sensation (5% to 7%), hypesthesia (1% to 2%), myalgia (1% to 2%), myasthenia (up to 2%)

Miscellaneous: Neck/throat/jaw pain (4% to 10%), diaphoresis (up to 3%), allergic reaction (up to 1%)

<1% Agitation, akathisia, alkaline phosphatase increase, amnesia, anorexia, anxiety, apathy, apnea, appetite increased, arrhythmia, arthritis, ataxia, back pain, bradycardia, bronchitis, bronchospasm, bruising, cerebral ischemia, chills, constipation, cyanosis, cystitis, depression, diplopia, dry eyes, dysmenorrhea, dystonia, ear pain, edema, emotional lability, eosinophilia, epistaxis, esophagitis, extrasystole, euphoria, eye pain, facial edema, fever, gastritis, gastroenteritis, hallucinations, hematemesis, hematuria, hiccups, hyperacusis, hyperesthesia, hyperglycemia, hyperkinesias, hypertension, hypertensive crisis, hypertonia, hypotonia, insomnia, irritability, lacrimation, laryngitis, leg cramps, leukopenia, liver function abnormality, malaise, melena, miscarriage, pancreatitis, parosmia, photosensitivity, polyuria, postural hypotension, pruritus, QT prolongation, rash, syncope, tachycardia, tenosynovitis, tetany, thirst, thrombocytopenia, thrombophlebitis, tinnitus, tongue edema, twitching, ulcer, urinary frequency, urinary urgency, urticaria, voice alteration, yawning

Postmarketing and/or case reports: Angina pectoris, coronary artery vasospasm, MI, myocardial ischemia

Events related to other serotonin 5-HT_{1D} receptor agonists: Cerebral hemorrhage, stroke, subarachnoid hemorrhage, peripheral vascular ischemia, colonic ischemia, ventricular fibrillation

Warnings/Precautions Indicated only in patient populations with a clear diagnosis of migraine; not for prophylactic treatment of migraine headaches.

Drug Interactions Substrate of CYP1A2

Increased Effect/Toxicity: Ergot-containing drugs may lead to vasospasm; cimetidine, MAO inhibitors, oral contraceptives, propranolol increase levels of zolmitriptan; concurrent use with SSRIs and sibutramine may lead to serotonin syndrome.

Dietary/Ethanol/Herb Considerations Ethanol: Avoid or limit use; may increase CNS toxicity and cause or worsen headaches.

Pharmacodynamics/Kinetics

Onset of action: 0.5-1 hour

Absorption: Well absorbed

Distribution: V_d: 7 L/kg

Protein binding: 25%

Metabolism: Converted to an active N-desmethyl metabolite (2-6 times more potent than zolmitriptan)

Half-life elimination: 2.8-3.7 hours

Bioavailability: 40%

Time to peak, serum: Tablet: 1.5 hours; Orally-disintegrating tablet: 3 hours

Excretion: Urine (~60% to 65% total dose); feces (30% to 40%)

Pregnancy Risk Factor C

Generic Available No

Zoloft® *see* Sertraline *on page 1216*

Zolpidem (zole PI dem)

U.S. Brand Names Ambien®

Canadian Brand Names Ambien®

Pharmacologic Category Hypnotic, Nonbenzodiazepine

Synonyms Zolpidem Tartrate

Use Short-term treatment of insomnia

Local Anesthetic/Vasoconstrictor Precautions No information available to require special precautions

Effects on Dental Treatment No significant effects or complications reported

Restrictions C-IV

Dosage Duration of therapy should be limited to 7-10 days.

Adults: Oral: 10 mg immediately before bedtime; maximum dose: 10 mg
Elderly: 5 mg immediately before bedtime
Hemodialysis: Not dialyzable
Dosing adjustment in hepatic impairment: Decrease dose to 5 mg

Mechanism of Action Structurally dissimilar to benzodiazepine, however, has much or all of its actions explained by its effects on benzodiazepine (BZD) receptors, especially the omega-1 receptor (with a high affinity ratio of the alpha 1/alpha 5 subunits); retains hypnotic and much of the anxiolytic properties of the BZD, but has reduced effects on skeletal muscle and seizure threshold.

Other Adverse Effects

1% to 10%:
- Cardiovascular: Palpitations
- Central nervous system: Headache, drowsiness, dizziness, lethargy, lightheadedness, depression, abnormal dreams, amnesia
- Dermatologic: Rash
- Gastrointestinal: Nausea, diarrhea, xerostomia, constipation
- Respiratory: Sinusitis, pharyngitis

<1% (Limited to important or life-threatening): Confusion, depression, falls, impaired concentration, manic reaction, tremor, vomiting

Drug Interactions Substrate of CYP1A2, 2C8/9, 2C19, 2D6, **3A4**

Increased Effect/Toxicity: Use of zolpidem in combination with other centrally-acting drugs may produce additive CNS depression. Concurrent use of drugs which inhibit cytochrome P450 3A4 (including erythromycin, clarithromycin, diltiazem, itraconazole, ketoconazole, nefazodone, and verapamil) may increase the levels of zolpidem.

Decreased Effect: Rifampin may reduce levels and effect of zolpidem. Other enzyme inducers may have a similar effect.

Dietary/Ethanol/Herb Considerations

Ethanol: Avoid use; may increase CNS depression.
Food: Grapefruit juice may increase serum levels.
Herb/Nutraceutical: Avoid gotu kola, kava, SAMe, and valerian; may increase CNS depression. Avoid St John's wort; may decrease serum concentration and increase CNS depression.

Pharmacodynamics/Kinetics

Onset of action: 30 minutes
Duration: 6-8 hours
Absorption: Rapid
Distribution: Very low amounts enter breast milk
Protein binding: 92%
Metabolism: Hepatic to inactive metabolites
Half-life elimination: 2-2.6 hours; Cirrhosis: Up to 9.9 hours

Pregnancy Risk Factor B

Generic Available No

Zolpidem Tartrate *see* Zolpidem *on page 1413*
Zometa® *see* Zoledronic Acid *on page 1410*
Zomig® *see* Zolmitriptan *on page 1411*
Zomig-ZMT™ *see* Zolmitriptan *on page 1411*
Zonalon® *see* Doxepin *on page 471*
Zone-A® *see* Pramoxine and Hydrocortisone *on page 1106*
Zone-A Forte® *see* Pramoxine and Hydrocortisone *on page 1106*
Zonegran® *see* Zonisamide *on page 1413*

Zonisamide (zoe NIS a mide)

U.S. Brand Names Zonegran®

Canadian Brand Names Zonegran®

Pharmacologic Category Anticonvulsant, Miscellaneous

Use Adjunct treatment of partial seizures in children >16 years of age and adults with epilepsy

Local Anesthetic/Vasoconstrictor Precautions No information available to require special precautions

Effects on Dental Treatment 2%: Xerostomia, abnormal taste

(Continued)

Zonisamide *(Continued)*

Dosage Oral:

Children >16 years and Adults: Adjunctive treatment of partial seizures: Initial: 100 mg/day; dose may be increased to 200 mg/day after 2 weeks. Further dosage increases to 300 mg/day and 400 mg/day can then be made with a minimum of 2 weeks between adjustments, in order to reach steady state at each dosage level. Doses of up to 600 mg/day have been studied, however, there is no evidence of increased response with doses above 400 mg/day.

Elderly: Data from clinical trials is insufficient for patients >65 years; begin dosing at the low end of the dosing range.

Dosing adjustment in renal/hepatic impairment: Slower titration and frequent monitoring are required; do not use if Cl_{cr} <50 mL/minute

Mechanism of Action The exact mechanism of action is not known. May stabilize neuronal membranes and suppress neuronal hypersynchronization through action at sodium and calcium channels. Does not affect GABA activity.

Other Adverse Effects Adjunctive Therapy: Frequencies noted in patients receiving other anticonvulsants:

>10%:

Central nervous system: Somnolence (17%), dizziness (13%)

Gastrointestinal: Anorexia (13%)

1% to 10%:

Central nervous system: Headache (10%), agitation/irritability (9%), fatigue (8%), tiredness (7%), ataxia (6%), confusion (6%), decreased concentration (6%), memory impairment (6%), depression (6%), insomnia (6%), speech disorders (5%), mental slowing (4%), anxiety (3%), nervousness (2%), schizophrenic/schizophreniform behavior (2%), difficulty in verbal expression (2%), status epilepticus (1%), tremor (1%), convulsion (1%), hyperesthesia (1%), incoordination (1%)

Dermatologic: Rash (3%), bruising (2%), pruritus (1%)

Gastrointestinal: Nausea (9%), abdominal pain (6%), diarrhea (5%), dyspepsia (3%), weight loss (3%), constipation (2%), vomiting (1%)

Neuromuscular & skeletal: Paresthesia (4%), weakness (1%), abnormal gait (1%)

Ocular: Diplopia (6%), nystagmus (4%), amblyopia (1%)

Otic: Tinnitus (1%)

Respiratory: Rhinitis (2%), pharyngitis (1%), increased cough (1%)

Miscellaneous: Flu-like syndrome (4%) accidental injury (1%)

<1%: Flank pain, malaise, abnormal dreams, vertigo, movement disorder, hypotonia, euphoria, chest pain, **facial edema, palpitations, tachycardia**, vascular insufficiency, hypotension, hypertension, syncope, bradycardia, peripheral edema, edema, cerebrovascular accident, maculopapular rash, acne, alopecia, dry skin, eczema, urticaria, hirsutism, pustular rash, vesiculobullous rash, dehydration, decreased libido, amenorrhea, flatulence, **gingivitis, gum hyperplasia, gastritis, gastroenteritis, stomatitis, glossitis,** melena, ulcerative stomatitis, gastroduodenal ulcer, dysphagia, weight gain, urinary frequency, dysuria, urinary incontinence, impotence, urinary retention, urinary urgency, polyuria, nocturia, rectal hemorrhage, gum hemorrhage, leukopenia, anemia, cholelithiasis, thrombophlebitis, neck rigidity, leg cramps, myalgia, myasthenia, arthralgia, arthritis, hypertonia, neuropathy, twitching, hyperkinesia, dysarthria, peripheral neuritis, paresthesia, increased reflexes, allergic reaction, lymphadenopathy, immunodeficiency, thirst, diaphoresis, parosmia, conjunctivitis, visual field defect, glaucoma, deafness, hematuria, dyspnea, dystonia, encephalopathy, atrial fibrillation, heart failure, ventricular extrasystoles, petechia, hypoglycemia, hyponatremia, gynecomastia, mastitis, menorrhagia, cholangitis, hematemesis, colitis, duodenitis, esophagitis, fecal incontinence, oral ulceration, enuresis, bladder pain, bladder calculus, thrombocytopenia, microcytic anemia, cholecystitis, cholestatic jaundice, increased AST (SGOT), increased ALT (SGPT), circumoral paresthesia, dyskinesia, facial paralysis, hypokinesia, myoclonus, lupus erythematosus, increased lactic dehydrogenase, oculogyric crisis, photophobia, iritis, albuminuria, pulmonary embolus, apnea, hemoptysis

Postmarketing and/or case reports: Agranulocytosis, aplastic anemia, BUN increased, hyperthermia, kidney stones, oligohydrosis, serum creatinine increased, serum alkaline phosphatase increased, Stevens-Johnson syndrome, toxic epidermal necrolysis

Drug Interactions Substrate of CYP2C19, **3A4**

Increased Effect/Toxicity: Sedative effects may be additive with other CNS depressants; monitor for increased effect; includes barbiturates, benzodiazepines, narcotic analgesics, ethanol, and other sedative agents. Serum level and/or toxicity of zonisamide may be increased by CYP3A4 inhibitors; inhibitors include amiodarone, cimetidine, clarithromycin, erythromycin, delavirdine, diltiazem, dirithromycin, disulfiram, fluoxetine, fluvoxamine, indinavir, itraconazole, ketoconazole, metronidazole, nefazodone, nevirapine, propoxyphene, quinupristin-dalfopristin, ritonavir, saquinavir, verapamil, zafirlukast, zileuton; monitor for increased response.

Decreased Effect: Zonisamide did NOT affect steady state levels of carbamazepine, phenytoin, or valproate; zonisamide half-life is decreased by carbamazepine, phenytoin, phenobarbital, and valproate. Enzyme inducers may increase the metabolism of zonisamide, reducing its effectiveness (ie, phenytoin, carbamazepine, phenobarbital, and rifampin).

Dietary/Ethanol/Herb Considerations

Ethanol: Avoid use; may increase CNS depression.

Food: May be taken with food; delays time to maximum concentration, but does not affect bioavailability. Avoid grapefruit products; may increase serum concentration/toxicity.

Herb/Nutraceutical: Avoid gotu kola, kava, SAMe, St John's wort, and valerian; may increase CNS depression.

Pharmacodynamics/Kinetics

Distribution: V_d: 1.45 L/kg

Protein binding: 40%

Metabolism: Hepatic via CYP3A4; forms N-acetyl zonisamide and 2-sulfamoylacetyl phenol (SMAP)

Half-life elimination: 63 hours

Time to peak: 2-6 hours

Excretion: Urine (62%, 35% as unchanged drug, 65% as metabolites); feces (3%)

Pregnancy Risk Factor C

Generic Available No

Zopiclone (ZOE pi clone)

Canadian Brand Names Alti-Zopiclone; Apo®-Zopiclone; Gen-Zopiclone; Imovane®; Nu-Zopiclone; Rhovane®

Pharmacologic Category Hypnotic, Nonbenzodiazepine

Use Symptomatic relief of transient and short-term insomnia

Local Anesthetic/Vasoconstrictor Precautions No information available to require special precautions

Effects on Dental Treatment No significant effects or complications reported

Dosage Oral (administer just before bedtime):

Adults: 5-7.5 mg

Patients with chronic respiratory insufficiency: 3.75 mg; may increase up to 7.5 mg with caution in appropriate cases

Elderly: Initial: 3.75 mg; may increase to 5-7.5 mg

Dosing adjustment in hepatic impairment: 3.75 mg; may increase up to 7.5 mg with caution in appropriate cases

Mechanism of Action Zopiclone is a cyclopyrrolone derivative and has a pharmacological profile similar to benzodiazepines. Zopiclone reduces sleep latency, increases duration of sleep, and decreases the number of nocturnal awakenings.

Other Adverse Effects Frequency not defined:

Cardiovascular: Palpitations

Central nervous system: Drowsiness, somnolence, dizziness, confusion, anterograde amnesia, chills, memory impairment, euphoria, nightmares, agitation, anxiety, nervousness, hostility, depression, asthenia, speech abnormalities, headache

Dermatological: Rash, spots on skin

Endocrine & metabolic: Anorexia; libido decreased; alkaline phosphatase, ALT, and AST increased; appetite increased

Gastrointestinal: Constipation, coated tongue, diarrhea, xerostomia, dyspepsia, halitosis, nausea, taste alteration (bitter taste, common), vomiting

Neuromuscular & skeletal: Hypotonia, impaired coordination, limb heaviness, muscle spasms, paresthesia, tremors

Ocular: Amblyopia

Respiratory: Dyspnea

Miscellaneous: Diaphoresis

Drug Interactions Substrate of **CYP2C8/9, 3A4**

Increased Effect/Toxicity: Zopiclone may produce additive CNS depressant effects when coadministered with ethanol; sedatives, antihistamines, anticonvulsants, or psychotropic medications. Inhibitors of cytochrome P450 may increase serum concentrations/effect of zopiclone.

Dietary/Ethanol/Herb Considerations

Ethanol: Avoid use; may increase CNS depression.

Food: Avoid grapefruit products; may increase effect/toxicity.

Herb/Nutraceutical: Avoid gotu kola, kava, SAMe, and valerian; may increase CNS depression. Avoid St John's wort; may decrease serum concentration and increase CNS depression.

Pharmacodynamics/Kinetics

Absorption: Elderly: 75% to 94%

Distribution: Rapidly from vascular compartment

Protein binding: ~45%

Metabolism: Extensively hepatic

Half-life elimination: 5 hours; Elderly: 7 hours; Hepatic impairment: 11.9 hours

Time to peak, serum: <2 hours; Hepatic impairment: 3.5 hours

(Continued)

Zopiclone *(Continued)*

Excretion: Urine (75%); feces (16%)

Pregnancy Risk Factor Not assigned; similar agents rated D

Generic Available Yes

ZORprin® *see* Aspirin *on page 131*

Zostrix® [OTC] *see* Capsaicin *on page 238*

Zostrix®-HP [OTC] *see* Capsaicin *on page 238*

Zosyn® *see* Piperacillin and Tazobactam Sodium *on page 1088*

Zovia™ *see* Combination Hormonal Contraceptives *on page 368*

Zovirax® *see* Acyclovir *on page 42*

Zyban® *see* BuPROPion *on page 209*

Zydone® *see* Hydrocodone and Acetaminophen *on page 678*

Zyflo™ *see* Zileuton *on page 1408*

Zyloprim® *see* Allopurinol *on page 57*

Zymase® [DSC] *see* Pancrelipase *on page 1030*

Zyprexa® *see* Olanzapine *on page 996*

Zyprexa® Zydis® *see* Olanzapine *on page 996*

Zyrtec® *see* Cetirizine *on page 289*

Zyrtec-D 12 Hour™ *see* Cetirizine and Pseudoephedrine *on page 290*

Zyvox™ *see* Linezolid *on page 809*

NATURAL PRODUCTS: HERBAL AND DIETARY SUPPLEMENTS

Medical problem: " I have a toothache."
2000 BC response: "Here, eat this root."
1000 AD: "That root is heathen; here, say this prayer."
1850 AD: "That prayer is superstitious; here, drink this potion."
1940 AD: "That potion is snake oil; here, swallow this pill."
1985 AD: "That pill is ineffective; here, take this new antibiotic."
2000 AD: "That antibiotic is artificial; here, eat this root."
Adapted from an anonymous Internet communication.

INTRODUCTION

For centuries, Eastern and Western civilizations have attributed a large number of medical uses to plants and herbs. Over time, modern scientific methodologies have emerged from some of these remedies. Conversely, some of these agents have fallen into less popularity as more medical knowledge has evolved. In spite of this dichotomy, herbal and natural therapies for treatment of common medical ailments have become exceedingly popular. In America, people consistently seek out natural products that may be able to offset some perceived ailment or assist in the prevention of an ailment. One area of particular interest to those individuals using herbal or natural remedies has commonly been weight loss. There are numerous systemic considerations when some of the natural products that have been attributed weight loss powers are utilized. Many of these products are sold under the blanket of dietary supplements and, therefore, have avoided some of the more stringent Food and Drug Administration legislation. However, in 1994, that legislation was modified to include herbs, vitamins, minerals, and amino acids that may be taken as dietary supplements and the federal guidelines were further modified in 1999. This information must be made available to patients taking these types of products.

The real concern lies in the fact that health claims need not be approved by the FDA, but advertisements must include a disclaimer saying that the product has not yet been fully evaluated. Claims of medicinal use/value are often drawn from popular use, not necessarily from scientific studies. Safety is a concern when these agents are taken in combination with other prescription drugs due to the medical risk which might result. Many of these natural products may have real medicinal value but caution on the part of the dental clinician is prudent. It is impossible to cover all of the natural products, therefore, this chapter has been limited to some of the most popular dietary and herbal supplements and natural remedies used by patients you might treat and what we know about the effects of some of these agents on the body's various systems. For each of the natural products described in this section, potential/suspected drug interactions have been compiled from:

- anecdotal reports,
- scientific studies (when available), and
- any known similarities of pharmacologic effects with prescription and OTC drugs.

Most drug interactions between prescription and OTC medications and natural products have not been subject to exhaustive investigation. Readers are encouraged to consult current and comprehensive references, as well as the evolving medical literature on these interactions, for additional data. An extensive reading list is provided for further research.

ALPHABETICAL LISTING OF NATURAL PRODUCTS

Aloe

Synonyms Aloe Barbadensis; Aloe Capensis; Aloe vera; Cape

Use Analgesic, antibacterial, antifungal, antiviral, anti-inflammatory, emollient/moisturizer, laxative, wound-healing and hypoglycemic agent; topical treatment of minor burns, cuts, and skin irritations, including irritant and roentgen dermatitis; oral rinse for gums and soft tissue; juice taken internally for digestive disorders (eg, constipation, peptic ulcers, irritable bowel syndrome) and as a blood purifier; root ingested for colic; gel used in many cosmetic and pharmaceutical formulations

Effects on Bleeding None reported

Local Anesthetic/Vasoconstrictor Precautions No information available to require special precautions

Dosage

Oral: Drink 4-8 oz/day 100% aloe vera juice plain or mixed with juice; may be used as a rinse to gargle with and swallow

Topical: Apply gel 3-5 times/day to affected area (fresh gel from plant is best as some compounds break down quickly)

Per Commission E: Constipation: 50-200 mg aloe latex (residue left after liquid from gel evaporated) taken as liquid or capsule once daily for up to 10 days

Mechanism of Action/Effect The thin, clear, gel found inside the cactus-like leaves contains barbaloin (a glycoside of anthraquinone origin), bradykinase (a protease inhibitor), emodin, mannans, tannins, volatile oils, calcium, sodium, potassium, manganese, magnesium, iron, lecithin zinc, and aloin. Aloin is a harsh, bitter-tasting substance which acts as a local irritant in the GI tract and is responsible for aloe's laxative properties. When aloe juice is taken internally, it has a protective and healing effect on the digestive system by increasing lubrication and peristaltic action in the colon; mannans (a class of compounds) are thought to stimulate wound healing. Studies indicate that aloe may also lower blood sugar levels and act as a restorative agent in the liver by purifying the blood. Topical application is therapeutic in a wide variety of soft tissue injuries as it penetrates injured tissues and dilates capillaries, thereby increasing blood flow to the injury. It prevents progressive dermal ischemia following burns, frostbite, and electrical injuries; has antithromboxane activity, yet maintains prostaglandin ratio without causing injured blood vessels to collapse.

Adverse Reactions Frequency not defined:

Central nervous system: Catharsis

Dermatologic: Contact dermatitis (allergic)

Endocrine & metabolic: Hypokalemia, electrolyte imbalance

Gastrointestinal: Abdominal cramps, diarrhea, nausea, vomiting

Renal: Albuminuria, hematuria (may cause red discoloration of urine), proteinuria

Contraindications Pregnancy and lactation (oral ingestion only); injection (illegal in U.S. and have caused the deaths of several people)

Warnings Use with caution in diabetics and those taking hypoglycemic agents or insulin; may lower blood sugar. Some juice products may have high sodium content. Some wound healing may be delayed when administered topically. May alter GI absorption of other herbs or drugs. Avoid other herbs with hypoglycemic or laxative properties (see below). Chronic ingestion of juice may lead to electrolyte abnormalities, especially potassium (if not using as laxative, look for juice products that do not contain the chemical anthranoids responsible for laxative properties); should not be used as a laxative for >2 weeks.

Potential/Suspected Interactions Increased Effect/Toxicity:

Herbs with hypoglycemic properties: Alfalfa, bilberry, bitter melon, burdock, celery, damiana, fenugreek, garcinia, garlic, ginger, ginseng (American), gymnema, marshmallow, stinging nettle

Herbs with laxative properties: Cascara, eyebright, plantain, psyllium, rhubarb, senna, yellow dock

Alpha-Lipoic Acid

Synonyms Alpha-lipoate; Lipoic Acid; Thioctic acid

Use Antioxidant; treatment of diabetes, diabetic neuropathy, glaucoma; prevention of cataracts and neurologic disorders including stroke

Effects on Bleeding None reported

Local Anesthetic/Vasoconstrictor Precautions No information available to require special precautions

Dosage Oral: Range: 20-600 mg/day; Common dosage: 25-50 mg twice daily

Stage II open angle glaucoma: 150 mg/day (studies showed significant improvement after 2 months)

Mechanism of Action/Effect Sulfur-containing cofactor for pyruvate dehydrogenase (PDH) and alpha-ketoglutarate dehydrogenase; one of the most potent antioxidants and is metabolized to dihydrolipoic acid (DHLA), which also has antioxidant properties. It is fat- and water-soluble and may improve recycling of other antioxidants (eg, coenzyme Q10, glutathione, vitamins C and E). This antioxidant activity may limit development of diabetic complications by increasing muscle cell glucose uptake and insulin sensitivity in (type 2 diabetics), increasing neuronal blood flow and distal nerve conduction, improving glucose utilization and regeneration of glutathione, and reducing oxidative stress. In HIV-infected individuals, it is useful in blocking activation of NF-kappa B (required for HIV virus transcription) and improving T-helper lymphocytes and T-helper/suppressor cell ratio.

Adverse Reactions Frequency not defined: Dermatologic: Rash

Warnings Use with caution in individuals predisposed to hypoglycemia including those receiving antidiabetic agents.

Potential/Suspected Interactions Increased Effect/Toxicity:

Insulin and oral hypoglycemics

Herbs with hypoglycemic properties: Alfalfa, aloe, bilberry, bitter melon, burdock, celery, damiana, fenugreek, garcinia, garlic, ginger, ginseng (American), gymnema, marshmallow, stinging nettle

Herbs with estrogenic activity: Black cohosh, dong quai, evening primrose

Androstenedione

Synonyms Andro

Use Androgenic, anabolic; Athletic performance and libido enhancement; believed to facilitate faster recovery from exercise, increase strength, and promote muscle development in response to training (studies inconclusive)

Effects on Bleeding None reported

Local Anesthetic/Vasoconstrictor Precautions No information available to require special precautions

Dosage Adults: Oral: 50-100 mg/day (usually about 1 hour before exercising)

Mechanism of Action/Effect A weak androgenic steroid hormone produced through natural gonadal and adrenal synthesis; precursor to testosterone and estrone (elevates serum testosterone from 15% to 300%) with androgenic and anabolic properties

Adverse Reactions Frequency not defined:

Cardiovascular: **Hypertension**

Central nervous system: **Aggressive behavior**, cerebrovascular accident, depression, euphoria, **psychosis**

Dermatologic: Acne, edema, exacerbation of psoriasis, hirsutism (increase in pubic hair growth), hypertrichosis, pruritus

Endocrine & metabolic: Amenorrhea, breast enlargement, breast soreness, clitoral enlargement, gynecomastia, hirsutism, hypercalcemia, hypoprolactinemia, increased libido, infertility (males), virilism

Gastrointestinal: **GI irritation, nausea, vomiting**

Genitourinary: Azoospermia, benign prostatic hyperplasia (BPA), bladder irritability, clitoral enlargement, epididymitis, impotence, testicular atrophy, oligospermia, priapism, prostatic carcinoma

Hematologic: Leukopenia or neutropenia (agranulocytosis, granulocytopenia), polycythemia

Hepatic: Aminotransferase level elevation (asymptomatic), cholestatic hepatitis, cholestatic jaundice, hepatic dysfunction, hepatic necrosis (especially with water-based oral preparations), hepatocellular carcinoma, jaundice

Neuromuscular & skeletal: Piloerection

Miscellaneous: Hypersensitivity reactions

Contraindications Hypertension

Warnings Use with caution in individuals with CHF, prostate conditions, or hormone-sensitive tumors. The FDA requires specific labeling noting that it "contains steroid hormones that may cause breast enlargement, testicular shrinkage, and infertility in males, and increased facial/body hair, voice-deepening, and clitoral enlargement in females." Avoid herbs with hypertensive properties (see below).

Potential/Suspected Interactions

Increased Effect/Toxicity:

Androgenic drugs and estrogens

Herbs with hypertensive properties: Bayberry, blue cohosh, cayenne, ephedra, ginger, ginseng , kola nut (caffeine), licorice

Decreased Effect: Requires cobalt, calcium, and zinc for conversion to testosterone; maintain selenium required for excretion of excess

Astragalus

Synonyms *Astragalus membranaceus*; Milk Vetch

Use Adaptogen, antibacterial, diuretic, immunostimulant/immunosupportive, radioprotective, vasodilator; treatment of cancer (adjunct to chemotherapy/radiation), hepatitis, peripheral vascular diseases, respiratory infections; disease resistance, stamina, tissue oxygenation; promotes adrenal cortical function

Unlabeled/Investigational: Treatment of HIV/AIDS; antiaging

Effects on Bleeding None reported

Local Anesthetic/Vasoconstrictor Precautions No information available to require special precautions

(Continued)

Astragalus *(Continued)*

Dosage Oral:

Children: 1/3 of adult dose

Adults: 20-500 mg 4 times/day (standardized to 0.5% glycosides and 70% polysaccharides per dose); Typical dose: 400 mg twice daily; Acute symptoms: 500 mg every 3 hours

Tea: 9-30 g dried root steeped in boiling water for 15 minutes; drink 3 cups/day

Tincture: 30 drops 3 times/day

Mechanism of Action/Effect Contains bioflavonoids, choline, isoflavones, polysaccharides (including astragalan B) saponins, and triterpenoids (including astragalosides I-VIII); astragalan B binds to cholesterol on outer membranes of viruses, allowing the immune system to attack by destabilizing and weakening the invader. Animal studies have shown that astragalan B controls bacterial infections and protects against many toxins. Saponins and triterpenoids have structural similarity to steroid hormone precursors and appear to increase adrenal activity. Polysaccharides stimulate natural killer (NK) cells, augment T-cell function, and increase interferon production; administration has been shown to increase phagocytosis by reticuloendothelial cells, decrease T-suppressor cell function, and improve T-killer cell function; may decrease cyclophosphamide-induced immune suppression; stabilizes heart rhythms

Warnings Use with caution in individuals with acute infection, especially when fever is present.

Potential/Suspected Interactions

Increased Effect/Toxicity: May enhance effects of immune stimulants

Decreased Effect: May limit effects of immunosuppressants

Bifidobacterium bifidum / Lactobacillus acidophilus

Use Antidiarrheal, digestive aid; treatment of GI complaints.

B. bifidum: Maintenance of anaerobic microflora in the colon; treatment of Crohn's disease, diarrhea, ulcerative colitis

L. acidophilus: Recolonization of the GI tract with beneficial bacteria during and after antibiotic use; treatment of constipation, infant diarrhea, lactose intolerance

Effects on Bleeding None reported

Local Anesthetic/Vasoconstrictor Precautions No information available to require special precautions

Dosage Oral: 5-10 billion colony forming units (CFU)/day [dairy free] (refrigerate to maintain optimum potency)

Mechanism of Action/Effect Natural components of colonic flora used to facilitate recolonization with benign symbiotic organisms; promotes vitamin K synthesis and absorption

Adverse Reactions No known toxicity or serious side effect

Potential/Suspected Interactions Antibiotics eliminate *B. bifidum* and *L. acidophilus*

Bilberry

Synonyms *Vaccinium myrtillus*

Use Anticoagulant, antioxidant; treatment of ophthalmic disorders (cataracts, diabetic retinopathy, day/night blindness, diminished visual acuity, macular degeneration, myopia) and vascular disorders (phlebitis, varicose veins); helps maintain capillary integrity and reduce hyperpermeability

Effects on Bleeding May see increased bleeding due to inhibition of platelet aggregation

Local Anesthetic/Vasoconstrictor Precautions No information available to require special precautions

Dosage Oral: 80 mg 2-3 times/day

Mechanism of Action/Effect Inhibits a variety of inflammatory mediators, including histamine, proteases, leukotrienes, and prostaglandins; may decrease capillary permeability and inhibit platelet aggregation

Contraindications Active bleeding (eg, intracranial bleeding, peptic ulcer)

Warnings Use with caution in diabetics (may lower blood sugar), individuals with a history of bleeding, hemostatic or drug-related hemostatic disorders, those taking anticoagulants (eg, aspirin or aspirin-containing products, NSAIDs, and warfarin) or antiplatelet agents (eg, ticlopidine, clopidogrel, and dipyridamole), hypoglycemic agents or insulin. Avoid other herbs with anticoagulant/antiplatelet and/or hypoglycemic properties (see below). May alter absorption of calcium, copper, magnesium, and zinc due to tannins. Discontinue at least 14 days prior to dental or surgical procedures.

Potential/Suspected Interactions Increased Effect/Toxicity:

Anticoagulant or antiplatelet agents and insulin or oral hypoglycemics

Herbs with anticoagulant/antiplatelet properties: Alfalfa, anise, bladderwrack, bromelain, cat's claw, celery, coleus, cordyceps, dong quai, evening primrose, fenugreek, feverfew, garlic, ginger, ginkgo biloba, ginseng (American/Panax/Siberian), grape seed, green tea, guggul, horse chestnut seed, horseradish, licorice, prickly ash, red clover, reishi, sweet clover, turmeric, white willow

Herbs with hypoglycemic properties: Alfalfa, aloe, bitter melon, burdock, celery, damiana, fenugreek, garcinia, garlic, ginger, ginseng (American), gymnema, marshmallow, stinging nettle

Black Cohosh

Synonyms *Cimicifuga racemosa*

Use Analgesic, anti-inflammatory, phytoestrogenic; treatment of rheumatoid arthritis, mild depression, vasomotor symptoms of menopause and premenstrual syndrome (PMS)

Effects on Bleeding None reported

Local Anesthetic/Vasoconstrictor Precautions No information available to require special precautions

Dosage Oral: 20-40 mg twice daily (standardized to contain 1 mg triterpenes per dose)

Mechanism of Action/Effect Active components are cimicifugosides (reported to affect hypothalamus/pituitary function) and isoflavones (eg, formononetin); also contains triterpene glycosides (eg, acetin and 27-deoxyactein), aromatic and fatty acids, starches, sugars, resins, small amounts of salicylic acid, and tannins; phytoestrogenic compounds mimic the body's natural estrogen but have not been associated with the adverse effects of synthetic estrogen. Further clinical trials are needed to determine whether black cohosh has significant estrogenic actions in the body.

Adverse Reactions Frequency not defined (high doses):

Cardiovascular: **Hypotension**

Central nervous system: **Headache**

Gastrointestinal: **Nausea, vomiting**

Contraindications History of endometrial cancer or estrogen-dependent tumors, lactation, pregnancy (may stimulate uterine contractions)

Warnings Use with caution in individuals taking hormonal contraceptives or receiving hormone replacement therapy (HRT), those with endometrial cancer, history of estrogen-dependent tumors, hypotension, thromboembolic disease, stroke, or salicylate allergy (unknown whether amount of salicylic acid may affect platelet aggregation or have other effects associated with salicylates). Monitor serum hormone levels after 6 months of therapy. Avoid other hypotensive or phytoestrogenic herbs (see below).

Potential/Suspected Interactions Increased Effect:

Antihypertensive agents, hormonal contraceptives, hormone replacement therapy (HRT), sedatives

Herbs with hypotensive properties: Aconite, arnica, baneberry, bryony, California poppy, choke cherry, coleus, golden seal, green (false) hellebore, hawthorn, immortal, Indian tobacco, jaborandi, mistletoe, night blooming cereus, pasque flower, pleurisy root, quinine, shepherd's purse

Phytoestrogenic herbs: Alfalfa, blood root, hops, kudzu, licorice, pomegranate, red clover, soybean, thyme, yucca

Bromelain

Synonyms *Anas comosus*

Use Anticoagulant, anti-inflammatory, digestive aid; treatment of arthritis, dyspepsia, sinusitis

Effects on Bleeding May cause increased bleeding due to inhibition of platelet aggregation

Local Anesthetic/Vasoconstrictor Precautions No information available to require special precautions

Dosage Oral:

Digestive enzyme: 500 mg 3 times/day with meals

Inflammation: 1000 mg twice daily either 1 hour before or 2 hours after meals

Mechanism of Action/Effect Inhibits the enzyme, thromboxane synthetase, which converts prostaglandin H_2 into proinflammatory prostaglandins and thromboxanes; early reports found ingesting bromelain to be beneficial in inflammatory conditions (arthritis) but research using enteric-coated bromelain at low dosages reported no benefit (studies inconclusive)

Contraindications Active bleeding (eg, peptic ulcer, intracranial bleeding)

Warnings Use with caution in individuals with cardiovascular disease (eg, CHF, hypertension), GI ulceration, history of bleeding, hemostatic or drug-related hemostatic disorders, those taking anticoagulants (eg, aspirin or aspirin-containing products, NSAIDs, warfarin), or antiplatelet agents (eg, ticlopidine, clopidogrel, dipyridamole). Avoid other herbs with anticoagulant/antiplatelet properties (see below). Discontinue at least 14 days prior to dental or surgical procedures.

Potential/Suspected Interactions Increased Effect/Toxicity:

Anticoagulant or antiplatelet agents

Herbs with anticoagulant/antiplatelet properties: Alfalfa, anise, bilberry, bladderwrack, cat's claw, celery, coleus, cordyceps, dong quai, evening primrose, fenugreek, feverfew, garlic, ginger, ginkgo biloba, ginseng (American/Panax/Siberian), grape seed, green tea, guggul, horse chestnut seed, horseradish, licorice, prickly ash, red clover, reishi, sweet clover, turmeric, white willow

Calendula

Synonyms *Calendula officinalis*

Use Analgesic, anti-inflammatory, antimicrobial (antibacterial, antifungal, antiviral), antiprotozoal, antiseptic, antispasmodic, immunostimulant, wound-healing agent; treatment of minor burns, cuts, and other skin irritation

Effects on Bleeding None reported

Local Anesthetic/Vasoconstrictor Precautions No information available to require special precautions

Dosage Topical: Apply to affected area as needed

Mechanism of Action/Effect Stimulates phagocytosis and increases granulation

Warnings Use with caution in individuals with plant allergies.

Carnitine

Synonyms L-Carnitine

Use Treatment of CHF, hyperlipidemia, male infertility; athletic performance enhancement, weight loss

Effects on Bleeding None reported

Local Anesthetic/Vasoconstrictor Precautions No information available to require special precautions

Dosage Oral: ODA: 500-2000 mg/day in divided doses

Mechanism of Action/Effect Normally synthesized in humans from two amino acids, methionine and lysine, physiologically, participates in the transport of long-chain fatty acids across mitochondrial membranes to allow energy production; assists in the oxidation of branched-chain amino acids (a substrate for muscle during stress) and ketones when necessary; may lower serum cholesterol and triglycerides; claimed to improve efficiency of energy production in muscle tissue, including the myocardium. Improved energy generation has been proposed to improve cardiac performance and increase energy and endurance.

Potential/Suspected Interactions Decreased Effect: Depleted by valproic acid and zidovudine

Cat's Claw

Synonyms *Uncaria tomentosa*

Use Anticoagulant, anti-inflammatory, antimicrobial (antibacterial, antifungal, antiviral), antiplatelet, antioxidant, immunosupportive; treatment of allergies and minor infections or inflammatory conditions

Effects on Bleeding May cause increased bleeding due to inhibition of platelet aggregation

Local Anesthetic/Vasoconstrictor Precautions No information available to require special precautions

Dosage 250-1000 mg 3 times/day (standardized to contain ≥3% pentacyclic oxindole alkaloids and ≤0.06% tetracyclic oxindole alkaloids per dose)

Mechanism of Action/Effect Unclear due to the number of potentially active components; immunomodulatory and anti-inflammatory activity may be derived from multiple components. Several glycosides are reported to stimulate phagocytosis. Isopteridine is claimed to have immunostimulatory properties. Triterpenoid alkaloids and quinovic acid glycosides may inhibit replication of some DNA viruses. In animal studies, sterols have demonstrated anti-inflammatory activity, while glycosidic components may reduce inflammation and edema. Rhynchophylline may inhibit platelet aggregation and thrombus formation. Proanthocyanidins (PCOs) appear to be potent antioxidants, improve capillary fragility, and inhibit platelet-activating factor (PAF).

Contraindications Active bleeding (eg, intracranial bleeding, peptic ulcer), pregnancy

Warnings Use with caution in individuals taking anticoagulants (eg, aspirin or aspirin-containing products, NSAIDs, warfarin) or antiplatelet agents (eg, clopidogrel, dipyridamole, ticlopidine), therapeutic immunosuppression or I.V. immunoglobulin therapy (eg, transplant recipients), those with a history of bleeding, and hemostatic or drug-related hemostatic disorders. Avoid other herbs with anticoagulant/antiplatelet properties (see below). Discontinue at least 14 days prior to dental or surgical procedures.

Potential/Suspected Interactions Increased Effect:

Anticoagulant or antiplatelet agents, immunosuppressant therapy, and IV immunoglobulin therapy

Herbs with anticoagulant/antiplatelet properties: Alfalfa, anise, bilberry, bladderwrack, bromelain, celery, coleus, cordyceps, dong quai, evening primrose, fenugreek, feverfew, garlic, ginger, ginkgo biloba, ginseng (American/Panax/Siberian), grape seed, green tea, guggul, horse chestnut seed, horseradish, licorice, prickly ash, red clover, reishi, sweet clover, turmeric, white willow

Cayenne

Related Information

Capsaicin *on page 238*

Synonyms *Capsicum annuum*; *Capsicum frutescens*

Use Analgesic, anti-inflammatory, digestive stimulant, sympathomimetic; treatment of arthritis (osteo and rheumatoid), diabetic neuropathy, postmastectomy pain syndrome, postherpetic neuralgia, pruritus, psoriasis; appetite suppressant, bronchial relaxation, cardiovascular circulatory support, decongestant

Effects on Bleeding None reported

Local Anesthetic/Vasoconstrictor Precautions No information available to require special precautions

Dosage

Oral: 400 mg 3 times/day (standardized to contain ≥0.25% capsaicin per dose)

Topical: Apply as directed by manufacturer's labeling

Mechanism of Action/Effect Contains a resinous and pungent substance known as capsaicin which increases mucosal blood flow and/or vascular permeability and may inhibit gastric motility and activate duodenal motility. Capsaicin selectively activates certain populations of unmyelinated primary afferent sensory neurons (type "C"); many positive cardiovascular effects are due to its excitation of a distinct population of these neurons in the vagus nerve. Gastric and duodenal mucosa are believed to contain capsaicin-sensitive areas that, when stimulated by capsaicin, protect against acid and drug-induced ulcers.

Adverse Reactions Frequency not defined:

Cardiovascular: **Hypertension, increased heart rate, vasoconstriction**

Central nervous system: Insomnia

High doses:

Central nervous system: **Dizziness, headache, hyperactivity, irritability, tremor**

Gastrointestinal: Anorexia, **xerostomia**

Contraindications Anticoagulant or antiplatelet agents, cardiovascular disease (eg, arrhythmias, hypertension), diabetes, hyperthyroidism, pregnancy, psychiatric disorders

Warnings Use with caution in individuals with GI ulceration, hypertension, and those taking MAO inhibitors. May alter GI absorption of other herbs or drugs; avoid other herbs with hypertensive or sympathomimetic properties (see below).

Potential/Suspected Interactions Increased Effect/Toxicity:

Anticoagulant or antiplatelet agents, and MAO inhibitors (due to increased catecholamine secretion), stimulants (eg, OTC decongestants);

Herbs with anticoagulant/antiplatelet properties: Alfalfa, anise, bilberry, bladderwrack, bromelain, cat's claw, celery, coleus, cordyceps, dong quai, evening primrose, fenugreek, feverfew, garlic, ginger, ginkgo biloba, ginseng (American/Panax/Siberian), grape seed, green tea, guggul, horse chestnut seed, horseradish, licorice, prickly ash, red clover, reishi, sweet clover, turmeric, white willow

Herbs with hypertensive properties: Bayberry, blue cohosh, ephedra, ginger, ginseng (American), kola nut (caffeine), licorice

Herbs with sympathomimetic properties: Calamus, ephedra, Fu-tse (Fo-tzu), kola nut (caffeine), guarana, night blooming cereus, peyote (mescal buttons), scotch broom tops, Syrian rue, yellow jasmine, yohimbe

Decreased Effect: Antihypertensives and salicylates

Chamomile

Synonyms *Matricaria chamomilla*; *Matricaria recutita*

Use Antibacterial, anti-inflammatory, antispasmodic, antiulcer agent, anxiolytic, appetite stimulant, carminative, digestive aid, sedative (mild); treatment of eczema and psoriasis, hemorrhoids, inflammatory skin conditions, indigestion and irritable bowel syndrome (IBS), insomnia, leg ulcers, mastitis, premenstrual syndrome (PMS)

Effects on Bleeding None reported

Local Anesthetic/Vasoconstrictor Precautions No information available to require special precautions

Dosage Oral: 400-1600 mg/day in divided doses (standardized to contain 1% apigenin and 0.5% essential oil per dose)

Liquid extract: 1-4 mL 3 times/day

Rinse: Gargle with liquid extract 2-3 times/day as needed

Tea: ±3 g dried flowers steeped in ±150 mL boiling water for 5-10 minutes; drink 3-4 times/day

Topical: Apply to affected area as needed

Mechanism of Action/Effect Contains many active compounds; principle components are the volatile oil, alpha bisabolol which is responsible for the antispasmotic and anti-inflammatory effect, and the flavonoid, apifenin, which provides the anti-anxiety effect; topical ointments containing alpha bisabolol have been reported to be more effective than hydrocortisone in the treatment of inflammatory skin conditions

Adverse Reactions Frequency not defined:

Dermatologic: Contact dermatitis (rare)

Gastrointestinal: **Emesis** (dried flower buds), GI upset (high doses)

Respiratory: **Nasal congestion, sneezing**

Miscellaneous: **Anaphylaxis, hypersensitivity** (atopic individuals)

(Continued)

Chamomile (Continued)

Contraindications Hypersensitivity to pollen from asters, chrysanthemums, daisies, feverfew, ragweed, or sunflowers; lactation and pregnancy

Warnings Use with caution in individuals with allergies and asthma (cross sensitivity may occur in those with allergies to asters, chrysanthemums, daisies, feverfew, sunflowers, or ragweed), and those taking anticoagulants, antiplatelets, and sedatives. Avoid other herbs with allergenic, anticoagulant, or antiplatelet properties (see below).

Potential/Suspected Interactions Increased Effect:

Anticoagulant/antiplatelet agents (coumarin-type anticoagulants with high doses), anxiolytics, barbiturates, benzodiazepines, CNS depressants, sedatives

Allergenic herbs: Bittersweet, devil's dung, echinacea, feverfew, flaxseed, garlic, ginseng, gotu kola, male fern, propolis, yucca

Herbs with anticoagulant/antiplatelet properties: Alfalfa, anise, bilberry, bladderwrack, bromelain, cat's claw, celery, coleus, cordyceps, dong quai, evening primrose, fenugreek, feverfew, garlic, ginger, ginkgo biloba, ginseng (American/Panax/Siberian), grape seed, green tea, guggul, horse chestnut seed, horseradish, licorice, prickly ash, red clover, reishi, sweet clover, turmeric, white willow

Chasteberry

Synonyms Chastetree; *Vitex agnus-castus*

Use Treatment of acne vulgaris, amenorrhea, corpus luteum insufficiency, endometriosis, hyperprolactinemia, lactation insufficiency, menopausal symptoms, premenstrual syndrome [PMS]

Effects on Bleeding None reported

Local Anesthetic/Vasoconstrictor Precautions No information available to require special precautions

Dosage Oral: 400 mg/day in the morning on an empty stomach (standardized to contain 0.5% agnuside and 0.6% aucubin per dose)

Mechanism of Action/Effect Reported to have a significant effect on pituitary function; demonstrates progesterone-like action; may stimulate luteinizing hormone (LH) and inhibit follicle-stimulating hormone (FSH)

Contraindications Lactation and pregnancy (based on case reports of uterine stimulation and emmenagogue effects)

Warnings Use with caution in individuals taking hormonal contraceptives or receiving hormone replacement therapy (HRT). Avoid other phytoprogestogenic herbs (see below).

Potential/Suspected Interactions Increased Effect/Toxicity:

Dopamine antagonists (eg, antipsychotics, levodopa, metoclopramide), hormonal contraceptives, and hormone replacement therapy (HRT)

Phytoprogestogenic herbs: Blood root, oregano, yucca

Chondroitin Sulfate

Use Treatment of osteoarthritis

Effects on Bleeding None reported

Local Anesthetic/Vasoconstrictor Precautions No information available to require special precautions

Dosage Oral: 300-1500 mg/day

Mechanism of Action/Effect Reported to act synergistically with glucosamine to support maintenance of strong, healthy cartilage and joint function (studies inconclusive); inhibits synovial enzymes, elastase and hyaluronidase, which may contribute to cartilage destruction and loss of joint function

Warnings No known toxicity or serious side effects

Chromium

Use Treatment of hyper- and hypoglycemia, hyperlipidemia, hypercholesterolemia, obesity

Effects on Bleeding None reported

Local Anesthetic/Vasoconstrictor Precautions No information available to require special precautions

Dosage Oral: 50-600 mcg/day

Mechanism of Action/Effect In its trivalent form, chromium picolinate (the only active form of chromium), appears to increase insulin sensitivity, improve glucose transport into cells, and improve lipid profile by decreasing total cholesterol and triglycerides, increasing the "good" high-density lipoprotein (HDL). The mechanism of action could include one or more of the following: Enhancing beta cell activity in the pancreas and insulin binding to target tissues, increasing the number of insulin receptors, promoting activation of insulin-receptor tyrosine dinase activity. Picolinic acid causes notable changes in brain chemicals (dopamine, norepinephrine, and serotonin).

Adverse Reactions Frequency not defined:

Central nervous system: Cognitive impairment

Gastrointestinal: Changes in appetite, flatulence, loose stools

Hematologic: Anemia (isolated reports)

Renal: Renal failure

Contraindications Behavioral disorders

Potential/Suspected Interactions Drugs that may affect blood sugar levels (eg, beta blockers, insulin, oral hypoglycemics, thiazides)

Coenzyme Q_{10}

Synonyms CoQ_{10}; Ubiquinone

Use Antioxidant; treatment of angina, breast cancer, cardiovascular diseases (eg, CHF), chronic fatigue syndrome, diabetes, hypertension, muscular dystrophy, obesity, periodontal disease

Effects on Bleeding None reported

Local Anesthetic/Vasoconstrictor Precautions No information available to require special precautions

Dosage Oral: 30-200 mg/day

Breast cancer, cardiovascular disease, and diabetes: >300 mg/day (per case reports)

Mechanism of Action/Effect Involved in ATP generation, the primary source of energy in human physiology; functions as a lipid-soluble antioxidant, providing protection against free radical damage within mitochondria

Warnings Avoid other agents with hypoglycemic properties (see below).

Potential/Suspected Interactions

Increased Effect: Antidiabetic agents

Herbs with hypoglycemic properties: Alfalfa, aloe, bilberry, bitter melon, burdock, celery, damiana, fenugreek, garcinia, garlic, ginger, ginseng (American), gymnema, marshmallow, stinging nettle

Decreased Effect: May decrease response to warfarin; potential of decreased effect with beta blockers, biguanides, chlorpromazine, clonidine, diazoxide, haloperidol, HMG-C_oA reductase inhibitors, hydralazine, methyldopa, sulfonylureas, thiazide diuretics, and tricyclic antidepressants

Cranberry

Synonyms *Vaccinium macrocarpon*

Use Treatment of urinary tract infection and prevention of nephrolithiasis

Effects on Bleeding None reported

Local Anesthetic/Vasoconstrictor Precautions No information available to require special precautions

Dosage Oral: 100% cranberry juice 300-400 mg twice daily or 8-16 oz/day

Mechanism of Action/Effect Current research indicates that a cranberry-derived glycoprotein inhibits *E. coli* adherence to the epithelial cells of the urinary tract.

Creatine

Use Athletic performance enhancement, energy production, and protein synthesis for muscle building

Effects on Bleeding None reported

Local Anesthetic/Vasoconstrictor Precautions No information available to require special precautions

Dosage Oral: Loading dose: 10-20 g/day in divided doses for 1 week; Maintenance: 5 g/day

Mechanism of Action/Effect A naturally occurring crystalline molecule that includes atoms of carbon, hydrogen, nitrogen, and oxygen; enhances formation of polyamines, a powerful growth promoting substance; promotes protein synthesis for quick energy; combines with phosphate to form phosphocreatine released in muscle contraction

Potential/Suspected Interactions Decreased Effect: Caffeine may block effects

Dehydroepiandrosterone

Synonyms DHEA

Use Antiaging; treatment of depression, diabetes, fatigue, lupus

Effects on Bleeding None reported

Local Anesthetic/Vasoconstrictor Precautions No information available to require special precautions

Dosage Oral: 5-50 mg/day; 100 mg/day sometimes used in elderly

Mechanism of Action/Effect Precursor for synthesis of >50 additional hormones (eg, estrogen, testosterone); secreted by adrenal glands; may increase circulating testosterone levels; stimulates production of insulin growth factor-1 (IGF-1), a hormone which enhances insulin sensitivity, energy production, anabolic metabolism, and muscle growth

Adverse Reactions No known toxicity or serious side effects; no long-term studies conducted

Contraindications History of breast or prostate cancer

Warnings Use with caution in individuals with diabetes, hepatic dysfunction, or those predisposed to hypoglycemia (monitor blood glucose and dosage of antidiabetic agents). Avoid other agents with hypoglycemic properties.

(Continued)

Dehydroepiandrosterone *(Continued)*

Potential/Suspected Interactions Increased Effect/Toxicity:

Androgens, corticosteroids, hormonal contraceptives, hormone replacement therapy (HRT), insulin, oral hypoglycemic agents, and testosterone

Herbs with hypoglycemic properties: Alfalfa, aloe, bilberry, bitter melon, burdock, celery, damiana, fenugreek, garcinia, garlic, ginger, ginseng (American), gymnema, marshmallow, stinging nettle

Devil's Claw

Synonyms *Harpagophytum procumbens*

Use Anti-inflammatory, cardiotonic; treatment of back pain, gout, osteoarthritis, and other inflammatory conditions

Effects on Bleeding May see increased bleeding due to inhibition of platelet aggregation

Local Anesthetic/Vasoconstrictor Precautions No information available to require special precautions

Dosage Oral: 100-200 m 1-2 times/day (standardized to contain 5% harpagosides per dose)

Mechanism of Action/Effect Reportedly improves joint mobility and reduces pain and swelling in arthritis (may be more effective for osteoarthritis and chronic symptoms compared to rheumatoid and acute symptoms). Anti-inflammatory activity has reported for constituents, harpagoside and beta sitosterol; therapeutic effect comparable to phenylbutazone (studies inconclusive); may have chronotropic and inotropic effects

Adverse Reactions Frequency not defined:

Cardiovascular: Cardiomegaly, cardiomyopathy, **hypertension, palpitations, tachycardia**, vasculitis, **vasoconstriction**

Central nervous system: **Agitation, anxiety, auditory and visual hallucination, CNS-stimulating effects, excitation, fear, headache**, insomnia, **irritability, nervousness, psychosis, restlessness**, sympathetic storm, **tension**

Endocrine & metabolic: Hypokalemia

Gastrointestinal: Anorexia, **nausea**

Hepatic: Aminotransferase level elevation (asymptomatic)

Neuromuscular & skeletal: **Tremors**, weakness

Contraindications Active bleeding (eg, intracranial bleeding, peptic ulcer), GI disorders, lactation, pregnancy (may stimulate uterine contractions)

Warnings Use with caution in individuals with history of bleeding, hemostatic or drug-related hemostatic disorders, and those taking anticoagulants (eg, aspirin or aspirin-containing products, NSAIDs, warfarin) or antiplatelet agents (eg, clopidogrel, dipyridamole, ticlopidine), antiarrhythmic agents, or cardiac glycosides (eg, digoxin). Avoid herbs with anticoagulant/antiplatelet properties (see below). Discontinue at least 14 days prior to dental or surgical procedures.

Potential/Suspected Interactions Increased Effect:

Antiarrhythmics or cardiac glycosides and anticoagulant or antiplatelet agents

Herbs with anticoagulant/antiplatelet properties: Alfalfa, anise, bilberry, bladderwrack, bromelain, cat's claw, celery, coleus, cordyceps, dong quai, evening primrose, fenugreek, feverfew, garlic, ginger, ginkgo biloba, ginseng (American/Panax/Siberian), grape seed, green tea, guggul, horse chestnut seed, horseradish, licorice, prickly ash, red clover, reishi, sweet clover, turmeric, white willow

Docosahexaenoic Acid

Synonyms DHA

Use Treatment of Alzheimer's disease, attention deficit disorder (ADD) and attention deficit hyperactivity disorder (ADHD), Crohn's disease, diabetes, eczema and psoriasis, hypertension, hypertriglyceridemia, and rheumatoid arthritis; coronary heart disease risk reduction

Effects on Bleeding None reported

Local Anesthetic/Vasoconstrictor Precautions No information available to require special precautions

Dosage Oral: 125-250 mg 1-2 times/day

Mechanism of Action/Effect A long-chain, unsaturated, omega-3 fatty acid critical in the development of infants' brains and retinas; highly concentrated in synaptosomes in the brain (the region where nerve cells communicate with each other), photoreceptors (the portion of the retina that receives light stimulation), the cerebral cortex, and the mitochondria. Alpha-linolenic acid (ALA) is the precursor for the other omega-3 fatty acids, however, it is estimated that only a small percentage gets converted to DHA; the primary dietary source of DHA is from cold water or oily fish (herring, mackerel, salmon, sardines, and tuna).

Warnings Use caution with individuals taking anticoagulants (eg, aspirin or aspirin-containing products, NSAIDs, warfarin) or antiplatelet agents (eg, clopidogrel, dipyridamole, ticlopidine), insulin or oral hypoglycemics. Avoid herbs with anticoagulant/antiplatelet properties (see below); may intensify the blood-thinning effect

Potential/Suspected Interactions Increased Effect:

Anticoagulant or antiplatelet agents

Herbs with anticoagulant/antiplatelet properties: Alfalfa, anise, bilberry, bladderwrack, bromelain, cat's claw, celery, coleus, cordyceps, dong quai, evening primrose, fenugreek, feverfew, garlic, ginger, ginkgo biloba, ginseng (American/Panax/Siberian), grape seed, green tea, guggul, horse chestnut seed, horseradish, licorice, prickly ash, red clover, reishi, sweet clover, turmeric, white willow

Dong Quai

Synonyms *Angelica sinensis*; Chinese angelica

Use Anabolic, anticoagulant; treatment of amenorrhea, anemia, dysmenorrhea, hypertension, menopausal symptoms, premenstrual syndrome (PMS); female vitality

Effects on Bleeding Has potential for decreasing platelet aggregation and may increase bleeding

Local Anesthetic/Vasoconstrictor Precautions No information available to require special precautions

Dosage Adults: Oral: 200 mg twice daily (standardized to contain 0.8% to 1.1% ligustilide per dose)

Mechanism of Action/Effect Reported to cause vasodilation; may have hematopoietic properties; rich in phytoestrogens, which may demonstrate similar pharmacological effects, but are less potent than pure estrogenic compounds

Contraindications Active bleeding (eg, peptic ulcer, intracranial bleeding), prolonged exposure to sunlight or other sources of ultraviolet radiation (eg, tanning booths)

Warnings May alter hemostasis, potentiate effects of warfarin, and/or cause photosensitization; use with caution in lactation, pregnancy, cardiovascular or cerebrovascular disease, endometrial cancer, estrogen-dependent tumors, hemostatic or drug-related hemostatic disorders, history of bleeding, hypotension, stroke, thromboembolic disease, and individuals taking anticoagulants (eg, aspirin or aspirin-containing products, NSAIDs, warfarin), antiplatelet agents (eg, clopidogrel, dipyridamole, ticlopidine), antihypertensive medications, hormonal contraceptives or hormone replacement therapy (HRT), or steroids. Avoid other herbs with anabolic, anticoagulant, or antiplatelet properties (see below). Discontinue at least 14 days prior to dental or surgical procedures.

Potential/Suspected Interactions Increased Effect/Toxicity:

Anticoagulant or antiplatelet agents, antihypertensives, hormonal contraceptives, hormone replacement therapy (HRT), photosensitizing agents

Anabolic herbs: Devil's club, ginseng (American/Asian/Siberian), muira puama, sarsparilla, suma, tribulus, wild yam

Herbs with anticoagulant/antiplatelet properties: Alfalfa, anise, bilberry, bladderwrack, bromelain, cat's claw, celery, coleus, cordyceps, evening primrose, fenugreek, feverfew, garlic, ginger, ginkgo biloba, ginseng (American/Panax/Siberian), grape seed, green tea, guggul, horse chestnut seed, horseradish, licorice, prickly ash, red clover, reishi, sweet clover, turmeric, white willow

Echinacea

Synonyms American Coneflower; Black Susans; Comb Flower; *Echinacea angustifolia*; *Echinacea purpurea*; Indian Head; Purple Coneflower; Scury Root; Snakeroot

Use Antibacterial, antihyaluronidase, anti-infective, anti-inflammatory, antiviral, immunostimulant, wound-healing agent; treatment of arthritis, chronic skin complaints, cold, flu, sore throat, tonsillitis, minor upper respiratory tract infections, urinary tract infections

Effects on Bleeding None reported

Local Anesthetic/Vasoconstrictor Precautions No information available to require special precautions

Dosage In addition to forms listed below, there are some products designed to be applied topically; refer to product labeling to ensure formulation is used correctly. Continuous use should not exceed 8 weeks; not to exceed 10 days in immunosuppressed individuals or acute infection therapy. If used for prophylaxis, cycle 3 weeks on and 1 week off.

Oral (with food):

Capsule, tablet, or tea: 500 mg to 2 g, 3 times/day for 1 day, then 250 mg 4 times/day (standardized to contain 4% sesquiterpene esters per dose)

Expressed juice of fresh herb: 6-9 mL/day (per Commission E)

Liquid extract: 0.25-1 mL 3 times/day

Tincture: 1-2 mL 3 times/day

Topical: Apply to affected areas as needed

Mechanism of Action/Effect Stimulates cytokines, TNF-alfa, and interferons; caffeic acid glycosides and isolutylamides associated with the plant can also cause immune stimulation (leukocyte phagocytosis and T-cell activation)

Adverse Reactions Frequency not defined:

Dermatologic: Allergic reactions (rare; none known for oral and external formulations per Commission E)

Gastrointestinal: **Tingling sensation of tongue**

(Continued)

Echinacea (Continued)

Miscellaneous: Immunosuppression (use >6-8 weeks)

Contraindications Hypersensitivity to asters, chamomile, chrysanthemums, daisies, feverfew, ragweed, sunflowers; autoimmune diseases such as collagen vascular disease (lupus, RA), HIV or AIDS, MS, tuberculosis; immunosuppressants; pregnancy (only parenteral administration per Commission E)

Warnings Use as a preventative treatment should be discouraged; may alter immunosuppression; long-term use may cause immunosuppression. Individuals allergic to asters, chamomile, chrysanthemums, daisies, feverfew, sunflowers, or ragweed may display cross-allergy potential (rare but severe); avoid other allergenic herbs (see below). Use with caution in individuals with renal impairment.

Potential/Suspected Interactions

Increased Effect/Toxicity:

Allergenic herbs: Bittersweet, chamomile, devil's dung, echinacea, feverfew, flaxseed, garlic, ginseng, gotu kola, male fern, propolis, yucca

Herbs with anticoagulant/antiplatelet properties: Alfalfa, anise, bilberry, bladderwrack, bromelain, cat's claw, celery, coleus, cordyceps, dong quai, evening primrose, fenugreek, feverfew, garlic, ginkgo biloba, ginseng (American/Panax/Siberian), grape seed, green tea, guggul, horse chestnut seed, horseradish, licorice, prickly ash, red clover, reishi, sweet clover, turmeric, white willow

Decreased Effect: Corticosteroids and immunosuppressants; depletes potassium

Ephedra

Related Information

Ephedrine *on page 499*

Synonyms *Ephedra sinica*

Use Appetite-suppressant, stimulant, sympathomimetic (potent), thermogenic, thyroid-stimulant; treatment of allergies, arthritis, asthma, bronchitis, edema, fever, hay fever, headache, obesity, urticaria; euphoria

Effects on Bleeding None reported

Local Anesthetic/Vasoconstrictor Precautions Has potential to interact with epinephrine and levonordefrin to result in increased BP; use vasoconstrictor with caution

Dosage not to exceed 8 mg of total ephedrine alkaloids per dose or <24 mg in 24 hours; per Commission E, herb preparation corresponds to 15-30 mg total alkaloid (calculated as ephedrine)

Adults: Oral:

E. sinica extracts (with 10% alkaloid content): 125-250 mg 3 times/day

Tea: Steep 1 heaping teaspoon in 240 mL of boiling water for 10 minutes (equivalent to 15-30 mg of ephedrine)

Mechanism of Action/Effect Active constituent is ephedrine; stimulates alpha-, $beta_1$-, and $beta_2$-adrenergic receptors and the release of norepinephrine; its activity on the sympathetic nervous system causes vasoconstriction and cardiac stimulation resulting in a temporary rise in both systolic and diastolic BP; causes mydriasis and produces bronchial muscle relaxation; contains the alkaloids, ephedrine and pseudoephedrine, which are routinely isolated and used in OTC products as decongestants

Adverse Reactions Frequency not defined:

Cardiovascular: **Hypertension, increased heart rate, vasoconstriction**

Central nervous system: Insomnia

High doses:

Central nervous system: **Dizziness, headache**, hyperactivity, insomnia, **irritability, tremor**

Gastrointestinal: Anorexia, **increased peristalsis, xerostomia**

Contraindications Anticoagulant or antiplatelet agents, cardiovascular disease (eg, arrhythmias, hypertension), children, diabetes, hyperthyroidism, MAO inhibitors, pregnancy, psychiatric disorders

Per Commission E: Anxiety, glaucoma, hypertension, impaired cerebral circulation, pheochromocytoma, prostate adenoma (with residual urine accumulation), thyrotoxicosis

Warnings Product labeling contains the following AHPA warning as of March 1994: "Seek advice from two health care professionals prior to use if you are pregnant or nursing, or if you have high BP, heart or thyroid disease, diabetes, difficulty in urination due to prostate enlargement, or if taking two MAO inhibitors or any other prescription drug. Reduce or discontinue use if nervousness, tremor, sleeplessness, loss of appetite, or nausea occur. Not intended for use by person <18 years of age. Keep out of reach of children."

Also use caution in individuals with diabetes (elevates blood glucose), osteoporosis, renal impairment (including nephrolithiasis) and those taking OTC stimulants (eg, caffeine, decongestants). May alter GI absorption of other herbs or drugs; avoid other herbs with hypertensive, thyroid-stimulating, or sympathomimetic properties (see below).

Potential/Suspected Interactions Increased Effect:

Antiarrhythmics, beta-blockers, cardiac glycosides, calcium channel blockers, OTC stimulants, sympathomimetic or thyroid medications

Secale alkaloid derivatives or oxytocin: Development of hypertension

Per Commission E: Guanethidine and MAO inhibitors potentiate ephedra's sympathomimetic effect

Herbs with hypertensive properties: Bayberry, blue cohosh, cayenne, ginger, ginseng (American), kola nut (caffeine), licorice

Thyroid-stimulating herbs: Fu-tse (Fo-tzu), gotu kola, mustard, yohimbe

Evening Primrose

Synonyms Evening Primrose Oil; *Oenothera biennis*

Use Anticoagulant, anti-inflammatory, hormone stimulant; treatment of atopic eczema and psoriasis, attention deficit disorder (ADD) and attention deficit hyperactivity disorder (ADHD), dermatitis, diabetic neuropathy, endometriosis, hyperglycemia, irritable bowel syndrome (IBS), multiple sclerosis (MS), omega-6 fatty acid supplementation, premenstrual syndrome (PMS), menopausal symptoms, rheumatoid arthritis

Effects on Bleeding May see increased bleeding due to inhibition of platelet aggregation

Local Anesthetic/Vasoconstrictor Precautions No information available to require special precautions

Dosage Oral: 500 mg to 8 g/day (standardized to contain 8% to 9% gamma-linolenic acid (GLA) and ≤72% linoleic acid (LA) per dose)

Mechanism of Action/Effect Contains high amounts of gamma-linolenic acid (GLA), and essential omega-6 fatty acid which reportedly stimulates hormone synthesis and reduces generation of arachidonic acid metabolites in short-term use, improving symptoms of various inflammatory and immune conditions

Contraindications Active bleeding (may inhibit platelet aggregation), anticonvulsant or antipsychotic agents, seizure disorders (may lower seizure threshold), schizophrenia

Warnings Use with caution in individuals with a history of bleeding, hemostatic or drug-related hemostatic disorders, those taking anticoagulants (eg, aspirin or aspirin-containing products, NSAIDs, warfarin) or antiplatelet agents (eg, clopidogrel, dipyridamole, ticlopidine). Avoid other herbs with anticoagulant/antiplatelet properties (see below). Discontinue at least 14 days prior to dental or surgical procedures.

Potential/Suspected Interactions Increased Effect/Toxicity:

Anticoagulant or antiplatelet agents, anticonvulsants, phenothiazines, and other drugs which lower seizure threshold

Herbs with anticoagulant/antiplatelet properties: Alfalfa, anise, bilberry, bladderwrack, bromelain, cat's claw, celery, coleus, cordyceps, dong quai, fenugreek, feverfew, garlic, ginger, ginkgo biloba, ginseng (American/Panax/Siberian), grape seed, green tea, guggul, horse chestnut seed, horseradish, licorice, prickly ash, red clover, reishi, sweet clover, turmeric, white willow

Feverfew

Synonyms Altamisa; Bachelor's Button; Featherfew; Featherfoil; Nosebleed; *Tanacetum parthenium*; Wild Quinine

Use Anticoagulant/anti-inflammatory, antiprostaglandin, antispasmodic, digestive aid, emmenagogue, sedative; prophylaxis and treatment of migraine headaches and rheumatoid arthritis; treatment of fever, hypertension, premenstrual syndrome (PMS), tinnitus

Effects on Bleeding May see increased bleeding due to inhibition of platelet aggregation

Local Anesthetic/Vasoconstrictor Precautions No information available to require special precautions

Dosage Oral (standardized to contain 0.2% parthenolide per dose): 125 mg once or twice daily

Inflammation and rheumatoid arthritis: 100-250 mg/day

Mechanism of Action/Effect Active ingredient is parthenolide (~0.2% concentration), a serotonin antagonist; reported to inhibit leukotrinenes, prostaglandins, thromboxanes and platelet aggregation; may have spasmolytic activity

Adverse Reactions

10%:

Gastrointestinal: **Bleeding gums** (within 3 days)

Frequency not defined:

Central nervous system (upon discontinuation): **Headache**, insomnia, **nervousness**

Dermatologic: Contact dermatitis

Gastrointestinal: Abdominal pain, **loss of taste, oral ulcerations, nausea, vomiting**

Neuromuscular & skeletal (upon discontinuation): Still joints

(Continued)

Feverfew *(Continued)*

Contraindications Active bleeding (eg, intracranial bleeding, peptic ulcer), children <2 years of age; hypersensitivity to asters, chrysanthemums, daisies, sunflowers, chamomile, feverfew, or ragweed pollens; lactation and pregnancy

Warnings Use with caution in individuals with a history of bleeding, hemostatic disorders or drug-related hemostatic problems, and those taking anticoagulants (eg, aspirin or aspirin-containing products, NSAIDs, warfarin), antiplatelet agents (eg, clopidogrel, dipyridamole, ticlopidine), or medications with serotonergic properties. Abrupt discontinuation may increase migraine frequency. May alter absorption of calcium, copper, magnesium, and zinc due to tannins. Avoid other herbs with allergenic, anticoagulant, or antiplatelet properties (see below). Discontinue at least 14 days prior to dental or surgical procedures.

Potential/Suspected Interactions Increased Effect/Toxicity:

Anticoagulant or antiplatelet agents

Allergenic herbs: Bittersweet, chamomile, devil's dung, echinacea, flaxseed, garlic, ginseng, gotu kola, male fern, propolis, yucca

Herbs with anticoagulant/antiplatelet properties: Alfalfa, anise, bilberry, bladderwrack, bromelain, cat's claw, celery, coleus, cordyceps, dong quai, evening primrose, fenugreek, garlic, ginkgo biloba, ginseng (American/Panax/Siberian), grape seed, green tea, guggul, horse chestnut seed, horseradish, licorice, prickly ash, red clover, reishi, sweet clover, turmeric, white willow

Fish Oils

Use Antiatherogenic, anticoagulant/antiplatelet, anti-inflammatory; prevention and treatment of cardiovascular diseases; treatment of arteriosclerosis, arthritis, Crohn's disease, diabetes, dyslipidemia, dysmenorrhea, eczema and psoriasis, glaucoma, hypercholesterolemia, hypertension, hypertriglyceridemia; memory enhancement

Effects on Bleeding None reported

Local Anesthetic/Vasoconstrictor Precautions No information available to require special precautions

Dosage Oral: 750 mg 2-3 times/day

Mechanism of Action/Effect Source of eicosapentaenoic acid (EPA) and docosahexaenoic acid (DHA), omega-3 fatty acids which are necessary for the production of cellular membranes, hormones, and nerve tissue; EPA is converted into the series 3 prostaglandins, which have anti-inflammatory activity; although the body synthesizes these fats from alpha-linolenic acid (ALA), conversion in many people is inefficient (most people are deficient in omega-3 fatty acids); prevents atherosclerotic plaque formation

Warnings Use caution with individuals taking anticoagulants (eg, aspirin or aspirin-containing products, NSAIDs, warfarin) or antiplatelet agents (eg, clopidogrel, dipyridamole, ticlopidine), insulin or oral hypoglycemics. Avoid herbs with anticoagulant/antiplatelet properties (see below); may intensify the blood-thinning effect.

Potential/Suspected Interactions Increased Effect/Toxicity:

Anticoagulant or antiplatelet agents and insulin or oral hypoglycemics

Herbs with anticoagulant/antiplatelet properties: Alfalfa, anise, bilberry, bladderwrack, bromelain, cat's claw, celery, coleus, cordyceps, dong quai, evening primrose, fenugreek, feverfew, garlic, ginger, ginkgo biloba, ginseng (American/Panax/Siberian), grape seed, green tea, guggul, horse chestnut seed, horseradish, licorice, prickly ash, red clover, reishi, sweet clover, turmeric, white willow

Flaxseed Oil

Synonyms ALA; Alpha-linolenic Acid

Use Antioxidant, antiatherogenic; treatment of eczema and psoriasis, hypertension, hypercholesterolemia, hypertriglyceridemia; contains 3 times more omega-3 than omega-6 and may be used to help reverse the imbalance between omega-3 and omega-6 (estimated optimal ratio between omega-3 and omega-6 fatty acids is about 1:4 and ratio for many in U.S. is 1:20 to 1:30)

Effects on Bleeding None reported

Local Anesthetic/Vasoconstrictor Precautions No information available to require special precautions

Dosage Oral: 1 Tbsp/day (contains ~58% to 60% omega-3 fatty acid) [available in capsules; must be refrigerated]

Mechanism of Action/Effect The richest source of alpha-linolenic acid (ALA), which contains approximately 58% to 60% omega-3 fatty acids and 18% to 20% omega-6 fatty acids; prevents atherosclerotic plaque formation and plays a critical role in the transport and oxidation of cholesterol; precursor for the omega-3 fatty acids, eicosapentaenoic acid (EPA) and docosahexaenoic acid (DHA), which are an integral part of the production of cellular membranes, hormones, and nerve tissue; EPA is converted into the series 3 prostaglandins, which have anti-inflammatory activity

Contraindications Hypersensitivity to flaxseed, flaxseed oil or any member of the flax plant (*Linaceae*) family

Warnings Use with caution in individuals with plant allergies, those taking anticoagulants (eg, aspirin or aspirin-containing products, NSAIDs, warfarin) or antiplatelet agents (eg, clopidogrel, dipyridamole, ticlopidine), insulin or oral hypoglycemics. Avoid herbs with allergenic, anticoagulant, or antiplatelet properties (see below); may intensify the blood-thinning effect

Potential/Suspected Interactions Increased Effect/Toxicity:

Allergenic herbs: Bittersweet, chamomile, devil's dung, echinacea, feverfew, garlic, ginseng, gotu kola, male fern, propolis, yucca

Anticoagulant or antiplatelet agents and insulin or oral hypoglycemics

Herbs with anticoagulant/antiplatelet properties: Alfalfa, anise, bilberry, bladderwrack, bromelain, cat's claw, celery, coleus, cordyceps, dong quai, evening primrose, fenugreek, feverfew, garlic, ginger, ginkgo biloba, ginseng (American/Panax/Siberian), grape seed, green tea, guggul, horse chestnut seed, horseradish, licorice, prickly ash, red clover, reishi, sweet clover, turmeric, white willow

Garlic

Synonyms *Allium savitum*; Comphor of the Poor; Nectar of the Gods; Poor Mans Treacle; Rustic Treacle; Stinking Rose

Use Antibiotic, anticoagulant/antiplatelet (potent), anti-inflammatory, antioxidant (aged extract improves benefits), antitumor agent, immunosupportive; treatment of hypercholesterolemia, hypertension, hypertriglyceridemia, hypoglycemia; may decrease thrombosis

Effects on Bleeding May see increased bleeding due to potent platelet inhibition

Local Anesthetic/Vasoconstrictor Precautions No information available to require special precautions

Dosage Onset of cholesterol-lowering and hypotensive effects may require months.

Adults: Oral: 400 mg 2-3 times/day (equivalent to 1200 mg of fresh garlic or 10 mg of allicin standardized to contain 4 mg of total allicin potential (TAP) per dose) **or** 600 mg of aged extract 1-3 times/day (standardized to contain 1 mg/g S-allyl cysteine (SAC) per dose)

Cardiovascular benefits: -0.25-1 g/kg or 1-4 cloves/day (in divided doses) in an 80 kg individual

Mechanism of Action/Effect May decrease LDL cholesterol and increase HDL cholesterol, decrease blood glucose levels and triglycerides, increase fibrinolytic activity, and decrease thrombosis; crushed bulb converts to allicin, which may have antioxidant activity. Ajoene, a byproduct of allicin, is potent platelet inhibitor. Per Commission E, antibiotic property is ~1% as active as penicillin.

Adverse Reactions Frequency not defined:

Dermatologic: Eczema, immunologic contact urticaria, skin blistering, systemic contact dermatitis

Gastrointestinal: Changes in intestinal flora (rare per Commission E), GI upset (>5 cloves)

Ocular: Lacrimation

Respiratory: **Asthma** (inhalation of garlic dust)

Miscellaneous: Allergic reactions (rare); change in odor of skin and breath (per Commission E)

Contraindications Active bleeding (eg, intracranial bleeding, peptic ulcer) and pregnancy

Warnings Use with caution in diabetics (may lower blood sugar), individuals taking anticoagulants (eg, aspirin or aspirin-containing products, NSAIDs, warfarin), antihypertensives, antiplatelet agents (eg, clopidogrel, dipyridamole, ticlopidine), hypoglycemic agents or insulin, hypolipidemic agents, and those with a history of bleeding, hemostatic or drug-related hemostatic disorders; may cause GI distress in sensitive individuals. Avoid other herbs with allergenic, anticoagulant/antiplatelet, hypoglycemic, or hypolipidemic properties (see below). Discontinue at least 14 days prior to dental or surgical procedures.

Potential/Suspected Interactions

Increased Effect:

Anticoagulant/antiplatelet agents, antihypertensives, hypoglycemic agents and insulin, amphotericin B (against *Cryptococcus neoformans*)

Allergenic herbs: Bittersweet, chamomile, devil's dung, echinacea, feverfew, flaxseed, ginseng, gotu kola, male fern, propolis, yucca

Herbs with anticoagulant/antiplatelet properties: Alfalfa, anise, bilberry, bladderwrack, bromelain, cat's claw, celery, coleus, cordyceps, dong quai, evening primrose, fenugreek, feverfew, ginger, ginkgo biloba, ginseng (American/Panax/Siberian), grape seed, green tea, guggul, horse chestnut seed, horseradish, licorice, prickly ash, red clover, reishi, sweet clover, turmeric, white willow

Herbs with hypoglycemic properties: Alfalfa, aloe, bilberry, bitter melon, burdock, celery, damiana, fenugreek, garcinia, ginger, ginseng (American), gymnema, marshmallow, stinging nettle

Herbs with hypolipidemic properties: Alfalfa, artichoke, blue cohosh, fenugreek, ginger, guggul, gymnema, plantain, skullcap, myrrh, tansy, red yeast rice

Decreased Effect: May reduce iodine uptake

Ginger

Synonyms *Zingiber officinale*

Use Analgesic, anticoagulant, antiemetic (lack of sedative effects is advantageous over other antiemetics), anti-inflammatory (musculoskeletal), digestive aid; treatment of amenorrhea (Chinese remedy), arthritis, colds, culinary herb, dyspepsia, flu, headaches, motion sickness, nausea/vomiting (eg, from chemotherapy/radiation)

Effects on Bleeding Very high doses may inhibit platelet aggregation.

Local Anesthetic/Vasoconstrictor Precautions No information available to require special precautions

Dosage Oral:

Digestive aid or prevention of motion sickness: 250 mg of ginger root powder 3-4 times/day with food (standardized to contain 4% volatile oils or 5% 6-gingerol and 6-shogaol per dose)

Per Commission E: 2-4 g/day or equivalent preparations

Ale/tea: 8 oz of ginger ale contains ~1 g; I cup tea contains ~250 mg

Mechanism of Action/Effect Unknown; antiemetic activity believed to be due to shogaol documented to be comparable to several antiemetic medications, having local effects in the GI tract and/or activity in CNS;. gingerol shown to stimulate gastric secretions and peristalsis; ginger may decrease nausea associated with radiation and chemotherapy and is claimed to be superior to antihistamines for motion sickness due to lack of sedative effects. It may increase GI motility and and thus block nausea feedback from the GI tract; decreases gastric-emptying delays associated with cisplatin; may delay coagulation due to effect on platelet-activating factor and inhibit platelet aggregation (very high doses); may have cardiotonic activity; appears to decrease prostaglandin synthesis

Adverse Reactions Frequency not defined:

Central nervous system: Depression (high doses)

Gastrointestinal: **Increased salivation**

Contraindications Active bleeding (eg, intracranial bleeding, peptic ulcer) and gallstones (per Commission E)

Warnings Use with caution in diabetics, individuals with a history of bleeding, hemostatic or drug-related hemostatic disorders, those taking anticoagulants (eg, aspirin or aspirin-containing products, NSAIDs, warfarin), antiplatelet agents (eg, clopidogrel, dipyridamole, ticlopidine), cardiac glycosides (eg, digoxin), hypolipidemic agents, hypoglycemic agents, or insulin. Has cardioactive constituents; avoid large and/or prolonged doses. Avoid other herbs with anticoagulant/antiplatelet, hypertensive, hyperlipidemic, or hypoglycemic properties (see below). Discontinue at least 14 days prior to dental or surgical procedures.

Potential/Suspected Interactions Increased Effect/Toxicity:

Anticoagulant or antiplatelet agents, antihypertensives, chemotherapy agents, cisplatin (decreases gastric emptying delays), insulin, oral hypoglycemics

Herbs with anticoagulant/antiplatelet properties: Alfalfa, anise, bilberry, bladderwrack, bromelain, cat's claw, celery, coleus, cordyceps, dong quai, evening primrose, fenugreek, feverfew, garlic, ginkgo biloba, ginseng (American/Panax/Siberian), grape seed, green tea, guggul, horse chestnut seed, horseradish, licorice, prickly ash, red clover, reishi, sweet clover, turmeric, white willow

Herbs with hypertensive properties: Bayberry, blue cohosh, cayenne, ephedra, ginseng (American), kola nut (caffeine), licorice

Herbs with hypoglycemic properties: Alfalfa, aloe, bilberry, bitter melon, burdock, celery, damiana, fenugreek, garcinia, garlic, ginseng (American), gymnema, marshmallow, stinging nettle

Herbs with hypolipidemic properties: Alfalfa, artichoke, blue cohosh, fenugreek, garlic, guggul, gymnema, plantain, skullcap, myrrh, tansy, red yeast rice

Ginkgo Biloba

Synonyms BN-52063; EGb; GBE; ginkgold; Ginkgopowder; Ginkogink; Kaveri; Kew Tree; Maidenhair Tree; Oriental Plum Tree; Rökan; Silver Apricot; Superginkgo; Tanakan; Tanakene; Tebonin; Tramisal; Valverde; Vasan; Vital

Use Anticoagulant/antiplatelet, antioxidant

Per Commission E: Treatment of primary degenerative dementia, vascular dementia, and demential syndromes (eg, memory deficit), depressive emotional conditions, headache, and tinnitus

Treatment of Alzheimer's disease, arterial insufficiency and intermittent claudication (European remedy), cerebral vascular disease (dementia), macular degeneration, resistant depression, traumatic brain injury, tinnitus, visual disorders, vertigo of vascular origin

Effects on Bleeding May see increased bleeding due to inhibition of platelet aggregation; antagonizes platelet activating factor (PAF)

Local Anesthetic/Vasoconstrictor Precautions No information available to require special precautions

Dosage May require 1-2 months of use for therapeutic effect (elderly: 1 month)

Oral (administer with food):

40-80 mg twice daily to 3 times/day (standardized to contain 24% to 27% ginkgo flavone glycosides and 6% to 7% triterpenes per dose); Maximum dose: 360 mg/day

Cerebral ischemia: 120 mg/day extract in 2-3 divided doses (standardized to contain 24% flavonoid-glycoside extract and 6% terpene glycosides)

Mechanism of Action/Effect Extract contains terpenoids and flavonoids reported to inactivate oxygen-free radicals; causes vasodilation and inhibits platelet aggregation; CNS effects may be due to 4-O-methylpyridoxine (an antipyridoxine compound). Reported to increase peripheral blood flow; can increase alpha waves and decrease slow potentials in EEG.

Adverse Reactions Frequency not defined:

Cardiovascular: Bilateral subdural hematomas, **palpitations**

Central nervous system: **Dizziness, headache (rare, per Commission E), restlessness, seizures (in children)**

Dermatologic: Allergic skin reactions (rare, per Commission E), cheilitis, urticaria

Gastrointestinal: Diarrhea, GI upset (rare, per Commission E), **nausea**, proctitis, **stomatitis, vomiting**

Hematologic: Hyphema

Contraindications Active bleeding (eg, intracranial bleeding, peptic ulcer) or clotting disorders, anticoagulants or antiplatelet agents, hypersensitivity to ginkgo biloba preparations (per Commission E), MAO inhibitors, pregnancy, vasodilators

Warnings Use with caution in individuals with a history of bleeding, hemostatic drug-related hemostatic disorders, those taking anticoagulants (eg, aspirin or aspirin-containing products, NSAIDs, warfarin) or antiplatelet agents (eg, clopidogrel, dipyridamole, ticlopidine), and MAO inhibitors. Cross reactivity for contact dermatitis (due to fruit pulp) exists with poison ivy and poison oak; may last for 10 days (washing skin within 10 minutes may prevent reaction or topical corticosteroids may be helpful). Fruit pulp contains ginkolic acids which are allergens (seeds are not sensitizing). Admit individuals with neurologic abnormalities after ingestion or ingestions >2 pieces of fruit; pyridoxine may be useful after ingestion of ginkgo seeds or kernels. Avoid other herbs with anticoagulant/antiplatelet properties (see below). Discontinue at least 2-3 weeks prior to surgery; use with caution following recent surgery or trauma.

Potential/Suspected Interactions

Increased Effect/Toxicity:

Anticoagulant/antiplatelet agents and MAO inhibitors

Herbs with anticoagulant/antiplatelet properties: Alfalfa, anise, bilberry, bladderwrack, bromelain, cat's claw, celery, coleus, cordyceps, dong quai, evening primrose, fenugreek, feverfew, garlic, ginger, ginseng (American/Panax/Siberian), grape seed, green tea, guggul, horse chestnut seed, horseradish, licorice, prickly ash, red clover, reishi, sweet clover, turmeric, white willow

Decreased Effect: Anticonvulsants, fluoxetine (may reverse genital anesthesia and diminished sexual desire induced by drug)

Ginseng, Panax

Synonyms Asian Ginseng; *Panax ginseng*

Use Adaptogen, adrenal tonic, anticoagulant, cardiotonic, hormone stimulant, immunostimulant; support in chemotherapy and radiation (decreases weight loss), postsurgical recovery (stabilize white blood cell counts), endurance

Effects on Bleeding May have antiplatelet effects

Local Anesthetic/Vasoconstrictor Precautions Has potential to interact with epinephrine and levonordefrin to result in increased BP; use vasoconstrictor with caution.

Dosage Oral:

Per Commission E: 1-2 g of dried root or equivalent preparations; for maximum benefit, cycle 4 weeks on, 2 weeks off.

100-600 mg/day in divided doses (standardized to contain a minimum of 5% ginsenosides per dose)

Herbal tea: ~1.75 g; 0.5-2 g/day

Mechanism of Action/Effect Ginsenosides, the active agent, stimulate secretion of adrenocorticotropic hormone (ACTH), leading to production of increased release of adrenal hormones (eg, cortisol) and are believed to act via hormone receptors in the hypothalamus, pituitary glands, and other tissues. Panax ginseng may have CNS stimulant and estrogen-like effect; reported to have immunostimulating effects on the reticuloendothelial system. Diols, specific triterpenoid saponins, contribute to sedative and antihypertensive properties; triols reportedly increase BP and function as CNS stimulants. Low doses increase BP while high doses exhibit a hypotensive effect.

Adverse Reactions Frequency not defined:

Endocrine & metabolic: Mastalgia (prolonged or high dose)

Genitourinary: Vaginal breakthrough bleeding

Signs/symptoms of Ginseng Abuse Syndrome:

Cardiovascular: **Hypertension, palpitations, and tachycardia** (in sensitive individuals, after prolonged use, or at high doses)

(Continued)

Ginseng, Panax *(Continued)*

Central nervous system: Insomnia, **nervousness**
Dermatologic: Eruptions
Gastrointestinal: Diarrhea

Contraindications Active bleeding (may alter hemostasis), acute infection, lactation, pregnancy, renal failure

Warnings Use with caution in elderly or individuals with cardiovascular disease (eg, hypertension), history of bleeding, hemostatic or drug-related hemostatic disorders, and those receiving anticoagulants (eg, aspirin or aspirin-containing products, NSAIDs, warfarin) or antiplatelet agents (eg, clopidogrel, dipyridamole, ticlopidine), hormonal contraceptives, MAO inhibitors, stimulants (eg, OTC decongestants, caffeine), and those receiving hormonal replacement therapy (HRT). May cause "Ginseng Abuse Syndrome"; monitor for signs/symptoms (see Adverse Reactions). Avoid other herbs with allergenic, anticoagulant/antiplatelet or hypertensive properties (see below). Discontinue at least 14 days prior to dental or surgical procedures.

Potential/Suspected Interactions

Increased Effect/Toxicity:

Anticoagulant or antiplatelet agents, CNS stimulants, chemotherapy agents, diuretics (eg, furosemide), MAO inhibitors, stimulants (eg, caffeine, decongestants), sympathomimetics

Allergenic herbs: Bittersweet, chamomile, devil's dung, echinacea, feverfew, flaxseed, garlic, gotu kola, male fern, propolis, yucca

Herbs with anticoagulant/antiplatelet properties: Alfalfa, anise, bilberry, bladderwrack, bromelain, cat's claw, celery, coleus, cordyceps, dong quai, evening primrose, fenugreek, feverfew, garlic, ginger, ginkgo biloba, grape seed, green tea, guggul, horse chestnut seed, horseradish, licorice, prickly ash, red clover, reishi, sweet clover, turmeric, white willow

Herbs with hypertensive properties: Bayberry, blue cohosh, cayenne, ephedra, ginger, kola nut (caffeine), licorice

Decreased Effect: Antihypertensive agents, cardiac glycosides (eg, digoxin), hormonal contraceptives, and hormone replacement therapy (HRT)

Ginseng, Siberian

Synonyms *Eleutherococcus senticosus*; Siberian Ginseng

Use Adaptogen, anticoagulant, antiviral, immunosupportive; treatment of arteriosclerosis, chronic inflammatory disease, diabetes, hypertension; adaptation to stress, athletic performance enhancement, energy production

Effects on Bleeding May have antiplatelet effects

Local Anesthetic/Vasoconstrictor Precautions Has potential to interact with epinephrine and levonordefrin to result in increased BP; use vasoconstrictors with caution

Dosage For maximum benefit, cycle 4 weeks on, 2 weeks off.

Oral: 100-200 mg twice daily (standardized to contain 0.8% eleutherosides B and E per dose)

Mechanism of Action/Effect Full mechanism unknown; different from Asian and Panax varieties; similar to Panax in adaptogenic and protective action but without stimulant properties; increases messenger and ribosomal RNA synthesis, lipolysis, and muscle efficiency while protecting glycogen and creatinine phosphate; reported to increase efficiency of natural killer cells and enhance the body's ability to decrease toxicity of certain drugs and pollutants

Adverse Reactions

Frequency not defined:

Endocrine & metabolic: Mastalgia (prolonged or high dose)
Genitourinary: Vaginal breakthrough bleeding

Signs/symptoms of Ginseng Abuse Syndrome:

Cardiovascular: **Hypertension, palpitations, and tachycardia** (in sensitive individuals, after prolonged use, or at high doses)
Central nervous system: Insomnia, **irritability, nervousness**
Dermatologic: Eruptions
Gastrointestinal: Diarrhea

Contraindications Active bleeding (may alter hemostasis); high doses during acute phases of infection (especially when high fever is present)

Warnings Use with caution in the elderly or individuals with cardiovascular disease (eg, CHF, hypertension), history of bleeding, hemostatic or drug-related hemostatic disorders, those taking anticoagulants (eg, aspirin or aspirin-containing products, NSAIDs, warfarin) or antiplatelet agents (eg, clopidogrel, dipyridamole, ticlopidine), antihypertensive agents, digoxin, hexobarbital, hypoglycemic agents or insulin, and steroids. Extensive or prolonged use may heighten estrogenic activity. Avoid other herbs with allergenic, anabolic, anticoagulant/antiplatelet, or hypertensive properties (see below). Discontinue at least 14 days prior to dental or surgical procedures.

Potential/Suspected Interactions

Increased Effect/Toxicity:

Anticoagulant or antiplatelet agents, antihypertensives, barbiturates, digoxin, insulin, oral hypoglycemics, stimulants (eg, OTC decongestants, caffeine)

Allergenic herbs: Bittersweet, chamomile, devil's dung, echinacea, feverfew, flaxseed, garlic, gotu kola, male fern, propolis, yucca

Anabolic herbs: Devil's club, dong quai, ginseng (American/Asian), muira puama, sarsparilla, suma, tribulus, wild yam

Herbs with anticoagulant/antiplatelet properties: Alfalfa, anise, bilberry, bladderwrack, bromelain, cat's claw, celery, coleus, cordyceps, dong quai, evening primrose, fenugreek, feverfew, garlic, ginger, ginkgo biloba, grape seed, green tea, guggul, horse chestnut seed, horseradish, licorice, prickly ash, red clover, reishi, sweet clover, turmeric, white willow

Herbs with hypertensive properties: Bayberry, blue cohosh, cayenne, ephedra, ginger, kola nut (caffeine), licorice

Decreased Effect: May shorten duration of certain sedatives

Glucosamine

Synonyms Glucosamine Hydrochloride; Glucosamine Sulfate

Use Treatment of bursitis, gout, osteoarthritis, rheumatoid arthritis, tendonitis

Effects on Bleeding None reported

Local Anesthetic/Vasoconstrictor Precautions No information available to require special precautions

Dosage Oral: 500 mg sulfate 3 times/day

Mechanism of Action/Effect An amino sugar which is a key component in the synthesis of proteoglycans, a group of proteins found in cartilage; these are negatively charged and attract water so they can produce synovial fluid in the joints. The theory is that supplying the body with these precursors replenishes important synovial fluid and lead to production of new cartilage. Glucosamine also appears to inhibit cartilage-destroying enzymes (eg, collagenase and phospholipase A2), thus stopping the degenerative processes of osteoarthritis. A third mechanism may be glucosamine's ability to prevent production of damaging superoxide radicals, which may lead to cartilage destruction.

Adverse Reactions Frequency not defined: Gastrointestinal: Flatulence, **nausea**

Warnings Use with caution in diabetics (may cause insulin resistance) and those taking oral anticoagulants (may increase effect). Avoid other herbs with hyperglycemic properties (see Drug Interactions).

Potential/Suspected Interactions Increased Effect: Oral anticoagulants, insulin or oral hypoglycemics

Herbs with anticoagulant/antiplatelet properties: Alfalfa, anise, bilberry, bladderwrack, bromelain, cat's claw, celery, coleus, cordyceps, dong quai, evening primrose, fenugreek, feverfew, garlic, ginger, ginkgo biloba, ginseng (American/Panax/Siberian), grape seed, green tea, guggul, horse chestnut seed, horseradish, licorice, prickly ash, red clover, reishi, sweet clover, turmeric, white willow

Herbs with hyperglycemic properties: Elecampane, ginseng (American), gotu kola

Golden Seal

Synonyms Eye Balm; Eye Root; *Hydrastis canadensis*; Indian Eye; Jaundice Root; Orange Root; Turmeric Root; Yellow Indian Paint; Yellow Root

Use Antibacterial, antifungal, anti-inflammatory, coagulant; treatment of bronchitis, cystitis, gastritis, infectious diarrhea, inflammation of mucosal membranes, hemorrhoids, postpartum hemorrhage

Effects on Bleeding None reported

Local Anesthetic/Vasoconstrictor Precautions No information available to require special precautions

Dosage Oral: 250 mg 2-4 times/day (standardized to contain 10% alkaloids or 2.5% berberine and 1.5% to 5% hydrastine per dose)

Root: 0.5-1 g 3 times/day

Solid form: 5-10 grains

Mechanism of Action/Effect Contains the alkaloids, hydrastine (4%) and berberine (6%), which at higher doses can cause vasoconstriction, hypertension, and mucosal irritation; berberine can produce hypotension

Adverse Reactions Frequency not defined (high doses):

Cardiovascular: **Hyper- or hypotension**, myocardial damage

Central nervous system: **CNS depression, delirium, hallucinations, hyper-reflexia, stimulation/agitation, seizures**

Gastrointestinal: Diarrhea, **mouth and throat irritation, nausea, vomiting**

Neuromuscular & skeletal: Extremity numbness

Respiratory: **Respiratory failure**

Contraindications Lactation and pregnancy, hypertension, glaucoma, diabetes, history of stroke, heart disease

Warnings Efficacy not established in clinical studies. High doses (2-3 g) may cause hypotension or GI distress; toxic doses (18 g) reported to induce CNS depression. Overdose associated with myocardial damage and respiratory failure; extended use of high doses associated with delirium, GI disorders, hallucinations, and neuroexcitation. May alter liver enzymes. Use with caution in individuals with history of bleeding, hemostatic or drug-related hemostatic disorders, hypotension, those taking anticoagulants (aspirin or aspirin-containing products, NSAIDs, and warfarin)

(Continued)

Golden Seal *(Continued)*

or antiplatelet agents (ticlopidine, clopidogrel, and dipyridamole). Avoid other herbs with coagulant or hypotensive properties (see below).

Potential/Suspected Interactions Increased Effect/Toxicity:

Antihypertensive agents, vasoconstrictors

Coagulant herbs: Agrimony, mistletoe, yarrow

Herbs with hypotensive properties: Aconite, arnica, baneberry, black cohosh, bryony, California poppy, choke cherry, coleus, green (false) hellebore, hawthorn, immortal, Indian tobacco, jaborandi, mistletoe, night blooming cereus, pasque flower, pleurisy root, quinine, shepherd's purse

Decreased Effect: Vitamin B

Gotu Kola

Synonyms *Centella asiatica*

Use Diuretic (mild), sedative (high doses), thermogenic, thyroid-stimulant, wound-healing agent; treatment of hemorrhoids, hypertension, poor circulation, psoriasis, tumors, varicose veins, venous insufficiency, and wounds from infection, inflammation, trauma, or surgery (scar reduction); memory enhancement; modulation/support of connective tissue synthesis; Ayurvedic medicine uses for revitalizing nerves and brain cells; Eastern healers use for emotional disorders (eg, depression) thought to be rooted in physical problems; alcoholic extract was used to treat leprosy in Western medicine

Effects on Bleeding None reported

Local Anesthetic/Vasoconstrictor Precautions No information available to require special precautions

Dosage

Infusion: 600 mg

Oral: 50-250 mg 2-3 times/day (standardized to contain 10% to 30% asiaticosides and 2% to 4% triterpenes per dose)

Topical: Apply a 0.2% to 0.4% preparation to wound areas 2-3 times/day

Mechanism of Action/Effect Extract contains asiaticoside, an active component of *C. asiatica*, in which a trisaccharide moiety is linked to the aglycone asiatic acid; madecassol, the other triterpenoid derivative is used as an ingredient in scar-reducing products. The wound-healing and vascular effects are mostly due to these triterpene saponins and their sapogenins. Many studies found *C. asiatica* acts on certain cells of the epidermis to promote keratinization in areas of infection and stimulates the reticuloendothelial system; reported to increase superoxide dismutase (SOD) and glutathione peroxidase while decreasing lipid peroxide levels. Topical administration improves tissue healing (skin, connective tissue, lymph, and mucous membranes) and may also stabilize connective tissue growth in scleroderma; reportedly stimulates synthesis of hyaluronidase and chondroitin sulfate in connective tissue

Adverse Reactions Frequency not defined:

Cardiovascular: **Increased heart rate**

Central nervous system: Insomnia

Gastrointestinal: **Increased peristalsis**

Dermatologic: Dermatitis (topical application)

Contraindications Pregnancy

Warnings Advise caution when driving or operating machinery; large doses may be sedating. Use with caution in individuals taking sedatives (eg, anxiolytics, benzodiazepines); effects may be additive with other CNS depressants. Topical administration may cause contact dermatitis in sensitive individuals. High or prolonged doses may elevate cholesterol levels. Avoid other allergenic, hyperglycemic, or thyroid-stimulating herbs (see below).

Potential/Suspected Interactions Increased Effect/Toxicity:

Anxiolytics, other CNS depressants, and sedatives (eg, benzodiazepines)

Allergenic herbs: Bittersweet, chamomile, devil's dung, echinacea, feverfew, flaxseed, garlic, ginseng, male fern, propolis, yucca

Herbs with hyperglycemic properties: Elecampane and ginseng (American)

Thyroid-stimulating herbs: Fu-tse (Fo-tzu), ephedra, mustard, yohimbe

Grapefruit Seed

Synonyms *Citrus paradisi*; GSE

Use Antibiotic, antimycotic, antiparasitic, antiprotozoan, antimicrobial (antibacterial, antifungal, antiviral), disinfectant, immunostimulant; treatment of GI complaints, herpes, various bacterial and fungal infections (eg, *Candida albicans*, *Salmonella*), inflammatory conditions of the gums, parasites; facial cleanser, water disinfectant

Effects on Bleeding None reported

Local Anesthetic/Vasoconstrictor Precautions No information available to require special precautions

Dosage Oral:

100 mg 1-3 times/day with food

Drops: 5-10 drops 2-3 times/day

Rinse: 5-10 drops 2-3 times/say; dilute in water, swish, and expectorate

Mechanism of Action/Effect Extract is in a highly acidic liquid rich in polyphenolic compounds (eg, apigenin, campherol glycoside, hesperidin, naringin, neohesperidin, poncirin, rutinoside, quercitin) and seems to exert its antimicrobial activity in the cytoplasmic membrane of bacteria by altering cell membrane with a dose-dependent inhibition of cellular respiration; effective against 800 various viruses and species of bacteria and about 100 types of fungi without damaging friendly intestinal bacteria; disinfectant effect and lack of bacterial resistance is believed to be due to the flavonoids

Contraindications Allergy to grapefruit; astemizole, cisapride, and terfenadine

Warnings GSE is not the equivalent of grapefruit juice but since grapefruit juice/pulp has been associated with the inhibition of drug metabolism via cytochrome P450 isoenzyme 3A4 (CYP3A4), resulting in a number of drug interactions, it is reasonable to avoid the concurrent use of grapefruit seed extract in individuals receiving astemizole, cisapride, terfenadine and other medications metabolized by this pathway.

Potential/Suspected Interactions Nonsedating antihistamines, concurrent use of medications metabolized by CYP3A4 (interaction reported with grapefruit juice)

Grape Seed

Synonyms *Vitis vinifera*

Use Anticoagulant/antiplatelet, anti-inflammatory, antioxidant (potent); treatment of allergies and asthma, arterial/venous insufficiency (capillary fragility, intermittent claudication, poor circulation, varicose veins); improves peripheral circulation

Effects on Bleeding May see increase in bleeding due to inhibition of platelet aggregation

Local Anesthetic/Vasoconstrictor Precautions No information available to require special precautions

Dosage Oral: 25-100 mg 1-3 times/day (standardized to contain 40% to 80% proanthocyanidins or 95% polyphenols or a procyanidolic value >95% per dose)

Mechanism of Action/Effect Contains proanthocyanidins reported to neutralize many free radicals, including hydroxyl, lipid peroxides, and iron-induced lipid peroxidation; antioxidant properties are believed to block lipid peroxidation, which stabilizes cell membranes. Proanthocyanidins inhibit destruction of collagen (possibly by stabilizing 1-antitrypsin), which inhibits destructive enzymes such as elastin and hyaluronic acid. Stabilization of collagen allows red blood cells to traverse the capillaries and prevent fluid exudation. Anti-inflammatory activity is due to inhibition of mediators, such as histamine and prostaglandins.

Contraindications Active bleeding; may inhibit platelet aggregation. use with caution in individuals with drug-related hemostatic problems, hemostatic disorders, or history of bleeding, and individuals taking anticoagulants including aspirin, aspirin-containing products, NSAIDs, warfarin, or antiplatelet agents (eg, clopidogrel, dipyridamole, ticlopidine). Discontinue use at least 14 days before dental or surgical procedures.

Warnings Use with caution in individuals with history of bleeding, hemostatic or drug-related hemostatic problems, those taking anticoagulants (eg, aspirin or aspirin-containing products, NSAIDs, warfarin) or antiplatelet agents (eg, clopidogrel, dipyridamole, ticlopidine). Avoid other herbs with anticoagulant/antiplatelet properties (see below). May alter absorption of calcium, copper, magnesium, and zinc due to tannins. Discontinue use at least 14 days before dental or surgical procedures.

Potential/Suspected Interactions Increased Effect/Toxicity:

Anticoagulant or antiplatelet agents, xanthine oxidase inhibitors (*In vitro* studies indicate may increase toxicity of methotrexate)

Herbs with anticoagulant/antiplatelet properties: Alfalfa, anise, bilberry, bladderwrack, bromelain, cat's claw, celery, coleus, cordyceps, dong quai, evening primrose, fenugreek, feverfew, garlic, ginger, ginkgo biloba, ginseng (American/Panax/Siberian), green tea, guggul, horse chestnut seed, horseradish, licorice, prickly ash, red clover, reishi, sweet clover, turmeric, white willow

Green Tea

Synonyms *Camellia sinensis*

Use Antibacterial, anticarcinogen, antioxidant, astringent, anticoagulant/antiplatelet, antifungal, antiviral, diuretic, immunosupportive; prophylaxis and treatment of cancer, cardiovascular disease, hypercholesterolemia

Effects on Bleeding May see increased bleeding due to inhibition of platelet aggregation

Local Anesthetic/Vasoconstrictor Precautions No information available to require special precautions

Dosage Recommend decaffeinated products; there are more drug interactions with high doses of caffeine-containing products.

Oral: 250-500 mg/day (standardize to contain 50% to 97% polyphenols per dose, providing ≥50% epigallocatechin-3-gallate)

Mechanism of Action/Effect Reportedly protects against oxidative damage to cells and tissues; demonstrated to increase HDL cholesterol, decrease LDL cholesterol and triglycerides, block peroxidation of LDL, inhibit formation of thromboxane

(Continued)

Green Tea *(Continued)*

formation, and block platelet aggregation; human studies have noted improvement in prognosis of some forms of breast cancer

Adverse Reactions Frequency not defined (refers to caffeinated products):

Cardiovascular: **Palpitations, tachycardia**

Central nervous system: **Insomnia, nervousness**

Gastrointestinal: Decreased appetite, **gastric irritation**

Contraindications Active bleeding (eg, peptic ulcer, intracerebral bleeding)

Warnings Use caffeinated products with caution in individuals with cardiovascular disease, peptic ulcer, and those taking other stimulants (eg, decongestants). Use with caution in individuals with a history of bleeding, hemostatic or drug-related hemostatic disorders, those taking anticoagulants (aspirin or aspirin-containing products, NSAIDs, warfarin) or antiplatelet agents (eg, ticlopidine, clopidogrel, dipyridamole). Addition of milk to any tea may significantly lower antioxidant potential. May alter absorption of calcium, copper, magnesium, and zinc due to tannins. Avoid other herbs with anticoagulant/antiplatelet properties (see below). Discontinue at least 14 days prior to dental or surgical procedures.

Potential/Suspected Interactions Increased Effect/Toxicity:

Anticoagulant or antiplatelet agents, theophylline; reported to enhance doxorubicin's inhibitory effects on tumor growth

Drugs which interact with high doses of caffeine-containing green tea products: Acid and MAO inhibitors, anticoagulant or antiplatelet agents, barbiturates, beta blockers, CNS stimulants, fluconazole, hormonal contraceptives or hormone replacement therapy, phenobarbital, phenytoin, quinidine, quinolones, sympathomimetics, theophylline, sedatives, verapamil

Herbs with anticoagulant/antiplatelet properties: Alfalfa, anise, bilberry, bladderwrack, bromelain, cat's claw, celery, coleus, cordyceps, dong quai, evening primrose, fenugreek, feverfew, garlic, ginger, ginkgo biloba, ginseng (American/Panax/Siberian), grape seed, guggul, horse chestnut seed, horseradish, licorice, prickly ash, red clover, reishi, sweet clover, turmeric, white willow

Hawthorn

Synonyms *Crataegus laevigata*; *Crataegus monogyna*; *Crataegus oxyacantha*; *Crataegus pinnatifida*; English Hawthorn; Haw; Maybush; Whitehorn

Use Cardiotonic, sedative, vasodilator; treatment of cardiovascular abnormalities (eg, arrhythmia, angina, CHF, hyper- or hypotension, peripheral vascular diseases, tachycardia); used synergistically with digoxin (Europe)

Effects on Bleeding None reported

Local Anesthetic/Vasoconstrictor Precautions No information available to require special precautions

Dosage Oral: 250 mg 1-3 times/day (standardized to contain ≥2% vitexin-2-O-rhamnoside or minimum of 10% to 20% procyanidins per dose)

Per Commission E: 160-900 mg native water-ethanol extract (ethanol 45% v/v or methanol 70% v/v, drug-extract ratio: 4-7:1, with defined flavonoid or procyanidin content), corresponding to 30-168.7 mg procyanidins, calculated as epicatechin, or 3.5-19.8 mg flavonoids, calculated as hyperoside in accordance with DAB 10 [German pharmacopoeia #10] in 2 or 3 individual doses; duration of administration: 6 weeks minimum

Mechanism of Action/Effect Contains catechin, epicatechin, and flavonoids, which may be cardioprotective and have vasodilatory properties; dilates coronary vessels

Adverse Reactions Frequency not defined:

Cardiovascular: **Bradycardia, hyper- or hypotension**

Central nervous system: Depression, fatigue

Dermatologic: Rash

Gastrointestinal: **Nausea**

Contraindications Lactation and pregnancy

Warnings Use with caution in individuals taking ACE inhibitors and antihypertensive agents (may lower BP further). Avoid other herbs with hypotensive properties (see below).

Potential/Suspected Interactions Increased Effect:

ACE inhibitors, antiarrhythmics, antihypertensives, cardiac glycosides (eg, digoxin)

Herbs with hypotensive properties: Aconite, arnica, baneberry, black cohosh, bryony, California poppy, choke cherry, coleus, golden seal, green (false) hellebore, immortal, Indian tobacco, jaborandi, mistletoe, night blooming cereus, pasque flower, pleurisy root, quinine, shepherd's purse

Horse Chestnut

Synonyms *Aesculus hippocastanum*

Use Analgesic, anticoagulant/antiplatelet, anti-inflammatory, cardiotonic, sedative, wound-healing agent; treatment of varicose veins, hemorrhoids, other venous insufficiencies, deep vein thrombosis, lower extremity edema

Effects on Bleeding Inhibits platelet aggregation; may see increased bleeding

Local Anesthetic/Vasoconstrictor Precautions No information available to require special precautions

Dosage

Oral: 300 mg 1-2 times/day (standardized to contain 50 mg escin per dose)

Topical: Apply 2% escin gel 1-2 times/day to affected area

Mechanism of Action/Effect Contains flavonoids, sterols, tannins, saponin, and escin (seed) which promotes circulation in the veins; reported to support collagen structures; anti-inflammatory activity may be related to quercetin's reported ability to inhibit cyclo-oxygenase and lipoxygenase, enzymes which form inflammatory prostaglandins and leukotrienes. Quercetin is also an inhibitor of phosphodiesterase; correlated with cardiotonic, hypotensive, spasmolytic, and sedative actions.

Adverse Reactions Frequency not defined:

Cardiovascular: **Vasodilation, decreased heart rate**

Gastrointestinal: **Increased peristalsis**, dyspepsia

Respiratory: **Bronchial constriction**

High dose:

Cardiovascular: **Flushing, hypotension**

Central nervous system: **Headache**

Ocular: Decreased visual acuity

Respiratory: **Asthmatic attack**

Miscellaneous: **Sweating**

Contraindications Active bleeding (eg, intracranial bleeding, peptic ulcer), asthma, bethanechol, carbachol, coronary insufficiency, hyperthyroidism, lactation, metoclopramide, pilocarpine, pregnancy

Warnings Use with caution in individuals with a history of bleeding, hemostatic or drug-related hemostatic disorders, hepatic or renal impairment, and those taking anticoagulants (eg, aspirin or aspirin-containing products, NSAIDs, warfarin) or antiplatelets (eg, clopidogrel, dipyridamole, ticlopidine). Avoid other herbs with anticoagulant/antiplatelet or parasympathomimetic properties (see below). May alter GI absorption of other herbs, minerals, or drugs (especially calcium, copper, magnesium, and zinc) due to tannins. Discontinue at least 14 days prior to dental or surgical procedures.

Potential/Suspected Interactions Increased Effect/Toxicity:

Anticoagulant or antiplatelet agents

Herbs with anticoagulant/antiplatelet properties: Alfalfa, anise, bilberry, bladderwrack, bromelain, cat's claw, celery, coleus, cordyceps, dong quai, evening primrose, fenugreek, feverfew, garlic, ginger, ginkgo biloba, ginseng (American/Panax/Siberian), grape seed, green tea, guggul, horseradish, licorice, prickly ash, red clover, reishi, sweet clover, turmeric, white willow

Herbs with parasympathomimetic properties: Bittersweet, blood root, blue flag, bryony, dogbane, dogwood, false/green hellebore, huperzineA, immortal, jaborandi, leptandra, pasque flower, pink root, pleurisy root, pokeweed, senega snakeroot, wahoo, yohimbe

HuperzineA

Synonyms *Huperzia serrata*

Use Acetylcholinesterase inhibitor; treatment of senile dementia and Alzheimer's disease

Effects on Bleeding None reported

Local Anesthetic/Vasoconstrictor Precautions No information available to require special precautions

Dosage Oral: 50 mcg 1-3 times/day

Mechanism of Action/Effect Purified huperzineA keeps AChE from breaking down into acetylcholine.

Adverse Reactions Frequency not defined:

Cardiovascular: **Vasodilation, decreased heart rate**

Gastrointestinal: Increased peristalsis, dyspepsia

Respiratory: **Bronchial constriction**

High dose:

Cardiovascular: **Flushing, hypotension**

Central nervous system: **Headache**

Ocular: Decreased visual acuity

Respiratory: **Asthmatic attack**

Miscellaneous: **Sweating**

Contraindications Active bleeding (eg, intracranial bleeding, peptic ulcer), asthma, bethanechol, carbachol, coronary insufficiency, hyperthyroidism, metoclopramide, pilocarpine

Warnings Use with caution in individuals taking AChE inhibitors (eg, donepezil or tacrine). Avoid cholinergic drugs and other herbs with parasympathomimetic properties (see below).

Potential/Suspected Interactions Increased Effect/Toxicity:

Acetylcholinesterase inhibitors (donepezil, tacrine)

Herbs with parasympathomimetic properties: Bittersweet, blood root, blue flag, bryony, dogbane, dogwood, false/green hellebore, horse chestnut, immortal,

(Continued)

HuperzineA *(Continued)*

jaborandi, leptandra, pasque flower, pink root, pleurisy root, pokeweed, senega snakeroot, wahoo, yohimbe

Kava

Synonyms Awa; Kava Kava; Kew; *Piper methysticum*; Tonga

Use Anxiolytic, diuretic, sedative; treatment of insomnia, nervous anxiety, postischemic episodes, stress; skeletal muscle relaxation

Effects on Bleeding None reported

Local Anesthetic/Vasoconstrictor Precautions No information available to require special precautions

Dosage

Oral: 100-250 mg 1-3 times/day (standardized to contain 60-120 kavalactones per dose)

Per Commission E: Herb and preparations equivalent to 60-120 mg kavalactones

Mechanism of Action/Effect Extract contains alpha-pyrones and may possess central dopaminergic antagonistic properties.

Adverse Reactions Frequency not defined:

Central nervous system: Depression (prolonged use), euphoria, **somnolence**

Neuromuscular & skeletal: Muscle weakness

Dermatologic: Allergic skin reactions (rare); temporary discoloration of hair, nails, and skin

Ocular: Visual disturbances (pupil enlargement and oculomotor equilibrium disturbance reported)

Contraindications Parkinson's disease (reported to cause dopamine antagonism)

Per Commission E: Endogenous depression and pregnancy

Warnings The FDA Center for Food Safety and Applied Nutrition (CFSAN) notified healthcare professionals and consumers of the potential risk of severe liver associated with the use of kava-containing dietary supplements. Recently, more than 20 cases of hepatitis, cirrhosis, and liver failure have been reported in Europe, with at least one individual requiring a liver transplant. Given these reports, individuals with hepatic impairment or those taking drugs which can affect the liver, should consult a physician before using supplements containing kava. Physicians are urged to closely evaluate these individuals for potential liver complications. Discontinue if yellow discoloration of skin, hair, or nails occurs (temporary; caused by extended continuous use). Accommodative disturbances (eg, enlargement of the pupils and disturbances of the oculomotor equilibrium) have been described.

Use with caution in individuals taking antianxiety or antidepressant agents, diuretics, hypnotic or sedative agents, alprazolam, or alcohol. May cause sedation; advise caution when driving or operating heavy machinery. Long-term use has resulted in rash. Avoid other herbs with diuretic properties (see below). Discontinue if depression occurs (per Commission E, should not be used >3 months without medical supervision).

Potential/Suspected Interactions Increased Effect/Toxicity:

Alprazolam (coma), barbiturates, CNS depressants, diuretics, psychopharmacological agents

Herbs with diuretic properties: Artichoke, celery seed, corn silk, couchgrass, dandelion, elder flower, horsetail, juniper berry, shepherd's purse, uva ursi, yarrow

Licorice

Synonyms Glycocome; Glycyrrhiza glabra; Lakriment Neu; Liquorice; Sweet Root; Ulgastrin Neo

Use Adaptogen, adrenocorticotropic, antidote, anti-inflammatory, antimicrobial (antibacterial, antifungal, antiviral), antioxidant, antispasmodic, antitussive, detoxification agent, emollient, emmenagogue (high doses), expectorant, immunostimulant, laxative (mild), phytoestrogenic; treatment of abdominal pain, Addison's disease, adrenal insufficiency, age spots, arthritis, asthma, atherosclerosis, benign prostatic hyperplasia (BPH), bronchitis, burns, cancer, candidiasis, carbuncle, chronic gastritis, circulatory disorders, colic, colitis, cold/flu, constipation, contact dermatitis, cough, debility, diabetes, diphtheria, diverticulosis, dizziness, dropsy, duodenal ulcer, dyspepsia, excessive thirst, fever, gastric ulcer, gastritis, hay fever, heart palpitation, heartburn, hemorrhoids, hypercholesterolemia, hyperglycemia, hypotension, inflammation, irritable bowel syndrome (IBS), laryngitis, liver disorders, malaria, menopausal symptoms, menstrual cramps, nausea, peptic ulcer, poisoning (eg, ethanol, atropine, chloral hydrate, cocaine, snakebite), pharyngitis, polyuria, rheumatism, rash, sore throat, stress, tetanus, vertigo; adjunct in long-term cortisone treatment

Per Commission E: GI ulceration, upper/lower respiratory tract infections; foodstuff in candy, chewing gum, chewing tobacco, and cough preparations

Effects on Bleeding None reported

Local Anesthetic/Vasoconstrictor Precautions No information available to require special precautions

Dosage Oral: <250-500 mg 3 times/day (standardized to contain 20% glycyrrhizinic acid per dose)

Liquid extract (dried root): 15-30 drops 3 times/day in juice

Deglycyrrhizinated licorice: Chew 250 mg 3 times/day (standardized to contain ≤2% glycyrrhizin per dose) 1 hour before or 2 hours after meals and at bedtime

Candy twists (2-4) contain 100 g licorice (equivalent to 700 mg of glycyrrhizinic acid); Toxic: 2-3 twists/day for 2-4 weeks

Catarrhs of upper respiratory tract (per Commission E): 5-15 g root/day (equivalent to 200-600 mg glycyrrhizin) or 0.5-1 g juice

Gastric/duodenal ulcers: 1.5-3 g juice

Mechanism of Action/Effect Reportedly inhibits adrenal and thymic atrophy in addition to leukotriene and prostaglandin synthesis; reported to have demulcent and weak phytoestrogenic activity; stimulates the adrenocortical axis and production of mucus, which may cause symptomatic improvements

Adverse Reactions Frequency not defined:

Cardiovascular: Edema, **hypertension**

Central nervous system: **Headache, seizures**, tetany

Endocrine & metabolic: Amenorrhea, distal sodium reabsorption, hypokalemia, hypomagnesemia, hyponatremia, potassium loss

Gastrointestinal: Intestinal dilatation (ileus)

Neuromuscular & skeletal: Carpopedal spasms, myopathy, rhabdomyolysis

Ocular: Bilateral ptosis

Renal: Myoglobinuria

Contraindications Cardiovascular disease (eg, arrhythmias, hypertension), diuretics, edema, hepatic or renal disorders, hypernatremia, hypokalemia, lactation, laxatives, nausea or vomiting, obesity (due to possible mineralocorticoid effects from glycyrrhizin content), penicillin, renal impairment; Per Commission E: Hypertonia and pregnancy

Warnings Use caution in diabetics, individuals with plant allergies, hypertension, and those taking antihypertensive agents, cardiac glycosides, corticosteroids, diuretics, hormonal contraceptives, laxatives, nitrofurantoin, or receiving hormone replacement therapy (HRT). Avoid other herbs that may be aldosterone synergistic (eg, horehound), hypertensive, or phytoestrogenic (see below).

Potential/Suspected Interactions

Increased Effect/Toxicity:

Cortisol half-life and progesterone; concomitant use of furosemide can exacerbate hypokalemia; licorice can antagonize the effects of spironolactone

Per Commission E: At daily dosages of glycyrrhizin >100 mg: Potassium loss due to other drugs (eg, thiazide diuretics) can be increased causing increased sensitivity to digitalis glycosides.

On prolonged use and with higher doses, mineral corticoid effects may occur in the form of sodium and water retention; in potassium loss, accompanied by edema, hypertension, and hypokalemia; in rare cases, myoglobinuria

Herbs with anticoagulant/antiplatelet properties: Alfalfa, anise, bilberry, bladderwrack, bromelain, cat's claw, celery, coleus, cordyceps, dong quai, evening primrose, fenugreek, feverfew, garlic, ginger, ginkgo biloba, ginseng (American/Panax/Siberian), grape seed, green tea, guggul, horse chestnut seed, horseradish, prickly ash, red clover, reishi, sweet clover, turmeric, white willow

Herbs with hypertensive properties: Bayberry, blue cohosh, cayenne, ephedra, ginger, ginseng (American), kola nut (caffeine)

Phytoestrogenic herbs: Alfalfa, black cohosh, blood root, hops, kudzu, pomegranate, red clover, soybean, thyme, yucca

Decreased Effect: Barbiturates, cocaine, ephedrine, epinephrine, nicotine, pilocarpine, strychnine, tetrodoxine, and urethane through glucuronic-like conjugation action

Lutein

Use Antioxidant; treatment of cataracts and macular degeneration

Effects on Bleeding None reported

Local Anesthetic/Vasoconstrictor Precautions No information available to require special precautions

Dosage Oral: 2-6 mg/day

Mechanism of Action/Effect A carotenoid present in high concentrations in the central portion of the macula, a highly sensitive area of the retina; within the eye, this pigment filters out blue light and has been claimed to prevent macular degeneration. It protects the visual structures from oxygen free radicals and singlet oxygen, strengthens capillaries, and protects the vessels responsible for nutrient supply to this region

Lycopene

Use Treatment of atherosclerosis, macular degeneration; prevention of cancer (especially prostate)

Effects on Bleeding None reported

Local Anesthetic/Vasoconstrictor Precautions No information available to require special precautions

(Continued)

Lycopene *(Continued)*

Dosage Oral: 5 mg 1-3 times/day

Mechanism of Action/Effect A carotenoid which function as natural pigment and antioxidant; supplementation reported to protect against macular degeneration, atherosclerosis, and several types of cancer (eg, prostate cancer); functions as a free radical scavenger which may prevent oxidative damage to subcellular components, protecting from degenerative changes and carcinogenesis

Mastic

Synonyms *Pistacia lentiscus*

Use Antibacterial; treatment of dyspepsia, gastric and duodenal ulcers, halitosis

Effects on Bleeding None reported

Local Anesthetic/Vasoconstrictor Precautions No information available to require special precautions

Dosage Oral: 1000-3000 mg/day in divided doses

Mechanism of Action/Effect Exact mechanism unknown; extract reduces stomach secretions and damage to stomach lining; reported to kill *H. pylori* bacteria, possibly by altering its structure and making it more susceptible to the immune system

Melaleuca Oil

Synonyms *Melaleuca alternifolia*; Tea Tree Oil

Use Analgesic, anti-inflammatory, antibacterial, antifungal, antiseptic, antiviral, disinfectant, immunosupportive, wound-healing agent; treatment of acne, allergy and cold symptoms, minor bruises/burns/cuts, dental plaque, gum inflammation, insect bites, eczema and psoriasis, fungal infections (eg, athlete's foot, oral thrush), hair lice, herpes, muscle pain, respiratory tract infections (eg, bronchitis), toothache, warts; aromatherapy, facial skin toner, household disinfectant (to remove dust mites and lice from laundry), insect repellent, massage oil

Effects on Bleeding None reported

Local Anesthetic/Vasoconstrictor Precautions No information available to require special precautions

Dosage Essential oil should be standardized to contain at least 30% terpinen 4-01 and 15% cineole.

Household disinfectant: 1% solution in laundry water

Inhalant (decongestant, facial toner): Up to 8 drops to be inhaled on handkerchief or pillow case or 5 drops in steaming water

Topical:
- Children: Toxic ≤5 mL
- Adults: <10 mL
  - Eczema and psoriasis: 10 drops in hot bath water
  - Oral rinse: Up to 10 drops in warm water
  - Massage oil: Diluted in carrier oil 1:40 (about 8 drops per tablespoon or 50 drops per 100 mL)
  - Minor skin irritations: 1 drop undiluted oil applied directly to problem area

Mechanism of Action/Effect Unclear; a complex chemical substance consisting of approximately 50 compounds; it is the strongest natural antiseptic, 4-5 times more potent than household disinfectants but can be used daily without damage to surrounding skin; consists of plant terpenes, pinenes, and cineole

Adverse Reactions Frequency not defined:

Central nervous system: CNS depression

Dermatologic: Rash (rare)

Contraindications Oral ingestion; undiluted oil on infants <1 year of age or during pregnancy

Warnings Contains cineole; may cause rash in sensitive individuals if applied directly to skin undiluted. Store in dark glass bottle; may react badly with some polymer plastics.

Melatonin

Use Antioxidant; treatment of sleep disorders (eg, jet lag, insomnia, neurologic problems, shift work), aging, cancer; supports immune system

Effects on Bleeding None reported

Local Anesthetic/Vasoconstrictor Precautions No information available to require special precautions

Dosage Sleep disturbances: Oral: 0.3-5 mg/day; to be taken in the evening

Mechanism of Action/Effect Hormone responsible for regulating the body's circadian rhythm and sleep patterns; receptors are found in blood cells, brain, gut, and ovaries. Release is prompted by darkness and inhibited by light. Secretion appears to peak during childhood, and declines gradually through adolescence and adulthood. Antioxidant properties may also assist in regulating cardiovascular and reproductive function.

Adverse Reactions Frequency not defined: Central nervous system: **Drowsiness, fatigue, headache, irritability, sedation**

Contraindications Immune disorders, lactation, pregnancy

Warnings Avoid agents that may cause additional CNS depression (see below).

Potential/Suspected Interactions Increased Effect/Toxicity:

Hypnotics, sedatives, or other drugs that induce drowsiness (eg, benzodiazepines, narcotics); CNS depressants (prescription, supplements such as 5-HTP)

Herbs with sedative properties: Gotu kola, kava, SAMe, St John's wort, and valerian

Methyl Sulfonyl Methane

Synonyms Dimethyl Sulfone; $DMSO_2$; MSM

Use Analgesic, anti-inflammatory; treatment of interstitial cystitis, lupus, and osteoarthritis

Effects on Bleeding None reported

Local Anesthetic/Vasoconstrictor Precautions No information available to require special precautions

Dosage Oral: 2000-6000 mg/day

Mechanism of Action/Effect Source of biological sulfur, derived from dimethyl sulfoxide (DMSO); roughly 15% of DMSO is converted metabolically to dimethyl sulfone ($DMSO_2$), another name for MSM. It is an important component of connective tissues, enzymes, hormones, proteins and is required for hepatic detoxification. Pain relief may be due to inhibition of pain impulses along type C nerve fibers, increased blood flow, and reduced muscular spasm.

Milk Thistle

Synonyms *Silybum marianum*

Use Antidote (Death Cap mushroom), antioxidant (hepatoprotective, including drug toxicities); treatment of acute/chronic hepatitis, jaundice, and stimulation of bile secretion/cholagogue

Effects on Bleeding None reported

Local Anesthetic/Vasoconstrictor Precautions No information available to require special precautions

Dosage Oral: 80-120 mg 1-3 times/day (standardized to contain 80% silymarin per dose)

Mechanism of Action/Effect Reported to inhibit inflammatory effects of leukotrienes which could contribute to hepatic damage and be hepatoprotective against acetaminophen, ethanol, psychotropics (eg, butyrophenones, phenothiazines), and other drugs that modify hepatic function. Activity is derived from silymarin, which is composed of three primary flavonoids (silybin, silydianin, and silychristin); silymarin reportedly alters the composition of hepatocytes, limiting entry of hepatotoxins. Silymarin stimulates hepatic regeneration, protein synthesis and increases hepatic glutathione by over 35%. Glutathione is an important antioxidant in detoxification reactions, acting as an important sulfhydryl donor in detoxification reactions.

Nicotinamide Adenine Dinucleotide

Synonyms Coenzyme 1; NADH

Use Treatment of chronic fatigue, Parkinson's disease; increases stamina and energy

Effects on Bleeding None reported

Local Anesthetic/Vasoconstrictor Precautions No information available to require special precautions

Dosage Oral: 2.5-5 mg 1-4 times/day

Mechanism of Action/Effect An essential coenzyme in the production of energy in the mitochondria; facilitates DNA-repair mechanisms and stimulates the production of adrenaline and dopamine

Passion Flower

Synonyms *Passiflora* spp

Use Sedative

Effects on Bleeding None reported

Local Anesthetic/Vasoconstrictor Precautions No information available to require special precautions

Dosage Oral (standardized to contain 3.5% isovitexin per dose):

Anxiety: 100 mg 2-3 times/day

Insomnia: 200 mg at bedtime

Mechanism of Action/Effect The constituents, maltol and ethylmaltol, have been shown to produce CNS sedation and reduce spontaneous motor activity (low doses) in laboratory animals. In humans, it may be effective combined with other sedative and antianxiety herbs, such as valerian. These effects may be due to synergism or the potential binding of passion flower constituents to benzodiazepine receptors *in vivo.*

Warnings Advise caution when driving or operating heavy machinery. Use with caution in individuals taking antianxiety agents or antidepressants and other sedatives; reported in animal studies to increase sleeping time induced by hexobarbital.

Potential/Suspected Interactions Increased Effect/Toxicity:

Antidepressants, anxiolytics, barbiturates, sedatives

(Continued)

Passion Flower *(Continued)*

Herbs with sedative properties: Gotu kola, kava, SAMe, St John's wort, and valerian

Red Yeast Rice

Synonyms *Monascus purpureus*

Use Antibiotic, anti-inflammatory, antioxidant, HMG-CoA reductase inhibitor; treatment of hypercholesterolemia, hypertension, hypertriglyceridemia

Effects on Bleeding None reported

Local Anesthetic/Vasoconstrictor Precautions No information available to require special precautions

Dosage Oral: 1200 mg twice daily (standardized to 0.4% total HMG-Coa reductase inhibitors per dose)

Mechanism of Action/Effect Special form of vitamin E; contains eight compounds with HMG-CoA reductase inhibitory activity; some forms contain large amounts of monacolin K, a natural substance closely related to lovastatin but not identical. Red yeast rice contains additional food-derived accessory factors and seems to be more effective than isolated, purified lovastatin.

Adverse Reactions Frequency not defined: Gastrointestinal: GI upset

Contraindications Active bleeding (eg, intracranial bleeding, peptic ulcer), alcoholics (>1-2 drinks/day), children and individuals <20 years of age, history or risk of hepatic disease, hypersensitivity to rice or yeast, lactation and pregnancy (or if trying to become pregnant), organ transplant recipients, recent major surgery, serious disease or infection

Warnings Use with caution in individuals with a history of bleeding, hemostatic or drug-related hemostatic disorders, and those taking anticoagulants (eg, aspirin or aspirin-containing products, NSAIDs, warfarin) or antiplatelet agents (eg, clopidogrel, dipyridamole, ticlopidine), cyclosporine, erythromycin, itraconazole, niacin, HMG-CoA reductase inhibitors (associated with rare but serious adverse effects, including hepatic and skeletal muscle disorders), and other hyperlipidemic agents. Avoid other herbs with hyperlipidemic properties (see below). Discontinue at the first sign of hepatic dysfunction; discontinue at least 14 days prior to dental or surgical procedures.

Potential/Suspected Interactions Increased Effect/Toxicity:

Anticoagulant and antiplatelet agents, HMG-CoA reductase inhibitors and other cholesterol-lowering agents, clofibrate, cyclosporine, erythromycin, fenofibrate, gemfibrozil, itraconazole, ketoconazole, niacin

Herbs with anticoagulant/antiplatelet properties: Alfalfa, anise, bilberry, bladderwrack, bromelain, cat's claw, celery, coleus, cordyceps, dong quai, evening primrose, fenugreek, feverfew, garlic, ginger, ginkgo biloba, ginseng (American/Panax/Siberian), grape seed, green tea, guggul, horse chestnut seed, horseradish, licorice, prickly ash, red clover, reishi, sweet clover, turmeric, white willow

SAMe

Synonyms S-adenosylmethionine

Use Treatment of depression

Effects on Bleeding None reported

Local Anesthetic/Vasoconstrictor Precautions No information available to require special precautions

Dosage Oral: 400-1600 mg/day

Mechanism of Action/Effect Not defined; functions as a cofactor in many synthetic pathways

Adverse Reactions Frequency not defined:

Central nervous system: **Restlessness**

Gastrointestinal: **Nausea, xerostomia**

Contraindications Active bleeding (eg, intracranial bleeding, peptic ulcer)

Warnings Use caution when combining with other antidepressants, tryptophan, or 5-HTP; ineffective in the treatment of depressive symptoms associated with bipolar disorder

Potential/Suspected Interactions Increased Effect/Toxicity: MAO inhibitors, tricyclic antidepressants, or SSRIs; may potentiate the antidepressant effects of 5-HTP, tryptophan, and St John's wort

Sassafras Oil

Synonyms *Laurus Sassafras*; *Sassafras albidum*; *Sassafras radix*; *Sassafras varifolium*; *Sassafrax*

Use Demulcent; treatment of inflammation of the eyes, insect bites, rheumatic pain; used in the past as a flavoring for beer, sauces, and tea

Effects on Bleeding None reported

Local Anesthetic/Vasoconstrictor Precautions No information available to require special precautions

Dosage Adults: Topical: 1-5 drops in distilled water

Mechanism of Action/Effect Contains safrole (up to 80%), one of the heaviest of the volatile oils chemically found to be the methylene ether of allyl-dioxibenene; safrole is slowly absorbed from the alimentary canal, escapes the lungs unaltered, and through the kidneys oxidized into piperonalic acid; inhibits liver microsomal enzymes and its metabolite may cause hepatic tumors

Adverse Reactions Frequency not defined: Dermatologic: Contact dermatitis, **diaphoresis**

Contraindications Ingestion considered unsafe by the FDA; banned in food by FDA since 1960

Warnings Ingestion can result in poisoning or death (dose-dependent). Sassafras tea can contain as much as 200 mg (3 mg/kg) of safrole; emesis (within 30 minutes) can be considered for ingestion >5 mL (considered lethal).

Saw Palmetto

Synonyms Palmetto Scrub; *Sabal serrulata*; *Sabasilis serrulatae*; *Serenoa repens*

Use Antiandrogen, anti-inflammatory; treatment of benign prostatic hyperplasia (BPH)

Effects on Bleeding None reported

Local Anesthetic/Vasoconstrictor Precautions No information available to require special precautions

Dosage Adults: Oral: 0.5-1 g dried fruit 3 times/day **or** 160 mg twice daily (standardized to contain at least 80% to 90% fatty acids and sterols per dose)

Mechanism of Action/Effect Liposterolic extract of berries may inhibit the enzymes 5α-reductase, along with cyclo-oxygenase and 5-lipoxygenase; does not reduce prostatic enlargement but may help increase urinary flow.

Adverse Reactions Frequency not defined:

Central nervous system: **Headache**

Endocrine & metabolic: Gynecomastia

Gastrointestinal: Stomach problems (rare, per Commission E)

Contraindications Hormone replacement therapy (HRT), lactation, pregnancy, prostate medications

Warnings Not FDA approved; use with caution in individuals on alpha-adrenergic blocking agents and finasteride.

Potential/Suspected Interactions Increased Effect/Toxicity: Alpha-adrenergic blocking agents, finasteride, hormone replacement therapy (HRT), prostate medications

Schisandra

Synonyms *Schizandra chinensis*

Use Adaptogen, anti-inflammatory, antioxidant, antitussive, hepatoprotective, immunostimulant; treatment of cancer, chronic diarrhea, cough, diabetes, diaphoresis, fatigue, hepatitis; adjunct support for chemotherapy and radiation, detoxification, energy production, health tonic

Effects on Bleeding None reported

Local Anesthetic/Vasoconstrictor Precautions No information available to require special precautions

Dosage Oral: 100 mg twice daily (standardized to contain at least 9% schisandrins per dose)

Mechanism of Action/Effect Reported to lower serum glutamic-pyruvic transaminase (SGPT) concentration, a liver enzyme found in blood when liver damage is present; stimulates hepatic glycogen synthesis and protein synthesis and increases microsomal enzyme activity

Contraindications Pregnancy (due to uterine stimulation)

Warnings May alter metabolism of many drugs; use with caution in individuals taking calcium channel blockers.

Potential/Suspected Interactions Cytochrome P450 enzyme induction may alter metabolism of many drugs (calcium channel blockers noted to be decreased). Cardioprotective action reported during administration of doxorubicin.

Shark Cartilage

Use Treatment of cancer, osteoarthritis, and rheumatoid arthritis

Effects on Bleeding None reported

Local Anesthetic/Vasoconstrictor Precautions No information available to require special precautions

Dosage

Oral: Dosage range: 3000 mg 3 times/day, taken 20 minutes before meals

Rectal: Retention enemas; 15-20 g/day

Mechanism of Action/Effect A mixture of glycosaminoglycans (GAGs), including chondroitin sulfate; contains antiangiogenesis factors which inhibit the growth of new blood vessels and may prevent tumors from developing the network of blood vessels they need to supply them with nutrients

Soy Isoflavones

Synonyms Isoflavones

Use Estrogenic (weak); treatment of bone loss, hypercholesterolemia, menopausal symptoms

Effects on Bleeding None reported

Local Anesthetic/Vasoconstrictor Precautions No information available to require special precautions

Dosage Oral: 500-1000 mg soy extract daily

Mechanism of Action/Effect Contains plant-derived estrogenic compounds (potency estimated to be only 1/1000 to 1/100,000 that of estradiol); claimed to inhibit bone reabsorption in postmenopausal women; reported to lower serum lipids, including LDL cholesterol and triglycerides, along with increases in HDL cholesterol

Contraindications History of estrogenic tumors (eg, endometrial or breast cancer)

Warnings May alter response to hormone replacement therapy; use with caution in individuals with history of thromboembolism or stroke

Potential/Suspected Interactions Increased Effect/Toxicity: Estrogen-containing medications, hormonal contraceptives, hormone replacement therapy (HRT)

St John's Wort

Synonyms Amber Touch-and-Feel; Goatweed; *Hypercium perforatum*; Klamath Weed; Rosin Rose

Use Antibacterial, anti-inflammatory, antiviral (high doses), anxiolytic, wound-healing agent; treatment of AIDS (popular due to possible antiretroviral activity), anxiety and stress, insomnia; mild to moderate depression; bruises, muscle soreness, and sprains; vitiligo

Per Commission E: Psychovegetative disorders, depressive moods, anxiety and/or nervous unrest; oily preparations for dyspeptic complaints; oily preparations externally for treatment of post-therapy of acute and contused injuries, myalgia, first degree burns

Effects on Bleeding None reported

Local Anesthetic/Vasoconstrictor Precautions No information available to require special precautions

Dosage

Oral: 300 mg 3 times/day (standardized to contain 0.3% to 0.5% hypericin and/or 3% to 5% hyperforin per dose); minimum of 4-6 weeks therapy recommended

Topical: Apply oil extract to bruises and use for muscle soreness and sprains

Mechanism of Action/Effect Active ingredients are xanthones, flavonoids (hypericin) which can act as MAO inhibitors (although *in vitro* activity is minimal); majority of activity appears to be related to GABA modulation; may also be related to dopamine, serotonin, norepinephrine modulation

Adverse Reactions Frequency not defined:

Cardiovascular: **Tachycardia**

Dermatologic: Photosensitization (especially in fair-skinned persons per Commission E)

Gastrointestinal: GI upset

Contraindications Children <2 years of age, indinavir, therapeutic immunosuppressants, stimulants, SSRIs, antidepressants, digoxin, endogenous depression, pregnancy

Warnings May be photosensitizing; use caution with drugs metabolized by CYP3A3/4 and tyramine-containing foods (eg, cheese, wine). Use with caution in individuals taking antidepressants, cardiac glycosides, MAO inhibitors, narcotics, reserpine, stimulants, and SSRIs. High does may elevate LFTs (reversible). May alter absorption of calcium, copper, magnesium, and zinc due to tannins. Interacts with many drugs, see below.

Potential/Suspected Interactions

Increased Effect/Toxicity: SSRIs or other antidepressants, tetracycline (photosensitivity)

Decreased Effect: Appears to induce CYP3A3/4 enzymes, potentially reducing effect of many medications (eg, ritonavir, MAO inhibitors, levodopa, 5-hydroxytryptophan, diltiazem, nicardipine, verapamil, etoposide, paclitaxel, vinblastine, vincristine, glucocorticoids, dextromethorphan, ephedrine, lithium, meperidine, pseudoephedrine, selegiline, yohimbine, and ACE inhibitors)

Turmeric

Synonyms *Curcuma longa*

Use Anti-inflammatory, antioxidant, antiplatelet, antirheumatic; treatment of rheumatoid arthritis and other inflammatory conditions, hypercholesterolemia, and hyperlipidemia

Effects on Bleeding May see increased bleeding due to inhibition of platelet aggregation

Local Anesthetic/Vasoconstrictor Precautions No information available to require special precautions

Dosage Oral: 300 mg 3 times/day with meals (standardized to contain 95% curcuminoids per dose)

Mechanism of Action/Effect Anti-inflammatory activity claimed to be comparable to NSAIDs in treatment of rheumatoid arthritis. Antioxidant activity is associated with phenolic fraction, curcuminoids, which also inhibit leukotrienes and prostaglandin synthesis. Curcuminoids reportedly lowered the levels of blood lipid peroxides; may decrease LDL cholesterol and total cholesterol, while increasing HDL cholesterol.

Contraindications Active bleeding (eg, intracranial bleeding, peptic ulcer), biliary obstruction

Warnings Use with caution in individuals with history of bleeding, hemostatic or drug-related hemostatic disorders, and those taking anticoagulants (eg, aspirin or aspirin-containing products, NSAIDs, warfarin) or antiplatelet agents (eg, clopidogrel, dipyridamole, ticlopidine). Discontinue at least 14 days prior to dental or surgical procedures.

Potential/Suspected Interactions Increased Effect/Toxicity:

Anticoagulant/antiplatelet agents and antihyperlipidemics

Herbs with anticoagulant/antiplatelet properties: Alfalfa, anise, bilberry, bladderwrack, bromelain, cat's claw, celery, coleus, cordyceps, dong quai, evening primrose, fenugreek, feverfew, garlic, ginger, ginkgo biloba, ginseng (American/Panax/Siberian), grape seed, green tea, guggul, horse chestnut seed, horseradish, licorice, prickly ash, red clover, reishi, sweet clover, white willow

Uva Ursi

Synonyms *Arctostaphylos uva-ursi*; Bearberry

Use Analgesic, antiseptic, astringent, diuretic; treatment and prevention of urinary tract infections; prevention of kidney stones; treatment of bladder infections, urethritis, and a variety of renal disorders (eg, cystitis, nephritis, nephrolithiasis)

Effects on Bleeding None reported

Local Anesthetic/Vasoconstrictor Precautions No information available to require special precautions

Dosage Oral: 100-200 mg/day (standardized to contain 10% to 25% arbutin per dose)

Mechanism of Action/Effect A potent urinary antiseptic with an astringent effect on the lower digestive tract, reducing general intestinal irritation; contains arbutin, a phenolic glycoside that demonstrates analgesic and antiseptic properties in the urinary tract similar to phenazopyridine; disinfectant properties are most prominent in alkaline urine. Constituents of whole plant preparations are believed to enhance efficacy by contributing to urinary alkalinization. Arbutin is destroyed in the GI tract but additional plant components block its degradation and enhance absorption when whole plant preparations are ingested.

Adverse Reactions Frequency not defined (high doses):

Central nervous system: **Convulsions**

Gastrointestinal: **Vomiting**

Contraindications Lactation and pregnancy, renal failure; use >7-10 days

Warnings May cause green-brown discoloration of urine; may alter GI absorption of other herbs, minerals, or drugs (especially calcium, copper, magnesium, and zinc) due to tannins. Use caution with individuals taking diuretics; avoid other herbs with diuretic properties (see below).

Potential/Suspected Interactions May alter absorption of other herbs, minerals, or drugs.

Increased Effect/Toxicity: Herbs with diuretic properties: Artichoke, celery seed, corn silk, couchgrass, dandelion, elder flower, horsetail, juniper berry, kava, shepherd's purse, yarrow

Decreased Effect: Has decreased effect in acidic urine; drinking water with 1 tsp baking soda prior to use may promote conversion of hydroquinones to their active form.

Valerian

Synonyms Radix; Red Valerian; *Valeriana edulis*; *Valeriana wallichi*

Use Antispasmotic, anxiolytic, sedative (mild); treatment of anxiety and panic attacks, headache, intestinal cramps, nervous tension during PMS and menopause, restless motor syndrome and muscle spasms, sleep disorders (eg, insomnia, jet lag)

Per Commission E: Treatment of sleep disorders based on nervous conditions, restlessness

Effects on Bleeding None reported

Local Anesthetic/Vasoconstrictor Precautions No information available to require special precautions

Dosage Oral: 200 mg 1-4 times/day (standardized to contain 0.8% to 1% valerenic acids per dose)

Dried root: 0.3-1 g

Sedative: 1-3 g (1-3 mL of tincture)

Mechanism of Action/Effect May affect neurotransmitter levels (serotonin, GABA, and norepinephrine)

(Continued)

Valerian *(Continued)*

Adverse Reactions Frequency not defined:

Cardiovascular: **Cardiac disturbances** (unspecified)

Central nervous system: Fatigue, **lightheadedness, restlessness**

Gastrointestinal: **Nausea**

Neuromuscular & skeletal: **Tremor**

Ocular: Blurred vision

Contraindications Children <3 years of age

Warnings Advise caution when driving or operating heavy machinery. Use only valepotriate and baldrinal-free supplements in children <12 years of age due to potential mutagenic properties. Use with caution in individuals taking antianxiety or antidepressant agents, antipsychotics, histamines, and hypnotics/sedatives. Avoid herbs with sedative properties (see below).

Potential/Suspected Interactions Increased Effect/Toxicity:

Antianxiety or antidepressant agents, antipsychotics, antihistamines, barbiturates, other CNS depressants (not synergistic with alcohol), hypnotics/sedatives

Herbs with sedative properties: Gotu kola, kava, SAMe, St John's wort, and valerian

Vanadium

Use Treatment of type 1 and type 2 diabetes

Effects on Bleeding None reported

Local Anesthetic/Vasoconstrictor Precautions No information available to require special precautions

Dosage Oral: RDI: 250 mcg 1-3 times/day

Mechanism of Action/Effect Reported to be a cofactor in nicotinamide adenine dinucleotide phosphate (NADPH) oxidation reactions, lipoprotein lipase activity, amino acid transport, and hematopoiesis; may augment glucose regulation

Adverse Reactions No dietary toxicity or serious side effects have been reported, however, industrial exposure has resulted in toxicity.

Warnings May alter glucose regulation; use with caution in diabetics, those predisposed to hypoglycemia, or taking hypoglycemic agents (eg, insulin). Monitor blood sugar and dosage of these agents; may require adjustment (should be carefully coordinated among the individual's healthcare providers).

Potential/Suspected Interactions Increased Effect:

Oral hypoglycemics, insulin

Herbs with hypoglycemic properties: Alfalfa, aloe, bilberry, bitter melon, burdock, celery, damiana, fenugreek, garcinia, garlic, ginger, ginseng (American), gymnema, marshmallow, stinging nettle

Wild Yam

Synonyms *Dioscorea villosa*

Use Anti-inflammatory, antispasmodic, cholagogue, diuretic (high doses), expectorant (high doses); treatment of diverticulitis, dysmenorrhea, intestinal colic, menopausal symptoms, nausea, premenstrual syndrome (PMS), rheumatic and other inflammatory conditions; female vitality

Effects on Bleeding None reported

Local Anesthetic/Vasoconstrictor Precautions No information available to require special precautions

Dosage Adults:

Oral: 250 mg 1-3 times/day (standardized to contain 10% diosgenin per dose)

Liquid extract: 2-4 mL/day

Tea: 1-2 teaspoons root steeped in 1 cup boiling water for 15 minutes; drink 3 times/day

Topical: Apply as directed

Mechanism of Action/Effect Primarily used for its spasmolytic properties; appears to decrease spasm in the large intestine and uterus; contains the steroidal saponin, diosgenin, but the plant itself is devoid of estrogen and progesterone. Anti-inflammatory action is believed to be due to an affinity for steroid receptors shown by the steroidal saponins present in the plant.

Adverse Reactions Frequency not defined: Gastrointestinal: **Emesis** (high doses), GI upset (sensitive individuals)

Contraindications Estrogen, progesterone, hormonal contraceptives, hormone replacement therapy (HRT), history of endometrial cancer or estrogen-dependent tumors

Warnings Use with caution in individuals with a history of stroke or thromboembolic disease and those taking steroids, hormonal contraceptives, or receiving hormone replacement therapy (HRT). Use in children, or women during lactation or pregnancy is not recommended. Overdose may result in poisoning. Avoid other anabolic herbs (see below).

Potential/Suspected Interactions Increased Effect:

Androgens, estrogens, hormonal contraceptives, hormone replacement therapy (HRT), steroids

Anabolic herbs: Devil's club, dong quai, ginseng (American/Asian/Siberian), muira puama, sarsparilla, suma, tribulus

Herbs with estrogenic properties: Black cohosh, dong quai, and evening primrose

Yohimbe

Related Information

Yohimbine *on page 1401*

Synonyms Johimbe; *Pausinystalia yohimbe*; Yohimbehe cortex

Use Anesthetic (local), antiatherogenic, antiviral, aphrodesiac, stimulant, sympathomimetic, thermogenic, vasodilator, vasopressomimetic; treatment of angina pectoris, arteriosclerosis, exhaustion, male erectile dysfunction

Effects on Bleeding None reported

Local Anesthetic/Vasoconstrictor Precautions Has potential to interact with epinephrine and levonordefrin to result in increased BP; use vasoconstrictor with caution

Dosage Adults: Oral: 500-750 mg twice daily

Mechanism of Action/Effect Alkaloid which contains several other psychoactive alkaloids believed to have an effect similar to yohimbine; has CNS, respiratory, and thyroid stimulatory activity; blocks peripheral 5-HT receptors and prevents accumulation of lipid-containing plaques on innermost layers of arteries; has selective alpha$_2$ adrenergic blocking properties; aphrodisiac activity may be due to enlargement of the vasculature in the genitals, increase of nerve impulses to genital tissue, and an increased transmission of reflex excitability in the sacral region of the spinal cord; may have MAO inhibitor activity

Adverse Reactions Frequency not defined:

Cardiovascular: **Cardiac failure, hypertension, tachycardia, vasoconstriction**

Central nervous system: Insomnia

Gastrointestinal: **Increased peristalsis**, dyspepsia

High doses:

Cardiovascular: **Hypotension**

Central nervous system: **Dizziness, headache, hyperactivity, irritability, psychosis, tremor**

Gastrointestinal: Anorexia, **xerostomia**

Ocular: Decreased visual acuity

Respiratory: **Asthmatic attack**

Miscellaneous: **Sweating**

Contraindications Alpha$_2$-blockers, anticoagulant or antiplatelet agents, antidepressants, asthma, bethanechol, carbachol, cardiovascular disease (eg, arrhythmias, hypertension), chronic inflammation of genitalia, chronic prostatitis, diabetes, hyperthyroidism, MAO inhibitors, metoclopramide, pilocarpine, pregnancy, psychiatric disorders

Warnings Toxic doses may trigger cardiac failure, hypotension, and psychosis. Use with caution in individuals with diabetes, GI ulceration, or osteoporosis. Avoid other herbs with hypertensive, parasympathomimetic, sympathomimetic, thyroid-stimulating, or vasopressomimetic properties (see below).

Potential/Suspected Interactions Antihypertensives; may cause both hyper- and hypotension (dose-dependent)

Increased Effect/Toxicity:

Alpha$_2$ blockers, MAO inhibitors, naloxone, other sympathomimetics, tricyclic antidepressants

Herbs with hypertensive properties: Bayberry, blue cohosh, cayenne, ephedra, ginger, ginseng, kola nut (caffeine), licorice

Herbs with parasympathomimetic properties: Bittersweet, blood root, blue flag, bryony, dogbane, dogwood, false/green hellebore, horse chestnut, huperzineA, immortal, jaborandi, leptandra, pasque flower, pink root, pleurisy root, pokeweed, senega snakeroot, wahoo

Herbs with sympathomimetic properties: Calamus, cayenne, ephedra, Fu-tse (Fo-tzu), guarana, kola nut (caffeine), night blooming cereus, peyote (mescal buttons), scotch broom tops, Syrian rue, yellow jasmine

Thyroid-stimulating herbs: Fu-tse (Fo-tzu), gotu kola, ephedra, mustard

Herbs with vasopressomimetic properties: Goat's head, peyote (mescal buttons)

EFFECTS ON VARIOUS SYSTEMS

CARDIOVASCULAR SYSTEM

CONGESTIVE HEART FAILURE

(Diuretics, Xanthine derivatives, Licorice, Ginseng, Aconite)

Alisma plantago, bearberry (*Arctostaphylos uva-ursi*), buchu (*Barosma betulina*), couch grass, dandelion, horsetail rush, juniper, licorice, and xanthine derivatives exert varying degrees of diuretic action. Many patients with congestive heart failure (CHF) are already taking a diuretic medication. By taking products containing one or more of these components, patients already on diuretic medications may increase their risk for dehydration.

Ginseng and licorice can potentially worsen congestive heart failure and edema by causing fluid retention. Aconite has varying effects on the heart that itself could lead to heart failure. Patients with CHF should be advised to consult with their healthcare provider before using products containing any of these components.

HYPERTENSION/HYPOTENSION

(Diuretics, Ginkgo biloba, Ginseng, Hawthorn, Ma-huang, Xanthine derivatives)

The stimulant properties of ginseng and ma-huang could worsen pre-existing hypertension. Elevated blood pressure has been reported as a side effect of ginseng. Although ma-huang contains ephedrine, a known vasoconstrictor, ma-huang's effect on blood pressure varies between individuals. Ma-huang can cause hypotension or hypertension. Due to its unpredictable effects, patients with pre-existing hypertension should use caution when using natural products containing ma-huang. Providers should caution patients with labile hypertension against the use of ginseng.

The diuretic effect of xanthine derivatives and other diuretic components could increase the effects of antihypertensive medications, increasing the risk for hypotension. Hawthorn and ginkgo biloba can cause vasodilation increasing the hypotensive effects of antihypertensive medication. Patients susceptible to hypotension or patients taking antihypertensive medication should use caution when taking products containing xanthine derivatives or diuretics. Patients with pre-existing hypertension or hypotension who wish to use products containing these components should be closely monitored by a healthcare professional for changes in blood pressure control.

ARRHYTHMIAS

(Ginseng)

It has been reported that ginseng may increase the risk of arrhythmias, although it is unclear whether this effect is due to the actual ingredient (ginseng) or other possible impurities. Patients at risk for arrhythmias should be cautioned against the use of products containing ginseng without first consulting with their healthcare provider.

CENTRAL NERVOUS SYSTEM

(Aconite, Ginseng, Xanthine derivatives)

Aconite and hawthorn have potentially sedating effects, and aconite also contains various alkaloids and traces of ephedrine. Some documented central nervous system (CNS) effects of aconite include sedation, vertigo, and incoordination. Hawthorn has been reported to exert a depressive effect on the CNS leading to sedation.

Ginseng, ma-huang, and xanthine derivatives can exert a stimulant effect on the central nervous system. Some of the CNS effects of ginseng include nervousness, insomnia, and euphoria. The action of ma-huang is due to the presence of ephedrine and pseudoephedrine. Ma-huang exerts a stimulant action on the CNS similar to decongestant/weight loss products (Dexatrim®, etc) thus causing nervousness, insomnia, and anxiety. Kola nut, green tea, guarana, and yerba mate contain varying amounts of caffeine, a xanthine derivative. Stimulant properties exerted by these herbs are expected to be comparable to those of caffeine, including insomnia, nervousness, and anxiety.

Products containing aconite and hawthorn should be used with caution in patients with known history of depression, vertigo, or syncope. Ginseng or xanthine derivatives should be avoided in patients with history of insomnia or anxiety. Use of natural products with these components may contribute to a worsening of a patient's pre-existing medical condition. Patients taking CNS-active medications should avoid or use extreme caution when using preparations containing any of the above components. These components may interact directly or indirectly with CNS-active medications causing an increase or decrease in overall effect.

ENDOCRINE SYSTEM

DIABETES MELLITUS

(Chromium, Glucomannan, Ginseng, Hawthorn, Ma-huang, Periploca, Spirulina)

Ma-huang and spirulina both may increase glucose levels. This could cause a decrease in glucose control, thereby, increasing a patient's risk for hyperglycemia. Patients with diabetes or glucose intolerance should avoid using ma-huang and spirulina containing products.

Chromium, ginseng, glucomannan, periploca (*gymneme sylvestre*), and hawthorn should be used with caution in patients being treated for diabetes. These ingredients may reduce glucose levels increasing the risk for hypoglycemia in patients who are already taking a hypoglycemic agent. Patients with diabetes who wish to use products containing these ingredients should be closely monitored for fluctuations in blood glucose levels.

GASTROINTESTINAL SYSTEM

PEPTIC ULCER DISEASE

(Betaine Hydrochloride, White Willow)

Betaine hydrochloride is a source of hydrochloric acid. The acid released from betaine hydrochloride could aggravate an existing ulcer. White willow, like aspirin, contains salicylates.

Aspirin has been known to induce gastric damage by direct irritation on the gastric mucosa and by an indirect systemic effect. As a result, patients with a history of peptic ulcer disease or gastritis are informed to avoid use of aspirin and other salicylate derivatives. These precautions should also apply to white willow. Patients with a history of peptic ulcer disease or gastritis should not use products containing white willow or betaine hydrochloride as either could exacerbate ulcers.

INFLAMMATORY BOWEL DISEASE

(Cascara Sagrada, Senna, Dandelion)

Cascara sagrada and senna are stimulant laxatives. Their laxative effect is exerted by stimulation of peristalsis in the colon and by inhibition of water and electrolyte secretion. The laxative effect produced by these herbs could induce an exacerbation of inflammatory bowel disease. Patients with a history of inflammatory bowel disease should avoid using products containing cascara sagrada or senna, and use caution when taking products containing dandelion which may also have a laxative effect.

OBSTRUCTION/ILEUS

(Glucomannan, Kelp, Psyllium)

Glucomannan, kelp, and psyllium act as bulk laxatives. In the presence of water, bulk laxatives swell or form a viscous solution adding extra bulk in the gastrointestinal tract. The resulting mass is thought to stimulate peristalsis. In the presence of an ileus, these laxatives could cause an obstruction.

If sufficient water is not consumed when taking a bulk laxative, a semisolid mass can form resulting in an obstruction. Any patient who wishes to take a natural product containing kelp, psyllium, or glucomannan should drink sufficient water to decrease the risk of obstruction. This may be of concern in particular disease states such as CHF or other cases where excess fluid intake may influence the existing disease presentation. Patients with a suspected obstruction or ileus should avoid using products containing kelp, psyllium, or glucomannan without consent of their primary healthcare provider.

HEMATOLOGIC SYSTEM

ANTICOAGULATION THERAPY & COAGULATION DISORDERS

(Horsetail Rush, Ginseng, Ginkgo Biloba, Guarana, White Willow)

Horsetail rush, ginseng, ginkgo biloba, guarana, and white willow can potentially affect platelet aggregation and bleeding time. Ginkgo biloba, ginseng, guarana, and white willow inhibit platelet aggregation resulting in an increase in bleeding time. Horsetail

(Continued)

EFFECTS ON VARIOUS SYSTEMS *(Continued)*

rush, on the other hand, may decrease bleeding time. Patients with coagulation disorders or patients on anticoagulation therapy may be sensitive to the effects on coagulation by these components and should, therefore, avoid use of products containing any of these components.

OTHER

PHENYLKETONURIA

(Aspartame, Spirulina)

Patients with phenylketonuria should not use products containing aspartame or spirulina. Aspartame, a common artificial sweetener, is metabolized to phenylalanine, while spirulina contains phenylalanine.

GOUT

(Diuretics, White Willow)

Patients with a history of gout should avoid using natural products containing components with diuretic action or white willow. By increasing urine output, ingredients with diuretic action may concentrate uric acid in the blood increasing the risk of gout in these patients. White willow, like aspirin, may inhibit excretion of urate resulting in an increase in uric acid concentration. The increase in urate levels could cause precipitation of uric acid resulting in an exacerbation of gout.

ORAL MEDICINE TOPICS

PART I:

DENTAL MANAGEMENT AND THERAPEUTIC CONSIDERATIONS IN MEDICALLY-COMPROMISED PATIENTS

This first part of the chapter focuses on common medical conditions and their associated drug therapies with which the dentist must be familiar. Patient profiles with commonly associated drug regimens are described.

TABLE OF CONTENTS

Cardiovascular Diseases 1456
Gastrointestinal Disorders 1474
Respiratory Diseases 1476
Endocrine Disorders and Pregnancy 1479
HIV Infection and AIDS 1482
Rheumatoid Arthritis, Osteoarthritis, and Osteoporosis 1488
Nonviral Infectious Diseases 1493
Antibiotic Prophylaxis - Preprocedural Guidelines for Dental Patients 1507
Systemic Viral Diseases 1517

CARDIOVASCULAR DISEASES

Cardiovascular disease is the most prevalent human disease affecting over 60 million Americans and this group of diseases accounts >50% of all deaths in the United States. Surgical and pharmacological therapy have resulted in many cardiovascular patients living healthy and profitable lives. Consequently, patients presenting to the dental office may require treatment planning modifications related to the medical management of their cardiovascular disease. For the purposes of this text, we will cover coronary artery disease (CAD) including angina pectoris and myocardial infarction, cardiac arrhythmias, heart failure, and hypertension.

CARDIOVASCULAR DRUGS AND DENTAL CONSIDERATIONS

Some of the drug listings are redundant because the drugs are used to treat more than one cardiovascular disorder. As a convenience to the reader, each table has been constructed as a stand alone listing of drugs for the given disorder. The dental implications of these cardiovascular drugs are listed in Tables 8 and 9. Each of these 2 tables is a consolidation of the drugs from Tables 1-7. The more frequent cardiovascular, respiratory, and central nervous system adverse reactions which you may see in the dental patient are described in Table 8 *on page 1469*. Table 9 *on page 1472* describes the effects on dental treatment reported for these drugs. It is suggested that the reader use Tables 8 and 9 to check for potential effects which could occur in the medicated cardiovascular dental patients.

CORONARY ARTERY DISEASE

Any long-term decrease in the delivery of oxygen to the heart muscle can lead to the condition ischemic heart disease. Often arteriosclerosis and atherosclerosis result in a narrowing of the coronary vessels' lumina and are the most common causes of vascular ischemic heart disease. Other causes such as previous infarct, mitral valve regurgitation, and ruptured septa may also lead to ischemia in the heart muscle. The two most common major conditions that result from ischemic heart disease are angina pectoris and myocardial infarction. Sudden death, a third category, can likewise result from ischemia.

To the physician, the most common presenting sign or symptom of ischemic heart disease is chest pain. This chest pain can be of a transient nature as in angina pectoris or the result of a myocardial infarction. It is now believed that sudden death represents a separate occurrence that essentially involves the development of a lethal cardiac arrhythmia or coronary artery spasm leading to an acute shutdown of the heart muscle blood supply. Risk factors in patients for coronary atherosclerosis include cigarette smoking, elevated blood lipids, hypertension, as well as diabetes mellitus, age, and gender (male).

Coronary artery disease (CAD) is the cause of about half of all deaths in the United States. CAD has been shown to be correlated with the levels of plasma cholesterol and/or triacylglycerol-containing lipoprotein particles. Primary prevention focuses on averting the development of CAD. In contrast, secondary prevention of (CAD) focuses on therapies to reduce morbidity and mortality in patients with clinically documented CAD.

Lipid-lowering and cardioprotective drugs provide significant risk-reducing benefits in the secondary prevention of CAD. By reducing the levels of total and low density cholesterol through the inhibition of hydroxymethylglutaryl coenzyme A (HMG-CoA) reductase, statin drugs significantly improve survival. Cardioprotective drug therapy includes antiplatelet/anticoagulant agents to inhibit platelet adhesion, aggregation and blood coagulation; beta-blockers to lower heart rate, contractility and blood pressure; and the angiotensin-converting enzyme (ACE) inhibitors to lower peripheral resistance and workload. For a listing of these drugs, see Table 1 on following page.

Table 1.
DRUGS USED IN THE TREATMENT OF CAD

Reduction of Total and Low-Density Cholesterol Levels

Bile Acid Sequestrant

Colesevelam *on page 365*

HMG-CoA Reductase Inhibitors

Fluvastatin *on page 603*
Lovastatin *on page 828*
Pravastatin *on page 1106*
Simvastatin *on page 1223*
Atorvastatin *on page 140*

Fibrate Group

Clofibrate *on page 347*
Fenofibrate *on page 561*
Gemfibrozil *on page 631*

Bile Acid Resins

Cholestyramine *on page 318*
Colestipol *on page 365*

Nicotinic Acid

Cardioprotective Therapy

Antiplatelet/Anticoagulant Agents

Aspirin *on page 131*
Clopidogrel *on page 353*
Ticlopidine *on page 1307*
Warfarin *on page 1397*

Beta-Adrenergic Receptor Blockers

Atenolol *on page 137*
Metoprolol *on page 901*
Propranolol *on page 1139*

Angiotensin-Converting Enzyme (ACE) Inhibitors

Captopril *on page 238*
Enalapril *on page 492*
Fosinopril *on page 616*
Lisinopril *on page 813*
Ramipril *on page 1166*

ANGINA PECTORIS

(EMPHASIS ON UNSTABLE ANGINA)

Numerous physiologic triggers can initiate the rupture of plaque in coronary blood vessels. Rupture leads to the activation, adhesion and aggregation of platelets, and the activation of the clotting cascade, resulting in the formation of occlusive thrombus. If this process leads to the complete occlusion of the artery, acute myocardial infarction with ST-segment elevation occurs. Alternatively, if the process leads to severe stenosis and the artery remains patent, unstable angina occurs. Triggers which induce unstable angina include physical exertion, mechanical stress due to an increase in cardiac contractility, pulse rate, blood pressure, and vasoconstriction.

Unstable angina accounts for more than 1 million hospital admissions annually. In 1989, Braunwald devised a classification system according to the severity of the clinical manifestations of angina. These manifestations are defined as acute angina while at rest (within the 48 hours before presentation), subacute angina while at rest (within the previous month but not within the 48 hours before presentation), or new onset of accelerated (progressively more severe) angina. The system also classifies angina according to the clinical circumstances in which unstable angina develops, defined as either angina in the presence or absence of other conditions (ie, fever, hypoxia, tachycardia, thyrotoxicosis) and whether or not ECG abnormalities are present. Recently, the term "acute coronary syndrome" has been used to describe the range of conditions that includes unstable angina, non-Q-wave myocardial infarction, and Q-wave myocardial infarction.

Pharmacologic therapy to treat unstable angina includes antiplatelet drugs, antithrombin therapy, and conventional antianginal therapy with beta-blockers, nitrates, and calcium channel blockers. These drug groups and selected agents are listed in Table 2 on following page.

CARDIOVASCULAR DISEASES *(Continued)*

Table 2.
DRUGS USED TO MANAGE UNSTABLE ANGINA

Antiplatelet Drugs
- Aspirin *on page 131*
- Clopidogrel *on page 353*
- Ticlopidine *on page 1307*
- **Glycoprotein IIb/IIIa Receptor Antagonists**
  - Abciximab *on page 23*
  - Eptifibatide *on page 507*
  - Tirofiban *on page 1313*

Antithrombin Drugs
- **Indirect Thrombin Inhibitors**
  - Unfractionated heparin (Heparin) *on page 662*
  - Low molecular weight heparins
    - Dalteparin *on page 394*
    - Enoxaparin *on page 495*
    - Tinzaparin *on page 1311*
- **Direct Thrombin Inhibitors**
  - Lepirudin *on page 781*
  - Argatroban *on page 120*
- **Dicumarols**
  - Warfarin *on page 1397*

Conventional Antianginal Drugs
- **Beta-Blockers**
  - Atenolol *on page 137*
  - Bisoprolol *on page 188*
  - Carteolol *on page 254*
  - Nadolol *on page 943*
  - Propranolol *on page 1139*
- **Nitrates**
  - Isosorbide Dinitrate *on page 750*
  - Isosorbide Mononitrate *on page 751*
  - Nitroglycerin *on page 981*
- **Calcium Channel Blockers**
  - Diltiazem *on page 447*
  - Nifedipine *on page 973*
  - Verapamil *on page 1382*

Antiplatelet Drugs

Aspirin reduces platelet aggregation by blocking platelet cyclo-oxygenase through irreversible acetylation. This action prevents the formation of thromboxane A_2. A number of studies have confirmed that aspirin reduces the risk of death from cardiac causes and fatal and nonfatal myocardial infarction by approximately 50% to 70% in patients presenting with unstable angina. Ticlopidine is a second-line alternative to aspirin in the treatment of unstable angina and is also used as adjunctive therapy with aspirin to prevent thrombosis after placement of intracoronary stents. Ticlopidine blocks ADP-mediated platelet aggregation. Clopidogrel inhibits platelet aggregation by affecting the ADP-dependent activation of the glycoprotein IIb/IIIa complex. Clopidogrel is chemically related to ticlopidine, but has fewer side effects.

Platelet Glycoprotein IIb/IIIa Receptor Antagonists

Antagonists of glycoprotein IIb/IIIa, a receptor on the platelet for adhesive proteins, inhibit the final common pathway involved in adhesion, activation and aggregation. Presently, there exist three classes of inhibitors. One class is murine-human chimeric antibodies of which abciximab is the prototype. The other two classes are the synthetic peptide forms (eg, eptifibatide) and the synthetic nonpeptide forms (eg, tirofiban). These agents, in combination with heparin and aspirin, have been used to treat unstable angina, significantly reducing the incidence of death or myocardial infarction.

Antithrombin Drugs

Unfractionated heparin, in combination with aspirin, is used to treat unstable angina. Unfractionated heparin consists of polysaccharide chains which bind to antithrombin III, causing a conformational change that accelerates the inhibition of thrombin and factor Xa. Unfractionated heparin is therefore an indirect thrombin inhibitor. Unfractionated heparin can only be administered intravenously. Low-molecular-weight heparins (LMWH) have a more predictable pharmacokinetic profile than the unfractionated heparin and can be administered subcutaneously. These heparins have a mechanism of action and use similar to unfractionated heparin.

The direct antithrombins decrease thrombin activity in a manner independent of any actions on antithrombin III. Two such direct antithrombins are lepirudin (also known as recombinant hirudin) and argatroban. These agents are highly specific, direct thrombin inhibitor with each molecule capable of binding to one molecule of thrombin and inhibiting its thrombogenic activity. Direct antithrombins are used for the prevention or reduction of ischemic complications associated with unstable angina.

Warfarin (Coumadin®) elicits its anticoagulant effect by interfering with the hepatic synthesis of vitamin K-dependent coagulation factors II, VII, IX, and X. Although warfarin appears to be somewhat effective after myocardial infarction in preventing death or recurrent myocardial infarction, its effectiveness in the treatment of acute coronary syndrome is questionable. Combination therapy with aspirin and heparin followed by warfarin has resulted in reduced incidence of recurrent angina, myocardial infarction, death, or all three at 14 days as compared with aspirin alone. In contrast, another study however failed to show any additional benefit in the treatment of acute coronary syndrome using a combination of aspirin and warfarin compared to aspirin alone.

Conventional Antianginal Therapy: Beta-Blockers, Nitrates, Calcium Channel Blockers

Current thinking is that there is a definite link between unstable angina and acute myocardial infarction. In this regard, beta-blockers are currently recommended as first-line agents in all acute coronary syndromes. A meta-analysis of studies involving 4700 patients with unstable angina demonstrated a 13% reduction in the risk of myocardial infarction among patients treated with beta-blockers. The various preparations of beta-blockers appear to have equal efficacy. The effects of beta-blockers are thought to be due to their ability to decrease myocardial oxygen demand.

Nitrates, such as nitroglycerin, are widely used in the management of unstable angina. Nitrates elicit a number of effects including a reduction in oxygen demand, arteriolar vasodilation, augmentation of collateral coronary blood flow and frequency of coronary vasospasm. Intravenous nitroglycerin is one of the first line therapies for unstable angina because of the ease of dose titration and the rapid resolution of effects. Continuous nitrate therapy with oral and transdermal patch preparations has resulted in tolerance to the beneficial effects of nitrates. A 6- to 8-hour daily nitrate-free interval will minimize the tolerance phenomenon. Also, supplemental use of vitamin C appears to prevent nitrate tolerance.

Calcium channel blockers such as nifedipine, verapamil, and diltiazem cause coronary vasodilation and reduced blood pressure. Because of these actions, the calcium channel blockers were thought to be a drug group which could be effective in the treatment of unstable angina. However, a meta analysis of studies in which patients with unstable angina were treated with calcium channel blockers found no effect of the drugs on the incidence of death or myocardial infarction. More recently, it has been shown that treatment with diltiazem and verapamil may result in increased survival and reduced rates of reinfarction in patients with acute coronary syndrome. Current thinking suggests that calcium channel blockers should be used in patients in whom beta-blockers are contraindicated or in those with refractory symptoms after treatments with aspirin, nitrates, or beta-blockers.

Dental Management

The dental management of the patient with angina pectoris may include sedation techniques for complicated procedures (see "Patients Requiring Sedation" *on page 1565*), to limit the extent of procedures, and to limit the use of local anesthesia containing 1:100,000 epinephrine to two capsules. Anesthesia without a vasoconstrictor might also be selected. The appropriate use of a vasoconstrictor in anesthesia, however, should be weighed against the necessity to maximize anesthesia. Complete history and appropriate referral and consultation with the patient's physician for those patients who are known to be at risk for angina pectoris is recommended.

MYOCARDIAL INFARCTION

Myocardial infarction is the leading cause of death in the United States. It is an acute irreversible ischemic event that produces an area of myocardial necrosis in the heart tissue. If a patient has a previous history of myocardial infarction, he/she may be taking a variety of drugs (ie, antihypertensives, lipid lowering drugs, ACE inhibitors, and antianginal medications) to not only prevent a second infarct, but to treat the long-term associated ischemic heart disease. Postmyocardial infarction patients are often taking anticoagulants such as warfarin and antiplatelet agents such as aspirin. Consultation with the prescribing physician by the dentist is necessary prior to invasive procedures. Temporary dose reduction may allow the dentist to proceed with very invasive procedures. Most procedures, however, can be accomplished without changing the anticoagulant therapy at all, using local hemostasis techniques.

Aspirin *on page 131*
Warfarin *on page 1397*

CARDIOVASCULAR DISEASES *(Continued)*

Thrombolytic drugs, that might dissolve hemostatic plugs, may also be given on a short-term basis immediately following an infarct and include:

Alteplase *on page 65*
Reteplase *on page 1174*
Streptokinase *on page 1243*
Tenecteplase *on page 1273*

Alteplase [tissue plasminogen activator (TPA)] is also currently in use for acute myocardial infarction. Following myocardial infarction and rehabilitation, outpatients may be placed on anticoagulants (such as coumadin), diuretics, beta-adrenergic blockers, ACE inhibitors to reduce blood pressure, and calcium channel blockers. Depending on the presence or absence of continued angina pectoris, patients may also be taking nitrates, beta-blockers, or calcium channel blockers as indicated for treatment of angina.

BETA-ADRENERGIC BLOCKING AGENTS CATEGORIZED ACCORDING TO SPECIFIC PROPERTIES

Alpha-Adrenergic Blocking Activity

Labetalol *on page 769*

Intrinsic Sympathomimetic Activity

Acebutolol *on page 25*
Pindolol *on page 1085*

Long Duration of Action and Fewer CNS Effects

Acebutolol *on page 25*
Atenolol *on page 137*
Betaxolol *on page 180*
Nadolol *on page 943*

Beta$_1$-Receptor Selectivity

Acebutolol *on page 25*
Atenolol *on page 137*
Metoprolol *on page 901*

Non-Selective (blocks both beta$_1$- and beta$_2$-receptors)

Betaxolol *on page 180*
Labetalol *on page 769*
Nadolol *on page 943*
Pindolol *on page 1085*
Propranolol *on page 1139*
Timolol *on page 1309*

ARRHYTHMIAS

Abnormal cardiac rhythm can develop spontaneously and survivors of a myocardial infarction are often left with an arrhythmia. An arrhythmia is any alteration or disturbance in the normal rate, rhythm, or conduction through the cardiac tissue. This is known as a cardiac arrhythmia. Abnormalities in rhythm can occur in either the atria or the ventricles. Various valvular deformities, drug effects, and chemical derangements can initiate arrhythmias. These arrhythmias can be a slowing of the heart rate (<60 beats/minute) as defined in bradycardia or tachycardia resulting in a rapid heart beat (usually >150 beats/minute). The dentist will encounter a variety of treatments for management of arrhythmias. Usually, underlying causes such as reduced cardiac output, hypertension, and irregular ventricular beats will require treatment. Pacemaker therapy is also sometimes used. Indwelling pacemakers may require supplementation with antibiotics, and consultation with the physician is certainly appropriate. Sinus tachycardia is often treated with drugs such as:

Propranolol *on page 1139*
Quinidine *on page 1158*

Beta-blockers are often used to slow cardiac rate and diazepam may be helpful when anxiety is a contributing factor in arrhythmia. When atrial flutter and atrial fibrillation are diagnosed, drug therapy is usually required.

Digitoxin *on page 440*
Digoxin *on page 441*

Atrial fibrillation (AF) is an arrhythmia characterized by multiple electrical activations in the atria resulting in scattered and disorganized depolarization and repolarization of the myocardium. Atrial contraction can lead to an irregular and rapid rate of ventricular contraction. The prevalence of atrial fibrillation within the US population ranges between 1% and 4%, with the incidence increasing with age. It is often associated with rheumatic valvular disease and nonvalvular conditions including coronary artery disease and hypertension. Coronary artery disease is present in about one-half of the patients with atrial fibrillation. Atrial fibrillation is a major risk factor for systemic and cerebral embolism. It is thought that thrombi develop as a result of stasis in the dilated left atrium and is dislodged by sudden changes in cardiac rhythm. About 10% of all strokes in patients >60 years of age are caused by atrial fibrillation.

The cornerstones of drug therapy for atrial fibrillation are the restoration and maintenance of a normal sinus rhythm through the use of antiarrhythmic drugs, ventricular rate control through the use of beta-blockers, digitalis drugs or calcium channel blockers, and stroke prevention through the use of anticoagulants.

Antiarrhythmic Drugs

Cardiac rhythm is conducted through the sinoatrial (SA) and atrioventricular (AV) nodes, bundle branches, and Purkinje fibers. Electrical impulses are transmitted within this system by the opening and closing of sodium and potassium channels. Antiarrhythmic drugs are classified by which channel they act upon, a classification known as Vaughan Williams after the author of the published paper. The Class I agents act primarily on sodium channels, and the Class III agents act on potassium channels. In addition, there are subclassifications within the Class I agents according to effects of the drug on conduction and refractoriness within the Purkinje and ventricular tissues. Class IA agents show moderate depression of conduction and prolongation of repolarization. Class IB agents show modest depression of conduction and shortening of repolarization. Class IC agents show marked depression of conduction and mild or no effect on repolarization. Class IA and IC agents are effective in the treatment of atrial fibrillation. Class IB agents (ie, lidocaine, phenytoin) are not used to treat atrial fibrillation, but are effective in treating ventricular arrhythmias. Class II drugs are the beta-adrenergic blocking drugs and Class IV are the calcium channel blockers. Table 3 lists the drugs and the categories used to treat atrial fibrillation.

Table 3.
DRUGS USED IN THE TREATMENT OF ATRIAL FIBRILLATION

Class I Antiarrhythmic Agents

- Disopyramide *on page 458*
- Flecainide *on page 574*
- Moricizine *on page 931*
- Procainamide *on page 1119*
- Propafenone *on page 1130*
- Quinidine *on page 1158*

Class II Antiarrhythmic Agents (Beta-Adrenergic Blockers)

Cardioselective (Beta$_1$-Receptor Block only)

- Acebutolol *on page 25*
- Atenolol *on page 137*
- Betaxolol *on page 180*
- Metoprolol *on page 901*

Noncardioselective (Beta$_1$- and Beta$_2$-Receptor Block)

- Nadolol *on page 943*
- Penbutolol *on page 1045*
- Pindolol *on page 1085*
- Propranolol *on page 1139*
- Timolol *on page 1309*

Class III Antiarrhythmic Agents

- Amiodarone *on page 80*
- Dofetilide *on page 464*
- Ibutilide *on page 706*
- Sotalol *on page 1235*

Class IV Antiarrhythmic Agents (Calcium Channel Blockers)

- Diltiazem *on page 447*
- Verapamil *on page 1382*

Miscellaneous Agents

- Digitalis
- Anticoagulants
  - Aspirin *on page 131*
  - Warfarin *on page 1397*

*Source: USP DI, Volumes I and II, Update, April, 1998.

Restoring and Maintaining Normal Sinus Rhythm

Cardioversion induced by drugs can usually restore sinus rhythm in patients with atrial fibrillation. Class I drugs (moricizine), Class IA drugs (disopyramide, procainamide, quinidine), Class IC drugs (flecainide, propafenone), and Class III antiarrhythmics (amiodarone, sotalol) are all effective in restoring normal sinus rhythm. Success rates may vary greatly and are complicated by the high rate of spontaneous conversion. The drugs used for pharmacologic conversion are also used to maintain sinus rhythm.

CARDIOVASCULAR DISEASES *(Continued)*

Ventricular Rate Control

It is accepted practice to treat patients with medication when the resting ventricular rate is >110 beats/minute. Digoxin, calcium channel blockers, and beta-adrenergic blockers are used in the regulation of ventricular rate. Digoxin increases the vagal tone to the AV node, calcium channel blockers slow the AV nodal conduction, and the beta-adrenergic blocking drugs decrease the sympathetic activation of the AV nodal conduction.

Stroke Prevention

Reports from stroke prevention trials indicate that patients with atrial fibrillation incurred a 4% annual risk of stroke if not treated. Also, patients with heart failure or coronary heart diseases were three times more likely to have a stroke than those without risk factors. Anticoagulation therapy with warfarin reduced the stroke risk by 64%. Warfarin was found to be more effective than aspirin in all age groups in the Stroke Prevention in Atrial Fibrillation II Trial. To achieve optimal levels of anticoagulation with the lowest incidence of bleeding, the INR (international normalized ratio) is usually maintained between 2 and 3. For patients <60 years of age with atrial fibrillation and having no other risk factors, no anticoagulant therapy is needed. Aspirin (325 mg daily) is recommended for those patients >60 years of age.

ANTICOAGULANT THERAPY

Many patients with ischemic heart disease, atherosclerosis, and those with atrial fibrillation are also frequently placed on anticoagulants such as Coumadin® (See Myocardial Infarction *on page 1459*).

Large numbers of patients are receiving oral anticoagulation therapy. The dental clinician is often faced with the decision as to how to manage these patients prior to invasive dental procedures. Key factors regarding the patient receiving anticoagulant therapy include: What is the bleeding risk of the procedure planned?, what are the clotting risks (ie, can the medication management be safely altered)?, and what is the patient's current anticoagulant therapy level in terms of bleeding measurements (ie, laboratory evaluations) and their prognosis? The International Normalized Ratio, or INR, is one of the most common coagulation values sought. The INR should be determined the day of the procedure if there is a high risk of bleeding.

Most patients receiving anticoagulant therapy are on one of two regimens. Warfarin, under the name Coumadin®, is the most common long-term outpatient anticoagulant given. Many patients, however, are also on aspirin products to achieve some level of anticoagulation. The mechanisms of the action of these two drugs are different and it is important that the clinician be aware of the appropriate tests and the appropriate time relative to treatment selection.

Partial thromboplastin time and bleeding time (IVY) are appropriate measures for platelet dysfunction. Aspirin, ticlopidine (Ticlid®), and other new drugs, such as Clopidogrel (Plavix®), are actually considered antiplatelet drugs, whereas oral Coumadin® is considered an oral anticoagulant. Aspirin works by inhibiting cyclo-oxygenase which is an enzyme involved in the platelet system associated with clot formation. As little as one aspirin (300 mg dose) can result in an alteration in this enzyme pathway. Although aspirin is cleared from the circulation very quickly (within 15-30 minutes), the effect on the life of the platelet may last up to 7-10 days. Therefore, the clinician planning an extensive invasive procedure on patients with antiplatelet therapy may wish to consider a change prior to one week before the invasive treatment. However, most routine dental procedures can be accomplished with no change in these medications using aggressive local hemostasis efforts and prudent treatment planning.

The effects of Coumadin® on the coagulation within patients, occur by way of the vitamin K-dependent clotting mechanism and are generally monitored by measuring the prothrombin time known as the PT. Often to prevent venous thrombosis, a patient will be maintained at approximately 1.5 times their normal prothrombin time. Other anticoagulant goals such as prevention of arterial thromboembolism, as in patients with artificial heart valves, may require 2-2.5 times the normal prothrombin time. It is important for the clinician to obtain not only the accurate PT but also the International Normalized Ratio (INR) for the patient. This ratio is calculated by dividing the patient's PT by the mean normal PT for the laboratory, which is determined by using the International Sensitivity Index (ISI) to adjust for the lab's reagents.

The response to oral anticoagulants varies greatly in patients and should be monitored regularly. The dental clinician planning an invasive procedure should consider not only what the patient can tell them from a historical point-of-view, but also when the last monitoring test was performed. In general, most dental procedures can be performed in patients that are 1.5 times normal or less. Most researchers suggest that 2.5 times normal poses little risk in most dental patients and procedures, but these values may be misleading unless the INR is also determined. When in doubt, the prudent dental clinician would consult with the patient's physician and obtain current prothrombin time and INR in order to evaluate fully and plan for his patients. The clinician is referred to the excellent review: Herman WW, Konzelman JL, and Sutley SH, "Current Perspectives on

Dental Patients Receiving Coumadin Anticoagulant Therapy," *J Am Dent Assoc*, 1997, 128:327-35.

Coumadin®-like Anticoagulants

Dicumarol *on page 433*
Warfarin *on page 1397*

Platelet Aggregation Inhibitors

Aspirin *on page 131*
Clopidogrel *on page 353*
Eptifibatide *on page 507*
Ticlopidine *on page 1307*
Tirofiban *on page 1313*

Anticoagulant, Other

Lepirudin *on page 781*

Antiplatelet Agent

Aspirin and Dipyridamole *on page 135*

Although not used specifically for this purpose, numerous herbal medicines and natural dietary supplements have been associated with inhibition of platelet aggregation or other anticoagulation effects, and therefore may lead to increased bleeding during invasive dental procedures. Current reports include bilberry, bromelain, cat's claw, devil's claw, dong quai, evening primrose, feverfew, garlic (irreversible inhibition), ginger (only at very high doses), ginkgo biloba, ginseng, grape seed, green tea, horse chestnut, and turmeric.

The basis for anticoagulation therapy is that mitral stenosis may be the result of the long-term arrhythmia and there is concern over the possibility of stroke. Ventricular dysrhythmias are often treated with drugs such as quinidine, procainamide, lidocaine, and beta-adrenergic agents. Quinidine is used for selected arrhythmias. Lidocaine is often used when there are ventricular dysrhythmias. Procainamide (Pronestyl®) is an alternative agent.

Over the past three decades, there has been an increasing use of drugs that relate to the clotting mechanism in patients. These drugs have included the widespread use of aspirin as well as an increasing use of the anticoagulant found in warfarin or Coumadin®. Also, there has been increasing evidence that more patients have a gastrointestinal sensitivity to aspirin. Therefore, alternative analgesics such as acetaminophen and the NSAID products have expanded in utilization tremendously. These factors resulted in numerous potential drug interactions that, until now, have been thought to be quite innocuous. The use of acetaminophen, which is primarily for analgesic and antipyretic properties, has increased dramatically. The drug is available as an over-the-counter medication for a wide range of nonspecific conditions and, in fact, in the United States, acetaminophen is the most frequently ingested medication.

Regarding dental management patients that are already taking warfarin, the use of analgesics is implicated as a potential source of drug interaction. In a recent article by Hayek in *JAMA*, it was found that patients taking warfarin for anticoagulation identified the use of dangerously elevated INRs and the fact was discovered that they concomitantly had been taking acetaminophen (not necessarily with their physician's recommendation). The study of the international normalized ratio (INR) in these patients has indicated that additional factors independently influence the INR, as well as the potential interaction with acetaminophen. Potential effects on the INR are greatest in patients taking acetaminophen at high doses over a protracted time period. Short term pain management with acetaminophen poses little risk. These factors included advanced malignancy, patients who did not take their warfarin properly (therefore, took more than was necessary), changes in oral intake of liquids or solids, acute diarrhea leading to dehydration, alcohol consumption, and vitamin K intake. The mechanisms of these augmenting factors for enhancement of the INR are that the cytochrome P450 system, present in the liver, is also affected by changes in metabolism associated with these factors. For instance, the metabolism of alcohol in the liver alters its ability to manage the CYP450 enzyme system necessary for warfarin, therefore, enhancing its presence and potentially increasing the half-life of warfarin. As oral intake of nutrients declines in patients with either diarrhea or reduced intake of liquids and/or solids, absorption of vitamin K is reduced and the vitamin K dependent system of metabolism of warfarin changes, therefore increasing warfarin blood levels. These factors, along with the liver metabolism of acetaminophen, have resulted in the increased concern that patients, who may be taking acetaminophen as an analgesic or for other reasons, may be at risk for enhancing or elevating, inadvertently, their anticoagulation effect of warfarin. The dentist should be aware of this potential interaction in prescribing any drug containing acetaminophen or in recommending that a patient use an analgesic for relief of even mild pain on a prolonged basis. Therefore, the dentist must be concerned with these factors and is referred to the discussion in the Pain Management section *on page 1524* for more consideration (adapted from *JAMA*, March 4, 1998, Vol 279, No 9).

Acetaminophen *on page 27*

CARDIOVASCULAR DISEASES *(Continued)*

HEART FAILURE

Heart failure is a condition in which the heart is unable to pump sufficient blood to meet the needs of the body. It is caused by impaired ability of the cardiac muscle to contract or by an increased workload imposed on the heart. Most frequently, the underlying cause of heart failure is coronary artery disease. Other contributory causes include hypertension, diabetes, idiopathic dilated cardiomyopathy, and valvular heart disease. It is estimated that heart failure affects approximately 5 million Americans. The New York Heart Association functional classification is regarded as the standard measure to describe the severity of a patient's symptom. Class I is characterized by having no limitation of physical activity. There is no dyspnea, fatigue, palpitations, or angina with ordinary physical activity. There is no objective evidence of cardiovascular dysfunction. Class II includes those patients having slight limitation of physical activity. These patients experience fatigue, palpitations, dyspnea, or angina with ordinary physical activity, but are comfortable at rest. There is evidence of minimal cardiovascular dysfunction. Class III is characterized by marked limitation of activity. Less than ordinary physical activity causes fatigue, palpitations, dyspnea, or angina, but patients are comfortable at rest. There is objective evidence of moderately severe cardiovascular dysfunction. Class IV is characterized by the inability to carry out any physical activity without discomfort. Symptoms of heart failure or anginal syndrome may be present even at rest, and any physical activity undertaken increases discomfort. There is objective evidence of severe cardiovascular dysfunction. Drug classes and the specific agents used to treat heart failure are listed in Table 4.

Table 4.
DRUGS USED IN THE TREATMENT OF HEART FAILURE

Angiotensin-Converting Enzyme Inhibitors (ACE)*
- Benazepril *on page 166*
- Captopril *on page 238*
- Enalapril *on page 492*
- Fosinopril *on page 616*
- Lisinopril *on page 813*
- Perindopril Ethumine *on page 1060*
- Quinapril *on page 1156*
- Ramipril *on page 1166*
- Trandolapril *on page 1331*

Diuretics

Thiazides
- Hydrochlorothiazide *on page 675*

Loop Diuretics
- Furosemide *on page 622*

Potassium-Sparing Agents
- Spironolactone *on page 1240*

Digitalis Glycosides
- Digoxin *on page 441*
- Digitoxin *on page 440*

Beta-Adrenergic Receptor Blockers
- Bisoprolol *on page 188*
- Carvedilol *on page 256*
- Metoprolol *on page 901*

Catecholamines
- Dobutamine *on page 460*
- Dopamine

Supplemental Agents

Direct-Acting Vasodilators
- Hydralazine *on page 673*
- Nitroglycerin *on page 981*
- Nitroprusside *on page 982*

Phosphodiesterase Inhibitors
- Inamrinone *on page 716*
- Milrinone *on page 914*

*Regarded as the cornerstone of treatment of heart failure and should be used routinely and early in all patients.

From USP DI, Volumes I and II, Update, December 1998.

Drug Classes and Specific Agents Used to Treat Heart Failure

Angiotensin-converting enzyme (ACE) inhibitors reduce left ventricular volume and filling pressure while decreasing total peripheral resistance. They induce cardiac output (modestly) and natriuresis. ACE inhibitors are usually used in all patients with heart failure if no contraindication or intolerance exists. This group of drugs is considered the cornerstone of treatment and are used routinely and early if pharmacologic treatment is indicated.

Diuretics increase sodium chloride and water excretion resulting in reduction of preload, thus relieving the symptoms of pulmonary congestion associated with heart failure. They may also reduce myocardial oxygen demand. The thiazides, loop diuretics, and potassium-sparing agents are all useful in reducing preload by way of their diuretic actions.

Digitalis glycosides have been used in the treatment of heart failure for more than 200 years. Digitalis drugs increase cardiac output by a direct positive inotropic action on the myocardium. This increased cardiac output results in decreased venous pressure, reduced heart size, and diminished compensatory tachycardia.

Beta-adrenergic receptor blocking drugs (beta-blockers) are used in the treatment of heart failure because of their beneficial effect in reducing mortality. A meta-analysis of randomized clinical trials showed that the beta-blockers significantly reduced all causes of cardiac-related deaths, with carvedilol (Coreg®) showing the greatest efficacy. The overall risk of death was reduced by over 30%.

Other drugs used in the treatment of heart failure are referred to as supplemental agents. The direct-acting vasodilators reduce excessive vasoconstriction and reduce workload of the failing heart. The catecholamines and phosphodiesterase inhibitors are alternative agents with positive inotropic effects, are effective for short-term therapy, and have not been demonstrated to prolong life during long-term therapy.

Treatment of arrhythmias often can result in oral manifestations including oral ulcerations with drugs such as procainamide, lupus-like lesions, as well as xerostomia.

HYPERTENSION

In the United States, almost 50 million adults, 25-74 years of age, have hypertension. Hypertension is defined as systolic blood pressure ≥140 mm Hg, and/or diastolic pressure >90 mm Hg. People with blood pressure above normal are considered at increased risk of developing damage to the heart, kidney, brain, and eyes, resulting in premature morbidity and mortality. Individuals with high normal blood pressure (systolic blood pressure of 130-139 mm Hg and diastolic blood pressure of 85-89 mm Hg) should be monitored and encouraged to reduce blood pressure by nondrug measures which include weight control, restriction of sodium and alcohol, and participation in an exercise program. Stage 1 hypertension is blood pressure of 140-159/90-99 mm Hg. If the desired blood pressure is not achieved with nondrug measures within 6 months in patients with stage 1 hypertension (without target organ disease and/or clinical cardiovascular disease), pharmacologic therapy is suggested.

The suggested initial goals of drug therapy are the maintenance of an arterial pressure of ≤140/90 mm Hg with concurrent control of other modifiable cardiovascular risk factors. Further reduction to 130/85 mm Hg should be pursued if cardiovascular and cerebrovascular function is not compromised. The Hypertension Optimal Treatment (HOT) randomized trial using patients 50-80 years of age found that the lowest incidence of major cardiovascular events and the lowest risk of cardiovascular mortality occurred at a mean diastolic blood pressure of 82.6 and 86.5 mm Hg respectively.

Table 5.
CLASSIFICATION OF BLOOD PRESSURE FOR ADULTS ≥18 YEARS OF AGE*

Category	Systolic (mm Hg)		Diastolic (mm Hg)
Optimal†	<120	and	<80
Normal	<130	and	<85
High-Normal	130-139	or	85-89
Hypertension‡			
Stage 1	140-159	or	90-99
Stage 2	160-179	or	100-109
Stage 3	≥180	or	≥110

*Not taking antihypertensive drugs and not acutely ill. When systolic and diastolic blood pressures fall into different categories, the higher category should be selected to classify the individual's blood pressure status. For example, 160/92 mm Hg should be classified as stage 2 hypertension, and 174/120 mm Hg should be classified as stage 3 hypertension. Isolated systolic hypertension is defined as SBP of 140 mm Hg or greater and DBP below 90 mm Hg and staged appropriately (ie, 170/82 mm Hg is defined as stage 2 isolated systolic hypertension). In addition to classifying stages of hypertension on the basis of average blood pressure levels, clinicians should specify presence or absence of target organ disease and additional risk factors. The specificity is important for risk classification and treatment.

†Optimal blood pressure with respect to cardiovascular risk is below 120/80 mm Hg. However, unusually low readings should be evaluated for clinical significance.

‡Based on the average of two or more readings taken at each of two or more visits after an initial screening.

CARDIOVASCULAR DISEASES *(Continued)*

Table 6. RECOMMENDATIONS FOR FOLLOW-UP BASED ON INITIAL BLOOD PRESSURE MEASUREMENTS FOR ADULTS

Initial Blood Pressure (mm Hg)*		Follow-Up Recommended†
Systolic	Diastolic	
<130	<85	Recheck in 2 years
130-139	85-89	Recheck in 1 year‡
140-159	90-99	Confirm within 2 months‡
160-179	100-109	Evaluate or refer to source of care within 1 month
≥180	≥110	Evaluate or refer to source of care immediately or within 1 week depending on clinical situation

*If systolic and diastolic categories are different, follow recommendations for shorter time follow-up (eg, 160/86 mm Hg should be evaluated or referred to source of care within 1 month).

†Modify the scheduling of follow-up according to reliable information about past blood pressure measurements, other cardiovascular risk factors, or target organ disease.

‡Provide advice about lifestyle modifications.

CLASSES OF DRUGS USED IN THE TREATMENT OF HYPERTENSION

- Diuretics
- Beta-adrenergic receptor blocking agents (beta-blockers)
- Alpha$_1$-adrenergic receptor blocking agents (alpha$_1$-blockers)
- Agents which have both alpha- and beta-adrenergic blocking properties (alpha-/beta-blockers)
- Angiotensin-converting enzyme (ACE) inhibitors
- Angiotensin II receptor blockers
- Calcium channel blocking agents
- Supplemental agents such as central-acting alpha$_2$-adrenergic receptor agonists and direct-acting peripheral vasodilators.

Table 7 lists the drug categories and representative agents used to treat hypertension. Combination drugs are now available to supply several classes of these drugs.

Table 7. DRUG CATEGORIES AND REPRESENTATIVE AGENTS USED IN THE TREATMENT OF HYPERTENSION*

Diuretics

Thiazide Types

Bendroflumethiazide *on page 168*
Chlorothiazide *on page 304*
Chlorthalidone *on page 315*
Hydrochlorothiazide *on page 675*
Indapamide *on page 716*
Methyclothiazide *on page 890*
Metolazone *on page 900*
Polythiazide *on page 1097*
Trichlormethiazide *on page 1347*

Loops

Bumetanide *on page 204*
Ethacrynic Acid *on page 538*
Furosemide *on page 622*
Torsemide *on page 1327*

Potassium-Sparing

Amiloride *on page 75*
Spironolactone *on page 1240*
Triamterene *on page 1344*

Potassium-Sparing Combinations

Hydrochlorothiazide and Spironolactone *on page 677*
Hydrochlorothiazide and Triamterene *on page 677*

Beta-Blockers

Cardioselective

Acebutolol *on page 25*
Atenolol *on page 137*
Betaxolol *on page 180*
Bisoprolol *on page 188*
Metoprolol *on page 901*
Sotalol *on page 1235*

(continued)

Noncardioselective

Carteolol *on page 254*
Carvedilol *on page 256*
Nadolol *on page 943*
Penbutolol *on page 1045*
Pindolol *on page 1085*
Propranolol *on page 1139*
Timolol *on page 1309*

Alpha$_1$-Blocker

Doxazosin *on page 470*
Guanadrel *on page 654*
Prazosin *on page 1108*
Reserpine *on page 1173*
Terazosin *on page 1276*

Alpha-/Beta-Blocker

Carvedilol *on page 256*
Labetalol *on page 769*

Angiotensin-Converting Enzyme (ACE) Inhibitors

Benazepril *on page 166*
Captopril *on page 238*
Enalapril *on page 492*
Fosinopril *on page 616*
Lisinopril *on page 813*
Moexipril *on page 926*
Quinapril *on page 1156*
Ramipril *on page 1166*
Trandolapril *on page 1331*

Angiotensin-Converting Enzyme (ACE) Inhibitor/Diuretic Combination

Captopril and Hydrochlorothiazide *on page 240*
Enalapril and Hydrochlorothiazide *on page 494*
Lisinopril and Hydrochlorothiazide *on page 814*

Angiotensin II Receptor Blockers

Candesartan *on page 232*
Eprosartan *on page 506*
Irbesartan *on page 739*
Losartan *on page 825*
Telmisartan *on page 1269*
Valsartan *on page 1374*

Angiotensin II Receptor Blocker/Diuretic Combination

Candesartan + HCTZ *on page 232*
Irbesartan + HCTZ *on page 232*
Valsartan/HCTZ + HCTZ *on page 1374*

Calcium Channel Blockers

Amlodipine *on page 87*
Bepridil *on page 174*
Diltiazem *on page 447*
Felodipine *on page 560*
Isradipine *on page 754*
Nicardipine *on page 969*
Nifedipine *on page 973*
Nisoldipine *on page 977*
Verapamil *on page 1382*

Supplemental Agents

Central-Acting Alpha$_2$-Agonist

Clonidine *on page 351*
Guanabenz *on page 654*
Guanfacine *on page 655*
Methyldopa *on page 891*

Direct-Acting Peripheral Vasodilator

Hydralazine *on page 673*
Minoxidil *on page 917*

*Source: USP DI, Volumes I and II, Update, November 1998.

CARDIOVASCULAR DISEASES *(Continued)*

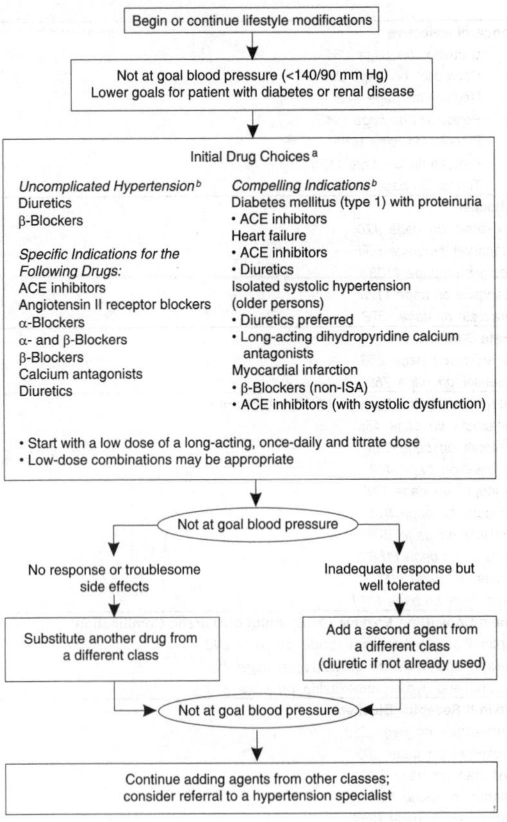

[a] Unless contraindicated. ACE indicates angiotensin-converting enzyme; ISA, intrinsic sympathomimetic activity.

[b] Based on randomized controlled trials.

Begin or continue lifestyle modifications
Not at goal blood pressure (<140/90 mm Hg)
Lower goals for patient with diabetes or renal disease
Initial Drug Choices[a]
Uncomplicated Hypertension[b]
Diuretics
β-Blockers
Specific Indications for the Following Drugs:
ACE inhibitors
Angiotensin II receptor blockers
α-Blockers
α- and β-Blockers
β-Blockers
Calcium antagonists
Diuretics
Compelling Indications[b]
Diabetes mellitus (type 1) with proteinuria
• ACE inhibitors
Heart failure
• ACE inhibitors
• Diuretics
Isolated systolic hypertension (older persons)
• Diuretics preferred
• Long-acting dihydropyridine calcium antagonists
Myocardial infarction
• β-Blockers (non-ISA)
• ACE inhibitors (with systolic dysfunction)
• Start with a low dose of a long-acting, once-daily and titrate dose
• Low-dose combinations may be appropriate
Not at goal blood pressure
No response or troublesome side effects
Inadequate response but well tolerated
Substitute another drug from a different class
Add a second agent from a different class (diuretic if not already used)
Not at goal blood pressure
Continue adding agents from other classes; consider referral to a hypertension specialist

Adapted from "The Sixth Report of the Joint National Committee on Prevention, Detection, Evaluation, and Treatment of High Blood Pressure," Arch Intern Med, 1997, 157(21):2413-46.

Current Thinking Regarding Antihypertensive Drug Selection

Medications in the first eight categories in Table 7 were held to be equally effective in two large-scale studies reported in the *New England Journal of Medicine* and the *Journal of the American Medical Association*, and that any of the medications could be used initially for monotherapy. According to the Sixth Report of the Joint National Committee on Prevention, Detection, Evaluation, and Treatment of High Blood Pressure (JNC VI), diuretics or beta-blockers are recommended as initial therapy for uncomplicated hypertension. If a diuretic is selected as initial therapy, a thiazide diuretic is preferred in patients with normal renal function. If necessary, potassium replacement or concurrent treatment with a potassium-sparing agent may prevent hypokalemia. Loop diuretics are used in patients with impaired renal function or who cannot tolerate thiazides. Diuretics are well tolerated and inexpensive. They are considered the drugs of choice for treating isolated systolic hypertension in the elderly.

Beta-blockers are the agents of choice in patients with coronary artery disease or supraventricular arrhythmia, and in young patients with hyperdynamic circulation. Beta-blockers are alternatives for initial therapy and are more effective in Caucasian patients than in African-American patients. Beta-blockers are not considered first choice drugs in elderly patients with uncomplicated hypertension. The beta-blocking drug carvedilol also selectively blocks alpha$_1$ receptors and has been shown to reduce mortality in hypertensive patients.

Alpha$_1$-adrenergic blocking agents can be used as initial therapy. The alpha$_1$-blocking agent prazosin and related drugs have an added advantage in treating hypertensive patients with coexisting hyperlipidemia since these medications seem to have beneficial effects on lipid levels. Selective blockade of the post-synaptic alpha$_1$-receptors by prazosin and related agents reduces peripheral vascular resistance and systemic blood pressure. In addition, all alpha$_1$-adrenergic blocking agents relieve symptoms of benign prostatic hyperplasia.

ACE inhibitors are the preferred drugs for patients with coexisting heart failure. They are useful as initial therapy in hypertensive patients with kidney damage or diabetes mellitus with proteinuria, and in Caucasian patients. No clinically relevant differences have been found among the available ACE inhibitors. The ACE inhibitors are well tolerated by young, physically active patients, and the elderly. The most common adverse effect of the ACE inhibitors is dry cough. Angiotensin II receptor blockers produce hemodynamic effects similar to ACE inhibitors while avoiding dry cough. These agents are similar to the ACE inhibitors in potency and are useful for initial therapy.

Calcium channel blocking agents are effective as initial therapy in both African-American and Caucasian patients, and are well tolerated by the elderly. These agents inhibit entry of calcium ion into cardiac cells and smooth muscle cells of the coronary and systemic vasculature. Nifedipine (Procardia®) and amlodipine (Norvasc®) are more potent as peripheral vasodilators than diltiazem (Cardizem®). Long-acting formulations of the calcium channel blockers have been shown to be very safe despite some earlier reports that short-acting calcium channel blockers were associated with a 60% increase in heart attacks among hypertensive patients given a short-acting calcium antagonist.

Supplemental antihypertensive agents include the central-acting alpha$_2$ agonists and direct-acting vasodilators. These agents are less commonly prescribed for initial therapy because of the impressive effectiveness of the other drug groups. Clonidine (Catapres®) lowers blood pressure by activating inhibitory alpha$_2$ receptors in the CNS, thus reducing sympathetic outflow. It lowers both supine and standing blood pressure by reducing total peripheral resistance. Hydralazine (Apresoline®) reduces blood pressure by directly relaxing arteriolar smooth muscle. Hydralazine is given orally for the management of chronic hypertension, usually with a diuretic and a beta-blocker.

The most common oral side effects of the management of the hypertensive patient are related to the antihypertensive drug therapy. A dry sore mouth can be caused by diuretics and central-acting adrenergic inhibitors. Occasionally, lichenoid reactions can occur in patients taking quinidine and methyldopa. The thiazides are occasionally also implicated. Lupus-like face rashes can be seen in patients taking calcium channel blockers as well as documented in Calcium Channel Blockers & Gingival Hyperplasia *on page 1598* of the Appendix.

Table 8.
CARDIOVASCULAR / RESPIRATORY / NERVOUS SYSTEM EFFECTS CAUSED BY DRUGS USED FOR CARDIOVASCULAR DISORDERS*

Agent	Incidence	Adverse Effect
Alpha$_1$-Blocker		
Prazosin (Minipress®)	*More frequent*	Orthostatic hypotension, dizziness
	Less frequent	Heart Palpitations
	Rare	Angina
Alpha-/Beta-Blocker		
Carvedilol (Coreg®)	*More frequent*	Bradycardia, postural hypotension, dizziness
	Rare	A-V block, hypertension, hypotension, palpitations, vertigo, nervousness, asthma
Angiotensin-Converting Enzyme (ACE) Inhibitors		
Benazepril (Lotensin®)	*Less frequent*	Dizziness, insomnia, headache
	Rare	Hypotension, bronchitis
Captopril (Capoten®)	*Less frequent*	Tachycardia, insomnia, transient cough, dizziness, headache
	Rare	Hypotension
Enalapril (Vasotec®)	*Less frequent*	Chest pain, palpitations, tachycardia, syncope, dizziness, dyspnea
	Rare	Angina pectoris, asthma
Fosinopril (Monopril®)	*Less frequent*	Orthostatic hypotension, dizziness, cough, headache Syncope, insomnia
	Rare	
Lisinopril (Prinivil®)	*Less frequent*	Hypotension, dizziness
	Rare	Angina pectoris, orthostatic hypotension, rhythm disturbances, tachycardia
Moexipril (Univasc®)	*Less frequent*	Hypotension, peripheral edema, headache, dizziness, fatigue, cough, pharyngitis, upper respiratory infection, sinusitis
	Rare	Chest pain, myocardial infarction, palpitations, arrhythmias, syncope, CVA, orthostatic hypotension, dyspnea, bronchospasm
Perindopril (Aceon®)	*Less frequent*	Headache, dizziness, cough†
	Rare	Hypotension
Quinapril (Accupril®)	*Less frequent*	Hypotension, dizziness, headache, cough
	Rare	Orthostatic hypotension, angina, insomnia
Ramipril (Altace®)	*Less frequent*	Tachycardia, dizziness, headache, cough
	Rare	Hypotension

CARDIOVASCULAR DISEASES *(Continued)*

Agent	Incidence	Adverse Effect
Trandolapril (Mavrik®)	*Less frequent* *Rare*	Tachycardia, headache, dizziness, cough‡ Hypotension
Angiotensin-Converting Enzyme Inhibitor/Diuretic Combination		
Captopril/HCTZ (Capozide®)	*Less frequent* *Rare*	Tachycardia, palpitations, chest pain, dizziness Hypotension
Angiotensin II Receptor Blockers		
Candesartan (Atacand®)	*Less frequent* *Rare*	Chest pain, flushing Myocardial infarction, tachycardia, angina, palpitations, dyspnea
Losartan (Cozaar®)	*Less frequent* *Rare*	Hypotension without reflex tachycardia, dizziness Orthostatic hypotension, angina, A-V block (second degree), CVA, palpitations, tachycardia, sinus bradycardia, flushing, dyspnea
Angiotensin II Receptor Blocker/Diuretic Combination		
Candesartan (Atacand HCT™) + HCTZ	*Less frequent* *Rare*	Chest pain, flushing Myocardial infarction, tachycardia, angina, palpitations, dyspnea
Irbesartan/HCTZ (Avalide®)		Effects unavailable
Valsartan/HCTZ (Diovan HCT®)		Effects unavailable
Antiplatelet/Anticoagulant Agents		
Abciximab (ReoPro®)	*More frequent* *Less frequent*	Hypotension, pain Bradycardia
Aspirin	*Less frequent or Rare*	Anaphylactoid reaction, bronchospastic allergic reaction
Clopidogrel (Plavix®)	*Less frequent*	Chest pain, edema, hypertension, headache, dizziness, depression, fatigue, dyspnea, rhinitis, bronchitis, coughing, upper respiratory infection, syncope, palpitations, cardiac failure, paresthesia, vertigo, atrial fibrillation, neuralgia
Eptifibatide (Integrilin®)	*More frequent*	Hypotension, bleeding
Ticlopidine (Ticlid®)	*Less frequent* *Rare*	Dizziness Peripheral neuropathy, angioedema, vasculitis, allergic pneumonitis
Tirofiban (Aggrastat®)	*More frequent* *Less frequent*	Bleeding Bradycardia, dizziness, headache
Warfarin (Coumadin®)	*Less frequent* *Rare*	Hemoptysis Fever, purple toes syndrome
Beta-Blockers		
Acebutolol (Sectral®)	*Less frequent* *Rare*	Chest pain, bradycardia, hypotension, dizziness, dyspepsia, dyspnea Ventricular arrhythmias
Atenolol (Tenormin®)	*Less frequent* *Rare*	Bradycardia, hypotension, chest pain, dizziness, dyspepsia, dyspnea Ventricular arrhythmias
Betaxolol (Kerlone®)	*Less frequent* *Rare*	Bradycardia, palpitations, dizziness Chest pain
Bisoprolol (Zebeta®)	*More frequent* *Less frequent*	Lethargy Hypotension, chest pain, bradycardia, headache, dizziness, insomnia, cough
Labetalol (Normodyne®, Trandate®)	*Less frequent* *Rare*	Orthostatic hypotension, dizziness, nasal congestion Bradycardia, chest pain
Metoprolol (Lopressor®)	*More frequent* *Less frequent* *Rare*	Dizziness Bradycardia, heartburn, wheezing Chest pain, confusion
Nadolol (Corgard®)	*More frequent* *Less frequent* *Rare*	Bradycardia Dizziness, dyspepsia, wheezing Congestive heart failure, orthostatic hypotension, confusion, paresthesia
Penbutolol (Levatol®)	*Less frequent* *Rare*	Congestive heart failure, dizziness Bradycardia, chest pain, hypotension, confusion
Pindolol (Visken®)	*More frequent* *Less frequent*	Dizziness Congestive heart failure, dyspnea
Propranolol (Inderal®)	*More frequent* *Less frequent* *Rare*	Bradycardia Congestive heart failure, dizziness, wheezing Chest pain, hypotension, bronchospasm
Timolol (Blocadren®)	*Less frequent* *Rare*	Bradycardia, dizziness, dyspnea Chest pain, congestive heart failure

Agent	Incidence	Adverse Effect
Calcium Channel Blockers		
Amlodipine (Norvasc®)	*Less frequent* *Rare*	Palpitations, dizziness, dyspnea Hypotension, bradycardia, arrhythmias
Diltiazem (Cardizem®)	*Less frequent* *Rare*	Bradycardia, dizziness Dyspepsia, paresthesia, tremor
Nifedipine (Procardia®)	*More frequent* *Less frequent* *Rare*	Flushing, dizziness Palpitations, hypotension, dyspnea Tachycardia, syncope
Verapamil (Calan®)	*Less frequent* *Rare*	Bradycardia, congestive heart failure, hypotension Chest pain, hypotension (excessive)
Class I Antiarrhythmics		
Disopyramide (Norpace®)	*More frequent* *Less frequent* *Rare*	Exacerbation of angina pectoris, dizziness Hypotension, hypertension, tachycardia, dyspnea Syncope, flushing, hyperventilation
Flecainide (Tambocor™)	*More frequent* *Less frequent* *Rare*	Dizziness, dyspnea Palpitations, chest pain, tachycardia, tremor Bradycardia, nervousness, paresthesia
Procainimide (Pronestyl®)	*Less frequent* *Rare*	Tachycardia, dizziness, lightheadedness Hypotension, confusion, disorientation
Propafenone (Rythmol®)	*More frequent* *Less frequent* *Rare*	Dizziness Palpitations, angina, bradycardia, loss of balance, dyspepsia, dyspnea Paresthesia
Quinidine (Quinaglute®)	*Less frequent* *Rare*	Hypotension, syncope, lightheadedness, wheezing Confusion, vertigo, angina, edema
Class III Antiarrhythmics		
Amiodarone (Cordarone®)	*More frequent* *Less frequent* *Rare*	Dizziness, tremor, paresthesia, dyspnea Congestive heart failure, bradycardia, tachycardia Hypotension
Sotalol (Betapace®)	*More frequent* *Less frequent* *Rare*	Bradycardia, chest pain, palpitations, fatigue, dizziness, lightheadedness, dyspnea CHF, hypotension, proarrhythmia, syncope, reduced peripheral circulation, edema, asthma, upper respiratory problems Diaphoresis, clouded sensorium, fever, lack of coordination
Digitalis Glycosides		
Digoxin (Lanoxicaps®, Lanoxin®) Digitoxin	*Rare*	Atrial tachycardia, sinus bradycardia, ventricular fibrillation, vertigo
Diuretics		
Thiazide type	*Rare*	Hypotension
Loops	*More frequent*	Orthostatic hypotension, dizziness
Potassium-sparing	*Less frequent* *Rare*	Hypotension, bradycardia, dizziness Flushing
Potassium-sparing combination	*Rare*	Dizziness
HMG-CoA Reductase Inhibitors		
Atorvastatin Fluvastatin Lovastatin Pravastatin Simvastatin	*Less frequent*	Headache, dizziness
Nitrates		
Nitroglycerins	*More frequent* *Rare*	Postural hypotension, flushing, headache, dizziness Reflex tachycardia, bradycardia, arrhythmia
Supplemental Drugs for Heart Failure		
Inamrinone	*Less frequent*	Arrhythmia, chest pain
Dobutamine (Dobutrex®)	*Less frequent* *Rare*	Tachycardia, chest pain Headache, dyspnea
Hydralazine	*More frequent* *Less frequent* *Rare*	Tachycardia, headache Hypotension, nasal congestion Edema, dizziness
Milrinone (Primacor®)	*More frequent* *Less frequent*	Arrhythmias Chest pain
Nitroprusside sodium (Nitropress®)	*Less frequent*	Palpitations, headache

CARDIOVASCULAR DISEASES *(Continued)*

Agent	Incidence	Adverse Effect
Supplemental Drugs for Hypertension		
Central-Acting Alpha$_2$-Agonists		
Clonidine (Catapres®)	*More frequent*	Dizziness
	Less frequent	Orthostatic hypotension, nervousness/agitation
	Rare	Palpitations, tachycardia, bradycardia, congestive heart failure
Direct-Acting		
Hydralazine	*More frequent*	Tachycardia, headache
	Less frequent	Hypotension, nasal congestion
	Rare	Edema, dizziness

Legend: % of Incidence: More frequent = >10%, Less frequent = 1% to 10%, Rare = <1%

*Source: Professional package insert for individual agents or United States Pharmacopeial Dispensing Information. *Drug Information for the Health Care Professional*, Vol I, 19th ed, Rockville, MD: The United States Pharmacopeial Convention, Inc, 1999.

†Incidence greater in women 3:1.

‡More frequent in women.

Table 9.
CARDIOVASCULAR DRUGS DENTAL DRUG INTERACTIONS AND EFFECTS ON DENTAL TREATMENT

Agent	Effect
Alpha$_1$-Blocker	
Prazosin (Minipress®)	Significant orthostatic hypotension a possibility; monitor patient when getting out of dental chair; significant dry mouth in up to 10% of patients.
Alpha-/Beta-Blocker	
Carvedilol (Coreg®)	See Nonselective Beta-Blockers
ACE Inhibitors	The NSAID indomethacin reduces the hypotensive effects of ACE inhibitors. Effects of other NSAIDs such as ibuprofen not considered significant.
Angiotensin-Converting Enzyme Inhibitor/Diuretic Combination	
Captopril/HCTZ (Capozide®)	No effect or complications on dental treatment reported.
Angiotensin II Receptor Blockers	
Candesartan (Atacand®)	No effect or complications on dental treatment reported.
Losartan (Cozaar®)	
Antiplatelet/Anticoagulant Agents	
Aspirin	May cause a reduction in the serum levels of NSAIDs if they are used to manage post-operative pain.
Clopidogrel (Plavix®)	If a patient is to undergo elective surgery and an antiplatelet effect is not desired, clopidogrel should be discontinued 7 days prior to surgery.
Eptifibatide (Integrilin®)	Bleeding may occur while patient is medicated with eptifibatide; platelet function is restored in about 4 hours following discontinuation.
Warfarin (Coumadin®)	Signs of warfarin overdose may first appear as bleeding from gingival tissue; consultation with prescribing physician is advisable prior to surgery to determine temporary dose reduction or withdrawal of medication.
Beta-Blockers	
Cardioselective	Cardioselective beta-blockers (ie, atenolol) have no effect or complications on dental treatment reported.
Noncardioselective	Any of the noncardioselective beta-blockers (ie, nadolol, penbutolol, pindolol, propranolol, timolol) may enhance the pressor response to vasoconstrictor epinephrine resulting in hypertension and reflex bradycardia. Although not reported, it is assumed that similar effects could be caused with levonordefrin (Neo-Cobefrin®). Use either vasoconstrictor with caution in hypertensive patients medicated with noncardioselective beta-adrenergic blockers.
Calcium Channel Blockers	Cause gingival hyperplasia in approximately 1% of the general population taking these drugs. There have been fewer reports with diltiazem and amlodipine than with other CBs such as nifedipine. The hyperplasia will usually disappear with cessation of drug therapy. Consultation with the physician is suggested
Class I Antiarrhythmics	
Disopyramide (Norpace®)	Increased serum levels and toxicity with erythromycin. High incidence of anticholinergic effect manifested as dry mouth and throat.
Flecainide (Tambocor™)	No effects or complications on dental treatment reported.

Procainimide (Pronestyl®)	Systemic lupus-like syndrome has been reported resulting in joint pain and swelling, pains with breathing, skin rash.
Propafenone (Rythmol®)	Greater than 10 % experience significantly reduced salivary flow; taste disturbance, bitter or metallic taste
Quinidine (Quinaglute®)	Secondary anticholinergic effects may decrease salivary flow, especially in middle-aged and elderly patients; known to contribute to caries, periodontal disease, and oral candidiasis.
Class III Antiarrhythmics	
Amiodarone	Bitter or metallic taste has been reported.
Digitalis Glycosides	Use vasoconstrictor with caution due to risk of cardiac arrhythmias. Sensitive gag reflex induced by digitalis drugs may cause difficulty in taking dental impressions.
Diuretics	
Thiazide type	No effects or complications on dental treatment reported.
Loops	NSAIDs may increase chloride and tubular water reuptake to counter-act loop type diuretics.
Potassium-sparing	No effects or complications on dental treatment reported.
Potassium-sparing combination	No effects or complications on dental treatment reported.
HMG-CoA Reductase Inhibitors	Concurrent use of erythromycin, clarithromycin, and some of the statin drugs may result in rhabdomyolysis.
Nitrates	No effects or complications on dental treatment reported.
Supplemental Drugs for Heart Failure	
Inamrinone Milrinone (Primacor®)	No effects or complications on dental treatment reported
Supplemental Drugs for Hypertension	
Central-Acting Alpha$_2$-Agonists	
Clonidine (Catapres®)	Greater than 10% of patients experience significant dry mouth.
Direct-Acting	
Hydralazine	No effect or complications on dental treatment reported.

GASTROINTESTINAL DISORDERS

The oral cavity and related structures comprise the first part of the gastrointestinal tract. Diseases affecting the oral cavity are often reflected in GI disturbances. In addition, the oral cavity may indeed reflect diseases of the GI tract, including ulcers, polyps, and liver and gallbladder diseases. The first oral condition that may reflect or be reflected in GI disturbances is that of taste. Typically, complaints of taste abnormalities are presented to the dentist. The sweet, saline, sour, and bitter taste sensations all vary in quality and intensity and are affected by the olfactory system. Often, anemic conditions are reflected in changes in the tongue, resulting in taste aberrations.

Gastric and duodenal ulcers represent the primary diseases that can reflect themselves in the oral cavity. Gastric reflux and problems with food metabolism often present as acid erosions to the teeth and occasionally, changes in the mucosal surface as well. Patients may be encountered that may be identified, upon diagnosis, as harboring the organism *Helicobacter pylori.* Treatment with antibiotics can oftentimes aid in correcting the ulcerative disease.

Gastric Acid Secretion Inhibitor

Lansoprazole *on page 777*
Omeprazole *on page 999*
Pantaprazole *on page 1031*

Histamine H_2 Antagonist

Cimetidine *on page 326*
Famotidine *on page 556*
Nizatidine *on page 984*
Ranitidine Hydrochloride *on page 1168*

Proton Pump Inhibitors

Lansoprazole *on page 777*
Omeprazole *on page 999*
Pantaprazole *on page 1031*

The oral aspects of gastrointestinal disease are often nonspecific and are related to the patient's gastric reflux problems. Intestinal polyps occasionally present as part of the "Peutz-Jeghers Syndrome", resulting in pigmented areas of the peri-oral region that resemble freckles. The astute dentist will need to differentiate these from melanin pigmentation, while at the same time encouraging the patient to perhaps seek evaluation for an intestinal disorder.

Diseases of the liver and gallbladder system are complex. Most of the disorders that the dentist is interested in are covered in the section on systemic viral disease*on page 1517.* All of the new drugs, including interferons, are mentioned in this section.

Multiple Drug Regimens for the Treatment of *H. pylori* Infection

Drug	Dosages	Duration of Therapy
H_2-receptor antagonist[1]	Any one given at appropriate dose	4 weeks
plus		
Bismuth *on page 186*	525 mg 4 times/day	2 weeks
plus		
Metronidazole *on page 902*	250 mg 4 times/day	2 weeks
plus		
Tetracycline *on page 1286*	500 mg 4 times/day	2 weeks
Proton pump inhibitor[1]	Esomeprazole 40 mg once daily	10 days
plus		
Clarithromycin *on page 337*	500 mg twice daily	10 days
plus		
Amoxicillin *on page 93*	1000 mg twice daily	10 days
Proton pump inhibitor[1]	Lansoprazole 30 mg twice daily or Omeprazole 20 mg twice daily	10-14 days
plus		
Clarithromycin *on page 337*	500 mg twice daily	10-14 days
plus		
Amoxicillin *on page 93*	1000 mg twice daily	10-14 days
Proton pump inhibitor[1]	Rabeprazole 20 mg twice daily	7 days
plus		
Clarithromycin *on page 337*	500 mg twice daily	7 days
plus		
Amoxicillin *on page 93*	1000 mg twice daily	7 days
Proton pump inhibitor	Lansoprazole 30 mg twice daily or Omeprazole 20 mg twice daily	2 weeks
plus		
Clarithromycin *on page 337*	500 mg twice daily	2 weeks
plus		
Metronidazole *on page 902*	500 mg twice daily	2 weeks
Proton pump inhibitor	Lansoprazole 30 mg once daily or Omeprazole 20 mg once daily	2 weeks
plus		
Bismuth *on page 186*	525 mg 4 times/day	2 weeks
plus		
Metronidazole *on page 902*	500 mg 3 times/day	2 weeks
plus		
Tetracycline *on page 1286*	500 mg 4 times/day	2 weeks

[1]FDA-approved regimen

Modified from Howden CS and Hunt RH, "Guidelines for the Management of *Helicobacter pylori* Infection," *AJG*, 1998, 93:2336.

RESPIRATORY DISEASES

Diseases of the respiratory system put dental patients at increased risk in the dental office because of their decreased pulmonary reserve, the medications they may be taking, drug interactions between these medications, medications the dentist may prescribe, and in some patients with infectious respiratory diseases, a risk of disease transmission.

The respiratory system consists of the nasal cavity, the nasopharynx, the trachea, and the components of the lung including, of course, the bronchi, the bronchioles, and the alveoli. The diseases that affect the lungs and the respiratory system can be separated by location of affected tissue. Diseases that affect the lower respiratory tract are often chronic, although infections can also occur. Three major diseases that affect the lower respiratory tract are often encountered in the medical history for dental patients. These include chronic bronchitis, emphysema, and asthma. Diseases that affect the upper respiratory tract are usually of the infectious nature and include sinusitis and the common cold. The upper respiratory tract infections may also include a wide variety of nonspecific infections, most of which are also caused by viruses. Influenza produces upper respiratory type symptoms and is often caused by orthomyxoviruses. Herpangina is caused by the Coxsackie type viruses and results in upper respiratory infections in addition to pharyngitis or sore throat. One serious condition, known as croup, has been associated with *Haemophilus influenzae* infections. Other more serious infections might include respiratory syncytial virus, adenoviruses, and parainfluenza viruses.

The respiratory symptoms that are often encountered in both upper respiratory and lower respiratory disorders include cough, dyspnea (difficulty in breathing), the production of sputum, hemoptysis (coughing up blood), a wheeze, and occasionally chest pain. One additional symptom, orthopnea (difficulty in breathing when lying down) is often used by the dentist to assist in evaluating the patient with the condition, pulmonary edema. This condition results from either respiratory disease or congestive heart failure.

No effective drug treatments are available for the management of many of the upper respiratory tract viral infections. However, amantadine (sold under the brand name Symmetrel®) is a synthetic drug given orally (200 mg/day) and has been found to be effective against some strains of influenza. Treatment other than for influenza includes supportive care products available over the counter. These might include antihistamines for symptomatic relief of the upper respiratory congestion, antibiotics to combat secondary bacterial infections, and in severe cases, fluids when patients have become dehydrated during the illness (see Therapeutic Category Index for selection). The treatment of herpangina may include management of the painful ulcerations of the oropharynx. The dentist may become involved in managing these lesions in a similar way to those seen in other acute viral infections (see Viral Infection section).

SINUSITIS

Sinusitis also represents an upper respiratory infection that often comes under the purview of the practicing dentist. Acute sinusitis characterized by nasal obstruction, fever, chills, and midface head pain may be encountered by the dentist and discovered as part of a differential work-up for other facial or dental pain. Chronic sinusitis may likewise produce similar dental symptoms. Dental drugs of choice may include ephedrine or nasal drops, antihistamines, and analgesics. These drugs sometimes require supplementation with antibiotics. Most commonly, broad spectrum antibiotics, such as ampicillin, are prescribed. These are often combined with antral lavage to re-establish drainage from the sinus area. Surgical intervention such as a Caldwell-Luc procedure opening into the sinus is rarely necessary and many of the second generation antibiotics such as cephalosporins are used successfully in treating the acute and chronic sinusitis patient (see "Antibiotic Prophylaxis" *on page 1507*).

Gatifloxacin *on page 628*
Moxifloxacin *on page 935*

LOWER RESPIRATORY DISEASES

Lower respiratory tract diseases, including asthma, chronic bronchitis, and emphysema are often identified in dental patients. Asthma is an intermittent respiratory disorder that produces recurrent bronchial smooth muscle spasm, inflammation, swelling of the bronchial mucosa, and hypersecretion of mucus. The incidence of childhood asthma appears to be increasing and may be related to the presence of pollutants such as sulfur dioxide and indoor cigarette smoke. The end result is widespread narrowing of the airways and decreased ventilation with increased airway resistance, especially to expiration. Asthmatic patients often suffer from asthmatic attacks when stimulated by respiratory tract infections, exercise, and cold air. Medications such as aspirin and some nonsteroidal anti-inflammatory agents as well as cholinergic and beta-adrenergic blocking drugs, can also trigger asthmatic attacks in addition to chemicals, smoke, and emotional anxiety.

The classical chronic obstructive pulmonary diseases (COPD) of chronic bronchitis and emphysema are both characterized by chronic airflow obstructions during normal ventilatory efforts. They often occur in combination in the same patient and their treatment is similar. One common finding is that the patient is often a smoker. The dentist can play a role in reinforcement of smoking cessation in patients with chronic respiratory diseases.

Treatments include a variety of drugs depending on the severity of the symptoms and the respiratory compromise upon full respiratory evaluation. Patients who are having acute and chronic obstructive pulmonary attacks may be susceptible to infection and antibiotics such as penicillin, ampicillin, tetracycline, or trimethoprim-sulfamethoxazole are often used to eradicate susceptible infective organisms. Corticosteroids, as well as a wide variety of respiratory stimulants, are available in inhalant and/or oral forms. In patients using inhalant medication, oral candidiasis is occasionally encountered.

Amantadine *on page 70*
Analgesics *on page 1643*
Antibiotics *on page 1644*
Antihistamines *on page 1650*
Decongestants *on page 1658*
Epinephrine *on page 499*
Gatifloxacin *on page 628*
Moxifloxacin *on page 935*

SPECIFIC DRUGS USED IN THE TREATMENT OF CHRONIC RESPIRATORY CONDITIONS

Beta$_2$-Selective Agonists

Albuterol *on page 48*
Bitolterol *on page 189*
Isoetharine *on page 747*
Metaproterenol *on page 873*
Pirbuterol *on page 1090*
Salmeterol *on page 1205*
Terbutaline *on page 1278*

Methylxanthines

Aminophylline *on page 78*
Theophylline *on page 1291*

Mast Cell Stabilizer

Cromolyn Sodium *on page 375*
Nedocromil Sodium *on page 957*

Corticosteroids

Beclomethasone *on page 163*
Dexamethasone *on page 413*
Flunisolide *on page 582*
Fluticasone *on page 599*
Mometasone Furoate *on page 928*
Prednisone *on page 1112*
Triamcinolone *on page 1341*

Anticholinergics

Ipratropium *on page 737*

Leukotriene Receptor Antagonists

Montelukast *on page 929*
Zafirlukast *on page 1402*

5-Lipoxygenase Inhibitors

Zileuton *on page 1408*

Other respiratory diseases include tuberculosis and sarcoidosis which are considered to be restrictive granulomatous respiratory diseases. Tuberculosis is covered in "Nonviral Infectious Diseases" *on page 1493*. Sarcoidosis is a condition that at one time was thought to be similar to tuberculosis, however, it is a multisystem disorder of unknown origin which has as a characteristic lymphocytic and mononuclear phagocytic accumulation in epithelioid granulomas within the lung. It occurs worldwide but shows a slight increased prevalence in temperate climates. The treatment of sarcoidosis is usually one that corresponds to its usually benign course, however, many patients are placed on corticosteroids at the level of 40-60 mg of prednisone daily. This treatment is continued for a protracted period of time. As in any disease requiring steroid therapy, consideration of adrenal suppression is necessary. Alteration of steroid dosage prior to stressful dental procedures may be necessary, usually increasing the steroid dosage prior to and during the stressful procedures and then gradually returning the patient to the original dosage over several days. Many dentists prefer to use the Medrol® Dosepak®, however, consultation with the patient's physician regarding dose selection is always advised. Even in the absence of evidence of adrenal suppression, consultation with the prescribing physician for appropriate dosing and timing of procedures is advisable.

Prednisone *on page 1112*

RESPIRATORY DISEASES *(Continued)*

RELATIVE POTENCY OF ENDOGENOUS AND SYNTHETIC CORTICOSTEROIDS

Agent	Equivalent Dose (mg)
Short-Acting (8-12 h)	
Cortisol	20
Cortisone	25
Intermediate-Acting (18-36 h)	
Prednisolone	5
Prednisone	5
Methylprednisolone (Medrol®)	4
Triamcinolone	4
Long-Acting (36-54 h)	
Betamethasone	0.75
Dexamethasone	0.75

Potential drug interactions for the respiratory disease patient exist. An acute sensitivity to aspirin-containing drugs and some of the nonsteroidal anti-inflammatory drugs is a threat for the asthmatic patient. Barbiturates and narcotics may occasionally precipitate asthmatic attacks as well. Erythromycin, clarithromycin, and ketoconazole are contraindicated in patients who are taking theophylline due to potential enhancement of theophylline toxicity. Patients that are taking steroid preparations as part of their respiratory therapy may require alteration in dosing prior to stressful dental procedures. The physician should be consulted.

Barbiturates *on page 1655*
Clarithromycin *on page 337*
Erythromycin *on page 512*
Ketoconazole *on page 762*

ENDOCRINE DISORDERS AND PREGNANCY

The human endocrine system manages metabolism and homeostasis. Numerous glandular tissues produce hormones that act in broad reactions with tissues throughout the body. Cells in various organ systems may be sensitive to the hormone, or they release, in reaction to the hormone, a second hormone that acts directly on another organ. Diseases of the endocrine system may have importance in dentistry. For the purposes of this section, we will limit our discussion to diseases of the thyroid tissues, diabetes mellitus, and conditions requiring the administration of synthetic hormones, and pregnancy.

THYROID

Thyroid diseases can be classified into conditions that cause the thyroid to be overactive (hyperthyroidism) and those that cause the thyroid to be underactive (hypothyroidism). Clinical signs and symptoms associated with hyperthyroidism may include goiter, heat intolerance, tremor, weight loss, diarrhea, and hyperactivity. Thyroid hormone production can be tested by TSH levels and additional screens may include radioactive iodine uptake or a pre-T_4 (tetraiodothyronine, thyroxine) assay or iodine index or total serum T_3 (triiodothyronine). The results of thyroid function tests may be altered by ingestion of antithyroid drugs such as propylthiouracil, estrogen-containing drugs, and organic and inorganic iodides. When a diagnosis of hyperthyroidism has been made, treatment usually begins with antithyroid drugs which may include propranolol coupled with radioactive iodides as well as surgical procedures to reduce thyroid tissue. Generally, the beta-blockers are used to control cardiovascular effects of excessive T_4. Propylthiouracil or methimazole are the most common antithyroid drugs used. The dentist should be aware that epinephrine is definitely contraindicated in patients with uncontrolled hyperthyroidism.

Diseases and conditions associated with hypothyroidism may include bradycardia, drowsiness, cold intolerance, thick dry skin, and constipation. Generally, hypothyroidism is treated with replacement thyroid hormone until a euthyroid state is achieved. Various preparations are available, the most common is levothyroxine, commonly known as Synthroid® or Levothroid®, and is generally the drug of choice for thyroid replacement therapy.

Drugs to Treat Hypothyroidism

Levothyroxine *on page 800*
Liothyronine *on page 810*
Liotrix *on page 811*
Thyroid *on page 1303*

Drugs to Treat Hyperthyroidism

Methimazole *on page 880*
Potassium Iodide *on page 1101*
Propranolol *on page 1139*
Propylthiouracil *on page 1142*

DIABETES

Diabetes mellitus refers to a condition of prolonged hyperglycemia associated with either abnormal production or lack of production of insulin. Commonly known as Type 1 diabetes, insulin-dependent diabetes (IDDM) is a condition where there are absent or deficient levels of circulating insulin therefore triggering tissue reactions associated with prolonged hyperglycemia. The kidney's attempt to excrete the excess glucose and the organs that do not receive adequate glucose essentially are damaged. Small vessels and arterial vessels in the eye, kidney, and brain are usually at the greatest risk. Generally, blood sugar levels between 70-120 mg/dL are considered to be normal. Inadequate insulin levels allow glucose to rise to greater than the renal threshold which is 180 mg/dL, and such elevations prolonged lead to organ damage.

The goals of treatment of the diabetic are to maintain metabolic control of the blood glucose levels and to reduce the morbid effects of periodic hyperglycemia. Insulin therapy is the primary mechanism to attain management of consistent insulin levels. Insulin preparations are categorized according to their duration of action. Generally, NPH or intermediate-acting insulin and long-acting insulin can be used in combination with short-acting or regular insulin to maintain levels consistent throughout the day.

In Type 2 or noninsulin-dependent diabetes (NIDDM), the receptor for insulin in the tissues is generally down regulated and the glucose, therefore, is not utilized at an appropriate rate. There is perhaps a stronger genetic basis for noninsulin-dependent diabetes than for Type 1. Treatment of the diabetes Type 2 patient is generally directed toward early nonpharmacologic intervention, mainly weight reduction, moderate exercise, and lower plasma-glucose concentrations. Oral hypoglycemic agents as seen in the list below are often used to maintain blood sugar levels. Thirty percent of Type 2

ENDOCRINE DISORDERS AND PREGNANCY *(Continued)*

diabetics require insulin, as well as, oral hypoglycemics in order to manage their diabetes. Generally, the two classes of oral hypoglycemics are the sulfonylureas and the biguanides. The sulfonylureas are prescribed more frequently and they stimulate beta cell production of insulin, increase glucose utilization, and tend to normalize glucose metabolism in the liver. The uncontrolled diabetic may represent a challenge to the dental practitioner.

Glycosylated hemoglobin or glycol-hemoglobin assays have emerged as a "gold standard" by which glycemic control is measured in diabetic patients. The test does not rely on the patient's ability to monitor their daily blood glucose levels and is not influenced by acute changes in blood glucose or by the interval since the last meal. Glyco-hemoglobin is formed when glucose reacts with hemoglobin A in the blood and is composed of several fractions. Numerous assay methods have been developed, however, they vary in their precision. Dental clinicians are advised to be aware of the laboratory's particular standardization procedures when requesting glycosylated hemoglobin values. One major advantage of the glycosylated hemoglobin assay is that it provides an overview of the level of glucose in the life span of the red blood cell population in the patient, and therefore is a measure of overall glycemic control for the previous six to twelve weeks. Thus, clinicians use glycosylated hemoglobin values to determine whether their patient is under good control, on average. These assays have less value in medication dosing decisions. Blood glucose monitoring methods are actually better in that respect. The values of glycosylated hemoglobin are expressed as a percentage of the total hemoglobin in the red blood cell population and a normal value is considered to be <6%. The goal is generally for diabetic patients to remain at <7% and values >8% would constitute a worrisome signal. Medical conditions such as anemias or any red blood cell disease, numerous levels of myelosuppression, or pregnancy can artificially lower glycosylated hemoglobin values.

See Insulin Preparations (various products) *on page 723*

Oral Hypoglycemic Agents

Acarbose *on page 24*
Acetohexamide *on page 38*
Chlorpropamide *on page 314*
Glimepiride *on page 637*
Glipizide *on page 638*
Glyburide *on page 642*
Glyburide and Metformin *on page 643*
Metformin *on page 874*
Miglitol *on page 913*
Repaglinide *on page 1172*
Tolazamide *on page 1318*
Tolbutamide *on page 1319*

Adjunct Therapy

Metoclopramide *on page 898*

Oral manifestations of uncontrolled diabetes might include abnormal neutrophil function resulting in a poor response to periodontal pathogens. Increased risk of gingivitis and periodontitis in these patients is common. Candidiasis is a frequent occurrence. Denture sore mouth may be more prominent and poor wound healing following extractions may be one of the complications encountered.

HORMONAL THERAPY

Two uses of hormonal supplementation include oral contraceptives and estrogen replacement therapy. Drugs used for contraception interfere with fertility by inhibiting release of follicle stimulating hormone, luteinizing hormone, and by preventing ovulation. There are few oral side effects; however, moderate gingivitis, similar to that seen during pregnancy, has been reported. The dentist should be aware that decreased effect of oral contraceptives has been reported with most antibiotics (see individual monographs for specific details). It is therefore recommended that dental professionals, when prescribing antibiotics to oral contraceptive users, advise them of this interaction and suggest consulting their physician for additional barrier contraception during antibiotic therapy.

The combination estradiol cypionate and medroxyprogesterone acetate has recently been approved. It is a single monthly injection and has similar warnings and guidelines. However, it's use with antibiotics have not been firmly established. Therefore, discussion/consultation with the patient's OB/GYN physician is indicated.

Drugs commonly encountered include:

Combination Hormonal Contraceptives *on page 368*
Estradiol *on page 521*
Estradiol Cypionate and Medroxyprogesterone Acetate *on page 523*

Levonorgestrel *on page 797*
Medroxyprogesterone Acetate *on page 849*
Mestranol and Norethindrone *on page 871*
Norethindrone *on page 986*
Norgestrel *on page 988*

Estrogens or derivatives are usually prescribed as replacement therapy following menopause or cyclic irregularities and to inhibit osteoporosis. The following list of drugs may interact with antidepressants and barbiturates. New tissue-specific estrogens like Evista® may help with the problem of osteoporosis.

Estrogens (Conjugated/Equine) *on page 529*
Estrogens (Conjugated A/Synthetic) *on page 528*
Estrogens (Esterified) *on page 533*
Estrogens (Conjugated/Equine) and Medroxyprogesterone *on page 531*
Estrogens (Esterified) and Methyltestosterone *on page 534*
Estrone *on page 535*
Estropipate *on page 536*
Ethinyl Estradiol *on page 541*
Raloxifene *on page 1165*

PREGNANCY

Normal endocrine and physiologic functions are altered during pregnancy. Endogenous estrogens and progesterone increase and placental hormones are secreted. Thyroid stimulating hormone and growth hormone also increase. Cardiovascular changes can result and increased blood volume can lead to blood pressure elevations and transient heart murmurs. Generally, in a normal pregnancy, oral gingival changes will be limited to gingivitis. Alteration of treatment plans might include limiting administration of all drugs to emergency procedures only during the first and third trimesters and medical consultation regarding the patients' status for all elective procedures. Limiting dental care throughout pregnancy to preventive procedures is not unreasonable. The effects on dental treatment of the "morning after pill" (Plan B® and PREVEN®) and the abortifacient, mifepristone *on page 912*, have not been documented at this time.

HIV INFECTION AND AIDS

Human immunodeficiency virus (HIV) represents agents HIV-1 and HIV-2 that produce a devastating systemic disease. The virus causes disease by leading to elevated risk of infections in patients and, from our experience over the last 18 years, there clearly are oral manifestations associated with these patients. Also, there has been a revolution in infection control in our dental offices over the last two decades due to our expanding knowledge of this infectious agent. Infection control practices (see "Infectious Disease Information" *on page 1601*) have been elevated to include all of the infectious agents with which dentists often come into contact. These might include in addition to HIV, hepatitis viruses (of which the serotypes include A, B, C, D, E, F, and G), the herpes viruses; sexually transmitted diseases such as syphilis, gonorrhea, papillomavirus, all of which are covered elsewhere in this book.

Acquired immunodeficiency syndrome (AIDS) has been recognized since early 1981 as a unique clinical syndrome manifest by opportunistic infections or by neoplasms complicating the underlying defect in the cellular immune system. These defects are now known to be brought on by infection and pathogenesis with human immunodeficiency virus 1 or 2 (HIV-1 is the predominant serotype identified). The major cellular defect brought on by infection with HIV is a depletion of T-cells, primarily the sub-type, T-helper cells, known as CD4+ cells. Over these years, our knowledge regarding HIV infection and the oral manifestations often associated with patients with HIV or AIDS, has increased dramatically. Populations of individuals known to be at high risk of HIV transmission include homosexuals, intravenous drug abuse patients, transfusion recipients, patients with other sexually transmitted diseases, and patients practicing promiscuous sex.

The definitions of AIDS have also evolved over this period of time. The natural history of HIV infection along with some of the oral manifestations can be reviewed in Table 1. The risk of developing these opportunistic infections increases as the patient progresses to AIDS.

Table 1.
NATURAL HISTORY OF HIV INFECTION/ORAL MANIFESTATIONS

Time From Transmission (Average)	Observation	CD4 Cell Count
0	Viral transmissions	Normal: 1000 (±500/mm^3)
2-4 weeks	Self-limited infectious mononucleosis-like illness with fever, rash, leukopenia, mucocutaneous ulcerations (mouth, genitals, etc), thrush	Transient decrease
6-12 weeks	Seroconversion (rarely requires ≥3 months for seroconversion)	Normal
0-8 years	Healthy/asymptomatic HIV infection; peripheral/persistent generalized lymphadenopathy; HPV, thrush, OHL; RAU, periodontal diseases, salivary gland diseases; dermatitis	≥500/mm^3 gradual reduction with average decrease of 50-80/mm^3/year
4-8 years	Early symptomatic HIV infection previously called (AIDS-related complex): Thrush, vaginal candidiasis (persistent, frequent and/or severe), cervical dysplasia/CA Hodgkin's lymphoma, B-cell lymphoma, oral hairy leukoplakia, salivary gland diseases, ITP, xerostomia, dermatitis, shingles; RAU, herpes simplex, HPV, bacterial infections, periodontal diseases, molluscum contagiosum, other physical symptoms: fever, weight loss, fatigue	≥300-500/mm^3
6-10 years	AIDS: Wasting syndrome, *Candida* esophagitis, Kaposi's sarcoma, HIV-associated dementia, disseminated *M. avium*, Hodgkin's or B-cell lymphoma, herpes simplex >30 days; PCP; cryptococcal meningitis, other systemic fungal infections; CMV	<200/mm^3

Natural history indicates course of HIV infection in absence of antiretroviral treatment. Adapted from Bartlett JG, "A Guide to HIV Care from the AIDS Care Program of the Johns Hopkins Medical Institutions," 2nd ed.

PCP -*Pneumocystis carinii* pneumonia; ITP -idiopathic thrombocytopenia purpura; HPV - human papilloma virus; OHL - oral hairy leukoplakia; RAU - recurrent aphthous ulcer

Patients with HIV infection and/or AIDS are seen in dental offices throughout the country. In general, it is the dentist's obligation to treat HIV individuals including patients of record and other patients who may seek treatment when the office is accepting new patients. These patients are protected under the Americans with Disabilities Act and the dentist has an obligation as described. Two excellent publications, one by the American Dental Association and the other by the American Academy of Oral Medicine, outline the dentist's responsibility as well as a very detailed explanation of dental management protocols for HIV patients. These protocols, however, are evolving just as our knowledge of HIV has evolved. New drugs and their interactions present the dentist with continuous need for updates regarding the appropriate management of HIV patients. Diagnostic tests, including determining viral load in combination with the CD4 status, now are used to modify a patient's treatment in ways that allow them to remain relatively illness-free for longer periods of time. This places more of a responsibility on the dental practice team to be aware of drug changes, of new drugs, and of the appropriate oral management in such patients.

Our knowledge of AIDS allows us to properly treat these patients while protecting ourselves, our staff, and other patients in the office. All types of infectious disease require consistent practices in our dental offices known as Universal Precautions (see Infectious Disease Information *on page 1601*). The office team that utilizes these precautions appropriately is well protected against passage of infectious agents. These agents include sexually transmitted disease agents, the highly virulent hepatitis viruses, and the less virulent but always worrisome HIV. In general, an office that is practicing universal precautions is one that is considered safe for patients and staff. Throughout this spectrum, HIV is placed somewhere in the middle in terms of infection risk in the dental office. Other sexually transmitted diseases and infectious diseases such as tuberculosis represent a greater threat to the dentist than HIV itself. However, due to the grave danger of HIV infection, many of our precautions have been instituted to assist the dentist in protecting himself, his staff, and other patients in situations where the office may be involved in treating a patient that is HIV positive.

As in the management of all medically compromised patients, the appropriate care of HIV patients begins with a complete and thorough history. This history must allow the dentist to identify risk factors in the development of HIV as well as identify those patients known to be HIV positive. Knowledge of all medications prescribed to patients at risk is also important.

The current antiretroviral therapy used to treat patients with HIV infection and/or AIDS includes three primary classifications of drugs. These are the nucleoside analogs, protease inhibitors, and the non-nucleoside/nucleotide analogs (analogs refers to chemicals that can substitute competitively for naturally produced cell components such as found in DNA, RNA, or proteins). The newest drugs include several nucleoside analogs, abacavir (Ziagen®), subprotease inhibitors, amprenavir, and several non-nucleoside analogs, efavirenz (Sustiva®) and adefovir. Finding the perfect "cocktail" of anti-HIV medications still eludes clinicians. This is partly due to the fact that therapies are still too novel and the patient's years too few to study. Numerous recently published studies have indicated that combinations of drugs are far better than individual drug therapy. Several of these studies have looked at two drug combinations particularly between nucleoside analogs in combination with protease inhibitors. The newer drugs (non-nucleoside analogs) have added the possibility of a triple cocktail. Recently several studies indicated that this three-drug combination may be the best in managing HIV infection.

When HIV was first discovered, the efforts for monitoring HIV infection focused on the CD4 blood levels and the ratios between the helper cells, suppressor cells within the patient's immune system. These markers were used to indicate success or failure of drug therapies as patients moved through HIV pathogenesis toward AIDS. More recently, however, the advent of protease inhibitors has allowed clinicians to monitor the actual presence of viral RNA within the patient and the term viral load has become the focus of therapy monitoring. The availability of better therapies and our rapidly expanding knowledge of molecular biology of the HIV virus have created new opportunities to control the AIDS epidemic. Cases can be monitored quite closely looking at the number of copy units or virions within the patient's bloodstream as an indication in combination with other infections and/or declining or increasing CD4 numbers to establish prognostic values for the patient's success. Long-term survival of patients infected with HIV has been accomplished by monitoring and adjusting therapy to these numbers.

Comprehensive coordinated approaches, that have been advocated by researchers, have sought to establish national standards for HIV reporting, greater access to effective newly approved medications, improved access to individual physicians treating HIV patients, and continued protection of patient's privacy. These goals allow the reporting of studies that suggest that combination therapies, some of which have been tried in less controlled individual patient treatments, may prove useful in larger populations of HIV-infected individuals. As these studies are reported, the dental clinician should be aware that patients' drug therapies change rapidly, various combinations may be tried, and the side effects and interactions as described in the chapter on drug interactions and the CYP system will also emerge. The dentist must be aware of these potential interactions with seemingly innocuous drugs such as clarithromycin, erythromycin, and some of the sedative drugs that a dentist may utilize in their practice as well as some of the analgesics. These drug interactions may be the most important part of monitoring that the dentist provides in helping to manage a situation. Some of the antiviral drugs more commonly used for HIV, AIDS, Asymptomatic, CD4 <500, and the newer drugs (ie, protease inhibitors, nucleoside analogs, and non-nucleoside nucleotide analogs) are listed in Table 2 on following page.

HIV INFECTION AND AIDS *(Continued)*

Table 2. CATEGORIES OF ANTIRETROVIRAL DRUGS

Nucleoside Analogs	Protease Inhibitors	Non-Nucleoside/Nucleotide Analogs
Zidovudine	Saquinavir	Nevirapine
(Retrovir®, AZT, SDV)	(Invirase®)	(Viramune®)
Didanosine	Ritonavir	Delavirdine
(Videx®, ddi)	(Norvir®)	(Rescriptor®)
Zalcitabine	Indinavir	Efavirenz
(Hivid®, ddc)	(Crixivan®)	(Sustiva®)
Stavudine	Nelfinavir	Adefovir
(Zerit®, d4T)	(Viracept®)	(HepSera™)
Lamivudine	Amprenavir	
(Epivir®)	(Agenerase®)	
Abacavir		
(Ziagen®)		

The presence of other infections is an important part of the health history. Appropriate medical consultation may be mandated after a health history in order to accomplish a complete evaluation of the patients at risk. Uniformity in the taking of a history from a patient is the dentist's best plan for all patients so that no selectivity or discrimination can be implicated.

An appropriate review of symptoms may also identify oral and systemic conditions that may be present in aggressive HIV disease. Medical physical examination may reveal pre-existing or developing intra- or extra-oral signs/symptoms of progressive disease. Aggressive herpes simplex, herpes zoster, papillomavirus, Kaposi's sarcoma or lymphoma are among the disorders that might be identified. In addition to these, intra-oral examination may raise suspicion regarding fungal infections, angular cheilitis, squamous cell carcinoma, and recurrent aphthous ulcers. The dentist should be vigilant in all patients regardless of HIV risk.

It will always be up to the dental practitioner to determine whether testing for HIV should be recommended following the history and physical examination of a new patient. Because of the severe psychological implications of learning of HIV positivity for a patient, the dentist should be aware that there are appropriate referral sites where psychological counseling and appropriate discrete testing for the patient is available. The dentist's office should have these sites available for referral should the patient be interested. Candid discussions, however, with the patient regarding risk factors and/or other signs or symptoms in their history and physical condition that may indicate a higher HIV risk than the normal population, should be an area the dentist feels comfortable in broaching with any new patient. Oftentimes, it is appropriate to recommend testing for other infectious diseases should risk factors be present. For example, testing for hepatitis B may be appropriate for the patient and along with this the dentist could recommend that the patient consider HIV testing. Because of the legal issues involved, anonymity for HIV testing may be appropriate and it is always up to the patient to follow the doctor's recommendations.

When a patient has either given a positive history of knowing that they are HIV positive or it has been determined after referral for consultation, the dentist should be aware of the AIDS-defining illnesses. Of course, current medical status and drug therapy that the patient may be undergoing is of equal importance. The dentist, through medical consultation and regular follow-up with the patient's physician, should be made aware of the CD4 count (Table 3), the viral load, and the drugs that the patient is taking. The presence of other AIDS-defining illnesses as well as complications, such as higher risk of endocarditis and the risk of other systemic infections such as tuberculosis, are extremely important for the dentist. These may make an impact on the dental treatment plan in terms of the selection of preprocedural antibiotics or the use of oral medications to treat opportunistic infections in or around the oral cavity.

Table 3. CD4+ LYMPHOCYTE COUNT AND PERCENTAGE AS RELATED TO THE RISK OF OPPORTUNISTIC INFECTION

CD4+ Cells/mm^3	CD4+ Percentage*	Risk of Opportunistic Infection
>600	32-60	No increased risk
400-500	<29	Initial immune suppression
200-400	14-28	Appearance of opportunistic infections, some may be major
<200	<14	Severe immune suppression. AIDS diagnosis. Major opportunistic infections. Although variable, prognosis for surviving greater than 3 years is poor
<50	—	Although variable, prognosis for surviving greater than 1 year is poor

*Several studies have suggested that the CD4+ percentage demonstrates less variability between measurements, as compared to the absolute CD4+ cell count. CD4+ percentages may therefore give a clearer impression of the course of disease.

Adapted from Glick M and Silverman S, "Dental Management of HIV-Infected Patients," *J Am Dent Assoc* (Supplement to Reviewers), 1995.

AIDS-defining illnesses such as candidiasis, recurrent pneumonia, or lymphoma are clearly important to the dentist. Chemotherapy that might be being given to the patient for treatment for any or all of these disorders can have implications in terms of the patient's response to simple dental procedures.

Drug therapies have become complex in the treatment of HIV/AIDS. Because of the moderate successes with protease inhibitors and the drug combination therapies, more patients are living longer and receiving more dental care throughout their lives. Drug therapies are often tailored to the current CD4 count in combination with the viral load. In general, patients with high CD4 counts are usually at lower risk for complications in the dental office than patients with low CD4 counts. However, the presence of a high viral load with or without a stable CD4 count may be indicative or a more rapid progression of the HIV/AIDS disease process than had previously been thought. Patients with a high viral load and a declining CD4 count are considered to have the greatest risk and the poorest prognosis of all the groups.

Other organ damage, such as liver compromise potentially leading to bleeding disorders, can be found as the disease progresses to AIDS. Liver dysfunction may be related to pre-existing hepatic diseases due to previous infection with a hepatitis virus such as hepatitis B or other drug toxicities associated with the treatment of AIDS. The dentist must have available current prothrombin and partial thromboplastin times (PT and PTT) in order to accurately evaluate any risk of bleeding abnormality. Platelet count and liver function studies are also important. Potential drug interactions include some antibiotics, as well as any anticoagulating drugs, which may be contraindicated in such patients. It may be necessary to avoid nonsteroidal anti-inflammatory drugs as well as aspirin. (See the introductory text "Pharmacology of Drug Metabolism and Interactions" *on page 18*).

The use of preprocedural antibiotics is another issue in the HIV patient. As the absolute neutrophil count declines during the progression of AIDS, the use of antibiotics as a preprocedural step prior to dental care may be necessary. If protracted treatment plans are necessary, the dentist should receive updated information as the patient receives such from their physician. It is always important that the dentist have current CD4 counts, viral load assay, as well as liver function studies, AST and ALT, and bleeding indicators including platelet count, PT, and PTT. If any other existing conditions such as cardiac involvement or joint prostheses are involved, antibiotic coverage may also be necessary. However, these determinations are no different than in the non-HIV population and this subject is covered in "Preprocedural Antibiotic Prophylaxis Guidelines for Dental Patients" *on page 1507*. Use the table of Normal Blood Values *on page 1618* as a general guideline for provision of dental care.

The consideration of current blood values is important in long-term care of any medically compromised patient and in particular the HIV-positive patient. Preventive dental care is likewise valuable in these patients, however, the dentist's approach should be no different than as with all patients. See Table 4 for oral lesions commonly associated with HIV disease and a brief description of their usual treatment. The clinician is referred to other sections of the text for more detailed descriptions of these common oral lesions. Other important parts of the text that may be useful for the dentist include the office protocol for universal precautions *on page 1601* and the Frequently Asked Questions at the end of this chapter. The clinician should also be aware that several of the protease inhibitors have now been associated with drug interactions. Some of these drug interactions include therapies that the dentist may be utilizing. The basis for these drug interactions with protease inhibitors is the inhibition of cytochrome P450 isoforms, which are important in normal liver function and metabolism of drugs. A detailed description of the mechanisms of inhibition can be found in "Pharmacology of Drug Metabolism and Interactions" *on page 18*, as well as a table illustrating some known drug interactions with antiviral therapy and drugs commonly prescribed in the dental office. The metabolism of these drugs could be affected by the patient's antiviral therapy. Please

HIV INFECTION AND AIDS *(Continued)*

see the section on selected references for more information on management of HIV patients.

Table 4. ORAL LESIONS COMMONLY SEEN IN HIV/AIDS

Condition	Management
Oral candidiasis	See "Oral Fungal Infections" *on page 1542*
Angular cheilitis	See "Oral Fungal Infections" *on page 1542*
Oral hairy leukoplakia	See "Systemic Viral Diseases" *on page 1517*
Periodontal diseases	See "Oral Bacterial Infections" *on page 1531*
Linear gingivitis	
Ulcerative periodontitis	
Herpes simplex	Acyclovir - see "Systemic Viral Diseases" *on page 1517*
Herpes zoster	Acyclovir - see "Systemic Viral Diseases" *on page 1517*
Chronic aphthous ulceration	Palliation / Thalidomide (Thalomid®)
Salivary gland disease	Referral
Human papillomavirus	Laser / Surgical excision
Kaposi's sarcoma	See "Antibiotic Prophylaxis" *on page 1507*; Biopsy / Laser
Non-Hodgkin's lymphoma	Biopsy / Referral
Tuberculosis	Referral

Dapsone *on page 399*
Delavirdine *on page 405*
Didanosine *on page 434*
Indinavir *on page 718*
Lamivudine *on page 773*
Lopinavir and Ritonavir *on page 820*
Nelfinavir *on page 959*
Ritonavir *on page 1188*
Stavudine *on page 1242*
Thalidomide *on page 1289*
Tenofovir *on page 1275*
Zalcitabine *on page 1403*
Zidovudine *on page 1406*
Zidovudine and Lamivudine *on page 1407*

FREQUENTLY ASKED QUESTIONS

How does one get AIDS, aside from having unprotected sex?

Our current knowledge about the immunodeficiency virus is that it is carried via semen, contaminated needles, blood products, transfusion products not tested, and potentially in other fluids of the body. Patients at highest risk include I.V. drug abusers, those receiving multiple transfusions with blood that has not been screened for HIV, or patients practicing unprotected sex with multiple partners, where the history of the partner may not be as clear as the patient would like.

Are patients safe from AIDS or HIV infection when they present to the dentist office?

Our current knowledge indicates that the answer is an unequivocal yes. The patient is protected because dental offices are practicing universal precautions using antimicrobial handwashing agents, gloves, face masks, eye protection, special clothing, aerosol control, and instrument soaking and autoclaving. All of these procedures stop potential transmission to a new patient, as well as, allow for easy disposal of contaminated office supplies for elimination of microbes by an antimicrobial technique, should they be contaminated through treatment of another patient. These precautions are mandated by OSHA requirements and covered in Universal Precautions in the Appendix.

What is the most common opportunistic infection that HIV-positive patients suffer that may be important in dentistry?

The most common opportunistic infection important to dentistry is oral candidiasis. This disease can present as white plaques, red areas, or angular cheilitis occurring at the corners of the mouth. Management of such lesions is appropriate by the dentist and is described in this handbook (see Oral Fungal Infections *on page 1542*). Other oral complications include HIV-associated periodontal disease, as well as the other conditions outlined in Table 4. Of great concern to the dentist is the risk of tuberculosis. In many HIV-positive patients, tuberculosis has become a serious, life-threatening opportunistic infection. The dentist should be aware that appropriate referral for anyone showing such respiratory signs and symptoms would be prudent.

Can one patient infect another through unprotected sex if the other patient has tested negative for HIV?

Yes, there is always the possibility that a sexual partner may be in the early window of time when plasma viremia is not at a detectable level. The antibody response to plasma viremia may be slightly delayed and diagnostic testing may not indicate HIV positivity. This window of time represents a period when the patient may be infectious but not show up yet on normal diagnostic testing.

Can HIV be passed by oral fluids?

As our knowledge about HIV has evolved, we have thought that HIV is inactivated in saliva by an agent possibly associated with secretory leukocyte protease inhibitors known as SLPI. There is, however, a current resurgence in our interest in oral transmission because some research indicates that in moderate to advanced periodontal lesions or other oral lesions where there is tissue damage, the presence of a serous exudate may increase the risk of transmission. The dentist should be aware of this ongoing research and attempt to renew knowledge regularly so that any future breakthroughs will be noted.

RHEUMATOID ARTHRITIS, OSTEOARTHRITIS, AND OSTEOPOROSIS

RA AND OSTEOARTHRITIS MANAGEMENT

Arthritis and its variations represent the most common chronic musculoskeletal disorders of man. The conditions can essentially be divided into rheumatoid, osteoarthritic, and polyarthritic presentations. Differences in age of onset and joint involvement exist and it is now currently believed that the diagnosis of each may be less clear than previously thought. These autoinflammatory diseases have now been shown to affect young and old alike. Criteria for a diagnosis of rheumatoid arthritis include a positive serologic test for rheumatoid factor, subcutaneous nodules, affected joints on opposite sides of the body, and clear radiographic changes. The hematologic picture includes moderate normocytic hypochromic anemia, mild leukocytosis, and mild thrombocytopenia. During acute inflammatory periods, C-reactive protein is elevated and IgG and IgM (rheumatoid factors) can be detected. Osteoarthritis lacks these diagnostic features.

Other systemic conditions, such as systemic lupus erythematosus and Sjögren's syndrome, are often found simultaneously with some of the arthritic conditions. The treatment of arthritis includes the use of slow-acting and rapid-acting anti-inflammatory agents ranging from the gold salts to aspirin (see following listings). Long-term usage of these drugs can lead to numerous adverse effects including bone marrow suppression, platelet suppression, and oral ulcerations. The dentist should be aware that steroids (usually prednisone) are often prescribed along with the listed drugs and are often used in dosages sufficient to induce adrenal suppression. Adjustment of dosing prior to invasive dental procedures may be indicated along with consultation with the managing physician. Alteration of steroid dosage prior to stressful dental procedures may be necessary, usually increasing the steroid dosage prior to and during the stressful procedures and then gradually returning the patient to the original dosage over several days. Even in the absence of evidence of adrenal suppression, consultation with the prescribing physician for appropriate dosing and timing of procedures is advisable.

Gold Salts

Auranofin *on page 147*
Aurothioglucose *on page 148*

Metabolic Inhibitor

Leflunomide *on page 779*
Methotrexate *on page 884*

Immunomodulator

Etanercept *on page 537*

Nonsteroidal Anti-inflammatory Agents

Aminosalicylic Acid
Choline Magnesium Trisalicylate *on page 319*
Choline Salicylate *on page 319*
Diclofenac *on page 429*
Diflunisal *on page 438*
Etodolac *on page 547*
Fenoprofen *on page 563*
Flurbiprofen *on page 596*
Ibuprofen *on page 703*
Indomethacin *on page 719*
Ketoprofen *on page 763*
Ketorolac *on page 765*
Magnesium Salicylate *on page 837*
Meclofenamate *on page 848*
Mefenamic Acid *on page 851*
Nabumetone *on page 941*
Naproxen *on page 953*
Oxaprozin *on page 1010*
Piroxicam *on page 1090*
Salsalate *on page 1206*
Sulindac *on page 1257*
Tolmetin *on page 1321*

COX-2 Inhibitor NSAID

Celecoxib *on page 281*
Rofecoxib *on page 1194*
Valdecoxib *on page 1368*

Combination NSAID Product to Prevent GI Distress

Diclofenac and Misoprostol *on page 431*

Salicylates

Aspirin *on page 131*
Choline Magnesium Trisalicylate *on page 319*
Salsalate *on page 1206*

Other

Hydroxychloroquine *on page 694*
Prednisone *on page 1112*

ANTI-INFLAMMATORY AGENTS USED IN THE TREATMENT OF RA AND OSTEOARTHRITIS

Drug	Adverse Effects
SLOW-ACTING	
GOLD SALTS	
Aurothioglucose; Auranofin; Gold Sodium Thiomalate	GI intolerance, diarrhea; leukopenia, thrombocytopenia, and/or anemia; skin and oral eruptions; possible nephrotoxicity and hepatotoxicity
METABOLIC INHIBITOR	
Leflunomide (Arava™)	Diarrhea, respiratory tract infection
Methotrexate	Oral ulcerations, leukopenia
IMMUNOMODULATOR	
Etanercept (Enbrel®)	Headache, respiratory tract infection, positive ANA
OTHER	
Hydroxychloroquine (Plaquenil®)	Usually mild and reversible; ophthalmic complications
Prednisone	Insomnia, nervousness, indigestion, increased appetite
RAPID-ACTING	
SALICYLATES	
Aspirin	Inhibition of platelet aggregation; gastrointestinal (GI) irritation, ulceration, and bleeding; tinnitus; teratogenicity
Choline magnesium salicylate (Trilisate®)	GI irritation and ulceration, weakness, skin rash, hemolytic anemia, troubled breathing
Salsalate	
OTHER NONSTEROIDAL ANTI-INFLAMMATORY DRUGS	
Diclofenac (Cataflam®, Voltaren®); Diflunisal (Dolobid®); Etodolac (Lodine®); Fenoprofen calcium (Nalfon®); Flurbiprofen sodium (Ansaid®); Ibuprofen (Motrin®); Indomethacin (Indocin®); Ketoprofen; Ketorolac tromethamine (Toradol®); Meclofenamate; Nabumetone (Relafen®); Naproxen (Naprosyn®); Oxaprozin (Daypro®); Piroxicam (Feldene®); Salsalate (Mono-Gesic®, Salflex®); Sulindac (Clinoril®); Tolmetin (Tolectin®)	GI irritation, ulceration, and bleeding; inhibition of platelet aggregation; displacement of protein-bound drugs (eg, oral anticoagulants, sulfonamides, and sulfonylureas); headache; vertigo; mucocutaneous rash or ulceration; parotid enlargement
COX-2 INHIBITOR NSAID	
Celecoxib (Celebrex®) Rofecoxib (Vioxx®) Valdecoxib (Bextra®)	Headache, dyspepsia, upper respiratory tract infection, sinusitis
COMBINATION NSAID PRODUCT TO PREVENT GI DISTRESS	
Diclofenac and Misoprostol (Arthrotec®)	Inhibition of platelet aggregation; displacement of protein-bound drugs (eg, oral anticoagulants, sulfonamides, and sulfonylureas); headache; vertigo; mucocutaneous rash or ulceration; parotid enlargement; diarrhea

OSTEOPOROSIS MANAGEMENT

PREVALENCE

Osteoporosis effects 25 million Americans of which 80% are women; 27% of American women >80 years of age have osteopenia and 70% of American women >80 years of age have osteoporosis.

CONSEQUENCES

1.3 million bone fractures annually (low impact/nontraumatic) and pain, pulmonary insufficiency, decreased quality of life, and economic costs; >250,000 hip fractures per year with a 20% mortality rate.

RHEUMATOID ARTHRITIS, OSTEOARTHRITIS, AND OSTEOPOROSIS *(Continued)*

RISK FACTORS

Advanced age, female, chronic renal disease, hyperparathyroidism, Cushing's disease, hypogonadism/anorexia, hyperprolactinemia, cancer, large and prolonged dose heparin or glucocorticoids, anticonvulsants, hyperthyroidism (current or history, or excessive thyroid supplements), sedentary, excessive exercise, early menopause, oophorectomy without hormone replacement, excessive aluminum-containing antacid, smoking, methotrexate.

DIAGNOSIS/MONITORING

DXA bone density, history of fracture (low impact or nontraumatic), compressed vertebrae, decreased height, hump-back appearance. Osteomark™ urine assay measures bone breakdown fragments and may help assess therapy response earlier than DXA but diagnostic value is uncertain as Osteomark™ does not reveal extent of bone loss. Bone markers may be tested to evaluate effectiveness of antiresorptive urine therapy.

PREVENTION

1. Adequate dietary calcium (eg, dairy products)
2. Vitamin D (eg, fortified dairy products, cod, fatty fish)
3. Weight-bearing exercise (eg, walking) as tolerated
4. Calcium supplement of 1000-1500 mg elemental calcium daily (divided in 500 mg increments); women >65 years on estrogen replacement therapy supplement 1000 mg elemental calcium; women >65 not receiving estrogens and men >55 years supplement 1500 mg elemental calcium. To minimize constipation add fiber and start with 500 mg/day for several months, then increase to 500 mg twice daily taken at different times than fiber. Chewable and liquid products are available. Calcium carbonate is given with food to enhance bioavailability. Calcium citrate may be given without regards to meals.
   - Contraindications: Hypercalcemia, ventricular fibrillation
   - Side effects: Constipation, anorexia
   - Drug interactions: Fiber, tetracycline, iron supplement, minerals
5. Vitamin D Supplement: 400-800 units daily (often satisfied by 1-2 multivitamins or fortified milk) in addition to calcium or a combined calcium and vitamin D supplement and/or >15 minutes direct sunlight/day. Some elderly, especially with significant renal or liver disease cannot metabolize (activate) vitamin D and require calcitriol 0.25 mcg orally twice daily or adjusted per serum calcium level, the active form of vitamin D; can check 1,25 OH vitamin D level to confirm need for calcitriol.
   - Contraindications: Hypercalcemia (weakness, headache, drowsiness, nausea, diarrhea), hypercalciuria and renal stones
   - Side effects (uncommon): Hypercalcemia (see above)
   - Monitor 24-hour urine and serum calcium if using >1000 units/day
6. Estrogen: Especially useful if bone density <80% of average plus symptoms of estrogen deficiency or cardiac disease. Bone density increases over 1-2 years then plateaus. This is considered 1st line therapy unless contraindicated due to medicinal history (see below) or risk:benefit assessment which leads to decision to avoid HRT (hormone replacement therapy). **Note:** Estrogens should not be used to prevent coronary heart disease.
   - Contraindications: Pregnancy, breast or estrogen-dependent cancer, undiagnosed abnormal genital bleeding, active thrombophlebitis, or history of thromboembolism during previous estrogen or oral contraceptive therapy or pregnancy. Pretreatment mammogram, gynecological exam are advised along with routine breast exam because of an increased risk of breast cancer with long-term use.
   - Dose: Conjugated estrogen of 0.625 mg/day or its equivalent (continuous therapy preferred).
   - Side effects: Vaginal spotting/bleeding, nausea, vomiting, breast tenderness/enlargement, amenorrheic with extended use.
     Initiate therapy slowly (side effects are more common and severe in women without estrogen for many years). Administer with medroxyprogesterone acetate (MPA) 2.5-5 mg daily, or another oral progesterone, in women with uterus (unopposed estrogen can cause endometrial cancer). MPA can increase vaginal bleeding, increase weight, edema, mood changes.
   - Drug Interactions: May increase corticosteroid effect, monitor for need to decrease corticosteroid dose.

7. Selective estrogen receptor modulators: Selective-estrogen receptor modulators (SERMs) are nonsteroidal modulators of estrogen-receptor mediated reactions. The key difference between these agents and estrogen replacement therapies is the potential to exert tissue specific effects. Due to their chemical differences, these agents retain some of estrogen's beneficial effects on bone metabolism and lipid levels, but differ in their actions on breast and endometrial tissues, potentially limiting adverse effects related to nonspecific hormone stimulation. Among the SERMs, tamoxifen retains stimulatory effects in endometrial tissue, while raloxifene does not stimulate endometrial or breast tissue, limiting the potential for endometrial or breast cancer related to this agent. Raloxifene is the only SERM which has been approved by the FDA for osteoporosis prevention.

   It should be noted that the effects on bone observed with SERMs appear to be less than that observed with estrogen replacement. In one study, the effect of raloxifene on hip bone mineral density was approximately half of that observed with conjugated estrogens. In addition, the effects on lipid profiles are less than with estrogen replacement. Finally, SERMs do not block the vasomotor effects observed with menopause, which may limit compliance with therapy. As with estrogen replacement, reloxifene has been associated with an increased risk of thromboembolism and is contraindicated in patients with a history of thromboembolic disease.

8. Estradiol, as well as various combination therapies, including ethinyl estradiol with norethindrone (Femhrt®) and ethinyl with norgestimate (Ortho-Prefest™), have been approved for the prevention of osteoporosis.

TREATMENT

1. Calcium, vitamin D, exercise, and estrogen: As above
2. Bisphosphonates:

   Consider if patient is intolerant of, or refuses estrogen or it is contraindicated, especially if severe osteoporosis (ie, ≥2.5 standard deviations below average young adult bone density, T-score, or history of low impact or nontraumatic fracture). Increasing bone density of hip and spine observed for at least 3 years (ie, no plateau as seen with estrogen).

   Contraindications: Hypocalcemia, not advised if existing gastrointestinal disorders (eg, esophageal disorders such as reflux, sensitive stomach).

   – Alendronate (Fosamax®): Dose: 10 mg once daily or 70 mg/week (treatment dose for osteoporosis; not recommended if creatinine clearance <35 mL/minute). Osteopenia: 5 mg per day or 35 mg/week for prevention.

   – Risedronate (Actonel®: Dose: 5 mg daily or 35 mg/week for treatment or prevention

   Take before breakfast on an empty stomach with 6-8 ounces tap water (not mineral water, coffee, or juice) and remain upright or raise head of bed for bedridden patients at least 30 degree angle for at least 30 minutes (otherwise may cause ulcerative esophagitis) before eating or drinking.

   Therapy with calcium and vitamin D is advised, but must be given at a different time of day than alendronate.

   - Side effects (well tolerated): Difficulty swallowing, heartburn, abdominal discomfort, nausea (GI side effects increase with aspirin products), arthralgia/myalgia, constipation, diarrhea, headache, esophagitis.
   - Drug interactions: None known to date.

3. Etidronate: Not FDA approved for postmenopausal osteoporosis and can decrease the quality of bone formation, therefore, change to alendronate.
4. Calcitonin (nasal; Miacalcin®): Indicated if estrogen refused, intolerant, or contraindicated. Potential analgesic effect.

   - Contraindications: Hypersensitivity to salmon protein or gelatin diluent; 1 spray (200 units) into 1 nostril daily (alternate right and left nostril daily); 5 days on and 2 days off is also effective; alternate day administration not effective. If used only for pain, can decrease dose once pain is controlled.
   - Side effects (few): Nasal dryness and irritation (periodically inspect); adequate dietary or supplemental calcium + vitamin D is essential.

   Subcutaneous route (100 units daily): Many side effects (eg, nausea, flushing, anorexia) and the discomfort/inconvenience of injection.

5. Fall prevention: Minimize psychoactive and cardiovascular drugs (monitor BP for orthostasis), give diuretics early in the day, environmental safety check.

RHEUMATOID ARTHRITIS, OSTEOARTHRITIS, AND OSTEOPOROSIS *(Continued)*

	% Elemental Calcium	Elemental Calcium
Calcium gluconate (various)	9	500 mg = 45 mg
Calcium glubionate (Neo-Calglucon®)	6.5	1.8 g = 115 g/5 mL
Calcium lactate (various)	13	325 mg = 42.25 mg
Calcium citrate (Citrical®)	21	950 mg = 200 mg
Effervescent tabs (Citrical Liquitab®)		2376 mg = 500 mg
Calcium acetate		
Phos-Ex 250®	25	1000 mg = 250 mg
Phos-Lo®		667 mg = 169 mg
Tricalcium phosphate (Posture®)	39	1565.2 mg = 600 mg
Calcium carbonate		
Tums®	40	1.2 g = 500 mg
Oscal-500® oral suspension		1.2 g/5 mL = 500 mg
Caltrate 600®		1.5 g = 600 mg

References

Ashworth L, "Focus on Alendronate. A Nonhormonal Option for the Treatment of Osteoporosis in Postmenopausal Women," *Formulary*, 1996, 31:23-30.

Johnson SR, "Should Older Women Use Estrogen Replacement," *J Am Geriatr Soc*, 1996, 44:89-90.

Liberman UA, Weiss SR, and Brool J, "Effect of Oral Alendronate on Bone-Mineral Density and the Incidence of Fracture in Postmenopausal Osteoporosis," *N Engl J Med*, 1995, 333:1437-43.

"New Drugs for Osteoporosis," *Med Lett Drugs Ther*, 1996, 38:1-3.

NIH Consensus Development Panel on Optimal Calcium Intake, *JAMA*, 1994, 272:1942-8.

NONVIRAL INFECTIOUS DISEASES

TUBERCULOSIS

Tuberculosis is caused by the organism *Mycobacterium tuberculosis* as well as a variety of other mycobacteria including *M. bovis, M. avium-intracellulare,* and *M. kansasii.* Diagnosis of tuberculosis can be made from a skin test and a positive chest x-ray as well as acid-fast smears of cultures from respiratory secretions. Nucleic acid probes and polymerase chain reaction (PCR) to identify nucleic acid of *M. tuberculosis* have recently become useful.

The treatment of tuberculosis is based on the general principle that multiple drugs should reduce infectivity within 2 weeks and that failures in therapy may be due to noncompliance with the long-term regimens necessary. General treatment regimens last 6-12 months.

Isoniazid-resistant and multidrug-resistant mycobacterial infections have become an increasingly significant problem in recent years. TB as an opportunistic disease in HIV-positive patients has also risen. Combination drug therapy has always been popular in TB management and the advent of new antibiotics has not diminished this need.

ANTITUBERCULOSIS DRUGS

Bactericidal Agents

Capreomycin *on page 237*
*Isoniazid *on page 748*
Kanamycin *on page 759*
*Pyrazinamide *on page 1150*
Rifabutin *on page 1179*
*Rifampin *on page 1180*
*Streptomycin *on page 1245*

Bacteriostatic Agents

Cycloserine *on page 383*
*Ethambutol *on page 539*
Ethionamide *on page 542*
Aminosalicyllic Acid

*Drugs of Choice

TESTING

Tuberculin Skin Test Recommendations[1]

Children for whom immediate skin testing is indicated:

- Contacts of persons with confirmed or suspected infectious tuberculosis (contact investigation); this includes children identified as contacts of family members or associates in jail or prison in the last 5 years
- Children with radiographic or clinical findings suggesting tuberculosis
- Children immigrating from endemic countries (eg, Asia, Middle East, Africa, Latin America)
- Children with travel histories to endemic countries and/or significant contact with indigenous persons from such countries

Children who should be tested annually for tuberculosis[2]:

- Children infected with HIV or living in household with HIV-infected persons
- Incarcerated adolescents

Children who should be tested every 2-3 years[2]:

- Children exposed to the following individuals: HIV-infected, homeless, residents of nursing homes, institutionalized adolescents or adults, users of illicit drugs, incarcerated adolescents or adults, and migrant farm workers. Foster children with exposure to adults in the preceding high-risk groups are included.

Children who should be considered for tuberculin skin testing at ages 4-6 and 11-16 years:

- Children whose parents immigrated (with unknown tuberculin skin test status) from regions of the world with high prevalence of tuberculosis; continued potential exposure by travel to the endemic areas and/or household contact with persons from the endemic areas (with unknown tuberculin skin test status) should be an indication for repeat tuberculin skin testing
- Children without specific risk factors who reside in high-prevalence areas; in general, a high-risk neighborhood or community does not mean an entire city is at high risk; rates in any area of the city may vary by neighborhood, or even from block to block; physicians should be aware of these patterns in determining the likelihood of exposure; public health officials or local tuberculosis experts should help clinicians identify areas that have appreciable tuberculosis rates

NONVIRAL INFECTIOUS DISEASES *(Continued)*

Children at increased risk of progression of infection to disease: Those with other medical risk factors, including diabetes mellitus, chronic renal failure, malnutrition, and congenital or acquired immunodeficiencies deserve special consideration. Without recent exposure, these persons are not at increased risk of acquiring tuberculosis infection. Underlying immune deficiencies associated with these conditions theoretically would enhance the possibility for progression to severe disease. Initial histories of potential exposure to tuberculosis should be included on all of these patients. If these histories or local epidemiologic factors suggest a possibility of exposure, immediate and periodic tuberculin skin testing should be considered. An initial Mantoux tuberculin skin test should be performed before initiation of immunosuppressive therapy in any child with an underlying condition that necessitates immunosuppressive therapy.

[1]BCG immunization is not a contraindication to tuberculin skin testing.

[2]Initial tuberculin skin testing is at the time of diagnosis or circumstance, beginning as early as at age 3 months.

Changes From Prior Recommendations on Tuberculin Testing and Treatment of Latent Tuberculosis Infection (LTBI)

Tuberculin Testing

- Emphasis on targeted tuberculin testing among persons at high risk for recent LTBI or with clinical conditions that increase the risk for tuberculosis (TB), regardless of age; testing is discouraged among persons at lower risk.
- For patients with organ transplant and other immunosuppressed patients (eg, persons receiving the equivalent of ≥15 mg/day prednisone for 1 month or more), 5 mm of induration rather than 10 mm of induration as a cut-off level for tuberculin positivity.
- A tuberculin skin test conversion is defined as an increase of ≥10 mm of induration within a 2-year period, regardless of age.

Treatment of Latent Tuberculosis Infection

- For HIV-negative persons, isoniazid given for 9 months is preferred over 6-month regimens.
- For HIV-positive persons and those with fibrotic lesions on chest x-ray consistent with previous TB, isoniazid should be given for 9 months instead of 12 months.
- For HIV-negative and HIV-positive persons, rifampin and pyrazinamide should be given for 2 months.
- For HIV-negative and HIV-positive persons, rifampin should be given for 4 months.

Clinical and Laboratory Monitoring

- Routine baseline and follow-up laboratory monitoring can be eliminated in most persons with LTBI, except for those with HIV infection, pregnant women (or those in the immediate postpartum period), and persons with chronic liver disease or those who use alcohol regularly.
- Emphasis on clinical monitoring for signs and symptoms of possible adverse effects, with prompt evaluation and changes in treatment, as indicated.

Modified from *MMWR Morb Mortal Wkly Rep*, 2000, 49(RR-6).

Criteria for Tuberculin Positivity, by Risk Group

Reaction ≥5 mm of Induration	Reaction ≥10 mm of Induration	Reaction ≥15 mm of Induration
HIV-positive persons	Recent immigrants (ie, within the last 5 years) from high prevalence countries	Persons with no risk factors for TB
Recent contacts of tuberculosis (TB) case patients	Injection drug users	
Fibrotic changes on chest radiograph consistent with prior TB	Residents and employees[1] of the following high risk congregate settings: prisons and jails, nursing homes and other long-term facilities for the elderly, hospitals and other healthcare facilities, residential facilities for patients with AIDS, and homeless shelters	
Patients with organ transplant and other immunosuppressed patients (receiving the equivalent of ≥15 mg/day of prednisone for 1 month of more)[2]	Mycobacteriology laboratory personnel	
	Persons with the following clinical conditions that place them at high risk: silicosis, diabetes mellitus, chronic renal failure, some hematologic disorders (eg, leukemias and lymphomas), other specific malignancies (eg, carcinoma of the head or neck and lung), weight loss of ≥10% of ideal body weight, gastrectomy, and jejunoileal bypass	
	Children <4 years of age or infants, children, and adolescents exposed to adults at high-risk	

[1]For persons who are otherwise at low risk and are tested at the start of employment, a reaction of ≥15 mm induration is considered positive.

[2]Risk of TB in patients treated with corticosteroids increases with higher dose and longer duration.

Modified from *MMWR Morb Mortal Wkly Rep*, 2000, 49(RR-6).

Recommendations, Rankings, and Performance Indicators for Treatment of Patients With Tuberculosis (TB)

Recommendation	Ranking[1] (Evidence)[2]	Performance Indicator
Obtain bacteriologic confirmation and susceptibility testing for patients with TB or suspected of having TB	A (II)	90% of adults with or suspected of having TB have 3 cultures for mycobacteria obtained before initiation of antituberculosis therapy (50% of children 0-12 y)
Place persons with suspected or confirmed smear-positive pulmonary or laryngeal TB in respiratory isolation until noninfectious	A (II)	90% of persons with sputum smear-positive TB remain in respiratory isolation until smear converts to negative
Begin treatment of patients with confirmed or suspected TB disease with one of the following drug combinations, depending on local resistance patterns: INH + RIF + PZA **or** INH + RIF + PZA + EMB **or** INH + RIF + PZA + SM	A (III)	90% of all patients with TB are started on INH + RIF + PZA + EMB or SM in geographic areas where >4% of TB isolates are resistant to INH
Report each case of TB promptly to the local public health department	A (III)	100% of persons with active TB are reported to the local public health department within 1 week of diagnosis
Perform HIV testing for all patients with TB	A (III)	80% of all patients with TB have HIV status determined within 2 months of a diagnosis of TB
Treat patients with TB caused by a susceptible organism for 6 months, using an ATS/CDC-approved regimen	A (I)	90% of all patients with TB complete 6 months of therapy with 12 months of beginning treatment
Re-evaluate patients with TB who are smear positive at 3 months for possible nonadherence or infection with drug-resistant bacilli	A (III)	90% of all patients with TB who are smear positive at 3 months have sputum culture/susceptibility testing performed within 1 month of the 3-month visit
Add ≥2 new antituberculosis agents when TB treatment failure is suspected	A (II)	100% of patients with TB with suspected treatment failure are prescribed ≥2 new antituberculosis agents
Perform tuberculin skin testing on all patients with a history of ≥1 of the following: HIV infection, I.V. drug use, homelessness, incarceration, or contact with a person with pulmonary TB	A (II)	80% of persons in the indicated population groups receive tuberculin skin test and return for reading
Administer treatment for latent TB infection to all persons with latent TB infection, unless it can be documented that they received such treatment previously	A (I)	75% of patients with positive tuberculin skin tests who are candidates for treatment for latent TB infection complete a course of therapy within 12 months of initiation

Adapted from the Infectious Diseases Society of America, *Clinical Infectious Diseases,* 2000, 31:633-9.

Note: ATS/CDC = American Thoracic Society and Centers for Disease Control and Prevention; EMB = ethambutol; INH = isoniazid; PZA = pyrazinamide; RIF = rifampin; SM = streptomycin.

[1]Strength of recommendation: A = preferred; B = acceptable alternative; C = offer when A and B cannot be given.

[2]Quality of evidence: I = randomized clinical trial data; II = data from clinical trials that are not randomized or were conducted in other populations; III = expert opinion.

NONVIRAL INFECTIOUS DISEASES *(Continued)*

PROPHYLAXIS

Specific Circumstances/ Organism	Comments	Regimen
Category I. Exposure (Household members and other close contacts of potentially infectious cases) (Exposee tuberculin test negative)[1]		
Neonate	Rx essential	INH (10 mg/kg/d) for 3 months, then repeat tuberculin test (TBnT). If mother's smear negative and infant's TBnT negative and chest x-ray (CXR) are normal, stop INH. In the United Kingdom, BCG is then given (*Lancet*, 1990, 2:1479), unless mother is HIV-positive. If infant's repeat TBnT is positive and/or CXR abnormal (hilar adenopathy and/or infiltrate), administer INH + RIF (10-20 mg/kg/d) (or streptomycin) for a total of 6 months. If mother is being treated, separation from mother is not indicated.
Children <5 y	Rx indicated	As for neonate first 3 months. If repeat TBnT is negative, stop. If repeat TBnT is positive, continue INH for a total of 9 months. If INH is not given initially, repeat TBnT at 3 months; if positive, treat with INH for 9 months (see Category II below).
Older children and adults	No Rx	Repeat TBnT at 3 months, if positive, treat with INH for 6 months (see Category II below)
Category II. Infection Without Disease (Positive tuberculin test)[1]		
Regardless of age (see INH Preventive Therapy)	Rx indicated	INH (5 mg/kg/d, maximum: 300 mg/d for adults, 10 mg/kg/d not to exceed 300 mg/d for children). Results with 6 months of treatment are nearly as effective as 12 months (65% vs 75% reduction in disease). *Am Thoracic Society* (6 months), *Am Acad Pediatrics*, 1991 (9 months). If CXR is abnormal, treat for 12 months. In HIV-positive patient, treatment for a minimum of 12 months, some suggest longer. Monitor transaminases monthly (*MMWR Morb Mortal Wkly Rep* 1989, 38:247).
Age <35 y	Rx indicated	Reanalysis of earlier studies favors INH prophylaxis for 6 months (if INH-related hepatitis case fatality rate is <1% and TB case fatality is ≥6.7%, which appears to be the case, monitor transaminases monthly (*Arch Int Med*, 1990, 150:2517).
INH-resistant organisms likely	Rx indicated	Data on efficacy of alternative regimens is currently lacking. Regimens include ETB + RIF daily for 6 months. PZA + RIF daily for 2 months, then INH + RIF daily until sensitivities from index case (if available) known, then if INH-CR, discontinue INH and continue RIF for 9 months, otherwise INH + RIF for 9 months (this latter is *Am Acad Pediatrics*, 1991 recommendation).
INH + RIF resistant organisms likely	Rx indicated	Efficacy of alternative regimens is unknown; PZA (25-30 mg/kg/d P.O.) + ETB (15-25 mg/kg/d P.O.) (at 25 mg/kg ETB, monitoring for retrobulbar neuritis required), for 6 months unless HIV-positive, then 12 months; PZA + ciprofloxacin (750 mg P.O. bid) or ofloxacin (400 mg P.O. bid) x 6-12 months *(MMWR Morb Mortal Wkly Rep*, 1992, 41(RR11):68).

INH = isoniazid; RIF = rifampin; KM = kanamycin; ETB = ethambutol.
SM = streptomycin; CXR = chest x-ray; Rx = treatment.
See also guidelines for interpreting PPD in "Skin Testing for Delayed Hypersensitivity."
[1]Tuberculin test (TBnT). The standard is the Mantoux test, 5 TU PPD in 0.1 mL diluent stabilized with Tween 80. Read at 48-72 hours measuring maximum diameter of induration. A reaction ≥5 mm is defined as positive in the following: positive HIV or risk factors, recent close case contacts, CXR consistent with healed TBc. ≥10 mm is positive in foreign-born in countries of high prevalence, injection drug users, low income populations, nursing home residents, patients with medical conditions which increase risk (see above, preventive treatment). ≥15 mm is positive in all others (*Am Rev Resp Dis*, 1990, 142:725). Two-stage TBnT: Use in individuals to be tested regularly (ie, healthcare workers). TBn reactivity may decrease over time but be boosted by skin testing. If unrecognized, individual may be incorrectly diagnosed as recent converter. If first TBnT is reactive but <10 mm, repeat 5 TU in 1 week, if then ≥10 mm = positive, not recent conversion (*Am Rev Resp Dis*, 1979, 119:587).

TREATMENT

Recommended Treatment Regimens for Drug-Susceptible Tuberculosis in Infants, Children, and Adolescents

Infection or Disease Category	Regimen	Remarks
Latent tuberculosis infection (positive skin test, no disease):		If daily therapy is not possible, therapy twice a week directly observed therapy may be used for 9 months. HIV-infected children should be treated for 9-12 months.
• Isoniazid-susceptible	9 months of isoniazid once daily	
• Isoniazid-resistant	6 months of rifampin once daily	
• Isoniazid-rifampin-resistant[1]	Consult a tuberculosis specialist	
Pulmonary	**6-Month Regimens** 2 months of isoniazid, rifampin, and pyrazinamide once daily, followed by 4 months of isoniazid and rifampin daily	If possible drug resistance is a concern (see text), another drug (ethambutol or streptomycin) is added to the initial 3-drug therapy until drug susceptibilities are determined.
	OR 2 months of isoniazid, rifampin, and pyrazinamide daily, followed by 4 months of isoniazid and rifampin twice a week	Drugs can be given 2 or 3 times per week under direct observation in the initial phase if nonadherence is likely.
	9-Month Alternative Regimens (for hilar adenopathy only) 9 months of isoniazid and rifampin once daily **OR** 1 month of isoniazid and rifampin once daily, followed by 8 months of isoniazid and rifampin twice a week	Regimens consisting of 6 months of isoniazid and rifampin once daily, and 1 month of isoniazid and rifampin once daily, followed by 5 months of isoniazid and rifampin directly observed therapy twice a week, have been successful in areas where drug resistance is rare.
Extrapulmonary meningitis, disseminated (miliary), bone/joint disease	2 months of isoniazid, rifampin, pyrazinamide, and streptomycin once daily, followed by 7-10 months of isoniazid and rifampin once daily (9-12 months total)	Streptomycin is given with initial therapy until drug susceptibility is known.
	OR 2 months of isoniazid, rifampin, pyrazinamide, and streptomycin once daily, followed by 7-10 months of isoniazid and rifampin twice a week (9-12 months total)	For patients who may have acquired tuberculosis in geographic areas where resistance to streptomycin is common, capreomycin (15-30 mg/kg/d) or kanamycin (15-30 mg/kg/d) may be used instead of streptomycin.
Other (eg, cervical lymphadenopathy)	Same as for pulmonary disease	See Pulmonary.

[1]Duration of therapy is longer in HIV-infected persons and additional drugs may be indicated.

Adapted from "Report of the Committee on Infectious Diseases," *2000 Red Book®*, 25th ed.

Commonly Used Drugs for the Treatment of Tuberculosis in Infants, Children, and Adolescents

Drugs	Dosage Forms	Daily Dose (mg/kg/d)	Twice a Week Dose (mg/kg per dose)	Maximum Dose	Adverse Reactions
Ethambutol	Tablets 100 mg 400 mg	15-25	50	2.5 g	Optic neuritis (usually reversible), decreased visual acuity, decreased red-green color discrimination, gastrointestinal disturbances, hypersensitivity
Isoniazid[1]	Scored tablets 100 mg 300 mg Syrup 10 mg/mL	10-15[2]	20-30	Daily, 300 mg Twice a week, 900 mg	Mild hepatic enzyme elevation, hepatitis,[2] peripheral neuritis, hypersensitivity
Pyrazinamide[1]	Scored tablets 500 mg	20-40	50	2 g	Hepatotoxicity, hyperuricemia

NONVIRAL INFECTIOUS DISEASES *(Continued)*

Commonly Used Drugs for the Treatment of Tuberculosis in Infants, Children, and Adolescents *(continued)*

Drugs	Dosage Forms	Daily Dose (mg/kg/d)	Twice a Week Dose (mg/kg per dose)	Maximum Dose	Adverse Reactions
Rifampin[1]	Capsules 150 mg 300 mg Syrup formulated in syrup from capsules	10-20	10-20	600 mg	Orange discoloration of secretions/urine, staining contact lenses, vomiting, hepatitis, flu-like reaction, and thrombocytopenia; may render birth-control pills ineffective
Streptomycin (I.M. administration)	Vials 1 g 4 g	20-40	20-40	1 g	Auditory and vestibular toxicity, nephrotoxicity, rash

[1]Rifamate® is a capsule containing 150 mg of isoniazid and 300 mg of rifampin. Two capsules provide the usual adult (>50 kg body weight) daily doses of each drug. Rifater® is a capsule containing 50 mg of isoniazid, 120 mg of rifampin, and 300 mg of pyrazinamide.

[2]When isoniazid in a dosage exceeding 10 mg/kg/day is used in combination with rifampin, the incidence of hepatotoxicity may be increased.

Adapted from "Report of the Committee on Infectious Diseases," *2000 Red Book®*, 25th ed.

Rifampin is a bactericidal agent. It is metabolized by the liver and affects the pharmacokinetics of many other drugs, affecting their serum concentrations. Mycobacterium tuberculosis, initially resistant to rifampin, remains relatively uncommon in most areas of the United States. Rifampin is excreted in bile and urine and can cause orange urine, sweat and tears. It can also cause discoloration of soft contact lenses and render oral contraceptives ineffective. Hepatotoxicity occurs rarely. Blood dyscrasia accompanied by influenza-like symptoms can occur if doses are taken sporadically.

Less Commonly Used Drugs for Treatment of Drug-Resistant Tuberculosis in Infants, Children, and Adolescents[1]

Drugs	Dosage Forms	Daily Dose (mg/kg/d)	Maximum Dose	Adverse Reactions
Capreomycin	Vials 1 g	15-30 I.M.	1 g	Ototoxicity, nephrotoxicity
Ciprofloxacin[2]	Tablets 250 mg 500 mg 750 mg	Adults 500-1500 mg total per day (twice daily)	1.5 g	Theoretical effect on growing cartilage, gastrointestinal tract disturbances, rash, headache
Cycloserine	Capsules 250 mg	10-20	1 g	Psychosis, personality changes, seizures, rash
Ethionamide	Tablets 250 mg	15-20 given in 2-3 divided doses	1 g	Gastrointestinal tract disturbances, hepatotoxicity, hypersensitive reactions
Kanamycin	Vials 75 mg/2 mL 500 mg/2 mL 1 g/3 mL	15-30 I.M.	1 g	Auditory and vestibular toxic effects, nephrotoxicity
Levofloxacin[2]	Tablets 250 mg 500 mg Vials 25 mg/mL	Adults 500-1000 mg once daily	1 g	Theoretical effect on growing cartilage, gastrointestinal tract disturbances, rash, headache
Ofloxacin[2]	Tablets 200 mg 300 mg 400 mg	Adults 400-800 mg total per day (twice daily)	0.8 g	Theoretical effect on growing cartilage, gastrointestinal tract disturbances, rash, headache
Para-amino salicylic acid (PAS)	Tablets 500 mg	200-300 (3-4 times/day)	10 g	Gastrointestinal tract disturbances, hypersensitivity, hepatotoxicity

[1]These drugs should be used in consultation with a specialist in tuberculosis.

[2]Fluoroquinolones are not currently approved for use in persons <18 years; their use in younger patients necessitates assessment of the potential risks and benefits.

Adapted from "Report of the Committee on Infectious Diseases," *2000 Red Book®*, 25th ed.

TB Drugs in Special Situations

Drug	Pregnancy	CNS TB Disease	Renal Insufficiency
Isoniazid	Safe	Good penetration	Normal clearance
Rifampin	Safe	Fair penetration Penetrates inflamed meninges (10% to 20%)	Normal clearance
Pyrazinamide	Avoid	Good penetration	Clearance reduced Decrease dose or prolong interval
Ethambutol	Safe	Penetrates inflamed meninges only (4% to 64%)	Clearance reduced Decrease dose or prolong interval
Streptomycin	Avoid	Penetrates inflamed meninges only	Clearance reduced Decrease dose or prolong interval
Capreomycin	Avoid	Penetrates inflamed meninges only	Clearance reduced Decrease dose or prolong interval
Kanamycin	Avoid	Penetrates inflamed meninges only	Clearance reduced Decrease dose or prolong interval
Ethionamide	Do not use	Good penetration	Normal clearance
Para-aminosalicylic acid	Safe	Penetrates inflamed meninges only (10% to 50%)	Incomplete data on clearance
Cycloserine	Avoid	Good penetration	Clearance reduced Decrease dose or prolong interval
Ciprofloxacin	Do not use	Fair penetration (5% to 10%) Penetrates inflamed meninges (50% to 90%)	Clearance reduced Decrease dose or prolong interval
Ofloxacin	Do not use	Fair penetration (5% to 10%) Penetrates inflamed meninges (50% to 90%)	Clearance reduced Decrease dose or prolong interval
Amikacin	Avoid	Penetrates inflamed meninges only	Clearance reduced Decrease dose or prolong interval
Clofazimine	Avoid	Penetration unknown	Clearance probably normal

Safe = the drug has not been demonstrated to have teratogenic effects.

Avoid = data on the drug's safety are limited, or the drug is associated with mild malformations (as in the aminoglycosides).

Do not use = studies show an association between the drug and premature labor, congenital malformations, or teratogenicity.

NONVIRAL INFECTIOUS DISEASES *(Continued)*

Recommendations for Coadministering Different Antiretroviral Drugs With the Antimycobacterial Drugs Rifabutin and Rifampin

Antiretroviral	Use in Combination with Rifabutin	Use in Combination with Rifampin	Comments
Saquinavir[1]			
Hard-gel capsules (HGC)	Possibly[2], if antiretroviral regimen also includes ritonavir	Possibly, if antiretroviral regimen also includes ritonavir	Coadministration of saquinavir SGC with usual-dose rifabutin (300 mg/day or 2-3 times/week) is a possibility. However, the pharmacokinetic data and clinical experience for this combination are limited.
Soft-gel capsules (SGC)	Probably[3]	Possibly, if antiretroviral regimen also includes ritonavir	The combination of saquinavir SGC or saquinavir HGC and ritonavir, coadministered with 1) usual-dose rifampin (600 mg/day or 2-3 times/week), or 2) reduced-dose rifabutin (150 mg 2-3 times/week) is a possibility. However, the pharmacokinetic data and clinical experience for these combinations are limited. Coadministration of saquinavir or saquinavir SGC with rifampin is not recommended because rifampin markedly decreases concentrations of saquinavir.
Ritonavir	Probably	Probably	If the combination of ritonavir and rifabutin is used, then a substantially reduced-dose rifabutin regimen (150 mg 2-3 times/week) is recommended. Coadministration of ritonavir with usual-dose rifampin (600 mg/day or 2-3 times/week) is a possibility, though pharmacokinetic data and clinical experience are limited.
Indinavir	Yes	No	There is limited, but favorable, clinical experience with coadministration of indinavir[4] with a reduced daily dose of rifabutin (150 mg) or with the usual dose of rifabutin (300 mg 2-3 times/week). Coadministration of indinavir with rifampin is not recommended because rifampin markedly decreases concentrations of indinavir.
Nelfinavir	Yes	No	There is limited, but favorable, clinical experience with coadministration of nelfinavir[5] with a reduced daily dose of rifabutin (150 mg) or with the usual dose of rifabutin (300 mg 2-3 times/week). Coadministration of nelfinavir with rifampin is not recommended because rifampin markedly decreases concentrations of nelfinavir.
Amprenavir	Yes	No	Coadministration of amprenavir with a reduced daily dose of rifabutin (150 mg) or with the usual dose of rifabutin (300 mg 2-3 times/week) is a possibility, but there is no published clinical experience. Coadministration of amprenavir with rifampin is not recommended because rifampin markedly decreases concentrations of amprenavir.

Recommendations for Coadministering Different Antiretroviral Drugs With the Antimycobacterial Drugs Rifabutin and Rifampin *(continued)*

Antiretroviral	Use in Combination with Rifabutin	Use in Combination with Rifampin	Comments
Nevirapine	Yes	Possibly	Coadministration of nevirapine with usual-dose rifabutin (300 mg/day or 2-3 times/week) is a possibility based on pharmacokinetic study data. However, there is no published clinical experience for this combination. Data are insufficient to assess whether dose adjustments are necessary when rifampin is coadministered with nevirapine. Therefore, rifampin and nevirapine should be used only in combination if clearly indicated and with careful monitoring.
Delavirdine	No	No	Contraindicated because of the marked decrease in concentrations of delavirdine when administered with either rifabutin or rifampin.
Efavirenz	Probably	Probably	Coadministration of efavirenz with increased-dose rifabutin (450 mg/day or 600 mg/day, or 600 mg 2-3 times/week) is a possibility, though there is no published clinical experience. Coadministration of efavirenz[6] with usual-dose rifampin (600 mg/day or 2-3 times/week) is a possibility, though there is no published clinical experience.

[1]Usual recommended doses are 400 mg twice daily for each of these protease inhibitors and 400 mg of ritonavir.

[2]Despite limited data and clinical experience, the use of this combination is potentially successful.

[3]Based on available data and clinical experience, the successful use of this combination is likely.

[4] Usual recommended dose is 800 mg every 8 hours; some experts recommend increasing the indinavir dose to 1000 mg every 8 hours if indinavir is used in combination with rifabutin.

[5]Usual recommended dose is 750 mg 3 times/day or 1250 mg twice daily; some experts recommend increasing the nelfinavir dose to 1000 mg if the 3-times/day dosing is used and nelfinavir is used in combination with rifabutin.

[6]Usual recommended dose is 600 mg/day; some experts recommend increasing the efavirenz dose to 800 mg/day if efavirenz is used in combination with rifampin.

Updated March 2000 from www.hivatis.org -"Updated Guidelines for the Use of Rifabutin or Rifampin for the Treatment and Prevention of Tuberculosis Among HIV-Infected Patients Taking Protease Inhibitors or Non-nucleoside Reverse Transcriptase Inhibitors," *MMWR*, March 10, 2000, 49(09):185-9.

Recommended Drug Regimens for Treatment of Latent Tuberculosis (TB) Infection in Adults

Drug	Interval and Duration	Comments	Rating[1] (Evidence)[2] HIV⁻	HIV⁺
Isoniazid	Daily for 9 months[3,4]	In HIV-infected patients, isoniazid may be administered concurrently with nucleoside reverse transcriptase inhibitors (NRTIs), protease inhibitors, or non-nucleoside reverse transcriptase inhibitors (NNRTIs)	A (II)	A (II)
	Twice weekly for 9 months[3,4]	Directly observed therapy (DOT) must be used with twice-weekly dosing	B (II)	B (II)
Isoniazid	Daily for 6 months[4]	Not indicated for HIV-infected persons, those with fibrotic lesions on chest radiographs, or children	B (I)	C (I)
	Twice weekly for 6 months[4]	DOT must be used with twice-weekly dosing	B (II)	C (I)
Rifampin plus pyrazinamide	Daily for 2 months	May also be offered to persons who are contacts of pyrazinamide patients with isoniazid-resistant, rifampin-susceptible TB In HIV-infected persons, protease inhibitors or NNRTIs should generally not be administered concurrently with rifampin; rifabutin can be used as an alternative for patients treated with indinavir, nelfinavir, amprenavir, ritonavir, or efavirenz, and possibly with nevirapine or soft-gel saquinavir[5]	B (II)	A (II)

NONVIRAL INFECTIOUS DISEASES *(Continued)*

Recommended Drug Regimens for Treatment of Latent Tuberculosis (TB) Infection in Adults *(continued)*

Drug	Interval and Duration	Comments	Rating[1] (Evidence)[2] HIV⁻	HIV⁺
	Twice weekly for 2-3 months	DOT must be used with twice-weekly dosing	C (II)	C (I)
Rifampin	Daily for 4 months	For persons who cannot tolerate pyrazinamide For persons who are contacts of patients with isoniazid-resistant rifampin-susceptible TB who cannot tolerate pyrazinamide	B (II)	B (III)

[1]Strength of recommendation: A = preferred; B = acceptable alternative; C = offer when A and B cannot be given.

[2]Quality of evidence: I = randomized clinical trial data; II = data from clinical trials that are not randomized or were conducted in other populations; III = expert opinion.

[3]Recommended regimen for children <18 years of age.

[4]Recommended regimens for pregnant women. Some experts would use rifampin and pyrazinamide for 2 months as an alternative regimen for HIV-infected pregnant women, although pyrazinamide should be avoided during the first trimester.

[5]Rifabutin should not be used with hard-gel saquinavir or delavirdine. When used with other protease inhibitors or NNRTIs, dose adjustment of rifabutin may be required.

Modified from *MMWR Morb Mortal Wkly Rep*, 2000, 49(RR-6).

SEXUALLY-TRANSMITTED DISEASES

Sexually transmitted diseases (STDs) represent a group of infectious diseases that include bacterial, fungal, and viral etiologies. Several related infections are covered elsewhere. Gonorrhea and syphilis will be covered here.

The management of a patient with a STD begins with identification. Paramount to the correct management of patients with a history of gonorrhea or syphilis is when the condition was diagnosed, how and with what agent it was treated, did the condition recur, and are there any residual signs and symptoms potentially indicating active or recurrent disease. With universal precautions, the patient with *Neisseria gonorrhoea* or *Treponema pallidum* infection poses little threat to the dentist; however, diagnosis of oral lesions may be problematic. Gonococcal pharyngitis, primary syphilitic lesions (chancre), secondary syphilitic lesions (mucous patch), and tertiary lesions (gumma) may be identified by the dentist.

Drugs used in treatment of gonorrhea/syphilis include:

- Cefixime *on page 268*
- Ceftriaxone *on page 278*
- Ciprofloxacin *on page 328*
- Doxycycline (alternate) *on page 476*
- Ofloxacin *on page 995*
- Penicillin G Benzathine *on page 1047*
- Penicillin G, Parenteral, Aqueous *on page 1049*
- Spectinomycin (alternate) *on page 1239*

The drugs listed above are often used alone or in stepped regimens, particularly when there is concomitant *Chlamydia* infection or when there is evidence of disseminated disease. The proper treatment for syphilis depends on the state of the disease.

Current treatment regimens for syphilis include:

1°, 2°, early latent (<1 y)	Benzathine penicillin G I.M.: 2-4 million units x 1 (alternate doxycycline)
Latent (>1 y), gumma, or cardiovascular	As above but once weekly for 3 weeks
Neurosyphilis	Aqueous penicillin G I.V.: 12-24 million units/day for 14 days

Type or Stage	Drug of Choice	Alternatives
CHLAMYDIAL INFECTION AND RELATED CLINICAL SYNDROMES[1]		
Urethritis, cervicitis, conjunctivitis, or proctitis (except lymphogranuloma venereum)		
	Azithromycin 1 g oral once **or** Doxycycline[2,3] 100 mg oral bid x 7 d	Ofloxacin[3] 300 mg oral bid x 7 d **or** Erythromycin[4] 500 mg oral qid x 7 d **or** Erythromycin ethylsuccinate 800 mg oral qid x 7 d **or** Levofloxacin 500 mg oral qd x 7 d
Recurrent/persistent		
	Metronidazole 2 g oral **plus** Erythromycin 500 mg oral qid x 7 d **or** Erythromycin ethylsuccinate 800 mg oral qid x 7 d	
Infection in pregnancy		
	Amoxicillin 500 mg oral tid x 7 d **or** Erythromycin[4] 500 mg oral qid x 7 d	Azithromycin[5] 1 g oral once **or** Erythromycin base 250 mg oral qid x 14 d **or** Erythromycin ethylsuccinate 800 mg oral qid x 7 d **or** Erythromycin ethylsuccinate 400 mg oral qid x 14 d
Neonatal		
Ophthalmia	Erythromycin (base or ethylsuccinate) 12.5 mg/kg oral qid x 10-14 d	
Pneumonia	Erythromycin (base or ethylsuccinate) 12.5 mg/kg oral or I.V. qid x 14 d	
Lymphogranuloma venereum		
	Doxycycline[2,3] 100 mg oral bid x 21 d	Erythromycin[4] 500 mg oral qid x 21 d
GONORRHEA[6]		
Urethral, cervical, rectal, or pharyngeal		
	Cefixime 400 mg oral once **or** Ceftriaxone 125 mg I.M. once **or** Ciprofloxacin[3] 500 mg oral once **or** Ofloxacin[3] 400 mg oral once **plus** (if chlamydial infection is not ruled out) Azithromycin 1 g oral once **or** Doxycycline 100 mg oral bid x 7 d	Spectinomycin 2 g I.M. once[7] **or** Lomefloxacin 400 mg oral once **or** Norfloxacin 800 mg oral once **or** Gatifloxacin 400 mg oral once
Disseminated gonococcal infection		
	Ceftriaxone 1 g I.M. or I.V. q24h	Cefotaxime 1 g I.V. q8h **or** Ceftizoxime 1 g I.V. q8h **or** **For persons allergic to β-lactam drugs:** Ciprofloxacin 500 mg I.V. q12h **or** Levofloxacin 250 mg I.V. once daily **or** Ofloxacin 400 mg I.V. q12h **or** Spectinomycin 2 g I.M. q12h All regimens should be continued for 24-48 hours after improvement begins, at which time therapy may be switched to one of the following regimens to complete a full week of antimicrobial therapy: Cefixime 400 mg oral bid **or** Ciprofloxacin 500 mg oral bid **or** Levofloxacin 500 mg oral once daily **or** Ofloxacin 400 mg oral bid
Gonococcal meningitis and endocarditis		
	Ceftriaxone 1-2 g I.V. q12h	

NONVIRAL INFECTIOUS DISEASES *(Continued)*

Type or Stage	Drug of Choice	Alternatives
EPIDIDYMITIS		
Most likely caused by enteric organisms, or in patients allergic to cephalosporins and/or tetracyclines		
	Ofloxacin 300 mg bid x 10 d **or** Levofloxacin 500 mg oral once daily x 10 d	
Most likely caused by gonorrhea or chlamydial		
	Ceftriaxone 250 mg I.M. once **followed by** Doxycycline[2] 100 mg oral bid x 10 d	
PELVIC INFLAMMATORY DISEASE		
– Inpatients	**Parenteral Regimen A** Cefotetan 2 g I.V. q12h **or** Cefoxitin 2 g I.V. q6h **plus** Doxycycline 100 mg oral or I.V. q12h (see Note) **Parenteral Regimen B** Clindamycin 900 mg I.V. q8h **plus** Gentamicin loading dose I.V. or I.M. (2 mg/kg of body weight) followed by maintenance dose (1.5 mg/kg) q8h. Single daily dosing may be substituted. **Note:** Because of pain associated with infusion, doxycycline should be administered orally when possible, even when the patient is hospitalized. Both oral and I.V. administration of doxycycline provide similar bioavailability. Parenteral therapy may be discontinued 24 hours after a patient improves clinically, and oral therapy with doxycycline (100 mg twice daily) should continue to complete 14 days of therapy. When tubo-ovarian abscess is present, many healthcare providers use clindamycin or metronidazole with doxycycline for continued therapy rather than doxycycline alone, because it provides more effective anaerobic coverage.	Ofloxacin 400 mg I.V. q12h **or** Levofloxacin 500 mg I.V. once daily **with or without** Metronidazole 500 mg I.V. q8h **or** Ampicillin/sulbactam 3 g I.V. q6h **plus** Doxycycline 100 mg oral or I.V. q12h
– Outpatients	**Regimen A** Ofloxacin 400 mg oral bid x 14 d **or** Levofloxacin 500 mg oral once daily x 14 d **with or without** Metronidazole 500 mg oral bid x 14 d **Regimen B** Ceftriaxone 250 mg I.M. once **or** Cefoxitin 2 g I.M. once and Probenecid 1 g oral once administered concurrently **or** Other parenteral 3rd generation cephalosporin (eg, ceftizoxime or cefotaxime) **plus** Doxycycline 100 mg oral bid x 14 d **with or without** Metronidazole 500 mg oral bid x 14 d If the healthcare provider prescribes outpatient oral or parenteral therapy, a follow-up examination should be performed within 72 hours using the criteria for clinical improvement described previously. If the patient has not improved, hospitalization for parenteral therapy and further evaluation are recommended.	

Type or Stage	Drug of Choice	Alternatives
VAGINAL INFECTION		
Trichomoniasis		
	Metronidazole 2 g oral once	Metronidazole 500 mg oral bid x 7 d
Bacterial vaginosis		
	Metronidazole 500 mg oral bid x 7 d **or** Metronidazole gel 0.75% 5 g intravaginally once or twice daily x 5 d **or** Clindamycin 2% cream 5 g intravaginally qhs x 3-7 d	Clindamycin 100 g intravaginally at bedtime x 3 d **or** Clindamycin 300 mg oral bid x 7 d **or** Metronidazole 2 g oral once[8]
Vulvovaginal candidiasis		
	Intravaginal butoconazole, clotrimazole, miconazole, terconazole, or tioconazole[9] **or** Fluconazole 150 mg oral once	Nystatin 100,000 unit vaginal tablet once daily x 14 d
SYPHILIS		
Early (primary, secondary, or latent <1 y)		
	Penicillin G benzathine 2.4 million units I.M. once[10]	Doxycycline[3] 100 mg oral bid x 14 d **or** Tetracycline 500 mg oral qid x 24 d
Late (>1 year's duration, cardiovascular, gumma, late-latent)		
	Penicillin G benzathine 2.4 million units I.M. weekly x 3 wk	Doxycycline[3] 100 mg oral bid x 4 wk
Neurosyphilis[11]		
	Penicillin G 3-4 million units I.V. q4h x 10-14 d	Penicillin G procaine 2.4 million units I.M. daily, **plus** Probenecid 500 mg qid oral, both x 10-14 d
Congenital		
	Penicillin G 50,000 units/kg I.V. q8-12h (q12h during first 7 d of life, then q8h for total of 10 d) **or** Penicillin G procaine 50,000 units/kg I.M. daily for 10 d	
CHANCROID[12]		
	Azithromycin 1 g oral once **or** Ceftriaxone 250 mg I.M. once **or** Ciprofloxacin[3] 500 mg oral bid x 3 d **or** Erythromycin[4] 500 mg oral qid x 7 d	
GENITAL HERPES		
First episode		
	Acyclovir 400 mg oral tid x 7-10 d[13] **or** Famciclovir 250 mg oral tid x 7-10 d **or** Valacyclovir 1 g oral bid x 7-10 d	Acyclovir 200 mg oral 5 times/d x 7-10 d[13]
Recurrent[14]		
	Acyclovir 400 mg oral tid x 5 d **or** Famciclovir 125 mg oral bid x 5 d **or** Valacyclovir 500 mg oral bid x 5 d	Acyclovir 200 mg orally 5 times/day for 5 d **or** Acyclovir 800 mg oral bid x 5 d
Severe (hospitalized patients)		
	Acyclovir 5-10 mg/kg I.V. q8h x 5-7 d	
Suppression of recurrence[15]		
	Valacyclovir 500 mg - 1 g once daily[16] **or** Acyclovir 400 mg oral bid **or** Famciclovir 250 mg oral bid	
GRANULOMA INGUINALE		
	TMP-SMZ 1 double-strength tablet oral bid for a minimum of 3 wk **or** Doxycycline 100 oral bid for a minimum of 3 wk	Ciprofloxacin 750 mg oral bid for a minimum of 3 wk **or** Erythromycin base 500 mg oral qid for a minimum of 3 wk **or** Azithromycin 1 g oral once per week for minimum of 3 weeks

NONVIRAL INFECTIOUS DISEASES *(Continued)*

[1]Related clinical syndromes include nonchlamydial nongonococcal urethritis and cervicitis.
[2]Or tetracycline 500 mg oral qid or minocycline 100 mg oral bid.
[3]Contraindicated in pregnancy.
[4]Erythromycin estolate is contraindicated in pregnancy.
[5]Safety in pregnancy not established.
[6]All patients should also receive a course of treatment effective for *Chlamydia*.
[7]Recommended only for use during pregnancy in patients allergic to beta-lactams. Not effective for pharyngeal infection.
[8]Higher relapse rate with single dose, but useful for patients who may not comply with multiple-dose therapy.
[9]For preparations and dosage of topical products, see *Medical Letter*, 36:81,1994; single-dose therapy is not recommended.
[10]Some experts recommend repeating this regimen after 7 days, especially in patients with HIV infection.
[11]Patients allergic to penicillin should be desensitized.
[12]All regimens, especially single-dose ceftriaxone, are less effective in HIV-infected patients.
[13]For first-episode proctitis, use acyclovir 800 mg oral tid or 400 mg oral 5 times/day.
[14]Antiviral therapy is variably effective for treatment of recurrences; only effective if started early.
[15]Preventive treatment should be discontinued for 1-2 months once a year to reassess the frequency of recurrence.
[16]Use 500 mg qd in patients with <10 recurrences per year and 500 mg bid or 1 g daily in patients with ≥10 recurrences per year.

Adapted from "Sexually Transmitted Diseases Treatment Guidelines 2002," *MMWR Morb Mortal Wkly Rep*, 2002, 51(RR-6).

ANTIBIOTIC PROPHYLAXIS

PREPROCEDURAL GUIDELINES FOR DENTAL PATIENTS

INTRODUCTION

In dental practice the clinician is often confronted with a decision to prescribe antibiotics. The focus of this chapter is on the use of antibiotics as a preprocedural treatment in the prevention of adverse infectious sequelae in the two most commonly encountered situations: prevention of endocarditis and prosthetic implants.

The criteria for preprocedural decisions begins with patient evaluation. An accurate and complete medical history is always the initial basis for any prescriptive treatments on the part of the dentist. These prescriptive treatments can include ordering appropriate laboratory tests, referral to the patient's physician for consultation, or immediate decision to prescribe preprocedural antibiotics. The dentist should also be aware that antibiotic coverage of the patient might be appropriate due to diseases that are covered elsewhere in this text, such as human immunodeficiency virus, cavernous thrombosis, undiagnosed or uncontrolled diabetes, lupus, renal failure, and periods of neutropenia as are often associated with cancer chemotherapy. In these instances, medical consultation is almost always necessary in making antibiotic decisions in order to tailor the treatment and dosing to the individual patient's needs.

Note: The ADA Council on Scientific Affairs recently restated the dentist's responsibility when prescribing antibiotics to oral contraceptive users (*JADA*, 2002, 133:880). It is recommended that dental professionals advise these patients to consult their physician for additional barrier contraception due to potential reduction in the efficacy of oral contraceptives from antibiotic interaction.

All tables or figures in this chapter were adapted from the ADA Advisory Statement: "Antibiotic Prophylaxis for Dental Patients With Total Joint Replacement," *J Am Dent Assoc*, 1997, 128:1004-8 or from Dajani AS, Taubert KA, Wilson W, et al, "Prevention of Bacterial Endocarditis. Recommendations by the American Heart Association," *JAMA*, 1997, 7(22):1794-801.

PREVENTION OF BACTERIAL ENDOCARDITIS

Guidelines for the prevention of bacterial endocarditis have been updated by the American Heart Association with approval by the Council of Scientific Affairs of the American Dental Association. These guidelines supercede those issued and published in 1990. They were developed to more clearly define the situations of antibiotic use, to reduce costs to the patient, to reduce gastrointestinal adverse effects, and to improve patient compliance. Highlights of the current recommendations are shown in Table 1 and the specific antibiotic regimens are listed in Table 2 and further illustrated in Figure 1.

Amoxicillin is an amino-type penicillin with an extended spectrum of antibacterial action compared to penicillin VK. The pharmacology of amoxicillin as a dental antibiotic has been reviewed previously in *General Dentistry*. The suggested regimen for standard general prophylaxis is a dose of 2 g 1 hour before the procedure. A follow-up dose is no longer necessary. This dose of amoxicillin is lower than the previous dosing regimen of 3 g 1 hour before the procedure and then 1.5 g 6 hours after the initial dose. Dajani, et al, stated that the 2 g dose of amoxicillin resulted in adequate serum levels for several hours making the second dose unnecessary, both because of a prolonged serum level of amoxicillin above the minimal inhibitory concentration for oral streptococci, and an inhibitory activity of 6-14 hours by amoxicillin against streptococci. The new pediatric dose is 50 mg/kg orally 1 hour before the procedure and not to exceed the adult dose. Amoxicillin is available in capsules (250 mg and 500 mg), chewable tablets (125 mg, 200 mg, 250 mg, 400 mg), and liquid suspension (400 mg/5 mL). The retail cost of generic capsules and tablets ranges from 20-30 cents each and suspension is approximately $12 per 100 mL.

The dentist should be vigilant in reviewing literature for updates. The guidelines for antibiotic prophylaxis continue to be reviewed and it is likely that additional modifications to the recommendations will be published in the near future.

ANTIBIOTIC PROPHYLAXIS *(Continued)*

Table 1.
HIGHLIGHTS OF THE NEWEST GUIDELINES FOR ENDOCARDITIS PREVENTION

No.	Change From Old Guidelines
1.	Oral initial dosing for amoxicillin reduced to 2 g
2.	Follow-up antibiotic dose is no longer recommended
3.	Erythromycin is no longer recommended for penicillin-allergic patients
4.	Clindamycin and other alternatives have been recommended to replace the erythromycin regimens
5.	Clearer guidelines for prophylaxis decisions for patients with mitral valve prolapse have been developed

For individuals unable to take oral medications, intramuscular or intravenous ampicillin is recommended for both adults and children (Table 2). It is to be given 30 minutes before the procedure at the same doses used for the oral amoxicillin medication. Ampicillin is also an amino-type penicillin having an antibacterial spectrum similar to amoxicillin. Ampicillin is not absorbed from the gastrointestinal tract as effectively as amoxicillin and, therefore, is not recommended for oral use.

Table 2. PROPHYLACTIC REGIMENS FOR BACTERIAL ENDOCARDITIS FOR DENTAL PROCEDURES

Situation	Agent	Regimen*
Standard general prophylaxis	Amoxicillin *on page 93*	Adults: 2 g orally 1 hour before procedure Children: 50 mg/kg orally 1 hour before procedure
Unable to take oral medications	Ampicillin *on page 103*	Adults: 2 g I.M. or I.V. within 30 minutes before procedure Children: 50 mg/kg I.M. or I.V. within 30 minutes before procedure
Allergic to penicillin	Clindamycin *on page 341* or	Adults: 600 mg orally 1 hour before procedure Children: 20 mg/kg orally 1 hour before procedure
	Cephalexin *on page 285* or Cefadroxil *on page 261*	Adults: 2 g orally 1 hour before procedure Children: 50 mg/kg orally 1 hour before procedure
	Azithromycin *on page 153* or Clarithromycin *on page 337*	Adults: 500 mg orally 1 hour before procedure Children: 15 mg/kg orally 1 hour before procedure
Allergic to penicillin and unable to take oral medications	Clindamycin *on page 341* or	Adults: 600 mg I.V. within 30 minutes before procedure Children: 20 mg/kg I.V. within 30 minutes before procedure
	Cefazolin *on page 263*	Adults: 1 g I.M. or I.V. within 30 minutes before procedure Children: 25 mg/kg I.M. or I.V. within 30 minutes before procedure

*Total children's dose should not exceed adult dose.

Note: Cephalosporins should not be used in individuals with immediate-type hypersensitivity reaction (urticaria, angioedema, or anaphylaxis) to penicillins

Individuals who are allergic to the penicillins such as amoxicillin or ampicillin should be treated with an alternate antibiotic. The new guidelines have suggested a number of alternate agents including clindamycin, cephalosporins, azithromycin, and clarithromycin. Clindamycin (Cleocin®) occupies an important niche in dentistry as a useful and effective antibiotic and it was a recommended alternative agent for the prevention of bacterial endocarditis in the previous guidelines. In the new guidelines, the oral adult dose is 600 mg 1 hour before the procedure. A follow-up dose is not necessary. Clindamycin is available as 300 mg capsules; thus 2 capsules will provide the recommended dose. The children's oral dose for clindamycin is 20 mg/kg 1 hour before the procedure. Clindamycin is available as pediatric-flavored granules for oral solution. When reconstituted with water, each bottle yields a solution containing 75 mg/5 mL. Intravenous clindamycin is recommended in adults and children who are allergic to penicillin and unable to take oral medications. Refer to Table 2 for the intravenous doses of clindamycin.

Clindamycin was developed in the 1960s as a semisynthetic derivative of lincomycin which was found in the soil organism, *Streptomyces lincolnensis*, near Lincoln, Nebraska. It is commercially available as the hydrochloride salt to improve solubility in the gastrointestinal tract. Clindamycin is antibacterial against most aerobic Gram-positive cocci including staphylococci and streptococci, and against many types of anaerobic

Gram-negative and Gram-positive organisms. It has been used over the years in dentistry as an alternative to penicillin and erythromycins for the treatment of oral-facial infections. For a review, see Wynn and Bergman.

The mechanism of antibacterial action of clindamycin is the same as erythromycin. It inhibits protein synthesis in susceptible bacteria resulting in the inhibition of bacterial growth and replication. Following oral administration of a single dose of clindamycin (150 mg, 300 mg, or 600 mg) on an empty stomach, 90% of the dose is rapidly absorbed into the bloodstream and peak serum concentrations are attained within 45-80 minutes. Administration with food does not markedly impair absorption into the bloodstream. Clindamycin serum levels exceed the minimum inhibitory concentration (MIC) for bacterial growth for at least 6 hours after the recommended dose of 600 mg. The serum half-life is 2-3 hours.

Adverse effects of clindamycin after a single dose are virtually nonexistent. Although it is estimated that 1% of patients taking clindamycin will develop symptoms of pseudomembranous colitis, these symptoms usually develop after 9-14 days of clindamycin therapy. These symptoms have never been reported in patients taking an acute dose for the prevention of endocarditis.

In lieu of clindamycin, penicillin-allergic individuals may receive cephalexin (Keflex®) or cefadroxil (Duricef®) provided that they have not had an immediate-type sensitivity reaction such as anaphylaxis, urticaria, or angioedema to penicillins. These antibiotics are first-generation cephalosporins having an antibacterial spectrum of action similar to amoxicillin and ampicillin. They elicit a bactericidal action by inhibiting cell wall synthesis in susceptible bacteria. The recommended adult prophylaxis dose for either of these drugs is 2 g 1 hour before the procedure. Again, no follow-up dose is needed. The children's oral dose for cephalexin and cefadroxil is 50 mg/kg 1 hour before the procedure. Cephalexin is supplied as capsules (250 mg and 500 mg) and tablets (250 mg, 500 mg, 1 g). Cefadroxil is supplied as 500 mg capsules and 1 g tablets. Both antibiotics are available in the form of powder for oral suspension at concentrations of 125 mg and 250 mg (cefadroxil also available as 500 mg/5 mL).

For those individuals (adults and children) allergic to penicillin and unable to take oral medicines, parenteral cefazolin (Ancef®) may be used provided that they do not have the sensitivities described previously and footnoted in Table 2. Cefazolin is also a first-generation cephalosporin. Please note that the parenteral cefazolin can be given I.M. or I.V. Refer to Table 2 for the adult and children's doses of parenteral cefazolin.

Azithromycin (Zithromax®) and clarithromycin (Biaxin®) are members of the erythromycin-class of antibiotics known as the macrolides. The pharmacology of these drugs has been reviewed previously in *General Dentistry*. The erythromycins have been available for use in dentistry and medicine since the mid 1950s. Azithromycin and clarithromycin represent the first additions to this class in >40 years. The adult prophylactic dose for either drug is 500 mg 1 hour before the procedure with no follow-up dose. The pediatric prophylactic dose of azithromycin and clarithromycin is 15 mg/kg orally 1 hour before the procedure. Although the erythromycin family of drugs are known to inhibit the hepatic metabolism of theophylline and carbamazepine to enhance their effects, azithromycin has not been shown to affect the liver metabolism of these drugs.

Azithromycin is well absorbed from the gastrointestinal tract and is extensively taken up from the circulation into tissues with a slow release from those tissues. It reaches peak serum levels in 2-4 hours and serum half-life is 68 hours. Zithromax® is supplied as 250 mg (retail cost ranges from $7-$8 each) and 600 mg tablets (approximately $15 each). It is also available for oral suspension, supplied as single-dose packets containing 1 g each (approximately $60 for 3 packets). Azithromycin is not yet available as a generic drug.

Clarithromycin (Biaxin®) achieves peak plasma concentrations in 3 hours and maintains effective serum concentrations over a 12-hour period. Reports indicate that it probably interacts with theophylline and carbamazepine by elevating the plasma concentrations of the two drugs. Biaxin® is supplied as 250 mg and 500 mg tablets (retail cost approximately $4 each) and 500 mg extended release tablets (approximately $5 each). It is also available as suspension, supplied as 125 mg/100 mL and 125 mg/50 mL (approximately $20 per 50 mL). Clarithromycin is not yet available as a generic drug.

Amoxicillin *on page 93*
Ampicillin *on page 103*
Azithromycin *on page 153*
Cefadroxil *on page 261*
Cefazolin *on page 263*
Cephalexin *on page 285*
Clarithromycin *on page 337*
Clindamycin *on page 341*

Clinical Considerations for Dentistry

See Figure 1 algorithm at the end of this chapter.

The clinician should review carefully those detailed dental procedures in Table 3 to determine those treatment conditions where prophylaxis is, or is not, recommended. In

ANTIBIOTIC PROPHYLAXIS *(Continued)*

general, in patients with cardiac conditions where prophylaxis is recommended (Table 4), invasive dental procedures where bleeding is likely to be induced from hard or soft tissues (Table 3) should be preceded by antibiotic coverage (Table 2). Clearly, the production of significant bacteremia during a dental procedure is the major risk factor. Patients with a suspicious history of a cardiac condition who are in need of an immediate dental procedure should be prophylaxed with an appropriate antibiotic prior to the procedure(s) until medical evaluation has been completed and the risk level determined. If unanticipated bleeding develops during a procedure in an at-risk patient, appropriate antibiotics should be given immediately. The efficacy of this action is based on animal studies and is possibly effective ≤ 2 hours after the bacteremia.

Table 3. DENTAL PROCEDURES AND PREPROCEDURAL ANTIBIOTICS

Endocarditis or Prosthesis Prophylaxis Recommended Due to Likely Significant Bacteremia*
Dental extractions
Periodontal procedures including surgery, subgingival placement of antibiotic fibers/strips, scaling and root planing, probing, recall maintenance
Dental implant placement and reimplantation of avulsed teeth
Endodontic (root canal) instrumentation or surgery only beyond the apex
Initial placement of orthodontic bands but not brackets
Intraligamentary local anesthetic injections
Prophylactic cleaning of teeth or implants where bleeding is anticipated
Endocarditis Prophylaxis Not Recommended Due to Usually Insignificant Bacteremia
Restorative dentistry† (operative and prosthodontic) with or without retraction cord‡
Local anesthetic injections (nonintraligamentary)
Intracanal endodontic treatment; postplacement and build-up‡
Placement of rubber dam‡
Postoperative suture removal
Placement of removable prosthodontic/orthodontic appliances
Oral impressions‡
Fluoride treatments
Taking of oral radiographs
Orthodontic appliance adjustment
Shedding of primary teeth
‡In general, the presence of moderate to severe gingival inflammation may elevate these procedures to a higher risk of bacteremia.

*Prophylaxis is recommended for patients with high- and moderate-risk cardiac as well as high-risk prosthesis conditions

†This includes restoration of decayed teeth and replacement of missing teeth

‡Clinical judgment may indicate antibiotic use in any circumstances that may create significant bleeding.

Patients with moderate to advanced gingival inflammatory disease and/or periodontitis should be considered at greater risk of bacteremia. However, the ongoing daily risk of self-induced bacteremia in these patients is currently thought to be minimal as compared to the bacteremia during dental procedures. The clinician may wish to consider the use of a preprocedural antimicrobial rinse in addition to antibiotic prophylaxis and, of course, efforts should always focus on improving periodontal health during dental care. If a series of dental procedures is planned, the clinician must judge whether an interval between procedures, requiring prophylaxis, should be scheduled. The literature supports 9- to 14-day intervals as ideal to minimize the risk of emergence of resistant organisms. Since serum levels of the standard amoxicillin dose may be adequate for 6-14 hours depending on the specific organism challenge, the clinician may have to consider the efficacy of a second dose if multiple procedures are planned over the course of a single day.

Table 4. CARDIAC CONDITIONS PREDISPOSING TO ENDOCARDITIS

Endocarditis Prophylaxis Recommended
High-Risk Category
Prosthetic cardiac valves, including bioprosthetic and homograft valves
Previous bacterial endocarditis
Complex cyanotic congenital heart disease (eg, single ventricle states, transposition of the great arteries, tetralogy of Fallot)
Surgically constructed systemic pulmonary shunts or conduits
Moderate-Risk Category
Most other congenital cardiac malformations (other than above and below)
Acquired valvar dysfunction (eg, rheumatic heart disease)
Hypertrophic cardiomyopathy
Mitral valve prolapse with valvar regurgitation and/or thickened leaflets*
Endocarditis Prophylaxis Not Recommended
Negligible-Risk Category (no greater risk than the general population)
Isolated secundum atrial septal defect
Surgical repair of atrial septal defect, ventricular septal defect, or patent ductus arteriosus (without residual defects beyond 6 mo)
Previous coronary artery bypass graft surgery
Mitral valve prolapse without valvar regurgitation
Physiologic, functional, or innocent heart murmurs
Previous Kawasaki disease without valvar dysfunction
Previous rheumatic fever without valvar dysfunction
Cardiac pacemakers (intravascular and epicardial) and implanted defibrillators
***Specific risk for patients with a history of fenfluramine or dexfenfluramine (fen-phen or Redux®) use, has not been determined. Such patients should have medical evaluation for potential cardiac damage, as currently recommended by the FDA.**

For patients with suspected or confirmed mitral valve prolapse (MVP), the risk of infection as well as other complications such as tachycardia, syncope, congestive heart failure, or progressive regurgitation are variable. The risk depends on age and severity of MVP. The decision to recommend prophylaxis in such patients is oftentimes controversial but it is generally agreed that the determination of regurgitation is the most predictive (see Algorithm Figure 2 at the end of this chapter). Therefore, patients with MVP with mitral regurgitation require prophylaxis. If the regurgitation is undetermined and the patient is in need of an immediate procedure, then prophylaxis should be given in any case and the patient referred for further evaluation. If echocardiographic or Doppler studies demonstrate regurgitation, then prophylaxis would be recommended routinely. If no regurgitation can be demonstrated by these studies, then MVP alone does not require prophylaxis.

PREPROCEDURAL ANTIBIOTICS FOR PROSTHETIC IMPLANTS

A significant number of dental patients have had total joint replacements or other implanted prosthetic devices. Prior to performing dental procedures that might induce bacteremia, the dentist must consider the use of antibiotic prophylaxis in these patients. Until recently, only the American Heart Association had taken a formal stance on implanted devices by suggesting guidelines for the use of antibiotic prophylaxis in patients with prosthetic heart valves. These guidelines and the recent guidelines for prevention of bacterial endocarditis have been published in *General Dentistry*.

The use of antibiotics in patients with other prosthetic devices, including total joint replacements has remained controversial because of several issues. Late infections of implanted prosthetic devices have rarely been associated with microbial organisms of oral origin. Secondly, since late infections in such patients are often not reported, data is lacking to substantiate or refute this potential. Also, there is general acceptance that patients with acute infections at distant sites such as the oral cavity may be at greater risk of infection of an implanted prosthetic device. Periodontal disease has been implicated as a distant site infection. Since antibiotics are associated with allergies and other adverse reactions, and because the frequent use of antibiotics may lead to emergence of resistant organisms, any perceived benefit of antibiotic prophylaxis must always be weighed against known risks of toxicity, allergy, or potential microbial resistance.

Recently, an advisory group made up of representatives from the American Dental Association and the American Academy of Orthopaedic Surgeons published a statement in the *Journal of the American Dental Association* on the use of antibiotics prior to dental procedures in patients with total joint replacements. The statement concluded that antibiotic prophylaxis should not be prescribed routinely for most dental patients with total joint replacements or for any patients with pins, plates, and screws. However, in an attempt to base the guidelines on available scientific evidence, the advisory group stated that certain patients may be potential risks for joint infection thus justifying the use of prophylactic antibiotics. Those conditions considered by the advisory group to be associated

ANTIBIOTIC PROPHYLAXIS *(Continued)*

with potential elevated risk of joint infections are listed in Table 5. The dentist should carefully review the patient's history to ensure identification of those medical problems leading to potential elevated risks of joint infections as listed in Table 5. Where appropriate, medical consultation with the patient's internist or orthopedist may be prudent to assist in this determination. The orthopedist should be queried specifically, as to the status of the joint prosthesis itself.

Table 5. PATIENTS WITH POTENTIAL ELEVATED RISK OF JOINT INFECTION

Inflammatory arthropathies: Rheumatoid arthritis, systemic lupus erythematosus
Disease-, drug-, or radiation-induced immunosuppression
Insulin-dependent diabetes
First 2 years following joint replacement
Previous prosthetic joint infections
Patients with acute infections at a distant site
Hemophilia

Patients who present with elevated risks of joint infections, in which the dentist is going to perform any procedures associated with a high risk of bacteremia, need to receive preprocedural antibiotics. Those dental procedures associated with high risk of bacteremia are listed in Table 3. Patients undergoing dental procedures involving low risk of bacteremia, probably do not require premedication even though the patient may be in the category of elevated risk of joint infections. Patients with an acute oral infection or moderate to severe gingival inflammation and/or periodontitis must be considered at higher risk for bacteremia during dental procedures than those without active dental disease. In these patients, as in all patients, the dental clinician should aggressively treat these oral conditions striving for optimum oral health. The listing of low bacteremia risks in Table 3 may need to be reconsidered, depending on the patient's oral health.

ANTIBIOTIC REGIMENS

The antibiotic prophylaxis regimens as suggested by the advisory panel are listed in Table 6. These regimens are not exactly the same as those listed in Table 2 (for prevention of endocarditis) and must be reviewed carefully to avoid confusion. Cephalexin, cephradine, or amoxicillin may be used in patients not allergic to penicillin. The selected antibiotic is given as a single 2 g dose 1 hour before the procedure. A follow-up dose is not recommended. Cephalexin (Keflex®) and amoxicillin have been described earlier in this chapter. Cephradine (Velosef®) is a first-generation cephalosporin-type antibiotic effective against anaerobic bacteria and aerobic Gram-positive bacteria. It is used in medicine predominantly to treat infections of the bones and joints, infections of the lower respiratory tract, urinary tract, and skin and soft tissues.

Parenteral cefazolin (Ancef®) or ampicillin are the recommended antibiotics for those patients unable to take oral medications; see Table 6 for doses. Cefazolin is a first-generation cephalosporin effective against anaerobes and aerobic Gram-positive bacteria. Ampicillin is an aminopenicillin described earlier. For patients allergic to penicillin, clindamycin is the recommended antibiotic of choice. Clindamycin is active against aerobic and anaerobic streptococci, most staphylococci, the *Bacteroides*, and the *Actinomyces* families of bacteria. The recommended oral and parenteral doses of clindamycin in the joint prosthetic patient are listed in Table 6.

Table 6. ANTIBIOTIC REGIMENS FOR PATIENTS WITH PROSTHETIC IMPLANTS

Patients not allergic to penicillin:	Cephalexin, cephradine, or amoxicillin:	2 g orally 1 hour prior to the procedure
Patients not allergic to penicillin and unable to take oral medications:	Cefazolin: or Ampicillin:	1 g I.M. or I.V. 1 hour prior to the procedure 2 g I.M. or I.V. 1 hour prior to the procedure
Patients allergic to penicillin:	Clindamycin:	600 mg orally 1 hour prior to dental procedure
Patients allergic to penicillin and unable to take oral medications:	Clindamycin:	600 mg I.V. 1 hour prior to the procedure

Amoxicillin *on page 93*
Ampicillin *on page 103*
Cefazolin *on page 263*
Cephalexin *on page 285*
Cephradine *on page 288*
Clindamycin *on page 341*

Clinical Considerations for Dentistry

See Algorithm Figure 3 at the end of this chapter.

The frequency of postinsertion infections in patients who have undergone total joint replacement or prosthetic device placement is variable. The most common cause of infection with all devices is found to be from contamination at the time of surgical insertions. The presence of an acute distant infection at a site other than the joint, however, appears to be a risk factor for late infection of these devices. The rationale by the American Dental Association and the American Academy of Orthopedic Surgeons in their advisory statement has been to provide guidelines to minimize the use of antibiotics to the first 2 years following total joint replacement. As more data are collected, these recommendations may be revised. However, it is thought to be prudent for the dental clinician to fully evaluate all patients with respect to history and or physical findings prior to determining the risk.

If a procedure considered to be low risk for bacteremia is performed in a patient at risk for joint complications, and inadvertent bleeding occurs, then an appropriate antibiotic should be given immediately. Although this is not ideal, animal studies suggest that it may be useful. Likewise, in patients where concern exists over joint complications and a medical consultation cannot be immediately obtained, the patient should be treated as though antibiotic coverage is necessary until such time that an appropriate consultation can be completed. The presence of an acute oral infection, in addition to any pre-existing dental conditions, may increase the risk of late infection at the prosthetic joint. Even though most late joint infections are caused by *Staphylococcus* sp, the risk of bacteremia involving another organism, predominant in an acute infection, may increase the risk of joint infection.

The dentist may also need to consider the question of multiple procedures over a period of time. Procedures planned over a period of several days would best be rescheduled at intervals of 9-14 days. The risk of emergence of resistant organisms in patients receiving multiple short-term doses of antibiotics has been shown to be greater than those receiving antibiotics over longer intervals of time.

FREQUENTLY ASKED QUESTIONS

Can erythromycin still be used to prevent bacterial endocarditis in dental patients?

If the clinician has successfully used erythromycin in the past, this form of prophylaxis can be continued using the regimen included in the recommendation of 1990. Erythromycin has, however, been excluded for the vast majority of patients due to gastric upset.

If the patient is presently taking antibiotics for some other ailment, is prophylaxis still necessary?

If a patient is already taking antibiotics for another condition, prophylaxis should be accomplished with a drug from another class. For example, in the patient who is not allergic to penicillin who is taking erythromycin for a medical condition such as mycoplasma infection, amoxicillin would be the drug of choice for prophylaxis. Also, in the penicillin-allergic patient taking clindamycin, prophylaxis would best be accomplished with azithromycin or clarithromycin. The new guidelines restated the position that doses of antibiotics for prevention of recurrence of rheumatic fever are thought to be inadequate to prevent bacterial endocarditis and prophylaxis should be accomplished with the full dose of a drug from another class.

Can clindamycin be used safely in patients with gastrointestinal disorders?

If a patient has a history of inflammatory bowel disease and is allergic to penicillin, azithromycin or clarithromycin should be selected over clindamycin. In patients with a negative history of inflammatory bowel disease, clindamycin has not been shown to induce colitis following a single-dose administration.

Why do the suggested drug regimens for patients with joint prostheses resemble so closely the regimens for the prevention of bacterial endocarditis?

Bacteremia is the predisposing risk factor for the development of endocarditis in those patients at risk due to a cardiac condition. Likewise, the potential of bacteremia during dental procedures is considered to be the risk factor in some late joint prostheses infections, even though this risk is presumed to be much lower.

How do we determine those patients who have had joint replacement complications?

Patients who have had complications during the initial placement of a total joint would be those who had infection following placement, those with recurrent pain, or those who have had previous joint replacement failures. If the patient reports even minor complications, a medical consultation with the orthopedist would be the most appropriate action for the dentist.

ANTIBIOTIC PROPHYLAXIS *(Continued)*

Is prophylaxis required in patients with pins, screws, or plates often used in orthopedic repairs?

There is currently no evidence supporting use of antibiotics following the placement of pins, plates, or screws. Breast implants, dental implants, and implanted lenses in the eye following cataract surgery are also all thought to be at minimal risk for infection following dental procedures. Therefore, no antibiotic prophylaxis is recommended in these situations. There is, however, some evidence indicating elevated risk of infection following some types of penile implants and some vascular access devices, used during chemotherapy. It is recommended that the dentist discuss such patients with the physician prior to determining the need for antibiotics.

What should I do if medical consultation results in a recommendation that differs from the published guidelines endorsed by the American Dental Association?

The dentist is ultimately responsible for treatment recommendations. Ideally, by communicating with the physician, a consensus can be achieved that is either in agreement with the guidelines or is based on other established medical reasoning.

What is the best antibiotic modality for treating dental infections?

Penicillin is still the drug of choice for treatment of infections in and around the oral cavity. Phenoxy-methyl penicillin (Pen VK®) has long been the most commonly selected antibiotic. In penicillin-allergic individuals, erythromycin may be an appropriate consideration. If another drug is sought, clindamycin prescribed 300 mg as a loading dose followed by 150 mg 4 times/day would be an appropriate regimen for a dental infection. In general, if there is no response to Pen VK®, then Augmentin® may be a good alternative in the nonpenicillin-allergic patient because of its slightly altered spectrum. Recommendations would include that the patient should take the drug with food.

Is there cross-allergenicity between the cephalosporins and penicillin?

The incidence of cross-allergenicity is 5% to 8% in the overall population. If a patient has demonstrated a Type I hypersensitivity reaction to penicillin, namely urticaria or anaphylaxis, then this incidence would increase to 20%.

Is there definitely an interaction between contraception agents and antibiotics?

There are well founded interactions between contraceptives and antibiotics. The best instructions that a patient could be given by their dentist are that should an antibiotic be necessary and the dentist is aware that the patient is on contraceptives, and if the patient is using chemical contraceptives, the patient should seriously consider additional means of contraception during the antibiotic management.

Are antibiotics necessary in diabetic patients?

In the management of diabetes, control of the diabetic status is the key factor relative to all morbidity issues. If a patient is well controlled, then antibiotics will likely not be necessary. However, in patients where the control is questionable or where they have recently been given a different drug regimen for their diabetes or if they are being titrated to an appropriate level of either insulin or oral hypoglycemic agents during these periods of time, the dentist might consider preprocedural antibiotics to be efficacious.

Do nonsteroidal anti-inflammatory drugs interfere with blood pressure medication?

At the current time there is no clear evidence that NSAIDs interfere with any of the blood pressure medications that are currently in use.

Is a patient who has taken phentermine at risk for cardiac problems just like a patient who took "fen-phen"?

No, there is often confusion with these drug names. "Fen-phen" referred to a combined use of fenfluramine and phentermine and it is this combination that has led to the FDA statement (see Table 4). The single drug phentermine has not been implicated in this current concern over cardiac complications.

Figure 1
Preprocedural Dental Action Plan for Patients With a History Indicative of Elevated Endocarditis Risk

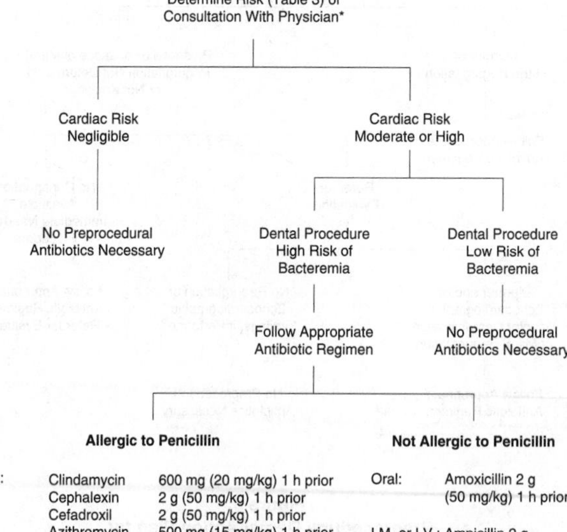

Allergic to Penicillin

Oral:	Clindamycin	600 mg (20 mg/kg) 1 h prior
	Cephalexin	2 g (50 mg/kg) 1 h prior
	Cefadroxil	2 g (50 mg/kg) 1 h prior
	Azithromycin	500 mg (15 mg/kg) 1 h prior
	Clarithromycin	500 mg (15 mg/kg) 1 h prior
I.V.:	Clindamycin	600 mg (20 mg/kg) 30 min prior
I.M. or I.V.:	Cefazolin	1 g (25 mg/kg) 30 min prior

Not Allergic to Penicillin

Oral:	Amoxicillin 2 g (50 mg/kg) 1 h prior
I.M. or I.V.:	Ampicillin 2 g (50 mg/kg) 30 min prior

Dosages for children are in parentheses and should never exceed adult dose. Cephalosporins should be avoided in patients with previous Type I hypersensitivity reactions to penicillin due to some evidence of cross allergenicity.

* For Emergency Dental Care, the clinician should attempt phone consultation. If unable to contact patient's physician or determine risk, the patient should be treated as though there is moderate or high risk of cardiac complication and follow the algorithm.

ANTIBIOTIC PROPHYLAXIS *(Continued)*

Figure 2
Patient With Suspected Mitral Valve Prolapse

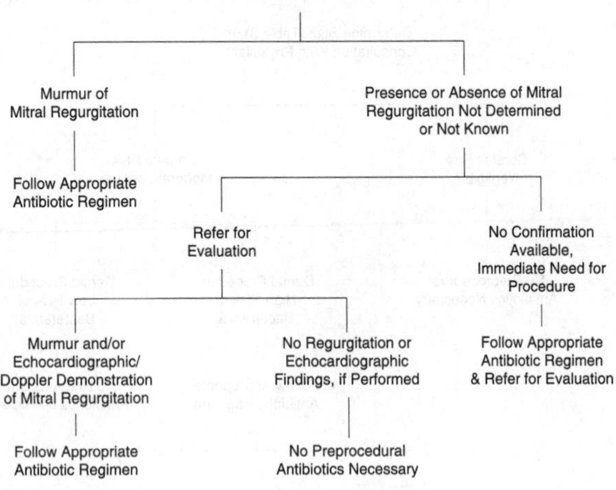

Figure 3
Preprocedural Dental Action Plan for Patients With Prosthetic Implants

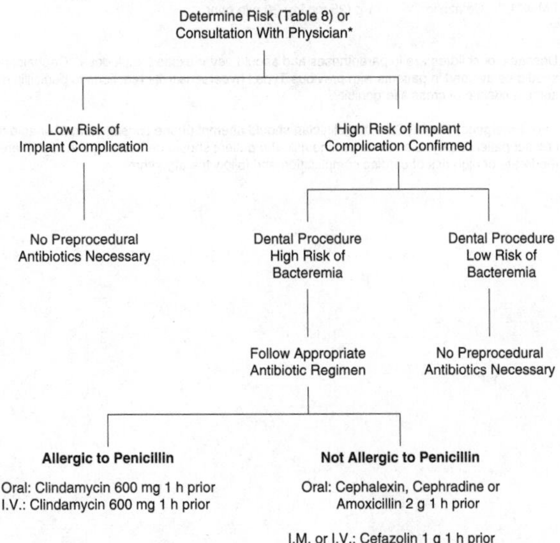

Allergic to Penicillin

Oral: Clindamycin 600 mg 1 h prior
I.V.: Clindamycin 600 mg 1 h prior

Not Allergic to Penicillin

Oral: Cephalexin, Cephradine or Amoxicillin 2 g 1 h prior

I.M. or I.V.: Cefazolin 1 g 1 h prior
Ampicillin 2 g 1 h prior

Cephalosporins should be avoided in patients with previous Type I hypersensitivity reactions to penicillin due to some evidence of cross allergenicity.

*For Emergency Dental Care the clinician should attempt phone consultation. If unable to contact patient's physician or determine risk, the patient should be treated as though there is high risk of implant complication and follow the algorithm.

SYSTEMIC VIRAL DISEASES

HEPATITIS

The hepatitis viruses are a group of DNA and RNA viruses that produce symptoms associated with inflammation of the liver. Currently, hepatitis A through G have been identified by immunological testing; however, hepatitis A through E have received most attention in terms of disease identification. Recently, however, there has been increased interest in hepatitis viruses F and G, particularly as relate to healthcare professionals. Our knowledge is expanding rapidly in this area and the clinician should be alert to changes in the literature that might update their knowledge. Hepatitis F, for instance, remains a diagnosis of exclusion effectively being non-A, B, C, D, E, or G. Whereas, hepatitis G has serologic testing available, however, not commercially at this time. Research evaluations of various antibody and RT-PCR tests for hepatitis G are under development at this time.

Signs and symptoms of viral hepatitis in general are quite variable. Patients infected may range from asymptomatic to experiencing flu-like symptoms only. In addition, fever, nausea, joint muscle pain, jaundice, and hepatomegaly along with abdominal pain can result from infection with one of the hepatitis viruses. The virus also can create an acute or chronic infection. Usually following these early symptoms or the asymptomatic period, the patient may recover or may go on to develop chronic liver dysfunction. Liver dysfunction may be represented primarily by changes in liver function tests known as LFTs and these primarily include aspartate aminotransferase known as AST and alanine aminotransferase known as ALT. In addition, for A, B, C, D, and E there are serologic tests for either antigen, antibody, or both. Of hepatitis A through G, five forms have both acute and chronic forms whereas A and E appear to only create acute disease. There are differences in the way clinicians may approach a known postexposure to one of the hepatitis viruses. In many instances, gamma globulin may be used, however, the indications for gamma globulin as a drug limit their use to several of the viruses only. The dental clinician should be aware that the gastroenterologist may choose to give gamma globulin off-label.

Hepatitis A

Hepatitis A virus is an enteric virus that is a member of the Picornavirus family along with Coxsackie viruses and poliovirus. Previously known as infectious hepatitis, hepatitis A has been detected in humans for centuries. It causes acute hepatitis, often transmitted by oral-fecal contamination and having an incubation period of approximately 30 days. Typically, constitutional symptoms are present and jaundice may occur. Drug therapy that the dentist may encounter in a patient being treated for hepatitis A would primarily include immunoglobulin. Hepatitis A vaccine (inactivated) is an FDA-approved vaccine indicated in the prevention of contracting hepatitis A in exposed or high-risk individuals. Candidates at high risk for HAV infection include persons traveling internationally to highly endemic areas, individuals with chronic liver disease, individuals engaging in high-risk sexual behavior, illicit drug users, persons with high-risk occupational exposure, hemophiliacs or other persons receiving blood products, pediatric populations, and food handlers in high-risk environments. Two formulations of hepatitis A vaccine are available, Havrix® and VAQTA®. Each is administered as an injection in the deltoid region and both are available in pediatric and adult dosages. For additional information, refer to Hepatitis A Vaccine *on page 665.*

Hepatitis B

Hepatitis B virus is previously known as serum hepatitis and has particular trophism for liver cells. Hepatitis B virus causes both acute and chronic disease in susceptible patients. The incubation period is often long and the diagnosis might be made by serologic markers even in the absence of symptoms. No drug therapy for acute hepatitis B is known; however, chronic hepatitis has recently been successfully treated with alfa-interferon. There are vaccines available for hepatitis A and B. See Hepatitis A Inactivated and Hepatitis B (Recombinant) Vaccine *on page 664.*

Hepatitis C

Hepatitis C virus was described in 1988 and has been formerly classified as non-A/non-B. It is clear that hepatitis C represents a high percentage of the transfusion-associated hepatitis that is seen. Treatment of acute hepatitis C infection is generally supportive. Interferon Alfa-2a therapy has been used with some success recently and interferon-alfa may be beneficial with hepatitis C related chronic hepatitis.

SYSTEMIC VIRAL DISEASES *(Continued)*

Hepatitis D

Hepatitis D, previously known as the delta agent, is a virus that is incomplete in that it requires previous infection with hepatitis B in order to be manifested. Currently, no antiviral therapy is effective against hepatitis D.

Hepatitis E

Hepatitis E virus is an RNA virus that represents a proportion of the previously classified non-A/non-B diagnoses. There is currently no antiviral therapy against hepatitis E.

Hepatitis F

Hepatitis F, as was mentioned, remains a diagnosis of exclusion. There are no known immunological tests available for identification of hepatitis F at present and currently the Centers for Disease Control have not come out with specific guidelines or recommendations. It is thought, however, that hepatitis F is a bloodborne virus and it has been used as a diagnosis in several cases of post-transfusion hepatitis.

Hepatitis G

Hepatitis G virus (HGV) is the newest hepatitis and is also assumed to be a bloodborne virus. Similar in family to hepatitis C, it is thought to occur concomitantly with hepatitis C and appears to be even more prevalent in some blood donors than hepatitis C. Occupational transmission of HGV is currently under study (see the references for updated information) and currently there are no specific CDC recommendations for postexposure to an HGV individual as the testing for identification remains experimental.

Hepatitis A Vaccine *on page 665*
Hepatitis A Inactivated and Hepatitis B (Recombinant) Vaccine *on page 664*
Hepatitis B Immune Globulin *on page 666*
Hepatitis B Vaccine *on page 666*
Immune Globulin, Intramuscular *on page 713*
Immune Globulin, Intravenous *on page 714*
Interferon Alfa-2a *on page 726*
Peginterferon Alfa-2b *on page 1042*

TYPES OF HEPATITIS VIRUS

Features	A	B	C	D	E	F	G
Incubation Period	2-6 wks	8-24 wks	2-52 wks	3-13 wks	3-6 wks	Unknown	Unknown
Onset	Abrupt	Insidious	Insidious	Abrupt	Abrupt	Insidious	Insidious
Symptoms							
Jaundice	Adults: 70% to 80%; Children: 10%	25%	25%	Varies	Unknown	Unknown	Unknown
Asymptomatic patients	Adults: 50%; Children: Most	~75%	~75%	Rare	Rare	Common	Common
Routes of Transmission							
Fecal/Oral	Yes	No	No	No	Yes	Unknown	Unknown
Parenteral	Rare	Yes	Yes	Yes	No		
Sexual	No	Yes	Possible	Yes	No		
Perinatal	No	Yes	Possible	Possible	No		
Water/Food	Yes	No	No	No	Yes		
Sequelae (% of patients)							
Chronic state	No	Adults: 6% to 10%; Children: 25% to 50%; Infants: 70% to 90%	>75%	10% to 15%	No	Unknown	Likely
Case-Fatality Rate	0.6%	1.4%	1% to 2%	30%	1% to 2% Pregnant women: 20%	Unknown	Unknown

PRE-EXPOSURE RISK FACTORS FOR HEPATITIS B

Healthcare factors:

Healthcare workers*

Special patient groups (eg, adolescents, infants born to HB_sAg–positive mothers, military personnel, etc)

Hemodialysis patients†

Recipients of certain blood products‡

Lifestyle factors:

Homosexual and bisexual men

Intravenous drug abusers

Heterosexually active persons with multiple sexual partners or recently acquired sexually transmitted diseases

Environmental factors:

Household and sexual contacts of HBV carriers

Prison inmates

Clients and staff of institutions for the mentally handicapped

Residents, immigrants and refugees from areas with endemic HBV infection

International travelers at increased risk of acquiring HBV infection

*The risk of hepatitis B virus (HBV) infection for healthcare workers varies both between hospitals and within hospitals. Hepatitis B vaccination is recommended for all healthcare workers with blood exposure.

†Hemodialysis patients often respond poorly to hepatitis B vaccination; higher vaccine doses or increased number of doses are required. A special formulation of one vaccine is now available for such persons (Recombivax HB®, 40 mcg/mL). The anti-HB_s (antibody to hepatitis B surface antigen) response of such persons should be tested after they are vaccinated, and those who have not responded should be revaccinated with 1-3 additional doses.

Patients with chronic renal disease should be vaccinated as early as possible, ideally before they require hemodialysis. In addition, their anti- HB_s levels should be monitored at 6- to 12-month intervals to assess the need for revaccination.

‡Patients with hemophilia should be immunized subcutaneously, not intramuscularly.

POSTEXPOSURE PROPHYLAXIS FOR HEPATITIS B*

Exposure	Hepatitis B Immune Globulin	Hepatitis B Vaccine
Perinatal	0.5 mL I.M. within 12 hours of birth	0.5 mL† I.M. within 12 hours of birth (no later than 7 days), and at 1 and 6 months‡; test for HB_sAg and anti-HB_s at 12-15 months
Sexual	0.06 mL/kg I.M. within 14 days of sexual contact; a second dose should be given if the index patient remains HB_sAg-positive after 3 months and hepatitis B vaccine was not given initially	1 mL I.M. at 0, 1, and 6 months for homosexual and bisexual men and regular sexual contacts of persons with acute and chronic hepatitis B
Percutaneous; exposed person unvaccinated		
Source known HB_sAg-positive	0.06 mL/kg I.M. within 24 hours	1 mL I.M. within 7 days, and at 1 and 6 months§
Source known, HB_sAg status not known	Test source for HB_sAg; if source is positive, give exposed person 0.06 mL/kg I.M. once within 7 days	1 mL I.M. within 7 days, and at 1 and 6 months§
Source not tested or unknown	Nothing required	1 mL I.M. within 7 days, and at 1 and 6 months
Percutaneous; exposed person vaccinated		
Source known HB_sAg-positive	Test exposed person for anti-HB_s¶. If titer is protective, nothing is required; if titer is not protective, give 0.06 mL/kg within 24 hours	Review vaccination status#
Source known, HB_sAg status not known	Test source for HB_sAg and exposed person for anti-HB_s. If source is HB_sAg-negative, or if source is HB_sAg-positive but anti-HB_s titer is protective, nothing is required. If source is HB_sAg-positive and anti-HB_s titer is not protective or if exposed person is a known nonresponder, give 0.06 mL/kg I.M. within 24 hours. A second dose of hepatitis B immune globulin can be given 1 month later if a booster dose of hepatitis B vaccine is not given.	Review vaccination status#

SYSTEMIC VIRAL DISEASES *(Continued)*

POSTEXPOSURE PROPHYLAXIS FOR HEPATITIS B* *(continued)*

Exposure	Hepatitis B Immune Globulin	Hepatitis B Vaccine
Source not tested or unknown	Test exposed person for anti-HB_s. If anti-HB_s titer is protective, nothing is required. If anti-HB_s titer is not protective, 0.06 mL/kg may be given along with a booster dose of hepatitis B vaccine.	Review vaccination status#

*HB_sAg = hepatitis B surface antigen; anti-HB_s = antibody to hepatitis B surface antigen; I.M. = intramuscularly; SRU = standard ratio units.

†Each 0.5 mL dose of plasma-derived hepatitis B vaccine contains 10 mcg of HB_sAg; each 0.5 mL dose of recombinant hepatitis B vaccine contains 5 mcg or 10 mcg of HB_sAg.

‡If hepatitis B immune globulin and hepatitis B vaccine are given simultaneously, they should be given at separate sites.

§If hepatitis B vaccine is not given, a second dose of hepatitis B immune globulin should be given 1 month later.

¶Anti-HB_s titers <10 SRU by radioimmunoassay or negative by enzyme immunoassay indicate lack of protection. Testing the exposed person for anti-HB_s is not necessary if a protective level of antibody has been shown within the previous 24 months.

#If the exposed person has not completed a three-dose series of hepatitis B vaccine, the series should be completed. Test the exposed person for anti-HB_s. If the antibody level is protective, nothing is required. If an adequate antibody response in the past is shown on retesting to have declined to an inadequate level, a booster dose (1 mL) of hepatitis B vaccine should be given. If the exposed person has inadequate antibody or is a known nonresponder to vaccination, a booster dose can be given along with one dose of hepatitis B immune globulin.

HERPES

The herpes viruses not only represent a topic of specific interest to the dentist due to oral manifestations, but are widespread as systemic infections. Herpes simplex virus is also of interest because of its central nervous system infections and its relationship as one of the viral infections commonly found in AIDS patients. Oral herpes infections will be covered elsewhere. Treatment of herpes simplex primary infection includes acyclovir. Ganciclovir is an alternative drug and foscarnet is also occasionally used. Epstein-Barr virus is a member of the herpesvirus family and produces syndromes important in dentistry, including infectious mononucleosis with the commonly found oral pharyngitis and petechial hemorrhages, as well as being the causative agent of Burkitt's lymphoma. The relationship between Epstein-Barr virus to oral hairy leukoplakia in AIDS patients has not been shown to be one of cause and effect; however, the presence of Epstein-Barr in these lesions is consistent. Currently, there is no accepted treatment for Epstein-Barr virus, although acyclovir has been shown in *in vitro* studies to have some efficacy. Varicella-zoster virus is another member of the herpesvirus family and is the causative agent of two clinical entities, chickenpox and shingles or herpes zoster. Oral manifestations of both chickenpox and herpes zoster include vesicular eruptions often leading to confluent mucosal ulcerations. Acyclovir is the drug of choice for treatment of herpes zoster infections.

There are other herpes viruses that produce disease in man and animals. These viruses have no specific treatment, therefore, incidence is thought to be less common than those mentioned and the specific treatment is not determined at present. The role of some of these viruses in concomitant infection with the HIV and other coinfection viruses is still under study.

ANTIVIRALS

AGENTS OF ESTABLISHED EFFECTIVENESS

Viral Infection	Drug
Cytomegalovirus	
Retinitis	Ganciclovir Foscarnet
Pneumonia	Ganciclovir
Hepatitis viruses	
Chronic hepatitis A & B	Hepatitis A Inactivated & Hepatitis B (Recombinant) vaccine
Chronic hepatitis C	Interferon Alfa-2a
Chronic hepatitis B	Interferon Alfa-2b Peginterferon Alfa-2b
Herpes simplex virus	
Orofacial herpes	
First episode	Acyclovir*
Recurrence	Acyclovir* Penciclovir*
Genital herpes	
First episode	Acyclovir
Recurrence	Acyclovir
Suppression	Acyclovir
Encephalitis	Acyclovir
Mucocutaneous disease in immunocompromised	Acyclovir
Neonatal	Acyclovir
Keratoconjunctivitis	Trifluridine Vidarabine
Influenza A virus	Amantadine Oseltamivir Rimantadine Zanamivir
Papillomavirus	
Condyloma acuminatum	Interferon Alfa-2b Imiquimod (Aldara™): (use for oral lesions is under study)
Respiratory syncytial virus	Ribavirin
Varicella-zoster virus	
Varicella in normal children	Acyclovir
Varicella in immunocompromised	Acyclovir
Herpes zoster in immunocompromised	Acyclovir
Herpes zoster in normal hosts	Acyclovir Famciclovir Valacyclovir

*Although acyclovir is often used for these infections, penciclovir is specifically approved for herpes labialis. The clinician is referred to the monographs for more discussion.

Acyclovir *on page 42*
Amantadine *on page 70*
Atovaquone *on page 142*
Cidofovir *on page 323*
Famciclovir *on page 555*
Fomivirsen *on page 611*
Foscarnet *on page 613*
Ganciclovir *on page 626*
Hepatitis B Immune Globulin *on page 666*
Imiquimod *on page 713*
Immune Globulin, Intramuscular *on page 713*
Interferon Alfa-2a *on page 726*
Interferon Alfa-2b *on page 727*
Interferon Alfa-n3 *on page 731*
Oseltamivir *on page 1006*
Penciclovir *on page 1046*
Rifabutin *on page 1179*
Rimantadine *on page 1185*
Trifluridine *on page 1350*
Valacyclovir *on page 1367*
Vidarabine *on page 1384*
Zanamivir *on page 1405*

ORAL MEDICINE TOPICS

PART II:

DENTAL MANAGEMENT AND THERAPEUTIC CONSIDERATIONS IN PATIENTS WITH SPECIFIC ORAL CONDITIONS AND OTHER MEDICINE TOPICS

This second part of the chapter focuses on therapies the dentist may choose to prescribe for patients suffering from oral disease or who are in need of special care. Some overlap between these sections has resulted from systemic conditions that have oral manifestations and vice-versa. Cross-references to the descriptions and the monographs for individual drugs described elsewhere in this handbook allow for easy retrieval of information. Example prescriptions of selected drug therapies for each condition are presented so that the clinician can evaluate alternate approaches to treatment, since there is seldom a single drug of choice.

Drug prescriptions shown represent prototype drugs and popular prescriptions and are examples only. The pharmacologic category index is available for cross-referencing if alternatives and additional drugs are sought.

TABLE OF CONTENTS

Oral Pain 1524

Oral Bacterial Infections 1531

Periodontal Diseases 1540

Oral Fungal Infections 1542

Oral Viral Infections 1545

Oral Nonviral Soft Tissue Ulcerations or Erosions 1549

Dentin Hypersensitivity, High Caries Index, and Xerostomia 1553

Management of Sialorrhea 1555

Temporomandibular Dysfunction (TMD) 1562

Patients Requiring Sedation 1565

Management of Patients Undergoing Cancer Therapy 1567

ORAL PAIN

PAIN PREVENTION

For the dental patient, the prevention of pain aids in relieving anxiety and reduces the probability of stress during dental care. For the practitioner, dental procedures can be accomplished more efficiently in a "painless" situation. Appropriate selection and use of local anesthetics is one of the foundations for success in this arena. Local anesthetics listed below include drugs for the most commonly confronted dental procedures. Ester anesthetics are no longer available in dose form for dental injections, and historically had a higher incidence of allergic manifestations due to the formation of the metabolic byproduct, para-aminobenzoic acid. Articaine, which has an ester side chain, is rapidly metabolized to a non-PABA acid and, hence, functions as an amide and has a low allergic potential. The amides, in general, have an almost negligible allergic rate, and only one well-documented case of amide allergy has been reported by Seng, et al. Although injectable diphenhydramine (Benadryl®) has been used in an attempt to provide anesthesia in patients allergic to all the local anesthetics, it is no longer recommended in this context. The vehicle for injectable diphenhydramine can cause tissue necrosis.

The potential interaction between acetaminophen and warfarin has been recently raised in the literature. The cytochrome P450 system of drug metabolism for these vitamin K dependent metabolic pathways has raised the possibility that prolonged use of acetaminophen may inadvertently enhance, to dangerous levels, the anticoagulation effect of warfarin. As monitored by the INR, the effects of these drugs may be one and one-half to two times greater than as expected from the warfarin dosage alone. This potential interaction could be of importance in selecting an analgesic/antipyretic drug for the dental patient.

LOCAL ANESTHETICS

Articaine and Epinephrine [U.S.] *on page 125*

Articaine and Epinephrine [Canada] *on page 124*

Bupivacaine *on page 205*

Bupivacaine and Epinephrine *on page 207*

Chloroprocaine *on page 302*

Etidocaine and Epinephrine *on page 545*

Levobupivacaine *on page 789*

Lidocaine and Epinephrine *on page 804*

Lidocaine *on page 801*

Lidocaine (Transoral) *on page 807*

Mepivacaine Dental Anesthetic *on page 863*

Mepivacaine and Levonordefrin *on page 862*

Prilocaine *on page 1114*

Prilocaine and Epinephrine *on page 1116*

Ropivacaine *on page 1198*

Tetracaine *on page 1284*

Tetracaine and Dextrose *on page 1285*

The selection of a vasoconstrictor with the local anesthetic must be based on the length of the procedure to be performed, the patient's medical status (epinephrine is contraindicated in patients with uncontrolled hyperthyroidism), and the need for hemorrhage control. The following table lists some of the common drugs with their duration of action. Transoral patches with lidocaine are now available (DentiPatch®) and the new long-acting amide injectable, Ropivacaine (Naropin®) may be useful for postoperative pain management.

DENTAL ANESTHETICS
(Average Duration by Route)

Product	Infiltration	Inferior Alveolar Block
Articaine HCl 4% and epinephrine 1:100,000	60 minutes	60 minutes
Carbocaine® HCl 2% with Neo-Cobefrin® 1:20,000 (mepivacaine HCl and levonordefrin)	50 minutes	60-75 minutes
Duranest® Injection (etidocaine)	5-10 hours	5-10 hours
Citanest® Plain 4% (prilocaine)	20 minutes	2.5 hours
Citanest Forte® with Epinephrine (prilocaine with epinephrine)	2.25 hours	3 hours
Lidocaine HCl 2% and epinephrine 1:100,000	60 minutes	90 minutes
Marcaine® HCl 0.5% with epinephrine 1:200,000 (bupivacaine and epinephrine)	60 minutes	5-7 hours

The use of articaine 4% with epinephrine 1:100,000 solution for mandibular blocks has been associated occasionally with parasthesia. (*J Am Dent Assoc*, 2001, 132(2):177-85.)

The use of preinjection topical anesthetics can assist in pain prevention (see also "Oral Viral Infections" *on page 1545* and "Oral Nonviral Soft Tissue Ulcerations or Erosions" *on page 1549*). Some clinicians are also using EMLA® (eutectic mixture of local anesthetic with lidocaine and prilocaine) as a topical. Skin patch available by Astra not currently approved for oral use.

Benzocaine *on page 169*

Lidocaine *on page 801*

Lidocaine Transoral *on page 807*

Tetracaine *on page 1284*

PAIN MANAGEMENT

The patient with existing acute or chronic oral pain requires appropriate treatment and sensitivity on the part of the dentist, all for the purpose of achieving relief from the oral source of pain. Pain can be divided into mild, moderate, and severe levels and requires a subjective assessment by the dentist based on knowledge of the dental procedures to be performed, the presenting signs and symptoms of the patient, and the realization that most dental procedures are invasive often leading to pain once the patient has left the dental office. The practitioner must be aware that the treatment of the source of the pain is usually the best management. If infection is present, treatment of the infection will directly alleviate the patient's discomfort. However, a patient who is not in pain tends to heal better and it is wise to adequately cover the patient for any residual or recurrent discomfort suffered. Likewise, many of the procedures that the dentist performs have pain associated with them. Much of this pain occurs after leaving the dentist office due to an inflammatory process or a healing process that has been initiated. It is difficult to assign specific pain levels (mild, moderate, or severe) for specific procedures; however, the dentist should use his or her prescribing capacity judiciously so that overmedication is avoided.

The following categories of drugs and appropriate example prescriptions for each follow. These include management of mild pain with aspirin products, acetaminophen, and some of the nonsteroidal noninflammatory agents. Management of moderate pain includes codeine, Vicodin®, Vicodin ES®, Lorcet® 10/650; and Motrin® in the 800 mg dosage. Severe pain may require treatment with Percodan®, Percocet®, or Demerol®. All prescription pain preparations should be closely monitored for efficacy and discontinued if the pain persists or requires a higher level formulation.

The chronic pain patient represents a particular challenge for the practitioner. Some additional drugs that may be useful in managing the patient with chronic pain of neuropathic origin are covered in the temporomandibular dysfunction section *on page 1562.* It is always incumbent on the practitioner to reevaluate the diagnosis, source of pain, and treatment, whenever prolonged use of analgesics (narcotic or non-narcotic) is contemplated. Drugs such as Dilaudid® are not recommended for management of dental pain in most states.

Narcotic analgesics can be used on a short-term basis or intermittently in combination with non-narcotic therapy in the chronic pain patient. Judicious prescribing, monitoring, and maintenance by the practitioner is imperative, particularly whenever considering the use of a narcotic analgesic due to the abuse and addiction liabilities.

ORAL PAIN *(Continued)*

MILD PAIN

Acetaminophen *on page 27*

Aspirin (various products) *on page 131*

Diflunisal *on page 438*

Ibuprofen *on page 703*

Ketoprofen *on page 763*

Naproxen *on page 953*

OVER-THE-COUNTER PRESCRIPTION EXAMPLES

Rx

Aspirin 325 mg

Disp: To be determined by practitioner

Sig: Take 2-3 tablets every 4 hours

Rx

Ibuprofen 200 mg

Disp: To be determined by practitioner

Sig: Take 2-3 tablets every 4 hours, not to exceed 16 tablets in 24 hours

Note: Ibuprofen is available over-the-counter as Motrin IB®, Advil®, Nuprin®, and many other brands in 200 mg tablets.

Note: NSAIDs should **never** be taken together, nor should they be combined with aspirin. NSAIDs have anti-inflammatory effects as well as analgesics. An allergy to aspirin constitutes a contradiction to all the new NSAIDs. Aspirin and the NSAIDs may increase post-treatment bleeding.

Note: Use with caution in patients with CHF, hypertension, decreased renal or hepatic function, history of GI disease, or those receiving anticoagulants; withhold for at least 4-6 half-lives prior to surgical or dental procedures

Rx

Acetaminophen 325 mg

Disp: To be determined by practitioner

Sig: Take 2-3 tablets every 4 hours

Note: Products include: Tylenol® and many others.

Note: Acetaminophen can be given if patient has allergy, bleeding problems, or stomach upset secondary to aspirin or NSAIDs.

Rx

Aleve® 220 mg

Disp: To be determined by practitioner

Sig: 1-2 tablets every 8 hours

Ingredient: Naproxen sodium

Rx

Orudis KT® 12.5 mg

Disp: To be determined by practitioner

Sig: 1-2 tablets every 8 hours

Ingredient: Ketoprofen

PRESCRIPTION ONLY EXAMPLES

Rx

Ketoprofen 25 mg

Disp: To be determined by practitioner

Sig: 1-2 tablets every 8 hours

Rx

Dolobid® 500 mg

Disp: 16 tablets

Sig: Take 2 tablets initially, then 1 tablet every 8-12 hours as needed for pain

Ingredient: Diflunisal

MODERATE/MODERATELY SEVERE PAIN

Aspirin and Codeine *on page 134*

Dihydrocodeine Compound *on page 444*

Hydrocodone and Acetaminophen *on page 678*

Hydrocodone and Ibuprofen *on page 684*

Acetaminophen and Tramadol *on page 32*

Ibuprofen (various products) *on page 703*

A new class of NSAIDs has been approved and indicated in the treatment of arthritis, COX-2 inhibitors (celecoxib, Celebrex®; rofecoxib, Vioxx®). Rofecoxib (Vioxx®) is indicated for use in short-term oral pain management. Celecoxib (Celebrex®) has recently been approved for use in oral pain management. Valdecoxib (Bextra®) is a COX-2 inhibitor also recently indicated for acute pain but its use in dental management is still under evaluation.

The following is a guideline to use when prescribing codeine with either aspirin or acetaminophen (Tylenol®):

Codeine No. 2 = codeine 15 mg

Codeine No. 3 = codeine 30 mg

Codeine No. 4 = codeine 60 mg

Example: ASA No. 3 = aspirin 325 mg + codeine 30 mg

PRESCRIPTION EXAMPLES

Not Controlled:

Rx

Motrin® 800 mg*
Disp: 16 tablets
Sig: Take 1 tablet 3 times/day as needed for pain

Ingredient: Ibuprofen

Note: May be taken up to 4 times/day for more severe pain.

***Note:** Also available as 600 mg

Rx

Ultracet™
Disp: 36 tablets
Sig: Take 2 tablets every 4-6 hours as needed for pain, not to exceed 8 tablets in 24 hours

Ingredients: Acetaminophen 325 mg and tramadol 37.5 mg

ORAL PAIN *(Continued)*

Controlled:

Rx	
	Tylenol® No. 3*
	Disp: 16 tablets
	Sig: Take 1 tablet every 4 hours as needed for pain

Ingredients: Acetaminophen and codeine

***Note:** Also available as #2 and #4

Rx	
	Synalgos® DC
	Disp: 16 capsules
	Sig: Take 1 capsule every 4 hours as needed for pain

Ingredients: Dihydrocodeine 16 mg, aspirin 356.4 mg, and caffeine 30 mg

Rx	
	Vicodin®
	Disp: 16 tablets
	Sig: Take 1 tablet every 4 hours as needed for pain

Ingredients: Hydrocodone 5 mg and acetaminophen 500 mg

Note: Available as Vicodin ES®; take 1 tablet every 8-12 hours

Rx	
	Lortab® 5 mg
	Disp: 16 tablets
	Sig: Take 1 or 2 tablets every 4 hours as needed for pain, not to exceed 8 tablets in 24 hours

Ingredients: Hydrocodone 5 mg and acetaminophen 500 mg

Rx	
	Darvocet–N 100®
	Disp: 36 tablets
	Sig: Take 1 tablet every 4 hours as needed for pain, not to exceed 6 tablets in 24 hours

Ingredients: Propoxyphene 100 mg and acetaminophen 650 mg

Rx		
	Vicoprofen®	
	Disp: 16 tablets	
	Sig: Take 1-2 tablets every 4-6 hours as needed for pain	No Refills

Ingredients: Hydrocodone 7.5 mg and ibuprofen 200 mg

HYDROCODONE PRODUCTS

Available hydrocodone oral products are listed in the following table and are scheduled as C-III controlled substances, indicating that prescriptions may either be oral or written. Thus, the prescriber may call–in a prescription to the pharmacy for any of these hydrocodone products. All the formulations are combined with acetaminophen except for Vicoprofen®, which contains ibuprofen, and Lortab® ASA and Damason–P®, which all contain aspirin. Most of these brand name drugs are available generically and the pharmacist will dispense the generic equivalent if available, unless the prescriber indicates otherwise.

HYDROCODONE ANALGESIC COMBINATION ORAL PRODUCTS (All Products DEA Schedule C-III)

Hydrocodone is available under numerous brand names with varying dosages and in combination with aspirin or ibuprofen.					
Hydrocodone Bitartrate	**Acetaminophen (APAP*)**	**Other**	**Brand Name**	**Generic Available**	**Form**
2.5 mg	500 mg	–	Lortab® 2.5/500	Yes	Tablet
5 mg	400 mg	–	Zydone®	No	Tablet
5 mg	500 mg	–	Vicodin®; Dolagesic®; Hy-Phen®; Hydrocet®; Anexsia® 5/500; Lortab®5/500	Yes	Tablet
5 mg	500 mg	–	Polygesic®; Lorcet-HD®	Yes	Capsule
7.5 mg	400 mg	–	Zydone®	No	Tablet
7.5 mg	500 mg	–	Lortab® 7.5/500	Yes	Tablet
7.5 mg	650 mg	–	Anexsia® 7.5/650; Lorcet Plus®	Yes	Tablet
7.5 mg	750 mg	–	Vicodin ES®	Yes	Tablet
10 mg	400 mg	–	Zydone®	No	Tablet
10 mg	325 mg	–	Norco®	No	Tablet
10 mg	500 mg	–	Lortab® 10/500	Yes	Tablet
10 mg	650 mg	–	Lorcet®	Yes	Tablet
10 mg	660 mg	–	Vicodin HP®; Anexsia® 10/660	Yes	Tablet
10 mg	750 mg		Maxidone™	No	Tablet
7.5 mg/15 mL	500 mg/15 mL	–	Lortab® Elixir	Yes	Elixir
5 mg	–	Aspirin 500 mg	Lortab® ASA; Damason–P®	Yes	Tablet
7.5 mg	–	Ibuprofen 200 mg	Vicoprofen®	No	Tablet

*APAP is the common acronym for acetaminophen and is the abbreviation of the chemical name N-acetylparaminophenol.

The following are the usual adult doses of the hydrocodone oral products as listed by the most recent edition of the Drug Information for the Health Care Professional (USPDI).

1 or 2 tablets containing 2.5 mg of hydrocodone and 500 mg of acetaminophen every 4-6 hours; or

1 tablet containing 5 mg of hydrocodone and 500 mg acetaminophen every 4-6 hours as needed, with dosage being increased to 2 tablets every 6 hours, if necessary; or

1 capsule containing 5 mg of hydrocodone and 500 mg of acetaminophen every 4-6 hours as needed, with dosage being increased to 2 capsules every 6 hours if necessary; or

1 tablet containing 7.5 mg hydrocodone and 650 mg of acetaminophen every 4-6 hours as needed, with dosage being increased to 2 tablets every 6 hours if necessary; or

1 tablet containing 7.5 mg hydrocodone and 750 mg of acetaminophen every 4-6 hours as needed; or

1 tablet containing 10 mg of hydrocodone and 650 mg acetaminophen every 4-6 hours as needed.

For the elixir (Lortab®), the recommended dose is 1 tablespoonful every 4-6 hours when necessary for pain.

For the aspirin products (Lortab® ASA and Damason-P®), the recommended dose is 1 or 2 tablets every 4-6 hours as needed.

For the ibuprofen product (Vicoprofen®), the recommended dose is 1 or 2 tablets every 4-6 hours as needed. The manufacturer recommends that the maximum dose of Vicoprofen® should not exceed 5 tablets in 24 hours.

The usual adult prescribing limits for the combination hydrocodone-acetaminophen products is up to 40 mg of hydrocodone and up to 4000 mg (4 g) of acetaminophen in a 24-hour period.

ORAL PAIN *(Continued)*

SEVERE PAIN

Meperidine *on page 858*

Oxycodone *on page 1017*

Oxycodone and Acetaminophen *on page 1018*

Oxycodone and Aspirin *on page 1020*

Oxycodone is available in a variety of dosages and combinations under numerous brand names. A new combination of Oxycodone hydrochloride with ibuprofen has been used in Phase III clinical trials at Forest Laboratories and is currently awaiting approval.

PRESCRIPTION EXAMPLES

Rx

Demerol® 50 mg*

Disp: 16 tablets

Sig: Take 1 tablet every 4 hours as needed for pain — No Refills

Ingredient: Meperidine

***Note:** Triplicate prescription required in some states.

Rx

Roxicodone™ 5 mg*

Disp: 24 tablets

Sig: Take 1 tablet every 6 hours as needed for pain — No Refills

Ingredient: Oxycodone

***Note:** Some formulations available as controlled release.

Rx

Percodan®*

Disp: 16 tablets

Sig: Take 1 tablet every 4 hours as needed for pain — No Refills

Ingredients: Oxycodone 4.88 mg and aspirin 325 mg

***Note:** Triplicate prescription required in some states.

Note: See monograph *on page 1020* for contraindications and precautions for aspirin or narcotic medications.

Rx

Percocet® tablets or Tylox® capsules*

Disp: 16 tablets or capsules

Sig: Take 1 tablet every 4 hours as needed for pain — No Refills

Ingredients: Oxycodone 5 mg and acetaminophen 325 mg (Tylox® contains acetaminophen 500 mg)

***Note:** Triplicate prescription required in some states.

ORAL BACTERIAL INFECTIONS

Dental infection can occur for any number of reasons, primarily involving pulpal and periodontal infections. Secondary infections of the soft tissues as well as sinus infections pose special treatment challenges. The drugs of choice in treating most oral infections have been selected because of their efficacy in providing adequate blood levels for delivery to the oral tissues and their proven usefulness in managing dental infections. Penicillin remains the primary drug for treatment of dental infections of pulpal origin. The management of soft tissue infections may require the use of additional drugs.

OROFACIAL INFECTIONS

The basis of all infections is the successful multiplication of a microbial pathogen on or within a host. The pathogen is usually defined as any microorganism that has the capacity to cause disease. If the pathogen is bacterial in nature, antibiotic therapy is often indicated.

DIFFERENTIAL DIAGNOSIS OF ODONTOGENIC INFECTIONS

In choosing the appropriate antibiotic for therapy of a given infection, a number of important factors must be considered. First, the identity of the organism must be known. In odontogenic infections involving dental or periodontal structures, this is seldom the case. Secondly, accurate information regarding antibiotic susceptibility is required. Again, unless the organism has been identified, this is not possible. And thirdly, host factors must be taken into account, in terms of ability to absorb an antibiotic, to achieve appropriate host response. When clinical evidence of cellulitis or odontogenic infection has been found and the cardinal signs of swelling, inflammation, pain, and perhaps fever are present, the selection by the clinician of the appropriate antibiotic agent may lead to eradication.

CAUSES OF ODONTOGENIC INFECTIONS

Most acute orofacial infections are of odontogenic origin. Dental caries, resulting in infection of dental pulp, is the leading cause of odontogenic infection.

The major causative organisms involved in dental caries have been identified as members of the viridans (alpha-hemolytic) streptococci and include *Streptococcus mutans, Streptococcus sobrinus,* and *Streptococcus milleri.* Once the bacteria have breached the enamel they invade the dentin and eventually the dental pulp. An inflammatory reaction occurs in the pulp tissue resulting in necrosis and a lower tissue oxidation-reduction potential. At this point, the bacterial flora changes from predominantly aerobic to a more obligate anaerobic flora. The anaerobic gram-positive cocci *(Peptostreptococcus* species), and the anaerobic gram-negative rods, including *Bacteroides, Prevotella, Porphyromonas,* and *Fusobacterium* are most frequently present. An abscess usually forms at the apex of the involved tooth resulting in destruction of bone. Depending on the effectiveness of the host resistance and the virulence of the bacteria, the infection may spread through the marrow spaces, perforate the cortical plate, and enter the surrounding soft tissues.

The other major source of odontogenic infection arises from the anaerobic bacterial flora that inhabits the periodontal and supporting structures of the teeth. The most important potential pathogenic anaerobes within these structures are *Actinobacillus actinomycetemcomitans, Prevotella intermedius, Porphyromonas gingivalis, Fusobacterium nucleatum,* and *Eikenella corrodens.*

Most odontogenic infections (70%) have mixed aerobic and anaerobic flora. Pure aerobic infections are much less common and comprise ~5% incidence. Pure anaerobic infections make up the remaining 25% of odontogenic infections. Clinical correlates suggest that early odontogenic infections are characterized by rapid spreading and cellulitis with the absence of abscess formation. The bacteria are predominantly aerobic with gram-positive, alpha-hemolytic streptococci *(S. viridans)* the predominant pathogen. As the infection matures and becomes more severe, the microbial flora becomes a mix of aerobes and anaerobes. The anaerobes present are determined by the characteristic flora associated with the site of origin, whether it be pulpal or periodontal. Finally, as the infectious process becomes controlled by host defenses, the flora becomes primarily anaerobic. For example, Lewis and MacFarlane found a predominance of facultative oral streptococci in the early infections (<3 days of symptoms) with the later predominance of obligate anaerobes.

In a review of severe odontogenic infections, it was reported that Brook, et al, observed that 50% of odontogenic deep facial space infections yielded anaerobic bacteria only. Also, 44% of these infections yielded a mix of aerobic and anaerobic flora. The results of a study published in 1998 by Sakamoto, et al, were also described in the review. The study confirmed that odontogenic infections usually result from a synergistic interaction among several bacterial species and usually consist of an oral streptococcus and an oral anaerobic gram-negative rod. Sakamoto and his group reported a high level of the *Streptococcus milleri* group of aerobic gram-positive cocci, and high levels of oral

ORAL BACTERIAL INFECTIONS *(Continued)*

anaerobes, including the *Peptostreptococcus* species and the *Prevotella, Porphyromonas,* and *Fusobacterium* species.

Oral streptococci, especially of the *Streptococcus milleri* group, can invade soft tissues initially, thus preparing an environment conducive to growth of anaerobic bacteria. Obligate oral anaerobes are dependent on nutrients synthesized by the aerobes. Thus the anaerobes appear approximately 3 days after onset of symptoms. Early infections are thus caused primarily by the aerobic streptococci (exquisitely sensitive to penicillin) and late infections are caused by the anaerobes (frequently resistant to penicillin).

It appears logical, as Flynn has noted, to separate infections presenting early in their course from those presenting later when selecting empiric antibiotics of choice for odontogenic infections.

If the patient is not allergic to penicillin, penicillin VK still remains the empiric antibiotic of first choice to treat mild or early odontogenic infections (see Table 1). In penicillin allergy, clindamycin clearly remains the alternative antibiotic for treatment of mild or early infections. Secondary alternative antibiotics still recognized as useful in these conditions are cephalexin (Keflex®), or other first generation cephalosporins available in oral dose forms. The first generation cephalosporins can be used in both penicillin-allergic and nonallergic patients, providing that the penicillin allergy is not the anaphylactoid type.

PENICILLIN VK

The spectrum of antibacterial action of penicillin VK is consistent with most of the organisms identified in odontogenic infections (see Table 2). Penicillin VK is a beta-lactam antibiotic, as are all the penicillins and cephalosporins, and is bactericidal against gram-positive cocci and the major pathogens of mixed anaerobic infections. It elicits virtually no adverse effects in the absence of allergy and is relatively low in cost. Adverse drug reactions occurring in >10% of patients include mild diarrhea, nausea, and oral candidiasis. To treat odontogenic infections and other orofacial infections, the usual dose for adults and children >12 years of age is 500 mg every 6 hours for at least 7 days (see Table 4). The daily dose for children ≤12 years of age is 25-50 mg/kg of body weight in divided doses every 6-8 hours (see Table 4). The patient must be instructed to take the penicillin continuously for the duration of therapy.

After oral dosing, penicillin VK achieves peak serum levels within 1 hour. Penicillin VK may be given with meals, however, blood concentrations may be slightly higher when penicillin is given on an empty stomach. The preferred dosing is 1 hour before meals or 2 hours after meals to ensure maximum serum levels. Penicillin VK diffuses into most body tissues, including oral tissues, soon after dosing. Hepatic metabolism accounts for <30% of the elimination of penicillins. Elimination is primarily renal. The nonmetabolized penicillin is excreted largely unchanged in the urine by glomerular filtration and active tubular secretion. Penicillins cross the placenta and are distributed in breast milk. Penicillin VK, like all beta-lactam antibiotics, causes death of bacteria by inhibiting synthesis of the bacterial cell wall during cell division. This action is dependent on the ability of penicillins to reach and bind to penicillin-binding proteins (PBPs) located on the inner membrane of the bacterial cell wall. PBPs (which include transpeptidases, carboxypeptidases, and endopeptidases) are enzymes that are involved in the terminal stages of assembling and reshaping the bacterial cell wall during growth. Penicillins and beta-lactams bind to and inactivate PBPs resulting in lysis of the cell due to weakening of the cell wall.

Penicillin VK is considered a "narrow spectrum" antibiotic. This class of antibiotics produces less alteration of normal microflora thereby reducing the incidence of superinfection. Also, its bactericidal action will reduce the numbers of microorganisms resulting in less reliance on host-phagocyte mechanisms for eradication of the pathogen.

Among patients, 0.7% to 10% are allergic to penicillins. There is no evidence that any single penicillin derivative differs from others in terms of incidence or severity when administered orally. About 85% of allergic reactions associated with penicillin VK are delayed and take >2 days to develop. This allergic response manifests as skin rashes characterized as erythema and bullous eruptions. This type of allergic reaction is mild, reversible, and usually responds to concurrent antihistamine therapy, such as diphenhydramine (Benadryl®). Severe reactions of angioedema have occurred, characterized by marked swelling of the lips, tongue, face, and periorbital tissues. Patients with a history of penicillin allergy must never be given penicillin VK for treatment of infections. The alternative antibiotic is clindamycin. If the allergy is the delayed type and not the anaphylactoid type, a first generation cephalosporin may be used as an alternate antibiotic.

CLINDAMYCIN

In the event of penicillin allergy, clindamycin is clearly an alternative of choice in treating mild or early odontogenic infections (see Table 1). It is highly effective against almost all oral pathogens. Clindamycin is active against most aerobic gram-positive cocci, including staphylococci, *S. pneumoniae*, other streptococci, and anaerobic gram-negative and gram-positive organisms, including bacteroides (see Table 3). Clindamycin is not effective against mycoplasma or gram-negative aerobes. It inhibits protein synthesis in bacteria through binding to the 50 S subunit of bacterial ribosomes. Clindamycin has bacteriostatic actions at low concentrations, but is known to elicit bactericidal effects against susceptible bacteria at higher concentrations of drug at the site of infection.

The usual adult oral dose of clindamycin to treat orofacial infections of odontogenic origin is 150-450 mg every 6 hours for 7-10 days. The usual daily oral dose for children is 8-25 mg/kg in 3-4 equally divided doses (see Table 4).

Following oral administration of a 150 mg or a 300 mg dose on an empty stomach, 90% of the dose is rapidly absorbed into the bloodstream and peak serum concentrations are attained in 45-60 minutes. Administration with food does not markedly impair absorption into the bloodstream. Clindamycin serum levels exceed the minimum inhibitory concentration for bacterial growth for at least 6 hours after the recommended doses. The serum half-life is 2-3 hours. Clindamycin is distributed effectively to most body tissues, including saliva and bone. Its small molecular weight enables it to more readily enter bacterial cytoplasm and to penetrate bone. It is partially metabolized in the liver to active and inactive metabolites and is excreted in the urine, bile, and feces.

Adverse effects caused by clindamycin can include abdominal pain, nausea, vomiting, and diarrhea. Hypersensitivity reactions are rare, but have resulted in skin rash. Approximately 1% of clindamycin users develop pseudomembranous colitis characterized by severe diarrhea, abdominal cramps, and excretion of blood or mucus in the stools. The mechanism is disruption of normal bacterial flora of the colon, which leads to colonization of the bacterium *Clostridium difficile*. This bacterium releases endotoxins that cause mucosal damage and inflammation. Symptoms usually develop 2-9 days after initiation of therapy, but may not occur until several weeks after taking the drug. If significant diarrhea develops, clindamycin therapy should be discontinued immediately. Theoretically, any antibiotic can cause antibiotic-associated colitis and clindamycin probably has an undeserved reputation associated with this condition.

Sandor, et al, also notes that odontogenic infections are typically polymicrobial and that anaerobes outnumber aerobes by at least four-fold. The penicillins have historically been used as the first-line therapy in these cases, but increasing rates of resistance have lowered their usefulness. Bacterial resistance to penicillins is predominantly achieved through production of beta-lactamases. Clindamycin, because of its relatively broad spectrum of activity and resistance to beta-lactamase degradation, is an attractive first-line therapy in treatment of odontogenic infections.

FIRST GENERATION CEPHALOSPORINS

Antibiotics of this class, which are available in oral dosage forms, include cefadroxil (Duricef®), cephalexin (Keflex®), and cephradine (Velosef®). The first generation cephalosporins are alternates to penicillin VK in the treatment of odontogenic infections based on bactericidal effectiveness against the oral streptococci. These drugs are most active against gram-positive cocci, but are not very active against many anaerobes. First generation cephalosporins are indicated as alternatives in early infections because they are effective in killing the aerobes. First generation cephalosporins are active against gram-positive staphylococci and streptococci, but not enterococci. They are active against many gram-negative aerobic bacilli, including *E. coli, Klebsiella,* and *Proteus mirabilis.* They are inactive against methicillin-resistant *S. aureus* and penicillin-resistant *S. pneumoniae.* The gram-negative aerobic cocci, *Moraxella catarrhalis,* portrays variable sensitivity to first generation cephalosporins.

Cephalexin (Keflex®) is the first generation cephalosporin often used to treat odontogenic infections. The usual adult dose is 250-1000 mg every 6 hours with a maximum of 4 g/day. Children's dose is 25-50 mg/kg/day in divided doses every 6 hours; for severe infections: 50-100 mg/kg/day in divided doses every 6 hours with a maximum dose of 3 g/day (see Table 4).

Cephalexin (Keflex®) causes diarrhea in about 1% to 10% of patients. About 90% of the cephalexin is excreted unchanged in urine.

SECOND GENERATION CEPHALOSPORINS

The second generation cephalosporins such as cefaclor (Ceclor®) have better activity against some of the anaerobes including some *Bacteroides, Peptococcus,* and *Peptostreptococcus* species. Cefaclor (Ceclor®) and cefuroxime (Ceftin®) have been used to treat early stage infections. These antibiotics have the advantage of twice-a-day dosing. The usual oral adult dose of cefaclor is 250-500 mg every 8 hours (or daily dose can be given in 2 divided doses) for at least 7 days. Children's dose is 20-40 mg/kg/day divided every 8-12 hours with a maximum dose of 2 g/day. The usual adult oral dose of cefuroxime is 250-500 mg twice daily. Children's dose is 20 mg/kg/day (maximum 500 mg/day) in 2 divided doses.

The cephalosporins inhibit bacterial cell wall synthesis by binding to one or more of the penicillin-binding proteins (PBPs), which in turn inhibits the final transpeptidation step of peptidoglycan synthesis in bacterial cell walls, thus inhibiting cell wall biosynthesis. Bacteria eventually lyse due to ongoing activity of cell wall autolytic enzymes while cell wall assembly is arrested.

ORAL BACTERIAL INFECTIONS *(Continued)*

BACTERIAL RESISTANCE TO ANTIBIOTICS

If a patient with an early stage odontogenic infection does not respond to penicillin VK within 24-36 hours, it is evidence of the presence of resistant bacteria. Bacterial resistance to the penicillins is predominantly achieved through the production of beta-lactamase. A switch to beta-lactamase-stable antibiotics should be made. For example, Kuriyama, et al, reported that past beta-lactam administration increases the emergence of beta-lactamase-producing bacteria and that beta-lactamase-stable antibiotics should be prescribed to patients with unresolved infections who have received beta-lactams. These include either clindamycin or amoxicillin/clavulanic acid (Augmentin®). Doses are listed in Table 4.

In the past, all *S. viridans* species were uniformly susceptible to beta-lactam antibiotics. However, over the years, there has been a significant increase in resistant strains. Resistance may also be due to alteration of penicillin-binding proteins. Consequently, drugs which combine a beta-lactam antibiotic with a beta-lactamase inhibitor, such as amoxicillin/clavulanic acid (Augmentin®), may no longer be more effective than the penicillin VK alone. In these situations, clindamycin is the recommended alternate antibiotic.

Evidence suggests that empirical use of penicillin VK as the first-line drug in treating early odontogenic infections is still the best way to ensure the minimal production of resistant bacteria to other classes of antibiotics, since any overuse of clindamycin or amoxicillin/clavulanic acid (Augmentin®) is minimized in these situations. There is concern that overuse of clindamycin could contribute to development of clindamycin-resistant pathogens.

In late odontogenic infections, it is suggested that clindamycin be considered the first-line antibiotic to treat these infections. The dose of clindamycin would be the same as that used to treat early infections (see Table 4). In these infections, anaerobic bacteria usually predominate. Since penicillin spectrum includes anaerobes, penicillin VK is also useful as an empiric drug of first choice in these infections. It has been reported, however, that the penicillin resistance rate among patients with serious and late infections is in the 35% to 50% range. Therefore, if penicillin is the drug of first choice and the patient does not respond within 24-36 hours, a resistant pathogen should be suspected and a switch to clindamycin be made. Clindamycin, because of its relatively broad spectrum of activity and resistance to beta-lactamase degradation, is an attractive first-line therapy in the treatment of these infections. Another alternative is to add a second drug to the penicillin (eg, metronidazole [Flagyl®]). Consequently, for those infections not responding to treatment with penicillin, the addition of a second drug (eg, metronidazole), not a beta-lactam or macrolide, is likely to be more effective. Bacterial resistance to metronidazole is very rare. The metronidazole dose is listed in Table 4.

Nonionized metronidazole is readily taken up by anaerobic organisms. Its selectivity for anaerobic bacteria is a result of the ability of these organisms to reduce metronidazole to its active form within the bacterial cell. The electron transport proteins necessary for this reaction are found only in anaerobic bacteria. Reduced metronidazole then disrupts DNA's helical structure, thereby inhibiting bacterial nucleic acid synthesis leading to death of the organism. Consequently, metronidazole is not effective against gram-positive aerobic cocci and most *Actinomyces, Lactobacillus,* and *Proprionibacterium* species. Since most odontogenic infections are mixed aerobic and anaerobic, metronidazole should rarely be used as a single agent. Alternatively, one can switch to a beta-lactamase resistant drug (eg, amoxicillin/clavulanic acid [Augmentin®]). The beta-lactamase resistant penicillins including methicillin, oxacillin, cloxacillin, dicloxacillin, and nafcillin, are only effective against gram-positive cocci and have no activity against anaerobes, hence, should not be used to treat the late stage odontogenic infections.

RESISTANCE IN ODONTOGENIC INFECTIONS

Recently, there has been an alarming increase in the incidence of resistant bacterial isolates in odontogenic infections. Many anaerobic bacteria have developed resistance to beta-lactam antibiotics via production of beta-lactamase enzymes. These include several species of *Prevotella, Porphyromonas, Fusobacterium nucleatum,* and *Campylobacter gracilus. Fusobacterium,* especially in combination with *S. viridans* species, has been associated with severe odontogenic infections. Often, they are resistant to macrolides. Clindamycin is the empiric drug of first choice in these patients.

SEVERE INFECTIONS

In patients hospitalized for severe odontogenic infections, I.V. antibiotics are indicated and clindamycin is the clear empiric antibiotic of choice. Alternative antibiotics include an I.V. combination of penicillin and metronidazole or I.V. ampicillin-sulbactam (Unasyn®). Clindamycin, I.V. cephalosporins (if penicillin allergy is not the anaphylactoid type), and ciprofloxacin have been used in patients allergic to penicillins. Flynn notes that *Eikenella corrodens*, an occasional oral pathogen, is resistant to clindamycin. Ciprofloxacin is an excellent antibiotic for this organism.

ERYTHROMYCIN, CLARITHROMYCIN, AND AZITHROMYCIN

In the past, erythromycins were considered highly effective antibiotics for treating odontogenic infections, especially in penicillin allergy. At the present time, however, the current high resistance rates of both oral streptococci and oral anaerobes have rendered the entire macrolide family of antibiotics obsolete for odontogenic infections. Montgomery has noted that resistance develops rapidly to macrolides and there may be cross-resistance between erythromycin and newer macrolides, particularly among streptococci and staphylococci. Hardee has stated that erythromycin is no longer very useful because of resistant pathogens. The antibacterial spectrum of the erythromycin family is similar to penicillin VK. Erythromycins are effective against streptococcus, staphylococcus, and gram-negative aerobes, such as *H. influenzae, M. catarrhalis, N. gonorrhoeae, Bordetella pertussis,* and *Legionella pneumophilia.* Erythromycins are considered narrow spectrum antibiotics.

Both azithromycin and clarithromycin have been used to treat acute odontogenic infections. This is because of the following spectrum of actions: Clarithromycin shows good activity against many gram-positive and gram-negative aerobic and anaerobic organisms. It is active against methicillin-sensitive *S. aureus* and most streptococcus species. *S. aureus* strains resistant to erythromycin are resistant to clarithromycin. Clarithromycin is active against *H. influenzae.* It is similar to erythromycin in effectiveness against anaerobic gram-positive cocci and *Bacteroides sp.* Clarithromycin has been suggested as an alternative antibiotic if the prescriber wants to give an antibiotic from the macrolide family (see Table 3). The recommended oral adult dose is 500 mg twice daily for 7 days.

Azithromycin is active against staphylococci, including *S. aureus* and *S. epidermidis*, as well as streptococci, such as *S. pyogenes* and *S. pneumoniae.* Erythromycin-resistant strains of staphylococcus, enterococcus, and streptococcus, including methicillin-resistant *S. aureus*, are also resistant to azithromycin. It has excellent activity against *H. influenzae.* Inhibition of anaerobes, such as *Clostridium perfringens*, is better with azithromycin than with erythromycin. Inhibition of *Bacteroides fragilis* and other bacteroides species by azithromycin is comparable to erythromycin. Both azithromycin and clarithromycin are presently recommended as alternatives in the prophylactic regimen for prevention of bacterial endocarditis.

AMOXICILLIN

Some clinicians select amoxicillin over penicillin VK as the penicillin of choice to empirically treat odontogenic infections. Except for coverage of *Haemophilus influenzae* in acute sinus and otitis media infections, amoxicillin does not offer any advantage over penicillin VK for treatment of odontogenic infections. It is less effective than penicillin VK for aerobic gram-positive cocci, and similar to penicillin for coverage of anaerobes. Although it does provide coverage against gram-negative enteric bacteria, this is not needed to treat odontogenic infections, except in immunosuppressed patients where these organisms may be present. If one adheres to the principle of using the most effective narrow spectrum antibiotic, amoxicillin should not be favored over penicillin VK.

Note: The ADA Council on Scientific Affairs recently published a review on the subject of antibiotic interaction with oral contraceptives in which a clear statement of the dental professional's responsibility was made. In essence, it was concluded that in any situation where a dentist is planning to prescribe a course of antibiotics, alternative/additional means of contraception should be recommended to the oral contraceptive users. Specifically, patients should be told about the potential for antibiotics to lower the usefulness of oral contraceptives and advised to consult their physician about nonhormonal contraceptive techniques while continuing their oral contraceptive regimen. Even though there is minimal scientific data supporting this position, the risk of possible unwanted pregnancies warrants this simple approach for professionals licensed to prescribe antibiotics (*JADA*, 2002, 133:880).

The following tables have been adapted from Wynn RL, Bergman SA, Meiller TF, et al. "Antibiotics in Treating Orofacial Infections of Odontogenic Origin," *Gen Dent*, 2001, 47(3): 238-52.

Amoxicillin and Clavulanate Potassium *on page 95*
Amoxicillin Trihydrate *on page 93*
Cephalexin *on page 285*
Ceftibuten *on page 276*
Cefditoren *on page 265*
Chlorpheniramine *on page 307*
Chlorhexidine *on page 300*
Clarithromycin *on page 337*
Clindamycin *on page 341*
Dicloxacillin *on page 432*
Erythromycin *on page 512*
Gatifloxacin *on page 628*
Loratadine and Pseudoephedrine *on page 823*
Metronidazole *on page 902*
Mouthwash, Antiseptic *on page 934*
Moxifloxacin *on page 935*

ORAL BACTERIAL INFECTIONS *(Continued)*

Oxymetazoline *on page 1022*
Penicillin V Potassium *on page 1051*
Pseudoephedrine *on page 1146*
Tetracycline *on page 1286*

Table 1.
EMPIRIC ANTIBIOTICS OF CHOICE FOR ODONTOGENIC INFECTIONS

Type of Infection	Antibiotic of Choice
Early (first 3 days of symptoms)	Penicillin VK
	Clindamycin
	Cephalexin (or other first generation cephalosporin)*
No improvement in 24-36 hours	Beta-lactamase-stable antibiotic: Clindamycin or amoxicillin / clavulanic acid
Penicillin allergy	Clindamycin
	Cephalexin (if penicillin allergy is not anaphylactoid type)
	Clarithromycin (Biaxin®)†
Late (>3 days)	Clindamycin
	Penicillin VK-metronidazole
Penicillin allergy	Clindamycin

*For better patient compliance, second generation cephalosporins (cefaclor; cefuroxime) at twice daily dosing have been used; see text.

†A macrolide useful in patients allergic to penicillin, given as twice daily dosing for better patient compliance; see text.

Table 2.
PENICILLIN VK: ANTIBACTERIAL SPECTRUM

Gram-positive cocci	**Oral anaerobes**
Streptococci	*Bacteroides*
Nonresistant staphylococci*	*Porphyromonas*
Pneumococci	*Prevotella*
	Peptococci
Gram-negative cocci	Peptostreptococci
Neisseria meningitides	*Actinomyces*
Neisseria gonorrhoeae	*Veillonella*
	Eubacterium
Gram-positive rods	*Eikenella*
Bacillus	*Capnocytophaga*
Corynebacterium	*Campylobacter*
Clostridium	*Fusobacterium*
	Others

*Nonresistant staphylococcus represents a small portion of community-acquired strains of *S. aureus* (5% to 15%). Most strains of *S. aureus* and *S. epidermidis* produce beta-lactamases, which destroy penicillins.

Table 3.
CLINDAMYCIN: ANTIBACTERIAL SPECTRUM*

Gram-Positive Cocci	Anaerobes†
Streptococci‡	Gram-negative bacilli
S. aureus¶	*Bacteroides* species including *B. fragilis*
Penicillinase and nonpenicillinase-producing staphylococcus	*B. melaninogenicus*
	Fusobacterium species
S. epidermidis	Gram-positive nonsporeforming bacilli
Pneumococci	*Propionibacterium*
	Eubacterium
	Actinomyces species
	Gram-positive cocci
	Peptococcus
	Peptostreptococcus
	Microaerophilic streptococci

**In vitro* activity against isolates; information from manufacturer's package insert

†*Clostridia* are more resistant than most anaerobes to clindamycin. Most *Clostridium perfringens* are susceptible but *C. sporogens* and *C. tertium* are frequently resistant.

‡Except *S. faecalis*

¶Some staph strains originally resistant to erythromycin rapidly develop resistance to clindamycin.

Table 4.
ORAL DOSE RANGES OF ANTIBIOTICS USEFUL IN TREATING ODONTOGENIC INFECTIONS*

Clinicians must select specific dose and regimen from ranges available to be prescribed based on clinical judgment		
Antibiotic	**Dosage**	
	Children	**Adults**
Penicillin VK	≤12 years: 25-50 mg/kg body weight in equally divided doses q6-8h for at least 7 days; maximum dose: 3 g/day	>12 years: 500 mg q6h for at least 7 days
Clindamycin	8-25 mg/kg in 3-4 equally divided doses	150-450 mg q6h for at least 7 days; maximum dose: 1.8 g/day
Cephalexin (Keflex®)	25-50 mg/kg/d in divided doses q6h severe infection: 50-100 mg/kg/d in divided doses q6h; maximum dose: 3 g/24 h	250-1000 mg q6h; maximum dose: 4 g/day
Amoxicillin/ clavulanic acid (Augmentin®)	<40 kg: 20-40 mg (amoxicillin)/kg/d in divided doses q8h >40 kg: 250-500 mg q8h or 875 mg q12h for at least 7 days; maximum dose 2 g/day	>40 kg: 250-500 mg q8h or 875 mg q12h for at least 7 days; maximum dose: 2 g/day
Metronidazole (Flagyl®)		500 mg q6-8h for 7-10 days; maximum dose: 4 g/day

*For doses of other antibiotics, see monographs

PRESCRIPTION EXAMPLES FOR ODONTOGENIC INFECTIONS

Penicillins are often prescribed with a double or triple loading dose initially, then followed by the courses described in the examples below. Clinicians should refer to Table 4 (above) for dose ranges or see individual monographs for specific information.

Rx

Augmentin® 250, 500, or 875 mg

Disp: Appropriate quantity for 7-10 days

Sig: Take 1 tablet 3 times/day for 250 or 500 mg; twice daily for 875 mg

Ingredients: Amoxicillin trihydrate 500 mg and clavulanate potassium 125 mg

Note: Amoxicillin alone may also be prescribed (same dosing for 250 mg and 500 mg)

Rx

Cephalexin 250 mg

Disp: 28 capsules

Sig: Take 1 capsule 4 times/day

Rx

Clindamycin 300 mg

Disp: 28 capsules

Sig: Take 1 capsule every 6 hours

Rx

Metronidazole 500 mg

Disp: 40 tablets

Sig: Take 1 tablet 4 times/day

Rx

Penicillin V potassium 500 mg

Disp: 28 tablets

Sig: Take 1 tablet 4 times/day

ORAL BACTERIAL INFECTIONS *(Continued)*

SINUS INFECTION TREATMENT

Sinus infections represent a common condition which may present with confounding dental complaints. Treatment is sometimes instituted by the dentist, but due to the often chronic and recurrent nature of sinus infections, early involvement of an otolaryngologist is advised. These infections may require antibiotics of varying spectrum as well as requiring the management of sinus congestion. Although amoxicillin is usually adequate, many otolaryngologists go directly to Augmentin®. Second-generation cephalosporins and clarithromycin are sometimes used depending on the chronicity of the problem.

PRESCRIPTION EXAMPLES FOR SINUS INFECTIONS

The selected antibiotic should be used with a nasal decongestant and possibly an antihistamine.

Antibiotics:

Rx

Amoxicillin 500 mg
Disp: 21 capsules or tablets
Sig: Take 1 capsule 3 times/day

OR

Rx

Augmentin® 250, 500, or 875 mg
Disp: Appropriate quantity for 7-10 days
Sig: Take 1 tablet 3 times/day for 250 or 500 mg; twice daily for 875 mg

Ingredients: Amoxicillin trihydrate 500 mg and clavulanate potassium 125 mg

AND

Decongestants/Antihistamine:

Rx

Afrin® Nasal Spray (OTC)
Disp: 15 mL
Sig: Spray once in each nostril every 6-8 hours for no more than 3 days

Ingredient: Oxymetazoline

OR

Rx

Sudafed® 60 mg tablets (OTC)
Disp: 30 tablets
Sig: Take 1 tablet every 4-6 hours as needed for congestion

Ingredient: Pseudoephedrine

AND

Rx

Chlor-Trimeton® 4 mg (OTC)
Disp: 14 tablets
Sig: Take 1 tablet twice daily

Ingredient: Chlorpheniramine

FREQUENTLY ASKED QUESTIONS

What is the best antibiotic modality for treating dental infections?

Penicillin is still the drug of choice for treatment of infections in and around the oral cavity. Phenoxy-methyl penicillin (Pen VK) long has been the most commonly selected antibiotic. In penicillin-allergic individuals, erythromycin may be an appropriate consideration. If another drug is sought, clindamycin prescribed 300 mg as a loading dose followed by 150 mg 4 times/day would be an appropriate regimen for a dental infection. In general, if there is no response to Pen VK, then Augmentin® may be a good alternative in the nonpenicillin-allergic patient because of its slightly altered spectrum. Recommendations would include that the patient should take the drug with food.

Is there cross-allergenicity between the cephalosporins and penicillin?

The incidence of cross-allergenicity is 5% to 8% in the overall population. If a patient has demonstrated a Type I hypersensitivity reaction to penicillin, namely urticaria or anaphylaxis, then this incidence would increase to 20%.

Is there definitely an interaction between contraception agents and antibiotics?

There are well founded interactions between contraceptives and antibiotics. The best instructions that a patient could be given by their dentist are that should an antibiotic be necessary and the dentist is aware that the patient is on contraceptives, and if the patient is using chemical contraceptives, the patient should seriously consider additional means of contraception during the antibiotic management.

Are antibiotics necessary in diabetic patients?

In the management of diabetes, control of the diabetic status is the key factor relative to all morbidity issues. If a patient is well controlled, then antibiotics will likely not be necessary. However, in patients where the control is questionable or where they have recently been given a different drug regimen for their diabetes or if they are being titrated to an appropriate level of either insulin or oral hypoglycemic agents during these periods of time, the dentist might consider preprocedural antibiotics to be efficacious.

Do nonsteroidal anti-inflammatory drugs interfere with blood pressure medication?

At the current time there is no clear evidence that NSAIDs interfere with any of the blood pressure medications that are currently in usage.

PERIODONTAL DISEASES

Periodontal diseases are common to mankind affecting, according to some epidemiologic studies, greater than 80% of the worldwide population. The conditions refer primarily to diseases that are caused by accumulations of dental plaque and the subsequent immune response of the host to the bacteria and toxins present in this plaque. Although most of the organisms that have been implicated in advanced periodontal diseases are anaerobic in nature, some aerobes contribute by either coaggregation with the anaerobic species or direct involvement with specific disease types.

Periodontal condition, as a group of diseases, affects the soft tissues supporting the teeth (ie, gingiva) leading to the term gingivitis or inflammation of gingival structures and those conditions that affect the bone and ligament supporting the teeth (ie, periodontitis) resulting from the infection and/or inflammation of these structures. Diseases of the periodontia can be further subdivided into various types including adult periodontitis, early onset periodontitis, prepubertal periodontitis, and rapidly progressing periodontitis. In addition, specific conditions associated with predisposing immunodeficiency disease, such as those found in HIV-infected patients, create further subclassifications of the periodontal diseases, some of which are covered in those chapters associated with those conditions.

It is well accepted that control of most periodontal diseases requires, at the very minimum, appropriate mechanical cleansing of the dentition and the supporting structures by the patient. These efforts include brushing, some type of interdental cleaning, preferably with either floss or other aids, as well as appropriate sulcular cleaning usually with a brush.

Following appropriate dental treatment by the general dental practitioner and/or the periodontist, aids to these efforts by the patient might include the use of chemical agents to assist in the control of the periodontal diseases, or to prevent periodontal diseases. There are many available chemical agents on the market, only some of which are approved by the American Dental Association. Several have been tested utilizing guidelines published in 1986 by the American Dental Association for assessment of agents that claim efficacy in the management of periodontal diseases. These chemical agents include chlorhexidine (Peridex®, PerioGard®), which are bisbiguanides and benzalkonium chloride, which is a quarternary compound. Chlorhexidine, in various concentrations, has shown efficacy in reducing plaque and gingivitis in patients with short-term utilization. Some side effects include staining of the dentition which is reversible by dental prophylaxis. Chlorhexidine demonstrates the concept of substantivity, indicating that after its use, it has a continued effect in reducing the ability of plaque to form. It has been shown to be useful in a variety of periodontal conditions including acute necrotizing ulcerative gingivitis and healing studies. Some disturbances in taste and accumulation of calculus have been reported, however, chlorhexidine is the most applicable chemical agent of the bisbiguanides that has been studied to date.

Other chemical agents available as mouthwashes include the phenol compound Listerine Antiseptic®. These compounds are primarily restricted to prototype agents; the first to be approved by the ADA being Listerine Antiseptic®. Listerine Antiseptic® has been shown to be effective against plaque and gingivitis in long-term studies and comparable to chlorhexidine in these long-term investigations. However, chlorhexidine performs better than Listerine Antiseptic® in short-term investigations. Triclosan, the chemical agent found in the toothpaste Total®, has been recently approved by the FDA and is an aid in the prevention of gingivitis. Antiplaque activity of triclosan is enhanced with the addition of zinc citrate and there are no serious side effects to the use of triclosan. Sanguinarine is a principle herbal extract used for antiplaque activity. It is an alkyloid from the plant *Sanguinaria canadensis* and has some antimicrobial properties perhaps due to its enzyme activity. Zinc citrate and zinc chloride have often been added to toothpastes as well as enzymes such as mucinase, mutanase, and dextrinase which have demonstrated varying results in studies. Some commercial anionic surfactants are available on the market which include aminoalcohols and the agent Plax® which essentially is comprised of sodium thiosulfate as a surfactant. Recent studies have shown Plax® to have some efficacy when it is added to triclosan.

Long-term use of prescription medications, including antibiotics, is seldom recommended and is not in any way a substitute for general dental/periodontal therapies. As adjunctive therapy, however, benefit has been shown and the new formulations of doxycycline (Periostat® and Atridox™), are recommended for long-term or repetitive treatments. It should be noted that the manufacturer's claims indicate that Periostat® functions as a collagenase inhibitor not as an antibiotic at recommended low doses for long-term therapy. Atridox™, however, functions as an antibiotic and is not recommended for constant long-term therapy, but rather in repetitive applications as necessary. Prescription medications used in efforts to treat periodontal diseases have historically included the use of antibiotics such as tetracycline although complications with use with young patients have often precluded their prescription. Doxycycline is often preferred to tetracycline in low doses. This broad-spectrum bacteriostatic agent has shown efficacy against a wide variety of bacterial organisms found in periodontal disease. Minocycline slow-release (Arestin™) has recently been approved.

The drug metronidazole is a nitromidazole. It is an agent that was originally used in treatment of protozoan infections and some anaerobic bacteria. It is bactericidal and has a good absorption and distribution throughout the body. The studies using metronidazole have suggested that it has a variety of uses in periodontal treatment and can be used as adjunct in both acute necrotizing ulcerative gingivitis and has specific efficacy against spirochetes, bacteria, and some *Porphyromonas* species. Clindamycin is a derivative of vancomycin and has been useful in treatment of suppurative periodontal lesions. However, long-term use is precluded by its complicating toxicities associated with colitis and gastrointestinal problems.

Research has also shown that various combination therapies of metronidazole and tetracycline for juvenile periodontitis and metronidazole with amoxicillin for rapidly progressive disease can be useful. The use of other prescription drugs including nonsteroidal anti-inflammatory, as well as other antibacterial agents, have been under study. Effects on prostaglandins of NSAIDs may indirectly slow periodontal disease progression. New research is currently underway in this regard. Perhaps, in combination therapy with some of the antibiotics, these drugs may assist in reducing the patient's immune response or inflammatory response to the presence of disease-causing bacteria.

Of greatest interest has been the improvement in technology for delivery of chemical agents to the periodontally-diseased site. These systems include biodegradable gelatins and biodegradable chips that can be placed under the gingiva and deliver antibacterial agents directly to the site as an adjunct to periodontal treatment. The initial therapy of mechanical debridement by the periodontal therapist is essential prior to using any chemical agent, and the dentist should be aware that the development of newer agents does not substitute for appropriate periodontal therapy and maintenance. The trade names of the gelatin chips and subgingival delivery systems include Periochip®, Atridox®, and Periostat®.

In addition to the periodontal therapy, consideration of the patient's pre-existing or developing medical conditions are important in the management of the periodontal patient. Several diseases illustrate these points most acutely. The reader is referred to the chapters on Diabetes, Cardiovascular Disease, Pregnancy, Respiratory Disease, HIV, and Cancer Chemotherapy. It has long been accepted that uncontrolled diabetes may predispose to periodontal lesions. Now, under current investigation is the hypothesis that pre-existing periodontal diseases may make it more difficult for a diabetic patient to come under control. In addition, the inflammatory response and immune challenge that is ongoing in periodontal disease appears to be implicated in the development of coronary artery disease as well as an increased risk of myocardial infarction and/or stroke. The accumulation of intra-arterial plaques appears enhanced by the presence of the inflammatory response often seen systemically in patients suffering with periodontal disease. The American Heart Association is currently considering recommendations regarding antibiotic prophylaxis in patients with cardiovascular disease. In addition, the clinician is referred to the section on preprocedural antibiotics in the text for a consideration of antibiotic usage in patients that may be at risk for infective endocarditis. Other conditions including pregnancy and respiratory diseases such as COPD, HIV, and cancer therapy must be considered in the overall view of periodontal diseases. The reader is referred to the sections within the text.

Amoxicillin *on page 93*
Minocycline *on page 916*
Benzalkonium chloride *on page 169*
Chlorhexidine *on page 300*
Clindamycin *on page 341*
Doxycycline *on page 479*
Listerine Antiseptic® *on page 934*
Metronidazole *on page 902*
NSAIDs see Oral Pain section *on page 1524*
Tetracycline *on page 1286*
Triclosan and Fluorides *on page 1348*

Oral fungal infections can result from alteration in oral flora, immunosuppression, and underlying systemic diseases that may allow the overgrowth of these opportunistic organisms. These systemic conditions might include diabetes, long-term xerostomia, adrenal suppression, anemia, and chemotherapy-induced myelosuppression for the management of cancer. The use of oral inhalers that include steroids, such as Advair™ Diskus®, have been implicated in the enhancing of the risk of fungal overgrowth. Drugs of choice in treating fungal infections are amphotericin B, ciclopirox olamine, clotrimazole, itraconazole, ketoconazole, fluconazole, naftifine hydrochloride, nystatin, and oxiconazole. Patients being treated for fungal skin infections may also be using topical antifungal preparations coupled with a steroid such as triamcinolone. Clinical presentation might include pseudomembranous, atrophic, and hyperkeratotic forms. Fungus has also been implicated in denture stomatitis and symptomatic geographic tongue.

Nystatin (Mycostatin®) is effective topically in the treatment of candidal infections of the skin and mucous membrane. The drug is extremely well tolerated and appears to be nonsensitizing. In persons with denture stomatitis in which monilial organisms play at least a contributory role, it is important to soak the prosthesis overnight in a nystatin suspension. Nystatin ointment can be placed in the denture during the daytime much like a denture adhesive. Medication should be continued for at least 48 hours after disappearance of clinical signs in order to prevent relapse. Patients must be re-evaluated after 14 days of therapy. Predisposing systemic factors must be reconsidered if the oral fungal infection persists. Topical applications rely on contact of the drug with the lesions. Therefore, 4-5 times daily with a dissolving troche or pastille is appropriate. Concern over the presence of sugar in the troches and pastilles has led practitioners to sometimes prescribe the vaginal suppository formulation for off-labeled oral use.

Voriconazole (VFEND®) is indicated for treatment of serious fungal infections in patients intolerant of, or refractory to, other therapy.

Amphotericin B *on page 98*
Clotrimazole *on page 356*
Fluconazole *on page 576*
Ketoconazole *on page 762*
Nystatin *on page 992*
Nystatin and Triamcinolone *on page 992*
Voriconazole *on page 1395* tablet or injection

Note: Consider Peridex® oral rinse, or Listerine® antiseptic oral rinse for long-term control in immunosuppressed patients.

PRESCRIPTION EXAMPLES

Rx

Mycostatin® pastilles

Disp: 70 pastilles

Sig: Dissolve 1 tablet in mouth until gone, 4-5 times/day for 14 days

Ingredient: 200,000 units of nystatin per tablet

Note: Pastille is more effective than oral suspension due to prolonged contact.

Rx

Mycostatin® oral suspension

Disp: 60 mL (2 oz)

Sig: Use 1 teaspoonful 4-5 times/day; rinse and hold in mouth as long as possible before swallowing or spitting out (2 minutes); do not eat or drink for 30 minutes following application

Ingredients: Nystatin 100,000 units/mL; vehicle contains 50% sucrose and not more than 1% alcohol

Rx

Mycostatin® ointment or cream

Disp: 15 g or 30 g tube

Sig: Apply liberally to affected areas 4-5 times/day; do not eat or drink for 30 minutes after application

Ingredients:

Cream: 100,000 units nystatin per g, aqueous vanishing cream base

Ointment: 100,000 units nystatin per g, polyethylene, and mineral oil gel base

Note: Denture wearers should apply to dentures prior to each insertion; for edentulous patients, Mycostatin® powder (15 g) can also be prescribed to be sprinkled on dentures.

OR

Rx

Mycelex® troche 10 mg

Disp: 70 tablets

Sig: Dissolve 1 tablet in mouth 5 times/day

Ingredient: Clotrimazole

Note: Tablets contain sucrose, risk of caries with prolonged use (>3 months); care must be exercised in diabetic patients.

Rx

Fungizone® oral suspension 100mg/mL

Disp: 50 mL

Sig: 1 mL; swish and swallow 4 times/day between meals

Ingredient: Amphotericin B (Conventional)

Note: Although the manufacturer has discontinued the solution formulation, prescriptions are being filled until the supply is exhausted. A lozenge formulation (10 mg amphotericin B per oz) is currently being manufactured and marketed in other countries but is not available in the U.S. at this time.

MANAGEMENT OF FUNGAL INFECTIONS REQUIRING SYSTEMIC MEDICATION

If the patient is refractory to topical treatment, consideration of a systemic route might include Diflucan® or Nizoral®. Also, when the patient cannot tolerate topical therapy, ketoconazole (Nizoral®) is an effective, well tolerated, systematic drug for mucocutaneous candidiasis. Concern over liver function and possible drug interactions must be considered.

PRESCRIPTION EXAMPLES

Rx

Nizoral® 200 mg

Disp: 10 or 28 tablets

Sig: Take 1 tablet/day for 10-14 days

Ingredient: Ketoconazole

Note: To be used if *Candida* infection does not respond to mycostatin; potential for liver toxicity; liver function should be monitored with long-term use (>3 weeks)

ORAL FUNGAL INFECTIONS *(Continued)*

Rx

Diflucan® 100 mg

Disp: 15 tablets

Sig: Take 2 tablets the first day and 1 tablet/day for 10-14 days

Ingredient: Fluconazole

MANAGEMENT OF ANGULAR CHEILITIS

Angular cheilitis may represent the clinical manifestation of a multitude of etiologic factors. Cheilitis-like lesions may result from local habits, from a decrease in the intermaxillary space, or from nutritional deficiency. More commonly, angular cheilitis represents a mixed infection coupled with an inflammatory response involving *Candida albicans* and other organisms. The drug of choice is now formulated to contain nystatin and triamcinolone and the effect is excellent.

PRESCRIPTION EXAMPLE

Rx

Mycolog®–II cream

Disp: 15 g tube

Sig: Apply to affected area after each meal and before bedtime

Ingredients: Nystatin 100,000 units and triamcinolone acetonide 0.1%

ORAL VIRAL INFECTIONS

Oral viral infections are most commonly caused by herpes simplex viruses and Coxsackie viruses. Oral pharyngeal infections and upper respiratory infections are commonly caused by the Coxsackie group A viruses. Soft tissue viral infections, on the other hand, are most often caused by the herpes simplex viruses. Herpes zoster or varicella-zoster virus, which is one of the herpes family of viruses, can likewise cause similar viral eruptions involving the mucosa.

The diagnosis of an acute viral infection is one that begins by ruling out bacterial etiology and having an awareness of the presenting signs and symptoms associated with viral infection. Acute onset and vesicular eruption on the soft tissues generally favors a diagnosis of viral infection. Unfortunately, vesicles do not remain for a great length of time in the oral cavity; therefore, the short-lived vesicles rupture leaving ulcerated bases as the only indication of their presence. These ulcers, however, are generally small in size and only when left unmanaged, coalesce to form larger, irregular ulcerations. Distinction should be made between the commonly occurring intraoral ulcers (aphthous ulcerations) which do not have a viral etiology and the lesions associated with intraoral herpes. The management of an oral viral infection may be palliative for the most part; however, with the advent of acyclovir we now have a family of drugs that can assist in managing primary and secondary infection. Human *Papillomavirus* is implicated in a number of oral lesions, the most common of which is *Condyloma acuminatum.* Recently, Aldara® has been approved for genital warts; oral use is under study.

It should be noted that herpes can present as a primary infection (gingivostomatitis), recurrent lip lesions (herpes labialis), and intraoral ulcers (recurrent intraoral herpes), involving the oral and perioral tissues. Primary infection is a systemic infection that leads to acute gingivostomatitis involving multiple tissues of the buccal mucosa, lips, tongue, floor of the mouth, and the gingiva. Treatment of primary infections utilizes acyclovir in combination with supportive care. Topical anesthetic used in combination with Benadryl® 0.5% in a saline vehicle was found to be an effective oral rinse in the symptomatic treatment of primary herpetic gingivostomatitis; however, Dyclone® is no longer available. Other agents for symptomatic and supportive treatment include commercially available elixir of Benadryl®, Xylocaine® viscous, Orajel® (OTC), and antibiotics to prevent secondary infections. Systemic supportive therapy should include forced fluids, high concentration protein, vitamin and mineral food supplements, and rest.

Antivirals

Abreva™(OTC) *on page 463*
Acyclovir *on page 42*
Imiquimod *on page 713*
Lysine® (OTC) *on page 832*
Nelfinavir *on page 959*
Penciclovir *on page 1046*
Vidarabine *on page 1384*
Valacyclovir *on page 1367*

Supportive Therapy

Diphenhydramine *on page 451*
Lidocaine *on page 801*

Prevention of Secondary Bacterial Infection

Penicillin V Potassium *on page 1051*

ORAL VIRAL INFECTIONS *(Continued)*

PRIMARY INFECTION

PRESCRIPTION EXAMPLE

Rx

Zovirax® 200 mg

Disp: 70 capsules

Sig: Take 1 capsule every 4 hours for 2 weeks, not to exceed 5 in 24 hours

Ingredient: Acyclovir

SUPPORTIVE CARE FOR PAIN AND PREVENTION OF SECONDARY INFECTION

Primary infections often become secondarily infected with bacteria, requiring antibiotics. Dietary supplement may be necessary. Options are presented due to variability in patient compliance and response.

PRESCRIPTION EXAMPLES

Rx

Benadryl® elixir 12.5 mg/5 mL

Disp: 4 oz bottle

Sig: Rinse with 1 teaspoonful for 2 minutes before each meal

Ingredient: Diphenhydramine

Rx

Benadryl® elixir 12.5 mg/5 mL with Kaopectate®, 50% mixture by volume

Disp: 8 oz

Sig: Rinse with 1 teaspoonful every 2 hours

Ingredients: Diphenhydramine and attapulgite

Rx

Xylocaine® viscous 2%

Disp: 450 mL bottle

Sig: Swish with 1 tablespoon 4 times/day and spit out

Ingredient: Lidocaine

Rx

Meritene®

Disp: 1 lb can (plain, chocolate, eggnog flavors)

Sig: Take 3 servings/day; prepare as indicated on can

Ingredient: Protein/vitamin/mineral food supplement

RECURRENT HERPETIC INFECTIONS

Following this primary infection, the herpesvirus remains latent until such time as it has the opportunity to recur. The etiology of this latent period and the degree of viral shedding present during latency is currently under study; however, it is thought that some trigger in the mucosa or the skin causes the virus to begin to replicate. This process may involve Langerhans cells which are immunocompetent antigen-presenting cells resident in all epidermal surfaces. The virus replication then leads to eruptions in tissues surrounding the mouth. The most common form of recurrence is the lip lesion or herpes labialis, however, intraoral recurrent herpes also occurs with some frequency. Prevention of recurrences has been attempted with lysine (OTC) 500-1000 mg/day but response has been variable. Herpes zoster outbreaks can involve the oral and facial tissues although this is uncommon. Valacyclovir is the drug of choice.

Water-soluble bioflavonoid-ascorbic acid complex, now available as Peridin-C®, may be helpful in reducing the signs and symptoms associated with recurrent herpes simplex virus infections. As with all agents used, the therapy is more effective when instituted in the early prodromal stage of the disease process.

PREVENTION PRESCRIPTION EXAMPLES

Rx

Lysine (OTC) 500 mg

Sig: Take 2 tablets/day as preventive; increase to 4 tablets/day if prodrome or recurrence begins

Rx

Citrus bioflavonoids and ascorbic acid tablets 400 mg (Peridin-C®)

Disp: 10 tablets

Sig: Take 2 tablets at once, then 1 tablet 3 times/day for 3 days

Where a recurrence is usually precipitated by exposure to sunlight, the lesion may be prevented by the application to the area of a sunscreen, with a high skin protection factor (SPF) in the range of 10-15.

PRESCRIPTION EXAMPLE

Rx

PreSun® (OTC) 15 sunscreen lotion

Disp: 4 fluid oz

Sig: Apply to susceptible area 1 hour before sun exposure

TREATMENT

Acyclovir (Zovirax®) and vidarabine (Vira-A®) possess antiviral activity against herpes simplex types 1 and 2. Historically, ophthalmic ointments were used topically to treat recurrent mucosal and skin lesions. These do not penetrate well on the skin lesions, thereby providing questionable relief of symptoms. If recommended, use should be closely monitored. Penciclovir, an active metabolite of famciclovir, has been specifically approved in a cream for treatment of recurrent herpes lesions. Valacyclovir has recently been approved for treatment of herpes labialis (see monograph for dosing). The FDA has also approved acyclovir cream for treatment of herpes labialis in adults and adolescents but the product is currently under regulatory review (check www.biovail for status). Biovail Corporation has acquired exclusive marketing and distribution rights for Zovirax® ointment and cream from the manufacturer, GlaxoSmithKline.

PRESCRIPTION EXAMPLES

Rx

Zovirax® ointment 5%

Disp: 15 g tube

Sig: Apply thin layer to lesions 6 times/day for 7 days

Ingredient: Acyclovir 50 mg (per g)

ORAL VIRAL INFECTIONS *(Continued)*

Rx
Zovirax® 200 mg
Disp: 70 capsules
Sig: Take 1 capsule every 4 hours for 2 weeks, up to 5 capsules within 24 hours

Ingredient: Acyclovir 200 mg

Rx
Denavir™
Disp: 2 g tube
Sig: Apply locally every 2 hours, during waking hours, for 4 days

Ingredient: Penciclovir 1%

Note: Denavir™ is approved for use in treating recurrent herpes labialis.

Rx
Abreva™ (OTC) cream
Sig: Apply locally as directed 5 times/day

Ingredient: Docosanol 10%

PRESCRIPTION EXAMPLE FOR HERPES ZOSTER

Rx
Valtrex®
Sig: Take 2 caplets 3 times/day for 7 days

Ingredient: Valacyclovir 500 mg

Note: Reevaluate after 7 days; may require dose reduction in patients with altered renal function, consult with patient's physician(s).

ORAL NONVIRAL SOFT TISSUE ULCERATIONS OR EROSIONS

RECURRENT APHTHOUS STOMATITIS

Kenalog® in Orabase is indicated for the temporary relief of symptoms associated with infrequent recurrences of minor aphthous lesions and ulcerative lesions resulting from trauma. More severe forms of recurrent aphthous stomatitis may be treated with an oral suspension of tetracycline. The agent appears to reduce the duration of symptoms and decrease the rate of recurrence by reducing secondary bacterial infection. Its use is contraindicated during the last half of pregnancy, infancy, and childhood to the age of 8 years. *Lactobacillus acidophilus* preparations (Bacid®, Lactinex®) are occasionally effective for reducing the frequency and severity of the lesions. Debacterol® has recently been approved. Patients with long-standing history of recurrent aphthous stomatitis should be evaluated for iron, folic acid, and vitamin B_{12} deficiencies. Regular use of Listerine® antiseptic has been shown in clinical trials to reduce the severity, duration, and frequency of aphthous stomatitis. Debacterol® has recently been approved. Chlorhexidine oral rinses 20 mL for 30 seconds 2-3 times/day have also demonstrated efficacy in reducing the duration of aphthae. With both of these products, however, patient intolerance of the burning from the alcohol content is of concern. Viractin® has been approved for symptomatic relief. Immunocompromised patients such as those with AIDS may have severe ulcer recurrences and the drug thalidomide has been approved for these patients.

Amlexanox *on page 87*
Attapulgite *on page 146*
Chlorhexidine *on page 300*
Clobetasol *on page 345*
Dexamethasone *on page 413*
Diphenhydramine *on page 451*
Fluocinonide ointment with Orabase *on page 585*
Debacterol® *on page 1257*
Lactobacillus acidophilus and *Lactobacillus bulgaricus* *on page 772*
Metronidazole *on page 902*
Mouthwash, Antiseptic *on page 934*
Prednisone *on page 1112*
Tetracaine *on page 1284*
Tetracycline liquid *on page 1286*
Thalidomide *on page 1289*
Triamcinolone Acetonide Dental Paste *on page 1344*

PRESCRIPTION EXAMPLES FOR MINOR APHTHAE, BURNING TONGUE SYNDROME, GEOGRAPHIC TONGUE, MILD FORMS OF ORAL LICHEN PLANUS

Rx

Listerine® antiseptic (OTC)

Sig: 20 mL for 30 seconds twice daily

Ingredients: Thymol 0.064%, eucalyptus 0.092%, methyl salicylate 0.060%, menthol 0.042%, and alcohol 26.9%

Rx

Peridex® oral rinse

Disp: 1 bottle

Sig: 20 mL for 30 seconds 3 times/day

Ingredients: Chlorhexidine gluconate 0.12% and alcohol 11.6%

ORAL NONVIRAL SOFT TISSUE ULCERATIONS OR EROSIONS *(Continued)*

Rx

PerioGard® oral rinse

Disp: 1 bottle

Sig: 20 mL for 30 seconds 3 times/day

Ingredients: Chlorhexidine gluconate 0.12% and alcohol 11.6%

Rx

Tetracycline capsules 250 mg

Disp: 40 capsules

Sig: Suspend contents of 1 capsule in a teaspoonful of water; rinse for 2 minutes 4 times/day and swallow

Note: Also available as liquid (125 mg/5 mL), which is convenient to use; swish 5 mL for 2 minutes 4 times/day

Rx

Kenalog® in Orabase 0.1%

Disp: 5 g tube

Sig: Coat the lesion with a film after each meal and at bedtime

Ingredient: Triamcinolone

Rx

Benadryl® elixir 12.5 mg/5 mL

Disp: 4 oz bottle

Sig: Rinse with 1 teaspoonful for 2 minutes before each meal and swallow

Ingredient: Diphenhydramine

Note: Elixir of Benadryl®, a potent antihistamine, is used in the oral cavity primarily as a mild topical anesthetic agent for the symptomatic relief of certain allergic deficiencies which should be ruled out as possible etiologies for the oral condition under treatment. It is often used alone and in solutions with agents such as Kaopectate® or Maalox® to assist in coating the oral mucosa. Benadryl® is also available in capsules.

Rx

Benadryl® syrup (mix 50/50) with Kaopectate®*

Disp: 8 oz total

Sig: Rinse with 2 teaspoons as needed to relieve pain or burning (use after meals)

Ingredient: Diphenhydramine and attapulgite

***Note:** May be mixed with Maalox® if constipation is a problem.

Rx

Lidex® ointment mixed 50/50 with Orabase®

Disp: 30 g total

Sig: Apply thin layer to oral lesions 4-6 times/day

Ingredient: Fluocinonide 0.05%

Note: To be used for oral inflammatory lesions that do not respond to Kenalog® in Orabase®.

EROSIVE LICHEN PLANUS AND MAJOR APHTHAE

Elixir of dexamethasone (Decadron®), a potent anti-inflammatory agent, is used topically in the management of acute episodes of erosive lichen planus and major aphthae. Continued supervision of the patient during treatment is essential and the dentist must be aware that treatment of any secondary infections such as fungal overgrowth may be essential in gaining control of the erosive lesions.

PRESCRIPTION EXAMPLE

Rx

Decadron® elixir 0.5 mg/5 mL

Disp: 100 mL bottle

Sig: Rinse with 1 teaspoonful for 2 minutes 4 times/day; do not swallow

Ingredient: Dexamethasone

Note: Other regimens altering topical and systemic uptake including swish-and-swallow can be designed by the dentist depending upon the severity and usual duration of the lesions.

For severe cases and when the oropharynx is involved, some practitioners have the patient swallow after a 2-minute rinse.

Allergy	Benadryl®
Aphthous	Benadryl®/Maalox® (compounded prescription) Benadryl®/Kaopectate® (compounded prescription) Lidex® in Orabase (compounded prescription) Kenalog® in Orabase Tetracycline mouth rinse
Oral inflammatory disease	Lidex® in Orabase (compounded prescription) Kenalog® in Orabase Prednisone Temovate® cream

The use of long-term steroids is always a concern due to possible adrenal suppression. If systemic steroids are contemplated for a protracted time, medical consultation is advisable.

PRESCRIPTION EXAMPLE FOR SYSTEMIC STEROID

Rx

Prednisone 5 mg

Disp: 60 tablets

Sig: Take 4 tablets in morning with food and 4 tablets at noon with food for 4 day, then decrease the total number of tablets by 1 each day until down to zero

Note: Medrol® (methylprednisolone) dose packs (2-60 mg/day) are an alternative choice; see Methylprednisolone *on page 895*

PRESCRIPTION EXAMPLE FOR HIGH POTENCY TOPICAL CORTICOSTEROID

Rx

Temovate® cream 0.05%

Disp: 15 g tube

Sig: Apply locally 4-6 times/day

Ingredient: Clobetasol

ORAL NONVIRAL SOFT TISSUE ULCERATIONS OR EROSIONS *(Continued)*

NECROTIZING ULCERATING PERIODONTITIS (HIV Periodontal Disease)

Initial Treatment *(In-Office)*

Gentle debridement
Note: Ensure patient has no iodine allergies

Betadine® rinse *on page 1104*

At-Home Treatment

Listerine® antiseptic rinse (20 mL for 30 seconds twice daily)
Peridex® rinse *on page 300*
Metronidazole (Flagyl®) 7-10 days *on page 902*

Follow-Up Therapy

Proper dental cleaning, including scaling and root planing (repeat as needed)
Continue Peridex® and Listerine® rinse (indefinitely)

DENTIN HYPERSENSITIVITY, HIGH CARIES INDEX, AND XEROSTOMIA

DENTIN HYPERSENSITIVITY

Suggested steps in resolving dentin hypersensitivity when a thorough exam has ruled-out any other source for the problem:

Treatment Steps

- Home treatment with a desensitizing toothpaste containing potassium nitrate (used to brush teeth as well as a thin layer applied, each night for 2 weeks)
- If needed, in office potassium oxalate (Protect® by Butler) and/or in office fluoride iontophoresis
- If sensitivity is still not tolerable to the patient, consider pumice then dentin adhesive and unfilled resin or composite restoration overlaying a glass ionomer base

Home Products (all contain nitrate as active ingredient):

Promise®
Denquel®
Sensodyne®

Dentifrice Products *on page 1619*

Other major brand name companies have added ingredients to their dentifrice product lines that also make hypersensitivity claims.

ANTICARIES AGENTS

Fluoride (Gel 0.4%, Rinse 0.05%) *on page 586*

New toothpastes with triclosan such as Colgate Total® show promise for combined treatment/prevention of caries, plaque, and gingivitis. The use of 5% sodium fluoride varnishes (Duraflor® and Duraphat®) have been encouraged by cariologists for the prevention of decay in persons of high-risk populations.

FLUORIDES

Used for the prevention of demineralization of the tooth structure secondary to xerostomia. For patients with long-term or permanent xerostomia, daily application is accomplished using custom applicator trays, such as omnivac. Patients with porcelain crowns should use a neutral pH fluoride (see Fluoride monograph *on page 586*). Final selection of a fluoride product and/or saliva replacement/stimulant product must be based on patient comfort, taste, and ultimately, compliance. Experience has demonstrated that, often times, patients must try various combinations to achieve the greatest effect and their highest comfort levels. The presence of mucositis during cancer management complicates the clinician's selection of products.

See also Oral Rinse Products *on page 1634*

OVER-THE-COUNTER (OTC) PRODUCTS

Form	Brand Name	Strength / Size
Gel, topical (stannous fluoride)	Gel-Kam® (cinnamon, fruit, mint flavors)	0.4% [0.1%] (65 g, 105 g, 122 g)
	Gel-Tin® (lime, grape, cinnamon, raspberry, mint, orange flavors)	0.4% [0.1%] (60 g, 120 g)
	Stop® (grape, cinnamon, bubblegum, piña colada, mint flavors)	0.4% [0.1%] (60 g, 120 g)
Rinse, topical (as sodium)	ACT®, Fluorigard®	0.05% [0.02%] (90 mL, 180 mL, 300 mL, 360 mL, 480 mL)
	Listermint® with Fluoride	0.02% [0.01%] (180 mL, 300 mL, 360 mL, 480 mL, 540 mL, 720 mL, 960 mL, 1740 mL)

DENTIN HYPERSENSITIVITY, HIGH CARIES INDEX, AND XEROSTOMIA *(Continued)*

PRESCRIPTION ONLY (Rx) PRODUCTS

Form	Brand Name	Strength / Size
Drops, oral (as sodium)	Fluoritab®, Flura-Drops®	0.275 mg/drop [0.125 mg/drop]
		0.55 mg/drop [0.25 mg/drop] (22.8 mL, 24 mL)
	Karidium®, Luride®	0.275 mg/drop [0.125 mg/drop] (30 mL, 60 mL)
	Pediaflor®	1.1 mg/mL [0.5 mg/mL] (50 mL)
Gel-Drops	Thera-Flur® (lime flavor), Thera-Flur-N®	1.1% [0.55%] (24 mL)
Gel, topical		
Acidulated phosphate fluoride	Minute-Gel® (spearmint, strawberry, grape, apple-cinnamon, cherry cola, bubblegum flavors)	1.23% (480 mL)
Sodium fluoride	Karigel® (orange flavor)	1.1% [0.5%]
	Karigel®-N	1.1% [0.5%]
	PreviDent® (mint, berry, cherry, fruit sherbet flavors)	1.1% [0.5%] (24 g, 30 g, 60 g, 120 g, 130 g, 250 g)
Lozenge (as sodium)	Flura-Loz® (raspberry flavor)	2.2 mg [1 mg]
Rinse, topical (as sodium)	Fluorinse®, Point-Two®	0.2% [0.09%] (240 mL, 480 mL, 3780 mL)
Solution, oral (as sodium)	Phos-Flur® (cherry, cinnamon, grape, wintergreen flavors)	0.44 mg/mL [0.2 mg/mL] (250 mL, 500 mL, 3780 mL)
Tablet (as sodium)		1.1 mg [0.5 mg]; 2.2 mg [1 mg]
Chewable	Fluor-A-Day®	0.55 mg [0.25 mg]
	Fluor-A-Day®, Fluoritab®, Luride® Lozi-Tab®, Pharmaflur®	1.1 mg [0.5 mg]
	Fluor-A-Day®, Fluoritab®, Karidium®, Luride® Lozi-Tab®, Luride®-SF Lozi-Tab®, Pharmaflur®	2.2 mg [1 mg]
Oral	Flura®, Karidium®	2.2 mg [1 mg]
Varnish	Duraflor®, Duraphat®	5% [50 mg/mL] (10 mL)

Tables copied from Newland, JR, Meiller, TF, Wynn, RL, et al, *Oral Soft Tissue Diseases,* 2nd ed, Hudson (Cleveland), OH: Lexi-Comp, Inc, 2002.

ANTIPLAQUE AGENTS

PRESCRIPTION EXAMPLES

Rx

Listerine® antiseptic mouthwash (OTC)

Sig: 20 mL, swish for 30 seconds twice daily

Ingredients: Thymol 0.064%, eucalyptus 0.092%, methyl salicylate 0.060%, menthol 0.042%, and alcohol 26.9%

Rx

Peridex® oral rinse

Disp: 3 times 16 oz

Sig: $^{1}/_{2}$ oz, swish for 30 seconds 2-3 times/day

Ingredients: Chlorhexidine gluconate 0.12% and alcohol 11.6%

Rx

PerioGard® oral rinse

Disp 3 times 16 oz

Sig: $^{1}/_{2}$ oz, swish for 30 seconds 2-3 times/day

Ingredients: Chlorhexidine gluconate 0.12% and alcohol 11.6%

Note: Peridex® may stain teeth yellow to brown (removable with dental cleaning), temporarily alter taste, and increase the deposition of calculus (reversible).

Chlorhexidine (Peridex®) *on page 300*

MANAGEMENT OF SIALORRHEA

In patients suffering with medical conditions that result in hypersalivation, the dentist may determine that it is appropriate to use an atropine sulfate medication to achieve a dry field for dental procedures or to reduce excessive drooling. Currently there is one ADA approved medication sold under the name of Sal-Tropine™. See Atropine Sulfate Dental Tablets *on page 145*

XEROSTOMIA

Xerostomia refers to the subjective sensation of a dry mouth. Numerous factors can play a role in the patient's perception of dry mouth. Changes in salivary function caused by drugs, surgical intervention, or treatment of cancer are among the leading causes of xerostomia. Other factors including aging, smoking, mouth breathing, and the immune complex of disorders, Sjögren's syndrome, can also be implicated in a patient's perception of xerostomia. Human immunodeficiency virus (HIV) may produce xerostomia when viral changes in salivary glands are present. Xerostomia affects women more frequently than men and is also more common in older individuals. Some alteration in salivary function naturally occurs with age, but it is extremely difficult to quantify the effects. Xerostomia and salivary gland hypofunction in the elderly population are contributory to deterioration in the quality of life.

Once a diagnosis of xerostomia or salivary gland hypofunction is made and possible causes confirmed, treatment for the condition usually involves management of the underlying disease and avoidance of unnecessary medications. In addition, good hydration is essential and water is the drink of choice. Also, the use of artificial saliva substitutes, selected chewing gums, and/or toothpastes formulated to treat xerostomia, is often warranted. In more difficult cases, such as patients receiving radiotherapy for cancer of the head and neck regions or patients with Sjögren's syndrome, systemic cholinergic stimulants may be administered if no contraindications exist.

CLINICAL PRODUCT USE

Because of the complex nature of xerostomia, management by the dental clinician is difficult. Treatment success is also difficult to assess and is often unsatisfactory. The salivary stimulants, pilocarpine and cevimeline, may aid in some conditions but are only approved for use as sialogogues in patients receiving radiotherapy and in Sjögren's patients, specifically as described above. Artificial salivas are available as over-the-counter products and represent the potential for continuous application by the patient to achieve comfort for their xerostomic condition.

The role of the clinician in attempting treatment of dry mouth is to first achieve a differential diagnosis and to ensure that other conditions are not simultaneously present. For example, many patients suffer burning mouth syndrome or painful oral tissues with no obvious etiology accompanying dry mouth. Also, higher caries incidence may be associated with changes in salivary flow. As previously mentioned, Sjögren's syndrome represents an immune complex of disorders that can affect the eyes, oral tissues, and other organ systems. The reader is referred to current oral pathology or oral medicine text for review of signs and symptoms of Sjögren's syndrome.

Treatment of cancer often leads to dry mouth. Surgical intervention removing salivary tissue due to the presence of a salivary gland tumor results in loss of salivary function. Also, many of the chemotherapeutic agents produce transitory changes in salivary flow, such that the patient may perceive a dry mouth during chemotherapy. Most notably related to salivary dysfunction is the use of radiation regimens to head and neck tissues. Tumors in or about salivary gland tissue, the oral cavity, and oropharynx are most notably sensitive to radiation therapy and subsequent dry mouth. In the head and neck, therapeutic radiation is commonly used in treatment of squamous cell carcinomas and lymphomas. The radiation level necessary to destroy malignant cells ranges from 40-70 Gy. Salivary tissue is extremely sensitive to radiation changes. Radiation dosages >30 Gy are sufficient to permanently change salivary function. In addition to the mucositis and subsequent secondary infection by fungal colonization or viral exacerbation, oral tissues can become exceptionally dry due to the effects of radiation on salivary glands. In fact, permanent damage to salivary gland tissue within the beam path produces significant levels of xerostomia in most patients. Some recovery may be noted by the patient. Most often, the effects are permanent and even progressive as the radiation dosage increases.

Artificial salivas do not produce any protectant or stimulation of the salivary gland. The use of pilocarpine and cevimeline as salivary stimulants in pre-emptive treatment, as well

DENTIN HYPERSENSITIVITY, HIGH CARIES INDEX, AND XEROSTOMIA *(Continued)*

as postradiation treatment, have been shown to have some efficacy in management of dry mouth. The success rate, however, still is often unsatisfactory and post-treatment management by the dentist usually requires fluoride supplements to prevent radiation-induced caries due to dry mouth. Also, management of dry mouth through patient use of the artificial salivary gel, solutions and sprays, or other over-the-counter products for dry mouth (eg, chewing gum, toothpaste, mouthwash, swab-sticks) is highly recommended. The use of pilocarpine or cevimeline should only be considered by the dentist in consultation with the managing physician. The oftentimes severe and widespread cholinergic side effects of pilocarpine and cevimeline mandate close monitoring of the patient.

The use of artificial salivary substitutes is less problematic for the dentist. The dentist should, in considering selection of a drug, base his or her decision on patient compliance and comfort. Salivary substitutes presently on the market may have some benefit in terms of electrolyte balance and salivary consistency. However, the ultimate decision needs to be based on patients' taste, their willingness to use the medication ad libitum, and improvement in their comfort related to dry mouth. Many of the drugs are pH balanced to reduce additional risk of dental demineralization or caries. Oftentimes, the dentist must try numerous medications, one at a time, prior to finding one which gives the patient some comfort. Another gauge of acceptability is to investigate whether the artificial saliva substitute has the American Dental Association's seal of approval. Most of the currently accepted saliva substitute products have been evaluated by the ADA.

In general, considerations that the clinician might use in a prescribed regimen would be that saliva substitutes are meant to be used regularly throughout the day by the patient to achieve comfort during meals, reduce tissue abrasion, and prevent salivary stagnation on teeth. Other than these, there are no specific recommendations for patients. Recommendations by the dentist need to be tailored to the patient's acceptance. Salivary substitutes may provide an allergic potential in patients who are sensitive to some of the preservatives present in artificial saliva products. In addition to this allergic potential, there is a risk of microbial contamination by placement of the salivary substitute container in close contact with the oral cavity.

Patient education regarding the use of saliva substitutes is also part of the clinical approach. The patient with chronic xerostomia should be educated about regular professional care, high performance in dental hygiene, the need to re-evaluate oral soft tissue pathology, and any changes that might occur long term. In patients with severe xerostomia, artificial salivary medications should be given in combination with topical fluoride treatment programs designed by the dentist to reduce caries.

PRODUCTS AND DRUGS TO TREAT DRY MOUTH

Medication	Manufacturer and Phone Number	Product Type	Manufacturer's Description	Indication	Ingredients	Directions for Use	Form and Availability
ARTIFICIAL SALIVAS (OTC)							
Moi-Stir® Moistening Solution	Kingswood Laboratories, Inc (800) 968-7772	Pump spray	Saliva supplement for moistening of mouth and mucosal area	Nontherapeutic treatment of dry mouth; intended for comfort only	Water, sorbitol, sodium carboxymethylcellulose, methylparaben, propylparaben, potassium chloride, sodium chloride, flavoring	Spray directly into mouth as necessary to treat drying conditions	4 oz spray bottle; order directly from manufacturer or various distributors
MouthKote® Oral Moisturizer	Parnell Pharmaceuticals, Inc (800) 457-4276	Aqueous solution	Pleasant lemon-lime-flavored oral moisturizer to lubricate and protect oral tissue	Treats the discomfort of oral dryness caused by medications, disease, surgery, irradiation, aging	Water, xylitol, sorbitol, yerba santa, citric acid, ascorbic acid, flavor, sodium benzoate, sodium saccharin	Swirl 1 or 2 teaspoonfuls in mouth for 8-10 seconds; swallow or spit out; shake well before using	2 oz and 8 oz bottles; available at drugstores or order directly from manufacturer
BreathTech™ Plaque Fighter Mouth Spray	Omnii Oral Pharmaceuticals (800) 445-3386	Pump dispenser	Plaque inhibitor in vanilla-mint flavor for breath malodor or reduced salivary flow	Treats the discomfort of oral dryness	Microdent® patented plaque-inhibitor formula	Spray directly into mouth; spread over teeth and tissue with tongue	18 mL pump dispenser; order directly from manufacturer
Optimoist™ Oral Moisturizer	Colgate Oral Pharmaceuticals (800) 225-3756	Oral moisturizer, aqueous solution	Pleasant tasting saliva substitute for instant relief of dry mouth and throat without demineralizing tooth enamel	Treats the discomfort of oral dryness	Deionized water, xylitol, calcium phosphate monobasic, citric acid, sodium hydroxide, sodium benzoate, flavoring, acesulfame potassium, hydroxyethylcellulose, polysorbate 20 and sodium monofluorophosphate (fluoride concentration is 2 parts per million)	Spray directly into mouth to relieve dry mouth discomfort; may be swallowed or expectorated; use as needed	2 oz and 12 oz bottles; available at mass merchandise stores, food stores, and drugstores

DENTIN HYPERSENSITIVITY, HIGH CARIES INDEX, AND XEROSTOMIA *(Continued)*

PRODUCTS AND DRUGS TO TREAT DRY MOUTH *(continued)*

Medication	Manufacturer and Phone Number	Product Type	Manufacturer's Description	Indication	Ingredients	Directions for Use	Form and Availability
Biotene® OralBalance® Mouth Moisturizing Gel	Laclede Professional Products, Inc (800) 922-5856	Gel	Sugar-free oral lubricant; relieves dry mouth symptoms up to 8 hours; soothes and protects oral tissue to promote healing; helps to inhibit harmful bacteria; improves retention under dentures	Relieves symptoms of dry mouth: burning, itching, cotton palate, sore tissue swallowing difficulties	Contains the "Biotene®" protective salivary enzyme system Active: Glucose oxidase (2000 units), lactoperoxidase (3000 units), lysozyme (5 mg), lactoferrin (5 mg) Other: Hydrogenated starch, xylitol, hydroxyethyl cellulose, glycerate polyhydrate, aloe vera	Using a clean fingertip, apply a 1" ribbon of gel on tongue; add additional amount of gel on other dry; use as needed	1.4 oz tube; available at mass merchandise stores, food stores, and drugstores
Salivart® Synthetic Saliva, Aqueous Solution	Gebauer Co (800) 321-9348	Aerosol aqueous spray	Oral moisturizer for patients with reduced salivary flow	Replacement therapy for patients complaining of xerostomia	Sodium carboxymethylcellulose, sorbitol, sodium chloride, potassium chloride, calcium chloride dihydrate, magnesium chloride hexahydrate, potassium phosphate dibasic, purified water, nitrogen (propellant)	Spray directly into mouth or throat for 1-2 seconds; use as needed	2.48 fl oz (75 g); available at most drugstores or directly from manufacturer
OTHER DRY MOUTH PRODUCTS (OTC)							
Biotene® Dry Mouth Gum	Laclede Professional Products, Inc (800) 922-9348	Chewing gum	Sugar-free; helps stimulate saliva flow; fights cause/effect of bad breath; reduces plaque	Treats oral dryness	Active: Lactoperoxidase (0.11 Units), glucose oxidase (0.15 Units) Other: Sorbitol, gum base, xylitol, hydrogenated glucose, potassium thiocyanate	Chew 1 or 2 pieces; use as needed	Each package contains 17 pieces; available at drugstores or directly from manufacturer
Biotene® Dry Mouth Toothpaste	Laclede Professional Products, Inc (800) 922-9348	Toothpaste	Reduces harmful bacteria which cause cavities, periodontal disease, and oral infections	Use in place of regular toothpaste for dry mouth	Active: Lactoperoxidase (15,000 Units), glucose oxidase (10,000 Units), lysozyme (16 mg), sodium monofluorophosphate Other: Sorbitol, glycerin, calcium pyrophosphate, hydrated silica, xylitol, isoceteth-20, cellulose gum, flavoring, sodium benzoate, beta-d-glucose, potassium thiocyanate	Use in place of regular toothpaste; rinse toothbrush before applying; brush for 2 minutes; rinse lightly	4.5 oz tube; available at drugstores or directly from manufacturer

PRODUCTS AND DRUGS TO TREAT DRY MOUTH *(continued)*

Medication	Manufacturer and Phone Number	Product Type	Manufacturer's Description	Indication	Ingredients	Directions for Use	Form and Availability
Biotene® Gentle Mouthwash	Laclede Professional Products, Inc (800) 922-9348	Mouthwash	Alcohol-free; strong antibacterial formula neutralizes mouth odors; soothes as it cleans to protect teeth and oral tissue	Treats dry mouth or oral irritations	Lysozyme, lactoferrin, glucose oxidase, lactoperoxidase	Use 15 mL (1 tablespoonful); swish thoroughly for 30 seconds and spit out; for dry throat, sip 1 tablespoonful of mouthwash 2-3 times/day	Available at drugstores or directly from manufacturer
Moi-Stir® Oral Swabsticks	Kingswood Laboratories, Inc (800) 968-7772	Swabsticks	Lubricates and moistens mouth and mucosal area	Lubricates and moistens mouth and mucosal area	Water, sorbitol, sodium carboxymethylcellulose, methylparaben, propylparaben, potassium chloride, sodium chloride, flavoring	Gently swab all intraoral surfaces of mouth, gums, tongue, palate, buccal mucosa, gingival, teeth, and lips where uncomfortable dryness exists	3 swabsticks/packet, 100 packets/case; order directly from manufacturer or from various distributors.
CHOLINERGIC SALIVARY STIMULANTS (Rx)							
Cevimeline (Evoxac®)	Snow Brand Pharmaceuticals (800) 475-6473			Treats symptoms of dry mouth in patients with Sjögren's syndrome	Active: Cevimeline 30 mg Other: Lactose monohydrate, hydroxypropyl cellulose, magnesium stearate	1 capsule (30 mg) 3 times/day	30 mg capsules
Pilocarpine (Salagen®)	MGI Pharmaceuticals, Inc (800) 562-5580			Treats xerostomia caused by radiation therapy in patients with head/neck cancer, Sjögren's syndrome	Active: Pilocarpine 5 mg Other: Carnauba wax, hydroxypropyl methylcellulose, iron oxide, microcrystalline cellulose, stearic acid, titanium dioxide	1-2 tablets (5 mg) 3-4 times/day, not to exceed 30 mg/day	5 mg tablets

DENTIN HYPERSENSITIVITY, HIGH CARIES INDEX, AND XEROSTOMIA *(Continued)*

CHOLINERGIC SALIVARY STIMULANTS (PRESCRIPTION ONLY)

Pilocarpine (Dental)(Salagen® *on page 1081*), approved in 1994, and cevimeline (Evoxac® *on page 292*), approved in 2000, are cholinergic drugs which stimulate salivary flow. They stimulate muscarinic-type acetylcholine receptors in salivary glands within the parasympathetic division of the autonomic nervous system, causing an increase in serous-type saliva. Thus, they are considered cholinergic, muscarinic-type (parasympathomimetic) drugs. Due to significant side effects caused by these drugs, they are available by prescription only.

Pilocarpine (Salagen®) is indicated for the treatment of xerostomia caused by radiation therapy in patients with head and neck cancer and xerostomia in patients suffering from Sjögren's syndrome. The usual adult dosage is 1-2 tablets (5 mg) 3-4 times/day, not to exceed 30 mg/day. Patients should be treated for a minimum of 90 days for optimum effect. The most frequent adverse side effect is perspiration, which occurs in about 30% of patients who use 5 mg 3 times/day. Other adverse effects (in about 10% of patients) are nausea, rhinitis, chills, frequent urination, dizziness, headache, lacrimation, and pharyngitis. Salagen® is contraindicated for patients with uncontrolled asthma and narrow-angle glaucoma.

The salivary-stimulative effects of oral pilocarpine have been documented since the late 1960s and 1970s. Pilocarpine has been documented to overcome xerostomia from different causes. More recent studies confirm its effectiveness in improving salivary flow in patients undergoing irradiation therapy for head and neck cancer. A capstone study by Johnson, et al, reported the effects of pilocarpine in 208 irradiation patients at 39 different treatment sites. Salagen®, at a dose of 5 mg 3 times/day, improved salivation in 44% of patients, compared with 25% in the placebo group. They concluded that treatment with pilocarpine (Salagen®) produced the best overall outcome with respect to saliva production and relief of symptoms of xerostomia in patients undergoing irradiation therapy.

Additional studies have been published showing the effectiveness of pilocarpine (Salagen®) in stimulating salivary flow in patients suffering from Sjögren's syndrome and the FDA has recently approved the use of Salagen® for this indication.

Recent reports suggest that pre-emptive use of pilocarpine may be effective in protecting salivary glands during therapeutic irradiation; further studies are needed to confirm this. As of this publication date, the use of pilocarpine has not been approved to treat xerostomia induced by chronic medication. Pilocarpine could be used as a sialagogue for individuals with xerostomia induced by antidepressants and other medications. However, the potential for serious drug interactions is a concern and more studies are needed to clarify the safety and effectiveness of pilocarpine when given in the presence of other medications.

Cevimeline (Evoxac®) is indicated for treatment of symptoms of dry mouth in patients with Sjögren's syndrome. The usual dosage in adults is 1 capsule (30 mg) 3 times/day. Cevimeline (Evoxac®) is supplied in 30 mg capsules. Some adverse effects reported for Evoxac® include increased sweating (19%), rhinitis (11%), sinusitis (12%), and upper respiratory infection (11%). Evoxac® is contraindicated for patients with uncontrolled asthma, narrow-angle glaucoma, acute iritis, and other conditions where miosis is undesirable.

OTHER DRUGS IMPLICATED IN XEROSTOMIA

>10%	1% to 10%
Alprazolam	Acrivastine and Pseudoephedrine
Amitriptyline hydrochloride	Albuterol
Amoxapine	Amantadine hydrochloride
Anisotropine methylbromide	Amphetamine sulfate
Atropine sulfate	Astemizole (withdrawn from market)
Belladonna and Opium	Azatadine maleate
Benztropine mesylate	Beclomethasone dipropionate
Bupropion	Bepridil hydrochloride
Chlordiazepoxide	Bitolterol mesylate
Clomipramine hydrochloride	Brompheniramine maleate
Clonazepam	Carbinoxamine and Pseudoephedrine
Clonidine	Chlorpheniramine maleate
Clorazepate dipotassium	Clemastine fumarate
Cyclobenzaprine	Clozapine
Desipramine hydrochloride	Cromolyn sodium
Diazepam	Cyproheptadine hydrochloride
Dicyclomine hydrochloride	Dexchlorpheniramine maleate
Diphenoxylate and Atropine	Dextroamphetamine sulfate
Doxepin hydrochloride	Dimenhydrinate
Ergotamine	Diphenhydramine hydrochloride
Estazolam	Disopyramide phosphate
Flavoxate	Doxazosin
Flurazepam hydrochloride	Dronabinol
Glycopyrrolate	Ephedrine sulfate
Guanabenz acetate	Flumazenil
Guanfacine hydrochloride	Fluvoxamine
Hyoscyamine sulfate	Gabapentin
Interferon Alfa-2a	Guaifenesin and Codeine
Interferon Alfa-2b	Guanadrel sulfate
Interferon Alfa-N3	Guanethidine sulfate
Ipratropium bromide	Hydroxyzine
Isoproterenol	Hyoscyamine, Atropine, Scopolamine, and Phenobarbital
Isotretinoin	Imipramine
Loratadine	Isoetharine
Lorazepam	Levocabastine hydrochloride
Loxapine	Levodopa
Maprotiline hydrochloride	Levodopa and Carbidopa
Methscopolamine bromide	Levorphanol tartrate
Molindone hydrochloride	Meclizine hydrochloride
Nabilone	Meperidine hydrochloride
Nefazodone	Methadone hydrochloride
Oxybutynin chloride	Methamphetamine hydrochloride
Oxazepam	Methyldopa
Paroxetine	Metoclopramide
Phenelzine sulfate	Morphine sulfate
Prochlorperazine	Nortriptyline hydrochloride
Propafenone hydrochloride	Ondansetron
Protriptyline hydrochloride	Oxycodone and Acetaminophen
Quazepam	Oxycodone and Aspirin
Reserpine	Pentazocine
Selegiline hydrochloride	Phenylpropanolamine hydrochloride
Temazepam	Prazosin hydrochloride
Thiethylperazine maleate	Promethazine hydrochloride
Trihexyphenidyl hydrochloride	Propoxyphene
Trimipramine maleate	Pseudoephedrine
Venlafaxine	Risperidone
	Sertraline hydrochloride
	Terazosin
	Terbutaline sulfate

TEMPOROMANDIBULAR DYSFUNCTION (TMD)

Temporomandibular dysfunction comprises a broad spectrum of signs and symptoms. Although TMD presents in patterns, diagnosis is often difficult. Evaluation and treatment is time-intensive and no single therapy or drug regimen has been shown to be universally beneficial.

The thorough diagnostician should perform a screening examination for the temporomandibular joint on all patients. Ideally, a baseline maximum mandibular opening along with lateral and protrusive movement evaluation should be performed. Secondly, the joint area should be palpated and an adequate exam of the muscles of mastication and the muscles of the neck and shoulders should be made. These muscle would include the elevators of the mandible (masseter, internal pterygoid, and temporalis); the depressors of the mandible (including the external pterygoid and digastric); extrusive muscles (including the temporalis and digastric), and protrusive muscles (including the external and internal pterygoids). These muscles also account for lateral movement of the mandible. The clinician should also be alert to indicators of dysfunction, primarily a history of pain with jaw function, chronic history of joint noise (although this can often be misinterpreted), pain in the muscles of the neck, limited jaw movement, pain in the actual muscles of mastication, and headache or even earache. The signs and symptoms are extremely variable and the clinician should be alert for any or all of these areas of interest. Because of the complexity of both evaluation and diagnosis, the general dentist often finds it too time consuming to spend the countless hours evaluating and treating the temporomandibular dysfunction patient. Therefore, oral medicine specialists trained in temporomandibular evaluation and treatment often accept referrals for the management of these complicated patients.

The Oral Medicine specialist in TMD management, the physical therapist interested in head and neck pain, and the Oral and Maxillofacial surgeon will all work together with the referring general dentist to accomplish successful patient treatment. Table 1 lists the wide variety of treatment alternatives available to the team. Depending on the diagnosis, one or more of the therapies might be selected. For organic diseases of the joint not responding to nonsurgical approaches, a wide variety of surgical techniques are available (Table 2).

ACUTE TMD

Acute TMD oftentimes presents alone or as an episode during a chronic pattern of signs and symptoms. Trauma, such as a blow to the chin or the side of the face, can result in acute TMD. Occasionally, similar symptoms will follow a lengthy wide open mouth dental procedure.

The condition usually presents as continuous deep pain in the TMJ. If edema is present in the joint, the condyle sometimes can be displaced which will cause abnormal occlusion of the posterior teeth on the affected side. The diagnosis is usually based on the history and clinical presentation. Management of the patient includes:

1. Restriction of all mandibular movement to function in a pain-free range of motion
2. Soft diet
3. NSAIDs (eg, Anaprox® DS 1 tablet every 12 hours for 7-10 days)
4. Moist heat applications to the affected area for 15-20 minutes, 4-6 times/day
5. Consideration of a muscle relaxant, such as Methocarbamol (Robaxin®) *on page 881*, adult patient of average height/weight, two (500 mg) tablets at bedtime; daytime dose can be tailored to patient

Additional therapies could include referral to a physical therapist for ultrasound therapy 2-4 times/week and a single injection of steroid in the joint space. A team approach with an oral maxillofacial surgeon for this procedure may be helpful. Spray and stretch with Fluori-methane® is often helpful for rapid relief of trismus.

Dichlorodifluoromethane and Trichloromonofluoromethane *on page 428*

CHRONIC TMD

Following diagnosis which is often problematic, the most common therapeutic modalities include:

- Explaining the problem to the patient
- Recommending a soft diet:
  - diet should consist of soft foods (eg, eggs, yogurt, casseroles, soup, ground meat)
  - avoid chewing gum, salads, large sandwiches, and hard fruit
- Reducing stress; moist heat application 4-6 times/day for 15-20 minutes coupled with a monitored exercise program will be beneficial. Usually, working with a physical therapist is ideal.
- Medications include analgesics, anti-inflammatories, tranquilizers, and muscle relaxants

MEDICATION OPTIONS

Most commonly used medication (NSAIDs)

Choline Magnesium Trisalicylate *on page 319*
Choline Salicylate *on page 319*
Diclofenac *on page 429*
Diflunisal *on page 438*
Etodolac *on page 547*
Fenoprofen *on page 563*
Flurbiprofen *on page 596*
Ibuprofen *on page 703*
Indomethacin *on page 719*
Ketoprofen *on page 763*
Ketorolac *on page 765*
Magnesium Salicylate *on page 837*
Meclofenamate *on page 848*
Mefenamic Acid *on page 851*
Nabumetone *on page 941*
Naproxen *on page 953*
Oxaprozin *on page 1010*
Piroxicam *on page 1090*
Salsalate *on page 1206*
Sulindac *on page 1257*
Tolmetin *on page 1321*

Tranquilizers and muscle relaxants, when used appropriately, can provide excellent adjunctive therapy. These drugs should be primarily used for a short period of time to manage acute pain. In low dosages, amitriptyline is often used to treat chronic pain and occasionally migraine headache. Two new drugs similar to the prototype drug, amitriptyline, have recently been approved for use in adults only, for treatment of acute migraine with or without aura: Almotriptan malate (Axert™ [tablets]; Pharmacia Corp) and frovatriptan succinate (Frova™ [tablets]; Elan). Selective serotonin reuptake inhibitors (SSRIs) are sometimes used in the management of chronic neuropathic pain, particularly in patients not responding to amitriptyline. Recently, gabapentin (Neurontin®) has been approved for chronic pain. Problems of inducing bruxism with SSRIs, however, have been reported and may preclude their use. Clinicians attempting to evaluate any patient with bruxism or involuntary muscle movement, who is simultaneously being treated with an SSRI, should be aware of this potential association.

See individual monographs for dosing instructions.

Common minor tranquilizers include:

Alprazolam *on page 61*
Diazepam *on page 424*
Lorazepam *on page 824*

Chronic neuropathic pain management:

Amitriptyline *on page 83*
Carbamazepine *on page 241*
Gabapentin *on page 624*

Acute migraine management:

Almotriptan *on page 59*
Frovatriptan *on page 620*
Rizatriptan *on page 1193*

TEMPOROMANDIBULAR DYSFUNCTION (TMD) *(Continued)*

Common muscle relaxants include:

Chlorzoxazone *on page 316*

Cyclobenzaprine *on page 379*

Methocarbamol *on page 881*

Orphenadrine *on page 1005*

Note: Muscle relaxants and tranquilizers should generally be prescribed with an analgesic or NSAID to relieve pain as well.

Narcotic analgesics can be used on a short-term basis or intermittently in combination with non-narcotic therapy in the chronic pain patient. Judicious prescribing, monitoring, and maintenance by the practitioner is imperative whenever considering the use of narcotic analgesics due to the abuse and addiction liabilities.

Table 1.
TMD - NONSURGICAL THERAPIES

1. Moist heat and cold spray
2. Injections in muscle trigger areas (procaine)
3. Exercises (passive, active)
4. Medications
   a. Muscle relaxants
   b. Minerals
   c. Multiple vitamins (Ca, B_6, B_{12})
5. Orthopedic craniomandibular repositioning appliance (splints)
6. Biofeedback, acupuncture
7. Physiotherapy: TMJ muscle therapy
8. Myofunctional therapy
9. TENS (transcutaneous electrical neural stimulation), Myo-Monitor
10. Dental therapy
    a. Equilibration (coronoplasty)
    b. Restoring occlusion to proper vertical dimension of maxilla to mandible by orthodontics, dental restorative procedures, orthognathic surgery, permanent splint, or any combination of these

Table 2.
TMD - SURGICAL THERAPIES

1. Cortisone injection into joint (with local anesthetic)
2. Bony and/or fibrous ankylosis: requires surgery (osteoarthrotomy with prosthetic appliance)
3. Chronic subluxation: requires surgery, depending on problem (possibly eminectomy and/or prosthetic implant)
4. Osteoarthritis: requires surgery, depending on problem
   a. Arthroplasty with implant
   b. Meniscectomy with implant
   c. Arthroplasty with repair of disc and/or implant
   d. Implant with Silastic insert
5. Rheumatoid arthritis
   a. Arthroplasty with implant with Silastic insert
   b. "Total" TMJ replacement
6. Tumors: require osteoarthrotomy — removal of tumor and restoring of joint when possible
7. Chronic disc displacement: requires repair of disc and possible removal of bone from condyle

PATIENTS REQUIRING SEDATION

Anxiety constitutes the most frequently found psychiatric problem in the general population. Anxiety can range from simple phobias to severe debilitating anxiety disorders. Functional results of this anxiety can, therefore, range from simple avoidance of dental procedures to panic attacks when confronting stressful situations such as seen in some patients regarding dental visits. Many patients claim to be anxious over dental care when in reality they simply have not been managed with modern techniques of local anesthesia, the availability of sedation, or the caring dental practitioner.

The dentist may detect anxiety in patients during the treatment planning evaluation phase of the care. The anxious person may appear overly alert, may lean forward in the dental chair during conversation or may appear concerned over time, possibly using this as a guise to require that they cut short their dental visit. Anxious persons may also show signs of being nervous by demonstrating sweating, tension in their muscles including their temporomandibular musculature, or they may complain of being tired due to an inability to obtain an adequate night's sleep.

The management of such patients requires a methodical approach to relaxing the patient, discussing their dental needs, and then planning, along with the patient the best way to accomplish dental treatment in the presence of their fears, both real or imagined. Consideration may be given to sedation to assist with managing the patient. This sedation can be oral or parenteral, or inhalation in the case of nitrous oxide. The dentist must be adequately trained in administering the sedative of choice, as well as in monitoring the patient during the sedated procedures. Numerous medications are available to achieve the level of sedation usually necessary in the dental office: Valium®, Ativan®, Xanax®, Vistaril®, Serax®, and BuSpar® represent a few. BuSpar® is soon to be available as a transdermal patch. These oral sedatives can be given prior to dental visits as outlined in the following prescriptions. They have the advantage of allowing the patient a good night's sleep prior to the day of the procedures and providing on-the-spot sedation during the procedures. Nitrous oxide represents an in the office administered sedative that is relatively safe, but requires additional training and carefully planned monitoring protocols of any auxiliary personnel during the inhalation procedures. Both the oral and the inhalation techniques can, however, be applied in a very useful manner to manage the anxious patient in the dental office.

Alprazolam *on page 61*

Buspirone *on page 211*

Diazepam *on page 424*

Hydroxyzine *on page 697*

Lorazepam *on page 824*

Nitrous Oxide *on page 983*

Oxazepam *on page 1011*

Triazolam *on page 1345*

Note: Although various sedatives have been used for preprocedure sedation, no specific regimens or protocols have been established. Guidelines for use are still under study.

Fluoxetine *on page 589*

Fluvoxamine *on page 605*

Paroxetine *on page 1036*

Sertraline *on page 1216*

PRESCRIPTION EXAMPLES

Rx

Valium® 5 mg*

Disp: 6 tablets

Sig: Take 1 tablet in evening before going to bed and 1 tablet 1 hour before appointment

Ingredient: Diazepam

***Note:** Also available as 2 mg and 10 mg

PATIENTS REQUIRING SEDATION *(Continued)*

Rx

Ativan® 1 mg*

Disp: 4 tablets

Sig: Take 2 tablets in evening before going to bed and 2 tablets 1 hour before appointment

Ingredient: Lorazepam

***Note:** Also available as 0.5 mg and 2 mg

Rx

Xanax® 0.5 mg

Disp: 4 tablets

Sig: Take 1 tablet in evening before going to bed and 1 tablet 1 hour before appointment

Ingredient: Alprazolam

Rx

Vistaril® 25 mg

Disp: 16 capsules

Sig: Take 2 capsules in evening before going to bed and 2 capsules 1 hour before appointment

Ingredient: Hydroxyzine

Rx

Halcion® 0.25 mg

Disp: 4 tablets

Sig: Take 1 tablet in evening before going to bed and 1 tablet 1 hour before appointment

Ingredient: Triazolam

Rx

Serax® 10 mg

Disp: 2 capsules

Sig: Take 1 capsule before bed and 1 capsule 30 minutes before appointment.

Ingredient: Oxazepam

MANAGEMENT OF PATIENTS UNDERGOING CANCER THERAPY

CANCER PATIENT DENTAL PROTOCOL

The objective in treatment of a patient with cancer is eradication of the disease. Oral complications, such as mucosal ulceration, xerostomia, bleeding, and infections can cause significant morbidity and may compromise systemic treatment of the patient. With proper oral evaluation before systemic treatment, many of the complications can be minimized or prevented.

MUCOSITIS

Normal oral mucosa acts as a barrier against chemical and food irritants and oral microorganisms. Disruption of the mucosal barrier can therefore lead to secondary infection, increased pain, delayed healing, and decreased nutritional intake.

Mucositis is inflammation of the mucous membranes. It is a common reaction to chemotherapy and radiation therapy. It is first seen as an erythematous patch. The mucosal epithelium becomes thin as a result of the killing of the rapidly dividing basal layer mucosal cells. Seven to ten days after cytoreduction chemotherapy and between 1000 cGy and 3000 cGy of radiation to the head and neck, mucosal tissues begin to desquamate and eventually develop into frank ulcerations. The mucosal integrity is broken and is secondarily infected by normal oral flora. The resultant ulcerations can also act as a portal of entry for pathogenic organisms into the patient's bloodstream and may lead to systemic infections. These ulcerations often force interruption of therapy.

Certain chemotherapeutic agents, such as 5-fluorouracil, methotrexate, and doxorubicin, are more commonly associated with the development of oral mucositis. Treatment of oral mucositis is mainly palliative, but steps should be taken to minimize secondary pathogenic infections. Culture and sensitivity data should be obtained to select appropriate therapy for the bacterial, viral, or fungal organisms found.

Prevention of radiation mucositis is difficult. Stents can be constructed to prevent irradiation of uninvolved tissues. The use of multiple ports and fractionation of therapy into smaller doses over a longer period of time can reduce the severity. Fractured restorations, sharp teeth, and ill-fitted prostheses can damage soft tissues and lead to additional interruption of mucosal barriers. Correction of these problems before radiation therapy can diminish these complications.

CHEMOTHERAPY

Chemotherapy for neoplasia also frequently results in oral complications. Infections and mucositis are the most common complications seen in patients receiving chemotherapy. Also occurring frequently are pain, altered nutrition, and xerostomia, which can significantly affect the quality of life.

RADIATION CARIES

Dental caries that sometimes follows radiation therapy is called radiation caries. It usually develops in the cervical region of the teeth adjacent to the gingiva, often affecting many teeth. It is secondary to the damage done to the salivary glands and is initiated by dental plaque, but its rapid progress is due to changes in saliva. In addition to the diminution in the amount of saliva, both the salivary pH and buffering capacity are diminished, which decreases anticaries activity of saliva. Oral bacteria also change with xerostomia leading to the increase in caries activity.

SALIVARY CHANGES

Chemotherapy is not thought to directly alter salivary flow, but alterations in taste and subjective sensations of dry mouth are relatively common complaints. Patients with mucositis and graft-vs-host disease following bone marrow or stem cell transplantation often demonstrate signs and symptoms of xerostomia. Radiation does directly affect salivary production. Radiation to the salivary glands produces fibrosis and alters the production of saliva. If all the major salivary glands are in the field, the decrease in saliva can be dramatic and the serous portion of the glands seems to be most severely affected. The saliva produced is increased in viscosity, which contributes to food retention and increased plaque formation. These xerostomic patients have difficulty in managing a normal diet. Normal saliva also has bacteriostatic properties that are diminished in these patients.

The dental management recommendations for patients undergoing chemotherapy, bone marrow transplantation, and/or radiation therapy for the treatment of cancer are based primarily on clinical observations. The following protocols will provide a conservative, consistent approach to the dental management of patients undergoing chemotherapy or bone marrow transplantation. Many of the cancer chemotherapy drugs produce oral side effects including mucositis, oral ulceration, dry mouth, acute infections, and taste aberrations. Cancer drugs include antibiotics, alkylating agents, antimetabolites, DNA inhibitors, hormones, and cytokines.

MANAGEMENT OF PATIENTS UNDERGOING CANCER THERAPY *(Continued)*

All patients undergoing chemotherapy or bone marrow transplantation for malignant disease should have the following baseline:

A. Panoramic radiograph

B. Dental consultation and examination

C. Dental prophylaxis and cleaning (if the neutrophil count is >1500/mm^3 and the platelet count is >50,000/mm^3)

- Prophylaxis and cleaning will be deferred if the patient's neutrophil count is <1500 and the platelet count is <50,000. Oral hygiene recommendations will be made. These levels are arbitrary guidelines and the dentist should consider the patient's oral condition and planned procedure relative to hemorrhage and level of bacteremia.

D. Oral Hygiene: Patients should be encouraged to follow normal hygiene procedures. Addition of a chlorhexidine mouth rinse such as Peridex® or PerioGard® *on page 300* is usually helpful. If the patient develops oral mucositis, tolerance of such alcohol-based products may be limited.

E. If the patient develops mucositis, bacterial, viral, and fungal cultures should be obtained. Sucralfate suspension in either a pharmacy-prepared form or Carafate® suspension, as well as Benadryl® *on page 451* or Xylocaine® viscous *on page 801* can assist in helping the patient to tolerate food. Patients may also require systemic analgesics for pain relief depending on the presence of mucositis. Positive fungal cultures may require a nystatin swish-and-swallow prescription or the selection of another antifungal agent (see Oral Fungal Infections *on page 1542*).

F. The determination of performing dental procedures must be based on the goal of preventing infection during periods of neutropenia. Timing of procedures must be coordinated with the patient's hematologic status.

G. If oral surgery is required, at least 7-10 days of healing should be allowed before the anticipated date of bone marrow suppression (eg, ANC <1000/mm^3 and/or platelet count of 50,000/mm^3).

H. Daily use of topical fluorides is recommended for those who have received radiation therapy to the head and neck region involving salivary glands. Any patients with prolonged xerostomia subsequent to graft-vs-host disease and/or chemotherapy can also be considered for fluoride supplement. Use the fluoride-containing mouthwashes (Act®, Fluorigard®, etc) each night before going to sleep; swish, hold 1-2 minutes, spit out or use prescription fluorides (gels or rinses); apply daily for 1-4 minutes as directed; if mouth is sore (mucositis), use flavorless/colorless gels (Thera-Flur®, Gel-Kam®). Improvement in salivary flow following radiation therapy to the head and neck has been noted with Salagen® *on page 1080* or Evoxac™ *on page 292*. Custom trays can be produced by the clinician for the patient's home use using heat-formed materials such as omnivac.

Benzonatate *on page 171*
Cevimeline *on page 292*
Chlorhexidine *on page 300*
Diphenhydramine *on page 451*
Lidocaine *on page 801*
Pilocarpine (Dental) *on page 1081*
Povidone-Iodine *on page 1104*
Sucralfate *on page 1247*

PRESCRIPTION EXAMPLES

Rx

Peridex® or PerioGard® oral rinse

Disp: 3 bottles

Sig: 20 mL for 30 seconds 3 times/day; swish and expectorate

Ingredient: Chlorhexidine gluconate 0.12% and alcohol 11.6%

Rx

Xylocaine® viscous 2%

Disp: 450 mL bottles

Sig: 1 tablespoonful; swish 4 times/day

Ingredient: Lidocaine

Rx

Betadine® mouthwash

Disp: 6 oz bottle

Sig: 1 tablespoonful, rinse 4 times/day; do not swallow

Ingredient: Povidone iodine 0.8%

Rx

Mycostatin® oral suspension

Disp: 60 mL bottle

Sig: 2 mL 4 times/day; hold in mouth for 2 minutes and swallow

Ingredient: Nystatin 100,000 units/mL

Note: When the oral mucous membranes are especially sensitive, nystatin "popsicles" can be made by adding 2 mL of nystatin oral suspension to the water in ice cube trays.

Rx

Tessalon Perles®

Disp: 50

Sig: Squeeze contents of capsule and apply to lesion

Ingredient: Benzonatate

Note: Tessalon Perles® have been used ad lib to provide relief in painful mucositis.

ORAL CARE PRODUCTS

BACTERIAL PLAQUE CONTROL

Patients should use an extra soft bristle toothbrush and dental floss for removal of plaque. Sponge/foam sticks and lemon-glycerine swabs do not adequately remove bacterial plaque.

PRESCRIPTION EXAMPLE

Rx

Ultra Suave® toothbrush

Biotene Supersoft® toothbrush

Note: Chlorhexidine 0.12% (Peridex® or other preparations available in Canada and Europe) may be used to assist with bacterial plaque control.

CHOLINERGIC AGENTS

See Products for Xerostomia *on page 1553*

Used for the treatment of xerostomia caused by radiation therapy in patients with head and neck cancer and from Sjögren's syndrome

Cevimeline *on page 292*
Pilocarpine (Dental) *on page 1081*

FLUORIDES

See Fluorides *on page 1553* in the Dentin Hypersensitivity, High Caries Index, and Xerostomia section.

Used for the prevention of demineralization of the tooth structure secondary to xerostomia. For patients with long-term or permanent xerostomia, daily application is accomplished using custom gel applicator trays, such as omnivac. Patients with porcelain crowns should use a neutral pH fluoride (see Fluoride monograph *on page 586*). Final selection of a fluoride product and/or saliva replacement/stimulant product must be based on patient comfort, taste, and ultimately, compliance. Experience has demonstrated that, often times, patients must try various combinations to achieve the greatest effect and their highest comfort levels. The presence of mucositis during cancer management complicates the clinician's selection of products.

MANAGEMENT OF PATIENTS UNDERGOING CANCER THERAPY *(Continued)*

SALIVA SUBSTITUTES

See Products for Xerostomia *on page 1553*

ORAL AND LIP MOISTURIZERS/LUBRICANTS

See Mouth Pain, Cold Sore, and Canker Sore Products *on page 1630*

Note: Water-based gels should first be used to provide moisture to dry oral tissues.

Surgi-Lube®
K-Y Jelly®
Oral Balance®
Mouth Moisturizer®

PALLIATION OF PAIN

See Mouth Pain, Cold Sore, and Canker Sore Products *on page 1630*

Note: Palliative pain preparations should be monitored for efficacy.

- For relief of pain associated with isolated ulcerations, topical anesthetic and protective preparations may be used.
  - Orabase-B® with 20% benzocaine *on page 169*
- For generalized oral pain:
  - Chloraseptic Spray® (OTC) anesthetic spray without alcohol *on page 1068*
  - Ulcer-Ease® anesthetic/analgesic mouthrinse
  - Xylocaine® 2% viscous *on page 801*
    Note: May anesthetize swallowing mechanism and cause aspiration of food; caution patient against using too close to eating; lack of sensation may also allow patient to damage intact mucosa
  - Tantum Mouthrinse® (benzydamine hydrochloride); may be diluted as required
    Note: Available only in Canada and Europe

PATIENT PREPARED PALLIATIVE MIXTURES

Coating agents:

Maalox® *on page 69*
Mylanta® *on page 69*
Kaopectate® *on page 146*

These products can be mixed with Benadryl® elixir (50:50):

Diphenhydramine (Benadryl®) *on page 451*

Mouth Pain, Cold Sore, and Canker Sore Products *on page 1630*

Topical anesthetics (diphenhydramine chloride):

Benadryl® elixir or Benylin® cough syrup *on page 451*

Note: Choose product with lowest alcohol and sucrose content; ask pharmacist for assistance

PHARMACY PREPARATIONS

A pharmacist may also prepare the following solutions for relief of generalized oral pain:

Benadryl-Lidocaine Solution

Diphenhydramine injectable 1.5 mL (50 mg/mL) *on page 451*
Xylocaine viscous 2% (45 mL) *on page 801*
Magnesium aluminum hydroxide solution (45 mL)

Swish and hold 1 teaspoonful in mouth for 30 seconds; do not use too close to eating

Rx

Carafate suspension 1 g/10 mL

Disp: 420 mL

Sig: 1 teaspoonful; swish and hold in mouth for 30 seconds

Ingredient: Sucralfate

ORAL MEDICINE TOPICS

PART III:
OTHER ORAL MEDICINE TOPICS

TABLE OF CONTENTS

Dentist's Role in Recognizing Domestic Violence 1572

Chemical Dependency and Smoking Cessation 1574

Animal and Human Bites Guidelines 1580

Dental Office Emergencies 1582

Suggested Readings 1587

DENTIST'S ROLE IN RECOGNIZING DOMESTIC VIOLENCE

Recognition of the signs and symptoms of domestic violence is becoming an important topic for dental and medical professionals throughout the world. Unfortunately, statistics related to domestic abuse of women and children appear to be on the rise, perhaps, in part, due to this increased recognition.

Some statistics are indeed staggering. In the United States, a woman or child is physically abused every five to fifteen seconds. In fact, violence is cited as one of the common causes of emergency room admissions for women 15-44 years of age. Furthermore, 50,000 deaths occur annually, which are attributable to violence in the form of homicide or suicide.

The dentist is in a unique position to recognize many of the signs and symptoms of domestic violence, including child abuse and neglect. The dentist's responsibilities and professional role in this arena are not clear in all states. However, each professional has the responsibility to understand the current state laws regarding the reporting of domestic violence, child abuse, and/or neglect within his/her state. Many states have existing codes defining the role of the professional in these regards. The overall problem of domestic violence, including child abuse, neglect, and other forms of abuse are indeed public health issues. The costs of domestic violence, such as medical, dental, psychiatric, hospital, and emergency care fees are borne to a great extent by the community in addition to the individual.

Domestic abuse is defined as "controlling behavior." Although this often includes physical injury, the primary focus of domestic abuse is one person being in control of another person, making that person do something against his/her will. Women are often abused both physically and mentally in relationships that have existed for many years. Children are often the focus of domestic violence; however, the pattern for an entire family's abuse may be present. Abuse comes in many forms and many victims do not even realize that abuse is occurring. Some victims simply "chalk it up" to things that happen within families. Abuse can include the following: battery and physical assault, such as throwing objects, pushing, hitting, slapping, kicking, or attacking with a weapon; sexual assault including the abuser forcing sexual activities upon another; and, psychological abuse, such as forcing a victim to perform degrading or humiliating acts, threatening harm to a female or male partner or child, or destroying valued possessions of another. Verbal abuse can also be included; however, the psychological forms of abuse are very difficult to ascertain and the signs and symptoms may be difficult to separate from other psychological traits. Abuse tends to have a cyclic pattern, often where a partner, or the controlling individual within the domestic situation, is extremely friendly, intimate, and a good household member. However, due to unknown reasons, as tension develops, family violence often erupts. Once battering has begun, it often increases in frequency and in severity with time. Early recognition by those around the domestic situation can often prevent serious effects. However, until physical violence becomes part of the domestic abuse situation, recognition is usually difficult.

Since nearly 65% of abuse cases (where physical injury is involved) involve injury to the head, neck, or mouth, dental professionals are in a unique position to detect and perhaps, if appropriate in their state, report suspected abuse. In children, these percentages are even higher. Much of our information and beliefs about domestic abuse stem from our knowledge regarding the dental professional in the arena of child abuse and neglect. Being wards of adults, children are vulnerable. Child abuse includes any act that is nonaccidental, endangering or impairing a child's safety or emotional health. Types of child abuse would include physical abuse, emotional abuse and neglect, including health care neglect. Any child suffering from an emotional injury, including sexual abuse or neglect, should be brought to the attention of the social welfare system. Occasionally, "Munchausen syndrome," which is defined as the guardians fabricating or inducing illness in the child, can be observed. Intentional poisoning and safety neglect are also included.

From a medical point-of-view, neglect is much more difficult to determine than abuse. The role of the dentist may be in defining the state of normal and customary pediatric health within a locality. However, due to parents and families moving about the country, sometimes one standard may not be appropriate for all locations.

To detect abuse, or to detect domestic patterns of abuse in the family, the medical or dental professional must be aware of several key behavioral indicators: when the child or adult in question avoids eye contact, is wary of their guardian or spouse, demonstrates fear of touch, or dramatic mood changes. Reports of any history of suicide attempts or running away would also be indicators. Any unexplained injury or injuries that are inconsistent with explanation, including delays in seeking care for such an injury, could represent an abusive situation. The guardian or spouse may also give specific indicators. When it is determined that they cannot explain the injury or that the explanation offered is inconsistent or changes, abuse may be suspected. Nonspecific indicators might include hostile or aggressive behavior or if the queried individual wants to go to a different practitioner when the questioning becomes too intense.

The principles of head-neck examination for the dentist are important and include gathering an overall visual impression of general cleanliness, dress, and stature and examining for any specific physical indicators such as bruises, welts, bite marks, abrasions, lacerations, or other injuries to the head or neck. Contusions or bruises represent the highest percentage of abuse injuries to the young child. The extremely young child or infant often suffers fractures, which fall to second place in terms of incidence as the child matures. In the adult, fractures are much less common. The dentist needs to document the location since often this represents the characteristic that may be difficult for the person to explain. Common areas for injuries include the bony eminences over the knees, shins, and elbows, but could also be on the face, including the zygomatic arch and the chin. Burns are more rare but represent one of the most serious types of injuries. Intraoral injuries including trauma to the oral mucosa, tooth fractures, palatal lesions, ecchymoses, and fractures represent serious evidence of domestic or child abuse. Physical indicators of sexual abuse may not be obvious to the dentist, however, bruising of the hard palate or other evidence of sexual dysfunction may sometimes be found.

The dentist has the responsibility to document from a forensic point-of-view the characteristics that are observed. If necessary, evidence including impressions for bite marks or photographs to document unexplained injuries to the head, neck, and face may be necessary. The legal liability for the dentist is determined by the state laws governing the dental practice. The dental practitioner's failure to diagnose child abuse and neglect is another consideration which goes along with ethical and legal considerations. In the area of child abuse, the states are generally much more clear than they are regarding spousal abuse or overall domestic violence. The dentist has a responsibility to refer a patient for a second opinion if there are concerns that abuse is taking place. Unfortunately, there is no uniformity in the state laws regarding either the responsibility for reporting adult domestic violence or abuse, nor is there uniformity in protecting the health professional by reporting, in good faith, abuse situations. When spousal abuse or other domestic violence is suspected, the definitions become even less clear. They are very similar in ambiguity to those that are faced by the professional regarding neglect as opposed to direct physical or mental abuse. The American Dental Association code is clear on principles and ethics regarding professional conduct regarding the responsibility for recognition of child abuse. They are much less clear on spousal or other abuse and it is likely that in the future as some consistency is noted between and among the various state laws, the ADA Council will undoubtedly take a position.

It is clearly up to the individual states to take the lead in establishing strict guidelines for recognition and reporting of domestic abuse, including protection under the "good faith" statutes for the practitioner. Rules and regulations regarding malicious reporting should also be better defined by the states. The national position is difficult to define because of the extreme variation among states. Dentists are encouraged to use their best judgement in proceeding in any situation of domestic abuse. They should primarily know their state laws and join in the discussion of the topic so that appropriate state actions and formation of legal codes can be undertaken.

CHEMICAL DEPENDENCY AND SMOKING CESSATION

INTRODUCTION

As long as history has been recorded, every society has used drugs that alter mood, thought, and feeling. In addition, pharmacological advances sometimes have been paralleled by physical as well as unfortunate behavioral dependence on agents initially consumed for therapeutic purposes.

In 1986, the American Dental Association passed a policy statement recognizing chemical dependency as a disease. In recognizing this disease, the Association mandated that dentists have a responsibility to include questions relating to a history of chemical dependency, or more broadly, substance abused in their health history questionnaire. A positive response may require the dentist to alter the treatment plan for the patient's dental care. This includes patients who are actively abusing alcohol, drugs, or patients who are in recovery. The use and abuse of drugs is not a topic that is usually found in the dental curriculum. Information about substance abuse is usually gleaned from newspapers, magazines, or just hearsay.

This chapter reviews street drugs, where they come from, signs and symptoms of the drug abuser, and some of the dental implications of treating patients actively using or in recovery from these substances. There are many books devoted to this topic that provide greater detail. The intent is to provide an overview of some of the most prevalent drugs, how patients abusing these drugs may influence dental treatment, and how to recognize some signs and symptoms of use and withdrawal.

Street drugs, like other drugs, can come from various sources. They may be derived from natural sources (ie, morphine and codeine). They may be semisynthetic, that is a natural product is chemically modified to produce another molecule (ie, morphine conversion to heroin). Street drugs may also be synthetic with no natural origin.

BENZODIAZEPINES AND OTHER NONALCOHOL SEDATIVES

Benzodiazepines are the most commonly prescribed drugs worldwide. These drugs are used mainly for treatment of anxiety disorders and, in some instances, insomnia. Even though they are used in high quantities throughout the world, intentional abuse is not that common. These drugs, however, have the ability to induce a strong physical dependency on the use of the medication. As tolerance builds up to the drug, the physical dependency increases dramatically. Unlike street drugs, where addiction is a primary consideration, the overuse of benzodiazepine lies in their ability to induce physical dependency. When these drugs are taken for several weeks, there is relatively little tolerance induced. However, after several months, the proportion of patients who become tolerant increases and reducing the dose or stopping the medication produces severe withdrawal symptoms.

Benzodiazepine Withdrawal Symptoms	
Craving for benzodiazepines	Irritability
Anxiety	Sleep disturbances

It is extremely difficult for the physician to distinguish between the withdrawal symptoms and the reappearance of the myriad anxiety symptoms that cause the drug to be prescribed initially. Many patients increase their dose over time because tolerance develops to at least the sedative effects of the drug. The antianxiety benefits of the benzodiazepines continue to occur long after tolerance to the sedating effects. Patients often take these drugs for many years with relatively few ill effects other than the risk of withdrawal. The dentist should be keenly aware of the signs and symptoms and the historical pattern in patients taking benzodiazepines.

BARBITURATES AND NONBENZODIAZEPINE SEDATIVES

The use of barbiturates as sedative medications has declined over the years due to the increased safety and efficacy of benzodiazepines. Abuse problems with barbiturates resemble those with benzodiazepines in many ways. Drugs in this category are frequently prescribed as hypnotics for patients complaining of insomnia. The physician should, therefore, be aware of the problems that can develop when the hypnotic agent is withdrawn. The underlying problem that has lead to the insomnia is not treated directly by the use of barbiturates and the patient seeking a sleep medication may have altered ability to sleep normally because of the medication. The withdrawal symptoms for the barbiturates are similar to the benzodiazepine sedatives.

ALCOHOL

The chronic use of alcohol, as well as that of other sedatives, is associated with the development of depression. The risk of suicide among alcoholics is one of the highest of any diagnostic category. Cognitive deficits have been reported in alcoholics tested while sober. These deficits usually improve after weeks to months of abstinence. More severe recent memory impairment is associated with specific brain damage caused by nutritional deficiencies common in alcoholics.

Alcohol is toxic to many organ systems. As a result, the medical complications of alcohol abuse and dependence include liver disease, cardiovascular disease, endocrine and gastrointestinal effects, and malnutrition, in addition to CNS dysfunctions. Ethanol readily crosses the placental barrier, producing the *fetal alcohol syndrome*, a major cause of mental retardation.

Alcohol Withdrawal Syndrome Signs and Symptoms	
Alcohol craving	Hypertension
Tremor, irritability	Sweating
Nausea	Perceptual distortion
Sleep disturbance	Seizures (12-48 hours after last drink)
Tachycardia	
Delirium tremens (rare in uncomplicated withdrawal):	
Severe agitation	Tachycardia
Confusion	Nausea, diarrhea
Visual hallucinations	Dilated pupils
Fever, profuse sweating	

NICOTINE

Cigarette (nicotine) addiction is influenced by multiple variables. Nicotine itself produces reinforcement; users compare nicotine to stimulants such as cocaine or amphetamine, although its effects are of lower magnitude.

Nicotine is absorbed readily through the skin, mucous membranes, and of course, through the lungs. The pulmonary route produces discernible central nervous system effects in as little as 7 seconds. Thus, each puff produces some discrete reinforcement. With 10 puffs per cigarette, the 1 pack per day smoker reinforces the habit 200 times daily. The timing, setting, situation, and preparation all become associated repetitively with the effects of nicotine.

Nicotine has both stimulant and depressant actions. The smoker feels alert, yet there is some muscle relaxation. Nicotine activates the nucleus accumbens reward system in the brain. Increased extracellular dopamine has been found in this region after nicotine injections in rats. Nicotine affects other systems as well, including the release of endogenous opioids and glucocorticoids.

Nicotine Withdrawal Syndrome Signs and Symptoms	
Irritability, impatience, hostility	Restlessness
Anxiety	Decreased heart rate
Dysphoric or depressed mood	Increased appetite or weight gain
Difficulty concentrating	

Medications to assist users in breaking a nicotine habit:

Bupropion *on page 209*

Nicotine *on page 971*

SMOKING CESSATION PRODUCTS

Several years ago, the journal, *Science*, stated that approximately 80% of smokers say they want to quit, but each year <1 in 10 actually succeed. Nicotine transdermal delivery preparations (or nicotine patches) were approved by the U.S. Food and Drug Administration in 1992 as aids to smoking cessation for the relief of nicotine withdrawal symptoms. Four preparations were approved simultaneously: Habitrol®, Nicoderm®, Nicotrol®, and ProStep®. These products differ in how much nicotine is released and whether they provide a 24- or 16-hour release time.

Studies are still being reported on the effectiveness of nicotine patches on smoking cessation. Most previous studies had good entry criteria including definition of the Fagerstrom score. Dr Fred Cowan of Oregon Health Sciences University described these Fagerstrom criteria in a previous report on nicotine substitutes in AGD *Impact*. Abstinence of smoking cessation has usually been assessed by self-report, measurement of carbon monoxide in breath, and plasma or urine nicotine products.

In numerous protocols, percentages of study subjects who abstained from smoking after 3-10 weeks of patch treatment with nicotine compared to placebo, have never exceeded 40%. After the initial assessment, six studies continued to follow the study subjects through 24-52 weeks of patch treatment. The results were even poorer with <25%

CHEMICAL DEPENDENCY AND SMOKING CESSATION *(Continued)*

sustained success. A review of these and additional studies, reveals some general conclusions regarding the effectiveness of nicotine patches in smoking cessation. In every study, many smokers abstained after treatment with placebo patches; nicotine treatment was initially more effective than placebo; and improved abstinence rates were more marked in the short term (10 weeks) than in the long term (52 weeks). Subjects undergoing smoking cessation trials tended to gain weight irrespective of whether placebo or nicotine patches were worn. Patients often favor the nicotine polacrilex gum (Nicorette®) which releases nicotine into the blood stream via the oral mucosa.

Data are now available from smoking cessation studies carried out in general medical practices. The effectiveness of nicotine patch substitution under these conditions is similar to the results described above. Most patch systems and gum are now available as over-the-counter products; only Habitrol® remains prescription. Practitioners and patients should remain skeptical since these aids appear to work best only when supplemented with psychological counseling and a single-minded effort on the part of the patient. New products (eg, Zyban®) are now also being marketed as smoking cessation aids. These drugs are norepinephrine serotonin reuptake inhibitors and their action directly affects the craving for tobacco.

OPIATES

The opiates are most often called narcotics. The most common opiate found on the street is heroin. Heroin is the diacetyl derivative of morphine which is extracted from opium. Although commercial production of morphine involves extraction from the dried opium plant which grows in many parts of the world, some areas still harvest opium by making slits in the unripened seed pod. The pod secretes a white, viscous material which upon contact with the air turns a blackish-brown color. It is this off-white material that is called opium. The opium is then dried and smoked or processed to yield morphine and codeine. Actually, the raw opium contains several chemicals that are used medicinally or commercially. Much (approximately 50%) of morphine is converted chemically into heroin which finds its way into the United States and then on the street. Heroin is a Schedule I drug and as such has no acceptable use in the United States today. In fact, possession is a violation of the Controlled Substances Act of 1970. The majority of the heroin found on the streets is from Southeast Asia and can be as concentrated as 100%.

The heroin user goes through many phases once the drug has been administered. When administered intravenously, the user initially feels a "rush" often described as an "orgasmic rush". This initial feeling is most likely due to the release of histamine resulting in cutaneous vasodilation, itching, and a flushed appearance. Shortly after this "rush" the user becomes euphoric. This euphoric stage often called "stoned" or being "high" lasts approximately 3-4 hours. During this stage, the user is lethargic, slow to react to stimuli, speech is slurred, pain reaction threshold is elevated, he/she exhibits xerostomia, slowed heart rate, and the pupils may be constricted. Following the "high", the abuser is "straight" for about 2 hours, with no tell-tale signs of abuse. Approximately 6-8 hours following the last injection of heroin, the user begins to experience a runny nose, lacrimation, and abdominal muscle cramps as he/she begins the withdrawal from the drug. During this stage and the one that follows, the person may become agitated as he/she develops anxiety about where the next "hit" will come from. The withdrawal signs and symptoms become more intense. For the next 3 days, the abuser begins to sweat profusely in combination with cutaneous vasoconstriction. The skin becomes cold and clammy, hence the term "cold turkey". Tachycardia, pupillary dilation, diarrhea, and salivation occur for 3 days following the last injection. Withdrawal signs and symptoms may last longer than the average of 3 days or they may be more abrupt.

Opioid Withdrawal Signs and Symptoms

Symptoms	Signs
Regular Withdrawal	
Craving for opioids	Pupillary dilation
Restlessness, irritability	Sweating
Increased sensitivity to pain	Piloerection ("gooseflesh")
Nausea, cramps	Tachycardia
Muscle aches	Vomiting, diarrhea
Dysphoric mood	Increased blood pressure
Insomnia, anxiety	Yawning
	Fever
Protracted Withdrawal	
Anxiety	Cyclic changes in weight, pupil size, respiratory center sensitivity
Insomnia	
Drug craving	

Many patients who have been abusing opiates for any length of time will exhibit multiple carious lesions, particularly class V lesions. This increased caries rate is probably a result of the heroin-induced xerostomia, high intake of sweets, and lack of daily oral hygiene. Patients who are recovering from heroin or any opiate addiction should not be given any kind of opiate analgesic, whether it be for sedation or as a postoperative analgesic because of the increased chance of relapse. The nonsteroidal anti-inflammatory drugs (NSAIDs) should be used to control any postoperative discomfort. Patients who admit to a past history of intravenous heroin use, or any intravenous drug for that matter, are at higher risk for subacute bacterial endocarditis (SBE), HIV disease, and hepatitis but with the exception of postoperative analgesia should present no special problem for dental care.

OxyContin®, a synthetic opiate, has gained popularity as a street drug in recent years. The drug manufacturer has tried to salvage its name, however, OxyContin® is one of the most widely abused pain medications in use today. It is an excellent analgesic, widely used and is, therefore, available for abuse potential. As with the other opiates, clinical signs and symptoms that the dentist should recognize are consistent with opiate addiction and usage.

MARIJUANA

The number one most abused illegal drug by high school students today is marijuana. Marijuana is a plant that grows throughout the world, but is particularly suited for a warm, humid environment. There are three species of plant but the two most frequently cited are *Cannabis sativa* and *Cannabis indica*. All species possess a female and male plant. Although approximately 450 chemicals have been isolated from the plant, the major psychoactive ingredient is delta-9-tetrahydrocannabinol (THC). Of these 450 chemicals, there are approximately 23 psychoactive chemicals, THC being the most abundant. The highest concentration of THC is found in the bud of the female plant. The concentration of THC varies according to growing conditions and location on the plant but has increased from approximately 2% to 3% in marijuana sold in the 1950s to approximately 30% sold on the streets today. Marijuana can be smoked in cigarettes (joints), pipes, water pipes (bongs), or baked in brownies, cakes, etc, and then ingested. However, smoking marijuana is more efficient and the "high" has a quicker onset. Marijuana is a Schedule I drug but has been promoted as a medicinal for the treatment of glaucoma, for increasing appetite in patients who have HIV disease, and to prevent the nausea associated with cancer chemotherapy. In response to this request, the FDA approved dronabinol (Marinol®), a synthetic THC and placed this drug in Schedule II to be prescribed by physicians for the indicated medical conditions.

Dronabinol *on page 480*

An individual under the influence of marijuana may exhibit no signs or symptoms of intoxication. The pharmacologic effects are dose-dependent and depend to a large extent on the set and setting of the intoxicated individual. As the dose of THC increases, the person experiences euphoria or a state of well-being, often referred to as "mellowing out". Everything becomes comical, problems disappear, and their appetite for snack foods increases. This is called the "munchies". The marijuana produces time and spatial distortion, which contribute, as the dose increases, to a dysphoria characterized by paranoia and fear. Although there has never been a death reported from marijuana overdose, certainly the higher doses may produce such bizarre circumstances as to increase the chances of accidental death. THC is fat soluble. Daily consumption of marijuana will result in THC being stored in body fat which will result in detectable amounts of THC being found in the urine for as long as 60 days in some cases.

Marijuana Withdrawal Syndrome Signs and Symptoms	
Restlessness	Restlessness
Irritability	Sleep EEG disturbance
Mild agitation	Nausea, cramping
Insomnia	

Because of anxiety associated with dental visits, marijuana would be the most likely drug, after alcohol, to be used when coming to the dental office. But, unlike alcohol, marijuana may not produce any detectable odor on the breath nor signs of intoxication. Fortunately, local anesthetics, analgesics, and antibiotics used by the general dentist do not interact with marijuana. The major concern with the marijuana-intoxicated patient is a failure to follow directions while in the chair, and the inability to follow postoperative instructions.

COCAINE

Cocaine, referred to on the street as "snow", "nose candy", "girl", and many other euphemisms, has created an epidemic. This drug is like no other local anesthetic. Known for about the last 2000 years, cocaine has been used and abused by politicians, scientists, farmers, warriors, and of course, on the street. Cocaine is derived from the leaves of a plant called *Erythroxylon coca* which grows in South America. Ninety percent of the world's supply of cocaine originates in Peru, Bolivia, and Colombia. At last estimate, the United States consumes 75% of the world's supply. The plant grows to a height of

CHEMICAL DEPENDENCY AND SMOKING CESSATION *(Continued)*

approximately 4 feet and produces a red berry. Farmers go through the fields stripping the leaves from the plant three times a year. During the working day, the farmers chew the coca leaves to suppress appetite and fight the fatigue of working the fields. The leaves are transported to a laboratory site where the cocaine is extracted by a process called maceration. It takes approximately 7-8 pounds of leaves to produce 1 ounce of cocaine.

On the streets of the United States, cocaine can be found in two forms – one is the hydrochloride salt which can be "snorted" or dissolved in water and injected intravenously, the other is the free base form which can be smoked and is sometimes referred to as "crack", "rock", or "free base". It is called crack because it cracks or pops when large pieces are smoked. It is called rock because it is hard and difficult to break into smaller pieces. The most popular method of administration of cocaine is "snorting" in which small amounts of cocaine hydrochloride are divided into segments or "lines" and any straw-like device can be used to inhale one or more lines of the cocaine into the nose. Although cocaine does not reach the lungs, enough cocaine is absorbed through nasal mucosa to provide a "high" within 3-5 minutes. Rock or crack, on the other hand, is heated and inhaled from any device available. This form of cocaine does reach the lungs and provides a much faster onset of action as well as a more intense stimulation. There are dangers to the user with any form of cocaine. Undoubtedly, the most dangerous form is the intravenous route.

Cocaine Withdrawal Signs and Symptoms	
Dysphoria, depression	Cocaine craving
Sleepiness, fatigue	Bradycardia

The cocaine user, regardless of how the cocaine was administered, presents a potential life-threatening situation in the dental operatory. The patient under the influence of cocaine could be compared to a car going 100 miles per hour. Blood pressure is elevated and heart rate is likely increased. Use of a local anesthetic with epinephrine in such a patient may result in a medical emergency. Such patients can be identified by jitteriness, irritability, talkativeness, tremors, and short abrupt speech patterns. These same signs and symptoms may also be seen in a normal dental patient with preoperative dental anxiety; therefore, the dentist must be particularly alert to identify the potential cocaine abuser. If a patient is suspected, they should never be given a local anesthetic with vasoconstrictor for fear of exacerbating cocaine-induced sympathetic response. Life-threatening episodes of cardiac arrhythmias and hypertensive crises have been reported when local anesthetic with vasoconstrictor was administered to a patient under the influence of cocaine. No local anesthetic used by any dentist can interfere with, nor test positive for cocaine in any urine testing screen. Therefore, the dentist need not be concerned with any false drug use accusations associated with dental anesthesia.

PSYCHEDELIC AGENTS

Perceptual distortions that include hallucinations, illusions, and disorders of thinking such as paranoia can be produced by toxic doses of many drugs. These phenomena also may be seen during toxic withdrawal from sedatives such as alcohol. There are, however, certain drugs that have as their primary effect the production of perception, thought, or mood disturbances at low doses with minimal effects on memory and orientation. These are commonly called *hallucinogenic drugs*, but their use does not always result in frank hallucinations.

Ecstasy (MDMA) and Phenylethylamines (MDA): MDA and MDMA have stimulant, as well as, psychedelic effects and produce degeneration of serotonergic nerve cells and axons. While nerve degeneration has not been well-demonstrated in human beings, the potential remains. Thus, there is possible neurotoxicity with overuse of these drugs. Ecstasy became popular during the 1980s on college campuses and it is still recommended by some psychotherapists as an aid to the process of therapy, although very little controlled data is available. Acute effects are dose-dependent and include dry mouth, jaw clinching, muscle aches, and tachycardia. At higher doses, effects include agitation, hyperthermia, panic attacks, and visual hallucinations. Frequent, repeated use of psychedelic drugs is unusual and, therefore, tolerance is not commonly seen. However, tolerance does develop to the behavioral effects of various psychedelic drugs, and after numerous doses, the tendency towards behavioral tolerance can be observed.

Lysergic Acid Diethylamide (LSD): LSD is the most potent hallucinogenic drug and produces significant psychedelic effects with a total dose of as little as 25-50 mcg. This drug is over 3000 times more potent than mescaline. It is sold on the illicit market in a variety of forms, as a tablet, capsule, sugar cube, or on blotting paper, a popular contemporary system involving postage stamp-sized papers impregnated with varying doses of LSD (≥50-300 mcg). A majority of street samples sold as LSD actually do contain LSD, while mushrooms and other botanicals sold as sources of psilocybin and other psychedelics have a low probability of containing the advertised hallucinogenics. Adverse effects which may affect treatment include visual and auditory hallucinations, tachycardia, psychosis, fear, tremors, delirium, hyperglycemia, fever, sweating, flushing, euphoria, hypertonia, nausea, vomiting, coma, seizures, tachypnea, and respiratory arrest.

Phencyclidine (PCP): Although PCP is illegal, it is easily manufactured and deserves special mention because of its widespread availability. PCP was originally developed as an anesthetic in the 1950s and later abandoned because of a high frequency of postoperative delirium with hallucinations. It was classed as a dissociative anesthetic because, in the anesthetized state, the patient remains conscious with staring gaze, flat facies, and rigid muscles. It was discovered as a drug of abuse in the 1970s, first in oral form as tablets or capsules, and then in a smoked version, enabling better control over the dose. The white crystal-like powder can also be snorted or injected. Street names include Angel Dust, Elephant Tranquilizers, Hog, Killer Weed, PCP, Peace Pills, and Rocket Fuel. Its pharmacological effects are different from LSD; small amounts act as a stimulant, speeding up body functions. Speech, muscle coordination, and vision are affected; sense of touch and pain are dulled; and body movements are slowed. Effects include increased heart rate and blood pressure, flushing, sweating, dizziness, and numbness. With large doses, effects include drowsiness, convulsions, coma, and may also cause death from repeated convulsions, heart and lung failure, or ruptured blood vessels in the brain.

INHALANTS

Anesthetic gases such as nitrous oxide or halothane are sometimes used as intoxicants by medical personnel. Nitrous oxide also is abused by food service employees because it is supplied for use as a propellant in disposable aluminum minitanks for whipping cream canisters. Nitrous oxide produces euphoria and analgesia and then loss of consciousness. Compulsive use and chronic toxicity rarely are reported, but there are obvious risks of overdose associated with the abuse of this anesthetic. Chronic use has been reported to cause peripheral neuropathy.

OTHER

Sodium Oxybate (Xyrem®): This drug is marketed for treatment of cataplexy in patients with narcolepsy and is in the pharmacologic category of CNS depressants. Known on the street as GHB, its illegal use has been associated with "date-rape" activity. Street names include Liquid Ecstasy, Liquid X, Liquid E, Georgia Home Boy, Grievous Bodily Harm, G-Riffick, Soap, Scoop, Salty Water, Somatomax, and Organic Quaalude. There are no specific oral signs and symptoms, however, the dentist should be aware of patients showing signs of CNS depression, as with all other drugs in this class.

Flunitrazepam (Rohypnol®): This drug is a benzodiazepine with sedative and hypnotic properties. It is not currently marketed in the U.S. but is used as a sedative in Europe. Known on the street as Roofies, La Rocha, Ruffies, Coma Capsules, Roche, Rope, R-2, Roofenol, Roachies, and Rib, the white tablets can be taken orally, smoked, or snorted. Florida reported the first case of abuse and subsequent cases have been found primarily in Western and Southern states, although abuse in the U.S. and Europe is growing due to its euphoric-effect and low street price ($1-$3/tablet). It is often abused in combination with heroin, marijuana, ethanol, cocaine, or methamphetamine which has proven to be fatal in many cases. In one study, 14 of 40 descendants who died from heroin overdose were found to be positive for flunitrazepam.

The dental team should be alert to the signs and symptoms of drug abuse and withdrawal. Further reading is recommended.

ANIMAL AND HUMAN BITES GUIDELINES

The dentist is often confronted with early management of animal and human bites. The following protocols may assist in appropriate care and referral.

WOUND MANAGEMENT

Irrigation: Critically important; irrigate all penetration wounds using 20 mL syringe, 19-gauge needle and >250 mL 1% povidone-iodine solution. This method will reduce wound infection by a factor of 20. When there is high risk of rabies, use viricidal 1% benzalkonium chloride in addition to the 1% povidone-iodine. Irrigate wound with normal saline after antiseptic irrigation.

Debridement: Remove all crushed or devitalized tissue remaining after irrigation; minimize removal on face and over thin skin areas or anywhere you would create a worse situation than the bite itself already has; do not extend puncture wounds surgically — rather, manage them with irrigation and antibiotics.

Suturing: Close most dog bites if <8 hours (<12 hours on face); do not routinely close puncture wounds, or deep or severe bites on the hands or feet, as these are at highest risk for infection. Cat and human bites should not be sutured unless cosmetically important. Wound edge freshening, where feasible, reduces infection; minimize sutures in the wound and use monofilament on the surface.

Immobilization: Critical in all hand wounds; important for infected extremities.

Hospitalization/I.V. Antibiotics: Admit for I.V. antibiotics all significant human bites to the hand, especially closed fist injuries, and bites involving penetration of the bone or joint (a high index of suspicion is needed). Consider I.V. antibiotics for significant established wound infections with cellulitis or lymphangitis, any infected bite on the hand, any infected cat bite, and any infection in an immunocompromised or asplenic patient. Outpatient treatment with I.V. antibiotics may be possible in selected cases by consulting with infectious disease.

LABORATORY ASSESSMENT

Gram's Stain: Not useful prior to onset of clinically apparent infection; examination of purulent material may show a predominant organism in established infection, aiding antibiotic selection; not warranted unless results will change your treatment.

Culture: Not useful or cost-effective prior to onset of clinically apparent infection.

X-ray: Whenever you suspect bony involvement, especially in craniofacial dog bites in very small children or severe bite/crush in an extremity; cat bites with their long needle-like teeth may cause osteomyelitis or a septic joint, especially in the hand or wrist.

IMMUNIZATIONS

Tetanus: All bite wounds are contaminated. If not immunized in last 5 years, or if not current in a child, give DPT, DT, Td, or TT as indicated. For absent or incomplete primary immunization, give 250 units tetanus immune globulin (TIG) in addition.

Rabies: In the U.S. 30,000 persons are treated each year in an attempt to prevent 1-5 cases. Domestic animals should be quarantined for 10 days to prove need for prophylaxis. High-risk animal bites (85% of cases = bat, skunk, raccoon) usually receive treatment consisting of:

- human rabies immune globulin (HRIG): 20 units/kg I.M. (unless previously immunized with HDCV)
- human diploid cell vaccine (HDCV): 1 mL I.M. on days 0, 3, 7, 14, and 28 (unless previously immunized with HDCV - then give only first 2 doses)

Rabies Immune Globulin, Human *on page 1164*
Rabies Virus Vaccine *on page 1164*
Tetanus Immune Globulin, Human *on page 1283*

BITE WOUNDS AND PROPHYLACTIC ANTIBIOTICS

Parenteral vs Oral: If warranted, consider an initial I.V. dose to rapidly establish effective serum levels, especially if high risk, delayed treatment, or if patient reliability is poor.

Dog Bite:

1. Rarely get infected (~5%)
2. Infecting organisms: Staph coag negative, staph coag positive, alpha strep, diphtheroids, beta strep, *Pseudomonas aeruginosa*, gamma strep, *Pasteurella multocida*
3. Prophylactic antibiotics are seldom indicated. Consider for high risk wounds such as distal extremity puncture wounds, severe crush injury, bites occurring in cosmetically sensitive areas (eg, face), or in immunocompromised or asplenic patients.

Cat Bite:

1. Often get infected (~25% to 50%)
2. Infecting organisms: *Pasteurella multocida* (first 24 hours), coag positive staph, anaerobic cocci (after first 24 hours)
3. Prophylactic antibiotics are indicated in all cases.

Human Bite:

1. Intermediate infection rate (~15% to 20%)
2. Infecting organisms: Coag positive staph α, β, γ strep, *Haemophilus*, *Eikenella corrodens*, anaerobic streptococci, *Fusobacterium*, *Veillonella*, bacteroides.
3. Prophylactic antibiotics are indicated in almost all cases except superficial injuries.

Amoxicillin *on page 93*
Amoxicillin and Clavulanate Potassium *on page 95*
Cefazolin *on page 263*
Cefotetan *on page 272*
Ceftriaxone *on page 278*
Clindamycin *on page 341*
Doxycycline *on page 476*
Imipenem/Cilastatin *on page 709*
Trimethoprim and Sulfamethoxazole *on page 1253*

BITE WOUND ANTIBIOTIC REGIMENS

	Dog Bite	Cat Bite	Human Bite
Prophylactic Antibiotics			
Prophylaxis	No routine prophylaxis, consider if involves face or hand, or immunosuppressed or asplenic patients	Routine prophylaxis	Routine prophylaxis
Prophylactic antibiotic	Amoxicillin	Amoxicillin	Amoxicillin
Penicillin allergy	Doxycycline if >10 y or co-trimoxazole	Doxycycline if >10 y or co-trimoxazole	Doxycycline if >10 y or erythromycin and cephalexin*
Outpatient Oral Antibiotic Treatment (mild to moderate infection)			
Established infection	Amoxicillin and clavulanic acid	Amoxicillin and clavulanic acid	Amoxicillin and clavulanic acid
Penicillin allergy (mild infection only)	Doxycycline if >10 y	Doxycycline if >10 y	Cephalexin* or clindamycin
Outpatient Parenteral Antibiotic Treatment (moderate infections – single-drug regimens)			
	Ceftriaxone	Ceftriaxone	Cefotetan
Inpatient Parenteral Antibiotic Treatment			
Established infection	Ampicillin + cefazolin	Ampicillin + cefazolin	Ampicillin + clindamycin
Penicillin allergy	Cefazolin*	Ceftriaxone*	Cefotetan* or imipenem
Duration of Prophylactic and Treatment Regimens			
Prophylaxis: 5 days			
Treatment: 10-14 days			

*Contraindicated if history of immediate hypersensitivity reaction (anaphylaxis) to penicillin.

DENTAL OFFICE EMERGENCIES

All dentists would like to avoid the problems associated with managing dental office medical emergencies. As practitioners, we cannot be certain that these situations will not occur. It is hoped that with preparation, most if not all dental office emergencies can be avoided.

The American Dental Association's publication on dental therapeutics describes the incidence of medical emergencies in the dental office. Most of the problems that the dentist encounters are not life-threatening, but any emergency can become serious if not properly managed. If the dentist and dental office personnel can identify the signs and symptoms of a developing potential office emergency, many emergencies can be aborted and treated within the dental office.

Occasionally, life-threatening office emergencies occur and it is incumbent upon the dentist to be well prepared, to not only evaluate, but to act to stabilize, activate EMS, and manage/refer these patients to an appropriate medical facility for more definitive emergency care.

THIS CHAPTER PRESENTS ONLY THE MOST BASIC GUIDELINES FOR ANY OFFICE EMERGENCY. SPECIFIC PROTOCOLS CAN BE FOUND IN OUR COMPANION MANUAL: *Dental Office Medical Emergencies, A Manual of Office Response Protocols,* 1st ed (revised), Hudson, OH: Lexi-Comp, Inc, 2000.

In addition, a recent statement update from the American Dental Association on Scientific Affairs has been published in the March 2002 Journal of the American Dental Association (Vol 133, pp. 364-5). Briefly, it states: Though rare, life-threatening medical emergencies occasionally occur in the dental office. Recently, the American Dental Association on Scientific Affairs published a preparedness statement to update its preexisting statements on the subject.

Preparedness to recognize and appropriately manage medical emergencies in the dental environment includes the following:

- Current basic life support certification for all office staff
- Didactic and clinical courses in emergency medicine
- Periodic office emergency drills
- Telephone numbers of EMS or other appropriately trained health care providers
- Emergency drug kit and equipment and knowledge to properly use all items

HISTORY AND PHYSICAL EXAMINATION

The best tool to reduce the risk of a medical emergency occurring in the dental office is the patient's history and record. The dentist should collect adequate information to establish a complete baseline history on all new patients and an adequate updated history on all recall or patients returning to the office.

History and physical examination on all new patients should include:

- Baseline history
- Medications
- Past/current medical conditions
- Allergies
- Need for and results of medical consultation
- Baseline vital signs – pulse, blood pressure, respirations, temperature

Having this information available in the patient record in a format that is easily accessible by trained dental office personnel, allows quick reference of baseline values should a medical emergency occur during the delivery of dental care.

In today's dental practice, some clinicians believe that patient care has become more complicated due to increased use of over-the-counter and prescription medications, as well as the increased complexity of medical diagnoses and management. Other clinicians believe that technological and medical care advances have actually simplified patient care. For the most part, patients seeking elective dental care are adequately managed medically. Patients often appear to have complications based on history, but may be quite stable. New patients and patients with dental emergencies require special attention on the part of the practitioner. It is incumbent upon the dentist to be able to adequately evaluate complete histories and the current medical status of patients, so patients can be assessed for any potential risk while undergoing dental procedures. Each dental office should design a history format that works best for them.

Obtaining the history is usually the first and often the most important interaction with any new patient and with any patient of record that is being re-evaluated after a period of time. Many techniques can be used when addressing sensitive or complicated medical information. Most commonly, the medical history addresses major medical problems in the form of a questionnaire; it follows a review-of-systems format in addressing other symptomatology, which might be present, but remains undiagnosed to-date. This style is often supplemented with a narrative description by the interviewer. Regardless of the technique used, all dental office personnel should be familiar with how to access the information and should have adequate medical knowledge to alert the dentist to any known pre-existing conditions.

A review of current medications must also be included. The review must include home remedies, nonprescription drugs, vitamins or dietary supplements, and medications not prescribed to the patient (but available from friends or relatives) that may have been used by the patient. Doses and frequency of use are important. Drugs that have known associations with some medical emergencies are described with each protocol.

Certain drug classes are associated with potential dental office medical emergencies. Syncope can be caused by alpha$_1$-adrenergic receptor blockers (used to treat hypertension), nitroglycerin, some tricyclic antidepressants, and those antipsychotics which inhibit dopamine type 2 receptors and block alpha$_1$-adrenergic receptors (ie, clozapine). Orthostatic or postural hypotension can also be caused by medication in these drug classes. In addition, this condition has occurred in patients taking angiotensin-converting enzyme (ACE) inhibitors, calcium channel blockers, or beta-adrenergic receptor blockers for hypertension. Hypoglycemia is associated with the oral antidiabetic drugs. These associations are not always obvious, but the dentist should be attentive to the increased risk when patients are taking drugs in these therapeutic categories.

Allergies must be covered in some detail so the dentist is made aware of any known pre-existing allergies, either to environmental agents or medications. Medical reactions or toxicities in the dental office can result in serious life-threatening symptoms. Recognizing any predisposing history may allow the dentist to avoid these interactions or recognize them should they occur. Previous substance abuse might predispose the patient to drug reactions, and untoward medical response, during the delivery of dental care.

If the past history and general state of health, as well as the current physical evaluation, determines that a patient requires medical consultation, this should be noted in the patient's record. The reason for the consultation and the outcome should be clearly indicated in the record so the dentist is aware of the result of such consultation at each subsequent visit. This readiness may reduce risk.

As part of the normal physical examination that the dentist provides for each new patient and each recall patient, vital signs should be recorded. In most instances, these procedures are limited to measurements of pulse and blood pressure; however, in instances where any predisposing conditions might warrant or suggest more detailed evaluation, baseline respiratory rate and temperature might also be recorded. These data should be available and readily accessible in each patient's record so that, should an office emergency occur, the dental office personnel can compare the status during the emergency with the baseline data.

Elaborate schemes are available in oral medicine texts that assign risk by a variety of classifications. One method is to use the American Society of Anesthesiologists classification scheme to evaluate whether a patient's pre-existing medical condition places them at high risk during the delivery of anesthesia. Another mechanism is to assign the risk of dental procedures based on an analysis of pre-existing medical conditions matched with the complexity of the planned dental procedure. This protocol takes into account the potential invasiveness of the dental procedure. Simple procedures in complicated patients may have low total risk, whereas complex procedures in simple patients may place the patient at significant risk for an office emergency. Each dental practitioner should design or adapt a patient analysis plan for their own office.

EQUIPMENT

The dental office should be adequately equipped to not only deliver routine care to each new patient and each returning patient, but also should be set up for appropriate management and stabilization of any potential office emergency. This requires that each patient and treatment area should be equipped with a minimum of a blood pressure cuff and a stethoscope. The office should also have available:

- Appropriately-sized blood pressure cuffs
- Tourniquets
- Stethoscopes
- First-aid kits
- Emergency number call list
- Emergency cabinet
- Oxygen tank (size E portable with low flow regulator)
- Nasal cannula
- Masks (non-rebreather and a bag-valve mask [Ambu®])
- Syringes (intramuscular: I.M. 3 cc disposable, subcutaneous: S.C. tuberculin)

The emergency call list should be properly posted so office personnel need not search other operatories or the reception area for such information. Centrally located emergency cabinets, which include tourniquets, emergency medical care drugs, instruments, and supplies, are essential.

DENTAL OFFICE EMERGENCIES *(Continued)*

DENTAL OFFICE EMERGENCY DRUGS

Protocols should be established for most office emergencies. Recognition and rapid diagnosis lead to appropriate management. Major drugs usually available in the emergency drug cabinet are listed below.

Albuterol *on page 48*
Ammonia Spirit, Aromatic *on page 89*
Dexamethasone *on page 413*
(Alternative is Solu-Cortef® Mix-O-Vials for I.M.; has a longer shelf life)
Diazepam *on page 424*
Diphenhydramine *on page 451*
Epinephrine *on page 499*
(AnaKit® includes preloaded Tubex® syringes, which have measured dosing in increments)
Flumazenil *on page 581*
Glucose *on page 641*
(Emergency kit should also have oral carbohydrate source, such as Glutose 15™ oral gel and injectable glucagon)
Hydrocortisone *on page 688*
Morphine *on page 931*
Naloxone *on page 949*
Nitroglycerin *on page 981*
Oxygen *on page 1022*

Drug cabinet supplies should be in dose forms which the dentist is comfortable administering. Typical routes of administration could include oral (eg, diphenhydramine), inhalation (eg, albuterol), intramuscular/I.M. (eg, hydrocortisone), subcutaneous/S.C. (eg, epinephrine), or intravenous/I.V. (eg, epinephrine). Sublingual/S.L. injection can be substituted for some I.V. administrations in situations (ie, anaphylaxis) where a drug such as epinephrine may be life-saving. Oral mucosal absorption (eg, nitroglycerin) is also useful.

STAFF TRAINING

Office personnel, including the dentist, dental hygienists, and dental assistants, should all be trained in measurement of vital signs. Primarily, this includes measurement of pulse and evaluation of blood pressure. Proper technique for evaluating vital signs is necessary so information is accurate, and in the event of an emergency situation, ongoing measurements could be made by assisting personnel. The dentist should be able to provide this training to new employees, however, continuing education courses in proper techniques are available.

Dental office personnel should all be trained in basic life support first-aid, although the dentist is ultimately in charge of delivering care to either patient or personnel. Each office member should be aware of basic principles for management of nonlife-threatening injuries. All office personnel should be trained in cardiopulmonary resuscitation (CPR) or basic life support (BLS). Training courses are readily available through the American Heart Association and/or hospital facilities in most areas. Training should include not only basic initial training, but also renewal of skills should be a requirement for continued employment. One to two years is a reasonable time for updating such skills in cardiopulmonary resuscitation. Applicable state requirements or recommendations should be reviewed.

GENERAL PRINCIPLES OF RECOGNITION

As a practicing dentist, you should be familiar with:

- Altered states or loss of consciousness
- Cardiovascular emergencies (often associated with chest pain), including heart attack and stroke
- Respiratory emergencies, including asthmatic bronchospasm and obstruction
- Allergic reactions, including signs of anaphylaxis
- Other potential emergencies:
  - Diabetes, including acute hypo- and hyperglycemic states/reactions
  - Acute neurologic disturbances, including convulsive disorders such as epilepsy, stress-induced panic attacks, and acute headaches
  - Abdominal distress, including the abdominal disorders and diseases classified as acute (sudden onset) abdominal distress
  - Communicable diseases, including the major bacteria- and virus-induced illnesses of our society

Although symptoms can be very specific, detecting medical emergencies usually means recognizing some general changes in the state of the patient:

- Acute changes in affect or consciousness
- Sudden onset of pain, anywhere in the body
- Feelings of fever and chills
- Tight feeling in the chest
- Difficulty in expiration or inspiration
- Choking
- Dizziness or feelings of faintness
- Numbness or tingling sensations

The dental practitioner must be familiar with several basic diagnostic signs that should be compared to baseline measurements in the patient's record:

- Pulse rate and character — remember that a pulse rate >120 or <50 beats per minute can indicate a true emergency for the adult patient
- Blood pressure — a systolic pressure <70 may indicate shock and pressures >200/100 may present a hypertensive crisis (pre-CVA)
- Breathing rate and character — a true emergency may exist when the adult patient's respirations are >30 per minute
- Skin temperature, condition, and color
- Diaphoresis — often associated with anxiety, but can indicate ischemia
- Pupil size, equality, and response
- Color of the lips, tongue, earlobes, and nailbeds
- Breath odors
- Muscular activity — spasms and paralysis or weakness such as seen in ischemic attacks or CVA
- Bleeding or discharges from the body

ALL PRACTITIONERS MUST BE PREPARED TO CARRY OUT A BASIC PLAN FOR STABILIZATION

These steps are the basic action plan for stabilization in every office emergency. They should be activated within the first seconds following recognition of any developing problem. Sometimes, based on the initial recognition signs, activation of the emergency medical system (EMS) will occur immediately, usually by calling 911 (if available in your area). If the dentist is unsure of the underlying reason for the medical emergency or does not feel adequately trained, then basic life support (BLS) procedures should be the extent of the treatment until the emergency medical team arrives.

BASIC ACTION PLAN FOR STABILIZATION

PATIENT PLACEMENT	→ **UPRIGHT / SEMI-RECLINING?**
	→ **SUPINE?**
	→ **TRENDELENBURG (FEET UP, HEAD DOWN)*?**
AIRWAY AND BREATHING	→ **IS THE AIRWAY OPEN?**
	→ **CLEAR OF OBSTRUCTIONS?**
	→ **IS THE PATIENT BREATHING ON THEIR OWN?**
	→ **DOES THE SITUATION REQUIRE OXYGEN TO INCREASE PERFUSION?**
	→ **ACTIVATE CPR IF NECESSARY**
CIRCULATION	→ **MONITOR PULSE**
	→ **PROCEED WITH CPR, IF APPROPRIATE**

DENTAL OFFICE EMERGENCIES *(Continued)*

ADDITIONAL MANAGEMENT†

→ **ALWAYS CONSIDER ACTIVATING EMS IMMEDIATELY**

→ **CONTINUALLY OBSERVE, MONITOR VITAL SIGNS, AND EVALUATE FOR ANY SIGNS OF RECOVERY OR DETERIORATION**

→ **ASSIGN SOMEONE IN THE OFFICE TO QUICKLY RE-EVALUATE PATIENT'S HISTORY AND RECORD FOR CLUES TO THE CAUSE OF THE INCIDENT OR DRUGS THE PATIENT MAY BE TAKING**

→ **DETERMINE, IF POSSIBLE, THE TENTATIVE MEDICAL CONDITION CAUSING THE SYMPTOMS**

→ **DELIVER SPECIFIC CARE IF APPROPRIATE**

→ **BE PREPARED TO ACTIVATE EMS CALL FOR ASSISTANCE IF PATIENT'S CONDITION DETERIORATES**

→ **ALWAYS CONSIDER THE NEED FOR FOLLOW-UP MEDICAL EVALUATION AS PATIENT RECOVERS**

*Trendelenburg's position is a supine position which is inclined at an angle so that the pelvis and legs are slightly higher than the head.

†Although these management suggestions are essentially the same for each of the protocols, the order and specific care will vary.

SUGGESTED READINGS

ANTIBIOTICS IN TREATMENT OF ODONTOGENIC INFECTIONS

Doern GV, Ferraro MJ, Breuggemann AB, et al, "Emergence of High Rates of Antimicrobial Resistance Among Viridans Group Streptococci in the United States," *Antimicrob Agents Chemother,* 1996, 40(4):891-84.

Flynn TR, "The Swollen Face. Severe Odontogenic Infections," *Emerg Med Clin North Am,* 2000, 18(3):481-519.

Hardee WM, "Tried-and-True Medication," *Practical Endodontics,* 1997, 7(5):38.

Johnson BS, "Principles and Practice of Antibiotic Therapy," *Infect Dis Clin North Am,* 1999, 13(4):851-70.

Kuriyama T, Nakagawa K, Karasawa T, et al, "Past Administration of Beta-lactam Antibiotics and Increase in the Emergence of Beta-lactamase-producing Bacteria in Patients With Orofacial Odontogenic Infections," *Oral Surg Oral Med Oral Path Oral Radiol Endod,* 2000, 89(2):186-92.

Lee CY, "Management of Odontogenic Infections With Microbial, Anatomic and Antibiotic Considerations," *Hawaii Dent J,* 1993, 24(8):8-11.

Mandell GM, Bennett JE, Douglas GR, et al, eds, *Mandell, Douglas, and Bennett's Principles and Practice of Infectious Disease,* 5th ed, Philadelphia, PA: Churchill Livingstone, Inc, 2000, 2567-8.

Montgomery EH, "Antimicrobial Agents in the Prevention and Treatment of Infection," *Pharmacology and Therapeutics for Dentistry,* 4th ed, Yagiela JA, Neidle EA, Dowd FJ, eds, St. Louis, MO: Mosby-Year Book, Inc, 1998, 637.

Palacios E and Valvassori G, "Deep Facial Infection of Odontogenic Origin," *Ear Nose Throat J,* 2001, 80(1):15.

Storoe W, Haug RH, and Lillich TT, "The Changing Face of Odontogenic Infections," *J Oral Maxillofac Surg,* 2001, 59(7):739-48

Wynn RL and Bergman SA, "Antibiotics and Their Use in the Treatment of Orofacial Infections, Part I," *Gen Dent,* 1994, 42(5):398, 400-2.

Wynn RL and Bergman SA, "Antibiotics and Their Use in the Treatment of Orofacial Infections, Part II," *Gen Dent,* 1994, 42(6):498-502.

Wynn RL and Bergman SA, Meiller TF, et al, "Antibiotics in Treating Oral-Facial Infections of Odontogenic Origin," *Gen Dent,* 2001, 47(3):238-52.

CANCER

Al-Balawi SA and Nwoku AL, "Management of Oral Cancer in a Tertiary Care Hospital," *Saudi Med J,* 2002, 23(2):156-9.

Carl W, "Oral Complications of Local and Systemic Cancer Treatment," *Curr Opin Oncol,* 1995, 7(4):320-4.

Chambers MS, Toth BB, Martin JW, et al, "Oral and Dental Management of the Cancer Patient: Prevention and Treatment of Complications," *Support Care Cancer,* 1995, 3(3):168-75.

Dutton JM, Graham SM, and Hoffman HT, "Metastatic Cancer to the Floor of Mouth: The Lingual Lymph Nodes, "*Head Neck,* 2002 24(4):401-5.

Flaitz CM, "Persistent White Lesion of the Lateral Tongue," *Am J Dent,* 2001, 14(6):402-3.

Gellrich NC, Schramm A, Bockmann R, et al, "Follow-Up in Patients With Oral Cancer," *J Oral Maxillofac Surg,* 2002, 60(4):380-6.

Hobson RS and Clark JD, "Management of the Orthodontic Patient at Risk From Infective Endocarditis," *Br Dent J,* 1995, 179(2):48.

Jullien JA, Downer MC, Zakrzewska JM, et al, "Evaluation of a Screening Test for the Early Detection of Oral Cancer and Precancer," *Community Dent Health,* 1995, 12(1):3-7.

Messer NC, Yant WR, and Archer RD, "Developing Provider Partnerships in the Detection of Oral Cancer and the Prevention of Smokeless Tobacco Use," *Md Med J,* 1995, 44(10):788-91.

Takinami S, Yahata H, Kanoshima A, et al, "Hepatocellular Carcinoma Metastatic to the Mandible," *Oral Surg Oral Med Oral Pathol Oral Radiol Endod,* 1995, 79(5):649-54.

Vigneswaran N, Tilashalski K, Rodu B, et al, "Tobacco Use and Cancer. A Reappraisal," *Oral Surg Oral Med Oral Pathol Oral Radiol Endod,* 1995, 80(2):178-82.

Weaver RG, Whittaker L, Valachovic RW, et al, "Tobacco Control and Prevention Effort in Dental Education," *J Dent Educ,* 2002, 66(3):426-9.

CARDIOVASCULAR

"Adjusted-Dose Warfarin Versus Low-Intensity, Fixed-Dose Warfarin Plus Aspirin for High-Risk Patients With Atrial Fibrillation: Stroke Prevention in Atrial Fibrillation III Randomized Clinical Trial," *Lancet,* 1996, 348(9028):633-8.

American Heart Association, "Heart and Stroke Facts: 1996 Statistical Supplement," Dallas, Texas: National Center of the American Heart Association, 1996, 15.

Ayala C, Croft JB, Greenlund KJ, et al, "Sex Differences in US Mortality Rates for Stroke and Stroke Subtypes by Race/Ethnicity and Age, 1995-1998," *Stroke,* 2002, 33(5):1197-201.

Frazier OH, "Mechanical Circulatory Support: New Advances, New Pumps, New Ideas," *Semin Thorac Cardiovasc Surg,* 2002, 14(2):178-86.

Garcia R, "Floss or Die: The Link Between Oral Health and Cardiac Disease," *Harv Dent Bull,* 1998, 7(2):16-7.

SUGGESTED READINGS *(Continued)*

Gilligan DM, Ellenbogen KA, and Epstein AE, "The Management of Atrial Fibrillation," *Am J Med*, 1996, 101:413-21.

Giuliani ER, Gersh BJ, McGoon MD, et al, *Mayo Clinic Practice of Cardiology*, 3rd ed, St Louis, MO: Mosby-Year Book, Inc, 1996, 1698-814.

Glick M, "Screening for Traditional Risk Factors for Cardiovascular Disease: A Review for Oral Health Care Providers," *J Am Dent Assoc*, 2002, 133(3):291-300.

Hansson L, Zanchetti A, Carruthers SG, et al, "Effects of Intensive Blood Pressure Lowering and Low-Dose Aspirin in Patients With Hypertension: Principal Results of the Hypertension Optimal Treatment (HOT) Randomized Trial. HOT Study Group," *Lancet*, 1998, 351:1755-62.

Heidenreich PA, Lee TT, and Massie BM, "Effect of Beta-Blockade on Mortality in Patients With Heart Failure: A Meta-analysis of Randomized Clinical Trials," *J Am Coll Cardiol*, 1997, 30(1):27-34.

Hylek EM, Skates SJ, Sheehan MA, et al, "An Analysis of the Lowest Effective Intensity of Prophylactic Coagulation for Patients With Nonrheumatic Atrial Fibrillation," *N Engl J Med*, 1996, 335:540-6.

Kannel WB, "Blood Pressure as a Cardiovascular Risk Factor. Prevention and Treatment," *JAMA*, 1996, 275:1571-6.

Kaplan NM, "Hypertension and Diabetes," *J Hum Hypertens*, 2002, 16(Suppl 1):S56-60.

Kaplan NM, "Perspectives on the New JNC VI Guidelines for the Treatment of Hypertension," *Formulary*, 1997, 32:1224-31.

Kerpen SJ, Kerpen HO, and Sachs SA, "Mitral Valve Prolapse: A Significant Cardiac Defect in the Development of Infective Endocarditis," *Spec Care Dentist*, 1984, 4(4):158-9.

Lopaschuk GD, "Metabolic Abnormalities in the Diabetic Heart," *Heart Fail Rev*, 2002, 7(2):149-59.

Morley J, Marinchak R, Rials SJ, et al, "Atrial Fibrillation, Anticoagulation, and Stroke," *Am J Cardiol*, 1996, 77:38A-44A.

Reyes AJ, "Diuretics in the Treatment of Patients who Present Congestive Heart Failure and Hypertension," *J Hum Hypertens*, 2002, 16(Suppl 1):S104-13.

"The Sixth Report of the Joint National Committee on Prevention, Detection, Evaluation, and Treatment of High Blood Pressure (JNC VI)," *Arch Intern Med*, 1997, 157:2413-46.

CHEMICAL DEPENDENCY AND SMOKING CESSATION

Abelin T, Buehler A, Muller P, et al, "Controlled Trial of Transdermal Nicotine Patch in Tobacco Withdrawal," *Lancet*, 1989, 1(8628):7-10.

Alterman AI, Droba M, Antelo RE, et al, "Amantadine May Facilitate Detoxification of Cocaine Addicts," *Drug Alcohol Depend*, 1992, 31(1):19-29.

Ciancio SG, ed, *ADA Guide to Dental Therapeutics*, 1st ed, Chicago, IL: ADA Publishing Co, 1998.

Fiester S, Goldstein M, Resnick M, et al, "Practice Guideline for the Treatment of Patients With Nicotine Dependence," *Am J Psych*, 1996, 15(Suppl 10):31.

Gelskey SC, "Tobacco-Use Cessation Programs and Policies at the University of Manitoba's Faculty of Dentistry," *J Can Dent Assoc*, 2001, 67(3):145-8.

Herkenham MA, "Localization of Cannabinoid Receptors in Brain: Relationship to Motor and Reward Systems," *Biological Basis of Substance Abuse*, Korenman SG and Barchas JD, eds, New York, NY: Oxford University Press, 1993, 187-200.

Kausch O and McCormick RA, "Suicide Prevalence in Chemical Dependency Programs: Preliminary Data from a National Sample, and an Examination of Risk Factors," *J Subst Abuse Treat*, 2002, 22(2):97-102.

Kreek MJ, "Rationale for Maintenance Pharmacotherapy of Opiate Dependence," O'Brien CP and Barchas JD, eds, *Addictive States*, New York, NY: Raven Press, 1992, 205-30.

Leshner AI, "Molecular Mechanisms of Cocaine Addiction," *N Engl J Med*, 1996, 335(2):128-9.

Mendelson JH and Mello NK, "Management of Cocaine Abuse and Dependence," *N Engl J Med*, 1996, 334(15):965-72.

O'Brien CP, "Drug Addiction and Drug Abuse," *The Pharmacological Basis of Therapeutics*, 9th ed, Molinoff PB and Ruddon R, eds, New York, NY: McGraw-Hill, 1996, 557-77.

O'Brien CP, "Treatment of Alcoholism as a Chronic Disorder," *Toward a Molecular Basis of Alcohol Use and Abuse*, Jansson B, Jornvall H, Rydberg U, et al, eds, Basel, Switzerland: Birkhauser Verlag, 1994, Vol 71, EXS, 349-59.

Ostroff JS, Hay JL, Primavera LH, et al, "Motivating Smoking Cessation Among Dental Patients: Smokers' Interest in Biomarker Testing for Susceptibility to Tobacco-Related Cancers," *Nicotine Tob Res*, 1999, 1(4):347-55.

Ostrowski DJ and DeNelsky GY, "Pharmacologic Management of Patients Using Smoking Cessation Aids," *Dental Clin North Am*, 1996, 40(3):779-801.

Schydlower M, "Adolescent Substance Use and Abuse: Current Issues," *Tex Med*, 2002, 98(2):31-5.

Self DW, Barnhart WJ, Lehman DA, et al, "Opposite Modulation of Cocaine-Seeking Behavior by D1- and D2-Like Dopamine Receptor Agonists," *Science*, 1996, 271(5255):1586-9.

The Smoking Cessation Clinical Practice Guideline Panel and Staff, The Agency for Health Care Policy and Research Smoking Cessation Clinical Practice Guideline, *JAMA*, 1996, 275(1):1270-80.

Tomar SL, "Dentistry's Role in Tobacco Control," *J Am Dent Assoc*, 200, 132 (Suppl):S30-35.

Weisner C, Mertens J, Tam T, et al, "Factors Affecting the Initiation of Substance Abuse Treatment in Managed Care," *Addiction*, 2001, 96(5):705-16.

DENTIST'S ROLE IN RECOGNIZING DOMESTIC ABUSE

World Wide Web Sites

American Academy of Pediatrics — http://www.aap.org
American College of Emergency Physicians — http://www.acep.org
American Dental Association — http://www.ada.org
National Clearinghouse on Child Abuse and Neglect Information — http://www.calib.com/nccanch
National Data Archive on Child Abuse and Neglect — http://www.ndacan.cornell.edu
Prevent Child Abuse America (formerly National Committee to Prevent Child Abuse) — http://www.childabuse.org
University of Medicine and Dentistry - New Jersey — http://www.umdnj.edu/~baum/famvio.htm
USDHHS Agency of Children and Families — http://www.acf.dhhs.gov

Toll-Free Hotlines

Bureau of Indian Affairs Federal Hotline — 800-633-5155
Child Abuse Hotlines (24-Hour) — 800-4-ACHILD
Covenant House Nineline — 800-999-9999
National Family Violence Helpline — 800-222-2000

Books and Journal Articles (available at a local library or through interlibrary loan)

Besharov DJ, *Recognizing Child Abuse*, New York, NY, Free Press, 1990.

Chiodo GT, Tolle SW, and Tilden VP, "The Dentist and Family Violence," *Gen Dent*, 1998, 46(1):20-5.

Davidhizar R, Dowd S, and Giger JN, "Recognizing Abuse in Culturally Diverse Clients," *Health Care Superv*, 1998, 17(2):10-20.

Domestic Violence: A Directory of Protocols for Health Care Providers, Children's Safety Network, Newton, MA: Education Development Center, Inc, 1992.

Erickson MJ, Hill TD, and Siegel RM, "Barriers to Domestic Violence Screening in the Pediatric Setting," *Pediatrics*, 2001, 108(1):98-102.

"Health and Human Rights: A Call to Action on the 50th Anniversary of the Universal Declaration of Human Rights. The Writing Group for the Consortium for Health and Human Rights," *JAMA*, 1998, 280(5).

LaCerva V, *Pathways to Peace: Forty Steps to a Less Violent America*, Tesuque, NM: Heartsongs Publications, 1996.

McDowell JD, Kassebaum DK, and Stromboe SE, "Recognizing and Reporting Victims of Domestic Violence," *J Am Dent Assoc*, 1992, 123(9):44-50.

Mouden LD and Bross DC, "Legal Issues Affecting Dentistry's Role in Preventing Child Abuse and Neglect," *J Am Dent Assoc*, 1995, 126(8):1173-80.

"Protecting Children From Abuse and Neglect," Center for the Future of Children, The David and Lucille Packard Foundation, *The Future of Children*, 1998, 8(1):1-142. (Electronic version: http://www.futureofchildren.org)

Reece RM, *Child Abuse: Medical Diagnosis and Management*, Philadelphia, PA: Lea and Febiger, 1994.

Rupp RP, "Conditions to Be Considered in the Differential Diagnosis of Child Abuse and Neglect," *Gen Dent*, 1998, 46(1):96-9.

Salber PR and Talliaferro EH, *The Physicians' Guide to Domestic Violence: How to Ask the Right Questions and Recognize Abuse...Another Way to Save a Life*, Volcano, CA: Volcano Press, 1995.

Silva C, McFarlane J, Socken K, et al, "Symptoms of Post-Traumatic Stress Disorder in Abused Women in a Primary Care Setting," *J Women's Health*, 1997, 6:543-52.

Sweet D, "Recognizing and Intervening in Domestic Violence: Proactive Role for Dentistry," *Medscape Womens Health*, 1996, 1(6):3.

Watts C and Zimmerman C, "Violence Against Women: Global Scope and Magnitude," *Lancet*, 2002, 359(9313):1232-7.

DIAGNOSIS AND MANAGEMENT OF PAIN

Brown RS, Hinderstein B, Reynolds DC, et al, "Using Anesthetic Localization to Diagnose Oral and Dental Pain," *J Am Dent Assoc*, 1995, 126(5):633-4, 637-41.

Denson DD and Katz JA, "Nonsteroidal Anti-inflammatory Agents," *Practical Management of Pain*, 2nd ed, PP Raj, ed, St Louis, MO: Mosby Year Book, 1992.

Henry G, "Postoperative Pain Experience With Flurbiprofen and Acetaminophen With Codeine," *J Dent Res*, 1992, 71:952.

Jaffe JH and Martin WR, "Opioid Analgesic and Antagonists," *The Pharmacological Basis of Therapeutics*, 8th ed, Gilman AG, Rall TW, Nies AD, et al, eds, New York, NY: Maxwell Pergamon MacMillan Publishing, 1990.

Kalso E and Vainio A, "Morphine and Oxycodone Hydrochloride in the Management of Cancer Pain," *Clin Pharmacol Ther*, 1990, 47(5):639-46.

McQuay H, Carroll D, Jadad AR, et al, "Anticonvulsant Drugs for Management of Pain: A Systemic Review," *BMJ*, 1995, 311(7012):1047-52.

Robertson S, Goodell H, and Wolff HG, "The Teeth as a Source of Headache and Other Pain," *Arch Neurol Psychiatry*, 1947, 57:277.

SUGGESTED READINGS *(Continued)*

Sandler NA, Ziccardi V, and Ochs M, "Differential Diagnosis of Jaw Pain in the Elderly," *J Am Dent Assoc* 1995, 126(9):1263-72.

Seng GF, Kraus K, Cartwright G, et al, "Confirmed Allergic Reactions to Amide Local Anesthetics," *Gen Dent*, 1996, 44(1):52-4.

Stoller EP, Gilbert GH, Pyle MA, et al, "Coping With Tooth Pain: A Qualitative Study of Lay Management Strategies and Professional Consultation," *Spec Care Dentist*, 2001, 21(6):208-15.

Wright EF and Schiffman EL, "Treatment Alternatives for Patients With Masticatory Myofascial Pain," *J Am Dent Assoc*, 1995, 126(7):1030-9.

HIV INFECTION AND AIDS

Alsakka H, "Dental Management of HIV/AIDS Patients," *Northwest Dent*, 2001, 80(3):33-4.

Center for Disease Control (CDC), CfDC, "Update: AIDS Cases in Males Who Have Sex With Males," *MMWR Morb Mortal Wkly Rep*, 1995, 44(29):401-2.

Center for Disease Control (CDC), CfDC, "First 500,000 AIDS Cases," *MMWR Morb Mortal Wkly Rep*, 1995, 44(46):849-53.

Center for Disease Control (CDC), CfDC, "Update: HIV Exposures in HCWs," *MMWR Morb Mortal Wkly Rep*, 1995, 44(50):929.

Center for Disease Control (CDC), CfDCaP, "Recommended Infection-Control Practices for Dentistry," *MMWR Morb Mortal Wkly Rep*, 1993, 42(RR-8).

Glick M, *Clinicians Guide to Treatment of HIV-Infected Patients*, Academy of Oral Medicine, 1996.

Greenspan D, Greenspan JS, Schiodt M, et al, *AIDS and the Mouth*, Munksgaard, Copenhagen, 1990.

Greenspan JS and Greenspan D, "Oral Manifestations of HIV Infection," *The Proceedings of the Second International Workshop*, Chicago, IL: Quintessence Publishing Co, 1995.

Lyles AM, "What the Dentist Should Know About a Patient With HIV/AIDS," *J Calif Dent Assoc*, 2001, 29(2):158-69.

"Oral Health Care for Adults With HIV Infection," New York, NY: AIDS Institute, New York State Department of Health, 1993.

Ryder MI, "Periodontal Management of HIV-infected Patients."*Periodontol 2000*, 2000, 23:85-93.

Silverman S, *Color Atlas of Oral Manifestations of AIDS*, 2nd ed, St Louis, MO: Mosby, 1996.

Squassi A, Khaszki C, Blanco B, et al, "Relation Between Demographic and Epidemiological Characteristics and Permanency Under a Dental Health Care Program for HIV Infected Patients," *Acta Odontol Latinoam*, 1998, 11(1):3-13.

NATURAL PRODUCTS: HERBAL AND DIETARY SUPPLEMENTS

1995 Martindale - The Extra Pharmacopoeia, Vol 86, Roy Pharm Soc, GB, 1996.

Blumenthal M, Goldberg A, Gruenwald J, et al, *German Commission E Monographs: Therapeutic Monographs on Medicinal Plants for Human Use*, Austin, TX: American Botanical Council, 1997.

Cohan RP and Jacobsen PL, "Herbal Supplements: Considerations in Dental Practice," *J Calif Dent Assoc*, 2000, 28(8):600-10.

D'Arcy PF, "Adverse Reactions and Interactions With Herbal Medicines: Part 1. Adverse Reactions," *Adverse Drug Reaction Toxicol Rev*, 1991, 10(4):189-208.

D'Arcy PF, McEmay JC, and Welling PG, *Mechanisms of Drug Interactions*, New York, NY: Springer-Verlag, 1996.

DeSmet PA, "Health Risks of Herbal Remedies," *Drug Saf*, 1995, 13(2):81-93.

Ernst E and DeSmet PA, "Risks Associated With Complementary Therapies," *Meyler's Side Effects of Drugs*, 13th ed, Dukes MN ed, New York, NY: Elsevier Science, 1996.

Heber D, Yip I, Ashley JM, et al, "Cholesterol-lowering Effects of a Proprietary Chinese Red Yeast Rice Dietary Supplement," *Am J Clin Nutr*, 1999, 69:231-6.

Keller K, "Therapeutic Use of Herbal Drugs and Their Potential Toxicity, Problems and Results of the Revision of Herbal Medicines in the EEC," *Proceedings of the 3rd International Conference on Pharmacopoeias and Quality Control of Drugs*, Rome, November, 1992, published in Bologna, Fondazione Rhone-Poulenc Rorer per le Scienze Mediche, 1993.

McGuffin M, Hobbs C, Upton R, et al, *American Herbal Product Association's Botanical Safety Handbook: Guidelines for the Safe Use and Labeling for Herbs of Commerce*, Boca Raton, FL: CRC Press, 1997.

Mistry MG and Mays DA, "Precautions Against Global Use of Natural Products for Weight Loss: A Review of Active Ingredients and Issues Concerning Concomitant Disease States," *Therapeutic Perspectives*, 1996, 10(1):2.

Moynihan P, "The British Nutrition Foundation Oral Task Force Report - Issues Relevant to Dental Health Professionals," *Br Dent J*, 2000, 188(6):308-12.

ORAL INFECTIONS

Caufield PW and Griffen AL, "Dental Caries. An Infectious and Transmissible Disease," *Pediatr Clin North Am*, 2000, 47(5):1001-19.

Chow AW, "Infections of the Oral Cavity, Neck, and Head," *Principles and Practice of Infectious Diseases*, 4th ed, Mandell GL, Bennett JE, Dolin R, eds, New York, NY: Churchill Livingstone, 1995, 593-605.

Dajani A, Taubert K, Ferrieri P, et al, "Treatment of Acute Streptococcal Pharyngitis and Prevention of Rheumatic Fever: A Statement for Health Professionals," *Pediatrics*, 1995, 96(4):758-64.

Diz Dios P, Ocampo Hermida A, Miralles Alvarez C, et al, "Fluconazole-Resistant Oral Candidiasis in HIV-Infected Patients," *AIDS*, 1995, 9(7):809-10.

Dobson RL, "Antimicrobial Therapy for Cutaneous Infections," *J Am Acad Dermatol*, 1990, 22(5):871-3.

Goldberg MH and Topazian R, "Odontogenic Infections and Deep Facial Space Infections of Dental Origin," *Oral and Maxillofacial Infections*, 3rd ed, Philadelphia, PA: WB Saunders, 1994, 232-6.

Lewis MA, Parkhurst CL, Douglas CW, et al, "Prevalence of Penicillin Resistant Bacteria in Acute Suppurative Oral Infection," *J Antimicrob Chemother*, 1995, 35(6):785-91.

Muzyka BC and Glick M, "A Review of Oral Fungal Infections and Appropriate Therapy," *J Am Dent Assoc*, 1995, 126(1):63-72.

Shay K, "Infectious Complications of Dental and Periodontal Diseases in the Elderly Population," *Clin Infect Dis*, 2002, 34(9):1215-23.

Sykes LM and Sukha A, " Potential Risk of Serious Oral Infections in the Diabetic Patient: a Clinical Report," *J Prosthet Dent*, 2001, 86(6):569-73.

ORAL LEUKOPLAKIA

Barker JN, Mitra RS, Griffiths CE, et al, "Keratinocytes as Initiators of Inflammation," *Lancet*, 1991, 337(8735):211-4.

Boehncke WH, Kellner I, Konter U, et al, "Differential Expression of Adhesion Molecules on Infiltrating Cells in Inflammatory Dermatoses," *J Am Acad Dermatol*, 1992, 26(6):907-13.

Corso B, Eversole LR, and Hutt-Fletcher L, "Hairy Leukoplakia: Epstein-Barr Virus Receptors on Oral Keratinocyte Plasma Membranes," *Oral Surg Oral Med Oral Pathol*, 1989, 67(4):416-21.

Flaitz CM, "Persistent White Lesion of the Lateral Tongue," *Am J Dent*, 2001, 14(6):402-3.

Greenspan D, Greenspan JS, Overby G, et al, "Risk Factors for Rapid Progression From Hairy Leukoplakia to AIDS: A Nested Case-Control Study, *J Acquir Immune Defic Syndr*, 1991, 4(7):652-8.

McGuff HS, Otto RA, and Aufdemorte TB, "Clinical Warning Signs and Symptoms of Head and Neck Cancer," *Tex Dent J*, 2000, 117(6):14-9.

Regezi JA, Stewart JC, Lloyd RV, et al, "Immunohistochemical Staining of Langerhans Cells and Macrophages in Oral Lichen Planus," *Oral Surg Oral Med Oral Pathol*, 1985, 60(4):396-402.

Sciubba JJ, "Oral Leukoplakia," *Crit Rev Oral Biol Med*, 1995, 6(2):147-60.

Sciubba JJ, "Oral Precancer and Cancer: Etiology, Clinical Presentation, Diagnosis, and Management," *Compend Contin Educ Dent* 2000, 21(10A):892-8, 900-2.

ORAL SOFT TISSUE DISEASES

Antenucci EL, "Integration of Lasers Into a Soft Tissue Management Program," *Dent Clin North Am*, 2000, 44(4):811-9.

Delaney JE and Keels MA, "Pediatric Oral Pathology. Soft Tissue and Periodontal Conditions," *Pediatr Clin North Am*, 2000, 47(5):1125-47.

Goupil MT, "Occupational Health and Safety Emergencies," *Dent Clin North Am*, 1995, 39(3):637-47.

Haddad AJ, Avon SL, Clokie CM, et al, "Nodular Fasciitis in the Oral Cavity," *J Can Dent Assoc*, 2001, 67(11):664-7.

MacPhail LA, Greenspan D, Greenspan JS, et al, "Recurrent Aphthous Ulcers in Association With HIV Infection. Diagnosis and Treatment," *Oral Surg Oral Med Oral Pathol*, 1992, 73(3):283-8.

Meiller TF, Kutcher MJ, Overholser CD, et al, "Effect of an Antimicrobial Mouthrinse on Recurrent Aphthous Ulcerations," *Oral Surg Oral Med Oral Pathol*, 1991, 72(4):425-9.

Moncarz V, Ulmansky M, and Lustmann J, "Lichen Planus: Exploring Its Malignant Potential," *J Am Dent Assoc*, 1993, 124(3):102-8.

Rodu B and Mattingly G, "Oral Mucosal Ulcers: Diagnosis and Management," *J Am Dent Assoc*, 1992, 123(10):83-6.

Van Dis ML and Vincent SD, "Diagnosis and Management of Autoimmune and Idiopathic Mucosal Diseases," *Dent Clin North Am*, 1992, 36(4):897-917.

Vincent SD and Lilly GE, "Clinical, Historic, and Therapeutic Features of Aphthous Stomatitis. Literature Review and Open Clinical Trial Employing Steroids," *Oral Surg, Oral Med, Oral Pathol*, 1992, 74(1):79-86.

Wactawski-Wende J, " Periodontal Diseases and Osteoporosis: Association and Mechanisms, "*Ann Periodontol*, 2001, (1):197-208.

ORAL VIRAL DISEASES

Balfour HH, Rotbart HA, Feldman S, et al, "Acyclovir Treatment of Varicella in Otherwise Healthy Adolescents. The Collaborative Acyclovir Varicella Study Group," *J Pediatr*, 1992, 120(4):627-33.

Chang Y, Cesarman E, Pessin MS, et al, "Identification of Herpesvirus-Like DNA Sequences in AIDS-Associated Kaposi's Sarcoma," *Science*, 1994, 266(5192):1865-9.

Farquharson A, Ajagbe O, and Brown RS, "Differential Diagnosis of Severe Recurrent Oral Ulceration," *Dent Today*, 2002, 21(3):74-9.

SUGGESTED READINGS *(Continued)*

Ficarra G and Shillitoe EJ, "HIV-Related Infections of the Oral Cavity," *Oral Biol Med*, 1992, 3(3):207-31.

Moore TO, Moore AY, Carrasco D, et al, "Human Papillomavirus, Smoking, and Cancer," *J Cutan Med Surg*, 2001, 5(4):323-8.

Skegg DC, "Oral Contraceptives, Parity, and Cervical Cancer," *Lancet*, 2002, 359(9312):1080-1.

Spruance SL, Stewart JC, Rowe NH, et al, "Treatment of Recurrent Herpes Simplex Labialis With Oral Acyclovir," *J Infect Dis*, 1990, 161(2):185-90.

Woldeamanuel Y and Abate D, "Characterization of *Candida albicans* Isolates from the Oral Cavity of HIV-Positive Patients," *Ethiop Med J*, 1998, 36(4):235-43.

PERIODONTAL DISEASE

Bollen CM and Quirynen M, "Microbiological Response to Mechanical Treatment in Combination With Adjunctive Therapy. A Review of the Literature," *J Periodontol*, 1996, 67(11):1143-58.

Brecx M, Netuschil L, Reichart B, et al, "Efficacy of Listerine®, Meridol®, and Chlorhexidine Mouthrinses on Plaque, Gingivitis, and Plaque Bacteria Vitality," *J Clin Periodontol*, 1990, 17(1):292-7.

Ciancio SG, "Medications as Risk Factors for Periodontal Disease," *J Periodontol*, 1996, 67(Suppl 10):S1055-9.

Crout RJ, Lee HM, Schroeder K, et al, "The Cyclic Regimen of Low-Dose Doxycycline for Adult Periodontitis. A Preliminary Study," *J Periodontol*, 1996, 67(5):506-14.

DePaola LG, Overholser CD, Meiller TF, et al, "Chemotherapeutic Inhibition of Supragingival Dental Plaque and Gingivitis Development," *J Clin Periodontol*, 1989, 16(1):311-5.

Desvarieux M, "Periodontal Disease, Race, and Vascular Disease," *Compend Contin Educ Dent*, 2001, 22(3):34-41.

Elter JR, White BA, Gaynes BN, et al, "Relationship of Clinical Depression to Periodontal Treatment Outcome," *J Periodontol*, 2002, 73(4):441-9.

Genco RJ, "Current View of Risk Factors for Periodontal Diseases," *J Periodontol*, 1996, 67(Suppl 10):S1041-9.

Graves DT, Jiang Y, and Genco C, "Periodontal Disease: Bacterial Virulence Factors, Host Response and Impact on Systemic Health," *Curr Opin Infect Dis*, 2000, 13(3):227-232.

Greenstein G and Hart TC, "Clinical Utility of a Genetic Susceptibility Test for Severe Chronic Periodontitis: A Critical Evaluation," *J Am Dent Assoc*, 2002, 133(4):452-9.

Hitzig C, Charbit Y, Bitton C, et al, "Topical Metronidazole as an Adjunct to Subgingival Debridement in the Treatment of Chronic Periodontitis," *J Clin Periodontol*, 1994, 21(2):146-51.

Kjaerheim V, Skaare A, Barkvoll P, et al, "Antiplaque, Antibacterial, and Anti-inflammatory Properties of Triclosan Mouthrinses in Combination With Zinc Citrate or Polyvinylmethylether Maleic Acid (PVM-MA) Copolymer," *Eur J Oral Sci*, 1996, 104(5-6):529-34.

Loesche WJ, Giordano J, Soehren S, et al, "Nonsurgical Treatment of Patients With Periodontal Disease," *Oral Surg, Oral Med Oral Pathol*, 1996, 81(5):533-43.

Michalowicz BS, Pihlstrom BL, Drisko CL, et al, "Evaluation of Periodontal Treatments Using Controlled-Release Tetracycline Fibers: Maintenance Response," *J Periodontol*, 1995, 66(8):708-15.

Landry RG and Jean M, "Periodontal Screening and Recording (PSR) Index: Precursors, Utility and Limitations in a Clinical Setting," *Int Dent J*, 2002, 52(1):35-40.

Mealey BL, "Diabetes and Periodontal Disease: Two Sides of a Coin," *Compend Contin Educ Dent*, 2000, 21(11):943-6, 948, 950, passim.

Moseley R, Waddington RJ, and Embery G, "Hyaluronan and Its Potential Role in Periodontal Healing," *Dent Update*, 2002, 29(3):144-8.

Palomo F, Wantland L, Sanchez A, et al, "The Effect of Three Commercially Available Dentifrices Containing Triclosan on Supragingival Plaque Formation and Gingivitis: A Six Month Clinical Study," *Int Dent J*, 1994, 44(I Suppl 1):75-81.

Pavici MJ, van Winkelhoff AJ, Steures NH, et al, "Microbiological and Clinical Effects of Metronidazole and Amoxicillin in *Actinobacillus actinomycetemcomitans*-Associated Periodontitis. A 2-Year Evaluation," *J Clin Periodontol*, 1994, 21(2):107-12.

Ross NM, Mankodi SM, Mostler KL, et al, "Effects of Rinsing Time on Antiplaque-Antigingivitis Efficacy of Listerine®, *J Clin Periodontol*, 1993, 20(1):279-81.

Seymour RA and Heasman PA, "Tetracyclines in the Management of Periodontal Diseases. A Review," *J Clin Periodontol*, 1995, 22(1):22-35.

Seymour RA and Heasman PA, "Pharmacological Control of Periodontal Disease. II. Antimicrobial Agents," *J Dent*, 1995, 23(1):5-14.

Slots J and Ting M, "Systemic Antibiotics in the Treatment of Periodontal Disease," *Periodontol 2000*, 2002, 28:106-76.

PERIODONTOLOGY

Listgarten MA, "Pathogenesis of Periodontitis," *J Clin Periodontol*, 1986, 13(5):418-30.

Loesche WJ, Syed SA, Laughon BE, et al, "The Bacteriology of Acute Necrotizing Ulcerative Gingivitis," *J Periodontol*, 1982, 53(4):223-30.

PHARMACOLOGY OF DRUG METABOLISM AND INTERACTIONS

DeVane CL, "Pharmacogenetics and Drug Metabolism of Newer Antidepressant Agents," *J Clin Psychiatry*, 1994, 55(Suppl 12):38-45.

Hupp WS, " Seizure Disorders," *Oral Surg Oral Med Oral Pathol Oral Radiol Endod*, 2001, 92(6):593-6.

Ketter TA, Flockhart DA, Post RM, et al, "The Emerging Role of Cytochrome P450 3A in Psychopharmacology,"*J Clin Psychopharmacol*, 1995, 15(6):387-98.

Michalets EL, "Update: Clinically Significant Cytochrome P450 Drug Interactions," *Pharmacotherapy*, 1998, 18(1):84-112.

Moore PA, "Dental Therapeutic Indications for the Newer Long-Acting Macrolide Antibiotics," *J Am Dent Assoc*, 1999, 130(9):1341-3.

Nemeroff CB, DeVane CL, and Pollock BG, "Newer Antidepressants and the Cytochrome P450 System," *Am J Psychiatry*, 1996, 153(3):311-20.

Schmider J, Greenblatt DJ, von Moltke LL, et al, "Relationship of *In Vitro* Data on Drug Metabolism to *In Vivo* Pharmacokinetics and Drug Interactions: Implications for Diazepam Disposition in Humans," *J Clin Psychopharmacol*, 1996, 16(4):267-72.

Watkins PB, "Role of Cytochrome P450 in Drug Metabolism and Hepatotoxicity," *Semin Liver Dis*, 1990, 10(4):235-50.

Weinberg MA and Fine JB, "The Importance of Drug Interactions in Dental Practice," *Dent Today*, 2001, 20(9):88-93.

PREPROCEDURAL ANTIBIOTICS

"Advisory Statement. Antibiotic Prophylaxis for Dental Patients With Total Joint Replacement. American Dental Association; American Academy of Orthopaedic Surgeons," *J Am Dent Assoc*, 1997, 128(7):1004-8.

Bartzokas CA, Johnson R, Jane M, et al, "Relation Between Mouth and Haematogenous Infection in Total Joint Replacements," *BMJ*, 1994, 309(6953):506-8.

Berney P and Francioli P, "Successful Prophylaxis of Experimental Streptococcal Endocarditis With Single-Dose Amoxicillin Administered After Bacterial Challenge," *J Infect Dis*, 1990, 161(2):281-5.

Brause BD, "Infections Associated With Prosthetic Joints," *Clin Rheum Dis*, 1986, 12(2):523-36.

Chenoweth CE and Burket JS, "Antimicrobial Prophylaxis: Principles and Practice," *Formulary*, 1997, 32:692-708.

Ching DW, Gould IM, Rennie JA, et al, "Prevention of Late Haematogenous Infection in Major Prosthetic Joints," *J Antimicrob Chemother*, 1989, 23(5):676-80.

Clauzel AM, Visier S, and Michel FB, "Efficacy and Safety of Azithromycin in Lower Respiratory Tract Infections," *Eur Respir J*, 1990, 3(Suppl 10):S89.

Clemens JD and Ransohoff DF, "A Quantitative Assessment of Predental Antibiotic Prophylaxis for Patients With Mitral-Valve Prolapse," *J Chron Dis*, 1984, 37(7):531-44.

Dajani AS, Taubert KA, Wilson W, et al, "Prevention of Bacterial Endocarditis. Recommendations by the American Heart Association," *JAMA*, 1997, 277(22):1794-801.

Doern GV, Ferraro MJ, Brueggemann AB, et al, "Emergence of High Rates of Antimicrobial Resistance Among Viridans Group Streptococci in the United States," *Antimicrob Agents Chemother*, 1996, 40(4):891-4.

Durack DT, "Antibiotics for Prevention of Endocarditis During Dentistry: Time to Scale Back?" *Ann Intern Med*, 1998, 129(10):829-31.

Durack DT, "Prevention of Infective Endocarditis," *N Engl J Med*, 1995, 332(1):38-44.

Fluckiger U, Francioli P, Blaser J, et al, "Role of Amoxicillin Serum Levels for Successful Prophylaxis of Experimental Endocarditis Due to Tolerant Streptococci," *J Infect Dis*, 1994, 169(6):1397-400.

Hanssen AD, Osmon DR, and Nelson CL, "Prevention of Deep Prosthetic Joint Infection," *J Bone Joint Surg*, 1996, 78:458-71.

Little J, "The American Heart Association's Guidelines for the Prevention of Bacterial Endocarditis: A Critical Review," *Gen Dent*, 1998, 46:508-15.

"Risks for and Prevention of Infective Endocarditis," *Cardiology Clinics - Diagnosis and Management of Infective Endocarditis*, Child JS, ed, Philadelphia, PA: WB Saunders Co, 1996, 14:327-43.

Sale L, "Some Tragic Results Following Extraction of Teeth. II." *J Am Dent Assoc*, 1939, 26:1647-51.

Strom BL, Abrutyn E, Berlin JA, et al, "Dental and Cardiac Risk Factors for Infective Endocarditis. A Population-Based, Case-Control Study," *Ann Intern Med*, 1998, 129(10):761-9.

Strom BL, Abrutyn E, Berlin JA, et al, "Prophylactic Antibiotics to Prevent Infective Endocarditis? Relative Risks Reassessed," *J Investig Med*, 1996, 44:229.

Wahl M, "Myths of Dental-Induced Prosthetic Joint Infections," *Clin Infect Dis*, 1995, 20(5):1420-5.

Wynn RL, "Amoxicillin Update," *Gen Dent*, 1991, 39(5):322, 324, 326.

Wynn RL and Bergman SA, "Antibiotics and Their Use in the Treatment of Orofacial Infections, Part I," *Gen Dent*, 1994, 42(5): 398, 400, 402.

Wynn RL, "New Erythromycins," *Gen Dent*, 1996, 44(4):304-7.

Wynn RL, Meiller TF, and Crossley HL, "New Guidelines for the Prevention of Bacterial Endocarditis. American Heart Association," *Gen Dent*, 1997, 45(5):426-8, 430-4.

TEMPOROMANDIBULAR DYSFUNCTION

Amir I, Hermesh H, and Gavish A, "Bruxism Secondary to Antipsychotic Drug Exposure: A Positive Response to Propranolol," *Clin Neuropharmacol*, 1997, 20(1):86-9.

SUGGESTED READINGS *(Continued)*

Becker IM, "Occlusion as a Causative Factor in TMD. Scientific Basis to Occlusal Therapy," *NY State Dent J*, 1995, 61(9):54-7.

Bell WE, *Temporomandibular Disorders: Classification Diagnosis, Management*, 3rd ed, Chicago IL: Year Book Medical Publishers, 1990.

Bostwick JM and Jaffee MS, "Buspirone as an Antidote to SSRI-Induced Bruxism in 4 Cases," *J Clin Psychiatry*, 1999, 60(12):857-60.

Brown ES and Hong SC, "Antidepressant-Induced Bruxism Successfully Treated With Gabapentin," *J Am Dent Assoc*, 1999, 130(10):1467-9.

Carlson CR, Bertrand PM, Ehrlich AD, et al, "Physical Self-Regulation Training for the Management of Temporomandibular Disorders," *J Orofac Pain*, 2001, 15(1):47-55.

Canavan D and Gratt BM, "Electronic Thermography for the Assessment of Mild and Moderate Temporomandibular Joint Dysfunction," *Oral Surg Oral Med Oral Pathol Oral Radiol Endod*, 1995, 79(6):778-86.

Clark GT and Takeuchi H, "Temporomandibular Dysfunction, Chromic Orofacial Pain and Oral Motor Disorders in the 21st Century," *J Calif Dent Assoc*, 1995, 23(4):44-6, 48-50.

Dos Santos J Jr, "Supportive Conservative Therapies for Temporomandibular Disorders," *Dent Clin North Am*, 1995, 39(2):459-77.

Felicio CM, Mazzetto MO, and Perri Angote Dos Santos C, "Masticatory Behavior in Individuals With Temporomandibular Disorders," *Minerva Stomatol*, 2002, 51(4):111-20.

Gerber PE and Lynd LD, "Selective Serotonin Reuptake Inhibitor-Induced Movement Disorders," *Ann Pharmacother*, 1998, 32(6):692-8.

Maini S, Osborne JE, Fadl HM, et al, "Temporomandibular Joint Dysfunction Following Tonsillectomy," *Clin Otolaryngol*, 2002, 27(1):57-60.

Nicolakis P, Erdogmus B, Kopf A, et al, "Effectiveness of Exercise Therapy in Patients With Myofascial Pain Dysfunction Syndrome," *J Oral Rehabil*, 2002, 29(4):362-8.

Okeson JP, "Occlusion and Functional Disorders of the Masticatory System," *Dent Clin North Am*, 1995, 39(2):285-300.

Quinn JH, "Mandibular Exercises to Control Bruxism and Deviation Problems," *Cranio*, 1995, 13(1):30-4.

Schiffman E, Haley D, Baker C, et al, "Diagnostic Criteria for Screening Headache Patients for Temporomandibular Disorders," *Headache*, 1995, 35(3):121-4.

Thayer T, "Acupuncture TMD and Facial Pain," *SAAD Dig*, 2001, 18(3):3-7.

XEROSTOMIA

American Dental Association. ADA Guide to Dental Therapeutics, 2nd ed, Chicago, IL: ADA Publishing Co, Inc, 2001.

"Cevimeline (Evoxac) for Dry Mouth," *Med Lett Drugs Ther,* 2000, 42(1084):70.

Fox PC, Atkinson JC, Macynski AA, et al, "Pilocarpine Treatment of Salivary Gland Hypofunction and Dry Mouth (Xerostomia)," *Arch Intern Med,* 1991, 151(6):1149-52.

Johnson JT, Ferretti GA, Nethery WJ, et al, "Oral Pilocarpine for Post-Irradiation Xerostomia in Patients With Head and Neck Cancer," *N Eng J Med,* 1993, 329(6):390-5.

Johnstone PA, Niemtzow RC, and Riffenburgh RH, "Acupuncture for Xerostomia: Clinical Update," *Cancer*, 2002, 94(4):1151-6.

Nusair S and Rubinow A, "The Use of Oral Pilocarpine in Xerostomia and Sjögren's Syndrome," *Semin Arthritis Rheum,* 1999, 28(6):360-7.

Rhodus NL and Schuh MJ, "Effects of Pilocarpine on Salivary Flow in Patients With Sjögren's Syndrome," *Oral Surg Oral Med Oral Pathol,* 1991, 72(5):545-9.

Sanchez-Guerrero J, Aguirre-Garcia E, Perez-Dosal MR, et al, "The Wafer Test: A Semi-Quantitative Test to Screen for Xerostomia," *Rheumatology (Oxford)*, 2002, 41(4):381-9.

Ship JA, Pillemer SR, and Baum BJ, "Xerostomia and the Geriatric Patient," *J Am Geriatr Soc*, 2002, 50(3):535-43.

Sugerman PB and Barber MT, "Patient Selection for Endosseous Dental Implants: Oral and Systemic Considerations," *Int J Oral Maxillofac Implants*, 2002, 17(2):191-201.

Taylor SE and Miller EG, "Pre-emptive Pharmacologic Intervention in Radiation-Induced Salivary Dysfunction," *Proc Soc Exp Biol Med,* 1999, 221(1):14-26.

Tenovuo J, "Clinical Applications of Antimicrobial Host Proteins Lactoperoxidase, Lysozyme and Lactoferrin in Xerostomia: Efficacy and Safety," *Oral Dis*, 2002, 8(1):23-9.

Wray D, Lowe GD, Dagg JH, et al, *Textbook of General and Oral Medicine,* London, England: Churchill Livingstone, 1999.

Wynn RL, Meiller TF, and Crossley HL, *Drug Information Handbook for Dentistry,* 6th ed, Hudson (Cleveland), OH: Lexi-Comp, Inc, 2000.

Valdez IH, Wolff A, Atkinson JC, et al, "Use of Pilocarpine During Head and Neck Radiation Therapy to Reduce Xerostomia and Salivary Dysfunction," *Cancer,* 1993, 71(5):1848-51.

APPENDIX

TABLE OF CONTENTS

Standard Conversions

Apothecary/Metric Conversions 1596
Pounds/Kilograms Conversion 1597

Calcium Channel Blockers & Gingival Hyperplasia

Some General Observations of CCB-Induced GH 1598
Calcium Channel Blockers 1600

Infectious Disease Information

Occupational Exposure to Bloodborne Pathogens (Standard/Universal Precautions) 1601
Immunizations (Vaccines) 1612

Laboratory Values

Normal Blood Values 1618

Over-the-Counter Dental Products

Dentifrice Products 1619
Denture Adhesive Products 1628
Denture Cleanser Products 1629
Mouth Pain, Cold Sore, and Canker Sore Products 1630
Oral Rinse Products 1634

Miscellaneous

Top 50 Prescribed Drugs in 2002 1636
Adult Multivitamin Products 1637
Vitamin B Complex Combination Products 1640

STANDARD CONVERSIONS

APOTHECARY/METRIC CONVERSIONS

Approximate Liquid Measures

Basic equivalent: 1 fluid ounce = 30 mL

Examples:

1 gallon .... 3800 mL
1 quart .... 960 mL
1 pint .... 480 mL
8 fluid ounces .... 240 mL
4 fluid ounces .... 120 mL

15 minims .... 1 mL
10 minims .... 0.6 mL
1 gallon ..... 128 fluid ounces
1 quart .... 32 fluid ounces
1 pint .... 16 fluid ounces

Approximate Household Equivalents

1 teaspoonful .... 5 mL
1 tablespoonful .... 15 mL

Weights

Basic equivalents:

1 ounce = 30 g
15 grains = 1 g

Examples:

4 ounces .... 120 g
2 ounces .... 60 g
10 grains .... 600 mg
7 1/2 grains .... 500 mg
1 grain .... 60 mg

1/100 grain ....600 mcg
1/150 grain ....400 mcg
1/200 grain ....300 mcg
16 ounces........... 1 pound

Metric Conversions

Basic equivalents:

1 g .... 1000 mg
1 mg ....1000 mcg

Examples:

5 g .... 5000 mg
0.5 g............... 500 mg
0.05 g............... 50 mg

5 mg..............5000 mcg
0.5 mg ....500 mcg
0.05 mg .... 50 mcg

Exact Equivalents

1 g	=	15.43 grains (gr)	0.1 mg	=	1/600 gr
1 mL	=	16.23 minims	0.12 mg	=	1/500 gr
1 minim	=	0.06 mL	0.15 mg	=	1/400 gr
1 gr	=	64.8 mg	0.2 mg	=	1/300 gr
1 pint (pt)	=	473.2 mL	0.3 mg	=	1/200 gr
1 oz	=	28.35 g	0.4 mg	=	1/150 gr
1 lb	=	453.6 g	0.5 mg	=	1/120 gr
1 kg	=	2.2 lbs	0.6 mg	=	1/100 gr
1 qt	=	946.4 mL	0.8 mg	=	1/80 gr
			1 mg	=	1/65 gr

Solids*

1/4 grain	=	15 mg
1/2 grain	=	30 mg
1 grain	=	60 mg
1 1/2 grains	=	90 mg
5 grains	=	300 mg
10 grains	=	600 mg

*Use exact equivalents for compounding and calculations requiring a high degree of accuracy.

Pounds/Kilograms Conversion

1 pound = 0.45359 kilograms
1 kilogram = 2.2 pounds

lb	=	kg	lb	=	kg	lb	=	kg
1		0.45	70		31.75	140		63.50
5		2.27	75		34.02	145		65.77
10		4.54	80		36.29	150		68.04
15		6.80	85		38.56	155		70.31
20		9.07	90		40.82	160		72.58
25		11.34	95		43.09	165		74.84
30		13.61	100		45.36	170		77.11
35		15.88	105		47.63	175		79.38
40		18.14	110		49.90	180		81.65
45		20.41	115		52.16	185		83.92
50		22.68	120		54.43	190		86.18
55		24.95	125		56.70	195		88.45
60		27.22	130		58.91	200		90.72
65		29.48	135		61.24			

CALCIUM CHANNEL BLOCKERS AND GINGIVAL HYPERPLASIA

Drug	FDA Approval	Cases Cited in Literature
Amlodipine (Norvasc®)	1992	3
Bepridil (Vascor®)	1993	0
Diltiazem (Cardizem®, Dilacor®)	1982	>20
Felodipine (Plendil®)	1992	1
Isradipine (DynaCirc®)	1991	1
Nicardipine (Cardene®)	1989	0
Nifedipine (Adalat®, Procardia®)	1982	>120
Nimodipine (Nimotop®)	1989	0
Nisoldipine (Sular®)	1995	0
Nitrendipine[1] (Baypress®)		1
Verapamil (Calan®, Isoptin®, Verelan®)	1982	7

[1]Not yet approved for use in the United States.

SOME GENERAL OBSERVATIONS OF CCB-INDUCED GH

Calcium channel blockers (CCBs) are well known to cause gingival enlargement. In the early 1990s, it was thought that this class of drugs caused a true hyperplasia of the gingiva. Current thinking is that the term "hyperplasia" is inappropriate since the drug-induced effect results in an increase in extracellular tissue volume rather than an increase in the number of cells. Most of the reported cases of CCB-induced gingival enlargement have involved patients >50 years of age taking CCBs for postmyocardial infarction syndrome, angina pain, essential hypertension, and Raynaud's syndrome. Nifedipine (Procardia®) is associated with the highest number of reported cases in the literature, followed by diltiazem (Cardizem®). Depending on the CCB in question, gingival enlargement has appeared any time between 1-24 months after daily dosing. Discontinuance of the CCB usually results in complete disappearance or marked regression of symptoms, with symptoms reappearing upon remedication. The time required after drug discontinuance for marked regression of enlargement has been 1 week. Complete disappearance of all symptoms usually takes 2 months. If gingivectomy is performed and the drug retained or resumed, the gingival enlargement can recur. Only when the CCB is discontinued or a switch to a non-CCB occurs, will the gingivectomy usually be successful. One study of Nishikawa et al, showed that if nifedipine could not be discontinued, gingival enlargement did not recur after gingivectomy when extensive plaque control was carried out. If the CCB is changed to another class of cardiovascular drug, the enlargement will probably regress and disappear. A switch to another CCB, however, will probably result in continued gingival enlargement. For example, Giustiniani et al, reported disappearance of symptoms within 15 days after discontinuance of verapamil, with recurrence of symptoms after resumption with diltiazem. One case report described a nonsurgical management of a patient presenting with nifedipine-induced gingival overgrowth. Establishment and maintenance of a considerably improved standard of plaque control led to complete resolution of the overgrowth without recurrence, even though the medication dose was increased. The reader is referred to the review of 1991 for descriptive clinical and histological findings of CCB-induced gingival enlargement. A more recent review has been authorized by Silverstein et al, and published in 1997.

Two reports described the prevalence of amlodipine (Norvasc®)-induced gingival overgrowth. The study by Ellis et al, examined a sample of patients taking 1 of 3 CCBs who were drawn from a community-based population in northeastern England. Out of 911 patients, 442 were taking nifedipine, 181 amlodipine, and 186 diltiazem. In addition, 102 control subjects were included. It was found that 6.3% of subjects taking nifedipine were seen to have significant overgrowth, which was significantly greater than the overgrowth seen with the other two drug groups or the control group. The prevalence of gingival overgrowth induced by amlodipine or diltiazem was not significantly different compared to the control group. This study concluded that the prevalence of significant gingival overgrowth related to CCBs was low. Also, males were 3 times as likely as females to develop significant overgrowth.

In a second study by Jorgensen, a large group of patients taking amlodipine was studied in order to determine the prevalence of, what he called, "gingival hyperplasia". Out of 150 dentate patients who volunteered to undergo a screening examination, mild hyperplasia was found in 5 patients (3.3%). This was significantly less than rates reported for patients taking nifedipine and not significantly different from rates reported in control groups of cardiac patients not taking CCBs. Jorgensen concluded that amlodipine, at a dose of 5 mg daily, did not induce gingival hyperplasia.

There have been reports of verapamil-induced gingival enlargement in the literature with at least 7 cases listed in the review by this author. The prevalence of verapamil-induced enlargement, however, has not been investigated.

References

Bullon P, Machuca G, Armas JR, et al, "The Gingival Inflammatory Infiltrate in Cardiac Patients Treated With Calcium Antagonists," *J Clin Periodontol*, 2001, 28(10):897-903.

Ciantar M, "Nifedipine-Induced Gingival Overgrowth: Remission Following Nonsurgical Therapy," *Dent Update*, 1997, 45(4):371-6.

Desai P and Silver JG, "Drug-Induced Gingival Enlargements," *J Can Dent Assoc*, 1998, 64(4):263-8.

Ellis JS, Seymour RA, Steele JG, et al, "Prevalence of Gingival Overgrowth Induced by Calcium Channel Blockers: A Community-Based Study," *J Periodontol*, 1999, 70(1):63-7.

Giustiniani S, Robestelli della Cuna F, and Marieni M, "Hyperplastic Gingivitis During Diltiazem Therapy," *Int J Cardiol*, 1987, 15(2):247-9.

Hood KA, "Drug-Induced Gingival Hyperplasia in Transplant Recipients," *Prog Transplant*, 2002, 12(1):17-21.

Jorgensen MG, "Prevalence of Amlodipine-Related Gingival Hyperplasia, *J Periodontol*, 1997, 68(7):676-8.

Missouris GG, Kalaitzidis RG, Cappuccio FP, et al, "Gingival Hyperplasia Caused by Calcium Channel Blockers," *J Hum Hypertens.* , 2000, 14(2):155-6.

Nishikawa S, Tada H, Hamasaki A, et al, "Nifedipine-Induced Gingival Hyperplasia: A Clinical and *In Vitro* Study," *J Periodontol*, 1991, 62(1):30-5.

Silverstein LH, Garnick JJ, Szikman M, et al, "Medication-Induced Gingival Enlargement: A Clinical Review," *Gen Dent*, 1997, 45(4):371-6.

Wynn RL, "Calcium Channel Blockers and Gingival Hyperplasia," *Gen Dent*, 1991, 39(4):240-3.

Wynn RL, "Update on Calcium Channel Blocker-Induced Gingival Hyperplasia," *Gen Dent*, 1995, 43(3):218-20, 222.

CALCIUM CHANNEL BLOCKERS

Comparative Pharmacokinetics

Agent	Bioavailability (%)	Protein Binding (%)	Onset (min)	Peak (h)	Half-Life (h)	Volume of Distribution	Route of Metabolism	Route of Excretion
Dihydropyridines								
Nifedipine (prototype) (Adalat® CC, Procardia®/Procardia XL®)	Immediate/sustained release 45-70/86	92-98	20	Immediate/ sustained release 0.5/6	2-5	ND	Liver, inactive metabolites	60%-80% urine, feces, bile
Amlodipine (Norvasc®)	52-88	97	6 h	6-9	33.8	21 L/kg	Liver, inactive metabolites, not a significant first-pass metabolism/presystemic metabolism	Bile, gut wall
Felodipine (Plendil®)	10-25	>99	3-5 h	2.5-5	10-36	10.3 L/kg	Liver, inactive metabolites, extensive metabolism by several pathways including cytochrome P450, extensive first-pass metabolism/presystemic metabolism	70% urine, 10% feces
Isradipine (DynaCirc®)	15-24	97	120	0.5-2.5	8	2.9 L/kg	Liver, inactive metabolites, extensive first-pass metabolism	90% urine, 10% feces
Nicardipine (Cardene®)	35	>95	20	0.5-2	2-4	ND	Liver, saturable first-pass metabolism	60% urine, 35% feces
Nimodipine (Nimotop®)	13	>95	ND	≤1	1-2	0.43 L/kg	Liver, inactive metabolites, high first-pass metabolism	Urine
Nisoldipine (Sular®)	4-8	>99	ND	6-12	7-12	4-5 L/kg	Liver, 1 active metabolite (10%), presystemic metabolism	70%-75% kidney, 6%-12% feces
Phenylalkylamines								
Verapamil (prototype) (Calan®, Isoptin®)	20-35	83-92	30	1-2.2	3-7	4.5-7 L/kg	Liver	70% urine, 16% feces
Benzothiazepines								
Diltiazem (prototype) (Cardizem®/Cardizem® CD, Dilacor® XR)	40-67	70-80	30-60	Immediate/ sustained release 2-3/6-11	Immediate/ sustained release 3.5-6/5-7	ND	Liver; drugs which inhibit/induce hepatic microsomal enzymes may alter disposition	Urine
Miscellaneous								
Bepridil (Vascor®)	59	>99	60	2-3	24	ND	Liver	70% urine, 22% feces

OCCUPATIONAL EXPOSURE TO BLOODBORNE PATHOGENS (STANDARD/ UNIVERSAL PRECAUTIONS)

OVERVIEW AND REGULATORY CONSIDERATIONS

Every healthcare employee, from nurse to housekeeper, has some (albeit small) risk of exposure to HIV and other viral agents such as hepatitis B and Jakob-Creutzfeldt agent. The incidence of HIV-1 transmission associated with a percutaneous exposure to blood from an HIV-1 infected patient is approximately 0.3% per exposure.[1] In 1989, it was estimated that 12,000 United States healthcare workers acquired hepatitis B annually.[2] An understanding of the appropriate procedures, responsibilities, and risks inherent in the collection and handling of patient specimens is necessary for safe practice and is required by Occupational Safety and Health Administration (OSHA) regulations.

The Occupational Safety and Health Administration published its "Final Rule on Occupational Exposure to Bloodborne Pathogens" in the Federal Register on December 6, 1991. OSHA has chosen to follow the Center for Disease Control (CDC) definition of universal precautions. The Final Rule provides full legal force to universal precautions and requires employers and employees to treat blood and certain body fluids as if they were infectious. The Final Rule mandates that healthcare workers must avoid parenteral contact and must avoid splattering blood or other potentially infectious material on their skin, hair, eyes, mouth, mucous membranes, or on their personal clothing. Hazard abatement strategies must be used to protect the workers. Such plans typically include, but are not limited to, the following:

- safe handling of sharp items ("sharps") and disposal of such into puncture resistant containers
- gloves required for employees handling items soiled with blood or equipment contaminated by blood or other body fluids
- provisions of protective clothing when more extensive contact with blood or body fluids may be anticipated (eg, surgery, autopsy, or deliveries)
- resuscitation equipment to reduce necessity for mouth to mouth resuscitation
- restriction of HIV- or hepatitis B-exposed employees to noninvasive procedures

OSHA has specifically defined the following terms: **Occupational exposure** means reasonably anticipated skin, eye mucous membrane, or parenteral contact with blood or other potentially infectious materials that may result from the performance of an employee's duties. **Other potentially infectious materials** are human body fluids including semen, vaginal secretions, cerebrospinal fluid, synovial fluid, pleural fluid, pericardial fluid, peritoneal fluid, amniotic fluid, saliva in dental procedures, and body fluids that are visibly contaminated with blood, and all body fluids in situations where it is difficult or impossible to differentiate between body fluids; any unfixed tissue or organ (other than intact skin) from a human (living or dead); and HIV-containing cell or tissue cultures, organ cultures, and HIV- or HBV-containing culture medium or other solutions, and blood, organs, or other tissues from experimental animals infected with HIV or HBV. An **exposure incident** involves specific eye, mouth, other mucous membrane, nonintact skin, or parenteral contact with blood or other potentially infectious materials that results from the performance of an employee's duties.[3] It is important to understand that some exposures may go unrecognized despite the strictest precautions.

A written Exposure Control Plan is required. Employers must provide copies of the plan to employees and to OSHA upon request. Compliance with OSHA rules may be accomplished by the following methods.

- **Universal precautions (UPs)** means that all human blood and certain body fluids are treated as if known to be infectious for HIV, HBV, and other bloodborne pathogens. UPs do not apply to feces, nasal secretions, saliva, sputum, sweat, tears, urine, or vomitus unless they contain visible blood.
- **Engineering controls (ECs)** are physical devices which reduce or remove hazards from the workplace by eliminating or minimizing hazards or by isolating the worker from exposure. Engineering control devices include sharps disposal containers, self-resheathing syringes, etc.
- **Work practice controls (WPCs)** are practices and procedures that reduce the likelihood of exposure to hazards by altering the way in which a task is performed. Specific examples are the prohibition of two-handed recapping of needles, prohibition of storing food alongside potentially contaminated material, discouragement of pipetting fluids by mouth, encouraging handwashing after removal of gloves, safe handling of contaminated sharps, and appropriate use of sharps containers.
- **Personal protective equipment (PPE)** is specialized clothing or equipment worn to provide protection from occupational exposure. PPE includes gloves, gowns, laboratory coats (the type and characteristics will depend upon the task and degree of exposure anticipated), face shields or masks, and eye protection. Surgical caps or hoods and/or shoe covers or boots are required in instances in

OCCUPATIONAL EXPOSURE TO BLOODBORNE PATHOGENS (STANDARD/UNIVERSAL PRECAUTIONS) *(Continued)*

which gross contamination can reasonably be anticipated (eg, autopsies, orthopedic surgery). If PPE is penetrated by blood or any contaminated material, the item must be removed immediately or as soon as feasible. **The employer must provide and launder or dispose of all PPE at no cost to the employee.** Gloves must be worn when there is a reasonable anticipation of hand contact with potentially infectious material, including a patient's mucous membranes or nonintact skin. Disposable gloves must be changed as soon as possible after they become torn or punctured. Hands must be washed after gloves are removed. OSHA has revised the PPE standards, effective July 5, 1994, to include the requirement that the employer certify in writing that it has conducted a hazard assessment of the workplace to determine whether hazards are present that will necessitate the use of PPE. Also, verification that the employee has received and understood the PPE training is required.[4]

Housekeeping protocols: OSHA requires that all bins, cans, and similar receptacles, intended for reuse which have a reasonable likelihood for becoming contaminated, be inspected and decontaminated immediately or as soon as feasible upon visible contamination and on a regularly scheduled basis. Broken glass that may be contaminated must not be picked up directly with the hands. Mechanical means (eg, brush, dust pan, tongs, or forceps) must be used. Broken glass must be placed in a proper sharps container.

Employers are responsible for teaching appropriate clean-up procedures for the work area and personal protective equipment. A 1:10 dilution of household bleach is a popular and effective disinfectant. It is prudent for employers to maintain signatures or initials of employees who have been properly educated. If one does not have written proof of education of universal precautions teaching, then by OSHA standards, such education never happened.

Pre-exposure and postexposure protocols: OSHA's Final Rule includes the provision that employees, who are exposed to contamination, be offered the hepatitis B vaccine at no cost to the employee. Employees may decline; however, a declination form must be signed. The employee must be offered free vaccine if he/she changes his/her mind. Vaccination to prevent the transmission of hepatitis B in the healthcare setting is widely regarded as sound practice.[5] In the event of exposure, a confidential medical evaluation and follow-up must be offered at no cost to the employee. Follow-up must include collection and testing of blood from the source individual for HBV and HIV if permitted by state law if a blood sample is available. If a postexposure specimen must be specially drawn, the individual's consent is usually required. Some states may not require consent for testing of patient blood after accidental exposure. One must refer to state and/or local guidelines for proper guidance.

The employee follow-up must also include appropriate postexposure prophylaxis, counseling, and evaluation of reported illnesses. The employee has the right to decline baseline blood collection and/or testing. If the employee gives consent for the collection but not the testing, the sample must be preserved for 90 days in the event that the employee changes his/her mind within that time. Confidentiality related to blood testing must be ensured. **The employer does not have the right to know the results** of the testing of either the source individual or the exposed employee.

MANAGEMENT OF HEALTHCARE WORKER EXPOSURES TO HBV, HCV, AND HIV

Likelihood of transmission of HIV-1 from occupational exposure is 0.2% per parenteral exposure (eg, needlestick) to blood from HIV infected patients. Factors that increase risk for occupational transmission include advanced stages of HIV in source patient, hollow bore needle puncture, a poor state of health or inexperience of healthcare worker (HCW). After first aid is initiated, the healthcare worker should report exposure to a supervisor and to the institution's occupational medical service for evaluation. All parenteral exposures should be treated equally until they can be evaluated by the occupational medicine service, who will then determine the actual risk of exposure. Counselling regarding risk of exposure, antiviral prophylaxis, plans for follow up, exposure prevention, sexual activity, and providing emotional support and response to concerns are necessary to support the exposed healthcare worker. Additional information should be provided to healthcare workers who are pregnant or planning to become pregnant.

Immediate actions include aggressive first aid at the puncture site (eg, scrubbing site with povidone-iodine solution or soap and water for 10 minutes) or at mucus membrane site (eg, saline irrigation of eye for 15 minutes), followed by immediate reporting to the hospital's occupational medical service where a thorough investigation should be performed, including identification of the source, type of exposure, volume of inoculum, timing of exposure, extent of injury, appropriateness of first aid, as well as psychological status of the healthcare worker. HIV serologies should be performed on the healthcare worker and HIV risk counselling should begin at this point. Although the data are not clear, antiviral prophylaxis may be offered to healthcare workers who are parenterally or mucous membrane exposed. If used, antiretroviral prophylaxis should be initiated within 1-2 hours after exposure.

Factors to Consider in Assessing the Need for Follow-up of Occupational Exposures

- **Type of exposure**
  - Percutaneous injury
  - Mucous membrane exposure
  - Nonintact skin exposure
  - Bites resulting in blood exposure to either person involved
- **Type and amount of fluid/tissue**
  - Blood
  - Fluids containing blood
  - Potentially infectious fluid or tissue (semen; vaginal secretions; and cerebrospinal, synovial, pleural, peritoneal, pericardial, and amniotic fluids)
  - Direct contact with concentrated virus
- **Infectious status of source**
  - Presence of HB_sAg
  - Presence of HCV antibody
  - Presence of HIV antibody
- **Susceptibility of exposed person**
  - Hepatitis B vaccine and vaccine response status
  - HBV, HCV, HIV immune status

Evaluation of Occupational Exposure Sources

Known sources

- Test known sources for HB_sAg, anti-HCV, and HIV antibody
  - Direct virus assays for routine screening of source patients are **not** recommended
  - Consider using a rapid HIV-antibody test
  - If the source person is **not** infected with a bloodborne pathogen, baseline testing or further follow-up of the exposed person is **not** necessary
- For sources whose infection status remains unknown (eg, the source person refuses testing), consider medical diagnoses, clinical symptoms, and history of risk behaviors
- Do not test discarded needles for bloodborne pathogens

Unknown sources

- For unknown sources, evaluate the likelihood of exposure to a source at high risk for infection
  - Consider the likelihood of bloodborne pathogen infection among patients in the exposure setting

OCCUPATIONAL EXPOSURE TO BLOODBORNE PATHOGENS (STANDARD/UNIVERSAL PRECAUTIONS) *(Continued)*

Recommended Postexposure Prophylaxis for Exposure to Hepatitis B Virus

Vaccination and Antibody Response Status of Exposed Workers[1]	Treatment		
	Source HB_sAg[2]-Positive	**Source HB_sAg[2] -Negative**	**Source Unknown or Not Available for Testing**
Unvaccinated	HBIG[3] x 1 and initiate HB vaccine series[4]	Initiate HB vaccine series	Initiate HB vaccine series
Previously vaccinated			
Known responder[5]	No treatment	No treatment	No treatment
Known nonresponder[6]	HBIG x 1 and initiate revaccination or HBIG x 2[7]	No treatment	If known high risk source, treat as if source was HB_sAg-positive
Antibody response unknown	Test exposed person for anti-HB_s[8] 1. If adequate,[5] no treatment is necessary 2. If inadequate,[6] administer HBIG x 1 and vaccine booster	No treatment	Test exposed person for anti-HB_s 1. If adequate,[4] no treatment is necessary 2. If inadequate,[4] administer vaccine booster and recheck titer in 1-2 months

[1]Persons who have previously been infected with HBV are immune to reinfection and do not require postexposure prophylaxis.

[2]Hepatitis B surface antigen.

[3]Hepatitis B immune globulin; dose is 0.06 mL/kg intramuscularly.

[4]Hepatitis B vaccine.

[5]A responder is a person with adequate levels of serum antibody to HB_sAg (ie, anti-HB_s ≥10 mIU/mL).

[6]A nonresponder is a person with inadequate response to vaccination (ie, serum anti-HB_s <10 mIU/mL).

[7]The option of giving one dose of HBIG and reinitiating the vaccine series is preferred for nonresponders who have not completed a second 3-dose vaccine series. For persons who previously completed a second vaccine series but failed to respond, two doses of HBIG are preferred.

[8]Antibody to HB_sAg.

Recommended HIV Postexposure Prophylaxis for Percutaneous Injuries

Exposure Type	Infection Status of Source				
	HIV-Positive Class 1[1]	HIV-Positive Class 2[1]	Unknown HIV Status[2]	Unknown Source[3]	HIV-Negative
Less severe[4]	Recommend basic 2-drug PEP	Recommend expanded 3-drug PEP	Generally, no PEP warranted; however, consider basic 2-drug PEP[5] for source with HIV risk factors[6]	Generally, no PEP warranted; however, consider basic 2 drug PEP[5] in settings where exposure to HIV-infected persons is likely	No PEP warranted
More severe[7]	Recommend expanded 3-drug PEP	Recommend expanded 3-drug PEP	Generally, no PEP warranted; however consider basic 2-drug PEP[5] for source with HIV risk factors[6]	Generally, no PEP warranted; however, consider basic 2 drug PEP[5] in settings where exposure to HIV-infected persons is likely	No PEP warranted

[1]HIV-Positive, Class 1 – asymptomatic HIV infection or known low viral load (eg, <1500 RNA copies/mL). HIV-Positive Class 2 – symptomatic HIV infection, AIDS, acute seroconversion, or known high viral load. If drug resistance is a concern, obtain expert consultation. Initiation of postexposure prophylaxis (PEP) should not be delayed pending expert consultation, and, because expert consultation alone cannot substitute for face-to-face counseling, resources should be available to provide immediate evaluation and follow-up care for all exposures.

[2]Source of unknown HIV status (eg, deceased source person with no samples available for HIV testing).

[3]Unknown source (eg, a needle from a sharps disposal container).

[4]Less severe (eg, solid needle and superficial injury).

[5]The designation "consider PEP" indicates the PEP is optional and should be based on an individualized decision between the exposed person and the treating clinician.

[6]If PEP is offered and taken and the source is later determined to be HIV-negative, PEP should be discontinued.

[7]More severe (eg, large-bore hollow needle, deep puncture, visible blood on device, or needle used in patient's artery or vein).

OCCUPATIONAL EXPOSURE TO BLOODBORNE PATHOGENS (STANDARD/UNIVERSAL PRECAUTIONS) *(Continued)*

Recommended HIV Postexposure Prophylaxis for Mucous Membrane Exposures and Nonintact Skin[1] Exposures

Exposure Type	Infection Status of Source				
	HIV-Positive Class 1[2]	HIV-Positive Class 2[2]	Unknown HIV Status[3]	Unknown Source[4]	HIV-Negative
Small volume[5]	Consider basic 2-drug PEP[6]	Recommend basic 2-drug PEP	Generally, no PEP warranted; however, consider basic 2-drug PEP[6] for source with HIV risk factors[7]	Generally, no PEP warranted; however, consider basic 2-drug PEP[6] in settings where exposure to HIV-infected persons is likely	No PEP warranted
Large volume[8]	Recommend basic 2-drug PE	Recommend expanded 3-drug PEP	Generally, no PEP warranted; however consider basic 2-drug PEP[6] for source with HIV risk factors[7]	Generally, no PEP warranted; however, consider basic 2-drug PEP[6] in settings where exposure to HIV-infected persons is likely	No PEP warranted

[1]For skin exposures, follow-up is indicated only if there is evidence of compromised skin integrity (eg, dermatitis, abrasion, or open wound).

[2]HIV-Positive, Class 1 – asymptomatic HIV infection or known low viral load (eg, <1500 RNA copies/mL). HIV-Positive Class 2 – symptomatic HIV infection, AIDS, acute seroconversion, or known high viral load. If drug resistance is a concern, obtain expert consultation. Initiation of postexposure prophylaxis (PEP) should not be delayed pending expert consultation, and, because expert consultation alone cannot substitute for face-to-face counseling, resources should be available to provide immediate evaluation and follow-up care for all exposures.

[3]Source of unknown HIV status (eg, deceased source person with no samples available for HIV testing).

[4]Unknown source (eg, splash from inappropriately disposed blood).

[5]Small volume (eg, a few drops).

[6]The designation "consider PEP" indicates the PEP is optional and should be based on an individualized decision between the exposed person and the treating clinician.

[7]If PEP is offered and taken and the source is later determined to be HIV-negative, PEP should be discontinued.

[8]Large volume (eg, major blood splash).

Situations for Which Expert[1] Consultation for HIV Postexposure Prophylaxis Is Advised

- **Delayed (ie, later than 24-36 hours) exposure report**
  - The interval after which there is no benefit from postexposure prophylaxis (PEP) is undefined
- **Unknown source (eg, needle in sharps disposal container or laundry)**
  - Decide use of PEP on a case-by-case basis
  - Consider the severity of the exposure and the epidemiologic likelihood of HIV exposure
  - Do not test needles or sharp instruments for HIV
- **Known or suspected pregnancy in the exposed person**
  - Does not preclude the use of optimal PEP regimens
  - Do not deny PEP solely on the basis of pregnancy
- **Resistance of the source virus to antiretroviral agents**
  - Influence of drug resistance on transmission risk is unknown
  - Selection of drugs to which the source person's virus is unlikely to be resistant is recommended, if the source person's virus is unknown or suspected to be resistant to ≥1 of the drugs considered for the PEP regimen
  - Resistance testing of the source person's virus at the time of the exposure is not recommended
- **Toxicity of the initial PEP regimen**
  - Adverse symptoms, such as nausea and diarrhea, are common with PEP
  - Symptoms can often be managed without changing the PEP regimen by prescribing antimotility and/or antiemetic agents
  - Modification of dose intervals (ie, administering a lower dose of drug more frequently throughout the day, as recommended by the manufacturer), in other situations, might help alleviate symptoms

[1]Local experts and/or the National Clinicians' Postexposure Prophylaxis Hotline (PEPline 1-888-448-4911).

OCCUPATIONAL EXPOSURE TO BLOODBORNE PATHOGENS (STANDARD/UNIVERSAL PRECAUTIONS) *(Continued)*

Occupational Exposure Management Resources

National Clinicians' Postexposure Prophylaxis Hotline (PEPline) Run by University of California-San Francisco/San Francisco General Hospital staff; supported by the Health Resources and Services Administration Ryan White CARE Act, HIV/AIDS Bureau, AIDS Education and Training Centers, and CDC	Phone: (888) 448-4911 Internet: http://www.ucsf.edu/hivcntr
Needlestick! A website to help clinicians manage and document occupational blood and body fluid exposures. Developed and maintained by the University of California, Los Angeles (UCLA), Emergency Medicine Center, UCLA School of Medicine, and funded in part by CDC and the Agency for Healthcare Research and Quality.	Internet: http://www.needlestick.mednet.ucla.edu
Hepatitis Hotline	Phone: (888) 443-7232 Internet: http://www.cdc.gov/hepatitis
Reporting to CDC: Occupationally acquired HIV infections and failures of PEP	Phone: (800) 893-0485
HIV Antiretroviral Pregnancy Registry	Phone: (800) 258-4263 Fax: (800) 800-1052 Address: 1410 Commonwealth Drive, Suite 215 Wilmington, NC 28405 Internet: http://www.glaxowellcome.com/preg_reg/antiretroviral
Food and Drug Administration Report unusual or severe toxicity to antiretroviral agents	Phone: (800) 332-1088 Address: MedWatch HF-2, FDA 5600 Fishers Lane Rockville, MD 20857 Internet: http://www.fda.gov/medwatch
HIV/AIDS Treatment Information Service	Internet: http://www.aidsinfo.nih.gov

Management of Occupational Blood Exposures

Provide immediate care to the exposure site

- Wash wounds and skin with soap and water
- Flush mucous membranes with water

Determine risk associated with exposure by:

- Type of fluid (eg, blood, visibly bloody fluid, other potentially infectious fluid or tissue, and concentrated virus)
- Type of exposure (ie, percutaneous injury, mucous membrane or nonintact skin exposure, and bites resulting in blood exposure)

Evaluate exposure source

- Assess the risk of infection using available information
- Test known sources for HB_sAg, anti-HCV, and HIV antibody (consider using rapid testing)
- For unknown sources, assess risk of exposure to HBV, HCV, or HIV infection
- Do not test discarded needle or syringes for virus contamination

Evaluate the exposed person

- Assess immune status for HBV infection (ie, by history of hepatitis B vaccination and vaccine response)

Give PEP for exposures posing risk of infection transmission

- HBV: See Recommended Postexposure Prophylaxis for Exposure to Hepatitis B Virus Table
- HCV: PEP not recommended
- HIV: See Recommended HIV Postexposure Prophylaxis for Percutaneous Injuries Table and Recommended HIV Postexposure Prophylaxis for Mucous Membrane Exposures and Nonintact Skin Exposures Table
  - Initiate PEP as soon as possible, preferably within hours of exposure
  - Offer pregnancy testing to all women of childbearing age not known to be pregnant
  - Seek expert consultation if viral resistance is suspected
  - Administer PEP for 4 weeks if tolerated

Perform follow-up testing and provide counseling

- Advise exposed persons to seek medical evaluation for any acute illness occurring during follow-up

HBV exposures

- Perform follow-up anti-HB_s testing in persons who receive hepatitis B vaccine
  - Test for anti-HB_s 1-2 months after last dose of vaccine
  - Anti-HB_s response to vaccine cannot be ascertained if HBIG was received in the previous 3-4 months

HCV exposures

- Perform baseline and follow-up testing for anti-HCV and alanine aminotransferase (ALT) 4-6 months after exposures
- Perform HCV RNA at 4-6 months if earlier diagnosis of HCV infection is desired
- Confirm repeatedly reactive anti-HCV enzyme immunoassays (EIAs) with supplemental tests

HIV exposures

- Perform HIV antibody testing for at least 6 months postexposure (eg, at baseline, 6 weeks, 3 months, and 6 months)
- Perform HIV antibody testing if illness compatible with an acute retroviral syndrome occurs
- Advise exposed persons to use precautions to prevent secondary transmission during the follow-up period
- Evaluate exposed persons taking PEP within 72 hours after exposure and monitor for drug toxicity for at least 2 weeks

OCCUPATIONAL EXPOSURE TO BLOODBORNE PATHOGENS (STANDARD/UNIVERSAL PRECAUTIONS) *(Continued)*

Basic and Expanded HIV Postexposure Prophylaxis Regimens

Basic Regimens

- Zidovudine (Retrovir™; ZDV; AZT) + Lamivudine (Epivir™; 3TC); available as Combivir™
  - ZDV: 600 mg daily, in two or three divided doses, and
  - 3TC: 150 mg twice daily

Alternative Basic Regimens

- Lamivudine (3TC) + Stavudine (Zerit™; d4T)
  - 3TC: 150 mg twice daily, and
  - d4T: 40 mg twice daily (if body weight is <60 kg, 30 mg twice daily)
- Didanosine (Videx™, chewable/dispersible buffered tablet; Videx™ EC, delayed-release capsule; ddI) + Stavudine (d4T)
  - ddI: 400 mg daily on an empty stomach (if body weight is <60 kg, 125 mg twice daily)
  - d4T: 40 mg twice daily (if body weight is <60 kg, 30 mg twice daily)

Expanded Regimen

Basic regimen plus one of the following:

- Indinavir (Crixivan™; IDV)
  - 800 mg every 8 hours, on an empty stomach
- Nelfinavir (Viracept™; NFV)
  - 750 mg three times daily, with meals or snack, or
  - 1250 mg twice daily, with meals or snack
- Efavirenz (Sustiva™; EFV)
  - 600 mg daily, at bedtime
  - Should not be used during pregnancy because of concerns about teratogenicity
- Abacavir (Ziagen™; ABC); available at Trizivir™, a combination of ZDV, 3TC, and ABC
  - 300 mg twice daily

Antiretroviral Agents for Use at PEP Only With Expert Consultation

- Ritonavir (Norvir™; RTV)
- Amprenavir (Agenerase™; AMP)
- Delavirdine (Rescriptor™; DLV)
- Lopinavir/Ritonavir (Kaletra™)
  - 400/100 mg twice daily

Antiretroviral Agents Generally Not Recommended for Use as PEP

- Nevirapine (Viramune™; NVP)
  - 200 mg daily for 2 weeks, then 200 mg twice daily

HAZARDOUS COMMUNICATION

Communication regarding the dangers of bloodborne infections through the use of labels, signs, information, and education is required. Storage locations (eg, refrigerators and freezers, waste containers) that are used to store, dispose of, transport, or ship blood or other potentially infectious materials require labels. The label background must be red or bright orange with the biohazard design and the word biohazard in a contrasting color. The label must be part of the container or affixed to the container by permanent means.

Education provided by a qualified and knowledgeable instructor is mandated. The sessions for employees must include:

- accessible copies of the regulation
- general epidemiology of bloodborne diseases
- modes of bloodborne pathogen transmission
- an explanation of the exposure control plan and a means to obtain copies of the written plan
- an explanation of the tasks and activities that may involve exposure
- the use of exposure prevention methods and their limitations (eg, engineering controls, work practices, personal protective equipment)
- information on the types, proper use, location, removal, handling, decontamination, and disposal of personal protective equipment)
- an explanation of the basis for selection of personal protective equipment
- information on the HBV vaccine, including information on its efficacy, safety, and method of administration and the benefits of being vaccinated (ie, the employee must understand that the vaccine and vaccination will be offered free of charge)
- information on the appropriate actions to take and persons to contact in an emergency involving exposure to blood or other potentially infectious materials
- an explanation of the procedure to follow if an exposure incident occurs, including the method of reporting the incident
- information on the postexposure evaluation and follow-up that the employer is required to provide for the employee following an exposure incident

- an explanation of the signs, labels, and color coding
- an interactive question-and-answer period

RECORD KEEPING

The OSHA Final Rule requires that the employer maintain both education and medical records. The medical records must be kept confidential and be maintained for the duration of employment plus 30 years. They must contain a copy of the employee's HBV vaccination status and postexposure incident information. Education records must be maintained for 3 years from the date the program was given.

OSHA has the authority to conduct inspections without notice. Penalties for cited violation may be assessed as follows:

Serious violations. In this situation, there is a substantial probability of death or serious physical harm, and the employer knew, or should have known, of the hazard. A violation of this type carries a mandatory penalty of up to $7000 for each violation.

Other-than-serious violations. The violation is unlikely to result in death or serious physical harm. This type of violation carries a discretionary penalty of up to $7000 for each violation.

Willful violations. These are violations committed knowingly or intentionally by the employer and have penalties of up to $70,000 per violation with a minimum of $5000 per violation. If an employee dies as a result of a willful violation, the responsible party, if convicted, may receive a personal fine of up to $250,000 and/or a 6-month jail term. A corporation may be fined $500,000.

Large fines frequently follow visits to laboratories, physicians' offices, and healthcare facilities by OSHA Compliance Safety and Health Offices (CSHOS). Regulations are vigorously enforced. A working knowledge of the final rule and implementation of appropriate policies and practices is imperative for all those involved in the collection and analysis of medical specimens.

Effectiveness of universal precautions in averting exposure to potentially infectious materials has been documented.[7] Compliance with appropriate rules, procedures, and policies, including reporting exposure incidents, is a matter of personal professionalism and prudent self-preservation.

Footnotes

1. Henderson DK, Fahey BJ, Willy M, et al, "Risk for Occupational Transmission of Human Immunodeficiency Virus Type 1 (HIV-1) Associated With Clinical Exposures. A Prospective Evaluation," *Ann Intern Med*, 1990, 113(10):740-6.
2. Niu MT and Margolis HS, "Moving Into a New Era of Government Regulation: Provisions for Hepatitis B Vaccine in the Workplace, *Clin Lab Manage Rev*, 1989, 3:336-40.
3. Bruning LM, "The Bloodborne Pathogens Final Rule — Understanding the Regulation," *AORN Journal*, 1993, 57(2):439-40.
4. "Rules and Regulations," *Federal Register*, 1994, 59(66):16360-3.
5. Schaffner W, Gardner P, and Gross PA, "Hepatitis B Immunization Strategies: Expanding the Target," *Ann Intern Med*, 1993, 118(4):308-9.
6. Fahey BJ, Beekmann SE, Schmitt JM, et al, "Managing Occupational Exposures to HIV-1 in the Healthcare Workplace," *Infect Control Hosp Epidemiol*, 1993, 14(7):405-12.
7. Wong ES, Stotka JL, Chinchilli VM, et al, "Are Universal Precautions Effective in Reducing the Number of Occupational Exposures Among Healthcare Workers?" *JAMA*, 1991, 265(9):1123-8.

References

Buehler JW and Ward JW, "A New Definition for AIDS Surveillance," *Ann Intern Med*, 1993, 118(5):390-2.

Brown JW and Blackwell H, "Complying With the New OSHA Regs, Part 1: Teaching Your Staff About Biosafety," *MLO*, 1992, 24(4)24-8. Part 2: "Safety Protocols No Lab Can Ignore," 1992, 24(5):27-9. Part 3: "Compiling Employee Safety Records That Will Satisfy OSHA," 1992, 24(6):45-8.

Department of Labor, Occupational Safety and Health Administration, "Occupational Exposure to Bloodborne Pathogens; Final Rule (29 CFR Part 1910.1030), "*Federal Register*, December 6, 1991, 64004-182.

Gold JW, "HIV-1 Infection: Diagnosis and Management," *Med Clin North Am*, 1992, 76(1):1-18.

"Hepatitis B Virus: A Comprehensive Strategy for Eliminating Transmission in the United States Through Universal Childhood Vaccination," Recommendations of the Immunization Practices Advisory Committee (ACIP), *MMWR Morb Mortal Wkly Rep*, 1991, 40(RR-13):1-25.

"Mortality Attributable to HIV Infection/AIDS — United States", *MMWR Morb Mortal Wkly Rep*, 1991, 40(3):41-4.

National Committee for Clinical Laboratory Standards, "Protection of Laboratory Workers From Infectious Disease Transmitted by Blood, Body Fluids, and Tissue," NCCLS Document M29-T, Villanova, PA: NCCLS, 1989, 9(1).

"Nosocomial Transmission of Hepatitis B Virus Associated With a Spring-Loaded Fingerstick Device — California," *MMWR Morb Mortal Wkly Rep*, 1990, 39(35):610-3.

Polish LB, Shapiro CN, Bauer F, et al, "Nosocomial Transmission of Hepatitis B Virus Associated With the Use of a Spring-Loaded Fingerstick Device," *N Engl J Med*, 1992, 326(11):721-5.

"Recommendations for Preventing Transmission of Human Immunodeficiency Virus and Hepatitis B Virus to Patients During Exposure-Prone Invasive Procedures," *MMWR Morb Mortal Wkly Rep*, 1991, 40(RR-8):1-9.

"Update: Acquired Immunodeficiency Syndrome — United States," *MMWR Morb Mortal Wkly Rep*, 1992, 41(26):463-8.

"Update: Transmission of HIV Infection During an Invasive Dental Procedure — Florida," *MMWR Morb Mortal Wkly Rep*, 1991, 40(2):21-7, 33.

"Update: Universal Precautions for Prevention of Transmission of Human Immunodeficiency Virus, Hepatitis B Virus, and Other Bloodborne Pathogens in Healthcare Settings," *MMWR Morb Mortal Wkly Rep*, 1988, 37(24):377-82, 387-8.

"U.S. Public Health Service Guidelines for the Management of Occupational Exposures to HBV, HCV, and HIV and Recommendations for Postexposure Prophylaxis," *MMWR Morb Mortal Wkly Rep*, 2001, 50(RR-11).

IMMUNIZATIONS[1] (VACCINES)

Vaccine	Use
Anthrax Vaccine (Adsorbed)[2] BioThrax™	Used for individuals who may come in contact with animal products which come from anthrax endemic areas and may be contaminated with *Bacillus anthracis* spores and for high-risk persons such as veterinarians and other handling potentially infected animals; Department of Defense is implementing an anthrax vaccination program for active duty and reserve personnel against the biological warfare agent anthrax
BCG Vaccine TheraCys®; TICE® BCG	Bladder instillation of vaccine as immunotherapy for treatment of bladder cancer (TheraCys®; TICE® BCG). BCG vaccine is not routinely recommended for use in the U.S. for prevention of tuberculosis. BCG should be administered with caution to persons in groups at high risk for HIV infection or persons know to be severely immunocompromised. Although limited data suggests that the vaccine may be safe for use in asymptomatic children infected with HIV, BCG vaccination is not recommended for HIV infected adults or for persons with symptomatic disease. Vaccination should be restricted to persons at exceptionally high risk for tuberculosis infection. HIV infected persons thought to be infected with *Mycobacterium tuberculosis* should be strongly recommended for tuberculosis preventive therapy.
Cholera Vaccine Mutacol Berna® (Canada)	Primary immunization for cholera prophylaxis. The World Health Organization no longer recommends cholera vaccination for travel to or from cholera-endemic areas. Some countries may still require evidence of a complete primary series or a booster dose given within 6 months of arrival. Vaccination should not be considered as an alternative to continued careful selection of foods and water. Ideally, cholera and yellow fever vaccines should be administered at least 3 weeks apart.
Diphtheria, Tetanus Toxoids, and Acellular Pertussis Vaccine Daptacel™; Infanrix®; Tripedia®	Active immunization against diphtheria, tetanus, and pertussis from age 6 weeks through seventh birthday
Diphtheria, Tetanus Toxoids, Acellular Pertussis Vaccine and *Haemophilus influenzae* b Conjugate Vaccine (Combined) TriHIBit®	Active immunization of children 15-18 months of age for prevention of diphtheria, tetanus, pertussis, and invasive disease caused by *H. influenzae* type b
Diphtheria, Tetanus Toxoids, Acellular Pertussis, Hepatitis B (Recombinant), and Poliovirus (Inactivated) Vaccine Pediarix™	Combination vaccine for the active immunization against diphtheria, tetanus, pertussis, hepatitis B virus (all known subtypes), and poliomyelitis (caused by poliovirus types 1, 2, and 3)

Vaccine	Use
Haemophilus b Conjugate Vaccine ActHIB®; HibTITER®; PedvaxHIB®	Routine immunization of children 2 months to 5 years of age against invasive disease caused by *H. influenzae* type b. Nonimmunized children ≥5 years of age with a chronic illness known to be associated with increased risk of *Haemophilus influenzae* type b disease, specifically, persons with anatomic or functional asplenia or sickle cell anemia or those who have undergone splenectomy, should receive Hib vaccine, as well as adults with specific dysfunction or certain complement deficiencies who are at especially high risk of *H. influenzae* type b infection (HIV-infected adults); patients with Hodgkin's disease or other hematologic neoplasms and immunosuppression (vaccinated at least 2 weeks before the initiation of chemotherapy or 3 months after the end of chemotherapy). *Haemophilus* b conjugate vaccines are not indicated for prevention of bronchitis or other infections due to *H. influenzae* in adults.
Hepatitis A Vaccine Havrix®; VAQTA®	For populations desiring protection against hepatitis A or for populations at high risk of exposure to hepatitis A virus (travelers to developing countries, household and sexual contacts of persons infected with hepatitis A), child day care employees, illicit drug users, patients with chronic liver disease, male homosexuals, institutional workers (eg, institutions for the mentally and physically handicapped persons, prisons, etc), and healthcare workers who may be exposed to hepatitis A virus (eg, laboratory employees); protection lasts for approximately 15 years
Hepatitis A (Inactivated) and Hepatitis B (Recombinant) Vaccine Twinrix®	Active immunization against disease caused by hepatitis A virus and hepatitis B virus (all known subtypes) in populations desiring protection against or at high risk of exposure to these viruses. Populations include travelers to areas of intermediate/high endemicity for both HAV and HBV; those at increased risk of HBV infection due to behavioral or occupational factors; patients with chronic liver disease; laboratory workers who handle live HAV and HBV; healthcare workers, police, and other personnel who render firstaid or medical assistance; workers who come in contact with sewage; employees of day care centers and correctional facilities; patients/staff of hemodialysis units; male homosexuals; patients frequently receiving blood products; military personnel; users of injectable illicit drugs; close household contacts of patients with hepatitis A and hepatitis B infection.
Hepatitis B Immune Globulin BayHepB™; Nabi-HB®	Provide prophylactic passive immunity to hepatitis B infection to those individuals exposed; newborns of mothers known to be hepatitis B surface antigen positive; hepatitis B immune globulin is not indicated for treatment of active hepatitis B infections and is ineffective in the treatment of chronic active hepatitis B infection
Hepatitis B Vaccine Engerix-B®; Recombivax HB®	Immunization against infection caused by all known subtypes of hepatitis B virus, in individuals considered at high risk of potential exposure to hepatitis B virus or HB_sAg-positive materials.
Immune Globulin (Intramuscular) BayGam®	Household and sexual contacts of persons with hepatitis A, measles, varicella, and possibly rubella; travelers to high-risk areas outside tourist routes; staff, attendees, and parents of diapered attendees in day-care center outbreaks. For travelers, IG is not an alternative to careful selection of foods and water; immune globulin can interfere with the antibody response to parenterally administered live virus vaccines. Frequent travelers should be tested for hepatitis A antibody, immune hemolytic anemia, and neutropenia (with TTP, I.V. route is usually used).
Influenza Virus Vaccine FluShield®; Fluvirin®; Fluzone®	Provide active immunity to influenza virus strains contained in the vaccine; for high-risk persons, previous year vaccines do not prevent present year influenza. Those at risk for influenza injection include persons ≥65 years of age; institutionalized patients; persons of any age with chronic disorders of pulmonary and/or cardiovascular system; persons who have required medical follow-up following hospitalization for other chronic diseases such as diabetes, renal disease, immunodepressive disorders, etc; and travelers, especially those at risk. Children and teenagers (6 months to 18 years) who are receiving long-term aspirin therapy and, therefore, may be at risk for developing Reye's syndrome after influenza.

IMMUNIZATIONS[1] (VACCINES) *(Continued)*

Vaccine	Use
Japanese Encephalitis Virus Vaccine (Inactivated) JE-VAX®	Active immunization against Japanese encephalitis for persons 1 year of age and older who plan to spend 1 month or more in endemic areas in Asia, especially persons traveling during the transmission season or visiting rural areas. Consider vaccination for shorter trips to epidemic areas or extensive outdoor activities in rural endemic areas. Elderly (>55 years of age) individuals should be considered for vaccination, since they have increased risk of developing symptomatic illness after infection. Those planning travel to or residence in endemic areas should consult the Travel Advisory Service (Central Campus) for specific advice.
Measles, Mumps, and Rubella Vaccines (Combined) M-M-R® II	Measles, mumps, and rubella prophylaxis
Measles Virus Vaccine (Live) Attenuvax®	Immunization for adults born after 1957 without documentation of live vaccine on or after first birthday, physician-diagnosed measles, or laboratory evidence of immunity should be vaccinated, ideally with two doses of vaccine separated by no less than 1 month. For those previously vaccinated with one dose of measles vaccine, revaccination is recommended for students entering colleges and other institutions of higher education, for healthcare workers at the time of employment, and for international travelers who visit endemic areas.
Meningococcal Polysaccharide Vaccine (Groups A, C, Y, and W-135) Menomune®-A/C/Y/W-135	Immunization of persons 2 years of age and older in epidemic or endemic areas as might be determined in a population delineated by neighborhood, school, dormitory, or other reasonable boundary. The prevalent serogroup in such a situation should match a serogroup in the vaccine. Individuals at particular high-risk include persons with terminal component complement deficiencies and those with anatomic or function asplenia. For use with travelers visiting areas of a country that are recognized as having hyperendemic or epidemic meningococcal disease. Vaccinations should be considered for household or institutional contacts of persons with meningococcal disease as an adjunct to appropriate antibiotic chemoprophylaxis as well as medical and laboratory personnel at risk of exposure to meningococcal disease.
Mumps Virus Vaccine (Live/Attenuated) Mumpsvax®	Mumps prophylaxis by promoting active immunity **Note:** Trivalent measles-mumps-rubella (M-M-R® II) vaccine is the preferred agent for most children and many adults. Persons born prior to 1957 are generally considered immune and need not be vaccinated.
Plague Vaccine	Vaccinate selected travelers to countries where avoidance of rodents and fleas is impossible; laboratory and field personnel working with *Yersinia pestis* organisms possibly resistant to antimicrobials; those engaged in *Yersinia pestis* aerosol experiments or in field operations in areas with enzootic plague where regular exposure to potentially infected wild rodents, rabbits, or their fleas cannot be prevented. Prophylactic antibiotics may be indicated following definite exposure, whether or not the exposed persons have been vaccinated.
Pneumococcal Conjugate Vaccine (7-Valent) Prevnar®	Immunization of infants and toddlers against active disease caused by *Streptococcus pneumoniae* due to serotypes included in the vaccine
Pneumococcal Polysaccharide Vaccine (Polyvalent) Pneumovax® 23; Pneumo 23™	For children >2 years of age and adults who are at increased risk of pneumococcal disease and its complications because of underlying health conditions; older adults, including all those ≥65 years of age

Vaccine	Use
Poliovirus Vaccine (Inactivated) IPOL®	AAP recommends three poliomyelitis vaccines schedules: OPV-only, IPV-only and sequential IPV-OPV. Inactivated poliovirus vaccine contains three types of poliovirus grown either in monkey kidney or human diploid cells and inactivated with formaldehyde. IPV is of enhanced potency and is highly immunogenic. OPV schedule ONLY is recommended when parents or providers who prefer not to have the child receive the additional injections needed if IPV were to be used, for infants and children starting vaccination regimens after 6 months of age in whom an accelerated schedule is necessary to complete immunizations, an OPV-only regimen will minimize the number of injections required at each visit. In populations with low vaccination rates, OPV may be preferred in order to expedite implementation of the routine childhood immunization schedule. IPV schedule ONLY is recommended for immunocompromised persons and their household contacts (OPV would be contraindicated); for infants and children in which an adult household member is know to be inadequately vaccinated against poliomyelitis, because unimmunized adults are at increased risk of vaccine-associated paralytic poliomyelitis (VAPP); when the number of injections is not likely to decrease compliance and when IPV is preferred by healthcare providers or parents or other caregivers. IPV Primary immunization is also recommended for unvaccinated adults because the risk of VAPP after OPV is slightly higher in adults than in children. Sequential IPV/OPV schedule is recommended to reduce the total number of injections required to reduce the risk of VAPP while maintaining optimal intestinal immunity, especially for travelers to areas where poliovirus is still endemic. The rationale of sequential use of IPV and OPV is that two doses of IPV induce sufficient humoral immunity to prevent VAPP in recipients from subsequent administration of OPV, given to induce optimal intestinal immunity as well as to sustain humoral immunity.
Rabies Immune Globulin (Human) BayRab®; Imogam®	Part of postexposure prophylaxis of persons with rabies exposure who lack a history of pre-exposure or postexposure prophylaxis with rabies vaccine or a recently documented neutralizing antibody response to previous rabies vaccination. It is preferable to give RIG with the first dose of vaccine, but it can be given up to 8 days after vaccination.
Rabies Virus Vaccine Imovax® Rabies	Pre-exposure rabies immunization for high-risk persons; postexposure antirabies immunization along with local treatment and immune globulin
Rh_o(D) Immune Globulin BayRho-D® Full-Dose; BayRh-D® Mini-Dose; RhoGAM®; WinRho SDF®	Suppression of Rh isoimmunization: Use in the following situations when an Rh_o(D)-negative individual is exposed to Rh_o(D)-positive blood: During delivery of an Rh_o(D)-positive infant; abortion; amniocentesis; chorionic villus sampling; ruptured tubal pregnancy; abdominal trauma; transplacental hemorrhage. Used when the mother is Rh_o(D) negative, the father of the child is either Rh_o(D) positive or Rho(D) unknown, the baby is either either Rh_o(D) positive or Rho(D) unknown. Transfusion: Suppression of Rh isoimmunization in Rh_o(D)-negative female children and female adults in their childbearing years transfused with Rh_o(D) antigen-positive RBCs or blood components containing Rh_o(D) antigen-positive RBCs. Treatment of idiopathic thrombocytopenic purpura (ITP): Used in the following nonsplenectomized Rh_o(D) positive individuals: Children with acute or chronic ITP, adults with chronic ITP, children and adults with ITP secondary to HIV infection
Respiratory Synctial Virus Immune Globulin RespiGam®	Orphan drug: Prevention of serious lower respiratory infection caused by respiratory syncytial virus (RSV) in children <24 months of age with bronchopulmonary dysplasia (BPD) or a history of premature birth (35 weeks gestation)

IMMUNIZATIONS[1] (VACCINES) *(Continued)*

Vaccine	Use
Rubella Virus Vaccine (Live) Meruvax® II	Selective active immunization against rubella; vaccination is routinely recommended for persons from 12 months of age to puberty. All adults, both male and female, lacking documentation of live vaccine on or after first birthday, or laboratory evidence of immunity (particularly women of childbearing age and young adults who work in or congregate in hospitals, colleges, and on military bases) should be vaccinated. Susceptible travelers should be vaccinated. **Note:** Trivalent measles-mumps-rubella (M-M-R® II) vaccine is the preferred agent for most children and many adults. Persons born prior to 1957 are generally considered immune and need not be vaccinated.
Smallpox Vaccine[3] Dryvax®	Active immunization agains vaccinia virus, the causative agent of smallpox. The ACIP recommends vaccination of laboratory workers at risk of exposure from cultures or contaminated animals which may be a source of vaccinia or related Orthopoxviruses capable of causing infections in humans (monkeypox, cowpox, or variola). Revaccination is recommended every 10 years. The Armed Forces recommend vaccination of certain personnel categories.
Tetanus Antitoxin	Tetanus prophylaxis or treatment of active tetanus only when tetanus immune globulin (TIG) is not available. Tetanus immune globulin (Hyper-Tet®) is the preferred tetanus immunoglobulin for the treatment of active tetanus. May be given concomitantly with tetanus toxoid adsorbed when immediate treatment is required, but active immunization is desirable.
Tetanus Immune Globulin (Human) (BayTet™)	Passive immunization against tetanus; tetanus immune globulin is preferred over tetanus antitoxin for treatment of active tetanus; part of the management of an unclean wound in a person whose history of previous receipt of tetanus toxoid is unknown or who has received less than three doses of tetanus toxoid; elderly may require TIG more often than younger patients with tetanus infection due to declining antibody titers with age
Tetanus Toxoid (Adsorbed)	Selective induction of active immunity against tetanus in selected patients. **Note:** Tetanus and diphtheria toxoids for adult use (Td) is the preferred immunizing agent for most adults and for children after 7 years of age. Young children should receive trivalent DTwP or DTaP (diphtheria/tetanus/ pertussis – whole cell or acellular), as part of their childhood immunization program, unless pertussis is contraindicated, then TD is warranted.
Tetanus Toxoid (Fluid)	Detection of delayed hypersensitivity and assessment of cell-mediated immunity; active immunization against tetanus in the rare adult or child who is allergic to the aluminum adjuvant (a product containing adsorbed tetanus toxoid is preferred)
Typhoid Vaccine Typhim Vi®; Vivotif Berna®	**Parenteral:** Promotes active immunity to typhoid fever for patients intimately exposed to a typhoid carrier or foreign travel to a typhoid fever endemic area. **Oral:** Immunize children older than 6 years and adults who expect intimate exposure of or household contact with typhoid fever, travelers to areas of the world with a risk of exposure to typhoid fever, and workers in microbiology laboratories with expected frequent contact with *S. typhi.* **Typhoid vaccine:** Live, attenuated TY21a typhoid vaccine should not be administered to immunocompromised persons, including those known to be infected with HIV. Parenteral inactivated vaccine is a theoretically safer alternative for this group.
Varicella Virus Vaccine Varivax®	The American Association of Pediatrics recommends that the chickenpox vaccine should be given to all healthy children between 12 months and 18 years. children between 12 months and 13 years who have not been immunized or who have not had chickenpox should receive 1 vaccination while children 13-18 years of age require 2 vaccinations 4-8 weeks apart. The vaccine has been added to the childhood immunization schedule for infants 12-28 months of age and children 11-12 years of age who have not been vaccinated previously or who have not had the disease. It is recommended to be given with the measles, mumps, and rubella (MMR) vaccine.

Vaccine	Use
Varicella-Zoster Immune Globulin (Human)	Passive immunization of susceptible immunodeficient patients after exposure to varicella. Most effective if begun within 72 hours of exposure. There is no evidence that VZIG modifies established varicella-zoster infections. **Restrict administration to:** Patients with neoplastic disease (leukemia, lymphoma); congenital or acquired immunodeficiency; immunosuppressive therapy with steroids, antimetabolites, or other immunosuppressive treatment regimens; newborns or mothers who had onset of chickenpox within 5 days before delivery or within 48 hours after delivery; premature infant (≥28 weeks gestation) whose mother has no history of chickenpox; premature infants (<28 weeks gestation or ≤1000 g VZIG) regardless of maternal history. **One of the following types of exposure to chickenpox or zoster patients may warrant administration:** Continuous household contact; playmate contact (>1 hour play indoors); hospital contact (in same 2-4 bedroom or adjacent beds in a large ward or prolonged face-to-face contact with an infectious staff member of patient); susceptible to varicella-zoster; age <15 years (administer to immunocompromised adolescents and adults and to other older patients on an individual basis). An acceptable alternative to VZIG prophylaxis is to treat varicella, if it occurs, with high-dose I.V. acyclovir.
Yellow Fever Vaccine YF-VAX®	Vaccinate selected persons traveling or living in areas where yellow fever infection exists.

[1]Contact Poison Control Center.

[2]Not commercially available in the U.S.; presently, all anthrax vaccine lots are owned by the U.S. Department of Defense. The Centers for Disease Control (CDC) does not currently recommend routine vaccination of the general public.

[3]Recommendations for use in response to bioterrorism are regularly updated by the CDC, and may be found at www.cdc.gov.

NORMAL BLOOD VALUES

Test	Range of Normal Values
Complete blood count (CBC)	
White blood cells	4,500-11,000
Red blood cells (male)	4.6-6.2 x 10^6 μL
Red blood cells (female)	4.2-5.4 x 10^6 μL
Platelets	150,000-450,000
Hematocrit (male)	40% to 54%
Hematocrit (female)	38% to 47%
Hemoglobin (male)	13.5-18 g/dL
Hemoglobin (female)	12-16 g/dL
Mean corpuscular volume (MCV)	80-96 μm^3
Mean corpuscular hemoglobin (MCH)	27-31 pg
Mean corpuscular hemoglobin concentration (MCHC)	32% to 36%
Differential white blood cell count (%)	
Segmented neutrophils	56
Bands	3.0
Eosinophils	2.7
Basophils	0.3
Lymphocytes	34.0
Monocytes	4.0
Hemostasis	
Bleeding time (BT)	2-8 minutes
Prothrombin time (PT)	10-13 seconds
Activated partial thromboplastin time (aPTT)	25-35 seconds
Serum chemistry	
Glucose (fasting)	70-110 mg/dL
Blood urea nitrogen (BUN)	8-23 mg/dL
Creatinine (male)	0.1-0.4 mg/dL
Creatinine (female)	0.2-0.7 mg/dL
Bilirubin, indirect (unconjugated)	0.3 mg/dL
Bilirubin, direct (conjugated)	0.1-1 mg/dL
Calcium	9.2-11 mg/dL
Magnesium	1.8-3 mg/dL
Phosphorus	2.3-4.7 mg/dL
Serum electrolytes	
Sodium (Na^+)	136-142 mEq/L
Potassium (K^+)	3.8-5 mEq/L
Chloride (Cl^-)	95-103 mEq/L
Bicarbonate (HCO_3^-)	21-28 mmol/L
Serum enzymes	
Alkaline phosphatase	20-130 IU/L
Alanine aminotransferase (ALT) (formerly called SGPT)	4-36 units/L
Aspartate aminotransferase (AST) (formerly called SGOT)	8-33 units/L
Amylase	16-120 Somogyi units/dL
Creatine kinase (CK) (male)	55-170 units/L
Creatine kinase (CK) (female)	30-135 units/L

DENTIFRICE PRODUCTS

Brand Name	Abrasive Ingredient	Therapeutic Ingredient	Foaming Agent
Aim® Baking Soda Gel	Hydrated silica, sodium bicarbonate	Sodium monofluorophosphate 0.7% (fluoride 0.14%)	Sodium lauryl sulfate
	Other Ingredients: Sorbitol and related polyols, water, glycerin, SD alcohol 38B, flavor, cellulose gum, sodium saccharin, blue #1, yellow #10		
Aim® Extra Strength Gel	Hydrated silica	Sodium monofluorophosphate 1.2%	Sodium lauryl sulfate
	Other Ingredients: Sorbitol, water, PEG-32, SD alcohol 38B, flavor, cellulose gum, sodium saccharin, sodium benzoate, blue #1, yellow #10		
Aim® Regular Strength	Hydrated silica	Sodium monofluorophosphate 0.8% (fluoride 0.14%)	Sodium lauryl sulfate
	Other Ingredients: Sorbitol and other related polyols, water, glycerin, SD alcohol 38B, flavor, cellulose gum, sodium saccharin, blue #1, yellow #10		
Aim® Tartar Control Gel	Hydrated silica	Sodium monofluorophosphate 0.8% (fluoride 0.14%)	Sodium lauryl sulfate
	Other Ingredients: Sorbitol and related polyols, water, glycerin, zinc citrate trihydrate, SD alcohol 38B, flavor, cellulose gum, sodium saccharin, blue #1, yellow #10		
Aquafresh® Baking Soda Toothpaste	Calcium carbonate, hydrated silica, sodium bicarbonate	Sodium monofluorophosphate	Sodium lauryl sulfate
	Other Ingredients: Calcium carrageenan, cellulose gum, colors, flavor, glycerin, PEG-8, sodium benzoate, sodium saccharin, sorbitol, titanium dioxide, water		
Aquafresh® Extra Fresh Toothpaste*	Hydrated silica, calcium carbonate	Sodium monofluorophosphate	Sodium lauryl sulfate
	Other Ingredients: Sorbitol, water, glycerin, PEG-8, titanium dioxide, cellulose gum, flavor, sodium saccharin, sodium benzoate, calcium carrageenan, colors		
Aquafresh® for Kids Toothpaste*	Hydrated silica, calcium carbonate	Sodium monofluorophosphate	Sodium lauryl sulfate
	Other Ingredients: Sorbitol, water, glycerin, PEG-8, titanium dioxide, cellulose gum, flavor, sodium saccharin, calcium carrageenan, sodium benzoate, colors		
Aquafresh® Gum Care Toothpaste	Hydrated silica, calcium carbonate	Sodium monofluorophosphate	Sodium lauryl sulfate
	Other Ingredients: Calcium carrageenan, cellulose gum, colors, flavor, PEG-8, sodium benzoate, sodium saccharin, sorbitol, titanium dioxide, water		
Aquafresh® Sensitive Toothpaste	Hydrated silica	Potassium nitrate, sodium fluoride	Sodium lauryl sulfate
	Other Ingredients: Colors, flavor, glycerin, sodium benzoate, sodium saccharin, sorbitol, titanium dioxide, water, xanthan gum		
Aquafresh® Tartar Control Toothpaste*	Hydrated silica	Sodium fluoride	Sodium lauryl sulfate
	Other Ingredients: Tetrapotassium pyrophosphate, tetrasodium pyrophosphate, sorbitol, glycerin, PEG-8, flavor, xanthan gum, sodium saccharin, sodium benzoate, colors, titanium dioxide, water		
Aquafresh® Triple Protection Toothpaste*	Hydrated silica, calcium carbonate	Sodium monofluorophosphate	Sodium lauryl sulfate
	Other Ingredients: PEG-8, sorbitol, cellulose gum, sodium benzoate, titanium dioxide, calcium carrageenan, flavor, sodium saccharin, colors, water		
Aquafresh® Whitening Gel or Toothpaste	Hydrated silica	Sodium fluoride	Sodium lauryl sulfate
	Other Ingredients: Colors, flavor, glycerin, PEG-8, sodium benzoate, sodium hydroxide, sodium saccharin, sodium tripolyphosphate, sorbitol, titanium dioxide, water, xanthan gum		
Biotene® Antibacterial Dry Mouth Toothpaste	Hydrated silica, calcium pyrophosphate	Lactoperoxidase, glucose oxidase, lysozyme, sodium monofluorophosphate (0.76%)	
	Other Ingredients: Sorbitol, glycerin, xylitol, isoceteth-20, cellulose gum, flavor, sodium benzoate, beta-d-glucose, potassium thiocyanate		

DENTIFRICE PRODUCTS *(Continued)*

Brand Name	Abrasive Ingredient	Therapeutic Ingredient	Foaming Agent
Close-Up® Baking Soda Toothpaste (mint)	Hydrated silica, sodium bicarbonate	Sodium monofluorophosphate 0.79% (fluoride 0.15%)	Sodium lauryl sulfate
	Other Ingredients: Sorbitol and related polyols, water, glycerin, SD alcohol 38B, flavor, cellulose gum, sodium saccharin, sodium benzoate, red #33, red #40, titanium dioxide		
Close-Up® Classic Red Gel	Hydrated silica	Sodium monofluorophosphate 0.8% (fluoride 0.14%)	Sodium lauryl sulfate
	Other Ingredients: Sorbitol and related polyols, water, glycerin, SD alcohol 38B, flavor, cellulose gum, sodium saccharin, sodium chloride, red #33, red #40		
Close-Up® Cool Mint Gel	Hydrated silica	Sodium monofluorophosphate 0.79% (fluoride 0.15%)	Sodium lauryl sulfate
	Other Ingredients: Sorbitol, water, glycerin, SD alcohol 38B, flavor, cellulose gum, sodium saccharin, polysorbate 20, blue #1, mica, red #33, titanium dioxide		
Close-Up® Original Red Whitening Toothpaste	Hydrated silica	Sodium monofluorophosphate 0.8% (fluoride 0.14%)	Sodium lauryl sulfate
	Other Ingredients: Sorbitol and related polyols, water, glycerin, SD alcohol 38B, flavor, cellulose gum, sodium saccharin, sodium chloride, red #30 lake, titanium dioxide, blue #1		
Close-Up® Tartar Control Gel (mint)	Hydrated silica	Sodium monofluorophosphate 0.79% (fluoride 0.15%)	Sodium lauryl sulfate
	Other Ingredients: Sorbitol and related polyols, water, glycerin, zinc citrate trihydrate, SD alcohol 38B, flavor, cellulose gum, sodium saccharin, red #33, red #40, **caffeine free**		
Close-Up® Tartar Control Whitening Toothpaste	Hydrated silica	Sodium monofluorophosphate 0.8% (fluoride 0.14%)	Sodium lauryl sulfate
	Other Ingredients: Sorbitol and related polypols, water, glycerin, SD alcohol 38B, flavor, zinc citrate trihydrate, cellulose gum, sodium saccharin, titanium dioxide, blue #1, yellow #10		
Colgate® Baking Soda & Peroxide Tartar Control Toothpaste*	Hydrated silica, sodium bicarbonate	Sodium monofluorophosphate 0.76%	Sodium lauryl sulfate
	Other Ingredients: Glycerin, propylene glycol, water, pentasodium triphosphate, tetrasodium pyrophosphate, titanium dioxide, flavor, sodium hydroxide, calcium peroxide, sodium saccharin, carrageenan, cellulose gum, FD&C blue #1, D&C yellow #10		
Colgate® Baking Soda & Peroxide Whitening Toothpaste*	Hydrated silica, sodium bicarbonate, aluminum oxide	Sodium monofluorophosphate 0.76%	Sodium lauryl sulfate
	Other Ingredients: Glycerin, polypylene glycol, water, pentasodium triphosphate, tetrasodium pyrophosphate, titanium dioxide, flavor, sodium hydroxide, calcium peroxide, sodium saccharin, carrageenan, cellulose gum, **dietetically sucrose free**		
Colgate® Baking Soda Tartar Control Gel or Toothpaste	Hydrated silica, sodium bicarbonate	Sodium fluoride 0.243%	Sodium lauryl sulfate
	Other Ingredients: Glycerin, tetrasodium pyrophosphate, PVM/MA copolymer, cellulose gum, flavor, sodium saccharin, sodium hydroxide, titanium dioxide (paste), FD&C blue #1, D&C yellow #10 (gel), **dietetically sucrose free**		
Colgate® Junior Gel*	Hydrated silica	Sodium fluoride 0.243%	Sodium lauryl sulfate
	Other Ingredients: Sorbitol, water, PEG-12, flavor, tetrasodium pyrophosphate, cellulose gum, sodium saccharin, mica, titanium dioxide, colorants, **dietetically sucrose free**		
Colgate® Platinum™ Whitening Toothpaste*	Silica, aluminum oxide	Sodium monofluorophosphate	Sodium lauryl sulfate
	Other Ingredients: Water, hydrated silica, sorbitol, glycerin, PEG-12, tetrapotassium pyrophosphate, PVM/MA copolymer, flavor, sodium hydroxide, sodium saccharin, titanium dioxide		
Colgate® Platinum™ Whitening with Baking Soda Toothpaste*	Sodium bicarbonate, aluminum oxide	Sodium monofluorophosphate 0.76%	Sodium lauryl sulfate
	Other Ingredients: Water, glycerin, PEG-12, tetrapotassium pyrophosphate, PVM/MA copolymer, flavor, sodium hydroxide, sodium saccharin, titanium dioxide, cellulose gum		

Brand Name	Abrasive Ingredient	Therapeutic Ingredient	Foaming Agent
Colgate® Sensitive Maximum Strength Toothpaste	Hydrated silica, sodium bicarbonate	Potassium nitrate 5%, stannous fluoride 0.45%	Sodium lauryl sulfate
	Other Ingredients: Glycerin and/or sorbitol, water, PEG-40 castor oil, PEG-12, poloxamer 407, sodium citrate, flavor, titanium dioxide, sodium hydroxide, cellulose gum, xanthan gum, sodium saccharin, stannous chloride, citric acid, tetrasodium pyrophosphate, FD&C Blue No. 1		
Colgate® Sensitive Plus Whitening	Hydrated silica, Sodium bicarbonate	Potassium nitrate 5% antisensitivity (FDA required amount), Stannous Fluoride 0.45% (0.15% w/v fluoride ion)	Sodium lauryl sulfate
	Other Ingredients: Glycerin and/or sorbitol, water, PEG-40 castor oil, PEG-12, poloxamer 405, sodium citrate, flavor, titanium dioxide, sodium hydroxide, cellulose gum, xanthan gum, sodium saccharin, stannous chloride, citric acid, tetrasodium pyrophosphate, mica, FD&C blue No.1, D&C yellow No. 10		
Colgate® Tartar Control Micro Cleansing Gel or Toothpaste*	Hydrated silica	Sodium fluoride 0.243%	Sodium lauryl sulfate
	Other Ingredients: Water, sorbitol, glycerin, PEG-12, tetrasodium pyrophosphate, PVM/MA copolymer, cellulose gum, flavor, sodium hydroxide, titanium dioxide, sodium saccharin, carrageenan, **dietetically sucrose free**		
Colgate® Tartar Control Plus Whitening	Hydrated silica, aluminum oxide	Sodium monofluorophosphate 0.76%	Sodium lauryl sulfate
	Other Ingredients: Water, sorbitol, glycerin, pentasodium triphosphate, tetrasodium pyrophosphate, PVM/MA copolymer, cellulose gum, flavor, sodium hydroxide, titanium dioxide, sodium saccharin, carrageenan		
Colgate® Toothpaste*	Dicalcium phosphate dihydrate	Sodium monofluorophosphate 0.76%	Sodium lauryl sulfate
	Other Ingredients: Glycerin, cellulose gum, tetrasodium pyrophosphate, sodium saccharin, flavor, **dietetically sucrose free**		
Colgate Total® Toothpaste	Hydrated silica	Sodium fluoride 0.243%, triclosan 0.3%	Sodium lauryl sulfate
	Other Ingredients: Water, glycerin, sorbitol, PVM/MA copolymer, cellulose gum, flavor, sodium hydroxide, propylene glycol, carrageenan, sodium saccharin, titanium dioxide		
Colgate Total® Fresh Stripe Toothpaste	Hydrated silica	Sodium fluoride 0.243%, triclosan 0.3%	Sodium lauryl sulfate
	Other Ingredients: Water, glycerin, sorbitol, PVM/MA copolymer, cellulose gum, flavor, sodium hydroxide, propylene glycol, carrageenan, sodium saccharin, mica, titanium dioxide, FD&C blue #1, D&C yellow #10		
Colgate® Winterfresh Gel*	Hydrated silica	Sodium fluoride 0.243%	Sodium lauryl sulfate
	Other Ingredients: Sorbitol, water, PEG-12, flavor, tetrasodium pyrophosphate, cellulose gum, sodium saccharin, FD&C blue #1, **dietetically sucrose free**		
Crest® Baking Soda Tartar Protection Gel or Toothpaste (mint)*	Hydrated silica, sodium bicarbonate	Sodium fluoride 0.243%	Sodium lauryl sulfate
	Other Ingredients: Water, glycerin, sorbitol, tetrasodium pyrophosphate, PEG-6, flavor, cellulose gum, sodium saccharin, titanium dioxide (paste), FD&C blue #1 (gel), disodium pyrophosphate, tetrapotassium pyrophosphate, carbomer 956, xanthan gum, FD&C yellow #5 (gel)		
Crest® Cavity Protection with Baking Soda Gel or Toothpaste (mint)*	Hydrated silica, sodium bicarbonate	Sodium fluoride 0.243%	Sodium lauryl sulfate
	Other Ingredients: Sorbitol, water, glycerin, sodium carbonate, flavor, cellulose gum, sodium saccharin, titanium dioxide (paste), FD&C blue #1 (gel)		
Crest® Cavity Protection Gel (cool mint)*	Hydrated silica	Sodium fluoride 0.243%	Sodium lauryl sulfate
	Other Ingredients: Sorbitol, water, trisodium phosphate, flavor, sodium phosphate, xanthan gum, sodium saccharin, carbomer 956, FD&C blue #1, carbomer 940A		

DENTIFRICE PRODUCTS *(Continued)*

Brand Name	Abrasive Ingredient	Therapeutic Ingredient	Foaming Agent
Crest® Cavity Protection Toothpaste* (icy mint or regular)	Hydrated silica	Sodium fluoride 0.243%	Sodium lauryl sulfate
	Other Ingredients: Sorbitol, water, glycerin (mint), trisodium phosphate, flavor, sodium phosphate, cellulose gum (mint), xanthan gum (regular), sodium saccharin, carbomer 956, titanium dioxide, FD&C blue #1. carbomer 940A		
Crest® Extra Whitening Gel or Toothpaste	Hydrated silica	Sodium fluoride 0.15%	Sodium lauryl sulfate, poloxamer 407
	Other Ingredients: Sorbitol, water, glycerin, tetrasodium pyrophosphate, sodium carbonate, carboxymethylcellulose sodium, titanium dioxide, carnauba wax, sodium saccharin, flavor, FD&C blue #1, FD&C yellow #5, PEG-6, sodium bicarbonate†		
Crest® for Kids Cavity Protection Gel	Hydrated silica	Sodium fluoride 0.243%	Sodium lauryl sulfate
	Other Ingredients: Sorbitol, water, trisodium phosphate, sodium phosphate, xanthan gum, flavor, sodium saccharin, carbomer 956, mica, titanium dioxide, FD&C blue #1		
Crest® Gum Care Gel or Toothpaste	Hydrated silica	Stannous fluoride 0.454%	Sodium lauryl sulfate
	Other Ingredients: Sorbitol, water, stannous chloride, titanium dioxide (paste), flavor, sodium hydroxide, sodium saccharin, sodium carrageenan, FD&C blue #1 (gel), sodium gluconate, hydroxyethylcellulose		
Crest® Multicare Gel or Toothpaste (cool mint, fresh mint)	Hydrated silica, sodium bicarbonate	Sodium fluoride 0.243%	Sodium lauryl sulfate
	Other Ingredients: Tetrasodium pyrophosphate, xylitol, water, glycerin, PEG-6, poloxamer 407, sodium carbonate, flavor, cellulose gum, xanthan gum, sodium saccharin, titanium dioxide, FD&C blue #1, FD&C yellow #5 (cool mint)		
Crest® Sensitivity Protection Toothpaste* (mild mint)	Hydrated silica	Potassium nitrate 5%, sodium fluoride 0.15%	Sodium lauryl sulfate
	Other Ingredients: Water, glycerin, sorbitol, trisodium phosphate, cellulose gum, flavor, xanthan gum, sodium saccharin, titanium dioxide, **dye free**		
Crest® Tartar Protection Gel* (fresh mint, smooth mint)		Sodium fluoride 0.243%	Sodium lauryl sulfate
	Other Ingredients: Water, sorbitol, glycerin, tetrapotassium pyrophosphate, PEG-6, disodium pyrophosphate, tetrasodium pyrophosphate, flavor, xanthan gum, sodium saccharin, carbomer 956, FD&C blue #1, FD&C yellow #5 (smooth mint)		
Crest® Tartar Protection Toothpaste* (original flavor)	Silica	Sodium fluoride 0.243%	Sodium lauryl sulfate
	Other Ingredients: Water, sorbitol, glycerin, tetrapotassium pyrophosphate, PEG-6, disodium pyrophosphate, tetrasodium pyrophosphate, flavor, xanthan gum, sodium saccharin, carbomer 956, titanium dioxide, FD&C blue #1		
Crest® Whitening Plus Scope®	Hydrated silica	Sodium fluoride 0.243% (0.15% w/v fluoride ion)	Sodium lauryl sulfate
	Other ingredients: Water, sorbitol, glycerin, tetrapotassium pyrophosphate, PEG-6, disodium pyrophosphate, tetrasodium pyrophosphate, flavor, alcohol (1.14%), xanthan gum, sodium saccharin, carbomer 956, polysorbate 80, sodium benzoate, cetylpyridinium chloride, benzoic acid, domiphen bromide (.0002 w/v%)		
Dr. Tichenor's Toothpaste	Hydrated silica	Sodium fluoride	Sodium lauryl sulfate
	Other Ingredients: Water, glycerin, sorbitol, insoluble sodium metaphosphate, peppermint oil, cellulose gum, sodium saccharin, sodium phosphate, titanium dioxide, magnesium aluminum silicate, **dye free**		
Enamelon® All-Family Toothpaste	Hydrated silica	Sodium fluoride (fluoride 0.14%)	Sodium lauryl sulfate
	Other Ingredients: Water, glycerin, sorbitol, monoammonium phosphate, calcium sulfate, xanthan gum, flavor, PEG-60 hydrogenated castor oil, sodium saccharin, ammonium chloride, cellulose gum, titanium dioxide, magnesium chloride, methylparaben, propylparaben, FD&C blue #1		

Brand Name	Abrasive Ingredient	Therapeutic Ingredient	Foaming Agent
First Teeth™ Baby Gel		Lactoperoxidase 0.7 units/g, lactoferrin, glucose oxidase	Sodium lauryl sulfate
	Other Ingredients: Water, glycerin, sorbitol, pectin, xylitol, flavor, aloe vera, propylene glycol		
Fluoride Foam™*‡	**Ingredients:** Fluoride 1.23% (from sodium fluoride and hydrogen fluoride), water, phosphoric acid, poloxamer, sodium saccharin, flavor		
Fluorigard® Anti-Cavity Liquid*‡	**Ingredients:** Sodium fluoride 0.05%, ethyl alcohol, pluronic F108 and F127, sweetener, flavor, glycerin, sorbitol, preservatives, **dye free**, **gluten free**		
Gleem® Toothpaste	Hydrated silica	Sodium fluoride 0.243%	Sodium lauryl sulfate
	Other Ingredients: Sorbitol, water, trisodium phosphate, flavors, sodium phosphate, xanthan gum, sodium saccharin, carbomer 956, titanium dioxide, **dye free**		
Listerine® Essential Care Gel	Hydrated silica	Anticavity: Sodium monofluorophosphate 0.76% (0.13% W/V fluoride ion Antiplaque/ Antigingivitis: Eucalyptol 0.738%, menthol 0.340%, methyl salicylate 0.480%, thymol 0.511%	Sodium lauryl sulfate
	Other Ingredients: Water, sorbitol, glycerin, flavors, cellulose gum, sodium saccharin, phosphoric acid, FD&C blue #1, D&C yellow #10, sodium phosphate, benzoic acid, PEG-32, and xanthan gum		
Listerine® Gel or Toothpaste (cool mint)	Hydrated silica	Sodium monofluorophosphate	Sodium lauryl sulfate
	Other Ingredients: Water, sorbitol, glycerin, flavors, cellulose gum, sodium saccharin, phosphoric acid, FD&C blue #1, D&C yellow #10, sodium phosphate, benzoic acid, titanium dioxide (paste), xanthan gum		
Listerine® Tartar Control Gel or Toothpaste (cool mint)	Hydrated silica	Sodium fluoride	Sodium lauryl sulfate
	Other Ingredients: Water, sorbitol, glycerin, PEG-32, flavor, cellulose gum, sodium saccharin, tetrapotassium pyrophosphate, FD&C blue #1, D&C yellow #10, titanium dioxide (paste)		
Mentadent® Advanced Whitening Gel or Toothpaste	Hydrated silica, sodium bicarbonate	Sodium fluoride 0.15%	Sodium lauryl sulfate, hydrogen peroxide
	Other Ingredients: Zinc citrate trihydrate, water, sorbitol, glycerin, poloxamer 407, PEG-32, SD alcohol 38B, flavor, cellulose gum, sodium saccharin, phosphoric acid, blue #1, titanium dioxide		
Mentadent® Gum Care Gel or Toothpaste	Hydrated silica, sodium bicarbonate	Sodium fluoride 0.24% (fluoride 0.15%)	Sodium lauryl sulfate, hydrogen peroxide
	Other Ingredients: Zinc citrate trihydrate (1.8%), water, sorbitol, glycerin, poloxamer 407, PEG-32, SD alcohol 38B, flavor, cellulose gum, sodium saccharin, menthol, methyl salicylate, phosphoric acid, green #3, titanium dioxide		
Mentadent® Tartar Control Gel or Toothpaste	Hydrated silica, sodium bicarbonate	Sodium fluoride 0.24%	Sodium lauryl sulfate, hydrogen peroxide
	Other Ingredients: Water, sorbitol, glycerin, poloxamer 407, PEG-32, zinc citrate, SD alcohol 38B, flavor, cellulose gum, sodium saccharin, phosphoric acid, blue #1, titanium dioxide, menthol		
Mentadent® with Baking Soda & Peroxide Gel or Toothpaste*	Hydrated silica, sodium bicarbonate	Sodium fluoride 0.24% (fluoride 0.15%)	Sodium lauryl sulfate, hydrogen peroxide
	Other Ingredients: Water, sorbitol, glycerin, poloxamer 407, PEG-32, SD alcohol 38B, flavor, cellulose gum, sodium saccharin, phosphoric acid, blue #1, titanium dioxide		
My First Colgate® Gel*	Hydrated silica	Sodium fluoride 0.243%	Sodium lauryl sulfate
	Other Ingredients: Water, sorbitol, PEG-12, flavor, tetrasodium pyrophosphate, cellulose gum, sodium saccharin, FD&C red #40, D&C red #33, **dietetically sucrose free**		
Natural White® Toothpaste	Hydrated silica	Sodium fluoride	Sodium lauryl sulfate
	Other Ingredients: Sorbitol, water, glycerin, sodium benzoate, titanium dioxide, flavor, cellulose gum, **dietetically sucrose free**		

DENTIFRICE PRODUCTS *(Continued)*

Brand Name	Abrasive Ingredient	Therapeutic Ingredient	Foaming Agent
Natural White® Baking Soda Toothpaste	Calcium carbonate	Sodium monofluorophosphate	Sodium lauryl sulfate
	Other Ingredients: Sorbitol, water, glycerin, sodium bicarbonate†, carrageenan, natural flavor, **dietetically sucrose free**		
Natural White® Fights Plaque Toothpaste	Hydrated silica	Sodium fluoride	Sodium lauryl sulfate
	Other Ingredients: Sorbitol, water, glycerin, sodium benzoate, titanium dioxide, flavor, cellulose gum, **dietetically sucrose free**		
Natural White® Sensitive Toothpaste	Hydrated silica	Sodium monofluorophosphate, potassium nitrate	Sodium lauryl sulfate
	Other Ingredients: Sorbitol, water, glycerin, flavor, FD&C red #40, sodium benzoate, titanium dioxide, sodium saccharin, **dietetically sucrose free**		
Natural White® Tartar Control Toothpaste	Hydrated silica	Sodium fluoride	Sodium lauryl sulfate
	Other Ingredients: Sorbitol, water, glycerin, xanthan gum, tetrapotassium pyrophosphate, titanium dioxide, cellulose gum, flavor, sodium benzoate, FD&C blue #1, D&C yellow #10, **dietetically sucrose free**		
Natural White® with Peroxide Gel		Hydrogen peroxide	
	Other Ingredients: Water, glycerin, flavor, dipotassium phosphate, sodium saccharin, phosphoric acid, poloxamer, **dietetically sucrose free**		
Orajel® Baby Tooth & Gum Cleanser Gel			
	Other Ingredients: Poloxamer 407 (2%), simethicone (0.12%), Microdent, carboxymethylcellulose, sodium, citric acid, flavor, glycerin, methylparaben, potassium sorbate, propylene glycol, propylparaben, water, sodium saccharin, sorbitol, **fluoride free**		
Orajel® Gold Sensitive Teeth Gel for Adults	Hydrated silica	Potassium nitrate 5%, sodium monofluorophosphate 0.2%	Sodium lauryl sulfate
	Other Ingredients: FD&C blue #1, flavor, glycerin, sodium lauroyl sarcosinate, sodium saccharin, sorbitol, xanthan gum		
Pearl Drops® Toothpolish Paste	Hydrated silica, calcium pyrophosphate, dicalcium phosphate, aluminum hydroxide	Sodium monofluorophosphate	Sodium lauryl sulfate
	Other Ingredients: Water, sorbitol, glycerin, PEG-12, flavor, cellulose gum, trisodium phosphate, sodium phosphate, sodium saccharin, **dietetically sucrose free, dye free**		
Pearl Drops® Toothpolish Gel	Hydrated silica	Sodium monofluorophosphate	Sodium lauryl sulfate
	Other Ingredients: Sorbitol, water, glycerin, PEG-12, flavor, cellulose gum, sodium saccharin, FD&C blue #1, FD&C yellow #10, **dietetically sucrose free**		
Pearl Drops® Whitening Extra Strength Paste	Hydrated silica, calcium pyrophosphate, dicalcium phosphate	Sodium monofluorophosphate	Sodium lauryl sulfate
	Other Ingredients: Water, sorbitol, glycerin, PEG-12, flavor, cellulose gum, trisodium phosphate, sodium phosphate, sodium saccharin, titanium dioxide, **dietetically sucrose free, dye free**		
Pearl Drops® Whitening Gel (icy cool mint)	Hydrated silica	Sodium monofluorophosphate	Sodium lauryl sulfate
	Other Ingredients: Sorbitol, water, glycerin, PEG-12, flavor, cellulose gum, sodium saccharin, FD&C blue #1, FD&C yellow #10, **dietetically sucrose free**		
Pepsodent® Baking Soda Toothpaste	Hydrated silica	Sodium monofluorophosphate 0.8% (fluoride (0.14%)	Sodium lauryl sulfate
	Other Ingredients: Sorbitol, water, sodium bicarbonate†, PEG-32, SD alcohol 38B, flavor, cellulose gum, sodium saccharin, titanium dioxide		
Pepsodent® Original Toothpaste	Hydrated silica	Sodium monofluorophosphate 0.8% (fluoride 0.14%)	Sodium lauryl sulfate
	Other Ingredients: Sorbitol and related polyols, water, glycerin, SD alcohol 38B, flavor, cellulose gum, sodium saccharin, titanium dioxide		

Brand Name	Abrasive Ingredient	Therapeutic Ingredient	Foaming Agent
Pepsodent® Tartar Control Toothpaste	Hydrated silica	Sodium monofluorophosphate 0.8% (fluoride 0.14%)	Sodium lauryl sulfate
	Other Ingredients: Sorbitol and related polyols, water, glycerin, SD alcohol 38B, zinc citrate trihydrate, flavor, cellulose gum, sodium saccharin, titanium dioxide, blue #1, yellow #1		
Pete & Pam™ Gel (premeasured strips)	Hydrated silica	Sodium monofluorophosphate 0.76%	Sodium lauryl sarcosinate
	Other Ingredients: Sorbitol, water, glycerin, xanthan gum, polysorbate 20, sodium benzoate, pluronic P84, FD&C blue #1, FD&C red #33, FD&C yellow #5, flavor, xylitol		
Promise® Toothpaste	Dicalcium phosphate	Potassium nitrate, sodium monofluorophosphate	Sodium lauryl sulfate
	Other Ingredients: Water, hydroxyethylcellulose, flavor, sodium saccharin, methylparaben, propylparaben, D&C yellow #10, FD&C blue #1, glycerin, sorbitol, silicon dioxide, **dietetically sucrose free**		
Reach Act Adult Anti-Cavity Treatment Liquid (cinnamon, mint)‡	**Ingredients:** Sodium fluoride 0.05%, cetylpyridinium chloride, D&C red #33 (cinnamon), EDTA calcium disodium, FD&C yellow #5, flavor, glycerin, monobasic sodium phosphate, dibasic sodium phosphate, poloxamer 407, polysorbate 80 (cinnamon), polysorbate 20 (mint), propylene glycol, sodium benzoate, sodium saccharin, water, FD&C green #3 (mint), menthol (mint), methyl salicylate (mint), potassium sorbate (mint), **alcohol free**		
Reach Act for Kids*‡	**Ingredients:** Sodium fluoride 0.05%, cetylpyridinium chloride, D&C red #33, EDTA calcium disodium, flavor, glycerin, monobasic sodium phosphate, dibasic sodium phosphate, poloxamer 407, polysorbate 80, propylene glycol, sodium benzoate, sodium saccharin, water, **alcohol free**		
Rembrandt® Age-Defying Adult Toothpaste (original or mint)	Dicalcium orthophosphate, soft silica	Sodium monofluorophosphate (fluoride 0.15%)	
	Other Ingredients: Trihydroxy propane, perhydrol urea, aluminum oxide, acetylated pectins, sodium citrate, iridium, papain, carboxyl polymethylene, saccharin, propylene glycol, flavor		
Rembrandt® Age-Defying Adult Formula Mouthwash‡	**Ingredients:** Sodium fluoride 0.05%, water, glycerin, hydrogen peroxide solution, sodium citrate, polyoxyl 40 hydrogenated castor oil, flavor, cocamidopropyl betaine, citric acid, sodium benzoate, sodium saccharin, sodium hydroxide, **alcohol free**		
Rembrandt® Daily Whitening Gel	Silica	Sodium monofluorophosphate (fluoride 0.15%)	Carbamide peroxide, sodium lauryl sulfate
	Other Ingredients: Glycerin, sodium citrate, carbopol, triethanolamine, flavor		
Rembrandt® Naturals Toothpaste	Silica	0.15% fluoride ion from sodium monofluorophosphate wt/vol%	None
	Other ingredients: Water (artesian springs), dicalcium phosphate (from monetite, a mineral), glycerine (by-product of vegetable soap), xylitol (from birch trees), cocamidopropyl betaine (from coconut), flavor (spearmint, peppermint, other natural sources), sodium citrate (from citrus fruit), stevia (from stevia plant), papain (from papaya plant), sodium carrageenan (from seaweed), citric acid and vitamin C (from citrus fruit), ginkgo extract, raspberry leaf extract. Also available containing aloe vera and echinacea or papaya and ginseng.		
Rembrandt® Whitening Baking Soda Toothpaste	Sodium bicarbonate, silica	Sodium monofluorophosphate (fluoride 0.15%)	Sodium lauryl sulfate
	Other Ingredients: Glycerin, sorbitol, alumina, water, sodium citrate, sodium carrageenan, papain, flavor, sodium hydroxide, FD&C blue #1, sodium saccharin		
Rembrandt® Whitening Canker Sore Prevention Toothpaste	Dicalcium phosphate, silica	Sodium monofluorophosphate (fluoride 0.15%)	
	Other Ingredients: Water, glycerin, xylitol, sodium citrate, natural flavors, sodium carrageenan, papain, citric acid, **dye free**		
Rembrandt® Whitening Natural Toothpaste	Dicalcium phosphate, silica	Sodium monofluorophosphate	
	Other Ingredients: Water, glycerin, xylitol, sodium citrate, natural flavors, sodium carrageenan, papain, citric acid, **dye free**		

DENTIFRICE PRODUCTS *(Continued)*

Brand Name	Abrasive Ingredient	Therapeutic Ingredient	Foaming Agent
Rembrandt® Whitening Sensitive Toothpaste	Dicalcium phosphate dihydrate	Potassium nitrate 5%, sodium monofluorophosphate 0.76%	Sodium lauryl sulfate
	Other Ingredients: Glycerin, sorbitol, water, alumina, papain, sodium citrate, flavor, carboxymethylcellulose sodium, sodium saccharin, methylparaben, FD&C red #40, citric acid		
Rembrandt® Whitening Toothpaste (mint or original)	Dicalcium phosphate dihydrate	Sodium monofluorophosphate 0.76%	Sodium lauryl sulfate
	Other Ingredients: Glycerin, sorbitol, water, alumina, sodium citrate, flavor, sodium carrageenan, papain, sodium saccharin, methylparaben, citric acid, FD&C blue #1, FD&C yellow #5		
Revelation® Toothpowder	Calcium carbonate		Vegetable soap powder
	Other Ingredients: Methyl salicylate, menthol, **dye free**		
Sensodyne® Baking Soda Toothpaste	Sodium bicarbonate, silica	Potassium nitrate, sodium fluoride	Sodium lauryl sulfate
	Other Ingredients: Water, glycerin, flavor, hydroxyethylcellulose, titanium dioxide, sodium saccharin, **dietetically sucrose free, dye free**		
Sensodyne® Cool Gel	Silica	Potassium nitrate, sodium fluoride	Sodium methyl cocoyl taurate
	Other Ingredients: Water, sorbitol, glycerin, sodium carboxymethylcellulose, flavor, sodium saccharin, FD&C blue #1, trisodium phosphate, **dietetically sucrose free**		
Sensodyne® Extra Whitening Toothpaste	Silica	Potassium nitrate, sodium monofluorophosphate	Sodium lauryl sulfate
	Other Ingredients: Water, flavor, glycerin, PEG-12, PEG-75, sodium carbonate, sodium saccharin, titanium dioxide, calcium peroxide, **dietetically sucrose free**		
Sensodyne® Tartar Control Toothpaste	Hydrated silica, silica, sodium bicarbonate	Potassium nitrate, sodium fluoride	Cocamidopropyl betaine
	Other Ingredients: Cellulose gum, flavor, glycerin, sodium saccharin, tetrasodium pyrophosphate, titanium dioxide, water		
Sensodyne® Toothpaste* (fresh mint)	Dicalcium phosphate	Potassium nitrate, sodium monofluorophosphate	Sodium lauryl sulfate
	Other Ingredients: Water, glycerin, sorbitol, hydroxmethylcellulose, flavor, sodium saccharin, methylparaben, propylparaben, D&C yellow #10, FD&C blue #1, silicon dioxide, **dietetically sucrose free**		
Sensodyne® Toothpaste (original)	Silica	Potassium nitrate, sodium fluoride	Sodium methyl cocoyl taurate
	Other Ingredients: Water, glycerin, sorbitol, cellulose gum, titanium dioxide, sodium saccharin, flavor, D&C red #28, trisodium phosphate		
Slimer® Gel*	Hydrated silica	Sodium fluoride 0.15%	
	Other Ingredients: Sorbitol, water, glycerin, PEG-32, flavor, ethyl alcohol, propylene glycol, glyceryl triacetate, cellulose gum, sodium saccharin, sodium benzoate, FD&C blue #1, FD&C red #33, **dietetically sucrose free**		
Thermodent Toothpaste	Diatomaceous earth, silica	Strontium chloride hexahydrate	Sodium methyl cocoyl taurate
	Other Ingredients: Sorbitol, glycerin, titanium dioxide, guar gum, PEG-40 stearate, hydroxyethylcellulose, flavor, preservative, water		
Tom's® Natural Baking Soda with Propolis & Myrrh Toothpaste	Calcium carbonate, sodium bicarbonate		Sodium lauryl sulfate
	Other Ingredients: Glycerin, water, carrageenan, peppermint oil, myrrh, propolis, **fluoride free**		
Tom's® Natural Baking Soda, Calcium, and Fluoride Toothpaste	Calcium carbonate, sodium bicarbonate	Sodium monofluorophosphate	Sodium lauryl sulfate
	Other Ingredients: Glycerin, water, carrageenan, peppermint oil, xylitol		
Tom's® Natural Calcium and Fluoride Toothpaste*	Calcium carbonate	Sodium monofluorophosphate	Sodium lauryl sulfate
	Other Ingredients: Glycerin; water; carrageenan; xylitol (spearmint); cinnamon, fennel oil, or spearmint; peppermint oil (cinnamon, spearmint)		
Tom's® Natural Calcium and Fluoride Toothpaste	Calcium carbonate, hydrated silica	Sodium monofluorophosphate	Sodium lauryl sulfate
	Other Ingredients: Glycerin, water, carrageenan, xylitol, natural wintergreen oil		

Brand Name	Abrasive Ingredient	Therapeutic Ingredient	Foaming Agent
Tom's® Natural for Children with Calcium and Fluoride Toothpaste	Calcium carbonate, hydrated silica	Sodium monofluorophosphate	Sodium lauryl sulfate
	Other Ingredients: Glycerin, fruit extracts, carrageenan, water		
Tom's® Natural with Propolis and Myrrh Toothpaste	Calcium carbonate		Sodium lauryl sulfate
	Other Ingredients: Glycerin; water; carrageenan; spearmint, peppermint, cassia, or fennel oil; propolis; myrrh, **fluoride free**		
Ultra Brite® Baking Soda & Peroxide Toothpaste	Hydrated silica, sodium bicarbonate	Sodium monofluorophosphate 0.76%	Sodium lauryl sulfate
	Other Ingredients: Glycerin, water, propylene glycol, cellulose gum, flavor, sodium saccharin, titanium dioxide, sodium hydroxide, calcium peroxide, carrageenan, **dietetically sucrose free**		
Ultra Brite® Gel	Hydrated silica	Sodium monofluorophosphate 0.76%	Sodium lauryl sulfate
	Other Ingredients: Sorbitol, water, PEG-12, flavor, cellulose gum, sodium saccharin, FD&C blue #1, D&C red #33		
Ultra Brite® Toothpaste	Hydrated silica, alumina	Sodium monofluorophosphate 0.76%	Sodium lauryl sulfate
	Other Ingredients: Glycerin, cellulose gum, sorbitol, carrageenan gum, titanium dioxide, sodium saccharin, flavor, tetrasodium pyrophosphate, **dietetically sucrose free**		
Viadent® Fluoride Gel	Hydrated silica	Sodium monofluorophosphate 0.8%	Sodium lauryl sulfate
	Other Ingredients: Sodium saccharin, zinc chloride, teaberry flavor, sodium carboxymethylcellulose, sorbitol, sanguinaria extract		
Viadent® Fluoride Toothpaste	Hydrated silica	Sodium monofluorophosphate 0.8%	Sodium lauryl sulfate
	Other Ingredients: Sorbitol, titanium dioxide, carboxymethylcellulose, flavor, sodium saccharin, citric acid, zinc chloride, anhydrous sanguinaria extract, citric acid		
Viadent® Original Toothpaste	Dicalcium phosphate		Sodium lauryl sulfate
	Other Ingredients: Glycerin, sorbitol, titanium dioxide, zinc chloride, carrageenan, flavor, sodium saccharin, citric acid, sanguinaria extract, **fluoride free**		
Vince Tooth Powder	Calcium carbonate, sodium carbonate, tricalcium phosphate		
	Other Ingredients: Sodium alum, sodium perborate monohydrate, magnesium trisilicate, sodium saccharin, flavor, D&C red		

*Carries American Dental Association (ADA) seal indicating safety and efficacy.

†Sodium bicarbonate can also be considered an abrasive.

‡Topical fluoride product

Adapted with permission from *Nonprescription Products: Formulations & Features, Companion to the Handbook of Nonprescription Drugs*, 11th ed,, Washington, DC, American Pharmaceutical Association, 1998, 344-58.

DENTURE ADHESIVE PRODUCTS

Brand Name	Product Form / Ingredients
Confident®	**Cream** / Carboxymethylcellulose gum 32%, ethylene oxide polymer 13%, petrolatum, liquid petrolatum, propylparaben
Cushion Grip®	**Gel** / Alcohol 26.2%, triacetin, polyvinyl acetate
Dentlock®	**Powder** / Karaya gum
Dentrol®	**Liquid** / Carboxymethylcellulose sodium, ethylene oxide polymer, mineral oil, polyethylene, flavor, propylparaben
Denturite®	**Liquid** / Butyl phthalyl butyl glycolate, vinyl acetate, SDA alcohol **Powder** / Polyethyl methacrylate polymer
Effergrip®*	**Cream** / Carboxymethylcellulose sodium, polyvinyl methyl ether maleic acid calcium sodium double salt, color, flavor, preservatives, vehicle
Ezo® Cushions	**Pad** / Paraffin wax, cotton
Fixodent®	**Cream** / Carboxymethylcellulose sodium, calcium zinc gantrez (PVA/MA copolymer), mineral oil, petrolatum, color **Powder** / Carboxymethylcellulose sodium, calcium zinc gantrez (PVM/MA copolymer), peppermint oil
Fixodent® Extra Hold	**Powder** / Carboxymethylcellulose sodium, calcium zinc gantrez (PVA/MA copolymer), peppermint oil
Fixodent® Free	**Cream** / Carboxymethylcellulose sodium, calcium zinc gantrez (PVM/MA copolymer), mineral oil, petrolatum
Fixodent® Fresh	**Cream** / Carboxymethylcellulose sodium, calcium zinc gantrez (PVM/MA copolymer), mineral oil, petrolatum, color, peppermint flavor
Orafix® Special	**Cream** / Carboxymethylcellulose sodium, calcium/sodium polyvinyl methyl ether anhydride copolymer, polyvinyl pyrolidone
Orafix® Ultra	**Cream** / Polyvinyl methyl ether copolymer, carboxymethylcellulose
Plasti-Liner®	**Strip** / Polyethyl methacrylate polymer, butyl phthalyl butyl glycolate, triacetin
Poli-Grip®	**Cream** / Carboxymethylcellulose sodium gum 32%, ethylene oxide polymer 13%, petrolatum 36.7%, liquid petrolatum, propylparaben, flavor, dye
Poli-Grip® Free	**Cream** / Carboxymethylcellulose sodium, methyl vinyl ether maleic acid salt, petrolatum, mineral oil
Poli-Grip® Super	**Cream** / Carboxymethylcellulose sodium, methyl vinyl ether maleic acid salt copolymer, petrolatum, mineral oil, flavor, dye **Powder** / Carboxymethylcellulose sodium, methyl vinyl ether maleic salt copolymer, flavor
Poli-Grip® Ultra Fresh	**Cream** / Carboxymethylcellulose sodium, methyl vinyl ether maleic acid salt copolymer, petrolatum, mineral oil, flavor, dye
Polident® Dentu-Grip	**Powder** / Carboxymethylcellulose gum 49%, methyl vinyl ether maleic acid salt copolymer, flavor
Quik-Fix®	**Liquid** / Methyl methacrylate monomer, hydroxyethyl methacrylate monomer, color stable concentrate, triacetin **Powder** / Polyethyl methacrylate polymer
Sea-Bond®	**Pad** / Ethylene oxide polymer, sodium alginate
Snug® Cushion	**Sponge** / Acrylate resin, propylene glycol monolaurate
Wernet's®	**Powder** / Karaya gum 94.6%, water-soluble ethylene oxide polymer 5%, flavor

*Carries American Dental Association (ADA) seal indicating safety and efficacy.

Adapted with permission from *Nonprescription Products: Formulations & Features, Companion to the Handbook of Nonprescription Drugs*, 11th ed,, Washington, DC, American Pharmaceutical Association, 1998, 358-9.

DENTURE CLEANSER PRODUCTS

Brand Name	Product Form / Ingredients
Ban-A-Stain®	**Liquid** / Phosphoric acid 25%, deionized water, methylparaben, xanthan gum, alkyl phenoxy polyethoxy ethanol, oil of cassis, FD&C red #40, imidurea
Dentu-Creme®	**Paste** / Dicalcium phosphate dihydrate, propylene glycol, calcium carbonate, sodium lauryl sulfate, glycerin, aluminum silicate, hydroxyethylcellulose, flavor, magnesium aluminum silicate, sodium saccharin, methylparaben, propylparaben, water. FD&C blue #1
Efferdent® Antibacterial*	**Tablet** / Potassium monopersulfate, sodium carbonate, sodium perborate, sodium bicarbonate, fragrance, colors
Efferdent® Plus	**Tablet** / Potassium monopersulfate, sodium perborate, sodium bicarbonate, fragrance, colors, (including FD&C yellow #5), sodium saccharin, chelating agents, detergents
Efferdent®, 2 Layer	**Tablet** / Potassium monopersulfate, sodium bicarbonate, sodium carbonate, detergents, fragrance, colors, sodium saccharin, chelating agents
Stain Away® Plus	**Powder** / Effervescent, high-oxygenating powder (at the time of publication, the manufacturer had not responded to a request for ingredients of this product)

* Carries American Dental Association (ADA) seal indicating safety and efficacy.

Adapted with permission from *Nonprescription Products: Formulations & Features, Companion to the Handbook of Nonprescription Drugs*, 11th ed,, Washington, DC, American Pharmaceutical Association, 1998, 357.

MOUTH PAIN, COLD SORE, AND CANKER SORE PRODUCTS

Brand Name	Anesthetic/ Analgesic	Other Ingredients
Abreva™ [OTC]		**Cream**: Docosanol 10%, benzyl alcohol, light mineral oil, propylene glycol, purified water, sucrose distearate, sucrose stearate
Anbesol® Baby Gel (grape, original)	Benzocaine 7.5%	Benzoic acid (grape), carbomer 934P, D&C red #33, EDTA disodium, FD&C blue #1 (grape), flavor (grape), glycerin, methylparaben (grape), PEG, propylparaben (grape), saccharin, purified water, clove oil (original)
Anbesol® Gel or Liquid	Benzocaine 6.3% (gel), 6.4% (liquid); phenol 0.5%	**Gel**: Alcohol 70%, glycerin, carbomer 934P, D&C red #33, D&C yellow #10, FD&C blue #1, FD&C yellow #6, flavor, camphor **Liquid:** Alcohol 70%, potassium iodide, povidone iodine, camphor, menthol, glycerin
Anbesol® Maximum Strength Gel or Liquid	Benzocaine 20%	Alcohol 60%, carbomer 934P (gel), D&C yellow #10, FD&C blue #1, FD&C red #40, flavor, PEG, saccharin
Baby® Gumz	Benzocaine 10%	PEG 8 and 32, **alcohol free, dietetically sucrose free**
Benzodent® Denture Analgesic Ointment*	Benzocaine 20%	8-hydroxyquinoline sulfate, petrolatum, sodium carboxymethycellulose, color, eugenol
Blistex® Lip Medex Ointment	Camphor 1%, menthol 1%, phenol 0.5%	Petrolatum, cocoa butter, flavor, lanolin, mixed waxes, oil of cloves
Blistex® Medicated Ointment	Menthol 0.6%, camphor 0.5%, phenol 0.5%	Water, mixed waxes, mineral oil, petrolatum, lanolin
Campho-Phenique® Cold Sore Gel†	Camphor 10.8%, phenol 4.7%	Eucalyptus oil, colloidal silicon dioxide, glycerin, light mineral oil, **alcohol free**
Cankaid® Liquid		Carbamide peroxide 10%‡, citric acid monohydrate, sodium citrate, dihydrate, EDTA disodium
Carmex Lip Balm Ointment	Menthol, camphor, salicylic acid, phenol	Alum, fragrance, petrolatum, lanolin, cocoa butter, wax, **alcohol free**, **dye free**, **gluten free**, **dietetically sucrose free**
Chap Stick® Medicated Lip Balm (stick, ointment)	Camphor 1%, menthol 0.6%, phenol 0.5%	**Stick:** Petrolatum 41%, paraffin wax, mineral oil, cocoa butter, 2-octyl dodecanol, arachidyl propionate, polyphenylmethylsiloxane 556, white wax, isopropyl lanolate, carnauba wax, isopropyl myristate, lanolin, fragrance, methylparaben, propylparaben, oleyl alcohol, cetyl alcohol **Ointment**: Petrolatum (jar 60%, tube 67%), microcrystalline wax, mineral oil, cocoa butter, lanolin, paraffin war (jar), fragrance, methylparaben, propylparaben
Dent's® Double-Action Kit (tablets, drops)	Benzocaine 20% (drops), acetaminophen 325 mg (tablet)	**Drops:** Denatured alcohol 74%, chlorobutanol anhydrous 0.09%, propylene glycol, FD&C red #40, eugenol

Brand Name	Anesthetic/ Analgesic	Other Ingredients
Dent's® Extra Strength Toothache Gum	Benzocaine 20%	Petrolatum, cotton and wax base, beeswax, FD&C red #40 aluminum lake, eugenol
Dent's® Maxi-Strength Toothache Treatment Drops	Benzocaine 20%	Denatured alcohol 74%, chlorobutanol anhydrous 0.09%, propylene glycol, FD&C red #40, eugenol
Dent-Zel-Ite® Oral Mucosal Analgesic Liquid	Benzocaine 5%, camphor	Alcohol 81%, wintergreen, glycerin, **dye free**
Dent-Zel-Ite® Temporary Dental Filling Liquid	Camphor	Alcohol 56.18%, sandarac gum, methyl salicylate
Dent-Zel-Ite® Toothache Relief Drops	Eugenol 85%, camphor	Alcohol 13.5%, wintergreen
Dentapaine® Gel	Benzocaine 20%	Glycerin, oil of cloves, sodium saccharin, methylparaben, PEG 400 and 4000, water, **alcohol free, dye free, gluten free, dietetically sucrose free**
Dr. Hand's® Teething Gel or Lotion	Menthol	SD alcohol 38B (gel 10%, lotion 11%), sterilized water, carbomer 940, witch hazel, polysorbate 80, sodium hydroxide, simethicone, D&C red #33, FD&C red #3
Gly-Oxide® Liquid		Carbamide peroxide 10%‡, citric acid, flavor, glycerin, propylene glycol, sodium stannate, water
Herpecin-L® Cold Sore Lip Balm Stick†		Padimate O 7%, allantoin 0.5%, titanium dioxide, beeswax, cetyl esters, flavor, octyldodecanol, paraffin, petrolatum, sesame oil, vitamins B_6, C, and E
Hurricaine® Aerosol* (wild cherry)	Benzocaine 20%	PEG, saccharin, flavor, alcohol, **dye free, gluten free, sulfite free**
Hurricaine® Gel* (wild cherry, pina colada, watermelon)	Benzocaine 20%	PEG, saccharin, flavor, **alcohol free, dye free, gluten free, sulfite free**
Hurricaine® Liquid* (wild cherry, pina colada)	Benzocaine 20%	PEG, saccharin, flavor, **alcohol free, dye free, gluten free, dietetically sucrose free**
Kank-A® Professional Strength Liquid*	Benzocaine 20%	Benzoin tincture compound, cetylpyridinium chloride, ethylcellulose, SD alcohol 24%, dimethyl isosorbide, castor oil, flavor, tannic acid, propylene glycol, saccharin, benzyl alcohol
Lip-Ex® Ointment	Phenol, camphor, salicylic acid, menthol	Petrolatum, cherry flavor
Lipmagik® Liquid	Benzocaine 6.3%, phenol 0.5%	Alcohol 70%, **dye free**, **sulfite free, gluten free**
Little Teethers® Oral Pain Relief Gel	Benzocaine 7.5%	Carbomer, glycerin, flavor, potassium sorbate, acesulfame K, PEGs, **alcohol free, dye free, dietetically sodium free, dietetically sucrose free**
Medadyne® Liquid	Benzocaine 10%, menthol, camphor, benzyl alcohol	Benzalkonium chloride, tannic acid, flavor, SD alcohol, thymol
Numzident® Adult Strength Gel	Benzocaine 10%	PEG-8, glycerin, PEG-75, sodium saccharin, purified water, flavor
Numzit® Teething Gel	Benzocaine 7.5%	PEG-8, PEG-75, sodium saccharin, clove oil, peppermint oil, purified water

MOUTH PAIN, COLD SORE, AND CANKER SORE PRODUCTS *(Continued)*

Brand Name	Anesthetic/ Analgesic	Other Ingredients
Orabase® Baby Gel*	Benzocaine 7.5%	Glycerin, PEG, carbopol, preservative, sweetener, flavor, **alcohol free**
Orabase® Gel	Benzocaine 15%	Ethanol, propylene glycol, ethylcellulose, tannic acid, salicylic acid, flavor, sodium saccharin
Orabase® Lip Cream	Benzocaine 5%, menthol 0.5%, camphor, phenol	Allantoin 1%, carboxymethylcellulose sodium, veegum, Tween 80, phenonip, PEG, biopure, talc, kaolin, lanolin, petrolatum, oil of clove, hydrated silica, **alcohol free**
Orabase® Plain Paste*		Pectin, gelatin, carboxymethylcellulose sodium, polyethylene, mineral oil, flavor, preservative, guar, tragacanth, **alcohol free**
Orabase-B® with Benzocaine Paste*	Benzocaine 20%	Plasticized hydrocarbon gel, guar, carboxymethylcellulose, tragacanth, pectin, preservatives, flavor, **alcohol free**
Oragesic Solution	Benzyl alcohol 2%, menthol	Water, sorbitol, polysorbate 20, sodium chloride, yerba santa, saccharin, flavor, **sulfite free**
Orajel® Baby Gel or Liquid	Benzocaine 7.5%	**Gel:** FD&C red #40, flavor, glycerin, PEGs, sodium saccharin, sorbic acid, sorbitol, **alcohol free** **Liquid:** Not applicable
Orajel® Baby Nighttime Gel	Benzocaine 10%	FD&C red #40, flavor, glycerin, PEGs, sodium saccharin, sorbic acid, sorbitol, **alcohol free**
Orajel® CoverMed Cream (tinted light, medium)	Dyclonine HCl 1%	Allantoin 0.5%
Orajel® Denture Gel	Benzocaine 20%	Cellulose gum, gelatin, menthol, methyl salicylate, pectin, plasticized hydrocarbon gel, PEG, sodium saccharin
Orajel® Maximum Strength Gel	Benzocaine 20%	Clove oil, flavor, PEGs, sodium saccharin, sorbic acid
Orajel® Mouth-Aid Gel or Liquid	Benzocaine 20%	**Gel**: Zinc chloride 0.1%, benzalkonium chloride 0.02%. allantoin, carbomer, EDTA disodium, peppermint oil, PEG, polysorbate 60, propyl gallate, propylene glycol, purified water, povidone, sodium saccharin, sorbic acid, stearyl alcohol **Liquid:** Ethyl alcohol 44.2%
Orajel® PM Cream	Benzocaine 20%	
Orajel® Periostatic Spot Treatment Oral Cleanser		Carbamide peroxide 15%‡, citric acid, EDTA disodium, flavor, methylparaben, PEG, purified water, sodium chloride, sodium saccharin
Orajel® Periostatic Super Cleaning Oral Rinse		Hydrogen peroxide 1.5%‡, ethyl alcohol 4%
Orajel® Regular Strength Gel	Benzocaine 10%	Clove oil, flavor, PEGs, sodium saccharin, sorbic acid
Peroxyl® Hygienic Dental Rinse		Hydrogen peroxide 1.5%‡, alcohol 5%, pluronic F108, sorbitol, sodium saccharin, dye, polysorbate 20, mint flavor, **gluten free**, **sulfite free**

Brand Name	Anesthetic/ Analgesic	Other Ingredients
Peroxyl® Oral Spot Treatment Gel		Hydrogen peroxide 1.5%‡, ethyl alcohol 5%, pluronic F108, sorbitol, sodium saccharin, dye, polysorbate 20, mint flavor, dye, pluronic F127, **gluten free, dietetically sucrose free**
Proxigel® Gel†	Menthol	Carbamide peroxide 10%‡, glycerin, carbomer, phosphoric acid, triethanolamine, flavor, **dye free, gluten free, dietetically sucrose free**
Red Cross® Canker Sore Medication Ointment†	Benzocaine 20%, phenol	Carbomer 974P, mineral oil, petrolatum, propylparaben
Red Cross® Toothache Medication Drops	Eugenol 85%	Sesame oil
Retre-Gel®†	Benzocaine 5%, menthol 1%	Glycerin 20%
Tanac® Medicated Gel	Dyclonine HCl 1%	Allantoin 0.5%
Tanac® No Sting Liquid	Benzocaine 10%	Benzalkonium chloride 0.125%, saccharin
Zilactin® Gel	Benzyl alcohol 10%	**Gluten free**
Zilactin® Baby Gel	Benzocaine 10%	**Alcohol free, dye free, gluten free**
Zilactin®-B Gel	Benzocaine 10%	**Gluten free**
Zilactin®-L Liquid	Lidocaine 2.5%	**Gluten free**

*Carries American Dental Association (ADA) seal indicating safety and efficacy

†Agent for cold sore treatment only

‡Agent for debridement or wound cleansing

Adapted with permission from *Nonprescription Products: Formulations & Features, Companion to the Handbook of Nonprescription Drugs*, 11th ed,, Washington, DC, American Pharmaceutical Association, 1998, 338-40.

ORAL RINSE PRODUCTS

Brand Name	Antiseptic	Other Ingredients
Astring-O-Sol® Liquid	SD alcohol 38B 75.6%, methyl salicylate	Water, myrrh extract, zinc chloride, citric acid
Betadine® Mouthwash/Gargle	Alcohol 8.8%	Povidone-iodine 0.5%, glycerin, sodium saccharin, flavor
Biotene® Mouthwash	Lysozyme (6 mg), lactoferrin (6 mg) glucose oxidase (4000 units)	Water, xylitol, hydrogenated starch, propylene glycol, hydroxyethylcellulose, aloe vera, natural peppermint, poloxamer 407, calcium lactate, zinc gluconate, sodium benzoate, benzoic acid
Cepacol® Mouthwash/Gargle	Alcohol 14%, cetylpyridinium chloride 0.05%	EDTA disodium, color, flavor, glycerin, polysorbate 80, saccharin, sodium biphosphate, sodium phosphate, water, **gluten free, dietetically sucrose free**
Cepacol® Mouthwash/Gargle (mint)	Alcohol 14.5%, cetylpyridinium chloride 0.5%	Color, flavor, glucono delta-lactone, glycerin, poloxamer 407, sodium saccharin, sodium gluconate, water, **gluten free, dietetically sucrose free**
Dr. Tichenor's® Antiseptic Liquid	SDA alcohol 38B 70%	Oil of peppermint, extract of arnica, water, **dye free, gluten free**
Listerine®* Liquid	Alcohol 26.9%, eucalyptol 0.092%, thymol 0.064%, methyl salicylate 0.06%, menthol 0.042%	Benzoic acid, poloxamer 407, caramel, water, sodium benzoate
Listerine®* Liquid (freshburst, cool mint)	Alcohol 21.6%, eucalyptol 0.092%, thymol 0.064%, methyl salicylate 0.06%, menthol 0.042%	Water, sorbitol solution, poloxamer 407, benzoic acid, flavor, sodium saccharin, sodium citrate, citric acid, FD&C green #3, D&C yellow #10 (freshburst)
Mentadent® Mouthwash (cool mint, fresh mint)	Alcohol 10%	Water, sorbitol, sodium bicarbonate, hydrogen peroxide, poloxamer 407, sodium lauryl sulfate, flavor, polysorbate 20, methyl salicylate (cool mint), sodium saccharin, phosphoric acid, blue #1, yellow #5 (cool mint)
Plax® Advanced Formula (mint sensation)	Alcohol 8.7%	Water, sorbitol solution, tetrasodium pyrophosphate, benzoic acid, flavor, poloxamer 407, sodium benzoate, sodium lauryl sulfate, sodium saccharin, xanthan gum, FD&C blue #1
Plax® Advanced Formula (original, SoftMINT)	Alcohol 8.7%	Sodium lauryl sulfate, water, sorbitol solution, sodium benzoate, tetrasodium pyrophosphate, benzoic acid, poloxamer 407, sodium saccharin, flavor (SoftMINT), xanthan gum (SoftMINT), flavor enhancer (SoftMINT), FD&C blue #1 (SoftMINT), FD&C yellow #5 (SoftMINT)

Brand Name	Antiseptic	Other Ingredients
Rembrandt® Naturals Mouthwash		Spring water, glycerin, xylitol, sodium citrate, vitamin C, stevia, citric acid, dicalcium phosphate, cocamidopropyl betain, flavor, ginkgo extract, raspberry leaf extract, alcohol free. Also available with papaya and ginseng or aloe and echinacea
S.T. 37® Solution	Hexylresorcinol 0.1%	Glycerin, propylene glycol, citric acid, EDTA disodium, sodium bisulfite, sodium citrate
Scope® Baking Soda	SD alcohol 38F 9.9%, cetylpyridinium chloride, domiphen bromide	Sorbitol, sodium bicarbonate, sodium saccharin, flavor
Scope® (cool peppermint)	SD alcohol 38F 14%, cetylpyridinium chloride, domiphen bromide	Purified water, glycerin, poloxamer 407, sodium saccharin, sodium benzoate, N-ethylmethylcarboxamide, benzoic acid, FD&C blue #1, flavor
Targon® Smokers' Mouthwash (clean taste)	SDA alcohol 38B 15.6%	Water, glycerin, polyoxyl 40 hydrogenated caster oil, sodium lauryl sulfate, dibasic sodium phosphate, benzoic acid, sodium saccharin, caramel powder, **dietetically sucrose free**
Targon® Smokers' Mouthwash (original)	SDA alcohol 38B 16%	Water, sodium saccharin, sodium benzoate, glycerin, sodium lauryl sulfate, FD&C green #3, FD&C yellow #5, polyoxyl 40 hydrogenated castor oil, **dietetically sucrose free**
Tom's of Maine® Natural Mouthwash (cinnamon, original)	Menthol	Water, glycerin, aloe vera juice, witch hazel, poloxamer 335, spearmint oil, ascorbic acid, **alcohol free**

*Carries American Dental Association (ADA) seal indicating safety and efficacy

Note: SD alcohol refers to "specially denatured" alcohol

Adapted with permission from *Nonprescription Products: Formulations & Features, Companion to the Handbook of Nonprescription Drugs*, 11th ed,, Washington, DC, American Pharmaceutical Association, 1998, 341-2.

TOP 50 MOST PRESCRIBED DRUGS IN 2002*

1. Hydrocodone/acetaminophen
2. Lipitor®
3. Synthroid®
4. Atenolol
5. Amoxicillin
6. Premarin® tabs
7. Furosemide, oral
8. Norvasc®
9. Albuterol (aerosol)
10. Alprazolam
11. Hydrochlorothiazide
12. Zoloft®
13. Paxil®
14. Propoxyphene-N/APAP
15. Zithromax® Z-PAK®
16. Cephalexin
17. Zocor®
18. Prevacid®
19. Ibuprofen
20. Celebrex®
21. Triamterene/HCTZ
22. Levoxyl®
23. Ortho Tri-Cyclen®
24. Allegra®
25. Prednisone, oral
26. Toprol-XL®
27. Acetaminophen/codeine
28. Celexa™
29. Prilosec®
30. Fluoxetine
31. Vioxx®
32. Ambien®
33. Zyrtec®
34. Metoprolol tartrate
35. Lorazepam
36. Fosamax®
37. Metformin
38. Claritin®
39. Trimox®
40. Viagra®
41. Ranitidine HCl
42. Amitriptyline
43. Augmentin®
44. Wellbutrin SR®
45. Neurontin®
46. Prempro™
47. Lisinopril
48. Effexor® XR
49. Zestril®
50. Pravachol®

*Based on units dispensed in U.S.
Source: Verispan Scott-Levin, SPA

ADULT MULTIVITAMIN PRODUCTS

Product	A (int. units)	B_1 (mg)	B_2 (mg)	B_6 (mg)	B_{12} (mcg)	C (mg)	D (int. units)	E (int. units)	Additional Information
Liquid									
Centrum® [OTC] (per 15 mL)	2500	1.5	1.7	2	6	60	400	30	Biotin 300 mcg, Cr 25 mcg, Fe 9 mg, iodine 150 mcg, Mn 2 mg, Mo 25 mg, niacin 20 mg, pantothenic acid 10 mg, Zn 3 mg; alcohol 5.4%, sodium benzoate (240 mL)
Geritol® Tonic [OTC] (per 15 mL)		2.5	2.5	0.5					Chlorine bitartrate 50 mg, Fe 18 mg, methionine 25 mg, niacin 50 mg, pantothenic acid 2 mg; sugars 7 g, alcohol 12%, benzoic acid (120 mL, 360 mL)
Iberet® [OTC] (per 5 mL)		1.2	1.35	0.925	5.63	33.8			Fe 23.6 mg, niacin 6.8 mg, pantothenic acid 2.4 mg; alcohol (240 mL)
Iberet®-500 [OTC] (per 5 mL)		1.2	1.35	0.925	5.63	125			Fe 23.6 mg, niacin 6.8 mg, pantothenic acid 2.4 mg; alcohol (240 mL)
Vi-Daylin® [OTC] (per 5 mL)	2500	1.05	1.2	1.05	4.5	60	400	15	Niacin 13.5 mg; alcohol <0.5%, benzoic acid; lemon/orange flavor (240 mL, 480 mL)
Vi-Daylin® + Iron [OTC] (per 5 mL)	2500	1.05	1.2	1.05	4.5	60	400	15	Fe 10 mg, niacin 13.5 mg; alcohol <0.5%, benzoic acid; lemon/orange flavor (240 mL, 480 mL)
Caplet									
Theragran® Heart Right™ [OTC]	5000	3	3.4	16	30	120	400	400	Alpha-carotene, beta-carotene, biotin 30 mcg, Ca 55 mg, Cr 50 mcg, cryptoxanthin, Cu 1.5 mg, Fe 4 mg, folic acid as folate 0.6 mg, iodine 150 mcg, lutein, lycopene, Mg 150 mg, Mn 2 mg, Mo 75 mcg, niacin 20 mg, pantothenic acid 10 mg, Se 70 mcg, vit K 14 mcg, zeaxanthin, Zn 15 mg
Theragran-M® Advanced Formula [OTC]	5000	3	3.4	6	12	90	400	60	Biotin 30 mcg, boron 150 mcg, Ca 40 mg, chloride 7.5 mg, Cr 50 mcg, Cu 2 mg, Fe 9 mg, folic acid 0.4 mg, iodine 150 mcg, Mg 100 mg, Mn 2 mg, Mo 75 mcg, niacin 20 mg, nickel 5 mcg, pantothenic acid 10 mg, phosphorus 31 mg, potassium 7.5 mg, Se 70 mcg, silicon 2 mg, tin 10 mcg, vanadium 10 mcg, vit K 28 mcg, Zn 15 mg
Capsule									
Vicon Forte®	8000	10	5	2	10	150		50	Folic acid 1 mg, Mg 70 mg, Mn 4 mg, niacinamide 25 mg, Zn 80 mg
Vicon Plus® [OTC]	3400	9.3	4.6	1.5		140		45	Mg 5 mg, Mn 1 mg, niacin 24 mg, pantothenic acid 11 mg, Zn 10 mg
Vitacon Forte	8000	10	5	2	10	150		50	Folic acid 1 mg, Mg 70 mg, Mn 4 mg, niacinamide 25 mg, Zn 80 mg

ADULT MULTIVITAMIN PRODUCTS *(Continued)*

(continued)

Product	A (int. units)	B_1 (mg)	B_2 (mg)	B_6 (mg)	B_{12} (mcg)	C (mg)	D (int. units)	E (int. units)	Additional Information
Tablet									
Centrum® [OTC]	5000	1.5	1.7	2	6	60	400	30	Biotin 30 mcg, boron 150 mcg, Ca 162 mg, chloride 72 mg, Cr 120 mcg, Cu 2 mg, Fe 18 mg, folic acid 0.4 mg, iodine 150 mcg, lutein 250 mcg, Mg 100 mg, Mn 2 mg, Mo 75 mcg, niacin 20 mg, nickel 5 mcg, pantothenic acid 10 mg, phosphorus 109 mg, potassium 80 mg, Se 20 mcg, silicon 2 mg, tin 10 mcg, vanadium 10 mcg, vit K 25 mcg, Zn 15 mg
Centrum® Performance™ [OTC]	5000	4.5	5.1	6	18	120	400	60	Biotin 40 mcg, boron 60 mcg, chloride 72 mg, folic acid 0.4 mg, Ca 100 mg, Cr 120 mcg, Cu 2 mg, Fe 18 mg, ginkgo biloba leaf 60 mg, ginseng root 50 mg, iodine 150 mcg, Mg 40 mg, Mn 4 mg, Mo 75 mcg, niacin 40 mg, nickel 5 mcg, pantothenic acid 10 mg, phosphorus 48 mg, potassium 80 mg, Se 70 mcg, silicon 4 mg, tin 10 mcg, vanadium 10 mcg, vit K 25 mcg, Zn 15 mg
Centrum® Silver® [OTC]	5000	1.5	1.7	3	25	60	400	45	Biotin 30 mcg, boron 150 mcg, Ca 200 mg, chloride 72 mg, Cr 150 mcg, Cu 2 mg, folic acid 0.4 mg, iodine 150 mcg, lutein 250 mcg, Mg 100 mg, Mn 2 mg, Mo 75 mcg, niacin 20 mg, nickel 5 mcg, pantothenic acid 10 mg, phosphorus 48 mg, potassium 80 mg, Se 20 mcg, silicon 2 mg, vanadium 10 mcg, vit K 10 mcg, Zn 15 mg
Iberet®-500 [OTC]		4.96	5.4	3.7	22.5	500			Fe 95 mg (controlled release), niacin 27.2 mg, pantothenic acid 8.28 mg, sodium 65 mg
Iberet-Folic-500® [OTC]		6	6	5	25	500			Fe 105 mg (controlled release), folic acid 0.8 mg, niacinamde 30 mg, pantothenic acid 10 mg
One-A-Day® 50 Plus Formula [OTC]	5000	4.5	3.4	6	30	120	400	60	Biotin 30 mcg, Ca 120 mg, chloride 34 mg, Cr 180 mcg, Cu 2 mg, folic acid 0.4 mg, iodine 150 mcg, Mg 100 mg, Mn 4 mg, Mo 93.75 mcg, niacin 20 mg, pantothenic acid 15 mg, potassium 37.5 mg, Se 150 mcg, vit K 20 mcg, Zn 22.5 mg
One-A-Day® Active Formula [OTC]	5000	4.5	5.1	6	18	120	400	60	American ginseng 55 mg, biotin 40 mcg, boron 150 mcg, Ca 110 mg, chloride 180 mg, Cr 100 mcg, Cu 2 mg, Fe 9 mg, folic acid 0.4 mg, iodine 150 mcg, Mg 40 mg, Mn 2 mg, Mo 25 mcg, niacin 40 mg, nickel 5 mcg, pantothenic acid 10 mg, phosphorus 48 mg, potassium 200 mg, Se 45 mcg, silicon 6 mg, tin 10 mcg, vanadium 10 mcg, vit K 25 mcg, Zn 15 mg
One-A-Day® Essential Formula [OTC]	5000	1.5	1.7	2	6	60	400	30	Folic acid 0.4 mg, niacin 20 mg, pantothenic acid 10 mg

(continued)

Product	A (int. units)	B_1 (mg)	B_2 (mg)	B_6 (mg)	B_{12} (mcg)	C (mg)	D (int. units)	E (int. units)	Additional Information
One-A-Day® Maximum Formula [OTC]	5000	1.5	1.7	2	6	60	400	30	Biotin 30 mcg, boron 150 mcg, Ca 162 mg, chloride 72 mg, Cr 65 mcg, Cu 2 mg, Fe 18 mg, folic acid 0.4 mg, iodine 150 mcg, Mg 100 mg, Mn 3.5 mg, Mo 160 mcg, niacin 20 mg, nickel 5 mcg, pantothenic acid 10 mg, phosphorus 109 mg, potassium 80 mg, Se 20 mcg, silicon 2 mg, tin 10 mcg, vanadium 10 mcg, vit K 25 mcg, Zn 15 mg
One-A-Day® Men's Formula [OTC]	5000	2.25	2.55	3	9	90	400	45	Chloride 34 mg, Cr 150 mcg, Cu 2 mg, folic acid 0.4 mg, iodine 150 mcg, Mg 100 mg, Mn 3.5 mg, Mo 42 mcg, niacin 20 mg, pantothenic acid 10 mg, potassium 37.5 mg, Se 87.5 mcg, Zn 15 mg
One-A-Day® Today [OTC]	3000	1.1	1.7	3	18	75	400	33	Biotin 30 mcg, Ca 240 mg, Cr 120 mcg, Cu 2 mg, folic acid 0.4 mg, Mg 120 mg, Mn 2 mg, niacin 14 mg, pantothenic acid 5 mg, potassium 100 mg, Se 70 mcg, soy extract 10 mg, vit K 20 mcg, Zn 15 mg
One-A-Day® Women's Formula [OTC]	2500	1.5	1.7	2	6	60	400	30	Ca 450 mg, Fe 18 mg, folic acid 0.4 mg, Mg 50 mg, niacin 10 mg, pantothenic acid 5 mg, Zn 15 mg
Tablet, Chewable									
Centrum® [OTC]	5000	1.5	1.7	2	6	60	400	30	Biotin 45 mcg, Ca 108 mg, Cr 20 mcg, Cu 2 mg, Fe 18 mg, folic acid 0.4 mg, iodine 150 mcg, Mg 40 mg, Mn 1 mg, Mo 20 mcg, niacin 20 mg, pantothenic acid 10 mg, Zn 15 mg

Legend: Ca = calcium, Cr = chromium, Cu = copper, Fe = iron, Mg = magnesium, Mn = manganese, Mo = molybdenum, Se = selenium, Zn = zinc.

VITAMIN B COMPLEX COMBINATION PRODUCTS

Product	B_1 (mg)	B_2 (mg)	B_6 (mg)	B_{12} (mcg)	C (mg)	E (int. units)	Additional Information
Caplet							
Allbee® with C [OTC]	15	10.2	5		300		Niacinamide 50 mg, pantothenic acid 10 mg
Allbee® C-800 [OTC]	15	17	25	12	800	45	Niacinamide 100 mg, pantothenic acid 25 mg
Allbee® C-800 + Iron [OTC]	15	17	25	12	800	45	Fe 27 mg, folic acid 0.4 mcg, niacinamide 100 mg, pantothenic acid 25 mg
Liquid							
Apatate® [OTC] (per 5 mL) [OTC]	15		0.5	25			Cherry flavor (120 mL)
Gevrabon® [OTC] (per 30 mL) [OTC]	5	2.5	1	1			Choline 10 mg, Fe 15 mg, iodine 100 mcg, Mg 2 mg, Mn 2 mg, niacinamide 60 mg, pantothenic acid 10 mg, Zn 2 mg; alcohol, benzoic acid; sherry wine flavor (480 mL)
Softgel							
Nephrocaps®	1.5	1.7	10	6	100		Biotin 150 mcg, folic acid 1 mcg, niacinamide 20 mg, pantothenic acid 5 mg
Tablet							
Diatx™	1.5	1.5	50		60		Biotin 300 mcg, cobalamin 1 mg, folacin 5 mg, niacinamide 20 mg, pantothenic acid 10 mg [dye free, lactose free, sugar free]
DiatxFe™	1.5	1.5	50		60		Biotin 300 mcg, cobalamin 1 mg, ferrous fumarate 304 mg, folacin 5 mg, niacinamide 20 mg, pantothenic acid 10 mg [dye free, lactose free, sugar free]
NephPlex® Rx	1.5	1.7	10	6	60		Biotin 300 mcg, folic acid 1 mg, niacinamide 20 mg, pantothenic acid 10 mg, zinc 12.5 mg
Nephro-Vite®	1.5	1.7	10	6	60		Biotin 300 mcg, folic acid 0.8 mcg, niacinamide 20 mg, pantothenic acid 10 mg
Nephro-Vite® Rx	1.5	1.7	10	6	60		Biotin 300 mcg, folic acid 1 mcg, niacinamide 20 mg, pantothenic acid 10 mg
Nephron FA®	1.5	1.7	10	6	40		Biotin 300 mcg, docusate sodium 75 mg, ferrous fumarate 200 mg, folic acid 1 mg, pantothenic acid 10 mg
Stresstabs® B-Complex [OTC]	10	10	5	12	500	30	Biotin 45 mcg, folic acid 0.4 mcg, niacinamide 100 mg, pantothenic acid 20 mg
Stresstabs® B-Complex + Iron [OTC]	10	10	5	12	500	30	Biotin 45 mcg, Fe 18 mg, folic acid 0.4 mcg, niacinamide 100 mg, pantothenic acid 20 mg
Stresstabs® B-Complex + Zinc [OTC]	10	10	5	12	500	30	Biotin 45 mcg, Cu 3 mg, folic acid 0.4 mcg, niacinamide 100 mg, pantothenic acid 20 mg, Zn 23.9 mg
Surbex-T® [OTC]	15	10	5	10	500		Ca 20 mg, niacinamide 100 mg
Z-Bec® [OTC]	15	10.2	10	6	600	45	Niacinamide 100 mg, pantothenic acid 25 mg, Zn 22.5 mg
Tablet, Chewable							
Apatate® [OTC]	15		0.5	25			Cherry flavor

Legend: Ca = calcium, Cu = copper, Fe = iron, Mg = magnesium, Mn = manganese, Zn = zinc.

PHARMACOLOGIC CATEGORY INDEX

ABORTIFACIENT

Carboprost Tromethamine 250
Dinoprostone 450
Mifepristone 912

ACETYLCHOLINESTERASE INHIBITOR

Physostigmine 1078

ACETYLCHOLINESTERASE INHIBITOR (CENTRAL)

Donepezil 467
Rivastigmine 1192
Tacrine 1260

ACNE PRODUCTS

Adapalene 44

ADRENERGIC AGONIST AGENT

Carbinoxamine and Pseudoephedrine 247
DOBUTamine 460
Epinephrine 499
Epinephrine (Racemic) and Aluminum Potassium Sulfate 501
Isoetharine 747
Oxymetazoline 1022
Phenylephrine and Zinc Sulfate 1073
Propylhexedrine 1142
Tetrahydrozoline 1288

ADRENERGIC AGONIST AGENT, OPHTHALMIC

Hydroxyamphetamine and Tropicamide 694

ALDEHYDE DEHYDROGENASE INHIBITOR

Disulfiram 459

ALKALINIZING AGENT

Citric Acid, Sodium Citrate, and Potassium Citrate 335
Potassium Citrate 1100
Potassium Citrate and Citric Acid 1101
Sodium Bicarbonate 1227
Sodium Citrate and Citric Acid 1230
Tromethamine 1360

ALPHA-ADRENERGIC INHIBITOR

Methyldopa 891

ALPHA/BETA AGONIST

Acetaminophen and Pseudoephedrine 31
Dipivefrin 455
Ephedrine 499
Epinephrine 499
Epinephrine (Racemic) 500
Epinephrine (Racemic) and Aluminum Potassium Sulfate 501
Norepinephrine 985
Phenylephrine 1071
Pseudoephedrine 1146
Triprolidine and Pseudoephedrine 1356

5 ALPHA-REDUCTASE INHIBITOR

Dutasteride 484
Finasteride 572

ALPHA$_1$ AGONIST

Midodrine 911
Naphazoline 952

ALPHA$_1$ BLOCKER

Doxazosin 470
Phenoxybenzamine 1068
Phentolamine 1070
Prazosin 1108
Tamsulosin 1266
Terazosin 1276

ALPHA$_1$ BLOCKER, OPHTHALMIC

Dapiprazole 399

ALPHA$_2$-ADRENERGIC AGONIST

Clonidine 351
Dexmedetomidine 416
Guanabenz 654
Guanfacine 655
Tizanidine 1314

ALPHA$_2$ AGONIST, OPHTHALMIC

Apraclonidine 118
Brimonidine 197

AMEBICIDE

Iodoquinol 735
Metronidazole 902
Paromomycin 1035

AMINOQUINOLINE (ANTIMALARIAL)

Chloroquine 303
Hydroxychloroquine 694
Primaquine 1117

5-AMINOSALICYLIC ACID DERIVATIVE

Mesalamine 869
Olsalazine 999

Sulfasalazine 1254

AMMONIUM DETOXICANT
Lactulose 772
Neomycin 961

ANABOLIC STEROID
Oxymetholone 1023
Stanozolol 1241

ANALGESIC COMBINATION (NARCOTIC)
Belladonna and Opium 164
Butalbital, Acetaminophen, Caffeine, and Codeine 215
Butalbital, Aspirin, Caffeine, and Codeine 217
Hydrocodone and Acetaminophen 678
Hydrocodone and Aspirin 680
Meperidine and Promethazine 860
Pentazocine Combinations 1054
Propoxyphene and Acetaminophen 1136
Propoxyphene and Aspirin 1137

ANALGESIC, NARCOTIC
Acetaminophen and Codeine 29
Alfentanil 55
Aspirin and Codeine 134
Buprenorphine 208
Butorphanol 218
Codeine 361
Dihydrocodeine, Aspirin, and Caffeine 444
Fentanyl 565
Hydrocodone and Ibuprofen 684
Hydromorphone 691
Levomethadyl Acetate Hydrochloride 796
Levorphanol 799
Meperidine 858
Methadone 876
Morphine Sulfate 931
Nalbuphine 946
Opium Tincture 1002
Oxycodone 1017
Oxycodone and Acetaminophen 1018
Oxycodone and Aspirin 1020
Oxymorphone 1024
Paregoric 1034
Pentazocine 1054
Propoxyphene 1135
Remifentanil 1171
Sufentanil 1248

ANALGESIC, MISCELLANEOUS
Acetaminophen 27
Acetaminophen and Diphenhydramine 30
Acetaminophen and Pseudoephedrine 31
Acetaminophen and Tramadol 32
Acetaminophen, Aspirin, and Caffeine 34
Acetaminophen, Chlorpheniramine, and Pseudoephedrine 35
Acetaminophen, Isometheptene, and Dichloralphenazone 36

ANALGESIC, NON-NARCOTIC
Acetaminophen and Phenyltoloxamine 31
Acetaminophen and Tramadol 32
Methotrimeprazine 887
Tramadol 1329

ANALGESIC, TOPICAL
Capsaicin 238
Dichlorodifluoromethane and Trichloromonofluoromethane 428
Lidocaine 801
Triethanolamine Salicylate 1348

ANALGESIC, URINARY
Pentosan Polysulfate Sodium 1056
Phenazopyridine 1064

ANDROGEN
Danazol 397
Fluoxymesterone 592
MethylTESTOSTERone 897
Nandrolone 951
Oxandrolone 1009
Testolactone 1281
Testosterone 1281

ANESTHETIC/CORTICOSTEROID
Lidocaine and Hydrocortisone 805
Pramoxine and Hydrocortisone 1106

ANGIOTENSIN-CONVERTING ENZYME (ACE) INHIBITOR
Benazepril 166
Captopril 238
Cilazapril 324
Enalapril 492
Fosinopril 616
Lisinopril 813
Moexipril 926
Perindopril Erbumine 1060
(Continued)

ANGIOTENSIN-CONVERTING ENZYME (ACE) INHIBITOR *(Continued)*
Quinapril . . . 1156
Quinapril and Hydrochlorothiazide . . . 1158
Ramipril . . . 1166
Trandolapril . . . 1331

ANGIOTENSIN II RECEPTOR BLOCKER
Candesartan . . . 232
Eprosartan . . . 506
Irbesartan . . . 739
Losartan . . . 825
Olmesartan . . . 997
Telmisartan . . . 1269
Valsartan . . . 1374

ANGIOTENSIN II RECEPTOR BLOCKER COMBINATION
Candesartan and Hydrochlorothiazide . . . 234
Telmisartan and Hydrochlorothiazide . . . 1270

ANOREXIANT
Benzphetamine . . . 172
Diethylpropion . . . 436
Mazindol . . . 843
Phendimetrazine . . . 1064
Phentermine . . . 1069
Sibutramine . . . 1219

ANTACID
Aluminum Hydroxide . . . 68
Aluminum Hydroxide and Magnesium Carbonate . . . 68
Aluminum Hydroxide and Magnesium Hydroxide . . . 69
Aluminum Hydroxide and Magnesium Trisilicate . . . 69
Aluminum Hydroxide, Magnesium Hydroxide, and Simethicone . . . 69
Calcium Carbonate and Simethicone . . . 224
Famotidine, Calcium Carbonate, and Magnesium Hydroxide . . . 557
Magaldrate and Simethicone . . . 833
Magnesium Hydroxide . . . 835
Sodium Bicarbonate . . . 1227

ANTHELMINTIC
Albendazole . . . 47
Ivermectin . . . 757
Mebendazole . . . 846
Piperazine . . . 1089
Praziquantel . . . 1108
Pyrantel Pamoate . . . 1150
Thiabendazole . . . 1294

ANTIANXIETY AGENT, MISCELLANEOUS
Aspirin and Meprobamate . . . 136
BusPIRone . . . 211
Meprobamate . . . 864

ANTIARRHYTHMIC AGENT, CLASS I
Moricizine . . . 931

ANTIARRHYTHMIC AGENT, CLASS IA
Disopyramide . . . 458
Procainamide . . . 1119
Quinidine . . . 1158

ANTIARRHYTHMIC AGENT, CLASS IB
Lidocaine . . . 801
Mexiletine . . . 905
Phenytoin . . . 1073
Tocainide . . . 1317

ANTIARRHYTHMIC AGENT, CLASS IC
Flecainide . . . 574
Propafenone . . . 1130

ANTIARRHYTHMIC AGENT, CLASS II
Acebutolol . . . 25
Esmolol . . . 518
Propranolol . . . 1139
Sotalol . . . 1235

ANTIARRHYTHMIC AGENT, CLASS III
Amiodarone . . . 80
Bretylium . . . 196
Dofetilide . . . 464
Ibutilide . . . 706
Sotalol . . . 1235

ANTIARRHYTHMIC AGENT, CLASS IV
Adenosine . . . 45
Digitoxin . . . 440
Digoxin . . . 441
Verapamil . . . 1382

ANTIBACTERIAL, DENTAL
Tetracycline Periodontal Fibers . . . 1287
Triclosan and Fluoride . . . 1348

ANTIBIOTIC, AMINOGLYCOSIDE
Amikacin . . . 74
Gentamicin . . . 634

Kanamycin 759
Neomycin 961
Streptomycin 1245
Tobramycin 1315

ANTIBIOTIC, CARBACEPHEM
Loracarbef 821

ANTIBIOTIC, CARBAPENEM
Ertapenem 511
Imipenem and Cilastatin 709
Meropenem 867

ANTIBIOTIC, CEPHALOSPORIN
Cefditoren 265

ANTIBIOTIC, CEPHALOSPORIN (FIRST GENERATION)
Cefadroxil 261
Cefazolin 263
Cephalexin 285
Cephalothin 286
Cephapirin 287
Cephradine 288

ANTIBIOTIC, CEPHALOSPORIN (SECOND GENERATION)
Cefaclor 260
Cefamandole 263
Cefonicid 269
Cefotetan 272
Cefoxitin 272
Cefprozil 275
Cefuroxime 279

ANTIBIOTIC, CEPHALOSPORIN (THIRD GENERATION)
Cefdinir 265
Cefixime 268
Cefoperazone 270
Cefotaxime 271
Cefpodoxime 273
Ceftazidime 275
Ceftibuten 276
Ceftizoxime 277
Ceftriaxone 278

ANTIBIOTIC, CEPHALOSPORIN (FOURTH GENERATION)
Cefepime 267

ANTIBIOTIC/CORTICOSTEROID, OPHTHALMIC
Neomycin and Dexamethasone 961
Neomycin, Polymyxin B, and Dexamethasone 962
Neomycin, Polymyxin B, and Hydrocortisone 963
Neomycin, Polymyxin B, and Prednisolone 963
Oxytetracycline and Hydrocortisone 1025
Prednisolone and Gentamicin 1112
Sulfacetamide and Fluorometholone 1250
Sulfacetamide and Prednisolone 1250
Tobramycin and Dexamethasone 1317

ANTIBIOTIC/CORTICOSTEROID, OTIC
Ciprofloxacin and Hydrocortisone 331
Colistin, Neomycin, and Hydrocortisone 367
Neomycin, Polymyxin B, and Hydrocortisone 963

ANTIBIOTIC, IRRIGATION
Polymyxin B 1095

ANTIBIOTIC, MACROLIDE
Azithromycin 153
Clarithromycin 337
Dirithromycin 457
Erythromycin 512
Erythromycin and Sulfisoxazole 516
Lincomycin 808
Spiramycin 1239
Troleandomycin 1359

ANTIBIOTIC, MACROLIDE COMBINATION
Erythromycin and Sulfisoxazole 516

ANTIBIOTIC, OPHTHALMIC
Bacitracin 156
Bacitracin and Polymyxin B 157
Bacitracin, Neomycin, and Polymyxin B 157
Bacitracin, Neomycin, Polymyxin B, and Hydrocortisone 158
Chloramphenicol 297
Chloramphenicol and Prednisolone 299
Chloramphenicol, Polymyxin B, and Hydrocortisone 299
Ciprofloxacin 328
Erythromycin 512
Gentamicin 634
Mercuric Oxide 867
Neomycin, Polymyxin B, and Gramicidin 963
Oxytetracycline and Polymyxin B 1025
Povidone-Iodine 1104
Silver Nitrate 1221
Sulfacetamide 1249
Tetracycline 1286
(Continued)

ANTIBIOTIC, OPHTHALMIC *(Continued)*

Tobramycin 1315
Trimethoprim and Polymyxin B 1353

ANTIBIOTIC, ORAL RINSE

Chlorhexidine Gluconate 300

ANTIBIOTIC, OTIC

Aluminum Acetate and Acetic Acid 67
Bacitracin, Neomycin, Polymyxin B, and Hydrocortisone 158
Chloramphenicol 297
Oxytetracycline and Polymyxin B 1025

ANTIBIOTIC, OXAZOLIDINONE

Linezolid 809

ANTIBIOTIC, PENICILLIN

Amoxicillin 93
Amoxicillin and Clavulanate Potassium 95
Ampicillin 103
Ampicillin and Sulbactam 104
Carbenicillin 245
Cloxacillin 357
Dicloxacillin 432
Nafcillin 945
Oxacillin 1007
Penicillin G Benzathine 1047
Penicillin G Benzathine and Penicillin G Procaine 1048
Penicillin G (Parenteral/Aqueous) 1049
Penicillin G Procaine 1050
Penicillin V Potassium 1051
Piperacillin 1087
Piperacillin and Tazobactam Sodium 1088
Ticarcillin 1305
Ticarcillin and Clavulanate Potassium 1306

ANTIBIOTIC, QUINOLONE

Cinoxacin 327
Ciprofloxacin 328
Gatifloxacin 628
Levofloxacin 794
Lomefloxacin 817
Moxifloxacin 935
Nalidixic Acid 947
Norfloxacin 987
Ofloxacin 995
Sparfloxacin 1238
Trovafloxacin/Alatrofloxacin 1361

ANTIBIOTIC, STREPTOGRAMIN

Quinupristin and Dalfopristin 1161

ANTIBIOTIC, SULFONAMIDE DERIVATIVE

Erythromycin and Sulfisoxazole 516
Sulfacetamide 1249
SulfaDIAZINE 1251
Sulfamethoxazole and Trimethoprim 1253
SulfiSOXAZOLE 1256

ANTIBIOTIC, TETRACYCLINE DERIVATIVE

Bismuth, Metronidazole, and Tetracycline 187
Demeclocycline 406
Doxycycline 476
Doxycycline Hyclate Periodontal Extended-Release Liquid 479
Doxycycline Subantimicrobial 480
Minocycline 915
Minocycline Hydrochloride Periodontal Microspheres 916
Oxytetracycline 1024
Tetracycline 1286

ANTIBIOTIC, TOPICAL

Bacitracin 156
Bacitracin and Polymyxin B 157
Bacitracin, Neomycin, and Polymyxin B 157
Bacitracin, Neomycin, Polymyxin B, and Hydrocortisone 158
Bacitracin, Neomycin, Polymyxin B, and Lidocaine 158
Benzalkonium Chloride 169
Benzoin 171
Chlorhexidine Gluconate 300
Erythromycin 512
Gentamicin 634
Gentian Violet 636
Hexachlorophene 669
Mafenide 832
Metronidazole 902
Mupirocin 937
Neomycin 961
Neomycin and Polymyxin B 962
Oxychlorosene 1017
Povidone-Iodine 1104
Silver Nitrate 1221
Silver Sulfadiazine 1222
Tetracycline 1286
Thimerosal 1296

ANTIBIOTIC, VAGINAL
Povidone-Iodine . . . 1104
Sulfabenzamide, Sulfacetamide, and Sulfathiazole . . . 1249

ANTIBIOTIC, MISCELLANEOUS
Aztreonam . . . 155
Bacitracin . . . 156
Capreomycin . . . 237
Chloramphenicol . . . 297
Clindamycin . . . 341
Colistimethate . . . 366
CycloSERINE . . . 383
Dapsone . . . 399
Fosfomycin . . . 615
Methenamine . . . 879
Methenamine, Sodium Biphosphate, Phenyl Salicylate, Methylene Blue, and Hyoscyamine . . . 880
Metronidazole . . . 902
Nitrofurantoin . . . 980
Pentamidine . . . 1052
Polymyxin B . . . 1095
Rifabutin . . . 1179
Rifampin . . . 1180
Rifampin and Isoniazid . . . 1181
Rifampin, Isoniazid, and Pyrazinamide . . . 1182
Spectinomycin . . . 1239
Sulfamethoxazole and Trimethoprim . . . 1253
Trimethoprim . . . 1352
Vancomycin . . . 1376

ANTICHOLINERGIC/ADRENERGIC AGONIST
Phenylephrine and Scopolamine . . . 1072

ANTICHOLINERGIC AGENT
Atropine . . . 144
Atropine Sulfate Dental Tablets . . . 145
Benztropine . . . 173
Biperiden . . . 185
Dicyclomine . . . 433
Glycopyrrolate . . . 645
Hyoscyamine . . . 699
Hyoscyamine, Atropine, Scopolamine, and Phenobarbital . . . 700
Hyoscyamine, Atropine, Scopolamine, Kaolin, and Pectin . . . 701
Hyoscyamine, Atropine, Scopolamine, Kaolin, Pectin, and Opium . . . 701
Ipratropium . . . 737
Mepenzolate . . . 858
Methscopolamine . . . 888
Procyclidine . . . 1125
Propantheline . . . 1132
Scopolamine . . . 1210
Tolterodine . . . 1322
Trihexyphenidyl . . . 1351
Trimethobenzamide . . . 1352

ANTICHOLINERGIC AGENT, OPHTHALMIC
Atropine . . . 144
Cyclopentolate . . . 380
Homatropine . . . 670

ANTICOAGULANT
Antithrombin III . . . 117
Danaparoid . . . 395
Heparin . . . 662

ANTICOAGULANT, COUMARIN DERIVATIVE
Dicumarol . . . 433
Warfarin . . . 1397

ANTICOAGULANT, INDANEDIONE
Anisindione . . . 110

ANTICOAGULANT, THROMBIN INHIBITOR
Argatroban . . . 120
Lepirudin . . . 781

ANTICONVULSANT, BARBITURATE
Pentobarbital . . . 1055
Phenobarbital . . . 1066
Thiopental . . . 1297

ANTICONVULSANT, HYDANTOIN
Ethotoin . . . 544
Fosphenytoin . . . 618
Phenytoin . . . 1073

ANTICONVULSANT, OXAZOLIDINEDIONE
Trimethadione . . . 1351

ANTICONVULSANT, SUCCINIMIDE
Ethosuximide . . . 543
Methsuximide . . . 889

ANTICONVULSANT, MISCELLANEOUS
AcetaZOLAMIDE . . . 37
Carbamazepine . . . 241
Felbamate . . . 558
Gabapentin . . . 624

(Continued)

ANTICONVULSANT, MISCELLANEOUS *(Continued)*

Lamotrigine . . . 774
Levetiracetam . . . 787
Oxcarbazepine . . . 1012
Primidone . . . 1118
Tiagabine . . . 1304
Topiramate . . . 1324
Valproic Acid and Derivatives . . . 1371
Vigabatrin . . . 1385
Zonisamide . . . 1413

ANTICYSTINE AGENT

Cysteamine . . . 388

ANTIDEPRESSANT, ALPHA-2 ANTAGONIST

Mirtazapine . . . 919

ANTIDEPRESSANT, DOPAMINE-REUPTAKE INHIBITOR

BuPROPion . . . 209

ANTIDEPRESSANT, MONOAMINE OXIDASE INHIBITOR

Isocarboxazid . . . 747
Phenelzine . . . 1065
Selegiline . . . 1213
Tranylcypromine . . . 1334

ANTIDEPRESSANT, SELECTIVE SEROTONIN REUPTAKE INHIBITOR

Citalopram . . . 334
Escitalopram . . . 516
Fluoxetine . . . 589
Fluvoxamine . . . 605
Paroxetine . . . 1036
Sertraline . . . 1216

ANTIDEPRESSANT, SEROTONIN/NOREPINEPHRINE REUPTAKE INHIBITOR

Venlafaxine . . . 1380

ANTIDEPRESSANT, SEROTONIN REUPTAKE INHIBITOR/ANTAGONIST

Nefazodone . . . 957
Trazodone . . . 1336

ANTIDEPRESSANT, TETRACYCLIC

Maprotiline . . . 841

ANTIDEPRESSANT, TRICYCLIC (SECONDARY AMINE)

Amoxapine . . . 91
Desipramine . . . 408
Nortriptyline . . . 989
Protriptyline . . . 1145

ANTIDEPRESSANT, TRICYCLIC (TERTIARY AMINE)

Amitriptyline . . . 83
Amitriptyline and Chlordiazepoxide . . . 85
Amitriptyline and Perphenazine . . . 85
ClomiPRAMINE . . . 349
Doxepin . . . 471
Imipramine . . . 711
Trimipramine . . . 1354

ANTIDIABETIC AGENT, ALPHA-GLUCOSIDASE INHIBITOR

Acarbose . . . 24
Miglitol . . . 913

ANTIDIABETIC AGENT, BIGUANIDE

Glipizide and Metformin . . . 639
Glyburide and Metformin . . . 643
Metformin . . . 874
Rosiglitazone and Metformin . . . 1200

ANTIDIABETIC AGENT, INSULIN

Insulin Preparations . . . 723

ANTIDIABETIC AGENT, SULFONYLUREA

AcetoHEXAMIDE . . . 38
ChlorproPAMIDE . . . 314
Glimepiride . . . 637
GlipiZIDE . . . 638
Glipizide and Metformin . . . 639
GlyBURIDE . . . 642
Glyburide and Metformin . . . 643
TOLAZamide . . . 1318
TOLBUTamide . . . 1319

ANTIDIABETIC AGENT, THIAZOLIDINEDIONE

Pioglitazone . . . 1086
Rosiglitazone . . . 1199
Rosiglitazone and Metformin . . . 1200

ANTIDIABETIC AGENT, MISCELLANEOUS

Repaglinide . . . 1172

ANTIDIARRHEAL

Attapulgite . . . 146
Bismuth . . . 186
Bismuth, Metronidazole, and Tetracycline . . . 187
Calcium Polycarbophil . . . 228
Charcoal . . . 294
Difenoxin and Atropine . . . 437

Diphenoxylate and Atropine 453
Hyoscyamine, Atropine, Scopolamine, Kaolin, and Pectin 701
Hyoscyamine, Atropine, Scopolamine, Kaolin, Pectin, and Opium 701
Kaolin and Pectin 760
Lactobacillus acidophilus and *Lactobacillus bulgaricus* 772
Loperamide 819
Octreotide 993
Opium Tincture 1002
Psyllium 1149

ANTIDIURETIC HORMONE ANALOG
Vasopressin 1379

ANTIDOTE
Acetylcysteine 40
Aluminum Hydroxide 68
Amifostine 73
Amyl Nitrite 107
Atropine 144
Calcitonin 222
Charcoal 294
Deferoxamine 404
Digoxin Immune Fab 443
Dimercaprol 449
Epinephrine 499
Epinephrine and Chlorpheniramine Insect Sting Kit 500
Flumazenil 581
Fomepizole 609
Glucagon 640
Insulin Preparations 723
Ipecac Syrup 736
Leucovorin 783
Nalmefene 948
Naloxone 949
Naltrexone 950
Pamidronate 1029
Protamine Sulfate 1144
Sodium Thiosulfate 1233

ANTIEMETIC
Dexamethasone 413
Dolasetron 465
Dronabinol 480
Droperidol 481
HydrOXYzine 697
Meclizine 847
Phosphorated Carbohydrate Solution 1078
Promethazine 1127
Thiethylperazine 1295
Trimethobenzamide 1352

ANTIFLATULENT
Aluminum Hydroxide, Magnesium Hydroxide, and Simethicone 69
Calcium Carbonate and Simethicone 224
Charcoal 294
Magaldrate and Simethicone 833
Simethicone 1222

ANTIFUNGAL AGENT, OPHTHALMIC
Natamycin 956

ANTIFUNGAL AGENT, ORAL
Fluconazole 576
Flucytosine 578
Griseofulvin 649
Itraconazole 755
Ketoconazole 762
Terbinafine 1277
Voriconazole 1395

ANTIFUNGAL AGENT, ORAL NONABSORBED
Clotrimazole 356
Nystatin 992

ANTIFUNGAL AGENT, PARENTERAL
Amphotericin B Cholesteryl Sulfate Complex 97
Amphotericin B (Conventional) 98
Amphotericin B (Lipid Complex) 100
Amphotericin B (Liposomal) 101
Caspofungin 258
Fluconazole 576
Voriconazole 1395

ANTIFUNGAL AGENT, TOPICAL
Amphotericin B (Conventional) 98
Betamethasone and Clotrimazole 179
Butenafine 217
Carbol-Fuchsin Solution 248
Ciclopirox 322
Clotrimazole 356
Econazole 486
Gentian Violet 636
Iodoquinol and Hydrocortisone 736
Ketoconazole 762
Miconazole 906

(Continued)

ANTIFUNGAL AGENT, TOPICAL *(Continued)*

Naftifine 946
Nystatin 992
Nystatin and Triamcinolone 992
Oxiconazole 1014
Sulconazole 1249
Terbinafine 1277
Tolnaftate 1322
Triacetin 1340
Undecylenic Acid and Derivatives 1365

ANTIFUNGAL AGENT, VAGINAL

Butoconazole 218
Clotrimazole 356
Miconazole 906
Nystatin 992
Terconazole 1279
Tioconazole 1312

ANTIGONADOTROPIC AGENT

Cetrorelix 291
Ganirelix 628

ANTIGOUT AGENT

Colchicine and Probenecid 364

ANTIHEMOPHILIC AGENT

Antihemophilic Factor (Human) 113
Antihemophilic Factor (Porcine) 114
Antihemophilic Factor (Recombinant) 115
Anti-inhibitor Coagulant Complex 116
Desmopressin 410
Factor IX Complex (Human) 553
Factor VIIa (Recombinant) 554
Tranexamic Acid 1333

ANTIHISTAMINE

Acetaminophen, Chlorpheniramine, and Pseudoephedrine 35
Acetaminophen, Dextromethorphan, and Pseudoephedrine 35
Acrivastine and Pseudoephedrine 41
Azatadine 149
Azelastine 151
Cetirizine 289
Chlorpheniramine 307
Clemastine 340
Cyclizine 379
Cyproheptadine 387
Dexchlorpheniramine 416
DimenhyDRINATE 449
DiphenhydrAMINE 451
HydrOXYzine 697
Meclizine 847
Olopatadine 998
Phenindamine 1066
Tripelennamine 1356
Triprolidine and Pseudoephedrine 1356

ANTIHISTAMINE/ANALGESIC

Chlorpheniramine and Acetaminophen 308

ANTIHISTAMINE/ANTITUSSIVE

Bromodiphenhydramine and Codeine 200
Carbetapentane and Chlorpheniramine 245
Hydrocodone and Chlorpheniramine 682
Promethazine and Codeine 1129
Promethazine and Dextromethorphan 1129

ANTIHISTAMINE/DECONGESTANT/ANTICHOLINERGIC

Chlorpheniramine, Phenylephrine, and Methscopolamine 310

ANTIHISTAMINE/DECONGESTANT/ANTITUSSIVE

Carbinoxamine, Pseudoephedrine, and Dextromethorphan 247
Chlorpheniramine, Ephedrine, Phenylephrine, and Carbetapentane 309
Chlorpheniramine, Phenylephrine, and Dextromethorphan 309
Chlorpheniramine, Pseudoephedrine, and Codeine 311
Promethazine, Phenylephrine, and Codeine 1130
Triprolidine, Pseudoephedrine, and Codeine 1357

ANTIHISTAMINE/DECONGESTANT/ANTITUSSIVE/EXPECTORANT

Chlorpheniramine, Phenylephrine, Codeine, and Potassium Iodide 311

ANTIHISTAMINE/DECONGESTANT COMBINATION

Azatadine and Pseudoephedrine 150
Brompheniramine and Pseudoephedrine 201
Cetirizine and Pseudoephedrine 290
Chlorpheniramine and Phenylephrine 308
Chlorpheniramine and Pseudoephedrine 308
Chlorpheniramine, Phenylephrine, and Phenyltoloxamine 311
Chlorpheniramine, Pyrilamine, and Phenylephrine 312
Dexbrompheniramine and Pseudoephedrine 415
Diphenhydramine and Pseudoephedrine 453
Fexofenadine and Pseudoephedrine 570
Loratadine and Pseudoephedrine 823
Promethazine and Phenylephrine 1129

ANTIHISTAMINE, H_1 BLOCKER

Carbinoxamine and Pseudoephedrine . . . 247

ANTIHISTAMINE, H_1 BLOCKER, OPHTHALMIC

Ketotifen . . . 768
Levocabastine . . . 791

ANTIHISTAMINE, NONSEDATING

Desloratadine . . . 410
Fexofenadine . . . 569
Loratadine . . . 822

ANTIHYPERTENSIVE

Diazoxide . . . 427
Eplerenone . . . 502
Oxprenolol . . . 1014
Quinapril and Hydrochlorothiazide . . . 1158

ANTIHYPERTENSIVE AGENT COMBINATION

Amlodipine and Benazepril . . . 89
Atenolol and Chlorthalidone . . . 138
Benazepril and Hydrochlorothiazide . . . 167
Bisoprolol and Hydrochlorothiazide . . . 189
Captopril and Hydrochlorothiazide . . . 240
Chlorothiazide and Methyldopa . . . 305
Chlorothiazide and Reserpine . . . 306
Clonidine and Chlorthalidone . . . 353
Enalapril and Felodipine . . . 494
Enalapril and Hydrochlorothiazide . . . 494
Fosinopril and Hydrochlorothiazide . . . 617
Hydralazine and Hydrochlorothiazide . . . 675
Hydralazine, Hydrochlorothiazide, and Reserpine . . . 675
Hydrochlorothiazide and Spironolactone . . . 677
Hydrochlorothiazide and Triamterene . . . 677
Irbesartan and Hydrochlorothiazide . . . 740
Lisinopril and Hydrochlorothiazide . . . 814
Losartan and Hydrochlorothiazide . . . 827
Methyclothiazide and Deserpidine . . . 890
Methyldopa and Hydrochlorothiazide . . . 892
Moexipril and Hydrochlorothiazide . . . 927
Prazosin and Polythiazide . . . 1109
Propranolol and Hydrochlorothiazide . . . 1142
Telmisartan and Hydrochlorothiazide . . . 1270
Trandolapril and Verapamil . . . 1332
Valsartan and Hydrochlorothiazide . . . 1375

ANTIHYPOGLYCEMIC AGENT

Diazoxide . . . 427
Glucose (Instant) . . . 641

ANTI-INFLAMMATORY AGENT

Colchicine and Probenecid . . . 364
Dexamethasone . . . 413
Triamcinolone Acetonide Dental Paste . . . 1344

ANTI-INFLAMMATORY AGENT, OPHTHALMIC

Dexamethasone . . . 413

ANTI-INFLAMMATORY, LOCALLY APPLIED

Amlexanox . . . 87

ANTILIPEMIC AGENT, 2-AZETIDINONE

Ezetimibe . . . 553

ANTILIPEMIC AGENT, BILE ACID SEQUESTRANT

Cholestyramine Resin . . . 318
Colesevelam . . . 365
Colestipol . . . 365

ANTILIPEMIC AGENT, FIBRIC ACID

Clofibrate . . . 347
Fenofibrate . . . 561
Gemfibrozil . . . 631

ANTILIPEMIC AGENT, HMG-COA REDUCTASE INHIBITOR

Atorvastatin . . . 140
Fluvastatin . . . 603
Lovastatin . . . 828
Niacin and Lovastatin . . . 968
Pravastatin . . . 1106
Rosuvastatin . . . 1201
Simvastatin . . . 1223

ANTILIPEMIC AGENT, MISCELLANEOUS

Niacin . . . 967
Niacin and Lovastatin . . . 968

ANTIMALARIAL AGENT

Atovaquone and Proguanil . . . 143
Halofantrine . . . 658
Mefloquine . . . 852
Pyrimethamine . . . 1152
Quinine . . . 1160
Sulfadoxine and Pyrimethamine . . . 1252

ANTIMICROBIAL MOUTH RINSE

Mouthwash (Antiseptic) . . . 934

ANTIMIGRAINE AGENT

Frovatriptan . . . 620

ANTINEOPLASTIC AGENT, ALKYLATING AGENT

Busulfan . . . 212
Carboplatin . . . 248
Carmustine . . . 253
Chlorambucil . . . 296
Cisplatin . . . 332
Cyclophosphamide . . . 381
Dacarbazine . . . 391
Estramustine . . . 527
Ifosfamide . . . 707
Lomustine . . . 818
Melphalan . . . 855
Oxaliplatin . . . 1008
Procarbazine . . . 1122
Streptozocin . . . 1246
Temozolomide . . . 1272
Thiotepa . . . 1300

ANTINEOPLASTIC AGENT, ANTHRACYCLINE

DAUNOrubicin Citrate (Liposomal) . . . 402
DAUNOrubicin Hydrochloride . . . 402
DOXOrubicin . . . 473
DOXOrubicin (Liposomal) . . . 475
Epirubicin . . . 501
Idarubicin . . . 706
Valrubicin . . . 1374

ANTINEOPLASTIC AGENT, ANTIANDROGEN

Bicalutamide . . . 183
Flutamide . . . 598
Nilutamide . . . 975

ANTINEOPLASTIC AGENT, ANTIBIOTIC

Bleomycin . . . 190
Dactinomycin . . . 393
Mitomycin . . . 921
Mitoxantrone . . . 923
Pentostatin . . . 1057

ANTINEOPLASTIC AGENT, ANTIMETABOLITE

Capecitabine . . . 235
Cladribine . . . 336
Cytarabine . . . 389
Cytarabine (Liposomal) . . . 390
Floxuridine . . . 576
Fludarabine . . . 579
Fluorouracil . . . 588
Gemcitabine . . . 630
Hydroxyurea . . . 696
Mercaptopurine . . . 866
Methotrexate . . . 884
Thioguanine . . . 1296

ANTINEOPLASTIC AGENT, AROMATASE INHIBITOR

Letrozole . . . 782

ANTINEOPLASTIC AGENT, ESTROGEN RECEPTOR ANTAGONIST

Fulvestrant . . . 621
Tamoxifen . . . 1264
Toremifene . . . 1326

ANTINEOPLASTIC AGENT, HORMONE ANTAGONIST

Mifepristone . . . 912

ANTINEOPLASTIC AGENT, MONOCLONAL ANTIBODY

Alemtuzumab . . . 52
Gemtuzumab Ozogamicin . . . 632
Ibritumomab . . . 702
Rituximab . . . 1190

ANTINEOPLASTIC AGENT, NATURAL SOURCE (PLANT) DERIVATIVE

Docetaxel . . . 461
Irinotecan . . . 740
Paclitaxel . . . 1026
Topotecan . . . 1325
VinBLAStine . . . 1386
VinCRIStine . . . 1387
Vinorelbine . . . 1389

ANTINEOPLASTIC AGENT, PODOPHYLLOTOXIN DERIVATIVE

Etoposide . . . 549
Etoposide Phosphate . . . 551

ANTINEOPLASTIC AGENT, MISCELLANEOUS

Alitretinoin . . . 57
Altretamine . . . 66
Aminoglutethimide . . . 77
Anastrozole . . . 109
Asparaginase . . . 129
Azacitidine . . . 149
Bexarotene . . . 182
Denileukin Diftitox . . . 407
Exemestane . . . 552

Goserelin . . . 647
Leuprolide . . . 784
Megestrol . . . 853
Mitotane . . . 922
Pegaspargase . . . 1039
Porfimer . . . 1098
Teniposide . . . 1274
Tretinoin (Oral) . . . 1338
Trimetrexate Glucuronate . . . 1354

ANTIPARASITIC AGENT, TOPICAL
Lindane . . . 809
Permethrin . . . 1062
Pyrethrins and Piperonyl Butoxide . . . 1151

ANTI-PARKINSON'S AGENT, ANTICHOLINERGIC
Benztropine . . . 173
Biperiden . . . 185
Orphenadrine . . . 1005
Procyclidine . . . 1125
Trihexyphenidyl . . . 1351

ANTI-PARKINSON'S AGENT, COMT INHIBITOR
Entacapone . . . 497
Tolcapone . . . 1320

ANTI-PARKINSON'S AGENT, DOPAMINE AGONIST
Amantadine . . . 70
Bromocriptine . . . 199
Carbidopa . . . 246
Levodopa . . . 792
Levodopa and Carbidopa . . . 793
Pergolide . . . 1059
Pramipexole . . . 1105
Ropinirole . . . 1196

ANTI-PARKINSON'S AGENT, MAO TYPE B INHIBITOR
Selegiline . . . 1213

ANTIPLAQUE AGENT
Mouthwash (Antiseptic) . . . 934

ANTIPLATELET AGENT
Aspirin and Dipyridamole . . . 135
Cilostazol . . . 325
Clopidogrel . . . 353
Dipyridamole . . . 456
Ticlopidine . . . 1307

ANTIPLATELET AGENT, GLYCOPROTEIN IIB/IIIA INHIBITOR
Abciximab . . . 23
Eptifibatide . . . 507
Tirofiban . . . 1313

ANTIPROGESTIN
Mifepristone . . . 912

ANTIPROTOZOAL
Atovaquone . . . 142
Eflornithine . . . 489
Furazolidone . . . 622
Metronidazole . . . 902
Nitazoxanide . . . 978

ANTIPSORIATIC AGENT
Anthralin . . . 111

ANTIPSYCHOTIC AGENT, BENZISOXAZOLE
Risperidone . . . 1187

ANTIPSYCHOTIC AGENT, BUTYROPHENONE
Droperidol . . . 481
Haloperidol . . . 659

ANTIPSYCHOTIC AGENT, DIBENZODIAZEPINE
Clozapine . . . 358

ANTIPSYCHOTIC AGENT, DIBENZOTHIAZEPINE
Quetiapine . . . 1155

ANTIPSYCHOTIC AGENT, DIBENZOXAZEPINE
Loxapine . . . 829

ANTIPSYCHOTIC AGENT, DIHYDOINDOLINE
Molindone . . . 927

ANTIPSYCHOTIC AGENT, DIPHENYLBUTYLPERIDINE
Pimozide . . . 1083

ANTIPSYCHOTIC AGENT, PHENOTHIAZINE, ALIPHATIC
ChlorproMAZINE . . . 312

ANTIPSYCHOTIC AGENT, PHENOTHIAZINE, PIPERAZINE
Amitriptyline and Perphenazine . . . 85
Fluphenazine . . . 593
Perphenazine . . . 1062
Prochlorperazine . . . 1123
Trifluoperazine . . . 1349

ANTIPSYCHOTIC AGENT, PHENOTHIAZINE, PIPERIDINE
Mesoridazine . . . 870
(Continued)

ANTIPSYCHOTIC AGENT, PHENOTHIAZINE, PIPERIDINE *(Continued)*
Thioridazine 1298

ANTIPSYCHOTIC AGENT, QUINOLONE
Aripiprazole 122

ANTIPSYCHOTIC AGENT, THIENOBENZODIAZEPINE
Olanzapine 996

ANTIPSYCHOTIC AGENT, THIOXANTHENE DERIVATIVE
Thiothixene 1301

ANTIRETROVIRAL AGENT, FUSION PROTEIN INHIBITOR
Enfuvirtide 495

ANTIRETROVIRAL AGENT, PROTEASE INHIBITOR
Amprenavir 105
Indinavir 718
Lopinavir and Ritonavir 820
Nelfinavir 959
Ritonavir 1188
Saquinavir 1207

ANTIRETROVIRAL AGENT, REVERSE TRANSCRIPTASE INHIBITOR (NON-NUCLEOSIDE)
Delavirdine 405
Efavirenz 488
Nevirapine 965

ANTIRETROVIRAL AGENT, REVERSE TRANSCRIPTASE INHIBITOR (NUCLEOSIDE)
Abacavir 22
Abacavir, Lamivudine, and Zidovudine 23
Adefovir 44
Didanosine 434
Lamivudine 773
Stavudine 1242
Zalcitabine 1403
Zidovudine 1406
Zidovudine and Lamivudine 1407

ANTIRETROVIRAL AGENT, REVERSE TRANSCRIPTASE INHIBITOR (NUCLEOTIDE)
Tenofovir 1275

ANTIRHEUMATIC, DISEASE MODIFYING
Anakinra 108
Etanercept 537
Infliximab 721
Leflunomide 779

ANTISPASMODIC AGENT, GASTROINTESTINAL
Atropine 144
Clidinium and Chlordiazepoxide 341
Hyoscyamine, Atropine, Scopolamine, and Phenobarbital 700
Mepenzolate 858

ANTISPASMODIC AGENT, URINARY
Belladonna and Opium 164
Flavoxate 573
Oxybutynin 1016

ANTITHYROID AGENT
Methimazole 880
Potassium Iodide 1101
Propylthiouracil 1142

ANTITRYPSIN DEFICIENCY AGENT
Alpha$_1$-Proteinase Inhibitor 61

ANTITUBERCULAR AGENT
Capreomycin 237
CycloSERINE 383
Ethambutol 539
Ethionamide 542
Isoniazid 748
Pyrazinamide 1150
Rifabutin 1179
Rifampin 1180
Rifapentine 1182
Streptomycin 1245

ANTITUSSIVE
Acetaminophen, Dextromethorphan, and Pseudoephedrine 35
Benzonatate 171
Codeine 361
Dextromethorphan 423
Guaifenesin and Codeine 650
Guaifenesin and Dextromethorphan 651
Hydrocodone and Homatropine 684

ANTITUSSIVE/DECONGESTANT
Hydrocodone, Chlorpheniramine, Phenylephrine, Acetaminophen, and Caffeine 686
Pseudoephedrine and Dextromethorphan 1147

ANTITUSSIVE/DECONGESTANT/EXPECTORANT
Guaifenesin, Pseudoephedrine, and Codeine 653
Guaifenesin, Pseudoephedrine, and Dextromethorphan 653

Hydrocodone, Pseudoephedrine, and Guaifenesin . . . 687

ANTITUSSIVE/EXPECTORANT
Hydrocodone and Guaifenesin . . . 683

ANTIVIRAL AGENT
Acyclovir . . . 42
Amantadine . . . 70
Cidofovir . . . 323
Famciclovir . . . 555
Foscarnet . . . 613
Ganciclovir . . . 626
Interferon Alfa-2b and Ribavirin . . . 730
Oseltamivir . . . 1006
Penciclovir . . . 1046
Ribavirin . . . 1176
Rimantadine . . . 1185
Valganciclovir . . . 1370
Zanamivir . . . 1405

ANTIVIRAL AGENT, OPHTHALMIC
Fomivirsen . . . 611
Trifluridine . . . 1350
Vidarabine . . . 1384

ANTIVIRAL AGENT, ORAL
Valacyclovir . . . 1367

ANTIVIRAL AGENT, TOPICAL
Docosanol . . . 463

APHTHOUS ULCER TREATMENT AGENT
Sulfonated Phenolics in Aqueous Solution . . . 1257

APPETITE STIMULANT
Dronabinol . . . 480

ASTRINGENT
Aluminum Chloride . . . 67
Epinephrine (Racemic) and Aluminum Potassium Sulfate . . . 501

BARBITURATE
Amobarbital . . . 90
Amobarbital and Secobarbital . . . 91
Butabarbital Sodium . . . 213
Butalbital, Acetaminophen, and Caffeine . . . 214
Butalbital, Acetaminophen, Caffeine, and Codeine . . . 215
Butalbital, Aspirin, and Caffeine . . . 216
Butalbital, Aspirin, Caffeine, and Codeine . . . 217
Mephobarbital . . . 860
Methohexital . . . 882
Pentobarbital . . . 1055
Phenobarbital . . . 1066
Primidone . . . 1118
Secobarbital . . . 1212
Thiopental . . . 1297

BENZODIAZEPINE
Alprazolam . . . 61
Amitriptyline and Chlordiazepoxide . . . 85
Bromazepam . . . 199
Chlordiazepoxide . . . 299
Clidinium and Chlordiazepoxide . . . 341
Clobazam . . . 344
Clonazepam . . . 350
Clorazepate . . . 355
Diazepam . . . 424
Estazolam . . . 521
Flunitrazepam . . . 583
Flurazepam . . . 595
Lorazepam . . . 824
Midazolam . . . 908
Oxazepam . . . 1011
Quazepam . . . 1154
Temazepam . . . 1271
Triazolam . . . 1345

BETA-ADRENERGIC BLOCKER, NONCARDIOSELECTIVE
Oxprenolol . . . 1014

BETA BLOCKER, BETA$_1$ SELECTIVE
Atenolol . . . 137
Betaxolol . . . 180
Bisoprolol . . . 188
Esmolol . . . 518
Levobetaxolol . . . 788
Metoprolol . . . 901

BETA BLOCKER, NONSELECTIVE
Levobunolol . . . 789
Metipranolol . . . 898
Nadolol . . . 943
Propranolol . . . 1139
Sotalol . . . 1235
Timolol . . . 1309

BETA BLOCKER WITH ALPHA-BLOCKING ACTIVITY
Carvedilol 256
Labetalol 769

BETA BLOCKER WITH INTRINSIC SYMPATHOMIMETIC ACTIVITY
Acebutolol 25
Carteolol 254
Penbutolol 1045
Pindolol 1085

BETA$_1$/BETA$_2$ AGONIST
Isoproterenol 749

BETA$_2$ AGONIST
Albuterol 48
Bitolterol 189
Fenoterol 564
Fluticasone and Salmeterol 601
Formoterol 612
Levalbuterol 786
Metaproterenol 873
Pirbuterol 1090
Salmeterol 1205
Terbutaline 1278

BILE ACID
Chenodiol 295

BIOLOGICAL, MISCELLANEOUS
Glatiramer Acetate 636

BIOLOGICAL RESPONSE MODULATOR
Aldesleukin 50
BCG Vaccine 161
Oprelvekin 1003

BISPHOSPHONATE DERIVATIVE
Alendronate 54
Etidronate Disodium 546
Pamidronate 1029
Risedronate 1186
Tiludronate 1309
Zoledronic Acid 1410

BLOOD MODIFIERS
Hemin 661
Pentastarch 1053

BLOOD PRODUCT DERIVATIVE
Antihemophilic Factor (Human) 113
Anti-inhibitor Coagulant Complex 116
Antithrombin III 117
Aprotinin 119
Factor IX Complex (Human) 553
Factor VIIa (Recombinant) 554

BLOOD VISCOSITY REDUCER AGENT
Pentoxifylline 1058

BRONCHODILATOR
Epinephrine 499
Ipratropium and Albuterol 738

CALCIUM CHANNEL BLOCKER
Amlodipine 87
Bepridil 174
Diltiazem 447
Felodipine 560
Isradipine 754
NiCARdipine 969
NIFEdipine 973
Nimodipine 976
Nisoldipine 977
Verapamil 1382

CALCIUM SALT
Calcium Citrate 224
Calcium Glubionate 225
Calcium Gluceptate 226
Calcium Lactate 227
Calcium Phosphate (Tribasic) 227

CALORIC AGENT
Fat Emulsion 558

CARBONIC ANHYDRASE INHIBITOR
AcetaZOLAMIDE 37
Brinzolamide 198
Dichlorphenamide 428
Dorzolamide 468
Methazolamide 878

CARDIAC GLYCOSIDE
Digoxin 441

CARDIOPROTECTANT
Dexrazoxane 419

CATHARTIC
Phosphate Supplements . . . 1076
Polyethylene Glycol-Electrolyte Solution . . . 1094

CAUTERIZING AGENT, TOPICAL
Silver Nitrate . . . 1221

CENTRAL NERVOUS SYSTEM DEPRESSANT
Sodium Oxybate . . . 1231

CENTRAL NERVOUS SYSTEM STIMULANT
Dexmethylphenidate . . . 417
Methylphenidate . . . 893

CHELATING AGENT
Edetate Calcium Disodium . . . 486
Edetate Disodium . . . 488
Penicillamine . . . 1046

CHOLINERGIC AGONIST
Acetylcholine . . . 39
Ambenonium . . . 72
Bethanechol . . . 181
Carbachol . . . 241
Cevimeline . . . 292
Pilocarpine . . . 1080
Pilocarpine (Dental) . . . 1081

COLCHICINE
Colchicine . . . 363

COLONY STIMULATING FACTOR
Darbepoetin Alfa . . . 400
Epoetin Alfa . . . 503
Filgrastim . . . 571
Pegfilgrastim . . . 1040
Sargramostim . . . 1209

CONTRACEPTIVE
Combination Hormonal Contraceptives . . . 368
Estradiol and Medroxyprogesterone . . . 523
Levonorgestrel . . . 797
MedroxyPROGESTERone . . . 849
Mestranol and Norethindrone . . . 871
Norethindrone . . . 986
Norgestrel . . . 988

CORTICOSTEROID, ADRENAL
Triamcinolone . . . 1341

CORTICOSTEROID, INHALANT (ORAL)
Beclomethasone . . . 163
Budesonide . . . 202
Flunisolide . . . 582
Fluticasone . . . 599
Fluticasone and Salmeterol . . . 601
Triamcinolone . . . 1341

CORTICOSTEROID, NASAL
Beclomethasone . . . 163
Budesonide . . . 202
Dexamethasone . . . 413
Flunisolide . . . 582
Fluticasone . . . 599
Mometasone Furoate . . . 928
Triamcinolone . . . 1341

CORTICOSTEROID, OPHTHALMIC
Bacitracin, Neomycin, Polymyxin B, and Hydrocortisone . . . 158
Chloramphenicol and Prednisolone . . . 299
Chloramphenicol, Polymyxin B, and Hydrocortisone . . . 299
Dexamethasone . . . 413
Fluorometholone . . . 587
Loteprednol . . . 827
Medrysone . . . 850
PrednisoLONE . . . 1110
Rimexolone . . . 1185

CORTICOSTEROID, OTIC
Bacitracin, Neomycin, Polymyxin B, and Hydrocortisone . . . 158

CORTICOSTEROID, RECTAL
Hydrocortisone . . . 688

CORTICOSTEROID, SYSTEMIC
Betamethasone . . . 177
Budesonide . . . 202
Corticotropin . . . 372
Cortisone Acetate . . . 373
Dexamethasone . . . 413
Fludrocortisone . . . 580
Hydrocortisone . . . 688
MethylPREDNISolone . . . 895
PrednisoLONE . . . 1110
PredniSONE . . . 1112
Triamcinolone . . . 1341

CORTICOSTEROID, TOPICAL
Alclometasone . . . 49
Amcinonide . . . 72
Bacitracin, Neomycin, Polymyxin B, and Hydrocortisone . . . 158
Betamethasone . . . 177
Betamethasone and Clotrimazole . . . 179
Clobetasol . . . 345
Clocortolone . . . 345
Desonide . . . 412
Desoximetasone . . . 412
Dexamethasone . . . 413
Diflorasone . . . 438
Fluocinolone . . . 584
Fluocinolone, Hydroquinone, and Tretinoin . . . 585
Fluocinonide . . . 585
Flurandrenolide . . . 594
Fluticasone . . . 599
Halcinonide . . . 657
Halobetasol . . . 658
Hydrocortisone . . . 688
Iodoquinol and Hydrocortisone . . . 736
Mometasone Furoate . . . 928
Nystatin and Triamcinolone . . . 992
Prednicarbate . . . 1110
Triamcinolone . . . 1341
Triamcinolone Acetonide Dental Paste . . . 1344
Urea and Hydrocortisone . . . 1365

CORTICOSTEROID, TOPICAL (MEDIUM POTENCY)
Fluticasone . . . 599

COUGH PREPARATION
Guaifenesin and Codeine . . . 650
Guaifenesin and Dextromethorphan . . . 651

DECONGESTANT
Carbinoxamine and Pseudoephedrine . . . 247
Guaifenesin and Phenylephrine . . . 652
Guaifenesin and Pseudoephedrine . . . 652

DECONGESTANT/ANALGESIC
Pseudoephedrine and Ibuprofen . . . 1148

DENTAL GASES
Nitrous Oxide . . . 983
Oxygen . . . 1022

DEPIGMENTING AGENT
Fluocinolone, Hydroquinone, and Tretinoin . . . 585
Hydroquinone . . . 693

DIAGNOSTIC AGENT
Adenosine . . . 45
Arginine . . . 121
Benzylpenicilloyl-polylysine . . . 174
Cosyntropin . . . 374
Glucagon . . . 640
Indocyanine Green . . . 719
Proparacaine and Fluorescein . . . 1133
Protirelin . . . 1144
Secretin . . . 1213
Sermorelin Acetate . . . 1215
Sincalide . . . 1225
Skin Test Antigens (Multiple) . . . 1227
Thyrotropin Alpha . . . 1304
Tuberculin Tests . . . 1362

DIETARY SUPPLEMENT
Cysteine . . . 388
Glucose Polymers . . . 641
Levocarnitine . . . 791
Lysine . . . 832
Medium Chain Triglycerides . . . 849
Methionine . . . 881

DISINFECTANT, ANTIBACTERIAL, TOPICAL
Sodium Hypochlorite Solution . . . 1231

DIURETIC, CARBONIC ANHYDRASE INHIBITOR
AcetaZOLAMIDE . . . 37
Dichlorphenamide . . . 428
Methazolamide . . . 878

DIURETIC, COMBINATION
Amiloride and Hydrochlorothiazide . . . 76

DIURETIC, LOOP
Bumetanide . . . 204
Ethacrynic Acid . . . 538
Furosemide . . . 622
Torsemide . . . 1327

DIURETIC, OSMOTIC
Urea . . . 1365

DIURETIC, POTASSIUM SPARING
Amiloride . . . 75

Hydrochlorothiazide and Triamterene ... 677
Spironolactone ... 1240
Triamterene ... 1344

DIURETIC, THIAZIDE
Bendroflumethiazide ... 168
Chlorothiazide ... 304
Chlorthalidone ... 315
Hydrochlorothiazide ... 675
Hydrochlorothiazide and Triamterene ... 677
Methyclothiazide ... 890
Polythiazide ... 1097
Quinapril and Hydrochlorothiazide ... 1158
Trichlormethiazide ... 1347

DIURETIC, THIAZIDE-RELATED
Indapamide ... 716
Metolazone ... 900

DIURETIC, MISCELLANEOUS
Caffeine and Sodium Benzoate ... 221

DOPAMINE AGONIST
Fenoldopam ... 562

ELECTROLYTE SUPPLEMENT
Calcium Supplements ... 229
Magnesium Supplements ... 837
Potassium Supplements ... 1102
Zinc Supplements ... 1410

ELECTROLYTE SUPPLEMENT, ORAL
Magnesium L-aspartate Hydrochloride ... 836
Phosphate Supplements ... 1076
Potassium Supplements ... 1102
Sodium Bicarbonate ... 1227
Sodium Chloride ... 1229

ELECTROLYTE SUPPLEMENT, PARENTERAL
Ammonium Chloride ... 89
Calcium Supplements ... 229
Phosphate Supplements ... 1076
Potassium Acetate ... 1099
Potassium Supplements ... 1102
Sodium Bicarbonate ... 1227
Sodium Chloride ... 1229

ENDOTHELIN ANTAGONIST
Bosentan ... 192

ENZYME
Alglucerase ... 56
Chymopapain ... 322
Dornase Alfa ... 467
Imiglucerase ... 709
Lactase ... 771
Pancreatin ... 1030
Pancrelipase ... 1030
Pegademase Bovine ... 1038
Rasburicase ... 1169

ENZYME, GASTROINTESTINAL
Sacrosidase ... 1203

ENZYME, TOPICAL DEBRIDEMENT
Collagenase ... 367

ENZYME, URATE-OXIDASE (RECOMBINANT)
Rasburicase ... 1169

ERGOT DERIVATIVE
Belladonna, Phenobarbital, and Ergotamine ... 165
Bromocriptine ... 199
Cabergoline ... 220
Dihydroergotamine ... 445
Ergoloid Mesylates ... 509
Ergonovine ... 509
Ergotamine ... 510
Methylergonovine ... 892
Methysergide ... 897
Pergolide ... 1059

ESTROGEN AND PROGESTIN COMBINATION
Combination Hormonal Contraceptives ... 368
Estradiol and Norgestimate ... 526
Mestranol and Norethindrone ... 871

ESTROGEN DERIVATIVE
Diethylstilbestrol ... 437
Estradiol ... 521
Estradiol and Norethindrone ... 525
Estradiol and Testosterone ... 527
Estrogens (Conjugated A/Synthetic) ... 528
Estrogens (Conjugated/Equine) ... 529
Estrogens (Conjugated/Equine) and Medroxyprogesterone ... 531
Estrogens (Esterified) ... 533
Estrogens (Esterified) and Methyltestosterone ... 534
Estrone ... 535
(Continued)

ESTROGEN DERIVATIVE *(Continued)*
Estropipate . . . 536
Ethinyl Estradiol . . . 541

EXPECTORANT
Guaifenesin . . . 650
Guaifenesin and Codeine . . . 650
Guaifenesin and Dextromethorphan . . . 651
Guaifenesin and Phenylephrine . . . 652
Guaifenesin and Pseudoephedrine . . . 652
Potassium Iodide . . . 1101
Terpin Hydrate and Codeine . . . 1281

FACTOR XA INHIBITOR
Fondaparinux . . . 611

FALSE NEUROTRANSMITTER
Guanadrel . . . 654

FLUORIDE
Fluoride . . . 586

GALLSTONE DISSOLUTION AGENT
Ursodiol . . . 1366

GANGLIONIC BLOCKING AGENT
Mecamylamine . . . 846

GASTROINTESTINAL AGENT, PROKINETIC
Cisapride . . . 332
Metoclopramide . . . 898

GASTROINTESTINAL AGENT, STIMULANT
Dexpanthenol . . . 418

GASTROINTESTINAL AGENT, MISCELLANEOUS
Chlorophyll . . . 302
Glutamic Acid . . . 641
Infliximab . . . 721
Saliva Substitute . . . 1205
Sucralfate . . . 1247

GENERAL ANESTHETIC
Etomidate . . . 549
Fentanyl . . . 565
Ketamine . . . 761
Nitrous Oxide . . . 983
Propofol . . . 1133
Sufentanil . . . 1248
Thiopental . . . 1297

GENITOURINARY IRRIGANT
Sorbitol . . . 1234

GLUTAMATE INHIBITOR
Riluzole . . . 1184

GOLD COMPOUND
Auranofin . . . 147
Aurothioglucose . . . 148
Gold Sodium Thiomalate . . . 646

GONADOTROPIN
Chorionic Gonadotropin (Recombinant) . . . 321
Follitropins . . . 607
Menotropins . . . 857

GONADOTROPIN RELEASING HORMONE ANALOG
Goserelin . . . 647

GROWTH FACTOR
Darbepoetin Alfa . . . 400

GROWTH FACTOR, PLATELET-DERIVED
Becaplermin . . . 162

GROWTH HORMONE
Human Growth Hormone . . . 671
Sermorelin Acetate . . . 1215

HEMOSTATIC AGENT
Aminocaproic Acid . . . 76
Aprotinin . . . 119
Cellulose (Oxidized) . . . 284
Cellulose (Oxidized/Regenerated) . . . 284
Collagen (Absorbable) . . . 367
Desmopressin . . . 410
Fibrin Sealant Kit . . . 570
Gelatin (Absorbable) . . . 630
Microfibrillar Collagen Hemostat . . . 907
Thrombin (Topical) . . . 1302

HERB
Aloe . . . 1420
Astragalus . . . 1421
Bilberry . . . 1422
Black Cohosh . . . 1423
Bromelain . . . 1423
Calendula . . . 1424
Cat's Claw . . . 1424

Cayenne 1424
Chamomile 1425
Chasteberry 1426
Cranberry 1427
Devil's Claw 1428
Dong Quai 1429
Echinacea 1429
Ephedra 1430
Evening Primrose 1431
Feverfew 1431
Garlic 1433
Ginger 1434
Ginkgo Biloba 1434
Ginseng, Panax 1435
Ginseng, Siberian 1436
Golden Seal 1437
Gotu Kola 1438
Grapefruit Seed 1438
Grape Seed 1439
Green Tea 1439
Hawthorn 1440
Horse Chestnut 1440
HuperzineA 1441
Kava 1442
Licorice 1442
Mastic 1444
Melaleuca Oil 1444
Milk Thistle 1445
Passion Flower 1445
Red Yeast Rice 1446
Sassafras Oil 1446
Saw Palmetto 1447
Schisandra 1447
St John's Wort 1448
Turmeric 1448
Uva Ursi 1449
Valerian 1449
Wild Yam 1450
Yohimbe 1451

HISTAMINE H_2 ANTAGONIST
Cimetidine 326
Famotidine 556
Famotidine, Calcium Carbonate, and Magnesium Hydroxide 557
Nizatidine 984
Ranitidine 1168

HOMOCYSTINURIA, TREATMENT AGENT
Betaine Anhydrous 177

HORMONE, POSTERIOR PITUITARY
Nafarelin 944
Vasopressin 1379

HUMAN GROWTH FACTOR
Oprelvekin 1003

4-HYDROXYPHENYLPYRUVATE DIOXYGENASE INHIBITOR
Nitisinone 979

HYPNOTIC, NONBENZODIAZEPINE
Zaleplon 1404
Zolpidem 1413
Zopiclone 1415

HYPNOTIC, MISCELLANEOUS
Chloral Hydrate 295

IMMUNE GLOBULIN
Hepatitis B Immune Globulin 666
Immune Globulin (Intramuscular) 713
Immune Globulin (Intravenous) 714
Rabies Immune Globulin (Human) 1164
Rh_o(D) Immune Globulin 1175
Tetanus Immune Globulin (Human) 1283
Varicella-Zoster Immune Globulin (Human) 1378

IMMUNE MODULATOR
Levamisole 786

IMMUNOSUPPRESSANT AGENT
Azathioprine 150
CycloSPORINE 383
Daclizumab 392
Lymphocyte Immune Globulin 831
Muromonab-CD3 938
Mycophenolate 939
Pimecrolimus 1083
Sirolimus 1225
Tacrolimus 1261
Thalidomide 1289

IMPOTENCY AGENT
Yohimbine 1401

INTERFERON
Interferon Alfa-2a 726
Interferon Alfa-2b 727
Interferon Alfa-2b and Ribavirin 730
Interferon Alfa-n3 731
Interferon Beta-1a 732
Interferon Beta-1b 733
Interferon Gamma-1b 734
Peginterferon Alfa-2a 1040
Peginterferon Alfa-2b 1042

INTERLEUKIN-1 RECEPTOR ANTAGONIST
Anakinra 108

IRON SALT
Ferric Gluconate 568
Ferrous Sulfate and Ascorbic Acid 569
Iron Dextran Complex 743
Iron Sucrose 744
Iron Supplements 745
Polysaccharide-Iron Complex 1096

KERATOLYTIC AGENT
Anthralin 111
Cantharidin 234
Podofilox 1093
Podophyllum Resin 1093
Salicylic Acid 1204
Tazarotene 1267
Trichloroacetic Acid 1347
Urea 1365

LAXATIVE
Glycerin 644
Magnesium Hydroxide and Mineral Oil 836
Malt Soup Extract 841
Methylcellulose 891

LAXATIVE, BOWEL EVACUANT
Phosphate Supplements 1076
Polyethylene Glycol-Electrolyte Solution 1094

LAXATIVE, BULK-PRODUCING
Calcium Polycarbophil 228
Psyllium 1149

LAXATIVE, SALINE
Magnesium Citrate 834

LAXATIVE, STIMULANT
Bisacodyl 186
Cascara 258
Senna 1215

LAXATIVE/STOOL SOFTENER
Docusate and Casanthranol 464

LAXATIVE, MISCELLANEOUS
Castor Oil 259
Lactulose 772
Sorbitol 1234

LEPROSTATIC AGENT
Clofazimine 346

LEUKOTRIENE RECEPTOR ANTAGONIST
Montelukast 929
Zafirlukast 1402

LIPASE INHIBITOR
Orlistat 1004

5-LIPOXYGENASE INHIBITOR
Zileuton 1408

LITHIUM
Lithium 815

LOCAL ANESTHETIC
Articaine Hydrochloride and Epinephrine (Canada) 124
Articaine Hydrochloride and Epinephrine (U.S.) 125
Benzocaine 169
Benzocaine, Butyl Aminobenzoate, Tetracaine, and Benzalkonium Chloride 170
Benzocaine, Gelatin, Pectin, and Sodium Carboxymethylcellulose 171
Bupivacaine 205
Bupivacaine and Epinephrine 207
Cetylpyridinium 292
Cetylpyridinium and Benzocaine 292
Chloroprocaine 302
Cocaine 360
Dibucaine 427
Ethyl Chloride 544
Ethyl Chloride and Dichlorotetrafluoroethane 545
Etidocaine and Epinephrine 545
Hexylresorcinol 670
Levobupivacaine 789
Lidocaine 801
Lidocaine and Epinephrine 804

Lidocaine and Prilocaine . . . 806
Mepivacaine . . . 861
Mepivacaine and Levonordefrin . . . 862
Mepivacaine Dental Anesthetic . . . 863
Pramoxine . . . 1105
Prilocaine . . . 1114
Prilocaine and Epinephrine . . . 1116
Procaine . . . 1121
Proparacaine and Fluorescein . . . 1133
Ropivacaine . . . 1198
Tetracaine . . . 1284
Tetracaine and Dextrose . . . 1285

LOCAL ANESTHETIC, DENTAL

Articaine Hydrochloride and Epinephrine (Canada) . . . 124
Articaine Hydrochloride and Epinephrine (U.S.) . . . 125
Benzocaine . . . 169
Benzocaine, Butyl Aminobenzoate, Tetracaine, and Benzalkonium Chloride . . . 170
Benzocaine, Gelatin, Pectin, and Sodium Carboxymethylcellulose . . . 171
Bupivacaine and Epinephrine . . . 207
Dibucaine . . . 427
Etidocaine and Epinephrine . . . 545
Lidocaine and Epinephrine . . . 804
Lidocaine and Prilocaine . . . 806
Lidocaine (Transoral) . . . 807
Mepivacaine and Levonordefrin . . . 862
Mepivacaine Dental Anesthetic . . . 863
Prilocaine . . . 1114
Prilocaine and Epinephrine . . . 1116
Tetracaine . . . 1284

LOCAL ANESTHETIC, OPHTHALMIC

Proparacaine . . . 1132

LOCAL ANESTHETIC, TRANSORAL

Lidocaine (Transoral) . . . 807

LOW MOLECULAR WEIGHT HEPARIN

Dalteparin . . . 394
Enoxaparin . . . 495
Tinzaparin . . . 1311

LUBRICANT, OCULAR

Sodium Chloride . . . 1229

LUNG SURFACTANT

Beractant . . . 176
Calfactant . . . 232
Colfosceril Palmitate . . . 366
Poractant Alfa . . . 1097

LUTEINIZING HORMONE-RELEASING HORMONE ANALOG

Goserelin . . . 647
Leuprolide . . . 784
Nafarelin . . . 944
Triptorelin . . . 1358

MAGNESIUM SALT

Magnesium Chloride . . . 833
Magnesium Citrate . . . 834
Magnesium Gluconate . . . 834
Magnesium Hydroxide . . . 835

MAST CELL STABILIZER

Cromolyn Sodium . . . 375
Lodoxamide . . . 816
Nedocromil . . . 957
Pemirolast . . . 1044

MINERAL, ORAL

Iron Supplements . . . 745
Zinc Supplements . . . 1410

MINERAL (ORAL/TOPICAL)

Fluoride . . . 586
Triclosan and Fluoride . . . 1348

MINERAL, PARENTERAL

Iron Supplements . . . 745
Zinc Supplements . . . 1410

MONOCLONAL ANTIBODY

Alefacept . . . 52
Basiliximab . . . 160
Infliximab . . . 721
Palivizumab . . . 1028
Trastuzumab . . . 1335

MUCOLYTIC AGENT

Acetylcysteine . . . 40

NATRIURETIC PEPTIDE, B-TYPE, HUMAN

Nesiritide . . . 964

NEURAMINIDASE INHIBITOR

Oseltamivir . . . 1006
Zanamivir . . . 1405

NEUROMUSCULAR BLOCKER AGENT, TOXIN
Botulinum Toxin Type A . . . 193
Botulinum Toxin Type B . . . 195

NONSTEROIDAL ANTI-INFLAMMATORY AGENT (NSAID), ORAL
Aminosalicylic Acid . . . 79

NONSTEROIDAL ANTI-INFLAMMATORY DRUG (NSAID)
Diclofenac . . . 429
Diclofenac and Misoprostol . . . 431
Diflunisal . . . 438
Etodolac . . . 547
Fenoprofen . . . 563
Flurbiprofen . . . 596
Ibuprofen . . . 703
Indomethacin . . . 719
Ketoprofen . . . 763
Ketorolac . . . 765
Meclofenamate . . . 848
Mefenamic Acid . . . 851
Meloxicam . . . 854
Nabumetone . . . 941
Naproxen . . . 953
Oxaprozin . . . 1010
Piroxicam . . . 1090
Sulindac . . . 1257
Tolmetin . . . 1321

NONSTEROIDAL ANTI-INFLAMMATORY DRUG (NSAID), COX-2 SELECTIVE
Celecoxib . . . 281
Rofecoxib . . . 1194
Valdecoxib . . . 1368

NOREPINEPHRINE REUPTAKE INHIBITOR, SELECTIVE
Atomoxetine . . . 139

OPHTHALMIC AGENT, ANTIGLAUCOMA
AcetaZOLAMIDE . . . 37
Brimonidine . . . 197
Brinzolamide . . . 198
Carbachol . . . 241
Carteolol . . . 254
Cyclopentolate and Phenylephrine . . . 381
Dichlorphenamide . . . 428
Dipivefrin . . . 455
Dorzolamide . . . 468
Echothiophate Iodide . . . 485
Latanoprost . . . 778
Levobetaxolol . . . 788
Levobunolol . . . 789
Methazolamide . . . 878
Metipranolol . . . 898
Phenylephrine . . . 1071
Physostigmine . . . 1078
Pilocarpine . . . 1080
Timolol . . . 1309

OPHTHALMIC AGENT, MIOTIC
Acetylcholine . . . 39
Carbachol . . . 241
Echothiophate Iodide . . . 485
Pilocarpine . . . 1080

OPHTHALMIC AGENT, MYDRIATIC
Atropine . . . 144
Homatropine . . . 670
Phenylephrine . . . 1071
Tropicamide . . . 1360

OPHTHALMIC AGENT, TOXIN
Botulinum Toxin Type A . . . 193

OPHTHALMIC AGENT, VASOCONSTRICTOR
Dipivefrin . . . 455
Naphazoline . . . 952
Naphazoline and Antazoline . . . 952
Naphazoline and Pheniramine . . . 953
Tetrahydrozoline . . . 1288

OPHTHALMIC AGENT, VISCOELASTIC
Chondroitin Sulfate and Sodium Hyaluronate . . . 320
Sodium Hyaluronate . . . 1230

OPHTHALMIC AGENT, MISCELLANEOUS
Artificial Tears . . . 128
Balanced Salt Solution . . . 160
Bimatoprost . . . 184
Carboxymethylcellulose . . . 251
Glycerin . . . 644
Hydroxypropyl Cellulose . . . 695
Hydroxypropyl Methylcellulose . . . 696
Olopatadine . . . 998
Pemirolast . . . 1044

OTIC AGENT, ANALGESIC
Antipyrine and Benzocaine . . . 116

OTIC AGENT, ANTI-INFECTIVE
Acetic Acid, Propylene Glycol Diacetate, and Hydrocortisone . . . 38
m-Cresyl Acetate . . . 844

OTIC AGENT, CERUMENOLYTIC
Antipyrine and Benzocaine . . . 116
Carbamide Peroxide . . . 244
Triethanolamine Polypeptide Oleate-Condensate . . . 1348

OVULATION STIMULATOR
Chorionic Gonadotropin (Human) . . . 320
Chorionic Gonadotropin (Recombinant) . . . 321
ClomiPHENE . . . 348
Follitropins . . . 607
Menotropins . . . 857

OXYTOCIC AGENT
Oxytocin . . . 1026

PARATHYROID HORMONE ANALOG
Teriparatide . . . 1280

PEDICULOCIDE
Lindane . . . 809
Pyrethrins and Piperonyl Butoxide . . . 1151

PHARMACEUTICAL AID
Boric Acid . . . 191
Phenol . . . 1068

PHOSPHATE BINDER
Sevelamer . . . 1218

PHOSPHODIESTERASE ENZYME INHIBITOR
Cilostazol . . . 325
Inamrinone . . . 716
Milrinone . . . 914
Sildenafil . . . 1220

PHOSPHOLIPASE A_2 INHIBITOR
Anagrelide . . . 108

PHOTOSENSITIZING AGENT, TOPICAL
Aminolevulinic Acid . . . 77

PLASMA VOLUME EXPANDER
Dextran . . . 419
Dextran 1 . . . 420

PLASMA VOLUME EXPANDER, COLLOID
Hetastarch . . . 669

PROGESTIN
MedroxyPROGESTERone . . . 849
Megestrol . . . 853
Norethindrone . . . 986
Progesterone . . . 1125

PROSTAGLANDIN
Alprostadil . . . 63
Carboprost Tromethamine . . . 250
Diclofenac and Misoprostol . . . 431
Dinoprostone . . . 450
Epoprostenol . . . 505
Misoprostol . . . 920

PROSTAGLANDIN, OPHTHALMIC
Latanoprost . . . 778
Travoprost . . . 1336

PROTECTANT, TOPICAL
Trypsin, Balsam Peru, and Castor Oil . . . 1362

PROTEIN C (ACTIVATED)
Drotrecogin Alfa . . . 483

PROTON PUMP INHIBITOR
Esomeprazole . . . 519
Lansoprazole . . . 777
Omeprazole . . . 999
Pantoprazole . . . 1031
Rabeprazole . . . 1162

PSORALEN
Methoxsalen . . . 888

RADIOPAQUE AGENTS
Radiological/Contrast Media (Nonionic) . . . 1165

RADIOPHARMACEUTICAL
Ibritumomab . . . 702

RAUWOLFIA ALKALOID
Rauwolfia Serpentina . . . 1170
Reserpine . . . 1173

RECOMBINANT HUMAN ERYTHROPOIETIN
Darbepoetin Alfa . . . 400

RESPIRATORY STIMULANT
Ammonia Spirit (Aromatic) . . . 89
Doxapram . . . 469

RETINOIC ACID DERIVATIVE

Fluocinolone, Hydroquinone, and Tretinoin . . . 585
Isotretinoin . . . 752
Mequinol and Tretinoin . . . 865
Tretinoin (Topical) . . . 1340

SALICYLATE

Aminosalicylic Acid . . . 79
Aspirin . . . 131
Choline Magnesium Trisalicylate . . . 319
Choline Salicylate . . . 319
Magnesium Salicylate . . . 837
Salsalate . . . 1206
Triethanolamine Salicylate . . . 1348

SALIVARY STIMULANT

Pilocarpine (Dental) . . . 1081

SCABICIDAL AGENT

Crotamiton . . . 376
Lindane . . . 809
Permethrin . . . 1062

SCLEROSING AGENT

Ethanolamine Oleate . . . 540
Morrhuate Sodium . . . 934

SEDATIVE

Dexmedetomidine . . . 416

SELECTIVE 5-HT_3 RECEPTOR ANTAGONIST

Alosetron . . . 60
Dolasetron . . . 465
Granisetron . . . 648
Ondansetron . . . 1000

SELECTIVE ALDOSTERONE BLOCKER

Eplerenone . . . 502

SELECTIVE ESTROGEN RECEPTOR MODULATOR (SERM)

Raloxifene . . . 1165

SEROTONIN 5-$HT_{1B, 1D}$ RECEPTOR AGONIST

Eletriptan . . . 490
Frovatriptan . . . 620

SEROTONIN 5-HT_{1D} RECEPTOR AGONIST

Almotriptan . . . 59
Naratriptan . . . 955
Rizatriptan . . . 1193
Sumatriptan . . . 1258
Zolmitriptan . . . 1411

SEROTONIN 5-HT_4 RECEPTOR AGONIST

Tegaserod . . . 1268

SHAMPOO, PEDICULOCIDE

Pyrethrins and Piperonyl Butoxide . . . 1151

SKELETAL MUSCLE RELAXANT

Baclofen . . . 158
Carisoprodol . . . 251
Carisoprodol and Aspirin . . . 252
Carisoprodol, Aspirin, and Codeine . . . 252
Chlorphenesin . . . 306
Chlorzoxazone . . . 316
Cyclobenzaprine . . . 379
Dantrolene . . . 398
Metaxalone . . . 874
Methocarbamol . . . 881
Orphenadrine . . . 1005
Orphenadrine, Aspirin, and Caffeine . . . 1005

SKIN AND MUCOUS MEMBRANE AGENT

Imiquimod . . . 713
Maltodextrin . . . 840
Sodium Hyaluronate . . . 1230

SMOKING CESSATION AID

BuPROPion . . . 209
Nicotine . . . 971

SODIUM SALT

Sodium Chloride . . . 1229

SOMATOSTATIN ANALOG

Octreotide . . . 993

SPERMICIDE

Nonoxynol 9 . . . 985

STIMULANT

Dextroamphetamine . . . 420
Dextroamphetamine and Amphetamine . . . 422
Doxapram . . . 469
Methamphetamine . . . 877
Modafinil . . . 924
Pemoline . . . 1044

STOOL SOFTENER
Docusate . . . 463
SYMPATHOMIMETIC
Isoetharine . . . 747
THEOPHYLLINE DERIVATIVE
Aminophylline . . . 78
Dyphylline . . . 485
Theophylline . . . 1291
Theophylline and Guaifenesin . . . 1293
THROMBOLYTIC AGENT
Alteplase . . . 65
Reteplase . . . 1174
Streptokinase . . . 1243
Tenecteplase . . . 1273
THYROID PRODUCT
Levothyroxine . . . 800
Liothyronine . . . 810
Liotrix . . . 811
Thyroid . . . 1303
TOPICAL SKIN PRODUCT
Aluminum Sulfate and Calcium Acetate . . . 70
Aminolevulinic Acid . . . 77
Becaplermin . . . 162
Bentoquatam . . . 168
Benzoin . . . 171
Benzoyl Peroxide . . . 171
Benzoyl Peroxide and Hydrocortisone . . . 172
Boric Acid . . . 191
Calcipotriene . . . 222
Camphor and Phenol . . . 232
Capsaicin . . . 238
Chloroxine . . . 306
Clindamycin and Benzoyl Peroxide . . . 343
Coal Tar . . . 359
Coal Tar and Salicylic Acid . . . 359
Coal Tar, Lanolin, and Mineral Oil . . . 360
Dexpanthenol . . . 418
Doxepin . . . 471
Eflornithine . . . 489
Erythromycin . . . 512
Erythromycin and Benzoyl Peroxide . . . 515
Imiquimod . . . 713
Iodine . . . 735
Lactic Acid and Ammonium Hydroxide . . . 771
Lactic Acid and Sodium-PCA . . . 771
Lanolin, Cetyl Alcohol, Glycerin, Petrolatum, and Mineral Oil . . . 776
Merbromin . . . 866
Minoxidil . . . 917
Monobenzone . . . 929
Neomycin, Polymyxin B, and Hydrocortisone . . . 963
Pimecrolimus . . . 1083
Podofilox . . . 1093
Povidone-Iodine . . . 1104
Pyrithione Zinc . . . 1154
Tacrolimus . . . 1261
Triethanolamine Salicylate . . . 1348
Urea . . . 1365
Vitamin A and Vitamin D . . . 1392
Zinc Gelatin . . . 1409
Zinc Oxide . . . 1409
TOPICAL SKIN PRODUCT, ACNE
Azelaic Acid . . . 151
Benzoyl Peroxide . . . 171
Benzoyl Peroxide and Hydrocortisone . . . 172
Clindamycin and Benzoyl Peroxide . . . 343
Erythromycin . . . 512
Erythromycin and Benzoyl Peroxide . . . 515
TOPICAL SKIN PRODUCT, ANTIBACTERIAL
Silver Nitrate . . . 1221
TOXOID
Tetanus Toxoid (Adsorbed) . . . 1283
Tetanus Toxoid (Fluid) . . . 1284
TRACE ELEMENT
Zinc Chloride . . . 1409
Zinc Supplements . . . 1410
TRACE ELEMENT, PARENTERAL
Selenium . . . 1214
Trace Metals . . . 1328
TYROSINE HYDROXYLASE INHIBITOR
Metyrosine . . . 905
UREA CYCLE DISORDER (UCD) TREATMENT AGENT
Sodium Phenylbutyrate . . . 1233
URICOSURIC AGENT
Colchicine and Probenecid . . . 364
(Continued)

URICOSURIC AGENT *(Continued)*

Probenecid . . . 1119
Sulfinpyrazone . . . 1255

URINARY ACIDIFYING AGENT

Ammonium Chloride . . . 89
Potassium Acid Phosphate . . . 1100

URINARY TRACT PRODUCT

Acetohydroxamic Acid . . . 39
Cellulose Sodium Phosphate . . . 284
Citric Acid Bladder Mixture . . . 335
Cysteamine . . . 388
Tiopronin . . . 1313

VACCINE

Anthrax Vaccine (Adsorbed) . . . 112
BCG Vaccine . . . 161
Cholera Vaccine . . . 317
Diphtheria, Tetanus Toxoids, Acellular Pertussis, Hepatitis B (Recombinant), and Poliovirus (Inactivated) Vaccine . . . 454
Haemophilus b Conjugate Vaccine . . . 656
Hepatitis A (Inactivated) and Hepatitis B (Recombinant) Vaccine . . . 664
Hepatitis A Vaccine . . . 665
Hepatitis B Vaccine . . . 666
Influenza Virus Vaccine . . . 722
Japanese Encephalitis Virus Vaccine (Inactivated) . . . 758
Meningococcal Polysaccharide Vaccine (Groups A, C, Y, and W-135) . . . 856
Mumps Virus Vaccine (Live/Attenuated) . . . 937
Pneumococcal Conjugate Vaccine (7-Valent) . . . 1091
Poliovirus Vaccine (Inactivated) . . . 1093
Rabies Virus Vaccine . . . 1164
Rubella Virus Vaccine (Live) . . . 1202
Typhoid Vaccine . . . 1363

VACCINE, LIVE VIRUS

Measles, Mumps, and Rubella Vaccines (Combined) . . . 844
Measles Virus Vaccine (Live) . . . 845

VASOCONSTRICTOR

Epinephrine . . . 499
Epinephrine (Racemic) . . . 500
Epinephrine (Racemic) and Aluminum Potassium Sulfate . . . 501
Oxymetazoline . . . 1022

VASOCONSTRICTOR, NASAL

Xylometazoline . . . 1401

VASODILATOR

Amyl Nitrite . . . 107
Cyclandelate . . . 378
Dipyridamole . . . 456
Ethaverine . . . 541
HydrALAZINE . . . 673
Isosorbide Dinitrate . . . 750
Isosorbide Mononitrate . . . 751
Isoxsuprine . . . 753
Minoxidil . . . 917
Nesiritide . . . 964
Nitroglycerin . . . 981
Nitroprusside . . . 982
Papaverine . . . 1033
Treprostinil . . . 1337

VASODILATOR, PERIPHERAL

Nylidrin . . . 991

VASODILATOR, PULMONARY

Nitric Oxide . . . 979

VASOPRESSIN ANALOG, SYNTHETIC

Desmopressin . . . 410

VITAMIN

Ferrous Sulfate and Ascorbic Acid . . . 569
Folic Acid, Cyanocobalamin, and Pyridoxine . . . 607
Vitamins (Multiple/Oral) . . . 1394

VITAMIN A DERIVATIVE

Mequinol and Tretinoin . . . 865

VITAMIN D ANALOG

Calcifediol . . . 221
Calcipotriene . . . 222
Calcitriol . . . 223
Cholecalciferol . . . 317
Dihydrotachysterol . . . 446
Doxercalciferol . . . 472
Ergocalciferol . . . 508
Paricalcitol . . . 1034

VITAMIN, FAT SOLUBLE

Beta-Carotene . . . 176
Phytonadione . . . 1079
Vitamin A . . . 1390
Vitamin E . . . 1393

VITAMIN, TOPICAL

Mequinol and Tretinoin 865

VITAMIN, WATER SOLUBLE

Ascorbic Acid 128
Cyanocobalamin 377
Folic Acid 606
Hydroxocobalamin 693
Leucovorin 783
Niacin 967
Niacinamide 968
Pantothenic Acid 1033
Pyridoxine 1152
Riboflavin 1178
Thiamine 1295
Vitamin B Complex 1392
Vitamin B Complex and Vitamin C 1392
Vitamin B Complex, Vitamin C, and Folic Acid 1393

XANTHINE OXIDASE INHIBITOR

Allopurinol 57

ALPHABETICAL INDEX

A200® Lice [OTC] *see* Permethrin . . . 1062
A-200® Maximum Strength [OTC] *see* Pyrethrins and Piperonyl Butoxide . . . 1151
A and D® Ointment [OTC] *see* Vitamin A and Vitamin D . . . 1392
Abacavir . . . 22
Abacavir, Lamivudine, and Zidovudine . . . 23
Abbreviations, Acronyms, and Symbols Used in Medical Orders . . . 13
ABCD *see* Amphotericin B Cholesteryl Sulfate Complex . . . 97
Abciximab . . . 23
Abelcet® *see* Amphotericin B (Lipid Complex) . . . 100
Abenol® *see* Acetaminophen . . . 27
Abilify™ *see* Aripiprazole . . . 122
ABLC *see* Amphotericin B (Lipid Complex) . . . 100
Abreva® [OTC] *see* Docosanol . . . 463
Absorbable Cotton *see* Cellulose (Oxidized) . . . 284
Absorbable Gelatin Sponge *see* Gelatin (Absorbable) . . . 630
Absorbine Jr.® Antifungal [OTC] *see* Tolnaftate . . . 1322
Acanol *see* Loperamide . . . 819
Acarbose . . . 24
A-Caro-25® *see* Beta-Carotene . . . 176
Accolate® *see* Zafirlukast . . . 1402
AccuNeb™ *see* Albuterol . . . 48
Accupril® *see* Quinapril . . . 1156
Accuretic™ *see* Quinapril and Hydrochlorothiazide . . . 1158
Accutane® *see* Isotretinoin . . . 752
Ac-De® *see* Dactinomycin . . . 393
ACE *see* Captopril . . . 238
Acebutolol . . . 25
Acebutolol Hydrochloride *see* Acebutolol . . . 25
Aceon® *see* Perindopril Erbumine . . . 1060
Acephen® [OTC] *see* Acetaminophen . . . 27
Acetadiazol® *see* AcetaZOLAMIDE . . . 37
Acetaminophen . . . 27
Acetaminophen and Chlorpheniramine *see* Chlorpheniramine and Acetaminophen . . . 308
Acetaminophen and Codeine . . . 29
Acetaminophen and Diphenhydramine . . . 30
Acetaminophen and Hydrocodone *see* Hydrocodone and Acetaminophen . . . 678
Acetaminophen and Oxycodone *see* Oxycodone and Acetaminophen . . . 1018
Acetaminophen and Phenyltoloxamine . . . 31
Acetaminophen and Pseudoephedrine . . . 31
Acetaminophen and Tramadol . . . 32
Acetaminophen, Aspirin, and Caffeine . . . 34
Acetaminophen, Butalbital, and Caffeine *see* Butalbital, Acetaminophen, and Caffeine . . . 214
Acetaminophen, Caffeine, Codeine, and Butalbital *see* Butalbital, Acetaminophen, Caffeine, and Codeine . . . 215
Acetaminophen, Caffeine, Hydrocodone, Chlorpheniramine, and Phenylephrine *see* Hydrocodone, Chlorpheniramine, Phenylephrine, Acetaminophen, and Caffeine . . . 686
Acetaminophen, Chlorpheniramine, and Pseudoephedrine . . . 35
Acetaminophen, Dextromethorphan, and Pseudoephedrine . . . 35
Acetaminophen, Dichloralphenazone, and Isometheptene *see* Acetaminophen, Isometheptene, and Dichloralphenazone . . . 36
Acetaminophen, Isometheptene, and Dichloralphenazone . . . 36
Acetaminophen, Pseudoephedrine, and Chlorpheniramine *see* Acetaminophen, Chlorpheniramine, and Pseudoephedrine . . . 35
Acetasol® HC *see* Acetic Acid, Propylene Glycol Diacetate, and Hydrocortisone . . . 38
AcetaZOLAMIDE . . . 37
Acetic Acid and Aluminum Acetate Otic *see* Aluminum Acetate and Acetic Acid . . . 67
Acetic Acid, Hydrocortisone, and Propylene Glycol Diacetate *see* Acetic Acid, Propylene Glycol Diacetate, and Hydrocortisone . . . 38
Acetic Acid, Propylene Glycol Diacetate, and Hydrocortisone . . . 38
AcetoHEXAMIDE . . . 38
Acetohydroxamic Acid . . . 39
Acetoxyl® *see* Benzoyl Peroxide . . . 171
Acetoxymethylprogesterone *see* MedroxyPROGESTERone . . . 849
Acetylcholine . . . 39
Acetylcholine Chloride *see* Acetylcholine . . . 39
Acetylcysteine . . . 40
Acetylcysteine Sodium *see* Acetylcysteine . . . 40
Acetylsalicylic Acid *see* Aspirin . . . 131
Achromycin® [DSC] *see* Tetracycline . . . 1286
Aciclovir *see* Acyclovir . . . 42
Acidulated Phosphate Fluoride *see* Fluoride . . . 586
Acifur® *see* Acyclovir . . . 42
Acilac *see* Lactulose . . . 772
Acimox® *see* Amoxicillin . . . 93
Aciphex® *see* Rabeprazole . . . 1162
Aclimafel® *see* Amoxicillin . . . 93
Acloral® *see* Ranitidine . . . 1168
Aclovate® *see* Alclometasone . . . 49
Acrivastine and Pseudoephedrine . . . 41
Acromicina *see* Tetracycline . . . 1286
Acroxil® *see* Amoxicillin . . . 93
ACT *see* Dactinomycin . . . 393
ACT® [OTC] *see* Fluoride . . . 586
Act-D *see* Dactinomycin . . . 393
ACTH *see* Corticotropin . . . 372
Acthar® *see* Corticotropin . . . 372
ActHIB® *see* *Haemophilus* b Conjugate Vaccine . . . 656
Acticin® *see* Permethrin . . . 1062
Actidose® [OTC] *see* Charcoal . . . 294
Actidose-Aqua® [OTC] *see* Charcoal . . . 294

Actifed® *see* Triprolidine and Pseudoephedrine . . . 1356
Actifed® Cold and Allergy [OTC] *see* Triprolidine and Pseudoephedrine . . . 1356
Actigall® *see* Ursodiol . . . 1366
Actilyse® *see* Alteplase . . . 65
Actimmune® *see* Interferon Gamma-1b . . . 734
Actinomycin *see* Dactinomycin . . . 393
Actinomycin Cl *see* Dactinomycin . . . 393
Actinomycin D *see* Dactinomycin . . . 393
Actiq® *see* Fentanyl . . . 565
Actisite® *see* Tetracycline Periodontal Fibers . . . 1287
Activase® *see* Alteplase . . . 65
Activase® rt-PA *see* Alteplase . . . 65
Activated Carbon *see* Charcoal . . . 294
Activated Charcoal *see* Charcoal . . . 294
Activated Dimethicone *see* Simethicone . . . 1222
Activated Ergosterol *see* Ergocalciferol . . . 508
Activated Methylpolysiloxane *see* Simethicone . . . 1222
Activated Protein C, Human, Recombinant *see* Drotrecogin Alfa . . . 483
Activella™ *see* Estradiol and Norethindrone . . . 525
Actonel® *see* Risedronate . . . 1186
Actos® *see* Pioglitazone . . . 1086
ACU-dyne® [OTC] *see* Povidone-Iodine . . . 1104
Acular® *see* Ketorolac . . . 765
Acularen® *see* Ketorolac . . . 765
Acular® PF *see* Ketorolac . . . 765
Acupril® *see* Quinapril . . . 1156
ACV *see* Acyclovir . . . 42
Acycloguanosine *see* Acyclovir . . . 42
Acyclovir . . . 42
Adaferin® *see* Adapalene . . . 44
Adagen® *see* Pegademase Bovine . . . 1038
Adalat® *see* NIFEdipine . . . 973
Adalat® CC *see* NIFEdipine . . . 973
Adalat® Oros *see* NIFEdipine . . . 973
Adalat® Retard *see* NIFEdipine . . . 973
Adalat® XL® *see* NIFEdipine . . . 973
Adalken® *see* Penicillamine . . . 1046
Adamantanamine Hydrochloride *see* Amantadine . . . 70
Adapalene . . . 44
Adderall® *see* Dextroamphetamine and Amphetamine . . . 422
Adderall XR™ *see* Dextroamphetamine and Amphetamine . . . 422
Adecur® *see* Terazosin . . . 1276
Adefovir . . . 44
Adefovir Dipivoxil *see* Adefovir . . . 44
Adel® *see* Clarithromycin . . . 337
Adena a Ungena *see* Vidarabine . . . 1384
Adenine Arabinoside *see* Vidarabine . . . 1384
Adenocard® *see* Adenosine . . . 45
Adenoscan® *see* Adenosine . . . 45
Adenosine . . . 45
ADH *see* Vasopressin . . . 1379
Adipex-P® *see* Phentermine . . . 1069
Adoxa™ *see* Doxycycline . . . 476
ADR *see* DOXOrubicin . . . 473
Adrenalin® (Dental) *see* Epinephrine . . . 499
Adrenocorticotropic Hormone *see* Corticotropin . . . 372
Adria *see* DOXOrubicin . . . 473
Adriamycin® *see* DOXOrubicin . . . 473
Adriamycin PFS® *see* DOXOrubicin . . . 473
Adriamycin RDF® *see* DOXOrubicin . . . 473
Adriblastina® *see* DOXOrubicin . . . 473
Adrucil® *see* Fluorouracil . . . 588
Adsorbent Charcoal *see* Charcoal . . . 294
Advair™ Diskus® *see* Fluticasone and Salmeterol . . . 601
Advantage 24™ *see* Nonoxynol 9 . . . 985
Advantage-S™ [OTC] *see* Nonoxynol 9 . . . 985
Advicor™ *see* Niacin and Lovastatin . . . 968
Advil® *see* Ibuprofen . . . 703
Advil® Children's [OTC] *see* Ibuprofen . . . 703
Advil® Cold, Children's [OTC] *see* Pseudoephedrine and Ibuprofen . . . 1148
Advil® Cold & Sinus *see* Pseudoephedrine and Ibuprofen . . . 1148
Advil® Infants' Concentrated Drops [OTC] *see* Ibuprofen . . . 703
Advil® Junior [OTC] *see* Ibuprofen . . . 703
Advil® Migraine [OTC] *see* Ibuprofen . . . 703
Aerius® *see* Desloratadine . . . 410
Aerobec *see* Beclomethasone . . . 163
AeroBid® *see* Flunisolide . . . 582
AeroBid®-M *see* Flunisolide . . . 582
Aesculus hippocastanum *see* Horse Chestnut . . . 1440
Afazol Grin® *see* Naphazoline . . . 952
Afrin® [OTC] *see* Oxymetazoline . . . 1022
Afrin® Extra Moisturizing [OTC] *see* Oxymetazoline . . . 1022
Afrin® Original [OTC] *see* Oxymetazoline . . . 1022
Afrin® Severe Congestion [OTC] *see* Oxymetazoline . . . 1022
Afrin® Sinus [OTC] *see* Oxymetazoline . . . 1022
Aftate® Antifungal [OTC] *see* Tolnaftate . . . 1322
Afungil® *see* Fluconazole . . . 576
A.f. Valdecasas® *see* Folic Acid . . . 606
Agenerase® *see* Amprenavir . . . 105
Aggrastat® *see* Tirofiban . . . 1313

Aggrenox® *see* Aspirin and Dipyridamole . . . 135
$AgNO_3$ *see* Silver Nitrate . . . 1221
Agoral® Maximum Strength Laxative [OTC] *see* Senna . . . 1215
Agrastat® *see* Tirofiban . . . 1313
Agrylin® *see* Anagrelide . . . 108
AHA *see* Acetohydroxamic Acid . . . 39
AHF (Human) *see* Antihemophilic Factor (Human) . . . 113
AHF (Porcine) *see* Antihemophilic Factor (Porcine) . . . 114
AHF (Recombinant) *see* Antihemophilic Factor (Recombinant) . . . 115
A-hydroCort® *see* Hydrocortisone . . . 688
Airomir *see* Albuterol . . . 48
Akacin® *see* Amikacin . . . 74
AK-Con™ *see* Naphazoline . . . 952
AK-Dilate® *see* Phenylephrine . . . 1071
Akineton® *see* Biperiden . . . 185
AK-Nefrin® *see* Phenylephrine . . . 1071
Akne-Mycin® *see* Erythromycin . . . 512
Akorazol® *see* Ketoconazole . . . 762
AK-Pentolate® *see* Cyclopentolate . . . 380
AK-Poly-Bac® *see* Bacitracin and Polymyxin B . . . 157
AK-Pred® *see* PrednisoLONE . . . 1110
AK-Spore® H.C. [DSC] *see* Bacitracin, Neomycin, Polymyxin B, and Hydrocortisone . . . 158
AK-Sulf® *see* Sulfacetamide . . . 1249
AK-T-Caine™ *see* Tetracaine . . . 1284
AKTob® *see* Tobramycin . . . 1315
AK-Tracin® *see* Bacitracin . . . 156
AK-Trol® *see* Neomycin, Polymyxin B, and Dexamethasone . . . 962
Akwa Tears® [OTC] *see* Artificial Tears . . . 128
ALA *see* Flaxseed Oil . . . 1432
Alamast™ *see* Pemirolast . . . 1044
Alatrofloxacin Mesylate *see* Trovafloxacin/Alatrofloxacin . . . 1361
Alavert™ [OTC] *see* Loratadine . . . 822
Albalon® *see* Naphazoline . . . 952
Albalon®-A Liquifilm *see* Naphazoline and Antazoline . . . 952
Albendazole . . . 47
Albenza® *see* Albendazole . . . 47
Albert® Docusate *see* Docusate . . . 463
Albert® Glyburide *see* GlyBURIDE . . . 642
Albert® Pentoxifylline *see* Pentoxifylline . . . 1058
Alboral® *see* Diazepam . . . 424
Albuterol . . . 48
Albuterol and Ipratropium *see* Ipratropium and Albuterol . . . 738
Alcaine® *see* Proparacaine . . . 1132
Alclometasone . . . 49
Alclometasone Dipropionate *see* Alclometasone . . . 49
Alcomicin® *see* Gentamicin . . . 634
Aldactazide® *see* Hydrochlorothiazide and Spironolactone . . . 677
Aldactazide 25® *see* Hydrochlorothiazide and Spironolactone . . . 677
Aldactazide 50® *see* Hydrochlorothiazide and Spironolactone . . . 677
Aldactone® *see* Spironolactone . . . 1240
Aldara™ *see* Imiquimod . . . 713
Aldesleukin . . . 50
Aldoclor® *see* Chlorothiazide and Methyldopa . . . 305
Aldomet® *see* Methyldopa . . . 891
Aldoril® *see* Methyldopa and Hydrochlorothiazide . . . 892
Aldoril® D *see* Methyldopa and Hydrochlorothiazide . . . 892
Alefacept . . . 52
Alemtuzumab . . . 52
Alendronate . . . 54
Alendronate Sodium *see* Alendronate . . . 54
Alepsal *see* Phenobarbital . . . 1066
Aler-Dryl [OTC] *see* DiphenhydrAMINE . . . 451
Alertec® *see* Modafinil . . . 924
Alesse® *see* Combination Hormonal Contraceptives . . . 368
Aleve® [OTC] *see* Naproxen . . . 953
Alfenta® *see* Alfentanil . . . 55
Alfentanil . . . 55
Alfentanil Hydrochloride *see* Alfentanil . . . 55
Alferon® N *see* Interferon Alfa-n3 . . . 731
Alfotax *see* Cefotaxime . . . 271
Algidol® *see* Ibuprofen . . . 703
Algitrin® *see* Acetaminophen . . . 27
Alglucerase . . . 56
Alidol® *see* Ketorolac . . . 765
Alin® *see* Dexamethasone . . . 413
Alin Depot® *see* Dexamethasone . . . 413
Alinia™ *see* Nitazoxanide . . . 978
Alitretinoin . . . 57
Alka-Mints® [OTC] *see* Calcium Supplements . . . 229
Alka-Seltzer® Gas Relief [OTC] *see* Simethicone . . . 1222
Alka-Seltzer Plus® Cold and Sinus [OTC] *see* Acetaminophen and Pseudoephedrine . . . 31
Alka-Seltzer® Plus Cold Liqui-Gels® [OTC] *see* Acetaminophen, Chlorpheniramine, and Pseudoephedrine . . . 35
Alka-Seltzer® Plus Flu Liqui-Gels® [OTC] *see* Acetaminophen, Dextromethorphan, and Pseudoephedrine . . . 35
Alkeran® *see* Melphalan . . . 855
Allbee® With C [OTC] *see* Vitamin B Complex and Vitamin C . . . 1392
Allegra® *see* Fexofenadine . . . 569
Allegra-D® *see* Fexofenadine and Pseudoephedrine . . . 570
Aller-Chlor® [OTC] *see* Chlorpheniramine . . . 307

Allerdryl® *see* DiphenhydrAMINE 451
Allerest® Maximum Strength [OTC] *see* Chlorpheniramine and Pseudoephedrine 308
Allerfrim® [OTC] *see* Triprolidine and Pseudoephedrine 1356
Allergen® *see* Antipyrine and Benzocaine 116
AllerMax® [OTC] *see* DiphenhydrAMINE 451
Allernix *see* DiphenhydrAMINE 451
Allerphed® [OTC] *see* Triprolidine and Pseudoephedrine 1356
Allersol® *see* Naphazoline 952
Allium savitum see Garlic 1433
Allopurinol 57
Allopurinol Sodium Injection *see* Allopurinol 57
All-*trans*-Retinoic Acid *see* Tretinoin (Oral) 1338
Almora® [OTC] *see* Magnesium Supplements 837
Almora® [OTC], Mag G® [OTC] *see* Magnesium Gluconate 834
Almotriptan 59
Alocril™ *see* Nedocromil 957
Aloe 1420
Aloe Barbadensis *see* Aloe 1420
Aloe Capensis *see* Aloe 1420
Aloe vera *see* Aloe 1420
Aloe Vesta® 2-n-1 Antifungal [OTC] *see* Miconazole 906
Aloid® *see* Miconazole 906
Alomide® *see* Lodoxamide 816
Alophen® [OTC] *see* Bisacodyl 186
Aloprim™ *see* Allopurinol 57
Alora® *see* Estradiol 521
Alosetron 60
Alpha$_1$-PI *see* Alpha$_1$-Proteinase Inhibitor 61
Alpha$_1$-Proteinase Inhibitor 61
Alpha$_1$-Proteinase Inhibitor, Human *see* Alpha$_1$-Proteinase Inhibitor 61
Alpha-Dextrano“40” *see* Dextran 419
Alphagan™ *see* Brimonidine 197
Alphagan® P *see* Brimonidine 197
Alpha-linolenic Acid *see* Flaxseed Oil 1432
Alpha-lipoate *see* Alpha-Lipoic Acid 1420
Alpha-Lipoic Acid 1420
Alphanate® *see* Antihemophilic Factor (Human) 113
Alphaquin HP *see* Hydroquinone 693
Alphatrex® *see* Betamethasone 177
Alprazolam 61
Alprazolam Intensol® *see* Alprazolam 61
Alprostadil 63
Alrex® *see* Loteprednol 827
Altace® *see* Ramipril 1166
Altamisa *see* Feverfew 1431
Altamist [OTC] *see* Sodium Chloride 1229
Alteplase 65
Alteplase, Recombinant *see* Alteplase 65
Alteplase, Tissue Plasminogen Activator, Recombinant *see* Alteplase 65
Alter H2® *see* Ranitidine 1168
ALternaGel® [OTC] *see* Aluminum Hydroxide 68
Alti-Acyclovir *see* Acyclovir 42
Alti-Alprazolam *see* Alprazolam 61
Alti-Amiodarone *see* Amiodarone 80
Alti-Amoxi-Clav® *see* Amoxicillin and Clavulanate Potassium 95
Alti-Azathioprine *see* Azathioprine 150
Alti-Captopril *see* Captopril 238
Alti-Clindamycin *see* Clindamycin 341
Alti-Clobazam *see* Clobazam 344
Alti-Clonazepam *see* Clonazepam 350
Alti-Desipramine *see* Desipramine 408
Alti-Diltiazem CD *see* Diltiazem 447
Alti-Divalproex *see* Valproic Acid and Derivatives 1371
Alti-Doxazosin *see* Doxazosin 470
Alti-Flunisolide *see* Flunisolide 582
Alti-Fluoxetine *see* Fluoxetine 589
Alti-Flurbiprofen *see* Flurbiprofen 596
Alti-Fluvoxamine *see* Fluvoxamine 605
Alti-Ipratropium *see* Ipratropium 737
Alti-Metformin *see* Metformin 874
Alti-Minocycline *see* Minocycline 915
Alti-MPA *see* MedroxyPROGESTERone 849
Altinac™ *see* Tretinoin (Topical) 1340
Alti-Nadolol *see* Nadolol 943
Alti-Nortriptyline *see* Nortriptyline 989
Alti-Ranitidine *see* Ranitidine 1168
Alti-Salbutamol *see* Albuterol 48
Alti-Sotalol *see* Sotalol 1235
Alti-Sulfasalazine *see* Sulfasalazine 1254
Alti-Terazosin *see* Terazosin 1276
Alti-Ticlopidine *see* Ticlopidine 1307
Alti-Timolol *see* Timolol 1309
Alti-Trazodone *see* Trazodone 1336
Alti-Verapamil *see* Verapamil 1382
Alti-Zopiclone *see* Zopiclone 1415
Altocor™ *see* Lovastatin 828
Altretamine 66
Altruline® *see* Sertraline 1216
Alu-Cap® [OTC] *see* Aluminum Hydroxide 68
Aluminum Acetate and Acetic Acid 67

Aluminum Chloride . . . 67
Aluminum Hydroxide . . . 68
Aluminum Hydroxide and Magnesium Carbonate . . . 68
Aluminum Hydroxide and Magnesium Hydroxide . . . 69
Aluminum Hydroxide and Magnesium Trisilicate . . . 69
Aluminum Hydroxide, Magnesium Hydroxide, and Simethicone . . . 69
Aluminum Sucrose Sulfate, Basic *see* Sucralfate . . . 1247
Aluminum Sulfate and Calcium Acetate . . . 70
Alupent® *see* Metaproterenol . . . 873
Alustra™ *see* Hydroquinone . . . 693
Alu-Tab® [OTC] *see* Aluminum Hydroxide . . . 68
Alvidina® *see* Ranitidine . . . 1168
Amantadine . . . 70
Amantadine Hydrochloride *see* Amantadine . . . 70
Amaryl® *see* Glimepiride . . . 637
Amatine® *see* Midodrine . . . 911
Ambenonium . . . 72
Ambenonium Chloride *see* Ambenonium . . . 72
Amber Touch-and-Feel *see* St John's Wort . . . 1448
Ambien® *see* Zolpidem . . . 1413
AmBisome® *see* Amphotericin B (Liposomal) . . . 101
Ambotetra *see* Tetracycline . . . 1286
Amcinonide . . . 72
Ameblin® *see* Metronidazole . . . 902
Amerge® *see* Naratriptan . . . 955
Americaine® [OTC] *see* Benzocaine . . . 169
Americaine® Anesthetic Lubricant *see* Benzocaine . . . 169
American Coneflower *see Echinacea* . . . 1429
A-Methapred® *see* MethylPREDNISolone . . . 895
Amethocaine Hydrochloride *see* Tetracaine . . . 1284
Amethopterin *see* Methotrexate . . . 884
Ametop™ *see* Tetracaine . . . 1284
Amevive® *see* Alefacept . . . 52
Amfepramone *see* Diethylpropion . . . 436
Amibid LA *see* Guaifenesin . . . 650
Amicar® *see* Aminocaproic Acid . . . 76
Amidate® *see* Etomidate . . . 549
Amifostine . . . 73
Amigesic® *see* Salsalate . . . 1206
Amikacin . . . 74
Amikacin Sulfate *see* Amikacin . . . 74
Amikafur® *see* Amikacin . . . 74
Amikalem® *see* Amikacin . . . 74
Amikason's® *see* Amikacin . . . 74
Amikayect® *see* Amikacin . . . 74
Amikin® *see* Amikacin . . . 74
Amiloride . . . 75
Amiloride and Hydrochlorothiazide . . . 76
Amiloride Hydrochloride *see* Amiloride . . . 75
2-Amino-6-Mercaptopurine *see* Thioguanine . . . 1296
2-Amino-6-Trifluoromethoxy-benzothiazole *see* Riluzole . . . 1184
Aminobenzylpenicillin *see* Ampicillin . . . 103
Aminocaproic Acid . . . 76
Amino-Cerv™ *see* Urea . . . 1365
Aminoglutethimide . . . 77
Aminolevulinic Acid . . . 77
Aminolevulinic Acid Hydrochloride *see* Aminolevulinic Acid . . . 77
Aminophylline . . . 78
Aminosalicylate Sodium *see* Aminosalicylic Acid . . . 79
Aminosalicylic Acid . . . 79
4-Aminosalicylic Acid *see* Aminosalicylic Acid . . . 79
5-Aminosalicylic Acid *see* Mesalamine . . . 869
Aminoxin® [OTC] *see* Pyridoxine . . . 1152
Amiodarone . . . 80
Amiodarone Hydrochloride *see* Amiodarone . . . 80
Amipaque® *see* Radiological/Contrast Media (Nonionic) . . . 1165
Ami-Tex PSE *see* Guaifenesin and Pseudoephedrine . . . 652
Amitone® [OTC] *see* Calcium Supplements . . . 229
Amitriptyline . . . 83
Amitriptyline and Chlordiazepoxide . . . 85
Amitriptyline and Perphenazine . . . 85
Amitriptyline Hydrochloride *see* Amitriptyline . . . 83
A.M.K.® *see* Amikacin . . . 74
AmLactin® [OTC] *see* Lactic Acid and Ammonium Hydroxide . . . 771
Amlexanox . . . 87
Amlodipine . . . 87
Amlodipine and Benazepril . . . 89
Ammens® Medicated Deodorant [OTC] *see* Zinc Oxide . . . 1409
Ammonapse *see* Sodium Phenylbutyrate . . . 1233
Ammonia Spirit (Aromatic) . . . 89
Ammonium Chloride . . . 89
Ammonium Lactate *see* Lactic Acid and Ammonium Hydroxide . . . 771
Amnesteen™ *see* Isotretinoin . . . 752
Amobarbital . . . 90
Amobarbital and Secobarbital . . . 91
Amoxapine . . . 91
Amoxicillin . . . 93
Amoxicillin and Clavulanate Potassium . . . 95
Amoxicillin and Clavulanic Acid *see* Amoxicillin and Clavulanate Potassium . . . 95
Amoxicillin Trihydrate *see* Amoxicillin . . . 93

Amoxifur® *see* Amoxicillin . . . 93
Amoxil® *see* Amoxicillin . . . 93
Amoxinovag® *see* Amoxicillin . . . 93
Amoxisol® *see* Amoxicillin . . . 93
Amoxycillin *see* Amoxicillin . . . 93
Amphetamine and Dextroamphetamine *see* Dextroamphetamine and Amphetamine . . . 422
Amphocin® *see* Amphotericin B (Conventional) . . . 98
Amphojel® *see* Aluminum Hydroxide . . . 68
Amphotec® *see* Amphotericin B Cholesteryl Sulfate Complex . . . 97
Amphotericin B Cholesteryl Sulfate Complex . . . 97
Amphotericin B Colloidal Dispersion *see* Amphotericin B Cholesteryl Sulfate Complex . . . 97
Amphotericin B (Conventional) . . . 98
Amphotericin B Desoxycholate *see* Amphotericin B (Conventional) . . . 98
Amphotericin B (Lipid Complex) . . . 100
Amphotericin B (Liposomal) . . . 101
Ampicillin . . . 103
Ampicillin and Sulbactam . . . 104
Ampicillin Sodium *see* Ampicillin . . . 103
Ampicillin Trihydrate *see* Ampicillin . . . 103
Ampliron® *see* Amoxicillin . . . 93
Amprenavir . . . 105
AMPT *see* Metyrosine . . . 905
Amrinone *see* Inamrinone . . . 716
Amrinone Lactate *see* Inamrinone . . . 716
Amyl Nitrite . . . 107
Amylobarbitone *see* Amobarbital . . . 90
Amytal® *see* Amobarbital . . . 90
Anacin PM Aspirin Free [OTC] *see* Acetaminophen and Diphenhydramine . . . 30
Anadrol® *see* Oxymetholone . . . 1023
Anafranil® *see* ClomiPRAMINE . . . 349
Anagrelide . . . 108
Anagrelide Hydrochloride *see* Anagrelide . . . 108
Anakinra . . . 108
Ana-Kit® *see* Epinephrine and Chlorpheniramine Insect Sting Kit . . . 500
Analfin® *see* Morphine Sulfate . . . 931
Analphen *see* Acetaminophen . . . 27
Analpram-HC® *see* Pramoxine and Hydrocortisone . . . 1106
Anamine® [OTC] *see* Chlorpheniramine and Pseudoephedrine . . . 308
Anandron® *see* Nilutamide . . . 975
Anapenil *see* Penicillin V Potassium . . . 1051
Anaplex® [OTC] *see* Chlorpheniramine and Pseudoephedrine . . . 308
Anaprox® *see* Naproxen . . . 953
Anaprox® DS *see* Naproxen . . . 953
Anapsique® *see* Amitriptyline . . . 83
Anas comosus *see* Bromelain . . . 1423
Anaspaz® *see* Hyoscyamine . . . 699
Anastrozole . . . 109
Anatuss LA *see* Guaifenesin and Pseudoephedrine . . . 652
Anbesol® [OTC] *see* Benzocaine . . . 169
Anbesol® Baby *see* Benzocaine . . . 169
Anbesol® Maximum Strength [OTC] *see* Benzocaine . . . 169
Ancef® *see* Cefazolin . . . 263
Ancobon® *see* Flucytosine . . . 578
Andehist DM NR Drops *see* Carbinoxamine, Pseudoephedrine, and Dextromethorphan . . . 247
Andehist NR Drops *see* Carbinoxamine and Pseudoephedrine . . . 247
Andehist NR Syrup *see* Brompheniramine and Pseudoephedrine . . . 201
Andox® *see* Acetaminophen . . . 27
Andriol® *see* Testosterone . . . 1281
Andro *see* Androstenedione . . . 1421
Androderm® *see* Testosterone . . . 1281
AndroGel® *see* Testosterone . . . 1281
Android® *see* MethylTESTOSTERone . . . 897
Andropository *see* Testosterone . . . 1281
Androstenedione . . . 1421
Androxicam® *see* Piroxicam . . . 1090
Anestacon® *see* Lidocaine . . . 801
Aneurine Hydrochloride *see* Thiamine . . . 1295
Anexate® *see* Flumazenil . . . 581
Anexsia® *see* Hydrocodone and Acetaminophen . . . 678
Angelica sinensis *see* Dong Quai . . . 1429
Angiotrofin® *see* Diltiazem . . . 447
Angiotrofin A.P. *see* Diltiazem . . . 447
Angiotrofin Retard *see* Diltiazem . . . 447
Anglix® *see* Nitroglycerin . . . 981
Anglopen® *see* Ampicillin . . . 103
Animal and Human Bites Guidelines . . . 1580
Anisindione . . . 110
Anistal® *see* Ranitidine . . . 1168
Anitrim *see* Sulfamethoxazole and Trimethoprim . . . 1253
Ansaid® *see* Flurbiprofen . . . 596
Ansamycin *see* Rifabutin . . . 1179
Antabuse® *see* Disulfiram . . . 459
Antagon® *see* Ganirelix . . . 628
Antalgin® *see* Indomethacin . . . 719
Antalgin® Dialicels *see* Indomethacin . . . 719
Antazoline and Naphazoline *see* Naphazoline and Antazoline . . . 952
Antepsin *see* Sucralfate . . . 1247
Anthra-Derm® *see* Anthralin . . . 111
Anthraforte® *see* Anthralin . . . 111
Anthralin . . . 111

Anthranol® *see* Anthralin . . . 111
Anthrascalp® *see* Anthralin . . . 111
Anthrax Vaccine (Adsorbed) . . . 112
AntibiOtic® Ear *see* Neomycin, Polymyxin B, and Hydrocortisone . . . 963
Antibiotic Prophylaxis, Preprocedural Guidelines for Dental Patients . . . 1507
Antidigoxin Fab Fragments, Ovine *see* Digoxin Immune Fab . . . 443
Antidiuretic Hormone *see* Vasopressin . . . 1379
Antihemophilic Factor (Human) . . . 113
Antihemophilic Factor (Porcine) . . . 114
Antihemophilic Factor (Recombinant) . . . 115
Antihist-1® [OTC] *see* Clemastine . . . 340
Anti-inhibitor Coagulant Complex . . . 116
Antiphlogistine Rub A-535 No Odour *see* Triethanolamine Salicylate . . . 1348
Antiphogistine Rub A-535 Capsaicin *see* Capsaicin . . . 238
Antiplaque Agents . . . 1554
Antipyrine and Benzocaine . . . 116
Antithrombin III . . . 117
Antithymocyte Globulin (Equine) *see* Lymphocyte Immune Globulin . . . 831
Antithymocyte Immunoglobulin *see* Lymphocyte Immune Globulin . . . 831
Antivert® *see* Meclizine . . . 847
Antizol® *see* Fomepizole . . . 609
Anucort-HC® *see* Hydrocortisone . . . 688
Anusol-HC® *see* Hydrocortisone . . . 688
Anusol® HC-1 [OTC] *see* Hydrocortisone . . . 688
Anusol® Ointment [OTC] *see* Pramoxine . . . 1105
Anzemet® *see* Dolasetron . . . 465
3-A Ofteno® *see* Diclofenac . . . 429
APAP *see* Acetaminophen . . . 27
APAP and Tramadol *see* Acetaminophen and Tramadol . . . 32
Apatate® [OTC] *see* Vitamin B Complex . . . 1392
Aphedrid™ [OTC] *see* Triprolidine and Pseudoephedrine . . . 1356
Aphrodyne® *see* Yohimbine . . . 1401
Aphthasol™ *see* Amlexanox . . . 87
A.P.L.® *see* Chorionic Gonadotropin (Human) . . . 320
Aplisol® *see* Tuberculin Tests . . . 1362
Aplonidine *see* Apraclonidine . . . 118
Apo®-Acebutolol *see* Acebutolol . . . 25
Apo®-Acetaminophen *see* Acetaminophen . . . 27
Apo®-Acetazolamide *see* AcetaZOLAMIDE . . . 37
Apo®-Acyclovir *see* Acyclovir . . . 42
Apo®-Allopurinol *see* Allopurinol . . . 57
Apo®-Alpraz *see* Alprazolam . . . 61
Apo®-Amilzide *see* Amiloride and Hydrochlorothiazide . . . 76
Apo®-Amitriptyline *see* Amitriptyline . . . 83
Apo®-Amoxi *see* Amoxicillin . . . 93
Apo®-Amoxi-Clav *see* Amoxicillin and Clavulanate Potassium . . . 95
Apo®-Ampi *see* Ampicillin . . . 103
Apo®-Atenol *see* Atenolol . . . 137
Apo®-Azathioprine *see* Azathioprine . . . 150
Apo®-Baclofen *see* Baclofen . . . 158
Apo®-Beclomethasone *see* Beclomethasone . . . 163
Apo®-Benztropine *see* Benztropine . . . 173
Apo®-Bisacodyl *see* Bisacodyl . . . 186
Apo®-Bromazepam *see* Bromazepam . . . 199
Apo® Bromocriptine *see* Bromocriptine . . . 199
Apo®-Buspirone *see* BusPIRone . . . 211
Apo®-Butorphanol *see* Butorphanol . . . 218
Apo®-Capto *see* Captopril . . . 238
Apo®-Carbamazepine *see* Carbamazepine . . . 241
Apo®-Carbamazepine CR *see* Carbamazepine . . . 241
Apo®-Cefaclor *see* Cefaclor . . . 260
Apo®-Cefadroxil *see* Cefadroxil . . . 261
Apo®-Cefuroxime *see* Cefuroxime . . . 279
Apo®-Cephalex *see* Cephalexin . . . 285
Apo®-Cetirizine *see* Cetirizine . . . 289
Apo®-Chlorax *see* Clidinium and Chlordiazepoxide . . . 341
Apo®-Chlordiazepoxide *see* Chlordiazepoxide . . . 299
Apo®-Chlorhexadine *see* Chlorhexidine Gluconate . . . 300
Apo®-Chlorpromazine *see* ChlorproMAZINE . . . 312
Apo®-Chlorpropamide *see* ChlorproPAMIDE . . . 314
Apo®-Chlorthalidone *see* Chlorthalidone . . . 315
Apo®-Cimetidine *see* Cimetidine . . . 326
Apo®-Clomipramine *see* ClomiPRAMINE . . . 349
Apo®-Clonazepam *see* Clonazepam . . . 350
Apo®-Clonidine *see* Clonidine . . . 351
Apo®-Clorazepate *see* Clorazepate . . . 355
Apo®-Cloxi *see* Cloxacillin . . . 357
Apo®-Cromolyn *see* Cromolyn Sodium . . . 375
Apo®-Cyclobenzaprine *see* Cyclobenzaprine . . . 379
Apo®-Desipramine *see* Desipramine . . . 408
Apo®-Desmopressin *see* Desmopressin . . . 410
Apo®-Diazepam *see* Diazepam . . . 424
Apo®-Diclo *see* Diclofenac . . . 429
Apo®-Diclo Rapide *see* Diclofenac . . . 429
Apo®-Diclo SR *see* Diclofenac . . . 429
Apo®-Diflunisal *see* Diflunisal . . . 438
Apo®-Diltiaz *see* Diltiazem . . . 447
Apo®-Diltiaz CD *see* Diltiazem . . . 447
Apo®-Diltiaz SR *see* Diltiazem . . . 447
Apo®-Dimenhydrinate *see* DimenhyDRINATE . . . 449

Apo®-Dipivefrin *see* Dipivefrin 455
Apo®-Dipyridamole FC *see* Dipyridamole 456
Apo®-Divalproex *see* Valproic Acid and Derivatives 1371
Apo®-Doxazosin *see* Doxazosin 470
Apo®-Doxepin *see* Doxepin 471
Apo®-Doxy *see* Doxycycline 476
Apo®-Doxy Tabs *see* Doxycycline 476
Apo®-Erythro Base *see* Erythromycin 512
Apo®-Erythro E-C *see* Erythromycin 512
Apo®-Erythro-ES *see* Erythromycin 512
Apo®-Erythro-S *see* Erythromycin 512
Apo®-Etodolac *see* Etodolac 547
Apo®-Famotidine *see* Famotidine 556
Apo®-Fenofibrate *see* Fenofibrate 561
Apo®-Feno-Micro *see* Fenofibrate 561
Apo®-Ferrous Gluconate *see* Iron Supplements 745
Apo®-Ferrous Sulfate *see* Iron Supplements 745
Apo®-Fluconazole *see* Fluconazole 576
Apo®-Flunisolide *see* Flunisolide 582
Apo®-Fluoxetine *see* Fluoxetine 589
Apo®-Fluphenazine *see* Fluphenazine 593
Apo®-Fluphenazine Decanoate *see* Fluphenazine 593
Apo®-Flurazepam *see* Flurazepam 595
Apo®-Flurbiprofen *see* Flurbiprofen 596
Apo®-Flutamide *see* Flutamide 598
Apo®-Fluvoxamine *see* Fluvoxamine 605
Apo®-Folic *see* Folic Acid 606
Apo®-Furosemide *see* Furosemide 622
Apo®-Gabapentin *see* Gabapentin 624
Apo®-Gain *see* Minoxidil 917
Apo®-Gemfibrozil *see* Gemfibrozil 631
Apo®-Glyburide *see* GlyBURIDE 642
Apo®-Haloperidol *see* Haloperidol 659
Apo®-Haloperidol LA *see* Haloperidol 659
Apo®-Hydralazine *see* HydrALAZINE 673
Apo®-Hydro *see* Hydrochlorothiazide 675
Apo®-Hydroxyzine *see* HydrOXYzine 697
Apo®-Ibuprofen *see* Ibuprofen 703
Apo®-Imipramine *see* Imipramine 711
Apo®-Indapamide *see* Indapamide 716
Apo®-Indomethacin *see* Indomethacin 719
Apo®-Ipravent *see* Ipratropium 737
Apo®-ISDN *see* Isosorbide Dinitrate 750
Apo®-Keto *see* Ketoprofen 763
Apo®-Ketoconazole *see* Ketoconazole 762
Apo®-Keto-E *see* Ketoprofen 763
Apo®-Ketorolac *see* Ketorolac 765
Apo®-Ketorolac Injectable *see* Ketorolac 765
Apo®-Keto SR *see* Ketoprofen 763
Apo®-Ketotifen *see* Ketotifen 768
Apo®-Labetalol *see* Labetalol 769
Apo®-Lactulose *see* Lactulose 772
Apo®-Levobunolol *see* Levobunolol 789
Apo®-Levocarb *see* Levodopa and Carbidopa 793
Apo®-Lisinopril *see* Lisinopril 813
Apo®-Lithium *see* Lithium 815
Apo®-Loperamide *see* Loperamide 819
Apo®-Loratadine *see* Loratadine 822
Apo®-Lorazepam *see* Lorazepam 824
Apo®-Lovastatin *see* Lovastatin 828
Apo®-Loxapine *see* Loxapine 829
Apo®-Mefenamic *see* Mefenamic Acid 851
Apo®-Megestrol *see* Megestrol 853
Apo®-Metformin *see* Metformin 874
Apo®-Methazide *see* Methyldopa and Hydrochlorothiazide 892
Apo®-Methazolamide *see* Methazolamide 878
Apo®-Methoprazine *see* Methotrimeprazine 887
Apo®-Methotrexate *see* Methotrexate 884
Apo®-Methyldopa *see* Methyldopa 891
Apo®-Metoclop *see* Metoclopramide 898
Apo®-Metoprolol *see* Metoprolol 901
Apo®-Metronidazole *see* Metronidazole 902
Apo®-Midazolam *see* Midazolam 908
Apo®-Minocycline *see* Minocycline 915
Apo®-Misoprostol *see* Misoprostol 920
Apo®-Nabumetone *see* Nabumetone 941
Apo®-Nadol *see* Nadolol 943
Apo®-Napro-Na *see* Naproxen 953
Apo®-Napro-Na DS *see* Naproxen 953
Apo®-Naproxen *see* Naproxen 953
Apo®-Naproxen SR *see* Naproxen 953
Apo®-Nefazodone *see* Nefazodone 957
Apo®-Nifed *see* NIFEdipine 973
Apo®-Nifed PA *see* NIFEdipine 973
Apo®-Nitrofurantoin *see* Nitrofurantoin 980
Apo®-Nizatidine *see* Nizatidine 984
Apo®-Norflox *see* Norfloxacin 987
Apo®-Nortriptyline *see* Nortriptyline 989
Apo®-Oflox *see* Ofloxacin 995
Apo®-Oxaprozin *see* Oxaprozin 1010

Apo®-Oxazepam *see* Oxazepam . . . 1011
Apo®-Pentoxifylline SR *see* Pentoxifylline . . . 1058
Apo®-Pen VK *see* Penicillin V Potassium . . . 1051
Apo®-Perphenazine *see* Perphenazine . . . 1062
Apo®-Pindol *see* Pindolol . . . 1085
Apo®-Piroxicam *see* Piroxicam . . . 1090
Apo®-Pravastatin *see* Pravastatin . . . 1106
Apo®-Prazo *see* Prazosin . . . 1108
Apo®-Prednisone *see* PredniSONE . . . 1112
Apo®-Primidone *see* Primidone . . . 1118
Apo®-Procainamide *see* Procainamide . . . 1119
Apo®-Prochlorperazine *see* Prochlorperazine . . . 1123
Apo®-Propafenone *see* Propafenone . . . 1130
Apo®-Propranolol *see* Propranolol . . . 1139
Apo®-Quin-G *see* Quinidine . . . 1158
Apo®-Quinidine *see* Quinidine . . . 1158
Apo®-Ranitidine *see* Ranitidine . . . 1168
Apo®-Salvent *see* Albuterol . . . 48
Apo®-Selegiline *see* Selegiline . . . 1213
Apo®-Sertraline *see* Sertraline . . . 1216
Apo®-Sotalol *see* Sotalol . . . 1235
Apo®-Sucralate *see* Sucralfate . . . 1247
Apo®-Sulfatrim *see* Sulfamethoxazole and Trimethoprim . . . 1253
Apo®-Sulfinpyrazone *see* Sulfinpyrazone . . . 1255
Apo®-Sulin *see* Sulindac . . . 1257
Apo®-Tamox *see* Tamoxifen . . . 1264
Apo®-Temazepam *see* Temazepam . . . 1271
Apo®-Terazosin *see* Terazosin . . . 1276
Apo®-Terbinafine *see* Terbinafine . . . 1277
Apo®-Tetra *see* Tetracycline . . . 1286
Apo®-Theo LA *see* Theophylline . . . 1291
Apo®-Thioridazine *see* Thioridazine . . . 1298
Apo®-Ticlopidine *see* Ticlopidine . . . 1307
Apo®-Timol *see* Timolol . . . 1309
Apo®-Timop *see* Timolol . . . 1309
Apo®-Tolbutamide *see* TOLBUTamide . . . 1319
Apo®-Trazodone *see* Trazodone . . . 1336
Apo®-Trazodone D *see* Trazodone . . . 1336
Apo®-Triazide *see* Hydrochlorothiazide and Triamterene . . . 677
Apo®-Triazo *see* Triazolam . . . 1345
Apo®-Trifluoperazine *see* Trifluoperazine . . . 1349
Apo®-Trihex *see* Trihexyphenidyl . . . 1351
Apo®-Trimethoprim *see* Trimethoprim . . . 1352
Apo®-Trimip *see* Trimipramine . . . 1354
Apo®-Verap *see* Verapamil . . . 1382
Apo®-Warfarin *see* Warfarin . . . 1397
Apo®-Zidovudine *see* Zidovudine . . . 1406
Apo®-Zopiclone *see* Zopiclone . . . 1415
APPG *see* Penicillin G Procaine . . . 1050
Apraclonidine . . . 118
Apraclonidine Hydrochloride *see* Apraclonidine . . . 118
Apresazide® [DSC] *see* Hydralazine and Hydrochlorothiazide . . . 675
Apresolina *see* HydrALAZINE . . . 673
Apresoline® *see* HydrALAZINE . . . 673
Apri® *see* Combination Hormonal Contraceptives . . . 368
Aprodine® [OTC] *see* Triprolidine and Pseudoephedrine . . . 1356
Aprotinin . . . 119
Aprovel® *see* Irbesartan . . . 739
Aquacare® [OTC] *see* Urea . . . 1365
Aquachloral® Supprettes® *see* Chloral Hydrate . . . 295
Aquacort® *see* Hydrocortisone . . . 688
Aqua Gem E® [OTC] *see* Vitamin E . . . 1393
Aqua Lube Plus [OTC] *see* Nonoxynol 9 . . . 985
AquaMEPHYTON® *see* Phytonadione . . . 1079
Aquanil HC® *see* Hydrocortisone . . . 688
Aquaphilic® With Carbamide [OTC] *see* Urea . . . 1365
AquaSite® [OTC] *see* Artificial Tears . . . 128
Aquasol A® *see* Vitamin A . . . 1390
Aquasol E® [OTC] *see* Vitamin E . . . 1393
Aquatab® *see* Guaifenesin and Pseudoephedrine . . . 652
Aquatab® C *see* Guaifenesin, Pseudoephedrine, and Dextromethorphan . . . 653
Aquatab® D Dose Pack *see* Guaifenesin and Pseudoephedrine . . . 652
Aquatab® DM *see* Guaifenesin and Dextromethorphan . . . 651
Aquatensen® *see* Methyclothiazide . . . 890
Aquazide® H *see* Hydrochlorothiazide . . . 675
Aqueous Procaine Penicillin G *see* Penicillin G Procaine . . . 1050
Aqueous Testosterone *see* Testosterone . . . 1281
Ara-A *see* Vidarabine . . . 1384
Arabinofuranosyladenine *see* Vidarabine . . . 1384
Arabinosylcytosine *see* Cytarabine . . . 389
Ara-C *see* Cytarabine . . . 389
Aralen® *see* Chloroquine . . . 303
Aralen® Phosphate *see* Chloroquine . . . 303
Aranesp™ *see* Darbepoetin Alfa . . . 400
Arava™ *see* Leflunomide . . . 779
Arctostaphylos uva-ursi *see* Uva Ursi . . . 1449
Ardine® *see* Amoxicillin . . . 93
Aredia® *see* Pamidronate . . . 1029
Arestin™ *see* Minocycline Hydrochloride Periodontal Microspheres . . . 916
Argatroban . . . 120

Arginine . . . 121
Arginine Hydrochloride *see* Arginine . . . 121
8-Arginine Vasopressin *see* Vasopressin . . . 1379
Aricept® *see* Donepezil . . . 467
Arimidex® *see* Anastrozole . . . 109
Aripiprazole . . . 122
Aristocort® *see* Triamcinolone . . . 1341
Aristocort® A *see* Triamcinolone . . . 1341
Aristocort® Forte *see* Triamcinolone . . . 1341
Aristospan® *see* Triamcinolone . . . 1341
Arixtra® *see* Fondaparinux . . . 611
Arlidin® *see* Nylidrin . . . 991
Armour® Thyroid *see* Thyroid . . . 1303
Aromasin® *see* Exemestane . . . 552
Aropax® *see* Paroxetine . . . 1036
Arovit *see* Vitamin A . . . 1390
Arthropan® [OTC] *see* Choline Salicylate . . . 319
Arthrotec® *see* Diclofenac and Misoprostol . . . 431
Articaine Hydrochloride and Epinephrine *see* Articaine Hydrochloride and Epinephrine (Canada) . . . 124
Articaine Hydrochloride and Epinephrine [Dental] *see* Articaine Hydrochloride and Epinephrine (U.S.) . . . 125
Articaine Hydrochloride and Epinephrine (Canada) . . . 124
Articaine Hydrochloride and Epinephrine (U.S.) . . . 125
Artificial Tears . . . 128
Artinor® *see* Piroxicam . . . 1090
Artosin *see* TOLBUTamide . . . 1319
Artrenac® *see* Diclofenac . . . 429
Artron® *see* Naproxen . . . 953
Artyflam *see* Piroxicam . . . 1090
ASA *see* Aspirin . . . 131
5-ASA *see* Mesalamine . . . 869
ASA 500® *see* Aspirin . . . 131
Asacol® *see* Mesalamine . . . 869
Asaphen *see* Aspirin . . . 131
Asaphen E.C. *see* Aspirin . . . 131
Ascorbic Acid . . . 128
Ascorbic Acid and Ferrous Sulfate *see* Ferrous Sulfate and Ascorbic Acid . . . 569
Ascriptin® [OTC] *see* Aspirin . . . 131
Ascriptin® Arthritis Pain [OTC] *see* Aspirin . . . 131
Ascriptin® Enteric [OTC] *see* Aspirin . . . 131
Ascriptin® Extra Strength [OTC] *see* Aspirin . . . 131
Asendin® [DSC] *see* Amoxapine . . . 91
Asian Ginseng *see* Ginseng, Panax . . . 1435
Asparaginase . . . 129
Aspercin [OTC] *see* Aspirin . . . 131
Aspercin Extra [OTC] *see* Aspirin . . . 131
Aspergum® [OTC] *see* Aspirin . . . 131
Aspirin . . . 131
Aspirin, Acetaminophen, and Caffeine *see* Acetaminophen, Aspirin, and Caffeine . . . 34
Aspirin and Carisoprodol *see* Carisoprodol and Aspirin . . . 252
Aspirin and Codeine . . . 134
Aspirin and Dipyridamole . . . 135
Aspirin and Hydrocodone *see* Hydrocodone and Aspirin . . . 680
Aspirin and Meprobamate . . . 136
Aspirin and Oxycodone *see* Oxycodone and Aspirin . . . 1020
Aspirina Protect® *see* Aspirin . . . 131
Aspirin, Caffeine and Acetaminophen *see* Acetaminophen, Aspirin, and Caffeine . . . 34
Aspirin, Caffeine, and Butalbital *see* Butalbital, Aspirin, and Caffeine . . . 216
Aspirin, Carisoprodol, and Codeine *see* Carisoprodol, Aspirin, and Codeine . . . 252
Aspirin Free Anacin® Maximum Strength [OTC] *see* Acetaminophen . . . 27
Aspirin, Orphenadrine, and Caffeine *see* Orphenadrine, Aspirin, and Caffeine . . . 1005
Astelin® *see* Azelastine . . . 151
AsthmaNefrin® *see* Epinephrine (Racemic) . . . 500
Astracaine® *see* Articaine Hydrochloride and Epinephrine (Canada) . . . 124
Astracaine® Forte *see* Articaine Hydrochloride and Epinephrine (Canada) . . . 124
Astragalus . . . 1421
Astragalus membranaceus *see* Astragalus . . . 1421
Astramorph/PF™ *see* Morphine Sulfate . . . 931
Atacand® *see* Candesartan . . . 232
Atacand HCT™ *see* Candesartan and Hydrochlorothiazide . . . 234
Atacand® Plus *see* Candesartan and Hydrochlorothiazide . . . 234
Atarax® *see* HydrOXYzine . . . 697
Atasol® *see* Acetaminophen . . . 27
Atemperator-S® *see* Valproic Acid and Derivatives . . . 1371
Atenolol . . . 137
Atenolol and Chlorthalidone . . . 138
ATG *see* Lymphocyte Immune Globulin . . . 831
Atgam® *see* Lymphocyte Immune Globulin . . . 831
Athos® *see* Dextromethorphan . . . 423
Atiflan *see* Naproxen . . . 953
AT III *see* Antithrombin III . . . 117
Atiquim® *see* Naproxen . . . 953
Atisuril® *see* Allopurinol . . . 57
Ativan® *see* Lorazepam . . . 824
Atomoxetine . . . 139
Atomoxetine Hydrochloride *see* Atomoxetine . . . 139
Atorvastatin . . . 140
Atovaquone . . . 142
Atovaquone and Proguanil . . . 143

Atridox™ *see* Doxycycline Hyclate Periodontal Extended-Release Liquid . . . 479
Atromid-S® *see* Clofibrate . . . 347
Atropine . . . 144
Atropine and Difenoxin *see* Difenoxin and Atropine . . . 437
Atropine and Diphenoxylate *see* Diphenoxylate and Atropine . . . 453
Atropine-Care® *see* Atropine . . . 144
Atropine, Hyoscyamine, Scopolamine, and Phenobarbital *see* Hyoscyamine, Atropine, Scopolamine, and Phenobarbital . . . 700
Atropine Sulfate *see* Atropine . . . 144
Atropine Sulfate Dental Tablets . . . 145
Atropisol® *see* Atropine . . . 144
Atrovent® *see* Ipratropium . . . 737
A/T/S® *see* Erythromycin . . . 512
Attapulgite . . . 146
Attenuvax® *see* Measles Virus Vaccine (Live) . . . 845
Audifluor® *see* Fluoride . . . 586
Augmentin® *see* Amoxicillin and Clavulanate Potassium . . . 95
Augmentin ES-600™ *see* Amoxicillin and Clavulanate Potassium . . . 95
Augmentin XR™ *see* Amoxicillin and Clavulanate Potassium . . . 95
Auralgan® *see* Antipyrine and Benzocaine . . . 116
Auranofin . . . 147
Auro® Ear Drops [OTC] *see* Carbamide Peroxide . . . 244
Aurolate® *see* Gold Sodium Thiomalate . . . 646
Aurothioglucose . . . 148
Auroto® *see* Antipyrine and Benzocaine . . . 116
Autoplex® T *see* Anti-inhibitor Coagulant Complex . . . 116
AVA *see* Anthrax Vaccine (Adsorbed) . . . 112
Avagard™ [OTC] *see* Chlorhexidine Gluconate . . . 300
Avage™ *see* Tazarotene . . . 1267
Avalide® *see* Irbesartan and Hydrochlorothiazide . . . 740
Avandamet™ *see* Rosiglitazone and Metformin . . . 1200
Avandia® *see* Rosiglitazone . . . 1199
Avapro® *see* Irbesartan . . . 739
Avapro® HCT *see* Irbesartan and Hydrochlorothiazide . . . 740
Avaxim® *see* Hepatitis A Vaccine . . . 665
Avaxim®-Pediatric *see* Hepatitis A Vaccine . . . 665
Avelox® *see* Moxifloxacin . . . 935
Avelox® I.V. *see* Moxifloxacin . . . 935
Aventyl® *see* Nortriptyline . . . 989
Aventyl® HCl *see* Nortriptyline . . . 989
Aviane™ *see* Combination Hormonal Contraceptives . . . 368
A-Vicon *see* Vitamin A . . . 1390
Avinza™ *see* Morphine Sulfate . . . 931
Avita® *see* Tretinoin (Topical) . . . 1340
Avitene® *see* Microfibrillar Collagen Hemostat . . . 907
A-Vitex *see* Vitamin A . . . 1390
Avodart™ *see* Dutasteride . . . 484
Avonex® *see* Interferon Beta-1a . . . 732
Awa *see* Kava . . . 1442
Axert™ *see* Almotriptan . . . 59
Axid® *see* Nizatidine . . . 984
Axid® AR [OTC] *see* Nizatidine . . . 984
Axofor® *see* Hydroxocobalamin . . . 693
Aygestin® *see* Norethindrone . . . 986
Ayr® Baby Saline [OTC] *see* Sodium Chloride . . . 1229
Ayr® Saline [OTC] *see* Sodium Chloride . . . 1229
Ayr® Saline Mist [OTC] *see* Sodium Chloride . . . 1229
Az® *see* Azelastine . . . 151
Azacitidine . . . 149
AZA-CR *see* Azacitidine . . . 149
Azactam® *see* Aztreonam . . . 155
5-Azacytidine *see* Azacitidine . . . 149
Azanplus® *see* Ranitidine . . . 1168
Azantac® *see* Ranitidine . . . 1168
Azatadine . . . 149
Azatadine and Pseudoephedrine . . . 150
Azatadine Maleate *see* Azatadine . . . 149
Azathioprine . . . 150
Azathioprine Sodium *see* Azathioprine . . . 150
Azatrilem® *see* Azathioprine . . . 150
5-AZC *see* Azacitidine . . . 149
Azelaic Acid . . . 151
Azelastine . . . 151
Azelastine Hydrochloride *see* Azelastine . . . 151
Azelex® *see* Azelaic Acid . . . 151
Azidothymidine *see* Zidovudine . . . 1406
Azidothymidine, Abacavir, and Lamivudine *see* Abacavir, Lamivudine, and Zidovudine . . . 23
Azithromycin . . . 153
Azithromycin Dihydrate *see* Azithromycin . . . 153
Azitrocin® *see* Azithromycin . . . 153
Azmacort® *see* Triamcinolone . . . 1341
Azo-Gesic® [OTC] *see* Phenazopyridine . . . 1064
Azopt™ *see* Brinzolamide . . . 198
Azo-Standard® [OTC] *see* Phenazopyridine . . . 1064
Azo Wintomylon *see* Phenazopyridine . . . 1064
AZT™ *see* Zidovudine . . . 1406
AZT + 3TC *see* Zidovudine and Lamivudine . . . 1407
AZT, Abacavir, and Lamivudine *see* Abacavir, Lamivudine, and Zidovudine . . . 23
Azthreonam *see* Aztreonam . . . 155
Aztreonam . . . 155

Azulfidine® *see* Sulfasalazine 1254
Azulfidine® EN-tabs® *see* Sulfasalazine 1254
B 9273 *see* Alefacept 52
Babee® Cof Syrup [OTC] *see* Dextromethorphan 423
Babee® Teething® [OTC] *see* Benzocaine 169
Baby Gasz [OTC] *see* Simethicone 1222
BAC *see* Benzalkonium Chloride 169
Bachelor's Button *see* Feverfew 1431
Bacid® *see* *Lactobacillus acidophilus* and *Lactobacillus bulgaricus* 772
Baciguent® *see* Bacitracin 156
Baci-IM® *see* Bacitracin 156
Bacillus Calmette-Guérin (BCG) Live *see* BCG Vaccine 161
Bacitracin 156
Bacitracin and Polymyxin B 157
Bacitracin, Neomycin, and Polymyxin B 157
Bacitracin, Neomycin, Polymyxin B, and Hydrocortisone 158
Bacitracin, Neomycin, Polymyxin B, and Lidocaine 158
Baclofen 158
Bactelan *see* Sulfamethoxazole and Trimethoprim 1253
Bactilen® *see* Trimethoprim 1352
Bactiver® *see* Trimethoprim 1352
Bactocin® *see* Ofloxacin 995
BactoShield® CHG [OTC] *see* Chlorhexidine Gluconate 300
Bactrim™ *see* Sulfamethoxazole and Trimethoprim 1253
Bactrim® *see* Trimethoprim 1352
Bactrim™ DS *see* Sulfamethoxazole and Trimethoprim 1253
Bactroban® *see* Mupirocin 937
Bactroban® Nasal *see* Mupirocin 937
Bactropin® *see* Trimethoprim 1352
Baking Soda *see* Sodium Bicarbonate 1227
BAL *see* Dimercaprol 449
Balanced Salt Solution 160
Balcoran *see* Vancomycin 1376
BAL in Oil® *see* Dimercaprol 449
Balmex® [OTC] *see* Zinc Oxide 1409
Balminil® Decongestant *see* Pseudoephedrine 1146
Balminil DM D *see* Pseudoephedrine and Dextromethorphan 1147
Balminil DM + Decongestant + Expectorant *see* Guaifenesin, Pseudoephedrine, and Dextromethorphan 653
Balminil DM E *see* Guaifenesin and Dextromethorphan 651
Balminil Expectorant *see* Guaifenesin 650
Balnetar® *see* Coal Tar 359
Balnetar® [OTC] *see* Coal Tar, Lanolin, and Mineral Oil 360
Bancap HC® *see* Hydrocodone and Acetaminophen 678
Band-Aid® Hurt-Free™ Antiseptic Wash [OTC] *see* Lidocaine 801
Banophen® [OTC] *see* DiphenhydrAMINE 451
Basaljel® *see* Aluminum Hydroxide 68
Base Ointment *see* Zinc Oxide 1409
Basiliximab 160
Bateral® *see* Trimethoprim 1352
Batrizol *see* Sulfamethoxazole and Trimethoprim 1253
Batrizol® *see* Trimethoprim 1352
Bausch & Lomb® Computer Eye Drops [OTC] *see* Glycerin 644
Bayer® Aspirin [OTC] *see* Aspirin 131
Bayer® Aspirin Extra Strength [OTC] *see* Aspirin 131
Bayer® Aspirin Regimen Adult Low Strength [OTC] *see* Aspirin 131
Bayer® Aspirin Regimen Adult Low Strength with Calcium [OTC] *see* Aspirin 131
Bayer® Aspirin Regimen Children's [OTC] *see* Aspirin 131
Bayer® Aspirin Regimen Regular Strength [OTC] *see* Aspirin 131
Bayer® Plus Extra Strength [OTC] *see* Aspirin 131
BayGam® *see* Immune Globulin (Intramuscular) 713
BayHep B™ *see* Hepatitis B Immune Globulin 666
BayRab™ *see* Rabies Immune Globulin (Human) 1164
BayRho-D® Full-Dose *see* Rh_o(D) Immune Globulin 1175
BayRho-D® Mini-Dose *see* Rh_o(D) Immune Globulin 1175
BayTet™ *see* Tetanus Immune Globulin (Human) 1283
Baza® Antifungal [OTC] *see* Miconazole 906
Baza® Clear [OTC] *see* Vitamin A and Vitamin D 1392
B-Caro-T™ *see* Beta-Carotene 176
BCG, Live *see* BCG Vaccine 161
BCG Vaccine 161
BCNU *see* Carmustine 253
B-D™ Glucose [OTC] *see* Glucose (Instant) 641
Bearberry *see* Uva Ursi 1449
Bebulin® VH *see* Factor IX Complex (Human) 553
Becaplermin 162
Beclomethasone 163
Beclomethasone Dipropionate *see* Beclomethasone 163
Beclovent® [DSC] *see* Beclomethasone 163
Beconase® [DSC] *see* Beclomethasone 163
Beconase® AQ *see* Beclomethasone 163
Beconase Aqua *see* Beclomethasone 163
Becotide 100 *see* Beclomethasone 163
Becotide 250 *see* Beclomethasone 163
Becotide Aerosol *see* Beclomethasone 163
Behenyl Alcohol *see* Docosanol 463
Bekidiba Dex® *see* Dextromethorphan 423
Beknol *see* Benzonatate 171
Belladonna and Opium 164
Belladonna, Phenobarbital, and Ergotamine 165

Bellamine S *see* Belladonna, Phenobarbital, and Ergotamine 165
Bellergal® Spacetabs® *see* Belladonna, Phenobarbital, and Ergotamine 165
Bel-Phen-Ergot S® *see* Belladonna, Phenobarbital, and Ergotamine 165
Bel-Tabs *see* Belladonna, Phenobarbital, and Ergotamine 165
Benadon *see* Pyridoxine 1152
Benadryl® *see* DiphenhydrAMINE 451
Benadryl® Allergy [OTC] *see* DiphenhydrAMINE 451
Benadryl® Allergy and Sinus Fastmelt™ [OTC] *see* Diphenhydramine and Pseudoephedrine 453
Benadryl® Allergy/Decongestant [OTC] *see* Diphenhydramine and Pseudoephedrine 453
Benadryl® Children's Allergy and Cold Fastmelt™ [OTC] *see* Diphenhydramine and Pseudoephedrine 453
Benadryl® Children's Allergy and Sinus [OTC] *see* Diphenhydramine and Pseudoephedrine 453
Benadryl® Dye-Free Allergy [OTC] *see* DiphenhydrAMINE 451
Benadryl® Gel [OTC] *see* DiphenhydrAMINE 451
Benadryl® Gel Extra Strength [OTC] *see* DiphenhydrAMINE 451
Benadryl® Injection *see* DiphenhydrAMINE 451
Benaxima® *see* Cefotaxime 271
Benaxona® *see* Ceftriaxone 278
Benazepril 166
Benazepril and Amlodipine *see* Amlodipine and Benazepril 89
Benazepril and Hydrochlorothiazide 167
Benazepril Hydrochloride *see* Benazepril 166
Bencelin® *see* Penicillin G Benzathine 1047
Bendapar® *see* Albendazole 47
Bendroflumethiazide 168
Benecid® *see* Probenecid 1119
Benecid Probenecida Valdecasas *see* Probenecid 1119
Benemid [DSC] *see* Probenecid 1119
Benerva® *see* Thiamine 1295
Benicar™ *see* Olmesartan 997
Benoquin® *see* Monobenzone 929
Benoxyl® *see* Benzoyl Peroxide 171
Bentoquatam 168
Bentyl® *see* Dicyclomine 433
Bentylol® *see* Dicyclomine 433
Benuryl™ *see* Probenecid 1119
Benylin® 3.3 mg-D-E *see* Guaifenesin, Pseudoephedrine, and Codeine 653
Benylin® Adult [OTC] *see* Dextromethorphan 423
Benylin® DM-D *see* Pseudoephedrine and Dextromethorphan 1147
Benylin® DM-D-E *see* Guaifenesin, Pseudoephedrine, and Dextromethorphan 653
Benylin® DM-E *see* Guaifenesin and Dextromethorphan 651
Benylin® E Extra Strength *see* Guaifenesin 650
Benylin® Expectorant [OTC] *see* Guaifenesin and Dextromethorphan 651
Benylin® Pediatric [OTC] *see* Dextromethorphan 423
Benza® [OTC] *see* Benzalkonium Chloride 169
Benzac® *see* Benzoyl Peroxide 171
Benzac AC® *see* Benzoyl Peroxide 171
Benzac® AC Wash *see* Benzoyl Peroxide 171
BenzaClin® *see* Clindamycin and Benzoyl Peroxide 343
Benzac® W *see* Benzoyl Peroxide 171
Benzac W® Gel *see* Benzoyl Peroxide 171
Benzac W® Wash *see* Benzoyl Peroxide 171
Benzaderm® *see* Benzoyl Peroxide 171
Benzagel® *see* Benzoyl Peroxide 171
Benzagel® Wash *see* Benzoyl Peroxide 171
Benzalkonium Chloride 169
Benzamycin® *see* Erythromycin and Benzoyl Peroxide 515
Benzanil® *see* Penicillin G Benzathine 1047
Benzanil *see* Penicillin G (Parenteral/Aqueous) 1049
Benzashave® *see* Benzoyl Peroxide 171
Benzathine Benzylpenicillin *see* Penicillin G Benzathine 1047
Benzathine Penicillin G *see* Penicillin G Benzathine 1047
Benzedrex® [OTC] *see* Propylhexedrine 1142
Benzene Hexachloride *see* Lindane 809
Benzetacil® *see* Penicillin G Benzathine 1047
Benzhexol Hydrochloride *see* Trihexyphenidyl 1351
Benzilfan *see* Penicillin G Benzathine 1047
Benzmethyzin *see* Procarbazine 1122
Benzocaine 169
Benzocaine and Antipyrine *see* Antipyrine and Benzocaine 116
Benzocaine and Cetylpyridinium Chloride *see* Cetylpyridinium and Benzocaine 292
Benzocaine, Butyl Aminobenzoate, Tetracaine, and Benzalkonium Chloride 170
Benzocaine, Gelatin, Pectin, and Sodium Carboxymethylcellulose 171
Benzodent® [OTC] *see* Benzocaine 169
Benzoin 171
Benzonatate 171
Benzoyl Peroxide 171
Benzoyl Peroxide and Clindamycin *see* Clindamycin and Benzoyl Peroxide 343
Benzoyl Peroxide and Erythromycin *see* Erythromycin and Benzoyl Peroxide 515
Benzoyl Peroxide and Hydrocortisone 172
Benzphetamine 172
Benzphetamine Hydrochloride *see* Benzphetamine 172
Benztropine 173
Benztropine Mesylate *see* Benztropine 173
Benzylpenicillin Benzathine *see* Penicillin G Benzathine 1047
Benzylpenicillin Potassium *see* Penicillin G (Parenteral/Aqueous) 1049
Benzylpenicillin Sodium *see* Penicillin G (Parenteral/Aqueous) 1049
Benzylpenicilloyl-polylysine 174

Bepridil . . . 174
Bepridil Hydrochloride *see* Bepridil . . . 174
Beractant . . . 176
Berotec® *see* Fenoterol . . . 564
Beta-2® *see* Isoetharine . . . 747
Beta-Carotene . . . 176
Betaderm *see* Betamethasone . . . 177
Betadine® *see* Povidone-Iodine . . . 1104
Betadine® First Aid Antibiotics + Moisturizer [OTC] *see* Bacitracin and Polymyxin B . . . 157
Betadine® Ophthalmic *see* Povidone-Iodine . . . 1104
9-Beta-D-ribofuranosyladenine *see* Adenosine . . . 45
Betaferon® *see* Interferon Beta-1a . . . 732
Betaferon® *see* Interferon Beta-1b . . . 733
Betagan® *see* Levobunolol . . . 789
Betagan® Liquifilm® *see* Levobunolol . . . 789
Betaine Anhydrous . . . 177
Betaject™ *see* Betamethasone . . . 177
Betaloc® *see* Metoprolol . . . 901
Betaloc® Durules® *see* Metoprolol . . . 901
Betamethasone . . . 177
Betamethasone and Clotrimazole . . . 179
Betamethasone Dipropionate *see* Betamethasone . . . 177
Betamethasone Dipropionate, Augmented *see* Betamethasone . . . 177
Betamethasone Sodium Phosphate *see* Betamethasone . . . 177
Betamethasone Valerate *see* Betamethasone . . . 177
Betapace® *see* Sotalol . . . 1235
Betapace AF® *see* Sotalol . . . 1235
Betasept® [OTC] *see* Chlorhexidine Gluconate . . . 300
Betaseron® *see* Interferon Beta-1b . . . 733
Betatrex® *see* Betamethasone . . . 177
Beta-Val® *see* Betamethasone . . . 177
Betaxin® *see* Thiamine . . . 1295
Betaxolol . . . 180
Betaxolol Hydrochloride *see* Betaxolol . . . 180
Betaxon® *see* Levobetaxolol . . . 788
Bethanechol . . . 181
Bethanechol Chloride *see* Bethanechol . . . 181
Betimol® *see* Timolol . . . 1309
Betnesol® *see* Betamethasone . . . 177
Betnovate® *see* Betamethasone . . . 177
Betoptic® S *see* Betaxolol . . . 180
Bexarotene . . . 182
Bextra® *see* Valdecoxib . . . 1368
BG 9273 *see* Alefacept . . . 52
Biaxin® *see* Clarithromycin . . . 337
Biaxin® XL *see* Clarithromycin . . . 337
Bicalutamide . . . 183
Bicillin® C-R *see* Penicillin G Benzathine and Penicillin G Procaine . . . 1048
Bicillin® C-R 900/300 *see* Penicillin G Benzathine and Penicillin G Procaine . . . 1048
Bicillin® L-A *see* Penicillin G Benzathine . . . 1047
Bicitra® *see* Sodium Citrate and Citric Acid . . . 1230
Biclin® *see* Amikacin . . . 74
BiCNU® *see* Carmustine . . . 253
Bifidobacterium bifidum / Lactobacillus acidophilus . . . 1422
Bilberry . . . 1422
Bilem *see* Tamoxifen . . . 1264
Biltricide® *see* Praziquantel . . . 1108
Bimatoprost . . . 184
Binotal *see* Ampicillin . . . 103
Biocef *see* Cephalexin . . . 285
Biofed [OTC] *see* Pseudoephedrine . . . 1146
Biolon® *see* Sodium Hyaluronate . . . 1230
Bion® Tears [OTC] *see* Artificial Tears . . . 128
BioQuin® Durules™ *see* Quinidine . . . 1158
Biosint® *see* Cefotaxime . . . 271
Bio-Statin® *see* Nystatin . . . 992
BioThrax™ *see* Anthrax Vaccine (Adsorbed) . . . 112
Biperiden . . . 185
Biperiden Hydrochloride *see* Biperiden . . . 185
Biperiden Lactate *see* Biperiden . . . 185
Bisac-Evac™ [OTC] *see* Bisacodyl . . . 186
Bisacodyl . . . 186
Bisacodyl Uniserts® [OTC] *see* Bisacodyl . . . 186
Bishydroxycoumarin *see* Dicumarol . . . 433
Bismatrol *see* Bismuth . . . 186
Bismuth . . . 186
Bismuth, Metronidazole, and Tetracycline . . . 187
Bismuth Subgallate *see* Bismuth . . . 186
Bismuth Subsalicylate *see* Bismuth . . . 186
Bismuth Subsalicylate, Tetracycline, and Metronidazole *see* Bismuth, Metronidazole, and Tetracycline . . . 187
Bisoprolol . . . 188
Bisoprolol and Hydrochlorothiazide . . . 189
Bisoprolol Fumarate *see* Bisoprolol . . . 188
Bistropamide *see* Tropicamide . . . 1360
Bitolterol . . . 189
Bitolterol Mesylate *see* Bitolterol . . . 189
Black Cohosh . . . 1423
Black Susans *see* *Echinacea* . . . 1429
Bladuril® *see* Flavoxate . . . 573

Blanoxan® *see* Bleomycin . . . 190
Blastocarb® *see* Carboplatin . . . 248
Blastolem® *see* Cisplatin . . . 332
Blenoxane® *see* Bleomycin . . . 190
Bleo *see* Bleomycin . . . 190
Bleolem® *see* Bleomycin . . . 190
Bleomycin . . . 190
Bleomycin Sulfate *see* Bleomycin . . . 190
Bleph®-10 *see* Sulfacetamide . . . 1249
Blephamide® *see* Sulfacetamide and Prednisolone . . . 1250
BLM *see* Bleomycin . . . 190
Blocadren® *see* Timolol . . . 1309
Blocan *see* Cimetidine . . . 326
Blokium® *see* Atenolol . . . 137
Bluboro® [OTC] *see* Aluminum Sulfate and Calcium Acetate . . . 70
BMS 337039 *see* Aripiprazole . . . 122
BN-52063 *see* Ginkgo Biloba . . . 1434
Bonamine™ *see* Meclizine . . . 847
Bonine® [OTC] *see* Meclizine . . . 847
Bontril® *see* Phendimetrazine . . . 1064
Bontril PDM® *see* Phendimetrazine . . . 1064
Bontril® Slow-Release *see* Phendimetrazine . . . 1064
Boric Acid . . . 191
Bosentan . . . 192
B&O Supprettes® *see* Belladonna and Opium . . . 164
Botox® *see* Botulinum Toxin Type A . . . 193
Botox® Cosmetic *see* Botulinum Toxin Type A . . . 193
Botulinum Toxin Type A . . . 193
Botulinum Toxin Type B . . . 195
Boudreaux's® Butt Paste [OTC] *see* Zinc Oxide . . . 1409
Bovine Lung Surfactant *see* Beractant . . . 176
Braccoprial® *see* Pyrazinamide . . . 1150
Bravelle™ *see* Follitropins . . . 607
Braxan® *see* Amiodarone . . . 80
Breathe Right® Saline [OTC] *see* Sodium Chloride . . . 1229
Breonesin® [OTC] [DSC] *see* Guaifenesin . . . 650
Brethaire® [DSC] *see* Terbutaline . . . 1278
Brethine® *see* Terbutaline . . . 1278
Bretylium . . . 196
Bretylium Tosylate *see* Bretylium . . . 196
Brevibloc® *see* Esmolol . . . 518
Brevicon® *see* Combination Hormonal Contraceptives . . . 368
Brevital® *see* Methohexital . . . 882
Brevital® Sodium *see* Methohexital . . . 882
Brevoxyl® *see* Benzoyl Peroxide . . . 171
Brevoxyl® Cleansing *see* Benzoyl Peroxide . . . 171
Brevoxyl® Wash *see* Benzoyl Peroxide . . . 171
Brexicam® *see* Piroxicam . . . 1090
Bricanyl® [DSC] *see* Terbutaline . . . 1278
Brimonidine . . . 197
Brimonidine Tartrate *see* Brimonidine . . . 197
Brinzolamide . . . 198
Brioschi® [OTC] *see* Sodium Bicarbonate . . . 1227
Brispen *see* Dicloxacillin . . . 432
Bris Taxol® *see* Paclitaxel . . . 1026
British Anti-Lewisite *see* Dimercaprol . . . 449
Brofed® *see* Brompheniramine and Pseudoephedrine . . . 201
Bromanate® [OTC] *see* Brompheniramine and Pseudoephedrine . . . 201
Bromazepam . . . 199
Bromelain . . . 1423
Bromfed® [OTC] *see* Brompheniramine and Pseudoephedrine . . . 201
Bromfed-PD® [OTC] *see* Brompheniramine and Pseudoephedrine . . . 201
Bromfenex® *see* Brompheniramine and Pseudoephedrine . . . 201
Bromfenex® PD *see* Brompheniramine and Pseudoephedrine . . . 201
Bromocriptine . . . 199
Bromocriptine Mesylate *see* Bromocriptine . . . 199
Bromodiphenhydramine and Codeine . . . 200
Brompheniramine and Pseudoephedrine . . . 201
Broncho Saline® [OTC] *see* Sodium Chloride . . . 1229
Bronkometer® *see* Isoetharine . . . 747
Bronkosol® *see* Isoetharine . . . 747
Brontex® *see* Guaifenesin and Codeine . . . 650
BSS® *see* Balanced Salt Solution . . . 160
BSS® Plus *see* Balanced Salt Solution . . . 160
B-type Natriuretic Peptide (Human) *see* Nesiritide . . . 964
Budesonide . . . 202
Bufferin® [OTC] *see* Aspirin . . . 131
Bufferin® Arthritis Strength [OTC] *see* Aspirin . . . 131
Bufferin® Extra Strength [OTC] *see* Aspirin . . . 131
Bufigen® *see* Nalbuphine . . . 946
Bumedyl® *see* Bumetanide . . . 204
Bumetanide . . . 204
Bumex® *see* Bumetanide . . . 204
Buphenyl® *see* Sodium Phenylbutyrate . . . 1233
Bupivacaine . . . 205
Bupivacaine and Epinephrine . . . 207
Bupivacaine Hydrochloride *see* Bupivacaine . . . 205
Buprenex® *see* Buprenorphine . . . 208
Buprenorphine . . . 208
Buprenorphine Hydrochloride *see* Buprenorphine . . . 208

BuPROPion . . . 209
Burinex® see Bumetanide . . . 204
Burnamycin [OTC] see Lidocaine . . . 801
Burn Jel [OTC] see Lidocaine . . . 801
Burn-O-Jel [OTC] see Lidocaine . . . 801
Burow's Otic see Aluminum Acetate and Acetic Acid . . . 67
BuSpar® see BusPIRone . . . 211
Buspirex see BusPIRone . . . 211
BusPIRone . . . 211
Buspirone Hydrochloride see BusPIRone . . . 211
Busulfan . . . 212
Busulfex® see Busulfan . . . 212
Butabarbital Sodium . . . 213
Butacortelone see Ibuprofen . . . 703
Butalbital, Acetaminophen, and Caffeine . . . 214
Butalbital, Acetaminophen, Caffeine, and Codeine . . . 215
Butalbital, Aspirin, and Caffeine . . . 216
Butalbital, Aspirin, Caffeine, and Codeine . . . 217
Butalbital Compound see Butalbital, Aspirin, and Caffeine . . . 216
Butenafine . . . 217
Butenafine Hydrochloride see Butenafine . . . 217
Butisol Sodium® see Butabarbital Sodium . . . 213
Butoconazole . . . 218
Butoconazole Nitrate see Butoconazole . . . 218
Butorphanol . . . 218
Butorphanol Tartrate see Butorphanol . . . 218
Buvacaina® see Bupivacaine . . . 205
BW-430C see Lamotrigine . . . 774
C2B8 see Rituximab . . . 1190
C7E3 see Abciximab . . . 23
C8-CCK see Sincalide . . . 1225
311C90 see Zolmitriptan . . . 1411
C-500-GR™ [OTC] see Ascorbic Acid . . . 128
Cabergoline . . . 220
Caelyx® see DOXOrubicin (Liposomal) . . . 475
Cafergor® see Ergotamine . . . 510
Cafergot® see Ergotamine . . . 510
Caffeine, Acetaminophen, and Aspirin see Acetaminophen, Aspirin, and Caffeine . . . 34
Caffeine, Acetaminophen, Butalbital, and Codeine see Butalbital, Acetaminophen, Caffeine, and Codeine . . . 215
Caffeine and Sodium Benzoate . . . 221
Caffeine, Aspirin, and Acetaminophen see Acetaminophen, Aspirin, and Caffeine . . . 34
Caffeine, Hydrocodone, Chlorpheniramine, Phenylephrine, and Acetaminophen see Hydrocodone, Chlorpheniramine, Phenylephrine, Acetaminophen, and Caffeine . . . 686
Caffeine, Orphenadrine, and Aspirin see Orphenadrine, Aspirin, and Caffeine . . . 1005
Calan® see Verapamil . . . 1382
Calan® SR see Verapamil . . . 1382
Cal Carb-HD® [OTC] see Calcium Supplements . . . 229
Calcibind® see Cellulose Sodium Phosphate . . . 284
Calci-Chew™ [OTC] see Calcium Supplements . . . 229
Calciday-667® [OTC] see Calcium Supplements . . . 229
Calcifediol . . . 221
Calciferol™ see Ergocalciferol . . . 508
Calcijex™ see Calcitriol . . . 223
Calcimar® see Calcitonin . . . 222
Calci-Mix™ [OTC] see Calcium Supplements . . . 229
Calcipotriene . . . 222
Calcitonin . . . 222
Calcitonin (Salmon) see Calcitonin . . . 222
Cal-Citrate® 250 [OTC] see Calcium Citrate . . . 224
Cal-citrate® 250 [OTC] see Calcium Supplements . . . 229
Calcitriol . . . 223
Calcium Acetate see Calcium Supplements . . . 229
Calcium Acetate and Aluminum Sulfate see Aluminum Sulfate and Calcium Acetate . . . 70
Calcium Carbonate see Calcium Supplements . . . 229
Calcium Carbonate and Simethicone . . . 224
Calcium Carbonate, Magnesium Hydroxide, and Famotidine see Famotidine, Calcium Carbonate, and Magnesium Hydroxide . . . 557
Calcium Channel Blockers and Gingival Hyperplasia . . . 1598
Calcium Channel Blockers, Comparitive Pharmacokinetics . . . 1600
Calcium Chloride see Calcium Supplements . . . 229
Calcium Citrate . . . 224
Calcium Citrate see Calcium Supplements . . . 229
Calcium Disodium Edetate see Edetate Calcium Disodium . . . 486
Calcium Disodium Versenate® see Edetate Calcium Disodium . . . 486
Calcium EDTA see Edetate Calcium Disodium . . . 486
Calcium Glubionate . . . 225
Calcium Glubionate see Calcium Supplements . . . 229
Calcium Gluceptate . . . 226
Calcium Gluceptate see Calcium Supplements . . . 229
Calcium Gluconate see Calcium Supplements . . . 229
Calcium Lactate . . . 227
Calcium Lactate see Calcium Supplements . . . 229
Calcium Leucovorin see Leucovorin . . . 783
Calcium Pantothenate see Pantothenic Acid . . . 1033
Calcium Phosphate (Tribasic) . . . 227
Calcium Phosphate, Tribasic see Calcium Supplements . . . 229
Calcium Polycarbophil . . . 228
Calcium-Sandoz® see Calcium Glubionate . . . 225
Calcium Supplements . . . 229

CaldeCORT® [OTC] *see* Hydrocortisone ... 688
Calderol® *see* Calcifediol ... 221
Calendula ... 1424
Calendula officinalis *see* Calendula ... 1424
Calfactant ... 232
Calmylin with Codeine *see* Guaifenesin, Pseudoephedrine, and Codeine ... 653
Calphron® *see* Calcium Supplements ... 229
Cal-Plus® [OTC] *see* Calcium Supplements ... 229
Caltine® *see* Calcitonin ... 222
Caltrate® 600 [OTC] *see* Calcium Supplements ... 229
Caltrate, Jr.® [OTC] *see* Calcium Supplements ... 229
Camellia sinensis *see* Green Tea ... 1439
Camila™ *see* Norethindrone ... 986
Campath® *see* Alemtuzumab ... 52
Campath-1H *see* Alemtuzumab ... 52
Campho-Phenique® [OTC] *see* Camphor and Phenol ... 232
Camphor and Phenol ... 232
Camphorated Tincture of Opium *see* Paregoric ... 1034
Camptosar® *see* Irinotecan ... 740
Camptothecin-11 *see* Irinotecan ... 740
Canasa™ *see* Mesalamine ... 869
Cancidas® *see* Caspofungin ... 258
Candesartan ... 232
Candesartan and Hydrochlorothiazide ... 234
Candesartan Cilexetil *see* Candesartan ... 232
Candesartan Cilexetil and Hydrochlorothiazide *see* Candesartan and Hydrochlorothiazide ... 234
Candimon® *see* Clotrimazole ... 356
Candistatin® *see* Nystatin ... 992
Canef® *see* Fluvastatin ... 603
Canesten® Topical, Canesten® Vaginal *see* Clotrimazole ... 356
C. angustifolia *see* Senna ... 1215
Canthacur® *see* Cantharidin ... 234
Cantharidin ... 234
Cantharone® *see* Cantharidin ... 234
Cantil® *see* Mepenzolate ... 858
Capastat® Sulfate *see* Capreomycin ... 237
Cape *see* Aloe ... 1420
Capecitabine ... 235
Capex™ *see* Fluocinolone ... 584
Capital® and Codeine *see* Acetaminophen and Codeine ... 29
Capitral® *see* Captopril ... 238
Capitrol® *see* Chloroxine ... 306
Capoten® *see* Captopril ... 238
Capotena *see* Captopril ... 238
Capozide® *see* Captopril and Hydrochlorothiazide ... 240
Capreomycin ... 237
Capreomycin Sulfate *see* Capreomycin ... 237
Capsaicin ... 238
Capsicum annuum *see* Cayenne ... 1424
Capsicum frutescens *see* Cayenne ... 1424
Capsin® [OTC] *see* Capsaicin ... 238
Captopril ... 238
Captopril and Hydrochlorothiazide ... 240
Captral® *see* Captopril ... 238
Capzasin-P® [OTC] *see* Capsaicin ... 238
Carac™ *see* Fluorouracil ... 588
Carafate® *see* Sucralfate ... 1247
Carapres® *see* Clonidine ... 351
Carbac® *see* Loracarbef ... 821
Carbachol ... 241
Carbacholine *see* Carbachol ... 241
Carbamazepine ... 241
Carbamide *see* Urea ... 1365
Carbamide Peroxide ... 244
Carbamylcholine Chloride *see* Carbachol ... 241
Carbastat® *see* Carbachol ... 241
Carbatrol® *see* Carbamazepine ... 241
Carbaxefed DM RF *see* Carbinoxamine, Pseudoephedrine, and Dextromethorphan ... 247
Carbaxefed RF *see* Carbinoxamine and Pseudoephedrine ... 247
Carbazep® *see* Carbamazepine ... 241
Carbazina® *see* Carbamazepine ... 241
Carbecin Inyectable *see* Carbenicillin ... 245
Carbenicillin ... 245
Carbenicillin Indanyl Sodium *see* Carbenicillin ... 245
Carbetapentane and Chlorpheniramine ... 245
Carbetapentane Tannate and Chlorpheniramine Tannate *see* Carbetapentane and Chlorpheniramine ... 245
Carbidopa ... 246
Carbidopa and Levodopa *see* Levodopa and Carbidopa ... 793
Carbinoxamine and Pseudoephedrine ... 247
Carbinoxamine, Dextromethorphan, and Pseudoephedrine *see* Carbinoxamine, Pseudoephedrine, and Dextromethorphan ... 247
Carbinoxamine, Pseudoephedrine, and Dextromethorphan ... 247
Carbocaine® [DSC] *see* Mepivacaine ... 861
Carbocaine® 2% with Neo-Cobefrin® *see* Mepivacaine and Levonordefrin ... 862
Carbocaine® 3% *see* Mepivacaine Dental Anesthetic ... 863
Carbol-Fuchsin Solution ... 248
Carbolic Acid *see* Phenol ... 1068
Carbolit® *see* Lithium ... 815

Carbolith™ *see* Lithium . . . 815
Carboplat *see* Carboplatin . . . 248
Carboplatin . . . 248
Carboprost *see* Carboprost Tromethamine . . . 250
Carboprost Tromethamine . . . 250
Carboptic® *see* Carbachol . . . 241
Carbose D *see* Carboxymethylcellulose . . . 251
Carbotec® *see* Carboplatin . . . 248
Carboxymethylcellulose . . . 251
Carboxymethylcellulose Sodium *see* Carboxymethylcellulose . . . 251
Cardene® *see* NiCARdipine . . . 969
Cardene® I.V. *see* NiCARdipine . . . 969
Cardene® SR *see* NiCARdipine . . . 969
Cardinit® *see* Nitroglycerin . . . 981
Cardiorona *see* Amiodarone . . . 80
Cardiovascular Diseases . . . 1456
Cardipril® *see* Captopril . . . 238
Cardispan® *see* Levocarnitine . . . 791
Cardizem® *see* Diltiazem . . . 447
Cardizem® CD *see* Diltiazem . . . 447
Cardizem® LA *see* Diltiazem . . . 447
Cardizem® SR *see* Diltiazem . . . 447
Cardura® *see* Doxazosin . . . 470
Cardura-1™ *see* Doxazosin . . . 470
Cardura-2™ *see* Doxazosin . . . 470
Cardura-4™ *see* Doxazosin . . . 470
Carexan® *see* Itraconazole . . . 755
Carimune™ *see* Immune Globulin (Intravenous) . . . 714
Carindacillin *see* Carbenicillin . . . 245
Carisoprodate *see* Carisoprodol . . . 251
Carisoprodol . . . 251
Carisoprodol and Aspirin . . . 252
Carisoprodol, Aspirin, and Codeine . . . 252
Carmol® 10 [OTC] *see* Urea . . . 1365
Carmol® 20 [OTC] *see* Urea . . . 1365
Carmol® 40 *see* Urea . . . 1365
Carmol® Deep Cleaning *see* Urea . . . 1365
Carmol-HC® *see* Urea and Hydrocortisone . . . 1365
Carmol® Scalp *see* Sulfacetamide . . . 1249
Carmustine . . . 253
Carnitine . . . 1424
Carnitor® *see* Levocarnitine . . . 791
Carnotprim® *see* Metoclopramide . . . 898
Carnotprim Primperan® *see* Metoclopramide . . . 898
Carnotprim Primperan® Retard *see* Metoclopramide . . . 898
Carrington Antifungal [OTC] *see* Miconazole . . . 906
Carteolol . . . 254
Carteolol Hydrochloride *see* Carteolol . . . 254
Cartia XT™ *see* Diltiazem . . . 447
Cartrol® Oral *see* Carteolol . . . 254
Carvedilol . . . 256
Casanthranol and Docusate *see* Docusate and Casanthranol . . . 464
Cascara . . . 258
Cascara Sagrada *see* Cascara . . . 258
Casodex® *see* Bicalutamide . . . 183
Caspofungin . . . 258
Caspofungin Acetate *see* Caspofungin . . . 258
Cassia acutifolia *see* Senna . . . 1215
Castellani Paint *see* Carbol-Fuchsin Solution . . . 248
Castellani Paint Modified *see* Carbol-Fuchsin Solution . . . 248
Castor Oil . . . 259
Cataflam® *see* Diclofenac . . . 429
Cataflam Dispersible® *see* Diclofenac . . . 429
Catapres® *see* Clonidine . . . 351
Catapresan-100® *see* Clonidine . . . 351
Catapres-TTS®-1 *see* Clonidine . . . 351
Catapres-TTS®-2 *see* Clonidine . . . 351
Catapres-TTS®-3 *see* Clonidine . . . 351
Cathflo™ Activase® *see* Alteplase . . . 65
Cat's Claw . . . 1424
Cauteridol® *see* Ranitidine . . . 1168
Caverject® *see* Alprostadil . . . 63
Cayenne . . . 1424
CB-1348 *see* Chlorambucil . . . 296
CBDCA *see* Carboplatin . . . 248
CBZ *see* Carbamazepine . . . 241
CCNU *see* Lomustine . . . 818
2-CdA *see* Cladribine . . . 336
CDDP *see* Cisplatin . . . 332
Ceclor® *see* Cefaclor . . . 260
Ceclor® CD *see* Cefaclor . . . 260
Cecon® [OTC] *see* Ascorbic Acid . . . 128
Cedax® *see* Ceftibuten . . . 276
Cedocard®-SR *see* Isosorbide Dinitrate . . . 750
CeeNU® *see* Lomustine . . . 818
Cefaclor . . . 260
Cefadroxil . . . 261
Cefadroxil Monohydrate *see* Cefadroxil . . . 261
Cefadyl® *see* Cephapirin . . . 287
Cefamandole . . . 263

Cefamandole Nafate *see* Cefamandole . . . 263
Cefamezin *see* Cefazolin . . . 263
Cefamox® *see* Cefadroxil . . . 261
Cefaxim *see* Cefotaxime . . . 271
Cefaxona® *see* Ceftriaxone . . . 278
Cefazolin . . . 263
Cefazolin Sodium *see* Cefazolin . . . 263
Cefdinir . . . 265
Cefditoren . . . 265
Cefditoren Pivoxil *see* Cefditoren . . . 265
Cefepime . . . 267
Cefepime Hydrochloride *see* Cefepime . . . 267
Cefixime . . . 268
Cefizox® *see* Ceftizoxime . . . 277
Cefobid® *see* Cefoperazone . . . 270
Cefoclin *see* Cefotaxime . . . 271
Cefonicid . . . 269
Cefonicid Sodium *see* Cefonicid . . . 269
Cefoperazone . . . 270
Cefoperazone Sodium *see* Cefoperazone . . . 270
Cefotan® *see* Cefotetan . . . 272
Cefotaxime . . . 271
Cefotaxime Sodium *see* Cefotaxime . . . 271
Cefotetan . . . 272
Cefotetan Disodium *see* Cefotetan . . . 272
Cefoxitin . . . 272
Cefoxitin Sodium *see* Cefoxitin . . . 272
Cefpodoxime . . . 273
Cefpodoxime Proxetil *see* Cefpodoxime . . . 273
Cefprozil . . . 275
Cefradil® Claforan® *see* Cefotaxime . . . 271
Ceftazidime . . . 275
Ceftazim *see* Ceftazidime . . . 275
Ceftibuten . . . 276
Ceftin® *see* Cefuroxime . . . 279
Ceftizoxime . . . 277
Ceftizoxime Sodium *see* Ceftizoxime . . . 277
Ceftrex® *see* Ceftriaxone . . . 278
Ceftriaxone . . . 278
Ceftriaxone Sodium *see* Ceftriaxone . . . 278
Cefuracet® *see* Cefuroxime . . . 279
Cefuroxime . . . 279
Cefuroxime Axetil *see* Cefuroxime . . . 279
Cefuroxime Sodium *see* Cefuroxime . . . 279
Cefzil® *see* Cefprozil . . . 275
Celebrex® *see* Celecoxib . . . 281
Celecoxib . . . 281
Celek® 20 *see* Potassium Supplements . . . 1102
Celestoderm®-EV/2 *see* Betamethasone . . . 177
Celestoderm®-V *see* Betamethasone . . . 177
Celestone® *see* Betamethasone . . . 177
Celestone® Phosphate *see* Betamethasone . . . 177
Celestone® Soluspan® *see* Betamethasone . . . 177
Celexa™ *see* Citalopram . . . 334
CellCept® *see* Mycophenolate . . . 939
Cellufresh® [OTC] *see* Carboxymethylcellulose . . . 251
Cellulose (Oxidized) . . . 284
Cellulose (Oxidized/Regenerated) . . . 284
Cellulose Sodium Phosphate . . . 284
Celluvisc® [OTC] *see* Carboxymethylcellulose . . . 251
Celontin® *see* Methsuximide . . . 889
Cenestin® *see* Estrogens (Conjugated A/Synthetic) . . . 528
Cenestin *see* Estrogens (Conjugated/Equine) . . . 529
Centella asiatica see Gotu Kola . . . 1438
Centrum® [OTC] *see* Vitamins (Multiple/Oral) . . . 1394
Centrum® Performance™ [OTC] *see* Vitamins (Multiple/Oral) . . . 1394
Centrum® Silver® [OTC] *see* Vitamins (Multiple/Oral) . . . 1394
Cēpacol® Anesthetic Troches [OTC] *see* Cetylpyridinium and Benzocaine . . . 292
Cēpacol® Mouthwash/Gargle [OTC] *see* Cetylpyridinium . . . 292
Cēpacol Viractin® [OTC] *see* Tetracaine . . . 1284
Cēpastat® [OTC] *see* Phenol . . . 1068
Cēpastat® Extra Strength [OTC] *see* Phenol . . . 1068
Cephalexin . . . 285
Cephalexin Hydrochloride *see* Cephalexin . . . 285
Cephalexin Monohydrate *see* Cephalexin . . . 285
Cephalothin . . . 286
Cephalothin Sodium *see* Cephalothin . . . 286
Cephapirin . . . 287
Cephapirin Sodium *see* Cephapirin . . . 287
Cephradine . . . 288
Ceporex *see* Cephalexin . . . 285
Ceptaz® *see* Ceftazidime . . . 275
Cerebyx® *see* Fosphenytoin . . . 618
Ceredase® *see* Alglucerase . . . 56
Cerezyme® *see* Imiglucerase . . . 709
Cerose-DM® [OTC] *see* Chlorpheniramine, Phenylephrine, and Dextromethorphan . . . 309
Cerubidine® *see* DAUNOrubicin Hydrochloride . . . 402
Cerumenex® *see* Triethanolamine Polypeptide Oleate-Condensate . . . 1348
Cervidil® *see* Dinoprostone . . . 450
C.E.S. *see* Estrogens (Conjugated/Equine) . . . 529

Cesol® *see* Praziquantel . . . 1108
Cetacaine® *see* Benzocaine, Butyl Aminobenzoate, Tetracaine, and Benzalkonium Chloride . . . 170
Cetacort® *see* Hydrocortisone . . . 688
Cetafen® [OTC] *see* Acetaminophen . . . 27
Cetafen Extra® [OTC] *see* Acetaminophen . . . 27
Cetamide™ *see* Sulfacetamide . . . 1249
Ceta-Plus® *see* Hydrocodone and Acetaminophen . . . 678
Ceta Sulfa® *see* Sulfacetamide . . . 1249
Cetina *see* Chloramphenicol . . . 297
Cetirizine . . . 289
Cetirizine and Pseudoephedrine . . . 290
Cetirizine Hydrochloride *see* Cetirizine . . . 289
Cetirizine Hydrochloride and Pseudoephedrine Hydrochloride *see* Cetirizine and Pseudoephedrine . . . 290
Cetoxil® *see* Cefuroxime . . . 279
Cetrorelix . . . 291
Cetrorelix Acetate *see* Cetrorelix . . . 291
Cetrotide™ *see* Cetrorelix . . . 291
Cetylpyridinium . . . 292
Cetylpyridinium and Benzocaine . . . 292
Cetylpyridinium Chloride *see* Cetylpyridinium . . . 292
Cetylpyridinium Chloride and Benzocaine *see* Cetylpyridinium and Benzocaine . . . 292
Cevalin® *see* Ascorbic Acid . . . 128
Cevi-Bid® [OTC] *see* Ascorbic Acid . . . 128
Cevimeline . . . 292
Cevimeline Hydrochloride *see* Cevimeline . . . 292
Ce-Vi-Sol® *see* Ascorbic Acid . . . 128
CFDN *see* Cefdinir . . . 265
CG *see* Chorionic Gonadotropin (Human) . . . 320
CGP-42446 *see* Zoledronic Acid . . . 1410
C-Gram [OTC] *see* Ascorbic Acid . . . 128
Chamomile . . . 1425
Charcadole® *see* Charcoal . . . 294
Charcadole®, Aqueous *see* Charcoal . . . 294
Charcadole® TFS *see* Charcoal . . . 294
CharcoAid® [OTC] *see* Charcoal . . . 294
Charcoal . . . 294
Charcocaps® [OTC] *see* Charcoal . . . 294
Chasteberry . . . 1426
Chastetree *see* Chasteberry . . . 1426
Chemical Dependency and Smoking Cessation . . . 1574
Chenix® *see* Chenodiol . . . 295
Chenodeoxycholic Acid *see* Chenodiol . . . 295
Chenodiol . . . 295
Cheracol® *see* Guaifenesin and Codeine . . . 650
Cheracol® D [OTC] *see* Guaifenesin and Dextromethorphan . . . 651
Cheracol® Plus [OTC] *see* Guaifenesin and Dextromethorphan . . . 651
Cheratussin DAC *see* Guaifenesin, Pseudoephedrine, and Codeine . . . 653
Chiggerex® [OTC] *see* Benzocaine . . . 169
Chiggertox® [OTC] *see* Benzocaine . . . 169
Children's Dimetapp® Elixir Cold & Allergy [OTC] *see* Brompheniramine and Pseudoephedrine . . . 201
Children's Kaopectate® [DSC] [OTC] *see* Attapulgite . . . 146
Children's Kaopectate® (reformulation) [OTC] *see* Bismuth . . . 186
Children's Sudafed® Cough & Cold [OTC] *see* Pseudoephedrine and Dextromethorphan . . . 1147
Children's Tylenol® Cold [OTC] *see* Acetaminophen, Chlorpheniramine, and Pseudoephedrine . . . 35
Children's Tylenol® Sinus [OTC] *see* Acetaminophen and Pseudoephedrine . . . 31
Chinese angelica *see* Dong Quai . . . 1429
Chirocaine® *see* Levobupivacaine . . . 789
Chlo-Amine® [OTC] *see* Chlorpheniramine . . . 307
Chlorafed® [OTC] *see* Chlorpheniramine and Pseudoephedrine . . . 308
Chloral *see* Chloral Hydrate . . . 295
Chloral Hydrate . . . 295
Chlorambucil . . . 296
Chlorambucilum *see* Chlorambucil . . . 296
Chloraminophene *see* Chlorambucil . . . 296
Chloramphenicol . . . 297
Chloramphenicol and Prednisolone . . . 299
Chloramphenicol, Hydrocortisone, and Polymyxin B *see* Chloramphenicol, Polymyxin B, and Hydrocortisone . . . 299
Chloramphenicol, Polymyxin B, and Hydrocortisone . . . 299
ChloraPrep® [OTC] *see* Chlorhexidine Gluconate . . . 300
Chloraseptic® Gargle [OTC] *see* Phenol . . . 1068
Chloraseptic® Mouth Pain Spray [OTC] *see* Phenol . . . 1068
Chloraseptic® Rinse [OTC] *see* Phenol . . . 1068
Chloraseptic® Spray [OTC] *see* Phenol . . . 1068
Chloraseptic® Spray for Kids [OTC] *see* Phenol . . . 1068
Chlorbutinum *see* Chlorambucil . . . 296
Chlordiazepoxide . . . 299
Chlordiazepoxide and Amitriptyline *see* Amitriptyline and Chlordiazepoxide . . . 85
Chlordiazepoxide and Clidinium *see* Clidinium and Chlordiazepoxide . . . 341
Chloresium® [OTC] *see* Chlorophyll . . . 302
Chlorhexidine Gluconate . . . 300
2-Chlorodeoxyadenosine *see* Cladribine . . . 336
Chloroethane *see* Ethyl Chloride . . . 544
Chloromag® *see* Magnesium Chloride . . . 833
Chloromag® *see* Magnesium Supplements . . . 837

Chloromycetin® *see* Chloramphenicol . . . 297
Chlorophyll . . . 302
Chlorophyllin *see* Chlorophyll . . . 302
Chloroprocaine . . . 302
Chloroprocaine Hydrochloride *see* Chloroprocaine . . . 302
Chloroptic® *see* Chloramphenicol . . . 297
Chloroptic-P® *see* Chloramphenicol and Prednisolone . . . 299
Chloroquine . . . 303
Chloroquine Phosphate *see* Chloroquine . . . 303
Chlorostat® [OTC] *see* Chlorhexidine Gluconate . . . 300
Chlorothiazide . . . 304
Chlorothiazide and Methyldopa . . . 305
Chlorothiazide and Reserpine . . . 306
Chloroxine . . . 306
Chlorphenesin . . . 306
Chlorphenesin Carbamate *see* Chlorphenesin . . . 306
Chlorpheniramine . . . 307
Chlorpheniramine, Acetaminophen, and Pseudoephedrine *see* Acetaminophen, Chlorpheniramine, and Pseudoephedrine . . . 35
Chlorpheniramine and Acetaminophen . . . 308
Chlorpheniramine and Carbetapentane *see* Carbetapentane and Chlorpheniramine . . . 245
Chlorpheniramine and Hydrocodone *see* Hydrocodone and Chlorpheniramine . . . 682
Chlorpheniramine and Phenylephrine . . . 308
Chlorpheniramine and Pseudoephedrine . . . 308
Chlorpheniramine, Ephedrine, Phenylephrine, and Carbetapentane . . . 309
Chlorpheniramine, Hydrocodone, Phenylephrine, Acetaminophen, and Caffeine *see* Hydrocodone, Chlorpheniramine, Phenylephrine, Acetaminophen, and Caffeine . . . 686
Chlorpheniramine Maleate *see* Chlorpheniramine . . . 307
Chlorpheniramine, Phenylephrine, and Dextromethorphan . . . 309
Chlorpheniramine, Phenylephrine, and Methscopolamine . . . 310
Chlorpheniramine, Phenylephrine, and Phenyltoloxamine . . . 311
Chlorpheniramine, Phenylephrine, Codeine, and Potassium Iodide . . . 311
Chlorpheniramine, Pseudoephedrine, and Acetaminophen *see* Acetaminophen, Chlorpheniramine, and Pseudoephedrine . . . 35
Chlorpheniramine, Pseudoephedrine, and Codeine . . . 311
Chlorpheniramine, Pyrilamine, and Phenylephrine . . . 312
ChlorproMAZINE . . . 312
Chlorpromazine Hydrochloride *see* ChlorproMAZINE . . . 312
ChlorproPAMIDE . . . 314
Chlorthalidone . . . 315
Chlorthalidone and Atenolol *see* Atenolol and Chlorthalidone . . . 138
Chlorthalidone and Clonidine *see* Clonidine and Chlorthalidone . . . 353
Chlor-Trimeton® [OTC] *see* Chlorpheniramine . . . 307
Chlor-Trimeton® Allergy/Decongestant [OTC] *see* Chlorpheniramine and Pseudoephedrine . . . 308
Chlor-Tripolon® *see* Chlorpheniramine . . . 307
Chlor-Tripolon ND® *see* Loratadine and Pseudoephedrine . . . 823
Chlorzoxazone . . . 316
Cholac® *see* Lactulose . . . 772
Cholecalciferol . . . 317
Cholera Vaccine . . . 317
Cholestyramine Resin . . . 318
Choline Magnesium Trisalicylate . . . 319
Choline Salicylate . . . 319
Chondroitin Sulfate . . . 1426
Chondroitin Sulfate and Sodium Hyaluronate . . . 320
Chooz® [OTC] *see* Calcium Supplements . . . 229
Chorex® *see* Chorionic Gonadotropin (Human) . . . 320
Choriogonadotropin Alfa *see* Chorionic Gonadotropin (Recombinant) . . . 321
Chorionic Gonadotropin (Human) . . . 320
Chorionic Gonadotropin (Recombinant) . . . 321
Choron® *see* Chorionic Gonadotropin (Human) . . . 320
Chromium . . . 1426
Chromium *see* Trace Metals . . . 1328
Chronovera® *see* Verapamil . . . 1382
Chymodiactin® *see* Chymopapain . . . 322
Chymopapain . . . 322
Cicloferon® *see* Acyclovir . . . 42
Ciclopirox . . . 322
Ciclopirox Olamine *see* Ciclopirox . . . 322
Cidofovir . . . 323
Cilag® *see* Acetaminophen . . . 27
Cilazapril . . . 324
Cilazapril Monohydrate *see* Cilazapril . . . 324
Cilostazol . . . 325
Ciloxan® *see* Ciprofloxacin . . . 328
Cilpen® *see* Dicloxacillin . . . 432
Cimetase® *see* Cimetidine . . . 326
Cimetidine . . . 326
Cimetigal *see* Cimetidine . . . 326
Cimicifuga racemosa *see* Black Cohosh . . . 1423
Cimogal® *see* Ciprofloxacin . . . 328
Cinobac® *see* Cinoxacin . . . 327
Cinoxacin . . . 327
Cipro® *see* Ciprofloxacin . . . 328
Ciprobiotic® *see* Ciprofloxacin . . . 328
Ciproflox® *see* Ciprofloxacin . . . 328
Ciprofloxacin . . . 328
Ciprofloxacin and Hydrocortisone . . . 331
Ciprofloxacin Hydrochloride *see* Ciprofloxacin . . . 328

Ciprofur® *see* Ciprofloxacin . . . 328
Cipro® HC *see* Ciprofloxacin and Hydrocortisone . . . 331
Cipro® HC Otic *see* Ciprofloxacin and Hydrocortisone . . . 331
Ciproxina® *see* Ciprofloxacin . . . 328
Cipro® XR *see* Ciprofloxacin . . . 328
Cisapride . . . 332
Cisplatin . . . 332
13-*cis*-Retinoic Acid *see* Isotretinoin . . . 752
Cisticid® *see* Praziquantel . . . 1108
Citalgan® *see* Ibuprofen . . . 703
Citalopram . . . 334
Citalopram Hydrobromide *see* Citalopram . . . 334
Citanest® Forte *see* Prilocaine . . . 1114
Citanest® Forte *see* Prilocaine and Epinephrine . . . 1116
Citanest Octapressin® *see* Prilocaine . . . 1114
Citanest® Plain *see* Prilocaine . . . 1114
Citax *see* Immune Globulin (Intravenous) . . . 714
Citoken® Dixonal® *see* Piroxicam . . . 1090
Citomid® *see* VinCRIStine . . . 1387
Citracal® [OTC] *see* Calcium Citrate . . . 224
Citracal® [OTC] *see* Calcium Supplements . . . 229
Citrate of Magnesia *see* Magnesium Citrate . . . 834
Citrate of Magnesia (Magnesium Citrate) *see* Magnesium Supplements . . . 837
Citric Acid and d-gluconic Acid Irrigant *see* Citric Acid Bladder Mixture . . . 335
Citric Acid and Potassium Citrate *see* Potassium Citrate and Citric Acid . . . 1101
Citric Acid Bladder Mixture . . . 335
Citric Acid, Magnesium Hydroxycarbonate, D-Gluconic Acid, Magnesium Acid Citrate, and Calcium Carbonate *see* Citric Acid Bladder Mixture . . . 335
Citric Acid, Sodium Citrate, and Potassium Citrate . . . 335
Citro-Mag® *see* Magnesium Citrate . . . 834
Citrovorum Factor *see* Leucovorin . . . 783
Citrucel® [OTC] *see* Methylcellulose . . . 891
Citrus paradisi *see* Grapefruit Seed . . . 1438
CI-719 *see* Gemfibrozil . . . 631
CL184116 *see* Porfimer . . . 1098
Cla *see* Clarithromycin . . . 337
Cladribine . . . 336
Claforan® *see* Cefotaxime . . . 271
Clanda® *see* Vitamins (Multiple/Oral) . . . 1394
Clarinex® *see* Desloratadine . . . 410
Claripel™ *see* Hydroquinone . . . 693
Clarithromycin . . . 337
Claritin® *see* Loratadine . . . 822
Claritin® Allergic Decongestant *see* Oxymetazoline . . . 1022
Claritin-D® 12-Hour [OTC] *see* Loratadine and Pseudoephedrine . . . 823
Claritin-D® 24-Hour [OTC] *see* Loratadine and Pseudoephedrine . . . 823
Claritin® Extra *see* Loratadine and Pseudoephedrine . . . 823
Claritin® Kids *see* Loratadine . . . 822
Claritin® Liberator *see* Loratadine and Pseudoephedrine . . . 823
Clarityne® *see* Loratadine . . . 822
Clavulin® *see* Amoxicillin and Clavulanate Potassium . . . 95
Clear Eyes® [OTC] *see* Naphazoline . . . 952
Clear Eyes® ACR [OTC] *see* Naphazoline . . . 952
Clemastine . . . 340
Clemastine Fumarate *see* Clemastine . . . 340
Cleocin® *see* Clindamycin . . . 341
Cleocin HCl® *see* Clindamycin . . . 341
Cleocin Pediatric® *see* Clindamycin . . . 341
Cleocin Phosphate® *see* Clindamycin . . . 341
Cleocin T® *see* Clindamycin . . . 341
Clexane® *see* Enoxaparin . . . 495
Clidinium and Chlordiazepoxide . . . 341
Climacteron® *see* Estradiol and Testosterone . . . 527
Climaderm® *see* Estradiol . . . 521
Climara® *see* Estradiol . . . 521
Clinac™ BPO *see* Benzoyl Peroxide . . . 171
Clindagel™ *see* Clindamycin . . . 341
Clindamycin . . . 341
Clindamycin and Benzoyl Peroxide . . . 343
Clindamycin Hydrochloride *see* Clindamycin . . . 341
Clindamycin Phosphate *see* Clindamycin . . . 341
Clindazyn® *see* Clindamycin . . . 341
Clindets® *see* Clindamycin . . . 341
Clinoril® *see* Sulindac . . . 1257
Clobazam . . . 344
Clobetasol . . . 345
Clobetasol Propionate *see* Clobetasol . . . 345
Clocort™ *see* Hydrocortisone . . . 688
Clocortolone . . . 345
Clocortolone Pivalate *see* Clocortolone . . . 345
Clocream [OTC] *see* Vitamin A and Vitamin D . . . 1392
Cloderm® *see* Clocortolone . . . 345
Clofazimine . . . 346
Clofazimine Palmitate *see* Clofazimine . . . 346
Clofibrate . . . 347
Clomid® *see* ClomiPHENE . . . 348
ClomiPHENE . . . 348
Clomiphene Citrate *see* ClomiPHENE . . . 348
ClomiPRAMINE . . . 349
Clomipramine Hydrochloride *see* ClomiPRAMINE . . . 349

Clonapam *see* Clonazepam 350
Clonazepam 350
Clonidine 351
Clonidine and Chlorthalidone 353
Clonidine Hydrochloride *see* Clonidine 351
Clonodifen® *see* Diclofenac 429
Clopidogrel 353
Clopidogrel Bisulfate *see* Clopidogrel 353
Clopsine® *see* Clozapine 358
Clorafen® *see* Chloramphenicol 297
Cloramfeni® *see* Chloramphenicol 297
Cloran® *see* Chloramphenicol 297
Clorazepate 355
Clorazepate Dipotassium *see* Clorazepate 355
Clordil® *see* Chloramphenicol 297
Clorimet® *see* Metoclopramide 898
Clor-K-Zaf® *see* Potassium Supplements 1102
Clorpactin® WCS-90 [OTC] *see* Oxychlorosene 1017
Cloruro® De Potasio Kaliolite® *see* Potassium Supplements 1102
Clostedal® *see* Carbamazepine 241
Clotrimaderm *see* Clotrimazole 356
Clotrimazole 356
Clotrimazole and Betamethasone *see* Betamethasone and Clotrimazole 179
Cloxacillin 357
Cloxacillin Sodium *see* Cloxacillin 357
Cloxapen® *see* Cloxacillin 357
Clozapine 358
Clozaril® *see* Clozapine 358
CoActifed® *see* Triprolidine, Pseudoephedrine, and Codeine 1357
Coagulant Complex Inhibitor *see* Anti-inhibitor Coagulant Complex 116
Coagulation Factor VIIa *see* Factor VIIa (Recombinant) 554
Coal Tar 359
Coal Tar and Salicylic Acid 359
Coal Tar, Lanolin, and Mineral Oil 360
Coal Tar, Mineral Oil, and Lanolin *see* Coal Tar, Lanolin, and Mineral Oil 360
Cocaine 360
Cocaine Hydrochloride *see* Cocaine 360
Codafed® Expectorant *see* Guaifenesin, Pseudoephedrine, and Codeine 653
Codafed® Pediatric Expectorant *see* Guaifenesin, Pseudoephedrine, and Codeine 653
Codehist® DH *see* Chlorpheniramine, Pseudoephedrine, and Codeine 311
Codeine 361
Codeine, Acetaminophen, Butalbital, and Caffeine *see* Butalbital, Acetaminophen, Caffeine, and Codeine 215
Codeine and Acetaminophen *see* Acetaminophen and Codeine 29
Codeine and Aspirin *see* Aspirin and Codeine 134
Codeine and Bromodiphenhydramine *see* Bromodiphenhydramine and Codeine 200
Codeine and Butalbital Compound *see* Butalbital, Aspirin, Caffeine, and Codeine 217
Codeine and Guaifenesin *see* Guaifenesin and Codeine 650
Codeine and Promethazine *see* Promethazine and Codeine 1129
Codeine, Aspirin, and Carisoprodol *see* Carisoprodol, Aspirin, and Codeine 252
Codeine, Butalbital, Aspirin, and Caffeine *see* Butalbital, Aspirin, Caffeine, and Codeine . . 217
Codeine, Guaifenesin, and Pseudoephedrine *see* Guaifenesin, Pseudoephedrine, and Codeine 653
Codeine Phosphate *see* Codeine 361
Codeine, Promethazine, and Phenylephrine *see* Promethazine, Phenylephrine, and Codeine 1130
Codeine, Pseudoephedrine, and Triprolidine *see* Triprolidine, Pseudoephedrine, and Codeine 1357
Codeine Sulfate *see* Codeine 361
Codiclear® DH *see* Hydrocodone and Guaifenesin 683
Codimal-LA® [OTC] *see* Chlorpheniramine and Pseudoephedrine 308
Codimal-LA® Half [OTC] *see* Chlorpheniramine and Pseudoephedrine 308
Cod Liver Oil *see* Vitamin A and Vitamin D 1392
Coenzyme 1 *see* Nicotinamide Adenine Dinucleotide 1445
Coenzyme Q_{10} 1427
CO Fluoxetine *see* Fluoxetine 589
Cogentin® *see* Benztropine 173
Co-Gesic® *see* Hydrocodone and Acetaminophen 678
Cognex® *see* Tacrine 1260
Colace® [OTC] *see* Docusate 463
Colax-C® *see* Docusate 463
ColBenemid® [DSC] *see* Colchicine and Probenecid 364
Colchicine 363
Colchicine and Probenecid 364
Colchiquim® *see* Colchicine 363
Colchiquim-30 *see* Colchicine 363
Colesevelam 365
Colestid® *see* Colestipol 365
Colestipol 365
Colestipol Hydrochloride *see* Colestipol 365
Colfosceril Palmitate 366
Colgate Total® Toothpaste *see* Triclosan and Fluoride 1348
Colistimethate 366
Colistimethate Sodium *see* Colistimethate 366
Colistin, Neomycin, and Hydrocortisone 367
CollaCote® *see* Collagen (Absorbable) 367
Collagen *see* Microfibrillar Collagen Hemostat 907
Collagen (Absorbable) 367
Collagenase 367
CollaPlug® *see* Collagen (Absorbable) 367

CollaTape® *see* Collagen (Absorbable) . . . 367
Colo-Fresh™ [OTC] *see* Bismuth . . . 186
Columina *see* Cimetidine . . . 326
Coly-Mycin® M *see* Colistimethate . . . 366
Coly-Mycin® S Otic *see* Colistin, Neomycin, and Hydrocortisone . . . 367
Colyte® *see* Polyethylene Glycol-Electrolyte Solution . . . 1094
Combantrin™ *see* Pyrantel Pamoate . . . 1150
Comb Flower *see* *Echinacea* . . . 1429
Combination Hormonal Contraceptives . . . 368
CombiPatch® *see* Estradiol and Norethindrone . . . 525
Combipres® *see* Clonidine and Chlorthalidone . . . 353
Combivent® *see* Ipratropium and Albuterol . . . 738
Combivir® *see* Lamivudine . . . 773
Combivir® *see* Zidovudine . . . 1406
Combivir® *see* Zidovudine and Lamivudine . . . 1407
Comhist® *see* Chlorpheniramine, Phenylephrine, and Phenyltoloxamine . . . 311
Comhist® LA *see* Chlorpheniramine, Phenylephrine, and Phenyltoloxamine . . . 311
Commit™ [OTC] *see* Nicotine . . . 971
Compazine® *see* Prochlorperazine . . . 1123
Comphor of the Poor *see* Garlic . . . 1433
Complan *see* Vitamins (Multiple/Oral) . . . 1394
Compound E *see* Cortisone Acetate . . . 373
Compound F *see* Hydrocortisone . . . 688
Compound S *see* Zidovudine . . . 1406
Compound S, Abacavir, and Lamivudine *see* Abacavir, Lamivudine, and Zidovudine . . . 23
Compound W® [OTC] *see* Salicylic Acid . . . 1204
Compound W® One Step Wart Remover [OTC] *see* Salicylic Acid . . . 1204
Compoz® Nighttime Sleep Aid [OTC] *see* DiphenhydrAMINE . . . 451
Compro™ *see* Prochlorperazine . . . 1123
Comtan® *see* Entacapone . . . 497
Comtrex® Allergy-Sinus [OTC] *see* Acetaminophen, Chlorpheniramine, and Pseudoephedrine . . . 35
Comtrex® Non-Drowsy Cough and Cold [OTC] *see* Acetaminophen, Dextromethorphan, and Pseudoephedrine . . . 35
Conazol® *see* Ketoconazole . . . 762
Conceptrol® [OTC] *see* Nonoxynol 9 . . . 985
Concerta® *see* Methylphenidate . . . 893
Condyline™ *see* Podofilox . . . 1093
Condylox® *see* Podofilox . . . 1093
Congest *see* Estrogens (Conjugated/Equine) . . . 529
Congestac® *see* Guaifenesin and Pseudoephedrine . . . 652
Conjugated Estrogen and Methyltestosterone *see* Estrogens (Esterified) and Methyltestosterone . . . 534
Constilac® *see* Lactulose . . . 772
Constulose® *see* Lactulose . . . 772
Consupren *see* CycloSPORINE . . . 383
Contac® Cold 12 Hour Relief Non Drowsy *see* Pseudoephedrine . . . 1146
Contac® Cough, Cold and Flu Day & Night™ *see* Acetaminophen, Dextromethorphan, and Pseudoephedrine . . . 35
Contac® Severe Cold and Flu/Non-Drowsy [OTC] *see* Acetaminophen, Dextromethorphan, and Pseudoephedrine . . . 35
Controlip® *see* Fenofibrate . . . 561
Controlled Substances . . . 12
Copal® *see* Sulindac . . . 1257
Copaxone® *see* Glatiramer Acetate . . . 636
Copegus™ *see* Ribavirin . . . 1176
Copolymer-1 *see* Glatiramer Acetate . . . 636
Copper *see* Trace Metals . . . 1328
Co-Pyronil® 2 Pulvules® [OTC] *see* Chlorpheniramine and Pseudoephedrine . . . 308
CoQ_{10} *see* Coenzyme Q_{10} . . . 1427
Cordarone® *see* Amiodarone . . . 80
Cordran® *see* Flurandrenolide . . . 594
Cordran® SP *see* Flurandrenolide . . . 594
Coreg® *see* Carvedilol . . . 256
Corgard® *see* Nadolol . . . 943
Coricidin® [OTC] *see* Chlorpheniramine and Acetaminophen . . . 308
Corlopam® *see* Fenoldopam . . . 562
Cormax® *see* Clobetasol . . . 345
Corogal *see* NIFEdipine . . . 973
Coronex® *see* Isosorbide Dinitrate . . . 750
Corotrend® *see* NIFEdipine . . . 973
Corotrend Retard *see* NIFEdipine . . . 973
CortaGel® Maximum Strength [OTC] *see* Hydrocortisone . . . 688
Cortaid® Intensive Therapy [OTC] *see* Hydrocortisone . . . 688
Cortaid® Maximum Strength [OTC] *see* Hydrocortisone . . . 688
Cortaid® Sensitive Skin With Aloe [OTC] *see* Hydrocortisone . . . 688
Cortamed® *see* Hydrocortisone . . . 688
Cortate® *see* Hydrocortisone . . . 688
Cortef® *see* Hydrocortisone . . . 688
Cortenema® *see* Hydrocortisone . . . 688
Corticool® [OTC] *see* Hydrocortisone . . . 688
Corticotropin . . . 372
Corticotropin, Repository *see* Corticotropin . . . 372
Cortifoam® *see* Hydrocortisone . . . 688
Cortimyxin® *see* Neomycin and Polymyxin B . . . 962
Cortimyxin® *see* Neomycin, Polymyxin B, and Hydrocortisone . . . 963
Cortisol *see* Hydrocortisone . . . 688
Cortisone Acetate . . . 373
Cortisporin® *see* Bacitracin, Neomycin, Polymyxin B, and Hydrocortisone . . . 158
Cortisporin® *see* Neomycin, Polymyxin B, and Hydrocortisone . . . 963

Cortisporin® Cream *see* Neomycin, Polymyxin B, and Hydrocortisone . . . 963
Cortisporin® Ointment *see* Bacitracin, Neomycin, Polymyxin B, and Hydrocortisone . . . 158
Cortisporin® Ophthalmic *see* Neomycin, Polymyxin B, and Hydrocortisone . . . 963
Cortisporin® Otic *see* Neomycin, Polymyxin B, and Hydrocortisone . . . 963
Cortisporin®-TC Otic *see* Colistin, Neomycin, and Hydrocortisone . . . 367
Cortizone®-5 [OTC] *see* Hydrocortisone . . . 688
Cortizone®-10 Maximum Strength [OTC] *see* Hydrocortisone . . . 688
Cortizone®-10 Plus Maximum Strength [OTC] *see* Hydrocortisone . . . 688
Cortizone® 10 Quick Shot [OTC] *see* Hydrocortisone . . . 688
Cortizone® for Kids [OTC] *see* Hydrocortisone . . . 688
Cortoderm *see* Hydrocortisone . . . 688
Cortone® *see* Cortisone Acetate . . . 373
Cortrosyn® *see* Cosyntropin . . . 374
Corvert® *see* Ibutilide . . . 706
Coryphen® Codeine *see* Aspirin and Codeine . . . 134
Cosmegen® *see* Dactinomycin . . . 393
Cosyntropin . . . 374
Cotazym® *see* Pancrelipase . . . 1030
Co-Trimoxazole *see* Sulfamethoxazole and Trimethoprim . . . 1253
Coumadin® *see* Warfarin . . . 1397
Covera® *see* Verapamil . . . 1382
Covera-HS® *see* Verapamil . . . 1382
Coversyl® *see* Perindopril Erbumine . . . 1060
Cozaar® *see* Losartan . . . 825
CP-99,219-27 *see* Trovafloxacin/Alatrofloxacin . . . 1361
CPM *see* Cyclophosphamide . . . 381
CPT-11 *see* Irinotecan . . . 740
CPZ *see* ChlorproMAZINE . . . 312
Cranberry . . . 1427
Crataegus laevigata see Hawthorn . . . 1440
Crataegus monogyna see Hawthorn . . . 1440
Crataegus oxyacantha see Hawthorn . . . 1440
Crataegus pinnatifida see Hawthorn . . . 1440
Creatine . . . 1427
Credaxol® *see* Ranitidine . . . 1168
Crema Blanca® *see* Hydroquinone . . . 693
Crema Blanca Bustillos *see* Hydroquinone . . . 693
Cremosan® *see* Ketoconazole . . . 762
Creomulsion® Cough [OTC] *see* Dextromethorphan . . . 423
Creomulsion® for Children [OTC] *see* Dextromethorphan . . . 423
Creon® *see* Pancreatin . . . 1030
Creon® *see* Pancrelipase . . . 1030
Creon® 5 *see* Pancrelipase . . . 1030
Creon® 10 *see* Pancrelipase . . . 1030
Creon® 20 *see* Pancrelipase . . . 1030
Creon® 25 *see* Pancrelipase . . . 1030
Creo-Terpin® [OTC] *see* Dextromethorphan . . . 423
Crestor® *see* Rosuvastatin . . . 1201
Cresylate® *see* m-Cresyl Acetate . . . 844
Crinone® *see* Progesterone . . . 1125
Crinone® V *see* Progesterone . . . 1125
Critic-Aid Skin Care® [OTC] *see* Zinc Oxide . . . 1409
Crixivan® *see* Indinavir . . . 718
Crolom® *see* Cromolyn Sodium . . . 375
Cromoglycic Acid *see* Cromolyn Sodium . . . 375
Cromolyn Sodium . . . 375
Cronovera® *see* Verapamil . . . 1382
Crotamiton . . . 376
Crude Coal Tar *see* Coal Tar . . . 359
Cruex® [OTC] *see* Clotrimazole . . . 356
Cryocriptina *see* Bromocriptine . . . 199
Cryoperacid® *see* Loperamide . . . 819
Cryopril® *see* Captopril . . . 238
Cryosolona *see* MethylPREDNISolone . . . 895
Cryoval® *see* Valproic Acid and Derivatives . . . 1371
Cryoxifeno *see* Tamoxifen . . . 1264
Cryselle™ *see* Combination Hormonal Contraceptives . . . 368
Crystalline Penicillin *see* Penicillin G (Parenteral/Aqueous) . . . 1049
Crystal Violet *see* Gentian Violet . . . 636
Crystamine® *see* Cyanocobalamin . . . 377
Crysti 1000® *see* Cyanocobalamin . . . 377
Crystodigin® [DSC] *see* Digitoxin . . . 440
CSA *see* CycloSPORINE . . . 383
CSP *see* Cellulose Sodium Phosphate . . . 284
CTM *see* Chlorpheniramine . . . 307
CTX *see* Cyclophosphamide . . . 381
Cuprimine® *see* Penicillamine . . . 1046
Curcuma longa see Turmeric . . . 1448
Curosurf® *see* Poractant Alfa . . . 1097
Cutacelan® *see* Azelaic Acid . . . 151
Cutaclin® *see* Clindamycin . . . 341
Cutivate® *see* Fluticasone . . . 599
CyA *see* CycloSPORINE . . . 383
Cyanocobalamin . . . 377
Cyanocobalamin, Folic Acid, and Pyridoxine *see* Folic Acid, Cyanocobalamin, and Pyridoxine . . . 607
Cyanoject® *see* Cyanocobalamin . . . 377
Cyclandelate . . . 378
Cyclessa® *see* Combination Hormonal Contraceptives . . . 368
Cyclizine . . . 379

Cyclizine Hydrochloride *see* Cyclizine . . . 379
Cyclizine Lactate *see* Cyclizine . . . 379
Cyclobenzaprine . . . 379
Cyclobenzaprine Hydrochloride *see* Cyclobenzaprine . . . 379
Cyclocort® *see* Amcinonide . . . 72
Cyclogyl® *see* Cyclopentolate . . . 380
Cyclomen® *see* Danazol . . . 397
Cyclomydril® *see* Cyclopentolate and Phenylephrine . . . 381
Cyclopentolate . . . 380
Cyclopentolate and Phenylephrine . . . 381
Cyclopentolate Hydrochloride *see* Cyclopentolate . . . 380
Cyclophosphamide . . . 381
CycloSERINE . . . 383
Cyclosporin A *see* CycloSPORINE . . . 383
CycloSPORINE . . . 383
Cycrin® *see* MedroxyPROGESTERone . . . 849
Cyklokapron® *see* Tranexamic Acid . . . 1333
Cylert® *see* Pemoline . . . 1044
Cylex® [OTC] *see* Benzocaine . . . 169
Cymevene® *see* Ganciclovir . . . 626
Cyomin® *see* Cyanocobalamin . . . 377
Cyproheptadine . . . 387
Cyproheptadine Hydrochloride *see* Cyproheptadine . . . 387
Cystadane® *see* Betaine Anhydrous . . . 177
Cystagon® *see* Cysteamine . . . 388
Cysteamine . . . 388
Cysteamine Bitartrate *see* Cysteamine . . . 388
Cysteine . . . 388
Cysteine Hydrochloride *see* Cysteine . . . 388
Cystistat® *see* Sodium Hyaluronate . . . 1230
Cystospaz® *see* Hyoscyamine . . . 699
Cystospaz-M® *see* Hyoscyamine . . . 699
CYT *see* Cyclophosphamide . . . 381
Cytadren® *see* Aminoglutethimide . . . 77
Cytarabine . . . 389
Cytarabine Hydrochloride *see* Cytarabine . . . 389
Cytarabine (Liposomal) . . . 390
Cytomel® *see* Liothyronine . . . 810
Cytosar® *see* Cytarabine . . . 389
Cytosar-U® *see* Cytarabine . . . 389
Cytosine Arabinosine Hydrochloride *see* Cytarabine . . . 389
Cytotec® *see* Misoprostol . . . 920
Cytovene® *see* Ganciclovir . . . 626
Cytoxan® *see* Cyclophosphamide . . . 381
Cytra-2 *see* Sodium Citrate and Citric Acid . . . 1230
Cytra-3 *see* Citric Acid, Sodium Citrate, and Potassium Citrate . . . 335
Cytra-K *see* Potassium Citrate and Citric Acid . . . 1101
D_3 *see* Cholecalciferol . . . 317
D-3-Mercaptovaline *see* Penicillamine . . . 1046
d4T *see* Stavudine . . . 1242
Dabex® *see* Metformin . . . 874
Dacarbazine . . . 391
Daclizumab . . . 392
DACT *see* Dactinomycin . . . 393
Dactinomycin . . . 393
Dafloxen® *see* Naproxen . . . 953
D.A.II™ *see* Chlorpheniramine, Phenylephrine, and Methscopolamine . . . 310
Dairyaid® *see* Lactase . . . 771
Dakin's Solution *see* Sodium Hypochlorite Solution . . . 1231
Daktarin® *see* Miconazole . . . 906
Dalacin C® *see* Clindamycin . . . 341
Dalacin T® *see* Clindamycin . . . 341
Dalacin V® *see* Clindamycin . . . 341
Dalacin® Vaginal *see* Clindamycin . . . 341
Dalisol *see* Leucovorin . . . 783
Dallergy® *see* Chlorpheniramine, Phenylephrine, and Methscopolamine . . . 310
Dallergy-D® *see* Chlorpheniramine and Phenylephrine . . . 308
Dalmane® *see* Flurazepam . . . 595
d-Alpha Tocopherol *see* Vitamin E . . . 1393
Dalteparin . . . 394
Damason-P® *see* Hydrocodone and Aspirin . . . 680
Danaparoid . . . 395
Danaparoid Sodium *see* Danaparoid . . . 395
Danazol . . . 397
Danocrine® *see* Danazol . . . 397
Dantrium® *see* Dantrolene . . . 398
Dantrolene . . . 398
Dantrolene Sodium *see* Dantrolene . . . 398
Daonil® *see* GlyBURIDE . . . 642
Dapiprazole . . . 399
Dapiprazole Hydrochloride *see* Dapiprazole . . . 399
Dapsoderm-X® *see* Dapsone . . . 399
Dapsone . . . 399
Daranide® *see* Dichlorphenamide . . . 428
Daraprim® *see* Pyrimethamine . . . 1152
Darbepoetin Alfa . . . 400
Darvocet-N® 50 *see* Propoxyphene and Acetaminophen . . . 1136
Darvocet-N® 100 *see* Propoxyphene and Acetaminophen . . . 1136
Darvon® *see* Propoxyphene . . . 1135
Darvon® Compound-65 Pulvules® *see* Propoxyphene and Aspirin . . . 1137

Darvon-N® *see* Propoxyphene . . . 1135
Datril® *see* Acetaminophen . . . 27
Daunomycin *see* DAUNOrubicin Hydrochloride . . . 402
DAUNOrubicin Citrate (Liposomal) . . . 402
DAUNOrubicin Hydrochloride . . . 402
DaunoXome® *see* DAUNOrubicin Citrate (Liposomal) . . . 402
1-Day™ [OTC] *see* Tioconazole . . . 1312
Daypro® *see* Oxaprozin . . . 1010
Days® *see* Ibuprofen . . . 703
DCF *see* Pentostatin . . . 1057
DDAVP® *see* Desmopressin . . . 410
ddC *see* Zalcitabine . . . 1403
ddI *see* Didanosine . . . 434
1-Deamino-8-D-Arginine Vasopressin *see* Desmopressin . . . 410
Deavynfar *see* ChlorproPAMIDE . . . 314
Debacterol® *see* Sulfonated Phenolics in Aqueous Solution . . . 1257
Debrox® Otic [OTC] *see* Carbamide Peroxide . . . 244
Decadron® *see* Dexamethasone . . . 413
Decadronal® *see* Dexamethasone . . . 413
Decadron® Phosphate *see* Dexamethasone . . . 413
Deca-Durabolin® *see* Nandrolone . . . 951
Decaris® *see* Levamisole . . . 786
Declomycin® *see* Demeclocycline . . . 406
Decofed® [OTC] *see* Pseudoephedrine . . . 1146
Decohistine® DH *see* Chlorpheniramine, Pseudoephedrine, and Codeine . . . 311
Deconamine® [OTC] *see* Chlorpheniramine and Pseudoephedrine . . . 308
Deconamine® SR [OTC] *see* Chlorpheniramine and Pseudoephedrine . . . 308
Decongest *see* Xylometazoline . . . 1401
Deconsal® II *see* Guaifenesin and Pseudoephedrine . . . 652
Decorex *see* Dexamethasone . . . 413
Defen-LA® *see* Guaifenesin and Pseudoephedrine . . . 652
Deferoxamine . . . 404
Deferoxamine Mesylate *see* Deferoxamine . . . 404
Deflox® *see* Diclofenac . . . 429
Dehydral® *see* Methenamine . . . 879
Dehydrobenzperidol® *see* Droperidol . . . 481
Dehydroepiandrosterone . . . 1427
Del Aqua® *see* Benzoyl Peroxide . . . 171
Delatestryl® *see* Testosterone . . . 1281
Delavirdine . . . 405
Delestrogen® *see* Estradiol . . . 521
Delfen® [OTC] *see* Nonoxynol 9 . . . 985
Delsym® [OTC] *see* Dextromethorphan . . . 423
Delta-9-tetrahydro-cannabinol *see* Dronabinol . . . 480
Delta-9 THC *see* Dronabinol . . . 480
Deltacortisone *see* PredniSONE . . . 1112
Delta-D® *see* Cholecalciferol . . . 317
Deltadehydrocortisone *see* PredniSONE . . . 1112
Deltahydrocortisone *see* PrednisoLONE . . . 1110
Deltasone® *see* PredniSONE . . . 1112
Demadex® *see* Torsemide . . . 1327
Demeclocycline . . . 406
Demeclocycline Hydrochloride *see* Demeclocycline . . . 406
Demerol® *see* Meperidine . . . 858
4-demethoxydaunorubicin *see* Idarubicin . . . 706
Demethylchlortetracycline *see* Demeclocycline . . . 406
Demolox *see* Amoxapine . . . 91
Demser® *see* Metyrosine . . . 905
Demulen® *see* Combination Hormonal Contraceptives . . . 368
Denavir® *see* Penciclovir . . . 1046
Denileukin Diftitox . . . 407
Denorex® [OTC] *see* Coal Tar . . . 359
Dental Office Emergencies . . . 1582
Dentifrice Products . . . 1619
Dentin Hypersensitivity, High Caries Index, and Xerostomia . . . 1553
DentiPatch® *see* Lidocaine (Transoral) . . . 807
Dentist's Role in Recognizing Domestic Violence . . . 1572
Denture Adhesive Products . . . 1628
Denture Cleanser Products . . . 1629
Denvar® *see* Cefixime . . . 268
Deoxycoformycin *see* Pentostatin . . . 1057
2′-deoxycoformycin *see* Pentostatin . . . 1057
Depacon® *see* Valproic Acid and Derivatives . . . 1371
Depakene® *see* Valproic Acid and Derivatives . . . 1371
Depakote® Delayed Release *see* Valproic Acid and Derivatives . . . 1371
Depakote® ER *see* Valproic Acid and Derivatives . . . 1371
Depakote® Sprinkle® *see* Valproic Acid and Derivatives . . . 1371
Depen® *see* Penicillamine . . . 1046
DepoCyt™ *see* Cytarabine (Liposomal) . . . 390
Depo®-Estradiol *see* Estradiol . . . 521
Depo-Medrol® *see* MethylPREDNISolone . . . 895
Deponit® [DSC] *see* Nitroglycerin . . . 981
Depo-Prevera® *see* MedroxyPROGESTERone . . . 849
Depo-Provera® *see* MedroxyPROGESTERone . . . 849
Depo-Provera® Contraceptive *see* MedroxyPROGESTERone . . . 849
Depotest® 100 *see* Testosterone . . . 1281
Depo-Testadiol® *see* Estradiol and Testosterone . . . 527
Depo®-Testosterone *see* Testosterone . . . 1281
Deprenyl *see* Selegiline . . . 1213
Derifil® [OTC] *see* Chlorophyll . . . 302

Derma Keri® *see* Urea 1365
Dermalog® *see* Halcinonide 657
Dermarest Dricort® [OTC] *see* Hydrocortisone 688
Derma-Smoothe/FS® *see* Fluocinolone 584
Dermatop® *see* Prednicarbate 1110
Dermatovate® *see* Clobetasol 345
Dermazene® *see* Iodoquinol and Hydrocortisone 736
Dermazin™ *see* Silver Sulfadiazine 1222
Dermazole *see* Miconazole 906
Dermifun® *see* Miconazole 906
Dermoplast® *see* Urea 1365
Dermovate® *see* Clobetasol 345
Dermox® *see* Methoxsalen 888
Dermtex® HC [OTC] *see* Hydrocortisone 688
DES *see* Diethylstilbestrol 437
Description of Sections and Fields 8
Deserpidine and Methyclothiazide *see* Methyclothiazide and Deserpidine 890
Desferal® *see* Deferoxamine 404
Desiccated Thyroid *see* Thyroid 1303
Desipramine 408
Desipramine Hydrochloride *see* Desipramine 408
Desitin® [OTC] *see* Zinc Oxide 1409
Desitin® Creamy [OTC] *see* Zinc Oxide 1409
Desloratadine 410
Desmethylimipramine Hydrochloride *see* Desipramine 408
Desmopressin 410
Desmopressin Acetate *see* Desmopressin 410
Desocort® *see* Desonide 412
Desogen® *see* Combination Hormonal Contraceptives 368
Desonide 412
Desowen® *see* Desonide 412
Desoxi® *see* Desoximetasone 412
Desoximetasone 412
Desoxyephedrine Hydrochloride *see* Methamphetamine 877
Desoxyn® *see* Methamphetamine 877
Desoxyphenobarbital *see* Primidone 1118
Desparasil® *see* Piperazine 1089
Desquam-E™ *see* Benzoyl Peroxide 171
Desquam-X® *see* Benzoyl Peroxide 171
Desyrel® *see* Trazodone 1336
Detane® [OTC] *see* Benzocaine 169
Detrol® *see* Tolterodine 1322
Detrol® LA *see* Tolterodine 1322
Detrusitol® *see* Tolterodine 1322
Devil's Claw 1428
Devrom® *see* Bismuth 186
Dex4 Glucose [OTC] *see* Glucose (Instant) 641
Dexacidin® *see* Neomycin, Polymyxin B, and Dexamethasone 962
Dexacine™ *see* Neomycin, Polymyxin B, and Dexamethasone 962
Dexagrin® *see* Dexamethasone 413
Dexalone® [OTC] *see* Dextromethorphan 423
Dexamethasone 413
Dexamethasone Acetate *see* Dexamethasone 413
Dexamethasone and Neomycin *see* Neomycin and Dexamethasone 961
Dexamethasone and Tobramycin *see* Tobramycin and Dexamethasone 1317
Dexamethasone Intensol® *see* Dexamethasone 413
Dexamethasone, Neomycin, and Polymyxin B *see* Neomycin, Polymyxin B, and Dexamethasone 962
Dexamethasone Sodium Phosphate *see* Dexamethasone 413
Dexasone® *see* Dexamethasone 413
Dexasone® L.A. *see* Dexamethasone 413
Dexbrompheniramine and Pseudoephedrine 415
Dexchlorpheniramine 416
Dexchlorpheniramine Maleate *see* Dexchlorpheniramine 416
Dexedrine® *see* Dextroamphetamine 420
Dexferrum® *see* Iron Dextran Complex 743
Dexiron™ *see* Iron Dextran Complex 743
Dexmedetomidine 416
Dexmedetomidine Hydrochloride *see* Dexmedetomidine 416
Dexmethylphenidate 417
Dexmethylphenidate Hydrochloride *see* Dexmethylphenidate 417
DexPak® TaperPak® *see* Dexamethasone 413
Dexpanthenol 418
Dexrazoxane 419
Dextran 419
Dextran 1 420
Dextran 40 *see* Dextran 419
Dextran 70 *see* Dextran 419
Dextran, High Molecular Weight *see* Dextran 419
Dextran, Low Molecular Weight *see* Dextran 419
Dextroamphetamine 420
Dextroamphetamine and Amphetamine 422
Dextroamphetamine Sulfate *see* Dextroamphetamine 420
Dextromethorphan 423
Dextromethorphan, Acetaminophen, and Pseudoephedrine *see* Acetaminophen, Dextromethorphan, and Pseudoephedrine 35
Dextromethorphan and Guaifenesin *see* Guaifenesin and Dextromethorphan 651
Dextromethorphan and Promethazine *see* Promethazine and Dextromethorphan 1129
Dextromethorphan and Pseudoephedrine *see* Pseudoephedrine and Dextromethorphan 1147

Dextromethorphan, Carbinoxamine, and Pseudoephedrine *see* Carbinoxamine, Pseudoephedrine, and Dextromethorphan . . . 247
Dextromethorphan, Guaifenesin, and Pseudoephedrine *see* Guaifenesin, Pseudoephedrine, and Dextromethorphan . . . 653
Dextromethorphan, Pseudoephedrine, and Carbinoxamine *see* Carbinoxamine, Pseudoephedrine, and Dextromethorphan . . . 247
Dextropropoxyphene *see* Propoxyphene . . . 1135
Dextrose and Tetracaine *see* Tetracaine and Dextrose . . . 1285
Dextrose, Levulose and Phosphoric Acid *see* Phosphorated Carbohydrate Solution . . . 1078
Dextrostat® *see* Dextroamphetamine . . . 420
DFMO *see* Eflornithine . . . 489
DHA *see* Docosahexaenoic Acid . . . 1428
DHAD *see* Mitoxantrone . . . 923
DHE *see* Dihydroergotamine . . . 445
D.H.E. 45® *see* Dihydroergotamine . . . 445
DHEA *see* Dehydroepiandrosterone . . . 1427
DHPG Sodium *see* Ganciclovir . . . 626
DHS™ Sal [OTC] *see* Salicylic Acid . . . 1204
DHS® Tar [OTC] *see* Coal Tar . . . 359
DHS™ Zinc [OTC] *see* Pyrithione Zinc . . . 1154
DHT™ *see* Dihydrotachysterol . . . 446
DHT™ Intensol™ *see* Dihydrotachysterol . . . 446
Diaβeta® *see* GlyBURIDE . . . 642
Diabetic Tussin® DM [OTC] *see* Guaifenesin and Dextromethorphan . . . 651
Diabetic Tussin® DM Maximum Strength [OTC] *see* Guaifenesin and Dextromethorphan . . . 651
Diabetic Tussin® EX [OTC] *see* Guaifenesin . . . 650
Diabe-Tuss DM [OTC] *see* Dextromethorphan . . . 423
Diabinese® *see* ChlorproPAMIDE . . . 314
Dialume® [OTC] *see* Aluminum Hydroxide . . . 68
Diaminocyclohexane Oxalatoplatinum *see* Oxaliplatin . . . 1008
Diaminodiphenylsulfone *see* Dapsone . . . 399
Diamox® *see* AcetaZOLAMIDE . . . 37
Diamox Sequels® *see* AcetaZOLAMIDE . . . 37
Diarr-Eze *see* Loperamide . . . 819
Diasorb® [OTC] *see* Attapulgite . . . 146
Diastat® *see* Diazepam . . . 424
Diastat® Rectal Delivery System *see* Diazepam . . . 424
Diatex *see* Diazepam . . . 424
Diaval® *see* TOLBUTamide . . . 1319
Diazemuls® *see* Diazepam . . . 424
Diazepam . . . 424
Diazepam Intensol® *see* Diazepam . . . 424
Diazoxide . . . 427
Dibacilina *see* Ampicillin . . . 103
Dibaprim® *see* Trimethoprim . . . 1352
Dibasona® *see* Dexamethasone . . . 413
Dibenzyline® *see* Phenoxybenzamine . . . 1068
Dibucaine . . . 427
Dibufen® *see* Ibuprofen . . . 703
DIC *see* Dacarbazine . . . 391
Dicarbosil® [OTC] *see* Calcium Supplements . . . 229
Dichloralphenazone, Acetaminophen, and Isometheptene *see* Acetaminophen, Isometheptene, and Dichloralphenazone . . . 36
Dichloralphenazone, Isometheptene, and Acetaminophen *see* Acetaminophen, Isometheptene, and Dichloralphenazone . . . 36
Dichlorodifluoromethane and Trichloromonofluoromethane . . . 428
Dichlorotetrafluoroethane and Ethyl Chloride *see* Ethyl Chloride and Dichlorotetrafluoroethane . . . 545
Dichlorphenamide . . . 428
Dichysterol *see* Dihydrotachysterol . . . 446
Diclofenac . . . 429
Diclofenac and Misoprostol . . . 431
Diclofenac Potassium *see* Diclofenac . . . 429
Diclofenac Sodium *see* Diclofenac . . . 429
Diclofenamide *see* Dichlorphenamide . . . 428
Dicloran® *see* Diclofenac . . . 429
Diclotec *see* Diclofenac . . . 429
Diclotride® *see* Hydrochlorothiazide . . . 675
Dicloxacillin . . . 432
Dicloxacillin Sodium *see* Dicloxacillin . . . 432
Dicumarol . . . 433
Dicyclomine . . . 433
Dicyclomine Hydrochloride *see* Dicyclomine . . . 433
Dicycloverine Hydrochloride *see* Dicyclomine . . . 433
Didanosine . . . 434
Dideoxycytidine *see* Zalcitabine . . . 1403
Dideoxyinosine *see* Didanosine . . . 434
Didrex® *see* Benzphetamine . . . 172
Didronel® *see* Etidronate Disodium . . . 546
Diestet® *see* Mazindol . . . 843
Diethylpropion . . . 436
Diethylpropion Hydrochloride *see* Diethylpropion . . . 436
Diethylstilbestrol . . . 437
Diethylstilbestrol Diphosphate Sodium *see* Diethylstilbestrol . . . 437
Difenoxin and Atropine . . . 437
Differin® *see* Adapalene . . . 44
Diflorasone . . . 438
Diflorasone Diacetate *see* Diflorasone . . . 438
Diflucan® *see* Fluconazole . . . 576
Diflunisal . . . 438

Difoxacil® *see* Norfloxacin . . . 987
Digezanol® *see* Albendazole . . . 47
Digibind® *see* Digoxin Immune Fab . . . 443
DigiFab™ *see* Digoxin Immune Fab . . . 443
Digitek® *see* Digoxin . . . 441
Digitoxin . . . 440
Digoxin . . . 441
Digoxin CSD *see* Digoxin . . . 441
Digoxin Immune Fab . . . 443
Dihematoporphyrin Ether *see* Porfimer . . . 1098
Dihistine® DH *see* Chlorpheniramine, Pseudoephedrine, and Codeine . . . 311
Dihistine® Expectorant *see* Guaifenesin, Pseudoephedrine, and Codeine . . . 653
Dihydrocodeine, Aspirin, and Caffeine . . . 444
Dihydrocodeine Compound *see* Dihydrocodeine, Aspirin, and Caffeine . . . 444
Dihydroergotamine . . . 445
Dihydroergotamine Mesylate *see* Dihydroergotamine . . . 445
Dihydroergotoxine *see* Ergoloid Mesylates . . . 509
Dihydrogenated Ergot Alkaloids *see* Ergoloid Mesylates . . . 509
Dihydrohydroxycodeinone *see* Oxycodone . . . 1017
Dihydromorphinone *see* Hydromorphone . . . 691
Dihydrotachysterol . . . 446
1,25 Dihydroxycholecalciferol *see* Calcitriol . . . 223
Dihydroxypropyl Theophylline *see* Dyphylline . . . 485
Diiodohydroxyquin *see* Iodoquinol . . . 735
Dilacoran® *see* Verapamil . . . 1382
Dilacoran HTA *see* Verapamil . . . 1382
Dilacoran Retard *see* Verapamil . . . 1382
Dilacor® XR *see* Diltiazem . . . 447
Dilafed *see* NIFEdipine . . . 973
Dilantin® *see* Phenytoin . . . 1073
Dilatrate®-SR *see* Isosorbide Dinitrate . . . 750
Dilatrend® *see* Carvedilol . . . 256
Dilaudid® *see* Hydromorphone . . . 691
Dilaudid-HP® *see* Hydromorphone . . . 691
Dilaudid-HP-Plus® *see* Hydromorphone . . . 691
Dilaudid® Sterile Powder *see* Hydromorphone . . . 691
Dilaudid-XP® *see* Hydromorphone . . . 691
Dilor® *see* Dyphylline . . . 485
Diltia XT® *see* Diltiazem . . . 447
Diltiazem . . . 447
Diltiazem Hydrochloride *see* Diltiazem . . . 447
Dimantil *see* Warfarin . . . 1397
Dimefor® *see* Metformin . . . 874
DimenhyDRINATE . . . 449
Dimercaprol . . . 449
Dimetapp® 12-Hour Non-Drowsy Extentabs® [OTC] *see* Pseudoephedrine . . . 1146
Dimetapp® Decongestant [OTC] *see* Pseudoephedrine . . . 1146
β,β-Dimethylcysteine *see* Penicillamine . . . 1046
Dimethyl Sulfone *see* Methyl Sulfonyl Methane . . . 1445
Dimethyl Triazeno Imidazol Carboxamide *see* Dacarbazine . . . 391
Dimodan *see* Disopyramide . . . 458
Dinoprostone . . . 450
Diocaine® *see* Proparacaine . . . 1132
Diocarpine *see* Pilocarpine . . . 1080
Diochloram® *see* Chloramphenicol . . . 297
Diocto® [OTC] *see* Docusate . . . 463
Diocto C® [OTC] *see* Docusate and Casanthranol . . . 464
Dioctyl Calcium Sulfosuccinate *see* Docusate . . . 463
Dioctyl Sodium Sulfosuccinate *see* Docusate . . . 463
Diodex® *see* Dexamethasone . . . 413
Diodoquin® *see* Iodoquinol . . . 735
Diogent® *see* Gentamicin . . . 634
Diomycin® *see* Erythromycin . . . 512
Dionephrine® *see* Phenylephrine . . . 1071
Diopentolate® *see* Cyclopentolate . . . 380
Diopred® *see* PrednisoLONE . . . 1110
Dioptic's Atropine Solution *see* Atropine . . . 144
Dioptimyd® *see* Sulfacetamide and Prednisolone . . . 1250
Dioptrol® *see* Neomycin, Polymyxin B, and Dexamethasone . . . 962
Dioscorea villosa *see* Wild Yam . . . 1450
Diosulf™ *see* Sulfacetamide . . . 1249
Diotame® [OTC] *see* Bismuth . . . 186
Diotrope® *see* Tropicamide . . . 1360
Diovan® *see* Valsartan . . . 1374
Diovan HCT® *see* Valsartan and Hydrochlorothiazide . . . 1375
Diovol® *see* Aluminum Hydroxide and Magnesium Hydroxide . . . 69
Diovol® Ex *see* Aluminum Hydroxide and Magnesium Hydroxide . . . 69
Diovol Plus® *see* Aluminum Hydroxide, Magnesium Hydroxide, and Simethicone . . . 69
Dipalmitoylphosphatidylcholine *see* Colfosceril Palmitate . . . 366
Dipedyne *see* Zidovudine . . . 1406
Dipentum® *see* Olsalazine . . . 999
Diphen® [OTC] *see* DiphenhydrAMINE . . . 451
Diphen® AF [OTC] *see* DiphenhydrAMINE . . . 451
Diphen® Cough [OTC] *see* DiphenhydrAMINE . . . 451
Diphenhist [OTC] *see* DiphenhydrAMINE . . . 451
DiphenhydrAMINE . . . 451
Diphenhydramine and Acetaminophen *see* Acetaminophen and Diphenhydramine . . . 30
Diphenhydramine and Pseudoephedrine . . . 453
Diphenhydramine Hydrochloride *see* DiphenhydrAMINE . . . 451
Diphenoxylate and Atropine . . . 453

Diphenylhydantoin *see* Phenytoin 1073
Diphtheria and Tetanus Toxoids and Acellular Pertussis Adsorbed, Hepatitis B (Recombinant) and Inactivated Poliovirus Vaccine Combined *see* Diphtheria, Tetanus Toxoids, Acellular Pertussis, Hepatitis B (Recombinant), and Poliovirus (Inactivated) Vaccine 454
Diphtheria CRM_{197} Protein *see* Pneumococcal Conjugate Vaccine (7-Valent) 1091
Diphtheria CRM_{197} Protein Conjugate *see* *Haemophilus* b Conjugate Vaccine 656
Diphtheria, Tetanus Toxoids, Acellular Pertussis, Hepatitis B (Recombinant), and Poliovirus (Inactivated) Vaccine 454
Diphtheria, Tetanus Toxoids, and Acellular Pertussis Vaccine *see* Immunizations (Vaccines) 1612
Diphtheria, Tetanus Toxoids, and Acellular Pertussis Vaccine and *Haemophilus influenzae* b Conjugate Vaccine (Combined) *see* Immunizations (Vaccines) 1612
Diphtheria Toxoid Conjugate *see* *Haemophilus* b Conjugate Vaccine 656
Dipivalyl Epinephrine *see* Dipivefrin 455
Dipivefrin 455
Dipivefrin Hydrochloride *see* Dipivefrin 455
Diprivan® *see* Propofol 1133
Diprodol® *see* Ibuprofen 703
Diprolene® *see* Betamethasone 177
Diprolene® AF *see* Betamethasone 177
Diprolene® Glycol *see* Betamethasone 177
Dipropylacetic Acid *see* Valproic Acid and Derivatives 1371
Diprosone® [DSC] *see* Betamethasone 177
Dipyridamole 456
Dipyridamole and Aspirin *see* Aspirin and Dipyridamole 135
Dirinol *see* Dipyridamole 456
Dirithromycin 457
Disalcid® [DSC] *see* Salsalate 1206
Disalicylic Acid *see* Salsalate 1206
Disodium Cromoglycate *see* Cromolyn Sodium 375
d-Isoephedrine Hydrochloride *see* Pseudoephedrine 1146
Disopyramide 458
Disopyramide Phosphate *see* Disopyramide 458
Disulfiram 459
Dithioglycerol *see* Dimercaprol 449
Dithranol *see* Anthralin 111
Ditropan® *see* Oxybutynin 1016
Ditropan® XL *see* Oxybutynin 1016
Ditterolina® *see* Dicloxacillin 432
Diupres® *see* Chlorothiazide and Reserpine 306
Diuril® *see* Chlorothiazide 304
Divalproex Sodium *see* Valproic Acid and Derivatives 1371
Dixaparine *see* Heparin 662
Dixarit® *see* Clonidine 351
dl-Alpha Tocopherol *see* Vitamin E 1393
4-dmdr *see* Idarubicin 706
$DMSO_2$ *see* Methyl Sulfonyl Methane 1445
DNA-derived Humanized Monoclonal Antibody *see* Alemtuzumab 52
DNase *see* Dornase Alfa 467
DNR *see* DAUNOrubicin Hydrochloride 402
Doan's® [OTC] *see* Magnesium Salicylate 837
Doan's® Extra Strength [OTC] *see* Magnesium Salicylate 837
Dobuject® *see* DOBUTamine 460
DOBUTamine 460
Dobutamine Hydrochloride *see* DOBUTamine 460
Dobutrex® *see* DOBUTamine 460
Docetaxel 461
Docosahexaenoic Acid 1428
Docosanol 463
Docusate 463
Docusate and Casanthranol 464
Docusate Calcium *see* Docusate 463
Docusate Potassium *see* Docusate 463
Docusate Sodium *see* Docusate 463
Docusoft Plus™ [OTC] *see* Docusate and Casanthranol 464
Docusoft-S™ [OTC] *see* Docusate 463
Dofetilide 464
Dolac® *see* Ketorolac 765
Dolac Inyectable *see* Ketorolac 765
Dolac Oral *see* Ketorolac 765
Dolaren® *see* Diclofenac 429
Dolasetron 465
Dolasetron Mesylate *see* Dolasetron 465
Dolflam® *see* Diclofenac 429
Dolobid® *see* Diflunisal 438
Dolo Pangavit-D *see* Diclofenac 429
Dolophine® *see* Methadone 876
Dolorac™ [OTC] *see* Capsaicin 238
Dolotor® *see* Ketorolac 765
Dolzycam® *see* Piroxicam 1090
Domeboro® [OTC] *see* Aluminum Sulfate and Calcium Acetate 70
Dome Paste Bandage *see* Zinc Gelatin 1409
Donepezil 467
Dong Quai 1429
Donnapectolin-PG® *see* Hyoscyamine, Atropine, Scopolamine, Kaolin, Pectin, and Opium 701
Donnatal® *see* Hyoscyamine, Atropine, Scopolamine, and Phenobarbital 700
Dopar® *see* Levodopa 792
Dopram® *see* Doxapram 469

Doral® *see* Quazepam 1154
Dormicum® *see* Midazolam 908
Dornase Alfa 467
Doryx® *see* Doxycycline 476
Dorzolamide 468
Dorzolamide Hydrochloride *see* Dorzolamide 468
DOS® [OTC] *see* Docusate 463
DOSS *see* Docusate 463
Dostinex® *see* Cabergoline 220
Dovonex® *see* Calcipotriene 222
Doxapram 469
Doxapram Hydrochloride *see* Doxapram 469
Doxazosin 470
Doxepin 471
Doxepin Hydrochloride *see* Doxepin 471
Doxercalciferol 472
Doxidan® [OTC] *see* Docusate and Casanthranol 464
Doxil® *see* DOXOrubicin (Liposomal) 475
Doxolem® *see* DOXOrubicin 473
DOXOrubicin 473
Doxorubicin Hydrochloride *see* DOXOrubicin 473
Doxorubicin Hydrochloride (Liposomal) *see* DOXOrubicin (Liposomal) 475
DOXOrubicin (Liposomal) 475
Doxotec® *see* DOXOrubicin 473
Doxy-100® *see* Doxycycline 476
Doxycin *see* Doxycycline 476
Doxycycline 476
Doxycycline Calcium *see* Doxycycline 476
Doxycycline Hyclate *see* Doxycycline 476
Doxycycline Hyclate Periodontal Extended-Release Liquid 479
Doxycycline Monohydrate *see* Doxycycline 476
Doxycycline Subantimicrobial 480
Doxytec *see* Doxycycline 476
DPA *see* Valproic Acid and Derivatives 1371
DPE *see* Dipivefrin 455
D-Penicillamine *see* Penicillamine 1046
DPH *see* Phenytoin 1073
DPPC *see* Colfosceril Palmitate 366
Drafilyn® *see* Aminophylline 78
Dramamine® [OTC] *see* DimenhyDRINATE 449
Dramamine® Less Drowsy Formula [OTC] *see* Meclizine 847
Drenural® *see* Bumetanide 204
Driken *see* Iron Dextran Complex 743
Drisdol® *see* Ergocalciferol 508
Dristan® Long Lasting Nasal *see* Oxymetazoline 1022
Dristan® N.D. *see* Acetaminophen and Pseudoephedrine 31
Dristan® N.D., Extra Strength *see* Acetaminophen and Pseudoephedrine 31
Dristan® Sinus [OTC] *see* Pseudoephedrine and Ibuprofen 1148
Drithocreme® *see* Anthralin 111
Drithocreme® HP 1% *see* Anthralin 111
Dritho-Scalp® *see* Anthralin 111
Drixomed® *see* Dexbrompheniramine and Pseudoephedrine 415
Drixoral® *see* Dexbrompheniramine and Pseudoephedrine 415
Drixoral® Cold & Allergy [OTC] *see* Dexbrompheniramine and Pseudoephedrine 415
Drixoral® Nasal *see* Oxymetazoline 1022
Drixoral® ND *see* Pseudoephedrine 1146
Dronabinol 480
Droperidol 481
Drotrecogin Alfa 483
Drotrecogin Alfa, Activated *see* Drotrecogin Alfa 483
Droxia™ *see* Hydroxyurea 696
Dr. Scholl's® Callus Remover [OTC] *see* Salicylic Acid 1204
Dr. Scholl's® Clear Away [OTC] *see* Salicylic Acid 1204
DSCG *see* Cromolyn Sodium 375
D-S-S® [OTC] *see* Docusate 463
DSS With Casanthranol *see* Docusate and Casanthranol 464
DTIC *see* Dacarbazine 391
DTIC-Dome® *see* Dacarbazine 391
DTO *see* Opium Tincture 1002
Duac™ *see* Clindamycin and Benzoyl Peroxide 343
Dulcolan® *see* Bisacodyl 186
Dulcolax® *see* Bisacodyl 186
Dull-C® [OTC] *see* Ascorbic Acid 128
Duofilm® *see* Salicylic Acid 1204
Duoforte® 27 *see* Salicylic Acid 1204
DuoNeb™ *see* Ipratropium and Albuterol 738
DuoPlant® [DSC] [OTC] *see* Salicylic Acid 1204
DuP 753 *see* Losartan 825
Duplex® T [OTC] *see* Coal Tar 359
Durabolin® *see* Nandrolone 951
Duracef® *see* Cefadroxil 261
Duraclon™ *see* Clonidine 351
Duradoce® *see* Hydroxocobalamin 693
Duragesic® *see* Fentanyl 565
Duralith® *see* Lithium 815
Duralmor L.P.® *see* Morphine Sulfate 931
Duramist® Plus [OTC] *see* Oxymetazoline 1022
Duramorph® *see* Morphine Sulfate 931
Duranest® [DSC] *see* Etidocaine and Epinephrine 545
Durater® *see* Famotidine 556

Duration® [OTC] *see* Oxymetazoline . . . 1022
Duratuss™ *see* Guaifenesin and Pseudoephedrine . . . 652
Duratuss® DM *see* Guaifenesin and Dextromethorphan . . . 651
Duratuss-G® *see* Guaifenesin . . . 650
Duratuss™ GP *see* Guaifenesin and Pseudoephedrine . . . 652
Duratuss® HD *see* Hydrocodone, Pseudoephedrine, and Guaifenesin . . . 687
Dura-Vent®/DA *see* Chlorpheniramine, Phenylephrine, and Methscopolamine . . . 310
Duricef™ *see* Cefadroxil . . . 261
Durogesic® *see* Fentanyl . . . 565
Dutasteride . . . 484
Duvoid® *see* Bethanechol . . . 181
D-Vi-Sol® *see* Cholecalciferol . . . 317
Dyazide® *see* Hydrochlorothiazide and Triamterene . . . 677
Dycill® *see* Dicloxacillin . . . 432
Dymelor® [DSC] *see* AcetoHEXAMIDE . . . 38
Dynabac® *see* Dirithromycin . . . 457
Dynacin® *see* Minocycline . . . 915
DynaCirc® *see* Isradipine . . . 754
DynaCirc® CR *see* Isradipine . . . 754
DynaCirc SRO® *see* Isradipine . . . 754
Dyna-Hex® [OTC] *see* Chlorhexidine Gluconate . . . 300
Dyphylline . . . 485
Dyrenium® *see* Triamterene . . . 1344
E_2C and MPA *see* Estradiol and Medroxyprogesterone . . . 523
7E3 *see* Abciximab . . . 23
E2020 *see* Donepezil . . . 467
EarSol® HC *see* Hydrocortisone . . . 688
Easprin® *see* Aspirin . . . 131
Ecapresan *see* Captopril . . . 238
Ecaten® *see* Captopril . . . 238
Echinacea . . . 1429
Echinacea angustifolia see Echinacea . . . 1429
Echinacea purpurea see Echinacea . . . 1429
Echothiophate Iodide . . . 485
EC-Naprosyn® *see* Naproxen . . . 953
E. coli Asparaginase *see* Asparaginase . . . 129
Econazole . . . 486
Econazole Nitrate *see* Econazole . . . 486
Econopred® *see* PrednisoLONE . . . 1110
Econopred® Plus *see* PrednisoLONE . . . 1110
Ecostatin® *see* Econazole . . . 486
Ecostigmine Iodide *see* Echothiophate Iodide . . . 485
Ecotrin® *see* Aspirin . . . 131
Ecotrin® Low Adult Strength [OTC] *see* Aspirin . . . 131
Ecotrin® Maximum Strength [OTC] *see* Aspirin . . . 131
Ectaprim® *see* Sulfamethoxazole and Trimethoprim . . . 1253
Ectaprim® *see* Trimethoprim . . . 1352
Ectaprim®-F *see* Sulfamethoxazole and Trimethoprim . . . 1253
Ectosone *see* Betamethasone . . . 177
Ed A-Hist® *see* Chlorpheniramine and Phenylephrine . . . 308
Edathamil Disodium *see* Edetate Disodium . . . 488
Edecrin® *see* Ethacrynic Acid . . . 538
Edenol® *see* Furosemide . . . 622
Edetate Calcium Disodium . . . 486
Edetate Disodium . . . 488
Edex® *see* Alprostadil . . . 63
EDTA *see* Edetate Disodium . . . 488
E.E.S.® *see* Erythromycin . . . 512
Efavirenz . . . 488
Efexor® *see* Venlafaxine . . . 1380
Effer-K™ *see* Potassium Supplements . . . 1102
Effexor® *see* Venlafaxine . . . 1380
Effexor® XR *see* Venlafaxine . . . 1380
Eflone® *see* Fluorometholone . . . 587
Eflornithine . . . 489
Eflornithine Hydrochloride *see* Eflornithine . . . 489
Efudex® *see* Fluorouracil . . . 588
Efudix *see* Fluorouracil . . . 588
EGb *see* Ginkgo Biloba . . . 1434
E-Gems® [OTC] *see* Vitamin E . . . 1393
EHDP *see* Etidronate Disodium . . . 546
ELA-Max® [OTC] *see* Lidocaine . . . 801
ELA-Max® 5 [OTC] *see* Lidocaine . . . 801
Elantan® *see* Isosorbide Mononitrate . . . 751
Elavil® *see* Amitriptyline . . . 83
Eldepryl® *see* Selegiline . . . 1213
Eldopaque™ *see* Hydroquinone . . . 693
Eldopaque Forte® *see* Hydroquinone . . . 693
Eldoquin® [OTC] *see* Hydroquinone . . . 693
Eldoquin Forte® *see* Hydroquinone . . . 693
Electrolyte Lavage Solution *see* Polyethylene Glycol-Electrolyte Solution . . . 1094
Elequine® *see* Levofloxacin . . . 794
Eletriptan . . . 490
Eletriptan Hydrobromide *see* Eletriptan . . . 490
Eleutherococcus senticosus see Ginseng, Siberian . . . 1436
Elidel® *see* Pimecrolimus . . . 1083
Eligard™ *see* Leuprolide . . . 784
Elimite® *see* Permethrin . . . 1062
Elitek™ *see* Rasburicase . . . 1169
Elixophyllin® *see* Theophylline . . . 1291

Elixophyllin-GG® *see* Theophylline and Guaifenesin . . . 1293
Ellence® *see* Epirubicin . . . 501
Elmiron® *see* Pentosan Polysulfate Sodium . . . 1056
Elocom® *see* Mometasone Furoate . . . 928
Elocon® *see* Mometasone Furoate . . . 928
Eloxatin™ *see* Oxaliplatin . . . 1008
Elspar® *see* Asparaginase . . . 129
Eltor® *see* Pseudoephedrine . . . 1146
Eltroxin® *see* Levothyroxine . . . 800
Embeline™ E *see* Clobetasol . . . 345
Emcyt® *see* Estramustine . . . 527
Emetrol® [OTC] *see* Phosphorated Carbohydrate Solution . . . 1078
Emgel® *see* Erythromycin . . . 512
Emko® [OTC] *see* Nonoxynol 9 . . . 985
EMLA® *see* Lidocaine and Prilocaine . . . 806
Emo-Cort® *see* Hydrocortisone . . . 688
Emtec-30 *see* Acetaminophen and Codeine . . . 29
Emulsan 20% *see* Fat Emulsion . . . 558
Emulsoil® [OTC] *see* Castor Oil . . . 259
ENA 713 *see* Rivastigmine . . . 1192
Enaladil® *see* Enalapril . . . 492
Enalapril . . . 492
Enalapril and Felodipine . . . 494
Enalapril and Hydrochlorothiazide . . . 494
Enalaprilat *see* Enalapril . . . 492
Enalapril Maleate *see* Enalapril . . . 492
Enbrel® *see* Etanercept . . . 537
Encare® [OTC] *see* Nonoxynol 9 . . . 985
Endal® *see* Guaifenesin and Phenylephrine . . . 652
Endantadine® *see* Amantadine . . . 70
Endocet® *see* Oxycodone and Acetaminophen . . . 1018
Endocrine Disorders and Pregnancy . . . 1479
Endodan® *see* Oxycodone and Aspirin . . . 1020
Endo®-Levodopa/Carbidopa *see* Levodopa and Carbidopa . . . 793
Endoplus® *see* Albendazole . . . 47
Endrate® *see* Edetate Disodium . . . 488
Enduron® *see* Methyclothiazide . . . 890
Enduronyl® *see* Methyclothiazide and Deserpidine . . . 890
Enduronyl® Forte *see* Methyclothiazide and Deserpidine . . . 890
Ener-B® *see* Cyanocobalamin . . . 377
Enfuvirtide . . . 495
Engerix-B® *see* Hepatitis B Vaccine . . . 666
Engerix-B® and Havrix® *see* Hepatitis A (Inactivated) and Hepatitis B (Recombinant) Vaccine . . . 664
English Hawthorn *see* Hawthorn . . . 1440
Enhanced-potency Inactivated Poliovirus Vaccine *see* Poliovirus Vaccine (Inactivated) . . . 1093
Eni® *see* Ciprofloxacin . . . 328
Enoxaparin . . . 495
Enoxaparin Sodium *see* Enoxaparin . . . 495
Enpresse™ *see* Combination Hormonal Contraceptives . . . 368
Entacapone . . . 497
Entacyl® *see* Piperazine . . . 1089
Enterobacticel *see* Sulfamethoxazole and Trimethoprim . . . 1253
Enteropride *see* Cisapride . . . 332
Entertainer's Secret® [OTC] *see* Saliva Substitute . . . 1205
Entex® LA *see* Guaifenesin and Phenylephrine . . . 652
Entex® PSE *see* Guaifenesin and Pseudoephedrine . . . 652
Entocort® *see* Budesonide . . . 202
Entocort™ EC *see* Budesonide . . . 202
Entrophen® *see* Aspirin . . . 131
Entsol® [OTC] *see* Sodium Chloride . . . 1229
Enulose® *see* Lactulose . . . 772
Enzone® *see* Pramoxine and Hydrocortisone . . . 1106
Epamin® *see* Phenytoin . . . 1073
Epaxal Berna® *see* Hepatitis A Vaccine . . . 665
Ephedra . . . 1430
Ephedra sinica *see* Ephedra . . . 1430
Ephedrine . . . 499
Ephedrine Sulfate *see* Ephedrine . . . 499
Epidermal Thymocyte Activating Factor *see* Aldesleukin . . . 50
Epifoam® *see* Pramoxine and Hydrocortisone . . . 1106
Epilem® *see* Epirubicin . . . 501
Epinephrine . . . 499
Epinephrine and Chlorpheniramine Insect Sting Kit . . . 500
Epinephrine and Lidocaine *see* Lidocaine and Epinephrine . . . 804
Epinephrine (Racemic) . . . 500
Epinephrine (Racemic) and Aluminum Potassium Sulfate . . . 501
Epipodophyllotoxin *see* Etoposide . . . 549
Epirubicin . . . 501
Epitol® *see* Carbamazepine . . . 241
Epival® *see* Valproic Acid and Derivatives . . . 1371
Epival® ER *see* Valproic Acid and Derivatives . . . 1371
Epival® I.V. *see* Valproic Acid and Derivatives . . . 1371
Epivir® *see* Lamivudine . . . 773
Epivir-HBV® *see* Lamivudine . . . 773
Eplerenone . . . 502
EPO *see* Epoetin Alfa . . . 503
Epoetin Alfa . . . 503
Epogen® *see* Epoetin Alfa . . . 503
Epomax® *see* Epoetin Alfa . . . 503

Epoprostenol . . . 505
Epoprostenol Sodium *see* Epoprostenol . . . 505
Eprex® *see* Epoetin Alfa . . . 503
Eprosartan . . . 506
Epsom Salts (Magnesium Sulfate) *see* Magnesium Supplements . . . 837
EPT *see* Teniposide . . . 1274
Eptifibatide . . . 507
Equagesic® *see* Aspirin and Meprobamate . . . 136
Equalactin® Chewable Tablet [OTC] *see* Calcium Polycarbophil . . . 228
Equilet® [OTC] *see* Calcium Supplements . . . 229
Eranz® *see* Donepezil . . . 467
Ergamisol® *see* Levamisole . . . 786
Ergocaf *see* Ergotamine . . . 510
Ergocalciferol . . . 508
Ergoloid Mesylates . . . 509
Ergomar® *see* Ergotamine . . . 510
Ergometrine Maleate *see* Ergonovine . . . 509
Ergonovine . . . 509
Ergonovine Maleate *see* Ergonovine . . . 509
Ergotamine . . . 510
Ergotamine Tartrate *see* Ergotamine . . . 510
Ergotamine Tartrate and Caffeine *see* Ergotamine . . . 510
Ergotamine Tartrate, Belladonna, and Phenobarbital *see* Belladonna, Phenobarbital, and Ergotamine . . . 165
Eritroquim *see* Erythromycin . . . 512
E•R•O Ear [OTC] *see* Carbamide Peroxide . . . 244
Errin™ *see* Norethindrone . . . 986
Ertapenem . . . 511
Ertapenem Sodium *see* Ertapenem . . . 511
Erwinia Asparaginase *see* Asparaginase . . . 129
Erybid™ *see* Erythromycin . . . 512
Eryc® *see* Erythromycin . . . 512
Erycette® *see* Erythromycin . . . 512
Eryderm® *see* Erythromycin . . . 512
Erygel® *see* Erythromycin . . . 512
EryPed® *see* Erythromycin . . . 512
Ery-Tab® *see* Erythromycin . . . 512
Erythra-Derm™ *see* Erythromycin . . . 512
Erythrocin® *see* Erythromycin . . . 512
Erythromid® *see* Erythromycin . . . 512
Erythromycin . . . 512
Erythromycin and Benzoyl Peroxide . . . 515
Erythromycin and Sulfisoxazole . . . 516
Erythromycin Base *see* Erythromycin . . . 512
Erythromycin Estolate *see* Erythromycin . . . 512
Erythromycin Ethylsuccinate *see* Erythromycin . . . 512
Erythromycin Gluceptate *see* Erythromycin . . . 512
Erythromycin Lactobionate *see* Erythromycin . . . 512
Erythromycin Stearate *see* Erythromycin . . . 512
Erythropoiesis Stimulating Protein *see* Darbepoetin Alfa . . . 400
Erythropoietin *see* Epoetin Alfa . . . 503
Eryzole® *see* Erythromycin and Sulfisoxazole . . . 516
Escitalopram . . . 516
Escitalopram Oxalate *see* Escitalopram . . . 516
Esclim® *see* Estradiol . . . 521
Eserine® *see* Physostigmine . . . 1078
Eserine Salicylate *see* Physostigmine . . . 1078
Esgic® *see* Butalbital, Acetaminophen, and Caffeine . . . 214
Esgic-Plus™ *see* Butalbital, Acetaminophen, and Caffeine . . . 214
Eskalith® *see* Lithium . . . 815
Eskalith CR® *see* Lithium . . . 815
Eskazole® *see* Albendazole . . . 47
Esmolol . . . 518
Esmolol Hydrochloride *see* Esmolol . . . 518
Esomeprazole . . . 519
Esomeprazole Magnesium *see* Esomeprazole . . . 519
Esoterica® Regular [OTC] *see* Hydroquinone . . . 693
Especol® [OTC] *see* Phosphorated Carbohydrate Solution . . . 1078
Estar® *see* Coal Tar . . . 359
Estazolam . . . 521
Esteprim *see* Sulfamethoxazole and Trimethoprim . . . 1253
Esteprim® *see* Trimethoprim . . . 1352
Esterified Estrogen and Methyltestosterone *see* Estrogens (Esterified) and Methyltestosterone . . . 534
Esterified Estrogens *see* Estrogens (Esterified) . . . 533
Estinyl® *see* Ethinyl Estradiol . . . 541
Estrace® *see* Estradiol . . . 521
Estraderm® *see* Estradiol . . . 521
Estraderm TTS® *see* Estradiol . . . 521
Estradiol . . . 521
Estradiol and Medroxyprogesterone . . . 523
Estradiol and NGM *see* Estradiol and Norgestimate . . . 526
Estradiol and Norethindrone . . . 525
Estradiol and Norgestimate . . . 526
Estradiol and Testosterone . . . 527
Estradiol Cypionate *see* Estradiol . . . 521
Estradiol Cypionate and Medroxyprogesterone Acetate *see* Estradiol and Medroxyprogesterone . . . 523
Estradiol Cypionate and Testosterone Cypionate *see* Estradiol and Testosterone . . . 527
Estradiol Hemihydrate *see* Estradiol . . . 521

Estradiol Transdermal *see* Estradiol . . . 521
Estradiol Valerate *see* Estradiol . . . 521
Estradiol Valerate and Testosterone Enanthate *see* Estradiol and Testosterone . . . 527
Estradot® *see* Estradiol . . . 521
Estramustine . . . 527
Estramustine Phosphate Sodium *see* Estramustine . . . 527
Estratab® [DSC] *see* Estrogens (Esterified) . . . 533
Estratest® *see* Estrogens (Esterified) and Methyltestosterone . . . 534
Estratest® H.S. *see* Estrogens (Esterified) and Methyltestosterone . . . 534
Estring® *see* Estradiol . . . 521
Estrogel® *see* Estradiol . . . 521
Estrogenic Substance Aqueous *see* Estrone . . . 535
Estrogenic Substances, Conjugated *see* Estrogens (Conjugated/Equine) . . . 529
Estrogens (Conjugated A/Synthetic) . . . 528
Estrogens, Conjugated, A (Synthetic) *see* Estrogens (Conjugated A/Synthetic) . . . 528
Estrogens (Conjugated/Equine) . . . 529
Estrogens (Conjugated/Equine) and Medroxyprogesterone . . . 531
Estrogens (Esterified) . . . 533
Estrogens (Esterified) and Methyltestosterone . . . 534
Estrone . . . 535
Estropipate . . . 536
Estrostep® 21 [DSC] *see* Combination Hormonal Contraceptives . . . 368
Estrostep® Fe *see* Combination Hormonal Contraceptives . . . 368
ETAF *see* Aldesleukin . . . 50
Etanercept . . . 537
Ethacrynate Sodium *see* Ethacrynic Acid . . . 538
Ethacrynic Acid . . . 538
Ethambutol . . . 539
Ethambutol Hydrochloride *see* Ethambutol . . . 539
Ethamolin® *see* Ethanolamine Oleate . . . 540
ETH and C *see* Terpin Hydrate and Codeine . . . 1281
Ethanolamine Oleate . . . 540
Ethaverine . . . 541
Ethaverine Hydrochloride *see* Ethaverine . . . 541
Ethinyl Estradiol . . . 541
Ethinyl Estradiol and Desogestrel *see* Combination Hormonal Contraceptives . . . 368
Ethinyl Estradiol and Drospirenone *see* Combination Hormonal Contraceptives . . . 368
Ethinyl Estradiol and Ethynodiol Diacetate *see* Combination Hormonal Contraceptives . . . 368
Ethinyl Estradiol and Etonogestrel *see* Combination Hormonal Contraceptives . . . 368
Ethinyl Estradiol and Levonorgestrel *see* Combination Hormonal Contraceptives . . . 368
Ethinyl Estradiol and Norelgestromin *see* Combination Hormonal Contraceptives . . . 368
Ethinyl Estradiol and Norethindrone *see* Combination Hormonal Contraceptives . . . 368
Ethinyl Estradiol and Norgestimate *see* Combination Hormonal Contraceptives . . . 368
Ethinyl Estradiol and Norgestrel *see* Combination Hormonal Contraceptives . . . 368
Ethiofos *see* Amifostine . . . 73
Ethionamide . . . 542
Ethmozine® *see* Moricizine . . . 931
Ethosuximide . . . 543
Ethotoin . . . 544
Ethoxynaphthamido Penicillin Sodium *see* Nafcillin . . . 945
Ethyl Aminobenzoate *see* Benzocaine . . . 169
Ethyl Chloride . . . 544
Ethyl Chloride and Dichlorotetrafluoroethane . . . 545
Ethylphenylhydantoin *see* Ethotoin . . . 544
Ethyol® *see* Amifostine . . . 73
Etibi® *see* Ethambutol . . . 539
Etidocaine and Epinephrine . . . 545
Etidocaine Hydrochloride *see* Etidocaine and Epinephrine . . . 545
Etidronate Disodium . . . 546
Etodolac . . . 547
Etodolic Acid *see* Etodolac . . . 547
Etomidate . . . 549
Etopophos® *see* Etoposide Phosphate . . . 551
Etopos® *see* Etoposide . . . 549
Etopos *see* Etoposide Phosphate . . . 551
Etoposide . . . 549
Etoposide Phosphate . . . 551
Etrafon® *see* Amitriptyline and Perphenazine . . . 85
Eudal®-SR *see* Guaifenesin and Pseudoephedrine . . . 652
Euflex® *see* Flutamide . . . 598
Euglucon® *see* GlyBURIDE . . . 642
Eulexin® *see* Flutamide . . . 598
Eumetinex *see* Amoxicillin and Clavulanate Potassium . . . 95
Eurax® *see* Crotamiton . . . 376
Eurax® Topical *see* Crotamiton . . . 376
Eutirox *see* Levothyroxine . . . 800
Evac-U-Gen [OTC] *see* Senna . . . 1215
Evening Primrose . . . 1431
Evening Primrose Oil *see* Evening Primrose . . . 1431
Everone® 200 *see* Testosterone . . . 1281
Evista® *see* Raloxifene . . . 1165
Evoxac™ *see* Cevimeline . . . 292
Exact® Acne Medication [OTC] *see* Benzoyl Peroxide . . . 171
Excedrin® Extra Strength [OTC] *see* Acetaminophen, Aspirin, and Caffeine . . . 34
Excedrin® Migraine [OTC] *see* Acetaminophen, Aspirin, and Caffeine . . . 34
Excedrin® P.M. [OTC] *see* Acetaminophen and Diphenhydramine . . . 30
Exelderm® *see* Sulconazole . . . 1249
Exelon® *see* Rivastigmine . . . 1192
Exemestane . . . 552
ex-lax® [OTC] *see* Senna . . . 1215

ex-lax® Maximum Strength [OTC] *see* Senna 1215
Ex-Lax® Stool Softener [OTC] *see* Docusate 463
Exosurf® *see* Colfosceril Palmitate 366
Exosurf Neonatal® *see* Colfosceril Palmitate 366
Extendryl *see* Chlorpheniramine, Phenylephrine, and Methscopolamine 310
Extendryl JR *see* Chlorpheniramine, Phenylephrine, and Methscopolamine 310
Extendryl SR *see* Chlorpheniramine, Phenylephrine, and Methscopolamine 310
Eye Balm *see* Golden Seal 1437
Eye Root *see* Golden Seal 1437
Eye-Sine™ [OTC] *see* Tetrahydrozoline 1288
Eyestil *see* Sodium Hyaluronate 1230
Eye-Stream® *see* Balanced Salt Solution 160
Ezetimibe 553
F_3T *see* Trifluridine 1350
Facicam® *see* Piroxicam 1090
Factor IX Complex (Human) 553
Factor VIIa (Recombinant) 554
Factor VIII (Human) *see* Antihemophilic Factor (Human) 113
Factor VIII (Porcine) *see* Antihemophilic Factor (Porcine) 114
Factor VIII (Recombinant) *see* Antihemophilic Factor (Recombinant) 115
Famciclovir 555
Famotidine 556
Famotidine, Calcium Carbonate, and Magnesium Hydroxide 557
Famoxal® *see* Famotidine 556
Famvir® *see* Famciclovir 555
Fansidar® *see* Sulfadoxine and Pyrimethamine 1252
Faraxen *see* Naproxen 953
Fareston® *see* Toremifene 1326
Farmorubicin® *see* Epirubicin 501
Farmotex® *see* Famotidine 556
Faslodex® *see* Fulvestrant 621
Fat Emulsion 558
5-FC *see* Flucytosine 578
FC1157a *see* Toremifene 1326
FDA Pregnancy Categories 10
FDA Tall-Man Project 11
Featherfew *see* Feverfew 1431
Featherfoil *see* Feverfew 1431
Febrin® *see* Acetaminophen 27
Fedahist® [OTC] *see* Chlorpheniramine and Pseudoephedrine 308
Feen-A-Mint® [OTC] *see* Bisacodyl 186
Feiba® VH Immuno *see* Anti-inhibitor Coagulant Complex 116
Felbamate 558
Felbatol® *see* Felbamate 558
Feldene® *see* Piroxicam 1090
Feliberal® *see* Enalapril 492
Felodipine 560
Felodipine and Enalapril *see* Enalapril and Felodipine 494
Femara® *see* Letrozole 782
femhrt® *see* Combination Hormonal Contraceptives 368
Femilax™ [OTC] *see* Bisacodyl 186
Femiron® [OTC] *see* Iron Supplements 745
Femizol-M™ [OTC] *see* Miconazole 906
Femstal® *see* Butoconazole 218
Femstat® One *see* Butoconazole 218
Fenesin™ [DSC] *see* Guaifenesin 650
Fenesin™ DM *see* Guaifenesin and Dextromethorphan 651
Fenidantoin® *see* Phenytoin 1073
Fenitron® *see* Phenytoin 1073
Fenofibrate 561
Fenoldopam 562
Fenoldopam Mesylate *see* Fenoldopam 562
Fenoprofen 563
Fenoprofen Calcium *see* Fenoprofen 563
Fenoterol 564
Fenoterol Hydrobromide *see* Fenoterol 564
Fentanest® *see* Fentanyl 565
Fentanyl 565
Fentanyl Citrate *see* Fentanyl 565
Feostat® [OTC] *see* Iron Supplements 745
Feratab® [OTC] *see* Iron Supplements 745
Fer-Gen-Sol [OTC] *see* Iron Supplements 745
Fergon® [OTC] *see* Iron Supplements 745
Fer-In-Sol® [OTC] *see* Iron Supplements 745
Fer-Iron® [OTC] *see* Iron Supplements 745
Fermalac *see* *Lactobacillus acidophilus* and *Lactobacillus bulgaricus* 772
Fero-Grad 500® [OTC] *see* Ferrous Sulfate and Ascorbic Acid 569
Ferretts [OTC] *see* Iron Supplements 745
Ferric Gluconate 568
Ferrlecit® *see* Ferric Gluconate 568
Ferro-Sequels® [OTC] *see* Iron Supplements 745
Ferrous Fumarate *see* Iron Supplements 745
Ferrous Gluconate *see* Iron Supplements 745
Ferrous Salts *see* Iron Supplements 745
Ferrous Sulfate *see* Iron Supplements 745
Ferrous Sulfate and Ascorbic Acid 569
Fertinex® *see* Follitropins 607
Ferval® Ferroso *see* Iron Supplements 745
$FeSO_4$ (Ferrous Sulfate) *see* Iron Supplements 745
Fe-Tinic™ 150 [OTC] *see* Polysaccharide-Iron Complex 1096

Feverall® [OTC] *see* Acetaminophen . . . 27
Feverfew . . . 1431
Fexofenadine . . . 569
Fexofenadine and Pseudoephedrine . . . 570
Fexofenadine Hydrochloride *see* Fexofenadine . . . 569
Fiberall® *see* Psyllium . . . 1149
Fiberall® Chewable Tablet [OTC] *see* Calcium Polycarbophil . . . 228
FiberCon® Tablet [OTC] *see* Calcium Polycarbophil . . . 228
FiberEase™ [OTC] *see* Methylcellulose . . . 891
Fiber-Lax® Tablet [OTC] *see* Calcium Polycarbophil . . . 228
Fibrin Sealant Kit . . . 570
Filgrastim . . . 571
Finacea™ *see* Azelaic Acid . . . 151
Finasteride . . . 572
Findol® *see* Ketorolac . . . 765
Finevin® *see* Azelaic Acid . . . 151
Fioricet® *see* Butalbital, Acetaminophen, and Caffeine . . . 214
Fioricet® with Codeine *see* Butalbital, Acetaminophen, Caffeine, and Codeine . . . 215
Fiorinal® *see* Butalbital, Aspirin, and Caffeine . . . 216
Fiorinal®-C 1/2 *see* Butalbital, Aspirin, Caffeine, and Codeine . . . 217
Fiorinal®-C 1/4 *see* Butalbital, Aspirin, Caffeine, and Codeine . . . 217
Fiorinal® With Codeine *see* Butalbital, Aspirin, Caffeine, and Codeine . . . 217
Fisalamine *see* Mesalamine . . . 869
Fish Oils . . . 1432
Fisopred® *see* PrednisoLONE . . . 1110
Fixoten® *see* Pentoxifylline . . . 1058
FK506 *see* Tacrolimus . . . 1261
Flagenase® *see* Metronidazole . . . 902
Flagyl® *see* Metronidazole . . . 902
Flagyl ER® *see* Metronidazole . . . 902
Flamazine® *see* Silver Sulfadiazine . . . 1222
Flamicina® *see* Ampicillin . . . 103
Flanax® *see* Naproxen . . . 953
Flarex® *see* Fluorometholone . . . 587
Flatulex® [OTC] *see* Simethicone . . . 1222
Flavoxate . . . 573
Flavoxate Hydrochloride *see* Flavoxate . . . 573
Flaxseed Oil . . . 1432
Flebocortid *see* Hydrocortisone . . . 688
Flecainide . . . 574
Flecainide Acetate *see* Flecainide . . . 574
Fleet® Babylax® [OTC] *see* Glycerin . . . 644
Fleet® Bisacodyl Enema [OTC] *see* Bisacodyl . . . 186
Fleet® Enema [OTC] *see* Phosphate Supplements . . . 1076
Fleet® Glycerin Suppositories [OTC] *see* Glycerin . . . 644
Fleet® Glycerin Suppositories Maximum Strength [OTC] *see* Glycerin . . . 644
Fleet® Liquid Glycerin Suppositories [OTC] *see* Glycerin . . . 644
Fleet® Phospho®-Soda [OTC] *see* Phosphate Supplements . . . 1076
Fleet® Sof-Lax® [OTC] *see* Docusate . . . 463
Fleet® Sof-Lax® Overnight [OTC] *see* Docusate and Casanthranol . . . 464
Fleet® Stimulant Laxative [OTC] *see* Bisacodyl . . . 186
Flemoxon® *see* Amoxicillin . . . 93
Fletcher's® Castoria® [OTC] *see* Senna . . . 1215
Flexafen® *see* Ibuprofen . . . 703
Flexen *see* Naproxen . . . 953
Flexeril® *see* Cyclobenzaprine . . . 379
Flexitec *see* Cyclobenzaprine . . . 379
Flixonase® *see* Fluticasone . . . 599
Flixotide® *see* Fluticasone . . . 599
Flogen® *see* Naproxen . . . 953
Flogosan® *see* Piroxicam . . . 1090
Flolan® *see* Epoprostenol . . . 505
Flomax® *see* Tamsulosin . . . 1266
Flonase® *see* Fluticasone . . . 599
Florazole® ER *see* Metronidazole . . . 902
Florical® [OTC] *see* Calcium Supplements . . . 229
Florinef® *see* Fludrocortisone . . . 580
Florone® *see* Diflorasone . . . 438
Flovent® *see* Fluticasone . . . 599
Flovent® HFA *see* Fluticasone . . . 599
Flovent® Rotadisk® *see* Fluticasone . . . 599
Floxacin® *see* Norfloxacin . . . 987
Floxil® *see* Ofloxacin . . . 995
Floxin® *see* Ofloxacin . . . 995
Floxstat® *see* Ofloxacin . . . 995
Floxuridine . . . 576
Flubenisolone *see* Betamethasone . . . 177
Flucaine® *see* Proparacaine and Fluorescein . . . 1133
Fluconazole . . . 576
Flucytosine . . . 578
Fludara® *see* Fludarabine . . . 579
Fludarabine . . . 579
Fludarabine Phosphate *see* Fludarabine . . . 579
Fludrocortisone . . . 580
Fluken® *see* Flutamide . . . 598
Flulem® *see* Flutamide . . . 598
Flumadine® *see* Rimantadine . . . 1185
Flumazenil . . . 581
Flunisolide . . . 582
Flunitrazepam . . . 583

Fluocinolone . . . 584
Fluocinolone Acetonide *see* Fluocinolone . . . 584
Fluocinolone, Hydroquinone, and Tretinoin . . . 585
Fluocinonide . . . 585
Fluoderm *see* Fluocinolone . . . 584
Fluohydrisone Acetate *see* Fludrocortisone . . . 580
Fluohydrocortisone Acetate *see* Fludrocortisone . . . 580
Fluoracaine® *see* Proparacaine and Fluorescein . . . 1133
Fluor-A-Day [OTC] *see* Fluoride . . . 586
Fluoride . . . 586
Fluoride and Triclosan (Dental) *see* Triclosan and Fluoride . . . 1348
Fluorides . . . 1553
Fluorigard® [OTC] *see* Fluoride . . . 586
Fluori-Methane® *see* Dichlorodifluoromethane and Trichloromonofluoromethane . . . 428
Fluorinse® *see* Fluoride . . . 586
Fluorodeoxyuridine *see* Floxuridine . . . 576
9α-Fluorohydrocortisone Acetate *see* Fludrocortisone . . . 580
Fluorometholone . . . 587
Fluorometholone and Sulfacetamide *see* Sulfacetamide and Fluorometholone . . . 1250
Fluor-Op® *see* Fluorometholone . . . 587
Fluoroplex® *see* Fluorouracil . . . 588
Fluorouracil . . . 588
Fluoro-uracil *see* Fluorouracil . . . 588
5-Fluorouracil *see* Fluorouracil . . . 588
Fluotic® *see* Fluoride . . . 586
Fluoxac® *see* Fluoxetine . . . 589
Fluoxetine . . . 589
Fluoxetine Hydrochloride *see* Fluoxetine . . . 589
Fluoxymesterone . . . 592
Flupazine® *see* Trifluoperazine . . . 1349
Fluphenazine . . . 593
Fluphenazine Decanoate *see* Fluphenazine . . . 593
Fluphenazine Enanthate *see* Fluphenazine . . . 593
Fluphenazine Hydrochloride *see* Fluphenazine . . . 593
Flura-Drops® *see* Fluoride . . . 586
Flura-Loz® *see* Fluoride . . . 586
Flurandrenolide . . . 594
Flurandrenolone *see* Flurandrenolide . . . 594
Flurazepam . . . 595
Flurazepam Hydrochloride *see* Flurazepam . . . 595
Flurbiprofen . . . 596
Flurbiprofen Sodium *see* Flurbiprofen . . . 596
5-Flurocytosine *see* Flucytosine . . . 578
Fluro-Ethyl® *see* Ethyl Chloride and Dichlorotetrafluoroethane . . . 545
FluShield® *see* Influenza Virus Vaccine . . . 722
Flutamide . . . 598
Fluticasone . . . 599
Fluticasone and Salmeterol . . . 601
Fluticasone Propionate *see* Fluticasone . . . 599
Fluvastatin . . . 603
Fluviral S/F® *see* Influenza Virus Vaccine . . . 722
Fluvirin® *see* Influenza Virus Vaccine . . . 722
Fluvoxamine . . . 605
Fluzone® *see* Influenza Virus Vaccine . . . 722
Flynoken® *see* Folic Acid . . . 606
Flynoken A *see* Leucovorin . . . 783
FML® *see* Fluorometholone . . . 587
FML Forte® *see* Fluorometholone . . . 587
FML-S® *see* Sulfacetamide and Fluorometholone . . . 1250
Focalin™ *see* Dexmethylphenidate . . . 417
Foille® [OTC] *see* Benzocaine . . . 169
Foille® Medicated First Aid [OTC] *see* Benzocaine . . . 169
Foille® Plus [OTC] *see* Benzocaine . . . 169
Folacin *see* Folic Acid . . . 606
Folacin, Vitamin B_{12}, and Vitamin B_6 *see* Folic Acid, Cyanocobalamin, and Pyridoxine . . . 607
Folate *see* Folic Acid . . . 606
Folgard® [OTC] *see* Folic Acid, Cyanocobalamin, and Pyridoxine . . . 607
Folic Acid . . . 606
Folic Acid, Cyanocobalamin, and Pyridoxine . . . 607
Folinic Acid *see* Leucovorin . . . 783
Folitab *see* Folic Acid . . . 606
Follistim® *see* Follitropins . . . 607
Follitropin Alfa *see* Follitropins . . . 607
Follitropin Alpha *see* Follitropins . . . 607
Follitropin Beta *see* Follitropins . . . 607
Follitropins . . . 607
Foltx® *see* Folic Acid, Cyanocobalamin, and Pyridoxine . . . 607
Fomepizole . . . 609
Fomivirsen . . . 611
Fomivirsen Sodium *see* Fomivirsen . . . 611
Fondaparinux . . . 611
Fondaparinux Sodium *see* Fondaparinux . . . 611
Foradil® *see* Formoterol . . . 612
Foradil® Aerolizer™ *see* Formoterol . . . 612
Formoterol . . . 612
Formoterol Fumarate *see* Formoterol . . . 612
Formula E *see* Guaifenesin . . . 650
Formulation R™ [OTC] *see* Phenylephrine . . . 1071
Formulex® *see* Dicyclomine . . . 433
5-Formyl Tetrahydrofolate *see* Leucovorin . . . 783

Fortaz® *see* Ceftazidime . . . 275
Forteo™ *see* Teriparatide . . . 1280
Fortovase™ *see* Saquinavir . . . 1207
Fortum® *see* Ceftazidime . . . 275
Fosamax® *see* Alendronate . . . 54
Foscarnet . . . 613
Foscavir® *see* Foscarnet . . . 613
Fosfocil® *see* Fosfomycin . . . 615
Fosfomycin . . . 615
Fosfomycin Tromethamine *see* Fosfomycin . . . 615
Fosinopril . . . 616
Fosinopril and Hydrochlorothiazide . . . 617
Fosphenytoin . . . 618
Fosphenytoin Sodium *see* Fosphenytoin . . . 618
Fostex® 10% BPO [OTC] *see* Benzoyl Peroxide . . . 171
Fotexina® *see* Cefotaxime . . . 271
Fototar® [OTC] *see* Coal Tar . . . 359
Fragmin® *see* Dalteparin . . . 394
Freezone® [OTC] *see* Salicylic Acid . . . 1204
Fresenizol® *see* Metronidazole . . . 902
Fresofol® *see* Propofol . . . 1133
Frisium® *see* Clobazam . . . 344
Froben® *see* Flurbiprofen . . . 596
Froben-SR® *see* Flurbiprofen . . . 596
Frova® *see* Frovatriptan . . . 620
Frovatriptan . . . 620
Frovatriptan Succinate *see* Frovatriptan . . . 620
Froxal® *see* Cefuroxime . . . 279
Frusemide *see* Furosemide . . . 622
FS *see* Fibrin Sealant Kit . . . 570
5-FU *see* Fluorouracil . . . 588
FUDR® *see* Floxuridine . . . 576
Fulvestrant . . . 621
Fulvicin® P/G *see* Griseofulvin . . . 649
Fulvicin-U/F® *see* Griseofulvin . . . 649
Fulvina® P/G *see* Griseofulvin . . . 649
Fungi-Guard [OTC] *see* Tolnaftate . . . 1322
Fungi-Nail® [OTC] *see* Undecylenic Acid and Derivatives . . . 1365
Fungiquim *see* Miconazole . . . 906
Fungistat® *see* Terconazole . . . 1279
Fungistat Dual *see* Terconazole . . . 1279
Fungizone® *see* Amphotericin B (Conventional) . . . 98
Fung-O® [OTC] *see* Salicylic Acid . . . 1204
Fungoid® Tincture [OTC] *see* Miconazole . . . 906
Fungoral® *see* Ketoconazole . . . 762
Furadantin® *see* Nitrofurantoin . . . 980
Furadantina *see* Nitrofurantoin . . . 980
Furazolidone . . . 622
Furazosin *see* Prazosin . . . 1108
Furosemide . . . 622
Furoxona® *see* Furazolidone . . . 622
Furoxona Gotas *see* Furazolidone . . . 622
Furoxona Tabletas *see* Furazolidone . . . 622
Furoxone® *see* Furazolidone . . . 622
Fustaren® *see* Diclofenac . . . 429
Fustaren Retard *see* Diclofenac . . . 429
Fuxen® *see* Naproxen . . . 953
Fuxol® *see* Furazolidone . . . 622
Fuzeon™ *see* Enfuvirtide . . . 495
Gabapentin . . . 624
Gabitril® *see* Tiagabine . . . 1304
Gadoteridol *see* Radiological/Contrast Media (Nonionic) . . . 1165
Galecin® *see* Clindamycin . . . 341
Galedol® *see* Diclofenac . . . 429
Galidrin® *see* Ranitidine . . . 1168
Gamikal® *see* Amikacin . . . 74
Gamimune® N *see* Immune Globulin (Intravenous) . . . 714
Gamma Benzene Hexachloride *see* Lindane . . . 809
Gammagard® S/D *see* Immune Globulin (Intravenous) . . . 714
Gamma Globulin *see* Immune Globulin (Intramuscular) . . . 713
Gamma Hydroxybutyric Acid *see* Sodium Oxybate . . . 1231
Gammaphos *see* Amifostine . . . 73
Gammar®-P I.V. *see* Immune Globulin (Intravenous) . . . 714
Ganciclovir . . . 626
Ganirelix . . . 628
Ganirelix Acetate *see* Ganirelix . . . 628
Gani-Tuss® NR *see* Guaifenesin and Codeine . . . 650
Gantrisin® *see* SulfiSOXAZOLE . . . 1256
Garalen *see* Gentamicin . . . 634
Garamicina® *see* Gentamicin . . . 634
Garamycin® *see* Gentamicin . . . 634
Garlic . . . 1433
Gascop® *see* Albendazole . . . 47
Gastrec *see* Ranitidine . . . 1168
Gastrocrom® *see* Cromolyn Sodium . . . 375
Gastrointestinal Disorders . . . 1474
Gas-X® [OTC] *see* Simethicone . . . 1222
Gas-X® Extra Strength [OTC] *see* Simethicone . . . 1222
Gatifloxacin . . . 628
Gaviscon® Extra Strength [OTC] *see* Aluminum Hydroxide and Magnesium Carbonate . . . 68

Gaviscon® Liquid [OTC] *see* Aluminum Hydroxide and Magnesium Carbonate . . . 68
Gaviscon® Tablet [OTC] *see* Aluminum Hydroxide and Magnesium Trisilicate . . . 69
GBE *see* Ginkgo Biloba . . . 1434
G-CSF *see* Filgrastim . . . 571
G-CSF (PEG Conjugate) *see* Pegfilgrastim . . . 1040
GCV Sodium *see* Ganciclovir . . . 626
Gelatin (Absorbable) . . . 630
Gelclair™ *see* Maltodextrin . . . 840
Gelfilm® *see* Gelatin (Absorbable) . . . 630
Gelfoam® *see* Gelatin (Absorbable) . . . 630
Gel-Kam® [OTC] *see* Fluoride . . . 586
Gel-Kam® Rinse *see* Fluoride . . . 586
Gelucast® *see* Zinc Gelatin . . . 1409
Gelusil® *see* Aluminum Hydroxide and Magnesium Hydroxide . . . 69
Gelusil® Extra Strength *see* Aluminum Hydroxide and Magnesium Hydroxide . . . 69
Gemcitabine . . . 630
Gemcitabine Hydrochloride *see* Gemcitabine . . . 630
Gemfibrozil . . . 631
Gemtuzumab Ozogamicin . . . 632
Gemzar® *see* Gemcitabine . . . 630
Genac® [OTC] *see* Triprolidine and Pseudoephedrine . . . 1356
Gen-Acebutolol *see* Acebutolol . . . 25
Genaced [OTC] *see* Acetaminophen, Aspirin, and Caffeine . . . 34
Gen-Acyclovir *see* Acyclovir . . . 42
Genahist® [OTC] *see* DiphenhydrAMINE . . . 451
Gen-Alprazolam *see* Alprazolam . . . 61
Gen-Amiodarone *see* Amiodarone . . . 80
Gen-Amoxicillin *see* Amoxicillin . . . 93
Genapap® [OTC] *see* Acetaminophen . . . 27
Genapap® Children [OTC] *see* Acetaminophen . . . 27
Genapap® Extra Strength [OTC] *see* Acetaminophen . . . 27
Genapap® Infant [OTC] *see* Acetaminophen . . . 27
Genaphed® [OTC] *see* Pseudoephedrine . . . 1146
Genasal [OTC] *see* Oxymetazoline . . . 1022
Genasoft® [OTC] *see* Docusate . . . 463
Genasoft® Plus [OTC] *see* Docusate and Casanthranol . . . 464
Genasyme® [OTC] *see* Simethicone . . . 1222
Gen-Atenolol *see* Atenolol . . . 137
Genatuss DM® [OTC] *see* Guaifenesin and Dextromethorphan . . . 651
Gen-Azathioprine *see* Azathioprine . . . 150
Gen-Baclofen *see* Baclofen . . . 158
Gen-Beclo *see* Beclomethasone . . . 163
Gen-Bromazepam *see* Bromazepam . . . 199
Gen-Budesonide AQ *see* Budesonide . . . 202
Gen-Buspirone *see* BusPIRone . . . 211
Gencalc® 600 [OTC] *see* Calcium Supplements . . . 229
Gen-Captopril *see* Captopril . . . 238
Gen-Carbamazepine CR *see* Carbamazepine . . . 241
Gen-Cimetidine *see* Cimetidine . . . 326
Gen-Clobetasol *see* Clobetasol . . . 345
Gen-Clomipramine *see* ClomiPRAMINE . . . 349
Gen-Clonazepam *see* Clonazepam . . . 350
Gen-Cyclobenzaprine *see* Cyclobenzaprine . . . 379
Gen-Diltiazem *see* Diltiazem . . . 447
Gen-Diltiazem SR *see* Diltiazem . . . 447
Gen-Divalproex *see* Valproic Acid and Derivatives . . . 1371
Gen-Doxazosin *see* Doxazosin . . . 470
Genebs® [OTC] *see* Acetaminophen . . . 27
Genebs® Extra Strength [OTC] *see* Acetaminophen . . . 27
Genemicin® *see* Gentamicin . . . 634
Genenicina® *see* Gentamicin . . . 634
Generlac *see* Lactulose . . . 772
Genesec® [OTC] *see* Acetaminophen and Phenyltoloxamine . . . 31
Geneye® [OTC] *see* Tetrahydrozoline . . . 1288
Gen-Famotidine *see* Famotidine . . . 556
Gen-Fenofibrate Micro *see* Fenofibrate . . . 561
Genfiber® [OTC] *see* Psyllium . . . 1149
Gen-Fluoxetine *see* Fluoxetine . . . 589
Gen-Gemfibrozil *see* Gemfibrozil . . . 631
Gen-Glybe *see* GlyBURIDE . . . 642
Gengraf™ *see* CycloSPORINE . . . 383
Gen-Hydroxyurea *see* Hydroxyurea . . . 696
Gen-Indapamide *see* Indapamide . . . 716
Gen-Ipratropium *see* Ipratropium . . . 737
Genkova® *see* Gentamicin . . . 634
Gen-Lovastatin *see* Lovastatin . . . 828
Gen-Medroxy *see* MedroxyPROGESTERone . . . 849
Gen-Metformin *see* Metformin . . . 874
Gen-Minocycline *see* Minocycline . . . 915
Gen-Nabumetone *see* Nabumetone . . . 941
Gen-Naproxen EC *see* Naproxen . . . 953
Gen-Nitro *see* Nitroglycerin . . . 981
Gen-Nortriptyline *see* Nortriptyline . . . 989
Genoptic® *see* Gentamicin . . . 634
Genotropin® *see* Human Growth Hormone . . . 671
Genotropin Miniquick® *see* Human Growth Hormone . . . 671
Genoxal® *see* Cyclophosphamide . . . 381
Gen-Oxybutynin *see* Oxybutynin . . . 1016
Gen-Pindolol *see* Pindolol . . . 1085
Gen-Piroxicam *see* Piroxicam . . . 1090

Genpril® [OTC] *see* Ibuprofen . . . 703
Gen-Ranidine *see* Ranitidine . . . 1168
Genrex® *see* Gentamicin . . . 634
Gen-Salbutamol *see* Albuterol . . . 48
Gen-Selegiline *see* Selegiline . . . 1213
Gen-Sertraline *see* Sertraline . . . 1216
Gen-Sotalol *see* Sotalol . . . 1235
Gentabac® *see* Gentamicin . . . 634
Gentacidin® *see* Gentamicin . . . 634
Gentacin® *see* Gentamicin . . . 634
Genta Grin® *see* Gentamicin . . . 634
Gentak® *see* Gentamicin . . . 634
Gentamicin . . . 634
Gentamicin and Prednisolone *see* Prednisolone and Gentamicin . . . 1112
Gentamicin Sulfate *see* Gentamicin . . . 634
Gen-Tamoxifen *see* Tamoxifen . . . 1264
Gentarim® *see* Gentamicin . . . 634
Gentazaf® *see* Gentamicin . . . 634
GenTeal® [OTC] *see* Hydroxypropyl Methylcellulose . . . 696
GenTeal® Mild [OTC] *see* Hydroxypropyl Methylcellulose . . . 696
Gen-Temazepam *see* Temazepam . . . 1271
Gen-Terbinafine *see* Terbinafine . . . 1277
Gentian Violet . . . 636
Gen-Ticlopidine *see* Ticlopidine . . . 1307
Gen-Timolol *see* Timolol . . . 1309
Gentran® *see* Dextran . . . 419
Gen-Trazodone *see* Trazodone . . . 1336
Gen-Triazolam *see* Triazolam . . . 1345
Gen-Verapamil *see* Verapamil . . . 1382
Gen-Verapamil SR *see* Verapamil . . . 1382
Gen-Warfarin *see* Warfarin . . . 1397
Gen-Zopiclone *see* Zopiclone . . . 1415
Geocillin® *see* Carbenicillin . . . 245
Geref® *see* Sermorelin Acetate . . . 1215
Geref® Diagnostic *see* Sermorelin Acetate . . . 1215
Geritol® Tonic [OTC] *see* Vitamins (Multiple/Oral) . . . 1394
German Measles Vaccine *see* Rubella Virus Vaccine (Live) . . . 1202
Gevrabon® [OTC] *see* Vitamin B Complex . . . 1392
GG *see* Guaifenesin . . . 650
GHB *see* Sodium Oxybate . . . 1231
G.I.® *see* Gentamicin . . . 634
GI87084B *see* Remifentanil . . . 1171
Gimalxina® *see* Amoxicillin . . . 93
Ginedisc® *see* Estradiol . . . 521
Ginger . . . 1434
Gingi-Aid® Gingival Retraction Cord *see* Aluminum Chloride . . . 67
Gingi-Aid® Solution *see* Aluminum Chloride . . . 67
Ginkgo Biloba . . . 1434
ginkgold *see* Ginkgo Biloba . . . 1434
Ginkgopowder *see* Ginkgo Biloba . . . 1434
Ginkogink *see* Ginkgo Biloba . . . 1434
Ginseng, Panax . . . 1435
Ginseng, Siberian . . . 1436
Glatiramer Acetate . . . 636
Gliadel® *see* Carmustine . . . 253
Glibenclamide *see* GlyBURIDE . . . 642
Glibenil® *see* GlyBURIDE . . . 642
Glimepiride . . . 637
Glioten® *see* Enalapril . . . 492
GlipiZIDE . . . 638
Glipizide and Metformin . . . 639
Glipizide and Metformin Hydrochloride *see* Glipizide and Metformin . . . 639
GlucaGen® *see* Glucagon . . . 640
GlucaGen® Diagnostic Kit *see* Glucagon . . . 640
Glucagon . . . 640
Glucagon Diagnostic Kit *see* Glucagon . . . 640
Glucagon Emergency Kit *see* Glucagon . . . 640
Glucal® *see* GlyBURIDE . . . 642
Glucobay® *see* Acarbose . . . 24
Glucocerebrosidase *see* Alglucerase . . . 56
GlucoNorm® *see* Repaglinide . . . 1172
Glucophage® *see* Metformin . . . 874
Glucophage® Forte *see* Metformin . . . 874
Glucophage® XR *see* Metformin . . . 874
Glucosamine . . . 1437
Glucosamine Hydrochloride *see* Glucosamine . . . 1437
Glucosamine Sulfate *see* Glucosamine . . . 1437
Glucose *see* Glucose (Instant) . . . 641
Glucose (Instant) . . . 641
Glucose Polymers . . . 641
Glucotrol® *see* GlipiZIDE . . . 638
Glucotrol® XL *see* GlipiZIDE . . . 638
Glucovance® *see* Glyburide and Metformin . . . 643
Glucoven® *see* GlyBURIDE . . . 642
Glu-K® [OTC] *see* Potassium Supplements . . . 1102
Glupitel® *see* GlipiZIDE . . . 638
Glutamic Acid . . . 641
Glutamic Acid Hydrochloride *see* Glutamic Acid . . . 641
Glutol™ [OTC] *see* Glucose (Instant) . . . 641
Glutose™ [OTC] *see* Glucose (Instant) . . . 641

Glybenclamide *see* GlyBURIDE . . . 642
Glybenzcyclamide *see* GlyBURIDE . . . 642
GlyBURIDE . . . 642
Glyburide and Metformin . . . 643
Glyburide and Metformin Hydrochloride *see* Glyburide and Metformin . . . 643
Glycerin . . . 644
Glycerol *see* Glycerin . . . 644
Glycerol Guaiacolate *see* Guaifenesin . . . 650
Glycerol Triacetate *see* Triacetin . . . 1340
Glyceryl Trinitrate *see* Nitroglycerin . . . 981
Glycocome *see* Licorice . . . 1442
Glycon *see* Metformin . . . 874
Glycopyrrolate . . . 645
Glycopyrronium Bromide *see* Glycopyrrolate . . . 645
Glycyrrhiza glabra *see* Licorice . . . 1442
Glydiazinamide *see* GlipiZIDE . . . 638
Glynase® PresTab® *see* GlyBURIDE . . . 642
Gly-Oxide® Oral [OTC] *see* Carbamide Peroxide . . . 244
Glyquin® *see* Hydroquinone . . . 693
Glyset® *see* Miglitol . . . 913
Glytuss® [OTC] *see* Guaifenesin . . . 650
GM-CSF *see* Sargramostim . . . 1209
Goatweed *see* St John's Wort . . . 1448
Golden Seal . . . 1437
Gold Sodium Thiomalate . . . 646
GoLYTELY® *see* Polyethylene Glycol-Electrolyte Solution . . . 1094
Gonak™ [OTC] *see* Hydroxypropyl Methylcellulose . . . 696
Gonal-F® *see* Follitropins . . . 607
Gonic® *see* Chorionic Gonadotropin (Human) . . . 320
Gonioscopic Ophthalmic Solution *see* Hydroxypropyl Methylcellulose . . . 696
Goniosol® [OTC] *see* Hydroxypropyl Methylcellulose . . . 696
Goody's® Extra Strength Headache Powder [OTC] *see* Acetaminophen, Aspirin, and Caffeine . . . 34
Goody's PM® Powder *see* Acetaminophen and Diphenhydramine . . . 30
Gopten® *see* Trandolapril . . . 1331
Gordofilm® [OTC] *see* Salicylic Acid . . . 1204
Gormel® [OTC] *see* Urea . . . 1365
Goserelin . . . 647
Goserelin Acetate *see* Goserelin . . . 647
Gotu Kola . . . 1438
GP 47680 *see* Oxcarbazepine . . . 1012
G-Phed *see* Guaifenesin and Pseudoephedrine . . . 652
G-Phed-PD *see* Guaifenesin and Pseudoephedrine . . . 652
Gramicidin, Neomycin, and Polymyxin B *see* Neomycin, Polymyxin B, and Gramicidin . . . 963
Graneodin-B *see* Benzocaine . . . 169
Granisetron . . . 648
Granulex® *see* Trypsin, Balsam Peru, and Castor Oil . . . 1362
Granulocyte Colony Stimulating Factor *see* Filgrastim . . . 571
Granulocyte Colony Stimulating Factor (PEG Conjugate) *see* Pegfilgrastim . . . 1040
Granulocyte-Macrophage Colony Stimulating Factor *see* Sargramostim . . . 1209
Grapefruit Seed . . . 1438
Grape Seed . . . 1439
Graten® *see* Morphine Sulfate . . . 931
Gravol® *see* DimenhyDRINATE . . . 449
Green Tea . . . 1439
Grifulvin® V *see* Griseofulvin . . . 649
Griseofulvin . . . 649
Griseofulvin Microsize *see* Griseofulvin . . . 649
Griseofulvin Ultramicrosize *see* Griseofulvin . . . 649
Grisovin® *see* Griseofulvin . . . 649
Grisovin-FP *see* Griseofulvin . . . 649
Gris-PEG® *see* Griseofulvin . . . 649
Growth Hormone *see* Human Growth Hormone . . . 671
Grunicina® *see* Amoxicillin . . . 93
GSE *see* Grapefruit Seed . . . 1438
Guaifed® [OTC] *see* Guaifenesin and Pseudoephedrine . . . 652
Guaifed-PD® *see* Guaifenesin and Pseudoephedrine . . . 652
Guaifenesin . . . 650
Guaifenesin and Codeine . . . 650
Guaifenesin and Dextromethorphan . . . 651
Guaifenesin and Hydrocodone *see* Hydrocodone and Guaifenesin . . . 683
Guaifenesin and Phenylephrine . . . 652
Guaifenesin and Pseudoephedrine . . . 652
Guaifenesin and Theophylline *see* Theophylline and Guaifenesin . . . 1293
Guaifenesin, Hydrocodone, and Pseudoephedrine *see* Hydrocodone, Pseudoephedrine, and Guaifenesin . . . 687
Guaifenesin, Pseudoephedrine, and Codeine . . . 653
Guaifenesin, Pseudoephedrine, and Dextromethorphan . . . 653
Guaifenex® DM *see* Guaifenesin and Dextromethorphan . . . 651
Guaifenex® G *see* Guaifenesin . . . 650
Guaifenex® GP *see* Guaifenesin and Pseudoephedrine . . . 652
Guaifenex® LA *see* Guaifenesin . . . 650
Guaifenex® PSE *see* Guaifenesin and Pseudoephedrine . . . 652
Guaifen PSE *see* Guaifenesin and Pseudoephedrine . . . 652
Guaituss AC® *see* Guaifenesin and Codeine . . . 650
Guai-Vent™/PSE *see* Guaifenesin and Pseudoephedrine . . . 652
Guanabenz . . . 654
Guanabenz Acetate *see* Guanabenz . . . 654
Guanadrel . . . 654
Guanadrel Sulfate *see* Guanadrel . . . 654

Guanfacine . . . 655
Guanfacine Hydrochloride *see* Guanfacine . . . 655
Gugecin *see* Cinoxacin . . . 327
Guiatuss® [OTC] *see* Guaifenesin . . . 650
Guiatuss™ CF *see* Guaifenesin, Pseudoephedrine, and Dextromethorphan . . . 653
Guiatuss™ DAC® *see* Guaifenesin, Pseudoephedrine, and Codeine . . . 653
Guiatuss-DM® [OTC] *see* Guaifenesin and Dextromethorphan . . . 651
Gum Benjamin *see* Benzoin . . . 171
Gynazole-1™ *see* Butoconazole . . . 218
Gyne-Lotrimin® [OTC] *see* Clotrimazole . . . 356
Gyne-Lotrimin® 3 [OTC] *see* Clotrimazole . . . 356
Gynix® [OTC] *see* Clotrimazole . . . 356
Gyno-Daktarin *see* Miconazole . . . 906
Gyno-Daktarin V *see* Miconazole . . . 906
Gynodiol® *see* Estradiol . . . 521
Gynol II® [OTC] *see* Nonoxynol 9 . . . 985
Gyno-Myfungar® *see* Oxiconazole . . . 1014
Habitrol® *see* Nicotine . . . 971
Haemophilus b Conjugate Vaccine . . . 656
Haemophilus b Oligosaccharide Conjugate Vaccine *see Haemophilus* b Conjugate Vaccine . . . 656
Haemophilus b Polysaccharide Vaccine *see Haemophilus* b Conjugate Vaccine . . . 656
HAES-steril® *see* Hetastarch . . . 669
Halcinonide . . . 657
Halcion® *see* Triazolam . . . 1345
Haldol® *see* Haloperidol . . . 659
Haldol decanoas® *see* Haloperidol . . . 659
Haldol® Decanoate *see* Haloperidol . . . 659
Halfprin® [OTC] *see* Aspirin . . . 131
Halobetasol . . . 658
Halobetasol Propionate *see* Halobetasol . . . 658
Halofantrine . . . 658
Halofantrine Hydrochloride *see* Halofantrine . . . 658
Halog® *see* Halcinonide . . . 657
Halog®-E *see* Halcinonide . . . 657
Haloperidol . . . 659
Haloperidol Decanoate *see* Haloperidol . . . 659
Haloperidol Lactate *see* Haloperidol . . . 659
Haloperidol-LA Omega *see* Haloperidol . . . 659
Haloperidol Long Acting *see* Haloperidol . . . 659
Haloperil® *see* Haloperidol . . . 659
Halotestin® *see* Fluoxymesterone . . . 592
Halotussin® DAC *see* Guaifenesin, Pseudoephedrine, and Codeine . . . 653
Haltran® [OTC] *see* Ibuprofen . . . 703
Harpagophytum procumbens see Devil's Claw . . . 1428
Havrix™ *see* Hepatitis A Vaccine . . . 665
Havrix® and Engerix-B® *see* Hepatitis A (Inactivated) and Hepatitis B (Recombinant) Vaccine . . . 664
Haw *see* Hawthorn . . . 1440
Hawthorn . . . 1440
Hayfebrol® [OTC] *see* Chlorpheniramine and Pseudoephedrine . . . 308
HbCV *see Haemophilus* b Conjugate Vaccine . . . 656
HBIG *see* Hepatitis B Immune Globulin . . . 666
hBNP *see* Nesiritide . . . 964
25-HCC *see* Calcifediol . . . 221
hCG *see* Chorionic Gonadotropin (Human) . . . 320
HCTZ *see* Hydrochlorothiazide . . . 675
HCTZ and Telmisartan *see* Telmisartan and Hydrochlorothiazide . . . 1270
HDA® Toothache [OTC] *see* Benzocaine . . . 169
HDCV *see* Rabies Virus Vaccine . . . 1164
Head & Shoulders® Classic Clean [OTC] *see* Pyrithione Zinc . . . 1154
Head & Shoulders® Classic Clean 2-In-1 [OTC] *see* Pyrithione Zinc . . . 1154
Head & Shoulders® Dry Scalp Care [OTC] *see* Pyrithione Zinc . . . 1154
Head & Shoulders® Extra Fullness [OTC] *see* Pyrithione Zinc . . . 1154
Head & Shoulders® Refresh [OTC] *see* Pyrithione Zinc . . . 1154
Head & Shoulders® Smooth & Silky 2-In-1 [OTC] *see* Pyrithione Zinc . . . 1154
Healon® *see* Sodium Hyaluronate . . . 1230
Healon®5 *see* Sodium Hyaluronate . . . 1230
Healon® GV *see* Sodium Hyaluronate . . . 1230
Hectorol® *see* Doxercalciferol . . . 472
Helberina *see* Heparin . . . 662
Helidac® *see* Bismuth, Metronidazole, and Tetracycline . . . 187
Helistat® *see* Microfibrillar Collagen Hemostat . . . 907
Helixate® FS *see* Antihemophilic Factor (Recombinant) . . . 115
Helminzole *see* Mebendazole . . . 846
Hemabate™ *see* Carboprost Tromethamine . . . 250
Hemiacidrin *see* Citric Acid Bladder Mixture . . . 335
Hemin . . . 661
Hemobion® 200 *see* Iron Supplements . . . 745
Hemobion® 400 *see* Iron Supplements . . . 745
Hemocyte® [OTC] *see* Iron Supplements . . . 745
Hemodent® Gingival Retraction Cord *see* Aluminum Chloride . . . 67
Hemofil® M *see* Antihemophilic Factor (Human) . . . 113
Hemril-HC® *see* Hydrocortisone . . . 688
Henexal *see* Furosemide . . . 622
Hepalean® *see* Heparin . . . 662
Hepalean® Leo *see* Heparin . . . 662
Hepalean®-LOK *see* Heparin . . . 662
Heparin . . . 662
Heparin Calcium *see* Heparin . . . 662

Heparin Cofactor I *see* Antithrombin III . . . 117
Heparin Lock Flush *see* Heparin . . . 662
Heparin Sodium *see* Heparin . . . 662
Hepatitis A (Inactivated) and Hepatitis B (Recombinant) Vaccine . . . 664
Hepatitis A Vaccine . . . 665
Hepatitis B Immune Globulin . . . 666
Hepatitis B Inactivated Virus Vaccine (plasma derived) *see* Hepatitis B Vaccine . . . 666
Hepatitis B Inactivated Virus Vaccine (recombinant DNA) *see* Hepatitis B Vaccine . . . 666
Hepatitis B (Recombinant) and Hepatitis A Inactivated Vaccine *see* Hepatitis A (Inactivated) and Hepatitis B (Recombinant) Vaccine . . . 664
Hepatitis B Vaccine . . . 666
Hep-Lock® *see* Heparin . . . 662
Hepsera™ *see* Adefovir . . . 44
Heptovir® *see* Lamivudine . . . 773
Herceptin® *see* Trastuzumab . . . 1335
Herklin *see* Lindane . . . 809
Herklin Shampoo® *see* Lindane . . . 809
HES *see* Hetastarch . . . 669
Hespan® *see* Hetastarch . . . 669
Hetastarch . . . 669
Hexachlorocyclohexane *see* Lindane . . . 809
Hexachlorophene . . . 669
Hexalen® *see* Altretamine . . . 66
Hexamethylenetetramine *see* Methenamine . . . 879
Hexamethylmelamine *see* Altretamine . . . 66
Hexit™ *see* Lindane . . . 809
HEXM *see* Altretamine . . . 66
Hextend® *see* Hetastarch . . . 669
Hexylresorcinol . . . 670
Hibiclens® [OTC] *see* Chlorhexidine Gluconate . . . 300
Hibidil® 1:2000 *see* Chlorhexidine Gluconate . . . 300
Hib Polysaccharide Conjugate *see* *Haemophilus* b Conjugate Vaccine . . . 656
HibTITER® *see* *Haemophilus* b Conjugate Vaccine . . . 656
Hidantoina® *see* Phenytoin . . . 1073
Hidramox® *see* Amoxicillin . . . 93
Hidroquin® *see* Hydroquinone . . . 693
Higroton 50 *see* Chlorthalidone . . . 315
Hipocol® *see* Niacin . . . 967
Hipokinon® *see* Trihexyphenidyl . . . 1351
Hiprex® *see* Methenamine . . . 879
Histalet® [OTC] *see* Chlorpheniramine and Pseudoephedrine . . . 308
Histatab® Plus [OTC] *see* Chlorpheniramine and Phenylephrine . . . 308
Histor-D® *see* Chlorpheniramine and Phenylephrine . . . 308
Hi-Vegi-Lip® [OTC] *see* Pancreatin . . . 1030
Hivid® *see* Zalcitabine . . . 1403
HIV Infection and AIDS . . . 1482
HMG Massone® *see* Menotropins . . . 857
HMM *see* Altretamine . . . 66
HMS Liquifilm® *see* Medrysone . . . 850
Hold® DM [OTC] *see* Dextromethorphan . . . 423
Homatropine . . . 670
Homatropine and Hydrocodone *see* Hydrocodone and Homatropine . . . 684
Homatropine Hydrobromide *see* Homatropine . . . 670
Horse Antihuman Thymocyte Gamma Globulin *see* Lymphocyte Immune Globulin . . . 831
Horse Chestnut . . . 1440
H.P. Acthar® Gel *see* Corticotropin . . . 372
HTF919 *see* Tegaserod . . . 1268
Humalog® *see* Insulin Preparations . . . 723
Humalog® Mix 25™ *see* Insulin Preparations . . . 723
Humalog® Mix 75/25™ *see* Insulin Preparations . . . 723
Human Diploid Cell Cultures Rabies Vaccine *see* Rabies Virus Vaccine . . . 1164
Human Growth Hormone . . . 671
Humanized IgG1 Anti-CD52 Monoclonal Antibody *see* Alemtuzumab . . . 52
Human LFA-3/IgG(1) Fusion Protein *see* Alefacept . . . 52
Human Thyroid Stimulating Hormone *see* Thyrotropin Alpha . . . 1304
Humate-P® *see* Antihemophilic Factor (Human) . . . 113
Humatin® *see* Paromomycin . . . 1035
Humatrope® *see* Human Growth Hormone . . . 671
Humegon® *see* Chorionic Gonadotropin (Human) . . . 320
Humegon® *see* Menotropins . . . 857
Humibid® DM *see* Guaifenesin and Dextromethorphan . . . 651
Humibid® L.A. *see* Guaifenesin . . . 650
Humibid® Pediatric *see* Guaifenesin . . . 650
Humulin® *see* Insulin Preparations . . . 723
Humulin 20/80® *see* Insulin Preparations . . . 723
Humulin 30/70® *see* Insulin Preparations . . . 723
Humulin® 50/50 *see* Insulin Preparations . . . 723
Humulin® 70/30 *see* Insulin Preparations . . . 723
Humulin L® *see* Insulin Preparations . . . 723
Humulin N® *see* Insulin Preparations . . . 723
Humulin R® *see* Insulin Preparations . . . 723
Humulin® R (Concentrated) U-500 *see* Insulin Preparations . . . 723
Humulin® U *see* Insulin Preparations . . . 723
Huperzia serrata *see* HuperzineA . . . 1441
HuperzineA . . . 1441
Hurricaine® *see* Benzocaine . . . 169
HXM *see* Altretamine . . . 66
Hyalgan® *see* Sodium Hyaluronate . . . 1230
Hyaluronic Acid *see* Sodium Hyaluronate . . . 1230
Hyate:C® *see* Antihemophilic Factor (Porcine) . . . 114

Hycamptamine *see* Topotecan 1325
Hycamtin® *see* Topotecan 1325
Hycodan® *see* Hydrocodone and Homatropine 684
Hycomine® Compound *see* Hydrocodone, Chlorpheniramine, Phenylephrine, Acetaminophen, and Caffeine 686
Hycort™ *see* Hydrocortisone 688
Hycosin *see* Hydrocodone and Guaifenesin 683
Hycotuss® *see* Hydrocodone and Guaifenesin 683
Hydeltra T.B.A.® *see* PrednisoLONE 1110
Hydergine® *see* Ergoloid Mesylates 509
Hyderm *see* Hydrocortisone 688
HydrALAZINE 673
Hydralazine and Hydrochlorothiazide 675
Hydralazine Hydrochloride *see* HydrALAZINE 673
Hydralazine, Hydrochlorothiazide, and Reserpine 675
Hydramine® [OTC] *see* DiphenhydrAMINE 451
Hydramine® Cough [OTC] *see* DiphenhydrAMINE 451
Hydrastis canadensis *see* Golden Seal 1437
Hydrate® [DSC] *see* DimenhyDRINATE 449
Hydrated Chloral *see* Chloral Hydrate 295
Hydrea® *see* Hydroxyurea 696
Hydrisalic™ [OTC] *see* Salicylic Acid 1204
Hydrocet® *see* Hydrocodone and Acetaminophen 678
Hydrochlorothiazide 675
Hydrochlorothiazide and Amiloride *see* Amiloride and Hydrochlorothiazide 76
Hydrochlorothiazide and Benazepril *see* Benazepril and Hydrochlorothiazide 167
Hydrochlorothiazide and Bisoprolol *see* Bisoprolol and Hydrochlorothiazide 189
Hydrochlorothiazide and Captopril *see* Captopril and Hydrochlorothiazide 240
Hydrochlorothiazide and Enalapril *see* Enalapril and Hydrochlorothiazide 494
Hydrochlorothiazide and Fosinopril *see* Fosinopril and Hydrochlorothiazide 617
Hydrochlorothiazide and Hydralazine *see* Hydralazine and Hydrochlorothiazide 675
Hydrochlorothiazide and Irbesartan *see* Irbesartan and Hydrochlorothiazide 740
Hydrochlorothiazide and Lisinopril *see* Lisinopril and Hydrochlorothiazide 814
Hydrochlorothiazide and Losartan *see* Losartan and Hydrochlorothiazide 827
Hydrochlorothiazide and Methyldopa *see* Methyldopa and Hydrochlorothiazide 892
Hydrochlorothiazide and Moexipril *see* Moexipril and Hydrochlorothiazide 927
Hydrochlorothiazide and Propranolol *see* Propranolol and Hydrochlorothiazide 1142
Hydrochlorothiazide and Quinapril *see* Quinapril and Hydrochlorothiazide 1158
Hydrochlorothiazide and Spironolactone 677
Hydrochlorothiazide and Telmisartan *see* Telmisartan and Hydrochlorothiazide 1270
Hydrochlorothiazide and Triamterene 677
Hydrochlorothiazide and Valsartan *see* Valsartan and Hydrochlorothiazide 1375
Hydrochlorothiazide, Hydralazine, and Reserpine *see* Hydralazine, Hydrochlorothiazide, and Reserpine 675
Hydrocil® [OTC] *see* Psyllium 1149
Hydrocodone and Acetaminophen 678
Hydrocodone and Aspirin 680
Hydrocodone and Chlorpheniramine 682
Hydrocodone and Guaifenesin 683
Hydrocodone and Homatropine 684
Hydrocodone and Ibuprofen 684
Hydrocodone, Chlorpheniramine, Phenylephrine, Acetaminophen, and Caffeine 686
Hydrocodone, Pseudoephedrine, and Guaifenesin 687
Hydrocortisone 688
Hydrocortisone Acetate *see* Hydrocortisone 688
Hydrocortisone, Acetic Acid, and Propylene Glycol Diacetate *see* Acetic Acid, Propylene Glycol Diacetate, and Hydrocortisone 38
Hydrocortisone and Benzoyl Peroxide *see* Benzoyl Peroxide and Hydrocortisone 172
Hydrocortisone and Ciprofloxacin *see* Ciprofloxacin and Hydrocortisone 331
Hydrocortisone and Iodoquinol *see* Iodoquinol and Hydrocortisone 736
Hydrocortisone and Lidocaine *see* Lidocaine and Hydrocortisone 805
Hydrocortisone and Oxytetracycline *see* Oxytetracycline and Hydrocortisone 1025
Hydrocortisone and Pramoxine *see* Pramoxine and Hydrocortisone 1106
Hydrocortisone and Urea *see* Urea and Hydrocortisone 1365
Hydrocortisone, Bacitracin, Neomycin, and Polymyxin B *see* Bacitracin, Neomycin, Polymyxin B, and Hydrocortisone 158
Hydrocortisone Buteprate *see* Hydrocortisone 688
Hydrocortisone Butyrate *see* Hydrocortisone 688
Hydrocortisone, Chloramphenicol, and Polymyxin B *see* Chloramphenicol, Polymyxin B, and Hydrocortisone 299
Hydrocortisone, Colistin, and Neomycin *see* Colistin, Neomycin, and Hydrocortisone 367
Hydrocortisone Cypionate *see* Hydrocortisone 688
Hydrocortisone, Neomycin, and Polymyxin B *see* Neomycin, Polymyxin B, and Hydrocortisone 963
Hydrocortisone, Polymyxin B, and Chloramphenicol *see* Chloramphenicol, Polymyxin B, and Hydrocortisone 299
Hydrocortisone, Propylene Glycol Diacetate, and Acetic Acid *see* Acetic Acid, Propylene Glycol Diacetate, and Hydrocortisone 38
Hydrocortisone Sodium Phosphate *see* Hydrocortisone 688
Hydrocortisone Sodium Succinate *see* Hydrocortisone 688
Hydrocortisone Valerate *see* Hydrocortisone 688
Hydrocortone® *see* Hydrocortisone 688
Hydrocortone® Phosphate *see* Hydrocortisone 688
Hydrogesic® [DSC] *see* Hydrocodone and Acetaminophen 678
Hydromet® *see* Hydrocodone and Homatropine 684
Hydromorph Contin® *see* Hydromorphone 691
Hydromorphone 691
Hydromorphone HP *see* Hydromorphone 691
Hydromorphone Hydrochloride *see* Hydromorphone 691
Hydropane® *see* Hydrocodone and Homatropine 684

Hydroquinol *see* Hydroquinone . . . 693
Hydroquinone . . . 693
Hydroquinone, Fluocinolone Acetonide, and Tretinoin *see* Fluocinolone, Hydroquinone, and Tretinoin . . . 585
Hydro-Tussin™-CBX *see* Carbinoxamine and Pseudoephedrine . . . 247
Hydro-Tussin™ DM *see* Guaifenesin and Dextromethorphan . . . 651
Hydro-Tussin™ HD *see* Hydrocodone, Pseudoephedrine, and Guaifenesin . . . 687
Hydro-Tussin™ XP *see* Hydrocodone, Pseudoephedrine, and Guaifenesin . . . 687
HydroVal® *see* Hydrocortisone . . . 688
Hydroxocobalamin . . . 693
Hydroxyamphetamine and Tropicamide . . . 694
4-Hydroxybutyrate *see* Sodium Oxybate . . . 1231
Hydroxycarbamide *see* Hydroxyurea . . . 696
Hydroxychloroquine . . . 694
Hydroxychloroquine Sulfate *see* Hydroxychloroquine . . . 694
25-Hydroxycholecalciferol *see* Calcifediol . . . 221
Hydroxydaunomycin Hydrochloride *see* DOXOrubicin . . . 473
Hydroxyethylcellulose *see* Artificial Tears . . . 128
Hydroxyethyl Starch *see* Hetastarch . . . 669
Hydroxyldaunorubicin Hydrochloride *see* DOXOrubicin . . . 473
Hydroxypropyl Cellulose . . . 695
Hydroxypropyl Methylcellulose . . . 696
Hydroxyurea . . . 696
25-Hydroxyvitamin D_3 *see* Calcifediol . . . 221
HydrOXYzine . . . 697
Hydroxyzine Hydrochloride *see* HydrOXYzine . . . 697
Hydroxyzine Pamoate *see* HydrOXYzine . . . 697
Hygroton® [DSC] *see* Chlorthalidone . . . 315
Hylorel® *see* Guanadrel . . . 654
Hyoscine *see* Scopolamine . . . 1210
Hyoscyamine . . . 699
Hyoscyamine, Atropine, Scopolamine, and Phenobarbital . . . 700
Hyoscyamine, Atropine, Scopolamine, Kaolin, and Pectin . . . 701
Hyoscyamine, Atropine, Scopolamine, Kaolin, Pectin, and Opium . . . 701
Hyoscyamine, Methenamine, Sodium Biphosphate, Phenyl Salicylate, and Methylene Blue *see* Methenamine, Sodium Biphosphate, Phenyl Salicylate, Methylene Blue, and Hyoscyamine . . . 880
Hyoscyamine Sulfate *see* Hyoscyamine . . . 699
Hyosine *see* Hyoscyamine . . . 699
Hypercium perforatum see St John's Wort . . . 1448
Hyperstat® *see* Diazoxide . . . 427
Hyperstat I.V.® *see* Diazoxide . . . 427
HypoTears [OTC] *see* Artificial Tears . . . 128
HypoTears PF [OTC] *see* Artificial Tears . . . 128
Hyrexin-50® *see* DiphenhydrAMINE . . . 451
Hytakerol® *see* Dihydrotachysterol . . . 446
Hytinic® [OTC] *see* Polysaccharide-Iron Complex . . . 1096
Hytone® *see* Hydrocortisone . . . 688
Hytrin® *see* Terazosin . . . 1276
Hytuss® [OTC] *see* Guaifenesin . . . 650
Hytuss-2X® [OTC] *see* Guaifenesin . . . 650
Hyzaar® *see* Losartan and Hydrochlorothiazide . . . 827
Hyzaar® DS *see* Losartan and Hydrochlorothiazide . . . 827
Iberet® [OTC] *see* Vitamins (Multiple/Oral) . . . 1394
Iberet®-500 [OTC] *see* Vitamins (Multiple/Oral) . . . 1394
Iberet-Folic-500® *see* Vitamins (Multiple/Oral) . . . 1394
Ibidomide Hydrochloride *see* Labetalol . . . 769
Ibritumomab . . . 702
Ibritumomab Tiuxetan *see* Ibritumomab . . . 702
Ibuprofen . . . 703
Ibuprofen and Hydrocodone *see* Hydrocodone and Ibuprofen . . . 684
Ibuprofen and Pseudoephedrine *see* Pseudoephedrine and Ibuprofen . . . 1148
Ibu-Tab® *see* Ibuprofen . . . 703
Ibutilide . . . 706
Ibutilide Fumarate *see* Ibutilide . . . 706
IC-Green® *see* Indocyanine Green . . . 719
ICI 182,780 *see* Fulvestrant . . . 621
ICI 204, 219 *see* Zafirlukast . . . 1402
ICRF-187 *see* Dexrazoxane . . . 419
Idamycin® [DSC] *see* Idarubicin . . . 706
Idamycin PFS® *see* Idarubicin . . . 706
Idarubicin . . . 706
Idarubicin Hydrochloride *see* Idarubicin . . . 706
Idulamine® *see* Azatadine . . . 149
Ifa Norex® *see* Diethylpropion . . . 436
Ifa Reducing "S"® *see* Phentermine . . . 1069
Ifex® *see* Ifosfamide . . . 707
IFLrA *see* Interferon Alfa-2a . . . 726
Ifolem® *see* Ifosfamide . . . 707
Ifosfamide . . . 707
Ifoxan® *see* Ifosfamide . . . 707
IG *see* Immune Globulin (Intramuscular) . . . 713
IGIM *see* Immune Globulin (Intramuscular) . . . 713
Ikatin® *see* Gentamicin . . . 634
IL-1Ra *see* Anakinra . . . 108
IL-2 *see* Aldesleukin . . . 50
IL-11 *see* Oprelvekin . . . 1003
Iletin® II Pork *see* Insulin Preparations . . . 723
Iliadin® *see* Oxymetazoline . . . 1022
Ilosone® *see* Erythromycin . . . 512

Ilsatec® *see* Lansoprazole . . . 777
Imdur® *see* Isosorbide Mononitrate . . . 751
Imidazole Carboxamide *see* Dacarbazine . . . 391
Imiglucerase . . . 709
Imigran® *see* Sumatriptan . . . 1258
Imipemide *see* Imipenem and Cilastatin . . . 709
Imipenem and Cilastatin . . . 709
Imipramine . . . 711
Imipramine Hydrochloride *see* Imipramine . . . 711
Imipramine Pamoate *see* Imipramine . . . 711
Imiquimod . . . 713
Imitrex® *see* Sumatriptan . . . 1258
ImmuCyst® *see* BCG Vaccine . . . 161
Immune Globulin (Intramuscular) . . . 713
Immune Globulin (Intravenous) . . . 714
Immune Serum Globulin *see* Immune Globulin (Intramuscular) . . . 713
Immunizations (Vaccines) . . . 1612
Imodium® *see* Loperamide . . . 819
Imodium® A-D [OTC] *see* Loperamide . . . 819
Imogam® *see* Rabies Immune Globulin (Human) . . . 1164
Imogam® Rabies Pasteurized *see* Rabies Immune Globulin (Human) . . . 1164
Imot Ofteno *see* Timolol . . . 1309
Imovane® *see* Zopiclone . . . 1415
Imovax® Rabies *see* Rabies Virus Vaccine . . . 1164
Imuran® *see* Azathioprine . . . 150
In-111 Zevalin *see* Ibritumomab . . . 702
Inamrinone . . . 716
Inapsine® *see* Droperidol . . . 481
Indapamide . . . 716
Indarzona® *see* Dexamethasone . . . 413
Inderal® *see* Propranolol . . . 1139
Inderalici *see* Propranolol . . . 1139
Inderal®-LA *see* Propranolol . . . 1139
Inderide® *see* Propranolol and Hydrochlorothiazide . . . 1142
Indian Eye *see* Golden Seal . . . 1437
Indian Head *see* *Echinacea* . . . 1429
Indinavir . . . 718
Indocid® *see* Indomethacin . . . 719
Indocid® P.D.A. *see* Indomethacin . . . 719
Indocin® *see* Indomethacin . . . 719
Indocin® I.V. *see* Indomethacin . . . 719
Indocin® SR *see* Indomethacin . . . 719
Indocyanine Green . . . 719
Indo-Lemmon *see* Indomethacin . . . 719
Indometacin *see* Indomethacin . . . 719
Indomethacin . . . 719
Indomethacin Sodium Trihydrate *see* Indomethacin . . . 719
Indotec *see* Indomethacin . . . 719
INF-alpha 2 *see* Interferon Alfa-2b . . . 727
Infantaire [OTC] *see* Acetaminophen . . . 27
Infants Tylenol® Cold [OTC] *see* Acetaminophen and Pseudoephedrine . . . 31
Infants' Tylenol® Cold Plus Cough Concentrated Drops [OTC] *see* Acetaminophen, Dextromethorphan, and Pseudoephedrine . . . 35
Infasurf® *see* Calfactant . . . 232
INFeD® *see* Iron Dextran Complex . . . 743
Inflamase® Forte *see* PrednisoLONE . . . 1110
Inflamase® Mild *see* PrednisoLONE . . . 1110
Infliximab . . . 721
Infliximab, Recombinant *see* Infliximab . . . 721
Influenza Virus Vaccine . . . 722
Influenza Virus Vaccine (inactivated whole-virus) *see* Influenza Virus Vaccine . . . 722
Influenza Virus Vaccine (purified split-virus) *see* Influenza Virus Vaccine . . . 722
Influenza Virus Vaccine (purified surface antigen) *see* Influenza Virus Vaccine . . . 722
Influenza Virus Vaccine (split-virus) *see* Influenza Virus Vaccine . . . 722
Infufer® *see* Iron Dextran Complex . . . 743
Infumorph® *see* Morphine Sulfate . . . 931
INH *see* Isoniazid . . . 748
Inhepar *see* Heparin . . . 662
Inhibace® *see* Cilazapril . . . 324
Inhibitron® *see* Omeprazole . . . 999
Innohep® *see* Tinzaparin . . . 1311
INOmax® *see* Nitric Oxide . . . 979
Insogen® *see* ChlorproPAMIDE . . . 314
Inspiryl® *see* Albuterol . . . 48
Inspra™ *see* Eplerenone . . . 502
Insta-Glucose® [OTC] *see* Glucose (Instant) . . . 641
Insulina Lenta *see* Insulin Preparations . . . 723
Insulina NPH *see* Insulin Preparations . . . 723
Insulina Regular *see* Insulin Preparations . . . 723
Insulin Novolin 30/70® *see* Insulin Preparations . . . 723
Insulin Novolin L® *see* Insulin Preparations . . . 723
Insulin Novolin N® *see* Insulin Preparations . . . 723
Insulin Novolin R® *see* Insulin Preparations . . . 723
Insulin Preparations . . . 723
Intacglobin *see* Immune Globulin (Intravenous) . . . 714
Intal® *see* Cromolyn Sodium . . . 375
Integrilin® *see* Eptifibatide . . . 507
α-2-interferon *see* Interferon Alfa-2b . . . 727
Interferon Alfa-2a . . . 726
Interferon Alfa-2a (PEG Conjugate) *see* Peginterferon Alfa-2a . . . 1040

Interferon Alfa-2b . . . 727
Interferon Alfa-2b and Ribavirin . . . 730
Interferon Alfa-n3 . . . 731
Interferon Beta-1a . . . 732
Interferon Beta-1b . . . 733
Interferon Gamma-1b . . . 734
Interleukin-1 Receptor antagonist *see* Anakinra . . . 108
Interleukin-2 *see* Aldesleukin . . . 50
Interleukin-11 *see* Oprelvekin . . . 1003
Intralipid® *see* Fat Emulsion . . . 558
Intravenous Fat Emulsion *see* Fat Emulsion . . . 558
Intrifiban *see* Eptifibatide . . . 507
Intron® A *see* Interferon Alfa-2b . . . 727
Invanz® *see* Ertapenem . . . 511
Inversine® *see* Mecamylamine . . . 846
Invirase® *see* Saquinavir . . . 1207
Iodex [OTC] *see* Iodine . . . 735
Iodine . . . 735
Iodine *see* Trace Metals . . . 1328
Iodoflex™ *see* Iodine . . . 735
Iodopen® *see* Trace Metals . . . 1328
Iodoquinol . . . 735
Iodoquinol and Hydrocortisone . . . 736
Iodosorb® *see* Iodine . . . 735
Iohexol *see* Radiological/Contrast Media (Nonionic) . . . 1165
Ionamin® *see* Phentermine . . . 1069
Ionil® [OTC] *see* Salicylic Acid . . . 1204
Ionil Plus® *see* Salicylic Acid . . . 1204
Iopamidol *see* Radiological/Contrast Media (Nonionic) . . . 1165
Iopidine® *see* Apraclonidine . . . 118
Iosat™ [OTC] *see* Potassium Iodide . . . 1101
Ioversol *see* Radiological/Contrast Media (Nonionic) . . . 1165
Ipecac Syrup . . . 736
I-Pentolate® *see* Cyclopentolate . . . 380
IPM Wound Gel™ [OTC] *see* Sodium Hyaluronate . . . 1230
IPOL® *see* Poliovirus Vaccine (Inactivated) . . . 1093
Ipratropium . . . 737
Ipratropium and Albuterol . . . 738
Ipratropium Bromide *see* Ipratropium . . . 737
I-Prin [OTC] *see* Ibuprofen . . . 703
Iproveratril Hydrochloride *see* Verapamil . . . 1382
IPV *see* Poliovirus Vaccine (Inactivated) . . . 1093
Irbesartan . . . 739
Irbesartan and Hydrochlorothiazide . . . 740
Ircon® [OTC] *see* Iron Supplements . . . 745
Irinotecan . . . 740
Iron Dextran Complex . . . 743
Iron Sucrose . . . 744
Iron Sulfate (Ferrous Sulfate) *see* Iron Supplements . . . 745
Iron Supplements . . . 745
Isadol® *see* Zidovudine . . . 1406
Isavir® *see* Acyclovir . . . 42
ISD *see* Isosorbide Dinitrate . . . 750
ISDN *see* Isosorbide Dinitrate . . . 750
ISG *see* Immune Globulin (Intramuscular) . . . 713
ISMN *see* Isosorbide Mononitrate . . . 751
Ismo® *see* Isosorbide Mononitrate . . . 751
Isoamyl Nitrite *see* Amyl Nitrite . . . 107
Isobac *see* Sulfamethoxazole and Trimethoprim . . . 1253
Isobamate *see* Carisoprodol . . . 251
Isocarboxazid . . . 747
Isodine® *see* Povidone-Iodine . . . 1104
Isoetharine . . . 747
Isoetharine Hydrochloride *see* Isoetharine . . . 747
Isoetharine Mesylate *see* Isoetharine . . . 747
Isoflavones *see* Soy Isoflavones . . . 1448
Isoket® *see* Isosorbide Dinitrate . . . 750
Isometheptene, Acetaminophen, and Dichloralphenazone *see* Acetaminophen, Isometheptene, and Dichloralphenazone . . . 36
Isometheptene, Dichloralphenazone, and Acetaminophen *see* Acetaminophen, Isometheptene, and Dichloralphenazone . . . 36
Isoniazid . . . 748
Isoniazid and Rifampin *see* Rifampin and Isoniazid . . . 1181
Isoniazid, Rifampin, and Pyrazinamide *see* Rifampin, Isoniazid, and Pyrazinamide . . . 1182
Isonicotinic Acid Hydrazide *see* Isoniazid . . . 748
Isonipecaine Hydrochloride *see* Meperidine . . . 858
Isoprenaline Hydrochloride *see* Isoproterenol . . . 749
Isoproterenol . . . 749
Isoproterenol Hydrochloride *see* Isoproterenol . . . 749
Isoproterenol Sulfate *see* Isoproterenol . . . 749
Isoptin® *see* Verapamil . . . 1382
Isoptin® I.V. *see* Verapamil . . . 1382
Isoptin® SR *see* Verapamil . . . 1382
Isopto® Atropine *see* Atropine . . . 144
Isopto® Carbachol *see* Carbachol . . . 241
Isopto® Carpine *see* Pilocarpine . . . 1080
Isopto® Eserine *see* Physostigmine . . . 1078
Isopto® Homatropine *see* Homatropine . . . 670
Isopto® Hyoscine *see* Scopolamine . . . 1210
Isopto® Tears [OTC] *see* Artificial Tears . . . 128

Isopto® Tears [OTC] *see* Hydroxypropyl Methylcellulose . . . 696
Isorbid® *see* Isosorbide Dinitrate . . . 750
Isordil® *see* Isosorbide Dinitrate . . . 750
Isosorbide Dinitrate . . . 750
Isosorbide Mononitrate . . . 751
Isotamine® *see* Isoniazid . . . 748
Isotretinoin . . . 752
Isotrex® *see* Isotretinoin . . . 752
Isovue® *see* Radiological/Contrast Media (Nonionic) . . . 1165
Isox® *see* Itraconazole . . . 755
Isoxsuprine . . . 753
Isoxsuprine Hydrochloride *see* Isoxsuprine . . . 753
Isradipine . . . 754
Isuprel® *see* Isoproterenol . . . 749
Italnik® *see* Ciprofloxacin . . . 328
Itch-X® [OTC] *see* Pramoxine . . . 1105
Itraconazole . . . 755
Itranax® *see* Itraconazole . . . 755
Iveegam EN *see* Immune Globulin (Intravenous) . . . 714
Iveegam Immuno® *see* Immune Globulin (Intravenous) . . . 714
Ivermectin . . . 757
IVIG *see* Immune Globulin (Intravenous) . . . 714
IvyBlock® [OTC] *see* Bentoquatam . . . 168
Izadima® *see* Ceftazidime . . . 275
Japanese Encephalitis Virus Vaccine (Inactivated) . . . 758
Jaundice Root *see* Golden Seal . . . 1437
JE-VAX® *see* Japanese Encephalitis Virus Vaccine (Inactivated) . . . 758
Johimbe *see* Yohimbe . . . 1451
K+8 *see* Potassium Supplements . . . 1102
K+10 *see* Potassium Supplements . . . 1102
Kadian® *see* Morphine Sulfate . . . 931
Kala® [OTC] *see Lactobacillus acidophilus* and *Lactobacillus bulgaricus* . . . 772
Kaletra™ *see* Lopinavir and Ritonavir . . . 820
Kalmz [OTC] *see* Phosphorated Carbohydrate Solution . . . 1078
Kanamycin . . . 759
Kanamycin Sulfate *see* Kanamycin . . . 759
Kantrex® *see* Kanamycin . . . 759
Kaodene® NN [OTC] *see* Kaolin and Pectin . . . 760
Kaolin and Pectin . . . 760
Kaon-Cl-10® *see* Potassium Supplements . . . 1102
Kaon-Cl® 20 *see* Potassium Supplements . . . 1102
Kaopectate® *see* Attapulgite . . . 146
Kaopectate® [OTC] *see* Bismuth . . . 186
Kaopectate® Advanced Formula [DSC] [OTC] *see* Attapulgite . . . 146
Kaopectate® Extra Strength [OTC] *see* Bismuth . . . 186
Kaopectate® Maximum Strength Caplets [DSC] [OTC] *see* Attapulgite . . . 146
Kao-Spen® [OTC] *see* Kaolin and Pectin . . . 760
Kapanol® *see* Morphine Sulfate . . . 931
Kapectolin® [OTC] *see* Kaolin and Pectin . . . 760
Kapectolin PG® *see* Hyoscyamine, Atropine, Scopolamine, Kaolin, Pectin, and Opium . . . 701
Kariva™ *see* Combination Hormonal Contraceptives . . . 368
Kasmal® *see* Ketotifen . . . 768
Kava . . . 1442
Kava Kava *see* Kava . . . 1442
Kaveri *see* Ginkgo Biloba . . . 1434
Kay Ciel® *see* Potassium Supplements . . . 1102
K+ Care® *see* Potassium Supplements . . . 1102
K+ Care® ET *see* Potassium Supplements . . . 1102
KCl (Potassium Chloride) *see* Potassium Supplements . . . 1102
K-Dur® 10 *see* Potassium Supplements . . . 1102
K-Dur® 20 *see* Potassium Supplements . . . 1102
Keduril® *see* Ketoprofen . . . 763
Kedvil *see* Ibuprofen . . . 703
Keflex® *see* Cephalexin . . . 285
Keftab® *see* Cephalexin . . . 285
Kefurox® [DSC] *see* Cefuroxime . . . 279
Kefzol® [DSC] *see* Cefazolin . . . 263
Kelfiprim *see* Sulfamethoxazole and Trimethoprim . . . 1253
Kemadrin® *see* Procyclidine . . . 1125
Kenacort® *see* Triamcinolone . . . 1341
Kenalin® *see* Sulindac . . . 1257
Kenalog® *see* Triamcinolone . . . 1341
Kenalog-10® *see* Triamcinolone . . . 1341
Kenalog-40® *see* Triamcinolone . . . 1341
Kenalog® in Orabase *see* Triamcinolone . . . 1341
Kenalog® in Orabase® *see* Triamcinolone Acetonide Dental Paste . . . 1344
Kenamil *see* Zidovudine . . . 1406
Kenaprol *see* Metoprolol . . . 901
Kenoket® *see* Clonazepam . . . 350
Kenolan® *see* Captopril . . . 238
Kenopril® *see* Enalapril . . . 492
Kentadin® *see* Pentoxifylline . . . 1058
Kenzoflex® *see* Ciprofloxacin . . . 328
Keoxifene Hydrochloride *see* Raloxifene . . . 1165
Keppra® *see* Levetiracetam . . . 787
Keralyt® [OTC] *see* Salicylic Acid . . . 1204
Kerlone® *see* Betaxolol . . . 180
Ketalar® *see* Ketamine . . . 761
Ketalin® *see* Ketamine . . . 761
Ketamine . . . 761

Ketamine Hydrochloride *see* Ketamine 761
Ketoconazole 762
Ketoderm® *see* Ketoconazole 762
Ketoprofen 763
Ketorolac 765
Ketorolac Tromethamine *see* Ketorolac 765
Ketotifen 768
Ketotifen Fumarate *see* Ketotifen 768
Kew *see* Kava 1442
Kew Tree *see* Ginkgo Biloba 1434
Key-E® [OTC] *see* Vitamin E 1393
Key- E® Kaps [OTC] *see* Vitamin E 1393
KI *see* Potassium Iodide 1101
Kidkare Decongestant [OTC] *see* Pseudoephedrine 1146
Kidrolase® *see* Asparaginase 129
Kineret™ *see* Anakinra 108
Kinestase® *see* Cisapride 332
Kinevac® *see* Sincalide 1225
Klamath Weed *see* St John's Wort 1448
Klaricid® *see* Clarithromycin 337
Klaron® *see* Sulfacetamide 1249
Klean-Prep® *see* Polyethylene Glycol-Electrolyte Solution 1094
Klerist-D® [OTC] *see* Chlorpheniramine and Pseudoephedrine 308
Klonopin™ *see* Clonazepam 350
K-Lor™ *see* Potassium Supplements 1102
Klor-Con® *see* Potassium Supplements 1102
Klor-Con® 8 *see* Potassium Supplements 1102
Klor-Con® 10 *see* Potassium Supplements 1102
Klor-Con®/25 *see* Potassium Supplements 1102
Klor-Con®/EF *see* Potassium Supplements 1102
Klor-Con® M10 *see* Potassium Supplements 1102
Klor-Con® M20 *see* Potassium Supplements 1102
Klotrix® *see* Potassium Supplements 1102
Klyndaken® *see* Clindamycin 341
K-Lyte® *see* Potassium Citrate 1100
K-Lyte® *see* Potassium Supplements 1102
K-Lyte/Cl® *see* Potassium Supplements 1102
K-Lyte/Cl® 50 *see* Potassium Supplements 1102
K-Lyte® DS *see* Potassium Supplements 1102
Koāte®-DVI *see* Antihemophilic Factor (Human) 113
Kodet SE [OTC] *see* Pseudoephedrine 1146
Koffex DM-D *see* Pseudoephedrine and Dextromethorphan 1147
Koffex DM + Decongestant + Expectorant *see* Guaifenesin, Pseudoephedrine, and Dextromethorphan 653
Koffex DM-Expectorant *see* Guaifenesin and Dextromethorphan 651
Koffex Expectorant *see* Guaifenesin 650
Kogenate® *see* Antihemophilic Factor (Recombinant) 115
Kogenate® FS *see* Antihemophilic Factor (Recombinant) 115
Kolephrin® GG/DM [OTC] *see* Guaifenesin and Dextromethorphan 651
Konaderm® *see* Ketoconazole 762
Konakion® *see* Phytonadione 1079
Konsyl® [OTC] *see* Psyllium 1149
Konsyl-D® [OTC] *see* Psyllium 1149
Konsyl® Easy Mix [OTC] *see* Psyllium 1149
Konsyl® Orange [OTC] *see* Psyllium 1149
Koptin® *see* Kanamycin 759
K-Phos® MF *see* Phosphate Supplements 1076
K-Phos® Neutral *see* Phosphate Supplements 1076
K-Phos® No. 2 *see* Phosphate Supplements 1076
K-Phos® Original *see* Phosphate Supplements 1076
K-Phos® Original *see* Potassium Acid Phosphate 1100
K-Phos® Original *see* Potassium Supplements 1102
K-Profen® *see* Ketoprofen 763
Kristalose™ *see* Lactulose 772
K-Tab® *see* Potassium Supplements 1102
Kutrase® *see* Pancreatin 1030
Ku-Zyme® *see* Pancreatin 1030
Ku-Zyme® HP *see* Pancrelipase 1030
Kwelcof® *see* Hydrocodone and Guaifenesin 683
Kwellada-P™ *see* Permethrin 1062
Kytril® *see* Granisetron 648
L-3-Hydroxytyrosine *see* Levodopa 792
L-749,345 *see* Ertapenem 511
Labetalol 769
Labetalol Hydrochloride *see* Labetalol 769
Lac-Hydrin® *see* Lactic Acid and Ammonium Hydroxide 771
Laciken® *see* Acyclovir 42
LAClotion™ *see* Lactic Acid and Ammonium Hydroxide 771
Lacrisert® *see* Hydroxypropyl Cellulose 695
Lactaid® [OTC] *see* Lactase 771
Lactaid® Extra Strength [OTC] *see* Lactase 771
Lactaid® Ultra [OTC] *see* Lactase 771
Lactase 771
Lacteol® Fort *see* *Lactobacillus acidophilus* and *Lactobacillus bulgaricus* 772
Lactic Acid and Ammonium Hydroxide 771
Lactic Acid and Sodium-PCA 771
LactiCare® [OTC] *see* Lactic Acid and Sodium-PCA 771
LactiCare-HC® *see* Hydrocortisone 688
Lactinex® [OTC] *see* *Lactobacillus acidophilus* and *Lactobacillus bulgaricus* 772
Lactinol® *see* Lactic Acid and Sodium-PCA 771

Lactinol-E® *see* Lactic Acid and Sodium-PCA . . . 771
Lactobacillus acidophilus see Lactobacillus acidophilus and *Lactobacillus bulgaricus* . . . 772
Lactobacillus acidophilus and *Lactobacillus bulgaricus* . . . 772
Lactoflavin *see* Riboflavin . . . 1178
Lactrase® [OTC] *see* Lactase . . . 771
Lactulax® *see* Lactulose . . . 772
Lactulose . . . 772
Ladakamycin *see* Azacitidine . . . 149
Ladogal® *see* Danazol . . . 397
Lakriment Neu *see* Licorice . . . 1442
L-AmB *see* Amphotericin B (Liposomal) . . . 101
Lamictal® *see* Lamotrigine . . . 774
Lamisil® *see* Terbinafine . . . 1277
Lamisil® AT™ [OTC] *see* Terbinafine . . . 1277
Lamivudine . . . 773
Lamivudine, Abacavir, and Zidovudine *see* Abacavir, Lamivudine, and Zidovudine . . . 23
Lamivudine and Zidovudine *see* Zidovudine and Lamivudine . . . 1407
Lamotrigine . . . 774
Lampicin® *see* Ampicillin . . . 103
Lamprene® *see* Clofazimine . . . 346
Lanacane® [OTC] *see* Benzocaine . . . 169
Lanaphilic® [OTC] *see* Urea . . . 1365
Lanexat® *see* Flumazenil . . . 581
Lanolin, Cetyl Alcohol, Glycerin, Petrolatum, and Mineral Oil . . . 776
Lanolin, Coal Tar, and Mineral Oil *see* Coal Tar, Lanolin, and Mineral Oil . . . 360
Lanolin, Mineral Oil, and Coal Tar *see* Coal Tar, Lanolin, and Mineral Oil . . . 360
Lanoxicaps® *see* Digoxin . . . 441
Lanoxin® *see* Digoxin . . . 441
Lansoprazole . . . 777
Lantus® *see* Insulin Preparations . . . 723
Lanvis® *see* Thioguanine . . . 1296
Laracit® *see* Cytarabine . . . 389
Largactil® *see* ChlorproMAZINE . . . 312
L-Arginine *see* Arginine . . . 121
Lariam® *see* Mefloquine . . . 852
Larodopa® *see* Levodopa . . . 792
Lasix® *see* Furosemide . . . 622
Lasix® Special *see* Furosemide . . . 622
L-asparaginase *see* Asparaginase . . . 129
Lassar's Zinc Paste *see* Zinc Oxide . . . 1409
Lastet® *see* Etoposide . . . 549
Latanoprost . . . 778
Latotryd® *see* Erythromycin . . . 512
Lauricin® *see* Erythromycin . . . 512
Lauritran® *see* Erythromycin . . . 512
Laurus Sassafras see Sassafras Oil . . . 1446
Laxilose *see* Lactulose . . . 772
l-Bunolol Hydrochloride *see* Levobunolol . . . 789
L-Carnitine *see* Carnitine . . . 1424
L-Carnitine *see* Levocarnitine . . . 791
LCD *see* Coal Tar . . . 359
LCR *see* VinCRIStine . . . 1387
L-Deprenyl *see* Selegiline . . . 1213
L-Dopa *see* Levodopa . . . 792
Leche De Magnesia Normex *see* Magnesium Supplements . . . 837
Lectopam® *see* Bromazepam . . . 199
Ledercort *see* Triamcinolone . . . 1341
Ledermicina *see* Demeclocycline . . . 406
Lederpax *see* Erythromycin . . . 512
Ledertrexate® *see* Methotrexate . . . 884
Ledoxina® *see* Cyclophosphamide . . . 381
Leflunomide . . . 779
Legatrin PM® [OTC] *see* Acetaminophen and Diphenhydramine . . . 30
Lemblastine® *see* VinBLAStine . . . 1386
Lenoltec *see* Acetaminophen and Codeine . . . 29
Lenpryl® *see* Captopril . . . 238
Lente® Iletin® II *see* Insulin Preparations . . . 723
Lentopenil *see* Penicillin G (Parenteral/Aqueous) . . . 1049
Lepirudin . . . 781
Lepirudin (rDNA) *see* Lepirudin . . . 781
Leponex® *see* Clozapine . . . 358
Leptilan® *see* Valproic Acid and Derivatives . . . 1371
Leptopsique® *see* Perphenazine . . . 1062
Lertamine® *see* Loratadine . . . 822
Lertamine-D® *see* Pseudoephedrine . . . 1146
Lescol® *see* Fluvastatin . . . 603
Lescol® XL *see* Fluvastatin . . . 603
Lessina™ *see* Combination Hormonal Contraceptives . . . 368
Letrozole . . . 782
Leucomax® *see* Sargramostim . . . 1209
Leucovorin . . . 783
Leucovorin Calcium *see* Leucovorin . . . 783
Leukeran® *see* Chlorambucil . . . 296
Leukine™ *see* Sargramostim . . . 1209
Leunase® *see* Asparaginase . . . 129
Leuprolide . . . 784
Leuprolide Acetate *see* Leuprolide . . . 784
Leuprorelin *see* Leuprolide . . . 784
Leuprorelin Acetate *see* Leuprolide . . . 784
Leurocristine *see* VinCRIStine . . . 1387

Leustatin® *see* Cladribine . . . 336
Levalbuterol . . . 786
Levamisole . . . 786
Levamisole Hydrochloride *see* Levamisole . . . 786
Levaquin® *see* Levofloxacin . . . 794
Levarterenol Bitartrate *see* Norepinephrine . . . 985
Levate® *see* Amitriptyline . . . 83
Levatol® *see* Penbutolol . . . 1045
Levbid® *see* Hyoscyamine . . . 699
Levetiracetam . . . 787
Levlen® *see* Combination Hormonal Contraceptives . . . 368
Levlite™ *see* Combination Hormonal Contraceptives . . . 368
Levobetaxolol . . . 788
Levobunolol . . . 789
Levobunolol Hydrochloride *see* Levobunolol . . . 789
Levobupivacaine . . . 789
Levocabastine . . . 791
Levocabastine Hydrochloride *see* Levocabastine . . . 791
Levocarnitine . . . 791
Levocina® *see* Methotrimeprazine . . . 887
Levodopa . . . 792
Levodopa and Carbidopa . . . 793
Levo-Dromoran® *see* Levorphanol . . . 799
Levofloxacin . . . 794
Levomepromazine *see* Methotrimeprazine . . . 887
Levomethadyl Acetate Hydrochloride . . . 796
Levonorgestrel . . . 797
Levophed® *see* Norepinephrine . . . 985
Levora® *see* Combination Hormonal Contraceptives . . . 368
Levorphanol . . . 799
Levorphanol Tartrate *see* Levorphanol . . . 799
Levorphan Tartrate *see* Levorphanol . . . 799
Levothroid® *see* Levothyroxine . . . 800
Levothyroxine . . . 800
Levothyroxine Sodium *see* Levothyroxine . . . 800
Levoxyl® *see* Levothyroxine . . . 800
Levsin® *see* Hyoscyamine . . . 699
Levsinex® *see* Hyoscyamine . . . 699
Levsin/SL® *see* Hyoscyamine . . . 699
Levulan® *see* Aminolevulinic Acid . . . 77
Levulan® Kerastick™ *see* Aminolevulinic Acid . . . 77
Levulose, Dextrose and Phosphoric Acid *see* Phosphorated Carbohydrate Solution . . . 1078
Lexapro™ *see* Escitalopram . . . 516
Lexxel™ *see* Enalapril and Felodipine . . . 494
LFA-3/IgG(1) Fusion Protein, Human *see* Alefacept . . . 52
l-Hyoscyamine Sulfate *see* Hyoscyamine . . . 699
Librax® *see* Clidinium and Chlordiazepoxide . . . 341
Librium® *see* Chlordiazepoxide . . . 299
Licorice . . . 1442
LidaMantle® *see* Lidocaine . . . 801
Lida-Mantle HC® *see* Lidocaine and Hydrocortisone . . . 805
Lidemol® *see* Fluocinonide . . . 585
Lidex® *see* Fluocinonide . . . 585
Lidex-E® *see* Fluocinonide . . . 585
Lidocaine . . . 801
Lidocaine and Epinephrine . . . 804
Lidocaine and Hydrocortisone . . . 805
Lidocaine and Prilocaine . . . 806
Lidocaine Hydrochloride *see* Lidocaine . . . 801
Lidocaine (Transoral) . . . 807
Lidodan™ *see* Lidocaine . . . 801
Lidoderm® *see* Lidocaine . . . 801
LID-Pack® *see* Bacitracin and Polymyxin B . . . 157
Lifenac® *see* Diclofenac . . . 429
Lifenal *see* Diclofenac . . . 429
Lignocaine Hydrochloride *see* Lidocaine . . . 801
Limbitrol® *see* Amitriptyline and Chlordiazepoxide . . . 85
Limbitrol® DS *see* Amitriptyline and Chlordiazepoxide . . . 85
Lin-Amox *see* Amoxicillin . . . 93
Lin-Buspirone *see* BusPIRone . . . 211
Lincocin® *see* Lincomycin . . . 808
Lincomycin . . . 808
Lincomycin Hydrochloride *see* Lincomycin . . . 808
Lindane . . . 809
Linezolid . . . 809
Lin-Megestrol *see* Megestrol . . . 853
Lin-Nefazodone *see* Nefazodone . . . 957
Lin-Pravastatin *see* Pravastatin . . . 1106
Lin-Sotalol *see* Sotalol . . . 1235
Lioresal® *see* Baclofen . . . 158
Liotec *see* Baclofen . . . 158
Liothyronine . . . 810
Liothyronine Sodium *see* Liothyronine . . . 810
Liotrix . . . 811
Lipancreatin *see* Pancrelipase . . . 1030
Lipidil® *see* Fenofibrate . . . 561
Lipidil Micro® *see* Fenofibrate . . . 561
Lipidil Supra® *see* Fenofibrate . . . 561
Lipitor® *see* Atorvastatin . . . 140
Lipocin *see* Fat Emulsion . . . 558

Lipoic Acid *see* Alpha-Lipoic Acid . . . 1420
Liposyn® III *see* Fat Emulsion . . . 558
Lipram 4500 *see* Pancrelipase . . . 1030
Lipram-CR *see* Pancrelipase . . . 1030
Lipram-PN *see* Pancrelipase . . . 1030
Lipram-UL *see* Pancrelipase . . . 1030
Liquibid® *see* Guaifenesin . . . 650
Liquibid® 1200 *see* Guaifenesin . . . 650
Liquibid-D *see* Guaifenesin and Phenylephrine . . . 652
Liqui-Char® [OTC] *see* Charcoal . . . 294
Liquid Antidote *see* Charcoal . . . 294
Liquifilm® Tears [OTC] *see* Artificial Tears . . . 128
Liquiprin® for Children [OTC] *see* Acetaminophen . . . 27
Liquorice *see* Licorice . . . 1442
Liroken® *see* Diclofenac . . . 429
Lisinopril . . . 813
Lisinopril and Hydrochlorothiazide . . . 814
Lithane™ *see* Lithium . . . 815
Lithellm® 300 *see* Lithium . . . 815
Litheum® *see* Lithium . . . 815
Lithium . . . 815
Lithium Carbonate *see* Lithium . . . 815
Lithium Citrate *see* Lithium . . . 815
Lithobid® *see* Lithium . . . 815
Lithostat® *see* Acetohydroxamic Acid . . . 39
Livostin® *see* Levocabastine . . . 791
L-Lysine *see* Lysine . . . 832
L-Lysine Hydrochloride *see* Lysine . . . 832
LMD® *see* Dextran . . . 419
LNg 20 *see* Levonorgestrel . . . 797
LoCHOLEST® *see* Cholestyramine Resin . . . 318
LoCHOLEST® Light *see* Cholestyramine Resin . . . 318
Locoid® *see* Hydrocortisone . . . 688
Locoid Lipocream® *see* Hydrocortisone . . . 688
Lodimol *see* Dipyridamole . . . 456
Lodine® *see* Etodolac . . . 547
Lodine® Retard *see* Etodolac . . . 547
Lodine® XL *see* Etodolac . . . 547
Lodosyn® *see* Carbidopa . . . 246
Lodoxamide . . . 816
Lodoxamide Tromethamine *see* Lodoxamide . . . 816
Loestrin® *see* Combination Hormonal Contraceptives . . . 368
Loestrin® Fe *see* Combination Hormonal Contraceptives . . . 368
Logesic® *see* Diclofenac . . . 429
Logimax *see* Felodipine . . . 560
L-OHP *see* Oxaliplatin . . . 1008
Lomacin® *see* Lomefloxacin . . . 817
Lomefloxacin . . . 817
Lomefloxacin Hydrochloride *see* Lomefloxacin . . . 817
Lomine *see* Dicyclomine . . . 433
Lomocot® *see* Diphenoxylate and Atropine . . . 453
Lomotil® *see* Atropine . . . 144
Lomotil® *see* Diphenoxylate and Atropine . . . 453
Lomustine . . . 818
Loniten® *see* Minoxidil . . . 917
Lonox® *see* Diphenoxylate and Atropine . . . 453
Lo/Ovral® *see* Combination Hormonal Contraceptives . . . 368
Loperacap *see* Loperamide . . . 819
Loperamide . . . 819
Loperamide Hydrochloride *see* Loperamide . . . 819
Lopid® *see* Gemfibrozil . . . 631
Lopinavir *see* Lopinavir and Ritonavir . . . 820
Lopinavir and Ritonavir . . . 820
Lopremone *see* Protirelin . . . 1144
Lopresor® *see* Metoprolol . . . 901
Lopressor® *see* Metoprolol . . . 901
Loprox® *see* Ciclopirox . . . 322
Lorabid® *see* Loracarbef . . . 821
Loracarbef . . . 821
Loratadine . . . 822
Loratadine and Pseudoephedrine . . . 823
Lorazepam . . . 824
Lorazepam Intensol® *see* Lorazepam . . . 824
Lorcet® 10/650 *see* Hydrocodone and Acetaminophen . . . 678
Lorcet®-HD *see* Hydrocodone and Acetaminophen . . . 678
Lorcet® Plus *see* Hydrocodone and Acetaminophen . . . 678
Loroxide® [OTC] *see* Benzoyl Peroxide . . . 171
Lortab® *see* Hydrocodone and Acetaminophen . . . 678
Losartan . . . 825
Losartan and Hydrochlorothiazide . . . 827
Losartan Potassium *see* Losartan . . . 825
Losec® *see* Omeprazole . . . 999
Lotemax® *see* Loteprednol . . . 827
Lotensin® *see* Benazepril . . . 166
Lotensin® HCT *see* Benazepril and Hydrochlorothiazide . . . 167
Loteprednol . . . 827
Loteprednol Etabonate *see* Loteprednol . . . 827
Lotrel® *see* Amlodipine and Benazepril . . . 89
Lotrel® *see* Benazepril and Hydrochlorothiazide . . . 167
Lotriderm® *see* Betamethasone and Clotrimazole . . . 179

Lotrimin® *see* Clotrimazole . . . 356
Lotrimin® AF [OTC] *see* Clotrimazole . . . 356
Lotrimin AF® *see* Miconazole . . . 906
Lotrimin® AF Powder/Spray [OTC] *see* Miconazole . . . 906
Lotrimin® Ultra™ [OTC] *see* Butenafine . . . 217
Lotrisone® *see* Betamethasone and Clotrimazole . . . 179
Lotronex® *see* Alosetron . . . 60
Lovastatin . . . 828
Lovastatin and Niacin *see* Niacin and Lovastatin . . . 968
Lovenox® *see* Enoxaparin . . . 495
Lovenox® HP *see* Enoxaparin . . . 495
Lowadina *see* Loratadine . . . 822
Low-Ogestrel® *see* Combination Hormonal Contraceptives . . . 368
Loxapine . . . 829
Loxapine Hydrochloride *see* Loxapine . . . 829
Loxapine Succinate *see* Loxapine . . . 829
Loxitane® *see* Loxapine . . . 829
Loxitane® C *see* Loxapine . . . 829
Lozide® *see* Indapamide . . . 716
Lozi-Flur™ *see* Fluoride . . . 586
Lozol® *see* Indapamide . . . 716
L-PAM *see* Melphalan . . . 855
L-Sarcolysin *see* Melphalan . . . 855
LTG *see* Lamotrigine . . . 774
L-Thyroxine Sodium *see* Levothyroxine . . . 800
Lu-26-054 *see* Escitalopram . . . 516
Lubriderm® [OTC] *see* Lanolin, Cetyl Alcohol, Glycerin, Petrolatum, and Mineral Oil . . . 776
Lubriderm® Fragrance Free [OTC] *see* Lanolin, Cetyl Alcohol, Glycerin, Petrolatum, and Mineral Oil . . . 776
Lucrin *see* Leuprolide . . . 784
Lucrin Depot *see* Leuprolide . . . 784
Ludiomil® *see* Maprotiline . . . 841
Lufyllin® *see* Dyphylline . . . 485
Lugol's Solution *see* Potassium Iodide . . . 1101
Lumigan™ *see* Bimatoprost . . . 184
Luminal® Sodium *see* Phenobarbital . . . 1066
Lumitene™ *see* Beta-Carotene . . . 176
Lunelle™ *see* Estradiol and Medroxyprogesterone . . . 523
LupiCare™ Dandruff [OTC] *see* Salicylic Acid . . . 1204
LupiCare™ II Psoriasis [OTC] *see* Salicylic Acid . . . 1204
LupiCare™ Psoriasis [OTC] *see* Salicylic Acid . . . 1204
Lupron® *see* Leuprolide . . . 784
Lupron Depot® *see* Leuprolide . . . 784
Lupron Depot-Ped® *see* Leuprolide . . . 784
Lurdex® *see* Albendazole . . . 47
Luride® *see* Fluoride . . . 586
Luride® Lozi-Tab® *see* Fluoride . . . 586
Luritran® *see* Erythromycin . . . 512
Lustra® *see* Hydroquinone . . . 693
Lustra-AF™ *see* Hydroquinone . . . 693
Lutein . . . 1443
Luvox® *see* Fluvoxamine . . . 605
Luxiq™ *see* Betamethasone . . . 177
LY139603 *see* Atomoxetine . . . 139
LY170053 *see* Olanzapine . . . 996
Lycopene . . . 1443
Lyderm® *see* Fluocinonide . . . 585
Lydonide *see* Fluocinonide . . . 585
Lymphocyte Immune Globulin . . . 831
Lymphocyte Mitogenic Factor *see* Aldesleukin . . . 50
Lyposyn *see* Fat Emulsion . . . 558
Lysine . . . 832
Lysinyl [OTC] *see* Lysine . . . 832
Lysodren® *see* Mitotane . . . 922
Lyteprep™ *see* Polyethylene Glycol-Electrolyte Solution . . . 1094
Maalox® [OTC] *see* Aluminum Hydroxide and Magnesium Hydroxide . . . 69
Maalox® Fast Release Liquid [OTC] *see* Aluminum Hydroxide, Magnesium Hydroxide, and Simethicone . . . 69
Maalox® Max [OTC] *see* Aluminum Hydroxide, Magnesium Hydroxide, and Simethicone . . . 69
Maalox® TC (Therapeutic Concentrate) [OTC] *see* Aluminum Hydroxide and Magnesium Hydroxide . . . 69
Mabicrol® *see* Clarithromycin . . . 337
Mabthera® *see* Rituximab . . . 1190
MacroBID® *see* Nitrofurantoin . . . 980
Macrodantin® *see* Nitrofurantoin . . . 980
Macrodantina® *see* Nitrofurantoin . . . 980
Madel *see* Phenazopyridine . . . 1064
Mafenide . . . 832
Mafenide Acetate *see* Mafenide . . . 832
Magaldrate and Simethicone . . . 833
Mag Delay® [OTC] *see* Magnesium Chloride . . . 833
Mag Delay® [OTC] *see* Magnesium Supplements . . . 837
Mag G® [OTC] *see* Magnesium Supplements . . . 837
Mag-Gel® 600 *see* Magnesium Supplements . . . 837
Maginex™ [OTC] *see* Magnesium L-aspartate Hydrochloride . . . 836
Maginex™ *see* Magnesium Supplements . . . 837
Maginex™ DS [OTC] *see* Magnesium L-aspartate Hydrochloride . . . 836
Maginex™ DS *see* Magnesium Supplements . . . 837
Magnesia Magma *see* Magnesium Hydroxide . . . 835
Magnesia Magma (Magnesium Hydroxide) *see* Magnesium Supplements . . . 837

Magnesium Carbonate and Aluminum Hydroxide *see* Aluminum Hydroxide and Magnesium Carbonate . . . 68
Magnesium Chloride . . . 833
Magnesium Chloride *see* Magnesium Supplements . . . 837
Magnesium Citrate . . . 834
Magnesium Citrate *see* Magnesium Supplements . . . 837
Magnesium Gluconate . . . 834
Magnesium Gluconate *see* Magnesium Supplements . . . 837
Magnesium Hydroxide . . . 835
Magnesium Hydroxide *see* Magnesium Supplements . . . 837
Magnesium Hydroxide, Aluminum Hydroxide, and Simethicone *see* Aluminum Hydroxide, Magnesium Hydroxide, and Simethicone . . . 69
Magnesium Hydroxide and Aluminum Hydroxide *see* Aluminum Hydroxide and Magnesium Hydroxide . . . 69
Magnesium Hydroxide and Mineral Oil . . . 836
Magnesium Hydroxide and Mineral Oil Emulsion *see* Magnesium Supplements . . . 837
Magnesium Hydroxide, Famotidine, and Calcium Carbonate *see* Famotidine, Calcium Carbonate, and Magnesium Hydroxide . . . 557
Magnesium L-aspartate Hydrochloride . . . 836
Magnesium L-aspartate Hydrochloride *see* Magnesium Supplements . . . 837
Magnesium Oxide *see* Magnesium Supplements . . . 837
Magnesium Salicylate . . . 837
Magnesium Sulfate *see* Magnesium Supplements . . . 837
Magnesium Supplements . . . 837
Magnesium Trisilicate and Aluminum Hydroxide *see* Aluminum Hydroxide and Magnesium Trisilicate . . . 69
Magnidol® *see* Acetaminophen . . . 27
Magonate® [OTC] *see* Magnesium Gluconate . . . 834
Magonate® [OTC] *see* Magnesium Supplements . . . 837
Magonate® Sport [OTC] *see* Magnesium Gluconate . . . 834
Magonste® Sprot [OTC] *see* Magnesium Supplements . . . 837
Mag-Ox 400® [OTC] *see* Magnesium Supplements . . . 837
Mag-SR® [OTC] *see* Magnesium Chloride . . . 833
Mag-SR® [OTC] *see* Magnesium Supplements . . . 837
Magtrate® [OTC] *see* Magnesium Gluconate . . . 834
Magtrate® [OTC] *see* Magnesium Supplements . . . 837
MAH™ *see* Magnesium L-aspartate Hydrochloride . . . 836
Maidenhair Tree *see* Ginkgo Biloba . . . 1434
Malarone™ *see* Atovaquone and Proguanil . . . 143
Malival® *see* Indomethacin . . . 719
Malival AP *see* Indomethacin . . . 719
Mallamint® [OTC] *see* Calcium Supplements . . . 229
Maltodextrin . . . 840
Malt Soup Extract . . . 841
Maltsupex® [OTC] *see* Malt Soup Extract . . . 841
Management of Patients Undergoing Cancer Therapy . . . 1567
Management of Sialorrhea . . . 1555
Mandelamine® *see* Methenamine . . . 879
Mandol® [DSC] *see* Cefamandole . . . 263
Mandrake *see* Podophyllum Resin . . . 1093
Manganese *see* Trace Metals . . . 1328
Mantoux *see* Tuberculin Tests . . . 1362
Maolate® *see* Chlorphenesin . . . 306
Mapap® [OTC] *see* Acetaminophen . . . 27
Mapap® Children's [OTC] *see* Acetaminophen . . . 27
Mapap® Extra Strength [OTC] *see* Acetaminophen . . . 27
Mapap® Infants [OTC] *see* Acetaminophen . . . 27
Mapluxin® *see* Digoxin . . . 441
Maprotiline . . . 841
Maprotiline Hydrochloride *see* Maprotiline . . . 841
Marcaine® *see* Bupivacaine . . . 205
Marcaine® Spinal *see* Bupivacaine . . . 205
Marcaine® with Epinephrine *see* Bupivacaine and Epinephrine . . . 207
Marcillin® *see* Ampicillin . . . 103
Marezine® [OTC] *see* Cyclizine . . . 379
Margesic® H *see* Hydrocodone and Acetaminophen . . . 678
Marinol® *see* Dronabinol . . . 480
Marovilina® *see* Ampicillin . . . 103
Marplan® *see* Isocarboxazid . . . 747
Masflex® *see* Meloxicam . . . 854
Mastic . . . 1444
Matricaria chamomilla *see* Chamomile . . . 1425
Matricaria recutita *see* Chamomile . . . 1425
Matulane® *see* Procarbazine . . . 1122
Mavik® *see* Trandolapril . . . 1331
Maxair™ *see* Pirbuterol . . . 1090
Maxair™ Autohaler™ *see* Pirbuterol . . . 1090
Maxalt® *see* Rizatriptan . . . 1193
Maxalt-MLT® *see* Rizatriptan . . . 1193
Maxalt RPD™ *see* Rizatriptan . . . 1193
Maxaquin® *see* Lomefloxacin . . . 817
Maxidex® *see* Dexamethasone . . . 413
Maxidone™ *see* Hydrocodone and Acetaminophen . . . 678
Maxifed® *see* Guaifenesin and Pseudoephedrine . . . 652
Maxifed® DM *see* Guaifenesin, Pseudoephedrine, and Dextromethorphan . . . 653
Maxifed-G® *see* Guaifenesin and Pseudoephedrine . . . 652
Maxiflor® *see* Diflorasone . . . 438
Maxipime® *see* Cefepime . . . 267
Maxitrol® *see* Neomycin, Polymyxin B, and Dexamethasone . . . 962
Maxivate® *see* Betamethasone . . . 177

Maxtrim® *see* Trimethoprim . . . 1352
Maxzide® *see* Hydrochlorothiazide and Triamterene . . . 677
Maxzide®-25 *see* Hydrochlorothiazide and Triamterene . . . 677
May Apple *see* Podophyllum Resin . . . 1093
Maybush *see* Hawthorn . . . 1440
Mazanor® [DSC] *see* Mazindol . . . 843
Mazindol . . . 843
3M™ Cavilon™ Skin Cleanser [OTC] *see* Benzalkonium Chloride . . . 169
MCH *see* Microfibrillar Collagen Hemostat . . . 907
m-Cresyl Acetate . . . 844
MCT Oil® [OTC] *see* Medium Chain Triglycerides . . . 849
MDL 73,147EF *see* Dolasetron . . . 465
ME-500® *see* Methionine . . . 881
Measles, Mumps, and Rubella Vaccines (Combined) . . . 844
Measles Virus Vaccine (Live) . . . 845
Mebaral® *see* Mephobarbital . . . 860
Mebendazole . . . 846
Mebensole *see* Mebendazole . . . 846
Mecamylamine . . . 846
Mecamylamine Hydrochloride *see* Mecamylamine . . . 846
Meclizine . . . 847
Meclizine Hydrochloride *see* Meclizine . . . 847
Meclofenamate . . . 848
Meclofenamate Sodium *see* Meclofenamate . . . 848
Meclomen® *see* Meclofenamate . . . 848
Meclomid® *see* Metoclopramide . . . 898
Meclozine Hydrochloride *see* Meclizine . . . 847
Med-Diltiazem *see* Diltiazem . . . 447
Medicinal Carbon *see* Charcoal . . . 294
Medicinal Charcoal *see* Charcoal . . . 294
Medicone® [OTC] *see* Phenylephrine . . . 1071
Mediplast® [OTC] *see* Salicylic Acid . . . 1204
Medi-Synal [OTC] *see* Acetaminophen and Pseudoephedrine . . . 31
Medium Chain Triglycerides . . . 849
Medrol® *see* MethylPREDNISolone . . . 895
MedroxyPROGESTERone . . . 849
Medroxyprogesterone *see* MedroxyPROGESTERone . . . 849
Medroxyprogesterone Acetate and Estradiol Cypionate *see* Estradiol and Medroxyprogesterone . . . 523
Medroxyprogesterone and Estrogens (Conjugated) *see* Estrogens (Conjugated/Equine) and Medroxyprogesterone . . . 531
Medrysone . . . 850
Medsaplatin *see* Cisplatin . . . 332
Medsaposide *see* Etoposide . . . 549
Medsaposide *see* Etoposide Phosphate . . . 551
Medsavorin *see* Leucovorin . . . 783
Mefenamic Acid . . . 851
Mefloquine . . . 852
Mefloquine Hydrochloride *see* Mefloquine . . . 852
Mefoxin® *see* Cefoxitin . . . 272
Megace® *see* Megestrol . . . 853
Megace® OS *see* Megestrol . . . 853
Megadophilus® [OTC] *see* *Lactobacillus acidophilus* and *Lactobacillus bulgaricus* . . . 772
Megestrol . . . 853
Megestrol Acetate *see* Megestrol . . . 853
Meladinina® *see* Methoxsalen . . . 888
Melaleuca alternifolia *see* Melaleuca Oil . . . 1444
Melaleuca Oil . . . 1444
Melanex® *see* Hydroquinone . . . 693
Melatonin . . . 1444
Melfiat®: Obezine® *see* Phendimetrazine . . . 1064
Mellaril® *see* Thioridazine . . . 1298
Melleril® *see* Thioridazine . . . 1298
Meloxicam . . . 854
Melpaque HP® *see* Hydroquinone . . . 693
Melphalan . . . 855
Melquin-3® [OTC] *see* Hydroquinone . . . 693
Melquin HP® *see* Hydroquinone . . . 693
Menadol® [OTC] *see* Ibuprofen . . . 703
Menest® *see* Estrogens (Esterified) . . . 533
Meningococcal Polysaccharide Vaccine (Groups A, C, Y, and W-135) . . . 856
Menomune®-A/C/Y/W-135 *see* Meningococcal Polysaccharide Vaccine (Groups A, C, Y, and W-135) . . . 856
Menotropins . . . 857
Mentax® *see* Butenafine . . . 217
292 MEP® *see* Aspirin and Meprobamate . . . 136
Mepenzolate . . . 858
Mepenzolate Bromide *see* Mepenzolate . . . 858
Meperidine . . . 858
Meperidine and Promethazine . . . 860
Meperidine Hydrochloride *see* Meperidine . . . 858
Meperitab® *see* Meperidine . . . 858
Mephobarbital . . . 860
Mephyton® *see* Phytonadione . . . 1079
Mepivacaine . . . 861
Mepivacaine and Levonordefrin . . . 862
Mepivacaine Dental Anesthetic . . . 863
Mepivacaine Hydrochloride *see* Mepivacaine . . . 861
Meprobamate . . . 864
Meprobamate and Aspirin *see* Aspirin and Meprobamate . . . 136

Mepron® *see* Atovaquone . . . 142
Mequinol and Tretinoin . . . 865
Merbromin . . . 866
Mercaptopurine . . . 866
6-Mercaptopurine *see* Mercaptopurine . . . 866
Mercapturic Acid *see* Acetylcysteine . . . 40
Mercuric Oxide . . . 867
Mercurochrome® *see* Merbromin . . . 866
Meridia® *see* Sibutramine . . . 1219
Meropenem . . . 867
Merrem® *see* Meropenem . . . 867
Merrem® I.V. *see* Meropenem . . . 867
Mersol® [OTC] *see* Thimerosal . . . 1296
Merthiolate® [OTC] *see* Thimerosal . . . 1296
Meruvax® II *see* Rubella Virus Vaccine (Live) . . . 1202
Merxil® *see* Diclofenac . . . 429
Mesalamine . . . 869
Mesalazine *see* Mesalamine . . . 869
Mesasal® *see* Mesalamine . . . 869
M-Eslon® *see* Morphine Sulfate . . . 931
Mesoridazine . . . 870
Mesoridazine Besylate *see* Mesoridazine . . . 870
Mestranol and Norethindrone . . . 871
Metacortandralone *see* PrednisoLONE . . . 1110
Metadate® CD *see* Methylphenidate . . . 893
Metadate™ ER *see* Methylphenidate . . . 893
Metadol™ *see* Methadone . . . 876
Metaglip™ *see* Glipizide and Metformin . . . 639
Metahydrin® *see* Trichlormethiazide . . . 1347
Metamucil® *see* Psyllium . . . 1149
Metamucil® Smooth Texture [OTC] *see* Psyllium . . . 1149
Metaproterenol . . . 873
Metaproterenol Sulfate *see* Metaproterenol . . . 873
Metatensin® *see* Trichlormethiazide . . . 1347
Metaxalone . . . 874
Metformin . . . 874
Metformin and Glipizide *see* Glipizide and Metformin . . . 639
Metformin and Rosiglitazone *see* Rosiglitazone and Metformin . . . 1200
Metformin Hydrochloride *see* Metformin . . . 874
Metformin Hydrochloride and Rosiglitazone Maleate *see* Rosiglitazone and Metformin . . . 1200
Methadone . . . 876
Methadone Hydrochloride *see* Methadone . . . 876
Methadone Intensol™ *see* Methadone . . . 876
Methadose® *see* Methadone . . . 876
Methaminodiazepoxide Hydrochloride *see* Chlordiazepoxide . . . 299
Methamphetamine . . . 877
Methamphetamine Hydrochloride *see* Methamphetamine . . . 877
Methazolamide . . . 878
Methenamine . . . 879
Methenamine Hippurate *see* Methenamine . . . 879
Methenamine Mandelate *see* Methenamine . . . 879
Methenamine, Sodium Biphosphate, Phenyl Salicylate, Methylene Blue, and Hyoscyamine . . . 880
Methergine® *see* Methylergonovine . . . 892
Methimazole . . . 880
Methionine . . . 881
Methitest® *see* MethylTESTOSTERone . . . 897
Methocarbamol . . . 881
Methohexital . . . 882
Methohexital Sodium *see* Methohexital . . . 882
Methotrexate . . . 884
Methotrexate Sodium *see* Methotrexate . . . 884
Methotrimeprazine . . . 887
Methotrimeprazine Hydrochloride *see* Methotrimeprazine . . . 887
Methoxsalen . . . 888
Methoxypsoralen *see* Methoxsalen . . . 888
8-Methoxypsoralen *see* Methoxsalen . . . 888
Methscopolamine . . . 888
Methscopolamine Bromide *see* Methscopolamine . . . 888
Methsuximide . . . 889
Methyclothiazide . . . 890
Methyclothiazide and Deserpidine . . . 890
Methylacetoxyprogesterone *see* MedroxyPROGESTERone . . . 849
Methylcellulose . . . 891
Methyldopa . . . 891
Methyldopa and Chlorothiazide *see* Chlorothiazide and Methyldopa . . . 305
Methyldopa and Hydrochlorothiazide . . . 892
Methyldopate Hydrochloride *see* Methyldopa . . . 891
Methylene Blue, Methenamine, Sodium Biphosphate, Phenyl Salicylate, and Hyoscyamine *see* Methenamine, Sodium Biphosphate, Phenyl Salicylate, Methylene Blue, and Hyoscyamine . . . 880
Methylergometrine Maleate *see* Methylergonovine . . . 892
Methylergonovine . . . 892
Methylergonovine Maleate *see* Methylergonovine . . . 892
Methylin™ *see* Methylphenidate . . . 893
Methylin™ ER *see* Methylphenidate . . . 893
Methylmorphine *see* Codeine . . . 361
Methylphenidate . . . 893
Methylphenidate Hydrochloride *see* Methylphenidate . . . 893
Methylphenobarbital *see* Mephobarbital . . . 860

Methylphenyl Isoxazolyl Penicillin *see* Oxacillin 1007
Methylphytyl Napthoquinone *see* Phytonadione 1079
MethylPREDNISolone 895
6-α-Methylprednisolone *see* MethylPREDNISolone 895
Methylprednisolone Acetate *see* MethylPREDNISolone 895
Methylprednisolone Sodium Succinate *see* MethylPREDNISolone 895
4-Methylpyrazole *see* Fomepizole 609
Methylrosaniline Chloride *see* Gentian Violet 636
Methyl Sulfonyl Methane 1445
MethylTESTOSTERone 897
Methysergide 897
Methysergide Maleate *see* Methysergide 897
Meticorten® *see* PredniSONE 1112
Metipranolol 898
Metipranolol Hydrochloride *see* Metipranolol 898
Metoclopramide 898
Metolazone 900
Metoprolol 901
Metoprolol Tartrate *see* Metoprolol 901
Metoxiprim *see* Sulfamethoxazole and Trimethoprim 1253
Metoxiprim® *see* Trimethoprim 1352
Metrizamide *see* Radiological/Contrast Media (Nonionic) 1165
MetroCream® *see* Metronidazole 902
MetroGel® *see* Metronidazole 902
MetroGel-Vaginal® *see* Metronidazole 902
MetroLotion® *see* Metronidazole 902
Metronidazole 902
Metronidazole, Bismuth Subsalicylate, and Tetracycline *see* Bismuth, Metronidazole, and Tetracycline 187
Metronidazole Hydrochloride *see* Metronidazole 902
Metronidazole, Tetracycline, and Bismuth Subsalicylate *see* Bismuth, Metronidazole, and Tetracycline 187
Metyrosine 905
Mevacor® *see* Lovastatin 828
Mevinolin *see* Lovastatin 828
Mexiletine 905
Mexitil® *see* Mexiletine 905
MG217 Sal-Acid® [OTC] *see* Salicylic Acid 1204
Miacalcic® *see* Calcitonin 222
Miacalcin® *see* Calcitonin 222
Miacalcin® NS *see* Calcitonin 222
Micaderm® [OTC] *see* Miconazole 906
Micanol® *see* Anthralin 111
Micardis® *see* Telmisartan 1269
Micardis® HCT *see* Telmisartan and Hydrochlorothiazide 1270
Micardis® Plus *see* Telmisartan and Hydrochlorothiazide 1270
Micatin® *see* Miconazole 906
Miccil® *see* Bumetanide 204
Miconazole 906
Miconazole Nitrate *see* Miconazole 906
Micostatin® *see* Nystatin 992
Micostyl® *see* Econazole 486
Micozole *see* Miconazole 906
MICRhoGAM® *see* Rh_o(D) Immune Globulin 1175
Microfibrillar Collagen Hemostat 907
Microgestin™ Fe *see* Combination Hormonal Contraceptives 368
Micro-Guard® [OTC] *see* Miconazole 906
microK® *see* Potassium Supplements 1102
microK® 10 *see* Potassium Supplements 1102
Microlut® *see* Levonorgestrel 797
Micronase® *see* GlyBURIDE 642
microNefrin® *see* Epinephrine (Racemic) 500
Micronor® *see* Norethindrone 986
Microrgan® *see* Ciprofloxacin 328
Microtid *see* Ranitidine 1168
Microzide™ *see* Hydrochlorothiazide 675
Midamor® *see* Amiloride 75
Midazolam 908
Midazolam Hydrochloride *see* Midazolam 908
Midodrine 911
Midodrine Hydrochloride *see* Midodrine 911
Midol® Maximum Strength Cramp Formula [OTC] *see* Ibuprofen 703
Midotens *see* Labetalol 769
Midrin® *see* Acetaminophen, Isometheptene, and Dichloralphenazone 36
Mifeprex® *see* Mifepristone 912
Mifepristone 912
Miglitol 913
Migranal® *see* Dihydroergotamine 445
Migratine® *see* Acetaminophen, Isometheptene, and Dichloralphenazone 36
Mi-Ke-Son's® *see* Ketoconazole 762
Milezzol *see* Metronidazole 902
Milk of Magnesia *see* Magnesium Hydroxide 835
Milk of Magnesia (Magnesium Hydroxide) *see* Magnesium Supplements 837
Milk Thistle 1445
Milk Vetch *see* Astragalus 1421
Milophene® *see* ClomiPHENE 348
Milrinone 914
Milrinone Lactate *see* Milrinone 914
Miltown® *see* Meprobamate 864
Mineral Oil, Coal Tar, and Lanolin *see* Coal Tar, Lanolin, and Mineral Oil 360

Mineral Oil, Lanolin, and Coal Tar *see* Coal Tar, Lanolin, and Mineral Oil . . . 360
Mineral Oil, Petrolatum, Lanolin, Cetyl Alcohol, and Glycerin *see* Lanolin, Cetyl Alcohol, Glycerin, Petrolatum, and Mineral Oil . . . 776
Minidyne® [OTC] *see* Povidone-Iodine . . . 1104
Minim's Atropine Solution *see* Atropine . . . 144
Minim's Gentamicin 0.3% *see* Gentamicin . . . 634
Minipres® *see* Prazosin . . . 1108
Minipress™ *see* Prazosin . . . 1108
Minirin® *see* Desmopressin . . . 410
Minitran™ *see* Nitroglycerin . . . 981
Minizide® *see* Prazosin and Polythiazide . . . 1109
Minocin® *see* Minocycline . . . 915
Minocycline . . . 915
Minocycline Hydrochloride *see* Minocycline . . . 915
Minocycline Hydrochloride Periodontal Microspheres . . . 916
Minodiab® *see* GlipiZIDE . . . 638
Minofen® *see* Acetaminophen . . . 27
Minox *see* Minoxidil . . . 917
Minoxidil . . . 917
Mintezol® *see* Thiabendazole . . . 1294
Miochol®-E *see* Acetylcholine . . . 39
Miostat® *see* Carbachol . . . 241
Miradon® *see* Anisindione . . . 110
MiraLax™ *see* Polyethylene Glycol-Electrolyte Solution . . . 1094
Mirapex® *see* Pramipexole . . . 1105
Miraphen PSE *see* Guaifenesin and Pseudoephedrine . . . 652
Mircette® *see* Combination Hormonal Contraceptives . . . 368
Mirena® *see* Levonorgestrel . . . 797
Mirtazapine . . . 919
Misoprostol . . . 920
Misoprostol and Diclofenac *see* Diclofenac and Misoprostol . . . 431
Misostol *see* Mitoxantrone . . . 923
Mitocin® *see* Mitomycin . . . 921
Mitomycin . . . 921
Mitomycin-C *see* Mitomycin . . . 921
Mitotane . . . 922
Mitoxantrone . . . 923
Mitoxantrone Hydrochloride *see* Mitoxantrone . . . 923
Mitozytrex™ *see* Mitomycin . . . 921
Mitrazol™ [OTC] *see* Miconazole . . . 906
Mitroken® *see* Ciprofloxacin . . . 328
Mitrolan® Chewable Tablet [OTC] *see* Calcium Polycarbophil . . . 228
Mitroxone® [inj.] *see* Mitoxantrone . . . 923
MK383 *see* Tirofiban . . . 1313
MK462 *see* Rizatriptan . . . 1193
MK594 *see* Losartan . . . 825
MK-0826 *see* Ertapenem . . . 511
MMR *see* Measles, Mumps, and Rubella Vaccines (Combined) . . . 844
M-M-R® II *see* Measles, Mumps, and Rubella Vaccines (Combined) . . . 844
Moban® *see* Molindone . . . 927
MOBIC® *see* Meloxicam . . . 854
Mobicox® *see* Meloxicam . . . 854
Mobidin® [DSC] *see* Magnesium Salicylate . . . 837
Mobisyl® [OTC] *see* Triethanolamine Salicylate . . . 1348
Modafinil . . . 924
Modane® Bulk [OTC] *see* Psyllium . . . 1149
Modane Tablets® [OTC] *see* Bisacodyl . . . 186
Modecate® *see* Fluphenazine . . . 593
Modicon® *see* Combination Hormonal Contraceptives . . . 368
Modified Dakin's Solution *see* Sodium Hypochlorite Solution . . . 1231
Modified Shohl's Solution *see* Sodium Citrate and Citric Acid . . . 1230
Moditen® Enanthate *see* Fluphenazine . . . 593
Moditen® HCl *see* Fluphenazine . . . 593
Moducal® [OTC] *see* Glucose Polymers . . . 641
Moduret® *see* Amiloride and Hydrochlorothiazide . . . 76
Moduretic® *see* Amiloride and Hydrochlorothiazide . . . 76
Moexipril . . . 926
Moexipril and Hydrochlorothiazide . . . 927
Moexipril Hydrochloride *see* Moexipril . . . 926
Moi-Stir® [OTC] *see* Saliva Substitute . . . 1205
Moisture® Eyes [OTC] *see* Artificial Tears . . . 128
Moisture® Eyes PM [OTC] *see* Artificial Tears . . . 128
Molindone . . . 927
Molindone Hydrochloride *see* Molindone . . . 927
Mollifene® Ear Wax Removing Formula [OTC] *see* Carbamide Peroxide . . . 244
Molybdenum *see* Trace Metals . . . 1328
Molypen® *see* Trace Metals . . . 1328
MOM *see* Magnesium Hydroxide . . . 835
Momentum® [OTC] *see* Magnesium Salicylate . . . 837
Mometasone Furoate . . . 928
MOM (Magnesium Hydroxide) *see* Magnesium Supplements . . . 837
MOM/Mineral Oil Emulsion *see* Magnesium Hydroxide and Mineral Oil . . . 836
Monacolin K *see* Lovastatin . . . 828
Monarc® M *see* Antihemophilic Factor (Human) . . . 113
Monascus purpureus *see* Red Yeast Rice . . . 1446
Monistat® *see* Miconazole . . . 906
Monistat® 1 Combination Pack [OTC] *see* Miconazole . . . 906
Monistat® 3 [OTC] *see* Miconazole . . . 906
Monistat® 7 [OTC] *see* Miconazole . . . 906
Monistat-Derm® *see* Miconazole . . . 906

Monitan® *see* Acebutolol . . . 25
Monobenzone . . . 929
Monocid® [DSC] *see* Cefonicid . . . 269
Monocidur *see* Cefonicid . . . 269
Monoclate-P® *see* Antihemophilic Factor (Human) . . . 113
Monoclonal Antibody *see* Muromonab-CD3 . . . 938
Monocor® *see* Bisoprolol . . . 188
Monodox® *see* Doxycycline . . . 476
Monoethanolamine *see* Ethanolamine Oleate . . . 540
Mono-Gesic® *see* Salsalate . . . 1206
Monoket® *see* Isosorbide Mononitrate . . . 751
Mono Mack® *see* Isosorbide Mononitrate . . . 751
Monopril® *see* Fosinopril . . . 616
Monopril-HCT® *see* Fosinopril and Hydrochlorothiazide . . . 617
Montelukast . . . 929
Montelukast Sodium *see* Montelukast . . . 929
Monurol® *see* Fosfomycin . . . 615
8-MOP® *see* Methoxsalen . . . 888
More Attenuated Enders Strain *see* Measles Virus Vaccine (Live) . . . 845
MoreDophilus® [OTC] *see* *Lactobacillus acidophilus* and *Lactobacillus bulgaricus* . . . 772
Moricizine . . . 931
Moricizine Hydrochloride *see* Moricizine . . . 931
Morphine HP® *see* Morphine Sulfate . . . 931
Morphine LP® Epidural *see* Morphine Sulfate . . . 931
Morphine Sulfate . . . 931
Morrhuate Sodium . . . 934
Mosco® Corn and Callus Remover [OTC] *see* Salicylic Acid . . . 1204
M.O.S.-Sulfate® *see* Morphine Sulfate . . . 931
Motofen® *see* Difenoxin and Atropine . . . 437
Motrin® *see* Ibuprofen . . . 703
Motrin® (Children's) *see* Ibuprofen . . . 703
Motrin® Cold, Children's [OTC] *see* Pseudoephedrine and Ibuprofen . . . 1148
Motrin® IB [OTC] *see* Ibuprofen . . . 703
Motrin® Infants' [OTC] *see* Ibuprofen . . . 703
Motrin® Junior Strength [OTC] *see* Ibuprofen . . . 703
Motrin® Migraine Pain [OTC] *see* Ibuprofen . . . 703
Motrin® Sinus Headache [OTC] *see* Pseudoephedrine and Ibuprofen . . . 1148
Mouthkote® [OTC] *see* Saliva Substitute . . . 1205
Mouth Pain, Cold Sore, and Canker Sore Products . . . 1630
Mouthwash (Antiseptic) . . . 934
Moxifloxacin . . . 935
Moxifloxacin Hydrochloride *see* Moxifloxacin . . . 935
Moxilin® *see* Amoxicillin . . . 93
Moxlin® *see* Amoxicillin . . . 93
4-MP *see* Fomepizole . . . 609
6-MP *see* Mercaptopurine . . . 866
MPA and Estrogens (Conjugated) *see* Estrogens (Conjugated/Equine) and Medroxyprogesterone . . . 531
MS *see* Morphine Sulfate . . . 931
MS Contin® *see* Morphine Sulfate . . . 931
MS-IR® *see* Morphine Sulfate . . . 931
MSM *see* Methyl Sulfonyl Methane . . . 1445
MST Continus® *see* Morphine Sulfate . . . 931
MTC *see* Mitomycin . . . 921
M.T.E.-4® *see* Trace Metals . . . 1328
M.T.E.-5® *see* Trace Metals . . . 1328
M.T.E.-6® *see* Trace Metals . . . 1328
M.T.E.-7® *see* Trace Metals . . . 1328
MTX *see* Methotrexate . . . 884
Mucinex™ [OTC] *see* Guaifenesin . . . 650
Mucomyst® *see* Acetylcysteine . . . 40
Mucosil™ *see* Acetylcysteine . . . 40
Multidex® [OTC] *see* Maltodextrin . . . 840
Multiple Vitamins *see* Vitamins (Multiple/Oral) . . . 1394
Multitest® CMI *see* Skin Test Antigens (Multiple) . . . 1227
Multitrace™-4 *see* Trace Metals . . . 1328
Multitrace™-4 Neonatal *see* Trace Metals . . . 1328
Multitrace™-4 Pediatric *see* Trace Metals . . . 1328
Multitrace™-5 *see* Trace Metals . . . 1328
Mumps, Measles and Rubella Vaccines, Combined *see* Measles, Mumps, and Rubella Vaccines (Combined) . . . 844
Mumpsvax® *see* Mumps Virus Vaccine (Live/Attenuated) . . . 937
Mumps Virus Vaccine (Live/Attenuated) . . . 937
Munobal *see* Felodipine . . . 560
Mupiban *see* Mupirocin . . . 937
Mupirocin . . . 937
Mupirocin Calcium *see* Mupirocin . . . 937
Murine® Ear Drops [OTC] *see* Carbamide Peroxide . . . 244
Murine® Tears [OTC] *see* Artificial Tears . . . 128
Murine® Tears Plus [OTC] *see* Tetrahydrozoline . . . 1288
Muro 128® [OTC] *see* Sodium Chloride . . . 1229
Murocel® [OTC] *see* Artificial Tears . . . 128
Murocoll-2® *see* Phenylephrine and Scopolamine . . . 1072
Muromonab-CD3 . . . 938
Muse® *see* Alprostadil . . . 63
Muse® Pellet *see* Alprostadil . . . 63
Mutacol Berna® *see* Cholera Vaccine . . . 317
Mutamycin® *see* Mitomycin . . . 921
Myambutol® *see* Ethambutol . . . 539
Mycelex® *see* Clotrimazole . . . 356

Mycelex®-3 [OTC] *see* Butoconazole . . . 218
Mycelex®-3 *see* Clotrimazole . . . 356
Mycelex®-7 [OTC] *see* Clotrimazole . . . 356
Mycelex® Twin Pack [OTC] *see* Clotrimazole . . . 356
Myciguent [OTC] *see* Neomycin . . . 961
Mycil® *see* Chlorphenesin . . . 306
Mycinettes® [OTC] *see* Benzocaine . . . 169
Mycitracin® [OTC] *see* Bacitracin, Neomycin, and Polymyxin B . . . 157
Mycobutin® *see* Rifabutin . . . 1179
Mycodib® *see* Ketoconazole . . . 762
Mycolog®-II *see* Nystatin and Triamcinolone . . . 992
Myco-Nail [OTC] *see* Triacetin . . . 1340
Mycophenolate . . . 939
Mycophenolate Mofetil *see* Mycophenolate . . . 939
Mycostatin® *see* Nystatin . . . 992
Mydfrin® *see* Phenylephrine . . . 1071
Mydriacyl® *see* Tropicamide . . . 1360
Myfungar® *see* Oxiconazole . . . 1014
Mykrox® *see* Metolazone . . . 900
Mylanta™ *see* Aluminum Hydroxide and Magnesium Hydroxide . . . 69
Mylanta™ Double Strength *see* Aluminum Hydroxide, Magnesium Hydroxide, and Simethicone . . . 69
Mylanta™ Extra Strength *see* Aluminum Hydroxide, Magnesium Hydroxide, and Simethicone . . . 69
Mylanta® Extra Strength Liquid [OTC] *see* Aluminum Hydroxide, Magnesium Hydroxide, and Simethicone . . . 69
Mylanta® Gas [OTC] *see* Simethicone . . . 1222
Mylanta® Gas Maximum Strength [OTC] *see* Simethicone . . . 1222
Mylanta® Liquid [OTC] *see* Aluminum Hydroxide, Magnesium Hydroxide, and Simethicone . . . 69
Mylanta™ regular Strength *see* Aluminum Hydroxide, Magnesium Hydroxide, and Simethicone . . . 69
Myleran® *see* Busulfan . . . 212
Mylicon® Infants [OTC] *see* Simethicone . . . 1222
Mylocel™ *see* Hydroxyurea . . . 696
Mylotarg™ *see* Gemtuzumab Ozogamicin . . . 632
Myobloc® *see* Botulinum Toxin Type B . . . 195
Myochrysine® *see* Gold Sodium Thiomalate . . . 646
Myoflex® *see* Magnesium Salicylate . . . 837
Myoflex® *see* Triethanolamine Salicylate . . . 1348
Myotonachol® *see* Bethanechol . . . 181
Mysoline® *see* Primidone . . . 1118
Mytelase® *see* Ambenonium . . . 72
Mytrex® *see* Nystatin and Triamcinolone . . . 992
Mytussin® AC *see* Guaifenesin and Codeine . . . 650
Mytussin® DAC *see* Guaifenesin, Pseudoephedrine, and Codeine . . . 653
Mytussin® DM [OTC] *see* Guaifenesin and Dextromethorphan . . . 651
Nabi-HB® *see* Hepatitis B Immune Globulin . . . 666
Nabumetone . . . 941
NAC *see* Acetylcysteine . . . 40
N-Acetylcysteine *see* Acetylcysteine . . . 40
N-Acetyl-L-cysteine *see* Acetylcysteine . . . 40
N-Acetyl-P-Aminophenol *see* Acetaminophen . . . 27
NaCl *see* Sodium Chloride . . . 1229
NADH *see* Nicotinamide Adenine Dinucleotide . . . 1445
Nadib® *see* GlyBURIDE . . . 642
Nadolol . . . 943
Nadopen-V® *see* Penicillin V Potassium . . . 1051
Nafarelin . . . 944
Nafarelin Acetate *see* Nafarelin . . . 944
Nafcillin . . . 945
Nafcillin Sodium *see* Nafcillin . . . 945
Naftifine . . . 946
Naftifine Hydrochloride *see* Naftifine . . . 946
Naftin® *see* Naftifine . . . 946
$NaHCO_3$ *see* Sodium Bicarbonate . . . 1227
Nalbuphine . . . 946
Nalbuphine Hydrochloride *see* Nalbuphine . . . 946
Nalcrom® *see* Cromolyn Sodium . . . 375
Nalcryn® *see* Nalbuphine . . . 946
Nalfon® *see* Fenoprofen . . . 563
Nalidixic Acid . . . 947
Nalidixinic Acid *see* Nalidixic Acid . . . 947
Nallpen [DSC] *see* Nafcillin . . . 945
N-allylnoroxymorphine Hydrochloride *see* Naloxone . . . 949
Nalmefene . . . 948
Nalmefene Hydrochloride *see* Nalmefene . . . 948
Naloxone . . . 949
Naloxone Hydrochloride *see* Naloxone . . . 949
Naltrexone . . . 950
Naltrexone Hydrochloride *see* Naltrexone . . . 950
Nandrolone . . . 951
Nandrolone Decanoate *see* Nandrolone . . . 951
Nandrolone Phenpropionate *see* Nandrolone . . . 951
Naphazoline . . . 952
Naphazoline and Antazoline . . . 952
Naphazoline and Pheniramine . . . 953
Naphazoline Hydrochloride *see* Naphazoline . . . 952
Naphcon® [OTC] *see* Naphazoline . . . 952
Naphcon-A® [OTC] *see* Naphazoline and Pheniramine . . . 953

Naphcon Forte® *see* Naphazoline 952
Naprelan® *see* Naproxen 953
Naprodil® *see* Naproxen 953
Naprosyn® *see* Naproxen 953
Naproxen 953
Naproxen Sodium *see* Naproxen 953
Naqua® *see* Trichlormethiazide 1347
Naramig® *see* Naratriptan 955
Naratriptan 955
Naratriptan Hydrochloride *see* Naratriptan 955
Narcan® *see* Naloxone 949
Narcanti® *see* Naloxone 949
Nardil® *see* Phenelzine 1065
Naropin® *see* Ropivacaine 1198
Nasacort® *see* Triamcinolone 1341
Nasacort® AQ *see* Triamcinolone 1341
NāSal™ [OTC] *see* Sodium Chloride 1229
Nasalcrom® [OTC] *see* Cromolyn Sodium 375
Nasalide® *see* Flunisolide 582
Nasal Moist® [OTC] *see* Sodium Chloride 1229
Nasarel® *see* Flunisolide 582
Nascobal® *see* Cyanocobalamin 377
Nasonex® *see* Mometasone Furoate 928
Natacyn® *see* Natamycin 956
Natamycin 956
Natrecor® *see* Nesiritide 964
Natriuretic Peptide *see* Nesiritide 964
Natulan® *see* Procarbazine 1122
Natural Lung Surfactant *see* Beractant 176
Natural Products: Herbal and Dietary Supplements 1417
Nature's Tears® [OTC] *see* Artificial Tears 128
Nature-Throid® NT *see* Thyroid 1303
Naturetin® *see* Bendroflumethiazide 168
Nausetrol® [OTC] *see* Phosphorated Carbohydrate Solution 1078
Navane® *see* Thiothixene 1301
Navelbine® *see* Vinorelbine 1389
Naxen® *see* Naproxen 953
Naxifelar *see* Cephalexin 285
Naxil *see* Naproxen 953
Na-Zone® [OTC] *see* Sodium Chloride 1229
n-Docosanol *see* Docosanol 463
Nebcin® *see* Tobramycin 1315
NebuPent® *see* Pentamidine 1052
Necon® 0.5/35 *see* Combination Hormonal Contraceptives 368
Necon® 1/35 *see* Combination Hormonal Contraceptives 368
Necon® 1/50 *see* Mestranol and Norethindrone 871
Necon® 7/7/7 *see* Combination Hormonal Contraceptives 368
Necon® 10/11 *see* Combination Hormonal Contraceptives 368
Nectar of the Gods *see* Garlic 1433
Nedocromil 957
Nedocromil Sodium *see* Nedocromil 957
Nefazodone 957
Nefazodone Hydrochloride *see* Nefazodone 957
NegGram® *see* Nalidixic Acid 947
Nelfinavir 959
Nemasol® Sodium *see* Aminosalicylic Acid 79
Nembutal® *see* Pentobarbital 1055
Nembutal® Sodium *see* Pentobarbital 1055
Neobes® *see* Diethylpropion 436
Neo-Calglucon® [OTC] *see* Calcium Glubionate 225
Neo-Calglucon® [OTC] *see* Calcium Supplements 229
NeoCeuticals™ Acne Spot Treatment [OTC] *see* Salicylic Acid 1204
NeoDecadron® *see* Neomycin and Dexamethasone 961
Neodol® *see* Acetaminophen 27
Neodolito® *see* Acetaminophen 27
Neofomiral® *see* Fluconazole 576
Neo-Fradin™ *see* Neomycin 961
Neoloid® [OTC] *see* Castor Oil 259
Neomicol® *see* Miconazole 906
Neomycin 961
Neomycin and Dexamethasone 961
Neomycin and Polymyxin B 962
Neomycin, Bacitracin, and Polymyxin B *see* Bacitracin, Neomycin, and Polymyxin B 157
Neomycin, Bacitracin, Polymyxin B, and Hydrocortisone *see* Bacitracin, Neomycin, Polymyxin B, and Hydrocortisone 158
Neomycin, Colistin, and Hydrocortisone *see* Colistin, Neomycin, and Hydrocortisone 367
Neomycin, Polymyxin B, and Dexamethasone 962
Neomycin, Polymyxin B, and Gramicidin 963
Neomycin, Polymyxin B, and Hydrocortisone 963
Neomycin, Polymyxin B, and Prednisolone 963
Neomycin Sulfate *see* Neomycin 961
Neonatal Trace Metals *see* Trace Metals 1328
Neonaxil® *see* Naproxen 953
Neopulmonier® *see* Dextromethorphan 423
Neoral® *see* CycloSPORINE 383
Neo-Rx *see* Neomycin 961
Neosar® *see* Cyclophosphamide 381
Neosporin® *see* Neomycin, Polymyxin B, and Gramicidin 963
Neosporin® G.U. Irrigant *see* Neomycin and Polymyxin B 962
Neosporin® Irrigating Solution *see* Neomycin and Polymyxin B 962

Neosporin® Oftalmico *see* Neomycin, Polymyxin B, and Gramicidin 963
Neosporin® Ophthalmic Ointment *see* Bacitracin, Neomycin, and Polymyxin B 157
Neosporin® Ophthalmic Solution *see* Neomycin, Polymyxin B, and Gramicidin 963
Neosporin® Topical [OTC] *see* Bacitracin, Neomycin, and Polymyxin B 157
NeoStrata AHA [OTC] *see* Hydroquinone 693
NeoStrata® HQ *see* Hydroquinone 693
Neo-Synephrine® *see* Phenylephrine 1071
Neo-Synephrine® 12 Hour [OTC] *see* Oxymetazoline 1022
Neo-Synephrine® 12 Hour Extra Moisturizing [OTC] *see* Oxymetazoline 1022
Neo-Synephrine® Extra Strength [OTC] *see* Phenylephrine 1071
Neo-Synephrine® Mild [OTC] *see* Phenylephrine 1071
Neo-Synephrine® Ophthalmic *see* Phenylephrine 1071
Neo-Synephrine® Regular Strength [OTC] *see* Phenylephrine 1071
Neotopic® *see* Bacitracin, Neomycin, and Polymyxin B 157
Neotrace-4® *see* Trace Metals 1328
Nephro-Calci® [OTC] *see* Calcium Supplements 229
Nephrocaps® *see* Vitamin B Complex, Vitamin C, and Folic Acid 1393
Nephro-Fer® [OTC] *see* Iron Supplements 745
Neptazane® [DSC] *see* Methazolamide 878
Nesacaine® *see* Chloroprocaine 302
Nesacaine®-CE *see* Chloroprocaine 302
Nesacaine®-MPF *see* Chloroprocaine 302
Nesiritide 964
Neugal® *see* Ranitidine 1168
Neugeron® *see* Carbamazepine 241
Neulasta™ *see* Pegfilgrastim 1040
Neumega® *see* Oprelvekin 1003
Neupogen® *see* Filgrastim 571
Neurontin® *see* Gabapentin 624
Neurosine® *see* BusPIRone 211
Neut® *see* Sodium Bicarbonate 1227
NeutraCare® *see* Fluoride 586
NeutraGard® [OTC] *see* Fluoride 586
Neutra-Phos® [OTC] *see* Phosphate Supplements 1076
Neutra-Phos®-K [OTC] *see* Phosphate Supplements 1076
Neutrexin® *see* Trimetrexate Glucuronate 1354
Neutrogena® Acne Mask [OTC] *see* Benzoyl Peroxide 171
Neutrogena® Acne Wash [OTC] *see* Salicylic Acid 1204
Neutrogena® Body Clear™ [OTC] *see* Salicylic Acid 1204
Neutrogena® Clear Pore [OTC] *see* Salicylic Acid 1204
Neutrogena® Clear Pore Shine Control [OTC] *see* Salicylic Acid 1204
Neutrogena® Healthy Scalp [OTC] *see* Salicylic Acid 1204
Neutrogena® Maximum Strength T/Sal® [OTC] *see* Salicylic Acid 1204
Neutrogena® On The Spot® Acne Patch [OTC] *see* Salicylic Acid 1204
Neutrogena® On The Spot® Acne Treatment [OTC] *see* Benzoyl Peroxide 171
Neutrogena® T/Derm *see* Coal Tar 359
Neutrogena® T/Sal [OTC] *see* Coal Tar and Salicylic Acid 359
Nevirapine 965
Nexium® *see* Esomeprazole 519
Niacin 967
Niacinamide 968
Niacin and Lovastatin 968
Niacor® *see* Niacin 967
Niar® *see* Selegiline 1213
Niaspan® *see* Niacin 967
NiCARdipine 969
Nicardipine Hydrochloride *see* NiCARdipine 969
Nicoderm® *see* Nicotine 971
NicoDerm® CQ® [OTC] *see* Nicotine 971
Nicolan *see* Nicotine 971
Nicorette® *see* Nicotine 971
Nicorette® Plus *see* Nicotine 971
Nicotinamide *see* Niacinamide 968
Nicotinamide Adenine Dinucleotide 1445
Nicotine 971
Nicotinell TTS® *see* Nicotine 971
Nicotinex [OTC] *see* Niacin 967
Nicotinic Acid *see* Niacin 967
Nicotrol® *see* Nicotine 971
Nicotrol® Inhaler *see* Nicotine 971
Nicotrol® NS *see* Nicotine 971
Nicotrol® Patch [OTC] *see* Nicotine 971
Nidagel™ *see* Metronidazole 902
Nidrozol® *see* Metronidazole 902
Nifedical™ XL *see* NIFEdipine 973
NIFEdipine 973
Nifedipres® *see* NIFEdipine 973
Niferex® [OTC] *see* Polysaccharide-Iron Complex 1096
Niferex® 150 [OTC] *see* Polysaccharide-Iron Complex 1096
Nilandron® *see* Nilutamide 975
Nilstat *see* Nystatin 992
Nilutamide 975
Nimodipine 976
Nimotop® *see* Nimodipine 976
Nipent® *see* Pentostatin 1057
Nipride® *see* Nitroprusside 982
Nisoldipine 977
Nistaken® *see* Propafenone 1130
Nistaquim *see* Nystatin 992
Nitalapram *see* Citalopram 334

Nitazoxanide . . . 978
Nitisinone . . . 979
Nitradisc® *see* Nitroglycerin . . . 981
Nitrek® *see* Nitroglycerin . . . 981
Nitric Oxide . . . 979
Nitro-Bid® *see* Nitroglycerin . . . 981
Nitroderm TTS® *see* Nitroglycerin . . . 981
Nitro-Dur® *see* Nitroglycerin . . . 981
Nitrofurantoin . . . 980
Nitrogard® *see* Nitroglycerin . . . 981
Nitroglycerin . . . 981
Nitroglycerol *see* Nitroglycerin . . . 981
Nitrol® *see* Nitroglycerin . . . 981
Nitrolingual® *see* Nitroglycerin . . . 981
Nitropress® *see* Nitroprusside . . . 982
Nitroprusside . . . 982
Nitroprusside Sodium *see* Nitroprusside . . . 982
NitroQuick® *see* Nitroglycerin . . . 981
Nitrostat™ *see* Nitroglycerin . . . 981
Nitro-Tab® *see* Nitroglycerin . . . 981
NitroTime® *see* Nitroglycerin . . . 981
Nitrous Oxide . . . 983
Nivoflox® *see* Ciprofloxacin . . . 328
Nix® [OTC] *see* Permethrin . . . 1062
Nixal® *see* Naproxen . . . 953
Niyaplat *see* Cisplatin . . . 332
Nizatidine . . . 984
Nizoral® *see* Ketoconazole . . . 762
Nizoral® A-D [OTC] *see* Ketoconazole . . . 762
N-Methylhydrazine *see* Procarbazine . . . 1122
Nobligan® *see* Tramadol . . . 1329
Nolahist® [OTC] *see* Phenindamine . . . 1066
Nolvadex® *see* Tamoxifen . . . 1264
Nolvadex®-D *see* Tamoxifen . . . 1264
Nonoxynol 9 . . . 985
Nonviral Infectious Diseases . . . 1493
No Pain-HP® [OTC] *see* Capsaicin . . . 238
Noradrenaline *see* Norepinephrine . . . 985
Noradrenaline Acid Tartrate *see* Norepinephrine . . . 985
Norboral® *see* GlyBURIDE . . . 642
Norciden® *see* Danazol . . . 397
Norco® *see* Hydrocodone and Acetaminophen . . . 678
Nordeoxyguanosine *see* Ganciclovir . . . 626
Nordette® *see* Combination Hormonal Contraceptives . . . 368
Norditropin® *see* Human Growth Hormone . . . 671
Norditropin® Cartridges *see* Human Growth Hormone . . . 671
Norepinephrine . . . 985
Norepinephrine Bitartrate *see* Norepinephrine . . . 985
Norethindrone . . . 986
Norethindrone Acetate *see* Norethindrone . . . 986
Norethindrone and Estradiol *see* Estradiol and Norethindrone . . . 525
Norethindrone and Mestranol *see* Mestranol and Norethindrone . . . 871
Norethisterone *see* Norethindrone . . . 986
Norfenon® *see* Propafenone . . . 1130
Norflex™ *see* Orphenadrine . . . 1005
Norfloxacin . . . 987
Norfloxacine® *see* Norfloxacin . . . 987
Norgesic™ *see* Orphenadrine, Aspirin, and Caffeine . . . 1005
Norgesic™ Forte *see* Orphenadrine, Aspirin, and Caffeine . . . 1005
Norgestimate and Estradiol *see* Estradiol and Norgestimate . . . 526
Norgestrel . . . 988
Norinyl® 1+35 *see* Combination Hormonal Contraceptives . . . 368
Norinyl® 1+50 *see* Mestranol and Norethindrone . . . 871
Noritate® *see* Metronidazole . . . 902
Norlutate® *see* Norethindrone . . . 986
Normal Blood Values . . . 1618
Normal Saline *see* Sodium Chloride . . . 1229
Normodyne® *see* Labetalol . . . 769
Noroxin® *see* Norfloxacin . . . 987
Norpace® *see* Disopyramide . . . 458
Norpace® CR *see* Disopyramide . . . 458
Norplant® Implant *see* Levonorgestrel . . . 797
Norpramin® *see* Desipramine . . . 408
Norpril® *see* Enalapril . . . 492
Nor-QD® *see* Norethindrone . . . 986
Nortrel™ *see* Combination Hormonal Contraceptives . . . 368
Nortrel™ 7/7/7 *see* Combination Hormonal Contraceptives . . . 368
Nortriptyline . . . 989
Nortriptyline Hydrochloride *see* Nortriptyline . . . 989
Norvas® *see* Amlodipine . . . 87
Norvasc® *see* Amlodipine . . . 87
Norventyl *see* Nortriptyline . . . 989
Norvir® *see* Ritonavir . . . 1188
Norvir® SEC *see* Ritonavir . . . 1188
Nosebleed *see* Feverfew . . . 1431
Nositrol *see* Hydrocortisone . . . 688
Nostril® [OTC] *see* Phenylephrine . . . 1071
Nōstrilla® [OTC] *see* Oxymetazoline . . . 1022
Novacef *see* Cefixime . . . 268
Novahistex® DM Decongestant *see* Pseudoephedrine and Dextromethorphan . . . 1147

Novahistex® DM Decongestant Expectorant *see* Guaifenesin, Pseudoephedrine, and Dextromethorphan . . . 653
Novahistex® Expectorant with Decongestant *see* Guaifenesin and Pseudoephedrine . . . 652
Novahistine® DM Decongestant *see* Pseudoephedrine and Dextromethorphan . . . 1147
Novahistine® DM Decongestant Expectorant *see* Guaifenesin, Pseudoephedrine, and Dextromethorphan . . . 653
Novamilor *see* Amiloride and Hydrochlorothiazide . . . 76
Novamoxin® *see* Amoxicillin . . . 93
Novantrone® *see* Mitoxantrone . . . 923
Novarel™ *see* Chorionic Gonadotropin (Human) . . . 320
Novasen *see* Aspirin . . . 131
Novaxen® *see* Naproxen . . . 953
Noviken-N *see* NIFEdipine . . . 973
Novo-5 ASA *see* Mesalamine . . . 869
Novo-Acebutolol *see* Acebutolol . . . 25
Novo-Alprazol *see* Alprazolam . . . 61
Novo-Amiodarone *see* Amiodarone . . . 80
Novo-Ampicillin *see* Ampicillin . . . 103
Novo-Atenol *see* Atenolol . . . 137
Novo-AZT *see* Zidovudine . . . 1406
Novo-Bromazepam *see* Bromazepam . . . 199
Novo-Buspirone *see* BusPIRone . . . 211
Novocain® *see* Procaine . . . 1121
Novo-Captopril *see* Captopril . . . 238
Novo-Carbamaz *see* Carbamazepine . . . 241
Novo-Cefaclor *see* Cefaclor . . . 260
Novo-Cefadroxil *see* Cefadroxil . . . 261
Novo-Chlorpromazine *see* ChlorproMAZINE . . . 312
Novo-Cholamine *see* Cholestyramine Resin . . . 318
Novo-Cholamine Light *see* Cholestyramine Resin . . . 318
Novo-Cimetidine *see* Cimetidine . . . 326
Novo-Clobazam *see* Clobazam . . . 344
Novo-Clobetasol® *see* Clobetasol . . . 345
Novo-Clonazepam *see* Clonazepam . . . 350
Novo-Clonidine® *see* Clonidine . . . 351
Novo-Clopate® *see* Clorazepate . . . 355
Novo-Clopramine *see* ClomiPRAMINE . . . 349
Novo-Cloxin® *see* Cloxacillin . . . 357
Novo-Cycloprine® *see* Cyclobenzaprine . . . 379
Novo-Desipramine *see* Desipramine . . . 408
Novo-Difenac® *see* Diclofenac . . . 429
Novo-Difenac K *see* Diclofenac . . . 429
Novo-Difenac-SR® *see* Diclofenac . . . 429
Novo-Diflunisal *see* Diflunisal . . . 438
Novo-Digoxin *see* Digoxin . . . 441
Novo-Diltazem *see* Diltiazem . . . 447
Novo-Diltazem-CD *see* Diltiazem . . . 447
Novo-Diltazem SR *see* Diltiazem . . . 447
Novo-Dipiradol *see* Dipyridamole . . . 456
Novo-Divalproex *see* Valproic Acid and Derivatives . . . 1371
Novo-Doxazosin *see* Doxazosin . . . 470
Novo-Doxepin *see* Doxepin . . . 471
Novo-Doxylin *see* Doxycycline . . . 476
Novo-Famotidine *see* Famotidine . . . 556
Novo-Fenofibrate *see* Fenofibrate . . . 561
Novo-Fluoxetine *see* Fluoxetine . . . 589
Novo-Flurprofen *see* Flurbiprofen . . . 596
Novo-Flutamide *see* Flutamide . . . 598
Novo-Fluvoxamine *see* Fluvoxamine . . . 605
Novo-Furantoin *see* Nitrofurantoin . . . 980
Novo-Gabapentin *see* Gabapentin . . . 624
Novo-Gemfibrozil *see* Gemfibrozil . . . 631
Novo-Glyburide *see* GlyBURIDE . . . 642
Novo-Herklin 2000® *see* Permethrin . . . 1062
Novo-Hydrazide *see* Hydrochlorothiazide . . . 675
Novo-Hydroxyzin *see* HydrOXYzine . . . 697
Novo-Hylazin *see* HydrALAZINE . . . 673
Novo-Indapamide *see* Indapamide . . . 716
Novo-Ipramide *see* Ipratropium . . . 737
Novo-Keto *see* Ketoprofen . . . 763
Novo-Ketoconazole *see* Ketoconazole . . . 762
Novo-Keto-EC *see* Ketoprofen . . . 763
Novo-Ketorolac *see* Ketorolac . . . 765
Novo-Ketotifen *see* Ketotifen . . . 768
Novo-Levobunolol *see* Levobunolol . . . 789
Novo-Levocarbidopa *see* Levodopa and Carbidopa . . . 793
Novo-Lexin® *see* Cephalexin . . . 285
Novolin® 70/30 *see* Insulin Preparations . . . 723
Novolin® ge *see* Insulin Preparations . . . 723
Novolin® L *see* Insulin Preparations . . . 723
Novolin® N *see* Insulin Preparations . . . 723
Novolin® R *see* Insulin Preparations . . . 723
NovoLog® *see* Insulin Preparations . . . 723
NovoLog® Mix 70/30 *see* Insulin Preparations . . . 723
Novo-Loperamide *see* Loperamide . . . 819
Novo-Lorazepam® *see* Lorazepam . . . 824
Novo-Maprotiline *see* Maprotiline . . . 841
Novo-Medrone *see* MedroxyPROGESTERone . . . 849
Novo-Meprazine *see* Methotrimeprazine . . . 887
Novo-Mepro *see* Meprobamate . . . 864

Novo-Metformin *see* Metformin . . . 874
Novo-Methacin *see* Indomethacin . . . 719
Novo-Metoprolol *see* Metoprolol . . . 901
Novo-Mexiletine *see* Mexiletine . . . 905
Novo-Minocycline *see* Minocycline . . . 915
Novo-Misoprostol *see* Misoprostol . . . 920
Novo-Mucilax *see* Psyllium . . . 1149
Novo-Nadolol *see* Nadolol . . . 943
Novo-Naproc EC *see* Naproxen . . . 953
Novo-Naprox *see* Naproxen . . . 953
Novo-Naprox Sodium *see* Naproxen . . . 953
Novo-Naprox Sodium DS *see* Naproxen . . . 953
Novo-Naprox SR *see* Naproxen . . . 953
Novo-Nidazol *see* Metronidazole . . . 902
Novo-Nifedin *see* NIFEdipine . . . 973
Novo-Nizatidine *see* Nizatidine . . . 984
Novo-Norfloxacin *see* Norfloxacin . . . 987
Novo-Nortriptyline *see* Nortriptyline . . . 989
Novo-Oxybutynin *see* Oxybutynin . . . 1016
Novo-Pen-VK® *see* Penicillin V Potassium . . . 1051
Novo-Peridol *see* Haloperidol . . . 659
Novo-Pindol *see* Pindolol . . . 1085
Novo-Pirocam® *see* Piroxicam . . . 1090
Novo-Pravastatin *see* Pravastatin . . . 1106
Novo-Prazin *see* Prazosin . . . 1108
Novo-Prednisolone® *see* PrednisoLONE . . . 1110
Novo-Profen® *see* Ibuprofen . . . 703
Novo-Propamide *see* ChlorproPAMIDE . . . 314
Novoquin® *see* Ciprofloxacin . . . 328
Novo-Quinidin *see* Quinidine . . . 1158
Novo-Ranidine *see* Ranitidine . . . 1168
NovoRapid® *see* Insulin Preparations . . . 723
Novo-Selegiline *see* Selegiline . . . 1213
Novo-Sertraline *see* Sertraline . . . 1216
Novo-Seven® *see* Factor VIIa (Recombinant) . . . 554
Novo-Sorbide *see* Isosorbide Dinitrate . . . 750
Novo-Sotalol *see* Sotalol . . . 1235
Novo-Soxazole® *see* SulfiSOXAZOLE . . . 1256
Novo-Spiroton *see* Spironolactone . . . 1240
Novo-Spirozine *see* Hydrochlorothiazide and Spironolactone . . . 677
Novo-Sucralate *see* Sucralfate . . . 1247
Novo-Sundac *see* Sulindac . . . 1257
Novo-Tamoxifen *see* Tamoxifen . . . 1264
Novo-Temazepam *see* Temazepam . . . 1271
Novo-Terazosin *see* Terazosin . . . 1276
Novo-Terbinafine *see* Terbinafine . . . 1277
Novo-Tetra *see* Tetracycline . . . 1286
Novo-Theophyl SR *see* Theophylline . . . 1291
Novothyrox *see* Levothyroxine . . . 800
Novo-Trazodone *see* Trazodone . . . 1336
Novo-Triamzide *see* Hydrochlorothiazide and Triamterene . . . 677
Novo-Trifluzine *see* Trifluoperazine . . . 1349
Novo-Trimel *see* Sulfamethoxazole and Trimethoprim . . . 1253
Novo-Trimel D.S. *see* Sulfamethoxazole and Trimethoprim . . . 1253
Novo-Tripramine *see* Trimipramine . . . 1354
Novo-Veramil *see* Verapamil . . . 1382
Novo-Veramil SR *see* Verapamil . . . 1382
Novoxapram® *see* Oxazepam . . . 1011
Nozinan® *see* Methotrimeprazine . . . 887
Nozolon *see* Gentamicin . . . 634
NPH Iletin® II *see* Insulin Preparations . . . 723
NSC-3053 *see* Dactinomycin . . . 393
NSC-3088 *see* Chlorambucil . . . 296
NSC-13875 *see* Altretamine . . . 66
NSC-26271 *see* Cyclophosphamide . . . 381
NSC-102816 *see* Azacitidine . . . 149
NSC-106977 (*Erwinia*) *see* Asparaginase . . . 129
NSC-109229 (*E. coli*) *see* Asparaginase . . . 129
NSC-123127 *see* DOXOrubicin . . . 473
NSC-125066 *see* Bleomycin . . . 190
NSC-373364 *see* Aldesleukin . . . 50
NTG *see* Nitroglycerin . . . 981
NTZ *see* Nitazoxanide . . . 978
Nu-Acebutolol *see* Acebutolol . . . 25
Nu-Acyclovir *see* Acyclovir . . . 42
Nu-Alprax *see* Alprazolam . . . 61
Nu-Amilzide *see* Amiloride and Hydrochlorothiazide . . . 76
Nu-Amoxi *see* Amoxicillin . . . 93
Nu-Ampi *see* Ampicillin . . . 103
Nu-Atenol *see* Atenolol . . . 137
Nu-Baclo *see* Baclofen . . . 158
Nubain® *see* Nalbuphine . . . 946
Nu-Beclomethasone *see* Beclomethasone . . . 163
Nu-Bromazepam *see* Bromazepam . . . 199
Nu-Buspirone *see* BusPIRone . . . 211
Nu-Capto® *see* Captopril . . . 238
Nu-Carbamazepine® *see* Carbamazepine . . . 241
Nu-Cefaclor *see* Cefaclor . . . 260
Nu-Cephalex® *see* Cephalexin . . . 285
Nu-Cimet® *see* Cimetidine . . . 326

Nu-Clonazepam *see* Clonazepam . . . 350
Nu-Clonidine® *see* Clonidine . . . 351
Nu-Cloxi® *see* Cloxacillin . . . 357
Nucofed® Expectorant *see* Guaifenesin, Pseudoephedrine, and Codeine . . . 653
Nucofed® Pediatric Expectorant *see* Guaifenesin, Pseudoephedrine, and Codeine . . . 653
Nu-Cotrimox® *see* Sulfamethoxazole and Trimethoprim . . . 1253
Nucotuss® *see* Guaifenesin, Pseudoephedrine, and Codeine . . . 653
Nu-Cromolyn *see* Cromolyn Sodium . . . 375
Nu-Cyclobenzaprine *see* Cyclobenzaprine . . . 379
Nu-Desipramine *see* Desipramine . . . 408
Nu-Diclo *see* Diclofenac . . . 429
Nu-Diclo-SR *see* Diclofenac . . . 429
Nu-Diflunisal *see* Diflunisal . . . 438
Nu-Diltiaz *see* Diltiazem . . . 447
Nu-Diltiaz-CD *see* Diltiazem . . . 447
Nu-Divalproex *see* Valproic Acid and Derivatives . . . 1371
Nu-Doxycycline *see* Doxycycline . . . 476
Nu-Erythromycin-S *see* Erythromycin . . . 512
Nu-Famotidine *see* Famotidine . . . 556
Nu-Fenofibrate *see* Fenofibrate . . . 561
Nu-Fluoxetine *see* Fluoxetine . . . 589
Nu-Flurprofen *see* Flurbiprofen . . . 596
Nu-Fluvoxamine *see* Fluvoxamine . . . 605
Nu-Gemfibrozil *see* Gemfibrozil . . . 631
Nu-Glyburide *see* GlyBURIDE . . . 642
Nu-Hydral *see* HydrALAZINE . . . 673
Nu-Ibuprofen *see* Ibuprofen . . . 703
Nu-Indapamide *see* Indapamide . . . 716
Nu-Indo *see* Indomethacin . . . 719
Nu-Ipratropium *see* Ipratropium . . . 737
Nu-Iron® 150 [OTC] *see* Polysaccharide-Iron Complex . . . 1096
Nu-Ketoprofen *see* Ketoprofen . . . 763
Nu-Ketoprofen-E *see* Ketoprofen . . . 763
NuLev™ *see* Hyoscyamine . . . 699
Nu-Levocarb *see* Levodopa and Carbidopa . . . 793
Nullo® [OTC] *see* Chlorophyll . . . 302
Nu-Loraz *see* Lorazepam . . . 824
Nu-Loxapine *see* Loxapine . . . 829
NuLytely® *see* Polyethylene Glycol-Electrolyte Solution . . . 1094
Nu-Medopa *see* Methyldopa . . . 891
Nu-Mefenamic *see* Mefenamic Acid . . . 851
Nu-Megestrol *see* Megestrol . . . 853
Nu-Metformin *see* Metformin . . . 874
Nu-Metoclopramide *see* Metoclopramide . . . 898
Nu-Metop *see* Metoprolol . . . 901
Numorphan® *see* Oxymorphone . . . 1024
Nu-Naprox *see* Naproxen . . . 953
Nu-Nifed *see* NIFEdipine . . . 973
Nu-Nortriptyline *see* Nortriptyline . . . 989
Nu-Oxybutyn *see* Oxybutynin . . . 1016
Nu-Pentoxifylline SR *see* Pentoxifylline . . . 1058
Nu-Pen-VK® *see* Penicillin V Potassium . . . 1051
Nupercainal® [OTC] *see* Dibucaine . . . 427
Nupercainal® Hydrocortisone Cream [OTC] *see* Hydrocortisone . . . 688
Nu-Pindol *see* Pindolol . . . 1085
Nu-Pirox *see* Piroxicam . . . 1090
Nu-Prazo *see* Prazosin . . . 1108
Nu-Prochlor *see* Prochlorperazine . . . 1123
Nu-Propranolol *see* Propranolol . . . 1139
Nuquin HP® *see* Hydroquinone . . . 693
Nu-Ranit *see* Ranitidine . . . 1168
Nu-Selegiline *see* Selegiline . . . 1213
Nu-Sotalol *see* Sotalol . . . 1235
Nu-Sucralate *see* Sucralfate . . . 1247
Nu-Sulfinpyrazone *see* Sulfinpyrazone . . . 1255
Nu-Sundac *see* Sulindac . . . 1257
Nu-Tears® [OTC] *see* Artificial Tears . . . 128
Nu-Tears® II [OTC] *see* Artificial Tears . . . 128
Nu-Temazepam *see* Temazepam . . . 1271
Nu-Terazosin *see* Terazosin . . . 1276
Nu-Tetra *see* Tetracycline . . . 1286
Nu-Ticlopidine *see* Ticlopidine . . . 1307
Nu-Timolol *see* Timolol . . . 1309
Nutracort® *see* Hydrocortisone . . . 688
Nutraplus® [OTC] *see* Urea . . . 1365
Nu-Trazodone *see* Trazodone . . . 1336
Nu-Triazide *see* Hydrochlorothiazide and Triamterene . . . 677
Nu-Trimipramine *see* Trimipramine . . . 1354
Nutropin® *see* Human Growth Hormone . . . 671
Nutropin® AQ *see* Human Growth Hormone . . . 671
Nutropin Depot® *see* Human Growth Hormone . . . 671
Nutropine® *see* Human Growth Hormone . . . 671
NuvaRing® *see* Combination Hormonal Contraceptives . . . 368
Nu-Verap *see* Verapamil . . . 1382
Nu-Zopiclone *see* Zopiclone . . . 1415
Nyaderm *see* Nystatin . . . 992
Nydrazid® *see* Isoniazid . . . 748
Nylidrin . . . 991
Nystatin . . . 992
Nystatin and Triamcinolone . . . 992

Nystat-Rx® *see* Nystatin . . . 992
Nystop® *see* Nystatin . . . 992
Nytol® [OTC] *see* DiphenhydrAMINE . . . 451
Nytol® Extra Strength *see* DiphenhydrAMINE . . . 451
Nytol® Maximum Strength [OTC] *see* DiphenhydrAMINE . . . 451
Occlusal™ *see* Salicylic Acid . . . 1204
Occlusal®-HP [OTC] *see* Salicylic Acid . . . 1204
Occupational Exposure to Bloodborne Pathogens (Standard/Universal Precautions) . . . 1601
Ocean® [OTC] *see* Sodium Chloride . . . 1229
OCL® [DSC] *see* Polyethylene Glycol-Electrolyte Solution . . . 1094
Octostim® *see* Desmopressin . . . 410
Octreotide . . . 993
Octreotide Acetate *see* Octreotide . . . 993
Ocu-Chlor® *see* Chloramphenicol . . . 297
OcuClear® [OTC] [DSC] *see* Oxymetazoline . . . 1022
OcuCoat® [OTC] *see* Artificial Tears . . . 128
Ocucoat® *see* Hydroxypropyl Methylcellulose . . . 696
OcuCoat® PF [OTC] *see* Artificial Tears . . . 128
Ocufen™ *see* Flurbiprofen . . . 596
Ocuflox® *see* Ofloxacin . . . 995
Ocupress® Ophthalmic *see* Carteolol . . . 254
Ocusulf-10 *see* Sulfacetamide . . . 1249
Oenothera biennis see Evening Primrose . . . 1431
Oesclim® *see* Estradiol . . . 521
Oestrogel *see* Estradiol . . . 521
Ofloxacin . . . 995
Ogastro® *see* Lansoprazole . . . 777
Ogen® *see* Estropipate . . . 536
Ogestrel® *see* Combination Hormonal Contraceptives . . . 368
OGMT *see* Metyrosine . . . 905
OKT3 *see* Muromonab-CD3 . . . 938
Olanzapine . . . 996
Oleovitamin A *see* Vitamin A . . . 1390
Oleum Ricini *see* Castor Oil . . . 259
Olexin® *see* Omeprazole . . . 999
Olmesartan . . . 997
Olmesartan Medoxomil *see* Olmesartan . . . 997
Olopatadine . . . 998
Olsalazine . . . 999
Olsalazine Sodium *see* Olsalazine . . . 999
Olux® *see* Clobetasol . . . 345
Omeprazole . . . 999
Omifin *see* ClomiPHENE . . . 348
Omnicef® *see* Cefdinir . . . 265
Omnipaque® *see* Radiological/Contrast Media (Nonionic) . . . 1165
Omnipen® *see* Ampicillin . . . 103
Oncaspar® *see* Pegaspargase . . . 1039
Oncotice™ *see* BCG Vaccine . . . 161
Oncovin® *see* VinCRIStine . . . 1387
Ondansetron . . . 1000
Ondansetron Hydrochloride *see* Ondansetron . . . 1000
One-A-Day® 50 Plus Formula [OTC] *see* Vitamins (Multiple/Oral) . . . 1394
One-A-Day® Active Formula [OTC] *see* Vitamins (Multiple/Oral) . . . 1394
One-A -Day® Essential Formula [OTC] *see* Vitamins (Multiple/Oral) . . . 1394
One-A-Day® Maximum Formula [OTC] *see* Vitamins (Multiple/Oral) . . . 1394
One-A- Day® Men's Formula [OTC] *see* Vitamins (Multiple/Oral) . . . 1394
One-A-Day® Today [OTC] *see* Vitamins (Multiple/Oral) . . . 1394
One-A-Day® Women's Formula [OTC] *see* Vitamins (Multiple/Oral) . . . 1394
Onofin-K® *see* Ketoconazole . . . 762
ONTAK® *see* Denileukin Diftitox . . . 407
Onxol™ *see* Paclitaxel . . . 1026
Ony-Clear [OTC] *see* Benzalkonium Chloride . . . 169
OPC13013 *see* Cilostazol . . . 325
OPC-14597 *see* Aripiprazole . . . 122
OP-CCK *see* Sincalide . . . 1225
Opcon-A® [OTC] *see* Naphazoline and Pheniramine . . . 953
o,p'-DDD *see* Mitotane . . . 922
Operand® [OTC] *see* Povidone-Iodine . . . 1104
Ophthetic® *see* Proparacaine . . . 1132
Ophtho-Dipivefrin™ *see* Dipivefrin . . . 455
Ophtho-Tate® *see* PrednisoLONE . . . 1110
Opium and Belladonna *see* Belladonna and Opium . . . 164
Opium Tincture . . . 1002
Opium Tincture, Deodorized *see* Opium Tincture . . . 1002
Oprad® *see* Amikacin . . . 74
Oprelvekin . . . 1003
Opthaflox® *see* Ciprofloxacin . . . 328
Opthavir® *see* Acyclovir . . . 42
Optho-Bunolol® *see* Levobunolol . . . 789
Opticaine® *see* Tetracaine . . . 1284
Opticrom® *see* Cromolyn Sodium . . . 375
Opticyl® *see* Tropicamide . . . 1360
Optifree® *see* Pancreatin . . . 1030
Optigene® 3 [OTC] *see* Tetrahydrozoline . . . 1288
Optimine® *see* Azatadine . . . 149
Optimyxin® *see* Bacitracin and Polymyxin B . . . 157
Optimyxin Plus® *see* Bacitracin and Polymyxin B . . . 157
Optimyxin Plus® *see* Neomycin, Polymyxin B, and Gramicidin . . . 963
OptiPranolol® *see* Metipranolol . . . 898
Optiray® *see* Radiological/Contrast Media (Nonionic) . . . 1165

Optivar™ *see* Azelastine . . . 151
Optomicin® *see* Erythromycin . . . 512
Orabase®-B [OTC] *see* Benzocaine . . . 169
Orabase® With Benzocaine [OTC] *see* Benzocaine, Gelatin, Pectin, and Sodium Carboxymethylcellulose . . . 171
Oracit® *see* Sodium Citrate and Citric Acid . . . 1230
Oracort *see* Triamcinolone . . . 1341
Oracort® *see* Triamcinolone Acetonide Dental Paste . . . 1344
Orafer® *see* Iron Supplements . . . 745
Orajel® [OTC] *see* Benzocaine . . . 169
Orajel® Baby [OTC] *see* Benzocaine . . . 169
Orajel® Baby Nighttime [OTC] *see* Benzocaine . . . 169
Orajel® Maximum Strength [OTC] *see* Benzocaine . . . 169
Orajel® Perioseptic® [OTC] *see* Carbamide Peroxide . . . 244
Oral Bacterial Infections . . . 1531
Oral Fungal Infections . . . 1542
Oral Nonviral Soft Tissue Ulcerations or Erosions . . . 1549
Oral Pain . . . 1524
Oral Rinse Products . . . 1634
Oral Viral Infections . . . 1545
Oramorph SR® *see* Morphine Sulfate . . . 931
Orange Root *see* Golden Seal . . . 1437
Oranor® *see* Norfloxacin . . . 987
Oranyl [OTC] *see* Pseudoephedrine . . . 1146
Orap® *see* Pimozide . . . 1083
Orapred® *see* PrednisoLONE . . . 1110
OraRinse™ [OTC] *see* Maltodextrin . . . 840
Orasol® [OTC] *see* Benzocaine . . . 169
Orciprenaline Sulfate *see* Metaproterenol . . . 873
Orelox® *see* Cefpodoxime . . . 273
Oretic® *see* Hydrochlorothiazide . . . 675
Orfadin® *see* Nitisinone . . . 979
Orgalutran® *see* Ganirelix . . . 628
Organidin® NR *see* Guaifenesin . . . 650
Orgaran® [DSC] *see* Danaparoid . . . 395
Oriental Plum Tree *see* Ginkgo Biloba . . . 1434
Orinase Diagnostic® [DSC] *see* TOLBUTamide . . . 1319
ORLAAM® *see* Levomethadyl Acetate Hydrochloride . . . 796
Orlistat . . . 1004
Ornex® [OTC] *see* Acetaminophen and Pseudoephedrine . . . 31
Ornex® Maximum Strength [OTC] *see* Acetaminophen and Pseudoephedrine . . . 31
ORO-Clense *see* Chlorhexidine Gluconate . . . 300
Orphenace® *see* Orphenadrine . . . 1005
Orphenadrine . . . 1005
Orphenadrine, Aspirin, and Caffeine . . . 1005
Orphenadrine Citrate *see* Orphenadrine . . . 1005
Orphengesic *see* Orphenadrine, Aspirin, and Caffeine . . . 1005
Orphengesic Forte *see* Orphenadrine, Aspirin, and Caffeine . . . 1005
Ortho-Cept® *see* Combination Hormonal Contraceptives . . . 368
Orthoclone OKT® 3 *see* Muromonab-CD3 . . . 938
Ortho-Cyclen® Lo *see* Combination Hormonal Contraceptives . . . 368
Ortho-Est® *see* Estropipate . . . 536
Ortho Evra™ *see* Combination Hormonal Contraceptives . . . 368
Ortho-Novum® *see* Combination Hormonal Contraceptives . . . 368
Ortho-Novum® 1/50 *see* Mestranol and Norethindrone . . . 871
Ortho-Prefest® *see* Estradiol and Norgestimate . . . 526
Ortho Sprintec™ *see* Combination Hormonal Contraceptives . . . 368
Ortopsique® *see* Diazepam . . . 424
Orudis® [DSC] *see* Ketoprofen . . . 763
Orudis® KT [OTC] *see* Ketoprofen . . . 763
Orudis® SR *see* Ketoprofen . . . 763
Oruvail® *see* Ketoprofen . . . 763
Os-Cal® 500 [OTC] *see* Calcium Supplements . . . 229
Oseltamivir . . . 1006
Oseltamivir Phosphate *see* Oseltamivir . . . 1006
Oseum® *see* Calcitonin . . . 222
Osiren® *see* Omeprazole . . . 999
Osmoglyn® *see* Glycerin . . . 644
Osteral® *see* Piroxicam . . . 1090
Ostoforte® *see* Ergocalciferol . . . 508
Otic Domeboro® *see* Aluminum Acetate and Acetic Acid . . . 67
Otrivin® [OTC] [DSC] *see* Xylometazoline . . . 1401
Otrivin® Pediatric [OTC] [DSC] *see* Xylometazoline . . . 1401
Otrozol *see* Metronidazole . . . 902
Ovace™ *see* Sulfacetamide . . . 1249
Ovcon® *see* Combination Hormonal Contraceptives . . . 368
Ovidrel® *see* Chorionic Gonadotropin (Recombinant) . . . 321
Ovol® *see* Simethicone . . . 1222
Ovral® *see* Combination Hormonal Contraceptives . . . 368
Ovrette® *see* Norgestrel . . . 988
Oxacillin . . . 1007
Oxacillin Sodium *see* Oxacillin . . . 1007
Oxaliplatin . . . 1008
Oxandrin® *see* Oxandrolone . . . 1009
Oxandrolone . . . 1009
Oxaprozin . . . 1010
Oxazepam . . . 1011
Oxcarbazepine . . . 1012
Oxeze® Turbuhaler® *see* Formoterol . . . 612
Oxicanol® *see* Piroxicam . . . 1090

Oxiconazole . . . 1014
Oxiconazole Nitrate *see* Oxiconazole . . . 1014
Oxifungol® *see* Fluconazole . . . 576
Oxiken® *see* DOBUTamine . . . 460
Oxilapine Succinate *see* Loxapine . . . 829
Oxipor® VHC [OTC] *see* Coal Tar . . . 359
Oxis® *see* Formoterol . . . 612
Oxistat® *see* Oxiconazole . . . 1014
Oxitopisa *see* Oxytocin . . . 1026
Oxitraklin® *see* Oxytetracycline . . . 1024
Oxizole® *see* Oxiconazole . . . 1014
Oxpentifylline *see* Pentoxifylline . . . 1058
Oxpram® *see* Oxazepam . . . 1011
Oxprenolol . . . 1014
Oxprenolol Hydrochloride *see* Oxprenolol . . . 1014
Oxsoralen® *see* Methoxsalen . . . 888
Oxsoralen-Ultra™ *see* Methoxsalen . . . 888
Oxy 10® Balanced Medicated Face Wash [OTC] *see* Benzoyl Peroxide . . . 171
Oxy Balance® [OTC] *see* Salicylic Acid . . . 1204
Oxy® Balance Deep Pore [OTC] *see* Salicylic Acid . . . 1204
Oxybutynin . . . 1016
Oxybutynin Chloride *see* Oxybutynin . . . 1016
Oxycel® *see* Cellulose (Oxidized) . . . 284
Oxychlorosene . . . 1017
Oxychlorosene Sodium *see* Oxychlorosene . . . 1017
Oxycocet® *see* Oxycodone and Acetaminophen . . . 1018
Oxycodan® *see* Oxycodone and Aspirin . . . 1020
Oxycodone . . . 1017
Oxycodone and Acetaminophen . . . 1018
Oxycodone and Aspirin . . . 1020
Oxycodone Hydrochloride *see* Oxycodone . . . 1017
OxyContin® *see* Oxycodone . . . 1017
Oxyderm™ *see* Benzoyl Peroxide . . . 171
Oxydose™ *see* Oxycodone . . . 1017
OxyFast® *see* Oxycodone . . . 1017
Oxygen . . . 1022
OxyIR® *see* Oxycodone . . . 1017
Oxylin® *see* Oxymetazoline . . . 1022
Oxymetazoline . . . 1022
Oxymetazoline Hydrochloride *see* Oxymetazoline . . . 1022
Oxymetholone . . . 1023
Oxymorphone . . . 1024
Oxymorphone Hydrochloride *see* Oxymorphone . . . 1024
Oxytetracycline . . . 1024
Oxytetracycline and Hydrocortisone . . . 1025
Oxytetracycline and Polymyxin B . . . 1025
Oxytetracycline Hydrochloride *see* Oxytetracycline . . . 1024
Oxytocin . . . 1026
Oxytrol™ *see* Oxybutynin . . . 1016
Oyst-Cal 500 [OTC] *see* Calcium Supplements . . . 229
Oystercal® 500 *see* Calcium Supplements . . . 229
Ozoken *see* Omeprazole . . . 999
P-071 *see* Cetirizine . . . 289
Pacerone® *see* Amiodarone . . . 80
Pacis™ *see* BCG Vaccine . . . 161
Pacitran® *see* Diazepam . . . 424
Paclitaxel . . . 1026
Pactens® *see* Naproxen . . . 953
Pain-A-Lay® [OTC] *see* Phenol . . . 1068
Palafer® *see* Iron Supplements . . . 745
Palane® *see* Enalapril . . . 492
Palgic®-D *see* Carbinoxamine and Pseudoephedrine . . . 247
Palgic®-DS *see* Carbinoxamine and Pseudoephedrine . . . 247
Palivizumab . . . 1028
Palmer's® Skin Success Acne [OTC] *see* Benzoyl Peroxide . . . 171
Palmer's Skin Success Acne Cleanser [OTC] *see* Salicylic Acid . . . 1204
Palmer's® Skin Success Fade Cream™ [OTC] *see* Hydroquinone . . . 693
Palmetto Scrub *see* Saw Palmetto . . . 1447
Palmitate-A® [OTC] *see* Vitamin A . . . 1390
PALS® [OTC] *see* Chlorophyll . . . 302
Pamelor® *see* Nortriptyline . . . 989
Pamidronate . . . 1029
Pamidronate Disodium *see* Pamidronate . . . 1029
Pamine® *see* Methscopolamine . . . 888
p-Aminoclonidine *see* Apraclonidine . . . 118
Pan-2400™ [OTC] *see* Pancreatin . . . 1030
Panax ginseng *see* Ginseng, Panax . . . 1435
Pancof®-XP *see* Hydrocodone, Pseudoephedrine, and Guaifenesin . . . 687
Pancrease® *see* Pancreatin . . . 1030
Pancrease® *see* Pancrelipase . . . 1030
Pancrease® MT *see* Pancrelipase . . . 1030
Pancreatin . . . 1030
Pancreatin 4X [OTC] *see* Pancreatin . . . 1030
Pancreatin 8X [OTC] *see* Pancreatin . . . 1030
Pancrecarb MS® *see* Pancrelipase . . . 1030
Pancrelipase . . . 1030
Pandel® *see* Hydrocortisone . . . 688
Pangestyme™ CN *see* Pancrelipase . . . 1030
Pangestyme™ EC *see* Pancrelipase . . . 1030
Pangestyme™ MT *see* Pancrelipase . . . 1030

Pangestyme™ UL *see* Pancrelipase . . . 1030
Panglobulin® *see* Immune Globulin (Intravenous) . . . 714
Panhematin® *see* Hemin . . . 661
PanMist®-DM *see* Guaifenesin, Pseudoephedrine, and Dextromethorphan . . . 653
PanMist® Jr. *see* Guaifenesin and Pseudoephedrine . . . 652
PanMist® LA *see* Guaifenesin and Pseudoephedrine . . . 652
PanMist® S *see* Guaifenesin and Pseudoephedrine . . . 652
PanOxyl® *see* Benzoyl Peroxide . . . 171
PanOxyl®-AQ *see* Benzoyl Peroxide . . . 171
PanOxyl® Bar [OTC] *see* Benzoyl Peroxide . . . 171
Panretin™ *see* Alitretinoin . . . 57
Panthoderm® [OTC] *see* Dexpanthenol . . . 418
Panto™ IV *see* Pantoprazole . . . 1031
Pantoloc™ *see* Pantoprazole . . . 1031
Pantomicina® *see* Erythromycin . . . 512
Pantoprazole . . . 1031
Pantothenic Acid . . . 1033
Pantothenyl Alcohol *see* Dexpanthenol . . . 418
Pantozol® *see* Pantoprazole . . . 1031
Papaverine . . . 1033
Papaverine Hydrochloride *see* Papaverine . . . 1033
Para-Aminosalicylate Sodium *see* Aminosalicylic Acid . . . 79
Paracetamol *see* Acetaminophen . . . 27
Parafon Forte® *see* Chlorzoxazone . . . 316
Parafon Forte® DSC *see* Chlorzoxazone . . . 316
Paraplatin® *see* Carboplatin . . . 248
Paraplatin-AQ *see* Carboplatin . . . 248
Parathyroid Hormone (1-34) *see* Teriparatide . . . 1280
Para-Time S.R.® *see* Papaverine . . . 1033
Paraxin *see* Chloramphenicol . . . 297
Paregoric . . . 1034
Paremyd® *see* Hydroxyamphetamine and Tropicamide . . . 694
Paricalcitol . . . 1034
Pariet® *see* Rabeprazole . . . 1162
Pariprazole *see* Rabeprazole . . . 1162
Parlodel® *see* Bromocriptine . . . 199
Parnate® *see* Tranylcypromine . . . 1334
Paromomycin . . . 1035
Paromomycin Sulfate *see* Paromomycin . . . 1035
Paroxetine . . . 1036
Parvolex® *see* Acetylcysteine . . . 40
PAS *see* Aminosalicylic Acid . . . 79
Paser® *see* Aminosalicylic Acid . . . 79
Passiflora spp *see* Passion Flower . . . 1445
Passion Flower . . . 1445
Patanol® *see* Olopatadine . . . 998
Pathocil® *see* Dicloxacillin . . . 432
Patients Requiring Sedation . . . 1565
Pausinystalia yohimbe *see* Yohimbe . . . 1451
Pavabid® [DSC] *see* Papaverine . . . 1033
Paxil® *see* Paroxetine . . . 1036
Paxil® CR™ *see* Paroxetine . . . 1036
PBZ® *see* Tripelennamine . . . 1356
PBZ-SR® *see* Tripelennamine . . . 1356
PCA *see* Procainamide . . . 1119
PCE® *see* Erythromycin . . . 512
PCV7 *see* Pneumococcal Conjugate Vaccine (7-Valent) . . . 1091
Pebegal *see* Benzonatate . . . 171
Pectin and Kaolin *see* Kaolin and Pectin . . . 760
Pedameth® *see* Methionine . . . 881
PediaCare® Decongestant Infants [OTC] *see* Pseudoephedrine . . . 1146
Pediacare® Decongestant Plus Cough [OTC] *see* Pseudoephedrine and Dextromethorphan . . . 1147
Pediacare® Long Acting Cough Plus Cold [OTC] *see* Pseudoephedrine and Dextromethorphan . . . 1147
Pediacof® *see* Chlorpheniramine, Phenylephrine, Codeine, and Potassium Iodide . . . 311
Pediaflor® *see* Fluoride . . . 586
Pediamist® [OTC] *see* Sodium Chloride . . . 1229
Pediapred® *see* PrednisoLONE . . . 1110
Pediarix™ *see* Diphtheria, Tetanus Toxoids, Acellular Pertussis, Hepatitis B (Recombinant), and Poliovirus (Inactivated) Vaccine . . . 454
Pediatrix *see* Acetaminophen . . . 27
Pediazole® *see* Erythromycin and Sulfisoxazole . . . 516
Pedi-Boro® [OTC] *see* Aluminum Sulfate and Calcium Acetate . . . 70
Pedi-Dri® *see* Nystatin . . . 992
PediOtic® *see* Neomycin, Polymyxin B, and Hydrocortisone . . . 963
Pedisilk® [OTC] *see* Salicylic Acid . . . 1204
Pedituss® *see* Chlorpheniramine, Phenylephrine, Codeine, and Potassium Iodide . . . 311
Pedtrace-4® *see* Trace Metals . . . 1328
PedvaxHIB® *see* *Haemophilus* b Conjugate Vaccine . . . 656
Pegademase Bovine . . . 1038
Peganone® *see* Ethotoin . . . 544
Pegaspargase . . . 1039
Pegasys® *see* Peginterferon Alfa-2a . . . 1040
Pegfilgrastim . . . 1040
Peginterferon Alfa-2a . . . 1040
Peginterferon Alfa-2b . . . 1042
PEG-Intron® *see* Peginterferon Alfa-2b . . . 1042
PEG-L-asparaginase *see* Pegaspargase . . . 1039
PegLyte® *see* Polyethylene Glycol-Electrolyte Solution . . . 1094

Pegylated Interferon Alfa-2a *see* Peginterferon Alfa-2a 1040
PemADD® *see* Pemoline 1044
PemADD® CT *see* Pemoline 1044
Pemirolast 1044
Pemoline 1044
Penamox® *see* Amoxicillin 93
Penbutolol 1045
Penbutolol Sulfate *see* Penbutolol 1045
Penciclovir 1046
Penicil *see* Penicillin G Procaine 1050
Penicillamine 1046
Penicillin G Benzathine 1047
Penicillin G Benzathine and Penicillin G Procaine 1048
Penicillin G Benzathine and Procaine *see* Penicillin G Benzathine and Penicillin G Procaine 1048
Penicillin G (Parenteral/Aqueous) 1049
Penicillin G Potassium *see* Penicillin G (Parenteral/Aqueous) 1049
Penicillin G Procaine 1050
Penicillin G Procaine and Benzathine Combined *see* Penicillin G Benzathine and Penicillin G Procaine 1048
Penicillin G Procaine and Penicillin G Benzathine *see* Penicillin G Benzathine and Penicillin G Procaine 1048
Penicillin G Sodium *see* Penicillin G (Parenteral/Aqueous) 1049
Penicillin V Potassium 1051
Penicilloyl-polylysine *see* Benzylpenicilloyl-polylysine 174
Penipot *see* Penicillin G Procaine 1050
Penlac™ *see* Ciclopirox 322
Penprocilina *see* Penicillin G Procaine 1050
Penta/3B® *see* Vitamin B Complex 1392
Penta/3B®+C *see* Vitamin B Complex and Vitamin C 1392
Pentacarinat® *see* Pentamidine 1052
Pentam-300® *see* Pentamidine 1052
Pentamidine 1052
Pentamidine Isethionate *see* Pentamidine 1052
Pentamycetin® *see* Chloramphenicol 297
Pentasa® *see* Mesalamine 869
Pentaspan® *see* Pentastarch 1053
Pentastarch 1053
Penta-Triamterene HCTZ *see* Hydrochlorothiazide and Triamterene 677
Pentazocine 1054
Pentazocine Combinations 1054
Pentazocine Hydrochloride *see* Pentazocine 1054
Pentazocine Lactate *see* Pentazocine 1054
Pentobarbital 1055
Pentobarbital Sodium *see* Pentobarbital 1055
Pentosan Polysulfate Sodium 1056
Pentostatin 1057
Pentothal® *see* Thiopental 1297
Pentothal Sodico® *see* Thiopental 1297
Pentoxifylline 1058
Pentoxil® *see* Pentoxifylline 1058
Pentrax® [OTC] *see* Coal Tar 359
Pentrexyl *see* Ampicillin 103
Pen-Vi-K *see* Penicillin V Potassium 1051
Pen VK *see* Penicillin V Potassium 1051
Pepcid® *see* Famotidine 556
Pepcid AC® *see* Famotidine 556
Pepcid® Complete [OTC] *see* Famotidine, Calcium Carbonate, and Magnesium Hydroxide 557
Pepcidine® *see* Famotidine 556
Pepcid® I.V. *see* Famotidine 556
Pepevit® *see* Niacin 967
Pepto-Bismol® [OTC] *see* Bismuth 186
Pepto-Bismol® Maximum Strength [OTC] *see* Bismuth 186
Percocet® *see* Oxycodone and Acetaminophen 1018
Percocet® 2.5/325 *see* Oxycodone and Acetaminophen 1018
Percocet® 5/325 *see* Oxycodone and Acetaminophen 1018
Percocet® 7.5/325 *see* Oxycodone and Acetaminophen 1018
Percocet® 7.5/500 *see* Oxycodone and Acetaminophen 1018
Percocet® 10/325 *see* Oxycodone and Acetaminophen 1018
Percocet® 10/650 *see* Oxycodone and Acetaminophen 1018
Percocet®-Demi *see* Oxycodone and Acetaminophen 1018
Percodan® *see* Oxycodone and Aspirin 1020
Percodan®-Demi *see* Oxycodone and Aspirin 1020
Percogesic® [OTC] *see* Acetaminophen and Phenyltoloxamine 31
Percolone® [DSC] *see* Oxycodone 1017
Perdiem® Fiber Therapy [OTC] *see* Psyllium 1149
Pergolide 1059
Pergolide Mesylate *see* Pergolide 1059
Pergonal® *see* Menotropins 857
Periactin® *see* Cyproheptadine 387
Peri-Colace® [OTC] *see* Docusate and Casanthranol 464
Peridane® *see* Pentoxifylline 1058
Peridex® *see* Chlorhexidine Gluconate 300
Peridol *see* Haloperidol 659
Perindopril Erbumine 1060
PerioChip® *see* Chlorhexidine Gluconate 300
Periodontal Diseases 1540
PerioGard® *see* Chlorhexidine Gluconate 300
Periostat® *see* Doxycycline Subantimicrobial 480

Permapen® Isoject® *see* Penicillin G Benzathine 1047
Permax® *see* Pergolide 1059
Permethrin 1062
Perphenazine 1062
Perphenazine and Amitriptyline *see* Amitriptyline and Perphenazine 85
Persantine® *see* Dipyridamole 456
Pertussin® DM [OTC] *see* Dextromethorphan 423
Pestarin® *see* Rifampin 1180
Pethidine Hydrochloride *see* Meperidine 858
Pevaryl Lipogel® *see* Econazole 486
Pexicam® *see* Piroxicam 1090
PFA *see* Foscarnet 613
Pfizerpen® *see* Penicillin G (Parenteral/Aqueous) 1049
Pfizerpen-AS® *see* Penicillin G Procaine 1050
PGE_1 *see* Alprostadil 63
PGE_2 *see* Dinoprostone 450
PGI_2 *see* Epoprostenol 505
PGX *see* Epoprostenol 505
Phanasin [OTC] *see* Guaifenesin 650
Pharmacology of Drug Metabolism and Interactions 18
Pharmaflur® *see* Fluoride 586
Pharmaflur® 1.1 *see* Fluoride 586
Pharmorubicin® *see* Epirubicin 501
Phazyme™ *see* Simethicone 1222
Phazyme® Quick Dissolve [OTC] *see* Simethicone 1222
Phazyme® Ultra Strength [OTC] *see* Simethicone 1222
Phenaphen® With Codeine *see* Acetaminophen and Codeine 29
Phenazo™ *see* Phenazopyridine 1064
Phenazopyridine 1064
Phenazopyridine Hydrochloride *see* Phenazopyridine 1064
Phendimetrazine 1064
Phendimetrazine Tartrate *see* Phendimetrazine 1064
Phenelzine 1065
Phenelzine Sulfate *see* Phenelzine 1065
Phenergan® *see* Promethazine 1127
Phenergan® With Codeine *see* Promethazine and Codeine 1129
Phenindamine 1066
Phenindamine Tartrate *see* Phenindamine 1066
Pheniramine and Naphazoline *see* Naphazoline and Pheniramine 953
Phenobarbital 1066
Phenobarbital, Belladonna, and Ergotamine Tartrate *see* Belladonna, Phenobarbital, and Ergotamine 165
Phenobarbital, Hyoscyamine, Atropine, and Scopolamine *see* Hyoscyamine, Atropine, Scopolamine, and Phenobarbital 700
Phenobarbital Sodium *see* Phenobarbital 1066
Phenobarbitone *see* Phenobarbital 1066
Phenol 1068
Phenol and Camphor *see* Camphor and Phenol 232
Phenoptic® *see* Phenylephrine 1071
Phenoxybenzamine 1068
Phenoxybenzamine Hydrochloride *see* Phenoxybenzamine 1068
Phenoxymethyl Penicillin *see* Penicillin V Potassium 1051
Phentermine 1069
Phentermine Hydrochloride *see* Phentermine 1069
Phentolamine 1070
Phentolamine Mesylate *see* Phentolamine 1070
Phenylalanine Mustard *see* Melphalan 855
Phenylazo Diamino Pyridine Hydrochloride *see* Phenazopyridine 1064
Phenylephrine 1071
Phenylephrine and Chlorpheniramine *see* Chlorpheniramine and Phenylephrine 308
Phenylephrine and Cyclopentolate *see* Cyclopentolate and Phenylephrine 381
Phenylephrine and Guaifenesin *see* Guaifenesin and Phenylephrine 652
Phenylephrine and Promethazine *see* Promethazine and Phenylephrine 1129
Phenylephrine and Scopolamine 1072
Phenylephrine and Zinc Sulfate 1073
Phenylephrine Hydrochloride *see* Phenylephrine 1071
Phenylephrine, Hydrocodone, Chlorpheniramine, Acetaminophen, and Caffeine *see* Hydrocodone, Chlorpheniramine, Phenylephrine, Acetaminophen, and Caffeine 686
Phenylephrine, Promethazine, and Codeine *see* Promethazine, Phenylephrine, and Codeine 1130
Phenylethylmalonylurea *see* Phenobarbital 1066
Phenylgesic® [OTC] *see* Acetaminophen and Phenyltoloxamine 31
Phenylisohydantoin *see* Pemoline 1044
Phenyl Salicylate, Methenamine, Methylene Blue, Sodium Biphosphate, and Hyoscyamine *see* Methenamine, Sodium Biphosphate, Phenyl Salicylate, Methylene Blue, and Hyoscyamine 880
Phenyltoloxamine and Acetaminophen *see* Acetaminophen and Phenyltoloxamine 31
Phenytek™ *see* Phenytoin 1073
Phenytoin 1073
Phenytoin Sodium *see* Phenytoin 1073
Phenytoin Sodium, Extended *see* Phenytoin 1073
Phenytoin Sodium, Prompt *see* Phenytoin 1073
Phillips'® Milk of Magnesia [OTC] *see* Magnesium Hydroxide 835
Phillips'® Milk of Magnesia [OTC] *see* Magnesium Supplements 837
Phillips' M-O® [OTC] *see* Magnesium Hydroxide and Mineral Oil 836
Phillips' M-O® [OTC] *see* Magnesium Supplements 837
Phillips'® Stool Softener Laxative [OTC] *see* Docusate 463
pHisoHex® *see* Hexachlorophene 669
Phos-Flur® *see* Fluoride 586
Phos-Flur® Rinse [OTC] *see* Fluoride 586

PhosLo® *see* Calcium Supplements . . . 229
Phosphate Supplements . . . 1076
Phospholine Iodide® *see* Echothiophate Iodide . . . 485
Phosphonoformate *see* Foscarnet . . . 613
Phosphonoformic Acid *see* Foscarnet . . . 613
Phosphorated Carbohydrate Solution . . . 1078
Phosphoric Acid, Levulose and Dextrose *see* Phosphorated Carbohydrate Solution . . . 1078
Photofrin® *see* Porfimer . . . 1098
Phoxal-timolol *see* Timolol . . . 1309
p-Hydroxyampicillin *see* Amoxicillin . . . 93
Phyllocontin® *see* Aminophylline . . . 78
Phyllocontin®-350 *see* Aminophylline . . . 78
Phylloquinone *see* Phytonadione . . . 1079
Physostigmine . . . 1078
Physostigmine Salicylate *see* Physostigmine . . . 1078
Physostigmine Sulfate *see* Physostigmine . . . 1078
Phytomenadione *see* Phytonadione . . . 1079
Phytonadione . . . 1079
Pilocar® *see* Pilocarpine . . . 1080
Pilocarpine . . . 1080
Pilocarpine (Dental) . . . 1081
Pilocarpine Hydrochloride *see* Pilocarpine . . . 1080
Pilocarpine Nitrate *see* Pilocarpine . . . 1080
Pilogrin *see* Pilocarpine . . . 1080
Pilopine HS® *see* Pilocarpine . . . 1080
Piloptic® *see* Pilocarpine . . . 1080
Pima® *see* Potassium Iodide . . . 1101
Pimaricin *see* Natamycin . . . 956
Pimecrolimus . . . 1083
Pimozide . . . 1083
Pindolol . . . 1085
Pink Bismuth *see* Bismuth . . . 186
Pin-X® [OTC] *see* Pyrantel Pamoate . . . 1150
PIO *see* Pemoline . . . 1044
Pioglitazone . . . 1086
Piperacillin . . . 1087
Piperacillin and Tazobactam Sodium . . . 1088
Piperacillin Sodium *see* Piperacillin . . . 1087
Piperacillin Sodium and Tazobactam Sodium *see* Piperacillin and Tazobactam Sodium . . . 1088
Piperazine . . . 1089
Piperazine Citrate *see* Piperazine . . . 1089
Piperazine Estrone Sulfate *see* Estropipate . . . 536
Piper methysticum *see* Kava . . . 1442
Piperonyl Butoxide and Pyrethrins *see* Pyrethrins and Piperonyl Butoxide . . . 1151
Pipracil® *see* Piperacillin . . . 1087
Pirbuterol . . . 1090
Pirbuterol Acetate *see* Pirbuterol . . . 1090
Piroxan® *see* Piroxicam . . . 1090
Piroxen *see* Piroxicam . . . 1090
Piroxicam . . . 1090
Pisacaina® *see* Lidocaine . . . 801
Pisacaina *see* Lidocaine and Epinephrine . . . 804
p-Isobutylhydratropic Acid *see* Ibuprofen . . . 703
Pistacia lentiscus *see* Mastic . . . 1444
Pit *see* Oxytocin . . . 1026
Pitocin® *see* Oxytocin . . . 1026
Pitressin® *see* Vasopressin . . . 1379
Pitrex *see* Tolnaftate . . . 1322
Pix Carbonis *see* Coal Tar . . . 359
Plague Vaccine *see* Immunizations (Vaccines) . . . 1612
Plan B™ *see* Levonorgestrel . . . 797
Plantago Seed *see* Psyllium . . . 1149
Plantain Seed *see* Psyllium . . . 1149
Plaquenil® *see* Hydroxychloroquine . . . 694
Plasil® *see* Metoclopramide . . . 898
Platinol® *see* Cisplatin . . . 332
Platinol®-AQ *see* Cisplatin . . . 332
Plavix® *see* Clopidogrel . . . 353
Plegine® *see* Phendimetrazine . . . 1064
Plendil® *see* Felodipine . . . 560
Pletal® *see* Cilostazol . . . 325
PMPA *see* Tenofovir . . . 1275
PMS-Amantadine *see* Amantadine . . . 70
PMS-Amitriptyline *see* Amitriptyline . . . 83
PMS-Atenolol *see* Atenolol . . . 137
PMS-Baclofen *see* Baclofen . . . 158
PMS-Bethanechol *see* Bethanechol . . . 181
PMS-Bromocriptine *see* Bromocriptine . . . 199
PMS-Buspirone *see* BusPIRone . . . 211
PMS-Captopril® *see* Captopril . . . 238
PMS-Carbamazepine *see* Carbamazepine . . . 241
PMS-Cefaclor *see* Cefaclor . . . 260
PMS-Chloral Hydrate *see* Chloral Hydrate . . . 295
PMS-Cholestyramine *see* Cholestyramine Resin . . . 318
PMS-Cimetidine *see* Cimetidine . . . 326
PMS-Clobazam *see* Clobazam . . . 344
PMS-Clonazepam *see* Clonazepam . . . 350
PMS-Deferoxamine *see* Deferoxamine . . . 404
PMS-Desipramine *see* Desipramine . . . 408
PMS-Dexamethasone *see* Dexamethasone . . . 413

PMS-Dicitrate™ *see* Sodium Citrate and Citric Acid . . . 1230
PMS-Diclofenac *see* Diclofenac . . . 429
PMS-Diclofenac SR *see* Diclofenac . . . 429
PMS-Diphenhydramine *see* DiphenhydrAMINE . . . 451
PMS-Dipivefrin *see* Dipivefrin . . . 455
PMS-Docusate Calcium *see* Docusate . . . 463
PMS-Docusate Sodium *see* Docusate . . . 463
PMS-Erythromycin *see* Erythromycin . . . 512
PMS-Fenofibrate Micro *see* Fenofibrate . . . 561
PMS-Ferrous Sulfate *see* Iron Supplements . . . 745
PMS-Fluorometholone *see* Fluorometholone . . . 587
PMS-Fluoxetine *see* Fluoxetine . . . 589
PMS-Fluphenazine Decanoate *see* Fluphenazine . . . 593
PMS-Flutamide *see* Flutamide . . . 598
PMS-Fluvoxamine *see* Fluvoxamine . . . 605
PMS-Gabapentin *see* Gabapentin . . . 624
PMS-Gemfibrozil *see* Gemfibrozil . . . 631
PMS-Glyburide *see* GlyBURIDE . . . 642
PMS-Haloperidol LA *see* Haloperidol . . . 659
PMS-Hydromorphone *see* Hydromorphone . . . 691
PMS-Hydroxyzine *see* HydrOXYzine . . . 697
PMS-Indapamide *see* Indapamide . . . 716
PMS-Ipratropium *see* Ipratropium . . . 737
PMS-Isoniazid *see* Isoniazid . . . 748
PMS-Isosorbide *see* Isosorbide Dinitrate . . . 750
PMS-Lactulose *see* Lactulose . . . 772
PMS-Levobunolol *see* Levobunolol . . . 789
PMS-Lindane *see* Lindane . . . 809
PMS-Lithium Carbonate *see* Lithium . . . 815
PMS-Lithium Citrate *see* Lithium . . . 815
PMS-Loperamine *see* Loperamide . . . 819
PMS-Loxapine *see* Loxapine . . . 829
PMS-Mefenamic Acid *see* Mefenamic Acid . . . 851
PMS-Metformin *see* Metformin . . . 874
PMS-Methylphenidate *see* Methylphenidate . . . 893
PMS-Metoprolol *see* Metoprolol . . . 901
PMS-Minocycline *see* Minocycline . . . 915
PMS-Nizatidine *see* Nizatidine . . . 984
PMS-Norfloxacin *see* Norfloxacin . . . 987
PMS-Nortriptyline *see* Nortriptyline . . . 989
PMS-Nystatin *see* Nystatin . . . 992
PMS-Oxazepam *see* Oxazepam . . . 1011
PMS-Oxybutynin *see* Oxybutynin . . . 1016
PMS-Pindolol *see* Pindolol . . . 1085
PMS-Polytrimethoprim *see* Trimethoprim and Polymyxin B . . . 1353
PMS-Procyclidine *see* Procyclidine . . . 1125
PMS-Propranolol® *see* Propranolol . . . 1139
PMS-Pseudoephedrine *see* Pseudoephedrine . . . 1146
PMS-Ranitidine *see* Ranitidine . . . 1168
PMS-Salbutamol *see* Albuterol . . . 48
PMS-Sotalol *see* Sotalol . . . 1235
PMS-Sucralate *see* Sucralfate . . . 1247
PMS-Tamoxifen *see* Tamoxifen . . . 1264
PMS-Temazepam *see* Temazepam . . . 1271
PMS-Terazosin *see* Terazosin . . . 1276
PMS-Terbinafine *see* Terbinafine . . . 1277
PMS-Theophylline *see* Theophylline . . . 1291
PMS-Ticlopidine *see* Ticlopidine . . . 1307
PMS-Timolol *see* Timolol . . . 1309
PMS-Tobramycin *see* Tobramycin . . . 1315
PMS-Trazodone *see* Trazodone . . . 1336
PMS-Trifluoperazine *see* Trifluoperazine . . . 1349
PMS-Valproic Acid *see* Valproic Acid and Derivatives . . . 1371
PMS-Valproic Acid E.C. *see* Valproic Acid and Derivatives . . . 1371
PMS-Yohimbine *see* Yohimbine . . . 1401
Pneumococcal 7-Valent Conjugate Vaccine *see* Pneumococcal Conjugate Vaccine (7-Valent) . . . 1091
Pneumococcal Conjugate Vaccine (7-Valent) . . . 1091
Pneumococcal Polysaccharide Vaccine (Polyvalent) *see* Immunizations (Vaccines) . . . 1612
Pneumotussin® *see* Hydrocodone and Guaifenesin . . . 683
Podocon-25® *see* Podophyllum Resin . . . 1093
Podofilm® *see* Podophyllum Resin . . . 1093
Podofilox . . . 1093
Podophyllin *see* Podophyllum Resin . . . 1093
Podophyllum Resin . . . 1093
Polaramine® [DSC] *see* Dexchlorpheniramine . . . 416
Poliovirus Vaccine (Inactivated) . . . 1093
Polocaine® *see* Mepivacaine . . . 861
Polocaine® *see* Mepivacaine Dental Anesthetic . . . 863
Polocaine® 2% and Levonordefrin 1:20,000 *see* Mepivacaine and Levonordefrin . . . 862
Polocaine® MPF *see* Mepivacaine . . . 861
Polycidin® Ophthalmic Ointment *see* Bacitracin and Polymyxin B . . . 157
Polycitra® *see* Citric Acid, Sodium Citrate, and Potassium Citrate . . . 335
Polycitra® *see* Potassium Citrate . . . 1100
Polycitra®-K *see* Potassium Citrate and Citric Acid . . . 1101
Polycose® [OTC] *see* Glucose Polymers . . . 641
Polyethylene Glycol-Electrolyte Solution . . . 1094
Polygam® S/D *see* Immune Globulin (Intravenous) . . . 714
Polymox® *see* Amoxicillin . . . 93
Polymyxin B . . . 1095

Polymyxin B and Bacitracin *see* Bacitracin and Polymyxin B 157
Polymyxin B and Neomycin *see* Neomycin and Polymyxin B 962
Polymyxin B and Oxytetracycline *see* Oxytetracycline and Polymyxin B 1025
Polymyxin B and Trimethoprim *see* Trimethoprim and Polymyxin B 1353
Polymyxin B, Bacitracin, and Neomycin *see* Bacitracin, Neomycin, and Polymyxin B 157
Polymyxin B, Bacitracin, Neomycin, and Hydrocortisone *see* Bacitracin, Neomycin, Polymyxin B, and Hydrocortisone 158
Polymyxin B, Chloramphenicol, and Hydrocortisone *see* Chloramphenicol, Polymyxin B, and Hydrocortisone 299
Polymyxin B, Hydrocortisone, and Chloramphenicol *see* Chloramphenicol, Polymyxin B, and Hydrocortisone 299
Polymyxin B, Neomycin, and Dexamethasone *see* Neomycin, Polymyxin B, and Dexamethasone 962
Polymyxin B, Neomycin, and Gramicidin *see* Neomycin, Polymyxin B, and Gramicidin 963
Polymyxin B, Neomycin, and Hydrocortisone *see* Neomycin, Polymyxin B, and Hydrocortisone 963
Polymyxin B, Neomycin, and Prednisolone *see* Neomycin, Polymyxin B, and Prednisolone 963
Polymyxin B Sulfate *see* Polymyxin B 1095
Poly-Pred® *see* Neomycin, Polymyxin B, and Prednisolone 963
Poly-Rx *see* Polymyxin B 1095
Polysaccharide-Iron Complex 1096
Polysporin® Ophthalmic *see* Bacitracin and Polymyxin B 157
Polysporin® Topical [OTC] *see* Bacitracin and Polymyxin B 157
Polytar® [OTC] *see* Coal Tar 359
Polythiazide 1097
Polythiazide and Prazosin *see* Prazosin and Polythiazide 1109
Polytrim™ *see* Trimethoprim and Polymyxin B 1353
Polyvinyl Alcohol *see* Artificial Tears 128
Ponstan® *see* Mefenamic Acid 851
Ponstel® *see* Mefenamic Acid 851
Pontocaine® *see* Tetracaine 1284
Pontocaine® With Dextrose *see* Tetracaine and Dextrose 1285
Poor Mans Treacle *see* Garlic 1433
Poractant Alfa 1097
Porfimer 1098
Porfimer Sodium *see* Porfimer 1098
Portia™ *see* Combination Hormonal Contraceptives 368
Posipen® *see* Dicloxacillin 432
Post Peel Healing Balm [OTC] *see* Hydrocortisone 688
Posture® [OTC] *see* Calcium Phosphate (Tribasic) 227
Posture® [OTC] *see* Calcium Supplements 229
Potassium Acetate 1099
Potassium Acetate *see* Potassium Supplements 1102
Potassium Acetate, Potassium Bicarbonate, and Potassium Citrate *see* Potassium Supplements 1102
Potassium Acid Phosphate *see* Phosphate Supplements 1076
Potassium Acid Phosphate 1100
Potassium Acid Phosphate *see* Potassium Supplements 1102
Potassium Bicarbonate *see* Potassium Supplements 1102
Potassium Bicarbonate and Potassium Chloride *see* Potassium Supplements 1102
Potassium Bicarbonate and Potassium Citrate *see* Potassium Supplements 1102
Potassium Chloride *see* Potassium Supplements 1102
Potassium Citrate 1100
Potassium Citrate *see* Potassium Supplements 1102
Potassium Citrate and Citric Acid 1101
Potassium Citrate, Citric Acid, and Sodium Citrate *see* Citric Acid, Sodium Citrate, and Potassium Citrate 335
Potassium Citrate Mixture and Sodium Citrate *see* Citric Acid, Sodium Citrate, and Potassium Citrate 335
Potassium Gluconate *see* Potassium Supplements 1102
Potassium Iodide 1101
Potassium Phosphate *see* Phosphate Supplements 1076
Potassium Phosphate and Sodium Phosphate *see* Phosphate Supplements 1076
Potassium Supplements 1102
Povidone-Iodine 1104
PPD *see* Tuberculin Tests 1362
PPL *see* Benzylpenicilloyl-polylysine 174
PPS *see* Pentosan Polysulfate Sodium 1056
Pramidal® *see* Loperamide 819
Pramipexole 1105
Pramosone® *see* Pramoxine and Hydrocortisone 1106
Pramotil *see* Metoclopramide 898
Pramox® HC *see* Pramoxine and Hydrocortisone 1106
Pramoxine 1105
Pramoxine and Hydrocortisone 1106
Pramoxine Hydrochloride *see* Pramoxine 1105
Prandase® *see* Acarbose 24
Prandin® *see* Repaglinide 1172
Pravachol® *see* Pravastatin 1106
Pravacol® *see* Pravastatin 1106
Pravastatin 1106
Pravastatin Sodium *see* Pravastatin 1106
Prax® [OTC] *see* Pramoxine 1105
Praxel® *see* Paclitaxel 1026
Prazidec® *see* Omeprazole 999
Praziquantel 1108
Prazolit® *see* Omeprazole 999
Prazosin 1108
Prazosin and Polythiazide 1109

Prazosin Hydrochloride *see* Prazosin . . . 1108
Precaptil *see* Captopril . . . 238
Precedex™ *see* Dexmedetomidine . . . 416
Precose® *see* Acarbose . . . 24
Pred Forte® *see* PrednisoLONE . . . 1110
Pred-G® *see* Prednisolone and Gentamicin . . . 1112
Pred Mild® *see* PrednisoLONE . . . 1110
Prednicarbate . . . 1110
Prednidib® *see* PredniSONE . . . 1112
PrednisoLONE . . . 1110
Prednisolone Acetate *see* PrednisoLONE . . . 1110
Prednisolone Acetate, Ophthalmic *see* PrednisoLONE . . . 1110
Prednisolone and Chloramphenicol *see* Chloramphenicol and Prednisolone . . . 299
Prednisolone and Gentamicin . . . 1112
Prednisolone and Sulfacetamide *see* Sulfacetamide and Prednisolone . . . 1250
Prednisolone, Neomycin, and Polymyxin B *see* Neomycin, Polymyxin B, and Prednisolone . . . 963
Prednisolone Sodium Phosphate *see* PrednisoLONE . . . 1110
Prednisolone Sodium Phosphate, Ophthalmic *see* PrednisoLONE . . . 1110
PredniSONE . . . 1112
Prednisone Intensol™ *see* PredniSONE . . . 1112
Prefrin™ [DSC] *see* Phenylephrine . . . 1071
Pregnenedione *see* Progesterone . . . 1125
Pregnyl® *see* Chorionic Gonadotropin (Human) . . . 320
Prelone® *see* PrednisoLONE . . . 1110
Prelu-2® *see* Phendimetrazine . . . 1064
Premarin® *see* Estrogens (Conjugated/Equine) . . . 529
Premjact® [OTC] *see* Lidocaine . . . 801
Premphase® *see* Estrogens (Conjugated/Equine) and Medroxyprogesterone . . . 531
Premplus® *see* Estrogens (Conjugated/Equine) and Medroxyprogesterone . . . 531
Prempro™ *see* Estrogens (Conjugated/Equine) and Medroxyprogesterone . . . 531
Preparation H® Hydrocortisone [OTC] *see* Hydrocortisone . . . 688
Pre-Pen® *see* Benzylpenicilloyl-polylysine . . . 174
Prepidil® *see* Dinoprostone . . . 450
Prescription Writing . . . 13
Presoken *see* Diltiazem . . . 447
Presoquim *see* Diltiazem . . . 447
Pressyn® *see* Vasopressin . . . 1379
Pretz-D® [OTC] *see* Ephedrine . . . 499
Pretz® Irrigation [OTC] *see* Sodium Chloride . . . 1229
Prevacid® *see* Lansoprazole . . . 777
Prevalite® *see* Cholestyramine Resin . . . 318
PREVEN® *see* Combination Hormonal Contraceptives . . . 368
Prevex® B *see* Betamethasone . . . 177
Prevex® HC *see* Hydrocortisone . . . 688
PreviDent® *see* Fluoride . . . 586
PreviDent® 5000 Plus™ *see* Fluoride . . . 586
Prevnar® *see* Pneumococcal Conjugate Vaccine (7-Valent) . . . 1091
Priftin® *see* Rifapentine . . . 1182
Prilocaine . . . 1114
Prilocaine and Epinephrine . . . 1116
Prilocaine and Lidocaine *see* Lidocaine and Prilocaine . . . 806
Prilosec® *see* Omeprazole . . . 999
Primaclone *see* Primidone . . . 1118
Primacor® *see* Milrinone . . . 914
Primaquine . . . 1117
Primaquine Phosphate *see* Primaquine . . . 1117
Primaxin® *see* Imipenem and Cilastatin . . . 709
Primidone . . . 1118
Primsol® *see* Trimethoprim . . . 1352
Principen® *see* Ampicillin . . . 103
Princol® *see* Lincomycin . . . 808
Prinivil® *see* Lisinopril . . . 813
Prinzide® *see* Lisinopril and Hydrochlorothiazide . . . 814
Priorix™ *see* Measles, Mumps, and Rubella Vaccines (Combined) . . . 844
Pristinamycin *see* Quinupristin and Dalfopristin . . . 1161
Privine® [OTC] *see* Naphazoline . . . 952
ProAmatine® *see* Midodrine . . . 911
Proartinal® *see* Ibuprofen . . . 703
Probenecid . . . 1119
Probenecid and Colchicine *see* Colchicine and Probenecid . . . 364
Probiotica® [OTC] *see* *Lactobacillus acidophilus* and *Lactobacillus bulgaricus* . . . 772
Procainamide . . . 1119
Procainamide Hydrochloride *see* Procainamide . . . 1119
Procaine . . . 1121
Procaine Amide Hydrochloride *see* Procainamide . . . 1119
Procaine Benzylpenicillin *see* Penicillin G Procaine . . . 1050
Procaine Hydrochloride *see* Procaine . . . 1121
Procaine Penicillin G *see* Penicillin G Procaine . . . 1050
Procanbid® *see* Procainamide . . . 1119
Procan® SR *see* Procainamide . . . 1119
Procarbazine . . . 1122
Procarbazine Hydrochloride *see* Procarbazine . . . 1122
Procardia® *see* NIFEdipine . . . 973
Procardia XL® *see* NIFEdipine . . . 973
Procef® *see* Cefprozil . . . 275
Procephal® *see* Erythromycin . . . 512
Procetofene *see* Fenofibrate . . . 561
Prochieve™ *see* Progesterone . . . 1125
Prochlorperazine . . . 1123

Prochlorperazine Edisylate *see* Prochlorperazine 1123
Prochlorperazine Maleate *see* Prochlorperazine 1123
Procrit® *see* Epoetin Alfa 503
Proctocort® *see* Hydrocortisone 688
ProctoCream® HC *see* Hydrocortisone 688
Proctofene *see* Fenofibrate 561
ProctoFoam®-HC *see* Pramoxine and Hydrocortisone 1106
ProctoFoam® NS [OTC] *see* Pramoxine 1105
Proctosol-HC® *see* Hydrocortisone 688
Procyclid™ *see* Procyclidine 1125
Procyclidine 1125
Procyclidine Hydrochloride *see* Procyclidine 1125
Procytox® *see* Cyclophosphamide 381
Prodium® [OTC] *see* Phenazopyridine 1064
Profasi® *see* Chorionic Gonadotropin (Human) 320
Profasi® HP *see* Chorionic Gonadotropin (Human) 320
Profenid® *see* Ketoprofen 763
Profenid® 200 *see* Ketoprofen 763
Profenid®-IM *see* Ketoprofen 763
Profilnine® SD *see* Factor IX Complex (Human) 553
Proflavanol C™ *see* Ascorbic Acid 128
Progestasert® *see* Progesterone 1125
Progesterone 1125
Progestin *see* Progesterone 1125
Proglycem® *see* Diazoxide 427
Prograf® *see* Tacrolimus 1261
Proguanil and Atovaquone *see* Atovaquone and Proguanil 143
ProHance® *see* Radiological/Contrast Media (Nonionic) 1165
Proken M® *see* Metoprolol 901
Prolaken® *see* Metoprolol 901
Prolastin® *see* Alpha$_1$-Proteinase Inhibitor 61
Proleukin® *see* Aldesleukin 50
Prolex-D *see* Guaifenesin and Phenylephrine 652
Prolixin® *see* Fluphenazine 593
Prolixin Decanoate® *see* Fluphenazine 593
Prolixin Enanthate® [DSC] *see* Fluphenazine 593
Proloprim® *see* Trimethoprim 1352
Promatussin® DM *see* Promethazine and Dextromethorphan 1129
Promethazine 1127
Promethazine and Codeine 1129
Promethazine and Dextromethorphan 1129
Promethazine and Meperidine *see* Meperidine and Promethazine 860
Promethazine and Phenylephrine 1129
Promethazine Hydrochloride *see* Promethazine 1127
Promethazine, Phenylephrine, and Codeine 1130
Prometrium® *see* Progesterone 1125
Promit® *see* Dextran 1 420
Pronap-100® *see* Propoxyphene and Acetaminophen 1136
Pronaxil® *see* Naproxen 953
Pronestyl® *see* Procainamide 1119
Pronestyl-SR® *see* Procainamide 1119
Pronto® [OTC] *see* Pyrethrins and Piperonyl Butoxide 1151
Prontofort® *see* Tramadol 1329
Pronto® Lice Control *see* Pyrethrins and Piperonyl Butoxide 1151
Propaderm® *see* Beclomethasone 163
Propafenone 1130
Propafenone Hydrochloride *see* Propafenone 1130
Propanthel™ *see* Propantheline 1132
Propantheline 1132
Propantheline Bromide *see* Propantheline 1132
Propa pH [OTC] *see* Salicylic Acid 1204
Proparacaine 1132
Proparacaine and Fluorescein 1133
Proparacaine Hydrochloride *see* Proparacaine 1132
Proparin® *see* Heparin 662
Propecia® *see* Finasteride 572
Propeshia® *see* Finasteride 572
Propess® *see* Dinoprostone 450
Propine® *see* Dipivefrin 455
Proplex® T *see* Factor IX Complex (Human) 553
Propofol 1133
Propoxyphene 1135
Propoxyphene and Acetaminophen 1136
Propoxyphene and Aspirin 1137
Propoxyphene Hydrochloride *see* Propoxyphene 1135
Propoxyphene Hydrochloride and Acetaminophen *see* Propoxyphene and Acetaminophen 1136
Propoxyphene Hydrochloride and Aspirin *see* Propoxyphene and Aspirin 1137
Propoxyphene Napsylate *see* Propoxyphene 1135
Propoxyphene Napsylate and Acetaminophen *see* Propoxyphene and Acetaminophen 1136
Propoxyphene Napsylate and Aspirin *see* Propoxyphene and Aspirin 1137
Propranolol 1139
Propranolol and Hydrochlorothiazide 1142
Propranolol Hydrochloride *see* Propranolol 1139
Propranolol Intensol™ *see* Propranolol 1139
Propulsid® *see* Cisapride 332
Propylene Glycol Diacetate, Acetic Acid, and Hydrocortisone *see* Acetic Acid, Propylene Glycol Diacetate, and Hydrocortisone 38
Propylene Glycol Diacetate, Hydrocortisone, and Acetic Acid *see* Acetic Acid, Propylene Glycol Diacetate, and Hydrocortisone 38

Propylhexedrine . . . 1142
2-Propylpentanoic Acid *see* Valproic Acid and Derivatives . . . 1371
Propylthiouracil . . . 1142
Propyl-Thyracil® *see* Propylthiouracil . . . 1142
2-Propylvaleric Acid *see* Valproic Acid and Derivatives . . . 1371
Proscar® *see* Finasteride . . . 572
ProSom® *see* Estazolam . . . 521
Prostacyclin *see* Epoprostenol . . . 505
Prostaglandin E_1 *see* Alprostadil . . . 63
Prostaglandin E_2 *see* Dinoprostone . . . 450
Prostin E_2® *see* Dinoprostone . . . 450
Prostin® VR *see* Alprostadil . . . 63
Prostin VR Pediatric® *see* Alprostadil . . . 63
Protamine Sulfate . . . 1144
Protein C (Activated), Human, Recombinant *see* Drotrecogin Alfa . . . 483
Prothrombin Complex Concentrate *see* Factor IX Complex (Human) . . . 553
Protirelin . . . 1144
Protonix® *see* Pantoprazole . . . 1031
Protopic® *see* Tacrolimus . . . 1261
Protriptyline . . . 1145
Protriptyline Hydrochloride *see* Protriptyline . . . 1145
Protropin® *see* Human Growth Hormone . . . 671
Protropine® *see* Human Growth Hormone . . . 671
Proventil® *see* Albuterol . . . 48
Proventil® HFA *see* Albuterol . . . 48
Proventil® Repetabs® *see* Albuterol . . . 48
Provera® *see* MedroxyPROGESTERone . . . 849
Provigil® *see* Modafinil . . . 924
Proviodine *see* Povidone-Iodine . . . 1104
Provisc® *see* Sodium Hyaluronate . . . 1230
Proxigel® Oral [OTC] *see* Carbamide Peroxide . . . 244
Proxymetacaine *see* Proparacaine . . . 1132
Prozac® *see* Fluoxetine . . . 589
Prozac® Weekly™ *see* Fluoxetine . . . 589
Prozoladex *see* Goserelin . . . 647
PRP-D *see* *Haemophilus* b Conjugate Vaccine . . . 656
Prudoxin™ *see* Doxepin . . . 471
Prymaccone *see* Primaquine . . . 1117
Pseudoephedrine . . . 1146
Pseudoephedrine, Acetaminophen, and Chlorpheniramine *see* Acetaminophen, Chlorpheniramine, and Pseudoephedrine . . . 35
Pseudoephedrine, Acetaminophen, and Dextromethorphan *see* Acetaminophen, Dextromethorphan, and Pseudoephedrine . . . 35
Pseudoephedrine and Acetaminophen *see* Acetaminophen and Pseudoephedrine . . . 31
Pseudoephedrine and Acrivastine *see* Acrivastine and Pseudoephedrine . . . 41
Pseudoephedrine and Azatadine *see* Azatadine and Pseudoephedrine . . . 150
Pseudoephedrine and Brompheniramine *see* Brompheniramine and Pseudoephedrine . . . 201
Pseudoephedrine and Carbinoxamine *see* Carbinoxamine and Pseudoephedrine . . . 247
Pseudoephedrine and Chlorpheniramine *see* Chlorpheniramine and Pseudoephedrine . . . 308
Pseudoephedrine and Dexbrompheniramine *see* Dexbrompheniramine and Pseudoephedrine . . . 415
Pseudoephedrine and Dextromethorphan . . . 1147
Pseudoephedrine and Diphenhydramine *see* Diphenhydramine and Pseudoephedrine . . . 453
Pseudoephedrine and Fexofenadine *see* Fexofenadine and Pseudoephedrine . . . 570
Pseudoephedrine and Guaifenesin *see* Guaifenesin and Pseudoephedrine . . . 652
Pseudoephedrine and Ibuprofen . . . 1148
Pseudoephedrine and Loratadine *see* Loratadine and Pseudoephedrine . . . 823
Pseudoephedrine and Triprolidine *see* Triprolidine and Pseudoephedrine . . . 1356
Pseudoephedrine, Carbinoxamine, and Dextromethorphan *see* Carbinoxamine, Pseudoephedrine, and Dextromethorphan . . . 247
Pseudoephedrine, Chlorpheniramine, and Acetaminophen *see* Acetaminophen, Chlorpheniramine, and Pseudoephedrine . . . 35
Pseudoephedrine, Dextromethorphan, and Acetaminophen *see* Acetaminophen, Dextromethorphan, and Pseudoephedrine . . . 35
Pseudoephedrine, Dextromethorphan, and Carbinoxamine *see* Carbinoxamine, Pseudoephedrine, and Dextromethorphan . . . 247
Pseudoephedrine, Dextromethorphan, and Guaifenesin *see* Guaifenesin, Pseudoephedrine, and Dextromethorphan . . . 653
Pseudoephedrine, Guaifenesin, and Codeine *see* Guaifenesin, Pseudoephedrine, and Codeine . . . 653
Pseudoephedrine Hydrochloride *see* Pseudoephedrine . . . 1146
Pseudoephedrine Hydrochloride and Cetirizine Hydrochloride *see* Cetirizine and Pseudoephedrine . . . 290
Pseudoephedrine, Hydrocodone, and Guaifenesin *see* Hydrocodone, Pseudoephedrine, and Guaifenesin . . . 687
Pseudoephedrine Sulfate *see* Pseudoephedrine . . . 1146
Pseudoephedrine, Triprolidine, and Codeine Pseudoephedrine, Codeine, and Triprolidine *see* Triprolidine, Pseudoephedrine, and Codeine . . . 1357
Pseudofrin *see* Pseudoephedrine . . . 1146
Pseudo-Gest Plus® [OTC] *see* Chlorpheniramine and Pseudoephedrine . . . 308
Pseudo GG TR *see* Guaifenesin and Pseudoephedrine . . . 652
Pseudomonic Acid A *see* Mupirocin . . . 937
Pseudovent™, Pseudovent™-Ped *see* Guaifenesin and Pseudoephedrine . . . 652
P & S™ Liquid Phenol *see* Phenol . . . 1068
Psorcon® *see* Diflorasone . . . 438
Psorcon® e™ *see* Diflorasone . . . 438
psoriGel® [OTC] *see* Coal Tar . . . 359
P & S Plus® [OTC] *see* Coal Tar and Salicylic Acid . . . 359
Psyllium . . . 1149
Psyllium Hydrophilic Mucilloid *see* Psyllium . . . 1149

P.T.E.-4® *see* Trace Metals 1328
P.T.E.-5® *see* Trace Metals 1328
Pteroylglutamic Acid *see* Folic Acid 606
PTU *see* Propylthiouracil 1142
Pulmicort® *see* Budesonide 202
Pulmicort Respules™ *see* Budesonide 202
Pulmicort Turbuhaler® *see* Budesonide 202
Pulmophylline *see* Theophylline 1291
Pulmozyme® *see* Dornase Alfa 467
Pulsol® *see* Enalapril 492
Puralube® Tears [OTC] *see* Artificial Tears 128
Puregon™ *see* Follitropins 607
Purge® [OTC] *see* Castor Oil 259
Purinethol® *see* Mercaptopurine 866
Purple Coneflower *see* *Echinacea* 1429
PVF® K *see* Penicillin V Potassium 1051
Pyrantel Pamoate 1150
Pyrazinamide 1150
Pyrazinamide, Rifampin, and Isoniazid *see* Rifampin, Isoniazid, and Pyrazinamide 1182
Pyrazinoic Acid Amide *see* Pyrazinamide 1150
Pyrethrins and Piperonyl Butoxide 1151
Pyridium® *see* Phenazopyridine 1064
Pyridoxine 1152
Pyridoxine, Folic Acid, and Cyanocobalamin *see* Folic Acid, Cyanocobalamin, and Pyridoxine 607
Pyridoxine Hydrochloride *see* Pyridoxine 1152
Pyrimethamine 1152
Pyrimethamine and Sulfadoxine *see* Sulfadoxine and Pyrimethamine 1252
Pyrinyl Plus® [OTC] *see* Pyrethrins and Piperonyl Butoxide 1151
Pyrithione Zinc 1154
Quadrax® *see* Ibuprofen 703
Quaternium-18 Bentonite *see* Bentoquatam 168
Quazepam 1154
Quemicetina® *see* Chloramphenicol 297
Questran® *see* Cholestyramine Resin 318
Questran® Light *see* Cholestyramine Resin 318
Questran® Light Sugar Free *see* Cholestyramine Resin 318
Quetiapine 1155
Quetiapine Fumarate *see* Quetiapine 1155
Quibron® *see* Theophylline and Guaifenesin 1293
Quibron®-T *see* Theophylline 1291
Quibron®-T/SR *see* Theophylline 1291
Quilagen *see* Gentamicin 634
Quimocyclar *see* Tetracycline 1286
Quinaglute® Dura-Tabs® *see* Quinidine 1158
Quinalbarbitone Sodium *see* Secobarbital 1212
Quinapril 1156
Quinapril and Hydrochlorothiazide 1158
Quinapril Hydrochloride *see* Quinapril 1156
Quinate® *see* Quinidine 1158
Quinidex® Extentabs® *see* Quinidine 1158
Quinidine 1158
Quinidine Gluconate *see* Quinidine 1158
Quinidine Polygalacturonate *see* Quinidine 1158
Quinidine Sulfate *see* Quinidine 1158
Quini Durules® *see* Quinidine 1158
Quinine 1160
Quinine-Odan™ *see* Quinine 1160
Quinine Sulfate *see* Quinine 1160
Quinoflox® *see* Ciprofloxacin 328
Quinol *see* Hydroquinone 693
Quintasa® *see* Mesalamine 869
Quinupristin and Dalfopristin 1161
Quixin™ *see* Levofloxacin 794
QVAR™ *see* Beclomethasone 163
Rabeprazole 1162
Rabies Immune Globulin (Human) 1164
Rabies Virus Vaccine 1164
Racovel *see* Levodopa and Carbidopa 793
Radiological/Contrast Media (Nonionic) 1165
Radix *see* Valerian 1449
Raductil® *see* Sibutramine 1219
rAHF *see* Antihemophilic Factor (Recombinant) 115
R-albuterol *see* Levalbuterol 786
Raloxifene 1165
Raloxifene Hydrochloride *see* Raloxifene 1165
Ramace® *see* Ramipril 1166
Ramipril 1166
Randikan *see* Kanamycin 759
Ranifur® *see* Ranitidine 1168
Ranisen® *see* Ranitidine 1168
Ranitidine 1168
Ranitidine Hydrochloride *see* Ranitidine 1168
Rapamune® *see* Sirolimus 1225
Rapifen® *see* Alfentanil 55
Rasburicase 1169
Rastinon® *see* TOLBUTamide 1319
ratio-Acyclovir *see* Acyclovir 42
ratio-AmoxiClav *see* Amoxicillin and Clavulanate Potassium 95
ratio-Brimonidine *see* Brimonidine 197

ratio-Colchicine *see* Colchicine . . . 363
ratio-Diltiazem CD *see* Diltiazem . . . 447
ratio-Famotidine *see* Famotidine . . . 556
ratio-Glyburide *see* GlyBURIDE . . . 642
ratio-Inspra-Sal *see* Albuterol . . . 48
ratio-Lovastatin *see* Lovastatin . . . 828
ratio-Methotrexate *see* Methotrexate . . . 884
ratio-Morphine SR *see* Morphine Sulfate . . . 931
ratio-Pentoxifylline *see* Pentoxifylline . . . 1058
ratio-Salbutamol *see* Albuterol . . . 48
ratio-Sertraline *see* Sertraline . . . 1216
ratio-Theo-Bronc *see* Theophylline . . . 1291
Raudil® *see* Ranitidine . . . 1168
Rauwolfia Serpentina . . . 1170
Raxedin *see* Loperamide . . . 819
R & C™ II *see* Pyrethrins and Piperonyl Butoxide . . . 1151
R & C™ Shampoo/Conditioner *see* Pyrethrins and Piperonyl Butoxide . . . 1151
Reactine™ *see* Cetirizine . . . 289
Rea-Lo® [OTC] *see* Urea . . . 1365
ReAzo [OTC] *see* Phenazopyridine . . . 1064
Rebetol® *see* Ribavirin . . . 1176
Rebetron® *see* Interferon Alfa-2b and Ribavirin . . . 730
Rebif® *see* Interferon Beta-1a . . . 732
Recofol® *see* Propofol . . . 1133
Recombinant Hirudin *see* Lepirudin . . . 781
Recombinant Human Deoxyribonuclease *see* Dornase Alfa . . . 467
Recombinant Human Follicle Stimulating Hormone *see* Follitropins . . . 607
Recombinant Human Interleukin-11 *see* Oprelvekin . . . 1003
Recombinant Human Parathyroid Hormone (1-34) *see* Teriparatide . . . 1280
Recombinant Human Platelet-Derived Growth Factor B *see* Becaplermin . . . 162
Recombinant Interleukin-11 *see* Oprelvekin . . . 1003
Recombinant Plasminogen Activator *see* Reteplase . . . 1174
Recombinate™ *see* Antihemophilic Factor (Recombinant) . . . 115
Recombivax HB® *see* Hepatitis B Vaccine . . . 666
Redoxon® *see* Ascorbic Acid . . . 128
Redoxon® Forte *see* Ascorbic Acid . . . 128
Reductil® *see* Sibutramine . . . 1219
Redutemp® [OTC] *see* Acetaminophen . . . 27
Red Valerian *see* Valerian . . . 1449
Red Yeast Rice . . . 1446
Reese's® Pinworm Medicine [OTC] *see* Pyrantel Pamoate . . . 1150
ReFacto® *see* Antihemophilic Factor (Recombinant) . . . 115
Refludan® *see* Lepirudin . . . 781
Refresh® [OTC] *see* Artificial Tears . . . 128
Refresh® Plus [OTC] *see* Artificial Tears . . . 128
Refresh Plus™ *see* Carboxymethylcellulose . . . 251
Refresh® Tears [OTC] *see* Artificial Tears . . . 128
Refresh Tears™ *see* Carboxymethylcellulose . . . 251
Regaine® *see* Minoxidil . . . 917
Regitine® *see* Phentolamine . . . 1070
Reglan® *see* Metoclopramide . . . 898
Regranex® *see* Becaplermin . . . 162
Regulact® *see* Lactulose . . . 772
Regular Iletin® II *see* Insulin Preparations . . . 723
Regulex® *see* Docusate . . . 463
Reguloid® [OTC] *see* Psyllium . . . 1149
Rejuva-A® *see* Tretinoin (Topical) . . . 1340
Relafen™ *see* Nabumetone . . . 941
Relefact® TRH *see* Protirelin . . . 1144
Relenza® *see* Zanamivir . . . 1405
Relief® [OTC] *see* Phenylephrine . . . 1071
Relifex® *see* Nabumetone . . . 941
Relpax® *see* Eletriptan . . . 490
Remeron® *see* Mirtazapine . . . 919
Remeron SolTab® *see* Mirtazapine . . . 919
Remicade® *see* Infliximab . . . 721
Remifentanil . . . 1171
Remodulin™ *see* Treprostinil . . . 1337
Renacidin® *see* Citric Acid Bladder Mixture . . . 335
Renagel® *see* Sevelamer . . . 1218
Renedil® *see* Felodipine . . . 560
Renese® *see* Polythiazide . . . 1097
Renitec® *see* Enalapril . . . 492
Renova® *see* Tretinoin (Topical) . . . 1340
Rentamine® [OTC] *see* Chlorpheniramine, Ephedrine, Phenylephrine, and Carbetapentane . . . 309
Reopro™ *see* Abciximab . . . 23
Repaglinide . . . 1172
Repan® *see* Butalbital, Acetaminophen, and Caffeine . . . 214
Repronex® *see* Menotropins . . . 857
ReQuip™ *see* Ropinirole . . . 1196
Rescriptor® *see* Delavirdine . . . 405
Reserpine . . . 1173
Reserpine and Chlorothiazide *see* Chlorothiazide and Reserpine . . . 306
Reserpine, Hydralazine, and Hydrochlorothiazide *see* Hydralazine, Hydrochlorothiazide, and Reserpine . . . 675
Respa-1st® *see* Guaifenesin and Pseudoephedrine . . . 652
Respa® DM *see* Guaifenesin and Dextromethorphan . . . 651
Respa-GF® *see* Guaifenesin . . . 650
Respaire®-60 SR *see* Guaifenesin and Pseudoephedrine . . . 652

Respaire®-120 SR *see* Guaifenesin and Pseudoephedrine . . . 652
Respiratory Diseases . . . 1476
Respiratory Synctial Virus Immune Globulin *see* Immunizations (Vaccines) . . . 1612
Restasis™ *see* CycloSPORINE . . . 383
Restoril® *see* Temazepam . . . 1271
Retavase® *see* Reteplase . . . 1174
Reteplase . . . 1174
Retin-A® *see* Tretinoin (Topical) . . . 1340
Retin-A® Micro *see* Tretinoin (Topical) . . . 1340
Retinoic Acid *see* Tretinoin (Topical) . . . 1340
Retinova® *see* Tretinoin (Topical) . . . 1340
Retrovir® *see* Zidovudine . . . 1406
Retrovir AZT® *see* Zidovudine . . . 1406
Revapol® *see* Mebendazole . . . 846
Revex® *see* Nalmefene . . . 948
Rēv-Eyes™ *see* Dapiprazole . . . 399
ReVia® *see* Naltrexone . . . 950
Revitalose C-1000® *see* Ascorbic Acid . . . 128
rFSH-alpha *see* Follitropins . . . 607
rFSH-beta *see* Follitropins . . . 607
rFVIIa *see* Factor VIIa (Recombinant) . . . 554
R-Gel® [OTC] *see* Capsaicin . . . 238
R-Gene® *see* Arginine . . . 121
rGM-CSF *see* Sargramostim . . . 1209
r-hCG *see* Chorionic Gonadotropin (Recombinant) . . . 321
Rheomacrodex® *see* Dextran . . . 419
Rheumatoid Arthritis, Osteoarthritis, and Osteoporosis . . . 1488
Rheumatrex® *see* Methotrexate . . . 884
rhFSH-alpha *see* Follitropins . . . 607
rhFSH-beta *see* Follitropins . . . 607
rhIL-11 *see* Oprelvekin . . . 1003
Rhinalar® *see* Flunisolide . . . 582
Rhinatate® *see* Chlorpheniramine, Pyrilamine, and Phenylephrine . . . 312
Rhinocort® [DSC] *see* Budesonide . . . 202
Rhinocort® Aqua™ *see* Budesonide . . . 202
Rhinocort® Turbuhaler® *see* Budesonide . . . 202
Rhinosyn® [OTC] *see* Chlorpheniramine and Pseudoephedrine . . . 308
Rhinosyn-PD® [OTC] *see* Chlorpheniramine and Pseudoephedrine . . . 308
Rho-Clonazepam *see* Clonazepam . . . 350
Rhodacine® *see* Indomethacin . . . 719
Rh_o(D) Immune Globulin . . . 1175
Rhodis™ *see* Ketoprofen . . . 763
Rhodis-EC™ *see* Ketoprofen . . . 763
Rhodis SR™ *see* Ketoprofen . . . 763
RhoGAM® *see* Rh_o(D) Immune Globulin . . . 1175
Rho®-Loperamine *see* Loperamide . . . 819
Rho®-Metformin *see* Metformin . . . 874
Rho-Nitro *see* Nitroglycerin . . . 981
Rho®-Sotalol *see* Sotalol . . . 1235
Rhotral *see* Acebutolol . . . 25
Rhotrimine® *see* Trimipramine . . . 1354
Rhovane® *see* Zopiclone . . . 1415
Rhoxal-amiodarone *see* Amiodarone . . . 80
Rhoxal-atenolol *see* Atenolol . . . 137
Rhoxal-clozapine *see* Clozapine . . . 358
Rhoxal-cyclosporine *see* CycloSPORINE . . . 383
Rhoxal-diltiazem CD *see* Diltiazem . . . 447
Rhoxal-diltiazem SR *see* Diltiazem . . . 447
Rhoxal-famotidine *see* Famotidine . . . 556
Rhoxal-fluoxetine *see* Fluoxetine . . . 589
Rhoxal-metformin FC *see* Metformin . . . 874
Rhoxal-minocycline *see* Minocycline . . . 915
Rhoxal-nabumetone *see* Nabumetone . . . 941
Rhoxal-orphendrine *see* Orphenadrine . . . 1005
Rhoxal-oxaprozin *see* Oxaprozin . . . 1010
Rhoxal-ranitidine *see* Ranitidine . . . 1168
Rhoxal-salbutamol *see* Albuterol . . . 48
Rhoxal-sertraline *see* Sertraline . . . 1216
Rhoxal-ticlopidine *see* Ticlopidine . . . 1307
Rhoxal-valproic *see* Valproic Acid and Derivatives . . . 1371
rhPTH(1-34) *see* Teriparatide . . . 1280
rHuEPO-α *see* Epoetin Alfa . . . 503
Ribavirin . . . 1176
Ribavirin and Interferon Alfa-2b Combination Pack *see* Interferon Alfa-2b and Ribavirin . . . 730
Riboflavin . . . 1178
Ridaura® *see* Auranofin . . . 147
Ridene® *see* NiCARdipine . . . 969
RID® Maximum Strength [OTC] *see* Pyrethrins and Piperonyl Butoxide . . . 1151
RID® Mousse *see* Pyrethrins and Piperonyl Butoxide . . . 1151
Rid® Spray [OTC] *see* Permethrin . . . 1062
Rifabutin . . . 1179
Rifadin® *see* Rifampin . . . 1180
Rifamate® *see* Rifampin and Isoniazid . . . 1181
Rifampicin *see* Rifampin . . . 1180
Rifampin . . . 1180
Rifampin and Isoniazid . . . 1181
Rifampin, Isoniazid, and Pyrazinamide . . . 1182
Rifapentine . . . 1182
Rifater™ *see* Rifampin, Isoniazid, and Pyrazinamide . . . 1182
rIFN-A *see* Interferon Alfa-2a . . . 726

rIFN beta-1a *see* Interferon Beta-1a 732
rIFN beta-1b *see* Interferon Beta-1b 733
RIG *see* Rabies Immune Globulin (Human) 1164
rIL-11 *see* Oprelvekin 1003
Rilutek® *see* Riluzole 1184
Riluzole 1184
Rimactan® *see* Rifampin 1180
Rimactane® *see* Rifampin 1180
Rimantadine 1185
Rimantadine Hydrochloride *see* Rimantadine 1185
Rimexolone 1185
Rimsalin® *see* Lincomycin 808
Riopan Plus® [OTC] *see* Magaldrate and Simethicone 833
Riopan Plus® Double Strength [OTC] *see* Magaldrate and Simethicone 833
Riphenidate *see* Methylphenidate 893
Risedronate 1186
Risedronate Sodium *see* Risedronate 1186
Risperdal® *see* Risperidone 1187
Risperdal Consta™ [Investigational] *see* Risperidone 1187
Risperidone 1187
Ritalin® *see* Methylphenidate 893
Ritalin® LA *see* Methylphenidate 893
Ritalin® SR *see* Methylphenidate 893
Ritmolol® *see* Metoprolol 901
Ritonavir 1188
Rituxan® *see* Rituximab 1190
Rituximab 1190
Riva-Diclofenac *see* Diclofenac 429
Riva-Diclofenac-K *see* Diclofenac 429
Riva-Famotidine *see* Famotidine 556
Riva-Loperamine *see* Loperamide 819
Riva-Lorazepam *see* Lorazepam 824
Riva-Naproxen *see* Naproxen 953
Rivanase AQ *see* Beclomethasone 163
Riva-Norfloxacin *see* Norfloxacin 987
Rivastigmine 1192
Riva-Zide *see* Hydrochlorothiazide and Triamterene 677
Rivotril® *see* Clonazepam 350
Rizatriptan 1193
rLFN-α2 *see* Interferon Alfa-2b 727
RMS® *see* Morphine Sulfate 931
RO5-420 *see* Flunitrazepam 583
Roaccutan® *see* Isotretinoin 752
Robafen® AC *see* Guaifenesin and Codeine 650
Robaxin® *see* Methocarbamol 881
Robidrine® *see* Pseudoephedrine 1146
Robinul® *see* Glycopyrrolate 645
Robinul® Forte *see* Glycopyrrolate 645
Robitussin® *see* Guaifenesin 650
Robitussin® A-C [DSC] *see* Guaifenesin and Codeine 650
Robitussin® CF [OTC] *see* Guaifenesin, Pseudoephedrine, and Dextromethorphan 653
Robitussin® Childrens Cough & Cold *see* Pseudoephedrine and Dextromethorphan 1147
Robitussin® Cold and Congestion [OTC] *see* Guaifenesin, Pseudoephedrine, and Dextromethorphan 653
Robitussin® Cough and Cold Infant [OTC] *see* Guaifenesin, Pseudoephedrine, and Dextromethorphan 653
Robitussin® Cough & Cold® *see* Guaifenesin, Pseudoephedrine, and Dextromethorphan 653
Robitussin®-DAC [DSC] *see* Guaifenesin, Pseudoephedrine, and Codeine 653
Robitussin® DM *see* Guaifenesin and Dextromethorphan 651
Robitussin® Maximum Strength Cough [OTC] *see* Dextromethorphan 423
Robitussin® Maximum Strength Cough & Cold [OTC] *see* Pseudoephedrine and Dextromethorphan 1147
Robitussin-PE® [OTC] *see* Guaifenesin and Pseudoephedrine 652
Robitussin® Pediatric Cough [OTC] *see* Dextromethorphan 423
Robitussin® Pediatric Cough & Cold [OTC] *see* Pseudoephedrine and Dextromethorphan 1147
Robitussin® Severe Congestion [OTC] *see* Guaifenesin and Pseudoephedrine 652
Robitussin® Sugar Free Cough [OTC] *see* Guaifenesin and Dextromethorphan 651
Rocaltrol® *see* Calcitriol 223
Rocephin® *see* Ceftriaxone 278
Rofact™ *see* Rifampin 1180
Rofecoxib 1194
Roferon-A® *see* Interferon Alfa-2a 726
Rogaine® *see* Minoxidil 917
Rogaine® Extra Strength for Men [OTC] *see* Minoxidil 917
Rogaine® for Men [OTC] *see* Minoxidil 917
Rogaine® for Women [OTC] *see* Minoxidil 917
Rogal® *see* Piroxicam 1090
Rogitine® *see* Phentolamine 1070
Rohypnol *see* Flunitrazepam 583
Rökan *see* Ginkgo Biloba 1434
Rolaids® Calcium Rich [OTC] *see* Calcium Supplements 229
Rolatuss® Plain *see* Chlorpheniramine and Phenylephrine 308
Romazicon™ *see* Flumazenil 581
Romilar® *see* Dextromethorphan 423
Romilar® AC *see* Guaifenesin and Codeine 650
Romir® *see* Captopril 238
Romycin® *see* Erythromycin 512
Rondec®-DM Drops *see* Carbinoxamine, Pseudoephedrine, and Dextromethorphan 247
Rondec® Drops *see* Carbinoxamine and Pseudoephedrine 247

Rondec® Syrup *see* Brompheniramine and Pseudoephedrine . . . 201
Rondec® Tablets *see* Carbinoxamine and Pseudoephedrine . . . 247
Rondec-TR® *see* Carbinoxamine and Pseudoephedrine . . . 247
Ropinirole . . . 1196
Ropinirole Hydrochloride *see* Ropinirole . . . 1196
Ropivacaine . . . 1198
Ropivacaine Hydrochloride *see* Ropivacaine . . . 1198
Rosiglitazone . . . 1199
Rosiglitazone and Metformin . . . 1200
Rosiglitazone Maleate and Metformin Hydrochloride *see* Rosiglitazone and Metformin . . . 1200
Rosin Rose *see* St John's Wort . . . 1448
Rosuvastatin . . . 1201
Rosuvastatin Calcium *see* Rosuvastatin . . . 1201
Rovamycine® *see* Spiramycin . . . 1239
Rowasa® *see* Mesalamine . . . 869
Roxanol® *see* Morphine Sulfate . . . 931
Roxanol 100® *see* Morphine Sulfate . . . 931
Roxanol®-T *see* Morphine Sulfate . . . 931
Roxicet® *see* Oxycodone and Acetaminophen . . . 1018
Roxicet® 5/500 *see* Oxycodone and Acetaminophen . . . 1018
Roxicodone™ *see* Oxycodone . . . 1017
Roxicodone™ Intensol™ *see* Oxycodone . . . 1017
RP54274 *see* Riluzole . . . 1184
RP59500 *see* Quinupristin and Dalfopristin . . . 1161
r-PA *see* Reteplase . . . 1174
rPDGF-BB *see* Becaplermin . . . 162
R-Tannamine® *see* Chlorpheniramine, Pyrilamine, and Phenylephrine . . . 312
R-Tannate® *see* Chlorpheniramine, Pyrilamine, and Phenylephrine . . . 312
RTCA *see* Ribavirin . . . 1176
RU-486 *see* Mifepristone . . . 912
RU-38486 *see* Mifepristone . . . 912
Rubella, Measles and Mumps Vaccines, Combined *see* Measles, Mumps, and Rubella Vaccines (Combined) . . . 844
Rubella Virus Vaccine (Live) . . . 1202
Rubeola Vaccine *see* Measles Virus Vaccine (Live) . . . 845
Rubex® *see* DOXOrubicin . . . 473
Rubidomycin Hydrochloride *see* DAUNOrubicin Hydrochloride . . . 402
Rubilem® *see* DAUNOrubicin Hydrochloride . . . 402
Rum-K® *see* Potassium Supplements . . . 1102
Rustic Treacle *see* Garlic . . . 1433
Ru-Tuss® *see* Chlorpheniramine and Phenylephrine . . . 308
Ryna® [OTC] *see* Chlorpheniramine and Pseudoephedrine . . . 308
Ryna-C® *see* Chlorpheniramine, Pseudoephedrine, and Codeine . . . 311
Rynatan® Pediatric Suspension *see* Chlorpheniramine, Pyrilamine, and Phenylephrine . . . 312
Rynatan® Tablet *see* Azatadine and Pseudoephedrine . . . 150
Rynatuss® [OTC] *see* Chlorpheniramine, Ephedrine, Phenylephrine, and Carbetapentane . . . 309
Rynatuss® Pediatric Suspension [OTC] *see* Chlorpheniramine, Ephedrine, Phenylephrine, and Carbetapentane . . . 309
Rythmodan® *see* Disopyramide . . . 458
Rythmodan®-LA *see* Disopyramide . . . 458
Rythmol® *see* Propafenone . . . 1130
S-2® *see* Epinephrine (Racemic) . . . 500
Sabal serrulata see Saw Palmetto . . . 1447
Sabasilis serrulatae see Saw Palmetto . . . 1447
SAB-Gentamicin *see* Gentamicin . . . 634
Sabril® *see* Vigabatrin . . . 1385
Sacrosidase . . . 1203
S-adenosylmethionine *see* SAMe . . . 1446
Safe Tussin® 30 [OTC] *see* Guaifenesin and Dextromethorphan . . . 651
Safe Writing Practices . . . 17
Saizen® *see* Human Growth Hormone . . . 671
SalAc® [OTC] *see* Salicylic Acid . . . 1204
Sal-Acid® [OTC] *see* Salicylic Acid . . . 1204
Salactic® [OTC] *see* Salicylic Acid . . . 1204
Salagen® *see* Pilocarpine . . . 1080
Salagen® *see* Pilocarpine (Dental) . . . 1081
Salazopyrin® *see* Sulfasalazine . . . 1254
Salazopyrin En-Tabs® *see* Sulfasalazine . . . 1254
Salbu-2 *see* Albuterol . . . 48
Salbu-4 *see* Albuterol . . . 48
Salbulin *see* Albuterol . . . 48
Salbulin Autohaler® *see* Albuterol . . . 48
Salbutalan *see* Albuterol . . . 48
Salbutamol *see* Albuterol . . . 48
Salflex® *see* Salsalate . . . 1206
Salicylazosulfapyridine *see* Sulfasalazine . . . 1254
Salicylic Acid . . . 1204
Salicylic Acid and Coal Tar *see* Coal Tar and Salicylic Acid . . . 359
Salicylsalicylic Acid *see* Salsalate . . . 1206
SalineX® [OTC] *see* Sodium Chloride . . . 1229
Salivart® [OTC] *see* Saliva Substitute . . . 1205
Saliva Substitute . . . 1205
Saliva Substitute™ [OTC] *see* Saliva Substitute . . . 1205
Salix® [OTC] *see* Saliva Substitute . . . 1205
Salk Vaccine *see* Poliovirus Vaccine (Inactivated) . . . 1093
Salmeterol . . . 1205
Salmeterol and Fluticasone *see* Fluticasone and Salmeterol . . . 601
Salmeterol Xinafoate *see* Salmeterol . . . 1205
Salmocide® *see* Furazolidone . . . 622

Salofalk *see* Aminosalicylic Acid . . . 79
Salofalk® *see* Mesalamine . . . 869
Sal-Plant® [OTC] *see* Salicylic Acid . . . 1204
Salsalate . . . 1206
Salt *see* Sodium Chloride . . . 1229
Sal-Tropine™ *see* Atropine Sulfate Dental Tablets . . . 145
SAMe . . . 1446
Sandimmune® *see* CycloSPORINE . . . 383
Sandimmune® I.V. *see* CycloSPORINE . . . 383
Sandimmun Neoral® *see* CycloSPORINE . . . 383
Sandoglobulina® *see* Immune Globulin (Intravenous) . . . 714
Sandostatin® *see* Octreotide . . . 993
Sandostatina® *see* Octreotide . . . 993
Sandostatin LAR® *see* Octreotide . . . 993
Sani-Supp® [OTC] *see* Glycerin . . . 644
Sanorex® *see* Mazindol . . . 843
Sansert® [DSC] *see* Methysergide . . . 897
Santyl® *see* Collagenase . . . 367
Saquinavir . . . 1207
Saquinavir Mesylate *see* Saquinavir . . . 1207
Sarafem™ *see* Fluoxetine . . . 589
Sargramostim . . . 1209
Sarna® HC *see* Hydrocortisone . . . 688
Sarnol®-HC [OTC] *see* Hydrocortisone . . . 688
Sassafras albidum see Sassafras Oil . . . 1446
Sassafras Oil . . . 1446
Sassafras radix see Sassafras Oil . . . 1446
Sassafras varifolium see Sassafras Oil . . . 1446
Sassafrax see Sassafras Oil . . . 1446
Saw Palmetto . . . 1447
Scabisan® *see* Lindane . . . 809
Scabisan Shampoo *see* Lindane . . . 809
Scheinpharm B12 *see* Cyanocobalamin . . . 377
Schisandra . . . 1447
Schizandra chinensis see Schisandra . . . 1447
S-Citalopram *see* Escitalopram . . . 516
Scleromate™ *see* Morrhuate Sodium . . . 934
Scopace™ *see* Scopolamine . . . 1210
Scopolamine . . . 1210
Scopolamine and Phenylephrine *see* Phenylephrine and Scopolamine . . . 1072
Scopolamine Hydrobromide *see* Scopolamine . . . 1210
Scopolamine, Hyoscyamine, Atropine, and Phenobarbital *see* Hyoscyamine, Atropine, Scopolamine, and Phenobarbital . . . 700
Scot-Tussin DM® Cough Chasers [OTC] *see* Dextromethorphan . . . 423
Scot-Tussin® Sugar Free Expectorant [OTC] *see* Guaifenesin . . . 650
Scury Root *see Echinacea* . . . 1429
SDZ ENA 713 *see* Rivastigmine . . . 1192
SeaMist® [OTC] *see* Sodium Chloride . . . 1229
Seba-Gel™ *see* Benzoyl Peroxide . . . 171
Sebcur® *see* Salicylic Acid . . . 1204
Sebcur/T® *see* Coal Tar and Salicylic Acid . . . 359
Secobarbital . . . 1212
Secobarbital and Amobarbital *see* Amobarbital and Secobarbital . . . 91
Secobarbital Sodium *see* Secobarbital . . . 1212
Seconal® *see* Secobarbital . . . 1212
Secotex® *see* Tamsulosin . . . 1266
SecreFlo™ *see* Secretin . . . 1213
Secretin . . . 1213
Sectral® *see* Acebutolol . . . 25
Sedalito® *see* Acetaminophen . . . 27
Sefulken® *see* Diazoxide . . . 427
Selax® *see* Docusate . . . 463
Selectadril® *see* Metoprolol . . . 901
Selecto® *see* Pancreatin . . . 1030
Selectofen® *see* Diclofenac . . . 429
Selectofur® *see* Furosemide . . . 622
Selegil® *see* Metronidazole . . . 902
Selegiline . . . 1213
Selegiline Hydrochloride *see* Selegiline . . . 1213
Selenium . . . 1214
Selenium *see* Trace Metals . . . 1328
Selenium Sulfide *see* Selenium . . . 1214
Selepen® *see* Selenium . . . 1214
Selepen® *see* Trace Metals . . . 1328
Seloken® *see* Metoprolol . . . 901
Selopres *see* Metoprolol . . . 901
Semicid® [OTC] *see* Nonoxynol 9 . . . 985
Semprex®-D *see* Acrivastine and Pseudoephedrine . . . 41
Senexon® [OTC] *see* Senna . . . 1215
Senna . . . 1215
Senna Alexandria *see* Senna . . . 1215
Senna-Gen® [OTC] *see* Senna . . . 1215
Sennatural™ [OTC] *see* Senna . . . 1215
Senokot® [OTC] *see* Senna . . . 1215
Senokot® Children's [OTC] *see* Senna . . . 1215
SenokotXTRA® [OTC] *see* Senna . . . 1215
Sensibit® *see* Loratadine . . . 822
Sensorcaine® *see* Bupivacaine . . . 205
Sensorcaine®-MPF *see* Bupivacaine . . . 205
Sensorcaine® With Epinephrine *see* Bupivacaine and Epinephrine . . . 207

Septocaine™ *see* Articaine Hydrochloride and Epinephrine (U.S.) . . . 125
Septra® *see* Sulfamethoxazole and Trimethoprim . . . 1253
Septra® DS *see* Sulfamethoxazole and Trimethoprim . . . 1253
Septra® Injection *see* Sulfamethoxazole and Trimethoprim . . . 1253
Septrin® *see* Trimethoprim . . . 1352
Serax® *see* Oxazepam . . . 1011
Serenoa repens *see* Saw Palmetto . . . 1447
Serentil® *see* Mesoridazine . . . 870
Serevent® *see* Salmeterol . . . 1205
Serevent® Diskus® *see* Salmeterol . . . 1205
Sermorelin Acetate . . . 1215
Serocryptin® *see* Bromocriptine . . . 199
Seromycin® Pulvules® *see* CycloSERINE . . . 383
Serophene® *see* ClomiPHENE . . . 348
Seropram® *see* Citalopram . . . 334
Seroquel® *see* Quetiapine . . . 1155
Serostim® *see* Human Growth Hormone . . . 671
Serozide® *see* Etoposide . . . 549
Serozide® *see* Etoposide Phosphate . . . 551
Sertraline . . . 1216
Sertraline Hydrochloride *see* Sertraline . . . 1216
Serutan® [OTC] *see* Psyllium . . . 1149
Servamox® *see* Amoxicillin . . . 93
Servigenta® *see* Gentamicin . . . 634
Serviradine® *see* Ranitidine . . . 1168
Servitrim® *see* Trimethoprim . . . 1352
Servizol® *see* Metronidazole . . . 902
Serzone® *see* Nefazodone . . . 957
Serzone-5HT$_2$® *see* Nefazodone . . . 957
Sevelamer . . . 1218
Sevelamer Hydrochloride *see* Sevelamer . . . 1218
Sexually-Transmitted Diseases . . . 1502
Shark Cartilage . . . 1447
Shemol® *see* Timolol . . . 1309
Shur-Seal® [OTC] *see* Nonoxynol 9 . . . 985
Siberian Ginseng *see* Ginseng, Siberian . . . 1436
Sibutramine . . . 1219
Sibutramine Hydrochloride Monohydrate *see* Sibutramine . . . 1219
Sigafam® *see* Famotidine . . . 556
Siladryl® Allergy [OTC] *see* DiphenhydrAMINE . . . 451
Silafed® [OTC] *see* Triprolidine and Pseudoephedrine . . . 1356
Silapap® Children's [OTC] *see* Acetaminophen . . . 27
Silapap® Infants [OTC] *see* Acetaminophen . . . 27
Sildenafil . . . 1220
Silexin® [OTC] *see* Guaifenesin and Dextromethorphan . . . 651
Silfedrine Children's [OTC] *see* Pseudoephedrine . . . 1146
Silphen® [OTC] *see* DiphenhydrAMINE . . . 451
Silphen DM® [OTC] *see* Dextromethorphan . . . 423
Silvadene® *see* Silver Sulfadiazine . . . 1222
Silver Apricot *see* Ginkgo Biloba . . . 1434
Silver Nitrate . . . 1221
Silver Sulfadiazine . . . 1222
Silybum marianum *see* Milk Thistle . . . 1445
Simethicone . . . 1222
Simethicone, Aluminum Hydroxide, and Magnesium Hydroxide *see* Aluminum Hydroxide, Magnesium Hydroxide, and Simethicone . . . 69
Simethicone and Calcium Carbonate *see* Calcium Carbonate and Simethicone . . . 224
Simethicone and Magaldrate *see* Magaldrate and Simethicone . . . 833
Simply Cough™ [OTC] *see* Dextromethorphan . . . 423
Simply Saline™ [OTC] *see* Sodium Chloride . . . 1229
Simply Sleep® *see* DiphenhydrAMINE . . . 451
Simulect® *see* Basiliximab . . . 160
Simvastatin . . . 1223
Sinaplin® *see* Ampicillin . . . 103
Sincalide . . . 1225
Sinedol® *see* Acetaminophen . . . 27
Sinedol 500 *see* Acetaminophen . . . 27
Sinemet® *see* Levodopa and Carbidopa . . . 793
Sinemet® CR *see* Levodopa and Carbidopa . . . 793
Sinequan® *see* Doxepin . . . 471
Sinestron® *see* Lorazepam . . . 824
Singulair® *see* Montelukast . . . 929
Sinogan® *see* Methotrimeprazine . . . 887
Sinozzard® *see* Prazosin . . . 1108
Sinuberase® *see* *Lactobacillus acidophilus* and *Lactobacillus bulgaricus* . . . 772
Sinus-Relief® [OTC] *see* Acetaminophen and Pseudoephedrine . . . 31
Sinutab® Non Drowsy *see* Acetaminophen and Pseudoephedrine . . . 31
Sinutab® Sinus & Allergy *see* Acetaminophen, Chlorpheniramine, and Pseudoephedrine . . . 35
Sinutab® Sinus Allergy Maximum Strength [OTC] *see* Acetaminophen, Chlorpheniramine, and Pseudoephedrine . . . 35
Sinutab® Sinus Maximum Strength Without Drowsiness [OTC] *see* Acetaminophen and Pseudoephedrine . . . 31
Siquial® *see* Fluoxetine . . . 589
Sirdalud® *see* Tizanidine . . . 1314
Sirolimus . . . 1225
SK *see* Streptokinase . . . 1243
SK and F 104864 *see* Topotecan . . . 1325
Skelaxin® *see* Metaxalone . . . 874
Skelid® *see* Tiludronate . . . 1309
SKF 104864 *see* Topotecan . . . 1325

SKF 104864-A *see* Topotecan 1325
Skin Test Antigens (Multiple) 1227
Sleepinal® [OTC] *see* DiphenhydrAMINE 451
Slo-Bid® *see* Theophylline 1291
Slo-Niacin® [OTC] *see* Niacin 967
Slow FE® [OTC] *see* Iron Supplements 745
Slow-Mag® [OTC] *see* Magnesium Chloride 833
Slow-Mag® [OTC] *see* Magnesium Supplements 837
Slow-Trasicor® *see* Oxprenolol 1014
Smallpox Vaccine *see* Immunizations (Vaccines) 1612
Smelling Salts *see* Ammonia Spirit (Aromatic) 89
SMZ-TMP *see* Sulfamethoxazole and Trimethoprim 1253
Snakeroot *see* *Echinacea* 1429
Sodipental® *see* Thiopental 1297
Sodium 4-Hydroxybutyrate *see* Sodium Oxybate 1231
Sodium Acid Carbonate *see* Sodium Bicarbonate 1227
Sodium Benzoate and Caffeine *see* Caffeine and Sodium Benzoate 221
Sodium Bicarbonate 1227
Sodium Biphosphate, Methenamine, Methylene Blue, Phenyl Salicylate, and Hyoscyamine *see* Methenamine, Sodium Biphosphate, Phenyl Salicylate, Methylene Blue, and Hyoscyamine 880
Sodium Cellulose Phosphate *see* Cellulose Sodium Phosphate 284
Sodium Chloride 1229
Sodium Citrate and Citric Acid 1230
Sodium Citrate and Potassium Citrate Mixture *see* Citric Acid, Sodium Citrate, and Potassium Citrate 335
Sodium Citrate, Citric Acid, and Potassium Citrate *see* Citric Acid, Sodium Citrate, and Potassium Citrate 335
Sodium Edetate *see* Edetate Disodium 488
Sodium Etidronate *see* Etidronate Disodium 546
Sodium Ferric Gluconate *see* Ferric Gluconate 568
Sodium Fluoride *see* Fluoride 586
Sodium Hyaluronate 1230
Sodium Hyaluronate-Chrondroitin Sulfate *see* Chondroitin Sulfate and Sodium Hyaluronate 320
Sodium Hydrogen Carbonate *see* Sodium Bicarbonate 1227
Sodium Hypochlorite Solution 1231
Sodium *L*-Triiodothyronine *see* Liothyronine 810
Sodium Nafcillin *see* Nafcillin 945
Sodium Nitroferricyanide *see* Nitroprusside 982
Sodium Nitroprusside *see* Nitroprusside 982
Sodium Oxybate 1231
Sodium PAS *see* Aminosalicylic Acid 79
Sodium-PCA and Lactic Acid *see* Lactic Acid and Sodium-PCA 771
Sodium Phenylbutyrate 1233
Sodium Phosphate *see* Phosphate Supplements 1076
Sodium Sulamyd® *see* Sulfacetamide 1249
Sodium Sulfacetamide *see* Sulfacetamide 1249
Sodium Thiosulfate 1233
Soflax™ *see* Docusate 463
Solagé™ *see* Mequinol and Tretinoin 865
Solaquin® [OTC] *see* Hydroquinone 693
Solaquin Forte® *see* Hydroquinone 693
Solaraze™ *see* Diclofenac 429
Solarcaine® [OTC] *see* Benzocaine 169
Solarcaine® Aloe Extra Burn Relief [OTC] *see* Lidocaine 801
Solciclina® *see* Amoxicillin 93
Solganal® *see* Aurothioglucose 148
Soltric *see* Mebendazole 846
Solucaps® *see* Mazindol 843
Solu-Cortef® *see* Hydrocortisone 688
Solugel® *see* Benzoyl Peroxide 171
Solu-Medrol® *see* MethylPREDNISolone 895
Solurex® *see* Dexamethasone 413
Solurex L.A.® *see* Dexamethasone 413
Soluver® *see* Salicylic Acid 1204
Soluver® Plus *see* Salicylic Acid 1204
Soma® *see* Carisoprodol 251
Soma® Compound *see* Carisoprodol and Aspirin 252
Soma® Compound w/Codeine *see* Carisoprodol, Aspirin, and Codeine 252
Somatrem *see* Human Growth Hormone 671
Somatropin *see* Human Growth Hormone 671
Sominex® [OTC] *see* DiphenhydrAMINE 451
Sominex® Maximum Strength [OTC] *see* DiphenhydrAMINE 451
Sonata® *see* Zaleplon 1404
Sophipren Ofteno *see* PrednisoLONE 1110
Sophixin® *see* Ciprofloxacin 328
Sophixin Ofteno *see* Ciprofloxacin 328
Sorbitol 1234
Sorine® *see* Sotalol 1235
Sotacor® *see* Sotalol 1235
Sotalol 1235
Sotalol Hydrochloride *see* Sotalol 1235
Soy Isoflavones 1448
Spacol *see* Hyoscyamine 699
Spacol T/S *see* Hyoscyamine 699
Sparfloxacin 1238
Spectazole™ *see* Econazole 486
Spectinomycin 1239
Spectinomycin Hydrochloride *see* Spectinomycin 1239

Spectracef™ *see* Cefditoren 265
Spectrocin Plus® [OTC] *see* Bacitracin, Neomycin, Polymyxin B, and Lidocaine 158
SpectroGram 2™ *see* Chlorhexidine Gluconate 300
SpectroTar Skin Wash™ *see* Coal Tar 359
Spiramycin 1239
Spironolactone 1240
Spironolactone and Hydrochlorothiazide *see* Hydrochlorothiazide and Spironolactone 677
Sporanox® *see* Itraconazole 755
Sportscreme® [OTC] *see* Triethanolamine Salicylate 1348
SSD™ *see* Silver Sulfadiazine 1222
SSD® AF *see* Silver Sulfadiazine 1222
SSKI® *see* Potassium Iodide 1101
Stadol® *see* Butorphanol 218
Stadol® NS *see* Butorphanol 218
Stagesic® *see* Hydrocodone and Acetaminophen 678
Standard Conversions 1596
Stan-gard® *see* Fluoride 586
Stannous Fluoride *see* Fluoride 586
Stanozolol 1241
Starnoc® *see* Zaleplon 1404
Statex® *see* Morphine Sulfate 931
Staticin® *see* Erythromycin 512
Statobex® *see* Phendimetrazine 1064
Stat Touch 2 [OTC] [DSC] *see* Chlorhexidine Gluconate 300
Stavudine 1242
Stelazine® *see* Trifluoperazine 1349
Stemetil® *see* Prochlorperazine 1123
Stenox® *see* Fluoxymesterone 592
Sterapred® *see* PredniSONE 1112
Sterapred® DS *see* PredniSONE 1112
Stieva-A® *see* Tretinoin (Topical) 1340
Stieva-A® 0.025% *see* Tretinoin (Topical) 1340
Stilbestrol *see* Diethylstilbestrol 437
Stimate™ *see* Desmopressin 410
Stinking Rose *see* Garlic 1433
St John's Wort 1448
St. Joseph® Pain Reliever [OTC] *see* Aspirin 131
Stop® *see* Fluoride 586
Strattera™ *see* Atomoxetine 139
Streptase® *see* Streptokinase 1243
Streptokinase 1243
Streptomycin 1245
Streptomycin Sulfate *see* Streptomycin 1245
Streptozocin 1246
Stri-dex® [OTC] *see* Salicylic Acid 1204
Stri-dex® Body Focus [OTC] *see* Salicylic Acid 1204
Stri-dex® Facewipes To Go™ [OTC] *see* Salicylic Acid 1204
Stri-dex® Maximum Strength [OTC] *see* Salicylic Acid 1204
Strifon Forte® *see* Chlorzoxazone 316
Stromectol® *see* Ivermectin 757
Strong Iodine Solution *see* Potassium Iodide 1101
Sublimaze® *see* Fentanyl 565
Subutex® *see* Buprenorphine 208
Sucraid® *see* Sacrosidase 1203
Sucralfate 1247
Sucrets® Original [OTC] *see* Hexylresorcinol 670
Sudafed® [OTC] *see* Pseudoephedrine 1146
Sudafed® 12 Hour [OTC] *see* Pseudoephedrine 1146
Sudafed® 24 Hour [OTC] *see* Pseudoephedrine 1146
Sudafed® Children's [OTC] *see* Pseudoephedrine 1146
Sudafed® Cold & Allergy [OTC] *see* Chlorpheniramine and Pseudoephedrine 308
Sudafed® Cold and Sinus [OTC] *see* Acetaminophen and Pseudoephedrine 31
Sudafed® Cold & Cough Extra Strength *see* Acetaminophen, Dextromethorphan, and Pseudoephedrine 35
Sudafed® Decongestant *see* Pseudoephedrine 1146
Sudafed® Head Cold and Sinus Extra Strength *see* Acetaminophen and Pseudoephedrine 31
Sudafed® Severe Cold [OTC] *see* Acetaminophen, Dextromethorphan, and Pseudoephedrine 35
Sudafed® Sinus Advance *see* Pseudoephedrine and Ibuprofen 1148
Sudafed® Sinus Headache [OTC] *see* Acetaminophen and Pseudoephedrine 31
Sudodrin [OTC] *see* Pseudoephedrine 1146
Sufenta® *see* Sufentanil 1248
Sufentanil 1248
Sufentanil Citrate *see* Sufentanil 1248
Sufisal® *see* Pentoxifylline 1058
Sufortan® *see* Penicillamine 1046
Sufortanon® *see* Penicillamine 1046
Suggested Readings 1587
Suiflox® *see* Ciprofloxacin 328
Sular® *see* Nisoldipine 977
Sulbactam and Ampicillin *see* Ampicillin and Sulbactam 104
Sulconazole 1249
Sulconazole Nitrate *see* Sulconazole 1249
Sulcrate® *see* Sucralfate 1247
Sulcrate® Suspension Plus *see* Sucralfate 1247
Sulf-10® *see* Sulfacetamide 1249
Sulfabenzamide, Sulfacetamide, and Sulfathiazole 1249
Sulfacetamide 1249
Sulfacetamide and Fluorometholone 1250

Sulfacetamide and Prednisolone . . . 1250
Sulfacetamide Sodium *see* Sulfacetamide . . . 1249
Sulfacetamide Sodium and Prednisolone *see* Sulfacetamide and Prednisolone . . . 1250
SulfaDIAZINE . . . 1251
Sulfadoxine and Pyrimethamine . . . 1252
Sulfamethoxazole and Trimethoprim . . . 1253
Sulfamylon® *see* Mafenide . . . 832
Sulfasalazine . . . 1254
Sulfinpyrazone . . . 1255
SulfiSOXAZOLE . . . 1256
Sulfisoxazole Acetyl *see* SulfiSOXAZOLE . . . 1256
Sulfisoxazole and Erythromycin *see* Erythromycin and Sulfisoxazole . . . 516
Sulfizole® *see* SulfiSOXAZOLE . . . 1256
Sulfonated Phenolics in Aqueous Solution . . . 1257
Sulindac . . . 1257
Sulphafurazole *see* SulfiSOXAZOLE . . . 1256
Sumatriptan . . . 1258
Sumatriptan Succinate *see* Sumatriptan . . . 1258
Summer's Eve® Medicated Douche [OTC] *see* Povidone-Iodine . . . 1104
Summer's Eve® SpecialCare™ Medicated Anti-Itch Cream [OTC] *see* Hydrocortisone . . . 688
Sumycin® *see* Tetracycline . . . 1286
Supartz™ *see* Sodium Hyaluronate . . . 1230
Superdophilus® [OTC] *see Lactobacillus acidophilus* and *Lactobacillus bulgaricus* . . . 772
Superginkgo *see* Ginkgo Biloba . . . 1434
Supeudol® *see* Oxycodone . . . 1017
Suplasyn® *see* Sodium Hyaluronate . . . 1230
Suplena *see* Vitamins (Multiple/Oral) . . . 1394
Supositorios Senosiain® *see* Glycerin . . . 644
Supradol® *see* Ketorolac . . . 765
Supradol® *see* Naproxen . . . 953
Suprax® [DSC] *see* Cefixime . . . 268
Surbex-T® Filmtabs® [OTC] *see* Vitamin B Complex and Vitamin C . . . 1392
Surbex® With C Filmtabs® [OTC] *see* Vitamin B Complex and Vitamin C . . . 1392
Sureprin 81™ [OTC] *see* Aspirin . . . 131
Surfak® [OTC] *see* Docusate . . . 463
Surgicel® *see* Cellulose (Oxidized) . . . 284
Surgicel® Absorbable Hemostat *see* Cellulose (Oxidized/Regenerated) . . . 284
Surmontil® *see* Trimipramine . . . 1354
Survanta® *see* Beractant . . . 176
Sus-Phrine® (Dental) *see* Epinephrine . . . 499
Sustiva® *see* Efavirenz . . . 488
Su-Tuss®-HD *see* Hydrocodone, Pseudoephedrine, and Guaifenesin . . . 687
Sween Cream® [OTC] *see* Vitamin A and Vitamin D . . . 1392
Sweet Root *see* Licorice . . . 1442
Sydolil *see* Ergotamine . . . 510
Symax SL *see* Hyoscyamine . . . 699
Symax SR *see* Hyoscyamine . . . 699
Symmetrel® *see* Amantadine . . . 70
Synacthen *see* Cosyntropin . . . 374
Synagis® *see* Palivizumab . . . 1028
Synalar® *see* Fluocinolone . . . 584
Synalgos®-DC *see* Dihydrocodeine, Aspirin, and Caffeine . . . 444
Synarel® *see* Nafarelin . . . 944
Syn-Diltiazem® *see* Diltiazem . . . 447
Synercid® *see* Quinupristin and Dalfopristin . . . 1161
Syngestal *see* Norethindrone . . . 986
Synthetic Lung Surfactant *see* Colfosceril Palmitate . . . 366
Synthroid® *see* Levothyroxine . . . 800
Syntocinon® *see* Oxytocin . . . 1026
Syraprim *see* Sulfamethoxazole and Trimethoprim . . . 1253
Syscor® *see* Nisoldipine . . . 977
Systemic Viral Diseases . . . 1517
Systen® *see* Estradiol . . . 521
T_3 Sodium *see* Liothyronine . . . 810
T_3/T_4 Liotrix *see* Liotrix . . . 811
T_4 *see* Levothyroxine . . . 800
T-20 *see* Enfuvirtide . . . 495
Tabalon® *see* Ibuprofen . . . 703
642® Tablet *see* Propoxyphene . . . 1135
Tac™-3 [DSC] *see* Triamcinolone . . . 1341
Tacex® *see* Ceftriaxone . . . 278
Tacozin® *see* Piperacillin and Tazobactam Sodium . . . 1088
Tacrine . . . 1260
Tacrine Hydrochloride *see* Tacrine . . . 1260
Tacrolimus . . . 1261
Tafil® *see* Alprazolam . . . 61
Tagal® *see* Ceftazidime . . . 275
Tagamet® *see* Cimetidine . . . 326
Tagamet® HB *see* Cimetidine . . . 326
Tagamet® HB 200 [OTC] *see* Cimetidine . . . 326
Talacen® *see* Pentazocine Combinations . . . 1054
Taloken *see* Ceftazidime . . . 275
Talpramin® *see* Imipramine . . . 711
Talwin® *see* Pentazocine . . . 1054
Talwin® NX *see* Pentazocine . . . 1054
Tambocor™ *see* Flecainide . . . 574
Tamiflu® *see* Oseltamivir . . . 1006
Tamofen® *see* Tamoxifen . . . 1264
Tamoxan *see* Tamoxifen . . . 1264
Tamoxifen . . . 1264

Tamoxifen Citrate *see* Tamoxifen 1264
Tamsulosin 1266
Tamsulosin Hydrochloride *see* Tamsulosin 1266
Tanacetum parthenium see Feverfew 1431
Tanakan *see* Ginkgo Biloba 1434
Tanakene *see* Ginkgo Biloba 1434
Tandax® *see* Naproxen 953
Tannic-12 *see* Carbetapentane and Chlorpheniramine 245
Tannic-12 S *see* Carbetapentane and Chlorpheniramine 245
Tanoral® *see* Chlorpheniramine, Pyrilamine, and Phenylephrine 312
Tao® *see* Troleandomycin 1359
Tapazole® *see* Methimazole 880
Taporin® *see* Cefotaxime 271
Targel® *see* Coal Tar 359
Targretin® *see* Bexarotene 182
Tarka® *see* Trandolapril and Verapamil 1332
Tarka® *see* Verapamil 1382
Taro-Carbamazepine Chewable *see* Carbamazepine 241
Taro-Desoximetasone *see* Desoximetasone 412
Taro-Sone® *see* Betamethasone 177
Taro-Warfarin *see* Warfarin 1397
Tasedan® *see* Estazolam 521
Tasmar® *see* Tolcapone 1320
Tavanic® *see* Levofloxacin 794
Tavist® *see* Clemastine 340
Tavist®-1 [OTC] *see* Clemastine 340
Tavor® *see* Oxybutynin 1016
Taxifur® *see* Ceftazidime 275
Taxol® *see* Paclitaxel 1026
Taxotere® *see* Docetaxel 461
Taxus® *see* Tamoxifen 1264
Tazarotene 1267
Tazicef® *see* Ceftazidime 275
Tazidime® *see* Ceftazidime 275
Taziken® *see* Terbutaline 1278
Tazorac® *see* Tazarotene 1267
3TC® *see* Lamivudine 773
3TC, Abacavir, and Zidovudine *see* Abacavir, Lamivudine, and Zidovudine 23
T-Cell Growth Factor *see* Aldesleukin 50
TCGF *see* Aldesleukin 50
TCN *see* Tetracycline 1286
TDF *see* Tenofovir 1275
Teardrops® *see* Artificial Tears 128
Teargen® [OTC] *see* Artificial Tears 128
Teargen® II [OTC] *see* Artificial Tears 128
Tearisol® [OTC] *see* Artificial Tears 128
Tearisol® [OTC] *see* Hydroxypropyl Methylcellulose 696
Tears Again® [OTC] *see* Artificial Tears 128
Tears Naturale® [OTC] *see* Artificial Tears 128
Tears Naturale® Free [OTC] *see* Artificial Tears 128
Tears Naturale® II [OTC] *see* Artificial Tears 128
Tears Plus® [OTC] *see* Artificial Tears 128
Tears Renewed® [OTC] *see* Artificial Tears 128
Tea Tree Oil *see* Melaleuca Oil 1444
Tebonin *see* Ginkgo Biloba 1434
Tebrazid™ *see* Pyrazinamide 1150
Tecnal C 1/2 *see* Butalbital, Aspirin, Caffeine, and Codeine 217
Tecnal C 1/4 *see* Butalbital, Aspirin, Caffeine, and Codeine 217
Tecnofen® *see* Tamoxifen 1264
Tecnoplatin® *see* Cisplatin 332
Tecprazin *see* Praziquantel 1108
Teejel® *see* Choline Salicylate 319
Tegaserod 1268
Tegaserod Maleate *see* Tegaserod 1268
Tegretol® *see* Carbamazepine 241
Tegretol®-XR *see* Carbamazepine 241
Tegrin® Dandruff Shampoo [OTC] *see* Coal Tar 359
Telmisartan 1269
Telmisartan and HCTZ *see* Telmisartan and Hydrochlorothiazide 1270
Telmisartan and Hydrochlorothiazide 1270
Temazepam 1271
Temgesic® *see* Buprenorphine 208
Temodal™ *see* Temozolomide 1272
Temodar® *see* Temozolomide 1272
Temovate® *see* Clobetasol 345
Temovate E® *see* Clobetasol 345
Temozolomide 1272
Temperal® *see* Acetaminophen 27
Temporomandibular Dysfunction (TMD) 1562
Tempra® *see* Acetaminophen 27
Tenecteplase 1273
Tenex® *see* Guanfacine 655
Teniposide 1274
Tenofovir 1275
Tenofovir Disoproxil Fumarate *see* Tenofovir 1275
Tenolin *see* Atenolol 137
Tenoretic® *see* Atenolol and Chlorthalidone 138
Tenormin® *see* Atenolol 137
Tenuate® *see* Diethylpropion 436
Tenuate® Dospan® *see* Diethylpropion 436

Teolong® *see* Theophylline 1291
Tequin® *see* Gatifloxacin 628
Terazol® *see* Terconazole 1279
Terazol® 3 *see* Terconazole 1279
Terazol® 7 *see* Terconazole 1279
Terazosin 1276
Terbac® *see* Ceftriaxone 278
Terbinafine 1277
Terbinafine Hydrochloride *see* Terbinafine 1277
Terbutaline 1278
Terconazole 1279
Terfluzine *see* Trifluoperazine 1349
Teriparatide 1280
Termizol® *see* Ketoconazole 762
Terpin Hydrate and Codeine 1281
Terra-Cortril® [DSC] *see* Oxytetracycline and Hydrocortisone 1025
Terramicina® *see* Oxytetracycline 1024
Terramycin® *see* Oxytetracycline 1024
Terramycin® I.M. *see* Oxytetracycline 1024
Terramycin® w/Polymyxin B Ophthalmic *see* Oxytetracycline and Polymyxin B 1025
Terranumonyl *see* Tetracycline 1286
Tesalon® *see* Benzonatate 171
Teslac® *see* Testolactone 1281
TESPA *see* Thiotepa 1300
Tessalon® *see* Benzonatate 171
Testim™ *see* Testosterone 1281
Testoderm® *see* Testosterone 1281
Testoderm® TTS [DSC] *see* Testosterone 1281
Testoderm® with Adhesive *see* Testosterone 1281
Testolactone 1281
Testopel® *see* Testosterone 1281
Testosterone 1281
Testosterone and Estradiol *see* Estradiol and Testosterone 527
Testosterone Cypionate *see* Testosterone 1281
Testosterone Enanthate *see* Testosterone 1281
Testosterone Propionate *see* Testosterone 1281
Testred® *see* MethylTESTOSTERone 897
Tetanus Antitoxin *see* Immunizations (Vaccines) 1612
Tetanus Immune Globulin (Human) *see* Immunizations (Vaccines) 1612
Tetanus Immune Globulin (Human) 1283
Tetanus Toxoid (Adsorbed) *see* Immunizations (Vaccines) 1612
Tetanus Toxoid (Adsorbed) 1283
Tetanus Toxoid (Fluid) *see* Immunizations (Vaccines) 1612
Tetanus Toxoid (Fluid) 1284
Tetanus Toxoid Plain *see* Tetanus Toxoid (Fluid) 1284
Tetra-Atlantis® *see* Tetracycline 1286
Tetracaine 1284
Tetracaine and Dextrose 1285
Tetracaine Hydrochloride *see* Tetracaine 1284
Tetracaine Hydrochloride, Benzocaine Butyl Aminobenzoate, and Benzalkonium Chloride *see* Benzocaine, Butyl Aminobenzoate, Tetracaine, and Benzalkonium Chloride 170
Tetracosactide *see* Cosyntropin 374
Tetracycline 1286
Tetracycline, Bismuth Subsalicylate, and Metronidazole *see* Bismuth, Metronidazole, and Tetracycline 187
Tetracycline Hydrochloride *see* Tetracycline 1286
Tetracycline, Metronidazole, and Bismuth Subsalicylate *see* Bismuth, Metronidazole, and Tetracycline 187
Tetracycline Periodontal Fibers 1287
Tetrahydroaminoacrine *see* Tacrine 1260
Tetrahydrocannabinol *see* Dronabinol 480
Tetrahydrozoline 1288
Tetrahydrozoline Hydrochloride *see* Tetrahydrozoline 1288
Tetryzoline *see* Tetrahydrozoline 1288
Teveten® *see* Eprosartan 506
Texacort® *see* Hydrocortisone 688
Texate® *see* Methotrexate 884
TG *see* Thioguanine 1296
6-TG *see* Thioguanine 1296
T/Gel® [OTC] *see* Coal Tar 359
THA *see* Tacrine 1260
Thalidomide 1289
Thalitone® *see* Chlorthalidone 315
Thalomid® *see* Thalidomide 1289
THAM® *see* Tromethamine 1360
THC *see* Dronabinol 480
Theo-24® *see* Theophylline 1291
Theochron® *see* Theophylline 1291
Theochron® SR *see* Theophylline 1291
Theo-Dur® *see* Theophylline 1291
Theolair™ *see* Theophylline 1291
Theolair-SR® [DSC] *see* Theophylline 1291
Theolate *see* Theophylline and Guaifenesin 1293
Theophylline 1291
Theophylline and Guaifenesin 1293
Theophylline Anhydrous *see* Theophylline 1291
Theophylline Ethylenediamine *see* Aminophylline 78
Theracort® [OTC] *see* Hydrocortisone 688
TheraCys® *see* BCG Vaccine 161
Thera-Flu® Flu and Cold *see* Acetaminophen, Chlorpheniramine, and Pseudoephedrine 35

Thera-Flu® Non-Drowsy Flu, Cold and Cough [OTC] *see* Acetaminophen, Dextromethorphan, and Pseudoephedrine . . . 35
Thera-Flur-N® *see* Fluoride . . . 586
Theragran® Heart Right™ [OTC] *see* Vitamins (Multiple/Oral) . . . 1394
Theragran-M® Advanced Formula [OTC] *see* Vitamins (Multiple/Oral) . . . 1394
Theramycin Z® *see* Erythromycin . . . 512
Therapeutic Multivitamins *see* Vitamins (Multiple/Oral) . . . 1394
Thermazene® *see* Silver Sulfadiazine . . . 1222
Thiabendazole . . . 1294
Thiamazole *see* Methimazole . . . 880
Thiamilate® [OTC] *see* Thiamine . . . 1295
Thiamine . . . 1295
Thiamine Hydrochloride *see* Thiamine . . . 1295
Thiaminium Chloride Hydrochloride *see* Thiamine . . . 1295
Thiethylperazine . . . 1295
Thiethylperazine Maleate *see* Thiethylperazine . . . 1295
Thimerosal . . . 1296
Thioctic acid *see* Alpha-Lipoic Acid . . . 1420
Thioguanine . . . 1296
6-Thioguanine *see* Thioguanine . . . 1296
Thiola™ *see* Tiopronin . . . 1313
Thiopental . . . 1297
Thiopental Sodium *see* Thiopental . . . 1297
Thiophosphoramide *see* Thiotepa . . . 1300
Thioplex® *see* Thiotepa . . . 1300
Thioridazine . . . 1298
Thioridazine Hydrochloride *see* Thioridazine . . . 1298
Thioridazine Intensol™ *see* Thioridazine . . . 1298
Thiotepa . . . 1300
Thiothixene . . . 1301
Thorazine® *see* ChlorproMAZINE . . . 312
Thrombate III® *see* Antithrombin III . . . 117
Thrombin-JMI® *see* Thrombin (Topical) . . . 1302
Thrombin (Topical) . . . 1302
Thrombogen® *see* Thrombin (Topical) . . . 1302
Thrombostat™ *see* Thrombin (Topical) . . . 1302
Thymocyte Stimulating Factor *see* Aldesleukin . . . 50
Thyrel® TRH *see* Protirelin . . . 1144
Thyrogen® *see* Thyrotropin Alpha . . . 1304
Thyroid . . . 1303
Thyroid Extract *see* Thyroid . . . 1303
Thyroid USP *see* Thyroid . . . 1303
Thyrolar® *see* Liotrix . . . 811
Thyrotropin Alpha . . . 1304
Thyrotropin Releasing Hormone *see* Protirelin . . . 1144
Tiabendazole *see* Thiabendazole . . . 1294
Tiagabine . . . 1304
Tiagabine Hydrochloride *see* Tiagabine . . . 1304
Tiamol® *see* Fluocinonide . . . 585
Tiazac® *see* Diltiazem . . . 447
Ticar® *see* Ticarcillin . . . 1305
Ticarcillin . . . 1305
Ticarcillin and Clavulanate Potassium . . . 1306
Ticarcillin and Clavulanic Acid *see* Ticarcillin and Clavulanate Potassium . . . 1306
Ticarcillin Disodium *see* Ticarcillin . . . 1305
TICE® BCG *see* BCG Vaccine . . . 161
Ticlid® *see* Ticlopidine . . . 1307
Ticlopidine . . . 1307
Ticlopidine Hydrochloride *see* Ticlopidine . . . 1307
Tienam® *see* Imipenem and Cilastatin . . . 709
TIG *see* Tetanus Immune Globulin (Human) . . . 1283
Tigan® *see* Trimethobenzamide . . . 1352
Tikosyn™ *see* Dofetilide . . . 464
Tilade® *see* Nedocromil . . . 957
Tilazem® *see* Diltiazem . . . 447
Tiludronate . . . 1309
Tiludronate Disodium *see* Tiludronate . . . 1309
Tim-AK *see* Timolol . . . 1309
Timentin® *see* Ticarcillin . . . 1305
Timentin® *see* Ticarcillin and Clavulanate Potassium . . . 1306
Timolol . . . 1309
Timolol Hemihydrate *see* Timolol . . . 1309
Timolol Maleate *see* Timolol . . . 1309
Timoptic® *see* Timolol . . . 1309
Timoptic® OcuDose® *see* Timolol . . . 1309
Timoptic-XE® *see* Timolol . . . 1309
Timoptol® *see* Timolol . . . 1309
Timoptol® XE *see* Timolol . . . 1309
Tinactin® Antifungal [OTC] *see* Tolnaftate . . . 1322
Tinactin® Antifungal Jock Itch [OTC] *see* Tolnaftate . . . 1322
Tinaderm [OTC] *see* Tolnaftate . . . 1322
Tinamed® [OTC] *see* Salicylic Acid . . . 1204
TinBen® [OTC] *see* Benzoin . . . 171
Tine Test *see* Tuberculin Tests . . . 1362
Ting® [OTC] *see* Tolnaftate . . . 1322
Tiniazol® *see* Ketoconazole . . . 762
Tinzaparin . . . 1311
Tinzaparin Sodium *see* Tinzaparin . . . 1311
Tioconazole . . . 1312
Tioguanine *see* Thioguanine . . . 1296

Tiopronin . . . 1313
Tiotixene *see* Thiothixene . . . 1301
Tirocal® *see* Calcitriol . . . 223
Tirofiban . . . 1313
Tirofiban Hydrochloride *see* Tirofiban . . . 1313
Tiroidine *see* Levothyroxine . . . 800
Tiseb® [OTC] *see* Salicylic Acid . . . 1204
Tisit® [OTC] *see* Pyrethrins and Piperonyl Butoxide . . . 1151
Tisit® Blue Gel [OTC] *see* Pyrethrins and Piperonyl Butoxide . . . 1151
Tisseel® VH *see* Fibrin Sealant Kit . . . 570
Titralac® Plus Liquid [OTC] *see* Calcium Carbonate and Simethicone . . . 224
Ti-U-Lac® H *see* Urea and Hydrocortisone . . . 1365
Tizanidine . . . 1314
TMP *see* Trimethoprim . . . 1352
TMP-SMZ *see* Sulfamethoxazole and Trimethoprim . . . 1253
TNKase™ *see* Tenecteplase . . . 1273
TOBI® *see* Tobramycin . . . 1315
Tobra *see* Tobramycin . . . 1315
Tobradex® *see* Tobramycin and Dexamethasone . . . 1317
Tobramycin . . . 1315
Tobramycin and Dexamethasone . . . 1317
Tobramycin Sulfate *see* Tobramycin . . . 1315
Tobrex® *see* Tobramycin . . . 1315
Tocainide . . . 1317
Tocainide Hydrochloride *see* Tocainide . . . 1317
Tofranil® *see* Imipramine . . . 711
Tofranil-PM® *see* Imipramine . . . 711
TOLAZamide . . . 1318
TOLBUTamide . . . 1319
Tolbutamide Sodium *see* TOLBUTamide . . . 1319
Tolcapone . . . 1320
Tolectin® *see* Tolmetin . . . 1321
Tolectin® DS *see* Tolmetin . . . 1321
Tolinase® *see* TOLAZamide . . . 1318
Tolmetin . . . 1321
Tolmetin Sodium *see* Tolmetin . . . 1321
Tolnaftate . . . 1322
Tol-Tab® *see* TOLBUTamide . . . 1319
Tolterodine . . . 1322
Tolterodine Tartrate *see* Tolterodine . . . 1322
Tolu-Sed® DM [OTC] *see* Guaifenesin and Dextromethorphan . . . 651
Tomedar® *see* Temozolomide . . . 1272
Tomoxetine *see* Atomoxetine . . . 139
Tomycine™ *see* Tobramycin . . . 1315
Tondex® *see* Gentamicin . . . 634
Tonga *see* Kava . . . 1442
Tonocalcin® *see* Calcitonin . . . 222
Tonocard® *see* Tocainide . . . 1317
Top 50 Most Prescribed Drugs in 2002 . . . 1636
Topamax® *see* Topiramate . . . 1324
Top-Dal® *see* Loperamide . . . 819
Topicaine® [OTC] *see* Lidocaine . . . 801
Topicort® *see* Desoximetasone . . . 412
Topicort®-LP *see* Desoximetasone . . . 412
Topilene® *see* Betamethasone . . . 177
Topiramate . . . 1324
Topisone® *see* Betamethasone . . . 177
TOPO *see* Topotecan . . . 1325
Toposar® *see* Etoposide . . . 549
Topotecan . . . 1325
Topotecan Hydrochloride *see* Topotecan . . . 1325
Toprol-XL® *see* Metoprolol . . . 901
Topsyn® *see* Fluocinonide . . . 585
Toradol® *see* Ketorolac . . . 765
Toradol® IM *see* Ketorolac . . . 765
Torecan® *see* Thiethylperazine . . . 1295
Toremifene . . . 1326
Toremifene Citrate *see* Toremifene . . . 1326
Tornalate® [DSC] *see* Bitolterol . . . 189
Torsemide . . . 1327
Touro™ Allergy *see* Brompheniramine and Pseudoephedrine . . . 201
Touro™ CC *see* Guaifenesin, Pseudoephedrine, and Dextromethorphan . . . 653
Touro® DM *see* Guaifenesin and Dextromethorphan . . . 651
Touro Ex® *see* Guaifenesin . . . 650
Touro LA® *see* Guaifenesin and Pseudoephedrine . . . 652
tPA *see* Alteplase . . . 65
T-Phyl® *see* Theophylline . . . 1291
TPT *see* Topotecan . . . 1325
Trace Metals . . . 1328
Tracleer™ *see* Bosentan . . . 192
Tradol® *see* Tramadol . . . 1329
Tramadol . . . 1329
Tramadol Hydrochloride *see* Tramadol . . . 1329
Tramadol Hydrochloride and Acetaminophen *see* Acetaminophen and Tramadol . . . 32
Tramisal *see* Ginkgo Biloba . . . 1434
Trandate® *see* Labetalol . . . 769
Trandolapril . . . 1331
Trandolapril and Verapamil . . . 1332
Tranexamic Acid . . . 1333
Transamine Sulphate *see* Tranylcypromine . . . 1334

Transderm-Nitro® *see* Nitroglycerin . . . 981
Transderm Scōp® *see* Scopolamine . . . 1210
Transderm-V® *see* Scopolamine . . . 1210
Trans-Plantar® *see* Salicylic Acid . . . 1204
trans-Retinoic Acid *see* Tretinoin (Topical) . . . 1340
Trans-Ver-Sal® *see* Salicylic Acid . . . 1204
Tranxene® *see* Clorazepate . . . 355
Tranylcypromine . . . 1334
Tranylcypromine Sulfate *see* Tranylcypromine . . . 1334
Trasicor® *see* Oxprenolol . . . 1014
Trastuzumab . . . 1335
Trasylol® *see* Aprotinin . . . 119
Travatan® *see* Travoprost . . . 1336
Travoprost . . . 1336
Trazil® *see* Tobramycin . . . 1315
Trazil Ofteno/Ungena *see* Tobramycin . . . 1315
Trazodone . . . 1336
Trazodone Hydrochloride *see* Trazodone . . . 1336
Trecator®-SC *see* Ethionamide . . . 542
Trelstar™ Depot *see* Triptorelin . . . 1358
Trelstar™ LA *see* Triptorelin . . . 1358
Trental® *see* Pentoxifylline . . . 1058
Treprostinil . . . 1337
Treprostinil Sodium *see* Treprostinil . . . 1337
Tretinoin *see* Tretinoin (Oral) . . . 1338
Tretinoin *see* Tretinoin (Topical) . . . 1340
Tretinoin, Fluocinolone Acetonide, and Hydroquinone *see* Fluocinolone, Hydroquinone, and Tretinoin . . . 585
Tretinoin (Oral) . . . 1338
Tretinoin (Topical) . . . 1340
Trexall™ *see* Methotrexate . . . 884
TRH *see* Protirelin . . . 1144
Triacetin . . . 1340
Triacetyloleandomycin *see* Troleandomycin . . . 1359
Triacin-C® [DSC] *see* Triprolidine, Pseudoephedrine, and Codeine . . . 1357
Triaconazole *see* Terconazole . . . 1279
Triaderm *see* Triamcinolone . . . 1341
Triaken® *see* Ceftriaxone . . . 278
Triamcinolone . . . 1341
Triamcinolone Acetonide, Aerosol *see* Triamcinolone . . . 1341
Triamcinolone Acetonide Dental Paste . . . 1344
Triamcinolone Acetonide, Parenteral *see* Triamcinolone . . . 1341
Triamcinolone and Nystatin *see* Nystatin and Triamcinolone . . . 992
Triamcinolone Diacetate, Oral *see* Triamcinolone . . . 1341
Triamcinolone Diacetate, Parenteral *see* Triamcinolone . . . 1341
Triamcinolone Hexacetonide *see* Triamcinolone . . . 1341
Triamcinolone, Oral *see* Triamcinolone . . . 1341
Triaminic® Allergy Congestion *see* Pseudoephedrine . . . 1146
Triaminic® Cold & Allergy *see* Chlorpheniramine and Pseudoephedrine . . . 308
Triaminic® Sore Throat Formula [OTC] *see* Acetaminophen, Dextromethorphan, and Pseudoephedrine . . . 35
Triamsicort® *see* Triamcinolone . . . 1341
Triamterene . . . 1344
Triamterene and Hydrochlorothiazide *see* Hydrochlorothiazide and Triamterene . . . 677
Triatec-8 *see* Acetaminophen and Codeine . . . 29
Triatec-8 Strong *see* Acetaminophen and Codeine . . . 29
Triatec-30 *see* Acetaminophen and Codeine . . . 29
Triavil® *see* Amitriptyline and Perphenazine . . . 85
Triaz® *see* Benzoyl Peroxide . . . 171
Triaz® Cleanser *see* Benzoyl Peroxide . . . 171
Triazolam . . . 1345
Tribakin *see* Sulfamethoxazole and Trimethoprim . . . 1253
Tribakin® *see* Trimethoprim . . . 1352
Tribavirin *see* Ribavirin . . . 1176
Tricalcium Phosphate *see* Calcium Phosphate (Tribasic) . . . 227
Tri-Chlor® *see* Trichloroacetic Acid . . . 1347
Trichlorex® *see* Trichlormethiazide . . . 1347
Trichlormethiazide . . . 1347
Trichloroacetaldehyde Monohydrate *see* Chloral Hydrate . . . 295
Trichloroacetic Acid . . . 1347
Trichloromonofluoromethane and Dichlorodifluoromethane *see* Dichlorodifluoromethane and Trichloromonofluoromethane . . . 428
Triclosan and Fluoride . . . 1348
TriCor® *see* Fenofibrate . . . 561
Tricosal® *see* Choline Magnesium Trisalicylate . . . 319
Tri-Cyclen® *see* Combination Hormonal Contraceptives . . . 368
Triderm® *see* Triamcinolone . . . 1341
Tridesilon® *see* Desonide . . . 412
Tridione® *see* Trimethadione . . . 1351
Triethanolamine Polypeptide Oleate-Condensate . . . 1348
Triethanolamine Salicylate . . . 1348
Triethylenethiophosphoramide *see* Thiotepa . . . 1300
Trifluoperazine . . . 1349
Trifluoperazine Hydrochloride *see* Trifluoperazine . . . 1349
Trifluorothymidine *see* Trifluridine . . . 1350
Trifluridine . . . 1350
Triglycerides, Medium Chain *see* Medium Chain Triglycerides . . . 849
Trihexyphenidyl . . . 1351
Trihexyphenidyl Hydrochloride *see* Trihexyphenidyl . . . 1351
Tri-K® *see* Potassium Supplements . . . 1102

Trilafon® *see* Perphenazine 1062
Trileptal® *see* Oxcarbazepine 1012
Tri-Levlen® *see* Combination Hormonal Contraceptives 368
Trilisate® *see* Choline Magnesium Trisalicylate 319
Tri-Luma™ *see* Fluocinolone, Hydroquinone, and Tretinoin 585
Tri-Luma *see* Furazolidone 622
Trimesuxol *see* Sulfamethoxazole and Trimethoprim 1253
Trimethadione 1351
Trimethobenzamide 1352
Trimethobenzamide Hydrochloride *see* Trimethobenzamide 1352
Trimethoprim 1352
Trimethoprim and Polymyxin B 1353
Trimethoprim and Sulfamethoxazole *see* Sulfamethoxazole and Trimethoprim 1253
Trimetoger *see* Sulfamethoxazole and Trimethoprim 1253
Trimetoger® *see* Trimethoprim 1352
Trimetox *see* Sulfamethoxazole and Trimethoprim 1253
Trimetox® *see* Trimethoprim 1352
Trimetrexate Glucuronate 1354
Trimexazol® *see* Trimethoprim 1352
Trimexole-F® *see* Trimethoprim 1352
Trimipramine 1354
Trimipramine Maleate *see* Trimipramine 1354
Trimox® *see* Amoxicillin 93
Trimzol *see* Sulfamethoxazole and Trimethoprim 1253
Trinalin® *see* Azatadine and Pseudoephedrine 150
Tri-Nasal® *see* Triamcinolone 1341
Tri-Norinyl® *see* Combination Hormonal Contraceptives 368
Triostat® *see* Liothyronine 810
Triotann® *see* Chlorpheniramine, Pyrilamine, and Phenylephrine 312
Tripelennamine 1356
Tripelennamine Citrate *see* Tripelennamine 1356
Tripelennamine Hydrochloride *see* Tripelennamine 1356
Triphasil® *see* Combination Hormonal Contraceptives 368
Triple Antibiotic® *see* Bacitracin, Neomycin, and Polymyxin B 157
Triple Care® Antifungal [OTC] *see* Miconazole 906
Triple Sulfa *see* Sulfabenzamide, Sulfacetamide, and Sulfathiazole 1249
Triprolidine and Pseudoephedrine 1356
Triprolidine, Codeine, and Pseudoephedrine *see* Triprolidine, Pseudoephedrine, and Codeine 1357
Triprolidine, Pseudoephedrine, and Codeine 1357
Triprolidine, Pseudoephedrine, and Codeine, Triprolidine, and Pseudoephedrine *see* Triprolidine, Pseudoephedrine, and Codeine 1357
TripTone® [OTC] *see* DimenhyDRINATE 449
Triptorelin 1358
Triptorelin Pamoate *see* Triptorelin 1358
Tris Buffer *see* Tromethamine 1360
Tris(hydroxymethyl)aminomethane *see* Tromethamine 1360
Tri-Sudo® [OTC] *see* Triprolidine and Pseudoephedrine 1356
Tritace® *see* Ramipril 1166
Tri-Tannate® *see* Chlorpheniramine, Pyrilamine, and Phenylephrine 312
Tri-Tannate Plus® [OTC] *see* Chlorpheniramine, Ephedrine, Phenylephrine, and Carbetapentane 309
Trivagizole-3® *see* Clotrimazole 356
Trivora® *see* Combination Hormonal Contraceptives 368
Trixilem *see* DAUNOrubicin Hydrochloride 402
Trixilem® *see* Methotrexate 884
Triyotex® *see* Liothyronine 810
Trizivir® *see* Abacavir, Lamivudine, and Zidovudine 23
Trobicin® *see* Spectinomycin 1239
Trocaine® [OTC] *see* Benzocaine 169
Troleandomycin 1359
Tromethamine 1360
Tromigal *see* Erythromycin 512
Trompersantin *see* Dipyridamole 456
Tronolane® [OTC] *see* Pramoxine 1105
Tropicacyl® *see* Tropicamide 1360
Tropicamide 1360
Tropicamide and Hydroxyamphetamine *see* Hydroxyamphetamine and Tropicamide 694
Tropyn Z® *see* Atropine 144
Trovafloxacin/Alatrofloxacin 1361
Trovan® *see* Trovafloxacin/Alatrofloxacin 1361
Troxidone *see* Trimethadione 1351
Truphylline® *see* Aminophylline 78
Trusopt® *see* Dorzolamide 468
Trypsin, Balsam Peru, and Castor Oil 1362
Tryptanol® *see* Amitriptyline 83
TSH *see* Thyrotropin Alpha 1304
TSPA *see* Thiotepa 1300
TST *see* Tuberculin Tests 1362
T-Stat® *see* Erythromycin 512
Tuberculin Skin Test *see* Tuberculin Tests 1362
Tuberculin Tests 1362
Tuberculosis 1493
Tubersol® *see* Tuberculin Tests 1362
Tuinal® *see* Amobarbital and Secobarbital 91
Tukol® *see* Guaifenesin 650
Tums® [OTC] *see* Calcium Supplements 229
Tums® E-X Extra Strength Tablet [OTC] *see* Calcium Supplements 229
Tums® Ultra® [OTC] *see* Calcium Supplements 229
Turmeric 1448

Turmeric Root *see* Golden Seal . . . 1437
Tusical® *see* Benzonatate . . . 171
Tusitato® *see* Benzonatate . . . 171
Tussend® Expectorant *see* Hydrocodone, Pseudoephedrine, and Guaifenesin . . . 687
Tussi-12® *see* Carbetapentane and Chlorpheniramine . . . 245
Tussi-12 S™ *see* Carbetapentane and Chlorpheniramine . . . 245
Tussigon® *see* Hydrocodone and Homatropine . . . 684
Tussionex® *see* Hydrocodone and Chlorpheniramine . . . 682
Tussi-Organidin® DM NR *see* Guaifenesin and Dextromethorphan . . . 651
Tussi-Organidin® NR *see* Guaifenesin and Codeine . . . 650
Tussi-Organidin® S-NR *see* Guaifenesin and Codeine . . . 650
Tusstat® *see* DiphenhydrAMINE . . . 451
Twice-A-Day® [OTC] *see* Oxymetazoline . . . 1022
Twilite® [OTC] *see* DiphenhydrAMINE . . . 451
Twinrix® *see* Hepatitis A (Inactivated) and Hepatitis B (Recombinant) Vaccine . . . 664
Tylenol® [OTC] *see* Acetaminophen . . . 27
Tylenol® Allergy Sinus *see* Acetaminophen, Chlorpheniramine, and Pseudoephedrine . . . 35
Tylenol® Arthritis Pain [OTC] *see* Acetaminophen . . . 27
Tylenol® Children's [OTC] *see* Acetaminophen . . . 27
Tylenol® Cold *see* Acetaminophen, Chlorpheniramine, and Pseudoephedrine . . . 35
Tylenol® Cold *see* Acetaminophen, Dextromethorphan, and Pseudoephedrine . . . 35
Tylenol® Cold Non-Drowsy [OTC] *see* Acetaminophen, Dextromethorphan, and Pseudoephedrine . . . 35
Tylenol® Decongestant *see* Acetaminophen and Pseudoephedrine . . . 31
Tylenol® Extra Strength [OTC] *see* Acetaminophen . . . 27
Tylenol® Flu Non-Drowsy Maximum Strength [OTC] *see* Acetaminophen, Dextromethorphan, and Pseudoephedrine . . . 35
Tylenol® Infants [OTC] *see* Acetaminophen . . . 27
Tylenol® Junior Strength [OTC] *see* Acetaminophen . . . 27
Tylenol® PM Extra Strength [OTC] *see* Acetaminophen and Diphenhydramine . . . 30
Tylenol® Severe Allergy [OTC] *see* Acetaminophen and Diphenhydramine . . . 30
Tylenol® Sinus *see* Acetaminophen and Pseudoephedrine . . . 31
Tylenol® Sinus Non-Drowsy [OTC] *see* Acetaminophen and Pseudoephedrine . . . 31
Tylenol® Sore Throat [OTC] *see* Acetaminophen . . . 27
Tylenol® with Codeine *see* Acetaminophen and Codeine . . . 29
Tylex® *see* Acetaminophen . . . 27
Tylex 750 *see* Acetaminophen . . . 27
Tylex CD *see* Acetaminophen and Codeine . . . 29
Tylox® *see* Oxycodone and Acetaminophen . . . 1018
Typhim Vi® *see* Typhoid Vaccine . . . 1363
Typhoid Vaccine . . . 1363
Typhoid Vaccine Live Oral Ty21a *see* Typhoid Vaccine . . . 1363
Tyzine® *see* Tetrahydrozoline . . . 1288
Tyzine® Pediatric *see* Tetrahydrozoline . . . 1288
U-90152S *see* Delavirdine . . . 405
Ubiquinone *see* Coenzyme Q_{10} . . . 1427
UCB-P071 *see* Cetirizine . . . 289
UK 92480 *see* Sildenafil . . . 1220
UK109496 *see* Voriconazole . . . 1395
Ulcedin® *see* Ranitidine . . . 1168
Ulcedine *see* Cimetidine . . . 326
Ulcerease® [OTC] *see* Phenol . . . 1068
Ulgastrin Neo *see* Licorice . . . 1442
Ulpax® *see* Lansoprazole . . . 777
Ulsaven® *see* Ranitidine . . . 1168
Ulsen® *see* Omeprazole . . . 999
Ultiva® *see* Remifentanil . . . 1171
Ultracaine® DS *see* Articaine Hydrochloride and Epinephrine (Canada) . . . 124
Ultracaine® DS Forte *see* Articaine Hydrochloride and Epinephrine (Canada) . . . 124
Ultracef® *see* Ceftizoxime . . . 277
Ultracet™ *see* Acetaminophen and Tramadol . . . 32
Ultram® *see* Tramadol . . . 1329
Ultra Mide® *see* Urea . . . 1365
UltraMide 25™ *see* Urea . . . 1365
Ultramop™ *see* Methoxsalen . . . 888
Ultran® *see* Ranitidine . . . 1168
Ultraquin™ *see* Hydroquinone . . . 693
Ultrase® *see* Pancrelipase . . . 1030
Ultrase® MT *see* Pancrelipase . . . 1030
Ultra Tears® [OTC] *see* Artificial Tears . . . 128
Ultravate™ *see* Halobetasol . . . 658
Unamol *see* Cisapride . . . 332
Unasyn® *see* Ampicillin and Sulbactam . . . 104
Unasyna *see* Ampicillin and Sulbactam . . . 104
Unasyna Oral *see* Ampicillin and Sulbactam . . . 104
Uncaria tomentosa *see* Cat's Claw . . . 1424
Undecylenic Acid and Derivatives . . . 1365
Unidet® *see* Tolterodine . . . 1322
Uni-Dur® *see* Theophylline . . . 1291
Uni-Fed® [OTC] *see* Triprolidine and Pseudoephedrine . . . 1356
Unipen® *see* Nafcillin . . . 945
Uniphyl® *see* Theophylline . . . 1291
Uniphyl® SRT *see* Theophylline . . . 1291
Uniretic™ *see* Moexipril and Hydrochlorothiazide . . . 927
Unisom® Maximum Strength SleepGels® [OTC] *see* DiphenhydrAMINE . . . 451
Unithroid® *see* Levothyroxine . . . 800
Univasc® *see* Moexipril . . . 926
Univol® *see* Aluminum Hydroxide and Magnesium Hydroxide . . . 69
Unizuric 300 *see* Allopurinol . . . 57
Unna's Boot *see* Zinc Gelatin . . . 1409

Unna's Paste *see* Zinc Gelatin . . . 1409
Urasal® *see* Methenamine . . . 879
Urea . . . 1365
Urea and Hydrocortisone . . . 1365
Ureacin® [OTC] *see* Urea . . . 1365
Urea Peroxide *see* Carbamide Peroxide . . . 244
Ureaphil® [DSC] *see* Urea . . . 1365
Urecholine® *see* Bethanechol . . . 181
Uremol® *see* Urea . . . 1365
Uremol® HC *see* Urea and Hydrocortisone . . . 1365
Urex® *see* Methenamine . . . 879
Urimar-T *see* Methenamine, Sodium Biphosphate, Phenyl Salicylate, Methylene Blue, and Hyoscyamine . . . 880
Urimax® *see* Methenamine, Sodium Biphosphate, Phenyl Salicylate, Methylene Blue, and Hyoscyamine . . . 880
Urisec® *see* Urea . . . 1365
Urispas® *see* Flavoxate . . . 573
Uristat® [OTC] *see* Phenazopyridine . . . 1064
Urocit®-K *see* Potassium Citrate . . . 1100
Urocit®-K *see* Potassium Supplements . . . 1102
Urofollitropin *see* Follitropins . . . 607
Uro-KP-Neutral® *see* Phosphate Supplements . . . 1076
Uro-Mag® [OTC] *see* Magnesium Supplements . . . 837
Urovalidin *see* Phenazopyridine . . . 1064
Urso® *see* Ursodiol . . . 1366
Ursodeoxycholic Acid *see* Ursodiol . . . 1366
Ursodiol . . . 1366
Ursofalk® *see* Ursodiol . . . 1366
UTI Relief® [OTC] *see* Phenazopyridine . . . 1064
Utradol™ *see* Etodolac . . . 547
Utrogestan *see* Progesterone . . . 1125
Uvadex® *see* Methoxsalen . . . 888
Uva Ursi . . . 1449
Uvega® *see* Lidocaine . . . 801
Uvega *see* Lidocaine and Epinephrine . . . 804
Vaccinium macrocarpon *see* Cranberry . . . 1427
Vaccinium myrtillus *see* Bilberry . . . 1422
Vagifem® *see* Estradiol . . . 521
Vagi-Gard® [OTC] *see* Povidone-Iodine . . . 1104
Vagistat®-1 [OTC] *see* Tioconazole . . . 1312
Valacyclovir . . . 1367
Valacyclovir Hydrochloride *see* Valacyclovir . . . 1367
Valcyte™ *see* Valganciclovir . . . 1370
Valdecoxib . . . 1368
Valerian . . . 1449
Valeriana edulis *see* Valerian . . . 1449
Valeriana wallichi *see* Valerian . . . 1449
Valganciclovir . . . 1370
Valganciclovir Hydrochloride *see* Valganciclovir . . . 1370
Valisone® Scalp Lotion *see* Betamethasone . . . 177
Valium® *see* Diazepam . . . 424
Valorin [OTC] *see* Acetaminophen . . . 27
Valorin Extra [OTC] *see* Acetaminophen . . . 27
Valproate Semisodium *see* Valproic Acid and Derivatives . . . 1371
Valproate Sodium *see* Valproic Acid and Derivatives . . . 1371
Valproic Acid *see* Valproic Acid and Derivatives . . . 1371
Valproic Acid and Derivatives . . . 1371
Valprosid® *see* Valproic Acid and Derivatives . . . 1371
Valrubicin . . . 1374
Valsartan . . . 1374
Valsartan and Hydrochlorothiazide . . . 1375
Valstar® *see* Valrubicin . . . 1374
Valtaxin® *see* Valrubicin . . . 1374
Valtrex® *see* Valacyclovir . . . 1367
Valverde *see* Ginkgo Biloba . . . 1434
Vanadium . . . 1450
Vanamide™ *see* Urea . . . 1365
Vanatrip® *see* Amitriptyline . . . 83
Vancenase® AQ 84 mcg [DSC] *see* Beclomethasone . . . 163
Vancenase® Pockethaler® [DSC] *see* Beclomethasone . . . 163
Vanceril® *see* Beclomethasone . . . 163
Vancocin® *see* Vancomycin . . . 1376
Vancomycin . . . 1376
Vancomycin Hydrochloride *see* Vancomycin . . . 1376
Vaniqa™ *see* Eflornithine . . . 489
Vanmicina® *see* Vancomycin . . . 1376
Vanoxide-HC *see* Benzoyl Peroxide and Hydrocortisone . . . 172
Vanquish® Extra Strength Pain Reliever [OTC] *see* Acetaminophen, Aspirin, and Caffeine . . . 34
Van R Gingibraid® *see* Epinephrine (Racemic) and Aluminum Potassium Sulfate . . . 501
Vantin® *see* Cefpodoxime . . . 273
Vaponefrin® *see* Epinephrine (Racemic) . . . 500
VAQTA® *see* Hepatitis A Vaccine . . . 665
Varicella Virus Vaccine *see* Immunizations (Vaccines) . . . 1612
Varicella-Zoster Immune Globulin (Human) . . . 1378
Vasan *see* Ginkgo Biloba . . . 1434
Vascor® *see* Bepridil . . . 174
Vaseretic® *see* Enalapril and Hydrochlorothiazide . . . 494
Vasocidin® *see* Sulfacetamide and Prednisolone . . . 1250
VasoClear® [OTC] *see* Naphazoline . . . 952

Vasocon® *see* Naphazoline ... 952
Vasocon-A® *see* Naphazoline and Antazoline ... 952
Vasodilan® *see* Isoxsuprine ... 753
Vasofyl® *see* Pentoxifylline ... 1058
Vasopressin ... 1379
Vasopressin Tannate *see* Vasopressin ... 1379
Vasotec® *see* Enalapril ... 492
Vasotec® I.V. *see* Enalapril ... 492
Vatrix-S *see* Metronidazole ... 902
Vaxigrip® *see* Influenza Virus Vaccine ... 722
VCF™ [OTC] *see* Nonoxynol 9 ... 985
VCR *see* VinCRIStine ... 1387
V-Dec-M® *see* Guaifenesin and Pseudoephedrine ... 652
Vectrin® [DSC] *see* Minocycline ... 915
Veetids® *see* Penicillin V Potassium ... 1051
Veg-Pancreatin 4X [OTC] *see* Pancreatin ... 1030
Velban® *see* VinBLAStine ... 1386
Velosef® *see* Cephradine ... 288
Velosulin® BR (Buffered) *see* Insulin Preparations ... 723
Velsay *see* Naproxen ... 953
Venlafaxine ... 1380
Venofer® *see* Iron Sucrose ... 744
Venoglobulin®-S *see* Immune Globulin (Intravenous) ... 714
Ventisol® *see* Ketotifen ... 768
Ventolin® *see* Albuterol ... 48
Ventolin® Diskus *see* Albuterol ... 48
Ventolin® HFA *see* Albuterol ... 48
Ventrodisk *see* Albuterol ... 48
VePesid® *see* Etoposide ... 549
Veracef *see* Cephradine ... 288
Veraken *see* Verapamil ... 1382
Verapamil ... 1382
Verapamil and Trandolapril *see* Trandolapril and Verapamil ... 1332
Verapamil Hydrochloride *see* Verapamil ... 1382
Verdilac *see* Verapamil ... 1382
Verelan® *see* Verapamil ... 1382
Verelan® PM *see* Verapamil ... 1382
Vermicol® *see* Mebendazole ... 846
Vermidil® *see* Mebendazole ... 846
Vermin® *see* Mebendazole ... 846
Vermox® *see* Mebendazole ... 846
Verr-Canth™ *see* Cantharidin ... 234
Versacaps® *see* Guaifenesin and Pseudoephedrine ... 652
Versed® [DSC] *see* Midazolam ... 908
Versiclear™ *see* Sodium Thiosulfate ... 1233
Vertisal® *see* Metronidazole ... 902
Vesanoid® *see* Tretinoin (Oral) ... 1338
Vexol® *see* Rimexolone ... 1185
VFEND® *see* Voriconazole ... 1395
Viadur® *see* Leuprolide ... 784
Viagra® *see* Sildenafil ... 1220
Vibramicina® *see* Doxycycline ... 476
Vibramycin® *see* Doxycycline ... 476
Vibra-Tabs® *see* Doxycycline ... 476
Vicks® 44® Cough Relief [OTC] *see* Dextromethorphan ... 423
Vicks® 44D Cough & Head Congestion [OTC] *see* Pseudoephedrine and Dextromethorphan ... 1147
Vicks® 44E [OTC] *see* Guaifenesin and Dextromethorphan ... 651
Vicks® DayQuil® Cold and Flu Non-Drowsy [OTC] *see* Acetaminophen, Dextromethorphan, and Pseudoephedrine ... 35
Vicks® Pediatric Formula 44E [OTC] *see* Guaifenesin and Dextromethorphan ... 651
Vicks Sinex® 12 Hour Ultrafine Mist [OTC] *see* Oxymetazoline ... 1022
Vicks® Sinex® Nasal Spray [OTC] *see* Phenylephrine ... 1071
Vicks® Sinex® UltraFine Mist [OTC] *see* Phenylephrine ... 1071
Vicodin® *see* Hydrocodone and Acetaminophen ... 678
Vicodin® ES *see* Hydrocodone and Acetaminophen ... 678
Vicodin® HP *see* Hydrocodone and Acetaminophen ... 678
Vicodin Tuss® *see* Hydrocodone and Guaifenesin ... 683
Vicon Forte® *see* Vitamins (Multiple/Oral) ... 1394
Vicon Plus® [OTC] *see* Vitamins (Multiple/Oral) ... 1394
Vicoprofen® *see* Hydrocodone and Ibuprofen ... 684
Vidarabine ... 1384
Vidarabine Monohydrate *see* Vidarabine ... 1384
Vi-Daylin® + Iron Liquid [OTC] *see* Vitamins (Multiple/Oral) ... 1394
Vi-Daylin® Liquid [OTC] *see* Vitamins (Multiple/Oral) ... 1394
Videx® *see* Didanosine ... 434
Videx® EC *see* Didanosine ... 434
Vigabatrin ... 1385
Viken® *see* Cefotaxime ... 271
Vilona® *see* Ribavirin ... 1176
Vilona Pediatrica *see* Ribavirin ... 1176
VinBLAStine ... 1386
Vinblastine Sulfate *see* VinBLAStine ... 1386
Vincaleukoblastine *see* VinBLAStine ... 1386
Vincasar PFS® *see* VinCRIStine ... 1387
VinCRIStine ... 1387
Vincristine Sulfate *see* VinCRIStine ... 1387
Vinorelbine ... 1389
Vinorelbine Tartrate *see* Vinorelbine ... 1389
Vintec® *see* VinCRIStine ... 1387

Viokase® *see* Pancrelipase 1030
Viosterol *see* Ergocalciferol 508
Vioxx® *see* Rofecoxib 1194
Vira-A® [DSC] *see* Vidarabine 1384
Viracept® *see* Nelfinavir 959
Viramune® *see* Nevirapine 965
Virazide® *see* Ribavirin 1176
Virazole® *see* Ribavirin 1176
Viread™ *see* Tenofovir 1275
Virilon® *see* MethylTESTOSTERone 897
Virilon® IM *see* Testosterone 1281
Virlix® *see* Cetirizine 289
Viroptic® *see* Trifluridine 1350
Viscoat® *see* Chondroitin Sulfate and Sodium Hyaluronate 320
Visicol™ *see* Phosphate Supplements 1076
Visine® *see* Tetrahydrozoline 1288
Visine-A™ [OTC] *see* Naphazoline and Pheniramine 953
Visine A.D.® *see* Oxymetazoline 1022
Visine® Advanced Relief [OTC] *see* Tetrahydrozoline 1288
Visine® L.R. [OTC] *see* Oxymetazoline 1022
Visine® Original [OTC] *see* Tetrahydrozoline 1288
Visken® *see* Pindolol 1085
Vistaril® *see* HydrOXYzine 697
Vistide® *see* Cidofovir 323
Vi-Syneral *see* Vitamins (Multiple/Oral) 1394
Vita 3B *see* Vitamin B Complex 1392
Vita 3B+C *see* Vitamin B Complex and Vitamin C 1392
Vita-C® [OTC] *see* Ascorbic Acid 128
Vitacon Forte *see* Vitamins (Multiple/Oral) 1394
Vital *see* Ginkgo Biloba 1434
Vitamin A 1390
Vitamin A Acid *see* Tretinoin (Topical) 1340
Vitamin A and Vitamin D 1392
Vitamin B_1 *see* Thiamine 1295
Vitamin B_2 *see* Riboflavin 1178
Vitamin B_3 *see* Niacin 967
Vitamin B_3 *see* Niacinamide 968
Vitamin B_5 *see* Pantothenic Acid 1033
Vitamin B_6 *see* Pyridoxine 1152
Vitamin B_{12} *see* Cyanocobalamin 377
Vitamin B_{12} *see* Hydroxocobalamin 693
Vitamin B Complex 1392
Vitamin B Complex and Vitamin C 1392
Vitamin B Complex Combination Products 1640
Vitamin B Complex, Vitamin C, and Folic Acid 1393
Vitamin C *see* Ascorbic Acid 128
Vitamin D_2 *see* Ergocalciferol 508
Vitamin E 1393
Vitamin G *see* Riboflavin 1178
Vitamin K_1 *see* Phytonadione 1079
Vitamins (Multiple/Oral) 1394
Vitamins, Multiple (Oral) *see* Vitamins (Multiple/Oral) 1394
Vitamins, Multiple (Therapeutic) *see* Vitamins (Multiple/Oral) 1394
Vitamins, Multiple With Iron *see* Vitamins (Multiple/Oral) 1394
Vitelle™ Irospan® [OTC] *see* Ferrous Sulfate and Ascorbic Acid 569
Viternum® *see* Cyproheptadine 387
Vitex agnus-castus *see* Chasteberry 1426
Vitis vinifera *see* Grape Seed 1439
Vitrasert® *see* Ganciclovir 626
Vitravene™ *see* Fomivirsen 611
Vitrax® *see* Sodium Hyaluronate 1230
Vitussin *see* Hydrocodone and Guaifenesin 683
Vivactil® *see* Protriptyline 1145
Viva-Drops® [OTC] *see* Artificial Tears 128
Vivelle® *see* Estradiol 521
Vivelle-Dot® *see* Estradiol 521
Vivotif Berna® *see* Typhoid Vaccine 1363
VLB *see* VinBLAStine 1386
VM-26 *see* Teniposide 1274
Volfenac Gel® *see* Diclofenac 429
Volfenac Retard® *see* Diclofenac 429
Volmax® *see* Albuterol 48
Voltaren® *see* Diclofenac 429
Voltaren Emulgel® *see* Diclofenac 429
Voltaren Ophtha® *see* Diclofenac 429
Voltaren Ophthalmic® *see* Diclofenac 429
Voltaren Rapide® *see* Diclofenac 429
Voltaren®-XR *see* Diclofenac 429
Vomisin® *see* DimenhyDRINATE 449
Voriconazole 1395
VõSol® HC *see* Acetic Acid, Propylene Glycol Diacetate, and Hydrocortisone 38
VoSpire ER™ *see* Albuterol 48
VP-16 *see* Etoposide 549
VP-16-213 *see* Etoposide 549
Vp-Tec® *see* Etoposide 549
Vumon® *see* Teniposide 1274
V.V.S.® *see* Sulfabenzamide, Sulfacetamide, and Sulfathiazole 1249
Vytone® *see* Iodoquinol and Hydrocortisone 736
VZIG *see* Varicella-Zoster Immune Globulin (Human) 1378
Warfarin 1397

Warfarin Sodium *see* Warfarin 1397
Wartec® *see* Podofilox 1093
Wart-Off® Maximum Strength [OTC] *see* Salicylic Acid 1204
4-Way® Long Acting [OTC] *see* Oxymetazoline 1022
Waytrax *see* Ceftazidime 275
WelChol™ *see* Colesevelam 365
Wellbutrin® *see* BuPROPion 209
Wellbutrin SR® *see* BuPROPion 209
Wesmycin® *see* Tetracycline 1286
Westcort® *see* Hydrocortisone 688
Westhroid® *see* Thyroid 1303
Whitehorn *see* Hawthorn 1440
Whole Root Rauwolfia *see* Rauwolfia Serpentina 1170
Wigraine® *see* Ergotamine 510
Wild Quinine *see* Feverfew 1431
Wild Yam 1450
Winasorb *see* Acetaminophen 27
Winpred™ *see* PredniSONE 1112
WinRho SDF® *see* Rh_o(D) Immune Globulin 1175
Winstrol® *see* Stanozolol 1241
Wound Wash Saline™ [OTC] *see* Sodium Chloride 1229
WR-139013 *see* Chlorambucil 296
Wycillin® *see* Penicillin G Procaine 1050
Wytensin® *see* Guanabenz 654
Xalatan® *see* Latanoprost 778
Xalyn-Or® *see* Amoxicillin 93
Xanax® *see* Alprazolam 61
Xanax TS™ *see* Alprazolam 61
Xanax XR® *see* Alprazolam 61
Xeloda® *see* Capecitabine 235
Xenical® *see* Orlistat 1004
Xigris® *see* Drotrecogin Alfa 483
Xitocin® *see* Oxytocin 1026
Xopenex® *see* Levalbuterol 786
X-Prep® [OTC] *see* Senna 1215
X-Seb™ T [OTC] *see* Coal Tar and Salicylic Acid 359
Xylocaina® *see* Lidocaine 801
Xylocaina *see* Lidocaine and Epinephrine 804
Xylocaine® *see* Lidocaine 801
Xylocaine® MPF *see* Lidocaine 801
Xylocaine® MPF With Epinephrine *see* Lidocaine and Epinephrine 804
Xylocaine® Viscous *see* Lidocaine 801
Xylocaine® With Epinephrine *see* Lidocaine and Epinephrine 804
Xylocard® *see* Lidocaine 801
Xylometazoline 1401
Xylometazoline Hydrochloride *see* Xylometazoline 1401
Xyrem® *see* Sodium Oxybate 1231
Y-90 Zevalin *see* Ibritumomab 702
Yasmin® *see* Combination Hormonal Contraceptives 368
Yectamicina® *see* Gentamicin 634
Yectamid® *see* Amikacin 74
Yellow Fever Vaccine *see* Immunizations (Vaccines) 1612
Yellow Indian Paint *see* Golden Seal 1437
Yellow Mercuric Oxide *see* Mercuric Oxide 867
Yellow Root *see* Golden Seal 1437
Yocon® *see* Yohimbine 1401
Yodine® *see* Povidone-Iodine 1104
Yodoxin® *see* Iodoquinol 735
Yohimbe 1451
Yohimbehe cortex *see* Yohimbe 1451
Yohimbine 1401
Yohimbine Hydrochloride *see* Yohimbine 1401
Zaditen® *see* Ketotifen 768
Zaditor™ *see* Ketotifen 768
Zafimida® *see* Furosemide 622
Zafirlukast 1402
Zagam® *see* Sparfloxacin 1238
Zalcitabine 1403
Zaleplon 1404
Zamacort® *see* Triamcinolone 1341
Zamtirel *see* Salmeterol 1205
Zanaflex® *see* Tizanidine 1314
Zanamivir 1405
Zanosar® *see* Streptozocin 1246
Zantac® *see* Ranitidine 1168
Zantac 75® *see* Ranitidine 1168
Zapzyt® [OTC] *see* Benzoyl Peroxide 171
Zapzyt® Acne Wash [OTC] *see* Salicylic Acid 1204
Zapzyt® Pore Treatment [OTC] *see* Salicylic Acid 1204
Zarontin® *see* Ethosuximide 543
Zaroxolyn® *see* Metolazone 900
ZDV *see* Zidovudine 1406
ZDV, Abacavir, and Lamivudine *see* Abacavir, Lamivudine, and Zidovudine 23
Zeasorb®-AF [OTC] *see* Miconazole 906
Zebeta® *see* Bisoprolol 188
Zelnorm™ *see* Tegaserod 1268
Zemplar™ *see* Paricalcitol 1034
Zenapax® *see* Daclizumab 392
Zentel® *see* Albendazole 47
Zephiran® [OTC] *see* Benzalkonium Chloride 169

Zephrex® *see* Guaifenesin and Pseudoephedrine 652
Zephrex LA® *see* Guaifenesin and Pseudoephedrine 652
Zerit® *see* Stavudine 1242
Zestoretic® *see* Lisinopril and Hydrochlorothiazide 814
Zestril® *see* Lisinopril 813
Zetar® *see* Coal Tar 359
Zetia™ *see* Ezetimibe 553
Zevalin™ *see* Ibritumomab 702
Ziac™ *see* Bisoprolol and Hydrochlorothiazide 189
Ziagen® *see* Abacavir 22
Zidovudine 1406
Zidovudine, Abacavir, and Lamivudine *see* Abacavir, Lamivudine, and Zidovudine 23
Zidovudine and Lamivudine 1407
Zilactin® *see* Lidocaine 801
Zilactin®-B [OTC] *see* Benzocaine 169
Zilactin® Baby [OTC] *see* Benzocaine 169
Zilactin-L® [OTC] *see* Lidocaine 801
Zileuton 1408
Zinacef® *see* Cefuroxime 279
Zinc *see* Trace Metals 1328
Zinc Acetate *see* Zinc Supplements 1410
Zinc Chloride 1409
Zincfrin® [OTC] *see* Phenylephrine and Zinc Sulfate 1073
Zinc Gelatin 1409
Zinc Gelatin Boot *see* Zinc Gelatin 1409
Zincofax® *see* Zinc Oxide 1409
Zincon® [OTC] *see* Pyrithione Zinc 1154
Zinc Oxide 1409
Zinc Sulfate *see* Zinc Supplements 1410
Zinc Sulfate and Phenylephrine *see* Phenylephrine and Zinc Sulfate 1073
Zinc Supplements 1410
Zinc Undecylenate *see* Undecylenic Acid and Derivatives 1365
Zinecard® *see* Dexrazoxane 419
Zingiber officinale see Ginger 1434
Zinnat® *see* Cefuroxime 279
Zipra® *see* Ciprofloxacin 328
Zithromax® *see* Azithromycin 153
Z-Max® *see* Phentolamine 1070
ZNP® Bar [OTC] *see* Pyrithione Zinc 1154
ZNP Shampoo® *see* Pyrithione Zinc 1154
Zocor® *see* Simvastatin 1223
Zofran® *see* Ondansetron 1000
Zofran® ODT *see* Ondansetron 1000
Zoladex® *see* Goserelin 647
Zoladex® LA *see* Goserelin 647
Zoldan-A *see* Danazol 397
Zoledronate *see* Zoledronic Acid 1410
Zoledronic Acid 1410
Zolmitriptan 1411
Zoloft® *see* Sertraline 1216
Zolpidem 1413
Zolpidem Tartrate *see* Zolpidem 1413
Zometa® *see* Zoledronic Acid 1410
Zomig® *see* Zolmitriptan 1411
Zomig® Rapimelt *see* Zolmitriptan 1411
Zomig-ZMT™ *see* Zolmitriptan 1411
Zonal® *see* Fluconazole 576
Zonalon *see* Doxepin 471
Zone-A® *see* Pramoxine and Hydrocortisone 1106
Zone-A Forte® *see* Pramoxine and Hydrocortisone 1106
Zonegran® *see* Zonisamide 1413
Zonisamide 1413
Zopiclone 1415
Zorbenal-G *see* Tetracycline 1286
ZORprin® *see* Aspirin 131
Zostrix® *see* Capsaicin 238
Zostrix® H.P. *see* Capsaicin 238
Zosyn® *see* Piperacillin and Tazobactam Sodium 1088
Zovia™ *see* Combination Hormonal Contraceptives 368
Zovirax® *see* Acyclovir 42
Zovirax I.V.® *see* Acyclovir 42
Zurcal® *see* Pantoprazole 1031
Zyban® *see* BuPROPion 209
Zydone® *see* Hydrocodone and Acetaminophen 678
Zyflo™ *see* Zileuton 1408
Zyloprim® *see* Allopurinol 57
Zymase® [DSC] *see* Pancrelipase 1030
Zymerol *see* Cimetidine 326
Zyprexa® *see* Olanzapine 996
Zyprexa® Zydis® *see* Olanzapine 996
Zyrtec® *see* Cetirizine 289
Zyrtec-D 12 Hour™ *see* Cetirizine and Pseudoephedrine 290
Zyvox™ *see* Linezolid 809
Zyvoxam® *see* Linezolid 809

NOTES

NOTES

NOTES

NOTES

NOTES

NOTES

NOTES

NOTES

NOTES

NOTES

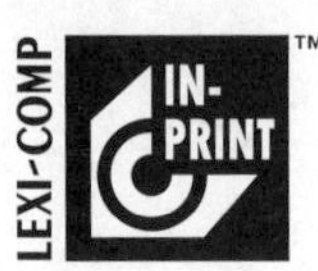

Other books offered by LEXI-COMP

DRUG INFORMATION HANDBOOK (International edition available)

by Charles Lacy, RPh, PharmD, FCSHP; Lora L. Armstrong, RPh, PharmD, BCPS; Morton P. Goldman, PharmD, BCPS; and Leonard L. Lance, RPh, BSPharm

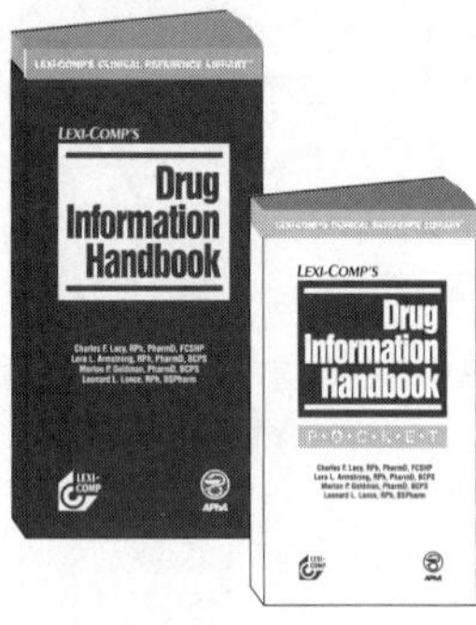

Specifically compiled and designed for the healthcare professional requiring quick access to concisely-stated comprehensive data concerning clinical use of medications.

The Drug Information Handbook is an ideal portable drug information resource, providing the reader with up to 34 key points of data concerning clinical use and dosing of the medication. Material provided in the Appendix section is recognized by many users to be, by itself, well worth the purchase of the handbook.

All medications found in the *Drug Information Handbook,* are included in the abridged *Pocket* edition (select fields were extracted to maintain portability).

PEDIATRIC DOSAGE HANDBOOK (International edition available)

by Carol K. Taketomo, PharmD; Jane Hurlburt Hodding, PharmD; and Donna M. Kraus, PharmD

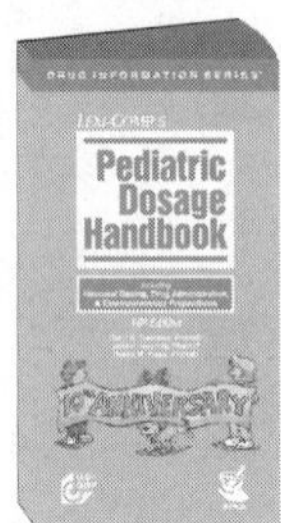

Special considerations must frequently be taken into account when dosing medications for the pediatric patient. This highly regarded quick reference handbook is a compilation of recommended pediatric doses based on current literature, as well as the practical experience of the authors and their many colleagues who work every day in the pediatric clinical setting.

Includes neonatal dosing, drug administration, and (in select monographs) extemporaneous preparations for medications used in pediatric medicine.

GERIATRIC DOSAGE HANDBOOK

by Todd P. Semla, PharmD, BCPS, FCCP; Judith L. Beizer, PharmD, FASCP; and Martin D. Higbee, PharmD, CGP

2000 "Book of the Year" — *American Journal of Nursing*

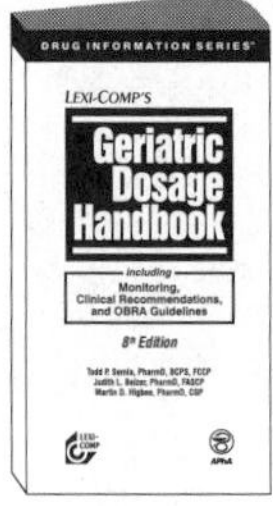

Many physiologic changes occur with aging, some of which affect the pharmacokinetics or pharmacodynamics of medications. Strong consideration should also be given to the effect of decreased renal or hepatic functions in the elderly, as well as the probability of the geriatric patient being on multiple drug regimens.

Healthcare professionals working with nursing homes and assisted living facilities will find the drug information contained in this handbook to be an invaluable source of helpful information.

An International Brand Name Index with names from 58 different countries is also included.

To order call toll free anywhere in the U.S.: 1-800-837-LEXI (5394)

Outside of the U.S. call: 330-650-6506 or online at www.lexi.com

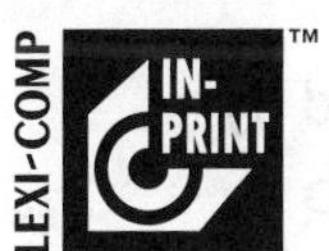

Other books offered by LEXI-COMP

DRUG INFORMATION HANDBOOK FOR THE ALLIED HEALTH PROFESSIONAL

by Leonard L. Lance, RPh, BSPharm; Charles Lacy, RPh, PharmD, FCSHP; Lora L. Armstrong, RPh, PharmD, BCPS; and Morton P. Goldman, PharmD, BCPS

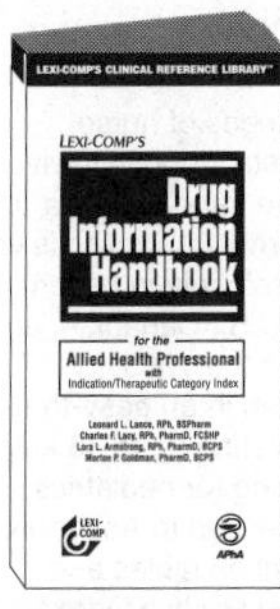

Working with clinical pharmacists, hospital pharmacy and therapeutics committees, and hospital drug information centers, the authors have assisted hundreds of hospitals in developing institution-specific formulary reference documentation.

The most current basic drug and medication data from those clinical settings have been reviewed, coalesced, and cross-referenced to create this unique handbook. The handbook offers quick access to abbreviated monographs for generic drugs.

This is a great tool for physician assistants, medical records personnel, medical transcriptionists and secretaries, pharmacy technicians, and other allied health professionals.

NATURAL THERAPEUTICS POCKET GUIDE

by Daniel L. Krinsky, RPh, MS; James B. LaValle, RPh, DHM, NMD, CCN; Ernest B. Hawkins, RPh, MS; Ross Pelton, RPh, PhD, CCN; Nancy Ashbrook Willis, BA, JD

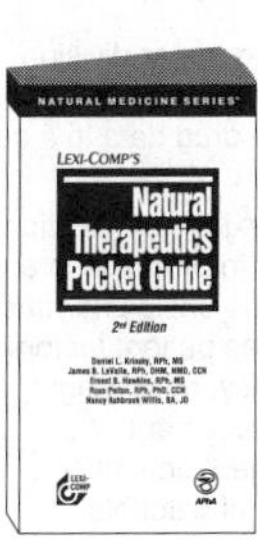

Provides condition-specific information on common uses of natural therapies. Each condition discussed includes the following: review of condition, decision tree, list of commonly recommended herbals, nutritional supplements, homeopathic remedies, lifestyle modifications, and special considerations.

Provides herbal/nutritional/nutraceutical monographs with over 10 fields including references, reported uses, dosage, pharmacology, toxicity, warnings & interactions, and cautions & contraindications.

The Appendix includes: drug-nutrient depletion, herb-drug interactions, drug-nutrient interaction, herbal medicine use in pediatrics, unsafe herbs, and reference of top herbals.

DRUG-INDUCED NUTRIENT DEPLETION HANDBOOK

by Ross Pelton, RPh, PhD, CCN; James B. LaValle, RPh, DHM, NMD, CCN; Ernest B. Hawkins, RPh, MS; Daniel L. Krinsky, RPh, MS

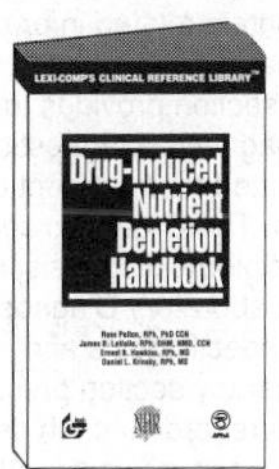

A complete and up-to-date listing of all drugs known to deplete the body of nutritional compounds.

This book is alphabetically organized and provides extensive cross-referencing to related information in the various sections of the book. Drug monographs identify the nutrients depleted and provide cross-references to the nutrient monographs for more detailed information on Effects of Depletion, Biological Function & Effect, Side Effects & Toxicity, RDA, Dosage Range, and Dietary Sources. This book also contains a Studies & Abstracts section, a valuable Appendix, and Alphabetical & Pharmacological Indexes.

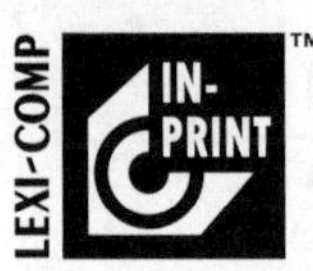

Other books offered by LEXI-COMP

DRUG INFORMATION HANDBOOK FOR ADVANCED PRACTICE NURSING

by Beatrice B. Turkoski, RN, PhD; Brenda R. Lance, RN, MSN; and Mark F. Bonfiglio, PharmD
Foreword by: Margaret A. Fitzgerald, MS, RN, CS-FNP

1999 "Book of the Year" — *American Journal of Nursing*
Advanced Practice Nursing Category

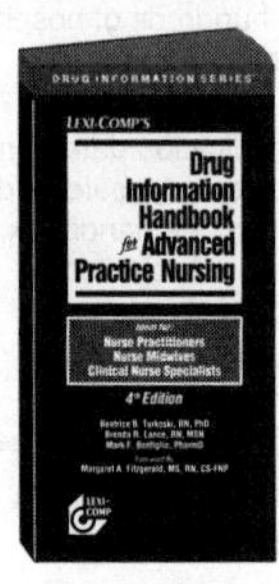

Designed specifically to meet the needs of nurse practitioners, clinical nurse specialists, nurse midwives, and graduate nursing students. The handbook is a unique resource for detailed, accurate information, which is vital to support the advanced practice nurse's role in patient drug therapy management. Over 4750 U.S., Canadian, and Mexican medications are covered in the 1000 monographs. Drug data is presented in an easy-to-use, alphabetically organized format covering up to 46 key points of information (including dosing for pediatrics, adults, and geriatrics). Cross-referenced to Appendix of over 230 pages of valuable comparison tables and additional information. Also included are two indexes, Pharmacologic Category and Controlled Substance, which facilitate comparison between agents.

DRUG INFORMATION HANDBOOK FOR NURSING

by Beatrice B. Turkoski, RN, PhD; Brenda R. Lance, RN, MSN; and Mark F. Bonfiglio, PharmD

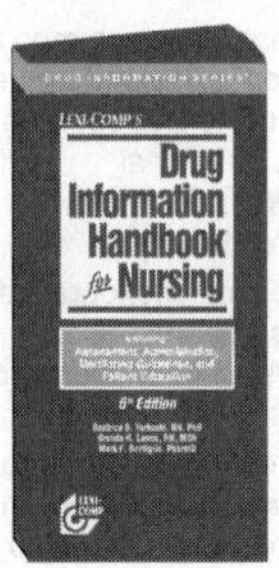

Registered Professional Nurses and upper-division nursing students involved with drug therapy will find this handbook provides quick access to drug data in a concise easy-to-use format.

Over 4000 U.S., Canadian, and Mexican medications are covered with up to 43 key points of information in each monograph. The handbook contains basic pharmacology concepts and nursing issues such as patient factors that influence drug therapy (ie, pregnancy, age, weight, etc) and general nursing issues (ie, assessment, administration, monitoring, and patient education). The Appendix contains over 230 pages of valuable information.

INFECTIOUS DISEASES HANDBOOK

by Carlos M. Isada, MD; Bernard L. Kasten Jr., MD; Morton P. Goldman, PharmD; Larry D. Gray, PhD; and Judith A. Aberg, MD

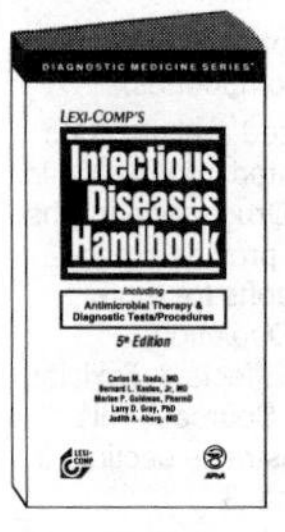

A four-in-one quick reference concerned with the identification and treatment of infectious diseases. Each of the four sections of the book contain related information and cross-referencing to one or more of the other three sections. The Disease Syndrome section provides the clinical presentation, differential diagnosis, diagnostic tests, and drug therapy recommended for treatment of more common infectious diseases. The Organism section presents the microbiology, epidemiology, diagnosis, and treatment of each organism. The Laboratory Diagnosis section describes performance of specific tests and procedures. The Antimicrobial Therapy section presents important facts and considerations regarding each drug recommended for specific diseases of organisms. Also contains an International Brand Name Index with names from 58 different countries.

To order call toll free anywhere in the U.S.: 1-800-837-LEXI (5394)

Outside of the U.S. call: 330-650-6506 or online at www.lexi.com

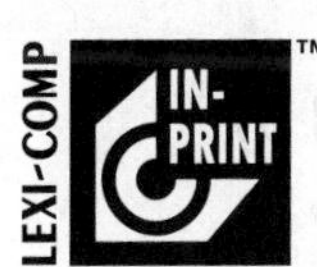

Other books offered by LEXI-COMP

ANESTHESIOLOGY & CRITICAL CARE DRUG HANDBOOK

by Andrew J. Donnelly, PharmD; Francesca E. Cunningham, PharmD; and Verna L. Baughman, MD

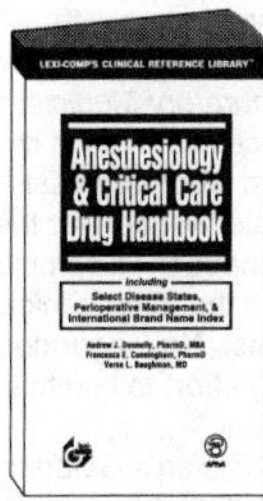

Contains the most commonly used drugs in the perioperative and critical care setting. This handbook also contains the following Special Issues and Topics: Allergic Reaction, Anesthesia for Cardiac Patients in Noncardiac Surgery, Anesthesia for Obstetric Patients in Nonobstetric Surgery, Anesthesia for Patients With Liver Disease, Chronic Pain Management, Chronic Renal Failure, Conscious Sedation, Perioperative Management of Patients on Antiseizure Medication, and Substance Abuse and Anesthesia.

The Appendix includes Abbreviations & Measurements, Anesthesiology Information, Assessment of Liver & Renal Function, Comparative Drug Charts, Infectious Disease-Prophylaxis & Treatment, Laboratory Values, Therapy Recommendations, Toxicology information, *and much more.*

International Brand Name Index with names from over 58 different countries is also included.

DRUG INFORMATION HANDBOOK FOR ONCOLOGY

by Dominic A. Solimando, Jr, MA; Linda R. Bressler, PharmD, BCOP; Polly E. Kintzel, PharmD, BCPS, BCOP; and Mark C. Geraci, PharmD, BCOP

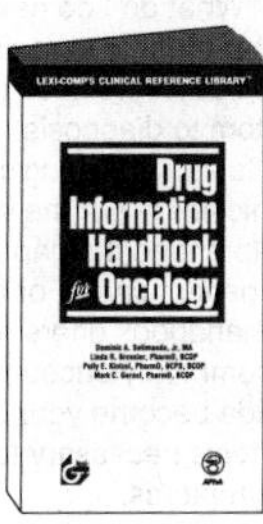

Presented in a concise and uniform format, this book contains the most comprehensive collection of oncology-related drug information available. Organized like a dictionary for ease of use, drugs can be found by looking up the *brand or generic name*!

This book contains individual monographs for both Antineoplastic Agents and Ancillary Medications.

The fields of information per monograph include: Use, U.S. Investigational, Bone Marrow/Blood Cell Transplantation, Vesicant, Emetic Potential. A Special Topics Section, Appendix, and Therapeutic Category & Key Word Index are valuable features to this book, as well.

DIAGNOSTIC PROCEDURE HANDBOOK by Frank Michota, MD

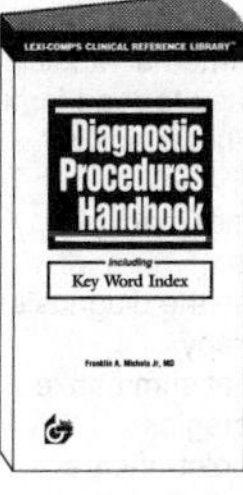

A comprehensive, yet concise, quick reference source for physicians, nurses, students, medical records personnel, or anyone needing quick access to diagnostic procedure information. This handbook is an excellent source of information in the following areas: allergy, rheumatology, and infectious disease; cardiology; computed tomography; diagnostic radiology; gastroenterology; invasive radiology; magnetic resonance imaging; nephrology, urology, and hematology; neurology; nuclear medicine; pulmonary function; pulmonary medicine and critical care; ultrasound; and women's health.

To order call toll free anywhere in the U.S.: 1-800-837-LEXI (5394)

Outside of the U.S. call: 330-650-6506 or online at www.lexi.com

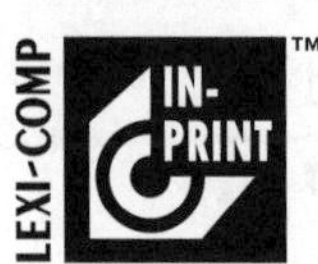

Other books offered by LEXI-COMP

CLINICIAN'S GUIDE TO LABORATORY MEDICINE —A Practical Approach

by Samir P. Desai, MD and Sana Isa-Pratt, MD

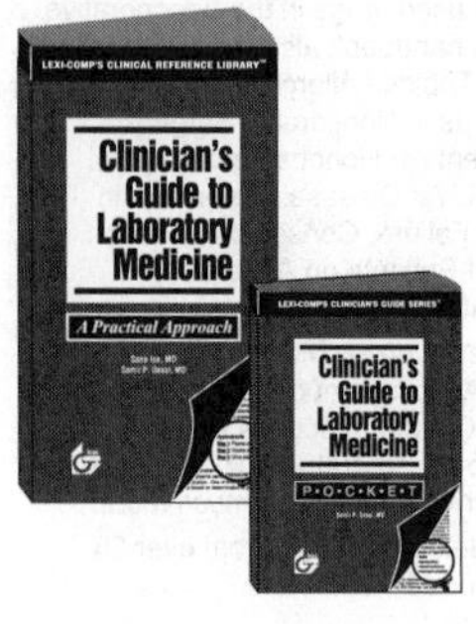

When faced with the patient presenting with abnormal laboratory tests, the clinician can now turn to the *Clinician's Guide to Laboratory Medicine: A Practical Approach.* This source is unique in its ability to lead the clinician from laboratory test abnormality to clinical diagnosis. Written for the busy clinician, this concise handbook will provide rapid answers to the questions that busy clinicians face in the care of their patients. No longer does the clinician have to struggle in an effort to find this information - *it's all here.*
Included is a **FREE** copy of *Clinician's Guide to Laboratory Medicine - Pocket.* Great to carry in your pocket! Perfect for use *"in the trenches".*

CLINICIAN'S GUIDE TO DIAGNOSIS—A Practical Approach

by Samir Desai, MD

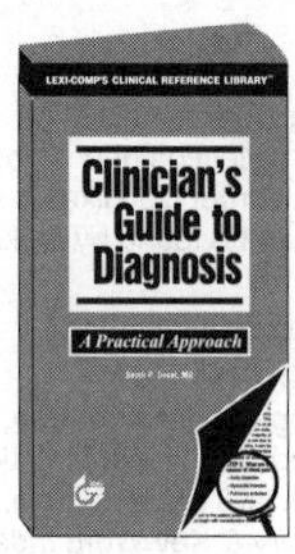

Symptoms are what prompt patients to seek medical care. In the evaluation of a patient's symptom, it is not unusual for healthcare professionals to ask "What do I do next?" This is precisely the question for which the *Clinician's Guide to Diagnosis: A Practical Approach* provides the answer. It will lead you from symptom to diagnosis through a series of steps designed to mimic the logical thought processes of seasoned clinicians. For the young clinician, this is an ideal book to help bridge the gap between the classroom and actual patient care. For the experienced clinician, this concise handbook offers rapid answers to the questions that are commonly encountered on a day-to-day basis. Let this guide become your companion, providing you with the tools necessary to tackle even the most challenging symptoms.

CLINICIAN'S GUIDE TO INTERNAL MEDICINE —A Practical Approach

by Samir P. Desai, MD

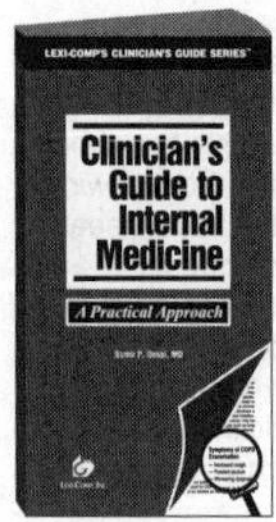

Provides quick access to essential information covering diagnosis, treatment, and management of commonly encountered patient problems in Internal Medicine.

- Up-to-date information in an easy-to-read format
- Clinically relevant information that is easily accessible
- Practical approaches that are not readily available in standard textbooks
- Algorithms to help you establish the diagnosis and select the appropriate therapy
- Numerous tables and boxes that summarize diagnostic and therapeutic strategies
- Ideal reference for use at the point-of-care

This is a reference companion that will provide you with the tools necessary to tackle even the most challenging problems in Internal Medicine.

To order call toll free anywhere in the U.S.: 1-800-837-LEXI (5394)

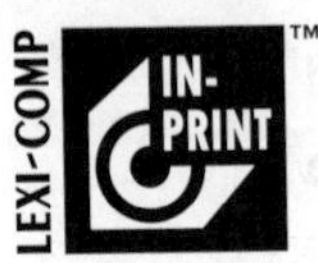

Other books offered by LEXI-COMP

DRUG INFORMATION HANDBOOK FOR PSYCHIATRY

by Matthew A. Fuller, PharmD and Martha Sajatovic, MD

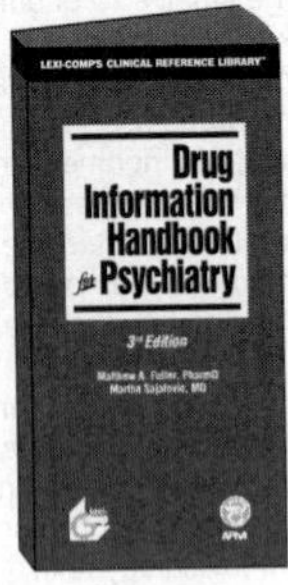

The source for comprehensive and clinically relevant drug information for the mental health professional. Alphabetically arranged by generic and brand name for ease-of-use. There are up to 35 key fields of information including these unique fields: "Effect on Mental Status" and "Effect on Psychiatric Treatment". A special topics/issues section includes psychiatric assessment, major psychiatric disorders, major classes of psychotropic medications, psychiatric emergencies, special populations, enhanced patient education information section, and DSM-IV classification. Also contains a valuable appendix section, Pharmacologic Index, and Alphabetical Index.

RATING SCALES IN MENTAL HEALTH

by Martha Sajatovic, MD and Luis F. Ramirez, MD

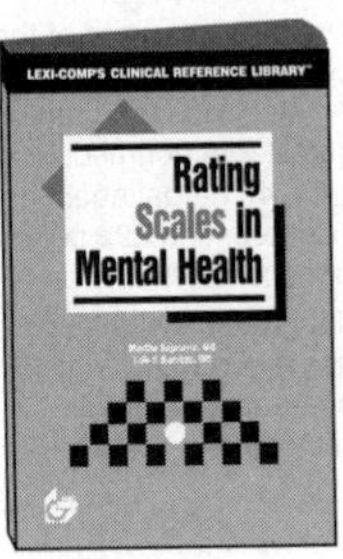

A basic guide to the rating scales in mental health, this is an ideal reference for psychiatrists, nurses, residents, psychologists, social workers, healthcare administrators, behavioral healthcare organizations, and outcome committees. It is designed to assist clinicians in determining the appropriate rating scale when assessing their client. A general concepts section provides text discussion on the use and history of rating scales, statistical evaluation, rating scale domains, and two clinical vignettes. Information on over 80 rating scales used in mental health organized in 6 categories. Appendix contains tables and charts in a quick reference format allowing clinicians to rapidly identify categories and characteristics of rating scales.

PSYCHOTROPIC DRUG INFORMATION HANDBOOK

by Matthew A. Fuller, PharmD and Martha Sajatovic, MD

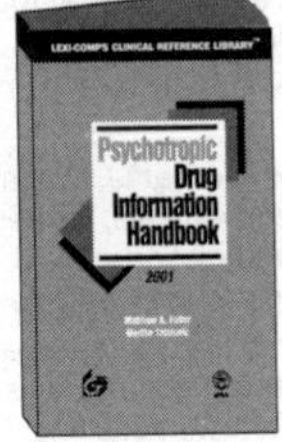

This portable, yet comprehensive guide to psychotropic drugs provides healthcare professionals with detailed information on use, drug interactions, pregnancy risk factors, warnings/precautions, adverse reactions, mechanism of action, and contraindications. Alphabetically organized by brand and generic name this concise handbook provides quick access to the information you need and includes patient education sheets on the psychotropic medications. It is the perfect pocket companion to the *Drug Information for Psychiatry*.

To order call toll free anywhere in the U.S.: 1-800-837-LEXI (5394)

Outside of the U.S. call: 330-650-6506 or online at www.lexi.com

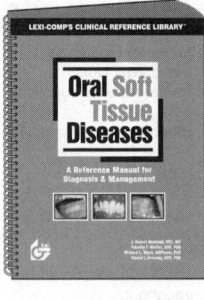

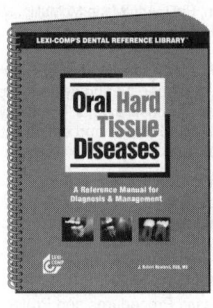

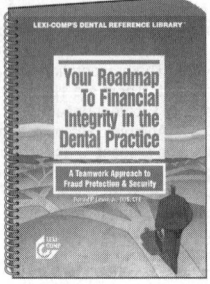

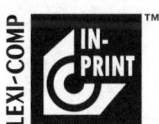

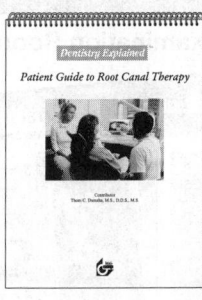

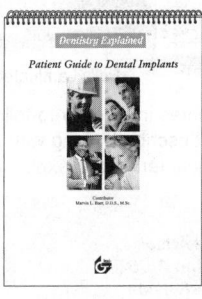

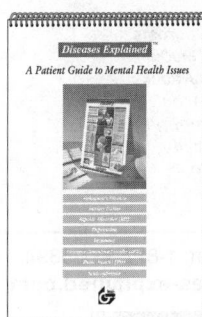

LEXI-COMP ON-HAND™

SOFTWARE LIBRARY

For Palm OS® and
Windows™ Powered Pocket PC Devices

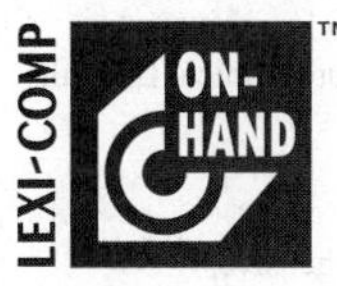

Lexi-Comp's handheld software solutions provide quick, portable access to clinical information needed at the point-of-care. Whether you need laboratory test or diagnostic procedure information, to validate a dose, or to check multiple medications and natural products for drug interactions, Lexi-Comp has the information you need in the palm of your hand. Lexi-Comp also provides advanced linking technology to allow you to hyperlink to related information topics within a title or to the same topic in another title for more extensive information. No longer will you have to exit 5MCC to look up a dose in Lexi-Drugs or lab test information in Lexi-Diagnostic Medicine — seamlessly link between all databases to **save valuable time**.

New Navigational Tools:

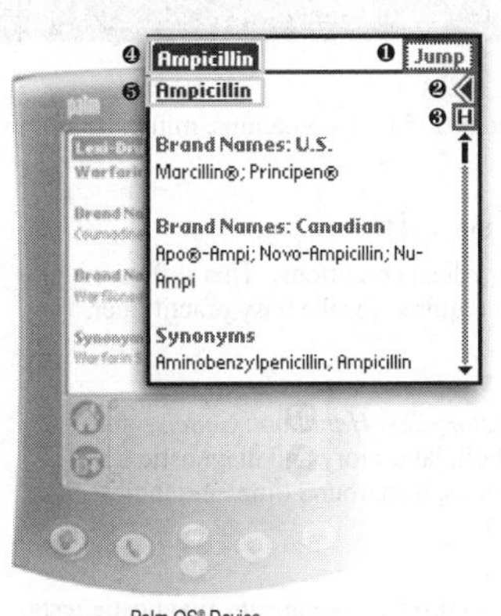

Palm OS® Device

❶ **"Jump"** provides a drop down list of available fields to easily navigate through information.

❷ **Back arrow** returns to the index from a monograph or to the "Installed Books" menu from the Index.

❸ **"H"** provides a linkable History to return to any of the last 12 Topics viewed during your session.

❹ **Title bar:** Tap the monograph or topic title bar to activate a menu to "Edit a Note" or return to the "Installed Books" menu.

❺ **Linking:** Link to another companion database by clicking the topic or monograph title link or within a database noted by various hyperlinked (colorized and underlined) text.

To order call toll free anywhere in the U.S.: 1-800-837-LEXI (5394)
Outside of the U.S. call: 330-650-6506 or online at www.lexi.com

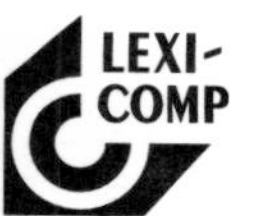

Lexi-Comp, Inc.
1100 Terex Road
Hudson, Ohio 44236

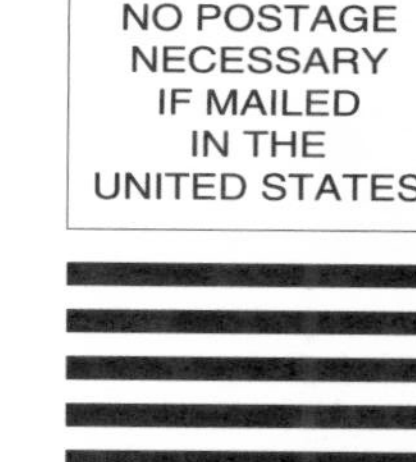

NO POSTAGE
NECESSARY
IF MAILED
IN THE
UNITED STATES

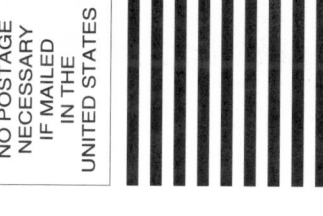

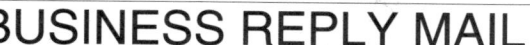

BUSINESS REPLY MAIL

FIRST-CLASS MAIL PERMIT NO 689 HUDSON, OH

POSTAGE WILL BE PAID BY ADDRESSEE

LEXI-COMP, INC.
1100 Terex Road
Hudson, OH 44236-9915